Equine Sports Medicine and Surgery

Content Strategist: *Robert Edwards, Penny Rudolph*
Content Development Specialist: *Catherine Jackson*
Project Manager: *Caroline Jones*
Designer/Design Direction: *Christian Bilbow*
Illustration Manager: *Jennifer Rose*
Illustrator: *Antbits*

Equine Sports Medicine and Surgery

Basic and clinical sciences of the equine athlete

Second Edition

Edited by

KENNETH W. HINCHCLIFF BVSc (Hons), MS, PhD, Diplomate ACVIM (Large Animal)
Dean and Professor, Faculty of Veterinary Science, University of Melbourne

ANDRIS J. KANEPS DVM, MS, PhD, Diplomate ACVS, Diplomate ACVSMR
Proprietor, Kaneps Equine Sports Medicine and Surgery

RAYMOND J. GEOR BVSc, MVSc, PhD, Diplomate ACVIM (Large Animal), Diplomate ACVSMR, Diplomate ACVN (Honorary)
Professor and Chairperson, Department of Large Animal Clinical Sciences, College of Veterinary Medicine, Michigan State University

SAUNDERS ELSEVIER

Edinburgh London New York Oxford Philadelphia St Louis Sydney Toronto 2014

SAUNDERS
ELSEVIER

First edition 2004
Second edition 2014
Reprinted 2014 (twice)

ISBN 978 0 7020 4771 8
eBook ISBN 978 0 7020 5422 8

British Library Cataloguing in Publication Data
A catalogue record for this book is available from the British Library

Library of Congress Cataloging in Publication Data
A catalog record for this book is available from the Library of Congress

Notices

Knowledge and best practice in this field are constantly changing. As new research and experience broaden our understanding, changes in research methods, professional practices, or medical treatment may become necessary.

Practitioners and researchers must always rely on their own experience and knowledge in evaluating and using any information, methods, compounds, or experiments described herein. In using such information or methods they should be mindful of their own safety and the safety of others, including parties for whom they have a professional responsibility.

With respect to any drug or pharmaceutical products identified, readers are advised to check the most current information provided (i) on procedures featured or (ii) by the manufacturer of each product to be administered, to verify the recommended dose or formula, the method and duration of administration, and contraindications. It is the responsibility of practitioners, relying on their own experience and knowledge of their patients, to make diagnoses, to determine dosages and the best treatment for each individual patient, and to take all appropriate safety precautions.

To the fullest extent of the law, neither the Publisher nor the authors, contributors, or editors, assume any liability for any injury and/or damage to persons or property as a matter of products liability, negligence or otherwise, or from any use or operation of any methods, products, instructions, or ideas contained in the material herein.

Printed in China

Contents

List of contributors

KATE ALLEN BVSc, PhD, CertEM (IntMed), Diplomate ACVSMR, MRCVS
Senior Lecturer in Equine Sports Medicine,
University of Bristol,
Bristol,
UK

BRIAN ANDERSON BVSc, MVSc, MANZCVSc, Diplomate ACVS
Surgeon and Partner,
Ballarat Veterinary Practice,
Ballarat,
Australia

TATIANA ART DVM, PhD, Diplomate ECEIM
Professor of Physiology,
Equine Sports Medicine Center,
Faculty of Veterinary Medicine,
University of Liège,
Liège,
Belgium

ERIC BARREY PhD, DVM
Research Director,
Unité de Biologie Intégrative des Adaptations à l'Exercice,
Genopole Evry, France;
Génétique Animale et Biologie Intégrative (GABI),
Jouy-en-Josas, France

LANCE H. BASSAGE II BA VMD
Assistant Professor of Large Animal Surgery,
University of Guelph,
Guelph,
Ontario,
Canada

WARWICK BAYLY BVSc (Hons), MS, PhD, Diplomate ACVIM
Provost and Executive Vice-President,
Washington State University, Pullman,
Washington,
USA

BRENDON BELL BVSc, MS, MANZCVSc
Staff Surgeon,
Southern Veterinary Centre,
Invercargill,
New Zealand

ANNA BERGH BSc(PT), DVM, PhD
Department of Anatomy,
Physiology and Biochemistry,
Swedish University of Agricultural Sciences,
Uppsala,
Sweden

ALICIA L. BERTONE DVM, PhD, Diplomate ACVS, ACVSMR
Professor,
Veterinary Medical Center,
The Ohio State University,
Columbus,
Ohio,
USA

HELEN L. BIRCH BSc, BSc(Ost), PhD
Institute of Orthopaedics and Musculoskeletal Science,
University College London,
London,
UK

LISA BODEN AB, BVSc, MANZCVSc, PhD, Diplomate ECVPH, MRCVS

Veterinary Epidemiologist,
School of Veterinary Medicine,
University of Glasgow,
Glasgow,
UK

ELIZABETH A. CARR DVM, PhD, Diplomate ACVIM, ACVECC

Associate Professor,
Large Animal Clinical Sciences,
College of Veterinary Medicine,
Michigan State University,
East Lansing,
Michigan,
USA

JON CHEETHAM VetMB, PhD, Diplomate ACVS

Department of Clinical Sciences,
College of Veterinary Medicine,
Cornell University,
Ithaca,
New York,
USA

LAURENT L. COUETIL DVM, PhD, Diplomate ACVIM

Professor,
Department of Veterinary Clinical Sciences,
Director,
Equine Research Programs,
Equine Sports Medicine Center,
College of Veterinary Medicine,
Purdue University,
West Lafayette,
Indiana,
USA

ANNE COUROUCÉ-MALBLANC DVM PhD Diplomate ECEIM

CISCO-ONIRIS,
Nantes Atlantic College of Veterinary Medicine,
Food Science and Engineering,
Nantes,
France

ALEXANDER J. DANIEL BVetMed MRCVS

Equine Surgery Resident,
Colorado State University,
Fort Collins,
Colorado,
USA

NORM G. DUCHARME DVM, MSc, Diplomate ACVS

Medical James Law Professor of Surgery,
Director of Equine and Farm Animals Hospital,
Department of Clinical Sciences,
College of Veterinary Medicine,
Cornell University,
Ithaca,
New York,
USA

PATRICIA M. ELLIS BVSc, MVSc, MANZCVSc, AM

Animal Health Consultant,
Victoria,
Australia

HOWARD H. ERICKSON DVM, PhD

Emeritus Professor,
College of Veterinary Medicine,
Kansas State University,
Manhattan,
Kansas,
USA

HILLARY FELDMANN BS

Department of Clinical Sciences,
Tufts Cummings School of Veterinary Medicine,
Tufts University,
North Grafton,
Massachussetts,
USA

JONATHAN H. FOREMAN DVM, MS, Diplomate ACVIM

Professor,
Associate Dean,
Veterinary Clinical Medicine,
University of Illinois,
Urbana,
Illinois,
USA

SAMANTHA FRANKLIN BVSc, PhD, MRCVS

School of Animal and Veterinary Science,
University of Adelaide,
Adelaide,
South Australia,
Australia

RAYMOND J. GEOR BVSc, MVSc, PhD, Diplomate ACVIM (Large Animal), ACVSMR, ACVN (Honorary)

Professor and Chairperson,
Department of Large Animal Clinical Sciences,
College of Veterinary Medicine,
Michigan State University,
East Lansing,
Michigan,
USA

CAROL GILLIS DVM, PhD, Diplomate ACVSMR

Practice Owner,
Equine Ultrasound and Sports Medicine,
Aiken,
South Carolina,
USA

AUDE GIRAUDET DVM

Practicien Hospitalier,
Clinique Equine,
ENVA,
Maisons-Alfort,
France

LESLEY GOFF PhD, MAnimSt (Anim Physio), MAppSc (Ex Sp Sc) GDipAppSc (Manip), BAPPSc (Physio)

Director,
Active Animal Physiotherapy and Hip Sport Spine Physiotherapy,
Toowoomba,
Queensland,
Australia;
Consultant Animal Physiotherapist,
Veterinary Medical Centre,
School of Veterinary Science,
Gatton Campus,
The University of Queensland,
Australia;
Honorary Lecturer,
School Of Veterinary Science,
Faculty of Health and Life Sciences,
University of Liverpool,
UK

LAURIE R. GOODRICH DVM, PhD, Diplomate ACVS

Associate Professor in Equine Surgery and Lameness,
Department of Clinical Sciences and Gail Holmes Equine Orthopaedic Research Center,
Colorado State University,
Fort Collins,
Colorado,
USA

ALLEN E. GOODSHIP BVSc, PhD, MRCVS

Director and Head of Centre,
Centre for Comparative and Clinical Anatomy,
University of Bristol,
Bristol;
Professor of Orthopaedic Sciences,
UCL Institute of Orthopaedics and Musculoskeletal Science and Royal National Orthopaedic Hospital,
Stanmore;
UCL Division of Surgery & Interventional Science,
London;
Honorary Professor,
Professor of Orthopaedic Science,
Royal Veterinary College,
London;
UK

JOANNE HARDY DVM, PhD, Diplomate ACVS, ACVECC

Clinical Associate Professor,
Large Animal Clinical Sciences,
Texas &M University,
College Station,
Texas,
USA

PATRICIA A. HARRIS MA, PhD, Diplomate ECVCN, VetMB, MRCVS

Director of Science for MARS Horsecare;
Head of Equine Studies Group,
Waltham Centre for Pet Nutrition,
Waltham-on-the-Wolds,
UK;
Adjunct Professor of Equine Studies,
Virginia Polytechnic Institute and State University,
USA;
Visiting Professor,
University of Liverpool,
UK;
Honorary Professor in Equine Nutrition,
University of Nottingham,
UK;
Adjunct Professor,
University of Queensland,
Australia

KEVIN K. HAUSSLER DVM, DC, PhD, Diplomate ACVSMR

Assistant Professor,
Department of Clinical Sciences,
College of Veterinary Medicine and Biomedical Sciences,
Colorado State University,
Fort Collins,
Colorado,
USA

KENNETH W. HINCHCLIFF BVSc, MS, PhD, Diplomate ACVIM

Professor and Dean,
Faculty of Veterinary Science,
University of Melbourne,
Melbourne,
Victoria,
Australia

TODD C. HOLBROOK DVM, DACVIM, Diplomate ACVSMR

Associate Professor of Equine Medicine,
Equine Section Chief,
Center for Veterinary Health Sciences,
Oklahoma State University,
Stillwater,
Oklahoma,
USA

SUSAN J. HOLCOMBE VMD, MS, PhD

Professor,
Large Animal Clinical Sciences,
Michigan State University,
East Lansing,
Michigan,
USA

JOHN A. E. HUBBELL DVM, MS

Professor,
Veterinary Clinical Sciences,
The Ohio State University,
Columbus,
Ohio,
USA

JO L. IRELAND BVMS, PhD, CertAVP(EM), MRCVS
Equine Epidemiologist,
Animal Health Trust,
Newmarket,
UK

LEO B. JEFFCOTT MA, BVetMed, PhD, DVSc, VetMedDR (h.c.), FRCVS
Professor Emeritus of Veterinary Science,
Faculty of Veterinary Science,
University of Sydney,
Australia

EDUARD JOSE-CUNILLERAS DVM, PhD, Diplomate ACVIM
Dept. Medicina i Cirurgia Animals,
Facultat de Veterinària,
Universitat Autònoma de Barcelona,
Barcelona,
Spain

ANDRIS J. KANEPS DVM, MS, PhD, Diplomate ACVS, ACVSMR
Proprietor,
Kaneps Equine Sports Medicine and Surgery,
Beverly,
Massachusetts,
USA

CHRISTOPHER E. KAWCAK DVM, PhD, Diplomate ACVS, ACVSMR
Professor,
Equine Orthopaedic Research Center,
College of Veterinary Medicine and Biomedical Sciences,
Colorado State University,
Fort Collins,
Colorado,
USA

KEVIN G. KEEGAN DVM, MS, Diplomate ACVS
Professor and Director,
E. Paige Laurie Endowed Program in Equine Lameness,
College of Veterinary Medicine,
University of Missouri,
Columbia,
Missouri,
USA

CARL A. KIRKER-HEAD MA,VetMB, MRCVS, Diplomate ACVS, ECVS
Marilyn M. Simpson Professor Director,
Orthopaedic Research Laboratory,
Tufts Cummings School of Veterianry Medicine,
North Grafton,
Massachusetts,
USA;
Adjunct Associate Professor,
Biomedical Engineering,
Tufts University,
Medford,
Massachusetts,
USA

JOANNE KRAMER DVM, Diplomate ACVS
Associate Teaching Professor,
Veterinary Medicine and Surgery,
University of Missouri,
Columbia,
Missouri,
USA

MICHAEL LINDINGER BSc, MSc, PhD
Associate Professor (retired),
Human Health and Nutritional Sciences,
University of Guelph,
Guelph,
Ontario;
Vice President,
Nutraceutical Alliance,
Guelph,
Ontario,
Canada

MIREIA LORENZO-FIGUERAS DVM, PhD
Professor,
Equine Medicine,
Surgery and Husbandry,
College of Veterinary Medicine and Husbandry,
Universidad Nacional Autónoma de México,
Mexico City,
Mexico

JONATHAN M. LUMSDEN BVSc, DipVetClinStud, MS, Diplomate ACVS
Partner and Surgeon,
Randwick Equine Centre,
Randwick,
New South Wales,
Australia

L. JILL McCUTCHEON DVM, PhD
Professor and Chair,
Pathobiology and Diagnostic Investigation,
Michigan State University,
East Lansing,
Michigan,
USA

CATHERINE M. MCGOWAN BVSc, MACVSc, DEIM, Diplomate ECEIM, PhD
Professor and Head of Equine Internal Medicine,
Faculty of Ageing and Chronic Disease,
University of Liverpool,
Wirral,
UK

KENNETH HARRINGTON MCKEEVER PhD FACSM
Professor,
Department of Animal Sciences,Rutgers – The State University of New Jersey,
New Brunswick,
New Jersey,
USA

ERICA C. MCKENZIE BSc, BVMS, PhD, Diplomate ACVIM, ACVSMR
Associate Professor,
Large Animal Medicine,
Department of Clinical Sciences,
Oregon State University,
Corvallis,
Oregon,
USA

OMAR MAHER DV, Diplomate ACVS, ACVSMR
Proprietor,
Atlantic Equine Services,
Dover,
New Hampshire and Wellington,
Florida,
USA

ALFRED M. MERRITT DVM, MS
Professor Emeritus,
Department of Large Animal Clinical Sciences,
College of Veterinary Medicine,
University of Florida,
Gainesville,
Florida,
USA

PAUL S. MORLEY DVM, Phd, Diplomate ACVIM
Professor of Epidemiology and Infection Control,
Director of Infection Control, James L. Voss Veterinary Teaching Hospital,
Colorado State University,
Fort Collins,
Colorado,
USA

RACHEL C. MURRAY MA, VetMB, MS, PhD, Diplomate ACVS
Senior Orthopedic Advisor,
Animal Health Trust,
Newmarket,
Suffolk,
UK

LAURA C. NATH BVSC(Hons), MVSc
Lecturer in Equine Medicine,
Faculty of Veterinary Science,
University of Melbourne,
Werribee,
Victoria,
Australia

BRAD B. NELSON DVM, MS
Equine Surgery Resident,
Gail Holmes Equine Orthopaedic Research Center,
Colorado State University,
Fort Collins,
Colorado,
USA

JORGE NIETO MVZ, PhD, Diplomate ACVS, ACVSMR
Professor,
Surgical and Radiological Sciences,
University of California,
Davis,
California,
USA

CHRISTOPHER B. O'SULLIVAN BVSc, DipVetClinStud, MS, Diplomate ACVS
Partner and Surgeon,
Randwick Equine Centre,
Randwick,
New South Wales,
Australia

TIM PARKIN BSc, BVSc, PhD, Diplomate ECVPH, FHEA, MRCVS
School of Veterinary Medicine,
University of Glasgow,
Glasgow,
UK

RICHARD J. PIERCY MA, VetMB, MS, PhD, Diplomate ACVIM, MRCVS
Associate,
Department of Veterinary and Clinical Science,
Royal Veterianry College,
London,
UK

ROB PILSWORTH MA, VetMB, CertVR, BSc(Hons), MRCVS
Associate,
Newmarket Equine Hospital,
Newmarket,
Suffolk,
UK;
Associate Lecturer,
School of Veterinary Medicine, University of Cambridge,
Cambridge,
UK

DAVID C. POOLE PhD DSc
Professor of Kinesiology,
Anatomy and Physiology,
Kansas State University,
Manhattan,
Kansas,
USA

NICOLA PUSTERLA DrMedVet, MedVet
Associate Professor,
Veterinary Medicine and Epidemiology,
School of Veterinary Medicine,
University of California,
Davis,
California,
USA

CHRISTOPHER M. RIGGS BSc BVSc, PhD, DEO, Diplomate ECVS, MRCVS

Head of Veterinary Clinical Services,
Department of Veterinary Clinical Services,
The Hong Kong Jockey Club,
Sha Tin,
Hong Kong

ANDREA RITMEESTER BVSc, MSc, Diplomate ACVS

Specialist Equine Surgeon,
Matamata Veterinary Services, Matamata,
New Zealand

JOSÉ-LUIS L. RIVERO DVM, PhD

Professor,
Comparative Anatomy and Pathological Anatomy,
University of Cordoba,
Faculty of Veterinary Sciences,
Cordoba,
Spain

CÉLINE ROBERT DVM, PhD

Université Paris-Est,
École Nationale Vétérinaire d'Alfort,
Unité d'Anatomie,
Maisons-Alfort,
France

COLIN C. SCHWARZWALD Prof.dr.med.vet., PhD, Diplomate ACVIM, ECEIM

Professor of Equine Internal Medicine,
Vetsuisse Faculty,
University of Zurich,
Zurich,
Switzerland

CHARLOTTE SINCLAIR BVSc, PhD, CertEP, CertES(Orth), FHEA, MRCVS

Equine Associate Veterinarian,
B&W Equine Group,
Willesley,
UK

ROGER K. W. SMITH MA, VetMB, PhD, DEO, Diplomate ECVS, MRCVS

Professor of Equine Orthopaedics,
Equine Medicine and Surgery Group,
The Royal Veterinary College,
Hatfield,
Hertfordshire,
UK

BRIAN D. STEWART BVSc, MBA

Head,
Equine Welfare and Veterinary Services,
Racing Victoria,
Victoria,
Australia

JOHANNES H. VAN DER KOLK DVM, PhD, Diplomate IECEIM

Head Section,
Equine Metabolic and Genetic Diseases,
Euregio Laboratory Services,
Maastricht,
Limburg,
The Netherlands

EMMANUELLE VAN ERCK-WESTERGREN DVM, PhD, Diplomate ECEIM

Equine Sports Medicine Practice,
Waterloo,
Belgium

GUNTHER VAN LOON DVM, PhD, Diplomate ECEIM, Ass Member ECVDI

Professor Doctor,
Large Animal Internal Medicine,
Ghent University,
Merelbeke,
Belgium

RENÉ VAN WEEREN DVM, PhD, Diplomate ECVS

Professor of Equine Musculoskeletal Biology,
Faculty of Veterinary Medicine,
University of Utrecht,
The Netherlands

DOMINIQUE VOTION DVM, PhD

Faculty of Veterinary Medicine,
University of Liège,
Liège,
Belgium

CHRIS WHITTON BVSc, FANZCVS, PhD

Associate Professor,
Equine Centre,
Faculty of Veterinary Science,
University of Melbourne,
Werribee,
Victoria,
Australia

LESLEY E. YOUNG BVSc, DVA, DVC, Diplomate ECEIM, PhD, MRCVS

Specialist Veterinary Cardiologist,
Specialist Equine Cardiology Services,
Newmarket,
Suffolk,
UK

Acknowledgments

The editors and contributors would like to thank the following contributors from the first edition of the book:

Dorothy M. Ainsworth
Laurie A. Beard
David Evans
Michael Hamlin
Seppo Hyyppä
Janene K. Kingston
Federico G. Latimer
Guy D. Lester
Rustin M. Moore
Nigel R. Perkins
A. Reeta Pösö
Sidney W. Ricketts
Katarina Schuback
Tracy A Turner
Honor A. Walesby
Keith L. Watkins

Preface

The cover of this, the second edition of 'Equine Sports Medicine and Surgery: Basic and clinical sciences of the equine athlete' depicts the use of horses in athletic endeavors in antiquity. The images are from the Parthenon Frieze and are part of the Elgin Marbles held in the British Museum. The images portray the close association between humans and horses, the sense of elation at winning an event astride a horse, and the important role that horses played in recreation, sport and war in ancient Greece. While fortunately horses are rarely, if ever, today subjected to the perils of war, they are used worldwide in competitive sports and for recreational riding. Although the very special relationship that riders have with their horses is no less intense today than in antiquity, our ability to ensure the health and wellbeing of our equine athletic companions is markedly improved. This is attributable in large part to burgeoning knowledge of the physiology of exercise and training – all aspects of which are covered in depth in this text. We now, after decades of intensive research, have a very thorough, although not complete, understanding of the physiologic processes that underlay the responses of horses to exercise and to physical conditioning.

The Parthenon Frieze depicts apparently healthy horses involved in athletic pursuits and indicates the importance of maintaining the health and well-being of horses in preparation for their participation in sport or recreation. Keeping athletic horses healthy and physically fit is a cornerstone of equine sports medicine and features prominently in this book, whether it be the appropriate nutritional support of athletes, prophylaxis of exercise-induced diseases, prevention of lameness, or modification of training regimens.

Another component of the Elgin Marbles, and one that captures the third strand of this text, is the head of a horse of Selene from the east pediment of the Parthenon sculptures (below). This work of art captures the very essence of the stress and fatigue of the mythical horse that has spent the night drawing the chariot of the Moon across the sky. The horse has all the hallmarks of an exhausted animal – the flared nostrils, the ears pinned back, the mouth open and the eyes bulging. This image captures the essence of the ill athletic horse and underscores our obligation to provide optimal medical and surgical care to our equine companions. Equine sports medicine and surgery is covered in detail and extensively in this text and is based wherever possible on sound research and evidence based medicine.

This book could not have been completed without the diligent efforts of our many collaborators and colleagues in equine exercise physiology and sports medicine and surgery. We are deeply appreciative of their efforts to contribute on short time frames a complete and up to date text. We hope that reading this book is both enjoyable and informative.

Sincerely,
K.W. Hinchcliff
A.J. Kaneps
R.J. Geor

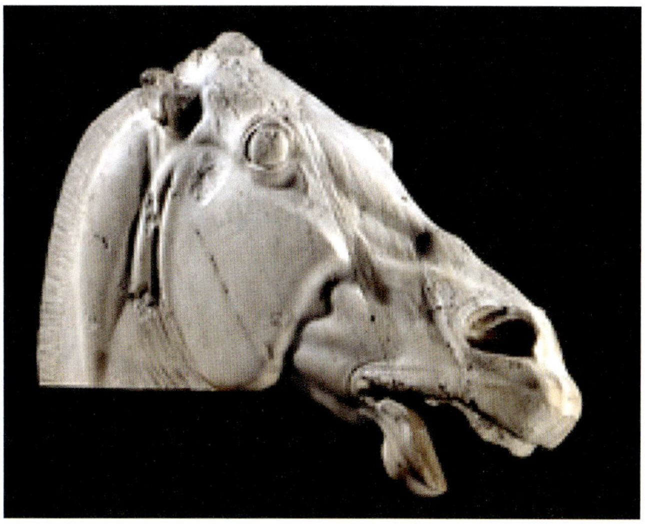

Image courtesy of Shutterstock.

section 1

Integrative physiology and exercise testing

The horse as an athlete

1

Kenneth W. Hinchcliff

CHAPTER CONTENTS

Origins of the horse

The horse is an extraordinary athlete, a characteristic that is the result of the evolution of horses as grazing animals on the ancient prairies of North America. Survival in these open lands was enhanced by speed to escape predators and endurance required to travel long distances in search of feed and water. These attributes are shared by prong horn antelopes (*Antilocapra americana*), another species that evolved on the prairies,[1] as well as black wildebeest (*Connochaetes gnou*), a South African herbivore.[2] The equid characteristics of speed and endurance were subsequently modified or enhanced by selective breeding by humans, resulting in the wide variety of breeds extant today.

While ancient horses, such as *Eohippus*, *Mesohippus* and *Equus ferus*, evolved on the prairies of North America, they became extinct in the Americas approximately 12 000 years ago, as did other endemic megafauna.[3] It appears that two clades of *Equus ferus*, the immediate progenitor of the modern horse, existed with one in North America becoming extinct and the other, which had a holartic distribution including Europe, evolving into the modern horse (*Equus caballus*).[3] Horses were returned to the Americas by European explorers, colonizers and missionaries after 1494.

Horses were domesticated as early as 4000 BCE (before current era) in Eastern Europe and the Eurasian steppes.[4] Archeological evidence of dental lesions consistent with use of a bit or bridle and biochemical evidence of storage of mare's milk and carcass products in ceramic cooking and food storage utensils provides clear demonstration of domestication of modern horses at this time.[4] Analysis of mitochondrial DNA and the Y chromosome of modern horses provides considerable evidence that horses were domesticated on more than one occasion and that this process involved introgression of wild females into the domestic population.[5,6] Przewalski's horse, with a karyotype of 2N = 66 chromosomes, is not a direct progenitor of the modern horse, with 64 chromosomes.[7]

Analysis of mitochondrial genomes and microsatellite markers provides compelling evidence that modern horses are derived from multiple matrilineal lineages from the extinct *Equus ferus*.[6] The earliest Ancestral Mare Mitogenome, from which all mitochondrial DNA in modern horses derive, is dated at approximately 153 000 years ago.[6] There were likely no fewer than 17 founding matrilineal lineages of modern horses, a situation that contrasts with domestication of other livestock species in which the modern population is based on a very small number of female founders.[6] In contrast, there is evidence based on analysis of sequence diversity in the Y chromosome of modern horses that only a small number of stallions were foundation stock for modern horses.[8] A plausible explanation is that modern horses were domesticated on more than one occasion and likely in the area of the Caspian Sea and, separately, in the geographically distant Iberian Peninsula, both areas of refugia of undomesticated horses during the Holocene when large areas of Europe were covered by dense forest (a habitat unsuitable for horses).[9] Domestication was likely achieved by breeding of a small number of founder stallions with both domesticated mares and mares caught from the wild. Societal factors also played a role in domestication of the horse as knowledge of how to do so lead different groups of people to undertake domestication of local horses resulting in multiple matrilineal lines.[5] The limited patrilineal lineages of horses could be a result of population bottlenecks or selective breeding to a small number of stallions during the demic spread of domesticated animals. [8]

Domesticated horses were selected and bred for certain traits, depending on the intended use, with the result that there are now many hundreds of breeds of horses.[10] Large heavy breeds of horses were bred for draft work, such as pulling ploughs, sleds or carts, or military work, such as the chargers that carried heavily armored knights into the battles of the middle ages. Lighter horses were bred for speed and endurance and were used for transportation, herding and sport. Thoroughbred racehorses run at high speed (18 m/s, 64 km/h) over distances of 800 to 5000 meters, Standardbred horses trot or pace at high speed for distances up to 3600 m, Quarter Horses sprint for 400 m or less at speed as high as 88 km/h, sometimes around figure of eight courses delineated by barrels (barrel racing), and Arabians trot or canter at speeds of up to 29 km/h for up to 160 km in a single day during endurance events (and over longer distances during multi-day races). In contrast, draft horses pull huge weights (1000 kg or more) short distances in pulling competitions, Warmbloods perform elegant, but demanding, dressage routines, and ponies pull lightly laden jinkers or buggies.

Large scale studies of SNP data from multiple breeds and large numbers of horses reveals the genetic relationships between breeds of horses (Fig. 1.1).[11] There is clear genomic evidence that selection has played a strong role in modifying both the genotype and phenotype of horses within breeds. This is best exemplified for Thoroughbred in which the emergence of a single nucleotide polymorphism for the myostatin gene can be clearly traced back to the influence of one or two key stallions. [12]The C/C and C/T polymorphisms of the MSTN gene (which encodes myostatin) are, compared to the T/T polymorphism, associated with superior athletic performance by Thoroughbred horses racing over short distances (<1600 m).[13] The presence of the C polymorphism was uncommon in Thoroughbreds before 1950 with the T allele being the most common ancestral allele[12]. The C allele was introduced into the Thoroughbred breed by a single female during the foundation of the breed, but was rare before it proliferated in the breed as a result of the success of offspring of Neartic and his son, Northern Dancer.[12] Northern Dancer was the most influential stallion of modern times and the success of his offspring in short to mid-distance races ensured the propagation of the C allele.[12] Amongst current Thoroughbred horses used for sprint racing (≤1400 m), over 90% are either C/C or C/T genotype with 70% of the alleles being C, indicating the effect of profound selection pressure for sprint racing on the distribution of this allele, and related genotypes, in Thoroughbreds.[12]

Limits to performance

A large number of physiological and anatomical features act in concert to endow the horse with extraordinary athletic capacity. Maximal athletic performance is dependent upon integrated functioning of these physiological and anatomical features.[14,15] However, there are limits to maximal performance of horses, and there is evidence that these limits have been reached or will soon be so, particularly for Thoroughbred and Standardbred racehorses.[16–18] The winning times for major Thoroughbred races have not improved significantly since approximately 1970 as is exemplified by the

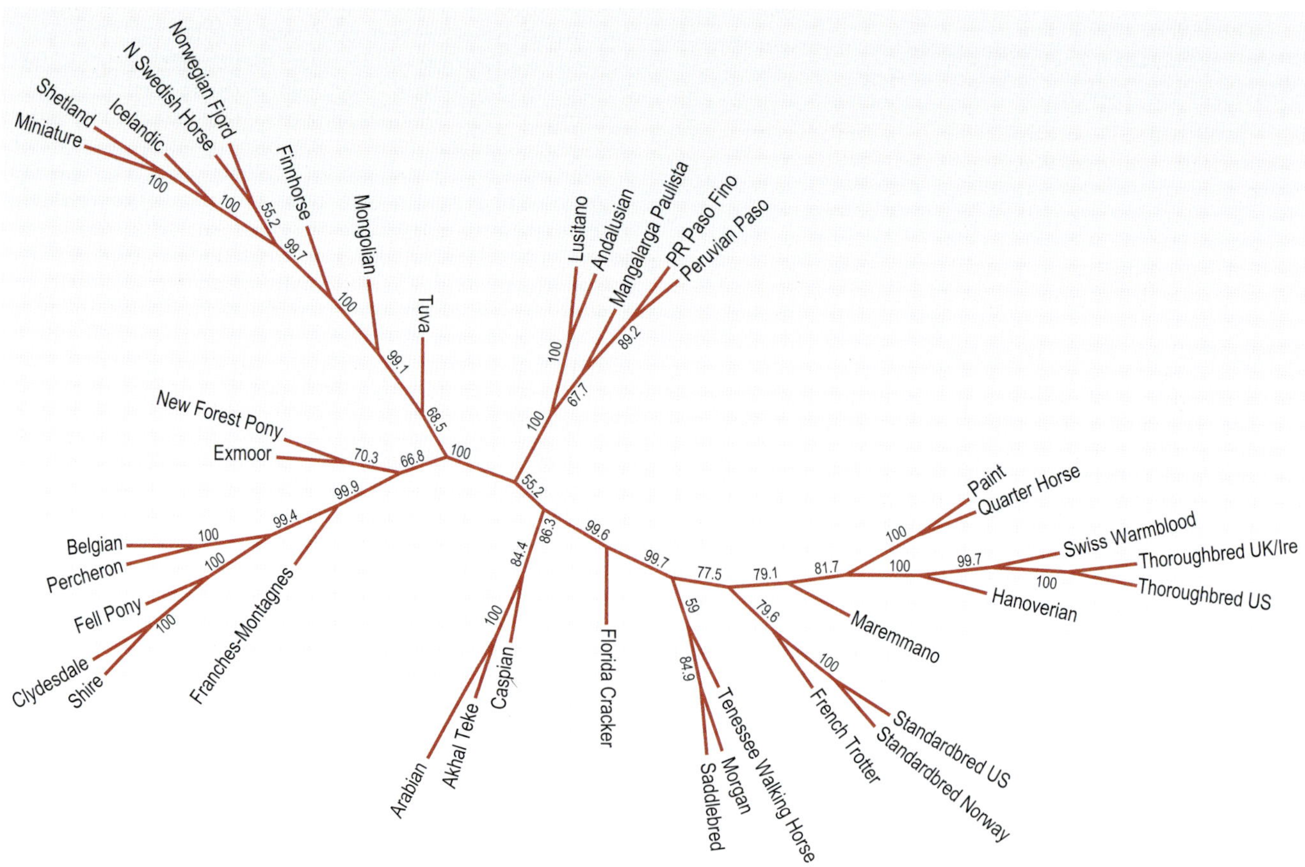

Fig 1.1 Genetic relationships amongst breeds of horses as determined by SNP analysis represented as a distance based, neighbor joining tree calculated from SNP frequencies in 38 horse populations.[11]

winning times for the Melbourne Cup, a 3200 m (two mile) race run every November in Melbourne, Australia (Fig. 1.2).

While it is hypothesized that winning times are a function of the size of the population available to compete in an event, in that the greater the number of animals or people available to compete, the more likely that one individual will excel.[16] However, analysis of the population statistics and winning times of Thoroughbred race horses does not provide evidence to support this hypothesis, with the maximal effect of population occurring at fewer than 10 000 horses.[16] The reasons for this plateau in winning times of Thoroughbreds is unclear. It might be that selective breeding has had its maximal effect in this closed population of horses originating from a small pool of ancestors and that in the absence of major developments in nutrition, management or health that there is no further genetic potential to increase speed.[16] Others disagree with this interpretation and provide evidence that there is sufficient genetic variation within Thoroughbreds to improve performance.[19]

The recent demonstration that genotype, and in particular a single nucleotide polymorphism (SNP) of the myostatin gene, of Thoroughbreds is associated with race performance provides evidence that there remains the capacity to improve further performance through selection.[12]

The situation differs somewhat with Standardbreds in which there has been a consistent reduction in race times and pace over recent times.[17,18] This improvement is presumably a result of one or more of strong selection pressure, improved training methods, or improved equipment and racing facilities.[17] The decrease in race time has been well documented for Swedish and Italian trotters.[17,18] The reduction is exponential and appears to be approaching an asymptote, which in 2001 was predicted to occur in 2015 [17] but which has not occurred for Italian trotters.[18]

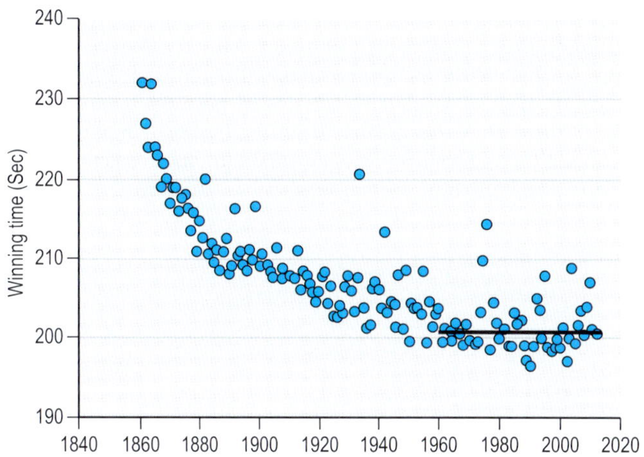

Fig 1.2 Winning times (seconds) for the Melbourne Cup, a race run over 3200 m (two miles) on the first Tuesday in November each year in Melbourne, Victoria, Australia. The green line represents the line of best fit for winning times for 1960–2012. There is no evidence of a decrease in winning times over this period (R = 0.004, P = 0.978).

Comparative physiology

Regardless of their size, provenance or intended use, all horses have in common an ability to perform physical activities, including running or jumping, at a level that surpasses that of most other animals of similar body size. The concept of body size is important as many physiological variables, and especially the maximum values of these variables, do not scale directly with body weight but often more closely scale to an exponent of body weight.[20] Commonly, exponents range between 0.68 and 0.75. This exponent is derived empirically from the measurement of variables such as maximum running speed or maximum rate of oxygen consumption ($\dot{V}O_{2max}$). Typically, when expressed as a one-to-one function of body weight (i.e. per kg), values for many variables are much higher for smaller mammals. The necessity to allometrically scale variables has fascinating physiological implications and interpretations.[20] However, direct comparison among species is to some extent specious from the point of view of depicting differences in physical capacity, given that the absolute values of these variables vary to such a large extent. Nonetheless, such comparisons are frequently made, if only to reinforce the magnitude of the maximal absolute values of these variables in the exercising horse (Table 1.1).

Table 1.1 Selected physiological variables of athletic and non-athletic species

SPECIES	BODY WEIGHT (kg)	SPEED* (km/h)	DURATION OF EXERCISE	$\dot{V}O_{2max}$ (ml O_2/kg/min)	HR* (bpm)	ENERGY EXPENDITURE PER DAY (kcal)
Thoroughbred racehorse	450	64 (max)	2 min	180–200	240 (max)	30 000
Endurance racehorse	400	15		180		38 000[a]
Steer	470			80		
Goat	32					
Greyhound	34	64 (max)	60 sec	Not reported	300*	2160
Sled dog	25	20	10 days	170	300	11 000
Human (Olympic class)	70	36 (max)	9.4 sec	85	220	7000[b]
Pronghorn antelope	32	65	10 min	300		

*During customary athletic activity. Max = maximum value. a = day of racing; b = Tour de France cyclists;
References:55, 56–58

The athletic capacity of horses is attributable to a number of physiological adaptations. In some cases these adaptations are not affected by training, for example lung size, whereas others change in response to training, for example blood volume.[21,22] The superior athletic ability of horses is attributable to their high maximal aerobic capacity, large intramuscular stores of energy substrates and in particular glycogen, high mitochondrial volume in muscle, the ability to increase oxygen carrying capacity of blood at the onset of exercise through splenic contraction, efficiency of gait, and efficient thermoregulation.

The maximal aerobic capacity ($\dot{V}O_{2max}$) of horses is approximately 2.6 times that of similarly sized cattle.[23] The larger aerobic capacity in horses is permitted by a larger maximum cardiac output and stroke volume and higher hemoglobin concentration.[23] Maximum heart rate is not different between horses and cattle. In addition to the cardiovascular differences between cattle and horses, horses also have lungs that are twice as large as those of cattle with gas exchange surfaces 1.6 times that of cattle.[24] Thus, horses have structural adaptations that enhance oxygenation of blood in the lungs, oxygen transport capacity of blood and the ability to deliver oxygen to tissues. The oxygen transport chain, from air to muscle, of horses is suited to transportation of the large volumes of oxygen required to support the high metabolic rate of strenuously exercising horses.

Substrate is required to support these high metabolic rates during exercise. Substrate to support exercise is either carbohydrate or fatty acids (Fig. 1.3).[25] Oxidation of fatty acids is limited and reaches maximal values in other species at a work intensity of approximately 40% to 60% of $\dot{V}O_{2max}$.[26,27] It is likely that a similar phenomenon occurs in horses. Additional work above this exercise intensity is fueled solely by oxidation of carbohydrates, predominantly glycogen.[28] Horses have high intramuscular concentrations of glycogen, as do other athletic species such as dogs.[29] Muscle concentrations of glycogen in horses are approximately 140 mmol per kg of muscle (wet weight) compared with 80–100 mmol/kg in humans.[30] High intramuscular concentrations of substrate are important for fueling muscle contractions during exercise. The flux of glucose from blood into muscle and subsequently to the mitochondria provides only a small amount (<10%) of the energy used during intense exercise,[31] likely because of limits to the rate of transportation of these compounds during exercise.[29] The presence of large amounts of readily available substrate in close proximity to mitochondria is therefore essential for horses to undertake strenuous exercise.

Mitochondria provide the energy for muscle contraction. The greater the quantity of mitochondria per unit of muscle weight, the greater is the oxidative capacity of muscle. Muscle of horses contains approximately twice the concentration of mitochondria as does muscle of cattle, a similarly sized animal but with a much lower aerobic capacity.[32] This greater aerobic capacity in muscle, when supported by adequate substrate availability and oxygen delivery, permits a higher whole animal maximal aerobic capacity.

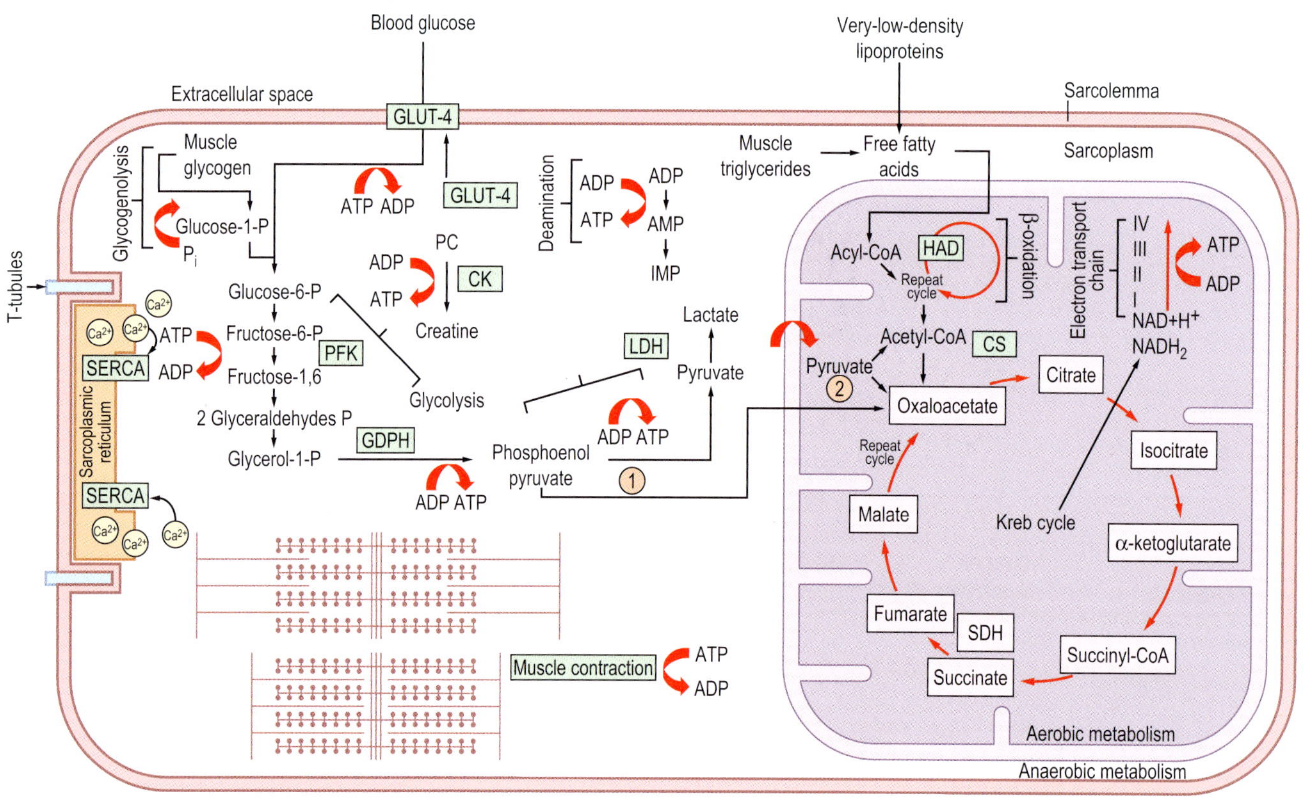

Fig 1.3 Schematic of substrate and oxygen flux demonstrating the integrated and sequential nature of many processes. Substrate supply to produce ATP that powers muscle contraction is through both lipid and carbohydrate. Carbohydrate is provided from muscle glycogen by phosphorylase or from glucose in blood. Important controlling hormones are glucagon, insulin and the catecholamines, in addition to control by local physicochemical factors. Lipid substrate is provided from both intramuscular and adipose tissues, with the former being more important during exercise. Ultimately carbon molecules are delivered to the mitochondria wherein they are oxidized to produce carbon dioxide, heat and work. Oxygen delivery to the mitochondria is dependent upon a chain of events leading from the atmospheric air to the mitochondria. Muscle contraction is associated with production of work, carbon dioxide, heat and lactate (under conditions of anaerobic metabolism).[25]

Reprinted from Votion, D.M., Navet, R., Lacombe, V.A., et al. 2007, Muscle energetics in exercising horses, Equine and Comparative Exercise Physiology, 4 (3–4); 105–118, with permission from Cambridge University Press.

Oxygen transport from the lungs to exercising muscle is achieved by circulation. In addition to cardiac output, oxygen delivery is limited by the oxygen carrying capacity of blood. Horses achieve rapid increases in the oxygen carrying capacity of blood by increasing hemoglobin concentration through splenic contraction. Splenic contraction in anticipation of exercise and during exercise increases the circulating red cell mass without concomitant increases in plasma volume.[33] The resulting increase in hemoglobin concentration increases the oxygen carrying capacity of arterial blood by up to 50% during intense exercise. The beneficial effect of this autoinfusion of red cells at the start of exercise is apparent in horses from which the spleen has been removed.[34–36] Splenectomized horses have lower hematocrits during exercise, altered systemic hemodynamics including lower right atrial and pulmonary artery pressures, and reduced capacity to perform strenuous exercise.

Energetically efficient gait is challenging for large animals because of the slow rate of contraction and low power output of their muscles.[37] However, the gait of horses is energetically efficient,[38] with the muscular work of galloping being halved by elastic storage of energy in muscle and tendon units.[39] For the forelimb, this use of stored energy and the subsequent catapult action mean that the biceps and brachiocephalicus muscles are less than one one-hundredth the size that they would need to be were there no use of stored energy.[37]

In summary, a large number of physiological and anatomical features act in concert to endow the horse with extraordinary athletic capacity. Optimal athletic performance is dependent upon optimal integrated functioning of these physiological and anatomical features.

Integrative physiology of exercise

The detailed responses of each body system to acute exercise and to repeated exercise (conditioning or training) are described in chapters throughout this book. These responses, although described in isolation for each body system, do not occur in isolation, but rather occur as a component of a complex and integrated response to exercise, the ultimate goal of which is to provide substrate for muscle contraction while maintaining homeostasis.

Exercise results in coordinated changes in almost all body systems. Fundamentally, exercise is associated with an increase in power output achieved by contraction of muscles. Contraction of muscles consumes adenosine triphosphate (ATP) and triggers an increase in metabolic rate to replace expended ATP. Increases in metabolic rate are dependent upon an adequate supply of substrate and, ultimately, oxygen. Energy production can be achieved for brief periods of time by anaerobic metabolism, but ultimately all energy production is linked to substrate oxidation and an adequate supply of oxygen.

Production of ATP during exercise is proximately dependent on supplies of substrate for oxidation and of oxygen. A schematic of factors influencing the supply of these fuels to muscle is depicted in Figure 1.1. The important concept is that there are a number of steps in the process or transport chain by which each of these products is delivered to the muscle cell. Because these processes are sequential and often non-duplicative, a limitation in one process or function will limit the rate of the whole system. In some cases these rate limiting steps may be modified by training, in which instance the rate of oxygen or substrate delivery will be increased, or may not be altered by training. The consequences of these differences are discussed below under 'Factors limiting performance'.

At the onset of exercise there is a coordinated response by a large number of body systems to increase fuel availability, maintain acid-base balance within acceptable limits, and limit body temperature. These responses include a large increase in flux of substrate, the nature of which depends on the intensity and duration of exercise. Increasing exercise intensity results in a greater proportion of total energy production being derived from carbohydrates in muscle (glycogen) and blood (glucose, either absorbed from the gastrointestinal tract or produced by the liver) than from fat.[40] The supply of these substrates is controlled by the hormonal responses to exercise, which include a reduction in blood insulin concentration and increases in blood catecholamine, cortisol and glucagon concentrations.[41] The net result is increased delivery of glucose to muscle from the blood as a result of increased hepatic glycolysis and gluconeogenesis. However, blood borne glucose provides only a small proportion (< 10%) of carbohydrate used during intense exercise, the remainder coming from intramuscular stores of glycogen.

Oxidation of substrate during exercise is dependent upon a nearly constant supply of oxygen. Oxygen delivery to the muscle is dependent upon optimal functioning of the respiratory and cardiovascular systems, which are described in detail in this text.[22,42] Increased oxygen delivery to muscle is achieved through increases in minute ventilation, alveolar ventilation, oxygen carrying capacity of blood (secondary to splenic contraction), and cardiac output. An increase in values of these variables with exercise is roughly dependent on the relative intensity of exercise.

Aerobic metabolism and anaerobic glycolysis result in the production of waste products principal among which are carbon dioxide and lactate. Carbon dioxide is produced by the aerobic metabolism of carbohydrate or fat. Produced in the mitochondria of metabolically active cells, it diffuses into the blood wherein it is transported either as dissolved carbon dioxide or as bicarbonate.[43] Transportation of the large amounts of carbon dioxide produced during exercise result in marked increases in venous partial pressure of carbon dioxide and venous blood bicarbonate concentrations.

Lactate, and associated H+, is produced during anaerobic metabolism. A 3 carbon monocarboxylate compound, lactate moves out of muscles and into other tissues by diffusion and by active transport by monocarboxylate transporters. Lactate is metabolized to carbon dioxide and water in well oxygenated metabolically active tissues, or is recycled to glucose and glycogen in the liver, kidney and inactive muscle cells.[40] The hydrogen ions produced during anaerobic metabolism are buffered by intracellular buffers including proteins and by extracellular buffers, the most quantitatively important of which is bicarbonate. Despite this buffering, intense exercise induces a pronounced acidosis and acidemia with decreases in arterial and mixed venous pH and base excess, decreases in arterial bicarbonate concentration and marked increases in carbon dioxide tension in venous blood. The acidosis associated with maximal exercise is severe and tolerable only for short periods of time. Resolution of the respiratory acidosis occurs within seconds to minutes of the cessation of exercise, whereas metabolic acidosis is slower to resolve taking 30–60 minutes.

Muscle contraction produces heat which if not effectively dissipated results in hyperthermia.[44] The heat generated by an exercising horse is sufficient to raise its body temperature by 3–5°C. If exercise is prolonged and not accompanied by effective heat dissipation, the rectal temperature may exceed 42°C, a temperature associated with markedly increased risk of heat shock and illness. Heat dissipation from horses is achieved by evaporation of sweat, evaporation of respiratory tract secretions and convective loss of heat in air moving over the horse's skin and respiratory membranes. Heat generated in muscle is transported by the blood to the skin and respiratory tract, from where it is lost into the ambient air.

Physiology of training

Training is essential for horses to compete effectively and safely. All equine athletes undergo some type of training regimen to prepare them for the rigors of competition. Training prepares the equine athlete for competition by inducing the physiological adaptations necessary to perform at a high level with minimal risk of injury, and by providing the appropriate behavioral and psychological factors essential for effective competition. In order to adequately prepare a horse for competition, the horse should regularly perform the type of activity that it will perform in competition at an intensity that will induce the physiological changes needed to permit optimal performance.

Repetitive exercise induces a multitude of physiological and anatomical adaptations in horses. The specific responses of each body system are dealt with in detail in the relevant sections of this book. However, there are a number of concepts that are common to many body systems.

The adaptive response

An important concept is that some physiological processes, functions or anatomical structures are malleable and able to adapt in response to the stresses and strains imposed by repetitive exercise. Collectively, induction of these adaptive responses to exercise is called training or conditioning. Strictly speaking, training refers to changes in behavior induced by certain practices whereas conditioning refers to the physical changes that occur in response to repetitive exercise. However, the terms are often used synonymously.

The adaptive responses induced by repetitive exercise act to reduce the effect of the strain induced by the physiological stressors associated with exercise. The body acts to minimize the disruption to homeostasis induced by exercise by increasing the capacity of the system to deal with the work imposed by exercise. For example, the stress of increased force production by muscle during exercise stimulates changes in muscle structure and function that act to reduce the stress on individual muscle fibers, while increasing the overall capacity of the muscle. This phenomenon is common to many, but not all, body systems and the cumulative effect is a change in body composition and capacity for physical work.

Mechanisms of training effects

Repetitive exercise (exercise training) results in a multitude of changes in the body at cellular, tissue, organ and whole organism level. At the most fundamental level, training occurs through increased production of proteins, both structural and functional proteins. Accumulation of metabolites and waste products is believed to induce increased transcription of DNA specific for proteins, including enzymes, that control rate limiting functions associated with these metabolites.[45] Characterization of the transcriptome from Thoroughbred horses before and after 10 months of training demonstrates a marked effect on training with increases in mRNA transcripts associated with mitochondrion, oxidative phosphorylation, and fatty acid metabolism and decreases in expression associated with structural genes including sarcoplasm, laminin complex and cytoskeleton.[45] Increased transcription, if associated with increased translation of mRNA to protein and appropriate post-translational events, results in production of more protein or of structurally different protein. For instance, the C/C polymorphism of the MSTN gene of Thoroughbred horses have the highest expression of mRNA for myostatin, compared to C/T and T/T genotypes, after training providing clear evidence of the association of genotype, gene expression and phenotype.[46] The expression of genes is also related to the intensity of exercise training, with the amount of transcription of different genes varying with the intensity of exercise during training.[47]

The increased quantity or activity of the enzymes then results in an increase in the maximal rate at which the metabolites can be processed or waste products eliminated. At an organ level these changes result in an increase in function, usually associated with increases in organ size.

Principles of training

For training to be effective in inducing the desired conditioning, there must be a degree of 'overreaching'. Overreaching refers to the performance of an activity at a sufficient intensity and duration to induce some strain into the organism. Without this strain, there will be no conditioning effect.

It is also important to recognize that training is task specific. The task for which conditioning is desired must be performed. A horse trained to compete in endurance events will be poorly trained for sprint racing. Given the specificity of training, there are three principles of training expressed for human exercise physiology:[48]

1. repetition
2. summation
3. duration.

To induce a training effect, there must be repetition of the training stimulus. The number of repetitions varies with the type and intensity of exercise. Summation refers to the total amount of work performed. To achieve some degree of overreaching, the total amount of work performed must be sufficient to induce some strain. If tasks are performed without sufficient time for substantial recovery between repetitions, then the total amount of work needed to achieve a training response may be lower than if recovery is allowed to occur.[48] Finally, the training stimulus must be of sufficient duration to induce an effect.

These principles of training must be used in a thoughtful and planned manner in order to induce the maximum training response while reducing the risk of injury. The art of training involves the judicious use of exercise of various intensities and durations in order to induce the optimal adaptations that will permit successful competition why preventing injury or occurrence of overtraining.

Overtraining

Overtraining is a well-recognized syndrome in human athletes in which increases or maintenance of training intensity are associated with decrements in performance.[49–51] Diagnosis of overtraining in humans is complicated by the absence of any one definitive test, although psychological profiles include evaluation of mood are the most specific indicators of overtraining.[49] The situation is even more complicated in horses for which psychological and mood evaluation is not available. Overtraining in horses is characterized by decrements in performance and maximal rate of oxygen consumption.[52,53] Specific aspects of overtraining are addressed in other sections of this book.

Factors limiting performance

Maximal performance involves the coordinated optimal functioning of almost all body systems. In most cases, maximal performance requires that these body systems operate at or close to their maximum capacity. Conceptually, this integrated maximal function may be viewed as a pipeline. The maximum overall flow through the pipe is limited by the narrowest segment of the pipe. This analogy is often employed for oxygen transport during exercise and the system is viewed as one of tuned resistors, with no one individual element limiting the capacity of the system.[54] While this analogy is appropriate for healthy animals, it may not be so for animals with performance limiting abnormalities, such as lameness or airway obstruction. In this instance, a single abnormality is sufficient to impair performance. Specific aspects of poor performance are dealt with elsewhere in this book.

For healthy horses, the actual performance limiting factor depends on the type of exercise and its duration. Standardbred or Thoroughbred racehorses running at top speed are likely limited by oxygen transport. In these animals, the malleable components of the oxygen transport chain (red cell mass, mitochondrial volume, muscle capillarity) have adapted to the extent that the capacity of these components approaches or exceeds the capacity of the non-malleable components, such as lung volume or tracheal diameter. A reduction in the capacity of the non-malleable component, for example a reduction in laryngeal diameter secondary to laryngeal hemiplegia, will reduce the capacity of the whole system. This has important consequences for a horse performing at maximal intensity. However, if the capacity of the non-malleable components exceeds those of the malleable components, then a reduction in capacity of the non-malleable component may not reduce performance, for instance in the case of a dressage horse with laryngeal hemiplegia. In this case, the disorder will likely not limit the physiological capacity of the horse to perform its task (although the associated respiratory noise may detract from the performance).

For other types of performance, other factors are limiting. Three day event horses may be limited by their capacity to thermoregulate, endurance horses by their capacity to maintain fluid and electrolyte homeostasis and draft horses by the strength of their muscles. Clearly, the factors limiting exercise capacity of horses varies with the type and duration of exercise. However, an understanding of what likely limits performance for each breed and use of horse is important to understanding not only the physiology of that form of exercise, but also in determining the likely causes of poor performance in animals with clinical disease.

References

1. Lindstedt SL, Hokanson JF, Wells DJ, Swain SD, Hoppeler H, Navarro V. Running energetics in the pronghorn antelope. Nature 1991;353:748–50.
2. Kohn TA, Curry JW, Noakes TD. Black wildebeest skeletal muscle exhibits high oxidative capacity and a high proportion of type IIx fibres. The Journal of experimental biology 2011;214:4041–7.
3. Weinstock J, Willerslev E, Sher A, et al. Evolution, Systematics, and Phylogeography of Pleistocene Horses in the New World: A Molecular Perspective. PLoS Biol 2005;3:e241.
4. Outram AK, Stear NA, Bendrey R, et al. The Earliest Horse Harnessing and Milking. Science 2009;323:1332–5.
5. Warmuth V, Eriksson A, Bower MA, et al. Reconstructing the origin and spread of horse domestication in the Eurasian steppe. Proceedings of the National Academy of Sciences 2012;109:8202–6.
6. Achilli A, Olivieri A, Soares P, et al. Mitochondrial genomes from modern horses reveal the major haplogroups that underwent domestication. Proceedings of the National Academy of Sciences 2012;109:2449–54.
7. Goto H, Ryder OA, Fisher AR, et al. A massively parallel sequencing approach uncovers ancient origins and high genetic variability of endangered Przewalski's horses. Genome Biology and Evolution 2011;3:1096–1106.
8. Lippold S, Knapp M, Kuznetsova T, et al. Discovery of lost diversity of paternal horse lineages using ancient DNA. Nature communications 2011;2:450.
9. Warmuth V, Eriksson A, Bower MA, et al. European domestic horses originated in two Holocene refugia. PloS one 2011;6:e18194.
10. Horse breeds of the world. International Museum of the Horse, 2013. (Accessed March 9, 2013, 2013, at http://imh.org/index.php/exhibits/online/horse-breeds-of-the-world.)
11. Petersen JL, Mickelson JR, Cothran EG, et al. Genetic diversity in the modern horse illustrated from genome-wide SNP data. PloS one 2013;8:e54997.
12. Bower MA, McGivney BA, Campana MG, et al. The genetic origin and history of speed in the Thoroughbred racehorse. Nat Commun 2012;3:643.
13. Hill EW, Fonseca RG, McGivney BA, Gu J, MacHugh DE, Katz LM. MSTN genotype (g. 66493737C/T) association with speed indices in Thoroughbred racehorses. Journal of Applied Physiology 2012;112:86–90.
14. Hinchcliff KW, Geor RJ. Integrative physiology of exercise. In: Hinchcliff KW, Kaneps A, Geor RJ, editors. Equine Sports Medicine and Surgery: Basic and clinical sciences of the equine athlete. London: WB Saunders; 2004; p. 3–8.
15. Evans DL. Physiology of equine performance and associated tests of function. Equine Veterinary Journal 2007;39:373.
16. Denny M. Limits to running speed in dogs, horses and humans. J Exp Biol 2008;211:3836–49.
17. Arnason T. Trends and asymptotic limits for racing speed in Standardbred trotters. Livestock production science 2001;72:135.
18. Pieramati C, Giontella A, Sarti F, Silvestrelli M. Assessments of limits for racing speed in the Italian trotter population. It J Anim Sci 2011;10:233–6.
19. Gaffney B, Cunningham E. Estimation of genetic trend in racing performance of Thoroughbred horses. Nature 1988;332:722–3.
20. Schmidt-Nielsen K. Scaling: Why is animal size so important? Cambridge: Cambridge University Press; 1984.
21. Jose-Cunilleras E, McKeever K. Body fluids and electrolytes: responses to exercise and training. In: Hinchcliff KW, Kaneps A, Geor RJ, editors. Equine Sports Medicine and Surgery: basic and clinical sciences of the equine athlete. London: Elsevier; 2013.
22. Art T. Lower respiratory system: responses to exercise and training. In: Hinchcliff KW, Kaneps A, Geor RJ, editors. Equine Sports Medicine and Surgery: basic and clinical sciences of the equine athlete. London: Elsevier; 2013.
23. Jones JH, Longworth KE, Lindholm A, et al. Oxygen transport during exercise in large mammals. I. Adaptive variation in oxygen demand. Journal of applied physiology (Bethesda Md: 1985) 1989;67:862–70.
24. Constantinopol M, Jones JH, Weibel ER, Taylor CR, Lindholm A, Karas RH. Oxygen transport during exercise in large mammals. II. Oxygen uptake by the pulmonary gas exchanger. Journal of applied physiology (Bethesda Md: 1985) 1989;67:871–8.
25. Votion D, Navet R, Lacombe V, et al. Muscle energetics in exercising horses. Equine and Comparative Exerc Physiol 2008;4:105–18.
26. Weber JM, Brichon G, Zwingelstein G, et al. Design of the oxygen and substrate pathways. IV. Partitioning energy provision from fatty acids. The Journal of experimental biology 1996;199 (Pt 8):1667–74.
27. Achten J, Gleeson, M, Jeukendrup, AE. Determination of the exercise intensity that elicits maximal fat oxidation. Med Sci Sports Exerc 2002;34:92–7.

28. Weber JM, Roberts TJ, Vock R, Weibel ER, Taylor CR. Design of the oxygen and substrate pathways. III. Partitioning energy provision from carbohydrates. The Journal of experimental biology 1996;199 (Pt 8):1659–66.
29. Weibel ER, Taylor CR, Weber JM, Vock R, Roberts T, Hoppeler H. Design of the oxygen and substrate pathways. VII. Different structural limits for oxygen and substrate supply to muscle mitochondria. J Exp Biol 1996;199:1699–709.
30. Essen-Gustavsson B, McMiken D, Karlstrom K, Lindholm A, Persson SDG. Muscular adaptations of horses during intense training and detraining. Equine Vet J 1989;21:27–33.
31. Geor R, Hinchcliff K, Sams R. Glucose infusion attenuates endogenous glucose production and enhances glucose use of horses during exercise. J Appl Physiol 2000;88:1765–76.
32. Kayar SR, Hoppeler H, Lindstedt SL, et al. Total muscle mitochondrial volume in relation to aerobic capacity of horses and steers. Pflugers Archiv : European journal of physiology 1989;413:343–7.
33. Persson SDG. On blood volume and working capacity of horses. Acta Physiol Scan 1967;Suppl. 19:9–189.
34. McKeever KH, Hinchcliff KW, Reed SM, Hamlin RL. Splenectomy alters blood-pressure response to incremental treadmill exercise in horses. Amer J Physiol 1993;265:R409–R13.
35. Persson SG, Ekman L, Lydin G, Tufvesson G. Circulatory effects of splenectomy in the horse. II. Effect on plasma volume and total and circulating red-cell volume. Zentralblatt fur Veterinarmedizin Reihe A 1973;20:456–68.
36. Persson SG, Lydin G. Circulatory effects of splenectomy in the horse. 3. Effect on pulse-work relationship. Zentralblatt fur Veterinarmedizin Reihe A 1973;20: 521–30.
37. Wilson A, Watson J, Lichtwark G. A catapult action for rapid limb protraction. Nature 2003;421:35–6.
38. Hoyt D, Taylor CR. Gait and energetics of locomotion in horses. Nature 1981;292:239–40.
39. Minetti A, Ardigo L, Reinach E, Saibene F. The relationship between mechanical work and energy expenditure of locomotion in horses. J Exp Biol 1999;202:2329–38.
40. Votion D. Metabolic responses to exercise and training. In: Hinchcliff KW, Kaneps A, Geor RJ, editors. Equine Sports Medicine and Surgery: basic and clinical sciences of the equine athlete. London: Elsevier; 2013.
41. Kolk VD. Endocrine function during exercise and responses to training. In: Hinchcliff KW, Kaneps A, Geor RJ, editors. Equine Sports Medicine and Surgery: basic and clinical sciences of the equine athlete. London: Elsevier; 2013.
42. Poole DC, Erickson HH. Cardiovascular responses to exercise and training. In: Hinchcliff KW, Kaneps A, Geor RJ, editors. Equine Sports Medicine and Surgery. London: Elsevier; 2013.
43. Lindinger M. Acid-base responses to exercise and training. In: Hinchcliff KW, Kaneps A, Geor RJ, editors. Equine Sports Medicine and Surgery: basic and clinical sciences of the equine athlete. London: Elsevier; 2013.
44. McCutcheon L, Geor RJ. Thermoregulation and heat stress. In: Hinchcliff KW, Kaneps A, Geor RJ, editors. Equine Sports Medicine and Surgery: basic and clinical sciences of the equine athlete. London: Elseveir; 2013.
45. McGivney BA, McGettigan PA, Browne JA, et al. Characterization of the equine skeletal muscle transcriptome identifies novel functional responses to exercise training. BMC genomics 2010;11: 398.
46. McGivney BA, Browne JA, Fonseca RG, et al. MSTN genotypes in Thoroughbred horses influence skeletal muscle gene expression and racetrack performance. Animal Genetics 2012;43:810–12.
47. Hill E, Eivers S, McGivney B, et al. Moderate and high intensity sprint exercise induce differential responses in COX4I2 and PDK4 gene expression in Thoroughbred horse skeletal muscle. Equine Veterinary Journal 2010;42:576–81.
48. Viru A, Viru M. Nature of training effects. In: Garrett W, Kirkendall D, editors. Exercise and Sport Science. Philadelphia: Lippincott, Williams and Wilkins; 2000. p. 67–95.
49. McKenzie DC. Markers of excessive exercise. Canadian journal of applied physiology/Revue canadienne de physiologie appliquee 1999;24:66–73.
50. Petibois C, Cazorla G, Poortmans J-R, Deleris G. Biochemical aspects of overtraining in endurance sports: a review. Sports Med 2002;32:867–78.
51. MCGowan CM, Whitworth DJ. Overtraining syndrome in horses. Comparative Exercise Physiology 2008;5:57–65.
52. Tyler C, Golland LC, Evans DL, Hodgson DR, Rose RJ. Changes in maximum oxygen uptake during prolonged training, overtraining and detraining in horses. Journal of Applied Physiology 1996;81:2244–9.
53. Hamlin M, Shearman J, Hopkins W. Changes in physiological parameters in overtrained Standardbred racehorses. Equin Vet J 2002;34:383–8.
54. Lindstedt SL, Wells DJ, Jones J, Hoppeler H, Thronson HAJ. Limitations to aerobic performance in animals: interaction of structure and demand. Int J Sports Med 1988;9:210–7.
55. Reynolds A, Reinhart G, Carey D, Simmerman D, Frank D, Kallfelz F. Effect of protein intake during training on biochemical and performance variables in sled dogs. Am J Vet Res 1999;60:795–99.
56. Lindstedt SL, Hokanson JF, Wells DJ, Swain SD, Hoppeler H, Navarro V. Running energetics in the pronghorn antelope. Nature 1991;353:748–50.
57. Hinchcliff K, Reinhart G, Burr J, Schreier C, Swenson R. Metabolizable energy intake and sustained energy expenditure of Alaskan sled dogs during heavy exertion in the cold. American Journal of Veterinary Research 1997;58:1457–62.
58. Hill R, Bloomberg M, Legrand-Defretin V, et al. Maintenance energy requirements and the effect of diet on performance in racing greyhounds. Am J Vet Res 2000;61:1566–73.

Laboratory exercise testing

2

Samantha Franklin Kate Allen

CHAPTER CONTENTS

Introduction

The treadmill has been used for the scientific study of horses for over 100 years. Early studies were focused on energy metabolism in working horses using a rudimentary treadmill.[1–4] However, during the war years, research declined and subsequently mechanization reduced the need for horses to be used in agriculture. It was not until the 1960s that there was resurgence in equine research, coinciding with increased use of horses for pleasure and sporting pursuits.

The first high-speed treadmill for equine use was developed in the 1960s in Stockholm, Sweden.[5,6] The research group there, under the leadership of Sune Persson, was responsible for many of the early studies in equine exercise physiology and until the 1980s this was the only center to have these facilities. However, since that time, the use of high-speed treadmills has increased dramatically and is now used in many institutions throughout the world for exercise testing of equine athletes.[7]

Several types of exercise test have been described.[8] *Performance exercise tests* are typically performed on the apparently healthy population to provide guidance for fitness improvement or as a basis for training athletes. They are also used in research to determine the effects of interventions on performance parameters. *Clinical exercise tests* are primarily used for individuals presenting with signs of poor performance or disease. The exercise test is generally used for diagnostic purposes.

Exercise testing can be performed in the laboratory or in the field and there are advantages and disadvantages to both types.

Field exercise tests can provide quantitative and objective measures of exercise performance within the performance or clinical disciplines and several authors have described exercise protocols for horses.[9–12] Field exercise tests enable the horse to be examined in the environment in which it normally competes, a key advantage over treadmill exercise testing. Furthermore, field exercise tests enable the horse to be examined whilst ridden and with tack modifications that may influence clinical findings.[13,14] However, exercise protocols are difficult to standardize and the types of tests that can be performed are more limited than those available in the laboratory. Field exercise testing is discussed in detail in Chapter 3.

Laboratory exercise tests are undertaken in a controlled environment with sophisticated instruments enabling greater precision and accuracy in the measurement of a larger number of physiological response variables. The benefits of treadmill exercise testing for both equine and human athletes are that exercise tests can be standardized and readily controlled, and a wide range of measurements can be made with no restriction on the size of the equipment. Because of this, laboratory exercise tests remain the preferred technique whenever feasible for human athletes.[8] Treadmill exercise testing will be the focus of this chapter.

Indications for laboratory exercise testing in horses

Laboratory or treadmill exercise testing has been used extensively for research and for clinical exercise testing. Treadmill exercise testing has formed the basis of our knowledge of equine exercise physiology to date. Studies have been performed, covering a wide range of aspects relating to equine exercise. Many have been published in the proceedings of the International Conference on Equine Exercise Physiology that was first established in 1982 and is held on a quadrennial basis. These proceedings provide a valuable resource for exercise physiologists, veterinary surgeons and veterinary students alike.

Treadmill exercise testing for clinical diagnostic purposes in poorly performing equine athletes was first described in the early 1990s[15,16] and is now routinely performed at many centers throughout the world. It is primarily used to assess the effect on performance of abnormalities found on the resting examination or to determine the reasons for reduced athletic capacity in horses in which no abnormality can be identified on resting examination. Abnormalities affecting the cardiovascular and respiratory systems may only be manifest during strenuous exercise due to the large reserves in the resting horse. It is well known that assessment of the upper respiratory tract (URT) at rest is frequently inaccurate at predicting the events that occur during exercise.[17–20] Also some cardiac arrhythmias and musculoskeletal disorders may only become evident during intense exercise.[21,22] Furthermore, poor performance is often multifactorial and hence it is important to perform a thorough examination of all body systems before, during and after exercise.[21,23–25]

In human athletics, exercise testing is used routinely to assess performance. Measurement of maximal oxygen uptake (VO_{2max}) and anaerobic threshold are critical in the assessment of performance capacity (26). Similarly, in horses, information related to the functional capacities of the cardiorespiratory and musculoskeletal systems are considered to be the most valuable when attempting to evaluate performance potential. Several studies have shown that a high VO_{2max} is associated with superior performance in racehorses.[27–29] Despite this, the use of treadmill exercise testing for performance prediction, in horses, is not commonplace. More recently there has been a move towards investigating genetic markers of performance in both human[30] and equine athletes.[31,32] In particular, genes that affect muscular capacity have proven to be promising.[33–37]

Preparation for exercise testing

Horse preparation

Ideally horses should be suitably fit for the assessment being undertaken. If unfit at the time of assessment, horses may not be able to exercise at a sufficiently high intensity that would be necessary to illicit abnormalities. Furthermore, it may not be possible to achieve exercise intensities that would be reached during competition. For racehorses, it is suggested that the horse should be in condition and prepared for the clinical exercise testing as if it were the date of a race.[38] However, yearlings have been tested on high-speed treadmills without apparent problems.[39–42]

Before commencing the exercise test, a thorough clinical examination of all body systems should be conducted in order to rule out obvious disease. It is important that horses are evaluated for lameness prior to exercise testing for two reasons. Firstly, lameness may be the reason for poor athletic performance and secondly, there is the potential to exacerbate any pre-existing lameness during high-speed exercise. Mild lameness is a common finding in racehorses referred for poor performance investigation[21,23] and it is often difficult to convince trainers or owners that the lameness might be the cause of the poor performance. Furthermore, as described previously, poor athletic performance is frequently multifactorial and hence it may be important to determine whether or not other conditions are contributing to the poor performance. In such cases it is important to carefully weigh up the potential advantages of performing a complete examination with the potential disadvantage of exacerbating the pre-existing lameness.

When performing treadmill exercise, it is recommended that horses be shod in order to prevent foot soreness. Friction associated with the movement of the foot against the treadmill belt results in heat build up and may lead to secondary foot problems in horses undergoing repeated exercise sessions.[43] It is not uncommon for loose shoes to come off during treadmill exercise resulting in a potential risk of injury to the horse or to any persons who may be positioned behind the treadmill. It is therefore important that shoes are checked before commencing exercise and any loose shoes removed and refitted. Studs should also be removed in order to reduce wear on the treadmill belt.

Treadmill instrumentation/equipment

A number of companies now manufacture high-speed equine treadmills throughout the world. The main requirements are the ability to incline to a slope of 10% (6°) and to reach speeds of 14–15 m/s, with rapid acceleration. Treadmills may be mounted in a pit in the ground or above ground and at least 4–5 m of space in front of, behind and on either side of the treadmill is needed to allow for equipment, personnel and to enable the horse to move on and off the treadmill.[43] It is thought that treadmills situated in the ground are safer.[43]

The room in which the treadmill is housed should ideally have full climatic control with large fans placed in front and overhead to prevent excessive hyperthermia during exercise (Fig. 2.1). It has

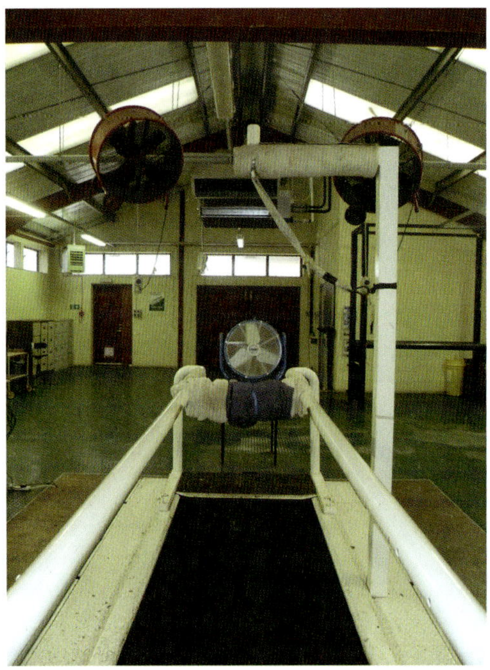

Fig 2.1 Sato high-speed treadmill with fans and air conditioning unit above and in front of horse. A safety harness, connected to an emergency stop is attached to a beam overhead.

been shown that horses undertaking treadmill exercise reach higher temperatures than horses exercising overground[44] and this is likely to reflect the reduced capacity for convective heat loss during treadmill exercise. Both the velocity and volume of air moved by the fans need to be taken into account. Air velocity should match that at which the horse is exercising and fans of at least 50 cm diameter are normally required to generate sufficient volume.[45]

The use of a safety harness, whilst not essential, is strongly recommended during exercise. This will ensure that horses do not come off the back of the treadmill should they stop suddenly. An emergency stop should also be available in order to stop the treadmill belt if the horse gets into difficulties. Finally, it is recommended that horses be fitted with boots in order to minimize the risk of injury to the limbs, particularly during training when they are not yet fully accustomed to treadmill exercise (Fig. 2.2). Overreach wounds and grazes to the limbs are the most common form of injury incurred during treadmill exercise.[46]

Acclimation to treadmill exercise

Although treadmill exercise may on first appearance seem alien, horses readily adapt to treadmill exercise, with less than 1% of tests abandoned because of behavioral issues.[43,46] It is recommended that horses undergo a period of training or acclimation before commencing exercise testing. The aim is to introduce the horse to exercising in a novel environment, improve coordination and hence reduce risk of injury and to reduce anxiety and excitement that might otherwise influence any physiological parameters being measured.

The most important part of the familiarization process is to have a competent horse handling team. When introducing a horse to the treadmill for the first time it is useful to have at least four people involved, including two handlers (one on each side). In addition, one person will be required to control the treadmill and an additional person may be required to encourage the horse to move forward (Fig. 2.3). During subsequent sessions one handler is likely to be sufficient. The protocol that we have used successfully at our center is as follows:

- The initial phase involves walking the horse onto the stationary treadmill and asking it to walk forwards and backwards repeatedly until it is accustomed to its surroundings and is used to starting and stopping on command.
- The horse is then removed from the treadmill and the treadmill is started, so that the horse becomes accustomed to the noise.
- Following this, the treadmill is stopped, the horse walked on to the treadmill and it is restarted with the horse in position. Once the horse is walking comfortably, the speed can be gradually increased.

When naïve horses are first introduced to treadmill exercise, they adapt a wide-based stance and typically lower the hindquarters and withers.[47] However, during the first two minutes a rapid adaptation occurs and by five minutes horses are able to stabilize their gaits.[47] During subsequent sessions, horses stabilize more quickly although there may be considerable variation between individuals.

The number of training sessions varies between clinics. Some perform acclimation runs over several days, whilst others do not perform extensive training prior to clinical exercise testing.[46] The number of acclimation runs performed will depend on the individual horse's ability to adapt to treadmill exercise, whether or not it has previously been exposed to treadmill exercise during routine training and the type of tests being performed.

Changes in behavioral responses and physiological parameters such as heart rate and plasma lactate concentrations occur following a period of acclimation and this is important to consider if you intend to make physiological measurements during the exercise test. King et al.[48] found that, in general, one acclimating run resulted in reasonably consistent submaximal heart rate and plasma lactate concentrations although there was significant inter-horse variation. Subjectively it was believed that most horses benefited from a second training run. Rose and Hodgson[49] reported that for reproducible results, at least four training runs were necessary. However, in another report, the same authors suggest that repeated treadmill exposure may have an adverse effect on acclimation, due

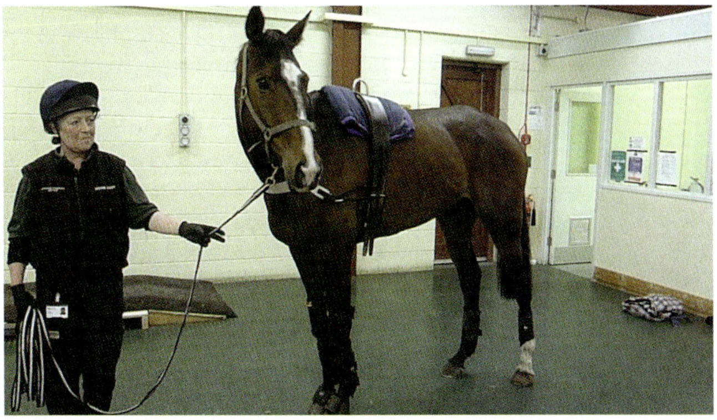

Fig 2.2 Horse and handler appropriately equipped for treadmill exercise. The horse wears surcingle (which gets attached to the treadmill safety harness) and breastplate, brushing boots, knee boots and overreach boots. Horses can be tested off the bridle or headcollar.

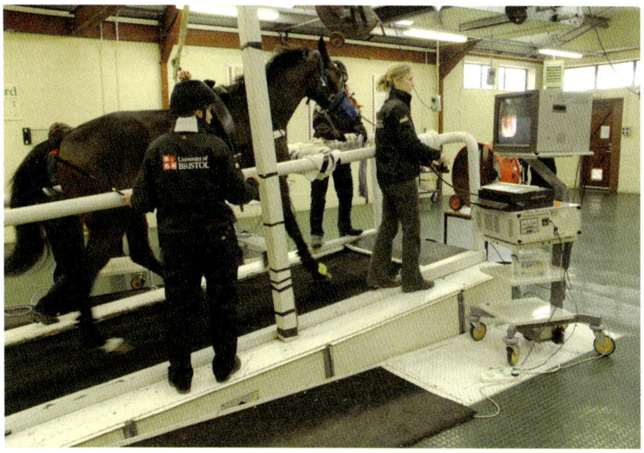

Fig 2.3 A Thoroughbred racehorse undergoing high-speed treadmill testing on a 10% incline. Equipment is positioned either side. In this instance there is one handler, one technician at the horses hindquarters to the left side manning the controls and one technician at the hindquarters on the right also encouraging the horse if required. One veterinary surgeon is performing the endoscopy and a second veterinary surgeon is on the other side of the horse, observing the horse's locomotion, the ECG recording and respiratory measurements. The horse is fitted with a respiratory mask in order to measure respiratory parameters on a breath-by-breath basis whilst upper airway endoscopy is performed concurrently.

to increased apprehension and excitement in anticipation of exercise.[48] We therefore recommend that horses receive two or three acclimation runs prior to exercise testing but that final decisions should be based on individual animal's ability to adapt to treadmill exercise. For horses that will be required to wear a respiratory mask during clinical exercise testing, a training session with the mask in place is recommended.

Treadmill safety

During any exercise at high-speed there is a potential risk of injury to the horse. A recent multicenter retrospective study investigated the risk of injury in 2305 horses undergoing treadmill exercise testing.[46] The risk of major injury (such as a fracture, tendon injury or severe myopathy) was 0.6%, whilst the risk of minor injury was 4.7%. Similarly, another report suggested that substantial injuries (e.g. tendon injuries) occurred in less than 1.5% horses and other injuries occur in less than 5% of horses.[43] These injury rates are, in fact, not dissimilar to those sustained during high-speed exercise during racing[50,51] and eventing.[52] Furthermore, in an earlier study in which comparisons were made between racehorses that were trained predominately on the track or on the treadmill, the treadmill group were perceived to have lower injury rates.[53]

Anecdotally, it has been suggested that horses may be at increased risk of tendon injury when exercising on a treadmill. However, in the study performed by Franklin et al.[46] there were only two cases of tendon injury following treadmill exercise. A previous study by Takahashi et al.[54] found that the peak forces in the superficial digital flexor tendon (SDFT) were lower during inclined running compared to the flat and hence uphill exercise (as is often performed on a treadmill) may reduce the risk of SDFT injury. Similarly, stress fractures were identified in only three horses. It has been found that bone strain is 75% less during gallop on a high-speed treadmill than that measured on a woodchip track.[55] Also, in human athletes, significantly higher tension and compression strains and strain rates have been measured in the tibia during overground running compared with treadmill running, suggesting that treadmill runners are in fact at a reduced risk of tibial stress fracture than overground runners.[56]

The most common injuries incurred by horses during treadmill exercise are due to abrasions and overreach injuries.[46] The risk of injury can be minimized by using an experienced handling team, providing adequate training before exercise testing, ensuring shoes are firmly fitted and that appropriate protective clothing, such as boots are fitted and making use of a safety harness.

Exercise test protocols

Whatever the reason for exercise testing, it is important that standardized procedures are followed so that data can be compared against subsequent tests for the same horse or with measurements from other horses of similar age and fitness level.

In human exercise testing, three factors are found to contribute to a good performance test[57] and these can also be applied to equine exercise testing:

1. validity: the protocol resembles the performance that is being simulated as closely as possible
2. reliability: the protocol provides a similar result from day to day when no intervention is used
3. sensitivity: the protocol is able to detect small but important changes in performance.

Validity of treadmill exercise testing

Clearly treadmill exercise testing will always struggle in terms of validity due to the lack of a rider and differences between treadmill and track surfaces. In fact, Evans[58] went as far as to state that attempts to design treadmill exercise tests to replicate competition conditions may be a fruitless endeavor. Several studies have shown that there are significant differences in locomotion and physiological responses between treadmill and overground exercise.[59] There are differences in stride and stance duration during treadmill locomotion,[60,61] likely associated with changes in belt velocity during hoof impact.[62] Furthermore, the energetic cost of locomotion is lower on the treadmill. Hence it is not surprising that many studies have found that both heart rates and blood lactate levels are lower in horses exercising on a level treadmill compared with exercise at the same speeds on the track.[44,63–65] These differences may be compensated for by increasing the treadmill speed by approximately 10%[64] or by increasing the incline by 2.4–3.7%.[63,66,67] In humans, it has been found that running on a 1% incline is more representative of the energy cost of running outdoors.[68] The increased cost of locomotion during outdoor running has been attributed to the need to overcome air resistance.[69] Other factors such as the stiffness of the treadmill itself may also influence the economic cost of locomotion.[70] For horses, it is necessary to increase the incline further to account for the lack of a rider or harness during treadmill exercise. Metabolic workload can be increased by increasing the load carried.[71] However, inclined running results in a much greater increase in metabolic rate than increasing the load.[71] The oxygen cost of running on a 10% incline has been calculated to be 2.5 times greater at any speed than running on the level.[72,73] During clinical exercise testing, inclines are commonly increased up to 10% making these tests more strenuous than routine field exercise tests.[74–76]

Treadmill reliability and sensitivity

Research in human athletes has shown that time-to-exhaustion exercise tests have a coefficient of variation (CV) of >10%, whereas time trials have been shown to have a CV of <5%. A sensitive protocol is one that is able to detect small changes in performance. The difference between finishing first and second in human sporting events is suggested to be <1%.[57] Therefore, it is important to be able to detect small changes with performance protocols. The repeatability/reliability of equine treadmill exercise tests is not well investigated. However, treadmill exercise testing has the advantage over field exercise testing in that it is much easier to standardize the exercise test. Factors such as treadmill speed, environmental conditions and the running surface can be replicated on multiple occasions. The reliability and sensitivity of treadmill exercise tests will depend to a greater extent on the reliability and sensitivity of the equipment being used to measure physiological parameters rather than the treadmill exercise protocol per se. Variability in measurements may also arise due to factors such as operator differences in the timing of measurements and the time taken to reach steady state values. Variables that depend on regression coefficients from the results of measurements made during submaximal exercise are likely to show increased variability compared to maximal values. Factors such as excitement and anticipation of exercise that cause release of adrenalin, may result in artificial increases in physiological parameters such as heart rate, blood lactate and PCV during submaximal exercise and hence adequate time for acclimation to treadmill exercise is important.

Several studies have been performed to assess the repeatability of measurements made during treadmill exercise tests. However, there are difficulties when making comparisons between papers as different measurements of variability are used. Measurements of HR_{max} have been found to have coefficients of variation between 0–7%.[15,77,78] A number of studies have examined the repeatability of VO_{2max} and values between 1 and 11% have been reported.[15,77–79] Studies examining the repeatability of blood lactate measurements have had conflicting results, with one study reporting a wide variability (21.4%) in peak blood lactate concentrations[15] whilst another study found only a 2–11% variability.[80]

Main types of exercise test protocols

Two main types of exercise testing protocols have been described in horses: The *incremental standardized exercise test* and the *high-speed single step exercise test*. Both are performed after an initial warm-up phase. The incremental exercise test was first described by Seeherman and Morris[15] and since that time this protocol has been adopted for clinical exercise testing. It involves the treadmill speed being increased typically every 60 sec (Table 2.1). Physiological measurements can be made at the end of each speed step in order to examine the relationship with speed. Depending on the requirements for the test, this protocol may be terminated at submaximal intensities or may be continued until the horse fatigues. The latter is important when determining maximal values of oxygen uptake and heart rate as well as for ruling out possible cardiorespiratory causes of poor performance.

During experimental trials and clinical exercise testing of Thoroughbred racehorses, tests are frequently performed on an inclined treadmill (up to 10%). This allows for exercise intensity to be increased without the need to attain excessively fast speeds.[15,84] A 10% slope provides a compromise between a steep slope that would be unrepresentative of track exercise and faster speeds that may compromise horse safety.[49] Inclined running does not appear to affect stride length or duration.[60,85,86] However, there are changes in hindlimb kinematics and muscles are recruited differently when exercising on a slope, because the hindlimbs have to carry more weight and provide greater propulsion.[86–88] Also, it has been shown that exercising on a 10% gradient results in significantly greater maximal values for cardiac output[89] and oxygen consumption,[90] and this should be taken into account when comparing results from different exercise trials.

It is acknowledged that the incremental exercise test does not reproduce racing conditions. Nevertheless this type of testing has been used extensively for clinical evaluation of racehorses. The number of steps completed and the total run time provide an index of performance capacity and degree of fitness. It has been argued that the incremental test may not be an accurate assessment of a racehorse exercising over sprint distances of a mile or less. Data analyzed at our center has indicated that National Hunt racehorses reached higher speed steps than flat racehorses during incremental step tests[91] confirming that this type of exercise test has a substantial stamina component and is appropriate for testing of horses that run over longer distances (>1 mile). However, since flat racehorses reach faster speeds during racing, a more appropriate test for sprinters would be to start the exercise test at close to maximal speeds and maintain this until the horse fatigues.[81] Several centers therefore use a high-speed single step exercise test for clinical exercise testing of sprint racehorses. Again, this may be performed on a level or inclined treadmill (Table 2.1). Speeds and distances for Thoroughbred and Standardbred racing are included in Table 2.2.

Table 2.2 Typical speeds and distances covered during racing

BREED (RACING TYPE)	DISTANCE	MEAN SPEED
[1]QH	302–402 m	70.7 km/h
[1]TB	402 m	65.5 km/h
[1]TB	1006 m	50.4 km/h
[2]TB flat	<1609 m	58 km/h
[2]TB flat	>1609 m	56 km/h
[2]TB NH	Up to 4022 m	50 km/h
[2]TB NH	>4022 m	48 km/h
[3,4]SB (pace)	1600 m[4]	45–49 km/h
[3,5]SB (trot)	2000–4400 m	45–48 km/h
[1]Arab	1006 m	46 km/h

[1]Nielsen et al 2006,[92] [2]Allen & Franklin 2010,[91] [3]Physick-Sheard, 1986,[93] [4]Soma et al. 2000,[94] [5]LeuLeu et al 2005.[95]
QH, Quarter Hose; TB, Thoroughbred; NH, National Hunt; SB, Standardbed.

Table 2.1 Exercise test protocols for clinical exercise testing in racehorses

EXERCISE TEST	INCLINE	TIME/ SPEED
*Incremental exercise test for Thoroughbred National Hunt and flat horses > 1 mile	10%	1 minute at 6, 8, and 10 m/s, followed by 1 m/s increases at 1 minute intervals until fatigue
*High-speed test for Thoroughbred flat, sprint horses	10%	Rapidly increase to 11–12 m/s, stay at this speed until fatigue
[1]High-speed test for Thoroughbred flat horses and Standardbreds	0–4%	Rapidly increase to 11–14.5 m/s, stay at this speed until fatigue
[2]Incremental exercise test for Standardbreds	0–4%	Three steps of 2–3 minutes each performed at speeds of 7.0, 9.0 and 10.5 or 11.0 m/s. Between each step horses recover for 1–2 minutes at walk (1.8 m/s) or trot (4.5 m/s).

*Typical exercise tests performed at the University of Bristol Equine Sports Medicine Centre.
[1]Data from Parente et al 1996;[81] Durando et al., 2002[82] and Strand et al 2012.[83]
[2]Data from Richard et al. 2010[75] and Courouce-Malblanc et al, 2000.[67]

For non-Thoroughbred racehorses, exercise tests tend to be performed at slower speeds and on a lower incline. The exact testing protocols vary. For Standardbreds or trotters, the incline is generally set lower (0–4%) than for Thoroughbred racehorses. This is because at high speeds, the energy cost of trotting is greater than that associated with galloping[96] and therefore a lower slope is needed to produce similar physiological responses to those experienced on the track, in comparison with gallopers.[67] Also, these horses may not be able to complete the exercise test if the incline is set at 4% or higher[67] or may break into non-racing gaits.[82] A typical incremental standardized exercise test for Standardbreds involves fewer steps of longer duration (2–3 minutes) with recovery periods, at walk or trot, between steps[46,67,75] whilst a single step high-speed test for these horses would involve them running at speeds of 11–14 m/s on the level or 8–11 m/s on a slight incline for a period of 3–5 minutes[82,83] (Table 2.1).

For other sport horses the exact protocol will depend on the discipline and the fitness of the horse. Again, it is important to recreate the conditions (speeds and distances) that would be encountered during competition. (Values for speed and distances encountered during international eventing are shown in Table 2.3). It is also important to note that for sport horses and harness racehorses it is necessary to recreate the degree of head and neck flexion that is incurred during exercise, especially when evaluating upper respiratory tract (URT) function, since poll flexion has been shown to be an important factor for inducing dynamic airway collapse in these horses.[14,83,97–99] During treadmill exercise, head and neck flexion can be imposed by the use of side reins or applying tension to long reins.

Selecting the optimal treadmill exercise test protocol

For experimental studies, the exercise protocol used will depend on the experimental design and the parameters of interest. When designing a clinical exercise test, a number of factors should be considered:

1. indication for performing the test
2. nature of competition/race
3. status of horse (breed, age, level of fitness, training history)
4. presenting complaint.

The exercise test should be structured and the protocol recorded so that the test can be repeated in the future allowing the effects of any subsequent interventions to be studied. For many situations the aim will be for the exercise test to be at least as strenuous as competition conditions. This is particularly important for those horses that only show signs of poor performance during racing. At the end of the test the veterinary surgeon needs to be confident that if no abnormality is seen under the test conditions, then no abnormality would be present under race conditions. Indeed we have found that incremental treadmill exercise tests had some benefits over field exercise testing since it is easier to perform a more strenuous test on the treadmill.[76,91] Consequently, a diagnosis of dorsal displacement of the soft palate was underestimated in horses undergoing overground endoscopy compared with those undergoing treadmill endoscopy.[76]

Table 2.3 Speeds and distances covered during FEI three-day eventing competitions (cross country phase)

LEVEL	AVERAGE SPEED	DISTANCE (M)
CCI*	520 mpm (~19 mph)	3640–4680
CCI**	550 mpm (~20 mph)	4400–5500
CCI***	570 mpm (~21 mph)	5130–6270
CCI****	570 mpm (~21 mph)	5700–6840

Measurements that can be made during treadmill exercise testing

A large number of measurements are possible during treadmill exercise testing and a comprehensive review has been provided by Evans.[100]

Measurements of performance capacity

Aerobic capacity – measurement of the maximal rate of oxygen consumption

Aerobic capacity can be measured by calculation of maximal oxygen consumption (VO_{2max}). Determination of VO_{2max} is one of the most commonly performed tests when assessing athletic performance in man, particularly for longer distance, endurance events.[26,101,102] As the distance increases, VO_{2max} becomes a more important predictor of performance.[101] However, other factors are also important including locomotor efficiency and the percentage of VO_{2max} that can be sustained during prolonged exercise.[103,104] In horses, VO_{2max} has been shown to be correlated with running speed in Thoroughbreds[27] and a higher VO_{2max} has been found in superior Standardbred racehorses compared with slower performing horses.[29] However, similar to findings in man, it is likely that many other factors also contribute to elite athletic performance.[28]

Maximal oxygen consumption is calculated during an incremental exercise test. Oxygen consumption (VO_2) increases linearly with speed up until VO_{2max}, which is defined as the point where no further increase in VO_2 is elicited despite further increases in speed (Fig. 2.4). Oxygen consumption can be measured in exercising horses using a number of methods; either through the use of open

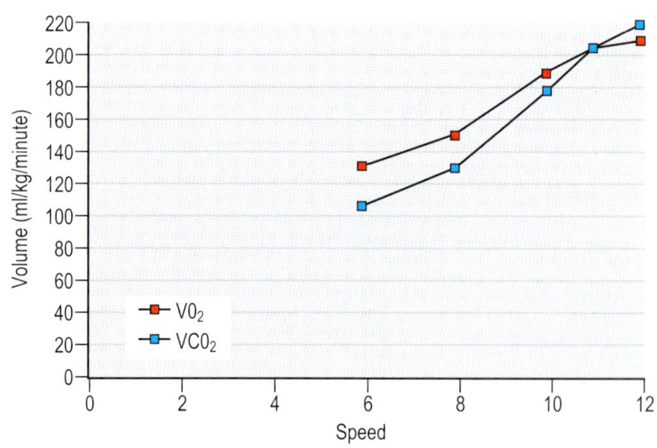

Fig 2.4 Oxygen uptake (VO_2) and carbon dioxide production (VCO_2) during exercise: Mean values from normal Thoroughbred horses undergoing exercise testing at the University of Bristol. Values were obtained with horses exercising on a 10% incline.

or biased flow systems[16,77,105] or breath-by-breath systems.[78,106,107] The latter have the advantage that they can also be used to measure ventilatory volumes and pulmonary mechanics. Maximal VO_2 values greater than 200 ml/kg/min have been measured in Thoroughbred racehorses.

Measurement of carbon dioxide production (VCO_2) is usually made concurrently with measurement of VO_2 (Fig. 2.4). Carbon dioxide production increases as a result of bicarbonate (HCO_3^-) buffering of hydrogen ions (H^+) produced from the dissociation of lactic acid. The gas exchange threshold (TGE) occurs at the point where VCO_2 starts to increase at a greater rate than VO_2, resulting in a deviation from linearity.[108] In humans, this is closely related to the lactate threshold (LT). However, in horses the TGE occurs after LT due to the enhanced buffering capacity in equine muscle by non-bicarbonate buffers.[109]

In some circumstances it may not be possible to measure oxygen consumption and hence other parameters may be useful in determining aerobic capacity. These include measurements of heart rate and blood lactate.

Heart rate

Measurement of heart rate during exercise is easy to perform using a heart rate monitor. Again there is a linear relationship between HR and speed, up until the maximal heart rate (HR_{max}) is achieved (Fig. 2.5). HR_{max} varies greatly between individuals and may be influenced by factors such as age, gender, breed and level of fitness.[110]

Although there is no correlation between VO_{2max} and HR_{max} per se, there is a close correlation between percentage of maximal heart rate and percentage of VO_{2max}.[111] The speed at which HR_{max} is reached (V_{HRmax}) is also significantly correlated with VO_{2max} and hence is a suitable measure of fitness in cases where VO_2 cannot be measured.[111] Individuals with the greatest athletic capacity will reach HR_{max} at the greatest speeds and a correlation has been shown between V_{HRmax} and race earnings.[112] Other parameters such as the velocity at a heart rate of 200 bpm (V_{200}) may be measured during submaximal exercise tests. However, these values are less useful predictors of maximal aerobic work capacity since HR_{max} is quite variable between individuals and hence horses may be exercising at quite different proportions of their HR_{max} at a set heart rate value.

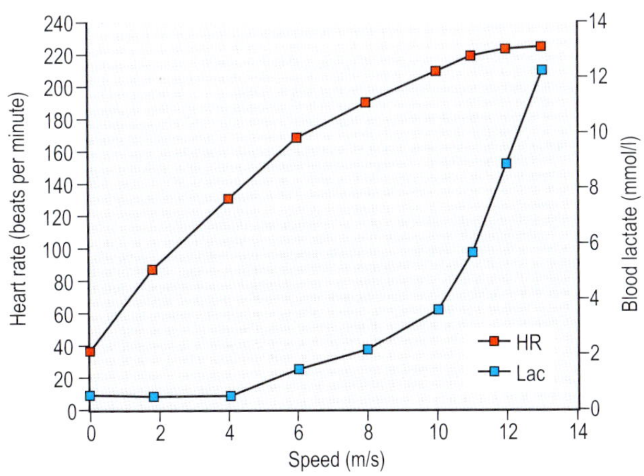

Fig 2.5 Heart rate and blood lactate responses to exercise. Mean data from Thoroughbred horses undergoing clinical exercise testing at the University of Bristol. Values were obtained with horses exercising on a 10% incline.

Blood lactate

Measurement of blood lactate concentrations can provide information relating to both the horse's aerobic and anaerobic capacity. Samples are usually taken by jugular venepuncture, into tubes containing fluoride-oxalate as an anticoagulant. A method for taking samples from the skin, using a lancet has also been described.[113] There are differences between whole blood and plasma lactate concentrations, with the plasma lactate concentration approximately 1.5 times greater than that of whole blood, although there is a large variation between individuals due to variable uptake of lactate by red blood cells.[114–116] Therefore it is recommended that whole blood be used for lactate measurements after exercise.[117] Samples can be analyzed using a bench top standard analyzer or a portable lactate meter. The latter are convenient for field studies but have a lower accuracy and are less suitable for scientific studies.[45,118]

Lactate is produced as a result of anaerobic muscle metabolism. At rest blood lactate levels are 0.5–1 mmol/l. The onset of blood lactate accumulation (OBLA) is considered to occur at the speed at which the horse's blood lactate concentration reaches 4 mmol/l (V_4). After this speed, a more rapid increase in blood lactate concentration is observed in response to further increases in speed as lactate production exceeds utilization. Determination of blood lactate curves and V_4 can be made from measurements taken during an incremental exercise test on the treadmill, with samples being taken during the last 10 seconds of each speed step (Fig. 2.5).

The OBLA or V_4 is also referred to as the lactate threshold or the aerobic-anaerobic threshold and is a useful indicator of aerobic capacity.[119,120] Several studies have confirmed that a high V_4 is associated with superior performance.[95,120,121] Also, plasma lactate concentrations following a submaximal exercise test have been found to be negatively correlated with performance.[80,122,123] It is likely that OBLA is far more important in 'stayers' and endurance athletes than in sprinters, due to the increased reliance of these horses on aerobic energy supply.[117]

Anaerobic capacity

The measurement of post-exercise lactate concentration gives an indication of anaerobic capacity[117] and in human athletes higher lactates are an indicator of superior sprinting ability.[124,125] Some equine studies have also found that blood lactate rises more rapidly and reaches higher concentrations in faster horses[27,126,127] and higher post-exercise blood lactate has been correlated with superior performance in Standardbred trotters.[128] There is also evidence that increased uptake of lactate into red blood cells is associated with superior performance.[128] It has been suggested that increased transport of lactate from the plasma into RBCs results in reduced plasma lactate levels, thereby facilitating lactate outflow from the muscles.[115] Individual variability in monocarboxylate transporters not only occurs in RBC membranes but also in muscle cells, greatly influencing lactate accumulation during exercise.[129] This may explain why some horses fatigue sooner than others.

Maximal blood lactate production is most repeatable after a standardized intense exercise test to fatigue rather than an incremental test.[125] Peak blood lactate concentrations in horses may reach levels in excess of 30 mmol/l after maximal exercise.[130,131] Depending on the intensity of exercise, peak lactate levels may not occur for 5–10 minutes after cessation of exercise due to efflux from muscle[132] and therefore the timing at which samples are taken is important. In general, it is recommended that samples are taken five minutes post-exercise.[117]

Estimation of anaerobic power is more complex than aerobic power. Aerobic power can be readily quantified by measurement of the rate of O_2 consumption and the stoichiometric knowledge that combustion of oxygen yields approximately 20.1 J/ml O_2 (STPD). Two methods have been described to estimate the net anaerobic energy utilization (NAEU) during exercise: the maximal accumulated O_2 deficit (MAOD) and the plasma lactate accumulation rate (PLAR). The MAOD technique calculates the deficit between the measured aerobic energy supplied and the total metabolic energy required during maximal exercise to fatigue, extrapolated from the measured submaximal VO_2.[72] The PLAR technique calculates the aerobic power equivalent of a given PLAR by calculating the ratio of their inverse changes when VO_{2max} is changed by altering the inspired O_2 fraction.[133] Ohmura et al.[134] compared these techniques and found that although they were highly correlated, $NAEU_{PLAR}$ was on average 40% greater than $NAEU_{AOD.}$ These authors suggested that MAOD may underestimate the total energy cost during high-speed galloping.

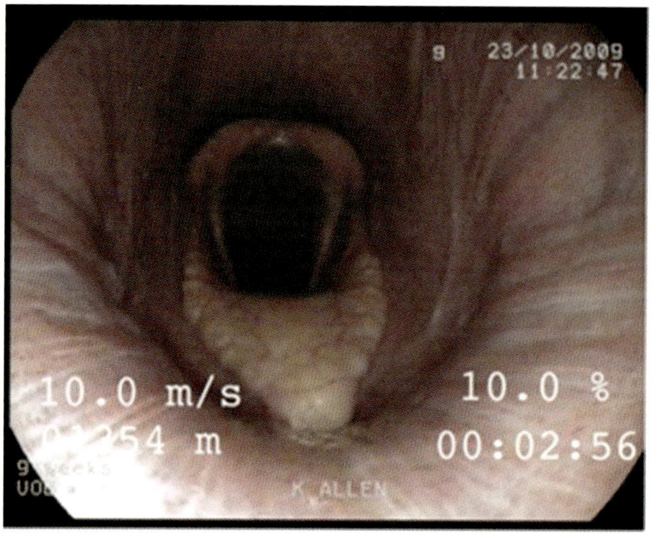

Fig 2.6 Configuration of the system so that performance data (speed, incline, distance, time) can be superimposed onto the endoscopic image.

Clinical exercise testing

Assessment of the respiratory tract

Endoscopic examination

Videoendoscopy of the URT is one of the most commonly performed clinical procedures during high-speed treadmill exercise (Fig. 2.3). It is now widely accepted that resting endoscopy is not necessarily a reliable indicator of events occurring during exercise.[17–20] This is because of the large differences in airflow rates and airway pressures that occur during exercise compared with at rest. A detailed description of the different forms of dynamic airway collapse that may occur during exercise is provided in Chapter 26.

Positioning of the endoscope is critical. If the endoscope is positioned too far caudally, it may not be possible to identify the presence of pharyngeal wall collapse or palatal instability. Whilst if positioned too far rostrally, it may be difficult to identify all the structures associated with the larynx (e.g. the vocal cords) and beyond (e.g. the cricotracheal membrane). Ideally, the tip of the endoscope should be positioned such that the tip of the epiglottis and a portion of the soft palate are clearly visible.[135] In Thoroughbred horses, this is approximately 40 cm from the nostril. It is also useful to overlay information relating to the exercise test on the endoscopic image, so that the timing of events within the upper airway can be clearly identified during subsequent review of the video-recording after the completion of the exercise test (Fig. 2.6).

Respiratory sound recording and analysis

Often respiratory sounds are measured concurrently with the videoendoscopy recording. This can be performed using a microphone placed in front of the horse's nostrils, either within a mask or attached to the bridle. The recording of respiratory sounds is useful to relate the sounds being reported by the owner or trainer with dynamic events occurring within the airway. Previously, there was some interest in the use of spectral analysis of respiratory sounds for the diagnosis of upper airway collapse[136–138] and repeated recordings have been used to measure changes in respiratory sounds following laryngeal surgery.[139,140] However, although it is possible to determine differences between conditions such as laryngeal hemiplegia and DDSP, the technique is not sufficiently sensitive to distinguish between different forms of inspiratory noise or horses with complex forms of dynamic collapse.

Respiratory function testing

Whilst videoendoscopy enables visualization of any dynamic airway collapse, it does not enable us to quantify the functional effects of an obstruction. It has been suggested that to definitively assess any respiratory limitation, it is necessary to measure upper airway mechanics.[141] Upper airway obstructions may result in an increase in the resistance along the URT, which may result in either reduced airflow or an increase in the trans-upper airway pressures required to maintain airflow.[142,143] Where airflow is reduced, the resulting hypoventilation may lead to decreased oxygen consumption, increased blood lactate concentration and exacerbation of arterial hypoxaemia and hypercapnia. Such findings have been confirmed in horses with experimentally induced and naturally occurring DDSP[25,144–146] and laryngeal hemiplegia.[147–156] Pharyngeal collapse is also associated with blood gas abnormalities although the effects on airflow have not been reported.[82]

Lower airway disease may also influence parameters measured during exercise despite horses having no obvious signs at rest. Horses with inflammatory airway disease (IAD) have been found to have increased blood lactate concentrations[25,157] and display more severe exercise-induced hypoxaemia[157,158] than healthy controls. These abnormalities may be further exacerbated in horses with a combination of upper and lower airway disorders.[24,25,158]

Methods of pulmonary function testing

Pulmonary function testing undoubtedly yields valuable information relating to the functional significance of respiratory disorders. However, its use has been limited during clinical exercise testing due to limited availability of the technology required. Most of the methods described are therefore used more commonly for research purposes.

A number of methods have been described for the measurement of ventilatory volumes and airflows using spirometry.[78,100,106,107,159] These are described in detail in Chapter 27. Currently, most systems are only suitable for use in a laboratory setting. The horse is required to wear a facemask in order to measure respiratory airflow on a breath-by-breath basis (Fig. 2.7). The measurement of airflow may be achieved through resistance or differential pressure pneumotachometers, ultrasonic transducers or pitot tubes that are incorporated within the face mask. The resulting data can be used to determine the tidal volume, breathing frequency, minute ventilation and peak inspiratory and expiratory flow rates. Tidal breathing flow volume loops (TBFVL) can also be constructed and may provide useful information relating to the degree of upper airway obstruction (Fig. 2.8).[142,146,160–164]

By combining ventilation measurements with expired gas concentrations, measured by mass spectrometry, it is possible to calculate VO_2 and VCO_2 as described previously. Furthermore, pulmonary and upper airway mechanics may be evaluated by making simultaneous measurements of airflow and airway or oesophageal pressures. This enables calculation of parameters such as work of breathing, total pulmonary resistance, upper airway resistance and dynamic lung compliance.[106,165]

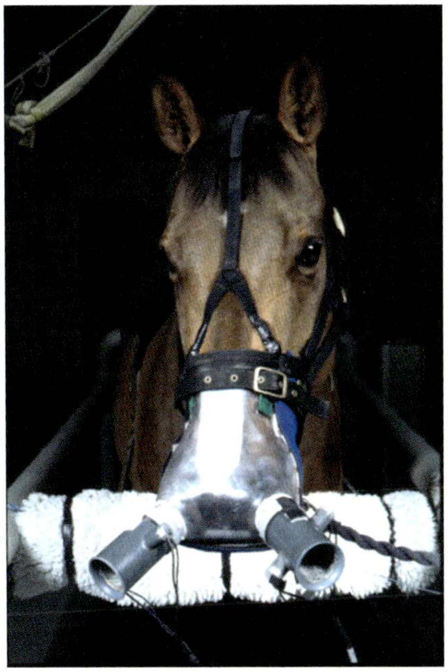

Fig 2.7 Horse fitted with facemask and ultrasonic flow transducers for measurement of respiratory parameters on a breath-by-breath basis.

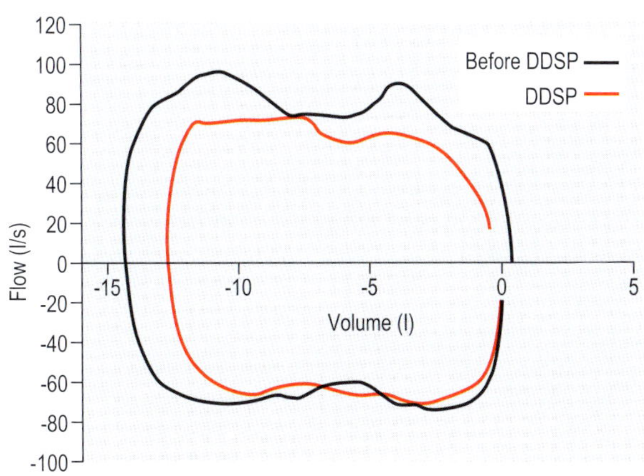

Fig 2.8 Tidal breathing flow volume loop before and during DDSP. Expiration is positive, inspiration is negative.

Measurement of blood gases

Measurement of venous blood gases reveals little or nothing concerning gas exchange during exercise. Measurement of arterial blood gases, however, is frequently performed during exercise in order to assess gas exchange and examine the extent of hypoxaemia and hypercapnia. It is important to draw samples whilst the horse is exercising since rapid changes occur once exercise has ceased and therefore arterial blood sampling immediately after exercise is usually of limited value. Whilst methods for arterial blood gas sampling during field exercise have been described,[166–168] this is generally not practical in the clinical setting and hence blood gas analysis is most commonly performed during treadmill exercise.

Collection of arterial blood is commonly performed via catheterization of the facial artery (Fig 2.9), although for research studies, catheterization of a translocated carotid artery may be performed. Sample collection must be performed anaerobically into heparinized syringes since, if air is introduced into the syringe, overestimation of O_2 and underestimation of CO_2 will occur. Samples should be stored on ice and analyzed promptly. Underestimation of blood gas values may also occur if the samples are not corrected for core body temperature.[169]

Unfortunately, interpretation of arterial blood gases is complicated by the fact that normal horses become hypoxaemic and hypercapnoeic during strenuous exercise. At rest, PaO_2 is approximately 100 mmHg and $PaCO_2$ is approx. 45 mmHg. During strenuous exercise, PaO_2 may decrease to 65–70 mmHg during strenuous exercise whilst $PaCO_2$ rises by 5–10 mmHg.[107,166,170] Hypoxaemia and hypercapnoea are more evident in trained horses and horses with a higher $\dot{V}O_{2max}$ when compared with less fit or less able athletes.[171,172] Therefore, it is important to make concurrent measurements of VO_{2max} in order to fully interpret blood gas data.

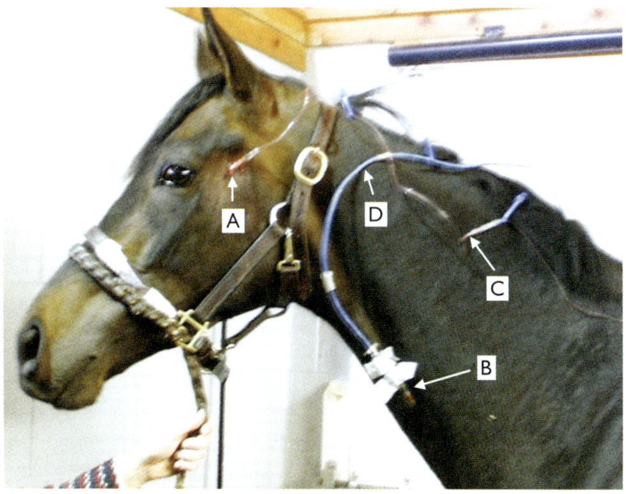

Fig 2.9 Catheter placement for evaluation of arterial blood during treadmill exercise. **(A)** 20-guage catheter secured with cyanoacrylate cement into the left transverse facial artery; **(B)** a thermocouple catheter passed via the left jugular vein; **(C)** catheter extension tubing to allow blood sampling during exercise; **(D)** thermocouple extension wire to allow recording of temperature signals from the sensor placed at the level of the right atrium.

Courtesy of E.K. Birks, M.M. Durando and B.B. Martin, Equine Sports Medicine and Surgery 1st Edition.

Assessment of the cardiovascular system

During clinical exercise tests, heart rate measurement is commonly performed and V_{HRmax} is a useful parameter to indicate the presence of a problem. However, it is not specific and lowered $V_{HR\ max}$ may occur for a number of reasons including lack of fitness, pain due to lameness and underlying respiratory or cardiac disease.[100] Post-exercise heart rate recovery may also be a useful indicator of an underlying problem or lack of fitness.[173]

In addition, to heart rate measurements electrocardiography is also commonly performed during treadmill exercise. One study has shown an association between cardiac arrhythmias and peak heart rate during exercise.[174] This suggests that during clinical exercise testing of horses suspected of having exercise-induced cardiac arrhythmias it is necessary to exercise the horse sufficiently strenuously that maximal heart rates are achieved. Exercise-induced arrhythmias, such as premature ventricular or supraventricular depolarizations and paroxysmal atrial fibrillation, are the most common arrhythmias detected during exercise. However, confirming a diagnosis of paroxysmal atrial fibrillation can be difficult due to the intermittent nature of the condition. Arrhythmias, due to supraventricular and ventricular premature depolarizations, are also frequently identified in the immediate recovery phase after exercise.[21,22,174–176] The significance of these findings remains uncertain, and may be related to changes in autonomic tone.[176,177]

Stress echocardiography may be performed immediately following treadmill exercise and has been suggested to potentially aid diagnosis of exercise-induced myocardial dysfunction.[178] However, heart rate declines rapidly after the cessation of exercise and it is important to acquire measurements quickly, preferably within 30–60 seconds whilst the heart rate remains elevated (>100 beats per minute).[178,179] Because of these difficulties, the development of pharmacological stress echocardiography is likely to supersede post treadmill stress echocardiography.

Assessment of the musculoskeletal system

The high-speed treadmill has been used widely for gait analysis and this is described in detail in Chapter 12 and Chapter 13. Treadmill exercise may also be useful for lameness assessment, particularly in those horses where lameness only occurs at high speeds or after an extended period of exercise such as Standardbred or endurance horses.[43]

Observation of lameness on the treadmill differs from that overground because the horse is stationary relative to the observer. This allows the horse to be viewed from all angles and offers some advantages. Video recordings can also be made for reviewing at a later date. As with overground lameness assessment, the most useful gaits to assess lameness are at the trot or pace due to the symmetrical nature of these gaits, which allows for easier observation of any gait abnormality.

Finally, one of the most common assessments of the musculoskeletal system involves the measurement of serum or plasma muscle enzymes (creatine kinase (CK) and aspartate aminotransferase (AST)) before and after treadmill exercise. This provides information relating to muscle damage and may be useful to identify individuals with subclinical myopathy. Various cut off criteria have been described in different studies. For muscle enzyme activities to be of pathological significance, they must be greater than those expected from the nature of the exercise and the fitness of the horse.[180] Both the type of exercise and level of conditioning affect post-exercise elevations in muscle enzymes, with higher levels found in unconditioned horses performing repeated submaximal exercise.[181] Increases in muscle enzymes also occur normally after strenuous exercise such as racing. However, in general there is only a 50% increase in values.[117] A recent review article suggested that values for CK taken 2– 6 hours after exercise should not exceed twice resting values and should return to baseline by 24 hours, whilst AST should not increase by more than 50% at any point.[182]

Conclusions

Historically, treadmill exercise testing has been widely used in equine exercise physiology research and for clinical evaluation of the poorly performing athlete. Recent advances in telemetric equipment have resulted in field exercise testing gaining in popularity. Nevertheless, treadmill exercise testing remains an important technique both for research and for clinical assessment of the equine athlete.

References

1. Zuntz N, Lehmann C. Untersuchungen uber den Stoffwechsel des Pferdes bei Ruhe und Arbeit. Landwirtsch Jahrb: Z Wiss Landwirthsch 1889;18:1–156.
2. Zuntz N. Praktische Folgenmgen aus den am Arbeitspferd ausgefuhrten Stoffwechselversuchen. Zschr Vetkde 1896;8:293–311.
3. Zuntz N, Hagemann O. Untersuchungen uber den Stoffwechsel des pferdes bei ruhe und arbeit. Landwirtsch Jahrb 1898;21(Suppl III):1–438.
4. Proctor RC, Jones MM, Brody S, et al. Energy expended by a horse at rest and at work. J Anim Sci 1934;1934:106–9.
5. Persson SGB. On blood volume and working capacity in horses. Acta Physiol Scand Suppl 1967;19:1–189.
6. Persson SGB. Blood volume, state of training and working capacity of racehorses. Equine Vet J 1968;1: 52–62.
7. Erickson H. History of horse-whims, teamboats, treadwheels and treadmills. Equine vet J Suppl 2006;36:83–7.
8. Cooper CB, Storer TW. In: Cooper CB, Storer TW, editors. Exercise testing and interpretation: A practical approach. Cambridge University Press; 2001.
9. Couroucе A. Field exercise testing for assessing fitness in French Standardbred Trotters. The Vet J 1999;157(2): 112–22.
10. Davie AJ, Evans DL. Blood lactate responses to submaximal field exercise tests in thoroughbred horses. The Vet J 2000;159:252–8.
11. Davie AJ, Priddle TL, Evans DL. Metabolic responses to submaximal field exercise tests and relationships with racing performance in pacing Standardbreds. Equine Vet J 2002;s34: 112–15.
12. van Erck E, Jakesova V, Lekeux P, et al. Field evaluation of poor performance in Standardbred Trotters. Pferdeheilkunde 2006;22:625–31.
13. Allen KJ, Hillyer MH, Terron-Canedo N, et al. Equitation and exercise factors affecting dynamic upper respiratory tract function: a review illustrated by case reports. Equine Vet Educ 2011;23: 361–8.
14. van Erck E. Dynamic respiratory videoendoscopy in ridden sport horses: effect of head flexion, riding and airway inflammation in 129 cases. Equine Vet J Suppl Suppl 2011;40:18–24.
15. Seeherman HJ, Morris EA. Methodology and repeatability of a standardised treadmill exercise test for clinical evaluation of fitness in horses. Equine Vet J Suppl 1990;20–5.
16. Morris. Application of clinical exercise testing for identification of respiratory fitness and disease in the equine athlete. Vet Clin North Am Equine Pract 1991;7: 383–401.

17. Kannegieter NJ, Dore ML. Endoscopy of the upper respiratory tract during treadmill exercise: a clinical study of 100 horses. Aust vet J 1995;72:101–7.
18. Parente EJ, Martin BB. Correlation between standing endoscopic examinations and those made during high-speed exercise in horses – 150 cases. Proc Am Ass Equine Practnrs 1995;41:170.
19. Tan RHH, Dowling BA, Dart AJ. High-sped treadmill videoendoscopic examination of the upper respiratory tract in the horse: The results of 291 clinical cases. The Vet J 2005;170:243–8.
20. Lane JG, Bladon B, Little DR, et al. Dynamic obstructions of the equine upper respiratory tract. Part 2: comparison of endoscopic findings at rest and during high-speed treadmill exercise of 600 Thoroughbred racehorses. Equine Vet J 2006;38:401–7.
21. Martin Jr BB, Reef VB, Parente EJ, et al. Causes of poor performance of horses during training, racing, or showing: 348 cases (1992–1996). J Am Vet Med Ass 2000;216:554–8.
22. Jose-Cunnileras E, Young LE, Newton JR, et al. Cardiac arrhythmias during and after treadmill exercise in poorly performing Thoroughbred racehorses. Equine Vet J Suppl 2006;36:163–70.
23. Morris EA, Seeherman HJ. Clinical evaluation of poor performance in the racehorse: the results of 275 evaluations. Equine Vet J 1991;23:169–74.
24. Courouce-Malblanc A, Pronost S, Fortier G, et al. Physiological measurements and upper and lower respiratory tract evaluation in French Standardbred Trotters during a standardised exercise test on the treadmill. Equine Vet J 2002;34(s34):402–7.
25. Courouce-Malblanc A, Deniau V, Rossignol F, et al. Physiological measurements and prevalence of lower airway diseases in Trotters with dorsal displacement of the soft palate. Equine Vet J 2010;42(s38):246–55.
26. Kenney WL, Hodgson JL. Variables predictive of performance in elite middle distance runners. Br J Sports Med 1985;19:207–9.
27. Harkins JD, Beadle RE, Kamerling SG. The correlation of running ability and physiological variables in Thoroughbred racehorses. Equine Vet J 1993;25: 53–60.
28. Hodgson DL, Rose RJ. Evaluation of performance potential. In: Hodgson DL, Rose RJ, editors. The athletic horse. Saunders; 1994. p. 231–41.
29. Gavreau GM, Staempfli H, McCutcheon LJ, et al. Comparison of aerobic capcity between racing standardbred horses. J Appl Physiol 1995;78:1447–51.
30. MacArthur DG, North KN. Genes and human elite athletic performance. Hum Genet 2005;116:331–9.
31. Barrey E. Genetics and genomics in equine exercise physiology: an overview of the new applications of molecular biology as positive and negative markers of performance and health. Equine Vet J 2010;42(s38):561–8.
32. Schröder W, Klostermann A, Distl O. Candidate genes for physical performance in the horse. The Vet J 2011;190:39–48.
33. Hill EW, Eivers SS, McGivney BA, et al. Moderate and high intensity sprint exercise induce differential responses in *COX4I2* and *PDK4* gene expression in Thoroughbred horse skeletal muscle. Equine Vet J 2010;42(s38):576–81.
34. Hill EW, McGivney BA, Gu J, et al. A genome-wide SNP-association study confirms a sequence variant (g.66493737C>T) in the equine *myostatin* (*MSTN*) gene as the most powerful predictor of optimum racing distance for Thoroughbred racehorses. BMC Genomics 2010;11:552.
35. Gu J, MacHugh DE, McGivney BA, et al. Association of sequence variants in *CKM* (creatine kinase, muscle) and *COX4I2* (cytochrome c oxidase, subunit 4, isoform 2) genes with racing performance in Thoroughbred horses. Equine Vet J 2010;42(s38):569–75.
36. Tozaki T, Miyake T, Kakoi H, et al. A genome-wide association study for racing performances in Thoroughbreds clarifies a candidate region near the *MSTN* gene. Anim Genet 2010;41(Suppl. 2):28–35.
37. Tozaki T, Hill EW, Hirota K, et al. A cohort study of racing performance in Japanese Thoroughbred racehorses using genome information on ECA18. Anim Genet 2012;43:42–52.
38. Parente E. Treadmill endoscopy. Equine Vet Educ 2004;16:250–4.
39. Rose RJ, Hendrickson DK, Knight PK. Clinical exercise testing in the normal Thoroughbred racehorse. Aust Vet J 1990;67:345–8.
40. Seeherman HJ, Morris EA. Comparison of yearling, two-year-old and adult Thoroughbreds using a standardised exercise test. Equine Vet J 1991;23: 175–84.
41. Hiraga A, Makato K, Kubo K, Sugano S. Effects of low intensity exercise during the breaking period on cardiopulmonary function in Thoroughbred yearlings. J Equine Sci 1997;8:21–4.
42. Ohmura H, Hiraga A, Matsui A, et al. Physiological responses of young Thoroughbreds during their first year of race training. Equine Vet J 2002;34(s34):140–6.
43. Martin Jr BB, Dyson SJ, Ross MW. Experiences using a high-speed treadmill to evaluate lameness. In: Ross MW, Dyson SJ, editors. Diagnosis and management of lameness in the horse. Elsevier Saunders; 2nd ed. 2011.
44. Nostell K, Funkquist P, Nyman G, et al. The physiological responses to simulated race tests on a track and on a treadmill in Standardbred trotters. Equine Vet J 2006;s36:123–7.
45. Marlin D, Nankervis K. Exercise testing. In: Equine exercise physiology. Blackwell Science; 2002. p. 233–4.
46. Franklin S, Barakzai S, Courouce-Malblanc A, et al. Assessment of the prevalence and types of injuries associated with high-speed treadmill exercise testing. Equine Vet J 2010;42(s38):70–5.
47. Buchner HHF, Savelberg HHCM, Schamhardt HC, et al. Habituation of horses to treadmill locomotion. Equine Vet J Suppl 1994;17:13–15.
48. King CM, Evans DL, Rose RJ. Acclimation to treadmill exercise. Equine Vet J Suppl 1995;18:453–6.
49. Rose RJ, Hodgson DR. Clinical exercise testing. In: Hodgson DL, Rose RJ, editors. The athletic horse. Saunders; 1994. p. 245–57.
50. Williams RB, Harkins LS, Hammond CJ, et al. Racehorse injuries, clinical problems and fatalities recorded on British racecourses from flat racing and National Hunt racing during 1996, 1997 and 1998. Equine vet J 2001;33: 478–86.
51. Pinchbeck GL, Clegg PD, Proudman CJ, et al. Horse injuries and racing practices in National Hunt racehorses in the UK: The results of a prospective cohort study. Vet J 2004;167:45–52.
52. Singer ER, Barnes J, Saxby F, et al. Injuries in the event horse: Training versus competition. The Vet J 2008;175:76–81.
53. Kobluk CN, Geor RJ, King VL, et al. A case control study of racing thoroughbreds conditioned on a high speed treadmill. J Equine Vet Sci 1996;16:511–13.
54. Takahashi T, Kasashima Y, Eto D, et al. Effect of uphill exercise on equine superficial digital flexor tendon forces at trot and canter. Equine Vet J 2006; 38(s36):435–9.
55. Nunamaker DM, Provost MW. Experiences using a high-speed treadmill to evaluate lameness. In: Ross MW, Dyson SJ, editors. Diagnosis and management of lameness in the horse. 2nd ed. Saunders; 2011. unpublished data, cited by Martin BB, Dyson SJ, Ross MW. 2003.
56. Milgram C, Finestone A, Segev S, et al. Are overground runners more likely to sustain ibial stress fracture? Br J Sports Med 2003;37:160–3.
57. Currell K, Jeukendrup AE. Validity, reliability and sensitivity of measures of

sporting performance. Sports Med 2008;38:297–316.
58. Evans D. Exercise testing in the field. In: Hinchcliff KW, Kaneps AJ, Geor RJ, editors. Equine sports medicine and surgery. Saunders; 2004. p. 19–31.
59. Sloet van Oldruitenborgh-Oosterbaan MM, Clayton HM. Advantages and disadvantages of track vs. treadmill tests. Equine Vet J Suppl 1999;30:645–7.
60. Barrey E, Galloux P, Auvinet B, et al. Stride characteristics of overground versus treadmill locomotion in the saddle horse. Acta Anat 1993;146:90–4.
61. Buchner HHF, Savelberg HHCM, Schamhardt HC, et al. Kinematics of treadmill vs overground locomotion in horses. Vet Quarterly 1994;16(suppl 2):s87–90.
62. Schamhardt HC, van den Bogert AJ, Lammertink JLMA. Power transfer from treadmill engine to athlete. Proc 8th Biennial Conference of the Canadian society of Biomechanics, Canada. 1994. p. 306–7.
63. Barrey E, Galloux P, Valette JP, et al. Determination of the optimal treadmill slope for reproducing the same cardiac response in saddle horses as overground exercise conditions. Vet Rec 1993;133:183–5.
64. Sloet van Oldruitenborgh-Oosterbaan MM, Barneveld A. Comparison of the workload of Dutch Warmblood horses ridden normally and on a treadmill. Vet Rec 1995;137:136–9.
65. Couroucе A, Geffroy O, Barrey E, et al. Comparison of exercise tests in French trotters under training track, racetrack and treadmill conditions. Equine Vet J Suppl 1999;30:528–32.
66. Galloux P, Valette JP, Barrey E, et al. Exercise tests in saddle horses. 1: comparison of step tests on a track and inclined treadmill. J Equine Vet Sci 1993;13:417–21.
67. Couroucе A, Corde R, Valette JP, et al. Comparison of some responses to exercise on the track and the treadmill: determination of the optimal treadmill incline. The Vet J 2000;159:57–63.
68. Jones AM, Doust AH. A 1% treadmill grade most accurately reflects the energetic cost of outdoor running. J Sports Sci 1996;14:321–7.
69. Davies CTM. Effects of wind assistance and resistance on the forward motion of a runner. J Appl Physiol 1980;48:702–9.
70. Jones JH, Ohmura H, Stanley SD, et al. Energetic cost of locomotion on different equine treadmills. Equine Vet J Suppl 2006;36:365–9.
71. Thornton J, Pagan J, Persson S. The oxygen cost of weight loading and inclined treadmill exercise in the horse. In: Gillespie JR, Robinson NE, editors. Equine exercise physiology, vol. 2. ICEEP Publications; 1987. p. 206–15.
72. Eaton MD, Evans DL, Hodgson DR, et al. Effect of treadmill incline and speed on metabolic rate during exercise in Thoroughbred horses. J Appl Physiol 1995;79:951–7.
73. Wickler SJ, Hoyt DF, Cogger EA, et al. Preferred speed and cost of transport: The effect of incline. J Exp Biol 2000;203:2195–200.
74. Van Erck E, Votion D-M, Serteyn D, et al. Evaluation of oxygen consumption during field exercise tests in Standardbred trotters. Equine Comp Exerc Physiol 2007;4:43–9.
75. Richard EA, Fortier GD, Pitel PH, et al. Sub-clinical diseases affecting performance in Standardbred trotters: diagnostic methods and predictive parameters. The Vet J 2010;184:282–9.
76. Allen KJ, Franklin SH. Comparisons of overground endoscopy and treadmill endoscopy in U.K. Thoroughbred racehorses. Equine Vet J 2010;42:186–91.
77. Evans DL, Rose RJ. Determination and repeatability of maximum oxygen uptake and other cardiorespiratory measurements in the exercising horse. Equine vet J 1988;20:94–8.
78. Curtis RA, Kusano K, Evans DL, et al. Reliability of cardiorespiratory measurements with a new ergospirometer during intense treadmill exercise in Thoroughbred horses. The Vet J 2005;169:223–31.
79. Franklin SH. Repeatability of the breath-by-breath system. In: PhD Thesis. University of Bristol; 2002. p. 228–30.
80. Evans DL, Harris RC, Snow DH. Correlation of racing performance with blood lactate and heart rate after exercise in Thoroughbred horses. Equine Vet J 1993;25:441–44.
81. Parente EJ. Testing methods for exercise intolerance in horses. Vet Clin N Am Equine Prac 1996;12:421–33.
82. Durando MM, Martin BB, Hammer EJ, et al. Dynamic upper airway changes and arterial blood gas parameters during treadmill exercise. Equine Vet J Suppl 2002;34:408–12.
83. Strand E, Fjordbakk CT, Sundberg K, et al. Relative prevalence of upper respiratory tract disorders in 2 breeds of harness racehorses (185 cases, 1998–2006). Equine Vet J 2012;44:518–23.
84. Eto D, Yamani S, Hiraga A, et al. Recruitment pattern of muscle fibre type during flat and sloped treadmill running in Thoroughbred horses. Equine Vet J Suppl 2006;36:349–53.
85. Kai M, Hiraga A, Kubo K, et al. Comparison of stride characteristics in a cantering horse on a flat and inclined treadmill. Equine Vet J Suppl 1997;23:76–9.
86. Robert C, Valette JP, Denoix JM. The effects of treadmill inclination and speed on the activity of two hindlimb muscles in the trotting horse. Equine Vet J 2000;32:312–17.
87. Sloet van Oldruitenborgh-Oosterbaan MM, Barneveld A, Scamhardt HC. Effects of treadmill inclination on kinematics of the trot in Dutch Warmblood horses. Equine Vet J Suppl 1997;24:353–8.
88. Hoyt DF, Molinari M, Wickler SJ, et al. Effect of trotting speed, load and incline on hindlimb stance-phase kinematics. Equine Vet J 2002;s34:330–6.
89. McDonough P, Kindig C, Hildreth TS, et al. Effect of body incline on cardiac performance. Equine Vet J 2002;s34:506–9.
90. McDonough P, Kindig CA, Ramsel C, et al. The effect of treadmill incline on maximal oxygen uptake, gas exchange and the metabolic response to exercise in the horse. Exp Physiol 2002;87:499–506.
91. Allen KJ, Franklin SH. Assessment of the exercise tests used during overground endoscopy in UK thoroughbred racehorses and how these may affect the diagnosis of dynamic upper respiratory tract obstructions. Equine Vet J Suppl 2010;38:587–91.
92. Nielsen BD, Turner KK, Ventura BA, et al. Racing speeds of Quarter horses, Thoroughbreds and Arabians. Equine Vet J 2006;38(s36):128–32.
93. Physick-Sheard PW. Career profile of the Canadian Standardbred II: Influence of age, gait and sex on number of races, money won and race times. Can J Vet Res 1986;50:457–70.
94. Soma LR, Birks EK, Uboh CE, et al. The effects of frusemide on racing times of Standardbred pacers. Equine Vet J 2000;32:334–40.
95. LeuLeu C, Cotrel C, Couroucе-Malblanc A. Relationships between physiological variables and race performance in French Standardbred trotters. Vet Rec 2005;156:339–42.
96. Hoyt DF, Taylor CR. Gait and the energetics of locomotion in horses. Nature 1981;292:239–40.
97. Franklin SH, Naylor JRJ, Lane JG. Videoendoscopic evaluation of the upper respiratory tract in 93 sport horses during exercise testing on a high-speed treadmill. Equine Vet J 2006;38(s36):540–5.
98. Davidson EJ, Martin BB, Boston RC, et al. Exercising upper respiratory videoendoscopic evaluation of 100 nonracing performance horses with abnormal respiratory noise and / or poor performance. Equine Vet J 2011;43:3–8.
99. Strand E, Hanche-Olsen S, Grønvold AMR, et al. Dynamic bilateral arytenoid and vocal fold collapse associated with

head flexion in 5 Norwegian Coldblooded Trotter racehorses. Equine Vet Educ 2004;16:242–50.
100. Evans DL. Physiology of equine performance and associated tests of function. Equine Vet J 2007;39:373–83.
101. Shaver LG. Maximal aerobic power and anaerobic work capacity prediction from various running performances of untrained collegemen. J Sports Med 1975;15:147–50.
102. Bassett DR, Howley ET. Limiting factors for maximum oxygen uptake and determinants of endurance performance. Med Sci Sports Exerc 2000;32:70–84.
103. Noakes TD. Implications of exercise testing for prediction of athletic performance: a contemporary perspective. Med Sci Sports Exerc 1988;20:319–30.
104. Noakes TD. Physiological models to understand exercise fatigue and the adaptations that predict or enhance athletic performance. Scand J Med Sci Sports 2000;10:123–45.
105. Bayly WM, Schultz DA, Hodgson DR, et al. Ventilatory responses of the horse to exercise: effect of gas collection systems. J Appl Physiol 1987;63:1210–17.
106. Art T, Anderson L, Woakes AJ, et al. Mechanics of breathing during strenuous exercise in thoroughbred horses. Resp Physiol 1990;82:279–94.
107. Butler PJ, Woakes AJ, Smale K, et al. Respiratory and cardiovascular adjustments during exercise of increasing intensity and during recovery in Thoroughbred racehorses. J Exp Biol 1993;179:159–80.
108. Wasserman K, Whip BJ, Koyal SN, et al. Anaerobic threshold and respiratory gas exchange during exercise. J Appl Physiol 1973;35:236–43.
109. McDonough P, Kindig CA, Erickson HH, et al. Mechanistic basis for gas exchange threshold in Thoroughbred horses. J Appl Physiol 2002;92:1499–505.
110. Vincent TL, Newton JR, Deaton CM, et al. Retrospective study of predictive variables for maximal heart rate (HRmax) in horses undergoing strenuous treadmill exercise. Equine Vet J 2006;38(s36):146–52.
111. Evans DL, Rose RJ. Maximum oxygen uptake in racehorses: changes with training state and prediction from submaximal cardiorespiratory measurements. In: Gillespie JR, Robinson NE, editors. Equine exercise physiology, vol. 2. Davis, Calif: ICEEP publications; 1987. p. 52–67.
112. Gramkow HL, Evans DL. Correlation of race earnings with velocity at maximal heart rate during a field exercise test in Thoroughbred racehorses. Equine Vet J Suppl 2006;36:118–22.
113. Kobayashi M. Simple lactate measurement in horses using a portable lactate analyzer with lancet skin puntures under field conditions. J Equine Sci 2007;18:5–11.
114. Rainger JE, Evans DL, Hodgson DR, et al. Distribution of lactate in plasma and erythrocytes during and after exercise in horses. Br Vet J 1995;151:299–310.
115. Pössö AR, Lampinen K, Rasanen L. Distribution of lactate between red blood cells and plasma after exercise. Equine Vet J Suppl 1995;18:231–4.
116. Koho NM, Väihkönen LK, Pösö AR. Lactate transport in red blood cells by monocarboxylate transporters. Equine Vet J Suppl 2002;34:555–9.
117. McGowan C. Clinical pathology in the racing horse: the role of clinical pathology in assessing fitness and performance in the racehorse. Vet Clin N Am Equine Prac 2008;24:405–21.
118. Evans DL, Golland LC. Accuracy of accusport for measurement of lactate concentrations in equine blood and plasma. Equine Vet J 1996;28:398–402.
119. Persson SGB. Evaluation of exercise tolerance and fitness in the performance horse. In: Snow DH, Persson SGB, Rose RJ, editors. Equine exercise physiology, vol. 1. Cambridge, UK: Granta Editions; 1983. p. 441–57.
120. Lindner AE. Relationships between racing times of Standardbreds and V4 and V200. J Anim Science 2010;88: 950–4.
121. Couroucе A, Chatard JC, Auvinet B. Estimation of performance potential of Standardbred trotters from blood lactate concentrations measured in field conditions. Equine Vet J 1997;29: 365–9.
122. Persson S, Ullberg L. Blood volume in relation to exercise tolerance in trotters. J Sth Afr Vet Med Ass 1974;45:293–9.
123. Ronéus N, Essén-Gustavsson B, Lindholm NA, et al. Plasma lactate response to submaximal and maximal exercise tests with training, and its relationship to performance and muscle characteristics in Standardbred trotters. Equine Vet J 1994;26:117–21.
124. Green S, Dawson B. Measurement of anaerobic capacities in humans. Definitions, limitations and unsolved problems. Sports Med 1993;15:312–27.
125. Weinstein Y, Bediz C, Dotan R, et al. Reliability of peak-lactate, heart rate, and plasma volume following the Wingate test. Med Sci Sports Exerc 1998;30:1456–60.
126. Saibene F, Conili G, Gavazzi P, et al. Maximal anaerobic (lactic) capacity and power of the horse. Equine Vet J 1985;17:130–2.
127. Bayly WM, Grant BD, Pearson RC. Lactate concentrations in Thoroughbred horses following maximal exercise under field conditions. In: Gillespie JR, Robinson NE, editors. Equine exercise physiology, vol. 2. Davis, CA: ICEEP Publications; 1987. p. 426–37.
128. Rasanen LA, Lampinen KJ, Poso AR. Responses of blood and plasma lactate and plasma purine concentrations to maximal exercise and their relation to performance in Standardbred trotters. Am J Vet Res 1995;56:1651–6.
129. Koho NM, Hyppä S, Pösö AR. Monocarboxylate transportes (MCT) as lactate carriers in equine muscle and red blood cells. Equine Vet J Suppl 2006; 36:354–8.
130. Harris PA, Marlin DJ, Snow DH. Metabolic responses to maximal exercise of 800 and 2000m in the Thoroughbred horse. J Appl physiol 1987;63(1):12–19.
131. Birks EK, Jones JH, Vandervort LJ, et al. Plasma lactate kinetics during exercise. In: Persson SGB, Lindholm A, Jeffcott LB. Equine exercise physiology, vol. 3. Davis, California: ICEEP Publications; 1991. p. 179–87.
132. Marlin DJ, Harris RC, Snow DH. Rates of blood lactate disappearance following exercise of different intensities. In: Persson SGB, Lindholm A, Jeffcott LB. Equine exercise physiology, vol. 3. Davis, California: ICEEP Publications; 1991. p. 188–95.
133. Ohmura H, Hiraga A, Jones JH. Method for quantifying net anaerobic power in exercising horses. Equine Vet J 2006; 38(s36):370–3.
134. Ohmura H, Mukai K, Takahashi T, et al. Comparison of net anaerobic energy utilisation estimated by plasma lactate accumulation rate and accumulated oxygen deficit in Thoroughbred horses. Equine Vet J Suppl 2010;38:62–9.
135. Franklin SH. Videoendoscopic examination during overground exercise. In: Auer JA, Stick JA, editors. Equine surgery. 4th ed. Elsevier; 2011. p. 540–2.
136. Attenburrow DP. Resonant frequency of the lateral ventricle and saccule and "whistling" In: Snow DH, Persson SGB, Rose RJ, editors. Equine exercise physiology. Cambridge: Granta editions; 1983. p. 27–32.
137. Derksen FJ, Holcombe SJ, Hartmann W, et al. Spectrum analysis of respiratory sounds in exercising horses with experimentally-induced laryngeal hempiplegia or dorsal displacement of the soft palate. Am J Vet Res 2001;62: 659–64.
138. Franklin SH, Usmar SG, Lane JG, et al. Spectral analysis of respiratory noise in horses with upper airway disorders. Equine Vet J 2003;35:264–8.
139. Brown JA, Derksen FJ, Stick JA, et al. Venticulocordectomy reduces respiratory noise in horses with laryngeal hemiplegia. Equine Vet J 2003;35:570–4.
140. Brown JA, Derksen FJ, Stick JA, et al. Effect of laryngoplasty on respiratory noise reduction in horses with laryngeal hemiplegia. Equine Vet J 2004;36: 420–5.

141. Kastner SBR, Weishaupt MA, Townsend HGG. Evaluation of the upper respiratory tract in the horse during treadmill exercise – a review. Part 1: endoscopy. Pferdeheilkunde 1998;14: 33–40.
142. Weishaupt. Upper airway mechanics. In: Ainsworth DM, McGorum BC, Viel L, et al, editors. Third World Equine Airways Symposium. Ithaca NY: International Veterinary Information Service; 2005.
143. Rakesh V, Ducharme NG, Cheetham J, et al. Implications of different degrees of arytenoid cartilage abduction on equine upper airway characteristics. Equine Vet J 2008;40:629–35.
144. Rehder RS, Ducharme NG, Hackett RP, et al. Measurement of upper airway pressures in exercising horses with dorsal displacement of the soft palate. Am J Vet Res 1995;56:269–74.
145. Holcombe SJ, Derksen FJ, Stick JA, et al. Effect of bilateral blockade of the pharyngeal branch of the vagus nerve on soft palate function in horses. Am J Vet Res 1998;59:504–8.
146. Franklin SH, Naylor JR, Lane JG. Effect of dorsal displacement of the soft palate on ventilation and airflow during high-intensity exercise. Equine Vet J Suppl 2002;34:379–83.
147. Dixon PM. Arterial blood gas values in horses with laryngeal paralysis. Equine Vet J 1982;14:246–8.
148. Derksen FJ, Stick JA, Scott EA, et al. Effect of laryngeal hemiplegia and laryngoplasty on airway flow mechanics in execising horses. Am J Vet Res 1986;47:16–20.
149. Williams WJ, Meagher DM, Pasce JR, et al. Effects of left recurrent laryngeal neurectomy, prosthetic laryngoplasty and subtotal arytenoidectomy on upper airway pressure during maximal exercise. Vet Surg 1990;19:136–42.
150. Williams JW, Meagher DM, Pascoe JR, et al. Upper airway function during maximal exercise in horses with obstructive upper airway lesions effect of surgical treatment. Vet Surg 1990;19:142–7.
151. Tate LP, Corbett WT, Bishop BJ, et al. Blood gas tensions, acid–base status, heart rates and venous profiles in exercising horses with laryngeal hemiplegia before and after corrective surgery. Vet Surg 1993;22:177–83.
152. Bayly WM, Grant BD, Modransky. Arterial blood gas tensions during exercise in a horse with laryngeal hemiplegia before and after corrective surgery. Res Vet Sci 1994;36:256–8.
153. Seeherman HJ, Ehrlich PJ, Morris EA. Physiological versus clinical consequences of left recurrent laryngeal neuropathy (LRLN). Equine Vet J Suppl 1995;18:7–12.
154. Ehrlich PJ, Seeherman HJ, Morris E, et al. The effect of reversible left recurrent laryngeal neuropathy on the metabolic cost of locomotion and peak aerobic power in Thoroughbred racehorses. Vet Surg 1995;24:36–48.
155. King CM, Evans DL, Rose RJ. Cardiorespiratory and metabolic responses to exercise in horses with various abnormalities of the upper respiratory tract. Equine Vet J 1994; 26:220–5.
156. Christley RM, Hodgson DR, Evans DL, et al. Cardiorespiratory responses to exercise in horses with different grades of idiopathic laryngeal hemiplegia. Equine Vet J 1997;29:6–10.
157. Couëtil LL, Denicola DB. Blood gas, plasma lactate, and bronchoalveolar lavage cytology analyzes in racehorses with respiratory disease. Equine Vet J 1999;30:77–82.
158. Sánchez A, Couëtil LL, Ward MP, et al. Effect of airway disease on blood gas exchange in racehorses. J Vet Intern Med 2005;19:87–92.
159. Marlin DJ, Roberts CA. Qualitative and quantitative assessment of respiratory airflow and pattern of breathing in exercising horses. Equine Vet Edu 1998;10:178–86.
160. Lumsden JM, Derksen FJ, Stick JA, et al. Use of flow-volume loops to evaluate upper airway obstruction in exercising Standardbreds. Am J Vet Res 1993;54:766–75.
161. Lumsden JM, Derksen FJ, Stick JA, et al. Evaluation of partial arytenoidectomy as a treatment for equine laryngeal hemiplegia. Equine Vet J 1994;26:125–9.
162. Guthrie AJ, Beadle RE, Bateman RD, et al. Characterisation of normal tidal breathing flow-volume loops for Thoroughbred horses. Vet Res Comm 1995;19:331–42.
163. Guthrie AJ, Beadle RE, Bateman RD, et al. The effects of three models of airway disease on tidal breathing flow-volume loops of Thoroughbred horses. Vet Res Comm 1995;19: 517–27.
164. Weishaupt MA, Vogt R, Fürst A, et al. Spirometric and endoscopic assessment of surgical treatment in horses with laryngeal hemiplegia. Havemeyer proc Equine recurrent laryngeal neuropathy 2004;81–3.
165. Art T, Lekeux P. A critical assessment of pulmonary function testing in exercising ponies. Vet Res Comm 1988;12:25–39.
166. Bayly WM, Grant BD, Breeze RG, et al. The effects of maximal exercise on acid-base balance and arterial blood gas tension in Thoroughbred horses. In: Snow DH, Persson SGB, Rose RJ, editors. Equine exercise physiology. Cambridge: Granta Editions; 1983. p. 401–7.
167. De Waal A, Littlejohn A, Potgieter GM, et al. An apparatus for collecting blood samples by radiotelemetry from horses during exercise. Vet Res Comm 1986;10: 65–72.
168. Littlejohn A, Snow DH. Circulatory, respiratory and metabolic responses in Thoroughbred horses during the first 400 meters of exercise. Eur J Appl Physiol 1988;58:307–14.
169. Jones JH, Taylor CR, Lindholm A, et al. Blood gas measurements during exercise: errors due to temperature correction. J Appl Physiol 1989;67:879–84.
170. Bayly WM, Hodgson DR, Schulz DA, et al. Exercise-induced hypercapnia in the horse. J Appl Physiol 1989;67: 1958–66.
171. Christley RM, Hodgson DR, Evans DL, et al. Effect of training on the development of exercise-induced arterial hypoxemia in horses. Am J Vet Res 1997;58:653–7.
172. Roberts CA, Marlin DJ, Lekeux P. The effects of training on ventilation and blood gases in exercising Thoroughbreds. Equine Vet J 1999;31:57–61.
173. Bitschnau C, Wiestner T, Trachsel DS, et al. Performance parameters and post exercise heart rate recovery in Warmblood sports horses of different performance levels. Equine Vet J Suppl 2010;38:17–22.
174. Ryan N, Marr CM, McGladdery AJ. Survey of cardiac arrhythmias during submaximal and maximal exercise in Thoroughbred racehorses. Equine Vet J 2005;37:265–8.
175. Barbesgaard L, Buhl R, Meldgaard C. Prevalence of exercise-associated arrhythmias in normal performing dressage horses. Equine vet J Suppl 2010;38:202–7.
176. Buhl R, Meldgaard C, Barbesgaard L. Cardiac arrhythmias in clinically healthy showjumping horses. Equine Vet J Suppl 2010;38:196–201.
177. Physick-Sheard PW, McGurrin MKJ. Ventricular arrhythmias during race recovery in Standardbred racehorses and associations with autonomic activity. J Vet Int Med 2010;24:1158–66.
178. Reef VB. Stress echocardiography and its role in performance assessment. Vet Clin N Am Equine Pract 2001;17:179–89.
179. Durando MM, Reef VB, Birks EK. Right ventricular pressure dynamics during exercise: relationship to stress echocardiography. Equine Vet J Suppl 2002b;34:472–7.
180. Harris PA, Snow DH, Greet TRC, et al. Some factors influencing plasma AST / CK activities in Thoroughbred racehorses. Equine Vet J 1990;22(s9):61–71.
181. Siciliano PD, Lawrence LM, Danielson K, et al. Effect of conditioning and exercise type on serum creatine kinase and aspartate aminotransferase activity. Equine Vet J Suppl 1995;18:243–7.
182. Keen J. Diagnosis and management of equine rhabdomyolysis. In Pract 2011;33:68–77.

Exercise testing in the field

3

Anne Couroucé-Malblanc   Emmanuelle van Erck-Westergren

CHAPTER CONTENTS

Introduction

Exercise testing is indicated for evaluation of a horse's physical condition as well as the investigation of poor athletic performance. Exercise tests are thus useful for the determination of the level of fitness, the assessment of progress made during training, and to evaluate if the horse has sufficient capacity to perform at an expected level. As all athletes respond in a different way to training, exercise testing may be used as an objective tool to validate or fine tune an individual preparation program. They also may enable detection of overreaching or overtraining. For veterinarians, exercise tests represent a useful tool to investigate cases of underperformance; the horse may be examined in real working conditions and exercise may reveal clinical signs not evident at rest. During a field exercise test, it is possible to measure simple and informative physiological parameters such as heart rate (HR), speed, or blood lactate concentration. These variables may be affected by subclinical disease and are helpful in determining which system (e.g. respiratory, cardiovascular) is responsible for limiting performance and to what degree.

Exercise tests can be conducted in a treadmill laboratory or in the field. There are advantages and disadvantages for both types of exercise test. An advantage of field studies is the conduct of tests in the environment likely to be used in competition. The surface, gaits and speeds used in a field test can be closely aligned to the demands faced during exercise in actual competition. Field tests also account for the effects of the rider, jockey, or driver, who in some instances may be the weakest link in the horse's performance. As field tests can be easily integrated into training sessions, it is possible to conduct multiple evaluations during a competitive season and thus enable a regular and rational follow-up of the horse. Of course, there may be difficulties in the standardization of field exercise tests as conditions may vary over time, according to climatic or other external conditions. To reduce the effect of extrinsic variations, field exercise tests should be repeated over time in similar conditions, i.e. on the same track, with the same rider.

This chapter describes techniques that have been used for field exercise tests in horses competing in different disciplines. The rationale for making the effort to perform field exercise tests is discussed. Limitations of treadmill exercise testing are also briefly described.

There have been many remarkable field studies that have, for example, measured the electrocardiogram, collected arterial blood and measured tracheal pressures in galloping horses. However, it is not the intention of this chapter to review in detail all such studies. The scope of this chapter will be limited mostly to field studies of cardiorespiratory function, and to the use of field studies to conduct fitness tests as well as to investigate poor performance in athletic horses of different equestrian disciplines.

Limitations of treadmill exercise testing

Most of the past publications on exercise physiology or poor performance relate to treadmill exercise testing. Although these studies have provided valuable information on the physiology of exercise and exercise-related pathological processes, treadmill exercise testing can be difficult to integrate into the management of an athletic horse. The use of a treadmill requires that the horse be transported to a facility with appropriate equipment. The necessary equipment is expensive to setup (e.g. purchase of a treadmill) and run given that a dedicated team of several experienced people is required for each test. Consequently, treadmill laboratories are usually limited to research facilities or large referral clinics. The use of a treadmill also may be wrongly perceived as dangerous. However, a recent multi-centered retrospective study has shown that the prevalence of treadmill-related accidents or injuries is low.[1]

The arguments for using high-speed treadmills to evaluate fitness and health of horses are obvious. The physical environment can be controlled, and the conduct of exercise tests with precise design is possible. The speeds and durations of each step of an exercise test are highly repeatable. There is also easy access to the horse at suitable times during and after exercise for cardiorespiratory measurements and blood collections. The necessity for an acclimation of horses prior to clinical exercise testing on a treadmill has been debated. Some performance testing laboratories do not acclimatize horses and others may apply up to three acclimation runs prior to testing.[2] Responses to acclimation runs are unpredictable in individual horses. Figure 3.1 illustrates the variability of HR and plasma lactate concentrations during treadmill exercise in horses that were given four treadmill tests on consecutive days.

Several studies have shown that physiologic responses to treadmill exercise do not replicate responses to field exercise. HR and plasma lactate concentrations in Standardbred horses pulling a 10 kilopond draught load were lower on the treadmill than on the racetrack.[3] It was also reported that HR and blood lactate in trotters were lower during exercise on a level treadmill than during exercise on a racetrack (Fig. 3.2).[4] HR were expressed as V200, the velocities (V) at which HR reached 200 beats per minute. Blood lactates were expressed as V4, the velocity at which blood lactate was 4 mmol/L. This value is sometimes referred to as VLA4. Stride frequency was lower and stride length was greater on the treadmill. Interestingly, this study also showed that there were no differences in any measurements on two sand tracks of 720 and 1250 m in length. A study of ridden Warmblood horses also found that HR and blood lactate concentrations were lower on a level treadmill at speeds of 6.5–9.4 m/s compared with exercise over ground.[5] The treadmill speed had to be increased by approximately 10% or the treadmill incline increased to 1–2% to elicit that same HR response observed in the field. Similar findings were found for HR and derived indices (V160 and V200) in endurance horses examined both on a racetrack and on a treadmill.[6]

Locomotion during treadmill exercise is quite different to that on the track. As a consequence, even if horses are given tasks on treadmills that produce similar HRs, their gaits may be quite dissimilar. Stride frequencies at identical trot and gallop speeds are greater on a racetrack.[7] Design of treadmill exercise tests to replicate field exercise therefore seems to be a fruitless endeavor.

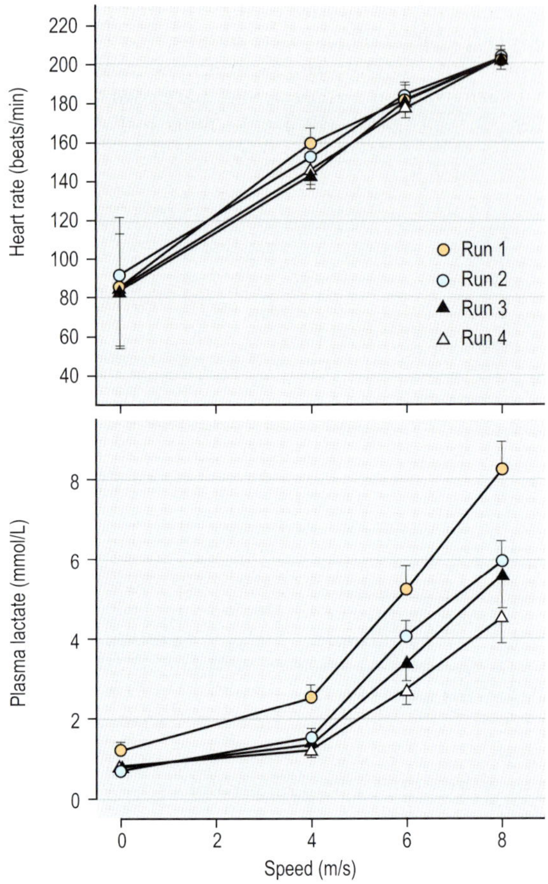

Fig 3.1 Heart rates and plasma lactate concentrations (mean ± SEM) during treadmill exercise in six race horses that had four sequential acclimating runs over a four-day period. Note the variability of heart rates during trotting at 4 m/s, and the high variability of plasma lactates at all velocities.

From King CM, Evans DL, Rose RJ. Acclimation to treadmill exercise. Equine Vet J. 1995; Suppl. 18:453–456. Reprinted with permission of the Equine Veterinary Journal.

Field exercise tests

In the field, HR and V during exercise and blood or plasma lactate concentration after exercise are the parameters that form the basis of an exercise test for athletic horses. However, other variables may be measured either during or after exercise, as described in the following sections. These include erythrocyte counts or packed cell volume (PCV), haematocrit (Ht), electrocardiogram (ECG), oxygen consumption (VO_2), investigation of respiratory noises, overground endoscopy and gait analysis.

An exercise test typically consists of several bouts of exercise after a warm-up, which may or may not be separated by a period of recovery. HR and V are usually measured during the exercise and blood samples may be collected following each step of the exercise test. Numerous testing procedures have been described for horses involved in different disciplines. Regardless of the discipline, field exercise test protocols should always be strictly defined in order to calculate meaningful fitness measurements and to limit variability (Box 3.1). Following standardized procedures is of great importance as the data derived from each test can be compared to subsequent tests for the same horse or with measurements from other horses of similar age and training status. Results may vary according to the methodology used and with factors such as number and duration of steps, resting time between steps and the degree of increment from one step to the next.

From the measured variables, HR, V and blood lactate concentration, derived parameters can be calculated to allow a comparison between the results of successive tests. HRs are usually expressed relative to a constant submaximal speed, such as V_{200}, the velocity at which heart rate is 200 bpm. However, expression of the V at lower HR is equally valid and some studies have used V140 and V170, although at such speeds, HR may be more markedly influenced by stress and vagal tone. To compare blood lactate values between horses, the V at a blood lactate concentration of 4 mmol/l (VLA4) has generally been used.[9,11,13–16] VLA4 is considered as a reference value for horses as it is a good predictor of aerobic capacity. A high value for VLA4 is an indication of a superior exercise capacity and is related to racing performance[17–20] As the horse increases fitness, VLA4 increases.

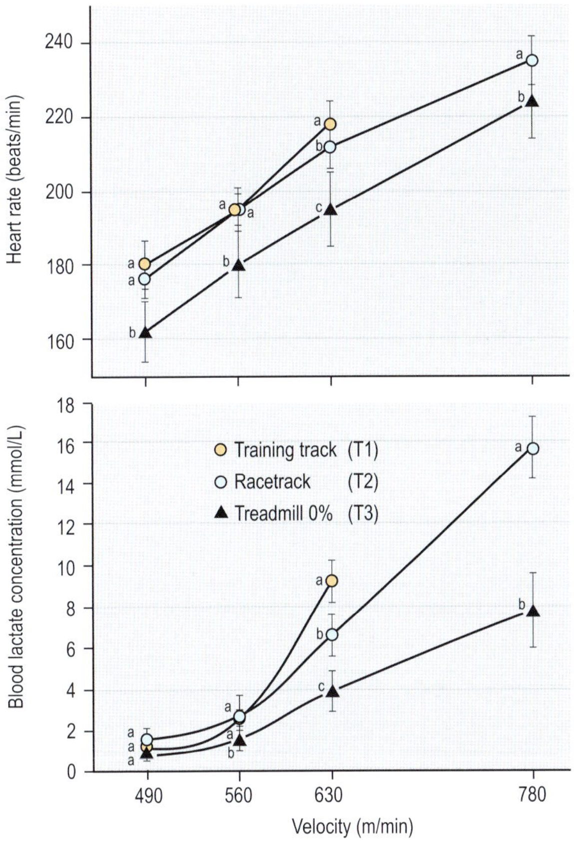

Fig 3.2 Mean ± SD heart rate (HR) and blood lactate concentrations in five French Standardbred trotters at three or four different speeds during exercise tests performed on two different tracks (T1, T2) and on a non-inclined treadmill (T3). At each velocity, values with a different letter are significantly different. The treadmill tests produced lower HRs abd blood lactate concentrations in most cases.
From Couroucé A, Geffroy O, Barrey E, et al. Comparison of exercise tests in French trotters under training track, racetrack and treadmill conditions. Equine Vet J. 1999; Suppl 30:528–531, with permission from the Equine Veterinary Journal.

Alternatively, the blood lactate response to a single episode of submaximal exercise can be used as a measure of fitness. This 'one-step' approach might be more applicable in field tests. It obviates the need for time-consuming, standardized multiple increments of speed as well as the need for multiple collections of blood via repeated venipuncture or a catheter secured in a jugular vein. The method also enables calculation of the HR–velocity relationships in field tests without use of protocols that necessitate strict adherence to steps of an exercise test at constant speed. Trainers may more readily adopt this technique because it does not necessitate changes to training schedules, and it can be incorporated into the usual daily training routine. It is important to refine field exercise tests so that they are easy to undertake.

The data obtained during an exercise test can be used to address several questions related to the fitness and performance capacity of a horse (Box 3.2). Ideally, measurement of HR, VO_2, and pulmonary ventilation is necessary to answer all of these questions. Nonetheless, blood lactate and HR measurements during or after suitable exercise tests can help with answers to questions 2–5 in Box 3.2. In the following sections, field exercise tests that have used HR and blood lactate measurements in a range of different disciplines will be described.

There are important principles to follow so that field fitness tests provide meaningful results. First, the test protocol should be simple. Multiple steps of increasing speeds of exercise are frequently used in treadmill testing and have been used in the field, but this type of exercise test may not be popular with trainers because of the time commitment and a perceived risk of injury. Exercise tests should be easy to implement, and not disrupt normal training schedules. It is possible to integrate an exercise test to a routine training session. Several features of the exercise test should be maintained, including consistency of:

1. warm-up routine prior to testing
2. rates and distances of acceleration during the exercise
3. test distances or times
4. speed during the exercise
5. time after exercise at which blood is collected
6. post-exercise activity
7. environmental conditions
8. track
9. rider, jockey, or driver.

Box 3.1 Important features in the design of an exercise test

1. Velocity should be controlled and maintained as constant as possible during each step of the exercise test.
2. The duration of each step should be sufficient to provide a steady-state HR and blood lactate response. Whereas 3–5 min seems to be necessary to reach a steady-state blood lactate concentration in human athletes, shorter steps may be possible in the horse.[8]
3. Because an efflux of lactate from muscle to blood occurs following exercise, a consistent rest period is essential between steps, unless the horse is working at submaximal levels and a stepwise accumulation of lactate an objective.
4. The responses of HR and blood lactate concentration to speed are dependent on age and training level of the horse.[9–12]

Box 3.2 Data collected during a field exercise test should address one or more of the following questions

1. Is the horse 'fit' for its next race, where fitness refers to a horse that is healthy and suitably trained?
2. Has the horse's fitness changed with recent training?
3. How does the fitness of horse A compare with horse B?
4. Does a horse with poor racing performance have suboptimal fitness?
5. Can an appropriate measure of fitness help with training of racehorses?
6. Does a horse with suboptimal or unexpectedly poor performance have a disease? Is there evidence of a cardiac or respiratory or other pathological limitation to performance?

Environmental conditions are an important consideration during field exercise testing.[21] HR and other variables were compared under high and low ambient temperature and relative humidity during a submaximal incremental field exercise test in horses tested in summer and in autumn. HR was measured continuously, the other variables at rest and immediately after 4 minutes of running at 3.5, 4.5 and 7.0 m/s, separated by three minute rest intervals, and after five and 10 minutes recovery. HR was significantly greater by a mean of 13 beats per minute during exercise in the hot versus cool conditions. It was concluded that differences in environmental conditions can affect assessment of exercise response. These factors must be considered when using fitness tests in the field. Sudden changes in environmental conditions might have considerable consequences for HR and blood lactate responses during exercise. The type and quality of a track is another consideration as track conditions have been shown to influence physiological variables measured and calculated during a standardized test.[16]

Racehorse trainers have been slow to adopt the use of field exercise tests. One explanation has been the difficulty in the design and implementation of exercise tests. Understandably, some trainers might also have reservations about adopting new techniques that could disrupt busy training schedules. However, many horse owners continue to be frustrated by a lack of information about the fitness and performance capacity of their horses and some types of exercise testing can easily be implemented in commercial training environments.

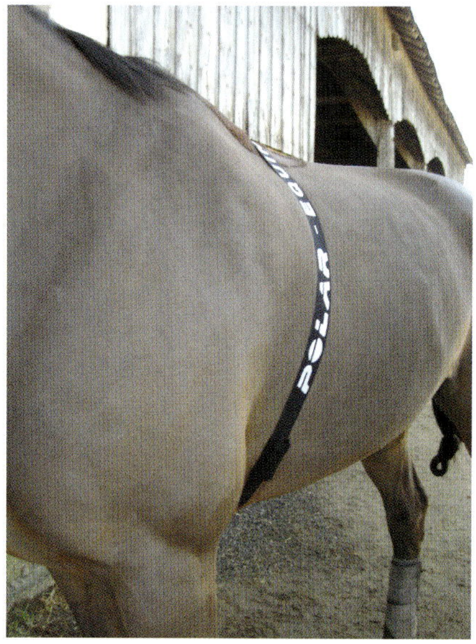

Fig 3.3 Polar girth strap that secures electrodes and a wearlink transmitter.
Photo courtesy of Anne Couroucé-Malblanc.

Measurements during field exercise tests

Heart rate

Telemetric electrocardiography was used widely in the 1960s and 1970s to study the HR and ECG of racehorses during exercise on racetracks.[22–27] Direct recording of the ECG with an on-board tape recorder was also used to assess HR during races.[28] These studies described typical HR responses during submaximal and maximal exercise in Thoroughbreds and Standardbreds. Studies of HR were also combined with telemetry of arterial blood pressure at speeds up to 800 m/min.[29] These studies were mostly descriptive, and did not focus on the design of the exercise tests.

The HR response to exercise is easily measured by means of electrodes placed in a thoracic girth strap (Polar, Finland) (Fig. 3.3) which is then placed under the saddle (Fig. 3.4). A coded and wireless transmitter placed on the girth transmits data to the HR meter which is either worn by the rider or placed on the saddle or on the sulky. Most of the heart rate meters record HR continuously and enable transfer of the data to a computer for analysis as shown in Figure 3.5 and Figure 3.6, which depict HR during exercise in two trotters. The exercise test consisted of three steps of 3 min at speeds of approximately 500, 580 and 660 m/min, with a brief period of walking between each step. When HR and V velocity are measured simultaneously (Fig. 3.6), it is possible to create a graph of the HR vs. speed relationship as shown in Figure 3.7. The graph also enables calculation of V200.

The HR response to exercise is linear between 120 and 210 bpm. Several factors can affect the HR/speed relationship including the geometry and length of the track, environmental conditions, training state[10,12,30] and disease[31–39] as well as the level of excitement.[36] However, the regression of HR to speed is repeatable when measured during standardized exercise.[8] In general, an increase in fitness results in an increase in V200 while loss of fitness, stress, cardiovascular and respiratory disease, lameness, and an increase in bodyweight could all cause a decrease in V200.[31–39] These factors should be considered when interpreting V200 values. Box 3.3 summarizes factors that may contribute to a higher than expected HR during submaximal exercise.

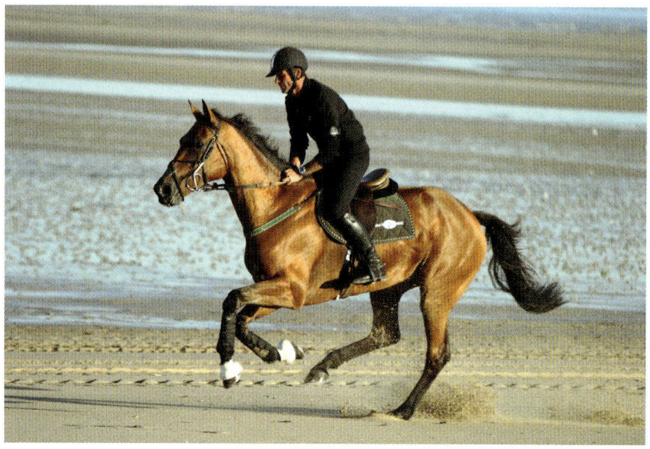

Fig 3.4 Horse equipped with a polar girth under the saddle. The rider is wearing a heart rate meter on his wrist and a GPS on his arm.
Photo courtesy of Barbara Conin.

In an excitable state, the slope of the regression line of HR on velocity is decreased because of high HRs during trotting.[36] V200 was thus falsely high. This finding emphasizes the need for careful observation of horses during field exercise tests, and for questioning of trainers and jockeys concerning the emotional state of the horse during exercise. If in doubt, calculation of V200 should be delayed until the horse has completed a test in a relaxed state. The correlation between 31 values of V200 measured on two consecutive days was 0.88.[36] The differences in V200 were in the range of 0–50 m/min. Precision of V200 measurements in the field would probably

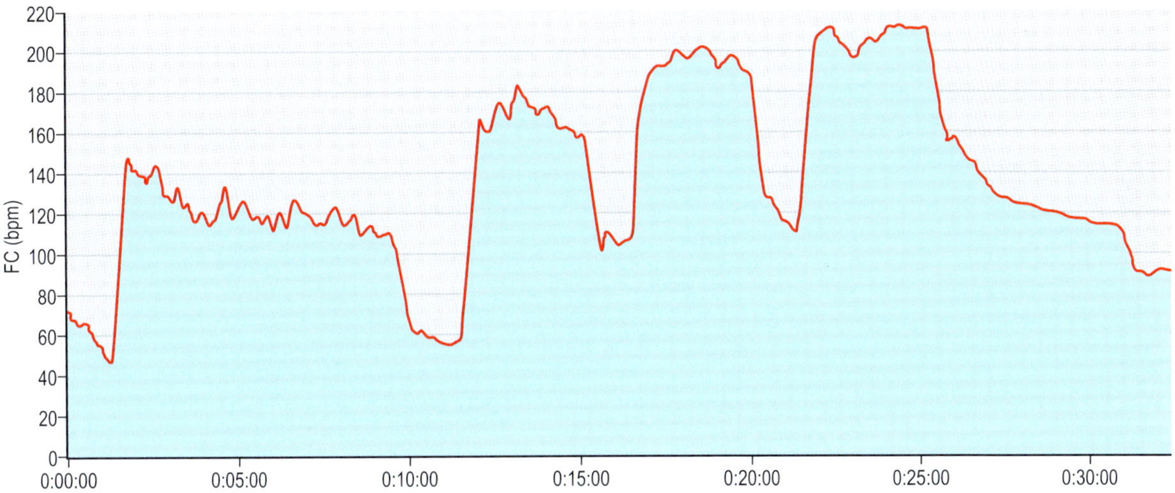

Fig 3.5 A heart rate tracing from a trotting horse during a standardized exercise test.

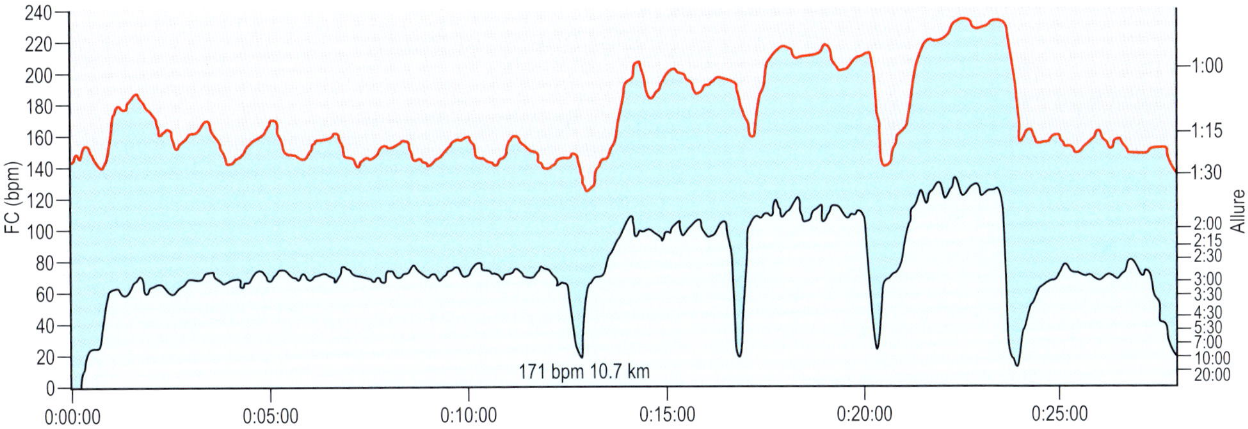

Fig 3.6 Heart rate and velocity measured during a standardized exercise test.

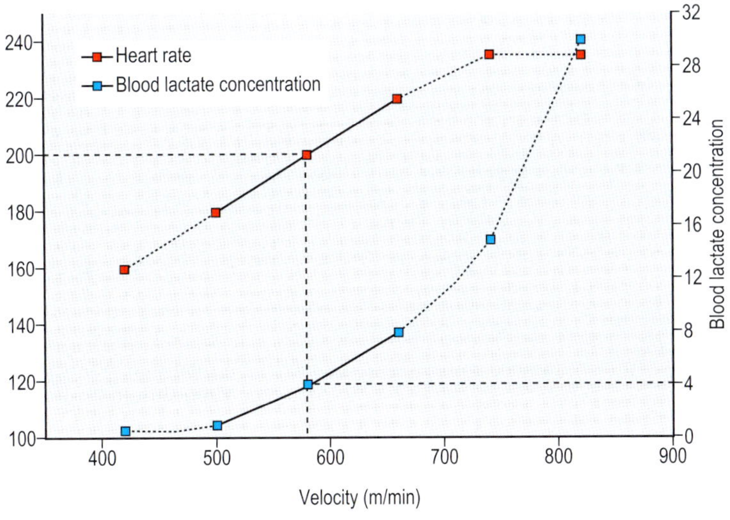

Fig 3.7 Linear regression between HR and velocity to measure V200 and exponential relationship between lactate and velocity to measure V4 or VLA4.[16]

Reprinted from Couroucé A. Field exercise testing for assessing fitness in French standardbred trotters. Vet J 1999; 157(2):112–122, with permission from Elsevier.

be increased by use of more than one exercise test, and inspection of scatter plots to discard obvious outliers. Figure 3.8 shows the effect of excitability on heart rates during trotting, and the effect on V200. High HRs in this study[36] were also associated with gait changes that were not 'smooth', and with phases of rapid acceleration.

V200 is also influenced by track type, with lower values on sand tracks than on grass or wood-chip surfaces. Interestingly, the V200 was not significantly different in horses ridden by light (55 kg) and heavy (70 kg) jockeys in a crossover study.[36] However, the mean V200 was 35 m/min higher with light jockeys, and it seems sensible to avoid large differences in rider weight when evaluating a horse in repeated tests over time. Age and training state also influence V200. In trotters, V200 was higher (641 ± 35 m/min) in horses aged six years or more when compared to horses aged 17 months (498 ± 39 m/min). The effects of growth and maturation as well as physical conditioning likely accounted for this difference in V200. In two-year-old Thoroughbred horses, mean V200 increased by approximately 65 m/min (10%) over a five-month training period (Fig. 3.9).[36] In French trotters, V200 increased with training over a six-month period. In two-year-old horses, the average increase in V200 was 40 m/min, while in horses above four years of age, the average increase in V200 was approximately 20 m/min.[12]

Comparison of data obtained from more than one exercise test (e.g. at periods during a training program) is most likely to give a trainer, veterinarian, or owner information that can help manage the horse's training program. No major decisions about a horse's fitness or health should be based on the results of a single exercise test. The finding of an unexpectedly high HR during an exercise test may or may not indicate a problem with fitness or health; however, a thorough evaluation is warranted to ascertain whether or not there is a new clinical or other condition that could explain the results. If there is some doubt concerning the validity of results in an individual exercise test, the test should be repeated.

Box 3.3 Factors that may contribute to a higher than expected heart rate response in horses during submaximal exercise

1. lameness or another painful condition
2. dehydration
3. exercise conducted in hot or hot and humid conditions
4. a loss of fitness, due to detraining or inappropriate training or overtraining
5. respiratory disease
6. cardiovascular disease or anemia
7. increased body mass, or a greater percentage of bodyweight as fat or water
8. a physiologically inferior horse, probably due to a relatively small heart
9. stress.

Electrocardiography

Telemetric ECG was first used in the 1960s, although wider clinical application during field exercise testing has only occurred during the last 10 years.[40–42] ECG measurement during a standardized exercise test is important for evaluation of poor performance because disturbances in cardiac rhythm may only manifest during exercise.[43] Previous studies have documented ECG responses to different types of exercise in clinically normal horses with no performance problems; review of these data is helpful for interpretation of ECG data in clinical cases.[40–42]

Blood or plasma lactate

Blood lactate concentration may be measured in blood samples obtained at the end of the exercise period; samples are typically

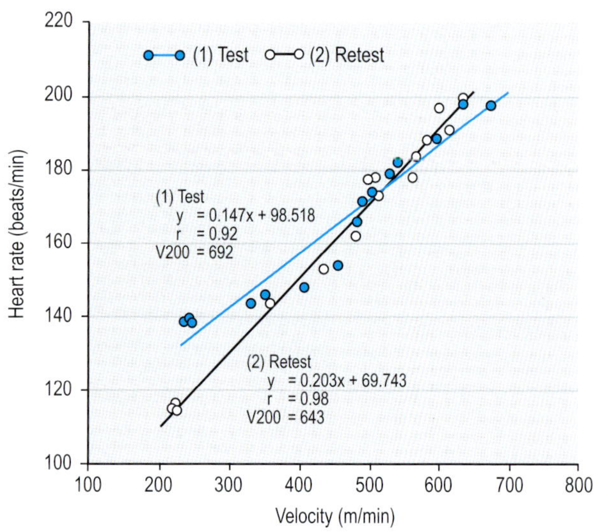

Fig 3.8 Relationships between heart rate and velocity in a Thoroughbred racehorse (1) exercising under field conditions after trotting in an excitable condition (blue symbols) and (2) when retested in a relaxed condition (white symbols). Note the pronounced increase in heart rates when trotting at 250 m/min in an excited condition. This effect has a marked influence of the slope of the line of best fit, which causes a false increase in V200.

From Kobayashi M, Kuribara K, Amada A. Application of V200 for evaluation of training effects in the young Thoroughbred under field conditions. Equine Vet J 1999; Suppl 30:159–162, with permission from the Equine Veterinary Journal.

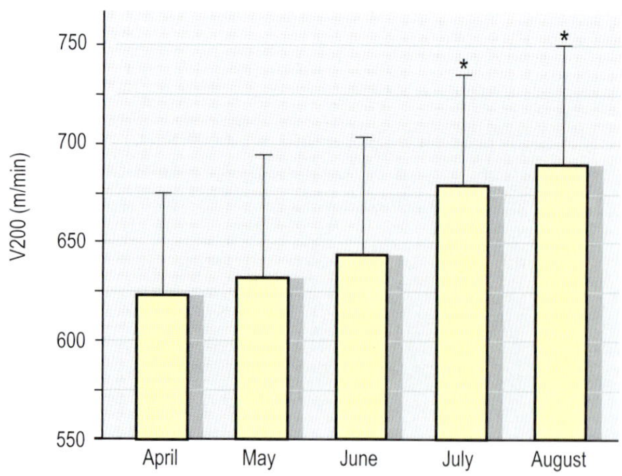

Fig 3.9 Changes in V200 (± SD) as training progressed from April to August in two-year-old Thoroughbreds.* Significantly different from April, May and June.

From Kobayashi M, Kuribara K, Amada A. Application of V200 for evaluation of training effects in the young Thoroughbred under field conditions. Equine Vet J 1999; Suppl 30:159–162, with permission from the Equine Veterinary Journal.

taken from a jugular vein and should be collected into tubes containing fluoride-oxalate as anticoagulant. Lactate is a product of muscular metabolism and accumulates in muscle and blood at high intensities of exercise. The concept of anaerobic threshold, extrapolated from the plotted curve of blood lactate concentration against speed, has been defined as the level of work just below that which results in the accumulation of lactate in blood.[44] The aerobic-anaerobic transition or onset of blood lactate accumulation (OBLA) has been defined empirically as 4 mmol/l blood lactate concentration.

Several factors, including the site of sample collection (e.g. venous vs. arterial), type of sample analyzed (whole blood vs. plasma), and method of sample preparation (e.g. addition of perchloric acid to the sample) will affect lactate concentrations and derived parameters such as VLA4 and VLA10.[45–49] Blood lactate is transported in plasma and RBC; the lactate concentration in whole blood is lower when compared to plasma due to the sequestration of some of the total lactate within RBC. Several rapid analysis/analyzer systems have been used for measurement of lactate in equine whole blood or plasma. One of the authors (ACM) has compared lactate measurements by the Accutrend Lactate, Ektachem and Boerhinger enzymatic techniques (n = 55 samples). In whole blood samples deproteinized by the addition of perchlotic acid, results obtained with the Accutrend were significantly higher (1.05 mmol/l ± 0.92) when compared to the Boehringer method. For plasma, there was no significant difference between measurements done with the Ektachem and the Accutrend. In another study, analysis with the Yellow Springs Instruments 2300 Stat Plus was found to be reliable for measurement of plasma lactate from 0–30 mmol/l. However, the TDx Lactic Acid Assay was deemed to be unsuitable for use with equine plasma due to greater variability in measurements.[50]

The VLA4 has been widely used to compare blood lactate responses between horses or in the same horse over time. Several studies have demonstrated a negative association between blood lactate responses and measures of racing performance. Evans et al[17] measured blood lactate in Thoroughbred horses at 2 and 5 min after an 800 m gallop and also during a submaximal exercise test on a 5% inclined treadmill, with results compared to retrospective racing performance as indicated by Timeform ratings. Blood lactate concentrations 2 and 5 min after treadmill exercise were significantly correlated ($r = -0.68$, $P < 0.01$) with Timeform.[17] In a small (n = 7) group of Swedish trotters, the first two horses to begin their racing career were the ones that had the lowest lactate concentration after submaximal tests. Leleu et al[18,20] showed that the VLA4 of good performing French trotters was significantly higher than in intermediate or poor performer horses.[20]

An increase in fitness results in an increase in VLA4. Loss of fitness, stress, respiratory disease and an increase in bodyweight could all cause a decrease in VLA4.[31–35] All these factors should be taken into account when interpreting individual values. The results of a study that measured VLA4 in 194 trotters that performed a total of 1105 standardized exercise tests on a sand racing track are presented in Table 3.1.[12] Growth and development, as well as physical conditioning, appears to influence VLA4. In two-year-old French trotters trained for six months, the mean increase in VLA4 was approximately 45 m/min, whereas in four-year-olds the average increase in VLA4 was 30 m/min.[12]

Underlying respiratory problems (upper airway disorders such as laryngeal hemiplegia as well as lower respiratory airway diseases such as inflammatory airway disease and/or exercise induces pulmonary hemorrhage) can limit oxygen exchange and may explain a higher than expected blood lactate concentration during exercise and thus a low VLA4.[51]

Table 3.1 VLA4, the velocity at which blood lactate concentration reaches 4 mmol/L, expressed in m/min according to age in 194 trotters that performed a total of 1105 standardized exercise tests on a sand racing track, 1250 m long[12]

AGE	MEAN VLA4 (EXPRESSED IN M/MIN) (±SD)
1	512 ± 21
2	551 ± 29
3	590 ± 41
4	611 ± 26
5	616 ± 26
6	626 ± 30

Red cell volume and hematocrit

Total red cell volume (RCV) is a major determinant of oxygen-carrying capacity. In horses, RCV has been measured by the Evans Blue dye dilution method when applied following mobilization of the splenic erythrocyte pool.[52,53] Total RCV relative to bodyweight was significantly correlated with maximal trotting speed over 1000 m in 35 Swedish trotters ($r = 0.68$, $P < 0.001$).[54] These results suggest that this measurement may be useful for assessment of performance capacity. However, measurement of total RCV by the dye dilution technique is not a simple procedure and cannot be readily applied in veterinary practice.

Hematocrit after maximal exercise, which ranges from 60 to 70%, was not correlated with Timeform rating in English Thoroughbreds[17] and does not appear to be valid measure of fitness or performance capacity. However, the hematocrit can be measured after maximal exercise if results of resting hematology suggest that a horse is anemic. Values should exceed 55% immediately after maximal exercise in trained Thoroughbreds. In Standardbred race horses, overtraining was associated with a decrease in PCV measured after a 2400 meter time trial at maximal speed. Mean values were 56% in control horses and 52% in overtrained horses.[55] Total RCV did not decrease during overtraining, so the decrease in hematocrit may have reflected the decrease in velocity of the horses during the time trial rather than a true decrease in the oxygen carrying capacity. A treadmill study also found that onset of overtraining was not associated with alterations in RCV.[56]

Measurement of oxygen consumption in field exercise

Oxygen consumption or uptake (VO_2) describes the rate of oxygen use in liters per minute, and is usually expressed relative to body mass. In human exercise physiology, the current gold standard for evaluating aerobic capacity is the measurement of the maximum rate of oxygen consumption (VO_{2max}). The VO_{2max} parameter integrates the efficiency and coordination between respiratory, cardiovascular and neuromuscular systems and thus yields both physiologic and metabolic information.[57] Measurements of VO_{2max} can be used to predict aerobic power and endurance performance in untrained human subjects. It is primarily limited by the maximal HR and cardiac stroke volume during exercise. A cardiac limit to performance can be best evaluated by measurement of oxygen pulse, the volume of oxygen ejected with each ventricular contraction. This measurement necessitates simultaneous measurement of VO_2 and HR during exercise. Rates of oxygen uptake during submaximal exercise will depend on gait, economy of locomotion, body mass, and other factors.

Determination of oxygen uptake necessitates measurements of air flow rates during breathing, and of oxygen and carbon dioxide concentrations in expired respiratory gas. The horse must wear a mask over its nose or face to enable these measurements, a technique referred to as *ergospirometry*. In horses during maximal exercise, respiratory rates often exceed 120 breaths per minute, with minute ventilation over 1500 L/min and peak flow rates of 30–40 L/s or more at each nostril. Measurement of breathing (minute ventilation) and expired gas concentrations during intense exercise in horses is obviously a considerable technical problem, especially in the field. In horses, most measurements of VO_2 have been performed during treadmill rather than overground exercise.

A landmark study of HR, pulmonary ventilation and VO_2 in two trotters was conducted in Russia.[58] A truck carried equipment beside the trotting horses as they completed a stepwise exercise test with peak speeds of 11 m/s. Notable findings during exercise at 11 m/s were tidal volumes of 17 L, pulmonary ventilation of 1200 L/min, and peak VO_2 of 64 L/min with a respiratory exchange ratio of 1.0. The horse plus vehicle approach to field ergospirometry was also used in a study of four Quarter Horses, one Appaloosa and one Thoroughbred at speeds ranging from 40 to 390 m/min, with and without a rider.[59] A tractor was used to pull a wagon, and on the wagon were the calorimeter and a gasoline generator. This study was conducted to enable calculation of the digestible energy intake needed to support the demands of exercise. Field ergospirometry was described in 23 riding horses at a walk, trot and gallop, using a pneumotachometer and an on-board oxygen sensor.[60] The key measurements of an ideal clinical exercise test were reported: HR, VO_2, pulmonary ventilation, ventilatory equivalent for oxygen, oxygen pulse and economy of locomotion. The synchrony of stride and locomotion was noted, as was the transitory effect of swallowing on breathing. The limitation of the performance of the pneumotachometer and response times of the oxygen sensor probably precluded measurements at maximal speeds.

Field ergospirometry and blood lactate measurements were conducted in 12 Warmbloods in order to calculate the relative contribution of aerobic and anaerobic metabolism to total energy output at speeds up to approximately 500 m/min.[61] Aliquots of expired gas were collected via tubes in the face mask, and the rider manipulated the bags that were used to collect the gas at each step of the exercise test. Oxygen debt was calculated from the oxygen uptake measurements made for 10 minutes after exercise, minus values before exercise. This value was referred to as the anaerobic contribution to energy output. It was reported that the percentages of energy expenditure that were anaerobic were 1%, 3%, 19%, and 30% at speeds of 100, 250, 350, and 530 m/min, respectively.

More recently, a portable breath-by-breath gas analyzer (Cosmed K4b2®) and mask (Equimask®) have been evaluated for the measurement of VO_2 in horses (Fig. 3.10).[62–63] The mask and associated turbines appear to result in additional ventilatory resistance and deadspace, with impairment to ventilation at high exercise levels. This may have imposed an excessive stress on the horses, preventing them from reaching maximal exertion.[64] Consequently, it has not been possible to determine VO_{2max} with this system. Votion et al[63] demonstrated the potential application of a portable ergospirometry system in ridden horses during submaximal field exercise tests. The authors suggested that the use of highly standardized field tests could allow interpretation of VO_2 in the absence of VO_{2max} attainment.[63]

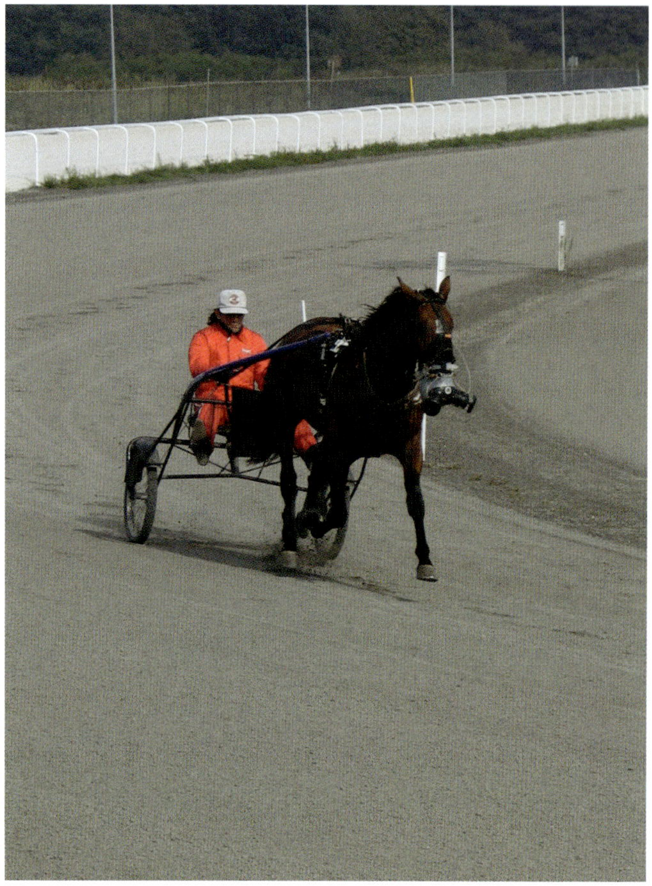

Fig 3.10 A horse equipped with a portable ergospirometer (Cosmed K4b2® / Equimask®) allowing breath-to-breath analysis of respired gases and VO_2 measurement in the field.

Coupling of measurements of heart rate, breathing (pulmonary ventilation) and VO_2 during field exercise will be a powerful technique for advancing knowledge in equine exercise physiology.

Gait analysis

Motion analysis techniques have been used in veterinary research for the assessment of normal and abnormal gait in horses since the late 19th century. Many of the studies involved capturing moving images in two dimensions and these techniques are still commonly used in field-based research and clinical practice. More advanced methods measure forces and motion in three dimensions. Stride characteristics (length, frequency, symmetry, regularity, dorsoventral displacement of the sternum and vertical, longitudinal and lateral activities measuring the amount of deceleration and acceleration along the 3 axis) can be routinely measured in field exercise tests by application of an accelerometric transducer.[65–69] These stride characteristics may be related to other variables such as VLA4 and V200,[67] oxygen consumption,[68] and respiratory strategy.[70]

Respiratory sound analysis during exercise

It has long been recognized that the production of abnormal respiratory sounds by horses during exercise is frequently associated with various upper airway obstructive conditions. Respiratory acoustic measurements have shown promise for the investigation of upper airway disorders in man and, more recently, in horses with experimentally-induced obstructions. Franklin et al[71] recorded respiratory sounds during exercise on the treadmill using an acoustically insulated subminiature omnidirectional microphone with a flat amplitude response between 50 and 13 kHz. Spectral analysis of the audio signal showed marked differences between control and clinically afflicted horses. Dorsal displacement of the soft palate was characterized by a narrow low frequency (20–80 Hz) peak during expiration. Horses with dynamic laryngeal collapse produced inspiratory sounds characterized by a broad band high frequency spectral component in the range 1.1–2.7 kHz. Spectral analysis of respiratory sounds in horses has potential as a diagnostic technique and this equipment may be used in the field.[71]

Endoscopy during exercise

Endoscopic examination of the upper airway during exercise enables diagnosis of obstructive disorders that may be undetectable or misdiagnosed when the examination is performed at rest.[72–75] Overground endoscopy allows evaluation of the upper airway under field conditions, with the horse ridden or driven and exercised in a manner comparable to competition. This examination is indicated for pre-purchase examinations and for the evaluation of horses that produce audible respiratory noise during exercise, exhibit poor performance, abnormal breathing or abnormal fatigue during or after exercise, or show abnormal behavior (e.g. head shaking) during riding. It is possible for upper airway obstruction to occur without generating a respiratory noise, especially in sport horses where air flow rates are lower than in racing horses and therefore less likely to produce excessive vibration of the upper airway structures. This examination may be coupled to other measurements during exertion (e.g. HR, V and lactate) as a means to determine whether or not the observed airway abnormality is contributing to performance limitation.

Overground endoscopy can be applied to all athletic disciplines.[76–81] In sport horses, ridden examination is particularly important as equitation-related maneuvers or movements have been shown to interfere with upper airway stability (Fig. 3.11). Rider intervention (described as the use of spurs, change of gait or short turns) as well as increased poll flexion seem to disrupt the rhythm of ventilation and induce an accentuation of upper airway instability.[81] This may explain why upper airway abnormalities (dorsal displacement of the soft palate, laryngeal collapse) are more frequently diagnosed in dressage horses than in show jumpers. These conditions were rarely associated with respiratory noise but could be associated with cough, head and neck extension (yanking of the reins), and reluctance to yield to the hand or flex the poll.[81]

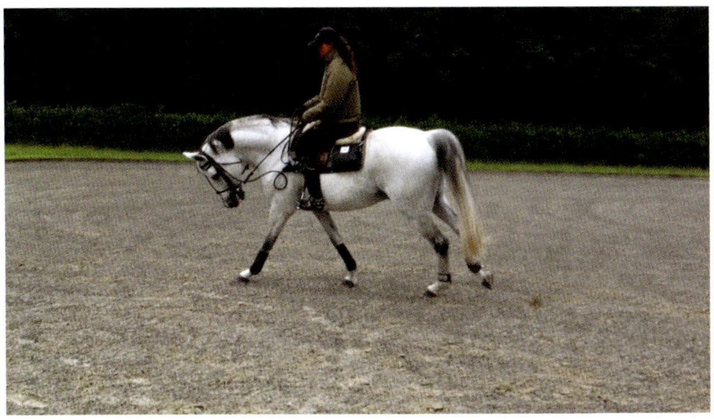

Fig 3.11 In sport horses, performing exercise endoscopy during ridden exercise is important as equitation and poll flexion may influence the stability of the upper airways and the diagnostic outcome.[81]

The prevalence of observed upper airway obstruction was higher in a population of sport horses examined during overground (track) exercise (82%) when compared to non-racing performance horses examined during treadmill running (72%).[82] Moreover, of the horses referred for poor performance, the percentage of horses diagnosed with an upper airway condition was higher in the field (70%) vs. treadmill (21%) study. The frequency of multiple airway abnormalities was higher (56%) in this field-based study in comparison to studies that performed upper airway endoscopy during treadmill exercise (~20%).[82–83] Although heterogeneity of the study populations may have explained some differences in results, the study by Davidson et al.[82] highlights the importance of examining horses under normal exercising conditions when an upper airway obstructive condition is suspected.

Field exercise tests in trotters and pacing horses

A review of exercise tests for French trotters concluded that track testing provided a more limited range of measurements than treadmill testing, but had the advantage of being performed in the horse's natural environment.[16] Various measurements such as HR during exercise and blood lactate concentration after exercise may be measured on the track, enabling calculation of physiological variables such as V200 and VLA4. Although VLA4 is calculated during submaximal intensity exercise, it is related to racing performance and seems to be the most important measurement to assess changes in fitness.[16] There is a significant influence of age and fitness on V200 and VLA4 in trotters.[24] The use of a graphical display of HR and blood lactate concentrations at different speeds of field exercise to calculate V200 and V4 in a trotting horse is illustrated in Figure 3.12.[16] This figure also shows the typical effect of training on the relationships; both curves shift to the right. Figure 3.13 shows the normal values for some HR and plasma lactate indices in relation to exercise velocity in trotters of various ages,[12] and the influence of training is described in Figure 3.14. The potential use of field exercise tests as an aid to the clinical evaluation of athletic horses is illustrated in Figure 3.15, which shows the effect of subclinical respiratory disease on HR and blood lactate concentrations during a submaximal field test in trotters.[16] It should be noted that blood lactate concentration is likely to be increased by excitement during the test, and by 'pulling', an inefficient gait due to effort expended against restraint by the driver. Results from exercise tests in which horses pull hard against a jockey or driver should be regarded with suspicion, and the test repeated.

Field tests with multiple speeds and blood collections have been conducted in Standardbred trotters and pacers to assess performance on the basis of HR and blood lactate measurements. A simple exercise test for pacing horses consisted of four steps of exercise over 1000 meters.[11] Speeds of each step were 450–550, 600–700, 700–800 and >800 m/min. The horse walked for 3–5 minutes between each of the four steps, with blood samples collected at the three minute mark during each recovery period. It was observed that superior horses had a lower blood lactate response to this exercise test. In a study of Swedish Standardbred trotters, 10 horses completed a track exercise test that consisted of five incremental heats at speeds of 9.1, 9.5, 10.0, 10.5, and 11.1 m/s over 1000 meters. A blood sample was

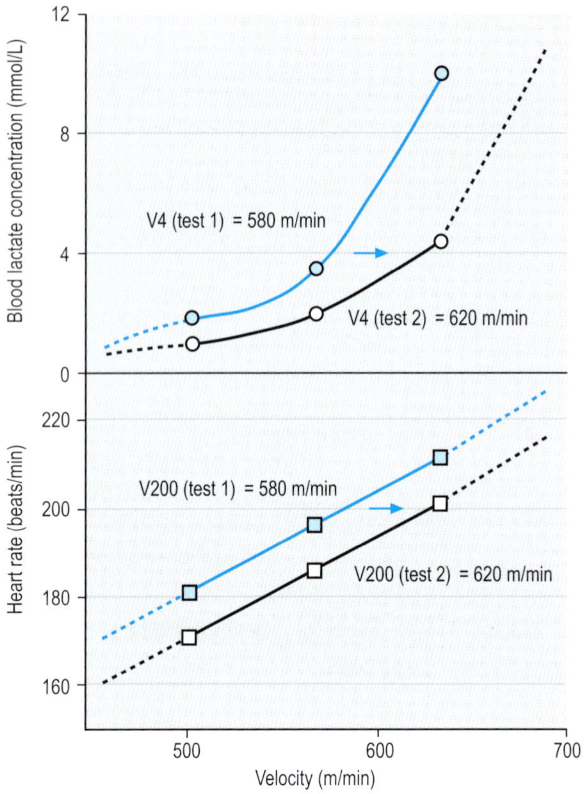

Fig 3.12 Heart rate and blood lactate concentrations related to velocity in a French trotter before (blue lines) and after (black lines) 6 weeks of training. There is a shift to the right with improved fitness. The heart rates and blood lactate concentrations during exercise at 500, 580 and 630 m/min are lower after training. V200 and V4 have increased.

Reprinted from Couroucé, A., Field exercise testing for assessing fitness in French standardbred trotters, Vet J, 1999; 157(2):112-122, with permission from Elsevier.

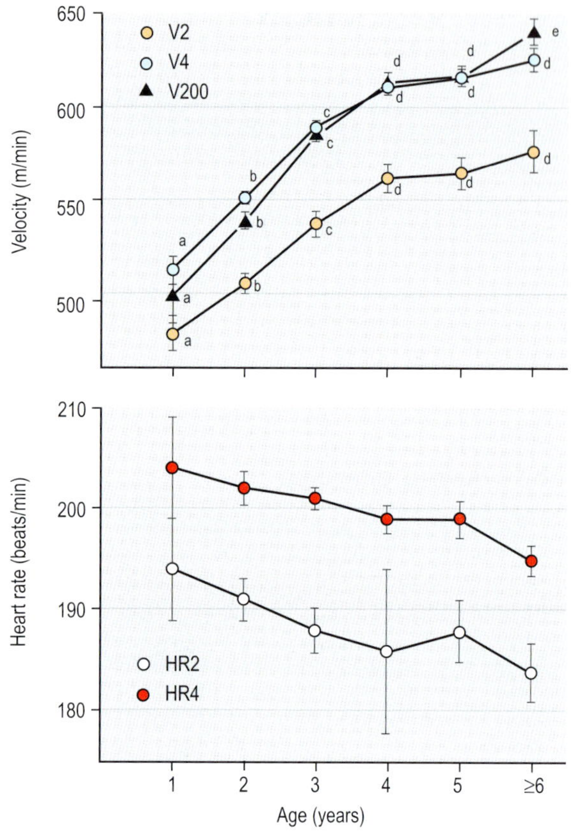

Fig 3.13 Mean and 95% confidence interval values for several indices of fitness in French Standardbred trotters of various ages. V2 and V4, velocities at which post-exercise blood lactate concentrations are 2 or 4 mmol/L; V200, velocity at which HR is 200 beats/min. HR2 and HR4 refer to heart rates at blood lactate concentrations of 2 and 4 mmol/L. Values with different letters at each age are significantly different ($P < 0.05$).

From Couroucé A., Chrétien M., Valette JP. Physiological variables measured under field conditions according to age and state of training in French standardbred trotters. Equine Vet J 2002; 34:91-97, with permission from the Equine Veterinary Journal.

drawn from the jugular vein for plasma lactate analysis immediately after each heat. The plasma lactate response to exercise differed between horses, but no correlation with an index of racing performance was detected in this small study population.[84] Van Erck et al[85] evaluated poor performance in Standardbreds with an exercise test that consisted of three bouts of 1500 m at increasing speeds with a recovery phase of 500 m between bouts. The fitness parameters VLA4 and V200 discriminated poor performers from healthy control horses, regardless of the cause of exercise intolerance.

A submaximal field exercise test consisting of two bouts of 1600 meters was used to assess fitness in Standardbred pacing horses in two stables (A and B).[86] Five minutes of rest or walking between runs was allowed. Performance indices were compiled for each horse: number of race starts, number of race wins, number of race placings (1, 2, or 3), and lifetime earnings. Regression analysis was conducted to describe the relationship between plasma lactate concentrations and speed for tests one, two, and pooled results. Using the regression equation, observed (measured) minus expected (predicted) (O – E) lactate concentrations for tests were calculated and plotted against performance indices to determine their relationship. The association between lactate and velocity for the two tests was best described by exponential equations. This study found no relationship in either stable between O – E and performance indices (number of race wins, number of race placings, lifetime earnings and average $/start) for test run one, two or pooled lactates. At one of the stables there was a significant association between VLA4 and log lifetime earnings ($r = 0.51$, $P = 0.05$) and log average $/start ($r = 0.54$, $P = 0.04$). There were no significant correlations at the other stable. It was concluded that a two-step determination method of VLA4 was a suitable method for studying limits to performance in pacing Standardbred racehorses. A major advantage of the technique used in this study was that the test was easily incorporated into the normal training routine. It was also noted that the correlations might be higher if studies of associations between fitness indices and performance included more horses with a wider range of racing abilities. Another limitation of such studies is that they do not include horses that have been discarded from training due to poor performance early in their racing career. More studies are needed on the variability in fitness of young, unraced horses. Does fitness in young unraced horses predict future racing performance? Is the rate of change in fitness equal in all horses when they are trained? Large-scale field studies may offer the best opportunities to investigate these questions.

Field exercise tests in Thoroughbreds

Heart rate measurements

A major difficulty with field exercise testing of galloping horses has been control of the exercise performed by the horse. However with the possibility of continuously and simultaneously recording speed and HR, there is less necessity for an absolute control of exercise speeds, as long as there are consistent rates of acceleration.[87] As for Standardbreds, V200 can also be calculated with an incremental field exercise test in Thoroughbred racehorses.[36] Commercial HR meters that log HR and V continuously and enable transfer of the data to a computer for analysis are suitable for this purpose.[87] More recently, telemetric units are able to transmit speed, ECG and HR recordings directly to smart-phones or tablet computers (Televet, Germany).

One exercise test designed for Thoroughbreds consisted of about 1000 m trotting at 250 m/min, followed by galloping at ~400, 460, 550, and 660 m/min for 600–800 m at each speed. Fine days and tracks in firm condition were used, and velocity was measured by stopwatch every 200 m of each step of the test. Mean HR and V were calculated for each 200 m section of the test. This exercise test was used to investigate the influence of rider and track conditions, repeatability of V200 measurements and the effects of training on V200.[36] Figure 3.16 shows the relationship between HR and V in one horse from this study.

The utility of V200 and speed at maximal HR (VHRmax) for evaluation of training-induced changes in fitness has been investigated in Thoroughbred racehorses.[87] These data were obtained by use of a GPS

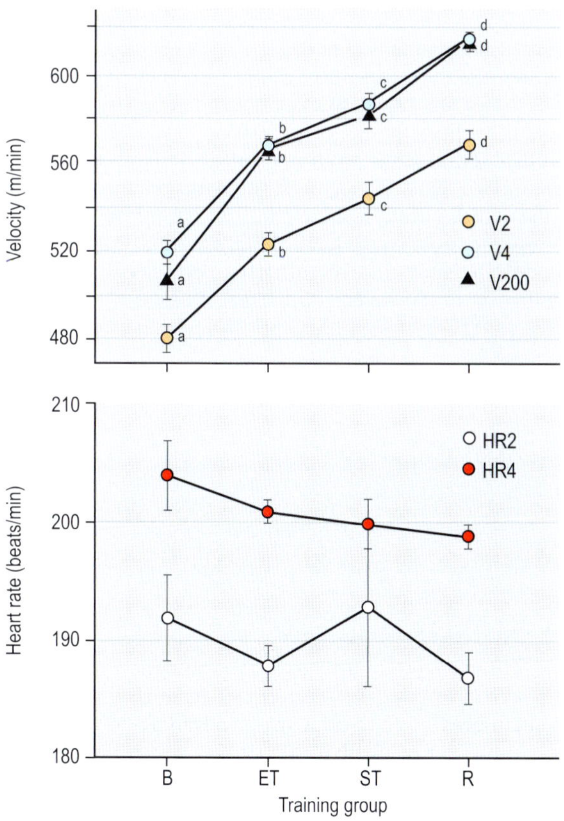

Fig 3.14 Mean and 95% confidence interval values for several indices of fitness in French Standardbred trotters of various ages. B, at beginning of training; ET, after endurance training; ST, after sprint training; R, when racing. At each age, values with different letters are significantly different ($P < 0.05$).

From Couroucé A, Chrétien M, Valette JP. Physiological variables measured under field conditions according to age and state of training in French Standardbred trotters. Equine Vet J 2002; 34:91–97, with permission from the Equine Veterinary Journal.

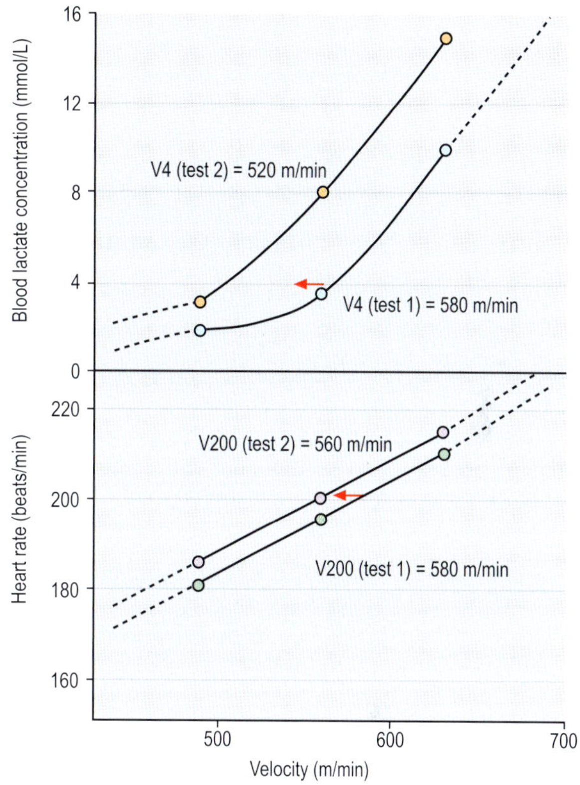

Fig 3.15 Heart rate and blood lactate concentrations related to velocity in a French trotter before (test 1) and after (test 2) six weeks of training, showing the influence of a subclinical respiratory infection. The heart rates and blood lactate concentrations during exercise at 500, 580 and 630 m/min are higher after training associated with the respiratory disease, and V200 and V4 have decreased.

Reprinted from Couroucé A. Field exercise testing for assessing fitness in French Standardbred trotters. Vet J 1999; 157(2):112–122, with permission from Elsevier.

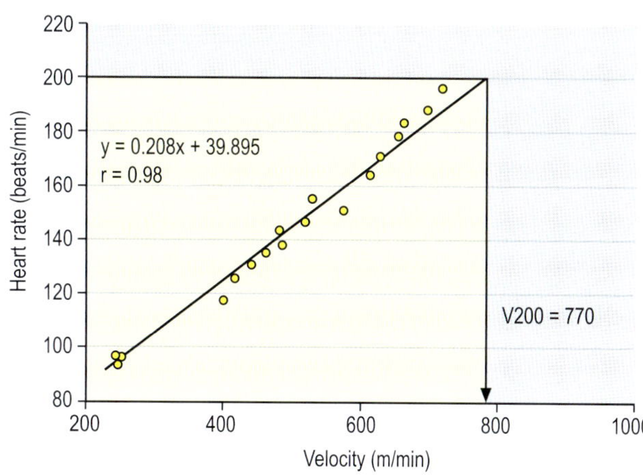

Fig 3.16 Relationship between heart rate and velocity in a Thoroughbred race horse exercising under field conditions.

From Kobayashi M, Kuribara K, Amada A. Application of V200 for evaluation of training effects in the young Thoroughbred under field conditions. Equine Vet J 1999; Suppl 30:159–162, with permission from the Equine Veterinary Journal.

and Polar HR meter with testing conducted at weeks 2 and 6 of 'fast' training. The measurements were made during a regular 'fast training session' rather than a standardized exercise test in order to avoid disruption of the training program. The results of this study indicated that VHRmax, V200 and HRmax were reliable measurements of fitness and that VHRmax and V200 both increased significantly with training. Additionally, this study demonstrated that it is possible to evaluate training responses in the context of routine exercise sessions, without the need for standardized exercise tests.

Blood lactate measurements

The conduct of racetrack exercise tests for measurement of VLA4 or VLA10 is especially problematic in Thoroughbreds because it is difficult to obtain constant track conditions and constant speeds during exercise. Moreover it may be dangerous to stop young Thoroughbreds on the track in order to draw blood samples. Measurement of the lactate responses to a single or pair of exercise bouts could be an alternative and more repeatable approach.

A standardized, two-step exercise test has been used to investigate the blood lactate-running speed relationship in nine Thoroughbred race horses.[88] Each horse completed a two-speed field test at intervals of 6–8 weeks to determine the running V that resulted in blood lactate concentrations of 4 (V(4)) and 12 mmol/L (V(12)). Changes of V(4) and V(12) between two consecutive tests were used to assess the effects of training history. The percentage of days with gallop workouts between two consecutive tests showed a significant correlation with changes in V(4) ($r = 0.71$, $P < 0.01$) and V(12) ($r = 0.56$, $P < 0.05$). The number of gallop workouts ($r = 0.60$, $P < 0.05$) and the total time of training ($r = 0.58$, $P < 0.05$) also correlated with the change of V(4). Furthermore the percentage of days without training was negatively correlated to changes of V(4) ($r = -0.75$, $P < 0.01$) and v(12) ($r = -0.56$, $P < 0.05$). These results imply that increases in fitness, as measured with the blood lactate response to submaximal exercise in a two-step field test, are more likely in Thoroughbred horses that have more galloping than trotting exercise, and have a higher number of gallops in a given time period. More days without training was associated with reduced fitness, and more training at higher speeds was associated with greater fitness.

An alternative approach is to determine the blood lactate concentration during a single bout of strenuous, submaximal exercise. An appropriate speed of the exercise must be chosen. The aim is to have an exercise test that is demanding for some horses, but achieved easily in others. Typical speeds for such tests are 800 meters in 65–70 seconds in a Standardbred horse,[11] and in 55–60 seconds in Thoroughbreds.[89] These speeds would need to be confirmed in an individual stable, because they will depend on the quality of horses being trained, and possibly on track size and surface conditions.

The use of a single blood lactate measurement after exercise has been validated as a measure of racing ability in Thoroughbred horses, and as a simple method of monitoring responses to treadmill training. A correlation coefficient of >0.6 was found between retrospective career racing performance in Thoroughbreds, and blood lactate concentration two minutes after treadmill exercise at 10 m/s.[17] During a treadmill training program, the blood lactate concentration after treadmill exercise at 9 m/s gradually decreased over nine weeks of training.[90] This response was similar to changes in VLA4. These results suggest that exercise tests with multiple steps may not be absolutely necessary for fitness evaluation in horses, and that measurement of the blood lactate concentration after a standardized, one-step test may suffice.

The feasibility of a one-step field test for assessment of fitness in Thoroughbred horses has been investigated.[89] Each horse completed a 1000 m warm-up at a slow trot of approximately 3–4 m/s prior to the test. Subsequently the horses completed an 800 m gallop with jockeys instructed to maintain a constant running speed in the range of 13 to 16 m/s. This range of speeds was selected to correspond with the speeds frequently used in training Thoroughbreds. The time for the 800 m and each of the four 200 m sections was obtained by stop-watch. All timing was conducted from the same position at each track by the same observer. Speed was determined from the total time for the 800 m gallop. At the completion of each gallop, the horse was trotted for 5 min, and then jugular venous blood was collected for measurement of blood lactate concentration.

After inspection of the scatter plots of the relationships between blood lactate concentration and velocity for data from each racetrack, regression analyzes were conducted to describe the line of best fit. Figure 3.17 shows the relationship between blood lactate after field exercise and exercise velocity on a sand racetrack in 21 trained Thoroughbred racehorses.[89] The variability of V during the exercise tests was expressed as the coefficient of variation (CV) of the times for the four 200 m sections of the exercise test. In horses tested more than once the result from the exercise test with the lowest CV was used in the regression analysis. Exercise tests were conducted at velocities in the range 13.2 to 15.9 m/s, and resulted in post-exercise blood lactate concentrations in the range 5.0 to 16.1 mmol/L. The mean speeds of the four consecutive 200 m sections of the exercise tests on the sand racetrack were 13.5, 14.6, 14.5, and 14.9 m/s. The jockeys were clearly unable to maintain a constant speed during the 800 m test.

A single step test that takes into account variability of V within a test, and is based on calculation of the difference between the measured and predicted lactate concentration, has potential application in field evaluations of fitness in Thoroughbred horses. Further studies are required to investigate whether the difference between the blood lactate response to exercise in an individual horse and the predicted concentration in a reference population is an accurate and reliable correlate of racing performance. Changes in this difference could also reflect changes in fitness over time.

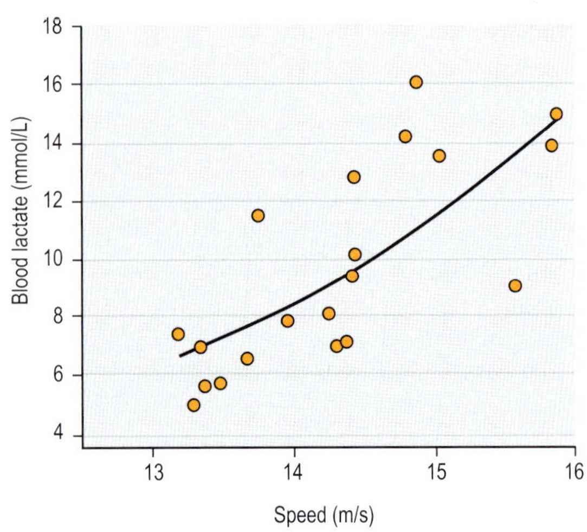

Fig 3.17 Relationship between blood lactate concentration (mmol/L) after field exercise and velocity (m/s) during an 800 m exercise test on a sand track in Thoroughbred horses.

Reprinted from Davie AJ, Evans DL. Blood lactate responses to submaximal field exercise tests in Thoroughbred horses. Vet J 2000; 159(3):252–258, with permission from Elsevier.

The use of the difference between the measured and predicted lactate concentration as an index of the lactate response to exercise obviates the need for strict control over the target speed during the conduct of a field exercise test. Potentially it could be possible to conduct tests at any speed in an appropriate range, and compare the measured lactate concentration with the predicted concentration based on the equation for the line of best fit. This approach enables horses to be tested at different speeds, and comparisons between individual responses to exercise can be based on the rating. Superior English Thoroughbred racehorses had a low blood lactate response to a single bout of exercise.[17] Therefore horses that consistently give a high 'rating' (that is, a high positive difference between measured and the predicted lactate concentration) could be expected to race poorly. Superior training in an individual horse should reduce the difference between measured and expected blood lactate concentrations.

The validity of results could be improved with some refinement of the technique. Accuracy and reliability of measurements could be improved if velocity did not vary during the exercise test. Anxiety or fear could also contribute to the variability, and these factors may not always be easy to recognize. The confounding effect of increases in speed may be more important in field tests that measure blood lactate concentration than in tests that measure HR, because the increase in speed can be related to the higher HR when the data are analyzed, as demonstrated in a study with Thoroughbred horses.[36]

A field exercise test with three steps was used with eight French Thoroughbred horses in France to investigate the use of HR measurements during and after track exercise as a suitable measure of changes in fitness.[91] The test consisted of a warm-up followed by three 3 min steps, one cantering and two galloping, followed by a recovery period. Heart rate was recorded during the entire test, and blood samples were taken during the 2 min rest periods following each step, and after the recovery period for the measurement of lactate concentrations. Fitness was described by the relationships between lactate concentrations, HR and V. The authors concluded that the efficiency score and the cardiac recovery index were good indicators of potential speed.

Field exercise tests in eventers

A number of protocols have been described for field exercise testing of eventing horses, either with steps of defined duration or defined distance.[92–94] Auvinet et al.[93] have used a test with six steps of 3 min each at speeds of 350 to 600 m/min, with a 50 m/min increase in speed from one step to the next and a 1 min recovery between the steps. Munoz et al.[91] described two test protocols: 1) a test with 4×1000 m steps at speeds from 400 to 700 m/min, with a 100 m/min increase in speed from one step to the next; and 2) a test with 3×1000 m steps at speeds between 400 to 600 m/min. In both tests a 5 min period of recovery at the walk was allowed between steps. Calculations of VLA2, VLA4, V150 and V200 were obtained from the linear and exponential relationships between V, HR and plasma lactate concentrations. Horses were divided into two groups according to their level of training; group designation was confirmed by evaluation of VLA2 and VLA4 data, with higher values in the better trained horses. A primary objective of these standardized exercise tests is to elicit blood/plasma lactate concentration >4 mmol/l and a HR >160 bpm at the end of the last step. In the study by Munoz et al.,[91] however, the three-step test (600 m/min during the last step) was not sufficient to elicit a blood lactate concentration >4 mmol/l. The VLA4 value was therefore calculated by extrapolation in the exponential equation that related V and plasma lactate concentrations; this extrapolation could lead to an overestimation of VLA4. In contrast, a study by Van Erck et al.[94] demonstrated that a three-step test can result in the desired peak of HR and blood/plasma lactate. These investigators used a 4 × 1000 m step test at speeds from 26.6 to 39.4 km/h (656 m/min) with a 1 min recovery period between steps. The horses reached a HR of, respectively, 160 ± 12, 174 ± 9, 197 ± 21 and 211 ± 22 bpm and a blood lactate concentration of 2.7 ± 0.7, 4.0 ± 1.1, 6.2 ± 2.1 and 11.2 ± 4.7 mmol/l.[94]

One should keep in mind that a standardized exercise test should be easy to perform by both horse and rider. Each step should be 2–3 min long, allowing 'steady-state' HR and blood lactate concentration to be achieved. Protocols with defined distances and in which the last step lasts less than 1 min 30 s may not be sufficient to provide reliable measurements. It is also recommended that these tests be performed on a flat track.

Field exercise tests in show jumpers and dressage horses

In dressage and show jumper horses, a primary goal of training programs is to improve the horse's stamina and movement (biomechanics). Field tests should be designed to enable assessment of fitness in relation to the demands of the sport. During competitions, even at middle-class level, show jumping efforts exceed the 'anaerobic threshold' and the evaluation of improvement in both aerobic and anaerobic metabolism is of interest.[95] In dressage, the physical requirements of a Grand Prix test include both low and high intensity work; however the low-intensity, slow speed exercise has been shown to account for 88% of the marks whereas movements performed in the faster gaits contributed only 12%.[96]

Assessment of fitness in Warmbloods during a field exercise test can be difficult because some horses are unable or unwilling to canter at higher speeds. Moreover, riders and trainers are usually unwilling to allow horses to perform very intense exercise between competitions. Finding an appropriate track may also be a problem as many sport horse stables are not equipped with a track suitable for cantering at higher speeds. Finding an acceptable compromise is essential to be able to reproduce the chosen standardized exercise test over time.

Although there are few publications relating to field exercising testing of sport horses, several protocols may be used routinely to assess the health and fitness of show jumpers and dressage horses. Some early work demonstrated high reproducibility of the HR versus V relationship in Warmbloods during standardized field tests run over the same 1000 m track.[97] As for racehorses, the relationship between HR and V was linear and evolved with age, activity type and level of training.[97] Given that these tests were conducted in the field, it was noteworthy that the scatter of HR values around the regression line was low (range: ± 3 to ± 4.9 bpm). Lactate measurements can be included in the testing protocol but a stepwise design should be used as lactate values obtained after a single effort may fail to detect training-induced changes or inter-individual differences when submaximal exercise is performed.[98]

A track test for Warmbloods that integrated HR, V and lactate measurements has been described.[99] The horses were submitted to a five-step incremental test over 1100 m on a sand track, with the last step at maximal exertion. There was an eight minute recovery at the walk after each step. The test was able to detect differences in lactate fitness parameters (V2, V4) between the saddle horses and a group of trained endurance horses; however, HR parameters did not differ between groups.

More recently, three different standardized exercise tests (SET) were compared for the evaluation of show jumpers after specific training programs.[100] The first test (SET1) was a stepwise incremental canter on a 850 m sand track (5 steps); the second (SET2) was a jumping test consisting of three runs over a series of 16 jumps placed on an elliptical track, with elevation of selected jumps from step to step; and the third test (SET3) comprised a show-jumping course with 11 jumps. In addition to HR and lactate measurements, the number of obstacles cleared was included as a performance criterion in SET2 and SET3. Based on lactate parameters, all tests succeeded in showing improvements in fitness over the six-week training period. However, only SET2 was able to highlight the benefits gained from the inclusion of fast sprint exercises into the training program. Moreover, SET2 detected a significant difference in the number of obstacle cleared before and after training. The integration of jumping protocols therefore appears to be useful for assessment of fitness and performance of show jumpers.

In addition to the evaluation of fitness conditioning, motion analysis may also be useful for objective assessment of progress in technical training. This methodology may be applied to field evaluation and has been described in dressage horses.[96]

Field exercise tests may also be applied in Warmbloods to diagnose subclinical diseases that impede performance. During a standardized exercise test executed at trot and canter in an indoor arena, Warmbloods suffering from upper and/ or lower respiratory disease or pathological cardiac arrhythmias during exercise display a higher rate of blood lactate accumulation when compared to healthy horses, even at low levels of exercise (personal observations). The assessment of HR is less useful when the horse is painful or suffers from lameness.

Field exercise tests in endurance horses

Interest in the sport of endurance racing has grown in the past decade and record average and peak racing speeds have been regularly broken in recent years. Given the high demands of endurance racing, adequate training is essential to ensure safe and successful competition. Although endurance exercise is essentially aerobic[102–103], endurance races also involve phases of anaerobic work[104] and exercise tests should take into consideration these physiological demands. Munoz et al[105] developed a field exercise test to investigate the adaptive response to endurance training of horses of different breeds over a period of 6 months.[105] The test consisted of a warm-up of 800 m at 0.7 km/h, and then steps at the following speeds and distances: 15 km/h for 1250 m, 20 km/h for 1670 m, 25 km/h for 2080 m, and 30 km/h for 2500 m. A 5 min active recovery (walk, trot) was included between each workload. This testing protocol demonstrated improvement in lactate-based parameters with training.

Fraipont et al[35] described a test that consisted of a warm-up phase of 10 minutes at walk then at trot, followed by three steps: 27 km at ~6 m/s (22 km/h), 1500m at ~7.5 m/s (27 km/h), and 1500m at ~8.8 m/s (32km/h). A recovery period at a slow-trot over 700m was allowed between each step and a recovery phase at walk of 10 min ended the test. The whole test lasted approximately 2 hours. The parameters measured were HR and V and blood was drawn between each step for measurements of lactate concentrations. The authors also compared the results of the field test to that of a standardized treadmill test. The field test was well accepted by the riders and the calculated fitness parameters V160, V200 and VLA4 enabled discrimination between two groups of horses racing at different levels. The use of continuous HR and speed recording from a GPS-based device facilitated determination of real-time HR, V and lactate relationships without use of strictly standardized speeds. It also proved to be more reliable than the treadmill test, as reproducible calculations of VLA4, V160 and V200 could not be obtained from treadmill tests in horses that had been acclimated to treadmill running.

The same test was used for evaluation of horses presented for poor performance (excluding elimination from races from known causes).[35] The field test enabled discrimination between healthy endurance horses and horses suffering from subclinical diseases (lameness, cardio-respiratory or muscular problems); specifically, VLA4, V160 and V200 were significantly lower in horses presented for poor performance and apparent subclinical disease (Table 3.2). This field exercise test is easily integrated into routine training sessions, increasing the acceptance from trainers and riders.

Measurements after exercise

Clinical evaluation of the horse after exercise is an important component of the overall assessment. The timing of measurements should be standardized and also interpreted in light of the exercise performed. Respiratory rate should return to resting within 60 min of the completion of exercise. The horse should also be examined for the presence of nasal discharge (e.g. blood or mucopurulent material). The HR decreases in two phases: the first phase, which lasts about 10 minutes, is characterized by a rapid decrease in HR. In healthy Standardbred trotters, HR is usually <85 bpm at 5 min after maximal exercise. The second phase is characterized by a slower rate of HR decline toward resting values.

Table 3.2 Mean (± SD) physiological variables obtained during standardized exercise tests in 11 control endurance horses, 18 intermediate performers, and 9 poor performers[35]

GROUND	GROUP	VLA4 (KM/H)	V200 (KM/H)	V160 (KM/H)
Treadmill	Control	31.7 ± 1.07	41.5 ± 6.44	26.3 ± 2.45
	Intermediate	30.2 ± 6.61	34.2 ± 5.19*	21.6 ± 5.17*
	Poor	25.1 ± 6.34*	33.6 ± 6.17*	21.9 ± 5.09
Racetrack	Control	33.8 ± 7.17	46.8 ± 7.35	30.4 ± 3.89
	Intermediate	30.1 ± 7.15	37.5 ± 6.31*	25.7 ± 4.37*
	Poor	24.5 ± 6.48*	36.3 ± 4.08*	24.9 ± 4.63*

*Significantly different from corresponding value in group 1 ($p < 0.05$).
VLA4, velocity at blood lactate concentration is 4 mmol/L; V160 and V200, velocity at which HR is 160 and 200 beats/min.

Blood samples also may be taken after exercise – soon after exercise for metabolic measurements and some hours after exercise for measurement of muscle enzyme (CK and AST) activities. Tests of the blood lactate response to submaximal exercise such as those described above are indications of endurance ability, or stamina. Measurements of VLA4 or VLA10 are unlikely to be highly correlated with the ability of a horse to accelerate at the start or finish of a race, or the ability of a horse to sprint 600–800 m.

High levels of 'anaerobic stress' are found in Thoroughbred horses after approximately 50 seconds of maximal field exercise.[26] After only 400 metres of field exercise near racing speeds the blood lactate concentration increased from less than 1.0 mmol/L to over 14 mmol/L,[106] values similar to concentrations found after races. This rapid increase in blood lactate concentration during maximal exercise also occurs in Standardbreds and polo horses.[107] Measurement of the blood lactate concentration after maximal exercise has been used to estimate anaerobic capacity, defined as the ability of an individual to resynthesize ATP via anaerobic metabolism. Markers of anaerobic metabolism in skeletal muscle include concentrations of plasma lactate and uric acid after maximal exercise.[108]

The blood lactate concentration after maximal exercise to fatigue does not change with submaximal treadmill exercise training,[90] or after high-intensity training.[109] As well, the blood lactate concentrations after maximal exercise were not correlated with race performance in trotters[110] or Thoroughbreds.[17] This measurement is therefore not a useful marker of fitness.

Relationships between racing performance and plasma lactate and uric acid concentrations after racing were investigated in pacing Standardbred racehorses.[111] Twenty horses were tested after races of 1760 meters and 28 horses after races over 2160 meters. Blood samples were taken 30–60 minutes before and eight and 30 minutes after a race. There were no significant differences between the race distances for prerace and eight minute post-race plasma lactates. Significant low correlations were obtained for plasma lactate concentration 8 minutes post-race and the number of race wins ($r = 0.29$, $P = 0.04$), number of race placings (first, second or third) ($r = 0.34$, $P = 0.02$) and lifetime earnings ($r = 0.29$, $P = 0.04$). There were no significant correlations between performance indices and plasma uric acid concentrations in races of 1760 meters. For races of 2160 meters, correlations were found between plasma uric acid concentration at eight minutes post-race and the number of race wins ($r = 0.37$, $P = 0.06$). As well, there was a significant correlation between uric acid concentration at eight minutes post-race and lifetime earnings ($r = 0.35$, $P = 0.07$). These results imply that only 10–15% of the variability in retrospective career performance in pacing Standardbreds can be explained by these metabolic markers of the muscle anaerobic response to racing. Blood or plasma lactate and uric acid responses to maximal exercise are not useful measures of fitness on their own, but they could be included in multifactorial studies.

A study of the relationships between racing performance and several physiologic measurements was also conducted in 25 Standardbred trotters.[84] Blood samples and muscle biopsies were obtained 5–10 minutes after racing. The biopsies were analyzed for fiber type composition and enzymatic profile and blood samples for plasma lactate and ammonia concentrations. Fiber type composition varied among horses (range 9–27% for type I, 32–54% for type IIA, and 27–46% for type IIB). Fiber type composition, muscle enzyme activities, plasma lactate and ammonia responses to racing were not correlated to a racing performance index.

The rate of accumulation of lactate in blood during maximal field exercise over distances up to 400 meters is closely related to speed in Standardbred, Thoroughbred and polo horses.[107] It was suggested that this lactate measurement could be a useful index of fitness. However, it is unlikely that any physiologic measurement after brief, maximal intensity exercise to estimate anaerobic capacity will be more closely correlated with fitness than a simple measurement of maximal speed during 40–50 seconds of exercise. In conclusion, the blood lactate response to maximal exercise has limited usefulness as a measure of fitness in horses. However, the blood lactate response to moderate, or submaximal speed exercise, expressed as VLA4 or another similar index, is a useful technique for differentiating poor performers and good performers, and for monitoring the changes in fitness during training programs.

Conclusion

Heart rate and blood lactate measurements during standardized field exercise tests are relevant to the management of athletic horses, whatever their discipline. These measurements can assist with performance prediction and evaluation of fitness changes, and can be used to alert veterinarians, owners and trainers to problems such as lameness and respiratory disease. More effort is needed to adapt new technologies and refine approaches to design of field exercise tests. It is unlikely that veterinarians, trainers or owners will be enthusiastic about equine fitness testing if the focus is not on simple approaches to field exercise tests. Simple tests and measuring the things that matter, is the approach in field studies in human sports laboratories, with emphasis on measurement of HR and blood lactate concentrations. Progress in technology transfer of applied exercise physiology might be greater if there was greater emphasis on field methods, using minimally invasive techniques. Every fitness test should answer a specific question, and results should be expressed in a way that helps a veterinarian, trainer or owner make more informed decisions about the training, fitness, health or management of horses.

A promising new technique for field fitness tests is the use of integrated HR and V measurements with differential GPS. Simultaneous logging of a horse's HR and speed is a powerful technique for field exercise tests. Automatic transmission of the data to a remote device will reduce the efforts required from the trainer or rider to communicate the horse's data and will improve the veterinarian's insight into the horse's workload, training and health status.

New partnerships between equine exercise scientists and biomedical engineers could also generate new technologies for field studies. For example, field studies of breath-by-breath respiratory gas flows, and field ergometry should be possible. The techniques for field ergomety have been developed for human athletes, and could be refined for use in horses. However, the technical challenge of reliably and accurately measuring respiratory flow rates of over 100 L/s in a horse galloping in the field at 1000 m/min has yet to be conquered. Field ergometry, coupled with measurements of HR, respiratory function and metabolic responses to exercise would enable new fundamental studies in many areas of equine exercise physiology. Descriptions of the metabolic and energetic demands of different athletic events would be possible, and design of appropriate training programs would be facilitated. As well, clinical exercise testing would be more likely to be adopted by trainers and owners. Such 'high tech' clinical exercise tests would contribute to greater knowledge concerning limits to performance in different events (such as anaerobic or aerobic capacity, and maximal rates of oxygen uptake). Greater rates of technology transfer to industry participants are likely if technical developments free researchers from the constraints and limitations of treadmill fitness tests.

With thanks to David Evans, who created the original chapter in the first edition.

References

1. Franklin SH, Barakzai SZ, Courouce-Malblanc A, et al. Investigation of the incidence and type of injuries associated with high-speed treadmill exercise testing. Equine Vet J Suppl 2010;38:70–5.
2. King CM, Evans DL, Rose RJ. Acclimation to treadmill exercise. Equine Vet J 1995;(Suppl. 18):453–6.
3. Gottlieb-Vedi M, Lindholm A. Comparison of Standardbred trotters exercising on a treadmill and a race track with identical draught resistances. Vet Rec 1997;140:525–8.
4. Couroucé A, Geffroy O, Barrey E, et al. Comparison of exercise tests in French trotters under training track, racetrack and treadmill conditions. Equine Vet J 1999;(Suppl 30):528–31.
5. Sloet van Oldruitenborgh-Osterbaan M, Barneveld A. Comparison of the workload of Dutch Warmblood horses ridden normally and on a treadmill. Vet Record 1995;137:136–9.
6. Fraipont A, Van Erck E, Ramery E, et al. Assessing fitness in endurance horses. Can Vet J 2012;53:311–14.
7. Barrey E, Galloux P, Valette JP, et al. Stride characteristics of overground versus treadmill locomotion in the saddle horse. Acta Anat 1993;146:90–4.
8. Evans DL, Rose RJ. Cardiovascular and respiratory responses in Thoroughbred horses during treadmill exercise. J Exp Biol 1988;134:397–408.
9. Persson SGB. Evaluation of exercise tolerance and fitness in the performance horse. In: Snow DH, Persson SGB, Rose RJ, editors. Equine exercise physiology. Cambridge: Granta publications; 1983. p. 441–57.
10. Thornton J, Essen-Gustavsson B, Lindholm A, et al. Effects of training and detraining on oxygen uptake, cardiac output, blood gas tensions, pH and lactate concentrations during and after exercise in the horse. In: Snow DH, Persson SGB, Rose RJ, editors. Equine exercise physiology. Cambridge: Granta publications; 1983. p. 470–86.
11. Wilson RG, Isler RB, Thornton JR. Heart rate, lactic acid production and speed during a standardised exercise test in Standarbred horses. In: Snow DH, Persson SGB, Rose RJ, editors. Equine exercise physiology. Cambridge: Granta Editions; 1983. p. 487–96.
12. Couroucé A, Chrétien M, Valette JP. Physiological variables measured under field conditions according to age and state of training in French Standardbred trotters. Equine Vet J 2002;34:91–7.
13. Lindholm A, Saltin B. The physiological and biochemical response of Standardbred horses to exercise of varying speed and duration. Acta Vet Scand 1974;15:310–24.
14. Harris MR, Morris EA, Seeherman HJ. Evaluation of the effects of a regular training program in two Thoroughbred yearling using an exercise stress test. Equine Vet Sci 1990;236–45.
15. Valette JP, Barrey E, Wolter R. Multivariate analysis of exercise parameters measured during and incremental treadmill test. In: Persson SGB, Lindholm A, Jeffcott LB, editors. Equine exercise physiology, vol. 3. Davis, California: ICEEP Publications; 1991. p. 337–42.
16. Couroucé A. Field exercise testing for assessing fitness in French Standardbred trotters. Vet J 1999;157:112–22.
17. Evans DL, Harris RC, Snow DH. Correlation of racing performance with blood lactate and heart rate in Thoroughbred horses. Equine Vet J 1993;25:441–5.
18. Roneus N, Essen-Gustavsson B, Lindholm A, et al. Plasma lactate response to submaximal and maximal exercise tests with training and its relationship to performance and muscle characteristics in Standardbred trotters. Equine Vet J 1994;26:117–21.
19. Couroucé A, Chatard JC, Auvinet B. Estimation of performance potential of Standardbred trotters from blood lactate concentrations measured in field conditions. Equine Vet J 1997;29:365–9.
20. Leleu C, Cotrel C, Couroucé-Malblanc A. Relationships between physiological variables and race performance in French Standardbred trotters. Vet Rec 2005;156:339–42.
21. Hargreaves BJ, Kronfeld DS, Naylor JRJ. Ambient temperature and relative humidity influenced packed cell volume, total plasma protein and other variables in horses during an incremental submaximal field exercise test. Equine Vet J 1999;31:314–18.
22. Banister EW, Purvis AD. Exercise electrocardiography in the horse by radiotelemetry. J Am Vet Med Assoc 1968;152:1004–8.
23. Marsland WP. Heart rate response to submaximal exercise in the Standardbred horse. J Appl Physiol 1968;24:98–101.
24. Asheim A, Knudsen O, Lindholm A, et al. Heart rates and blood lactate concentrations of Standardbred horses during training and racing. J Am Vet Med Assoc 1970;157:304–12.
25. Hall MC, Steel JD, Stewart GA. Cardiac monitoring during exercise tests in the horse. 2. Heart rate responses to exercise. Aust Vet J 1976;52:1–5.
26. Steel JD, Hall MC, Stewart GA. Cardiac monitoring during exercise tests in the horse. 3. Changes in the electrocardiogram during and after exercise. Aust Vet J 1976;52:6–10.
27. Senta T, Smetzer DL, Smith CR. Effects of exercise on certain electrocardiographic parameters and cardiac arrhythmias in the horse. A radiotelemetric study. Cornell Vet 1970;60:552–69.
28. Krzywanek H, Wittke G, Bayer A, et al. The heart rates of Thoroughbred horses during a race. Equine Vet J 1970;2:115–17.
29. Hörnicke H, Engelhardt WV, Ehrlein H-J. Effect of exercise on systemic blood pressure and heart rate in horses. Pflugers Arch 1977;372:95–9.
30. Foreman JH, Bayly WM, Grant BD, et al. Standardized exercise test and daily heart responses of Thoroughbreds undergoing conventional race training and detraining. Am J Vet Res 1990;51:914–20.
31. Morris E. Application of clinical exercise testing for identification of respiratory fitness and disease in the equine athlete. Vet Clin North Am Equine Pract 1991;7:383–401.
32. Erickson BK, Erickson HH, Sexton WL, et al. Performance evaluation and detection of injury during exercise training in the Quarter horse using a heart rate computer. In: Gillespie JR, Robinson NE, editors. Equine exercise physiology, vol. 2. Davis: ICEEP publications; 1987. p. 92–101.
33. Couroucé-Malblanc A, Pronost S, Fortier G, et al. Physiological measurements and upper and lower respiratory tract evaluation in French Standardbred Trotters during a standardised exercise test on the treadmill. In: Equine Exercise Physiology 6, Equine Vet J 2002;(Suppl. 34):402–7.
34. Richard EA, Fortier GD, Pitel PH, et al. Sub-clinical diseases affecting performance in Standardbred trotters: diagnostic methods and predictive parameters. Vet J 2010;184:282–9.
35. Fraipont A, van Erck E, Ramery E, et al. Subclinical diseases underlying poor performance in endurance horses: diagnostic methods and predictive tests. Vet Rec 2011;169:154.
36. Kobayashi M, Kuribara K, Amada A. Application of V200 for evaluation of training effects in the young Thoroughbred under field conditions. Equine Vet J 1999;(Suppl 30):159–62.
37. Serrano MG, Evans DL, Hodgson JL. Heart rate and blood lactate concentrations in a field fitness test for event horses. Aust Equine Vet 2001;19:154–61.
38. Hörnicke H, Weber M, Schweiker W. Pulmonary ventilation in Thoroughbred horses at maximum performance. In: Gillespie JR, Robinson NE, editors. Equine exercise physiology, vol. 2.

Davis, CA: ICEEP Publications; 1987. p. 216–24.
39. Pollmann U, Hörnicke H. Characteristics of respiratory airflow during exercise in horses with reduced performance due to pulmonary emphysema or bronchitis. In: Gillespie JR, Robinson NE, editors. Equine exercise physiology, vol. 2. Davis, CA: ICEEP Publications; 1987. p. 760–71.
40. Ryan N, Marr CM, McGladdery AJ. Survey of cardiac arrhythmias during submaximal and maximal exercise in Thoroughbred racehorses. Equine Vet J 2005;37:265–8.
41. Buhl R, Meldgaard C, Barbesgaard L. Cardiac arrhythmias in clinically healthy showjumping horses. Equine Vet J 2010;(Suppl. 38):196–201.
42. Barbesgaard L, Buhl R, Meldgaard C. Prevalence of exercise-associated arrhythmias in normal performing dressage horses. Equine Vet J 2010;(Suppl. 38):202–7.
43. Jose-Cunilleras E, Young LE, Newton JR, et al. Cardiac arrhythmias during and after treadmill exercise in poorly performing Thoroughbred racehorses. Equine Vet J 2006;36:163–70.
44. Wasserman K, Whipp BJ, Koyl SN, et al. Anaerobic threshold and respiratory gas exchange during exercise. J Appl Physiol 1973;35:226–43.
45. Lehnhard RA, Bartlett M, Roche BM, et al. Variations in lactate during a graded exercise test due to sampling location and method. Comp Exerc Physiol 2010;7:81–7.
46. Taylor LE, Ferrante PL, Wilson JA, et al. Arterial and mixed venous acid base status and strong ion difference during repeated sprints. Equine Vet J 1995;(Suppl. 18):326–30.
47. Miller-Graber P, Lawrence L, Foreman J, et al. Lactate, pyruvate and blood gases in the carotid artery, jugular vein and pulmonary artery during submaximal exercise. J Equine Vet Sci 1988;8:322–6.
48. Poso AR, Laampinen KJ, Rasanen LA. Distribution of lactate between red blood cells and plasma after exercise. Equine Vet J 1995;(Suppl. 18):231–4.
49. Ferrante PL, Taylor LE, Wilson JA, et al. Plasma and erythrocyte ion concentrations during exercise in Arabian horses. Equine Vet J 1995;(Suppl. 18):306–9.
50. Butudom P, Foreman JH, Kline KH, et al. Validation and comparison of two methods of measuring lactate in equine plasma. Equine Vet J 2010;38:155–60.
51. Couroucé-Malblanc A, Deniau V, Rossignol F, et al. Physiological measurements and prevalence of lower airway diseases in Trotters with dorsal displacement of the soft palate. Equine Vet J 2010;(Suppl. 38):246–55.
52. Persson SGB. On blood volume and working capacity in horses. Acta Vet Scand 1967;(Suppl 19):1–189.
53. Persson SGB, Essen-Gustavsson B, Lindholm A, et al. Cardiorespiratory and metabolic effects of training of Standardbred yearlings. In: Snow DH, Persson SGB, Rose RJ, editors. Equine exercise physiology. Cambridge: Granta publications; 1983. p. 458–69.
54. Persson SGB, Ullberg LE. Blood volume in relation to exercise tolerance in trotters. J South Afr Vet Assoc 1974;45: 293–9.
55. Hamlin MJ, Shearman JP, Hopkins WG. Changes in physiological parameters in overtrained Standardbred racehorses. Equine Vet J 2002;34:383–8.
56. Golland LC, Evans DL, McGowan CM, et al. Effects of overtraining on blood volumes in Standardbred racehorses. Vet J 2003;165:228–33.
57. Mitchell JH, Sproule BJ, Chapman CB. The physiological meaning of the maximal oxygen intake test. J Clin Invest 1958;37:538–47.
58. Karlsen GG, Nadaljak EA. Gas and energy exchange in breathing of trotters during exercise (in Russian). Konevodstvo I Konesport 1964;34:27–31.
59. Pagan JD, Hintz HF. Energy expenditure in horses during submaximal exercise. Proceedings of the 9th Equine Nutrition and Physiology Symposium 1985: 182–187.
60. Hörnicke H, Meixner R, Pollmann U. Respiration in exercising horses. In: Snow DH, Persson SGB, Rose RJ, editors. Equine exercise physiology. Cambridge: Granta Editions; 1983. p. 7–16.
61. Hanak J, Jahn P, Kabes R, et al. A field study of oxygen consumption and estimated energy expenditure in the exercising horse. Acta Vet Brno 2001;70: 133–9.
62. Art T, Duvivier DH, van Erck E, et al. Validation of a portable equine metabolic measurement system. Equine Vet J 2006;(Suppl. 36):557–61.
63. Votion DM, Caudron I, Lejeune J-P, et al. New perspective for field measurement of cardiorespiratory parameters in exercising horses. Pferdeheilkunde 2006;5:619–24.
64. Van Erck E, van Votion DM, Serteyn D, et al. Evaluation of oxygen consumption during field exercise tests in Standardbred trotters. Equine Comp Exerc Physiol 2007;4:43–9.
65. Barrey E, Evans SE, Evans DL, et al. Locomotion evaluation for racing Thoroughbreds. Equine Vet J 2001;(Suppl. 33):99–103.
66. Leleu C, Gloria E, Renault G, et al. Analysis of trotter gait on the track by accelerometry and image analysis. Equine Vet J 2002;(Suppl. 34):344–8.
67. Mottini V, Leleu C, Cotrel C. Harnessed vs. mounted Standardbreds on the track: changes in gait and physiological variables. Equine Vet J 2006;(Suppl. 36):468–72.
68. Cottin F, Metayer N, Goachet AG, et al. Oxygen consumption and gai variables of Arabian endurance horses measured during a field exercise test. Equine Vet J 2010;(Suppl 38):1–5.
69. Chateau H, Holden L, Robin D, et al. Biomechanical analysis of hoof landing and stride parameters in harness trotter horses running on different tracks of a sand beach (from wet to dry) and on an asphalt road. Equine Vet J 2010;(Suppl 38):488–95.
70. Cotrel C, Leleu C, Courouсé-Malblanc A. Locomotor and respiratory coupling: factors of variation in Standardbred Trotters in the field. Equine Vet J 2006;(Suppl. 36):562–6.
71. Franklin SH, Usmar SG, Lane JG, et al. Spectral analysis of respiratory noise in with upper airway disorders. Equine Vet J 2003;35:264–8.
72. Parente EJ, Martin BB. Correlation between standing endoscopic examination and those made during high-speed exercise in horses – 150 cases. Proc Am Ass Equine Pract 1995;41:170.
73. Ferrucci F, Zucca E, Croci C, et al. Rest and treadmill endoscopic findings in 87 race horses presented for poor performance. In: Lindner A, editor. The elite race and endurance horse, Conference on Equine Sports Medicine and Science (CESMAS). 2004. p. 133–6.
74. Tan RH, Dowling BA, Dart AJ. High-speed treadmill videoendoscopic examination of the upper-respiratory tract in the horse: the results of 291 clinical cases. Vet J 2005;170:243–8.
75. Lane JG, Bladon B, Little DRM, et al. Dynamic obstructions of the equine upper respiratory tract. Part 2: Comparison of endoscopic findings at rest and during high-speed treadmill exercise of 600 Thoroughbred racehorses. Equine Vet J 2006; 38:401–8.
76. Van Erck E, Frippiat T, Dupuis M-C, et al. Upper airway dynamic endoscopy: are track and treadmill observations comparable? In: Proc. 4th World Equine Airways Symposium. Berne, Switzerland. 2009. p. 254.
77. Allen KJ, Franklin SH. Comparisons of overground endoscopy and treadmill endoscopy in U.K. Thoroughbred racehorses. Equine Vet J 2010;42: 186–91.
78. Franklin SH, Burn JF, Allen KJ. Clinical trials using a telemetric endoscope for use during over-ground exercise: a preliminary study. Equine Vet J 2008;40:712–15.

79. Desmaizieres LM, Serraud N, Plainfossé B, et al. Dynamic endoscopy without treadmill in 68 performance Standadbred, Thoroughbred and saddle horses under natural training conditions. Equine Vet J 2009;41:347–52.
80. Pollock PJ, Reardon RJM, Parkin TDH, et al. Dynamic respiratory endoscopy in 67 Thoroughbred racehorses in training under normal ridden exercise conditions. Equine Vet J 2009;41: 354–60.
81. van Erck E. Dynamic respiratory videoendoscopy in ridden sport horses: effect of head flexion, riding and airway inflammation in 129 cases. Equine Vet J 2011;(Suppl. 40):18–24.
82. Davidson EJ, Martin BB, Boston RC, et al. Exercising upper respiratory videoendoscopic evaluation of 100 nonracing performance horses with abnormal respiratory noise and/or poor performance. Equine Vet J 2011;4:3–8.
83. Franklin SH, Naylor JRJ, Lane JG. Videoendoscopic evaluation of the upper respiratory tract in 93 sport horses during exercise testing on a high speed treadmill. Equine Exercise Physiology 7. Equine Vet J 2006; (Suppl. 36):540–5.
84. Roneus N, Essen-Gustavsson B, Lindholm A, et al. Muscle characteristics and plasma lactate and ammonia response after racing in Standardbred trotters: relation to performance. Equine Vet J 1999;31:170–3.
85. Van Erck E, Jakesova V, Lekeux P, et al. Field evaluation of poor performance in Standardbred trotters. Pferdeheilkunde 2006;22:625–31.
86. Davie AJ, Priddle TL, Evans DL. Metabolic responses to submaximal field exercise tests and relationships with racing performance in pacing Standardbreds. Equine Vet J 2002;(Suppl 34):112–15.
87. Vermeulen AD, Evans DL. Measurements of fitness in Thoroughbred racehorses using field studies of heart rate and velocity with a global positioning system. Equine Vet J 2006;38:113–17.
88. Vonwittke P, Lindner A, Deegen E, et al. Effects of training on blood lactate running speed relationship in Thoroughbred racehorses. J Appl Physiol 1994;77:298–302.
89. Davie AJ, Evans DL. Blood lactate responses to submaximal field exercise tests in Thoroughbred horses. Vet J 2000;159:252–8.
90. Evans DL, Rainger JE, Hodgson DR, et al. The effect of intensity and duration of training on blood lactate concentrations during and after exercise. Equine Vet J 1995;(Suppl 18):422–5.
91. Valette JP, Heiles PH, Wolter R. Multivariate analysis of exercise parameters measured during the training of Thoroughbred racehorses. Pferdeheilkunde 1996;12:470–3.
92. Muñoz A, Riber C, Santisteban R, et al. Investigation of standardized exercise tests according to fitness level for three day event horses. J Equine Vet Sci 1998;9:1–7.
93. Auvinet B, Galloux P, Michaux JM, et al. Test d'effort standardisé de terrain pour chevaux de concours complet d'équitation, Médecine et sports équestres, VIIème congrès des pays francophones, Saumur, 1989:432–63.
94. Van Erck E, de Moffarts B, Art T, et al. Evaluation de la condition sportive du cheval de concours complet sur le terrain, Proceedings des Journées AVEF, Angers, 2005:469.
95. Art T, Amory H, Desmecht D, et al. Effect of show jumping on heart rate, blood lactate and other plasma biochemical values. Equine Vet J 1990;(Suppl.):78–82.
96. Clayton HM. Time-motion analysis of the Canadian Equestrian Federation dressage tests. J Appl Physiol 1993;74: 2325–9.
97. Ehrlein H-J, Hörnicke H, Engelhardt WV, et al. Die Herzschlagfrequenz während standardisierter Belastung als Maß für die Leistungsfähigkeit von Pferden. Zentralbl Veterinärmed A 1973;20:188–208.
98. Gill J, Jablońska EM, Ziólkowska SM, et al. Influence of Differential Training on some Haematological and Metabolic Indices in Sport Horses before and after Exercise Trials. J Vet Med Ser A 1987;34:609–16.
99. Sloet-van Oldruitenborgh-Oosterbaan MM, Wensing T, Breukink HJ. Standardized exercise test on a track to evaluate fitness and training of saddle horses. In: Gillespie JR, Robinson NE, editors. Equine exercise physiology, vol. 2. Davis California: ICEEP Publications; 1987. p. 68–76.
100. Munk R. Effects of 3 different interval training programs on horses used for jumping. Evaluaation based on blood lactate concentration, heart rate, obstacle faults, technique and energy level while jumping. Fagdyrelaege verdrorende Hest, Final research paper 2010. https://www.ddd.dk/organisatorisk/fagdyrlaeger/heste/Hovedopgaver/Documents/2010/Rikke%20Munk%20Andersen.pdf.
101. Clayton HM. Time-motion analysis of the Canadian Equestrian Federation dressage tests. J Appl Physiol 1993;74: 2325–9.
102. Rose RJ, Ilkiw JE, Martin IC. Blood-gas, acid-base and haematological values in horses during an endurance ride. Equine Vet J 1979;11:56–9.
103. Lucke JN, Hall GM. Long distance exercise in the horse: Golden Horseshoe Ride 1978. Vet Rec 1980;106: 405–7.
104. Flaminio MJ, Gaughan EM, Gillespie JR. Exercise intolerance in endurance horses. Vet Clin North Am Equine Pract 1996;12:565–80.
105. Muñoz A, Riber C, Santisteban R, et al. Effect of training duration and exercise on blood-borne substrates, plasma lactate and enzyme concentrations in Andalusian, Anglo-Arabian and Arabian breeds. Equine Vet J Suppl 2002;34: 245–51.
106. Littlejohn A, Snow DH. Circulatory, respiratory and metabolic responses in Thoroughbred horses during the first 400 meters of exercise. Eur J Appl Physiol 1988;58:307–14.
107. Saibene F, Cortilli G, Gavazzi P, et al. Maximal anaerobic (lactic) capacity and power of the horse. Equine Vet J 1985;17:130–2.
108. Schuback K, Essen-Gustavsson B. Muscle anaerobic response to a maximal treadmill exercise test in Standardbred trotters. Equine Vet J 1998;30: 504–10.
109. Hinchcliff KW, Lauerdale MA, Dutson J, et al. High intensity exercise conditioning increases accumulated oxygen deficit of horses. Equine Vet J 2002;34:9–16.
110. Krzywanek H. Lactic acid concentrations and pH values in trotters after racing. J South Afr Vet Assoc 1974;45: 355–60.
111. Evans DL, Priddle TL, Davie AJ. Plasma lactate and uric acid responses to racing in pacing Standardbreds and relationships with performance. Equine Vet J 2002;(Suppl. 34):131–4.

Genetic basis of equine performance

4

Eric Barrey

CHAPTER CONTENTS

Introduction

Equine breeding selection has recently been developed for some breeds and uses of horses by applying quantitative genetic methods for calculating the heritability of the complex traits, such as performance in racing or sport competitions. Genetic indices are now calculated routinely in different horse breeds in order to select the best stallions and mares according to a breeding plan with a well-defined genetic objective. Other exercise variables and disease characteristics have been studied by the same type of quantitative genetic methods. With development of biotechnologies, equine molecular genetics has come of age. The equine mitochondrial genome was sequenced in 1994[1] and then partial genome sequencing was undertaken.[2–4] The recent sequencing of the entire equine genome by an international consortium[5] was the major genetic result that will impact all the other equine genomics in the near future. With the rapid progress in equine genetics, new applications in early evaluation of the potential for performance and the detection of disease markers are available. Many new biomolecular tools will change the way selection, disease diagnosis and choice of treatment in athletic horses are made. In human exercise physiology, the research project HERITAGE family study provided continuous new knowledge and data about the genes and quantitative trait loci (QTL) related to exercise activity, health and performance. The last update of the gene list validated by experimental studies revealed 214 autosomal genes and quantitative trait loci and seven others on the X chromosome.[6] Moreover, there are 18 mitochondrial genes that influence fitness and performance phenotypes. This important collection of genetic data related to exercise in humans demonstrates the great interest of studying equine genetics for performance evaluation and sports medicine applications.

The purpose of this chapter was to present the new development in equine genetics and genomics for performance evaluation and health markers after a review of the previous knowledge about the genetic components of the exercise performance traits obtained by quantitative genetics.

Genomics of performance

Genetic component of the performance traits: how to measure the heritability of the exercise variables and performance traits using phenotypic measurements

With the development of equine exercise physiology, more functional traits can be measured for early evaluation of exercise ability. The objective is to predict the level of performance that a young horse can reach by measuring some physiological characteristics during an exercise test. For breeding purposes, the heritability of each trait should be determined to know if it is useful for breeding selection. This chapter presents how to calculate the heritability and apply the method to some physiological and biomechanical traits that are related to exercise capacity and performance. Several exercise traits have been studied in different breeds: muscle fiber types, heart rate, blood lactate, conformation, gaits and jump style.

Heritability calculation in horse performance

Heritability estimates (h^2) of the exercise traits have been calculated in order to estimate the influence of genetic components and environment effects (i.e. non-genetic) on the variability of expression of the trait. More simply, heritability of a trait expresses the percentage of the parents' trait that could be transmitted to the offspring. This is a statistical result which is valid in a genetic population where it has been estimated from a sub-group of. Briefly, heritability is the ratio between genetic variance and the total variance including environmental effects. For each variable, the variance components are calculated using restricted maximum likelihood resolution (REML). The genetic variance is estimated by the following variance analysis model including fixed (known during the experiment) and random effects (unknown: Animal genetic effect and error). The total variability of the trait is equal to the sum of fixed effects (for example: age, height, track, breed) and the random Animal genetic effect:

$$Y_{ijklmn} = Age_i + Height_{ij} + Track_{ijk} + Breed_{ijkl} + \underline{Animal}_{ijklm} + \underline{error}_{ijklmn}$$

Thus, heritability (h^2) is given by:

$$h^2 = \text{Variance}\ (\underline{\text{Animal}}\ \text{effect}) \,/\, \text{Total variance}(Y)$$

Heritability values (h^2) of 0.4 indicate that 40% of the trait could be transmitted to the offspring by the mare and stallion. Forty percent represents a high percentage of genetic influence. Note that heritability estimates are valid only for the breed for which they were calculated and they should be recalculated periodically if there is an active breeding program going in the population. The heritabilities of the performance traits are used to calculate genetic index using best linear unbiased predictor method (BLUP) in sport horses in different countries[7]. Performance heritability estimates in racing and equestrian sports are: 0.15 to 0.55 for flat gallop racing, 0.28 for endurance racing, 0.17 to 0.26 for trot or pace racing, 0.05 to 0.28 for show jumping and three-day-eventing and 0.11 for dressage.[7–10] In addition, it was interesting to note that there is no or a weak negative genetic correlation between jumping ability and other sport performance. In show jumping, the longevity of the jumpers' career could be considered as one important trait of the performance and its heritability is rather low 0.10.[11] It has been studied in a large population of French saddle horses. Two main results were demonstrated: the younger the horse started competing, the longer it stayed in competition; the less success in competition, the greater was the chance for leaving competition, especially for horses without earnings. The risk to be removed from the competition is 1.45-fold higher for female than gelding, likely because of the use of females in breeding.

Muscle power and fiber composition in gluteus medius muscle

Myosin Heavy Chain percentages were measured in small muscle samples of 20–30 mg collected by microbiopsy under local anesthesia in Anglo-Arabian horses. The analysis of slow MHC I and fast MHC IIA and IIX was performed using monoclonal antibodies with an ELISA method.[12] The heritability of the percentage of fast MHC was 0.13 in Anglo-Arabian and 0.28 in Andalusian horses.[13] The relative area h^2 of the fast muscle fibres was 0.12 in Anglo-Arabian and 0.15–0.23 in Andalusian horses for fast and slow fibers, respectively. The capillary density heritability in Andalusian horses was 0.20. Their muscular trait heritabilities are rather low in comparison with Andalusian horses. The low heritabilies mean that the trait is genetically homogenous in the Anglo-arabian breed probably because the trait has been already selected for fast speed. The breeding selection on the muscular trait would be poorly efficient in this case.

The relationships with the performance should be taken into account. With a larger percentage of slow twitch fibers, Andalusian horses are more adapted for dressage and cattle work. A higher percentage of fast twitch fibers were observed in Anglo-Arabian performers in racing and jumping horses than in poor performers ($p < 0.05$). Anglo-Arabian horses are well adapted for competing in steeple-chase races and three-day-events where they required high muscular power.

Evaluation of cardiac and aerobic capacity

A group of more than 400 French trotters performed an exercise test at increasing speed. The heart rate and blood lactate were measured in order to determine the speed related changes of these variables. The speed eliciting 200 heart beats/min (V200) and a blood lactate concentration of 4 mmol/l (VLA4) were calculated. The V200 heritability was higher (0.46) than the VLA4 heritability (0.10) which was more influenced by the training effect.[14] For harness trotters, the VLA4 is less heritable but more correlated to performance than V200.[15] Breeding selection on V200 could be efficient to improve the sub-maximal heart rate capacity and thus aerobic capacity however the racing performance depends mainly on the ability to get a positive adaptation to training stimulation quantified by the VLA4 measurements.

Gait and jump tests

To measure kinetic and temporal variables of the walk, trot, gallop and jump the horses were equipped with the gait analysis system Equimetrix®.[16,17] A three axial accelerometer was attached with an elastic girth onto the sternum. This ensured that the transducer was held close to the horse's centre of gravity. The device recorded the dorso-ventral, medio-lateral and longitudinal acceleration of the horse during the exercise (Fig. 4.1). Gait tests in hand and free canter and jump tests provided gait variables which were used to calculate heritabilities in French saddle horses (Table 4.1 and Table 4.2). Heritabilities of the slow gaits such as walk and trot were lower that fast gaits such as canter and gallop. Heritabilities of canter, gallop and jumping variables, as with take-off impulse were rather high: 0.23 to 0.52.[18] For equestrian sport horses, the use of gait variables such as stride frequency, propulsion power and jump variables could be efficiently used both for early selection and breeding selection.

Conformation

Using a two-dimensional image analysis, it has been possible to measure French saddle horses and to calculate the heritability estimates of the main morphological traits. Conformation is poorly heritable in Selle Français horses and more heritable in Poney de Selle.[19] In the two breeds these conformation traits are poorly correlated to sport performance. However, in a review of the conformation heritabilties obtained by other methods (judge scoring and direct measurements) and in other breeds, the heritabilities are higher for height at withers ($h^2 = 0.25–0.89$) or body weight ($h^2 = 0.13–0.90$).[20]

Equine genetics and genomics come of age

The equine genome has been sequenced and annotated by an international consortium.[5] The task has been conducted by the Broad

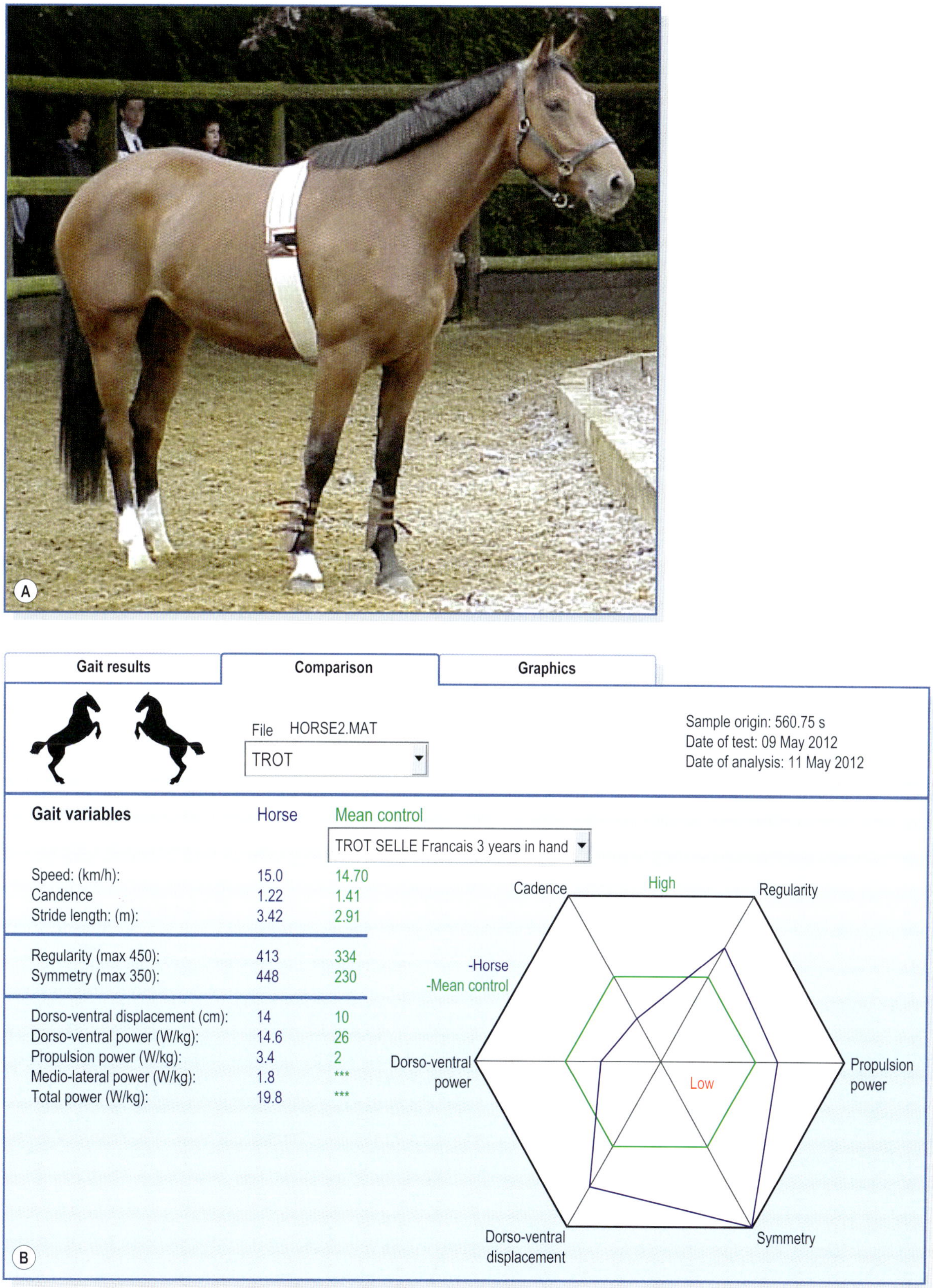

Fig 4.1 Horses equipped with the gait analysis device (Equimetrix ®) used to measure thousands of horses of different breeds to calculate heritability of the gait variables.

Reprinted from Barrey E, Galloux P (1997) Analysis of the equine jumping technique by accelerometry. Equine Vet. J. Suppl. *23, 45–49 with permission from the* Equine Veterinary Journal.

Table 4.1 Heritability (h^2) of the gait variables measured in French saddle horses. The walk and trot were recorded in hand and the canter under free condition. Heritability estimates for canter were higher than for walk and trot

GAIT VARIABLES	WALK h^2 (SE)	TROT h^2 (SE)	CANTER h^2 (SE)
Stride characteristics			
Speed	0	0.30 (0.14)	NA
Stride length	0	0.29 (0.13)	NA
Stride frequency	0	0.20 (0.15)	0.32 (0.19)
Dorsoventral motion			
Symmetry	0.10 (0.08)	0.12 (0.08)	NA
Regularity	0.10 (0.13)	0.12 (0.09)	NA
Displacement	0.16 (0.12)	0.14 (0.08)	NA
Dorsoventral activity	0.41 (0.12)	0.22 (0.10)	0.50 (0.13)
Gait rhythm	0.29 (0.10)	0.05 (0.07)	NA
Longitudinal motion			
Mean propulsion vector	0.19 (0.07)	0.20 (0.11)	NA
Propulsion duration	0.69 (0.13)	0.38 (0.15)	NA
Longitudinal activity	0	0.44 (0.14)	0.46 (0.20)

h^2: Heritability SE: standard error. NA: Non available data

Table 4.2 Heritabilities (h^2) of jump variables measured in French saddle horses and saddle pony. The jumps were recorded under free condition. Heritability for jump variables were higher than for walk or trot

TRAITS	HORSE	PONY
Approach strides	0.34	0.41
Take off force	0.23	0.43
Jump flight	0.30	0.42
Landing force	0.52	0.40

Institute Sequencing Platform (Cambridge, MA, USA). All the database is available online at: http://www.ncbi.nlm.nih.gov/genome/guide/horse/. Briefly, the equine genome includes 20 322 predicted protein-coding genes according to the annotation process made by alignments and comparisons with the human, mouse and dog genome. Transcriptomic analysis showed that 87% of 18 039 genes can be detected using expression microarrays designed with equine probes. In order to have markers along all the equine genome, a single nucleotide polymorphism (SNP) map was designed including a total 106 SNP candidates with an average density of 1 SNP/2 kilo base. A first genotyping array including 54K SNPs was designed and validated by using a panel of 14 horse breeds, Equus Przewalski and other related Perissodactyl species (zebras, asses, tapirs, and rhinoceros)[21]. It was possible to discriminate between 14 breeds by genotyping a set of 1007 SNP (Fig. 4.2). These important results allows one to produce new genetic investigations in various domains and to design new genomic tools such as single nucleotide polymorphism chips for genotyping studies and expression microarrays to analyze gene expression.

Gene expression and regulation determine most of the phenotype. The analysis of the cell transcriptome using DNA microarray provides qualitative and quantitative information about the up- and down-regulated pathways involved during exercise. The collected data are massive and complex and should be studied by sophisticated data mining methods in order to extract only the informative data. The first transcriptomic studies in exercising horses were performed in the blood leucocytes of performers and disqualified endurance horses[22] and in muscles of Thoroughbred racehorses in training.[23] The main results of these two studies are described in the following parts.

Using a genome-wide scan analysis study with microsatellites markers or more recently single nucleotide polymorphism (SNP) chips, it is now possible to identify some interesting genetic markers linked to some performance traits or health troubles. Some small variations of the gene sequences such as a single nucleotide polymorphism SNP can be detected and the association to interesting traits can be demonstrated by statistical tests. Then, if the genetic marker is close to an interesting candidate gene, it could be a way to discover the genetic determinism of a particular phenotype. Another application is to use the best informative SNP markers to genotype a subject in relationship with a specific phenotype.

Genomic applications in gallop and trot racing

Short time genomic response to exercise in Thoroughbreds

Two types of responses to exercise can be distinguished: immediate responses and long adaption. Immediate and delayed response to intense exercise could be observed at the genomic level in skeletal muscle. In training, repetitive exercise will stimulate a genomic

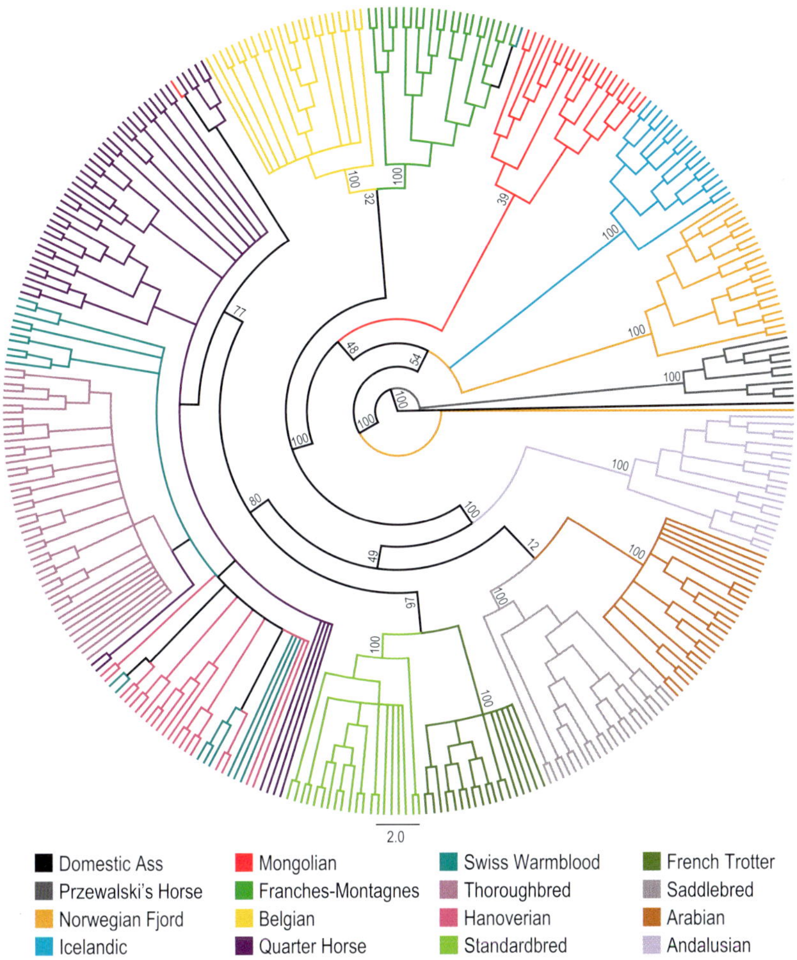

Fig 4.2 Phylogenetic tree of 14 horse breeds and Przewalski' horses using 46244 autosomal loci. *Reprinted from McCue ME, Bannasch DL, Petersen JL, Gurr J, Bailey E, et al. (2012) A High Density SNP Array for the Domestic Horse and Extant Perissodactyla: Utility for Association Mapping, Genetic Diversity, and Phylogeny Studies. PLoS Genet 8(1): e1002451 with permission.*

response during each exercise bout that will produce an adaptive response in the energetic pathway and organization of the heart and skeletal muscle fibers.

Exercise stimulates immediate early molecular responses as well as delayed responses during recovery, resulting in a return to homeostasis and enabling long-term adaptation.[23] Global gene expression occurring in equine skeletal muscle after exercise was explored using equine-specific cDNA microarrays to examine global mRNA expression in skeletal muscle from a cohort of eight Thoroughbred horses at three time points (before exercise, immediately afterexercise, and four hours after exercise) after a single bout of treadmill exercise. Skeletal muscle biopsies were taken from the gluteus medius before exercise, immediately after and four hours after exercise. While only two genes had increased expression after exercise ($P < 0.05$), by four hours after exercise 932 genes had increased ($P < 0.05$) and 562 genes had decreased expression ($P < 0.05$). Functional analysis of genes differentially expressed during the recovery phase (4 hours after exercise) revealed an over-representation of genes localized to the actin cytoskeleton and with functions in the MAPK signalling, focal adhesion, insulin signalling, mTOR signaling, p53 signalling and Type II diabetes mellitus pathways. After the exercise, there was an over-representation of genes involved in the stress response, metabolism and intracellular signalling. These findings suggest that protein synthesis, mechano-sensation and muscle remodeling contribute to skeletal muscle adaptation towards improved integrity and hypertrophy.

In order to assess the short term response to exercise at the muscular level of three-year-old Thoroughbreds, the gene expression of creatine kinase (CKM), two sub-units of the respiratory chain complex IV (cytochrome c oxidase subunit IV isoform 1 (COX4I1), cytochrome c oxidase subunit IV isoform 2 (COX4I2) and pyruvate dehydrogenase kinase (PDK4) were measured by quantitative real time PCR after exercise.[24] During high intensity sprint exercise, pyruvate dehydrogenase kinase (PDK4) was highly up-regulated in the gluteus medius muscle while during moderate intensity exercise on treadmill, one sub-unit of the respiratory complex IV was slightly down-regulated (COX4I2). PDK4 encodes a protein located in the matrix of the mitochondria and inhibits the pyruvate dehydrogenase complex by phosphorylating one of its subunits, thereby contributing to limit the glucose importation in mitochondria. Thus, PDK4 up-regulation after exercise increases beta-oxidation of fatty acids to acetyl-CoA as substrate for oxidative phosphorylation. This way, the pool of ATP can be efficiently restored.

Genotyping in Thoroughbreds for gallop racing ability

The high heritability estimate calculated for racing performance could suggest that a small number of genes have a major effect on the gallop racing ability. Thus, it has been proposed to look for genomic markers of these putative major genes. Using a genome-wide scan study with microsatellites markers or more recently single nucleotides polymorphism (SNP) chips, it is now possible to identify some interesting genes linked to the performance traits. Some small variations of the gene sequences such as a SNP can be detected and the association to interesting traits can be demonstrated by statistical tests. Then, if the genetic marker like a SNP is close to an interesting candidate gene, it could be a way to discover the genetic determinism of a particular phenotype like a disease or another trait. Another application is to use the best informative SNP markers to genotype a subject in relationship with a specific phenotype for breeding selection.

In a wide genome scan study of 112 Thoroughbred horses, some gene candidates related racing performance were identified by using 394 microsatellite markers.[25] These genes were close to the genetic markers and were mainly involved in the energetic metabolism and muscle strength and integrity. The genes identified were in the energetic pathway (ADHFE1, alcohol dehydrogenase; PDK4 pyruvate dehydrogenase kinase 4), mitochondrial respiration (MTFR1, mitochondrial fission regulator 1; COX cytochrome units), hypoxia (HIF1A), fatty acid oxidation (ACSS1, acyl-CoA synthetase short-chain family member 1), phosphoinositide-mediated signalling, insulin receptor signalling (PI3KR1), and muscular proteins (ACTA1, ACTN2, TNC).

Using the last genotyping technology based on SNP detection, three SNPs were detected as significant genetic markers of elite winner Thoroughbreds for the two genes: muscular creatine kinase (CKM) and a sub-unit of the respiratory chain complex IV (COX4I2).[26] Another association study identified two significant SNPs linked to the pyruvate dehydrogenase kinase (PDK4) variants which could confer a significant advantage in elite racing horses.[27] The pyruvate dehydrogenase kinase is involved in the regulation of the pyruvate dehydrogenase which catalyzes the reduction of Actely CoA in pyruvate.

Variants of the myostatin gene (MSTN) are associated with muscle hypertrophy phenotypes in a range of mammalian species, most notably cattle, dogs, mice, and humans. Myostatin gene is well known in animal production because several mutations have been identified to be responsible of muscle hypertrophy in cattle and pigs which is an advantage for meat production. However, the increase of muscle size due to these mutations does not improve the muscle strength. It has been demonstrated in vitro that MSTN knock-out increases the protein synthesis by activation of the Akt/mTOR pathway in mouse myotubes.[28] In fact, the protein translation initiation is improved in MSTN knock-out myotubes, which becomes larger than wild-type myotubes. Recently, it was demonstrated that the racing distance and speed ability in gallop racing were associated to significant SNP genotypes of myostatin gene in two different Thoroughbred populations in Ireland and Japan. In a sample of registered Thoroughbred horses, a novel MSTN single nucleotide polymorphism (g.66493737C/T SNP) was identified and was strongly associated with best race distance among elite racehorses.[29] The authors observed that the SNP C/C horses are suited to fast, short-distance races; C/T horses compete favourably in middle-distance races; and T/T horses have greater stamina for longer distance (Fig. 4.3). Evaluation of retrospective racecourse performance (n = 142) and stallion progeny performance predict that C/C and C/T horses are more likely to be successful two-year-old racehorses than T/T animals. This is the first SNP study which demonstrates a relationship between a racing performance trait and an SNP gene variability.

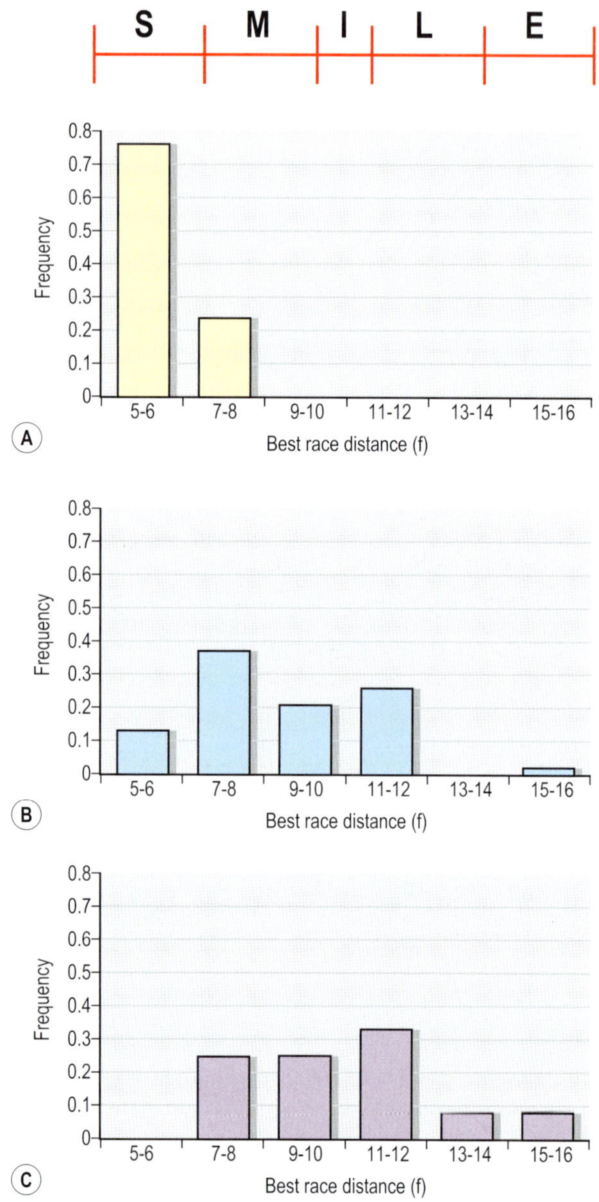

Fig 4.3 Distribution of C/C (yellow), C/T (blue) and T/T (purple) genotypes of the myostatin gene SNP in relationship with the racing distances (S-M-I-L-E) among 79 listed race winning Thoroughbreds (Hill et al. 2010). **(A)** The Thorougbreds genotyped C/C (yellow bars) are more adapted to race short distance (5–6 furlongs – 1000–1200 m). **(B)** The Thoroughbred genotyped C/T have middle distance racing ability. The International Federation of Horseracing Authorities recognizes five race distance categories S-M-I-L-E: Sprint (5–6.5 f, #1,300 m), Mile (6.51–9.49 f, 1,301–1,900 m), Intermediate (9.5–10.5 f, 1,901–2,112 m), Long (10.51–13.5 f, 2,114–2,716 m) and Extended (>13.51 f, >2,717 m); [Note: 1 furlong = 1/8 mile = 201.2 meters]. **(C)** On the other hand, the Thoroughbreds genotyped T/T (purple bars) are more adapted to race long distance gallop race (12–13 furlongs – 2400–2600 m).

A complimentary study demonstrated that the same MSTN single nucleotide polymorphism (g.66493737C/T SNP) is also linked to the maximum gallop speed variables measured in a sub-population of 85 Thoroughbreds.[30] For this trait, there is again a dose effect of the SNP genotype because it has been observed the faster horses have a C/C or C/T genotype. Among the fast horses, the horses having a C/C genotype could reach a higher peak speed measured during six seconds. Taken together the two studies demonstrated that the MSTN C/C variant might explain a good ability to sprint at high speed on short distance by providing a higher muscular power. Another MSTN SNPs study in Japan, revealed significant association between the body weight/withers height in Thoroughbreds and the genotype C/C at the same SNP locus g.66493737C>T.[31] The faster horses with a C/C genotype were significantly heavier per cm height than the other genotypes. The same result was observed both for males and females. Thus, it seems that Thoroughbred performers in short distance races should have a C/C gentotype at this locus of the myostatin which is linked to a high muscularity and low height showing compact conformation.

Gene mutation related to tölt and trot

A recent publication revealed a mutation of a gene involved gene expression regulation in the central nervous system that was linked to ability to perform a very specific gait the tölt. This is a four beat symmetric gait with small dorsoventral displacement which is faster than walk and more comfortable for the rider than trot. The tölt is observed in few breeds like in Icelandic horses and Paso Fino, for example. The mutation has been observed for first time in Icelandic horses who some families use the tölt and other not.[32] One allele of the mutation of this gene seems to be more frequent in the breeds more adapted for high speed trotting like Standardbred trotters and French trotters. It seems that this mutation could be related to poor coordination ability for high speed trot and could explain a higher risk of disqualification for trot irregularities.

Genotyping in show jumping

A first genome-wide association study for quantitative trait loci of show-jumping identified six significant SNPs on four chromosomes associated with jumping ability in 115 Warmblood Hanoverian stallions.[33] All together these SNPs could explain 54% of the total variability of the show-jumping performance of the horses. In addition, it was observed that the frequencies of the SNPs alleles were significantly influenced by the original animals of the breed. The percentage of genes inherited from Hanoverian, Holsteiner, Trakehner and Thoroughbred was taken into account for the statistical analysis and it was found that Holsteiner genes are more related to positive effects of the alleles for four SNPs. Finally, some candidate genes close to the significant SNPs were indentified using the human gene map of exercise adaptation:[6] *PAPSS2* on chromosome 1, *MYL2* on chromosome 8, *TRHR* on chromosome 9 and *GABPA* on chromosome 26 and other putative genes were *NRAP* on chromosome 1, and *TBX4* on chromosome 11. However, at this level of the knowledge, there is no explanation how these putative genes might influence the jumping performance.

Another genome-wide association study was performed in 908 French saddle horses competing in show jumping.[34] Preliminary results did not detect any significant SNP related to jumping performances. However, the SNP genomic data were better correlated to the performance index ($r^2 = 0.39$) than the genetic BLUP index ($r^2 = 0.36$). Among the population of jumpers, the different breeds especially Anglo-Arabian can be well discriminated from the French saddle horses by multivariate analysis using the SNPs as variables.

Gene expression in endurance racing

Gene expression related to physiological adaptations and metabolic disorders in endurance horses have been analyzed using cDNA microarrays.[22] In order to show that genes are modulated in leucocytes in relationship with performance and clinical status of the horses, gene expression in leucocytes, haematological and biochemical parameters were compared between successful and disqualified endurance horses. Blood samples were collected at rest and just after a 140–160 km endurance race in two groups of horses: 10 continuing successfully and 10 disqualified horses stopped at a vet-gate for metabolic disorders. Total RNA was extracted from the total blood cells, checked for purity, amplified and hybridized using mouse cDNA microarrays including 15 264 unique genes (equine microarray were not available in 2006). Differential gene expressions were studied by hybridization of each sample collected at the end of the race vs. the control sample collected before the race. Significant differences were observed in the haematology and biochemistry of the two groups. In the disqualified group, rhabdomyolysis was confirmed with CK 13,124 u/l and AST 1,242 u/l. The list of 726 (including 603 annotated genes) significant genes was filtered according to a high p-value cut-off ($P < 0.00001$). Among them, 130 genes were up-regulated (expression ratio>1.5) and 288 were down-regulated (<1/1.5). Analysis of variance revealed 62 genes differentially expressed ($P < 0.05$) in disqualified and successful horses. The expression levels of 28 and 50 genes were significantly correlated ($r > 0.75$) with CK and AST levels in the disqualified group, respectively. The gene ontology classification showed that more genes were up-regulated in the successful than in the disqualified horses. More genes were down-regulated in the disqualified horses (Fig. 4.4). Long distance exercise induced many significant gene modulations in leucocytes and many of them are involved in inflammation signaling. Some genes were expressed in relationship with the clinical phenotype observed in the disqualified horses: inflammation, rhabdomyolysis and haemolysis. Some of these genes could be interesting markers and/or candidates of poor performance or pathologies.

Another functional genomic study in peripheral blood mononuclear cells of endurance horses confirmed that immediately after the race many gene modulations related to inflammation and immunological response were observed in comparison with the rest condition before racing[35]. However, 24 hours after the race the gene modulations decreased and return to the rest level. The most significantly modulated genes belong to the following functions: inflammatory response (n = 129), cell death (n = 49), haematological system development and function (n = 160). Many genes coding for chemokines pathway were detected in the top 10 genes up-regulated: Interleukin 8 (IL8), Interleukin 18 (interferon-gamma-inducing factor, IL18), IL6-dependent DNA binding protein (IL6DBP), Interleukin 1 receptor type II (IL1R2), Suppressor of cytokine signalling 3, Chemokine (C-X-C motif) ligand 2 (CCR2). It has been demonstrated in another study that interleukin 6 (IL6) and IL6 receptor were significantly increased in trained endurance horses in comparison to sedentary mares.[36] The training response was an adaptation to control the physiological inflammation due to endurance exercise. Surprisingly in trained human athletes, IL6 increased significantly too but IL6 receptor was not up-regulated (Fig. 4.5).

Other genomics studies are going on in a large population of Arabian endurance horses which were considered as the best performers in this discipline probably because of there high running economy at canter speed.[37] The GenEndurance project conducted in France (2011–2014) will produce new knowledge about the relationships between the genotype of both nuclear and mitochondrial genomes, racing performances and phenotypes (morphology, gaits, biochemistry, functional genomics: www.genendurance.over-blog.com).

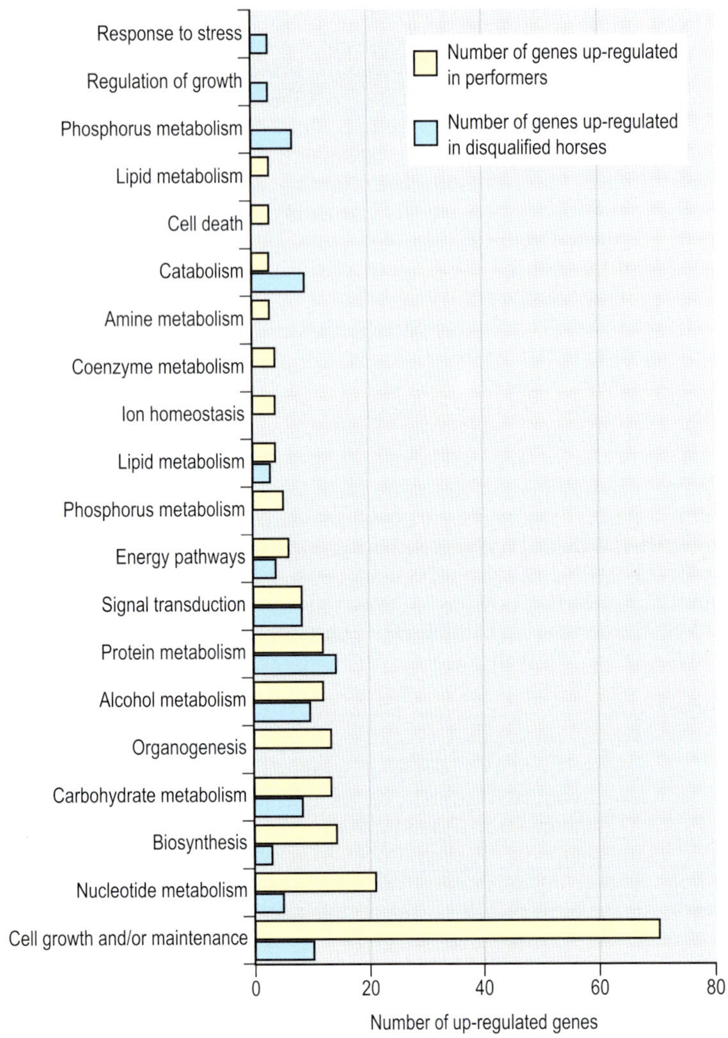

Fig 4.4 Gene ontology chart of the up-regulated genes in the blood leucocytes of the performer and disqualified horses for metabolic disorders in endurance races. There were more genes up-regulated in the performer horses and their functions are more related to synthesis and maintenance of the cell homeostasis. The genes were classified with DAVID software into functional categories according to the annotations derived from NCBI database.

Reprinted from Barrey E, Mucher E, Robert C, Amiot F, Gidrol X (2006) Gene expression profiling in blood cells of endurance horses completing competition or disqualified due to metabolic disorder. Equine Vet. J. Suppl. *36, 43–49, with permission from the* Equine Veterinary Journal.

Genomic applications in poor performance evaluation

Genotyping and gene expression disorders in myopathies

Using the genome database, comparative genomics and genome-wide scan results, it is now possible to identify the variability in some genes linked to disease phenotype such as polysaccharide storage myopathy (PSSM). Some small variations of the gene sequences, such as a single nucleotide polymorphism or SNP, can be related to the change of function of the gene in case of a mutation. By genotyping one identified SNP it is now possible to make a genetic diagnosis of PSSM and other diseases.

The polysaccharide storage myopathy (PSSM) is an equine glycogenosis (metabolic myopathy) related to an abnormal glycogen accumulation. In humans, 11 types of glycogenosis have been described, each containing several sub-types due to various gene mutations.[38] In horses, it has been firstly described in Quarter Horses[39] and then in other breeds: Spanish purebred horses, Belgian draft horses, Morgan, Arabian, Standardbred, Warmblooded horses, ponies and mules.[40–44]

The common clinical signs of PSSM are poor performance, back soreness, exercise intolerance, gait disorders, poor muscling, generalized muscle atrophy, rhabdomyolysis, spontaneous decumbency with inability to rise and episodic 'colic'. A PSSM phenotype can be characterized by histological demonstration in striated muscular fibers of an accumulation of some periodic acid Schiff (PAS)-positive amylase-resistant polysaccharides appearing ultrastructurally as glycogen-like particles.[45] In horses, a specific form of fatal glycogen storage disease was observed in a Quarter Horse foal where a nonsense mutation in codon 34 of the glycogen branching enzyme (GBE1) was identified.[46] This PSSM form can be compared to human glycogenosis type IV where several mutations and deletions explain the total or partial deficiency of the GBE1 gene.[38] In adult horses, a G-to-A mutation within the gene encoding glycogen synthase 1 (GYS1) has recently been observed in Quarter Horses and some Warmblooded horses[47–48] (Fig. 4.6). This mutation increases the glycogen synthase GYS1 activity which might partially explain the accumulation of glycogen in muscle. However, the abnormal structure of the synthetized glycogen could also be responsible.

The PSSM mutation was identified in horses from 17 different breeds. The prevalence of the GYS1 mutation in PSSM horses was high in Draft- (87%) and Quarter Horse related breeds (72%) and

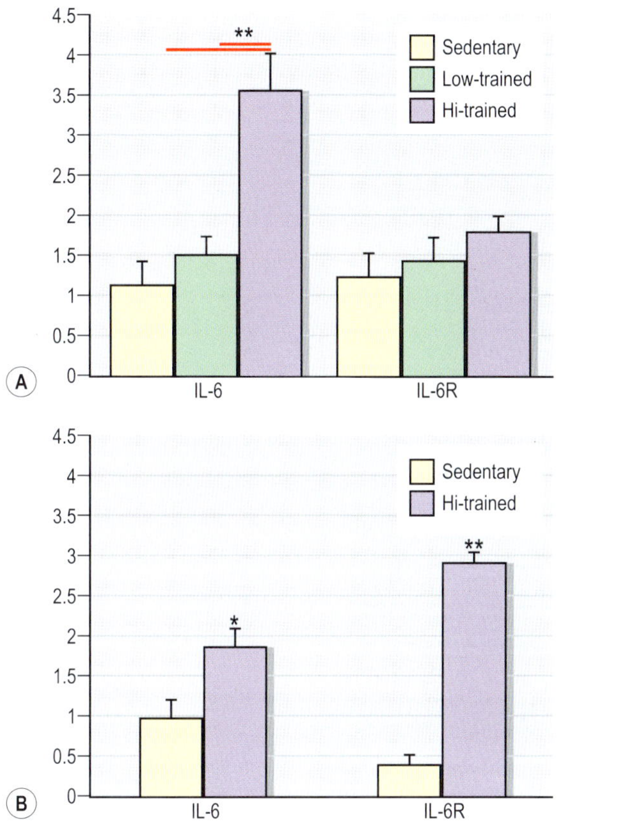

Fig 4.5 Interleukin-6 (IL-6) and its receptor IL-6R relative expression (in fold change) in human **(A)** and equine **(B)** in peripheral blood mononuclear cells in sedentary or trained subjects and horses. In humans, the IL-6 expression increases significantly (*$P < 0.05$, **$P < 0.001$) with the training response while in horses, both IL6 and it receptor expression increase significantly with training. The red lines represent significant differences to the Hi-trait.

Reprinted from Capomaccio S, Cappelli K, Spinsanti G, Mencarelli M, Muscettola M, Felicetti M, Verini Supplizi A, Bonifazi M (2011). Athletic humans and horses: comparative analysis of interleukin-6 (IL-6) and IL-6 receptor (IL-6R) expression in peripheral blood mononuclear cells in trained and untrained subjects at rest. BMC Physiol *21;11:3 with permission from Stefano Capomaccio.*

lower in Warmbloods (18%) and other light horse breeds (24%), when diagnosis was based on grade 2 diagnostic criteria. Overall, the PSSM mutation was present in 16% of grade 1 and 70% of grade 2 PSSM horses. False-positive diagnosis, as well as the possibility of a second glycogenosis in horses with neuromuscular disease, might explain the absence of the GYS1 mutation in horses diagnosed with excessive glycogen accumulation in muscle.

In some severe cases of PSSM, another gene mutation has been observed in the ryanodine receptor RYR1 responsible for an excess calcium release by the sarcoplasmic reticulum into the cytosol of the muscle fibers which suffers from contractures.[49] In addition to the clinical examination and muscular histology diagnosis, the genotyping of the genes GYS1 and RYR1 could be used to confirm the PSSM disease to establish a risk evaluation and to avoid the gene transmission to the offspring.

More recently, two myopathies were investigated by functional genomic analysis: polysaccharide storage myopathy (PSSM)[50] and recurrent exertional rhabdomyolysis (RER).[51] Several cases of myopathies have been observed in Norman Cob breed horses. Muscle histology examinations revealed that some families suffer from a polysaccharide storage myopathy (PSSM). It is assumed that a gene expression signature related to PSSM should be observed at the transcriptional level because the glycogen storage disease could also be linked to other dysfunctions in gene regulation. Thus, the functional genomic approach could be conducted in order to provide new knowledge about the metabolic disorders related to PSSM. It was proposed to explore the PSSM muscle fiber metabolic disorders by measuring gene expression in relationship with the histological phenotype.

Genotyping analysis of GYS1 mutation revealed two homozygous (AA) and five heterozygous (GA) PSSM horses. In the PSSM muscles, histological data revealed positive amylase resistant abnormal polysaccharides (PAS), inflammation, necrosis, and lipomatosis and active regeneration of fibers. Ultrastructural evaluation revealed a decrease of mitochondrial number and structural disorders. Extensive accumulation of an abnormal polysaccharide displaced and partially replaced mitochondria and myofibrils. The severity of the disease was higher in the two homozygous PSSM horses. Gene expression analysis revealed 129 genes significantly modulated ($P < 0.05$). The following genes were up-regulated over two-fold: IL18, CTSS, LUM, CD44, FN1, GST01. The most down-regulated genes were the following: mitochondrial tRNA, SLC2A2, PRKC alpha, VEGF alpha.

Data mining analysis showed that protein synthesis, apoptosis, cellular movement, growth and proliferation were the main cellular functions significantly associated with the modulated genes ($P < 0.05$). Several up-regulated genes, especially IL18, revealed a severe muscular inflammation in PSSM muscles. The up-regulation of glycogen synthase kinase-3 (GSK3B) under its active form could be responsible for glycogen synthase (GYS1) inhibition and hypoxia-inducible factor (HIF1A) destabilization (Fig. 4.7). The main disorders observed in PSSM muscles could be related to mitochondrial dysfunction, glycogenesis inhibition and the chronic hypoxia of the PSSM muscles.

The recurrent exertional rhabdomyolysis (RER) is a myopathy which is observed in a horse during exercise activity like a training session after a day of rest. The clinical signs observed are lumbar and back stiffness, reluctance to move and cramping, sweating, tachypnae, tachycardia. High creatine phosphokinase (CPK) activity is detected within 24 hours after the exercise and arginine succinyl-transaminase (AST) activity increases at least 48 hours after the rhabdomyolysis and remains high in case of recurrent rhabdomyolysis.

The terminology 'recurrent exertional rhabdomyolysis' (RER) has been proposed to define a chronic rhabdomyolysis observed in exercising Thoroughbreds with aberrant myofiber calcium regulation and caffeine-hypersensitive muscle.[52–54] Epidemiological studies reported a RER prevalence of about 5–10 % in Thoroughbreds during a racing season, with a recurrence of 17%.[55,56] In Warmblood horses, the polysaccharide storage myopathy (PSSM) prevalence is higher than RER according to a retrospective study of the cases presented at the University of Minnesota Neuromuscular Diagnostic Laboratory.[57] In Standardbreds[58] and French trotters[51,59] recurrent exertional rhabdomyolysis is one of the most common myopathies related to exercise.

In RER cases, some risk factors have been observed: young age, female, excitable behavior, high energetic diet and external risk factors such as cold temperature, humidity, return to work after a rest period. Some aspects of RER etiology have been identified such as the genetic component which has been demonstrated as an autosomal inheritance in Thoroughbred bloodlines of two affected sires.[60,61] An in vitro contracture test of the isolated RER muscle samples showed abnormal contracture under stimulation with potassium, halothane and caffeine, which demonstrated some

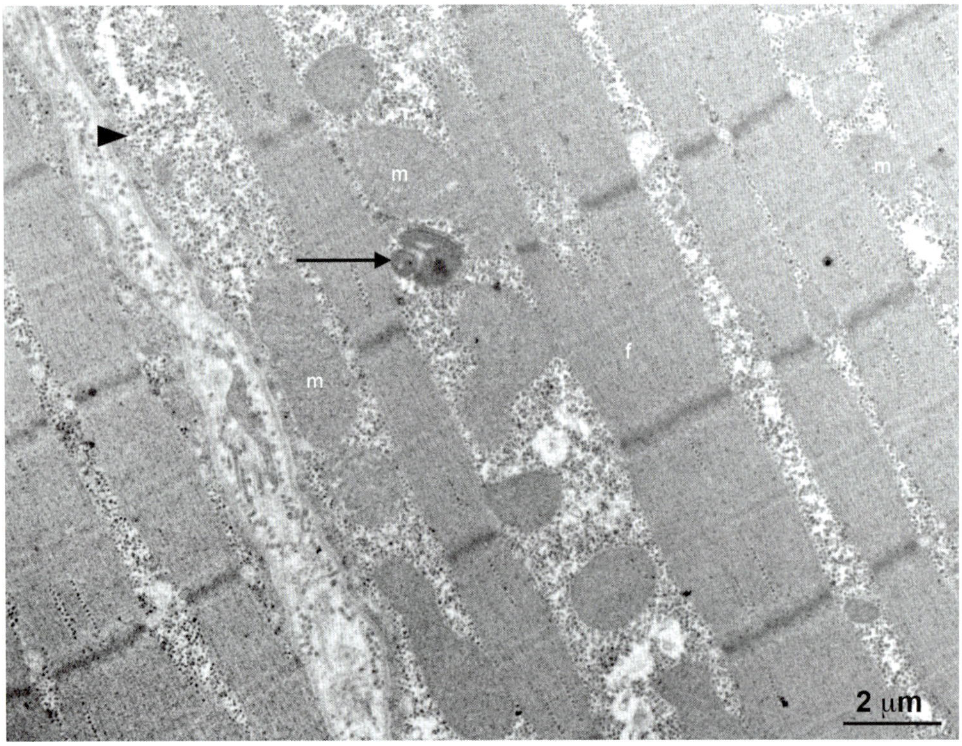

Fig 4.6 Muscular ultrastructure of longitudinal section from Norman cob horse affected by PSSM (homozygous AA for GYS1 c.926G>A mutation). We can observe a severe mitochondrial (m) and myofibrillar (f) loss due to abnormal accumulation of granular material (arrowhead) resembling glycogen. Some myelinic bodies (arrow) were present that demonstrated mitochondrial degeneration.
Reprinted from Barrey E, Mucher E, Jeansoule N, Larcher T, Guigand L, Herszberg B, Chaffaux S, Guérin G, Mata X, Benech P, Canale M, Alibert O, Maltere P, Gidrol X (2009) Gene expression profiling in equine polysaccharide storage myopathy revealed inflammation, glycogenesis inhibition, hypoxia and mitochondrial dysfunctions. BMC Vet. Res. *7, 5, 29.*

calcium regulation dysfunction.[52,53,62,63] Consequently, several candidate genes involved in calcium regulation such as RYR1, ATP2A1, CACNA1S were investigated and excluded as being associated with the disease.[64]

A first genome-wide association study was conducted in Thoroughbreds suffering from tying-up syndrome using microsatellites markers.[65] One strong hit was identified on chromosome 12 and another significant hit on chromosome 20. However, no candidate genes can be proposed at this time.

Having taken into account all the previous findings, we hypothesized that in RER muscle the calcium concentration regulation of one or several cellular compartments is no more under control and breaks the cytoplasmic calcium homeostasis. After the contraction, stimulated by calcium sarcoplasmic release, the cytoplasmic calcium should be actively pumped into the sarcoplasmic reticulum. If this process is disturbed, relaxation does not occur normally and the mechanical stress could be the cause of the myofiber injury.

A transcriptome analysis of muscle was conducted in horses suffering from recurrent exertional rhabdomyolysis.[66] Functional genomic data analysis revealed energetic pathway alterations and disruption in the cytosolic calcium regulation. The study compared the gene expression profile of RER vs. control muscles in the French Trotter to determine any metabolic or structural disruption. Gene expression analyzes were performed on the total RNA extracted from muscle biopsies collected in 15 French trotter horses, including 10 controls and five RER horses affected by tying-up with high plasmatic muscular enzyme activities. Microarray analyzes revealed 191 genes significantly modulated in RER vs. control muscles ($P < 0.05$). Many genes involved in fatty acid oxidation (CD36/FAT, SLC25A17), the Krebs cycle (SLC25A11, SLC25A12, MDH2) and the mitochondrial respiratory chain were severely down-regulated (tRNA, MT-ND5, MT-ND6, MT-COX1). According to the down-regulation of RYR1, SLC8A1/NCX1 and UCP2 and up-regulation of APP and HSPA5, the muscle fibre calcium homeostasis seemed to be greatly affected by an increased cytosolic calcium and a depletion of the sarcoplasmic reticulum calcium (Fig. 4.8). Gene expression analysis suggested an alteration of ATP synthesis, with severe mitochondrial dysfunction that could explain the disruption of cytosolic calcium homeostasis and inhibition of muscular relaxation.

MicroRNAs (miRNA) are small endogenous non-coding interfering RNA molecules (18–25 nucleotides) regarded as major regulators in eukaryotic gene expression. They play a role in developmental timing, cellular differentiation, signaling and apoptosis pathways. Recently, microRNAs were detected in equine muscle and blood and could be interesting markers of diseases in the near future.[67] The use of miRNA profile in tissues and blood for the disease diagnostic is under development in human oncology and it has been evaluated in myology.[68,69] In the major human myopathies, many miRNA (151) were up-regulated and only 28 were down-regulated among 428 miRNA measured in affected muscles.[70] Because of the central function of miRNAs in the proliferation and differentiation of the

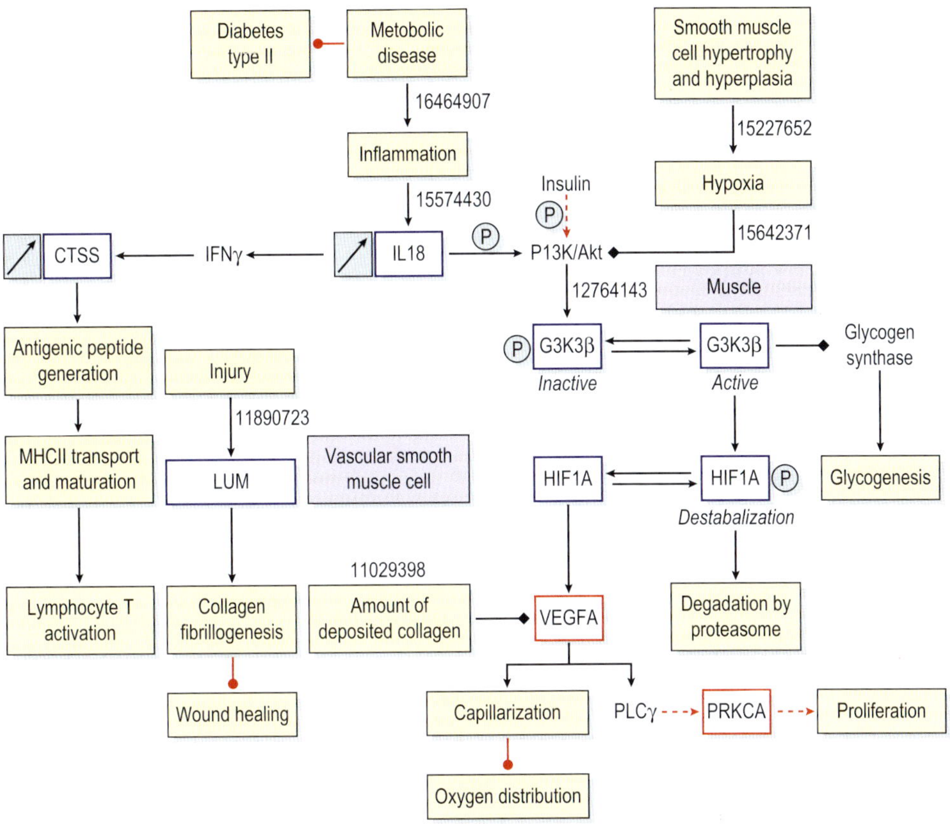

Fig 4.7 Relationships between inflammatory process, inhibition of glycogen synthase and hypoxia according to data mining analysis of PSSM transcriptomic results (Barrey et al. 2009). The up-regulation of the glycogen synthase kinase (GSK3β) under its active form was responsible for the glycogen synthase (GYS1) inhibition. The up-regulation of GSK3β has another effect on hypoxia and low capillarization of the PSSM muscle. Phosphorylation of GSK3β increases the HIF1α destabilization which is degraded in the proteosome. Consequently, the low expression of HIF1α down-regulates VEGFα expression which contributes to a poor capillarization and increases chronic hypoxia of the regenerated muscle fibers. The PubMed ID of the related publications found by the data mining analysis were indicated on the pathway.

myoblasts demonstrated in mice and humans, we assumed that they could be present in equine muscles and their expression profile could be related to the muscle status (Fig. 4.9). Several miRNA candidates (miR-1, 23, 30, 133, 181, 188, 195, 206, 339, 375) were significantly detected in the normal and diseased muscles and some other miRNAs in blood samples collected in PSSM cases.[67] This first study about muscular miRNAs profiles in equine myopathies indicated that it is possible to discriminate diseased from control horses according to their miRNA profile. The RER muscles showed a miRNA profile which could be related to the proliferation and differentiation regulation of the myoblasts activated after rhabdomyolysis. The RER miRNA profile was more contrasted and specific with several highly up-regulated miRNA (mir-133, mir-1, mir-23) than the PSSM miRNA profile (mir-195). Further investigations including more mirRNAs will be required to characterize the specificity and sensitivity of these new genomic biomarkers of myopathies both in muscle and blood samples.

Genotyping in osteochondrosis

Osteochondrosis is a major skeletal disorder in sport and racing horses. Several projects were started to identify genetic markers of this multifactorial joint disease affecting young horses. A first genome-wide scan detected quantitative trait loci (QTLs) for osteochondrosis (OC) and osteochondrosis dissecans (OCD) in horses.[71] The genetic marker set comprised 260 microsatellites. Data were collected from 211 Hanoverian Warmblood horses consisting of 14 paternal half-sib families. Traits used were OC (fetlock and/or hock joints affected), OCD (fetlock and/or hock joints affected), fetlock OC, fetlock OCD, hock OC, and hock OCD. Genome-wide significant loci were located on eight different equine chromosomes: 2, 3, 4, 5, 15, 16, 19, and 21. QTLs for fetlock OC and hock OC partly overlapped on the same chromosomes, indicating that these traits may be genetically related. QTLs reached the chromosome-wide significance level. Then, candidate genes should be investigated in theses significant loci using more accurate method.

In a second study, of 29 microsatellite markers distributed in chromosome, five were used to refine the map positions of the QTL already identified for OC in the fetlock.[72] Collagen type XXIV alpha 1 was identified as a potential functional candidate gene for the fetlock osteochondrosis. Another chromosome-wide linkage analysis revealed a new QTL on chromosome 18 for osteochondrosis in fetlock, hock, or both joints, as well as for osteochondrosis

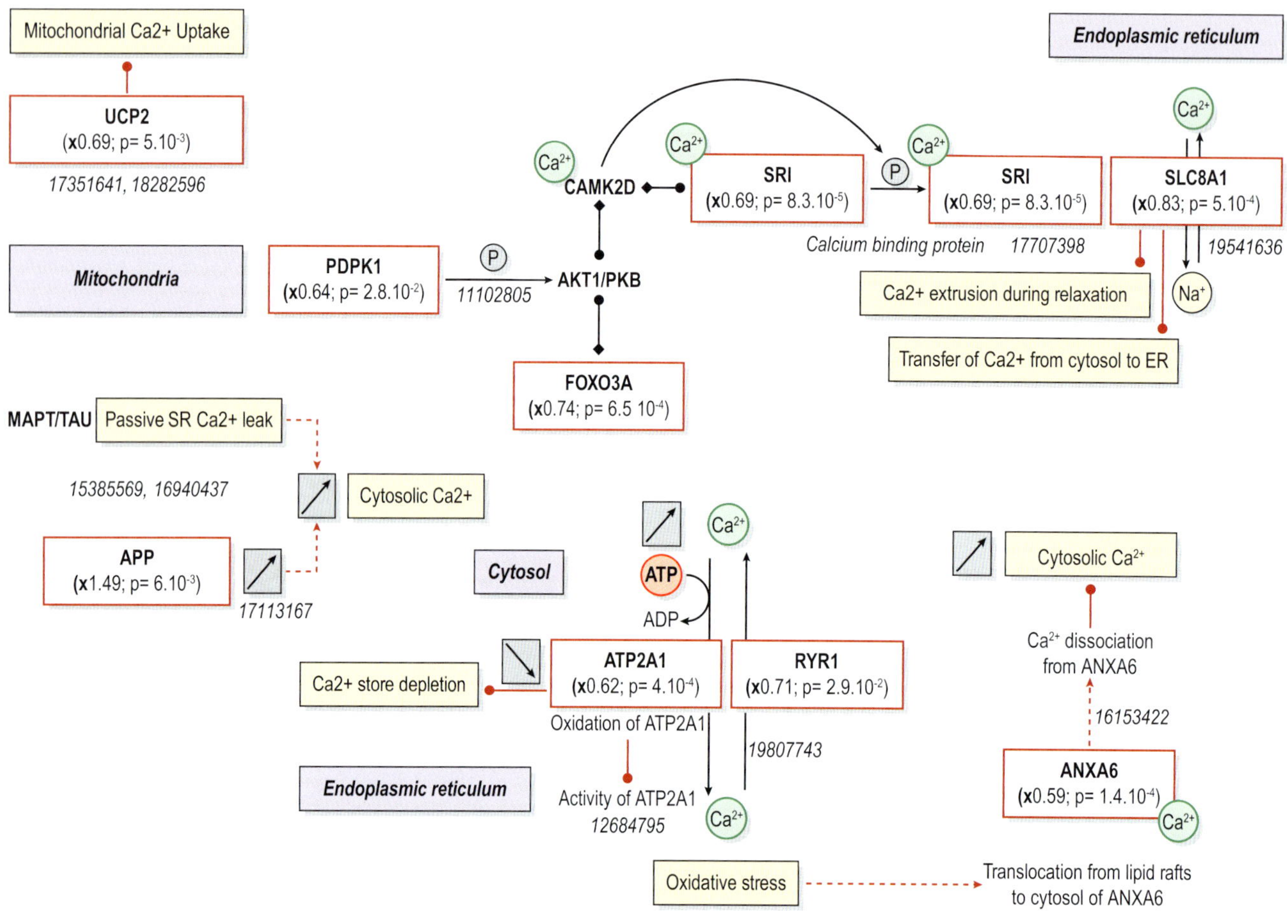

Fig 4.8 Disruption of calcium homeostasis towards increased levels of cytosolic Ca2+. Cytosolic calcium concentration should increase because of the sarcoplasmic reticulum passive leaks and active pumping inhibition (down-regulation of RYR1, SLC8A, up-regulation of APP), the inhibition of calcium mitochondrial sequestration by the uncoupling protein (down-regulation of UCP2 and PDPK1) and inhibition of the cellular membrane translocation (down-regulation of SLC8A1). The sarcoplasmic reticulum exhibited stress signals indicating a depletion of calcium store (down-regulation of ATP2A1, RYR1, ; up-regulation of APP). Signs and conventions used to describe the pathways are indicated figure 1: down-regulated genes were in red boxes with their normalized ratio and p-value. Up-regulated genes were in green boxes with their normalized ratio and p-value. The PubMed ID of the related publications found by the data mining analysis Predictsearch® are indicated on the figure by the numbers in black italic.

dissecans in hock joints.[73] Within this QTL for equine osteochondrosis, the parathyroid hormone 2 receptor gene could be identified as a positional candidate gene.

Other genome-wide association analyzes of osteochondrosis were conducted in Standardbred trotters. In Norwegian Standardbreds, the results obtained by genotyping 80 OCD cases *versus* 82 controls allowed to identify quantitative trait loci (QTL) associated with osteochondrosis dissecans (OCD) at the intermediate ridge of the distal tibia.[74] Several hits were detected on *Equus callabus* chromosome 5, 10, 27 and 28. Two SNPs on chromosome 10 represent the most significant hits ($p = 1.19 \times 10^{-5}$). The other genome-wide association study for osteochondrosis in French trotter horses was carried out in 98 sire families with 525 progeny.[75] Radiographic data were obtained from progeny using at least ten views. All radiographic findings were described by at least two veterinary experts in equine orthopaedics and severity indices (scores) were assigned based on the size and location of the lesion. The results showed one significant ($p < 5 \times 10^{-5}$) hit for general score of osteochondrosis on chromosome 13, two hits for hock joint on chromosome 3 and 14, and one hit for other joints except fetlock on chromosome 15. The hit on chromosome 3 was the most significant ($P = 3 \times 10^{-6}$). Interestingly, no common SNP was found between fetlock and hock joints. Moreover, the four SNPs significantly related to the general score of osteochondrosis were associated either to fetlock or hock osteochondrosis but never both of them. Thus, the two joints osteochondrosis could be induced by the alteration of two different gene combinations. The different genome-wide association studies conducted on osteochondrosis among the different breeds didn't detect any common QTLs which suggests that either a difficulty to characterize the osteochondrosis phenotypes or different diseases for each joint and/or each breed (Fig. 4.10). The chromosomes 5 and 15 were the only ones detected in at least two studies however their hits were different.

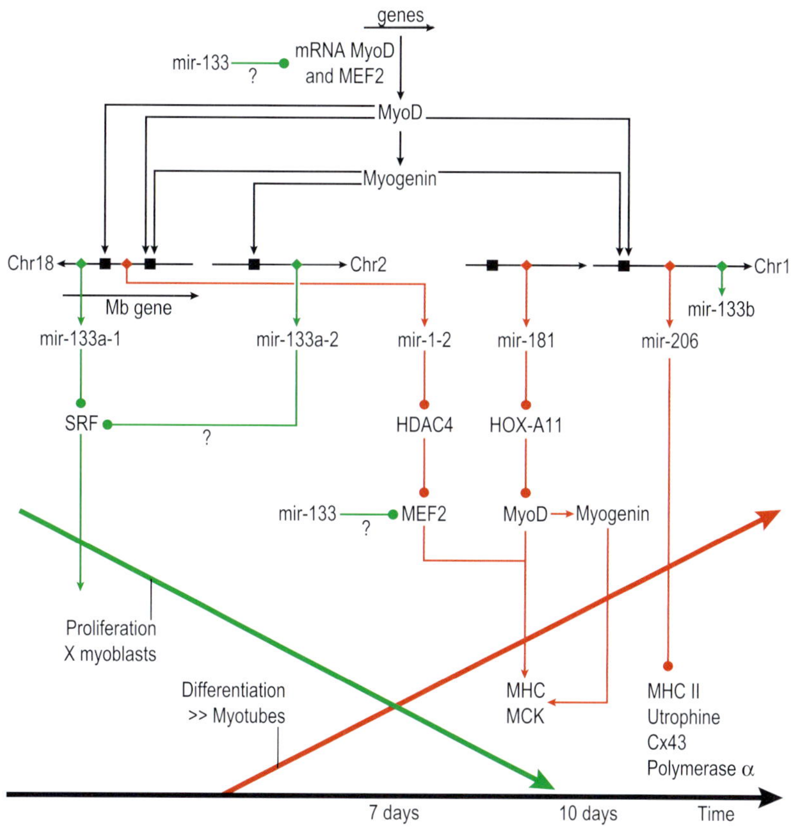

Fig 4.9 Overview of the knowledge of the miRNA functions in human myoblasts proliferation and differentiation. The mir-1, mir-133 and mir-181 have several isoforms indicated by different letters with one nucleotide differences.
Adapted from the data presented in Rao et al. (2006), Naguibneva et al. (2006), Chen et al. (2006) and McCarthy et al. (2007).

Genotyping in respiratory diseases

Upper airways obstruction syndrome causes poor performance because of the decrease of ventilation capacity during exercise. The recurrent laryngeal neuropathy (Fig. 4.11) is the main upper airways disease, but its exact etiology remains unknown. Genetic component has been suspected by the professionals however few data are available to demonstrate this hypothesis. The first genome-wide association study was conducted on 234 cases (196 Warmbloods, 20 trotters, 14 Thoroughbreds, and 4 draft horses), 228 breed-matched controls, and 69 parents that were genotyped using 54K SNP arrays.[76] Two SNP hits were identified in Warmbloods, respectively on chromosomes 21 ($p = 1.62 \times 10^{-6}$) and 31 ($p = 1.69 \times 10^{-5}$).

In lower airways diseases, chronic pulmonary obstructive disease or recurrent airways obstruction is on common pulmonary allergy in horses related to sensitization and exposure to moldy hay. Clinically the inspiration and expiration becomes noisy and more difficult even at rest and one can observe diaphragm efforts and poor exercise performance. A genome wide-scan study using few hundred microsatellites revealed two regions in chromosome 13 and 15 significantly associated to the disease ($p < 0.05$)[77]. Some interesting candidate genes as interleukins were suspected and should be further investigated.

Conclusion: genetic and genomic perspective in equine exercise

With the development of the genomic technologies many new applications will be available for the horse industry: identification of candidate genes responsible for diseases and performance, genotyping, diagnostic tools and treatments. The first genotype test for racing speed and distance ability is now available for potential early evaluation of horses used for flat racing. The diagnosis of PSSM myopathy by genotyping is routinely applied. Within five years, other genotyping methods will be available for early evaluation of performance and detection of the genetic basis of diseases enabling diagnosis and risk evaluation for disease such as osteochondrosis or respiratory diseases. New genomic treatments will be probably designed to treat some myopathies and metabolic diseases as it is now applied in humans. The drawback of the biotechnologies availability will be the potential illicit use for doping using gene modulators or transgenesis of key genes for examples. Hopefully, research projects are already going on to detect this new type of genomic doping both in humans and horses.

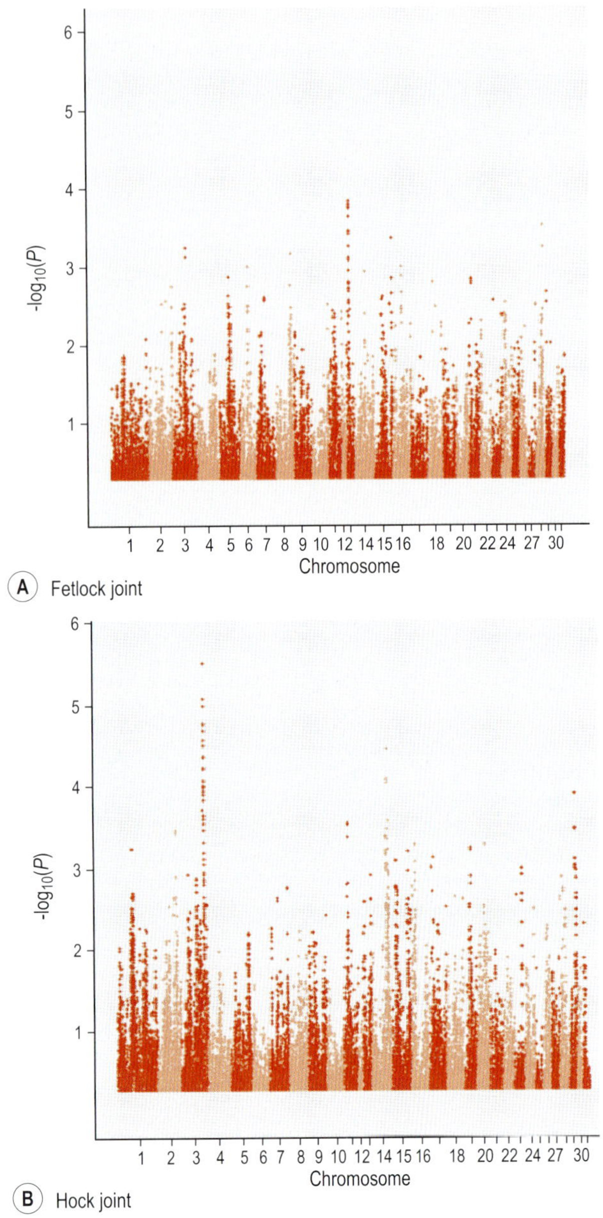

Fig 4.10 Detection of the SNPs of osteochondrosis of the fetlock (no significant SNP) and hock joints on chromosome 13 and 14 (significant SNP at p $5 < 10^{-5}$) in French trotters (n = 525). The Manhattan plots of –log10 of *P*-values displays the haplotype mixed-model test results at each SNP position on each chromosome.

Reprinted from Teyssèdre S, Dupuis MC, Guérin G, Schibler L, Denoix JM, Elsen JM, Ricard A (2011) Genome-wide association studies for osteochondrosis in French trotters. J Anim Sci. *Aug 12, with permission.*

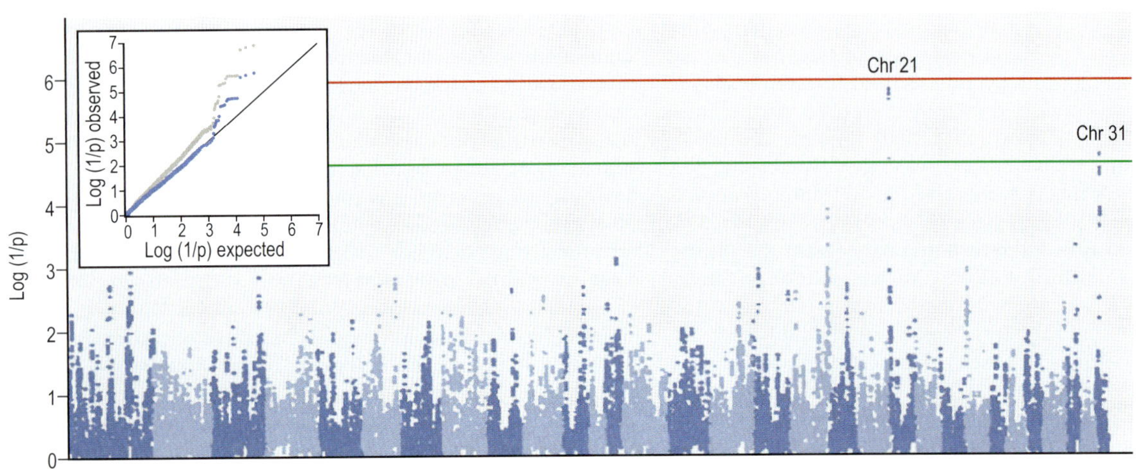

Fig 4.11 Genotyping results in 230 cases of recurrent laryngeal neuropathy. Two significant SNPs on chromosomes 21 ($p = 1.62 \times 10^{-6}$) and 31 ($p = 1.69 \times 10^{-5}$) in Warmblood horses.

Reprinted from Dupuis MC, Zhang Z, Druet T, Denoix JM, Charlier C, Lekeux P, Georges M. (2011) Results of a haplotype-based GWAS for recurrent laryngeal neuropathy in the horse. Mamm Genome *22 (9–10):613–20 with permission of Springer Science and Business Media.*

References

1. Xu X, Arnason U. The complete mitochondrial DNA sequence of the horse, Equus caballus: extensive heteroplasmy of the control region. Gene 1994;148:357–62.
2. Caetano AR, Shiue YL, Lyons LA, et al. A comparative gene map of the horse (Equus caballus). Genome Res 1999;9:1239–49.
3. Milenkovic D, Oustry-Vaiman A, Lear TL, et al. Cytogenetic localization of 136 genes in the horse: comparative mapping with the human genome. Mamm Genome 2002;13:524–34.
4. Chowdhary BP, Raudsepp T, Kata SR, et al. The first-generation whole-genome radiation hybrid map in the horse identifies conserved segments in human and mouse genomes. Genome Res 2003;13(4):742–51. Erratum in: Genome Res 13, 1258.
5. Wade CM, Giulotto E, Sigurdsson S, et al; Broad Institute Genome Sequencing Platform; Broad Institute Whole Genome Assembly Team. Genome sequence, comparative analysis, and population genetics of the domestic horse. Science 2009;326(5954):865–7.
6. Bray MS, Hagberg JM, Pérusse L, et al. The human gene map for performance and health-related fitness phenotypes: the 2006–2007 update. Med Sci Sports Exerc 2009;41:35–73.
7. Ricard A, Bruns E, Cunningham EP. Genetics of performance traits. In: Bowling AT, Ruvinsky A, editors. New York: CABI Publishing; 2000. p. 411–38.
8. Hintz RL. Genetics of Performance in the Horse. J Anim Sci 1980;51:582–94.
9. Langlois B. Heritability of racing ability in Thoroughbreds – a review. Livestock Prod Sci 1980;7:583–94.
10. Ricard A, Touvais M. genetic parameters of performance traits in horse endurance races. Livestock Sci 2007;110:118–25.
11. Ricard A, Blouin C. Genetic analysis of the longevity of French sport horses in jumping competition. J Anim Sci 2011;89:2988–94.
12. Barrey E, Valette JP, Jouglin M, et al. Heritability of percentage of fast myosin heavy chains in skeletal muscles and relationship with performance. Equine vet J Suppl 1999;30:289–92.
13. Rivero JL, Barrey E. Heritabilities and genetic and phenotypic parameters for gluteus medius muscle fibre type composition, fibre size and capillaries in purebred Spanish horses. Livestock Prod Sci 2001;72:233–41.
14. Barrey E, Courouce A, Langlois B, et al. Genetic component of exercise test parameters in French Trotters: first estimations. Conference on Equine Sports Medicine and Science by Arno Lindner (Ed). Cordoba, Spain, April 24th–26th, 1999. p. 219–24.
15. Leleu C, Cotrel C, Barrey E. Relationships between locomotor test and racing performances in Standardbreds. 54th Annual Meeting of the European Association for Animal Production, Horse Production, Rome, Italy, August 31–September 3, 2003, abstract H2.9.
16. Barrey E, Desliens F, Poirel D, et al. Early evaluation of dressage ability in different breeds. Equine vet J Suppl 2002c;34:319–24.
17. Barrey E, Galloux P. Analysis of the equine jumping technique by accelerometry. Equine vet J Suppl 1997;23:45–9.
18. Barrey E, Desliens F, Blouin C, et al. Heritabilities of gait characteristics: application for breeding in dressage. Conference on Equine Sports Medicine and Science 2002, "The Elite Dressage and Three-Day-Event horse", Lindner A. (Ed), 2002a. p. 91–5.
19. Barrey E, Desliens F, Blouin C, et al. (2002b). Mesures du modèle, des allures et du saut des étalons nationaux par la méthode Equimétrix. 27èmes Journées de la Recherche équine, Les Haras Nationaux, Paris, France, 27 février 2002, p. 157–76.
20. Saastamoinen and Barrey. The genetics of the horse: 16 conformation and physiological traits: their evaluation and heritability. In: Bowling AT, Ruvinsky A, editors. The genetics of the horse. Chapter 16: Conformation and physiological traits: their evaluation and heritability. New York: CABI Publishing; 2000. p. 441–72.
21. McCue ME, Bannasch DL, Petersen JL, et al. A High Density SNP Array for the Domestic Horse and Extant Perissodactyla: Utility for Association Mapping, Genetic Diversity, and Phylogeny Studies. PLoS Genet 2012;8(1):e1002451.
22. Barrey E, Mucher E, Robert C, et al. Gene expression profiling in blood cells of endurance horses completing competition or disqualified due to metabolic disorder. Equine vet J Suppl 2006;36:43–9.
23. McGivney BA, Eivers SS, MacHugh DE, et al. Transcriptional adaptations following exercise in Thoroughbred horse skeletal muscle highlights molecular mechanisms that lead to muscle hypertrophy. BMC Genomics 2009;30(10):638.
24. Hill EW, Eivers SS, McGivney BA, et al. Moderate and high intensity sprint exercise induce differential responses in COX4I2 and PDK4 gene expression in Thoroughbred horse skeletal muscle. Equine vet J 2010;42(Suppl. 38):576–81.
25. Gu J, Orr N, Park SD, et al. A Genome Scan for Positive Selection in Thoroughbred Horses. PLoS ONE 2009;4(6):e5767.
26. Gu J, MacHugh DE, McGivney BA, et al. Association of sequence variants in CKM (creatine kinase, muscle) and COX4I2 (cytochrome c oxidase, subunit 4, isoform 2) genes with racing performance in Thoroughbred horses. Equine vet J 2010;42(Suppl 38):569–75.
27. Hill EW, Gu J, McGivney BA, et al. Targets of selection in the Thoroughbred genome contain exercise-relevant gene SNPs associated with elite racecourse performance. Anim Genet 2010;41(Suppl. 2):56–63.
28. Rodriguez J, Vernus B, Toubiana M, et al. Myostatin inactivation increases myotube size through regulation of translational initiation machinery. J Cell Biochem 2011;112(12):3531–42.
29. Hill EW, Gu J, Eivers SS, et al. Sequence polymorphism in MSTN predicts sprinting ability and racing stamina in Thoroughbred horses. PLoS One 2010;5(1):e8645.
30. Hill EW, Fonseca RG, McGivney BA, et al. MSTN genotype (g.66493737C/T) association with speed indices in Thoroughbred racehorses. J Appl Physiol 2011.
31. Tozaki T, Sato F, Hill EW, et al. Sequence Variants at the myostatin Gene Locus Influence the Body Composition of Thoroughbred Horses. J Vet Med Sci 2011.
32. Andersson LS, Larhammar M, Memic F, et al. Mutations in DMRT3 affect locomotion in horses and spinal circuit function in mice. Nature 2012;488(7413):642–6. doi: 10.1038/nature11399.
33. Schröder W, Klostermann A, Stock KF, et al. A genome-wide association study for quantitative trait loci of show-jumping in Hanoverian Warmblood horses. Anim Genet 2011;43(4):392–400.
34. Ricard A, Legarra A, Meriaux JC, et al. Premiers résultats de l'évaluation génomique chez les chevaux de concours hippique. 38ème Journée de la Recherche Equine, Paris, 1st March, Abstract book, 2012. p. 17–23.
35. Capomaccio S, Cappelli K, Barrey E, et al. Microarray analysis after strenuous exercise in peripheral blood mononuclear cells of endurance horses. Anim Genet 2010;41(Suppl 2):166–75.
36. Capomaccio S, Cappelli K, Spinsanti G, et al. Athletic humans and horses: comparative analysis of interleukin-6 (IL-6) and IL-6 receptor (IL-6R) expression in peripheral blood mononuclear cells in trained and untrained subjects at rest. BMC Physiol 2011;21(11):3.
37. Cottin F, Metayer N, Goachet AG, et al. Oxygen consumption and gait variables of Arabian endurance horses measured

during a field exercise test. Equine vet J 2010;42(Suppl. 38):1–5.
38. Yoon SS. Glycogen storage disease: clinical, biochemichal and molecular heterogeneity. Seminar in Pediatric Neurology 2006;13:115–20.
39. Valberg SJ, Cardinet GH 3rd, Carlson GP, et al. Polysaccharide storage myopathy associated with recurrent exertional rhabdomyolysis in horses. Neuromusc Disord 1992;2:351–9.
40. Quiroz-Rothe E, Novales M, Aguilera-Tejero E, et al. Polysaccharide storage myopathy in the M. longissimus lumborum of showjumpers and dressage horses with back pain. Equine vet J 2002;34:171–6.
41. Valentine BA, Cooper BJ. Incidence of polysaccharide storage myopathy : necropsy study of 225 horses. Vet Pathol 2005;42:823–37.
42. McCue ME, Ribeiro WP, Valberg SJ. Prevalence of polysaccharide storage myopathy in horses with neuromuscular disorders. Equine vet J Suppl 2006;36:340–4.
43. McCue ME, Valberg SJ. Estimated prevalence of polysaccharide storage myopathy among overtly healthy Quarter Horses in the United States. J Am Vet Med Ass 2007;231:746–50.
44. McGowan CM, McGowan TW, Patterson-Kane JC. Prevalence of equine polysaccharide storage myopathy and other myopathies in two equine populations in the United Kingdom. Vet J 2009;180:330–6.
45. Firshman AM, Valberg SJ, Bender JB, et al. Comparison of histopathologic criteria and skeletal muscle fixation techniques for the diagnosis of polysaccharide storage myopathy in horses. Vet Pathol 2006;43:257–69.
46. Ward TL, Valberg SJ, Adelson DL, et al. Glycogen branching enzyme (GBE1) mutation causing equine glycogen storage disease IV. Mamm Genome 2004;15:570–7.
47. McCue ME, Valberg SJ, Miller MB, et al. Glycogen synthase (GYS1) mutation causes a novel skeletal muscle glycogenosis. Genomics 2008;91:458–66.
48. Herszberg B, McCue ME, Larcher T, et al. A GYS1 gene mutation is highly associated with polysaccharide storage myopathy in Cob Normand draught horses. Anim Genet 2009;40:94–6.
49. McCue ME, Valberg SJ, Jackson M, et al. Polysaccharide storage myopathy phenotype in quarter horse-related breeds is modified by the presence of an RYR1 mutation. Neuromuscul Disord 2009;19:37–43.
50. Barrey E, Mucher E, Jeansoule N, et al. Gene expression profiling in equine polysaccharide storage myopathy revealed inflammation, glycogenesis inhibition, hypoxia and mitochondrial dysfunctions. BMC Vet Res 2009;7(5):29.
51. Jayr L. Predisposition à la rhabdomyolyse d'effort chez le trotteur français: analyze génomique. Veterinary thesis ENV Alfort. Presented 24th september, 2009. p. 84.
52. Lentz LR, Valberg SJ, Balog EM, et al. Abnormal regulation of muscle contraction in horses with recurrent exertional rhabdomyolysis. Am J Vet Res 1999;60:992–9.
53. Lentz LR, Valberg SJ, Mickelson JR, et al. In vitro contractile responses and contracture testing of skeletal muscle from Quarter Horses with exertional rhabdomyolysis. J Vet Res 1999b;60: 684–8.
54. Piercy RJ, Rivero JL. Muscle disorders of equine athletes. In: Hinchcliff KW, Kaneps AJ, Geor RJ, et al, editors. Equine Sports Medicine and Surgery. 2004. p. 77–110.
55. MacLeay JM, Sorum SA, Valberg SJ, et al. Epidemiologic analysis of factors influencing exertional rhabdomyolysis in Thoroughbreds. Am J Vet Res 1999a;60:1562–6.
56. McGowan CM, Fordham T, Christley RM. Incidence and risk factors for exertional rhabdomyolysis in Thoroughbred racehorses in the United Kingdom. Vet Rec 2002;151:623–6.
57. Hunt LM, Valberg SJ, Steffenhagen K. et al. An epidemiological study of myopathies in Warmblood horses. Equine Vet J 2008;40:171–7.
58. Collinder E, Lindholm A, Rasmuson M. Genetic markers in Standardbred trotters susceptible to the rhabdomyolysis syndrome. Equine Vet J 1997;29:117–20.
59. Couroucé-Malblanc A, Deniau V, De Rancourt B. L'entraînement, la prophylaxie et le traitement des cas de myopathie à l'exercice. Pratique Vét Equine 2009;41:4–49.
60. MacLeay JM, Valberg SJ, Sorum SA, et al. Heritability of recurrent exertional rhabdomyolysis in Thoroughbred racehorses. Am J Vet Res 1999b;60:250–6.
61. Dranchak PK, Valberg SJ, Onan GW, et al. Inheritance of recurrent exertional rhabdomyolysis in Thoroughbreds. J Am Vet Med Ass 2005;227:762–7.
62. Ward TL, Valberg SJ, Gallant EM, et al. Calcium regulation by skeletal muscle membranes of horses with recurrent exertional rhabdomyolysis. Am J Vet Res 2000;61:242–7.
63. Lentz LR, Valberg SJ, Herold LV, et al. Myoplasmic calcium regulation in myotubes from horses with recurrent exertional rhabdomyolysis. Am J Vet Res 2002;63:1724–31.
64. Dranchak PK, Valberg SJ, Onan GW, et al. Exclusion of linkage of the RYR1, CACNA1S, and ATP2A1 genes to recurrent exertional rhabdomyolysis in Thoroughbreds. Am J Vet Res 2006;67:1395–400.
65. Tozaki T, Hirota K, Sugita S, et al. A genome-wide scan for tying-up syndrome in Japanese Thoroughbreds. Anim Genet 2010;41(Suppl 2):80–6.
66. Barrey E, Jayr L, Mucher E, et al. Transcriptome analysis of muscle in horses suffering from recurrent exertional rhabdomyolysis revealed energetic pathway alterations and disruption in the cytosolic calcium regulation. Anim Genet 2011. Epub: 27 SEP 2011.
67. Barrey E, Bonnamy B, Barrey E, et al. Muscular microRNA expressions in healthy and myopathic horses suffering from polysaccharide storage myopathy or recurrent exercise rhabdomyolysis. Equine vet J 2010;42(Suppl. 38):303–10.
68. Calin GA, Croce CM. MicroRNA signatures in human cancers. Nat Rev Cancer 2006;6(11):857–66.
69. Chen X, Ba Y, Ma L, et al. Characterization of microRNAs in serum: a novel class of biomarkers for diagnosis of cancer and other diseases. Cell Res 2008;18(10):983–4.
70. Eisenberg I, Eran A, Nishino I, et al. Distinctive patterns of microRNA expression in primary muscular disorders. Proc Natl Acad Sci USA 2007;104(43):17016–21.
71. Dierks C, Löhring K, Lampe V, et al. Genome-wide search for markers associated with osteochondrosis in Hanoverian Warmblood horses. Mamm Genome 2007;18:739–47.
72. Lampe V, Dierks C, Distl O. Refinement of a quantitative trait locus on equine chromosome 5 responsible for fetlock osteochondrosis in Hanoverian Warmblood horses. Anim Genet 2009a;40:553–5.
73. Lampe V, Dierks C, Komm K, et al. Identification of a new quantitative trait locus on equine chromosome 18 responsible for osteochondrosis in Hanoverian Warmblood horses. J Anim Sci 2009b;87:3477–81.
74. Lykkjen S, Dolvik NI, McCue ME, et al. Genome-wide association analysis of osteochondrosis of the tibiotarsal joint in Norwegian Standardbred trotters. Anim Genet 2010;41(Suppl 2):111–20.
75. Teyssèdre S, Dupuis MC, Guérin G, et al. Genome-wide association studies for osteochondrosis in French Trotters. J Anim Sci 2011.
76. Dupuis MC, Zhang Z, Druet T, et al. Results of a haplotype-based GWAS for recurrent laryngeal neuropathy in the horse. Mamm Genome 2011;22(9–10):613–20.
77. Swinburne JE, Bogle H, Klukowska-Rötzler J, et al. A whole-genome scan for recurrent airway obstruction in Warmblood sport horses indicates two positional candidate regions. Mamm Genome 2009;20(8):504–15.

section 2

Musculoskeletal system

Epidemiology of orthopedic diseases in athletic horses

5

Tim Parkin Lisa Boden

CHAPTER CONTENTS

Epidemiology

The goal of epidemiology is to identify multi-factorial causes of disease in populations and apply this knowledge to minimize the prevalence or impact of deleterious outcomes. In most species, the primary application of epidemiology is usually related to the control of infectious disease. Although there are obvious examples of infectious disease epidemiology applied to athletic horse populations (Equine Influenza,[1,2] Hendra Virus,[3] West Nile Virus,[4,5,6]) most epidemiological work in this area has focused on injury prevention and improving horse performance. The vast majority of this work has been conducted in Thoroughbred racehorses and as such most of this chapter will focus on that particular breed.

The racehorse

The majority of epidemiological research on orthopedic disease and injury has been conducted on Thoroughbred racehorses. This is not due to a greater importance being attached to this breed or a greater motivation of veterinarians and epidemiologists to address the particular problems faced by this breed. Rather, it is the greater availability of suitable and complete datasets which makes these types of studies feasible.

As far back as the 1960s and early 1970s, the equine veterinary community started describing racehorse injury and fatality at a population level: leg problems in racehorses,[7] sore shins,[8] third metacarpal (MCIII) and third metatarsal (MTIII) fractures,[9,10,11] carpal fractures[12,13] and equine fatalities during racing on British racecourses.[14] Since then, many case definitions have been used in the major epidemiological studies of racecourse injury or fatality. Choice of case definition within each study may be based on wider issues such as local or regional priorities or specific jurisdiction requests, but in most instances, case definition has typically been based on the limitations of data resolution (i.e. the level of detail contained within race reports). In early studies, this resulted in fairly broad case definitions. However, data recording has improved over time (possibly as a result of increased awareness of the importance of these data and developments in computational power). As a result, more recent studies have been able to describe and analyze the risk of specific injury types.

Risk of orthopedic disease, injury, or fatality in Thoroughbred racehorses

There are relatively few studies investigating the risk of orthopedic disease in the Thoroughbred.[15,16] Most descriptive studies have focused on the risk of musculoskeletal injury or fatality of Thoroughbreds during racing or training. In response to increased public cognizance of animal welfare issues, many of these studies have been driven by the racing industry in an effort to publicly demonstrate the impact of interventions to improve safety and minimize injury and fatality. For example, the risks associated with jump racing in Victoria, Australia were formally reviewed in 1994, 1998 and in 2002 in response to public demand for improved safety at jump races. It is important that these studies correctly report the level of risk (with both numerator and denominator) before an intervention is introduced, so that the impact of an intervention can be assessed appropriately. A reduction in the annual number of fatalities at a particular racecourse should not be regarded as good evidence of a safer racecourse unless the annual number of race starts over the same time period is also reported.

The risk of disease or injury is typically measured by prevalence, incidence risk, or incidence rate.[17,18,19] Prevalence describes the number of instances of disease in a defined population at a specific point in time without any distinction between recent (acute) and long established (chronic) cases. Incidence risk (synonym, cumulative incidence) is a measure of the average risk of developing the disease during a specific time period and is a proportion (and therefore a value between zero and 100%).[18] Mortality 'rates' are special measures of incidence used when the outcome is death.[17,18] Studies of racecourse injury or fatality typically report 'the number of events per 1000 starts'.[20,21,22,23,24,25,26,27] Incidence rate uses the number of new cases that occur in a defined population of animals over a specified period at risk.[17] This measure of risk is reported less frequently as it requires very detailed information on the time at risk. As such, it is best suited to studies of training injury where the number of events per 100 horse days (or months) in training (at risk) is reported.[28,29,30,31,32]

There are many more reports on the level of risk during racing than training, largely due to the availability of data. Within racing there are sufficient reports to enable the level of risk of fracture and soft tissue injury to be described separately.

The level of risk during racing

Risk of fracture (catastrophic or non-catastrophic fractures)

The risk of injury or fatality of Thoroughbred horses due to catastrophic musculoskeletal injury whilst racing varies within and between countries and also with race type. Since 1983, there have been multiple studies in North America, Great Britain and Australia that have described the risk of fatality due to catastrophic musculoskeletal injury in different race types: flat[33,34,35,36,37] and jump.[35,37]

In New York, between 1983 and 1985, there were 2.1 fracture injuries per 1000 starts on dirt tracks and 1.1 per 1000 starts on turf tracks.[33] In Kentucky, between 1992 and 1993, there were 1.4 catastrophic injuries per 1000 starts[34] and in California 1.7 fatalities per 1000 starts has been reported.[36] In the UK, between 1987 and 1993 there were 0.33 catastrophic fractures per 1000 flat racing starts, 1.4 catastrophic fractures per 1000 hurdle racing starts and 2.3 catastrophic fractures per 1000 steeplechase racing starts.[35] In Australia, the risk of serious musculoskeletal injury (resulting in euthanasia or a failure to return to racing for at least six months) on city tracks in Victoria was 0.6 per 1000 starts in flat races, 6.3 per 100 starts in hurdle races and 14.3 per 1000 starts in steeplechase races.[37]

Typically, the risk of injury in these studies has been calculated from veterinary reports on racing injuries (numerator) and centrally collected racing data on the number of starts (denominator) from different racing jurisdictions.[20,35] In some studies, the site of injury was identified in these veterinary reports. In those instances, the majority of musculoskeletal injuries were reported to have affected the bones of the distal forelimb. In North American studies, fractures of the proximal sesamoids were the most common injuries, followed by fractures of MCIII and carpal bones.[25,34,38] In the UK, lateral condylar fractures of MCIII were the most common racing injuries.[14,35,24] Differences between countries in the anatomic location of fractures may point to differences in the pathogenesis of different fracture types.

Other studies have initiated or used on-going post-mortem examinations to ensure accurate injury classification.[14,24,25,39,40] The cost of racecourse post-mortem examination programs often restricts their implementation, but unpublished data would suggest that in order to investigate accurate and precise case definitions, they are invaluable.[41] In 1990, the California Horse Racing Board (CHRB) requested that the California Veterinary Diagnostic Laboratory System carry out a post-mortem examination on all horses that die at California racecourses under the jurisdiction of the CHRB. The risk of catastrophic musculoskeletal injury (of which 88% (69/78) were fractures) was 1.7 per 1000 starts on these tracks.[26,36] Similar post mortem examination programs in the UK and Australia have subsequently highlighted the value of such examinations to enable the diagnosis of fracture at specific sites.[24,39] For example, in the UK, lateral condylar fractures of MCIII were most common in national hunt racing (from 0.28 per 1000 starts in hurdle racing to 0.96 per 1000 starts in national hunt flat racing), whereas proximal phalangeal fractures were most common in turf flat racing (0.16 per 1000 starts) and biaxial sesamoid fractures were most common in all-weather flat racing (0.39 per 1000 starts).[24] Continued collection of cases enabled the identification of risk factors for precise fracture definitions such as lateral condylar fracture of MCIII/MTIII.[42] In Victoria, Australia, the most common catastrophic musculoskeletal injury in horses submitted for post mortem examination was fracture of the MCIII or MTIII.[43] The second most common injury was the concurrent fracture of MCIII or MTIII and the proximal sesamoid bones and proximal phalanx. Although extremely costly and requiring a great deal of industry initiative and cooperation, further efforts to introduce routine post-mortem examinations in other jurisdictions should be encouraged.

Risk of soft tissue injury

There are fewer reports describing the level of risk of soft tissue injury during racing and all of these studies focus on tendon injuries.[20,22,44] The dearth of studies in this area of research is most likely due to lack of good quality data. Many soft tissue injuries do not require immediate euthanasia and may indeed only become clinically apparent once the horse has left the racecourse. As a result, these injuries may not be recorded by racecourse veterinarians and many of the estimates that are derived from racecourse reports are likely to be underestimates of the true level of risk. In Hong Kong, where detailed data on all racehorses in training and racing is recorded, Superficial Digital Flexor Tendon (SDFT) injury is the most common reason for horse retirements from racing (14%).[44] This highlights the importance of long-term soft tissue injury in curtailing the racing career of Thoroughbreds. In the USA, the earliest report on the frequency of soft tissue injury comes from work on 24 race courses where 0.9 and 0.6 severe tendon injuries per 1000 starts on dirt and turf tracks, respectively were reported.[45] These figures are comparable with later reports in the UK where the majority of races are on turf. The risk of injury to the suspensory ligament (SL) and superficial (SDFT) and deep digital flexor tendons (DDFT) together in the UK varied from 0.78 per 1000 starts in flat racing up to 9.12 per 1000 starts in steeplechase racing.[20] The majority of these injuries were likely to be associated with SDFT strain. In comparison, using data from 2000 to 2005 on the same UK racecourses, 0.55 SDFT strains per 1000 starts in flat racing, 6.6 per 1000 starts in hurdle racing and 8.0 per 1000 starts in steeplechase racing, were reported.[22]

The level of risk during training

The incidence risk or rate of injury during training is more difficult to quantify and compare. This is largely due to the use of different denominator data. These data cannot typically be obtained retrospectively as it is more common and appropriate to use the number of horse days or months at risk than number of race starts. Inconsistency arises because different studies use different definitions of a 'day at risk'. A horse on box rest is generally regarded as not being at risk of a training related fracture. But is a horse at risk when it is walking and trotting, cantering, or doing gallop-paced exercise?

Similarly how much more risk does a horse experience when galloping compared to cantering?

In the UK, the incidence rate of non-traumatic fractures per total days in training in flat racing horses was estimated at 1.15 per 100 horse months,[32] whereas in national hunt horses, the incidence rate was estimated as 1.5 per 100 horse months.[46] In the same national hunt population, 2.1 tendon and ligament injuries per 100 horse months were reported.[46] In New Zealand, incidence rates of 0.13 SDFT cases per 1,000 horse training days at risk and 0.12 suspensory apparatus (SA) cases per 1000 horse training days at risk were calculated.[29] In that study, SA included both soft tissue (suspensory ligament and distal sesamoidean ligament) and proximal sesamoid bone injuries. In Japan, forelimb superficial digital flexor tendonitis has been reported as being significantly more common than SL desmitis in training and racing Thoroughbred racehorses.[47] The prevalence of forelimb SDFT tendonitis and SL desmitis was 11.1% (1130 cases) and 3.61% (370 cases) of the population, respectively.

Different local industry conditions and study aims have resulted in the use of different measures of occurrence in these studies. Inevitably this makes meaningful comparisons between studies and jurisdictions extremely difficult. However, with rapid technological advances being made in the ability to collect and process more accurate training information it is not unreasonable to expect that incidence rates describing the number of events per 1000 meters of canter work or 1000 meters of gallop work, for example, will soon be reported. This will enable greater emphasis on the development of modifications to training schedules, specifically designed to minimize injury rates during the aspects of training and levels of work that present the greatest risk to the Thoroughbred.

Risk factor studies

Risk factor studies for orthopedic disease, injury and fatality in the racehorse are nearly always analytical, observational, retrospective, or prospective studies. The value of the animals, the nature of the risk factors and the undesirable outcome of severe injury or fatality mean that experimental studies are impractical, costly and in some instances, unethical. The observational nature of these studies means that veterinary clinicians and racehorse trainers should interpret results carefully as associations between risk factors and study outcomes (case definitions) are not necessarily causal in nature.

Much research has already focused on the identification of risk factors for musculoskeletal injury in the Thoroughbred horse. Case definitions that have predominated include fatality, musculoskeletal injury and fracture. Recent studies have also included tendon injury.[29,48] The majority of these risk factor studies have focused on flat racing.[23,26,34,38,49,50] In the UK,[51,52] Australia[37,53] and the USA,[54] risk factors for musculoskeletal injury or fatality in jump racing have been identified.

Risk factors can be classified as either extrinsic or intrinsic risk factors. Intrinsic risk factors may include horse breed, genetics, age and gender. Extrinsic risk factors may include environmental influences such as training regimens, prior race history, prior medical history, nutrition and horse management.

Intrinsic risk factors

Horse-level risk factors are likely to make an important contribution to the variation in the likelihood of injury or fatality. Some studies have attempted to investigate training regimens.[28,48,51] A history of previous injury has also been identified as a risk factor. However, few studies have investigated this explicitly. Reardon and colleagues[52] did identify an association between racecourse SDFT injury and previous racecourse SDFT injury, but this study did not include complete medical histories as data from training was not available.

Horse breed is also likely to be one of the most important factors with respect to prevalence of different injury types (although it may simply be a partial proxy measure of the use to which that horse is put, which in turn determines how it is trained). However, risk factors like horse breed or gender[36,50,55] are not readily modifiable and unlikely to be causal in their association with the outcome. The value of such findings is that they may provide insight into the pathogenesis of a particular injury type.

Extrinsic risk factors

Racing surface, exercise intensity and time off before return to exercise (after injury) are the most important risk factor themes that have emerged from current racehorse injury research.

Racing surface

Turf and 'all weather' tracks are different with respect to the risk of injury or fatality. In the UK[24] and the USA,[25] biaxial sesamoid fracture is the most common type of catastrophic fracture on all weather and dirt surfaces, respectively. In the UK, where the majority of racing is on turf, lateral condylar fractures of the third metacarpus are the most common type of fracture in national hunt racing and proximal phalangeal fractures predominate in turf flat racing.[24] New artificial surfaces are being introduced by a number of racing jurisdictions around the world in an effort to reduce the incidence of racing injuries (predominantly fractures). It is hoped that this will have the desired effect, but racecourse veterinarians should expect a change in the type of injuries encountered by horses racing on the new surfaces.

Exercise intensity

There is good evidence of the association between increased amounts of high-speed exercise and the risk of several musculoskeletal injury case definitions. This is unsurprising as the ability of bone to optimally adapt to its mechanical environment is well documented[56] and adaptation in the racehorse is principally influenced by the training schedule to which the horse is exposed. Structural changes to the distal condyles of MCIII and MTIII of horses in race training have been observed[57] and more specifically the subchondral bone of this region has been shown to undergo an adaptive response to high-speed exercise.[58] However, there is no consensus over the rate, distance or speeds at which that exercise is accumulated.[23,26,28,36,53]

There have also been several studies that have failed to identify significant associations between increased exercise distance and the risk of injury.[42,49,51] The bones of the horses which were doing no high-speed exercise in these studies may not have been optimally adapted to the loads they would experience under racing conditions and were therefore more likely to fracture.[42,51] It is also entirely possible that the associations between reduced or zero exercise and increased risk are an example of effect rather than cause. In other words, horses that are suffering sub-clinical injury are unable to train to the same extent as the rest of the population and it is the sub-clinical injury itself and not the reduced exercise that increases the likelihood of the severe final outcome. This is known as a 'healthy horse effect'. The potential for this effect may be more likely when studying soft tissue injuries. For example, SA or SDFT injury were more likely to occur in training preparations in New Zealand that included no starts[29] and horses that retired from racing due to SDFT injury in Hong Kong, had significantly reduced exercise intensity as much as six months prior to their last recorded episode of fast work.[48]

Risk of injury after rest

The epidemiological evidence for inappropriate lay-up periods is not as strong as that for increased exercise intensity. In the racehorse, some work has demonstrated that inappropriate rest periods can be detrimental. The hazardous length of time for a lay-up is believed to be between 30 and 90 days, based on the differing rates of osteoclastic and osteoblastic activity.[50,59] One study has found even longer inter-race intervals (>6 months) to pre-dispose to breakdown.[38] It is hypothesized that osteoclastic resorption may have taken place within this timeframe, but osteoblastic remodeling is not yet complete.[60] Horses returning to exercise before the remodeling process is complete (about three months) may have bones that are less able to withstand training load than before the lay-up period. Exercise is believed to suppress the resorption of bone, as the initial part of the reparative process, thus preventing a reduction in bone strength while the horse continues to train.[61] The problem with this and other studies investigating the risk of injury after rest is the lack of information on the exercise activity between races (i.e. in training). It is therefore difficult to be sure that the increase in risk was associated with changes in bone structure during a true lay-off period and not an effect of pre-existing injury that prevented an appearance on the racecourse at any earlier date.

Modifiable risk factors

Identification of modifiable risk factors is important, if epidemiological studies are to have an impact on the improvement of injury and fatality rates. Previous studies of racehorse injury and fatality have led to a range of recommended intervention strategies. These recommendations have included increasing moisture in the track surface,[20,37,42] modifications of track surface, structure and design,[62] utilization of pre-race inspections,[63] early detection of subclinical injuries through veterinarian examinations[64] and modifications of exercise speed and intensity.[28,36,51]

Despite the depth of epidemiological studies in this area, it is difficult to present a coherent, consistent view of important risk factors for orthopedic injury and fatality in racehorses. This is likely due to the different approaches to study design and data analysis, selection of the sampling frame and differences in racing jurisdictions and training regimens, which makes extrapolation of results from different studies, difficult if not impossible. However, if the end users (i.e. trainers, racecourse managers etc.) are not presented with a clear and consistent message it is unreasonable to expect them to implement major change to improve welfare.

Other athletic horses

It is only in recent years that descriptions of injuries in athletic breeds (other than the Thoroughbred) have been published. As a consequence, there is a significant degree of uncertainty about the true prevalence of fatal or non-fatal injury incurred during training or competition for these horses compared to Thoroughbred racehorses.

Osteochondrosis

In Standardbred trotters racing and training in Norway, osteochondrosis and osteochondral fragments have been recently described in some detail.[65] Tarsocrural and fetlock joints of 363 horses were examined radiographically. Almost 50% of horses (179/363) had no lesions identified. The most common site of OCD was the proximo-plantar attachment sites of the short sesamoidean ligaments to the proximal phalanx where 22.6% (82) of cases were identified. The other location demonstrating a significant number of lesions was the distal intermediate ridge of the tibia where 17.1% (62) of cases were identified. In this particular population and during the investigation of OCD, it is important to remember that it is common for multiple lesions to be apparent. Indeed, in this study 23% (85 horses) of the population had more than one lesion identified. This paper is useful in that it follows up the prevalence estimates with an analysis of the relationships between lesions in different locations. For example, OCD of the distal intermediate ridge and of the lateral trochlear ridge of the tibia were likely to be bilateral as were lesions of the metacarpo-phalangeal joint. This sort of extension to the usual reporting of prevalence estimates where statistical analysis is used to demonstrate significant associations between different sites within the same horse is recommended and will aid in the ability of clinicians to prognosticate when faced with different types of lesion.

Of 458 Quarter Horses intended for cutting, whose radiographs were examined as yearlings or two year olds, 304 of 438 (69%) and 202 of 454 (45%) had radiographic changes in the tarsi and stifle, respectively.[66] Changes in the metacarpo- (36%)/tarso- (44%) phalangeal joints were also commonly identified. Carpi were less frequently affected with only 7% of horses showing radiographic signs. More specifically, the medial femoral condyle in the stifle was the commonly affected location with 188 (41%) horses showing either uni- or bi-lateral changes at this site. Osteophytes were the most common change in the tarsus, affecting 201 (46%) horses, one-third of whom had bilateral osteophytes present. Some degree of lysis in the distal tarsal bones was present in 76 (17%) of horses and 54 (12%) horses had flattening of the medial trochlear ridge of the talus. Flattening of the sagittal ridge at the distal dorsal aspect of the third metatarsus (54 horses – 15%) and palmar supracondylar lysis in the fore fetlocks (47 horses – 13%), were the most common OCD changes in the fetlocks.[66]

The Breeding, Osteoarticular Status and Athletic Career (BOSAC) study conducted in Normandy in France has generated prevalence estimates of changes associated with developmental orthoaedic disease in Selle Français (French Warmblood), French trotter Standardbreds and Thoroughbreds.[16] Warmblood and Thoroughbred foals were mainly affected at the dorsal aspect of the hind fetlock (36% and 18%, respectively), the fore fetlock (32% and 18%, respectively), the femoro-patellar joint (28% and 15%, respectively) and the carpus (25% and 15%, respectively). Whereas Standarbreds were most commonly affected in the carpus (20%), plantar part of the hind fetlock (16%) and the proximal part of the hock (15%).

The work by van Grevenhoff and colleagues[67] in Dutch Warmbloods reported prevalence estimates of OCD at a number of different locations, also describing the severity of radiographic changes. Of 811 horses 39% had at least minimal changes (described as smoothly flattened and with obscure lucency but no fragmentation) in the femoro-patellar joint; 35% had at least minimal changes in the fetlock joint; and 31% had at least minimal changes in the tarso-crural joint. Within the femoro-patellar joint the trochlear groove was the predominant predilection site. Lesions in the fetlock were isolated to the proximal part of the sagittal ridge. The lateral trochlear of the talus, the sagittal ridge of distal tibia and the medial trochlear of the talus were the most commonly affected sites within the tarso-crural joint.

A recent genome wide association study of OCD in Thoroughbreds[15] identified that of 169 horses with surgical cases of OCD, the hock was affected in 56% of horses, the stifle was affected in 30% of cases and the fetlock was affected in 25% of cases. Several horses had OCD in multiple joints.

See Table 5.1 for a comparative ranking of the prevalence of OCD lesions at different sites in different breeds of sports horse.

Other injury types

An examination of more than 1000 records of horses that underwent veterinary examination at the Animal Health Trust (AHT) in Newmarket, UK,[68] was specifically aimed at identifying associations between the type of equestrian sport and anatomical site of injury. Comparisons between elite and non-elite horse athletes were investigated. Elite show-jumpers were most often seen with SL injuries whereas non-elite show-jumpers were most often seen with injuries located to the navicular bone or ligaments. In dressage horses, the SL was most often the cause of lameness in both elite and non-elite horses and in eventing horses, the distal phalanx and suspensory ligaments were most often affected. An interesting and statistically significant difference in the prevalence of SDFT injury was observed in elite and non-elite event horses, it being the site of injury in six times as many elite horses as non-elite horses. In flat racehorses the carpus, crus, pelvis and thoracolumbar region were most commonly affected, whereas in national hunt racehorses, the SL, thoracolumbar region and distal interphalangeal joints were the sites most often affected. Further detail on specific injury sites is provided[68] but it is also important to remember that the horse population used in this study is of a particular type and largely referral in nature. It may therefore be the case that a moderately different distribution of injuries is seen in first opinion practice of in different horse populations. Further detailed studies focusing on different types of equine athlete have been published since this study and these provide further details in different populations.

Dressage

In a study of dressage horses, which relied upon owner reports of injury and disease, 40% of horses were reported to have had a 'back problem', although 80% of these had not been diagnosed by a veterinary surgeon. Over the two year period to which the questionnaire referred, 24% of horses had been lame at some time. Forelimb lameness was most common, with 13% of horses reported to have had at least one episode of either uni- or bilateral forelimb lameness. The prevalence of hindlimb injury was approximately half of that (7% were reported to have had at least one episode of either uni- or bilateral hindlimb lameness). No further details were available on the exact anatomical location of these injuries.[69] However, this paper did go on to provide some useful estimates on the amount of time taken off training and lameness due to lameness. The median (range) time taken off training was three months (1–48 months) and time off competing was five months (1–57 months). There was also an indication that elite horses spent significantly more time off training that non-elite horses with lameness.

Endurance

The prevalence of different fracture types and locations in endurance horses has been described by Misheff and colleagues.[70] Although this was a small study, in more than 50% of cases (20/38), the third metacarpal/tarsal bone was the anatomical location of

Table 5.1 Comparative ranking of prevalence of OCD lesions at different sites in different breeds of sports horse.

		RANKING IN PREVALENCE OF PARTICULAR OCD CHANGES IN DIFFERENT BREEDS				
Joint	**Lesion or location of OCD change**	**Thoroughbred**	**Standardbred trotters**	**Quarter Horse used for cutting**	**Dutch Warmblood**	**Selle Français (French Warmblood)**
Hock	Not specified	1e				
	Distal intermediate ridge of the tibia		2a		3 = d	
	Osteophytes			1b		
	Lysis in distal tarsal bones			3b		
	Flattening of the lateral/ medial trochlear ridge of the talus			5b	3 = d	
Stifle	Not specified	2e				
	Medial femoral condyle			2b		
	Femoro-patellar joint	3 = c			1d	3c
Fetlock	Not specified	3e				
	Proximo-plantar phalanx		1a			
	Flattening of the dorsal ridge of the third metacarpus/-tarsus			4b	2d	
	Dorsal aspect of hind fetlock	1 = c				1c
	Dorsal aspect of the fore fetlock	1 = c				2c
Carpus	Not specified	3 = c				4c

1–5 represent the order of prevalence of OCD lesions in different locations in different breeds within the same reference (a–e). References: a = 65; b = 66; c = 16; d = 67; e = 15.

fracture and the vast majority of these fractures were lateral condylar fractures of the forelimb. Endurance horses train and race on a wide variety of surfaces. In this study, endurance horses sustained a number of fractures of the proximal phalanx (8/38). This was similar to racehorses training and racing on turf in the UK. However, unlike racehorses racing on dirt (in North America) or all weather surfaces (in the UK), fractures of the proximal sesamoid bones were not reported.[70] This potentially provides further evidence of the importance of surface type on the prevalence of different fracture types.

Eventing

In a comprehensive study of injuries in event horses, which included reports from 125 competitions (86% of all competitions in the UK in 2002), Singer and colleagues[71] calculated that 0.45% of starts returned from the cross country phase with an injury and that 79% of all injuries occurred during this part of the competition. The percent of cross-country starters that returned injured in different levels of one-day events increased as the difficulty of the event increased: Introductory – 0.06%; Pre-Novice – 0.22%; Novice – 0.5%; Intermediate – 0.66%; and Advanced – 2.09%. Of a total of 290 injuries the most commonly affected anatomical locations were the carpus (54 cases), the stifle (40 cases), the fore foot (33 cases), the third metacarpus (30 cases) and the gluteal (23 cases). The vast majority of injuries did not result in an obvious lameness and only 9% of injured horses had severe lameness. A total of 24 horses sustained an superficial or deep digital flexor tendon strain, 21 had unspecified trauma, 12 sustained a fracture and 11 horses sustained joint problem. Only 0.07% of cross-country starters sustained a severe injury that necessitated retirement or euthanasia.

An additional part of this study reported injuries sustained during training that prevented 137 of 403 (38%) horses entering competitions during 2003. These data were acquired through the use of a questionnaire, reflect owner reported diagnoses and also included a number of unspecified lamenesses or illnesses (23 cases). SL (12 cases – 9% of injuries) and SDFT injury (11 cases – 8% of injuries) were the most frequently reported sites of injury, followed by the foot (9 cases – 7% of injuries) and the back/shoulder/pelvis (9 cases – 7% of injuries).

Team roping

Team roping is a sport primarily conducted in North America which commonly involves two Quarter Horses, one for 'heading' and one 'heeling'. The heading horse carries a rider who ropes the head or a steer whereas the heeling horse carries a rider who ropes the hindlimbs of the steer. Interestingly a study by Dabareiner and colleagues[72] identified some significant differences in the types and locations of injuries sustained by horses used for the two different parts of the sport. Pain isolated to the navicular bone region (with or without tarsal osteoarthritis) was significantly more common in heading horses that heeling horses, whereas osteoarthritis of the metacarpo-phalangeal joint was significantly more common in healing horses than heading horses. Osteoarthritis of the carpus, soft tissue injury in the pastern region and SL body desmitis were all significantly more common in the heading horse than the healing horse. The description of the differences in the type of work undertaken by the two types of horse in this sport given by Dabareiner and colleagues,[72] is likely to be related to the different distribution of injuries and certainly may aid in the understanding of the pathogenesis and potentially prevention of the most common injury types.

Barrel racing

A related paper by the same authors[73] in horses used for barrel racing demonstrated further significant differences in the distribution of injuries in what was also a largely pure-bred Quarter Horse population. These horses compete around a number of barrels in a cloverleaf pattern race at high speeds and turn very abruptly. The predominant injury types that they incurred were forelimb foot pain, distal tarsal joint osteoarthritis and SL desmitis.

How does this information help?

Early identification of injuries, when clinical signs and associated pathology are mild, can help to preserve the career or indeed life of many sports horses. Information on the types and locations of likely injuries or diseases which are most common in different types of sports horse will enhance the clinicians ability to make those early diagnoses. The epidemiology of sports horse medicine and injury has, in the last few years, moved away from the identification of risk factors to the identification of the 'at-risk horse'. This is most apparent in the racehorse, the breed in which the majority of resources continues to be invested. Tranquille and colleagues[74] have identified significant differences in adaptation and pathology in bones with and without lateral condylar fracture that may be predictive of lateral condylar fracture of the third metacarpus.[74] Current work is attempting to identify bio- or genetic markers that will improve the predictive ability of geometric or pathological change by enabling the selection of horses that are more likely to be truly positive when identified as such by new screening tools.

References

1. Morton JM, Dups JN, Anthony ND, et al. Epidemic curve and hazard function for occurrence of clinical equine influenza in a closed population of horses at a 3-day event in southern Queensland, Australia, 2007. Aust Vet J 2011;89(Suppl. 1):86–8.
2. Dhand NK, Sergeant ES. Assessment of the proportion of under-reporting during the: 2007 equine influenza outbreak in New South Wales, Australia. Aust Vet J 2011;89(Suppl. 1):73–4.
3. Hess IM, Massey PD, Walker B, et al. Hendra virus: what do we know? N S W Public Health Bull 2011;22:118–22.
4. Trock SC, Meade BJ, Glaser AL, et al. West Nile virus outbreak among horses in New York Statem, 1999 and 2000. Emerg Infect Dis 2001;7(4): 745–7.
5. Ostlund EN, Crom RL, Pedersen DD, et al. Equine West Nile encephalitis. Emerg Infect Dis 2001;7(4):665–9.
6. Miszczak F, Legrand L, Balasuriya UB, et al. Emergence of novel equine arteritis virus (EAV) variants during persistent infection in the stallion: origin of the 2007 French EAV outbreak was linked to an EAV strain present in the semen of a persistently infected carrier stallion. Virology 2012;423(2): 165–74.
7. Montgomery T. Leg problems in racehorses. Vet Med Small Anim Clin 1965;60(11):1106–8.
8. Devas MB. Shin splints, or stress fractures of the metacarpal bone in horses, and shin soreness, or stress fractures of the tibia, in man. J Bone Joint Surg 1967;49: 310–13.
9. Lingard DR. Fissure fracture of the equine metatarsus. Vet Med Small Anim Clin 1969;64(10):895–8.

10. Cheney JA, Liou SY, Wheat JD. Cannon-bone fracture in the Thoroughbred racehorse. Med Biol Eng 1973;11(5):613–20.
11. Rooney JR. Distal condylar fractures of the cannon bone in the horse. Mod Vet Pract 1974;55(2):113–14.
12. Thrall DE, Lebel JL, O'Brien TR. A five-year survey of the incidence and location of equine carpal chip fractures. J Am Vet Med Assoc 1971;158(8):1366–8.
13. Wyburn RS, Goulden BE. Fractures of the equine carpus: a report on 57 cases. N Z Vet J 1974;22(8):133–42.
14. Vaughan LC, Mason BJE. A Clinico-pathological Study Of Racing Accidents In Horses. A Report Of A Study On Equine Fatal Accidents On Racecourses. London, United Kingdom: Horserace Betting Levy Board; 1976.
15. Corbin LJ, Blott SC, Swinburne JE, et al. a genome-wide association study of osteochondritis dissecans in the Thoroughbred. Mamm Genome 2012;23:294–303.
16. Lepeule J, Bareille N, Valette JP, et al. Developmental orthopaedic disease in limbs of foals: between-bred variations in the prevalence, location and severity at weaning. Animal 2008;2(2):284–91.
17. Martin SW, Meek AH, Willeberg P. Veterinary Epidemiology Principles and Methods. Ames, Iowa: Iowa State University Press; 1987. p. 53–8.
18. Thrusfield M. Veterinary Epidemiology. 2nd ed. Oxford: Blackwell Science Ltd.; 2005. p. 39–64.
19. Dohoo I, Martin W, Stryhn H. Measures of disease frequency. In: McPike SM, editor. Veterinary Epidemiologic Research. 1st ed. Charlottetown, Prince Edward Island: AVC Inc.; 2003. p. 65–83.
20. Williams RB, Harkins LS, Hammond CJ, et al. Racehorse injuries, clinical problems and fatalities recorded on British racecourses from flat racing and National Hunt racing during 1996, 1997 and 1998. Equine Vet J 2001;33(5):478–86.
21. Henley WE, Rogers K, Harkins L, et al. A comparison of survival models for assessing risk of racehorse fatality. Prev Vet Med 2006;74(1):3–20.
22. Parkin TDH, Rogers K, Stirk AJ, et al. Risk factors for tendon strain injury during racing in Great Britain. In: Proceedings of the 16th International Conference of Racing Analysts and Veterinarians. Tokyo, Japan, 21–27 October 2006. R and W Publications, Newmarket, UK, 2006. p. 104.
23. Boden LA, Anderson GA, Charles JA, et al. Risk factors for Thoroughbred racehorse fatality in flat starts in Victoria (1989–2004). Equine Vet J 2007;39(5): 430–7.
24. Parkin TDH, Clegg PD, French NP, et al. Risk of fatal distal limb fractures among Thoroughbreds involved in the five types of racing in the United Kingdom. Vet Rec 2004;154(16):493–7.
25. Johnson BJ, Stover SM, Daft BM, et al. Causes of death in racehorses over a 2 year period. Equine Vet J 1994;26(4):327–30.
26. Estberg L, Stover SM, Gardner IA, et al. Relationship between race start characteristics and risk of catastrophic injury in Thoroughbreds: 78 cases 1992. J Am Vet Med Assoc 1998;212(4):544–9.
27. Hernandez J, Hawkins DL, Scollay MC. Race-start characteristics and risk of catastrophic musculoskeletal injury in Thoroughbred racehorses. J Am Vet Med Assoc 2001;218:83–6.
28. Verheyen KLP, Newton JR, Price JS, et al. A case-control study of factors associated with pelvic and tibial stress fractures in Thoroughbred racehorses in training in the UK. Prev Vet Med 2006;74(1):21–35.
29. Perkins NR, Reid SWJ, Morris RS. Risk factors for injury to the superficial digital flexor tendon and suspensory apparatus in Thoroughbred racehorses. N Z Vet J 2005;53(3):184–92.
30. Cogger N, Perkins N, Hodgson DR, et al. Risk factors for musculoskeletal injuries in 2-year-old Thoroughbred racehorses. Prev Vet Med 2006;74(1):36–43.
31. Ely ER, Davis CS, Verheyen KLP, et al. Epidemiology of fractures and tendon injuries in National Hunt racehorses in training: preliminary findings. In: Proceedings of the 16th International Conference of Racing Analysts and Veterinarians. Tokyo, Japan 21–27 October 2006. R and W Publications, Newmarket, UK, 2006. p. 116.
32. Verheyen KLP, Wood JLN. Descriptive epidemiology of fractures occurring in British Thoroughbred racehorses in training. Equine Vet J 2004;36(2): 167–73.
33. Hill T, Carmichael D, Maylin G, et al. Track condition and racing injuries in Thoroughbred horses. Cornell Vet J 1986;76(4):361–79.
34. Peloso JG, Mundy GD, Cohen ND. Prevalence of and factors associated with musculoskeletal racing injuries of Thoroughbreds. J Am Vet Med Assoc 1994;204(4):620–6.
35. McKee SL. An update on racing fatalities in the UK. Equine Vet Educ 1995;7: 202–4.
36. Estberg L, Stover SM, Gardner IA, et al. Fatal musculoskeletal injuries incurred during racing and training in Thoroughbreds. J Am Vet Med Assoc 1996;208(1):92–6.
37. Bailey CJ, Reid SWJ, Hodgson DR, et al. Flat, hurdle and steeple racing: risk factors for musculoskeletal injury. Equine Vet J 1998;30(6):498–503.
38. Mohammed HO, Hill T, Lowe J. Risk factors associated with injuries in Thoroughbred horses. Equine Vet J 1991;23(6):445–8.
39. Boden LA, Charles JA, Slocombe RF, et al. Sudden death in racing Thoroughbreds in Victoria, Australia. Equine Vet J 2005;37(3):269–71.
40. Boden LA, Anderson GA, Charles JA, et al. Risk of fatality and causes of death of Thoroughbred horses associated with racing in Victoria, Australia: 1989–2004. Equine Vet J 2006;38(4):312–18.
41. Parkin TDH. Identification Of Risk Factors For Fatal Distal Limb Fracture In Racing Thoroughbreds. 2002 PhD thesis. United Kingdom: The University of Liverpool; 2002.
42. Parkin TDH, Clegg PD, French NP, et al. Risk factors for fatal lateral condylar fracture of the third metacarpus/metatarsus in UK racing. Equine Vet J 2005;37(3):192–9.
43. Boden LA. Determinants of Thoroughbred racehorse fatality in Victoria, Australia. 2006 PhD Thesis. Australia: The University of Melbourne; 2006.
44. Lam KH, Parkin TDH, Riggs CM, et al. Descriptive analysis of retirement of Thoroughbred racehorses due to tendon injuries at the Hong Kong Jockey Club (1992 to 2004). Equine Vet J 2007;39(2): 143–8.
45. Wilson JH, Robinson RA, Jenson RC. Equine soft tissue injuries associated with racing. Descriptive statistics from American racetracks. In: Rantanen NW, Hauser ML, editors. Proceedings of the 1996 Dubai International Equine Symposium. 27–30 March 1996. Dubai, UAE: Matthew R. Rantanen Design; 1996. p. 1–21.
46. Ely ER, Verheyen KL, Wood JLN. Fractures and tendon injuries in National Hunt horses in training in the UK: a pilot study. Equine Vet J 2004;36(4):365–7.
47. Kasashima Y, Takahashi T, Smith RK, et al. Prevalence of superficial digital flexor tendonitis and suspensory desmitis in Japanese Thoroughbred flat racehorses in 1999. Equine Vet J 2004;36(4): 346–50.
48. Lam KH, Parkin TDH, Riggs CM, et al. Tendon injuries in Thoroughbreds in Hong Kong – the value of detailed training data. Am J Vet Res 2007b;68: 1188–97.
49. Cohen ND, Berry SM, Peloso JG, et al. Association of high-speed exercise with racing injury in Thoroughbreds. J Am Vet Med Assoc 2000;216(8):1273–8.
50. Hernandez J, Hawkins DL, Scollay MC. Race-start characteristics and risk of catastrophic musculoskeletal injury in Thoroughbred racehorses. J Am Vet Med Assoc 2001;218:83–6.
51. Parkin TDH, Clegg PD, French NP, et al. Horse level risk factors for fatal distal limb fracture in racing Thoroughbreds in the UK. Equine Vet J 2004;36(6):513–19.

52. Reardon RJM, Boden LA, Mellor DJ, et al. Risk Factors for Superficial Digital Flexor Tendinopathy in Thoroughbred Racehorses in Hurdle Starts in the United Kingdom (2001–2009). Equine Vet J (in press).
53. Boden LA, Anderson GA, Charles JA, et al. Risk Factors for Fatality in Jump Starts in Victoria (1989–2004). Equine Vet J 2007;39(5):422–8.
54. Stephen JO, White NA, McCormick WH, et al. Risk factors and prevalence of injuries in horses during various types of steeplechase races. J Am Vet Med Assoc 2003;223(12):1788–90.
55. Takahashi T, Kasashima Y, Ueno Y. Association between race history and risk of superficial digital flexor tendon injury in Thoroughbred racehorses. J Am Vet Med Assoc 2004;225(1):90–3.
56. Riggs CM, Vaughan LC, Evans GP, et al. Mechanical implications of collagen fiber orientation in cortical bone of the equine radius. Anat Embryol (Berl) 1993;187(3):239–48.
57. Riggs CM, Whitehouse GH, Boyde A. Structural variation of the distal condyles of the third metacarpal and third metatarsal bones in the horse. Equine Vet J 1999;31(2);130–9.
58. Kawcak CE, McIlwraith CW, Norrdin RW, et al. Clinical effects of exercise on subchondral bone of carpal and metacarpophalangeal joints in horses. Am J Vet Res 2000;61(10):1252–8.
59. Carrier TK, Estberg L, Stover SM, et al. Association between long periods without high-speed workouts and risk of complete humeral or pelvic fracture in Thoroughbred racehorses: 54 cases (1991–1994). J Am Vet Med Assoc 1998;212(10):1582–7.
60. Pentecost RL, Murray RA, Brindley HH. Fatigue, insufficiency, and pathologic fractures. J Am Vet Med Assoc 1964;187: 1001–4.
61. Riggs CM. Fractures – a preventable hazard of racing Thoroughbreds? Vet J 2002;163(1):19–29.
62. Oikawa M, Ueda Y, Inada S, et al. Effect of restructuring a racetrack on the occurrence of racing injuries in Thoroughbred horses. J Equine Vet Sci 1994;14: 262–8.
63. Cohen ND, Mundy GD, Peloso JG, et al. Results of physical inspection before races and race-related characteristics and their association with musculoskeletal injuries in Thoroughbreds during races. J Am Vet Med Assoc 1999;215(5):654–61.
64. Hill AE, Carpenter TE, Gardner IA, et al. Evaluation of a stochastic Markov-chain model for the development of forelimb injuries in Thoroughbred racehorses. Am J Vet Res 2003;64(3):328–36.
65. Lykkjen S, Roed KH, Dolvik NI. Osteochondrosis and osteochondral fragments is Standardbred trotters: Prevalence and relationships. Equine Vet J 2011;44:332–8.
66. Contino EK, Park RD, McIlwraith CW. Prevalence of radiographic changes in yearling and 2-year old Quarter Horses intended for cutting. Equine Vet J 2011;44:185–95.
67. van Grevenhof EM, Ducro BJ, Van Weeren PR, et al. Prevalence of various radiographic manifestations of osteochondrosis and their correlations between and within joints in Dutch Warmblood horses. Equine Vet J 2009;41(1):11–16.
68. Murray RC, Dyson SJ, Tranquille C, Adams V. Association of type of sport and performance level with anatomical site of orthopaedic injury diagnosis. Equine Vet J 2006;(Suppl. 36):411–16.
69. Murray RC, Walters JM, Snart H, et al. Identification of risk factors for lameness in dressage horses. The Vet J 2010;184(1): 27–36.
70. Misheff MM, Alexander GR, Hirst GR. Management of fractures in endurance horses. Equine Vet Educ 2010;22(12):623–30.
71. Singer ER, Barnes J, Saxby F, Murray JK. Injuries in the event horse: training versus competition. The Vet J 2008;175(1):76–81.
72. Dabareiner RM, Cohen ND, Carter GK, et al. Lameness and poor performance in horses used for team roping: 118 cases (2000–2003). J Am Vet Med Assoc 2005a;226(10):1694–9.
73. Dabareiner RM, Cohen ND, Carter GK, et al. Musculoskeletal problems associated with lameness and poor performance among horses used for barrel racing: 118 cases (2000–2003). J Am Vet Med Assoc 2005b;227(10):1646–50.
74. Tranquille CA, Parkin TDH, Murray RC. MRI-detected adaptation and pathology in the distal condyles of the third metacarpus, associated with lateral condylar fracture in Thoroughbred racehorses. Equine Vet J (in press).

Muscle physiology: responses to exercise and training

6

José-Luis L. Rivero   Richard J. Piercy

CHAPTER CONTENTS

Muscular response to exercise

Overview

The horse's skeletal musculature is highly physically adapted: in particular, and relative to other species, it has a greater muscle mass relative to body weight, large intramuscular stores of energy substrates (glycogen in particular), a high global mitochondrial volume, a high proportion of fast-twitch muscle fibers with shortening velocities greater than would be expected for an animal of this size. With all these adaptations, a horse's locomotion is highly efficient.[1,2] Some of these muscular adaptations likely reflect functional specialization following selective breeding of animals for elite endurance, sprint and jumping capacities.[3] For example, in contrast to most mammals in which 30–40% of bodyweight consists of muscle, and in non-athletic horse breeds (~42%), skeletal muscle comprises more than half (~55%) of a mature Thoroughbred's bodyweight.[3]

Total muscle blood flow in horses exercising at an intensity when O_2 consumption is at a maximum ($\dot{V}O_{2max}$ 134 ± 2 mL/min/kg) has been estimated at 226 L/min, which represents approximately 78% of total cardiac output.[4] This exercise requires the integration of many different body systems under the control of the nervous system (Fig. 6.1). Metabolites and oxygen reach skeletal muscle fibers via the respiratory, cardiovascular, and hematologic systems; in turn muscle fibers produce energy in the form of adenosine triphosphate (ATP), which, via the contractile machinery, is converted into mechanical work. The structural arrangement of the musculoskeletal system provides the means with which to harness this energy, either moving the horse's limbs in a characteristic rhythmic pattern for each gait, or enabling diaphragm contraction, which contributes substantially to inspiratory effort.

Equine muscle is considerably heterogeneous, the diversity reflecting functional specialization and adaptive plasticity which has been studied extensively over the past 40 years. Muscle biopsy in particular has resulted in a greater understanding of the response of this tissue to exercise and training, and much of this work is summarized in previous reviews.[5–7] This chapter focuses specifically on new data obtained in the past decade, while assessing earlier studies from a later perspective.

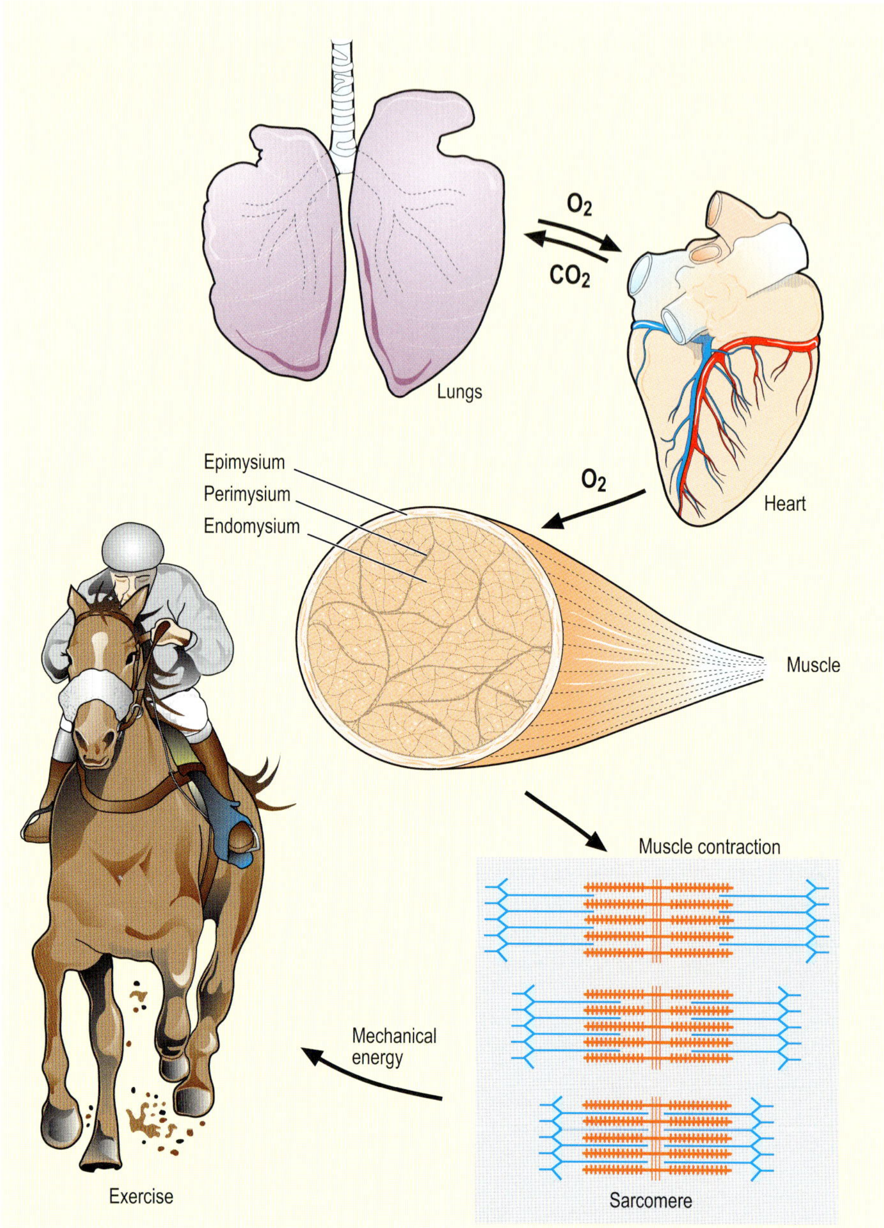

Fig 6.1 Interaction between the main body systems (respiratory, cardiovascular, hematologic and muscular) involved in exercise. In the sarcomere, the thick myofilaments/myosin) are red and the thin myofilaments (actin) are blue.

Methodology

Percutaneous needle biopsy technique

Equine muscle physiology research has centered on use of percutaneous needle biopsy (Fig. 6.2), a technique originally described for the M. gluteus medius by Lindholm & Piehl.[8] This is the heaviest muscle of the entire pelvic limb,[9] it is very active during exercise[10,11] and shows considerable adaptation to training.[5–7] However, care must be exercised in interpreting data from a single biopsy from this muscle, particularly given its heterogeneity.[12] Other locomotory muscles (e.g. semitendinosus, biceps femoris, longissimus lumborum, triceps brachii and cleidocephalicus) can also easily be biopsied using the same technique. Equine muscle biopsy samples for routine histologic are optimally shipped sealed in plastic containers and shipped on ice packs to be processed within 24 h and can thus be interpreted by the receiving laboratory with minimal artifact.[13] Samples intended for more specialized analysis, such as genomic or metabolic studies, might require more particular storage and transport conditions.

Muscle samples are useful for studies in vivo and in vitro using a range of morphologic, biochemical, physiologic, and molecular techniques. Muscle samples for histochemistry are frozen in isopentane pre-cooled in liquid nitrogen. Samples for biochemistry are immersed directly in liquid nitrogen. Samples for microarray expression are put in RNA stabilizer.[14] In addition, a portion of the sample may be directly fixed for electron microscopy, thereby allowing analysis of ultrastructure and measurement of capillary and mitochondrial density.[15] Biochemical and physiologic studies can also be made on dissected and skinned single fibers.[16,17]

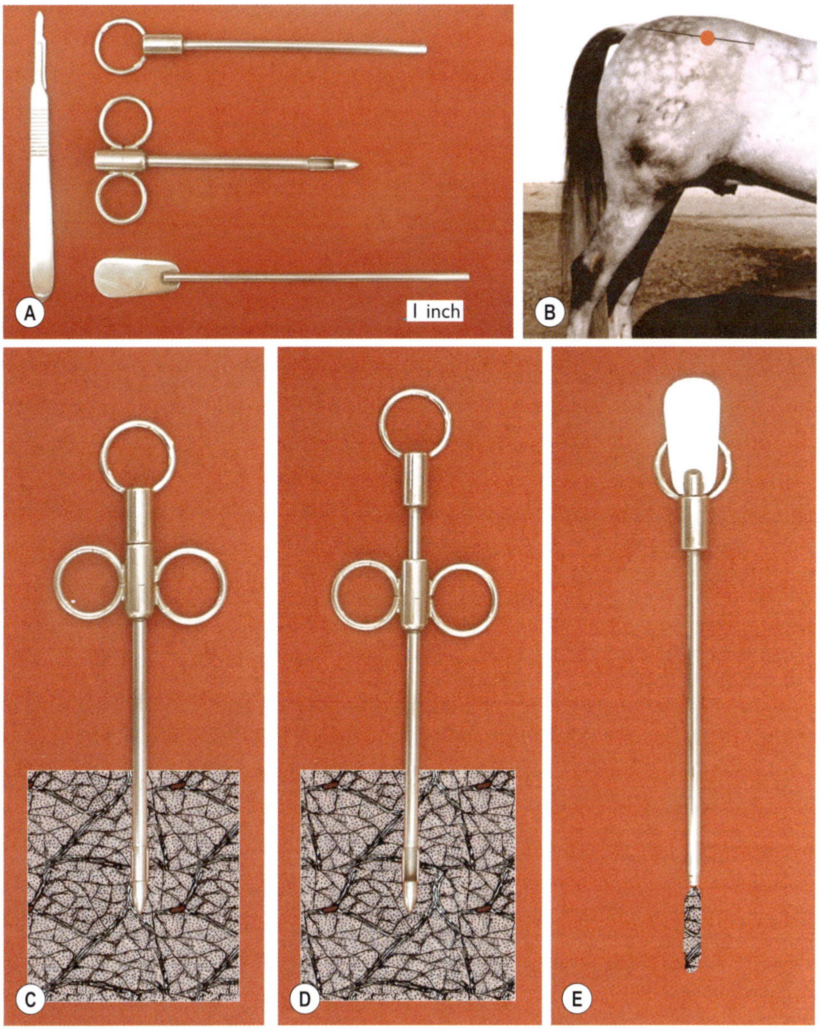

Fig 6.2 **(A)** Percutaneous muscle biopsy needle; this needle, which has an outer diameter of 6 mm, was modified with finger and thumb rings by Henckel.[170] **(B)** Site for the collection of biopsy specimens from the right gluteus medius muscle according to Lindholm & Piehl.[8] This fixed site is located one-third of the distance along a line running from the tuber coxae to the root of the tail. **(C–E)** An illustration of the various steps for the needle biopsy technique; **(C)** the needle biopsy, together with the internal cutting cylinder, is inserted into the muscle; **(D)** once within the muscle, the cutting cylinder is partially withdrawn so that the window is opened up, allowing muscle to enter the slot, and a piece is then cut by pushing down the internal cylinder; **(E)** between 50 and 150 mg of muscle tissue are usually acquired.

Several recent studies in endurance horses have used a minimally traumatic muscle 'microbiopsy' technique, which allows collection of enough tissue to evaluate cellular functions in exercised muscle.[18,19] Some heritable myopathies can also be diagnosed in horses with a similar minimally invasive method (see Chapter 7).[14]

Laboratory methods

Biochemical analysis of homogenized equine muscle samples has enabled the study of broad metabolic responses to exercise and metabolic adaptation to training (see reference[5] for a review) through analysis of selected muscle enzyme activities, their substrates, and intermediary metabolites. However, homogenization of samples prevents the differentiation of the various individual fiber types or the study of important morphologic features such as fiber size, capillary density, and myonuclear location. Some of these disadvantages can be overcome by analyzing single fibers biochemically.[20] Histochemical evaluation of muscle, combined with image analysis, has provided invaluable information about the contractile and metabolic properties of equine muscles, specifically regarding fiber types, oxidative and glycolytic capacities, fiber sizes, and capillary density. However, subjective visual assessment of qualitative histochemical reactions (Fig. 6.3A,B) has until recently limited the application of these methods.[21,22] In recent years, more objective and quantitative histochemical methods have been applied to equine muscle.[23]

Cellular and molecular diversity within equine muscle has also been addressed via study of myofibrillar and non-contractile proteins by immunohistochemistry,[23] gel electrophoresis,[24] a combination of both techniques,[25,26] enzyme-linked immunosorbent assay,[27] and multiple immunofluorescence labeling.[22] The past few years have seen the production of a considerable number of monoclonal antibodies that label contractile and non-contractile muscle isoproteins, some of which can be used effectively in immunohistochemical evaluation of horse muscle.[28,29] The technique's specificity provides, among other things, a more objective way to assess muscle fiber type (Fig. 6.3C).[22,30] Electrophoretic methods for the quantification of myosin isoforms have also been validated in the horse (Fig. 6.3D),[24] and immunoelectrophoresis has enabled the specific identification and relative quantitation of certain muscle-derived proteins.[27]

Molecular biology and genomic techniques have also been extensively applied to the field of equine muscle physiology.[31–38] Northern blotting, reverse transcription followed by polymerase chain reaction, in situ hybridization, and direct sequencing of muscle-specific genes provide the means with which to study the molecular and genetic diversity of muscle proteins at the transcript (mRNA) and cDNA levels; microarray technology enables a more global approach. Furthermore, given that during the early phase of fiber

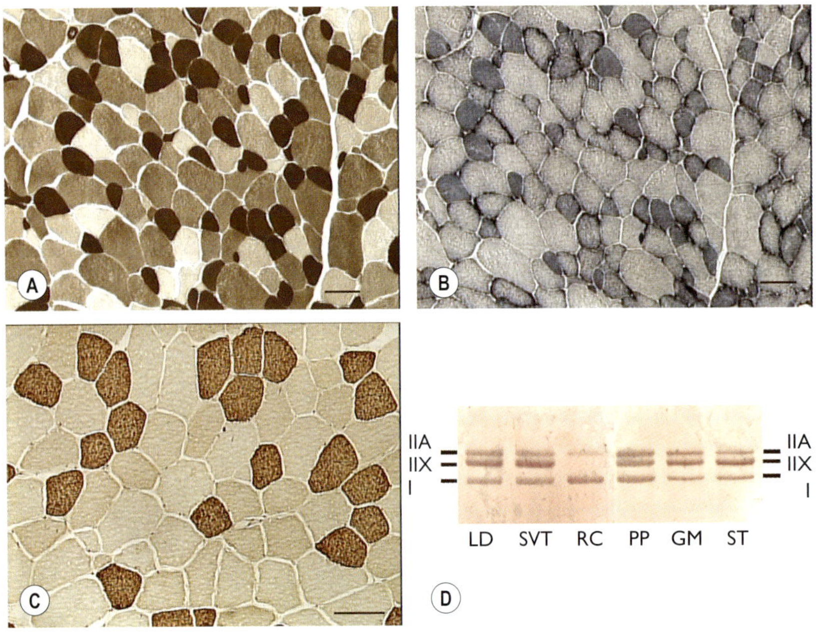

Fig 6.3 Illustration of three integrated approaches for investigating skeletal muscle samples in horses: histochemistry **(A, B)**, immunohistochemistry **(C)**, and gel electrophoresis **(D)**. **(A)** Transverse section of a gluteus medius muscle biopsy sample stained for demonstration of adenosine triphosphatase activity after acid pre-incubation (pH 4.4); the differential staining allows identification of the various fiber types. **(B)** Serial section of the previous sample stained to demonstrate succinate dehydrogenase activity; this histochemical stain is performed to examine the oxidative capacity of myofibers. **(C)** Transverse section of the same sample stained by immunohistochemistry with a monoclonal antibody to the β-slow (type I) myosin heavy chain isoform; this method enables more objective delineation of muscle fiber types than histochemistry. **(D)** Coomassie blue staining to show myosin heavy chain composition of whole-muscle extracts on 8% sodium dodecyl sulfate polyacrylamide gel electrophoresis; isoforms are identified as IIA, IIX, and I going from the slowest (highest) to the fastest band. LD, M. latissimus dorsi; SVT, M. serratus ventralis thoracis; RC, M. rhomboideus cervicis; PP, M. pectoralis profundus; GM, M. gluteus medius; ST, M. semitendinosus. Scales in A–C, 50 μm.

type transformation, isoform-specific mRNA is detectable some time before a change in the specific protein,[33] mRNA quantitation is useful for examining exercise and training effects on muscle composition and gene expression.[33] Furthermore, the recent sequencing of the equine genome by an international consortium was a major advance that will impact equine genomics in the near future. With this rapid progress, new applications in early performance evaluation and the detection of disease markers become available.[38] For example, expression profiling could be used to explore muscle metabolism changes related to exercise, training, pathology and illegal medication in horses.[35] Several candidate athletic-performance genes have been identified in the racehorse as principal responsible for fatty acid oxidation, muscle glycogen degradation, increased insulin sensitivity, muscle strength, muscle speed, and transport of lactate across membrane.[36,39–42]

Other techniques

In addition to cellular and molecular techniques, non-invasive analyzes such as nuclear magnetic resonance and electromyography,[43,44] are increasingly utilized to examine the effects of exercise and training on the neuromuscular system. Furthermore, combined electromyography, force plate, and gait analysis have applications for assessing muscle activation patterns during locomotion.[10,11,45,46] Data can be examined in terms of whole muscle architecture (the arrangement of muscle fibers within the whole muscle relative to the axis of muscle force generation) when evaluating biomechanically distinct functions.[47] Often attributes are described in terms of muscle belly and tendon length, muscle fascicle length, muscle fascicle pennation angle and physiological cross-sectional area.[46,48–51]

Muscle structure and function

Morphology

Development

Most skeletal muscles are derived from paraxial mesodermal tissue following its condensation into segmentally-arranged somites. Cells of certain lineages become compartmentalized within each somite as it differentiates; the dorsolateral compartment (known as the myotome) contains two subsets of myogenic precursor cells: the cells of one subset are destined to become the axial musculature, whereas cells of the other subset migrate into the periphery to form the muscles of the body wall and the limbs.[52] Myogenic precursor cells differentiate to form myoblasts and these fuse to become discrete populations of myotubes that subsequently fuse into myofibers,[53] while α-motor neurons establish neuromuscular junctions. Embryonic myogenesis shares many similarities with the regeneration of mature myofibers following injury, a subject that is covered in detail elsewhere (see Chapter 7).

Gross anatomy and muscle function

The two primary requirements of locomotor muscle are to support the center of mass and to move the limbs. During steady-state locomotion, metabolic energy is primarily required to support the body weight against gravity. This role is most effectively fulfilled by muscles with short, pennnate fibers, and long tendons, such as those found in the limbs of horses.[48,54] Yet locomotion in athletic horses is rarely steady-state: for example, gait is perturbed when accelerating from standing, running uphill or jumping over obstacles. During such activities, net muscle work must increase to raise either the kinetic or potential energy of the center of mass.[9] Muscles that are useful for doing work on the system have long, parallel fibers and limited in-series elastic tissue and are, in most cursors, primarily found in the proximal limb.[9,55] Thus, functional specialization of muscle architecture is seen in a wide range of animals in which proximal limb muscles are specialized for doing work and more distal limb muscles are specialized for economical generation of large forces.[9] Horses and other quadrupeds reveal further functional specialization between the limbs. When compared with proximal thoracic limb muscles, proximal pelvic limb muscles of the horse are larger in volume and have shorter fascicles, indicating that from an evolutionary perspective, pelvic limb muscles have sacrificed the ability to exert force over a wide range of motion, in order to produce large forces.[9,55,56] Muscle architecture has also been shown to vary between the same muscles in different breeds of horses. Thus, Quarter Horses inherently possess large strong pelvic limb muscles, with the potential to accelerate their body mass more rapidly than those of Arab horses[47] which are optimized to function with maximum economy rather than maximum power output.[51]

Equine locomotor muscles are mainly located proximally on the appendicular skeleton with their tendon located distally, which has the effect of reducing the weight of the lower limb and decreasing the energy necessary to overcome inertia when the limb swings back and forth. Equine natural gaits typically consists of stretch-shortening cycle exercises, in which lengthening (eccentric) and shortening (concentric) actions of the muscle-tendon complex in the limbs are repeated during each cycle.[45,57,58] During contractions, elastic energy is stored in tendons and intramuscular connective tissues during the lengthening (eccentric) phase of the cycle, and then reused and added to the active energy produced in the shortening (concentric) phase. Thus, the total force exerted across a muscle is the sum of active force generated by the contractile machinery and passive forces provided by elastic structures that are arranged either in parallel or in series with the contractile proteins in the muscle-tendon complex.[45,46,59] Consequently, movements of the distal limb are mainly passive and result from the release of elastic energy of the digital flexor tendons and suspensory ligament when the limb is unloaded.[57] However, while the equine interosseus muscle (suspensory ligament) has undergone a reduction of muscle content during its evolution, it still contains significant muscular components that likely contribute to limb stability and elastic storage of energy during locomotion.[49] Thoracic limb protraction is largely a passive process in horses[60] and thoracic limb protraction is likened to a catapult mechanism in which energy is stored relatively slowly in elastic tissues (the internal tendon of biceps brachii and lacertus fibrosus) during limb loading, but that is released rapidly when the toe leaves the ground, thereby rapidly protracting the limb. Furthermore, the equine biceps muscle-tendon unit acts as a tuneable spring and the contractile component functions to modulate the energy required to accelerate forelimb protraction at different speeds.[60] Tendon springs are particularly important in a cursorial quadruped like the horse, as they facilitate the exchange of kinetic potential and elastic strain energy and reduce the amount of work that muscles must perform in order to move the animal's limbs and center of mass. This effective utilization of elastic energy explains much of the admirable (superior) locomotor efficiency of horses, which consume rather less metabolic energy than would be expected based on the substantial energetic demands on this animal, particularly at fast gaits.[58] Moreover, metabolically-economical force production can also be increased through eccentric muscle contraction, where muscle length increases while active (developing contractile force) due to-externally applied forces.

In contrast, movements of the proximal limb result primarily from active muscular contraction and generally, most locomotor muscles are active during the propulsion stage of weight bearing in each limb.[11,45,61] Muscle activity, as measured by electromyography, is positively correlated with running speed, with muscles within the same group having significant differences in their activities when a horse exercises at constant speed.[11,61,62] Furthermore, different locomotor tasks, such as moving up or down gaits or changing speed, require adjustment of the amount of work that a muscle must perform to raise or lower, or to accelerate or decelerate the animal's centre of mass.[11,61,62]

Histology

More than 90% of a muscle is made up of myofibers, with the rest consisting of nerves, blood vessels and the fat and connective tissue that separates the individual fibers (endomysium), the fascicles (perimysium), and the whole muscle (epimysium; see Fig. 6.1). The connective tissue merges with both the origin and the insertion tendons of the muscle, as well as with internal tendons in compartmentalized muscles. Blood vessels and nerves course within the perimysium. Capillary arrangement in the skeletal muscle is optimized for oxygen delivery to tissue during exercise; usually several capillaries are located within close to the muscle fiber proximity, sometimes circumferentially but more often running parallel to each fiber.

Skeletal myofibers are typically elongated cells (generally believed to be between 30 and 100 mm in length) with tapered ends. Fibers vary from 10 to 100 μm in diameter and are multinucleated (Fig. 6.4A). Nuclei are normally located at the fiber's periphery in a subsarcolemmal position. Although the cytoplasm contains other organelles found in many cell types, it is largely occupied by the contractile apparatus, which consists of contractile proteins and their supportive structures all grouped together as myofibrils. In longitudinal sections, individual muscle fibers have numerous cross-striations (dark and light bands), orientated perpendicularly to the fiber's long axis (Fig. 6.4B). Lighter I bands alternate with darker A bands; within the I band there are dense striations called Z disks.

Ultrastructure

The repeating unit between two adjacent Z disks is known as a sarcomere, the unit of muscular contraction. Each sarcomere includes half the I band on each side of the A band (Fig. 6.4C,D). I bands contain only thin filaments (8 nm diameter), whereas A bands contain both thin and thick (15 nm diameter) filaments. Within the A band, the H band is defined as the central area where the thick filaments do not overlap with thin filaments (Fig. 6.4D). The central darker portion of the H band is designated as the M line (see Fig. 6.4D). Transverse section of the sarcomere at the overlapping zone between thick and thin filaments reveals each thick myofilament surrounded by thin myofilaments arranged in a hexagonal lattice (Fig. 6.4E). Muscle contraction occurs when (within each sarcomere), thin myofilaments slide over the thick myofilaments, bringing the adjacent Z disks closer together. Hence, upon contraction, the I band shortens and the H band starts to disappear.

Thick filaments contain myosin and other myosin-binding proteins. Sarcomeric myosins have two heads and a long tail and consist of two heavy chains and two pairs of light chains (Fig. 6.5A). The myosin head is the motor domain that contains the ATP-binding site, the actin-binding site and the myofibrillar ATPase enzyme. The major components of the thin filaments are tropomyosin, the troponin complex (consisting of three subunits: troponin C (TnC), troponin T (TnT) and troponin I (TnI)), and two helical

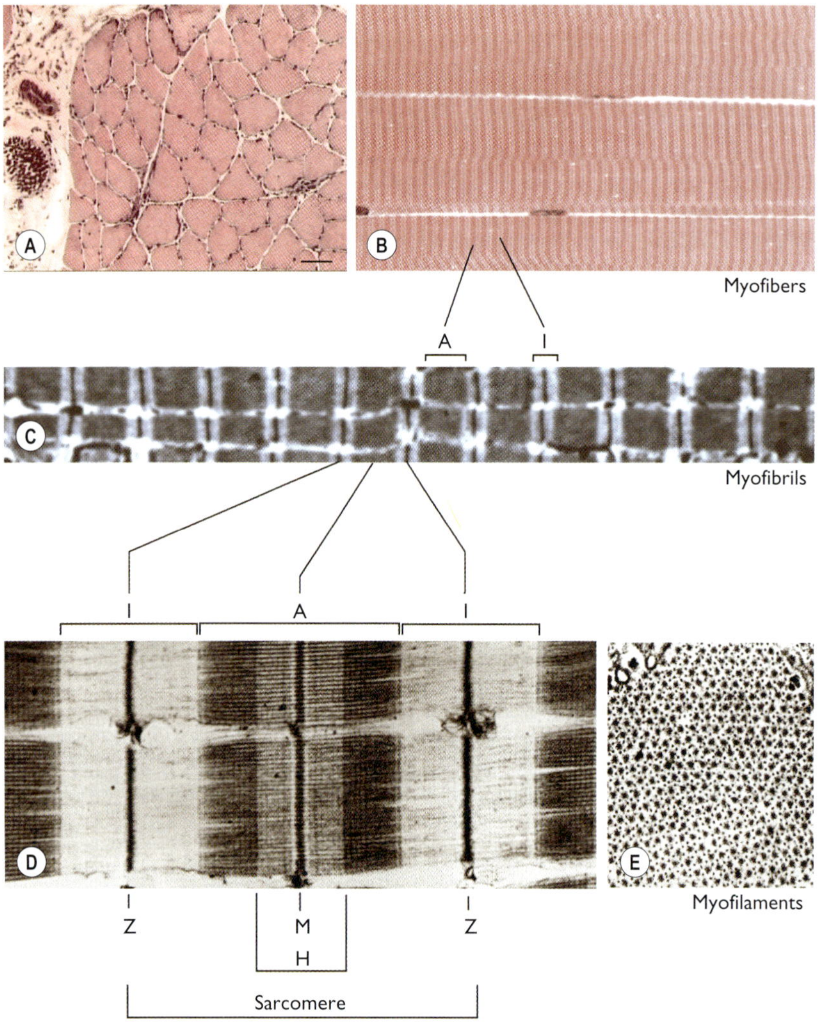

Fig 6.4 Organization of the contractile apparatus from the cellular to the molecular level. **(A)** Transverse section from a specimen of the M. sacrocaudalis dorsalis medialis stained by hematoxylin and eosin and examined by light microscopy; scale = 50 μm. **(B)** Longitudinal section from the same specimen with the same stain. **(C)** Striated aspect of myofibrils when observed by electron microscopy at very low magnification, showing Z disks, A bands, and I bands of sarcomeres. **(D)** Electron micrograph of longitudinal sectioned myofibrils at × 30 000 magnification. **(E)** Electron micrograph of transverse sections of one myofibril in the overlap zone (A band) between thick and thin myofilaments of sarcomere, illustrating the hexagonal arrangement of these filaments, × 150 000.

filamentous strands of actin (F-actin), made up of polymerized globular actin monomers (G-actin) (Fig. 6.5B). Elongated tropomyosin dimers lie within the major groove of the actin filament, spanning seven actin monomers; each troponin complex is also associated with a seven-actin repeat. The elongated NH_2-terminal of TnT extends for a considerable length from each tropomyosin molecule, spanning the gap between adjacent molecules.

Mitochondria are located beneath the sarcolemma and between myofibrils (Fig. 6.6, Fig. 6.7). This intimate relationship means that ATP produced during oxidative phosphorylation is readily available for the contractile machinery. Intramuscular substrates, such as glycogen and lipids, are also stored between the myofilaments and under the sarcolemma (see Fig. 6.7). Numerous other proteins, including myoglobin, glycolytic enzymes, and various intermediate filaments, are distributed throughout the cytoplasm.

The sarco(endo)plasmic reticulum (SR) of skeletal myofibers is an intracellular membranous system located between the myofibrils (see Fig. 6.6, Fig. 6.7), but which has no physical continuity with the external surface membrane (sarcolemma). Much of its tubular network is orientated longitudinally to the myofibrils. The SR contains, amongst other molecules, a large amount of a Ca^{2+}-ATPase enzyme, the protein calsequestrin, and the calcium release channel (ryanodine receptor or RYR1). At the AI junction of the sarcomere, the SR tubules become confluent and form terminal cisternae orientated perpendicularly to the long axis of the cell (Fig. 6.7D). Two adjacent cisternae are separated by a structure known as the T-tubule, which is a long tubular invagination of the sarcolemma communicating directly with the extracellular space. Together the three structures make up a triad (see Fig. 6.6, Fig. 6.7).

The motor end-plate (see Fig. 6.11B) is a specialized region on each fiber where the α-motor neuron interdigitates with the sarcolemma. The postsynaptic membrane of the motor end-plate contains numerous acetylcholine receptors. The remainder of the sarcolemma contains a variety of specific structural proteins, channels, pumps, and hormone receptors. Of note, myofibers have a cytoskeleton of various intermediate filament proteins that link the

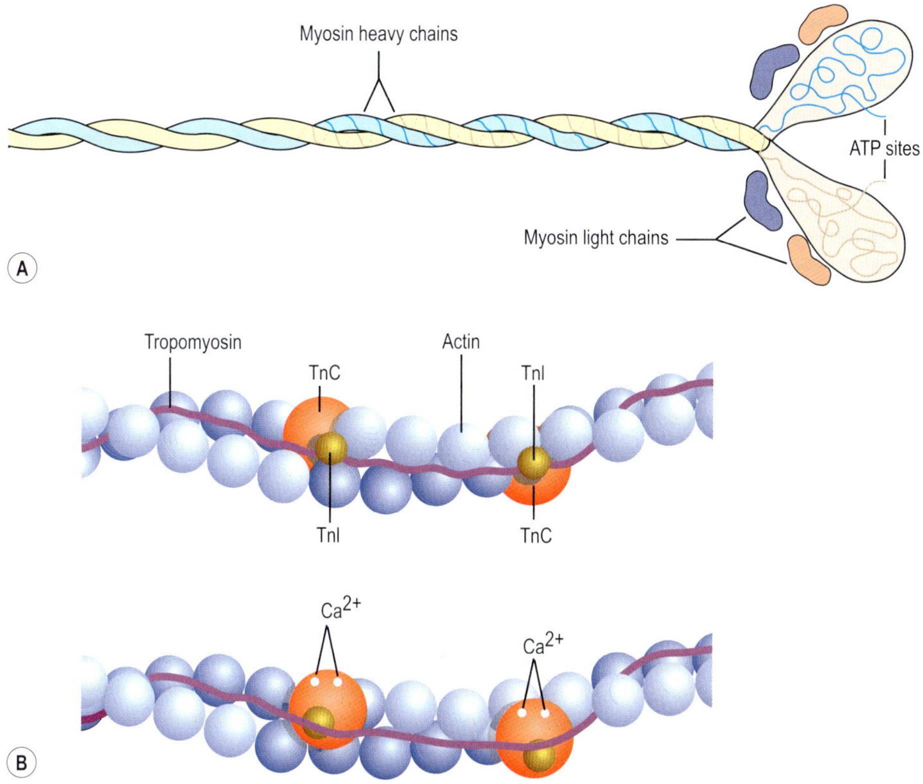

Fig 6.5 **(A)** Diagram of the myosin molecule illustrating the α-helical coiled-coil tail, the folding of each heavy chain to form a globular head, the site of ATP hydrolysis, and the location of the four myosin light chains (regulatory and essential). **(B)** Model of the troponin–tropomyosin–actin that make up the thin myofilaments, during muscle relaxation (above) and contraction (below). In the relaxed state, the inhibitory region of troponin (TnI, colored yellow) is attached to actin and tropomyosin, whereas troponin C (TnC, colored organge) is bound to Mg^{2+}. In this conformation, myosin cannot bind. In the contracted state, two Ca^{2+} ions bind to TnC, which in turn interacts with TnI. A conformational change to the troponin–tropomyosin complex exposes the myosin-binding sites, thereby allowing the power stroke to occur.

contractile apparatus with a complex of proteins at the sarcolemma, known as the dystrophin-associated complex (see Fig. 6.14), which itself provides a structural link with the extracellular matrix. Between the sarcolemma and the extracellular matrix is the basal lamina (Fig. 6.7E), which is generally closely apposed to the sarcolemma except where it leaves the sarcolemma to course over the surface of satellite cells (Fig. 6.8). Further information about satellite cells is available elsewhere (Chapter 7).

General muscle physiology

The motor unit

A motor unit consists of an α-motor neuron and the skeletal muscle fibers that it innervates (Fig. 6.9). Since each time an α-motor neuron fires, the entire motor unit contracts, coarser movements are generated in those muscles that have many muscle fibers making up motor units (such as the locomotor muscles) compared with those with few (such as the extrinsic eye muscles). Muscle fibers within one motor unit are generally all of the same histochemical type, but they are normally widely distributed between fibers from other motor units and therefore give rise to the characteristic checkerboard pattern that is apparent with certain histochemical stains (see Fig. 6.3A). Loss of this checkerboard pattern is evident in denervated muscle (Fig. 6.10A,B) where there may be selective loss and atrophy of fibers of one histochemical type (Fig. 6.10A), or in reinnervated muscle following disease or injury, by patterns of fiber grouping (Fig. 6.10C).[34,63] Large-diameter α-motor neurons innervate fast-twitch fibers, whereas smaller ones tend to innervate slow-twitch fibers.

Contractile force for a particular muscle is partly regulated by the rapidity of neuron discharge; muscle fibers contract with a twitch following a single discharge of a motor neuron, but sustained contraction (tetanus) results from repetitive neuron firing. The force of a contraction increases with the rate of discharge up to a maximum limit that is determined by the properties of the muscle. Furthermore, a process known as recruitment, which reflects the gradual inclusion of larger motor neurons as greater force is required, also regulates force (see below). Relatively weak and slow contractions required for maintenance of posture therefore involve small-diameter α-motor neurons and slow-twitch fiber types, whereas locomotion and rapid movements rely on recruitment of larger diameter α-motor neurons and fast-twitch fibers.

Muscle proprioception

Proprioception is the term given to the mechanism underlying the self-regulation of posture and movement through stimuli originating in sensory receptors embedded in joints, tendons, muscles, and the labyrinth of the ear. In skeletal muscles and tendons these receptors are known as spindles and Golgi tendon organs and each type has been characterized in the horse.[64] Signals derived within these sensory receptors are conveyed via a variety of well-defined reflex pathways that generate specific motor responses.

Muscle spindles consist of specialized intrafusal muscle fibers surrounded by a connective tissue capsule and lie parallel to regular

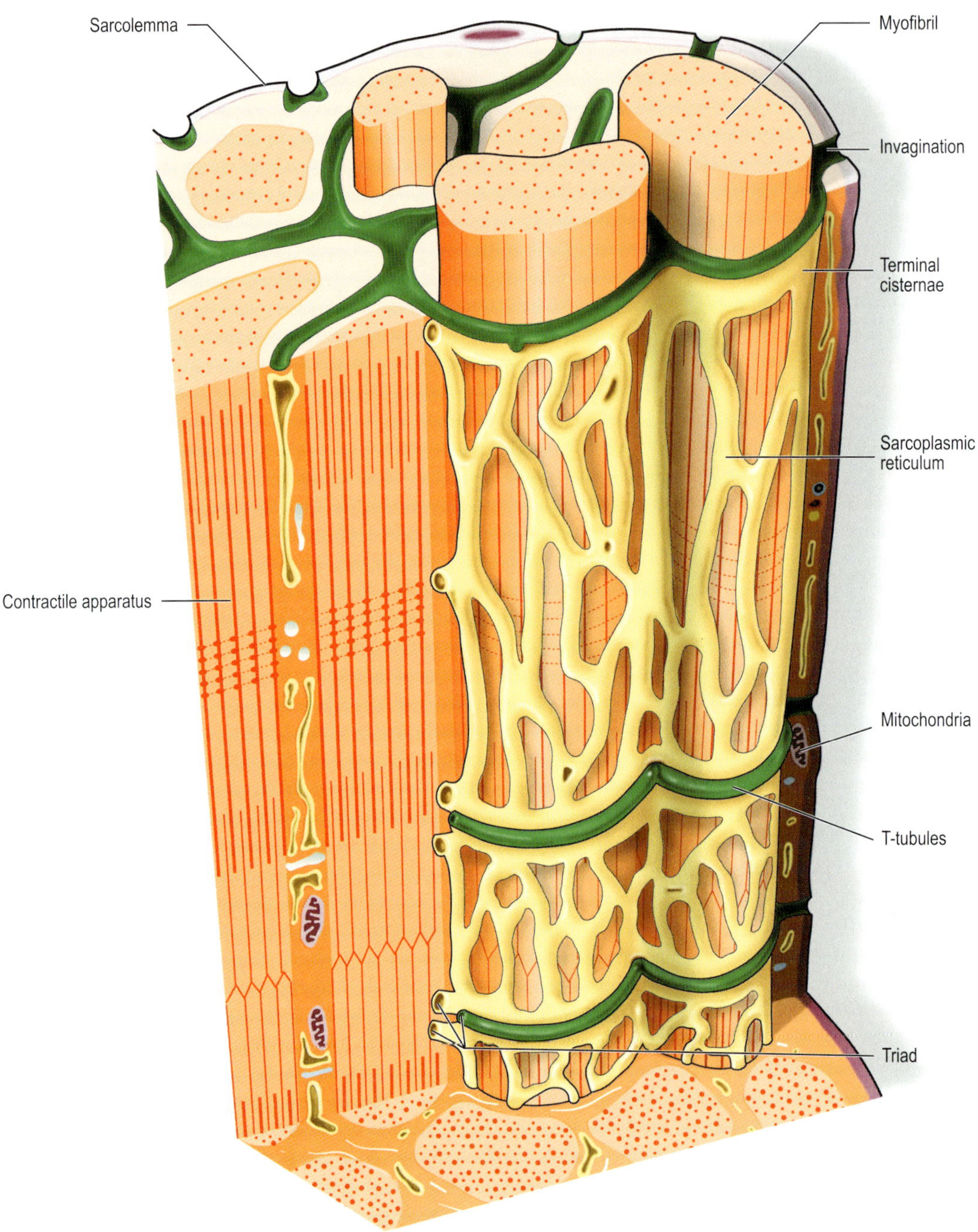

Fig 6.6 Diagrammatic representation of the internal structure of a muscle fiber. Myofibrils are surrounded by the net-like tubular sarcoplasmic reticulum (SR); the SR converges at the junction between A and I bands of sarcomeres to form terminal cisternae. Between each pair of terminal cisternae there is an invagination of the sarcolemma called the T-tubule. Together, the three structures make up a triad. Mitochondria are dispersed between myofibrils.

muscle fibers (Fig. 6.11A). Sensory nerves (type Ia and type II) terminate on the intrafusal fibers in specialized sensory endings and generate afferent signals that are relayed to the spinal cord via the dorsal horn. Type Ia nerves carry both dynamic (rate of stretch) and static (amount of stretch) afferent signals, whereas type II nerves sense only static muscle length. Motor innervation to the muscle spindle is provided by γ-motor neurons, which regulate the sensitivity of muscle spindles to muscle stretch. Golgi tendon organs are located within the connective tissues of tendons, joint capsules, and muscles. They lie in parallel with the direction of mechanical force that they measure and, from them, afferent type Ib fibers convey proprioceptive signals to the spinal cord.

Electrical and ionic properties of the sarcolemma

The sarcolemma maintains the interior of the fiber at a negative potential (the membrane potential) when compared to the extracellular fluid while the fiber is in a resting state. The negative potential is derived from the disequilibrium of ionic concentrations (mostly Na^+ and K^+) across the membrane and is generated partly by the

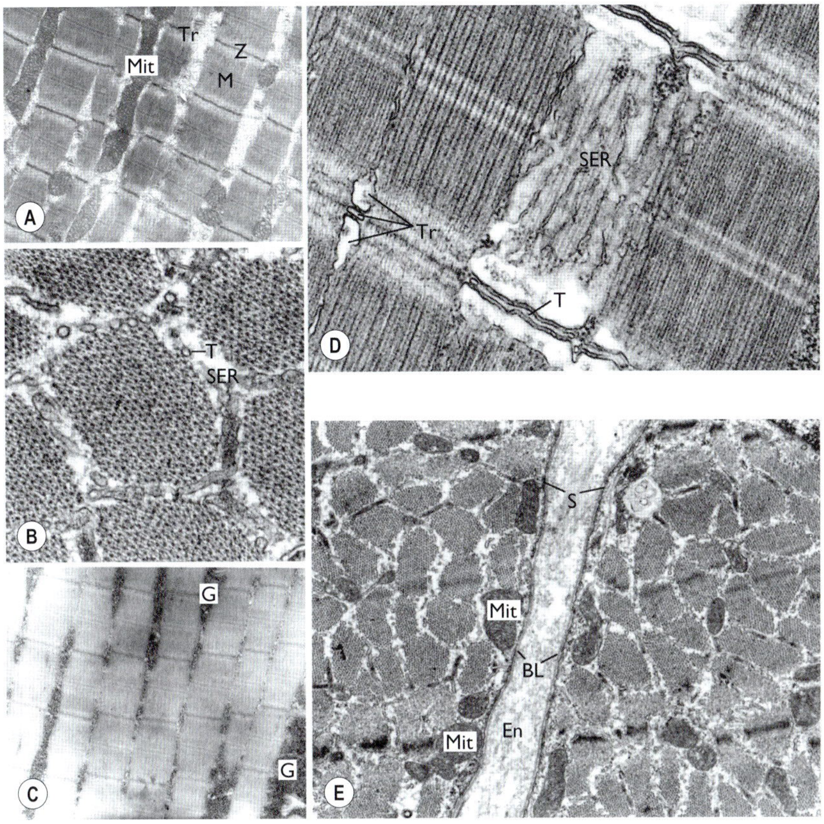

Fig 6.7 Ultrastructural appearance of equine skeletal muscle cells when observed by electron microscopy. **(A)** Type IIA myofiber sectioned longitudinally; note the straight and thin appearance of Z lines, M lines in the middle of each sarcomere, a triad (Tr), and abundant mitochondria (Mit) within the intermyofibrillar spaces. **(B)** Transverse sectioned myofibrils showing the arrangement of the sarco(endo)plasmic reticulum (SER) and T-tubules (T); magnification × 54 000. **(C)** Type IIX muscle (as determined by immunoelectron microscopy – not shown) fiber sectioned longitudinally; note the abundant glycogen granules (G); magnification × 25 312. **(D)** Electron micrograph of an equine sarcomere showing the arrangement of the sarco(endo)plasmic reticulum (SER), T-tubule (T), and a triad (Tr); magnification × 58 125. **(E)** Two adjacent equine myofibers sectioned transversely showing the sarcolemma (S) and the basal lamina (BL), interposed between the sarcolemma and the extracellular matrix of the endomysium (En); there are also abundant mitochondria (Mit) located beneath the sarcolemma and between myofibrils; magnification × 35 835.

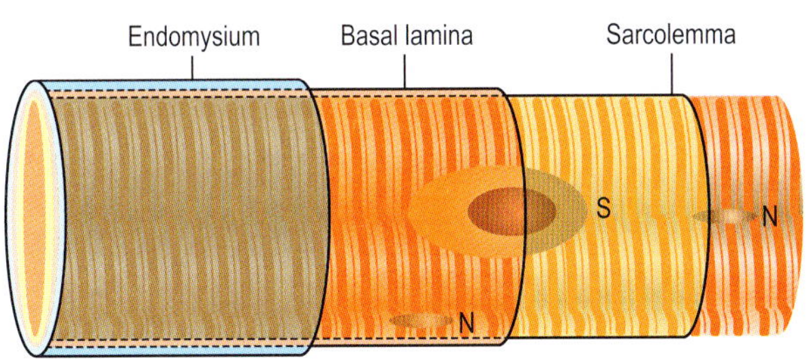

Fig 6.8 Diagram illustrating the relationship of a satellite cell (S) to the sarcolemma, basal lamina, and endomysium. N, myonucleus.

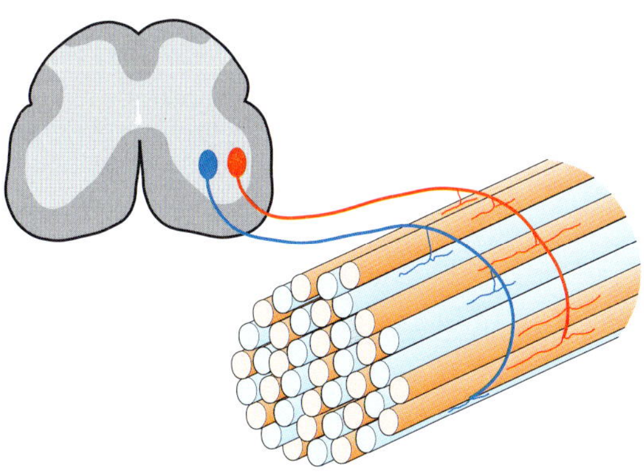

Fig 6.9 Diagram illustrating the organization of motor units. A motor neuron from the ventral horn of the spinal cord supplies the motor innervation to a group of muscle fibers with similar contractile and metabolic properties.

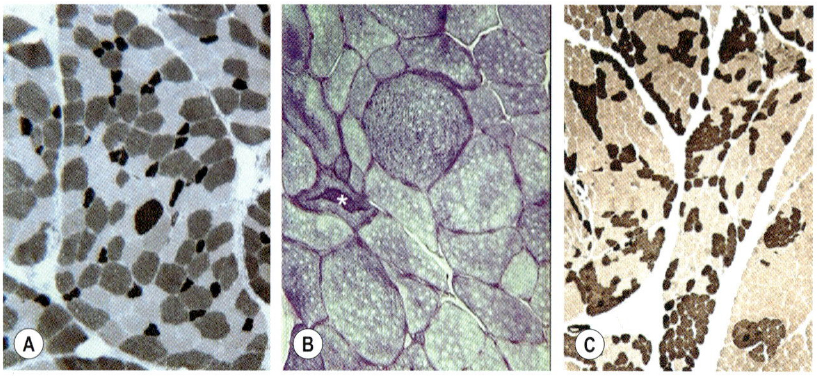

Fig 6.10 Histopathological evidence of neurogenic muscle atrophy in the horse. **(A)** Transverse section of the M. gluteus medius (7 cm depth) stained with ATPase at pH 4.5 from one horse with motor neuron disease; note the general, but particularly type I (black) fiber, atrophy. **(B)** Transverse section of the M. vastus lateralis stained with periodic acid–Schiff (PAS) from a horse with femoral nerve paralysis; the asterisk shows a fiber with a target structure in its center, suggesting reinnervation following denervation. **(C)** Transverse section of the M. cricoarytenoideus dorsalis stained with ATPase (pH 9.4) from a horse with recurrent laryngeal neuropathy showing disruption of the normal checkerboard pattern and fiber type grouping.

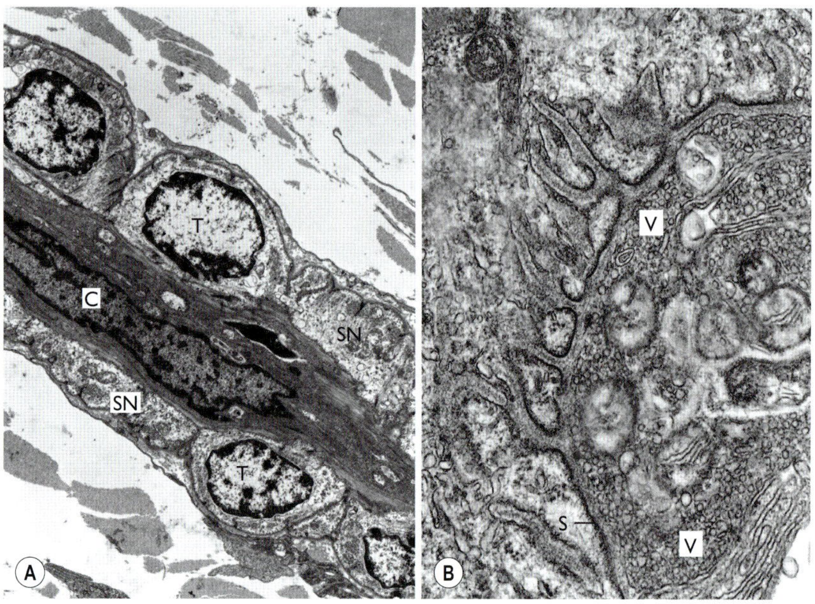

Fig 6.11 **(A)** Electron micrograph of an equine muscle spindle; sensory nerves (SN) appose the abundant teloglia cells (T) which are surrounded by an internal capillary (C); magnification × 37 125. **(B)** Electron micrograph of an equine myofiber showing the neuromuscular junction (end-plate) of the sarcolemma (S); note the clear (acetylcholine-containing) vesicles (V) in the pre-synaptic nerve terminal; magnification × 43 000.

action of the Na^+/K^+ ATPase pump, which extrudes three Na^+ ions for every two K^+ ions taken up. This results in the cytoplasm having a much higher K^+ concentration but much lower Na^+ concentration than the extracellular fluid. The remainder of the membrane potential is derived from the tendency of ions to diffuse down their electrochemical gradients across the semipermeable membrane.

Acetylcholine released from pre-synaptic nerve terminals at neuromuscular junctions (end-plates; Fig. 6.11B) binds to acetylcholine receptors and increases the conductance of the post-junctional membrane to Na^+ and K^+. The inward movement of Na^+ down its concentration gradient predominates, causing a transient depolarization (about 20 mV) in the end-plate, known as the end-plate potential. This depolarization is sufficient to activate sarcolemmal voltage-gated Na^+ channels – the channels that are mutated in hyperkalemic periodic paralysis. These Na^+ channels open, eliciting propagation of an action potential along the membrane. Following this, and in response to depolarization, voltage-gated K^+ channels open, resulting in the downswing of the action potential. The action potential therefore conducts rapidly along the sarcolemma in a wavelike fashion away from the neuromuscular junction.

Excitation–contraction coupling

Action potentials are conducted into the interior of muscle fibers via the T-tubules and there they activate voltage-gated channels known as dihydropyridine receptors (DHPR). Unlike in

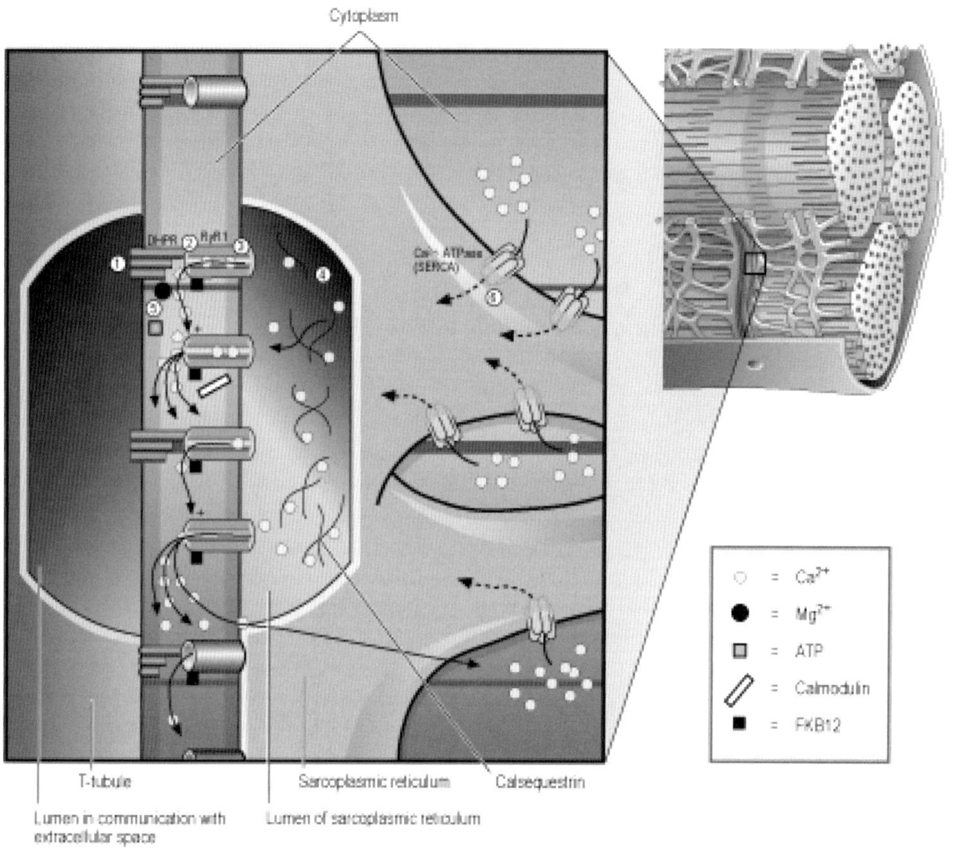

Fig 6.12 Depolarization of the T-tubule membrane during the action potential activates voltage-gated Ca^{2+} channels (1) (dihydropyridine receptors, DHPR) in the wall of the T-tubule. A mechanical link (2) with ryanodine receptors (RyR1) (3) located in the wall of the sarcoplasmic reticulum causes them to open and release calsequestrin-bound Ca^{2+} ions from the lumen of the SR (4). This Ca^{2+} stimulates further Ca^{2+} release via the calcium-induced calcium release mechanism. The process is modulated by other factors within the cytoplasm that include ATP, calmodulin, and Mg^{2+} (5). After release into the cytoplasm, calcium activates the contractile apparatus by binding to troponin-C (Fig. 6.13). Reuptake into the SR occurs via the Ca^{2+}-ATPase pumps (6).

cardiac muscle, very little calcium enters the muscle fiber from the extracellular space (via the DHPR).[65] Instead, a mechanical link between DHPR and the SR Ca^{2+} release channel (ryanodine receptor, RYR1) at the junctional feet of the triads causes release of calsequestrin-bound Ca^{2+} from the SR's interior (Fig. 6.12). A positive feedback loop, known as calcium-induced calcium release, is responsible for further activation of RYR1, with the result that the calcium concentration within the cytoplasm increases about 100-fold from a resting concentration of approximately 50 nM.[65] The anatomical location of the terminal cisternae results in Ca^{2+} being released adjacent to the overlapping contractile apparatus.

Binding of Ca^{2+} to high-affinity binding sites on troponin C causes a conformational change to the troponin–tropomyosin complex (see Fig. 6.5B). This results in the exposure of the myosin-binding sites on F-actin and allows the myosin globular head to attach as ATP is hydrolyzed, thus forming the crossbridge. Force generation and shortening of the sarcomere occur as a result of a conformational change of the myosin head. Adenosine diphosphate and inorganic phosphate are displaced by actin, which is followed by dissociation of the actin–myosin bridge due to the binding of ATP to myosin again. The crossbridge cycle continues while the cytoplasmic Ca^{2+} concentration remains high. Relaxation is achieved when the Ca^{2+} is resequestered within the SR via the action of the Ca^{2+}- ATPase pumps (see Fig. 6.13 for a summary).

Force transmission

The force that is generated in the crossbridge cycle is transmitted via the contractile apparatus to intermediate filament proteins that act to maintain and stabilize the muscle fiber's shape during contraction. These intermediate filaments provide a structural link first to the sarcolemma and then to the extracellular matrix via a group of proteins known as the dystrophin-associated protein complex (Fig. 6.14, Fig. 6.15).[66] Contractile forces are transmitted from each muscle fiber via the extracellular matrix and the connective tissues of tendons, and ultimately to the bones of the skeleton.

Oxygen availability

ATP replenishment in (predominantly) oxidative fibers requires a readily available source of oxygen that is provided by the O_2-binding heme protein known as myoglobin. The P_{50} for equine myoglobin (the PO_2 when it is 50% saturated) is about 2.4 mmHg at physiological temperatures and pH,[67] and therefore far to the left (lower) than the P_{50} of equine hemoglobin (23.8 mm/Hg) and close to the PO_2 of muscle cells. During exercise, oxygen demand rises dramatically, met by a 20–30 times increased blood flow through the muscle capillary beds.[4] Capillary dilation results partly from autonomic control and stretch imposed by the higher blood pressure, but also

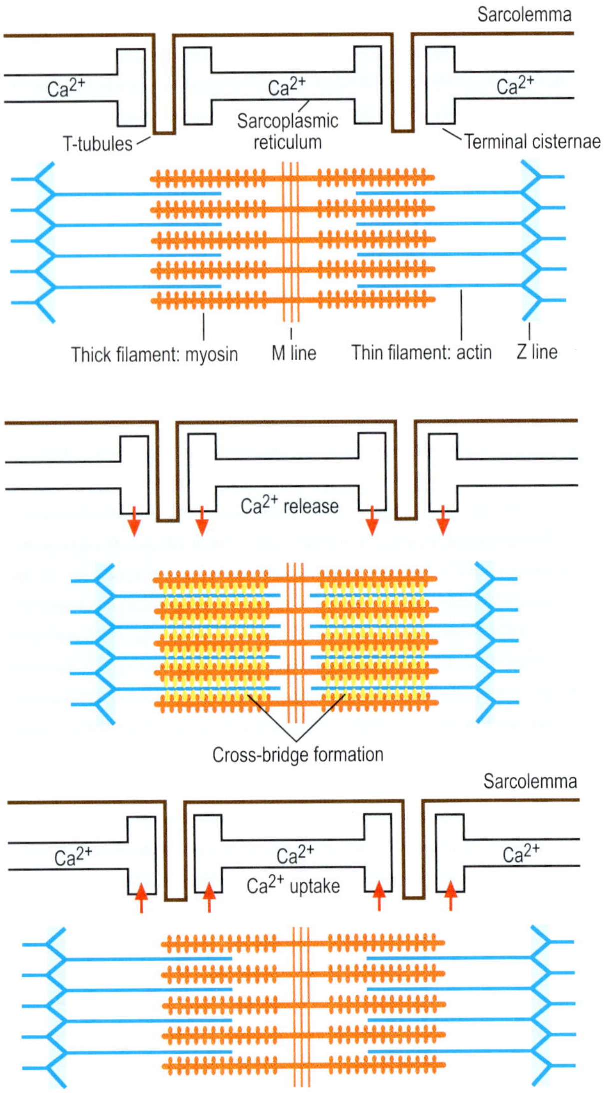

Fig 6.13 Diagram illustrating excitation–contraction coupling and the role of calcium in the contractile mechanism. (Top) Calcium (light blue) stored in the SR during the relaxed state of the muscle. (Middle) A wave of depolarization moves along the sarcolemma and alters the membrane potential of the T-tubules. The altered membrane potential culminates in movement of Ca^{2+} ions into the cytoplasm from the SR (see Fig. 6.12). Thin filament inhibition is removed, allowing the globular heads of myosin to interact with actin and form a crossbridge that results in shortening of the total length of sarcomere. (Bottom) Muscle relaxation is achieved when Ca^{2+} is pumped back into the SR.

follows the local production of vasoactive substances that include potassium, adenosine, and nitric oxide. The latter is produced by nitric oxide synthase, found both in the endothelium of the capillaries and bound to the dystrophin-associated protein complex within the contracting muscle fibers themselves (Fig. 6.16).

Energy provision for muscular functions

Muscles cannot contract without a biochemical source of energy provided by the cleavage of high-energy phosphate bonds within ATP. In addition to the normal cellular metabolic requirements and the energy needed for ion pumping up concentration gradients, ATP is required in the contractile crossbridge cycle; at the head of each myosin molecule, an ATP molecule is hydrolyzed, releasing energy (E) in a reaction catalyzed by the enzyme actomyosin ATPase:

$$ATP + H_2O \rightarrow ADP + Pi + H^+ + E$$

where ADP is adenosine diphosphate and Pi is inorganic phosphate.

Aerobic pathways

Within mitochondria, β-oxidation of free fatty acids (FFA), the tricarboxylic acid (TCA) cycle, and oxidative phosphorylation (via the electron transport chain) combine to produce ATP aerobically (Fig. 6.17). During the process, the coenzymes nicotinamide adenine dinucleotide (NAD) and flavin adenine dinucleotide (FAD) are reduced to $NADH_2$ and $FADH_2$, respectively. Subsequently, $NADH_2$ and $FADH_2$ are reoxidized to NAD and FAD via the electron-transport chain in which oxygen acts as the final hydrogen acceptor to form water. Oxygen dissolved within the cytoplasm and bound to myoglobin is rapidly used up and must be replenished; hence oxidative phosphorylation depends on a dense capillary network between muscle fibers (Fig. 6.18).

Acetyl-CoA is the substrate for the TCA cycle and its complete oxidation results in the formation of 12 ATP molecules. Acetyl-CoA is derived from pyruvate following anaerobic metabolism of glucose and glycogen within the cytoplasm (glycolysis) (see Fig. 6.17); at submaximal exercise intensities, most pyruvate produced via glycolysis is transported into mitochondria and is converted to acetyl-CoA, which enters the TCA cycle. Thirty-six molecules of ATP are produced in the complete breakdown of glucose via these pathways. However, acetyl-CoA is also derived from the oxidation of fatty acids, following their mobilization from the liver or adipose tissue. Beta-oxidation of FFA is highly efficient, as complete oxidation provides up to 146 molecules of ATP.

Anaerobic pathways

In addition to the pathways described above, additional anaerobic mechanisms exist for ATP replenishment in muscle. They can be divided into two different mechanisms. The first system involves high-energy phosphate transfer in the coupling of the creatine kinase (*i*), adenylate kinase (*ii*) and AMP deaminase (*iii*) enzyme systems:

1. ADP + phosphocreatine → ATP + creatine
2. ADP + ADP → ATP + AMP
3. AMP + H_2O → IMP + NH_3.

The enzymes that catalyze these reactions help buffer ATP concentrations at the expense of lowering the cellular concentration of phosphocreatine and free ADP, while increasing the concentrations of creatine, adenosine monophosphate (AMP) and inosine monophosphate (IMP). These reactions occur in active muscles at top speeds, but provide only a small amount of ATP for a few seconds. Deamination of adenosine nucleotides leads to the production of ammonia (NH_3), uric acid, and allantoin.[68]

The second anaerobic pathway involves glycolysis acting independently from the oxidative pathways. Glycolysis requires glucose-6-phosphate as a substrate, which may be derived from the phosphorylation of glucose by hexokinase or by the mobilization of stored intracellular glycogen that is metabolized first to glucose-1-phosphate via glycogenolysis (see Fig. 6.17) and then converted to glucose-6-phosphate. Blood glucose is transported across the sarcolemma by means of specific glucose transporters that include

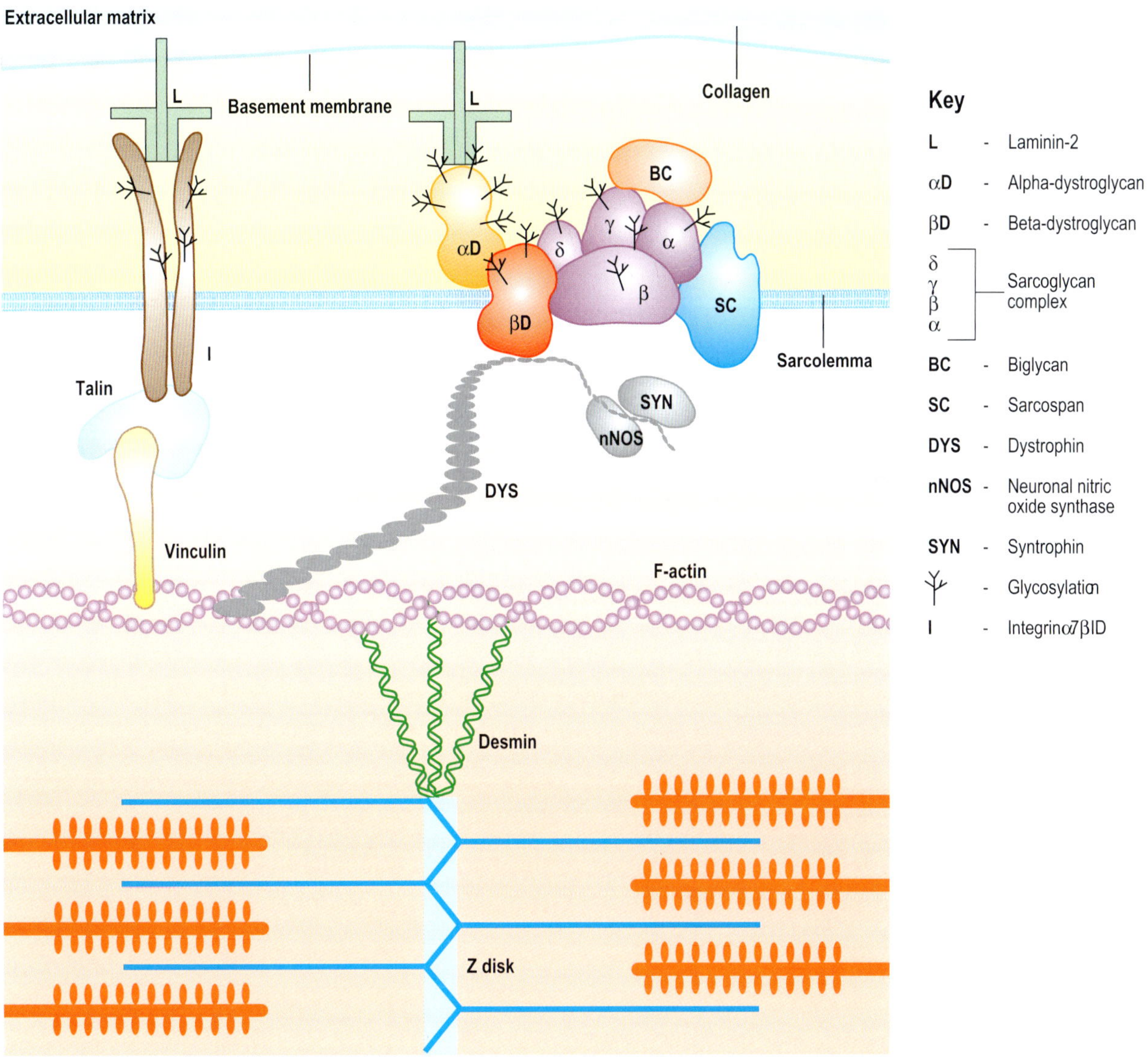

Fig 6.14 Interconnections between the contractile apparatus, the dystrophin-associated complex (DAC), and the extracellular matrix. Further structural support is provided by integrin molecules that span the sarcolemma. Note nNOS makes up part of the DAC. In addition to a structural role, the DAC likely has a role in cell signalling.

GLUT-1 and GLUT-4 (see Fig. 6.18).[69] GLUT-1 is normally located within the sarcolemma and provides basal glucose requirements; however, GLUT-4 receptors translocate to the sarcolemma in vesicles, in response to insulin or the demands of exercise (Fig. 6.19). The glycolytic pathways result in the formation of two pyruvate molecules that in the absence of oxygen are converted to lactate.

Integration of aerobic and anaerobic pathways

Aerobic production of ATP is a relatively slow but highly efficient process, while anaerobic pathways produce energy rapidly but relatively inefficiently. Although both pathways are generally active during exercise, the relative contribution within each muscle depends on the nature, intensity level and duration of the activity, the muscle's fiber-type composition, the availability of oxygen and substrates, and the relative concentrations of intermediary metabolites that may potentially activate or inhibit selected enzymes.[68] Hence, at the beginning of low-speed exercise when oxygen is abundant, energy production depends largely on metabolism of glycogen via aerobic pathways.[68] Within a few minutes, glucose and FFA concentrations rise in the blood and following 20–30% glycogen depletion, there is a shift towards β-oxidation of FFA[70] With higher energy demands, the muscle ATP/ADP ratio decreases, providing a stimulus for energy production via anaerobic mechanisms. The activity of the key regulatory glycolytic enzyme phosphofructokinase increases, causing greater production of pyruvate via glycolysis.

The point where the availability of oxygen becomes a limiting factor in oxidative phosphorylation is reflected by partial reoxidation of $NADH_2$, as more and more pyruvate is converted to lactate. As exercise intensity increases, the anaerobic pathway supplies a greater proportion of energy. The point when the increased rate of lactate production can be detected in the plasma is known as the anaerobic threshold. This threshold varies and depends on several factors including the muscle's fiber-type composition and the level

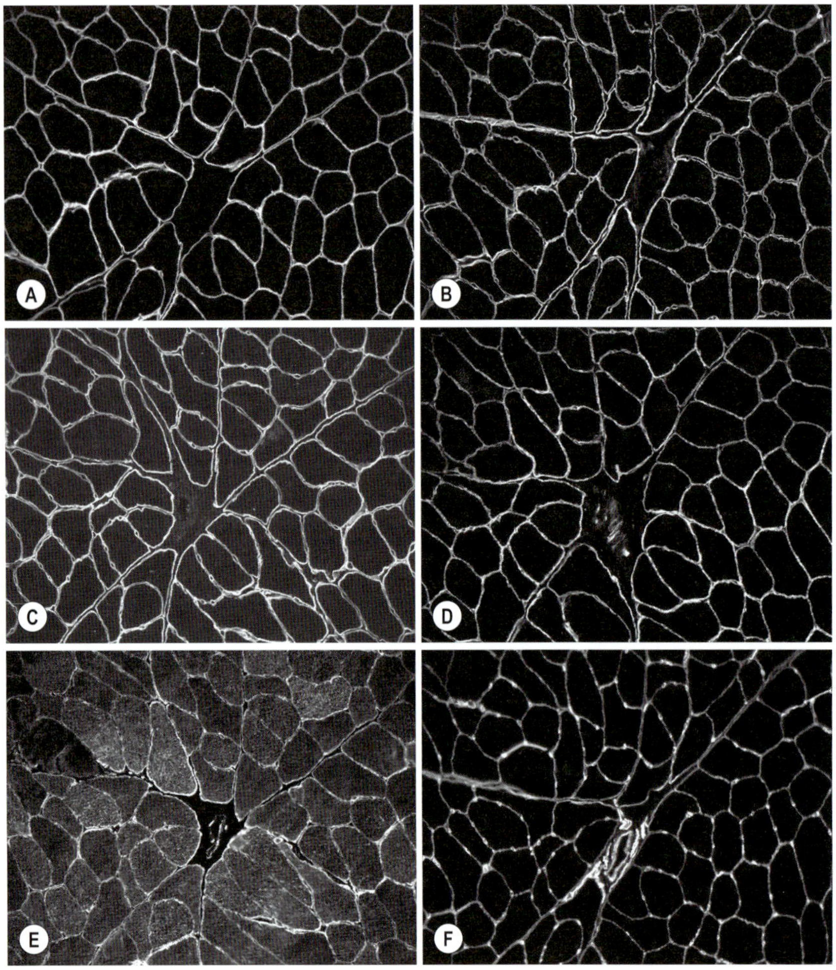

Fig 6.15 Immunofluorescence labeling of serial 7 μm sections from the gluteus medius muscle of a normal Thoroughbred, showing proteins that link the contractile apparatus to the extracellular matrix. **(A)** Beta dystroglycan; **(B)** laminin $\alpha 2$; **(C)** dystrophin; **(D)** integrin $\alpha 7\beta 1d$; **(E)** desmin; **(F)** collagen IV. Working clockwise from desmin **(E)**, contractile force is conveyed via dystrophin **(C)** to the dystrophin-associated complex **(A and B)** and ultimately to the extracellular matrix **(F)**. Integrin $\alpha 7\beta 1d$ likely also plays a structural role. Compare with Figure 6.14 and Figure 6.16. Note the capillaries located around each muscle fiber, and a central blood vessel that are also localized with the collagen IV antibody in **(F)**.

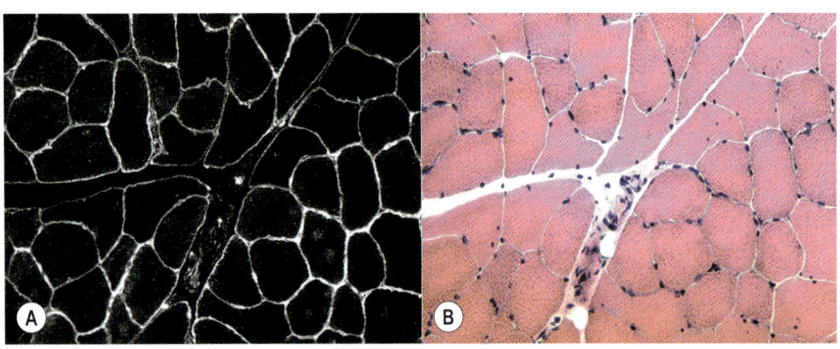

Fig 6.16 Serial 7 μm **(A)** and 10 μm **(B)** sections from the gluteus medius muscle of a normal Thoroughbred. (A) Immunofluorescence labeling of neuronal nitric oxide synthase (nNOS). **(B)** Hematoxylin and eosin stain. Note the sarcolemmal distribution of nNOS, and compare with Figure 6.14 and Figure 6.15.

Fig 6.17 Diagram summarizing the integration of metabolic pathways in muscle cells. Abbreviations: AC, aconitase; ACDH, acyl-CoA dehydrogenase; ADP, adenosine diphosphate; AMP, adenosine monophosphate; ATP, adenosine triphosphate; CAT, carnitine acyltransferase; CoA, coenzyme A; CS, citrate synthase; FAD, flavin adenine dinucleotide; FDP, fructose diphosphatase; FUM, fumarase; GP, glycogen phosphorylase; GS, glycogen synthetase; GTP, guanosine triphosphate; HADH, 3-hydroxyacyl-CoA dehydrogenase; HK, hexokinase; I, complex I; II, complex II; III, complex III; IDH, isocitrate dehydrogenase; IV, complex IV; KDH, ketoglutarate dehydrogenase; LDH, lactate dehydrogenase; LIPDH, lipoamide dehydrogenase; MDH, malate dehydrogenase; NAD, nicotinamide adenine dinucleotide; PbK, phosphorylase b kinase; PFK, phosphofructokinase; PGK, phosphoglyceratekinase; PGM, phosphoglyceratemutase; Pi, phosphate; PK, protein kinase; PPi, pyrophosphate; SDH, succinate dehydrogenase; V, complex V; UDP, uridine diphosphate; UTP, uridine triphosphate.

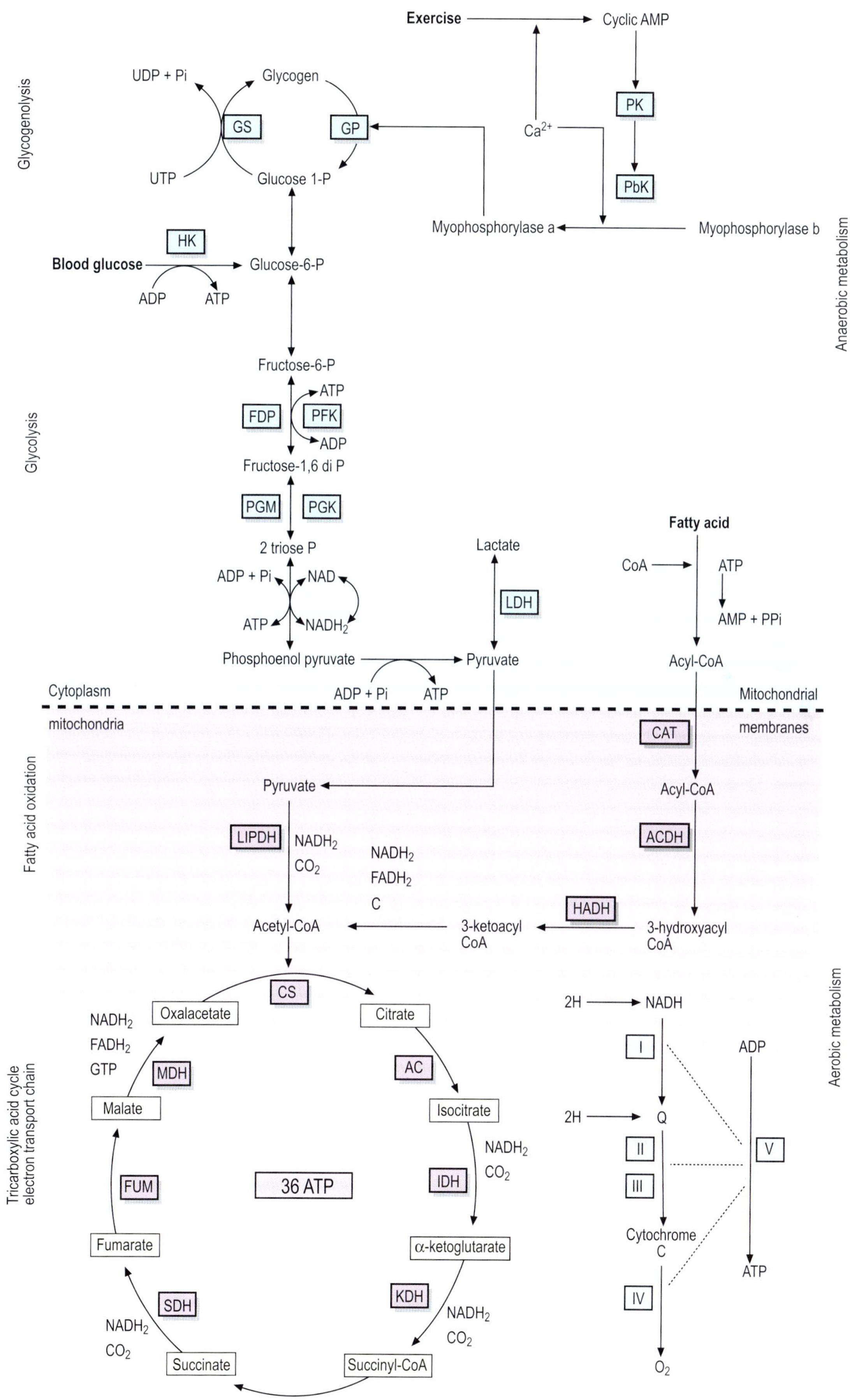
Exercise
Cyclic AMP
PK
PbK
Ca^{2+}
Myophosphorylase a
Myophosphorylase b
Glycogenolysis
UDP + Pi
Glycogen
GS
GP
UTP
Glucose 1-P
HK
Blood glucose
Glucose-6-P
ADP
ATP
Anaerobic metabolism
Glycolysis
Fructose-6-P
ATP
FDP
PFK
ADP
Fructose-1,6 di P
PGM
PGK
2 triose P
ADP + Pi
NAD
ATP
$NADH_2$
Phosphoenol pyruvate
Pyruvate
ADP + Pi
ATP
Lactate
LDH
Fatty acid
CoA
ATP
AMP + PPi
Acyl-CoA
Cytoplasm
mitochondria
Mitochondrial
membranes
CAT
Fatty acid oxidation
Pyruvate
Acyl-CoA
LIPDH
$NADH_2$
CO_2
$NADH_2$
$FADH_2$
C
ACDH
HADH
Acetyl-CoA
3-ketoacyl CoA
3-hydroxyacyl CoA
Tricarboxylic acid cycle electron transport chain
CS
Oxalacetate
Citrate
$NADH_2$
$FADH_2$
GTP
MDH
AC
Malate
Isocitrate
$NADH_2$
CO_2
FUM
36 ATP
IDH
Fumarate
α-ketoglutarate
SDH
KDH
$NADH_2$
CO_2
$NADH_2$
CO_2
Succinate
Succinyl-CoA
Aerobic metabolism
2H
NADH
I
ADP
2H
Q
II
V
III
Cytochrome C
ATP
IV
O_2

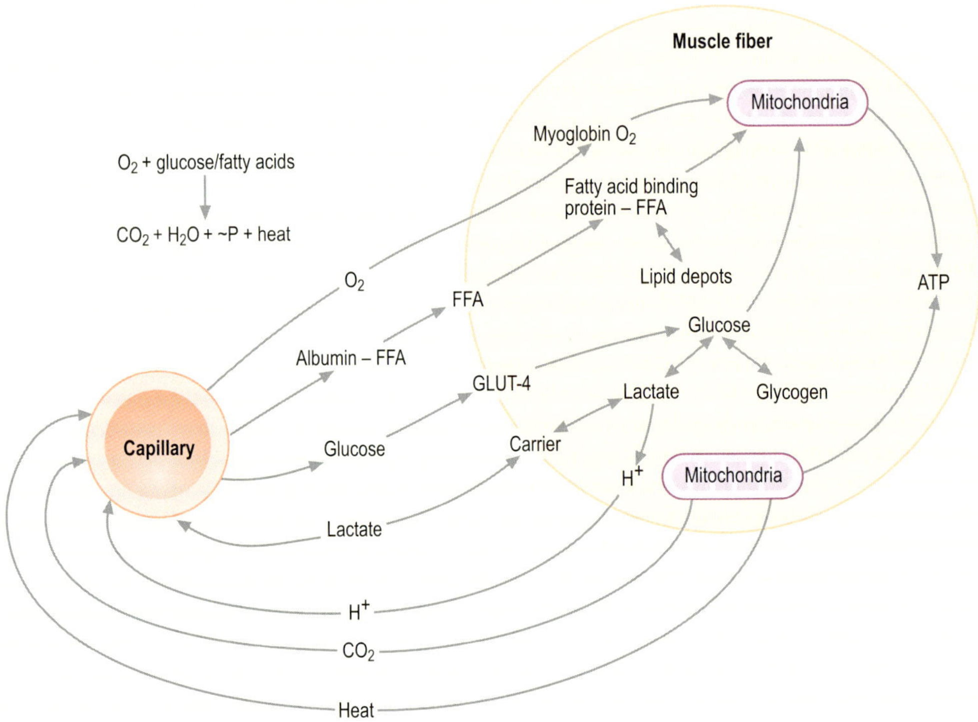

Fig 6.18 Diagram of intermediary steps involved in the transfer of substrates to and from skeletal muscle fibers. FFA, free fatty acids; GLUT-4, glucose transport protein 4.

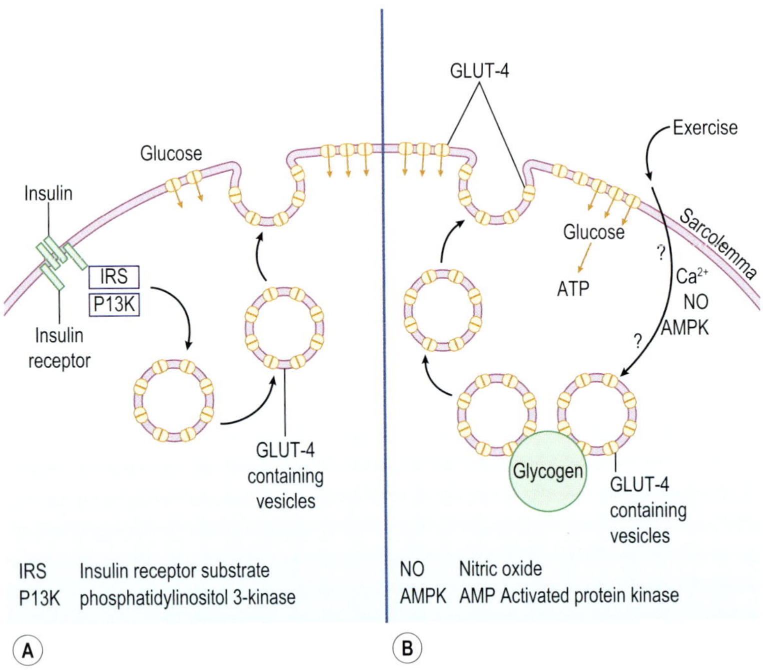

Fig 6.19 Diagrammatic representation of insulin-dependent translocation of vesicle-bound GLUT-4 receptors from the cytoplasm to the sarcolemma **(A)** and the similar translocation of GLUT-4 receptors in response to exercise **(B)**.

of fitness of the horse. Furthermore, diet plays an additional role; for example, a fat-rich diet promotes oxidative energy production via FFAs,[71] thereby increasing the oxidative capacity of muscle[72] and sparing glycogen.[72] However, other substrates also influence the pathways employed during energy production; for instance, energy production can be steered towards that derived from glucose by the provision of additional glucose during exercise.[73]

Muscle heterogeneity

The ability of muscle tissue to perform efficiently in spite of very different types of exercise of varying intensity and duration is mediated partly by overall nervous control. However, it is significantly enhanced by the heterogeneous fiber type composition of each muscle.

Muscle fiber types

Fiber type differentiation

There are important differences in the morphologic, physiologic, and biochemical properties of fibers both within and between muscles. These differences form the basis for the classification of fiber types. Better understanding of the expression patterns of groups of proteins within individual fibers has allowed refinement of fiber-type classification. For example, myofibrillar proteins exist as different isoforms encoded by separate genes that are expressed in a myofiber type-specific and coordinated manner.[74]

Fiber types can best be differentiated by analyzing the specific myosin heavy chain (MyHC) isoform(s) expressed by each fiber, since MyHC composition closely reflects each fiber's phenotype.[23] Three MyHC isoforms have been characterized in adult equine skeletal muscles at the protein,[27] mRNA,[31] and cDNA,[32] levels; they are designated as types I, IIA, and IIX[27] (or IID)[29] (henceforth IIX). The differential distribution of these MyHCs defines three pure fiber types containing a single isoform (types I, IIA, and IIX) and two hybrid fiber types coexpressing two isoforms (I+IIA and IIA + IIX (IIAX)) (Fig. 6.20). Hybrid IIAX fibers exist in equine locomotor muscles in significant numbers,[29,30] although the coexpression of IIA and IIX MyHCs at the protein level seems not to be reflected by cotranscription of the corresponding genes (Fig. 6.21).[33] This suggests that hybrids might represent fibers that are undergoing committed fiber type switching, towards the type corresponding to the mRNA currently being expressed, and that this conversion occurs in equine muscle not subjected to any specific training stimulus.[33]

Some studies have demonstrated either minimal (less than 0.6%)[75] or no expression of the MyHC-IIB isoform in locomotor muscles of the horse,[27,31–33] hence the fibers classified as type IIB in earlier studies are now more appropriately classified as type IIX. It remains unclear why the MyHC-IIB gene is only minimally (or not) expressed in various ungulates,[32] although it could be related to body size and muscle fiber length. As a muscle's maximum contraction velocity is proportional to the number of sarcomeres in series[76] and the MyHC-IIB isoform exhibits the fastest shortening velocity,[74] the expression of this isoform in the very long muscle fibers of the horse would, in theory, result in an extremely high contraction velocity. Nevertheless, some recent studies have demonstrated the expression of this isoform in the skeletal musculature of some other large mammals (pig and llama),[77,78] indicating that the expression (or lack) of this isoform is not only a reflection of body size.

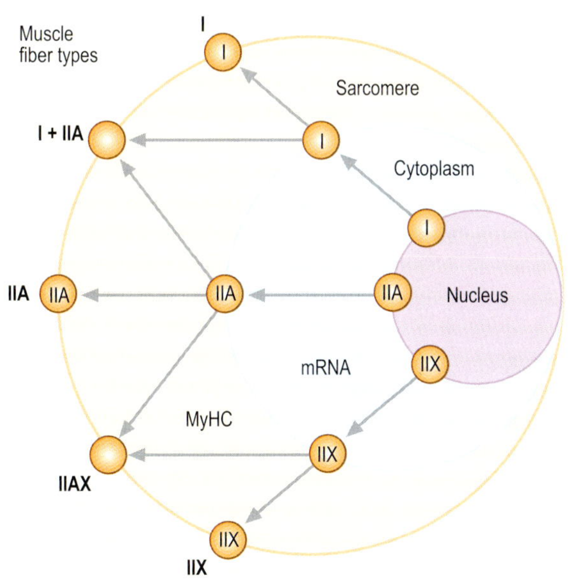

Fig 6.20 Diagram illustrating the relationship between muscle fiber phenotype and the regulation of gene expression for the separate myosin heavy chain isoforms in adult horse skeletal muscle. Horses only express three myosin heavy chain isoforms: one slow or type I and two fast termed type IIA and type IIX. The differential expression of these isoforms defines three major fiber types, each containing a single isoform (i.e. types I, IIA, and IIX) and two intermediate hybrid fiber populations containing either slow and fast IIA isoforms or the two fast isoforms.

Muscle fiber type properties

Certain important differences between the various equine skeletal muscle fiber types are illustrated in Figure 6.22 and summarized in Table 6.1. When studied in combination, these differences allow more objective delineation (Fig. 6.23) and represent the considerable interdependence of contractile, metabolic, and morphologic features. Type I fibers have a MyHC isoform that hydrolyzes ATP slowly, resulting in a slow crossbridge cycle. These fibers have a small cross-sectional area, a high number of capillaries and high oxidative capacity. However, their glycolytic capacity and glycogen content are relatively low. Together, these properties make type I fibers highly efficient and economical in producing slow repetitive movements and sustaining isometric force, but not significant power generators.

In contrast, type II fibers have MyHC isoforms that create fast crossbridge cycling and therefore develop force rapidly. Within the type II group, type IIX fibers have a maximal velocity of shortening that is three times higher than that of IIA fibers.[17] Overall, equine type II muscle fibers have a shortening velocity higher than expected in accordance with its increased body size.[17,76,79] Hence, IIX fibers are adapted for high power outputs for a limited time because they have a low oxidative capacity and limited oxygen availability (as reflected by their large cross-sectional area and relatively low capillary supply). Type IIA fibers, however, have a considerable number of both capillaries and mitochondria and rely on glycolytic and oxidative metabolism; they are therefore able to sustain high power outputs for longer than IIX fibers. Hybrid IIAX fibers are intermediate in their properties.[23] Although they are classified according to the MyHC composition, it is important to remember that the expression of other protein isoforms varies within muscle fibers, in each case with the isoform closely correlating with the fiber's function and with one another. Furthermore, fibers also differ with respect to other factors, such as the availability of high-energy phosphate,[80] GLUT-4 protein expression (Fig. 6.24), the calcium sensitivity of force production,[16] Ca^{2+}-ATPase content,[81] carnosine and taurine contents,[82] protein kinase C isoforms,[83] expression of splice variants of neuronal nitric oxide synthase,[84] expression of monocarboxylate transporters facilitating efflux of lactate from the muscle,[85,86] and expression of sarcoplasmic(endo)reticulum Ca^{2+}-ATPase, phospholamban and calcineurin.[23,87]

Muscle fiber recruitment

Although muscle can be separated into individual fiber types, the basic functional unit of skeletal muscle remains the motor unit (see section above on general muscle physiology). Motor units are commonly classified according to the MyHC profile of their constituent fibers (hence I, IIA, and IIX; Fig. 6.25). This is possible because fibers within a single motor unit show relatively homogeneous, although not identical, biochemical and histochemical properties.

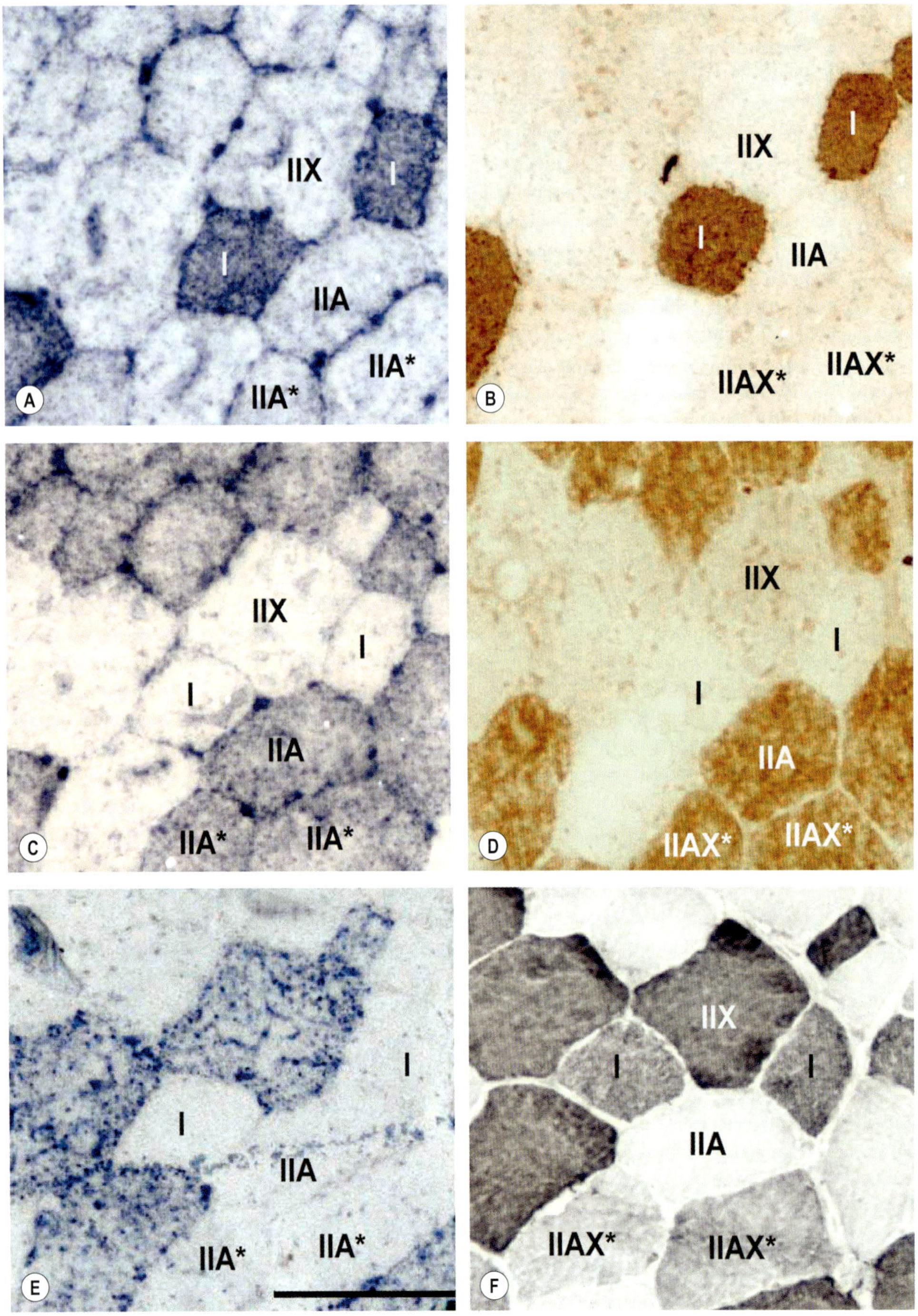

Fig 6.21 Serial cryosections of adult untrained M. gluteus medius showing identification of myofiber types by in situ hybridization using non-radioactive MyHC mRNA probes specific for type I **(A)**, type IIA **(B)**, and type IIX **(C)** isoforms; and immunohistochemistry with a number of monoclonal antibodies to specific MyHC isoproteins: 219 (**D**, anti-MyHC-I), 333 (**E**, anti-MyHC-IIA), and 412 (**F**, anti-MyHCs I plus IIX). Fiber types are identified according to the mRNA expression **(A–C)** or according to the protein expression (D–F). Two hybrid IIAX fibers at the protein level but expressing only type IIA mRNA are labelled with asterisks. Calibration bar, 100 μm.

Reprinted from Eizemaa, van den Burg MMM, de Jonge HW, et al. Journal of Histochemistry and Cytochemistry, 53(11) pp. 1383–90, ©2005. Reprinted by permission of SAGE Publishers.

Although the motor unit's structure, function, and hence role in motor control have been studied extensively in experimental animals, they have not been widely studied in larger mammals. However, specific muscle fiber type recruitment has been examined in horses by observing glycogen depletion patterns during and after exercise of varying intensity and duration (Fig. 6.26).[5] In horses, it appears that motor units are selectively recruited in a specific pattern that changes according to the gait, and to the intensity and duration of exercise.[88] For the maintenance of posture, only type I motor units are recruited. As intensity and duration of exercise increase, further motor units are recruited, in the rank order: I → IIA → IIAX → IIX.[88,89] Short duration with high intensity exercise, such as 4 min running at 100% $\dot{V}O_{2max}$ or 8 min running at 80% or 60% $\dot{V}O_{2max}$, is effective to stimulate type IIX and IIAX fibres.[89]

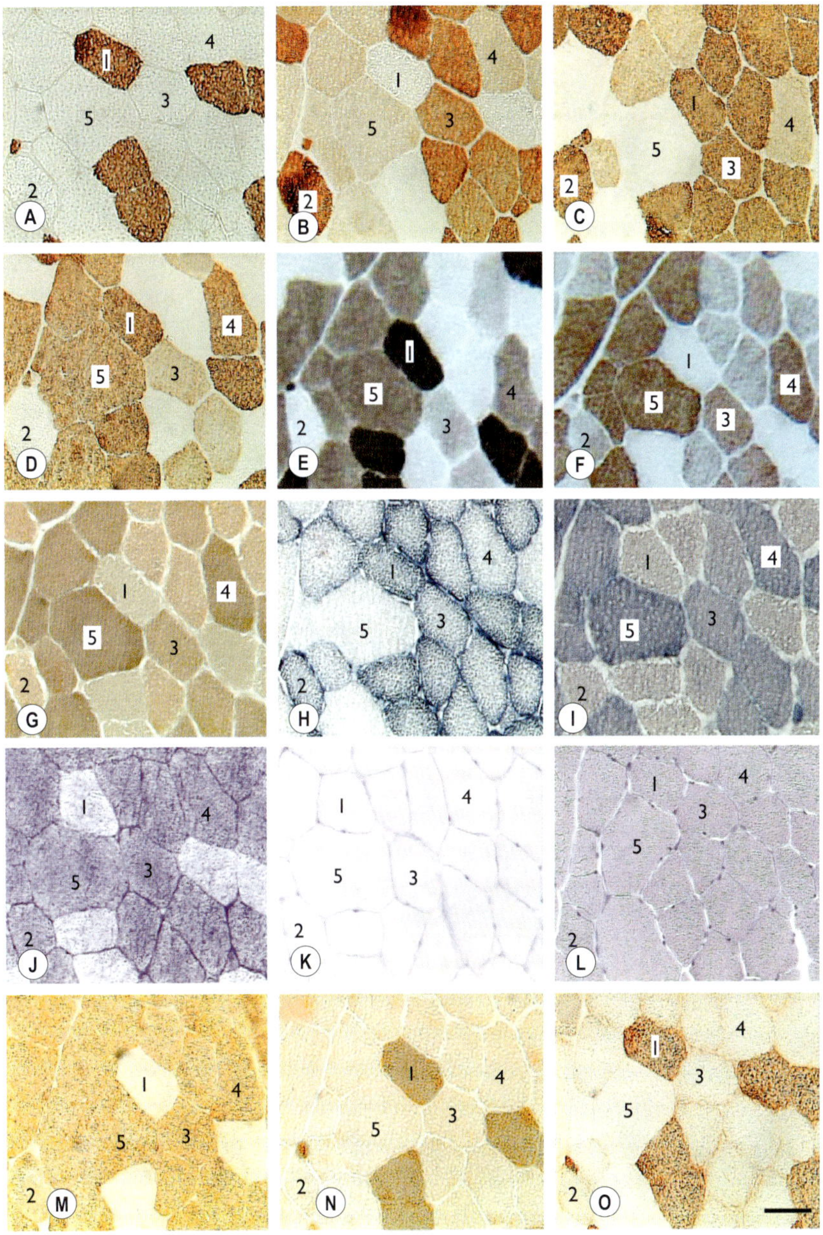

Fig 6.22 Serial cryosections of adult horse M. gluteus medius stained by immunohistochemistry, enzyme histochemistry, and histology. **(A–D)** Sections were stained with a number of monoclonal antibodies against specific myosin heavy chain (MyHC) isoforms: BA-D5 (**A**, anti-MyHC-b/slow), SC-71 (**B**, anti-MyHC-IIA), BF-35 (**C**, anti-MyHCs b/slow and IIA), and S5–8H2 (**D**, anti-MyHCs b/slow and IID/X). **(E–G)** Sections were assayed for myofibrillar actomyosin adenosine triphosphatase activity after acid (pH 4.4, **E**) and alkaline (pH 10.45, **F**) pre-incubations, and by Blanco and Sieck's quantitative histochemical procedure **(G)**.[89] **(H–I)** Sections assayed for succinate dehydrogenase and **(H)**, glycerol-3-phosphate dehydrogenase activities **(I)** and periodic acid–Schiff (PAS) for selective staining of glycogen **(J)**. **(K–L)** PAS with α-amylase digestion, for visualizing capillaries **(K)**, and hematoxylin and eosin for visualizing myonuclei **(L)**. **(M–O)** Sections were stained by immunohistochemistry with monoclonal antibodies to SR Ca^{2+}-ATPase (SERCA) isoforms and phospholamban: CaF2–5D2 (**M**, anti-SERCA1a), MA3–910 (**N**, anti-SERCA2a) and 05–205 (**O**, antiphospholamban). The fibers labeled 1, 2, 3, 4, and 5 are types I, IIA, IIAx, IlaX, and IIX, respectively. Calibration bar, 50 μm.

Muscle fiber type distribution between and within muscles

In horses, muscle fiber types are spatially distributed according to the general checkerboard pattern present in mixed muscles of many other species. However, this pattern is never completely random, since fast-glycolytic type IIX fibers are more common along the rim than in the center of individual fascicles (see Fig. 6.3A).[90] Fiber-type composition varies extensively between muscles depending largely on function.[91,92] For example, significant components of the thoracic limb musculature have a higher percentage of type I and IIA fibres and a significantly lower percentage of type IIX fibers than the pelvic limb muscles (Fig. 6.27A,B).[92] Variation is also seen between muscles belonging to the same synergic group. Differences in the metabolic properties of different muscles have also been reported in the horse.[93] For example, the low substrate concentrations and oxidative capacity of superficial digital flexor muscle compared to gluteus medius may predispose that muscle to catastrophic fatigue during maximal exercise.[93]

Significant regional variation in fiber composition within a muscle has also been reported in several horse muscles.[12,25,26,30,54,94] Most locomotory muscles have greater numbers of oxidative type I and type IIA fibers in the deep portions and a predominance of glycolytic type IIX in more superficial portions (Fig. 6.27C,D). This compartmentalization reflects the relationship between structure and function: the deeper regions appear best suited for posture maintenance and low-level, but longer duration muscular activity, whereas the more superficial regions are involved with short-duration, rapid propulsive force generation. In general, groups studying equine muscle physiology have formed conclusions based on data derived from a single biopsy sample site (see references[5-7] for review of relevant citations); however, it is apparent that this approach is too simplistic. Several studies by the first author's group (J-LR) for instance, have demonstrated a greater muscular response

Table 6.1 Quantitative fiber type features of equine skeletal muscle[1]

	MUSCLE FIBER TYPES[2]				
	I	**IIA**	**IIAx**	**IIaX**	**IIX**
No. of fibers	51	80	25	25	27
Anti-MyHC monoclonal antibodies[3]					
BA-D5 (OD)	0.60 ± 0.02 b		0.34 ± 0.02 a		
SC-71 (OD)	0.30 ± 0.02 a	0.52 ± 0.03 d	0.46 ± 0.02 c	0.34 ± 0.01 b	0.34 ± 0.01 b
BF-35 (OD)	0.47 ± 0.03 c	0.49 ± 0.03 d	0.46 ± 0.03 cd	0.36 ± 0.02 b	0.30 ± 0.02 a
S5-8H2 (OD)	0.44 ± 0.02 d	0.33 ± 0.01 a	0.37 ± 0.02 b	0.41 ± 0.01 c	0.41 ± 0.01 c
Myofibrillar ATPase activity[4]					
Ac-mATPase (OD)	0.77 ± 0.02 d	0.28 ± 0.03 a	0.34 ± 0.03 b	0.47 ± 0.02 c	0.50 ± 0.02 c
Alk-mATPase (OD)	0.27 ± 0.02 a	0.37 ± 0.03 b	0.46 ± 0.04 c	0.52 ± 0.02 d	0.54 ± 0.02 d
Qu-mATPase (OD/min)	0.30 ± 0.02 a	0.39 ± 0.02 b	0.42 ± 0.01 c	0.45 ± 0.01 d	0.51 ± 0.01 e
Metabolic properties[5]					
SDH (OD/min)	0.49 ± 0.02 d	0.46 ± 0.03 c	0.37 ± 0.02 b	0.34 ± 0.02 b	0.24 ± 0.03 a
GPD (OD/min)	0.33 ± 0.02 a	0.36 ± 0.03 b	0.41 ± 0.01 c	0.46 ± 0.01 d	0.47 ± 0.01 d
PAS (OD)	0.34 ± 0.02 a		0.45 ± 0.03 b		
Fiber size, capillaries, and myonuclei[6]					
CSA (μm^2)	3124 ± 723 a	3339 ± 763 b	4623 ± 807 c	5039 ± 1293 c	7635 ± 2930 d
cap/10^3 μm^2	2.06 ± 0.94 b	1.96 ± 0.57 b	1.60 ± 0.41 ab	1.38 ± 0.21 a	1.23 ± 1.07 a
nuc/10^3 μm^2	2.26 ± 0.65 b	2.32 ± 1.02 b	1.65 ± 0.36 ab	1.44 ± 0.78 a	1.11 ± 0.70 a
Anti-SERCA and PLB antibodies[7]					
CaF2–5D2 (OD)	0.33 ± 0.03 a		0.44 ± 0.03 b		
MA3–910 (OD)	0.48 ± 0.02 b		0.38 ± 0.03 a		
05–205 (OD)	0.54 ± 0.03 b		0.37 ± 0.02 a		

[1]Values are mean ± SE. Within a row, means with different letters are statistically different ($P < 0.05$), where a expresses the lowest value and e the highest. In the absence of significant differences between type II fibers, values are presented as pooled means for all type II fibers (n = 157 fibers). OD = optical density.
[2]Hybrid I+IIA fibers are not considered in this analysis; IIAx = hybrid fibers with a predominant myosin heavy chain type IIA content; IIaX = hybrid fibers with a predominant myosin heavy chain type IIX isoform.
[3]See Figure 6.22's legend for origins and specificities of antibodies.
[4]Ac-mATPase = myofibrillar ATPase after acid (pH 4.45) pre-incubation; Alk-ATPase = myofibrillar ATPase after alkaline (pH 10.45) pre-incubation; Qu-mATPase = quantitative myofibrillar ATPase activity (pH 7.6).
[5]SDH = succinate dehydrogenase activity; GPD = glycerol-3-phosphate dehydrogenase activity; PAS = periodic acid–Schiff.
[6]CSA = cross-sectional area; cap = number of capillaries; nuc = nuclear number.
[7]SERCA = sarco(endo)plasmic reticulum Ca^{2+}-ATPase; PLB = phospholamban; see [23] for sources and specificities of these antibodies.

to training in the deeper region of the M. gluteus medius compared with more superficial regions.[95–97]

Relationship to performance

Some studies in horses have shown that performance is correlated with selected muscle characteristics (see references[5–7] for reviews). Unsurprisingly, endurance capacity is correlated with (1) high percentages of type I and IIA fibers[98] and (2) high activities of oxidative enzymes,[99] whereas sprint capacity is correlated with high percentages of type II fibers.[100] It is therefore feasible to differentiate the endurance potential of horses based on the fiber type composition of certain muscles,[101] although different conclusions have been obtained in Thoroughbreds[94] and trotters.[102,103] Nevertheless, trotting speed is highly dependent on the ability of muscle to produce energy via anaerobic glycolysis.[102] Interestingly, some myofiber properties are correlated with kinematic profiles. For example, stride length and frequency are positively correlated with both the

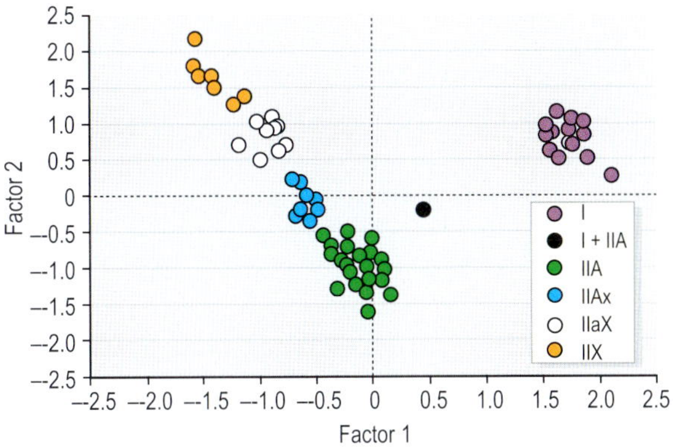

Fig 6.23 Principal component analysis of muscle fiber type features in a representative sample (n = 82 fibers) to show graphically the spatial discrimination of myosin heavy chain (MyHC)-based fiber types. This scatter plot shows the spatial distribution of a set of equine muscle fibers upon the basis of muscle variables included in Table 6.1; this analysis resulted in an optimal discrimination (100%) of all muscle fiber types; Factor 1 axis discriminates between type I (right) and type II (left) fibers, whereas Factor 2 axis discriminates type IIA (bottom) and IIX (top) fibers.

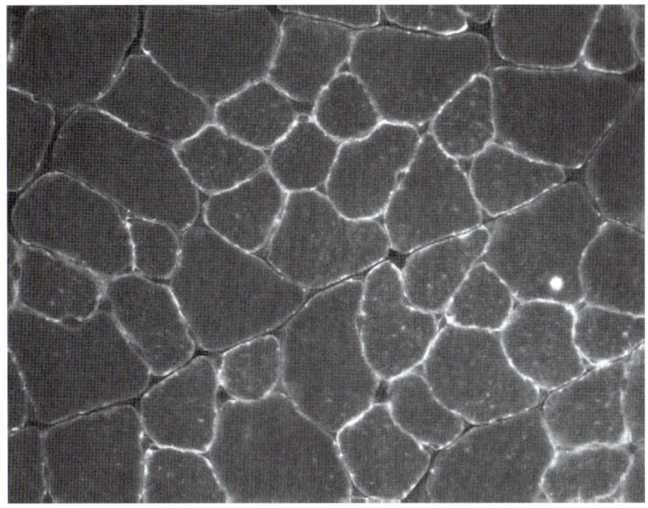

Fig 6.24 Transverse section of rat extensor digitorum muscle samples labeled by immunohistochemistry with a monoclonal antibody to GLUT-4 (glucose transport protein). Note the higher intensity of staining in the periphery of the smaller fibers (presumably types I and IIA) compared with the larger ones (presumably IIX and IIB).

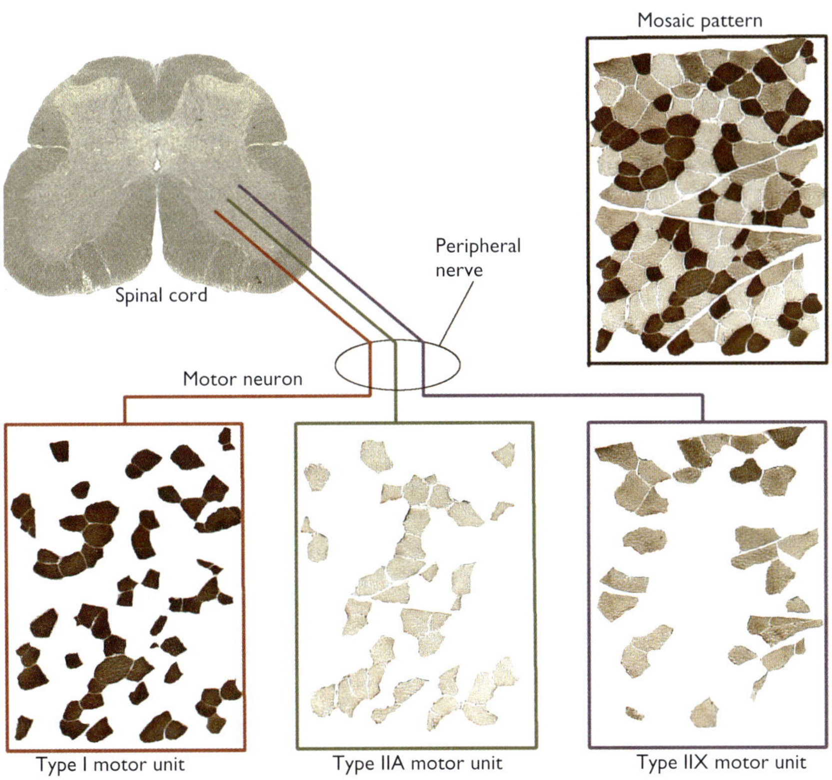

Fig 6.25 Diagram showing the spatial distribution of muscle fibers integrating three different motor units classified according to myosin heavy chain isoform expression as types I, IIA, and IIX. Note how muscle fibers within each motor unit are dispersed between those of others producing the characteristic mosaic or checkerboard distribution seen in transverse section.

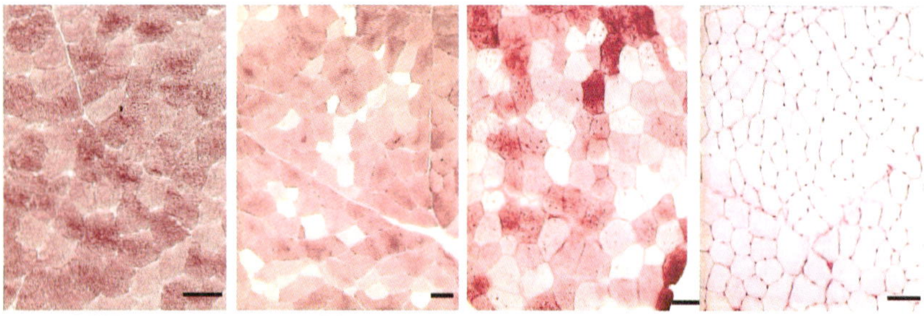

Fig 6.26 Transverse sections of gluteus medius muscle biopsies (6 cm depth) to show muscle glycogen depletion patterns in a horse competing in an endurance ride of 120 km. Note the increase in the number of myofibers without glycogen when the intensity and duration of the exercise increase. Bars, 75 μm.

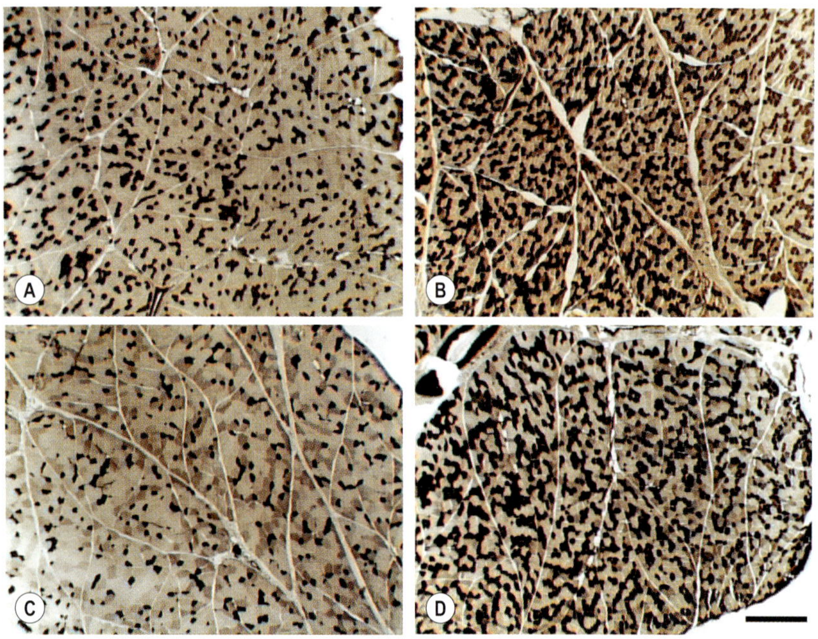

Fig 6.27 **(A, B)** Transverse sections stained for myofibrillar adenosine triphosphatase activity after acid pre-incubation (pH 4.4) demonstrating the differential muscle fiber type composition in two locomotor muscles with different functions: M. semitendinosus **(A)** vs M. rhomboideus cervicis **(B)**. Note the higher percentage of type I fibers (black staining) and the lower proportion of types IIA (white) and IIX fibers (gray) in the rhomboideus muscle compared with the semitendinosus muscle. **(C, D)** Transverse sections stained with myofibrillar adenosine triphosphatase activity after acid pre-incubation (pH 4.4) from two muscle samples removed from the equine gluteus medius muscle at two different sampling depths: 2 cm (C) vs 8 cm **(D)**. Note the higher percentage of type I fibers and the lower proportion of type IIX fibers in the deeper region of the muscle than in the superficial region. Scale bar, 1000 μm.

percentage of IIA fibers and fiber size, and the stance time of the stride is inversely correlated with the percentage of IIX fibers and fiber diameter.[104] Furthermore, certain primary muscular adaptations to training occur with concomitant modifications in the temporal characteristics of the trot.[104]

Control and regulation

Myogenic factors

Multiple factors, both myogenic and non-myogenic in origin, regulate the expression of proteins that comprise the various muscle-specific characteristics of each muscle fiber (Fig. 6.28) and, in combination, these factors also regulate the percentage of individual fiber types found within each muscle. During development and maturation, these factors change, resulting in significant changes in protein expression.[105] However, the myogenic lineage from which a muscle fiber develops generally defines its ultimate type.[74] All fibers during embryonic development express an embryonic MyHC isoform. At birth, some fibers are found to express type I MyHC; these are destined to become mature type I fibers in the adult. Other fibers express a neonatal MyHC isoform that is gradually replaced by either IIA or IIX, or both MyHCs; these subsequently become type II fibers in the adult. The α-cardiac MyHC isoform mRNA is also expressed in horse skeletal muscle,[29] but its transcript is only detectable at young age, indicating silencing of the gene around birth.[105]

The influence of genetic factors on equine muscle fiber types is clearly illustrated by dramatic variations observed between different breeds (Fig. 6.29)[91] and between separate bloodlines within the same breed.[6,7,106] Furthermore, there is a tendency for fiber type ratios (type I:type II) to be inherited.[100] Although equine muscle is already functional at birth, expression patterns of contractile and metabolic proteins show adaptation, depending on the MyHC fibre type.[87] During growth and maturation, muscle fibers continuously adapt their size and MyHC content at both the mRNA and protein level,[105] there is a gradual conversion of fast to slow phenotype that is especially pronounced in the first year postpartum[107], but that can continue until about 6 years of age or older.[108,109] Hybrid fibers play an important role in this process.[110] Interestingly, aged (20+ years) sedentary horses exhibit a shift in MyHC and metabolic profiles toward faster and more glycolytic phenotypes,[111,112] which explains some of the lower exercise capacity seen in the older horse.[112] The expression of other proteins such as monocarboxylate transporters and lactate dehydrogenase isoenzymes, also change as horses grow, suggesting that metabolism of

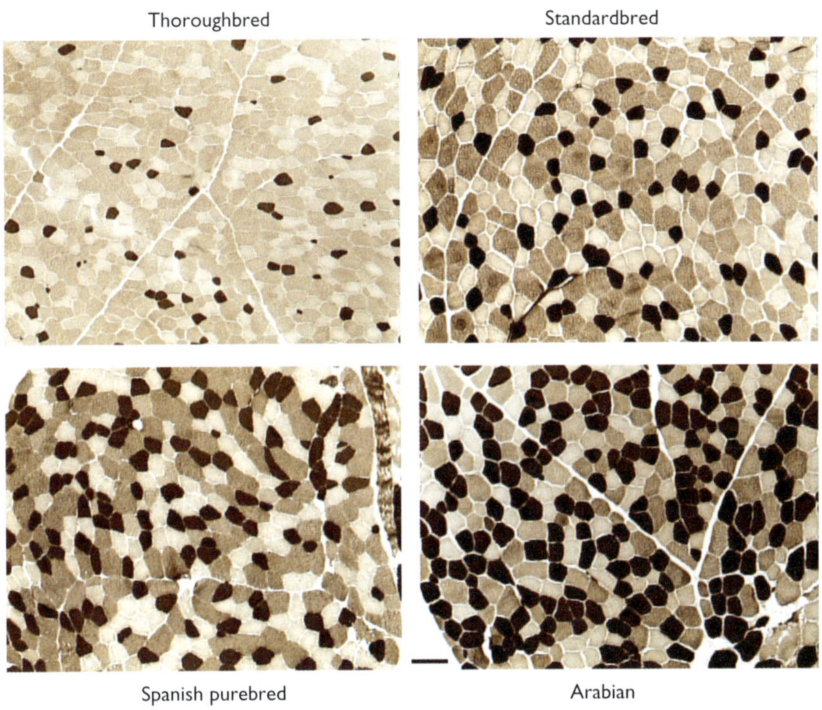

Fig 6.29 Transverse sections of M. gluteus medius specimens stained with myofibrillar adenosine triphosphatase after acid pre-incubation (pH 4.4), removed at the same depth, from four different breeds of athletic horse. Note how the percentage of type I (oxidative) fibers and the fiber size increase from the fastest breed (Thoroughbred) towards the slower, more endurance-suited breed (Arabian). Bar scale, 150 μm.

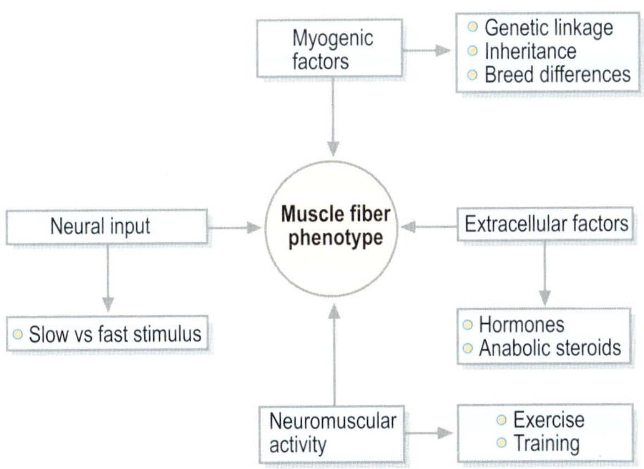

Fig 6.28 Schematic diagram summarizing regulation of muscle fiber type. Fiber type is determined by a combination of four factors: (*i*) the myogenic lineage from which the muscle fiber developed; (*ii*) the innervating motor neuron that regulates fiber type via activity pattern and basal activity and/or via other mediators such as neurotrophic factors; (*iii*) activity levels affected by exercise and training; and (*iv*) extracellular factors. The extracellular factors include hormones (e.g. thyroid hormone and growth hormone), growth factors (e.g. insulin-like growth factor), anabolic steroids, substrate availability (e.g. β-guanidinopropionic acid), and other unidentified factors (e.g. certain extracellular matrix proteins).

lactate increases with growth and maturation, accompanied by increased oxidative capacity.[113]

Non-myogenic factors

In addition to the underlying myogenic lineage, additional factors influence muscle fiber phenotype. Muscle fibers are syncytial (multinucleated), with their myonuclei arranged peripherally throughout the length of the fiber. The volume of cytoplasm associated with a single nucleus is known as the myonuclear domain.[114] Each individual nucleus therefore determines the expression of proteins within a particular cytoplasmic region. In horses, myonuclear domains of type I fibers are smaller than those of IIX fibers, but similar in size to those of IIA fibers (Fig. 6.30).[23,114] These observations are related to the different activity patterns of the various fiber types: the more active type I fibers have a higher rate of both protein synthesis and protein turnover than the less frequently recruited, faster fiber types. The myonuclear domain size of equine muscle fibers depends on fiber type population rather than mitochondrial enzyme activities.[114,115] However, myosin isoform expression is not the sole protein determining mynouclear domain size, and other protein systems, such as mitochondrial proteins may be also important determinants.[115]

Neural input also has a significant influence on muscle fiber growth and type (fast/slow, glycolytic/oxidative) through altered regulation of gene expression. This is convincingly demonstrated by dramatic changes observed in muscles after denervation (Fig. 6.10, Fig. 6.31).[34,63,116] Additional factors that are known to influence myofiber diversity include hormonal and drug (anabolic steroid)-induced changes, that might vary depending on the underlying fiber type.[117] For example, chronic administration of clenbuterol, a β_2-adrenoceptor agonist primarily used for treating some respiratory diseases in the horse, with and without exercise, results in a significant change in MyHC profile toward the faster phenotype,[118] although not affecting the Ca^{2+}-activated contractile characteristics of isolated myofibers.[119] Of particular interest, and as discussed in the sections that follow, neuromuscular (contractile) activity associated with exercise and training has a significant impact on fiber type adaptation and the expression of fiber-specific protein isoforms. Neuromuscular electrical stimulation is used in horses to increase or maintain muscle strength during rehabilitation. However, no significant effects of this stimulus on fiber type characteristics and muscle enzyme activities have been found in horses.[120]

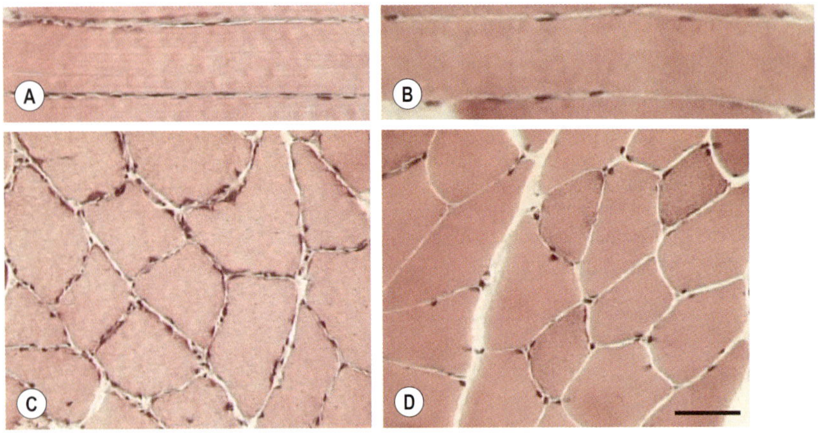

Fig 6.30 Representative images of longitudinal **(A and B)** and transverse **(C and D)** sections stained with hematoxylin and eosin of a muscle containing predominantly slow fibers (type I) (M. sacrocaudalis dorsalis medialis, **A and C**) compared with a muscle containing predominantly fast-contracting (type II) fibers (superficial region of the M. longissimus lumborum, **B and D**). Note the higher myonuclear number in the fibers from the slow-contracting muscle compared with the fast-contracting muscle. Scale bar, 50 μm.

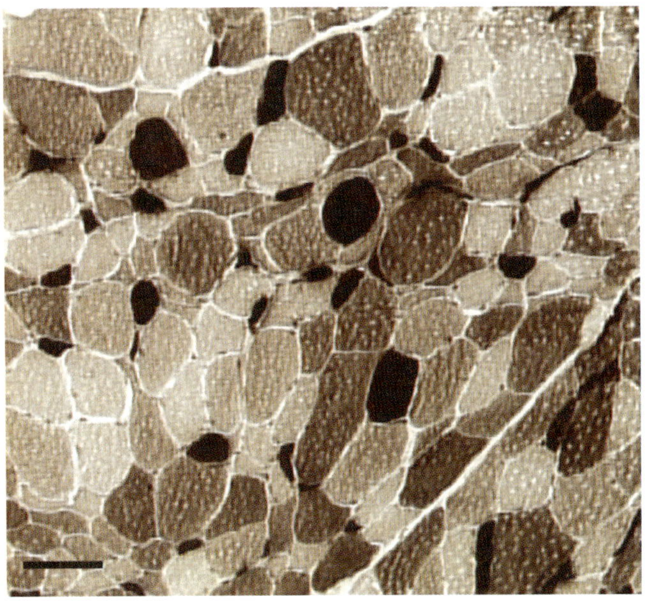

Fig 6.31 Transverse section of a M. vastus lateralis muscle sample from a horse with denervation atrophy (femoral nerve paralysis) stained with myofibrillar adenosine triphosphatase after acid pre-incubation. Note selective angular atrophy of some type I (black) and type IIA (white) fibers, while other type I and IIA fibers presumably belonging to other motor units are of normal size. Bar, 50 μm.

Responses to exercise

When aerobic metabolism can meet energy demands (during submaximal exercise), oxygen uptake correlates with increasing speed. However, the slope of the linear relationship varies according to the load, incline, track surface, and ambient temperature. At a certain point, energy demand outstrips oxygen uptake and the shortfall must be met by anaerobic metabolism. Muscle fatigue can occur during either aerobic or anaerobic exercise; in the following sections, we consider the major metabolic changes that occur within muscle that are believed to contribute to the development of fatigue.

Aerobic exercise

Muscle and liver glycogenolysis begins soon after the start of aerobic exercise. Glucose derived from the liver is subsequently transported into myofibers to join the glycolytic cascade via glucose-6-phosphate formation (see Fig. 6.17). However, although elevated glucose-6-phosphate concentrations have been detected after submaximal exercise in horses, circulating epinephrine (adrenaline) released during exercise stimulates the release of FFAs from adipose tissue, liver stores or both, which partially inhibit glucose utilization during moderate-intensity exercise.[121] Nevertheless, during prolonged submaximal exercise, blood glucose can still account for up to 25% of the total energy output.[68] This reliance on glucose, derived mainly from the liver, results in an early sparing of muscle glycogen. As energy demands increase, higher rates of pyruvate oxidation tend to cause a further shift towards FFA β-oxidation. The overall effect is that muscle glycogenolysis declines over time during aerobic exercise, whereas FFA oxidation increases.[70]

Although lipids are the predominant fuel utilized during prolonged submaximal exercise, fatigue occurs long before the complete utilization of lipid stores.[5] At submaximal workloads, fatigue has been associated with intramuscular glycogen depletion (Fig. 6.32)[68] because FFA oxidation cannot produce sufficient ATP without a source of pyruvate. During prolonged activity, glycogen depletion patterns occur in parallel with the progressive recruitment of fiber types, i.e. occurring initially in type I fibers, then in IIA, and finally in glycolytic IIX (see Fig. 6.26). This depletion (at least during submaximal long term exercise) affects the acid-soluble form of glycogen (macroglycogen) to a greater extent than the acid-insoluble form (proglycogen).[122] Muscular fatigue then does not occur at the same time in all fibers but in a progressive manner that results in gradual compromise to performance. Following exercise, glycogen replenishment occurs in the reverse order (i.e. IIX → IIA → I) and can take up to 72 hours.[117,123] If the time between exercise sessions during training is too short, the recovery period will be inadequate for complete restoration of muscle glycogen.[123] A faster replenishment of muscle glycogen stores can be obtained in the horse with certain feeding strategies[124] or with intravenous glucose supplementation,[125] oral acetate supplementation,[126] and postexercise rehydratation using a hypotonic electrolyte solution.[127] However, although ingestion of starch-rich meals after exercise increases glucose kinetics, it fails to enhance muscle glycogen replenishment in horses.[128] The apparently slower rate of glycogen synthesis after exercise in horses in comparison with other species likely reflects the lack of increased GLUT-4 expression reported by some authors after grain feeding and exercise,[129] as well as with a lack of post-exercise increase in insulin sensitivity.[130] Nevertheless, strenuous exercise causes an increase in total content of GLUT-4 protein in skeletal muscle: an increase that is attenuated by replenishing muscle glycogen stores through glucose infusion.[131] However,

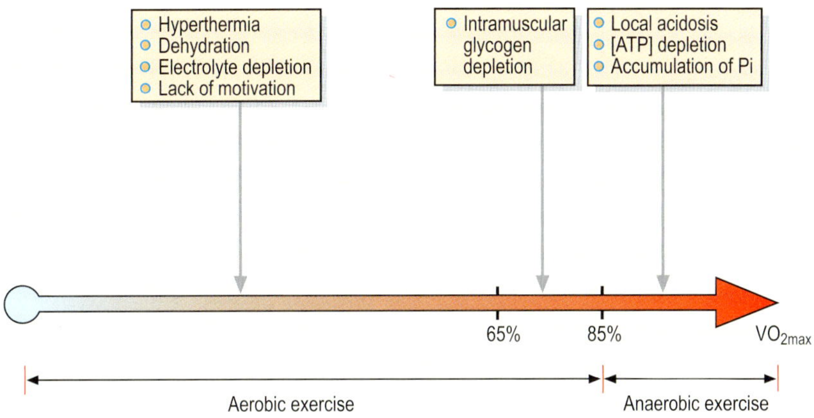

Fig 6.32 Schematic diagram summarizing the main causes of fatigue during or after exercise of different intensity and duration. Intramuscular glycogen depletion is considered to be the main cause of fatigue during aerobic exercise (workloads between 65% and 85% of $\dot{V}O_{2max}$). At lower exercise intensities however, hyperthermia, fluid and electrolyte depletion, and poor motivation have been suggested to be the primary factors in initiating fatigue. Causes of fatigue during supramaximal anaerobic exercise include local acidosis, ATP depletion, and accumulation of pyrophosphates (Pi).

although glycogen depletion appears to play a major role in fatigue onset during aerobic exercise, a variety of other factors is also implicated, including AMP deamination, hyperthermia, dehydration, electrolyte depletion, and lack of motivation.[132] The onset of fatigue itself is hard to assess objectively but evidence suggests that electromyography can be useful in the experimental setting.[43]

Aerobic exercise in the horse is also associated with decreased serum[122] and muscle[133] branched-chain amino acid concentrations, and the oral administration of a protein/amino acid supplement within 1 h after exercise increases intramuscular amino acid pools.[133] Also, administration of amino acids following exercise accelerates the rate of synthesis of muscle protein, and this effect is enhanced when combined with glucose, because of increasing insulin secretion or a decreased requirement for amino acids for energy.[134]

Additionally, increased oxygen utilization during exercise results in proportional increases in reactive oxygen species (ROS) production, potentially causing oxidative stress, a state where increased generation of ROS overwhelms body antioxidant protection, resulting in lipid, protein, and DNA damage.[135] Intense endurance exercise in horses also induces an increase of the muscle activity of the strong oxidant enzyme myeloperoxidase.[18] In response to oxidative stress, cells synthesize heat shock proteins in protective homeostatic responses.[135,136] However, a moderate bout of aerobic exercise in horses, though associated with mild muscle damage and potentially mild oxidative stress, failed to induce this defense mechanism,[137] perhaps because acidosis rather than energy depletion, appears to be the instigator of this response after long-term moderate-intensity exercise.[135] Recent studies have suggested that alpha-lipoic acid supplementation can enhance muscle protection through a decreased exercise-induced oxidative stress in skeletal muscle.[138,139]

Anaerobic exercise

The functional demands imposed by high-intensity exercise require the recruitment of most motor units within a given muscle, while intramuscular glycogen and blood glucose act as the predominant fuels to replenish ATP during anaerobic glycolysis. Some ATP is derived from the deamination of adenosine nucleotides; however, in contrast to aerobic metabolism, there is relatively little reliance on FFA oxidation. The effects of high-intensity exercise on horse skeletal muscle and development of fatigue have been comprehensively reviewed by Snow & Valberg.[5] Further research has confirmed many previous observations and provided new insight on mechanisms underlying the onset of fatigue.

Lactate accumulation and pH decline

Limitations imposed by oxidative metabolism result in more pyruvate (the end-product of glycolysis) being converted to lactate rather than acetyl-CoA; in the process, NAD is used to regenerate more ATP. As a consequence, muscle lactate concentrations increase during anaerobic exercise.[102,103,140] This rise is correlated with the proportion of type II fibers within muscles.[141] Initially, intracellular lactate accumulation is removed from the cell by active transport into the blood (Fig. 6.18, Fig. 6.33). Thus, monocarboxylate transporters facilitate the transport of lactate across the sarcolemma.[142] Saturation of this mechanism results in a sudden exponential rise in intracellular lactate accumulation known as the anaerobic threshold, that generally occurs when the plasma lactate concentration reaches about 4 mmol/L. Recent studies support the view that lactate transport activity in muscles varies between fibers (as with red blood cells).[142,143] These studies are consistent with suggestion that exercise performance is enhanced when glycolytic muscle has an improved ability to remove cellular lactate from within the contracting myofibers.[144]

The rise in intracellular lactate, together with free H^+ ions, significantly lowers the cytoplasmic pH, a factor believed to be the major cause of fatigue during anaerobic exercise (see Fig. 6.32).[68] Muscle pH can decline to as low as 6.25–6.50 and lead to impairment of both structure and function; for example, abnormal mitochondrial and SR ultrastructure has been documented in horses that exhibit fatigue during maximal exercise.[145] Low pH also leads to dysfunction of the excitation–contraction coupling mechanism, through impairment of SR calcium release via RYR1 channels, and decreased reuptake of calcium into the SR during relaxation.[146] Additionally, low pH inhibits the glycolytic enzyme phosphofructokinase, thereby diminishing ATP production.[141]

A fall in cytoplasmic pH is partially overcome by a buffering system within myofibers (see Fig. 6.33). Dynamic buffering of H^+ occurs during the hydrolysis of phosphocreatine in reactions catalyzed by creatine kinase and by glutamine synthetase; static physicochemical buffering is provided by various proteins, bicarbonate, inorganic phosphate, and carnosine.[141,145] Race horses have a higher muscle buffering capacity than humans, thought to be associated with their myofibers having high carnosine concentrations.[82] Muscle carnosine content appears to be influenced by β-alanine bioavailability and is greatest in glycolytic IIX fibers.[82]

Nucleotide depletion

Since initial observations by Snow and co-workers,[147] numerous studies confirm a decline in muscle ATP concentration during

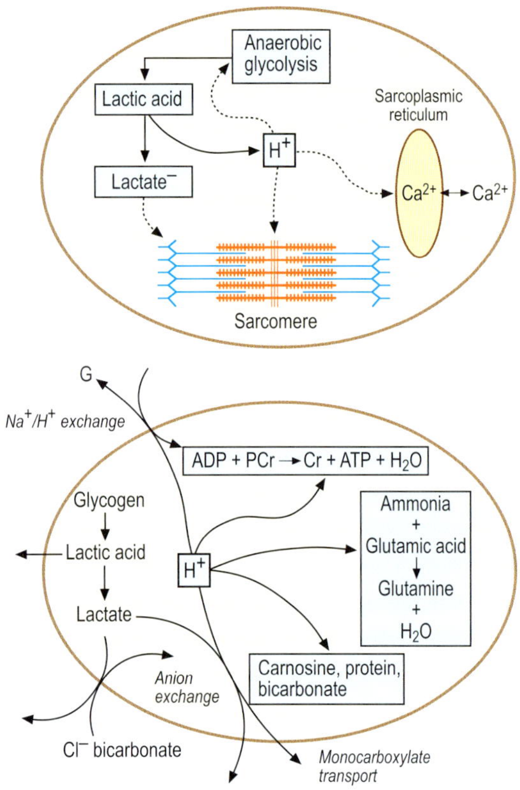

Fig 6.33 Schematic diagrams illustrating intramuscular acidosis and buffering capacity of muscle (according to [214]). (Top) Performance inhibition (dotted arrows) caused by the accumulation of protons and lactate anions. (Bottom) Diagram summarizing the major regulatory mechanisms that control intramuscular pH (explained in[214]).
PCr, phosphocreatine; Cr, creatine.

anaerobic exercise,[20,80,102] suggesting that ATP regeneration might be insufficient to meet energy demands.[82] Depletion of muscle ATP concentration has also been implicated as a primary cause of fatigue during maximal effort in horses,[68] and a correlation between muscle nucleotide stores after racing and performance has recently been reported.[80] The fall in ATP occurs in parallel with a rise in IMP concentration,[80,147] the latter being a particularly prominent response in equine muscle due to high underlying AMP deaminase activity. High concentrations of IMP within muscle therefore act as a marker for depletion of total nucleotide stores, given that reamination of IMP to ADP and finally restoration of ATP is a slow process that may take up to an hour.[148] ATP depletion, and formation of IMP within muscles working maximally, are closely correlated with the production of ammonia,[103,140] uric acid[147] and allantoin,[68] all of which may be detected in the plasma. Theoretically, low levels of ATP in some fibers would impair the optimal functioning of all ATP-dependent muscular processes. However, because nucleotide depletion occurs concurrently with a rise in muscle lactate and free H^+ concentrations,[80] it is still unclear which of these mechanisms plays the more significant role in the development of fatigue.

Glycogen depletion

Muscle glycogen concentration declines rapidly during maximal exercise[141,147] to an extent that varies between 30% and 50% of initial concentrations depending on the number and frequency of exercise bouts.[148] Glycogen depletion occurs most rapidly in the glycolytic low oxidative IIX fibers simultaneously with lactate production.[5] Although glycogen depletion is not considered to be a major factor contributing to fatigue during anaerobic exercise,[68] its depletion is associated with diminished anaerobic power generation and hence the capacity for high-intensity exercise.[149]

Other muscular changes

Other factors, though not necessarily contributing directly to fatigue, result in reduced performance and are reviewed by Snow & Valberg[5] and include increased intracellular potassium concentration, a stoichiometrically altered proportion of free carnitine and acetylcarnitine, increased formation of alanine from pyruvate, and significant changes in the free intracellular amino acid pool.[5,150,151] Additional factors that are implicated include a reduction in calcium SR uptake through decreased Ca^{2+}-ATPase activity, increased Na^+/K^+ ATPase concentration,[81,152] and a rise in muscle temperature that occurs during high-intensity exercise.[146] High intensity exercise also results in a transient increase in the expression of inflammatory cytokines in muscle and blood.[153]

Molecular responses to exercise in muscle

Recent studies have shown that different exercise protocols elicit variable transcriptional responses in key exercise-relevant genes in equine skeletal muscle due to variation in metabolic demand.[154–156] Overall, these studies reveal novel genes and mechanisms that are temporarily expressed following exercise and provide new information about the early and late molecular responses to exercise in the equine skeletal muscle transcriptome. For example, in a study characterizing global mRNA expression profiles in equine skeletal muscle using an equine-specific microarray platform, only two genes had increased expression immediately after exercise; however, four hours after end of exercise 932 genes had increased and 562 genes had decreased expression.[154] Functional analysis of genes differentially expressed during this recovery phase revealed an over-representation of genes localized to the actin cytoskeleton, with functions relating to MAPK signaling, focal adhesion, insulin signaling, mTOR signaling, p53 signaling and pathways relevant to type II diabetes mellitus.[154] Immediately after exercise, there was over-expression of genes involved in the stress response, metabolism and intracellular signaling.[154] Together, these findings suggest that protein synthesis, mechanosensation and muscle remodeling contribute to skeletal muscle adaptation towards improved integrity and hypertrophy.

Muscular responses to training

Overview

The adaptation of equine skeletal muscle during training is largely mediated by the structural and functional plasticity of myofibers. These long-term adaptations occur independently from the immediate or short-term physiologic responses to either aerobic or anaerobic exercise and are associated with altered rates and regulation of transcription of specific genes and consequently, a change in the amount or specific isoform of proteins expressed within individual fibers.

Depending on the nature (type, frequency, intensity, and duration) of the stimulus (exercise training), the adaptive response can take the form of: (*i*) hypertrophy, when myofibers increase in size but otherwise retain their basal structural, physiologic, and biochemical properties; or (*ii*) remodeling without hypertrophy, where myofibers do not enlarge but acquire markedly different enzymatic and structural characteristics, often accompanied by changes in the microvasculature; or (*iii*) a mixed response, i.e. remodeling in conjunction with hypertrophy (Fig. 6.34). Furthermore, the modality and amplitude of the response depend significantly on the basal muscle profile before training[157] because the increased contractile activity that is associated with training induces a change towards slow and oxidative muscle profiles. Hence fast-twitch fibers (and therefore muscles that contain a higher proportion of glycolytic fibers) can show a relatively greater training adaptation than slow-twitch fibers. This response is particularly prominent in young, inactive[158] and aged, sedentary horses,[159] which have a high percentage of glycolytic (low oxidative) pure IIX fibers (Fig. 6.35A,B), in contrast to active mature horses, which have muscle fiber type profiles that are more oxidative (Fig. 6.35C,D). Although it can be hard to differentiate altered fiber properties caused by growth and training, specific training effects have been delineated in growing foals,[106,107,160] and young horses.[96,97,158,161–163] Thus, the muscular response to training at an early age can be interpreted with knowledge of muscle characteristics.[106] Overall, muscular adaptations with training have important physiological implications that influence power generation, shortening velocity and resistance to fatigue.[164]

Muscular adaptations to training

Muscle fiber size

The effects of training on equine muscle fiber size are still controversial. In general, the adaptive response of equine skeletal muscle to early and long-term exercise training takes the form of remodeling with minimal, if any, muscle fiber hypertrophy (see references[5,164] for reviews). However, specific muscle fiber hypertrophy can be stimulated with bursts of high-resistance muscle activity.[15,96,97,165] Weight bearing, as a form of progressive-resistance exercise training, has been investigated in ponies for improving strength, and resulted in increased muscle power, muscle size, and increased (though not statistically significant) type II fiber cross-sectional area, without parallel changes in MyHC composition.[165] Six months of conventional jump training in competitive show-jumpers also induced a selective hypertrophy of type II fibers, with minimal switching between myofiber phenotypes.[164] Other longitudinal studies have also reported significant and early (less than three months) increases in the mean cross-sectional areas of type I and/or IIA fibers after training,[15,75,95,97,104,158,166–168] a result also noted in horses less than a year of age.[160] A marked and generalized fiber hypertrophy (~50%) was documented in endurance-trained Arabians performing moderate-intensity exercise (~80% of $\dot{V}O_{2max}$) of long duration (50–80 minutes per day), four days/week for three months.[168]

In Thoroughbred racehorses, exercises of short-moderate duration (5–15 min) and high-intensity (velocities eliciting a blood lactate concentration of 4 mmol/l) applied for only three weeks can induce fiber type hypertrophy.[169] Even though a fiber transition occurs towards more oxidative fibers (IIX → IIA → I) with normally smaller cross-sectional area (see Table 6.1), the hypertrophy may represent either the new fibers retaining size characteristics of their previous type, or generalized increased protein production (or both). In contrast, other studies of Standardbreds and Thoroughbreds reveal minimal changes[21,170,171] or even a reduction in fiber cross-sectional area.[161,172–174] These observations are hard to reconcile with the prominent increase in muscle mass, especially in the hindquarters, generally observed in horses after most training programs.[7,128,165] When considered together, the only explanation for an increase in muscle mass, despite either no change or a reduction in fiber size, is a parallel increase in the number of muscle fibers (hyperplasia), as previously demonstrated in humans.[175] Several recent studies indicate that horses in training have increased

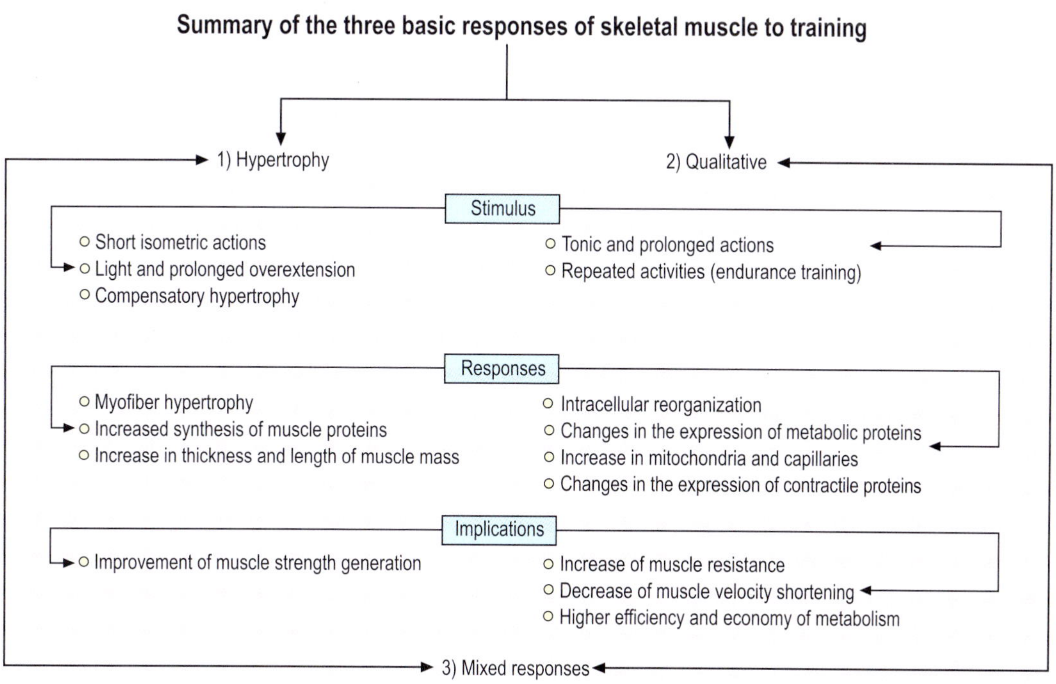

Fig 6.34 Summary of the three basic responses of skeletal muscle to training: (*i*) hypertrophy, (*ii*) remodeling without hypertrophy, and (*iii*) remodeling with hypertrophy. Possible stimuli and the nature of the responses and physiological implications are indicated.

rates of muscle protein synthesis in response to high-protein diets.[176–179]

Muscle fiber type transitions

Muscle fiber type distribution and MyHC composition are strongly influenced by training (Fig. 6.36, Fig. 6.37). Endurance training studies in horses reveal (by myofibrillar ATPase histochemistry, immunohistochemistry and electrophoresis), increases in the fraction of both type IIA and type IIAX fibers and a concomitant decrease in the proportion of IIX fibers.[15,75,84,86,95–97,104,158,159,168,169,172,173,180–183] Thus, a tendency towards increased percentages of type IIA fibres found in Thoroughbred racehorses has been attributed to training effects.[92] In addition, several endurance training studies in horses reveal fiber transitions beyond type IIA fibers: i.e. an increase in hybrid I+IIA fibers and pure type I fibers.[95,96,170] Fiber type transitions during resistance training appear to resemble qualitatively, those observed in endurance training. Hence, strength training in horses results in both increased IIA : IIX fiber ratio[164] and, when training is long enough, the I : II fiber ratio.[97] Similarly, sprint training in horses results in increased numbers of type IIA and decreased numbers of type IIX fibers, with a corresponding change in their respective MyHC content.[75,169,174,183] In contrast to endurance and strength training, a specific decrease of type I fibers has been reported as an early, and probably transitory, response to high-intensity training.[174]

When these various training studies are considered in combination, it is reasonable to assume that fiber type transitions occur in

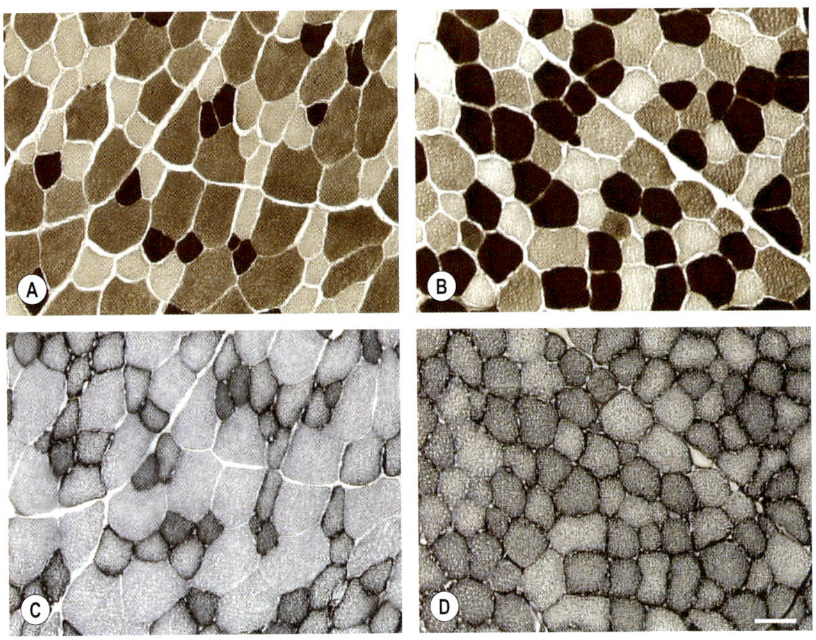

Fig 6.35 Transverse serial sections of gluteus medius muscle biopsies stained with myofibrillar ATPase after acid pre-incubation at pH 4.45 **(A and B)** and succinate dehydrogenase **(C and D)** in a young adult (3-year-old) and untrained Andalusian **horse (A and C)**, and in an adult and regularly trained (10-year-old) Andalusian horse **(B and D)**. Note that the young animal has a lower proportion of type I fibers and a higher percentage of low-oxidative type IIX fibers than the adult horse; furthermore, differences in fiber size are much more pronounced in the young animal than in the adult. This therefore may explain the broader range of adaptive responses to training in young unfit horses than in adults or regularly trained animals. Bar, 50 μm.

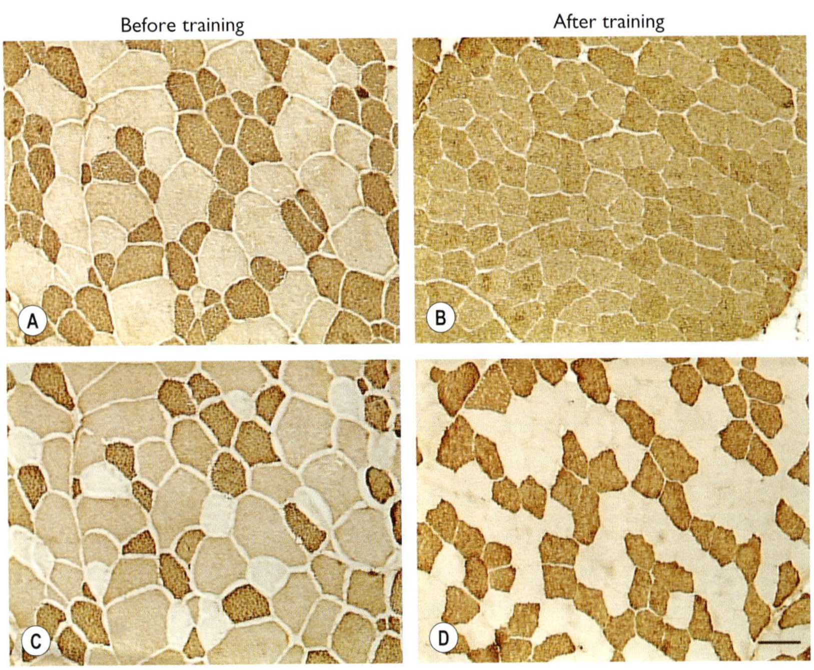

Fig 6.36 Transverse serial sections of M. gluteus medius biopsies (depth, 6 cm) of the same horse before **(A and C)** and after **(B and D)** a long-term endurance training program (nine months in total). **(A and B)** Sections are stained by immunohistochemistry with a monoclonal antibody to types I or IIA myosin heavy chain isoforms; note that almost all muscle fibers express either or both of these isoforms after training. **(C and D)** The same sections stained by immunohistochemistry with a monoclonal antibody specific to type IIA myosin heavy chain isoform; note the significant increase in the number of fibers expressing this isoform after nine months of training. Scale, 50 μm. Details of the training program are described in the study by Serrano et al.[96]

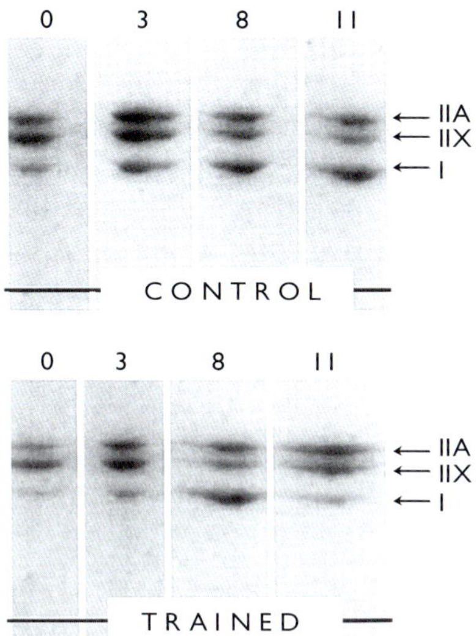

Fig 6.37 Eight percent sodium dodecyl sulfate polyacrylamide gel electrophoresis of muscle samples from the gluteus medius muscle of a control horse (upper row) and a trained horse (bottom row) throughout an experiment to investigate the effects of prolonged endurance exercise training and detraining program. 0, pre-training; 3 and 8, after three and eight months of training; 11, after a further three months of detraining. More details of the experiment in reference.[97] The three myosin heavy chain isoforms are identified as I, IIA, and IIX. Note the effect of training on the relative densities of the I and IIX bands, indicating a fiber type transition in the order IIX → IIA → I.

a graded and orderly sequential manner and typically change from faster, more glycolytic fibers to slower and more oxidative fiber types, i.e. IIX → IIAX → IIA → IIA+I → I.[157] A dose–response relationship between the duration (in total) of the training program and the magnitude of induced changes has recently been demonstrated at the molecular level.[96,97] This relationship can be explained more readily in terms of a threshold for the type IIX → IIA transition during the early phase of training, and then a further threshold for the type IIA → type I transition. Thus, a single fiber is capable of a complete fast-to-slow transformation in response to a sufficiently long physiological training stimulus. Finally, although many reports describe the training response shown by muscle fibers in terms of the MyHC component, it is important to remember that many other protein isoforms of the sarcomere (such as the regulatory proteins of the thin filaments) and the calcium regulatory proteins of the SR change in parallel.[184]

Metabolic changes and increased capillary density

Perhaps the most commonly detected and earliest muscular adaptation to training is an increase in the activity of enzymes of aerobic metabolism, such as selected enzymes of the TCA cycle, the electron transport chain and fat oxidation.[75,86,96,99,108,158–160,185–187] These changes are associated with increased mitochondrial and capillary densities (Fig. 6.38),[15,95,169,181,188,189] the latter response promoting improved oxygen diffusion and more expeditious removal of waste products (such as CO_2).

The activities of key anaerobic enzymes, such as phosphofructokinase and lactate dehydrogenase, either do not change or decrease following training.[75,96,99,187,190] However, high-intensity training (~80–100% of $\dot{V}O_{2max}$, 5 minutes × 2, 5 days/week for 12–16 weeks)

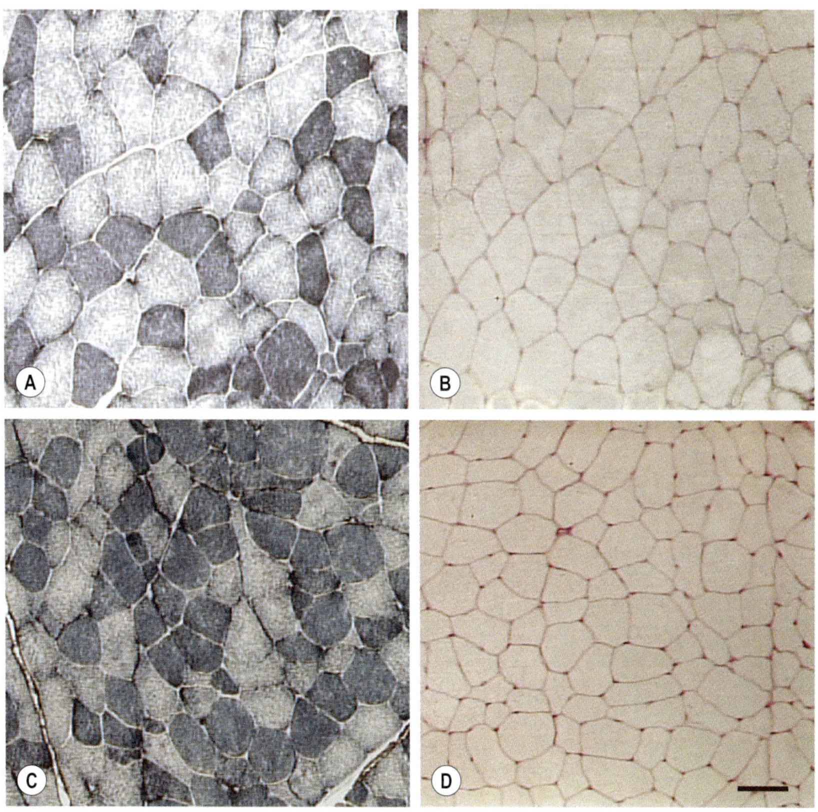

Fig 6.38 Transverse serial sections of muscle biopsy samples from the M. gluteus medius from the same horse taken before **(A and B)** and after **(C and D)** nine months of prolonged endurance training. **(A and C)** Sections are stained with succinate dehydrogenase to demonstrate the oxidative capacity of individual muscle fibers; note the increase in the number of fibers with dark staining after training. **(B and D)** Sections are stained with the α-amylase PAS to visualize capillaries; note the increased capillary density (e.g. number of capillaries per mm^2) after the training program. Scale, 75 μm.

for both young and adult Thoroughbreds did result in increased glycolytic phosphofructokinase enzyme activity.[191] Histochemical assessment of glycerol-3-phosphate dehydrogenase enzyme activity, an enzyme well correlated with other glycolytic enzymes, was also increased by exercise that consisted of alternating days of either high-intensity, short-duration (~100–140% of the speed that results in a blood lactate of 4 mmol/L (or V4) for 15 minutes) exercise or moderate-intensity, long-duration (~65% of V4, 60–90 minutes) exercise for a total of five weeks.[174] However, the activity of this enzyme did not change in adolescent Thoroughbreds after several conditioning programs of varying intensities and durations.[169]

Although training also causes increased AMP deaminase activity along with that of other purine nucleotide cycle enzymes, such as creatine kinase, the concentration of total nucleotide stores is usually not affected by training (discussed in reference[5]). Nevertheless, moderate-intensity (~55% of $\dot{V}O_{2max}$) and long-duration (60 minutes, over ~13–14 km) exercise for 10 consecutive days, increases muscle phosphocreatine concentration and reduces muscle creatine content at the point of fatigue.[190]

Training also results in a modest increase in muscle glycogen storage[96,104,171,186,192] that may well be associated with reduced activities of glycolytic enzymes, since the capacity to mobilize endogenous glycogen is partially influenced by the absolute activity of anaerobic enzymes expressed within muscle fibers.[5] In experimental animals, training increases the sensitivity of glucose uptake across the sarcolemma via increased GLUT-4 expression.[193] In horses, moderate-intensity exercise training increases middle gluteal muscle GLUT-4 protein content and glycogen synthase activity, and enhances whole body insulin sensitivity.[194–196] Thus, regular physical activity can mitigate risk of several disease conditions associated with insulin resistance in the horse.[195] The transfer of FFAs from the vascular to the intracellular compartment is also enhanced with endurance training, and is promoted by increased extracellular (interstitial) albumin concentration.[197] Finally, evaluation of the proteome of Standardbred horses at different stages of training involved structural changes towards a higher oxidative capacity, increased capacity to take up long-chain fatty acids, and a greater dependency on glycogen storage.[198]

Physiological adaptations and buffering capacity

Training has significant effects on the electrical and ionic membrane properties of equine skeletal muscle.[199–202] Short-term exercise training of moderate intensity results in an increase in the density of Na^+/K^+-ATPase pumps measured by ouabain-binding assays, together with attenuation in K^+ efflux from working muscles during high-intensity exercise.[199,200] Although the physiologic implication of these training-induced adaptations is unclear, enhanced ionic control at the sarcolemma may result in myofibers that are better able to respond to the rate of motor neuron discharge. Additional responses following physical conditioning include increased SR calcium uptake (Ca^{2+}-ATPase activity) and an attenuation of the exercise-induced decline of calcium uptake.

Several studies have reported an increase in buffering capacity of equine skeletal muscle after a few weeks of sprint training[181] and after prolonged (34 weeks) training.[186] This increase can be due to (*i*) increased incorporation of myofiber protein, (*ii*) increased creatine phosphate concentration, or (*iii*) higher muscle carnosine concentrations,[141] although with regard to the latter, no differences in carnosine concentration were found in muscle from either trained or untrained Thoroughbreds.[203] Recent results suggest that the content of lactate transporters increases after high-intensity training (3 min at 90–110% of $\dot{V}O_{2max}$ for 18 weeks) in skeletal muscle of Thoroughbred racehorses.[187]

Other training consequences

Training increases the expression of heat shock proteins,[135] and splice variants of neuronal nitric oxide synthase,[84] which protect muscle cells from exercise-induced oxidative stress. Furthermore, the reported apoptosis that occurs in trained equine skeletal muscle[204] probably promotes the work/recovery/rebound/supercompensation cycle, when unconditioned muscle cells undergo programmed cell death, to be replaced by new, stronger cells. In fact, training attenuates exercise-induced ultrastructural damage in equine skeletal muscle,[159] probably via a parallel fiber type transition, myofiber hypertrophy or increased satellite cell activation (or perhaps all three).

Overtraining

Overtraining is a syndrome that has been recognized as a cause of poor performance in racehorses over the course of both high-intensity and prolonged (more than four months) training.[15,186,205,206] However, clinical signs of overtraining are accompanied by relatively few characteristic changes in skeletal muscle. In the study by Tyler and associates,[15] overtraining caused significant type IIA fiber atrophy (~8%), a decrease in type IIA: IIX mATPase fiber ratio, and increased mitochondrial volume in type I (~16%) and type II (~39%) fibers, accompanied by an increase in $\dot{V}O_{2max}$ (~8%). As a

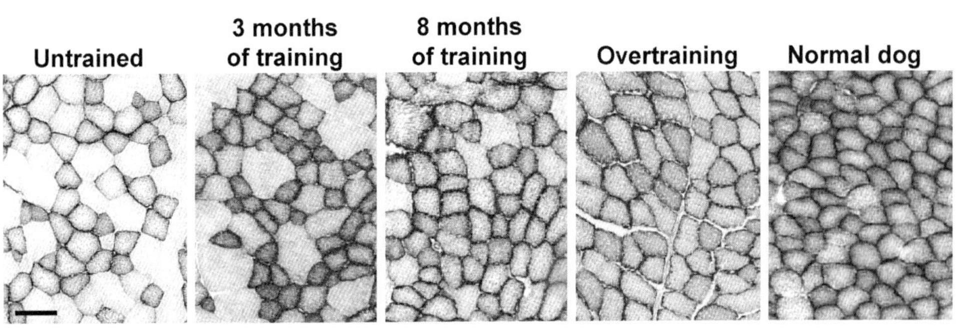

Fig 6.39 Cryosections of the M. gluteus medius stained for succinate dehydrogenase activity to demonstrate the oxidative capacity of individual myofibers of an endurance horse with clinical signs of overtraining due to heavy overload and prolonged (more than one year) training. Microphotograph is compared with equivalent images of muscles samples from untrained and trained horses and with a sample, also from the M. gluteus medius, of an untrained dog. Note the more uniform staining pattern in muscle from the overtrained horse in comparison with the untrained and trained horse samples, a pattern that is somewhat similar to that seen in normal canine muscle. Bar scale, 50 μm.

consequence, muscle fibers of overtrained horses are generally highly oxidative (Fig. 6.39). Additional metabolic adaptation of overtrained muscle includes ATP depletion[205] and reduced resting glycogen concentration,[186] though this latter finding may relate to delayed glycogen replenishment seen in normal horses, particularly given that glycogen utilization during exercise itself is not influenced by overtraining.[186] In overtrained horses, quantitative needle electromyography results in a significant increment of motor unit activation despite a 19% decrease in performance.[44] In addition to structural changes observed in the proteome of Standardbred horses associated with normal training, intensified training (overtraining) leads to additional protein changes.[198] For example, alpha-1-titrypsin is found in serum increased after intensified training but not after normal training.[198] This protein might thus be considered as a marker of overtraining in horses.

Detraining

Maintenance of the trained muscle signature during inactivity is more prolonged in horses than other athletic species, lasting throughout 5–6 weeks of inactivity,[15,171,173] although not beyond 12 weeks.[27,95,96] Researchers have suggested that expression of the MyHC-IIX gene constitutes a default setting that may be altered (decreased) by chronic increased contractile activity (i.e. training), and compensated for by increased expression of MyHC-IIA.[207] In line with this hypothesis is the observation that a return to sedentary activity levels following a prolonged endurance training period, normalizes the expression of MyHC-IIX, via a slow-to-fast fiber type transformation in the order I → IIA → IIX (see Fig. 6.37).[96] These detraining-induced changes in MyHC phenotype parallel a reversion of the muscle's size and return of the muscle's metabolic and capillary characteristics to pre-training levels.[96] In summary, fiber sizes decrease, together with a decline in mitochondrial density, aerobic enzyme activities and glycogen content, and normalization of anaerobic enzyme activities. Expression of lactate transporters (increased after 18 weeks of high-intensity training) also returns to the pretraining level after six weeks of detraining.[187]

Possible mechanisms underlying muscular adaptations to training

Skeletal muscle responds to altered functional demands by specific quantitative and/or qualitative alterations in gene expression (Fig. 6.40), provided the stimuli are of sufficient magnitude and duration.[184] Repeated or persistent elevation of neuromuscular activity (i.e. during exercise and training) induces a series of concerted changes in gene expression, evoking either myofiber hypertrophy or myofiber remodeling, or both. In general, exercise training in horses results in coordinate changes in the gene expression of functional groups of genes related to metabolism, oxidative phosphorylation and muscle structure.[208]

Recent data have highlighted the roles of genes responsible for the regulation of oxygen-dependent metabolism, glucose metabolism and fatty acid utilization in equine skeletal muscle adaptation to exercise training.[155] Myofiber hypertrophy is generally characterized by a coordinated increase in abundance (per fiber) of most protein constituents. To some extent this process includes the selective and transient activation of specific genes immediately following the onset of work overload. The major events underlying muscle hypertrophy however, involve a general and non-specific augmentation of protein synthesis within cells. Remodeling of myofiber phenotype, with minimal or no hypertrophy, is the typical muscular response to prolonged training in the horse.[96] During this type of adaptation, myofibers undergo striking reorganization, with selective activation and repression of many genes, and switching between different myofibrillar isoproteins occurring in a graded and orderly sequential manner.[184] These changes occur in parallel, but not simultaneously over time, and correspond to the changes observed in enzymatic profiles, cytosolic proteins, and membrane receptors and transporters.

The complexity and pleiotropic nature of the physical and metabolic stimuli presented to myofibers during contraction that ultimately results in altered gene regulation were reviewed by Williams & Neufer.[209] Acetylcholine released from motor neurons, and other signaling molecules of neural origin, bind to cell surface receptors on myofibers, triggering intracellular events that may be linked to altered gene expression (Fig. 6.41). Additional signals are probably derived from contraction-induced mechanical stress perturbing the sarcolemma and extracellular matrix, thus exerting tension via intermediate filaments on the cytoskeleton, organelles, and nucleus. Changes in the intracellular concentrations of ions and metabolites

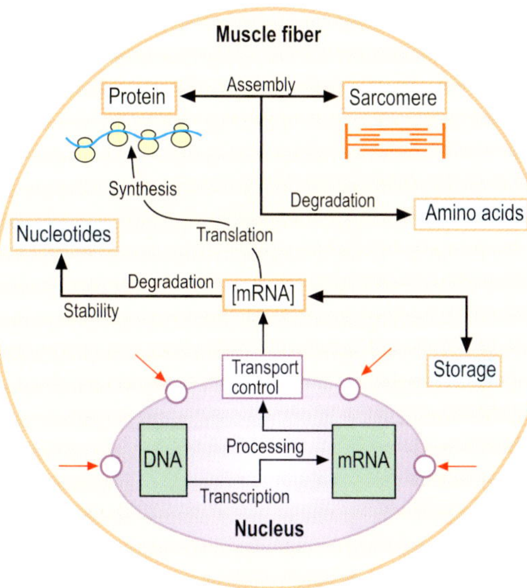

Fig 6.40 Schematic diagram showing different steps in the regulation of gene expression in skeletal muscle associated with increased contractile activity.

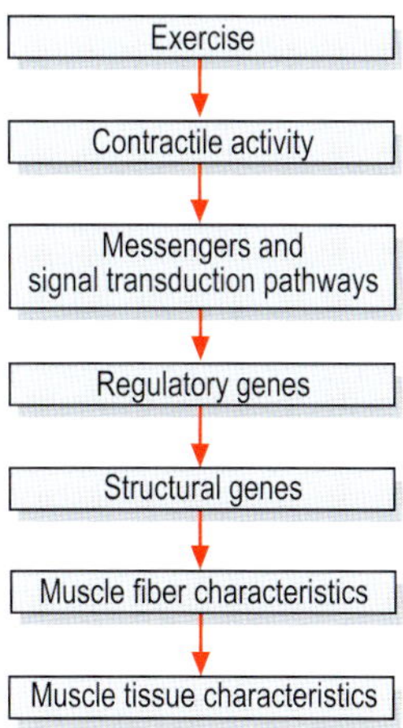

Fig 6.41 Steps in the cascade of events by which exercise and increased neuromuscular activity lead to physiologically relevant changes in the characteristics of skeletal muscle.

during repeated muscle contraction are also implicated in the activation of signaling pathways. These signals include intracellular calcium, hydrogen ions produced during anaerobic exercise, the marked reduction in phosphorylation potential of the adenylate system ([ATP]/[ADP_{free}]), a depletion of the redox state (NADH/NAD), and hypoxia. Among all these factors, an imbalance between energy requirement and energy supply is possibly the most important signal that triggers appropriate adjustment of contractile and metabolic protein expression.[210] Finally, recent years have seen significant advances in our understanding of the signaling mechanism by which the information contained in specific action potential patterns alters transcription within muscle fiber nuclei.[211] Specific genes known to undergo altered expression following contractile activity include those encoding sarcomeric and cytosolic proteins and enzymes of the glycolytic pathway, TCA cycle, electron transport chain, and fat oxidation. Additionally, signals inducing the expression of proteins derived from mitochondrial genes are coordinated with the activation of the various nuclear genes that encode mitochondrial proteins.

The factors that promote angiogenesis in skeletal muscle in response to training have not been clarified, although they may be related to a chronic increase in muscle capillary blood flow and the corresponding endothelial shear stress, as well as increased capillary wall tension.[212] Hudlicka and colleagues speculated that endothelial stress may disturb the luminal surface, resulting in the release of bound proteases that damage the basement membrane and contribute to an increase in basic fibroblast growth factor release.[212] Subsequently, growth factors may enhance vascular growth and satellite cell proliferation.[213] Still unclear, however, is the influence of training intensity and duration on neovascularization and the mechanisms that underlie the increase seen in intramuscular substrates in response to long-term endurance training. These latter adaptations may be related to either (*i*) increased glucose and FFA availability (via GLUT-4 and albumin respectively), (*ii*) a lower utilization of these substrates for energy production, or (*iii*) possible artifacts imposed by experimental design (i.e. they might be a reflection of increased dietary intake of soluble starches and fat from a parallel change in diet in horses in training).

Implications of training-induced changes to the physiologic response to exercise

The main physiologic consequence of increased muscle mass in response to training is to produce a muscle with a greater peak force capacity, because force output is proportional to total cross-sectional area of the fiber mass recruited. At slow speeds, this adaptation has an impact on gait, causing a marked reduction of both stance time and stride duration.[104] This adaptation significantly affects the performance of showjumpers via enhanced power output from the hindquarters.[164] Furthermore, because increased power output results in a greater ability to accelerate and increase stride length, these training adaptations (strength rather than endurance) are important for racehorses competing over short distances.[5] However, enhanced power through training comes with the cost of a corresponding decline in aerobic potential, because the increased mass of recruited fibers and concomitant rise in ATP utilization occur simultaneously with a relative inability of oxygen to diffuse into the larger fibers.[173]

From a physiologic standpoint, remodeling of myofiber phenotype with minimal or with no hypertrophy in response to training, produces a muscle that is much more resistant to fatigue but with decreased maximal shortening velocity, the former corresponding to each myofiber's increased oxidative capacity, and the latter to the increased expression of slow MyHC and other contractile protein isoforms.[17] In a similar but reciprocal fashion to that described for strength training, some conventional training programs of young racehorses, produce a decrease in the size of type II fibers[174] and a corresponding decline of both speed and force of contraction. Clearly a balance must be acquired at a level deemed most appropriate for the intended use of the horse (see below).

Following endurance training, exercise at submaximal intensity is facilitated by optimal delivery of oxygen and blood-borne substrates, early activation of oxidative metabolism with low utilization of endogenous carbohydrates, and increased reliance on fat oxidation as an energy source. The increased oxidative capacity observed in skeletal muscle after training occurs concurrently with increased maximum oxygen uptake[15] and a significant reduction in the net rate of muscle glycogenolysis and anaerobic metabolism.[190] As a consequence, in the trained state, the speed at which a horse begins to accumulate lactate increases gradually (i.e. there is a delay in the onset of lactate accumulation and ATP depletion).[68,162,163] This is accompanied by enhanced muscle buffering capacity and more efficient excitation–contraction coupling. Hence, collectively, endurance may be enhanced by a wide variety of related factors that delay the onset of fatigue during anaerobic exercise. Although relative sparing of muscle glycogen underlies the delay in fatigue onset during this type of exercise in the trained state, it is likely that all the metabolic adaptations summarized above combine to increase endurance.

Although controversial, then, it is clear from extensive scientific literature that equine skeletal muscle has considerable potential to adapt during training, and overall, that these adaptations have important functional implications affecting stamina, strength and speed (Table 6.2). Ideally therefore, conditioning programs of athletic horses should promote characteristics that optimize equilibrium between these physiological traits. While interpreting Table 6.2, first note that certain changes occur together, whereas others occur independently. For example, reduced intrinsic muscle shortening velocity, occurs together with increased endurance capacity following IIX → IIA fiber transition, whereas increased aerobic muscle enzyme activities are never associated with decreased mitochondrial volume. Second, note that certain changes precede others; for instance, aerobic metabolic adaptation occurs prior to any structural adaptation. Thus significant increases in muscle glycogen concentration occur after only 10 consecutive days of training,[190] whilst a significant degree of type II → type I fiber type conversion needs much longer (8 months).[96] Third, adaptations are cumulative and dose-dependent,[169,183] but there is an upper limit above which further adaptations do not occur, even when the stimulus continues.[15] Most relevant training adaptations, then, occur in the first 3–4 months; prolonging training beyond this period – although improving aerobic capacity – reduces anaerobic capacity and has no effect on strength.[164] Simultaneously, the risk of overtraining increases. Finally, certain adaptations to training are reversible, tending to return to the pre-training situation when the stimulus is stopped.

The response of equine muscle to training therefore depends on two sets of factors: (*i*) the basal status of the muscle (determined by the breed, age, sex, and level of fitness of the horse), and (*ii*) the stimulus applied (i.e. type, intensity, duration, frequency, and volume of the training exercise). Unfortunately, little is known about the relative influence of most of these factors. For example, only a few studies compare muscular adaptations that occur with different training programs. Of these, two studies (with contradictory results) examine the influence of different exercise intensity,[181,185] and others have examined the combined influence of intensity and

Table 6.2 Summary of main muscular adaptations to training reported in horses and their functional significance for endurance, strength, and speed

	PHYSIOLOGICAL TRAIT			
MUSCULAR ADAPTATIONS	**STAMINA**	**STRENGTH**	**SPEED**	**REFERENCES**
Morphological adaptations				
Muscle fiber hypertrophy	–	+ + +	+	15, 75, 95, 96, 104, 158, 160, 163, 165–168
Muscle fiber atrophy	+	– – –	–	161, 172–174
Increased number of capillaries	+ + +	nc	nc	15, 96, 181, 188
Increased mitochondrial volume	+ + +	nc	nc	15
Increased myonuclear density	nc	+ + +	nc	Not reported in horses
Metabolic adaptations				
Increased aerobic muscle enzyme activities	+ + +	nc	nc	75, 96, 99, 108, 158–160, 185, 186
Increased glucose and fatty acid transport	+ + +	nc	nc	193, 194, 197
Increased muscle [glycogen] and its sparing during exercise	+ + +	nc	nc	96, 171, 174, 186, 192
Increased muscle [triglycerides]	+ + +	nc	nc	96
Decreased post-exercise muscle [lactate]	+ + +	nc	nc	68, 162, 163
Increased anaerobic muscle enzymes	nc	nc	+ + +	158, 174, 191
Decreased anaerobic muscle enzymes	nc	nc	– – –	75, 96, 99, 190
Increased muscle [high energy phosphate]	nc	nc	+ + +	190
Increased muscle buffering capacity	+	nc	+ + +	68, 162, 163
Contractile adaptations				
Unidirectional IIX→IIA→I fiber type (MyHC isoform) transition	+	nc	– – –	15, 75, 84, 95–97
Bidirectional IIX→IIA→I fiber type (MyHC isoform) transition	+	nc	– – –	174
Increase of IIA:IIX fiber type (MyHC isoform) ratio	+	nc	– – –	172, 173, 180–182
Increase of I:IIA fiber type (MyHC isoform) ratio	+	nc	– – –	97
Increase of IIA:I fiber type (MyHC isoform) ratio	–	nc	+ + +	174

+ + + and – – – = primary implication (positive and negative, respectively) towards the particular characteristic; + and – = secondary implication (positive and negative, respectively); nc = no contribution to the particular characteristic.

duration.[169,183,192] One of these latter studies concluded that low-intensity exercise (~50% of V4) for long duration (45 minutes) was, after six weeks, more effective in improving aerobic capacity exercise than high-intensity exercise (~100% of V4) of moderate duration (25 minutes). In adolescent Thoroughbreds, the short-term training-induced up-regulation of MyHC IIA isoform and down-regulation of MyHC-IIX isoform are more dependent on intensity than duration of exercise. However, protocols with exercise of moderate intensity and long duration can induce MyHC changes similar to those promoted by programs with exercise of higher intensities.[183] As previously noted, exercise of 5–15 min at v4 is necessary to enhance strength-related muscle adaptation in Thoroughbreds.[169]

From the comparative analyzes of several well-documented experimental studies (Table 6.3) it seems that moderate- to high-intensity (~80–100% of $\dot{V}O_{2max}$) exercise of short duration (5–10 minutes) improves both stamina and strength in racehorses following 12–16 weeks of training,[15,75,169] whereas anaerobic capacity can only be increased in the short to mid-term (up to 16 weeks), by introducing supramaximal intensity exercise(~100–150% of either $\dot{V}O_{2max}$ or V4) of short (two minutes) to moderate (15 minutes) duration.[158,174,191] Interestingly, adaptation occurs more readily in younger (~2-year-old) than in mature racehorses; for instance, muscle adaptations compatible with a combination of improved stamina, strength and speed were reported in young Thoroughbreds following exercise of high (~100% of $\dot{V}O_{2max}$) to very high (~165% of $\dot{V}O_{2max}$) intensity and short duration or distance (1.6–5.3 minutes; 1600–3600 meters) five days/week for 16 weeks.[158]

In general though, it seems clear that improved stamina through enhanced aerobic capacity is the most common response of equine skeletal muscle to training, regardless of either the basal status of the muscle or the exercise-training program. Given that many equestrian disciplines, including Thoroughbred racing, are largely aerobic in nature, this underlies the likely benefit of training to the equine athlete.

Table 6.3 Physiological implications of muscular adaptations in various training programs scientifically evaluated in horses

HORSES			CONDITIONING PROTOCOL			FUNCTIONAL SIGNIFICANCE			
BREED	**AGE**	**INTENSITY**	**DURATION (DISTANCE)**	**FREQUENCY**	**VOLUME**	**STAMINA**	**STRENGTH**	**SPEED**	**REFERENCE**
Thoroughbred	4–8 yr	~55% $\dot{V}O_{2max}$	60 min (~13–14 km)	Daily	10 days	+	ni	–	190
Thoroughbred	2–9 yr	~80% $\dot{V}O_{2max}$	3 min (1500 m) × 2	6 d/wk	6 wk	+	ni	–	181
Thoroughbred	5–7 yr	~80–100% $\dot{V}O_{2max}$	5 min (×2)	5 d/wk	12 wk	ne	ni	+ +	191
Thoroughbred	2–3 yr	~100–165% $\dot{V}O_{2max}$	1.6–5.3 min (1600–3200 m)	5 d/wk	16 wk	+ +	+	–	75
Thoroughbred	2 yr	~100–165% $\dot{V}O_{2max}$	1.6–5.3 min (1600–3200 m)	5 d/wk	16 wk	+ +	+	+	158
Standardbred	3–5 yr	~60–100% $\dot{V}O_{2max}$	6–12.5 min (~3–9 km)	5 d/wk	16 wk 32 wk	+ + + +	+ + +	ne –	15
Standardbred	2 yr	~100–140% V4 ~65% V4	15 min 60–90 min	2nd day 2nd day	5 wk	+	–	+	174
Arab	8.6 yr	~80% V4	50–80 min (~10–20 km)	3 d/wk	12 wk	+	+ + +	–	168
Andalusian	~4 yr	~25–30% V4 ~50–60% V4	45–60 min 75–120 min	5 d/wk	12 wk 32 wk	+ + + +	+ +	– –	96

Intensity is expressed as a fraction of either $\dot{V}O_{2max}$ (velocity at maximal aerobic capacity) or V4 (velocity inducing a blood lactate concentration of 4 mmol/L). The symbols + and – indicate that either the muscular adaptations to training had positive or negative effect respectively towards the particular characteristic; the number of symbols is proportional to the magnitude of the adaptation; ne = no effect; ni = not investigated.

References

1. Hinchcliff KW, Geor RJ. Integrative physiology of exercise. In: Hinchcliff KW, Kaneps AJ, Geor RJ, editors. Equine sports medicine and surgery. Basic and clinical sicences of the equine athlete. 1st ed. Edinburgh: Saunders; 2004. p. 3–8.
2. Rivero JL. Plyometric training for the development of strength in humans: principle and practice for its application in horses. In: Lindner A, editor. Applied equine nutrition and training. Wageningen: Wageningen Press; 2009. p. 139–68.
3. Kearns CF, McKeever KH, Abe T. Overview of horse body composition and muscle architecture: implications for performance. Vet J 2002;164:224–34.
4. Armstrong RB, Essen-Gustavsson B, Hoppeler H, et al. O2 delivery at VO2max and oxidative capacity in muscles of standardbred horses. J Appl Physiol 1992;73:2274–82.
5. Snow DH, Valberg SJ. Muscle anatomy, physiology and adaptations to exercise and training. In: Hodgson DR, Rose RJ, editors. The athletic horse: principles and practice of equine sports medicine. Philadelphia: Saunders; 1994. p. 145–79.
6. Rivero JL, Piercy RJ. Muscle physiology: responses to exercise and training. In: Hinchcliff KW, Kaneps AJ, Geor RJ, editors. Equine sports medicine and surgery. Basic and clinical sciences of the equine athlete. Edinburgh: Saunders; 2004. p. 45–76.
7. Rivero JL, Piercy RJ. Muscle physiology: responss to exercise and training. In: Hinchcliff KW, Geor RJ, Kaneps AJ, editors. Equine exercise physiology. The sicence of exercise in the athletic horse. Edinburg: Saunders Elsevier; 2008. p. 30–80.
8. Lindholm A, Piehl K. Fibre composition, enzyme activity and concentrations of metabolites and electrolytes in muscles of standardbred horses. Acta Vet Scand 1974;15:287–309.
9. Payne RC, Hutchinson JR, Robilliard JJ, et al. Functional specialisation of pelvic limb anatomy in horses (Equus caballus). J Anat 2005;206:557–74.
10. Robert C, Valette JP, Degueurce C, et al. Correlation between surface electromyography and kinematics of the hindlimb of horses at trot on a treadmill. Cells Tissues Organs 1999;165:113–22.
11. Crook TC, Wilson A, Hodson-Tole E. The effect of treadmill speed and gradient on equine hindlimb muscle activity. Equine Vet J 2010;42(Suppl. 38):412–16.
12. Lopez-Rivero JL, Serrano AL, Diz AM, et al. Variability of muscle fibre composition and fibre size in the horse gluteus medius: an enzyme-histochemical and morphometric study. J Anat 1992;181(Pt 1):1–10.
13. Stanley RL, Maile C, Piercy RJ. Storage-associated artefact in equine muscle biopsy samples. Equine Vet J 2009;41:82–6.
14. Barrey E, Bonnamy B, Barrey EJ, et al. Muscular microRNA expressions in healthy and myopathic horses suffering from polysaccharide storage myopathy or recurrent exertional rhabdomyolysis. Equine Vet J 2010;42(Suppl. 38): 303–10.
15. Tyler CM, Golland LC, Evans DL, et al. Skeletal muscle adaptations to prolonged training, overtraining and detraining in horses. Pflugers Arch 1998;436:391–7.
16. Mlekoday JA, Mickelson JR, Valberg SJ, et al. Calcium sensitivity of force production and myofibrillar ATPase activity in muscles from Thoroughbreds with recurrent exertional rhabdomyolysis. Am J Vet Res 2001;62: 1647–52.
17. Rome LC, Sosnicki AA, Goble DO. Maximum velocity of shortening of three fibre types from horse soleus muscle: implications for scaling with body size. J Physiol 1990;431:173–85.
18. Franck T, Votion DM, Ceusters J, et al. Specific immuno-extraction followed by enzymatic detection (SIEFED) of myeloperoxidase and mitochondrial complex I in muscular microbiopsies: preliminary results in endurance horses. Equine Vet J 2010;42(Suppl. 38): 296–302.
19. Votion DM, Fraipont A, Goachet AG, et al. Alterations in mitochondrial respiratory function in response to endurance training and endurance racing. Equine Vet J 2010;42(Suppl. 38): 268–74.
20. Harris DB, Harris RC, Wilson AM, et al. ATP loss with exercise in muscle fibres of the gluteus medius of the thoroughbred horse. Res Vet Sci 1997;63:231–7.
21. Rivero JL, Talmadge RJ, Edgerton VR. Correlation between myofibrillar ATPase activity and myosin heavy chain composition in equine skeletal muscle and the influence of training. Anat Rec 1996;246:195–207.
22. Tulloch LK, Perkins JD, Piercy RJ. Multiple immunofluorescence labelling enables simultaneous identification of all mature fibre types in a single equine skeletal muscle cryosection. Equine Vet J 2011;43:500–3.
23. Quiroz-Rothe E, Rivero JL. Co-ordinated expression of contractile and non-contractile features of control equine muscle fibre types characterised by immunostaining of myosin heavy chains. Histochem Cell Biol 2001;116:299–312.
24. Rivero JL, Talmadge RJ, Edgerton VR. A sensitive electrophoretic method for the quantification of myosin heavy chain isoforms in horse skeletal muscle: histochemical and immunocytochemical verifications. Electrophoresis 1997;18:1967–72.
25. Hermanson JW, Hegemann-Monachelli MT, Daaod MJ, et al. Correlation of myosin isoforms with anatomical divisions in equine musculus biceps brachii. Acta Anat (Basel) 1991;141: 369–76.
26. Serrano AL, Petrie JL, Rivero JL, et al. Myosin isoforms and muscle fiber characteristics in equine gluteus medius muscle. Anat Rec 1996;244:444–51.
27. Rivero JL, Serrano AL, Barrey E, et al. Analysis of myosin heavy chains at the protein level in horse skeletal muscle. J Muscle Res Cell Motil 1999;20:211–21.
28. Rivero JL, Talmadge RJ, Edgerton VR. Myosin heavy chain isoforms in adult equine skeletal muscle: an immunohistochemical and electrophoretic study. Anat Rec 1996;246:185–94.
29. Dingboom EG, Dijkstra G, Enzerink E, et al. Postnatal muscle fibre composition of the gluteus medius muscle of Dutch Warmblood foals; maturation and the influence of exercise. Equine Vet J Suppl 1999; 95–100.
30. Linnane L, Serrano AL, Rivero JL. Distribution of fast myosin heavy chain-based muscle fibres in the gluteus medius of untrained horses: mismatch between antigenic and ATPase determinants. J Anat 1999;194(Pt 3):363–72.
31. Eizema K, van den Burg M, Kiri A, et al. Differential expression of equine myosin heavy-chain mRNA and protein isoforms in a limb muscle. J Histochem Cytochem 2003;51:1207–16.
32. Chikuni K, Muroya S, Nakajima I. Absence of the functional Myosin heavy chain 2b isoform in equine skeletal muscles. Zoolog Sci 2004;21:589–96.
33. Eizema K, van den Burg MM, de Jonge HW, et al. Myosin heavy chain isoforms in equine gluteus medius muscle: comparison of mRNA and protein expression profiles. J Histochem Cytochem 2005;53:1383–90.
34. Adreani CM, Li ZB, Lehar M, et al. Myosin heavy chain composition in normal and atrophic equine laryngeal muscle. Vet Pathol 2006;43:881–9.
35. Mucher E, Jayr L, Rossignol F, et al. Gene expression profiling in equine

muscle tissues using mouse cDNA microarrays. Equine Vet J Suppl 2006;359–64.
36. Gu J, Orr N, Park SD, et al. A genome scan for positive selection in thoroughbred horses. PLoS One 2009;4:e5767.
37. Ichibangase T, Imai K. Application of fluorogenic derivatization-liquid chromatography-tandem mass spectrometric proteome method to skeletal muscle proteins in fast Thoroughbred horses. J Proteome Res 2009;8:2129–34.
38. Barrey E. Reviewe: Genetics and genomics in equine exercise physiology: an overview of the new applications of molecular biology as positive and negative markers of performance and health. Equine Vet J 2010;42(Suppl. 38):561–8.
39. Reeben M, Koho NM, Raekallio M, et al. MCT1 and CD147 gene polymorphisms in standardbred horses. Equine Vet J Suppl 2006;322–5.
40. Hill EW, Fonseca RG, McGivney BA, et al. MSTN genotype (g.66493737C/T) association with speed indices in Thoroughbred racehorses. J Appl Physiol 2012;112:86–90.
41. Nam GH, Ahn K, Bae JH, et al. Genomic structure and expression analyzes of the PYGM gene in the thoroughbred horse. Zoolog Sci 2011;28:276–80.
42. Mata X, Vaiman A, Ducasse A, et al. Genomic structure, polymorphism and expression of the horse alpha-actinin-3 gene. Gene 2012;491:20–4.
43. Cheung TK, Warren LK, Lawrence LM, et al. Electromyographic activity of the long digital extensor muscle in the exercising Thoroughbred horse. Equine Vet J 1998;30:251–5.
44. Wijnberg ID, van Dam KG, Graaf-Roelfsema E, et al. (Over)training effects on quantitative electromyography and muscle enzyme activities in standardbred horses. J Appl Physiol 2008;105:1746–53.
45. Butcher MT, Hermanson JW, Ducharme NG, et al. Superficial digital flexor tendon lesions in racehorses as a sequela to muscle fatigue: a preliminary study. Equine Vet J 2007;39:540–5.
46. Butcher MT, Chase PB, Hermanson JW, et al. Contractile properties of muscle fibers from the deep and superficial digital flexors of horses. Am J Physiol Regul Integr Comp Physiol 2010;299:R996–R1005.
47. Crook TC, Cruickshank SE, McGowan CM, et al. Comparative anatomy and muscle architecture of selected hind limb muscles in the Quarter Horse and Arab. J Anat 2008;212:144–52.
48. Brown NA, Kawcak CE, McIlwraith CW, et al. Architectural properties of distal forelimb muscles in horses, Equus caballus. J Morphol 2003;258:106–14.
49. Soffler C, Hermanson JW. Muscular design in the equine interosseus muscle. J Morphol 2006;267:696–704.
50. Parsons KJ, Pfau T, Wilson AM. High-speed gallop locomotion in the thoroughbred racehorse. I. The effect of incline on stride parameters. J Exp Biol 2008;211:935–44.
51. Crook TC, Cruickshank SE, McGowan CM, et al. A comparison of the moment arms of pelvic limb muscles in horses bred for acceleration (Quarter Horse) and endurance (Arab). J Anat 2010;217:26–37.
52. Buscher D, Izpisua Belmonte JC. Muscle development during vertebrate limb outgrowth. Cell Tissue Res 1999;296:131–9.
53. Draeger A, Weeds AG, Fitzsimons RB. Primary, secondary and tertiary myotubes in developing skeletal muscle: a new approach to the analysis of human myogenesis. J Neurol Sci 1987;81:19–43.
54. Hermanson JW. Architecture and the division of labor in the extensor carpi radialis muscle of horses. Acta Anat (Basel) 1997;159:127–35.
55. Payne RC, Veenman P, Wilson AM. The role of the extrinsic thoracic limb muscles in equine locomotion. J Anat 2005;206:193–204.
56. Watson JC, Wilson AM. Muscle architecture of biceps brachii, triceps brachii and supraspinatus in the horse. J Anat 2007;210:32–40.
57. Wilson AM, McGuigan MP, Su A, et al. Horses damp the spring in their step. Nature 2001;414:895–9.
58. Bobbert MF, Santamaria S. Contribution of the forelimbs and hindlimbs of the horse to mechanical energy changes in jumping. J Exp Biol 2005;208: 249–60.
59. Swanstrom MD, Zarucco L, Stover SM, et al. Passive and active mechanical properties of the superficial and deep digital flexor muscles in the forelimbs of anesthetized Thoroughbred horses. J Biomech 2005;38:579–86.
60. Lichtwark GA, Watson JC, Mavrommatis S, et al. Intensity of activation and timing of deactivation modulate elastic energy storage and release in a pennate muscle and account for gait-specific initiation of limb protraction in the horse. J Exp Biol 2009;212:2454–63.
61. Hoyt DF, Wickler SJ, Biewener AA, et al. In vivo muscle function vs speed. I. Muscle strain in relation to length change of the muscle-tendon unit. J Exp Biol 2005;208:1175–90.
62. Wickler SJ, Hoyt DF, Biewener AA, et al. In vivo muscle function vs speed. II. Muscle function trotting up an incline. J Exp Biol 2005;208:1191–200.
63. Rhee HS, Steel CM, Derksen FJ, et al. Immunohistochemical analysis of laryngeal muscles in normal horses and horses with subclinical recurrent laryngeal neuropathy. J Histochem Cytochem 2009;57:787–800.
64. Meyers RA, Hermanson JW. Horse soleus muscle: postural sensor or vestigial structure? Anat Rec A Discov Mol Cell Evol Biol 2006;288:1068–76.
65. Berchtold MW, Brinkmeier H, Muntener M. Calcium ion in skeletal muscle: its crucial role for muscle function, plasticity, and disease. Physiol Rev 2000;80:1215–65.
66. Ehmsen J, Poon E, Davies K. The dystrophin-associated protein complex. J Cell Sci 2002;115:2801–3.
67. Schenkman KA, Marble DR, Burns DH, et al. Myoglobin oxygen dissociation by multiwavelength spectroscopy. J Appl Physiol 1997;82:86–92.
68. Valberg SJ. Muscular causes of exercise intolerance in horses. Vet Clin North Am Equine Pract 1996;12:495–515.
69. Manso Filho HC, McKeever KH, Gordon ME, et al. Novel findings regarding Glut-4 expression in adipose tissue and muscle in horses – a preliminary report. Vet J 2007;174:565–9.
70. Davie AJ, Evans DL, Hodgson DR, et al. Effects of muscle glycogen depletion on some metabolic and physiological responses to submaximal treadmill exercise. Can J Vet Res 1999;63:241–7.
71. Orme CE, Harris RC, Marlin DJ, et al. Metabolic adaptation to fat-supplemented diet by the thoroughbred horse. Br J Nutr 1997;78:443–58.
72. Geelen SN, Blazquez C, Geelen MJ, et al. High fat intake lowers hepatic fatty acid synthesis and raises fatty acid oxidation in aerobic muscle in Shetland ponies. Br J Nutr 2001;86:31–6.
73. Geor RJ, Hinchcliff KW, Sams RA. Glucose infusion attenuates endogenous glucose production and enhances glucose use of horses during exercise. J Appl Physiol 2000;88:1765–76.
74. Schiaffino S, Reggiani C. Molecular diversity of myofibrillar proteins: gene regulation and functional significance. Physiol Rev 1996;76:371–423.
75. Miyata H, Sugiura T, Kai M, et al. Muscle adaptation of Thoroughbred racehorses trained on a flat or sloped track. Am J Vet Res 1999;60:1536–9.
76. Li M, Marx JO, Larsson L. There is no slowing of motility speed with increased body size in rat, human, horse and rhinoceros independent on temperature and skeletal muscle myosin isoform. Acta Physiol (Oxf) 2011;202:671–81.
77. Graziotti GH, Rios CM, Rivero JL. Evidence for three fast myosin heavy chain isoforms in type II skeletal muscle fibers in the adult llama (Lama glama). J Histochem Cytochem 2001;49: 1033–44.

78. Quiroz-Rothe E, Rivero JL. Coordinated expression of myosin heavy chains, metabolic enzymes, and morphological features of porcine skeletal muscle fiber types. Microsc Res Tech 2004;65:43–61.
79. Marx JO, Olsson MC, Larsson L. Scaling of skeletal muscle shortening velocity in mammals representing a 100,000-fold difference in body size. Pflugers Arch 2006;452:222–30.
80. Essen-Gustavsson B, Roneus N, Poso AR. Metabolic response in skeletal muscle fibres of standardbred trotters after racing. Comp Biochem Physiol B Biochem Mol Biol 1997;117:431–6.
81. Suwannachot P, Verkleij CB, Van Weeren PR, et al. Ca2+ ATPase in Dutch Warmblood foals compared with Na+, K+ ATPase: intermuscular differences and the effect of exercise. J Vet Med A Physiol Pathol Clin Med 2003;50:385–90.
82. Sewell DA, Harris RC, Marlin DJ, et al. Estimation of the carnosine content of different fibre types in the middle gluteal muscle of the thoroughbred horse. J Physiol 1992;455:447–53.
83. van Ginneken MM, Keizer HA, Wijnberg ID, et al. Immunohistochemical identification and fiber type specific localization of protein kinase C isoforms in equine skeletal muscle. Am J Vet Res 2004;65:69–73.
84. Gondim FJ, Modolo LV, Campos GE, et al. Neuronal nitric oxide synthase is heterogeneously distributed in equine myofibers and highly expressed in endurance trained horses. Can J Vet Res 2005;69:46–52.
85. Mykkanen AK, Hyyppa S, Poso AR, et al. Immunohistochemical analysis of MCT1 and CD147 in equine skeletal muscle fibres. Res Vet Sci 2010;89:432–7.
86. Revold T, Mykkanen AK, Karlstrom K, et al. Effects of training on equine muscle fibres and monocarboxylate transporters in young Coldblooded Trotters. Equine Vet J 2010;42(Suppl. 38):289–95.
87. Eizema K, van der Wal DE, van den Burg MM, et al. Differential expression of calcineurin and SR Ca2+ handling proteins in equine muscle fibers during early postnatal growth. J Histochem Cytochem 2007;55:247–54.
88. Eto D, Yamano S, Hiraga A, et al. Recruitment pattern of muscle fibre type during flat and sloped treadmill running in thoroughbred horses. Equine Vet J Suppl 2006;349–53.
89. Yamano S, Eto D, Hiraga A, et al. Recruitment pattern of muscle fibre type during high intensity exercise (60–100% VO2max) in thoroughbred horses. Res Vet Sci 2006;80:109–15.
90. Grotmol S, Totland GK, Kryvi H, et al. Spatial distribution of fiber types within skeletal muscle fascicles from Standardbred horses. Anat Rec 2002;268:131–6.
91. Snow DH, Guy PS. Muscle fibre type composition of a number of limb muscles in different types of horse. Res Vet Sci 1980;28:137–44.
92. Kawai M, Minami Y, Sayama Y, et al. Muscle fiber population and biochemical properties of whole body muscles in Thoroughbred horses. Anat Rec (Hoboken) 2009;292:1663–9.
93. Borgia LA, Valberg SJ, Essen-Gustavsson B. Differences in the metabolic properties of gluteus medius and superficial digital flexor muscles and the effect of water treadmill training in the horse. Equine Vet J 2010;42(Suppl. 38):665–70.
94. Sewell DA, Harris RC, Marlin DJ. Skeletal muscle characteristics in 2 year-old race-trained thoroughbred horses. Comp Biochem Physiol Comp Physiol 1994;108:87–96.
95. Rivero JL, Ruz MC, Serrano AL, et al. Effects of a 3 month endurance training programme on skeletal muscle histochemistry in Andalusian, Arabian and Anglo-Arabian horses. Equine Vet J 1995;27:51–9.
96. Serrano AL, Quiroz-Rothe E, Rivero JL. Early and long-term changes of equine skeletal muscle in response to endurance training and detraining. Pflugers Arch 2000;441:263–74.
97. Serrano AL, Rivero JL. Myosin heavy chain profile of equine gluteus medius muscle following prolonged draught-exercise training and detraining. J Muscle Res Cell Motil 2000;21:235–45.
98. Rivero JL, Serrano AL, Henckel P, et al. Muscle fiber type composition and fiber size in successfully and unsuccessfully endurance-raced horses. J Appl Physiol 1993;75:1758–66.
99. Rivero JL, Serrano AL, Henckel P. Activities of selected aerobic and anaerobic enzymes in the gluteus medius muscle of endurance horses with different performance records. Vet Rec 1995;137:187–92.
100. Barrey E, Valette JP, Jouglin M, et al. Heritability of percentage of fast myosin heavy chains in skeletal muscles and relationship with performance. Equine Vet J Suppl 1999;30:289–92.
101. Rivero JL, Henckel P. Muscle biopsy index for discriminating between endurance horses with different performance records. Res Vet Sci 1996;61:49–54.
102. Roneus N, Essen-Gustavsson B. Skeletal muscle characteristics and metabolic response to exercise in young standardbreds. Am J Vet Res 1997;58:167–70.
103. Roneus N, Essen-Gustavsson B, Lindholm A, et al. Muscle characteristics and plasma lactate and ammonia response after racing in Standardbred trotters: relation to performance. Equine Vet J 1999;31:170–3.
104. Rivero JL, Serrano AL, Quiroz-Rothe E, et al. Coordinated changes of kinematics and muscle fibre properties with prolonged endurance training. Equine Vet J Suppl 2001;104–8.
105. Eizema K, van der Wal DE, van den Burg MM, et al. Myosin heavy chain fibre type composition in foals: analyzes at the mRNA and protein level. Equine Vet J Suppl 2006;316–21.
106. Rietbroek NJ, Dingboom EG, Everts ME. Muscle characteristics of dutch Warmblood foals with different genetic background at ages 6 and 12 months. Equine Vet J Suppl 2006;326–9.
107. Dingboom EG, van Oudheusden H, Eizema K, et al. Changes in fibre type composition of gluteus medius and semitendinosus muscles of Dutch Warmblood foals and the effect of exercise during the first year postpartum. Equine Vet J 2002;34:177–83.
108. Roneus M, Lindholm A, Asheim A. Muscle characteristics in Thoroughbreds of different ages and sexes. Equine Vet J 1991;23:207–10.
109. Rivero JL, Galisteo AM, Aguera E, et al. Skeletal muscle histochemistry in male and female Andalusian and Arabian horses of different ages. Res Vet Sci 1993;54:160–9.
110. Yamano S, Eto D, Kasashima Y, et al. Evaluation of developmental changes in the coexpression of myosin heavy chains and metabolic properties of equine skeletal muscle fibers. Am J Vet Res 2005;66:401–5.
111. Lehnhard RA, McKeever KH, Kearns CF, et al. Myosin heavy chain profiles and body composition are different in old versus young Standardbred mares. Vet J 2004;167:59–66.
112. Kim JS, Hinchcliff KW, Yamaguchi M, et al. Age-related changes in metabolic properties of equine skeletal muscle associated with muscle plasticity. Vet J 2005;169:397–403.
113. Kitaoka Y, Hoshino D, Mukai K, et al. Effect of growth on monocarboxylate transporters and indicators of energy metabolism in the gluteus medius muscle of Thoroughbreds. Am J Vet Res 2011;72:1107–11.
114. Kawai M, Kuwano A, Hiraga A, et al. Relationships between myonuclear domain size and fibre properties in the muscles of Thoroughbred horses. Equine Vet J 2010;42(Suppl. 38):311–6.
115. Liu JX, Hoglund AS, Karlsson P, et al. Myonuclear domain size and myosin isoform expression in muscle fibres from mammals representing a 100,000-fold difference in body size. Exp Physiol 2009;94:117–29.

116. Palencia P, Quiroz-Rothe E, Rivero JL. New insights into the skeletal muscle phenotype of equine motor neuron disease: a quantitative approach. Acta Neuropathol 2005;109:272–84.
117. Hyyppa S, Karvonen U, Rasanen LA, et al. Androgen receptors and skeletal muscle composition in trotters treated with nandrolone laureate. Zentralbl Veterinarmed A 1997;44:481–91.
118. Beekley MD, Ideus JM, Brechue WF, et al. Chronic clenbuterol administration alters myosin heavy chain composition in standardbred mares. Vet J 2003;165:234–9.
119. Plant DR, Kearns CF, McKeever KH, et al. Therapeutic clenbuterol treatment does not alter Ca2+ sensitivity of permeabilized fast muscle fibres from exercise trained or untrained horses. J Muscle Res Cell Motil 2003;24:471–6.
120. Bergh A, Nordlof H, Essen-Gustavsson B. Evaluation of neuromuscular electrical stimulation on fibre characteristics and oxidative capacity in equine skeletal muscles. Equine Vet J 2010;42(Suppl. 38):671–5.
121. Geor RJ, Hinchcliff KW, McCutcheon LJ, et al. Epinephrine inhibits exogenous glucose utilization in exercising horses. J Appl Physiol 2000;88:1777–90.
122. Essen-Gustavsson B, Jensen-Waern M. Effect of an endurance race on muscle amino acids, pro- and macroglycogen and triglycerides. Equine Vet J Suppl 2002;209–13.
123. Brojer J, Holm S, Jonasson R, et al. Synthesis of proglycogen and macroglycogen in skeletal muscle of standardbred trotters after intermittent exercise. Equine Vet J Suppl 2006;335–9.
124. Waller AP, Lindinger MI. Nutritional aspects of post exercise skeletal muscle glycogen synthesis in horses: a comparative review. Equine Vet J 2010;42:274–81.
125. Geor RJ, Larsen L, Waterfall HL, et al. Route of carbohydrate administration affects early post exercise muscle glycogen storage in horses. Equine Vet J Suppl 2006;590–5.
126. Waller AP, Geor RJ, Spriet LL, et al. Oral acetate supplementation after prolonged moderate intensity exercise enhances early muscle glycogen resynthesis in horses. Exp Physiol 2009;94:888–98.
127. Waller AP, Heigenhauser GJ, Geor RJ, et al. Fluid and electrolyte supplementation after prolonged moderate-intensity exercise enhances muscle glycogen resynthesis in Standardbred horses. J Appl Physiol 2009;106:91–100.
128. Jose-Cunilleras E, Hinchcliff KW, Lacombe VA, et al. Ingestion of starch-rich meals after exercise increases glucose kinetics but fails to enhance muscle glycogen replenishment in horses. Vet J 2006;171:468–77.
129. Nout YS, Hinchcliff KW, Jose-Cunilleras E, et al. Effect of moderate exercise immediately followed by induced hyperglycemia on gene expression and content of the glucose transporter-4 protein in skeletal muscles of horses. Am J Vet Res 2003;64:1401–8.
130. Pratt SE, Geor RJ, Spriet LL, et al. Time course of insulin sensitivity and skeletal muscle glycogen synthase activity after a single bout of exercise in horses. J Appl Physiol 2007;103:1063–9.
131. Jose-Cunilleras E, Hayes KA, Toribio RE, et al. Expression of equine glucose transporter type 4 in skeletal muscle after glycogen-depleting exercise. Am J Vet Res 2005;66:379–85.
132. Lacombe VA, Hinchcliff KW, Devor ST. Effects of exercise and glucose administration on content of insulin-sensitive glucose transporter in equine skeletal muscle. Am J Vet Res 2003;64:1500–6.
133. van den Hoven R, Bauer A, Hackl S, et al. Changes in intramuscular amino acid levels in submaximally exercised horses – a pilot study. J Anim Physiol Anim Nutr (Berl) 2010;94:455–64.
134. Matsui A, Ohmura H, Asai Y, et al. Effect of amino acid and glucose administration following exercise on the turnover of muscle protein in the hindlimb femoral region of thoroughbreds. Equine Vet J Suppl 2006;611–16.
135. Kinnunen S, Hyyppa S, Lappalainen J, et al. Exercise-induced oxidative stress and muscle stress protein responses in trotters. Eur J Appl Physiol 2005;93:496–501.
136. van Ginneken MM, de Graaf-Roelfsema E, Keizer HA, et al. Effect of exercise on activation of the p38 mitogen-activated protein kinase pathway, c-Jun NH2 terminal kinase, and heat shock protein 27 in equine skeletal muscle. Am J Vet Res 2006;67:837–44.
137. Powers SK, Locke, Demirel HA. Exercise, heat shock proteins, and myocardial protection from I-R injury. Med Sci Sports Exerc 2001;33:386–92.
138. Kinnunen S, Hyyppa S, Oksala N, et al. alpha-Lipoic acid supplementation enhances heat shock protein production and decreases post exercise lactic acid concentrations in exercised standardbred trotters. Res Vet Sci 2009;87:462–7.
139. Kinnunen S, Oksala N, Hyyppa S, et al. alpha-Lipoic acid modulates thiol antioxidant defenses and attenuates exercise-induced oxidative stress in standardbred trotters. Free Radic Res 2009;43:697–705.
140. Poso AR, Eklund-Uusitalo S, Hyyppa S, et al. Induction of heat shock protein 72 mRNA in skeletal muscle by exercise and training. Equine Vet J Suppl 2002;214–18.
141. Gottlieb-Vedi M, Essen-Gustavsson B, Thornell LE, et al. A comparison of the ultrastructure and metabolic response of the skeletal muscle of horses performing intense treadmill exercise at 20 and 35 degrees C. Zentralbl Veterinarmed A 1999;46:209–18.
142. Koho NM, Hyyppa S, Poso AR. Monocarboxylate transporters (MCT) as lactate carriers in equine muscle and red blood cells. Equine Vet J Suppl 2006;354–8.
143. Koho NM, Mykkanen AK, Reeben M, et al. Sequence variations and two levels of MCT1 and CD147 expression in red blood cells and gluteus muscle of horses. Gene 2012;491:65–70.
144. Lindinger MI. Lactate: metabolic fuel or poison for racehorses? Exp Physiol 2011;96:261.
145. McCutcheon LJ, Byrd SK, Hodgson DR. Ultrastructural changes in skeletal muscle after fatiguing exercise. J Appl Physiol 1992;72:1111–17.
146. Vaihkonen LK, Heinonen OJ, Hyyppa S, et al. Lactate-transport activity in RBCs of trained and untrained individuals from four racing species. Am J Physiol Regul Integr Comp Physiol 2001;281:R19–24.
147. Snow DH, Harris RC, Gash SP. Metabolic response of equine muscle to intermittent maximal exercise. J Appl Physiol 1985;58:1689–97.
148. Dunnett M, Harris RC. Influence of oral beta-alanine and L-histidine supplementation on the carnosine content of the gluteus medius. Equine Vet J Suppl 1999;30:499–504.
149. Lacombe VA, Hinchcliff KW, Geor RJ, et al. Muscle glycogen depletion and subsequent replenishment affect anaerobic capacity of horses. J Appl Physiol 2001;91:1782–90.
150. King N, Suleiman MS. Effect of regular training on the myocardial and plasma concentrations of taurine and alpha-amino acids in thoroughbred horses. Amino Acids 1998;15:241–51.
151. Westermann CM, Dorland B, de Sain-van der Velden MG, et al. Plasma acylcarnitine and fatty acid profiles during exercise and training in Standardbreds. Am J Vet Res 2008;69:1469–75.
152. van den Burg MM, Eizema K, de Graaf-Roelfsema E, et al. Effects of acute exercise and long-term exercise on total Na+,K+ -ATPase content and Na+,K+ -ATPase isoform expression profile in equine muscle. Am J Vet Res 2009;70:895–901.
153. Liburt NR, Adams AA, Betancourt A, et al. Exercise-induced increases in inflammatory cytokines in muscle and blood of horses. Equine Vet J 2010;42(Suppl. 38):280–8.

154. McGivney BA, Eivers SS, MacHugh DE, et al. Transcriptional adaptations following exercise in thoroughbred horse skeletal muscle highlights molecular mechanisms that lead to muscle hypertrophy. BMC Genomics 2009;10:638.
155. Eivers SS, McGivney BA, Fonseca RG, et al. Alterations in oxidative gene expression in equine skeletal muscle following exercise and training. Physiol Genomics 2010;40:83–93.
156. Hill EW, Eivers SS, McGivney BA, et al. Moderate and high intensity sprint exercise induce differential responses in COX4I2 and PDK4 gene expression in Thoroughbred horse skeletal muscle. Equine Vet J 2010;42(Suppl. 38): 576–81.
157. Pette D, Staron RS. Mammalian skeletal muscle fiber type transitions. Int Rev Cytol 1997;170:143–223.
158. Yamano S, Eto D, Sugiura T, et al. Effect of growth and training on muscle adaptation in Thoroughbred horses. Am J Vet Res 2002;63:1408–12.
159. Kim JS, Hinchcliff KW, Yamaguchi M, et al. Exercise training increases oxidative capacity and attenuates exercise-induced ultrastructural damage in skeletal muscle of aged horses. J Appl Physiol 2005;98:334–42.
160. Eto D, Yamano S, Kasashima Y, et al. Effect of controlled exercise on middle gluteal muscle fibre composition in Thoroughbred foals. Equine Vet J 2003; 35:676–80.
161. Roneus M, Essen-Gustavsson B, Lindholm A, et al. Skeletal muscle characteristics in young trained and untrained standardbred trotters. Equine Vet J 1992;24:292–4.
162. Roneus N, Essen-Gustavsson B, Lindholm A, et al. Plasma lactate response to submaximal and maximal exercise tests with training, and its relationship to performance and muscle characteristics in standardbred trotters. Equine Vet J 1994;26:117–21.
163. Rivero JL, Serrano AL. Skeletal myosin heavy chain composition and carriage training. Equine Vet J Suppl 1999;30: 318–23.
164. Rivero JL. A scientific background for skeletal muscle conditioning in equine practice. J Vet Med A Physiol Pathol Clin Med 2007;54:321–32.
165. Heck RW, McKeever KH, Alway SE, et al. Resistance training-induced increases in muscle mass and performance in ponies. Med Sci Sports Exerc 1996;28: 877–83.
166. Gottlieb M, Essen-Gustavsson B, Lindholm A, et al. Effects of a draft-loaded interval-training program on skeletal muscle in the horse. J Appl Physiol 1989;67:570–7.
167. Lopez-Rivero JL, Aguera E, Monterde JG, et al. Skeletal muscle fiber size in untrained and endurance-trained horses. Am J Vet Res 1992;53:847–50.
168. D'Angelis FH, Ferraz GC, Boleli IC, et al. Aerobic training, but not creatine supplementation, alters the gluteus medius muscle. J Anim Sci 2005;83:579–85.
169. Rivero JL, Ruz A, Marti-Korff S, et al. Effects of intensity and duration of exercise on muscular responses to training of thoroughbred racehorses. J Appl Physiol 2007;102:1871–82.
170. Henckel P. Training and growth induced changes in the middle gluteal muscle of young Standardbred trotters. Equine Vet J 1983;15:134–40.
171. Foreman JH, Bayly WM, Allen JR, et al. Muscle responses of thoroughbreds to conventional race training and detraining. Am J Vet Res 1990;51: 909–13.
172. Essen-Gustavsson B, Lindholm A. Muscle fibre characteristics of active and inactive standardbred horses. Equine Vet J 1985;17:434–8.
173. Essen-Gustavsson B, McMiken D, Karlstrom K, et al. Muscular adaptation of horses during intensive training and detraining. Equine Vet J 1989;21:27–33.
174. Rivero JL, Sporleder HP, Quiroz-Rothe E, et al. Oral L-carnitine combined with training promotes changes in skeletal muscle. Equine Vet J Suppl 2002;269–74.
175. Sjostrom M, Lexell J, Eriksson A, et al. Evidence of fibre hyperplasia in human skeletal muscles from healthy young men? A left-right comparison of the fibre number in whole anterior tibialis muscles. Eur J Appl Physiol Occup Physiol 1991;62:301–4.
176. Graham-Thiers PM, Kronfeld DS. Amino acid supplementation improves muscle mass in aged and young horses. J Anim Sci 2005;83:2783–8.
177. Essen-Gustavsson B, Connysson M, Jansson A. Effects of crude protein intake from forage-only diets on muscle amino acids and glycogen levels in horses in training. Equine Vet J 2010;42(Suppl. 38):341–6.
178. Urschel KL, Escobar J, McCutcheon LJ, et al. Effect of feeding a high-protein diet following an 18-hour period of feed withholding on mammalian target of rapamycin-dependent signaling in skeletal muscle of mature horses. Am J Vet Res 2011;72:248–55.
179. Tozaki T, Sato F, Hill EW, et al. Sequence Variants at the myostatin Gene Locus Influence the Body Composition of Thoroughbred Horses. J Vet Med Sci 2012;73:1617–24.
180. Lopez-Rivero JL, Morales-Lopez JL, Galisteo AM, et al. Muscle fibre type composition in untrained and endurance-trained Andalusian and Arab horses. Equine Vet J 1991;23:91–3.
181. Sinha AK, Ray SP, Rose RJ. Effect of constant load training on skeletal muscle histochemistry of thoroughbred horses. Res Vet Sci 1993;54:147–59.
182. Rivero JL. Muscle biopsy as a tool for assessing muscular adaptation to training in horses. Am J Vet Res 1996;57:1412–6.
183. Rivero JL, Ruz A, Marti-Korfft S, et al. Contribution of exercise intensity and duration to training-linked myosin transitions in thoroughbreds. Equine Vet J Suppl 2006;311–15.
184. Pette D. Training effects on the contractile apparatus. Acta Physiol Scand 1998;162:367–76.
185. Eaton MD, Hodgson DR, Evans DL, et al. Effects of low- and moderate-intensity training on metabolic responses to exercise in thoroughbreds. Equine Vet J Suppl 1999;30:521–7.
186. McGowan CM, Golland LC, Evans DL, et al. Effects of prolonged training, overtraining and detraining on skeletal muscle metabolites and enzymes. Equine Vet J Suppl 2002;257–63.
187. Kitaoka Y, Masuda H, Mukai K, et al. Effect of training and detraining on monocarboxylate transporter (MCT) 1 and MCT4 in Thoroughbred horses. Exp Physiol 2011;96:348–55.
188. Misumi K, Sakamoto H, Shimizu R. Changes in skeletal muscle composition in response to swimming training for young horses. J Vet Med Sci 1995;57: 959–61.
189. Rietbroek NJ, Dingboom EG, Schuurman SO, et al. Effect of exercise on development of capillary supply and oxidative capacity in skeletal muscle of horses. Am J Vet Res 2007;68:1226–31.
190. Geor RJ, McCutcheon LJ, Shen H. Muscular and metabolic responses to moderate-intensity short-term training. Equine Vet J Suppl 1999;30:311–17.
191. Eto D, Yamano S, Mukai K, et al. Effect of high intensity training on anaerobic capacity of middle gluteal muscle in Thoroughbred horses. Res Vet Sci 2004;76:139–44.
192. Gansen S, Lindner A, Marx S, et al. Effects of conditioning horses with lactate-guided exercise on muscle glycogen content. Equine Vet J Suppl 1999;30:329–31.
193. Rodnick KJ, Henriksen EJ, James DE, et al. Exercise training, glucose transporters, and glucose transport in rat skeletal muscles. Am J Physiol 1992;262:C9–14.
194. McCutcheon LJ, Geor RJ, Hinchcliff KW. Changes in skeletal muscle GLUT4 content and muscle membrane glucose transport following 6 weeks of exercise training. Equine Vet J Suppl 2002; 199–204.
195. Stewart-Hunt L, Geor RJ, McCutcheon LJ. Effects of short-term training on

insulin sensitivity and skeletal muscle glucose metabolism in standardbred horses. Equine Vet J Suppl 2006;226–32.

196. Stewart-Hunt L, Pratt-Phillips S, McCutcheon LJ, et al. Dietary energy source and physical conditioning affect insulin sensitivity and skeletal muscle glucose metabolism in horses. Equine Vet J 2010;42(Suppl. 38):355–60.

197. Heilig A, Pette D. Albumin in rabbit skeletal muscle. Origin, distribution and regulation by contractile activity. Eur J Biochem 1988;171:503–8.

198. Bouwman FG, van Ginneken MM, Noben JP, et al. Differential expression of equine muscle biopsy proteins during normal training and intensified training in young standardbred horses using proteomics technology. Comp Biochem Physiol Part D Genomics Proteomics 2010;5:55–64.

199. Suwannachot P, Verkleij CB, Weijs WA, et al. Effects of training on the concentration of Na+, K+-ATPase in foal muscle. Equine Vet J Suppl 1999;101–5.

200. Suwannachot P, Verkleij CB, Kocsis S, et al. Specificity and reversibility of the training effects on the concentration of Na+,K+-Atpase in foal skeletal muscle. Equine Vet J 2001;33:250–5.

201. Suwannachot P, Joosten BJ, Klarenbeek A, et al. Effects of training on potassium homeostasis during exercise and skeletal muscle Na+,K(+)-ATPase concentration in young adult and middle-aged Dutch Warmblood horses. Am J Vet Res 2005;66:1252–8.

202. Rietbroek NJ, Dingboom EG, Joosten BJ, et al. Effect of show jumping training on the development of locomotory muscle in young horses. Am J Vet Res 2007;68:1232–8.

203. Marlin DJ, Harris RC, Gash SP, et al. Carnosine content of the middle gluteal muscle in thoroughbred horses with relation to age, sex and training. Comp Biochem Physiol A Comp Physiol 1989;93:629–32.

204. Boffi FM, Cittar J, Balskus G, et al. Training-induced apoptosis in skeletal muscle. Equine Vet J Suppl 2002;275–8.

205. Bruin G, Kuipers H, Keizer HA, et al. Adaptation and overtraining in horses subjected to increasing training loads. J Appl Physiol 1994;76:1908–13.

206. Rivero JL, van Breda E, Rogers CW, et al. Unexplained underperformance syndrome in sport horses: classification, potential causes and recognition. Equine Vet J 2008;40:611–18.

207. Goldspink G, Scutt A, Loughna PT, et al. Gene expression in skeletal muscle in response to stretch and force generation. Am J Physiol 1992;262: R356–63.

208. McGivney BA, McGettigan PA, Browne JA, et al. Characterization of the equine skeletal muscle transcriptome identifies novel functional responses to exercise training. BMC Genomics 2010;11:398.

209. Williams RS, Neufer PD. Regulation of gene expression in skeletal muscle by contractile activity. In: Rowell LB, Shepherd JT, editors. Handbook of physiology: integration of motor, circulatory, respiratory and metabolic control during exercise. Bethesda, MD: American Physiological Society; 1996. p. 1124–50.

210. Green HJ, Dusterhoft S, Dux L, et al. Metabolite patterns related to exhaustion, recovery and transformation of chronically stimulated rabbit fast-twitch muscle. Pflugers Arch 1992;420:359–66.

211. Yan Z, Serrano AL, Schiaffino S, et al. Regulatory elements governing transcription in specialized myofiber subtypes. J Biol Chem 2001;276: 17361–6.

212. Hudlicka O, Brown M, Egginton S. Angiogenesis in skeletal and cardiac muscle. Physiol Rev 1992;72:369–417.

213. Morrow NG, Kraus WE, Moore JW, et al. Increased expression of fibroblast growth factors in a rabbit skeletal muscle model of exercise conditioning. J Clin Invest 1990;85:1816–20.

214. Hyyppa S, Poso AR. Fluid, electrolyte, and acid-base responses to exercise in racehorses. Vet Clin North Am Equine Pract 1998;14:121–36.

Muscle disorders of equine athletes

7

Richard J. Piercy José-Luis L. Rivero

CHAPTER CONTENTS

Introduction

Veterinarians have long recognized muscle diseases of athletic horses, but only recently have there been significant advances in our understanding of the etiopathogenesis underlying these disorders. These achievements can be attributed to various factors including:

- recognition of similarities between human and equine muscle diseases
- greater awareness that muscle has a limited range of responses despite different mechanisms of injury
- subdivision of diseases based on breed susceptibility and histopathology, and
- the application of genomic, genetic, molecular and cellular investigative techniques.

Future developments should lead to more accurate diagnostic tests and better treatments, thereby enabling the veterinarian to provide an improved service, while benefiting from a more clinically rewarding experience.

General response of muscle to trauma and disease

Muscle tissue has a limited range of responses to different insults whether traumatic, ischemic, exercise-induced or due to underlying disease. Cell membrane damage causes abnormal ion fluxes and osmotic imbalance that rapidly perturbs fiber homeostasis. Normally the resting myoplasmic Ca^{2+} concentration is maintained at a concentration that is 60–100 times lower than that of the extracellular fluid (Chapter 6). Membrane damage allows Ca^{2+} to enter the cytoplasm from the interstitium, causing activation of destructive cellular proteases and inhibition of mitochondrial respiration.[1,2] Necrotic cell death is often associated with inflammatory responses including the chemotaxis of neutrophils and macrophages and collagen deposition. However, in certain muscle diseases, fibers die without marked inflammatory responses in which case cell death can be due to apoptosis.[3]

Muscle's remarkable regenerative capacity is usually associated with a characteristic sequence (Fig. 7.1). Following injury, ruptured myofibers retract, forming a gap between the stumps and allowing access for inflammatory cells via capillaries.[4] Contraction bands – condensations of cytoskeletal and sarcomeric material – plug the myofiber stumps and prevent further damage prior to plasma membrane repair.[5,6] Satellite cells, a subpopulation of adult skeletal muscle stem cells[7] that are normally relatively undifferentiated, quiescent and located between the myofiber's sarcolemma and its basement membrane (Fig. 7.2), are responsible for regeneration. Growth factors cause satellite cell activation, division and differentiation within 24 hours.[8] The cells migrate into the damaged region and over a period of about five days, fuse to form multinucleated myotubes (often within the basal lamina of the damaged fiber).[9] As the proteins of the myofilaments mature, myotubes gradually differentiate into myofibers,[5] a process taking several months, during which histopathology reveals immature fibers of variable sizes and with internally-located nuclei (Fig. 7.3).[10] Basement membrane damage results in more extensive fibrosis that can impede reinnervation and revascularization and hence regeneration.[9] Scarring

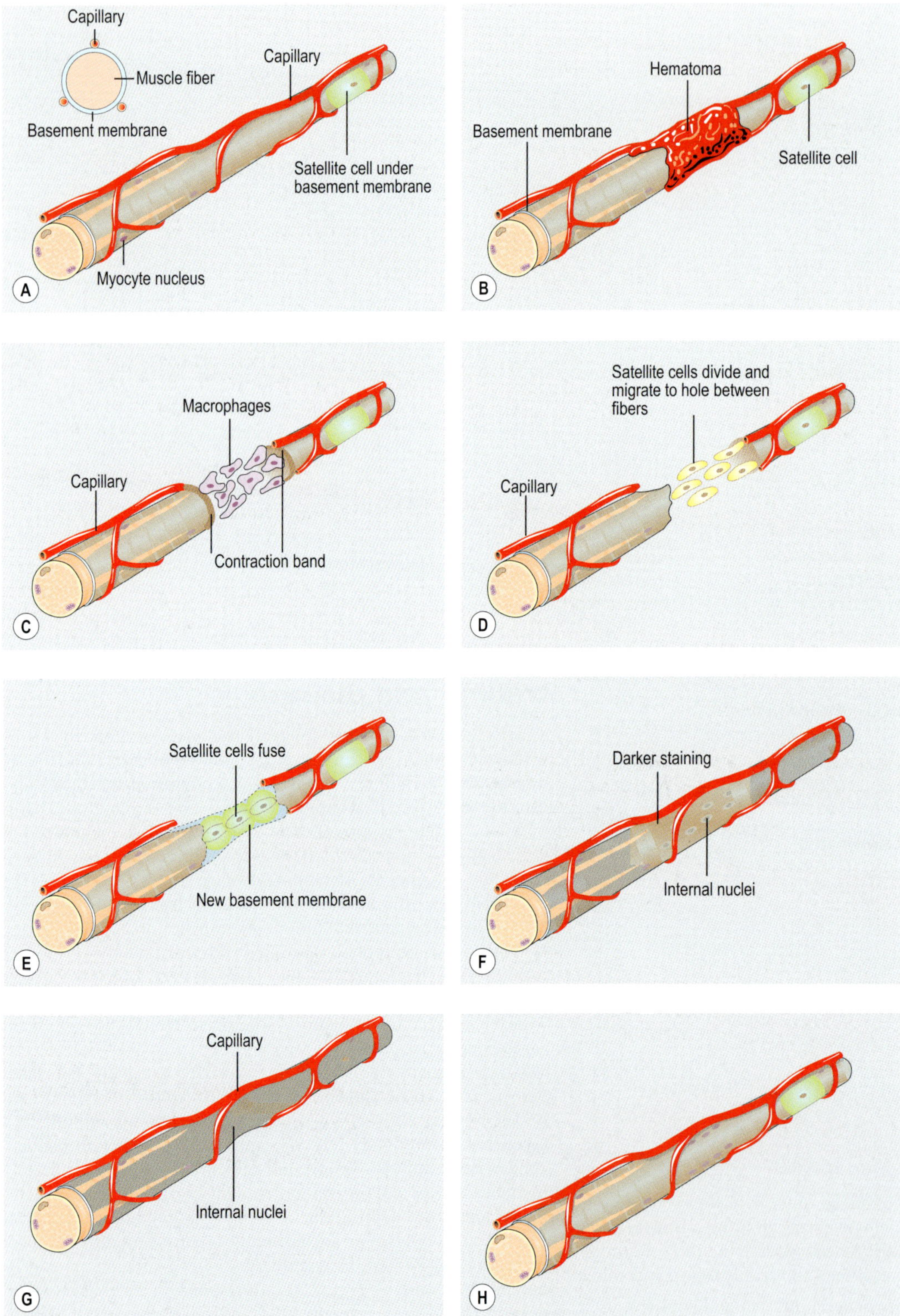

Fig 7.1 Repair and regeneration in muscle following damage and disease. **(A)** Normal muscle fiber surrounded by a basement membrane that covers the occasional satellite cell together with a rich network of capillaries. **(B)** Damage causes myofiber disruption that might or might not involve the basement membrane and hematoma formation, depending on severity of injury. **(C)** Myofiber stumps retract and the ends become plugged with the contraction band, made of sarcomeric proteins. Macrophages migrate into the (remnants of the) basement membrane cylinder within the first 24 hours and engulf and remove damaged tissue. **(D)** Satellite cells become activated (12–24 hours following injury), proliferate, differentiate into myoblasts and migrate to the damaged region. By days 2–3, satellite cells align and bridge the gap, fusing between the fiber stumps **(E)**. The process continues over the next week as narrower, more differentiated myotubes with internally located nuclei form **(F)** followed by more mature myotubes **(G)**. Nuclei return to the normal subsarcolemmal location over several months **(H)**.

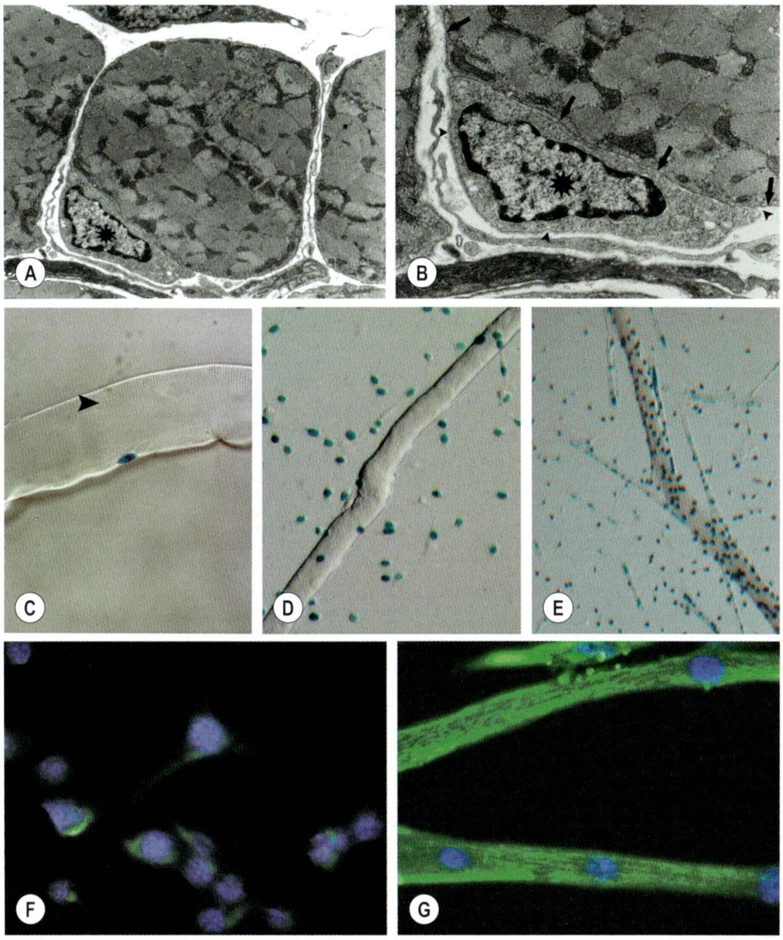

Fig 7.2 Satellite cells in vivo and in vitro. **(A)** Satellite cell in situ on the sarcolemmal surface of a nine-day-old B10 mouse muscle fiber. Notice the patchwork-like distribution of myofibrils in the muscle fiber and the satellite cell nucleus marked with an asterisk. **(B)** Higher power view of the satellite cell from **(A)** showing the sarcolemma (arrows) and the basement membrane (arrowheads). **(C)** Single muscle fiber in culture following its isolation from a transgenic mouse that expresses lacZ (blue staining) in satellite cell nuclei in response to Myf5 transcription factor expression; notice the fiber striations and the unlabeled subsarcolemmal myonuclei (arrowhead). **(D)** Single fiber from a transgenic mouse (as in C) following several days in culture. Notice the proliferation of satellite cells. **(E)** Following several further days in culture, satellite cells begin to fuse into myotubes. **(F)** H2K myoblasts in culture labeled with a monoclonal antibody to the muscle-specific protein, desmin (green); nuclei are stained blue with the chromosomal DNA marker 4,6-diamidino-2-phenylindoledihydrochloride hydrate (DAPI). **(G)** H2K cells as in **(F)** following their differentiation and fusion into myotubes.
A & B courtesy of Dr Susan Brown, C, D & E courtesy of Dr Peter Zammit, Imperial College of Science Technology and Medicine, UK.

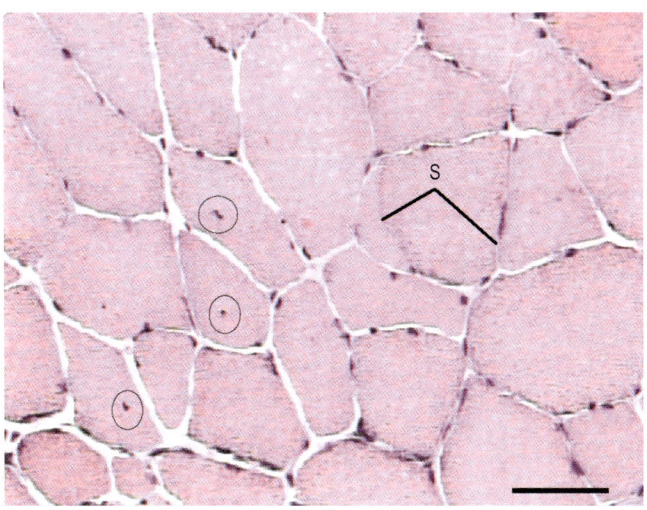

Fig 7.3 Hematoxylin and eosin transverse section from a M. gluteus medius biopsy from a horse with idiopathic recurrent exertional rhabdomyolysis. A few fibers have internalized nuclei (circled), and signs of fiber splitting (S) are evident.

might hinder action potential proliferation; however, this is overcome by sprouts from nearby axons piercing interposed scar tissue and creating new neuromuscular junctions (Fig. 7.4).[9]

Muscle damage caused by trauma, strains and tears

- Muscle damage caused by strains or tears is common in athletic horses.
- The site of damage dictates the signs that can include lameness or back stiffness.
- Plasma CK and AST activities can be mildly elevated.
- Ultrasound, thermography and scintigraphy can aid diagnosis.
- Rest and non-steroidal anti-inflammatory drugs often bring full return to function.

Recognition

History and presenting complaint

Delay in the onset of inflammation after trauma might complicate the history, but pain can be evident in showjumpers and eventers (both prone to lumbar and gluteal strain) as unwillingness to jump or turn sharply[11] or in other animals as mild to moderate lameness

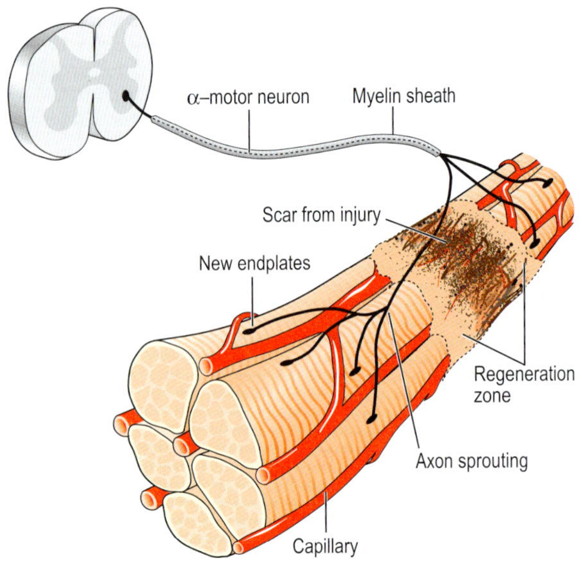

Fig 7.4 Diagrammatic representation of resprouting of an alpha motor neuron after injury to a group of myofibers. Axon sprouts penetrate interposed scar tissue forming new end-plates, thereby reinnervating the myofiber stumps.

or stiffness. Generally, injuries occur during exercise but severe muscle damage can follow prolonged recumbency or direct trauma.[12–14]

Physical examination

In acute stages, palpation reveals painful muscles with focal heat, swelling and edema. Trauma, secondary to impact injury, can be associated with overlying skin damage. In more chronic cases, an organizing hematoma, a scar, or both might be palpable. Certain lacerations and muscle tears can manifest as an abnormally held limb, unusual gait or an inability to bear weight.[14,15]

Special examination

Radiography can rule out bony abnormalities such as avulsion fractures. Thermography, scintigraphy and ultrasound can aid diagnosis and lesion localization and help assess healing.[16–18]

Laboratory examination

Plasma muscle enzyme activities can be moderately increased in the early stages.

Diagnostic confirmation

In some cases establishing a definitive diagnosis can be difficult, but confirmation is aided by ruling out skeletal injury.

Treatment and prognosis

Therapeutic aims

Minimizing further damage, while allowing for the repair and regeneration of the damaged muscle and providing analgesia are critical.

Therapy

Adequate rest followed by gradual return to exercise is essential. Severe injuries might require immobilization in casts or splints. Non-steroidal anti-inflammatory drugs (NSAIDs) (e.g. phenylbutazone 4.4mg/kg i.v. or p.o. q 12 h for one day followed by 2.2mg/kg p.o. q 12 h for several days; or flunixin meglumine 0.5–1.1mg/kg i.v. or p.o. q 12 h or q 24 h) provide analgesia and might reduce fibrosis. Massage, electrical stimulation and swimming might also speed recovery.

Prognosis

The prognosis for most muscle strains and tears is good, although fibrosis can cause mechanical lameness.[19] When this is severe, or where tearing occurs near the myotendinous junction, the prognosis for return to full function becomes guarded.

Prevention

Although traumatic injuries are hard to prevent, exercise-induced injuries are probably less likely when exercise schedules are intensified gradually.

Exertional rhabdomyolysis syndrome

- Both acquired and inherited forms of exertional rhabdomyolysis exist.
- Disease severity ranges from subclinical to life threatening.
- During an episode, plasma CK and AST activities are moderately to markedly elevated but they can return to normal between episodes.
- In severe cases, myoglobinuria can cause renal tubular damage and acute renal failure.
- In acute, severe cases, rest and intravenously-administered isotonic fluids and analgesics form the mainstays of treatment.
- Depending on breed, muscle biopsy, genetic testing, or both are indicated in an animal with a history of multiple episodes.
- Overexertion is likely a common cause of acquired disease.
- A common genetic cause in multiple breeds, known as polysaccharide storage myopathy type 1 (PSSM1), is associated with an autosomal dominant, gain of function mutation in the skeletal muscle glycogen synthase gene.
- Separate, but likely inherited disorder(s), occur in Thoroughbreds, Standardbreds and several other breeds.
- Environmental influences probably modify the phenotype in genetically-susceptible animals.
- Dietary and exercise management can prevent recurrence in many horses.

There are many historical, somewhat speculative reports suggesting different possible causes of equine exertional rhabdomyolysis (ER).[20] A large number of causes of this disease in horses is unsurprising given the numerous acquired and inherited forms in humans.[21,22] However, since certain types of equine ER have underlying genetic causes, the intermittent and varying severity of phenotype in these animals can be explained by the influence of modifying genes and environmental factors; factors that in the past were determined to be the primary etiology (Fig. 7.5). Episodes of rhabdomyolysis not generally associated with exercise can be of toxic, infectious, immune-mediated or iatrogenic origin (Fig. 7.5) and are not included in this chapter but are discussed in detail in reviews or other medicine texts.[23]

The recent identification of certain specific forms of ER means that classification for some cases is based on underlying

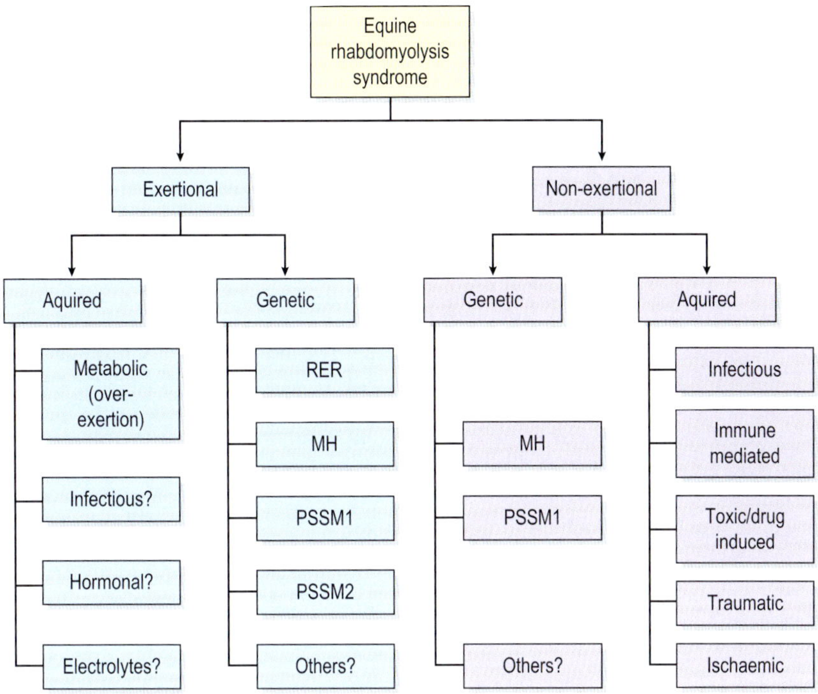

Fig 7.5 Diagrammatic representation of the various forms of rhabdomyolysis recognized in horses. Both exertional and non-exertional forms exist and there is some overlap between them. Note that some of the potential acquired forms of rhabdomyolysis could themselves be modifying factors for rhabdomyolysis in a horse with an underlying genetic problem. Those causes marked '?', remain largely speculative.

etiopathogenesis. In the text that follows, the clinical sections are written in a manner aimed at the investigation of a case with unknown etiology, when there are generally two presentations. The first is that of an animal with acute signs requiring emergency medical treatment. The second scenario is a clinically-normal horse with a history of several episodes of ER or a history of poor performance. The clinical investigation and management for each situation differ, even though the underlying cause might be the same. Specific diseases within this syndrome are considered in the etiology and pathogenesis sections.

Recognition

History and presenting complaint

In horses with acute exertional rhabdomyolysis, often the history includes recent exercise and sometimes training or management changes. The complaint can vary from a mild, stilted gait to severe stiffness, sweating or recumbency.[24] However, most animals are only mildly or moderately affected.

Some horses will present as apparently clinically normal, but with histories compatible with recurring episodes of post-exercise stiffness or gait changes, that might previously have been classified as muscle-related by appropriate biochemical testing. Frequently, there is no good explanation for the rhabdomyolysis and owners believe that some underlying factor is responsible. Some horses present with histories of poor performance.[25]

Physical examination

Although most horses are clinically normal between episodes, during an episode horses can show varying clinical signs. Mildly or moderately affected animals are tachycardic, with firm, painful pelvic limb, epaxial and gluteal musculature causing gait stiffness.[24] In some, pain localization can be difficult or pain is manifest in other ways: male horses, for example, sometimes posture to urinate[26] and other horses exhibit colic. Pigmenturia might be evident, especially in more severe cases (Fig. 7.6). These animals are often extremely painful, tachycardic, hyperthermic and tachypneic; they sweat profusely and can be totally unwilling or unable to move.[24] These horses have widespread muscle involvement and can become recumbent. The worst affected animals can show signs compatible with underlying shock and disseminated intravascular coagulation.

Laboratory examination

Blood sampling

Routine clinicopathologic changes in mild cases, during or immediately following an episode, usually consist solely of elevations in the plasma activities of the muscle-derived enzymes creatine kinase (CK) and aspartate aminotransferase (AST). Enzyme activity can be normal in horses between disease episodes, even when significant underlying muscle lesions are present.[27]

Plasma CK activity is the most convenient and specific marker of acute muscle damage and peaks at 4–6 hours following muscle damage and (unless the damage continues) starts to decline, with a half-life of approximately 12 hours (Fig. 7.7).[28] AST activity peaks about 24 hours after an episode and can remain elevated for several days to weeks.[13,26] Although both CK and AST activities rise in proportion to the degree of muscle damage, they do not always reflect the severity as assessed clinically or the prognosis. A high plasma AST activity without a concomitant elevation in plasma CK activity can indicate that muscle damage has occurred within preceding weeks. However, given that AST is not a specific marker for muscle disease, careful evaluation of the hemogram and biochemistry profile, and if necessary, further tests, are indicated to rule out hepatocellular disease.

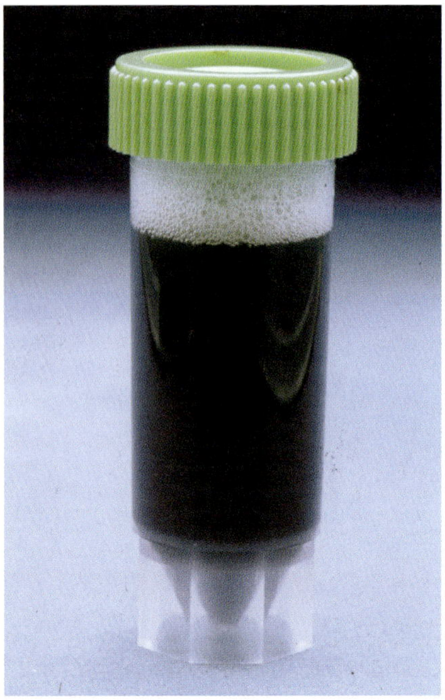

Fig 7.6 Urine containing myoglobin (brown discoloration) from a horse with severe rhabdomyolysis (plasma CK activity > 700 000IU/L).

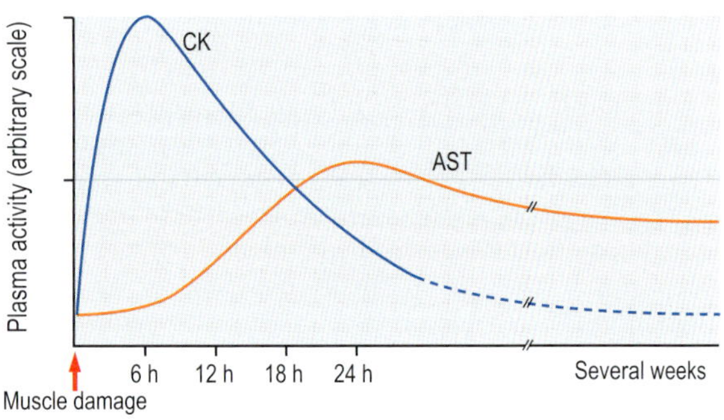

Fig 7.7 Diagrammatic representation of changes to serum CK and AST activity following an acute brief episode of rhabdomyolysis.

Other markers, sometimes used experimentally to assess muscle damage, such as serum myoglobin concentration or aldolase, LDH and carbonic anhydrase III activities, offer few if any clinical advantages over the measurement of CK and AST.

During disease episodes, more severe cases have additional less-specific abnormalities. Hyperkalemia can reflect the release of potassium from damaged muscle fibers. The hematocrit and total protein can rise due to intracompartmental fluid shifts. High serum creatinine concentration suggests the possibility of acute renal failure. Complex acid-base abnormalities are sometimes present as the usual hypochloremic metabolic alkalosis[29] shifts to metabolic acidosis if shock ensues. Widespread hematological and biochemical abnormalities are evident in terminal cases.

Exercise testing

An exercise test combined with blood sampling can be helpful in confirming an underlying muscle disorder in horses with no recent clinical or clinicopathological evidence of ongoing muscle damage and in animals under investigation for poor performance; exercise is however potentially dangerous in ER-susceptible animals so caution and sound clinical judgment is critical. Exercise testing is contraindicated in animals with current clinical or biochemical evidence of recent muscle damage and is unlikely to provide informative clinical information in an animal in which several episodes of ER have already been identified.

Ideally, a positive test should provoke a subclinical episode of rhabdomyolysis that can be detected via a rise in CK activity between pre- and 4h post-exercise serum samples or in AST activity between pre- and 24h samples. Titrating the amount and type of exercise can be difficult, but should be based on the horse's history and level of fitness. Bouts of maximal exercise appear less likely to precipitate episodes in Thoroughbreds with recurrent exertional rhabdomyolysis (RER),[30,31] and generally, 10–20 minutes of moderate exercise (trot and canter) on a longe line or a treadmill is considered appropriate. The sensitivity and specificity of exercise tests have not been evaluated however and the intermittent nature of the disease can result in a negative test in a susceptible animal. Furthermore, it remains unclear whether the same exercise testing protocol is appropriate for identification of all forms of ER since types or duration of exercise have not been compared in horses with different underlying disorders. Disparity among horses with results of exercise testing is revealed by studies in different breeds with the same underlying disorder: the rise in serum CK activity detected in Belgian and Percheron draught horses with PSSM1 after moderate exercise was greater in homozygotes than heterozygotes but there was considerable overlap between the groups (range of CK rise in both groups 21% to 826%).[27] In a separate study, the mean rise in CK activity in exercised Haflinger heterozygotes with PSSM1 was approximately 40%.[32] Importantly, in neither study was there a rise in CK or AST activity after exercise in unaffected horses.[27,32] Consequently, even modest rises in CK or AST after exercise should be considered as potentially relevant.

Plasma vitamin E and selenium

Most ER-susceptible horses are not deficient in vitamin E or selenium, but measuring plasma vitamin E and selenium concentrations (and/or glutathione peroxidase activities) might demonstrate deficiencies in animals on poor planes of nutrition or from selenium-deficient areas. Low anti-oxidant concentrations measured during or following a disease episode could be a consequence of the disease, rather than the cause.

Urinalysis

A urine sample collected early following a disease episode might, with microscopic examination, reveal urinary casts, a useful indicator of tubular necrosis and impending acute renal failure prior to the plasma creatinine concentration rising. Reagent strip analysis of urine does not differentiate myoglobin from hemoglobin, so specific assays are required to determine the cause of any pigmenturia. However, measurement of urinary myoglobin concentration is not usually necessary in an animal with significantly elevated serum muscle enzyme activities. Mild pigmenturia is a normal finding in some horses following high-intensity exercise.[33]

Electrolyte clearance ratios

Urinary clearance ratios are calculated to assess whole-body electrolyte status and renal function and historically, were used to evaluate horses with histories of ER.[34] Electrolytes and creatinine concentrations are measured in a urine (free catch or catheterized) and serum sample from the same animal. Ratios determined following collection of a single urine sample give similar results to those obtained with a 24-hour pooled (volumetric) urine sample, except for magnesium,[35] but accurate measurement requires urinary acidification (e.g. addition of concentrated nitric or hydrochloric acid)[35,36] to dissolve any suspended crystals. Horses should not eat between collection of the samples.[37]

The fractional clearance for each electrolyte ($FC_{(electrolyte)}$), is calculated as follows:[38]

$$FC_{(electrolyte)}\% = \frac{[electrolyte]_{urine}}{[electrolyte]_{plasma}} \times \frac{[creatinine]_{plasma}}{[creatinine]_{urine}} \times 100$$

where the square brackets represent the concentration (the acidification dilution factor should be factored in). There are wide variations for normal values in veterinary literature,[36,38–41] probably from differences in management, sampling and analysis. Normal ranges for FC(sodium) have been reported as 0.04–0.52%; for potassium, 35–80%; for chloride, 0.7–2.1%; and for phosphate, 0–0.2%.[34]

The calculation of electrolyte clearance ratios during an episode of ER can help evaluate renal function,[38] but should not be used to determine whether electrolyte imbalances were responsible for precipitating the attack. Furthermore, identification of wide daily fluctuations in clearance ratios in the same horse, despite standardized management, casts serious doubt on the test's interpretation or relevance.[39,41]

Muscle biopsy

Depending on the breed (see genetic testing below), muscle biopsy is often indicated in an animal with several unexplained episodes of ER (Fig. 7.8). The closed Bergstrom technique is described in Chapter 6; however although this method is useful in the research setting where samples can be handled rapidly, it is often preferable to collect an open biopsy in the clinical setting, since larger samples can be obtained that are less prone to drying artifact. The biopsy site is based on the physical examination, but epaxial, gluteal and semimembranosus muscles are most commonly chosen for exertional myopathies.[42] Ideally, a fresh muscle sample should be snap-frozen immediately in isopentane cooled in liquid nitrogen,[10] but since this is not usually practical, a compromise is necessary. Good results can be obtained when a sample is sent overnight to a specialist laboratory provided it is packaged appropriately.[43] Details regarding an appropriate sampling method follow in Box 7.1.

Histopathological examination and interpretation is compromised in samples that are exposed to excessive saline or that are submitted at ambient temperature;[43]consequently samples are best submitted in a sealed dry plastic container, without saline-moistened gauzes, and kept chilled (not frozen) on ice packs and sent in a polystyrene (Styrofoam) box. Formalin fixation, though more convenient, is unsuitable for histochemical investigation and leads to more artifact;[44] it does allow morphological assessment however, and has enabled a diagnosis to be reached in cases of polysaccharide storage myopathy (PSSM).[45]

Genetic testing

Genetic testing is available for detection of specific mutations associated with PSSM1 and malignant hyperthermia (MH) (see sections on etiology). Blood samples (in EDTA) or hair plucks containing the roots should be submitted to specialist laboratories. Since pretest probability for disease-associated mutations is higher in certain breeds, genetic testing is recommended before more invasive testing (for example muscle biopsy) in some animals (Fig.7.8).

For both PSSM1 and MH, founder mutations have been disseminated within and between breeds so testing for specific mutations is prudent. However, note that these genetic tests only identify each specific mutation. The current available tests would not rule out the

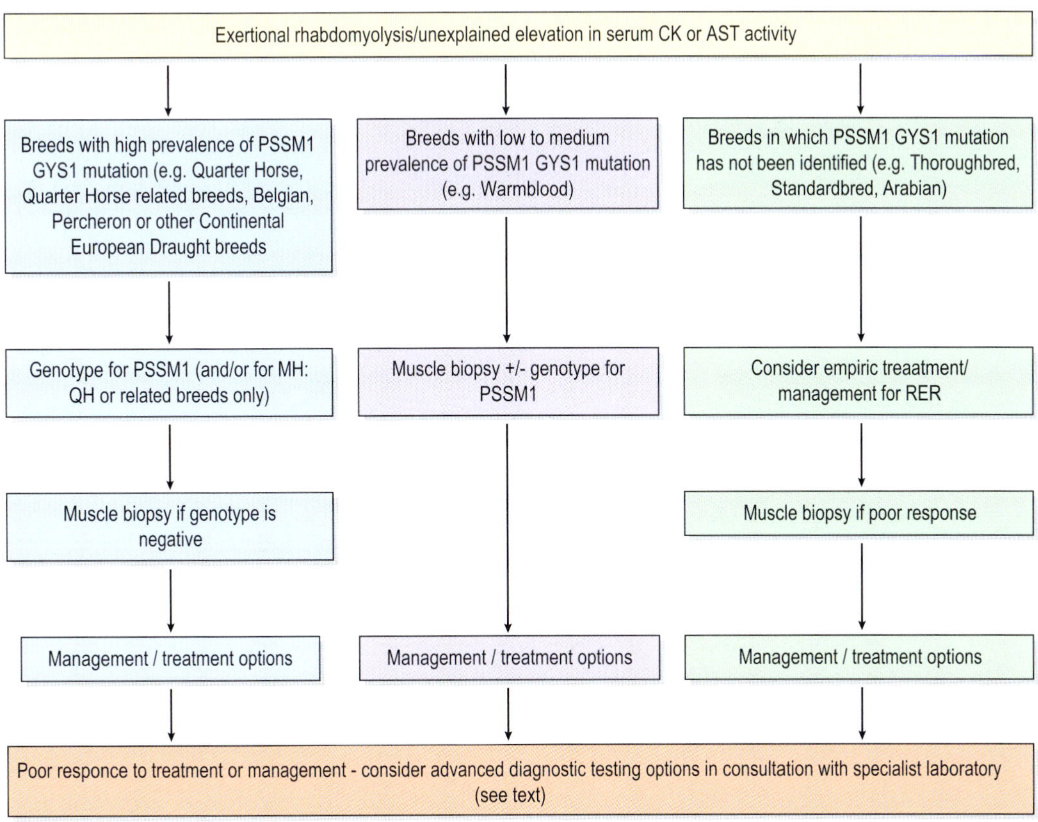

Fig 7.8 Flow diagram illustrating a suggested approach to horses with exertional rhabdomyolysis or unexplained or persistent elevations in serum muscle enzyme activities. Note that the approach differs between breeds.

existence of different mutations in the same genes, which occur commonly in humans with related phenotypes.

Scintigraphy

The history, clinical signs and clinicopathologic investigation (see below) are usually sufficient to establish a diagnosis of ER but scintigraphy can be helpful to localize muscle involvement in certain cases.[16] Alternatively scintigraphy can suggest an underlying muscle problem where instead a skeletal disorder was suspected (Fig.7.9).

Box 7.1 Sampling method

Required items:

Drugs for sedation
Local anesthetic
Sterile gloves
Scalpel
Forcep
Small Gelpi retractor
Needle holders
Suture material/staples
Chilled 0.9% sterile saline
Sterile gauze swabs
Screw top container x2
10% buffered formalin (10–20 ml)
Ice packs
Polystyrene (Styrofoam) box
Card and pins

Method

1. Contact the specialist laboratory and organize same day or overnight courier service prior to sampling. Avoid shipping over the weekend.
2. Sedate horse and prepare skin for sterile surgery.
3. Inject subcutaneously up to 10 ml of local anesthetic, taking care to avoid direct injection into the muscle layer.
4. Dampen several sterile gauzes with chilled sterile saline, squeeze them very tightly so they remain slightly damp but not wet, and lay them flat. If they are too wet, the sample is ruined. This step is not required if an assistant is available.
5. Make a 4cm incision (in the same orientation as the muscle fibers) in the skin and subcutaneous tissue, exposing the underlying muscle belly. Separate with Gelpi retractor.
6. Make 2 parallel incisions (3 cm) in the muscle parallel to the muscle fibers, about 1 cm apart.
7. Then, while holding the incised muscle proximally, incise the proximal region and carefully undermine the strip (1cm depth). Finally incise distally. The muscle will contract as it is incised.
8. Carefully place the muscle sample on the damp gauze, and fold the top layer of gauze over it to prevent it drying. Alternatively, and preferably, pass the sample to an assistant who should proceed immediately with step 11 below, or place the sample in a plastic container on ice (without the dampened gauze).
9. Close dead space completely and close subcutaneous layer. Note: a thorough closure reduces chance of dehiscence.
10. Suture or staple skin.
11. Divide muscle into two pieces by cutting cleanly 1cm along the 3 cm dimension. Pin the smaller piece (1 cm^3) at either end onto card and place in 10% buffered formalin in a screw top container. There should be at least 20 times the volume of formalin.
12. Taking care not to compress the remaining sample (2x1x1cm), remove it from the gauze, and place on the inside surface of a screw top plastic container (on its own). DO NOT INCLUDE THE WET GAUZE AS THIS RUINS THE SAMPLE.
13. Place both containers in a polystyrene (Styrofoam) box containing ice packs. Take care not to place the containers directly against the icepacks (the muscle itself must not freeze). Instead, provide some insulation (e.g. cotton wool).
14. Complete appropriate submission forms, seal the box and submit by courier or hand deliver.

Additional tests

Additional tests are often recommended in human patients with unexplained ER. Depending on the clinical presentation, and histopathology, these can include specific enzyme histochemistry or immunohistochemistry, electron microscopy, in vitro contracture testing of muscle strips, assessment of urine organic acid concentrations, analysis of plasma acyl carnitine profiles, measurement of plasma lactate and pyruvate concentrations before and after exercise, respiratory chain complex activity measurement, testing for fatty acid oxidation defects or specific DNA sequencing. Clinicians should contact a specialist laboratory to discuss more advanced testing if routine investigation has previously been unrewarding or if there has not been a good response to treatment or management changes (Fig. 7.8).

Necropsy examination

Histopathological assessment often reveals widespread muscle involvement, even in non-locomotor muscles. Occasionally there can be focal muscle involvement so a wide selection of muscles should be sampled, including several epaxial muscles, thoracic and pelvic limb locomotor muscles and psoas muscle. Lesions in muscle can indicate acute disease or provide evidence of an ongoing or chronic underlying problem (see sections on pathology below). Unfortunately, formalin fixation of muscle substantially

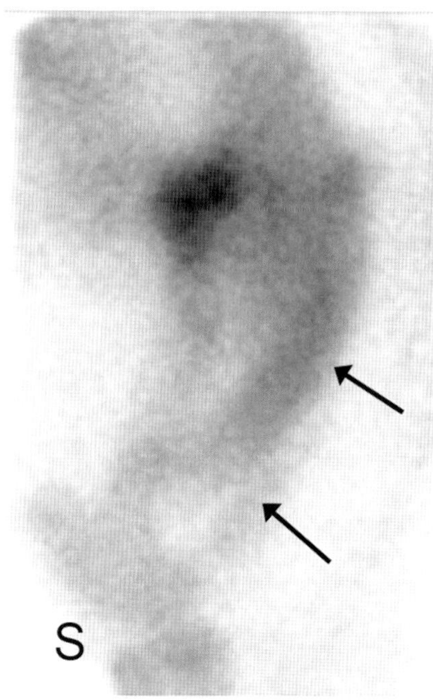

Fig 7.9 Scintigraphic image (bone phase) of lateral aspect of proximal pelvic limb and stifle (S) of a Thoroughbred horse that presented with unexplained pelvic limb lameness, revealing increased radiopharmaceutical uptake (arrows) in hamstring musculature. Signs are compatible with recurrent exertional rhabdomyolysis (RER) and were confirmed by muscle biopsy. Similar scintigraphic abnormalities can also be seen in the gluteal musculature in some affected horses.

limits the histopathological examination and any future diagnostic modalities.

Diagnostic confirmation

In the acute form, ER syndrome can be confused with colic, laminitis, tetanus, hyperkalemic periodic paralysis and some cardiac arrhythmias. Usually these disorders are readily distinguishable by additional signs, specific tests and the lack of significantly elevated serum muscle enzyme activities. However, in animals with raised CK or AST activities, it is important not to overlook the possibility of two separate (unrelated) disorders occurring in the same animal, given the high prevalence of specific forms of ER within certain breeds. For example, some forms of ER are more likely encountered following time off, or during investigation for a separate injury or disease: in these cases, clinical judgment is necessary to determine the primary, clinically-relevant problem. Similarly, coincidence, rather than direct association, was proposed as an explanation for a previously suggested,[46] but now refuted, link between Shivers syndrome and PSSM in susceptible animals.[47] Occasionally, sedentary horses present with classic signs of rhabdomyolysis with markedly elevated serum muscle enzyme activities. In these animals, underlying genetic susceptibility more usually associated with exertional forms of the disease is possible, because other events such as stress can precipitate attacks. Toxic, infectious or immune-mediated muscle diseases should also be considered.[23,42,48,49]

Treatment and prognosis

Therapeutic aims

In an animal with acute, ongoing rhabdomyolysis, the therapeutic goals are to minimize further muscle damage, to prevent myoglobin-induced kidney injury by establishing and maintaining diuresis, to correct underlying systemic metabolic or cardiovascular abnormalities and provide analgesia. Early and prompt treatment is essential to maximize the chances of recovery.[50]

Therapy

Management

While clinical signs of pain or stiffness remain, exercise should be stopped and the horse rested in a deep-bedded stall. In mildly-affected animals, slow hand-walking is sometimes recommended. Most horses subsequently benefit from turn out and mild exercise when clinical signs have resolved, even when plasma CK and AST activities remain elevated.

Fluid therapy

Mildly affected animals – when vital signs are close to normal – can recover from an acute episode without intravenous administration of isotonic fluids. However, they should be monitored for signs of deterioration. In moderate to more severe cases, however (even in those without pigmenturia), establishing diuresis and preventing or treating hypovolemia is the priority because myoglobin is nephrotoxic. Large volumes of isotonic fluids are usually effective (0.9% NaCl or lactated Ringer's solution infused intravenously at 100–150mL/kg/24h). Urine should be alkalinized, however, the addition of sodium bicarbonate to fluids is rarely necessary,[29] and only indicated in a horse with metabolic acidosis when the urine remains acidic despite fluid therapy, because myoglobin is significantly more nephrotoxic when in acidic urine.[51]

In rare cases, isotonic electrolyte solutions, even when administered rapidly intravenously, cannot compensate for the worsening hypovolemia. This state is reflected by a climbing heart rate and hematocrit, accompanied by steady or occasionally falling total plasma protein and serum albumin concentrations, as widespread muscle lysis and associated inflammation, allow water and proteins to leave the vasculature and enter the interstitium and damaged muscle fibers. These animals often die despite intensive therapy.

Diuretics

If there is little or no urine production during appropriate intravenous administration of fluids to acutely affected animals, attempts should be made to invoke diuresis. Furosemide (frusemide) is generally effective (0.5–1mg/kg i.v. or i.m. q 12 h). Careful monitoring and adjustment of fluid rates are essential to ensure that diuresis does not cause or exacerbate hypovolemia. Diuretics should not be administered to animals that are not concomitantly receiving fluid therapy.

Analgesia

In mild to moderate acute cases, NSAID (e.g. phenylbutazone 4.4mg/kg i.v. or p.o. q 12h for one day followed by 2.2mg/kg p.o. q 12h for several days; or flunixin meglumine 0.5–1.1mg/kg i.v. or p.o. q 12–24h) medication is all that is necessary; however, clinicians should monitor renal function given the drugs' nephrotoxicity. In severe cases, more potent analgesics such as butorphanol (0.1mg/kg i.v. or i.m. q 4–6h) can be required. In the worst cases the pain is very difficult to relieve.

Other therapies

Traditionally, acepromazine (0.04–0.11mg/kg i.v. or i.m. q 8h) has been advocated for its vasodilatory effects within the musculature; however, it should be used with caution in hypovolemic animals. Corticosteroids (e.g. dexamethasone 0.02mg/kg i.v. q 24 h for 1–2 days) are sometimes used to stabilize membranes or for anti-inflammatory effects. Neither medication has been shown to be efficacious.

Dantrolene, a drug that limits release of Ca2+ from the sarcoplasmic reticulum (SR) by antagonising the skeletal muscle ryanodine receptor (RYR1),[52] has been used in the acute stages of idiopathic rhabdomyolysis[53] but pharmacokinetic studies[54,55] suggest that the dose and the frequency of administration were unlikely to have resulted in beneficial drug concentrations based on those required to effect a response in humans.[56] Refer to the section on prevention (below) for a discussion of use of dantrolene for ER prophylaxis.

Prognosis

The prognosis for most horses with mild to moderate acute episodes of ER is good for recovery, but horses with an underlying genetic susceptibility are prone to future episodes. For severely affected horses in shock, the prognosis is poor. Many horses that develop acute renal failure recover, if treated early.

The long term prognosis for successful athletic function varies, depending on the etiology and whether appropriate management and prophylaxis are instituted. Future athletic function can be compromised in animals with substantial underlying muscle lesions, however many horses with inherited forms of ER compete successfully: indeed evidence suggests that certain forms of ER are associated with underlying improved athletic performance.[57]

Prevention

The association of a disease with a considerable number of anecdotal preventative treatments usually reflects the treatments' questionable or limited efficacies and current and historical inability to establish the precise etiology. Such is the case for the prophylaxis of ER where a wide variety of putative preventive treatments exists,[58] with only a few having been scrutinized objectively. Much of this confusion likely relates to the fact that ER in horses has multiple etiologies and that therefore one treatment is unlikely to be effective for all forms of the disorder.

Diet

Despite apparent differences in etiology and pathogenesis,[59] the substitution of a proportion of dietary calories derived from soluble carbohydrate, with additional fat, reduces the severity of episodes of ER via poorly understood mechanisms in both Thoroughbreds with RER[60] and horses with PSSM1.[61]

High-carbohydrate diets lead to more severe muscle damage in horses with RER,[30,60] while high-fat diets are protective.[60] Though unexplained, one possibility is that a high-fat diet can result in the stabilization of sarcolemmal membranes but the rapidity of the protective response[60] suggests that this is unlikely. High-fat diets have a calming effect on horses[62] and are associated with lower plasma cortisol concentrations during exercise.[63] Since stress has been associated with RER in Thoroughbreds,[58] this dietary calming effect could explain the rapid prophylactic efficacy of high-fat diets in RER.[64] Stress is also associated with ER in Standardbred horses:[57] consequently, though not yet tested experimentally, similar dietary adjustment might also be beneficial in this breed.

There is conflicting evidence as to whether low-carbohydrate (high-fat) diets reduce the excessive glycogen accumulation in muscle in horses with PSSM.[65,66] However, since glycogen synthase activity (and therefore glycogen synthesis) in muscle is increased by glucose-6 phosphate,[67] which itself rises in muscle during hyperglycemia,[68] diets high in soluble carbohydrates and simple sugars are probably best avoided in horses with PSSM1. Dietary adjustments of this kind reduce the severity of myopathy in PSSM1-affected animals.[69]

Most studies have investigated the beneficial effect of diets that contain approximately 20% fat, together with a reduction in soluble carbohydrate (grain) intake.[60] Increased fat in the diet can be achieved by the addition of vegetable oil (up to approximately 1g/kg bodyweight per day or 1.1mL/kg bodyweight per day). Rice bran (15–20% fat) can also be used as a substitute source in animals that find the oil unpalatable or a combination can be suitable in some animals.[70] Forage intake should be at least 1% of bodyweight, but fast-growing lush pastures and high-quality sweet hays should be avoided in horses with PSSM1.[71]

Horses should be introduced to higher fat diets over several weeks and the dietary intake of minerals and vitamins should meet current recommendations.[72] In particular, owners should ensure that the calcium: phosphorus ratio in the diet is adequate, as rice bran and high-fiber products contain excessive phosphorus relative to calcium. There are several high-fat, low soluble-carbohydrate feeds that are commercially available. Unfortunately, trainer compliance within racing yards is sometimes hard to achieve, because of concern that Thoroughbred horses in training lose condition on diets designed for management of ER.

Finally, it is important to remember that the efficacy of dietary adjustment has only been established in RER and PSSM1 and that horses with other forms of ER, or idiopathic disorders, might not respond. Indeed, in ER-affected humans with fatty acid metabolism defects, low fat and high carbohydrate diets are sometimes recommended.[73] Consequently, further diagnostic investigation might be warranted in horses that do not respond as expected to widely-accepted dietary changes.

Exercise

Evidence suggests that a regular daily exercise program with changes introduced gradually, and preferably daily access to pasture or turnout, reduces the severity of disease in horses with RER or PSSM1.[58,61,74]

Electrolyte therapy

Although electrolyte supplementation is appropriate in animals that have been identified as deficient by specific testing, it is unlikely to be of benefit in most horses. There is no valid rationale for the once popular administration of sodium bicarbonate to Thoroughbred horses with RER to prevent episodes, because most affected animals do not have underlying acid-base disorders prior to exercise and become alkalotic during exercise.[29,60]

Lactate modifiers

Supplements or medications designed to reduce lactate accumulation, for example dichloroacetic acid, have not been evaluated experimentally, and are not recommended in Thoroughbreds with RER, since lactic acidosis is not a precipitating factor.[29,60]

Dantrolene

Although dantrolene administration has been associated with causing paresis in some horses at high doses (4mg/kg IV[54] and 9mg/kg PO,[75]) manifest as muscle trembling or prolonged recumbency, some experimental evidence[76,77] supports its use in RER prophylaxis in Thoroughbred horses. As it has a short half life, administration should be 1.7–4 hours before exercise to ensure peak plasma concentrations at the time of exercise;[54,55] published and anecdotal reports suggest that a dose of 1–3 mg/kg PO)[76] can be beneficial. An early report suggested that feed restriction is necessary to optimize bioavailability,[76] however more recent data suggests that feed withdrawal is unnecessary: indeed it can adversely affect drug absorption.[78] A low (approximately 1mg/kg) dose was undetectable in horse urine after 168 hours (7 days).[55]

Oral dantrolene, as prophylaxis for ER has not been tested in breeds other than Thorougbreds, or in disorders other then RER, but epidemiological evidence suggests that it could be beneficial, particularly in breeds where the disease etiology is suspected to be similar or identical to the Thoroughbred disorder, RER.[57]

Antioxidant supplementation

Studies reveal that vitamin E or selenium supplementation enhances plasma anti-oxidant capacity and can reduce oxidative stress[79] but there is no good evidence that either can reduce exercise-associated increases in CK or AST activity, or the frequency or severity of episodes of ER.[80,81] There is evidence that supports an owner placebo effect, rather than any beneficial effect of anti-oxidant supplementation in horses with various perceived muscle-related problems.[82] Despite this, vitamin E (1–6 IU/kg/day alpha-tocopherol) and selenium (1–2mg/day) supplementation in food are probably indicated when deficiencies have been confirmed.

Etiology, pathophysiology and pathology

Although reaching a diagnosis of ER is not usually difficult, categorizing the disease according to the etiology can be much harder. Both acquired and inherited causes should be considered in an animal with acute signs whereas in a horse that presents following multiple episodes, underlying genetic predisposition is more likely. Certain acquired causes can be obvious from the history (e.g. overexertion) and specific genetic testing can identify other forms. Unfortunately, many cases contribute to a large idiopathic category, a situation in common with the diagnosis of human ER.[21,22] Continued use of muscle biopsy, other tests, and more research is likely better to categorize ER-associated disorders in horses in the future.

Acquired causes

Overexertion

Extreme or unaccustomed exercise predisposes some horses to rhabdomyolysis, as it does in human military recruits.[83] Muscle damage in such cases can include a combination of physical damage incurred during excessive eccentric contractions, metabolic exhaustion and oxidative injury.

Eccentric contraction

Delayed-onset muscle soreness in humans is associated with damage caused by excessive eccentric contractions (contraction during muscle lengthening).[84] Stiffness and pain, usually experienced 1–2 days following such exercise, is initially most evident at the myotendinous junction and then spreads throughout the muscle. Although the mechanism is poorly understood, there are prominent signs of damage within a muscle following eccentric contractions that include disruption of sarcomeres and damage to the excitation-contraction coupling mechanism and the sarcolemma.[85] This damage is reflected by (sometimes considerable) elevations in serum muscle enzyme activities[86,87] and triggers a local inflammatory response accompanied by edema and the sensitization of nociceptors.[84]

Whether horses experience this syndrome is unknown. Exercising horses are most likely to encounter eccentric contractions during downhill exercise and jumping. Given that muscle damage in humans generally occurs when the type or extent of eccentric contractions are unaccustomed and that adaptation occurs with training,[85] it seems sensible to introduce horses gradually to these types of exercise.

Metabolic exhaustion

Exceeding the level of training either by excessive endurance exercise or overexertion when galloping is a common cause of acute ER in horses.[88] Exhaustion during endurance exercise results in heat retention, fluid and electrolyte loss, acid-base imbalance and intramuscular glycogen depletion.[89] Although the causes are numerous and likely involve electrolyte imbalances and hyperthermia, in certain cases a presumed underlying factor is the deficiency of ATP, which results in an inability to maintain ion homeostasis. In turn, a corresponding rise in intracellular calcium concentration precedes the final common pathways, leading to muscle fiber death described at the beginning of this chapter.

Oxidative injury

Increased oxygen utilized during exercise leads to proportionate increases in free radical production (Fig. 7.10).[90] Free radicals are widely believed to cause post-exercise stiffness and fatigue in muscle, through several deleterious mechanisms that include the peroxidation of lipid membranes. Cell damage is normally minimized by the action of a complex cascade of free radical scavengers and antioxidants, including vitamin E and the selenium-dependent enzyme, glutathione peroxidase. When antioxidants fail to quench free radicals sufficiently, the body is subjected to so-called 'oxidative stress'.[90]

Exercise-induced oxidative stress occurs in horses, particularly when ambient temperature and humidity are high,[91] but most studies fail to provide evidence supporting a role for oxidative stress in exercise-associated sarcolemmal damage.[80,81,92] Furthermore, if oxidant damage played an important role in horses with ER, one might expect deficiencies (through excessive consumption) to be encountered commonly in ER-susceptible animals, but this is not the case in either ER-prone Arabians[93] or Belgian horses with PSSM1.[27] Indeed, in one study, higher serum and muscle vitamin E concentrations and serum glutathione peroxidase activities were detected in ER-susceptible Standardbreds compared with controls, although supplementation could not be ruled out as a cause of these higher concentrations.[94]

In adult horses, vitamin E or selenium deficiency has been associated with nutritional myodegeneration (white muscle disease) of the masseter muscle[95] and was implicated in horses with rhabdomyolysis, colic and myocardial disease.[96] In growing foals, nutritional myodegeneration is characterized histopathologically by changes that are sometimes seen in horses with ER.[97] However, such changes likely reflect the general response of muscle to cycles of degeneration and regeneration, rather than damage caused specifically by oxidative stress.

There is therefore no good evidence that oxidative stress plays a primary role in ER, particularly given the apparent high incidence of the disorder in horses on excellent planes of nutrition. Despite this, during conditions likely to result in significant oxidative stress, such as very strenuous or prolonged exercise, antioxidant deficiencies might exacerbate muscle damage caused by other mechanisms. Horses from selenium-deficient regions or animals on poor diets that are denied access to green pasture are most at risk.

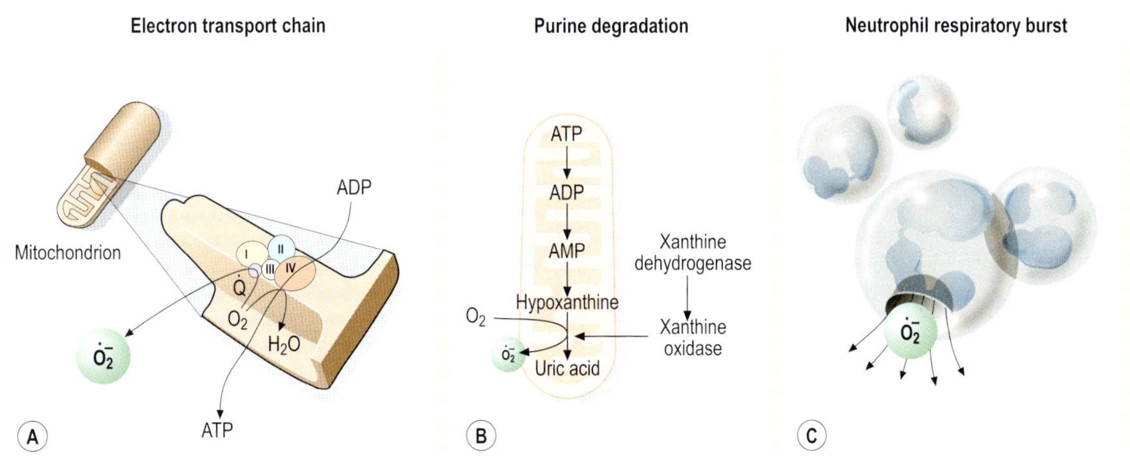

Fig 7.10 Diagrammatic representation of free radical formation via the electron transport chain in mitochondria **(A)**, via hypoxanthine degradation after ischemia **(B)** and during the neutrophil respiratory burst **(C)**.

Electrolyte imbalance

Published and anecdotal reports of improvement following correction of electrolyte clearance ratios underlie historical interest in this area.[34] In a group of 38 ER-susceptible Thoroughbreds, about a third had potassium clearance ratios of less than 30% or low chloride clearance.[98] These differences could potentially reflect differences in the handling of electrolytes by ER-susceptible animals but Thoroughbred horses prone to ER exhibit the same dietary-induced alterations to electrolyte clearance ratios as normal animals.[35]

Much attention has been directed at potassium, because low muscle potassium concentrations can precipitate rhabdomyolysis in other species.[99] Erythrocyte potassium concentration has been measured in attempts to investigate whole-body potassium stores: results indicate both low[100] and normal[98] erythrocyte potassium in horses with ER. However, the significance of either study is questionable given that erythrocyte potassium concentrations do not correlate with muscle or plasma potassium concentrations in horses.[98,101,102] Compared with normal animals, lower dry weight muscle potassium concentrations were detected in ER-susceptible horses.[98] However, characteristic muscle histopathological changes, seen in humans with potassium deficiency,[99] are generally not observed in muscle from horses with ER so it is hard to draw conclusions about the importance of potassium in causing or exacerbating ER in horses.

The primary influence of altered electrolyte status as a cause of ER is better studied prospectively in normal horses, rather than retrospectively in horses known to be susceptible to the disorder. In comparison with controls, normal Thoroughbreds administered furosemide (frusemide) and sodium bicarbonate developed lower plasma calcium, chloride, magnesium and potassium concentrations. Following exercise, serum CK activity was significantly higher in the treated group,[103] though results were skewed by two of the six animals, that could have had an underlying primary genetic susceptibility. Consequently, as with other factors, it is possible that electrolyte imbalance can modify the phenotype of a genetically-susceptible animal.

Hormonal influence

In experimental animal models, sex hormones influence the degree of disruption and inflammatory response to injury in skeletal muscle. For instance, estrogen protects muscle from injury induced by eccentric contractions and ischemia-reperfusion injury.[104] It is intriguing therefore that many studies of RER report a higher incidence in female horses compared with males.[57,58,105–109] No correlation has been found between the stage of the estrus cycle and plasma CK activities in Thoroughbreds in training,[110] suggesting that a direct association of female sex hormones with ER is unlikely. As yet, therefore, the higher incidence of ER in females remains unexplained. No association with sex is seen in PSSM1 (see below).[61]

Hypothyroidism is associated with subclinical elevations of serum CK activity and rarely causes ER in humans.[111,112] Although a cause of poor performance in horses,[113] hypothyroidism has not been associated with ER in horses.[59,114–116] Other signs associated with hypothyroidism in horses, such as alopecia, lethargy and excessive fat accumulation,[117,118] are not typical of ER-susceptible horses and, given its rarity, it is unlikely that hypothyroidism is associated with ER in most animals.

Infectious causes

Equine herpes virus 1 (EHV1) infection was proposed as causing an outbreak of ER in a training yard, where several horses seroconverted to the virus.[119] Equine influenza virus (EIV) has also been diagnosed by seroconversion as the potential cause of certain equine myopathies.[106] Both EIV and EHV1 infections are common in groups of young race horses and although the acute-phase response to viral infection can cause transient arthralgia and myalgia, and therefore stiffness, rhabdomyolysis is not a common feature of these diseases.

Inherited causes: recurrent exertional rhabdomyolysis

Etiology and pathogenesis

Recurring episodes of ER are common in various breeds and with other ER-related disorders such as PSSM1 (below), but the term 'recurrent exertional rhabdomyolysis' (RER) is applied to a presumed inherited[120] disorder of Thoroughbreds that are affected intermittently with episodes of ER, often without any clear inciting cause. Though possibly a result of an inherited trait from a common ancestral founder animal, it should not be assumed that a disorder with the same etiology is shared by all Thoroughbreds with intermittent bouts of ER, particularly given the potential acquired causes discussed above. Furthermore, it remains unclear whether this disease is unique to Thoroughbreds: certain similarities in vivo and in vitro suggest that other breeds, such as Standardbreds, and some Warmbloods, might share a similar, if not identical disorder.[57,74,107] Although episodes of RER are associated with time away from training, and are themselves a welfare issue, intriguingly, ER-susceptible racing Standardbreds outperform matched controls, leading researchers to speculate that breeders have inadvertently selected for the RER trait[57] as occurred in Quarter Horses with hyperkalaemic periodic paralysis (HYPP).[121]

There is in vitro evidence of underlying kinetic abnormalities of muscle in RER-susceptible Thoroughbreds: muscle from susceptible animals contracts more rapidly than normal muscle in vitro than does muscle from unaffected horses.[107] Furthermore, authors have detected abnormal relaxation, though they disagree as to whether relaxation is hastened or slowed.[107,122] The SR Ca2+- ATPase (SERCA) pump is a major determinant of muscle relaxation, but this pump's activity is normal in extracted SR vesicles from horses with RER,[123] suggesting that RER in Thoroughbred horses is not associated with abnormal SR Ca2+ uptake.

Speculation that ER might be related to a defect in calcium regulation[124,125] was strengthened by a report of elevated resting intracellular calcium concentrations in muscle from ER-susceptible horses.[53] However, resting calcium concentration in cultured equine myotubes (muscle cells) from Thoroughbreds with RER is no different to that of control cells.[126] Disparity in results from these studies could reflect differences in case selection, active disease processes (with a secondary rise in myoplasmic calcium) in the former study, or inability of the cell culture system to detect differences when compared to mature muscle.

Muscle strips examined in vitro from some Standardbreds and Thoroughbreds that are susceptible to ER are hypersensitive to agents that induce calcium release from the SR (Fig. 7.11) such as caffeine, a potent activator of the skeletal muscle sarcoplasmic reticulum calcium release channel (ryanodine receptor; RYR1).[107,122] In contrast, caffeine-hypersensitivity is not a feature of muscle from horses with PSSM (see below).[59,127] Caffeine was traditionally used to identify humans that are susceptible to malignant hyperthermia (MH) when stressed or under halothane anesthesia, because lower caffeine concentrations elicit contraction in biopsied strips of muscle from subjects with MH compared to that of normal subjects.[128–130] In pigs, dogs, horses (see below) and in most humans, MH is associated with mutations in the gene encoding RYR1,[130–132] but abnormal RYR1- ligand binding, detected in vesicles prepared

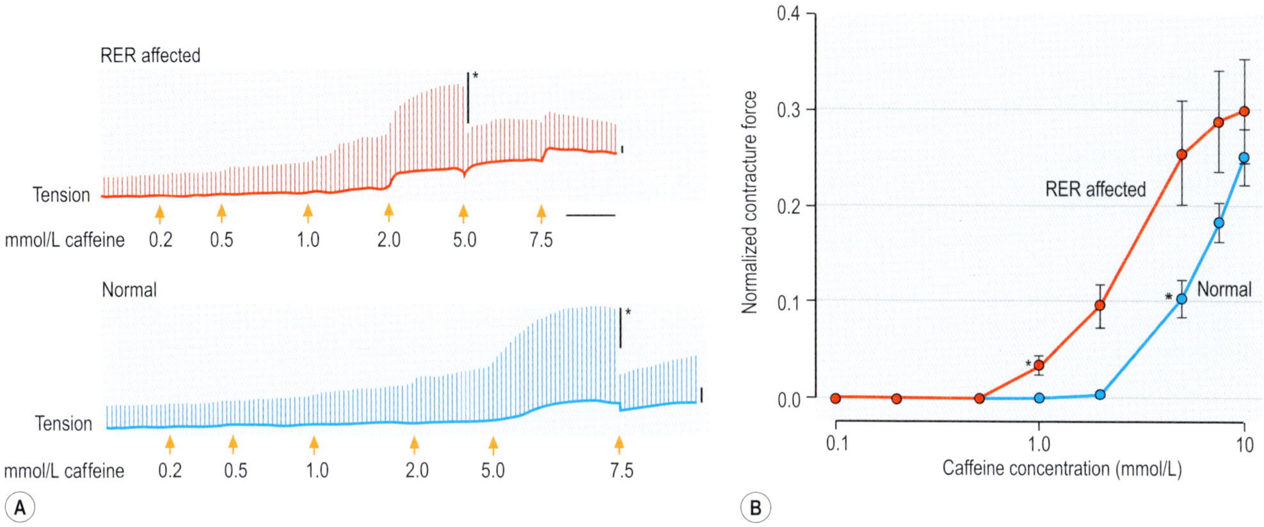

Fig 7.11 Tension (baseline) record for a caffeine contracture experiment performed on isolated intercostal muscle preparations from a normal horse and a Thoroughbred with RER. Twitches (vertical deflections) were elicited via electrical stimulation at 0.05Hz and caffeine was added to the bathing solution as indicated by the arrows to obtain the final concentration as noted. Horizontal bar = 5min; heavy left vertical bar = 0.5N/cm; heavy right vertical bar = 1.0N/cm.2 Asterisk = recorder gain change. Notice that caffeine elicits a change in baseline tension in muscle from the RER-affected horse at between 1 and 2mmol/L caffeine, whereas the baseline does not change until the bathing solution contains 5.0mmol/L caffeine for the control muscle. **(B)** Contracture force versus caffeine concentration for muscle bundles from clinically normal horses (n = 12; blue line) and RER(c)-affected horses (n = 10; red line). Contracture force was normalized to the preceding tetanus for both groups. Asterisks show force of contracture thresholds > 0 at 1.0mmol/L and 5.0mmol/L caffeine for RER-affected and clinically normal horses respectively.

Reprinted from Lentz LR, Valberg SJ, Balog EM, et al. Abnormal regulation of muscle contraction in horses with recurrent exertional rhabdomyolysis. Am J Vet Res 1999;60:992–9, with permission from the American Journal of Veterinary Research, http://avmajournals.avma.org/loi/ajvr.

from the muscle of MH pigs,[133] is not a feature of similar vesicles that are prepared from horses with RER.[123] Furthermore, muscle from RER-susceptible Thoroughbreds is not hypersensitive to 4chloro-m-cresol, a RYR1 agonist with higher specificity than caffeine.[126]

Caffeine-hypersensitive muscle is not exclusively found in human MH patients with RYR1 mutations: the same abnormality is reported in MH patients with mutations in other genes, such as the gene that encodes the alpha1-subunit of the L-type voltage-sensitive calcium channel (dihydropyridine receptor; DHPR).[134] At least three more genes are implicated in human MH.[135] Linkage analysis has effectively ruled out mutations in RYR1, DHPR and SERCA in RER-susceptible Thoroughbred horses.[136]

Recent work suggests that increased caffeine sensitivity of SR calcium release, detectable in cultured equine myotubes from MH-susceptible horses (see below), is not detectable in virally transducted,[137] cultured, skin-derived muscle cells from Thoroughbred horses with RER,[138] further suggesting that the RER-pathogenesis is not closely related to MH. Further, given that characteristic clinical and histopathologic features seen in various human myopathies caused by mutations in proteins involved with SR calcium release or excitation-contraction coupling are not seen in muscle from horses with RER,[139–141] any calcium homeostasis defect in RER could involve other cellular processes, or be a consequence, rather than the cause of the disorder. Abnormalities of the contractile apparatus could explain some of the in vitro caffeine sensitivity results in mature muscle from RER horses; however, when compared with normal horses, there was no difference in myofibrillar calcium sensitivity or ATPase activity.[142] Finally, given that muscle from some humans with different types of myopathy can be hypersensitive to caffeine,[143] Thoroughbreds might have an unrelated disorder.

Epidemiology

Studies indicate that between 4.9% and 6.7% of racing Thoroughbreds can be affected by RER during a single season[58,109] with the disorder reportedly inherited as an autosomal dominant trait with variable expression.[120,144] Subjective impression that RER occurs more frequently in young fillies has been confirmed by several studies.[58,109,116] Additionally, researchers found that Thoroughbreds that were nervous or lame were more likely to develop episodes of rhabdomyolysis.[58,145] Another study that examined ER in polo ponies in the UK and the US also found a high incidence,[145] particularly in animals with an excitable temperament. In both Thoroughbreds and polo ponies, the disease resulted in significant time away from training or competing.[58,109,145] Similar risk factors are reported in Standardbreds, in particular, a higher disease-associated susceptibility in females and in horses with a nervous temperament.[57]

Genomic studies

There are several reports of studies at the genome level where researchers have attempted to define genetic loci associated with RER-susceptibility.[108] These range from an early study in Standardbreds,[108] and more recent studies in Thoroughbreds.[146,147] As yet there is no consensus between research groups as to genomic regions implicated in RER, perhaps reflecting difficulties in accurately defining the disease or control phenotype (due to variable penetrance and co-existence of separate disorders), the influence of modifying genes, differences between populations of horses in different geographical locations or a combination of these factors.

Pathology

Histopathological lesions of many idiopathic cases and RER are highly variable and depend on severity and the time between the biopsy and the last bout of rhabdomyolysis (Figs 7.12) but muscle from most horses with RER, when biopsied between episodes, has low grade, non-specific features – typically scattered fibers with internalized nuclei and excessive variation in fiber size.

Mild inflammation, with hypercontracted and swollen fibers, interstitial edema and occasionally hemorrhage is seen after single episodes of acute rhabdomyolysis and during the first 24–48 hours after a new episode in animals with histories of recurring episodes (Fig. 7.12A). In this latter group, there can be hyaline degeneration, edema, scattered swollen fibers, fiber fragmentation, necrosis and macrophage infiltration and signs of regeneration (occasional fibroblasts with large nuclei and prominent nucleoli, myotubes and basophilic fibers and mature fibers with internalised nuclei) within the same section. Additionally, in severe chronic cases, fibrosis and fat infiltration or substitution are occasionally seen (Fig. 7.12E,F).[24,148–150] Fast-twitch (type 2X) fibers are usually most severely affected. Scattered fibers with subsarcolemmal and/or intracytoplasmic masses, possibly of calcium, are occasionally present (Fig. 7.12G). Other signs of regeneration, such as whorled fibers and fiber splitting (Fig. 7.12H) can be observed.

Common electron microscopic lesions found in many idiopathic cases and RER include non-specific changes such as myofibrillar disruption with loss of contractile material, streaming, or poorly aligned Z disks, dilated SR, enlarged and rounded mitochondria with dilated matrices and degenerated cristae, macrophage infiltration and increased granular deposits of glycogen(Fig. 7.13).[31]

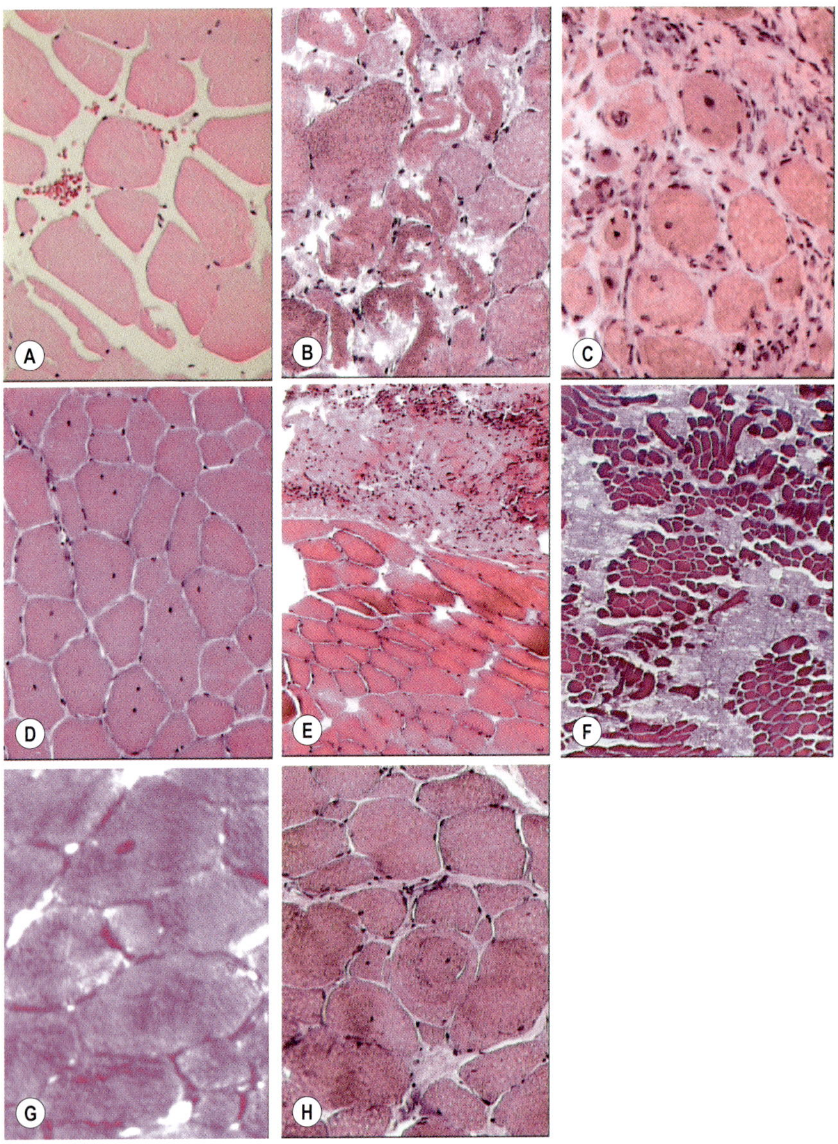

Fig 7.12 Transverse sections stained with hematoxylin and eosin of the pelvic limb and epaxial musculature of horses with idiopathic RER. **(A)** Several large, rounded and hypercontracted fibers are shown with diffuse interstitial edema and abundant hemorrhage. **(B)** Focal hyaline degeneration of type II fibers. **(C)** Severe myopathic changes characterized by increased fiber size variability, hypercontraction and degeneration, macrophage infiltration and abundant fibroblasts with large nuclei and prominent nucleoli. **(D)** Mature fibers with internalized nuclei that have regenerated following damage within the previous 1–2 months. **(E)** A scar is shown in the top of this frame, indicating ineffective muscle repair in an animal after recurrent rhabdomyolytic episodes. **(F)** Extensive ineffective muscle repair with massive loss of myofibers and replacement by connective tissue. **(G)** A fiber (top) with an intracytoplasmic mass, probably an aggregate of intracellular calcium. **(H)** Signs of regeneration including a whorled fiber towards the center.

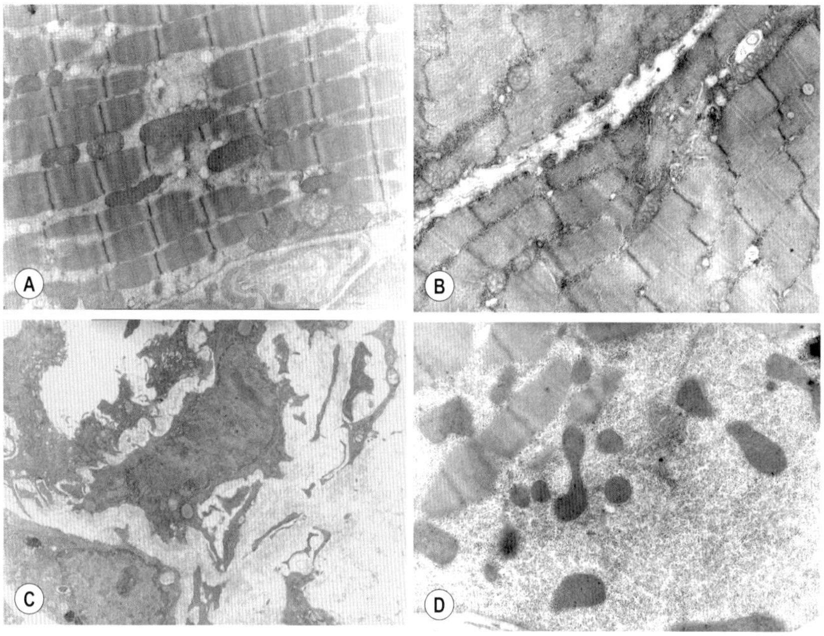

Fig 7.13 Electron micrographs of muscle from horses with idiopathic recurrent ER. **(A)** Myofibrillar degeneration with loss of contractile material, dilated terminal cisternae and swollen mitochondria with different electrodensities and abnormal cristae; x16,800. **(B)** Loss of myofibrillar architecture with abundant Z-line streaming; x22,400. **(C)** Macrophage infiltration; x11,200. **(D)** Loss of contractile material with abundant glycogen; x25,200.
Courtesy of Drs Sucre and Finol from the Universidad Central de Venezuela.

Malignant hyperthermia

Malignant hyperthermia (MH)-like reactions have been reported in several breeds of horse during or following anesthesia.[124,151–153] and in 2004, researchers identified a heterozygous non-synonymous polymorphism – a suspected mutation (R2454G) in RYR1 in Quarter Horses that died when anesthetized with halothane.[154] Subsequently, the same autosomal dominant mutation was reported in further halter Quarter Horses with histories of sudden death, rhabdomyolysis, muscle rigidity and persistent increases in serum muscle enzyme activities.[155] Cultured muscle cells derived from affected horses are hypersensitive to caffeine when compared with control cells (unlike cells cultured from horses with RER).[138] The disorder is associated with non-specific muscle histopathological changes and can be identified by genetic testing from whole blood (in EDTA) or hair root plucks.[156] This founder mutation has been reported in Quarter Horses and Paint horses[157] but not in other breeds of horse: given that there are reports of other equine breeds with MH, it is probable that additional RYR1 mutations are present in certain breeds or that mutations occur sporadically in some horses, as in humans.

Polysaccharide storage myopathy type 1 (PSSM1)

Since the first detailed report of PSSM in Quarter Horses,[158] a histopathologically-comparable disease was recognized in other breeds.[159–163] Classically, horses were diagnosed on the basis of either excessive amylase-sensitive glycogen or the presence of amylase-resistant polysaccharide in periodic acid schiff stained muscle sections.[44] Excessive glycogen and abnormal polysaccharide accumulation are seen in several human muscle diseases known as glycogenoses, many of which are caused by abnormal regulation or deficiencies of glycolytic or glycogenolytic enzymes; others are idiopathic or caused by lysosomal dysfunction.[164] Early experiments suggested that lactate production was impaired in Quarter Horses with PSSM[158,165]similar to humans with glycogenolytic or glycolytic enzyme deficiencies.[166] However, subsequent experiments using more stringent exercise tests demonstrated normal or exaggerated lactate production.[167] Affected Quarter Horses did not have detectable abnormalities in either glycolytic enzyme activities or their regulation,[158,168] and their oxidative metabolism appeared functional since they were able to maintain low plasma lactate concentrations during long-term submaximal exercise.[167]

Glycogen is a branched, three-dimensional molecule formed by the enzyme glycogen synthase that adds straight 1–4 glucose (actually uridine diphosphate glucose) linkages, and branching enzyme, which adds 1–6 linkages after every seventh molecule (Fig. 7.14). Abnormal polyglucosan accumulates in tissues of humans with branching enzyme deficiency,[169] a fatal disease identified in Quarter Horse foals.[170]

In 2008, researchers identified a single missense mutation (R309H) in the skeletal muscle glycogen synthase gene (*GYS1*) in PSSM-affected Quarter Horses[171]. This specific mutation is more prevalent in Halter Quarter Horses than other types.[172] Subsequently, the same mutation was reported in numerous breeds around the world with the prevalence being particularly high in certain continental European draught breeds.[32,173–178] Although affected horses often have histories of exertional rhabdomyolysis, in many animals the disease is subclinical and in some it is associated with other clinical signs (such as muscle atrophy and paresis).[179] In addition, genetic testing revealed that some ER-affected horses with similar histopathological myopathic changes, including excessive normal glycogen or amylase-resistant polysaccharide, do not have the same mutation,[178,180] indicating that these horses have one or more separate disorders. Currently horses with the *GYS1* mutation are described as having PSSM type 1 (PSSM1) whereas horses with muscle histopathological features that are compatible with a

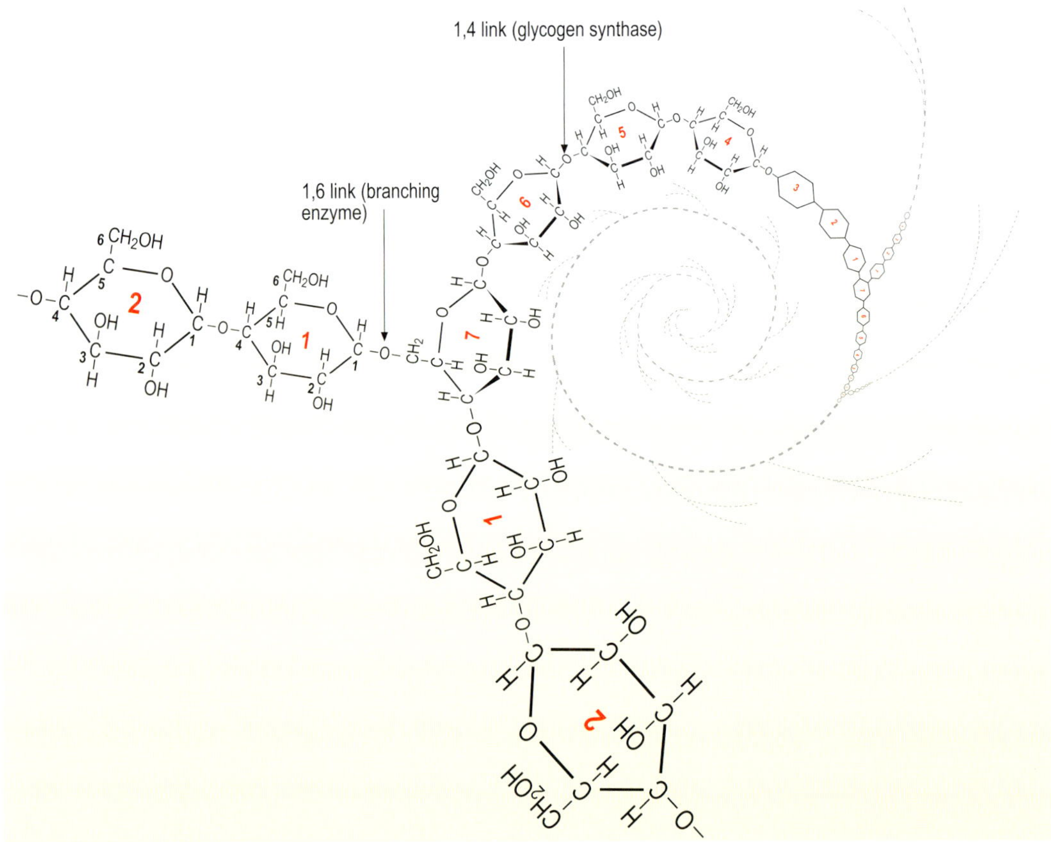

Fig 7.14 Diagrammatic representation of the three-dimensional structure of glycogen. Note that glycogen is composed of chains of UDP-glucose molecules joined enzymatically via 1–4 linkages (glycogen synthase) and 1–6 linkages (branching enzyme).

glycogenosis but without the R309H *GYS1* mutation, are described as having PSSM2 (see below).[178,180]

Pathogenesis

The mechanism(s) that lead to rhabdomyolysis in PSSM1 remain unclear. Several studies evaluating pathogenesis were conducted prior to the identification of the genetic cause and might therefore have included horses with separate disorders. Nonetheless, given the high prevalence of the *GYS1* mutation in certain breeds, it is reasonable to assume that most previous reports on pathogenesis of PSSM, apply to PSSM1.[181]

Glycogen synthase activity is higher in muscle from PSSM1-affected horses than in muscle from control horses.[171] Without a concomitant rise in branching enzyme activity, the higher glycogen synthase: branching enzyme ratio, likely results in a tendency to form polysaccharide with an abnormal filamentous structure (polyglucosan). Typically, this material accumulates as animals age[182], with amylase-resistant inclusions being first found at three years in affected Quarter Horses, even though biochemical evidence of an underlying myopathy and enhanced insulin sensitivity were present from a much younger age.[183] Consequently, excessive glycogen and polyglucosan accumulation can occur independently from any underlying susceptibility to rhabdomyolysis. Evidence supporting an underlying metabolic defect is to be found in a study that revealed increased inosine monophoshate (IMP; an intermediate byproduct of purine metabolism) concentrations in single muscle fibers and whole muscle of exercised horses with PSSM when compared to controls.[184] However, there is an association between underlying pathological changes (sub-sarcolemmal vacuolation and polysaccharide accumulation) and subclinically-raised CK and AST activity in affected horses, suggesting that physical disruption of myofiber architecture might also contribute to the phenotype.[27,178]

Various human glycogenoses affect tissues other than skeletal muscle, including the heart.[164,185]However, of nine draught horses examined, amylase-resistant polysaccharide was identified in the otherwise histologically normal myocardium of only one Belgian horse with PSSM.[162] Furthermore, cardiac arrhythmias were not detected in a separate group of Belgian and Percheron PSSM1-affected draught horses, even though a few animals had mild and subclinical elevations in cardiac troponinI.[186] Neither Quarter Horses nor Belgian or Percheron draught horses with PSSM1 have overt cardiac disease.[158,186]

Phenotypic variation

Homozygote horses with PSSM1 are more severely affected than heterozygotes, revealing incomplete dominance of the R309H mutation and explaining some of the variation in phenotypic severity between horses.[27] Nonetheless, there are other factors that influence phenotype which can include the breed. For example, affected Quarter Horses and Belgian draught horses differ metabolically: compared with normal animals, Quarter Horses with PSSM cleared glucose from plasma more rapidly after its intravenous injection (Fig. 7.15) and had reduced peak plasma glucose concentrations after oral carbohydrate intake.[187,188] Insulin sensitivity was not however detected in Belgian draught horses with PSSM.[189] Differences between breeds likely reflect the genetic background: for example, some phenotypic variation might result from the underlying fiber-type profiles of the major muscle groups. The influence of modifying genes is also revealed by evidence showing that PSSM1-affected horses that carry an additional mutation in RYR1 (associated with MH – see above) – are more severely affected.[157] The influence of diet on the phenotype is discussed in the treatment and management sections above.

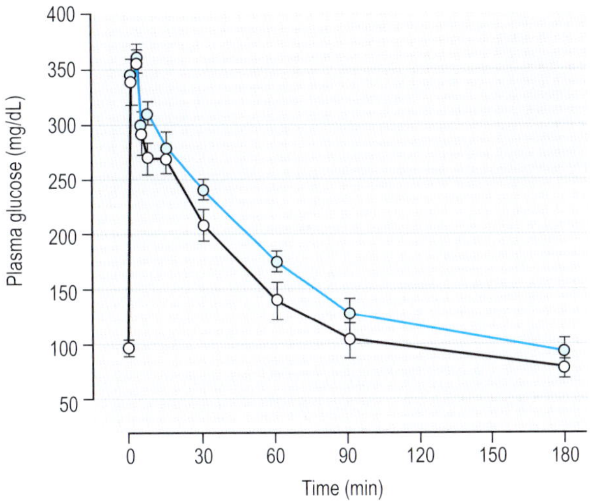

Fig 7.15 Mean plasma glucose concentrations in six horses with PSSM (black line) and 10 healthy control horses (blue line) immediately before (time 0) and at various times after i.v. glucose injection. Glucose concentration from 0 to 180 minutes was significantly ($P < 0.001$) lower in horses with PSSM than in controls. Bars represent SEM.

Reprinted from de la Corte FD, Valberg SJ, MacLeay JM, Williamson SE, Mickelson JR. Glucose uptake in horses with polysaccharide storage myopathy. Am J Vet Res 1999;60:458–462, with permission from the American Journal of Veterinary Research, http://avmajournals.avma.org/loi/ajvr.

Pathology

Horses with PSSM1 have many of the same non-specific myopathic changes discussed under the RER subheading, reflecting the general disease processes explained at the beginning of this chapter. Additional histopathologic changes associated with PSSM1[27,44,158,159,182,190] include: (a) a heterogeneous distribution of periodic acid-Schiff (PAS) stained intrafibrillar glycogen with subsarcolemmal, but non-membrane bound vacuoles; (b) PAS-positive inclusions; and (c) alpha-amylase-resistant PAS-positive inclusions (i.e. consistent with abnormal polysaccharide or polyglucosan) (Fig. 7.16). The PAS-positive and alpha-amylase-resistant inclusions are typically observed in type II fibers, do not stain with ATPase and SDH histochemistry, and have a slight eosinophilic light blue appearance with hematoxylin and eosin stains, magenta to dark blue with PAS and magenta with alpha-amylase-PAS (Fig. 7.16). The morphology of these inclusions, as multiple intracytoplasmic 'lakes', or more confluent accumulations totally or partially replacing the fiber in transverse section, or both, is consistent with similar changes recognized in formalin-fixed, paraffin-embedded muscle from affected animals.[44]

Pathological features of PSSM can also be detected by electron microscopy (Fig. 7.17). Muscle damage is usually extensive and consists of numerous fibers containing varying degrees of myofibrillar disruption and both loss and disruption of contractile material, characterized by irregular myofibrils and striation patterns. Filamentous material consisting of disrupted contractile proteins and polysaccharide are present amongst excessive granular glycogen.[160,180,191]

Polysaccharide storage myopathy type 2 (PSSM2)

Some horses with histories of ER and histopathological features consistent with PSSM do not carry the R309H *GYS1* mutation associated with PSSM1[171] suggesting that at least one further disorder of glycogenosis or glycolysis occurs in horses.[178,180] In one study, age at presentation for these animals was younger than for horses with PSSM1.[180] The genetic defect(s) have not yet been identified in these animals and currently, this disorder(s), termed PSSM2, is best diagnosed by muscle biopsy.[178,180] Unfortunately, recommendations for treatment and management of these horses, loosely based on recommendations for RER and PSSM1, remain largely speculative.

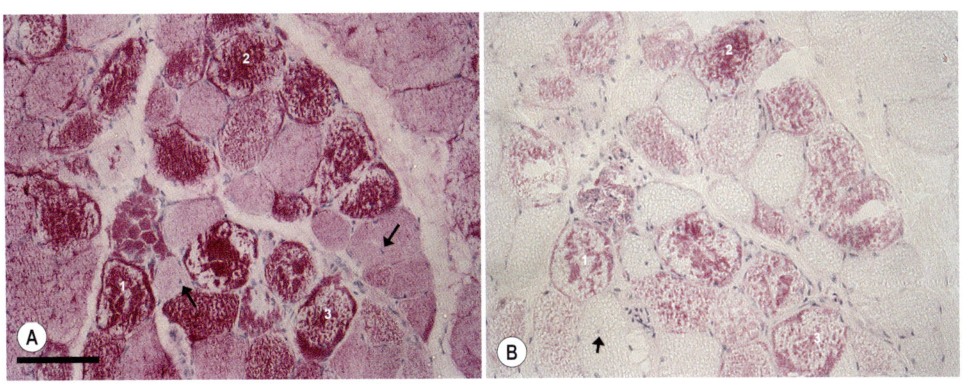

Fig 7.16 Serial fresh-frozen semimembranosus muscle sample sections from a 10 year old Connemara x Welsh Cob mare with intermittent exertional rhabdomyolysis. **(A)** Periodic Acid Schiff stain; **(B)** – amylase-pretreated Periodic Acid Schiff stain. Note that dense alpha crystalline polysaccharide material remains following enzymatic digestion (for example fibers labeled 1, 2 and 3 in each image), compared with fibers with more normal appearing glycogen (pink stain). Also note the internalized nuclei (arrows) revealing previous evidence of degeneration followed by regeneration. The horse was confirmed as having type 1 polysaccharide storage myopathy on the basis of genotyping. Nuclei are stained blue. Scale bar = 50 μm.

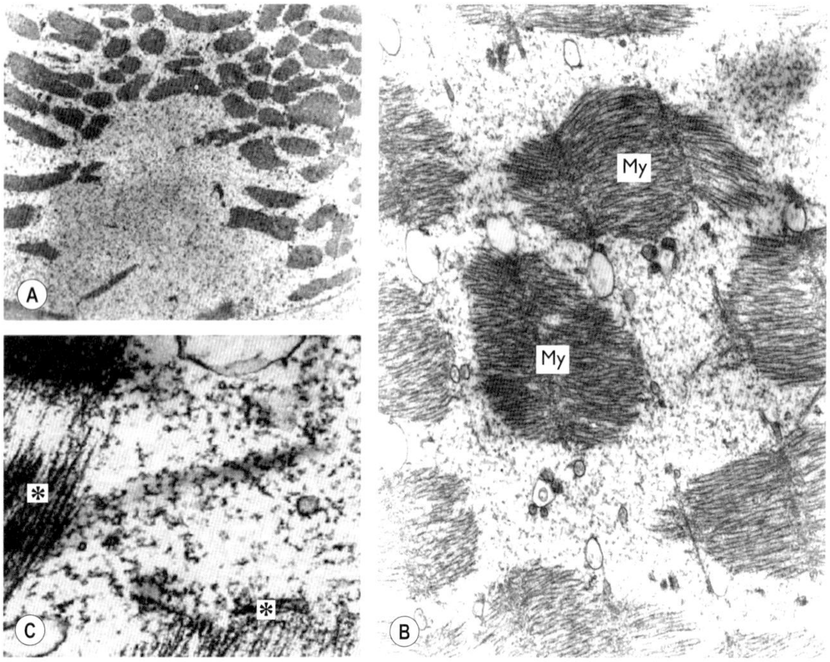

Fig 7.17 Transmission electron micrographs of M. longissimus lumborum biopsies from horses with polysaccharide storage myopathy (PSSM). **(A)** A large intracytoplasmic irregular aggregate of granular material is distributed between myofibrils with massive disruption of their normal arrangement (' 20000). At higher magnifications (**B**; x37000) the inclusions appear to consist of b-particles of glycogen disrupting myofibrils (My) and (**C**; x65000) large aggregates of filamentous material (asterisks).

Hyperkalemic periodic paralysis

- Genetic disorder seen in Quarter Horses and related breeds descended from the stallion Impressive.
- It is caused by a mutation in the alpha subunit of the skeletal muscle sodium channel.
- Autosomal dominant inheritance.
- Homozygotes are more severely affected than heterozygotes.
- Signs vary from subclinical to severe.
- Paresis is the predominant physical sign, although muscle spasm and fasciculation can occur.
- Life-threatening complications include cardiac arrhythmias secondary to hyperkalemia and asphyxiation due to laryngospasm.
- Prophylactic dietary and therapeutic management can reduce the frequency and severity of attacks.

Recognition

History and presenting complaint

Hyperkalemic periodic paralysis (HYPP) manifests as episodes that occur intermittently, last several minutes to hours, and are more common in young adults or foals. Between episodes, horses do not exhibit clinical signs though electromyographic abnormalities can be detected. Affected horses typically have a phenotype characterized by highly developed and defined skeletal musculature, particularly over the pelvis. Episodes often follow sleep or can be precipitated by stress, cold weather and sometimes exercise.[192] Evidence suggests that the condition is recognized more commonly in young males[193–195] although this has not been confirmed experimentally.

Physical examination

Clinical signs vary, with homozygotes being more severely affected than heterozygotes. Myotonia is often brief or not apparent; however, third eyelid protrusion is sometimes seen along with spasm of certain facial muscles and, more commonly, muscle fasciculation.[196] Laryngeal or pharyngeal spasm can occur, causing pharyngitis, dysphagia and occasionally severe dyspnea.[197] These signs are more common in young homozygous foals,[197] but in adults can present as abnormal respiratory noise during exercise.[198] More characteristic, especially in older horses, are signs of paresis, such as swaying or buckling, a stilted gait, dog sitting, collapse or recumbency.[196] Respiratory muscle weakness and increased muscular effort can be manifest as shallow tachypnea and sweating. Horses remain alert, responsive and do not present signs of pain.[192,196] Death, if it occurs, can follow the dyspnea associated with laryngospasm or, more commonly, cardiac arrhythmia (ventricular fibrillation) due to underlying hyperkalemia;[199,200] horses that are under, or recovering from anesthesia, appear particularly at risk of episodes of the disease.[201–203]

Special examinations

Electrocardiography

Consistent with hyperkalemia, during episodes, the ECG reveals smaller, wider P waves, increased amplitude of T waves and widening of QRS complexes.[195,204–206] Between episodes the ECG is normal.[195]

Endoscopy

Endoscopy can reveal pharyngeal collapse and edema, dorsal displacement of the soft palate, bilateral laryngeal paresis and persistent opening of the guttural pouch ostia.[192,198]

Electromyography

Electromyography reveals abnormalities such as doublets and characteristic myotonic discharges between and during disease episodes (Fig. 7.18).[207]

Laboratory examination

Serum biochemistry

During an episode, clinical pathological changes usually, but not always,[193,202,208] include hyperkalemia (5.5–12mEq/L).[195,196] Elevated

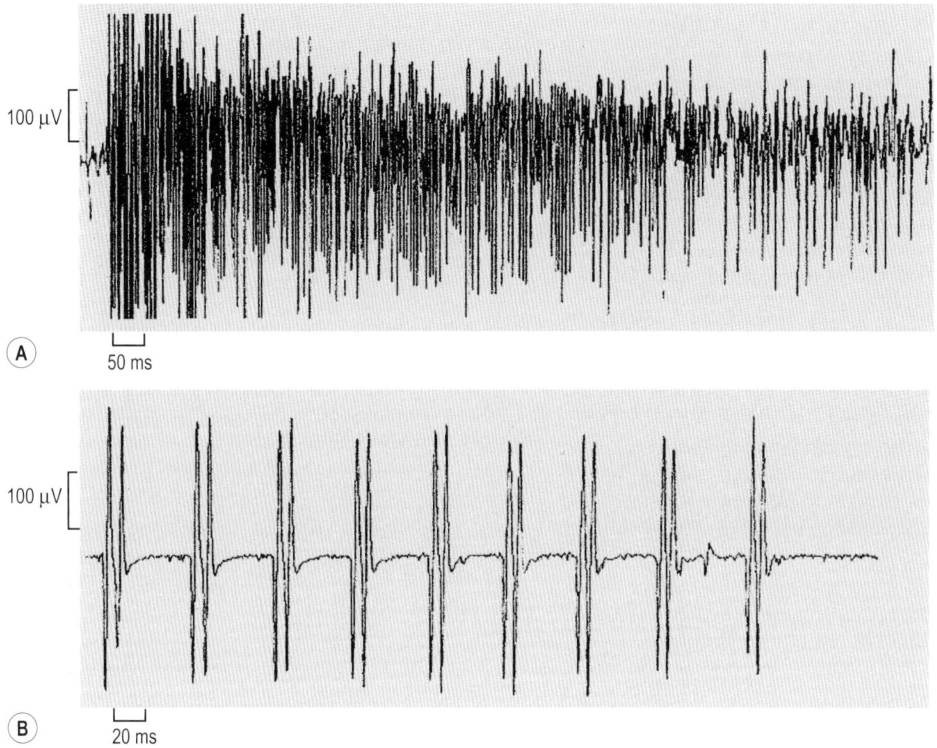

Fig 7.18 Electromyographic features of HYPP-affected muscle. **(A)** Myotonic discharges and **(B)** trains of doublets recorded in an HYPP-affected horse while clinically normal.

total serum protein concentration (7.0–9.0mg/dL) suggests fluid compartmental shifts.[195,209] Serum CK and AST activities are normal to moderately elevated.[195,210]

Muscle biopsy

Muscle biopsy is not normally indicated and is often histologically normal, but can reveal centrally located vacuoles in type II fibers, excessive fiber size variation, occasional internalized nuclei, moth-eaten fibers, connective tissue proliferation and fiber degeneration.[194,195,211] Electron microscopy reveals distension and proliferation of the SR and copious networks of transverse tubules.[192]

Diagnostic confirmation

The differential diagnosis includes colic, ER, laminitis, cardiac disease, tetanus, botulism, seizures and upper airway obstruction. Myotonic discharges, observed during EMG examination, are also seen in the rare disorders known as myotonic dystrophy and myotonia congenita (see later sections).[212–215] Recognition of paresis and muscle fasciculations in combination with hyperkalemia in an Impressive-related Quarter Horse or related breed, should leave little doubt that the animal has HYPP. Hyperkalemia itself, though not always present, can be due to other causes such as recent exercise, a hemolyzed blood sample or, more rarely, renal failure.

Diagnostic confirmation via the potentially fatal potassium chloride challenge test[192,195,196,216] was rendered obsolete with the advent of genotyping. Electromyography, a useful ancillary test with a reported sensitivity of 90%,[217] can support the diagnosis before DNA test results are available. Abnormal EMG signals can be detected both during and between episodes and in HYPP-positive horses undergoing treatment.[217,218]

Definitive diagnosis can only be achieved by mutational analysis of the sodium channel alpha subunit gene, which determines an animal as heterozygous or homozygous. Any sample containing DNA (for example, tissues removed at necropsy) could be used but whole blood (in EDTA) or a plucked hair sample (containing roots) is preferred. The American Quarter Horse Association recommends testing foals born to unclassified parents; those related to Impressive are identified with their established genotype on registration certificates. Note that a horse can be heterozygous for HYPP but display weakness and collapse for some other reason and that the genetic test only identifies the single specific mutation seen in all horses to date with HYPP.[219] Many different sodium channel mutations have been identified in humans with HYPP so full sequencing of the entire sodium channel gene should be considered in animals (especially other breeds) with classic HYPP clinical signs, diagnostic testing and clinicopathology, if the common founder mutation has been ruled out.

Treatment and prognosis

Therapeutic aims

Therapy is aimed at systemic abnormalities, specifically the life-threatening hyperkalemia and, if present, the dyspnea.

Therapy

Mild cases require stall rest or hand walking together with grain or a sweet-feed meal or orally-administered corn syrup.[196] Horses should be observed closely for worsening signs. More severely affected animals with prominent paresis or auscultable cardiac arrhythmia require aggressive medical therapy. Severe dyspnea can require emergency tracheotomy.

Emergency treatment during an attack

Slow intravenous administration of calcium gluconate diluted in isotonic fluids (0.2–0.4mL/kg of 23% calcium gluconate in 2 L of 5% dextrose) raises membrane threshold potential, reducing the likelihood of an action potential despite the muscle cells' relatively depolarized state; it similarly protects cardiomyocytes.[192,203]

Intravenous administration of potassium-free fluids containing dextrose triggers insulin release and hence facilitates movement of glucose and potassium into cells. Intravenous administration of insulin has been advocated but should be done in combination with administration of dextrose-containing fluids to avoid hypoglycemia; a dose of 0.05IU/kg has been used.[203] A mild alkalosis from sodium bicarbonate administration should also promote intracellular potassium movement. One author recommends 0.9% NaCl, containing 0.5–1mL/kg 1.3% NaHCO3 and 0.5–1mL/kg 50% dextrose.[196] Other treatments aimed at reducing hyperkalemia include beta-adrenergic agonists[192,220] to stimulate the Na/K ATPase pump, which reduces the resting membrane potential. These drugs are rarely necessary though, and could increase the risk of cardiac arrhythmia.

Phenytoin ameliorates skeletal muscle signs probably by altering sodium channel activity through the influence of cytoplasmic free fatty acids;[221,222] however, serum phenytoin concentrations should be monitored. Note that phenytoin does not reduce serum potassium concentrations[199] and is not usually required.

Prognosis

Most mildly to moderately affected animals will respond well but if hyperkalemia is severe and not treated promptly, sudden cardiac death can occur. Asphyxiation is possible in cases with laryngospasm as is aspiration pneumonia, particularly in nursing foals. Evidence suggests that in many animals the signs can be controlled successfully, but given the underlying genetic abnormality, horses remain susceptible for life.

Prevention

Management and dietary changes

Horses that have repeated attacks often benefit from long-term management changes and prophylaxis. In some cases a change in diet and avoidance of the cold and stressful events such as transportation, can suffice.

Feed modification reduces the number of attacks.[193] Many horses do well when maintained principally at pasture but when not practical, they should always have access to hay, and concentrate feed should be divided and given several times daily. High potassium-containing forages such as brome hay and alfalfa should be avoided, as should canola and soybean oil, molasses and certain potassium-containing mineral supplements. Late bloom timothy hay, sugar beet pulp and barley or oats are suitable alternatives, although calcium supplementation can be required to ensure appropriate calcium : phosphorus ratios.[223]

Prophylaxis

Acetazolamide (2–4mg/kg q 12–14 h p.o.), a carbonic anhydrase inhibitor, is widely used in horses. It prevents attacks induced by experimental potassium challenge[224] and anecdotal evidence suggests that the drug is useful in the field.[196,210] Carbonic anhydrase inhibition in renal proximal convoluted tubules decreases reabsorption of sodium ions via an indirect inactivation of luminal H+-Na+ antiporters, thereby enhancing sodium for potassium exchange in the distal tubules and promoting potassium excretion.[225] However, some have doubted this explanation for acetazolamide's efficacy, suggesting that other mechanisms, such as the stimulation of insulin secretion, might be involved.[192,226,227] Other potassium-wasting diuretics, such as hydrochlorothiazide, have also been tried in horses but experience is limited.[228]

Etiology and pathophysiology

A disease resembling human HYPP was reported in Quarter Horses in the mid 1980s[229,230] but the etiology of human HYPP was then unknown. In the early 1990s, several groups confirmed that human HYPP is caused by mutations in a gene encoding the alpha subunit of a sodium channel expressed only in skeletal muscle.[231,232] Linkage of equine HYPP to a single locus[233] and identification of a single base pair substitution in the equine sodium channel alpha subunit gene quickly followed.[121] Unlike in humans, in equine HYPP all identified cases to date have the same mutation,[219] the substitution of a cytosine for a guanine residue, causing the amino acid phenylalanine to be replaced by leucine in the cytoplasmic end of the IVS3 transmembrane domain (Fig. 7.19, Fig. 7.20) of the encoded 260kDa protein.[121]

As in the human disorder, equine HYPP is inherited in autosomal dominant fashion.[209,234] The different severity of homozygotes

Human	V G W N I F D F V V V I L S I V G L A L S D L I	*Homo sapiens*
Horse	V G W N I F D F V V V I L S I V G L A L S D L I	*Equus caballus*
Horse HYPP	V G W N I L D F V V V I L S I V G L A L S D L I	*Equus caballus* (HYPP)
Rabbit	I G W N I F D F V V V I L S I V G M F L A E L I	*Oryctolagus cuniculus*
Mouse	I G W N I F D F V V V I L S I V G L A L S D L I	*Mus musculus*
Rat	I G W N I F D F V V V I L S I V G L A L S D L I	*Rattus norvegicus*
Bony fish	N G W N I F D F I V V I L S I A G T M L S D I I	*Takifugu pardalis*
Tunicate	N P W N V F D F I V V I L S V V G S T M N E V I	*Halocynthia roretzi*
Mosquito	E P W N L F D F V V V I L S I L G L V L S D I I	*Anopheles gambiae*
Mollusc	E P W N I F D F V V V V L S I L G I A L S D I I	*Loligo opalescens*
Newt	I G W N V F D F V V V I L S I V G M F L S E I I	*Cynops pyrrhogaster*

Fig 7.19 Comparison of IVS3 amino acid sequences of various species. Standard single letter codes for each amino acid are used and amino acids with similar properties are shown with the same background color; hence polar-negative amino acids are red, polar-neutral amino acids are green, non-polar aliphatic amino acids are white and non-polar aromatic amino acids are purple. Glycine and proline tend to have structural properties in biological membranes and are colored brown. Note the significant conservation of either amino acid sequence or amino acid type within the structural domain between species. Such conservation usually reflects the functional and structural importance of the region to the protein. Also note the replacement of phenylalanine (F) by leucine (L) (circled in red), in horses with HYPP.

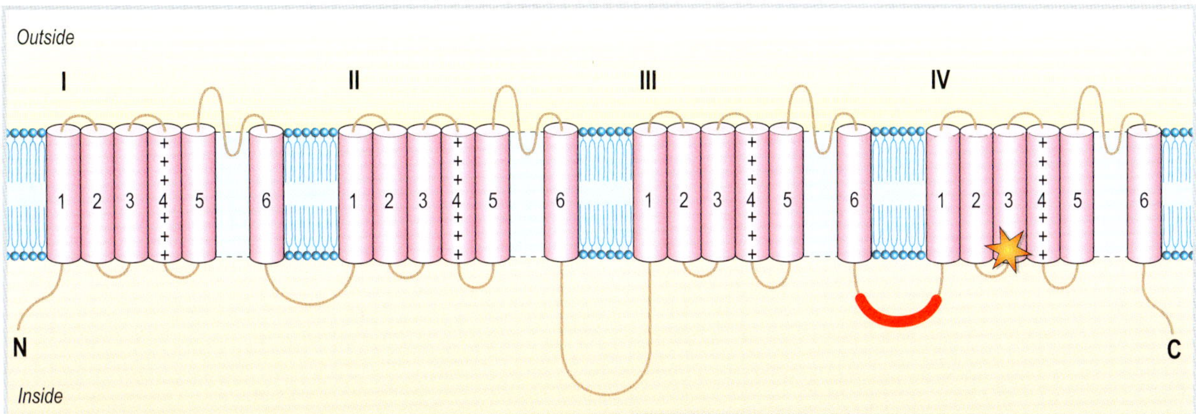

Domains labeled **I–IV**

Hydrophobic transmembrane segments labeled 1–6

Phe–Leu mutation in domain IV S_3 close to intracellular surface

Fig 7.20 Diagrammatic representation of the equine sodium channel alpha-subunit. The protein contains four domains (I–IV), each containing six transmembrane hydrophobic segments (1–6) that combine to form a channel in the sarcolemma. Segment 4 in each domain contains a high density of charged amino acids that participate in sensing voltage changes across the sarcolemma. The phenylalanine to leucine mutation is located close to the cytoplasmic surface of segment 3 in domain IV (asterisk). The spanning region between III-S6 and IV-S1 is believed to participate in channel inactivation (colored red).

compared to heterozygotes is a reflection of the codominance of the mutated and wild-type alleles. As with many diseases, phenotypic severity varies among heterozygotes, perhaps due to the modifying influence of other genes or environmental effects. One group has reported a correlation of disease severity with the ratio of mRNA from affected: wild-type (unaffected) alleles,[235] although this finding has not been confirmed at the protein level.

Transient myotonia

The skeletal muscle sodium channel associated with HYPP lies in the sarcolemmal (and T-tubule) membrane and allows sodium to enter the fiber during action potential conduction (see Chapter 6). In vitro studies demonstrate dysfunctional inactivation of the mutant channel and an increased open probability, hence abnormal influx of sodium while at rest (Fig. 7.21).[236,237] Although individual fibers vary, in HYPP, the resting potential is higher (less negative) than normal.[238] Blocking sodium channels in HYPP muscle with tetrodotoxin returns the membrane potential towards normal (more polarized) but has no effect on the resting potential in normal muscle.[238] The closer proximity to the threshold potential in HYPP muscle results in more readily-elicited action potentials, explaining the transient myotonia and muscle fasciculations. Fibers from younger horses with HYPP have higher resting potentials than older horses and muscle cooling raises the resting potential. These observations explain the higher incidence of HYPP episodes in young horses and during cold weather.[238]

Paresis

Following rapid depolarization of the action potential, sodium channels normally close in response to the now positive membrane potential. In addition, voltage-gated potassium channels open, allowing potassium to leave the muscle fiber and return it to its resting potential. Failure of mutant sodium channels to inactivate, prevents repetitive trains of action potentials[236,239] (required for Ca^{2+} release), causing the paresis that is the predominant sign in affected horses.

Hyperkalemia can be both the consequence and the cause of an attack

Most horses are hyperkalemic during or immediately after an episode, probably due to voltage-gated potassium channels remaining open, allowing continual potassium efflux. Hyperkalemia itself raises the fiber resting potential and promotes an open sodium channel configuration, thereby exacerbating the condition[240,241] or, as demonstrated by the formerly used potassium challenge test, precipitating an attack. Spontaneous recovery often follows attacks, perhaps as a result of the kidneys' correcting the hyperkalemia or a local rise in muscle temperature.[196]

Muscle hypertrophy

Horses with HYPP typically have hypertrophied muscles and this favorable trait in halter classes likely resulted in the maintenance and propagation of the mutation in the gene pool until a rule change by the American Quarter Horse Association.[218] The mechanism causing the hypertrophy is not understood, but can relate to myotonia-induced muscle protein synthesis.

Exercise intolerance

Experiments show that despite the hypertrophic muscles, horses with HYPP have reduced exercise tolerance compared with normal animals and produce relatively more lactate during exercise.[242] Even when paresis or muscle fasciculations are absent, exercised homozygotes exhibit intermittent laryngospasm, pharyngeal collapse, hypoxia, hypercapnia and ventricular premature contractions.[243]

Epidemiology

The spontaneous mutation that first occurred in Impressive (born 1969) spread via line breeding throughout the Quarter Horse population (Fig. 7.22). Dominant inheritance has led to cases in Quarter Horse-related breeds such as Appaloosas, American paint

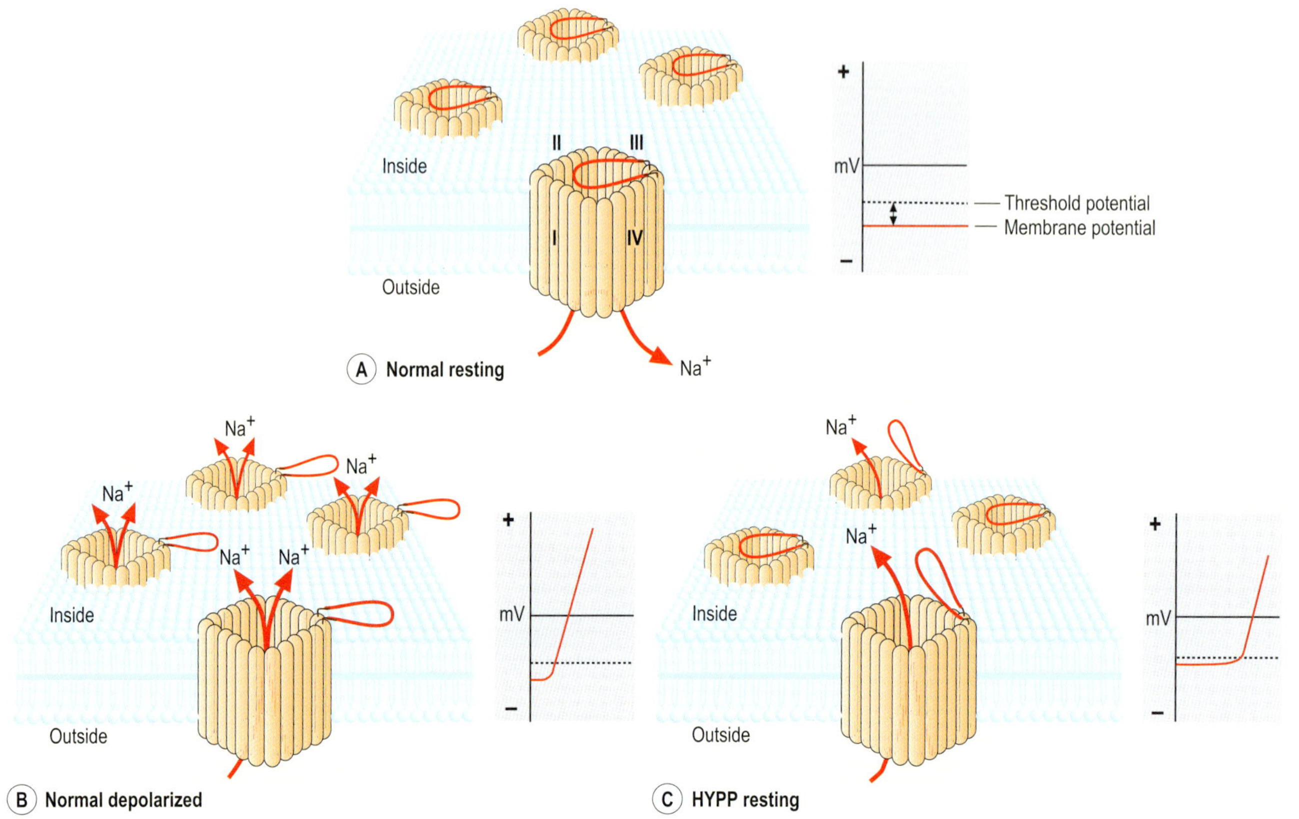

Fig 7.21 Diagrammatic explanation for the pathophysiology of HYPP. In a normal resting muscle cell, sodium channels are inactive and closed and the resting potential lies some way below the threshold potential **(A)**. A regional change in voltage activates sodium channels, causing them to open, allowing sodium to enter the fiber (the upswing of the action potential) **(B)**. In muscle fibers from horses with HYPP, some sodium channels have abnormal inactivation and remain open, despite the fibers resting state. Sodium can enter the fiber down its concentration gradient. This results in the fiber's resting potential being close to the threshold potential **(C)** and hence more readily elicited action potentials.

horses and crosses. Within the US in 2009, the overall HYPP allele frequency (proportion of mutant alleles within all alleles in a population) was estimated to be 0.8% in Quarter Horses and 2.5% in paint horses.[172] However the mutation remains highly prevalent within halter Quarter Horses.[172] Although seen predominantly in North America, HYPP has also been reported in Impressive-descended Quarter Horses in Australia.[205]

Myotonia

- Equine myotonia is rare.
- In New Forest ponies, the disorder (Myotonia congenita) has been associated with a mutation in the gene encoding the sarcolemmal chloride channel (CLCN1).
- Percussion dimpling and prolonged muscle contractions are present from an early age.
- Electromyography reveals frequent myotonic discharges.
- No successful treatment or prophylaxis has been reported.

Although horses with HYPP can exhibit (usually transient) myotonia, several case reports describe more prolonged myotonia. As in HYPP, previously recognized cases were probably associated with mutations in genes encoding sarcolemmal ion channels,[214] and recently a specific mutation have been identified.[215] In humans, the phenotype varies depending on the channel involved and the mutation, but there is considerable overlap. Early literature combined equine myotonia with myotonic dystrophy but on close evaluation of the disease descriptions, it was clear that at least two myotonia-causing disorders occur in horses.

Recognition

History and presenting complaint

Gait abnormalities and stiffness that are worst following a period of rest can be apparent early in life.[214] Some affected animals can collapse.[215]

Physical examination

Examination reveals symmetrical muscle hypertrophy and muscle percussion causes localized spasm and prolonged dimpling.[214,215] Clinical signs in horses with myotonia do not deteriorate significantly with time.

Special examinations

Electromyography

Changes are similar to those observed in HYPP (Fig. 7.18).[214,215]

Muscle biopsy

Histopathological evaluation of muscle samples will likely be normal or show mild myopathic changes including excessive fiber size variation and occasional internally-located nuclei.[215]

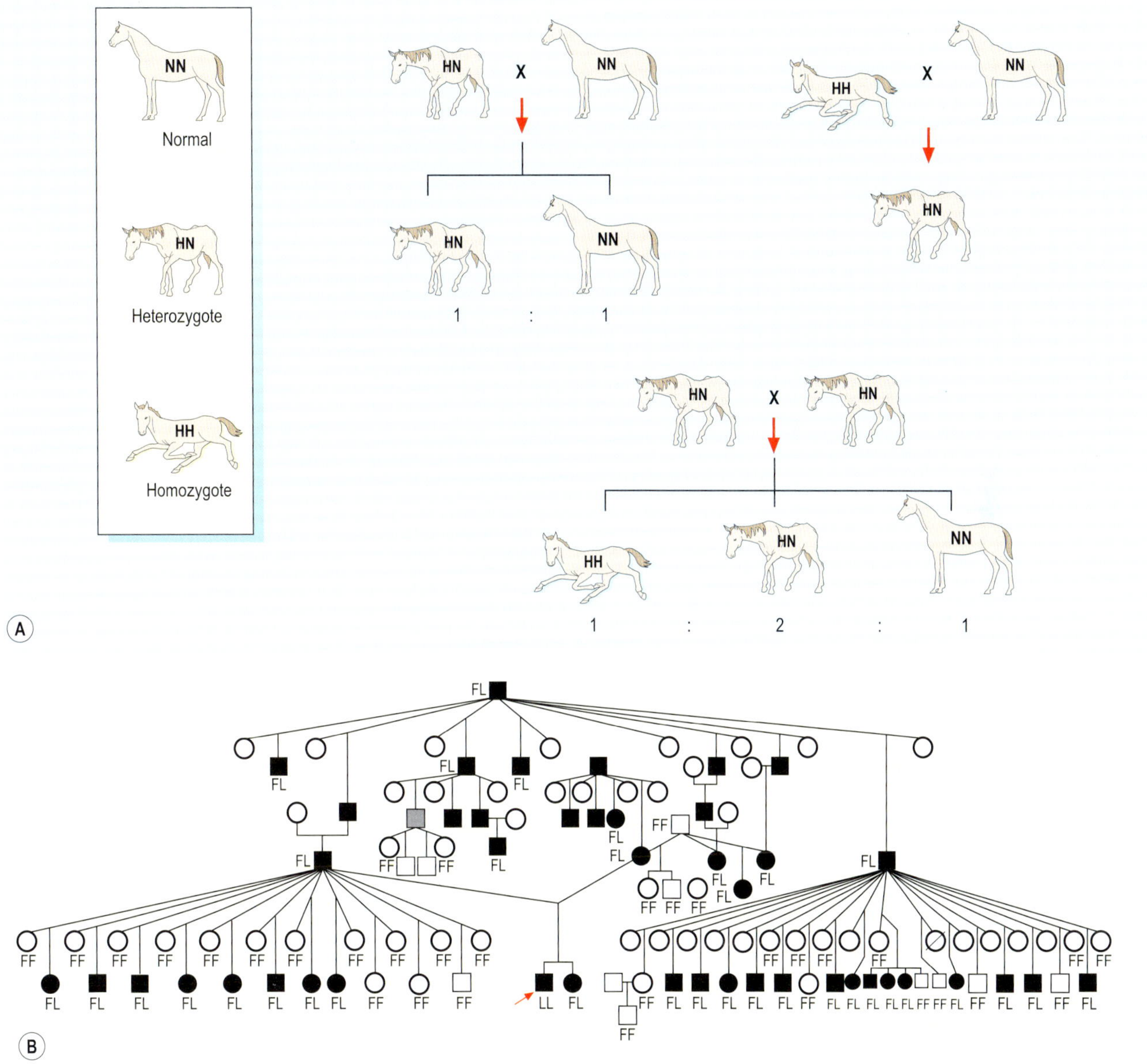

Fig 7.22 **(A)** Diagrammatic representation of matings between horses with HYPP and normal animals. **(B)** HYPP Quarter Horse pedigree. Horses are shown typed for the normal allele of the sodium channel (phenylalanine (F)) and the allele that causes HYPP (leucine (L)) in the sodium channel region IVS3. A homozygous affected horse is indicated by an arrow. The horse represented by a gray symbol has an unknown status. Squares represent males and circles represent females. Black symbols represent horses with the HYPP phenotype and open symbols represent normal horses.

Reprinted by permission from Macmillan Publishers Ltd, Nature Genetics, © 1992 from Rudolph JA, Spier SJ, Byrns G, et al. Periodic paralysis in Quarter Horses: a sodium channel mutation disseminated by selective breeding, 1992;2:144–147, http://www.nature.com/ng/index.html.

Diagnostic confirmation

The main differential is myotonic dystrophy, which is characterized by severe muscle histopathological changes, endocrine abnormalities and progressive clinical signs. Certain mutations in the human sarcolemmal sodium channel alpha subunit gene are manifest as myotonia rather than periodic paralysis: direct sequencing, rather than the routine HYPP DNA test would be required for definitive diagnosis of a sodium channel disorder in affected horses. Candidate gene sequencing, or testing for a specific mutation in other ion channels (e.g. chloride channel) would be appropriate in some cases.[215]

Treatment and prognosis

There are no reports of successful treatment. The prognosis for athletic function is poor but the prognosis for life can be fair.[214]

Etiology and pathophysiology

Clinical descriptions and comparison with human diseases suggest that a sarcolemmal chloride channel (CLCN1) mutation probably accounted for a single report of equine myotonia in a Thoroughbred filly in the USA;[214] consequently, and in parallel with the related human disease, this specific equine disorder is best termed

Myotonia congenita. In 2012, researchers identified the first (homozygous recessive) missense mutation (D592A) in the equine skeletal muscle chloride channel within a single family of New Forest ponies.[215] Clinical signs can be explained by reduced muscle chloride conductance that causes membrane potential to rise, resulting in membrane hyperexcitability and hence myotonia.[232]

Myotonic dystrophy

- Myotonic dystrophy is rare and probably has an underlying genetic cause.
- Percussion dimpling and prolonged muscle contractions are early signs.
- Horses with myotonic dystrophy can develop tendon contractures, kyphoscoliosis and endocrine anomalies.
- Electromyography reveals myotonic discharges in certain muscles.
- Muscle histopathology reveals moderate to severe dystrophic changes.
- Successful treatment has not been reported and euthanasia can be necessary.

Recognition

History and presenting complaint

Horses are usually presented early in life with stiff gaits and prolonged contraction of certain muscles.

Physical examination

Animals are alert and responsive, with marked muscular hypertrophy particularly in the gluteal region and pelvic limbs. Percussion dimpling is readily elicited in many animals and prolonged contraction can follow spontaneous or induced movements (Fig. 7.23A, B). Paresis, manifest as knuckling or stumbling, can also be seen. Signs can progress to include tendon contractures, kyphoscoliosis, a pendulous abdomen, colic and, in males, testicular atrophy.[212,213]

Special examination

Electromyography

Myotonic discharges are common in some but not all muscles, as are high-frequency electrical bursts during needle insertion, movement or following percussion.[212,213] Motor unit potentials in the thoracic paraspinal muscles of one animal were polyphasic and reduced in amplitude, but normal in the gastrocnemius.[213]

Laboratory examination

Hematology and biochemistry

Hematology and biochemistry values can become abnormal with age.[244] Serum CK and AST activities have been reported to be both normal and raised in affected horses. Some animals have endocrine abnormalities.[212,213]

Muscle biopsy

Mild to severe dystrophic changes such as fiber-size variation and fiber-type grouping, increased perimyseal and endomyseal connective tissue, necrosis with inflammatory cell infiltration, internally-located nuclei and whorled fibers are seen (Fig. 7.24). There can be selective type I muscle fiber hypertrophy with moth-eaten fibers and ring bands.[211–213,244–246]

Diagnostic confirmation

The main differentials are equine myotonia or HYPP (see above). Additional clinical signs, genetic testing and muscle biopsy will aid in the diseases' differentiation.

Treatment and prognosis

There are no reports of successful treatment.

Prevention

Owners should be advised with regard to breeding affected or related animals, as the disorder is likely genetic in origin.

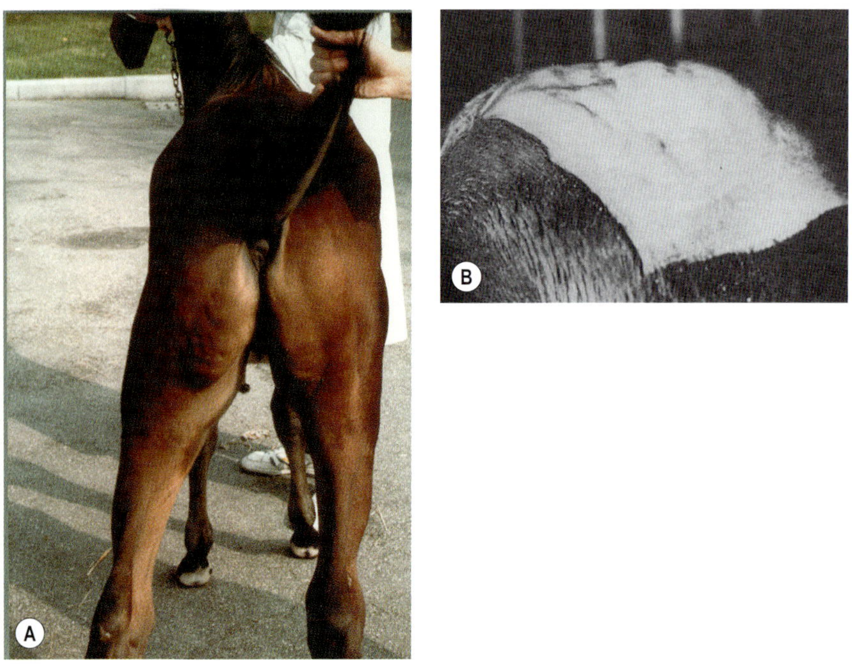

Fig 7.23 Spontaneous contraction and dimpling of hindlimb muscles of a five-month-old colt of Anglo-Arab-Sardinian descent with myotonic dystrophy (courtesy of Prof Pascale Montagna, University of Bologna, Italy). **(B)** Percussion dimpling following clipping in the gluteal musculature of a one-month-old Quarter Horse colt with myotonic dystrophy.
Fig. 7.23B reprinted from Reed SR, Hegreberg GA, Bayley WM, et al. Progressive myotonia in foals resembling human dystrophia myotonica. Muscle and Nerve. 1988;11:291–6, © 1988 John Wiley and Sons, Inc.

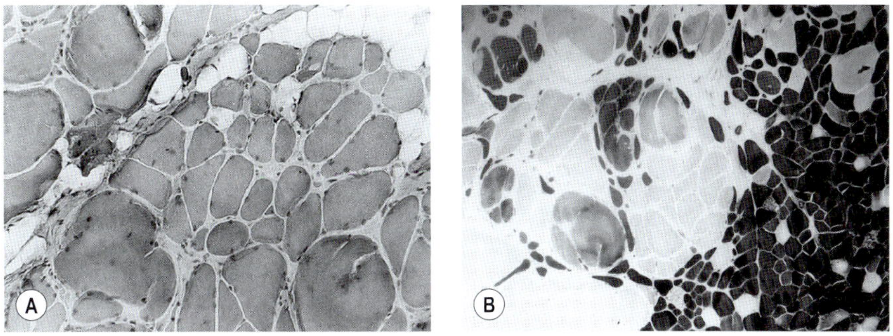

Fig 7.24 **(A)** Transverse section of gluteus medius muscle from a horse with myotonic dystrophy stained with hematoxylin and eosin. Note the fiber size variability, extensive perimysial connective tissue and internalized nuclei. **(B)** ATPase staining at alkaline pH. Note the marked variation in fiber size with type I hypertrophy and fiber type grouping. *Courtesy of Prof Mario Cipone, University of Bologna, Italy.*

Etiology and pathogenesis

The etiology and pathogenesis have not been established in horses. There are two main forms of inherited myotonic dystrophy in people, one of which is caused by a heterozygous trinucleotide expansion (CTG)n in the 3-primed untranslated region of the dystrophica myotonica protein kinase gene (*DMPK*).[247] A second form is caused by a heterozygous expansion of a CCTG repeat in intron 1 of the zinc finger protein-9 gene (*ZNF9*).[248] The mutations likely result in aberrant splicing of other genes: one in particular, amphiphysin 2 (*BIN1*) which is implicated in T tubule maintenance, is miss-spliced in both forms.[249] In humans, in addition to the muscle defects, endocrine disorders including hyperinsulinemia and hypogonadism and cataracts are common.[250,251]

Epidemiology

The condition has been reported in Quarter Horses and in a horse of Anglo-Arab-Sardinian descent.[212,213,244]

Mitochondrial myopathy

- Rare cause of severe exercise intolerance.
- Light exercise causes pronounced lactic acidemia.
- Diagnosis is achieved via muscle biopsy and measurement of mitochondrial enzyme activities.
- Reduced activity of mitochondrial enzyme complexes are probably associated with mitochondrial or genomic DNA mutations.
- There is no treatment and prognosis is poor.

Recognition

History and presenting complaint

The most likely history will include severe exercise intolerance. Mitochondrial myopathies in people are associated with exercise-induced myalgia and cramps.[252]

Physical examination

In the reported case, the Arabian horse appeared normal at rest.[253] However, human patients frequently have additional cardiac and central nervous system involvement.[254]

Special examination

Exercise test

Light exercise resulted in stiff, short strides, profuse sweating and metabolic acidosis due to marked lactic acidemia (Fig. 7.25). Oxygen consumption was reduced, but PVO2 increased. The horse was unable to exercise for more than 6 minutes and recovery was prolonged.[253]

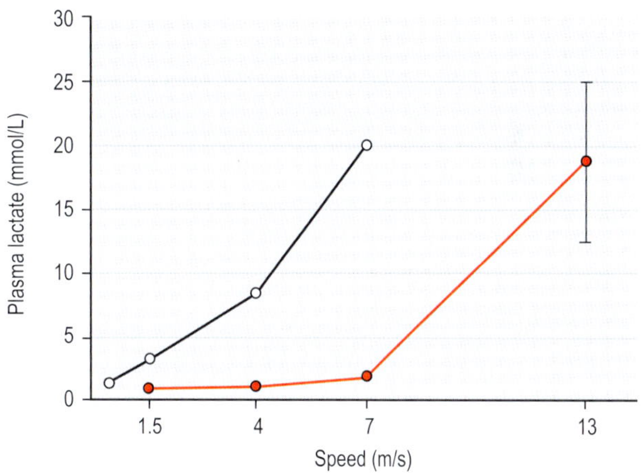

Fig 7.25 Graph showing rise in plasma lactate concentration in a control horse (red line) and in a horse with a mitochondrial myopathy (black line) according to the speed of the treadmill. Notice that the affected horse produces large amounts of lactate even at slow treadmill speeds. *Reprinted from Valberg SJ, Carlson GP, Cardinet GH et al. Skeletal muscle and mitochondrial myopathy as a cause of exercise intolerance in a horse. Muscle and Nerve 2004;17:305–312. © 2004 John Wiley and Sons, Inc.*

Laboratory examinations

Hematology and biochemistry

Routine hematology and biochemistry analysis, including CK activity, was normal in the reported horse at rest.[253] However, given the multiple systems involvement in humans,[254] other cases could have various different abnormalities.

Muscle biopsy

Mild myopathic changes can be evident. In humans, classic findings include intense red-staining subsarcolemmal deposits of mitochondria in a few fibers revealed with modified Gomori's trichrome stain – so-called 'ragged red fibers'. However, normal trained horses have abundant subsarcolemmal mitochondria, which can appear similar. Histochemical staining of NADH-dehydrogenase (complex I), succinate dehydrogenase (complex II) and cytochrome oxidase (complex IV)[10] can be abnormal, suggesting respiratory chain enzyme dysfunction (Fig. 7.26). Electron microscopy can reveal

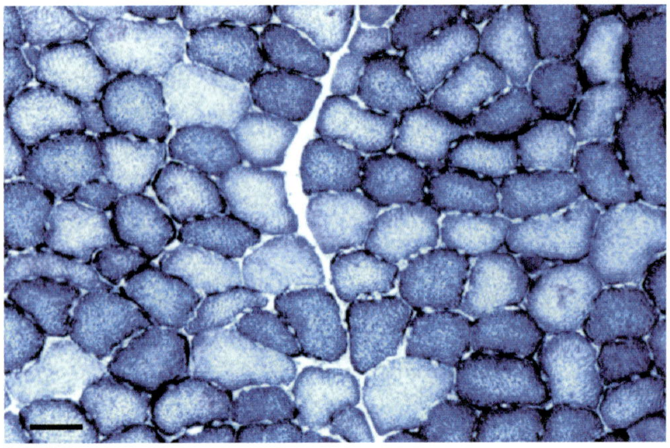

Fig 7.26 Light microscopic transverse section of gluteus medius muscle stained with nicotinamide adenine dinucleotide tetrazolium reductase from an Arabian horse with suspected mitochondrial myopathy. Note the dark staining (mitochondria), particularly towards the rim of many myofibers, including the paler glycolytic fibers.

extensive subsarcolemmal and intermyofibrillar mitochondria with distorted or concentric cristae.[253]

Biochemical analysis of mitochondrial oxidative enzymes

Mitochondrial electron transport system enzyme activities are analyzed in mitochondrial preparations from affected muscle. The following enzyme activities should be measured by a specialist laboratory and compared with controls; in the reported horse, complex I enzyme activities were significantly reduced.[253]

Citrate synthase	(matrix enzyme)
NADH-dehydrogenase	(complex I)
Rotenone-sensitive NADH – cytochrome-c-reductase	(complex I and III)
Succinate – cytochrome-c-reductase	(complex II and III)
Succinate dehydrogenase	(complex II)
Cytochrome oxidase	(complex IV)
ATP-synthase	(complex V)

Diagnostic confirmation

Other much more common causes of exercise intolerance should be ruled out before diagnosing mitochondrial myopathy. In their absence, severe exercise intolerance and unusually pronounced exercise-induced lactic acidemia should prompt muscle histopathological investigation and measurement of mitochondrial enzyme activities. Mutational analysis of mitochondrial or genomic DNA enables definitive diagnosis in humans: the complete equine mtDNA sequence is available.[255]

Treatment and prognosis

The prognosis depends on the degree of respiratory chain compromise, but is likely to be poor as there is no treatment. Affected animals are very unlikely to be athletic.[253]

Etiology and pathophysiology

Etiology

The respiratory chain enzyme complexes that produce ATP during oxidative phosphorylation are located in the folded cristae of the inner mitochondrial membranes (Fig. 7.27). In humans, the proteins that make up complex II are encoded by genomic DNA, whereas the other complexes are encoded by genes in both genomic DNA and mtDNA,[254] hence mitochondrial myopathies can be caused by mutations in either.

Pathophysiology

Mutations in mtDNA occur spontaneously or are inherited from the mother, because mitochondria are maternally derived. Within individuals, different tissues can contain normal and mutated mitochondria in varying amounts (heteroplasmy). If sufficient normal mitochondria exist, oxidative phosphorylation defects go unrecognized, but they become evident in tissues when mutated mtDNA predominates, especially when ATP requirements are high, as in muscle. In muscle, defective oxidative phosphorylation results in greater emphasis on anaerobic glycolysis for energy production and correspondingly, a rise in lactate production. In humans, mitochondrial diseases often affect multiple systems, although post-mitotic tissues, such as the central nervous system and muscle, are overrepresented, probably because of inability to select against abnormal mitochondria in affected cells.[254]

Fibrotic myopathy

- Mechanical pelvic limb lameness characterized by the foot abruptly slapping the ground at the end of the anterior phase.
- Congenital and acquired forms have been recognized.
- Most horses have a history of trauma to the affected limb.
- A fibrotic mass might be palpable in the semitendinosus or other hamstring muscles.
- Transection of the mass or tibial insertion tenotomy results in return to normal function in some horses.

Recognition

History and presenting complaint

Horses present with unilateral or occasionally bilateral pelvic limb lameness. There might be a history of injury, trauma or intramuscular injection in the affected limb.[274]

Physical examination

The mechanical lameness, which does not respond to analgesics, is most obvious at the walk or slow trot and is characterized by a sudden cessation of the anterior phase of the stride, with the hoof abruptly slapping the ground. At faster gaits the lameness can disappear. Taut muscles containing a firm, fibrous is often palpable in the bellies or myotendinous junctions of the semitendinosus (most commonly), but also the semimembranosus, biceps femoris and gracilis muscles (Fig. 7.28).[19,256–259]

Special examination

Ultrasound can help locate sites of fibrosis[18,260] and radiography can identify ossification.[19,256] Electromyography in some cases might suggest denervation that can be confirmed by muscle biopsy.[261]

Diagnostic confirmation

Other causes of pelvic limb lameness should be considered. Mild stringhalt is sometimes confused with fibrotic myopathy but stringhalt is associated with abnormal sudden flexion of the limb. In most cases of fibrotic myopathy the gait is pathognomonic.

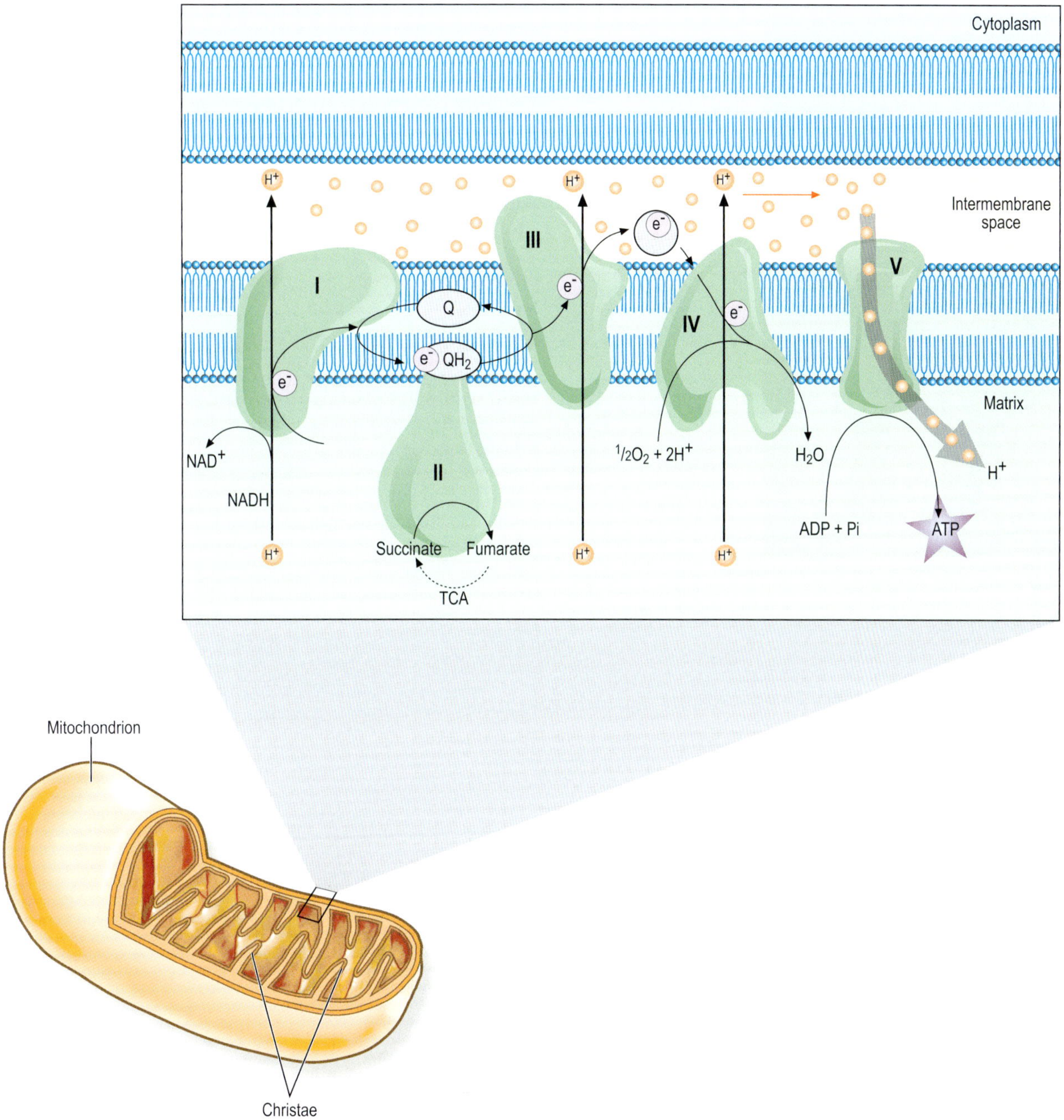

Fig 7.27 Diagrammatic representation of the mitochondrial electron transport system in mitochondria. The enzyme components of each complex are located in the inner membrane. Protons accumulate in the intermembrane space and their energy is harnessed to regenerate ATP (via ATP synthase). Q = ubiquinone.

Treatment and prognosis

Therapeutic aims

The main aim is to restore the normal mechanical function of the limb.

Surgery

Transection[258,259] or excision[256] of the fibrotic mass or tenotomy of the tibial insertion of the semitendinosus muscle are described.[19,262]

Muscle transection

Although usually performed under general anesthesia, transection of the fibrotic mass using a bistoury knife has been performed in the standing horse under local anesthesia. Post-surgery drainage is maintained with a Penrose drain inserted through a second incision, ventral to the first, and healing occurs via second intention. Light exercise is resumed the day after surgery.[48,258]

Tibial insertion tenotomy under general anesthesia

The tendon of insertion of the semitendinosus muscle is palpated medially (with the horse in lateral recumbency and the affected limb down), caudodistal to the femorotibial joint (Fig. 7.29). The tendon is exposed and transected following vertical skin incision caudal to the medial saphenous vein. Closure is routine and tension sutures are placed in the skin. Residual healing occurs via second intention if dehiscence occurs. Mild exercise is

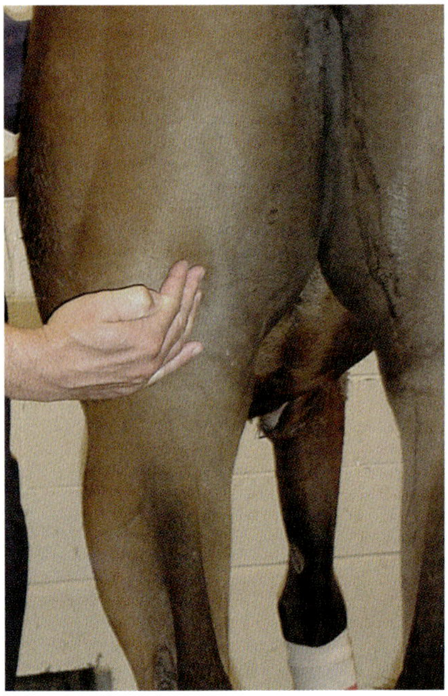

Fig 7.28 Palpating the hamstring musculature for evidence of fibrotic myopathy.

recommended two weeks postoperatively with full exercise allowed after six weeks.[19,263]

Analgesia

Treatment consists of NSAIDs (e.g. 2–3 mg/kg phenylbutazone i.v., q 12h p.o.) postoperatively for 2–3 days.

Prognosis

Tenotomy is reported to result in fewer complications and have greater success.[19,256] Results depend on which muscles are affected and are reportedly better when only the semitendinosus muscle is involved.[262]

Etiology and pathophysiology

This disorder is seen worldwide in athletic horses and is often associated with trauma during work (particularly Quarter Horses) or injury from fences or ropes. Fibrosis following intramuscular injection has also been described[256] as has denervation atrophy (e.g. sciatic nerve entrapment following fracture of the greater trochanter).[261] In young animals, the disorder can be congenital.[19]

The hamstring musculature supports the stifle during the early stance phase of the gait cycle, enhances propulsion in the late phase and controls the limb's momentum during the swing phase of the stride. Limited range of movement imposed by fibrotic muscle causes an abrupt termination of the swing phase.

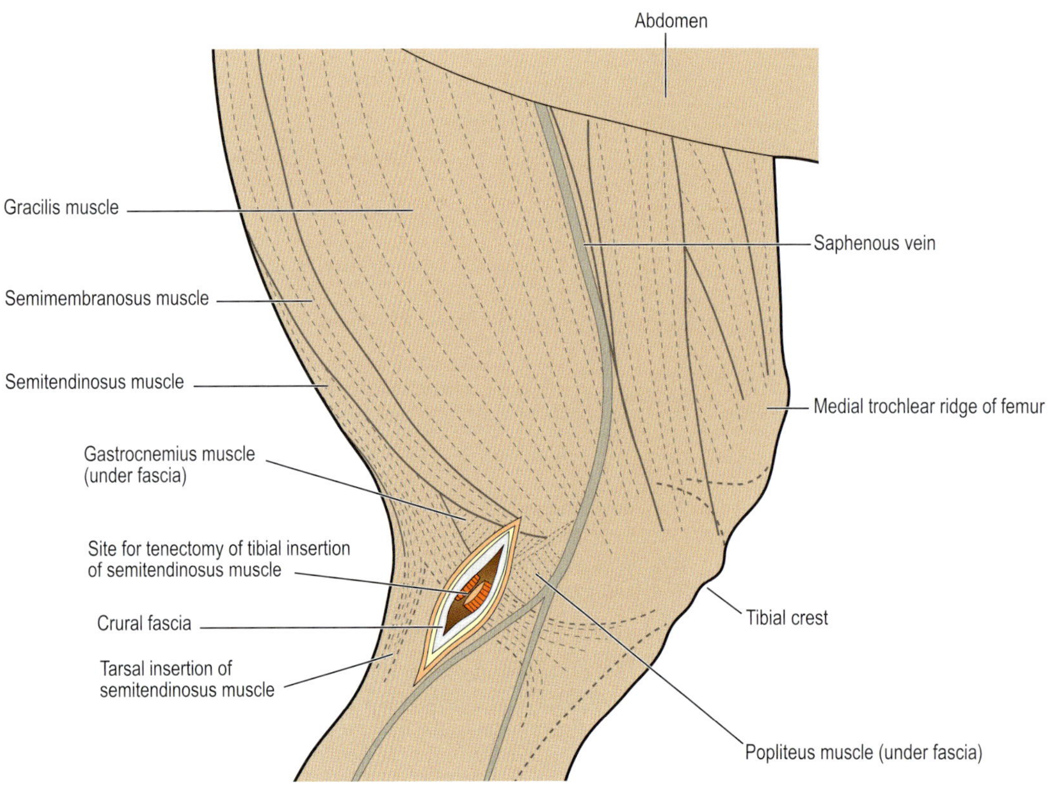

Fig 7.29 Diagrammatic representation of the medial aspect of the pelvic limb showing the semitendinosus tibial insertion tenotomy site with regional anatomy.

References

1. Gissel H, Clausen T. Excitation-induced Ca2+ influx and skeletal muscle cell damage. Acta Physiol Scand 2001;171: 327–34.
2. Belcastro AN, Shewchuk LD, Raj DA. Exercise-induced muscle injury: a calpain hypothesis. Mol Cell Biochem 1998;179:135–45.
3. Sandri M, Carraro U. Apoptosis of skeletal muscles during development and disease. Int J Biochem Cell Biol 1999;31:1373–90.
4. Tidball JG. Inflammatory cell response to acute muscle injury. Med Sci Sports Exerc 1995;27:1022–32.
5. Hurme T, Kalimo H, Lehto M, et al. Healing of skeletal muscle injury: an ultrastructural and immunohistochemical study. Med Sci Sports Exerc 1991;23:801–10.
6. Grounds MD. Muscle regeneration: molecular aspects and therapeutic implications. Curr Opin Neurol 1999;12:535–43.
7. Zammit P, Beauchamp J. The skeletal muscle satellite cell: stem cell or son of stem cell? Differentiation 2001;68: 193–204.
8. Rantanen J, Hurme T, Lukka R, et al. Satellite cell proliferation and the expression of myogenin and desmin in regenerating skeletal muscle: evidence for two different populations of satellite cells. Lab Invest 1995;72:341–7.
9. Kaariainen M, Jarvinen T, Jarvinen M, et al. Relation between myofibers and connective tissue during muscle injury repair. Scand J Med Sci Sports 2000;10: 332–7.
10. Dubowitz V, Sewry C, Fitzsimons R. Muscle Biospy: A Practical Approach. 2nd ed. London: Balliere Tindall; 1985.
11. Rivero JL, Letelier AI, editors. Skeletal muscle profile of show jumpers: physiological and pathological considerations. Conference on Equine sports medicine and science. Dortmund: Gestalt manufaktur GmbH; 2000.
12. Sprinkle F, Swerczek T, Ward Crowe M. Gastrocnemius muscle rupture and hemorrhage in foals. Equine Pract 1985;7:10–17.
13. Harris P, Mayhew I. Musculoskeletal disease. In: Reed S, Bayley W, editors. Equine internal medicine. Philadelphia: W.B. Saunders; 1998. p. 384–5.
14. Schneider J, Guffy M, Leipold H. Ruptured flexor muscles in a neonatal foal. Equine Pract 1986;8:11–15.
15. Stashak T. Serratus ventralis rupture. In: Stashak T, editor. Adams' Lameness in horses. 4th ed. Philadelphia: Lea and Febiger; 1987. p. 693–4.
16. Morris E, Seeherman HJ, O'Callaghan MW, et al. Scintigraphic identification of skeletal muscle damage in horses 24 hours after strenuous exercise. Equine Vet J 1991;23:347–52.
17. Eddy AL, Van Hoogmoed LM, Snyder JR. The role of thermography in the management of equine lameness. Vet J 2001;162:172–81.
18. Reef VB. Equine diagnostic ultrasound. Philadelphia: W.B. Saunders; 1998. p. 143–9.
19. Bramlage LR, Reed SM, Embertson RM. Semitendinosus tenotomy for treatment of fibrotic myopathy in the horse. J Am Vet Med Assoc 1985;186:565–7.
20. Gibson JS, Ellory JC. More theories than facts: equine rhabdomyolysis. Equine Vet J 1993;25:327–8.
21. Warren JD, Blumbergs PC, Thompson PD. Rhabdomyolysis: a review. Muscle Nerve 2002;25:332–47.
22. Landau ME, Kenney K, Deuster P, et al. Exertional rhabdomyolysis: a clinical review with a focus on genetic influences. J Clin Neuromuscul Dis 2012;13:122–36.
23. Aleman M. A review of equine muscle disorders. Neuromuscul Disord 2008;18:277–87.
24. McEwen SA, Hulland TJ. Histochemical and morphometric evaluation of skeletal muscle from horses with exertional rhabdomyolysis (tying-up). Vet Pathol 1986;23:400–10.
25. Martin BB Jr , Reef VB, Parente EJ, et al. Causes of poor performance of horses during training, racing, or showing: 348 cases (1992–1996). J Am Vet Med Assoc 2000;216:554–8.
26. Snow DH, Valberg SJ. Muscle Anatomy, Physiology, and Adaptions to Exercise and Training. In: DR H, RJ R, editors. The Athletic horse: principals and practice of equine sports medicine. Philadelphia: W.B. Saunders; 1994. p. 169.
27. Naylor RJ, Livesey L, Schumacher J, et al. Allele copy number and underlying pathology are associated with subclinical severity in equine type 1 polysaccharide storage myopathy (PSSM1). PloS One; In press. 2012.
28. Toutain PL, Lassourd V, Costes G, et al. A non-invasive and quantitative method for the study of tissue injury caused by intramuscular injection of drugs in horses. J Vet Pharmacol Ther 1995;18:226–35.
29. Koterba A, Carlson GP. Acid base and electrolyte alterations in horses with exertional rhabdomyolysis. J Am Vet Med Assoc 1982;180:303–6.
30. MacLeay JM, Valberg SJ, Pagan JD, et al. Effect of ration and exercise on plasma creatine kinase activity and lactate concentration in Thoroughbred horses with recurrent exertional rhabdomyolysis. Am J Vet Res 2000;61:1390–5.
31. Valberg S, Jonsson L, Lindholm A, et al. Muscle histopathology and plasma aspartate aminotransferase, creatine kinase and myoglobin changes with exercise in horses with recurrent exertional rhabdomyolysis. Equine Vet J 1993;25:11–16.
32. Schwarz B, Ertl R, Zimmer S, et al. Estimated prevalence of the GYS-1 mutation in healthy Austrian Haflingers. Vet Rec 2011;169:583.
33. Schott 2nd HC, Hodgson DR, Bayly WM. Haematuria, pigmenturia and proteinuria in exercising horses. Equine Vet J 1995;27:67–72.
34. Harris P, Colles C. The use of creatinine clearance ratios in the prevention of equine rhabdomyolysis: a report of four cases. Equine Vet J 1988;20:459–63.
35. McKenzie EC, Valberg SJ, Godden SM, et al. Plasma and urine electrolyte and mineral concentrations in Thoroughbred horses with recurrent exertional rhabdomyolysis after consumption of diets varying in cation-anion balance. Am J Vet Res 2002;63:1053–60.
36. Toribio RE, Kohn CW, Chew DJ, et al. Comparison of serum parathyroid hormone and ionized calcium and magnesium concentrations and fractional urinary clearance of calcium and phosphorus in healthy horses and horses with enterocolitis. Am J Vet Res 2001;62:938–47.
37. Clarke LL, Argenzio RA, Roberts MC. Effect of meal feeding on plasma volume and urinary electrolyte clearance in ponies. Am J Vet Res 1990;51:571–6.
38. Kohn CW, Chew DJ. Laboratory diagnosis and characterization of renal disease in horses. Vet Clin North Am Equine Pract 1987;3:585–615.
39. McKenzie EC, Valberg SJ, Godden SM, et al. Comparison of volumetric urine collection versus single-sample urine collection in horses consuming diets varying in cation–anion balance. Am J Vet Res 2003;64:284–91.
40. Kohn CW, Strasser SL. 24-hour renal clearance and excretion of endogenous substances in the mare. Am J Vet Res 1986;47:1332–7.
41. Morris DD, Divers TJ, Whitlock RH. Renal clearance and fractional excretion of electrolytes over a 24-hour period in horses. Am J Vet Res 1984;45:2431–5.
42. Valberg SJ. Spinal muscle pathology. Vet Clin North Am Equine Pract 1999;15:87–96, vi–vii.
43. Stanley RL, Maile C, Piercy RJ. Storage-associated artefact in equine muscle biopsy samples. Equine Vet J 2009;41:82–6.
44. Firshman AM, Valberg SJ, Bender JB, et al. Comparison of histopathologic criteria and skeletal muscle fixation

techniques for the diagnosis of polysaccharide storage myopathy in horses. Vet Pathol 2006;43:257–69.
45. Valentine B, Divers TJ, DJ M, et al. Muscle biopsy diagnosis of equine motor neuron disease and equine polysaccharide storage myopathy. Eq Vet Educ 1998;10:42–50.
46. Valentine B, De Lahunta A, Divers TJ, et al. Clinical and pathologic findings in two draft horses with progressive weakness, and abnormal gait characteristic of shivers syndrome. J Am Vet Med Assoc 1999;215:1661–5.
47. Firshman AM, Baird JD, Valberg SJ. Prevalences and clinical signs of polysaccharide storage myopathy and shivers in Belgian draft horses. J Am Vet Med Assoc 2005;227:1958–64.
48. Hodgson DR. Diseases of muscle. In: Colahan P, editor. Equine medicine and surgery. 5th ed. St Louis, Missouri: Mosby, Inc; 1999. p. 1489–90.
49. Westermann CM, Dorland L, Votion DM, et al. Acquired multiple Acyl-CoA dehydrogenase deficiency in 10 horses with atypical myopathy. Neuromuscul Disord 2008;18:355–64.
50. Andrews FM. Acute rhabdomyolysis. Vet Clin North Am Equine Pract 1994;10:567–73.
51. Moore KP, Holt SG, Patel RP, et al. A causative role for redox cycling of myoglobin and its inhibition by alkalinization in the pathogenesis and treatment of rhabdomyolysis-induced renal failure. J Biol Chem 1998;273:31731–7.
52. Fruen BR, Mickelson JR, Louis CF. Dantrolene inhibition of sarcoplasmic reticulum Ca2+ release by direct and specific action at skeletal muscle ryanodine receptors. J Biol Chem 1997;272:26965–71.
53. Lopez JR, Linares N, Cordovez G, et al. Elevated myoplasmic calcium in exercise-induced equine rhabdomyolysis. Pflugers Arch 1995;430:293–5.
54. Court MH, Engelking LR, Dodman NH, et al. Pharmacokinetics of dantrolene sodium in horses. J Vet Pharmacol Ther 1987;10:218–26.
55. DiMaio Knych HK, Arthur RM, Taylor A, et al. Pharmacokinetics and metabolism of dantrolene in horses. J Vet Pharmacol Ther 2011;34:238–46.
56. Beech J. Chronic exertional rhabdomyolysis. Vet Clin North Am Equine Pract 1997;13:145–68.
57. Isgren CM, Upjohn MM, Fernandez-Fuente M, et al. Epidemiology of exertional rhabdomyolysis susceptibility in standardbred horses reveals associated risk factors and underlying enhanced performance. PLoS One 2010;5:e11594.
58. MacLeay JM, Sorum SA, Valberg SJ, et al. Epidemiologic analysis of factors influencing exertional rhabdomyolysis in Thoroughbreds. Am J Vet Res 1999;60:1562–6.
59. Valberg S, Mickelson J, Gallant E, et al. Exertional Rhabdomyolysis in Quarterhorses and Thoroughbreds: one syndrome, multiple aetiologies. Equine Veterinary Jounal supp 1999;30:533–8.
60. McKenzie EC, Valberg SJ, Godden SM, et al. Effect of dietary starch, fat, and bicarbonate content on exercise responses and serum creatine kinase activity in equine recurrent exertional rhabdomyolysis. J Vet Intern Med 2003;17:693–701.
61. Firshman AM, Valberg SJ, Bender JB, et al. Epidemiologic characteristics and management of polysaccharide storage myopathy in Quarter Horses. Am J Vet Res 2003;64:1319–27.
62. Holland JL, Kronfeld DS, Meacham TN. Behavior of horses is affected by soy lecithin and corn oil in the diet. J Anim Sci 1996;74:1252–5.
63. Crandell KG, Pagan JD, Harris P, et al. A comparison of grain, oil and beet pulp as energy sources for the exercised horse. Equine Vet J Suppl 1999;30: 485–9.
64. McKenzie E, Valberg S, Godden S, et al. Effect of dietary starch, fat and bicarbonate content on exercise responses and serum creatine kinase activity in equine recurrent exertional rhabdomyolysis. Am J Vet Res In Press.
65. Valentine B, Reynolds A, Wakshlag J, et al. Muscle Glycogen, Myopathy, and Diet. World Eq Vet Review 1997;2: 27–31.
66. De La Corte F, Valberg SJ, MacLeay JM. The effect of feeding a fat supplement to horses with polysaccharide storage myopathy. World Eq Vet Review 1999;4: 12–19.
67. Bouskila M, Hunter RW, Ibrahim AF, et al. Allosteric regulation of glycogen synthase controls glycogen synthesis in muscle. Cell Metab 2010;12:456–66.
68. Sugden MC, Holness MJ, Fryer LG. Differential regulation of glycogen synthase by insulin and glucose in vivo in skeletal muscles of the rat. Am J Physiol 1997;273:E479–487.
69. Ribeiro WP, Valberg SJ, Pagan JD, et al. The effect of varying dietary starch and fat content on serum creatine kinase activity and substrate availability in equine polysaccharide storage myopathy. J Vet Intern Med 2004;18: 887–94.
70. Valentine BA, Van Saun RJ, Thompson KN, et al. Role of dietary carbohydrate and fat in horses with equine polysaccharide storage myopathy. J Am Vet Med Assoc 2001;219:1537–44.
71. Borgia L, Valberg S, McCue M, et al. Glycaemic and insulinaemic responses to feeding hay with different non-structural carbohydrate content in control and polysaccharide storage myopathy-affected horses. J Anim Physiol Anim Nutr (Berl). 2011;95: 798–807.
72. Committee on Nutrient Requirements of Horses NRC. Nutrient Requirements of Horses. 6th revised edition ed. Washington D.C.: The National Academies Press; 2007.
73. Spiekerkoetter U, Lindner M, Santer R, et al. Treatment recommendations in long-chain fatty acid oxidation defects: consensus from a workshop. J Inherit Metab Dis 2009;32:498–505.
74. Hunt LM, Valberg SJ, Steffenhagen K, et al. An epidemiological study of myopathies in Warmblood horses. Equine Vet J 2008;40:171–7.
75. Valverde A, Boyd CJ, Dyson DH, et al. Prophylactic use of dantrolene associated with prolonged postanesthetic recumbency in a horse. J Am Vet Med Assoc 1990;197:1051–3.
76. McKenzie EC, Valberg SJ, Godden SM, et al. Effect of oral administration of dantrolene sodium on serum creatine kinase activity after exercise in horses with recurrent exertional rhabdomyolysis. Am J Vet Res 2004;65:74–9.
77. Edwards JG, Newtont JR, Ramzan PH, et al. The efficacy of dantrolene sodium in controlling exertional rhabdomyolysis in the Thoroughbred racehorse. Equine Vet J 2003;35:707–11.
78. McKenzie EC, Garrett RL, Payton ME, et al. Effect of feed restriction on plasma dantrolene concentrations in horses. Equine Vet J Suppl 2010:613–17.
79. Avellini L, Chiaradia E, Gaiti A. Effect of exercise training, selenium and vitamin E on some free radical scavengers in horses (Equus caballus). Comp Biochem Physiol B Biochem Mol Biol 1999;123:147–54.
80. White A, Estrada M, Walker K, et al. Role of exercise and ascorbate on plasma antioxidant capacity in thoroughbred race horses. Comp Biochem Physiol A Mol Integr Physiol 2001;128:99–104.
81. Siciliano PD, Parker AL, Lawrence LM. Effect of dietary vitamin E supplementation on the integrity of skeletal muscle in exercised horses. J Anim Sci 1997;75:1553–60.
82. Kienzle E, Freismuth A, Reusch A. Double-blind placebo-controlled vitamin E or selenium supplementation of sport horses with unspecified muscle problems. An example of the potential of placebos. J Nutr 2006;136:2045S–7S.
83. Hill OT, Wahi MM, Carter 3rd R, et al. Rhabdomyolysis in the US Active Duty Army, 2004–2006. Med Sci Sports Exerc 2012;44:442–9.
84. MacIntyre DL, Reid WD, McKenzie DC. Delayed muscle soreness. The inflammatory response to muscle injury

and its clinical implications. Sports Med 1995;20:24–40.

85. Proske U, Morgan DL. Muscle damage from eccentric exercise: mechanism, mechanical signs, adaptation and clinical applications. J Physiol 2001;537:333–45.

86. Sayers SP, Clarkson PM, Rouzier PA, et al. Adverse events associated with eccentric exercise protocols: six case studies. Med Sci Sports Exerc 1999;31:1697–702.

87. Sayers SP, Clarkson P, Patel JJ. Metabolic response to light exercise after exercise-induced rhabdomyolysis. Eur J Appl Physiol 2002;86:280–2.

88. Snow DH, Valberg SJ. Muscle Anatomy, Physiology, and Adaptions to Exercise and Training. In: Hodgson DR, Rose RJ, editors. The Athletic Horse: principles and practice of equine sports medicine. Philadelphia: W.B. Saunders Company; 1994. p. 145–79.

89. Foreman JH. The exhausted horse syndrome. Vet Clin North Am Equine Pract 1998;14:205–19.

90. Powers SK, Nelson WB, Hudson MB. Exercise-induced oxidative stress in humans: cause and consequences. Free Radic Biol Med 2011;51:942–50.

91. Mills PC, Smith NC, Casas I, et al. Effects of exercise intensity and environmental stress on indices of oxidative stress and iron homeostasis during exercise in the horse. Eur J Appl Physiol 1996;74:60–6.

92. Brady PS, Ku PK, Ullrey DE. Lack of effect of selenium supplementation on the response of the equine erythrocyte glutathione system and plasma enzymes to exercise. J Anim Sci 1978;47:492–6.

93. El-Deeb WM, El-Bahr SM. Investigation of selected biochemical indicators of Equine Rhabdomyolysis in Arabian horses: pro-inflammatory cytokines and oxidative stress markers. Vet Res Commun 2010;34:677–89.

94. Roneus B, Hakkarainen J. Vitamin E in serum and skeletal muscle tissue and blood glutathione peroxidase activity from horses with the azoturia-tying-up syndrome. Acta Vet Scand 1985;26:425–7.

95. Step DL, Divers TJ, Cooper B, et al. Severe masseter myonecrosis in a horse. J Am Vet Med Assoc 1991;198:117–19.

96. Owen RR, Moore JN, Hopkins JB, et al. Dystrophic myodegeneration in adult horses. J Am Vet Med Assoc 1977;171:343–9.

97. Lofstedt J. White muscle disease of foals. Vet Clin North Am Equine Pract 1997;13:169–85.

98. Beech J, Lindborg S, Braund KG. Potassium concentrations in muscle, plasma and erythrocytes and urinary fractional excretion in normal horses and those with chronic intermittent exercise-associated rhabdomyolysis. Res Vet Sci 1993;55:43–51.

99. Shintani S, Shiigai T, Tsukagoshi H. Marked hypokalemic rhabdomyolysis with myoglobinuria due to diuretic treatment. Eur Neurol 1991;31:396–8.

100. Bain FT, Merritt AM. Decreased erythrocyte potassium concentration associated with exercise-related myopathy in horses. Journal of the American Veterinary Medical Association 1990;196:1259–61.

101. Johnson PJ, Goetz TE, Foreman JH, et al. Effect of whole-body potassium depletion on plasma, erythrocyte, and middle gluteal muscle potassium concentration of healthy, adult horses. Am J Vet Res 1991;52:1676–83.

102. Muylle E, Van den Hende C, Nuytten J, et al. Potassium concentration in equine red blood cells: normal values and correlation with potassium levels in plasma. Equine Vet J 1984;16:447–9.

103. Freestone JF, Gossett K, Carlson GP, et al. Exercise induced alterations in the serum muscle enzymes, erythrocyte potassium and plasma constituents following feed withdrawal or furosemide and sodium bicarbonate administration in the horse. J Vet Intern Med 1991;5:40–6.

104. Tiidus PM. Oestrogen and sex influence on muscle damage and inflammation: evidence from animal models. Curr Opin Clin Nutr Metab Care 2001;4:509–13.

105. Harris PA. The equine rhabdomyolysis syndrome in the United Kingdom: epidemiological and clinical descriptive information. Br Vet J 1991;147:373–84.

106. Freestone JF, Carlson GR. Muscle disorders in the horse: a retrospective study. Equine Vet J 1991;23:86–90.

107. Beech J, Lindborg S, Fletcher JE, et al. Caffeine contractures, twitch characteristics and the threshold for Ca(2+)-induced Ca2+ release in skeletal muscle from horses with chronic intermittent rhabdomyolysis. Res Vet Sci 1993;54:110–17.

108. Collinder E, Lindholm A, Rasmuson M. Genetic markers in standardbred trotters susceptible to the rhabdomyolysis syndrome. Equine Vet J 1997;29:117–20.

109. McGowan CM, Fordham T, Christley RM. Incidence and risk factors for exertional rhabdomyolysis in thoroughbred racehorses in the United Kingdom. Vet Rec 2002;151:623–6.

110. Frauenfelder HC, Rossdale PD, Ricketts SW, et al. Changes in serum muscle enzyme levels associated with training schedules and stage of the oestrous cycle in Thoroughbred racehorses. Equine Vet J 1986;18:371–4.

111. Beyer IW, Karmali R, Demeester-Mirkine N, et al. Serum creatine kinase levels in overt and subclinical hypothyroidism. Thyroid 1998;8:1029–31.

112. Lochmuller H, Reimers CD, Fischer P, et al. Exercise-induced myalgia in hypothyroidism. Clin Investig 1993;71: 999–1001.

113. Foreman JH. Metabolic causes of equine exercise intolerance. Vet Clin North Am Equine Pract 1996;12:537–54.

114. Valberg S, Jonsson L, Lindholm A, et al. Muscle histopathology and plasma aspartate aminotransferase, creatine kinase and myoglobin changes with exercise in horses with recurrent exertional rhabdomyolysis [published erratum appears in Equine Vet J 1993 May;25(3):255] [see comments]. Equine Vet J 1993;25:11–16.

115. Waldron-Mease E. Hypothyroidism and myopathy in racing. Thoroughbreds and Standardbreds J Equine Med Surg 1979;3:124–8.

116. Harris PA, Snow DH, Greet TR, et al. Some factors influencing plasma AST/CK activities in thoroughbred racehorses. Equine Vet J Suppl 1990:66–71.

117. Lowe JE, Baldwin BH, Foote RH, et al. Equine hypothyroidism: the long term effects of thyroidectomy on metabolism and growth in mares and stallions. Cornell Vet 1974;64:276–95.

118. Stanley O, Hillidge CJ. Alopecia associated with hypothyroidism in a horse. Equine Vet J 1982;14:165–7.

119. Harris PA. An outbreak of the equine rhabdomyolysis syndrome in a racing yard. Vet Rec 1990;127:468–70.

120. Dranchak PK, Valberg SJ, Onan GW, et al. Inheritance of recurrent exertional rhabdomyolysis in thoroughbreds. J Am Vet Med Assoc 2005;227:762–7.

121. Rudolph JA, Spier SJ, Byrns G, et al. Periodic paralysis in quarter horses: a sodium channel mutation disseminated by selective breeding. Nat Genet 1992;2:144–7.

122. Lentz LR, Valberg SJ, Balog EM, et al. Abnormal regulation of muscle contraction in horses with recurrent exertional rhabdomyolysis. Am J Vet Res 1999;60:992–9.

123. Ward TL, Valberg SJ, Gallant EM, et al. Calcium regulation by skeletal muscle membranes of horses with recurrent exertional rhabdomyolysis. Am J Vet Res 2000;61:242–7.

124. Hildebrand SV, Arpin D, Cardinet 3rd G. Contracture test and histologic and histochemical analyzes of muscle biopsy specimens from horses with exertional rhabdomyolysis. J Am Vet Med Assoc 1990;196:1077–83.

125. Hodgson DR. Exercise-associated myopathy: is calcium the culprit? Equine Vet J 1993;25:1–3.

126. Lentz LR, Valberg SJ, Herold LV, et al. Myoplasmic calcium regulation in

myotubes from horses with recurrent exertional rhabdomyolysis. Am J Vet Res 2002;63:1724–31.

127. Lentz LR, Valberg SJ, Mickelson JR, et al. In vitro contractile responses and contracture testing of skeletal muscle from Quarter Horses with exertional rhabdomyolysis. Am J Vet Res 1999;60:684–8.

128. Allen GC, Fletcher JE, Huggins FJ, et al. Caffeine and halothane contracture testing in swine using the recommendations of the North American Malignant Hyperthermia Group. Anesthesiology 1990;72:71–6.

129. Bina S, Karan SM, Lojeski EW, et al. Prolonging viability of swine muscle biopsy specimens in malignant hyperthermia testing. Anesth Analg 2001;93:781–6.

130. Roberts MC, Mickelson JR, Patterson EE, et al. Autosomal dominant canine malignant hyperthermia is caused by a mutation in the gene encoding the skeletal muscle calcium release channel (RYR1). Anesthesiology 2001;95:716–25.

131. Fujii J, Otsu K, Zorzato F, et al. Identification of a mutation in porcine ryanodine receptor associated with malignant hyperthermia. Science 1991;253:448–51.

132. Lanner JT, Georgiou DK, Joshi AD, et al. Ryanodine receptors: structure, expression, molecular details, and function in calcium release. Cold Spring Harb Perspect Biol 2010;2:a003996.

133. Mickelson JR, Gallant EM, Litterer LA, et al. Abnormal sarcoplasmic reticulum ryanodine receptor in malignant hyperthermia. J Biol Chem 1988;263:9310–15.

134. Monnier N, Procaccio V, Stieglitz P, et al. Malignant-hyperthermia susceptibility is associated with a mutation of the alpha 1-subunit of the human dihydropyridine-sensitive L-type voltage-dependent calcium-channel receptor in skeletal muscle. Am J Hum Genet 1997;60:1316–25.

135. Jurkat-Rott K, McCarthy T, Lehmann-Horn F. Genetics and pathogenesis of malignant hyperthermia. Muscle Nerve 2000;23:4–17.

136. Dranchak PK, Valberg SJ, Onan GW, et al. Exclusion of linkage of the RYR1, CACNA1S, and ATP2A1 genes to recurrent exertional rhabdomyolysis in Thoroughbreds. Am J Vet Res 2006;67:1395–400.

137. Fernandez-Fuente M, Ames EG, Wagner ML, et al. Assessment of the transformation of equine skin-derived fibroblasts to multinucleated skeletal myotubes following lentiviral-induced expression of equine myogenic differentiation 1. Am J Vet Res 2008;69:1637–45.

138. Fernandez-Fuente M, Terracciano C, Brown S, et al. Caffeine sensitivity of sarcoplasmic reticulum calcium release in virally transduced skin-derived myotubes from Thoroughbred horses with recurrent exertional rhabdomyolysis. Under Review 2013.

139. Valberg SJ. Spinal muscle pathology. Veterinary Clinics of North America – Equine Practice 1999;15:87–96.

140. Tilgen N, Zorzato F, Halliger-Keller B, et al. Identification of four novel mutations in the C-terminal membrane spanning domain of the ryanodine receptor 1: association with central core disease and alteration of calcium homeostasis. Hum Mol Genet 2001;10:2879–87.

141. Zhou H, Treves S, Jungbluth H, et al. RYR1 gene genotype-phenotype and functional correlative studies in central core disease and multi-minicore myopathy. Neuromuscular Disorders 2005;15:680–1.

142. Mlekoday JA, Mickelson JR, Valberg SJ, et al. Calcium sensitivity of force production and myofibrillar ATPase activity in muscles from Thoroughbreds with recurrent exertional rhabdomyolysis. Am J Vet Res 2001;62:1647–52.

143. Peluso A, Bianchini A. Malignant hyperthermia susceptibility in patients with Duchenne's muscular dystrophy. Can J Anaesth 1992;39:1117–18.

144. MacLeay JM, Valberg SJ, Sorum SA, et al. Heritability of recurrent exertional rhabdomyolysis in Thoroughbred racehorses. Am J Vet Res 1999;60:250–6.

145. McGowan CM, Posner RE, Christley RM. Incidence of exertional rhabdomyolysis in polo horses in the USA and the United Kingdom in the 1999/2000 season. Vet Rec 2002;150:535–7.

146. Fritz KL, McCue ME, Valberg SJ, et al. Genetic mapping of recurrent exertional rhabdomyolysis in a population of North American Thoroughbreds. Anim Genet 2012.

147. Tozaki T, Hirota K, Sugita S, et al. A genome-wide scan for tying-up syndrome in Japanese Thoroughbreds. Anim Genet 2010;41(Suppl. 2):80–6.

148. Lindholm A, Johansson HE, Kjaersgaard P. Acute rhabdomyolysis ('tying-up') in standardbred horses. A morphological and biochemical study. Acta Vet Scand 1974;15:325–39.

149. Meijer AE, van den Hoven R, Wensing T, et al. [Histochemical changes in skeletal muscles of racehorses susceptible to rhabdomyolysis after exertion. II. Later myopathological and regeneration phenomena]. Acta Histochem 1989;87:13–21.

150. Meijer AE, van den Hoven R, Wensing T, et al. [Histochemical changes in skeletal muscles of racehorses susceptible to rhabdomyolysis after exertion. I. Early myopathological changes]. Acta Histochem 1989;87:1–11.

151. Waldron-Mease E, Klein LV, Rosenberg H, et al. Malignant hyperthermia in a halothane-anesthetized horse. J Am Vet Med Assoc 1981;179:896–8.

152. Manley SV, Kelly AB, Hodgson D. Malignant hyperthermia-like reactions in three anesthetized horses. J Am Vet Med Assoc 1983;183:85–9.

153. Klein L, Ailes N, Fackelman GE, et al. Postanesthetic equine myopathy suggestive of malignant hyperthermia. A case report. Vet Surg 1989;18:479–82.

154. Aleman M, Riehl J, Aldridge BM, et al. Association of a mutation in the ryanodine receptor 1 gene with equine malignant hyperthermia. Muscle Nerve 2004;30:356–65.

155. Aleman M, Nieto JE, Magdesian KG. Malignant hyperthermia associated with ryanodine receptor 1 (C7360G) mutation in Quarter Horses. J Vet Intern Med 2009;23:329–34.

156. Nieto JE, Aleman M. A rapid detection method for the ryanodine receptor 1 (C7360G) mutation in Quarter Horses. J Vet Intern Med 2009;23:619–22.

157. McCue ME, Valberg SJ, Jackson M, et al. Polysaccharide storage myopathy phenotype in quarter horse-related breeds is modified by the presence of an RYR1 mutation. Neuromuscul Disord 2009;19:37–43.

158. Valberg SJ, Cardinet 3rd GH, Carlson GP, et al. Polysaccharide storage myopathy associated with recurrent exertional rhabdomyolysis in horses. Neuromuscul Disord 1992;2:351–9.

159. Quiroz-Rothe E, Novales M, Aguilera-Tejero E, et al. Polysaccharide storage myopathy in the M. longissimus lumborum of showjumpers and dressage horses with back pain. Equine Vet J 2002;34:171–6.

160. Valentine BA, Credille KM, Lavoie JP, et al. Severe polysaccharide storage myopathy in Belgian and Percheron draught horses. Equine Vet J 1997;29:220–5.

161. Valentine BA, McDonough SP, Chang YF, et al. Polysaccharide storage myopathy in Morgan, Arabian, and Standardbred related horses and Welsh-cross ponies. Vet Pathol 2000;37:193–6.

162. Valentine BA, Habecker PL, Patterson JS, et al. Incidence of polysaccharide storage myopathy in draft horse-related breeds: a necropsy study of 37 horses and a mule. J Vet Diagn Invest 2001;13:63–8.

163. McGowan CM, Menzies-Gow NJ, McDiarmid AM, et al. Four cases of equine polysaccharide storage myopathy

in the United Kingdom. Vet Rec 2003;152:109–12.
164. DiMauro S, Lamperti C. Muscle glycogenoses. Muscle Nerve 2001;24: 984–99.
165. Valberg S, Jones J, Smith B, et al. Limitations to performance caused by skeletal muscle enzyme deficiencies. Equine Vet J Suppl 1995;18:205–8.
166. DiMauro S, Tsujino S, Shanske S, et al. Biochemistry and molecular genetics of human glycogenoses: an overview. Muscle Nerve 1995;3:S10–17.
167. Valberg SJ, Macleay JM, Billstrom JA, et al. Skeletal muscle metabolic response to exercise in horses with 'tying-up' due to polysaccharide storage myopathy. Equine Vet J 1999;31:43–7.
168. Valberg SJ, Townsend D, Mickelson JR. Skeletal muscle glycolytic capacity and phosphofructokinase regulation in horses with polysaccharide storage myopathy. Am J Vet Res 1998;59:782–5.
169. Bao Y, Kishnani P, Wu JY, et al. Hepatic and neuromuscular forms of glycogen storage disease type IV caused by mutations in the same glycogen-branching enzyme gene. J Clin Invest 1996;97:941–8.
170. Valberg SJ, Ward TL, Rush B, et al. Glycogen branching enzyme deficiency in quarter horse foals. J Vet Intern Med 2001;15:572–80.
171. McCue ME, Valberg SJ, Miller MB, et al. Glycogen synthase (GYS1) mutation causes a novel skeletal muscle glycogenosis. Genomics 2008;91: 458–66.
172. Tryon RC, Penedo MC, McCue ME, et al. Evaluation of allele frequencies of inherited disease genes in subgroups of American Quarter Horses. J Am Vet Med Assoc 2009;234:120–5.
173. Baird JD, Valberg SJ, Anderson SM, et al. Presence of the glycogen synthase 1 (GYS1) mutation causing type 1 polysaccharide storage myopathy in continental European draught horse breeds. Vet Rec 2010;167:781–4.
174. Herszberg B, McCue ME, Larcher T, et al. A GYS1 gene mutation is highly associated with polysaccharide storage myopathy in Cob Normand draught horses. Anim Genet 2009;40:94–6.
175. McCue ME, Anderson SM, Valberg SJ, et al. Estimated prevalence of the Type 1 Polysaccharide Storage Myopathy mutation in selected North American and European breeds. Anim Genet 2010;41(Suppl. 2):145–9.
176. McCue ME, Valberg SJ. Estimated prevalence of polysaccharide storage myopathy among overtly healthy Quarter Horses in the United States. J Am Vet Med Assoc 2007;231:746–50.
177. McCue ME, Valberg SJ, Lucio M, et al. Glycogen synthase 1 (GYS1) mutation in diverse breeds with polysaccharide storage myopathy. J Vet Intern Med 2008;22:1228–33.
178. Stanley RL, McCue ME, Valberg SJ, et al. A glycogen synthase 1 mutation associated with equine polysaccharide storage myopathy and exertional rhabdomyolysis occurs in a variety of UK breeds. Equine Vet J 2009;41: 597–601.
179. McCue ME, Ribeiro WP, Valberg SJ. Prevalence of polysaccharide storage myopathy in horses with neuromuscular disorders. Equine Vet J Suppl 2006: 340–4.
180. McCue ME, Armien AG, Lucio M, et al. Comparative skeletal muscle histopathologic and ultrastructural features in two forms of polysaccharide storage myopathy in horses. Vet Pathol 2009;46:1281–91.
181. Valberg SJ, McCue ME, Mickelson JR. The Interplay of Genetics, Exercise, and Nutrition in Polysaccharide Storage Myopathy. Journal of Equine Veterinary Science 2011;31:205–10.
182. Valentine BA, Cooper BJ. Development of polyglucosan inclusions in skeletal muscle. Neuromuscul Disord 2006;16: 603–7.
183. De La Corte FD, Valberg SJ, MacLeay JM, et al. Developmental onset of polysaccharide storage myopathy in 4 Quarter Horse foals. J Vet Intern Med 2002;16:581–7.
184. Annandale EJ, Valberg SJ, Essen-Gustavsson B. Effects of submaximal exercise on adenine nucleotide concentrations in skeletal muscle fibers of horses with polysaccharide storage myopathy. Am J Vet Res 2005;66: 839–45.
185. Guertl B, Noehammer C, Hoefler G. Metabolic cardiomyopathies. Int J Exp Pathol 2000;81:349–72.
186. Naylor RJ, Luis-Fuentes V, Livesey L, et al. Evaluation of cardiac phenotype in horses with type 1 polysaccharide storage myopathy (PSSM1). J Vet Intern Med 2012;In press.
187. De La Corte FD, Valberg SJ, MacLeay JM, et al. Glucose uptake in horses with polysaccharide storage myopathy. Am J Vet Res 1999;60:458–62.
188. De La Corte FD, Valberg SJ, Mickelson JR, et al. Blood glucose clearance after feeding and exercise in polysaccharide storage myopathy. Equine Vet J Suppl 1999;30:324–8.
189. Firshman AM, Valberg SJ, Baird JD, et al. Insulin sensitivity in Belgian horses with polysaccharide storage myopathy. Am J Vet Res 2008;69: 818–23.
190. Valentine BA, Flint TH, Fischer KA. Ubiquitin expression in muscle from horses with polysaccharide storage myopathy. Vet Pathol 2006;43:270–5.
191. Larcher T, Herszberg B, Molon-Noblot S, et al. Polysaccharide storage myopathy in Cob Normand draft horses. Vet Pathol 2008;45:154–8.
192. Meyer TS, Fedde MR, Cox JH, et al. Hyperkalaemic periodic paralysis in horses: a review. Equine Vet J 1999;31:362–7.
193. Reynolds J, Potter G, Greene L, et al. Genetic-diet interactions in the hyperkalemic periodic paralysis syndrome in Quarter horses fed varying amounts of potassium. J Equine vet Sci 1998;18:591–600.
194. Cox J, DeBowes R. Episodic weakness caused by hyperkalemic periodic paralysis in horses. Comp cont Educ pract Vet 1990;12:83–8.
195. Spier SJ, Carlson GP, Holliday TA, et al. Hyperkalemic periodic paralysis in horses. J Am Vet Med Assoc 1990;197: 1009–17.
196. Naylor JM. Hyperkalemic periodic paralysis. Vet Clin North Am Equine Pract 1997;13:129–44.
197. Guglick MA, MacAllister CG, Breazile JE. Laryngospasm, dysphagia, and emaciation associated with hyperkalemic periodic paralysis in a horse. J Am Vet Med Assoc 1996;209: 115–17.
198. Carr EA, Spier SJ, Kortz GD, et al. Laryngeal and pharyngeal dysfunction in horses homozygous for hyperkalemic periodic paralysis. J Am Vet Med Assoc 1996;209:798–803.
199. Beech J, Fletcher JE, Tripolitis L, et al. Effects of phenytoin in two myotonic horses with hyperkalemic periodic paralysis. Muscle Nerve 1992;15: 932–6.
200. Glazier DB, Littledike ET, Evans RD. Electrocardiographic changes in induced hyperkalemia in ponies. Am J Vet Res 1982;43:1934–7.
201. Cornick JL, Seahorn TL, Hartsfield SM. Hyperthermia during isoflurane anaesthesia in a horse with suspected hyperkalaemic periodic paralysis. Equine Vet J 1994;26:511–14.
202. Robertson SA, Green SL, Carter SW, et al. Postanesthetic recumbency associated with hyperkalemic periodic paralysis in a quarter horse. J Am Vet Med Assoc 1992;201:1209–12.
203. Pang DS, Panizzi L, Paterson JM. Successful treatment of hyperkalaemic periodic paralysis in a horse during isoflurane anaesthesia. Vet Anaesth Analg 2011;38:113–20.
204. Castex AM, Bertone JJ. ECG of the month. Sinus tachycardia and hyperkalemia in a horse. J Am Vet Med Assoc 1989;194:654–5.
205. Church S. Hyperkalaemic periodic paralysis in Australian quarter horses. Aust Vet J 1995;72:314–16.
206. Beech J, Lindborg S. Prophylactic efficacy of phenytoin, acetazolamide and hydrochlorothiazide in horses with

hyperkalaemic periodic paralysis. Res Vet Sci 1995;59:95–101.
207. Naylor JM, Robinson JA, Crichlow EC, et al. Inheritance of myotonic discharges in American quarter horses and the relationship to hyperkalemic periodic paralysis. Can J Vet Res 1992;56:62–6.
208. Stewart RH, Bertone JJ, Yvorchuk-St. Jean K, et al. Possible normokalemic variant of hyperkalemic periodic paralysis in two horses. J Am Vet Med Assoc 1993;203:421–4.
209. Spier SJ, Carlson GP, Harrold D, et al. Genetic study of hyperkalemic periodic paralysis in horses. J Am Vet Med Assoc 1993;202:933–7.
210. Traub-Dargatz JL, Ingram JT, Stashak TS, et al. Respiratory stridor associated with polymyopathy suspected to be hyperkalemic periodic paralysis in four quarter horse foals. J Am Vet Med Assoc 1992;201:85–9.
211. Andrews FM, Reed SM, Johnson GC. Muscle biopsy in the horse: its indications, techniques and complications. Veterinary Medicine US: Equine Practice 1993:357–65.
212. Reed SM, Hegreberg GA, Bayly WM, et al. Progressive myotonia in foals resembling human dystrophia myotonica. Muscle Nerve 1988;11: 291–6.
213. Montagna P, Liguori R, Monari L, et al. Equine muscular dystrophy with myotonia. Clin Neurophysiol 2001;112: 294–9.
214. Steinberg S, Botelho S. Myotonia in a horse. Science 1962;137:979–80.
215. Wijnberg ID, Owczarek-Lipska M, Sacchetto R, et al. A missense mutation in the skeletal muscle chloride channel 1 (CLCN1) as candidate causal mutation for congenital myotonia in a New Forest pony. Neuromuscul Disord 2012;22:361–7.
216. Naylor JM, Jones V, Berry SL. Clinical syndrome and diagnosis of hyperkalaemic periodic paralysis in quarter horses. Equine Vet J 1993;25: 227–32.
217. Robinson JA, Naylor JM, Crichlow EC. Use of electromyography for the diagnosis of equine hyperkalemic periodic paresis. Can J Vet Res 1990;54:495–500.
218. Naylor JM. Selection of quarter horses affected with hyperkalemic periodic paralysis by show judges. J Am Vet Med Assoc 1994;204:926–8.
219. Bowling AT, Byrns G, Spier S. Evidence for a single pedigree source of the hyperkalemic periodic paralysis susceptibility gene in quarter horses. Anim Genet 1996;27:279–81.
220. Bendheim PE, Reale EO, Berg BO. beta-Adrenergic treatment of hyperkalemic periodic paralysis. Neurology 1985;35:746–9.
221. Fletcher JE, Erwin K, Beech J. Phenytoin increases specific triacylglycerol fatty esters in skeletal muscle from horses with hyperkalemic periodic paralysis. Biochim Biophys Acta 1993;1168: 292–8.
222. Yudkowsky ML, Beech J, Fletcher JE. Phenytoin alters transcript levels of hormone-sensitive lipase in muscle from horses with hyperkalemic periodic paralysis. Arch Biochem Biophys 1998;358:264–70.
223. Duren S. Feeding management of horses with hyperkalemic periodic paralysis. World Equine Vet Res 1998;3:5–8.
224. Cox J, editor. Response of normal and acetazolamide treated horses to oral potassium chloride challenge. American College of Veterinary Medicine; 1988.
225. Rose B, Post T, Narins R. Clinical Physiology of Acid-Base and Electrolyte Disorders. 5th ed. New York: McGraw-Hill Professional Publishing; 2000.
226. Hoskins B. Studies on the mechanism of action of acetazolamide in the prophylaxis of hyperkalemic periodic paralysis. Life Sci 1977;20:343–9.
227. Alberts MK, Clarke CR, MacAllister CG, et al. Pharmacokinetics of acetazolimide after intravenous and oral administration in horses. Am J Vet Res 2000;61:965–8.
228. Smith CA. Hyperkalemic periodic paralysis presents medical and ethical challenge. J Am Vet Med Assoc 1993;202:1203–9.
229. Cox J, editor. An episodic weakness in four horses associated with intermittent serum hyperkalemia and the similarity of the disease to hyperkalemic periodic paralysis in man. American Association of Equine Practitioners; 1985.
230. Steiss J, Naylor JR. Episodic muscle tremors in a quarter horse: Resemblance to hyperkalemic periodic paralysis. Can Vet J 1986;27:332.
231. Cannon SC. Ion-channel defects and aberrant excitability in myotonia and periodic paralysis. Trends Neurosci 1996;19:3–10.
232. Hoffman EP. Voltage-gated ion channelopathies: inherited disorders caused by abnormal sodium, chloride, and calcium regulation in skeletal muscle. Annu Rev Med 1995;46:431–41.
233. Rudolph JA, Spier SJ, Byrns G, et al. Linkage of hyperkalaemic periodic paralysis in quarter horses to the horse adult skeletal muscle sodium channel gene. Anim Genet 1992;23:241–50.
234. Naylor JM, Robinson JA, Bertone J. Familial incidence of hyperkalemic periodic paralysis in quarter horses. J Am Vet Med Assoc 1992;200:340–3.
235. Zhou J, Spier SJ, Beech J, et al. Pathophysiology of sodium channelopathies: correlation of normal/ mutant mRNA ratios with clinical phenotype in dominantly inherited periodic paralysis. Hum Mol Genet 1994;3:1599–603.
236. Hanna WJ, Tsushima RG, Sah R, et al. The equine periodic paralysis Na+ channel mutation alters molecular transitions between the open and inactivated states. J Physiol (Lond) 1996;497:349–64.
237. Cannon SC, Hayward LJ, Beech J, et al. Sodium channel inactivation is impaired in equine hyperkalemic periodic paralysis. J Neurophysiol 1995;73:1892–9.
238. Pickar JG, Spier SJ, Snyder JR, et al. Altered ionic permeability in skeletal muscle from horses with hyperkalemic periodic paralysis. Am J Physiol 1991;260:C926–933.
239. Lehmann-Horn F, Iaizzo PA, Hatt H, et al. Altered gating and conductance of Na+ channels in hyperkalemic periodic paralysis. Pflugers Arch 1991;418:297–9.
240. Cannon SC, Brown RH Jr, Corey DP. A sodium channel defect in hyperkalemic periodic paralysis: potassium-induced failure of inactivation. Neuron 1991;6:619–26.
241. Ricker K, Camacho LM, Grafe P, et al. Adynamia episodica hereditaria: what causes the weakness? Muscle Nerve 1989;12:883–91.
242. Steele D, Naylor JM. Hyperkalemic periodic paralysis, plasma lactate and exercise tolerance. J Equine vet Sci 1996;202:933–7.
243. Maxson-Sage A, Parente EJ, Beech J, et al. Effect of high-intensity exercise on arterial blood gas tensions and upper airway and cardiac function in clinically normal quarter horses and horses heterozygous and homozygous for hyperkalemic periodic paralysis. Am J Vet Res 1998;59:615–18.
244. Jamison JM, Baird JD, Smith-Maxie LL, et al. A congenital form of myotonia with dystrophic changes in a quarterhorse. Equine Vet J 1987;19:353–8.
245. Hegreberg GA, Reed SM. Skeletal muscle changes associated with equine myotonic dystrophy. Acta Neuropathol (Berl) 1990;80:426–31.
246. Andrews FM, Spurgeon TL, Reed SM. Histochemical changes in skeletal muscles of four male horses with neuromuscular disease. Am J Vet Res 1986;47:2078–83.
247. Brook JD, McCurrach ME, Harley HG, et al. Molecular basis of myotonic dystrophy: expansion of a trinucleotide (CTG) repeat at the 3′ end of a transcript encoding a protein kinase family member. Cell 1992;69:385.
248. Todd PK, Paulson HL. RNA-mediated neurodegeneration in repeat expansion disorders. Ann Neurol 2010;67:291–300.

249. Fugier C, Klein AF, Hammer C, et al. Misregulated alternative splicing of BIN1 is associated with T tubule alterations and muscle weakness in myotonic dystrophy. Nat Med 2011;17:720–5.
250. Johansson A, Carlstrom K, Ahren B, et al. Abnormal cytokine and adrenocortical hormone regulation in myotonic dystrophy. J Clin Endocrinol Metab 2000;85:3169–76.
251. Mastrogiacomo I, Pagani E, Novelli G, et al. Male hypogonadism in myotonic dystrophy is related to (CTG)n triplet mutation. J Endocrinol Invest 1994;17: 381–3.
252. DiMauro S, Bonilla E, Davidson M, et al. Mitochondria in neuromuscular disorders. Biochim Biophys Acta 1998;1366:199–210.
253. Valberg SJ, Carlson GP, Cardinet 3rd GH, et al. Skeletal muscle mitochondrial myopathy as a cause of exercise intolerance in a horse. Muscle Nerve 1994;17:305–12.
254. Larsson NG, Oldfors A. Mitochondrial myopathies. Acta Physiol Scand 2001;171:385–93.
255. Xu X, Arnason U. The complete mitochondrial DNA sequence of the horse, Equus caballus: extensive heteroplasmy of the control region. Gene 1994;148:357–62.
256. Turner AS, Trotter GW. Fibrotic myopathy in the horse. J Am Vet Med Assoc 1984;184:335–8.
257. Bishop R. Fibrotic myopathy in the gracilis muscle of a horse. Vet Med Small Anim Clin 1972;67:270.
258. Irwin DH, Howell DW. Fibrotic myopathy, haematomas and scar tissue in the gaskin area of the thoroughbred. J S Afr Vet Assoc 1981;52:65–6.
259. Dabareiner RM, Schmitz DG, Honnas CM, et al. Gracilis muscle injury as a cause of lameness in two horses. J Am Vet Med Assoc 2004;224:1630–3, 1605–36.
260. Walmsley EA, Steel CM, Richardson JL, et al. Muscle strain injuries of the hindlimb in eight horses: diagnostic imaging, management and outcomes. Aust Vet J 2010;88:313–21.
261. Valentine BA, Rousselle SD, Sams AE, et al. Denervation atrophy in three horses with fibrotic myopathy. J Am Vet Med Assoc 1994;205: 332–6.
262. Gomez-Villamandos R, Santisteban J, Ruiz I, et al. Tenotomy of the tibial insertion of the semitendinosus muscle of two horses with fibrotic myopathy. Vet Rec 1995;136:67–8.
263. McIlwraith W, Robertson J. McIlwraith & Turner's equine surgery: advanced techniques. Sect. Surgery for fibrotic myopathy 1998.

8 Skeletal physiology: responses to exercise and training

Charlotte Sinclair Helen L. Birch Roger K.W. Smith Allen E. Goodship

CHAPTER CONTENTS

Introduction

Role of the skeleton

The main role of the mammalian skeleton is to provide structural support and a means of locomotion using jointed bones stabilized and moved by ligaments, tendons and muscles. In addition, the bony skeleton provides protection for vital organs and a reservoir of minerals. The components of the skeleton have evolved to optimize posture and locomotion for the lifestyle of individual species such that the type of joints and position of muscle and tendon attachment relative to lever arms and fulcra provide an optimal mechanical advantage. In addition, the skeleton has evolved to provide maximum strength with minimal mass. The skeleton comprises a series of morphologically distinct elements; the bones. The shape and size of these individual bones are determined by genetic and functional factors to provide an appropriate structure for functional demands with a low risk of failure and without incurring excess energy expenditure. The demands for energetic efficiency are greater in animals evolved for high-speed locomotion, such as horses.

The horse has not only evolved to become a high-speed animal, but has also been the subject of selective breeding as an elite animal athlete. The Thoroughbred racehorse is a prime example of selection for speed. However, it has been suggested that this selection process has reached its limit as classic race speeds in Thoroughbred horses have not increased in the last 40–60 years.[1] The Thoroughbred has arisen from a somewhat limited gene pool and this may have resulted in a plateau of performance[2] in contrast to the performance of human athletes in which records are broken almost year on year. However, an alternative explanation is that training methods to condition racehorses have not developed to optimize the capacity of the adaptive responses of the musculoskeletal system. In human athletics, the application of sports science has undoubtedly contributed to the enhancement of performances over recent years. Equine sports science is not yet developed or applied to the same extent. In addition, many training systems continue to be based on empirical and traditional methods.

The skeleton has the capacity to respond to changes in mechanical loading in the short term and can, therefore, optimize for energetic efficiency in relation to changes in mechanical demands. There is a need not only to understand these mechanisms in general, but to apply the information to training regimens for equine athletes.

Epidemiology of skeletal injuries

There are many factors that influence the risk of fractures in horses. The majority of research has focused on racehorses. In racehorses, the type of surface is influential on the type of fracture that occurs. For example, on all-weather and dirt tracks, bi-axial proximal sesamoid bone fractures are most common, whereas in horses jumping on turf tracks, lateral condylar fractures of the third metacarpal bone are most common, and in flat turf races, proximal phalanx fractures are most common.[3]

In the UK, the catastrophic fracture rate per 1000 starts was 0.33 in flat races, 1.4 in hurdling, and 2.3 in steeple chasing.[3] Track conditions have also been shown to affect the risk of fracture with risk increasing on turf as the conditions become softer, and on dirt tracks the risk increased when the tracks became 'muddier'.[4] However, conversely others found that risk of fracture increased with firmer turf.[5]

In racehorses in training, the risk of non-traumatic (i.e. spontaneous) fracture in horses that are in flat race training was 1.15 per 100 horse months in training and 1.5 in national hunt (jump) training. An increased risk of fracture was found in horses that had more days in training following a 60 day non-racing period (i.e. lay-off) and the distance exercised in the two months prior to fracture were correlated with increased risk of condylar fractures. The odds of condylar fracture increased by 0.3% per day for every additional day that the horse was in training since the 60 day non-racing period.[3] The risk of condylar fracture increased by 4% for each extra furlong that the horse was exercised at a 'fast pace'. Horses that suffered fractures were those that had had been in training for longer, had higher exercise intensities and completed more races compared to controls.[3]

A further study showed that horses were at increased risk of fracture if they either exceeded 44 km at canter (<14 m/s) or 6 km at gallop (>14 m/sec) in a 30 day period. Increasing the distance cantered up to 50 km in a 30 day period further increased the risk of tibial and pelvic stress fractures. Distal limb fracture has been shown to be at higher risk in horses that do no fast work compared to those doing 4–10 furlongs of fast work per week. Hence, short periods of high intensity exercise may be protective against fracture by stimulating appropriate adaptation of the bone. A 30–90 day rest period has been shown to be detrimental. However, interpreting rest periods is difficult as the horse may have been rested due to an existing injury that increases the risk of future injury, or the lack of stimulation to the bone may be responsible for increasing osteoclastic activity and thus weakening the bone.[3] Also the training protocol following a rest period may influence adaptation and related fracture risk.

The conformation of the individual horse has shown to influence predisposition to fractures in Thoroughbred racehorses. For example long pasterns are associated with increased risk of forelimb fracture, and carpal valgus decreases the risk of carpal fracture.[6] In racehorses in training, gender and age were not shown to significantly affect fracture rate, whereas there was a significant difference in risk between trainers. The overall incidence of fracture for horses in National Hunt training was 1.1/100 horse months.[7] Foals born to primiparous mares are at less risk of fracture than those of multiparous mares and the rate of fracture also decreased with increasing dam age.[8] Thus early skeletal development can potentially affect the risk of fracture later in life.

There is less documentation of the incidence of fractures in other equestrian disciplines. In event horses, a study demonstrated that in over 60 000 cross-country starts during 'eventing' there were 0.12 per 1000 starts of fracture or 'bone injury' recorded which is dramatically lower than those described above for racing.[9]

In general, there has been a significant lag between scientific advances in the understanding of mechanisms controlling functional adaptation of bone and translation to changes in the training methods used in the equine world in general and in the horseracing industry in particular. No doubt some of the biologic mechanisms controlling adaptation of bone to its functional environment could and should be applied to the conditioning of equine athletes. It is also probable that the empirical traditional methods of training do incorporate some scientific principles as a consequence of many years of experience and these may inform research programs to validate the methods used.

Design of the equine skeleton

The equine skeleton is a refinement of the basic mammalian pattern. The horse is an unguligrade (hoofed) animal and a member of the order Perissodactyla (odd toed), standing on the hoof of the third digit. The major muscle masses of the limbs are positioned proximally to reduce the energy required to move the limb as it swings backward and forward in cursorial locomotion. Bone mass is also minimized at the distal extremities and safety margins decrease toward the distal extremity of the limbs, which may explain why the incidence of fractures in racehorses is higher in the distal bones than those located proximally.[10]

Selection for high-speed gait is also reflected in the morphology of the equine skeleton. The lever arms at the elbow and hock result in small muscle contractions producing fast extensive movement of the lower limb segments. These skeletal refinements in the elite equine athlete are basically a fine tuning of the general pattern. Analysis of skeletal conformation has been used to assess the level of performance in several different types of horse. Elite show jumpers and dressage horses were found to have larger hock angles and more sloping scapulas than other horses[11], while another study found that in Quarter Horses the ability to generate greater torque at the hip and stifle joint was due to a greater muscle physiological cross-sectional area rather than longer moment arms.[12] However, these systems have not yet been perfected to identify potential winners at an early age. Interestingly, a recent study of the skeleton of the great racehorse Eclipse has shown that his skeleton was 'average' in all respects.[13]

The ability to train elite equine athletes must result from a sound understanding of many aspects of the biology of the horse, from the cell and molecular level to that of the whole animal. One of the most important systems in relation to performance is the musculoskeletal system, and bone, as the major structural support tissue, is one of the most critical aspects.

Bone as a tissue

Bone as a tissue is a member of the family of connective tissues which are characterized by a large amount of extracellular matrix (ECM) and relatively few cells. The ECM in the case of bone is a composite of an organic, predominantly collagenous component and an inorganic hydroxyapatite component.

Bone matrix molecular composition

As with all connective tissue matrices, there is a high proportion of water in bone tissue in the order of 20%, depending upon the type of bone. The remaining dry weight of bone comprises approximately 65% inorganic mineral, largely hydroxyapatite, and 35% organic material. The organic component of bone is predominantly the fibrous protein collagen, imparting high tensile strength. The inorganic hydroxyapatite imparts high compressive strength.

Bone mineral

Hydroxyapatite consists of predominantly calcium and phosphate in a hexagonal crystal system and has the formula $Ca_{10}(PO_4)_6(OH)_2$. The hydroxyl ion can be replaced by fluoride, chloride or carbonate. The deposition of calcium and phosphate into hydroxyapatite occurs initially by nucleation of extracellular, lipid bilayer-enclosed microstructures (matrix vesicles) released by cells but ultimately requires collagen fibrils.[14] The normal process of mineral precipitation is primarily dependent on extracellular phosphate concentration, with calcium playing a secondary role.[15] Mineralization is inhibited by molecular crystal inhibitors such as pyrophosphate (PPi) which binds to the hydroxyapatite crystals preventing phosphate ion incorporation.[16] Inactivation of tissue nonspecific alkaline phosphatase (TNAP); an enzyme that is able to hydrolyse PPi, reduces tissue mineralization.[14] Other inhibitors of nucleation include matrix Gla protein (MGP) and osteocalcin, both calcium binding proteins.[15] Mineralization depends on the balance between inhibitors and promoters of crystal formation.

Organic matrix

The organic matrix is predominantly (>90%) type I collagen together with a small proportion of minor collagens including types III, V, XI and XIII and non-collagenous proteins. Type I collagen is a fibril forming collagen. The collagen molecule, known as tropocollagen, is formed from three polypeptide chains. Two identical $\alpha 1$ polypeptide chains and one $\alpha 2$ chain form a right handed triple helix. The initial collagen molecule is synthesized as a procollagen precursor and the propeptides are cleaved from the ends of the molecule before collagen is able to assemble into fibrils. A more detailed description of the collagen molecule and fibrillogensis is given in Chapter 9.

The non-collagenous proteins make up <10% of the organic component. Proteoglycans form about 10% of the non-collagenous ECM protein. Most of the proteoglycans in immature bone are large chondroitin sulphate containing proteoglycans, as in cartilage, but as the bone matures these are replaced with the small proteoglycans, decorin and biglycan. Biglycan and decorin associate with collagen fibrils and are therefore implicated in control of fibril diameters and mineral deposition in bone[17] in addition to binding growth factors such as TGF-β.[18]

The γ-carboxyglutamic acid containing proteins, osteocalcin (OCN) and matrix Gla protein (MGP), are present in bone and are inhibitors of mineralization. OCN is a bone specific protein while MGP is present in most tissues[19] and may play a role in prevention of extra-osseous mineralization.[15] The glycoproteins osteonectin, fibronectin and thrombospondin are all found in bone. Osteonectin forms ~ 15% of the non-collagenous protein and is thought to be a nucleator in collagen-mediated mineralization.[20] Fibronectin is involved in cell adhesion and may also be involved in mechanosignaling.[21] Thrombospondin promotes bone formation by bringing matrix components closer together.[18] The sialoproteins (bone sialoprotein and osteopontin) form about 15% of non-collagenous ECM protein.[18] Bone sialoprotein promotes cell attachment, is osteoconductive (encourages bone deposition), osteoinductive (promotes recruitment and stimulation of bone forming cells)[22] and plays a role as a nucleator of mineralization.[23] Osteopontin, expressed by bone cells, chondrocytes and fibroblasts may be involved in recruitment of cells for fracture healing and remodeling of bone.[24] α2 Heremans-Schmid glycoprotein (AHSG) accounts for about 20% of the non-collagenous ECM protein. However AHSG is synthesized by the liver and 40% localizes to bone.[25] AHSG is a chemo attractant for monocytes and may serve in the recruitment of osteoclast precursors.[26]

Bone cells

Adult bone tissue comprises three major populations of cells, each with a specific functional role but with both cell-to-cell interactions and also cell-matrix interactions. It is the coordinated interaction of the activities of these cell populations that optimizes the morphology of bones in relation to changing mechanical demands. Understanding these mechanisms and applying the principles to training regimens has the potential to improve performance and minimize injury in conditioning of equine athletes.

Osteoblasts

These cells are derived from local lining cells. Osteoblast differentiation results from activation of β-catenin through Wnt signaling by the Wnt co-receptors, low-density lipoprotein receptor-related proteins 5 and 6 (LRP5, LRP6) and Frizzled.[27] The flattened mononuclear cells become plump when activated and synthesize bone matrix in the form of osteoid (Fig. 8.1). The osteoid then becomes mineralized over a period of weeks to form bone matrix. In rapidly forming surfaces some osteoblasts are entrapped in their own matrix and these then become osteocytes (Fig. 8.2). The osteoblasts communicate with osteoclasts and enable activation of osteoclasts to allow bone resorption. Osteoblasts also produce colony-stimulating factor that increases numbers of pre-osteoclasts from mononuclear precursors in the bone marrow and also osteoclast activation factor that activates the pre-osteoclasts and initiates resorption of bone matrix (Fig. 8.3).

Osteoclasts

These cells are derived from circulating monocytes. They are multinucleate cells (Fig. 8.3) which, when activated, reside on a bone surface with a ruffled border to isolate the local environment between the cell and the bone surface. The perimeter of the cell membrane forms a seal against the underlying bone involving adhesion molecules, the integrins to isolate the local environment beneath the cell which is then lowered in pH by an active proton pump generating hydrogen ions.[28] The pH falls to around 2–3 and the bone matrix and embedded osteocytes are resorbed, forming a resorption pit, and the resorption products are trafficked through

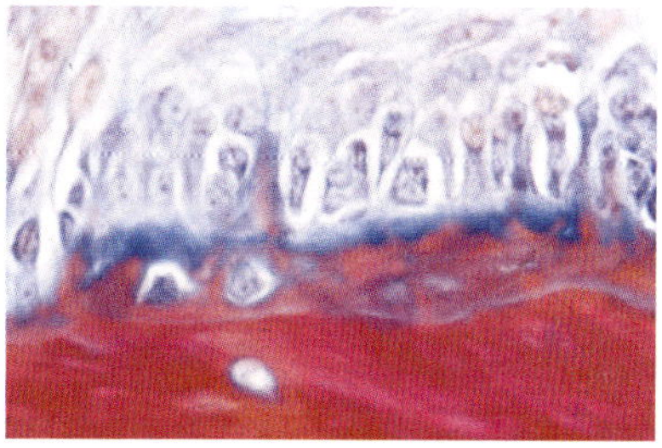

Fig 8.1 A photomicrograph of bone showing the bone-forming cells called 'osteoblasts'. The blue staining matrix is the precalcified osteoid. Cells can be seen becoming entrapped in matrix to become osteocytes.

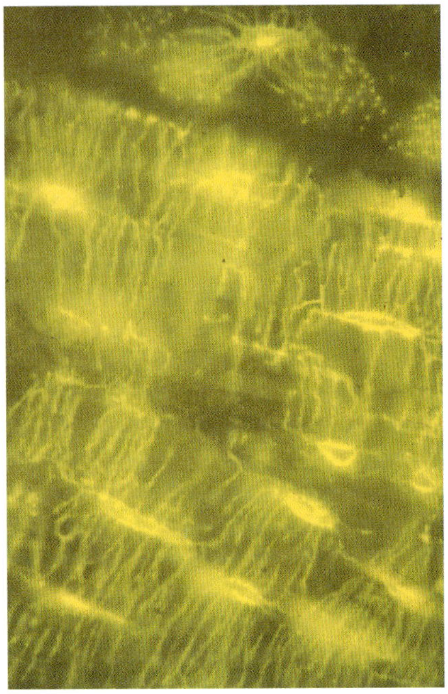

Fig 8.2 Bone cells – osteocytes entrapped within bone matrix showing communication via cytoplasmic processes within canaliculi.

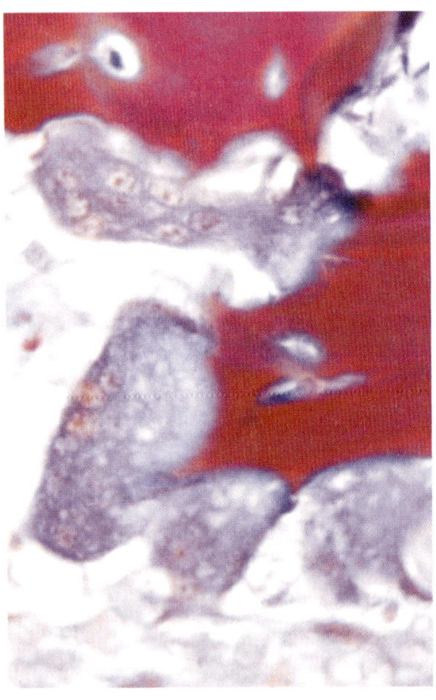

Fig 8.3 A photomicrograph showing bone resorption by osteoclasts.

the cell.[29] This process is regulated by the osteoblasts (see below), which in turn communicate with the third population of cell; the osteocytes. The bone-resorbing osteoclasts are also influenced directly by some specific hormones such as calcitonin.

Osteocytes

These cells arise from osteoblasts that become trapped in the bone matrix within lacunae. They are cells with many long cytoplasmic processes within small tunnels in the matrix called canaliculi (Fig. 8.2). Processes from adjacent cells connect by means of gap junctions allowing cell-to-cell communication. Work by Skerry and co-workers has identified that the neurotransmitter glutamate is involved in osteocyte cell signaling.[30] This transmitter also operates in the central nervous system, where complex interneuronal signaling occurs. The presence of such a signaling mechanism among osteocyte bone cells provides supporting evidence that this population of cells plays a role in the overall perception of mechanical environment on a bone and co-ordinates an appropriate response to ensure optimal bone size and architecture.

The osteocytes and their cell processes are surrounded by extracellular fluid. The mechanical loading of a bone results in deformation and movement of this extracellular fluid within the matrix around the cells. Extracellular fluid contains ions and the movement of this ionic fluid with respect to the charged surfaces of the matrix induces electrical potentials. These electrical charges are referred to as 'streaming potentials' which are also thought to influence the cell activity and provide a putative mechanotransduction pathway.[31, 32] The gap junctions linking cell communication are also modulated in number by mechanical loading of bone and thus may play a role in regulation of bone form in response to functional demands.[33]

The networks of osteocytes also communicate with the surface lining cells and osteoblasts. Thus the integration of the cell populations by the osteoblasts provides a complex but extremely sensitive mechanism to enable bone mass and architecture to be optimized for the changing mechanical demands throughout life.

Lining cells

Quiescent bone surfaces are covered by lining cells which have the capacity to respond to both mechanical and biological signals and are activated to change shape into plump, metabolically active osteoblasts. These cells are found in the osteogenic layer of the periosteum or endosteum; these membranes comprise a deep cellular layer and a more superficial fibrous layer (Fig. 8.4). Some pluripotent cells have been demonstrated in the osteogenic cellular layer and these have been shown to have the capacity to differentiate into other connective tissues such as cartilage. There is currently considerable interest in the various types of pluripotent cells in the adult as a source of 'stem' cells that play a role in tissue regeneration. These quiescent lining cells are activated by mechanical or hormonal stimuli to generate a bone-forming front of metabolically functional osteoblasts involved in a modeling or remodeling process to maintain or restructure the matrix. The bone lining cells are thought to have a specific role in coupling bone resorption to bone formation[34] and it has been suggested that this is by physically defining bone remodeling compartments.[35]

Intercellular communication between bone cells

The activity of bone producing cells and bone resorbing cells must be balanced under normal conditions to maintain the integrity of the skeleton. The coupling of bone resorption and subsequent bone formation has been shown to involve a receptor on the osteoblast cell membrane known as receptor activator of nuclear factor κβ ligand (RANKL) which binds to RANK present on the surface of pre-osteoclasts and induces activation of the intracellular cascades to activate the osteoclasts. The RANKL can also bind to a protein called osteoprotegerin (OPG), which is stimulated by canonical Wnt signaling.[36] OPG prevents binding with and activation of osteoclasts. Thus a regulation of coupling of these cells and associated amounts of bone resorption and formation is effected by this system (Fig. 8.5).[37, 38] More recent work has shown that RANKL is also expressed by mature osteocytes and this expression is necessary for normal bone structure[39, 40] as deletion of the RANKL gene in mice results in excess bone formation. It is not clear at present how osteocytes embedded within the matrix make contact with osteoclast precursor cells.[41] Factors that increase RANKL expression are important and, in less mature osteoblasts, include parathyroid hormone (PTH), parathyroid hormone-related protein (PTHrP), 1,25-dihydroxyvitamin D_3 and oncostatin M.[41] In mature osteocytes, apoptosis[42] and the protein sclerostin may stimulate RANKL production.[43]

The osteoblasts can also secrete collagenase, an enzyme that removes the surface layer of osteoid, unmineralized bone matrix, on bone surfaces and allows osteoclasts access to the bone matrix. Hormonal influences on calcium metabolism and bone resorption act indirectly on receptors on the osteoblast which in turn regulates osteoclast recruitment and activity. Thus the osteoblast is central to the control of the bone modeling and remodeling process. Boyde et al used in vitro systems to measure bone resorption activity of osteoclasts and also to show the interactions between osteoblasts and osteoclasts.[44]

The pro-inflammatory cytokine interleukin-33 (IL-33) is a newly identified factor produced by osteoblasts that inhibits osteoclast formation in vitro.[45, 46] A study has demonstrated that mice deficient in the IL-33 receptor demonstrated increased osteoclast formation and low bone mass.[46]

The regulation of bone resorption and bone formation also relies on coupling factors released from osteoclasts that influence the bone forming osteoblast cells. Examples are cardiotrophin-1 that stimulates bone formation[47] and the recently identified Semaphorin 4D which inhibits bone formation in female mice.[48, 49]

Furthermore, factors released by osteocytes can influence osteoblast activity. Sclerostin, a protein released by osteocytes, is an inhibitor of bone formation and is of interest because of its potential therapeutic potential in treating osteoporosis in humans. However sclerostin mRNA and protein has been identified in other non-bone sites[41] including the adult human aortic intima[41] where it is suspected to inhibit aortic calcification. Sclerostin is up-regulated by calcitonin[50] and inhibited by factors that stimulate bone formation such as prostaglandin E2[51], oncostatin M and cardiotrophin-1.[52]

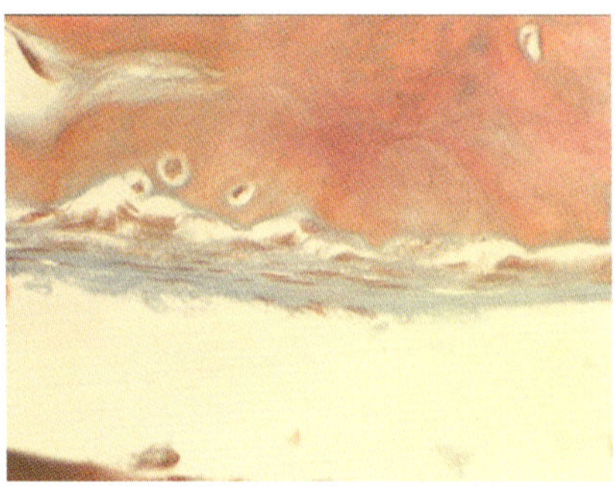

Fig 8.4 Lining cells on a bone surface – periosteum, comprising a fibrous outer layer and an osteogenic or cambium inner layer of cells.

Bone ultra-structure

As a composite material, bone matrix is anisotropic and the architecture of the matrix in relation to the osteocytes forms the basic unit of structure, termed the lamella. The architecture of the lamellae can be observed under polarized light microscopy as the collagen is a birefringent material. The architecture of these bone lamellae in different geometrical arrangements forms the basis of the different histological types of bone. Concentric circumferential lamellae form osteons and when these are formed in the original development of the bone they are termed 'primary osteons'. A similar architecture is also seen in the secondary osteons that are formed to repair damage such as micro-cracks or infill porosities within the cortex. Lamellae formed around vascular networks or plexi result in laminar or the less regular plexiform bone often seen in ungulates like the horse (Fig. 8.6). This type of bone allows very rapid increases in cross-sectional area with later consolidation.[10] Lamellar bone can also form circumferential lamella on the entire periosteal and endosteal surfaces of individual bones (Fig. 8.7).

In embryological development and in the early stages of fracture repair a rapidly forming bone with irregular lamellae, coarse collagen fibers and large osteocyte lacunae is seen. This is called 'woven' bone and is rapidly remodeled to the various types of organized lamellar bone, such as primary and secondary osteonal bone, previously termed 'Haversian' bone (Fig. 8.8).

Bone morphology has been related to the mechanical loading requirements of different specific bones. For example, the orientation of collagen fibers in the cranial and caudal cortices of the radius reflects the mechanical requirements of this bone. Strain gauge studies have shown that this bone is loaded in both compression and bending with principal tensile strains aligned with the long axis

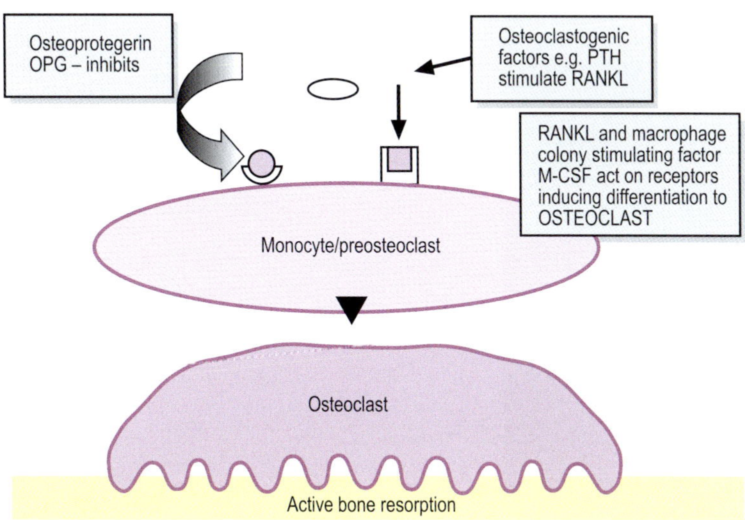

Fig 8.5 Coupling of the bone remodeling cycle.

of the bone in the cranial cortex and principal compressive strains aligned to the long axis in the caudal cortex.[53] The arrangement of collagen fibers in relation to this pattern of loading has been demonstrated by Riggs et al.[54] This has been supported by a comprehensive analysis of matrix morphology in the equine radius[55], in which the analysis of primary bone and bone within secondary osteones of the cranial and caudal cortices of the radius were arranged appropriately to optimize for the pattern of functional loading. This study also confirmed a predominant longitudinal arrangement of collagen fibers in the cranial cortex of this bone, to resist the functional tensile strains at this location. Any consistent changes in the magnitude and pattern of loading induce a modeling response in which the bone cell activity will modify the matrix to maintain the optimization of the overall bone architecture in relation to the new prevailing loading conditions. Matrix, and embedded osteocytes, can be removed by osteoclasts and new matrix formed by osteoblasts. This coupled cellular activity allows bone as both a material and structure to be changed in terms of mass and distribution throughout life.

Material properties

The material properties of bone matrix as a composite material vary and are largely related to the degree of mineralization, particularly with respect to modulus of elasticity. Bone such as the tympanic bulla, with a very high mineral volume fraction and density, has a high modulus eminently suitable for conduction of sound, whereas deer antler is low in mineral content and has a low modulus, again appropriate to avoid fracture in its role in fighting. Bone matrix is an anisotropic brittle elastic material and the elastic modulus is related to the level of mineralization. The influence of mineralization on material properties has also been evaluated during growth and maturation. In immature horses the level of mineralization is low and increases to a higher level with maturation to adult equine bone. With development and increased mineralization there is a significant correlation with changes in mechanical properties; it is suggested that such changes may be measured non-invasively using ultrasound transmission systems. This would provide the potential to monitor material properties of bone during growth and possibly during training.[56] More recently bone microindentation testing has been used to give a direct measure of bone mechanical properties at the tissue level.[57] This technique involves applying a number of cycles of load to the bone using a very small probe which is capable of passing through the skin and can be used in vivo. The probe creates microscopic fractures giving information about a bone's ability to resist macroscopic failure.

The material properties and morphology of specific bones determine the structural properties of the individual skeletal elements. Thus changes in the mechanical competence of bones as structures

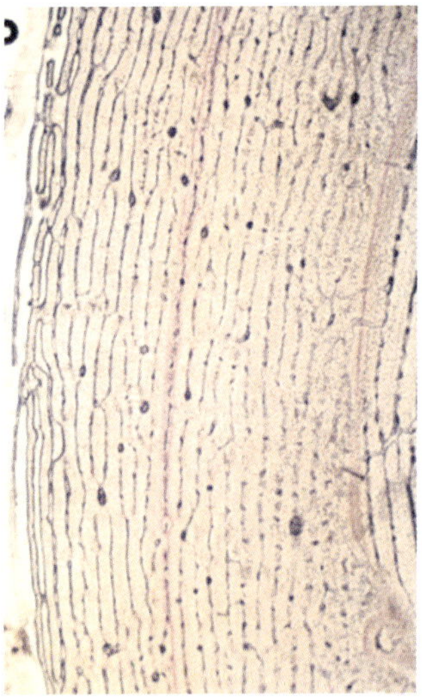

Fig 8.6 Photomicrograph of a transverse section of laminar bone.

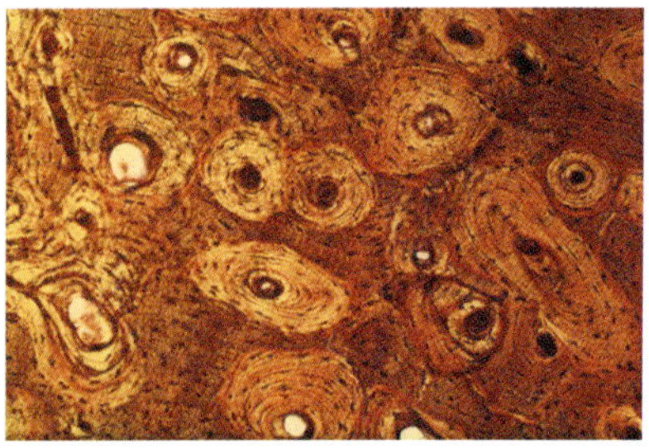

Fig 8.8 Photomicrograph of a transverse section of highly remodeled secondary osteonal cortical bone.

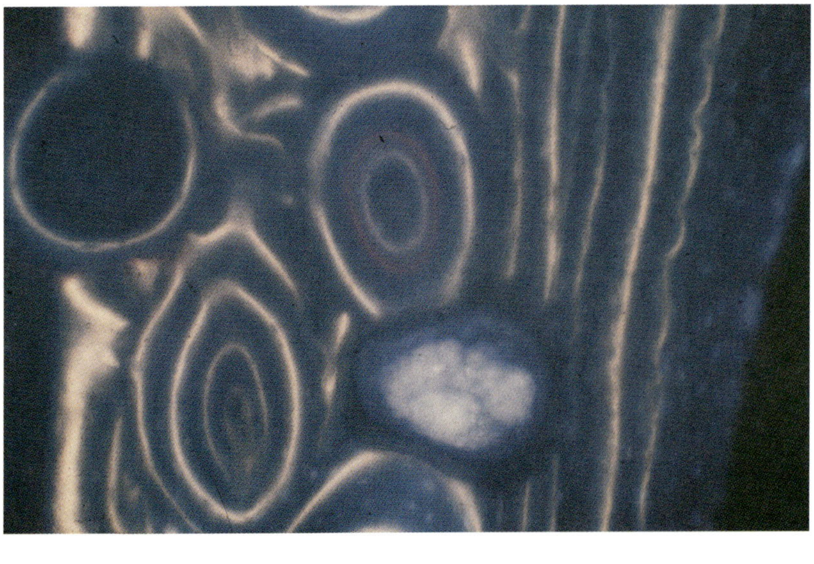

Fig 8.7 Photomicrograph of a transverse section of cortical bone to show secondary osteons at different stages of formation in the process of remodeling and endosteal circumferential lamellar bone.

may be a consequence of either changes in the material properties of the constituent tissue or an alteration in the structural distribution of the material in relation to the magnitude and distribution of the loads applied at a particular time. The dynamic nature of bone tissue provides the ability to optimize structure in response to changes in matrix material properties.

Mechanical characteristics

Bone tissue as a material contributes to the mechanical characteristics of the individual skeletal elements. The architectural arrangement of the material is predominantly related to the general functional requirements of the particular skeletal elements. In the long bones the diaphysis is tubular to resist the functional loading patterns of bending and torsion. In engineering terms, these loading patterns can be sustained with maximum strength and minimal material by tubular structures with the material distributed at a distance from the neutral axis. For example, if a solid beam is subjected to bending, one surface will experience tensile stresses and the opposite surface compression stresses. At some plane between these two surfaces there will be neither tensile nor compressive stresses (the neutral axis), thus no material is required in this region. When bone tissue organizes into the components of the skeleton, its structure is based on optimization of energetic efficiency. Thus to minimize the mass of material, bone is not present in the medullary cavity (Fig. 8.9). The relative thickness of the cortices also reflects the loading patterns of a particular bone. These changes may be measured using radiographic and ultrasound transmission techniques.[58]

At the extremities of the long bones and in short bones the functional loads are predominantly those of axial compression. This is reflected in a different architecture with a thin cortical shell supported by internal cancellous bone (Fig. 8.10). The plates and rods of bone are termed trabecula and formed of aligned bone lamellae (Fig. 8.11). These rods and plates are not randomly arranged but strategically placed in relation to the trajectories of principal compressive and tensile stresses. In the cancellous bone of the epiphyses, underlying the articular surfaces of the synovial joints, the trabecula are orthogonal (perpendicular) to the articular surface. This architecture of the plates and rods again allows the use of minimal material to provide maximum strength and minimize energy requirements for locomotion. In short bones that are loaded predominantly in compression, the internal structure is of strategically arranged bony trabecula. Some short bones, such as the calcaneus, are subjected to bending moments. The internal cancellous architecture reflects this with arcades of trabecular bone arranged orthogonally to resist the principal compressive and tensile stresses. Nature reflects the calculated stress-related bracing seen in some engineering structures such as the Fairbairn crane in which the loading and principal stresses resemble those of the femur (Fig. 8.12).

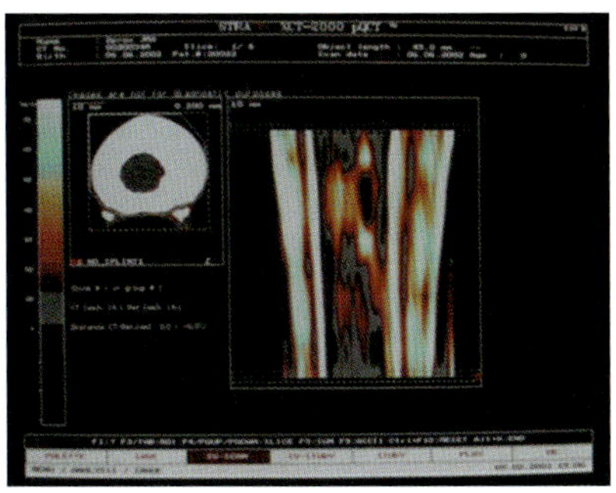

Fig 8.9 Data from a pqCT scan of an equine MC3 bone to show the variation in cortical thickness and the presence of the medullary cavity as the region of the 'neutral axis'.

The increased diameter of the bones in the regions of the epiphyses and the presence of subchondral trabecular bone act both to reduce stresses on the articular cartilage and provide a compliant structure to absorb impact loads. Thus any changes in the compliance of the trabecular bone will influence the loading of the overlying cartilage and can indirectly induce changes in the articular cartilage.

Bone as a structure/organ

Adult bone form is determined by a combination of genetic and environmental influences. Fell demonstrated that certain anatomic features of the developing skeleton are formed as a consequence of

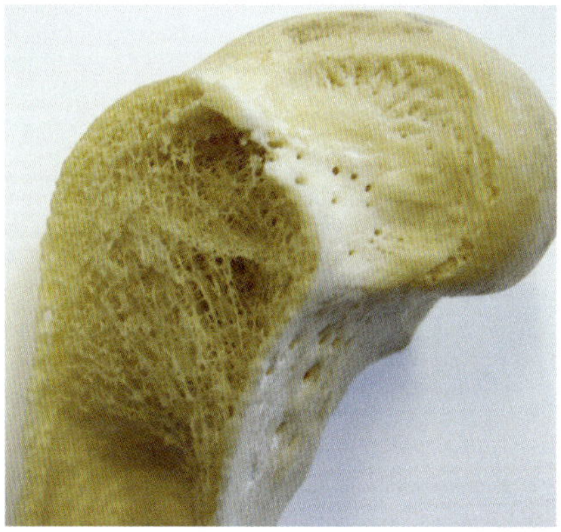

Fig 8.10 Photograph of the metaphysis and epiphysis of a long bone sectioned longitudinally to show the cortical shell supported by internal cancellous spongy bone.

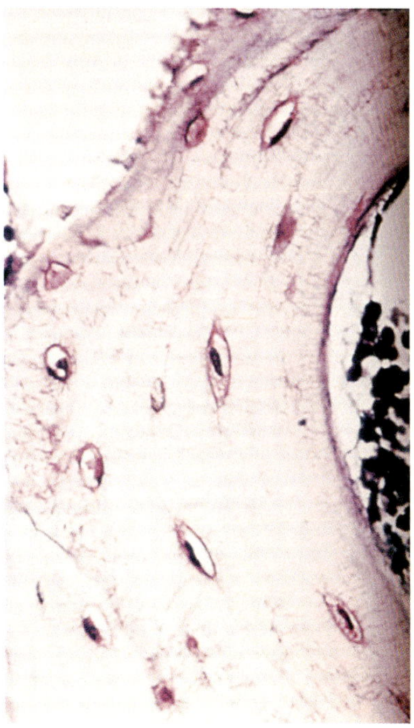

Fig 8.11 Photomicrograph of histological section of a bone trabeculum to show lamellar bone structure.

inherent genetic control whereas others require a functional loading to form.[59] An elegant study by Chalmers investigated the development of a mouse femur implanted into the spleen when at the cartilage anlage (precursor) stage of development.[60] This cartilaginous bone precursor developed into a bone with the basic form of the femur but lacked the architectural refinements seen in the normal adult mouse femur. The refinements, such as a waisted femoral neck, cortical thickness and trabecular architecture, are induced as a consequence of functional loading and are determined by the prevailing loading conditions (Fig. 8.13). There is a dynamic interaction between the loads imposed on the skeleton and the morphology of the bones at any point in time throughout life. It is therefore important to appreciate these interactions in order to condition the skeleton for the demands of athletic performance and to understand the modes and mechanisms of failure.

Skeletal development

Growth

Ossification

The skeleton is developed both pre- and post-natally. The majority of the bones of the skeleton, particularly the appendicular skeleton, are pre-formed as miniature replicas in hyaline cartilage. This has the advantage of enabling rapid three-dimensional growth. The material and structural properties of hyaline cartilage are adequate to support the low level of loading prevailing in utero. In preparation for the postnatal changes in loading with gravitational and muscular forces, a more appropriate material must replace the hyaline cartilage. This is accomplished by vascular invasion, calcification and removal of cartilage and replacement with lamellar bone. This process is endochondral ossification. In a few sites of the skeleton, for instance the bones of the vault of the skull, bone is formed by direct ossification of a fibrous type I collagen scaffold. This process is intramembranous ossification.

The bones associated with locomotion are formed by both endochondral and intramembranous ossification. This allows simultaneous longitudinal and circumferential growth of the bones.

Endochondral ossification

The initial vascular invasion of the cartilage replica occurs in the midshaft. In this region the chondrocytes within the lacunae undergo hypertrophy and the extracellular matrix becomes calcified. It is now thought that the endothelial cell invasion occurs in the non-calcified territorial and pericellular matrices following cell death[59] and that cell death in the growth plate occurs through an apoptotic pathway.[61] The calcified cartilaginous matrix is then removed by chondroclasts derived from vascular cells and replaced by woven and then lamellar bone. These spicules of bone become strategically organized and form the cancellous bone structure of the metaphysis, termed the primary spongiosa. In human growth this has been suggested by Byers et al as a critical component of the growth process and the development of the mineralization of the primary spongiosa may be of importance in relation to bone-altering disease in later life.[62] These authors also suggest that the secondary spongiosa retains a constant bone mineral volume throughout development. Thus in the developing horse the mechanical loading from exercise during growth and maturation could affect the level of mineralization of the primary spongiosa.

Simultaneously with the longitudinal growth, the fibrous layer covering the replica bone, the perichondrium, initiates ossification

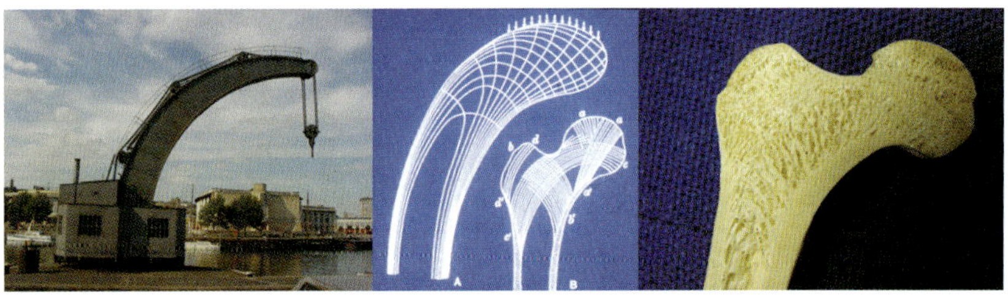

Fig 8.12 Comparison of the structure and stress distribution of the Fairbairn crane and proximal femur.

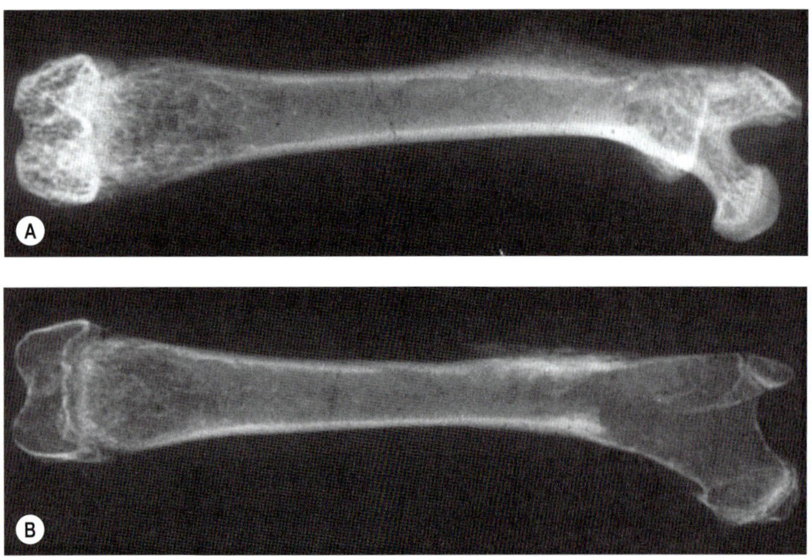

Fig 8.13 Radiographs of mouse femora, showing the adaptations to functional environment **(A)** from the basic genetic template **(B)**.
Adapted from Chalmers et al 1962.[60]

of the fibrous tissue and forms a cuff of bone which develops to form cortices of the tubular diaphysis. This process forms the 'primary' ossification center and is followed by further vascular invasion at one or both ends of the developing bone to form secondary ossification centers. The secondary ossification centers are separated from the primary center by plates of hyaline cartilage known as the growth plate or physis. This process allows for both circumferential and longitudinal growth and enlargement of the bone. The longitudinal growth occurs by utilizing the interstitial growth potential of hyaline cartilage in the proliferative zone of the growth plate. The physis has a distinct structural pattern relating to specific functional activities. The epiphyseal side of the plate is characterized by a resting zone of randomly arranged cells within an extracellular matrix. These cells give rise to the zone of proliferation in which the chondrocyte population is actively dividing. These cells then align into palisades extending toward the metaphysis, with the cells closest to the metaphysis showing hypertrophy of the lacunae. In this zone of hypertrophy the matrix becomes calcified and is removed by chondroclasts. Osteoblasts then deposit woven bone on the calcified cartilage scaffold. This tissue is rapidly remodeled to lamellar bone and forms the trabecular rods and plates of the spongiosa that support the metaphyseal cortex. The width of the physis is increased by appositional growth from the overlying perichondrium. The physis can be described as a discoid physis contributing to the increase in longitudinal growth and width of the metaphysis. The epiphysis also acts as a spheroid physis to increase the size of the epiphysis by radial growth. The early articular cartilage is thick and arranged in a similar pattern to the physeal plate with the proliferating chondrocytes close to the articular surface and a radial arrangement of palisades toward the center of the epiphysis (Fig. 8.14). The secondary ossification centers and spheroid physes form the cancellous bone that supports the articular cartilage. Abnormalities in the process of ossification can lead to specific orthopedic conditions such as angular deviations of the limbs and osteochondral dysplasias.

The limited thickness of the physis in normal animals allows growth without excessive deformation of the cartilage which would result in angular deformations of the growing bone. In some conditions where ossification is inhibited and the cartilaginous component of the physis increases in thickness, limb deformities occur during growth. A classic example is dietary rickets. Rapid growth can also result in angular deformities of the long bones.

Intramembranous ossification

As the bones increase in length there is also an increase in overall width of the metaphysis and diaphysis of the bone, accomplished by appositional bone growth on the periosteal surface. In the developing bone a cuff of periosteal bone is formed. The periosteum comprises an outer fibrous layer and an inner osteogenic 'cambium' layer. In this osteogenic layer cells differentiate into osteoblasts which deposit osteoid directly onto collagen type I fibers. This process ultimately forms lamellar bone. In ungulates the type of lamellar bone formed is laminar or plexiform bone. This primary vascular bone is capable of a rapid increase in cross-sectional area. In this type of bone a rapid appositional growth occurs with subsequent infilling of lamellae within the laminae of the vascular network.[63] Thus bone growth occurs to the age of skeletal maturity by means of these two processes.

Modeling and remodeling

During the processes of both bone growth and adaptation to changes in loading, the shape or architecture of the bone is changed by cellular activity to remove and form bone. Unlike cartilage, bone cannot increase in size by interstitial growth; only by these processes of removal and formation of bone surfaces can the relative proportions of curvatures and the positions of tuberosities be maintained. Changes in shape result from removal and formation of bone at the same time but at different locations; this process is termed modeling and allows changes in three-dimensional tissue space (Fig. 8.15).

Modeling is determined both by growth and by mechanical loading. As a long bone increases in length the flared metaphysis is narrowed into the diaphysis by bone resorption on the periosteal surface and bone formation on the endosteal surface. In the diaphyseal region increase in bone width during growth occurs by periosteal appositional growth and endosteal bone resorption (Fig. 8.16).

Within the bone matrix microdamage can occur as a consequence of repeated loading cycles. Repetitive loading in many inert materials results in accumulation of microdamage and ultimately, the gross fracture of the structure. Although bone is a structural material, it is living and there are cell-to-cell and cell-to-matrix interactions. Thus changes in matrix can initiate cellular responses to maintain and adjust the matrix. Microdamage is a stimulus to induce osteoclastic resorption of the damaged matrix followed by deposition of lamellar bone by osteoblasts. Osteocytes undergo apoptosis in response to microdamage[64] which imitates bone resorption through the release of soluble signaling molecules.[65, 66] This dynamic repair process occurs throughout life and during normal functional loading of the skeleton. It is termed remodeling and involves the resorption and removal of bone at the same site but at different points in time (Fig. 8.7). Bone that is formed in remodeling is called secondary bone. These secondary osteons continue to increase in level of mineralization for several weeks after formation of the osteon has been completed. The secondary bone is not as strong as primary bone but is stronger than the damaged matrix. The remodeling process results in the formation of 'secondary osteons'. The initial resorption is affected by a cutting cone of osteoclasts traveling longitudinally within the cortical bone, followed by lining osteoblasts that secrete the new circumferential lamellar bone with entrapment of osteoblasts within the matrix to become the osteocytes within the circumferential lamellae (Fig. 8.17). A glycoprotein layer is formed between the newly formed secondary osteon and the adjacent bone tissue which forms the cement line.

Bones as structures

Individual bones have specific morphologic features related to their functional contribution to the skeleton as a whole. The types of bones can be divided broadly into long bones, such as the femur, humerus, radius, tibia and the metacarpal/tarsal bones, short bones, such as the carpal, tarsal and distal phalangeal bones, and flat bones, such as the scapula, and some bones of the skull and pelvis. In addition, some bones are not directly involved in the structural support of the body but contribute to the mechanical arrangements of tendons in facilitating the change in direction of tensile forces. These bones, often associated with tendons, are the sesamoid bones, of which the patella, proximal and distal (navicular) sesamoids are examples.

The long bones can be divided into regions: the epiphyses, metaphyses and diaphysis. These regions show different morphologic arrangements of the bone tissue. The epiphyseal and metaphyseal regions comprise a thin cortical shell of compact bone supported by internal cancellous bone, sometimes termed spongy or trabecular bone. This internal arrangement of bone tissue comprises plates and rods of bone with spaces or cancelli filled with marrow or fat. The bone tissue in these areas often shows a definite pattern of

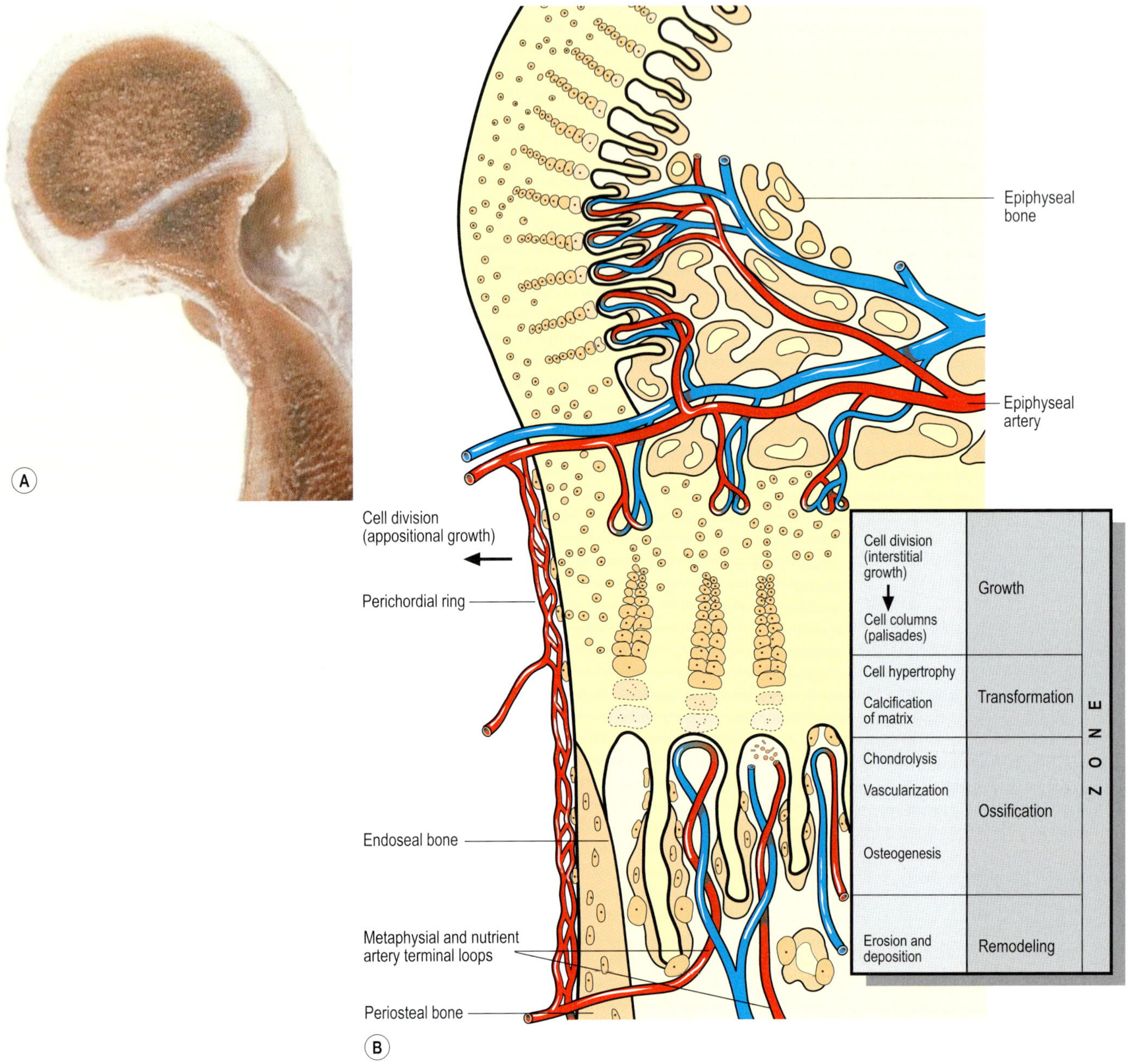

Fig 8.14 **(A)** The growing spheroid and discoid physes in an immature growing long bone sectioned longitudinally. **(B)** Diagram to show the arrangement of palisades in the two physes.

trabecular arcades. This arrangement of internal spongy bone is also seen in the short bones. The geometric pattern is particularly noticeable on radiographs and especially those of the proximal femur and calcaneus (Fig. 8.18).

The internal structure of spongy bone has been of interest to scientists, engineers and surgeons since the time of Galileo. In the 1890s comparisons were made between the pattern of cancellous bone and analysis of stress trajectories in engineering structures. The proximal region of the femur with the femoral neck and head is loaded in a manner very similar to that in engineering structures like the Fairbairn crane and the trabecular architecture reflects the lines of principal tensile and compressive stresses calculated for these structures (see Fig. 8.12).

Recent developments in technology have allowed the distribution of principal strains to be measured in the living skeleton and the data from such studies have provided supporting evidence that these bone trabeculae are strategically placed to optimize the strength of the structure with minimal mass of tissue. In animals this is important to reduce the energetic cost of locomotion. The thickness and structural density of trabecular bone also reflect the magnitude of the loads taken in that region of the bone. This has been shown in training studies; for example, the trabeculae in the dorsal region of the third and radial carpal bones are thicker than those in the more palmar regions in horses that have been trained for peak athletic performance. These observations can be used in diagnosis of bony changes related to mechanical loading of the

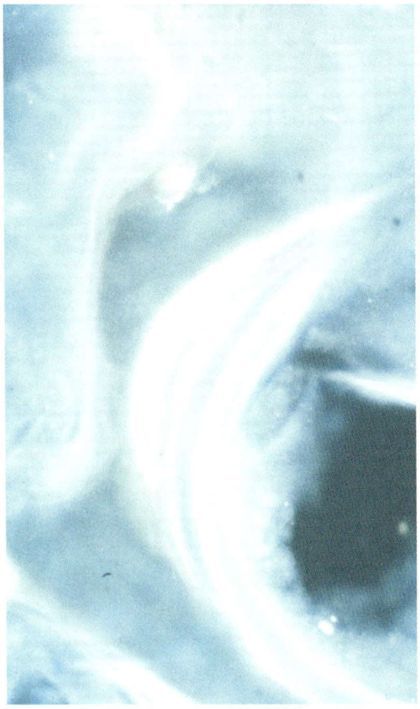

Fig 8.15 Photomicrograph of a fluorochrome-labeled section of trabecular bone, showing apposition on one surface indicating a modeling change in architecture.

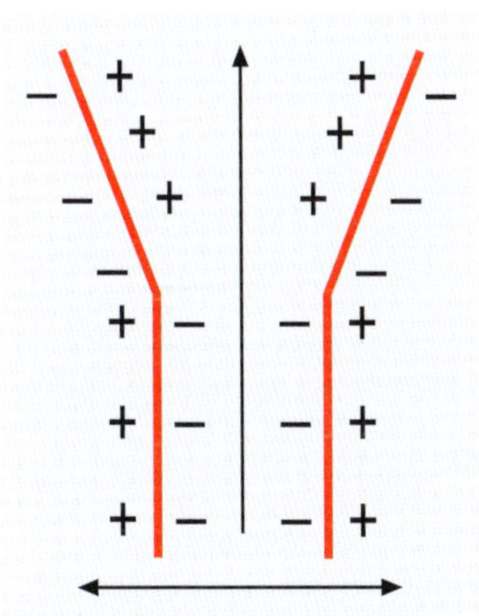

Fig 8.16 Diagram of modeling changes at metaphysis and diaphysis during growth.

skeleton. The site-specific changes, such as those in the carpal bones, are often found to be related to predilection sites of skeletal injury and pathology so knowledge of these interactions can enhance diagnostic and prognostic clinical skills.

The arrangement of bone tissue in the diaphyseal region of long bones is markedly different. This region is similar to a tube, hence the term tubular bone. The wall of the tube comprises compact cortical bone, of differing thickness, and a medullary cavity containing blood vessels, marrow and fat. This arrangement of bone reflects a different mechanical loading pattern; whereas in the short bones the loads are predominantly compressive loads, in the long bones spanned by tendons and ligaments there are large bending and torsional moments in addition to compressive loading.

Again, the biologic drive is to reduce the energetic costs of locomotion, whilst ensuring adequate structural strength to avoid failure during physiologic loading levels. In engineering design these requirements to provide maximum strength in bending and torsion using a minimal mass of material are met by a wide-diameter, thin-walled tube. This essentially places the material at the greatest distance from the neutral axis, where there are neither tensile nor compressive stresses. In long bones the medullary cavity represents the average neutral axis relative to the loading pattern of the bone. Thus strength is maximized and mass minimized to reduce the energy costs associated with moving the limb. In animals evolved for high-speed locomotion there is a high biologic drive to

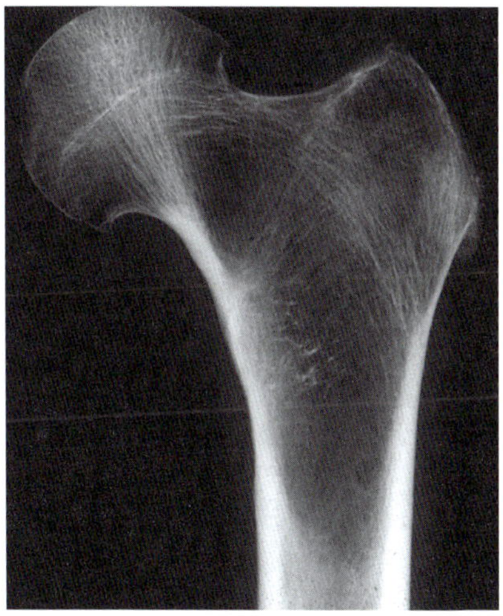

Fig 8.18 Radiograph of the proximal human femur to show trabecular arcades.

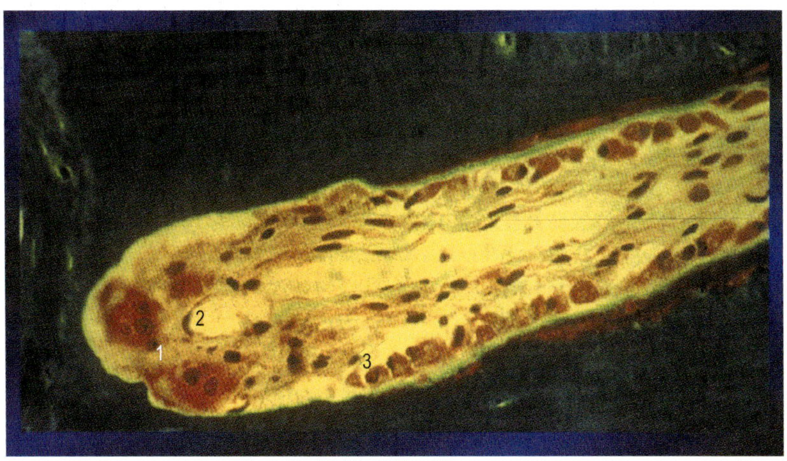

Fig 8.17 A 'cutting cone' of osteoclasts (1) followed by a blood capillary (2) and osteoblasts (3) infilling with circumferential lamellae to form a secondary osteon.

reduce energy costs. In engineering structures, the material type, mass and distribution all contribute to the ability of the structure to resist functional loads. However, to allow for occasional overload a safety margin is normally incorporated into the design, such that the structure will not fail as a consequence of occasional overload. Studies have shown that the skeleton also incorporates a safety margin although this is not uniform in relation to skeletal location. The neck of the femur in humans is known to be able to withstand about five times bodyweight. The disadvantage of a safety margin is the additional mass of material. This becomes significant in the more distal regions of the limb since additional mass increases the momentum of the swinging limb and this in turn would result in a significantly increased energy requirement in decelerating and accelerating the limb, particularly in high-speed equine athletes. Currey, analyzing data from Vaughan and Mason, showed that a higher incidence of fractures during racing occurred in the more distal bones of the limb and hypothesized that this could be explained by a lower safety margin in the more distal limb bones.[67]

Although the diaphysis of long bones is essentially tubular, the distribution of bone in terms of cortical thickness may be non-uniform around the circumference of the bone. This reflects different levels of resistance to bending in different planes and the associated distribution of bone mass.

Factors controlling shape and size

Genetic influences

Both between species and within species, the variation in the specific geometry of individual bones is a consequence of two main factors. First, a genetic component that will control a basic bone mass. Second, a response to prevailing mechanical conditions which will modify the basic genetic pattern in relation to both the magnitude and the distribution of loads applied to the particular bone. Furthermore genetic factors also determine the response to a specific loading regime. The genotype for a polymorphism in IL-6 gene promoter determined whether femoral cortical area increased or decreased following a 10 week training program in human subjects, supporting a fundamental role for IL-6 in the regulation of bone mass and bone remodeling.[68]

Disuse will result in a tendency toward the genetic basic bone mass. Abnormal loading will induce a concomitant abnormality in the size and shape of the bone. Chalmers in 1962 demonstrated these controlling factors by transplantation of the cartilage precursor of the mouse femur to the spleen, where it developed with adequate blood supply but devoid of mechanical input.[60] Although the basic shape of a femur could be recognized, this bone lacked the refinements in both mass and architecture exhibited by the normal functionally located bone in littermates (see Fig. 8.13). Further evidence that certain anatomic features of specific bones were genetically predetermined and others were formed as a consequence of local stimuli was provided by Fell using isolated limb buds from developing embryos in organ culture.[59] Genetic modification of a basic anatomic skeletal pattern is often seen in relation to attaining specific conformation for either visual or functional requirements.

Even within specific breeds of horse certain genetic strains are evident and linked to differences in bone mass and architecture. Other factors influenced by selective breeding, which could be described as genetic modification, such as muscle mass, may have an indirect influence on bone mass as a consequence of increased levels of mechanical loading of the bones. As both a tissue and a structure, bone has the property of functional adaptation.

Environmental influences

Other factors such as nutrition and hormonal environment may also influence the ability of a bone to attain the full genetic potential. However, one of the most potent environmental influences on bone mass and architecture is the prevailing mechanical environment.

Functional loading of bone refines the inherent genetic form. The levels of mechanical input can vary throughout life with an associated response in terms of skeletal adaptation.

Both during growth and maturation and in the skeletally mature adult, bone responds to mechanical loading. The relationship of the pathophysiology of functional adaptation to training and conditioning regimens in general and in the horse in particular is important in maximizing performance and minimizing skeletal injury (see Chapter 22). In determining the aspects of functional loading that influence the bone cell populations and consequently are important in controlling the architecture of the skeleton, it was essential to be able to quantify the functional environment of the skeleton.

Although techniques were available to measure strains on cadaveric bone, using photoelastic coatings, stress coat and electronic strain gauges, it had not been possible to quantify the effects of loads on the living skeleton until the cyanoacrylate tissue adhesives became available. In the early 1970s Lanyon and Smith[69] and van Cochran[70] made the first measurements of strain in the living skeleton. The ability to bond foil rosette strain gauges to living bone allowed both the magnitude and distribution of the principal strains on the surfaces of a number of bones to be measured during activities such as locomotion. From these measurements it was possible to determine the loading patterns of different specific bones. For example, the radius in quadrupeds is loaded in bending with principal tensile strain aligned to the long axis of the bone on the cranial cortex and principal compressive strain aligned to the long axis of the bone on the caudal cortex[54], whereas the tibia showed a significant component of torsional loading.[71] The physiologic loading pattern of these long bones can be used in determining the appropriate fixation methods to treat fractures in these bones.

Strain distributions on the surface of bones with defined internal trabecular arcades again provide confirmatory data to show the strategic alignment of the trabeculae of spongy bone with the directions of principal tensile and compressive strains.[72] This technique increased the understanding of the response of bone to changes in mechanical demands, a mechanism called functional adaptation.

Functional adaptation of bone

General principles

The bony skeleton provides structural support for the body throughout life and also enables locomotion by virtue of the linked skeletal elements forming a system of rigid levers upon which forces can be exerted by muscles through tendons and ligaments. Articulations between the individual bones allow energetically efficient movement. The basic genetically determined bone mass is optimized for energetic efficiency and to accommodate the loads imposed. Thus throughout life as the activities change, the process of functional adaptation enables the appropriate adjustments to be made to the mass and architecture of the skeleton. The biologic signals that induce bone cell activity and control the adaptive process are related to the deformation of the tissue as a consequence of the loads applied by muscles and gravity. Recent work has identified some of the genes that are regulated in response to mechanical load and the time sequence for the response.[73] Deformation is termed 'strain' and is the change in length in relation to the original length (Fig. 8.19). Although the response of bone to mechanical loading has been known for some time, the ability to quantify imposed changes in mechanical environment of the skeleton and relate these to the consequent biologic response of the bone has only been possible using the technique of in vivo strain measurement.

Dynamic strain similarity

By applying strain gauges to the living skeleton of a variety of species, from fish through reptiles, birds and mammals, including the horse and human, the level of bone deformation during peak physiologic activity has been shown to be remarkably similar.[74] Thus it was hypothesized that bone had evolved in this wide range of species to optimize to a threshold level of deformation, sometimes likened to a thermostat and termed a 'mechanostat', irrespective of histological structure. A simple strain-controlled feedback loop was proposed. If an increase in loading resulted in an elevated strain above the threshold value, this triggered the bone cell populations to synthesize bone matrix to increase the mass of bone and thus for the new loading conditions to reduce the increased levels of deformation back to the threshold values. In the event of a decrease in loading and consequent level of deformation, the bone cells would respond by activating a net bone resorption and decrease bone mass.

Optimization of mass and architecture (Wolff's concepts)

In the event of a persistent change in the normal pattern of loading, the bone strain patterns would be altered and this persistent change in strain distribution would initiate a redistribution of bone through a modeling response to alter the architecture of the bone as a structure. Such changes may involve structural optimization by changes in both the distribution and mass of bone to withstand the new loading environment.

Early studies in which the strain on the skeleton was increased and an adaptive response was evoked supported the theory of a strain control feedback mechanism. The characteristics of the mechanical osteogenic stimulus were elucidated by a series of studies in which bones were subjected to known strain characteristics and the consequent osteogenic response was measured. These studies were of two basic types: those in which a defined mechanical regimen was imposed on a bone following surgical intervention and those in which an exercise regimen was applied to the intact skeleton. Increased loading of parts of the skeleton induced by removal of adjacent bone or by attachment of loading devices to isolated bones allowed the imposition of a specific strain environment. The early studies inducing increased loading by removal of an adjacent bone and consequent overloading of the remaining ones by normal locomotion demonstrated an adaptive response to increase the overall cross-sectional area and thus restore the strain levels to the functional optimal values, thus supporting one of Wolff's hypotheses.[75, 76]

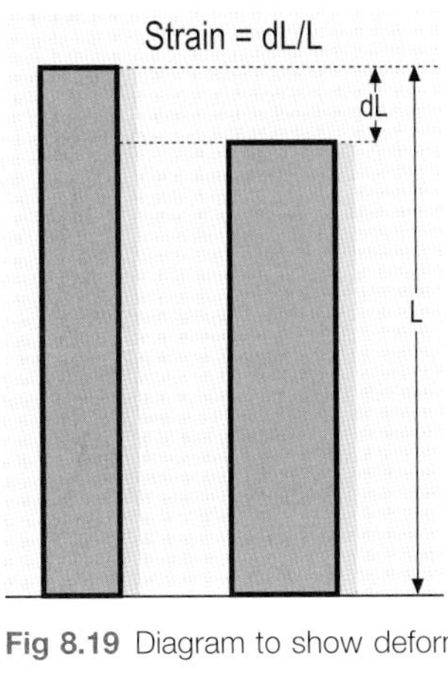

Fig 8.19 Diagram to show deformation or 'strain'.

Osteogenic mechanical stimuli

The nature of the mechanical stimulus that elicited an osteogenic response was investigated by a more controlled study of specific mechanical variables and their influence on adjustment of bone mass and architecture.

Such studies involved the use of implants attached to the bone and used to impose controlled mechanical stimulation. These experiments elucidated some of the osteogenic aspects of the strain environment. During normal strain distributions, such as those occurring during walking, the level of osteogenic response, in terms of increased cross-sectional area of bone, to imposed strains was found to show a high correlation with the rate of bone deformation.[76] This suggests that training using a normal type of exercise requires a high loading rate to elicit an osteogenic response. A more refined method of studying the exact nature of mechanical signals that stimulate bone formations was developed by using isolated segments of bone. Ideally an organ culture might be used for such studies but culture of bone is difficult in terms of culturing a significant mass of true ossified tissue and the absence of the hormonal regulation and its interaction with mechanical cues precludes such models.

Using isolated bone models in vivo, it was possible to define in a more specific manner the strain characteristics that induced bone formation.[77] The effect of numbers of cycles of loading applied on a daily basis was investigated, together with the effect of magnitude of the imposed strain. It was shown that there was a 'dose-response' effect with strains below the normal physiologic threshold inducing bone resorption and a consequent decrease in cross-sectional area and those above the physiologic threshold showing an increase related to strain magnitude. From these experimental studies a number of mathematical models were derived in which it appeared that there was a window of strain magnitude that retained bone mass with neither resorption nor formation. This was termed the 'lazy zone'.[78] Strain magnitudes outside this zone induced either bone resorption or bone formation. Interestingly, Rubin and Lanyon investigated the relationship between the number of loading cycles imposed on a daily basis and the resultant effect on bone mass in terms of bone mineral content and cross-sectional area.[77] This work showed that a maximal effect on bone mass could be attained with only 36 cycles of loading at 0.5Hz each day. Any additional cyclical loading did not attain a greater effect on bone mineral density or cross-sectional area. Bone mass was shown to be maintained with as few as four loading cycles per day, whereas complete cessation of loading resulted in a decrease in bone, predominantly by endosteal resorption leading to a reduced cortical thickness, together with some increase in cortical porosity. This study suggests that short periods of osteogenic cyclical deformation can induce a maximal adaptive response. In terms of conditioning bone in equine athletes this might be interpreted as a short period of daily trotting. The stimulus appears to require cyclical deformation as the application of constant load did not induce bone adaptation.[79]

Hillam and Skerry developed a non-invasive method of loading the rat forearm and used this model to demonstrate that mechanical loading could modify the normal modeling patterns seen during growth.[80] A short period of cyclical loading changed a bone resorption surface to a bone-forming surface. The applied loading induced an aberrant strain distribution. This model was also used by Mason et al in determining the gene activation patterns associated with mechanical loading and putative signaling molecules in the transduction and integration of mechanically induced bone remodeling.[81] Forwood and Turner used a similar approach by applying a bending moment to the rat tibia and confirmed the response to high strain rate cyclical deformation in a mammalian model. This suggests the principles can be extrapolated to other species, including the horse.[82]

Thus the principles of these findings have implications for the training of young horses using a diverse exercise regimen. Perhaps on the basis of this evidence, horses that are used for competitive events that involve movements outside the natural range on a frequent basis should be introduced to such exercises at an early age when the architecture of the skeleton could be influenced to adapt to these loading demands and thus resist damage and failure in adulthood. Events such as jumping, dressage, trotting, racing and pacing may be candidates for such practice. However, any training regimens must be introduced over an adequate time period with a graded increase to accommodate adaptation and avoid damage.

Rate of adaptation

Adaptation to loading in bone can be initiated by short periods of cyclical loading. Therefore, to prolong this type of exercise or to introduce long periods of such exercise too rapidly, particularly on a hard surface, may lead to induction of microcracks and ultimately the gross fracture of the bone. Damage even to the delicate internal architecture of the trabecular bone with subsequent stiffening, particularly of subchondral regions, may reduce the absorption of high impact loads and inflict damage upon the overlying articular cartilage (Fig. 8.20).[83] Mechanical factors may thus initiate a cascade of events leading to osteoarthritis. The joint must be considered as an organ and changes to one component tissue or structure will impact on the whole joint.[84] Interestingly, Chen et al observed differences in heel strike transients between races with different incidence of osteoarthritis so it is possible that conformation may influence the transmission of impact transients in equine limbs and predispose to degenerative joint disease. This localized adaptive hypertrophy of trabecular bone can be seen following imposed exercise regimens, for instance the dorsal regions of the third and radial carpal bones.[85] Furthermore, with an osteogenic exercise regimen given for only a short period each day, these localized bone changes occur extremely rapidly.[86] This localized change in loading can induce a change in both bone and cartilage, the osteochondral unit. Increased exercise in the adult horse results in a thickening of the trabecula of the subchondral bone, a thickening of the subchondral plate and a thickening of both the calcified and hyaline layers of the overlying articular cartilage.[87] Experimental studies have also shown the sensitivity of cancellous bone to changes in mechanical loading and these data can be indirectly related to training methods in the horse.[88]

These morphological changes result in a change to the mechanical properties of the microstructure which can be measured by indentation techniques[89] and micromechanical testing of single trabeculae.[90] The adaptation within a bone in relation to a very specific pathway of load transmission through the bones of the skeleton is seen particularly well in the carpal bones where significant differences are found between the dorsal and palmar regions of these bones. Long-term loading with associated stiffening of the bone in the dorsal region may relate to the common occurrence of cartilage fibrillation and breakdown in this region.

Microdamage

If the exercise training is based upon a structured increase in duration of short periods of exercise that induces high bone strain, the bone will adapt and the physiologic adaptation will condition the bone for athletic exercise rather than a pathophysiologic response leading to micro-damage and stress-fractures which can lead to catastrophic fractures (see Chapter 22).

Microcracks

Accumulation of microcracking within the bone matrix results in a remodeling response in which the secondary bone has inferior properties to primary bone. Crack formation is seen as a fractal pattern of matrix damage (Fig. 8.21). Microcracks have been demonstrated in several species of athletic individuals such as the horse[91, 92] and the racing greyhound.[93] Cracks can be observed by bulk staining the bone prior to histological sectioning in order to confirm that the cracks are not processing artefacts. The cracks can be seen as stained defects within the matrix (Fig. 8.21). When the level of magnification is increased these defects in the bone matrix can be seen to continue at an ultrastructural level (Fig. 8.22). This damage to bone matrix through which the delicate processes of the osteocytes pass can potentially alter the interaction between cell and matrix and cell-to cell communication. Processes such as generation of streaming potentials by movement of ionic fuid through the macro-, micro- and nanoporosities of bone will be altered. These changes may be the cause of the known response to microdamage such as apoptosis and osteonal remodeling. Experimental studies using the non-invasively loaded rat antebrachium have demonstrated that a rapid application of osteogenic cyclical loading will lead to a change in structural stiffness, indicating a plastic postyield

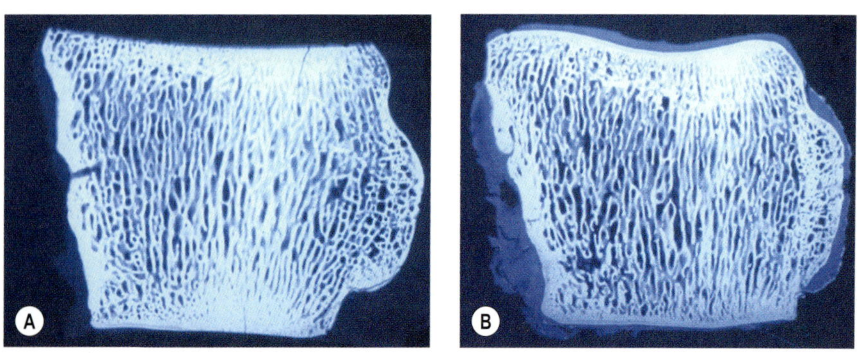

Fig 8.20 Photomicroradiograph to show localized adaptive hypertrophy of trabecular and subchondral bone to imposed exercise **(A)** compared to control **(B)**.

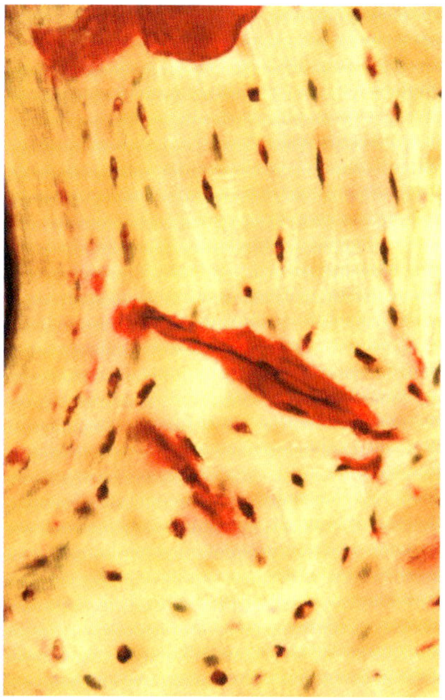

Fig 8.21 Photomicrograph of a section of cortical bone stained to show a microcrack within the matrix.

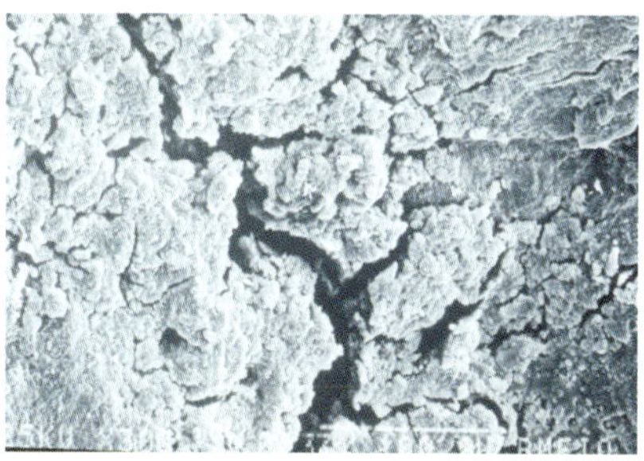

Fig 8.22 Scanning electron micrograph of a microcrack in bone matrix, showing the fractal pattern of damage.

deformation of the bone. The bone will fracture if such loading is continued. However, if bones treated in this way are examined histologically a short time after loading has stopped, an increased porosity is seen as osteoclastic cutting cones target the intracortical damage. A predominance of secondary osteons is found on examination after a longer period of time.

Once primary bone has been remodeled, the bone type has been permanently changed. These changes, seen in the experimental model used by Bentolila et al[94], are closely related to those seen in studies on the induction of sore/bucked shins using a high volume of high strain rate exercise.[94] The effect on subsequent adaptation and failure of highly remodeled bones compared to those in which a gradual adaptation of primary bone has been induced is not really known. Epidemiological studies on race track fractures and relation to training methods are few. One such study by Wood et al[95] has shown that certain types of training regimens are associated with a higher odds risk of fatal failure related to commencement of training at an earlier age. Short bursts of high-speed training in the months before racing reduces the fracture risk.[96] This appears to agree with marker data showing increased bone formation with short periods of fast work.[97] Also Boston and Nunamaker[98] report the advantages of short-distance breezing rather than long-distance gallops in reducing 'bucked shins'.

Osteocyte apoptosis

In addition to the overt fracture of the matrix that occurs with microdamage, there is an effect of this type of loading-induced damage on the cellular component of the bone tissue. Microdamage within bone has been shown to induce osteocyte apoptosis which results in the release of osteoclastogenic factors thus induce bone resorption and 'targeted remodeling'.[99] Interestingly, estrogen treatment also modulates osteocyte apoptosis.[100] Observations by Ehrlich et al that mechanical cues to bone cells are mediated through the estrogen receptor may explain this commonly observed response.[101]

Remodeling

The consequence of exercise-mediated microdamage through a rapid imposition of cyclical mechanical loading is seen either as overt fracture or, more often, as an increase in formation of secondary osteons to limit crack propagation and replace damaged matrix. However, secondary bone has been shown to be inferior in terms of material properties and may compromise mechanical properties of the bone as a structure.

Thus the avoidance of undue secondary osteon formation may prevent the reduction of the mechanical properties of the overall bone structure. Controlled osteogenic exercise during training would induce a more gradual adaptive response and increase the bone mass with minimal damage of the matrix, thus preserving the mechanical properties of the skeletal structure and reducing the risk of catastrophic failure. Training regimens that appear to optimize bone adaptation without matrix damage comprise short periods of high-intensity exercise (see fracture epidemiology section).

In physiologic loading, exercise at a high rate of deformation was found to be a potent osteogenic stimulus.[86, 98] However, strain distributions that differed from those experienced during normal physiologic activities may elicit osteogenic responses at subphysiologic strain magnitudes. It has been suggested that these represent an 'error' signal which, if only imposed occasionally, does not lead to modeling changes; however, a repeated imposition of these unusual strain distributions can induce structural changes in bone architecture. An example is seen in the serving arms of professional tennis players where bone mass can be approximately 30% higher than the non-serving arm.[102] Thus an abnormal gait, particularly if inducing high strain rates, will induce an osteogenic response.

In the horse the level of bone deformation increases as a function of locomotor speed. Thus, as the speed of the walk increases so too does the level of bone deformation. This is also seen in the trot, with an extended trot leading to abnormally high rates of bone strain. In the horse, as speed increases there is normally a change in gait which is controlled by energy efficiency drives; the levels of oxygen increase with speed but there is an optimal speed at each gait for oxygen utilization. At speeds beyond the optimal, the utilization of oxygen becomes less efficient and this leads to a gait transition and further optimal levels of oxygen utilization for the new gait.[103] In addition, at the gait transition the level of bone deformation is reduced.[104] This may represent a means of controlling bone mass and also reducing damage due to fatigue loading of bone.

Safety factors and site-specific fracture incidence

As with most structures, the skeleton can withstand occasional overloads. In designing a structure such as a bridge there is a built-in safety factor to accommodate unforeseen overload. The level of overdesign is related to a balance between risk of overload and cost of materials. The architecture of the skeleton has been shown to follow very similar principles to those seen in engineering of structures. An excess of material would minimize risk of structural failure but carry a high cost in terms of energy requirements.

Gross fractures

As with any structure, a single overload can result in a monotonic failure. Since bone exhibits functional adaptation the mass and architecture are adapted to meet the prevailing magnitude and distribution of load. However, a single excessive load that is greater than the given safety factor will result in failure. The type of failure in terms of damage of the structure at a gross and microscopic level will depend upon the energy and velocity of crack propagation.

When the bones are subjected to load distributions different from those to which the bone has adapted, failure can occur at much lower levels. This type of failure may be seen when limb movements are uncoordinated such as during recovery from anesthesia or at the end of periods of strenuous activity when muscles are fatigued and limbs loaded asymmetrically.[105] The risk of fracture may also be increased if a new type of exercise is introduced suddenly without an appropriate period of training for both muscle and bone adaptation.

Monitoring of skeletal responses to training

The ability to make an objective study on the monitoring of adaptive changes in the skeleton to training requires two components. First, the ability to define and quantify the training input and second, to measure the effect on the bones of the skeleton directly or indirectly. Even in the laboratory these are difficult to achieve; in field studies direct measurements such as radiography, scintigraphy and DXA/CT scanning are not practical. Therefore, indirect assessments of bone modeling and remodeling are being developed. Blood markers have been used both in controlled studies and in commercial training facilities. In studies using controlled exercise regimens it is possible to relate these to changes in marker levels and to evaluate factors such as seasonal, age and gender-related effects. GPRS technology is now readily available to record precise data regarding the distances, gradients and speeds of training of horses.

Markers of bone adaptation

In a controlled exercise study over one year in two year-old Thoroughbreds, the effects of the exercise on two biochemical markers of bone formation were determined. These markers were the carboxy-terminal propeptide of type I collagen (CTX-I) and the bone-specific alkaline phosphatase. In addition, one potential marker of bone resorption, the pyridinoline cross-linked telopeptide domain of type I collagen (ICTP), was also monitored. In both the low and high intensity exercised groups there was a significant reduction in marker levels over the year. This is expected as a normal age-related change. However, it was encouraging that the pattern of reduction differed between groups in a way that indicated an increase in bone turnover in the high intensity trained group.[106] Subsequent work in two and three-year-old Thoroughbreds has shown that serum bone biomarkers (osteocalcin, C-terminal procollagen peptide (PICP), ICTP and CTX-I) did not predict the occurrence of fractures. However this study involved sampling each horse once, and the authors suggest that serial serum sampling may have a better predictive value for fractures.[107]

Serum COMP levels have been shown to be significantly increased in horses with carpal osteochondral fractures however this test is not predictive of injury so is of limited clinical relevance.[108] Further research is required into potential biological markers to predict fractures.

Direct monitoring of skeletal adaptation

There is a need for effective non-invasive methods to monitor both bone quality and skeletal integrity during development and in both athletic training and competition.

Dual energy X-ray absorptiometry (DXA)

Dual energy x-ray absorptiometry is considered the method of choice for evaluating bone mineral density in humans. DXA uses x-rays of two energy levels that that are absorbed by either bone or soft tissue. In humans it is possible to relate individual scan data to population values and provide a fracture risk score. The disadvantage in relation to monitoring of equine skeletal responses to training is the need to anesthetize the horse together with the limited area that can be scanned.

Radiographic techniques

Radiography can be used to visualize some direct responses of the skeleton to increased or decreased mechanical demands. Changes in the architecture and radiographic density of bones can be used to monitor the competence of the skeleton. Standardized positioning and the use of a calibration step wedge allows standardization of exposure by optical digitization, which may then allow a determination of relative bone density in relation to responses to applied training or conditioning regimens. Radiologic methods have been used to assess functional adaptation to exercise in the equine skeleton and a radiographic index has been used to assess the changes in shape of the third metacarpal bone in response to training. Studies have been performed to define the limitations and level of accuracy of this technique that indicated acceptable accuracy providing alignment of the limb, cassette and X-ray machine is accurate. These findings suggest that the radiographic index can be used to measure MC3 bone shape using relatively simple and widely available technology.[109]

Radiography is not a sensitive method of monitoring bone mineral density as a 30–40% alteration is required before it becomes evident on survey radiographs.[110] Computer assisted image analysis software (CAIAS) based on gray-level analysis of digital radiographs of equine bone specimens has recently been investigated. The results of the study showed that mean grey value from digital radiographs correlated highly with bone mineral density and thus may be an alternative to DEXA scanning.[111]

Peripheral quantitative computed tomography (pqCT)

pqCT is used to measure volumetric bone mineral density and bone geometry. A two-dimensional image showing bone mineral density distributions may be generated and quantitative information on cortical cross-sectional area and second moment of area can be provided (see Fig. 8.9). Thus the effects of training could be monitored in relation to specific regimens. The disadvantage of this technique at present is that the machine is fragile and the horse has to be anesthetized. Also the aperture of the machine is limited and thus only small peripheral limb segments can be assessed. For experimental studies and in young horses, this technique can provide considerable useful data on the response of specific distal limb bones to imposed exercise.

Nuclear scintigraphy

Attaching a radioisotope to a bisphosphonate and administering it intravenously results in uptake by osteoclasts and thus areas of active bone modeling or remodeling can be radiolabeled. By imaging with a gamma camera these active sites can be located in the living skeleton at specific points in time. Although used predominantly for diagnostic purposes, this technique can identify site-specific skeletal responses to exercise or mechanical loading and has been used for this purpose in humans.

Magnetic resonance imaging (MRI)

MRI provides a much more comprehensive evaluation of bone remodeling compared to radiography and provides 'physiological' information e.g. it can detect 'bone oedema' and subtle bone mineral densification. Standing MRI can be used to detect changes within the distal metacarpal/metatarsal bones and proximal phalanx that may precede gross fracture (Fig. 8.23). Due to continuous improvements in motion correction software, MRI can be used to evaluate the equine distal limb in the standing sedated horse using a low-field (0.27T) open magnet. Focal necrosis of the palmarodistal third metacarpal bone may represent bone necrosis, accumulation of proteinaceous fluid, cartilage thickening and infolding of sub-chondral bone.[112] The area of necrosis is typically surrounded by a low signal area due to increased bone mineral densification and deceased medullary fat content.[112] Proximal phalanx fractures were originally assumed to result from a single over-load rather than repetitive trauma, however there is now evidence that there could be an element of stress remodeling. Sub-chondral bone trauma in the sagittal groove of the proximal phalanx can also be detected with MRI prior in the absence of a radiographically detectable fracture line. These changes are likely secondary to repetitive trauma, sclerosis and mircofracture.[113] MRI may become the gold standard in the diagnosis of lameness localized to the MCP /MTP joint when radiography is inconclusive.[114]

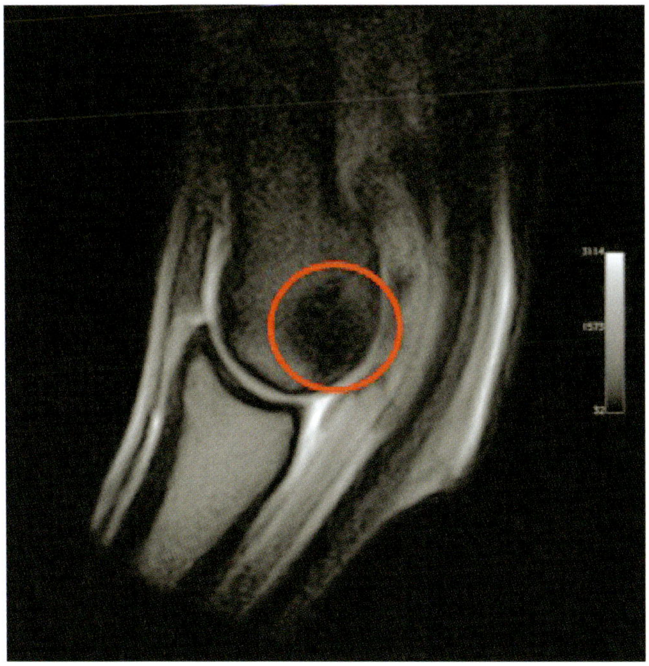

Fig 8.23 Low-field standing T2* GRE sagittal MR image of the metacarpophalangeal joint an elite event horse with densification (sclerosis) of the condyles of the third metacarpus which was also evident on T1 images.

Training strategies to condition the skeleton of the equine athlete

Age-related changes in the skeleton

In a study on fatigue strength, Nunamaker et al measured surface bone strains on the third metacarpal bone of young and old North American Thoroughbred horses to determine the mechanisms involved in fatigue failure of bone leading to fracture.[115] They found greater levels of strain (deformation) at the gallop in the young horses with almost a 40% reduction in strain in the older horses. The significance of this is that the fatigue failure point of a bone depends upon both the magnitude of the deformation and the number of loading cycles to the failure point. Thus if the strain magnitude is reduced there can be a greater number of cycles of deformation prior to failure. In addition, since bone is a dynamic tissue that responds to mechanical deformation, the bone architecture as a structure can be modeled to reduce the bone strain at high loads.

These authors suggest that changes in shape of the third metacarpal bone during growth and maturity may represent a mechanism to reduce strain and mitigate fatigue failure. The high incidence of fatigue failure as seen in 'bucked shins' in young horses subjected to exercise that induces high strains over short periods of time would support this hypothesis. Interestingly, Nunamaker et al also investigated breed differences in the incidence of 'bucked shins', hypothesizing that there might be a breed difference in the material properties of the bone matrix leading to a difference in the fatigue failure patterns.[116] They determined fatigue properties in the bone material of the third metacarpal bone in Thoroughbred and Standardbred horses. No significant differences were found in the mechanical properties of the bone. This may suggest that other factors such as the training methods and type of loading affect the incidence between these two breeds. Perhaps this is indicative that imposed mechanical events, even within a breed of horse, can influence the incidence of such conditions. An understanding of the pathobiology and material properties of bone could be used to determine the appropriate age and exercise regimen to minimize such injuries.

Exercise during development

Exercise in young Thoroughbreds has been shown to result in an increased in radius and tibia strength compared to non-exercised horses. This increase in strength was attributed to an increase in bone size as opposed to higher bone mineral density or cortical thickness.[117] However, most of the training and conditioning of equine athletes occurs after skeletal maturity. In some cases, such as training of racehorses, the period of training is relatively short and the ongoing training is also limited to short periods. The training methods are largely empirical based on a traditional approach rather than advances in the science underlying training.

Recently a number of studies have been investigating the concept of introducing conditioning for athletic performance during the period of postnatal growth and development. This approach imposed the distribution of mechanical loads associated with the athletic activity at a time when modeling processes are active in forming the functionally related aspects of skeletal structure. Thus optimization of primary bone development can be attained in relation to the loading patterns that will be experienced during athletic activity. There is some evidence that bone strain can be reduced with gait transition, decreasing by 42% at the trot/canter transition.[104] Thus in activities where gait changes are suppressed as a component of the particular athletic activity, for example in dressage and in racing trotters and pacers, the high strains at high speeds may predispose to microdamage when introduced in the adult. Whereas if these patterns of gait are introduced gradually during the growth and modeling phase of skeletal development, then appropriate skeletal architecture can be attained with lower risk of damage. This, combined with the incremental increases in training load during development, will also increase skeletal mass and may reduce the strain magnitudes that would occur if training is introduced after skeletal development, and thus minimize injuries.

Changes in foot balance in foals have also been shown to induce strain changes of up to 40% reduction in medial metacarpal compressive strains and 100% increase in lateral compressive strains. However, these were found to return to normal distributions after a period of time.[118] As discussed previously, bone adapts to increased strain and changed strain distribution, so a return to normal strain at a local site may reflect an adaptation resulting from changes in mass and distribution of bone. In this study changes in bone mass or architecture as a consequence of the changed loading were not reported. This adaptation to abnormal loading during growth may result in an abnormal architecture of the bone with possible implications for other skeletal components such as joints in later life. Therefore, attention to exercise type, intensity and foot balance during growth and development should optimize the skeleton for athletic activity in the adult. The concept may also apply to other skeletal tissues in which the process of growth can be modified by early conditioning.

Conclusion

Horses as equine athletes must be conditioned and trained to optimize the whole animal for the particular type of athletic activity. An extremely high proportion of all injuries in the equine athlete in general and in the racehorse in particular are associated with the musculoskeletal system. Within musculoskeletal injuries, fractures and bone-related pathology account for a great proportion. Bone both as a tissue and structure is acutely responsive to mechanical loading and thus can be conditioned to withstand the applied loads. In order to maximize performance and minimize injury it is important to appreciate the pathobiology of functional adaptation of bone. This together with appropriate monitoring can enable owners, trainers and veterinarians to apply the science underlying functional adaptation to the training of specific equine athletes, thus improving equine welfare.

References

1. Denny MW. Limits to running speed in dogs, horses and humans. The Journal of experimental biology 2008;211(Pt 24): 3836–49. Epub 2008/12/02.
2. Hill WG. Why aren't horses faster? Nature 1988;332(6166):678. Epub 1988/04/21.
3. Parkin TD. Epidemiology of racetrack injuries in racehorses. The Veterinary clinics of North America Equine practice 2008;24(1):1–19. Epub 2008/03/04.
4. Oikawa M, Kusunose R. Fractures sustained by racehorses in Japan during flat racing with special reference to track condition and racing time. Vet J 2005;170(3):369–74. Epub 2005/11/04.
5. Parkin TD, Clegg PD, French NP, et al. Race- and course-level risk factors for fatal distal limb fracture in racing Thoroughbreds. Equine veterinary journal 2004;36(6):521–6. Epub 2004/10/06.
6. Anderson TM, McIlwraith CW, Douay P. The role of conformation in musculoskeletal problems in the racing Thoroughbred. Equine veterinary journal 2004;36(7):571–5. Epub 2004/12/08.
7. Ely ER, Avella CS, Price JS, et al. Descriptive epidemiology of fracture, tendon and suspensory ligament injuries in National Hunt racehorses in training. Equine veterinary journal 2009;41(4):372–8. Epub 2009/07/01.
8. Verheyen KL, Price JS, Wood JL. Fracture rate in Thoroughbred racehorses is affected by dam age and parity. Vet J 2007;174(2):295–301. Epub 2006/09/26.
9. Singer ER, Barnes J, Saxby F, et al. Injuries in the event horse: training versus competition. Vet J 2008;175(1): 76–81. Epub 2007/01/06.
10. Currey JD. Ontogenetic changes in compact bone material properties. In: Cowin SC, editor. Bone Biomechanics Handbook. London: CRC Press; 2001.
11. Holmstrom M, Magnusson LE, Philipsson J. Variation in conformation of Swedish warmblood horses and conformational characteristics of elite sport horses. Equine veterinary journal 1990;22(3):186–93. Epub 1990/05/01.
12. Crook TC, Cruickshank SE, McGowan CM, et al. A comparison of the moment arms of pelvic limb muscles in horses bred for acceleration (Quarter Horse) and endurance (Arab). Journal of anatomy 2010;217(1):26–37. Epub 2010/05/25.
13. Briggs H. 'Averageness' key to great racehorses. BBC News Website 2006; Available from: http://news.bbc.co.uk/1/hi/sci/tech/4815378.stm.
14. Allori AC, Sailon AM, Warren SM. Biological basis of bone formation, remodeling, and repair-part II: extracellular matrix. Tissue engineering Part B, Reviews 2008;14(3):275–83. Epub 2009/02/03.
15. Murshed M, Harmey D, Millan JL, et al. Unique coexpression in osteoblasts of broadly expressed genes accounts for the spatial restriction of ECM mineralization to bone. Genes & development 2005;19(9):1093–104. Epub 2005/04/19.
16. Fleisch H, Bisaz S. Mechanism of calcification: inhibitory role of pyrophosphate. Nature 1962;195:911. Epub 1962/09/01.
17. Blumenthal NC, Posner AS, Silverman LD, et al. Effect of proteoglycans on in vitro hydroxyapatite formation. Calcified tissue international 1979;27(1):75–82. Epub 1979/03/13.
18. Gehron Robey P. The biochemistry of bone. Endocrinology and metabolism clinics of North America 1989;18(4):858–902. Epub 1989/12/01.
19. Fraser JD, Price PA. Lung, heart, and kidney express high levels of mRNA for the vitamin K-dependent matrix Gla protein. Implications for the possible functions of matrix Gla protein and for the tissue distribution of the gamma-carboxylase. The Journal of biological chemistry 1988;263(23):11033–6. Epub 1988/08/15.
20. Fisher LW, Termine JD. Noncollagenous proteins influencing the local mechanisms of calcification. Clinical orthopaedics and related research 1985(200):362–85. Epub 1985/11/01.
21. Ingber DE. Cellular mechanotransduction: putting all the pieces together again. FASEB journal: official publication of the Federation of American Societies for Experimental Biology 2006;20(7):811–27. Epub 2006/05/06.
22. Gordon JA, Tye CE, Sampaio AV, et al. Bone sialoprotein expression enhances osteoblast differentiation and matrix mineralization in vitro. Bone 2007;41(3):462–73. Epub 2007/06/19.
23. Tye CE, Rattray KR, Warner KJ, et al. Delineation of the hydroxyapatite-nucleating domains of bone

sialoprotein. The Journal of biological chemistry 2003;278(10):7949–55. Epub 2002/12/21.
24. Sandberg MM, Aro HT, Vuorio EI. Gene expression during bone repair. Clinical orthopaedics and related research 1993(289):292–312. Epub 1993/04/01.
25. Triffitt JT, Owen ME, Ashton BA, et al. Plasma disappearance of rabbit alpha2HS-glycoprotein and its uptake by bone tissue. Calcified tissue research 1978;26(2):155–61. Epub 1978/12/08.
26. Malone JD, Richards M. alpha 2HS glycoprotein is chemotactic for mononuclear phagocytes. Journal of cellular physiology 1987;132(1):118–24. Epub 1987/07/01.
27. Crockett JC, Rogers MJ, Coxon FP, et al. Bone remodelling at a glance. Journal of cell science 2011;124(Pt 7):991–8. Epub 2011/03/16.
28. Vaananen HK, Horton M. The osteoclast clear zone is a specialized cell-extracellular matrix adhesion structure. Journal of cell science 1995;108(Pt 8):2729–32. Epub 1995/08/01.
29. Nesbitt SA, Horton MA. Trafficking of matrix collagens through bone-resorbing osteoclasts. Science 1997; 276(5310):266–9. Epub 1997/04/11.
30. Skerry TM. The role of glutamate in the regulation of bone mass and architecture. Journal of musculoskeletal & neuronal interactions 2008;8(2):166–73. Epub 2008/07/16.
31. Cochran GV, Wu DD, Lee BY, et al. Streaming potentials in gap osteotomy callus and adjacent cortex. A pilot study. Clinical orthopaedics and related research 1997(337):291–301. Epub 1997/04/01.
32. Cowin SC, Weinbaum S, Zeng Y. A case for bone canaliculi as the anatomical site of strain generated potentials. Journal of biomechanics 1995;28(11): 1281–97. Epub 1995/11/01.
33. Donahue HJ. Gap junctions and biophysical regulation of bone cell differentiation. Bone 2000;26(5):417–22. Epub 2000/04/25.
34. Everts V, Delaisse JM, Korper W, et al. The bone lining cell: its role in cleaning Howship's lacunae and initiating bone formation. Journal of bone and mineral research: the official journal of the American Society for Bone and Mineral Research 2002;17(1):77–90. Epub 2002/01/05.
35. Andersen TL, Sondergaard TE, Skorzynska KE, et al. A physical mechanism for coupling bone resorption and formation in adult human bone. The American journal of pathology 2009;174(1):239–47. Epub 2008/12/20.
36. Glass 2nd DA, Bialek P, Ahn JD, et al. Canonical Wnt signaling in differentiated osteoblasts controls osteoclast differentiation. Developmental cell 2005;8(5): 751–64. Epub 2005/05/04.
37. Teitelbaum SL. Bone resorption by osteoclasts. Science 2000;289(5484): 1504–8. Epub 2000/09/01.
38. Chambers TJ. Regulation of the differentiation and function of osteoclasts. The Journal of pathology 2000;192(1):4–13. Epub 2000/08/22.
39. Nakashima T, Hayashi M, Fukunaga T, et al. Evidence for osteocyte regulation of bone homeostasis through RANKL expression. Nature medicine 2011;17(10):1231–4. Epub 2011/09/13.
40. Xiong J, Onal M, Jilka RL, et al. Matrix-embedded cells control osteoclast formation. Nature medicine 2011;17(10):1235–41. Epub 2011/09/13.
41. Sims NA, Walsh NC. Intercellular cross-talk among bone cells: new factors and pathways. Current osteoporosis reports 2012;10(2):109–17. Epub 2012/03/20.
42. Tatsumi S, Ishii K, Amizuka N, et al. Targeted ablation of osteocytes induces osteoporosis with defective mechanotransduction. Cell metabolism 2007;5(6):464–75. Epub 2007/06/07.
43. Wijenayaka AR, Kogawa M, Lim HP, et al. Sclerostin stimulates osteocyte support of osteoclast activity by a RANKL-dependent pathway. PloS one 2011;6(10):e25900. Epub 2011/10/13.
44. Boyde A, Dillon CE, Jones SJ. Measurement of osteoclastic resorption pits with a tandem scanning microscope. Journal of microscopy 1990;158(Pt 2):261–5. Epub 1990/05/01.
45. Saleh H, Eeles D, Hodge JM, et al. Interleukin-33, a target of parathyroid hormone and oncostatin m, increases osteoblastic matrix mineral deposition and inhibits osteoclast formation in vitro. Endocrinology 2011;152(5):1911–22. Epub 2011/03/03.
46. Schulze J, Bickert T, Beil FT, et al. Interleukin-33 is expressed in differentiated osteoblasts and blocks osteoclast formation from bone marrow precursor cells. Journal of bone and mineral research: the official journal of the American Society for Bone and Mineral Research 2011;26(4):704–17. Epub 2010/10/13.
47. Walker EC, McGregor NE, Poulton IJ, et al. Cardiotrophin-1 is an osteoclast-derived stimulus of bone formation required for normal bone remodeling. Journal of bone and mineral research: the official journal of the American Society for Bone and Mineral Research 2008;23(12):2025–32. Epub 2008/07/31.
48. Negishi-Koga T, Shinohara M, Komatsu N, et al. Suppression of bone formation by osteoclastic expression of semaphorin 4D. Nature medicine 2011;17(11):1473–80. Epub 2011/10/25.
49. Dacquin R, Domenget C, Kumanogoh A, et al. Control of bone resorption by semaphorin 4D is dependent on ovarian function. PloS one 2011;6(10):e26627. Epub 2011/11/03.
50. Gooi JH, Pompolo S, Karsdal MA, et al. Calcitonin impairs the anabolic effect of PTH in young rats and stimulates expression of sclerostin by osteocytes. Bone 2010;46(6):1486–97. Epub 2010/03/02.
51. Genetos DC, Yellowley CE, Loots GG. Prostaglandin E2 signals through PTGER2 to regulate sclerostin expression. PloS one 2011;6(3):e17772. Epub 2011/03/26.
52. Walker EC, McGregor NE, Poulton IJ, et al. Oncostatin M promotes bone formation independently of resorption when signaling through leukemia inhibitory factor receptor in mice. The Journal of clinical investigation 2010;120(2):582–92. Epub 2010/01/07.
53. Biewener AA, Thomason J, Goodship A, et al. Bone stress in the horse forelimb during locomotion at different gaits: a comparison of two experimental methods. Journal of biomechanics 1983;16(8):565–76. Epub 1983/01/01.
54. Riggs CM, Vaughan LC, Evans GP, et al. Mechanical implications of collagen fibre orientation in cortical bone of the equine radius. Anatomy and embryology 1993;187(3):239–48. Epub 1993/03/01.
55. Mason MW, Skedros JG, Bloebaum RD. Evidence of strain-mode-related cortical adaptation in the diaphysis of the horse radius. Bone 1995;17(3):229–37. Epub 1995/09/01.
56. Bigot G, Bouzidi A, Rumelhart C, et al. Evolution during growth of the mechanical properties of the cortical bone in equine cannon-bones. Medical engineering & physics 1996;18(1):79–87. Epub 1996/01/01.
57. Diez-Perez A, Guerri R, Nogues X, et al. Microindentation for in vivo measurement of bone tissue mechanical properties in humans. Journal of bone and mineral research: the official journal of the American Society for Bone and Mineral Research 2010;25(8):1877–85. Epub 2010/03/05.
58. Davies HM. Dorsal metacarpal cortex ultrasound speed and bone size and shape. Equine veterinary journal Supplement 2002(34):337–9. Epub 2002/10/31.
59. Fell HB. skeletal development in tissue culture. In: Bourne GW, editor. The biochemistry and physiology of bone. London: Academic Press; 1956.
60. Chalmers J, Ray RD. The growth of transplanted foetal bones in different immunological environments. Journal of Bone and Joint Surgery 1962;44B:149–64.

61. Adams CS, Shapiro IM. The fate of the terminally differentiated chondrocyte: evidence for microenvironmental regulation of chondrocyte apoptosis. Critical reviews in oral biology and medicine: an official publication of the American Association of Oral Biologists 2002;13(6):465–73. Epub 2002/12/25.
62. Byers S, Moore AJ, Byard RW, et al. Quantitative histomorphometric analysis of the human growth plate from birth to adolescence. Bone 2000;27(4):495–501. Epub 2000/10/18.
63. Currey JD. Differences in the blood supply of bone of different histological types. Quarterly Journal of Microscopical Science 1960;101:351.
64. Verborgt O, Gibson GJ, Schaffler MB. Loss of osteocyte integrity in association with microdamage and bone remodeling after fatigue in vivo. Journal of bone and mineral research: the official journal of the American Society for Bone and Mineral Research 2000;15(1):60–7. Epub 2000/01/26.
65. Al-Dujaili SA, Lau E, Al-Dujaili H, et al. Apoptotic osteocytes regulate osteoclast precursor recruitment and differentiation in vitro. Journal of cellular biochemistry 2011;112(9):2412–23. Epub 2011/05/04.
66. Shandala T, Shen Ng Y, Hopwood B, et al. The role of osteocyte apoptosis in cancer chemotherapy-induced bone loss. Journal of cellular physiology 2012;227(7):2889–97. Epub 2011/09/23.
67. Vaughan LC, Mason BJE. A Clinico-pathological Study Of Racing Accidents In Horses. A Report Of A Study On Equine Fatal Accidents On Racecourses. London: Horserace Betting Levy Board; 1976.
68. Dhamrait SS, James L, Brull DJ, et al. Cortical bone resorption during exercise is interleukin-6 genotype-dependent. European journal of applied physiology 2003;89(1):21–5. Epub 2003/03/11.
69. Lanyon LE, Smith RN. Bone strain in the tibia during normal quadrupedal locomotion. Acta orthopaedica Scandinavica 1970;41(3):238–48. Epub 1970/01/01.
70. Van Cochran GB. A method for direct recording of electromechanical data from skeletal bone in living animals. Journal of biomechanics 1974;7(6):563–5. Epub 1974/11/01.
71. Hartman W, Schamhardt HC, Lammertink JL, et al. Bone strain in the equine tibia: an in vivo strain gauge analysis. American journal of veterinary research 1984;45(5):880–4. Epub 1984/05/01.
72. Lanyon LE. Experimental support for the trajectorial theory of bone structure. The Journal of bone and joint surgery British volume 1974;56(1):160–6. Epub 1974/02/01.
73. Mantila Roosa SM, Liu Y, Turner CH. Gene expression patterns in bone following mechanical loading. Journal of bone and mineral research: the official journal of the American Society for Bone and Mineral Research 2011;26(1):100–12. Epub 2010/07/27.
74. Rubin CT, Lanyon LE. Dynamic strain similarity in vertebrates; an alternative to allometric limb bone scaling. Journal of theoretical biology 1984;107(2): 321–7. Epub 1984/03/21.
75. Goodship AE, Lanyon LE, McFie H. Functional adaptation of bone to increased stress. An experimental study. The Journal of bone and joint surgery American volume 1979;61(4):539–46. Epub 1979/06/01.
76. Lanyon LE, Goodship AE, Pye CJ, et al. Mechanically adaptive bone remodelling. Journal of biomechanics 1982;15(3):141–54. Epub 1982/01/01.
77. Rubin CT, Lanyon LE. Regulation of bone formation by applied dynamic loads. The Journal of bone and joint surgery American volume 1984;66(3): 397–402. Epub 1984/03/01.
78. Prendergast PJ, Taylor D. Prediction of bone adaptation using damage accumulation. Journal of biomechanics 1994;27(8):1067–76. Epub 1994/08/01.
79. Lanyon LE, Rubin CT. Static vs dynamic loads as an influence on bone remodelling. Journal of biomechanics 1984;17(12):897–905. Epub 1984/01/01.
80. Hillam RA, Skerry TM. Inhibition of bone resorption and stimulation of formation by mechanical loading of the modeling rat ulna in vivo. Journal of bone and mineral research: the official journal of the American Society for Bone and Mineral Research 1995;10(5):683–9. Epub 1995/05/01.
81. Mason DJ, Hillam RA, Skerry TM. Constitutive in vivo mRNA expression by osteocytes of beta-actin, osteocalcin, connexin-43, IGF-I, c-fos and c-jun, but not TNF-alpha nor tartrate-resistant acid phosphatase. Journal of bone and mineral research: the official journal of the American Society for Bone and Mineral Research 1996;11(3):350–7. Epub 1996/03/01.
82. Forwood MR, Turner CH. Skeletal adaptations to mechanical usage: results from tibial loading studies in rats. Bone 1995;17(4 Suppl):197S–205S. Epub 1995/10/01.
83. Boyde A, Jones SJ, Radcliffe, R, et al. Non-explosive fracture in a cannon bone: A case report. Journal of Scanning Microscopies 1997;19(3):209–11.
84. Radin EL, Burr DB, Caterson B, et al. Mechanical determinants of osteoarthrosis. Seminars in arthritis and rheumatism 1991;21(3 Suppl 2):12–21. Epub 1991/12/01.
85. Firth EC, Delahunt J, Wichtel JW, et al. Galloping exercise induces regional changes in bone density within the third and radial carpal bones of Thoroughbred horses. Equine veterinary journal 1999;31(2):111–15. Epub 1999/04/23.
86. Firth EC, Goodship AE, Delahunt J, et al. Osteoinductive response in the dorsal aspect of the carpus of young thoroughbreds in training occurs within months. Equine veterinary journal Supplement 1999;30:552–4. Epub 2000/02/05.
87. Murray RC, Whitton RC, Vedi S, et al. The effect of training on the calcified zone of equine middle carpal articular cartilage. Equine veterinary journal Supplement 1999;30:274–8. Epub 2000/02/05.
88. Iwamoto J, Yeh JK, Aloia JF. Differential effect of treadmill exercise on three cancellous bone sites in the young growing rat. Bone 1999;24(3):163–9. Epub 1999/03/11.
89. Murray RC, Vedi S, Birch HL, et al. Subchondral bone thickness, hardness and remodelling are influenced by short-term exercise in a site-specific manner. Journal of orthopaedic research: official publication of the Orthopaedic Research Society 2001;19(6):1035–42. Epub 2002/01/10.
90. Bini F, Marinozzi A, Marinozzi F, et al. Microtensile measurements of single trabeculae stiffness in human femur. Journal of biomechanics 2002;35(11):1515–19. Epub 2002/11/05.
91. Reilly GC, Currey JD. The development of microcracking and failure in bone depends on the loading mode to which it is adapted. The Journal of experimental biology 1999;202(Pt 5): 543–52. Epub 1999/02/04.
92. Fleck C, Eifler D. Deformation behaviour and damage accumulation of cortical bone specimens from the equine tibia under cyclic loading. Journal of biomechanics 2003;36(2):179–89. Epub 2003/01/28.
93. Tomlin JL, Lawes TJ, Blunn GW, et al. Fractographic examination of racing greyhound central (navicular) tarsal bone failure surfaces using scanning electron microscopy. Calcified tissue international 2000;67(3):260–6. Epub 2000/08/24.
94. Bentolila V, Boyce TM, Fyhrie DP, et al. Intracortical remodeling in adult rat long bones after fatigue loading. Bone 1998;23(3):275–81. Epub 1998/09/16.
95. Verheyen K, Price J, Lanyon L, et al. Exercise distance and speed affect the risk of fracture in racehorses. Bone 2006;39(6):1322–30. Epub 2006/08/24.
96. Parkin TD, Clegg PD, French NP, et al. Risk factors for fatal lateral condylar fracture of the third metacarpus/

metatarsus in UK racing. Equine veterinary journal 2005;37(3):192–9. Epub 2005/05/17.

97. Jackson BF, Lonnell C, Verheyen KL, et al. Biochemical markers of bone metabolism and risk of dorsal metacarpal disease in 2-year-old Thoroughbreds. Equine veterinary journal 2005;37(1):87–91. Epub 2005/01/18.
98. Boston RC, Nunamaker DM. Gait and speed as exercise components of risk factors associated with onset of fatigue injury of the third metacarpal bone in 2-year-old Thoroughbred racehorses. American journal of veterinary research 2000;61(6):602–8. Epub 2000/06/13.
99. Kennedy OD, Herman BC, Laudier DM, et al. Activation of resorption in fatigue-loaded bone involves both apoptosis and active pro-osteoclastogenic signaling by distinct osteocyte populations. Bone 2012;50(5):1115–22. Epub 2012/02/22.
100. Tomkinson A, Gevers EF, Wit JM, et al. The role of estrogen in the control of rat osteocyte apoptosis. Journal of bone and mineral research: the official journal of the American Society for Bone and Mineral Research 1998;13(8):1243–50. Epub 1998/08/26.
101. Ehrlich PJ, Noble BS, Jessop HL, et al. The effect of in vivo mechanical loading on estrogen receptor alpha expression in rat ulnar osteocytes. Journal of bone and mineral research: the official journal of the American Society for Bone and Mineral Research 2002;17(9):1646–55. Epub 2002/09/05.
102. Jones HH, Priest JD, Hayes WC, et al. Humeral hypertrophy in response to exercise. The Journal of bone and joint surgery American volume 1977;59(2):204–8. Epub 1977/03/01.
103. Hoyt DF, Taylor CR. Gait and the energetics of locomotion in horses. Nature 1981;292:239–40.
104. Rubin CT, Lanyon LE. Limb mechanics as a function of speed and gait: a study of functional strains in the radius and tibia of horse and dog. The Journal of experimental biology 1982;101:187–211. Epub 1982/12/01.
105. Milgrom C, Radeva-Petrova DR, Finestone A, et al. The effect of muscle fatigue on in vivo tibial strains. Journal of biomechanics 2007;40(4):845–50. Epub 2006/05/10.
106. Price JS, Jackson B, Eastell R, et al. The response of the skeleton to physical training: a biochemical study in horses. Bone 1995;17(3):221–7. Epub 1995/09/01.
107. Jackson BF, Dyson PK, Lonnell C, et al. Bone biomarkers and risk of fracture in two- and three-year-old Thoroughbreds. Equine veterinary journal 2009;41(4):410–13. Epub 2009/07/01.
108. Skioldebrand E, Heinegard D, Eloranta ML, et al. Enhanced concentration of COMP (cartilage oligomeric matrix protein) in osteochondral fractures from racing Thoroughbreds. Journal of orthopaedic research: official publication of the Orthopaedic Research Society 2005;23(1):156–63. Epub 2004/12/21.
109. Walter LJ, Davies HM. Analysis of a radiographic technique for measurement of equine metacarpal bone shape. Equine veterinary journal Supplement 2001(33):141–4. Epub 2001/11/28.
110. Butler JA, Colles CM, Dyson, SJ, et al. General principles. Clinical Radiology of the Horse Third ed. Chichester, UK: John Wiley & Sons; 2008.
111. Vaccaro C, Busetto R, Bernardini D, et al. Accuracy and precision of computer-assisted analysis of bone density via conventional and digital radiography in relation to dual-energy x-ray absorptiometry. American journal of veterinary research 2012;73(3):381–4. Epub 2012/03/01.
112. Tranquille CA, Parkin TD, Murray RC. Magnetic resonance imaging-detected adaptation and pathology in the distal condyles of the third metacarpus, associated with lateral condylar fracture in Thoroughbred racehorses. Equine veterinary journal 2012. Epub 2012/01/20.
113. Dyson S, Nagy A, Murray R. Clinical and diagnostic imaging findings in horses with subchondral bone trauma of the sagittal groove of the proximal phalanx. Veterinary radiology & ultrasound: the official journal of the American College of Veterinary Radiology and the International Veterinary Radiology Association 2011;52(6):596–604. Epub 2011/08/13.
114. Powell SE. Low-field standing magnetic resonance imaging findings of the metacarpo/metatarsophalangeal joint of racing Thoroughbreds with lameness localised to the region: a retrospective study of 131 horses. Equine veterinary journal 2012;44(2):169–77. Epub 2011/06/24.
115. Nunamaker DM, Butterweck DM, Provost MT. Fatigue fractures in thoroughbred racehorses: relationships with age, peak bone strain, and training. Journal of orthopaedic research: official publication of the Orthopaedic Research Society 1990;8(4):604–11. Epub 1990/07/01.
116. Nunamaker DM, Butterweck DM, Black J. In vitro comparison of Thoroughbred and Standardbred racehorses with regard to local fatigue failure of the third metacarpal bone. American journal of veterinary research 1991;52(1):97–100. Epub 1991/01/01.
117. Nicholson CL, Firth EC. Assessment of bone response to conditioning exercise in the radius and tibia of young thoroughbred horses using pQCT. Journal of musculoskeletal & neuronal interactions 2010;10(3):199–206. Epub 2010/09/03.
118. Firth EC, Schamhardt HC, Hartman W. Measurements of bone strain in foals with altered foot balance. American journal of veterinary research 1988;49(2):261–5. Epub 1988/02/01.

Tendon and ligament physiology

9

Helen L. Birch   Charlotte Sinclair   Allen E. Goodship   Roger K.W. Smith

CHAPTER CONTENTS

Introduction

Definition and role of tendons and ligaments

Tendons and ligaments are soft connective tissues that form part of the skeletal system. The distinction between tendons and ligaments is an anatomic one; tendons join muscle to bone whereas ligaments join bone to bone. In terms of their biomechanical, ultra-structural and matrix compositional properties however, the two structures are similar and investigations have revealed an overlap of properties resulting in a continuum from 'pure' tendon to 'pure' ligament.[1]

In connecting muscle to bone, tendons have been considered rather inert force-transmitting structures that are involved in the movement of joints. While this positioning function is important, certain tendons in cursorial animals have developed another more specialized role acting as springs to store energy for efficient locomotion.[2] This is particularly true in the horse, where the tendinous structures on the palmar aspect of the metacarpal region, particularly the superficial digital flexor tendon (SDFT) and the musculus interosseous medius tendon (suspensory ligament; SL), act to support the hyper-extended metacarpophalangeal joint during weight bearing (Fig. 9.1), releasing energy when the limb is protracted. Hence, at fast gaits, the horse effectively bounces up and down on springs, similar to a child's pogo stick thereby decreasing the energy required for high speed locomotion.[3] As further modifications to this role, the digital flexor tendons have accessory ligaments (AL), which attach the tendon directly to bone providing a direct bone-to-bone tendinous connection (Fig. 9.2) when under full weight bearing so further reducing the requirement for muscular exertion.

It would be expected that these energy storing tendons have mechanical characteristics suited for this function as a spring, while tendons with a less specialized positional role (e.g. human digital flexor tendons and the common digital extensor tendon (CDET) of the horse) require different characteristics. Indeed up to a two-fold difference in material stiffness has been found between the equine SDFT and CDET indicating differences in molecular composition and organization.[4]

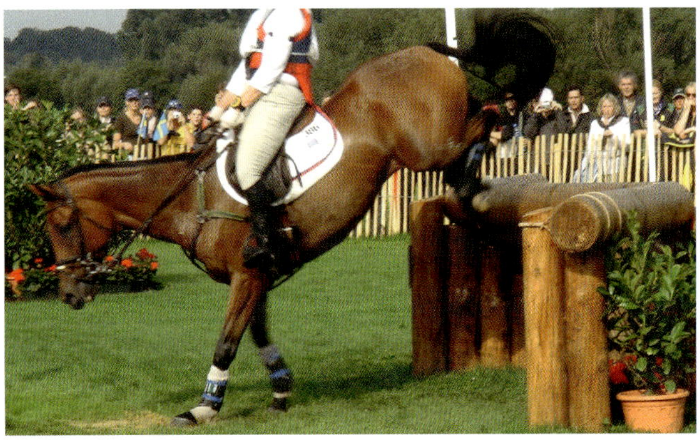

Fig 9.1 Hyperextension of the metacarpophalangeal joint under weight bearing.

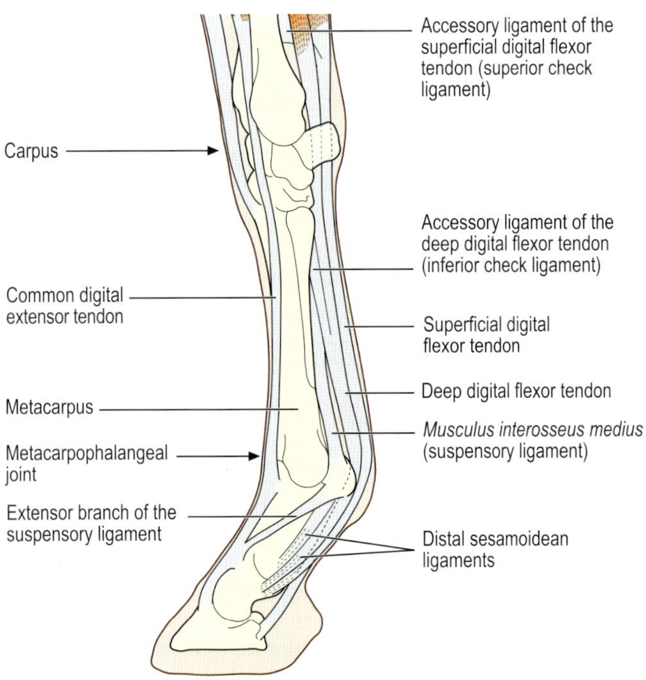

Fig 9.2 Topographical anatomy of the distal limb of the horse.
Adapted from Adam's Lameness in horses, 3rd edn. This material is reproduced with permission of John Wiley & Sons, Inc.

Ligaments also show a degree of specialization. Peri-articular ligaments have a similar composition to tendons and other ligaments (SL, AL), but are anatomically more complex. These ligaments have multiple bundles of fascicles that frequently spiral and are taut and relaxed at different joint positions. In addition to their role in providing support for the joint, they also provide proprioceptive information. The fibrous joint capsule is usually closely associated with these peri-articular ligaments and functions in a similar way. Consequently, fibrous joint capsule could also be considered a ligament.

Incidence of injury

Strain-induced injury of the tendons and ligaments is the most common orthopedic injury in athletic animals, be they equine or human. Increased risk of certain injuries has been associated with both discipline and competition. For example, in elite event horses (intermediate level and above) there is a significantly increased risk of SDFT injuries; in elite show jumpers (grade A and above) there is a significantly increased risk of both SDFT and DDFT injuries; in elite (advanced-medium and above) and non-elite dressage horses there is an increased risk of hindlimb suspensory injury.[5]

Epidemiologic surveys of race horse injuries sustained at UK race tracks between 1996 and 1998 showed that of all limb injuries (82% of all incidents), almost one-half (46%) were due to flexor tendon and/or SL injuries.[6] As observed clinically, this study confirmed that these injuries were much more common in older horses racing over jumps (steeplechasers or hurdlers) than in younger race horses racing on the flat. Furthermore, the data from these flat races correlated well with previous data published from studies in the USA (0.760 per 1000 starts in 1992).[7] However, this epidemiologic data, being obtained from only those injuries occurring during racing, represents only the tip of the iceberg. Evaluation of a cohort of National Hunt racehorses in training revealed a prevalence of SDFT pathology detected using ultrasonography of 24% (n = 148), with a non-significant variation between yards of 10–40%.[8] Older horses had a significantly higher prevalence of SDFT pathology compared to younger horses, and horses with tendinopathy were more likely to suffer an acute injury compared to horses with no evidence of pathology. The rate of tendon and ligament injury in 1223 National Hunt racehorses in training was shown to be 1.9/100 horse months, however this varied significantly between trainers.[9] Of these injuries 89% were SDFT injuries with the remainder being suspensory injuries. Interestingly, the incidence of Achilles tendinopathy in man has doubled in incidence in Europe in the last 10 years, believed to be associated with greater levels of exercise and increased longevity.[10]

SDFT injury has been shown to account for the cause of 14% of racehorse retirements in Hong Kong and was the single most common reason for retirement.[11] It is interesting that ponies rarely suffer from superficial digital flexor tendinopathy, although they do have a relatively high incidence of desmitis of the accessory ligament of the DDFT.

Structure of tendon

Anatomical arrangement of the muscle-tendon-bone unit

The horse has evolved a number of mechanisms to allow for high speed locomotion. The distal part of the limb is elongated and has reduced the number of phalanges to a single digit (with vestigial digits, the splint bones either side of the third metacarpus). The musculature in the limb of the horse is proximally positioned to minimize the weight of the distal limb. This enables the horse to achieve efficient high speed locomotion through increased stride length and reduced energetics of limb protraction. As a consequence, the tendons associated with these muscles have to be long to traverse the joints on which they act; the digital flexor tendons, for example, are some 45 cm in length.

A single digit has resulted in a simplified tendon and ligament anatomy (see Fig. 9.2). The distal fore and hind limb has an arrangement of three structures on the palmar aspect; the SDFT and DDFT with their associated accessory ligaments, and the SL which serve to support the hyperextended metacarpo- or metatarsophalangeal joint. On the dorsal aspect are two or three digital extensor tendons, which function only to extend the distal limb during protraction. Hence the loads experienced by these tendon groups are very different; the extensor tendons experience only low loads while the palmar tissues are subjected to high loads of weight bearing (7–10kN on the SDFT).[12]

The horse has further adapted the basic muscle-tendon-bone unit in order to withstand the high weight-bearing loads and to allow the palmar soft tissue structures to act as an elastic unit for energy storage and efficient locomotion. Thus, the SDF muscle has a large amount of connective tissue within it in addition to the accessory ligament (accessory ligament of the SDFT; proximal, or superior, check ligament) that 'bypasses' the muscle belly to insert on the distal radius. These two adaptations allow the musculotendinous unit to withstand greater loads than would be possible by the muscle itself. The SL has taken this adaptation even further; it was originally derived from a muscle and still contains a variable amount of muscle within its mid and proximal regions. The SL could therefore be classified as a structure in which the tendon component has replaced the muscular tissue. However, its cellular morphology more closely resembles a ligament and, in the absence of a significant muscle belly, is usually classified as a ligament.

Despite large amounts of connective tissue, the muscle belly of the SDFT is not redundant although its proposed role is different from the classical function of flexing the limb. The muscle fibers are short (2–6 mm) and not capable of contributing to limb flexion or 'tuning' the spring-like mechanism.[3] However it has been shown that the SDF muscle belly is capable of dampening high-frequency vibrations in the limb, which are generated when the foot is placed on the ground at high speeds.[3] These high frequency vibrations could cause fatigue damage to the tendon.

As another protective mechanism, the digital flexor tendons are contained within synovial sheaths in regions where they pass over high motion joints (the carpal sheath proximally and the digital sheath distally). While these structures protect the tendons from shear damage, they appear to limit the ability of the tendons to heal. This may be because they are bathed in a synovial environment and also because the thick surrounding layer (paratenon) of extra-synovial tendon is absent within the confines of a tendon sheath. The paratenon is believed to be important in supplying fibroblasts capable of repairing tendon after injury.

Tendon as a structure

Tendon, although an example of a dense regular connective tissue, as a structure can be considered an organ. The seemingly homogeneous appearance on initial gross inspection disguises the fact that tendon is composed of a complex arrangement of tendon cells and extracellular matrix proteins, alongside blood vessels, lymphatic vessels and nerves.

The blood vessels are an important supplier of nutrients for the tendon cells. Intra-tendinous blood supply emanates from the musculo-tendinous junction, the osseous insertion (enthesis) and blood vessels entering the tendon via mesotenon attachments within tendon sheaths or the paratenon. Another potential source of nutrients is the synovial fluid within the tendon sheath. The relevant importance of these components depends on the tendon and tendon site. For the metacarpal region of the SDFT, a study has suggested that the intra-tendinous supply from the myotendinous junction and enthesis is the most important, as necrosis was only achieved by ligation of the intratendinous blood vessels whereas stripping the paratenon had no effect.[13]

The blood flow in the SDFT has been recorded between 1 and 2 mL/min/100g[14, 15] which is of similar magnitude to that within resting skeletal muscle.[16] Blood flow has been shown to increase two-fold with exercise,[15] although this can be delayed in horses that have not been trained. Injury caused an even greater increase in blood flow (>300%), which has been recorded in both limbs of a horse with clinically unilateral tendinitis, suggesting bilateral nature of tendon disease.

Tendon as a connective tissue

Tendon tissue originates from the mesenchyme and is composed of a large amount of extracellular matrix and a relatively sparse population of fibroblast-like cells. The matrix component is mainly composed of the fibrous protein collagen which forms a regular parallel arrangement along the tensional axis of the tendon.

Tendon cells

Tendon cells are known as tenocytes and these reside between the parallel aligned collagen fibers. Tenocytes are unlikely to be a uniform population of cells because they differ considerably in nuclear morphology on light microscopy and when grown in culture. Previous descriptions have described three types based on nuclear morphology[17, 18] although a fourth type is evident within the endotenon tissue (see Fig. 9.3 and Table 9.1), and in other species, the synovial cells lining the outside of the tendon are differentiated from those within the tendon.[19]

Unlike bone, the function of these cell types is not known but their location, morphology and presence in young or adult tendon suggest functions which are activity based and these are reflected in the type classification (Table 9.1). A study on SDFT and CDET tissue sections has shown that immature horses have tenocytes with a rounder nuclei than adult horses and a greater tenocyte density than the adult horses.[18] This study also found that tenocyte density was higher in the SDFT than the CDET.

The tenoctyes are responsible for synthesizing and degrading the matrix components and gene expression studies on equine tendon tissue have shown a pattern of expression that reflects the composition of the tendon tissue.[20] The actual synthetic activity of these different cell types is unknown, however the turnover of the non-collagenous component is much more rapid than the collagen component[21] in equine tendons supporting the theory that plumper cell nuclei, such as those seen in the endotenon, are more active than the thin elongated nuclei located between the collagen fibers.

Work performed on laboratory animals[22] and equine tendons[23] has shown that tenocytes have a large number of cytoplasmic extensions (Fig. 9.4), which connect to neighboring cells via gap junctions. Gap junctions allow the passage of small molecules to move between the cytoplasm of neighboring cells. The transmembrane proteins forming these channels are known as connexins (Cx) of which there are different forms. Connexin 32 (Cx32) and Connexin 43 (Cx 43) in equine tendon have been shown to be location specific, with Cx32 occurring only between cells in the same row and

Table 9.1 Types of cells within tendon and ligament based on nuclear morphology and location.

CELL CLASSIFICATION	TYPE	NUCLEAR MORPHOLOGY	LOCATION
I	'Resting'	Spindle-shaped nuclei lying between collagen fibers	Within the tensional region of all adult tendons
II	'Active'	Cigar-shaped nuclei lying between collagen fibers	Within young tendon and both young and adult ligaments
III	'Chondrocytic'	Round nuclei	In compressed regions of tendons and areas of chondroid metaplasia
IV	'Precursor'	Round nuclei with prominent nucleoli	Endotendon

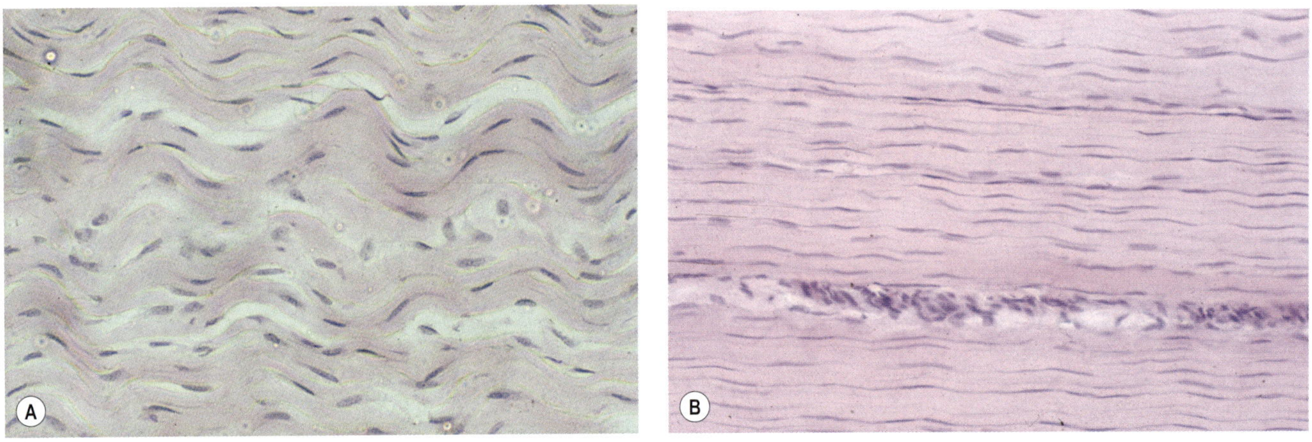

Fig 9.3 H&E histologic sections showing the different morphologies of tenocyte nuclei in young **(A)** and mature **(B)** equine tendon. Note the large numbers of cell nuclei within the endotendon in the mature tendon.

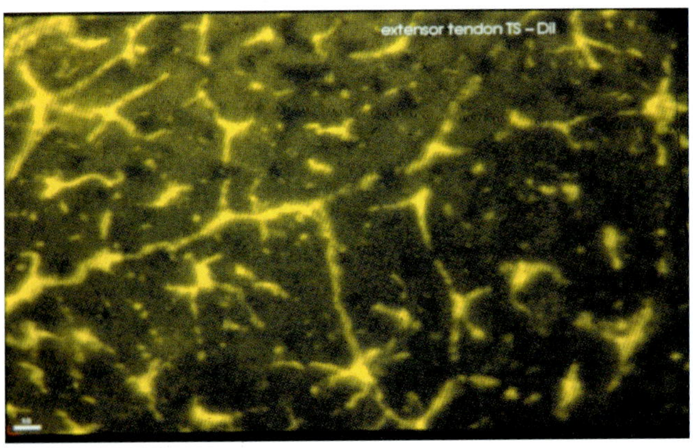

Fig 9.4 Transverse section through equine CDET. Cells are stained with a fluorescent membrane dye (DiI) showing transverse cytoplasmic extensions connecting cells in neighboring rows.

Cx43 occurring between cells in the same row and adjacent rows.[23] This three-dimensional network provides an efficient system for mechanotransduction, similar to that occurring between osteocytes in bone.

Following the surge of interest in stem cell therapy, tendon has been shown to possess an innate population of progenitor cells.[24] These progenitor cells have stem cell characteristics of clonogenicity, multipotency and self-renewal capacity and reside in a unique niche organized by the proteoglycans biglycan and fibromodulin. More recently tendon progenitor cells have been isolated from human[25] and equine[26] tendons.

Tendon matrix

As the cellular component of tendon is small, the functional properties of tendon rely on the extracellular matrix. This is determined, in turn, by both the composition and, equally importantly, the arrangement of these proteins within the matrix. It is constructed from a series of increasingly sized subunits into a hierarchic arrangement (Fig. 9.5).

Molecular composition

Water content

Tendon is predominantly composed of water, which makes-up approximately two-thirds of the weight of the tissue. The presence of this water is fundamental to maintaining the elasticity of the tissue because dehydration results in an increase in stiffness and tendons containing less water tend to be stiffer.[27] Tendon has been shown to exhibit strain-induced flow of ionized fluids (streaming potentials) when subjected to mechanical stress.[28] These fluid movements could provide a mechanism for mechanotransduction, whereby mechanical forces on the tendon influence the metabolic activity of the tenocytes. Furthermore, it has recently been shown that the change in electrical resistance is proportional to tendon strain leading to the suggestion that tendon electric properties could be used as an in vivo strain sensor.[29]

Collagen component

The remaining third of the content of tendon (the dry weight) is predominantly composed of type I collagen. This protein is a major component of all connective tissues. Each type I collagen molecule is assembled within the golgi apparatus of the cell from two α1(I) polypeptide chains and one α2(I) polypeptide chain, forming a right-handed triple super-helix. The initial product is a procollagen molecule with non-helical N and C terminal extensions (propeptides). These individual collagen molecules are assembled by cleavage of their propeptides at the N and C terminal ends by specific N- and C- proteinases, either after secretion into the immediate pericellular environment[30] or intracellularly.[31] This results in a tropocollagen molecule that is 285 nm long and 1.4 nm wide. These molecules are then assembled into collagen fibrils in a highly organized fashion, each collagen molecule staggered relative to its neighbor by a quarter length. This results in a gap and overlap region (D-period) that is responsible for giving the banded pattern seen in electron microscopy. Five collagen molecules make up a subunit of the collagen fibril (Fig. 9.6). Although collagen molecules will spontaneously self-assemble, other proteins play a role in orchestrating this assembly (see below).

Collagen molecules are stabilized within the fibril by the formation of covalent cross-links between lysine and hydroxylysine residues mediated by the enzyme lysyl oxidase.[32] Lysyl oxidase converts lysine and hydroxylysine residues in the telopeptide region into aldehydes. Lysine aldehydes and hydroxylysine aldehydes undergo

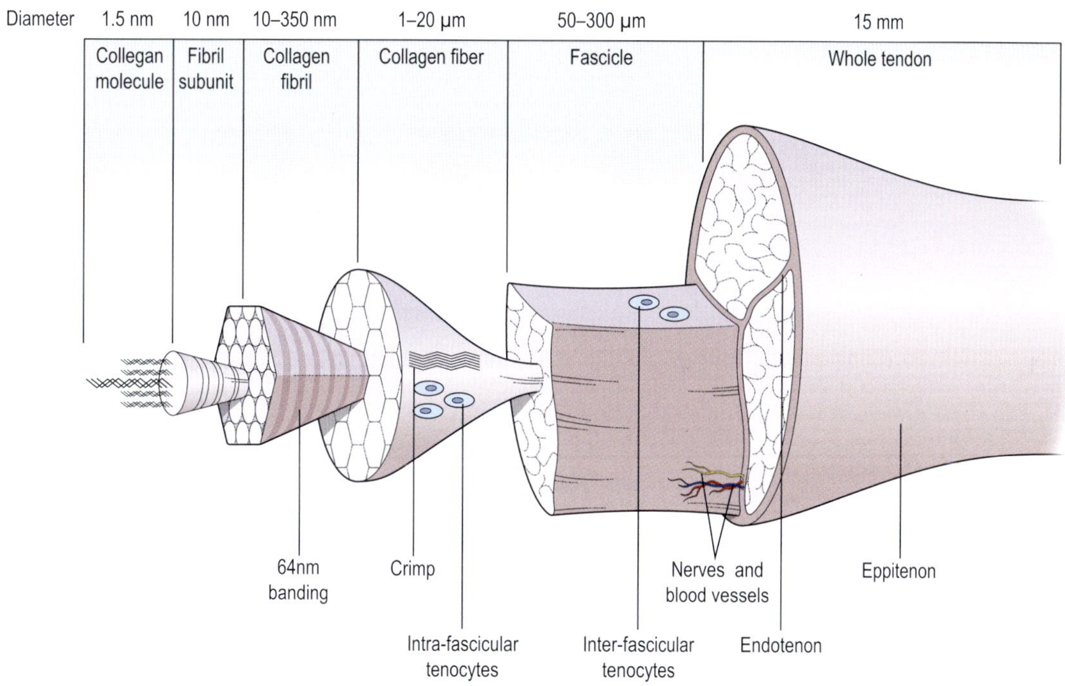

Fig 9.5 Hierarchic arrangement of collagen in tendon.
Reproduced from Thorpe et al. 2010.[119]

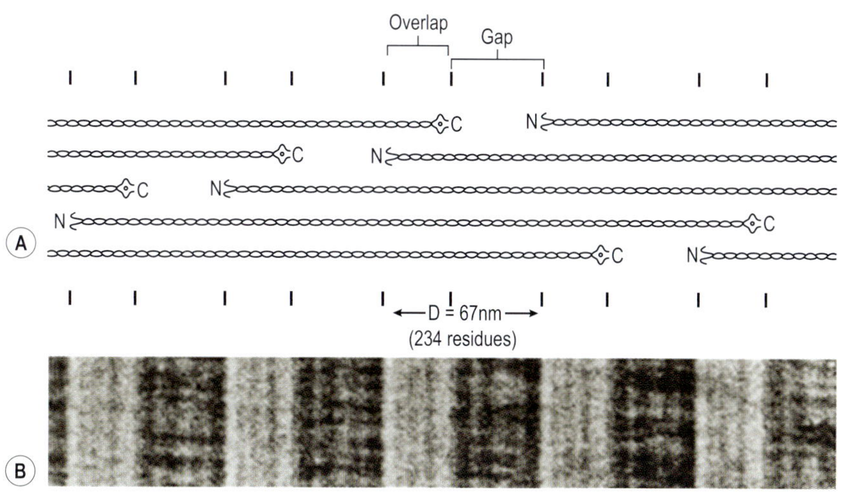

Fig 9.6 Axial structure of D-periodic collagen fibrils. **(A)** Schematic representation of the axial packing arrangement of triple-helical collagen molecules in a fibril. **(B)** Collagen fibril negatively stained showing repeating dark and light zones, produced by preferential stain penetration into regions of lowest packing (the gap regions).
Reproduced with permission from Kadler, KE, Holmes, DF, Trotter, JA, Chapman, JA, 1996, Collagen fibril formation, Biochem J, 316 (pt1), 1–11. © the Biochemical Society.[120]

a spontaneous reaction with lysine or hydroxylysine residues in the helical region of neighbouring molecules to form the immature bivalent cross-links. These immature cross-links undergo further spontaneous reactions to form mature trivalent pyridinoline and pyrrole cross-links. The type of crosslink formed depends on the degree of lysine hydroxylation in the helical part of the molecule and non-helical telopeptide region. Extensive hydroxylation of lysine residues throughout the collagen molecule results in the formation of hydroxylysyl-pyridinoline (HL-Pyr). In the equine SDFT, HL-Pyr is the predominant lysyl oxidase mediated mature crosslink.[33] In tissues where less hydroxylation of the helical or telopeptide lysine residues occurs, the mature cross-links lysyl-pyridinoline (L-Pyr) and pyrrole form, respectively.

A variety of minor collagens, including the fibril forming collagens, type III, type V and type XI; the fibril associated collagens with interrupted triple helices, type XII and type XIV and the beaded filament collagen type VI are present in small amounts in tendon.

Non-collagenous components

While 80% of the dry weight of tendon is composed of collagen, the remaining 20% (5–6% of the wet weight of the tendon) is comprised of a wide variety of non-collagenous proteins including proteoglycans and glycoproteins. Although these are only a small component of the tissue, they are vital for the organization and function of the tissue.

Proteoglycans consist of a central protein core with O-linked glycosaminoglycan side-chains. The extracellular matrix proteoglycans can be divided into two classes; the large proteoglycans (such as aggrecan, the large proteoglycan of cartilage, and the soft tissue equivalent, versican) and the small leucine-rich proteoglycans (such as decorin, biglycan, fibromodulin, lumican and keratocan) all of which are present in tendon.[34] The large proteoglycans have numerous highly sulfated glycosaminoglycan side-chains, which hold water and therefore are present where the tendon has to resist compression. Aggrecan is also present in the tensional region of tendon however there appear to be differences in the GAG side chains suggesting a different physiological function of aggrecan in this region.[34] The small proteoglycans are closely associated with the collagen fibrils and are believed to regulate collagen fibril diameters. Knock-out of the decorin gene in mice resulted in large, irregular sized collagen fibrils believed to be caused by un-regulated lateral fusion and this was associated with weak and fragile skin.[35] A more recent study has shown that reduced decorin increases the material stiffness of patellar tendon in mice but does not change fibril diameters suggesting that decorin influences mechanical properties in a way that cannot be explained completely by collagen fibrillogenesis.[36] Fibromodulin knock-out mice showed paradoxically smaller collagen fibrils but also a compensatory increase in another small proteoglycan, lumican, which binds to the collagen molecule at the same site to fibromodulin[37], demonstrating that many of these small proteoglycans can 'cross-function'.

During growth of the digital flexor tendons, one of the most abundant proteins is the glycoprotein cartilage oligomeric matrix protein (COMP). There are only low levels of this protein in tendon at birth but it accumulates during growth within the digital flexor tendons with the highest levels achieved in the tensional region of the SDFT at skeletal maturity in the horse (at approximately two years of age) of approximately 10 mg/g wet weight.[38] This equates to approximately 30 mg/g dry weight or approximately 1% of the wet weight. After the period of growth, however, levels of COMP in the tensional, but not the compressed, region of the SDFT fall.

COMP binds to fibrillar collagens (including type I) via a zinc-dependent mechanism.[39] Each COMP molecule can bind to five collagen molecules possibly for assembly into a collagen fibril, once the fibril is formed COMP is displaced. Recent studies have shown that COMP can accelerate collagen fibrillogenesis in vitro and it is possible that this protein acts more as an organizational molecule rather than in a structural role.[40] Correspondingly, the highest levels are present during the growth of the tendon when matrix is being synthesized and levels fall after skeletal maturity when there is little change in the structural properties of the tendon. It has been suggested that the more COMP synthesized during growth, the stronger the resulting tendon and this is supported by the finding that mechanical properties of SDFT at skeletal maturity demonstrate a significant positive relationship to COMP levels.[41]

Other proteins

Small amounts of the protein elastin and other components of elastic fibres can be found in varying amounts in tendon and ligament and these appear to be localized to between the collagen fascicles.[42, 43] The glycoprotein lubricin has also been found in tendon in an inter-fascicular location where it facilitates sliding between fascicles[44, 45] and on the surface of tendon in both intra- and extra-synovial locations.[46] Other proteins expressed by tendon cells include thrombospondin 4, tenascin-C, and tenomodulin which have been used to identify a tendon cell phenotype.[47]

Morphology

Collagen fibrils are assembled in a longitudinally oriented pattern into increasingly larger subunits, which ultimately form the whole tendon (Fig. 9.5). The precise arrangement of at each sub level of the hierarchal arrangement has an influence on the mechanical properties of the final tendon structure and is therefore vital for tendon function.

Ultra-structural morphology

The quarter staggered arrangement of collagen molecules during fibrillogenesis results in micro-fibril structures which group together to form fibrils. The collagen fibrils in tendon follow an essentially straight path, as opposed to the right-handed helical course taken by fibrils in tissues such as skin.[48] However scanning electron microscopy studies have shown that collagen fibrils in tendon show 'knots' or fibrillar crimps. These 'knots' are formed as the fibrils first twist leftwards, changing their plane of running, and then bent sharply also changing the direction of coursing.[49] The fibrillar crimp functions as a biological hinge opening when tensional load is applied and recoiling when load is removed.[49] Transverse sections viewed under an electron microscope show the collagen fibrils as electron dense circular structures of varying sizes. The distribution of collagen fibril diameters can be determined from these sections, as well as assessment of the mass average diameter, which takes into account the relative proportion of the area taken up by different-sized fibrils. The adult SDFT has a bimodal distribution of fibrils with large numbers of small fibrils and lower numbers of large-diameter fibrils[50] (Fig. 9.7). Furthermore, there are differences between tendons, with the DDFT having fewer small-diameter and greater numbers of large-diameter fibrils.[51] The size of the collagen fibrils shows a significant correlation with the stiffness of the tendon tissue; larger fibrils resulting in a stiffer tissue.[27]

Micro- and macro-structural morphology

Collagen fibrils group together to form fibers which have a diameter of approximately 10 µm. The fibrillar crimps align resulting in the

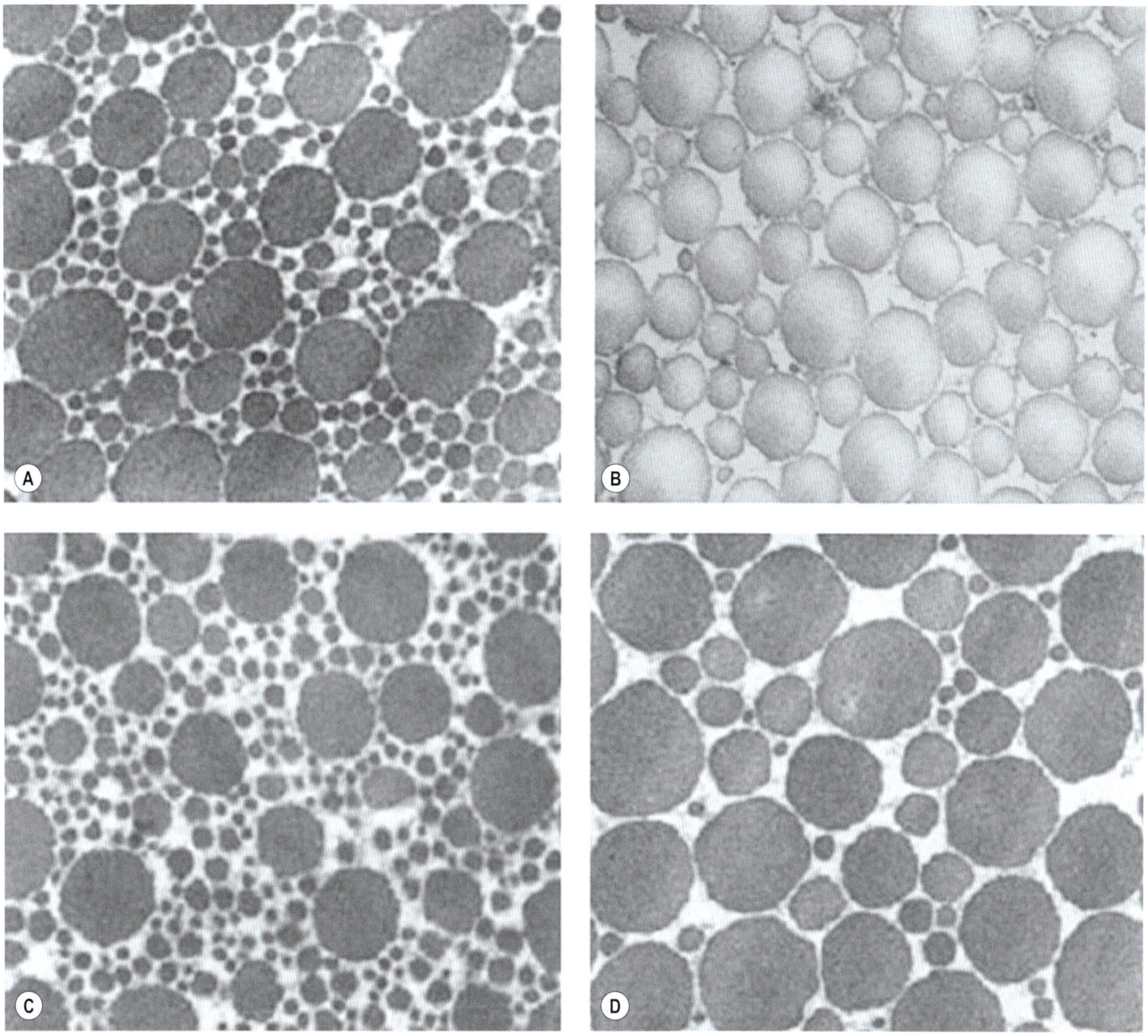

Fig 9.7 Collagen fibril morphology in **(A)** the superficial digital flexor tendon, **(B)** the deep digital flexor tendon, **(C)** the suspensory ligament, and **(D)** the common digital extensor tendon. Note the similarities of the primary supporters of the metacarpophalangeal joint (superficial digital flexor tendon), and the positional tendon (common digital extensor tendon) with the deep digital flexor tendon.

waveform seen in longitudinal tendon histologic sections at the fiber level (Fig. 9.3). When viewed under polarized light, crimp results in alternating light and dark bands. Crimp can be described by its angle and length and these change as the animal ages (see below). Collagen fibres group together to form sub-fascicles and sub-fascicles assemble to form fascicles which finally come together to form the whole tendon (Fig. 9.8). The tendon is surrounded by a thin connective tissue membrane known as the epitenon, which continues into the tendon surrounding the fascicles where it is known as the endotenon.

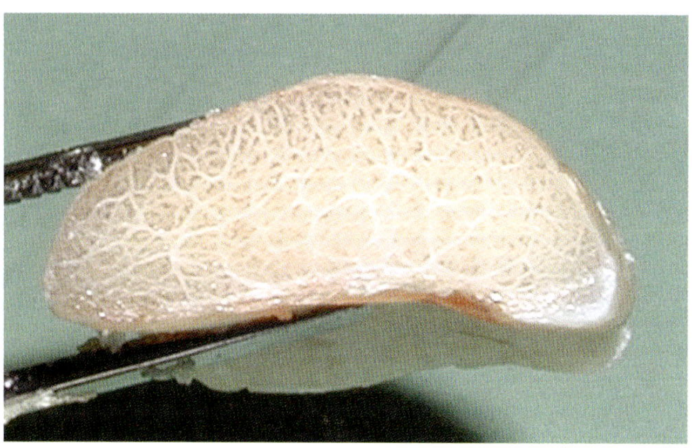

Fig 9.8 The cut surface of the superficial digital flexor tendon (SDFT), showing the fascicular arrangement.

Functional characteristics of tendon

Tendon and ligaments transmit forces to move the equine skeleton, or for support of the distal limb in the case of the digital flexor tendons, or, as ligaments, to maintain joint integrity. At heel strike, the loads rise the quickest in the soft tissue structures primarily supporting the metacarpo-phalangeal joint; the SDFT and the SL. High-frequency transients are also a feature of the early phase of weight bearing in these tendons. The load in the deep digital flexor tendon is slower to rise, which may help to explain why the SDFT and SL are the most prone to injury.

Load/deformation characteristics

The biomechanical properties of a tendon can be defined in vitro by its structural (as an organ) or material (as a tissue) properties. To establish these data, tendons can be recovered from cadavers and pulled to failure in a material testing machine. Anchoring of the tendon ends is problematical as final rupture often occurs at the tendon-clamp interface, which can result in artificially low values. Furthermore, data varies depending on a number of factors including rate of loading. Thus, comparisons between data sets performed in different ways should be made with caution.

In vitro loading experiments generate a load-deformation curve from which the structural properties of ultimate tensile strength (kN) and stiffness (N/mm) can be derived (see Fig. 9.9). There are four regions to the curve:

1. The 'toe' region, where there is non-linear stretch to the tendon. This has been associated with the elimination of the crimp pattern of the collagen fibers. More recent work suggests that fascicle sliding also contributes significantly to initial elongation at low loads.[52]
2. Linear deformation is the area of the curve from which the stiffness is determined (load divided by deformation for the linear portion of the curve). The mechanism for this elongation is thought to arise from elongation of the collagen fibrils, fibrillar crimp straightening and/or sliding of fibrils and fibers relative to one another. Fiber sliding appears to provide the major mechanism enabling tendon fascicle extension within rat-tail tendon[53] and equine SDFT.[54]
3. The yield region represents irreversible lengthening of the tendon, arising from slippage of collagen fibrils, fibers or fascicles.
4. Rupture, where the stress-strain curve falls quickly to zero as the collagen structures sequentially rupture.

Knowing the cross-sectional area of the tendon and its length, the stress (force per unit area) can be plotted against strain (change in length over original length), from which the material properties of ultimate tensile stress (N/mm2) and Young's modulus of elasticity (E; MPa) can be calculated. As both the cross-sectional area and original length are assumed to be constant, the stress-strain curve has a similar shape to the load-deformation.

Ultimate tensile strength and stress

The ultimate tensile strength for the equine SDFT (rupturing at the mid-metacarpal region) in the horse is approximately 12 kN or 1.2 tonnes.[52] The approximate ultimate tensile stress is 100MPa for the equine SDFT[52], which agrees well with previously documented figures for other species (45–125MPa).[55, 56]

Ultimate tensile strain

Equine SDFT strains of 16.6% have been recorded in vivo at gallop[57] while values of around 25% have been reported before the tendon ruptures in vitro.[27, 52] However, the ultimate tensile strain reflects only the final strain before rupture and includes that yield portion of the stress-strain curve that represents irreversible damage to the tendon tissue. In addition, the ultimate tensile strain may not be constant along the length of the SDFT in vitro[58] Work has demonstrated that the normal strains in the digital flexor tendons in vivo (in ponies) are in the region of 2–4% at the walk and 4–6% at the trot.[59] Riemersma and colleagues[59] also noted that different results were obtained in vivo to in vitro, thereby indicating caution in the interpretation of in vitro measurements.

Hysteresis

Tendon is a viscoelastic tissue and as such, its response to mechanical loading is time and history dependent. The property known as hysteresis is demonstrated by the difference in the stress-strain relationship when the tendon is loaded compared to when it is unloaded (Fig. 9.10). The area between these two curves represents the energy lost during the loading cycle. This is usually about 5% in equine tendons. Much of this energy is lost as heat and is responsible for the rise in temperature within the tendon core associated

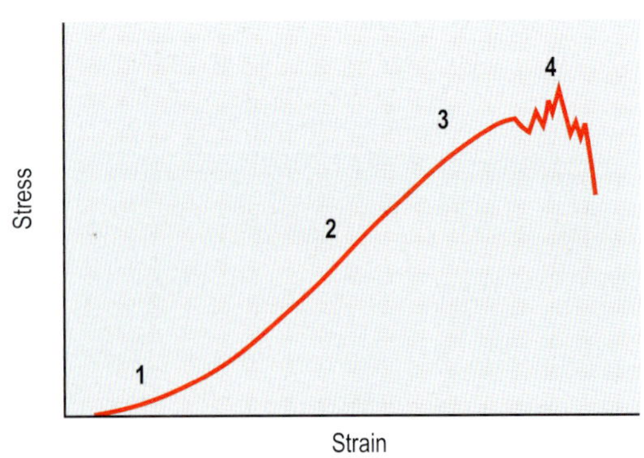

Fig 9.9 Stress-strain curve for tendon. Zone 1 refers to the toe region, thought to be associated with the elimination of crimp; zone 2 to the linear phase from which the elastic modulus is calculated; zone 3 to the yield point after which irreversible damage occurs; and zone 4 to where individual tendon fibers rupture leading to complete failure. *Courtesy of Goodship, AE, Birch, HL, Wilson, AM, 1994, The pathobiology and repair of tendon and ligament injury, 10: 323–349, The Veterinary Clinics of North America: Equine Practice, with permission from Elsevier.*

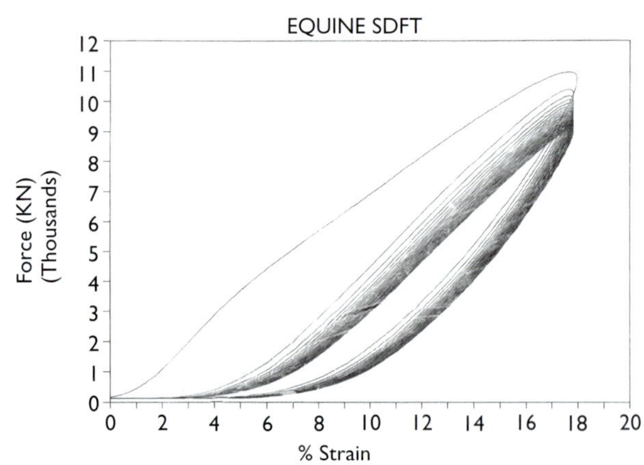

Fig 9.10 The effect of repeated loading and unloading of tendon. The loading and unloading curves are different resulting in a loss of energy (hysteresis). Repeated loading shifts the curve to the right (conditioning).

with repeated loading (as in an exercising horse).[60] These temperatures can rise to as high as 46 °C, which is potentially damaging to either tendon matrix or tenocytes. However, tenocytes recovered from the center of equine SDFT remain viable when subjected to rises in temperature of this magnitude, whereas fibroblasts from other locations do not.[61] This property is also present in fetal tenocytes, which suggests that the tendon has an inherent genetic adaptation to this physical process.

Conditioning

The viscoelastic properties of tendon are demonstrated by movement of the stress-strain curve to the left or right (Fig. 9.10). Repeated loading results in shifting of the curve to the right (i.e. the tendon becomes less stiff), a process known as conditioning. This change is recoverable but significant resting time is necessary. This property, however, has been demonstrated in vitro and may not reflect the normal behavior in vivo.

Contribution of tendon mechanics to the energetics of locomotion

Tendon loading under weight-bearing is essentially a passive process and energy is stored in the extension of the tendon. The energy stored in the tendon is represented by the area under the stress-strain curve. To allow this energy to be returned in a usable form, the rate of unloading needs to be tuned to stride frequency; as a result the SDFT is subjected to relatively high strains. The failure strain of the SDFT in vitro is 25% while in vivo strain levels of up to 16% at the gallop have been recorded (see above). This demonstrate that the high efficiency comes at a cost; there is little tolerance in the system and the tendon is prone to overstrain injury. Consequently, any small deterioration in the mechanical properties would have a significant effect on the risk of tendon injury.

The tendon returns energy with an efficiency of approximately 93%[62], which provides considerable energy-saving for the horse. Predicted efficiencies of locomotion in the horse at different gaits calculated from the energy expenditure required for limb and trunk movement and the movement of the horse, and the energy production by the muscles (which have an efficiency of approximately 30%) shows an efficiency of greater than 100% at the gallop. This discrepancy is due to the energy-storage capacities of the locomotor soft tissues, in particular the SDFT and SL. Thus, these structures are critical to the optimum efficiency of equine locomotion.

Tendon-specific differences in structure, composition and mechanical properties

Tendons with different functional requirements differ in their mechanical properties as a result of differences in composition and organization of the extracellular matrix components.[27] In addition, tendons differ along their length; for example where compressive forces are applied to the tendons as they change direction around the palmar aspect of the metacarpophalangeal joint, there is an accumulation of those matrix proteins most suited to resisting that compression. Thus, the tendon has a fibrocartilage-like composition in this region.[63, 64]

The properties of the tendon as a structure are governed by tendon size and the properties of the tendon tissue (material properties). The energy storing SDFT has a significantly lower elastic modulus and ultimate tensile stress than the positional CDET, while the strain at peak stress is greater in the SDFT than in the CDET.[52] Interestingly these differences in elastic modulus and failure stress are not apparent at the fascicle level and fascicles from the SDFT fail at a lower strain than those from the CDET.[52] This suggests that the ability of the SDFT to deform relatively large amounts stems from the interfascicular matrix.

Clear differences can be seen in the molecular composition between the energy storing SDFT and positional CDET. The SDFT has a higher water content, higher glycosaminoglycan content and higher cellularity than the CDET. The collagen crosslink profiles are distinct; the predominant mature crosslink detected in the SDFT was hydroxylysylpyridinoline (HP) however levels of HP were low in the CDET; the main crosslink found here being histidinohydroxymesodesmosine (HHMD).[27] A dramatic difference is also seen in the COMP content. Both tendons have similarly low levels at birth but there is a dramatic rise in COMP levels in the SDFT to ten times the levels at birth, while levels in the CDET do not alter.[65]

Despite a higher cellularity, recent work[21] suggests that the SDFT has a lower collagen turnover rate than the CDET. A collagen half-life of 200 years for the SDFT was significantly higher than that for the CDET (34 years). However the half-life of non-collagenous protein was 2 years in the SDFT and was significantly lower than the value of 3.5 years measured for the CDET, in agreement with a more influential role of the interfascicular matrix in the energy storing tendon.

Age and exercise effects on tendon pathophysiology

With preceding tendon degeneration proposed as an important factor in the initiation of equine SDFT tendinopathy, investigations have concentrated on changes occurring within the tendon matrix associated with aging and exercise. The importance of these factors on tendon physiology has been supported by epidemiologic studies in both horses (SDFT tendinopathy)[7, 8] and man (Achilles tendinopathy).[10]

A combination of in vivo and post-mortem studies on 'normal' horses, both domesticated (trained) and feral (untrained), and analyzes of tendons from a number of experimental exercise studies has shone new light onto the influence of both exercise and aging on equine tendon. These studies have investigated mechanical, morphological (ultrasonographic and histologic), ultrastructural, compositional, and metabolic changes in association with aging and exercise in equine tendon. The effects of these two factors have been found to be different between immature (growing) and mature (adult) tendon. The age at which equine digital flexor tendon matures is estimated at approximately two years of age based on these studies.

Mature (adult) tendon

Mechanical changes

There is a large variation in mechanical properties between individuals; more than two-fold for ultimate tensile strength[17] so that alterations in both structural and material properties are difficult to determine. In vitro testing from a large number of horses has not demonstrated a decrease in ultimate tensile stress with age.[66] Previous studies in humans have failed to show a clear reduction in tendon material properties with increasing age.[67–69] The effect of exercise on the mechanical properties of tendon and ligament are variable, although much of this variation may be due to different ages and species used. Recent work however has shown a stiffening of the fascicular interface with ageing in the equine SDFT (Thorpe, personal communication).

Morphological changes

The crimp pattern of equine SDFT was found to reduce in both angle and length with age.[70,71] Furthermore, the imposition of exercise resulted in an accelerated loss of this crimp in a heterogeneous manner; the central region of the tendon was disproportionately affected.[72] This may help to explain the occurrence of central 'core' lesions seen clinically as the central fascicles, having less crimp, straighten first and are therefore loaded preferentially, becoming the first ones to rupture.[70]

Other studies have assessed the change in fascicle pattern with aging and training. One study found a significant reduction in the number of fascicles in the SDFT with a thickening of the interfascicular (endotenon) tissue with aging[73] while more recent work suggests tighter packing of the fascicles with ageing (Thorpe, personal communication).

The effect of exercise on the cross-sectional area of tendon has shown inconsistent results. Ultrasonographic and gross cross-sectional measurements during experimental treadmill exercise in young adult horses failed to show any significant change with exercise over and above that caused by growth in digital flexor tendons.[74] In contrast, the common digital extensor tendon did show a significant increase with exercise[74], confirming similar findings in exercise studies on mini-pigs.[75] Another study, following cross-sectional area changes with the onset of training showed a significant increase.[76] However, two of the seven horses followed developed evidence of clinical tendon injury and so it is difficult to relate such increases in cross-sectional area to either adaptation or injury.

Ultrastructural changes

Collagen fibril diameters, calculated using transmission electron microscopy, in the adult SDFT in horses show a biphasic distribution, with a large number of small (40 nm) fibrils and a low number, but broader range, of large fibrils, while very old tendons have a more unimodal distribution characteristic of fetal and newborn tendon.[50] The bimodal distribution was unaffected by a short-term (4.5 months) experimental treadmill exercise program in two-year-old horses,[77] but there was a shift to smaller diameter collagen fibrils in the longer term study (18 months) where the horses were over three years of age[78] (Fig. 9.11). This effect was believed to be due to the disruption of large fibrils rather than the formation of new ones as the collagen content and 'age' (as determined by non-enzymatic glycation) were unaltered.[79]

Compositional changes

Collagen content varies little with age and exercise but the non-collagenous component of tendon is much more labile. Analysis of tendons from a wide range of ages, together with those from experimental exercise studies has shown a decrease in glycosaminoglycan (GAG) levels with exercise,[79] and a decrease with age in the CDET.[21] This is in contrast to the central discolored regions seen as an occasional coincidental finding at post-mortem, which contain increased GAG levels[80] suggestive of scar tissue formation. GAGs are part of proteoglycan molecules but vary in amount between different proteoglycan species. Thus, the small proteoglycans of tensile tendon contain only one or two side-chains of GAGs while the large proteoglycans, more characteristic of areas of tendon under compression (e.g. where the digital flexor tendons change direction at the level of the metacarpophalangeal joints contain large numbers of GAG side-chains. Thus, changes in GAG levels within tendon probably reflect more changes in the large, rather than small, proteoglycan species.

Another non-collagenous protein, COMP, which is abundant within the digital flexor tendons of horses, shows marked changes with age and exercise. Levels are low at birth but rapidly increase with tendon growth during the first two years of life. Once maturity is reached, which is at approximately two years in tendon, levels

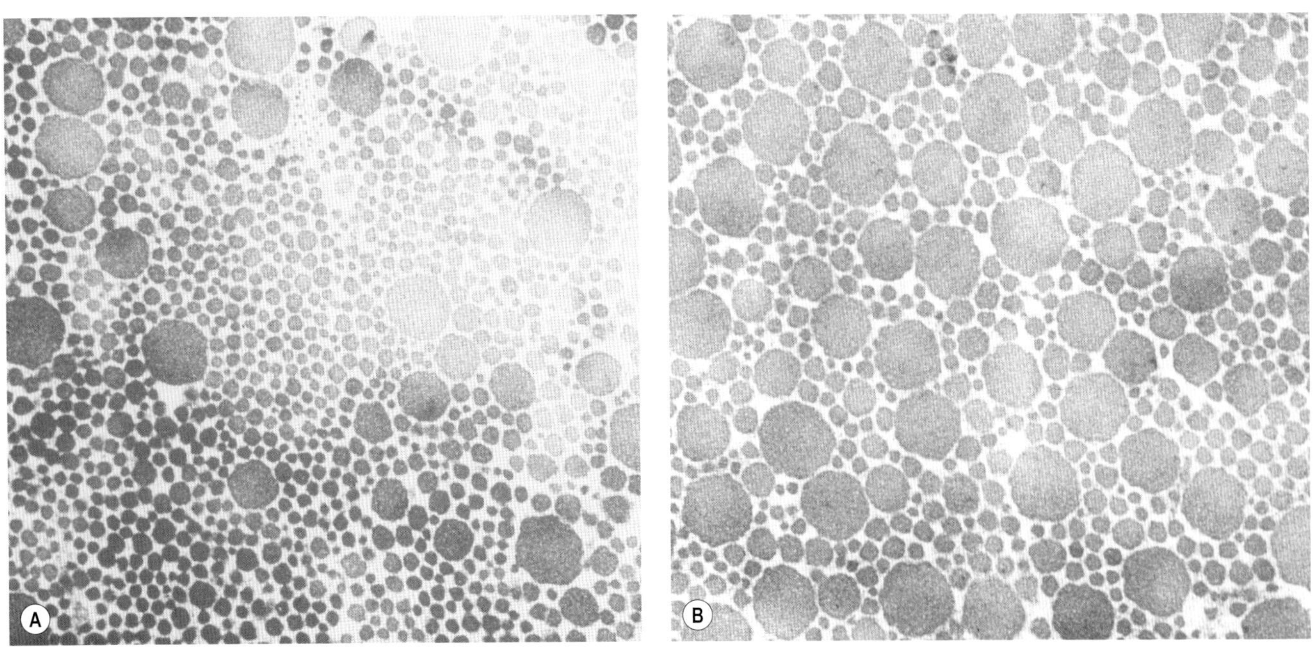

Fig 9.11 Transmission electron microscopy of superficial digital flexor tendon in three-year-old Thoroughbreds after 18 months of treadmill exercise **(A)**, compared with controls that received only walking exercise **(B)**. Exercise has induced a greater number of small-diameter fibrils.
Courtesy of the Equine Veterinary Journal, reproduced with permission.

rapidly decline but only within the tensile (metacarpal) regions of the digital flexor tendons.[38] The superimposition of exercise at this time, results in increased loss of COMP from this area of the tendon.[77] In contrast, levels of COMP within the low loaded tendons, such as the common digital extensor tendon are also low at birth but do not alter significantly with growth and aging[65] although exercise did alter levels in immature tendon (see below).

Although collagen content varies little with age, there are marked alterations at the molecular level which are likely to impact on functional characteristics. Tissue fluorescence, a non-specific marker of glycation, increases with age in the SDFT and the CDET.[21] Pentosidine levels also show a positive correlation with horse age, demonstrating that glycation results in the formation of advanced glycation end-product crosslinks.[21] Increasing horse age was also found to result in an increase in the crosslink lysylpyridinoline suggesting changes in the lysine hydroxylation in ageing tendons.[21]

Metabolic changes

Studies investigating the distribution of the growth factor, TGF-β, a potent anabolic growth factor and stimulus for COMP synthesis in vitro has demonstrated reduction in the presence of the three isoforms of TGF-β after skeletal maturity, although TGF- β1, believed to be most associated with scar tissue formation in wound healing, remains prominent within the interfascicular (endotenon) tissue where age-associated changes occur.[81]

These findings have resulted in the hypothesis that the tensile region of the digital flexor tendons of the horse lose their ability to adapt to exercise after skeletal maturity and both age and exercise provoke degeneration in the tendon matrix, characterized by a loss in non-collagenous proteins. In support of this hypothesis, analysis of matrix gene expression in bovine digital flexor tendons has shown prominent matrix gene expression at birth and during growth but a complete absence of gene expression in the tensile (but not compressed) regions.[82] However more recent data have shown this not to the case in equine flexor tendons where gene expression for all major matrix proteins (e.g. col1A1, decorin, COMP) and matrix degrading enzymes (MMP1, MMP13, MMP3) is detected in the tensional regions of the SDFT and CDET and furthermore, levels of expression do not decline with increasing age.[20] In this study, markers of collagen synthesis and degradation were present in the tendon matrix demonstrating expression is translated into protein.

Investigations into the synthetic response by equine tenocytes to mechanical load (biaxial stretch) and growth factors (TGF-β) in vitro have demonstrated little response to mechanical load alone.[83] TGF-β has a major effect on protein synthesis and, when combined with mechanical load, is synergistic. However, tenocytes recovered from aged flexor tendons demonstrate a small, but significant, reduced response to combined load and TGF-β.[83] Interestingly, PCR analysis of TGF-β gene expression showed no growth factor expression after birth, except when the tendon was injured, suggesting that the tendon TGF-β stores are fixed and limited at birth.[81] This suggests that the failure of an adaptive response in adult tendon is potentially due to a combination of the absence of growth factors and a reduced ability of the cell to respond to increased levels of growth factors.

Mechanisms of strain-induced degeneration

The close association between age and exercise suggests that number of loading cycles is important. It is logical to presume that the highest loading rates are likely to be the most damaging, so the amount of time spent at the fastest gaits (canter and gallop) where strains can reach 16% with an initial strain rate of up to 200%/s are likely to be the most contributory for degeneration. To combat these deleterious effects of exercise, it has been proposed that the muscle of the SDFT primarily acts to fix the origin of the tendon and dampen the potentially harmful high frequency vibrations.[3]

The actual mechanism for the degeneration of the tendon is currently unknown although there are several possibilities. These mechanisms can be either physical or metabolic processes. The physical energy imparted to the tendon under weight-bearing load can produce direct damage to the matrix by disrupting tendon ultrastructure. An indirect physical effect of weight bearing is via the energy lost through hysteresis. This results in a temperature rise within the center of the tendon.[60] While the tenocytes in the superficial digital flexor tendon have been shown to be resistant to these temperature rises[61], this temperature could still be damaging to matrix proteins.

Loading cycles can induce cellular activity with potentially the release of proteolytic enzymes. Work in vitro has shown that cyclical loading of equine SDFT explants reduces their mechanical strength and that explants from older horses are more susceptible.[84] Viable cells and active MMPs were shown to be necessary to produce the weakening effect of cyclical loading suggesting that it is an active cell-mediated process.[84] Recent work has shown that ageing results in an accumulation of partially cleaved collagen in the matrix suggesting that increased susceptibility to injury in older individuals results from an inability to remove partially degraded collagen from the matrix leading to reduced mechanical competence.[21] Further work is necessary to elucidate the mechanisms of soft tissue degeneration so that preventative strategies can be developed.

Immature (growing) tendon

Although there appeared to be a failure in adaptive response to exercise in mature digital flexor tendon in the studies outlined above, is this also the case in immature tendon? Three studies have addressed this question; the first involving three different exercise regimes (box rest, box rest with enforced exercise (training), and pasture exercise) in Warmblood foals from six weeks to five months of age[85]; the second an increasing amount of treadmill exercise in Thoroughbred foals from six weeks to 15 months of age[86] and the third enforced exercise on grass in Thoroughbred foals from 21 days to 18 months of age.[87]

Mechanical changes

In the Warmblood study[88], foals kept at pasture had significantly stronger tendons structurally at five months of age than the other two groups largely due to the development of a larger cross-sectional area (see below) as the ultimate tensile stress at rupture (material property) was not different between groups. By 11 months of age, after all three groups had received a six-month period of low-level exercise, the differences between groups were largely no longer present.

Morphological changes

The study by Kasashima and colleagues[86] documented a significant increase in the rate of increase in cross-sectional area of the superficial digital flexor tendon with treadmill exercise administered for only a small period each day in addition to pasture exercise. Interestingly, the variation in tendon cross-sectional area between limbs increased in both exercise and control groups towards the end of the study. In the other Thoroughbred study by Moffat et al.[87] there was no difference in tendon CSA between groups. In the study on Warmblood foals[88], the cross-sectional area was significantly larger at five months of age in the foals kept on pasture in comparison to those maintained on box rest or box rest with small bouts of enforced intense exercise. These differences were no longer significant at 11 months after all three groups had received a similar level of low-level exercise for six months.

Ultrastructural changes

Fetal and newborn equine SDFT has a uniform fibril size of moderate diameter (i.e. not universally small).[50] During growth, a bimodal distribution of fibril sizes, with the largest number of small (~40 nm) diameter fibrils and lower numbers of large fibrils (>200 nm in diameter) becomes apparent within the first year of life. These small fibrils may represent either new collagen fibrils waiting to be incorporated into larger fibrils, different collagen (type III has universally smaller fibril diameters than type I) or the disruption of larger diameter fibrils. This change in fibril diameter distribution appears to be influenced by loading and exercise, as different exercise regimes given to foals altered the time at which the small fibrils appeared.[89] Pasture exercise resulted in the most rapid appearance, with a predominance of small fibrils present by five months of age. Foals maintained in a box had a delayed onset of this 'adult' phenotype.

In comparison, treadmill exercise given to foals from six weeks to 15 months of age failed to alter the fibril diameter distribution between controls and exercised foals[90], although these foals also had access to pasture exercise, which may have been sufficient to induce the bimodal distribution of fibrils.

Compositional changes

Five-month-old foals given pasture exercise, box rest, or box rest with enforced exercise (training) from seven days of age, demonstrated changes in molecular composition with respect to exercise.[91] Both COMP and polysulphated GAG levels were lowest in the training group, suggesting that this exercise regimen was detrimental to tendon development. After normalizing the exercise across all groups for a further 6 months, there was only limited ability for the tendons to recover, although there were changes associated with growth, in particular increases in hyaluronic acid and COMP. Thus, early exercise is potentially the most important determinant of tendon development. In keeping with this, COMP levels have been found to be exquisitely sensitive to loading in vivo early in life. COMP failed to accumulate in the digital flexor tendons of an 11-week-old foal that had been non-weight-bearing on one limb for six weeks. This effect was not marked if the period of non-weight-bearing occurred after COMP had accumulated within the digital flexor tendons.[38]

In contrast, in the exercise study performed by Kasashima and colleagues[90], COMP levels were not altered in the SDFT, although significant rises were induced in the CDET. It may be that the load 'history' over the 15 months of exercise was not sufficiently different between the two groups to induce a significant change in the digital flexor tendons.

Metabolic changes

The investigations described above suggest that tendon is able to respond to exercise during growth although the response appears to be dependent on the exercise regimes. In the study using Warmblood foals[91], pasture (constant) exercise appeared to produce a better quality tendon than that resulting from either box rest (limited, low level, exercise) or enforced exercise with box rest (limited, but high level, exercise). Some, but not complete, recovery appeared to be possible between five and 11 months when the animals were allowed low-level free exercise. This study also confirmed that the 'window of opportunity' for tendon adaptation appeared to be early in the life of the animal.

The minimal changes induced by additional, albeit small, amounts of treadmill exercise suggested that the natural exercise level at pasture may be optimal for tendon development. Certainly, the gamboling activities of foals at pasture would appear to be ideally suited for high strain rate controlled loading of the digital flexor tendons (Fig. 9.12). It may be that both time and intensity 'windows of opportunity' exist above or past which further augmentation of tendon properties cannot be achieved.

Tendon injury and repair

Pathogenesis of tendon injury

Tendons and ligaments can be injured in one of two ways; overstrain or percutaneous penetration/laceration. The latter will not be considered further in this chapter. Overstrain injuries are believed to occur by one of two mechanisms. They can result from a sudden overloading of the structure, which overwhelms its resistive strength. This type of injury is probably the mechanism for most ligament and some DDFT injuries in the horse. However, for the most common strain-induced injuries in the horse, involving the palmar soft tissue structures of the metacarpal region, the clinical injury is believed to be preceded by a phase of degeneration. The evidence for this preceding degeneration is based on four observations:

1. The identification of 'asymptomatic' lesions, both grossly and microscopically, in post-mortem studies of normal horses.[17,92] Care, however, should be made in distinguishing gross central discolorations in otherwise normal tendons from changes which are more likely to represent early clinical injury than the preceding degeneration. Many of these 'asymptomatic' lesions can now be identified ultrasonographically[8] (Fig. 9.13).
2. Many, if not all, clinical strain-induced tendinopathies are bilateral with one limb more severely affected than the other. Careful ultrasonographic examination will reveal changes in the contralateral limb in many cases. In those seemingly

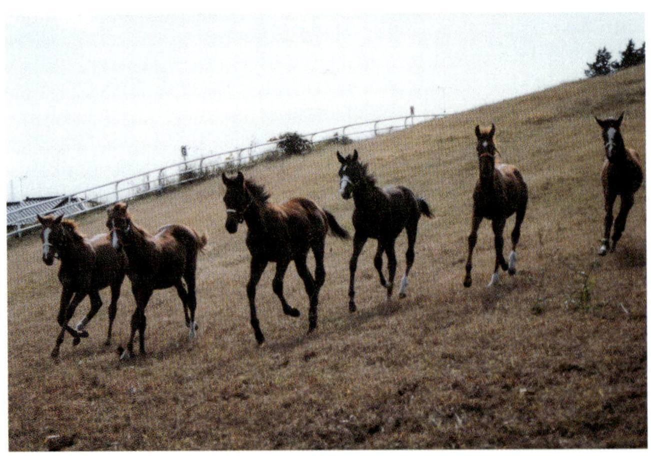

Fig 9.12 Gamboling activity of foals at pasture may be ideally suited to the development of tendons.
Courtesy of Dr Yoshinori Kasashima, Japan Racing Association.

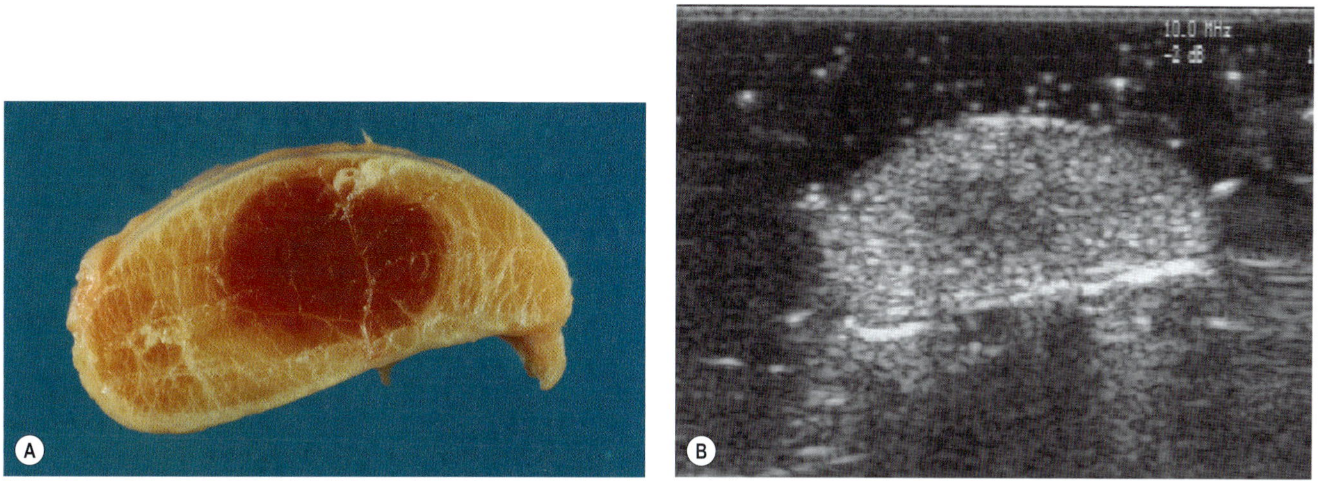

Fig 9.13 (A) Central discolored region of 'asymptomatic' superficial digital flexor tendon (SDFT) – these 'lesions' are probably more representative of subtle clinical injury than the degenerative stage of tendinitis because they can be visualized ultrasonographically in a water bath as core lesions characteristic of clinical injury **(B)**.

unilateral cases, blood-flow studies have demonstrated increases in the 'normal' contralateral tendon, which would suggest that it is not totally unaffected.[15]

3. Epidemiologic studies have demonstrated close associations between age and exercise, and tendon injury.[6, 8]
4. Following on from these epidemiologic observations, experimental investigations have demonstrated evidence of degeneration associated with a synergistic action of both age and exercise (see above).[77, 93]

Thus, degeneration is usually the first phase of tendinopathy. This can be likened to 'molecular inflammation'[94] which does not provoke a repair process, as after clinical injury, but rather progressively weakens the tendon. Any change in the structural properties of the tendon does not have to be great as the tendon is already operating close to its tolerance limit. Clinical injury occurs when the highest stresses encountered by the tendon overwhelm its structural integrity, resulting in irreversible damage. Once this occurs, the damage created induces a repair process characterized by inflammation followed by fibroplasia (scar tissue formation).

This process allows the incorporation of risk factors that have been identified for tendinitis. These risk factors act to increase the peak loads on the SDFT, thereby increasing the risk of structural disruption. One of the most important factors is the speed of the horse. The faster the horse is going, the greater the risk of tendinitis.[6] Thus, hard going is associated with tendinitis as it increases the speed of the horse and also increases the peak impact loading.[6] Slower surfaces (including soft going) tend to be protective. Other factors, such as the weight the horse is carrying, fatigue, and the shoeing, can all influence peak tendon loads in this way. Low heels was thought to be protective of tendinitis as this conformation tends to increase the load in the DDFT, a secondary supporter of the metacarpophalangeal joint, thereby reducing the support necessary from the SDFT and SL. However, as the highest loading in the DDFT is towards the end of the weight-bearing phase, this may not have an influence on the initial high level loading of the SDFT at the onset of weight bearing.

Once the peak load on the tendon overcomes its structural strength, there is physical disruption to the tendon matrix. This varies in degree from fibrillar slippage to fibrillar rupture and, in some cases, complete separation of tendon tissue. This damage initiates a reparative sequence of events not dissimilar to that in other soft tissues, such as skin, which is characterized by phases of inflammation, followed by fibroplasia, which results in the replacement of normal tendon tissue with scar. With the formation of abundant scar tissue, the healed tendon becomes strong but it is functionally inferior to normal tendon. As a structure, healed tendon is stiffer than normal tendon, which compromises the tendon function and predisposes to re-injury, often at sites adjacent to the original injury.[95]

Gross damage and mechanical failure

With the advent of clinical injury, the extent of the damage to the matrix varies from disruption of individual fibers/fascicles to fiber ruptures and ultimately failure of the entire tendon. This damage can be focal or generalized and one of the more common manifestations of superficial digital flexor tendinitis is a centrally located region of injury (so-called 'core' lesion seen ultrasonographically; Fig. 9.14), usually with the most severe level being just below the mid-metacarpal region but also extending throughout most of the length of the metacarpal extrasynovial tendon. Regions of the SDFT enclosed within a tendon sheath (carpal sheath proximally; digital sheath distally) are usually much less severely affected, although this can be relatively more common when the metacarpal region has been previously injured.

Desmitis of the accessory ligament of the DDFT can occur as an isolated injury or in conjunction with superficial digital flexor tendinitis. Its pathogenesis is therefore more related to the SDFT than the DDFT to which it attaches. While ponies rarely suffer strain-induced tendinopathy, they do have a relatively high incidence of desmitis of the accessory ligament of the DDFT.

The SL can fail at any site along its length, although certain areas are more common in horses used in different disciplines. Thus, race horses tend to suffer lesions of the body (and branches) of the SL, while sports horses more frequently have pathology centered within the proximal or branch regions of the ligament.

In contrast to the SDFT and SL, the deep digital flexor tendon (DDFT) is most frequently injured within the digital sheath. It is not known whether these injuries have a preceding phase of tendon degeneration but many are potentially due to single loading cycles which induce overstrain damage. Consequently, bilateral pathology is rarer. Two manifestations are seen clinically. The first arises within

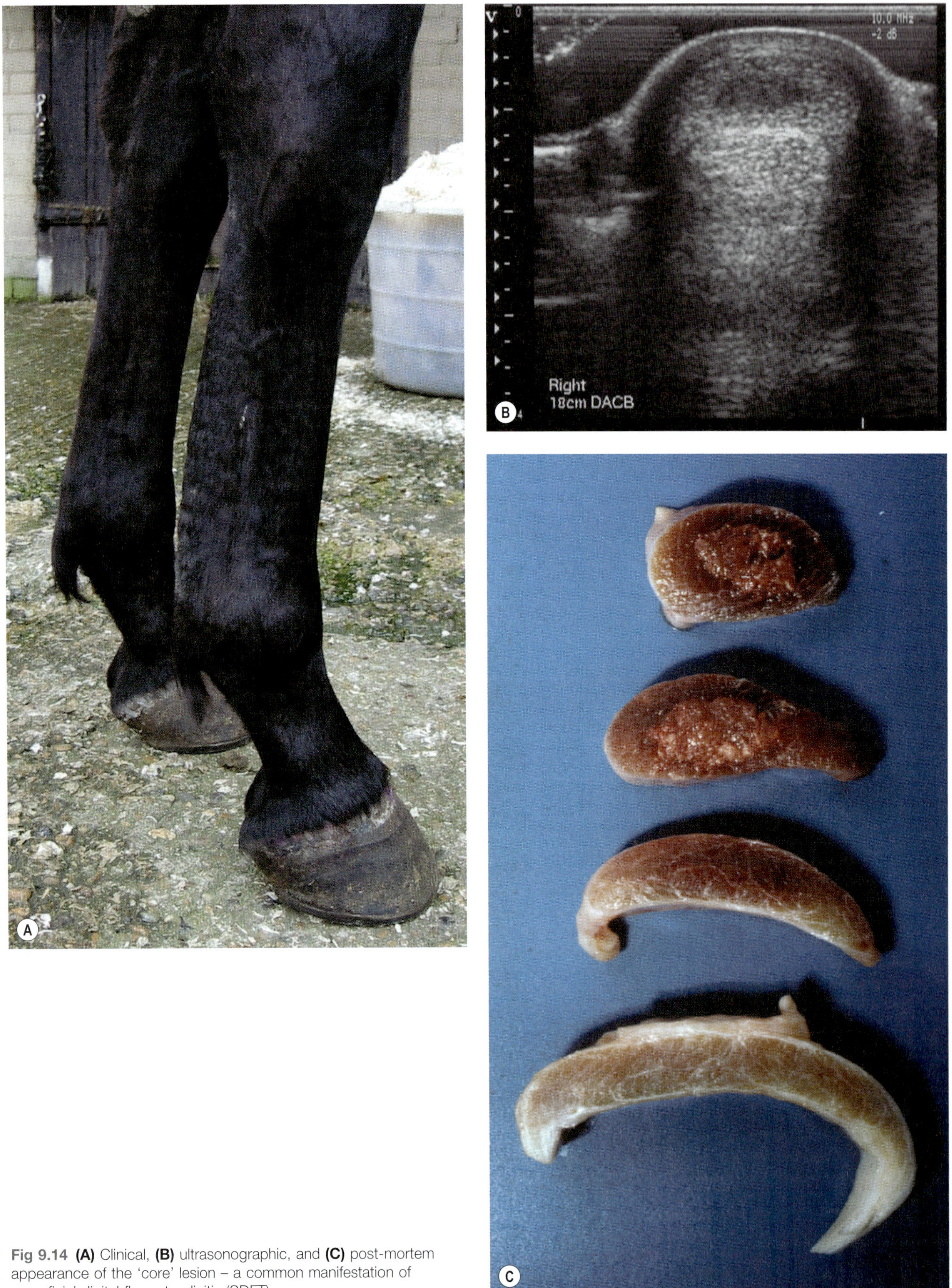

Fig 9.14 (A) Clinical, **(B)** ultrasonographic, and **(C)** post-mortem appearance of the 'core' lesion – a common manifestation of superficial digital flexor tendinitis (SDFT).

the substance of the tendon (although it may extend to the borders of the tendon), which is similar to other clinical manifestations of tendinitis. The second arises at the medial or lateral borders of the tendon, usually in the region of the metacarpo/metatarsophalangeal joint, with no, or limited, involvement of the internal substance of the tendon. These tendon 'tears' are thought to arise from 'bursting' pressures within the tendon when the metacarpo/ metatarsophalangeal joint is overextended.

Other tendons can suffer from strain-induced injury, although much less commonly than that affecting the palmar soft tissue structures of the metacarpus. Ligament injuries tend to occur when the joint they span is loaded inappropriately to result in a degree of subluxation.

Repair processes in tendon

Once the tendon suffers clinical injury with disruption of the tendon matrix, there is intratendinous hemorrhage initially, usually followed rapidly by a pronounced inflammatory reaction. This inflammatory reaction results in an increase in blood flow, the development of edema, infiltration of neutrophils, macrophages and monocytes, and the release of proteolytic enzymes. While this is the earliest stage of repair, designed to remove damaged tendon tissue, the response is usually excessive, causing further damage to the tendon. This inflammatory phase is usually short lived but, within a few days, the reparative phase of repair begins. This results in a pronounced angiogenic response and the synthesis of scar tissue. This tissue has a different composition to tendon, having a higher ratio of collagen types III/I (~50% cf. 10% for normal tendon;[96]) and higher levels of glycosaminoglycans.[80]

The reparative phase of tendon healing merges with the remodeling phase when there is a gradual, but incomplete replacement of collagen type III to I as the scar tissue matures.[97] The new collagen fibrils become thicker and cross-linked. Even mature scar tissue tends to be less stiff as a material than tendon, but because large amounts are formed, the scarred tendon often becomes stiffer as a structure than the original tendon.[95]

Diagnosis

Diagnosis of tendon injury is usually based on history (frequently a preceding bout of intense exercise) and the development of the signs of inflammation (pain, heat, swelling and lameness) over the affected structure (Fig. 9.14). Lameness may not always be present and tends to be related to the degree of inflammation rather than the degree of damage. In many cases, however, the onset of clinical tendinitis is associated with severe lameness.

The posture of the limb may be altered depending on the structure damaged and the severity of the injury. In the case of severe superficial digital flexor tendinitis, resting metacarpophalangeal joint angle may be normal because of the action of the other supporters of this joint (SL and DDFT). However, when loading on the limb increases (e.g. when the contralateral limb is raised), the affected limb shows greater than normal overextension of the metacarpophalangeal joint. Severe damage to the SL will have greater effect on metacarpophalangeal joint extension.

For more subtle cases, careful palpation of the tendons in the limb should be made both with the limb weight bearing and raised. Careful attention should be made to pain response, subtle enlargement and consistency of the structure (soft after recent injury; firm after healing). The horse must be relaxed so that muscle activity does not tense the tendons and make them appear artificially firm. Careful visual assessment of 'bowing' of the palmar contour of the metacarpal region can help to identify subtle superficial digital flexor tendinitis.

Clinical examination, however, may not detect the most subtle injuries and assessment of the severity is limited by clinical examination alone. As prognosis is most dependent on the severity of the initial injury, it is prudent to evaluate the damaged area ultrasonographically and this is best carried out 4–7 days after the onset of the injury as many lesions expand during the initial few days. Modern ultrasound machines with a 7.5–14 MHz linear transducer produce excellent quality images of the flexor tendons and SL (see Chapter 20). While the metacarpal region can be evaluated ultrasonographically without clipping the hair, it is recommended to prepare the limb by clipping and washing (with a surgical scrub and spirit) to give the best-quality images. The horse should be standing square and both transverse and longitudinal images obtained in a methodical fashion throughout the length of the region containing the injured tendon. For the metacarpal region, the area is divided up into seven levels or zones, each with characteristic anatomy. Alternatively, the distance between the transducer and the accessory carpal bone can be recorded. The palmar soft tissue structures of the metacarpus can be evaluated satisfactorily from the palmar aspect of the limb, except for the SL branches which should also be evaluated from the medial and lateral aspects of the limb. Both limbs should always be examined as many cases of strain-induced tendon injury have bilateral components but with one limb more severely affected than the other.

Acute tendon pathology is manifest ultrasonographically by enlargement, hypoechogenicity (focal, e.g. 'core' lesion; see Fig. 9.14, or generalized), reduced striated pattern in the longitudinal images, and changes in shape, margin, or position. In contrast to normal tendons, natural repair is characterized by a detectable Doppler signal when the tendon is not loaded.[98] Chronic tendinopathy is associated with variable enlargement and echogenicity (often heterogeneous), and a reduced irregular striated pattern indicative of fibrosis.

Markers of tendon injury

When a tendon is injured, proteins are released from the tendon into either a surrounding synovial fluid (for intrathecal injuries) and/or the blood (for extrathecal injuries). It is potentially possible to detect these released proteins in either tendon sheath synovial fluid or blood which could then be used as a molecular marker of tendon disease.

The development of a specific assay for a molecular marker of tendon injury relies on one of two different approaches. One alternative is to identify a protein which is specific for tendon tissue and released into the bloodstream following injury. Studies on the molecular composition of tendon using 2D gel electrophoresis (Smith & Heinegard, personal communication) have demonstrated that there are many similarities between the proteins present in cartilage and tendon and few, if any, specific for tendon tissue, making this approach less viable at present.

The second alternative is to identify a protein that is not specific to tendon but whose distribution is restricted and/or whose fragmentation with injury is specific for tendon injury. One such protein is COMP, which has a restricted distribution to tendon, ligament, cartilage, intervertebral disk, and meniscus. Furthermore, COMP is particularly abundant in young mid-metacarpal SDFT, the area most prone to injury. After skeletal maturity, the natural decrease in COMP levels within the metacarpal region of the SDFT can be accelerated by exercise.[77] These findings suggest that it might be a useful indicator of tendon damage if, once it is released from the metacarpal region of the SDFT, it gains access to the bloodstream and can subsequently be assayed. COMP is not significantly absorbed by the peripheral lymph nodes (cf. proteoglycan fragments; Frazer et al, unpublished data) and COMP fragments are found in the serum in humans.[99] While studies in man have demonstrated that COMP has potential usefulness as a marker of joint disease[100], assay of the total amount of COMP in serum showed no significant alterations in COMP levels with tendon disease[99], although there were significant increases associated with the commencement of training (Smith and Bathe, unpublished data). This assay quantifies COMP using a polyclonal antiserum that recognizes a number of epitopes on the COMP molecule. There is a normal significant background level of COMP in the serum (1–2 mg/mL), possibly representing the normal turnover of COMP from all tissues containing the protein. Certainly there are considerably higher levels of total COMP in the serum of growing horses compared to adults[99], when COMP is being accumulated in the tissues. In addition, damage to cartilage in joint disease also contributes to the 'pool' of COMP in the serum and is therefore responsible for a reduction in the sensitivity of the assay for tendon disease itself.

However, COMP levels in digital sheath synovial fluid in horses with intrasynovial tendon injury demonstrated significant rises.[101] We know from previous studies that there is <1/100 the level of COMP in the digital sheath capsule[38], so that rises observed in the digital sheath synovial fluid (approximately four times normal levels) suggest that COMP is lost from the intrasynovial tendon rather than the digital sheath. The COMP released within the digital sheath synovial fluid is composed of fragments which have been identified on SDS-PAGE after partial purification with ion exchange chromatography. This fragmentation pattern is different from that described for human joint diseases[99, 100], although may not be in the horse. These fragments represent ideal candidates for markers of tendon disease. Assay of these fragments, not normally present, would potentially enable a very sensitive assay to be developed.

In addition to proteins released after injury being useful for the detection of tendon damage, the healing process can also potentially be monitored using markers of protein synthesis. While serological markers of collagen synthesis (e.g. propeptide of collagen type I; PICP) were thought to be relatively specific for bone remodeling, recent studies have demonstrated significant rises of PICP following tendon injury.[102] Further work is necessary to determine if this molecular marker will be useful for the monitoring of tendon repair.

Review of current treatment strategies

Over the years, many treatment modalities have been tried with most showing equivocal or even deleterious effects. From our knowledge of the phases of tendon healing, the following have at least a rationale for treating tendinitis.[103]

Acute (inflammatory) phase

Physical therapy (rest, application of cold, and compression with bandaging) is the most important aspect of early management where the goal is to minimize inflammation and limit the action of proteolytic enzymes that continue to destroy tendon tissue (see Chapter 25). Pharmacologic interventions include short-acting steroids within the first 24–48h (later application can inhibit the second phase of fibroplasia) and the use of polysulfated glycosaminoglycans, which have been shown to inhibit prostaglandin E2 production in vitro.[104] The intra-lesional use of steroids should be avoided as this has been associated, at least with depot preparations, with intratendinous calcification. Surgical treatment at this stage includes percutaneous tendon splitting, which has been shown to accelerate the resolution of the 'core' lesion seen ultrasonographically.[105] This can be done with a scalpel or, less invasively, performed with needle puncture, when it can be combined with intratendinous polysulfated glycosaminoglycan therapy. Desmotomy of the accessory ligament of the SDFT, often performed concurrently with percutaneous tendon splitting early on in the disease process, is suggested to reduce peak strains on the SDFT by bringing the superficial digital flexor muscle into play.[106] However, although initial data suggested a beneficial effect[107], this has not been confirmed in other studies and has been suggested to contribute to a higher incidence of suspensory desmitis after its use.[108]

Subacute (fibroblastic) phase

Early and progressive mobilization and regular ultrasonographic monitoring aims to improve the quality of the forming scar tissue is the goal of this phase. If the cross-sectional area of the healing tendon increases by more than 10%, the exercise level should be reduced. The quality of the longitudinal fiber pattern when the animal returns to full work has been linked with the overall prognosis.[109] In an attempt to improve the quality of the scar tissue, b-aminoproprionitrile fumarate (BAPTEN; no longer marketed for the treatment of tendon injuries) has been injected intratendinously 30–90 days after injury.[109] This drug inhibits lysyl oxidase, the enzyme that cross-links collagen molecules. In preventing the formation of cross-links, it is believed that collagen fibers will form with better longitudinal alignment under the stimulus of controlled exercise. When the drug wears off, cross-linking occurs and the scar increases in strength. Clinical trials in the USA indicated a benefit in the more severe cases.

Other drugs, such as sodium hyaluronate, have been used both intratendinously and peritendinously but studies have shown equivocal results. Some benefit in reducing adhesion formation in intrathecal tendon injuries has been demonstrated experimentally.[110]

Newer treatments aimed at regenerating rather than repairing tendon represent the best hope for the future. Anabolic growth factors, such as IGF-1[111], recombinant equine growth hormone[112], and TGF-β have been tried empirically or in a collagenase model of tendon injury, but not comprehensively evaluated in the clinical situation, making interpretation of the benefits of these agents difficult. An important factor in assessing these new treatments is that they do actually generate tendon-like tissue rather than just increasing the amount of scar tissue produced, which will still compromise the outcome. For example platelet rich plasma (PRP) (plasma with at least twice the concentration of normal plasma) can be recovered using centrifugation or gravity filtration from autologous blood. PRP is a rich source of growth factors that can stimulate cell proliferation and matrix synthesis, including platelet derived growth factor (PDGF), TGF-β and vascular endothelial growth factor (VEGF).

The use of autologous intra-lesional mesencymal stem cell therapy offers the opportunity for regeneration of tendon or ligament rather than repair. MSCs have the potential to differentiate into tenocytes and to regenerate matrix thus creating a repair that is superior to scar tissue formation. A recent study demonstrated that in a population of 105 National Hunt racehorses treated with intra-lesional MSC therapy for SDF tendinitis that the re-injury rate after 3 years was 27%, which is significantly lower that the re-injury rates previously reported for SDF tendinitis treated with conventional therapy and analyzed in the same way.[113] Thus the use of mesenchymal stem cells (recovered from bone marrow) is one of the most exciting new developments [114,115] although much work is still necessary to determine their effectiveness.

Chronic (remodeling) phase

A controlled ascending exercise program with regular ultrasonographic examinations encourages the further optimization of the scar tissue. In addition, ultrasound can enable the detection of early signs of re-injury to minimize the risk of catastrophic re-injury. Other methods aimed at preventing re-injury include desmotomy of the accessory ligament of the SDFT (see 'Acute phase' treatments) and the use of boots capable of providing significant support to the metacarpophalangeal joint. Traditional bandages fail to provide sufficient support under weight-bearing load, while novel designed boots have been shown to do so and potentially may help to prevent re-injury[116] (Fig. 9.15).

Specific therapies

Some tendon and ligament injuries have specific therapies in addition to those outlined above. DDFT tears within the digital flexor tendon sheath (DFTS) or navicular bursa, manica flexoria tears within the DFTS, and SL tears into the metacarpo/ metatarsophalangeal joint are best treated by tenoscopic / bursoscopic/ arthroscopic debridement. The outcome of hindlimb, but not forelimb, proximal suspensory desmitis appears to be improved (from 13% to 43%) by the use of extracorporeal shock wave therapy.[117, 118] For those cases of hindlimb proximal suspensory desmitis (PSLD) also failing to respond to shock wave therapy, surgical neurectomy of the deep branch of the lateral plantar nerve combined with transection of the fascia overlying the proximal suspensory ligament provides an additional rational management technique. Both these latter two treatments are consistent with the hypothesis that hindlimb proximal suspensory desmitis is an example of a compartmental syndrome, unlike the forelimb (which carries a considerably better prognosis with conservative management alone). It has been shown that the prognosis for horses with hindlimb PSLD with normal conformation to return to full work for at least one year after DBLPN and fasciotomy is 78% whereas horses with a 'straight hock conformation' or hyperextension of the metatarsophalangeal joint had a worse prognosis with 44% remaining in full work for at least one year post-surgery.[5]

Current concepts in prevention of tendinitis in the equine athlete

Strategies for the prevention of equine tendinitis

With the limitation of our ability with current treatments to return a horse with tendinitis to full work without danger of re-injury, prevention of the injury has to be considered as the most appropriate strategy. From our understanding of tendon physiology described in the preceding sections, four broad approaches for prevention can be considered.

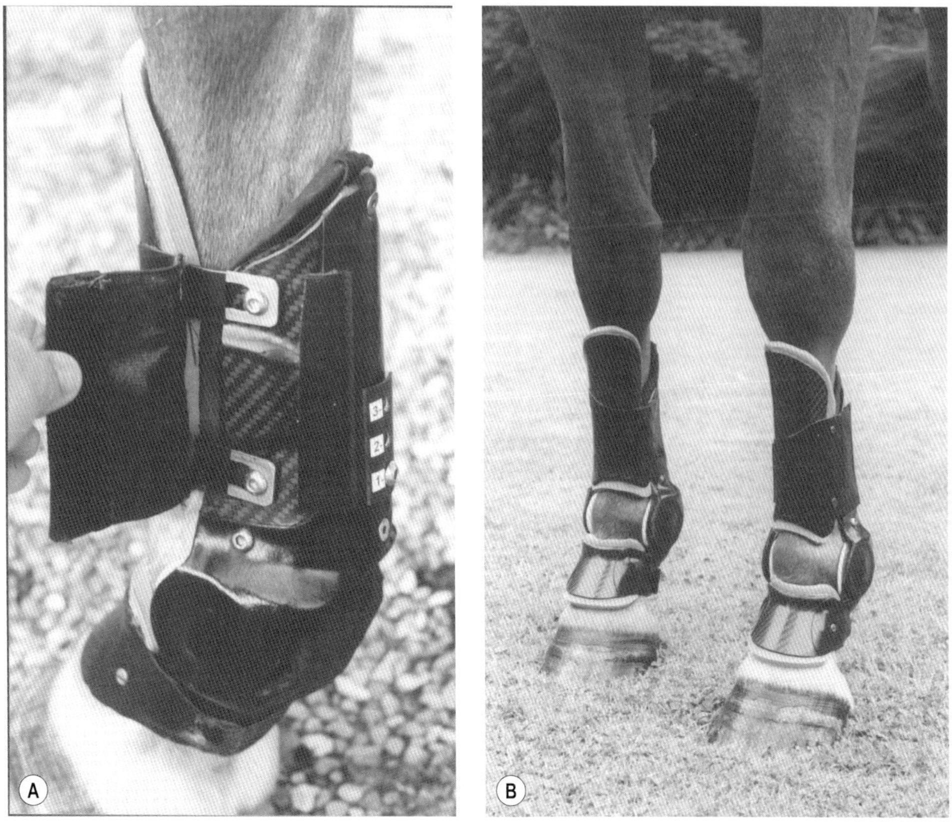

Fig 9.15 (A, B) Dalmar support boot capable of being used in the exercising horse and able to provide significant support to the metacarpophalangeal joint, unlike traditional bandages. This may provide a method of minimizing re-injury after rehabilitation.
Courtesy of the Equine Veterinary Journal, reproduced with permission.

Maximize the quality of the tendon prior to skeletal maturity

There is a large variation in the strength of the SDFT in a population of horses. Some of this variation may be due to specific genes. Either breeding out, or identifying horses with those genetic variants associated with a genetic susceptibility to tendinitis, would potentially lower the incidence of tendon injury. However, while the concept is simple, its achievement is considerably more difficult.

Skeletal tissues are much more able to adapt to the loads placed on them when they are immature and growing. This is certainly true for bone and muscle and we believe it to also be the case in tendon. Thus, carefully tailored exercise regimes during growth (0–2 years of age) would potentially improve the 'quality' of the tendon and minimize the effects of degeneration induced by training and racing after skeletal maturity (approximately two years of age in the horse) (Fig. 9.16). These exercise regimes must be within the 'windows of opportunity' of the right time and the right level. Growing tendon is also more susceptible to injury so these 'conditioning' programs have to induce adaptation suitable for subsequent racing without causing injury. However, the optimal property of equine tendon still needs to be determined. Probably the most important characteristic would be fatigue resistance and, for any exercise regime in immature animals to be effective, it must demonstrate a reduction of tendon injuries within the subsequent athletic careers. The answers to these questions are not known but studies are underway to assess the effects of early exercise on musculoskeletal development.

Reduce the degeneration after skeletal maturity

Studies are turning towards investigating the mechanisms of aging in soft tissues, which may give therapeutic options for intervening in the aging process. At present, the only advice that can be given in this area is to avoid training solely aimed at the tendon in the adult horse. This will serve only to advance the rate of degeneration, which has to be considered an inevitable consequence of athleticism. Some forms of exercise may be more provocative of degeneration than others, but, at present, these are not known. However, high loading (i.e. fast speeds) is likely to be the most damaging.

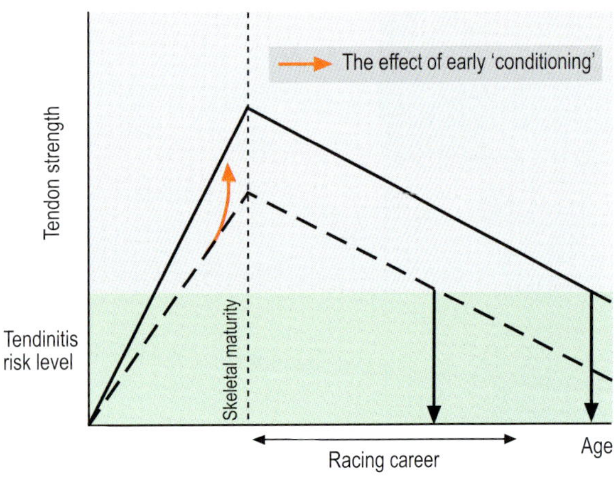

Fig 9.16 Hypothetical response of tendons to the early introduction of exercise. The two lines refer to two different horses – one that develops poor-quality tendon during growth (dashed line) and one that develops good-quality tendon (solid line). Both accumulate damage within the tendon associated with post-skeletal exercise and aging, which inevitably and progressively weakens the tendon. However, in the former, this weakening precedes the individual to clinical tendinitis within its racing career, whereas the latter is able to survive its racing career without suffering such injury. The imposition of 'appropriate' conditioning exercise during growth is hypothesized to improve the quality of the growing tendon, resulting in an individual more resistant to subsequent injury.

Courtesy of the Journal of Comparative Biochemistry and Physiology, reproduced with permission.

Reduce the risk factors for tendinitis

The initiation of clinical tendinitis is provoked by sudden peak forces that overcome the strength of the (degenerated) tendon. This can obviously occur at any time, including out at pasture, but it is obviously most likely when the horse is loading its tendon maximally. This occurs when the horse is running fastest (hence the best horses are potentially more prone to tendon injury). Ground surface (which affects the horse's speed), fatigue (e.g. after longer races or in unfit horses), jumping, shoeing, and weight are all examples of factors that can increase the peak loading on the tendon and hence are risk factors for tendon injury. Some of these are avoidable but others are a consequence of racing and not easily altered.

Early detection

This is not really a prevention strategy, as, by definition, a degree of tendon injury will already have occurred. However, if tendon injury can be detected very early, it is possible to prevent progression to more severe disease. Obviously, careful clinical inspection is vital in this area, but this is rather insensitive.

Ultrasonography has been the mainstay of tendon imaging and has advanced our knowledge and capabilities for management considerably. Ultrasonographic technology is still advancing and new machines have even better resolution. However, they are still relatively insensitive for predicting injury and the ideal time for a return to full work in the chronic stages. Ultrasonography at three monthly intervals was shown not to be a sensitive method of predicting tendon injury[8] although ultrasound is useful to identify at risk animals through the detection of pre-existing injury. This may be useful when a horse enters training for athletic activity since pre-existing injury is the highest risk factor for future injury.[8]

Future techniques in this area may rely on molecular markers of tendon injury. Fragments of proteins within the tendon, which are released with injury, can potentially be assayed for in the blood, which would give a practical test that would provide useful diagnostic, management, and prognostic information.

Recommendations for training of immature and mature animals

Pasture exercise early in life is essential for the development of digital flexor tendon that is likely to be most resistant to injury during adulthood. Additional imposed exercise may be able to augment this effect, but the tendon is also more susceptible to injury at this age and so exercise levels have to be chosen with care. In addition, what about the other skeletal tissues? How do they respond to these exercise regimes? It would be pointless to develop a training regime beneficial for tendon but harmful to other tissues, such as bone and joints. However, different skeletal tissues mature at different times, thus potentially allowing different time 'windows of opportunity' for different tissues. We would suggest that tendon, ligament, and possibly cartilage are most responsive in the first year of life, while bone is more responsive at the yearling stage.

After skeletal maturity, training will have no effect on tendon adaptation and therefore training should be directed at muscular, respiratory, and cardiovascular fitness rather than the tendon.

References

1. Rumian AP, Wallace AL, Birch HL. Tendons and ligaments are anatomically distinct but overlap in molecular and morphological features – a comparative study in an ovine model. Journal of orthopaedic research: official publication of the Orthopaedic Research Society 2007;25(4):458–64. Epub 2007/01/06.
2. Alexander RM. Tendon elasticity and muscle function. Comparative biochemistry and physiology Part A, Molecular & integrative physiology 2002;133(4):1001–11. Epub 2002/12/18.
3. Wilson AM, McGuigan MP, Su A, et al. Horses damp the spring in their step. Nature 2001;414(6866):895–9. Epub 2002/01/10.
4. Batson EL, Paramour RJ, Smith TJ, et al. Are the material properties and matrix composition of equine flexor and extensor tendons determined by their functions? Equine veterinary journal 2003;35(3):314–18. Epub 2003/05/21.
5. Murray RC, Dyson SJ, Tranquille C, et al. Association of type of sport and performance level with anatomical site of orthopaedic injury diagnosis. Equine veterinary journal Supplement 2006(36):411–16. Epub 2007/04/04.
6. Williams RB, Harkins LS, Hammond CJ, et al. Racehorse injuries, clinical problems and fatalities recorded on British racecourses from flat racing and National Hunt racing during 1996, 1997 and 1998. Equine veterinary journal 2001;33(5):478–86. Epub 2001/09/18.
7. Wilson JH, Robinson RA, Jensen RC, et al., editors. Equine soft tissue injuries associated with racing: descriptive statistics from American racetracks. Dubai: Dubai Equine International Symposium; 1996.
8. Avella CS, Ely ER, Verheyen KL, et al. Ultrasonographic assessment of the superficial digital flexor tendons of National Hunt racehorses in training over two racing seasons. Equine veterinary journal 2009;41(5):449–54. Epub 2009/08/01.
9. Ely ER, Avella CS, Price JS, et al. Descriptive epidemiology of fracture, tendon and suspensory ligament injuries in National Hunt racehorses in training. Equine veterinary journal 2009;41(4):372–8. Epub 2009/07/01.
10. Maffulli N, Waterston SW, Squair J, et al. Changing incidence of Achilles tendon rupture in Scotland: a 15-year study. Clinical journal of sport medicine: official journal of the Canadian Academy of Sport Medicine 1999;9(3):157–60. Epub 1999/10/08.
11. Lam KH, Parkin TD, Riggs CM, et al. Descriptive analysis of retirement of Thoroughbred racehorses due to tendon injuries at the Hong Kong Jockey Club (1992–2004). Equine veterinary journal 2007;39(2):143–8. Epub 2007/03/24.
12. McGuigan MP, Wilson AM. The effect of gait and digital flexor muscle activation on limb compliance in the forelimb of the horse Equus caballus. The Journal of experimental biology 2003;206(Pt 8): 1325–36. Epub 2003/03/08.
13. Kraus-Hansen AE, Fackelman GE, Becker C, et al. Preliminary studies on the vascular anatomy of the equine superficial digital flexor tendon. Equine veterinary journal 1992;24(1):46–51. Epub 1992/01/01.
14. Stromberg B. The normal and diseased superficial flexor tendon in race horses. A morphologic and physiologic investigation. Acta radiologica Supplementum 1971;305:1–94. Epub 1971/01/01.
15. Jones AJ. Normal and diseased equine digital flexor tendon: blood flow, biochemical and serological studies. University of London; 1993.
16. Lassen NA, Lindbjerg J, Munck O. Measurement of Blood-Flow through Skeletal Muscle by Intramuscular Injection of Xenon-133. Lancet 1964;1(7335):686–9. Epub 1964/03/28.
17. Goodship AE, Birch HL, Wilson AM. The pathobiology and repair of tendon and ligament injury. The Veterinary clinics of North America Equine practice 1994;10(2):323–49. Epub 1994/08/01.
18. Stanley RL, Goodship AE, Edwards B, et al. Effects of exercise on tenocyte cellularity and tenocyte nuclear morphology in immature and mature equine digital tendons. Equine veterinary journal 2008;40(2):141–6. Epub 2007/12/21.
19. Banes AJ, Donlon K, Link GW, et al. Cell populations of tendon: a simplified method for isolation of synovial cells and internal fibroblasts: confirmation of origin and biologic properties. Journal of orthopaedic research: official publication of the Orthopaedic Research Society 1988;6(1):83–94. Epub 1988/01/01.
20. Thorpe C. Extracellular matrix synthesis and degradation in functionally distinct tendons. PhD thesis, University college London; 2010.
21. Thorpe CT, Streeter I, Pinchbeck GL, et al. Aspartic acid racemization and collagen degradation markers reveal an accumulation of damage in tendon collagen that is enhanced with aging. The Journal of biological chemistry 2010;285(21):15674–81. Epub 2010/03/24.
22. McNeilly CM, Banes AJ, Benjamin M, et al. Tendon cells in vivo form a three dimensional network of cell processes linked by gap junctions. Journal of anatomy 1996;189(Pt 3):593–600. Epub 1996/12/01.
23. Stanley RL, Fleck RA, Becker DL, et al. Gap junction protein expression and cellularity: comparison of immature and adult equine digital tendons. Journal of anatomy 2007;211(3):325–34. Epub 2007/09/13.
24. Bi Y, Ehirchiou D, Kilts TM, et al. Identification of tendon stem/progenitor cells and the role of the extracellular matrix in their niche. Nature medicine 2007;13(10):1219–27. Epub 2007/09/11.
25. Lee WY, Lui PP, Rui YF. Hypoxia-mediated efficient expansion of human tendon-derived stem cells in vitro. Tissue Eng Part A 2012;18(5–6):484–98. Epub 2011/09/29.
26. Lovati AB, Corradetti B, Lange Consiglio A, et al. Characterization and differentiation of equine tendon-derived progenitor cells. Journal of biological regulators and homeostatic agents 2011;25(2 Suppl):S75–84. Epub 2011/12/08.
27. Birch HL. Tendon matrix composition and turnover in relation to functional requirements. International journal of experimental pathology 2007;88(4):241–8. Epub 2007/08/19.
28. Chen CT, McCabe RP, Grodzinsky AJ, et al. Transient and cyclic responses of strain-generated potential in rabbit patellar tendon are frequency and pH dependent. Journal of biomechanical engineering 2000;122(5):465–70. Epub 2000/11/25.
29. West CR, Bowden AE. Using Tendon Inherent Electric Properties to Consistently Track Induced Mechanical Strain. Annals of biomedical engineering 2012. Epub 2012/02/09.
30. Birk DE, Trelstad RL. Fibroblasts create compartments in the extracellular space where collagen polymerizes into fibrils and fibrils associate into bundles. Annals of the New York Academy of Sciences 1985;460:258–66. Epub 1985/01/01.
31. Canty EG, Lu Y, Meadows RS, et al. Coalignment of plasma membrane channels and protrusions (fibripositors) specifies the parallelism of tendon. The Journal of cell biology 2004;165(4): 553–63. Epub 2004/05/26.
32. Bailey AJ, Paul RG, Knott L. Mechanisms of maturation and ageing of collagen. Mechanisms of ageing and development 1998;106(1–2):1–56. Epub 1999/01/12.
33. Thorpe CT, Stark RJ, Goodship AE, et al. Mechanical properties of the equine superficial digital flexor tendon relate to specific collagen cross-link levels. Equine veterinary journal Supplement 2010(38):538–43. Epub 2011/05/27.

34. Rees SG, Dent CM, Caterson B. Metabolism of proteoglycans in tendon. Scandinavian journal of medicine & science in sports 2009;19(4):470–8. Epub 2009/05/09.
35. Danielson KG, Baribault H, Holmes DF, et al. Targeted disruption of decorin leads to abnormal collagen fibril morphology and skin fragility. The Journal of cell biology 1997;136(3):729–43. Epub 1997/02/10.
36. Dourte LM, Pathmanathan L, Jawad AF, et al. Influence of decorin on the mechanical, compositional, and structural properties of the mouse patellar tendon. Journal of biomechanical engineering 2012;134(3):031005. Epub 2012/04/10.
37. Svensson L, Aszodi A, Reinholt FP, et al. Fibromodulin-null mice have abnormal collagen fibrils, tissue organization, and altered lumican deposition in tendon. The Journal of biological chemistry 1999;274(14):9636–47. Epub 1999/03/27.
38. Smith RK, Zunino L, Webbon PM, et al. The distribution of cartilage oligomeric matrix protein (COMP) in tendon and its variation with tendon site, age and load. Matrix biology: journal of the International Society for Matrix Biology 1997;16(5):255–71. Epub 1998/03/21.
39. Rosenberg K, Olsson H, Morgelin M, et al. Cartilage oligomeric matrix protein shows high affinity zinc-dependent interaction with triple helical collagen. The Journal of biological chemistry 1998;273(32):20397–403. Epub 1998/08/01.
40. Halasz K, Kassner A, Morgelin M, et al. COMP acts as a catalyst in collagen fibrillogenesis. The Journal of biological chemistry 2007;282(43):31166–73. Epub 2007/08/25.
41. Smith RK, Gerard M, Dowling B, et al. Correlation of cartilage oligomeric matrix protein (COMP) levels in equine tendon with mechanical properties: a proposed role for COMP in determining function-specific mechanical characteristics of locomotor tendons. Equine veterinary journal Supplement 2002(34):241–4. Epub 2002/10/31.
42. Smith KD, Vaughan-Thomas A, Spiller DG, et al. The organisation of elastin and fibrillins 1 and 2 in the cruciate ligament complex. Journal of anatomy 2011;218(6):600–7. Epub 2011/04/07.
43. Ritty TM, Ditsios K, Starcher BC. Distribution of the elastic fiber and associated proteins in flexor tendon reflects function. The Anatomical record 2002;268(4):430–40. Epub 2002/11/07.
44. Funakoshi T, Schmid T, Hsu HP, et al. Lubricin distribution in the goat infraspinatus tendon: a basis for interfascicular lubrication. The Journal of bone and joint surgery American volume 2008;90(4):803–14. Epub 2008/04/03.
45. Kohrs RT, Zhao C, Sun YL, et al. Tendon fascicle gliding in wild type, heterozygous, and lubricin knockout mice. Journal of orthopaedic research: official publication of the Orthopaedic Research Society 2011;29(3):384–9. Epub 2010/10/05.
46. Sun Y, Berger EJ, Zhao C, et al. Expression and mapping of lubricin in canine flexor tendon. Journal of orthopaedic research: official publication of the Orthopaedic Research Society 2006;24(9):1861–8. Epub 2006/07/26.
47. Jelinsky SA, Archambault J, Li L, et al. Tendon-selective genes identified from rat and human musculoskeletal tissues. Journal of orthopaedic research: official publication of the Orthopaedic Research Society 2010;28(3):289–97. Epub 2009/09/26.
48. Franchi M, Raspanti M, Dell'Orbo C, et al. Different crimp patterns in collagen fibrils relate to the subfibrillar arrangement. Connective tissue research 2008;49(2):85–91. Epub 2008/04/03.
49. Franchi M, Ottani V, Stagni R, et al. Tendon and ligament fibrillar crimps give rise to left-handed helices of collagen fibrils in both planar and helical crimps. Journal of anatomy 2010;216(3):301–9. Epub 2010/01/15.
50. Parry DA, Craig AS, Barnes GR. Tendon and ligament from the horse: an ultrastructural study of collagen fibrils and elastic fibres as a function of age. Proc R Soc Lond B Biol Sci 1978; 203(1152):293–303. Epub 1978/12/18.
51. Patterson-Kane JC, Parry DA, Birch HL, et al. An age-related study of morphology and cross-link composition of collagen fibrils in the digital flexor tendons of young thoroughbred horses. Connective tissue research 1997;36(3):253–60. Epub 1997/01/01.
52. Chavaunne T. Thorpe CPU, Helen L. Birch, Peter D. Clegg, Hazel R.C. Screen. Specialisation of tendon mechanical properties results from inter-fascicular differences. 2012.
53. Screen HR, Lee DA, Bader DL, et al. An investigation into the effects of the hierarchical structure of tendon fascicles on micromechanical properties. Proceedings of the Institution of Mechanical Engineers Part H, Journal of engineering in medicine 2004;218(2):109–19. Epub 2004/05/01.
54. Thorpe CTB, Screen HR, et al., editors. The micro-structural response of tendon fascicles to applied strain is altered with ageing. Barcelona, Spain: Osteoarthritis Research Society International; 2012.
55. Viidik A. Tensile strength properties of Achilles tendon systems in trained and untrained rabbits. Acta orthopaedica Scandinavica 1969;40(2):261–72. Epub 1969/01/01.
56. Woo SL. Mechanical properties of tendons and ligaments. I. Quasi-static and nonlinear viscoelastic properties. Biorheology 1982;19(3):385–96. Epub 1982/01/01.
57. Stephens PR, Nunamaker DM, Butterweck DM. Application of a Hall-effect transducer for measurement of tendon strains in horses. American journal of veterinary research 1989;50(7):1089–95. Epub 1989/07/01.
58. Crevier N, Pourcelot P, Denoix JM, et al. Segmental variations of in vitro mechanical properties in equine superficial digital flexor tendons. American journal of veterinary research 1996;57(8):1111–17. Epub 1996/08/01.
59. Riemersma DJ, van den Bogert AJ, Jansen MO, et al. Tendon strain in the forelimbs as a function of gait and ground characteristics and in vitro limb loading in ponies. Equine veterinary journal 1996;28(2):133–8. Epub 1996/03/01.
60. Wilson AM, Goodship AE. Exercise-induced hyperthermia as a possible mechanism for tendon degeneration. Journal of biomechanics 1994;27(7):899–905. Epub 1994/07/01.
61. Birch HL, Wilson AM, Goodship AE. The effect of exercise-induced localised hyperthermia on tendon cell survival. The Journal of experimental biology 1997;200(Pt 11):1703–8. Epub 1997/06/01.
62. Minetti AE, Ardig OL, Reinach E, et al. The relationship between mechanical work and energy expenditure of locomotion in horses. The Journal of experimental biology 1999;202(Pt 17):2329–38. Epub 1999/08/10.
63. Evanko SP, Vogel KG. Ultrastructure and proteoglycan composition in the developing fibrocartilaginous region of bovine tendon. Matrix 1990;10(6):420–36. Epub 1990/12/01.
64. Vogel KG, Koob TJ. Structural specialization in tendons under compression. International review of cytology 1989;115:267–93. Epub 1989/01/01.
65. Batson EL, Smith RKW, Patterson-Kane JC, et al., editors. Postnatal development initiates rapid tendon speciþc structural changes associated with a dramatic increase in cartilage oligomeric matrix protein (COMP). Transactions of the 49th Annual Meeting of the Orthopedic Research Society; 2003.
66. Birch HLS, Lawes TJ, et al., editors. Mechanical properties of equine ßexor tendons show symmetry between right and left forelimbs within individuals but a wide variation in strength and stiffness between individuals. Patras, Greece: XVIIth FECTS Meeting; 2000.

67. Carroll CC, Dickinson JM, Haus JM, et al. Influence of aging on the in vivo properties of human patellar tendon. J Appl Physiol 2008;105(6):1907–15. Epub 2008/10/18.
68. Faria A, Gabriel R, Abrantes J, et al. Biomechanical properties of the triceps surae muscle-tendon unit in young and postmenopausal women. Clin Biomech (Bristol, Avon) 2011;26(5):523–8. Epub 2011/02/01.
69. Kubo K, Kanehisa H, Miyatani M, et al. Effect of low-load resistance training on the tendon properties in middle-aged and elderly women. Acta physiologica Scandinavica 2003;178(1):25–32. Epub 2003/04/26.
70. Wilmink J, Wilson AM, Goodship AE. Functional significance of the morphology and micromechanics of collagen fibres in relation to partial rupture of the superficial digital flexor tendon in racehorses. Research in veterinary science 1992;53(3):354–9. Epub 1992/11/01.
71. Patterson-Kane JC, Firth EC, Goodship AE, et al. Age-related differences in collagen crimp patterns in the superficial digital flexor tendon core region of untrained horses. Australian veterinary journal 1997;75(1):39–44. Epub 1997/01/01.
72. Patterson-Kane JC, Wilson AM, Firth EC, et al. Exercise-related alterations in crimp morphology in the central regions of superficial digital flexor tendons from young thoroughbreds: a controlled study. Equine veterinary journal 1998;30(1):61–4. Epub 1998/02/12.
73. Gillis C, Pool RR, Meagher DM, et al. Effect of maturation and aging on the histomorphometric and biochemical characteristics of equine superficial digital flexor tendon. American journal of veterinary research 1997;58(4):425–30. Epub 1997/04/01.
74. Birch HL, McLaughlin L, Smith RK, et al. Treadmill exercise-induced tendon hypertrophy: assessment of tendons with different mechanical functions. Equine veterinary journal Supplement 1999;30:222–6. Epub 2000/02/05.
75. Woo SL, Ritter MA, Amiel D, et al. The biomechanical and biochemical properties of swine tendons – long term effects of exercise on the digital extensors. Connective tissue research 1980;7(3):177–83. Epub 1980/01/01.
76. Gillis CL, Meagher DM, Pool RR, et al. Ultrasonographically detected changes in equine superficial digital flexor tendons during the first months of race training. American journal of veterinary research 1993;54(11):1797–802. Epub 1993/11/01.
77. Smith RK, Birch H, Patterson-Kane J, et al. Should equine athletes commence training during skeletal development?: changes in tendon matrix associated with development, ageing, function and exercise. Equine veterinary journal Supplement 1999;30:201–9. Epub 2000/02/05.
78. Patterson-Kane JC, Wilson AM, Firth EC, et al. Comparison of collagen fibril populations in the superficial digital flexor tendons of exercised and nonexercised thoroughbreds. Equine veterinary journal 1997;29(2):121–5. Epub 1997/03/01.
79. Birch HL, Wilson AM, Goodship AE. Physical activity: does long-term, high-intensity exercise in horses result in tendon degeneration? J Appl Physiol 2008;105(6):1927–33. Epub 2008/10/04.
80. Birch HL, Bailey AJ, Goodship AE. Macroscopic 'degeneration' of equine superficial digital flexor tendon is accompanied by a change in extracellular matrix composition. Equine veterinary journal 1998;30(6):534–9. Epub 1998/12/09.
81. Cauvin ERJ. An investigation into the roles of transforming growth factor-beta (TGFb) in the development, adaptation and repair of equine tendons. University of London; 2001.
82. Perez-Castro AV, Vogel KG. In situ expression of collagen and proteoglycan genes during development of fibrocartilage in bovine deep flexor tendon. Journal of orthopaedic research: official publication of the Orthopaedic Research Society 1999;17(1):139–48. Epub 1999/03/12.
83. Goodman SA, May SA, Heinegard D, et al. Tenocyte response to cyclical strain and transforming growth factor beta is dependent upon age and site of origin. Biorheology 2004;41(5):613–28. Epub 2004/10/13.
84. Dudhia J, Scott CM, Draper ER, et al. Aging enhances a mechanically-induced reduction in tendon strength by an active process involving matrix metalloproteinase activity. Aging cell 2007;6(4):547–56. Epub 2007/06/21.
85. van Weeren PR, Barneveld A. Study design to evaluate the influence of exercise on the development of the musculoskeletal system of foals up to age 11 months. Equine veterinary journal Supplement 1999(31):4–8. Epub 2000/09/22.
86. Kasashima Y, Smith RK, Birch HL, et al. Exercise-induced tendon hypertrophy: cross-sectional area changes during growth are influenced by exercise. Equine veterinary journal Supplement 2002(34):264–8. Epub 2002/10/31.
87. Moffat PA, Firth EC, Rogers CW, et al. The influence of exercise during growth on ultrasonographic parameters of the superficial digital flexor tendon of young Thoroughbred horses. Equine veterinary journal 2008;40(2):136–40. Epub 2007/12/21.
88. Cherdchutham W, Meershoek LS, van Weeren PR, et al. Effects of exercise on biomechanical properties of the superficial digital flexor tendon in foals. American journal of veterinary research 2001;62(12):1859–64. Epub 2002/01/05.
89. Cherdchutham W, Becker CK, Spek ER, et al. Effects of exercise on the diameter of collagen fibrils in the central core and periphery of the superficial digital flexor tendon in foals. American journal of veterinary research 2001;62(10):1563–70. Epub 2001/10/11.
90. Kasashima Y, Takahashi T, Birch HL, et al. Can exercise modulate the maturation of functionally different immature tendons in the horse? J Appl Physiol 2008;104(2):416–22. Epub 2007/12/15.
91. Cherdchutham W, Becker C, Smith RK, et al. Age-related changes and effect of exercise on the molecular composition of immature equine superficial digital flexor tendons. Equine veterinary journal Supplement 1999(31):86–94. Epub 2000/09/22.
92. Webbon PM. A post mortem study of equine digital flexor tendons. Equine veterinary journal 1977;9(2):61–7. Epub 1977/04/01.
93. Smith RK, Birch HL, Goodman S, et al. The influence of ageing and exercise on tendon growth and degeneration – hypotheses for the initiation and prevention of strain-induced tendinopathies. Comparative biochemistry and physiology Part A, Molecular & integrative physiology 2002;133(4):1039–50. Epub 2002/12/18.
94. Tsuzaki M, Guyton G, Garrett W, et al. IL-1 beta induces COX2, MMP-1, -3 and -13, ADAMTS-4, IL-1 beta and IL-6 in human tendon cells. Journal of orthopaedic research: official publication of the Orthopaedic Research Society 2003;21(2):256–64. Epub 2003/02/06.
95. Crevier-Denoix N, Collobert C, Pourcelot P, et al. Mechanical properties of pathological equine superficial digital flexor tendons. Equine veterinary journal Supplement 1997(23):23–6. Epub 1997/05/01.
96. Birch HL, Bailey JV, Bailey AJ, et al. Age-related changes to the molecular and cellular components of equine flexor tendons. Equine veterinary journal 1999;31(5):391–6. Epub 1999/10/03.
97. Watkins JP, Auer JA, Gay S, et al. Healing of surgically created defects in the equine superficial digital flexor tendon: collagen-type transformation and tissue morphologic reorganization. American journal of veterinary

research 1985;46(10):2091–6. Epub 1985/10/01.

98. Kristoffersen M, Ohberg L, Johnston C, et al. Neovascularisation in chronic tendon injuries detected with colour Doppler ultrasound in horse and man: implications for research and treatment. Knee surgery, sports traumatology, arthroscopy: official journal of the ESSKA 2005;13(6):505–8. Epub 2005/05/03.
99. Saxne T, Heinegard D. Cartilage oligomeric matrix protein: a novel marker of cartilage turnover detectable in synovial fluid and blood. British journal of rheumatology 1992;31(9): 583–91. Epub 1992/09/01.
100. Neidhart M, Hauser N, Paulsson M, et al. Small fragments of cartilage oligomeric matrix protein in synovial fluid and serum as markers for cartilage degradation. British journal of rheumatology 1997;36(11):1151–60. Epub 1997/12/24.
101. Smith MR, Wright IM, Minshall GJ, et al. Increased cartilage oligomeric matrix protein concentrations in equine digital flexor tendon sheath synovial fluid predicts intrathecal tendon damage. Veterinary surgery: VS 2011;40(1):54–8. Epub 2010/11/17.
102. Jackson BE, Smith RK, Price JS. A molecular marker of type I collagen metabolism reflects changes in connective tissue remodelling associated with injury to the equine superficial digital flexor tendon. Equine veterinary journal 2003;35(2):211–13. Epub 2003/03/18.
103. Dowling BA, Dart AJ, Hodgson DR, et al. Superficial digital flexor tendonitis in the horse. Equine veterinary journal 2000;32(5):369–78. Epub 2000/10/19.
104. Frean SP, Lees P. Effects of polysulfated glycosaminoglycan and hyaluronan on prostaglandin E2 production by cultured equine synoviocytes. American journal of veterinary research 2000; 61(5):499–505. Epub 2000/05/10.
105. Henninger R, Bramlage LR, Schneider, R, editors. Short term effects of superior check ligament desmotomy and percutaneous tendon splitting as a treatment of acute tendinitis. American Association of Equine Practitioners; 1990.
106. Bramlage LR, editor. Superior check ligament desmotomy as a treatment for superþcial digital ßexor tendinitis. American Association of Equine Practitioners; 1986.
107. Bramlage LR, Rantanen NW, Genovese RL, et al, editors. Long term effects of surgical treatment of superþcial digital ßexor tendinitis by superior check ligament desmotomy. American Association of Equine Practitioners; 1988.
108. Gibson KT, Burbidge HM, Pfeiffer DU. Superficial digital flexor tendonitis in thoroughbred race horses: outcome following non-surgical treatment and superior check desmotomy. Australian veterinary journal 1997;75(9):631–5. Epub 1997/11/05.
109. Reef VB, Genovese RL, Davis WM, editors. Initial long term results of horses with superficial digital flexor tendinitis treated with intralesional beta-aminoproprionitrile fumarate. American Association of Equine Practitioners; 1997.
110. Gaughan EM, Nixon AJ, Krook LP, et al. Effects of sodium hyaluronate on tendon healing and adhesion formation in horses. American journal of veterinary research 1991;52(5):764–73. Epub 1991/05/01.
111. Dahlgren LA, van der Meulen MC, Bertram JE, et al. Insulin-like growth factor-I improves cellular and molecular aspects of healing in a collagenase-induced model of flexor tendinitis. Journal of orthopaedic research: official publication of the Orthopaedic Research Society 2002;20(5):910–19. Epub 2002/10/18.
112. Dowling BA, Dart AJ, Hodgson DR, et al. Recombinant equine growth hormone does not affect the in vitro biomechanical properties of equine superficial digital flexor tendon. Veterinary surgery: VS 2002;31(4): 325–30. Epub 2002/07/03.
113. Godwin EE, Young NJ, Dudhia J, et al. Implantation of bone marrow-derived mesenchymal stem cells demonstrates improved outcome in horses with overstrain injury of the superficial digital flexor tendon. Equine veterinary journal 2012;44(1):25–32. Epub 2011/05/28.
114. Herthel DJ, editor. Enhanced suspensory ligament healing in 100 horses by stem cells and other bone marrow components. American Association of Equine Practitioners; 2001.
115. Smith RK, Korda M, Blunn GW, et al. Isolation and implantation of autologous equine mesenchymal stem cells from bone marrow into the superficial digital flexor tendon as a potential novel treatment. Equine veterinary journal 2003;35(1):99–102. Epub 2003/01/30.
116. Smith RK, McGuigan MP, Hyde JT, et al. In vitro evaluation of nonrigid support systems for the equine metacarpophalangeal joint. Equine veterinary journal 2002;34(7):726–31. Epub 2002/11/29.
117. Dyson SJ, editor. Proximal suspensory desmitis in the forelimb and the hindlimb. American Association of Equine Practitioners; 2000.
118. Crowe OM, Dyson SJ, Wright IM, et al. Treatment of chronic or recurrent proximal suspensory desmitis using radial pressure wave therapy in the horse. Equine veterinary journal 2004;36(4):313–16. Epub 2004/05/28.
119. Thorpe CT, Clegg PD, Birch HL. A review of tendon injury: why is the equine superficial digital flexor tendon most at risk? Equine veterinary journal 2010;42(2):174–80. Epub 2010/02/17.
120. Kadler KE, Holmes DF, Trotter JA, et al. Collagen fibril formation. The Biochemical journal 1996;316(Pt 1): 1–11. Epub 1996/05/15.

Biomechanics of locomotion in the athletic horse

10

Eric Barrey

CHAPTER CONTENTS

Introduction

The horse is a super athlete who often suffers from injuries of its locomotor apparatus because of human management errors (nutrition, training, shoeing, and breeding), bad environmental conditions (tracks, weather) and/or an unfavorable constitution (limb conformation, genetics). In stables specialized in gallop racing, about 53% to 68% of the wastage in racehorses is due to lamenesses.[1,2] This economic disaster justifies the great effort now being put into equine locomotion research, including clinical applications and techniques for preventing lameness. Economic constraints also favor the development of early performance evaluation in order to improve the training and selection of young horses. This chapter presents a review on equine locomotion and the applications of gait analysis. Current knowledge concerning the equine locomotion variables in various sporting disciplines and the influence of training are discussed. Finally, a survey of the practical applications of equine gait analysis will be presented.

Locomotion analysis

The body of the horse is composed of a set of rigid segments articulated one to another. Consequently, the body of the horse follows exactly the same mechanical laws as a series of inanimate objects (Fig. 10.1). However, these laws need to be applied carefully because the mechanical equations which determine the motions of a set of articulated body segments are much more complicated than those that determine the motion of a single inanimate object like a bullet. There are two complimentary methods for studying the body in motion: kinetics and kinematics.

- *Kinetics or dynamics* studies the cause of the motion, which can be explained by the force applied to the body, its mass distribution and its dimensions. Kinetics is concerned with forces, energy, and work which are also in relation to kinematic variables such as acceleration and velocity. Acceleration can be directly measured by specific sensors. However, acceleration is defined as an instantaneous change of velocity (i.e. the derivative of the velocity against time). Consequently, it can be deduced from velocity data obtained in kinematics by the displacement measurements.

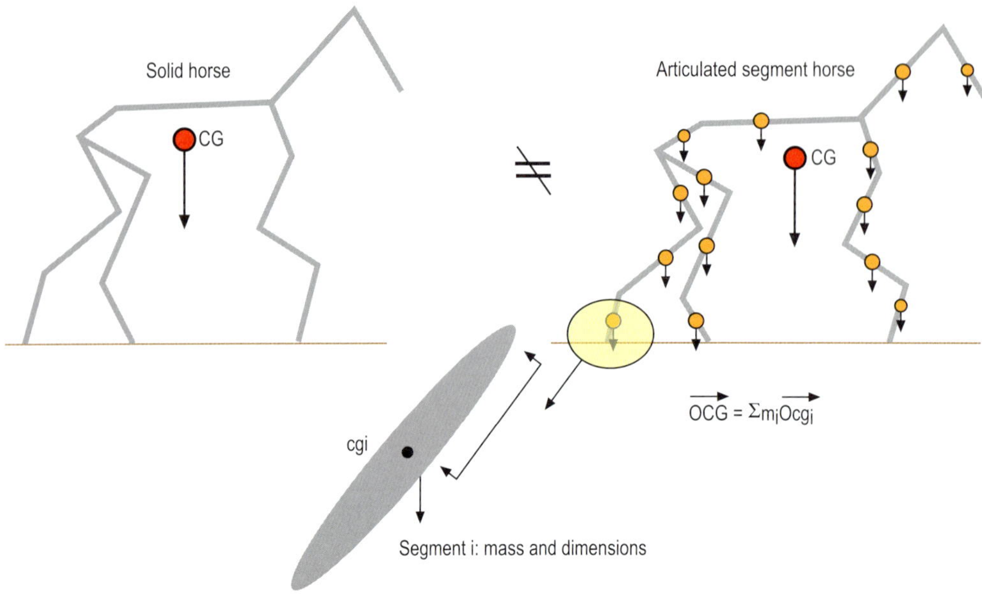

$\overrightarrow{OCG} = \Sigma m_i \overrightarrow{Ocg_i}$

Fig 10.1 A horse mechanical model composed of articulated body segments. It is very different from a mechanical model with only one solid segment. For each segment (i) of the body, the center of gravity (cg_i) and the moment of inertia can be calculated. The location of the general center of gravity (CG) of the horse can be calculated by considering the mass and the coordinates of each center of gravity segment.

- *Kinematics* studies the changes in the position of the body segments in space during a specified time. The motions are described quantitatively by linear and angular variables which relate time, displacement, velocity and acceleration. No reference is made in kinematics to the cause of motion. The kinematic approach is more commonly employed, probably because it is easier to measure and visualize some displacements or velocities than to measure and imagine some forces, moments or accelerations applied to the body.

Kinematic analysis

The use of chronophotography was first developed by Muybridge and Marey for animal locomotion analysis. Currently new technology, using high-speed cameras (16 mm–500 images/s), is used for example to film the locomotion of Standardbred horses from a camera car under track conditions.[3] Markers are used which are composed of small white spots or half spheres glued onto the skin over standard anatomical locations (Fig. 10.2A).[4,5] They are intended to indicate the approximate instantaneous center of rotation of the joint.[6,7] However, the skin displacements over the skeleton during the locomotion generate some artifacts especially in the proximal joints.[8,9]

The processing of the film for collecting the joint marker coordinates is undertaken using a computer. This is a relatively time-consuming task, but many time and linear characteristics of the strides can be obtained for describing individual gait variations. With the improvement of the video camera sensors (CCD) many professional high-speed video cameras (100–2000 images/s) and home video cameras (PAL or NTSC Standard: 25–30 images/s or 50–60 frames/s) can be employed for locomotion analysis. The video signal can be treated by a video interface in order to digitize the images which are then analyzed by the appropriate software to collect semi-automatically or automatically the marker coordinates in space and time.[10] A more sophisticated motion analysis system uses active markers which consist of photodiodes (modified Cartesian Optoelectronic Dynamic Anthropometer CODA-3). The advantage of this system is its good resolution (0.2–2.6 mm) in three dimensions, high recording frequency (300 Hz) and the automatic tracking possibilities of the active markers.[11] The main disadvantage is that the subject needs to be equipped with many photodiodes connected to wires.

Most equine locomotion studies show two-dimensional motion analysis, but some systems including four or more video cameras make it possible to reconstruct the motion in three dimensions and to analyze the limb motions of both sides.[12,13] One limit of these sophisticated gait analysis systems is the restricted field of view. This is only about five meters which corresponds to several walking strides or one trotting stride. In order to analyze sporting exercise in a wider field (up to 30 m), a camera panning technique has been developed and has been used to study gait parameters in dressage and jumping horses.[10,14,15] This technique can be used for the kinematic analysis of athletic locomotion under real exercise conditions (Fig. 10.2B).

After filming, the operator needs to track manually, semi-automatically or automatically, the coordinates of the markers on each image of the film. In most of the systems, the tracking phase is a long task because there are a lot of images to analyze and as the markers are not always easy to detect automatically, manual supervision is required. Nowadays, the use of specific algorithms such as direct linear transform (DLT) is an efficient way to automatically determine the trajectory of the markers. This makes it possible to use these systems for practical applications such as lameness quantification or athletic gait evaluation.

After collecting the coordinates of the markers, the linear and angular velocities can be obtained by computing the first derivative of the trajectories and angles with respect to time. If the filming image frequency is high, the second order derivative of a trajectory or angular variations with respect to time using appropriate smoothing and filtering techniques provides linear and angular acceleration data. The advantage of kinematics methods is that you can obtain all the kinematic parameters (displacement, velocity, and linear

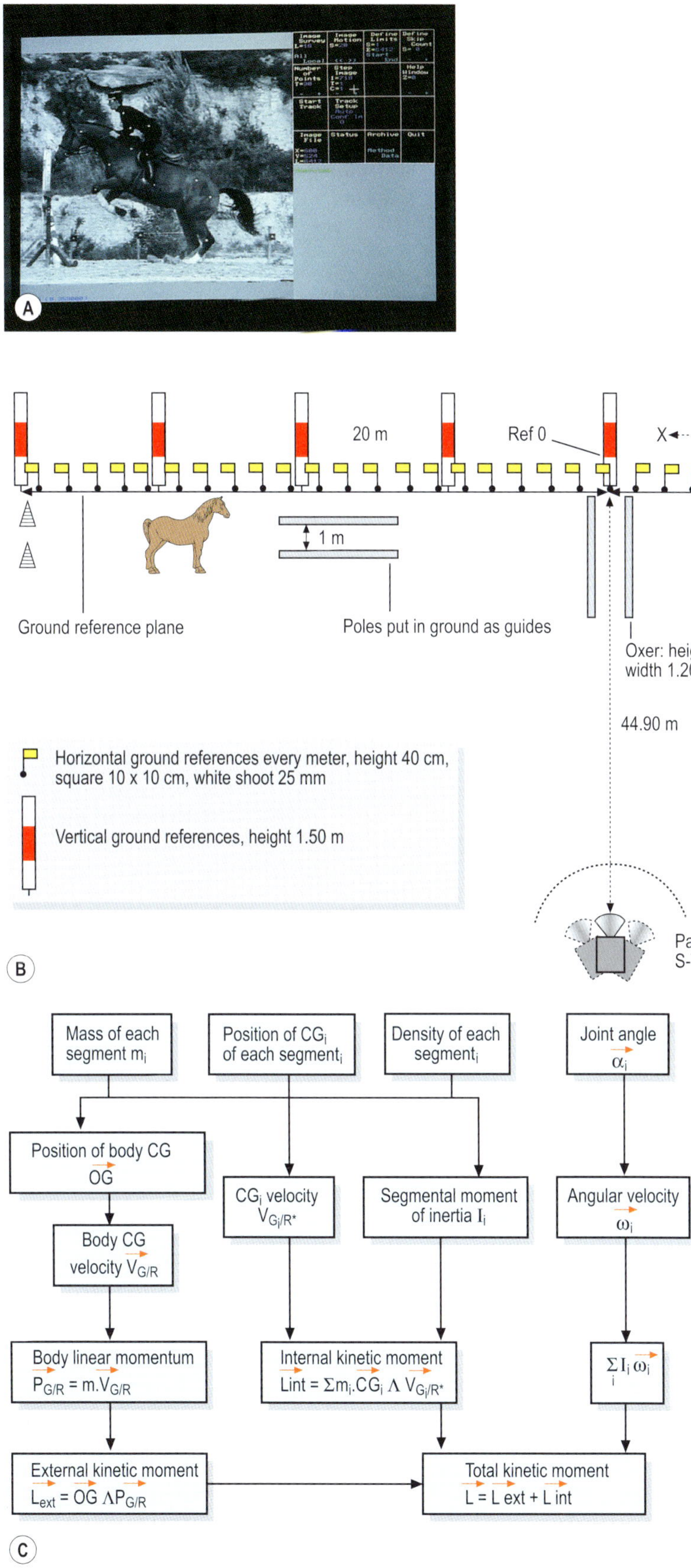

Fig 10.2 Example of two-dimensional kinematic study of jumping horse.
(A) One image extracted from the video film. It shows the horse and rider equiped with white anatomical markers. These markers are used to identify the location of each joint on each image.
(B) Film recording procedure for a panning camera system. This method allowed filming and analyzing the motion on a large field (30 m), as in jumping exercise. A set of ground references were placed parallel to the horse trajectory.
(C) Data analysis procedure to compute the center of gravity (CG) and total kinetic moment (L). After tracking the markers of each joint, the coordinates data were used to calculate the center of gravity (CG_i) of each segments, the velocity (Vg_i), the moment of inertia (I_i), the angles (α_i), the angular velocity (ω_i) and the external and internal kinetic moment.

acceleration, angle of rotation, angular velocity and angular acceleration) of the identified segments. If the center of gravity and the moment of inertia of each segment can be determined by measuring their mass distribution and their dimensions, it is possible to calculate the kinetic parameters (forces and kinetic moment), which determine the motion of each segment, from the kinematic data. Finally, the kinetic energy can be estimated for each segment and for the whole body in motion. Several methods have been described to estimate the location of center of gravity and the moment of inertia of each segment (Fig. 10.2C).[15,16,17]

Kinetic analysis

Another approach to the study of the biomechanics of locomotion is to measure either the external forces applied to the body or the accelerations of the center of gravity of the body segments. Marey (1873) was the first author to use a pressure sensor attached to the ground surface of a horse shoe and accelerometers attached to the limbs to measure the hoof ground contact durations at the various gaits.[18] All the sensors measured forces using pneumatic principles. The variations in pressure generated by the various transducers were recorded by tracing curves with a portable pneumotachograph.

Ground reaction forces

Modern sensor technology is much improved and is capable of making accurate measurements over a large range of conditions. However, the measurement principles have remained identical. The external forces are measured using electronic force sensors which record the ground reaction forces when the hooves are in contact with the ground. The sensors can be installed either on the ground in a force plate device or in a shoe attached to the hoof.[19] The force plates can provide the force amplitude and orientation (vector coordinates in three dimensions, Fig. 10.3), the coordinates of the point of application of the force and the moment value at this point.[20] The accuracy of this type of device is usually good but the sensitive surface is rather small (about 0.5 m^2) and a visual control of the hoof trajectory is required.

In human biomechanics, the treadmill has been used to measure vertical ground reaction forces in standardized exercise conditions. In equine biomechanics, vertical ground reaction forces were measured for all four limbs simultaneously with the treadmill integrated force measuring system [21] (Fig. 10.4). After collecting reference data on warmblood horses walking and trotting [22], it has been used for dressage gait analysis and lameness evaluation in standardized conditions of speed, hardiness of the ground, environment.[23, 24]

In order to measure the ground reaction forces during various exercises, several authors have developed hoof force shoes including one or several force sensors (Fig. 10.5).[18,25–29] Depending on their design, these devices can give between one and three components of the ground reaction forces and the point of application. They are generally less accurate than the force plate and their main disadvantage is the additional weight and thickness of the special shoe. Recently, another indirect ambulatory technique of ground reaction force evaluation was proposed using strain gauges glued onto the hoof wall. After the training of the appropriate artificial neural networks, the ground reaction forces can be estimated from the hoof wall deformations.[30]

Acceleration analysis

Acceleration analysis is a kinetic method which measures instantaneous change of velocity which is produced by applying a force on a solid during the same duration. Acceleration measurements are performed using small sensors (accelerometers) which should be firmly attached to the body segment under study. These sensors are made of a small suspended mass giving a signal which is proportional to the acceleration.

A sudden change in velocity can give a high acceleration or deceleration (decrease of acceleration) even if the displacement is small. The acceleration vector is proportional to the resultant force applied to the body's center of gravity and its measurement provides a convenient way to study the kinetics of a body in motion. In order to analyze horse locomotion, the accelerometer should be placed as near as possible to the body center of gravity. The caudal part of the sternum between the right and left pectoralis ascendens muscles at the level of the girth provides a good compromise between transducer stability and closeness to the horse's center of gravity (about 65 cm dorsocaudally at the gallop). The acceleration signal is transmitted to a PC or recorded with a small data logger placed in the saddle pad (Fig. 10.6A). The first application of this gait analysis system (Equimetrix TM) was used for evaluation of harnessed trotters and then for sport and racing horses.[31] The acceleration signal, such as dorsoventral acceleration at the trot, could be treated by signal analysis procedures in order to extract the dynamic and temporal stride variables such as stride frequency, regularity, symmetry and power in the three axes (Fig. 10.6B). Calculating the double integral of the linear acceleration makes it possible to find kinematic variables (linear or angular displacement) such as the instantaneous displacement of the saddle in space.[32] Several examples of gait variables calculated from acceleration data will be presented in the following paragraphs.

Acceleration measurements could also be employed for analyzing the energy characteristics of shocks and vibrations which are transient in the hoof.[33–35] An accelerometer could be fixed on the hoof wall in order to measure the maximal deceleration of the hoof impact on the ground and the vibration frequency (Fig. 10.7). The influence of horse shoes and ground surface characteristics could be studied using this method.

The main advantage of using an accelerometric transducer is the simplicity of the measuring technique. It can easily be used under field conditions. The main limitation is that the measurements are given with respect to a set of body axes and consequently it is not easy to calculate the acceleration, velocity or displacement values with respect to a set of ground axes.

Conditions of gait measurements: treadmill exercise vs. ground exercise

Under laboratory conditions it is possible to study the locomotion of horses running on an experimental track or on a treadmill. The latter provides an excellent means of controlling the regularity of the gaits because the velocity and slope of the treadmill belt are entirely fixed by the operator. In order to analyze the gait of a horse without stress, some pre-experimental exercise sessions are required to accustom it to this unusual exercise condition.[36] The horse adapts rapidly at the trot, and stride measurements can be undertaken beginning at the third session. For the walk, many stride parameters are not stable even after the 9th training session. Within a session, a minimum of five minutes of walking or trotting is required to reach a steady state of locomotion.

Many fundamental locomotion studies have been performed on commercially available high speed treadmills, since the development of the first installation of this type of machine at the Swedish University of Agricultural Science in Uppsala.[37] At the beginning of human treadmill use, it was suggested that locomotion on a treadmill would be exactly the same as on the ground.[38] This hypothesis

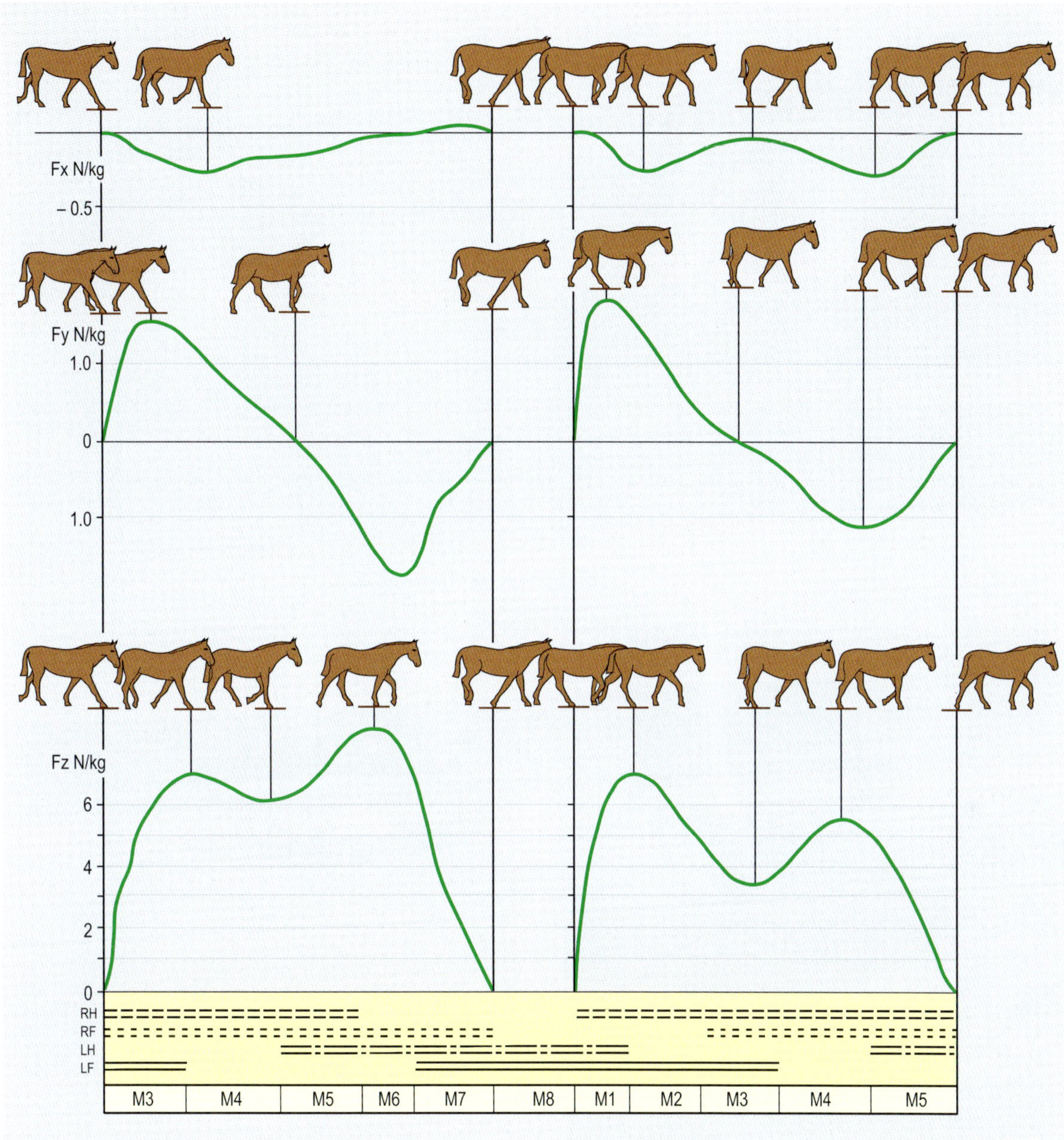

Fig 10.3 Limb positioning at the time of characteristic ground reaction force amplitudes of the right fore and hindlimbs of a clinically sound Dutch Warmblood horse at normal walk. The phase of the concurrently loaded limbs are presented in a bar diagram.

Reprinted from Schamhardt HC, Merkens HW, van Osch GJVM. Ground reaction force analysis of horses ridden at the walk and trot. In: Persson SGB, Lindholm A, Jeffcott LB, eds. Equine Exercise Physiology. 3rd edn., ed . Davis: ICEEP publications; 1991:120–127, with permission from the ICEEP.

did not take into account the fact that the human body is not a rigid body system but an articulated set of segments. In horses, it was demonstrated experimentally that the stride parameters are modified in flat and inclined exercise at trot and canter.[39] At the same speed, the stride frequency was lower on the treadmill and the stride length was longer than in over ground conditions (Fig. 10.8A). The exercise on a flat treadmill generated lower cardiac and blood lactate responses than exercise on the track at the same velocities.[39,40] In trotters tested under two training tracks and treadmill conditions, there were no significant differences in locomotor and physiological variables between tracks but the treadmill had the same influence as in saddle horses.[41] In order to reproduce approximately the same energetic exercise on a treadmill, it was found that a treadmill incline of 3.5% gives the same heart rate response as in over ground condition (Fig. 10.8B).

The mechanical reasons for these differences are not entirely known today but some explanations have been suggested by the experimental and theoretical results. The treadmill belt is driven by the motor and it helps the horse limbs to go back (Fig. 10.9). The speed of the treadmill belt fluctuates in relationship to the hoof impact on the belt.[30] The total kinetic energy of human runners filmed at the same speed on a flat track and treadmill was calculated using the kinematic data (all the body segments taken into account). It was found that the total kinetic energy was reduced by a factor of 10 on the treadmill compared to on the track.[42] This difference was mainly explained by a reduction of the kinetic energy of each limb

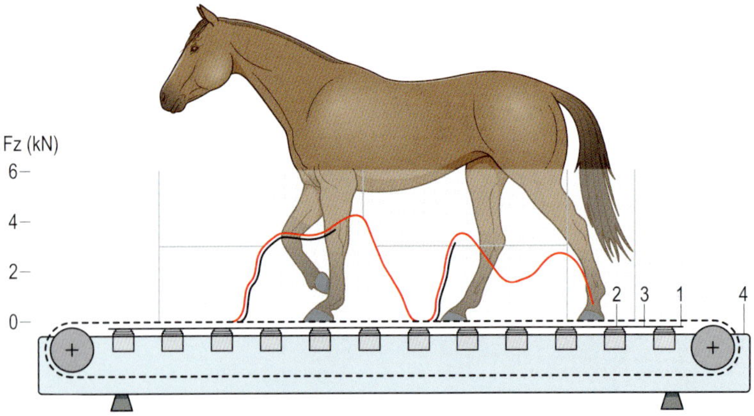

Fig 10.4 Illustration of the overhead and cross-sectional lateral views of treadmill-integrated force measuring system. This instrumented treadmill is capable of determining the vertical ground reaction forces and the hoof positions during stance phase of all limbs simultaneously. Note: Fz, vertical ground reaction force in kilo-newton; R1–R9, piezoelectric force sensors of the right side of the treadmill.

Reprinted from Weishaupt MA, Hogg HP, Wiestner T, Denoth J, Stüssi E, Auer JA. Instrumented treadmill for measuring vertical ground reaction forces in horses. Am J Vet Res. 2002; 63(4):520–527,with permission from the American Journal of Veterinary Research, http://avmajournals.avma.org/loi/ajvr.

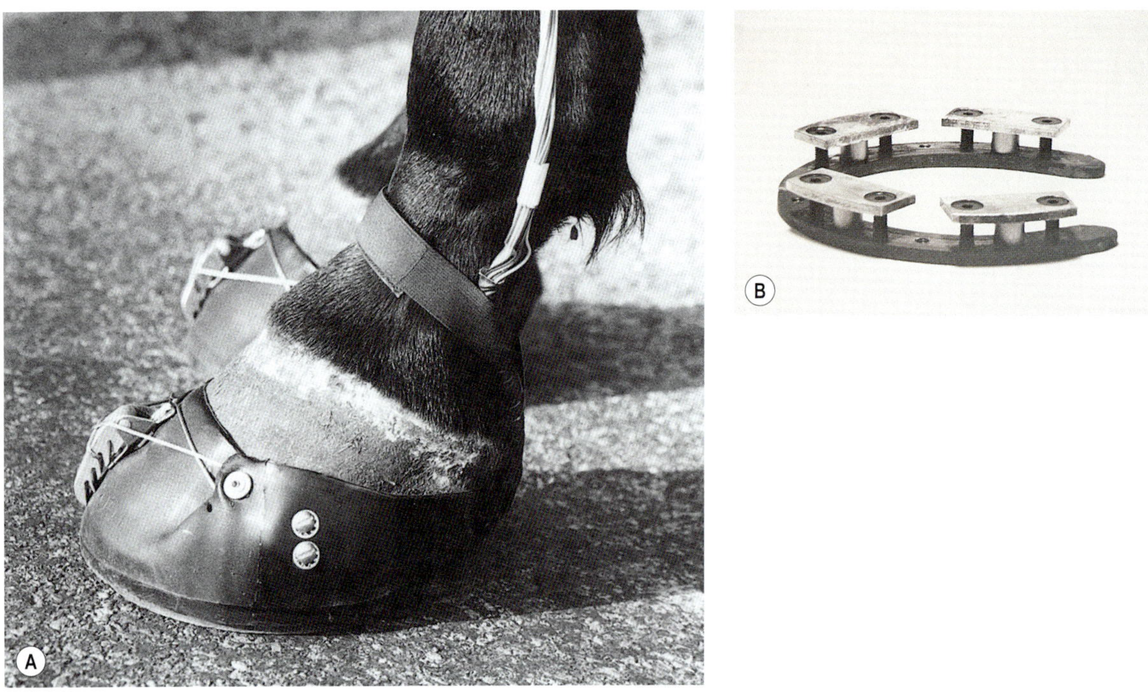

Fig 10.5 Horse shoe for measuring vertical ground reaction forces **(A)**. The hoof was supported by four force transducers (strain gauges Wheatstone bridge) in order to measure hoof force distribution between heels, quarters and toe **(B)**.

Reprinted from Barrey E. Investigation of the vertical hoof force distribution in the equine forelimb with an instrumented horseboot. Equine Vet J 1990; (suppl 9):35–38, with permission from the Equine Veterinary Journal.

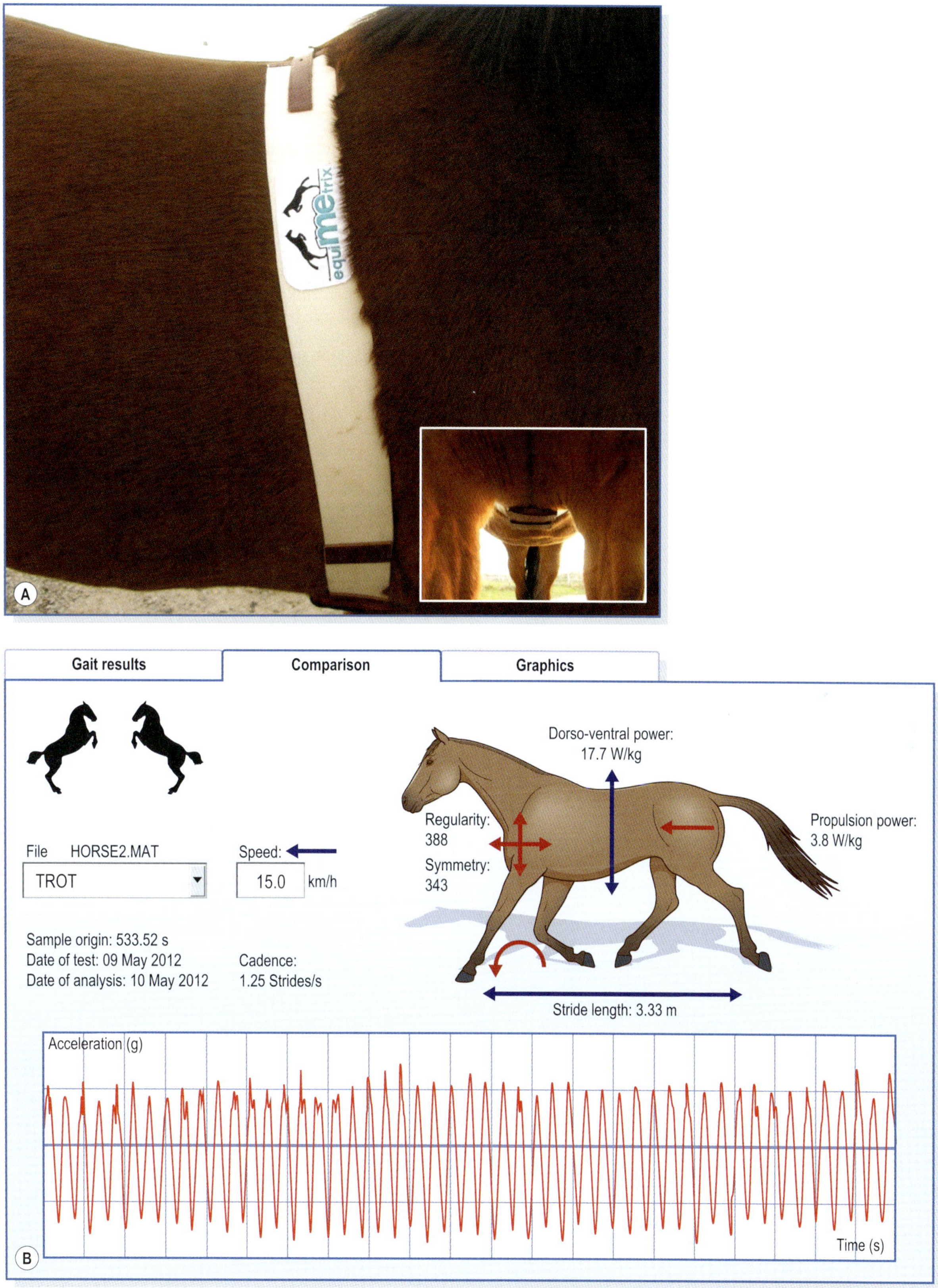

Fig 10.6 Accelerometric gait analysis system Equimetrix™ (Barrey et al. 1994).
(A) Three dimensional accelerometers are fixed on the sternum by an elastic belt or the girth of the saddle. The accelerations are recorded continuously during the exercise. Then, the software calculates gait variables such as stride frequency, regularity, symmetry and power in the longitudinal, dorso-ventral and latero-medial axes.
(B) Example of gait analysis results calculated at the trot. The peaks correspond to the maximum loading of the diagonal. The valleys correspond to the suspension phases. The results can be compared to reference values of different breeds, age and ability.

and arm segment, which moved with a lower amplitude around the total body center of gravity on the treadmill as compared to under track conditions. However, these results cannot be extrapolated to the horse because the measurements and calculations do not relate to quadrupedal locomotion.

At a slow trot, a 6% inclination of the treadmill tends to increase the stride duration and significantly increases the stance duration of the forelimbs and hind limbs.[43] Kinematic analysis has confirmed that the hind limbs generated higher propulsion work on the inclined, rather than flat, treadmill. The inclination of the treadmill did not change the stride length nor did it change the stance, swing and stride duration in a cantering Thoroughbred.[44]

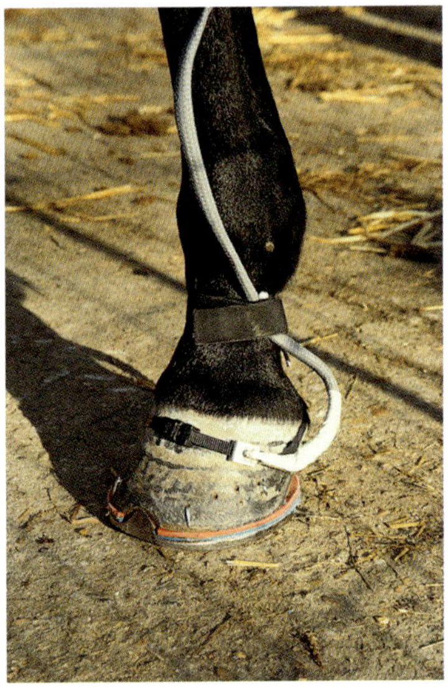

Fig 10.7 Accelerometer fixed on the hoof to study the shocks and vibrations of the hoof after impact on the ground. The influence of the ground surface and the shoe on the shock damping was studied using this transducer.
Barrey et al. 1991, 1993.

Response to exercise: velocity-related changes in gaits and stride characteristics

Gait terminology and definitions of stride characteristics

Gait variety and complexity have always created difficulties when it is necessary to choose adequate terminology to describe the locomotor phenomenon. Some efforts have been made to define a standard terminology for use in describing equine locomotion.[45–47] A *gait* can be defined as a complex and strictly coordinated rhythmic and automatic movement of the limbs and the entire body of the animal which result in the production of progressive movements. A two, three or four beat gait corresponds to the number of hoof impacts that can be heard during a stride of trot, canter and gallop,

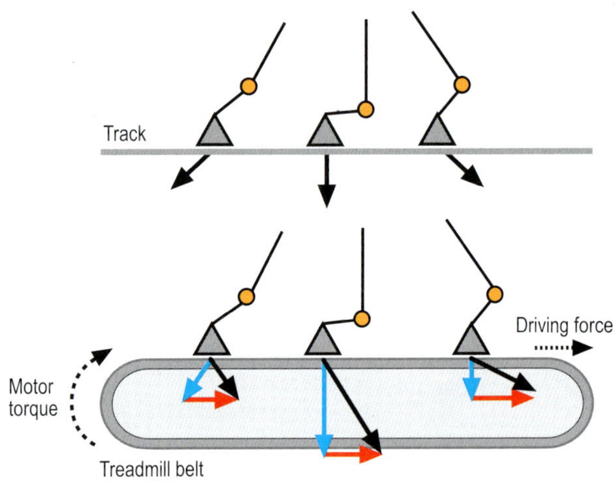

Fig 10.9 Schematic diagram of hoof force differences in overground and treadmill locomotion. The additional force of the treadmill motor acts on the hoof. It could explain the decrease of work, increase of stride length observed in treadmill exercise.

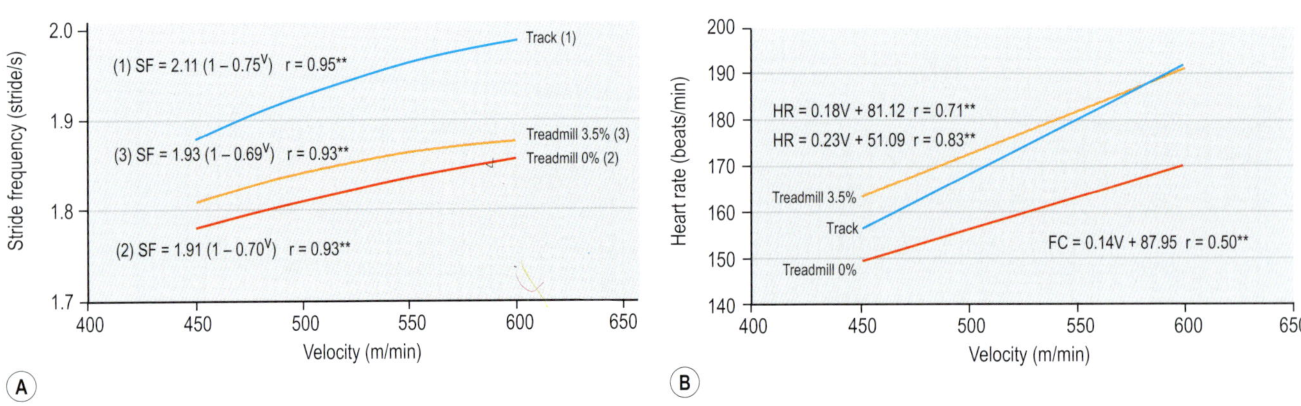

Fig 10.8 Comparison of the stride frequency **(A)** and heart rate **(B)** of horses galloping of track, flat treadmill and 3.5% inclined treadmill. At the same velocity, the stride frequency is lower on the treadmill (i.e. stride length longer) than on the track. The heart rate response is the same on track and 3.5% inclined treadmill.
Barrey et al. 1993.

respectively. The sounds are related to the footfall sequence of the gait but small asynchrony cannot be detected audibly. To describe the footfall sequence of each gait, it is useful to name the four limbs: right forelimb (RF), left forelimb (LF), right hindlimb (RH) and left hindlimb (LH). Many methods have been proposed to describe more precisely in time and space the limb movements: drawings, chronophotograpies, stick bar (Fig. 10.10), phase and pie diagrams.[18, 48–50]

The stride is defined as a full cycle of limb motion. Since the pattern is repeated, the beginning of the stride can be at any point in the pattern and the end of that stride at the same place in the beginning of the next pattern. A complete limb cycle includes a stance phase when the limb is in contact with the ground, a swing phase when the limb is not in contact with the ground and a suspension phase when none of the hooves is in contact with the ground. The stride duration is composed of the stride stance phase (total duration of ground contact) plus the suspension phase. It is also equal to the sum of the stance and swing phase duration of one limb. The stride frequency corresponds to the number of strides performed per unit of time. The stride frequency is equal to the inverse of stride duration and it is usually expressed in stride/s or in hertz (Hz).

During a unipodal stance phase, only one limb is in contact with the ground as in the gallop. One fore and hind limb can be synchronized in two different ways:

1. During a diagonal stance phase, for example at the trot, a hind limb and the contralateral forelimb are in contact with the ground at the same time. The left diagonal is composed of the left forelimb and right hindlimb; the right diagonal is composed of the right forelimb and left hindlimb.
2. During a lateral stance phase, for example at the pace, the hindlimb and forelimb of the same side are in contact with the ground at the same time.

When the fore and hind limbs hit the ground non-synchronously during a lateral or a diagonal stance phase, the time elapsed between the hindlimb and forelimb contact is called the advanced placement. It is positive if the hindlimb hits the ground first. Similarly, the advanced lift-off can be measured between the hooves at lift off from the ground.

The stride length corresponds to the distance between two successive hoof placements of the same limb. Overreach or overtrack is defined as the distance between the hindlimb imprint and the ipsilateral forelimb imprint. It can be positive or negative if the imprint of the hindlimb is in front of the forelimb imprint (positive) or behind it (negative).

The number of lines defined by the successive hoof imprints on the ground defines the number of tracks. This qualitative information characterizes the transverse motion of the gait. If the horse locomotion is slow and straight, there should be two tracks because the forefeet are exactly in the same line as the ipsilateral hind feet. In some dressage exercises such as 'shoulder in', 'haunches-in', quarters-in', 'quarters-out' or 'half pass' the horse can use 2–4 tracks. During the examination of a hind limb lameness three or four tracks can be observed and usually the lame hindlimb follows one of the median tracks. A harness racehorse at the fast trot usually shows four tracks with the two hindlimbs most abaxial.

Variety of gaits

Main characteristics of the equine gaits are described in Table 10.1 Within each gait are continuous variations from slow speed with a collected gait to higher speed with an extended gait. Two types of gait can be distinguished by the symmetry of the limb movement sequence with respect to time and the median plane of the horse:

- *symmetric gaits*: walk, trot, toelt and pace
- *asymmetric gaits*: canter, transverse and rotary gallop.

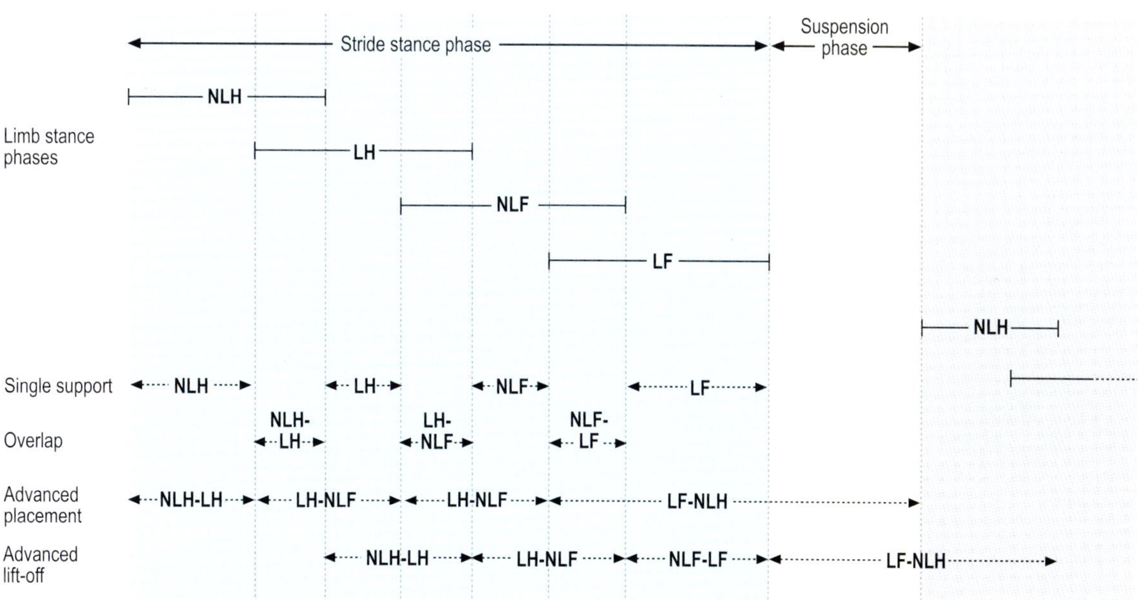

Fig 10.10 Example of temporal stride variables at the gallop. Bars indicate the stance phase of the limbs: NLH non-lead hindlimb, LH lead hindlimb, NLF non-lead forelimb, LF lead forelimb.

Reprinted from Clayton HM. Termiology for the description of equine jumping kinematics. J Equine Vet Sci 1989;9:341–348, with permission from Elsevier.

Table 10.1 Gait characteristics

CLASSIFICATION	GAIT	GAIT VARIATIONS	FOOTFALL SEQUENCE	RHYTHM (beat/ stride)	TYPE OF SYMMETRY	SPEED (m/s)	STRIDE LENGTH (m)	STRIDE FREQUENCY (stride/s)	LIMB STANCE PHASE (s or % stride)	SUSPENSION PHASE (s or % stride)
Symmetric gaits	Walk	Collected, medium, extended	RH,RF,LH,LF	4	Right/left bipedal	1.2–1.8	1.5–1.9	0.8–1.1	65–75%	0
	Toelt = Paso		RH,RF,LH,LF	4	Right/left lateral	3.4–5.3	1.7–2.3	2.23–2.36	40–55%	0
	Trot	Piaffe, passage, collected, medium, extended, flying trot	RH-LF, Susp., LH-RF, Susp.	2	Right/left diagonal	2.8–14.2	1.8–5.9	0.9–2.52	26–53%	0–9%
	Pace		RH-RF, Susp., LH-LF, Susp.	2	Right/left lateral	9.1–16.0	4.5–6.3	1.8–2.4	0.130–0.138s	0.081–0.094s
Asymmetric gaits	Canter	Collected, medium, extended, disunited	Trail.H,Lead.H-Trail.F,Lead.F, Susp.	3	Asymmetry with a phase lag between limb pairs	2.9–9	1.9–4.6	1.6–2.0	0.28–0.30s	0–0.013s
	Gallop	Transverse, rotary	Transverse: Trail.H,Lead.H, Trail.F,Lead.F, Susp.	4	Asymmetry with a phase lag between limb pairs	9–20	4.5–7.2	2.27–2.92	0.085–0.09s	0.063–0.114s 16–28%

Several methods have been proposed to classify the gaits according to their temporal characteristics. The continuum of symmetric gaits was described by a diagram proposed by Hildebrand.[51] The stance duration of the hindlimb was plotted against the lateral advanced placement. On the x-axis, the stance duration of the hindlimb indicates if the gait is walked (no suspension phase) or run (two suspension phases). On the y-axis, the lateral advanced placement quantifies the asynchrony or the phase lag of the lateral fore and hind limbs. The two beat gaits are up and down the diagram and the four beat gaits are in the middle part of the diagram. Another diagram has been proposed for illustrating the diagonal gaits by plotting the hind stance phase duration against the diagonal advanced placement.[52]

Another method based on a series of coupled oscillators has been proposed to describe and simulate both symmetric and asymmetric gaits. This model also has the advantage of describing the gait transitions and unique gaits like 'aubin' and 'traquenard'. The model uses four coupled oscillators which simulate the cyclical patterns of the four limb movements. By using five methods of coupling the oscillators, it was possible to generate all types of equine gaits. This type of functional model can be useful to understand the locomotor control which includes rhythmic pattern generators.

Symmetric gaits

Walk

The walk is a four beat gait with a large overlap time between stance phases of the limbs. This is the slowest equine gait but probably one of the more complex because of overlap and lag phase variability. During lameness examination, the variability of stride regularity and symmetry measured at the walk was higher than at the trot.[53] In dressage horses, the speed of the walk increases from the collected walk (1.37 m/s) to the extended walk (1.82 m/s) and simultaneously there is a small increase in stride frequency.[54] The change in speed was primarily the result of lengthening of the stride by increasing the over-tracking distance. Even in horses trained for dressage, the regular four beat rhythm of the footfall was observed in only one of the six horses measured.

Toelt

Icelandic and Paso fino breeds exhibit a four beat symmetric lateral gait. This gait can be called 'toelt', 'paso', 'rack', 'fox-trot' or 'slow gait'. The toelt is comfortable for the rider because the amplitude of the dorsoventral displacement is lower than at the trot. The speed ranges between 1.7 to 2.3 m/s and the natural gait transition for a toelter is walk-toelt-canter.

Trot

The slow trot is a two beat symmetric diagonal gait. Among the normal variations of the trot of saddle horses, the speed of the gait increases from collected to extended trot. Passage and piaffe are two dressage exercises derived from collected trot. However, their temporal variables are different as it has been shown in the dressage finalists at the Olympic Games in Barcelona.[52] The stride duration is longer (i.e. slower stride frequency) for piaffe (1.08 s) and passage (1.09 s) than for collected trot (0.84). For most of the other temporal variables, collected trot and passage were very similar except for the suspension phase which was shorter in passage. A positive diagonal advanced placement measured at the collected trot was observed in the elite dressage horses.[52, 55] This means that the hindlimb hits the ground about 20–30 ms before the diagonal forelimb.

In harness trotters, the trot is so extended that it can reach a maximum speed of 14.2 m/s with a maximum stride frequency of 2.52 strides/s and a maximum stride length of 5.92 m.[56] The diagonal sequence is usually affected and this particular gait is named the flying-trot. It is a four beat gait because there is an asynchrony of the impact and/or lift off of the diagonal.[57] In most cases the hindlimb touches the ground first (a positive advanced placement). The dissociation at lift off is greater than at impact.

Various trot irregularities can occur during a harness race and the horse can be disqualified by the gait judges. At the aubin, the forelimbs gallop and the hindlimbs trot while at the traquenard, the forelimbs trot and the hindlimbs gallop. A trotter is also disqualified if it breaks into a pace or gallop. With increasing speed the stride length increases linearly but the interference between the hindlimb and the lateral forelimb becomes a limiting factor. A large overreach of the hindlimbs can be performed only if the hindlimbs follow two lateral tracks (track abaxial to the forelimbs) during the swing phase.

Pace

This lateral symmetric gait is used in harness racing mainly in North America and Australia. The maximum speed can be faster than at the flying trot. It is also a four beat-gait at high speeds with dissociation of lateral symmetry at impact and lift off. The hindlimb hits the ground before the ipsilateral forelimb. This lateral advanced placement of the hindlimb is about 26–30 m/s. In comparison with the flying trot there is less limb interference because the lateral sequence avoids any contact between the ipsilateral limbs. Consequently, there are fewer coordination difficulties and it is easier for the horse to increase stride length. This difference may explain the faster speed records obtained by pacers (9.4–16.0 m/s) than by trotters (11.8–14.2 m/s).

Asymmetric gaits: canter and gallop

Canter and gallop refer to the same gait at increasing speed: the canter is a three-beat gait at slow speed and the gallop is a four-beat gait at a higher speed. At the canter, the diagonal stance phase is synchronized while at the gallop the footfalls of the diagonal limbs are dissociated. The first hindlimb hits the ground before the diagonal forelimb at the gallop. The gallop is the fastest equine gait and is used by racing horses such as Thoroughbreds and Quarter Horses.

These two gaits are composed of asymmetric movements of the hind and fore limbs. Because of this asymmetry, each limb is referred to differently: the lead limb is the last one of the limb pairs to leave the ground. The contralateral limb is called the non-lead limb or trailing limb. Consequently, there are two possible symmetric footfall sequences: right lead canter and left lead canter, and similarly, right lead gallop and left lead gallop. In free conditions the horse prefers to canter or gallop on the right lead to go into a right curve. If it is cantering on the right lead before going into a left curve, the horse will probably change the lead limb to maintain balance.

The lead change is the transition between right lead canter and the left lead canter footfalls sequence. It is commonly accomplished by initially having the horse change the order of hindlimb placements and then the forelimb placements. However, in dressage the rider can elicit the canter lead change during the suspension phase. Racing horses change leads 8 or more times per mile to avoid excessive muscular fatigue due to asymmetric work of the limbs and also to minimize the centrifugal forces as they accommodate to the curve.[58]

At the gallop, there are two types of footfall sequences: the transverse gallop and the rotary gallop. The transverse gallop is more frequently used by the horse than the rotary gallop. Rotary gallop may be used briefly under some circumstances, for example after a lead change or when muscular fatigue occurs during a racing gallop. A disunited canter occurs with the same footfall sequence as a rotary gallop except that the stance phase of the diagonal is synchronized. It can be observed for a few strides after a bad lead change in dressage or following a jump.

The jump is a unique gallop stride where the airborne phase is a long dissociation of the diagonal. The footfalls of the jump stride are: Trail-H, Lead-H at take off and Trail-F, Lead-F at landing. At take-off, the hindlimb stance phase is more synchronized than in a normal gallop stride to provide a powerful push-off. The footfalls of the forelimbs at landing are not synchronized.[59] A lead change can take place during the airborne phase and in this case the change of forelimb placement order takes place before those of the hindlimbs. A disunited canter can be observed after the jump if the lead change of the hindlimbs does not occur immediately after the landing phase.

Gait transitions

For increasing its velocity, the horse can switch gait from walk to trot and from trot to canter and then extend the canter to gallop. Each gait can also be extended by changing the spatial and temporal characteristics of the strides. From a dynamic point of view, a gait transition can be characterized by a gait change with non-stationary motions of the limbs. Periodicity and rhythm of the limb motions change suddenly. Gait transition is one of the most difficult basic exercises in dressage where specific coordination should be learned during training exercise.

There is little information about gait transitions in the scientific literature. The footfall sequence of various gait transitions has been described by Marey and Lenoble du Teil.[18,50] One kinematic study described four types of footfall sequences observed in dressage horses during the walk-trot transition.[60] One accelerometric study described the instantaneous changes of stride frequency and dorsoventral activity during all types of transitions recorded in competitons.[61]

From an energetic point of view, it appears that each equid has a preferred speed for the trot to gallop transition and this particular speed is related to an optimal metabolic cost of running.[62] However, another experiment demonstrated that the trot-gallop transition is triggered when the peak of ground reaction force reaches a critical level of about 1 to 1.25 times the body weight (Fig. 10.11).[63] Carrying additional weight reduced the speed of trot-gallop transition.

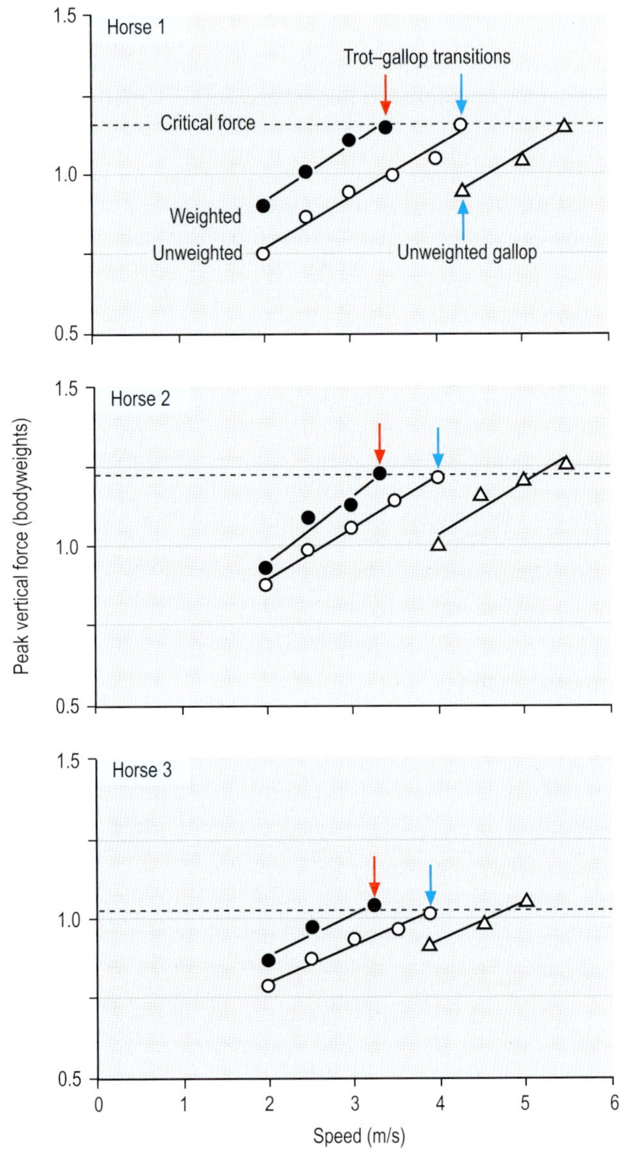

Fig 10.11 Gait transition determinism. When the horses carried weights, they switched to a gallop at a lower speed but essentially the same critical level of forces as when they did not carry weights. By switching to a gallop, the peak ground reaction force was reduced by an average of 14%. The open circles and triangles denote unweighted trotting and galloping, respectively, and the closed circles denote weighted trotting. The plotted values are the average of the peak forces under each of the four limbs. The lines are linear leastsquares regressions.

Reprinted from Farley CT, Taylor CR. A mechanical trigger for the trot-gallop transition in horses. Science 1991;253:306–308. Reprinted with permission from AAAS.

Velocity related changes in stride characteristics

For increasing the speed at a particular gait, the amplitude of the steps becomes larger and the duration of the limb cycle is reduced in order to repeat the limb movements more frequently. Stride frequency (SF) and stride length (SL) are the two main components of gait speed. The mean speed (V) can be estimated by the product of stride frequency by stride length: $V = SF \times SL$. The velocity-related changes in stride parameters have been studied in many horse breeds and disciplines. Stride length increases linearly with the speed of the gait. Stride frequency increases non-linearly and more slowly.[5,64,65] For a quick increase of running velocity such as that occurring at the start of a gallop race, stride frequency reaches its maximum value first to produce the acceleration, while the maximum stride length slowly reaches its maximum value.[66]

In Thoroughbred racehorses, the fatigue effect on stride characteristics increases the overlap time between the lead hind limb and the non-lead forelimb, the stride duration and the suspension phase duration.[67] The compliance of the track surface also can influence the stride parameters when the horse is trotting or galloping at high speed. At the gallop, stride duration tends to be reduced on a harder track surface.[37] There is a slight increase in stride duration on wood-fiber tracks in comparison with turf tracks at the same speed. When the rider stimulated the horse with a stick, a reduction in stride length and an increase in stride frequency corresponding to a reduction of the forelimb stance phase duration were observed. However, velocity was not significantly influenced.[68]

Most of the kinetic and temporal stride variables were influenced by the velocity of the gallop. Stride frequency, stride length and diagonal dissociation increased linearly with velocity. Velocity was primarily increased by the increase in stride length and then by stride frequency. Increase in stride length is mainly explained by the lengthening of the diagonal and airborne phases of the stride.[65] The overlap duration of the diagonal decreased linearly to about 50 ms as the galloping speed increases.[58, 69] In order to increase gallop stride length, the movements of the hindlimbs and forelimbs are dissociated and length between the footfalls of the diagonal increases. The time elapsed between forelimbs midstance phases and between hindlimbs midstance phases is kept constant and independent from velocity.[65]

Respiratory coupling at trot, canter and gallop

Some relationships have been established between stride parameters and other physiological variables. At the canter and gallop, the respiratory and limb cycle are synchronized. Inspiration starts from the beginning of the suspension phase and ends at the beginning of the non-lead forelimb stance phase. Expiration then occurs during the stance phase of the non-lead and lead forelimbs (Fig. 10.12).[70] Expiration is facilitated by compression of the rib cage during weight bearing of the forelimbs. This functional coupling might be a limiting factor for ventilation at maximal exercise intensity. At the walk, trot and pace there is not a consistent coupling of locomotion and the respiratory cycle. At a trot, the ratio between locomotor and respiratory frequency ranged between one and three with respect to the speed, the duration of exercise and the breed.[71,72] The same type of low-level coupling was observed at a pace where the ratio between stride and respiratory frequency was 1 to 1.5.[73]

Muscle fiber characteristics and locomotion

The relationship between stride parameters and muscle fiber composition was studied in Standardbreds at high speed.[74] The stride length and frequency were extrapolated at a speed of V200 or V = 9m/s. The stride length is positively correlated with the percentages of type I fiber (aerobic slow twitch) and type IIA (aero-anaerobic fast twitch) and negatively correlated with the percentages of fiber type IIB (anaerobic fast twitch). The stride frequency was positively correlated with only the percentage of type IIA fiber. However, in another study the opposite result was found: a negative correlation between the stance duration of young trotters and the percentage of type IIB fibers.[75] For race trotters the force-velocity relationship for skeletal muscles implied in limb protraction and retraction might be an important limiting factor of maximal stride frequency.[58] In Andalusian horses, there is no significant correlation between the stance duration and the fiber type percentages. However, the diameter of fibers was negatively correlated with stance duration.[76] The propulsive force during the stance phase might be higher with larger fibers, especially of type I.

During a treadmill exercise test, blood lactate concentration and heart rate at high speed seem to be more correlated to stride length than to stride frequency.[74, 77] This finding confirms that the high speed which elicited a cardiac and metabolic response is primarily explained by an increase in stride length. Furthermore, the velocity relating to change of stride frequency is not linear and consequently decreases the coefficient of correlation. In ponies tested on the track, stride frequency was more correlated to blood lactate concentration and heart rate than to stride length, which is more limited in this animal.[40]

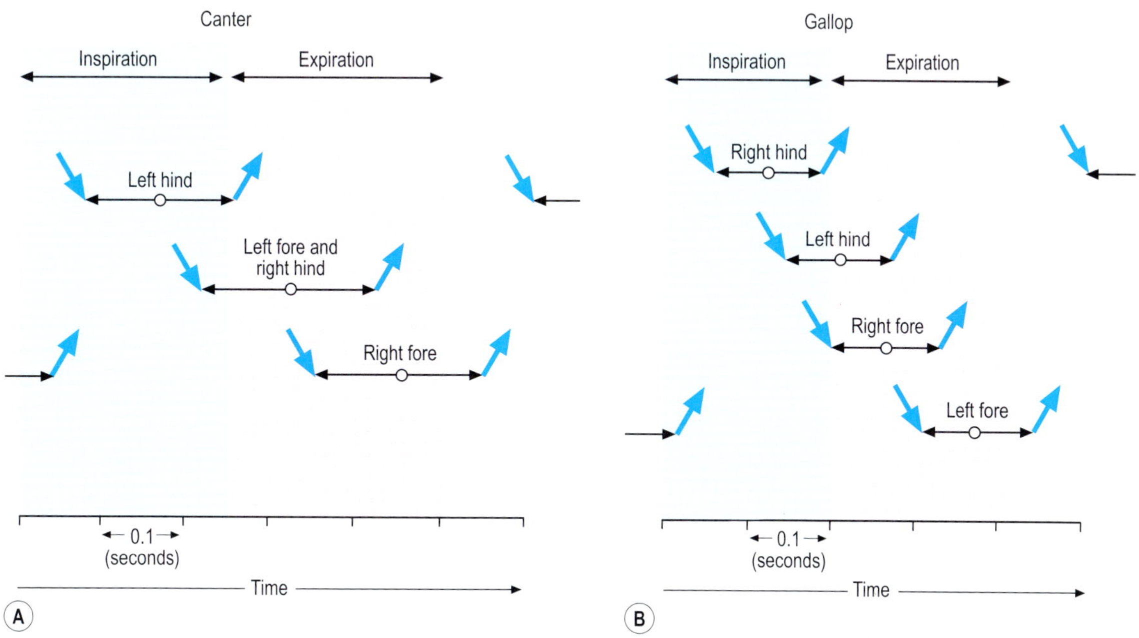

Fig 10.12 Schematic diagram showing the relationship between the timing of the events of the respiratory cycle and the timing of the events in the cycle of limb movement when a normal horse is cantering **(A)** or galloping **(B)** leading with the right forelimb. The distances (x) reprent the periods of ground contact of the feet.

Reprinted from Attenburrow DP. Time relationship between the respiratory cycle and limb cycle in the horse. Equine Vet J 1982;14:69–72, with permission from the Equine Veterinary Journal.

Response to training: influence of age and training on locomotor variables

Gait development in foals and yearling

Gait patterns are influenced by the age of the horse, but little is known about gait development. The relationship between conformation and stride variables in foals aged 6–8 months has been reported. Speed increases were achieved by longer stride length in heavier foals and higher stride frequency in taller foals.[5] The elbow, carpal and fetlock joint angle flexions were the most significant differences between the foals.[78] The stride and stance duration increased with age but the swing duration and pro-retraction angle were consistent. The joint angle patterns recorded at four and 26 months were nearly similar. The good correlations of some of the kinematic parameters measured in foals and adults make it possible to predict the gait quality of adult horses.[79]

Training effects

According to several studies, some of the gait characteristics can be also modified after a training period. However, little is known about the training effect, because little data from longitudinal studies are available. In one study, after 70 days of dressage and jumping training, the stance duration of the hind limb decreased, its flexion increased and its maximal protraction occurred earlier. In addition, the protraction and retraction range of the forelimb decreased, and the stride duration was unchanged. After the same period, the horses which had been left in pasture showed other locomotion modifications. They had a longer swing and stride duration and the range of the forelimb movement was larger.[80]

In racehorses, the training influence has been investigated in Standardbreds and Thoroughbreds. After three years of training, the following changes in the trotting strides were observed: the stride length, the stride duration and swing phase increased.[57] Another study on Standardbreds trained on a treadmill did not show any change in temporal or linear stride variables after five month of training. In gallop racing, a stride duration and stride length increase was found.[67] After eight weeks of a high intensity training regime on a treadmill, the stance phase duration of the Thoroughbred gallop stride was reduced by 8–20%.[81]

Dressage horses should be trained to improve their coordination, their suppleness and their gait collection. Collection of the gait means that the forward movement becomes more upward movement and the stride frequency slows down. A group of horses competing in dressage has been tested from four to seven years of age to determine the training related changes in locomotion variables. The changes of the trot were more pronounced than the changes in the walk and gallop (Table 10.2). At the trot, the stride frequency decreases between five and six years old. During the same time, walk and gallop stride frequency remains the same. At the trot, dorsoventral displacement increases after the first year of training. The increase of dorsoventral activity with age corresponded to an increase of muscular power and an increase of the dorsoventral displacement with collected gaits. Stride regularity and symmetry increases in early training and then decreases after six years of age.

Applications of equine gait analysis

Gait tests for breeding

Early jumping evaluation

Free jumping tests are often used in the performance test for early evaluation of three-year-old horses. These tests are useful for selection of stallions and mares for breeding, and to select potential performance horses. Gallop, take-off, jump path and landing characteristics were measured during a free jumping test using Equimetrix system. Heritabilities of these jump measurements were calculated in French saddle horses to determine the use of breeding criteria (see Chapter 4). The heritabilities of jumping characteristics are moderate to high ($h^2 = 0.21–0.64$) and can be used efficiently in making decisions on selection of bloodlines for breeding.

Basic gait characteristics of the young dressage horses

Gait and conformation test information is useful in making breeding plans and to more accurately identify young horses with good dressage potential. Gait characteristics may be measured early in a horse's under saddle training. Walk and trot may be measured earlier in hand. Several studies were conducted in France and Germany to measure gait and conformation variables in three-year-old horses presented in a performance test.[82, 83] The relationships between these measurements and the judge's scores were analyzed. The locomotor profile of the future dressage horses should have the following gait characteristics:

Table 10.2 Changes in trot variables with the stage of training in dressage horses

	4 YEARS	5 YEARS	6 YEARS	7 YEARS AND OLDER
Stride frequency (stride/s)	1.34 a	1.32 a	1.26 b	1.27 b
Stride regularity (/200)	186 a	185 a	185 a	179 b
Dorsoventral activity (g^2/Hz or W/kg)	7.8	8.3	8.7	10.4
Longitudinal activity (g^2/Hz or W/kg)	1.14	1.62	1.55	2.1
Propulsion acceleration vector (g)	2.3	2.2	1.4	3
Dorsoventral displacement (m)	0.11 a	0.13 b	0.13 b	0.13 b

Means followed by different letters are significantly different at $P < 0.05$.

- walk: large vertical limb displacement and propulsion activity, high regularity
- trot: slow cadence, large vertical displacement, high regularity, large propulsion activity
- gallop: three-beat gallop with high regularity, slow cadence and good propulsion activity.

Horses having these basic gait characteristics obtain better scores in performance tests and they have better performance during the first year of dressage competition.

The three-year-old German horses evaluated had gait characteristics more advantageously adapted for dressage competition. The results obtained in the best German horses tested could be considered as a reference standard for dressage breeding. Purebred Spanish horses should be considered as a reference standard for collected gaits used in farm work and classical dressage. Specific conformation and gait characteristics in German breeds may explain their higher level of success in dressage competition.[84] For dressage performance, the trot characteristics and its variations are very important because they form the basis of passage and piaffe, movements which are performed at the upper levels of dressage competition.

According to the FEI standards, the trot should be a two beat gait with free, active and regular steps. Regularity and elasticity of the steps and engagement of the hind quarters are important qualities of the trot. The same cadence and rhythm should be maintained during trot variations. The trot characteristics of the German horses were consistent with the FEI standards: slow stride frequency, high regularity, large dorsoventral displacement and activity. Activity is considered good when the horse displays elasticity and good propulsion (Table 10.3). Spanish horses have a shorter stride length, higher stride frequency and lower dorsoventral displacement and activity than German horses. Spanish horses exhibited elevated movements (large flexion of carpus and tarsus) rather than extended movements of the limbs. It has been shown that Purebred Spanish horses had larger elbow and carpus angular range than Dutch Warmblood horses.[85] Spanish and German groups have high propulsion and longitudinal activity which should be an advantage for collecting the trot to passage and piaffe. Spanish groups exhibited gaits with lower regularity than the German group but this could be explained by the lower training level of the Spanish horses at this age. Traditionally, Purebred Spanish horses are broken to ride at the age of four years instead of two to three years for German horses.

The mean heritability of dressage performance was rather low ($h^2 = 0.04$ to 0.27) as reported by several authors because non-genetic effects like training have a large influence on outcome.[86–88] Consequently, early selection using gait tests could be more efficient than selection based on performance results. Moderate and high heritabilities have been found for trot and gallop variables such as stride length, stride frequency, dorsoventral displacement, and propulsion variables (see Chapter 4).[83] Some of the gait variables such as stride frequency, dorsoventral and longitudinal activity which have moderate to high heritability could be used for improving gait collection ability by genetic selection. Most of the trot variables had a moderate to high heritability (mean heritability $h^2 = 0.24$). The trot characteristics are very important for dressage ability and should be used for early selection at two or three years old. Slow stride frequency, high dorsoventral activity and high propulsion vector and longitudinal activity are the trot characteristics required for performing in dressage. Gallop variables are highly heritable (mean heritability $h^2 = 0.43$) and could be also used for genetic selection. Slow stride frequency and high longitudinal activity are required. Walk heritabilities were rather low (mean heritability $h^2 = 0.15$) except for vertical activity, longitudinal propulsion and percentage of four-beat walk which were highly heritable. The low heritabilities could be explained because the walk is a complex gait which could be modified by many environmental factors.

Table 10.3 Comparison of the trot characteristics measured by the Equimetrix system in three groups of breeds used for dressage: German horses (Hannoverian, Westphalian, Oldenburger), purebred Spanish horses and French saddle horses

TROT CHARACTERISTICS	GER	SF	PRE
Speed (m/s)	3.97 a	4.24 a	3.18 b
Stride length (m)	2.98 a	3.02 a	2.31 b
Stride frequency (stride/s)	1.33 a	1.40 b	1.38 b
Stride symmetry (%)	97	97	96
Stride regularity (/200)	185 a	182 a	174 b
Dorsoventral displacement (10^{-2} cm)	13 a	10 b	10 b
Dorsoventral activity (g^2/Hz or W/kg)	24.33 a	22.01 a	19.76 ab
Percentage of 2-beat rhythm (%)	89 ab	90 a	87 b
Propulsion acceleration vector (g)	8.49 a	7.39 b	9.22 a
Propulsion duration (%)	26 a	29 b	29 b
Longitudinal activity (g^2/Hz or W/kg)	2.35 a	1.43 b	2.42 a

GER Hannoverian + Oldenburger + Westphalian
SF Selle Français
PRE Pura Raza Espaniola
Means followed by different letters are significantly different at $P < 0.05$.

Specific locomotion in racing and equestrian sports

Galloping race

Maximum gallop velocity is primarily determined by stride length. An increase in this component is obtained by decreasing the overlap duration of the lead hind limb and nonlead forelimb stance phase.[58] The movements of the hind limbs and forelimbs are dissociated and the length between the footfalls of the diagonal increases. Overlap time of the diagonal decreases linearly down to about 50 ms as galloping speed increases.[68,69] In poorly performing Thoroughbreds tested on an inclined treadmill (10% slope) at a maximum velocity of 12 m/s, stride length and velocity at maximum heart rate were the variables that were most highly correlated to running speed.[89]

The racing career of a Thoroughbred is short, and the number of racing opportunities is limited. To maximize an individual horse's potential for winning, it should be entered in races appropriate for its racing ability. To help make optimal decisions about entering horses in a profile may be developed for each horse while in early training. The profile should include indicators of the animal's speed, endurance, preferred track conditions, and locomotor variables that help determine these characteristics. Locomotor variables of the racing gallop while at maximal speed can only be obtained on a race track because the temporal stride variables should be natural. On a high speed treadmill maximal speed is limited to14–15 m/s and the biomechanics of locomotion are modified by the driven belt.[39] However, the physiological variables such as respiratory parameters are more accurately measured on an inclined treadmill at submaximal speed.[89]

A gallop test has been designed to determine the locomotor profile of Thoroughbreds. The gallop test is part of normal 'fast work' training, is easy to perform and provides locomotor variables to evaluate the racing capacity of Thoroughbreds in training. This test may be used for early evaluation of young horses as soon as they can gallop close to maximal speed on a race track. The results characterize the gallop and could assist the trainer in planning the training and racing program of the horse. Several gait variables were related to race performance which was evaluated by the percentage of wins, placings and the logarithm of average earnings per start. The best performers had a higher stride frequency, stride regularity and diagonal dissociation. Stride length increase described most of the velocity increase but was negatively correlated with performance. Horses that appeared to be better adapted for short racing distances had higher stride frequency but longer ground contact duration which provided more time for propulsion. It has been found that suspension duration (suspension duration = stride duration − ground contact duration) decreased at maximal velocities greater than 13–14 m/s.[69] A quick gallop acceleration at the start of the race is achieved initially by a high rate of stride frequency increase and then by stride lengthening.[66] During a race, a gallop acceleration is required at the finish to win. Consequently, horses that can increase their stride frequency to the highest value have a better chance to win. A locomotor test performed in harnessed trotters on a track confirmed that the best race performances were obtained by horses that had the highest maximal stride frequency and a long stride length.[56]

These findings suggest that good racehorses are able to trot or gallop at high speed using an optimal stride length and that they can accelerate by increasing their stride frequency in order to finish the race. The best performers reached high stride frequencies of 2.52 strides/s at trot and 2.81 strides/s at the gallop. However, stride length is negatively correlated with performance but stride frequency is positively correlated. Because of pendulum mechanics of the body, maximal stride frequency is dependent on the height of the horse (length of the limbs), weight distribution of the limbs (moment of inertia), elasticity of the limbs and rib cage (module of elasticity) and the percentage of fast-twitch muscle fibers (forces). Increased propulsive activity produced a much greater velocity. Dorsoventral loading of the limbs was increased at high speed probably because of the large effect of kinetic energy of the body. Dorsoventral displacement of the thorax decreased linearly with velocity and minimized the potential energy changes of the center of gravity which reduced the energy expenditure of locomotion. At the fastest speed, horses reached the 'wheel gallop' by lowering and keeping their center of gravity at the same height during the entire stride, even the suspension phase. The 'wheel gallop' is optimized to produce maximum energy for propulsive work in the longitudinal axis and avoid energy wastage for vertical oscillations of the body. Energy cost of the gallop increases as stride regularity decreases. This may make regularity of the stride one of the limiting factors which determines maximum galloping speed. Regularity was affected by the increase in speed as it has been found in harness trotters and it is highly correlated with racing performance.[31]

Harness racing

In order to measure gait variables during training sessions on a race track, an mobile gait analysis system has been used in harness trotters.[41,56] Good trotters have a short stance phase duration with a longer stance phase in the hind limbs than in the forelimbs.[90] A locomotor test performed in race trotters on a track confirmed that the best race performances were obtained by trotters that had the highest maximal stride frequency and a long stride length.[56] These findings suggest that good race trotters are able to trot at high speed using an optimal stride length and that they can accelerate by increasing their stride frequency in order to finish the race.

Show jumping

During the 1988 Seoul Olympic Games, the kinematics of jumping over a high and wide obstacle (oxer) were analyzed in 29 horses and the relationship to the total penalty score was studied.[91] Fewer total penalties were associated with lower velocities during the jump strides, closer take-off hindlimb placements and closer landing forelimb placements. Another study on elite horses jumping a high vertical fence demonstrated that the push-off produced by the hind limbs at take-off was associated with the mechanical energy required for clearing the fence.[92] The action of the forelimbs should be limited to positioning the horse's body into proper orientation with the jump before the final push-off of the hind limbs. A more vertical component of the initial velocity was observed in the horses that successfully cleared a wide water jump (4.5 m).[93] The angle of the velocity (vector) relative to the horizontal was 15° in a successful jump compared to 12° in an unsuccessful jump and the vertical component of the velocity was about 0.5 m/s greater in a successful rather than an unsuccessful jump. This initial velocity was generated by the impulse of the hind limbs and determined the ballistic flight characteristics of the body.

These kinematic findings agree with another study which showed that poor jumpers had a lower acceleration peak of the hindlimb at take-off than good jumpers.[94] Poor jumpers brake too much with the forelimbs at take-off impulse and the hindlimbs produce an acceleration which is too weak for clearing the fence. This force is one of the main factors affecting a successful jump because it determines the ballistic flight of the center of gravity and also the characteristics of the body rotation over the obstacle during the airborne phase. The moment of inertia and its influence on body rotation was also studied in a group of jumping horses but no consistent relationship with the level of performance was found.[94] More penalties were recorded for horses that cantered at a low stride frequency (lower or equal to 1.76 stride/s) and suddenly reduced their stride frequency at take-off.

Dressage

In dressage the horse should easily execute complex exercises, gait variations and gait transitions while maintaining his equilibrium and suppleness. This discipline requires a high level of locomotor control of the horse by the rider which is achieved progressively through exercise and collecting the gaits. A horse's ability for collection is one of the main limiting factors for dressage because it is impossible to execute the more complex exercises correctly in competition without having attained good basic collection of the gaits. The collected gaits have been extensively described in kinematic studies.[54, 55, 95, 96]

The trot

Among the normal variations of the trot in saddle horses, the speed of the gait and the stride length increase from collected, to medium and to extended trot. A slow stride frequency including a long swing phase is required for good trot quality. The time elapsing between hindlimb contact and diagonal forelimb contact defines the diagonal advanced placement and should be positive and high at the trot. The horse should place its hindlimbs as far as possible under itself. A large amplitude of vertical displacement of the body during collected trot is desired in the dressage horse. Vertical displacement of the trot is obtained through the storage of elastic strain energy in the fetlock, hock, stifle and pelvis. For extending the trot, having an inclined scapula (a steeper angle to the scapula) and the amplitude of the elbow joint appeared as important factors. The horses judged to have a good trot should have large degree of flexion in the elbow and carpal joints at the beginning of the swing phase of the stride. A positive diagonal advanced placement measured at the collected trot was observed in elite dressage horses.[52, 97] In these elite horses the hindlimb contacts the ground about 20–30 m/s before the diagonal forelimb. This advanced foot placement could be a means for the hindlimbs to push-off earlier during the stance phase.

The degree of collection at the trot could also be measured by the acceleration components of the body. Horses equipped with the Equimetrix gait analysis system in a dressage test were recorded at all trot variations and passage. With increasing collection at the trot, the vertical component of acceleration increased.[83] At the same time, the forward component of acceleration decreased. This indicates that propulsion power in dressage horses is used to increase vertical displacement instead of longitudinal displacement.

The passage and piaffe

Passage and piaffe are two dressage exercises derived from the collected trot but the kinetics of each are quite different. Differences in the temporal variables has been demonstrated in kinetic analyzes of the dressage finalists at the Olympic Games in Barcelona.[52] Stride duration is longer (i.e. stride frequency is slower) for piaffe (1.08 s) and passage (1.09 s) than for the collected trot (0.84). For most of the other temporal variables, collected trot and passage were very similar except for the suspension phase which was shorter in passage.

Specific kinetics of passage and piaffe were analyzed on experienced horses using the Equimétrix gait analysis system. Mean dorsoventral and longitudinal acceleration vectors were measured during the exercise. At the passage, the mean acceleration vector shows that the largest component of propulsion is dorsoventral instead of longitudinal as it is in the extended or working trot. The high collection of passage transforms forward propulsion into upward propulsion. The greatest propulsive activity in passage is from the forelimbs, while the hindlimbs provide for braking.

At the piaffe, the amplitude of dorsoventral acceleration during the stance phase is lower than at the passage because the amplitude of dorsoventral displacement is reduced. Hindlimbs have greater braking activity to avoid forward movement of the body. The forelimbs have moderate dorsoventral propulsion. The same type of results were observed in a horse at the piaffe with a force plate.[98] However, at the passage the longitudinal ground reaction force of the hindlimbs was higher than in the forelimbs.

The canter

At slow speed the canter is a three-beat gait. At the canter, the diagonal stance phase is synchronized while at the gallop the footfalls of the diagonal are dissociated. The speed of the canter increases from collected, to working, medium and extended canter by increasing stride length. While stride length increases, stride frequency remains nearly constant.[95] Stride length increase is due to increase of diagonal step length and distance covered during suspension.

Relationships between the total dressage competition score and canter characteristics in Olympic dressage horses revealed that the best horses were able to extend their canter strides by increasing their stride length without changing their stride frequency.[99] For Three-day-event horses at the Olympic Games, extended canter stride length and velocity were positively associated with points awarded by judges. However, non-finishers of the event had higher extended canter stride lengths and velocities in the dressage phase than finishers.[100]

The lead change is the transition between the footfall sequences of two different canter leads. Normally the hindlimb sequence changes first, then the front limb sequence. In dressage the rider can elicit the canter lead change during the suspension phase. In a bad lead change, the change in forelimb placements occurs before the change of the hindlimbs, resulting in a disunited canter, which may be observed for several strides. The canter during the two and one tempi lead change is slow (3.35–3.95 m/s) with a short stride length (2.08–2.44 m) and a stride frequency of 1.62 strides/s.[101] Two tempi changes result in a change in the canter lead every-other-stride and one tempi changes result in canter lead changes on every stride.

During the canter pirouette, the canter footfall sequence is altered. The cadence is reduced from 1.58 stride/s at the collected canter to 1.13 stride/s.[96] The diagonal support is entirely dissociated and there is no suspension phase.

The walk

In dressage horses, the speed of the walk increases from the collected walk (1.37 m/s) to the extended walk (1.82 m/s) and simultaneously there is a little increase in stride frequency.[54] The speed change was mainly the result of the stride lengthening by increasing the over-tracking distance. Even in horses trained for dressage, the regular four beat rhythm of the footfall was observed only in one of the six horses evaluated. The stride regularity could be assessed by dorsoventral acceleration recording. Extended walk has a more regular pattern than collected walk where the footfall sequence is slightly disturbed by the actions of the rider. Elite dressage horses usually have a very regular acceleration pattern at the walk. This is a signature of a high level of coordination and stability in the rhythm of footfall sequence.

Gait transitions

A study of transitions from trot-to-walk showed a positive correlation between a higher level of training and a 'clean' transition without a short intermediate step.[60] The combination of gait analysis by accelerometric measurement and wavelet analysis allowed quantification of some of the temporal and kinetic characteristics of gait transitions.[61] Transition duration, dorsoventral activity and frequency were specific of each transition. Training improved smoothness of braking deceleration and frequency changes with a longer transition duration.

The transition duration increased significantly with training for trot-walk, canter-halt and canter-trot transitions. The lengthening of the transition duration allowed a slow decrease of stride frequency (canter-trot transition) and a smooth decrease of vertical activity (canter-halt and trot-halt transition). The rider adapted his technique to locomotion and training level of the horse. By lengthening transition duration, experienced horses could perform a smooth deceleration. In contrast, young horses could not adequately prepare their gait transition and suddenly brake their forward motion, which produced a high peak of deceleration. The amplitude of frequency change during the gait transition decreased with training for all transitions especially for canter-halt and trot-walk transition.

Effects of head-neck position and reins on the gaits

The head-neck position is one of the components of the gait collection related to the back attitude and hindlimb propulsion. Different types of reins are used by the trainers to modify the head-neck attitude in sport horses (Fig. 10.13). The effects of three types of reins on the gaits were studied in horses walking and trotting in a circular walker.[103] The effects of the Chambon, rubber bands and Back lift™ were tested by using two Equimetrix™ accelerometric devices simultaneously located at the sternum and sacrum. Many kinetic modifications of the gaits were detected mainly in the forelimbs and few in the hindlimbs. The three types of reins increased the propulsion activity of the forelimbs at walk and/or trot. Only the Chambon increased the hindlimbs propulsion power at walk and forelimbs dorsoventral power at the trot. The Back lift increased the dorsoventral power of the forelimbs both at walk and trot. The effects of head-neck position on the ground reaction force and interlimb coordination were also studied under the control of a rider on the force instrumented treadmill[21]. There is no impressive modification in load distribution between forelimbs and hindlimbs caused by the change in head-neck position[102]. The extreme neck elevation shortened forelimb stance phase duration, reduced the forelimb impulse and increased peaks of vertical ground reaction force both in fore- and hindlimbs (Fig. 10.14). A low head-neck position decreased the overreach distance.

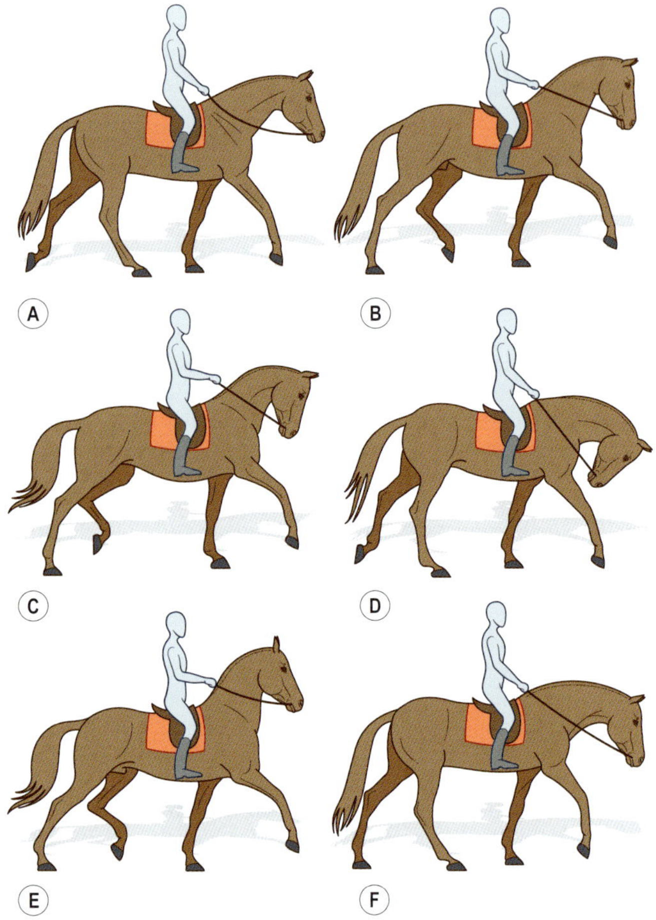

Fig 10.14 Six head-neck positions studied in the dressage horses ridden at walk and trot on a treadmill. Reprinted from Weishaupt MA, Wiestner T, von Peinen K, Waldern N, Roepstorff L, van Weeren R, Meyer H, Johnston C. Effect of head and neck position on vertical ground reaction forces and interlimb coordination in the dressage horse ridden at walk and trot on a treadmill.

Three-day eventing

The analysis of the gallop stride characteristics of three-day event horses during the steeplechase of the Seoul Olympic Games revealed optimal values for successful performance. The optimal stride length should range between 1.85 and 2.05 m while the optimal velocity should range between 13 and 14.3 m/s.[104]

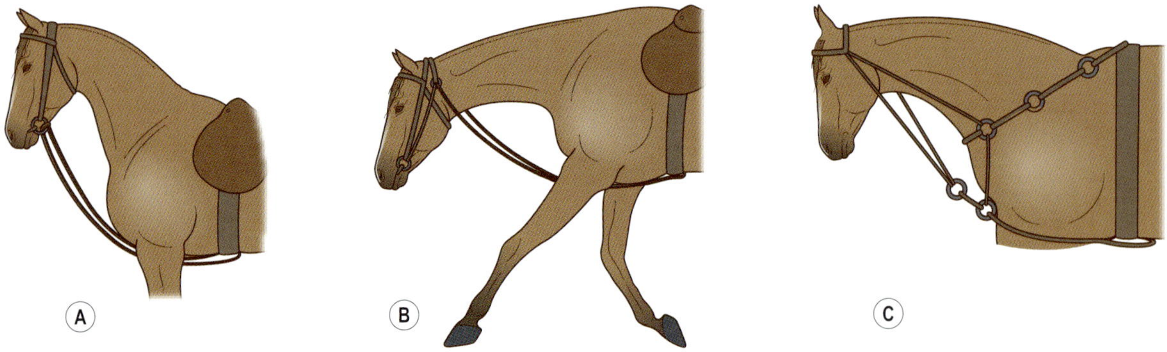

Fig 10.13 The kinetic gait effects of three types of reins were studied: **(A)** Rubber bands **(B)** Chambon **(C)** Back lift™. Reprinted from Biau S, Couve O, Lemaire S, Barrey E. The effect of reins on kinetic variables of locomotion.

Biomechanics of the hoof and lameness prevention in the athletic horses

Effects of the track

The kinetics of hoof impact is an interesting subject for lameness prevention because a relationship between repeated exposure to shock and the onset of chronic injuries has been established in human medicine and in animal models[105]. The shoes and the track surface can be designed in order to minimize hoof shock intensity especially for race and show jumping horses which undergo very large hoof decelerations at high speeds and landing, respectively. Hoof shock and vibration acceleration measurements after the moment of impact on the ground were used for testing the influence of the track surface on shock and vibration intensity of hoof impact at the trot.[33] The shock of deceleration can reach 707 m/s^2 on asphalt and 31 m/s^2 on sawdust mixed with sand. The subsequent transient vibrations have frequencies between 592 Hz and 41 Hz, respectively. The stiffness of the track surface directly influences these mechanical parameters and should be controlled to minimize vibration damage. In horses, as in human athletes, damping hoof impact with visco-elastic shoes and a soft track surface is useful to prevent overuse injuries of the distal joints.

Improvements in race track designs and surfaces for racehorses exemplify the application of research for the betterment of horses and the racing industry. The limb kinematic studies on Standardbreds trotting on various types of race tracks (length, curves) made it possible to propose some recommendations regarding the ideal geometry for race tracks (Fig. 10.15).[106, 107] The most important factor affecting comfort is the total length of the track which determine the curve length and their inclination to avoid any load disequilibrium between the lateral and medial sides of the limbs.

Effects of shoeing

Many shoeing techniques are available but any assumption concerning their effects on hoof biomechanics should be verified experimentally by locomotion analysis studies. The limb kinematics of six sound horses was studied at trot in hand to determine the effect of long toes and acute hoof angles.[108] In this study, no lengthening of the trotting strides was observed after reducing the hoof angle about 10° from the normal value. However, this hoof angle change resulted in toe-first impact and prolonged breakover, both of which are potentially disadvantageous for athletic performance and may predispose the horse to injury. In another study, the effect of acute angulations of the hind hooves showed some changes in the limb

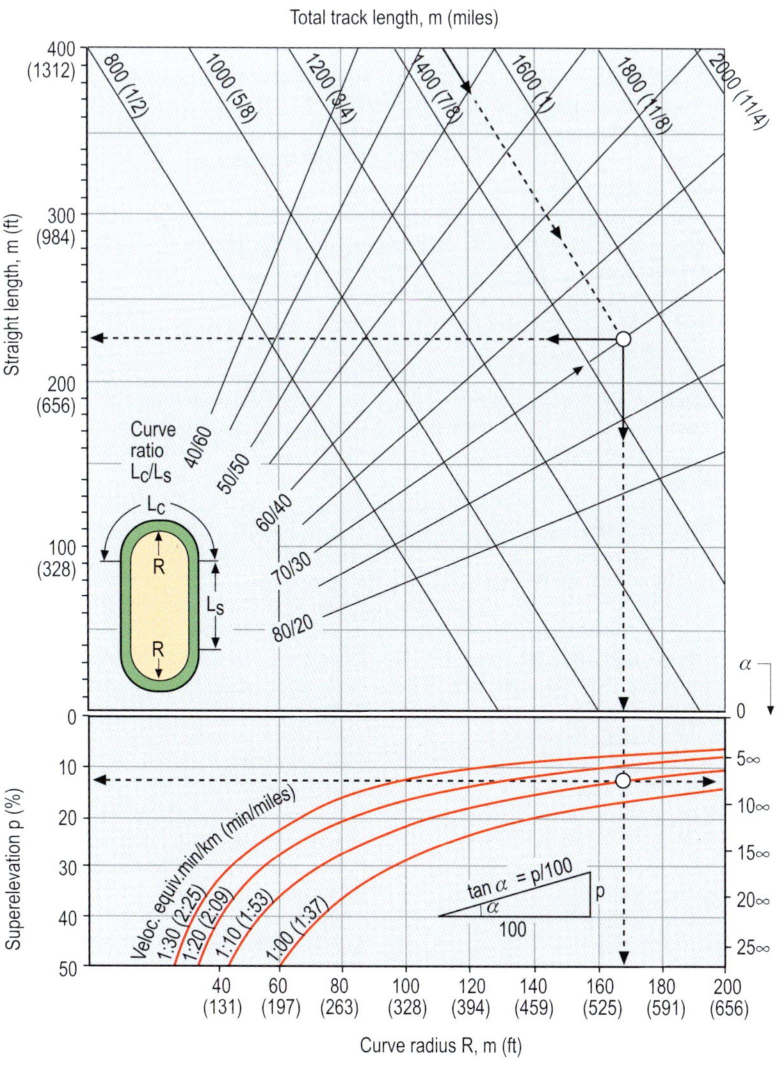

Fig 10.15 Relationship between the geometric characteristics of a track with semicircular curves. Examples: given a track length of 1500 m and a curve ratio (ratio of curve length to straight length) of 70/30. From these data, the length of each straight is read as 225 m and the curve radius as 167 m. For a velocity equivalent of 1:10 min/km the superelevation of the curve is read off on the scale as approximately 12.5 per cent or 7 degrees.

Reprinted from Fredricson I, Dalin G, Drevemo S, Hjerten G. A biotechnical approach to the geometric design of racetracks. Equine Vet J 1975;7:91–96, with permission from the Equine Veterinary Journal.

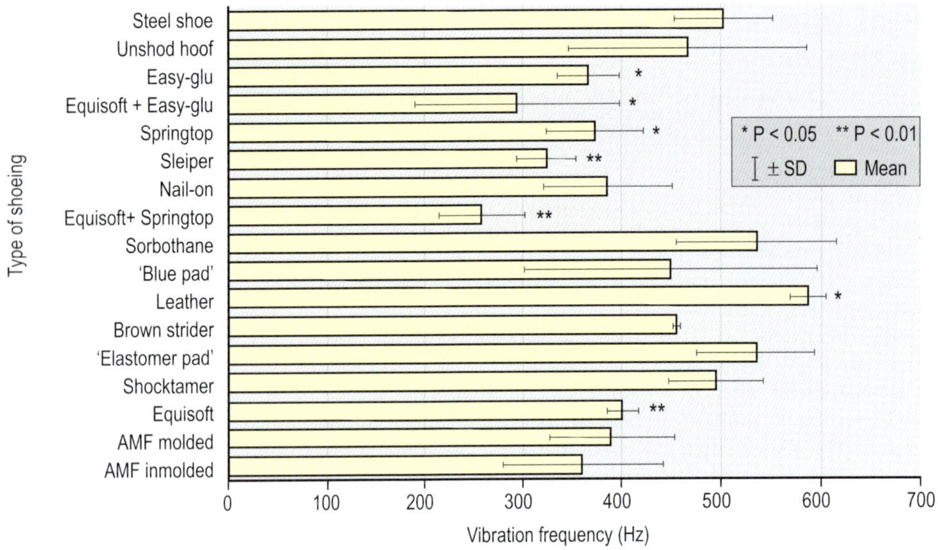

Fig 10.16 Comparison of the hoof vibration recorded by an accelerometer at the trot on an asphalt road with different types of shoeing (shoe and pads). A better damping of the hoof vibrations after impact was observed with light shoes and soft pads.

Reprinted from Benoit E, Barrey E, Regnault JC, Brochet JL. Comparison of the damping effect of different shoeing by the measurement of hoof acceleration. Acta Anat 1993; 146:109–113.

coordination which could be interesting for reducing limb interference. The hind hoof breakover can be prolonged and the lift off of the hind limbs delayed, which could prevent interference with the ipsilateral forelimb.

Hoof shock and vibration acceleration measurements after the moment of impact on the ground were used to investigate the damping capacity of various hoof pads and shoes.[34] Compared to the reference steel shoe, shock reduction was higher for light shoes made of a polymer and/or aluminum alloy which had lower stiffness values and density than steel (Fig. 10.16). The use of visco-elastic pads contributed to shock reduction and attenuated the high frequency vibrations up to 75%.

Damping hoof impact with visco-elastic shoes and a soft track surface is useful to prevent orthopedic overuse injuries of the distal joints. The shock damping potential of the track surface has much higher effect than those of the shoes but when the track surface is too hard, the use of damping shoes is highly recommended for horses.

References

1. Jeffcott LB, Rossdale PD, Freestone J, et al. An assessment of wastage in Thoroughbred racing from conception to 4 years of age. Equine Vet J 1982;14: 185–98.
2. Rossdale PD, Hopes R, Wingfield Digby NJ, et al. Epidemiological study of wastage among racehorses 1982 and 1983. Vet Rec 1985;11: 66–9.
3. Fredricson I, Drevemo S, Dalin G, et al. The application of high-speed cinematography for the quantitative analysis of equine locomotion. Equine Vet J 1980;12:54–9.
4. Langlois B, Froideveaux J, Lamarche L, et al. Analyze des liaisons entre la morphologie et l'aptitude au gallop, au trot et au saut d'obstacles chez le cheval. Annales de Génétique et de Sélection Animale 1978;10:443–74.
5. Leach DH, Cymbaluk NF. Relationship between stride length, stride frequency, velocity and morphometrics of foals. Am J Vet Res 1986;47:2090–7.
6. Leach DH, Dyson S. Instant centres of rotation of equine limb joints and their relationship to standard skin marker locations. Equine Vet J; 1988(suppl 6): 113–19.
7. Schamhardt HC, van den Bogert AJ, Hartman W. Measurement techniques in animal locomotion analysis. Acta Anat 1993;146:123–9.
8. van Weeren PR, van den Bogert AJ, Barneveld A. A quantitative analysis of skin displacement in the trotting horse. Equine Vet J 1990;(suppl 9):101–9.
9. van Weeren PR, van den Bogert AJ, Barneveld A. Quantification of skin displacement in the proximal parts of the limbs of the walking horse. Equine Vet J 1990;(suppl 9):110–18.
10. Drevemo S, Johnston CJ. The use of a panning camera technique in equine kinematic analysis. Equine Vet J 1993;(suppl 17):39–43.
11. van Weeren PR, van den Bogert AJ, Barneveld A, et al. The role of the reciprocal apparatus in the hind limb of the horse investigated by a modified CODA-3 optoelectronic kinematic analysis system. Equine Vet J 1990;(suppl 9):95–100.
12. Peloso JG, Stick JA, Soutas-Lttle RW, et al. Computer assisted three dimensional gait analysis of amphotericin-induced carpal lameness in horses. Am J Vet Res 1993;54: 535–1543.
13. Degeurce C, Dietrich G, Pourcelot P, et al. Three dimensional kinematic technique for evaluation of horse locomotion in outdoor conditions. Medical and Biological Engineering and Computing 1996;34:1–4.
14. Holmström M, Fredricson I. High speed cinematographic gait analysis in riding horses. Proc. 43th European Association for Animal Production – Horse commission H 1 1992:540–1.
15. Galloux P, Barrey E. Components of the total kinetic moment in jumping horses. Equine Vet J 1997;(suppl 23): 41–4.

16. Springings EJ, Leach DH. Standardised technique for determining the center of gravity of body and limb segments of horses. Equine Vet J 1986;18: 43–9.
17. Kubo K, Sakai T, Sakuraoka H, Ishii Segmental body weight, volume, mass center in Thoroughbreds horses. J Equine Sci 1992;3:149–55.
18. Marey EJ. In: Marey EJ, editor. La machine animale: locomotion terrestre et aérienne. 2nd ed. Coll. Bibliothèque Science Internationale, Paris: Librairie Gerner Baillere et Cie; 1873. p. 145–86.
19. Pratt GW, O'Connor JT. A relationship between gait and breakdown in the horse. Am J Vet Res 1978;39: 249–53.
20. Schamhardt HC, Merkens HW, van Osch GJVM. Ground reaction force analysis of horses ridden at the walk and trot. In: Persson SGB, Lindholm A, Jeffcott LB, editors. Equine Exercise Physiology. 3rd ed. Davis: ICEEP publications; 1991. p. 120–7.
21. Weishaupt MA, Hogg HP, Wiestner T, et al. Instrumented treadmill for measuring vertical ground reaction forces in horses. Am J Vet Res 2002; 63(4):520–7.
22. Weishaupt MA, Hogg HP, Auer JA, et al. Velocity-dependent changes of time, force and spatial parameters in Warmblood horses walking and trotting on a treadmill. Equine Vet J 2010;42(Suppl 38):530–7.
23. Weishaupt MA, Wiestner T, Hogg HP, et al. Assessment of gait irregularities in the horse: eye vs. gait analysis. Equine Vet J 2001;(suppl 33): 135–40.
24. Weishaupt MA, Wiestner T, Hogg HP, et al. Compensatory load redistribution of horses with induced weightbearing hindlimb lameness trotting on a treadmill. Equine Vet J 2004;36(8): 727–33.
25. Björck G. Studies on the draught force of horse: development of a method using strain gauges for measuring between hoof and ground. Acta Agri Scan 1958;(suppl 4).
26. Frederick Jr FH, Henderson JM. Impact force measurement using preloaded transducers. Am J Vet Res 1970;31: 2279–83.
27. Ratzlaff MH, Grant, BD, Frame JM, et al. Locomotor force of gallopping horses. In: Gillespie JR, Robinson RE, editors. On Equine Exercise Physiology 2. Davis: ICEEP Publications; 1987. p. 574–86.
28. Barrey E. Investigation of the vertical hoof force distribution in the equine forelimb with an instrumented horseboot. Equine Vet J 1990;(suppl 9): 35–8.
29. Roepstorff L, Drevemo S. Concept of a force-measuring horseshoe. Acta Anat 1993;146:114–19.
30. Savelberg HCM, Vostenbosch MATM, Kamman EH, et al. The effect of intra-stride speed variation on treadmill locomotion. Proc. 2nd World congress of Biomechanics; 1994.
31. Barrey E, Hermelin M, Vaudelin JL, et al. Utilisation of an accelerometric device in equine gait analysis. Equine Vet J 1994;(suppl 17):7–12.
32. Galloux P, Richard N, Dronka T, et al. Analysis of equine gait using three-dimensional accelerometers fixed on the saddle. Equine Vet J 1994;(suppl 17): 44–7.
33. Barrey E, Landjerit B, Wolter R. Shock and vibration during the hoof impact on different track surfaces. In: Persson SGB, Lindholm A, Jeffcott L, editors. Equine Exercise Physiology 3. Davis: ICEEP publications; 1991. p. 97–106.
34. Benoit E, Barrey E, Regnault JC, et al. Comparison of the damping effect of different shoeing by the measurement of hoof acceleration. Acta Anat 1993;146:109–13.
35. Burns TE, Clayton HM. Classification of the temporal kinematics of the canter pirouette and collected canter. Equine Vet J 1997;(suppl 23):58–61.
36. Buchner HHF, Savelberg HCM, Schamhardt HC, et al. Habituation of horses to treadmill locomotion. Equine Vet J 1994;(suppl 17):13–15.
37. Fredricson I, Drevemo S, Dalin G, et al. Treadmill for equine locomotion analysis. Equine Vet J 1983;15: 111–15.
38. van Igen Schenau GJ. Some fundamental aspects of biomechanics of overground versus treadmill locomotion. Med Sci Sports Exerc 1980;12:257–61.
39. Barrey E, Galloux P, Valette JP, et al. Stride characteristics of overground versus treadmill locomotion in the saddle horse. Acta Anat (Basel) 1993;146(2–3):90–4.
40. Valette JP, Barrey E, Wolter R. Influence des deux composantes de la vitesse (fréquence et longueur des foulées) sur le métabolisme énergétique musculaire chez le poney, Annale de Zootechnie 1990;39:187–92.
41. Couroucé A, Geoffroy O, Barrey E, et al. Comparison of exercise tests in French trotters under training track and treadmill conditions. Equine Vet J 1999;(suppl 30):528–32.
42. Duboy J, Junqua A, Lacouture P. Vers le réexamen d'autres tests d'aptitude physique. In: Mécanique humaine. Paris: Revue EPS; 1994. p. 157–9.
43. Sloet van Oldruitenborgh-Oosterbaan MM, Barneveld A, Schamhardt HC. Effect of treadmill inclination on kinematics of the trot in Dutch Warmblood horses. Equine Vet J 1997;(suppl 23), 71–5.
44. Kai M, Hiraga A, Kubo K, et al. Comparison of stride characteristics in a cantering horse on a flat and inclined treadmill. Equine Vet J 1997;(suppl 23), 76–9.
45. Leach DH. Locomotion analysis technology for evalution of lameness in horses. Equine Vet J 1983;19:97–9.
46. Clayton HM. Termiology for the description of equine jumping kinematics. J Equine Vet Sci 1989;9:341–8.
47. Leach DH. Recomended terminology for researchers in locomotion and biomechanics of quadrupedal animals. Acta Anat 1993;146:130–6.
48. Muybridge E. Muybridge's complete human and animal locomotion vol. 3 (Republication of Animal Locomotion). New York: Dover Publication; 1887.
49. Marey Etienne-Jules, Pagès C. Analyze cinématique de la locomotion du cheval. Comptes rendus hebdomadaires des séances de l'Académie des Sciences 1886;103:538–47.
50. Lenoble du Teil. Les allures du cheval dévoilées par la méthode expérimentale. Paris and Nancy: Berger Levrault; 1893. p. 192–211.
51. Hildebrand M. Symmetrical gaits of horses. Science 1965;191:701–8.
52. Clayton H. Classification of collected trot, passage and piaffe based on temporal variables. Equine Vet J 1997;(suppl 23):54–7.
53. Barrey E, Desbrosse F. Lameness detection using an accelerometric device. Pferdeheilkunde 1996;12, 617–22.
54. Clayton HM. Comparison of the stride kinematics of the collected, medium and extended walks in horses. Am J Vet Res 1995;56, 849–52.
55. Holmström M, Fredricson I, Drevemo S. Biokinematic effect of collection in the elite dressage horse trot. In: Quantitative studies on conformation and trotting gaits in the Swedish Warmblood riding horse. Thesis, Dösjebro (SW): Hippo Vet AB; 1994. p. V1–7.
56. Barrey E, Auvinet B, Couroucé A. (1995). Gait evaluation of race trotters using an accelerometric device. Equine Vet J 1995;(suppl 18):156–60.
57. Drevemo S, Dalin G, Fredricson I, et al. Equine locomotion 3: the reproducibility of gait in Standardbred trotters. Equine Vet J 1980;12:71–3.
58. Leach DH. Locomotion of the athletic horse. In: Gillespie JR, Robinson NE, editors. Equine Exercise Physiology 2.

Davis: ICEEP publications; 1987. p. 516–35.
59. Leach DH, Ormrod K, Clayton HM. Standardised terminology for the description and analysis of equine locomotion. Equine Vet J 1984;16:522–8.
60. Argue CK, Clayton HM. A preliminary study of transitions between the walk and trot in dressage horses. Acta Anat 1993;146(2–3):179–82.
61. Biau S, Lemaire S, Barrey E. Analysis of gait transitions in dressage horses using wavelet analysis of dorsoventral acceleration. Pferdeheilkunde 2002;4: 343–50.
62. Hoyt DF, Taylor CR. Gait and energetics of locomotion in horses. Nature 1981;292:239.
63. Farley CT, Taylor CR. A mechanical trigger for the trot-gallop transition in horses. Science 1991;253:306–8.
64. Dusek J, Ehrlein HJ, von Engelhardt W, et al. Beziehungen zwischen trittlange, trittfrequenz und geschwindigkeit bei Pferden. Zeitschrift fur Tierzuechtung und Zuechtungsbiologie 1970;87: 177–88.
65. Ishii K, Amano K, Sakuraoka H. Kinetics analysis of horse gait. Bulletin of Equine Research Institue 1989;26: 1–9.
66. Hiraga A, Yamanobe A, Kubo K. Relationships between stride length, stride frequency, step length and velocity at the start dash in a racehorse. J Equine Sci 1994;5: 127–30.
67. Leach DH, Springings EJ. Gait fatigue in the racing Thoroughbred. J Equine Med Surg 1979;3:436–43.
68. Deuel NR, Lawrence LM. Effect of urging by the rider on equine gallop stride limb contacts. Proc. 10th Equine Nutrition and Physiology Symposium; 1987. p. 487–92.
69. Hellander J, Fredricson I, Hertén G, et al.Galloppaktion I – Basala gangartsvariabler i relation till hästens hastighet. Svensk Veterinärtidning 1983;35(Suppl.3):75–82.
70. Attenburrow DP. Time relationship between the respiratory cycle and limb cycle in the horse. Equine Vet J 1982;14:69–72.
71. Hörnicke H, Meixner R, Pollmam U. Respiration in exercising horses. In: Snow DH, Persson SGB, Rose RJ, editors. Equine Exercise Physiology. Cambridge: Granta Editions; 1987. p. 7–16.
72. Art T, Desmecht D, Amory H, et al. Synchronization of locomotion and repiration in trotting ponies. J Am Vet Med Assoc 1990;37:95–103.
73. Evans DL, Silverman EB, Hodgson DR, et al. Gait and respiration in Standardbred horses when pacing and galloping. Res Vet Sci 1994;57: 233–9.
74. Persson SGB, Essen-Gustavsson B, Lindholm A. Energy profile and locomotor pattern of trotting on an inclined treadmill, In: Persson SGB, Lindholm A, Jeffcott LB, editors. Equine Exercise Physiology 3. Davis: ICEEP publications; 1991. p. 231–8.
75. Roneus N, Essen-Gustavsson B, Johnston C, et al. Lactate response to maximal exercise on the track: relation to muscle characteristics and kinematic variables. Equine Vet J 1995;(suppl 18): 191–4.
76. Rivero J.-LL, Clayton HM. The potential role of the muscle in kinematic characteristics, Pferdeheilkunde 1996;12:635–40.
77. Valette JP, Barrey E, Auvinet B, et al. Comparison of track and treadmill exercise tests in saddle horses: a preliminary report, Annale de Zootechnie 1992;41:129–35.
78. Back W, van den Bogert AJ, van Weeren PR, et al. (1993). Quantification of the locomotion of Dutch Warmblood foals. Acta Anat 1993;146:141–7.
79. Back W, Barneveld A, Schamhardt HC, et al. Longitudinal development of the kinematics of 4-, 10-, 18- and 26-month-old Dutch Warmblood horses. Equine Vet J 1994;(suppl 17): 3–6.
80. Back W, Barneveld A, Bruin G, et al. Kinematic detection of superior gait quality in young trotting Warmbloods. Vet Q 1994;16:S91–96.
81. Corley JM, Goodship AE. Treadmill training induced changes to some kinematic variables measured at the canter in Thoroughbred fillies. Equine Vet J 1994;(suppl 17): 20–4.
82. Barrey E, Holmström M, Biau S, et al. A new type of early performance test: gait and conformation measurements in 3 years old horses. Proceedings of 50th of European Association of Animal Production; 1999.
83. Barrey E, Biau S. Locomotion of dressage horses. Proceedings of Conference of Equine Sport Medicine and Applied Science; 2002.
84. Barrey E, Desliens F, Blouin C, et al. Mesures du modèle, des allures et du saut des étalons nationaux par la méthode Equimétrix. In Proceedings of '28ème Journée d'étude', Les Haras nationaux (Ed); 2002. p. 157–76.
85. Galisteo AM, Vivo J, Cano MR, et al. Differences between breeds (Dutch warmblood vs Andalusian Purebred) in forelimb kinematics. J Equine Sci 1997;8:43–7.
86. Langlois B. (1980) Estimation de la valeur génétique des chevaux de sport d'après les sommes gagnées dans les compétitions équestres françaises. Ann Génet Sel Anim 1980;12:15–31.
87. Bruns E. Estimation of the breeding value of stallions from the tournament performance of their offspring. Livest Prod Sci 1981;8:465–73.
88. Huizinga HA, Van der Meij GJW. (1989) Estimated parameters of performance in jumping and dressage competition of the Dutch Warmblood horses. Livest Prod Sci 1989;21:333–45.
89. Rose RJ, King CM, Evans DL, et al. Indices of exercise capacity in horses presented for poor racing performance. Equine Vet J 1995; (suppl 18):418–21.
90. Bayer A. (1973). Bewegungsanalyzen an Trabrennpferden mit Hilfe der Ungulographie, Zentralblatt fur Veterinarmedizin reihe A 1973;20:209–21.
91. Deuel NR, Park J. Kinelatic analysis of jumping sequences of olympic show jumping horses. In: Persson SGB, Lindholm A, Jeffcott LB, editors. Equine Exercise Physiology 3. Davis: ICEEP publications; 1991. p. 158–66.
92. van den Bogert AJ, Janssen MO, Deuel NR. Kinematics of the hind limb push-off in elite show jumping horses. Equine Vet J 1994;(suppl 17): 80–6.
93. Clayton HM, Colborne GR, Burns T. Kinematic analysis of successful and unsuccessful attempts to clear a water jump. Equine Vet J 1995;(suppl 18):166–9.
94. Barrey E, Galloux P. Analysis of the jumping technique by accelerometry. Equine Vet J 1997;(suppl 23):45–9.
95. Clayton HM. Comparison of the collected, working, medium and extended canters. Equine Vet J 1994;(suppl 17):16–19.
96. Burns TE, Clayton HM. Comparison of the temporal kinematics of the canter pirouette and collected canter. Equine Vet J 1997;(suppl 23):58–61.
97. Holmström M, Fredricson I, Drevemo S. Biokinematic differences between riding horses judged as good and poor at the trot. Equine Vet J 1994;(suppl 17): 51–6.
98. Clayton HM. Performance in equestrian sport. In: Back W, Clayton H, editors. Equine locomotion. London: Saunders; 2001. p. 211.
99. Deuel NR, Park J. The gait patterns of Olympic dressage horses. Int J Sport Biomech 1990;6:198–226.
100. Deuel NR. Dressage canter kinematics and performances in an Olympic three-day event. In: Proceedings of 46th Annual meeting of the European Association for Animal Production,

Horse commission H-2.3; 1995. p. 341.

101. Deuel NR, Park J. Canter lead change kinematics of superior Olympic dressage horses. J Equine Vet Sci 1990;10:287–98.

102. Biau S, Couve O, Lemaire S, et al. The effect of reins on kinetic variables of locomotion. Equine Vet J Suppl 2002;34:359–62.

103. Weishaupt MA, Wiestner T, von Peinen K, et al. Effect of head and neck position on vertical ground reaction forces and interlimb coordination in the dressage horse ridden at walk and trot on a treadmill. Equine Vet J Suppl 2006;36:387–92.

104. Deuel NR, Park J. Gallop kinematics of Olympic Three-day-event horses. Acta Anat 1993;146:168–74.

105. Radin EL, Martin RB, Burr DB, et al. Effects of mechanical loading on the tissues of the rabbit knee. J Orthop Res 1984;2:231–4.

106. Fredricson I, Dalin G, Drevemo S, et al. A biotechnical approach to the geometric design of racetracks. Equine Vet J 1975;7:91–6.

107. Drevemo S, Hjerten G. Evaluation of shock absorbing woodship layer on a harness race-track. In: Persson SGB, Lindholm A, Jeffcott LB, editors. Equine Exercise Physiology 3. Davis: ICEEP publications; 1991. p. 107–12.

108. Clayton HM. Comparison of the stride of trotting horses trimmed with a normal and a broken-back hoof axis. In Proceedings 33rd Annu Conv Am Assoc Equine Practnr 1987;289–299.

11 Joint physiology: responses to exercise and training

René van Weeren

CHAPTER CONTENTS

Introduction

The horse was domesticated around 3000 BC, probably in what is now Southern Russia.[1] From the beginning, the species had a special position. Unlike most other species that had been domesticated before, the horse was not to provide human beings with tangible products such as meat, milk or fur, but to serve mankind with its exceptionally developed locomotor system.

Until very recently, the horse held key positions in human society in the areas of warfare, agriculture and transport. Whereas all these traditional roles of the horse during the past five millennia have come to an end due to the introduction of the internal combustion engine and the subsequent mechanization of society, the horse has not become a zoo species, as feared by some in the early 1950s. It is the appeal of the species to humans that has helped the species to overcome the great dip after World War II and to celebrate a glorious comeback, now as a sports and leisure animal. Currently, horse riding is immensely popular. In France, equestrian sports are third popular in terms of numbers of active participants (after soccer and tennis), in the Netherlands they rank second (after soccer). It can be expected that equestrian activities will retain their attractiveness in the foreseeable future thanks to the individual bonds people tend to develop with horses, albeit equestrian activities are vulnerable to the economic environment. Apart from its use as a sports and leisure animal, the racing industry has, from its initiation in the late eighteenth century, also always maintained a certain number of horses for flat, hurdle and harness racing. The industry as a whole does not seem threatened, but changes in betting customs have their impact, which is most evident in harness racing.

The common denominator of all uses of the horse, whether in the past or in modern-day society, is that they are based on the species' very well developed locomotor system that has enabled the evolution from the less than two hands tall eohippus or *Hyracotherium*, which was a forest-dwelling browser relying on hiding for survival, to the approximately 15 hands tall *Equus Przewalski*, a grazing inhabitant of open savannahs and a typical example of a flight-and-fright animal that survives thanks to its locomotor performance. Given the prominent role of locomotion for the performance of the horse, it will be no surprise that disorders of the musculoskeletal system rank first in causes of wastage in the equine species. Most figures come from the racing industry[2], but also the relatively scarce data for sport horses point in the same direction.[3]

Of all musculoskeletal disorders, joint problems rank, depending on equestrian discipline, invariably first or second (after tendon injury) as a cause of loss of performance.[2,4] They are rarely as acute and dramatic as fractures, but their insidious onset and the inherently low regenerative capacity of (mature) articular cartilage makes them a major plague to the equine industry, which has large economical impact and is a severe welfare issue as well. There is an important parallel with human medicine. The importance of joint disease in man was already well recognized in the eighteenth century when William Hunter wrote his famous statement that *'ulcerated cartilage is universally allowed to be a very troublesome disease;*

that it admits of a cure with more difficulty than a carious bone; and that, when destroyed, it is never recovered'.[5] Chronic joint disorders, of which osteoarthritis (OA) is the most important, are a literally crippling problem in human health care and an important cause of loss of quality of life. Directly in parallel to the equine situation, joint disease is an important issue in human sports performance and therefore there is much interest in the effects of exercise and training on joint function, an area to which relatively much research effort has been dedicated in the past decades.

Where research into joint disorders has long focused on single tissues only (mainly articular cartilage), the current concept is that joints should be seen as organs where the constituting tissues (articular cartilage, subchondral bone, synovial membrane, synovial fluid and in some cases intra-articular ligaments or menisci) act together and proper joint homeostasis is the key element.[6] The effects of exercise and/or training on joints can be translated as changes in (mechanical) loading of joints, which will elicit responses from the tissues and hence affect joint homeostasis. The range of effects on both sides of the optimum is wide and goes from direct trauma to stress deprivation. The almost complete immutability of cartilage, as already alluded to by Hunter, is an important and specific feature. However, in young, growing individuals the plasticity of cartilage is considerably greater and this makes that discrimination should be made between the effects of exercise in full-grown adults and juvenile individuals. The potential long-term effects of (lack of) exercise in youngsters have received relatively much attention in the past years, both in horses and humans.

In the following chapter, first a synopsis will be presented of joint physiology, as elementary knowledge of this is fundamental to understanding the effects of exercise or training. Joint loading is intrinsically connected with proper joint development in juvenile individuals, for which reason a section on the effects of joint loading on immature cartilage will follow. The chapter ends with the effects of biomechanical loading on mature joints.

Principles of joint physiology

Diarthrodial joints flexibly interconnect parts of the skeleton, making deformation (and hence locomotion) of the body possible without losing the rigidity of the individual segments. To accomplish this task, joints have to meet challenging and sometimes even contradictory demands. They must absorb and transmit the heavy forces generated by locomotion just like the bony skeleton, but they must also enable smooth gliding of the bony ends over each other. The latter aspect not only requires specific capacities with respect to lubrication, but also high resistance to shear loading. Joints can be seen as the bearings of the body, parts that are known to be vulnerable and prone to failure in mechanical engineering.

Figure 11.1 is a schematic drawing of a diarthrodial joint, outlining its principal components: subchondral bone, cartilage, the joint capsule and synovial fluid. These components will be reviewed briefly in the following section. The emphasis will be on articular cartilage, which is the joint tissue with most morbidity and least regenerative capacity.

Subchondral bone

The subchondral bone supports the overlying cartilage and is connected with it through a layer of calcified cartilage. Typically, subchondral bone consists of a layer of compact bone directly adjacent to the layer of calcified cartilage and trabecular bone at greater distance from the joint cavity. This conformation has mechanical consequences: the compact subchondral plate provides firm support, but is rigid, while the trabecular component provides some elasticity. Sclerosis of the subchondral plate is one of the hallmarks of OA and it has been suggested that this might be a primary event in cartilage damage, rather than a sequel to it, which is the commonly held opinion.[7] Subchondral bone is, unlike cartilage, richly vascularized and has a well-developed nerve supply that plays a major role in pain perception in joint diseases.

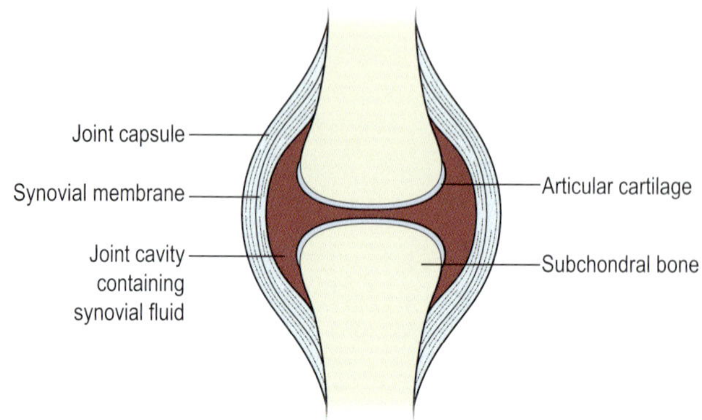

Fig 11.1 Schematic representation of a diarthrodial joint.
From: De Grauw JC, Molecular monitoring of equine joint homeostasis. Thesis, Utrecht University, 2010, with kind permission.

Cartilage

Articular cartilage has an important role in both the transmission and attenuation of forces generated by locomotion. This leads to seemingly contradicting requirements of both elasticity and great strength, for which Nature has provided a solution by conceiving an extracellular matrix (ECM) that consists of two principal components: collagen fibrils and proteoglycan aggregates.

The collagen fibrils consist of collagen type II molecules (3 α_1 chains in triple helix configuration) and form a three-dimensional arcade network.[8] The fibrils are anchored within the layer of calcified cartilage that is adjacent to the subchondral bone, then course perpendicular to this layer towards the joint surface to bend before reaching the surface, running tangentially to and directly under it, to close the arch by bending back again and returning perpendicularly to the calcified cartilage layer where they end (Fig. 11.2). Structural coherence and extra strength is provided by cross-links that connect the α_1 chains within the same collagen molecule and interconnect different collagen molecules and different collagen fibrils. The formation of cross-links is one of the so-called post-translational modifications of collagen and is the last chemical modification occurring during the formation of the primary collagen structure. There are various types of cross-links. Common covalent cross-links are the pyridinoline cross-links that form between lysyl and hydroxylysyl residues in the collagen network (lysylpyridinoline or LP cross-links and hydroxylysylpyridinoline or HP-cross-links respectively) in a largely irreversible process. They have a major influence on the structural and hence on the biomechanical characteristics of the collagen network.[9] A special category of cross-links is formed through the process of non-enzymatic glycation. Collagen molecules have an exceptionally long lifetime once incorporated into the ECM of cartilage, which makes them susceptible to the accumulation of advanced non-enzymatic glycation end products (AGEs) via the so-called Maillard reaction. This process results in increased cross-linking, such as pentosidine formation from lysine, sugar and arginine moieties. Pentosidine is one of the few Maillard cross-links

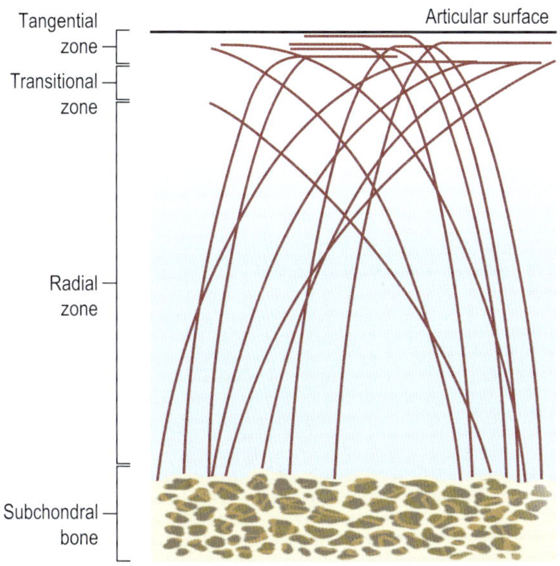

Fig 11.2 Schematic representation of the configuration of the collagen network within articular cartilage, showing the arcade-like structure originally described by Benninghoff (1925).
Redrawn from: Van Weeren and Firth: Vet Clin North Am Equine Pract ***24****, 153–175, 2008, with permission from Elsevier.*

of which the structure has been elucidated and can be used as a sensitive marker for the process of non-enzymatic glycation. As the accumulation of AGEs depends on the turnover rate of a protein or tissue, they can be used as a measure for the metabolic rate of that structure.[10]

The other main component of cartilage extracellular matrix is formed by proteoglycan aggregates, which are interspersed between the collagen fibrils and connected to them either directly or via hyaluronan (hyaluronic acid) molecules. Aggrecan is the most important of these aggregates. Aggrecan is a composite molecule, consisting of a core protein with large numbers of sulphated glycosaminoglycans (chondroitin sulphate and keratan sulphate) as side chains. The sulphate groups give these side chains a negative charge, making them hydrophilic. The combination of the swelling pressure that results from this hydrophilic character with the confinement due to the stiffness of the collagen network creates an intrinsic pressure within the ECM of articular cartilage that provides it with the unique combination of resilience under compression and resistance against tensional and shear forces.

Due to anatomical and geometric particularities, joints are not loaded evenly over their surface. Different areas are subject to different magnitudes and types of loading, such as low-level constant loading, intermittent loading, and very high impact loading. These variable loading conditions can only adequately be met by cartilage that possesses different mechanical properties in different sites.[11] This heterogeneity in biomechanical behaviour can only be accomplished through different biochemical and ultrastructural characteristics, which indeed have been shown to exist (Fig. 11.3).[12–16]

Cartilage not only displays 'horizontal' zonal heterogeneity over the surface, but also 'vertical' along its depth. The superficial layer is characterized by flattened chondrocytes, densely packed type II collagen fibrils running parallel to the surface, a relatively small amount of proteoglycans (PG) and high water content.[17] The middle or transitional zone has lower water content, more PG and a lower density of collagen fibrils that seem less organized because they form arches and thus do not run parallel, and rounded chondrocytes dispersed irregularly in the extracellular matrix. The deep zone has collagen fibrils that are oriented perpendicular to the articular surface (again running parallel to each other), the highest concentration of PG but the lowest percentage of water of any zone, and chondrocytes arranged in columns perpendicular to the subchondral bone.

Articular cartilage may seem to be a very static tissue, but it undergoes constant remodelling through anabolic and catabolic processes. The chondrocyte, as the only cell type found in normal articular cartilage, produces all ECM components. Collagen molecules are manufactured intracellularly in the form of pro-collagen and are subsequently extracellularly modified by enzymatic cleavage of the C- and N-terminal propeptides before being integrated in the collagen network. Degradation of ECM is effectuated by various proteinases, of which the matrix metalloproteinases (MMPs) and aggrecanases (members of the disintegrin and metalloproteinase with thrombospondin motifs (ADAMTS) gene family) are the most important. It is important to note that the two principal constituents of the cartilage ECM, collagens and proteoglycans, have very different turnover rates. Turnover time of proteoglycans is variable and ranges in mature individuals from approximately 300 days for overall turnover in canine articular cartilage to around 20 years for the long-lived globular hyaluronic acid binding domain of aggrecan in humans.[18] This may seem long, but collagen turnover times have been estimated to be up to 350 years in mature human cartilage.[19] Comparable data for the horse do not exist, but can be assumed to be in the same order of magnitude. It is this very low turnover rate and thus extremely limited repair capacity that lies at the basis of the famous observation by William Hunter cited earlier[5] and that makes OA in both humans and horses into a disease with an almost invariably poor long-term prognosis for performance.

Synovial membrane

The outer layer of the joint capsule consists of relatively stiff fibrous tissue. It serves mainly for mechanical stability and to host a great number of proprioceptive nerve endings that provide information on actual joint position to the brain. The inner layer of the capsule, which is the actual lining of the joint cavity, is two to three cells thick and has great influence on synovial fluid composition and hence on joint homeostasis. The synovial membrane contains two types of cells: type A macrophage-like synovial cells and type B synoviocytes or fibroblast-like synoviocytes that have the capacity to produce hyaluronan or hyaluronic acid, a non-sulphated glycosaminoglycan macromolecule that is both a major component of the cartilage extracellular matrix and a principal component of synovial fluid, determining to a large extent the viscosity of this fluid. Both cell types can produce large arrays of cytokines, growth factors and inflammatory mediators, especially in case of joint pathology. Unlike articular cartilage, the joint capsule is richly vascularized and is much more reactive to external stimuli than cartilage itself, giving the joint capsule and especially the synovial membrane a very important role in both the maintenance and aberrations of joint homeostasis.

Synovial fluid

The synovial membrane has no basement membrane or tight junctions. In fact, the cells are located within a loose and porous bed of collagen fibrils and other matrix proteins. This configuration allows the diffusion of all but the largest molecules (>10KDa) from the blood to the synovial cavity and synovial fluid (SF) can hence

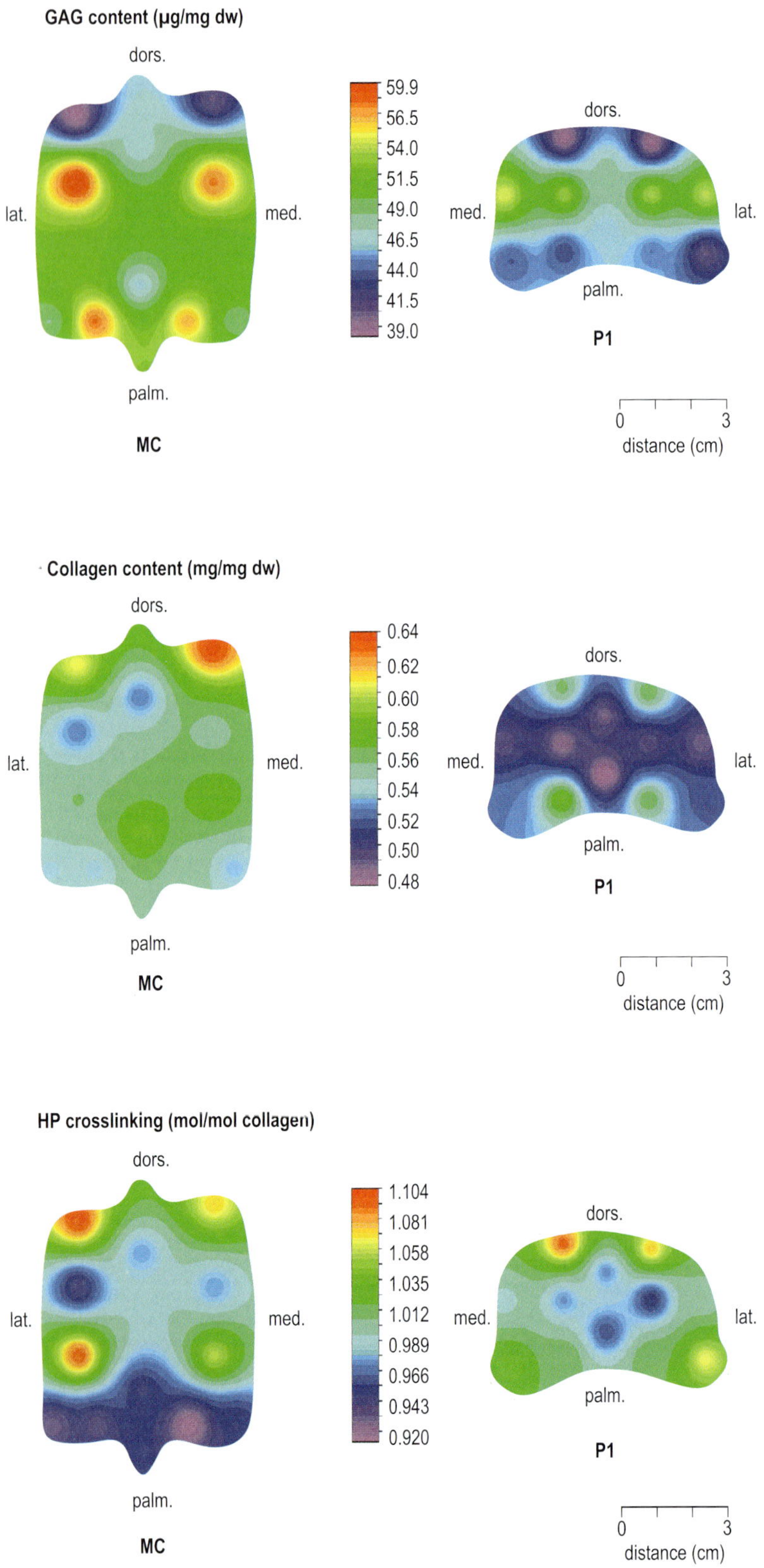

Fig 11.3 Distribution of glycosaminoglycan content (GAG), collagen content, and hydroxylysylpyridinoline (HP) cross-linking over the proximal articular surface of the proximal phalanx and the distal articular surface of the third metacarpal bone. Cm=centimeter; dors.=dorsal; GAG=glycosaminoglycan; HP=hydroxylysylpyridinoline; lat.=lateral; MC=distal third metacarpal bone; med.=medial; palm.=palmar; P1=proximal first phalanx.
From: Brama et al.*: Equine Veterinary Journal* ***33****, 26–32, 2001, with permission from the Equine Veterinary Journal.*

be seen as an ultrafiltrate of blood plasma, supplemented with hyaluronic acid and other products from the A and B type synoviocytes. This situation allows the supply with nutrients and the removal of waste products from the avascular cartilage. Synovial fluid is yellowish in color and highly viscous, due to the high hyaluronic acid content. The cellular component is limited, normally not surpassing 0.5 G/L, and consists mainly of lymphocytes and other bone marrow derived mononuclear cells. The SF can be seen as a mirror of joint homeostasis *par excellence*, as it bathes both tissue types that line the synovial cavity, articular cartilage and the synovial membrane. In case of an infringement of joint homeostasis, the synovial membrane is likely to respond first as the most reactive of the tissues and may produce a plethora of inflammatory mediators and cytokines, of which Tumour Necrosis Factor alpha (TNF-α) and Interleukin 1 beta (IL-1β) are known to be major players in joint disorders. Through their dispersion in the SF, these mediators affect the cartilage. The determination of the inflammatory profile of SF has received increased attention in recent years in the context of the quest for early detection of OA, as it now is widely accepted that also in this seemingly 'degenerative' disease, low-grade inflammation plays a crucial role too.[20] On the other hand, metabolic responses of the cartilage will be reflected in changes of in levels of products and by-products of proteoglycan and collagen metabolism, such as the proteoglycan marker CS846, and C2C and CPII as makers for collagen break-down and synthesis respectively.[21]

Loading the immature joint: crucial conditioning

So far, this chapter has described normal joint physiology and looked at the load-related topographical heterogeneity of cartilage. In the following paragraphs, first the physiological development of this topographical heterogeneity will be discussed, followed by an overview of the effects of biomechanical loading on both juvenile and mature articular cartilage.

The origins of topographical heterogeneity of articular cartilage

In theory, there are two possible origins of the topographical heterogeneity of articular cartilage: genetic predetermination or formation in the early juvenile period when cartilage metabolism is still high. The first indication for the latter option came from work by Little and Ghosh[22], who showed that proteoglycan content was identical over the entire joint surface in neonatal lambs, which is unlike the situation in adult sheep where there is topographical heterogeneity. Extensive work by Brama and co-authors showed that proteoglycan content and collagen, including post-translational modifications of collagen such as cross-links, were homogeneously distributed across the joint of the newborn foal as well. They called this neonatal situation the 'blank joint'.[23] Most of the topographical heterogeneity was already present at age five months, but HP cross-links (the most abundant pyridinoline cross-link in articular cartilage) did not reach a mature value until after 12 months.[12,23] Later, the underlying maturation process of articular cartilage in early life was indirectly confirmed using equine-specific cDNA micro-arrays. There was a distinct difference between neonatal and mature individuals in the expression of genes encoding matrix proteins and matrix modifying enzymes, with the former expressing more collagens, matrix-modifying enzymes and provisional matrix non-collagenous proteins and the latter showing a transition from growth to homeostasis and tissue function related to coping with shear and compressive forces.[24]

The changes during early life are not limited to the biochemical composition of the extracellular matrix. The arcade structure of the collagen network, as originally described by Benninghoff[8], is typical for mature cartilage, but not yet present in the newborn. Investigations using polarized light microscopy have shown that collagen fibril orientation is predominantly parallel to the joint surface and subchondral bone at birth to gradually change to the classic arcade structure after birth.[25]

Shaping the joint: the process of functional adaptation

The term 'functional adaptation' to describe the transition from a blank, neonatal joint to the mature joint featuring topograpraphical heterogeneity was coined by Brama et al.[23] The first evidence that biomechanical loading is the driving force in this process came from a study that was originally designed to study the influence of exercise on the developmental orthopaedic disease osteochondrosis. That study, commonly referred to by the acronym 'EXOC' (for exercise and osteochondrosis), used a group of 43 Warmblood foals, which was subdivided into three groups from the age of one week. One group (n = 14) was kept in box stalls for 24 hours per day; the second group (n = 14) was kept in identical box stalls, but was additionally subjected to exercise in the form of a number of short sprints during a restricted period, i.e. in this group high-intensity exercise was alternated with a sedentary lifestyle; the third group (n = 15) had free pasture exercise for 24 hours/day. These different exercise regimens were maintained until weaning at five months of age. Then, eight foals from each group were euthanized and their tissues harvested for a variety of analyzes. The remaining 19 foals were brought together in a single group and subjected to a moderate exercise regimen. These animals were euthanized at age 11 months and had their tissues analyzed to see if any difference that might have been provoked by the different exercise regimens during the first five months of their lives would be reversible or not. Figure 11.4 schematically depicts the experimental design of the experiment.

Topographical heterogeneity, which was expressed as a significant difference from zero of the ratio of two very differently loaded sites within the joint, developed in the pastured group and in the boxed/sprinted group alike. However, it failed to develop in the boxed foals. This was direct proof of the steering effect of biomechanical loading on the process of functional adaptation.[23] As expected, not only the cartilage responded, also the subchondral bone. At age five months, bone density in the third tarsal bone was about 25% less in the box-rested foals compared to the other two groups.[26] Also, calcium content and HP and LP cross-links increased significantly less over time in the subchondral bone of the proximal phalanx in box-rested foals.[27] However, the most interesting observation was that, where proteoglycans and also subchondral bone density

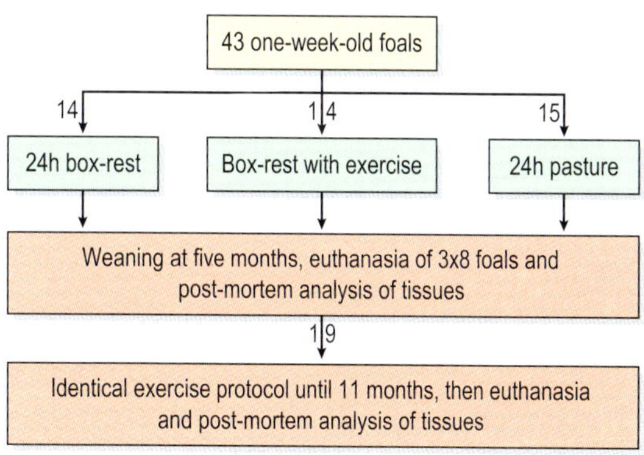

Fig 11.4 Experimental set-up of the EXOC study. Forty-three warmblood foals were divided into three different exercise groups at age one week. Exercise regimens consisted of either 24 hours/day box rest (N = 14), a similar sedentary protocol but with additional high-intensity sprinting exercise for 30 minutes per day (N = 14), or free pasture exercise (N = 15). After weaning at age five months, eight foals from each group were euthanized and their tissues harvested. The remaining 19 foals were housed together and given a moderate exercise regimen. These animals were euthanized at age 11 months.

became normal after the common training programme from 5 to 11 months with foals from all former exercise groups showing similar levels, collagen and other collagen-related parameters such as hydroxylysine remained abnormal. They failed to 'catch up' and to develop the topographical heterogeneity that is characteristic of mature individuals (Fig. 11.5).[23] Therefore, for collagen there seems to be a limited window in time when the process of functional adaptation can take place. It is very likely that, when the period of time when the collagen component of the ECM is still responsive to loading is not appropriately used, the joint will be left with inferior cartilage that is less resistant to life-long wear and tear and hence more susceptible to injury. This stresses the great importance of sufficient exercise in the early juvenile phase.

In the boxed/sprinted animals that had been subjected to a combination of short bouts of high-intensity exercise with a sedentary lifestyle the degree of development of topographical heterogeneity was comparable to the pastured animals, which were regarded as controls. However, culture experiments with chondrocytes harvested at age 11 months from animals from all former exercise groups showed that chondrocytes from the former box/sprinted group could not be stimulated to increase metabolic activity, in contrast to samples from both other groups. Apparently, there was a deleterious long-term effect of the combination of sedentary lifestyle with bouts of high intensity exercise, possibly because of a kind of cellular exhaustion that might be due to overstimulation during the first five months of life.[28] Analysis of serum markers (CPII and Ctx1) showed indirectly a negative effect on collagen turnover, compared to pastured foals.[29] Also in other tissues from these animals a negative effect of the combination of rest with bouts of high-intensity exercise could be detected.[30]

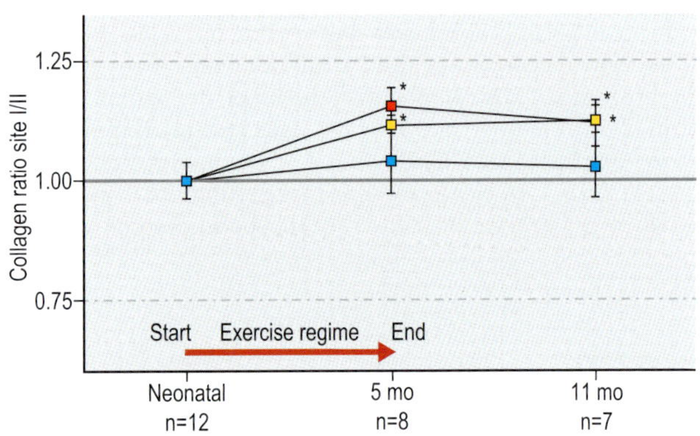

Fig 11.5 The influence of different exercise levels during the first five months after birth on the collagen ratio of two different sites of the proximal articular surface of the proximal phalanx. Site 1 at the medial dorsal margin of the joint surface is not loaded when standing still or in a slowly moving animal, but it is subject to high intermittent peak loading in overextended joints at high speeds and during jumping. Site 2 in the central fovea is continually loaded when the limb is weight-bearing, but experiences lower absolute forces than site 1. Values are given as mean ± standard error of the mean. (____: pasture exercise; _ _ _: box-rest with additional high-intensity exercise; -.-.-: box-rest). N = number of animals; *= p<0.01. Both groups that were exercised develop a site 1 / site 2 ratio that is significantly different from one in the first five months of life, *i.e.* develop topographical heterogeneity. The box rested animals do not develop this topographical heterogeneity and failed to compensate for this in the following six months when undergoing a moderate exercise regimen.
*From Brama et al., Equine Veterinary Journal **34**, 265–269, 2002, with permission from the Equine Veterinary Journal.*

Manipulating Mother Nature: conditioning the youngster through exercise

The Global Equine Research Alliance (GERA, a consortium of the equine orthopedic research groups from Massey University, Colorado State University, the Royal Veterinary College, and Utrecht University), conducted another large-scale study on the effect of early exercise on foals, which became known under the acronym GEXA. From the EXOC study the pasture group came out best in terms of conditioning of musculoskeletal tissues and this raised immediately the question whether it would be possible, through the combination of pasture exercise and superimposed on this additional exercise, to even better prepare the musculoskeletal system for future athletic performance. In the GEXA study 33 Thoroughbred foals were raised divided into two groups. One group (PASTEX, n = 15) had free pasture exercise all year round, in agreement with common New Zealand practice; the second group (CONDEX, n = 18) was raised under similar conditions, but also subjected to an additional exercise programme. The programme implied cantering and sprinting, increasing overall workload by a moderate, but significant, 30%.[31] At age 18 months, 12 animals (six from each group) were sacrificed for detailed tissue analyzes.

The differences in exercise load in the GEXA study were much less extreme than in the earlier EXOC study and less outspoken differences, if any, were to be expected. However, notwithstanding the only gradual difference in exercise load, several effects were observed. Biochemical and biomechanical analyzes of full thickness cartilage samples from the distal metacarpal bone showed site-related differences, but no exercise effect.[32] Also, the metabolic rate of chondrocytes (measured by ^{35}S-uptake) from third metacarpal cartilage was not different[33], and there was no exercise effect on the thickness of calcified cartilage of the distal metacarpal condyle.[34] However, exercised horses had more viable chondrocytes in the more heavily loaded sites compared to less loaded sites of the same metacarpal cartilage.[35] Further, a detailed study of contiguous 100μm thick slices taken from the proximal articular surface of the proximal phalanx down to the tidemark at differently loaded sites showed not only obvious site differences, but also exercise-related changes. There was no exercise effect on proteoglycan content, indicating that the exercise level had not been strenuous and confirming the earlier work[32,33], but the normal physiological increase in collagen at the site located at the joint margin was less in the CONDEX group.[36] This was interpreted as a precocious cessation of collagen remodelling at this site due to a load-induced speeding up of the normal maturation process. The collagen characteristics of similar slices from the same site in the metatarsophalangeal joint pointed in the same direction: in the CONDEX animals, hydroxylysine content, HP cross-links and pentosidine cross-links were all higher, which is indicative of advancement of the normal process of functional adaptation.[37] The increased pentosidine levels in the CONDEX animals are of particular interest, because they indicate a lower metabolic activity in this group, confirming an advanced degree of maturation compared to the PASTEX animals.

Additional evidence for this exercise-induced difference in maturation rate came from ultrastructural studies. The parallelism index (PI, a measure of the degree to which the collagen fibrils are aligned to each other) and orientation index (OI, a measure of the average angle of collagen fibrils with respect to the articular surface) were measured using polarized light microscopy. Parallelism index was higher in CONDEX animals, which was again indicative of advanced maturation.[38] An interesting supplementary observation was that the orientation of collagen fibrils in the deep zone of the cartilage was less perpendicular to the layer of calcified cartilage than expected. This was explained as an adaptation of the direction of collagen fibres to the high shear forces in the equine metacarpophalangeal joint, which is a heavily loaded joint with an exceptionally high range of motion where an oblique insertion of the collagen fibres in the calcified cartilage layer may yield better resistance to shear than would a more perpendicular configuration. Based on this observation it was suggested that the Benninghoff arcade model might be more flexible than commonly thought and that local adaptation of fibril direction may lead to a predominantly non-perpendicular direction of the collagen fibrils in the deep zone of cartilage in certain joints.[38]

Evidence from other species

Most large-scale and long-term studies into the effect of exercise on the maturation process of the juvenile musculoskeletal system have been carried out in horses, but there is also evidence from other species that the exercise regimen at early age may affect cartilage properties and that this effect need not always be reversible. In a study in young Beagles, in which one of the hindlimbs was immobilized for 11 weeks, it was shown that GAG content may be reduced by almost 50% in the non weight-bearing limb. Cartilage thickness and GAG-content were increased in the contralateral limb.[39] When the study was repeated, but now followed by a 15-week rehabilitation programme, the normal situation appeared to be not fully restored. From this the authors concluded that immobilization of skeletally immature joints may affect cartilage development such that recovery is very slow or alterations are permanent.[40]

In humans a similar pattern is seen: physical activity was a significant explanatory factor for cartilage thickness at all sites investigated by MRI in children in a cross-sectional study, which led to the conclusion that *'the current evidence supports a prescription of vigorous physical activity for optimum joint development in children'*.[41]

There is thus compelling evidence that early exercise affects the tissues of the musculoskeletal system. However, very little is known about the long-term effects on orthopedic health. Too little exercise may be detrimental, but too much exercise may have negative effects as well. In a study in hamsters, animals having free access to a running wheel during the first three months of life showed differences in the collagen network organization at age five months, especially in the middle and deep zones. They had less OA than sedentary controls at age 12 months, but three months later the situation was reversed.[42]

On the brink of maturity: experimental evidence for the effects of exercise in young-adult horses

There are no large-scale experimental studies on the effects of exercise on cartilage from mature or elderly horses, but a substantial amount of work has been performed in two-year-old Thoroughbreds. These animals are still growing, be it at a much lower rate than foals, and therefore cannot be considered as fully skeletally mature yet. They could be classified as "young-adult".

In what is called the short-term Bristol study, two-year-old Thoroughbreds were subjected to a 19-week exercise regimen in which they galloped three times weekly on a treadmill, trotted in a mechanical horse walker also three times per week and were walked for 40 minutes six times weekly. The control group only received the walking exercise.[43,44] In the Massey University Grass Exercise Study (MUGES), a group of two-year-old Thoroughbreds was trained for 13 weeks on grass and sand tracks. After this, the musculoskeletal tissues were analyzed.[45]

In the Bristol study, cartilage from the proximal articular surface of the radial, intermediate and third carpal bone from exercised animals had a thicker calcified layer than from non-exercised animals, but the hyaline cartilage layer was similar in thickness.[43] Biomechanically the cartilage of the strenuously trained animals was less stiff, more fibrillated and with more chondrocyte clusters than the gentler trained animals, suggesting deterioration of cartilage due to strenuous exercise.[44] Also cartilage oligomeric matrix protein (COMP) distribution[46], subchondral bone thickness and hardness[47] and fibronectin[48] were influenced by exercise. When culturing cartilage to measure chondrocyte metabolic activity, proteoglycan synthesis rates were higher in the trained animals than in the controls, which confirmed the overall effect of strenuous exercise on the proteoglycan component of articular cartilage.[49] There were no overall effects on the collagen component of the extracellular matrix, but sites that are known to be predisposed to injury contained significantly less collagen in exercised horses. Strenuously exercised animals had also higher glycosaminoglycan content than horses from the gentler trained group. This was most marked in the cartilage from the dorsal radial and dorsal intermediate carpal surfaces, which are sites known to be heavily loaded during exercise.[16] In contrast to the Bristol study, in the MUGES study a significant increase in thickness of (hyaline) cartilage was seen in particular sites within the middle carpal joint after 13 weeks of training, in comparison to the pasture-raised controls.[50] The response of the tissue was thought to be adaptive and not degenerative in nature, because at these sites there was no patho-anatomical damage. Stiffness of the metacarpal condylar subarticular calcified tissue, measured by nano indentation, was not different between the exercised groups.[51] However, in the metacarpophalangeal (MCP) joints of the same animals wear lines and fibrillation were present and water content was increased while HP cross-links had fallen compared to the controls. These observations were interpreted as signs of loosening of the collagen network due to micro-damage.[52]

Loading the mature joint: the balance between maintenance and morbidity

The metacarpophalangeal joint is known to be the equine joint most susceptible to damage.[53] It is the MCP joint that, together with the carpal joint, has received most attention in terms of effect of exercise. This can to a large extent be explained by the high incidence of condylar fractures in the MCP joint and of third carpal bone slab fractures in the carpus in racehorses.

In mature horses the articular cartilage has lost its plasticity and cannot be conditioned further, but (subchondral) bone remains responsive to exercise according to Wolff's law[54] and a certain degree of loading is necessary for maintenance. Cast immobilization for seven weeks followed by a gradually increasing rehabilitation programme for eight weeks led to substantial loss of volumetric bone mineral density of subchondral bone that was not fully recovered during the rehab period.[55]

Too much exercise is more common in the equine industry than too little and the effect of loading may vary from avoidance of negative effects due to disuse to the infliction of severe overload-induced damage, depending on the type and intensity of exercise. Different types of high-intensity exercise were associated with different patterns of SCB thickness in tarsal joints[56], and exercise-induced microcracks are well-known to be the initial stages of condylar fractures of the metacarpus in racehorses.[57] Exercise may, apart from its effect on subchondral bone, also affect thickness of both the calcified and hyaline cartilage layer and increase the risk of osteochondral lesions.[58,59] Exercise-induced loading has been shown to decrease COMP content at intermittently highly loaded areas, whereas regular lower level loading promotes COMP synthesis and/or retention.[60] A similar negative effect of too much exercise was seen in an *ex vivo* study in which material from the dorsal radial facet of the third carpal bone, an area subjected to high contact stresses in galloping horses, was cultured.[61] The material came from horses having undergone a strenuous exercise regimen and in these animals a significant reduction in aggrecan synthesis and a concomitant increase in decorin synthesis could be determined compared to less vigorously trained controls. Based on these findings, it was suggested that this alteration in articular cartilage metabolism could be a predisposing factor for cartilage degeneration and OA at a later stage.

The overall metabolism-enhancing effect of exercise on articular cartilage has been studied indirectly in several studies focusing on a variety of potential biomarkers in serum or synovial fluid. Moderate to strenuous exercise led to increases in plasma GAG levels, and serum keratan sulphate and COMP.[62–64] Higher chondroitin sulphate peak chain lengths, but shorter hyaluronic acid chain lengths were found in exercised versus rested horses.[65] Another study confirmed the increase in proteoglycan markers in both serum and synovial fluid after exercise, and showed the same was true for a number of collagen markers.[66] Exercise increased prostaglandin E_2 content in synovial fluid[67], but moderate exercise did not affect MMP-1 activity.[68] There is a mutual interaction between synovial fluid and articular cartilage. The former is not just a reflection of the status of the latter, but may in itself influence cartilage metabolism. In fact, the effects of joint loading on cartilage are, at least in part, mediated by alterations in the synovial fluid. Cartilage explants cultured in post-exercise synovial fluid showed enhanced GAG synthesis and diminished release when compared to cultures using pre-exercise synovial fluid.[69]

An influence of exercise on articular cartilage has been demonstrated in other species than the horse as well. In young Beagle dogs, moderate loading levels tended to increase GAG production, while strenuous exercise led to GAG depletion in high-load areas.[70]

Conclusion

Articular cartilage is responsive to biomechanical loading and responsiveness is highest in the youngest individuals. There is now compelling evidence that the characteristic topographical heterogeneity in composition and ultrastructure of the extracellular matrix of mature cartilage is formed under the influence of loading, i.e. through physical exercise. The comparison with bone has been made and it has been suggested that the collagen network of juvenile animals that are in a phase of rapid growth responds to loading in a fashion similar to which trabecular bone is known to respond to exercise, a mechanism demonstrated more than a century ago by Julius Wolff.[54,71] However, there is a big difference with bone. Whereas bone will continue to respond to exercise throughout life, the collagen network can most probably do so only in the young, growing animal before the collagen remodelling rate falls to the extremely low level that is typical for mature individuals and is characterized by the very long collagen turnover times mentioned earlier. Indeed, where some studies have shown a response of the proteoglycan component of the ECM of cartilage to exercise in (young) adult horses, no adaptive response of collagen has ever been demonstrated in this age group. This makes the early juvenile period into the only window of opportunity to manipulate the collagen network through modification of loading, *i.e.* differences in exercise. Recent studies show that such manipulation is possible indeed and may either irreversibly delay the normal maturation process as a result of lack of sufficient exercise level, or accelerate maturation. Such advanced maturation will result in a different topographical pattern in animals subjected to additional exercise on top of the "gold standard" of free pasture exercise. There is thus good reason to believe that exercise at early age may indeed have long-lasting effects on the collagen matrix of articular cartilage. Therefore, the hypothesis that variations in exercise regimens of juvenile persons or animals may influence the risk for the development of degenerative joint diseases later in life seems to be true.[72] In practical terms, this may mean support the suggestion that athletic training of horses might better start earlier rather than later.[73] However, no definitive answer can be given yet about the possible beneficial effect of additional exercise. For this, long-term epidemiological studies are necessary to establish what the clinical effect is in terms of injury risk and/or performance over the entire career of the equine athlete of the permanent modifications in the make-up of articular cartilage that can be provoked by exercise at early age.

In mature joints both reduced loading and overloading have catabolic effects, which have most clinical impact on the cartilage component, as cartilage damage, irrespective whether it is due to joint overuse or prolonged disuse, is irreversible because of the very limited spontaneous repair capacity of articular cartilage.

References

1. Dunlop RH, Williams DJ, editors. Veterinary Medicine. An illustrated history. St. Louis: Mosby; 1996.
2. Williams RB, Harkins LS, Hammond CJ, et al. Racehorse injuries, clinical problems and fatalities recorded on British racecourses from flat racing and National Hunt racing during 1996, 1997 and 1998. Equine Vet J 2001;33:478–86.
3. Sloet van Oldruitenborgh-Oosterbaan MM, Genzel, W, van Weeren PR. A pilot study on factors influencing the career of Dutch sport horses. Equine Vet J 2010;(Suppl 38):28–32.
4. Murray RC, Dyson SJ, Tranquille C, et al. Association of type and sport and performance level with anatomical site of orthopaedic injury diagnosis. Equine Vet J 2006;(Suppl 36):411–16.
5. Hunter W. Of the structure and diseases of articulating cartilages. Proc R Soc London 1743;9:514–21.
6. Samuels J, Krasnokutsky S, Abramson SB. Osteoarthritis. A tale of three tissues. Bull NYU Hosp Joint Dis 2008;66:244–50.
7. Radin EL. Subchondral bone changes and cartilage damage. Equine Vet J 1999;31:94–5.
8. Benninghoff A. Form und Bau der Gelenkknorpel in ihren Beziehungen zur Funktion. Zweiter teil: Der Aufbau des Gelenkknorpels in seinen Beziehungen zur Funktion. Zsch Zelforsch Mikroskop Anat 1925;2:783–862.
9. Eyre DR, Wu JJ. Collagen structure and cartilage matrix integrity. J Rheumatol 1995;22:82–5.
10. Verzijl N, DeGroot J, Bank RA, et al. Age-related accumulation of the advanced glycation end product pentosidine in human articular cartilage aggrecan: The use of pentosidine levels as a quantitative measure of protein turnover. Matrix Biol 2001;20:409–17.
11. Herzog W, Federico S. Considerations on joint and articular cartilage mechanics. Biomech Mod Mechanobiol 2006;5:64–81.

12. Brama PA, Tekoppele JM, Bank RA, et al. Functional adaptation of equine articular cartilage: the formation of regional biochemical characteristics up to age one year. Equine Vet J 2000;32:217–21.
13. Brama PA, Tekoppele JM, Bank RA, et al.Topographical mapping of biochemical properties of articular cartilage in the equine fetlock joint. Equine Vet J 2000;32:19–26.
14. Brommer H, Brama PA, Laasanen MS, et al. Functional adaptation of articular cartilage from birth to maturity under the influence of loading: A biomechanical analysis. Equine Vet J 2005;37:148–54.
15. Palmer JL, Bertone AL, Mansour J, et al. Biomechanical properties of third carpal articular cartilage in exercised and nonexercised horses. J Orthop Res 1995;13:854–60.
16. Murray RC, Birch HL, Lakhani K, et al. Biochemical composition of equine carpal articular cartilage is influenced by short-term exercise in a site-specific manner. Osteoarthritis Cart 2001;9:625–32.
17. Aydelotte MN, Kuettner KE. Differences between sub-populations of cultured bovine articular chondrocytes. I. Morphology and cartilage matrix production. Connect Tissue Res 1988;18:205–22.
18. Maroudas A, Bayliss MT, Uchitel-Kraushansky N, et al. Aggrecan turnover in human articular cartilage: use of aspartic acid racemisation as a marker of molecular age. Arch Bioche. Biophys 1998;350:61–71.
19. Maroudas A, Palla G, Gilav E. Racemization of aspartic acid in human articular cartilage. Connect Tissue Res 1992;28:161–9.
20. Attur MG, Dave M, Akamatsu M, et al. Osteoarthritis or osteoarthrosis: the definition of inflammation becomes a semantic issue in the genomic era of molecular medicine. Osteoarthritis Cart 2002;10:1–4.
21. Van Weeren PR, Firth EC. Future tools for early diagnosis and monitoring of musculoskeletal injury: biomarkers and CT. Vet Cli. North Am Equine Practice 2008;24:153–75.
22. Little CB, Ghosh P. Variation in proteoglycan metabolism by articular chondrocytes in different joint regions is determined by post-natal mechanical loading. Osteoarthritis Cart 1997;5:49–62.
23. Brama PA, TeKoppele JM, Bank RA, et al. Development of biochemical heterogeneity of articular cartilage: influences of age and exercise. Equine Vet J 2002;34:265–9.
24. Mienaltowski MJ, Huang L, Stromberg AJ, et al. Differential gene expression associated with postnatal equine articular cartilage maturation. BMC Musculoskelet Disord 2008;9:149.
25. Van Turnhout MC, Haazeleger MB, Gijsen MA, et al. Quantitative description of collagen structure in the articular cartilage of the young and adult equine distal metacarpus. Anim Biol 2008;58:353–70.
26. Barneveld A, van Weeren PR. Early changes in the distal intertarsal joint of Dutch warmblood foals and the influence of exercise on bone density in the third tarsal bone. Equine Vet J 1999;(Suppl 31):67–73.
27. Brama PA, TeKoppele JM, Bank RA, et al. Biochemical development of subchondral bone from birth until age eleven months and the influence of physical activity. Equine Vet J 2002;34:143–9.
28. Van den Hoogen BM, van de Lest CH, van Weeren PR, et al. Effect of exercise on proteoglycan metabolism of articular cartilage in growing foals. Equine Vet J 1999;(Suppl 31):62–6.
29. Billinghurst RC, Brama PA, van Weeren PR, et al. Significant exercise-related changes in the serum levels of two biomarkers of collagen metabolism in young horses. Osteoarthritis Cart 2003;11:760–9.
30. Barneveld A, van Weeren PR. Conclusions regarding the influence of exercise on the development of the equine musculoskeletal system with special reference to osteochondrosis. Equine Vet J 1999;(Suppl 31):112–19.
31. Rogers CW, Firth EC, McIlwraith CW, et al. Evaluation of a new strategy to modulate skeletal development in Thoroughbred performance horses by imposing track-based exercise during growth. Equine Vet J 2008;40:111–18.
32. Nugent GE, Law AW, Wong EG, et al. Site- and exercise-related variation in structure and function of cartilage from equine distal metacarpal condyle. Osteoarthritis Cart 2004;12:826–33.
33. Kawcak CE, McIlwraith CW, Firth EC. Effects of early exercise on metacarpophalangeal joints in horses. Am J Vet Res 2009;71:405–11.
34. Doube M, Firth EC, Boyde A. Variations in articular cartilage by site and exercise in the 18-month-old equine metacarpal condyle. Osteoarthritis Cart 2007;15:1283–92.
35. Dykgraaf S, Firth EC, Rogers CW, et al. Effects of exercise on chondrocyte viability and subchondral bone sclerosis in the distal third metacarpal and metatarsal bones of young horses. Vet J 2008;178:53–61.
36. Brama PA, Holopainen J, van Weeren PR, et al. Influence of exercise and joint topography on depth-related spatial distribution of proteoglycan and collagen content in immature equine articular cartilage. Equine Vet J 2009;41:557–63.
37. Van Weeren PR, Firth EC, Brommer H, et al. Early exercise advances the maturation of glycosaminoglycans and collagen in the extracellular matrix of articular cartilage in the horse. Equine Vet J 2008;40:128–35.
38. Brama PA, Holopainen J, van Weeren PR, et al. The effect of loading on the organisation of the collagen network in juvenile equine cartilage. J Ort. Res 2009;27:1226–34.
39. Kiviranta I, Jurvelin J, Tammi M, et al. Weight bearing controls glycosaminoglycan concentration and articular cartilage thickness in the knee joints of young beagle dogs. Arthr Rheum 1987;30:801–9.
40. Kiviranta I, Tammi M, Jurvelin J, et al. Articular cartilage thickness and glycosaminoglycan distribution in the young canine knee joint after remobilization of the immobilized limb. J Orthop Res 1994;12:161–7.
41. Jones G, Bennell K, Cicuttini FM. Effect of physical activity on cartilage development in healthy kids. Br J Sports Med 2003;37:382–3.
42. Julkunen P, Halmesmäki EP, Livarinen J, et al. Effects of growth and exercise on composition, structural maturation and appearance of osteoarthritis in articular cartilage of hamsters. J Anat 2010;217:262–74.
43. Murray RC, Whitton RC, Vedi S, et al. The effect of training on the calcified zone of equine middle carpal articular cartilage. Equine Vet J 1999;(Suppl 30):274–8.
44. Murray RC, Zhu CF, Goodship AE, et al. Exercise affects the mechanical properties and histological appearance of equine articular cartilage. J Orthop Res 1999;17:725–31.
45. Firth EC, Rogers CW, Perkins NR, et al. Musculoskeletal responses of 2-year-old Thoroughbred horses to early training. 1. Study design and clinical, nutritional, radiological and histological observations. N Z Vet J 2004;52:261–71.
46. Murray RC, Smith RK, Henson FM, et al. The distribution of cartilage oligomeric matrix protein (COMP) in equine carpal articular cartilage and its variation with exercise and cartilage deterioration. Vet J 2001;162:121–8.
47. Murray RC, Vedi S, Birch HL, et al. Subchondral bone thickness, hardness and remodelling are influenced by short-term exercise in a site-specific manner. J Orthop Res 2001;19:1035–42.
48. Murray RC, Janicke HC, Henson FM, et al. Equine carpal articular cartilage fibronectin distribution associated with training, joint location and cartilage deterioration. Equine Vet J 2000;32:47–51.
49. Bird JL, Platt D, Wells T, et al. Exercise-induced changes in proteoglycan metabolism of equine articular cartilage. Equine vet J 2000;32:161–3.
50. Firth EC, Rogers CW. Musculoskeletal responses of 2-year-old Thoroughbred

horses to early training. 7. Bone and cartilage response in the carpus. N Z Vet J 2005;53:113–22.
51. Ferguson V, Bushby AJ, Firth EC, et al. Exercise does not affect stiffness and mineralisation of third metacarpal condylar subarticular calcified tissues in 2-year-old thoroughbred racehorses. Eur Cell Mater 2008;17:40–6.
52. Brama PA, Tekoppele JM, Bank RA, et al. The influence of strenuous exercise on collagen characteristics of articular cartilage in Thoroughbreds age 2 years. Equine Vet J 2000;32:551–4.
53. Kawcak CE, McIlwraith CW, Norrdin RW, et al. Clinical effects of exercise on subchondral bone and metacarpophalangeal joints in horses. Am J Vet Res 2000;61:1252–8.
54. Wolff J. Das Gesetz der Knochen. Berlin: Hirschwald; 1892.
55. Van Harreveld PD, Lillich JD, Kawcak CE, et al. Effects of immobilization followed by remobilization on mineral density, histomorphometric features, and formation of the bones of the metacarpophalangal joint in horses. Am J Vet Res 2002;63: 276–81.
56. Murray RC, Branch MV, Dyson SJ, et al. How does exercise intensity and type affect equine distal tarsal subchondral bone thickness? J Appl Physiol 2007;102:2194–200.
57. Muir P, Peterson AL, Sample SJ, et al. Exercise-induced metacarpophalangeal joint adaptation in the Thoroughbred racehorse. J Anat 2008;213:706–17.
58. Tranquille CA, Dyson SJ, Blunden AS, et al. Histopathological features of distal tarsal joint cartilage and subchondral bone in ridden and pasture-exercised horses. Am J Vet Res 2011;72:33–41.
59. Tranquille CA, Blunden AS, Dyson SJ, et al. Effect of exercise on thicknesses of mature hyaline cartilage, calcified cartilage, and subchondral bone of equine tarsi. Am J Vet Res 2009;70:1477–83.
60. Skiöldebrand E, Ekman S, Heinegård D, et al. Ultrastructural immunolocalization of cartilage oligomeric matrix protein (COMP) in the articular cartilage of the equine third carpal bone in trained and untrained horses. Res Vet Sci 2009;88:251–7.
61. Little CB, Ghosh P, Rose, R. The effect of strenuous versus moderate exercise on the metabolism of proteoglycans in articular cartilage from different weight-bearing regions of the equine third carpal bone. Osteoarthritis Cart 1997;5:161–72.
62. Calatroni A, Avenoso A, Feriazzo AM, et al. Transient increase with strenuous exercise of plasma levels of glycosaminoglycans in humans and horses. Connect Tissue Res 2008;49:416–25.
63. Helal IE, Misumi K, Tateno O, et al. Effect of exercise on serum concentration of cartilage oligomeric matrix protein in Thoroughbreds. Am J Vet Res 2007;68:134–40.
64. Okumura M, Kim GH, Tagami M, et al. Serum keratan sulphate as a cartilage metabolic marker in horses: the effect of exercise. J Vet Med A Physiol Pathol Clin Med 2002;49:195–7.
65. Brown MP, Trumble TN, Plaas AH, et al. Exercise and injury increase chondroitin sulfate chain length and decrease hyaluronan chain length in synovial fluid. Osteoarthritis Cart 2007;15:1318–25.
66. Frisbie DD, Al-Sobayil F, Billinghurst RC, et al. Changes in synovial fluid and serum biomarkers with exercise and early osteoarthritis in horses. Osteoarthritis Cart 2008;16:1196–204.
67. Van den Boom R, van de Lest CH, Bull S, et al. Influence of repeated arthrocentesis and exercise on synovial fluid concentrations of nitric oxide, prostaglandin E2 and glycosaminoglycans in healthy equine joints. Equine Vet J 2005;37:250–6.
68. Brama PA, van den Boom R, DeGroot J, et al. Collagenase-1 (MMP-1) activity in equine synovial fluid: influence of age, joint pathology, exercise and repeated arthrocentesis. Equine Vet J 2004;36:34–40.
69. Van den Hoogen BM, van de Lest CH, van Weeren, PR, et al. Loading-induced changes in synovial fluid affect cartilage metabolism. Br J Rheumatol 1998;37:671–6.
70. Kiviranta I, Tammi M, Jurvelin J, et al. Articular cartilage thickness and glycosaminoglycan distribution in the canine knee joint after strenuous running exercise. Clin Orthop Rel Res 1992;283:302–8.
71. Van Weeren PR, Brama PA. Equine joint disease in the light of new developments in articular cartilage research. Pferdeheilk 2003;19:336–44.
72. Helminen HJ, Hyttinen MM, Lammi MJ, et al. Regular joint loading in youth assists in the establishment and strengthening of the collagen network of articular cartilage and contributes to the prevention of osteoarthrosis later in life: A hypothesis. J Bone Min Metab 2000;18:245–257.
73. Smith RK, Birch H, Patterson-Kane J, et al. Should equine athletes commence training during skeletal development?: changes in tendon matrix associated with development, ageing, function and exercise. Equine Vet J 1999;(Suppl. 30):201–9.

Kinematics of lameness

12

Joanne Kramer Kevin G. Keegan

CHAPTER CONTENTS

Introduction

Lameness is a frequent problem in the horse and the ability to detect lameness by observing movement is a skill that must be acquired by the equine clinician. With practice and experience, equine clinicians develop this skill by recognizing how certain patterns of movement of the body and limbs correlate with lameness. However, there is no set of universally accepted rules about what to observe or how important different movements are in correctly evaluating lameness. We are all trained somewhat differently to identify lameness and this contributes to diversity in the developed skills of lameness recognition between equine clinicians.

It is not difficult to correctly detect and identify the affected limb in a lameness of moderate to severe intensity. There is little disagreement among equine clinicians and the diversity in our training poses little difficulty in these cases. However, when examining horses with intermittent lameness, lameness of mild intensity, or shifting-limb lameness, the diversity in our lameness training results in confusion, disagreement and, ultimately, disparate diagnoses. Even between skilled equine clinicians, inter-individual agreement for recognition of mild to moderate lameness and the designation of the correct lame limb have been shown to be poor or only marginally acceptable.[1–4] The success of treatments for various lameness conditions has traditionally been based on subjective evaluations, imprecise lameness scores computed by few individuals or broad classifications of recovery such as return to function. These evaluative techniques are all potentially influenced by numerous factors unrelated to lameness severity. It has also been demonstrated that evaluators can be biased towards judging improvement in lameness after diagnostic analgesia.[5] A more objective methodology to detect and quantify lameness would make lameness evaluations more scientific and thus more reliable. Additionally, objective methods may detect lameness earlier than subjective evaluation.[6,7]

Kinematic gait analysis is an objective measurement of body movement. In its traditional form, movement is captured with cameras and a quantitative analysis is performed. In a newer form, movement is captured using wireless technology. Real time objective kinematic evaluation can now readily be performed simultaneously with traditional subjective evaluation and used to enhance lameness examination.

Kinematic gait analysis is fundamentally practical because it is intuitive. When equine clinicians evaluate lameness in the field, they evaluate movement. We see movement (a kinematic measurement) directly. Force (a kinetic measurement) must be transduced for human perception. Therefore, what we learn about movement and how it changes with lameness can be described, taught and learned. Simultaneous objective and subjective evaluation thus can be used to improve our understanding and clinical detection of lameness.

Although movement compensation occurs with lameness during many gaits, the ideal gait for kinematic evaluation is the trot. The trot is a symmetrical gait with simultaneous contralateral forelimb and hindlimb placement in each half-cycle of the full stride. Vertical movement of the body is sinusoidal with equivalent amplitudes in each half-cycle. One of the most characteristic features of lameness is its tendency to upset the simple periodicity of normal movement.

This perturbation of movement is most easily appreciated at the trot against the normal background of symmetrical vertical movement. In addition, the total vertical movement of the trunk's center of gravity, and thus the resulting forces placed on the limbs during weight bearing, is greater during the trot than at a walk or canter.[8,9] Lameness exacerbated by weight bearing, which includes the majority of lameness in the horse, may therefore be more expressed at the trot than at a walk or canter. In this chapter the kinematic changes referred to as representative of lameness are those primarily observed and measured at the trot.

Methodology

The kinematic method used most frequently to study how a horse moves in response to lameness is to mark the horse in some way at important body positions and to capture the movement of these markers with high speed cameras. Recently, movement in response to lameness can be captured wirelessly with small inertial sensors attached to the horse's body.[10–13] Both methods take advantage of being able to capture movement at higher sampling rates than the human eye, which is only about 15–20 samples per second.[14] Thus, small changes in movement due to lameness that occur within millisecond durations can be reliably identified and recorded.

When cameras are used to capture the movement, in order to maintain spatial resolution of measurements, the area in which the movement to be captured will occur is limited. To track movement reliably in three dimensions at least two cameras are required. Each marker must be 'seen' in every frame of movement from at least two camera views, thus, line-of-site obstructions from overlapping body parts frequently require more than two cameras. Limited size of acceptable fields-of-view will allow collection of only 1–2 contiguous strides of movement. Multiple passes back and forth in front of the cameras are required to collect sufficient data for study. Movement from multiple contiguous strides can be collected by filming horses moving on a treadmill. Speed of locomotion can be precisely controlled on a treadmill, which is advantageous to limit variability in parameters used to measure lameness, but then the influence of treadmill locomotion on lameness must be considered.

Depending on the frame rate of the camera and the number of markers followed, the large amount of data generated requires computer-assisted processing and analysis. Substantial investment in time and money is required to setup, maintain and utilize computer-assisted kinematic gait analysis systems. Because of these limitations, using camera-based kinematic gait analysis to measure lameness in clinical cases is not likely to be widely adopted. Nevertheless, camera-based kinematic systems are uniquely positioned to be able to track multiple body parts, in all three dimensions, at high frame rates and sub-millimeter spatial resolution. These systems are indispensable for studying the biomechanics of movement in the horse and how this movement is related to lameness detection and evaluation. Much of what we know and will learn in the future about the biomechanics of movement related to lameness in the horse was and will be discovered by investigations utilizing camera-based kinematic gait analysis.

By contrast, when inertial sensors are used to capture the movement, the area in which the movement is to occur is limited only by the range of wireless transmission of data, which, depending on the unique combination of radio and battery technology used, can be quite long. The main advantage of inertial sensor systems over camera-based kinematics is the ability to collect data from multiple, contiguous strides from horses moving naturally overground. However, in comparison to camera-based kinematics, less movement information can be captured and transmitted. Increasing the number of sensors, the sampling rate of the sensors, and the analog to digital conversion rate (required for radio transmission) strains the radio's band width capability and battery size requirements. The ultimate size and weight of the body-mounted sensor is determined primarily by the radio and battery. Large, heavy sensors may influence movement. Without data logging, which is inconvenient for clinical use because data is not transmitted in real time, small sensors of low weight can only capture and transmit limited data in real time. The raw data from inertial sensors (acceleration, angular velocity) must also be converted to position and angle measurements in order to track trajectories of movement similar to camera-based systems. This conversion process is not error free and sophisticated error correction procedures must be implemented. Because of these limitations, kinematic systems utilizing inertial sensors are designed to sample movement from few locations on the horse's body. They are more useful for quantifying movement with known association to a specific intent, for example lameness, rather than as a general investigative tool into the biomechanics of movement in horses. There are commercially available body-mounted inertial sensors systems (such as the Lameness Locator®, Equinosis LLC, Columbia, MO 65211 and the Equimetrix®, Centaure-Metrix, Evry, France) designed specifically as an aid to standard, expert veterinary evaluation of lameness in horses (Fig. 12.1).

Kinematic parameters of importance for the detection of lameness

It is not the purpose of this chapter to exhaustively explain all the kinematic parameters of interest that have been studied, or that may be used by practitioners when visually assessing lameness. Much of what has been described in textbooks is subjective expert opinion. Text descriptions of how to visually identify lameness have at times conflicted with each other or have not been adequately described to allow for comparison. One only has to try to define and then reconcile the term 'hip hike' or 'pelvic hike', a frequent descriptor of hindlimb lameness in horses[15–17] with pelvic 'sinking' or excessive rotation towards the side of lameness that is described in other reports.[18,19] Some clinicians evaluate the 'head bob or nod' as greater upward movement of the head during the stance phase of the lame limb[15–17] and others evaluate it as less downward movement during the stance phase of the lame limb.[20] Some evaluate stride length and detect lameness when the length of stride or the caudal or cranial phase of the stride seems to be shortened or lengthened.[16,17] The shape of the hoof flight arc is said to be representative of lameness.[16] Joint angle excursions, during both the stance and swing phase of the stride, have been purported to be accurate indicators of lameness.[19–21] Objective evaluations have indicated that some of the parameters described above are either incorrect or insensitive.[22–25] In other cases when objective measurements of lameness are made we suspect that many clinicians are seeing the same alteration in movement but describing it differently.

Movement of the limbs or changes in joint angles within the limbs, which may be specific for certain types or causes of lameness, displays either high side-to-side variability or is difficult to 'see' from multiple vantage points. For completeness, descriptions of limb movement parameters that have objectively been shown to be sensitive indicators of lameness are summarized in Table 12.1. We leave it to the reader to decide whether these parameters are useful in detecting lameness in a standard clinical examination.

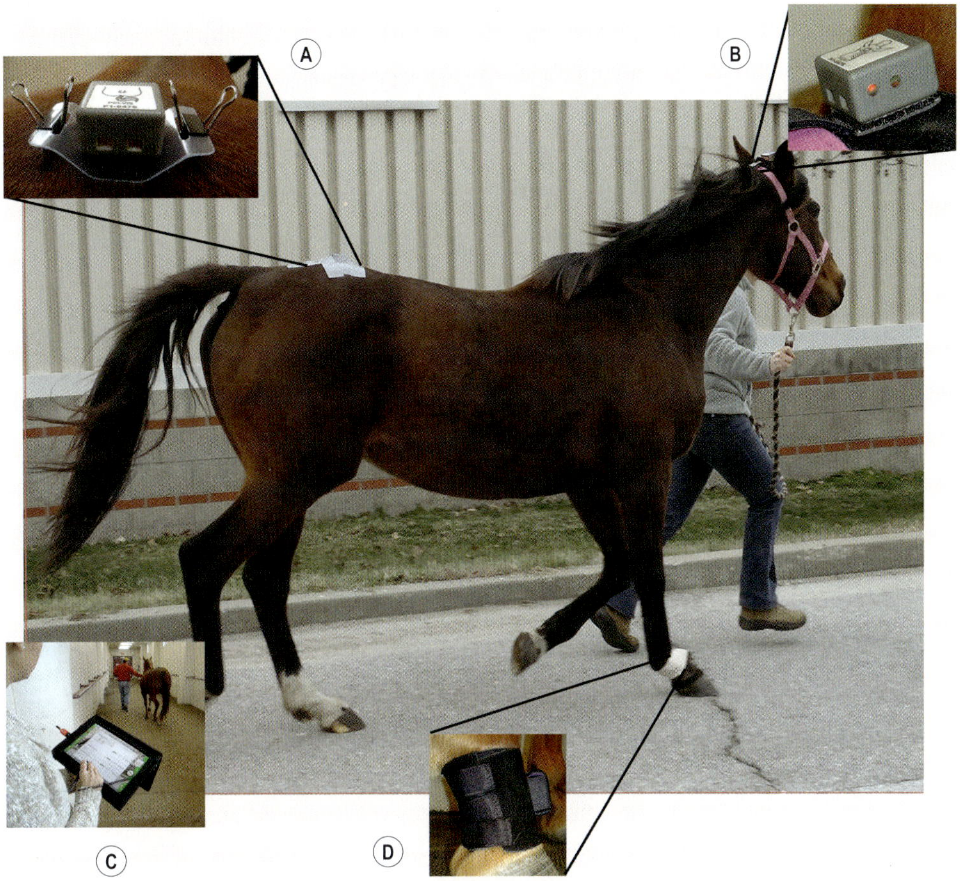

Fig 12.1 Body-mounted inertial sensor system for lameness detection and evaluation (Lameness Locator®, Equinosis LLC, Columbia, MO). **(A)** Uni-axial pelvic accelerometer attached with strip of 3M Dual Lock tape and pelvic clip (for long haired horses). **(B)** Uni-axial head accelerometer, attached to felt head bumper. **(C)** Data is transmitted live to a receiver attached to a tablet computer. **(D)** Uni-axial gyroscope in right forelimb pastern pouch.

Table 12.1 Kinematic parameters of limb movement with known association to lameness

PARAMETER	DESCRIPTION	INCREASE OR DECREASE WITH LAMENESS
Maximum fetlock joint extension	Palmar/planter angle of fetlock at midstance	Decreases[20,22–24,47–50]
Maximum coffin joint flexion	Dorsal angle of coffin joint at midstance	Decreases[20,22–24,49,50]
Maximum carpal joint extension	Palmar angle of carpus during midstance	Decreases[20,48,51]
Stance phase duration	Duration between lame hoof impact and breakover	Increases[20,23,47,52–54]
Hindlimb protraction	The extent to which the hindlimb swings forward before impact	Decreases[22,24]

In this chapter we have concentrated on describing head and pelvic motion as it relates to lameness in the horse. These are the generally-accepted and frequently-used motion parameters used by researchers and practitioners worldwide to evaluate lameness in horses. There is evidence to suggest that vertical movement of the torso, including the head, neck and pelvis, is the most sensitive indicator of lameness in horses.[18,25–30] All of the information necessary to detect lameness and identify it to the correct limb can be found in evaluation of vertical head and pelvic movement.

Kinematic evaluation of vertical head movement to detect and differentiate forelimb lameness

In the authors' opinion, vertical head position is the most applicable and accurate movement parameter for use in clinical examination of forelimb lameness. It can be evaluated equally from the front or side of the horse. It is frequently exacerbated and made more apparent at the beginning (when the horse is accelerating) and end (when the horse is decelerating) of a short trot and when lunging the horse in short circles. However, conditions sometimes arise that make evaluation using this parameter more difficult.

The asymmetrical nature of vertical head movement in some mild lameness conditions may not occur at every stride. As the intermittent nature of the lameness increases, the need to evaluate increasing numbers of strides becomes more important and the ability to detect overall asymmetric head movement becomes more difficult. In addition, extraneous head movement, especially in the curious or excitable horse in an unfamiliar environment, may obscure small perturbations in vertical head movement. It is especially important not to jump to conclusions after a few strides and instead try to determine the overall predominant head movement pattern before committing oneself to a final decision. Algorithms to remove extraneous vertical head movement have been described and can be used in objective analysis of vertical head movement to increase accuracy in detection of lameness.[27]

When the horse is trotting, its head moves up and down twice during a single stride. The head reaches a local maximum vertical position just before hoof contact of one forelimb and a local minimum vertical position near midstance of the same forelimb. Second local maximum and local minimum vertical positions are reached just before foot contact and at midstance of the other forelimb. In the sound horse the total vertical head excursions during the right and left forelimb stance phases are approximately equal; therefore, the local maximums and minimums are approximately the same heights relative to the ground.

Thus, the head moves up and down in a sinusoidal, temporally symmetrical pattern, with amplitude equivalent cycles corresponding to each half of the full stride cycle (Fig. 12.2). The familiar 'head nod', as an indicator of forelimb lameness in horses, is a disruption of this symmetrical movement. In most weight-bearing lameness conditions, the downward head movement during weight bearing of the painful limb is reduced compared to that in the sound limb (Fig. 12.3). With increasing severity of lameness, there is more reduction in the downward movement of the head (Fig. 12.4). With severe lameness, there may be no downward movement of the head during the stance phase of the lame limb and with very severe lameness the head may actually move upward during the stance phase of the lame limb.

For purposes of categorization, we have labeled lameness manifest by less downward movement of the head in the stance phase of the lame limb as impact lameness. Frequently in horses with impact lameness there is also more upward movement of the head immediately preceding lame limb stance, such that the head may actually still be moving upward at the moment of lame limb impact. This effectively reduces vertical force on the lame limb during the first half of stance. Consequently, with impact lameness, there is comparatively less upward movement of the head at the end of stance phase of the lame limb (Fig. 12.4). Most horses with weight-bearing forelimb lameness will display this pattern (impact). Sometimes during a clinical examination it is easier to appreciate the greater downward movement of the head during the stance phase of the normal or least lame forelimb. 'Down on sound' is an aphorism frequently used to describe this phenomenon.

Infrequently, horses with forelimb lameness will have greater upward movement of the head at the end and shortly following the stance phase of the lame forelimb. We have categorized this variant of head movement as indicative of pushoff, or end-of-stance, lameness (Fig. 12.5). Horses with pain occurring only in the second half of stance or during the breakover portion of stance may be more likely to exhibit this type of abnormal head movement, which could be described as 'up on bad' as opposed to 'down on sound'.

These vertical head movement patterns can be captured with a uni-axial accelerometer attached to the poll. Vertical accelerations in this location in most horses trotting are less than 10 g (1 g = 9.8 m/sec^2). Vertical accelerations are converted to relative vertical position and the 'down on sound' and 'up on bad' patterns can be quantified and related to lameness. In one commercially-available system the head movement pattern is shown in a ray plot, with the x-axis representing the measure MAXDIFFHEAD, or maximum

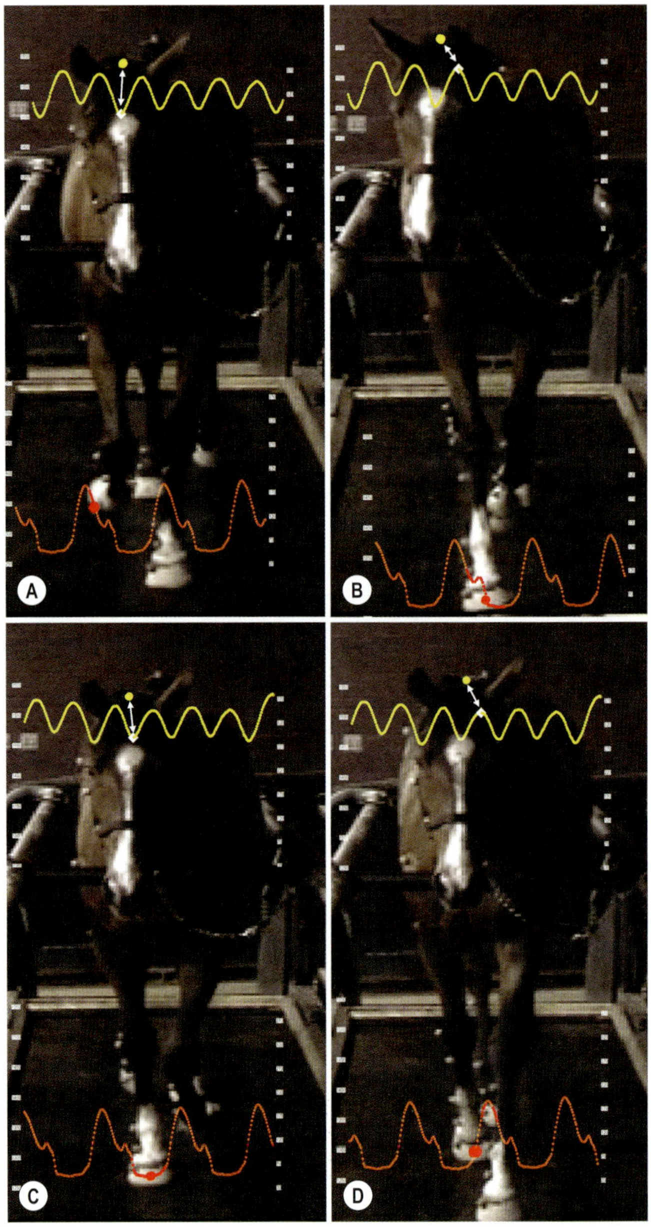

Fig 12.2 Video frames and graphs depicting vertical head and right forelimb foot movement in a sound trotting horse. **(A)** First vertical minimum at midstance of the left forelimb. Right forelimb is at midswing. **(B)** First vertical maximum just after lift-off of the left forelimb foot and just before impact of the right forelimb foot. **(C)** Second vertical minimum at midstance of the right forelimb. Left forelimb is at midswing. **(D)** Second vertical maximum just after lift-off of the right forelimb foot and just before impact of the left forelimb foot. Curves at the top of each video frame (yellow) are the vertical head position. Arrows indicate points on the curve corresponding to video frame shown. Curves at the bottom of each video frame (orange) are the vertical position of the right forelimb foot. Orange circles on curve indicate the points corresponding to the video frame shown. Head and right forelimb foot heights are not in same scale. Approximately three full strides are indicated by the curves.

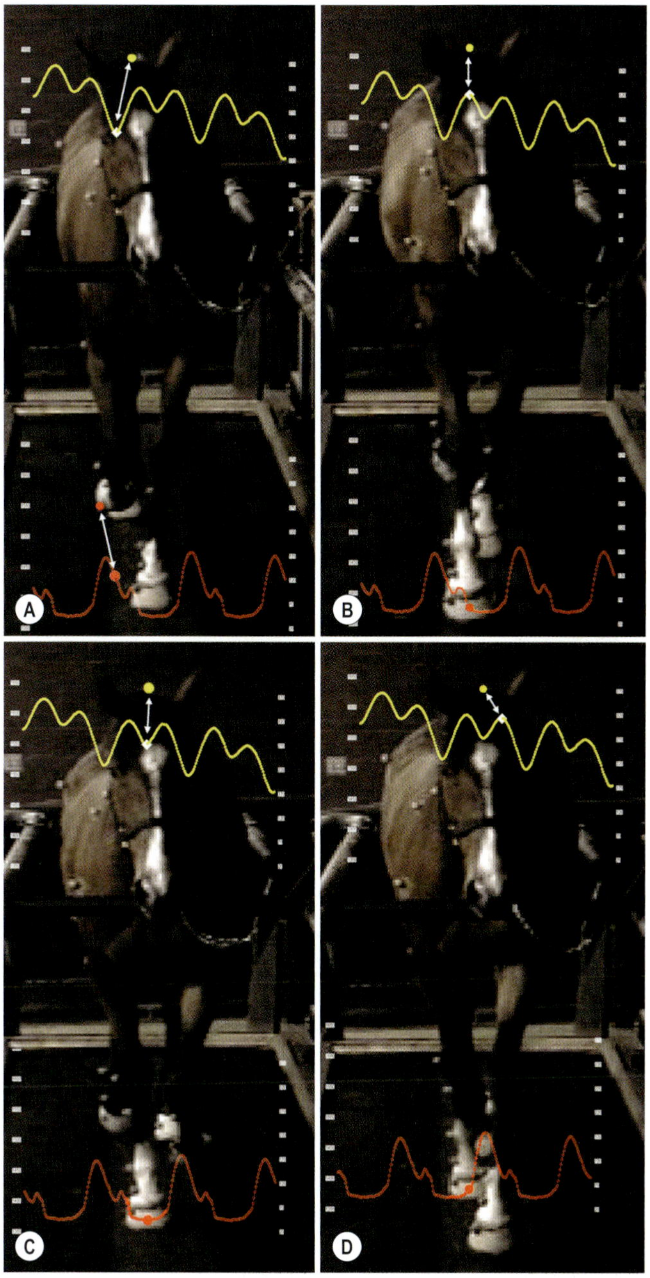

Fig 12.3 Video frames and graphs depicting vertical head and right forelimb foot movement in a trotting horse with a unilateral (right) impact induced forelimb lameness. **(A)** First vertical minimum is lowest at midstance of the left forelimb. Right forelimb is at midswing. **(B)** First vertical maximum just after lift-off of the left forelimb foot and just before impact of the right forelimb foot. **(C)** Second vertical minimum at midstance of the right forelimb. Left forelimb is at midswing. There is less downward movement of the head compared to the minimum in left forelimb stance. **(D)** Second vertical maximum just after lift-off of the right forelimb foot and just before impact of the left forelimb foot. Curves at the top of each video frame (yellow) are the vertical head position. Arrows indicate points on the curve corresponding to video frame shown. Curves at the bottom of each video frame (orange) are the vertical position of the right forelimb foot. Orange circles on curve indicate the points corresponding to the video frame shown. Head and right forelimb foot heights are not in same scale. Approximately three full strides are indicated by the curves.

vertical head height after right forelimb stance subtracted from maximum vertical head height after left forelimb stance, and the y-axis representing the measure MINDIFFHEAD, or minimum vertical head height during right forelimb stance subtracted from minimum vertical head height during left forelimb stance, both in units of millimeters. Right and left stance phases of the stride are determined using data from a simultaneously-sampled gyroscope attached to the dorsal surface of the right forelimb pastern. MAXDIFFHEAD and MINDIFFHEAD will be near zero in horses with perfect vertical head movement symmetry. With lameness MAXDIFFHEAD and MINDIFFHEAD will have increasingly positive or negative values (depending on side and type [impact or pushoff] of lameness). In this ray plot each stride is represented as a single line or ray. The length of each ray, which is the vector sum of MAXDIFFHEAD and MINDIFFHEAD, is proportional to the asymmetry of vertical head movement due to lameness. The direction into which the ray is pointing is indicative of the side and timing (impact through pushoff) of forelimb lameness. For example a horse with a right forelimb, impact lameness, will have a vertical head movement pattern that is strongly 'down on sound', but not 'up on bad', with positive values for MINDIFFHEAD and MAXDIFFHEAD. Strides with positive values of MINDIFFHEAD and MAXDIFFHEAD will 'point' into the first quadrant (upper right) on the ray plot.(Fig. 12.6) By contrast, a horse with a left forelimb, pushoff lameness, will have vertical head movement pattern that is 'down on sound', and 'up on bad', with positive values for MAXDIFFHEAD and negative values for MINDIFFHEAD. (Strides with negative values of MINDIFFHEAD and positive values of MAXDIFFHEAD will 'point' into the fourth quadrant (lower right) of the ray plot (Fig. 12.7). Threshold values for MINDIFFHEAD and MAXDIFFHEAD between 'sound' and 'lame' have been estimated by experimentation.[2,31]

Kinematic parameters used to detect and differentiate hindlimb lameness

Vertical pelvic movement

Analysis of pelvic movement is frequently used in the identification of hindlimb lameness and varying descriptions of how to do this have been published.[15–17,32–34] The pattern of vertical movement of the pelvis is similar to that of the head seen in trotting horses.[18] Vertical pelvic movement has a sinusoidal pattern with two cycles occurring during one complete stride. The first minimum height is reached during the middle of one of the limb's stance phase and the first maximum height at the end of this stance phase. A second symmetrical oscillation occurs during the stance phase of the contralateral limb (Fig. 12.8). Although extraneous vertical movement of the pelvis (unassociated with normal inertial changes due to mechanics of movement) does occur, its contribution to total vertical movement of the pelvis is much less than that seen in the head. However, as in the forelimb, algorithms can be applied to eliminate extraneous pelvic movement and evaluate only movement due to the biphasic vertical excursion.[28]

Unilateral hindlimb lameness changes the symmetry of pelvic movement.[13,18,24,28,32,35] During lameness the entire pelvis exhibits less lowering during the stance phase and less lifting at the end and following the stance phase of the lame limb (Fig. 12.9). These changes are proportional to the degree of lameness and may also reflect where in the phase of the stride the most pain is present. Severe hindlimb lameness may change the degree of symmetry to the extent that there is very little downward movement of the pelvis during the stance phase of the lame limb (Fig. 12.10).

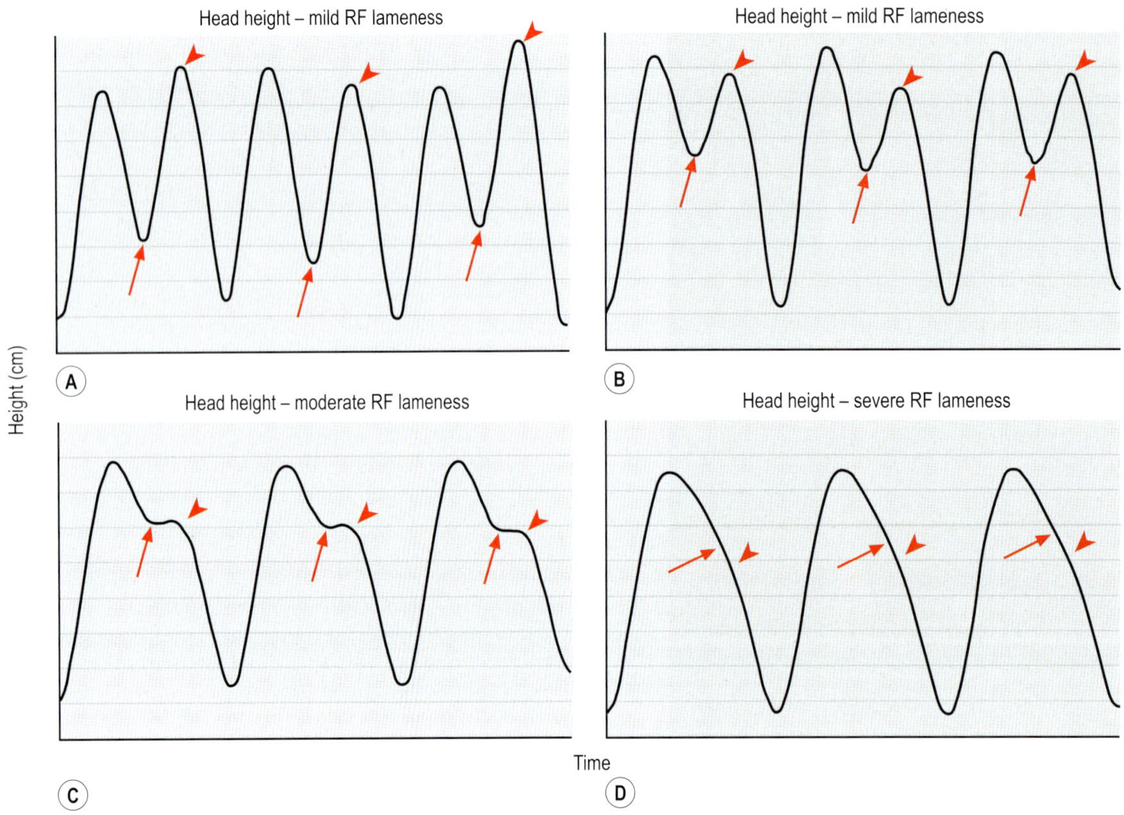

Fig 12.4 Vertical head movement asymmetry with increasing severity of forelimb lameness **(A–D)**. Amount of downward movement during the stance phase of the lame limb becomes less and less, until **(D)** minimum vertical position during stance phase of lame limb disappears. Arrows indicate approximate time of lame (right) forelimb midstance. Arrowheads indicate corresponding decreasing elevation of the head after the stance phase of the lame (right) forelimb.

Similar to the forelimb, vertical acceleration of the pelvis can be captured with a uni-axial accelerometer attached to the pelvis on the dorsal midline. Vertical accelerations can then be converted to relative vertical pelvic position and the movement pattern quantified. Similar to the MAXDIFFHEAD and MINDIFFHEAD in the forelimb, MAXDIFFPELVIS (the difference in the maximum pelvic position between right and left hindlimb pushoff) and MINDIFFPELVIS (the difference in the minimum pelvic position between right and left hindlimb stance phase) can be calculated. MAXDIFFPELVIS and MINDIFFPELVIS will be near 0 in horses with perfectly symmetrical vertical pelvic movement. Increasing amplitude of MAXDIFFPELVIS or MINDIFFPELVIS indicates vertical pelvic movement asymmetry. Horses with an impact lameness or greatest pain in the deceleratory phase of stance, should primarily display decreased downward movement of the pelvis during the lame limb's stance phase, increasing MINDIFFPELVIS (Fig. 12.11). Horses with a pushoff lameness or greatest pain in the acceleratory phase of the lame limb's stance phase should primarily display decreased upward movement of the pelvis at the end of and following the lame limb's stance phase, increasing MAXDIFFPELVIS (Fig. 12.12).[36]

Tuber coxae movement

Vertical movement of the tuber coxae is normally slightly asymmetric in time. The vertical movement of the tuber coxae has the same basic pattern as the entire pelvis, but the two oscillations are not completely symmetric. The first minimum height is reached during the middle of one limb's stance phase and first maximum height is reached at the end of this stance phase. The second oscillation occurs during and shortly following the stance phase of the contralateral hindlimb. However, the vertical movement of the tuber coxae is greater during and shortly after the stance phase of the contralateral hindlimb than that of the ipsilateral hindlimb. The tuber coxae reaches its lowest height at midstance and its maximum height just following the stance phase of the contralateral limb (Fig. 12.13). The asymmetrical movement of the tuber coxae has been attributed to rotational movements of the pelvis around the longitudinal axis of the vertebral column.[18,35] If the pelvis did not rotate, the pattern of vertical movements of both tuber coxae would be identical to each other and to the entire pelvis.

The degree of vertical tuber coxae movement asymmetry seen normally in the sound horse is exaggerated in the lame horse (Fig. 12.14). In lame horses, the tuber coxae of the lame limb has less downward movement during and less upward movement at the end and shortly following the stance phase of the lame limb. During the stance phase of the sound limb the contralateral tuber coxae has more downward movement during and more upward movement at the end and shortly following the stance phase of the sound limb. This increased upward movement after the stance phase of the sound limb may be what is referred to as 'hip hike'.

Clinically, tuber coxae movement has been described to be useful in the diagnosis of hindlimb lameness.[32] Because of pelvic rotation, total vertical movement of the tuber coxae is greater than total vertical pelvic movement and thus may be easier to observe. Total vertical movement of the tuber coxae is greater on the side of hindlimb lameness. This asymmetry in the amplitudes of left and right vertical

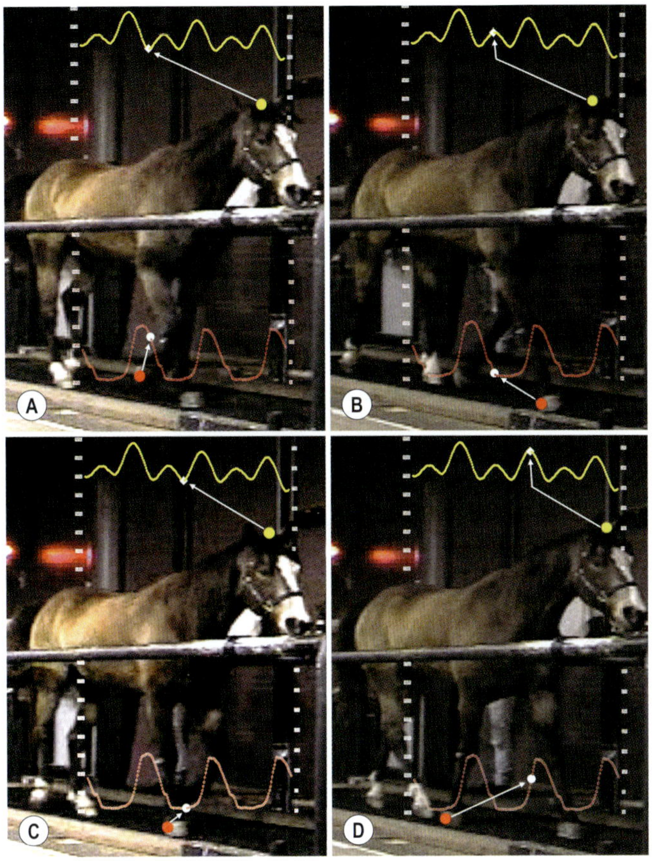

Fig 12.5 Video frames and graphs depicting vertical head and right forelimb foot movement in a trotting horse with a unilateral (right) pushoff forelimb lameness. **(A)** First vertical minimum at midstance of the left forelimb. Right forelimb is at midswing. **(B)** First vertical maximum just after lift-off of the left forelimb foot and just before impact of the right forelimb foot. **(C)** Second vertical minimum at midstance of the right forelimb. Left forelimb is at midswing. **(D)** Second vertical maximum just after lift-off of the right forelimb foot and just before impact of the left forelimb foot. Vertical head position is at the highest point in the stride. Curves at the top of each video frame (yellow) are the vertical head position. Arrows indicate points on the curve corresponding to video frame shown. Curves at the bottom of each video frame (orange) are the vertical position of the right forelimb foot. Arrows indicate points on curve corresponding to the video frame shown. Head and right forelimb foot heights are not in same scale. Approximately three full strides are indicated by the curves.

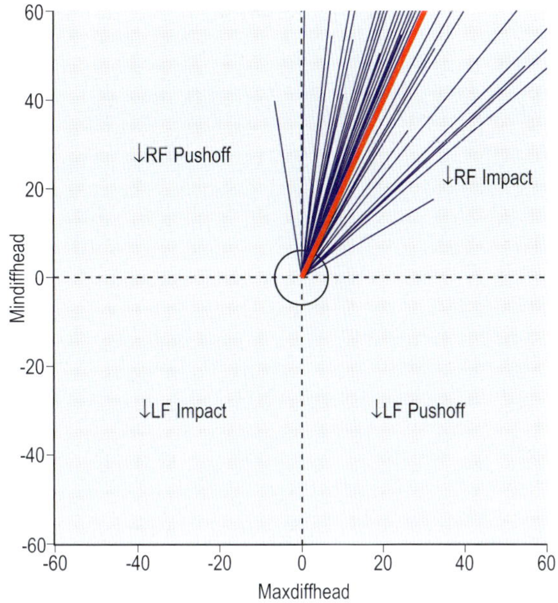

Fig 12.6 Right forelimb impact lameness. Forelimb ray plot from body-mounted inertial sensor system analysis. Each ray is a stride. Length of ray is proportional to asymmetry of vertical head movement. X-axis is MAXDIFFHEAD (mm). Y-axis is MINDIFFHEAD (mm). Horse with right forelimb impact lameness will have positive MAXDIFFHEAD and positive MINDIFFHEAD values.

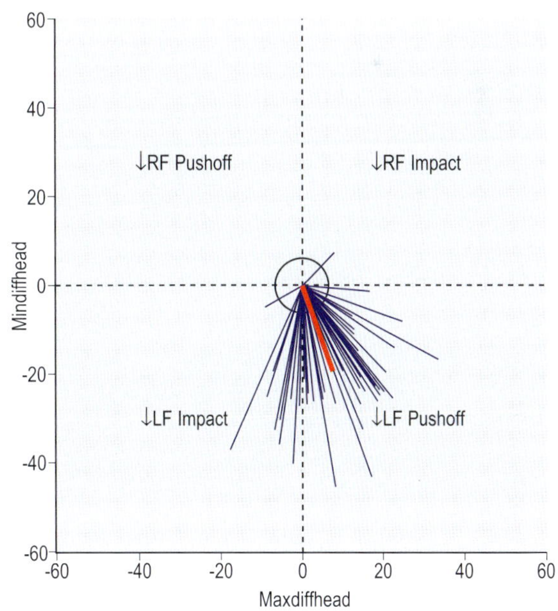

Fig 12.7 Left forelimb pushoff lameness. Forelimb ray plot from body-mounted inertial sensor system analysis. Each ray is a stride. Length of ray is proportional to asymmetry of vertical head movement. X-axis is MAXDIFFHEAD (mm). Y-axis is MINDIFFHEAD (mm). Horse with left forelimb pushoff lameness will have positive MAXDIFFHEAD and negative MINDIFFHEAD values.

tuber coxae movements has been measured and used to diagnose hindlimb lameness in horses.[13,18,19,24,32] One explanation for the exaggerated tuber coxae movement on the lame side has been offered by Buchner et al.[18] In a right hindlimb lameness, the right tuber coxae during right stance has mainly vertical movements. These excursions are enlarged during left stance by rotational movements in the spine. Exaggerated back rotation during the stance of the lame limb may reduce lifting effort during lame limb stance phase.

Although total vertical tuber coxae movement may be observed more easily than total vertical pelvic movement, observing only total vertical tuber coxae movement in some cases may be misleading. Individual horses have varying amounts of vertical tuber coxae movement asymmetry, likely due to different rotational flexibilities of the pelvis and vertebral columns. In some horses tuber coxae movement is primarily due to vertical movement of the trunk and is equally symmetrical as total vertical pelvic movement. In other horses with more significant pelvic rotational movement there is greater vertical tuber coxae movement asymmetry (Fig. 12.13). Mild asymmetries between right and left vertical tuber coxae movement have been identified in clinically sound horses,[19,35] suggesting that

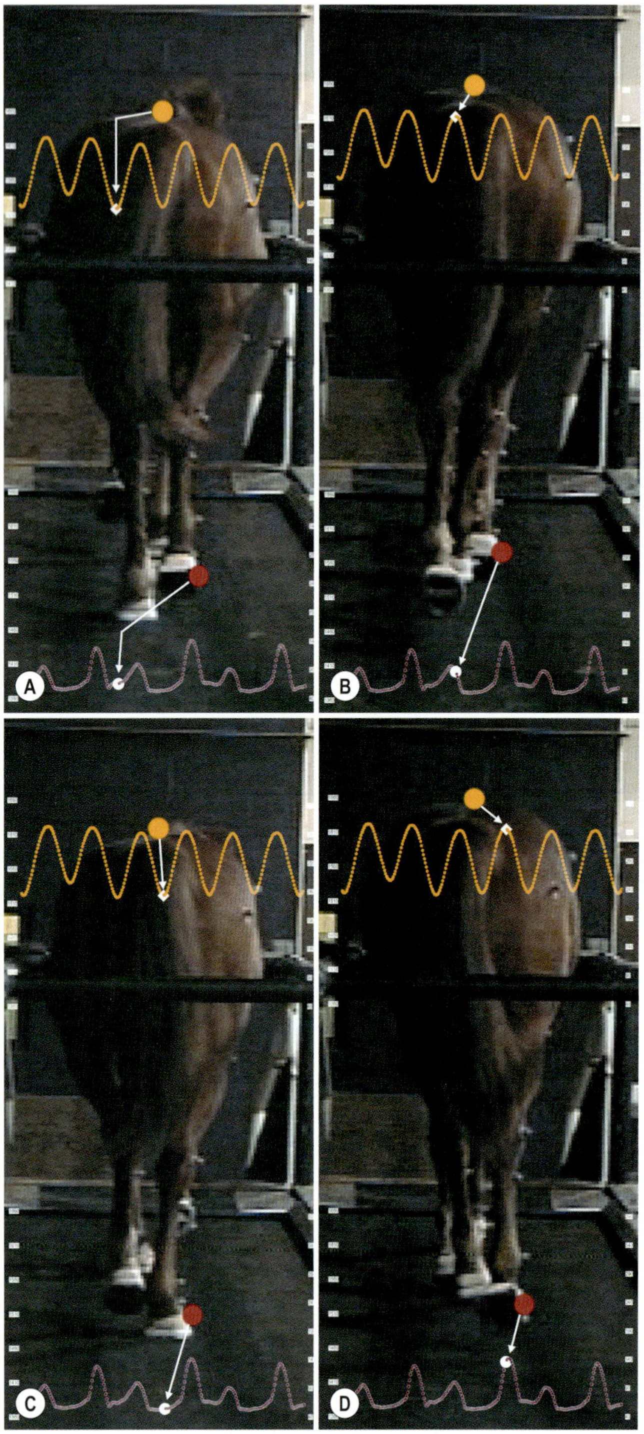

Fig 12.8 Video frames and graphs depicting vertical pelvic and right hindlimb foot movement in a sound trotting horse. **(A)** First vertical minimum at midstance of the left hindlimb. Right hindlimb is at midswing. **(B)** First vertical maximum just after lift-off of the left hindlimb foot and just before impact of the right hindlimb foot. **(C)** Second vertical minimum at midstance of the right hindlimb. Left hindlimb is at midswing. **(D)** Second vertical maximum just after lift-off of the right hindlimb foot and just before impact of the left hindlimb foot. Curves at the top of each video frame (yellow) are the vertical pelvic position. Arrows indicate points on the curve corresponding to video frame shown. Curves at the bottom of each video frame (orange) are the vertical position of the right hindlimb foot. Arrows indicate points on the curve corresponding to the video frame shown. Pelvic and right hindlimb foot heights are not in same scale. Approximately three full strides are indicated by the curves.

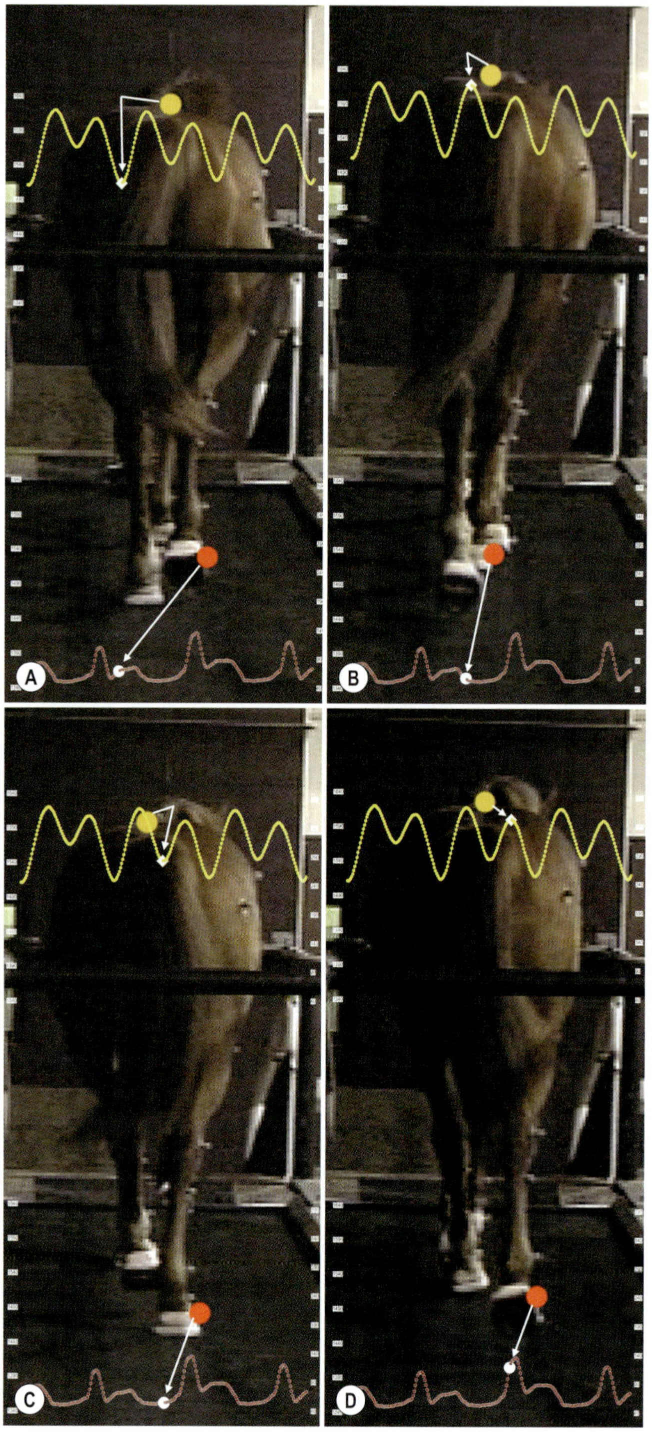

Fig 12.9 Video frames and graphs depicting vertical pelvic and right hindlimb foot movement in a trotting horse with an induced right hindlimb lameness. **(A)** First vertical minimum is lowest at midstance of the left hindlimb. Right hindlimb is at midswing. **(B)** First vertical maximum just after lift-off of the left hindlimb foot and just before impact of the right hindlimb foot. **(C)** Second vertical minimum at midstance of the right hindlimb. Left hindlimb is at midswing. There is less downward movement of the pelvis compared to vertical minimum at left hindlimb stance. **(D)** Second vertical maximum just after lift-off of the right hindlimb foot and just before impact of the left hindlimb foot. Curves at the top of each video frame (yellow) are the vertical pelvic position. Arrows indicate points on the curve corresponding to video frame shown. Curves at the bottom of each video frame (orange) are the vertical position of the right hindlimb foot. Arrows indicate points on the curve corresponding to the video frame shown. Pelvic and right hindlimb foot heights are not in same scale. Approximately three full strides are indicated by the curves.

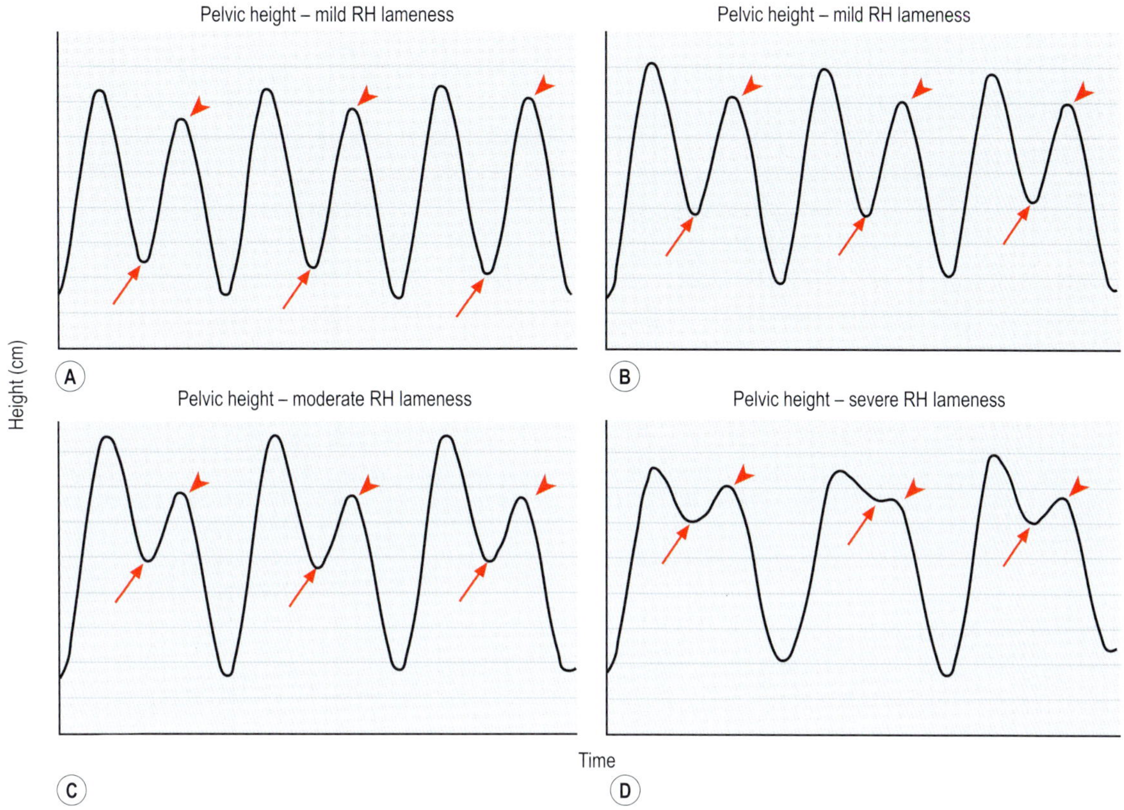

Fig 12.10 Vertical pelvic movement asymmetry with increasing severity of hindlimb lameness **(A–D)**. Amount of downward movement during the stance phase of the lame limb becomes less and less, until **(D)** minimum vertical position during stance phase of lame limb almost disappears. Arrows indicate approximate time of lame (right) hindlimb midstance. Arrowheads indicate corresponding decreasing elevation of the pelvis after the stance phase of the lame (right) hindlimb.

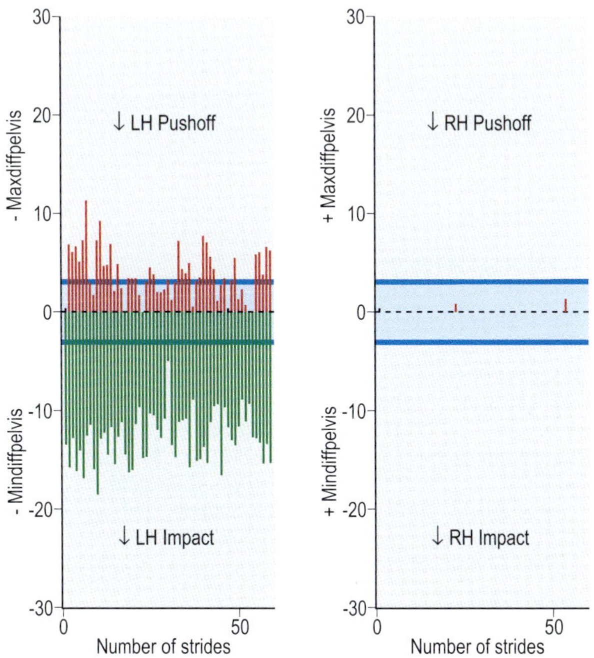

Fig 12.11 Left hindlimb impact lameness. Hindlimb ray plot from body-mounted inertial sensor system analysis. Length of rays (combined red and green) are proportional to asymmetry of vertical pelvic movement. Green rays directed down on left subplot indicate less impact of the left hindlimb (negative MINDIFFPELVIS).

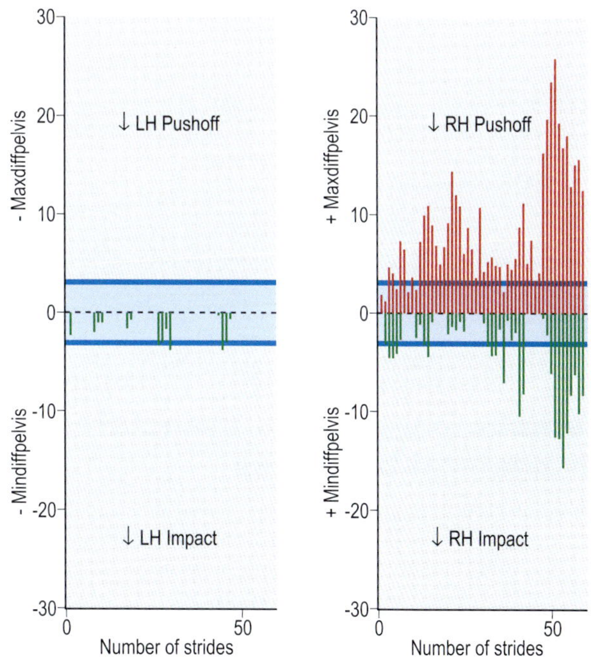

Fig 12.12 Right hindlimb pushoff lameness. Hindlimb ray plot from body-mounted inertial sensor system analysis. Length of rays (combined red and green) are proportional to asymmetry of vertical pelvic movement. Red rays directed up on right subplot indicate less pushoff on the right hindlimb (positive MAXDIFFPELVIS).

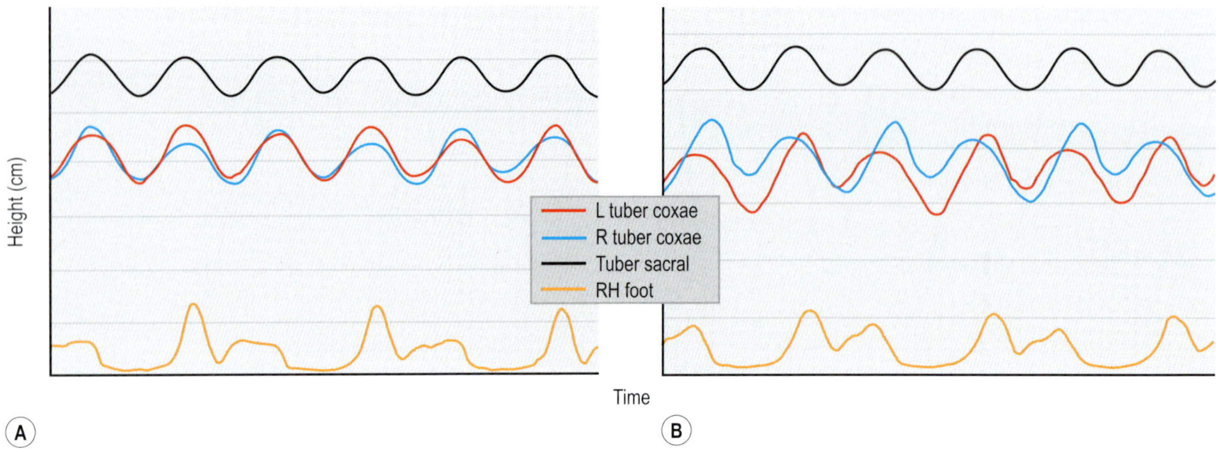

Fig 12.13 Vertical tuber coxae movement in two sound horses. Tuber sacral movement is symmetric. **(A)** In horse 1, vertical tuber coxae movement is only slightly asymmetric, indicating little pelvic rotation. **(B)** In horse 2, vertical tuber coxae movement is very asymmetric, indicating greater pelvic rotation.

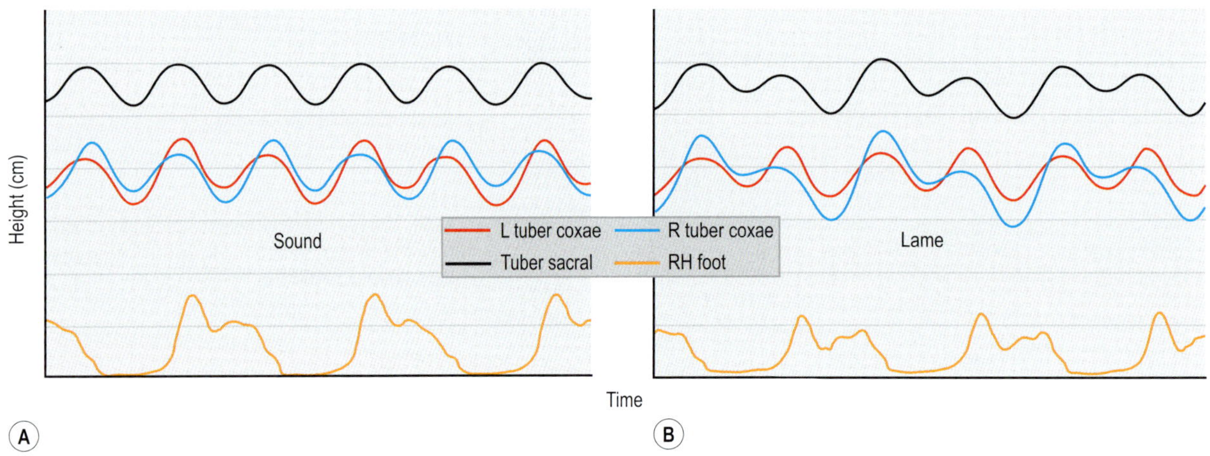

Fig 12.14 Vertical tuber coxae movement in **(A)** a sound horse and in **(B)** the same horse after induction of a right hindlimb lameness. Note the increased vertical movement asymmetry in the right tuber coxae after induction of lameness. Note also the development of asymmetry of vertical tuber sacral movement after induction of lameness.

the degree of acceptable asymmetry has not yet been determined. Horses with pre-existing pelvic shape asymmetry unassociated with lameness may also have fairly dramatic vertical tuber coxae movement.

Kinematic parameters associated with bilateral lameness

Many musculoskeletal problems in horses present as bilateral lameness. Common examples include navicular disease and distal tarsal degenerative joint disease. The evaluation of bilateral lameness is complicated by two factors. Symmetry of movement between the right and left sides of the body is maintained to some extent with bilateral lameness.[26,37] Often the magnitude of pain and dysfunction in one limb is only slightly more or less intense than in the similarly affected other side. Careful observation is necessary to detect the small differences in symmetry of movement between the affected sides. A second factor complicating the detection of bilateral lameness is the propensity for the lameness to shift sides during the lameness examination. In some cases of bilateral lameness, local, regional, or joint anesthesia may be used to temporarily reduce lameness on one side. Frequently, after local anesthesia of one limb, the lameness will become more unilateral, simplifying lameness detection. In other cases the source of lameness may not be amenable to local anesthesia, or the effects of local anesthetics may actually interfere with the detection of very mild changes in lameness.[38,39]

The characteristic stride described for a horse with a bilateral lameness is a short, stiff and shuffling or choppy gait.[17,33] Attempts to objectively measure changes in stride parameters during bilateral lameness have been made and described.[26,37] In one study utilizing a bilateral hoof-induced lameness model, horses exhibited some characteristic gait compensations. Fetlock extension decreased and a diagonal advanced placement (placing forelimbs earlier than hindlimbs) was initiated.[37]

Without pre-existing control data from a horse with bilateral lameness of equivalent severity between the right and left sides, diagnosis of lameness based upon kinematic parameters is challenging. Kinematic detection of such cases requires analysis of multiple stride sequences to evaluate the limb-shifting nature of the lameness and precise detection of subtle asymmetries between left and right sides. A database of kinematic evaluation of normal sound horses to establish accepted asymmetry measurements for relative comparison would also be needed.

Kinematic parameters in compensatory lameness

At the trot, horses with hindlimb lameness will frequently appear to have false, ipsilateral forelimb lameness (Fig. 12.15).[18,26,32,40,41] The hindlimb pain during weight bearing causes the horse to shift weight forward, towards the contralateral forelimb. The head moves down more when the contralateral forelimb is weight bearing. Comparatively, the head then moves down less when the ipsilateral forelimb is in stance. Sometimes rather mild primary hindlimb lameness, which may be difficult to appreciate, will cause a more apparent severe, but actually false, forelimb lameness on the ipsilateral side. Concentration on head movement and the 'down on sound' phenomenon, without looking closely at pelvic movement asymmetry, may wrongly conclude that a forelimb lameness is present. Because of this, some hindlimb lameness may be missed.

Conversely, at the trot sometimes horses with true forelimb lameness will appear to have false, hindlimb lameness (Fig. 12.16).[18,40,41] The forelimb pain causes the horse to shift weight backward, towards the contralateral hindlimb. The pelvis moves down more when the contralateral hindlimb is weight bearing. Comparatively, the pelvis moves down less when the ipsilateral hindlimb is in stance, making it seem like the horse is not landing on the ipsilateral hindlimb as hard as the contralateral hindlimb. However, when

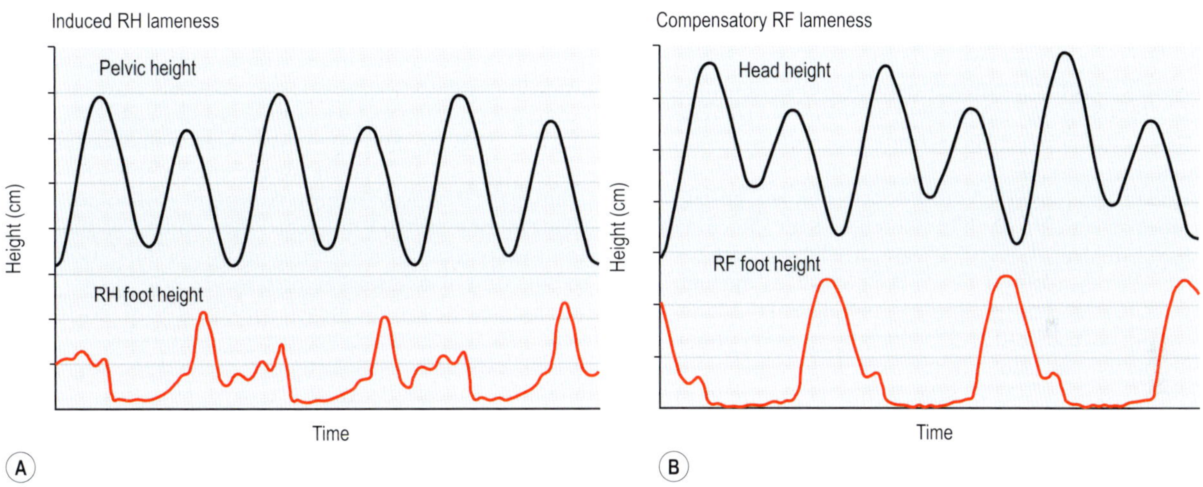

Fig 12.15 **(A)** Mild induced right hindlimb lameness causing a **(B)** moderate to severe compensatory right forelimb lameness. Notice less downward movement of the pelvis during the stance phase of the right hindlimb in **(A)** and less downward movement of the head during the stance phase of the right forelimb in **(B)**.

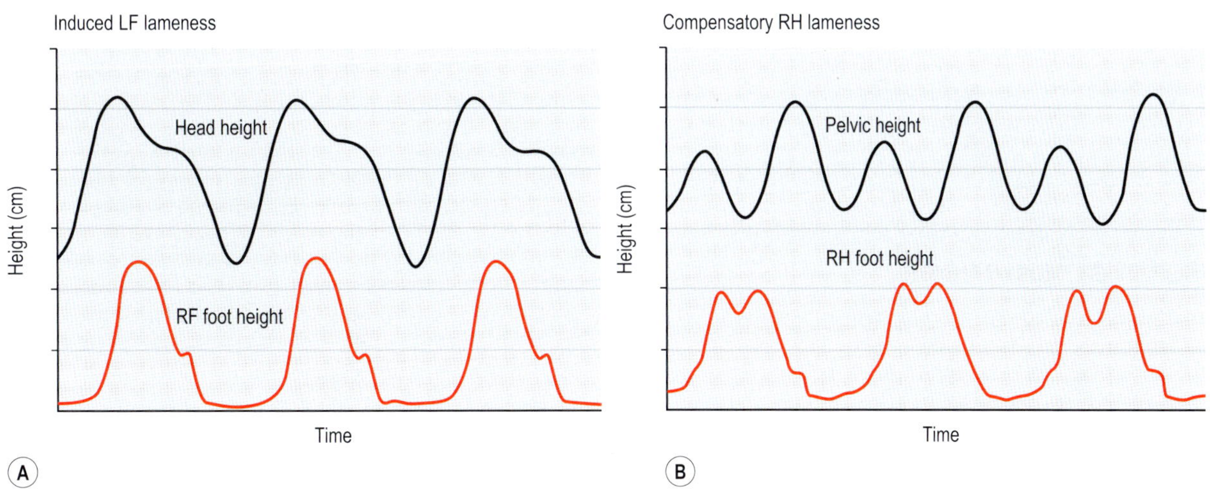

Fig 12.16 **(A)** Severe induced left forelimb lameness causing a **(B)** mild compensatory right hindlimb lameness. Notice less downward movement of the head during the swing phase of the right forelimb (stance phase of the left forelimb) in **(A)** and slightly less downward movement of the pelvis during the stance phase of the right hindlimb in **(B)**.

the horse is trotting in a straight line, it will usually pushoff the ipsilateral hindlimb harder, and the entire pelvis will rise and move forward more than the hindlimb that is weight bearing at the same time as the painful forelimb (the contralateral hindlimb). Comparatively, it seems that the pelvis does not rise as much when the horse pushes off the contralateral hindlimb. Thus, a horse with primary forelimb lameness will have vertical pelvic movements that mimic lameness on both hindlimbs, with less pelvic fall (an impact hindlimb lameness) on the ipsilateral hindlimb and less pelvic rise (a pushoff hindlimb lameness) on the contralateral hindlimb. Usually the primary forelimb lameness must be severe before these characteristic vertical pelvic movements are noticeable. Because of this, mistaking a hindlimb lameness for a true forelimb lameness does not occur often.

This relationship between compensatory movements in the opposite half of the body as a result of primary lameness is sometimes referred to as the 'Law of Sides'. The first part of the 'Law of Sides' asserts that an ipsilateral lameness is usually a primary hindlimb lameness. The second part of the 'Law of Sides' asserts that a contralateral lameness is usually a primary forelimb lameness. Because kinematic systems are capable of sampling movement at higher rates than the human eye, these compensatory patterns can be more easily found. Detecting a mild hindlimb lameness, which may be difficult to 'see' subjectively, with even a moderate apparent ipsilateral forelimb lameness, that is easy to 'see' subjectively, should at least cause the practitioner to pause and consider a primary hindlimb lameness (Fig. 12.17). Detecting less upward movement of the pelvis after pushoff of a hindlimb with a forelimb lameness that is contralateral should at least cause the practitioner to pause and consider that the lameness is likely a primary forelimb lameness (Fig. 12.18). An ipsilateral impact, contralateral hindlimb pushoff pattern can be helpful to find forelimb lameness in unruly horses that frequently and randomly toss their head while being lead at a trot on a lead shank by a handler. Vertical head movement pattern in some fresh, unruly, and generally misbehaving horses, can be so random and frequent as to render vertical head movement pattern analysis for lameness unreliable. The presence of compensatory vertical movement patterns of the pelvis are helpful in these situations.

Kinematic parameters during movement in a circle

Lameness, especially forelimb lameness, can become more pronounced when the horse is lunged in a circle. Small circles exacerbate lameness more than larger circles. Circling horses on hard ground especially aggravates hoof-related lameness and lameness caused by arthritis in the distal limb joints, most frequently on the inside limb. Circling on very soft ground is thought to aggravate lameness caused by tendon and/or suspensory ligament pain of the outside limb. When horses are trotting in a circle the torso is tilted towards the inside and the forces of torsion, compression and tension on the limbs are different than when trotting in a straight line.[42–45] The lateral surface of the inside limb and the medial surface of the outside limb experience increased compressive load and the medial surface of the inside limb and the lateral surface of the outside limb experience increased tensile load.

It is important to note that when the horse is lunging the torso is tilted. This causes the limb movements, joint angle changes, and the vertical and lateral excursion of the torso (head, neck and pelvis) during the stance and swing phases of the stride of the inside and outside limbs to be quite different. When trotting, vertical head excursion is commonly greatest during pushoff of the outside forelimb and the vertical excursion of the center of mass is commonly greatest during pushoff of the outside hindlimb. Thus, it is important to compare what is seen when the horse is lunging to the left to what is seen when the horse is lunging to the right. 'Seeing' and concluding that lameness exists after observing the horse lunging in only one direction is prone to error. This can be somewhat

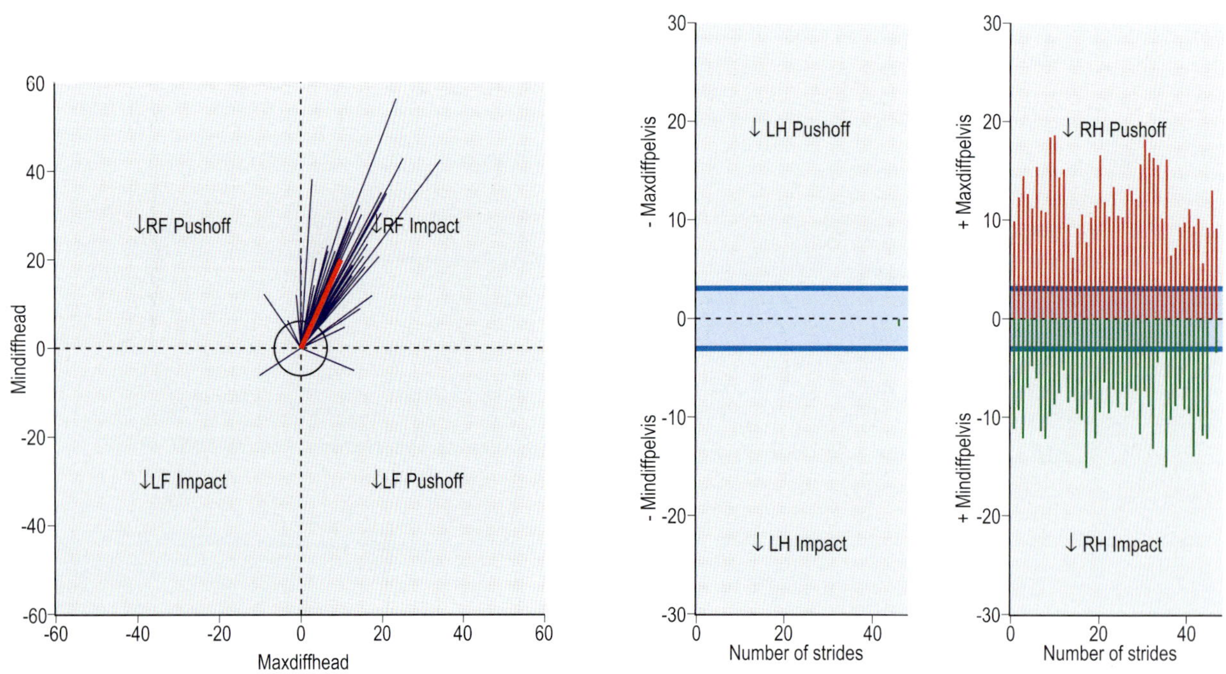

Fig 12.17 Inertial sensor system analysis displaying the 'First Law of Sides'. There is apparent ipsilateral lameness, in this case right hindlimb and right forelimb. The most likely explanation is a true right hindlimb lameness with an apparent, but false, right forelimb lameness.

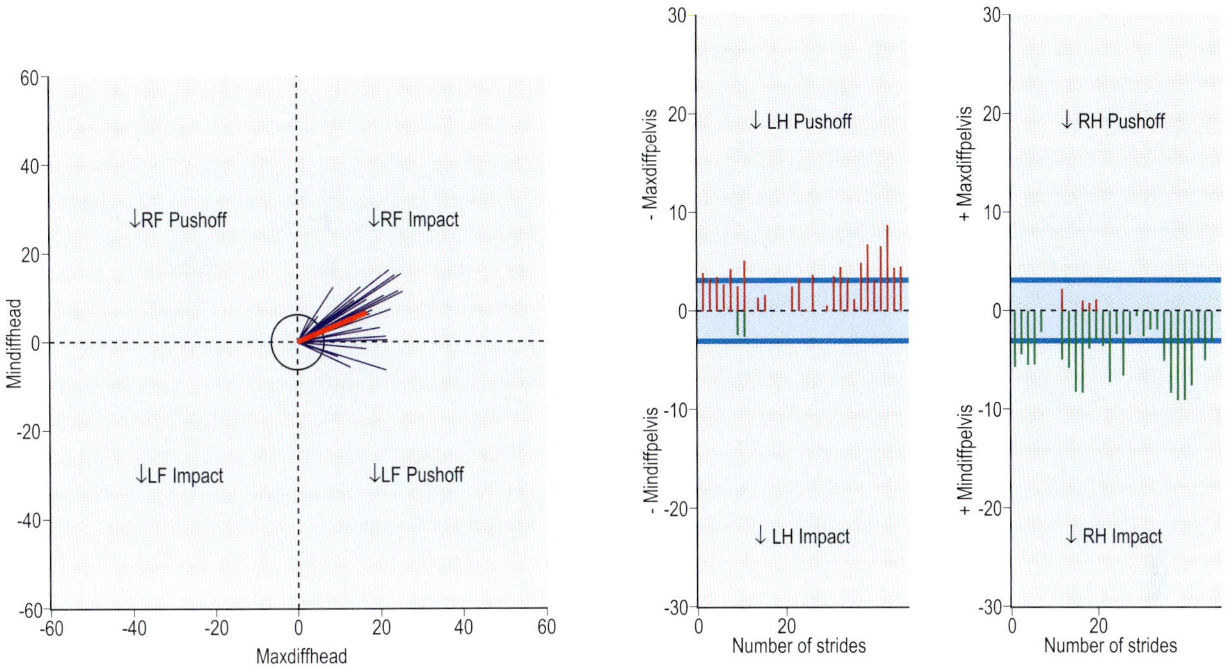

Fig 12.18 Inertial sensor system analysis displaying the 'Second Law of Sides'. There is an apparent right forelimb lameness with an apparent right hindlimb impact lameness and an apparent left hindlimb pushoff lameness. The most likely explanation is true right forelimb lameness with compensatory movement in the pelvis giving the appearance of hindlimb lameness. The compensatory movement in the pelvis mimicking a contralateral pushoff lameness is frequently most prominent.

confusing, however, in some horses that do not lunge regularly, or in horses that lunge in one direction easily but refuse to lunge in the other direction, or in horses that lunge in the other direction only with strong handler encouragement. Not all lameness conditions are exacerbated by lunging, some are masked and more difficult to see. Also, lunging large horses in tight circles on hard ground, especially when they may not be accustomed to such activity, may be uncomfortable, and an apparent inside limb lameness may be seen that is not clinically relevant. This is important to consider especially during pre-purchase evaluations.

Considerable effort has been expended documenting the effect of circling on the signals produced by inertial sensors attached to the head and midline torso in sound horses. The majority, but not all, horses will have asymmetric vertical head and torso movement. Expected patterns are somewhat dependent on surface characteristics. On soft and deep ground the horse will thrust its head upward (and toward the inside of the circle) during pushoff of the outside forelimb, and subsequently the head will fall further during the first half of stance in the inside forelimb. This gives the appearance of an outside forelimb pushoff lameness (negative MAXDIFFHEAD/positive MINDIFFHEAD when lunging to the left, and positive MAXDIFFHEAD/negative MINDIFFHEAD when lunging to the right, Fig. 12.19). Also, the horse will sink more into the ground on the outside hindlimb and, because the ground gives way, the pelvis will rise less after pushoff of the outside hindlimb. This gives the appearance of a combination of an outside hindlimb pushoff and an inside hindlimb impact lameness (positive MAXDIFFPELVIS/negative MINDIFFPELVIS when lunging to the left, and negative MAXDIFFPELVIS/positive MINDIFFPELVIS when lunging to the right, Fig. 12.19).

On hard and firm ground the head will fall and rise more on the outside forelimb, giving the appearance of an inside forelimb impact lameness (negative MAXDIFFHEAD/MINDIFFHEAD when lunging to the left, and a positive MAXDIFFHEAD/MINDIFFHEAD when lunging to the right). On hard and firm ground the pelvis will also rise and fall more on the outside hindlimb, giving the appearance of an inside (pushoff and impact) hindlimb lameness (negative MAXDIFFPELVIS/MINDIFFPELVIS when lunging to the left, and positive MAXDIFFPELVIS/MINDIFFPELVIS when lunging to the right. However, in a horse with lameness, unless the lameness is of equivalent severity on opposite sides when lunging in both directions, the degree of asymmetric head or pelvic motion in one direction compared to the other is still useful to detect and measure lameness.

Future directions for kinematic analysis of lameness in horses

Advances in technology are resulting in clinically useful kinematic evaluation techniques. Kinematic analysis has identified objective and specific changes in movement indicative of lameness. Understanding how we see these movement alterations is increasing.[46] This knowledge is improving our understanding and therefore teaching of normal and abnormal locomotion. With simultaneous objective and clinical examination techniques in realistic settings, the steepness of the learning curve in basic lameness evaluation is lessened and our ability to understand more about complex lameness evaluation is enhanced.

The majority of research and clinical investigations have focused on evaluation of the trot in a straight line. Limited evaluations of horses trotting in a circle have been performed.[42–45] Future work should include additional study of pelvic and head movement of lame horses trotting in a circle. Analysis of gaits other than a trot including the canter and gallop and the various movement patterns of gaited horses should also be pursued.

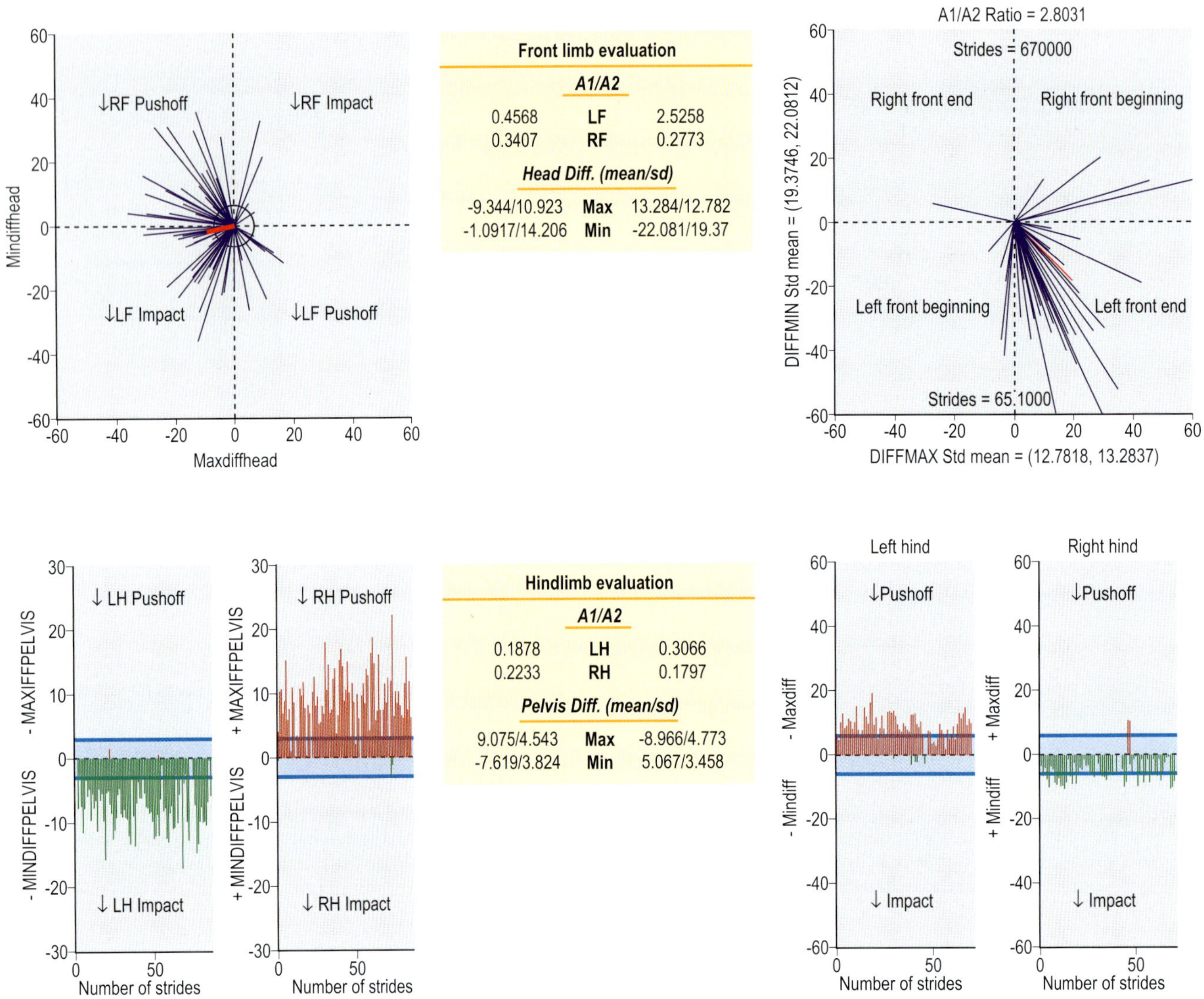

Fig 12.19 Inertial sensor system analysis displaying a normal, expected pattern of vertical head (upper subplots) and pelvis (lower subplots) movement in a sound horse while lunging to the left (left subplots) and then to the right (right subplots) on soft ground. Because of a combination of torso tilt and surface pliability the head will display an outside forelimb pushoff asymmetry and the pelvis will display a combination of outside hindlimb pushoff asymmetry and inside hindlimb impact asymmetry.

References

1. Keegan KG, Wilson DA, Wilson DJ, et al. Evaluation of mild lameness in horses trotting on a treadmill by clinicians and interns or residents and correlation of their assessments with kinematic gait analysis. American journal of veterinary research 1998;59(11):1370–7.
2. Keegan KG, Dent EV, Wilson DA, et al. Repeatability of subjective evaluation of lameness in horses. Equine veterinary journal 2010;42(2):92–7.
3. Fuller CJ, Bladon BM, Driver AJ, et al. The intra- and inter-assessor reliability of measurement of functional outcome by lameness scoring in horses. Vet J 2006; 171(2):281–6.
4. Hewetson M, Christley RM, Hunt ID, et al. Investigations of the reliability of observational gait analysis for the assessment of lameness in horses. The Veterinary record 2006;158(25): 852–7.
5. Arkell M, Archer RM, Guitian FJ, et al. Evidence of bias affecting the interpretation of the results of local anaesthetic nerve blocks when assessing lameness in horses. The Veterinary record 2006;159(11):346–9.
6. McCracken MJ, Lopes M, Kramer J, et al. Comparison of Inertial Sensor Based System and Traditional Lameness Exam. Chicago, IL: 2011 American College of Veterinary Surgeons Symposium; 2011 Nov 3–5, 2011; 2011. p. E37.
7. Ishihara A, Bertone AL, Rajala-Schultz PJ. Association between subjective lameness grade and kinetic gait parameters in horses with experimentally induced forelimb lameness. American journal of veterinary research 2005;66(10): 1805–15.
8. Nanua P, Waldron KJ. Energy comparison between trot, bound, and gallop using a simple model. J Biomech Eng 1995;117(4):466–73.
9. Rubin CT, Lanyon LE. Limb mechanics as a function of speed and gait: a study of functional strains in the radius and tibia of horse and dog. J Exp Biol 1982;101:187–211.
10. Keegan KG, Kramer J, Yonezawa Y, et al. Assessment of repeatability of a wireless, inertial sensor–based lameness evaluation system for horses. American

journal of veterinary research 2011;72(9):1156–63.

11. Keegan KG, Yonezawa Y, Pai PF, et al. Evaluation of a sensor-based system of motion analysis for detection and quantification of forelimb and hind limb lameness in horses. American journal of veterinary research 2004;65(5):665–70.
12. Church EE, Walker AM, Wilson AM, et al. Evaluation of discriminant analysis based on dorsoventral symmetry indices to quantify hindlimb lameness during over ground locomotion in the horse. Equine veterinary journal 2009;41(3): 304–8.
13. Pfau T, Robilliard JJ, Weller R, et al. Assessment of mild hindlimb lameness during over ground locomotion using linear discriminant analysis of inertial sensor data. Equine veterinary journal 2007;39(5):407–13.
14. Nasanen R, Ojanpaa H, Tanskanen T, et al. Estimation of temporal resolution of object identification in human vision. Exp Brain Res 2006;172(4):464–71.
15. Wilson DA, Keegan KG. Pathophysiology and diagnosis of musculoskeletal disease. The Horse, Diseases and Clinical Management 1995:607–58.
16. Baxter GM, Stashak TS. History, Visual Exam, Palpation and Manipulation. In: Baxter GM, editor. Adams and Stashak's lameness in horses. 6th ed. Oxford: Wiley Blackwell; 2011. p. 109–53.
17. Ross MW. Movement. In: Ross MW, Dyson SJ, editors. Diagnosis and management of lameness in the horse. 2nd ed. St. Louis: Elsevier Saunders; 2011. p. 64–80.
18. Buchner HH, Savelberg HH, Schamhardt HC, et al. Head and trunk movement adaptations in horses with experimentally induced fore- or hindlimb lameness. Equine veterinary journal 1996;28(1):71–6.
19. Kobluk CN, Schnurr D, Horney FD, et al. Use of high-speed cinematography and computer generated gait diagrams for the study of equine hindlimb kinematics. Equine veterinary journal 1989;21(1): 48–58.
20. Keegan KG, Wilson DA, Smith BK, et al. Changes in kinematic variables observed during pressure-induced forelimb lameness in adult horses trotting on a treadmill. American journal of veterinary research 2000;61(6):612–19.
21. Martinez-del Campo LJ, Kobluk CN, Greer N. The use of high-speed videography to generate angle-time and angle-angle diagrams for the study of equine locomotion. Vet Comp Orthop Trauma 1991;4:120–31.
22. Buchner HH, Savelberg HH, Schamhardt HC, et al. Limb movement adaptations in horses with experimentally induced fore- or hindlimb lameness. Equine veterinary journal 1996;28(1):63–70.
23. Keegan KG, Wilson DJ, Wilson DA, et al. Effects of anesthesia of the palmar digital nerves on kinematic gait analysis in horses with and without navicular disease. American journal of veterinary research 1997;58(3):218–23.
24. Kramer J, Keegan KG, Wilson DA, et al. Kinematics of the hind limb in trotting horses after induced lameness of the distal intertarsal and tarsometatarsal joints and intra-articular administration of anesthetic. American journal of veterinary research 2000;61(9):1031–6.
25. Peloso JG, Stick JA, Soutas-Little RW, et al. Computer-assisted three-dimensional gait analysis of amphotericin-induced carpal lameness in horses. American journal of veterinary research 1993;54(9):1535–43.
26. Pourcelot P, Audigie F, Degueurce C, et al. Kinematic symmetry index: a method for quantifying the horse locomotion symmetry using kinematic data. Vet Res 1997;28(6):525–38.
27. Keegan KG, Pai PF, Wilson DA, et al. Signal decomposition method of evaluating head movement to measure induced forelimb lameness in horses trotting on a treadmill. Equine veterinary journal 2001;33(5):446–51.
28. Kramer J, Keegan KG, Kelmer G, et al. Objective determination of pelvic movement during hind limb lameness by use of a signal decomposition method and pelvic height differences. American journal of veterinary research 2004;65(6):741–7.
29. Peham C, Scheidl M, Licka T. A method of signal processing in motion analysis of the trotting horse. J Biomech 1996;29(8):1111–14.
30. Audigie F, Pourcelot P, Degueurce C, et al. Fourier analysis of trunk displacements: a method to identify the lame limb in trotting horses. J Biomech 2002;35(9):1173–82.
31. Keegan KG, Macallister C, Wilson DA, et al. Validation of an inertial sensor system for evaluation of horses with bilateral forelimb lameness using the stationary force plate. American journal of veterinary research 2012;(In press).
32. May SA, Wyn-Jones G. Identification of hindleg lameness. Equine veterinary journal 1987;19(3):185–8.
33. Gough M, Munroe G. Decision making in the diagnosis and management of bone spavin in horses. In Practice 1998;20(5):252–9.
34. Dyson S. An approach to hindlimb lameness 2. Gait assessment, flexion tests and what to do next. In Practice 1997; 19(1):14.
35. Buchner F, Kastner J, Girtler D, et al. Quantification of hind limb lameness in the horse. Acta Anat (Basel) 1993; 146(2–3):196–9.
36. Keegan KG. Evidence-based lameness detection and quantification. Veterinary Clinics of North America, Equine Practice 2007;23(2):403–23.
37. Buchner HH, Savelberg HH, Schamhardt HC, et al. Bilateral lameness in horses–a kinematic study. Vet Q 1995;17(3): 103–5.
38. Drevemo S, Johnston C, Roepstorff L, et al. Nerve block and intra-articular anaesthesia of the forelimb in the sound horse. Equine Vet J Suppl 1999;30: 266–9.
39. Keg PR, Schamhardt HC, van Weeren PR, et al. The effect of diagnostic regional nerve blocks in the fore limb on the locomotion of clinically sound horses. Vet Q 1996;18 Suppl 2:S106–9.
40. Kelmer G, Keegan KG, Kramer J, et al. Computer-assisted kinematic evaluation of induced compensatory movements resembling lameness in horses trotting on a treadmill. American journal of veterinary research 2005;66(4):646–55.
41. Uhlir C, Licka T, Kubber P, et al. Compensatory movements of horses with a stance phase lameness. Equine Vet J Suppl 1997;(23):102–5.
42. Starke SD, Willems E, May SA, et al. Vertical head and trunk movement adaptations of sound horses trotting in a circle on a hard surface. Vet J. 2012; (In press).
43. Clayton HM, Sha DH. Head and body centre of mass movement in horses trotting on a circular path. Equine Vet J Suppl 2006;(36):462–7.
44. Hobbs SJ, Licka T, Polman R. The difference in kinematics of horses walking, trotting and cantering on a flat and banked 10 m circle. Equine veterinary journal 2011;43(6):686–94.
45. Walker AM, Wilson AM, Pfau T. Comparison of kinematic symmetry index calculations and the effects of straight and circular trotting. Equine veterinary journal 2010;42 (Suppl 38):482–7.
46. Parkes RS, Weller R, Groth AM, et al. Evidence of the development of 'domain-restricted' expertise in the recognition of asymmetric motion characteristics of hindlimb lameness in the horse. Equine veterinary journal 2009;41(2):112–17.
47. Keegan KG, Wilson DJ, Wilson DA, et al. Effects of balancing and shoeing of the forelimb feet on kinematic gait analysis in five horses with navicular disease. Journal of Equine Veterinary Science 1998;18(8):522–7.
48. Buchner HHF, editor. Limb movement pattern in forelimb and hindlimb lameness. 51st Annual Convention of the American Association of Equine Practitioners; Seattle, WA, USA, Dec 3–7, 2005:128–34.
49. Lanovaz JL, Clayton HM, Colborne GR, et al. Forelimb kinematics and net joint moments during the swing phase of the trot. Equine Vet J Suppl 1999;30:235–9.

50. Back W, Barneveld A, van Weeren PR, et al. Kinematic gait analysis in equine carpal lameness. Acta Anat (Basel) 1993;146(2–3):86–9.
51. Clayton HM, Theoret CL, Barber SM, et al. Effects of carpal synovectomy on stride kinematics of trotting horses. Veterinary and Comparative Orthopaedics and Traumatology 1998;11(2):80–4.
52. Weishaupt MA, Wiestner T, Hogg HP, et al. Compensatory load redistribution of horses with induced weightbearing hindlimb lameness trotting on a treadmill. Equine veterinary journal 2004;36(8):727–33.
53. Weishaupt MA, Wiestner T, Hogg HP, et al. Vertical ground reaction force-time histories of sound Warmblood horses trotting on a treadmill. Vet J 2004;168(3):304–11.
54. ChristovÃ£o FG, Barros RML, Martins CB, et al. Three-dimensional kinematic analysis of head and limb movements of lame and non-lame colts. Equine and Comparative Exercise Physiology 2007;4(01):31–6.

Diagnosis of lameness

13

Andris J. Kaneps

CHAPTER CONTENTS

Introduction

Lameness evaluation steps are as follows:

- history
- visual examination at rest
- in motion examination
- manipulations
- localization
- diagnostic imaging.

A horse without gait abnormalities should move in a balanced manner with all limb movements in equilibrium. If lameness is present, it is the examiner's task to identify the gait abnormality, its location, the likely causes and to recommend appropriate treatment. Evaluation of lameness requires an ability to visualize gait abnormalities, skill in applying techniques that localize the abnormality to a specific site, and obtaining and interpreting appropriate images of the site. These findings must be consolidated to determine a diagnosis.

Experience in observing and interpreting the equine gait is a hard fought and ongoing process. The science of gait evaluations (see Chapters 10 and 12) may help us understand how and why a horse moves in a particular fashion, but visualization by a trained and experienced examiner remains the basis for most lameness examinations.

History

A complete anamnesis of the horse presented for evaluation of lameness helps to narrow the list of differential diagnoses, determines the effect of previous treatment or shoeing protocols, and may help to narrow the focus of the examination. The signalment of the horse (age, sex, breed, and use of the horse) should be clearly elucidated. The list of potential diagnoses will be different for a two-year-old Warmblood horse in early training as opposed to a two-year-old Thoroughbred that has started three races.

Specific questions to ask during the history include:

1. **When was the lameness first noticed and how long has it been present?**
   Acute onset of lameness may indicate abnormalities such as severe subsolar bruising or osteochondral fracture. Prolonged, insidious onset of lameness may be due to wear-and-tear disorders such as navicular syndrome or bone spavin.
2. **Describe what was initially noticed.**
   Owners and trainers may make an incorrect interpretation of the initial signs of subtle lameness, but their interpretations may still be very useful. For example, a short and choppy forelimb gait associated with heel pain is often described by clients as 'sore in the shoulders' because of the shuffling gait. Also, advanced riders may notice subtle abnormalities in their horse's gait that may be extremely difficult to observe during the lameness examination. An example would be reluctance of a dressage horse to enter a round frame while being ridden.
3. **Under what circumstances is the lameness most obvious?**
   Lameness that is first evident when the horse comes out of the stall or early in an exercise period (when the horse is 'cold') may be associated with synovitis or arthritis. Lameness that decreases in severity as the horse warms up during exercise is also often associated with arthritis. Lameness that becomes more pronounced with longer periods of exercise may be indicative of tendon or ligament inflammation. The lameness may be more evident on different types of surfaces.

Deep footing may make soft tissue injuries more apparent, while very firm footing will cause greater concussion and may exacerbate lameness due to arthritis.

4. **Have any swellings or thickenings been observed?** Some effusions and soft tissue swellings may be transient. Joint effusion with carpal osteochondral fracture often is pronounced near the time of occurrence and then gradually subsides. Soft tissue swelling due to tendonitis is often observable for prolonged periods of time.
5. **Has the horse undergone any treatment for this condition?** For example, has the horse had rest, medication, change in level of use, or shoeing modifications.
6. **When was the horse last shod or trimmed?** Changes in hoof angle and paring of a thin sole may be a cause of transient lameness. Excessive wear of the hoof or shoes soon after a farrier visit may be indicative of a more severe gait abnormality.
7. **Is there any previous history of lameness?** Is this a new condition or a continuation of a previous injury?

Visual examination at rest

Before observing the horse in motion a careful appraisal of the horse's conformation and close visualization of the horse's stance and limbs should be made. Start by evaluating the horse from a distance to allow appreciation of its stance, general conformation, areas of swelling or atrophy and attitude. Evaluate wear patterns of the hoof or shoes. Closer inspection should always involve palpation of each limb in its entirety. Subtle effusion of the carpal joints and medial femorotibial joints may only be noticed with palpation. Swollen regions should be palpated to evaluate tissue temperature and the degree of sensitivity to deep palpation. A swelling that is sensitive to touch and is warmer than surrounding areas is likely undergoing active inflammation. A cold, insensitive swelling may be a lesion that has healed and is no longer actively inflamed.

The digital pulses should always be palpated at the level of the proximal sesamoid bones or in the pastern region of each distal limb. Elevated pulses are associated with injury or inflammation in the distal limb and may help localize the lesion to medial or lateral aspects of the limb.

Tendons and ligaments should be palpated with the limb in both weight bearing and flexed positions. Tendon sheath effusions are best evaluated with the limb bearing weight. When the limb is flexed the tendons and ligaments on the palmar or plantar surface are more easily defined and separated. Deep palpation of the mid- to proximal suspensory ligament often elicits some discomfort in the normal horse. Compare contralateral limbs if there is a concern regarding palpation sensitivity.[1]

In motion examination

Examination of the lame horse in motion is necessary to characterize the nature and intensity of the gait abnormality. The lameness should be graded using a consistent scale (Table 13.1).[2] Conducting the in motion examination in controlled surroundings will add consistency to the findings. The ideal location to examine a horse for lameness is a flat, firm surface where the horse may by jogged for 30 to 40 meters without encountering obstructions or distractions.[3] An asphalt surface has the advantage of allowing the examiner to both visualize and listen to the horse's footfalls. The sound of the lame limb impacting the surface will be diminished when compared to the unaffected contralateral limb. A common finding with subtle gait abnormalities may be the unaffected limb of a pair impacting the surface louder than the affected limb. Gait symmetry and footfalls are best evaluated at the walk and trot with the observer sighting along the longitudinal axis of the horse as it moves away and returns (Fig. 13.1).

A safe place to work the horse in a circle, preferably on a longe line, should be available (Fig. 13.2). The surface may be firm or on soft footing, but safe enough to permit circles from 10 to 20 meters in diameter without risk of the horse slipping. Horses with subtle gait abnormalities may need to be observed while being worked in normal tack. In select circumstances an examiner with sufficient

Table 13.1 Lameness grading scale

GRADE	LAMENESS GRADING SCALE (AFTER AMERICAN ASSOCIATION OF EQUINE PRACTITIONERS SCALE[2])
0	Lameness is not observed
1	Intermittent or inconsistent lameness at the trot that is difficult to discern under any circumstance
2	Lameness is difficult to observe at a walk or trot in a straight line, but is consistently apparent under special circumstances such as with manipulation longeing, or riding
3	Lameness is consistently observed at the trot under all conditions
4	Lameness is obvious with marked asymmetry of gait at the trot without manipulation.
5	Minimal or no weight bearing on the affected limb, horse is reluctant to move

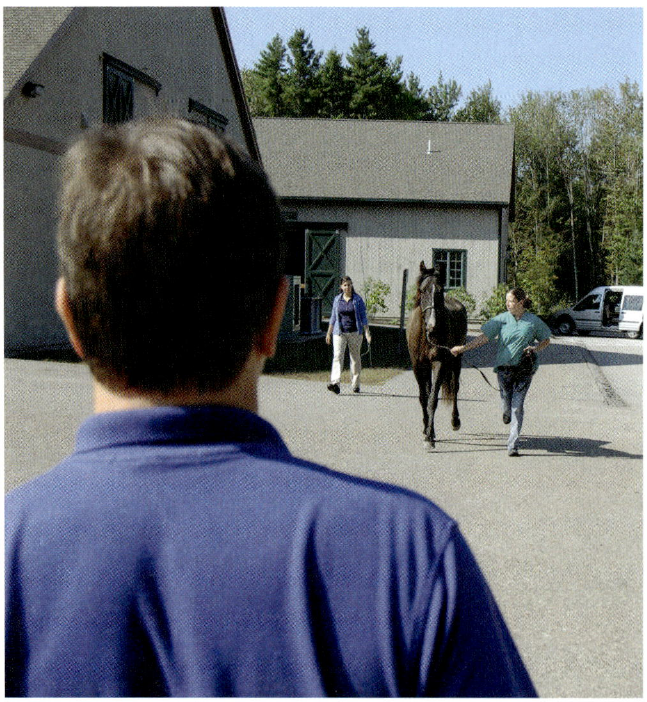

Fig 13.1 Initial lameness evaluation should be made on a hard surface and observing the horse along its longitudinal axis.

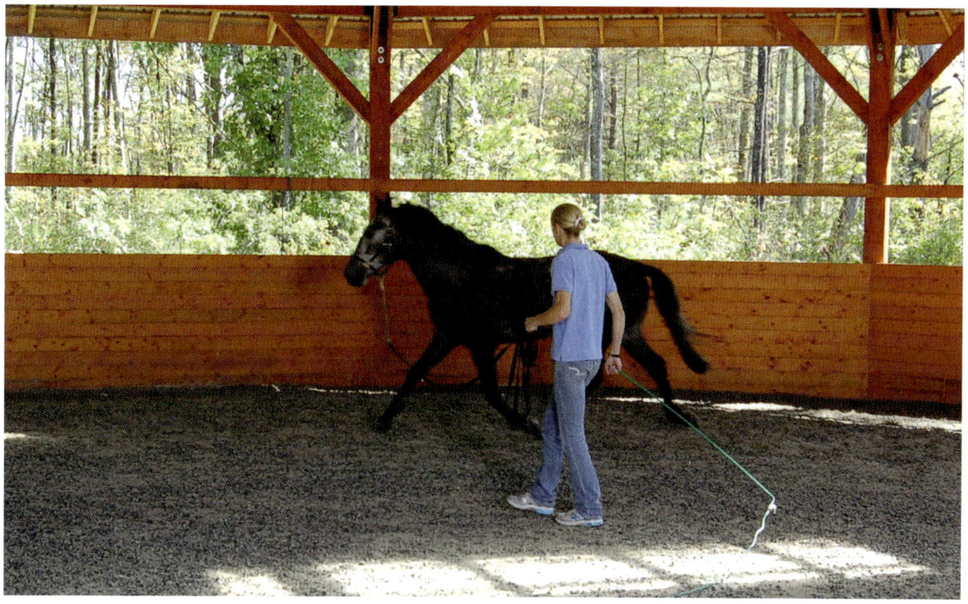

Fig 13.2 Evaluating lameness on the longe line may be used to exacerbate mild gait abnormalities and to determine how a horse performs during transitions of gait.

experience may find it useful to work or ride the horse. This is particularly useful in harness racehorses that only demonstrate their gait abnormalities at speed.

Watch the horse initially at a walk to evaluate footfall patterns and to familiarize the horse with the environment in which the examination will take place. Each foot should normally land heel first, then toe with the lateral and medial aspects of the hoof landing nearly equally in time.[4] Deviations from normal footfall may indicate dynamic imbalance of the limb that could be due to abnormalities of conformation, hoof shape, shoeing or due to pain. The swinging phase of the limb in a correctly conformed horse should be a straight track without any predilection to swinging-in or -out. Toe-in or toe-out conformations predispose the horse to swinging-out ('paddling') or swinging-in ('winging-in'), respectively.[3]

The trot is the most useful gait to evaluate lameness because it is a symmetrical, two-beat gait where diagonal limb pairs are simultaneously in the stance phase. The horse should be trotted at a comfortable, unhurried speed with the head allowed to move freely up and down. Subtle imbalances in gait may easily be missed if the examiner is not directly aligned with the center of the long axis of the horse (the vertebral column). The examiner should also observe the horse from the side as it trots by for characteristics of stride length and to determine if there is any toe dragging. Viewing the horse from the side at the trot may provide better evaluation of rear limb lameness.[5]

Lameness is evident to the observer as an asymmetry of the gait. Forelimb lameness is usually evident as a head bob: the head rises immediately prior to and during weight bearing of the lame limb. Conversely, the head drops as the sound limb contacts the ground and bears weight.[6] Stride length may also be altered by gait abnormalities. A shortened anterior phase to the stride (shuffling gait) may be associated with heel pain as the horse is reluctant to extend the affected limb and bear full weight on the heel.[3] This type of change in the stride may also occur due to pain during the swing phase of the gait, such as may be encountered with bicipital bursitis/tendonitis of the forelimb. Subtle forelimb lameness may only be evident as an unequal shift in weight with the unaffected limb bearing more weight than the lame limb. Such subtle weight shifts are best observed with the horse trotting directly toward the examiner.

Rear limb gait abnormalities may be evident as elevation of the hip (hip hike, gluteal rise), dropping of the hip (hip drop, gluteal drop), toe dragging and decreased stride length.[3] These responses to rear limb lameness are mechanisms the horse uses to avoid discomfort during various portions of the stride and are due to the nature of the abnormality. Elevation of the hip occurs when the horse shifts weight away from the lame limb during the weight bearing phase of the stride. Dropping of the hip occurs if pain is most acute during the posterior phase of the weight bearing portion of the stride. Often this movement is associated with abnormalities of the caudal/plantar aspect of the rear limb such as: suspensory desmitis, flexor tendonitis, desmitis of the distal suspensory apparatus, and injury to the semimembranosus/semitendinosus muscle group. Dragging of the toe is associated with reluctance to raise the limb during the swing phase of the stride and is usually associated with upper rear limb joint lameness such as bone spavin and abnormalities of the stifle or coxofemoral joints.

Stashak describes 'gluteal rise and use' as characteristics observed from the rear of the horse at the trot. Gluteal rise is observed during the swing phase of the stride and use is observed during weight bearing.[3] Three characteristics of rear limb lameness in relationship to the gluteals were described:

1. depressed gluteal rise and use is associated with upper rear limb (usually hip region) lameness,
2. symmetric gluteal rise, but decreased gluteal use, is seen in subtle rear limb lameness and is non-localizing, and
3. rapid increased gluteal rise with decreased gluteal use is found in horses with marked discomfort during weight bearing and is often associated with a noticeable head bob.[3]

During the trot, the pelvis normally rocks symmetrically from left to right in the sound horse when observed from the rear. In a study of induced right distal tarsal lameness, the right limb had greater vertical displacement of the tuber coxae than did the left (unaffected) limb, but the difference was not significant.[5] However, the ratio of left to right tuber coxae vertical displacement decreased

20% with the induction of distal tarsal lameness.[5] The change in ratio was evidence that tuber coxae asymmetric movement is a sensitive indicator of rear limb lameness at the trot.[5] A practical application of these findings is: when a rear limb lameness is observed at the trot from the rear of the horse, the tuber coxae of the lame limb usually has greater up-and-down motion compared to the tuber coxae of the sound limb.

Severe rear limb lameness (>grade 3) is often associated with a head bob. At the trot the rear limb and the contralateral forelimb are simultaneously in the same stride phase (working as a diagonal pair). If lameness of the rear limb is severe enough, as the affected limb contacts the ground the horse will shift weight forward (off of the lame rear limb) using his neck – resulting in an observable head drop as the contralateral forelimb enters the weight bearing phase of the stride. Kinematic analysis has found a measurable head bob with even mild rear limb lameness.[7] The examiner needs to be aware of this process as moderate to severe rear limb lameness may be confused with a lameness of the ipsilateral forelimb.[3,7]

When the examiner encounters difficulty in determining which limb is lame, it may be easier to determine 'which limb is sound'. At times it is simpler to visualize and/or hear which limb is bearing more weight (the sound limb). Manipulative tests should be used when lameness is subtle.

Manipulative tests and techniques

Manipulations that enhance or localize lameness include:

- work on the longe line
- hoof tester application
- flexion tests
- riding or working with tack
- rectal palpation.

Longe line

Most sport horses may be safely worked in a circle on a longe (lunge) line. Working the horse in a 10 to 20 meter diameter circle will put additional weight and stress on the innermost limbs and the medial aspect of the outermost limbs (Fig 13.2). The additional stress on the limbs helps the examiner identify subtle lamenesses and in some cases will help localize the region of soreness to a portion of the limb. A round pen of appropriate size may be similarly used.

Use of hoof testers

Hoof testers are squeezed on the sole and hoof capsule to determine if there are any sensitive areas present. Hoof tester pressure on normal hoof or sole does not result in a significant withdrawal response. If a sensitive area is found, the hoof tester pressure should be repeated to verify the finding, then pressure should be maintained for 20 to 30 seconds and the horse should be trotted off to determine if pressure on the sensitive area causes an exacerbation of the lameness. Significant sensitive areas should be closely evaluated by paring out the foot.

While using the hoof testers, the foot should also be evaluated for balance, general condition of the hoof and sole, and the degree of wear of shoes and hoof walls. Abnormalities such as: dished hoof, long toe, low heels, sheared heels, contracted heels, hoof cracks, thrush, flaky sole, hard sole, sole bruising, and white line disease should be noted. Percuss the hoof wall with the hoof tester or a hammer. Hollow-sounding areas may correspond to a deep abscess or hoof wall separation. Areas of pain on concussion may be indicative of a tightly clinched nail or a nail that has penetrated the sensitive laminae and is causing a local abscess.

Flexion tests

Flexion tests are used to apply stress or pressure on an anatomical region of the limb for a set period of time. Following the flexion period the horse is trotted off and observed for the effects of the test on gait. Recalling the baseline level of lameness during both trotting on the lead rope and on the longe line (if appropriate) is crucial to objectively evaluating the results of both flexion tests and diagnostic local anesthesia. The amount and duration of pressure applied may affect the outcome of flexion tests.[8] Consistency of application is also a key to correct interpretation of flexion tests. The flexion test, particularly of the distal limb, should not be over interpreted. More than 60 of 100 horses determined to be sound prior to application of manipulative tests had some degree of lameness evident after distal limb flexion.[9]

Each flexion test should be completed in anatomical pairs (for example: distal flexions of both fore limbs) with the sound limb flexed first. Tests should progress from the distal to proximal aspect of the limbs. Moderate and equal pressure should be applied for each flexion test. Consistency is improved by having the same individual perform all of the tests during an examination. One study found a 12% coefficient of variation between multiple distal forelimb flexion tests applied by one clinician and a 20% coefficient of variation between different clinicians.[10]

Flexion tests used for lameness evaluation are described in Table 13.2 and figures that demonstrate various manipulations are included (Fig. 13.3, Fig. 13.4, Fig. 13.5 and Fig.13.6). Results of flexion tests may be recorded as: *negative:* no change in lameness, *slight positive:* slight exacerbation of lameness following flexion that is noticed during only a portion of the trotting course, *moderate positive:* lameness is exacerbated while the horse is trotting away from the examiner, but not on the return and *severe positive:* marked exacerbation of lameness during the outbound and return portions of the trotting course.

Other aids to localizing lameness include rectal palpation of the pelvis for upper rear limb lameness, manipulations of the back (see Chapter 21), and working the horse in its given discipline with full tack. Working horses in circumstances that are similar to those when lameness is noticed by the owner or trainer is especially important for evaluation of subtle lamenesses or those that only occur under special circumstances.

Localization with diagnostic local analgesia

Diagnostic local analgesia ('nerve block') is performed to localize lameness. Important considerations are:

1. understanding the anatomy to provide accurate placement of the anesthetic,
2. being aware of different options for administering anesthetic to a site as clinical situations may dictate one technique over another, and
3. maintaining strict asepsis when penetrating synovial spaces.

Mepivacaine HCl 2% is the preferred local anesthetic for regional and joint analgesia in horses. Compared to lidocaine it is less irritating to tissues and has a comparable onset, yet a longer duration, of action.[11,12] Local anesthetics cause blockade of sodium channels that results in inhibition of nerve conduction.[13] The effectiveness of local anesthesia depends on local tissue pH (local anesthetics are

Table 13.2 Manipulative tests for lameness evaluation

SEQUENCE OF FLEXION TESTS	TECHNIQUE	DURATION OF TEST
FORELIMB:		
Distal limb	Stand to the front or side of the horse with the carpus relaxed. Grasp the toe with one hand using the other hand placed on the palmar aspect of the distal metacarpus as a fulcrum (Fig. 13.3A). Alternatively, stand in front of the horse and grasp the toe with both hands placing the dorsal aspect of the fetlock on your knees and flex the distal joints (Fig. 13.3B). Distal limb flexion stresses the metacarpophalangeal, proximal interphalangeal, and distal interphalangeal joints and the navicular region.	30 seconds
Carpus	Stand to the side of the horse, grasp the distal dorsal aspect of the metacarpus with one hand. Flex the carpus maximally. A full range of motion is evident when the palmar metacarpus contacts the caudal aspect of the antebrachium. The metacarpus may be adducted and abducted during flexion to provide more stress to the medial and lateral aspects of the joints.	30 seconds
Metacarpus	Direct pressure on the flexor tendons or suspensory ligament	30 seconds
Proximal forelimb	The shoulder and elbow are difficult to isolate. The bicipital bursa of the shoulder may be evaluated by applying direct pressure over the bicipital tendon at the point of the shoulder or by retracting the upper fore limb caudally to its full extent. The upper limb should be abducted and adducted to stress the medial and lateral support structures of the joints.	30–60 seconds
REAR LIMB:		
Distal rear limb	Techniques are similar to that used in the forelimb. Flexion is performed with the tarsus and stifle relaxed. See Figs. 13.4 A and B for two techniques.	30 seconds
Full rear limb	Also referred to as the 'spavin test'. This flexion test stresses all of the rear limb joints to some degree because of their connection via the reciprocal apparatus, however the tarsus and stifle joints are stressed more than others. The rear limb is grasped with both hands around the distal metatarsus and the full limb is flexed maximally (Fig. 13.5).	45 seconds
Stifle	This joint is stressed during application of the full limb flexion. The cruciate ligaments may be stressed by abruptly forcing the tibial crest caudally using a hand on the tibial crest while the horse is fully weight bearing on the limb. The medial collateral ligament of the stifle may be stressed by picking up the limb, grasping the mid-metatarsus and using placing the examiner's shoulder over the lateral aspect of the stifle. Abruptly abduct the distal limb using the examiner's shoulder as the fulcrum.	15–30 seconds
Coxofemoral joint	With the limb not bearing weight and nearly extended 'stir' the limb in an arc. An alternative method is to adduct the limb. For example: to stress the right coxofemoral joint stand on the horse's left, pick up the right rear limb while maintaining limb extension and pulling the distal limb to the horse's left side (Fig. 13.6).	30 seconds

much less effective in acid pH), accuracy of deposition, and the size of nerves being blocked (small, unmyelinated fibers are more sensitive than large, myelinated fibers).[13] The toxic dose is approximately 13 mg/kg (~6 mg/lb). Overdose of local anesthetics may result in heart block, bradycardia and convulsions.[14] Toxicity is usually only a concern in smaller animals. Onset of action for regional nerve blocks is 10 to 25 minutes with smaller diameter nerves desensitized earlier than larger nerves. Onset of intra-articular analgesia is 5 to 10 minutes with a gradual increase in analgesia over that time. Check the effects of the local anesthetic in most joints at 20 minutes and in complex joints such as the stifle in 30 minutes. Mepivacaine inhibits nerve sensation for 90 to 180 minutes.[13]

Strict aseptic techniques should always be followed when injecting joints or synovial structures. A fresh bottle of local anesthetic should always be used. The site to be injected may be clipped, but in a study of various methods of preparing the site of intra-articular injections, clipping of the site was not found to improve results of skin surface bacteriological cultures.[15] A 7 to 10 minute scrub with povidone-iodine or chlorhexidine should be made of the injection site. Immediately prior to injection the site should be carefully wiped with 70% isopropyl alcohol. The operator should wear sterile surgical gloves. Adequate assistance should be available for restraining the horse. The most painful portion of the injection is needle penetration of the skin and joint capsule. Confident, quick insertion of the needle in the correct anatomical site minimizes discomfort for the horse. A skin bleb of local anesthetic may be helpful in making the joint injection less uncomfortable to the horse, particularly when a larger gauge needle must be used.[16]

The sequence of diagnostic local analgesia begins with the most distal nerves being injected first and gradually working proximally until the lameness has been localized. Regional anesthesia usually results in less effective analgesia of intra-articular soreness than

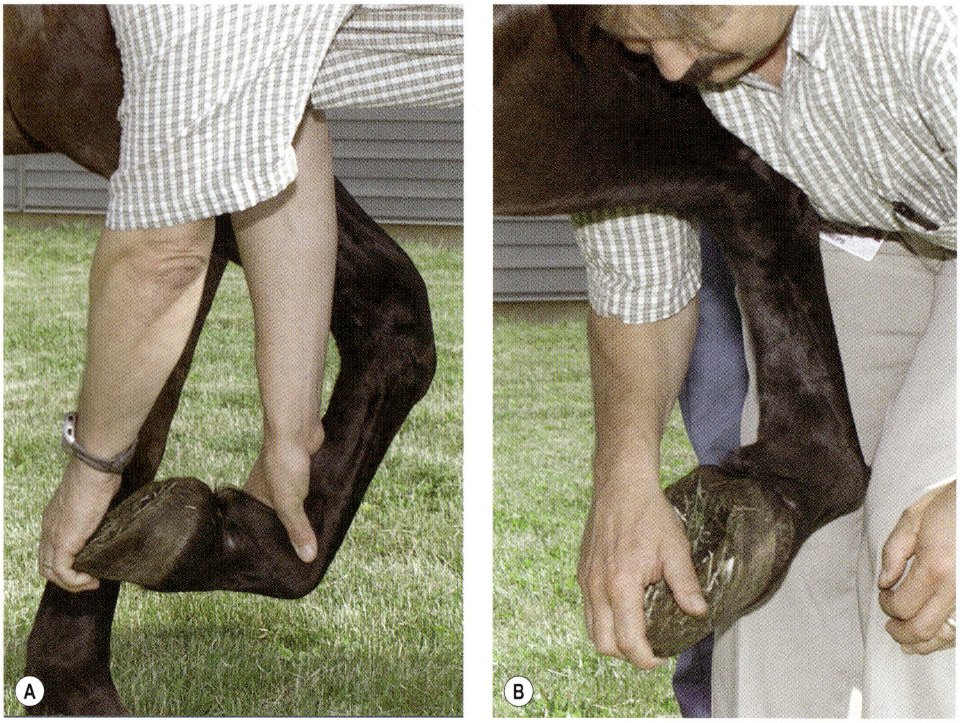

Fig 13.3 **(A)** Distal forelimb flexion using one hand as the fulcrum on the palmar aspect of the fetlock and one hand pulling on the toe of the hoof. **(B)** Distal forelimb flexion with the dorsal aspect of the fetlock resting on the operators knees and both hands used to pull on the toe. Excessive force during this manipulation may lead to false positive results.

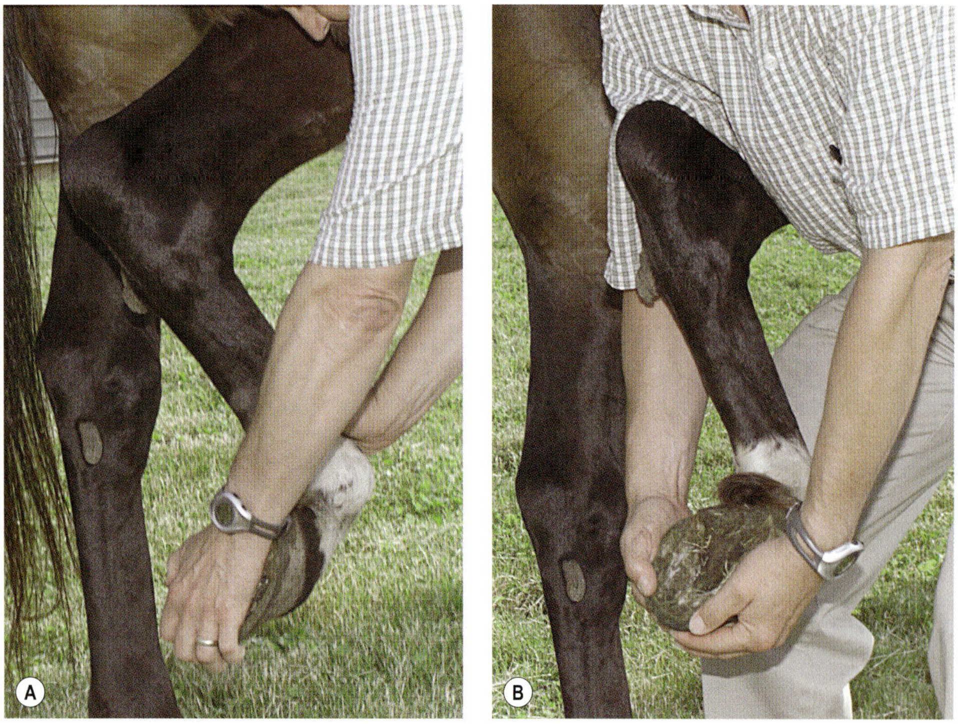

Fig 13.4 **(A)** Distal rear limb flexion with the limb nearly extended and one hand on the plantar aspect of the fetlock acting as the fulcrum and the other hand flexing at the toe of the hoof. **(B)** An alternative method of applying a distal rear limb flexion test by tucking the tuber calcis under the operators inside arm pit and using both hands to flex the toe.

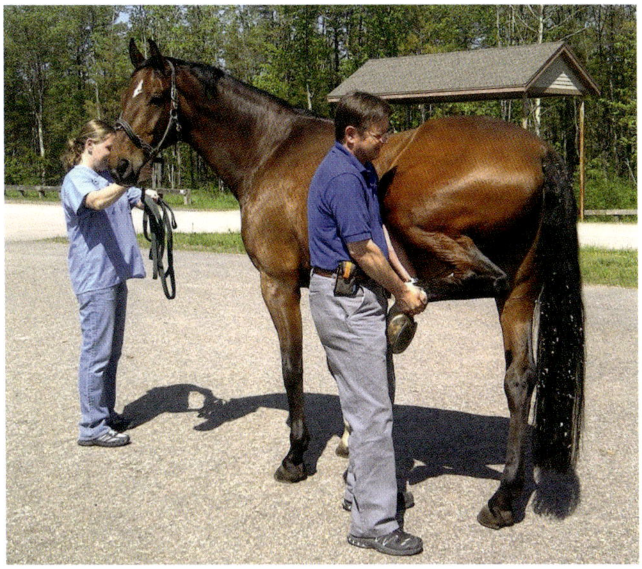

Fig 13.5 Full rear limb flexion demonstrating full range of motion. This manipulative test stresses all the joints of the rear limb, but especially the tarsus, stifle and coxofemoral joint.

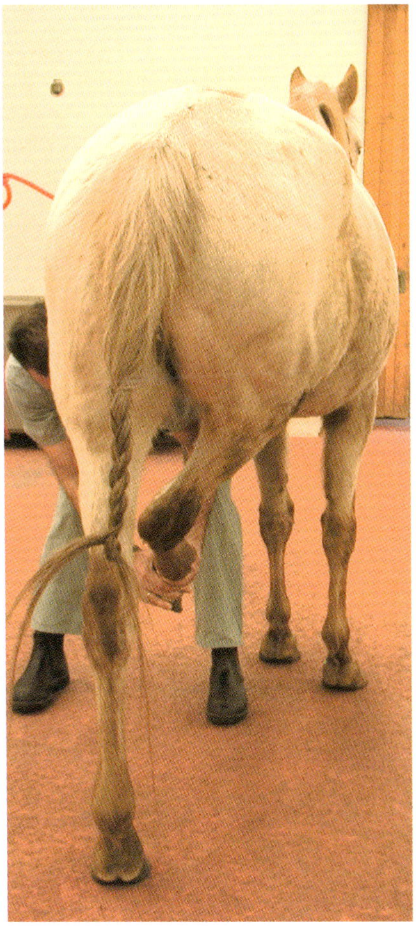

Fig 13.6 Manipulative test of the coxofemoral joint by adduction of the rear limb. An assistant can initially pick up the limb and hand it to the operator.

direct intra-articular anesthesia. If the lameness has been improved noticeably, but not completely, following regional nerve anesthesia, intra-articular anesthesia of the suspect joint should be conducted. Regional nerve blocks are described for the forelimb (Table 13.3) and rear limb (Table 13.4).

Intra-articular anesthesia

Navicular bursa

Strict asepsis must be adhered to at this site because of its close proximity to the ground and the attendant contaminants. An 18-ga, three inch (1.2 × 90 mm) spinal needle is advanced parallel to the bearing surface of the hoof until it contacts the flexor surface of the navicular bone. The needle should be aimed at a point one cm distal to the coronary band and midway between its most dorsal and palmar extent.[22] Correct placement of the needle should be confirmed with radiography or ultrasonography. Three to 5 mL of local anesthetic is injected.[23]

Comparing the results of navicular bursa, distal interphalangeal joint and palmar digital nerve local anesthesia may aid localization of distal limb lameness.[23] However, mepivacaine has been found to diffuse widely following injection in the distal equine limb, potentially confounding efforts to specifically localize the site of lameness.[26]

Distal interphalangeal joint

The distal interphalangeal (DIP) joint has a large dorsal pouch that is easily entered with a needle.[24] The joint may also be approached immediately cranial to the collateral cartilage.

Anesthetic injected in the DIP joint will desensitize other nearby structures. The proximal suspensory ligament of the navicular bone, distal extent of the palmar digital nerves, navicular bursa and impar ligaments are directly adjacent to palmar aspects of the DIP joint.[25] Thirty minutes after mepivacaine was injected in the DIP, local anesthetic concentrations sufficient to result in analgesia were found in the navicular bursa synovial fluid (10 of 10 horses) and in the medullary cavity of the navicular bone (six of 10 horses).[26] Mepivacaine diffused from the distal interphalangeal joint into the navicular bursa and vice versa in 25 of 25 joints evaluated.[26] Ten minutes following distal interphalangeal joint anesthesia lameness induced by tightening a set screw on the sole was resolved.[17]

Dorsal approach

This injection is best made with the horse fully weight bearing using a 20–18 ga, 1½ inch (0.9–1.2 × 40 mm) needle. The needle is placed on the dorsal midline, perpendicular to the second phalanx and enters the skin 2–2.5 cm proximal to the coronary band. Insert the needle to bone (the second phalanx) and withdraw slightly.[27] This technique usually causes less discomfort and is less likely to result in hemorrhage compared to the other dorsal techniques. For the alternative dorsal techniques the needle is inserted 1.5–2 cm proximal to the coronary band and a like distance lateral or medial to the extensor process of the distal phalanx and directed toward the extensor process.[16] The needle usually penetrates the skin approximately 1″ (25 mm) before entering the joint. Four to 6 mL of anesthetic is injected.

Hemorrhage often occurs from the coronary corium when the needle is withdrawn. Counter pressure and a light bandage will control any bleeding and help protect the region from contamination until the needle puncture seals.

Table 13.3 Forelimb diagnostic local analgesia

SEQUENCE OF DIAGNOSTIC LOCAL ANESTHESIA	ANATOMIC SITE OF INJECTION	REGION DESENSITIZED	NEEDLE SIZE AND ANESTHETIC VOLUME	ONSET OF ACTION
Palmar digital nerves (PDN)	Palmar aspect of pastern, immediately proximal to the collateral cartilages.	Palmar heel, entire sole	25–22 g × 1 inch 0.5–0.7 × 16 mm 1.5–2 ml/nerve.	10–15 minutes
Dorsal branch of PDN	Same as above, redirect needle dorsally approximately 1 inch (25 mm).	All structures within the hoof.	As above.	As above.
Abaxial sesamoid (palmar nerves)	Abaxial aspect of proximal sesamoid bones (may use either dorsal branch or abaxial sesamoid block).	All structures within the hoof and most of structures from mid-pastern distal.	25–22 g × 1 inch 0.5–0.7 × 16 mm 2–2.5 ml/nerve.	As above.
Low four-point (palmar nerves and palmar metacarpal nerves)	At the level of the distal aspect of MCII and MCIV (splint bones). Palmar nerves are injected subcutaneously between the suspensory branch and the deep digital flexor tendon immediately proximal to the digital sheath. Palmar metacarpal nerves are injected subcutaneously immediately dorsal and distal to the splint buttons.	Fetlock joint and all distal structures.	22 g × 1 inch 0.7 × 25 mm 4–5 ml per palmar nerve, 3 ml per palmar metacarpal nerve.	15 minutes
High four-point (palmar nerves and palmar metacarpal nerves)	At the most proximal aspect of the metacarpus that a palpable groove between the deep digital flexor tendon and suspensory ligament is palpable. The palmar nerves are injected in this groove. The palmar metacarpal nerves are injected by redirecting the needle to the axial surface of MCII and MCIV.	All structures distal to the point of injection. Inadvertent injection of the carpometacarpal joint may occur.[18]	22 g × 1 inch 0.7 × 25 mm 4–5 ml per palmar nerve, 3 ml per palmar metacarpal nerve.	15 minutes
Base of the accessory carpal bone	The lateral and medial palmar metacarpal and lateral palmar nerves lie together at a site between the flexor retinaculum and the carpal sheath at a point midway between the head of MCIV and the base of the accessory carpal bone and immediately distal to the accessoriometacarpal ligament. The medial palmar nerve is injected as previously described at the axial aspect of proximal MCII.[19]	All structures distal to the point of injection including the origin of the suspensory ligament. Inadvertent injection within the carpal canal may occur.[18]	22 g × 1 inch 0.7 × 25 mm 3–4 ml at base of accessory carpal bone, 3 ml at palmar metacarpal nerve.	15 minutes
Suspensory ligament origin	The needle is inserted directly into the origin of the suspensory ligament. A large needle is used to reduce the chance of breakage. (High four-point, base of accessory carpal and suspensory origin blocks may be interchanged depending on operator preference).	The entire suspensory ligament and structures distal to the injection point. Inadvertent injection within the ccarpometacarpal joint may occur.[18]	18 g × 1–1.5 inch 1.2 × 25–40 mm 4–6 ml	First check in 10 minutes, then again after 20 minutes.
Median/ulnar/ musculocutaneous	The median nerve is injected on the caudomedial aspect of the radius immediately distal to the pectoral muscle mass. The needle is partially removed and redirected subcutaneously to a point just cranial to the cephalic vein for the musculocutaneous nerve. The ulnar nerve is injected 25 mm deep to the skin at a point 6–8 cm proximal to the accessory carpal bone between the flexor carpi ulnaris and ulnaris lateralis muscles.	The entire limb distal to points of injection including the carpus, suspensory origin.	22–20 g × 1.5 inch 0.7–0.9 × 40 mm 6–8 ml at median nerve, 4–6 ml at musculocutaneous nerve, 4–6 ml at the ulnar nerve.	20–30 minutes

Table 13.4 Rear limb diagnostic analgesia

SEQUENCE OF DIAGNOSTIC LOCAL ANESTHESIA	ANATOMIC SITE OF INJECTION	REGION DESENSITIZED	NEEDLE SIZE AND ANESTHETIC VOLUME	ONSET OF ACTION
Plantar digital nerves (PDN)	Plantar aspect of pastern, immediately proximal to the collateral cartilages.	plantar heel, entire sole	25–22 g × 1 inch 0.5–0.7 × 16 mm 1.5–2 ml/nerve.	10–15 minutes
Dorsal branch of PDN	Same as above, redirect needle dorsally approximately 1 inch (25 mm).	All structures within the hoof.	As above	As above.
Abaxial sesamoid (plantar nerves)	Abaxial aspect of proximal sesamoid bones (may use either dorsal branch or abaxial sesamoid block).	All structures within the hoof and most of structures from mid-pastern distal.	25–22 g × 1 inch 0.5–0.7 × 16 mm 2–2.5 ml/nerve.	As above.
Low six-point (plantar, plantar metatarsal and dorsal metatarsal nerves)	At the level of the distal aspect of MTII and MTIV (splint bones). Plantar nerves are injected subcutaneously between the suspensory branch and the deep digital flexor tendon immediately proximal to the digital sheath. Plantar metatarsal nerves are injected subcutaneously immediately dorsal and distal to the splint buttons. Dorsal metatarsal nerves are injected immediately lateral and medial to the common extensor tendon.	Fetlock joint and all distal structures.	22 g × 1 inch 0.7 × 25 mm 4–5 ml per plantar nerve, 3 ml per plantar metatarsal nerve, 3 ml per dorsal metatarsal nerve.	15 minutes
High six-point (plantar, plantar metatarsal and dorsal metatarsal nerves)	At the most proximal aspect of the metatarsus that a palpable groove between the deep digital flexor tendon and suspensory ligament is palpable. The plantar nerves are injected in this groove. The plantar metatarsal nerves are injected by redirecting the needle to the axial surface of MTII and MTIV. Dorsal metatarsal nerves are injected immediately lateral and medial to the long digital extensor tendon.	All structures distal to the point of injection. Inadvertent injection within the tarsometatarsal joint may occur.[20]	22 g × 1 inch 0.7 × 25 mm 4–5 ml per plantar nerve, 3 ml per plantar metatarsal nerve, 3 ml per dorsal metatarsal nerve.	15 minutes
Suspensory ligament origin	The needle is inserted directly into the origin of the suspensory ligament. A large needle is used to reduce the chance of breakage. (High four-point, base of accessory carpal and suspensory origin blocks may be interchanged depending on operator preference).	The entire suspensory ligament and structures distal to the injection point. Inadvertent injection within the tarsometatarsal joint may occur.[20]	18 g × 1 – 1.5 inch 1.2 × 25-40 mm 4 – 6 ml	First check in 10 minutes, then again after 20 minutes.
Deep branch of lateral plantar nerve	The needle is inserted through the heavy fascia axial and 15 mm distal to the head of the fourth metatarsal bone and abaxial to the flexor tendons. It is directed toward the suspensory origin 1½ to 1 inch (13-25 mm). The limb is picked up with the stifle and distal limb flexed to relax the tension of the flexor tendons over the injection site.[21]	The entire suspensory ligament and lateral structures distal to the point of injection.	20 g × 1 inch 0.9 × 25 mm 4 ml	First check in 10 minutes, then again after 20 minutes.
Tibial/peroneal	The tibial nerve is injected subcutaneously on the medial aspect of the limb approximately 6 to 8 cm proximal to the tuber calcis and immediately deep to the calcaneal tendon. The peroneal nerves are injected on the lateral aspect of the tibia with the needle inserted between the muscle bellies of the lateral and long digital extensor muscles. Injections are made 25 mm deep to the skin (deep peroneal n.) and subcutaneously (superficial peroneal n.).	The entire limb distal to points of injection including the tarsus, suspensory origin.	20 g × 1.5 inch 0.9 × 40 mm 6-8 ml at tibial nerve, 4 ml at each peroneal nerve.	20 – 30 minutes.

Lateral approaches

Two dorsolateral approaches have been described with the needle inserted either cranial[28] or proximal[24] to the collateral cartilage. The most cranial extent of the collateral cartilages is palpated and the needle is inserted at that point approximately 1–2 cm proximal to the coronary band with the horse fully weight bearing. The needle is first inserted parallel to the bearing surface of the hoof, then immediately angled 30° distally and 30° toward the midline.

Needle placement proximal to the collateral cartilage may be performed with the horse non-weight bearing. The needle is inserted just proximal to the collateral cartilage midway between the dorsal and palmar aspect of the second phalanx and is directed along the palmar surface of the second phalanx by aiming at the center of the frog.[24]

Proximal interphalangeal joint

A dorsolateral or palmar approach may used to enter the proximal interphalangeal (PIP) joint. The dorsal approach is made with the horse weight bearing. A large palmar pouch of the PIP joint is readily entered with the limb non-weight bearing and with the distal joints flexed.[29]

Dorsal approach

The horse should be weight bearing for this approach. A 20-ga, 1½ inch (0.9 × 40 mm) needle is directed through the skin approximately 1–1½ cm distal to the distal eminence of the first phalanx and under the extensor tendon. Orient the needle parallel with the dorsal joint surface. Inject 4–5 mL of local anesthetic.[16]

Palmar approach

The limb should be picked up and held with the distal joints in moderate flexion. The palmar pouch of the PIP joint is bounded by the palmar first phalanx, the palmarodistal eminence of the first phalanx and the insertion of the lateral branch of the superficial digital flexor tendon. When the pastern is moderately flexed these structures form a 'V' on the palmar first phalanx. Retract the palmar digital neurovascular bundle that lies directly over the needle insertion site in a palmar direction using the operator's thumb. The needle is placed through the skin dorsal to the neurovascular bundle within the region of the distal 25% of the first phalanx and directed distally and toward midline. Joint fluid is commonly aspirated.[29]

Metacarpophalangeal/Metatarsophalangeal joint

The fetlock joint is commonly injected for diagnostic and therapeutic reasons. Three approaches may be used: dorsal, palmar/plantar pouch and palmar/plantar approach through the collateral sesamoidean ligament. The collateral sesamoidean ligament approach is best used if arthrocentesis is an objective because synovial fluid free of blood contamination is more readily obtained.[30] Administration of local anesthesia is most easily performed using the palmar/plantar pouch approach.

Palmar/plantar pouch

The approach is made with the horse weight bearing. The palmar/plantar pouch is bounded by the third metacarpus/metatarsus dorsally, distally by the apex of the sesamoid bone, and palmar/plantar by the suspensory ligament. A 20-ga, 1½ inch (0.9 × 40 mm) needle is inserted through the skin in the center of this site and directed distally and toward midline. Synovial fluid commonly will drip from the needle if effusion is present, but aspiration with a syringe often results in plugging of the needle with synovial tissue. Four to 6 mL of local anesthetic is injected.[16]

Dorsal approach

This approach should only be used if effusion is present because of the possibility of abrading joint cartilage with the needle. The horse should be weight bearing. The needle is placed from the lateral side into the proximal aspect of the dorsal joint capsule and directed toward midline and under the extensor tendon. Care should be taken to not abrade the sagittal ridge.[16]

Collateral ligament approach

The limb should be held up with the fetlock joint flexed. This procedure is facilitated by having an assistant hold the limb. The lateral palmar aspect of the distal metacarpal/metatarsal condyle and the dorsal surface of the proximal sesamoid bone are palpated. The collateral sesamoidean ligament may be rarely palpated. The neurovascular bundle over the abaxial surface of the sesamoid bone does not interfere with this approach because it is displaced palmar when the joint is flexed. The needle is inserted in the palpable space between the third metacarpus/metatarsus and the proximal sesamoid bone. Entry into the joint is easily determined because the needle may be inserted up to its hub.[30]

Carpal joints

The radiocarpal joint is always separate from the middle carpal and carpometacarpal joints, which always communicate.[31] Complete intra-articular anesthesia of the carpus requires injecting local anesthetic into the radiocarpal and middle carpal joints. The joints are traditionally injected with the limb flexed, but may also be injected with the horse weight bearing on the limb.

Dorsal approach

The limb is flexed and the joint spaces of the middle and radial carpal joints are easily palpated medial or lateral to the extensor carpi radialis tendon.[16] A 20 ga, 1–1½ inch (0.9 × 25–40 mm) needle is most often inserted medial to the extensor carpi radialis tendon. If the needle is inserted lateral to the extensor carpi radialis tendon, care must be taken to avoid the common digital extensor tendon and its sheath. The most common difficulty encountered when inserting the needle is penetrating into articular cartilage. To avoid this, visualize the plane of the carpal articular surfaces distal to the intended needle insertion site. Direct the needle parallel to the joint surfaces on insertion. Inject 10 mL of local anesthetic per joint.

Caudolateral approach

The carpal joints may also be injected with the horse weight bearing on the limb. By inducing slight carpal flexion, the joint spaces may be identified by palpation of the lateral aspect of the carpus. The radiocarpal joint is approached immediately cranial to the accessory carpal bone at roughly 50% of its proximal-distal length. The middle carpal joint is approached immediately cranial to the distal aspect of the accessory carpal bone.[32]

Cubital (elbow) joint

The cubital joint is injected on the lateral aspect of the limb just cranial to the lateral collateral ligament.[33] The joint space may be palpated in most horses by identifying the humeral condyle and tracing its margin. The procedure may be done with the horse standing or by having an assistant elevate the forelimb slightly to open the joint space dorsally.[33] An 18– 20 ga, 1½ inch (0.9–1.2 × 40 mm) needle is inserted perpendicular to the limb and 15–20 mL of local anesthetic is injected. An alternate approach may be used by inserting the needle on the cranial aspect of the olecranon at a point approximately 3 cm distal to its most proximal extent. The needle is directed distally and axially.[3]

Scapulohumeral (shoulder) joint

Craniolateral approach

This is the most common approach used to inject the scapulohumeral joint. Identify the cranial and caudal parts of the greater tubercle on the craniolateral aspect (point) of the shoulder. An intradermal bleb of anesthetic will facilitate insertion of the spinal needle. An 18-ga, 3½ inch (1.2 × 90 mm) spinal needle with a stylet is inserted in the notch between the cranial and caudal parts of the greater tubercle and directed slightly distally and toward the opposite tarsus (roughly a 30–40° angle to the long axis of the horse). The needle is inserted 2–3 inches (50–75 mm) to reach the joint. Synovial fluid is rarely aspirated to confirm the needle is within the joint. Injection of 10–20 mL of anesthetic with minimal resistance initially, followed by increased resistance as the joint fills, confirms that the needle is correctly positioned.[33] Excessive diffusion of local anesthetic into the surrounding tissues may cause temporary anesthesia of the suprascapular nerve. While this nerve is desensitized, the horse will lack use of the infraspinatus and supraspinatus muscles, which results in abaxial displacement of the shoulder during weight bearing. This may be avoided by injecting the minimum volume of anesthetic necessary to affect joint desensitization and by minimizing multiple needle punctures of the joint capsule.[3,33]

Lateral approach

A skin bleb of anesthetic may be placed immediately caudal to the infraspinatus tendon at the level of the proximal humerus. The needle is inserted immediately caudal to the infraspinatus tendon, roughly perpendicular to the long axis of the horse and directed slightly distally. The needle is inserted 1½ to 2 inches (40–50 mm) to enter the joint. Synovial fluid is more commonly obtained with this approach.[3]

Bicipital bursa

The bicipital bursa lies between the bicipital tendon and the dorsoproximal aspect of the humerus. The bursa is injected using an 18-ga, 1½ inch (1.2 × 40 mm) needle entering perpendicular to the skin at a point proximal to the deltoid tuberosity and distal to the proximal humeral tuberosity.[33] Ten to 15 mL of local anesthetic is injected.

Tarsal joints

It is commonly accepted that the tarsocrural (tibiotarsal) and proximal intertarsal (PIT) joints always communicate. Communication between the distal intertarsal (DIT) and tarsometatarsal (TMT) joints is reported to occur 8 to 38% of the time.[20,34,33] For accurate diagnosis or complete treatment of the distal tarsal joints separate injections must be made in the DIT and TMT joints.

Use of 22-ga (0.7 mm) needles with metal hubs facilitates injections of the distal tarsal joints, particularly when medications are being administered. The small needle size makes placement within the joint easier and the syringe is more securely seated in a metal than a plastic hub needle. The more secure syringe attachment decreases the inadvertent leakage of costly medications.

Tarsocrural (tibiotarsal) and proximal intertarsal joints

These joints communicate and are approached on the dorsomedial aspect of the proximal tarsus. An 18-20-ga, 1½ inch (0.9–1.2 × 40 mm) needle is inserted either lateral or medial to the medial saphenous vein at a point 1–3 cm distal to the medial malleolus.[16] Eight to 10 mL of local anesthetic is injected. If joint effusion is present, the needle may be inserted in the plantarolateral pouch of the tarsocrural joint.

Tarsometatarsal joint

The TMT joint may be injected from a plantarolateral or medial approach. The plantarolateral approach is the easiest method because the landmarks are readily palpated and the needle can usually be inserted securely into the joint. The site for plantarolateral injection is directly proximal to the head of the lateral splint bone (metatarsal IV). The plantar edge of the splint and the indentation at its head is identified. A 22–20-ga, 1 inch (0.7–0.9 × 25 mm) needle is directed toward the opposite fore limb and distally at approximately 10–15 degrees.[34] When correctly placed, the needle is inserted nearly to its hub and 3–4 mL of local anesthetic is injected.

No landmarks are palpable when injecting the TMT from the medial approach. The needle is inserted perpendicular to the medial surface of the tarsus approximately 1 cm distal to the DIT joint (see below). A 22-ga (0.7 mm) needle should be used and the joint is found by probing with the needle until it enters the joint.

Distal intertarsal joint

The DIT joint is injected by placing a 22-ga, 1 inch (0.7 × 25 mm) needle in a small space between the fused first and second tarsal bones, and the third and central tarsal bones. The space is immediately distal to the cunean tendon on the medial aspect of the tarsus. Firm digital pressure is necessary to identify the space. The needle is inserted perpendicular to the medial tarsal surface and some probing is often necessary to fall into the joint space.[35] If the needle doesn't enter the joint easily, inject 1–2 ml of local anesthetic subcutaneously. This will make repeated needle insertions more comfortable for the horse. Probing for the joint space often causes a burr to form on the needle tip, necessitating changing of the needle. Formation of a burr will be obvious because of the increased friction and rough feel of the needle during continued probing. Inject 3–4 mL of local anesthetic.

Stifle joints

The stifle includes three large volume joints: the femoropatellar, lateral femorotibial and medial femorotibial. The femoropatellar and medial femorotibial joints communicate in 60–80% of horses.[36,37] The lateral and medial femorotibial joints do not communicate under normal circumstances.[36] Each joint should be separately injected to assure complete analgesia of the stifle.[37]

Femoropatellar joint

Insert an 18-ga, 3½ inch (1.2 × 90 mm) spinal needle at the cranial aspect of the stifle between the middle and medial or middle and lateral patellar ligaments at a point approximately 2 cm proximal to the tibial crest with the limb fully weight bearing. Direct the needle slightly proximad to a depth of approximately 2-3 inches (50–75 mm). Synovial fluid is rarely aspirated using this approach, but entry into the joint is assumed when there is minimal resistance during injection of 30–50 mL of local anesthetic.

An alternative approach may be used to enter the lateral proximal pouch of the femoropatellar joint. With the limb fully weight bearing an 18-ga, 1½ inch (1.2 × 40 mm) needle is placed immediately caudal to the proximal aspect of the lateral trochlear ridge and the lateral patellar ligament. The needle is directed lateral to medial and somewhat distad. The insertion point is approximately 5 cm proximal to the lateral tibial condyle. This approach avoids abrasion of articular cartilage with the needle and facilitates aspiration of synovial fluid.[38]

Lateral and medial femorotibial joints

For needle placement in the lateral femorotibial joint have the limb fully weight bearing and identify the space between the proximal tibia and the distal trochlear ridge of the femur between the lateral patellar ligament and the lateral collateral ligament. The space is a small triangle of soft tissue that you may indent on digital palpation. An 18–20 ga, 1½ inch (0.9–1.2 × 40 mm) needle is inserted perpendicular to the skin and may be placed nearly to its hub.[32] Inject 15–20 mL of local anesthetic. The approach is similar for the medial femorotibial joint with the needle being placed between the medial patellar and medial collateral ligaments.

Coxofemoral joint

Accurately injecting local anesthetic into the coxofemoral joint is not easily accomplished. The landmarks may be difficult to palpate in heavily muscled horses and the joint is very distant to the insertion point of the needle. Ultrasound guided insertion of the needle provides assurance of correct placement.

The horse should be standing squarely in stocks and a bleb of local anesthetic in the skin should be placed at the needle insertion point. The paired eminences of the major trochanter of the femur lie on a line approximately two-thirds of the distance from the tuber coxae to the tuber ischium. The proximal aspect of the cranial part of the greater trochanter lies approximately 5 cm distal to the proximal extent of the caudal part. A 16-ga, 5–8 inch (1.5 mm × 15–20 cm) needle is inserted immediately proximal to the cranial part of the greater trochanter. The needle is directed in nearly a horizontal plane, slightly cranial and distal, toward the coxofemoral joint. The joint capsule is thick and may require vigorous pressure on the needle to penetrate. A volume of 20–40 mL of local anesthetic is injected.[33]

Digital flexor tendon sheath

The digital flexor tendon sheath (DFTS) may be injected through three approaches. Approaches for the forelimbs and hindlimbs are identical.

Entry at the proximal extent of the DFTS is readily made when there is effusion present. The proximal aspect of the sheath is palpated on the flexor tendons proximal to the fetlock joint. An 18– 20 ga, 1½ inch (0.9–1.2 × 40 mm) needle is inserted through the skin abaxial and parallel to the superficial and deep digital flexor tendons. Eight to 10 milliliters of local anesthetic is injected.

Axial sesamoid approach

The needle is inserted through the skin at the apex of the proximal sesamoid bone and directed distally between the bone's axial surface and the flexor tendons. The needle may also be placed in the skin at the middle of the proximal sesamoid bone between the bone's axial surface and the flexor tendons and directed toward the intersesamoidean region.[39] These approaches are facilitated by lifting the distal limb and flexing the fetlock joint. This will relax tension in the flexor tendons and allow more space for the needle.

Palmar/plantar aspect of pastern

If effusion is present within the DFTS at pastern level, the needle may be inserted perpendicular through the skin. Penetration is very shallow to avoid penetrating the flexor tendons.

Infusion of local anesthetic within the DFTS does not block pain originating from the sole, navicular bursa or distal interphalangeal joint.[40]

Imaging

When the lameness has been localized with manipulations and/or diagnostic local anesthesia, the region should have appropriate images obtained to allow a diagnosis of the lameness. Most often this would involve radiography or ultrasonography. Occasionally this may require nuclear scintigraphy, computed tomography, magnetic resonance imaging or thermography.

References

1. Denoix J-M. Diagnostic techniques for identification and documentation of tendon and ligament injuries. Vet Clin North Am Equine Pract 1994;10(2): 365–407.
2. Guide for veterinary service and judging of equestrian events. 4th ed. Lexington, KY: American Association Equine Practitioners; 1991. p. 19.
3. Stashak TS. Adams' Lameness in Horses. 5th ed. Philadelphia: Lippincott Williams Wilkins; 2002. p. 113–83, 664–680.
4. Back W, Schamhardt HC, Hartman W, et al. Kinematic differences between the distal portions of the forelimbs and hindlimbs of horses at the trot. Am J Vet Res 1995;56(11):1522–8.
5. Kramer J, Keegan KG, Wilson DA, et al. Kinematics of the hind limb in trotting horses after induced lameness of the distal intertarsal and tarsometatarsal joints and intra-articular administration of anesthetic. Am J Vet Res 2000;61(9): 1031–6.
6. Buchner HH, Savelberg HH, Schamhardt HC, et al. Limb movement adaptations in horses with experimentally induced fore-or hindlimb lameness. Equine Vet J 1996;28(1):63–70.
7. Buchner HH, Savelberg HH, Schamhardt HC, et al. Head and trunk movement adaptations in horses with experimentally induced fore- or hindlimb lameness. Equine Vet J 1996;28(1):71–6.
8. Keg PR, van Weeren PR, Back W, et al. Influence of the force applied and its period of application on the outcome of the flexion test of the distal forelimb of the horse. Vet Rec 1997;141(18): 463–6.
9. Busschers E, van Weeren PR. Use of the flexion test of the distal forelimb in the sound horse: repeatability and effect of age, gender, weight, height and fetlock range of motion. J Vet Med A Physiol Pathol Clin Med 2001;48(7):413–27.
10. Keg PR, van Weeren PR, Schamhardt HC, et al. Variations in the force applied to flexion tests of the distal limb of horses. Vet Rec 1997;141(17):435–8.
11. Specht TE, Nixon AJ, Moyer DJ. Equine synovia after an intra-articular injection of lidocaine or mepivacaine. Vet Surg 1988;17:42.
12. Moore DC, Bridenbaugh DL, Bridenbaugh PO, et al. Bupivacaine for peripheral nerve block: a comparison with mepivacaine, lidocaine and tetracaine. Anesthesiology 1970;32:462–3.
13. Mama KR, Steffey EP. Local anesthetics. In: Adams HR, editor. Veterinary Pharmacology and Therapeutics. 8th ed. Ames: Iowa State University Press; 2001. p. 343–59.

14. Riebold TW, Geiser DR, Goble DO. Large Animal Anesthesia: Principles and Techniques. 2nd ed. Ames: Iowa State University Press; 1995. p. 205–9.
15. Hague BA, Honnas CM, Simpson RB, et al. Evaluation of skin bacterial flora before and after aseptic preparation of clipped and nonclipped arthrocentesis sites in horses. Vet Surg 1997;26: 121–5.
16. Schmotzer WB, Timm KI. Local anesthetic techniques for diagnosis of lameness. Vet Clin North Am Equine Pract 1990;6(3):705–28.
17. Schumacher J, Steiger R, Schumacher J, et al. Effects of analgesia of the distal interphalangeal joint or palmar digital nerves on lameness caused by solar pain in horses. Vet Surg 2000;29:54–8.
18. Ford TS, Ross MW, Orsini PG. A comparison of methods for proximal palmar metacarpal analgesia in horses. Vet Surg 1989;18:146–50.
19. Wheat JD, Jones K. Selected techniques of regional anesthesia. Vet Clin North Am Large Animal Pract 1981;3:223–46.
20. Dyson SJ, Romero JM. An investigation of injection techniques for local analgesia of the equine distal tarsus and proximal metatarsus. Equine Vet J 1993;25(1):30–5.
21. Hughes TK, Eliashar E, Smith RK. In vitro evaluation of a single injection technique for diagnostic analgesia of the proximal suspensory ligament of the equine pelvic limb. Equine Vet J 2007;36(8):760–4.
22. Schramme MC, Boswell JC, Hamhougias K, et al. An in vitro study to compare 5 different techniques for injection of the navicular bursa in the horse. Equine Vet J 2000;32(3):263–7.
23. Dyson SJ, Kidd L. A comparison of responses to analgesia of the navicular bursa and intra-articular analgesia of the distal interphalangeal joint in 59 horses. Equine Vet J 1993;25(2):93–8.
24. Vazquez de Mercado R, Stover SM, Taylor KT, et al. Lateral approach for arthroentesis of the distal interphalangeal joint in horses. J Am Vet Med Assoc 1998;212(9):1413–8.
25. Bowker RM, Linder K, Van Wulfen KK, et al. Anatomy of the distal interphalangeal joint of the mature horse: relationships with navicular suspensory ligaments, sensory nerves and neurovascular bundle. Equine Vet J 1997;29:126–35.
26. Keegan KG, Wilson DA, Kreeger JM, et al. Local distribution of mepivacaine after distal interphalangeal joint injection in horses. Am J Vet Res 1996;57:422–6.
27. Gandini M. Comparison of three dorsal techniques for arthrocentesis of the distal interphalangeal joint in horses. J Am Vet Med Assoc 2007;231:254–8.
28. Moyer W, Carter GK. Techniques to facilitate intra-articular injection in equine joints. Proceedings Am Assoc Equine Practnr 1996;42:48–54.
29. Miller SM, Stover SM, Taylor KT, et al. Palmaroproximal approach for arthrocentesis of the proximal interphalangeal joint in horses. Equine Vet J 1996;28(5):376–80.
30. Misheff MM, Stover SM. A comparison of two techniques for arthrocentesis of the equine metacarpophalangeal joint. Equine Vet J 1991;23(4):273–6.
31. Ford TS, Ross MW, Orsini PG. Communication and boundaries of the middle carpal and carpometacarpal joints in horses. Am J Vet Res 1988;49:2161–4.
32. Kiely RG, McMullen W. Lateral arthrocentesis of the equine carpus. Equine Practice 1987;9:22.
33. Lewis RD. Techniques for arthrocentesis of equine shoulder, elbow, stifle and hip joints. Proceedings Am Assoc Equine Practnr 1996;42:55–63.
34. Sack WO, Orsini PG. Distal intertarsal and tarsometatarsal joints in the horse: communication and injection sites. J Am Vet Med Assoc 1981;179(4): 355–9.
35. Kraus-Hansen AE, Jann HW, Kerr DV, et al. Arthrographic analysis of communication between the tarsometatarsal and distal intertarsal joints of the horse. Vet Surg 1992;21(2):139–44.
36. Vacek JR, Ford TS, Honnas CM. Communication between the femoropatellar and medial and lateral femorotibial joints in horses. Am J Vet Res 1992;53(8):1431–4.
37. Reeves MJ, Trotter GW, Kainer RA. Anatomical and functional communications between the synovial sacs of the equine stifle joint. Eq Vet J 1991;23(3):215–18.
38. Hendrickson DA, Nixon AJ. Comparison of the cranial and a new lateral approach to the femoropatellar joint for aspiration and injection in horses. J Am Vet Med Assoc 1994;205(8): 1177–9.
39. Hassel, DM, Stover, SM, Yarbrough, TM, et al. Palmar-plantar axial sesamoidean approach to the digital flexor tendon sheath in horses. J Am Vet Med Ass 2000;217:1343–7.
40. Harper J, Schumacher J, Degraves F, et al. Effects of analgesia of the digital flexor tendon sheath on pain originating from the sole, distal interphalangeal joint or navicular bursa of horses. Equine Vet J 2007;39(6): 535–9.

Diseases of the foot

14

Andris J. Kaneps

CHAPTER CONTENTS

Introduction

A thorough examination and assessment of the equine foot forms an essential part of both the physical and lameness evaluation. Because foot problems are the most common cause of lameness in horses, the examiner must have an accurate knowledge of foot anatomy and must be willing to take a 'hands-on' approach to fully identify any problems the horse might be experiencing.

There are numerous causes of pain in the foot of the horse. These can be divided arbitrarily into:

1. conditions of the hoof wall and horn-producing tissues
2. conditions of the distal phalanx and
3. conditions of the heel region.

Anatomy

- The hoof capsule is comprised of tubular and intertubular keratin arranged as a laminated composite material.
- Ninety per cent of the energy imparted by foot strike is dissipated by the hoof capsule and its associated structures.
- The anatomy of the support structures within the hoof must be understood to appreciate the various sites that could cause distal limb lameness.

The hoof capsule not only provides strength but also supports the horse's skeletal column. In the horse, the tubular hoof of the wall is composed of hard keratin and is rich in disulphide bonds, so has great physical strength. The frog and the white zone are rich in sulfhydryl groups, but poor in disulphide bonds, and therefore have lower physical strength but greater elasticity. The strength, hardness, and insolubility of keratin are due to disulphide bonds between and within the molecules.

Two types of horn are produced from the coronary band. Tubular horn arises from cells surrounding papillae (finger-like projections from the coronary band) and become organized into thin, elongated, cylinders or tubules. In cross-section, the keratinocytes of individual hoof wall tubules are arranged around a central hollow medulla in nonpigmented concentric layers. The keratinocytes generated between the papillae mature into intertubular hoof, thus forming a keratin matrix in which tubules are embedded. The intertubular horn is formed at right angles to the tubular horn and bestows on the hoof wall the unique property of a mechanically stable, multidirectional, fiber-reinforced composite.

The corium is the region of the foot that nourishes the hoof-wall cells. There are several distinct zones, the coronary corium, lamellar corium, solar corium, and frog corium. The coronary corium fills the coronary groove and blends distally with the lamellar corium. Its inner surface is attached to the extensor tendon and the cartilages of the coffin bone by the subcutaneous tissue of the coronary cushion. Collectively the coronary corium and the germinal epidermal cells that produce the hoof wall are known as the coronary band. A feature of the coronary corium is the large numbers of hair-like papillae projecting from its surface.[1]

The innermost layer of the hoof wall and bars is named the stratum lamellatum after the 550–600 primary epidermal lamellae that project from its surface in parallel rows. Examination of the hoof capsule, with its contents removed, shows that the lamellae of the dorsal hoof wall are shaped like long, thin, rectangles approximately 7 mm wide and 50 mm long. One edge of the rectangle is incorporated into the tough, heavily keratinized hoof wall proper and the opposite end faces the outer surface of the coffin bone. The proximal end is curved and forms the curved shoulder of the coronary groove. The distal end merges with the sole and becomes part of the white zone visible at the ground surface of the hoof (white line).

The lamellae of the inner hoof wall are avascular and depend on capillaries in the microcirculation of the adjacent corium for nutrition. The lamellar corium covers the coffin bone. The primary function of the lamellar hoof is to suspend the coffin bone within the hoof capsule. The tips of the lamellae (both primary and secondary) all are oriented towards the distal phalanx, thus indicating the lines of tension to which the lamellar suspensory apparatus is subjected. The surface area of the equine inner hoof wall has been calculated to average 13.75 square feet (1.28 square meters). This large surface area for suspension of the coffin bone and the great compliance of the interdigitating lamellar architecture helps reduce stress and ensures even energy transfer during peak loading of the equine foot.

The supporting structures within the hoof include the collateral cartilages, digital cushion, digital extensor tendon, collateral ligaments of the distal interphalangeal joint, deep digital flexor tendon, collateral sesamoidean ligament, distal sesamoidean impar ligament.[2]

The collateral cartilages have considerable variation in anatomic details from horse to horse. They vary in thickness and degree of mineralization, but the heel portion is usually thinner than the more dorsal and distal portions. The cartilages are stabilized by ligaments that attach to the middle and distal phalanges, the navicular bone and to the collateral sesamoidean ligaments. A venous plexus lies on the abaxial surface of the cartilage.[2]

The digital cushion is an elastic tissue composed of collagen, elastin and adipose tissue. It lies between the frog and the deep digital flexor tendon at the heel of the foot and is responsible for shock absorption.[2]

The navicular bone is stabilized by:

1. the paired collateral sesamoidean ligaments which originate on the distal, abaxial and dorsal aspects of the first phalanx and insert on the abaxial surfaces of the second phalanx and the proximal border of the navicular bone
2. the distal sesamoidean impar ligament which originates on the distal border of the navicular bone and inserts on the flexor surface of the distal phalanx and
3. the distal extension of the deep digital flexor tendon that courses over the flexor surface of the navicular bone and inserts on the flexor surface of the distal phalanx. The distal border of the navicular bone also has synovial invaginations that contain blood vessels.[2]

The invaginations may be referred to as synovial channels or vascular channels and may become enlarged and irregular when navicular bone degenerative changes have occurred.

The distal interphalangeal joint shares an articulation with the dorsal surface of the navicular bone and is stabilized by collateral ligaments that originate on the distal abaxial surface of the middle phalanx and insert in the abaxial surface of the distal phalanx.[2] This joint has a dorsal and palmar pouch. The dorsal pouch extends proximally to the mid-portion of the middle phalanx. The palmar pouch is extensive and is closely associated with the palmar nerves, making desensitization of palmar structures of the foot with anatomic specificity problematic. [2, 3] The navicular bursa lies between the deep digital flexor tendon and the flexor surface of the navicular bone and has close association with the distal interphalangeal joint.

Examination of the distal limb

Size, shape, toe length, heel length, hoof pastern axis, and position of each foot relative to each limb and to each other are assessed with the horse standing quietly.[4–6] Hoof alignment is viewed from the dorsal and lateral aspect.[2] Most horses will have a hoof angle between 50 and 55°. Ideally, when the horse is standing square; the cannon bone, pastern, and hoof should have straight axial alignment as observed from the front. From the side, the hoof/pastern axis should be straight. The angle created by the dorsal hoof wall should be the same as the pastern angle and the heel angle should be within 5° of the toe angle.[7] Horses that have a low hoof angle compared to the pastern have a broken-back hoof/pastern axis (Fig. 14.1). This hoof conformation is also called 'long toe and low heel'. The opposite case is a steep hoof angle and sloping pastern which will have a broken-forward hoof/pastern axis. This hoof conformation may also be called 'club foot'.

Generally, the front hoof should be round or circular in shape, whereas the rear hoof is more triangular or pear-shaped. Front and rear hooves should be shaped like inverted cones. Both hooves should be evaluated for differences in length and width. Hooves of equal width and length tend to look circular but as hoof capsule length increases the width of the hoof wall in the quarters becomes

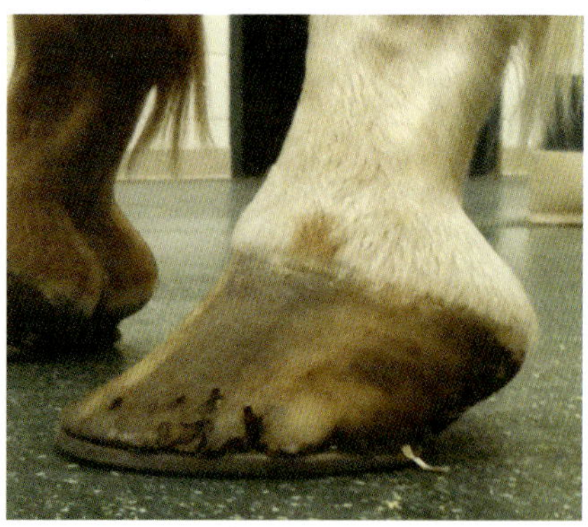

Fig 14.1 Long toe with underrun heels. Note how the bearing surface of the hoof and the caudal extent of the shoe is well cranial of the optimal position. Less heel stress would occur in this foot if the hoof was trimmed to bring the bars caudally and the shoe was set with its caudal aspect in line with the bulbs of the heel.

more upright and the stresses on the hoof will naturally be different. A normally balanced hoof should have a flat ground-bearing surface and the bearing surface should be perpendicular to the upper limb. The heels should be evaluated to determine if they provide sufficient support to the hoof and limb.

Observing the foot while the horse is walking will help determine the manner in which the horse lands and breaks over, as well as the path of the foot during the flight phase of the stride. Toe-first landing or excessively heel-first landing indicates either compensation for pain or dorsopalmar hoof imbalance. Similarly, medial or excessively lateral heel-quarter-first landing suggest either compensation for limb conformation or pain leading to mediolateral hoof imbalance. The flight of the foot during the stride is correlated with rotational deviation of the limb and imbalance of the foot. The horse that wings-in or 'dishes' is either toed-out or breaking over the inside toe. Conversely, the horse that paddles or wings-out is either toed-in or breaking over the outside toe.

Once the above observations have been made, the examiner needs to make a closer evaluation of the hoof. This evaluation needs to be performed first with the horse in weight-bearing position and then with the foot in non-weight-bearing position.

The pastern is palpated to determine if there is heat, pain, or swelling. More subtly, the examiner needs to palpate the bones and tendinous structures. The digital neurovascular bundle is palpated to evaluate the digital pulse and to determine if a neurectomy may have been perfomed. It is normal to feel a digital pulse but not a bounding pulse, which is abnormal and an indicator of foot inflammation. The strength of the pulse can be compared to other limbs if one is in doubt. A symmetrical abnormal pulse indicates generalized inflammation, whereas an asymmetric pulse indicates the inflammatory process on the side of the stronger pulse.

Palpation is continued to the coronary band. Abnormalities such as swelling, discharge, focal pain or heat, or absence of tissue (loss of sponginess or a 'trough') should be examined more closely. The examiner should feel that the hairline forms a smooth edge with the hoof capsule.

From the coronet, the examiner moves to the collateral cartilages where they are palpated and manipulated. The palmar and proximal edges should be easily defined. The thickness, density, and pliability of the cartilages need to be assessed. Palpation of this area will not only determine if there is any pain, but also can give an impression of the flexibility of the hoof. For instance, a very stiff inflexible collateral cartilage is associated with a narrow, upright hoof. On the other hand, flimsy cartilages are commonly seen in the hoof with collapsed heels and a narrow, convex frog.

The entire hoof wall must be examined for the presence of cracks, fissures, bulges, growth abnormalities, focal heat, wall loss, or breakage. A high percentage of quarter and heel cracks begin as small, very fine fissures at the coronet. They might extend less than 1 cm distally and are easily missed if this area is not examined carefully. These small fissures are a definite cause of foot pain and usually associated with deeper injury to the coronet and/or lamina below.

From this point it is natural to begin manipulating the foot in the non-weight-bearing position.[4] Begin by cleaning the bottom of the hoof and lightly paring away any debris that obscures visualization of the frog, sulci of the frog, sole, and white line if the horse is unshod. The frog should be examined for size, shape, and consistency, and to determine whether it is securely attached to the underlying tissue and its sulci (collateral and central). The frog should be resilient and rubbery, rather than hard and flaky, and the caudal two-thirds should be nearly level with the ground surface of the hoof wall. The frog should not be recessed deep into the sulci of the foot and nor should the frog be convex at its apex. The receded frog is often associated with upright narrow feet, whereas the convex frog is associated with weak and underrun heels.

The entire sole of the foot should be carefully examined for condition of the bars, fissures, punctures, consistency, discoloration (bruising), and the degree of concavity. The shape of the sole should be concave. A flat sole might signify either poor hoof conformation (a weak hoof) or distal coffin bone displacement. A convex (dropped) sole indicates a displaced coffin bone. The consistency (relative degree of stiffness) of the sole is determined using digital pressure as well as hoof testers. At this point it is necessary to evaluate the texture of the sole. By grasping the quarters with your fingers, the thumbs can be used to gently press on the sole. A sole that moves under this pressure is thin and there is little space between the coffin bone and the outside environment. On the other hand, if the sole does not move then the examiner knows there is at least some thickness and depth to the sole. True sole depth can be determined via radiography.

The white line (the junction between the sole and inner hoof capsule) is examined to determine its width and character. The white line is usually wider at the toe and gradually thins as it approaches the heels. It is best visualized following either light paring with the hoof knife or light rasping of the superficial portion of the sole margin. Hoof structures superficial to the white line are insensitive, while structures more central are considered sensitive. Widening of this area represents stress and separation of the laminar hoof wall from coronary hoof wall. The deeper the separation, the more severe the injury. This separation can be seen anywhere on the solar surface and indicates a bending force on the wall that is pulling the wall away from the coffin bone. Most frequently this separation is seen at the toe and is referred to as 'seedy toe' because it looks like small seeds could fit between the spaces created by the separation.

Digitally explore the heel bulbs for the presence of swelling, heat, pain, or separation at the coronet. The central sulcus of the frog should be examined and probed to determine its depth. Normally this should be a shallow depression of no more than a centimeter. If the sulcus is deeper it can be due to either very serious thrush or loss of structural support in heel bulbs (the heel bulbs can be distracted in opposite vertical directions).

Lightly support the limb at the metacarpus (metatarsus) and allow the foot to drop naturally. Position your line of vision so as to appreciate foot balance and levelness of the walls (see above). Examine the entire ground surface of the foot to determine the divisions of the hoof (toe, quarters, and heels) and their proportions (Fig. 14.2). Imagine a line drawn through the axial center of

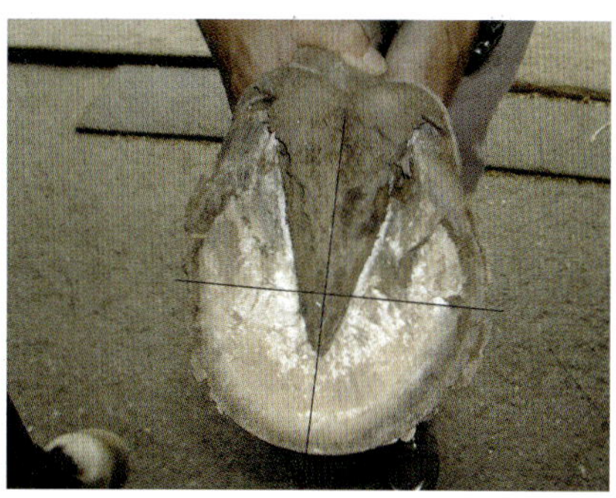

Fig 14.2 Solar surface of a foot prior to trimming. Lines have been drawn across the widest portion of the foot and sagittally. From this perspective the foot is in quite good balance. The dorsal and palmar portions of the foot are nearly equal. The half to the viewers right (lateral) is slightly larger than the half to the left (medial).

the limb, which transects the ground surface of the foot, and then determine the relative proportion of medial and lateral foot to this imaginary line. For example, a given foot may demonstrate a unilateral medial heel contraction in combination with a flared lateral quarter and toe (diagonal imbalance).

If the horse is shod, the exam should include the following additions.[4] Note the shoe type as well as the presence or absence of additions such as toe grabs, block heels, trailers, and so forth. Determine if abnormal shoe wear exists.

Objective assessment of hoof balance

As part of the overall evaluation of the horse an objective assessment of hoof balance is important.

Examination of lateral and dorsopalmar (plantar) radiographic projections of the hoof allows objective evaluation of hoof balance. The lateral radiograph should be evaluated for middle and distal phalanx alignment, which may reveal the presence of a broken-hoof axis (Fig. 14.3). In addition, the alignment between the distal phalanx and the hoof wall should be assessed. If the hoof wall and dorsal surface of the distal phalanx are not parallel the functional hoof angle can be determined by measuring the angle of the dorsal surface of the bone with the ground. The slope of the heels can be seen on the radiograph and evaluation is used to determine whether the heels are underrun.

The dorso-palmar radiographic projection should be assessed for joint alignment, medial and lateral hoof wall lengths, and foot symmetry (Fig. 14.4). Joint alignment is determined by examining the symmetry of the joint space. The hoof wall length can be measured directly from digital images.

Assessment of pain

Examine the horse in motion; watch the foot strike for each foot. Determine if the foot lands flat, heel or toe first, medial or lateral quarter first. The landing position of the individual foot relative to the vertical axis of the respective limb should be noted. Evaluate the path the individual foot takes from foot breakover to striking the ground. Always conduct this evaluation at the walk because this gait is sufficiently slow to permit the determination of fine movement error. Repeat the same process when viewing the horse from the side. The horse is then trotted (or paced) and visualized in the same manner. Circling the horse will often exacerbate foot problems.

Two manipulative tests should be performed: hoof tester examination and distal limb flexion. Two additional manipulations, hoof extension wedge test, and palmar hoof wedge test, may add more information.[8] A positive response to any of these tests is important but a negative response is equivocal and does not rule out any problem. Examine the foot systematically with hoof testers. Percussion utilizing a small hammer can also provide important information regarding pain in the hoof wall or sole.

The distal limb flexion test can exacerbate lameness if any of the three distal joints of the leg are affected by synovitis or osteoarthritis. A positive response could also be expected by any condition that causes induration of the tissues of the foot. This has been shown to be positive in over 95% of horses with foot pain.[8]

The hoof extension test is performed by elevating the toe with a block, holding the opposite limb, and trotting the horse away after 60 seconds. The palmar hoof wedge test is performed by placing the block under the palmar two-thirds of the frog and forcing the horse to stand on that foot. The test can be further modified so that the wedge can be placed under either heel to determine if the pressure there causes exacerbation of the lameness.

These tests allow the examiner to evaluate the horse's response to a particular stress. None has been shown to be pathognomonic for any particular cause of lameness.

Diagnostic analgesia

Regional analgesia will localize the region of pain. See Chapter 13 for details on local and intra-articular diagnostic anesthesia.

Imaging of the foot

After localization of the lameness to the foot imaging will be necessary to determine what pathology is present. Radiographic examination of the hoof requires a minimum of five radiographic views of each foot.[9] The views consist of a dorso-60°-proximal to palmarodistal (D60PrPD) of the navicular bone, a dorso-45°-proximal to palmarodistal (D45PrPD) of the distal phalanx, a lateral to medial projection, a horizontal dorsopalmar projection,

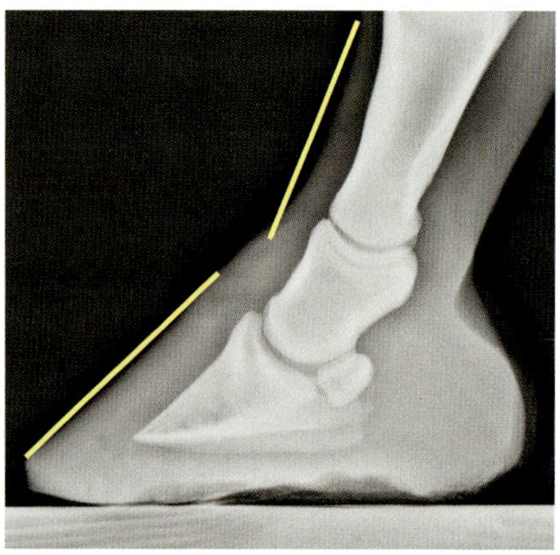

Fig 14.3 Lateral radiographic view of the distal limb with a broken-back hoof-pastern axis. The dorsal hoof angle (distal yellow line) has lower angle of slope than the higher angle of slope pastern (proximal dorsal line).

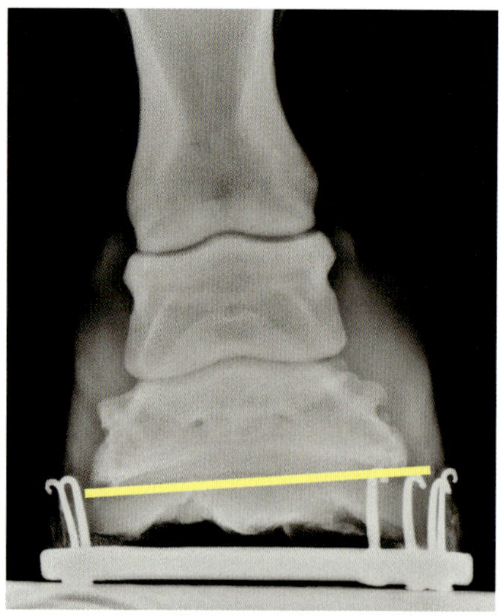

Fig 14.4 Dorsopalmar radiographic view of the distal limb with marked lateral-medial imbalance. The solar surface of the distal phalanx (yellow line) should be parallel to the shoe and ground surface.

and a palmaroproximal to palmarodistal navicular bone projection (navicular skyline). Digital imaging is the current standard for radiography and provides more detail than analog film/screen radiography, allows for manipulation of image window and level, and permits measurement of various aspects of conformation using DICOM image software.

Many structures within the hoof may be evaluated sonographically.[10] The collateral ligaments of the DIP joint can be clearly identified, as can the deep flexor insertion on the third phalanx, the distal deep flexor tendon, the impar ligament, and the navicular bursa (see Chapter 20).

The presence or absence of inflammation within the distal limb can be evaluated through the use of nuclear scintigraphy.[11]

Magnetic resonance imaging (MRI) has increased the understanding of the inter-relationships between soft tissues, bone and cartilage within the foot. To fully determine the cause of foot lameness, MRI must be considered for a horse with lameness that resolves with distal limb diagnostic analgesia and that has few abnormalities evident on a radiographic or sonographic study of the distal limb. MRI allows for high-detail imaging in multiple planes and is a particularly sensitive technique for soft tissue evaluation.[12,13] Imaging with fat suppressed MRI sequences also provides a degree of physiological understanding of the region. For example, fat suppressed MRI imaging may identify increased levels of fluid within bone, referred to as bone contusion or bone edema that cannot be identified with any other imaging technique.[14]

Diseases of the hoof wall

Hoof wall defects

- Lameness associated with hoof wall defects is due to irritation of the sensitive lamellae due to exposure, local infection or shearing of the unstable hoof capsule.
- Treatment should clean and stabilize the defect to permit healing from the coronary band.
- Healing of defects may require 5–10 months.

Recognition

History and presenting complaint

The horse is presented for evaluation of cracks, fissures or morphologic defects in the hoof wall. Lameness may or may not be a presenting complaint.

Physical examination

Defects should always be examined to determine their depth and size. Depth can be usually determined by probing the defect. If pain is elicited by probing the defect, then it involves sensitive tissue. A percussion hammer is useful to determine the size of defects that are not readily visible. Normal percussion of the hoof results in a crisp resonance, whereas hoof wall separated from its deeper structures has a dull resonance.

Defects at or near the coronary band should have the hair clipped from the coronary band. The coronary band then should be examined for injuries, wounds, splits, or other defects that would account for the abnormal hoof growth.

Diagnostic confirmation

Radiographs may be necessary to rule-out involvement of the distal phalanx or sensitive tissues of the foot and may identify gas or fluid in within the hoof.

Treatment and prognosis

Therapeutic aims

The first objective and most important goal of treatment is to eliminate or correct the problem that caused the hoof defect. If the underlying problem is not corrected recurrence should be expected.

Initial treatment is done to either stabilize a defect or prevent its further extension in the hoof capsule. Debridement of the defect is necessary to remove contamination of the hoof capsule and deeper laminae. Long-term support or protection of the affected region must be made, usually with appropriate shoeing and hoof capsule stabilization.

Therapy

Healing of these injuries is based on growth of new horn from the coronary band. These tissues do not heal side to side; therefore healing is slow, and may take 5–10 months. The defect must be stabilized to prevent the crack from expanding. This can be accomplished by application of a bar shoe that relieves pressure on the affected wall. The bar may be a full bar or a diagonal bar. Also, if the crack is near the heel, weight bearing to the heel can be reduced by floating the heel (Fig. 14.5). The affected heel is trimmed short enough to prevent contact with the shoe during weight bearing. The objective is to relieve shear forces across the defect, which may cause movement at the area of the crack. In addition, clips placed on either side of the defect will help prevent hoof expansion and, therefore, will further immobilize the crack. The crack may also be sutured or wired. In some cases a small metal plate can be screwed into the wall over the crack.

If the hoof crack does not extend from the ground to the coronary band, changes in the hoof wall may be made to prevent crack lengthening. Grooving the hoof wall perpendicular to the defect has the effect of deflecting stress away from the crack. Cracks that originate from the weight-bearing surface should be grooved at the most proximal aspect of the crack. Cracks that originate from the coronary band should be grooved at their distal aspect and in the shape of a V. Grooving will only be effective if the crack does not extend into sensitive tissues. Acrylic repair of a crack is a cosmetic and very successful method used to obliterate the crack and provide some level of immobilization. Sealing of a contaminated crack should not be done as it may lead to a local abscess.

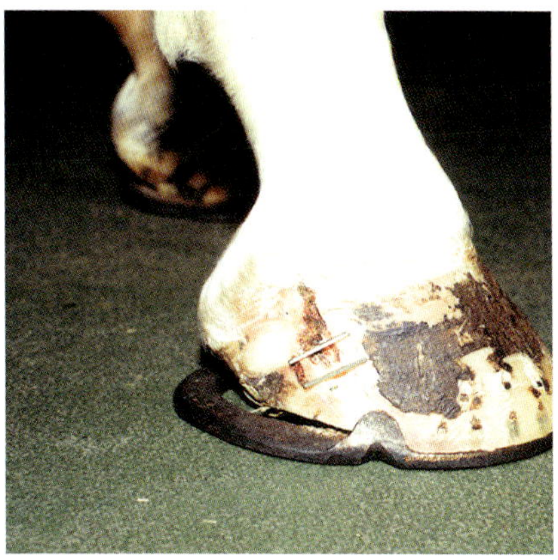

Fig 14.5 Repaired hoof crack with floated heel. The hoof crack has been debrided and stabilized with hoof staples. The foot has been shod with an egg bar shoe. A quarter clip is placed immediately dorsal to the hoof crack and the affected heel has been trimmed short enough to prevent contact with the shoe ('floated heel').

Because of their horizontal orientation hoof clefts do not lengthen as do cracks. However, clefts are much more likely to involve sensitive layers and cause lameness. The horn around the cleft should be removed to the depth of the cleft. Sufficient horn should be removed so there is no undermined horn. In many cases, this may require a partial resection of the hoof wall from the cleft to the weight-bearing surface; a rotary burr (Dremel tool) does an excellent job. After sufficient hoof wall is debrided, the underlying tissue should be inspected carefully.

Treatment of crumbling hoof may require wide debridement of hoof wall. As for a cleft, all undermined hoof wall should be removed. It should be removed until intact hoof wall is present around the edge of the debrided area. Again, the deep tissues must be carefully examined for necrotic tissue or contaminated debris.

Long-term support or protection of the defect is necessary to return the horse to use as soon as possible. This usually requires some type of repair to restore the integrity of the hoof wall. First, the area must be free of hemorrhage or sepsis. Controlling hemorrhage requires packing the bleeding area with gauze and wrapping the foot. Approximately one week is required to dry the hemorrhagic area and allow new horny growth over the area. Application of a 1% tincture of iodine to the horn in and around the defect will usually dry the area without desiccating it. If sepsis has occurred, or a foreign body has penetrated the hoof wall, it is necessary to soak the foot in a saturated solution of magnesium sulfate and povidone-iodine solution to eliminate the infection. It may be necessary to soak or poultice the foot for 7–10 days before the septic area is healed. An alternative to soaking is to pack the affected area with a magnesium sulfate paste or povidone-iodine ointment mixed with magnesium sulfate. This treatment is followed by application of tincture of iodine solution. A helpful hint to determine if infection is still present is to examine the area 24 h after application of iodine. The presence of moisture or exudate in or around the defect is indicative of continued active infection. Soaking should continue until the infection is resolved.

The hoof wall can be repaired after the defect has been adequately debrided and the hemorrhage/sepsis has been controlled. The hoof should be properly trimmed and balanced. In most cases, a bar shoe with clips should be applied. The hoof should be dry. Application of either acetone or alcohol to the outer layers of the horn is an excellent method to remove debris and dry the hoof. To aid retention of the repair material, the hoof wall around the defect may be beveled (undermined) for 6 mm (¼ inch) using a rotary hand burr. Some defects can be reinforced by wire laced across the gap. This not only helps immobilize the area but also adds substrate to which the repair material can bond. If the defect is not sutured, holes should be drilled from the normal hoof into the undermined area to allow penetration of repair material. The holes should be 0.5 to 1 cm apart.

There are numerous agents that are available for repair, including fiberglass, thin metal sheets, and acrylic/epoxy materials. The acrylic/epoxies are the most versatile materials. Modern hoof epoxies have biomechanical properties similar to normal hoof capsule, reducing the complications of hard, inflexible materials such as hoof capsule contraction. The material is mixed and applied to the defect and surrounding hoof wall. When sufficient time has elapsed to allow hardening of the material, excess acrylic is rasped away resulting in a cosmetic repair.

The horse should be re-examined at 4–8 week intervals. The shoe will need to be reset and in many cases the repair repeated until the hoof wall grows out. If the animal is active and competitive, the constant trauma may cause the repair to loosen. If the repair material loosens, it should be removed and the repair repeated.

Prognosis

The prognosis for healing of hoof wall defects is usually good to excellent. Given proper hoof care, adequate time, and proper follow-up care, the defect will heal. Large defects that have resulted from an inflammatory cause may have a tendency to recur because of damage to the laminae and loss of bonding between the hoof wall layers. However, if the hoof is kept shod and protected, further problems can be avoided.

Etiology and pathophysiology

Etiology

There are numerous causes of defects in the hoof. Careful examination of the hoof can often identify the probable cause, which must be eliminated before therapy will be effective. The first consideration is moisture; either excessive dryness or excessive moisture can result in defects. Dryness usually results in a brittle hoof that tends to crack when stressed. If the hoof is unprotected, large portions of hoof wall may break away at the weight-bearing edge. Conversely, excessive moisture can cause the hoof wall to crumble. This is probably due to a combination of a decay process caused by micro-organisms, a disruption of the normal horn tubules by the moisture, and stress on the hoof wall. This problem is usually characterized by hoof-wall crumbling, which starts at the weight-bearing surface. Examination of the wall reveals a hoof wall that is soft in nature at the area of crumbling. The hoof wall can easily be dislodged for several millimeters around the defect. The wall that is affected has little normal architecture and crumbles into a fine powder when pressure is applied.

Other contributing factors to defects include hoof conformation, balance, or improper shoe application. These problems can cause overloading of a portion of hoof wall and result in disruption of the integrity of horn. Defects resulting from speed work or work on uneven surfaces are also due to similar abnormal stresses.

Infection or foreign bodies in the hoof may also result in defects. Clefts and crumbling are the most common results of these factors. Clefts may result from either a separation of horn from the coronary band, as occurs with gravel, or from splitting of the hoof wall as a result of the inflammation associated with infection. Inflammation caused by infection disrupts the normal architecture of the hoof sufficiently to cause the wall to break or crumble under normal stress and usage.

Prevention

Prevention of hoof wall defects is best accomplished by regular farrier attention and early recognition and response to changes in hoof moisture (too dry, too wet). Hooves that are exposed to excessively moist conditions may benefit from application of sealing agents. Hooves that are extremely dry may be moisturized by simply allowing the paddock stock tank to overflow. The resulting muddy area will moisturize the hooves of horses that come to the water to drink. Horses that are in regular work and have a regular bath do not usually suffer from dry, cracked hooves. In fact, excessive hoof moisture remains a considerable problem in these horses.

Lacerations to the hoof and coronary band

- First aid should control hemorrhage and prevent further contamination.
- Damage to the corium may result in hoof wall defects.
- Deep wounds may affect synovial structures.
- Wounds that involve the hoof capsule will heal slowly by second intention.

Lacerations to the hoof causing loss of germinal tissue and either partial or complete avulsions of the hoof wall are not common injuries to the horse. When these injuries do occur, however, their management can be perplexing for the veterinarian.

Recognition

History and presenting complaint

Horses with hoof-wall lacerations are presented for distal limb injury that usually includes considerable hemorrhage and may include varying degrees of lameness. The horse may have been caught in wire or kicked through a solid partition.

Physical examination

Complete examination of the wound is necessary to determine the extent of the injury. Although the foot has as great a capacity for healing as any other tissue, the prognosis for return to full function is dependent on the severity of tissue destruction and the tissues involved. In most cases, adequate collateral circulation develops following injury.

Complete denervation of the foot by extensive damage to the digital nerve trunks may result in neurogenic degeneration and sloughing of the foot. Ironically, transection of the nerve, where damage has not been extensive, may aid recovery by reducing chronic pain associated with the injury.

Injuries that involve the corium of the foot should be inspected carefully. The corium is modified vascular tissue similar to the dermis, and is responsible for nutrition to the horny layers of the hoof. Damage to these structures often results in permanent defects in the coronary band and hoof. Injuries that cause avulsion or necrosis of corium will cause changes in horn production around the hoof. The absolute outcome must await regrowth of the hoof to assess these changes and how they may affect the horse.

Deep wounds that extend to the middle or distal phalanges cause additional complications. Hoof avulsions may involve all or part of the wing of the distal phalanx. In these cases, it is usually easiest to simply remove the fractured portion of the bone. However, wounds that damage the periosteum or collateral ligaments surrounding these bones may cause permanent lameness as a result of excessive calcification of soft tissues or joint instability. Associated soft tissue injuries such as these will not be apparent on initial radiographic examination and can only be anticipated after close examination of the wound. Once soft tissue support is damaged the veterinarian may have to wait 3–4 months to evaluate the final consequences of this type of deep injury.

Wounds that enter a synovial space (joint or tendon sheath) may respond favorably if appropriate therapy is initiated immediately. Small wounds into a joint may not be readily apparent, the only sign being synovial fluid leaking into the wound. Occasionally, serum is mistaken for joint fluid. Wounds of the foot usually heal over an extended period, resulting in increased expense and residual lameness due to the injury; permanent deformity is a distinct possibility.

Special examination

Radiographs of the affected region should be obtained to determine if skeletal injury accompanies the hoof laceration. If any doubt exists as to whether a synovial space has been entered, a needle is aseptically placed within the synovial structures in question, an attempt is made to obtain a fluid sample in EDTA and for bacterial culture, sterile crystalloid solution is injected under pressure and the wound is examined for the leakage of fluid. After obtaining fluid, it is prudent to inject antibacterial medication in the wound such as amikacin (250–500 mg). The fluid should be evaluated for cell count, total protein and a sample for cytology should be prepared. Arthrocentesis/tenocentesis may be performed under general anesthesia, if that is an option. Another method of testing for synovial structure involvement is to perform an arthrogram and determine if leakage of contrast media from the synovial space is evident on a radiograph.

Treatment and prognosis

Therapeutic aims

The principal goals of surgery are to optimize conditions for wound healing and to achieve the most favorable cosmetic and functional result. Sepsis must be controlled. The horse's hoof is not amenable to suturing and therefore wounds must heal by second intention.

Therapy

Therapy consists of surgical debridement, wound apposition and providing appropriate antibacterial medication to control sepsis. The foot should be prepared for aseptic surgery. The hoof wall, sole, and frog should be trimmed, pared, and rasped to remove any contamination that may reside in cracks or crevices. The hair from the fetlock distally should be clipped to allow surgical preparation of the entire foot and pastern area with an antiseptic scrub. Exposed tissues should be cleansed and irrigated with a physiologic saline solution.

Surgery may be performed on either a standing or an anesthetized patient. Standing surgery is performed with sedation and local anesthesia. However, this should be reserved for the most tractable of horses. It will also often require one person to hold the leg or to tie the leg up for surgery to be performed. General anesthesia provides optimal conditions to establish and maintain aseptic techniques, as well as optimizing the surgeon's ability to inspect the wound, obtain synovial fluid samples and to lavage and medicate synovial structures that have been invaded.

The goal of surgery is to optimize conditions for wound healing that will result in the most favorable cosmetic and functional result. The horse's hoof is not amenable to suturing and therefore wounds must heal by second intention. The most important factor in the management of these wounds is adequate debridement. Necrotic or severely damaged tissues and all foreign materials provide media for bacterial growth and impede wound healing. However, vital tissues such as nerves, arteries, and tendons should be salvaged, if possible. Complete wound excision is the simplest, most effective means of debridement. If this is not feasible, simple debridement of obviously devitalized tissue and foreign material combined with wound irrigation should be performed. Pulsating lavage is the most effective type of irrigation system.

If a synovial structure is opened or if it is suspected that a synovial cavity has been entered, the structure should be lavaged with copious amounts of sterile crystalloid solution (lactated Ringer's). The foot is a highly vascular structure and hemostasis is difficult. Hemostasis by ligation and electrocautery are usually not adequate. A temporary pressure bandage is usually necessary and will stop bleeding if left in place for 12 h. The initial bandage applied after surgical debridement should be moistened with sterile saline or an antimicrobial dressing over the wound and covered with an outer waterproof bandage.

Wounds of the hoof generally heal slowly, due in part to the high incidence of contamination. Subsequent wound infection can be minimized by proper cleaning, appropriate bandaging, and ensuring that enough help is available when changing the dressing (this usually requires two people). Contraction of hoof wounds is also minimal because of the inelasticity of the epithelial tissues and the fact that they are all attached to bone or rigid connective tissue. Thus, healing is the result of epithelialization and regeneration of connective tissue. All portions of corium can migrate and cover a healthy bed of granulation tissue. This process will be slow and may require 3–5 months.

Immobilization and protection of the wound are important considerations in the maintenance of the tissue environment achieved at surgery. A short limb cast that encases the hoof is usually the most effective method. The cast will not only immobilize the tissues and protect them from excess motion but will also serve as protection for the hoof from moisture and fecal contamination. On a long-term basis, a cast can be a much less expensive method of immobilization than daily bandage changes.

Ten to 14 days is the minimum duration suggested for cast immobilization. The cast should be maintained as long as necessary to provide a good initial healing (4–6 weeks if necessary). The cast needs to be monitored daily. If lameness, excessive heat, or odors develop, it should be removed. After cast removal, the hoof and laceration site should be stabilized using a bar shoe with clips or other methods to reduce motion during healing (Fig. 14.6).

Antibacterial medications are indicated during the acute phase of wound healing with traumatic wounds, when deep structures are involved, or when there has been severe tissue damage and loss. However, antibiotics should not be used in lieu of adequate surgical debridement, or without appropriate bacterial cultures and antibiotic sensitivity testing. Often the contamination in these cases involves multiple organisms, so the debrided deep tissues may be submitted for bacterial culture. Broad spectrum systemic antibacterial drugs should be used and modified based on bacterial culture and antibacterial sensitivity results. Regional limb perfusion and intra-synovial antibacterial administration are highly effective means to improve local tissue levels of medications to control sepsis.

Pain relief may be necessary postoperatively. Nonsteroidal anti-inflammatory drugs (NSAIDs) are recommended to reduce inflammation and to minimize the effects of unequal weight bearing on the unaffected limbs. For severe pain butorphanol administered in the muscle or via constant rate infusion should be considered.

As healing progresses, the hoof should be trimmed to remove excess horn. The hoof should have excess wall removed, the sole should be pared of scales, and the horn surrounding the wound should be kept even with the wound until complete keratinization of the wound has occurred.

The horse should not be allowed free exercise until keratinization is complete. Follow-up examination at 2–4 week intervals is usually adequate. Once keratinization is complete, corrective shoeing, acrylic remodeling, or simply cessation of bandaging is in order. This will have to continue until the hoof completely grows out. Usually this takes about 8–12 months.

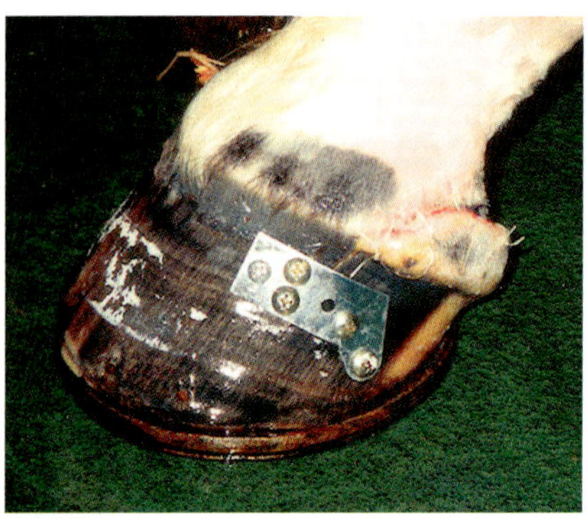

Fig 14.6 Repaired distal limb heel and hoof laceration stabilized with a shoe and metal plate secured to the hoof capsule with screws.

Prognosis

The prognosis for these injuries is generally good for soundness. However, a prognosis should be withheld until after adequate inspection of the wound has been made. The prognosis should be based on the duration of injury, the structures involved, the temperament of the horse, how adequately debridement can be achieved, and the structural integrity of the hoof after debridement

Sepsis within the hoof: subsolar abscess, laminar abscess, septic navicular bursitis

- Sepsis within the hoof is a primary differential diagnosis for non-weight-bearing lameness.
- Treatment must successfully approach, open, and drain the site of sepsis.
- Deep puncture wounds must be aggressively treated with parenteral and local antibiotics. Surgical debridement may be necessary.

Sepsis within the hoof capsule may be due to defects in the sole or hoof capsule, penetrating wounds. The treatment and prognosis for successful outcome depend on the location and duration of the abscess and response to initial therapy.

Recognition

History and presenting complaint

Lameness of acute onset that becomes more pronounced over several days is the primary presenting complaint for horses with sepsis within the hoof. Sole abscessation occurs more frequently when the weather changes from dry to wet conditions. The sole and white line become softer and more prone to penetration of contaminants. Penetrating wounds may cause abscessation at any site within the hoof.

Of particular concern are nails or other foreign bodies that penetrate in the caudal one-third of the foot. Contaminants that penetrate the caudal portion of the foot are readily sealed in by the elastic frog and digital cushion. Close proximity of the navicular bursa, distal interphalangeal joint, and tendon sheath make deep abscesses in the site difficult to drain and treat, with a high risk for extension of infection into these synovial spaces.

Physical examination

Lameness will vary from mild (grade 2 of 5) to non-weight-bearing (grade 5 of 5). The horse will often point with the affected foot and that distal limb will usually have a pronounced digital pulse. Application of hoof testers to the affected sole usually results in a very painful response directly over the abscess site. Examination of the sole may reveal a tract, site of foreign body penetration, soft and painful spot overlying the abscess or any combination of the above. If a foreign body is found, it should be left in place, if possible, until radiographs can be taken of the foot.

Special examination

Radiographs are warranted in nonresponsive cases of hoof sepsis to help identify sites of gas or fluid accumulation in the hoof or beneath the sole and to rule-out osteomyelitis or other causes of severe lameness of the distal limb (Fig. 14.7). Contrast-enhanced computed tomography may more clearly identify and delineate the extent of affected distal phalanx than radiography (Fig. 14.8). Imaging is not required for the great majority of feet suffering from routine sole abscessation.

If a foreign body remains within the foot, radiographs can be used to determine the depth of penetration and the most likely anatomical structures affected (Fig. 14. 9). If a tract is suspected to be due to a foreign body that has been removed, a contrast study of the foot will often provide similar information regarding location and depth of penetration.

If the foreign body penetrated the caudal one-third of the foot, it is imperative to determine if synovial structures have been invaded. Arthrocentesis of the distal interphalangeal joint, navicular bursa and the digital sheath may need to be done. Samples should be obtained for fluid analysis, cytology, and bacterial culture. These procedures are most easily accomplished with the horse under general anesthesia.

Diagnostic confirmation

The diagnosis is confirmed when the sole abscess is drained. Other differential diagnoses include deep penetrating wound to the foot, distal limb fracture, severe bruising of the sole, deep bruising of the sole that has become septic, laminar necrosis secondary to laminitis, keratoma, septic arthritis, and osteomyelitis.

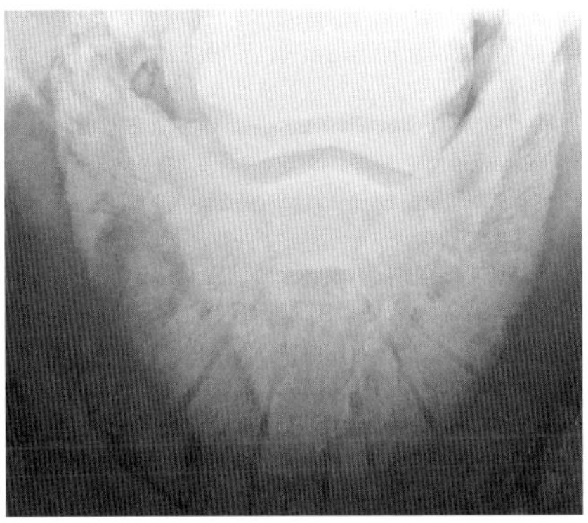

Fig 14.7 Dorsal oblique (D60Pr-PaDiO) radiographic view of a distal phalanx with suspect osteitis within the lateral portion of the bone. There is a history of chronic subsolar abscessation, drainage and severe lameness.

Treatment and prognosis

Therapeutic aims

A simple abscess should be opened to allow drainage and access of antiseptic solutions. Parenteral antibiotics are usually not necessary for simple abscesses. Horses with deep penetrating wounds of the foot should be treated with broad-spectrum antibiotics including regional limb perfusion, lavage of the affected synovial spaces, and may require exploration and debridement of the wound tract.

Therapy

The sole of the affected foot should be carefully pared to reveal clean, uniform sole. A combination of hoof tester and finger pressure may be use to localize the likely site of the abscess. If the horse is shod, the shoe must often be removed to afford evaluation of the sole margins and the white line, the most common sites for sole abscess. Tracts should be pared and followed in the painful region until the abscess is relieved or until on further paring the solar corium is revealed by a slight pink hue. A specialized hoof knife with a tightly curved tip, or a bone curette may be useful for following tracts through the sole. You may probe the suspect site of the abscess by inserting a 16 g needle into the site. If abscess material is encountered, the area should be pared out to open and drain the site. Most sole abscesses consist of a gray-colored, malodorous liquid that flows freely when the abscess cavity is breached during paring. Excessive paring may result in hemorrhage from the solar corium. The size of the sole opening used to drain the abscess and permit local treatment is quite small. Excessively large defects used to drain an abscess require prolonged healing time and protection with a sole pad.

If the abscess cannot be drained on the initial visit, verify tetanus status and poultice or soak the foot. Poulticing and soaking are done to soften the foot and draw out the abscess. Soaking is done by placing the foot in warm water with diluted povidone-iodine and a handful of Epsom's salts for 10 to 20 min once or twice daily. Agents appropriate for a foot poultice include a mixture of

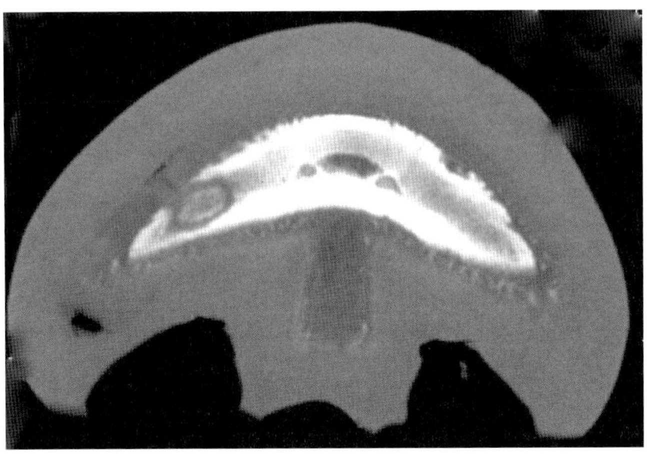

Fig 14.8 Frontal plane contrast-enhanced computed tomography of the distal phalanx in Fig. 14.7. The extent of the affected bone defect is now evident as a sequestrum.

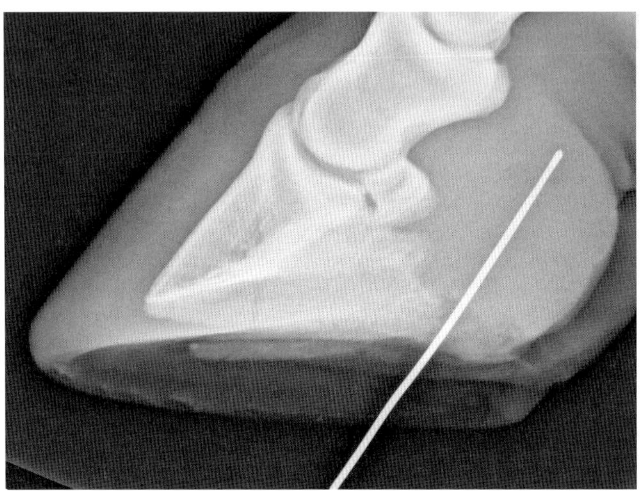

Fig 14.9 Lateral radiographic view of the distal limb of a horse that has stepped on a nail in the palmar one-third of the foot. The nail was removed and a probe was placed into the tract. The tract appears to be palmar to the major synovial structures of the heel region.

povidone-iodine solution and granular sugar, an ointment consisting of magnesium sulfate, methyl salicylate, and menthol (Magnapaste, The Butler Company, Columbus, OH) and Ichthammol (ammonium bituminosulfonate, 20%), an antiseptic emollient ointment. Another method of providing prolonged soaking of the foot is by using a bran mash poultice. Place a strong plastic bag that fits over the foot, add one handful of bran, a small handful of Epsom's salts. Add sufficient water to soak the bran and add povidone-iodine (approximately one part to 10 parts other constituents). Fit the bag with mixture over the foot and secure with gauze, elastic tape and duct tape. This poultice is changed every 24 h.

If the abscess was easily drained, apply a povidone-iodine-soaked gauze to the pared defect and protect the sole with a commercial protective boot or a bandage. Change the bandage daily for the first few days, then as needed to protect the foot. After the abscess is dry (as soon as 4–5 days or as long as two weeks) a shoe with a leather pad should be applied to protect the pared area. Systemic antibiotics are not administered in uncomplicated sole abscess cases. In all cases of hoof sepsis, tetanus status should be determined. If the horse has not been vaccinated within the previous 6-month period, reimmunization is indicated.

Deep sole abscesses that cannot be drained through the sole result in prolonged lameness and often break out at the coronary band of the hoof capsule or over the bulbs of the heels. If the abscess cannot be accessed from the sole or white line, radiographs may help localize the site. Radiographs will also determine if the distal phalanx has suffered osteomyelitis or osteitis due to the prolonged inflammation and infection. Rarely extensive, prolonged sole abscesses must be treated with localized, partial hoof or sole resection, and/or curettage of the distal phalanx.

More extensive treatment must be done in the case of a deep penetrating wound to the caudal one-third of the foot. At the first indication of a deep wound in this crucial location, the horse should be administered broad-spectrum parenteral antibiotics such as penicillin and gentamicin, or ceftiofur and gentamicin. Enhanced coverage for anaerobic organisms may be obtained by adding oral metronidazole to either protocol.

Because of the poor prognosis for horses that develop sepsis of the deep structures within the caudal aspect of the hoof, vigorous initial therapy is imperative. If the radiographic study confirms deep penetration in this critical zone the horse should be placed under general anesthesia to allow sampling and treating of the most at-risk structures: navicular bursa, distal interphalangeal joint, and the distal digital sheath.

If lameness is severe at presentation and a tract in the caudal foot is recognized surgical debridement is necessary via arthroscopy or by an open surgical approach (street nail procedure). This procedure requires cleansing and soaking of the foot in antiseptic solution, general anesthesia, arthroscopic evaluation of the distal digital sheath, navicular bursa and distal interphalangeal joint as indicated by the orientation of the foreign body and lavage of the synovial structures. The wound tract may be debrided using a motorized soft tissue resector or via hand tools.

Following debridement, the foot must have sterile bandage changes to prevent contamination. This process is facilitated by applying a hospital plate shoe to the foot.

Prognosis

Prognosis is usually excellent for return to complete soundness within two weeks for uncomplicated sole abscesses.

Deep penetrating wounds to the caudal aspect of the foot have a guarded to poor prognosis if they penetrate into the synovial structures. Treatment using the street nail procedure resulted in 32% of affected horses returning to soundness.[15] Using the arthroscopic approach resulted in 75% of treated horses returning to their intended use.[16]

Laminitis

- Bounding digital pulses, marked lameness, and postural efforts to shift weight from the affected feet characterize the signs of laminitis.
- Inciting causes include metabolic derangements, severe illness, and excessive weight bearing.
- Treatment must resolve the inciting cause, reduce inflammation, maintain blood flow, and prevent distal phalanx displacement.
- Trimming using radiographic control is necessary to return the hoof to function.
- Overall prognosis for soundness in most cases is favorable.

Laminitis is defined as inflammation of the pedal laminae, which provide the support between the hoof wall and distal phalanx. Numerous causes of the disease have been defined but the leading cause remains gastrointestinal disturbances. Although the condition primarily affects the foot, the disease is actually a systemic disease, which causes disturbances in most body systems. The disease can be arbitrarily divided into four phases: developmental, acute, chronic, and postchronic.

Recognition

History and presenting complaint

Horses presented with clinical signs of laminitis are always in the acute, chronic or postchronic phases of the disorder. Signs of acute laminitis include: bounding digital pulses, warm feet, and 'camped out' stance. This characteristic stance is an effort by the horse to shift weight bearing to the (usually) unaffected rear limbs. The severity of lameness relates to the severity of damage to the laminae. Pain and inflammation from ischemia to the secondary laminae is the direct cause of acute pain in laminitis. Horses with chronic laminitis are presented for misshapen hooves, seedy toe, chronic, recurring hoof abscessation, and chronic lameness.

The practitioner must be aware of potential inciting causes of laminitis. When a horse is exposed to a situation that may cause laminitis, preventive measures must be taken to minimize the adverse effects. The period of time between exposure to a situation that may cause laminitis and the onset of clinical signs is called the developmental or subclinical phase. Factors that may induce laminitis should be identified in the history and include: grain overload, colic, illness associated with endotoxemia, retained placenta, exhaustion and metabolic derangements, exposure to black walnut shavings, excessive ingestion of lush pasture grasses (grass founder), excessive concussion (road founder), equine metabolic syndrome, equine Cushing's syndrome (equine pituitary pars intermedia dysfunction), excessive weight bearing on a limb, and excessive ingestion of cold water.[13–17]

Physical examination

Horses with acute laminitis generally show varying levels of foot pain, often characterized by treading in place or a shifting limb lameness.[17,18] When severe pain is present in the forelimbs a characteristic 'walking-on-egg shells' gait is evident as the horse shifts weight to the rear limbs. Most commonly, both forelimbs are affected. All limbs may be affected in extraordinary cases. Unilateral limb involvement is usually found in the contralateral limb of horses that have non-weight-bearing lameness due to fracture or infection.[19] Digital pulses are generally increased and may be bounding in severe laminitis. Hoof tester sensitivity at the toe near the apex of the frog is usually marked. When rotation or distal displacement of the distal phalanx has occurred the sole will lose its normal concavity and a depression may be palpated at the coronary band. Imminent exposure of the distal phalanx or separation of the hoof capsule from the foot may be first recognized with serum weeping from the sole or coronary band, respectively.

Horses with chronic laminitis may have remodeling of the tip and dorsal border of the distal phalanx, solar margin fractures, and distal phalanx rotation evident on radiographic examination. Inadequate trimming may leave a dished hoof with long toes and severely underrun heels. Chronic abscessation of the hoof and coronary band associated with a wide and weakened white line is also commonly found in chronic laminitis cases.

Diagnostic confirmation

Diagnosis is based on physical signs and radiographic examination. The dorsal hoof wall and dorsal distal phalanx in the normal horse should be parallel and the space should measure <19 mm or <30% of the length of the distal phalanx measured from its tip to its articular surface at the navicular bone (Fig. 14.10).[20] Rotation is the most common displacement and is caused by disruption of dorsal laminar attachments and the pull of the deep digital flexor tendon (DDFT). Radiographic evaluation of distal phalanx displacement may help determine a prognosis. Prognosis has been reported to be good for horses with rotation <5.5°, but poor for rotation >11.5°.[21]

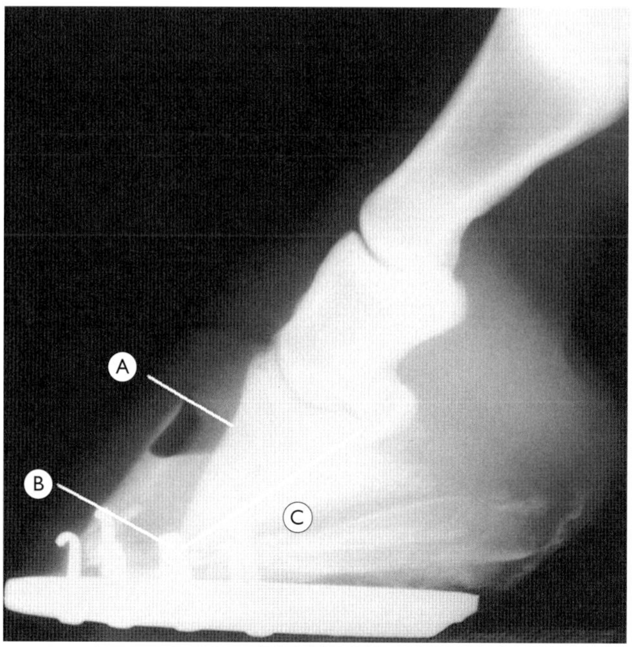

Fig 14.10 Radiographic measurement of distal phalanx displacement. This lateral radiographic projection of the distal phalanx has been marked to demonstrate two methods for measuring distal phalanx displacement. Measured distances: A, 24 mm; B, 30 mm; C, 54 mm. Normally, A and B should measure less than or equal to 19 mm and be equal values, indicative of parallelism of the dorsal distal phalanx with the dorsal hoof capsule. A and B should also be less than 30% of the measurement taken from the tip of the distal phalanx to the articulation with the navicular bone (C). In this case C/A = 44% and C/B = 55%. These values are indicative of severe distal phalanx displacement. A gas and fluid pocket indicative of lamellar necrosis is also found in the dorsal laminae.

Horses with distal displacement ('sinking') have a poor prognosis. Another study contradicted the aforementioned report and found no correlation between radiographically measured distal phalanx displacement and prognosis for resolution of laminitis.[18]

Venograms of the distal limb have been advocated to help determine prognosis.[22] The prognosis for successful treatment is enhanced when the vasculature of the coronary corium and dorsal laminae are visible during venography.

Differential diagnoses include deep abscess, distal phalanx or navicular bone fracture, septic tenosynovitis, or deep bruising. Most of these conditions commonly occur in a single limb, but laminitis most commonly occurs bilaterally except when caused by excessive weight bearing.

Treatment and prognosis

Therapeutic aims

The treatment objectives for laminitis include resolving the inciting cause, reducing inflammation, and supporting the structures of the foot to prevent displacement of the distal phalanx.

Treatment during the developmental phase is done to prevent the onset of clinically apparent laminitis or to reduce the potential adverse effects of exposure to inciting causes of laminitis.

The aims of treatment during the chronic phases of laminitis include supporting the distal phalanx to reduce further displacement and providing an environment where the distal phalanx, laminae and hoof capsule may re-establish a firm, stable bond. When all other significant hoof issues have been resolved, gradually returning distal phalanx to normal orientation with the ground surface is the ultimate goal.

Therapy

Treatment during the developmental and acute phases of laminitis includes appropriate therapy to resolve the inciting cause, cryotherapy to reduce destructive enzyme activity such as matrix metalloproteinases and provide analgesia, administration of anti-inflammatory medication and distal phalanx support.[23] In the developmental phase, successful treatment should prevent the laminar damage that results in distal phalanx displacement and the untoward sequellae, while treatment in the acute phase should reduce the adverse effects and extent of the damage.

Cryotherapy is a crucial part of treatment of laminitis in both the developmental and acute phases. In experimental models of carbohydrate overload constant ice water immersion has been demonstrated to reduce enzyme activity and pro-inflammatory cytokines and prevent the onset of severe pain associated with clinical laminitis.[23] An easy method to apply cryotherapy to distal limbs is by placing the foot within an empty 5 L fluid bag and taping it to the cannon bone. A second bag is pulled over the first and filled with ice (Fig. 14.11). In a study that measured laminar and digital venous temperatures and compared them between ice water immersion in a wader boot, ice bags as described above, and commercial gel cold pack wraps, the ice bag produced marked cooling (23.2°C lower than baseline), the wader boot produced the most profound cooling of the three methods (24.7°C lower than baseline with mean laminar temperatures of 9.8°C) and gel packs provided the least cooling (3.2°C lower than baseline). Digital venous temperature was closely correlated with laminar temperature.[24]

In horses that have been exposed to the inciting causes of laminitis, it is prudent to exclude all grains and concentrates from the diet until the outcome is evident. Cathartics are administered in grain or pasture overload. Mineral oil or water with Epsom's salts (up to 1 kg per 4 L water) may be administered via nasogastric intubation.

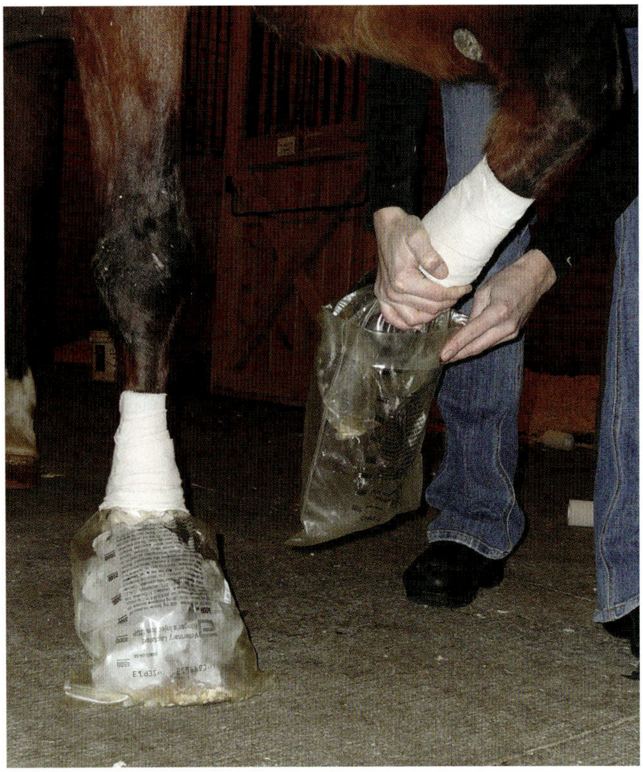

Fig 14.11 This method of applying ice to the distal limbs makes use of two fluid bags with ice between them. The inner bag protects the hoof and skin from excess moisture.

Gastric lavage may be performed within 2–6 h of overeating. Intravenous fluid and electrolyte therapy should be instituted in exhausted horses. Fractures and severe lameness should be treated to permit weight bearing in the affected limb as soon as possible.

If a severe illness, abdominal surgery, or other condition that may cause endotoxin release is present the horse should be administered hyperimmune serum and flunixin meglumine at the anti-endotoxic dose (2.5 mg/kg i.v., q 6 h).[22]

NSAIDs such as phenylbutazone (4.4–8.8 mg/kg/day), flunixin meglumine (1 mg/kg/day) or ketoprofen (2.2 mg/ kg/day) should be administered in all cases of laminitis. Phenylbutazone is most commonly used, yet ketoprofen may have a slightly better effect in select cases. Based on anecdotal reports, COX-specific NSAIDs such as firocoxib may not have as strong an analgesic effect as flunixin or phenylbutazone.[24] NSAIDs reduce prostaglandin and thromboxane production through inhibition of cyclo-oxygenase, decreasing inflammation associated with ischemia and thereby decreasing pain and promoting blood flow through small peripheral vessels by inhibiting platelet aggregation and thrombosis.

Dimethyl sulfoxide (DMSO) may be used to prevent reperfusion injury of the laminae. It acts as a free-radical scavenger and nonspecific anti-inflammatory agent.[25] DMSO is administered at 0.25–1.0 g/kg i.v. in saline or 5% dextrose solution at a concentration less than 20%. In acute laminitis treatment with DMSO is usually continued for three days.

Increasing blood flow to the laminae may be controversial with more recent information on the pathophysiology of laminitis.[23, 24] Blood flow may be enhanced with peripheral vasodilators and with medication that allows more flexibility of blood cells.[26, 27] Acepromazine maleate is an alpha-adrenergic antagonist and is administered at 0.03–0.06 mg/kg i.m. either q 6 h or q 8 h for 3–5 days, or until the horse improves. This drug is readily available in all practices and should be used at the first indication of laminitis. Isoxsuprine HCl is a beta- and alpha-adrenergic antagonist that is administered at 1.2 mg/kg p.o. q 12 h for indefinite periods. There is controversy regarding systemic availability of this drug via the oral route in horses and treatment effects should not be expected for days or weeks.[25] Pentoxifylline improves small vessel blood flow by rheologic mechanisms, increased flexibility of blood cells. Administer 8.4 mg/kg q12 h *per os*.[27] Small vessel blood flow may also be enhanced by administering antithrombotic or anticoagulant medications. Aspirin is very effective at inhibiting platelet aggregation and may be administered at 10–20 mg/kg p.o. every other day.[18] Heparin may be administered at a dosage of 40–80 units/kg SQ q 12 h.[28]

The distal phalanx must be supported in the developmental phase to prevent displacement and in the acute phase to also prevent or limit distal phalanx displacement. Initially simple gauze rolls taped over the frogs may be helpful. Lily Pads (Kentucky Blacksmith Supply, KY), fitted over the heel bulbs and frogs and secured with tape, may be a longer-term solution. Full sole support may be custom fitted using Scotchcast Custom Support Foam fiberglass cast padding tape (3 M Orthopedic Products, St Paul, MN), dental impression material, or common foam building insulation. These pads can be frequently reset to provide the most comfort in cases with rapidly changing sole contours. Commercially available soft-padded strap on hoof boots are another helpful option to provide sole support and comfort (Soft-Ride Equine Comfort Boots, Soft-Ride, Inc, Bacliff, TX USA). The boots are custom-sized, available with gel pad inserts of varying densities and are often available via overnight delivery (in North America). Deep sand footing is a simple method to maintain good sole contact and soft bedding.

Excessive tension of the DDFT is one of the factors responsible for distal phalanx rotation by increased strain and ultimate disruption of hoof lamellae. DDFT tension can be reduced through several methods. Special horse shoes have been developed to help reduce DDFT tension and to support the foot. The Ultimate Wedge shoe (Kentucky Blacksmith Supply, KY) raises the heel 20°, significantly reducing DDFT stress.[29] The Ovnicek shoe (Equine Digital Support System, Columbia Falls, MT) has several components that results in custom foot support and can be configured with a high heel wedge and styrofoam-like sole padding. A recent report has made the common practice of raising heel angle to reduce strain on the hoof lamellae controversial. When the heel angle was raised 15 degrees in an equine finite element model, dorsal lamellar strain increased between 1.3 and 3.8 times.[30]

A surgical alternative for reducing DDFT tension also exists. Tenotomy of the DDFT at mid-cannon bone or at the level of the heel bulbs has been used as a salvage method for nonresponsive cases of laminitis with severe or continued rotation and in some cases for treatment of peracute distal phalanx displacement.[31] Tenotomy at the mid-cannon level is a practical technique that may be performed under local anesthesia through a small stab incision. The limb is bandaged and the foot is supported with sole pads. An extended heel shoe or a shoe with a marked wedge pad is necessary to prevent subluxation of the distal interphalangeal joint. Response to tenotomy has been variable. In the successful case, the DDFT eventually heals, but scarring and adhesions may limit athletic use of the horse.

Chronic laminitis presents a variety of treatment challenges. Displacement of the distal phalanx usually occurs by rotation in the sagittal plane but may also involve complete distal phalanx displacement ('sinking'). The damaged lamellae also predispose the hoof to abscessation at both the sole and the coronary band. The displaced distal phalanx is predisposed to solar margin fractures, especially near the toe. In the most serious cases, complete slough of the hoof may occur or the distal phalanx may penetrate the sole. Management of these conditions requires long-term treatment with NSAIDs and repeated shoeing and trimming. Follow-up treatment should always involve the veterinarian, farrier, and horse owner. Decisions regarding continued support of the sole, easing of breakover, and correct trimming of heel and toe should be made using radiographs of the affected feet taken at intervals during recuperation.

In most cases of mild laminitis, gradual reshaping of the hoof capsule must be performed over several months to return the distal phalanx to the proper relationship with the ground surface and the hoof. This generally requires removing excess heel and excess toe. Trimming should result in gradual changes only and should be controlled by measurements and relationships made from lateral radiographs of the distal phalanx. In some cases more radical trimming changes may be indicated. The four-point trimming protocol as described by Ovnicek may help reduce DDFT tendon strain and the strain on the distal limb during breakover. By providing more surface area of contact with the ground surface the method may also reduce overall foot pain.

Prognosis

Most mild cases of laminitis respond to treatment in several days to weeks. Those that linger, have marked displacement of the distal phalanx, display increasing levels of severe pain or suddenly slough the hoof capsule may be candidates for euthanasia. The owner's strong desire for resolution of this devastating condition because of close emotional attachment to the horse must not override rational analysis of the horse's condition and humane aspects of continuing treatment. In most cases the horse should be euthanized when pain is unmanageable and the horse shows signs of anorexia, cachexia, or severe decubital ulcers. Most cases with distal phalanx penetration of the sole, sloughing of the hoof capsule, and recurrent deep abscessation of the sole or laminae should be euthanized. There are always exceptions, and quality of life for the horse should be a primary, although at times arbitrary and qualitative, concern.

Prognosis for resolution of laminitis is usually fair to good for horses with minimal distal phalanx displacement. Horses with marked displacement nearly always suffer more chronic hoof problems that may limit soundness. Horses with sinking displacement have a poor prognosis for survival, as do horses that slough the entire hoof or have penetration of the sole by the distal phalanx.

Prognostic indicators for laminitis were reported in a study from the UK.[32] Of 216 horses with laminitis: 162 (77%) became sound as athletes, 7 (3%) did not become completely sound, but survived and 42 (20%) horses were euthanized or died due to laminitis. The remaining five horses were euthanized and not treated. The most significant prognostic indicator was quantification of distal phalanx displacement from radiographs. Less significant prognostic indicators were the severity of lameness, distal phalanx rotation angles, the presence of dropped sole, and the number of feet affected.[32]

Etiology and pathophysiology

Etiology

The following conditions are associated with laminitis: excessive grain or lush pasture ingestion; endotoxemia associated with infectious diseases such as diarrhea, septicemia, or retained placenta; excessive metabolic stress associated with dehydration or overexertion; excessive weight bearing on a limb opposite one with a fracture or severe lameness; and management factors such as bedding with black walnut shavings, excessive obesity, and underconditioned horses worked excessively. Horse's with metabolic syndrome (insulin resistance) and equine Cushing's disease are predisposed to laminitis.

Pathophysiology

There is general agreement that laminitis is associated with circulatory disturbances at the level of the lamellae, but the specific nature of the changes continues to be under investigation.[17,18,26,33–37] Current research suggests that there is a period of lamellar vasodilatation during the developmental phase of laminitis [26,33,34] In experimental laminitis vasodilatation within the hoof was found from 12 to 32 h after carbohydrate overload.[33] The increased local blood flow may result in exposure of the lamellae to enzymes such as metalloproteinase-2 and metalloproteinase-9 (MMP-2 and MMP-9).[35] These enzymes are normally required to temporarily break the lamellar attachments as the keratinized hoof capsule grows and 'slides' along the dermal lamellae. In the normal hoof, inhibitor enzymes are present to control MMP activity, whereas the laminitic hoof lacks these inhibitors. Vasodilatation of the vessels in the lamellae carries the activated MMP enzymes to their site of action, the cytokines and free radicals associated with reperfusion then act on the lamellae and cause their destruction. A variety of inflammatory mediators such as chemokines, proinflammatory cytokines, COX-2 and endothelial adhesion molecules have increased expression in lamellar tissues obtained from experimental carbohydrate overload models of equine laminitis.[23] In hoof tissues from experimental acute and chronic carbohydrate-induced laminitis, high expression of endothelin-1 (ET-1) has also been identified.[37] The presence of ET-1 causes marked vasoconstriction, which leads to ischemia of the lamellar tissues. This potential cycle of vasodilatation, followed by vasoconstriction and the attendant breakdown of lamellar attachments, necrosis, and inflammation constitutes the vicious cycle that leads to pain, distal phalanx displacement, and the other physical signs of laminitis.

Prevention

Minimizing changes in diet, particularly changes in the amount of grain fed and controlling access to lush, new pasture grasses, will decrease the incidence of laminitis. Recognize that horses that have had a previous bout of laminitis are predisposed to having the problem again. When inciting causes of laminitis are present, preventive treatment should be instituted.

Diseases of the distal phalanx

Distal phalanx fractures

Distal phalangeal fractures can be classified into one of seven types (Fig. 14.12).[38–40] Type I is a non-articular fracture of the wing of the third phalanx. Type II fractures are articular wing fractures (Fig. 14.13). Type III fractures are sagittal and divide the bone nearly into equal halves. Type IV fractures comprise all extensor process fractures. Comminuted and irregular distal phalanx fractures are type V. Fractures of the solar margin are type VI (Fig. 14.14). Palmar process fractures are considered type VII (Fig. 14.15).[39]

Recognition

History and presenting complaint

Acute onset of grade 3–5 of 5 lameness is the primary presenting complaint for fractures of the distal phalanx. Often the inciting event is not seen but kicking in the stall or a miss-step followed by acute lameness may be reported. Young foals with distal phalanx palmar process fractures may be presented for evaluation of club-footed conformation that is accompanied by mild, short-term lameness.[41–43]

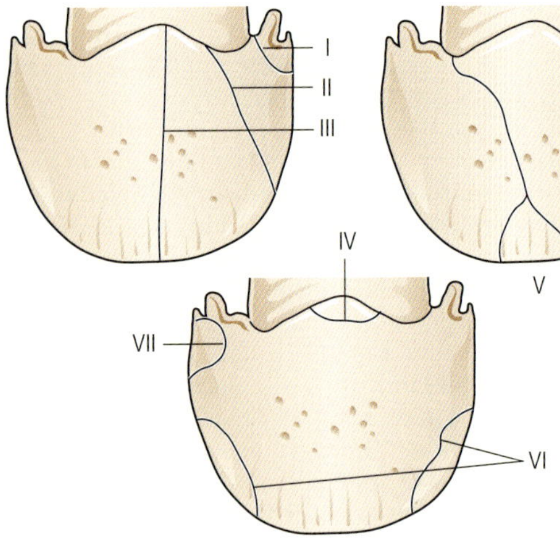

Fig 14.12 Diagrammatic representation of distal phalanx fractures. Type I: non-articular fracture of the wing; type II: non-sagittal fracture that enters the distal interphalangeal joint; type III: mid-sagittal, articular fracture from the extensor process to the solar margin; type IV: extensor process fracture; type V: comminuted or irregular fractures; type VI: fractures of the solar margin; type VII: non-articular fractures of the palmar process.

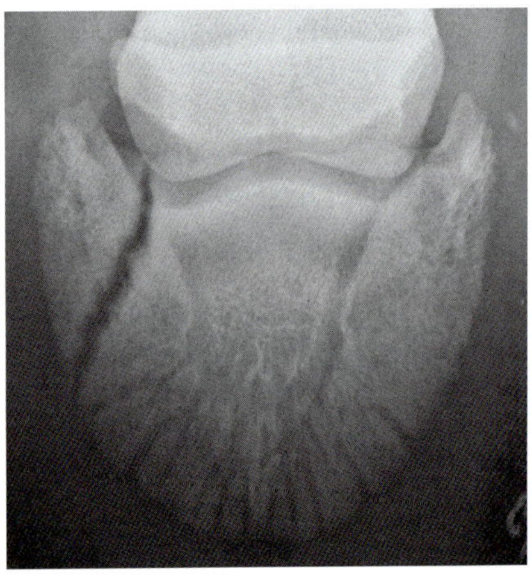

Fig 14.13 Dorsal oblique (D60Pr-PaDiO) radiographic view of the distal phalanx with a articular fracture (type II).

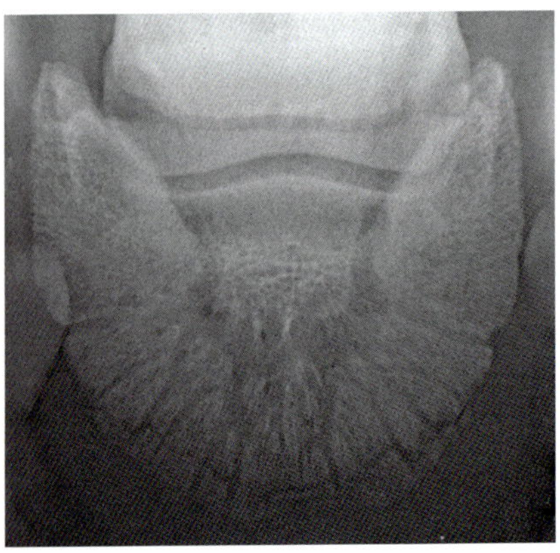

Fig 14.14 Dorsal oblique (D60Pr-PaDiO) radiographic view of the distal phalanx with dorsal solar margin fractures (type VI).

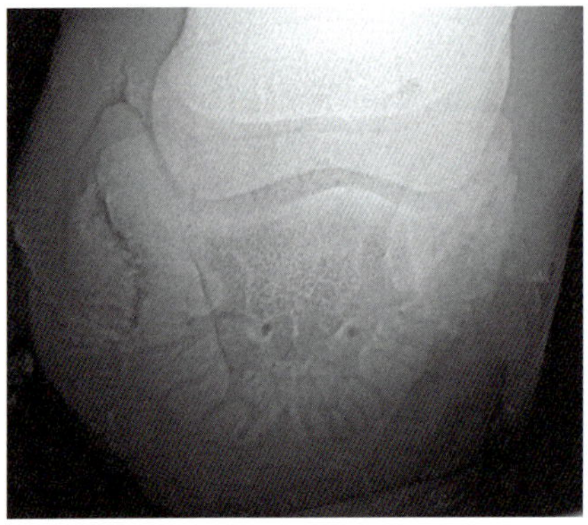

Fig 14.15 Dorsal oblique (D60Pr-PaDiO) radiographic view of the distal phalanx of a foal with non-articular palmar process fracture (type VII). Courtesy of Dr. B. Faramarzi, Western University College of Veterinary Medicine.

Physical examination

Lameness is usually accompanied by an increased digital pulse. Extensor process fractures are often accompanied by swelling over the coronary band. Hoof tester examination usually reveals marked pain over the entire hoof but especially over the fracture. Hoof percussion reveals sensitivity around the entire hoof but especially over the fracture. These two techniques can usually aid the practitioner in lining up for radiography in order to center the X-ray beam on the fracture.

Diagnostic confirmation

Radiographs are necessary to confirm the diagnosis. Usually at least four to five views should be made in order to examine the entire bone from several angles. The fracture may not be visible until lysis occurs along the fracture line, often for 10–14 days.[38] Nuclear scintigraphy and computed tomography are additional imaging methods to help recognize distal phalanx fractures.

Treatment and prognosis

Therapeutic aims

Sufficient stability and reduced activity must be provided for the affected foot to permit healing of the fracture.

Therapy

Fracture types I, II, III, and V are treated by therapeutic shoeing. A full bar shoe with quarter clips, full rim shoe, or certain glue-on shoes will immobilize the hoof capsule and effectively turn the hoof into a cast. Foals with any type of distal phalanx fracture should not be treated with a restrictive shoe because of the secondary complications that accompany hoof contracture. Foals under 1 year of age with these fractures usually respond favorably to stall or paddock confinement alone.[42–43]

Fracture types II, III, and IV may be repaired with lag screw fixation. This can be difficult because the fracture line cannot be visualized during surgery, therefore radiographic control during surgery is essential for a successful outcome. Also, the bone in the wings of the distal phalanx is porous and does not hold screws well.

Type IV fractures are best treated by surgical intervention. Small fragments are easily removed via arthroscopy. Larger fragments should be stabilized using lag screw fixation but can be removed completely via an arthrotomy. Neurectomy of the palmar digital nerve may be necessary to resolve chronic low-grade pain. Neurectomy is most effective for wing fractures but may reduce pain in all the fractures. It should not be performed if a palmar digital nerve block fails to substantially improve the lameness.

Prognosis

The prognosis for soundness of fracture types I and II is fair to good.[38] Fracture types III and IV have a guarded to fair prognosis due to the likelihood of distal interphalangeal arthritis. The prognosis for type V fractures due to trauma is good, yet prognosis for this type of fracture secondary to osteomyelitis is guarded. Type VI fractures have an excellent prognosis. In adults complete healing of distal phalanx fractures may require 9–12 months. All fractures in foals less than one year of age have a very good to excellent prognosis for soundness.[42,43]

Etiology and pathophysiology

Etiology

These fractures are usually caused by trauma. Pathological fractures of the distal phalanx may occur secondary to osteomyelitis. Improper shoeing, hard surfaces, stone bruises, infectious conditions, and nutritional deficiencies are all considered to be contributing factors.

Diseases of the navicular region

Navicular bone fractures

Navicular bone fractures are uncommon and can be classified into one of four types. These are simple sagittal fractures, comminuted fractures, avulsion fracture of the navicular suspensory ligament, and avulsion fractures of the impar ligament.

Recognition

History and presenting complaint

History, presenting complaint and physical signs for avulsion fractures of the navicular bone are the same as for other causes of palmar foot pain (see below). Complete navicular fractures will present with acute onset of severe lameness that may decrease somewhat over time.[44]

Physical examination

These fractures have pain referable to the navicular bone. They are usually acute and exhibit a grade III–V of V lameness. In most cases the horse is unwilling to place the heel of the affected foot on the ground. Marked pain over the navicular area is noted with hoof testers. Distal limb flexion markedly exacerbates the lameness.

Diagnostic confirmation

Conformation of navicular fracture is made by localizing the foot pain to the heel region and radiographic evidence of fracture (Fig. 14.16). Recognize that occasionally the navicular bone will develop with two (bipartite) or three (tripartite) ossification centers. If these centers do not bridge with mineralized bone, the navicular bone may appear to be fractured. Localization of pain to the heel region using diagnostic local anesthesia should rule-out separate ossification centers.

Treatment and prognosis

Therapeutic aims

Conventional therapy for navicular fractures is similar to that used for distal phalanx fractures. An alternative technique reduces DDFT and heel strain and is followed by a gradual exercise program to limit adhesions.

Therapy

Navicular bone fractures are usually treated conservatively. Surgical exposure of the site and internal fixation of the fracture is challenging, but has been reported. Therapy traditionally entails variable periods of rest with corrective trimming and shoeing to immobilize the hoof. Palmar digital neurectomy often is required after the fracture heals to increase soundness. However, the results of this type of therapy have been poor. The poor results are thought to be due in part to adhesion formation between the navicular bone and the deep flexor tendon.

An alternative technique may be used that reduces heel strain and returns the horse to controlled exercise sooner than conventional therapy.[45] Following the diagnosis of a navicular bone fracture, the affected hoof should be trimmed to its normal hoof pastern axis. The hoof is then shod with a shoe and wedge pads to elevate the heels 10–12° (Fig. 14.17). The objective is to prevent the navicular bone from having weight-bearing contact with the second phalanx and to decrease the strain on the deep flexor tendon. Proper elevation of the hoof can be confirmed through the use of a lateral radiograph.

The horse should be stall rested for the first 60 days, then short periods of handwalking (15 min daily) can begin. The shoe is reset every 4–6 weeks. At each reset the hoof is trimmed and the horse

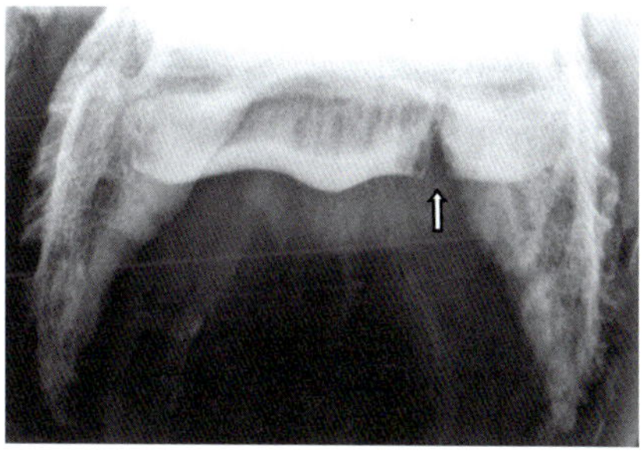

Fig 14.16 Navicular skyline (Pa45Pr-PaDiO) radiographic view with a complete sagittal plane fracture (arrow).

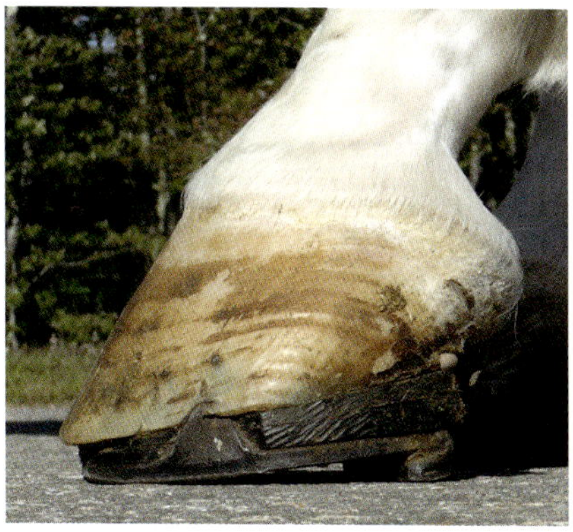

Fig 14.17 Raised heel shoe for conservative treatment of navicular bone fracture and navicular region soft tissue injuries.

is reshod with 2° less elevation. At the end of four months, when the horse is shod normally, an assessment of the degree of soundness is made. Navicular bursography or MRI can be utilized at the end of the four month period to assess the degree of adhesion formation. Four cases have been treated utilizing this method. Three horses had simple sagittal fractures of the navicular bone involving the forelimb and one had a comminuted fracture of a rear limb navicular bone. Upon initial presentation these horses were grade 3–5 of 5 lame. Typically, the fracture was noted radiographically as a clearly demarcated fracture with well-defined margins. The fracture line became less well defined within 30 days. This was presumably due to bone resorption. Mineralization around the fracture in each of these cases occurred but complete radiographic healing of the fracture did not occur in any case. However, the horse's lameness resolved after the four month treatment period. Two horses returned to competition, one as a gaited horse and the other is a multipurpose Arabian show horse. The other two horses are not lame and are being ridden.[45]

Complete navicular bone fractures often heal with a fibrous, rather than an osseous, union.[44] Avulsion fractures of the proximal or distal border of the navicular bone usually respond to treatment for palmar foot pain.

Prognosis

The prognosis for navicular fracture caused by trauma is guarded prognosis due to likelihood of secondary arthritis. Pathologic fractures due to infection have a grave prognosis.

Etiology and pathophysiology

Etiology

The etiology of navicular fractures is always traumatic but can be predisposed by either infection or chronic demineralization from navicular disease. Repetitive trauma that predisposes the foot to palmar heel pain may lead to avulsion fractures of the proximal or distal border of the navicular bone. The navicular bone may have more than one center of ossification, resulting in either a bipartite or tripartite bone.

Palmar foot pain

- Manipulative tests and diagnostic anesthesia often do not specifically identify the site of palmar heel pain.
- Shoeing goals for palmar heel pain: correcting hoof imbalance, improving heel support, easing breakover, and providing concussion protection.
- There are more than 15 specific causes of palmar heel pain.

Lameness in this region accounts for more than one-third of all chronic lameness in the horse.[5] It must be understood that diagnostic analgesia of the palmar digital nerves simply localizes the source of the pain the horse senses to the back of the foot and sole. It is important to identify as specifically as one can the pathological and clinical findings. This in turn will help the clinician make their best assessment of the problem, and recommend the most specific treatment.

Recognition

History and presenting complaint

Horses are presented for mild to moderate unilateral or bilateral forelimb lameness that is usually exacerbated in a circle. Quarter Horses, Thoroughbreds, Warmbloods, other Western stock-type horses and other breeds that compete over fences are predisposed to palmar heel pain. Subtle heel pain may be presented as a horse that no longer extends the forelimbs during the trot, resulting in a short, choppy or shuffling gait. Affected horses may stumble due to their preference to land toe first.

Physical examination

The examination should closely follow the guidelines presented earlier in this chapter. No diagnostic test is pathognomonic for navicular or palmar foot pain.[46] Distal limb flexion has been suggested by Turner to be of importance in the differentiation of navicular disease. In that study, 87.5% of the horses responded to this test.[46] When grouped according to diagnostic analgesia response, the navicular region pain (NRP) group that blocked to palmar digital, distal interphalangeal and navicular bursa analgesia injections was positive to distal limb flexion in 88% of the cases. The palmar foot pain (PFP) group that did not respond equally to the three injections was positive to distal limb flexion in 87% of horses. This indicates that the test is good for exacerbating pain in the palmar hoof but does not help in specific differentiation of the cause.

The frog wedge test is thought to exert pressure directly on the navicular bone similar to hoof testers but is thought to be more accurate because the horse's weight exerts the pressure rather than man-made pressure. The study found that 75% of the horses responded to this test.[46] But 76% were from the NRP group and 74% from PFP group again indicating no difference.

The toe wedge test was positive in 56%. This is higher than that reported by Wright.[47] However, the test was of no help in differentiating the source of pain; 55% were positive in the NRP group and 58% were positive in the PFP group.

Hoof tester examination over the frog is considered by some clinicians as the definitive test for navicular pain. However, hoof tester examination was found not only to be less sensitive than other manipulative tests for navicular pain but that other types of palmar foot pain were more likely to respond to the hoof tester examination over the frog than horses with navicular pain.[46,47]

The first step in the treatment of palmar hoof pain is accurate assessment of the pain and careful evaluation of hoof structure that may predispose to or cause the pain. The examination of the foot has been previously described in this chapter.

Typically, all causes of lameness in the palmar foot will be improved by at least 90% after perineural analgesia of the palmar digital nerves. Analgesia of the distal interphalangeal (DIP) joint and the navicular bursa are additional procedures that provide localizing information about palmar hoof pain. The pain relief by anesthesia of any of these three regions has been shown to overlap.[48] Further, identification of neuroreceptors for the navicular bone and navicular region have indicated how these other diagnostic techniques may help differentiate these clinical conditions. The DIP joint and navicular bursa do not communicate, and yet the response to local anesthesia injected into these synovial cavities is similar.[49] Both cavities have in common the navicular bone, the impar ligament, and the collateral sesamoidean ligament (proximal suspensory ligament of the navicular bone). The neuroreceptors for the navicular bone are in these two ligaments and can be anesthetized from either synovial cavity.[50] Furthermore, Bowker et al. have shown that the palmar digital nerve is in very close proximity to the medial and lateral limits of the bursa and that the nerve may be anesthetized at this level whenever the bursa is injected.[51]

Diagnostic confirmation

Radiographic examination is the imaging method most often used to assess osseous changes in the navicular bone. These changes with the exception of fractures are usually not pathognomonic but do provide insight into damage that has occurred to the foot.

Scintigraphy provides information on relative vascularity and rate of tissue metabolism. This is particularly useful in studying bone pathology and can help differentiate sites of injury in the foot. High-detail scintigraphy of the foot obtained using a skyline view can localize inflammation specifically to the navicular bone or to other structures in the palmar heel region.

Magnetic resonance imaging (MRI) has helped identify many specific causes for heel and distal limb pain. If diagnostic analgesia localizes pain to the foot and radiography is not consistent with the level of pain, MRI is indicated to further identify potentials lesions in the foot. Also, if initial treatment of the foot pain has been unrewarding, MRI is indicated (Fig. 14.18 and Fig. 14.19).[13]

It is clear that the diagnosis of navicular disease and palmar heel pain is facilitated by noting the response to diagnostic analgesia. However, as discussed earlier in this chapter, none of the diagnostic anesthesia procedures employed results in specific desensitization of a single anatomic site. The diagnostician must use physical findings, response to diagnostic anesthesia, and imaging to determine the specific diagnosis.

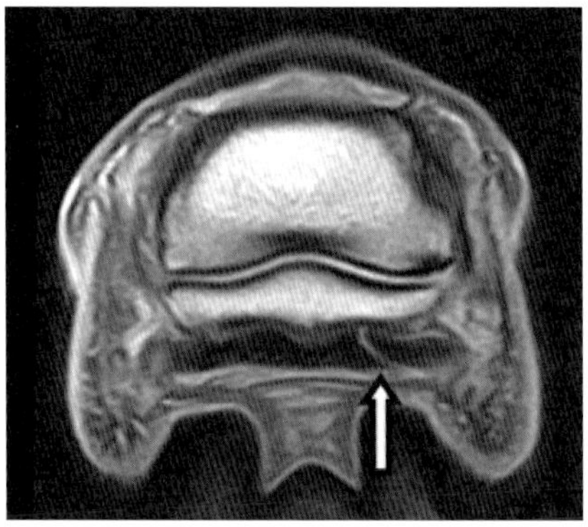

Fig 14.18 Transverse T1 sequence magnetic resonance image at the level of the navicular bone. A sagittal split in the lateral lobe of the deep digital flexor tendon is evident (arrow).

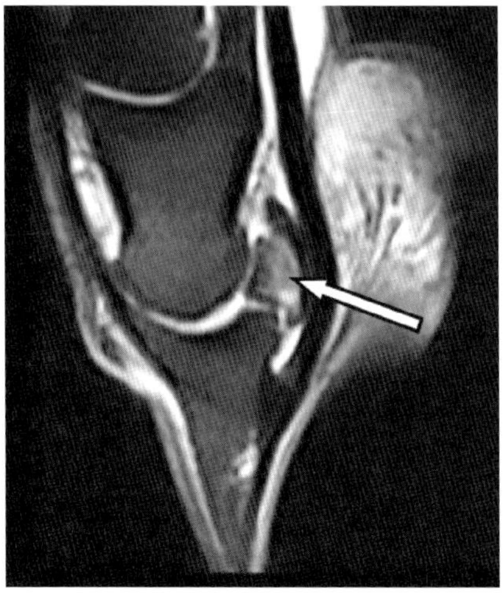

Fig 14.19 Sagittal STIR sequence magnetic resonance image with increased signal (more white) of the navicular bone (arrow) indicative of bone edema.

Treatment and prognosis

Therapeutic aims

Palmar heel pain is treated primarily by correcting hoof balance abnormalities, providing improved heel support, easing breakover and adding concussion protection to the foot. Anti-inflammatory medications and peripheral vasodilating agents can also be utilized, but often play a secondary roll to corrective shoeing in the treatment of this type of lameness. If soft tissue injuries are identified, arthroscopic debridement of deep digital flexor injuries may be indicated and regenerative medicine treatments such as platelet-rich plasma (PRP) or bone marrow derived stem cells may be injected within the lesions to facilitate healing (see Chapter 9).

Therapy

Treatment must be tailored specifically to the hoof characteristics and use of the horse. Corrective shoeing and anti-inflammatory medication are the basis of initial therapy.

The most successful approach to shoeing is that based on individual case needs rather than a standard formula. The following principles should be followed:

1. Correct any pre-existing problems of the hoof such as underrun heels, contracted heels, sheared heels, mismatched hoof angles, or broken hoof/pastern axis.
2. Trimming and shoeing must allow for use of all weight-bearing structures of the foot.
3. Allow for hoof expansion.
4. Facilitate break over.

The importance of a balanced foot in the treatment of equine lameness is well recognized. Six hoof balance abnormalities have been described: broken hoof axis, underrun heels, contracted heels, shear heels, mismatched hoof angles, and small feet. A broken hoof axis exists when the slopes of the pastern and hoof are not the same. This condition is further defined as broken-back, when the hoof angle is lower than the pastern angle, and as broken-forward when the hoof angle is steeper than the pastern angle. Underrun heels have been defined as angle of the heels of 5° less than the toe angle. Contracted heels were defined as frog width less than 67% of the frog length. Sheared heels have been defined as a disparity between the medial and lateral heel lengths of 0.5 cm or more.

One of the most difficult parameters to assess is the hoof's ability to expand. Expansion of the foot is necessary for optimal concussion protection. Protection from concussion also depends on an elastic frog/digital cushion and pliable collateral cartilages.[52] Applied clinical studies have shown that the frog size influences hoof expansion. A frog in contact with the shoe or ground surface provides more hoof expansion than a frog that has no contact.[53] Identification of a narrow, recessed frog should alert the clinician that steps need to be taken to promote hoof expansion. This may vary from simply ensuring proper heel support and not nailing the shoe palmar to the hoof quarters to encouraging hoof expansion through the use of swedged or slipper heels on the shoes.

As previously discussed, shoeing parameters must be individualized for each horse. However, in most horses with heel pain the following changes are made in most instances. Trim and balance the feet to eliminate hoof-pastern axis abnormalities and underrun heels. Lateromedial radiographs should be used to determine hoof/pastern axis and to assess improvement of the axis following shoeing (Fig. 14.3). Shoe the horse to raise the heels 2–3°, ease break over by rolling the toe, and provide heel support for horses with underrun heels. If necessary, the shoe may be set slightly palmar to the natural toe to set the break over point further palmar. Decrease concussion to the foot by providing more surface area of contact (wide-web) or padding. Horses with contracted heels may benefit from shoes that encourage heel expansion during weight bearing, such as swedged heel shoes (outside rim of shoe at the heels is slightly lower than the inside rim: during weight bearing the hoof is encouraged to 'slide out'), or shoes that are not nailed caudal to the quarters. These practices will decrease stress on the DDFT and pressure of the DDFT over the navicular bone. Effective shoe types include wide-web aluminum shoes (more concussion protection than steel, less weight on distal limb) and egg bar shoes (provide heel support). Egg bar shoes may be filled in with resilient sole packing material to increase the surface area of weight bearing and provide further concussion protection.

Inflammation is reduced by systemic administration of phenylbutazone (4.4 mg/kg daily) for up to 30 days. The DIP joint may also be medicated with triamcinolone (10 mg) and hyaluronic acid (HA; 20 mg). The intra-articular medication will treat coffin joint arthrosis directly, and also diffuse to navicular structures.[54]

Medication injected into the navicular bursa resulted in soundness for an average of seven months in 74% of horses treated.[55] The best response was in horses with navicular bursitis only. Treatment with HA or PSGAGs by intramuscular or intravenous routes is supportive and may prolong the interval between intra-synovial injections of medication.

Tiludronate is a bisphosphonate medication that is indicated for treatment of navicular disease and osteoarthritis. The drug reduces the bone resorption and modeling that occurs with degenerative changes in the navicular bone and other sites. A dose of 1 mg/kg is administered as an intravenous infusion, and followed up in two months with a second dose is effective in reducing navicular bone pain and edema. In a study evaluating efficacy of tiludronate for navicular pain, 0.5 mg/kg and 1 mg/kg doses were compared in horses with recent and chronic onset of navicular bone pain. The 1 mg/kg dose resulted in improvement and return to normal activity of 42% of horses at two months and 67% of horses at six months after the administration of one dose. The 0.5 mg/kg dose resulted in return to normal activity of 33% of horses at two months and 55% of horses at six months.[56] Tiludronate is also administered in horses that have bone edema identified with MRI imaging.

Surgical options for treatment of navicular syndrome and palmar heel pain include: tenoscopy/bursoscopy, navicular suspensory desmotomy and neurectomy. Arthroscopic tenoscopy/bursoscopy allows for direct visualization of tendon injuries and the opportunity to debride navicular bone flexor surface lesions, tendon lesions and adhesions.[57,58] Outcomes are improved following arthroscopic debridement of tendon lesions compared to medical treatment alone. For comparison, in horses with a deep digital flexor tendon lesion as the primary cause of lameness, 60% of horses returned to full work and soundness following arthroscopic surgery, while 28% resolved with medical treatment.[57,59]

Desmotomy of the collateral sesamoidean ligaments (CSL) had been historically indicated in horses not responding to medication and shoeing. The desmotomy involves transecting the ligaments near their origin on the distal abaxial aspect of the proximal phalanx at the level of the proximal interphalangeal joint. This results in less than complete release of the ligament as there are other attachments of the CSL to the abaxial surface of the middle phalanx. Seventy-six percent of horses treated with this technique were sound six months following surgery, with 43% sound at 36 months. Horses that were lame less than 10 months at the time of surgery were more likely to be sound than horses that were lame longer than 18 months.[60] A technique for transaction of the CSL immediately proximal to the navicular bone has been reported. This arthroscopically guided technique results in complete release of the ligament and has not been evaluated in clinical cases.[61]

Neurectomy is the last option for treatment. Complications may be expected in 30% of the horses following neurectomy and include incomplete denervation, regrowth of nerves, neuroma formation, unrecognized injury/abscess at the desensitized heels.[62] In a follow-up study of neurectomy, 74% of horses were sound one year after surgery with 63% sound two years after the procedure.[62]

Prognosis

Shoeing alone is a very effective method to treat heel pain and navicular syndrome. When correction is made within the first 10 months of lameness, up to 96% of horses are successfully treated. This is in contrast to when shoeing changes are not made until after one year of lameness, where only 56% of the cases have been successfully treated.[63] Addition of medications such as phenylbutazone also improve soundness of horses with palmar foot pain. Horses with multiple lesions in the heel region such as soft tissue injuries, damage to the flexor surface of the navicular bone and/or avulsion fragments at the distal border of the navicular bone have a poor prognosis for soundness with medical therapy.[64]

Etiology and pathophysiology

Etiology

Causes of heel pain are multifactorial. A combination of repeated overloading of the navicular bone and/or soft tissue support structures may results in desmitis, tendinitis or navicular bone degenerative changes.[65]

Pathophysiology

A unifying hypothesis for the cause of navicular disease which is based on pathologic findings has been described by Pool et al.[66] Changes associated with navicular syndrome are thought to be similar to degenerative joint disease found elsewhere in the horse. Repeated excessive biomechanical stresses on the flexor surface of the navicular bone result in fibrocartilage degeneration. Decreased shock absorption by the cartilage results in subchondral bone sclerosis. Defects in the cartilage may fill with granulation tissue, which can lead to adhesions between the navicular bone and DDFT. Inflammation associated with these degenerative changes causes excessive bone resorption, especially around synovial tissue attachments and may result in the increased synovial fossae of the distal border and medullary cysts seen on radiographic examinations.

Predisposing factors for lameness of the palmar heel region include faulty conformation such as long toe/ underrun heel, long sloping pastern, and small foot for large body mass. Horses used for jumping, or which are used frequently on hard footing, are also predisposed to this lameness.

Miscellaneous diseases of the distal limb

Underrun heels

Underrun heels have been defined as occurring when the angle at the heels is 5° less than the toe angle. Underrun heels are the most commonly encountered hoof abnormality (see Fig. 14.1). If left uncorrected, underrun heels can cause alterations in hoof-wall growth that can be very difficult to correct and it can predispose to lameness problems that range from bruised heels to navicular syndrome. In dealing with underrun heels it is important to assess several factors. The first is palmar hoof support. This is most easily assessed by radiography and observing where the heel ground contact is relative to the widest part of the hoof and relative to the navicular bone. It is generally accepted that at least half of the weight-bearing area of the foot should be palmar to the widest part of the foot. If this is not the case, the second assessment is of the orientation of the horn tubules in the heel region. With long-term hoof imbalance these tubules grow more horizontally. The proper position of the heels can be determined by either drawing a bisecting line through the metacarpus to the ground or by measuring the appropriate position on the radiograph. Where these lines contact the ground is the point where the heels should be. From a practical point, the heel-ground contact should be even with the base of the frog. Shoeing to achieve adequate heel support can frequently restore the foot health. In some cases, however, it requires rebuilding the heels with acrylics or urethanes and altering the stresses on the coronary band to get the heel growth to improve. Some cases if uncorrected for too long, simply cannot be corrected.

Upright hoof

The upright or 'club' hoof is another frequently encountered problem. Most veterinarians consider this to be a problem when the hoof angle exceeds 60°. However, a more important consideration is the hoof-pastern axis. This axis should form a straight line when the horse is standing square. When the pastern angle is less than the hoof angle, this causes a 'broken forward' hoof axis. The problem with this conformation is that in order to correct it, the hoof angle must be decreased. However, if the difference is more than 5°, the deep flexor tendon will not allow further correction.

This can lead to several problems, such as hoof capsule separation, toe bruising, and coffin joint inflammation. A number of correction possibilities exists. In horses less than two years of age, extensions are placed on the toe either by shoeing or the application of acrylics or urethanes. This will cause stretching of the deep flexor tendon and muscle and slowly allow the hoof to assume a normal conformation. A problem with this method is that the stretching can actually lead to tendon injury and in some cases cause the problem to become worse.

A unique approach that has merit especially in acute cases is the use of heel wedges and rest. Raising the heel reduces deep flexor tendon stress and rest will allow the flexor muscle and tendon to relax. Wedges are continued for approximately two weeks. The hoof may then be trimmed or shod in a normal position. If shoeing fails to correct the axis deviation correction of this problem can always be made by inferior check (accessory ligament of the DDFT) desmotomy. Transection of the check ligament permits elongation of the flexor tendon/muscle unit. Application of a corrective shoe or acrylic toe extension is usually performed at the time of surgery. Correction of the hoof abnormality is critical to the success of club-foot confirmation due to deep digital flexor tendon contracture.

Distal interphalangeal (coffin) joint arthrosis

Distal interphalangeal (DIP) joint arthrosis is a lameness referable to the distal limb and localized to the distal interphalangeal joint with no evident radiographic abnormalities. This lameness is commonly found in many performance horses, particularly racing Quarter Horses, polo ponies, and horses that compete over fences. Horses that respond to DIP joint anesthesia should be treated for inflammation of that joint. Treatment may include parenteral NSAID therapy but intra-articular therapy or specific joint therapy should be considered. Hyaluronan and corticosteroids are commonly injected within the DIP joint for treatment.

Occasionally, horses affected with DIP joint arthrosis also have a chronic broken forward hoof-pastern axis. Many of these cases appear to be mild flexural deformities. Because of the malarticulation of the second and distal phalanges, the joint may remain inflamed despite therapy. In these cases, inferior check desmotomy to allow correction of the broken forward axis has been a very useful method to correct the hoof-pastern axis.

Keratoma

Keratoma is a rare benign tumor produced by the keratin-producing cells of the coronary band. The tumor becomes a space-occupying mass that causes pressure necrosis of the soft tissues and distal phalanx resulting in lameness, and may cause drainage from the white line or coronary band. Differential diagnoses include distal phalanx fracture, deep sole abscess, 'gravel', or corn. The diagnosis is suggested by radiographs that show smooth, circumscribed lysis of the distal phalanx. Treatment is excision via an approach through the hoof wall or sole. The mass is reminiscent of an onion: it has many layers that must be peeled away.

Collateral cartilage: side bone, quittor

Side bone is normal mineralization of the collateral cartilages and occurs in most adult horses. Mineralization may be accelerated by local trauma and is more prevalent in draft horses. Lameness is rarely associated with side bone but excessive mineralization could interfere with expansion of the heels during weight bearing. Rarely, a portion of the mineralized collateral cartilage may fracture, causing significant lameness (Fig. 14.20).[67] Treatment involves stall or paddock confinement and shoeing to reduce expansion and contraction of the hoof capsule. Significant mineralization of collateral cartilages is associated with injury of the collateral ligaments of the distal interphalangeal joint.[68]

Quittor is infection and necrosis of the collateral cartilages, usually due to trauma. The horse has localized pain and swelling at the coronary band region of the heels and may have a draining tract. Treatment is excision of the affected cartilage.

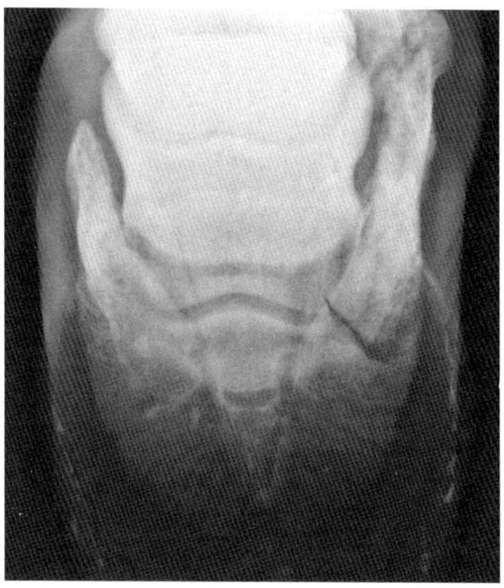

Fig 14.20 Dorsal oblique (D60Pr-PaDiO) radiographic view of the distal phalanx with a fracture evident at the base of the lateral collateral cartilage.

Thrush

Thrush is a degenerative condition of the frog and sulci due to excessive moisture, poor hoof hygiene, or filthy stabling conditions. It is characterized by a dark gray or black discharge around the frog, and poor-quality frog tissue. *Fusobacterium necrophorum* is frequently isolated from thrush-affected feet. Treatment consists of paring away affected tissue, cleaning the environment and providing dry bedding, and application of astringents. Simple cases respond well to daily application of povidone-iodine but formalin, phenol, strong tincture iodine, and copper sulfate have also been used alone or in varying combinations.

Canker

Canker is an uncommonly encountered chronic proliferation of the keratinized tissues of the sole and/or frog and is usually associated with poor foot hygiene (Fig. 14.21). Canker may initially appear similar to proliferative granulation tissue but the tissue usually becomes white in color, bleeds easily on manipulation, and has a bad odor. Purulent exudate is often admixed with the tissue. Lameness is usually present because the proliferative tissue is very sensitive. Differential diagnosis includes severe thrush, large 'corns', and extensive underrun sole abscess.

Treatment is difficult and involves debridement of the proliferative tissue, cleaning the foot surfaces and application of topical antibiotics and astringents. The proliferative tissue may be removed with electrocautery, laser, or with cryosurgery. Astringents such as 5% picric acid or 10% neutral buffered formalin solution may be applied to the tissue. Debridement of the tissue is gradually made manually or by applying a saturated solution of benzoyl peroxide dissolved in acetone daily until the excessive keratinized tissue is all debrided. Metronidazole tablets ground into a powder and applied to the tissues are effective at controlling the bacterial infection. Prognosis for successful treatment is always guarded.

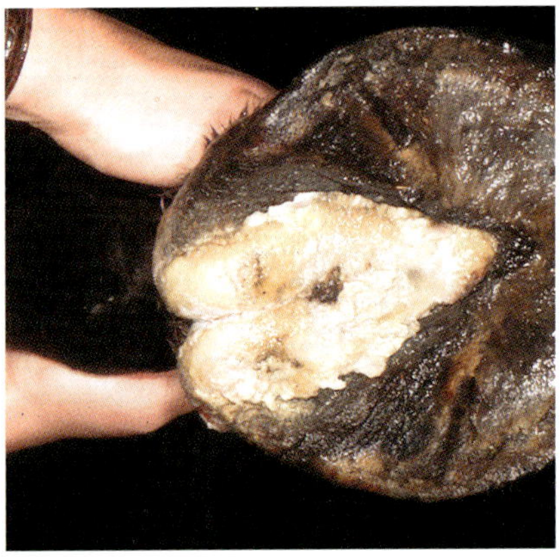

Fig 14.21 Palmar view of a foot with severe canker affecting the frog. The white tissue now comprising the frog is very friable and bleeds easily. The horse is lame because the tissue is very sensitive to pressure.

Corns

Corns are usually found in the front feet at the angle formed by the hoof wall and bars. Shoes left on too long or shoes that overlap the bars and frog too much and irritate these tissues are implicated in the formation of corns. Corns may be dry, moist or suppurating. The tissue often appears similar to proliferative granulation tissue, but is usually only found in a localized area at the heels. The tissue is usually quite sensitive to palpation. Treatment is similar to that used for canker, but usually does not require extensive tissue debridement.

Sole bruise

Sole bruises occur when vessels in the solar corium are traumatized and bleed. The hemorrhage is trapped with the solar tissues and causes varying degrees of lameness. Bruises are evident as discoloration of the affected sole that is painful to hoof tester application. Occasionally bruises will become contaminated and develop into a subsolar abscess.

Poor-fitting shoes, thin soles, and riding on hard terrain all are potential factors that contribute to solar bruising. Initial treatment is administration of NSAIDs, application of a foot poultice and removal of any inciting cause. Poor fitting or loose shoes should be removed. When the initial discomfort resolves the shoe should be reset. A full pad should also be used for feet with extensive bruising.

With thanks to Tracy A. Turner, who co-created the original chapter in the first edition.

References

1. Dyce KM, Sack WO, Wensing CJG, editors. Textbook of Veterinary Anatomy. 2nd ed. St. Louis: Saunders; 1996.
2. Bowker RM. Functional anatomy of the palmar aspect of the foot. In: Ross MW, Dyson SJ, editors. Lameness in the Horse. St. Louis: Elsevier; 2011.
3. Bowker RM, Linder K, Van Wulfen KK, et al. Anatomy of the distal interphalangeal joint of the mature horse: relationships with the navicular suspensory ligaments, sensory nerves and neurovasdcular bundle. Equine Vet J 1997;29(2):126–35.
4. Moyer W. Clinical examination of the equine foot. Vet Clin NAm Equine Pract 1989;5(1):29–46.
5. Balch O, White KK, Butler D. Factors involved in the balancing of equine hooves. J Am Vet Med Assoc 1991; 198(7):1980–9.
6. Turner TA. The art and frustration of hoof balance. Am Farriers J 2002;28(6): 1A–8A.
7. Turner TA. The use of hoof measurements for the objective assessment of hoof balance. Proc Am Assoc Equine Pract 1992;38:157–64.
8. Turner TA. Predictive value of diagnostic tests for navicular pain. Proc Am Assoc Equine Pract 1996;42:201–4.
9. Butler JA, Colles CM, Dyson SJ, et al. Clinical radiology of the horse. 3rd ed. London: Blackwell Scientific; 2008
10. Sage AM, Turner TA. Ultrasonography of the soft tissues of the equine foot. Eq Vet Educ 2002;4:278–83.
11. Dyson S, Murray R, Schramme M, et al. Magnetic resonance imaging of the equine foot: 15 horses. Equine Vet J. 2003;35(1):18–26.
12. Widmer WR, Buckwalter KA, Fessler JF, et al. Use of radiography, computed tomography and magnetic resonance imaging for evaluation of navicular syndrome in the horse. Vet Radiol Ultrasound 2000;41(2):108–16.
13. Dyson S, Murray R. Magnetic resonance imaging evaluation of 264 horses with foot pain: The podotrochlear apparatus, deep digital flexor tendon and collateral

ligaments of the distal interphalangeal joint. Equine Vet J 2007;39(4):340–3.

14. Busoni V, Heimann M, Trenteseaux J, et al. Magnetic resonance imaging findings in the equine deep digital flexor tendon and distal sesamoid bone in advanced navicular disease—an ex vivo study. Vet Radiol Ultrasound 2005;46(4):279–86.
15. Richardson GL, O'Brien TR, Pascoe JR, et al. Puncture wounds of the navicular bursa in 38 horses: a retrospective study. Vet Surg 1986;15:156–60.
16. Wright IM, Phillips TJ, Walmsley JP. Endoscopy of the navicular bursa: a new technique for treatment of contaminated and septic bursae. Equine Vet J 1999;31: 5–11.
17. Baxter GM. Acute laminitis. Vet Clin N Am Equine Pract 1994;10(3):627–42.
18. Hunt RJ. A retrospective evaluation of laminitis. Equine Vet J 1993;25:61–4.
19. Peloso JG, Cohen ND, Walker MA, et al. Case-control study of risk factors for development of laminitis in the contralateral limb in Equidae with unilateral lameness. J Am Vet Med Assoc 1996;209:1746–8.
20. Linford RL, O'Brien TR, Trout DR. Qualitative and morphometric radiographic findings in the distal phalanx and digital soft tissues of sound Thoroughbred racehorses. Am J Vet Res 1993;54:38–51.
21. Stick JS, Jann HW, Scott EA, et al. Pedal bone rotation as a prognostic sign in laminitic horses. J Am Vet Med Assoc 1982;180:251–3.
22. Hunt RJ. Diagnosing and treating chronic laminitis in horses. Vet Med 1996;91: 1025–32.
23. van Eps AW, Leise BS, Watts M, et al. Digital hypothermia inhibits early lamellar inflammatory signaling in the oligofructose laminitis model. Equine Vet J 2012;44(2):230–7.
24. Reesink HL, Divers TJ, Bookbinder LC, et al. 230Cryotherapy of the Equine Digit for the Treatment of Laminitis: Assessment of a Novel Method by Measuring Digital Venous Temperature. Proc Am Assoc Equine Pract 2010;56:149.
25. Blythe LL, Craig AM, Christensen JM, et al. Pharmacokinetic disposition of dimethyl sulfoxide administered intravenously to horses. Am J Vet Med Assoc 1986;47:1739–43.
26. Adair HS, Goble DO, Shires GM, et al. Evaluation of laser Doppler flowmetry for measuring coronary band and laminar microcirculatory blood flow in clinically normal horses. Am J Vet Res 1994;55:445–9.
27. Pollitt CC. Laminitis (Founder). In: Orsini JA, Divers TJ, editors. Equine Emergencies. 3rd ed. St. Louis: Saunders; 2008.
28. Cohen ND, Parson EM, Seahorn TL, et al. Prevalence and factors associated with laminitic horses with duodenitis/proximal jejunitis: 116 cases (1985–1991). J Am Vet Med Assoc 1994;204: 250–4.
29. Redden RF. 18° elevation of the heel as an aid to treating acute and chronic laminitis in the equine. Proc Am Assoc Equine Pract 1992;37:375–9.
30. Ramsey GD, Hunter PJ, Nash MP. The effect of hoof angle variations on dorsal lamellar load in the equine hoof. Equine Vet J 2001;43(5):536–42.
31. Hunt RJ, Allen D, Baxter GM, et al. Mid-metacarpal deep digital flexor tenotomy in the management of refractory laminitis in horses. Vet Surg 1991;20:15–20.
32. Cripps PJ, Eustace RA. Factors involved in the prognosis of equine laminitis in the UK. Equine Vet J 1999;31(5):433–42.
33. Pollitt CC, Davies CT. Equine laminitis: its development coincides with increased sublamellar blood flow. Equine Vet J (Suppl.) 1998;26:125–32.
34. Trout DR, Hornof WJ, Linford RL, et al. Scintigraphic evaluation of digital circulation during the developmental and acute phases of equine laminitis. Equine Vet J 1990;22(6):416–21.
35. Pollitt CC. Equine laminitis: a revised pathophysiology. Proc Am Assoc Equine Pract 1999;45:188–92.
36. Molyneux GS, Haller CJ, Mogg K, et al. The structure, innervation and location of arteriovenous anastomoses in the equine foot. Equine Vet J 1994;26(4): 305–12.
37. Katwa LC, Johnson PJ, Ganjam VK, et al. Expression of endothelin in equine laminitis. Equine Vet J 1999;31(3): 243–7.
38. Honnas CM, O'Brien TR, Linford RL. Distal phalanx fractures in horses: a survey of 274 horses with radiographic assessment of healing in 36 horses. Vet Radiol 1988;29:98–100.
39. Honnas CM, O'Brien TR, Linford RL. Solar margin fractures of the equine distal phalanx. Proc Am Assoc Equine Pract 1987;33:399–410.
40. Yovich JV. Fractures of the distal phalanx in the horse. Vet Clin N Am Equine Pract 1989;5(1):145–60.
41. Kaneps AJ, O'Brien TR, Redden RF, et al. Characterisation of osseous bodies of the distal phalanx of foals. Equine Vet J 1993;25:285–92.
42. Kaneps AJ, O'Brien TR, Willits NH, et al. Effect of hoof trimming on the occurrence of distal phalangeal palmar process fractures in foals. Equine Vet J (Suppl.) 1998;26:36–45.
43. Yovich JV, Stashak TS, DeBowes RM, et al. Fractures of the distal phalanx of the forelimb in eight foals. J Am Vet Med Assoc 1986;189(5):550–4.
44. Lillich JD, Ruggles AJ, Gabel AA, et al. Fracture of the distal sesamoid bone in horses: 17 cases (1982–1992). J Am Vet Med Assoc 1995;207:924–7.
45. Turner TA. How to treat navicular bone fractures. Proc Am Assoc Equine Pract 1997;43:370–1.
46. Turner TA. Predictive value of diagnostic tests for navicular pain. Proc Am Assoc Equine Pract 1996;42:201–4.
47. Wright IM. A study of 118 cases of navicular disease: clinical features. Equine Vet J 1993;25:488–92.
48. Dyson SJ, Kidd L. A comparison of responses to analgesia of the navicular bursa and intra-articular analgesia of the distal interphalangeal joint in 59 horses. Equine Vet J 1993;25:93–8.
49. Bowker RM, Linder K, VanWulfen KK et al. Distribution of local anesthetic injected into the distal interphalangeal joint and podotrochlear bursa: an experimental study. Pferdeheilkunde 1996;12:609–12.
50. Van Wulfen KK, Bowker RM. Evaluation of tachykinins and their receptors to determine sensory innervation in the dorsal hoof wall and insertion of the distal sesamoidean impar ligament and deep digital flexor tendon on the distal phalanx in healthy feet of horses. Am J Vet Res 2002;63(2):222–8.
51. Bowker RM, Linder K, Van Wulfen KK, et al. Anatomy of the distal interphalangeal joint of the mature horse: relationships with navicular suspensory ligaments, sensory nerves and neurovascular bundle. Equine Vet J 1997;29(2):126–35.
52. Bowker RM, Van Wulfen KK, Springer SE, et al. Functional anatomy of the cartilage of the distal phalanx and digital cushion in the equine foot and a hemodynamic flow hypothesis of energy dissipation. Am J Vet Res 1998;59(8):961–8.
53. Roepstorff L, Johnston C, Drevemo S. In vivo and in vitro heel expansion in relation to shoeing and frog pressure. Equine Vet J (Suppl.) 2001;33:54–7.
54. Boyce M, Malone ED, Anderson LB, et al. Evaluation of diffusion of triamcinolone acetonide from the distal interphalangeal joint into the navicular bursa in horses. Am J Vet Res. 2010;71(2): 169–75.
55. Bell CD, Howard RD, Taylor S, et al. Outcomes of Podotrochlear (navicular) bursa injections for signs of foot pain in horses evaluated via magnetic resonance imaging: 23 cases (2005–2007). J Am Vet Med Assoc 2009;234:920–5.
56. Denoix JM, Thibaud D, Riccio B. Tiludronate as a new therapeutic agent in the treatment of navicular disease: a double-blind placebo-controlled clinical trial. Equine Vet J 2003;35(4):407–13.
57. Smith MR, Wright IM, Smith RK. Endoscopic assessment and treatment of lesions of the deep digital flexor tendon in the navicular bursae of 20 lame horses. Equine Vet J 2007;39(1):18–24.

58. Schramme MC. Treatment of deep digital flexor tendinitis in the foot. Equine Vet Educ 2008;20(7):389–91.
59. Dyson S, Murray R, Schramme M. (2005) Lameness associated with foot pain: results of MRI in 199 horses (January 2001–December 2003) and response to treatment. Equine Vet J 2005;37:113–21.
60. Wright IM. A study of 118 cases of navicular disease: treatment by navicular suspensory desmotomy. Equine Vet J 1993;25:501–9.
61. Sarah N, Sampson SN, Robert K, et al. Evaluation of an arthroscopic approach for transection of the equine collateral sesamoidean ligament. Vet Surgery 2010;39(8):1011–20.
62. Jackman BR, Baxter GM, Doran RE, et al. Palmar digital neurectomy in horses: 57 cases 1984–1990. Vet Surg 1993;22: 285–8.
63. Turner TA. Diagnosis and treatment of navicular disease in horses. Vet Clin N Am Equine Pract 1989;5:131–43.
64. Gutierrez-Nibeyro SD, White NA, Werpy NM. Outcome of medical treatment for horses with foot pain: 56 cases. Equine Vet J 2010;42(8):680–5.
65. Dyson S, Murray R, Blunden T, et al. Current concepts of navicular disease. Equine Vet Educ 2006;18(1): 45–56.
66. Pool RR, Meagher DM, Stover SM. Pathophysiology of navicular disease. Vet Clin N Am Equine Pract 1989;5:109–29.
67. Dakin SG, Robson KE, Dyson SJ. Fractures of the ossified cartilages of the foot: 10 cases. Equine Vet Educ 2006;18: 120–8.
68. Dyson S, Brown V, Collins S, et al. Is there an association between ossification of the cartilages of the foot and collateral desmopathy of the distal interphalangeal joint or distal phalanx injury? Equine Vet J 2010;42(6):504–11.

Distal limb: fetlock and pastern

15

Alicia L. Bertone

CHAPTER CONTENTS

Introduction

The fetlock joint is a rotary joint that can exhibit the greatest range of motion of any equine joint, ranging from 120° of extension to 120° of flexion, particularly during athletic events such as racing or jumping (Fig. 15.1). This high degree of activity makes this joint particularly susceptible to exercise-induced wear and indeed, the fetlocks are commonly associated with injury and signs of degenerative joint disease. The pastern joint, by contrast, is a low range of motion joint exhibiting ~30° range of motion in the normal horse (Fig. 15.2). The pastern is less frequently afflicted with injury or degenerative wear than the fetlock, although its location just above the hoof and at the termination of the suspensory apparatus makes it vulnerable to high-impact, traumatic injury. Degenerative joint disease (high ringbone) frequently follows pastern joint injury. The combination of high-impact loading during sport performance and the distal location of these joints puts them at higher risk for fractures and breakdown.

Fractures of the fetlock joint

- Signs include acute lameness that often resolves in days, joint effusion and pain on flexion.
- Radiography confirms the diagnosis.
- Treatment is arthroscopic removal or internal fixation based on size and location of fragment.

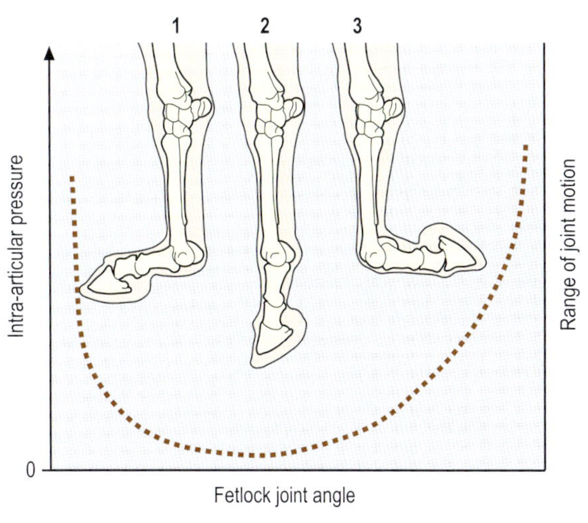

Fig 15.1 The wide range of joint motion and intra-articular pressures associated with the fetlock joint.

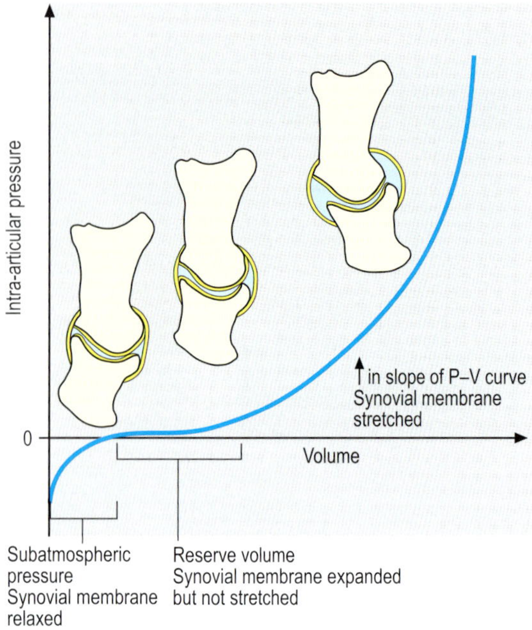

Fig 15.2 The low range of joint motion and intra-articular pressures associated with the pastern joint.

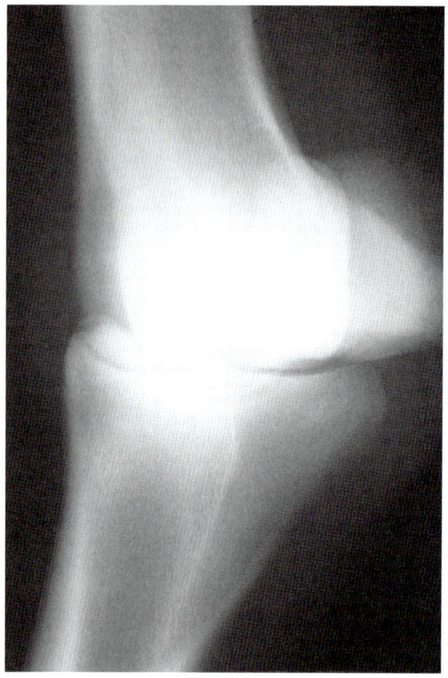

Fig 15.3 Dorsolateral to palmaromedial oblique radiograph of the fetlock joint demonstrating a typical dorsomedial eminence first phalanx osteochondral 'chip' fracture.

Osteochondral (chip) fractures

Recognition

History and presenting complaint

Most articular chip fractures of the fetlock are of the eminences of the proximal phalanx (P1) and are relatively common in the forelimb of the horse, particularly the sport horse (Fig. 15.3). In racehorses, the left forelimb and medial eminence are affected more often. Other less frequently occurring fractures of the fetlock include fractures of the palmar/plantar eminences which, if articular and small, can be successfully removed arthroscopically with a good prognosis (~70%) for return to performance. These fractures, however, may be associated with subluxation of the fetlock joint and/or disruption of a palmar/plantar osteochondrosis lesion.[1-3] Careful evaluation of the joint is indicated to identify this more complex injury which can include injury to the collateral ligaments and distal sesmoidean ligaments.

Palmar/plantar fractures of the proximal phalanx are uncommon and should not be confused with osteochondral fragmentation of this site in young growing horses.[3] Developmental osteochondral fragmentation of the caudal eminences of the proximal phalanx occurs in ~5% of Standardbreds and Thoroughbreds without clinical signs in most horses. Clinical signs can occur as a high-performance lameness in which case fragments can be arthroscopically removed. True fractures of the caudal eminences of the proximal phalanx usually cause lameness and soreness to direct pressure over the eminence. Developmental osteochondral fragmentation in this location should not induce pain to pressure.

Physical examination

Horses that sustain fetlock chip fractures develop clinical signs within hours after the injury. Clinical signs include fetlock joint effusion, pain on fetlock flexion and lameness at the trot. Soreness resolves within weeks with stall rest and anti-inflammatory medication. Chronic chip fractures are usually associated with generalized fetlock joint disease and may have capsular fibrosis, dorsal enlargement and reduced range of joint motion. Joint effusion, however, may or may not be present. Lameness may resolve with rest and return with athletic use.

Special examination

In chronic fractures of unknown contribution to a lameness, direct intra-articular fetlock anesthesia may be indicated to localize the soreness to the intra-articular structures. Resolution of the lameness with a fetlock block would support arthroscopic exploration and fragment removal.

Diagnostic confirmation

Diagnosis is confirmed with radiography, to include four views of the affected fetlock joint and the contralateral fetlock if surgery is to be considered. Osteochondral fragments are readily visible on the oblique radiographic views (see Fig. 15.3).

Nuclear scintigraphy can be used to distinguish fractures from incidental caudal eminence fragments.

Treatment and prognosis

Therapeutic aims

Osteochondral fragments are removed, usually with arthroscopy, to decrease painful synovitis and to prevent further degenerative joint disease.

Therapy

In horses with continued athletic expectations, acute fractures are preferably removed arthroscopically unless they are completely non-displaced. In non-displaced fractures a follow-up radiograph at 30 days is indicated as many of these fragments go on to displace and result in a non-union. In chronic chip fractures, other lesions commonly seen include proliferative synovitis of the dorsal metacarpal synovial pad (32% of which have chip fracture) and cartilage erosion of the metacarpal condyle.[4] Two to four months' rest is recommended before training is resumed depending on the degree of joint damage and cartilage debridement.

Fractures that continue to be a source of pain or are large enough to secure with a bone screw can be treated surgically. Injury to the collateral ligaments in conjunction with palmar/plantar fractures of the proximal phalanx should be supported by cast or support boot for 4–8 weeks to minimize joint laxity and osteoarthritis. Reconstruction of the ligament has been reported but is generally felt not to be necessary to regain use of the joint. Palmar/plantar eminence fracture healing is poor due to distraction by the distal sesmoidean ligament insertions and usually requires 4–6 months' rest.

Prognosis

The prognosis for return to athletic performance, including elite performance, is ~80% with arthroscopic surgery to remove fragments. Concomitant injuries to the fetlock lower the prognosis.[5–8]

Etiology and pathogenesis

Etiology

Concussion and overextension of the joint, exacerbated by fatigue, are factors in the production of these fractures and suspensory apparatus injury (Fig. 15.4). The overextension causes pinching of the dorsal eminences and dorsal metacarpal synovial pad.

Prevention

Incidence of fracture may be reduced by use of elastic bandages placed over the fetlock in a snug figure-of-eight configuration during hard workouts. The bandage absorbs some of the kinetic energy in the limb, thereby reducing the kinetic energy absorbed by the tissues supporting the fetlock.

Proximal sesamoid bone fractures

- Sesamoid fractures are most common in racehorses.
- Apical fractures occur most commonly, followed by basilar and midbody fractures.
- Treatment is excision for fragments less than one-third the size of the entire bone and internal fixation for larger fractures.
- Prognosis may be affected by suspensory branch desmitis.

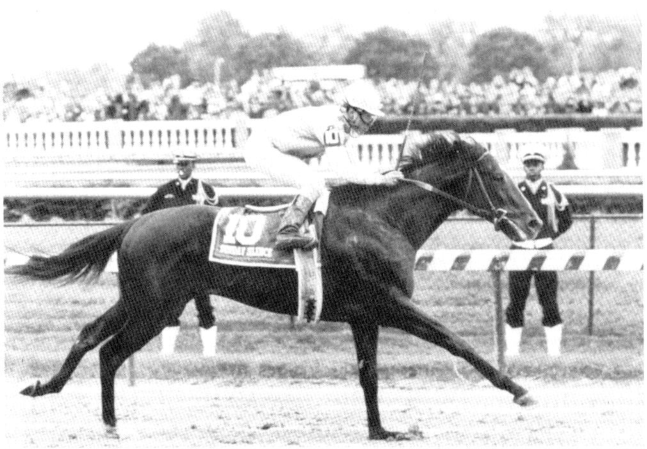

Fig 15.4 Finish-line photograph demonstrating the extreme dorsiflexion of the fetlock joint at the finish of the race with fatigue and maximal loading.

Fractures of the proximal sesamoid bones are a common fracture of the fetlock joint. Most are articular although non-articular (suspensory avulsion) fractures occur and can be distinguished by lack of joint effusion and firm swelling over the caudal aspect of the bone. Fetlock breakdown, including sesamoid fractures, is the most common fatal fracture in racing Thoroughbreds and Quarter Horses.[9] Sesamoid fractures are categorized as apical, abaxial (articular and non-articular), midbody, basilar (articular and non-articular), sagittal and comminuted.[10]

Sesamoid fractures are most common (53.4%) in two-year-old and then three-year-old (23%) racehorses. Apical sesamoid fractures are the most common, comprising over 88% of sesamoid fractures with an approximately equal distribution between the right and left limbs (Fig. 15.5). Apical fractures are frequently articular and singular, rarely comminuted and usually involve less than one-third of the bone.

Basilar fractures are more common in the Thoroughbred than the Standardbred, comprise 6% of sesamoid fractures in Standardbreds and represent an avulsion fracture associated with the distal sesamoidean ligaments. Basilar fractures are often comminuted into two pieces through a sagittal separation. These fractures can vary in size, from the smaller, triangular articular pieces to the larger fragments with a significant non-articular component.

Abaxial fractures appear to be more common in Thoroughbreds and Quarter Horses than in Standardbreds (3% of sesamoid fractures).[11,12] These can be difficult to diagnose and may require an additional tangential projection on the radiographic examination to identify their exact location or can be identified on the craniocaudal view.[13] Articular abaxial fractures will have joint effusion.

The midbody transverse fracture is seen most frequently in the Thoroughbred, older Standardbreds (mean age 6.5 years) and in young foals under two months of age. Most have a several millimeter gap and are distracted at the caudal surface. Fracture of both sesamoids usually results in complete loss of suspensory support and a 'dropped' fetlock (hyperextended during loading).[10]

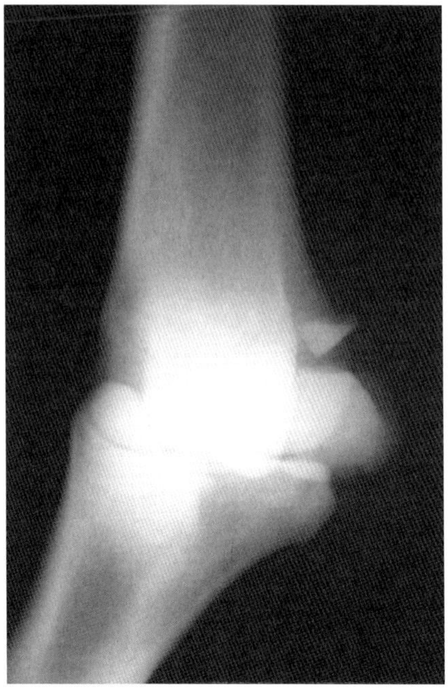

Fig 15.5 Oblique radiograph of a typical displaced apical sesamoid fracture. Recommended treatment is arthroscopic removal.

Recognition

History and presenting complaint

As with other fetlock fractures, horses become lame with joint effusion within hours of injury. Non-articular sesamoid fractures may not have joint effusion and swelling may be directly over the abaxial surface of the sesamoid.

Physical examination

Clinical signs include lameness which is very pronounced in acute stages. Associated suspensory desmitis may confuse the diagnosis if radiographs are not taken. The horse evidences pain when pressure is applied to the affected bone. After 1–2 weeks' rest, lameness at the walk and trot may not be obvious but joint effusion persists.

Diagnostic confirmation

Diagnosis is confirmed with radiography (see Fig. 15.5). Non-displaced fractures may be hard to see with plain radiography. The addition of the skyline projection of the abaxial surface of the sesamoid bone may help identify the exact location of fractures on the abaxial surface.[13] Suspicious but unconfirmed fractures should have a repeat radiograph taken after 2–4 weeks of stall rest or nuclear scintigraphy can be performed.

Treatment and prognosis

Therapeutic aims

Most fractures should be surgically removed, usually arthroscopically, for the fastest return to athletic function and soundness. Large fractures may be best treated with internal fixation. Stall rest may be satisfactory for incomplete sesamoid bone fractures.

Therapy

Preferred treatment for articular sesamoid fractures (apical, basilar or abaxial) of less than one-third of the bone is arthroscopic removal to provide the most rapid return to athletic use and least risk of degenerative joint disease and sesamoid reinjury. Stall rest (with or without soft cast or external coaptation) for 3–4 months may achieve fibrous or partial bony union, but management is prolonged, weakening of the bone is anticipated and continued soreness or refracture can occur due to failure of complete bony union.[12–17] Non-articular fractures can be removed, but conservative treatment is considered to produce similar outcomes and is generally recommended. Midbody transverse fractures affecting the middle third of the proximal sesamoid bones can be treated successfully with lag screw fixation or circumferential wiring to provide postoperative bone compression and immobilization.[13,18–21]

Fractures involving disruption of both sesamoid bones are a common cause of breakdown in speed horses.[9] Many of these horses are humanely euthanized due to compounding of the injury (disruption of the skin) or loss of vascular supply. Horses without an open injury and with immediate support to the limb with a support splint can be salvaged for breeding or retirement. The preferred management is appropriately timed surgical arthrodesis for the fastest return to comfort and to reduce the risk of contralateral laminitis from overloading[22] (see Fetlock luxation below). Fractures of the sesamoid can occur in conjunction with a condylar fracture of the metacarpus or metatarsus. This concomitant injury significantly reduces the prognosis for returning to sport athletics even with repair of the condylar fracture.[23] These sesamoid fractures are usually sagittal and axial from avulsion of the intersesmoidean ligament that occurs when the condylar fracture displaces. The fractures indicate significant soft tissue injury to the fetlock joint and degenerative joint disease is likely to develop.

Prognosis

The prognosis for most simple sesamoid fractures ranges from fair to excellent. Eighty-eight percent of Standardbreds with apical fractures,[24] 71% of Thoroughbred or Quarter Horse racehorses with abaxial fractures,[12] 50–60% of Thoroughbreds with basilar fractures[14,17] and 50–60% of Standardbreds with midbody fractures repaired by either lag screw fixation or circumferential wiring can return to racing.[18,19] Conservatively managed basilar or midbody fractures are most likely to develop significant degenerative joint disease and restricted range of joint motion. If both sesamoids are fractured, the prognosis is less favorable.

Etiology and pathogenesis

Etiology

Sesamoid fractures are a result of excessive forces within the bone, generated by the tension of the suspensory apparatus during loading and occasionally contributed by direct concussion with the ground during fatigue–fetlock 'rundown'[11,13,14,23] (see Fig. 15.4). The forelimbs are most frequently affected in flat racing, whereas the hindlimbs are more frequently affected in Standardbreds. Displaced fractures are common due to the pull of the suspensory ligament proximally and the distal sesamoidean ligaments distally.

Severe blunt trauma to the sesamoid bone can cause highly comminuted fractures. The fetlock can contact the ground in an athletic event or at the time of a uniaxial sesamoid fracture. Fractures caused by 'running down' or interference are most likely to also contain a wound.

Pathophysiology

Although the vascular pattern of sesamoid bones may be implicated in site selection of fractures as the orientation and distribution of vessels correspond to the configuration of apical fracture patterns,[25] the sesamoid fracture or the predisposition for sesamoid fracture has not been associated with the presence of sesamoiditis. Sesamoiditis describes a condition of sesamoid pain that demonstrates radiographic lucencies which parallel vascular channels seen radiographically.[25]

Prevention

Protective and support bandages for the fetlock can be worn during hard workouts to help prevent direct injury to the sesamoid and to reduce strain in the suspensory apparatus during loading. Appropriate training can result in strengthening and conditioning of the bone which is important to help prevent sesamoid fractures. Smooth racing surfaces may help prevent missteps.

Longitudinal fractures of the first phalanx

- Fractures may be complete or incomplete.
- Most fractures are treated with internal fixation.
- Some proximal incomplete fractures will heal with stall rest.

The first phalanx is prone to sagittal and, less commonly, frontal plane longitudinal fractures that occur during heavy exercise (Fig. 15.6). Almost all of these fractures are initiated at the articular surface of the fetlock joint and propagate distally.[26] Patterns of propagation for sagittal fractures include spiral fractures toward the pastern joint and/or lateral deviation toward the cortex (Fig. 15.7).

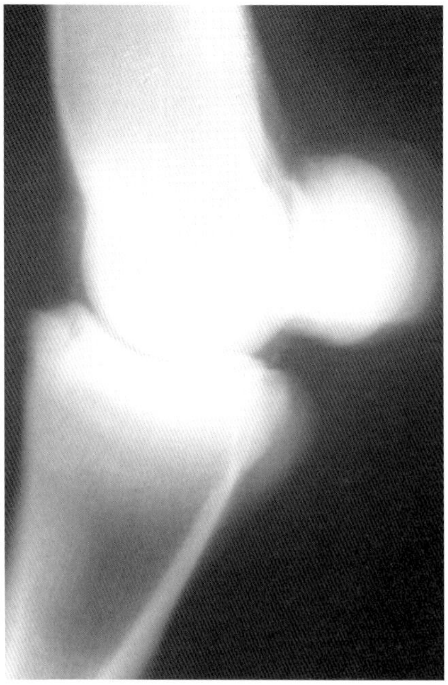

Fig 15.6 Lateral radiograph of a typical frontal plane dorsal first phalanx fracture.

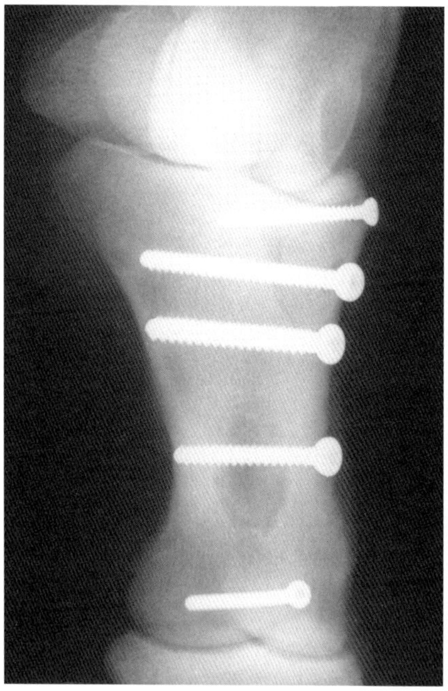

Fig 15.8 Lag screw repair of a comminuted first phalanx fracture. Frontal and sagittal fracture planes required fixation in multiple planes. The fracture was complete into the pastern joint.

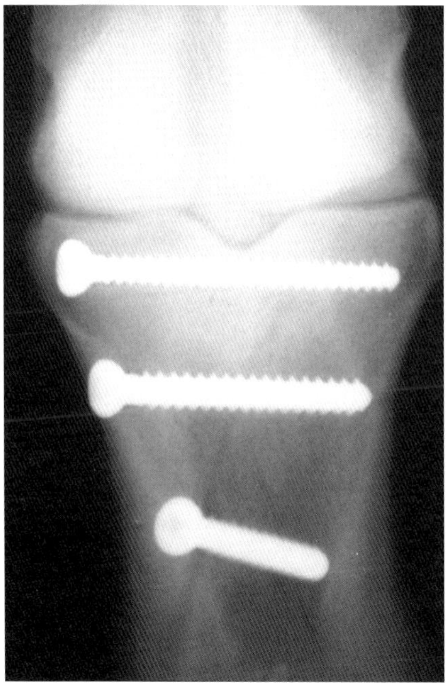

Fig 15.7 Craniocaudal radiograph of a recently repaired typical complete sagittal first phalanx fracture. The fracture originates near the sagittal groove and exits the lateral cortex.

If fractures extend into the pastern joint or exit the lateral cortex, they are considered complete. Many sagittal fractures are incomplete and propagate distally for varying distances, ranging from < 1 cm (short incomplete) to 5–6 cm (long incomplete) and ending just above the pastern joint.[27,28] Complete fractures can be displaced or non-displaced. Incomplete fractures are non-displaced or minimally displaced. A small proportion of sagittal fractures can also contain frontal plane fractures (Fig. 15.8). If this combination of fractures occurs, it is highly predisposed to displacement (comminution) since the sagittal ridge of the metacarpus/tarsus acts as a pile driver upon loading, even with the limb in a cast or splint. Securely positioning the limb vertically on the toe minimizes this effect.

A portion of these fractures will also have a third fracture plane (transverse or coronal) which commonly results in complete instability and displacement of the fragments (comminution). Displaced, comminuted fractures are categorized by the presence or absence of an intact strut of bone from the proximal metacarpal/tarsophalangeal joint to the proximal interphalangeal joint. Prognosis for successful surgical reconstruction is greater if an intact strut of bone is present due to the longitudinal support to prevent collapse and providing a secure anchor for reconstruction of fragments.[26]

Frontal single plane longitudinal fractures can occur in the first phalanx, but are much less common than sagittal fractures (see Fig. 15.6). Clinical signs, treatment and outcome are as for sagittal fractures.[29] If a frontal plane fracture is identified on a lateral radiograph, an additional sagittal plane fracture should be suspected and ruled out.

Recognition

History and presenting complaint

Most first phalanx fractures occur at racing speeds and therefore are closely associated with heavy workouts or competitive events. More severe fractures are associated with immediate lameness and rapid swelling (within minutes to hours).

Physical examination

Clinical signs of longitudinal fractures include lameness, which is immediate for all but the short incomplete fractures, fetlock joint effusion and pain on joint manipulation early after injury. Pain can be elicited by squeezing the P1 bone, particularly proximally. Lameness can resolve with stall rest within days to weeks with incomplete fractures, particularly short fractures, and local swelling may be imperceptible. Complete fractures usually result in a non-weight bearing lameness that persists and swelling in the pastern is present.

Special examination

A first phalanx fracture should be suspected in any competitive horse, particularly a racehorse, that is lame the day after the race and has fetlock joint effusion. The horse should not be jogged excessively or jogged following a nerve block to the distal limb as complete bone failure may occur.

Diagnostic confirmation

The diagnosis can usually be confirmed with a complete series of radiographs. Most fractures are evident on the craniocaudal view (sagittal fractures) or lateral view (frontal plane fractures). Acute non-displaced first phalanx fractures can be undetectable by radiography. If a high degree of suspicion for a first phalanx fracture persists due to clinical signs and history, the radiographs should be repeated in 2–4 weeks or a nuclear scan performed. Horses with a confirmed fracture should remain on stall rest with appropriate coaptation for the fracture configuration until surgery, if elected.

Treatment and prognosis

Therapeutic aims

The goals of therapy are to prevent worsening or displacement of an existing fracture with stall rest and coaptation and surgical treatment to provide immediate reduction and compression of the fracture. Internal fixation provides the most rapid healing and best joint alignment.

Therapy

Most sagittal and frontal plane first phalanx fractures are best treated with surgical lag screw compression if the fracture length on radiograph is > 1 cm[26–29] (see Fig. 15.7, Fig. 15.8). In non-displaced fractures, screws can be placed in lag fashion through small stab incisions. In displaced fractures an incision can improve exposure to ensure anatomic reduction prior to screw placement. Comminuted fractures that have lost an intact strut of bone support from the fetlock to the pastern joint are best treated ideally for several weeks with diverted loading through coaptative devices.[30] Positive profile transfixation pins in the metacarpus/tarsus supported with a cast or use of an external fixator apparatus have been successful in managing these fractures and can be used in the presence of open wounds.

Prognosis

The prognosis for return to athletic use following repair is good to excellent (> 70%) for non-comminuted, incomplete, non-displaced fractures and complete fractures that exit the lateral cortex.[26–28] The prognosis following repair for complete fractures that enter the pastern joint is lower (49%).[27] The prognosis for complete fractures is also good if surgical repair effectively compresses the fracture with minimal displacement in the pastern joint. Repair of displaced complete fractures or comminuted fractures can achieve pasture soundness and breeding soundness, but athletic soundness is usually compromised.

Etiology and pathogenesis

Etiology

Sagittal first phalanx fractures occur as the sagittal ridge of the metacarpal/tarsal condyle is loaded rapidly into the first phalanx during galloping (see Fig. 15.1). The shape of the bones and the rotation during movement create torsional forces within the bone, resulting in the classic spiraling fracture.

Pathophysiology

Preceding bone pathology is not necessary for this fracture to occur and it is considered a high-speed casualty.

Proximal sesamoiditis

- Lameness localized to the fetlock and suspensory branches.
- Radiographically apparent widened vascular channels in the sesamoid confirms the diagnosis.
- Reduced exercise level and time for bone remodeling are necessary.

Recognition

History and presenting complaint

Sesamoiditis is a condition characterized by pain and associated lameness located to the proximal sesamoid bones and attachment of the suspensory branches.

Physical examination

Pain, heat and inflammation are detected at the insertion of the suspensory ligament early in the disease, but usually marked lameness and limitations on performance occur without any clinically detectable signs.[31,32]

Lameness is usually obvious, particularly after exercise. Pain on pressure over the abaxial surface of the sesamoid bone and on fetlock flexion is typical. A distal metacarpal nerve block, but not an intra-articular fetlock block, will locate the lameness to the extra-articular structures of the fetlock. Additional diagnostic tests would include radiographs and ultrasound examination of the suspensory ligament.

Special examination

Primary disease of the suspensory ligament or distal sesamoidean ligament can accompany the bone pain and should be evaluated with diagnostic ultrasound.

Radiographs can reveal a range of changes from accelerated early remodeling response in the bones (increased size and number of vascular channels) to marked proliferation of bone along the abaxial margin of the sesamoid and increased bone density of the sesamoid. Some radiographic changes associated with chronic sesamoiditis are persistent and present in sound performing horses.

Nuclear scintigraphy usually demonstrates increased radiopharmaceutical uptake in the sesamoids of greater degree than bone remodeling associated with training and of lesser degree than sesamoid bone fracture.

Diagnostic confirmation

The diagnosis is confirmed with a combination of radiographic changes indicated above, lameness that locates to the fetlock area and fetlock lameness that does not locate intra-articularly with a fetlock joint block. Ultrasound examination of the suspensory ligament is often normal.

Treatment and prognosis

Therapeutic aims

The goal of therapy is to reduce bone pain so that a convalescent training program can be initiated to strengthen the bone. Bone remodeling will need to occur to permit the sesamoids to accommodate to the high-tensile strains of competitive sport without reinjury.

Therapy

Initial therapy is stall rest, anti-inflammatory and pain medication to eliminate lameness. With a convalescent exercise program, bone remodeling can conclude, heal the injury and suspensory strength be regained.

Treatment is palliative, including anti-inflammatory medications, physical and adjunctive therapy and supportive wraps in the acute phases. [31] Bisphosphonate therapy has been anticipated to assist with bone quality is sesamoiditis, but these medications have not yet been approved for use in horses in the United States.

X-ray and γ-ray radiation, laser heat application, shock wave therapy and a balanced mineral diet are considered by some to be valuable in this condition. Rest from athletic activities is necessary until soundness is achieved. A convalescent exercise program would include lower levels of exercise that would stimulate bone strengthening, but not induce pain or bone damage. Typical programs are prolonged, similar to suspensory ligament injuries (7–9 months). Pain can recur upon return to original levels of performance and may force retirement or a reduction in level of athletic competition.

Prognosis

The specific prognosis is case dependent and can range from poor for severe cases with concomitant suspensory ligament injury to good for cases with mild lameness and minimal radiographic changes.

Etiology and pathogenesis

Etiology

The etiology is considered to be excessive strain to the suspensory apparatus around the fetlock, including the sesamoid bones and the insertion of the suspensory ligament branches.

Pathophysiology

The intraosseous blood supply to the sesamoid bone enters through a series of abaxial vascular channels that correspond to the enlarged channels seen radiographically in sesamoiditis, indicating bone resorption. This may represent the initiation of the remodeling response to bone stress of training or may reflect an increase in blood flow due to inflammation and injury to the suspensory ligament, or both.[25] Sesamoid bone remodeling is a normal response to training and only if stresses exceed the capability to strengthen bone would microfracture and bone damage occur. Although radiographic vascular changes of bone remodeling were not associated with sesamoid fracture, the vascular structures course along known lines of fracture in adult racehorses. The sesamoid bones have an extensive sensory nerve supply that may explain bone pain associated with trabecular bone injury.[33]

Epidemiology

Sesamoiditis is observed frequently in racing horses and hunters and jumpers.[10]

Prevention

Appropriate training schedules to permit time for bone strengthening are helpful. A dietary cause has not been identified.

A separate condition of the axial border of the sesamoid bones, an osteomyelitis, has also been called sesamoiditis. Horses with axial sesamoid osteomyelitis are quite lame at the walk and radiographs reveal surface bone lysis at the attachment of the intersesamoidean ligament. The lesions and clinical signs suggest a septic condition in some animals but on histology infarction and necrosis predominate. Presumably an injury to the attachment of the intersesamoidean ligament and possibly seeding with bacteria from intra-articular injections may be associated with the condition. The prognosis for soundness with or without surgical debridement is poor.[34]

Rupture of the suspensory apparatus

- This injury is unique to the racehorse.
- Fractures of the sesamoid bones and/or suspensory ligament disruption occur.
- First aid splinting should be done to preserve soft tissues and the local blood supply.
- Surgery is done to stabilize the joint for salvage as a breeding animal.

Disruption of the suspensory apparatus is a common cause of acute breakdown in the racing Thoroughbred and frequently results in humane destruction of the animal.[9,22] Disruption can occur because of rupture of the suspensory ligament, fracture of both proximal sesamoid bones or avulsion of the distal sesamoidean ligaments. Due to the violent nature of these injuries, open fractures, fetlock joint luxation and loss of the vascular supply to the distal limb are associated complications. Successful treatment of these injuries requires immediate and appropriate emergency management of the horse, including sedation, possibly general anesthesia, ambulance service and limb stabilization. Commercial splints such as the Kimzey Leg Saver Splint (Kimzey Welding Works, Woodland, CA) have been designed for this purpose. Euthanasia may be chosen due to the extent of the injuries, risk of treatment failure, lack of sentimental or breeding value of the horse and cost of treatment.[22]

Recognition

History and presenting complaint

These injuries occur during maximal exercise and are immediately recognized by distortion of the distal limb and the inability of the horse to bear weight without collapse of the distal limb.

Physical examination

Immediate sedation or general anesthesia is recommended to gain control of the panicked horse for examination by palpation, radiography, ultrasound and Doppler ultrasound.

Special examination and diagnostic confirmation

The diagnosis is confirmed by observation (the fetlock drops to the ground upon loading), palpation and radiograph. Ultrasound evaluation can locate the sites of suspensory ligament failure and, with Doppler, assesses blood flow to the distal limb. The vascular supply is best evaluated after the horse has been treated for shock and the limb has been stabilized to over-ride initial vasoconstriction. Radiographic examination most often reveals the proximal displacement of the intact sesamoid bone (rupture of the distal sesamoidean ligaments) or proximal displacement of the apical portions of the fractured sesamoid bones (sesamoid fracture).

Treatment and prognosis

Therapeutic aims

The goal of treatment is to salvage the horse's life for breeding or as a retired pasture companion. Surgical fusion of the fetlock joint can be successful if limb blood supply is intact and infection can be prevented.

Therapy

If treatment is chosen, a splint should be maintained for 4–5 days prior to the selection of the final treatment to permit recovery from the shock and trauma and to define the extent of skin necrosis and loss of vascular supply accompanying the injury. The arthrodesis procedure should be undertaken at the optimal time and evaluation of the soft tissue injury and permanent deficit and risk of infection must be ascertained to properly predict the outcome with surgery.[22] Surgical treatment options include fetlock ankylosis supported by use of an external fixator placed on the foot and metacarpus to fix the position of the joint during healing[35] or arthrodesis with implants and bone graft to achieve a pain-free stable fusion of the fetlock joint.[10,22] For implants, the soft tissues should be intact and the risk of infection minimal. Treatment by surgical means is preferable to relieve extended loading on the contralateral limb. In conservative management, supporting limb laminitis and erosion of the sesamoid bones by casts and splints is a significant cause of failure.

Prognosis

The prognosis is grave for horses that also have open joint luxation, significant skin loss, loss of vascularity and open wounds. With the preselection and appropriate management of cases, the prognosis is good for pasture and breeding soundness. In one report, 60% of horses with fetlock arthrodesis fused the joint, survived and eventually had unrestricted activity.[22]

Etiology and pathogenesis

Etiology

Fetlock disruption occurs during racing or maximal exercise as a traumatic event.

Pathophysiology

Disruption of the suspensory apparatus is due to extreme overextension of the fetlock at high speeds and forces of loading. Pre-existing pathology of the bones or suspensory ligament is not a prerequisite for this injury to occur.

Epidemiology

Risk factors have been identified and include an abnormal finding in the suspensory ligament on pre-race inspection by a regulatory veterinarian[36] and racing with toe grabs.[37]

Prevention

Pulling horses with abnormal suspensory ligament findings from racing and maintenance of optimal track conditions will reduce the number of these catastrophic failures.

Fetlock luxation

Recognition

History and presenting complaint

Luxation of the fetlock is usually in the frontal plane and occurs during a high-impact injury, such as slipping, running into an object or catching the hoof under a board or in a hole. A collateral ligament ruptures, resulting in an obvious varus or valgus deformity of the limb.[38] The dislocation of the joint may be temporary and often replaces spontaneously or is reduced by an attendant.

Physical examination

After reduction, lameness may be minimal. Articular fractures of palmar/plantar eminence of the first phalanx may accompany the luxation[39] and can be avulsed several inches proximally. Medial to lateral laxity is present and the joint may be subluxated upon flexion. Swelling of the joint and torn soft tissues will locate over the injured side of the joint within hours. Persistent laxity can be palpated and presumably contributes to the chronic osteoarthritis that is often the sequela to this injury.[40]

Special examination

Reluxation can occur at any moment if the joint is not stabilized until the swelling and pain begin to protect the joint, so it is critical to restrict the horse's activity.

Diagnostic confirmation

The diagnosis is often made by the historical description of the limb deformity and manipulation of the fetlock. Radiographs should be taken to identify an avulsion fracture, intra-articular fractures or damage to the articular surface that has entered into the subchondral bone. Craniocaudal stress radiographs displacing the distal limb medially or laterally will identify more laxity to the fetlock joint than the contralateral joint, but is not necessary for a diagnosis (Fig. 15.9).

Treatment and prognosis

Therapeutic aims

The goal of therapy is to reduce the luxation and stabilize the limb to prevent reluxation and decrease the risk of osteoarthritis.

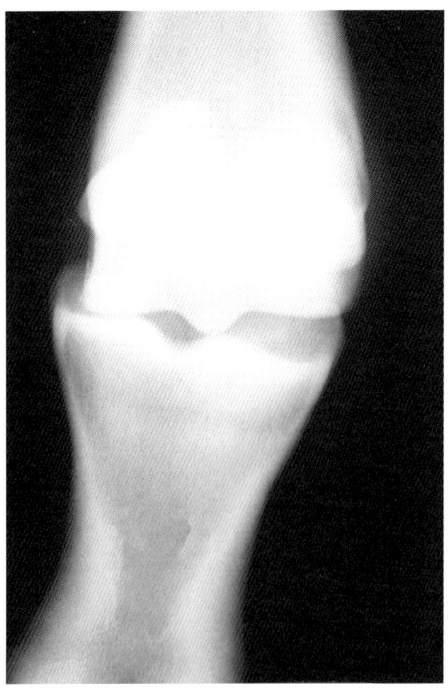

Fig 15.9 Stress radiograph demonstrating excessive joint laxity in the frontal plane, indicating rupture of the medial collateral ligament.

Therapy

Arthroscopic removal of articular fragments can be undertaken if the chances for athletic soundness are to be optimized. Reduction and immobilization for 4–6 weeks will result in fibrous restabilization of the joint and a good prognosis for light riding soundness. Surgical repair of the ligament is reported,[38,41] but is not universally accepted as an improvement over conservative coaptation. If osteoarthritis and permanent lameness occur as sequelae, a surgical arthrodesis can result in pasture soundness. In open fractures/luxations, external fixation may be necessary followed by bone grafting and stimulated joint fusion.

Prognosis

Closed luxations without fracture that are quickly reduced can result in soundness, although competitive athletic soundness is less likely. Most luxations result in some degree of osteoarthritis and lameness with exercise. Luxations with associated injuries, such as an open joint, additional fractures or disrupted vascular supply, would carry a less favorable prognosis.

Etiology and pathogenesis

Etiology

This injury is a sporadic, relatively random traumatic event.

Pathophysiology

Lateral and medial luxation of the fetlock joint is a recognized syndrome, affects all ages and breeds of horses and usually occurs during high-speed falls or collisions. Pre-existing joint disease or collateral ligament disease is not associated with injury.

Traumatic bone and cartilage impact injury to the fetlock and pastern joints

- Definitive diagnosis is via magnetic resonance imaging.
- Rule out is nondisplaced fracture.
- Treatment is aimed at rest and rehabilitation and cartilage restoration procedures where indicated.
- Traumatic synovitis/arthritis of the fetlock joint is one of the most common conditions in the equine athlete. The high range of rotary motion predisposes this joint to injury and wear.

Recognition

Sport horses are prone to impact injury to the lower limb and joints during elite competitive performance. Impact injury to the subchondral bone and articular cartilage can create significant lameness without radiographic evidence of injury or fracture. Magnetic resonance imaging (MRI) has permitted the identification of these injuries.

History and presenting complaint

Most horses present with the onset of lameness of one limb initially which worsens with exercise and duration. Most horses are in competition.

Physical examination

Clinical signs can include modest joint effusion and soreness to lower limb flexion, but the lameness is often remarkable considering the lack of radiographic findings or joint enlargement. Regional nerve blocks or joint blocks locate the lameness to the fetlock or pastern. With duration, the joints can stiffen.

Special examination

Radiographs are often normal until the condition becomes chronic and joint space narrowing begins to appear. Eventually degenerative joint disease (osteoarthritis) may be evident but radiographs can remain normal for months to years. Arthrocentesis and fluid cytology are often performed as the clinical signs are severe enough to warrant them and intra-articular steroid medication is commonly in the history, sometimes multiple administrations. MRI demonstrates bone signal intensity alterations that are frequently focal, subchondral and may be relatively small. MRI usually simultaneously demonstrates bone signal intensity alterations that correspond to the abnormal bone signal and may be 'dot' like [Fig. 15.10A–C and Fig. 15.11A–B].

Laboratory examination

Synovial fluid analysis may be normal or reveal a mild increase in protein concentration.

Diagnostic confirmation

The diagnosis is definitive if the lameness resolves with an intra-articular fetlock or pastern joint block, radiographs are normal, and MRI demonstrates focal subchondral bone signal alterations.

Treatment and prognosis

Therapeutic aims

Most primary traumatic impact injuries are treated with aggressive medical management is aimed at reducing joint pain and inflammation. Arthroscopic surgery to identify the extent of articular cartilage injury and permit restorative techniques such as concentrated bone marrow aspirate, microfracture or cell therapy may be of benefit (Fig. 15.12A–C).

Therapy

Early medical intervention and appropriate joint rest and physiotherapy similar to that described under traumatic synovitis are recommended. Additionally use of intra-articular autologous blood products such as autologous conditioned serum, platelet rich plasma and autologous protein solution, may support cartilage health and reduce joint pain. Arthroscopic surgery to perform articular cartilage debridement, microfracture of injured subchondral bone and apply cell therapy such as allogeneic juvenile chondrocyte transplantation can be performed [Fig. 15.12A–C].

Prognosis

The prognosis for impact trauma to bone and cartilage is not well known, but many horses have continued lameness that progresses and becomes severe. Many of these horses are euthanized once joint space narrowing is confirmed and chronic.

Etiology and pathogenesis

Etiology

Impact injury is presumed to occur during maximal performance exercise with direct crushing injury to cartilage and bone.

Pathophysiology

Microfracture of subchondral bone and adjacent cartilage lead to focal bone edema, hemorrhage and matrix disruption that results

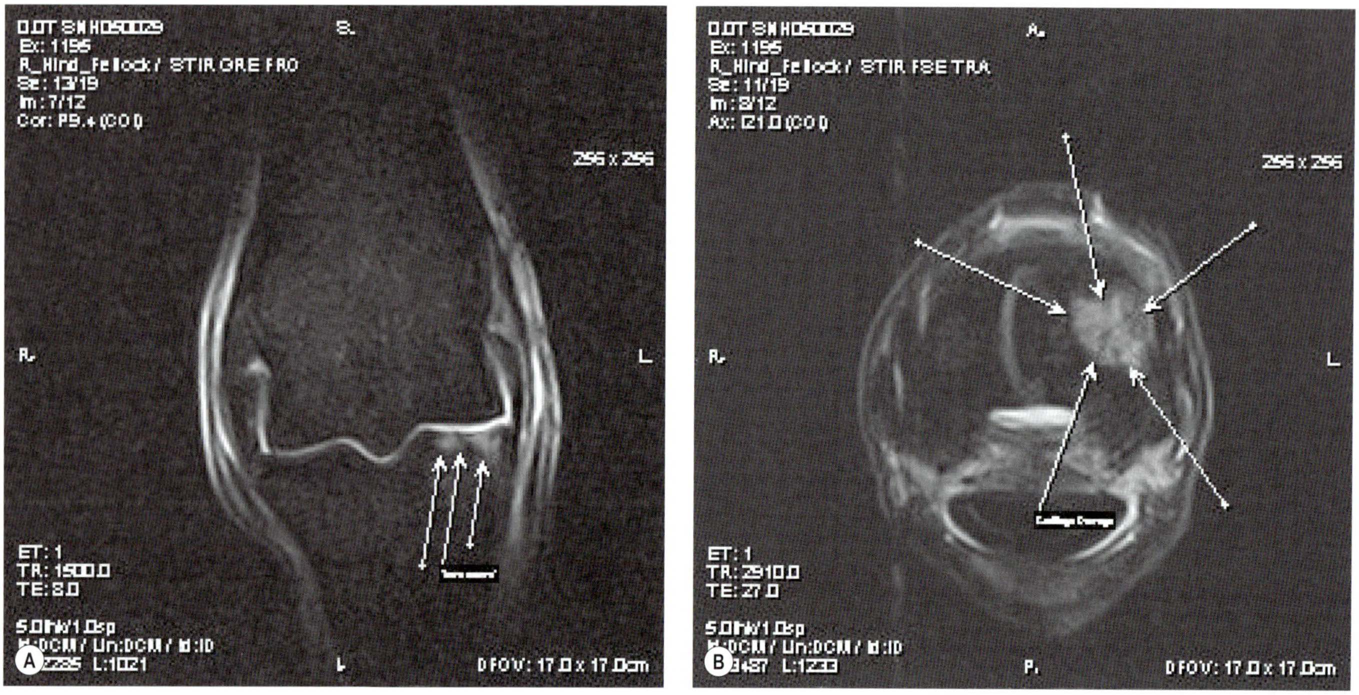

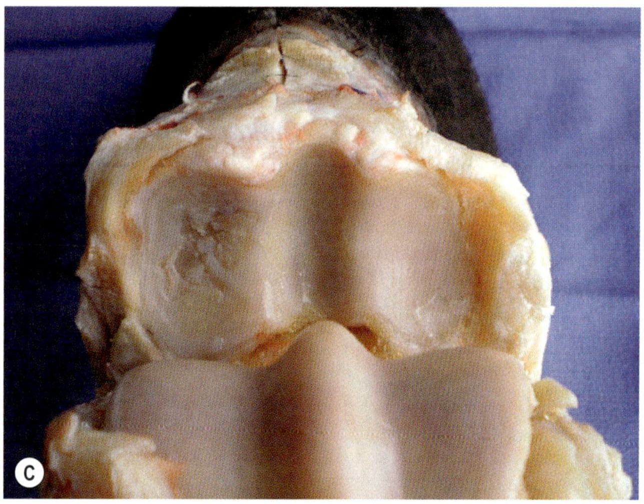

Fig 15.10 Frontal **(A)** and coronal **(B)** plane MR and gross **(C)** images of the proximal first phalanx of a hunter show horse with lameness noted at the walk for over eight months. Clinical signs started with joint effusion and lameness that responded to joint injection with steroids. Continued work worsened the lameness, rest did not improve the lameness, and MRI demonstrated abnormal subchondral bone intensity in the proximal medial first phalanx that corresponded to articular damage and abnormal bone at that site on necropsy. In that last four months radiographic narrowing of the joint space became apparent although subtle.

Photos courtesy of Cleveland Equine Clinic and Dr Matt Brokken.

is a focal change in the MRI signal. Progression to loss of cartilage can occur and joint space narrowing becomed identified.

Epidemiology

Horses identified with this problem have been jumping horses in competition mostly, although all sport horses would have potential to develop the injury.

Prevention

Avoidance of aggressive jumping, spinning and hard surfaces along with regular joint care can reduce the likelihood of this injury. The association with prior intra-articular steroid injections may suggest a weakening of the bone and cartilage, predisposing it to more permanent injury. A judicious training program following intra-articular steroid injections for lameness combined with decreasing the most forceful impacts on the joint are recommended to prevent these impact injuries.

Traumatic synovitis and capsulitis

- Definitive diagnosis is via intra-articular anesthesia.
- Rule out osteochondral fractures.
- Treatment reduces joint inflammation to prevent deterioration of cartilage.

Traumatic synovitis/arthritis of the fetlock joint is one of the most common conditions in the equine athlete. The high range of rotary motion predisposes this joint to injury and wear.

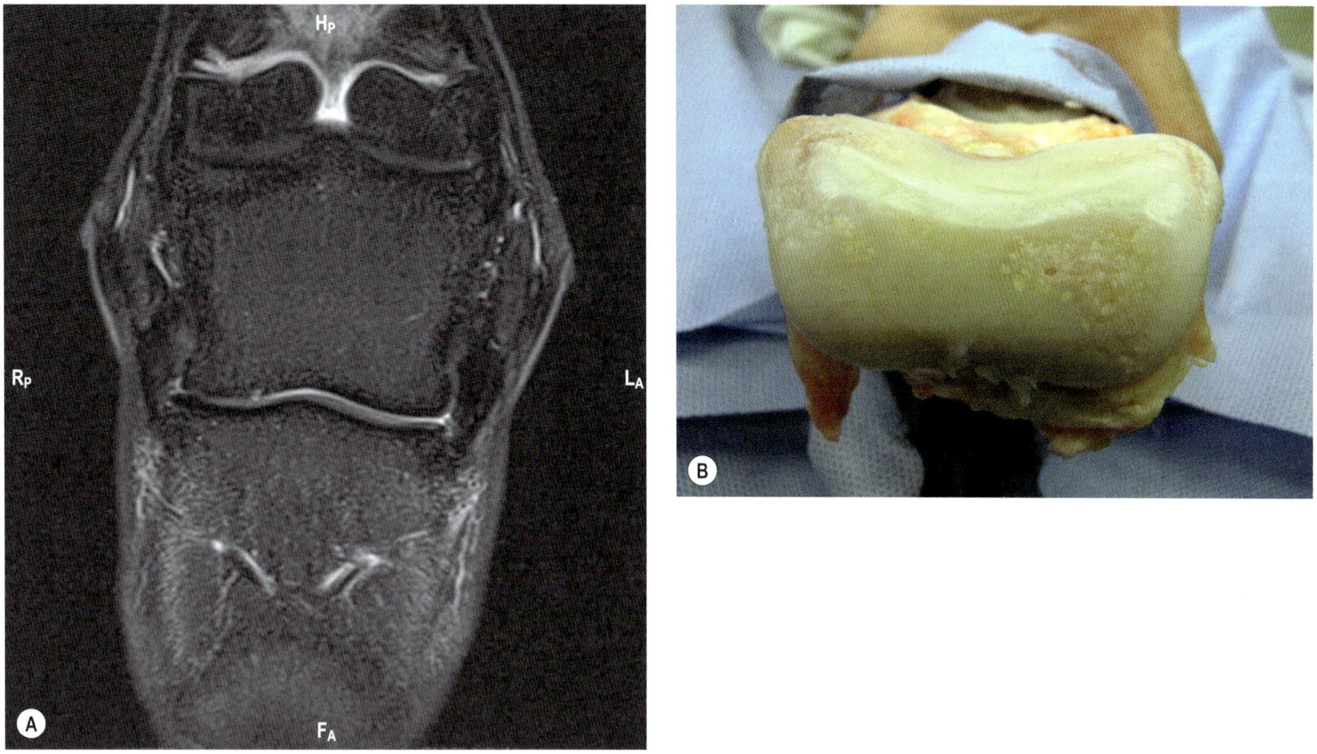

Fig 15.11 Frontal plane **(A)** and gross **(B)** images of a jumper show horse that has significant lameness that repeatably blocked to the coffin joint. Medical and shoeing therapies were exhausted without improvement. MR demonstrated a small focal subchondral bone lesion on the distal second phalanx as well as loss of MR intensity in the cartilage adjacent to the lesion. The necropsy demonstrates the classic appearance of these impact injuries with a cobblestone appearance to the cartilage and pits to the subchondral bone.
Photos courtesy of Dr Matt Brokken.

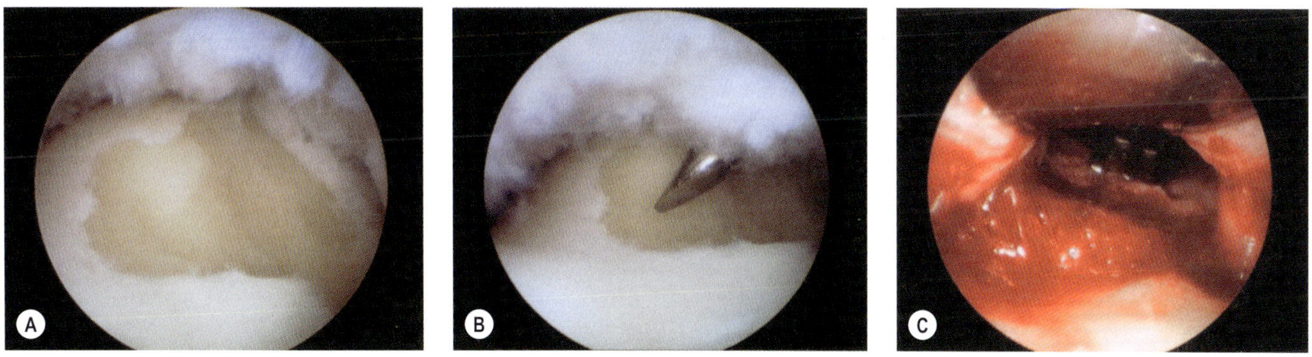

Fig 15.12 Arthroscopic photograph of the dorsal metacarpus that shows final debridement of a full-thickness articular cartilage injury **(A)**, microfracture procedure prior to **(B)**, and then after **(C)** the transplantation of 50 million juvenile chondrocytes engineered to produce bone morphogenetic protein 2 (In Clinical Trial, The Ohio State University, photos courtesy of Dr Alicia Bertone.) in platelet rich plasma glue. Cell therapy using chondrocytes or stem cells has been used experimentally as a cartilage restoration procedure.

Recognition

History and presenting complaint

Most horses present with the onset of lameness of one limb initially which may be intermittent and worse after exercise. A specific injury may have been noted.

Physical examination

Joint effusion, soreness to joint flexion and joint heat (detected by palpation or thermography) are the classic clinical signs.

Special examination

Radiographs are normal until the condition becomes chronic and degenerative joint disease (osteoarthritis) develops. Arthrocentesis and fluid cytology are often not performed as the clinical signs are not severe enough to warrant them; however, intra-articular and systemic joint medication is commonly used. If training is continued with the use of aggressive medical therapy, a proportion of these horses will develop proliferative synovitis (see next section), chip fractures and articular cartilage damage (erosion and scoring). Intermittent hemarthrosis may be detected with primary traumatic synovitis but often indicates injury to subchondral bone, such as chip fracture or cartilage elevation.

Laboratory examination

Synovial fluid analysis may be normal or reveal a mild increase in white blood cell count or protein concentration.

Diagnostic confirmation

The diagnosis is definitive if the lameness resolves with an intra-articular fetlock joint block, radiographs are normal and a synovitis or hemarthrosis is present on synovial fluid analysis.

Treatment and prognosis

Therapeutic aims

Most primary traumatic synovitis is mild, permitting continued training with medical management. Medical management is aimed at reducing joint pain and inflammation.

Therapy

Early medical intervention and appropriate joint rest and physiotherapy are critical to prevent loss of glycosaminoglycan from articular cartilage and permanent joint wear. Early loss of articular cartilage proteoglycan is reversible with medication and joint rest. Systemic hyaluronan and polysulfated glycosaminoglycans may be used to reduce joint inflammation and assist with protection of articular cartilage. Topical dimethylsulfoxide (DMSO) and hyperosmotic agents under plastic and supportive wraps assist with removal of joint edema and fluid accumulation. Nonsteroidal anti-inflammatory medication can reduce joint inflammation and should be used if close monitoring of the lameness is not critical. Long-term use of Non-steroidal anti-inflammatory drugs would require continued evaluation of the patient.

Prognosis

The prognosis for traumatic arthritis ranges from good for minor and first-time injuries to poor for severe or recurrent injuries. Early and less severe disease that is permitted joint rest to resolve the inflammation can often be managed. Traumatic arthritis can be progressive or result in degenerative joint disease.

Etiology and pathogenesis

Etiology

Traumatic arthritis usually begins as a strain to the joint during exercise that results in a joint bleed, pinching of the synovium and/or a cartilage erosion and secondary joint inflammation. Horses with high action and high-impact loading are the most susceptible.

Pathophysiology

Joint inflammation (synovitis) induced by a traumatic injury results in immediate swelling of the synovium and possible joint hemorrhage. Capillary leakage introduces fluid and white blood cells into the area of injury and increases blood flow locally. These cells release inflammatory mediators, such as interleukins, eicosanoids and nitric oxide that perpetuate the inflammation until healing occurs. The result is joint effusion, synovial hemorrhage and edema, an increased joint fluid white blood cell count and protein content and activation of joint pain (see Chapter 11).

Epidemiology

Horses at risk for traumatic synovitis are in active training with maximal performances on a regular schedule. This includes all racing breeds (Thoroughbred, Standardbred, Quarter Horse, Warmbloods) and types of racing competition (flat racing, barrel racing, cross-country, steeple chase); dressage horses; Western performance horses; hunters; jumpers; three-day competition; and show horses.

Prevention

Regular exercise, appropriate warm-up, conservative competitive schedules and judicious use of joint medications, particularly steroids and non-steroidal anti-inflammatory drugs, will reduce the risk of joint trauma and prolong joint health.

Proliferative (villonodular) synovitis

- Result of chronic joint inflammation.
- Radiographically evident as supracondylar lysis.
- Treatment is surgical resection of proliferative tissue if medical therapy fails.

Proliferative synovitis is a clinical condition in which chronic traumatic synovitis and continued exercise result in a painful thickening of the synovium, particularly in areas of compression trauma.[8,42–46]

Recognition

History and presenting complaint

Classic clinical presentation for chronic proliferative villonodular synovitis is joint effusion, decreased range of joint motion and soreness on joint flexion.

Physical examination

Enlargement at the dorsal fetlock is often visible and disproportionately large for the amount of palmar effusion. The joints may appear and palpate normally, however.

Special examination

Confirmation of enlargement of the pad is most easily obtained with dorsal metacarpophalangeal joint ultrasound. Normal dorsal fetlock pads measure <4 mm dorsal to palmar in a plane perpendicular to the mass surface. A typical enlarged pad in clinical disease measured 11 mm.[8] Proliferative synovitis is often bilateral and therefore comparative measurements of one limb to another may not be helpful. Diagnosis can also be made with contrast arthrography and at arthroscopy (Fig. 15.13). Joints should be radiographed prior to surgery to identify presence and extent of bone erosion, mineralization in the masses, degenerative joint disease and concomitant proximal phalanx chip fractures. In a recent report of 63 horses, 93% of joints demonstrated a concavity at the distal dorsal metacarpus and 32% had a first phalanx chip fracture[8] but these findings are not conclusively diagnostic for an enlarged dorsal pad. In severe cases, these masses can become locally invasive of bone and joint capsule, continuing expansion beyond normal joint structures, similar to benign tumors.

Laboratory examination

Synovial fluid analysis may be normal or indicative of mild to moderate synovitis.

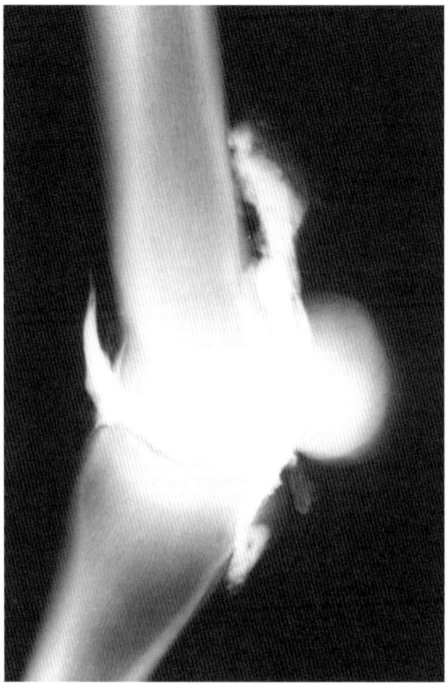

Fig 15.13 Contrast arthrogram of the fetlock joint demonstrating a space-occupying soft tissue mass in the dorsal and palmar joint recesses typical of proliferative synovitis.

Diagnostic confirmation

The presence of clinical signs, pain located to the fetlock joint and a measurably enlarged synovial pad confirm the diagnosis. Radiographic changes are supportive, but not always present, particularly in early disease.

Treatment and prognosis

Therapeutic aims

The goal of therapy is to reduce joint pain and inflammation and reduce the size of the dorsal synovial pad to prevent immediate recurrence on resuming exercise.

Therapy

Upon identification of an enlarged dorsal fetlock proliferative mass, initial therapy would include joint rest, all forms of adjunctive joint synovitis therapy and consideration of a short-acting intra-articular steroid. Intra-articular steroids are potent suppressors of angiogenesis and fibrosis and will reduce active inflammation. Short-acting steroids, such as soluble dexamethasone and hydrocortisone, may minimize the long-term corticosteroid influence on chondrocyte metabolism. Arthroscopic surgical mechanical or laser removal of the enlarged masses is indicated if any associated fractures are identified, if pain persists or at planned lay-off periods.[47] Surgery should be undertaken before signs are associated with bone changes, articular cartilage damage or degenerative joint disease.

Prognosis

Successful return to racing is reported in Thoroughbreds[8] and trotters[43] after surgical removal of the dorsal pad and intra-articular chip fractures. Proliferation of the pad can return despite surgical and medical management, but most horses are clinically improved with a longer performance career with surgical treatment.

Diffuse proliferative synovitis and capsulitis is also common in the fetlock joint and can be associated with chronic joint injection, joint damage and joint wear. Palpable joint soft tissue thickening and loss of joint range of motion are classic clinical findings and are commonly noted in retired jumpers and racehorses. Fibrosis of the joint capsule and loss of fine villous architecture are notable at arthroscopy. Diffuse synovectomy in these cases is probably of minimal benefit as restoration of normal villi is unlikely and loss of remaining villous architecture may be permanent. The loss of joint motion is permanent and may not be associated with lameness in retired horses.

Etiology and pathogenesis

Etiology

This condition is most commonly seen in Thoroughbred racehorses. High-impact joint use with extreme dorsiflexion causes direct mechanical trauma to the dorsal fetlock synovial pad between the metacarpal/tarsal condyle and the first phalanx.

Pathophysiology

Proliferative synovitis is a clinical condition in which chronic traumatic synovitis and continued exercise result in a painful thickening of the synovium, particularly in areas of compression trauma.[8,42–46] The most common location in the horse for this condition is the dorsal fibrous pad of the metacarpophalangeal joint. This pad is normally present at the dorsal reflection of the metacarpophalangeal joint directly under the broad, flat extensor tendon and associated joint capsule.[8] At hyperextension and maximal flexion, this pad is compressed and can result in intrasynovial hemorrhage, granulation tissue formation, fibrosis and mineralization. Pigment in the pad is often hemosiderin, but melanin has also been noted.

Epidemiology

The condition is typically progressive as joint trauma is continued with use.

Prevention

Early treatment and adequate rest early in the disease process may arrest the development or progression of this condition.

Developmental osteochondral fragments in the fetlock

Recognition

History and presenting complaint

Classic clinical presentation for metacarpo/tarsophalangeal osteochondral fragments is joint effusion, soreness on joint flexion after exercise and intermittent or no lameness.

Physical examination

The joints may appear and palpate normally, however, joint effusion is often detected.

Special examination

Confirmation of osteochondral fragmentation is made with radiography.

Laboratory examination

Synovial fluid analysis may be normal or indicative of mild to moderate synovitis.

Diagnostic confirmation

The presence of clinical signs, pain located to the fetlock joint and radiographic fragments are diagnositic for the condition.

Treatment and prognosis

Therapeutic aims

The goal of therapy is to reduce joint pain and inflammation, remove the fragments and remove accompanying fibrosis of the dorsal synovial pad.

Therapy

Upon identification of the osteochondral fragments, initial therapy would include joint rest, all forms of adjunctive joint synovitis therapy and consideration of arthroscopic surgical removal of the fragments.[47] Surgery should be undertaken before signs are associated with articular cartilage damage, lameness or degenerative joint disease.

Prognosis

Most horses with dorsoproximal proximal phalanx osteochondral fragmentation[47] or osteochondral fragmentation of in the synovial pad[48] are not lame at diagnosis. Horses with dorsal phalanx fragments that are seven years or older or with more than one fragment have an increased risk of lameness.[47] Presence of arthroscopic abnormalities correlated to larger synovial pad fragments, but the effect on prognosis was undefined.

Etiology and pathogenesis

Etiology

This condition is most commonly seen in Thoroughbred and Standardbred racehorses as well as Warmblood breeds. The presence in young horses without lameness and the frequent lack of other articular cartilage abnormality suggests the fragments are developmental.

Pathophysiology

Osteochondral fragmentation of the fetlock may have an inherited component, reflect delayed mineralization of the cartilage during growth and be influenced by trauma at the dorsal phalanx eminence.

Epidemiology

The fragments remain and are associated with lameness and articular cartilage abnormalities in older horses or horses with longer athletic careers.

Prevention

Prevention of the development of fragments is unknown, but removal is permanent.

Osteoarthritis of the fetlock (osselets)

Osteoarthritis is a chronic degenerative joint condition with the hallmark criteria of joint pain, articular cartilage degeneration, subchondral bone change, osteophyte production and loss of joint motion.[49] The fore fetlocks in athletic horses are probably the most commonly affected joint with this condition and therefore it is common bilaterally in geriatric horses, retired horses and exceptional athletes.

Recognition

History and presenting complaint

Lameness is insidious in onset, often bilateral with one limb less and later affected.

Physical examination

The gait is classically a stiff and shortened stride with an asymmetrical lameness. Lameness worsens on turns and after exercise. Joints are stiff, but may be minimally sore to forced flexion.

Laboratory examination

Standard synovial fluid analysis is often normal.

Diagnostic confirmation

The diagnosis is confirmed by the combination of clinical signs and radiographic evidence of osteophytes, subchondral bone sclerosis and narrowed joint space. Extent of cartilage degeneration can only be assessed by direct visualization arthroscopically or by magnetic resonance imaging.

Treatment and prognosis

Therapeutic aims

The goal of therapy is to relieve joint pain and improve joint use.

Therapy

Treatment of osteoarthritis includes medical therapy and regular joint motion exercises, both passive and active. Surgical debridement of frayed cartilage and exposed bone as well as copious joint lavage have been described to alleviate pain in people, but are palliative only. Use of hyaluronan, glycosamine, and autologous conditioned serum (Arthrex, Inc) products systemically or intra-articularly is advised as needed and as per manufacturer's recommendations. Intra-articular administration of an autologous protein solution product (Biomet, Inc.) can relieve lameness, joint pain, and joint swelling for weeks in clinical cases of osteoarthritis. This product contains growth factors that could be beneficial to articular cartilage.[50] Intra-articular steroids can be used on a limited basis to provide comfort or short durations of athletic use. Non-steroidal anti-inflammatory medication, such as phenylbutazone, is commonly needed in these horses to permit their turnout or restricted athletic use. Chronic use of non-steroidal anti-inflammatory medication is common for osteoarthritis and can alleviate pain and permit activity. Chronic use can be associated with complications such as oral and gastrointestinal ulcers so it should be titrated to the lowest dose possible and used intermittently. Regular exercise on a limited basis is critical to maintain joint comfort and improve quality of life.

Many other adjunctive therapies, such as heat application, passive joint flexion, swimming, etc. have been anecdotally described as effective.

Prognosis

The prognosis for resolution of osteoarthritis is poor because the cartilage degeneration is permanent. Disease-modifying drugs, such as interleukin-1 antagonists, are available for use in humans, but are costly and species specific.

Etiology and pathogenesis

Etiology

Chronic joint 'wear and tear' associated with athletic careers is typical in the sport horse.

Pathophysiology

Healthy joints can develop osteoarthritis with time and use. A predisposition to earlier and more severe osteoarthritis may exist and be related to prior joint injury, conformation and use.

Epidemiology

Osteoarthritis is seen more commonly in geriatric and career horses.

Prevention

Care of the joints during a horse's athletic career may help maintain joint health. Joint support wraps, judicious use of joint medications and immediate veterinary attention to joint injury are critical to containing the development and progression of osteoarthritis.

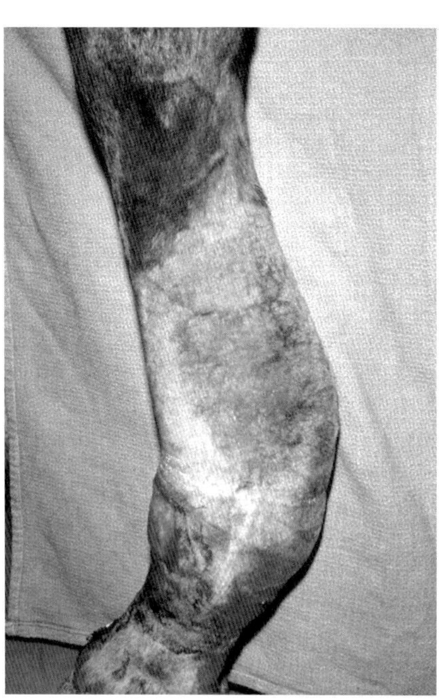

Fig 15.14 Chronic low superficial digital flexor tendinitis with interference at the annular ligament.

Fetlock annular ligament constriction

- Annular ligament constriction is usually secondary to chronic digital sheath synovitis or tendinitis or secondary to direct injury to the palmar/plantar annular ligament.
- Treatment of the primary cause is often insufficient.
- Annular ligament resection may be done using arthroscopy or via a percutaneous approach.

The fetlock annular ligament is a ~3 cm wide fascial band spanning the abaxial ridges of the sesamoid bones and strategically located to support the superficial and deep flexor tendons as they course around the back of the fetlock joint. Synovia from the digital sheath reflects on the deep surface of the ligament. Damage to the flexor tendons can result in swelling and pressure within the sheath.

Recognition

History and presenting complaint

The primary complaint is 'windpuffs' or swelling of the digital sheath. Lameness may or may not be evident initially.

Physical examination

The clinical signs include pain, restricted range of fetlock motion and ischemia to the tissues within the fetlock canal (tunnel syndrome). Once present, lameness is persistent and worsens with exercise. Lameness is characterized by a decreased extension of the fetlock during weight bearing and a shortened caudal phase to the stride. In the most severe cases the horse will be reluctant to place the heel on the ground.

The pathognomonic clinical sign of fetlock annular ligament constriction is swelling of the palmar/plantar soft tissues of the distal limb around the fetlock and a characteristic observable proximal border of the annular ligament ('notching') caused by annular ligament constriction. Typically, there will be distension of the digital sheath of the superficial and deep flexor tendons proximal to the annular ligament and thickening of the superficial flexor tendon (tendinitis) (Fig. 15.14).

In Warmblood horses with fetlock annular ligament constriction, nine had thickening of the annular ligament and tenosynovitis, three were dominated by distension of the sheath, three had superficial digital flexor tendon injury and one had marked synovial sheath proliferation.[51] In racehorses, superficial digital flexor tendinitis may be more commonly associated with fetlock annular ligament constriction.[52]

Special examination

Regional diagnostic anesthesia usually results in improvement after a metacarpal block. Direct anesthesia of the digital sheath incompletely alleviates pain. Radiographic evaluation should be performed but is often normal unless infection is a cause. In 38 cases of annular ligament constriction, six horses had proximal sesamoid bone abnormality and 12 had bone enthesiophytes at the attachment of the annular ligament (insertion desmopathy).[53]

Laboratory examination

Synovial fluid analysis of the sheath fluid and contrast radiography can be of value, but are usually limited in diagnostic value.

Diagnostic confirmation

Diagnostic ultrasound confirms the diagnosis and permits the differentiation of structures involved, including thickening of the annual ligament (> 2 mm thick), tears of the deep flexor tendon, sheath adhesions and proliferative tenosynovitis.

Treatment and prognosis

Therapeutic aims

The goal of therapy is to reduce the constriction of the annular ligament by either decreasing sheath effusion or releasing the ligament or both.

Therapy

Initial conservative treatment often includes an intrathecal injection of steroid to decrease sheath effusion. This is typically palliative and may further weaken or slow healing of injured tendinous structures. To relieve the constriction, the annular ligament is transected either percutaneously or endoscopically. Accessory ligament desmotomy of the superficial digital flexor tendon, tendon splitting, adhesiolysis and synovial resection to simultaneously treat tendinitis, tendon core lesions, adhesions and synovial proliferation, respectively, are indicated.[54–56] Limitations of open transection include incisional drainage and dehiscence, limited visibility as compared to tenoscopy, and greater soft tissue morbidity. Open transection may be necessary for tendon repair (Fig. 15.15).

Prognosis

If the primary etiology is desmitis of the palmar or plantar annular ligament and is not accompanied by extensive changes in the tendon (bowed tendon), the prognosis is good (84% returned to performance).[57,58] Middle aged to older riding horses with fibrosis and thickening of the annular ligament were less able to return to to athletic function (<50%) than horses with desmopathy alone. Bilateral or concurrent fore-and hindlimb injury had a negative effect on prognosis.[59] In Standardbreds in which annular ligament desmotomy was performed in addition to other surgical procedures for tendinitis improved and were able to race.[52] In horses with synovial masses or adhesions that were resected endoscopically at the time of annular ligament resection, the prognosis for athletic soundness was 72%.[56]

Etiology and pathogenesis

Etiology

Specific causes are usually trauma and/or infection (Fig. 15.16) and are associated with distal superficial digital flexor tendinitis (low bow) (see Fig. 15.14), fibrosis from wounds and tenosynovial adhesions and inflammation. The annular ligament may also be directly injured and thickened (desmitis) with the same constricting result. The fetlock annular ligament constriction syndrome is reduction in pain-free movement of the fetlock due to the movement of the structures within the fetlock canal. The result is persistent lameness.

Pathophysiology

Thickening of the ligament occurs through the process of fiber tearing and fibrosis.

Epidemiology

Desmitis of the fetlock annular ligament is diagnosed mainly in sport horses and less frequently in racehorses and histologic changes suggest it is traumatic in origin.[58,60] Excessive use of the hindlimbs, such as in jumpers and cross-country competitors, puts horses at increased risk.

Prevention

Protection of fetlock support structures, such as with support wraps and heel extension shoes, particularly in the hindlimbs, may decrease risk of injury.

Pastern joint injuries

Intra-articular fractures

The pastern joint is uncommonly involved in articular fractures, in comparison to other joints. Articular chip fractures can occur from the proximal dorsal eminences of the second phalanx (P2) and the palmar/plantar intereminence of P2 (Fig. 15.17).

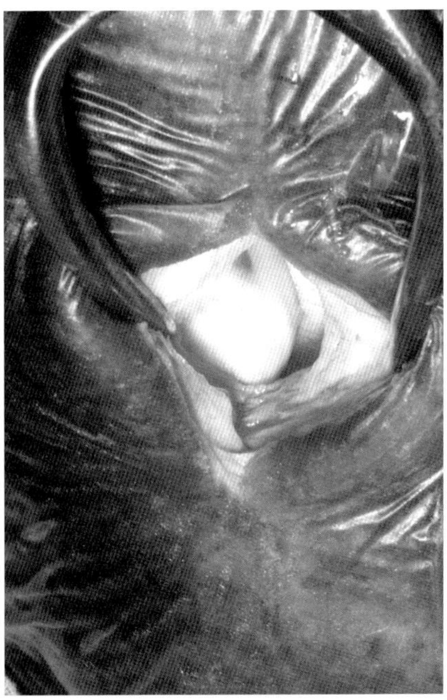

Fig 15.15 Open annular ligament transection revealing a chronic blunt end of the deep digital flexor tendon.

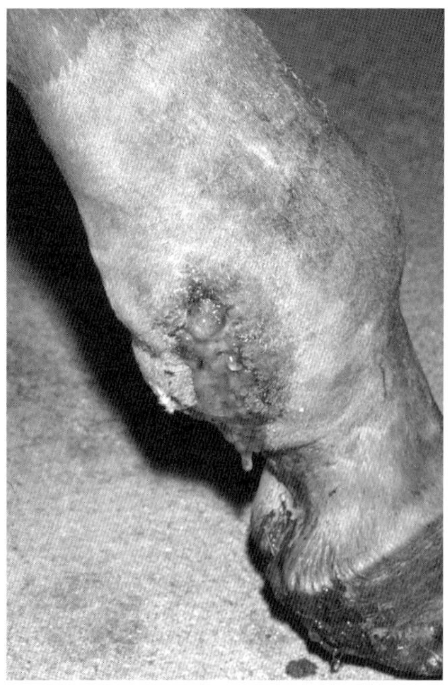

Fig 15.16 Infectious tenosynovitis and digital sheath swelling associated with annular ligament constriction.

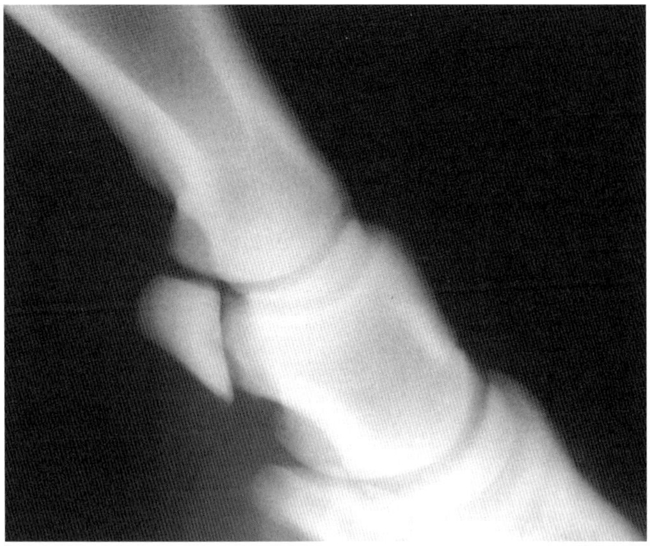

Fig 15.17 Typical biaxial palmar second phalanx eminence fracture.

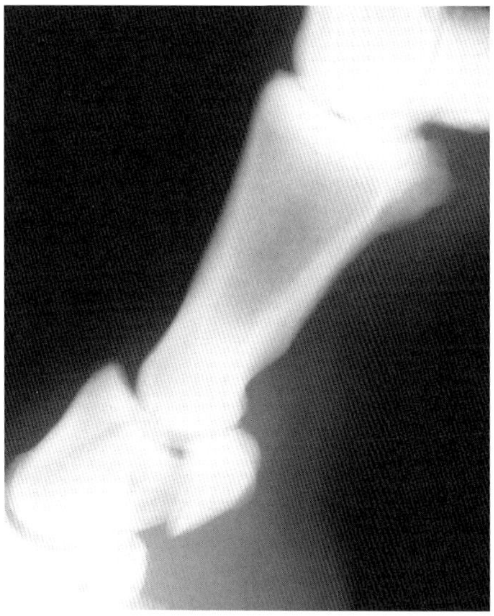

Fig 15.18 Typical comminuted second phalanx fracture.

Recognition

History and presenting complaint

These injuries are associated with acute onset of lameness and swelling at the pastern.

Physical examination

Lameness located to the distal limb with regional nerve blocks and visible pastern swelling are often present.

Diagnostic confirmation

Source of the lameness can be confirmed with direct pastern joint block but this is often not necessary in acute cases. Fractures are confirmed on radiographs.

Treatment and prognosis

Therapeutic aims

The goal of therapy is to eliminate or reduce the lameness due to the fracture. In many cases a pastern arthrodesis may ultimately be necessary for soundness.

Therapy

The smaller articular fragments are retrievable surgically by direct arthrotomy (dorsally) or arthroscopy (palmar/plantar pouch).[61] Unfortunately, degenerative joint disease is often a sequela because significant soft tissue injury is necessary to induce a fracture in such a stable joint. Disruption of the joint capsule frequently results in persistent thickening of the joint and chronic lameness due to osteoarthritis (high ringbone).

Immediate stabilization of the distal limb in splints or preferably casts is recommended to prevent collapse or displacement for comminuted fractures of the second phalanx (Fig. 15.18). Prognosis is dependent on the degree of displacement, particularly at the coffin joint. Surgical exposure of the coffin joint is not possible to aid in reduction, so prevention of distraction or displacement is strongly advised. Preferable treatment is surgical reduction, lag screw fixation and simultaneous plate arthrodesis of the pastern joint[62,63] (Fig. 15.19).

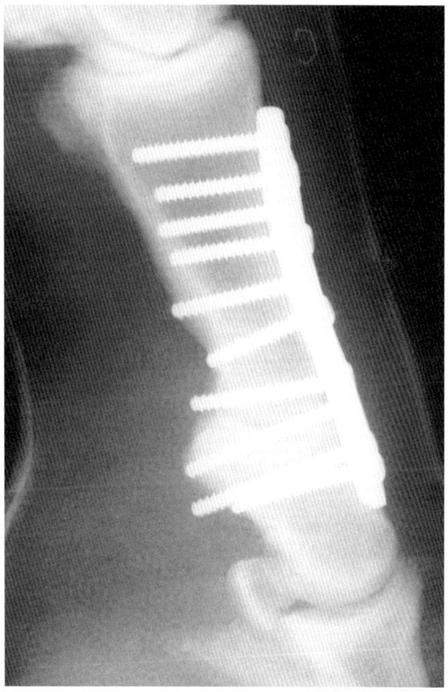

Fig 15.19 Surgical repair of a comminuted second phalanx fracture at two months postoperatively. Pastern arthrodesis and fracture fragment stabilization were performed simultaneously.

Caudal eminence traction fractures usually heal with a fibrous union. For athletic soundness, pastern arthrodesis is recommended either at the time of fracture or if soundness does not result with time. Reduction and direct lag screw fixation of the fragment is described, but osteoarthritis is often the sequela. Pastern arthrodesis is recommended (Fig. 15.20).

Prognosis

With surgery, prognosis for pasture or breeding soundness is good to excellent. Athletic soundness can be achieved with pastern arthrodesis if fractures did not enter the coffin joint. Prognosis for athletic soundness is guarded if the fracture entered the coffin joint. The prognosis for pasture or breeding soundness with conservative treatment is guarded to fair as horses remain lame for extended periods of time and healing is usually asymmetrical.

Etiology and pathogenesis

Etiology

Fractures of the second phalanx can occur at exercise, typically when the horse is turning on a supporting limb.

Pathophysiology

Pathophysiology is dependent on the type of second phalanx fracture. Larger caudal eminence fractures usually occur on the second phalanx, are often articular and can be biaxial. These fractures are distracted due to pull of the insertion of the collateral ligaments, flexor tendons and palmar annular ligaments.

Longitudinal and comminuted fractures of the second pastern bone are probably the most common fracture involving the pastern joint and can be catastrophic. Fractures of this short bone are high-energy injuries, usually from high-speed twists and turns with the foot planted. It is often reported that a loud 'pop' sound, like a gun going off, was heard and the horse was immediately non-weight bearing in the limb. Palpation can confirm the immediate pain, swelling and instability. Most P2 fractures are initiated at the pastern joint surface and spiral toward (incomplete) or into (complete) the distal interphalangeal joint (coffin joint). Fractures are often displaced and comminuted into five pieces in a classic pattern.[64]

Epidemiology

This injury may occur more commonly in Quarter Horses and jumpers, during slides, landings and turns.

Prevention

This injury is considered a sporadic and relatively random event that cannot be prevented.

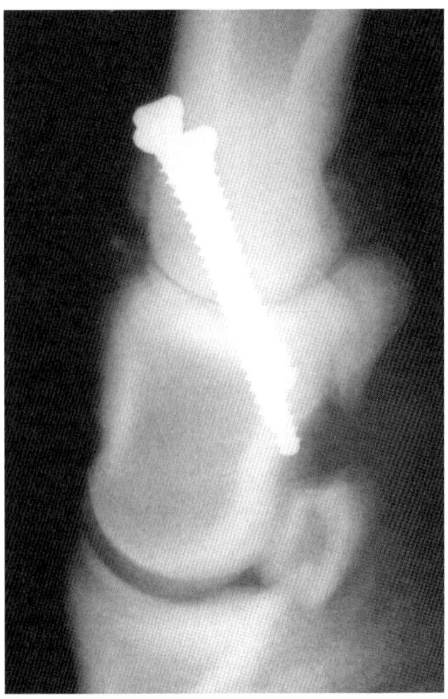

Fig 15.20 Triple lag screw pastern arthrodesis as treatment for a caudal eminence fracture.

Traumatic luxation/subluxation of the pastern joint

Traumatic luxation of the pastern joint usually occurs in front limbs with dorsal displacement of the first phalanx and is considered secondary to disruption of the insertion of the superficial digital flexor tendon and superficial distal sesamoidean ligament and palmar joint capsule[65] (Fig. 15.21). In the author's experience it is seen most commonly in event horses. This injury can appear similar to a fetlock breakdown injury in that the fetlock area drops upon weight bearing. However, closer observation reveals the distortion to the pastern with loading. The fetlock drops as the first phalanx moves dorsally. In complete luxations, similar complications can occur as with fetlock luxations. In subluxations, the pastern joint retains some stability although dorsal subluxation of the first phalanx is evident on palpation and radiograph.

Lameness depends on the degree of subluxation and disruption of the support structures of the pastern. Pastern arthrodesis is the treatment of choice as the outcome can be pasture and breeding soundness and possibly athletic soundness, depending on the extent of soft tissue injury to the flexor tendons. Use of strong implants and consideration of caudal joint wiring is recommended as the normal caudal support structures to the joint are disrupted. Repair should be approached in a similar manner to a fetlock luxation with loss of the caudal support structures.[22]

Pastern arthritis

Degenerative joint disease of the pastern joint is commonly called high ringbone or ringbone (Fig. 15.22).

Recognition

History and presenting complaint

Horses are typically lame in one limb with a spontaneous onset. A traumatic etiology is often inferred. The lameness persists and pastern joint enlargement, although often overlooked, may be noted by the owner.

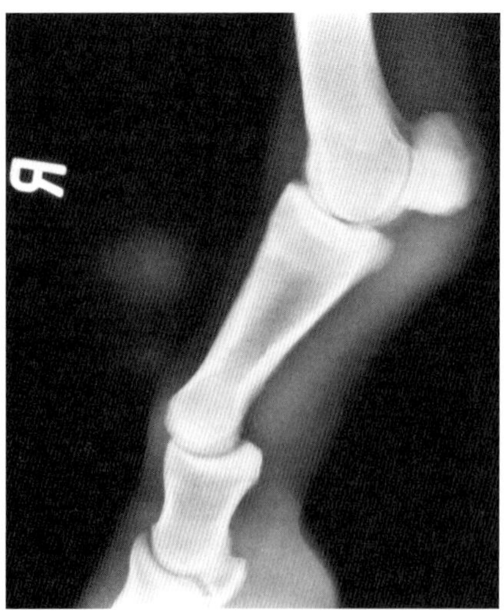

Fig 15.21 Pastern luxation with typical dorsal displacement.

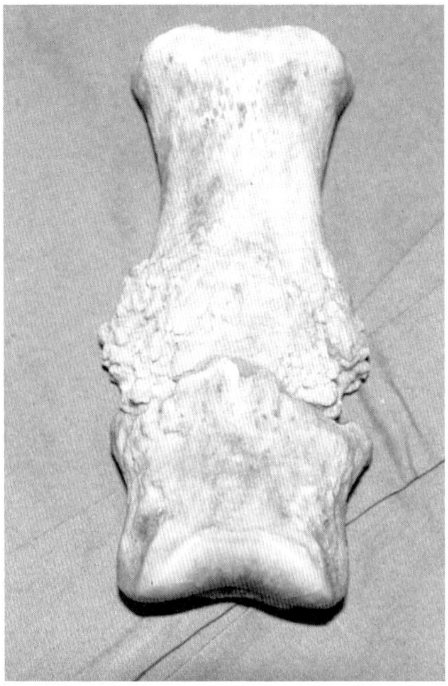

Fig 15.22 Degenerative joint disease of the pastern joint demonstrating bony proliferation and joint destruction typical of ringbone.

Physical examination

Pastern arthritis has a classic outward appearance of an enlarged, thickened pastern joint. Horses are lame often at the walk and are sore to flexion of the limb or joint.

Diagnostic confirmation

The diagnosis is confirmed by radiography demonstrating osteophytes, narrowing of the joint space and subchondral bone sclerosis (Fig. 15.23).

Treatment and prognosis

Therapeutic aims

The goal of therapy is to reduce pain and inflammation. To achieve athletic soundness, the joint must fuse.

Therapy

Treatment with joint therapies is less successful in the pastern due to the greater degree of lameness, but non-steroidal anti-inflammatory medication improves movement and gait. Intra-articular steroids may improve comfort but often do not result in athletic soundness. Rest does not result in joint fusion. Resolution of lameness can be achieved with surgical pastern arthrodesis. Current procedures with plates and screws usually produce fusion within six months, even in older horses (Fig. 15.24). Assuming the pastern was the sole source of lameness, complete athletic soundness can be expected in >80% of horses treated with surgical arthrodesis (Fig. 15.16). Current technique employs a combination of plates and screws for transarticular compression and stabilization.[66–69]

Prognosis

The prognosis is poor for soundness or fusion of the joint without surgical intervention. The pastern joint does not fuse on its own, even with extended time, in the author's experience.

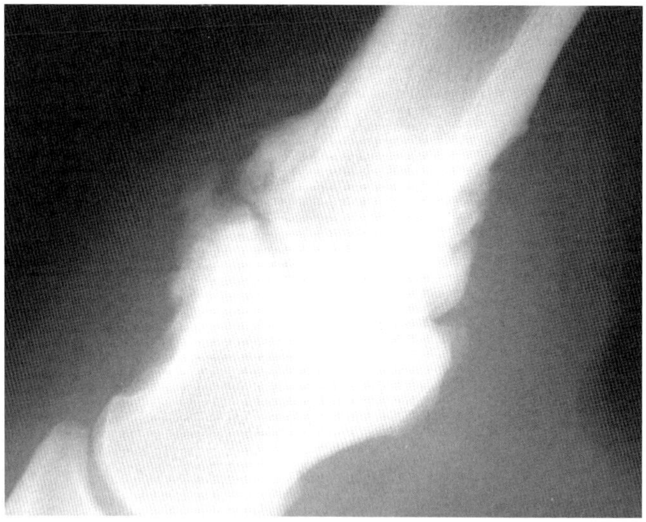

Fig 15.23 Lateral radiograph of a pastern joint with arthritis demonstrating joint space narrowing and severe osteophytosis.

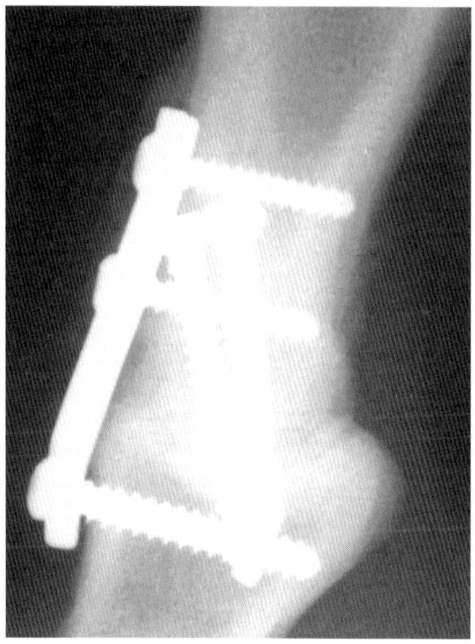

Fig 15.24 Recommended surgical technique for pastern arthrodesis for adult horses is a single plate and two transarticular compression screws.

Etiology and pathogenesis

Etiology

Trauma and/or repetitive use are common inciting causes.

Pathophysiology

Initial joint injury (fracture or sprain) results in joint inflammation and capsulitis. The process of persistent inflammation results in chronic joint destruction and degeneration.

Epidemiology

Although osteoarthritis of the pastern may not be as common as osteoarthritis of the fetlock, it is progressive and produces a greater degree of lameness in almost 100% of affected horses. Many horses with ringbone are lame at the walk and do not want to move around in pasture. Severe osteopenia of the affected limb and contralateral limb laminitis are complications of chronic ringbone.

Pastern osteochondrosis

Articular developmental orthopedic disease (osteochondrosis) occurs in the pastern joint.

Recognition

History and presenting complaint

Lameness may be acute in onset and associated with heavy exercise or an incident, such as a fall, suggesting a traumatic etiology.

Physical examination

Lameness and an enlarged pastern joint are the hallmark signs. Clinical signs occur most commonly in yearlings and become identical to osteoarthritis of the pastern (ringbone).

Diagnostic confirmation

Radiographs demonstrate cysts on the articular surface and irregularity to the articular surface (Fig. 15.25). Osteophytes may not be present early on in the disease. The condition is often bilateral and contralateral radiographs are indicated before surgical treatment is considered.

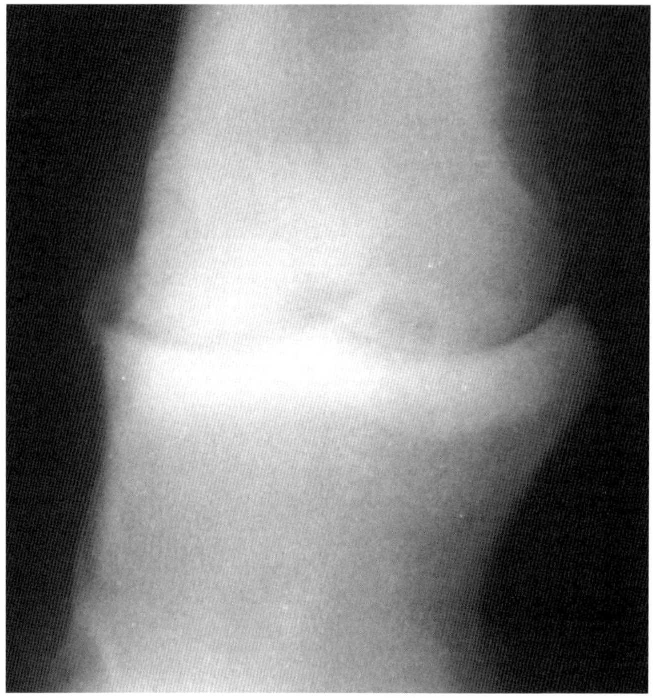

Fig 15.25 Radiograph of pastern osteochondrosis demonstrating articular cysts and joint destruction.

Treatment and prognosis

Therapeutic aims

The goal of therapy is to eliminate the lameness with joint fusion.

Therapy

Preferable treatment is surgical arthrodesis[70] as has been described for pastern arthritis.

Prognosis

In young horses, the possibility of full athletic soundness is excellent and fusion is relatively rapid (3–4 months). Left untreated, the joint will progress into osteoarthritis and lameness will persist.

Etiology and pathogenesis

Etiology

Osteochondrosis is part of a developmental orthopedic disease complex.

Pathophysiology

Endochondral ossification of articular cartilage is delayed or arrested, such that it forms abnormally. Articular cartilage flaps and cysts develop during growth, and joint pain and ultimately arthritis are a consequence.

Prevention

Although osteochondrosis has multifactorial risk factors, including high-energy diets, rapid growth and male gender, it is not possible to control the onset of clinical disease by controlling these factors. This is an active area of research.

References

1. Pettersson H, Ryden G. Avulsion fractures of the caudoproximal extremity of the first phalanx. Equine Vet J 1982;14(4):333–5.
2. Hubert J, Williams J, Moore RM. What is your diagnosis? Avulsion fracture of the medial plantar eminence of the first phalanx; subluxation of the metatarsophalangeal joint resulting from avulsion of the insertion of the medial collateral ligament. J Am Vet Med Assoc 1998;213(2):203–4.
3. Grondahl AM. Incidence and development of ununited proximoplantar tuberosity of the proximal phalanx in Standardbred trotters. Vet Rad Ultra 1992;33(1):18–26.
4. Dabareiner RM, White NA, Sullins KE. Metacarpophalangeal joint synovial pad fibrotic proliferation in 63 horses. Vet Surg 1996;25(3):199–206.
5. Yovich JV, McIlwraith CW. Arthroscopic surgery for osteochondral fractures of the proximal phalanx of the metacarpophalangeal and metatarsophalangeal (fetlock) joints in horses. J Am Vet Med Assoc 1986;188(3):273–9.
6. Kawcak CE, McIlwraith CW. Proximodorsal first phalanx osteochondral chip fragmentation in 336 horses. Equine Vet J 1994;26(5):392–6.
7. Colon JL, Bramlage LR, Hance SR, et al. Qualitative and quantitative documentation of the racing performance of 461 Thoroughbred racehorses after arthroscopic removal of dorsoproximal first phalanx osteochondral fractures (1986–1995). Equine Vet J 2000;32(6):475–81.
8. Elce YA, Richardson DW. Arthroscopic removal of dorsoproximal chip fractures of the proximal phalanx in standing horses. Vet Surg 2002;31(3):195–200.
9. Johnson BJ, Stover SM, Daft BM, et al. Causes of death in racehorses over a 2 year period. Equine Vet J 1994;26(4):327–30.
10. Bertone AL. The fetlock. In: Stashak TS, editor. Adams' lameness in horses, vol. 8. 5th ed. Philadelphia, PA: Lippincott,

Williams and Wilkins; 2002. p. 768–96.
11. Torre K, Motta M. Incidence and distribution of 369 proximal sesamoid bone fractures in 354 Standardbred horses (1984–1995). Equine Pract 1999;21(8):6–12.
12. Southwood LL, Trotter GW, McIlwraith CW. Arthroscopic removal of abaxial fracture fragments of the proximal sesamoid bones in horses: 47 cases (1989–1997). JAVMA 1998;213(7): 1016–21.
13. Bertone AL. Fractures of the proximal sesamoid bones. In: Nixon AJ, editor. Equine fracture repair, vol. 16. Philadelphia, PA: Saunders; 1996. p. 163–71.
14. Parente EJ, Richardson DW, Spencer P. Basal sesamoidean fractures in horses: 57 cases (1989–1991). JAVMA 1993; 202(8):1293–7.
15. Boure L, Marcoux M, Laverty S, et al. Use of electrocautery probes in arthroscopic removal of apical sesamoid fracture fragments in 18 Standardbred horses. Vet Surg 1999;28:226–32.
16. Malone ED, Anderson BH, Turner TA. Proximal sesamoid bone fracture following cast removal in two horses. Equine Vet J 1997;9:185–9.
17. Southwood LL, McIlwraith CW. Arthroscopic removal of fracture fragments involving a portion of the base of the proximal sesamoid bone in horses: 26 cases (1984–1997). JAVMA 2000;217(2):236–40.
18. Henninger RW, Bramlage LR, Schneider RK, et al. Lag screw and cancellous bone graft fixation of transverse proximal sesamoid bone fractures in horses: 25 cases (1983–1989). JAVMA 1991;199(5): 606–12.
19. Martin BB, Nunamaker DM, Evans LH, et al. Circumferential wiring of mid-body and large basilar fractures of the proximal sesamoid bone in 15 horses. Vet Surg 1991;20(1):9–14.
20. Woodie JB, Ruggles AJ, Litsky AS. In vitro biomechanical properties of 2 compression fixation methods for midbody proximal sesamoid bone fractures in horses. Vet Surg 2000;29(4):358–63.
21. Rothaug PG, Boston BC, Richardson DW, et al. A comparison of ultra-high-molecular weight polyethylene cable and stainless steel wire using two fixation techniques for repair of equine midbody sesamoid fractures: an in vitro biomechanical study. Vet Surg 2002; 31(5):445–54.
22. Bramlage LR. Fetlock arthrodesis. In: Nixon AJ, editor. Equine fracture repair, vol. 17. Philadelphia: Saunders; 1996. p. 172–8.
23. Bassage LH, Richardson DW. Longitudinal fractures of the condyles of the third metacarpal and metatarsal bones in racehorses: 224 cases (1986–1995). JAVMA 1998;212:1757–64.
24. Woodie JB, Ruggles AJ, Bertone AL, et al. Apical fracture of the proximal sesamoid bone in standardbred horses: 43 cases (1990–1996). JAVMA 1999;214(11): 1653–6.
25. Trumble TN, Arnoczky SP, Stick JA, et al. Clinical relevance of the microvasculature of the equine proximal sesamoid bone. Am J Vet Res 1995;56(6):720–4.
26. Markel MD, Richardson DW. Noncomminuted fractures of the proximal phalanx in 69 horses. J Am Vet Med Assoc 1985;186(6):573–9.
27. Holcombe SJ, Schneider RK, Bramlage LR, et al. Lag screw fixation of noncomminuted sagittal fractures of the proximal phalanx in racehorses: 59 cases (1973–1991). J Am Vet Med Assoc 1995;206(8):1195–9.
28. Tetens J, Ross MW, Lloyd JW. Comparison of racing performance before and after treatment of incomplete, midsagittal fractures of the proximal phalanx in standardbreds: 49 cases (1986–1992). J Am Vet Med Assoc 1997;210(1):82–6.
29. Dechant JE, MacDonald DG, Crawford WH. Repair of complete dorsal fracture of the proximal phalanx in two horses. Vet Surg 1998;27(5):445–9.
30. Schneider RK, Ratzlaff MC, White KK, et al. Effect of three types of half-limb casts on in vitro bone strain recorded from the third metacarpal bone and proximal phalanx in equine cadaver limbs. Am J Vet Res 1998;59(9):1188–93.
31. Grondahl AM, Gaustad G, Engeland A. Progression and association with lameness and racing performance of radiographic changes in the proximal sesamoid bones of young standardbred trotters. Equine Vet J 1994;26(2):152–5.
32. Clayton HM. Cinematographic analysis of the gait of lame horses II: chronic sesamoiditis. Equine Vet Sci 1986;6: 310–12.
33. Cornelissen BP. The proximal sesamoid bone of the horse; vascular and neurologic characteristics. Tijdschr Diergeneeskd 1998;123(12):375–80.
34. Wisner ER, O'Brien TR, Pool RR, et al. Osteomyelitis of the axial border of the proximal sesamoid bones in seven horses. Equine Vet J 1991;23(5):383–9.
35. Richardson DW, Nunamaker DM, Sigafoos RD. Use of an external skeletal fixation device and bone graft for arthrodesis of the metacarpophalangeal joint in horses. J Am Vet Med Assoc 1987;191(3):316–21.
36. Cohen ND, Peloso JG, Mundy GD, et al. Racing-related factors and results of prerace physical inspection and their association with musculoskeletal injuries incurred in thoroughbreds during races. J Am Vet Med Assoc 1997;211(4):454–63.
37. Kane AJ, Stover SM, Gardner IA, et al. Horseshoe characteristics as possible risk factors for fatal musculoskeletal injury of Thoroughbred racehorses. Am J Vet Res 1996;57(8):1147–52.
38. Yovich JV, Turner AS, Stashak TS, et al. Luxation of the metacarpophalangeal and metatarsophalangeal joints in horses. Equine Vet J 1987;19(4):295–8.
39. Hubert J, Williams J, Moore RM. What is your diagnosis? Avulsion fracture of the medial plantar eminence of the first phalanx; subluxation of the metatarsophalangeal joint resulting from avulsion of the insertion of the medial collateral ligament. J Am Vet Med Assoc 1998;213(2):203–4.
40. Simmon EJ, Bertone AL, Weisbrode SE. Instability-induced osteoarthritis in the metacarpophalangeal joint of horses. Am J Vet Res 1999;60(1):7–13.
41. van der Harst MR, Rijkenhuizen AB. The use of polypropylene mesh for treatment of ruptured collateral ligaments of the equine metatarsophalangeal joint: a report of 2 cases. Vet Q 2000;22(1): 57–60.
42. Vickers KL, Ross MW. Atypical villonodular synovitis in a horse. J Am Vet Med Assoc 1996;209(9):1602–3.
43. Roneus B, Andersson AM, Ekman S. Racing performance in standardbred trotters with chronic synovitis after partial arthroscopic synovectomy in the metacarpophalangeal, metatarsophalangeal and intercarpal (midcarpal) joints. Acta Vet Scand 1997;38(1):87–95.
44. Kannegieter NJ. Chronic proliferative synovitis of the equine metacarpophalangeal joint. Vet Rec 1990;127(1):8–10.
45. van Veenendaal JC, Moffatt RE. Soft tissue masses in the fetlock joint of horses. Aust Vet J 1980;56(11):533–6.
46. Murphy DJ, Nixon AJ. Arthroscopic laser extirpation of metacarpophalangeal synovial pad proliferation in eleven horses. Equine Vet J 2001;33(3):296–301.
47. Declerq J, Martens A, Maes D, et al. Dorsoproximal proximal phalanxosteochondral fragmentation in 117 Warmblood horses. Vet Comp Traumatol 2009;22(1):1–6.
48. Declerq J, Martens A, Bogaert L, et al. Osteochondral fragmentation in the synovial pad of the fetlock in Warmblood horses. Vet Surg 2008;37(7):613–18.
49. McIlwraith CW. Diseases of joints, ligaments and related structures. In: Stashak TS, editor. Adams' lameness in horses, vol. 7. 5th ed. Philadelphia, PA: Lippincott Williams and Wilkins; 2002. p. 533–43.
50. Bertone, et al. 2012 ACVS Symposium
51. Verschooten F, Picavet TM. Desmitis of the fetlock annular ligament in the horse. Equine Vet J 1986;18(2):138–42.

52. Hawkins JF, Ross MW. Transection of the accessory ligament of the superficial digital flexor muscle for the treatment of superficial digital flexor tendinitis in Standardbreds: 40 cases (1988–1992). J Am Vet Med Assoc 1995;206(5): 674–8.
53. Stanek C, Edinger H. Radiographic diagnosis of stricture of, or constriction by, the annular ligament of the equine fetlock. Pferdeheilkunde 1990;6(3): 125–8.
54. Bertone AL. Septic tenosynovitis. In: Dyson S, editor. Equine tendon injuries. Philadelphia, PA: Saunders; 1995. p. 163–77.
55. Fortier LA, Nixon AJ, Ducharme NG, et al. Tenoscopic examination and proximal annular ligament desmotomy for treatment of equine 'complex' digital sheath tenosynovitis. Vet Surg 1999;28(6):429–35.
56. Honnas CM, Schumacher J, Cohen ND, et al. Septic tenosynovitis in horses: 25 cases (1983–1989). J Am Vet Med Assoc 1991;199(11):1616–22.
57. Gerring EL, Webbon PM. Fetlock annular ligament desmotomy: a report of 24 cases. Equine Vet J 1984;16(2):113–16.
58. van den Berg MJ, Rijkenhuizen AB, Nemeth F, et al. The fetlock tunnel syndrome: a macroscopic and microscopic study. Vet Q 1995; 17(4):138–42.
59. Owen KR, Dyson SJ, Parkin TDH, et al. Retrospective study of palmar/plantar annular ligament injury in 71 horses: 2001–2006. Equine Vet J 2008;40(3): 237–44.
60. Dik KJ, van den Belt JM, Keg PR. Ultrasonographic evaluation of the fetlock annular ligament constriction in the horse. Equine Vet J 1991;23(4): 285–8.
61. Radcliffe RM, Cheetham J, Bezuidenhout AJ, et al. Arthroscopic removal of palmar/plantar osteochondral fragments from the proximal interphalangeal joint four. Vet Surg 2008;37(8):733–40.
62. Galuppo LD, Stover SM, Willits NH. A biomechanical comparison of double-plate and Y-plate fixation for comminuted equine second phalangeal fractures. Vet Surg 2000;29(2):152–62.
63. Crabill MR, Watkins JP, Schneider RK, et al. Double-plate fixation of comminuted fractures of the second phalanx in horses: 10 cases (1985–1993). J Am Vet Med Assoc 1995;207(11): 1458–61.
64. Rose PL, Seeherman H, O'Callaghan M. Computed tomographic evaluation of comminuted middle phalangeal fractures in the horse. Vet Radiol Ultrasound 1997;38(6):424–9.
65. Harrison LJ, May SA. Bilateral subluxation of the pastern joint in the forelimbs of a foal. Vet Rec 1992;131(4):68–70.
66. Schaer TP, Bramlage LR, Embertson RM, et al. Proximal interphalangeal arthrodesis in 22 horses. Equine Vet J 2001;33(4):360–5.
67. MacLellan KN, Crawford WH, MacDonald DG. Proximal interphalangeal joint arthrodesis in 34 horses using two parallel 5.5-mm cortical bone screws. Vet Surg 2001;30(5):454–9.
68. Watt BC, Edwards RB 3rd, Markel MD, et al. Arthrodesis of the equine proximal interphalangeal joint: a biomechanical comparison of three 4.5-mm and two 5.5-mm cortical screws. Vet Surg 2001;30(3): 287–94.
69. Watt BC, Edwards RB 3rd, Markel MD, et al. Arthrodesis of the equine proximal interphalangeal joint: a biomechanical comparison of two 7-hole 3.5-mm broad and two 5-hole 4.5-mm narrow dynamic compression plates. Vet Surg 2002;31(1):85–93.
70. Yovich JV, Stashak TS, Sullins KE. Bilateral pastern arthrodesis in a horse. Equine Vet J 1986;18(1):79–81.

Metacarpus/metatarsus

16

Lance H. Bassage II

CHAPTER CONTENTS

Dorsal metacarpal disease (the 'bucked shins' complex)

'Bucked shins' or dorsal metacarpal periostitis and dorsal cortical stress fractures of the third metacarpus (MC-III) are the two components of dorsal metacarpal disease (DMD). Over the last 2–3 decades, extensive investigation into the etiopathogenesis of the condition – including the role of the training regimen, track surface and shoeing techniques – has led to a far greater understanding of the syndrome of DMD and how to prevent it. However, despite these advances, 'bucked shins' and dorsal cortical stress fractures remain important problems in the racing industry. Points to note are:

- These problems are common in young Thoroughbreds and Quarter Horses in early race training.
- Bilateral dorsal metacarpal swelling, heat and pain, with stiffness/soreness or 'choppy-gaited' lameness are common symptoms.
- Acute onset may follow a high-speed workout ('breeze') or first race.
- Treatment involves anti-inflammatory therapy, rest and controlled exercise, and modified training.
- Prevention involves modification of the training regimen.
- Prognosis is generally very good to excellent and recurrence is rare in skeletally mature horses.
- Horses that develop clinical 'bucked shins' are at risk for dorsal cortical stress fractures in the future.

Recognition

History and presenting complaint

Horses with 'bucked shins' present with an acute onset of bilateral soft tissue swelling, heat and sensitivity over the dorsal aspect of the metacarpus, with an associated lameness or 'stiffness' immediately after a high-speed workout ('breeze') or race. Very often this is the first race or first speed work for the horse at near-racing distances. In some horses there may be a more gradual onset of these signs, with a marked exacerbation following the first race or a longer 'breeze', If training continues, the lameness typically worsens considerably, as opposed to the horse 'warming out of it'. The signs of 'bucked shins' are generally so specific that most experienced trainers can make a reliable diagnosis.

Physical examination

Horses with 'bucked shins' exhibit variable degrees of soft tissue swelling, heat and sensitivity on palpation over the dorsal diaphyses of MC-III. When viewing the metacarpi from the lateral aspect, there is often a distinct dorsal convexity. Firm digital pressure in this location will elicit a painful response. These signs are particularly pronounced in the acute stages, but after a period of rest and anti-inflammatory treatment, there is generally considerable improvement. The exceptions are horses that have progressed to the chronic or 'recurrent' category and have developed a marked periosteal reaction along with chronic inflammation and associated soft tissue swelling. Less commonly, a more focal area of swelling may be present at some point along the dorsal diaphysis,[1] which must be differentiated from a true stress fracture (see section below).

Lameness examination

Horses with acute 'bucked shins' typically exhibit a bilateral stiff or choppy forelimb gait at a trot (sometimes mimicking a foot or carpal lameness), but in those in which one metacarpus is more severely affected than the other, a distinct head nod may be evident. Lameness in these horses ranges from grade 1 to 3.[2] The most severely affected horses may acutely exhibit mild lameness at the walk. The severity of the lameness will vary greatly with the stage of the disease and the timing of the examination in relation to the last speed work.

Diagnostic confirmation

Diagnostic analgesia

Diagnostic analgesia is generally not necessary to localize the source of pain in a horse with acute 'bucked shins'. High palmar analgesia (high palmar nerve block) with a dorsal ring block in the proximal metacarpus can be helpful in confirming the location of pain in those horses with subacute or chronic 'bucked shins'.

Nuclear scintigraphy

Bone-phase (delayed-phase) nuclear scintigraphy classically reveals *diffuse* moderate-to-intense abnormal increased radiopharmaceutical uptake along the dorsal diaphyses of the affected MC-III[3] (Fig. 16.1).

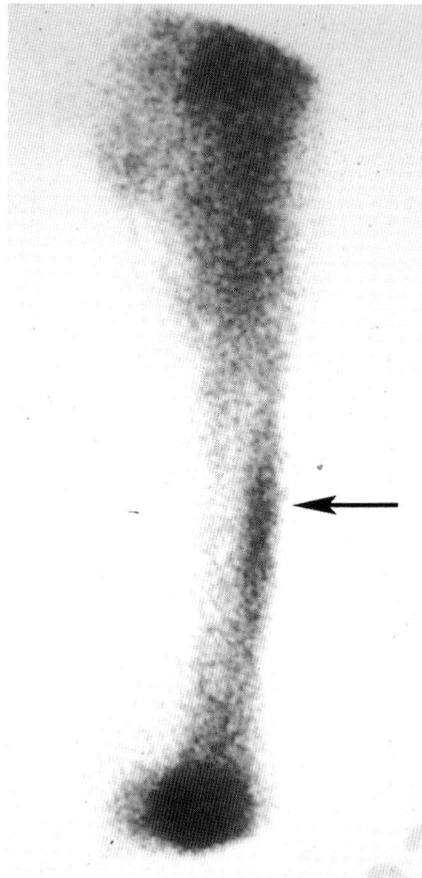

Fig 16.1 Lateral bone-phase scintigraphic image of the right metacarpus of a two-year-old Thoroughbred racehorse with clinical 'bucked shins'. Notice the diffuse moderate-to-intense abnormal increased radiopharmaceutical uptake along the dorsal diaphysis of MC-III (arrow).

Radiography

Radiographic findings vary with each case and the stage of disease. Radiographs in mildly affected horses or in the very early stages of the disease (subclinical) are often negative or equivocal for osseous abnormalities. In more severely affected horses, diffuse subperiosteal osteolytic change in combination with smooth, low-density periosteal proliferative reaction is typically seen along the dorsal and dorsomedial diaphysis of MC-III (Fig. 16.2). High-detail digital radiographs are superior for detecting the subtle abnormalities. Soft tissue swelling, when present, will also be evident radiographically in this location.

Thermography

Thermography in the hands of an *experienced* operator has been shown to be a valuable diagnostic aid for the detection of abnormalities in the metacarpi of racing Thoroughbreds, with up to 60% of two year olds in training exhibiting abnormal findings.[4]

Treatment and prognosis

Therapeutic aims

The goals of treatment for acute 'bucked shins' are two-fold: decrease or eliminate further excessive cyclic strains on MC-III and shift the balance from net bone resorption to net bone apposition, and reduce acute inflammation.

Therapy

Exercise restriction

The degree of exercise restriction depends on several factors, of which the severity of clinical signs, in conjunction with radiographic and/or scintigraphic findings, is the most important.

Initially, all horses diagnosed with acute 'bucked shins' should receive stall rest and hand grazing (no purposeful hand-walking exercise) until soft tissue swelling and pain on palpation of the dorsum of MC-III have subsided. A program of controlled exercise can begin. In horses without extensive periosteal new bone formation or other severe radiographic changes, 2 weeks of stall rest with daily hand-walking (10–15 minutes once or twice a day) are initially recommended. Once horses are sound at a trot in-hand then formal training can commence, ideally employing a modified exercise protocol (see below).

Horses with moderate-to-marked periosteal reaction and/or subperiosteal osteolytic change, along with moderate-to-intense abnormal increased radiopharmaceutical uptake scintigraphically, require a more extended period of rest and controlled exercise. Generally,

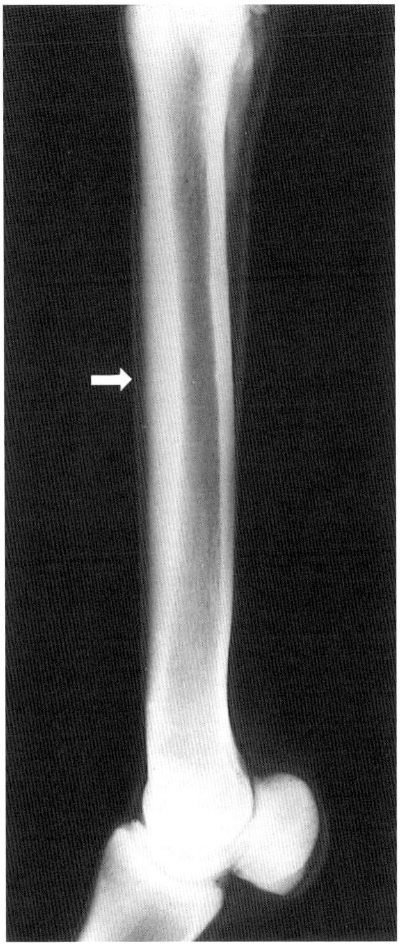

Fig 16.2 Lateral radiograph of the left metacarpus of a two-year-old Thoroughbred racehorse with clinical 'bucked shins'. Notice the diffuse low-density periosteal proliferative reaction and subperiosteal osteolysis along the dorsal diaphysis of MC-III (arrow).

this encompasses four weeks of hand-walking, followed by 4–8 weeks of turnout exercise in a small paddock or 'shed row' exercise daily. The duration and extent of exercise restriction is modified based on the specifics of each case. Horses with chronic or recurrent 'bucked shins' (i.e. those that have had several acute episodes with or without an appropriate period of convalescence) should be allowed a total of 90–120 days' rest and in many instances they are simply turned out for the remainder of the season and training is resumed the following year.

Follow-up radiographic and scintigraphic examinations can help guide the recommendations for resumption of training in those cases where this is economically feasible.

Anti-inflammatory therapy

Anti-inflammatory therapy should be initiated immediately in cases of acute 'bucked shins' and continue until signs of swelling and 'shin sensitivity' (pain) subside. Up to 30 minutes of cold hosing or icing, several times a day, along with bandaging, are generally effective. Anecdotally, application of a poultice or antiphlogistic dressing (e.g. Gel-o-cast®) for several days may also help decrease swelling.

The use of NSAIDs for their anti-inflammatory and analgesic effects in patients with inflammatory bone disorders is controversial in light of the gathering body of evidence that these drugs, when used chronically at high doses, may impair bone healing in horses.[5] However, it is this author's opinion that a brief period (i.e. a few days) of NSAID treatment during the acute stage of 'bucked shins' is warranted in horses with moderate-to-severe signs. Phenylbutazone or flunixin meglumine at standard doses is generally effective. Long-term NSAID treatment is contraindicated, in this author's opinion, for the reasons noted above.

Modified training protocol

The key to preventing 'bucked shins' is to stress the dorsal cortices of the developing metacarpi in such a way as to stimulate adaptation to the cyclic compressive loads under conditions that are similar to those experienced during a race, i.e. to train at racing speeds.[6] Traditional training strategies for flat-racing Thoroughbreds have employed a basic scheme of daily galloping exercise for extended distances (e.g. 1–2 miles) with speed work or 'breezes' at shorter distances (e.g. 2–6 furlongs) weekly to every third week. In immature (untrained) horses the timing (too infrequent) and distance (too long) of the high-speed work sets up a state of maladaptive remodeling in which bone resorption outpaces apposition and fibrous periosteal new bone predominates.[6] Eventually, this inferior bone develops microfractures and resulting inflammation, which manifests clinically as periostitis or 'bucked shins'.

To prevent or mitigate the potential for this vicious cycle, horses should be trained in such a way as to increase the frequency of high-strain cyclic compressive loading (high-speed exercise or 'breezes') and decrease the total distance at which they are galloped.[6] It is recommended that horses be worked at or near racing speed at least twice a week, initially at very short distances, for example one furlong. The distance of the speed work is increased gradually (e.g. adding one furlong every 1–2 weeks) and then as the horse is asked to go faster, the distance is reduced and the process repeated until the horse is conditioned to race. Throughout this process, daily galloping is limited,[6] for example to no more than one mile/day. Upon resumption of training, horses are continually monitored for signs of 'shin soreness', lameness or dorsal metacarpal swelling and exercise intensity should be modified accordingly.

Traditional or alternative therapies

Over the course of time, seemingly endless 'traditional' therapies or essentially 'home remedies' have been promoted for treating 'bucked shins', as well as the many other inflammatory lesions and injuries of racehorses. Many have gone by the wayside but a handful have persisted and remain in use today and other 'alternative' therapies continue to arise on almost a daily basis. The list includes: 'paints' (topical rubefacients), 'blisters' (chemical vesicants), 'pin firing' (thermocautery), 'freeze firing' (focal cryotherapy), electrostimulation, periosteal 'picking' (or 'needling') and extracorporeal shockwave therapy. Unfortunately, many of these modalities have not undergone the necessary scientific scrutiny to enable rational conclusions regarding their efficacy, and some may be contraindicated. Some of these adjunct therapies will be covered in detail in other chapters, and the interested reader is referred there.

Prognosis

The prognosis for the vast majority of horses with 'bucked shins' is generally very good if appropriate intervention is undertaken and adhered to. Recurrence is rare; however, a variable proportion of horses will experience repeated episodes or 'chronic' DMD. Horses not given adequate convalescence and those that have not had their training protocol modified (see above) are at high risk for recurrence. 'Bucked shins' is quite rare in older horses (>4 years of age)[7] once the immature bone has remodeled and changed its inertial properties in response to the demands of high-speed exercise. However, horses that have experienced clinical 'bucked shins' as two or three year olds are in the high-risk group for dorsal cortical stress fractures (see section below).[8]

Etiology and pathophysiology

The reader is referred to the chapters on skeletal physiology and repetitive strain injuries of the skeleton. See Chapter 8 and Chapter 22 for detailed discussions of this topic.

Epidemiology

Historically, DMD and, more specifically, 'bucked shins' have been and continue to be an extremely common problem in young flat-racing horses in early training. In the US, a prevalence of 65–70% in Thoroughbreds has been reported[12,13] and in Australia the prevalence has been estimated at 42–80%.[14–16] Similarly, estimates of 5–50% have been given for the prevalence in racing Quarter Horses in the US.[17] DMD also affects racing Arabians. In contrast, the incidence of DMD is comparatively low in the UK, with an estimate of 17% in young Thoroughbreds in one large study.[10] This difference could be attributed to a number of variables, but differences in training surface (predominantly grass in the UK and predominantly dirt in the US) are regarded by many to be a primary factor.[9]

In stark contrast is the very low incidence of DMD in Standardbred racehorses.[12] This has been attributed to differences in speed and gait between Standardbreds and Thoroughbreds, which result in different strains imposed on MC-III, and not to an inherent difference in bone material properties between the breeds.[18]

Prevention

The most effective way to prevent or decrease the incidence of 'bucked shins' is to modify the training scheme as outlined previously (see under Therapy). Essentially, this involves decreasing the daily distance worked at a gallop and increasing the frequency of short intervals of high-speed work or 'breezes'. The distance of the speed work is initially very short and is increased gradually.[19,20]

Different training surfaces may also affect the incidence of 'bucked shins'. Training on woodchip-based surfaces or grass appears to be superior to the traditional dirt of most tracks in the US.[9,10] For example, in one two-year study of Thoroughbred racehorses, 55.8% of those trained on dirt experienced 'bucked shins' compared to only 26.1% of those trained on a woodchip-based surface.[9] This study did not rigidly control for differences in training methods, however.

Prevention also involves close monitoring of the horse for signs of impending shin problems. Along with physical examination for shin soreness, thermography and scintigraphy are useful imaging modalities for screening high-risk horses. In one study, pre-race detection using physical examination to screen horses for signs of DMD resulted in reduction in post-race diagnoses of lameness attributable to DMD, and more predictable race results, on Thoroughbred tracks in Australia.[11] More recent work has demonstrated significant increases in biochemical markers of bone turnover in horses in early training that ultimately developed signs of DMD.[21] However, the use of these measurements in the clinical setting remains only theoretical at this point.

Dorsal cortical stress fractures of MC-III ('saucer fractures', metacarpal fatigue fractures)

- Fatigue fractures are seen in racing Thoroughbreds, Quarter Horses and Arabians.
- Horses experiencing previous 'bucked shins' are at high risk.
- Short, oblique, intracortical fracture are seen most commonly in the mid-diaphysis of the left MC-III (in Thoroughbreds in the US).
- Acute onset of moderate-to-severe lameness may follow high-speed work ('breeze') or a race.
- Fractures are often slow to heal and chronic or recurrent. Fractures are common if initially undiagnosed or mismanaged.
- Surgical treatment is preferred for the majority of fractures and involves osteostixis, screw fixation, or a combination of the two.
- Prognosis is generally very good for return to racing.
- New or recurrent fractures develop on occasion.

Recognition

History and presenting complaint

Horses with an acute dorsal cortical stress fracture of MC-III typically exhibit a moderate-to-severe lameness immediately following high-speed work ('breeze') or a race. Less commonly, the lameness will not be evident until several hours after the horse has 'cooled out'. Acutely, these horses are too lame to continue training. There is almost invariably a focal area of soft tissue swelling, focal periosteal irregularity and sensitivity at the fracture site along the dorsal aspect of MC-III.

Some horses have a history of low-grade, chronic or intermittent lameness on the affected limb for several weeks prior to the acute onset of a more severe lameness once overt fracture has occurred. Another subset develops signs of acute fracture upon resumption of training after a brief period of lay-up (a few to several weeks) for an unrelated illness or injury.

Some horses may become sound enough to train or even race after extended rest, but continue to be plagued by recurrent lameness and poor performance. This is a common scenario for those with chronic stress fractures that have gone undiagnosed. Almost all horses with dorsal cortical stress fractures of MC-III will have a history of clinical 'bucked shins' in the 6–12 months preceding the fracture.[20]

Physical examination

For horses with acute fracture, physical examination will classically reveal a focal area of soft tissue swelling along the dorsum of the metacarpus at the site of the fracture, with a corresponding bony 'knot' or periosteal irregularity (hard swelling or exostosis) along the dorsal or dorsolateral diaphysis of MC-III. Firm digital pressure at the fracture site will consistently elicit a painful response. These signs are less dramatic in horses with chronic or subacute fractures. Horses with multiple fractures may have signs more suggestive of 'bucked shins' (i.e. diffuse pain and swelling along the diaphysis). Fractures are almost always unilateral in Thoroughbreds (in contrast to 'bucked shins') and involve predominantly the left forelimb in the US.[22–25] Bilateral fractures occur, but are rare.

Lameness examination

Acutely, horses exhibit a moderate-to-severe lameness on the affected limb, which is typically grade 3–4.[2] Many are lame at a walk

fractures and other subtle pathology have been documented.[51] As such, these modalities, in clinics where available, are sometimes used to assess fracture configuration in the more complex cases – in particular medial condylar fractures – prior to surgical repair.

Treatment and prognosis

Therapeutic aims

The goals in treating condylar fractures are to reduce healing time and minimize the potential for further degenerative changes in the affected joint. Optimal anatomic reconstruction of the articular surface and stabilization of the fracture are the keys. When dealing with medial condylar fractures (and the rare lateral fracture that extends into the mid-diaphysis), prevention of a catastrophic fracture is also paramount.

Therapy

Emergency treatment

Horses with acute condylar fractures should be confined strictly to a stall. The majority of non-displaced or incomplete lateral condylar fractures can be managed by coaptation with a firm, padded bandage pending definitive treatment (see below). Horses with displaced lateral condylar fractures are initially best managed by more rigid coaptation with the distal limb in a neutral or 'equinus' position (oriented such that the metacarpus/metatarsus and digit are in line). This can be accomplished with a dorsally applied splint and bandage that extends from the toe to just distal to the carpus or tarsus (such as a Kimzey splint®). This type of coaptation is important until the full extent of the injury can be assessed to rule out concurrent suspensory apparatus pathology and to prevent further fracture displacement and damage to the fetlock joint.

Horses with short medial condylar fractures should at least be managed with a rigid heavily padded bandage (such as a Robert-Jones bandage), with the addition of splints a prudent option. In horses with radiographically identifiable fracture lines in the mid-diaphysis, dorsally and laterally applied splints in the forelimb (extending to the elbow) or plantar and lateral splints in the hind limb extending to the point of the hock are recommended. Rigid coaptation with a bandage and splints or application of a well-constructed full-limb cast should also be considered prior to transportation given the propensity for catastrophic failure.[44,47]

NSAIDs are administered as needed for analgesia.

Non-surgical management

In certain cases of short, incomplete condylar fractures, particularly those in which economic considerations preclude surgery, non-surgical treatment can result in a good outcome.[41,44,52] The distal limb is kept in a bandage for 2–3 weeks to help minimize any soft tissue swelling and to provide some support. NSAIDs are administered only as needed to provide analgesia. Generally, the majority of horses in this category are quite comfortable within a few days to a week or so following the injury. Horses initially should have 1–2 months of strict stall rest, followed by another 1–2 months of stall confinement with daily hand-walking exercise. Follow-up radiographs are repeated three months from the time of fracture and if healing is progressing well, exercise in the form of small paddock turnout can begin. Under ideal circumstances, fractures heal in approximately four months.

The major disadvantage of non-surgical treatment is the tendency for fractures to exhibit delayed healing at the articular surface.[41,52,53] Resumption of training should not commence until fractures have completely healed and this may take up to six months or longer in some horses treated non-surgically. However, in a small percentage of horses a gap or defect in the subchondral bone may persist indefinitely well beyond the point at which the fracture has healed, which can complicate the decision on when to resume training.

Surgical treatment of lateral condylar fractures

With the exceptions noted above, interfragmentary screw compression[35,54] is the treatment of choice for the majority of horses with lateral condylar fractures. Surgical treatment is imperative for all horses with displaced fractures, regardless of their intended future use. The severity of the degenerative joint disease that develops in horses with untreated displaced fractures, even within a few months, is crippling and horses that are not surgical candidates should be euthanized.

Surgery is performed with the horse in lateral recumbency under general anesthesia with the affected limb up. The limb is clipped and aseptically prepared from the foot to the carpus or tarsus and draped to allow access to the fetlock and distal metacarpus/metatarsus.Non-displaced fractures are compressed and stabilized using 4.5 mm or 5.5 mm cortex screws placed in lag fashion through stab incisions. The most distal screw is inserted first and should be centered in the epicondylar fossa. Screw position should be monitored radiographically or fluoroscopically throughout the procedure. Countersinking is not necessary for this screw since the contour of the bone at this level accepts the head of the screw. Given the density of the trabecular bone in this location, it is not necessary for this screw to engage or exit the trans (medial) cortex to achieve adequate holding power and compression. This avoids having the tip of the screw impinging on or irritating the medial collateral ligament.

Subsequent screws are placed proximally at 1.5–2.0 cm intervals and in contrast to the most distal screw, these holes must be countersunk (Fig. 16.9). Care should be taken not to place a screw too close to the apex (proximal extent) of complete fractures since this may cause fragmentation when the screw is tightened. Arthroscopic exploration of the joint is optional (unless chip fractures or other lesions are present), but this does allow thorough evaluation, which may identify radiographically occult pathology.

Displaced lateral condylar fractures must be reduced prior to screw compression. Different techniques can be employed depending on individual preferences and the degree of displacement. If the fracture is not more than a few days old, reduction can often be achieved under arthroscopic visualization while manipulating the limb and fragment. Alternatively, reduction can be monitored through a small incision near the apex of the fracture or through a small arthrotomy. Arthroscopy has the advantage of allowing thorough evaluation of the joint and some debridement of the fracture gap to facilitate reduction.

Fractures that are more chronic or any that require extensive debridement that cannot be accomplished arthroscopically must be reduced through a large dorsal arthrotomy. This incision is located over the fracture line and extends from the apex of the fracture to the distal insertion of the fetlock joint capsule on P1. Any blood clots, fibrin and bone fragments are cleaned from the fracture line and the fracture is then reduced.

Reduction is maintained with self-retaining bone reduction forceps. Alternatively, a 2 mm drill bit can be inserted through the fragment and into the parent bone to maintain reduction. Screws are inserted in a manner similar to that described for non-displaced fractures. Screw position and articular alignment are checked radiographically or fluoroscopically prior to closure and recovery from

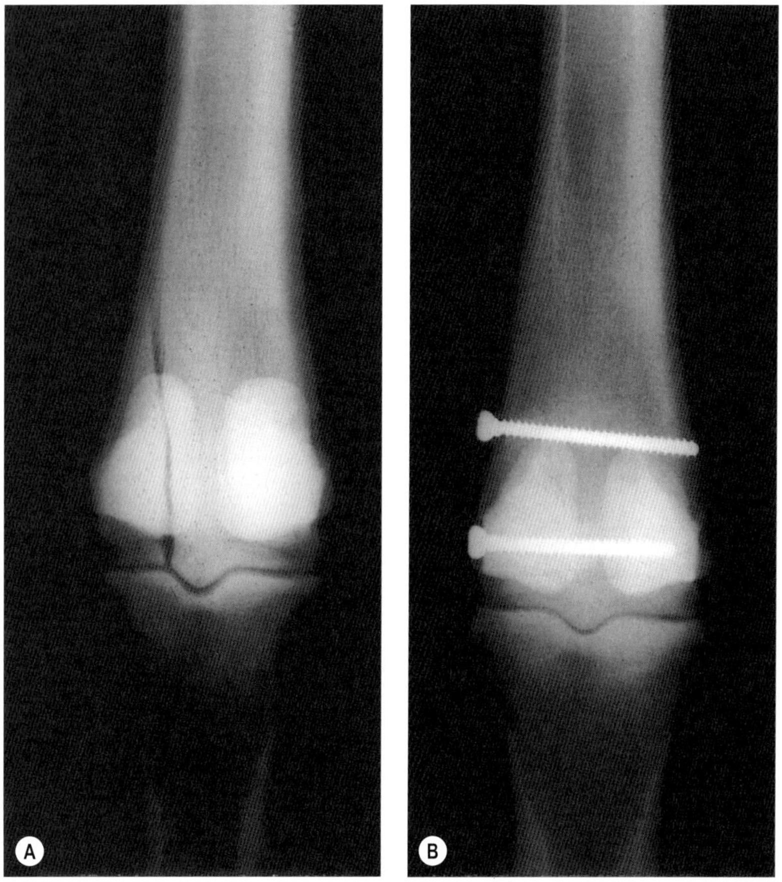

Fig 16.9 **(A)** Preoperative dorsopalmar radiograph of the metacarpophalangeal joint of a horse with an incomplete lateral condylar fracture. **(B)** Postoperative radiograph following interfragmentary screw compression using 4.5 mm cortical screws in lag fashion.

anesthesia. Failure to anatomically reconstruct the articular surface is an inexcusable technical error.

Stab incisions are closed with simple interrupted skin sutures using a 2-0 monofilament. Arthrotomies are closed in multiple layers, consisting of joint capsule/deep fascia, subcutaneous fascia and skin. A sterile dressing is applied to cover all incisions. Horses should be recovered from anesthesia in a half-limb fiberglass cast, although some surgeons do not customarily apply casts for horses with incomplete fractures. A customized compression boot (e.g. Farley boot®) is an alternative. Assistance during recovery in the form of head and tail ropes should be provided where feasible.

Casts or splints are removed within 24 hours of recovery and a firm, padded bandage is maintained for 2–3 weeks following surgery. NSAIDs are administered for a few days to provide analgesia and help decrease the inflammatory response in the joint. For the majority of horses antibiotics are limited to a single preoperative dose of an intravenous broad-spectrum antimicrobial or combination of antimicrobials. For horses undergoing an arthrotomy, antibiotic treatment is continued for 24–48 hours. Skin sutures are removed 10–14 days after surgery. Horses receive strict stall confinement for one month, followed by 1–2 months of stall rest with increasing daily hand-walking exercise. Follow-up radiographs are taken 2–3 months postoperatively and if healing is progressing satisfactorily, horses are allowed a minimum of 1–2 months of small paddock turnout before gradually resuming training.

Screw removal is not customarily recommended following repair of lateral condylar fractures. However, screw-associated pain in some horses upon resumption of high-speed exercise has historically been a concern. Subchondral bone reaction ('subchondral stiffening') or collateral ligament irritation, associated with the most distal screw, have been proposed as possible causes.[55,56] Another possible explanation is simply pain and lameness associated with degenerative joint disease or from an unrelated injury, with the screw being implicated as the cause. In the author's experience, screw-associated pain is very rare. Surgeons that advocate screw removal generally do so between three and four months following surgery. Others remove screws only when there is strong reason to suspect them to be causing problems. In any situation, this can usually be accomplished with the horse standing under sedation and using local anesthesia. Screws are identified (using radiographs if necessary) and removed through stab incisions. An additional two months of rest and controlled exercise are recommended before resuming hard training.

Surgical treatment: medial condylar fractures

'Short' medial condylar fractures (sagittally oriented fractures that do not extend proximal to the distal diaphysis) are repaired in a manner similar to that described for non-displaced lateral condylar fractures.

Medial condylar fractures that extend proximally in a spiral configuration are typically repaired by interfragmentary compression using 4.5 mm or 5.5 mm cortex screws in lag fashion. Some surgeons repair these fractures with screws placed entirely through individual stab incisions when a spiral configuration has been accurately confirmed preoperatively. In other cases, the diaphyseal component is approached through a long dorsal incision that splits the digital extensor tendons. With the latter approach, the periosteum is elevated and the fracture line inspected for any signs of radiographically inapparent comminution or mid-diaphyseal divergence of fracture lines. The most distal screws are inserted through separate stab incisions (as above) and subsequent screws are inserted perpendicular to the fracture plane at 2.0–2.5 cm intervals through the long dorsal incision. Application of a dorsal or dorsolaterally positioned dynamic compression plate (DCP) or locking compression plate (LCP) is an alternative to help minimize the potential for catastrophic failure (see below).[57]

Given the recognized risks of catastrophic fracture in these cases during recovery from general anesthesia some surgeons opt to perform surgery with the horse standing under local anesthesia.[58–60]

Care should be taken not to unnecessarily traumatize the splint bones, suspensory ligament or other soft tissues during drilling and tapping. Screw length and position should be monitored radiographically or fluoroscopically to ensure that they do not engage soft tissues or the splint bones. Similarly, screws that are placed through a fracture line can significantly weaken the bone and increase the risk for catastrophic fracture[54] and this should be avoided.

Long sagittally oriented fractures that exhibit mid-diaphyseal comminution or the so-called 'Y' configuration are at high risk for catastrophic failure, either preoperatively or in the early postoperative period. Fractures of this nature are almost exclusively seen in MT-III.[44,47] However, because of the potential adverse consequences, all medial condylar fractures should be regarded as having the possibility of catastrophic failure. These fractures should be treated with a combination of interfragmentary screw compression followed by application of a broad compression plate that spans the length of the bone.

Screws that compress the sagittal (distal) component are inserted through a combination of stab incisions (for the condylar screws) and through the long dorsal incision as previously described. Alternatively, plate screws inserted in lag fashion can be used to compress the fracture, although they will not be absolutely perpendicular to the fracture plane. A broad LCP or DCP of appropriate length is then applied along the dorsal or dorsolateral aspect of the bone, using 4.5 mm or 5.5 mm cortex screws and routine ASIF techniques. Again, care should be taken not to place a screw through a fracture line. Some surgeons apply an LCP in these cases using a minimally invasive approach with the plate and all screws inserted through stab incisions.[35]

The dorsal incision is closed routinely in multiple layers and stab incisions are closed with skin sutures. Unless a pool recovery system is available, horses with medial condylar fractures that have not been plated should be recovered from anesthesia in a full-limb cast and recovery should be assisted. A cast is also prudent for cases in which plates have been applied but the risks of a full-limb cast, particularly in the hind limbs, should be taken into consideration.

Postoperative care and exercise restriction are similar to that for lateral condylar fractures with a few exceptions. Hand-walking exercise does not begin until two months post-operatively in cases of spiral or long sagittal fracture. Antimicrobial treatment may be extended for an additional 24–48 hours in cases of plate application.

Horses that are intended to resume athletic careers must have plates and any independent screws placed in a dorsal-palmar/plantar direction removed prior to resumption of training. This is generally performed 3–4 months postoperatively under local anesthesia and is followed by an additional two months of convalescence.

Prognosis

The prognosis for horses with non-displaced lateral condylar fractures is generally very good. Results of retrospective studies indicate that 61–86% of Thoroughbreds with non-displaced fractures will race successfully following surgical treatment.[41,44,52,56,57] The prognosis for horses with displaced fractures is less favorable, with a reported range of 18–48% successfully returning to racing following surgical repair.[41,44,52,56,57] Fractures in the hind-limbs carry a more favorable prognosis, with 34% versus 76% of horses with complete fractures, and 79% versus 93% of horses with incomplete fractures of the front and hind-limbs, respectively, returning to racing in one study.[44]

Differences in prognosis between displaced and non-displaced fractures can be attributed to several factors, including a greater degree of articular and periarticular trauma associated with the original injury or with an open surgical approach, or technical errors during surgery for displaced fractures resulting in poor reduction and realignment of the articular surface.

The presence of a concurrent axial fracture of the proximal sesamoid (typically the lateral sesamoid) has also been shown to impart a poor prognosis for racing in Thoroughbreds with condylar fractures.[44]

Convalescent time (time from injury to first postoperative start) for horses with lateral condylar fractures generally ranges from 6–12 months, with an average of 8–9 months. This time is generally slightly shorter for non-displaced fractures and longer for horses with displaced fractures, but will vary considerably depending on the specifics of each case.

The propensity for catastrophic fractures to occur in horses with medial condylar fractures is now well recognized. The prevalence of this complication has been reported at 25–40% and can occur even up to several weeks following surgery if supplemental plate application is not utilized.[41,43,47] However, if catastrophic failure is not encountered, the prognosis for these horses to return to racing soundness is generally quite good following implant removal.[44,47,57] It should be noted that convalescent time for horses with medial condylar fractures tends to be longer than for those with fractures of the lateral condyles and has been attributed to a prolonged period of controlled exercise associated with implant removal.[44,57]

Etiology and pathophysiology

Etiology

There is convincing evidence that indicates condylar fractures are another form of fatigue fracture in horses associated with repetitive trauma, or cyclic strain, incurred during high-speed exercise (see Pathophysiology below).

Pathophysiology

Research focused on improving our understanding of the etiology and pathogenesis of condylar fractures is ongoing. It is recognized that condylar fractures originate in the palmar/plantar articular surface of the condyles of distal MC-III/MT-III.[41,46,52,61] In racehorses, the subchondral bone in the region of the condyles undergoes intense adaptive and maladaptive remodeling in response to the strains of high-speed exercise.[61–63] There is ample evidence, both grossly and histologically, of degenerative changes in the subchondral bone associated with lateral condylar fractures[64–67] (Fig. 16.10). These findings support the theory that condylar fractures are another manifestation of a cyclic fatigue injury, rather than an acute fracture in otherwise normal bone. However, it should be noted that a recent study by Firth and colleagues demonstrated morphologic abnormalities in the subchondral bone of the parasagittal groove in a small group of yearlings prior to entering race training, which suggests that the pathogenesis could involve a developmental component in some horses.[68]

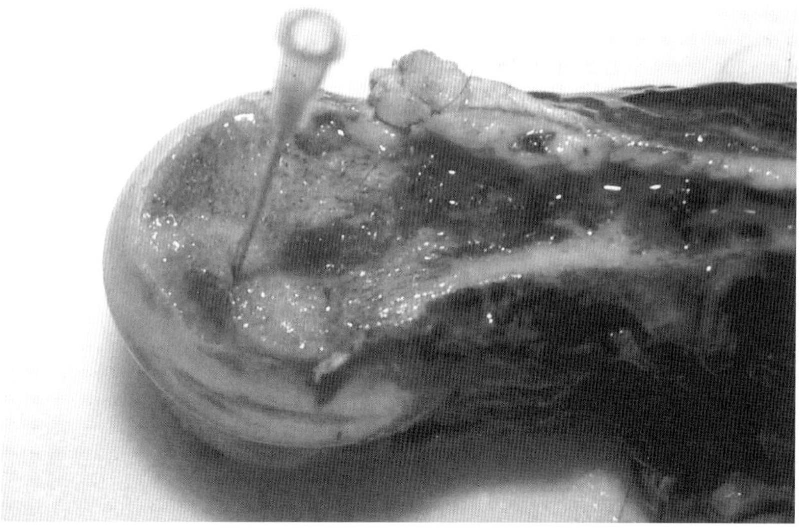

Fig 16.10 Post-mortem photograph of the lateral condyle of MC-III from a horse with a complete, displaced lateral condylar fracture. Notice the well-demarcated degenerative lesion in the subchondral bone in the palmar aspect of the condyle (needle).

In one of the earlier morphologic studies in Thoroughbred racehorses, Riggs et al (1999)[69] demonstrated that as training progresses, high-speed strains stimulate subchondral sclerosis in the palmar/plantar aspect of the condyles of MC-III/MT-III. This results in the development of a steep density gradient between the subchondral bone of the condyles and the adjacent sagittal ridge. The investigators proposed that this density gradient results in stress concentration in this region of MC-III/MT-III (the 'condylar groove'), which is the location of the majority of condylar fractures. A related post-mortem study demonstrated that small fissures develop first in the zone of calcified cartilage in this area.[70] When sufficient pathologic forces are generated on the condyle, overt fracture may then occur. Because the trabecular bone in the distal metaphyses is organized into sagittally oriented plates[71] – an adaptation to resist the strong bending loads applied in the dorsal-palmar/plantar direction – these fractures propagate in a characteristic sagittal configuration and course axially or abaxially depending on the location of the fracture (i.e. medial or lateral condyle).[70] For additional information on stress-related changes and injuries to bone see Chapter 8 and Chapter 22.

Epidemiology

Condylar fractures most commonly occur in young Thoroughbred racehorses, but they also occur in Standardbred, Quarter Horse and Arabian racehorses.[41,44,45,52] In one study in racing Thoroughbreds in Britain, condylar fractures and sagittal fractures of the first phalanx were the two most common fractures occurring during racing or race training, each accounting for approximately 15% of all fractures.[43] In another study in the US, approximately 20% of Thoroughbreds euthanized for musculoskeletal injury on California racetracks had lateral condylar fractures of MC-III.[42]

In Thoroughbreds, condylar fractures occur more frequently in the forelimbs, and lateral fractures are much more common than medial.[41,44,45,52,72] However, in Standardbreds there is a more even distribution between fore and hind-limbs and there may be a more equal distribution between lateral and medial fractures.[44] This difference in fracture distribution between the two breeds can presumably be attributed to biomechanical differences between the gallop or pace/trot. Among Standardbreds, pacers may be more commonly affected than trotters.[44]

Identification and elimination or reduction of risk factors associated with condylar fractures and other racing injuries has been and continues to be an intense area of interest. In particular, the quality and composition of training and racing surfaces, and the interactions of the hoof-shoe-track surface have received much attention. The depth of this topic is beyond the scope of this chapter, and interested readers are referred elsewhere for more information.

While numerous variables have been suspected or implicated, few *specific* definitive risk factors for condylar fracture have been identified. Several post-mortem epidemiologic studies on racing Thoroughbreds in the US have implicated shoes with toe grabs and poor dorsopalmar hoof balance (specifically long toe/low heel or 'underrun' heel conformation) as *potential* risk factors.[73,74] The results of at least one in vitro study have supported a suspicion long-held by some that suspensory ligament injury/weakness may predispose to condylar fracture.[75] The rate and volume of accumulated exercise in early training, and certain race characteristics have also been implicated as risk factors in a recent epidemiologic study of Thoroughbred racehorses in the UK.[76]

Prevention

In light of our understanding and recognition that the majority of condylar fractures are fatigue fractures (see Etiology and Pathophysiology above), early detection of pathologic changes in the subchondral bone of the distal metacarpus or metatarsus should, at least in theory, enable intervention prior to fracture. At present, bone-phase nuclear scintigraphy remains the most sensitive means for detecting maladaptive remodeling processes in the clinical setting.[61–64] However, the specificity of scintigraphy for identifying pre-fracture pathology vs. palmar osteochondral disease (POD) as a whole may be low.[77] Nonetheless, horses with abnormal increased radiopharmaceutical uptake in the distal palmar or plantar subchondral bone of MC-III/MT-III should be regarded as being at increased risk for condylar fracture, and modifications in training intensity would be warranted. Common sense would also dictate that horses with clinical signs of a problem in the fetlock joint be thoroughly evaluated.

Proliferative periostitis of the small metacarpal/metatarsal bones/ interosseous desmitis ('splints')

- Inflammatory lesions affect primarily young athletic horses of all breeds and uses.
- Splints are recognized as a focal area of firm, painful swelling along the shaft of the affected splint bone.
- Lesions on MC-II are most common, but all splint bones can be affected.
- Lameness is generally mild to moderate, with acute or insidious onset.
- Splints are caused by exercise-associated strain and tearing of the interosseous ligament with associated periostitis.
- They are also caused by external trauma and resulting primary periostitis.
- The majority respond to exercise restriction and anti-inflammatory therapy.
- Surgery is reserved for chronic or recalcitrant cases.
- Prognosis is generally favorable.

'Splints' are inflammatory lesions resulting from repetitive strain during exercise, or from external trauma, that affect the small metacarpal/metatarsal bones or splint bones (MC-II/IV, MT-II/IV), and are seen in all varieties of athletic horses.

Recognition

History and presenting complaint

Horses with 'splints' typically are presented with a mild-to-moderate lameness having either an acute or insidious onset. Many horses can continue training, albeit with impaired performance, while others must be taken out of work. Lameness may also be intermittent and quickly improve with rest, but recurs upon resumption of exercise if the lesion has not been allowed adequate time to heal. Whether or not lameness improves, worsens or remains static *during* exercise is also highly variable, but in most horses lameness worsens as exercise progresses.

In addition to lameness, the other chief complaint or clinical sign is a variable degree of focal swelling at the site of the lesion. Astute trainers or owners may also recognize the lesion to be painful on palpation. There is a subset of young horses that develop 'splints' without overt lameness and in these cases the cosmetic blemish is the primary concern.

Physical examination

A 'splint' is recognized as a focal swelling along the shaft of the affected bone that is smooth and firm to hard on palpation. In some cases, the swelling is located axially and the lesion can only be detected by palpation. Axially located 'splints' are most easily palpated with the limb held in flexion while running the fingers along the shaft of the splint.

There may be a single lesion or multiple lesions affecting the same bone but, overall, a single lesion is most common. Multiple lesions are most common on MC-II in young horses associated with early training. In this group, 'splints' are also commonly bilateral.

Horses exhibit variable degrees of pain on palpation of the 'splint'. Pain is most severe in the acute stages and does not always correlate well with the degree of swelling/exostosis. Chronic 'splints' or those that have healed clinically are not sensitive to palpation, but some horses react to firm skin pressure and this can give a false-positive response.

Open wounds or abrasions may be present over the lesion when the cause is external trauma.

Lameness examination

Lameness, when present, typically is mild to moderate (grade 1–3 of 5).[2] The majority of horses walk comfortably and only exhibit lameness during exercise. Acutely, most horses will exhibit lameness at a trot in-hand and the lameness tends to be exacerbated with the affected bone on the inside of a circle when working on a lunge line. Horses that are affected bilaterally may exhibit a 'choppy' or 'stiff' gait bilaterally and not a distinct 'head nod' or 'hip hike' per se. Firm digital pressure on the splint will often exacerbate the lameness.

Other horses are only affected when working at speed. Classic examples are the Standardbred racehorse that is bearing in or out, or is 'on a line' or 'getting over on a shaft', or the performance horse that will not take or maintain the appropriate lead.

Diagnostic confirmation

Diagnostic analgesia

High palmar/plantar analgesia (a 'high palmar/plantar block') will reduce lameness in horses with 'splints'. Selectively blocking just the medial or lateral nerves provides greater specificity. Local infiltration of anesthetic directly over the lesion is also an alternative method for localizing the site of pain. Local infiltration may be less effective if a substantial component of the pain is related to inflammation of the interosseous ligament and the anesthetic is deposited superficially (abaxially). The same is true if there is suspensory ligament impingement as a component of the lameness. In these horses a combination of successive blocks may be necessary to pinpoint the problem.

Scintigraphy

As with other inflammatory bone disorders, nuclear scintigraphy is a very sensitive method for detecting increased bone remodeling at the site of a 'splint'. It should be noted that the majority of acute 'splints' can be diagnosed on physical examination. Nuclear scintigraphy, like diagnostic analgesia, has its strongest application in ruling in or out other potential causes for lameness, as well as monitoring healing in exceptional cases.

Focal abnormal increased radiopharmaceutical uptake will vary from mild to intense, depending on the stage of disease (Fig. 16.11). As with many other conditions, scintigraphy will often be positive when radiographs are negative or equivocal in the acute stages. Scintigraphic activity also tends to persist after the lesions have healed clinically and therefore, results of physical/lameness examination, diagnostic analgesia, radiographs and clinical experience are necessary to formulate a therapeutic plan.

Radiographs

Radiographic abnormalities may not be evident with many acute 'splints', even in cases where considerable external swelling is present (see Pathophysiology below). For that reason, and because treatment for young horses in early athletic training is not necessarily modified based on radiographic findings, many clinicians do not recommend an initial set of radiographs in every case. However, radiographs are essential to rule out a fracture and to assess the nature and extent of any periosteal reaction – which is particularly

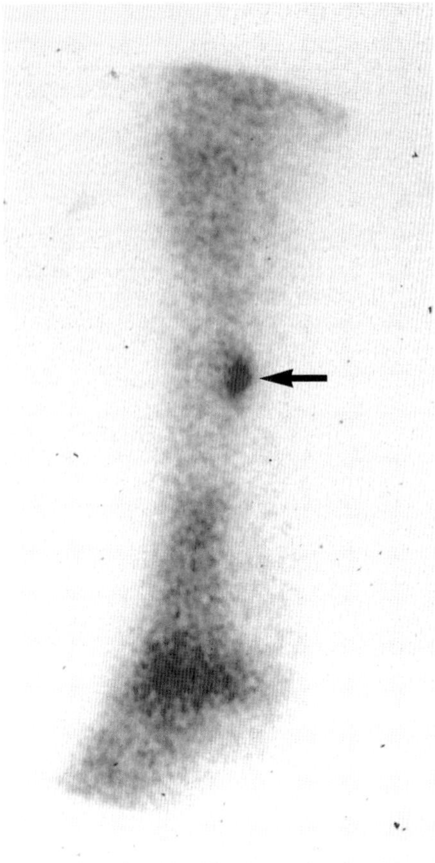

Fig 16.11 Lateral bone-phase scintigraphic image of the left metacarpus of a horse with an active proliferative periostitis lesion ('splint'). Notice the focal area of moderately intense abnormal increased radiopharmaceutical uptake affecting MC-IV (arrow).

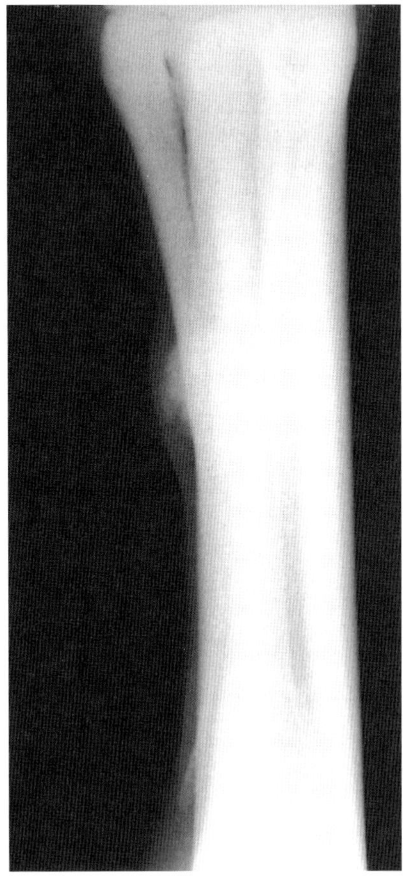

Fig 16.12 Dorsomedial-to-palmarolateral oblique radiograph of the left metacarpus of a horse with a proliferative periostitis lesion ('splint') affecting MC-II. Notice the exuberant irregular periosteal reaction, which is typical of lesions resulting from external trauma.

important in horses with chronic or recalcitrant 'splints', cases where lameness is profound, those with a large swelling/exostosis and certainly any with a draining wound.

Four views (lateral, dorsopalmar/plantar, DMPLO, DLPMO) of the affected metacarpus/metatarsus are recommended, although most information is obtained on the appropriate oblique view that isolates the affected bone(s). Lesions that are the result of internal trauma (exercise-associated cyclic strain) most commonly have a variable degree of focal, smooth periosteal reaction along the shaft of the affected splint bone. In addition, there may be evidence of subtle osteolytic change along the axial aspect of the bone (the region of the interosseous ligament) as well as subtle or mild proliferative and lytic changes in the underlying cannon bone. Lesions resulting from external trauma are more likely to have an irregular and exuberant periosteal reaction (Fig. 16.12). It is important to note that superimposition of normal and periosteal new bone can result in misdiagnosis of a fracture in some cases if radiographs are not interpreted carefully.

Ultrasound

A sonogram is important for evaluation of concurrent suspensory ligament pathology in cases with potential impingement on this structure by a large exostosis.

Computed Tomography and Magnetic Resonance Imaging

Advanced imaging techniques are rarely necessary to make an initial diagnosis in the vast majority of 'splints'. However, in select cases these modalities have demonstrated advantages for detecting pathologic change that is otherwise difficult or impossible to identify with radiography and ultrasound. In particular, MRI has proven useful for identifying adhesions between the suspensory ligament and metacarpal/metatarsal exostoses,[78] and lesions involving the interosseous ligament and associated insertions.[79]

Thermography

In the hands of an experienced operator, thermography can be useful in identifying active lesions.

Treatment and prognosis

Therapeutic aims

The goals of therapy for 'splints' are to reduce or eliminate the inciting cause, reduce inflammation, minimize the size of the exostosis and allow the lesion to become quiescent or 'set up' (see Pathophysiology below).

Therapy

Exercise restriction

The extent of exercise restriction varies with each case and depends on the duration and severity of clinical signs and, to some extent, the use of the horse and stage of training.

Most horses should be confined to a stall with exercise limited to daily hand-walking or small paddock confinement until lameness and the majority of the focal pain have subsided. In most cases this will be a period of 2–6 weeks. However, this will also vary depending on response to treatment. Exercise intensity is increased gradually and, as above, the specific protocol will vary with each case.

Anti-inflammatory treatment

As with exercise restriction the extent of anti-inflammatory treatment for 'splints' will vary with each case. Systemic and/or topical NSAID therapy is administered at standard doses for several days in most cases, or up to a few weeks in exceptional cases. As in other inflammatory disorders, long-term systemic NSAID treatment is becoming more controversial due to its potentially negative impact on bone healing. Promoting metacarpal/metatarsal fusion (see Pathophysiology) is desirable but how NSAIDs affect this process is unclear. NSAIDs, along with corticosteroids (see below), may be of greatest importance in minimizing the development of an exuberant exostosis.

Local cold therapy, in the form of cold hosing or icing (bucket or ice boot) administered for 20–30 minutes several times daily for several days in the acute stages, is also beneficial to reduce soft tissue swelling and inflammation in the affected tissues.

Local injection of corticosteroids can also be highly beneficial, particularly with respect to decreasing the fibrous and osseous proliferative response. Local injection of corticosteroids is particularly efficacious for managing lameness associated with 'splints' in horses whose competition schedules will not allow an extended period of lay-up.

Corrective shoeing

Corrective trimming and shoeing plays an important role in reducing or eliminating the tendency for interference when this form of external trauma is the cause of a 'splint'.

Boots and protective bandages

In cases in which interference is the primary cause, 'shin boots' or other protective wraps or bandages are helpful to prevent further trauma.

Surgery

The vast majority of 'splints' respond well to non-surgical management.[34,80] Refractory cases associated with chronic or recurrent lameness, cases with exuberant exostoses and suspected suspensory ligament impingement and those with osteitis associated with an open wound are appropriate candidates for surgery. Surgery is also occasionally undertaken to improve the cosmetic appearance of show horses.

Surgery involves either a partial ostectomy (osteotomy just proximal to the lesion with excision of the distal aspect of the splint bone) or surgical debridement of the exostosis with preservation of the bone. The option chosen depends on the nature and location of the lesion, the bone involved and in some cases the surgeon's preference. With the exception of MT-IV,[81] excision of more than the distal two-thirds to three-quarters of a splint bone will result in instability of the remaining proximal portion, which can lead to chronic lameness of various origins.[82] This is particularly true when dealing with MC-II. Therefore, when considering surgery for a large impinging exostosis affecting the proximal portion of a splint bone, debridement of the exostosis and preservation of the bone are appropriate.

Fortunately, 'splints' resulting from cyclic internal trauma (exercise-associated repetitive strain) that affect the proximal aspect of the bone rarely become chronic problems once allowed to 'set up' (formation of a stabilizing synostosis or fusion – see Pathophysiology), and surgical intervention is therefore not a consideration. 'Splints' of this nature that are most likely to result in chronic lameness generally affect the midshaft of the splint bone and in the author's opinion they are candidates for partial ostectomy.

Surgery is performed with the horse in lateral recumbency under general anesthesia. A tourniquet is helpful but not essential. The limb is clipped and aseptically prepared from midpastern to carpus/tarsus and draped to allow access to the full metacarpus/metatarsus. An incision is made directly over the splint bone and extends from a few centimeters proximal to the lesion to just distal to the distal aspect or 'button'. Sharp and blunt dissection is used to expose the portion of the bone to be excised. Care is taken to avoid trauma to the suspensory ligament and neurovascular structures in the area (particularly when dealing with MT-IV). A 6–12 mm osteotome and mallet are used to transect the splint bone just proximal to the lesion, at a 30–45° angle with the long axis of the bone (Fig. 16.13). The distal portion is then excised, beginning distally and working proximally. Mayo scissors can be used to cut the heavy fibrous tissue attached to the most distal aspect and then an osteotome or chisel and mallet are used to undermine and separate the more proximal portion from the cannon bone. The periosteum is removed with the

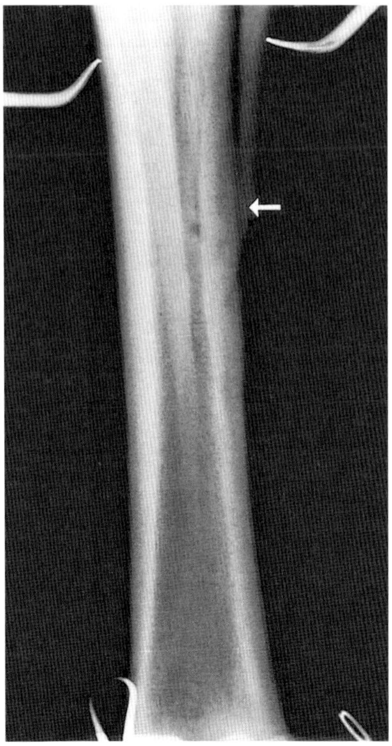

Fig 16.13 Intraoperative DMPLO radiograph of the right metacarpus following ostectomy of the distal portion of MC-II (arrow) in a horse with a chronic proliferative periostitis lesion ('splint').

bone. Remaining bone fragments and fibrous tissue are carefully debrided and a bone rasp is used to smooth the remaining proximal stump and cannon bone where needed. Excessive rasping or other trauma to the cannon bone should be avoided. The surgical field is lavaged copiously to remove small bone fragments. Intraoperative radiographs are helpful to identify small fragments that may not be readily seen. A Penrose drain is not essential, but does help prevent seroma formation in some cases. The wound is closed routinely in multiple layers and a dressing containing rolled or folded sterile gauze pads is applied over the incision to provide increased direct pressure and help minimize swelling and seroma formation prior to application of a padded bandage.

The surgical approach for debridement of a large exostosis is similar, but with a shorter incision centered over the lesion. After reflecting the soft tissues an osteotome (or chisel) and mallet are used to carefully separate the proliferative periosteal bone from the surfaces of the underlying splint and cannon bones. The periosteal bone is usually softer and more irregular than the normal cortical bone and in most cases is easily identified. All overlying periosteum is removed with the exostosis, taking care not to unnecessarily traumatize bone that is left behind. Any adhesions involving the suspensory ligament are carefully transected and the fibrous tissue excised using careful sharp dissection. Intraoperative radiographs may help identify foci of remaining periosteal new bone and bone debris. Lavage, closure and bandaging are similar to that for ostectomy.

Postoperatively, horses are treated with an NSAID for 3–7 days. Broad-spectrum antibiotics are initiated preoperatively and continued for 24–48 hours postoperatively. If excessive soft tissue swelling or a seroma develops, antibiotic treatment is continued at the discretion of the surgeon. Sutures are removed in 12–14 days and a bandage is maintained on the limb for 3–4 weeks to help minimize swelling. Horses are confined to a stall for 6–8 weeks, with light hand-walking exercise beginning after suture removal. Exercise intensity gradually increases over the ensuing 6–8 weeks. Early resumption of harder exercise predisposes horses to inflammation at the site of the ostectomy and sets up the possibility of chronic problems postoperatively.

Traditional and alternative therapies

Many of the numerous traditional therapeutic modalities mentioned in the section on 'bucked shins' continue to be used by some lay persons and veterinarians for treating 'splints'. As with 'bucked shins', the efficacy of these techniques for treating 'splints' has not been substantiated scientifically, but many clinicians remain strong advocates based on anecdotal evidence and personal experience. A detailed discussion of this topic is beyond the scope of this chapter. In addition to those modalities mentioned earlier, soft lasers, therapeutic ultrasound and magnet boots have been employed in the treatment of 'splints'.[80] The efficacy and scientific rationale of these treatments also remain controversial.

Prognosis

The prognosis for most horses with 'splints' is generally very good if appropriate intervention is undertaken and adhered to. This is particularly true for 'splints' that develop in young horses in early training. The majority of horses will recover and their athletic potential will not be impaired. Most chronic or recurrent problems develop in situations where the lesion initially goes undiagnosed or horses are not allowed an adequate time to heal and undergo fusion or synostosis (see Pathophysiology below).

'Splints' that develop in older horses, either from internal or external trauma, tend to take longer to heal and are more likely to fall into the chronic or recurrent category. Other exceptions are cases of chronic interference where repeated external trauma cannot be corrected or rare proliferative lesions that affect the very proximal aspect of the bone and contribute to problems with the carpometacarpal/tarsometatarsal joints.

The prognosis for athletic soundness following partial ostectomy is also generally fair to good if appropriate case selection, surgical technique and aftercare are adhered to.[83] Prognosis is guarded for horses undergoing proximal ostectomy, with or without supplemental stabilization of the remaining portion.[84] Recurrence of the exostosis following surgical debridement has been a recognized problem[80] and owners should be cautioned accordingly. Careful removal of the associated periosteum appears to minimize this complication.[85]

Etiology and pathophysiology

Etiology

'Splints' can be caused by internal or external trauma. Internal trauma is in the form of repetitive or cyclic strains incurred during exercise. External trauma is essentially blunt force or concussive trauma, resulting either from a kick or interference.

Pathophysiology

'Splints' caused by cyclic strains during exercise (internal trauma) are initiated by tearing and inflammation of the interosseous ligament and underlying periosteum of the cannon and splint bones. In immature horses the splint bones are mobile relative to the adjacent cannon bone. As such, during exercise, axial forces applied to the proximal aspect of the splint bones by the overlying carpal or tarsal bones result in strain and shearing of the interosseous ligament and periosteum. As exercise continues a focal desmitis and periostitis develop, which in turn results in the clinical signs of focal swelling and lameness. The swelling is initially a combination of soft tissue edema and fibrosis, and progresses to periosteal new bone or exostosis.

This type of 'splint' is most common in younger horses in early training and the small metacarpals, in particular MC-II, are most frequently affected. The small metacarpal bones have larger articulations with the overlying carpal bones, and more extensive soft tissue attachments, than do the small metatarsal bones. Functionally, it is assumed that the small metacarpal bones play a more important role in stabilizing the carpus and experience greater stresses during exercise than the small metatarsals.

Eventually, a synostosis between the splint and cannon bones develops at the site of a 'splint' – termed 'metacarpal fusion'[86] – and it is hypothesized that this results in stabilization and resistance to further strain and shear.[86] 'Splints' at this stage are said to have 'set up' and no longer appear to cause clinical problems. Given that metacarpal fusion has an estimated prevalence of over 95%, with 78% of horses over two-years-old having two or more sites of fusion,[86] it is reasonable to assume that the process is not always associated with an inflammatory reaction severe enough to produce clinical signs of 'splints' and, in fact, may be a normal adaptive process as the skeleton matures.

Poor conformation is also implicated as a risk factor for the development of 'splints',[53] presumably by exacerbating the shearing forces applied on the splint bones and interosseous ligament. Specifically offset or 'bench knees' appear to favor development of splints of MC-II.[53,86] Carpal or tarsal valgus or varus deformities may also potentiate the development of 'splints'.

In contrast to the above, 'splints' caused by external trauma begin as a primary focal periostitis/osteitis of the affected splint bone, although a primary interosseous desmitis may also be initiated by the event.[53] Exercise can aggravate and perpetuate this inflammatory process and presumably a secondary interosseous desmitis and periostitis of the cannon bone may result. Base narrow, toe-out conformation, which may exacerbate the tendency for interference – specifically trauma to the contralateral MC-II – has been suggested as one risk factor.[80]

Regardless of the underlying cause, if the exostosis becomes exuberant and projects axially a secondary, focal suspensory desmitis may develop in some cases. However, in the author's experience, this condition is uncommon but is more likely with the marked exostosis that tends to develop following external trauma.

Epidemiology

'Splints' resulting from cyclic strains associated with exercise are common in young performance horses of many breeds and uses. As previously mentioned, MC-II is the bone most commonly affected in this group, followed by MT-II, but the lateral splint bones (MC-IV, MT-IV) can certainly also be affected. Lesions are very commonly bilateral and multiple 'splints' affecting a single bone are not unusual, particularly on MC-II.

'Splints' are very common problems in racehorses of all breeds aged 2–4 years and, as with 'bucked shins', many trainers still consider them to be almost a 'rite of passage'. In performance horses other than racehorses, 'splints' can develop at any age but are common in those aged 3–10 years (young adults). 'Splints' also develop in weanling and yearling horses that are not in formal training and in the author's experience, these are frequently fast-growing or over-conditioned animals. Over-nutrition has been cited as an associated risk factor by others.[70]

'Splints' resulting from external trauma can affect horses of any age and involve any of the splint bones. Obviously, those resulting from interference are most likely to occur during performance and affect MC-II. However, this type of splint is also frequently seen on MT-IV resulting from a kick or contact with natural or manmade objects.

Prevention

In theory, with training modifications it should be possible to prevent or minimize the incidence of 'splints' that develop in young horses in early training as a result of cyclic trauma that exceeds the physiologic limits of the tissues and their capacity to adapt to the imposed stresses. In reality, it is impossible at this stage to outline a specific training regimen that would be appropriate for each breed and use of athletic horse. Early detection using physical examination and diagnostic imaging techniques such as thermography and scintigraphy, to then enable timely intervention, is a more realistic goal. Correction of gait abnormalities that predispose to interference should minimize the incidence of traumatic 'splints' in the individual horse. In horses with a tendency for interference, long-term use of shin boots or other protective wraps is also an option.

Fractures of the small metacarpal/metatarsal bones (splint bone fractures)

- Splint bone fractures occur in all types of performance horses.
- Fractures of the distal third are the most common type.
- Fractures of the middle and proximal aspect result from trauma associated with interference.
- Fractures of the head may be caused by torsional forces or be avulsions.
- Distal fractures are treated by surgical excision.
- Middle and proximal fractures are treated by excision or internal fixation.
- The prognosis is generally favorable for all fracture types.
- Concurrent suspensory desmitis is the limiting factor with distal fractures.

Splint bone fractures can occur during exercise or randomly as a result of some form of external trauma.[87] The following will deal exclusively with fractures that occur in athletic horses during performance. The most common in this category are fractures of the distal third. Others include fractures of the midshaft or proximal portion (head) resulting from interference, and oblique fractures of the head that may result from torsional forces or be avulsions associated with the extensive soft tissue attachments.

Recognition

History and presenting complaint

Acute lameness and swelling are the primary clinical signs of splint bone fractures.

Degree of lameness in horses with fractures of the distal portion is highly variable and may have an acute or more insidious onset. Most horses develop an acute lameness during or immediately after exercise. Lameness is generally mild to moderate. Many horses are able to resume exercise after a period of rest, but have lingering problems with low-grade lameness. Acutely, mild soft tissue swelling and sensitivity are usually present near the fracture site. Horses may have a history or clinical signs of suspensory desmitis. Some chronic distal fractures are incidental findings.

Lameness with fractures of the proximal portions of the splint bones is generally acute in onset, ranges from moderate to severe and generally persists despite rest. The majority of these horses are too lame to continue exercise. Soft tissue swelling ranges from mild to marked, and abrasions or wounds may be present.

Physical examination

Horses with distal splint bone fractures generally have very mild to moderate local soft tissue inflammation. The degree varies with the chronicity of the injury. Fractures that are more than a week or two old may have minimal residual associated swelling. Distal splint fractures have a high incidence of associated suspensory desmitis and therefore suspensory enlargement, most commonly of the associated branch, may also be present. Focal pain is common on firm palpation of the fracture site. If the fracture is chronic, a callus can often be palpated, along with instability if the distal tip or 'button' is pressed axially.

Variable degrees of soft tissue swelling and pain on palpation of the fracture site are the hallmarks of fractures of the more proximal portions of the splint bones. Open wounds or abrasions may be present if the fracture is the result of interference.

Lameness examination

Lameness in horses with splint bone fractures ranges from very mild to relatively severe and depends in great part on the type of fracture and the chronicity.

Horses with acute fractures of the distal aspect generally exhibit mild-to-moderate lameness at a trot and in some cases exhibit mild lameness at a walk (grade 1–4). Horses with chronic distal fractures generally exhibit only mild lameness at a trot, but performance is impaired at high speeds. Lameness may be exacerbated on a circle.

Lower limb ('fetlock') flexion may exacerbate the lameness, particularly if concurrent suspensory desmitis is present.

Horses with acute fractures of the middle and proximal portions of the splint bones generally exhibit severe lameness at a trot and many are markedly lame at a walk (grade 2–4 of 5). Lameness in chronic cases is highly variable. Lameness is exacerbated with the fractured bone on the inside of a circle in many horses. Carpal or tarsal flexion may be positive in horses with fractures affecting the head of the splint.

Diagnostic confirmation

Diagnostic analgesia

Diagnostic analgesia is rarely needed to definitively localize the source of pain in horses with most acute splint fractures. Diagnostic analgesia becomes important in the work-up of horses with chronic fractures involving either the distal aspect or the head of the splint, in which soft tissue swelling and lameness have improved considerably. In horses with distal splint fractures, response to low palmar/plantar analgesia is variable. High palmar/plantar analgesia will consistently be positive in all cases of splint bone fracture, with the exception of those involving the articular aspect, in which the response is variable. In these cases, intra-articular analgesia of the carpometacarpal (via the middle carpal joint) or tarsometatarsal joint will be positive or result in substantial improvement.

Scintigraphy

Nuclear scintigraphy is unnecessary for diagnosis of acute splint bone fractures. This modality is beneficial in the work-up of horses with chronic fractures when attempting to rule in or out other potential causes of lameness.

Radiography

Radiographs are necessary to confirm the diagnosis. Four views (lateral, dorsopalmar/plantar, DMPLO and DLPMO) of the full metacarpus/metatarsus are required. In cases of fractures involving the head of the bone (articular fractures) a full series of the associated carpus/tarsus is also warranted.

Ultrasonography

A sonogram should be performed to evaluate the suspensory ligament in cases where concurrent desmitis is suspected.

Treatment and prognosis

Therapeutic aims

Therapy for distal fractures is directed at eliminating a source of chronic irritation/inflammation. Goals of therapy for fractures involving the midshaft include minimizing the convalescent time and mitigating the tendency for development of delayed or non-union and formation of exuberant callus/exostosis. Goals in treating proximal fractures include promoting primary bone healing, preservation of the stability of the proximal portion and minimizing the potential for degenerative joint disease.

Therapy

First aid

Initial treatment for all splint bone fractures includes bandaging and anti-inflammatory therapy, as previously discussed for other metacarpal/metatarsal injuries. Horses should be confined to a stall pending decisions on definitive treatment. Wound care and antibiotics are administered as needed.

Treatment of distal fractures

There is no strong consensus on the most appropriate way to manage distal splint fractures. Many will heal or become quiescent as non-unions and no longer appear to cause problems.[88,89] Residual lameness/poor performance is generally attributed to chronic suspensory desmitis. However, because the distal portion of the splint bone is highly mobile, healing is often slow and associated with considerable callus (Fig. 16.14). The fragment and associated inflammation appear to cause chronic irritation in some horses. Surgical excision of the fragment reduces the convalescent period and eliminates the fracture as a continued cause for concern. Therefore, it is this author's opinion that *acute* or *clinically active* distal splint fractures are best treated by surgical excision.

Surgery is generally best performed under general anesthesia, but excision under local anesthesia is a viable alternative in some cases. The preparation and approach are similar to that described for splint ostectomy in the previous section, but the incision is considerably shorter. Fractures of the distal third involve the portion of the splint bone not attached to the interosseous ligament. Therefore, excision is relatively easy and can be performed with heavy scissors, again working from distal to proximal while grasping the 'button' to elevate it. The distal fragment, callus and a small segment of the proximal fragment (that involved with the callus), along with associated periosteum, are excised. A small osteotome or bone rongeur can be used for transecting the proximal fragment. Closure and bandaging are carried out in a routine manner.

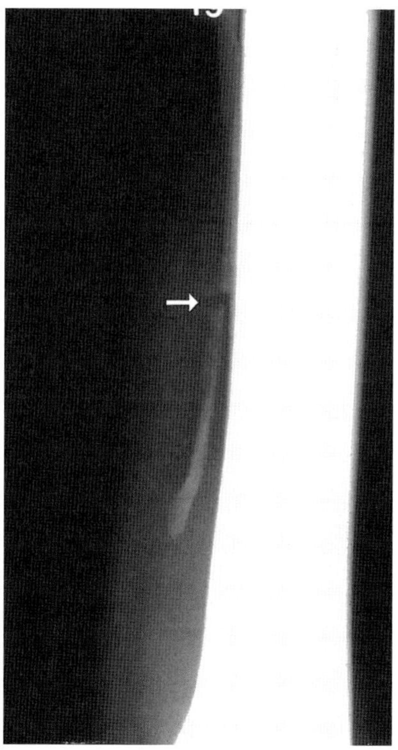

Fig 16.14 Dorsolateral-to-plantaromedial radiograph of the right metatarsus of a horse with a chronic fracture of the distal aspect of MT-IV. Notice the callus and evidence of non-union (arrow).

Aftercare involves 2–4 weeks of stall confinement with increasing daily hand-walking exercise, followed by 2–4 weeks of small paddock turnout or other form of light exercise. Exceptions are horses with concurrent suspensory desmitis, in which case rest and controlled exercise, and other adjunct therapy, are dictated by the extent of the ligamentous injury (see Chapter 20). A bandage is maintained for 2–3 weeks and sutures are removed 10–14 days postoperatively. NSAID and antibiotic treatment are at the discretion of the surgeon, but neither is required for an extended period.

Treatment of mid-body fractures

Mid-body fractures can be managed conservatively or surgically depending on the nature of the injury, use of the horse and any economic constraints. Because of motion at the fracture site, healing is often delayed and frequently results in exuberant callus or exostosis, along with chronic pain/lameness, which may be considered as another manifestation of proliferative periostitis/interosseous desmitis or 'splints' (Fig. 16.15). For that reason it is this author's opinion that the majority of these fractures should be treated surgically. Surgery involves partial ostectomy, and the technique and aftercare are similar to that described for managing chronic 'splints' in the previous section. Some surgeons prefer segmental ostectomy (leaving the proximal and distal segments intact), which can be less invasive and offers a prognosis comparable to partial ostectomy.[90]

Treatment for proximal fractures

The consequences of partial ostectomy alone for treating fractures of the proximal third of a splint bone are well recognized.[82] These fractures must be managed by either ostectomy with supplemental internal fixation to stabilize the remaining proximal portion or by primary repair using internal fixation. Failure to do so leads to loss of stability of the proximal portion and chronic lameness will result. The exception is MT-IV, in which the entire bone can be excised with a good outcome in many cases.[81]

With respect to fractures that occur during performance, the most common proximal splint fracture is an oblique fracture involving the head, most commonly MC-II (Fig. 16.16A). The fractures involve the articular aspect and are almost always displaced. Surgical repair involves open reduction and internal fixation using a small bone plate. An incision of appropriate length is centered over the proximal aspect of the bone along the palmaromedial or palmarolateral aspect of the limb. Sharp dissection is carefully carried out using a sharp elevator or scalpel to sever the heavy ligamentous attachments and expose the bone. The fracture line is debrided as needed to allow reduction. A 4–6 hole, narrow, 3.5 mm DCP is appropriately contoured and applied using 3.5 mm cortical screws. Screws should not engage the MC-III (Fig. 16.16B). Screws crossing the fracture line can be inserted in lag fashion but this may be difficult, depending on fragment width and fracture configuration, and is not essential if the fracture is well reduced. The incision is closed in multiple layers and a tight, padded bandage is securely applied.

Broad-spectrum antibiotics are administered for 24–48 hours and NSAIDs are administered for 3–5 days postoperatively. A bandage is maintained for 2–3 weeks and skin sutures are removed 12–14 days postoperatively. Horses are confined to a stall for two months. Daily hand-walking begins after suture removal. Exercise in a small paddock can begin at the two-month point. Implants are removed three months postoperatively. This can be performed under local or general anesthesia but because of the heavy soft tissue covering is easier under general anesthesia, particularly for implants in MC-II. Screws are removed through stab incisions and the plate is elevated and removed through a small incision over the distal end. An additional 4–6 weeks of limited exercise are allowed before resumption of training once fractures have healed radiographically.

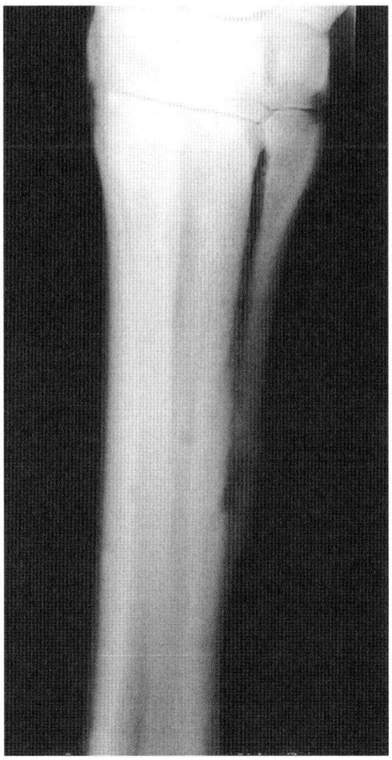

Fig 16.15 Dorsomedial-to-palmarolateral oblique radiograph of the right metacarpus of a horse with a chronic fracture of the mid-body of MC-II.

Prognosis

The prognosis for fractures involving the distal aspect of the splint bones is generally very good if there is no concurrent suspensory desmitis.[89,91] The prognosis for horses with suspensory ligament injury is directly related to the severity of the desmitis.

The prognosis following partial ostectomy for management of fractures of the mid-portion of the splint bones is fair to good and is similar to ostectomy for treatment of recalcitrant 'splints'.[92] In this author's experience, problems tend to arise if horses are not allowed an appropriate period of convalescence and training is resumed too quickly.

The prognosis for the oblique fractures involving the heads of the splint bones treated with internal fixation, in the author's experience, appears to be good but reports involving large numbers of this specific fracture type are lacking.

Etiology and pathophysiology

Etiology

Many distal splint fractures are associated with either axial compressive forces exerted through the proximal aspect of the bone or tension imparted by the attachments to the suspensory ligament.

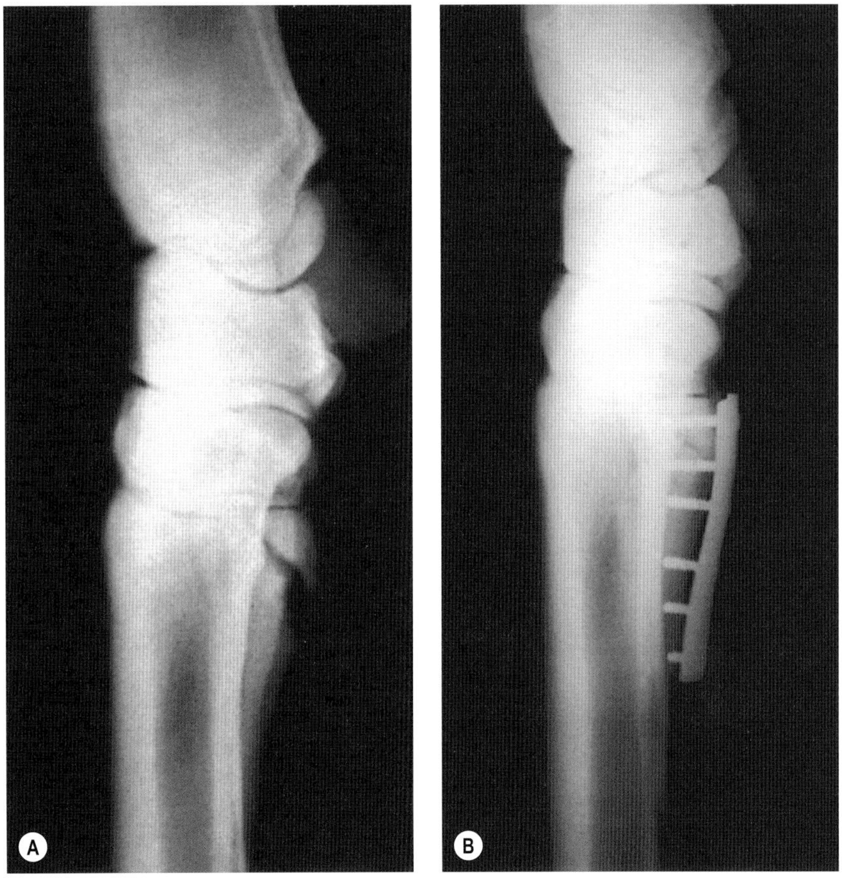

Fig 16.16 (A) Lateral radiograph of the proximal left metacarpus and carpus of a Thoroughbred racehorse that sustained an oblique fracture of the proximal portion of MC-II during a race. (B) Postoperative radiograph following open reduction and internal fixation using a 3.5 mm narrow dynamic compression plate. Note that screws do not engage MC-III.

Most fractures of the middle and proximal portions of the splint bones are the result of blunt external trauma. Some oblique fractures of the head of the splint bone, specifically MC-II, may be avulsion fractures or the result of internal torsional forces.

Pathophysiology

Unlike the middle and proximal portions of the splint bones, the distal portion is not tightly adhered to the cannon bone through the interosseous ligament. It is therefore relatively mobile and has fascial attachments to the adjacent branch of the suspensory ligament. During exercise, compressive axial forces on the bone in some cases, or in others flexion and extension of the fetlock joint with the associated elongation and retraction of the suspensory ligament, create cyclic strain on the distal splint bone. If this proceeds at a rate that exceeds the bone's ability to adapt, it weakens and eventually fracture occurs. However, fractures appear clinically as an acute injury. The inherent motion at this location commonly leads to delayed or non-union or healing with a considerable callus.

Enlargement of the suspensory branch, as occurs with desmitis, displaces the distal splint bone abaxially, which may exacerbate the strain on the bone. Local inflammation associated with the desmitis may also lead to osteitis and a predisposition to fracture. However, the temporal relationship between desmitis and fracture is not completely understood and fracture may precede desmitis in some cases.

Blunt trauma from interference in the mid-to-proximal portion of the splint generally results in a short oblique or transverse fracture, but comminuted fractures or fracture of a crescent-shaped fragment are also seen. On rare occasions these fractures are open. (Conversely, open fractures are very common in non-exercise related cases.) Strains exerted on the proximal aspect of the bone (see previous section on 'splints') invariably result in motion and healing with a large callus or exostosis.

Fractures of the head of the splint bone can result from blunt external trauma, but they are also suspected to result from torsional stresses during exercise[80] and in some cases maybe avulsions. In this author's opinion, the oblique fractures of the head of MC-II appear in many cases to be avulsion fractures that presumably occur during hyperextension of the carpus. In addition to the medial collateral ligament of the carpus, the flexor carpi radialis and extensor carpi obliquus muscles insert on the proximal aspect of MC-II.

Epidemiology

Distal splint fractures affect performance horses of all breeds and uses, but are particularly common in racehorses. Overall, distal splint fractures more commonly involve the forelimbs, with the exception of Standardbred racehorses. For comparison, in Thoroughbreds left MC-IV and right MC-II are the most commonly affected and in Standardbreds fractures of the left MT-II and right MT-IV are most common.[55,89,91] Distal splint fractures are unusual in immature horses (<2 years of age) and this is thought to be due to a decrease in pliability of the suspensory ligament and an increase in brittleness of the bone as horses age.[82,91] Younger horses are also not in formal athletic training.

Fractures of the middle and proximal portions resulting from interference are seen in all performance horses. Oblique fractures of the head caused by torsional strains during performance are most common in racehorses and jumpers.[80]

Prevention

The use of shin boots, and corrective trimming and shoeing to correct gait abnormalities, can minimize the incidence of splint fractures resulting from interference.

Many distal splint fractures are fatigue fractures and concurrent or pre-existing suspensory desmitis may contribute to the development of this injury. Early detection of prefecture pathology, using such modalities as thermography and nuclear scintigraphy, along with careful physical examination and recognition of subtle signs of soreness or lameness, should enable early intervention/prevention in some horses.

Stress remodeling ('stress reaction') and stress fracture (avulsion fracture) at the suspensory origin

- Stress reaction and stress fractures at the suspensory origin are two of the three components of the 'high suspensory syndrome'.
- Either disorder may exist as a primary, distinct entity or be associated with desmitis at the suspensory origin.
- Stress reaction affects all types of performance horses.
- Stress fractures are seen most commonly in racehorses.
- Pain on palpation of the suspensory origin, but few other overt clinical signs.
- Lameness may have gradual or sudden onset with stress reaction.
- Lameness typically has an acute onset with stress fracture.
- Scintigraphy plays an important role in the diagnosis.
- Treatment involves rest and controlled exercise for 2–6 months.
- Prognosis is generally favorable for either condition.

Stress remodeling or stress reaction, which can be thought of as an enthesitis, and stress or avulsion fractures at the origin of the suspensory ligament, along with desmitis of the suspensory origin, are the three components of the 'high suspensory syndrome'. This section will focus specifically on the primary osseous disorders and the reader is referred to Chapter 20 on suspensory desmitis for details on the primary ligamentous disorder. It is important to remember that although each condition can occur as a distinct injury, an element of both osseous and ligamentous pathology may exist in many cases.

Recognition

History and presenting complaint

Horses with stress reaction typically have a progressive lameness of insidious onset, but cases with apparent acute onset are also seen. Initially, lameness may be intermittent and improve or resolve with short-term rest. Eventually, lameness becomes persistent and worsens as exercise continues, rather than being a lameness that the horse 'warms out of'. In a subset of horses the condition only causes poor performance at peak exertion. An example would be Standardbred racehorses that 'bear in or out' (drift into the rail or away from the rail) or frequently break stride during a race.

Lameness in horses with stress fracture is typically acute in onset and is first evident during or shortly after high-speed or hard exercise. Most horses are too lame to continue training. Some horses have a history of low-grade or intermittent lameness (as above) prior to acute fracture.

Physical examination

There are very few overt physical abnormalities in horses with primary osseous disease at the suspensory origin. Soft tissue swelling is minimal or absent (unless concurrent suspensory desmitis is present). Some horses stand 'over' at the knee (slight carpal flexion at rest). Focal pain in the region of the suspensory origin is the primary sign. This is most easily assessed with the limb in flexion and with firm pressure applied by the thumb along the proximal palmar aspect of the metacarpus (or with fingers along the plantar metatarsus), while displacing the flexor tendons medially or laterally.

Lameness examination

Lameness in horses with stress reaction ranges from subtle to moderate – grades < 1–3 of 5. The condition may be present bilaterally, in which case an overt lameness may not be apparent and horses have a change in gait mechanics or loss of action. Lameness in horses with acute stress fracture is typically grade 2–4 of 5. Bilateral fractures are rare. Lameness with either condition may be exacerbated with firm pressure over the suspensory origin and often is more pronounced with the affected limb on the outside of a circle. Lameness may also be exacerbated on soft footing, but this is more consistent with cases of desmitis at the suspensory origin. Lameness with stress fracture may be exacerbated with carpal or tarsal flexion, but this is not consistent.

Diagnostic confirmation

Diagnostic analgesia

High palmar or high plantar analgesia will be positive in horses with pain at the suspensory origin. The proximal palmar metacarpus and plantar metatarsus are regions notorious for anatomic nuances that may contribute to misinterpretation of the response to local anesthetic injections.[93] Of chief concern are the distal palmar/plantar outpouchings of the carpometacarpal (CMC)/tarsometatarsal (TMT) joints and their close relationship with the suspensory origin.[94,95]

In the forelimb, a high lateral palmar nerve block[96,97] is the most specific perineural block for the suspensory origin and is therefore preferred to the traditional high palmar block (high 'four-point' block) or local infiltration of the suspensory origin (see Chapter 13).[98,99] A comparable technique in the hind limb involves blocking the deep branch of the lateral plantar nerve proximal to the metatarsus;[100] although the specificity of this block for proximal plantar metatarsal pain has been called into question by some.[101] In light of that, and because the distal plantar outpouchings of the TMT joint are less extensive than the CMC outpouchings (making inadvertent intra-articular (IA) injection less likely in the hind limb) a traditional high plantar block (high 'four-point' block) is still preferred by some clinicians. Nevertheless, this possibility (inadvertent IA injection), along with deposition of anesthetic in the tarsal sheath, must be recognized.[95,98]

Similarly, intra-articular injection of anesthetic in the middle carpal (and thus, CMC) or TMT joint can result in a false-positive diagnosis of articular pathology with bony disease at the suspensory origin.

Scintigraphy

Nuclear scintigraphy is invaluable in the diagnostic work-up of horses with suspected stress reaction or stress fracture at the suspensory origin.[102,103] The minimal overt clinical signs and potential for misinterpretation of diagnostic analgesia, along with the fact that radiographs are often negative or equivocal in the early stages of stress reaction, make this imaging modality particularly beneficial.

Bone-phase images will reveal focal, mild to intense, abnormal increased radiopharmaceutical uptake in the proximal palmar metacarpus/plantar metatarsus in horses with stress reaction. Uptake is typically moderate to intense in horses with acute stress fracture (Fig. 16.17).

Radiography

A full radiographic study of the proximal metacarpus/metatarsus should be obtained in all cases, but the most important views in horses with stress reaction or stress fracture are the dorsopalmar/plantar (DP) and lateral or flexed lateral. In the early or acute stages radiographs are often equivocal or may be negative, and correlation of lameness examination and scintigraphic findings is important.

Horses with stress reaction will exhibit varying degrees of trabecular bone sclerosis in the proximal palmar/plantar aspect of MC-III/MT-III at the suspensory origin. Careful evaluation may also reveal osteolytic change in the early stages in some cases. In the forelimbs this is most commonly medially and in the hind limbs the changes are most commonly laterally (associated with the respective heads of the bipartite suspensory origin). Endosteal proliferative reaction and/or enthesiophyte formation along the palmar/plantar cortex may also be present.

Stress fractures in this location typically appear as an inverted V- or U-shaped radiolucency on the DP view and are often seen as a small crescent-shaped fragment on the lateral or flexed lateral view. Endosteal callus may be identifiable on the lateral view.

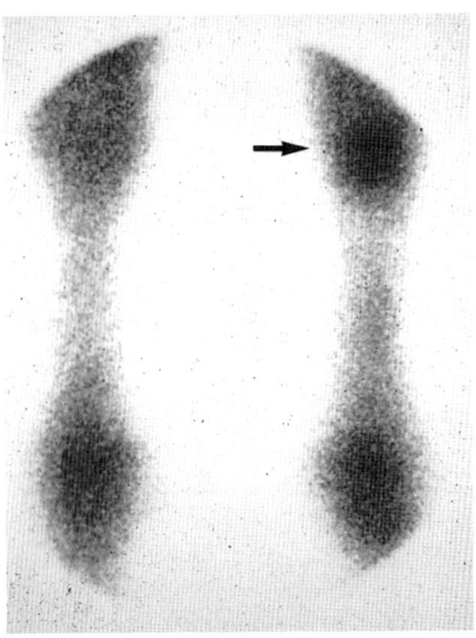

Fig 16.17 Dorsopalmar bone-phase scintigraphic image of the metacarpal and carpal regions of a horse. Notice the focal area of intense abnormal increased radiopharmaceutical uptake in the proximal left metacarpus associated with an avulsion fracture at the origin of the suspensory ligament (arrow).

Ultrasonography

A sonogram should be performed to assess the state of the suspensory ligament although, as previously mentioned, distinct changes indicative of active desmitis are inconsistent and frequently absent. Osseous abnormalities, including irregularity of the cortex or a separate avulsion fragment, may be identifiable.

Computed Tomography and Magnetic Resonance Imaging

As noted earlier, the advantages of CT and MRI over more conventional imaging modalities for diagnosis of musculoskeletal injuries in people and horses are well-recognized. With the exception of the digit, the proximal palmar metacarpus/plantar metatarsus is the anatomic location in horses in which CT and MRI have undergone the most investigation and clinical application to date. The use of these techniques in the diagnosis of primary ligamentous injury in this location will be covered elsewhere in this text. With respect to the osseous pathology, CT and MRI have demonstrated superiority compared to radiography for identifying exostoses and other entheseous change at the suspensory origin.[104,105] As such, in situations where it is logistically and economically feasible, a CT or MRI study should be given consideration for cases where additional information will facilitate a definitive diagnosis.

Thermography

In the hands of an experienced operator thermography may be useful for identifying inflammation at the suspensory origin.

Treatment and prognosis

Therapeutic aims

The goal of treatment is to reduce or eliminate strains on the affected area(s) and promote bone healing.

Therapy

Treatment for stress reaction at the suspensory origin involves anti-inflammatory therapy along with rest and controlled exercise, the specifics of which depend a great deal on the severity of the condition and the use and performance demands (i.e. competition schedule) of the horse. Local and systemic anti-inflammatory therapy, including local corticosteroid injection, is often effective in alleviating lameness associated with stress reaction in horses whose competition schedules will not allow an extended period of rest.

In general, horses should have stall confinement with daily hand-walking exercise until lameness at a trot in-hand has resolved. Exercise is then gradually increased. Time for recovery is highly variable, but a range of 2–6 months is typical. Follow-up scintigraphic examination can be used to monitor healing and enable a more informed recommendation on increases in exercise intensity. Sclerosis will persist after scintigraphic activity has resolved, and therefore radiographs are less helpful in monitoring healing.

Extracorporeal shockwave therapy (ESWT) has become popular with many clinicians for treating osseous and ligamentous pathology at the suspensory origin. Details of the possible mechanism(s) of action and the clinical applications of this modality are beyond the scope of this chapter, and will be covered elsewhere in the text. Suffice to say that apparent efficacy is based almost entirely on anecdotal information and collective personal experiences. Strong scientific evidence of beneficial or potentially beneficial effects in the horse is lacking. Results of investigations published in the respected literature to date are unimpressive and often contradictory, and therefore confusing. This author has very little personal experience to draw on. However, the reader should be aware that ESWT remains a potentially beneficial therapeutic option for this condition with apparently few serious associated complications when used appropriately.

Long toe/low heel conformation is often associated with this condition and may contribute to strain at the suspensory origin. Therefore, corrective trimming to shorten the toes to facilitate breakover may be helpful in these cases. Heel wedges (to elevate the heels) are contraindicated as they will actually increase suspensory ligament strain.[106]

Stress fractures usually heal readily in 3–4 months. Recommendations include 1 month of strict stall rest, followed by 1–2 months of stall confinement with daily hand-walking exercise and then 1–2 months of limited turnout in a small paddock. Follow-up radiographs (± scintigraphy) are taken at approximately 3–4 months to assess healing.

Prognosis

The prognosis for most horses with primary stress reaction or stress fracture at the suspensory origin is good if the condition has been allowed sufficient time to heal. The prognosis with concurrent desmitis at the suspensory origin is much more guarded, particularly in the hindlimbs, and therefore it is important to assess the suspensory ligament in these cases. (See Chapter 20 for details.)

Etiology and pathophysiology

Etiology

Stress reaction and stress fractures at the suspensory origin are cyclic fatigue injuries associated with repetitive strain.

Pathophysiology

Repeated hyperextension of the fetlock joint during exercise with associated cyclic strain on the suspensory ligament is believed to be the primary cause of these conditions. In the forelimbs, carpal hyperextension is also believed to be a contributing factor. As previously noted, long toe/low heel conformation may exacerbate the strain on the suspensory ligament. Stress reaction at the suspensory origin can be classified as an enthesitis resulting from tearing of Sharpey's fibers and associated inflammation of the underlying bone. Maladaptive remodeling and the onset of a stress fracture follow a pathogenesis similar to that of others and the reader is referred elsewhere for a detailed discussion. Stress fractures are most common in racehorses and it is presumably the high-speed cyclic strain that promotes the development of fracture in these cases. Stress fractures can be classified as a form of avulsion fracture.

Epidemiology

Stress reaction at the suspensory origin is seen in all types of performance horses. It appears to be most common in racehorses, eventers and show hunters or show jumpers.[102,103] Stress fractures at the suspensory origin are most commonly seen in racehorses.[102,103,106,107]

Prevention

Like other bone disorders associated with high-strain cyclic fatigue and/or maladaptive remodeling ('repetitive stress-induced bone disease'), prevention of stress reaction and stress fracture at the origin of the suspensory ligament, in theory, should involve both modification of the training regimen and early detection of the subclinical pathologic changes. In actuality, it is impossible to make a blanket recommendation on appropriate training schemes for all ages and uses of athletic horses. Detection of early pathologic changes using advanced diagnostic imaging modalities such as scintigraphy and thermography during the evaluation of horses at high risk for these conditions, or those exhibiting early clinical signs typical of pain at the suspensory origin, with subsequent modification in training intensity is a more realistic approach.

Long toe/low heel conformation exacerbates strain on the suspensory ligament. Therefore, corrective trimming and shoeing to improve hoof balance and shape is also important. However, elevating the heels with wedges and the use of egg bar shoes actually increases strain on the suspensory ligament[106] and their application in these horses should be avoided.

Other metacarpal/metatarsal injuries in performance horses

Proximal metacarpal/metatarsal fractures

This group consists of incomplete longitudinal fractures of the proximal palmar cortex of MC-III, dorsomedial articular fractures of proximal MC-III and dorsolateral articular fractures of proximal MT-III All of these fractures are relatively uncommon compared to other metacarpal/metatarsal injuries and are seen almost exclusively in racehorses. Recommended treatment for all is extended rest (3–6 months). The prognosis for the two metacarpal fracture types is generally good.[108–110] The prognosis for the dorsolateral articular fractures of proximal MT-III is more guarded.[111,112] This may be related to the association with osteoarthritis of the TMT joint.

Exostoses of the distal palmar/plantar aspect of the third metacarpus/metatarsus

This is an apparently uncommon or previously unrecognized phenomenon that was recently reported in a small group of horses.[113] These are irregular exostoses located at the junction of the distal and middle thirds of the cannon bone on the palmar/plantar aspect. They are presumed to be an enthesitis associated with the proximal attachment of the intersesamoidean ligament. Lameness, when present, is attributed to impingement and irritation of the overlying suspensory ligament. Prognosis appears to be favorable, but surgical debridement may be necessary in some cases to achieve full resolution.[113]

Transverse stress fractures of the distal third metacarpus

This is an uncommon fracture that is unique to Thoroughbred racehorses. Clinical signs are typical for other stress fractures. Unlike stress fractures of the dorsal cortex ('saucer fractures') there does not appear to be a predilection for left or right.[114] There is onset of relatively severe lameness after a race or high-speed training. Some horses have a history of chronic or vague lameness that suddenly worsens. Fractures are transversely oriented with slight dorsal-palmar obliquity, and are typically located in the distal metaphysis 2–4 cm proximal to the physeal scar. Unlike the more common dorsal cortical stress fractures they characteristically traverse the width of the bone, and may progress to a complete, unstable fracture in some cases. (Fig. 16.18) Because of that, rigid external coaptation should be considered for all cases once the diagnosis is made. Prognosis is favorable for incomplete or non-displaced fractures, but is guarded-to-poor if catastrophic failure occurs.[114]

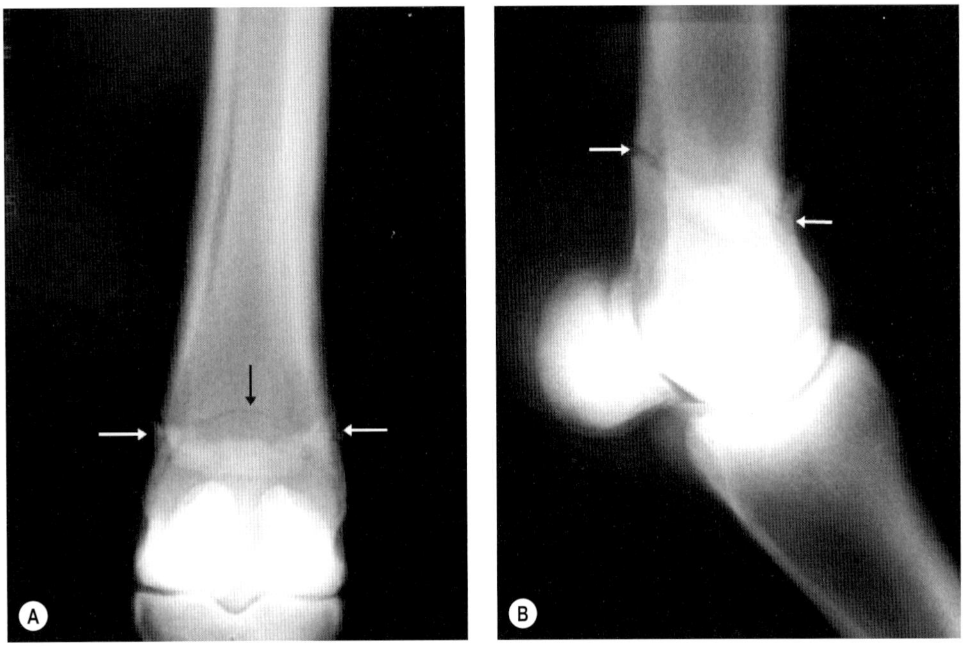

Fig 16.18 **(A)** Dorsopalmar and **(B)** lateral radiographs of the distal right metacarpus/metacarpophalangeal joint of a four-year-old Thoroughbred racehorse with an acute, complete, displaced transverse stress fracture of the distal metacarpus (arrows) demonstrating characteristic location and fracture configuration.

References

1. Goodman NL, Baker BK. Lameness diagnosis and treatment in the Quarter Horse racehorse. Vet Clin North Am Equine Pract 1990;6(1):85–108.
2. Swanson TD. Lameness grading system. In: Guide for veterinary service and judging of equestrian events. 3rd ed. Golden, CO: American Association of Equine Practitioners; 1984.
3. Koblik PD, Hornof WJ, Seeherman HJ. Scintigraphic appearance of stress-induced trauma of the dorsal cortex of the third metacarpal bone in racing Thoroughbred horses: 121 cases (1978–1986). J Am Vet Med Assoc 1988;192(3):390–5.
4. Turner TA, Pansch J, Wilson JH. Thermographic assessment of racing Thoroughbreds. Proceedings of the 47th Annual Convention of the American Association of Equine Practitioners; 2001. p. 344–6.
5. Rohde C, Anderson DE, Bertone AL, et al. Effects of phenylbutazone on bone activity and formation in horses. Am J Vet Res 2000;61(5):537–43.
6. Nunamaker DM, Provost MT. The bucked shin complex revisited. Proceedings of the 37th Annual Convention of the American Association of Equine Practitioners; 1992. p. 757–62.
7. Copelan RW. Incidence, location, and principles of treatment of stress fractures of the third metacarpal bone. Proceedings of the 25th Annual Convention of the American Association of Equine Practitioners; 1979. p. 159–62.
8. Nunamaker DM. The bucked shins complex. Proceedings of the 32nd Annual Convention of the American Association of Equine Practitioners; 1986. p. 457–60.
9. Moyer W, Spencer PA, Kallish M. Relative incidence of dorsal metacarpal disease in young Thoroughbred racehorses training on two different surfaces. Equine Vet J 1991;23(3): 166–8.
10. Jeffcott LB, Rossdale PD, Freestone J, et al. An assessment of wastage in Thoroughbred racing from conception to four years of age. Equine Vet J 1982;14:185–98.
11. Griffiths JB, Steel CM, Symons PJ, et al. Improving the predictability of performance by prerace detection of dorsal metacarpal disease in Thoroughbred racehorses. Aust Vet J 2000;78(7):466–7.
12. Norwood GL. The bucked shins complex in Thoroughbreds. Proceedings of the 24th Annual Convention of the American Association of Equine Practitioners; 1978. p. 319–36.
13. Stover SM, Pool RR, Morgan JP, et al. A review of bucked shins and metacarpal stress fractures in Thoroughbred racehorses. Proceedings of the 34th Annual Convention of the American Association of Equine Practitioners; 1988. p. 129–34.
14. Buckingham SHW, Jeffcott LB. Shin soreness: a survey of Thoroughbred trainers and racetrack veterinarians. Aust Equine Vet 1990;8:148–52.
15. Bailey CJ. Wastage in the racing industry – approaches to study. Proceedings of the Rural Industries Research and Development Corporation Epidemiology Workshop for Equine Research Workers; 1998. p. 43–52.
16. Jeffcott LB, McCarthy RN, Buckingham SHW, et al. Shin soreness in racehorses. University of Melbourne, Melbourne: Equine Clinical Research Unit, Department of Veterinary Science; 1991. p. 5–23.
17. Goodman NL. Quarter Horse racetrack practice. Proceedings of the 33rd Annual Convention of the American Association of Equine Practitioners; 1987;835–841.
18. Nunamaker DM, Butterweck DM, Black J. In vitro comparison of Thoroughbred and Standardbred racehorses with regard to local fatigue failure of the third metacarpal bone. Am J Vet Res 1991;52(1):97–100.
19. Verheyen KL, Henley WE, Price JS, Wood JL. Training-related factors associated with dorsometacarpal disease in young Thoroughbred racehorses in the UK. Equine Vet J 2005;37(5):442–8.

20. Nunamaker DM. Metacarpal stress fractures. In: Nixon AJ, editor. Equine fracture repair. Philadelphia, PA: Saunders; 1996. p. 195–9.
21. Jackson BF, Lonnell C, Verheyen KL, et al. Biochemical markers of bone metabolism and risk of dorsal metacarpal disease in 2-year-old Thoroughbreds. Equine Vet J 2005; 37(1):87–91.
22. Dallap BL, Bramlage LR, Embertson RM. Results of screw fixation combined with cortical drilling for treatment of dorsal cortical stress fractures of the third metacarpal bone in 56 Thoroughbred racehorses. Equine Vet J 1999;31(3):252–7.
23. Hanie EA, Sullins KE, White NA. Follow-up of 28 horses with third metacarpal unicortical stress fractures following treatment with osteostixis. Equine Vet J 1992;24(Suppl 11):4–9.
24. Cervantes C, Madison JB, Ackerman N, et al. Surgical treatment of dorsal cortical fractures of the third metacarpal bone in Thoroughbred racehorses: 53 cases (1985–1989). J Am Vet Med Assoc 1992;200(12):1997–2000.
25. Specht TE, Colahan PT. Osteostixis for incomplete cortical fracture of the third metacarpal bone – results in 11 horses. Vet Surg 1990;19(1):34–40.
26. Spurlock GH. Propagation of a dorsal cortical stress fracture of the third metacarpal bone in two horses. J Am Vet Med Assoc 1988;192(11):1587–9.
27. Watt BC, Foerner JJ, Haines GR. Incomplete oblique sagittal fractures of the dorsal cortex of the third metacarpal bone in six horses. Vet Surg 1998;27: 337–41.
28. Norwood GL, Haynes PF. Dorsal metacarpal disease. In: Mansmann RA, McAllister ES, editors. Equine medicine and surgery. 3rd ed. Santa Barbara, CA: American Veterinary Publications; 1982. p. 1110–14.
29. Specht TE, Miller GJ, Colahan PT. Effects of clustered drill holes on the breaking strength of the equine third metacarpal bone. Am J Vet Res 1990;51(8):1242–6.
30. Burstein AH, Currey J, Frankel VH, et al. Bone strength. The effect of screw holes. J Bone Joint Surg 1972;54-A:1143–56.
31. Williams JGP. Recalcitrant stress fracture: a case managed by drilling. Br J Sports Med 1979;13:84–5.
32. Richardson DW. Dorsal cortical fractures of the equine metacarpus. Comp Cont Educ Pract Vet 1984;6: 248–55.
33. Frost HM. The regional acceleratory phenomenon: a review. Henry Ford Hosp Med J 1983;31:3–9.
34. Bertone AL. The metacarpus and metatarsus. In: Baxter GM, editor. Adam's lameness in horses. 6th ed. Chichester, West Sussex, UK: Wiley-Blackwell; 2011. p. 621–59.
35. Richardson DW. Third metacarpal and metatarsal bones. In: Auer JA, Stick JA, editors. Equine surgery. 4th ed. St. Louis, MO: Elsevier; 2011. p. 1325–38.
36. Carter DR, Hayes WC. Compact bone fatigue damage: a microscopic examination. Clin Orthop 1977;127: 265–74.
37. Nunamaker DM, Butterweck DM, Provost MT. Fatigue fractures in Thoroughbred racehorses: relationships with age, peak bone strain, and training. J Orthop Res 1990;8:604–11.
38. Nunamaker DM, Butterweck DM, Provost MT. Some geometric properties of the third metacarpal bone: a comparison between the Thoroughbred and Standardbred racehorse. J Biomech 1989;22:129–34.
39. Stover SM, Sprayberry K, Pool RR, et al. Incomplete cortical fractures of the Thoroughbred third metacarpal bones. Trans Ann Vet Orth Soc Mtg 1988; 15:19.
40. Ferraro GL. Lameness diagnosis and treatment in the Thoroughbred racehorse. Vet Clin North Am Equine Pract 1990;6(1):147–78.
41. Ellis DR. Some observations on condylar fractures of the third metacarpus and third metatarsus in young Thoroughbreds. Equine Vet J 1994;26(3):178–83.
42. Johnson BJ, Stover SM, Daft BM, et al. Causes of death in racehorses over a 2-year period. Equine Vet J 1994;26(4): 327–30.
43. Bathe AP. 245 fractures in Thoroughbred racehorses: results of a 2-year prospective study in Newmarket. Proceedings of the 40th Annual Convention of the American Association of Equine Practitioners; 1994. p. 175–6.
44. Bassage LH, Richardson DW. Longitudinal fractures of the condyles of the third metacarpal and metatarsal bones in racehorses: 224 cases (1986–1995). J Am Vet Med Assoc 1998;212(11):1757–64.
45. Zekas LJ, Bramlage RM, Embertson RM, et al. Characterization of the type and location of fractures of the third metacarpal/metatarsal condyles in 135 horses in central Kentucky (1986–1994). Equine Vet J 1999;31(4):304–8.
46. Kawcak CE, Bramlage LR, Embertson RM. Diagnosis and management of incomplete fractures of the distal palmar aspect of the third metacarpal bone in five horses. J Am Vet Med Assoc 1995;206(3):335–7.
47. Richardson DW. Medial condylar fractures of the third metatarsal bone in horses. J Am Vet Med Assoc 1984;185(7):761–5.
48. Hornof WJ, O'Brien TR. Radiographic evaluation of the palmar aspect of the equine metacarpal condyles: a new projection. Vet Radiol 1980;21(4): 161–7.
49. Pilsworth RC, Hopes R, Greet TRC. A flexed dorso-palmar projection of the equine fetlock in demonstrating lesions of the distal third metacarpus. Vet Rec 1988;122:332–3.
50. Barclay WP, Foerner JJ, Phillips TN. Axial sesamoid injuries associated with lateral condylar fractures in horses. J Am Vet Med Assoc 1985;186(3): 278–9.
51. Morgan JW, Santschi EM, Zekas LJ, et al. Comparison of radiography and computed tomography to evaluate metacarpo/metatarsophalangeal joint pathology of paired limbs of thoroughbred racehorses with severe condylar fracture. Vet Surg 2006;35(7): 611–17.
52. Rick MC, O'Brien TR, Pool RR, et al. Condylar fractures of the third metacarpal bone and third metatarsal bone in 75 horses: radiographic features, treatments, and outcome. J Am Vet Med Assoc 1983;183(3):287–96.
53. Bertone AL. The metacarpus and metatarsus. In: Baxter GM, editor. Adam's lameness in horses. 6th ed. Chichester, West Sussex, UK: Wiley-Blackwell; 2011. p. 621–59.
54. Schneider RK, Jackman BR. Fractures of the third metacarpus and metatarsus. In: Nixon AJ, editor. Equine fracture repair. Philadelphia, PA: Saunders; 1996. p. 179–94.
55. Richardson DW. Third metacarpal/ metatarsal condylar fractures. In: White NA, Moore JN, editors. Current practice of equine surgery. Philadelphia, PA: JB Lippincott; 1990. p. 617–22.
56. Martin GS. Factors associated with racing performance of Thoroughbreds undergoing lag screw repair of condylar fractures of the third metacarpal or metatarsal bone. J Am Vet Med Assoc 2000;217(12):1870–7.
57. Zekas LJ, Bramlage LR, Embertson RM, et al. Results of treatment of 145 fractures of the third metacarpal/ metatarsal condyles in 135 horses (1986–1994). Equine Vet J 1999;31(4):309–13.
58. Wright IM, Smith MR. A lateral approach to the repair of propagating fractures of the medial condyle of the third metacarpal and metatarsal bone in 18 racehorses. Vet Surg 2009;38(6):689–95.
59. Smith LC, Greet TR, Bathe AP. A lateral approach for screw repair in lag fashion of spiral third metacarpal and metatarsal medial condylar fractures in horses. Vet Surg 2009;38(6):681–8.
60. Russell TM, Maclean AA. Standing surgical repair of propagating

metacarpal and metatarsal condylar fractures in racehorses. Equine Vet J 2006;38(5):423–7.

61. Ross MW. Scintigraphic and clinical findings in the standardbred metatarsophalangeal joint: 114 cases (1993–1995). Equine Vet J 1998;30(2): 131–8.
62. Martinelli MJ, Chambers MD, Baker GJ, et al. A retrospective study of increased bone scintigraphic uptake in the palmar-plantar fetlock and its relationship to performance: 50 horses (1989–1993). Proceedings of the 40th Annual Convention of the American Association of Equine.
63. Arthur RM, Constantinide D. Results of 428 nuclear scintigraphic examinations of the musculoskeletal system at a Thoroughbred racetrack. Proceedings of the 41st Annual Convention of the American Association of Equine Practitioners; 1995. p. 84–7.
64. Stover SM, Read DH, Johnson BJ, et al. Lateral condylar fracture histomorphology in racehorses. Proceedings of the 40th Annual Convention of the American Association of Equine Practitioners; 1994. p. 173.
65. Tranquille CA, Parkin TD, Murray RC. Magnetic resonance imaging-detected adaptation and pathology in the distal condyles of the third metacarpus, associated with lateral condylar fracture in Thoroughbred racehorses. Equine Vet J 2012 Jan 19 (Epub).
66. Whitton RC, Trope GD, Ghasem-Zadeh A, et al. Third metacarpal condylar fatigue fractures in equine athletes occur within previously modelled subchondral bone. Bone 2010;47(4):826–31.
67. Radtke CL, Danova NA, Scollay MC, et al. Macroscopic changes in the distal ends of the third metacarpal and metatarsal bones of Thoroughbred racehorses with condylar fractures. Am J Vet Res 2003;64(9):1110–16.
68. Firth EC, Doube M, Boyde A. Changes in mineralised tissue at the site of origin of condylar fracture are present before athletic training in Thoroughbred horses. N Z Vet J 2009;57(5):278–83.
69. Riggs CM, Whitehouse GH, Boyde A. Structural variation of the distal condyles of the third metacarpal and third metatarsal bones in the horse. Equine Vet J 1999;31(2):130–9.
70. Riggs CM, Whitehouse GH, Boyde A. Pathology of the distal condyles of the third metacarpal and third metatarsal bones of the horse. Equine Vet J 1999;31(2):140–8.
71. Boyde A, Haroon Y, Jones SJ, et al. Three dimensional structure of the distal condyles of the third metacarpal bone of the horse. Equine Vet J 1999;331(2):122–9.
72. Jacklin BD, Wright IM. Frequency distributions of 174 fractures of the distal condyles of the third metacarpal and metatarsal bones in 167 Thoroughbred racehorses (1999–2009). Equine Vet J 2012 Mar 12 (Epub).
73. Kane AJ, Stover SM, Gardner IA, et al. Horseshoe characteristics as possible risk factors for fatal musculoskeletal injury of Thoroughbred racehorses. Am J Vet Res 1996;57(8):1147–51.
74. Kane AJ, Stover SM, Gardner IA, et al. Hoof size, shape, and balance as possible risk factors for catastrophic musculoskeletal injury of Thoroughbred racehorses. Am J Vet Res 1998;59(12): 1545–52.
75. Le Jeune SS, Macdonald MH, Stover SM, et al. Biomechanical investigation of the association between suspensory ligament injury and lateral condylar fracture in thoroughbred racehorses. Vet Surg 2003;32(6):585–97.
76. Parkin TD, Clegg PD, French NP, et al. Risk factors for fatal lateral condylar fracture of the third metacarpus/metatarsus in UK racing. Equine Vet J 2005;37(3):192–9.
77. Trope GD, Anderson GA, Whitton RC. Patterns of scintigraphic uptake in the fetlock joint of Thoroughbred racehorses and the effect of increased radiopharmaceutical uptake in the distal metacarpal/tarsal condyle on performance. Equine Vet J 2011;43(5): 509–15.
78. Zubrod CJ, Schneider RK, Tucker RL. Use of magnetic resonance imaging to identify suspensory desmitis and adhesions between exostoses of the second metacarpal bone and the suspensory ligament in four horses. J Am Vet Med Assoc 2004;224(11): 1815–20.
79. Nagy A, Dyson S. Magnetic resonance imaging findings in the carpus and proximal metacarpal region of 50 lame horses. Equine Vet J 2012;44(2):163–8.
80. Ray C, Baxter GM. Splint bone injuries in horses. Comp Cont Educ Pract Vet 1995;17(5):723–30.
81. Baxter GM, Doran RE, Allen D. Complete excision of a fractured fourth metatarsal bone in eight horses. Vet Surg 1992;21(4):273–8.
82. Doran R. Fractures of the small metacarpal and metatarsal (splint) bones. In: Nixon AJ, editor. Equine fracture repair. Philadelphia, PA: Saunders; 1996. p. 200–7.
83. Bramlage LR, van Hoogmoed L, Embertson R, et al. Treatment of refractory exostoses of the midportion of the splint bones. Proceedings of the 43rd Annual Convention of the American Association of Equine Practitioners; 1997. p. 126–7.
84. Welling EK. Evaluation of the efficacy of surgical intervention on middle and proximal splint bone injuries in 95 Standardbred horses. Vet Surg 1993;22:293.
85. Barber SM, Caron J, Pharr J. Metatarsal/ metacarpal exostosis removal – a prospective study. Vet Surg 1987;16:82.
86. Les CM, Stover SM, Willits NH. Necropsy survey of metacarpal fusion in the horse. Am J Vet Res 1995;56(11): 1421–32.
87. Verschooten F, Gasthuys F, de Moor A. Distal splint bone fractures in the horse: an experimental and clinical study. Equine Vet J 1984;16(6):532–6.
88. du Preez P. Fractures of the small metacarpal and metatarsal bones (splint bones). Equine Vet Edu 1994; 6(5):279–83.
89. Jones RD, Fessier JF. Observations on small metacarpal and metatarsal fractures with or without associated suspensory desmitis in Standardbred horses. Can Vet J 1977;18(2):29–32.
90. Jenson PW, Gaughan EM, Lillich JD, et al. Segmental ostectomy of the second and fourth metacarpal and metatarsal bones in horses: 17 cases (1993–2002). J Am Vet Med Assoc 2004;224(2):271–4.
91. Bowman KF, Evans LH, Herring ME. Evaluation of surgical removal of fractured distal splint bones in the horse. Vet Surg 1982;11:116–20.
92. Bowman KF, Fackelman GE. Surgical treatment of complicated fractures of the splint bones in horses. Vet Surg 1982;11:121–4.
93. Dyson S. Some observations on lameness associated with pain in the proximal metacarpal region. Equine Vet J 1988;20(suppl 6):43–52.
94. Ford TS, Ross MW, Orsini PG. Communications and boundaries of the middle carpal and carpometacarpal joints in horses. Am J Vet Res 1988;49(12):2161–4.
95. Dyson SJ, Romero JM. An investigation of injection techniques for local analgesia of the equine distal tarsus and proximal metatarsus. Equine Vet J 1993;25(1):30–5.
96. Wheat JD, Jones K. Selected techniques of regional anesthesia. Vet Clin North Am Large An Pract 1981;3:223–46.
97. Castro FA, Schumacher JS, Pauwels F, et al. A new approach for perineural injection of the lateral palmar nerve in the horse. Vet Surg 2005;34(6): 539–42.
98. Ford TS, Ross MW, Orsini PG. A comparison of methods for proximal palmar metacarpal analgesia in horses. Vet Surg 1989;18(2):146–50.
99. Bassage LH, Ross MW. Diagnostic analgesia. In: Ross MW, Dyson SJ, editors. Diagnosis and management of lameness in the horse. 2nd ed. St. Louis, MO: Elsevier; 2011. p. 100–35.

100. Hughes TK, Eliashar E, Smith RK. In vitro evaluation of a single injection technique for diagnostic analgesia of the proximal suspensory ligament of the equine pelvic limb. Vet Surg 2007;36(8):760–4.
101. Labens R, Schramme MC, Robertson ID, et al. Clinical, magnetic resonance, and sonographic imaging findings in horses with proximal plantar metatarsal pain. Vet Radiol Ultrasound 2010;51(1): 11–18.
102. Pleasant RS, Baker GJ, Muhlbauer MC, et al. Stress reactions and stress fractures of the proximal palmar aspect of the third metacarpal bone in horses: 58 cases (1980–1990). J Am Vet Med Assoc 1992;201(12):1918–23.
103. Edwards RB, Ducharme NG, Fubini SL, et al. Scintigraphy for diagnosis of avulsions of the origin of the suspensory ligament in horses: 51 cases (1980–1993). J Am Vet Med Assoc 1995;207(5):608–11.
104. Launois MT, Vandeweerd JM, Perrin RA, et al. Use of computed tomography to diagnose new bone formation associated with desmitis of the proximal aspect of the suspensory ligament in third metacarpal or third metatarsal bones of three horses. J Am Vet Med Assoc 2009;234(4):514–18.
105. Coudry V, Denoix JM, Didierlaurent D, et al. Use of magnetic resonance imaging to diagnose the cause of proximal metacarpal pain in a standardbred trotter. Vet Rec 2008; 162(24):790–2.
106. Riemersma DJ, van den Bogert AJ, Jansen MO, et al. Influence of shoeing on ground reaction forces and tendon strains in the forelimbs of ponies. Equine Vet J 1996;28(2):126–32.
107. Bramlage LR, Gabel AA, Hackett RP. Avulsion fractures of the origin of the suspensory ligament in the horse. J Am Vet Med Assoc 1980;176(10):1004–10.
108. Ross MW, Ford TS, Orsini PG. Incomplete longitudinal fracture of the proximal palmar cortex of the third metacarpal bone in horses. Vet Surg 1988;17(2):82–6.
109. Ross MW, Martin BB. Dorsomedial articular fracture of the proximal aspect of the third metacarpal bone in Standardbred racehorses: seven cases (1978–1990). J Am Vet Med Assoc 1992;201(2):332–5.
110. Lloyd KCK, Koblik P, Ragle C, et al. Incomplete palmar fracture of the proximal extremity of the third metacarpal bone in horses: 10 cases (1981–1986). J Am Vet Med Assoc 1988;192(6):798–803.
111. Ross MW, Sponseller ML, Gill HE, et al. Articular fracture of the dorsoproximal aspect of the third metatarsal bone in five Standardbred racehorses. J Am Vet Med Assoc 1993;203(5):698–700.
112. Pilsworth RC. Incomplete fracture of the dorsal aspect of the proximal cortex of the third metatarsal bone as a cause of hind-limb lameness in the racing Thoroughbred: a review of three cases. Equine Vet J 1992;24(2):147–50.
113. Bertoni L, Forresu D, Coudry V, et al. Exostoses on the palmar or plantar aspect of the diaphysis of the third metacarpal or metatarsal bone in horses: 16 cases (2001–2010). J Am Vet Med Assoc 2012;240(6):740–7.
114. Ramzan PH. Transverse stress fracture of the distal diaphysis of the third metacarpus in six Thoroughbred racehorses. Equine Vet J 2009;41(6):602–5.

The Carpus

17

Alexander J. Daniel   Christopher E. Kawcak

CHAPTER CONTENTS

Introduction

Diseases of the carpus commonly affect racehorses, in which repeated stress from training and racing can lead to degradative changes within synovium, joint capsule, articular cartilage, subchondral bone and ligaments. These chronic changes often lead to acute problems ranging from synovitis to catastrophic injuries. Identification and prevention of the chronic processes and risk factors that lead to the development of clinical disease should be the ultimate goal. With advances in biomarkers, three dimensional imaging modalities such as computed tomography (CT) and magnetic resonance imaging (MRI) our understanding of disease processes has progressed. Consequently therapeutics have advanced and become more specified towards certain conditions which has had a profound effect on our ability to effectively treat conditions. In many instances, the clinical manifestation of carpal disease results in synovial effusion, pain on flexion with or without reduction in the range of motion of the limb and therefore additional testing is required to characterize disease. This can be achieved with radiographic imaging, ultrasound, three dimensional imaging (CT and MRI), biomarker analysis and diagnostic arthroscopy.

Carpal disease in racehorses is common and the lesions occur in consistent areas. This permits in-depth clinical study of carpal diseases, allowing practitioners to give an accurate prognosis for a particular injury based on these studies. Carpal injuries can also affect other types of equine athlete; however, these disease processes are usually manifested as acute, traumatic injuries which sometimes occur in uncommon areas of the carpus. In either situation, accurate diagnosis of these conditions is essential when determining the prognosis for these types of injuries however this has historically been difficult due to lack of sufficiently sized clinical studies.

Synovitis

- Variable lameness with synovial effusion.
- Radiographs are often unremarkable.
- Intra-articular medication is often effective for eliminating signs.
- Horses with synovitis often respond well to medical therapy.

Recognition

History and presenting complaint

Synovitis manifests as lameness associated with significant synovial effusion. Synovial effusion alone in young racehorses that are not showing lameness or training problems is not uncommon. However, the effusion may be significant if there is a history of training-associated problems or lameness with the horse.

Physical examination

Synovial effusion in the carpal joints can occur in both the dorsal and palmar aspects. Synovial effusion can be graded as mild, moderate or severe. Mild effusion is palpable on the dorsal aspect of the carpal joints, while severe is palpable effusion that can also be detected on the palmar aspect of the joint. It is typical to see pain with static flexion in horses with synovitis and focal pain on palpation can sometimes be appreciated in those with synovitis and other associated injuries leading to synovitis. Heat on palpation is not uncommon in horses with synovitis; however, the presence of topical medications and recent bandaging may influence surface heat.

Most horses with synovitis will be lame at the trot and, in carpal lameness in particular, wide movement of the forelimbs is appreciable. This wide movement occurs because horses with synovitis, and the resulting pain in the carpal joints, do not want to flex their carpi. Consequently, they will circumduct the limb, leading to a wide moving gait. Furthermore, in cases of carpal synovitis, it is quite common to see worsening of the lameness after flexion.

Special examination

Regional anesthesia of the carpus, although often unnecessary for diagnosis of synovitis, can be accomplished by performing a median and ulnar nerve block after perineural anesthesia below the carpus has been performed. Intra-articular anesthesia is usually not necessary to diagnose synovitis of the carpal joints but occasionally may be needed to confirm carpal disease and rule out other diseases in the limb. As an example, it may be prudent to block the carpal joints and eliminate the lameness there in order to document additional lameness in another area of the limb. Although carpal joint blocks have been described elsewhere, it is important to remember that the radiocarpal and intercarpal joints should be blocked separately. Radiographs are usually negative; however, good-quality radiographs in multiple views are necessary to rule out any small or subtle injuries. In many cases of primary synovitis, it is not uncommon to see soft tissue thickening or dorsal displacement of the fat pad on the dorsum of the carpus on the radiographs.

Advances in ultrasonographic examination of joints have given clinicians a better impression of soft tissue injuries. Because soft tissue injuries can lead to synovitis, documentation of capsular and synovial lining thickening and edema can help not only to diagnose the primary problem but also to monitor therapy over time. Ultrasound also allows the clinician to rule out extracapsular thickenings such as hygromas and synovial hernias. An in-depth review of ultrasonographic examination of joints has been documented.[1]

Synovial fluid can also be evaluated subjectively. It is not uncommon in cases of synovitis to see a watery, clear to light yellow fluid. In some cases, there is increased opacity and flocculants in the fluid. In cases such as this, laboratory examination of the synovial fluid may be necessary to rule out septic arthritis.

Laboratory examination

Synovial fluid analysis results can be variable in cases of synovitis although most white blood cell counts are less than 1000 cells/mm^3 and total protein concentrations are generally between 2.5 and 4.0 g/dL. Biomarker analysis often shows elevated concentrations of prostaglandin E2.[2]

Diagnostic confirmation

The lack of radiographic findings, which rules out osteochondral fragmentation and fracture, is often enough to lead to a diagnosis of synovitis, although a negative diagnostic arthroscopy is needed to completely rule out intra-articular ligament disease. It is often difficult to justify diagnostic arthroscopy in cases that are most likely synovitis compared to intra-articular ligament injury; therefore most veterinarians will monitor response to medical therapy. Refractory cases are then easier to justify as needing surgery as synovitis usually responds well to intra-articular medications. MRI is not required to make a diagnosis of synovitis although this condition is readily detectable when performed (Fig. 17.1).

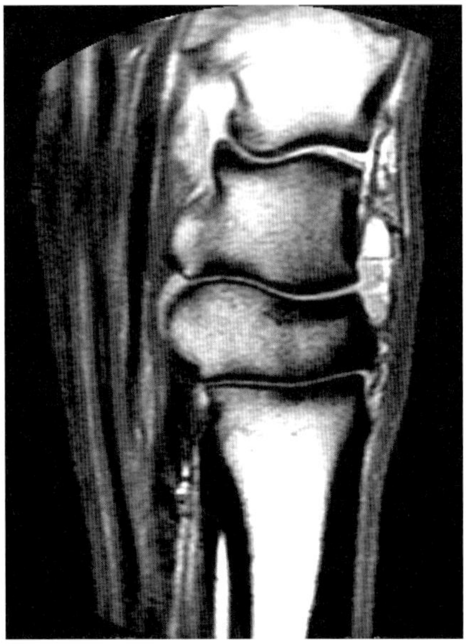

Fig 17.1 Proton density sagittal view of a right front carpus in a racing Quarter Horse. There is subchondral bone thickening of the third carpal bone and subtle subchondral thickening of the radiocarpal bone. The middle-carpal joint demonstrates mild synovitis with thickening of the joint capsule. These changes were considered normal physiological adaptation and lameness associated with this limb was localized distal to this region.

Images provided by Dr L.Goodrich.

Treatment and prognosis

Therapeutic aims

The goal of therapy is to provide timely, effective anti-inflammatory medications either systemically, locally or topically.

Therapy

Systemic anti-inflammatory medications, such as non-steroidal anti-inflammatory medications or intravenous hyaluronic acid, are the simplest forms of therapy which are often very effective for controlling synovitis. However, intra-articular anti-inflammatory medication in the form of corticosteroids and/or hyaluronic acid may be necessary to provide effective treatment. Interleukin-1 receptor antagonist protein (IRAP) or topical diclofenac sodium can also be used for refractory cases. Physical therapy methods such as ice, hydrotherapy, daily range of motion exercises and walking are often used in addition to medications. Intra-articular morphine (20 mg) with ropivacaine (20 mg) has been used in experimental settings to provide up to 24 hours of pain relief for acute cases of synovitis.[3]

Prognosis

The prognosis for synovitis is often excellent for resumption of athletic training with rapid, effective therapy barring predisposing conformational abnormalities, osteochondral disease or intra-articular ligament disease.

Etiology and pathophysiology

Acute injuries can lead to synovitis, but in racehorses, the chronic effects of training and racing can lead to failure of tissues to adapt properly to training. Early, chronic stress can lead to adaptive changes until a certain threshold is crossed, when degradative changes overcome adaptive changes. This can occur within any tissues. Conformational abnormalities can accelerate the degradative process due to high, focal stresses.

Epidemiology

As stated previously, young racehorses typically develop some form of synovitis early in their training. However, most cases of synovitis are secondary to a primary disease entity within the joint, such as osteochondral fragmentation or fracture. Conformational abnormalities especially offset and/or calf-kneed conformation can increase the chances of synovitis.

Prevention

Critical evaluation of conformation is essential as gross abnormalities in conformation may cause persistent abnormal loading and hence synovitis and ultimately osteoarthritis (OA). Careful monitoring during training is also essential as treatment and change in training early in cases of synovitis are helpful.

Capsulitis

- Capsulitis often results in joint capsule thickening.
- Restricted range of motion is common in cases of capsulitis.
- Enthesophytes are often seen on radiographs.
- Response to treatment is often variable.

Recognition

History and presenting complaint

Capsulitis can be caused by several disease processes so the history can be quite variable. For instance, it is not uncommon to see capsulitis in horses with a history of carpal disease such as osteochondral fractures, fragmentation or ligamentous injuries. However, capsulitis can also result from non-articular diseases, such as extracapsular ligament damage or capsular injury. In some cases, capsulitis can also occur because of acute injury, which may lead to edema and possibly fibrosis of the joint capsule. In some recurrent or unresponsive idiopathic synovitis cases, capsular thickening and scarring can also result. In most of these cases in athletes, the animal will fail to train and will have chronic unresponsive joint disease.

Physical examination

Horses with capsulitis typically show soft tissue thickening over the dorsal aspect of the carpus. However, the severity of effusion can be difficult to appreciate because of this thickening. Range of motion is often restricted and maximal flexion often results in a painful response. At the trot, these horses typically move wide and are often significantly worse after carpal flexion. Occasionally, pain on palpation will be apparent on the dorsal aspect of the carpus, especially in acute cases. Although capsular swelling is difficult to appreciate on the palmar aspect of the joint, horses with palmar capsular pain are extremely sensitive to carpal flexion.

Special examination

Horses with acute capsular changes may show no radiographic changes; however, those horses with capsular tearing, especially at the insertion of the capsule into the bone, will often show enthesophyte formation several weeks after injury. Enthesophytes can vary in severity and location; however, in most equine athletes, especially racehorses, enthesophyte formation on the dorsal aspect of the carpal bones is quite common (Fig. 17.2). Ultrasound examination of the joint capsule in horses with acute capsulitis will often show edema formation within the capsular tissues, and thickening of those tissues. Nuclear scintigraphy may also be helpful in some cases, especially in the vascular and soft tissue phases. CT examination may be of little use in these cases unless a primary osteochondral disease process is leading to the capsular change. As for synovitis, MRI is rarely needed to make a diagnosis of capsulitis but is often seen with this modality (Fig. 17.1).

Laboratory examination

Synovial fluid analysis in horses with capsular damage is often quite variable.

Diagnostic confirmation

As mentioned previously, radiographs are usually only suggestive of capsular changes. In particular, enthesophyte formation certainly indicates previous capsular insertional damage and peri-articular lysis may indicate acute inflammation at the insertion. Even though capsular damage can occur by itself, other intra-articular diseases must be ruled out, either by the special examinations mentioned above or, as in most cases by diagnostic arthroscopy.

Finally, capsulitis is sometimes diagnosed based on response to therapy. For instance, some cases of acute capsular tearing may respond well to intra-articular anti-inflammatory medications. Unlike secondary capsulitis, which occurs in response to other osteochondral diseases, primary capsular damage will usually respond to medical therapy. However, this is dependent upon the severity of damage.

Treatment and prognosis

Therapeutic aims

The principal therapeutic aim is to remove the primary disease. In cases of secondary capsular damage, the primary objective is to remove the intra-articular damage that is leading to capsulitis. Second, inflammation must be reduced by either systemic or intra-articular methods. Finally, because capsular disease often leads to scar tissue formation, methods that help restore function and range of motion are essential to decrease scar tissue formation. Effective regimens include passive range of motion, hypothermia/hydrotherapy, massage therapy and progressive increases in exercise in an attempt to restore full function to the joint.

Therapy

Arthroscopic removal or fixation of the primary problem is essential to overcoming capsular damage. Systemic and intra-articular anti-inflammatory medications and physical therapy, including passive range of motion, are also essential in dealing with capsular damage. Topical diclofenac cream is also an effective medication.

Prognosis

The prognosis in cases with capsular damage can be quite variable. In cases of acute, mild capsulitis or capsular damage, the prognosis is usually quite good with prompt identification of the disease process and therapy. However, severe cases of capsular damage can be quite limiting to the prognosis of an athlete and often require ongoing medical management to continue competing. Decreased range of motion and pain on flexion often hinder the horse's ability to use the limb properly. The prognosis for cases of secondary capsulitis or capsular damage is dependent on the severity and form of the primary disease process.

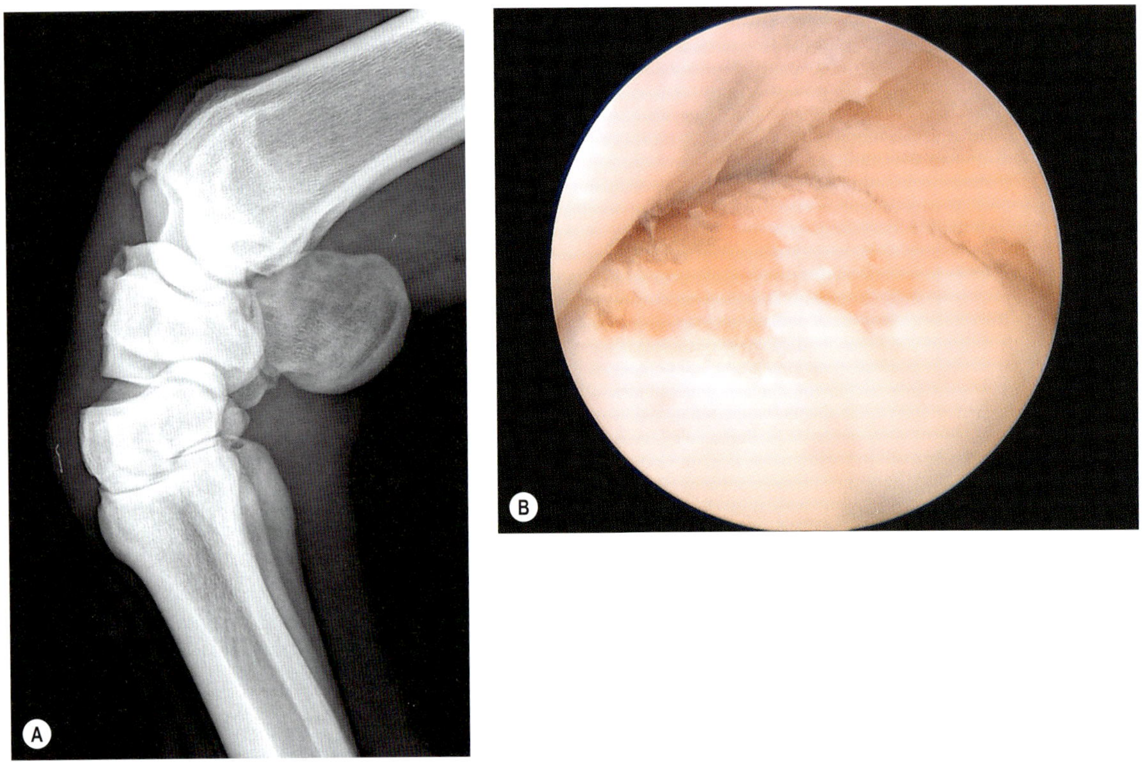

Fig 17.2 **(A)** Flexed lateral radiograph of a racing Quarter Horse with chronic lameness localized to the carpus. There is enthesophyte formation on the dorsal aspect of the intermediate carpal bone with multiple sites of osteochondral (OC) fragmentation on the proximal intermediate and proximal radiocarpal bones and the distal radius. **(B)** Arthroscopic view of the osseous and cartilaginous changes of the distomedial radius following surgical removal of OC fragments and micropicking of the distal radius. This horse was treated with intra-articular hyaluronic acid and triamcinolone at the time of suture removal.

Images provided by Dr C. Kawcak.

Etiology and pathophysiology

In most primary cases of capsular damage, an acute sprain type of injury is often the cause of the problem. However, as stated above, repetitive trauma to the joint capsule due to training and racing can lead to chronic changes in the joint capsule, and hence chronic capsulitis. Secondary forms of capsular damage often result from osteochondral damage elsewhere in the joint and failure to treat that primary disease promptly.

Epidemiology

It seems that most cases of carpal disease often result in some form of capsulitis. Only in those very acute cases of primary joint disease will capsulitis not be a factor. However, failure to treat promptly or a wait and see approach to carpal disease will most likely lead to some form of capsular disease. Capsulitis is common in racehorses and in retired racehorses which are used in other disciplines. In some of the latter cases, the primary osteochondral injury may not be treated because the horse is retired, and hence leads to capsulitis.

Prevention

When capsulitis is secondary, aggressive and prompt treatment of the primary cause is essential in order to prevent capsular damage and thickening. In some cases, failure to treat the primary problem often results in persistent capsular changes that often limit the prognosis of the animal, even though the primary disease may be mild or cured.

Osteochondral fragmentation (chip fracture)

- Chronic disease processes often lead to osteochondral fragmentation.
- Synovitis is a common feature of osteochondral fragmentation.
- Arthroscopy is the treatment of choice.
- The prognosis is dependent on the severity of articular cartilage erosion as well as the presence of palmar carpal fragments.

Recognition

History and presenting complaint

Most horses with osteochondral fragmentation appear to have a history of acute lameness isolated to the carpal joints. However, in some cases, especially in racehorses, synovial effusion or synovitis often precedes diagnosis of osteochondral fragmentation. Unusual traumatic events, e.g. recovery from anesthesia, can also be rare causes of osteochondral fragmentation.

Physical examination

Clinical signs in horses with osteochondral fragmentation are very similar to those in horses with synovitis.

Special examination

Radiographs are often diagnostic in cases of osteochondral fragmentation; however, radiographs often underestimate the severity of damage. CT examination has proven beneficial in diagnosing unusual cases of osteochondral fragmentation, as has MRI.

Laboratory examination

Standard synovial fluid analysis is not beneficial for identifying cases of osteochondral fragmentation. However, synovial fluid markers (specifically type II collagen degradation products) have been shown to increase following OC injury within the carpus and have also been correlated with the severity of injury.[4] Other biomarkers have also been shown to increase significantly above exercise related increases[5] including prostaglandin E2 concentrations which are raised in synovial fluid following OC fragmentation[2]. Although not commonly performed, monitoring of these may lend useful information regarding the severity of pathological changes to articular cartilage and the degree of the inflammatory response within the joint. Cartilage oligomeric matrix protein (COMP) has also been shown to be elevated in the urine of horses with osteochondral fragmentation with osteophyte production[6] and also in synovial fluid[7], but not in joints with osteoarthritis.[8]

Diagnostic confirmation

Diagnostic arthroscopy is by far the best means of characterizing osteochondral fragmentation, identifying any associated gross pathological changes to articular cartilage and also has the benefit of allowing for treatment of the disease. In most cases, standard radiographic projections of the carpus including flexed and skyline views, are used for confirmation of disease (Fig. 17.2). The palmar surface of the carpal bones must be closely examined on radiographs prior to surgery so that arthroscopic examination of this area is performed, if necessary (Fig. 17.3).

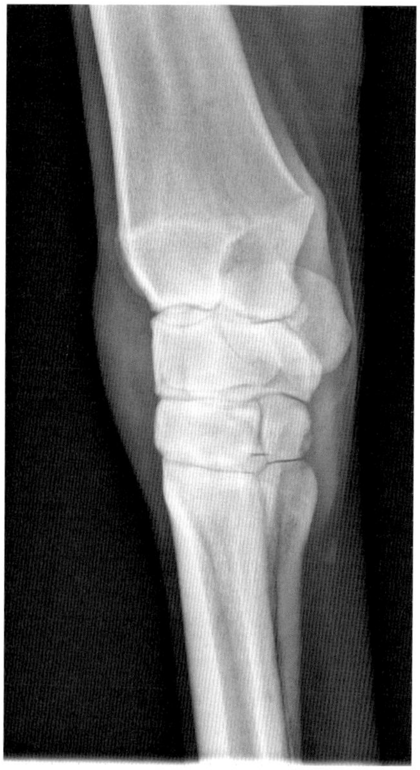

Fig 17.3 Dorsomedial-palmarolateral oblique radiograph of a carpus from a Warmblood eventer with acute signs of lameness, joint effusion and pain on flexion of the limb following a traumatic event to the carpus. There is an osteochondral fragment associated with the palmar lateral surface of the radiocarpal bone. This was arthroscopically removed via a palmar arthroscopic approach, there was no soft tissue trauma and the horse returned to full work. *Images provided by Dr W.McIlwraith.*

Treatment and prognosis

Therapeutic aims

Removal of the fragment is essential for restoring the joint to normal function. Accurate grading of articular cartilage lesions is also essential and, of course, much like all other cases, decreasing inflammation is also essential.

Therapy

Arthroscopic removal of the fragment and use of anti-inflammatory medications are necessary in treating these diseases. Furthermore, chondral supplementation, be it by intra-articular or systemic means, is also beneficial, especially in severe cases of osteochondral fragmentation. The authors also find physical therapy to be beneficial in these cases, to limit the amount of capsulitis that can accompany osteochondral fragmentation. Selected use of intra-articular triamcinolone acetonide with hyaluronic acid may also be of benefit in some cases.[9] Selective use of subchondral micropicking with mesenchymal stem cell therapy as an intra-articular injection may benefit cases with more severe cartilaginous degeneration.

Prognosis

The prognosis following arthroscopic removal of the osteochondral fragment varies with articular cartilage erosion severity. In particular, return to racing at equal to or better than before surgery was 71.1% for grade 1 lesions, 75% for grade 2 lesions, 53.2% for grade 3 lesions and 54% for grade 4 lesions.[10] Grade 4 lesions (which involve a significant loss of the subchondral bone) have also been repaired with 2.7 mm lag screw fixation with reported success of 68% return to racing.[11] In addition the presence of palmar carpal fragments with or without dorsal osteochondral fragmentation has a negative effect on prognosis. When present, these palmar fragments can be a continual source of inflammation and can themselves be associated with cartilaginous degeneration/loss[12] and removal should be attempted where possible.

Etiology and pathophysiology

Evaluation of post-mortem cases[9] has shown that most osteochondral fragments in racehorses are acute manifestations of chronic disease processes. In particular, most fragments occur in areas of stress-induced subchondral bone sclerosis, in which micro damage exceeds healing and acute fragmentation results. Although there is a healing response, as shown by the presence of granulation tissue at these sites, continued training ultimately results in fragmentation through the granulation tissue bed.

Epidemiology

Osteochondral fragmentation of the carpus is very common in racehorses, particularly in racing Quarter Horses, Thoroughbreds, and Standardbreds. However, in non-racing breeds, it is quite rare and when it does occur, it arises in unusual locations other than the dorsal aspect of the carpus.

Prevention

Again, there is no effective means of preventing osteochondral fragmentation in horses, especially in racehorses. However, subtle subchondral bone lysis on radiographic examination and persistent synovial effusion may be indicative of impending osteochondral fragmentation. In the future, the use of biomarkers may also prove beneficial in early identification of osteochondral fragmentation.

Osteochondral fracture (slab fracture)

- Horses with osteochondral fracture often present with significant acute lameness.
- Synovitis is a common sign of osteochondral fracture.
- Horses with osteochondral fracture are often very responsive to flexion.
- Radiographs are recommended prior to performing intra-articular anesthesia, which is often not required for diagnosis.

Recognition

History and presenting complaint

Acute, severe lameness often accompanies osteochondral fracture; however, some horses may not be lame acutely but rather may manifest severe lameness within 24 hours.

Physical examination

Horses with osteochondral fracture appear to be severely lame compared to horses with other disease processes within the carpus, and they are very responsive to carpal flexion. In some cases, the horse may actually resent even partial flexion of the carpus and the clinician must take care when performing the flexion test.

Special examination

The authors do not recommend intra-articular diagnostic analgesia in cases of severe carpal lameness with severe response to flexion. Instead, a complete series of radiographs is essential, including skyline and, in some cases, special views to highlight the fractures. CT and MRI are also valuable, especially in assessing those fractures that are not absolutely clear on radiographs. However, since both modalities require general anesthesia, it is recommended that the surgeon perform these imaging studies just prior to surgery so the fracture can be repaired to prevent further comminution that may occur during recovery.

Laboratory examination

There are no synovial fluid parameters that are specific for osteochondral fracture; however, hemorrhage into the joint is not uncommon.

Diagnostic confirmation

Radiographs and diagnostic arthroscopy are helpful to confirm the diagnosis. Visualization of the slab fracture in orthogonal planes helps to determine the treatment recommendation i.e. removal or internal fixation. Of note, sagittal slab fractures are best seen on a DL-PaMO view.

Treatment and prognosis

Therapeutic aims

The aim of therapy is to restore the articular surface to as normal congruence as possible and to provide axial support to the limb.

Therapy

Internal fixation or removal of the fracture fragment via arthroscopy are considered the treatments of choice. Only small fractures or fractures within the palmar aspects of the joints should be removed and usually only if they are not suited for screw placement. Since there is often significant articular cartilage loss, systemic and/or intra-articular chondro-protective agents are often used to treat associated articular cartilage damage. Mesenchymal stem cells may provide regenerative benefit to the cartilaginous surfaces as a part of the rehabilitation program.

Prognosis

In general, the prognosis for successful repair of intra-articular fractures is often poor, especially in racehorses; however, the prognosis for third carpal slab fractures is often dependent on the severity of articular cartilage erosion at the site. Incomplete non-displaced third carpal bone fractures have been treated with lag screw fixation in racing thoroughbreds with an 85% (11/13 cases) return to racing. In another study 7/7 horses treated with inter-fragmentary compression raced versus 8/9 horses treated by arthroscopic debridement alone and 7/16 treated by conservative management alone.[13]

Etiology and pathophysiology

Subchondral bone sclerosis is very common in cases of osteochondral fracture, indicating that these fractures may be the result of accumulated micro-damage.[14] Furthermore, the proximal portions of these fractures often have fibrous tissue within them, indicating that a chronic pathologic condition may exist prior to acute manifestation of the fracture.

Epidemiology

Osteochondral fractures are quite common in racehorses and occur most frequently within the radial fossa of the third carpal bone. Other fracture configurations can occur and fractures can occur within other bones of the carpus.

Prevention

As with the above disease entities, it is difficult to prevent osteochondral fracture. However, close monitoring of horses with persistent carpal disease is essential.

Desmopathy (intra-articular and extra-articular ligament disease)

- Effusion often persists in the face of medical therapy.
- Radiographs are often unremarkable.
- Magnetic resonance imaging and/or diagnostic arthroscopy is often required to establish a diagnosis.
- Fiber tearing is common in athletes and avulsion injuries are frequently associated.

Recognition

History and presenting complaint

There are no distinguishing historical characteristics for horses with desmitis of intra-articular ligaments.[15]

Physical examination

A retrospective study has shown that there are no distinguishing clinical characteristics for diagnosis of intra-articular ligament damage over other forms of carpal disease[15]. Most cases of intra-articular ligament damage present similar to cases of synovitis, which in an acute case, will show as synovial effusion.

Special examination

Radiographs can be negative (often when there is tearing of the medial palmar intercarpal ligament-MPICL) however in some cases of disease there are associated lytic areas e.g. adjacent to the attachment of the lateral palmar intercarpal ligament (LPICL). These lytic regions must be differentiated from subchondral bone cysts.[16] Dorsolateral-palmaromedial 45° oblique (DL-PaMO) and dorsopalmar (DP) views are most helpful for evaluation of ulnar carpal avulsions. Nuclear scintigraphy may show increased radiopharmaceutical uptake within the intercarpal area. CT examination has revealed stress reaction in the subchondral bone adjacent to intra-articular ligament sites, which may be indicative of damage at that site.[17] Ultrasound is useful for diagnosis of collateral ligament injuries along with stressed radiographs to demonstrate laxity when severe traumatic injury has occurred. Arthroscopy allows assessment of the dorsal surface of the MPICL and LPICL. MRI is the current gold standard for diagnosis for intra-articular ligamentous pathology if radiographs are suspicious and nuclear scintigraphy is suggestive.

Diagnostic confirmation

Although other diagnostic modalities exist, diagnostic arthroscopy is an excellent diagnostic and therapeutic tool, in that it not only allows characterization of the severity of damage but also aids in debridement of the torn ligament fibers and removal of avulsion fragments

Treatment and prognosis

Therapeutic aims

The primary therapeutic aim is to identify the diseased tissues and debride those torn ligamentous fibers. In cases of avulsion fracture, it is best to remove the avulsed portion of bone

Therapy

Arthroscopic debridement of tissue ends is essential for treatment of intra-articular desmitis and when avulsion injury is detected then fragments should be removed. Furthermore, anti-inflammatory medications and joint supplements may also be beneficial, as is physical therapy.

Prognosis

The prognosis for intra-articular ligament damage is based on the severity of damage and the presence of other lesions within the carpus, although generally prognosis is good. Following removal of LPICL avulsions fragments in one study, 20 of 22 horses returned to work.[18] Carpal collateral ligament desmopathy beyond mild injuries carry a poorer prognosis.[19]

Etiology and pathophysiology

It appears that intra-articular ligament damage is quite common as most horses older than one year have some form of tearing.[20] It has also been shown that larger ligaments show varying forms of damage at the ultrastructural level. Therefore, it appears that most of these cases are the result of chronic progressive damage, most likely due to training and racing. However, the gross changes have variable clinical effects on equine athletes.

Epidemiology

Reports have shown that hypertrophy of the dorsal medial intercarpal ligament is quite common and may not relate to clinical disease.[20] MPICL and LPICL desmopathy occur with 51% and 18.5% frequency respectively.[15] Additionally they may occur with concurrent osteochondral disease. In situations where other imaging has not provided and answer, MRI allows for differentiation between normal anatomical variation and pathological changes.

Prevention

There appears to be no effective means of preventing intra-articular ligament damage other than identifying the lesions at an early stage in order to prevent secondary joint changes that could lead to OA.

Catastrophic injury (breakdown)

- Catastrophic injury can result from chronic or acute disease processes.
- Catastrophic injuries are often life threatening.
- Aggressive first aid is often needed prior to surgical repair.
- Local and systemic stabilization of the horse is necessary.

Recognition

History and presenting complaint

Horses with catastrophic injuries of the carpus often show acute non-weight bearing lameness and axial instability at the carpal area.

Physical examination

Cases present as a non-weight bearing lameness, with generalized swelling around the carpus, significant instability of the carpal joints and loss of axial support.

Special examination

Standard radiographic examination is often diagnostic in identifying multiple carpal bone fractures and stressed views can highlight joint laxity. Individual or multiple bones can be involved as well as luxation or subluxation of bones or joints with or without compression fractures.

Laboratory examination

Laboratory examination is not diagnostic, as clinical signs are absolute in localizing this problem.

Diagnostic confirmation

Diagnostic confirmation is often via radiographs (Fig. 17.4).

Treatment and prognosis

Therapeutic aims

Systemic support of the animal is often essential, as most of these horses will present excited and hypotensive because of sweating. This often seems to be overlooked and acute treatment of systemic effects is critical, especially if the horse is to undergo surgical treatment. Local, effective, temporary stabilization of the carpus is also essential in promoting a good prognosis. This may also help with the horse's temperament in that localized stabilization may allow the horse some degree of weight bearing and have a calming effect. Acute stabilization entails both palmar and lateral support of the carpus via bandaging with splints.[21] Ultimate therapy or ultimate

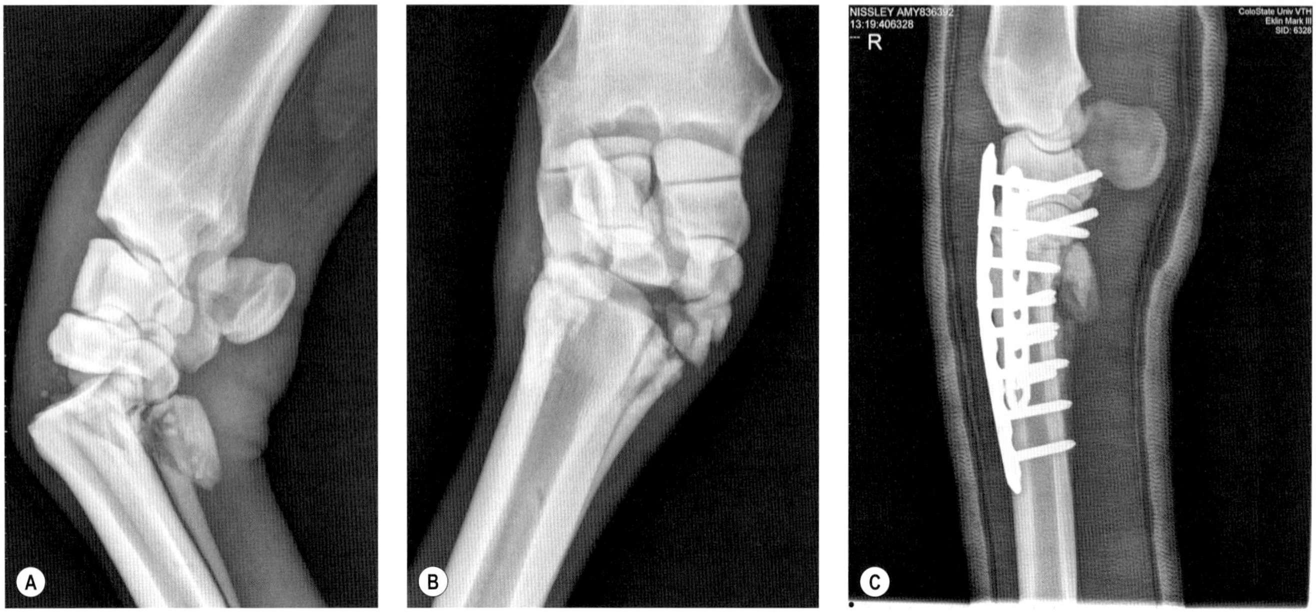

Fig 17.4 **(A)** Lateral radiograph of right front carpus with subluxation of the carpometacarpal joint, fracture of the second and fourth metacarpal bones and the fourth carpal bone. Multiple bone fragments can be seen within the joint space. **(B)** Dorsopalmar stressed radiograph demonstrating medial instability of the carpus with the same fractures as described in A. **(C)** Lateral radiograph taken two weeks after surgery following treatment by partial carpal arthrodesis. External coaption provided by a full limb cast. This horse remained sound at pasture following the surgery. Images provided by Dr B.Leise.

treatment for this condition will rely on surgical restoration of axial support.

Therapy

Again, aggressive first aid and sedation are essential for prompt treatment and transportation of the horse. Stabilization via splints is also essential to allow the horse some degree of comfort and to prevent further damage to the articular and peri-articular structures. Surgical reduction and internal fixation are often the definitive means of treatment for restoration of axial stability. However, the ultimate goal is pasture soundness for breeding animals. Conservative therapy has also been used in some of these cases, in which cast application, usually via a sleeve cast, has allowed for ankylosis of the joints to occur. Partial or pancarpal arthrodesis has also been used to salvage these horses for breeding[22] (Fig. 17.4).

Prognosis

The prognosis for athletic soundness in these horses is grave. However, prognosis for pasture soundness is often good with acute aggressive therapy. Accessory carpal bone fractures have been treated successfully with return to racing following surgery.[23]

Etiology and pathophysiology

Catastrophic injury of the carpus can result from either acute or chronic disease processes. As mentioned above, acute diseases can occur due to some sort of traumatic event e.g. a kick. However, some acute injuries may be a result of pain elsewhere in the animal that causes either overloading of that limb or abnormal use of the limb. Chronic disease processes can also lead to catastrophic injury of the carpus. In particular, slab fractures that go unrecognized, are not treated, or are compounded by an acute traumatic event, may lead not only to damage of the fracture portion but also to the surrounding bones.

Epidemiology

Catastrophic injury of the carpus is quite rare, especially in non-racing breeds.

Prevention

Again, there is no definitive means of preventing catastrophic injuries of the carpus but accurate diagnosis of early diseases may be helpful. However, especially in non-racing animals, acute injury to the carpus can occur with jumping or falling, thus limiting any means of prevention.

Stress-induced bone reaction (subchondral sclerosis)

- One sign is failure of subchondral bone to adapt to exercise.
- Response to intra-articular anesthesia is variable.
- Nuclear scintigraphy often shows mild to moderate increased radiopharmaceutical uptake.
- Radiographic findings are inconsistent.
- MRI is the gold standard for diagnosis.
- Early detection and decreased training are often necessary for successful treatment.

Recognition

History and presenting complaint

Horses with subchondral sclerosis that leads to clinical disease often present with a non-specific history of lameness or, more frequently, a decrease in performance.

Physical examination

Physical examination findings typically show signs of chronic carpal joint disease consisting of joint capsule thickening and pain on flexion. However, occasionally, those signs are not present.

Special examination

Most subchondral sclerosis is located in or begins from the medial aspect of the carpal bones.[24]

Radiographic findings when present include increased radio-opacity of bone caused by increased trabecular thickness, usually in the third carpal bone, with lysis on the proximal joint surface (Fig. 17.5). These findings are best seen on the dorsoproximal-dorsodistal oblique (skyline) projections. When intra-articular anesthesia has confirmed pain to originate from this region sclerosis has been attributed as the cause of lameness.[25,26]

Care must be taken not to over-interpret this finding as in many athletic horses, including Thoroughbred and Standardbred[26] race-horses, mild sclerosis is considered a normal physiologic change. Grading schemes have been described to correlate sclerotic changes with lameness.[26,27]

Nuclear scintigraphy is useful to confirm active stress-induced bone reaction as horses will have mild, moderate or severely increased radiopharmaceutical uptake in this area. Computed tomography can also help to confirm diagnosis seen as areas of intense subchondral bone thickening and lysis. Magnetic resonance imaging can also be used to view these changes (Fig. 17.1), and may be associated with osseous hyperintensity although, again, over interpretation of sclerosis should still be avoided.[28] MRI also provides information regarding the overlying articular cartilage which is often found damaged with the subchondral bone.[29]

Laboratory examination

There are no distinguishing changes in synovial fluid parameters that can lead to a diagnosis of subchondral bone stress reaction. However, early work using biochemical markers of bone turnover in synovial fluid and serum indicates that changes in osteocalcin may help to identify the change.

Diagnostic confirmation

Nuclear scintigraphy is often adequate to confirm diagnosis of subchondral stress reaction in the carpus. If a full series of radiographs are non-diagnostic (including skyline projections), MRI can be used to confirm subchondral sclerosis and helps differentiate from other conditions.

Treatment and prognosis

Therapeutic aims

The goal of therapy is to promote bone remodeling in the hope of re-establishing a more compliant subchondral bone. This can either be done through reduced training or by medication.

Therapy

Reduced training may help in re-establishing a more normal subchondral bone. The re-initiation of remodeling, including the osteoclastic function that occurs with rest, along with re-establishment of exercise may help to provide a more normal bone. However, prior to treatment, diagnostic arthroscopy may be needed if subchondral lysis has led to collapse of the overlying articular surface. In addition, arthroscopically guided micropicking may also help to stimulate blood flow into the area and thus reinitiate remodeling.

A few medications have also been recommended for this problem. Although not objectively established, isoxsuprine is thought to help in stimulating blood flow in bone. Bisphosphonates, which are used to control osteoporosis in humans have had beneficial effects on the subchondral bone plate in other joints of the horse and may be used more frequently for treatment of carpal subchondral bone sclerosis.[30] Topical liposomal diclofenac sodium cream has shown to reduced radial carpal bone sclerosis in an experimental setting.[31]

Prognosis

The prognosis for successfully treating subchondral stress reaction is dependent on the severity of the disease and the presence of articular cartilage collapse in the joint. The prognosis with articular

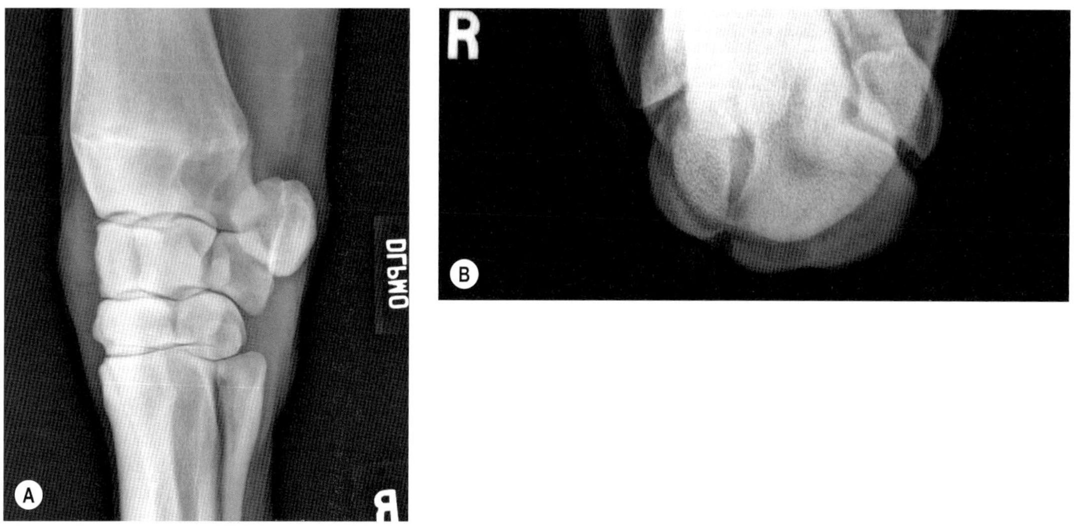

Fig 17.5 (A) Dorsolateral-palmaromedial 45° oblique radiograph of the carpus. There is a proximal radiocarpal bone osteochondral fragment present with moderate subchondral sclerosis of the 3rd carpal bone. **(B)** Proximodorsal-proximodistal (skyline) radiograph of the carpus highlighting the distal row of carpal bones. Subchondral sclerosis can be seen in the medial portion of the 3rd carpal bone.
Images provided by Dr K.Selburg.

cartilage collapse is dependent on the size of articular cartilage erosion and the depth of subchondral bone collapse.

Etiology and pathophysiology

The etiology of subchondral stress reaction has been identified as an inappropriate bone modeling response due to high loads experienced by the bone during exercise. This high stress may be due to faulty conformation or inappropriate use of the limb. However, although not objectively identified, inherent bone metabolism could be at fault. Regardless, the subchondral bone appears to model and thicken as normal with exercise[28], except that it models to the point of inducing ischemia in the subchondral bone plate, leading to subchondral bone death and degeneration.[14] This degeneration then leads to loss of support and collapse of the overlying articular cartilage.

Epidemiology

Stress-induced bone response is primarily a disease of young (2–3 year old) racehorses that are at the peak of bone modeling and remodeling. The radial facet of the third carpal bone is the primary area affected by the disease.

Prevention

Prevention of this disease is difficult as the onset is insidious and the disease progressive with training. Since there is no hallmark clinical sign of disease onset, nuclear scintigraphy may be the only method of identifying stress-induced bone reaction in its early phases and may also be helpful in monitoring its progression. Serum and synovial fluid biomarkers could prove useful in the early detection of this disease, and hence prevention of serious damage.

Osteoarthritis (degenerative joint disease, arthritis)

- OA is usually secondary to other disease processes.
- Diagnosis is based on clinical and radiographic signs.
- Radiographic changes include joint collapse and subchondral sclerosis and lysis.
- Treatment is aimed at management.

Recognition

History and presenting complaint

Most horses with osteoarthritis (OA) have a history of previous joint injury or disease. However, in some cases, the cause is unknown and the development of the disease is insidious. A specific condition of older (average 14 years old) Arabian horses affecting the carpometacarpal joint is described.[32]

Physical examination

Most horses with OA of the carpal joints show lameness, joint effusion, joint capsule thickening on palpation, and decreased range of motion that leads to pain in response to maximal flexion. Joint circumference and pressure algometry scores may be increased compared to the contra-lateral limb. Sometimes acquired conformational changes are present including medial collapse of the carpal joints, leading to carpal varus, or persistent flexing of the carpus, leading to carpal contracture.

Special examination

Radiographic findings are often mixed but can consist of osteophyte and enthesophyte formation, reduced joint space and a mixture of subchondral bone lysis and sclerosis. Nuclear scintigraphic findings are often mixed due to the chronic nature of the disease and the variable use of the limb. Computed tomographic findings often include variable subchondral bone sclerosis and lysis as well as the presence of osteophytes and enthesophytes. Loss of joint space can also be seen. High field (1.5T) MRI is the best diagnostic test to show loss of articular cartilage, which is the hallmark of OA.[29]

Laboratory examination

Synovial fluid varies in color and viscosity, but usually is thick, orange to red and cloudy. However, in some cases synovial fluid is impossible to obtain which gives the subjective impression of a dry joint. Work using biochemical markers[5] has shown progressive changes with OA, including reduced aggrecan and collagen content in synovial fluid and serum.

Diagnostic confirmation

Confirmation of the diagnosis is based on historical, physical examination and radiographic findings. The establishment of a chronic, progressive disease isolated to the carpus and the radiographic changes mentioned above often lead to a diagnosis.

Treatment and prognosis

Therapeutic aims

The therapeutic aims in treating OA are to realize that complete resolution of the disease is impossible and instead, management of the disease is needed. .Medical management is usually chosen over surgical debridement. In some severe cases, arthrodesis, either pancarpal or partial carpal arthrodesis is performed.

Therapy

The management of pain is varied based on the expected use of the horse, the severity of disease, the severity of compensatory pain and the individual horse's pain tolerance. Consequently several different management schemes must be tried before one can be selected. Pain management is often through the use of medications, supplements and/or physical therapy. Medications typically used include NSAIDs, systemic hyaluronic acid (HA) or polysulfated glycosaminoglycan (PSGAG) and/or intra-articular administration of corticosteroids and HA or PSGAG. A combination of these medications is often used. The most frequently used and most effective parenteral or oral NSAIDs include phenylbutazone and firocoxib.[33] In addition, it is common to use neutraceutical supplements to aid in management of pain, including orally administered glucosamine, chondroitin sulfates, hyaluronic acid and various herbs. Avocado and soybean unsaponifiable (ASU) extracts have been shown to have a significant disease modifying effect by increasing GAG synthesis[34] in experimentally induced OA.

Interleukin-1 receptor antagonist protein (IRAP) has also been shown to decrease pain and reduce cartilage degradation[35]. Extracorporeal shockwave therapy (ESWT) has been shown to improve lameness but with no disease modifying effect.[36,37] Topically applied liposomal diclofenac sodium cream has beneficial disease modifying effects.

If medical management of joint pain fails to work, then surgical fusion of the joint can be considered. In some cases, the increased likelihood of laminitis in the support limb often leads to the decision to perform surgery. Disease of the carpometacarpal joints justifies a partial carpal arthrodesis, or disease of the proximal joints warrants a pancarpal arthrodesis.

Prognosis

The prognosis for managing carpal pain due to OA is dependent on several factors, but mostly on the response to therapy. Identification of a management scheme is of the utmost importance in determining a prognosis for the owner and period in which various medications are tested is needed prior to committing to a prognosis. Furthermore, some horses fail to respond to treatment over time as the disease progresses and alteration of a prognosis is needed. OA of the carpometacarpal joints in older Arabian horses often fails to respond to medical therapy.[32] The prognosis for arthrodesis techniques is good for breeding animals.

Etiology and pathophysiology

The etiology of OA is varied but usually due to a primary traumatic or developmental disease. The severity of the initiating disease and the success of treatment often dictate the rate of progression of OA. Whether by progressive subchondral bone sclerosis, leading to thinning of articular cartilage, or by primary loss of articular cartilage, leading to subchondral bone sclerosis, the progressive nature of the changes in the joint at the osteochondral junction leads to pain.

Epidemiology

Osteoarthritis of the carpal joints occurs in all breeds and uses of horses, but is most common in the racehorse. Many retired racehorses that continue a career in another discipline run the risk of OA because of previous injury and continued athletic use. This seems to be the group of horses that require significant management for continued athletic function.

Prevention

Aggressive and prompt treatment of the primary problem and early identification of inherent problems that could lead to OA are needed in order to establish a management scheme early in the course of the disease.

Septic arthritis

- Failure to recognize open joint lacerations and punctures.
- Iatrogenic causes are not uncommon.
- Early identification is critical to successful treatment.
- Aggressive therapy is critical to successful treatment.
- Septicaemic foals often have associated joint sepsis.

Recognition

History and presenting complaint

Horses with septic arthritis often have a history of a laceration or joint injection, although cases of idiopathic joint sepsis have been reported. Horses with septic arthritis have acute-onset lameness and swelling of the limb.

Physical examination

Horses with septic arthritis are usually severely lame, although early detection may prevent this. They often have heat, pain and swelling in the area of the infected joint and may have cellulitis. They also may or may not have an elevated temperature. In cases of post injection sepsis, a reaction to the injected substances must be ruled out, although there is no absolute method of discerning injection reaction from sepsis.

Special examination

In the case of a laceration and potential joint contamination, remote injection of saline into the joint and visual confirmation of fluid flow out of the laceration documents contamination. A lack of flow out of a wound using this technique can occur if sepsis has been present for some time and partial healing of a puncture wound has occurred. Radiographic changes are sometimes seen, including focal or diffuse lysis of the bone and if present indicate concurrent osteomyelitis.

Laboratory examination

Synovial fluid analysis often shows white blood cell values greater than 3000 cells/mm^3 and total protein greater than 4 g/dL. Differential cell analysis reveals predominant neutrophils with variable toxic changes. Culture and sensitivity of the fluid is useful to guide therapy although treatment should begin prior to the results of this test.

Diagnostic confirmation

Remote saline injection and visualization at the laceration is the best confirmatory method for detecting joint contamination. In the carpus, lacerations on the dorsum of the carpus are common and injection into the palmar pouches is useful to confirm the diagnosis. For established sepsis, whether by laceration or iatrogenic injection, synovial fluid analysis is often confirmatory. However, reaction to injected medication is difficult to distinguish from sepsis and it is recommended to treat cases as septic.

Treatment and prognosis

Therapeutic aims

The aims of therapy are to reduce the bacterial load and fibrin accumulation in the joint, provide appropriate antibiotic therapy and reduce inflammation and pain in the joint. Total synovial nucleated cell count analysis can be helpful to monitor the response to treatment.

Therapy

Early recognition of septic arthritis and early and aggressive treatment are essential in successful management. This includes documenting the organism causing the infection, the use of systemic and intra-articular antibiotics with lavage and debridement of the joint. Regional limb perfusion with bactericidal antibiotics using the cephalic vein as an entry point can be helpful in the early phases of therapy.

In refractory cases, open or closed suction drainage is often needed and synovectomy may be needed if infection is felt to be harbored within the synovium. Curettage and debridement of osseous structures is indicated if osteomyelitis is identified with radiographs although radiographic changes often lag behind pathologic changes. Long-standing, refractory cases of septic arthritis may require arthrodesis through massive bone grafts and drains.

Prognosis

The prognosis for overcoming septic arthritis is good with early treatment. However, long-standing or refractory cases are less likely to recover or will recover with some form of limiting lameness especially if there is osseous involvement

Etiology and pathophysiology

Establishment of infection within a joint may be due to several factors. In the case of joint injections, the use of intra-articular polysulfated glycosaminoglycan has been shown to perpetuate infection if an aminoglycoside is not used. In addition, the basic nature of corticosteroids is to reduce inflammatory cell density in an area, hence limiting the joints ability to fight bacteria.

Epidemiology

Septic arthritis can occur in any horse, but is more common in athletic horses which are subjected to intra-articular medications.

Prevention

Strict adherence to aseptic injection techniques and early and rapid identification of open joint lacerations are needed in order to prevent septic arthritis.

Developmental orthopedic disease

- Angular limb deformity is a common form of DOD.
- Physitis can result from conformational abnormalities and rapid growth.
- Osteochondrosis is often in the form of subchondral cystic lesions.
- Nutritional and breeding management are the only forms of intervention.

Recognition

History and presenting complaint

Most horses with developmental orthopedic disease (DOD) of the carpus are young and tend to show signs of disease at various stages of development. Angular limb deformities tend to arise early or are acquired as the horse ages. Subchondral cystic lesions can occur within the cuboidal bones and manifest as carpal lameness.

Physical examination

Horses with subchondral cystic lesions of the carpus tend to show either chronic, progressive signs or acute signs. Foals are typically born with some form of carpal valgus, but should improve over time until fully grown. The challenge lies in recognizing normal angulation for a specific age.

Special examination

Radiographs are often the only modality needed to diagnose subchondral cystic lesions within the carpus. Computed tomographic studies have been used to plan for surgical debridement of cysts and to assess follow-up.[17]

Laboratory examination

Synovial fluid analyzes are often unhelpful in diagnosing DOD of the carpus; however, serum and synovial fluid biomarker analyzes have shown promise as indicated earlier in the chapter.

Diagnostic confirmation

Radiographs are often all that is necessary to diagnose DOD (Fig. 17.6).

Treatment and prognosis

Therapeutic aims

The primary aim is to correct the problem and then treat the resulting joint disease as described in previous sections.

Therapy

Arthroscopic examination and treatment of subchondral cystic lesions of the carpus are necessary. In addition, medical treatment of the resulting joint disease is needed.

Prognosis

Prognosis is dependent on the size of the lesion and the amount of articular cartilage erosion that is present within the joint. Fracture through a cyst or angular deviation caused by the presence of the cyst must be taken into consideration when formulating a prognosis. Yearlings with unilateral or bilateral carpal varus deformity treated with 4.5 mm transphyseal cortical screws have no decrease in racing sales or performance compared to unaffected age matched maternal siblings.[38] Due to the risk physeal closure and over-correction, the authors treat carpal valgus/varus deformities with screw and wire bridging surgeries.

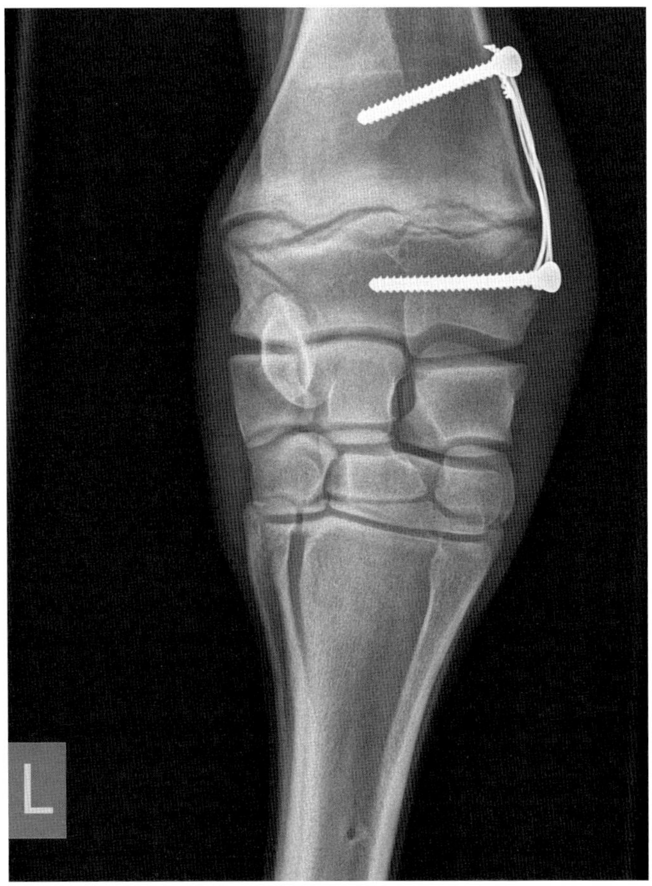

Fig 17.6 Dorsopalmar radiograph of a three-month-old foal with carpal valgus deformity treated with 4.5 mm cortical bone screws with cerclage wiring. Six weeks after this surgery, the valgus had corrected sufficiently and the screws and cerclage wires were removed.

Etiology and pathophysiology

The pathogenesis of DOD is complex and theoretical in some aspects. However, a few things have been proven clinically and experimentally. Trauma to the articular cartilage and subchondral bone has been shown experimentally to cause subchondral cystic lesions in the stifle.[39] The influence of body size and growth rate on the development of DOD has also been proposed, and supported in Warmbloods and Standardbreds, but again, these were shown in the tarsus and stifle.[40] Nutritional imbalances in minerals, energy and protein have also been suggested in the pathogenesis of DOD, as has heredity.[40] Because DOD manifestations other than angular limb deformity are rare in the carpus, there has been little clinical or experimental work done to gain information on the pathogenesis of disease.

Prevention

Nutrition is paramount to prevent DOD in horses. In particular, adequate energy, protein and mineral balance are critical. Furthermore, changes in feed should be gradual. It also appears that genetics may be a factor in DOD and should be considered when inquiring about a certain breeding pair. Some consider trauma to be a factor in the development of DOD and early training should be monitored closely.

Tenosynovitis of the carpal sheath

- Causes include:
  - osteochondroma of the distal radius
  - exotosis of the distal radial growth plate
  - tearing of the accessory ligament of the superficial digital flexor tendon
  - accessory carpal bone fracture
  - DDFT tearing including incomplete rupture and tearing of the the radial head
  - sepsis.
- Idiopathic hemorrhage is not uncommon.
- Lameness severity is variable.

Recognition

History and presenting complaint

Acute or chronic carpal sheath swelling is seen with this disease with variable degrees of lameness.

Physical examination

Carpal sheath swelling with variable lameness and variable response to flexion is often seen. In chronic cases of the disease, fibrosis may be appreciated medially, but little effusion may be present.

Special examination

Radiographs often reveal an osteochondroma or a re-active area at the physis. In some cases nothing is seen and ultrasound is needed to evaluate soft tissue structures. Hemorrhage into the sheath can be appreciated with ultrasound, as can fibrin and adhesion formation. Synoviocentesis confirms cases with sepsis of the sheath.

Laboratory examination

Synovial fluid analysis is often unremarkable, although in acute hemorrhagic conditions, bright red blood may be seen.

Diagnostic confirmation

Diagnostic confirmation is dependent on the disease process that is present. For instance, osteochondroma may be confirmed with radiographs, but deep digital flexor tendon tearing would be seen with ultrasound. It is not uncommon to see deep digital flexor tendon tearing secondary to osteochondroma formation, warranting ultrasound use when osteochondroma is diagnosed.

Treatment and prognosis

Therapeutic aims

Removal of the primary disease entity and treatment with anti-inflammatory medications are needed. However, with tendon damage, prolonged rest and gradual return to exercise are essential.

Therapy

Tenoscopic exploration of the sheath is often needed, especially in the case of osteochondroma removal. Debridement of deep digital flexor tendon fibers may also be carried out during tenoscopic examination. In addition, anti-inflammatory medications are useful and visco-supplementation may be indicated to prevent adhesion formation e.g. hyaluronic acid. Without the presence of an osteochondroma, drainage and injection of corticosteroids and hyaluronic acid may provide benefit.

Prognosis

Prognosis is often good for injuries to structures within the carpal canal. Of 11 horses with tearing of the radial head of the DDFT, all returned to work after tenoscopically assisted debridement of torn fibrils.[41] The prognosis for return to soundness is good following removal of exostosis of the caudal radial physis[42] and osteochondroma as well as flexor carpal retinaculum release for carpal canal syndrome.

Etiology and pathophysiology

The formation of an osteochondroma is thought to be due to the presence of residual physeal tissues within the area and subsequent endochondral bone formation. Hemorrhage into the carpal canal is thought to be a result of osteochondroma fracture, generalized trauma to structures within the sheath or idiopathic.

Epidemiology

In general, carpal canal diseases are rare and can occur in any breed or use of horse.

Prevention

No good form of prevention is available for carpal canal injuries, although removal of an osteochondroma is necessary to prevent chronic damage to the sheath and deep digital flexor tendon.

Periarticular disease

- Hygroma can lead to isolated dorsal swelling.
- Synovial hernia is evidenced by palpable swelling between the skin and a joint.
- Synovial fistula leads to effusion of two adjacent synovial structures.
- Synovial fistula often occurs with other lesions.

Recognition

History and presenting complaint

Horses with periarticular diseases of the carpus often present with a history of acute or chronic swelling in the carpal area. However, lameness is often absent with most of these diseases.

Physical examination

Horses with periarticular disease often show dorsal carpal swelling and in the case of synovial fistula formation, swelling may occur in two separate locations, such as two joints or a joint and an associated tendon sheath. Lameness may be absent, but in most cases of synovial fistula, other diseases such as osteochondral fragmentation or OA are present, which in themselves may cause lameness.

Special examination

Radiographs of the carpal area in horses with synovial hernia or hygroma formation are often unremarkable. In horses with synovial fistula formation, it is not uncommon to see radiographic signs of osteochondral fragmentation or OA. Intra-articular or intra-lesional injection of contrast agent often indicates the connection of the lesion to the joint. However, in some cases such as ganglion formation, the injection may need to be within the joint as a one-way valve may exist that would prevent passage of the contrast agent into the joint from the lesion.

Ultrasonographic examination can show the communication between a hernia and the joint, although the lack of visualization does not rule out its presence.

Laboratory examination

There are no laboratory tests that are helpful in diagnosing these lesions.

Diagnostic confirmation

Arthrographic documentation is often necessary to confirm the presence of these lesions. However, often lesions that communicate to a joint can be visualized arthroscopically.

Treatment and prognosis

Therapeutic aims

Removal of the inciting cause is often necessary.

Therapy

Anti-inflammatory medications and bandaging are often useful in resolving hygroma formation. However, persistence of the lesion occasionally results. Anecdotally, injection of contrast agents into the lesion has resulted in resolution in a few cases. However, surgical resection is sometimes needed and should be weighed against the presence of the existing lesion.

Synovial hernias are often only of cosmetic concern, but their removal is sometimes desired. Primary herniorrhaphy is needed to correct this problem, which requires the creation of an incision in the area. Again, the presence of the scar must be weighed against the cosmetic blemish of the existing hernia.

Treatment of intra-synovial fistula has been documented; however, other lesions, such as osteochondral fragmentation and fracture, should also be treated at the same time.

Prognosis

The prognosis for hygromas and hernias is good although a cosmetic blemish may persist. In the case of synovial fistula, the prognosis is dependent on the severity of the associated lesions.

Etiology and pathophysiology

Trauma is the primary etiology for these lesions.

Epidemiology

Hygroma formation is common although the others are not. Again, horses with dorsal carpal swelling should be monitored to see if they are prone to continual trauma.

Prevention

Early recognition and treatment of dorsal carpal swelling are essential to prevent persistent hygroma formation. Furthermore, careful observation of the animal may show that it persistently strikes the area during eating or play and a change in management during feeding or proximity to other animals may be needed.

Tenosynovitis of carpal extensor tendons

- Jumpers commonly exhibit this after hitting rails.
- Cross-country horses can acquire this from hitting fixed rails.
- Sepsis due to foreign bodies (e.g. thorns) is not uncommon.
- Medical or surgical therapy is often needed.

Recognition

History and presenting complaint

Acute or chronic swelling of the dorsal carpal area is often reported and in some cases, the swelling may represent cellulitis and severe lameness.

Physical examination

In non-septic cases, the swelling is localized to the extensor tendons dorsal and proximal to the carpus. There may or may not be associated lameness, but in most cases there is some discomfort with carpal flexion. In septic cases, a diffuse, painful swelling is present and the horse is usually severely lame.

Special examination

In some long-standing cases, periosteal reaction may be seen on the dorsum of the radius. However, in general, radiographs are often unremarkable. Ultrasonographic examination often shows the increased fluid within the sheath and damage to the extensor tendons.

Laboratory examination

Synovial fluid analysis is essential for confirming the presence of sepsis, but non-septic conditions are often unremarkable in their presentation.

Diagnostic confirmation

Synovial fluid is confirmatory for septic cases and ultrasound is confirmatory in most other cases.

Treatment and prognosis

Therapeutic aims

Non-septic conditions require anti-inflammatory treatments and rest for management of tissue changes. Septic conditions require surgical treatment, drainage and antimicrobial therapy.

Therapy

Anti-inflammatory medications are necessary in any case of tendon sheath swelling. In septic cases, tenoscopy, foreign body removal and debridement are indicated, as is antimicrobial treatment. Persistent cases may require open drainage. Surgical synovial debridement is indicated for persistent non-septic cases either via tenoscopy or via open surgical treatment with judicious resection of synovial proliferation[43] Viscosupplementation can be used to prevent adhesion formation in any case.

Prognosis

The prognosis is good for return to athletic soundness and although a cosmetic blemish may remain, the appearance can generally be improved. Presence of periosteal new bone on the cranio-distal ridge of the radius adjacent to the sheath does not appear to adversely affect prognosis.[43] Septic cases are dependent on the ability to overcome the infectious process.

Etiology and pathophysiology

Striking of the carpus on an object is often the cause of this syndrome and in septic cases, a foreign body is sometimes present.

Epidemiology

Traumatic events are usually the cause of tendon sheath swelling, so horses that are used for jumping, especially those that jump fixed structures, may be more at risk for developing the disease.

Prevention

There are no good preventive measures for this disease, except for early recognition of punctures or lacerations into the sheaths, and aggressive treatment once recognized.

References

1. Denoix J. Ultrasonographic examination in the diagnosis of joint disease. In: McIlwraith C, Trotter G, editor. Joint disease in the horse, vol. Philadelphia: Saunders; 1996. p. 165–202.
2. Frisbie DD, Kawcak CE, Baxter GM, et al. Effects of 6alpha-methylprednisolone acetate on an equine osteochondral fragment exercise model. Am J Vet Res 1998;59:1619–28.
3. Santos LC, de Moraes AN, Saito ME. Effects of intraarticular ropivacaine and morphine on lipopolysaccharide-induced synovitis in horses. Vet Anaesth Analg 2009;36:280–6.
4. Trumble TN, Scarbrough AB, Brown MP. Osteochondral injury increases type II collagen degradation products (C2C) in synovial fluid of Thoroughbred racehorses. Osteoarthritis Cartilage 2009;17:371–4.
5. Frisbie DD, Al-Sobayil F, Billinghurst RC, et al. Changes in synovial fluid and serum biomarkers with exercise and early osteoarthritis in horses. Osteoarthritis Cartilage 2008;16:1196–204.
6. Arai K, Tagami M, Hatazoe T, et al. Analysis of cartilage oligomeric matrix protein (COMP) in synovial fluid, serum and urine from 51 racehorses with carpal bone fracture. J Vet Med Sci 2008;70: 915–21.
7. Arai K, Misumi K, Carter SD, et al. Analysis of cartilage oligomeric matrix protein (COMP) degradation and synthesis in equine joint disease. Equine Vet J 2005;37:31–6.
8. Skioldebrand E, Heinegard D, Eloranta ML, et al. Enhanced concentration of COMP (cartilage oligomeric matrix protein) in osteochondral fractures from racing Thoroughbreds. J Orthop Res 2005;23:156–63.
9. Frisbie DD, Kawcak CE, Trotter GW, et al. Effects of triamcinolone acetonide on an in vivo equine osteochondral fragment exercise model. Equine Vet J 1997;29:349–59.
10. Mcilwraith CW, Yovich JV, Martin GS. Arthroscopic Surgery for the Treatment of Osteochondral Chip Fractures in the Equine Carpus. J Am Vet Med Assoc 1987;191:531–40.
11. Wright IM, Smith MR. The use of small (2.7 mm) screws for arthroscopically guided repair of carpal chip fractures. Equine Vet J 2011;43:270–9.
12. Getman LM, Southwood LL, Richardson DW. Palmar carpal osteochondral fragments in racehorses: 31 cases (1994–2004). J Am Vet Med Assoc 2006;228:1551–8.
13. Kraus BM, Ross MW, Boston RC. Surgical and nonsurgical management of sagittal slab fractures of the third carpal bone in racehorses: 32 cases (1991–2001). J Am Vet Med Assoc 2005;226:945–50.
14. Poole R. Pathologic manifestations of joint disease in the athletic horse. In: McIlwraith C, Trotter G, editor. Joint disease in the horse, vol. Philadelphia: Saunders; 1996. p. 87–104.
15. Whitton RC, Kannegieter NJ, Rose RJ. The intercarpal ligaments of the equine midcarpal joint, Part 3: Clinical observations in 32 racing horses with midcarpal joint disease. Vet Surg 1997;26:374–81.
16. Beinlich CP, Nixon AJ. Radiographic and pathologic characterization of lateral palmar intercarpal ligament avulsion fractures in the horse. Vet Radiol Ultrasound 2004;45:532–7.
17. Kawcak CFE, Herthel D, Sandler E. Clinical uses of computed tomography. In: Robinson EA, editor. Current therapy in equine medicine, vol. Philadelphia: Saunders; 2003.
18. Beinlich CP, Nixon AJ. Prevalence and response to surgical treatment of lateral palmar intercarpal ligament avulsion in horses: 37 cases (1990–2001). J Am Vet Med Assoc 2005;226:760–6.
19. Desmaizieres LM, Cauvin ER. Carpal collateral ligament desmopathy in three horses. Vet Rec 2005;157:197–201.
20. Whitton RC, Rose RJ. Postmortem lesions in the intercarpal ligaments of the equine midcarpal joint. Aust Vet J 1997;75: 746–50.
21. Bramlage L. First aid and transportation of fracture patients. In: Nixon AJ, editor. Equine fracture repair, vol. Philadelphia: Saunders; 1996. p. 36–42.
22. Carpenter RS, Goodrich LR, Baxter GM, et al. Locking compression plates for pancarpal arthrodesis in a Thoroughbred filly. Vet Surg 2008;37:508–14.
23. Munroe GA, Cauvin E. Surgical treatment of a comminuted articular fracture of the accessory carpal bone in a thoroughbred horse. Vet Rec 1997;141:47–9.
24. Nagy A, Dyson S. Magnetic resonance imaging findings in the carpus and proximal metacarpal region of 50 lame horses. Equine Vet J 2012;44:163–8.
25. Steel CM, Hopper BJ, Richardson JL, et al. Clinical findings, diagnosis, prevalence and predisposing factors for lameness localised to the middle carpal joint in young Standardbred racehorses. Equine Vet J 2006;38:152–7.
26. Hopper BJ, Steel C, Richardson JL, et al. Radiographic evaluation of sclerosis of the third carpal bone associated with exercise and the development of lameness in Standardbred racehorses. Equine Vet J 2004;36:441–6.

27. Uhlhorn H, Carlsten J. Retrospective study of subchondral sclerosis and lucency in the third carpal bone of Standardbred trotters. Equine Vet J 1999;31:500–5.
28. Nagy A, Dyson S. Magnetic resonance anatomy of the carpus of the horse described from images acquired from low-field and high-field magnets. Vet Radiol Ultrasound 2011;52:273–83.
29. Murray RC, Branch MV, Tranquille C, et al. Validation of magnetic resonance imaging for measurement of equine articular cartilage and subchondral bone thickness. Am J Vet Res 2005;66: 1999–2005.
30. Gough MR, Thibaud D, Smith RK. Tiludronate infusion in the treatment of bone spavin: a double blind placebo-controlled trial. Equine Vet J 2010;42: 381–7.
31. Frisbie DD, McIlwraith CW, Kawcak CE, et al. Evaluation of topically administered diclofenac liposomal cream for treatment of horses with experimentally induced osteoarthritis. Am J Vet Res 2009;70:210–15.
32. Malone ED, Les CM, Turner TA. Severe carpometacarpal osteoarthritis in older Arabian horses. Vet Surg 2003;32: 191–5.
33. Doucet MY, Bertone AL, Hendrickson D, et al. Comparison of efficacy and safety of paste formulations of firocoxib and phenylbutazone in horses with naturally occurring osteoarthritis. J Am Vet Med Assoc 2008;232:91–7.
34. Kawcak CE, Frisbie DD, McIlwraith CW, et al. Evaluation of avocado and soybean unsaponifiable extracts for treatment of horses with experimentally induced osteoarthritis. Am J Vet Res 2007;68: 598–604.
35. Frisbie DD, Ghivizzani SC, Robbins PD, et al. Treatment of experimental equine osteoarthritis by in vivo delivery of the equine interleukin-1 receptor antagonist gene. Gene Ther 2002;9: 12–20.
36. Frisbie DD, Kawcak CE, McIlwraith CW. Evaluation of the effect of extracorporeal shock wave treatment on experimentally induced osteoarthritis in middle carpal joints of horses. Am J Vet Res 2009;70: 449–54.
37. Kawcak CE, Frisbie DD, McIlwraith CW. Effects of extracorporeal shock wave therapy and polysulfated glycosaminoglycan treatment on subchondral bone, serum biomarkers, and synovial fluid biomarkers in horses with induced osteoarthritis. Am J Vet Res 2011;72:772–9.
38. Baker WT, Slone DE, Lynch TM, et al. Racing and sales performance after unilateral or bilateral single transphyseal screw insertion for varus angular limb deformities of the carpus in 53 thoroughbreds. Vet Surg 2011;40:124–8.
39. Ray CS, Baxter GM, McIlwraith CW, et al. Development of subchondral cystic lesions after articular cartilage and subchondral bone damage in young horses. Equine Vet J 1996;28:225–32.
40. Douglas J. Pathogenesis of osteochondrosis. In: Ross M, Dyson S, editor. Diagnosis and management of lameness in the horse, vol. Philadelphia: Saunders; 2003. p. 534–43.
41. Minshall GJ, Wright IM. Tenosynovitis of the carpal sheath of the digital flexor tendons associated with tears of the radial head of the deep digital flexor: observations in 11 horses. Equine Vet J 2012;44:76–80.
42. Nixon AJ, Schachter BL, Pool RR. Exostoses of the caudal perimeter of the radial physis as a cause of carpal synovial sheath tenosynovitis and lameness in horses: 10 cases (1999–2003). J Am Vet Med Assoc 2004;224:264–70.
43. Platt D, Wright IM. Chronic tenosynovitis of the carpal extensor tendon sheaths in 15 horses. Equine Vet J 1997;29:11–16.

18 Elbow and Shoulder

Brad B. Nelson   Laurie R. Goodrich

CHAPTER CONTENTS

Anatomy

The elbow joint is composed of the articulation between the distal humerus and the proximal radius and ulna. The joint undergoes a large range of motion; however, due to the soft tissue attachments and bone articulation, joint movement is restricted to the sagittal plane.[1,2] The humeral epicondyles articulate with the proximal aspect of the radius. Between the epicondyles is the olecranon fossa where the anconeal process from the olecranon interdigitates with the distal humerus. The olecranon tapers distally until it fuses (with maturity) with the caudal aspect of the radius. There is an intraosseus space that remains in the proximal portion of the antebrachium between the radius and ulna.[1] The collateral ligaments are present medially and laterally to prevent movement in the frontal plane. The medial collateral ligament is divided into the long, superficial portion and short, deep portion. The medial collateral ligament is also covered by the transverse pectoral muscle making palpation of this ligament more difficult than the lateral collateral ligament.[1] The muscles that aid in flexion of the joint consist of the biceps brachii and brachialis. The extensor muscles consist mostly of the triceps, but the tensor fasciae antebrachii and anconeus also have some importance for extending the elbow. The attachment of the triceps muscle group to the olecranon is the main source for extension of the elbow joint.[1]

Diagnosis of elbow disease is uncommon in the equine athlete, but can be due to developmental, traumatic, infectious, or non-septic inflammatory causes. Other causes of elbow lameness can be due to damage of the ligament and tendons in the region.[3]

The best approach to diagnosing elbow disease is with intra-articular blocks with 2% mepivicaine (See Chapter 13). The elbow joint can be anesthetized with the lateral, caudolateral, or caudal approaches. If the lateral approach is chosen and the needle inserted cranial to the lateral collateral ligament, verification of the needle within the joint should be confirmed as peri-articular deposition of the anesthetic has resulted in radial nerve paralysis.[4] Treatment for radial nerve paralysis is described later in this chapter. The lameness rarely resolves completely following the block but can improve to greater than 80%.[3] Flexion tests can be performed on the elbow by advancing the leg forward; this action simultaneously extends the shoulder joint.[3,5] These flexion tests may be hard to interpret as some horses may resent this test and are negative for elbow disease.

Radiographic examination of the elbow can be performed easily and can help evaluate for osteoarthritis, fractures, or osteochondrosis. Ultrasound can be helpful in visualizing the collateral ligaments and other surrounding soft tissue structures. Arthroscopic approaches of the elbow joint are well described, but its clinical usefulness is limited. Stress fractures may be visible radiographically, but may require nuclear scintigraphy in certain cases.

Ulnar/olecranon fractures

- Fractures of the ulna are relatively common in foals and adult horses.
- Olecranon fractures typically result from a direct kick or falling injuries and so therefore are commonly associated with an open wound.
- Diagnosis is typically with radiography or nuclear scintigraphy.
- Many different fracture configurations are possible and most are amenable to repair or successful conservative therapy.

Recognition

History and presenting complaint

Most horses with olecranon fractures have a history of a direct kick from another horse or are injuries sustained when falling. Horses typically present with an acute onset, severe lameness and, due to a lack of functional triceps, may have a dropped elbow appearance with an inability to extend the carpus.[6] (Fig. 18.1)

Physical examination

Clinical signs in horses with olecranon fractures may show a dropped elbow appearance, which is due to the lack of effective triceps function as this muscle attachment is to the fractured olecranon.[6] This dropped elbow appearance occurs with displaced or unstable fractures. These horses may display swelling around or near the point of the elbow and may be sensitive to palpation in this area depending upon the degree and configuration of the fracture.[3] Contrary to other horses with a dropped elbow appearance, such as those with complete humeral fractures or radial neuropathy, these horses may be able to bear weight on the limb (minimally displaced fractures). An open wound may also accompany these fractures, which may communicate with the elbow joint.

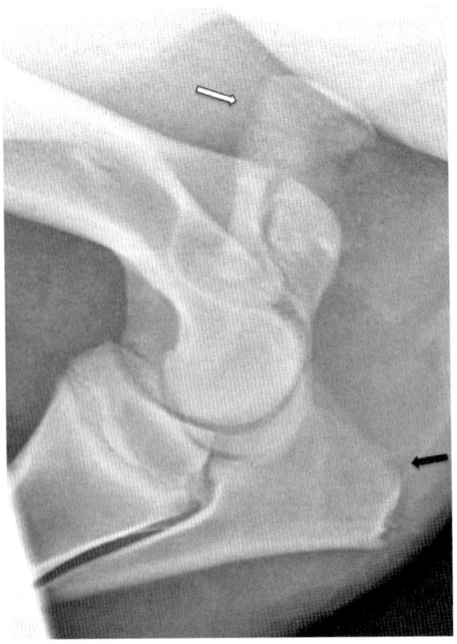

Fig 18.1 Complete and comminuted fracture of the olecranon. Notice the proximal aspect of the olecranon (white arrow) is displaced from the body of the olecranon (black arrow), which results in failure of the triceps apparatus.

Special examination

Latero-medial and cranio-caudal radiographic projections are recommended to assess the fracture configuration and to determine if there is an articular component. Once the fracture is identified, it can be classified. There have been different grading schemes reported, but the authors use the one described below.[7]

Classifications

- **Type 1a**: Fracture through the apophysis
- **Type 1b**: Articular fracture through the apophysis propagating through the metaphysis of the olecranon to the articular margin
- **Type 2**: Articular fracture through the olecranon ending into the elbow joint
- **Type 3**: Fracture through the olecranon (non-articular)
- **Type 4**: Comminuted fracture through the olecranon (articular or non-articular)
- **Type 5**: Oblique fracture through the olecranon distally (minimal articular involvement).

Laboratory examination

Synovial fluid analysis in fractures with an articular component may demonstrate non-septic inflammation; whereas, open fractures may demonstrate septic inflammation depending upon the time of fluid collection. Fluid analysis is not typically helpful aside from ruling out septic inflammation.

Diagnostic confirmation

Radiography is the most common way to confirm the diagnosis (Fig. 18.2). Nuclear scintigraphy may be useful in simple non-displaced fractures that are difficult to visualize radiographically. Computed tomography would be more useful for surgical planning; however, this is still not an easily accessible area to image in the adult horse due to the current gantry size in most available scanners.

Treatment and prognosis

Therapeutic aims

The main therapeutic goal is to restore the articular margin as quickly as possible to prevent secondary osteoarthritis. Infection in open fractures should be addressed. Fractures that are displaced, articular and disrupt the triceps apparatus warrant internal fixation.

Therapy

First aid to stabilize the fracture is indicated in cases where the horse is unable to bear weight on the limb. The leg should be bandaged and a full limb caudal splint from elbow to fetlock should be applied to lock the carpus in extension. Local wounds in open fractures should be clipped of hair and cleaned. Many of these horses become more comfortable with the splint applied. Displaced and articular fractures warrant internal fixation to restore the joint surface. Locking or Dynamic Compression Plates are typically used to repair these fractures.[8–10] Articular fractures that are not displaced have the potential to be treated conservatively. Non-displaced and non-articular fractures are typically treated conservatively with rest, but should frequently be re-evaluated to ensure the fracture has not become displaced.

Prognosis

A favorable prognosis can be achieved with most olecranon fractures. Non-displaced and non-articular fractures are the most amenable to conservative management. Type 5 and minimally

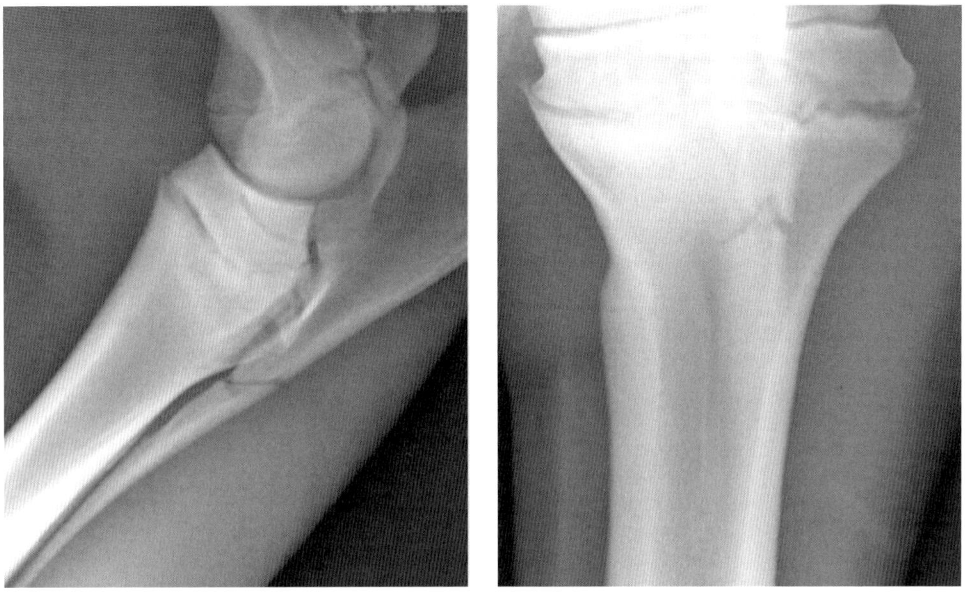

Fig 18.2 Short oblique ulna fracture. This ulnar fracture was diagnosed with radiography and not suspected to be articular nor disrupt the triceps apparatus. Notice the irregularity of the proximal radial physis. This foal was suspected to have damage to the physis concurrently.

displaced type 3 fractures can be treated conservatively successfully; whereas, other fracture configurations will typically require surgical treatment.[11–14]

Etiology and pathophysiology

These fractures result from direct trauma to the olecranon from a kick or fall.

Epidemiology

Olecranon fractures are relatively common when compared to other fractures in adult horses.

Prevention

Since these fractures are traumatic, there are no reported prevention strategies.

Radial fractures

- Radial fractures in horses are usually due to direct trauma to the area from a kick or a foal being stepped on.
- There are reported cases of radial stress fractures albeit rare.
- Diagnosis is best confirmed with radiography or in minimally displaced or incomplete fractures with nuclear scintigraphy.
- If the fracture can be treated conservatively, the prognosis is good.
- The prognosis for displaced radial fractures in adult horses is poor regardless of treatment.

Recognition

History and presenting complaint

Horses typically present following a history of direct trauma or acute, severe lameness. The severity of lameness will depend upon the degree of displacement of the fracture.[3,5,15] Complete, displaced fractures will result in a non-weight bearing lameness. A wound over the radius may be present and is commonly on the medial aspect of the limb due to decreased soft tissue coverage in this area.

Physical examination

Clinical signs in horses with radial fractures will depend upon the degree of displacement and can range from a walking lameness to non-weight bearing. In horses with displaced fractures, attempts at weight bearing usually result in deviation of the limb and many will stand with their carpus and fetlock joints flexed and the toe dragging. Most horses will have significant swelling over the site of fracture. Affected horses may also have a visible deviation in the limb or palpable crepitance. Since there is minimal soft tissue covering over the radius many of these fractures have an associated wound medially. Non-displaced or minimally displaced fractures can be harder to diagnose as horses will be severely lame, but palpable swelling, crepitus, or a wound may not be present to point the examiner to the radius.[15]

Special examination

Visual assessment of complete, displaced radial fractures is usually diagnostic; however, radiography is extremely helpful in determining the degree of comminution and the configuration of the fracture. Nuclear scintigraphy is helpful in cases of non-displaced or stress fractures of the radius.[3]

Diagnostic confirmation

Standard latero-medial and cranio-caudal radiographic views are the minimum required to evaluate the fracture, but oblique views and stress views may provide valuable information. Stress fractures or incomplete radial fractures can be diagnosed with radiography or nuclear scintigraphy. Trauma to the radius can also result in sequestration or osteomyelitis, which can be suspected with radiography and/or scintigraphy.[16] Computed tomography may be beneficial to fully characterize the fracture in foals with radial fractures, but the gantry size in most computed tomography scanners does not typically allow imaging of this area in the adult patient. Furthermore, since scanning requires general anesthesia substantial risk is encountered during anesthetic recovery unless the fracture is repaired with internal fixation. High-resolution ultrasound may be beneficial in locating breaks within the periosteum; however, the methods mentioned above are preferred.

Treatment and prognosis

Therapeutic aims

The main therapeutic goal is to return stability to the radius. External coaptation and local wound care in open fractures is crucial to prevent further soft tissue trauma to the area and to prevent the fracture from propagating.

Therapy

First aid therapy in displaced open fractures is to clip the open wound and thoroughly clean the area with dilute saline solution. Foreign material should be removed from the area and the leg should be bandaged to prevent further contamination. This is with a heavy bandage with a lateral splint that extends from the ground up to the withers and a caudal splint that extends from the ground to the olecranon.

In horses with non-displaced or incomplete fractures, conservative therapy is recommended. This entails strict stall confinement and cross-ties to prevent the horse from laying down. Horses that have incomplete fractures that are not cross tied have the potential of causing further displacement or propagation of the fracture due to the stresses placed on the limb when attempting to stand. This stall confinement is recommended for 3–4 months prior to attempting short handwalks with periodic radiographic assessment of fracture healing.[3] In cases that are not amenable to conservative management (displaced fractures), internal fixation with bone plates is required. Involvement of the fracture line into the elbow joint or a wound communicating with the joint must be ruled out to treat the horse conservatively.[16] Sequestration requires removal of the fragment. Osteomyelitis requires long-term antimicrobial therapy.

Prognosis

The prognosis of adult horses with complete radial fractures is poor. Although there have been successful attempts at internal fixation, oftentimes the internal fixation cannot withstand the forces applied to the radius. Although stronger locking plates are now available (5.5 broad), these can still be challenging fractures to internally stabilize due to secondary complications such as contralateral limb laminitis or implant infection. Conservatively treated horses with non-displaced fractures that strictly adhere to the stall confinement can have a good prognosis.[17] Horses with sequestration without fracture have a good prognosis and those with osteomyelitis can have a good prognosis following surgical debridement and long-term antimicrobial therapy.[16]

Etiology and pathophysiology

As previously mentioned, these fractures usually result from direct trauma and most are comminuted.[17] Potentially, radial stress fractures may propagate into complete, displaced fractures if not treated appropriately.

Epidemiology

Radial fractures in adult horses are relatively uncommon.

Prevention

Aside from avoiding the traumatic event there are no strategies to prevent radial fractures.

Septic elbow arthritis

- Septic arthritis of the elbow joint is almost always associated with a penetrating wound communicating with the elbow joint or recent history of joint injection.
- Affected horses typically have a severe lameness that may result within 7–10 days following a traumatic wound to the area.
- Definitive diagnosis is obtained with synovial fluid analysis.
- Radiographs are useful in ruling out concurrent osseous damage.
- In cases that are not treated aggressively, the long term prognosis is fair for soundness.

Recognition

History and presenting complaint

Horses with advanced sepsis in the elbow joint have a severe (grade 4 or 5) lameness, which is due to joint distention secondary to the inflammation. Acute injuries or those with open wounds into the joint will typically have a less severe lameness until the joint distention occurs. Horses that have had a recent injection into the elbow that become acutely lame should be considered septic until proven otherwise.

Physical examination

Horses with septic arthritis will have a severe lameness that may be variable depending upon the degree of infection. The limb may be warm to the touch and attempts at flexing or extending the elbow joint will typically result in pain. Palpable effusion within the elbow joint is possible; although unless severe it will be difficult to palpate.

Special examination

Radiographic examination can be beneficial in these cases to evaluate for osseous damage, secondary arthritic changes or osteomyelitis. Radiography is also recommended to rule out other causes of lameness in this area. Progressive radiographic arthritic changes are typically not encountered unless the cases are chronic.

Laboratory examination

Synovial fluid analysis is extremely beneficial in cases of septic arthritis. Nucleated cell counts will be greater than 2000 cells/uL and are typically greater than 10 000 cells/uL with a neutrophil differential of >90% with or without degeneration. Synovial fluid culture and sensitivity can be performed, but is frequently unrewarding.

Diagnostic confirmation

Synovial fluid analysis is the most beneficial test to evaluate for septic arthritis; however, radiography can also help rule out other causes of severe lameness in this area such as articular olecranon fractures.

Treatment and prognosis

Therapeutic aims

The main therapeutic goal is to remove the source of infection and fibrin within the joint and to prevent degeneration of cartilage and subsequent osteoarthritis.

Therapy

Removal of inflammatory cells and fibrin can be accomplished with lavage of the elbow joint under general anesthesia.

Through-and-through needle lavage can remove the source of infection and inflammatory mediators; however, advanced cases or those with gross contamination are better treated with arthroscopic lavage. Arthroscopic lavage not only provides a larger bore flush and facilitates removal of fibrin, but also provides a diagnostic view of the elbow joint. The horse should also be placed on systemic antibiotics and anti-inflammatory medications post-operatively.[5,18]

Prognosis

The prognosis will depend upon the degree of contamination and the chronicity of infection. Horses treated aggressively and early will have the best chance to prevent the onset of future osteoarthritis. Horses that develop osteoarthritis in the elbow joint are more difficult to manage than other joints.[3]

Etiology and pathophysiology

The cause of septic arthritis in adult horses is almost always a penetrating wound that communicates with the elbow joint or secondary to joint injection. Once infection is established within the joint, progressive accumulation of inflammatory cells and bacteria result in severe joint distention. The inflammatory cells and bacteria result in progressive damage of articular cartilage and septic inflammation. The progressive inflammation results in osteoarthritis. Hematogenous spread to the elbow joint can occur in neonates.

Epidemiology

Septic arthritis is an uncommon cause of lameness to the elbow region.

Prevention

Aside from preventing the trauma to the area and good husbandry in neonates, there are no prevention strategies. Strict aseptic technique should be adhered to for joint injections.

Osteoarthritis of the elbow joint

- Osteoarthritis in the elbow joint is an uncommon cause of lameness in adult horses.
- Osteoarthritis is typically secondary to degenerative or traumatic causes.
- Diagnosis is by intra-articular anesthesia of the elbow joint.
- Treatments consist of intra-articular and systemic anti-inflammatory medications.
- Management of osteoarthritis in the elbow joint is more difficult than other joints.
- Once diagnosed, lifetime treatment is typically required.

Recognition

History and presenting complaint

The horse typically presents for a unilateral forelimb lameness that varies from mild to moderate.[3,5]

Physical examination

Horses with elbow arthritis have variable grades of forelimb lameness. Unless a wound is present over the elbow, these horses are clinically difficult to differentiate from other causes of forelimb lameness without diagnostic analgesia. Palpable effusion may be present over the elbow joint, but this is typically difficult to determine.

Special examination

Flexion or extension tests of the elbow may help localize the lameness to this region. Horses with effusion in the elbow joint will typically have a positive response to flexion. Interpretation of these tests may be difficult since some normal horses resent this leg manipulation. Comparison to the contralateral limb is recommended. Intra-articular anesthesia will improve the lameness in these cases.[3,5]

Laboratory examination

Synovial fluid collected from the elbow joint in horses with osteoarthritis may demonstrate an increased nucleated cell count, but does not typically exceed 10 000 cells/uL and total protein will typically be less than 2.0 g/dL. Cytological differential cell counts will have a predominantly (>90%) mononuclear cell population.

Diagnostic confirmation

The best way to confirm the diagnosis is with radiography (Fig. 18.3). Periarticular osteophytes, enthesiophytes, subchondral lysis or sclerosis, and decreased joint space can confirm the diagnosis.

Treatment and prognosis

Therapeutic aims

Therapeutic strategies are aimed at decreasing the inflammation within the joint. Complete resolution should not be expected, as osteoarthritis is a progressive condition and in this joint can be difficult to manage.

Therapy

Therapies to treat osteoarthritis include: intra-articular corticosteroids, hyaluronan, polysulfated glycosaminoglycans or IRAP (see Chapter 23). Systemic joint therapies such as NSAIDs, hyaluronan,

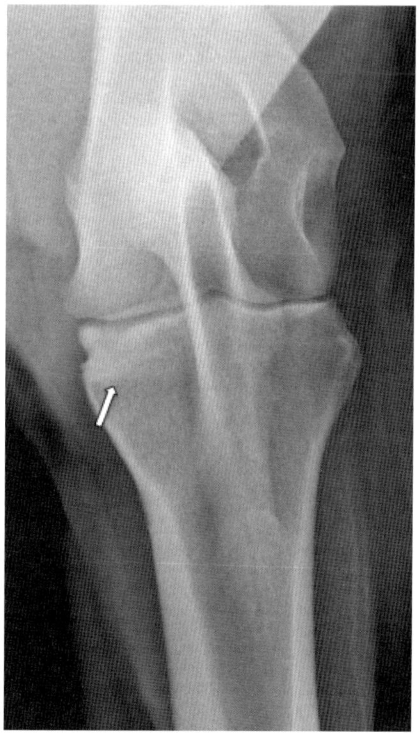

Fig 18.3 Mild osteoarthritis of the elbow joint. Notice the sclerosis within the proximal radius (white arrow).

and polysulfated glycosaminoglycans can also be explored for treatment. Numerous oral supplements are available to reduce inflammation, but the authors typically only recommend those that have undergone testing such as glucosamine and chondroitin sulfate, specifically brands such as Cosequin® ASU (Nutramax® Laboratories, Inc Edgewood, MD, USA) as they have been tested for their contents and studied in clinical trials. Significant disease modifying effects have not been demonstrated in horses although anectodal evidence of efficacy abounds. Topical medications such as 1% diclofenac sodium (Surpass® Boehringer Ingelheim Vetmedica, Inc. St. Joseph, MO, USA) has proven to have disease modifying effects in carpal joints with osteoarthritis and as such are frequently recommended to treat other joints with osteoarthritis.[19]

Prognosis

The prognosis for treating low-grade osteoarthritis is good with administration of the medications listed above; however, as this disease is progressive, these medications will ultimately become less effective over time. Prognosis is dependent upon the response to therapy, but cases with advanced radiographic changes will likely have a guarded prognosis for long term soundness. Overall osteoarthritis in this joint is more difficult to manage than in other joints.[3]

Etiology and pathophysiology

The insinuating cause of osteoarthritis is typically due to primary trauma, chronic use or secondary to developmental disease such as osteochondrosis. No matter how the process begins, inflammatory cytokines and thinning cartilage lead to progressive inflammation and pain within the joint.

Epidemiology

Elbow osteoarthritis is rare in the adult horse in cases that do not involve developmental disease. Older horses with long performance careers can develop osteoarthritis in this joint; however, it is more common to see osteoarthritis in other joints.[3,5]

Prevention

Early intervention to resolve the primary cause and persistent maintenance are required to prevent progression of the disease.

Olecranon bursitis

- Olecranon bursitis is also known as capped elbow, elbow hygroma, or shoe boil.
- It is typically as a result of trauma to the olecranon.
- The 'bursa' is not a normal anatomic structure, but forms from the trauma.
- The prognosis is excellent for soundness, but may be difficult to resolve.

Recognition

History and presenting complaint

Horses present with a swelling over the point of the elbow. The overlying skin may either be closed or open resulting in local infection. There is typically no lameness.[20,21]

Physical examination

Examination reveals a swelling over the point of the elbow that is not associated with the underlying bone (Fig. 18.4). The swelling is usually freely movable. Typically lameness is not present, even with infection. The non-septic swelling typically contains fluid, fibrous tissue or both.[21] If the skin is damaged it is possible that there may be a wound and associated local infection.

Special examination

Palpable and visible examination is typically diagnostic. Radiographs may be performed to determine if there is any olecranon involvement; however, this is typically not necessary in most cases. Cases where a penetrating trauma occurred near the olecranon, osteomyelitis may occur, but is rare.

Laboratory examination

Collection of hygroma fluid may be attempted, but does not provide further information unless it is septic.

Diagnostic confirmation

Visual examination and palpation is diagnostic. Cases with lameness or open wounds associated with the swelling warrant radiographs to rule out fractures or osteomyelitis of the olecranon.

Treatment and prognosis

Therapeutic aims

As this is typically a cosmetic blemish, most can be ignored; however, treatments can be explored to remove the swelling.

Therapy

If therapy is chosen, injections with corticosteroids, orgotein, dysprosium-165 or atropine have been reported.[20,21] Similarly injection of iodine or Lugol's solution has been reported to be successful.[3,21] Regardless of the product injected, most are unrewarding and/or require multiple injections to treat the condition. If there is an open wound, lavage with curettage of the 'bursal' lining can resolve the bursitis. The bursa may be surgically resected if the above methods fail to resolve the condition.

Prognosis

The prognosis for soundness is excellent. Unless surgical excision is performed, multiple treatments are typically required and may be frustrating to treat.

Etiology and pathophysiology

These typically form with pressure being placed on the olecranon either by the heels of the shoe when the horse is recumbent or due to trauma, which is why they have been historically referred to as 'shoe boils'. The resultant pressure leads to fluid accumulation underneath the skin. As the edema subsides, a fluid pocket remains. If the skin is irritated, an open wound may communicate with the 'bursa'.[21]

Epidemiology

Olecranon bursitis can occur in any breed or age of horse and is not uncommon.

Prevention

Horses can have boots placed over the shoes to prevent the rubbing over the olecranon.

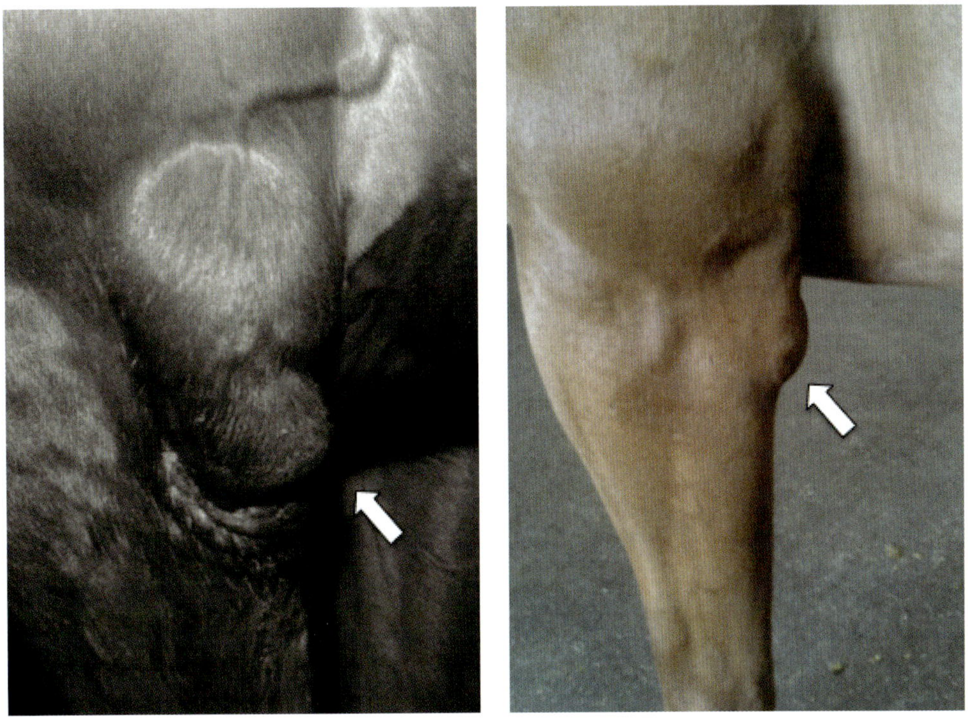

Fig 18.4 Olecranon bursitis. Notice the fluctuant swelling over the point of the elbow (white arrows) consistent with the condition in these two horses.
Left image: From Baxter, G.M., 2002, Management of Bursitis, in Equine Surgery, 4th edn, Auer, J.A., and Stick, J.A., eds, with permission from Elsevier.

Collateral ligament injury/luxation

- Collateral ligament injury typically occurs from trauma or a fall.
- Lateral collateral ligament tears are more common than medial collateral tears and are relatively uncommon.
- Diagnosis can be made using ultrasound.
- Prognosis depends upon the degree of the tear with partial thickness. A favorable prognosis can be expected in partial tears and those with complete tears and corresponding subluxation of the elbow joint have a guarded prognosis for return to use.

Recognition

History and presenting complaint

Horses present with a variable degree of lameness, but it is typically severe in the acute stages. The resultant lameness after this acute phase is dependent upon the degree of injury to the region if the elbow is destabilized.[3]

Physical examination

Horses will typically have a severe lameness and may have soft tissue swelling over the corresponding trauma. Abduction or adduction of the limb may provide a presumptive diagnosis; however without complete tearing the bone articulation between the humerus and the radius/ulna, the diagnosis may be difficult without imaging.[3]

Special examination

Ultrasound is the diagnostic method of choice for collateral ligament injuries. Radiography can be beneficial in cases where the ligament is completely torn, there are avulsion fragments or secondary osteoarthritis within the elbow joint.[22] Distraction views can be helpful in diagnosing the rupture (Fig. 18.5). Nuclear scintigraphy can be beneficial if ultrasound or radiographs fail to diagnose the condition due to the bone attachments of these ligaments to the lateral humeral epicondyle or the lateral radial tuberosity. Intra-articular analgesia may improve the lameness; however, if the tears are outside of the elbow joint, these may be negative.

Laboratory examination

There are no specific laboratory tests to diagnose the condition. Synovial fluid may demonstrate a non-septic inflammation if the joint has instability.

Diagnostic confirmation

Ultrasound is the most effective way to diagnose collateral ligament tears. Radiography with stressed views can help determine joint stability or confirm complete ligament rupture as well as evaluate for avulsion fragments or osteoarthritis.

Treatment and prognosis

Therapeutic aims

The goal of therapy is for the ligament to heal via rest with or without regenerative therapies.

Therapy

As there are no surgical procedures for treating these ligaments, healing is by second intention. Regenerative therapies such as bone marrow derived mesenchymal stem cells or platelet rich plasma may be beneficial in these cases.[23–25] Recheck ultrasound and lameness examinations should be performed periodically. The horse

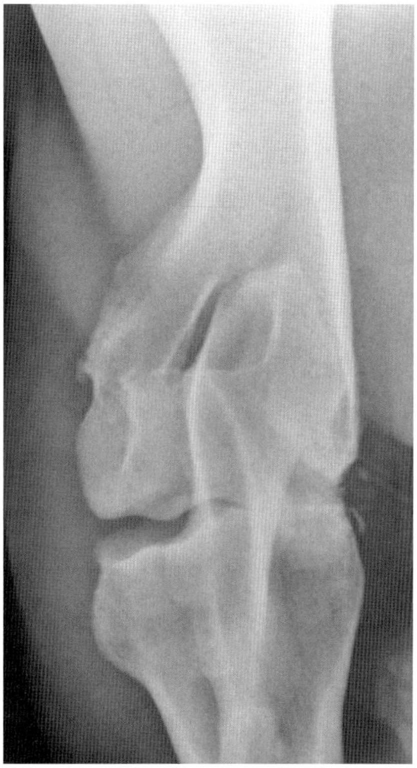

Fig 18.5 Lateral collateral ligament rupture. Notice the increased joint space on the lateral aspect of the limb compared to medially. Radiographic views with the limb distracted can allow for more consistent evidence of collateral ligament rupture. Also of note are the osseous fragments on the medial aspect of the limb. Ultrasound can also be very useful to evaluate the ligament.

should be kept under stall confinement for at least a few months depending upon the degree of damage and then can be gradually re-introduced to handwalking. The course of healing will depend upon the degree of damage, but can take upwards of six months to one year for complete healing. Rehabilitation depends on ultrasound appearance on recheck examinations.

Prognosis

The prognosis for return to use in partial collateral ligament injury is good; however, horses with secondary osteoarthritis or those that have subluxation of the elbow joint may have persistent osteoarthritis and thus have a more guarded prognosis.

Etiology and pathophysiology

The cause of these collateral ligament tears is due to trauma either from a direct kick or the horse getting the limb lodged in a fence. The resultant trauma can also result in subluxations or luxations of the elbow joint.[3]

Epidemiology

Collateral ligament injury is rare as well as subluxations of the elbow joint.

Prevention

There are no prevention strategies.

Radial nerve paralysis

- The radial nerve innervates the flexor muscles of the shoulder joint and extensors of the elbow, carpus, fetlock and interphalangeal joints.
- Injury can occur to this nerve when the limb is severely extended or abducted.
- Since the distal portion of the nerve courses along the lateral aspect of the elbow, direct kicks, or prolonged lateral recumbency can result in neuropathy.
- Diagnosis is the characteristic stance of a dropped elbow and inability for the horse to extend the carpus or digit. Fractures of the humerus/olecranon or brachial plexus avulsion should be ruled out.
- Treatment is with prolonged rest and splinting to allow the horse to bear weight on the limb.
- Prognosis is typically good.

Recognition

History and presenting complaint

Horses typically present secondary to elective surgery in lateral recumbency, or following a traumatic event such as a kick or humeral fracture.[26] Horses with radial neuropathy stand with a dropped elbow appearance and an inability to extend the carpus or other joints distally. Effected horses may attempt to stand, but will buckle on the limb. They are unable to plant their foot due to the requirement of the extensor muscles innervated from the radial nerve. When they attempt to walk they may exaggerate extension of their shoulder in attempts to place the foot.

Physical examination

Physical examination will reveal no apparent fractures (unless secondary to humeral/olecranon fracture). Unless there is physical trauma, there is typically no associated swelling, but there can be pain upon palpation of the limb and the horse will not be able to extend the carpus or fetlock.

Special examination

The visual assessment is typically diagnostic. Radiographs to rule out humeral and olecranon fractures should confirm this diagnosis. Electromyography can be performed on the triceps muscles to confirm neural damage and to rule out brachial plexus avulsion after 14 days; however, this degree of evaluation does not typically change therapy and many cases improve prior to 14 days.[27,28]

Laboratory examination

There are no specific laboratory examinations to differentiate this condition.

Diagnostic confirmation

The diagnosis is typically confirmed by visual examination with either a history of trauma or elective surgery. In some cases, radiographs of the humerus/olecranon are indicated to rule these conditions out. Electromyography may be useful.

Treatment and prognosis

Therapeutic aims

The goal of therapy is to correct the underlying problem and wait for return of nerve function.

Therapy

Therapy depends upon the cause of neuropathy. A caudal splint may be applied in cases where the horse cannot place their foot flatly on the ground to provide stability. The goal of the splint is to lock the carpus in extension, thus the splint should be applied caudally and extend from the fetlock to the olecranon or proximal radius. After these steps are taken rest is needed to allow nerve healing. The duration required depends upon the degree of damage to the nerve. Short-term compromise typically resolves more quickly than longer damage. More intensive damage to the nerve may result in triceps muscle atrophy. Electromyography can be performed approximately two weeks after injury to determine the degree of muscle damage.[28]

Prognosis

The prognosis is correlated to the cause of damage. Horses undergoing elective surgery in lateral recumbency typically have a good prognosis; whereas, those with soft tissue trauma or humeral fractures resulting in nerve transection are fair and poor respectively.[3,26]

Etiology and pathophysiology

The cause of radial neuropathy is due to direct trauma to the nerve or secondary to prolonged lateral recumbency. Increased pressure on the nerve results in perineural swelling and damage to the normal axonal conduction resulting in inhibited nerve function. These injuries are typically reversible and improve with time (neuropraxia). However, injuries to the axon and nerve sheath, which result in degeneration of the nerve (axonotmesis), typically have more permanent damage.[28]

Epidemiology

Radial neuropathy is a more common cause of nerve damage in horses. Most commonly this condition is encountered with lateral recumbency from general anesthesia, but can also occur from other scenarios which involve prolonged recumbency or trauma.

Prevention

Attempts to prevent this condition are made during positioning in lateral recumbency for elective surgery. The elbow area should be adequately padded and the limb pulled cranially to prevent excessive pressure over the nerve. This is especially important during anesthetic recovery since only 30 minutes of compression of the nerve may result in paresis/paralysis.[27]

Triceps myopathy

- Traumatic myopathies can occur following general anesthesia or direct trauma.
- The triceps muscles are usually firm and painful upon palpation.
- Elevated serum muscle enzymes with palpable firm triceps muscles provide a diagnosis.
- The prognosis is typically good.

Recognition

History and presenting complaint

Horses with myopathy of the triceps muscle group typically present following general anesthesia in lateral recumbency or with a history of direct trauma to the associated limb. Severity of lameness depends upon the degree of muscle involvement, but horses may be unable to stand or demonstrate severe lameness in the corresponding limb.

Physical examination

The severity of lameness will depend upon the degree of involvement. Palpation of the triceps muscle group may be firm and there may be some swelling. Horses may also appear to have a dropped elbow appearance and be reluctant to stand on the leg.[3,26] If severe muscle damage has occurred, myoglobinuria may be present.

Special examination

Horses with triceps myopathy will likely have no radiographic abnormalities. However, radiographs may be beneficial to rule out humeral or olecranon fractures in horses with a dropped elbow appearance or with an inability to bear weight on the limb. Ultrasound examination may not demonstrate any abnormalities aside from suggesting local muscle inflammation and possibly compartment-like syndrome.

Laboratory examination

Serum muscle enzymes (creatine kinase (CK) and/or aspartate aminotransferase (AST)) may be elevated. These muscle enzymes may not be elevated immediately following the insinuating event, but they will usually reach a peak within 4–6 hours.

Diagnostic confirmation

Palpation of the area along with corresponding history is typically diagnostic. Radiographs to rule out fracture and serum biochemistry profiles to evaluate muscle enzymes may be useful in some cases.

Treatment and prognosis

Therapeutic aims

Goals of therapy are to reduce anxiety and stress and to promote perfusion to the affected muscles.

Therapy

Pain management in the form of systemic NSAID therapy is indicated. Topical 1% diclofenac sodium (Surpass® Boehringer Ingelheim Vetmedica, Inc. St. Joseph, MO, USA) may also be useful. Affected horses may require acepromazine, butorphanol tartrate or other forms of sedation to reduce anxiety and stress. Horses with moderate to severe myopathy require intravenous fluid therapy with a balanced electrolyte solution to help prevent pigment nephropathy and maintain renal perfusion. Horses should remain standing to promote adequate perfusion to the affected muscles.[26]

Prognosis

The overall prognosis is good if affected cases are treated aggressively. If multiple muscle groups are affected or there is severe damage which could result in muscle fibrosis, the prognosis is worse. There are reported cases of persistent myopathy requiring humane euthanasia due to unresponsive treatment.[26]

Etiology and pathophysiology

In cases that were in lateral recumbency during general anesthesia, risk factors have been postulated to include positioning on the table, increased intracompartmental muscle pressure, length of the procedure, venous stasis and hypotension under anesthesia. Horses that do not have their lower leg pulled forward and padding of the other limbs can be predisposed to the condition. This occurs due to increased intracompartmental muscle pressure in affected muscle groups, which can also promote venous stasis. The longer periods under anesthesia can promote the condition as well as larger bodyweight. Although hypotension under general anesthesia has been suggested as a cause, there has been no statistical evidence to support this conclusion.[26]

Epidemiology

Studies have demonstrated that the incidence of post anesthetic myopathy/neuropathy is 0.63–0.9% of horses undergoing general anesthesia. In some studies, horses undergoing MRI under general anesthesia have a higher incidence.[26]

Prevention

When horses are placed in lateral recumbency, the dependent limb should be pulled forward and the other limbs padded to prevent undue pressure on the limbs. Even when these precautions are adhered to there are reported cases of myopathy. General anesthesia should be kept as short as possible especially in horses that have higher bodyweights.

Osteochondrosis, subchondral cystic lesion

- Osteochondrosis of the elbow is rare.
- Subchondral cystic lesions (SCL) are the most common developmental lesions encountered.

Recognition

History and presenting complaint

Horses are typically juvenile and have a low-grade forelimb lameness, but in some cases lameness can be severe. Since effusion is difficult to appreciate in the elbow joint, these horses typically do not present only for joint effusion.

Physical examination

Palpation will typically reveal no abnormalities and palpation of elbow joint effusion is difficult except in severely effusive cases. Lameness is typically low grade.

Special examination

Flexion of the elbow joint may elicit a painful response. Younger horses may resent this test making interpretation difficult. Intra-articular anesthesia of the elbow joint localizes the lameness. Radiography of the elbow can visualize the cystic lesions. The caudo-cranial view is typically the most beneficial. Radiographs are also useful to monitor for osteoarthritis.

Laboratory examination

Synovial fluid analysis can reveal non-septic inflammation; however, this test is typically unrewarding in providing a diagnosis.

Diagnostic confirmation

Radiography is the diagnostic method of choice (Fig. 18.6). Although more advanced imaging methods would be more sensitive, many times this region is not accessible with currently manufactured scanners.

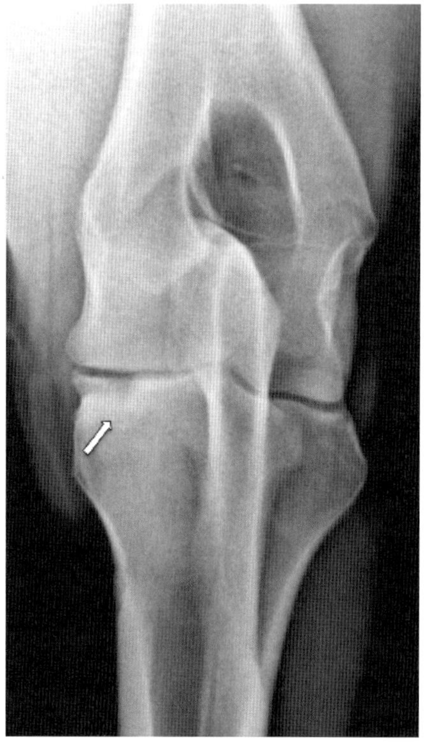

Fig 18.6 Osseous cyst of the proximal radius consistent with osteochondrosis. Notice the radiolucency in the subchondral bone and the surrounding sclerosis (white arrow) and the periarticular ostephyte on the radius

Treatment and prognosis

Therapeutic aims

The main goal is to prevent persistent inflammation in the elbow joint resulting in osteoarthritis.

Therapy

Intra-articular anti-inflammatory medications and hyaluronan can be useful in controlling the inflammation. Diagnostic arthroscopy may be used to evaluate the cartilage, determine the degree of damage and possibly access the cyst. However, due to the anatomy of the elbow joint, many of these lesions are not accessible from the joint surface and proximal radial cysts typically need to be accessed with preiarticular drilling (Fig. 18.7).

Prognosis

Intra-articular or systemic treatments can improve lameness. The prognosis is dependent upon the response to intra-articular medications or if the cyst can be accessed surgically. The long-term prognosis for medical and surgical treatment is typically unrewarding, especially in cases with secondary osteoarthritis at a young age.[3]

Etiology and pathophysiology

Osteochondrosis is a multi-factorial disease and is not completely understood. However, nutrition and genetics play a role in the disease. Failure of endochondral ossification results in separation between the articular cartilage and subchondral bone resulting in cyst formation.

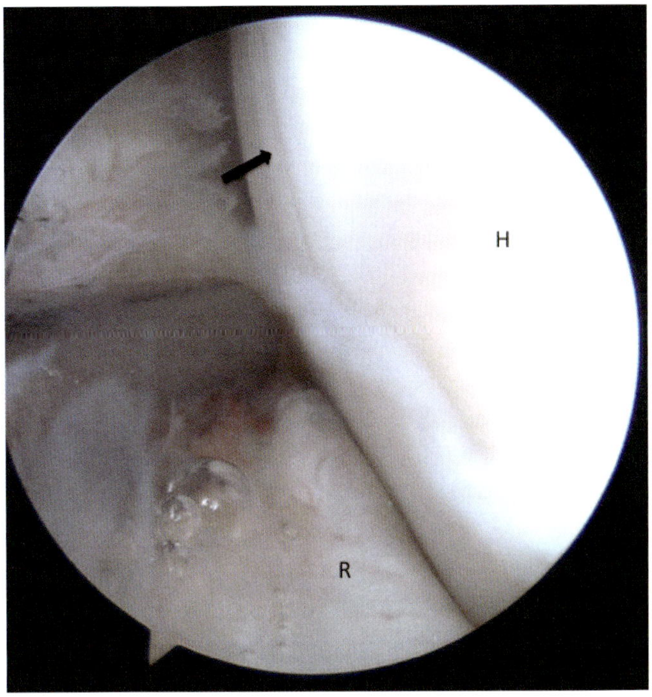

Fig 18.7 Arthroscopic view of the elbow joint. The radius (R) is on the bottom and the caudal aspect of the humeral epicondyle (H) is to the right. Arthroscopy diagnosed a cartilage score line (black arrow) on the humerus; however a large amount of the elbow joint cannot be accessed with arthroscopy, thus its application is limited. The horse also had an osseous cyst in the proximal radius that was not visible arthroscopically.

Epidemiology

With regard to osteochondrosis in horses, the elbow is a rare location for this disease to occur.[3]

Prevention

Prevention strategies are geared toward preventing rapid growth in the juvenile horse.

Shoulder

Anatomy

The shoulder joint is a high motion joint that operates predominantly in the sagittal plane. The shoulder joint is composed of the articulation between the distal scapula and the proximal humerus via the humeral head. The proximal humerus has protuberances labeled the greater and lesser tubercles, both of which have a cranial and caudal portion. The cranial portion of the greater tubercle is defined as the 'point of the shoulder'. Axially on the proximal portion of the humerus, there is an intermediate tubercle (between the greater and lesser tubercles) with intertubercular grooves separating this tubercle from the greater and lesser tubercles.[1] This provides the groove for the biceps brachii tendon. The biceps brachii tendon originates from the supraglenoid tubercle of the scapula, a common location for fracture. Surrounding the biceps tendon is the intertubercular (bicipital) bursa, which is typically a separate synovial compartment from the shoulder joint. The shoulder joint does not contain collateral ligaments as most other joints that operate in the sagittal plane. Instead, the lateral excursion of the joint is prevented by the infraspinatus muscle and to a lesser degree the supraspinatus muscle. The infraspinatus muscle is innervated by the suprascapular nerve, which courses dorsally over the supraglenoid tubercle. Scapular injury could damage this nerve or the brachial plexus resulting in neuropathy. Medial support is provided by the subscapularis and teres minor muscles. The scapula has a cartilaginous portion proximally that approaches the withers and the limb is attached by the serratus ventralis muscles to the axial skeleton.[1]

Many horse owners associate decreased cranial phase of the forelimb stride with 'shoulder lameness.' Even though horses with shoulder disease will have a decreased cranial phase of the stride it is not pathognomonic for shoulder disease and lameness of the shoulder region is rare. Many other sources of forelimb lameness can have a similar appearance. Horses with lameness in the carpal region may have secondary shoulder muscle strain.

Flexion tests of the shoulder may help point the clinician to this region, but the most effective way to evaluate for shoulder lameness is with intra-articular blocks .

Shoulder radiographs can be very beneficial in determining osteoarthritis, osteochondrosis, and intra-articular fractures. Positive or double contrast arthrography can be beneficial in outlining cyst-like lesions or subtle changes in the glenoid cavity. Ultrasonography is beneficial in determining soft tissue pathology such as bicipital tendonitis or bursitis. Nuclear scintigraphy is helpful in cases that have negative radiographs or have stress fractures of the humerus or scapula that are not distinct enough to be seen radiographically.[29,30] (See Fig. 18.8.)

Osteoarthritis

Osteoarthritis of the shoulder is an uncommon cause of lameness in the adult horse. The disease may be a result of chronic use, but may also be a sequella of intra-articular fracture, joint capsule tearing, or a developmental condition such as osteochondrosis.

Recognition

History and presenting complaint

Affected horses will have a variable lameness depending upon the severity, but is typically mild to moderate.

Physical examination

Palpation between the cranial and caudal portions of the greater tubercle may elicit pain depending upon the severity of osteoarthritis. Visible swelling is usually not present in this location even in the severe cases due to the degree of muscle coverage over the shoulder joint. The shoulder joint can be flexed by pulling the leg caudally.[30] Both palpation and the flexion tests needs to be interpreted with caution as some horses resent pressure over the shoulder and some are not accustomed to having the shoulder flexed and therefore may appear to have a positive response.

Special examination

Flexion of the shoulder may be suggestive of lameness in this location; however, intra-articular blocks will be the most specific test to confirm. Radiographs may reveal evidence of osteoarthritis. Lateromedial views are recommended. It is important to protract the limb forward to have the glenoid cavity superimposed over the trachea to better outline the joint.

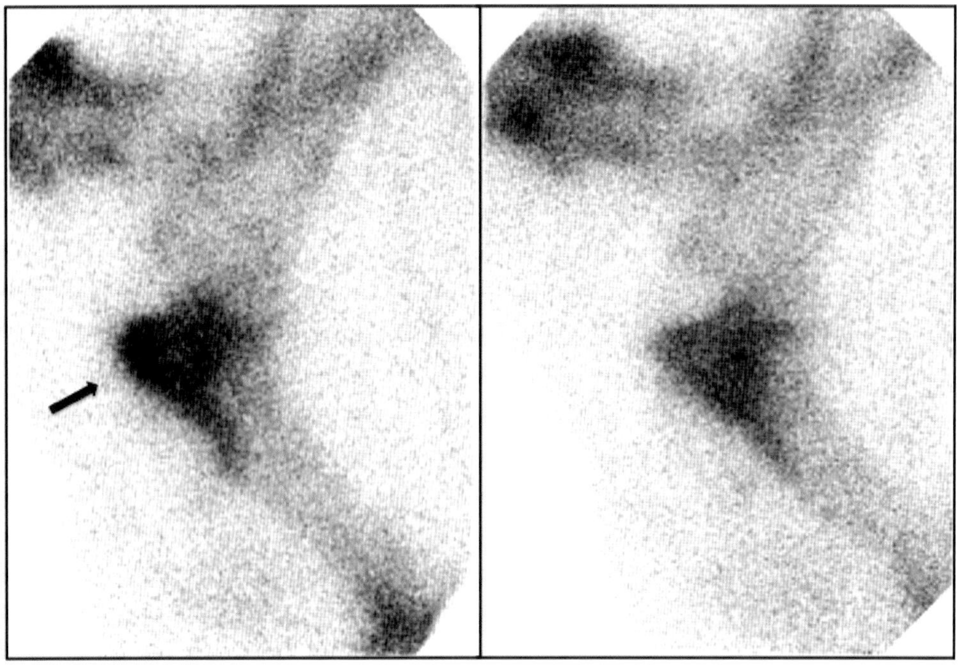

Fig 18.8 Nuclear scintigraphy of the shoulder. Notice the increased radiopharmaceutical uptake in the cranioproximal aspect of the humerus on the left image (black arrow). The right image is the contralateral shoulder of the same horse. This horse's lameness significantly improved to anesthesia of the bicipital bursa and an osteochondral fragment was diagnosed with bicipital bursoscopy. Radiographs prior to scintigraphy were unremarkable.

Laboratory examination

Although not routinely performed in cases with osteoarthritis, synovial fluid may have slightly increased total protein and nucleated cell counts. Synovial fluid analysis is not typically beneficial in diagnosing this condition.

Diagnostic confirmation

Radiographs of the affected shoulder may show evidence of osteoarthritis especially in the glenoid cavity (Fig. 18.9).

Treatment and prognosis

Therapeutic aims

The goal of treating osteoarthritis in the shoulder is similar to treating the disease in other joints. First addressing the insinuating cause followed by decreasing the inflammation within the joint.

Therapy

Therapies to treat osteoarthritis are the same as for the elbow. Topical 1% diclofenac sodium (Surpass®) has proven to have disease modifying effects in carpal joints with osteoarthritis and can be used over the shoulder joint expecting similar results.[19]

Prognosis

Since this is an uncommon cause of lameness there are not large controlled studies documenting treatment effectiveness. Also, since each horse responds differently, the prognosis is typically dependent upon the response to initial therapy and the severity of changes seen radiographically. Some authors report a decreased prognosis for long term soundness when treating arthritis in this joint compared to other joints.[3]

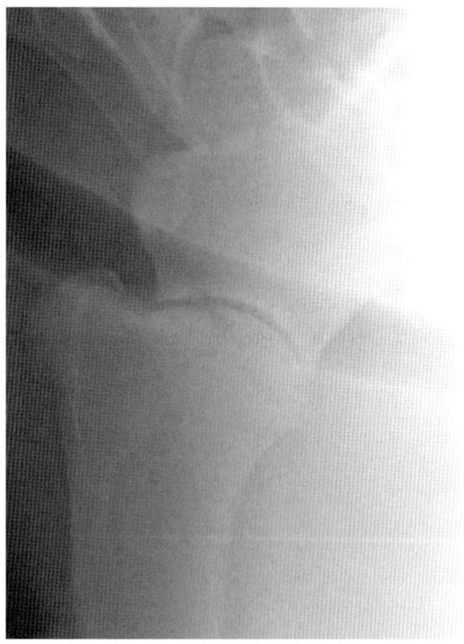

Fig 18.9 Mild osteoarthritis of the shoulder joint. Notice the very subtle osteophyte on the craniodistal aspect of the scapula suggestive of osteoarthritis.

Etiology and pathophysiology

The insinuating cause of osteoarthritis is typically due to primary trauma, chronic use or secondary to developmental disease such as osteochondrosis. No matter how the process begins, inflammatory cytokines and thinning cartilage lead to progressive inflammation within the joint.

Epidemiology

Osteoarthritis of the shoulder joint occurs uncommonly.

Prevention

Early detection and anti-inflammatory treatment is the best prevention strategy for further osteoarthritis.

Supraglenoid tubercle fracture

- These fractures typically result in communication with the shoulder joint.
- This portion of the scapula is the origin of the biceps brachii tendon.
- Treatment typically involves internal fixation or fragment removal.
- Prognosis of fragments removed or fixed surgically are good assuming no secondary osteoarthritis.

Recognition

History and presenting complaint

Horses with supraglenoid tubercle fractures typically have a history of trauma to the shoulder area. Initially horses will have a severe lameness, which appears to improve quickly. Since these horses improve dramatically after the initial trauma, a low-grade lameness may persist. Presentation can be after this chronic low-grade lameness does not improve with rest and/or with shoulder muscle atrophy.[3,31,32]

Physical examination

In the acute phase, swelling will usually be present and palpation over the area will elicit pain. In horses that present weeks following the initial trauma, there may not be a pronounced swelling nor significant pain when palpated. Pain upon palpation depends upon the degree of displacement or involvement with the shoulder joint.[29] Traction on the biceps tendon usually elicits pain. Muscle atrophy may also be present over the shoulder if the horse presents chronically. Since the suprascapular nerve courses dorsal to the supraglenoid tubercle and the radial nerve lies on the axial surface of the scapula, fractures may result in neuropathy.[29]

Special examination

Radiographs of the shoulder are typically diagnostic. Lateromedial, cranial 45° medial to caudolateral oblique or skyline views can be useful. The radiographic views are indicated to fully characterize the fracture. Some chronic cases will also demonstrate mineralization of the biceps tendon. Intra-articular blocks may not dramatically improve the lameness. Nuclear scintigraphy may be beneficial in cases with minimal displacement and negative radiographs; however, this is not a common requirement for diagnosis.

Laboratory examination

There are no effective laboratory tests to evaluate this condition.

Diagnostic confirmation

Radiographs are typically diagnostic in most cases (Fig. 18.10).

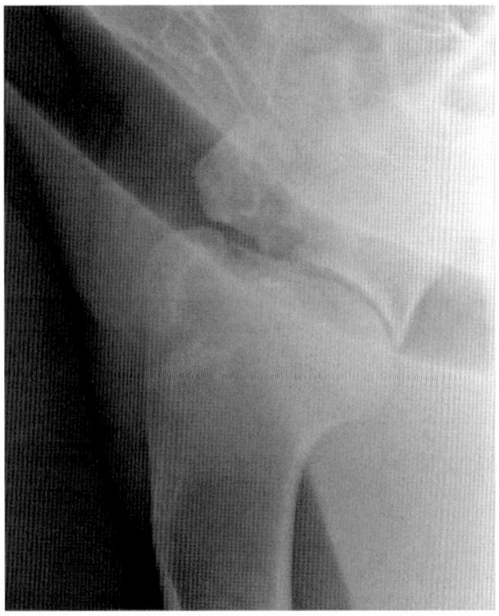

Fig 18.10 Supraglenoid tubercle fracture. In this case, diagnosis was delayed for weeks following the onset of lameness. Internal fixation was considered, but due to the chronicity of the fracture and callus formation removal of the fragment was performed under general anesthesia.

Treatment and prognosis

Therapeutic aims

Goals of therapy are to prevent secondary osteoarthritis if there is joint involvement.

Therapy

In cases with no articular involvement and minimally displaced fractures, conservative management can be elected. The horse should be restricted to stall rest for at least 3–4 months with periodic radiographic examination to ensure the fragment is not becoming a delayed or non-union fracture. Following this period the horse can gradually be reintroduced to handwalking although training will not be able to be resumed until 9–12 months (or greater) following the fracture depending upon the progress of healing.[3,29] Systemic NSAIDs are useful in this case to decrease the inflammation. Displaced fractures or those with articular involvement are amenable to surgery. Surgery will either consist of fragment removal or internal fixation with lag screws. The former is typically chosen in chronic cases due to the increased callus formation and internal fixation is not likely to provide anatomic reduction.[29,30] Acutely diagnosed lesions are amenable to internal fixation; however, the size of the fragment is also a factor and the piece may still be excised. Either surgery may include partial or complete transection of the biceps brachii tendon.[29,33]

Prognosis

The prognosis for those cases treated conservatively is good assuming no involvement of the shoulder joint has occurred. Conservative management in cases with displaced articular fractures has a guarded prognosis. A good prognosis can be expected in cases where the fragment has been removed (comminuted or displaced fragments). Internal fixation has had variable success; however, a good prognosis has been reported in these cases when combined with biceps brachii tenotomy and these horses returned to their intended use.[29,33] Prolonged articular fragments will likely have a decreased prognosis secondary to osteoarthritis regardless of treatment.

Etiology and pathophysiology

Supraglenoid tubercle fractures are typically the result of trauma to the cranial shoulder. Some have advocated the possibility of hyperflexion of the shoulder resulting in traction of the biceps tendon fracturing the supraglenoid tubercle where this tendon originates.[3]

Epidemiology

Fractures in this area are relatively common and are one of the most common types of scapular fractures.

Prevention

The only prevention strategy is to prevent the cause of trauma.

Scapular fractures

- Scapular fractures are an occasional cause of forelimb lameness.
- Fractures can occur along the body of the scapula, scapular spine, or supraglenoid tubercle.
- Stress fractures of the scapula are not uncommon in racing Thoroughbreds.

Recognition

History and presenting complaint

An acute severe forelimb lameness is typically encountered. Depending upon the degree of displacement, the horse may bear weight on the limb. An obvious deviation may be present in the shoulder region. A kick to the scapular region can also be a cause of fracture.

Physical examination

Palpation of the area will reveal swelling and an obvious deviation in the scapula in displaced fractures. Stress fractures or incomplete fractures may be more difficult to diagnose without imaging. Since there is considerable muscle mass surrounding the scapula, these fractures typically do not have external wounds unless it is from a direct trauma externally.[29]

Special examination

In cases with displaced fractures, diagnosis is not difficult and can be made without further imaging. Radiography can be beneficial in evaluating minimally displaced or stress fractures or to completely evaluate the fracture. Due to the large muscle mass and the inability for the radiography plate to fit in the axilla, proximal scapular fractures may be difficult to appreciate radiographically. Ultrasound may be a useful diagnostic aid with scapular fractures as well. Nuclear scintigraphy is useful in stress fractures or those in which initial radiographs fail to produce a diagnosis. Supraglenoid tubercle fractures are diagnosed with radiography and are described previously.

Laboratory examination

There are no laboratory tests to evaluate scapular fractures.

Diagnostic confirmation

Radiography typically provides a definitive diagnosis in incomplete or complete and minimally displaced fractures. However depending upon the equipment some horses can be difficult to image due to the large volume of soft tissue coverage. Those with displaced fractures typically do not require radiographs to definitively diagnose the condition; however, are typically performed to evaluate the configuration of the fracture. Nuclear scintigraphy is mostly beneficial for stress fractures.

Treatment and prognosis

Therapeutic aims

The goal with stress fractures is to provide adequate rest to allow for fracture healing.

Therapy

Horses with stress fractures should undergo 2–3 months of stall rest with a gradual increase in exercise and periodic monitoring of fracture healing.[3,29] Splinting and bandaging are not required due to the inability to stabilize the area; however, the considerable muscle mass protects the area. Fractures that do not involve the shoulder joint and are incomplete can also be treated conservatively with rest. Fractures involving the shoulder joint or complete fractures of the scapular body have a poor prognosis for conservative treatment and many are humanely euthanized. Foals may undergo internal fixation, but adult horses typically cannot be treated with this method. Treatment of supraglenoid tubercle fractures is described previously.

Prognosis

The prognosis of fractures treated conservatively has a favorable outcome for return to use (stress fractures, minimally displaced scapular body fractures). Those with complete displaced fractures have a poor prognosis regardless of treatment.

Etiology and pathophysiology

These fractures originate from trauma to the scapula. Stress fractures have the potential to propagate into complete fractures.

Epidemiology

Scapular fractures are an occasional cause of lameness and are observed in racing Thoroughbreds most commonly.

Prevention

There are no prevention strategies for scapular fractures.

Humeral fractures

- Fractures of the humerus occur occasionally in horses, and are more common in Thoroughbreds in race training.
- Horses that become acutely non-weight bearing should be suspected of these fractures.
- Stress fractures can propagate into complete fractures if an adequate course of rest is not completed.
- Common fracture sites in the humerus include the proximal tubercles, deltoid tuberosity, and the diaphysis/metaphysis. Fractures of the diaphysis/metaphysis are commonly on the medial aspect.

Recognition

History and presenting complaint

Horses will typically present with an acute severe lameness. The degree of lameness thereafter depends upon the fracture location and configuration. Those with stress fractures will typically show some minor improvement in lameness, but typically will not have associated swelling or deviation of the limb. Fracture configurations that are displaced and complete will have a more severe lameness, dropped elbow appearance and the horse may not be able to bear weight on the limb without buckling.[3,34]

Physical examination

Palpation of the humerus may or may not suggest fracture. In cases with stress fractures or minimally displaced fractures of the deltoid tuberosity may not have any palpable swelling.[3] Palpation of the fractured area will typically result in a painful response. There may be crepitus if a more complete fracture configuration is present. Most horses with any degree of humeral fracture will have lameness at a walk and in the acute phases very severe or even non-weight bearing.[34]

Special examination

Radiography must be undertaken to classify the fracture configuration. Multiple views are recommended (latero-medial, craniocaudal, and craniomedial to caudolateral oblique). This is especially important in cases with minimally displaced or stress fractures, as they will not appear on every radiographic view. Skyline (cranioproximal to craniodistal) views may be indicated in cases of tubercle fractures of the proximal humerus. Ultrasound can be useful in cases that have fractures of the proximal tubercles. Ultrasound may also be beneficial to outline soft tissue trauma such as biceps brachii tendonopathy; however, this damage is not as critical as the fractured humerus. Nuclear scintigraphy is very helpful in diagnosing stress fractures or non-displaced humeral fractures that do not appear to be present on radiographs.[3,35]

Diagnostic confirmation

Displaced humeral fractures are usually diagnosed with radiographs (Fig. 18.11). Fractures of the proximal tubercles (Fig. 18.12), deltoid tuberosity or the metaphyseal and diaphyseal portions of the humerus are all visible radiographically. Stress fractures can be also diagnosed with radiographs, but nuclear scintigraphy is very helpful in suggesting the condition. In cases where stress fractures are suspected, increased radiopharmaceutical uptake is typically present on the proximocaudal, distocranial or distocaudal aspects of the humerus, which corresponds to the common sites of fracture.[3,35]

Treatment and prognosis

Therapeutic aims

Goals of therapy are to maintain anatomical alignment while attempting to prevent further fracture propagation. If there is no displacement, the goals are to prevent the fracture from worsening.

Therapy

Stress fractures are best treated conservatively with stall rest for 3–4 months with a gradual increase in exercise. Stress fractures that are not diagnosed because the radiographs appear negative are at risk for propagating the fracture resulting in catastrophic injury. Fractures of the deltoid tuberosity that are non-displaced are treated conservatively with stall rest for 3–4 months. If this fracture is displaced or comminuted, internal fixation is recommended. Proximal tubercle fractures are treated based upon the degree of displacement, comminution and location (Fig. 18.13). If the fracture of the greater tubercle is complete arthroscopic evaluation of the

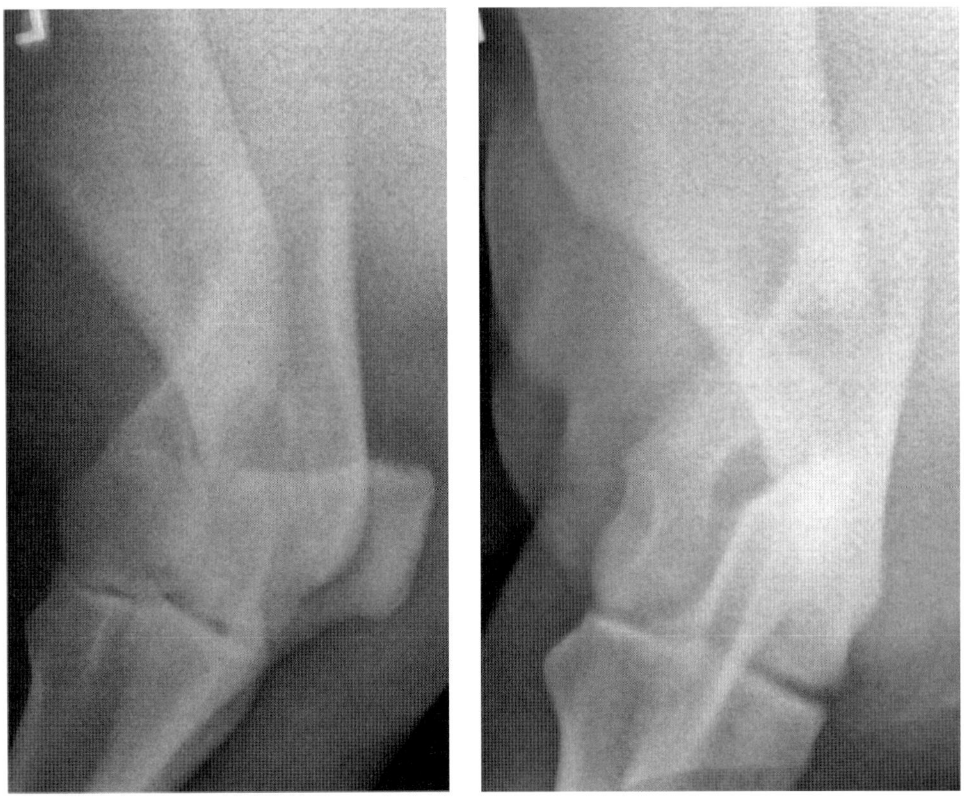

Fig 18.11 Complete long oblique displaced fracture of the humerus at the mid-diaphysis. These horses cannot be treated conservatively and unfortunately attempts at internal fixation are typically unsuccessful.

intertubercular bursa (bursoscopy) can be performed to remove fragments. The lesser tubercle cannot be approached with bursoscopy.[3] Displaced diaphyseal/metaphyseal fractures cannot be treated conservatively and would require internal fixation. However, these attempts typically fail in adult horses due to the adult horse's body weight and uncontrollable stresses placed upon the implants and fractured bone. As such, humane euthanasia is a reasonable option. Foals and juvenile horses with complete fractures treated with internal fixation can have a favorable outcome.

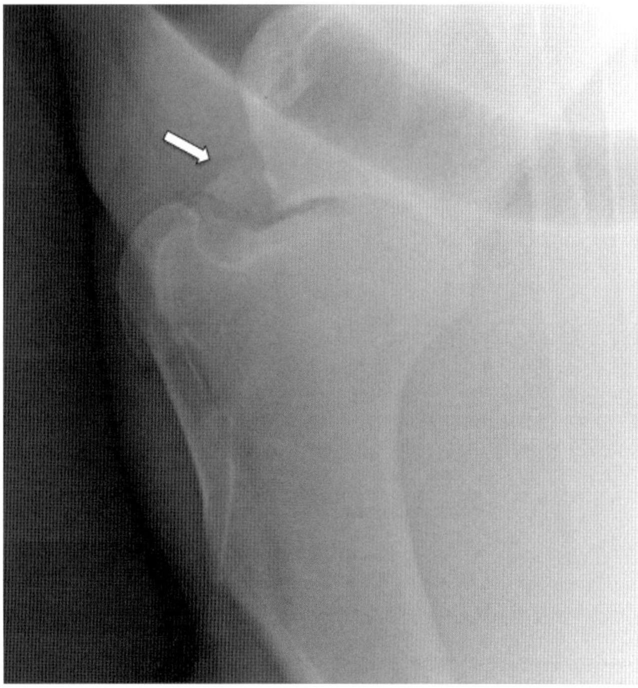

Fig 18.12 Fracture of the caudal portion of the greater humeral tubercle (white arrow).

Prognosis

Fractures of the deltoid tuberosity treated conservatively or with internal fixation have a good prognosis.[3] Stress fractures treated conservatively also have a good prognosis if given an adequate course of rest prior to return to work. Fractures of the greater or lesser tubercles typically have a good prognosis if severe disruption of the biceps tendon not encountered.[3] Diaphyseal or metaphyseal fractures typically do not have a good prognosis unless they are stress or non-displaced fractures that can be treated conservatively. Displaced fractures of the humerus in adult horses have a guarded prognosis. Foals treated with internal fixation can have a good prognosis with internal fixation.[3,29]

Etiology and pathophysiology

The cause of these fractures is typically due to trauma. In racing Thoroughbreds, stress fractures are not uncommon due to forces placed on this bone. These stress fractures can propagate into complete, displaced fractures if an adequate course of rest is not completed.[35]

Epidemiology

Stress fractures are relatively common in racing Thoroughbreds. The other causes of fracture are less common.

Prevention

As mentioned above with trauma being the cause, these fractures are difficult to prevent. However, if stress fractures are suspected, a

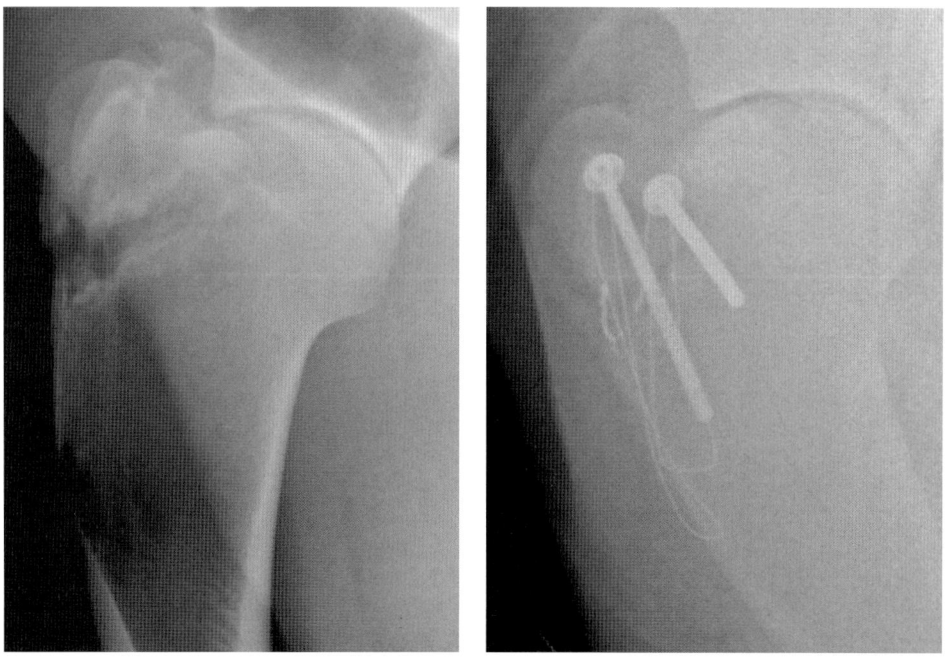

Fig 18.13 Fracture of the greater and intermediate tubercles of the humerus. The left image demonstrates the articular component of the fracture and without internal fixation, this horse would have persistent lameness in the shoulder joint. The right image is the post-operative view following internal fixation with lag screws and tension band wiring.

preventative course of rest should be performed or this condition ruled out to prevent complete fractures from occurring.

Bicipital bursitis (septic and non-septic)

- Although this structure is classified as a bursa, it is more similar to a tendon sheath.
- It can be caused by non-septic and septic inflammation.
- Treatment strategies are focused on eliminating the insinuating cause and decreasing the inflammation.
- Proximal humeral cyst-like lesions may be a concurrent cause of lameness.

Recognition

History and presenting complaint

Horses will typically present with a history of trauma to the area. They may appear to have a decreased cranial phase of the stride and an apparent lack of shoulder movement. In the septic cases, a penetrating wound may have occurred. More commonly, these cases will typically present as a forelimb lameness of variable degree. As the inflammation within the bursa increases, the horse may present for acute onset forelimb lameness.[3,21]

Physical examination

Palpation of the biceps brachii muscle and pulling it laterally or caudally will likely incite a strong response. Swelling may be present over the biceps brachii muscle or a penetrating wound near the point of the shoulder, but neither of these signs are always present. Flexion of the shoulder joint resulting in tension placed on the biceps brachii tendon will likely invoke a positive response and furthermore horses trotted off after flexion will likely be positive.[3,21,36] It is important to note that some normal horses are reluctant to palpation of the shoulder region so bilateral palpation should be performed to determine if the sensitivity is relevant.

Special examination

Ultrasound examination of the biceps brachii tendon and bicipital bursa can demonstrate effusion within the sheath that is typically present in cases with bursal inflammation. Abnormalities within the biceps tendon or peritendionus swelling may accompany the bursal inflammation. Radiographs of the shoulder region are helpful in ruling out other causes of severe lameness such as supraglenoid tubercle fractures. Moreover, radiographs can visualize mineralization within the biceps brachii tendon.[3,29] In addition to the typical latero-medial, cranio-caudal, and craniomedial to caudolateral oblique, a skyline (cranio-proximal to cranio-distal) view can better visualize the humeral tubercles and the groove where the biceps tendon is present. The bicipital bursa can be injected with local anesthetic to prove lameness is occurring from this location. If this condition is suspected based upon palpation, ultrasound of the area should be performed first so that the infusion of local anesthetic does not make the amount of fluid within the bursa hard to interpret. After the ultrasound examination, a needle can be placed under ultrasound guidance into the bursa and a sample of synovial fluid collected for fluid analysis. The local anesthetic can then be injected and the horse re-examined for lameness. If a penetrating wound is present in the region of the bicipital bursa, injecting the bursa with sterile saline or contrast material should be performed to determine if communication exists. Nuclear scintigraphy is an option for evaluating this area as the attachment of the bicipital tendon to the supraglenoid tubercle or irregularities along the cranio-proximal aspect of the humerus can demonstrate increased radiopharmaceutical uptake; however, the other imaging modalities listed above are the primary choices for evaluation. In the cases of osseous cyst-like lesions of the intertubercular groove, nuclear scintigraphy was used to localize the lameness, but the lesions were visible with radiographs.[37,38]

Laboratory examination

Synovial fluid analysis will demonstrate inflammation. In cases with non-septic bursitis, the nucleated cell differential will be predominantly mononuclear cells with a slightly increased nucleated cell count and/or total protein. Septic bursitis cases will have a predominantly neutrophil differential count with a much higher nucleated cell count (usually over 10 000 cells/uL and typically >30 000 cells/uL).

If synovial fluid suggests a septic etiology and there is no history of a penetrating wound to the area, some advocate collecting serum titers of Brucella abortus as there have been reported cases of this organism causing infection in the bicipital bursa in cases without history of a traumatic wound.[3]

Diagnostic confirmation

Confirmation of the diagnosis is typically due to absolving the lameness with intrasynovial anesthesia and/or synovial fluid analysis. Osseous cyst-like lesions are usually visible radiographically.[37,38]

Treatment and prognosis

Therapeutic aims

The goals of treatment are to decrease inflammation within the bursa. The etiology of inflammation will dictate the specific treatment plan.

Therapy

Cases with acute non-septic bursitis can be treated conservatively with rest, systemic NSAIDs and intrasynovial injection of corticosteroids and hyaluronan. The clinician should be confident that there is not an infectious cause of inflammation as the corticosteroids could perpetuate the infection in these cases. Chronic cases of non-septic bursitis may benefit from arthroscopic evaluation and treatment. Septic causes of bursitis should be treated as other synovial infections and lavaged with needles but ideally utilizing arthroscopy followed with local and systemic antibiotic therapy. Cases with osseous cyst-like lesions should be treated with intrasynovial corticosteroids and hyaluronan.

Prognosis

The prognosis for acute non-septic bursitis is good if no underlying tendonopathy exists. Chronic bursitis or those cases that do not respond to local anti-inflammatory therapy (i.e. corticosteroids) have a less favorable prognosis. Cases of septic bursitis have a good prognosis if addressed early and aggressively with lavage and antibiotic therapy. Septic cases treated conservatively or that are chronic have a poor prognosis.[20] Three of the five cases available for long-term follow up with osseous cyst-like lesions were all performing at their previous level of performance; although, another report describes a poor outcome.[37,38]

Etiology and pathophysiology

Trauma to the cranial aspect of the shoulder over the biceps brachii muscle is the most common reported cause of non-septic bicipital bursitis. As the bicipital bursa encompasses the origin of the bicipital brachii tendon, any damage/tearing of this structure could result in residual inflammation in the bursa. For example, horses that have hyperflexion of the shoulder joint, putting pressure on the biceps tendon could result in this condition. There are also reported congenital abnormalities of the lesser tubercle of the humerus (hypoplasia) that predispose the biceps tendon to move more medially from its normal location in the intertubercular groove.[39] This movement can result in inflammation within the encompassing bursa. There have also been reports of the bicipital bursa communicating with the shoulder joint, thus inflammation in one structure can translocate to the other. Osseous cyst-like lesions have been described as being similar to other osteochondrosis lesions, but are typically diagnosed in adult horses.[37] Septic causes are typically the result of a penetrating wound to the biceps region resulting in infection within the bicipital bursa. Other proposed causes include hematogenous spread, or septic arthritis of the shoulder joint.

Epidemiology

Bicipital bursitis is an uncommon cause of lameness and can occur in any age.[3]

Prevention

There are no effective prevention strategies.

Infraspinatus bursitis

- The infraspinatus bursa is located deep to the infraspinatous musculotendinous junction and superficial to the caudal eminence of the greater tubercle.
- The infraspinatus bursa is not visible with ultrasonography unless there is inflammation within the bursa.
- Other causes of shoulder lameness should be ruled out, especially within the shoulder joint and bicipital bursa.

Recognition

History and presenting complaint

Horses typically present with a history of penetrating trauma to the shoulder region. Affected horses will typically stand with the shoulder adducted and will have a forelimb lameness of varying degree.[3,21] Cases that are septic will have a severe lameness.

Physical examination

Palpation will likely elicit pain over the affected shoulder especially laterally over the insertion of the infraspinatus tendon on the caudal eminence of the greater tubercle of the humerus. Picking the leg up and adducting it will likely invoke a painful response as this engages pressure over the bursal region. Lameness examination under a trot will demonstrate a decreased cranial phase of the stride.[3,40]

Special examination

An ultrasound-guided aspirate of fluid should be collected (if present) and should be cytologically evaluated to determine the etiology of the inflammation. The needle is placed under ultrasound guidance to ensure it is correctly placed into the bursa. The ultrasound may also help suggest possible abnormalities within the tendon of the infraspinatus and may suggest a fracture line in the caudal eminence. Radiography is helpful to rule out fractures to the caudal eminence or other bone abnormalities within the shoulder joint.

Laboratory examination

Fluid collected from the bursa can help determine the degree of inflammation and etiology. Total protein and nucleated cell counts are typically elevated especially in septic cases. Nucleated cell differential counts in septic cases will be predominantly neutrophils versus monocytes in non-septic bursitis.[40]

Diagnostic confirmation

Diagnosis is confirmed with ultrasound-guided centesis and local anesthesia of the bursa.

Treatment and prognosis

Therapeutic aims

Goals of treatment are to reduce inflammation within the bursa. If the bursitis is due to sepsis, removal of the infected fibrin or contaminated debris is indicated.

Therapy

In cases with septic bursitis, the synovial cavity should undergo needle lavage. In subacute cases or cases with suspected gross contamination, lavage via arthroscopy is indicated. The bursa is small and triangulation within this structure is difficult.[30] Following lavage, intrasynovial injections with antibiotics as well as administered systemically is indicated. Early cases of non-septic bursitis are amenable to ultrasound-guided injections with corticosteroids and systemic NSAIDs. Chronic cases are treated similarly, but may require multiple injections. If damage to the caudal eminence of the greater tubercle is encountered, removal is indicated. In cases that have osteomyelitis of the caudal eminence, surgical debridement may be indicated.

Prognosis

There are very few cases reported involving prognosis of this condition. In a case series of three horses with septic bursitis, all returned to soundness following aggressive treatment with lavage and intrasynovial injections of antibiotics.[40]

Etiology and pathophysiology

Trauma to the shoulder is the most frequent reported cause of infraspinatus bursitis. If a penetrating trauma occurs, that may result in infection of the synovial cavity. Conversely non-penetrating trauma may result in local inflammation within the bursa.[30,40]

Epidemiology

Infraspinatus bursitis is a rare cause of shoulder lameness.

Prevention

As the cause is trauma, attempts to prevent this condition are difficult. If an acute bursitis is encountered, aggressive therapy will likely help prevent worsening of the disease and lameness.

Biceps brachii tendonitis

- Injury to the biceps brachii tendon is a rare cause of lameness.
- Tendonitis in the biceps brachii may be part of a syndrome that includes intertubercular bursitis and/or humeral osteitis.

Recognition

History and presenting complaint

Horses will typically present for a forelimb lameness with no other discerning characteristics of this condition.

Physical examination

Affected horses will typically resent palpation of the biceps tendon especially when it is grasped and retracted laterally.[29,36] These horses will typically react strongly. However, it must be taken into consideration that some horses resent palpation of this area and those with mild reactions may be difficult to interpret. Shoulder flexion will likely invoke some resentment by the horse and when trotted following this flexion test, the lameness will worsen. The severity of lameness is dependent upon the degree of damage to the tendon and associated inflammation within the intertubercular bursa and osteitis of the proximal humerus.[3]

Special examination

Intrasynovial anesthesia into the intertubercular bursa will typically improve the lameness; however, it may take upwards of 30 minutes prior to noticing an improvement and more severe tendonitis lesions may not demonstrate a significant improvement in the lameness.[3] Ultrasound examination of the area should include a detailed examination of both lobes of the biceps tendon to visualize any abnormalities within the fiber pattern or tears. The intertubercular bursa can simultaneously be evaluated for evidence of inflammation. Radiographs should also be performed on these cases to evaluate for potential humeral osteitis or mineralization within the biceps tendon. Nuclear scintigraphy may be beneficial in cases with humeral osteitis and where intrasynovial anesthesia and ultrasound fail to provide a diagnosis.

Laboratory examination

Synovial fluid collected from the intertubercular bursa may suggest inflammation within the bursa and accompanying tendon, but will not likely be of diagnostic value.

Diagnostic confirmation

While a strong reaction to palpation of the biceps brachii tendon may be suggestive, intrasynovial anesthesia into the intertubercular bursa with ultrasound examination are the most beneficial examinations to definitively diagnose this condition (Fig. 18.14).

Treatment and prognosis

Therapeutic aims

The goals of therapy are to remove the source of inflammation and pain within the biceps brachii tendon.

Therapy

Conservative therapy with NSAIDs is a potential treatment option in acute cases and may benefit from intrasynovial administration of hyaluronan and corticosteroids. In cases with a tear in the biceps tendon, large doses of intrasynovial corticosteroids are discouraged

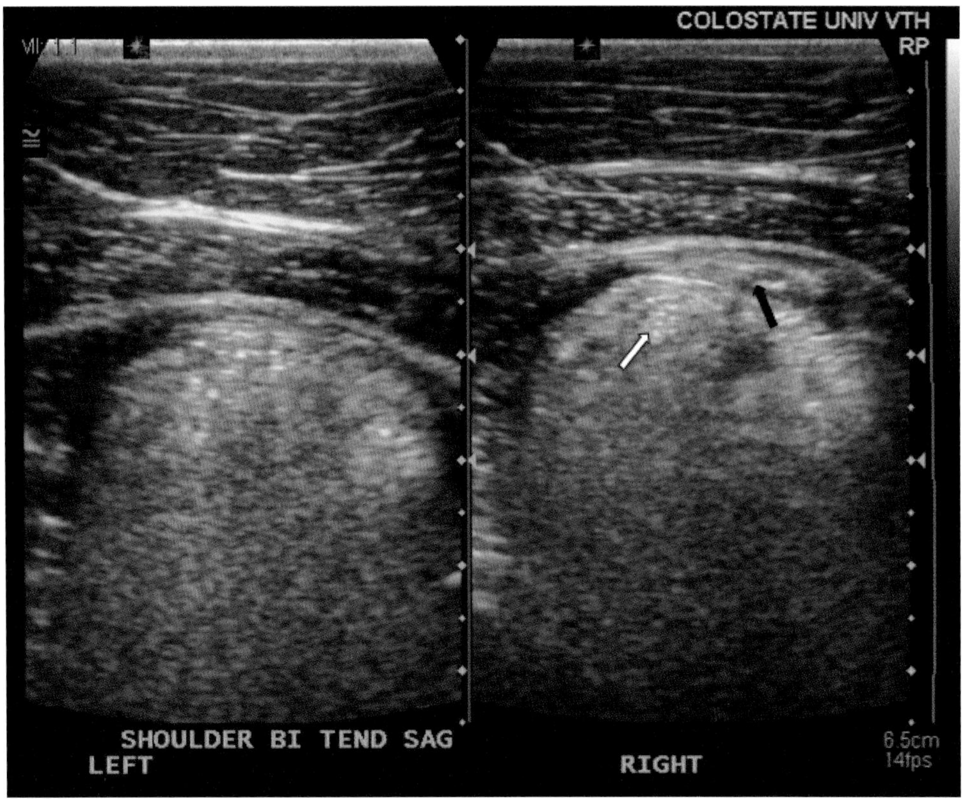

Fig 18.14 Biceps brachii tendonopathy. Notice the hypoechogenicity within the lobe of the biceps brachii tendon (white arrow) and the irregularity along the superficial aspect of the tendon (black arrow) on the right image. The same ultrasound image of the contralateral limb is on the left.

to prevent further trauma due to the profound anti-inflammatory response encountered with using this medication.[3] Chronic cases will likely require a combination of all these treatments most of which will need to be repeated. In chronic cases that do not respond to conservative therapy or in cases that have septic bursitis, surgical intervention in the form of biceps brachii tenotomy may be required.[29] Biologic therapies such as mesenchymal stem cells and platelet plasma may be considered.

Prognosis

The prognosis for return to use in acute cases treated promptly is fair. In chronic cases or those that do not respond to intrasynovial treatments, the prognosis is poor. Longer periods of inflammation lead to chronic enlargement of the biceps tendon, preventing the normal gliding surface over the cranioproximal humerus restricting normal ambulation.

Etiology and pathophysiology

The cause of biceps brachii tendonopathy is likely hyperextension of the elbow with hyperflexion of the shoulder. This action causes force to be placed on the tendon resulting tearing. Inflammation then ensues and can cause intertubercular bursitis. Depending upon the damage at the initial injury, there may be associated fractures or inflammation along the proximal humerus. Conversely, if a penetrating wound causes sepsis within the intertubercular bursa, the biceps tendon may secondarily develop inflammation or sepsis.

Epidemiology

Injury to the biceps brachii tendon is an uncommon cause of lameness.[3,29]

Prevention

There are no prevention strategies for this condition.

Suprascapular nerve paralysis/'Sweeny'

- The suprascapular nerve innervates the infraspinatus and supraspinatus, which provide lateral support to the shoulder.
- This condition needs to be differentiated from rupture of the infraspinatus musculature or brachial plexus injury, which can result in a similar gait.
- The suprascapular nerve courses dorsally over the supraglenoid tubercle of the scapula thus trauma to this area can result in this condition.

Recognition

History and presenting complaint

Horses typically present for abnormal gait in the shoulder with possible shoulder muscle atrophy. A history of shoulder trauma is also possible, but not typically witnessed by most clients at the time of injury. The clinical signs may not be present immediately following the trauma and may take weeks to be noticeable.

Physical examination

Affected horses will have an abnormal gait and stance by having the shoulder appear to dislocate laterally ('shoulder slip', Fig. 18.15). In chronic cases, muscle atrophy will be present over the infraspinatus and supraspinatus muscles making the scapular spine more apparent. There may be associated swelling due to the initial trauma. The degree of damage to the area is not a good indicator for the degree of recovery of the horse.[3,30,31]

Special examination

Electromyography can be performed on surrounding muscles after seven days following the injury to confirm the diagnosis. This technique can differentiate brachial plexus injury from suprascapular neuropathy.[28]

Laboratory examination

There are no specific laboratory tests for this condition.

Diagnostic confirmation

The gait is strongly suggestive of the condition; however, rupture of the infraspinatus tendon and brachial plexus avulsion should be ruled out. As mentioned above electromyography can also aid in diagnosis. Radiographs should be performed to rule out fractures of the scapula.

Treatment and prognosis

Therapeutic aims

The goals of therapy are to allow the inflammation around the nerve to decrease, while also treating the sequella of the initial trauma such as supraglenoid tubercle fractures.

Therapy

The main treatments are to provide the horse time to rest in hope of regaining normal nerve function.[41] Stall rest with systemic and topical NSAIDs is indicated. Systemic corticosteroids are sometimes utilized as well. If conservative therapy is not effective after three months, surgical decompression of the nerve can be performed. Even with rest if the nerve function returns, some residual muscle atrophy may persist. Surgical decompression has been advocated and may result in a faster recovery; however, due to the time required for nerve healing this will still take many months.[28,29]

Prognosis

The prognosis is good in cases that are treated conservatively; however, it can take an average of seven months to regain shoulder stability. In one study, 90% of 20 horses returned to previous use.[42] The prognosis is dependent upon the degree of damage to the nerve; however, there are no good tests to predict the final outcome. If there is no resolution after 12 months, re-innervation of the area is unlikely.[29]

Etiology and pathophysiology

The insinuating event is trauma to the shoulder and may also include scapular fracture. As a result the nerve is injured and inflammation disrupts the normal action potentials across the nerve (neuropraxia), thus preventing the innervated muscles from supporting the shoulder.

Epidemiology

Suprascapular nerve paralysis is uncommon.

Prevention

There are no prevention strategies.

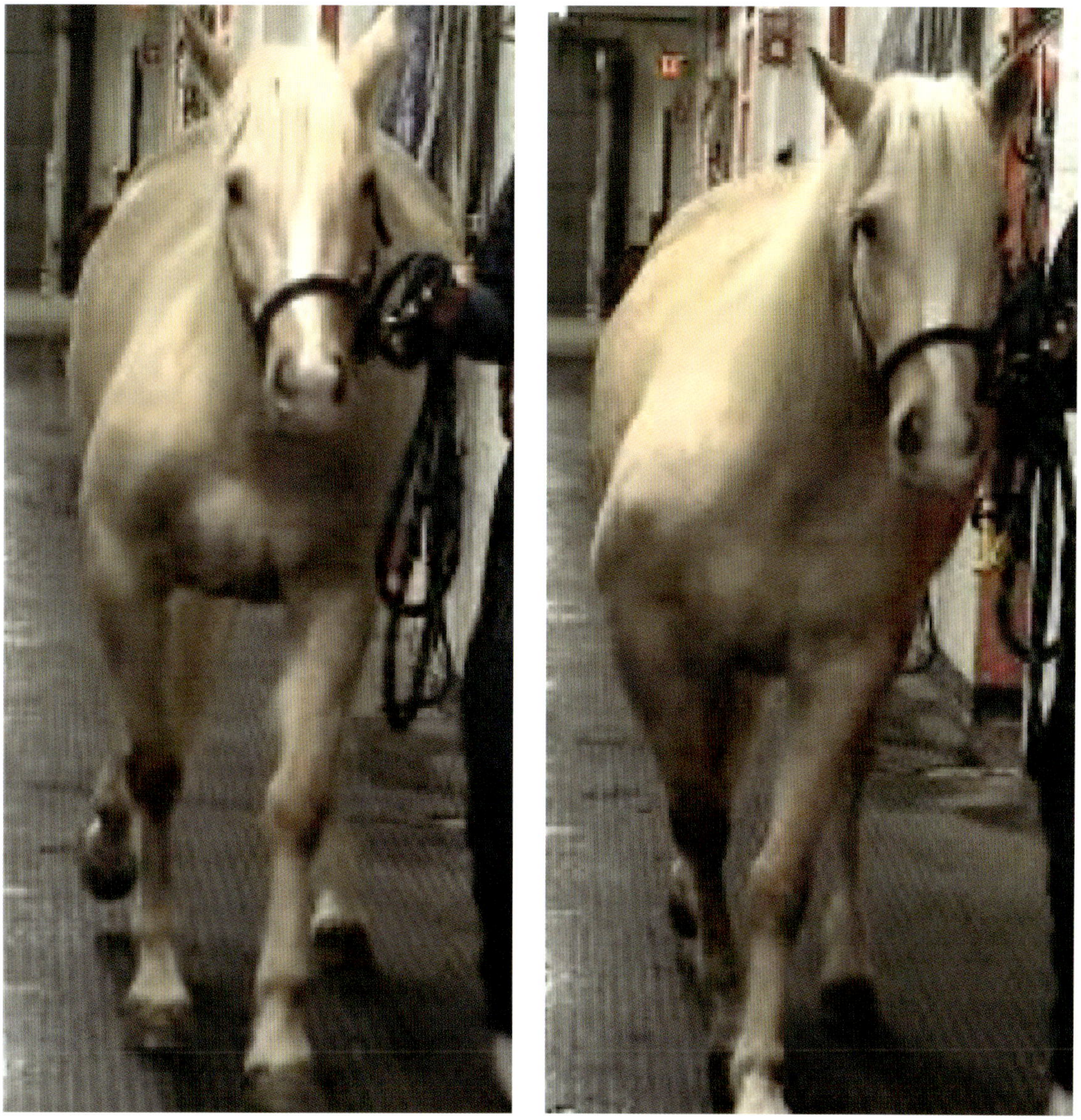

Fig 18.15 Suprascapular nerve paralysis 'Sweeny'. The left image shows the right forelimb immediately prior to the stance phase; whereas, the right image shows the limb under weight bearing. Notice the lateral excursion at the right shoulder.

Brachial plexus injury

- Brachial plexus injury is rare and secondary to trauma.
- Diagnosis is with clinical examination or electromyography.
- Treatment is typically conservative.

Recognition

History and presenting complaint

Horses typically present with lateral instability of the shoulder with or without muscle atrophy or an apparently severe forelimb lameness.[3]

Physical examination

Gait abnormalities are usually appreciated at a walk and may range from lateral shoulder instability to inability of the horse to bear weight on the affected limb (Fig. 18.16). Infraspinatus and supraspinatus muscle atrophy may be present.[3,27]

Special examination

Electromyography may help aid the diagnosis by determining the muscles affected.

Laboratory examination

There are no specific laboratory methods to diagnose injury to the brachial plexus.

Diagnostic confirmation

The diagnosis is typically presumptive based upon clinical examination, but electromyography may help aid the diagnosis. Post-mortem examination with histopathology may be required.

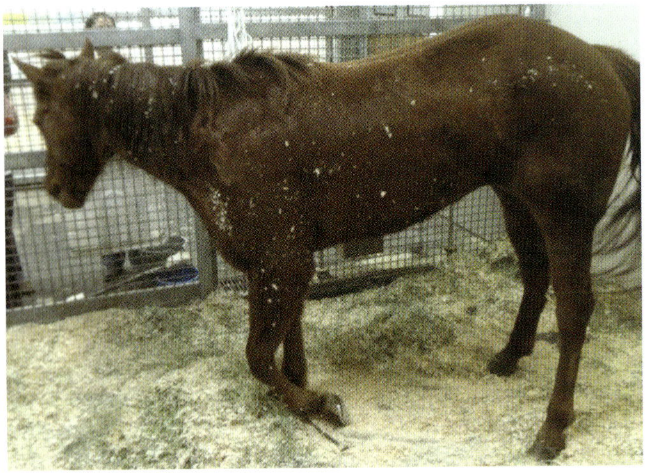

Fig 18.16 Brachial plexus injury. Injury to the brachial plexus can have a similar appearance to suprascapular nerve paralysis with affected horses having shoulder instability. This horse was initially treated conservatively with splinting and anti-inflammatory medications and after lack of improvement was humanely euthanized. Post-mortem examination revealed perineural swelling along the brachial plexus. Horses with radial nerve paralysis, humeral or olecranon fractures, or triceps myopathy may have a similar stance. These differential diagnoses in this horse were ruled out at post-mortem examination.

Treatment and prognosis

Therapeutic aims

Goals of treatment are rest and supportive care.

Therapy

Treatment is aimed as supportive care with rest and anti-inflammatory medications while nerve conduction is restored.

Prognosis

Prognosis will depend upon the severity of injury and the ability for nerve regeneration.

Etiology and pathophysiology

Injury to the brachial plexus results from trauma and resultant inflammation. Depending upon the severity of the damage perineural swelling can impede normal nerve conduction.

Epidemiology

Injury to the brachial plexus is rare.

Osteochondrosis

- Osteochondrosis is a developmental disease typically seen in younger horses.
- Osteochondrosis in this region can be difficult to manage and secondary osteoarthritis is common.

Recognition

History and presenting complaint

Horses are typically juvenile and present for a mild to moderate forelimb lameness.

Physical examination

Palpation of the shoulder region may elicit pain if moderate joint distention is present. Flexion of the stifle may result in a positive response. Chronically, some horses will develop shoulder muscle atrophy due to disuse.[30] Decreased cranial phase of the stride is typically present, but difficult to visualize differently from other causes of forelimb lameness.

Special examination

Radiography is the most effective way to evaluate the shoulder region for osteochondrosis and may demonstrate a cystic lesion within the glenoid or remodeling or flattening of the joint surface. Ultrasonography and nuclear scintigraphy are further options to evaluate these horses.[30]

Laboratory examination

Synovial fluid analysis will typically not be beneficial in ruling in or out this condition.

Diagnostic confirmation

Radiographs are typically diagnostic; however, contrast arthrography can be of benefit to better outline the glenoid cavity as well as determine the degree of detachment of cartilage on the humeral head.[29,43]

Treatment and prognosis

Therapeutic aims

The goal of therapy is to stop the progression of the lesion and reduce the inflammation within the joint.

Therapy

Treatment may consist of rest in horses not planned for an athletic career. Injection of the joint or arthroscopic surgery can be performed.[29,30]

Prognosis

The prognosis for most cases is guarded as osteoarthritis is typically present at the time of diagnosis. Mild to moderate osteochondrosis lesions can have a successful outcome if severe cartilage damage is not present.

Etiology and pathophysiology

Osteochondrosis is a multi-factorial disease of which is not completely understood. However, nutrition and genetics play a role in the disease. Failure of endochondral ossification results in separation between the articular cartilage and subchondral bone resulting in cyst formation.

Epidemiology

Osteochondrosis of the shoulder is not uncommon.[30]

Prevention

Prevention strategies are to prevent rapid growth and imbalanced nutrition.

References

1. Dyce KM, Sack WO, Wensing CJG. The forelimb of the horse. In: Dyce KM, Sack WO, Wensing CJG, editors. Textbook of veterinary anatomy. 3rd ed. Philadelphia, PA: Saunders; 2002. p. 571–7.
2. Garvican E, Clegg P. Clinical aspects of the equine shoulder and elbow joints. UK vet. Companion Anim 2008;13(5): 5–9.
3. Dyson SJ. The elbow, brachium, and shoulder. In: Ross MW, Dyson SJ, editors. Diagnosis and management of lameness in the horse. 2nd ed. St. Louis, MO: Saunders; 2011. p. 456–74.
4. Baxer GM, Stashak TS. Perineural and intrasynovial anesthesia. In: Baxter GM, editor. Adams and Stashaks Lameness in Horses. 6th ed. Ames, IA: Wiley-Blackwell; 2011. p. 173–202.
5. Hubert J, Stashak T. The antebrachium, elbow, and humerus. In: Baxter GM, editor. Adams and Stashaks Lameness in horses. 6th ed. Ames, IA: Wiley-Blackwell; 2011. p. 687–707.
6. Swor TM, Watkins JP, Bahr A, et al. Results of plate fixation of type 5 olecranon fractures in 20 horses. Equine Vet J 2006;38(1):30–4.
7. Donecker JM, Bramlage LR, Gabel AA. Retrospective analysis of 29 fractures of the olecranon process of the equine ulna. J Am Vet Med Assoc 1984;185:183,
8. Hanson,PD, Hartwig H, Markel MD. Comparison of three methods of ulnar fixation in horses. Vet Surg 1997;26: 165–71.
9. Jackson M, Kummar M, Auer J, et al. Treatment of type 2 and 4 olecranon fractures with locking compression plate osteosynthesis in horses: a prospective study (2002–2008). Vet Comp Orthop Traumatol 2011;24:57–61.
10. Levine DG, Richardson DW. Clinical use of the locking compression plate (LCP) in horses: a retrospective study of 31 cases (2004–2006). Equine Vet J 2007;39(5):401–6.
11. Swor TM, Watkins JP, Bahr A, et al. Results of plate fixation of type 1b olecranon fractures in 24 horses. Equine Vet J 2003;35(7):670–5.
12. Anderson DE, Allen D, DeBowes RD. Comminuted, articular fractures of the olecranon process in horses: 17 cases (1980 to 1990). Vet Comp Orthop Traumatol 1995;8(3):141–5.
13. Janicek JC, Rodgerson DH, Hunt RJ, et al. Racing prognosis of horses following surgically repaired olecranon fractures. Can Vet J 2006;47:241–5.
14. Wilson D, Riedesel E. Non-surgical management of ulnar fractures in the horse: a retrospective study of 43 cases. 1985;14:283,
15. Sanders-Shamis M, Bramlage LR, Gable AA. Radius fractures in the horse: A retrospective study of 47 cases. Equine Vet J 1986;18(6):432–7.
16. Swinebroad EL, Dabareiner RM, Swor TM, et al. Osteomyelitis secondary to trauma involving the proximal end of the radius in horses: five cases (1987–2001). J Am Vet Med Assoc 2003;223:486–91.
17. Watkins JP. Radius and Ulna. In: Auer JA, Stick JA, editors. Equine Surgery. St. Louis, MO: Saunders; 2011. p. 1363–78.
18. Dunkerley SC, Schumcher J, Marshall AE. Sepsis of the ulnaris lateralis bursa and elbow joint in a horse. J Am Vet Med Assoc 1996;208(8):1238–40.
19. Frisbie DD, McIlwraith CW, Kawcak CE, et al. Evaluation of topically administered diclofenac liposomal cream for treatment of horses with experimentally induced osteoarthritis. Am J Vet Res 2009;70(2):210–15.
20. Honnas CM, Schumacher J, McClure SR, et al. Treatment of olecranon bursitis in horses: 10 cases (1986–93). J Am Vet Med Assoc 1995;206(7):1022–6.
21. Baxter GM. Management of bursitis. In: Auer JA, Stick JA, editors. Equine Surgery. St. Louis, MO: Saunders; 2011. p. 1148–56.
22. Chopin J, Wright J, Melvill L, et al. Lateral collateral ligament avulsion of the humeroradial joint in a horse. Vet Radiol Ultrasound 1997;38:50.
23. Textor J. Autologous Biologic Treatment for Equine Musculoskeletal Injuries: Platelet-Rich Plasma and IL-1 Receptor Antagonist Protein. Vet Clin Equine 2011;27:275–98.
24. Boswell SG, Cole BJ, Sundman EA, et al. Platelet-rich plasma: a milieu of bioactive factors. Arthroscopy 2012;28:429–39.
25. Sundman EACB, Fortier LA. Growth Factor and Catabolic Cytokine Concentrations Are Influenced by the Cellular Composition of Platelet-Rich Plasma. Am J Sports Med 2011;39: 2135–40.
26. Franci P, Leece EA, Brearley JC. Post anesthetic myopathy/neuropathy in horses undergoing magnetic resonance imaging compare to horses undergoing surgery. Equine Vet J 2006;38(6): 497–501.
27. Cuvin E, Munroe GA, Mitsopoulos A. Peripheral neuropathy involving brachial plexus nerves in 2 horses. Equine vet. Educ 1993;5(2):90–4.
28. Mackay RJ. Peripheral Nerve Injury. In: Auer JA, Stick JA, editors. Equine Surgery. St. Louis, MO: Saunders; 2011. p. 720–7.
29. Fortier LA. Shoulder. In: Auer JA, Stick JA, editors. Equine Surgery. St. Louis, MO: Saunders; 2011. p. 1379–87.
30. Hubert J, Stashak T. The shoulder and scapula. In: Baxter GM, editor. Adams and Stashaks Lameness in horses. 6th ed. Ames, IA: Wiley-Blackwell; 2011. p. 708–24.
31. Pankowski RL, Grant BD, Dande R, et al. Fracture of the supraglenoid tubercle: Treatment and results in five horses. Vet Surg 1986;15(1):33–9.
32. Bleyaert HF, Sullins KE, White NA. Supraglenoid tubercle fractures in horses. Comp Cont Educ 1994;16(4):531–6.
33. Bleyaert HF, Madison JB. Complete biceps brachii tenotomy to facilitate internal fixation of supraglenoid tubercle fractures in three horses. Vet Surg 1999;28:48–53.
34. Mez JC, Dabareiner RM, Cole RC, et al. Fractures of the greater tubercle of the humerus in horses: 15 cases (1986–2004). J Am Vet Med Assoc 2007;230: 1350–5.
35. Stover S, Johnson B, Daft B, et al. An association between complete and incomplete stress fractures of the humerus in racehorses. Equine Vet J 1992;24:260,
36. Hawe C, McDiarmid AM. Tendonitis of the biceps brachii and intertubercular (bicipital) bursitis in a Thoroughbred racehorse. Equine Vet Educ 1999;11(2):60–2.
37. Little D, Redding WR, Gerard MP. Osseous cyst-like lesions of the lateral intertubercular groove of the proximal humerus: A report of 5 cases. Equine Vet Educ 2009;21(2):60–6.
38. Ramzan PHL. Osseous cyst-like lesion of the intermediate humeral tubercle of a horse. Vet Rec 2004;154:534–6.
39. Courdry V, Allen AK, Denoix JM. Congenital abnormalities of the bicipital apparatus in four mature horses. Equine Vet J 2005;37(3):272–5.
40. Whitcomb MB, le Jeune SS, MacDonald MM, et al. Disorders of the infraspinatus tendon and bursa in three horses. J Am Vet Med Assoc 2006;229(4):549–56.
41. Dutton D, Honnas C, Watkins J. Nonsurgical treatment of surascapular nerve injury in horses: 8 cases (1988–98). J Am Vet Med Assoc 1999;214:1657.
42. Schneider R, Bramlage LR. Suprascapular nerve injury horses. Compendium Contin Educ Vet Pract 1990;12:1783–9.
43. Nixon AJ, Spencer CP. Arthrography of the equine shoulder joint. Equine Vet J 1990;22:107.

19 Tarsus and stifle

Chris Whitton

CHAPTER CONTENTS

Introduction

The tarsus is an extremely complex joint made up of multiple articulations. Common problems in athletic horses include osteoarthritis of the distal tarsal joints, osteochondrosis of the tarsocrural joint and injury resulting from direct trauma to the boney prominences such as the calcaneus, sustentaculum tali, lateral malleolus and the head of the lateral splint bone.

The stifle joint is the largest in the horse. Uniquely it has an array of soft tissue structures that provide stability but are prone to injury and degeneration. Although positioned proximal in the limb, it may be subjected to direct trauma in horses that jump unforgiving obstacles, for example, eventers and hunters. It is also one of the more common joints affected by osteochondrosis, which may escape detection early in life and then present as a lameness problem in the athletic horse.

Tarsus

Anatomy

The equine tarsus has high-motion (tarsocrural) and low-motion (talocalcaneal, tarsometatarsal, centrodistal and talocalcaneal-centroquatral) joints. The distal tibia articulates with the medial and lateral trochlear ridges of the talus with its distal intermediate ridge lying within the trochlear groove in the tarsocrural joint (TC) (Fig. 19.1). This articulation provides for hock flexion and extension during locomotion. The proximoplantar aspect of the calcaneus projects plantar to the tibia and serves as the attachment of the gastrocnemius tendon (GT). The superficial digital flexor (SDF) tendon courses over the calcaneus on the plantar surface of the hock where it forms a fibrocartilagenous cap which has firm fascial attachments to the calcaneus to maintain its central position. The calcaneal and intertendinuous bursae surround these tendons at this level. The deep digital flexor (DDF) tendon lies within the tarsal sheath as it courses over the sustentaculum tali of the calcaneus. Distally, the talus and calcaneus articulate with the central tarsal bone and the proximal aspect of the fourth tarsal bone to form the talocalcaneal-centroquatral (proximal intertarsal, PIT) joint (Fig. 19.1). The central tarsal bone articulates distally with the third and fused first and second tarsal bones to form the centrodistal (distal intertarsal, DIT) joint. The tarsometatarsal joint (TMT) is the collective articulation of the fused first and second, third and fourth tarsal bones with the second, third and fourth metatarsal bones, respectively (Fig. 19.1).

This complex bony arrangement is held together by complex collateral ligaments.[1] The long lateral collateral ligament (CoL) originates proximally on the lateral tibial malleolus and courses distally to insert on to the calcaneus, fourth tarsal bone, talus and the fourth

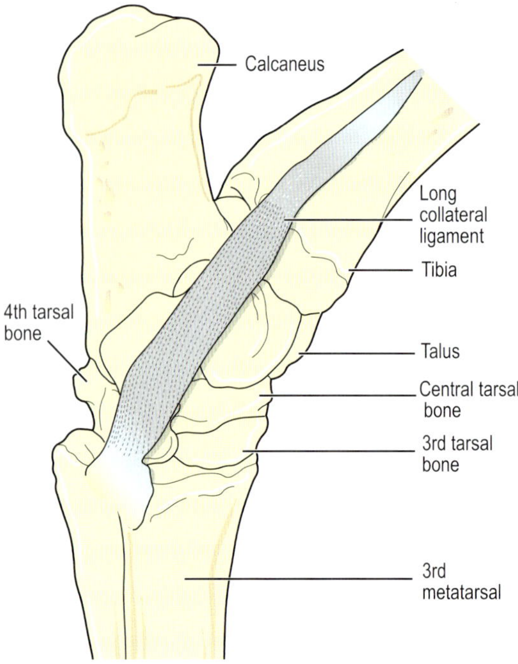

Fig 19.1 Lateral view of the right equine tarsus.

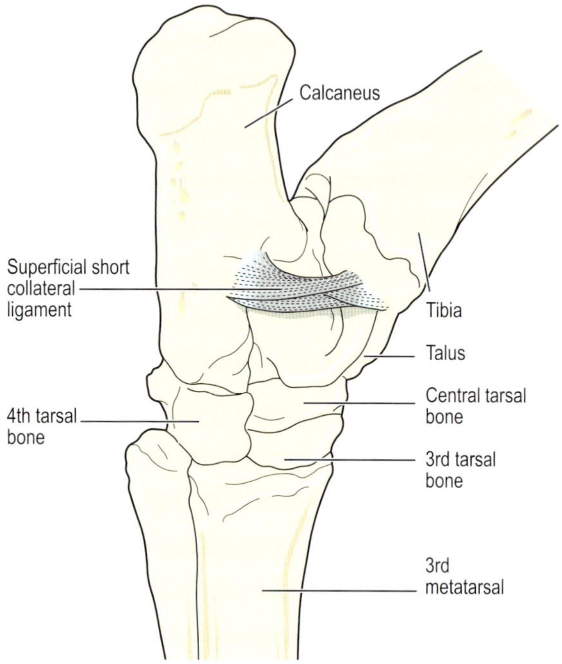

Fig 19.2 Lateral view of the right equine tarsus demonstrating the superficial short lateral collateral ligament.

and third metacarpal bones (Fig. 19.1). The long lateral CoL is loose in flexion and taut during extension of the tarsus. There are three short lateral CoLs; the superficial, middle and deep ligaments (Fig. 19.2, Fig. 19.3). All originate proximally on the lateral tibial malleolus and insert distally on the calcaneus (superficial) and talus (middle and deep). The lateral short CoLs are variably tight or loose during flexion or extension of the tarsus. The medial long CoL originates proximally at the medial tibial malleolus and inserts distally on the fused first and second tarsal bones and on the talus, central and third tarsal bones by two separate fiber bundles (Fig. 19.4). It is loose during TC joint flexion and tight during extension. The short medial CoL is made up of the superficial, middle and deep short medial CoLs (Fig. 19.5, Fig. 19.6, Fig. 19.7). They originate proximally on the medial tibial malleolus and insert distally on the deep fascia, fibrous joint capsule, sustentaculum tali and central tarsal bone. The medial short CoLs are variably tight or loose during flexion or extension of the tarsus, with the majority of the deep component remaining tight during the entire range of motion of the TC joint.[1]

The TC joint communicates with the PIT joint in most horses. Communication between the DIT and TMT joints has been reported to occur in between 26% to 38% of horses when the TMT joint is injected first.[2–4] Following the same injection, 34% of TMT joints would be expected to communicate with PIT and DIT joints.[3,4] Increasing the volume or pressure of injection of liquid agents does not increase the probability of communication, but will increase the amount of subcutaneous leakage of fluid.[2] The TMT and DIT joints may also communicate with the tarsal sheath, tendon of the tibialis cranialis and the subtarsal tissues near the origin of the suspensory ligament at the plantar surface of the third metacarpal bone.[2,4] Due to this variable communication between synovial structures of the tarsus, intrasynovial anesthesia or medication of the DIT or TMT joint cannot be accurately predicted to affect more

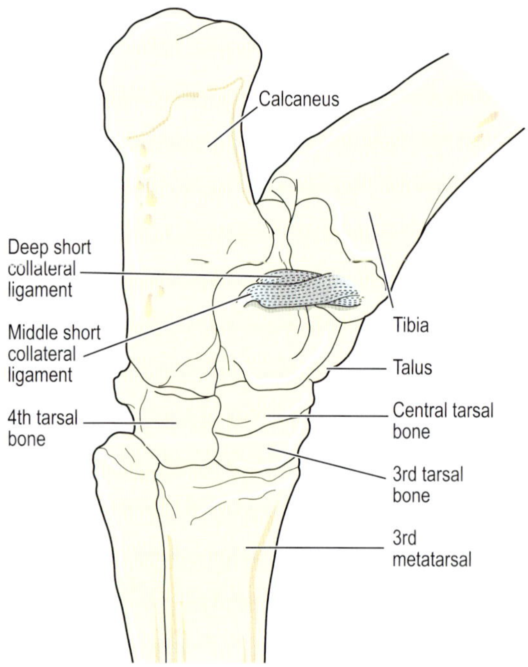

Fig 19.3 Lateral view of the right equine tarsus demonstrating the middle short lateral collateral ligament and deep short lateral collateral ligament.

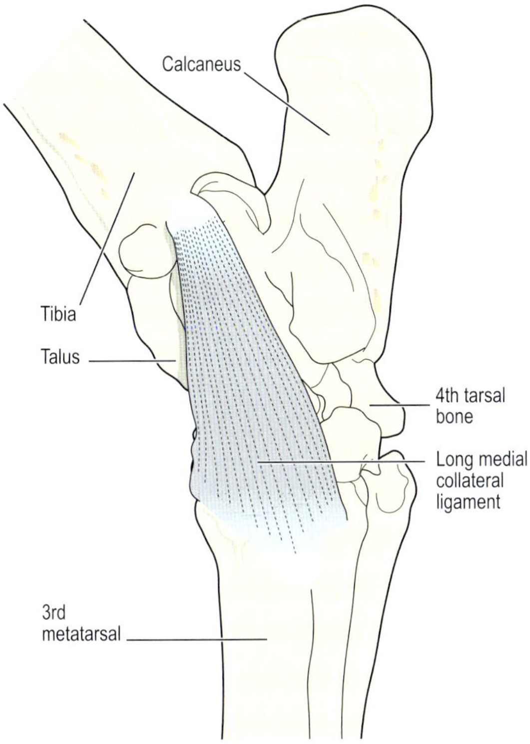

Fig 19.4 Medial view of the right equine tarsus demonstrating the long medial collateral ligament.

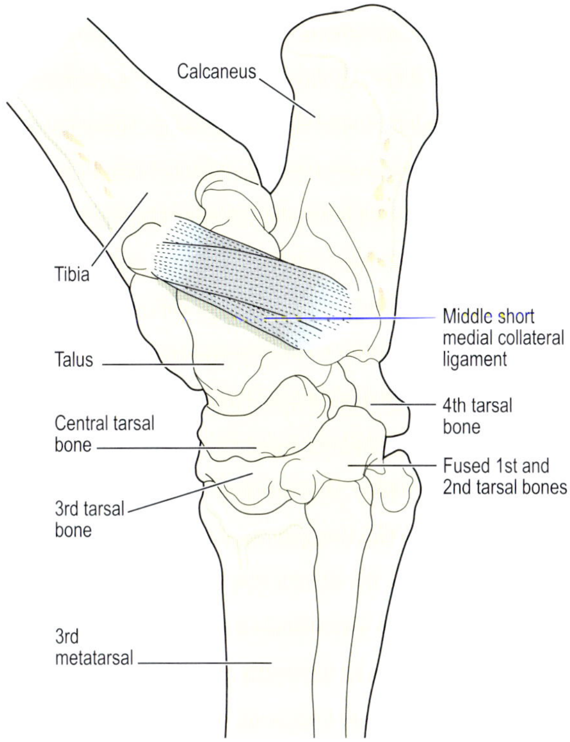

Fig 19.6 Medial view of the right equine tarsus demonstrating the middle short medial collateral ligament.

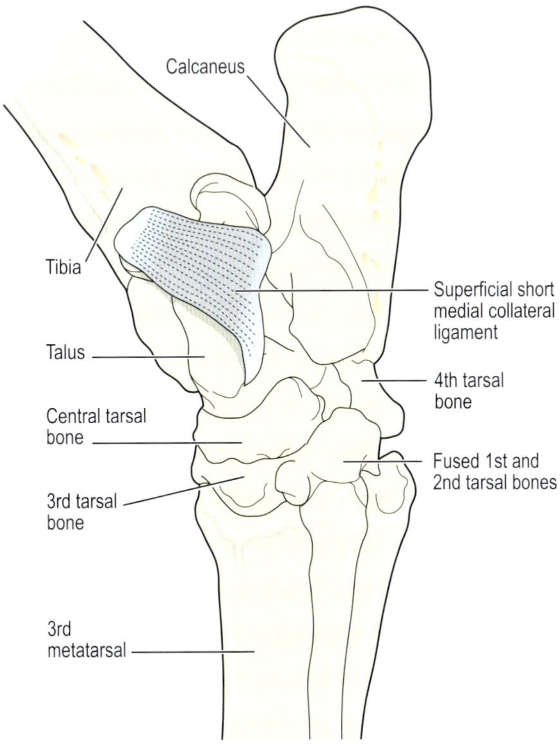

Figure 19.5 Medial view of the right equine tarsus demonstrating the superficial short medial collateral ligament.

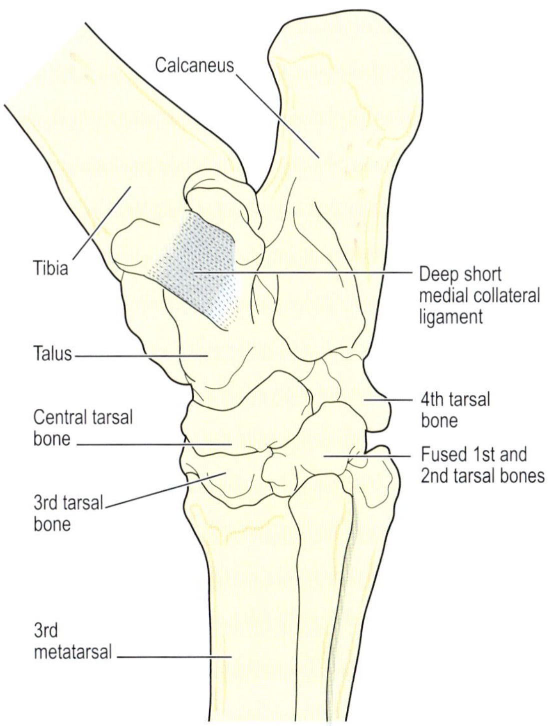

Fig 19.7 Medial view of the right equine tarsus demonstrating the deep short medial collateral ligament.

than a single compartment and may have an extrasynovial effect on the suspensory ligament, tarsal sheath or TC joint.

Swelling of the tarsal region is a common presentation. The three large synovial structures in the tarsal region that will present with fluid swellings are the TC joint, the tarsal sheath and the calcaneal bursa. These can readily be identified with knowledge of the anatomy of the region but if in doubt, ultrasound may assist. Extra synovial swelling may be observed with conditions such as peritarsal cellulitis, false thoroughpins (synoviocoele), plantar ligament desmitis and superficial digital flexor tendonitis.

Conditions of the tarsus that present with lameness and no swelling include osteoarthritis of the distal tarsal joints and insertional desmitis of the collateral ligaments.

Osteochondrosis

The TC joint is one of the most common sites of osteochondrosis lesions. Affected horses commonly present with joint effusion rather than lameness, which is usually absent or mild. Lesions may also be identified on survey radiographs when there may be no clinical signs. The cranial aspect of the distal intermediate ridge of the tibia is affected with the highest frequency, followed by the lateral trochlear ridge of the talus, the medial malleolus of the tibia and the medial trochlear ridge of the talus. Osteochondral fragments of the distal intermediate ridge of the tibia can remain clinically 'silent' in horses in training but suddenly result in swelling due to fragment loosening at any time. Trochlear ridge lesions are commonly associated with TC effusion.

Recognition

Physical examination

Cases with clinical osteochondrosis of the TC joint may have varying degrees of distension. Lameness varies from mild to moderate and hindlimb flexion is often positive. The lameness is characterized by reduced hock flexion during the swing phase of the stride which may result in a toe drag. Extended high-speed exercise or collected work where optimal hock flexion is required becomes more difficult for the athlete to perform. Affected Standardbreds may break gait at high speeds, lean on the shafts of the cart during high-speed exercise or pull away from the affected side, making it difficult to keep the horse in a straight line.

Diagnostic analgesia is rarely necessary for the diagnosis of osteochondrosis of the TC joint as effusion is nearly always present in cases with a blockable lameness. An intrasynovial block may be required to differentiate an osteochondrosis lesion from other possible causes of lameness.

Imaging

Complete radiographic evaluation of the affected and contralateral tarsi should be performed where osteochondrosis is suspected. These include the dorsoplantar, lateromedial, dorsolateral-plantaromedial and dorsomedial-plantarolateral obliques and a flexed lateromedial view. Osteochondral lesions of the distal intermediate ridge of the tibia and lateral trochlear ridge of the talus are best observed on the dorsomedial plantarolateral view (Fig. 19.8 and Fig. 19.9). Medial malleolus lesions are more difficult to observe and can be obscured by the medial trochlear ridge.[5] Angling a dorsoplantar view 10 degrees towards dorsolateral plantaromedial will help view the whole medial malleolus. Lesions of the distal intermediate ridge and medial malleolus of the tibia consist of

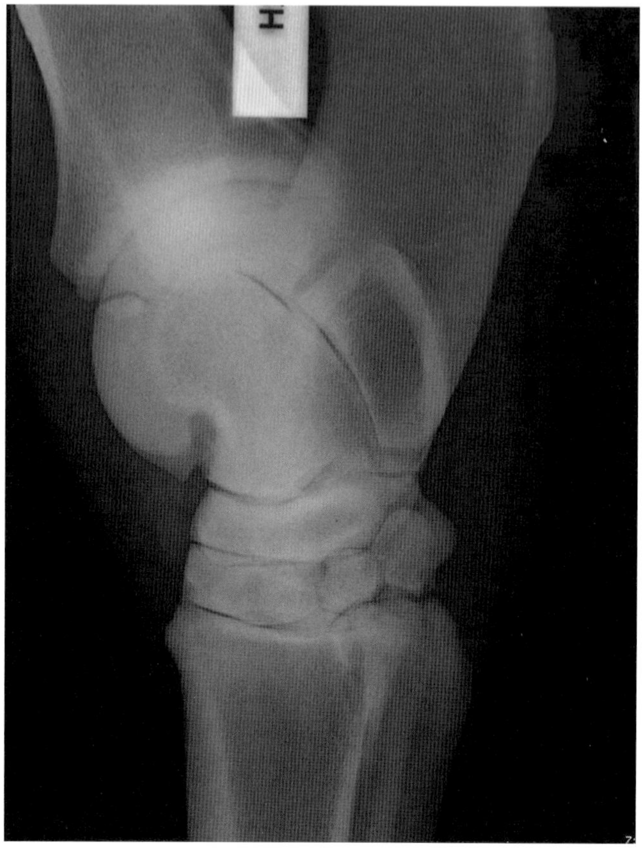

Fig 19.8 A lateromedial view of a tarsus from a two-year-old Standardbred with an osteochondral fragment of the distal intermediate ridge of the tibia.

variably sized osteochondral fragments still attached to the parent bone (Fig. 19.8). Lateral trochlear ridge lesions are usually lucent areas on the distal aspect of the ridge accompanied by overlying, variably sized osteochondral flaps (Fig. 19.9). The lesions can vary in size and depth and in some horses marked distal trochlear ridge osteochondral fragmentation may be the predominant radiographic finding. Horses may have radiographically inapparent osteochondral lesions of the trochlear ridges causing lameness and effusion. These may be imaged using ultrasound.[6,7]

Further diagnostic techniques are rarely indicated for the diagnosis of osteochondrosis of the TC joint however may be required where additional problems are suspected or the clinical picture is not typical of osteochondrosis. For example, intra-articular fractures including stress fractures may be difficult to observe radiographically and may partially or fully respond to intrasynovial analgesia. Scintigraphy would be useful in these circumstances. Joint swelling may also be due to sepsis and this can be differentiated using synovial fluid analysis. Therefore, where lameness is moderate to severe further diagnostic techniques should be considered.

Treatment and prognosis

Treatment

Arthroscopic debridement of osteochondral lesions is recommended for most cases of osteochondrosis where there is TC swelling provided the lesions are mature. Arthroscopy will allow a more

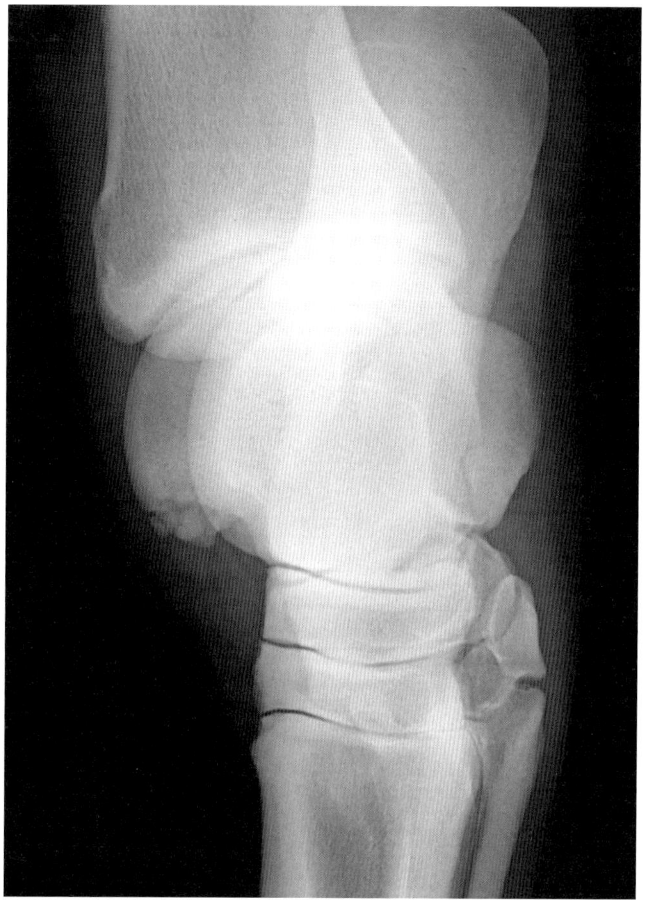

Fig 19.9 A dorsomedial plantarolateral view of a tarsus from a two-year-old Thoroughbred with fragmentation of the distal aspect of the lateral trochlear ridge.

complete assessment of the affected area and identify lesions that are radiographically silent. Conservative therapy may be appropriate for yearlings prior to complete development of lesions or cases without swelling or lameness. The aim of treatment is to remove the involved tissue and debride the surrounding area of all loose and unattached cartilage.[8] This will remove the stimulus for synovitis and minimize continued trauma to the affected area during high-speed exercise. In horses treated conservatively with rest or a reduction in the exercise schedule, the aim is to minimize disruption of the osteochondral lesion to allow healing by completion of endochondral ossification with increasing skeletal maturity or by fibrous attachment of the affected area to the parent bone.[9] This will increase stability of the lesion and minimize the development and progression of synovitis. It is difficult to predict how long it will take for conservative therapy to work and how effectively the lesion is ossified or anchored, as radiographic monitoring will usually reveal persistence of the lesion. Return to high-speed exercise may cause a recrudescence of the lameness, necessitating surgical therapy or a more prolonged rest period.[9]

Approaches for arthroscopic surgery of the tarsus are well described.[10] Bandaging and stall rest are continued for 2–3 weeks after surgery. Hand-walking can be started 10–14 days after surgery with limited turnout (paddock) initiated after 30–45 days, depending on the location of the osteochondrosis and extent of articular cartilage involvement. Horses with uncomplicated distal intermediate ridge lesions usually have a shorter convalescent time. Training is resumed after 90–120 days for most cases of TC osteochondrosis. Horses with extensive articular cartilage fibrillation or synovitis will usually benefit from an extended (5–6 months) interruption of strenuous activity. Single-dose intra-articular hyaluronic acid and corticosteroids may be beneficial in decreasing synovitis and reducing the catabolic effects of inflammation on the articular cartilage.

Conservative treatment entails rest or reduction in the exercise schedule for a variable period of time. The length of the rest period is somewhat arbitrary, but will be at least 60–120 days. The disadvantage of this approach is that surgery will be required if the lameness recurs when high-speed exercise is reinstated, thereby doubling the lay-off or time away from competition.

Prognosis

The prognosis for horses with OC of the TC joint is excellent if there is a favorable response to either surgical or conservative treatment. Horses treated conservatively may be less likely to have a prolonged athletic career, but the performance is usually comparable to unaffected horses while they are actually competing.[8] In young growing horses, lesions of the TC joint are less likely to spontaneously resolve than stifle lesions.[11] Horses treated conservatively or surgically are likely to race as successfully as unaffected horses of the same age, breed and use.[8,12] The size of the lesion or resolution of the effusion after surgery do not appear to be as reliable prognostic indicators for horses that undergo arthroscopic surgery for osteochondrosis of the distal intermediate ridge or medial malleolus of the tibia or the lateral trochlear ridge of the talus. Horses that have erosive articular cartilage lesions at the time of surgery have a guarded prognosis for athletic soundness.

Prevention

Osteochondrosis is a multifactorial disease so complete prevention is unlikely.[11] Genetic selection away from breeding lines predisposed to osteochondrosis is controversial because superior racing stock in some breeds may have a genetic predisposition for the disease. In cases of TC osteochondrosis, the prognosis for racing performance with treatment is good, making removal of these animals from the breeding pool unrealistic.

Etiology and pathophysiology

Osteochondrosis is a developmental disease characterized by disorders of the growing cartilage in the epiphysis and growth plates. The disease is multifactorial with genetic, nutritional (copper deficiency or zinc excess, calcium and phosphorus imbalance from feeding excess grain), metabolic (vitamin D deficiency) and endocrine (hypothyroidism) influences.[11,13–15] The predictable locations of many osteochondral articular lesions in the horse are sites where the developing articular cartilage or growth plates are thick, the vascular supply is tenuous and the biomechanical loads are high. Therefore, vascular and traumatic insults in these locations are probably very important in the expression of this disease in horses.[14,16,17] The ultimate expression of the disease is unpredictable but controlling some of these factors may help reduce the incidence of the disease in a particular area or farm.

Collateral ligament injuries

Injuries of the collateral ligaments of the tarsus may present as poor performance or chronic lameness often without localizing signs in racehorses, or as lameness, and swelling with or without limb angulation of sudden onset following trauma in any type of horse.

Recognition

Physical examination

Athletes with tarsal CoL injuries will present with a rear limb lameness of variable severity that worsens with exercise and can usually be markedly exacerbated by upper limb flexion.[18] There may be palpable swelling, thickening and pain of the soft tissues surrounding the affected structure. Effusion of the TC joint or tarsal sheath may be obvious. TC joint effusion has been reported as a consistent finding in Standardbred pacers with long CoL injuries.[18]

Horses with TC luxations will have marked periarticular swelling, crepitus and an obvious angular (valgus or varus) and rotational deformity of the tarsus at presentation.[19,20] Open tarsal luxations usually involve the synovial cavity of the affected joint and the articular cartilage can often be visualized through the wound. The limb should be carefully evaluated for concomitant structure involvement before proceeding with attempts at reduction and stabilization as the prognosis worsens with extensive soft tissue damage. Horses with intertarsal or TMT luxations may also present with an open wound, which makes the diagnosis straightforward.

These horses are usually toe touching the limb to the ground and the injury may not be readily apparent except for the obvious swelling around the tarsus. As the limb is manipulated or the horse moves the limb spontaneously, the cranial to caudal instability is easily appreciated. The calcaneus, reciprocal apparatus and suspensory ligament on the plantar surface of the limb limit these luxations to a cranial caudal plane. As the soft tissue swelling increases within hours of the injury, it will stabilize some of the laxity and the swinging movement may not be as appreciable. A high index of suspicion for a tarsal luxation is warranted for any horse with a sudden onset of severe lameness and swelling of the tarsus without a wound, especially if there are few or subtle bony changes radiographically to explain the degree of lameness.

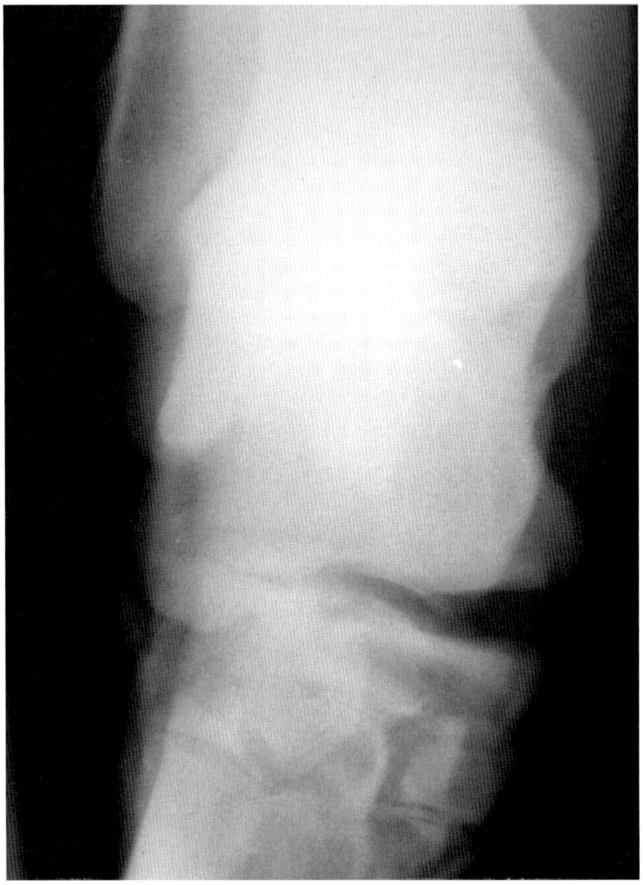

Fig 19.10 A stressed dorsopalmar radiograph of the tarsus of a horse with a severe medial collateral ligament injury and luxation of the PIT joint, demonstrating widening of the joint space.

Imaging

In horses with desmitis of the CoL tarsal radiographs may reveal enthesiophytes at the attachments of the CoL to the parent bone.[18] There may be dystrophic mineralization of the tissue evident in chronic cases and degenerative joint disease or collapse of the joint space(s) if there is long-standing instability present due to the CoL injury.

Tarsal radiographs of horses with intertarsal or TMT luxations may reveal a widened joint space dorsally at the affected site during the acute phase (Fig. 19.10). If the radiographs are taken with the foot on the ground or the soft tissue swelling has stabilized the joint (luxation is reduced), the radiographic diagnosis may not be obvious. Therefore, a stressed lateromedial radiographic view is recommended to identify this injury. The foot is lifted slightly off the ground by an assistant and pulled in a plantar direction to open the affected articulation dorsally and obtain an adequate image of the luxation (Fig. 19.10). The patient will often resent this manipulation, necessitating adequate restraint (sedation and/or lip chain).

The CoLs of the tarsus are easily accessible for ultrasonography. Their structure is complex making interpretation challenging but disruptions of the long components of the medial or lateral CoL are more readily diagnosed.[21–23] Collateral ligament injury is often associated with other soft tissue injuries of the tarsus so a complete ultrasound investigation of the area is important.[22] In horses with desmitis of the CoL tarsal radiographs may reveal enthesiophytes at the attachments of the CoL to the parent bone.[18,24] There may be dystrophic mineralization of the tissue evident in chronic cases and degenerative joint disease or collapse of the joint space(s) if there is long-standing instability present. The more superficial areas of the short portions of the CoLs and long plantar ligament can be adequately imaged.[21,22] Ultrasonographically there will be disruption of the fiber pattern, hypoechoic fluid accumulation within the ligament or hyperechoic deposition of fibrous or mineralized soft tissue, depending on the stage and extent of the injury. Pronounced periarticular soft tissue swelling may interfere with ultrasonographic imaging of these structures.

Perineural analgesia of the peroneal and tibial nerve should improve most lameness associated with CoL injuries of the tarsus. Nuclear scintigraphy in horses with tarsal CoL injuries will reveal a pattern of increased radioisotope uptake at the attachment of the CoL to the bone.[18] The pattern of uptake and its location will help identify the structure involved (long versus short CoL) and the degree of involvement (single versus multiple areas).[18] Scintigraphy is especially useful in horses with a subtle lameness localized to the hock where radiographic studies are inconclusive. Magnetic resonance imaging would be ideally suited for the diagnosis of CoL injuries of the tarsus in horses.[25,26]

Treatment and prognosis

Treatment

Horses with desmitis of the CoL need to be rested to allow the collagen in the ligament to be replaced and to organize along the lines of stress. Affected horses should have stall rest for the first 14–21 days after the injury, with a gradual resumption of hand-walking only (5–10 minutes twice a day) after that time. Systemic NSAID therapy, cold compresses or hydrotherapy and leg wraps are helpful in eliminating soft tissue swelling and restoring adequate circulation to the injured area. Continued activity with further ligament disruption will generate a pronounced fibrovascular response that will eventually fibrose in a disorganized manner, resulting in an architecturally weakened structure with little elasticity and poor function. This will interfere with joint movement and create a persistent mechanical or painful disruption of the gait.[18] These horses should be monitored ultrasonographically and with nuclear scintigraphy during their convalescence to evaluate ligament healing. Exercise intensity can be gradually increased when there is a significant reduction in the size of the original injury and increased tissue organization. This usually requires 3–6 months of rest. Swimming these patients may be beneficial before starting flat work to increase the strength of the tissues without loading them.

Prognosis

Patients with CoL injuries can return to full athletic use if these injuries are diagnosed early, treated aggressively and rehabilitated properly. Standardbred pacers have a good prognosis for racing as well or better after diagnosis (scintigraphy) and treatment (rest) of long CoL injuries. However, horses with extensive disruption that involves most of the cross or longitudinal section of the ligament(s) will usually not be able to return to rigorous athletic use, especially if mineralization or osteophyte production eventually interferes with joint function.[18]

Prevention

It is difficult to make recommendations on prevention of a relatively rare condition where risk factors are unknown. Treating any front limb lameness that may be forcing the horse to shift more weight on the rear limbs to get off the front leg(s) and maintaining a reasonable work/training schedule in light of the athletes age and level of conditioning may help reduce the frequency of these injuries.

Tarsal fractures or osteitis of the calcaneus or talus

Fractures of the bones of the tarsus may be traumatic or a result of fatigue in racehorses. The most common traumatic fracture is of the lateral malleollus. Direct blows may result in fractures of other tarsal bony prominences including the calcaneus, the sustentaculum tali, and the head of the fourth metatarsal bone. Fatigue fractures tend to occur dorsally affecting the proximal aspect of third metatarsal bone or the third tarsal bone.

Recognition

Presentation

Depending on the inciting cause, location and size of the fracture, there will be a sudden onset of a moderate to severe lameness following a traumatic episode (fall, kick or collision) or high-speed exercise.[27] The location and size of the fracture will determine the degree and location of any observed synovial effusion or periarticular swelling. Horses with the more common non-displaced fractures of the tarsus will usually exhibit a significant improvement in the degree of lameness at a walk or slow jog within a few days of the injury. Horses treated with NSAIDs may show an even more dramatic improvement while on the medication. A persistent draining tract may be present when the original trauma results in a break in the skin over the affected bone.

Physical examination

Horses with fractures of the malleolus, talus or calcaneus will often present with a moderate to severe lameness depending on the size of the fragment(s), duration of the condition and degree of synovial effusion of the TC joint, tarsal sheath or calcaneal bursa. Concurrent sepsis of a synovial structure will exacerbate the lameness.

There is usually some degree of soft tissue swelling, pain and crepitus localized over the area of the fracture. Horses with slab fractures of the central or third tarsal bone are usually very lame immediately after the injury, but improve considerably after a few days.[28,29] There is minimal swelling, crepitus or effusion associated with third tarsal bone fractures at presentation, but there may be effusion of the TC joint in horses with central tarsal bone fractures.[29] A painful response can often be elicited by deep palpation over the cranial or lateral surface of the affected joint.[29]

Horses with fractures of the calcaneus will usually present with effusion of the tarsal sheath and/or calcaneal bursa. There may be a wound near the calcaneus that can discharge clear synovial fluid or purulent material. The degree of lameness is variable depending on the location of the injury. Horses with osteomyelitis of the calcaneus, sustentaculum tali and/or sepsis of the tarsal sheath are usually very lame.[30]

Horses with stress fractures of the talus will usually present with a mild to moderate but persistent lameness of variable duration that worsens with high-speed exercise (pacing or trotting). Tibiotarsal joint effusion is usually present but not dramatic. Upper limb flexion will exacerbate the lameness and analgesia of the joint will relieve it considerably.

Intrasynovial anesthesia or tibial and peroneal nerve analgesia should provide considerable improvement in affected horses with most types of non-displaced tarsal fractures. This must be done with caution, because although fractures of the small tarsal bones rarely displace markedly, stress fractures elsewhere in the limb cannot be ruled out. Any equine athlete that presents for a lameness evaluation with a history of an acute onset of a severe lameness after work, with or without synovial effusion and having no obvious soft tissue swelling or crepitus on the limb, should be assumed to have a stress or non-displaced fracture that could be aggravated by an extended lameness examination. Radiographic imaging of suspect or frequently involved areas and nuclear scintigraphy (after 3–5 days) may be preferable to avoid further damage to an injured osseous structure(s), which could mean a treatable condition becoming the end of an athletic career.

Imaging

Lateral malleolus fractures are readily seen on the dorsoplantar radiographs (Fig. 19.11).[27,31] Oblique views may assist in determining whether the fragment is dorsal or plantar (Fig. 19.12). Ultrasound examination will also be helpful in locating the exact position of the fragment which is important for surgical planning (Fig. 19.13). The fragments are variably sized and the degree of surrounding osseous reaction is an indicator of duration.

Most slab fractures of the third or central tarsal bone are located in a frontal plane or on the craniolateral edge of the bone. Therefore, they are best imaged on the lateromedial or dorsomedial to plantarolateral oblique radiographic views.[28,29] Most are non-displaced and there is minimal dorsal or medial distraction of the slab. For this reason they may be difficult to observe with radiography.[32] They can be 4–8 mm thick and variably wide.[29]

Fragmentation of the calcaneus or sustentaculum tali can be difficult to image on conventional radiographic views if they are small and located on the dorsal, distal or axial surface of the bone. Those on the proximal, caudal and lateral surfaces are easier to identify

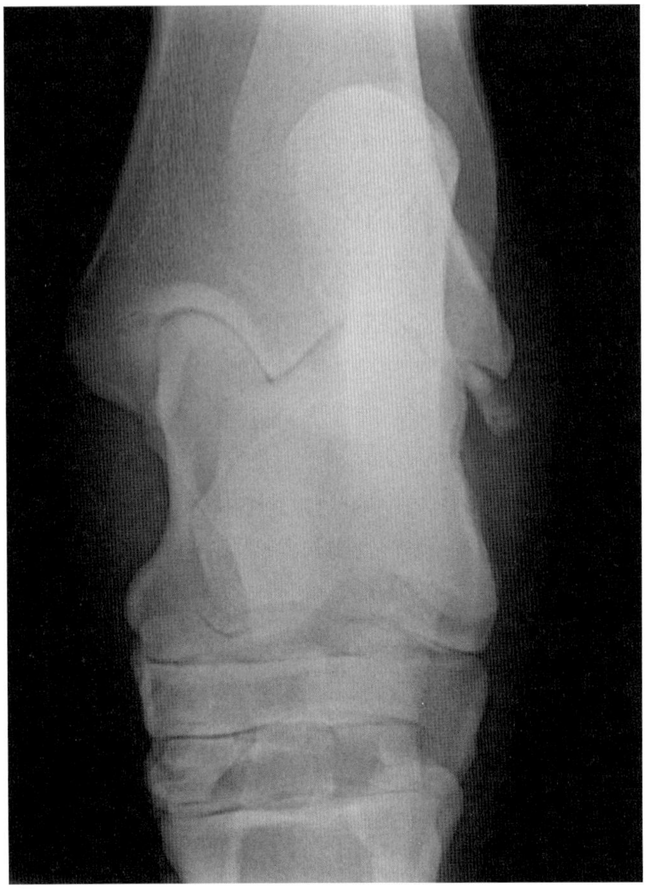

Fig 19.11 A dorsoplantar view of a tarsus from a three-year-old Thoroughbred with a displaced lateral malleolus fracture.

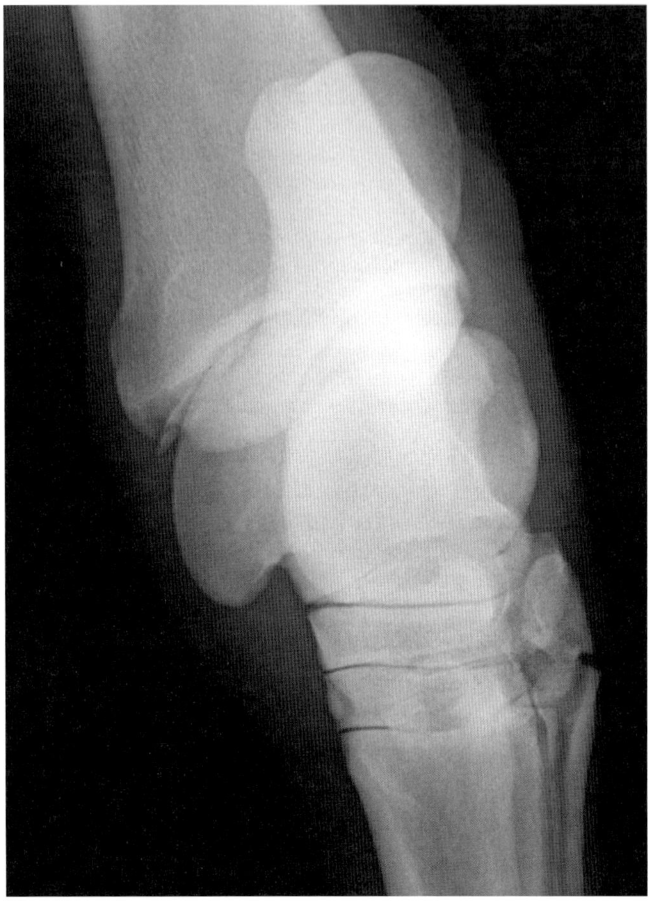

Fig 19.12 A dorsomedial plantarolateral view of the tarsus from the same horse in Fig. 19.11 showing the lateral malleolus fracture is located dorsally.

on conventional views. If axial or distal fragmentation of the calcaneus is suspected or there is distension of the tarsal sheath associated with a wound, a skyline (dorsoplantar to distoplantar) view of the plantar aspect of the tarsus should be obtained. Radiographically there may be marked lysis of the calcaneus or sustentaculum tali associated with bony fragments in horses with osteomyelitis and/or sequestrum formation (Fig. 19.14). Transverse fractures of the calcaneus are readily apparent on the lateromedial and oblique radiographic projections. These fractures are rare and will have a similar presentation to a horse with disruption of the reciprocal apparatus (dropped hock and hyperflexion of the limb during attempts at weight bearing). Ultrasound may be helpful to determine synovial cavity involvement in traumatic injuries to this area. The calcaneal bursa and tarsal sheath should be carefully examined for evidence of synovial thickening, intra-synovial gas or foreign bodies and echongenic material within the synovial space.

Osseous disruption of the talus can usually be seen on the conventional views of the tarsus. Large fractures are readily apparent, but distomedial fragments may be visible only on a skyline view of the plantar tarsus and there will be bony lysis when a septic process accompanies the injury within the tarsal sheath. Fractures affecting the trochlear ridges of the talus may be small and located distally on the ridge(s) or groove or they can involve a large portion of the articular surface with marked joint instability, pain and effusion (Fig. 19.15). Sagittal fractures of the talus can be difficult to observe and multiple of dorsoplantar views may be required to highlight the fracture line (Fig. 19.16). Scintigraphy will identify the site of the fracture if one is suspected (Fig. 19.17).

Standardbred horses with remodeling or stress fracture of the talus will often have a sclerotic area in the center of the talus, best projected on the weight-bearing lateromedial or flexed lateromedial view of the tarsus. The degree of sclerosis will depend on the duration and severity of the injury. Nuclear scintigraphy will reveal a very intense but focal area of radioisotope uptake in the talus on the lateromedial, flexed lateromedial and plantar views of the tarsus. Arthroscopic evaluation of the plantar aspect of the TC joint will often reveal mild proliferative synovitis, roughening of the distal plantar surface of the tibia and/or mild fibrillation or wear lines in the articular cartilage of the plantar surface of the trochlear ridges or groove of the talus.

More complex fractures of the talus or fractures of the fused first and second or fourth tarsal bone can be readily imaged on routine radiographic projections. Flexed lateromedial views will allow the calcaneus and sustentaculum tali to rotate distally, permitting better visualization of the proximoplantar aspect of the talus.

Laboratory examination

Where there is any evidence of a penetrating injury, cytologic evaluation of effusions from associated synovial spaces is critical to

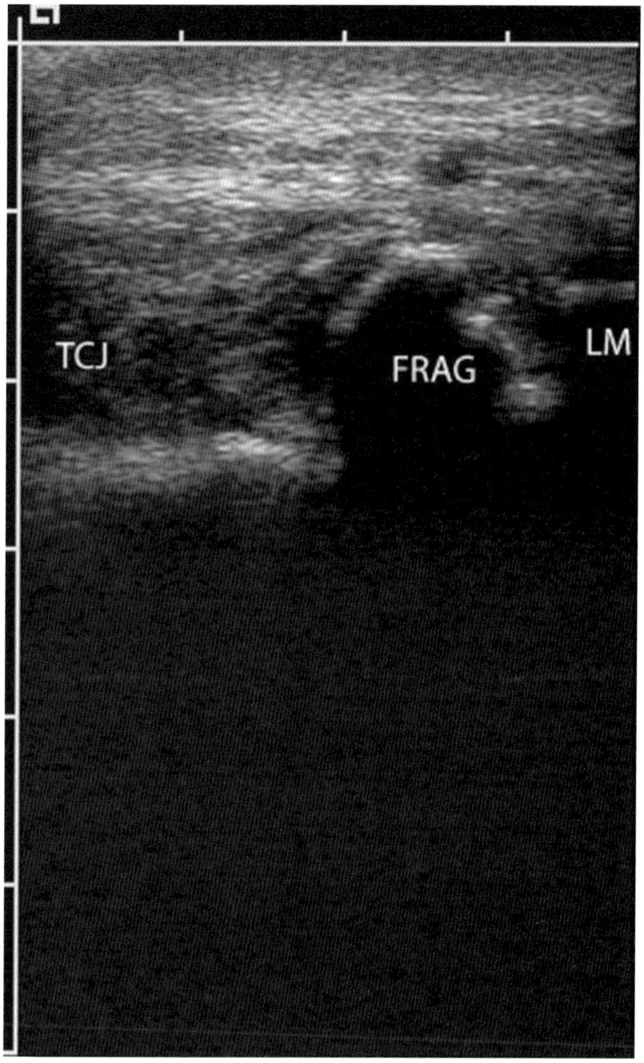

Fig 19.13 A longitudinal ultrasound view of the lateral aspect of the tarsocrural joint (TCJ). Proximal is to the right of the image. A lateral malleolus fracture fragment (FRAG) is shown distal to the lateral malleolus (LM). Ultrasound allows localisation of the fracture fragment which will assist surgical planning.

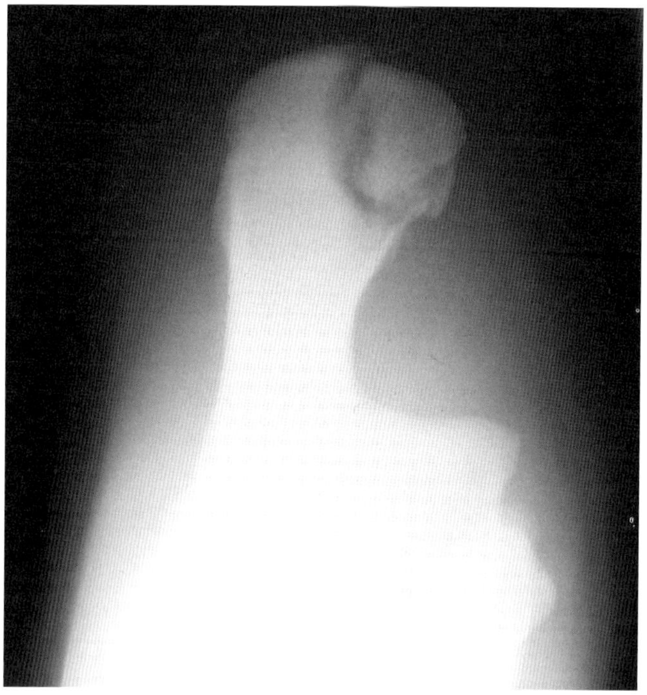

Fig 19.14 A skyline view of a calcaneus with a large medial fracture fragment resulting from direct trauma to the point of the hock.

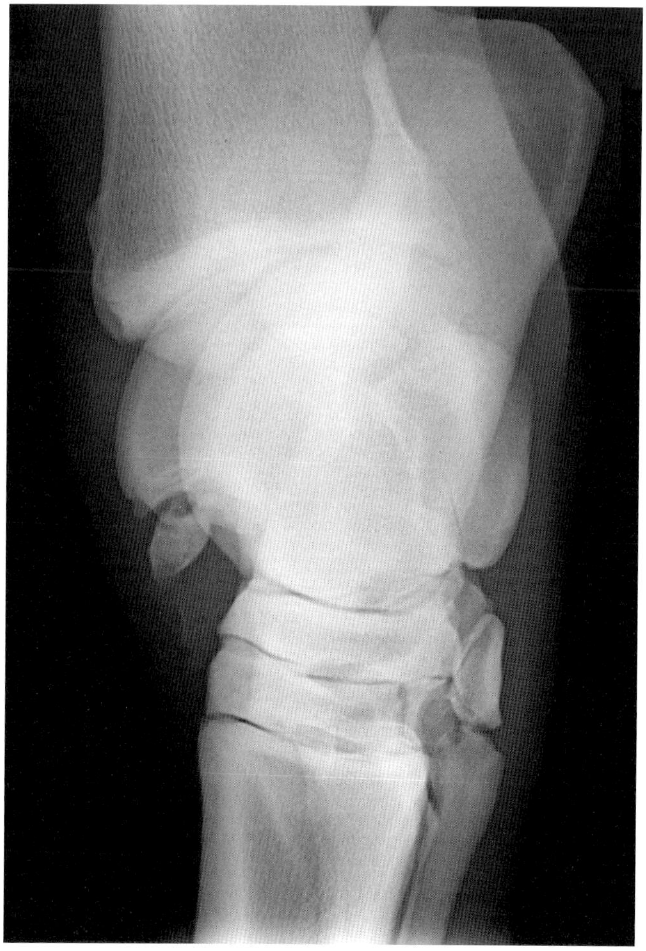

Fig 19.15 A dorsomedial plantarolateral view of a tarsus from a horse with a traumatic fracture of the distal aspect of the lateral trochlear ridge.

identify sepsis. With calcaneal fractures, fluid should be obtained from the calcaneal/intertendinous bursa. For sustentaculum tali fractures, the tarsal sheath should be sampled, and for fractures of the head of the fourth metatarsal bone, fluid from the TMT joint is required. Synovial fluid examination is less useful for differentiating fractures from osteochondrosis lesions although in acute fractures heamarthrosis may be observed.

Diagnosis

A definitive diagnosis can generally be made with appropriate radiographic views. However, scintigraphy may be required to identify non-displaced stress fractures and the addition of synovial fluid analysis will allow the diagnosis of associated synovial sepsis.

The major differential diagnosis is osteochondrosis, although these tend to occur at different sites with the occasional exception of distal trochlear ridge of the talus fractures.

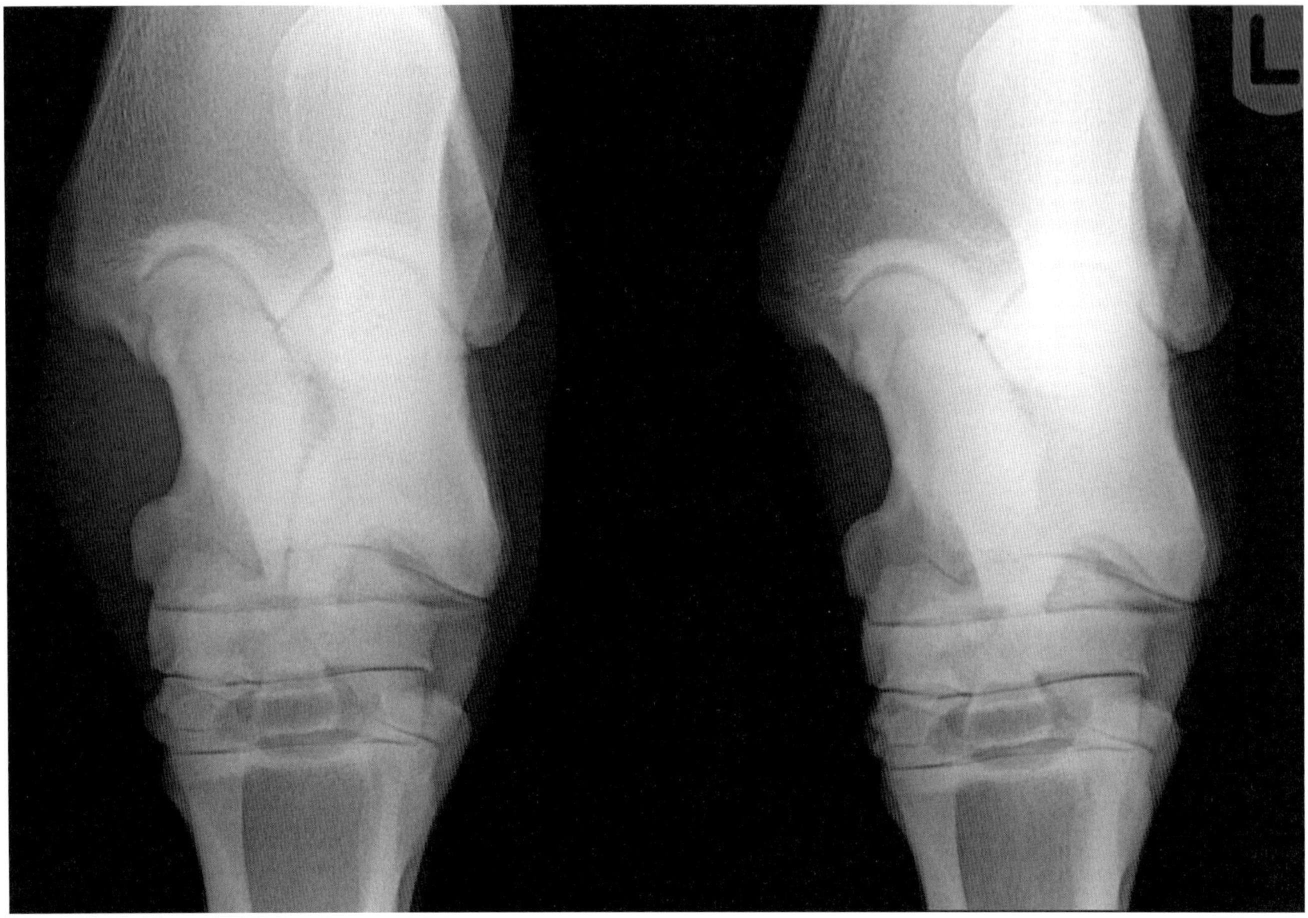

Fig 19.16 Two dorsoplantar radiographs of the tarsus of the same horse taken at slightly different angles. A sagittal fracture of the talus is visible on the left radiograph but difficult to see on the right radiograph demonstrating the importance of multiple views to identify these fractures.

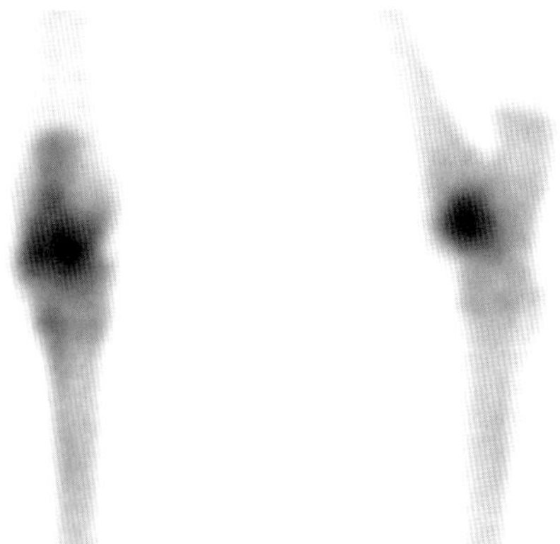

Fig 19.17 Plantar and lateral scintigraphic views of the tarsus of the same horse as in Fig. 19.16 showing intense uptake of radiopharmaceutical associated with a sagittal fracture of the talus.

Treatment and prognosis

Treatment

The therapeutic goal is to stabilize unstable structures, remove loose or devitalized bone or soft tissues, rid tissues of any infectious organisms and provide rest and support to allow adequate healing. Serial monitoring with radiographs or nuclear scintigraphy may be required to critically evaluate the rate and quality of the repair process.

Slab fractures of the third or central tarsal bone in racehorses can be managed both conservatively or with lag screw fixation.[29,33] Horses treated conservatively (stall rest) may develop osteoarthritis of the affected joint however many can successfully return to racing. This appears to be more common with third than with central tarsal bone fractures.[28,33–35] Standardbred racehorses tend to have a better prognosis for a return to racing following conservative treatment than Thoroughbred racehorses.[35]

The surgical technique requires general anesthesia and radiographic or fluoroscopic guidance for proper drill and screw placement.[29] These fractures can usually be repaired with a single 3.5 or 4.5 mm cortical screw or a cannulated screw system. The head of the cortical screw is usually not countersunk to reduce the probability of the fragment shattering when the implant is tightened. An incision over the affected joint to identify the center of the fragment and proximal and distal margins of the joint for proper screw placement will expedite surgery. It should minimize the risk of damage to the dorsal tarsal vessels that can occur when the surgery is done with needle guidance through stab incisions. The horses are assisted during recovery and confined to a stall for 4–6 weeks. Gradual introduction to hand-walking can begin at that time and return to training can occur 4–8 months after repair. Radiographic evaluation may be the best guide for increasing activity levels.

Lateral malleolus fractures should be treated surgically, especially in horses with synovial effusion and lameness.[27,31] Arthroscopic visualization will allow a thorough evaluation of the entire joint to assess the articular surface for damage, look for and remove any loose osteochondral fragments, inspect the fractured malleolus and flush debris out of the joint. The fracture fragment(s) can be removed arthroscopically, although this is a challenging procedure for large fragments that require extensive dissection of the short collateral ligaments.[27] Dorsal and plantar portals are often required. Alternatively, the fragment can be removed quickly and effectively through a dorsal arthrotomy centered over the fragment.[31] Careful dissection will prevent further damage to the long lateral CoL. If the fragment is large enough, where a considerable portion of the attachment of the long lateral CoL is involved, reduction and fixation with a lag screw (4.5 or 5.5 mm cortical screw) will be necessary. Removing these large fragments will cause further damage to the CoL and would perpetuate TC instability. Assisted recovery should be used with these horses to limit further damage to the CoL and avoid tarsal luxation and a short cast may be applied for recovery. Postoperatively, the limb is kept bandaged for 2–4 weeks to control swelling and reduce the effusion. In some horses, a residual amount of effusion will remain that appears to be inconsequential to future performance. Hand-walking can be initiated at 2–3 weeks after surgery and turnout in 4–6 weeks. Training can resume in 90–120 days depending on the resolution of the majority of the effusion and lameness and the degree of pre-existing damage to the long lateral CoL. If a lag screw fixation was performed, 6–8 months of rest will be required before resuming exercise to insure healing of the malleolus and CoL. Radiographs can be used to assess bony healing.

Fractures of the calcaneus can be treated conservatively or surgically. Fragmentation of the calcaneus or sustentaculum tali is usually accompanied by a soft tissue defect over the lesion and/or marked effusion of the tarsal sheath. Secondary sepsis of the tissue will be manifested as osteomyelitis of the calcaneus and/or sepsis of the tarsal sheath or calcaneal bursa, depending on the location of the wound or bony lesion.[30,36,37] Arthroscopic exploration of the calcaneal and intertendinous bursae or the tarsal sheath allows surgical debridement of fracture fragments and necrotic bone and any associated tendon injury and lavage.[38–40] Systemic and local administration of appropriate antibiotic based on culture and sensitivity results should be continued post surgery. When trying to salvage a horse for breeding, a midtarsal tenotomy or tenectomy of the DDF will decrease motion of the tendon within the sheath, reducing pain and remove infected tendon tissue.[30]

Fractures of the talus may be confined to the dorsal or plantar articular surfaces of the trochlear ridges or oriented sagittally in the intertrochlear groove. Fragments of the trochlear ridges can be removed arthroscopically. Stress fracture or remodeling of the talus as seen in pacing or trotting racehorses will respond to rest. Return to training recommendations are based on repeat scintigraphic evaluations. Non-displaced fractures of the talus can be repaired with lag screw fixation if the articular surface is minimally disrupted and there are pieces large enough where one or two cortical screws will adequately reduce and secure the fracture. The size of the implants and surgical approach are dictated by the location and configuration of the fracture. Comminuted fractures with complete collapse of the TC joint are not amenable to repair and these patients should be humanely destroyed. Casting may be necessary during recovery and the immediate postoperative period, but if the repair is well secured then assisted recovery should suffice. Removal of the implants is usually not necessary, but the return to athletic use will be influenced by the degree of articular involvement or damage to soft tissue structures such as the collateral or plantar ligaments. Sufficient bone, articular cartilage and soft tissue healing to allow return to work may require 4–8 months. Limited activity (hand-walking or turnout) can begin after 4–6 weeks of stall rest.

Fractures of the fused first and second or fourth tarsal bone are rare. Choice of therapy (conservative or surgical) will depend on the size of the fragment, location and articular involvement. Fractures or fragments that are minimally displaced will usually heal without surgical intervention. These tarsal bones are not subjected to the compressive forces that the third and central tarsal bones experience and conservative therapy may be sufficient for adequate healing. This approach may not be suitable for performance horses because a fibrous union with articular or periarticular degenerative changes could result in residual lameness during high-speed or rigorous exercise. Larger fragments may have to be removed or secured with lag screws. If the fracture is unstable or the articulation of the bone with the splint bone, central tarsal bone or talus is compromised, then an attempt at surgical repair is justified. Approach and choice of implant is determined by the size and location of the fragment(s). Convalescence and return to work are as described before.

Rehabilitation of the soft tissues as soon as possible after surgery will restore range of motion to the joint and decrease the morbidity associated with disuse and fibrosis. This may be as important as surgical therapies in bringing these athletes back to work. Range of motion exercises with the joint and swimming may be useful adjuncts to exercise regimens to rehabilitate periarticular soft tissues.

Prognosis

Due to the low numbers of many types of tarsal fractures reported, establishing a prognosis is challenging. A thorough assessment of the ligamentous, synovial cavity, articular and bony involvement is important. Horses with extensive damage to the CoL, SDF, fibrous joint capsule or articular cartilage have a poor prognosis for athletic use, even if a surgical procedure successfully removed fragmentation, secured loose fractures or resolved sepsis. Horses with fragmentation of the dorsodistal or very plantar aspect of the trochlear ridges, and fractures of the lateral malleolus, have a good prognosis for return to function with proper therapy. Standardbred racehorses with slab fractures of the third tarsal bone treated surgically or conservatively appear to have a good prognosis for return to racing but the prognosis of Thoroughbred racehorses is not so good when treated conservatively.[35] Horses with more complex injuries (transverse calcaneal or complete talus fractures) have a poor prospect for returning to high-level athletic activity.

Bone injuries with secondary synovial sepsis carry a guarded prognosis.[37,38,41] Aggressive treatment may salvage affected horses for non-athletic purposes. A rapid return of synovial fluid variables to normal levels suggests a better prognosis than those where they remain high at days 4–6.[41]

Prevention

There are no definitive recommendations that can be made to prevent these tarsal injuries. Most are traumatically induced from a sudden internal or external application of force that is difficult to predict or avoid. Stress fractures in young racehorses may be prevented by reducing distance work in favor of speed work may decrease the accumulation of microtrauma that can cause these injuries.

Etiology and pathophysiology

The etiology of these injuries is accumulated microtrauma (stress fractures in racehorses) or single event application of external (kick or collision) or internal (fall or slip) torque sufficient to disrupt the osseous and soft tissue structures.

Thoroughbred or other performance horses that have a wedge-shaped conformation of the craniolateral aspect of the third tarsal bone may be predisposed to sustaining a slab fracture of this bone during high-speed training or racing, by presumably concentrating compressive forces along the trough in the wedge.[42]

Osteoarthritis

Osteoarthritis of the distal tarsal joints can affect a wide range of equine athletes. Although common, this condition is often over diagnosed due to the frequent findings of a positive hindlimb flexion test and radiographic changes of the TMT and DIT joints. Due to the unreliability of radiographic changes for the diagnosis of osteoarthritis, it is essential that further diagnostics are performed and most cases will require diagnostic local analgesia to confirm the diagnosis. Foals with incomplete ossification of the central and third tarsal bones are predisposed to osteoarthritis when mature. Icelandic horses are also predisposed to osteoarthritis of the distal tarsal joints. Talocalacaneal (TCa) osteoarthritis is rare.

Recognition

Presentation

Osteoarthritis of the tarsus can affect athletes at a young age (in training) or at later stages of their athletic careers. Affected horses will present with a rear limb(s) lameness of variable severity and duration, and that has a variable response to rest. Poor performance may be the only sign in some horses. Affected athletes can sometimes warm out of the lameness after a short period of work or will get worse when they are forced to work vigorously with their rear limbs while in a collected posture (dressage or approaches to obstacles for jumping). This disease is often insidious in onset and some chronically affected horses will refuse to perform certain movements under tack and may even object vigorously by tail swishing, bucking, refusals at jumps and an unwillingness to take or stay in a particular leg lead.

Horses with talocalcaneal degenerative joint disease will commonly have a history of trauma preceding the lameness.

Physical examination

There is usually no external soft tissue swelling or effusion evident on the rear limb(s) and affected horses may have straight-legged or a tarsal valgus or varus conformation. The medial aspect of the intertarsal and TMT joints may appear thickened or have a boxed appearance in some horses. There is generally little pain on flexion of the tarsus but flexion tests are often positive.

The severity of the presenting lameness will vary dramatically, but often affected horses have decreased hock flexion (reduced arc during the swing phase often with a toe drag). When ridden in a collected fashion, the lameness will often become more apparent than when being trotted in hand or lunged.

Diagnostic analgesia is required in most cases to localize pain to the distal tarsus. Regional anesthesia involves performing tibial and peroneal nerve blocks following desensitization of the lower limb and proximal plantar metatarsus. This is not specific for the distal tarsal joints, however most problems of the larger synovial structures of the tarsus will result in easily identified effusion. The horse should be examined at 20 minutes post injection and further blocks should be delayed for one hour as sometimes the response is delayed. Intra-articular anesthesia of the distal tarsal joints is also not specific due to variable communications with a number of other structures but does localize pain to the region. The TMT and DIT joints communicate in approximately 26–35% of horses and anesthetic can also diffuse into the tarsal sheath or proximal intertarsal or TC joint after injection into the TMT joint space.[2–4] The proximal palmar metatarsus should be blocked prior to a TMT block because the plantar distal extensions of the synovial cavity run either side of the proximal suspensory ligament.[4] In cases with severe radiographic changes the response to intra-articular analgesia may be poor.

Imaging

Radiographs are difficult to interpret in isolation because many horses have mild radiographic changes where pain cannot be localized to the distal tarsal joints, whereas some horses with significant pain localized to this area have normal radiographs.[43] Based on MRI findings, radiography is unreliable for the detection of subchondral bone lesions, subchondral bone sclerosis and even fractures of the tarsal bones.[32] Radiographic changes that may be observed in association with osteoarthritis of the small tarsal joints include loss of joint space, periarticular osteophyte and enthesiophyte production and/or subchondral bone lysis (Fig. 19.18, Fig. 19.19). The disease may be localized to either the dorsomedial or the dorsolateral aspect of the joint(s). The radiographic changes, when present, are consistently seen on the lateromedial and dorsolateral to plantaromedial oblique projections. Horses with degenerative joint disease of the TCa joint will have radiographic evidence of bony lysis and sclerosis at the normally smooth contour of the articulation between the talus and calcaneus.

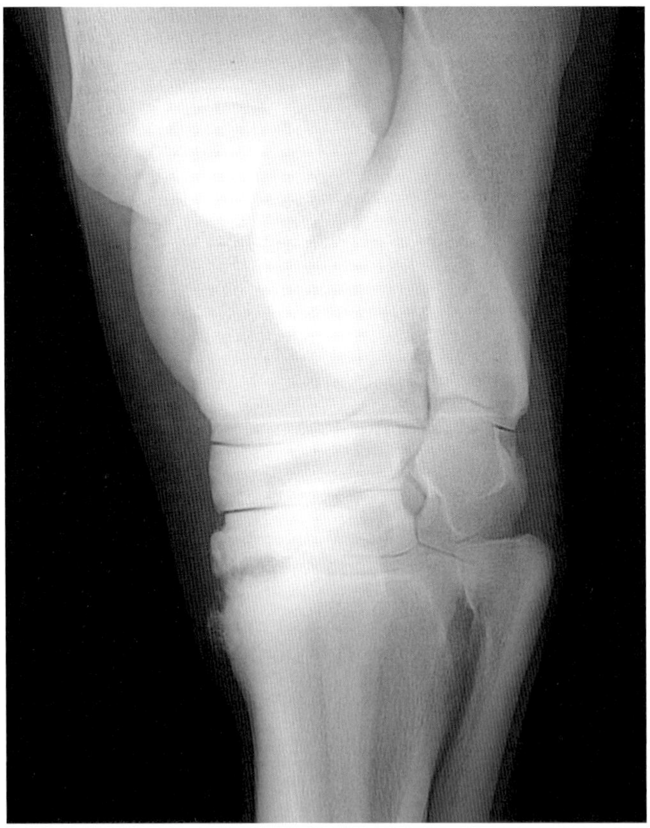

Fig 19.18 A dorsolateral plantaromedial view of the tarsus of a horse with osteoarthritis of the TMT joint. There is marked periarticular modeling and subchondral bone lysis.

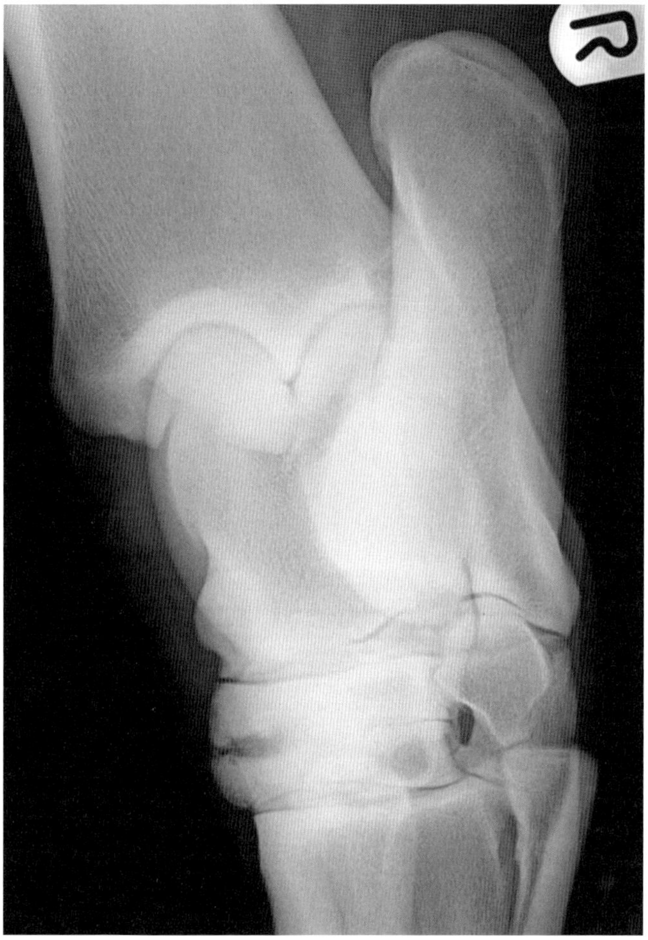

Fig 19.19 A dorsolateral plantaromedial view of the tarsus of a horse with osteoarthritis of the DIT joint. Subchondral bone lysis is observed on the medial aspect of the joint.

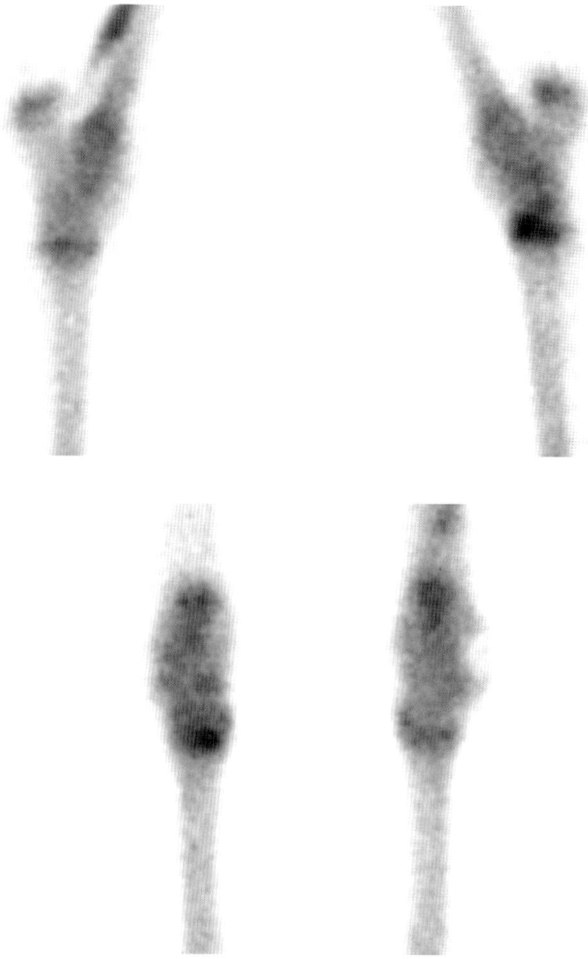

Fig 19.20 Lateral and plantar scintigraphic views of the tarsi of a horse with osteoarthritis of the distal tarsal joints. There is marked uptake of radiopharmaceutical in the left hind and mild increased uptake in the right hind associated with these joints.

Scintigraphy is useful to determine if subchondral bone is actively modeling or remodeling. In a high proportion of horses with distal tarsal joint pain, there is a loss of the normal pattern of uptake of radioisotope[44] and lesions detected with MRI can be identified with scintigraphy, albeit with less anatomical detail[32] (Fig. 19.20). It is important to note that the normal scintigraphic pattern is different for different breeds and disciplines.[45,46] Three dimensional imaging techniques such as CT and MRI are rarely necessary but allow more accurate assessment of subchondral bone thickness in various regions of the tarsus and more sensitive identification of subchondral bone changes such as subchondral cystic lesions.[47]

Standing MRI can be challenging due to excessive movement in some horses degrading the image, but if achievable provides more information than other techniques.[32] Subchondral bone plate thickness can be readily measured and increased signal may indicate subchondral bone damage.[48]

Diagnosis

Horses with proximal suspensory ligament disease may appear clinically similar to horses with tarsal disease, have a positive response to upper limb flexion and may also respond favorably to anesthesia of the TMT joint. Subtarsal analgesic techniques should be used to rule out proximal plantar metatarsal pain prior to performing an intra-articular TMT joint block.

If pain is localized to the region following exclusion of proximal plantar metacarpal pain and radiographic changes are not definitive, scintigraphy should be performed.

In horses with subtle lameness or poor performance, intra-articular medication may be administered as a treatment trial. The horse should be re-assessed at two weeks post injection.

Treatment and prognosis

Treatment

Medical therapy should be attempted initially and includes intra-articular or systemically administered anti-inflammatory medications. When medical therapy fails, arthrodesis of the affected joint may be considered.

Medical therapy for horses with osteoarthritis of the tarsus includes intra-articular or parenterally administered drugs (see Chapter 23).

Intra-articular corticosteroids (methylprednisolone, betamethasone, triamcinolone) are the most commonly used medical treatment for osteoarthritis of the distal tarsal joints. Approximately 60% of affected horses improve following intra-articular treatment, but treatment is considered successful in only 40% of horses as judged by their owners.[49] It is difficult to determine which horses will respond to intra-articular corticosteroids, although horses with more severe radiographic changes tend to respond less favorably.[43] They can be used alone or in combination with hyaluronate which may prolong the action of the corticosteroid. Intra-articular injection of the TMT joint alone may be attempted initially even if there is evidence that the CD joint is also affected as a good response is often achieved.[50] If there is a poor response, then both joints should be treated. Triamcinolone (6 mg/joint) or methylprednisilone (60–80 mg/joint) are most commonly used. When multiple joints are treated at one time, the dose for each joint should be decreased to keep the total dose at a safe level. The response and the duration of action are variable. If a good response is achieved for a reasonable period, then repeat injections are a good method of ongoing management.

Systemic administration of chondroprotective agents such as hyaluronate and polysulfated glycosaminoglycans are frequently used alone or in combination with intra-articular medication (see Chapter 23).

Modifications to the shoeing such as lateral extensions are often recommended for affected horses. The use of heel caulks or trailers may increase the rotational forces placed across the joint surfaces in horses during high-speed exercise, especially in Standardbreds. Avoiding their use may limit development and/or expression of the condition. In horses with sickle or cow hocks, attempts to induce breakover of the medial toe may be of benefit in limiting uneven loading of the joint surfaces.

Arthrodesis of the distal tarsal joints should be considered for cases of osteoarthritis that have not responded to conservative therapies. Due to the risk of significant complications, it is not recommended as a primary treatment. A number of techniques have been described. Chemical arthodesis is simpler and more economic than surgical fusion but the risks of adverse outcomes are higher. More recently lasers have been trialed to induce arthrodesis of these joints.

Sodium monoiodoacetate (MIA) has been most commonly used to achieve chemical fusion.[51–53] This chemical will induce cartilage necrosis which then leads to arthodesis. A single injection of 100–150 mg of filtered MIA administered intra-articularly is the most common method of treatment.[51,52,54] The joint space must be localized with radiographic guidance prior to injecton. Contrast arthrography is important to make sure there is no communication of these joints with the TC joint or the tarsal sheath. Even without evidence of communication TC synovitis has been observed following treatment and owners should be made aware of this possible complication. Extra-articular placement of the chemical will cause cellulitis and may lead to tissue necrosis with loss of some soft tissue coverage requiring prolonged wound therapy. Treated horses may be very uncomfortable for 12–36 hours after the procedure, requiring appropriate analgesia.[52,54] Hand-walking or light riding can be initiated in 7–10 days following the first injection.[52,53] There will be a radiographically evident narrowing of the joint space(s), but only about half the joints treated with a single injection of MIA will have evidence of fusion at six months.[54] Prolonged swelling, chronic pain and lameness have been reported after its use.[51,52] In the largest study of intra-articular MIA efficacy (104 horses), most ultimately successful cases were not sound at six months and only a third of horses were followed up long term (two years), of which 85% were sound.[52] Due to the risk of complications, and the limited evidence for efficacy, chemical arthrodesis with MIA should not be the first choice of therapy for most affected horses.

Arthrodesis of the distal tarsal joints using ethyl alcohol has been investigated in the horse.[55,56] Along with its tissue destructive properties which appear to induce arthrodesis, it induces neurolysis and therefore may provide prolonged pain relief. As with MIA care needs to be taken to avoid alcohol entering additional synovial cavities. Intra-articular injection of alcohol does not cause the pain associated with MIA injection.[55,56] Local swellings may occur but do not persist long term.[55,56] When used for treating osteoarthritis of the distal tarsal joints, success rates appear to be similar to that achieved with MIA but resolution of lameness may be more rapid in some horses.[55]

Surgical arthodesis techniques include drilling the joint spaces, internal fixation or laser ablation of cartilage. Limited drilling of the joint surfaces to focally remove articular cartilage is the most commonly used technique.[57] The cunean tendon is resected and the TMT and DIT joints are identified with radiographic guidance on their medial aspect. Using three separate 3.5 mm drill passes, each joint is drilled in a fan-shaped manner towards the lateral aspect. The tarsus is bandaged and the horse kept in a stall for 7–14 days at which time hand-walking is begun. Arthrodesis may take 6–9 months to complete and it is not uncommon for treated horses to be out of work for up to 12 months. A bony thickening of the medial aspect of the tarsus may develop.[57] Some horses may have a residual lameness despite apparent radiographic arthrodesis.

Arthrodesis using internal fixation techniques has also been described. These include a single 4.5 mm cortical lag screw placed from distal to proximal through the third metacarpal bone into the third and central tarsal bone, application of a fingerplate or a T-plate on the medial aspect of the tarsus with 3.5 or 4.5 mm cortical screws placed into the central and third tarsal and third metatarsal bones to bridge and compress the joints, and insertion of stainless steel cylinders.[57,58] It appears that use of a stabilizing implant on the medial aspect of the joint may reduce the number of horses in which failure of arthrodesis occurs when compared to drilling alone but it does not appear to reduce the convalescent period, which may be 6–12 months irrespective of procedure used.[57]

Arthrodesis using a diode laser has been used in experimental animals but it use in clinical cases has not been reported.[54] As the laser fiber is introduced via needles positioned in the joint spaces, the technique may be challenging in cases with advanced osteoarthritis. There is less postoperative morbidity following laser arthrodesis than either surgical drilling or MIA arthrodesis.[54]

Prognosis

The prognosis for athletic performance is guarded for most horses with osteoarthritis of the distal tarsal joints. Intra-articular medication is successful in approximately 40% of cases. Studies of arthrodesis techniques either use low numbers or suffer from poor inclusion criteria and the loss of a large proportion of horses to follow up making assessment of the prognosis for these treatments difficult.

Prevention

Prevention of this disease in horses is difficult as there are few studies of risk factors. In Icelandic horses modifiable risk factors such as exercise intensity and housing during winter have no effect on the development of osteoarthritis in the distal tarsal joints.[59]

Etiology and pathophysiology

Osteoarthritis is the end stage of many disease processes. Incomplete ossification of the tarsal bones in foals may result in abnormal tarsal bone conformation that predisposes horses to osteoarthritis of the distal tarsal joints. Trauma and synovial sepsis are other possible inciting causes and some breeds such as Icelandic horses are predisposed suggesting a genetic cause. However, in many cases a specific etiology is not identified.

Gastrocnemius, plantar ligament and superficial digital flexor tendon injuries of the tarsus

Tendon and ligament injuries of the palmar aspect of the tarsus are rare. Horses presenting with swelling of the plantar aspect of the tarsus should be investigated with careful palpation and ultrasound examination.

Recognition

Presentation

Gastrocnemius or superficical digitial flexor (SDF) tendinitis or plantar ligament desmitis will more often present with a chronic lameness of variable severity and less obvious swelling on the proximoplantar or plantar aspect of the hock.[60] These injuries can occur after high-speed exercise or after a fall or traumatic episode (collision or impact) during a competition. Tendinitis or dislocation of the SDF, tendinitis of the gastrocnemius or plantar ligament desmitis can be observed in horses competing in high-speed events or jumping disciplines.

Physical examination

Horses with tendinitis or dislocation of the SDF, tendinitis of the gastocnemius or plantar ligament desmitis will present with a mild to moderate lameness depending on the severity of the injury and duration of the condition. Where the SDF tendon is unstable over the point of the calcaneus, horses may present with a severe lameness initially. There may be diffuse swelling over the point of the hock or more discrete thickening of the SDF or gastrocnemius at the site of injury. The lameness evident at presentation is usually exacerbated by flexion of the upper limb. Luxation of the SDF may be difficult to identify initially due to swelling but once the swelling subsides the abnormal position of the tendon is more easily appreciated. The tendon may be observed to slip off the calcaneus when walking.

Diagnostic analgesia is generally not required for tendon injuries due to the presence of obvious swelling but may be helpful if lameness is more severe than expected or other areas of lameness are suspected.

Imaging

In cases of tendonitis ultrasound will reveal increased cross sectional area and variably sized areas of tendon or ligament hypoechogenicity associated with fiber disruption and fluid accumulation. Ultrasonographic examination of the SDF is useful in cases of luxation of the SDF to determine if there is associated disruption of the fibrocartilagenous cap. This will require resection to enable the tendon to stabilize in the luxated position.[61]

Routine radiographs of the tarsus (all standard views and a skyline) should be obtained to identify avulsions or fractures of the calcaneus or enthesiophytes at the insertions of these soft tissue structures. Nuclear scintigraphy may be useful in subtle cases with a more chronic duration.

Diagnosis

A combination of palpation and ultrasound examination is diagnostic in most cases.

Treatment and prognosis

Treatment

Cases of desmitis or tendinitis should initially be rested and treated with anti-inflammatory medications until the acute swelling has resolved, and then enter a controlled training program with regular ultrasound examination to monitor healing. This may require up to 6–12 months before full training can resume. Although there is limited evidence for any improvement in long term outcome, intralesional injection of stem cells or platelet rich plasma may be used initially to enhance healing.

Luxation of the SDF is usually treated conservatively. Surgical replacement and repair of the fibrous attachments is described but is not always successful and associated with complications. If the SDF tendon stabilizes in its new position, the horse will be sound. Intermittent luxation is more problematic and arthroscopic resection of the damaged figrocartilagenous cap of the tendon is required to allow the tendon to fully luxate and stabilize.[61]

Prognosis

Tendinitis of the gastrocnemius carries a guarded prognosis for future athletic performance. These injuries are often chronic when diagnosed and they can affect a significant portion of the tendon. The chronicity, extent and restriction of motion by the scar tissue will all combine to decrease the prognosis for athletic use.[60] Luxations of the SDF have a good prognosis once the tendon is stable in the new position.[61]

Prevention

There are few specific recommendations that can be made to prevent these injuries. Early recognition of athletes with gastrocnemius tendinitis may improve the prognosis by allowing adequate therapy (rest, rehabilitation, extracorporeal shock wave) to be instituted prior to the development of debilitating scar tissue, large defects and adhesions.

Peritarsal cellulitis

Infection of the subcutaneuous tissues surrounding in the tarsal region is an occasional severe problem in Thoroughbred racehorses.[62]

Recognition

Presentation

Affected horses present acutely with generalized swelling of the tarsus and marked lameness. Many have a fever or develop one within 24 hours of presentation.

Physical examination

Affected horses will have generalized swelling around the tarsus. If no analgesics have been administered, the horse will be severely lame and reluctant to flex the limb, although it may improve with walking. The affected area is often extremely painful to touch.

Imaging

Ultrasound is useful to localize abscesses and assess whether synovial structures are involved. Fluid collections within the tissues can be sampled for culture and sensitivity. Often there are synovial effusions due to the surrounding inflammation, but associated synovial infection is rare and synovial fluid will be anechoic. If there is any evidence of echogenicity within the synovial fluid, a sample should be collected. Ultrasound is essential to avoid passing a needle through an abscess and contaminating the synovial structure.

Diagnosis

The diagnosis is based on the clinical presentation and ultrasound examination. Radiographs may be required to differentiate other causes of severe lameness and tarsal swelling such as fractures. The causative organism will often be cultured from abscess fluid.

Treatment and prognosis

Treatment

Broad spectrum antibiotics should be commenced prior to obtaining culture and sensitivity results. Non-steroidal anti-inflammatories should be administered and forced walking exercise if helpful if lameness improves with walking. If abscesses develop, percutaneous drainage is beneficial.

Prognosis

Most cases of peritarsal cellulitis respond well to aggressive antibiotic and anti-inflammatory treatment. In rare cases, synovial structures or underlying bone becomes involved and these cases will have guarded prognosis.

Prevention

As the cause is not known it is difficult to give recommendations on how to prevent this condition.

Stifle

Anatomy

The stifle is separated into three compartments; the femoropatellar joint, and the lateral and medial femorotibial joints. Communication between these is variable with no communication in 17.5% of horses, all compartments communicating in 17.5% of horses and the femoropatellar and medial femorotibial communicating in the remainder (65%).[63] Swelling of the femoropatellar joint is readily detected dorsally between the patellar ligaments. Swelling of the medial femortibial joint occurs just proximal to the tibial plateau and cranial to the medial collateral ligament. Swelling of the lateral femortibial joint is not commonly detected due to the overlying musculature.

The joint is stabilized by a complex of ligaments. The three patellar ligaments continue the quadriceps apparatus distal to the patellar (Fig. 19.21). The cranial and caudal cruciate ligaments are extrasynovial located in the septum between the lateral and medial femorotibial joints (Fig. 19.21). Further soft tissues stabilizing the stifle include the lateral and medial collateral ligaments, and two menisci and their associated ligaments (Fig. 19.21).

Osteochondrosis of the stifle

The stifle is a common site for osteochondrosis in the horse. Osteochondral fragmentation and flap formation affects the lateral trochlear ridge, the medial trochlear ridge and the patella. Subchondral cystic lesions (SC) most commonly occur in the medial condyle of the femur.

Recognition

Presentation

With the widespread use of screening radiographs for yearling sales, clinical presentation of horses with osteochondrosis of the stifle is less common as the majority are identified prior to signs developing.[64] If detected early, horses with osteochondral fragmentation will present with swelling of the femoropatellar joint and mild or no lameness. In contrast, subchondral bone cysts present with lameness of varying severity, often moderate to severe.

Physical examination

Horses with clinically significant ostechondrosis of the trochlear ridges or patella have effusion of the femoropatellar joint and no or mild hindlimb lameness. As these are often young horses that may have received limited handling, manipulative tests can be difficult. There is generally little response to flexion, but flexion tests may be positive. If lameness is more marked, significant joint compromise is likely.

Horses with subchondral bone cysts may have effusion of the medial femorotibial joint and often mild effusion of the femoropatellar joint as well.

Diagnostic analgesia is rarely required for femoropatellar lesions due to the presence of obvious swelling. Swelling of the medial femorotibial joint can be more difficult to detect and diagnostic analgesia may therefore be required to localize the lameness. All three compartments should be blocked at once.

Diagnosis

Radiographs of the stifle are usually diagnostic for the condition although the full extent of the intra-articular pathology is not always evident and some mild lesions may be radiographically silent. In these cases ultrasonographic examination of the cartilage of the dorsal aspect of the trochlear ridges with the probe positioned between the patellar ligaments may reveal cartilage defects in the femoropatellar joint not visible radiographically.[65]

Both stifles should be radiographed, as the condition is commonly bilateral[66], even though the clinical signs or radiographic changes may be more obvious or severe on one limb. The lateromedial and oblique views are best suited to evaluate lesions of the lateral or medial trochlear ridge of the distal femur or rarely the patella (Fig. 19.22, Fig. 19.23). There may be subchondral lucencies or flattening of the subchondral bone, most commonly on the mid to distal aspect of the lateral trochlear ridge, but they can occur anywhere on either ridge (Fig. 19.22, Fig. 19.23). Mineralized or ossified cartilage fragments that are attached or loose can also be present along the articular margin of the trochlear ridges, trochlear groove or patella, either within the articular defects or loose distally in the joint. The radiographic appearance of osteochondrosis lesions will usually underestimate their severity. The caudocranial view will usually reveal the central location of the subchondral cyst of the medial femoral condyle (Fig. 19.24). An oblique caudolateral-craniomedial view or a flexed lateromedial view may allow better visualization of medial condylar cysts when limited power radiographic equipment is available and also shows the extent of joint surface involvement in the craniocaudal plane (Fig. 19.25). In long-standing cases of stifle OC, there may be radiographic evidence of osteoarthritis along the articular joint margins. Scintigraphy is useful for identifying SC lesions of the medial femoral condyle but caudal views are important as the lateral condyle attenuates the radiation in a lateral view.

Treatment and prognosis

Treatment

Osteochondral flaps or fragments should be debrided arthroscopically.[10,66]

Arthroscopic debridement has been used to treat subchondral bone cysts of the medial femorotibial joint.[67,68] Relatively poor success rates for this treatment have prompted the development of alternative treatments. Injection of corticosteroids into the soft tissue lining the cyst has shown some promise.[69] Although injection into the cyst can be performed under ultrasound guidance, accurate placement of the drug in the lining of the cyst is best achieved under

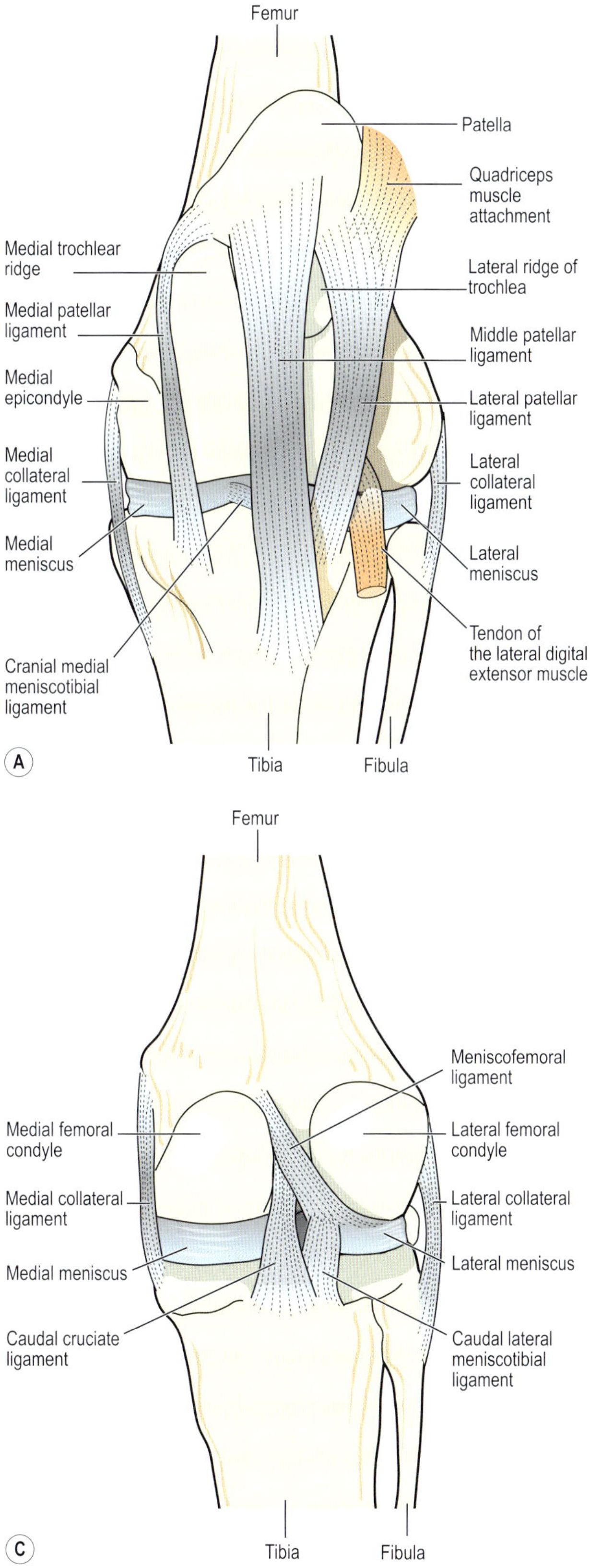

Fig 19.21 **(A)** Cranial aspect of the stifle joint. **(B)** Medial aspect of the stifle joint. **(C)** Caudal aspectof the stifle joint.

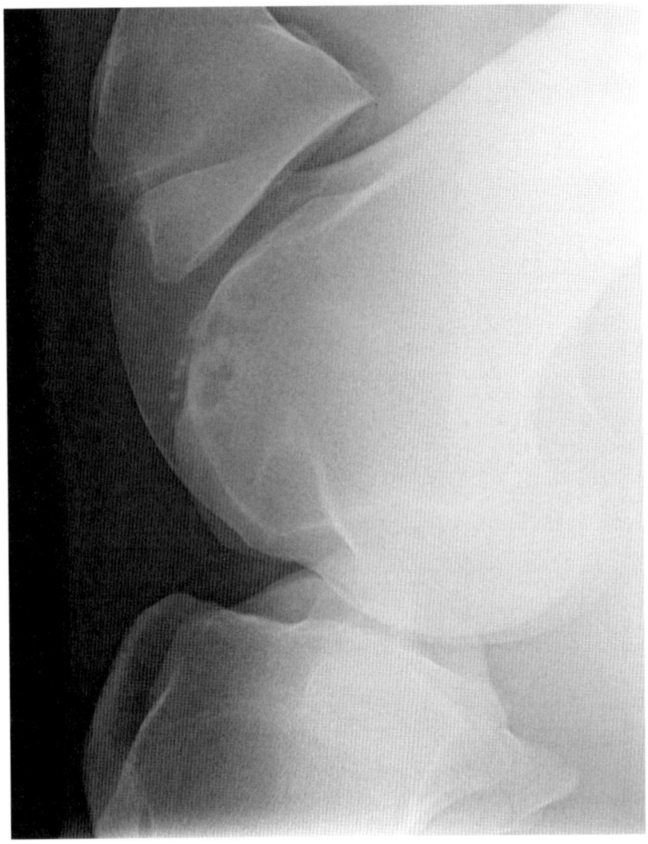

Fig 19.22 A lateromedial view of the stifle of a three-year-old Warmblood horse with an osteochondrosis lesion of the lateral trochlear ridge of the femur. There is lucency of the subchondral bone of the lateral trochlear ridge and osteochondral fragmentation of the proximal part of the ridge.

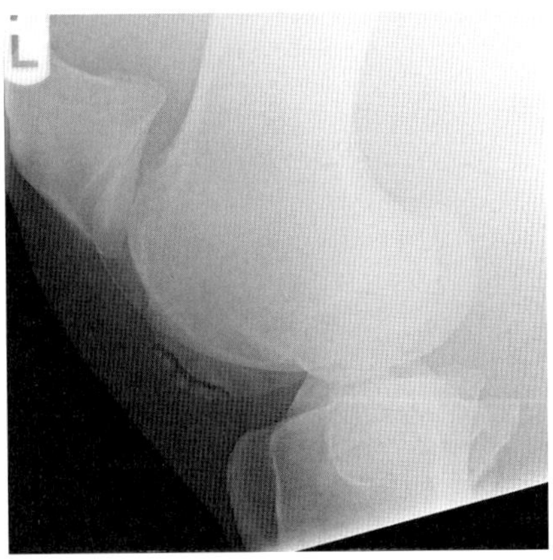

Fig 19.23 A caudolateral craniomedial view of the stifle of a mature Thoroughbred with an osteochondrosis lesion of the lateral trochlear ridge of the femur. The lateral trochlear ridge is irregular and there are multiple ostechondral fragments.

arthroscopic guidance. A similar success rate to surgical debridement has been reported however the return to work is quicker and the option of surgery remains if the treatment is unsuccessful.[69] Many cysts will persist radiographically, but this has no bearing on the success rate. Horses are rested for two weeks prior to beginning controlled walking exercise. If the lameness has resolved at 30 or 60 days, the horse can return to work.

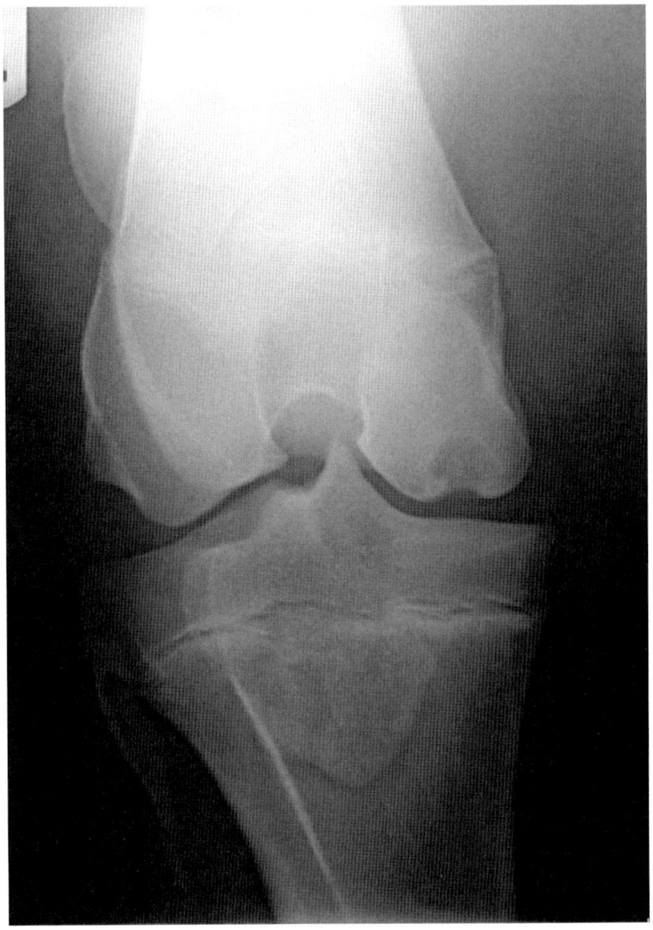

Fig 19.24 A caudocranial view of the stifle of a yearling Thoroughbred with a large subchondral bone cyst of the medial condyle of the femur.

Postoperative pain may be significant in horses with cystic lesions or large osteochondrosis lesions operated on bilaterally. Use of intra-articular mepivicaine or narcotics (morphine sulfate, 6–15 mg) at the conclusion of surgery will reduce articular pain and often will improve recovery from general anesthesia. Epidural analgesics in the immediate postoperative period may make pain management more effective. Stall confinement for 4–6 weeks is necessary and a gradual reintroduction to hand-walking started at 10–14 days. Gradual return to exercise after five months may be an option for horses with smaller lesions while those with extensive lesions may require 6–9 months of rest.

Postoperative use of anti-inflammatory and chondroprotective agents will decrease discomfort and may maximize the quality and quantity of repair tissue in the defect. Various methods have been used to fill the large defect left following debridement of subchondral cystic lesions however none have gained widespread use clinically.[70–72]

Conservative treatment of stifle osteochondrosis is suitable for OCD lesions in younger horses where lysis is the only radiographic sign, prior to fragmentation. Conservative treatment is also recommended for flattening or indentation of the medial femoral condyle. Horses treated conservatively should be rested for 6–8 months with frequent radiographic monitoring for progression of healing. Radiographic resolution of the lesions is usually very slow and incomplete. Often the initiation of exercise will exacerbate the lameness, requiring more aggressive surgical treatment. Conservative therapy

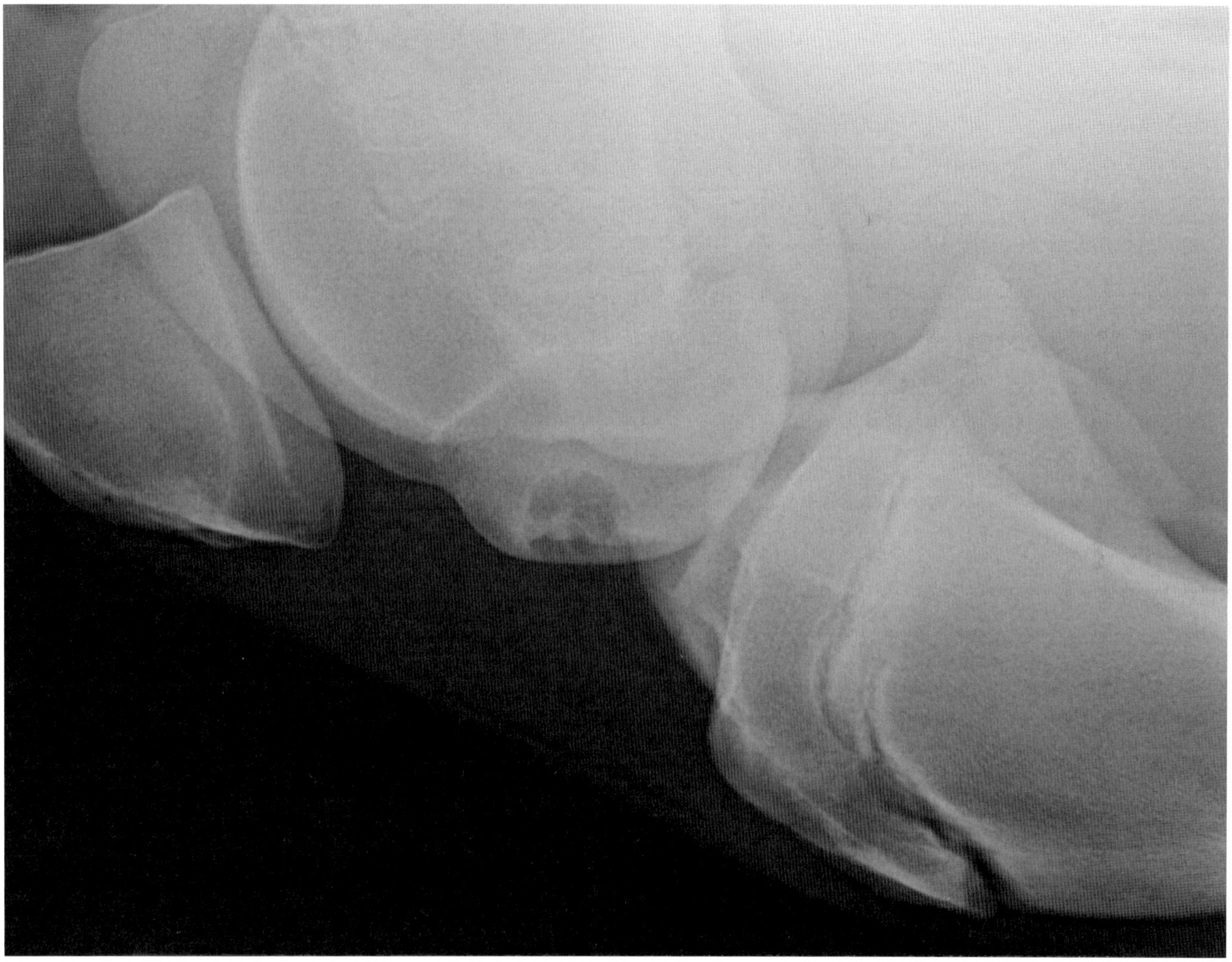

Fig 19.25 A flexed lateral view of the same horse as in Fig. 19.15 showing the craniocaudal extent of the subchondral bone cyst.

may result in loss of the early part of an athletic career if, after a prolonged lay-off, there is no radiographic or clinical improvement and surgery is then required.

Prognosis

Stifle OC carries a good prognosis for return to athletic activity in most horses with small defects treated arthroscopically.[67] The prognosis is more guarded in horses with femoral trochlear ridge lesions greater than 2 cm in length, and approximately 50% of horses with lesions greater than 4 cm are able to perform athletically.[66] Subchondral cysts of the stifle also have a guarded prognosis. Similar results have been achieved with intra-lesional injection of corticosteroids and with surgical debridement with approximately 60% of horses treated successfully.[67,69] Bilateral SC have a poorer prognosis than unilateral lesions.[69]

Prevention

Since the disease is multifactorial, complete prevention is unlikely. Maintaining balanced mineral (copper, zinc, calcium and phosphorus) levels in the diet and avoiding excessive grain feeding is recommended. Delaying rigorous training may reduce the incidence in horses that are skeletally immature and predisposed to traumatically induced subchondral bone damage and the development of growth cartilage defects.

Etiology and pathophysiology

Osteochondrosis is a developmental disease characterized by disorders of the growing cartilage in the epiphysis and growth plates.[11,13,14,73,74]

Epidemiology

The disease has worldwide distribution and varied breed predilection. The incidence of the disease may vary from one farm to another and between geographical areas, highlighting the multifactorial nature of the disease. It is a disease of young horses and is reported frequently in breeds used for speed events such as Standardbreds, Thoroughbreds, Warmbloods and Quarter Horses. Exercise in these breeds at a young age in conjunction with genetic or nutritional predispositions may account for its expression.

Stifle fractures

Fractures of the stifle generally follow direct trauma. This is most common in horses that jump unforgiving obstacles such as eventers and hunters. The patella, tibial crest and femoral trochlear ridges all project cranially and are therefore subject to fracture. These injuries will often have concurrent articular soft tissue or ligament injuries that will make diagnosis, treatment and rehabilitation very challenging. Prompt recognition, adequate case selection and excellent clinical therapy are important aspects of managing these injuries in adult horses to restore joint stability and function.

Recognition

Presentation

There is usually a history of an acute onset of severe lameness of a hindlimb after a fall or impact. Marked swelling, pain or crepitus over the cranial aspect of the stifle or proximal tibia of the affected limb is common. In horses with complete transverse patellar fractures, there may be an inability to maintain the stifle in extension during any attempt at weight bearing, with an obvious protrusion of the distal femoral trochlear ridges. Any attempt to manipulate the stifle will cause marked discomfort and palpation of the periarticular structures will reveal crepitation. There may be obvious soft tissue defects or contusions if the injury resulted from direct impact trauma. These soft tissue injuries need to be completely evaluated to determine if the soft tissues are viable and if communication with the underlying bone or joint is present. Open fractures with devitalized soft tissues will complicate therapy, minimize options and worsen the prognosis. If the fracture has an intra-articular component, the degree of femoropatellar and/or femorotibial effusion or hemorrhage will be readily palpable. Horses with distal patellar fragmentation usually present with less severe lameness, femoropatellar effusion and soft tissue swelling.[9,39,41,42]

Special examination

Intra-articular anesthesia or limb manipulations are not necessary in horses with complete sagittal, transverse or comminuted patellar fractures or those with tibial tuberosity or distal femoral fractures. The clinical presentation will usually localize the lameness to the stifle. Horses with distal patellar fragmentation or stress fractures will have a less obvious clinical presentation and intra-articular anesthesia or limb manipulations will be necessary.[75,76]

Radiographs of the stifle are necessary to make an accurate diagnosis, formulate a therapeutic plan and determine a prognosis. Transverse or comminuted patellar fractures are imaged on standard lateromedial, caudocranial and flexed lateromedial views. When sagittal patellar or medial patellar avulsion fractures are suspected, the dorsoproximal to dorsodistal (skyline) view (Fig. 19.26) is ideal for imaging the size of the fragments and the location of the fracture line.[75] The caudomedial to craniolateral and caudolateral to craniomedial oblique views are necessary to visualize bony fragments associated with distal patellar avulsions or fragmentation. Distomedial patellar fragmentation may be evident in horses after medial patellar ligament desmotomy was performed for treatment of intermittent upward fixation of the patella.[77] The flexed lateromedial or skyline view may be hard to obtain in painful horses. Sedation (detomidine 0.01–0.02 mg/kg i.v. and/or butorphanol 0.01–0.02 mg/kg i.v.) or intra-articular anesthesia may facilitate the manipulations necessary to obtain adequate images. Radiographic quality and completeness will affect preoperative planning and formulation of a prognosis. Tibial tuberosity or distal femoral fractures can be imaged on the lateromedial, caudocranial or oblique views. These radiographs should be carefully evaluated for any intra-articular component or fracture line propagation. Tibial tuberosity fractures may be confused with the active tibial tuberosity physis present in horses up to three or four years of age and in these cases the lateromedial radiograph of the opposite tibia should be used for comparison.[78,79]

Ultrasonography of the patellar ligaments and the CoL is indicated for all horses with patellar, tibial tuberosity or distal femoral

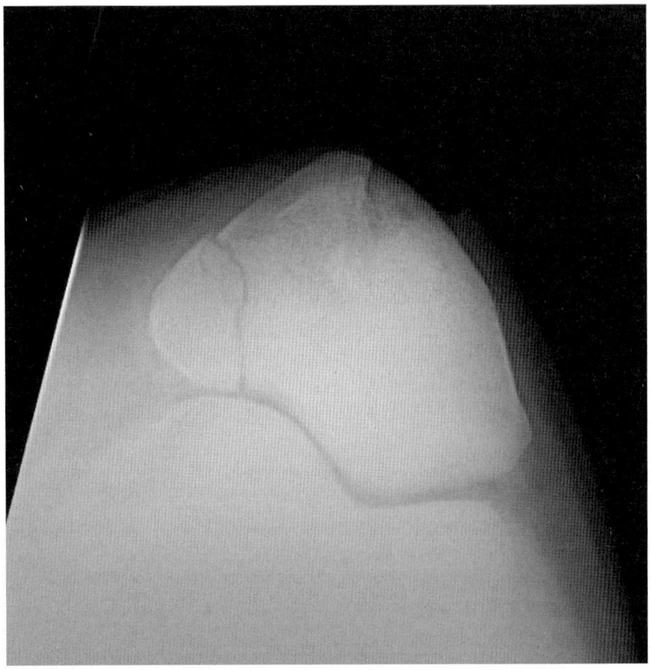

Fig 19.26 A dorsoproximal dorsodistal skyline view of the stifle of a 12-year-old eventer with a non-displaced fracture of the medial pole of the patella. These fractures are difficult to appreciate on other radiographic views.

fractures. These scans can be performed standing using a 7.5–15.0 MHz linear probe positioned directly over each structure. It is not uncommon to sustain concurrent ligament (patellar, CoL and CrL) or intra-articular soft tissue (MM and articular cartilage) injuries with these fractures.[76] Scintigraphy may be helpful in the diagnosis of incomplete stress fractures or traumatically induced osteitis of the patella, distal femur or proximal tibia.

Diagnosis

The clinical presentation and lameness evaluation will localize the source of lameness to the stifle. Diagnosis of these injuries is dependent on adequate and detailed radiographic studies of the stifle. Special views (skyline) are necessary when unusual fracture configurations are suspected (Fig. 19.26). Ultrasonographic evaluation will reveal concurrent soft tissue injuries. Accurate imaging is imperative to permit optimal therapeutic selection and prognosis.

Treatment and prognosis

Treatment

Before any therapy is attempted, a precise and accurate diagnosis of all affected bony or soft tissue structures is imperative. The therapeutic aim is to stabilize fractures amenable to internal fixation, remove any intra-articular fragments that cannot be reduced and stabilized but contribute little to joint stability and debride or remove any damaged soft tissues.[76,79,80]

Surgical treatment of sagittal patellar fractures involves removal of the smaller (usually medial) fragment. Small fragments can be removed arthroscopically.[81] Larger fragments may require an arthrotomy directly over the fragment in order to complete dissection of the soft tissue attachments.

Internal fixation of patellar fractures is reserved for fractures resulting in disruption of the quadriceps mechanism (transverse or comminuted). Conservative management of these will invariably fail and lead to persistent pain, osteoarthritis and joint fibrosis with contralateral limb breakdown. Transverse fractures can be stabilized using 5.5 mm cortical or 6.5 mm cancellous lag screws reinforced with a tension band of 16 or 18 gauge orthopedic wire to neutralize the pull of the quadriceps apparatus.[80] The aim of any surgical procedure is to restore continuity of the quadriceps mechanism and re-establish congruency of the joint surface. Assisted recovery from anesthesia is important to minimize disruption of the internal fixation and incisional dehiscence. After surgery, cross-tying the patient for 4–6 weeks will prevent recumbency and minimize incisional or orthopedic implant failure.

Non-displaced fractures may be diagnosed radiographically or with scintigraphy and can be treated conservatively with stall rest and cross-tying for 3–6 weeks. They should be serially radiographed to insure that the pull of the quadriceps does not displace the fracture during convalescence. Displaced fractures and those with an intra-articular component should be surgically repaired using a tension band principle to offset the pull of the quadriceps muscle through the middle patellar ligament.[79,82]

Large fractures with an intra-articular component can be repaired using a 4.5 mm broad dynamic compression plate (DCP) with 4.5 or 5.5 mm cortical screws.[78,79,83] The 5.5 mm screws have greater holding power and the broad DCP with the staggered screw hole configuration will reduce the probability of inducing horizontal fissures through the fractured tuberosity.[78] However, the 4.5 mm narrow DCP is more easily contoured to the cranial aspect of the tibia, thereby avoiding placement of the screws in one plane.[79,83] Alternatively, 4.5 or 5.5 mm cortical lag screws can be used with 16 or 18 gauge orthopedic wire in a tension band principle to secure smaller fractures.[78] Small non-displaced fragments can be treated conservatively to minimize disruption of the attachment of the middle patellar ligament to the tibia during attempts at surgical removal or the fragments can be carefully removed if they are unstable or causing lameness.[79] After surgery, horses should be assisted during the recovery and confined to a stall for 6–8 weeks.[78,79] Handwalking or exercise can be gradually introduced after radiographic evaluations of complete fracture healing.

Adult athletes with comminuted or over-riding distal femoral fractures that involve the diaphysis, metaphysis or femoral condyle(s) should be humanely destroyed.[84] The small or comminuted distal fragments are not usually large enough to permit secure fixation with orthopedic implants. Non-displaced distal femoral Salter-Harris physeal fractures that occur in young (18–20 months) horses will generally respond to conservative treatment and will usually heal in 8–12 weeks. Femoral condylar fragments that involve less than 25% of the caudal aspect of the condyle in an adult horse can be removed surgically via a caudal arthrotomy or arthroscopic approach.[85]

Prognosis

The prognosis for horses following removal of sagittal patellar fractures fragments is good with up to a third of the patellar being able to be removed without complications.[76,81] Follow up of large numbers of transverse patellar fractures has not been reported. Horses with significant comminution of the patella have a worse prognosis due to difficulty in re-establishment of joint congruity.

Horses with tibial tuberosity fractures that are non-displaced or displaced fractures that can be adequately reduced and secured at surgery have a favorable prognosis for return to athletic function if the implants and soft tissues remain intact during the recovery and early postoperative period. Horses in which significant disruption of either occurs postoperatively will have a poor prognosis for use or pain-free ambulation.[78,79]

Adult horses with femoral condylar fractures involving less than 25% of the condyle treated surgically (fragment removal) may be able to return to athletic use.[85] Those with non-displaced distal femoral physeal fractures have an excellent prognosis for full return to function if displacement or limb contracture does not occur.

Prevention

There is no effective way to prevent these athletic injuries. Attention to footing, conditioning and level of training in light of the degree of difficulty of the endeavor may reduce the possibility of an accident causing one of these injuries.

Etiology and pathophysiology

Patellar fractures in adult horses occur infrequently and are the result of a kick or collision with a fence or cross rail while jumping.[75] When the stifle is flexed (as in jumping), the patella is fixed in the trochlear groove, concentrating the force of the impact on the patella.

Tibial tuberosity fractures are caused by blunt or impact trauma to the cranial aspect of the dorsal tibia, which has little soft tissue coverage to dissipate any disruptive force applied directly to it. The physis of the tibial tuberosity does not completely ossify and fuse with the proximal tibial epiphysis until 2–3 years of age. The quadriceps muscle group attaches to the tibial tuberosity through the middle patellar ligament. This attachment may concentrate distractive forces during contraction or loading of the quadriceps apparatus.

Distal femoral fractures in adult horses are rare and traumatically induced after a kick or collision. There is often a marked amount of soft tissue trauma associated with these injuries.

Epidemiology

These injuries can occur in any type of athletic horse involved in a discipline in which a sudden loss of footing at high speed can occur or full-speed exercise around or over immovable objects is undertaken.

Meniscal injuries

The stifle is stabilized by a complex array of soft tissues. Soft tissue stifle injuries can cause lameness which, in the absence of swelling, may result in few radiographic changes and therefore be difficult to diagnose. Meniscal injuries are the most common soft tissue injury of the stifle.[86] They may occur due to an acute traumatic event but degeneration of menisci is also observed which may be the result of previously undiagnosed trauma or chronic instability.

Horses have a medial and lateral meniscus. Each cupped fibrocartilaginous meniscus functions to provide stability and congruency between the rounded femoral condyles and the flat tibial condyles at the femorotibial articulation (Fig. 19.21). Cranial and caudal attachments (meniscal ligaments) to the tibia maintain the menisci in position during locomotion (Fig. 19.21). The medial meniscus and medial CoL are firmly attached to each other.

Recognition

Presentation

Horses with meniscal injuries may present with an acute onset of moderate to severe unilateral hindlimb lameness. For more chronic cases the lameness may be milder. Occasionally lameness will be more insidious in onset and in some rare cases bilateral lameness may occur. Swelling has rarely been observed by riders, owners or trainers. Meniscal injury may accompany other soft tissue or bony injuries to the stifle.

Physical examination

Horses with injuries of the medial meniscus will generally have swelling on the medial aspect of the stifle. Detection of swelling may require careful palpation in many cases just proximal to the tibial crest and cranial to the medial collateral ligament with the horse standing square. Swelling of the lateral femorotibial joint is rarely detectable clinically. In the acute phase, many will resent limb flexion often abducting the limb in an exaggerated manner and full limb flexion tests will be positive. When trotting, reduced flexion in the swing phase may result in a consistent toe-drag. In horses with concurrent injury to the cranial cruciate ligament (CrL) the degree of stifle instability will be more pronounced.

Intra-articular anesthesia of all three stifle joint compartments will usually improve the lameness but the response is variable depending on the severity of the injury and additional extracapsular soft tissue or intra-articular cartilage structures involved.[87]

Imaging

Substantial medial meniscal tears will cause collapse of the medial femorotibial joint space on the caudocranial radiographic projection. Periarticular modeling and subchondral bone sclerosis will be observed radiographically in chronic cases. Modelling may also be observed on the cranial aspect of the intercondylar eminence of the tibia. Ultrasonography is essential for a complete examination of the stifle and allows visualization of a large proportion of the lateral and medial menisci.[88] A sensitivity of 79% and a specificity of 56% has been reported for the detection of meniscal tears.[89] Ultrasonography of the menisci can be performed with a linear or microconvex transducer along the cranial, lateral and medial aspects of the femorotibial joint.[88–90] Defects or injuries of the MM may be imaged as hypoechoic areas in the horn or ligament at the axial or cranial portion of the structure (Fig. 19.27). The scintigraphic appearance of the stifle of horses with meniscal tears is variable.[89] Arthroscopy allows direct examination of the cranial and caudal parts of the menisci although visualization of the whole meniscus, especially the caudal aspect of the lateral meniscus is limited.[88]

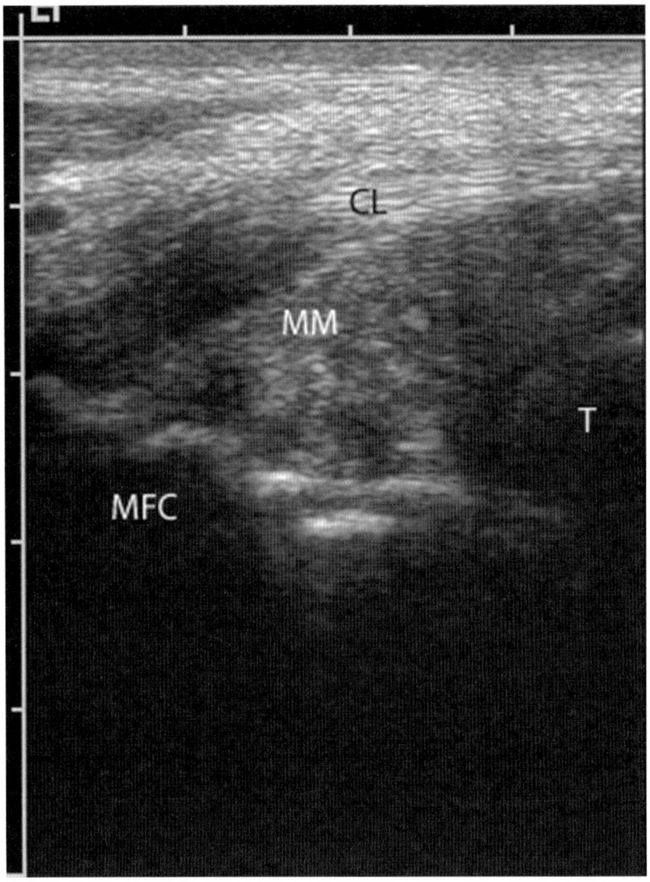

Fig 19.27 A longitudinal ultrasound view of a medial meniscus of a nine-year-old Warmblood horse with a meniscal injury. Proximal is to the left of the image. The meniscus (MM) lies deep to the collateral ligament (CL) and proximal to the tibia (T). It has irregular hypoechoic areas and the surface of the medial femoral condyle (MFC) is also irregular.

Diagnosis

Differential diagnoses include other causes of acute lameness originating from the stifle such as fractures, cruciate or patellar ligament injuries, and sepsis. Chronic injuries need to be differentiated from stifle lameness caused by subchondral bone cysts, synovitis and osteoarthritis secondary to instability or inflammation. The physical examination and the radiographic and ultrasonographic may be suggestive but definitive diagnosis requires arthroscopic visualization of the injury. Both the cranial and caudal pouches of the femorotibial joints need to be entered for a complete examination of the menisci.[87,91,92]

Treatment and prognosis

Treatment

Arthroscopic surgery of the femorotibial joints is essential to determine the extent of the injury as well as enabling treatment. The most appropriate treatment depends on the configuration of the tear. Loose or unstable tissue, usually at the cranial axial aspect of the meniscus, should be debrided.[87] Longer more abaxial tears may disappear from view under the femoral condyle making debridement challenging and the resulting defect extremely large (Fig. 19.28). For these cases, some method of repair is required. Two repair options include implantation of stems cells or intra-articular suturing, neither of which have been trialed in large numbers of affected horses. Stall rest for 4–8 weeks will minimize further damage to the MM and associated soft tissue. Systemic (NSAID and chondroprotectives) and/or intra-articular (hyaluronic acid and/or corticosteroids) therapy can be used to control the deleterious effects of synovitis on intra-articular structures.

Prognosis

Horses with lesions confined to the cranial ligament and cranial horn of the meniscus have a fair to good prognosis for returning to athletic competition following arthroscopic debridement and prolonged rest (6–9 months).[87] Athletes with large tears involving the body of the meniscus as it courses under the femoral condyle, complete avulsion of the cranial attachment and concurrent CoL or CrL damage have a poor prognosis for athletic use.[87]

Prevention

Because the majority of meniscal tears are a result of trauma prevention is difficult and involves reducing exposure to traumatic events.

Etiology and pathophysiology

Meniscal injuries can result from crushing forces when the femur rotates over the menisci with the leg in extension during high-speed athletic activities or a traumatic event such as a fall or kick.[93]

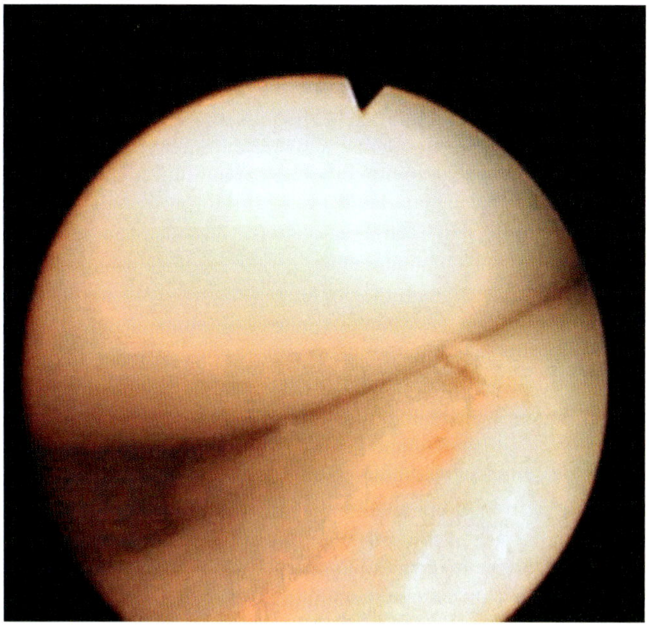

Fig 19.28 An arthroscopic view of the cranial pouch of the medial femortibial joint of the same horse as in Fig. 19.27 showing a tear extending longitudinally through the cranial meniscal ligament into the medial meniscus under the medial femoral condyle. This type of tear is not amenable to debridement and was treated by implantation of stem cells.

Meniscal injuries can occur following joint instability caused by cruciate ligament disruptions and may be a sequelae to a subchondral cystic lesion. Small lesions confined to the cranial horn or ligament of the meniscus may cause minimal stifle instability but the ensuing synovitis from the damaged soft tissue can cause chronic lameness and, if not treated in a timely fashion, shorten an athletic career. Extensive lesions involving the body of the meniscus or those that occur in conjunction with other soft tissue injuries will often end a career due to the resulting stifle instability.

Epidemiology

Meniscal injuries are more common in horses competing in jumping disciplines, participating in galloping events with sudden stops and turns or during a fall or traumatic event during a competition. Poor footing, extreme course difficulty and inadequate conditioning or talent may also be contributory.

Cruciate ligament injuries

Cranial cruciate ligament (CrL) injuries in horses usually involve the ligament rather than its bony insertions and are more common than caudal CrL injuries. Avulsion fractures at the attachments are less common and will generally occur in combination with the mid-body injury. The prognosis for cruciate ligament injury is poor.

Horses have paired (cranial and caudal) CrLs that are extrasynovial and located in the septum between the medial and lateral femorotibial joints (Fig. 19.21A). They provide stability to the stifle joint and limit cranial or caudal movements of the tibia or femur during locomotion. The CrLs are loaded maximally during stifle extension and the caudal CrL is axially rotated during stifle flexion.[94] During weight bearing the CrLs will limit rotation and forward displacement of the tibia and stabilize the medial aspect of the femorotibial joint.[94] Cranial CrL injuries are more common in horses and are often accompanied by other soft tissue injuries (CoL or MM).[87,95] Caudal CrL injuries may occur independently or may accompany cranial CrL injuries.[96]

Recognition

Presentation

Horses with a cranial CrL injury present with an acute onset of moderate to severe lameness and often have a history of a fall, loss of footing with a sudden forceful attempt to regain it or colliding with an immovable object.[75]

Physical examination

There is moderate to severe lameness characterized by non-weight bearing or toe-touching gait on the affected limb immediately following the injury. Over time the lameness may improve but the horse will remain reluctant to flex the stifle during the swing phase and will not completely load the tibia during the stance phase of the stride. Effusion of the medial femorotibial joint is usually discernible in acute cases but may resolve in more chronic cases. Flexion of the stifle will often be vigorously objected and will worsen the lameness.[75] Stifle instability and worsening of the lameness may be noted if the tibia is repeatedly rocked caudally while the horse is weight bearing (cruciate test). Crepitus or periarticular thickening is uncommon. Atrophy of the thigh and gluteal musculature is common in chronic cases with marked lameness.

Anesthesia of the medial and/or lateral femorotibial joint will often improve the lameness considerably.[95] However, with complete disruptions of the cranial CrL there will be a residual mechanical instability of the gait. In acute cases, intra-articular anesthesia is rarely necessary.

Imaging

Radiographs are often non-diagnostic because avulsion fractures at the attachments are rare.[97] Even when observed, fractures of the intercondylar eminence of the tibia are often not avulsion fractures and are therefore not specific for cruciate ligament injuries.[98,99] If a weight-bearing lateromedial projection can be obtained, cranial displacement of the proximal tibia relative to the distal femur may be present after complete cranial CrL disruptions. In chronic cases of CrL disruptions, radiographic evidence of degenerative joint disease will be present and mineralization of the damaged CrL may be seen.

Ultrasonographic imaging of a cranial CrL tear can be performed in the standing horse by directing a linear or curvilinear probe parallel and between the medial and middle patellar ligaments with the stifle fully flexed or from a craniolateral approach.[88,90] The tibial insertion of the ligament may not be visible.[88] This requires sedation and/or articular analgesia as many horses with CrL injuries resent this manipulation. Discontinuity of the fiber pattern or size of the structure is suggestive of injury to the cranial CrL. The caudal CrL may be imaged ultrasonographically from the caudal aspect of the femorotibial joint. Arthroscopic surgery will enable accurate evaluation of the CrL and other intra-articular structures.6 Magnetic resonance imaging or computed tomography would be ideally suited for the diagnosis and quantification of intra-articular soft tissue injuries of the equine stifle.

Diagnosis

The differential diagnoses include stifle fractures, soft tissue injuries (CrL, MM), hemorrhage or sepsis. Horses with acute cranial CrL disruptions are usually very lame. Arthroscopic findings are usually diagnostic.[68] Arthroscopic findings may include a variable amount of fiber disruption in the cranial and/or caudal CrL, tearing of the septum between the femorotibial joints, widening of the femorotibial joint space, and concurrent fractures of the intercondylar eminence of the tibia and meniscal injuries.[68]

Treatment and prognosis

Treatment

There are no effective surgical procedures available to reinforce or reconstruct the cranial CrL in horses, as there are in humans, dogs or cattle, due to anatomic differences, biomechanical demands and expectations for eventual outcome. In addition, horses with complete cranial CrL tears have other intra-articular soft tissue injuries that make any attempt at stabilization unrewarding. A craniomedial or craniolateral arthroscopic approach to the femorotibial joints will allow visualization of the CrL, articular septum and menisci.[68,87] Arthroscopic debridement of loose soft tissue associated with partial cranial CrL injuries and lavage to remove protein debris and inflammatory mediators may be effective in minimizing the deleterious effects of synovitis and enable some athletes to return to work. Small fracture fragments from the intercondylar eminence of the tibia can be removed but care must be taken to avoid further damage to the CrL or its attachment. Larger fragments involving the insertion of the cranial CrL can be secured to the parent bone using cortical screws.[98] Lag screw technique may be contraindicated as it could weaken the fragment, causing it to shatter when the implant is tightened.

Concurrent use of systemic and intra-articular anti-inflammatory or chondroprotective therapy after surgery is indicated. Complete rest (6–9 months) may increase the strength of the repair tissue in the cranial CrL. Hand-walking immediately after surgery is detrimental if any degree of instability is present. Swimming after 4–6 weeks of stall rest will allow the soft tissues to gain strength and increase the range of motion of the joint without loading the healing structures and exacerbating the instability.

Prognosis

The prognosis for future athletic soundness is guarded to poor due to the considerable stifle instability that results from CrL injuries. This will restrict pain-free locomotion and eventually lead to osteoarthritis. Horses with partial injuries without additional soft tissue injuries may return to light work, but return to more demanding disciplines like eventing, jumping or polo may not be a realistic expectation unless the degree of CrL fiber disruption is minimal and stifle stability is not affected. Horses that require constant analgesic or anti-inflammatory medication to remain in work should be retired from competition. Complete CrL tears usually carry a poor prognosis for even a sedentary pain-free life and euthanasia is a humane option.

Prevention

As with all traumatic injuries prevention is extremely difficult.

Etiology and pathophysiology

The cranial CrL is loaded maximally during stifle extension. Most cranial CrL injuries occur when the stifle is impacted or twisted during weight bearing, causing hyperextension.[75] During a fall, internal rotation of the tibia with the stifle fully flexed can exert enough force to tear the cranial CrL. Once disrupted, the stability of the stifle is adversely affected, making precise alignment of the femur and tibia impossible, leading to painful ambulation and degenerative joint disease. Since the CrLs are loaded maximally during stifle extension, most CrL injuries are mid-body tears.[94]

Collateral ligament injuries

The collateral ligaments (CoL) provide lateral and medial stabilization to the stifle (Fig. 19.21B, Fig. 19.21C). The medial CoL attaches to the medial meniscus (MM) at the joint space (Fig. 19.21A, Fig. 19.21B). Injuries to the medial CoL are more common in horses and may be associated with other soft tissue injuries within the stifle.[100]

Recognition

Presentation

Horses with medial CoL injuries will usually present with an acute onset of severe lameness after a traumatic event or fall or with milder lameness when the injury is more chronic.

Physical examination

There will be a variable amount of soft tissue swelling and pain on the medial aspect of the stifle. Chronic injuries may have palpable thickening of the medial CoL, particularly when compared to the unaffected side. Horses with major disruption of the medial CoL will have obvious stifle instability and resent manipulation of the joint. Horses with more subtle injuries will have shortened cranial phase of the stride with decreased stifle flexion and toe dragging on the affected side. Flexion of the proximal limb and a medial CoL stress test (abduction of the limb distal to the stifle) may exacerbate the lameness.

Special examination

Horses with incomplete disruptions of the medial CoL may partially improve after intra-articular analgesia of the medial femorotibial joint. Caudocranial stress radiographs revealing a widened medial joint space or an avulsion fracture of the distal femur or proximal tibia are diagnostic when complete disruptions are present. Chronic injuries may demonstrate a narrowed medial femorotibial joint space and multiple osteophytes or enthesiophytes on the medial aspect on the standard radiographic projections. Ultrasonography of the medial CoL and MM can identify the extent of structural disruption and fiber discontinuity.[88,90] The scans can be performed on the medial aspect of the femorotibial joint with horses standing using a 7.5–15 MHz linear probe (Fig. 19.27). The images should be obtained in a longitudinal and transverse orientation relative to the CoL.[88,90]

Diagnosis

Differential diagnoses include other causes of acute and severe lameness originating from the stifle such as fractures of the femur, patella or proximal tibia, cruciate or patellar ligament injuries, meniscal injuries, sepsis and traumatic patellar luxation. Chronic injuries need to be differentiated from stifle lameness caused by subchondral bone cysts, synovitis, meniscal injuries and osteoarthritis. A definitive diagnosis is based on instability identified on a stressed radiograph or during arthroscopic surgery or an abnormal appearance on ultrasonographic examination.[100] The presence of concurrent soft tissue injuries will also require ultrasound and/or arthroscopic examination.

Treatment and prognosis

Treatment

Stall rest and systemic NSAIDs, chondroprotective agents (polysulfated glycosaminoglycans or hyaluronic acid) and/or intra-articular anti-inflammatory therapy (hyaluronic acid and/or corticosteroids) may be beneficial in horses with acute but partial disruptions of the medial CoL. Intra-articular corticosteroids should be used judiciously as they may delay ligament healing. Arthroscopic debridement of meniscal abrasions or fibrillation may reduce intra-articular inflammation. Stall rest for 4–8 weeks followed by gradual increase in hand-walking for 8–12 weeks should be adequate, depending on the severity of the injury. The horse should be re-evaluated radiographically and ultrasonographically at 6–9 months for soft tissue healing and osteoarthritis before considering a return to athletic activity.

Prognosis

Horses with significant disruption of the medial CoL will respond poorly to attempts at surgical repair and the ensuing stifle instability and meniscal injury make the prognosis for athletic use or pain-free life very poor.[100] The prognosis for horses with subtle injuries is guarded for athletic use and good for life, depending on the severity of the original injury, the degree of stifle instability and whether degenerative joint disease develops. Horses competing in more demanding athletic disciplines have a very guarded prognosis for full return to function.

Prevention

Proper shoeing (caulks when traction is required), avoiding strenuous activity when footing is poor, not placing the horse in competitive events beyond its ability or degree of conditioning, as well as withdrawal from competition if fatigue ensues may help prevent these injuries. Demanding disciplines in horses that are poorly conditioned, lame or schooled improperly may predispose to injuries.

Etiology and pathophysiology

Medial CoL injuries are the result of intense lateral to medial bending stresses during exercise or during a fall. Loss of footing, striking an immovable object or placement of large rotational forces on the stifle during weight bearing can result in CoL injuries in equine athletes. The paired CoL stabilize the stifle medially and laterally and disruptions of the CoL in horses will cause joint instability, impeding ambulation or pain-free exercise. Medial CoL injuries will often involve the MM, adversely affecting joint function.

Epidemiology

Collateral ligament injuries of the stifle are seen more frequently in athletes that jump (event horses, steeplechasers and hunters) or those that participate in disciplines with sudden stops or turns (barrel racing and polo).

Patellar luxation

Patellar luxations in adult horses are usually the result of severe impact trauma from a fall or collision. Affected horses will present with severe lameness and an inability to fix their stifles in extension. Lateral luxations are more frequent.

Horses have three patellar ligaments (medial, middle and lateral). These attach the distal aspect of the patella to the proximal aspect of the tibia (Fig. 19.21). The medial patellar ligament will be pulled over the medial trochlear ridge of the femur when the stifle is locked in extension. Lateral patellar luxations are more common in horses because the large medial trochlear ridge, particularly in adults, usually prevents medial dislocation. Most luxations are congenital or hereditary and seen in miniature horse or pony foals. In adults or young horses, luxation is secondary to trauma or severe hypoplasia of the lateral trochlear ridge as a consequence of osteochondrosis.

Recognition

Presentation

Patellar luxations in adult horses present as an acute onset of severe lameness and swelling of the stifle following a traumatic episode.

Physical examination

There is a severe lameness with marked swelling of the involved stifle. Any attempt to fully bear weight on the leg will lead to an inability to fix the stifle in extension. The patella can usually be palpated laterally or may be displaced distally if the attachments of the quadriceps muscle have become detached from the proximal patella.[101] The horse will usually resent any attempt at limb manipulation or ambulation.

Special examination

Radiographs are usually diagnostic and will reveal the direction of the dislocation. The caudocranial, lateromedial or oblique views are diagnostic for either the more common lateral luxation or the infrequent distal luxation by evaluating the patella in relation to its normal anatomic position in the trochlear groove on the cranial aspect of the femur. A skyline (dorsoproximal to dorsodistal) view of the cranial distal femur will confirm the presence of an empty trochlear groove and the location of the displaced patella (Fig. 19.29). This view may be hard to obtain in a horse with an acute luxation that resists stifle manipulation. The radiographs should be closely evaluated for the presence of any patellar fragmentation, fractures or avulsions that can accompany the luxation. An attempt should be made to evaluate the integrity of the patellar ligaments and medial aspect of the stifle ultrasonographically.

Diagnosis

The differential diagnosis for acute onset of stifle swelling and severe lameness includes disruption of intra-articular soft tissue structures (CrL, menisci, CoL), fractures, hemorrhage, sepsis and cellulitis. The radiographic and physical examination findings are diagnostic for patellar luxation.

Treatment and prognosis

Treatment

Using heavy sedation and possibly a caudal epidural analgesic, the laterally luxated patella should be reduced manually by manipulating it proximally and medially with the horse standing. The manipulation may be difficult and if the horse is attempting to flex the limb while movement of the patella is being attempted, it will make reduction of the lateral luxation impossible. Reduction of the luxation under general anesthesia is generally easier but it will usually re-luxate when the horse attempts to stand and flexes the leg or contracts the quadriceps forcefully. If the luxation can be reduced standing, the horse should be cross-tied for 4–6 weeks to prevent recumbency and extreme joint flexion. Systemically administered analgesics and NSAIDs will help control discomfort and inflammation. Gradual introduction to hand-walking is instituted for another 12–16 weeks, allowing the extracapsular and patellar soft tissue support to adequately fibrose. Ultrasonographic and radiographic imaging should be performed before initiating work to insure complete healing of all the involved structures.

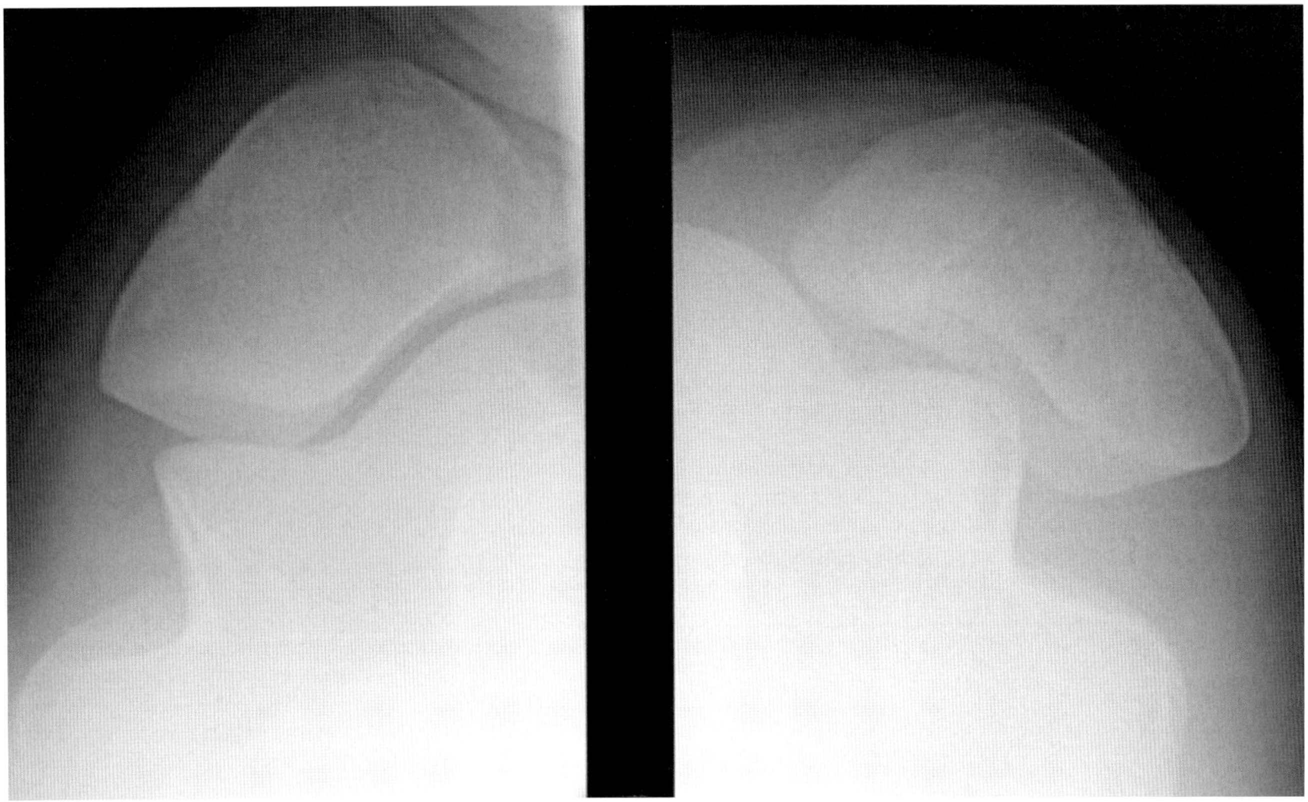

Fig 19.29 Dorsoproximal dorsodistal oblique views of the left (left image) and right stifle of a horse with luxation of the right patella. Both the right patella and the right lateral trochlear ridge have abnormal contours. The condition in this horse appeared to be congenital.

Prognosis

The prognosis for soundness is good if there are minimal concurrent injuries to the intra-articular soft tissue structures and the collateral or patellar ligaments. Marked periarticular fibrosis will worsen the prognosis for return to function and luxations accompanied by significant patellar fractures may be difficult to manage to achieve a successful outcome.[101]

Prevention

These injuries are usually unforeseen and generally not preventable. However, proper shoeing, schooling and conditioning and avoiding precarious footing conditions may help minimize their occurrence.

Etiology and pathophysiology

Patellar luxations are traumatically induced and are usually the result of a fall, collision with a solid object or a kick. A sudden forceful contraction of the quadriceps muscle group during strenuous activity may lead to disruption of their attachments to the proximal patella, predisposing to distal or lateral luxation.[101]

Epidemiology

This disease occurs infrequently and there are few predisposing factors.

Patellar ligament desmitis

Desmitis or tearing of the patellar ligaments in horses is a rare condition. It may be associated with intermittent upward fixation of the patellar or previous medial patellar ligament desmotomy.[102]

Recognition

Presentation

Patellar ligament injuries are most often identified in show jumpers but may affect horses used for other disciplines. These horses may present with an acute onset of lameness, but more commonly chronic lameness or poor performance. Lameness is generally mild to moderate and swelling around the ligaments is often mild or absent but will be more severe in cases of ligament rupture.[102]

Physical examination

There is usually mild effusion of the femoropatellar joint and palpable thickening of the affected ligament or surrounding soft tissues. The ligaments should be palpated both weight bearing and non-weight bearing.[102] The lameness will usually become worse after stifle flexion.

Intra-articular anesthesia of the femoropatellar joint may improve the lameness slightly due to diffusion of anesthetic around the ligament. The response is more dramatic if intra-articular injuries occur concurrently. Local infiltration of the area of the ligament with mepivicaine may also improve the lameness to some degree.

Imaging

Increased uptake of radiopharmaceutical at the tibial insertions of the ligaments has been observed in some horses.[102] Both modelling or fragmentation of the distal aspect of the patellar is observed in some cases radiographically.

Ultrasonographically, desmitis of the ligaments will appear as hypoechoic areas within the affected ligament. The ligaments may be thickened due to edema or scar tissue or have very reflective areas consistent with mineralization. Ultrasonographic evaluations should be performed with the horse weight bearing and the scans compared to the contralateral limb for ligament size and fiber uniformity (Fig. 19.30).[90]

Diagnosis

Patellar ligament desmitis must be differentiated from other causes of acute or chronic stifle lameness. A diagnosis is confirmed by ultrasound examination of the ligaments.[102]

Treatment and prognosis

Treatment

Affected horses should be rested with controlled exercise beginning at 6–12 weeks. Most horses will require at least six months of exercise at a reduced level. Healing of the ligament should be monitored ultrasonographically and return to work recommendations made on the basis of these findings.

Prognosis

Horses with desmitis, partial tears or small avulsion fractures of the patella have a guarded prognosis for return to working soundness.[102] Complete avulsion or tearing of the middle patellar ligament causes marked stifle instability and is generally unresponsive to treatment, making the prognosis for athletic soundness poor.[101,102]

Prevention

These injuries are infrequent and prevention is difficult.

Etiology and pathophysiology

Acute patellar ligament injuries are likely a result of trauma or a sudden forceful contraction of the quadriceps during a fall. The cause of chronic desmitis is unknown.

Epidemiology

Patellar ligament injuries appear to be more common in horses that jump such as show jumpers, eventers, or hunters.[102]

Upward fixation and chondromalacia of the patella

Upward fixation of the patella is usually intermittent but can become persistent. Fixation occurs when the medial patellar ligament remains engaged on the medial trochlear ridge during the swing phase of the stride. It is more common in younger horses and those with upright conformation. Poor quadriceps tone, due to disuse atrophy from injury, inactivity or neurological disease, predisposes to the condition. Chondromalacia of the patella can result

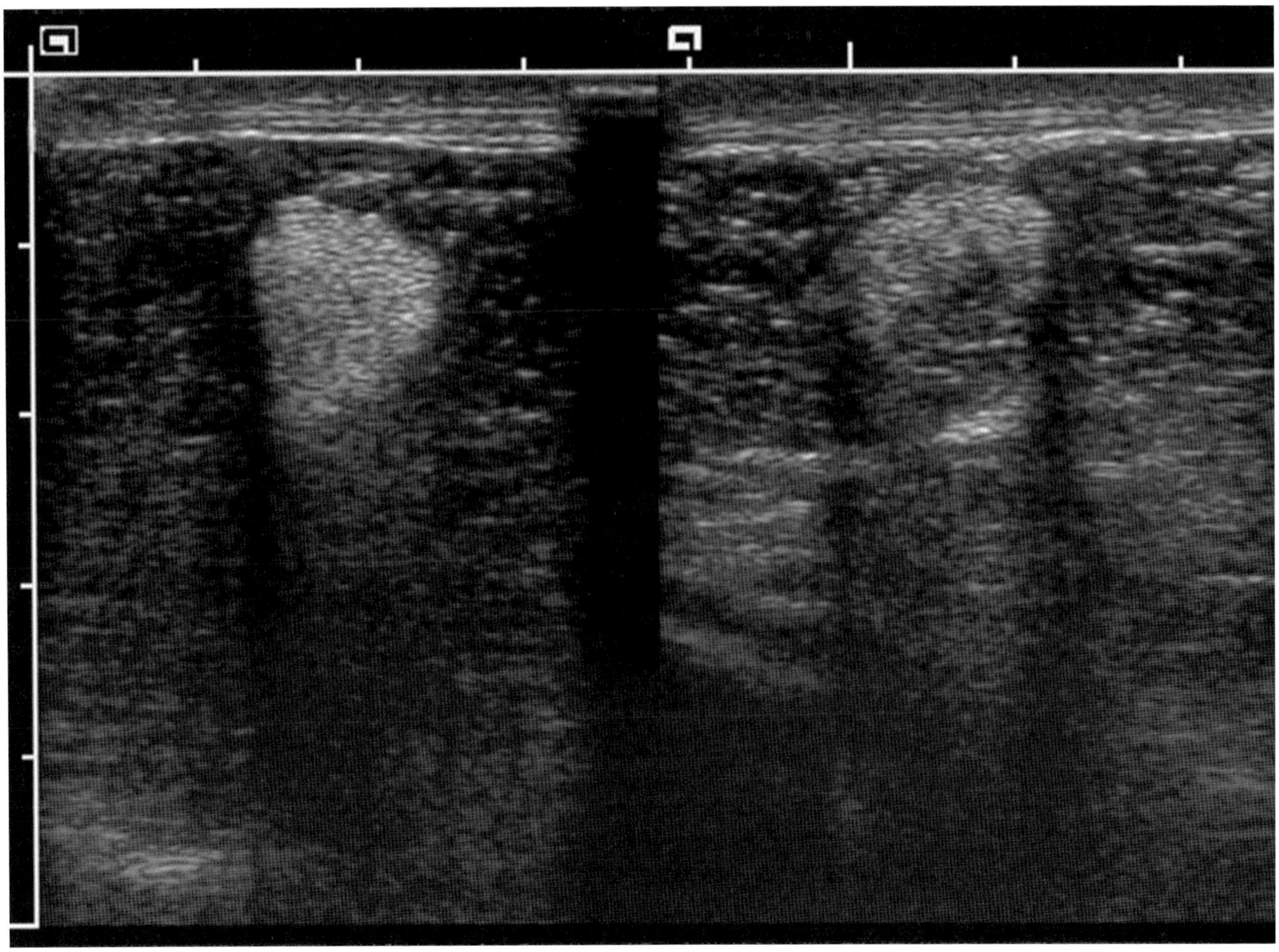

Fig 19.30 Dorsal transverse ultrasound views of the left (left side of image) and right middle patellar ligaments from a 15-year-old eventer. There is a large hypoechoic region in the right middle patellar ligament. Compare with the normal appearance of the left patellar ligament.

from instability or weakness of the quadriceps mechanism or patellar ligaments or as a complication of medial patellar desmotomy.

Recognition

Presention

The presenting complaint and history may entail only a change in gait with an exaggerated action to the cranial phase of the stride or complete inability to move the limb with the affected leg flexed in extension. In some routinely active athletes, there may be a history of a decline or cessation of their work schedule due to an injury or illness, leading to loss of muscle conditioning that will precipitate the condition once a higher level of activity is resumed. Horses with chondromalacia will present with a rear limb lameness of variable duration and severity.

Physical examination

Horses with persistent upward fixation of the patella will present with the affected limb(s) fixed in extension, with an inability to flex their stifle or hock. The distal limb joints can still be flexed. The condition will impede locomotion if bilateral and if unilateral, the horse may advance the affected limb by dragging it in extension. In some horses, excessive wearing of the toe in the affected limb(s) will be apparent. In some cases, backing the horse, manual pressure on the patella, or light sedation may disengage the patella. In many cases, it will recur within a short time. Most cases present as intermittent upward fixation with a prolonged posterior stance phase of the stride and a shortened or exaggerated swing phase which can be evident at every stride or only at variable intervals, depending on surface, incline or duration of exercise. Femoropatellar effusion and response to stifle manipulation and a favorable response to intra-articular anesthesia will be evident in horses with chondromalacia of the patella.

Special examination

The clinical presentation and history are usually diagnostic in most horses. Limb manipulation, intra-articular anesthesia or radiographs are usually unrewarding. If there is an obvious loss of muscle mass associated with the quadriceps or rear limbs, further diagnostic testing for neuromuscular diseases such as equine lower motor neuron disease, shivers, polysaccharide storage disease, or equine protozoal myelitis would be warranted. Young horses with intermittent upward fixation of the patella that present with an upright conformation, flexural contracture or stifle effusion should be evaluated radiographically to determine if there is an underlying developmental orthopedic disease predisposing to the condition. Horses with intermittent upward fixation of the patella may have radiographic evidence of chondromalacia of the patella. Chondromalacia may be the cause or result of upward fixation of the patella and may be a response to chronic inflammation or repeated trauma to the articular cartilage of the patella. The patella may have areas of radiographic lucency or bony proliferation. There may be radiographic evidence of distal medial patellar fragmentation if medial patellar ligament desmotomy was used for treatment of intermittent upward fixation of the patella.

Diagnosis

The principal differential diagnoses include stringhalt, fibrotic myopathy and shivers. Horses with stringhalt will usually have exaggerated hock and stifle flexion that is consistently present at every step and can be severe enough to cause the horse to hit the ventral aspect of the abdomen with the distal limb during walking. The stance phase of the stride in horses with stringhalt is usually normal or shortened. Stringhalt may be unilateral or bilateral, can occur as a herd outbreak and may be related to exposure to certain weeds (Hypochaeris radicata; dandelions), trauma or disease of the sciatic or peroneal nerves.[103] Horses with fibrotic myopathy have a pronounced and consistent interruption of the cranial or swing phase of the stride marked by a rapid caudal movement of the affected limb before it makes contact with the ground. The gait in this condition is characteristic and palpation of the semitendinosus and semimembranosus muscles will reveal the fibrotic component of these muscles that will not be apparent in horses with upward fixation of the patella. Shivers will usually present as an exaggerated flexion of the rear limb and quivering of the tail when the rear limbs are picked up or the horse is backing up or turning in a tight circle. It is often not so obvious when the horse is moving forward in a straight line and may be more common in draft-type horses.

Treatment and prognosis

Treatment

If there is an underlying cause, then its removal or treatment will help recovery or resolution of the upward fixation. In cases with marked atrophy of the quadriceps muscle due to neurological disease, identification and resolution of the neurological disease are necessary to restore muscle function and resolve the condition.

When a lack of muscle tone is present due to inactivity or reduced training schedule, these horses will usually benefit from a gradual reintroduction to work coupled with an increase in the intensity and frequency of exercise until the condition is no longer apparent. For severe cases, exercise regimens that include swimming, underwater treadmill or backing up will increase the strength of the quadriceps muscle group and minimize periods of complete weight bearing that often lead to upward fixation of the patella. As the horse improves, walking up and down a slope will further strengthen the muscles that control patellar movements.

Injection of sclerosing agents such as iodine into or surrounding the patellar ligaments or distal quadriceps has been used clinically to induce fibrosis of the periarticular connective tissue in an attempt to reduce the occurrence of patellar fixation. Injection of 2% iodine or ethanolamine oleate into the medial or middle patellar ligament in horses resulted in a significant accumulation of inflammatory cells and fibroplasia of the ligaments.[104] This fibrous reaction may result in contraction and stiffening of the ligaments and may be responsible for the clinical improvement observed when used in cases of intermittent upward fixation of the patella.[104]

Routine desmotomy of the medial patellar ligament for intermittent upward fixation of the patella is not recommended due to the potential, albeit rarely, of complications.[77,105–109] Desmotomy is indicated when the fixation is permanent and cannot be reduced by manipulation or sedation.[109] The procedure is performed in sedated standing horses under local anesthesia. In order to reduce the risk of complications horses should be box rested for two weeks and gradually returned to exercise over a further 6–12 weeks following surgery. Alternatively, splitting of the proximal third of the medial patellar ligament can resolve upward fixation with less risk of complications.[110] Originally described as being performed under general anesthesia with a number 15 blade this can be performed standing using an 18 gauge needle. The procedure results in a marked enlargement of the proximal third of the ligament which is thought to mechanically prevent upward fixation of the patellar.

Horses with chondromalacia of the patellar should be treated arthroscopically to remove intra-articular fragments and debride soft bone and loose articular cartilage.[111]

Prognosis

The prognosis for athletes with this condition is excellent as the majority will resolve with conditioning. For those that require surgery, the prognosis is also good and the complication rate low if well managed.[109] Those horses that develop chondromalacia of the patella respond well to arthroscopic debridment.[111]

Prevention

There is no general recommendation on preventing this condition in horses. Maintaining a consistent exercise program of adequate rigor for the particular discipline being pursued is usually all that is required. If predisposed athletes have been removed from training or active exercise for a period of time, an incremental approach to training will be helpful in limiting the disruption caused by this gait abnormality. Reducing or eliminating exercise in horses with a weak quadriceps mechanism and avoiding the indiscriminate use of medial patellar ligament desmotomy may prevent chondromalacia of the patella.

Etiology and pathophysiology

An upright conformation and developmental or orthopedic diseases causing pain during stifle flexion can precipitate the condition. Disuse atrophy or neurological dysfunction of the quadriceps muscle group, limiting the ability to disengage the patella from the medial trochlear ridge as the horse moves, is probably the most common cause for this condition. The condition will affect athletic performance by interfering with the normal range of motion of the stifle joint during locomotion.

Chronic trauma to the posterior aspect of the patella caused by stifle instability (idiopathic or iatrogenic) may lead to chondromalacia of the patella.

Epidemiology

The condition can affect any age and use of horse. It may be more common in younger horses or those with decreased quadriceps tone due to underlying disease or inactivity.

With thanks to Federico G. Latimer, who created the original chapter in the first edition.

References

1. Updike SJ. Functional anatomy of the equine tarsocrural collateral ligaments. Am J Vet Res 1984;45(5):867–74.
2. Kraus-Hansen AE, Jann HW, Kerr DV, et al. Arthrographic analysis of communication between the tarsometatarsal and distal intertarsal joints of the horse. Vet Surg 1992;21(2):139–44.
3. Bell BT, Baker GJ, Foreman JH, et al. In vivo investigation of communication between the distal intertarsal and tarsometatarsal joints in horses and ponies. Vet Surg 1993;22(4):289–92.
4. Dyson SJ, Romero JM. An investigation of injection techniques for local analgesia of the equine distal tarsus and proximal metatarsus. Equine Vet J 1993;25(1):30–5.
5. Relave F, Meulyzer M, Alexander K, et al. Comparison of radiography and ultrasonography to detect osteochondrosis lesions in the tarsocrural joint: a prospective study. Equine Vet J 2009;41(1):34–40.
6. Tomlinson JE, Redding WR, Sage A. Ultrasonographic evaluation of tarsocrural joint cartilage in normal adult horses. Vet Radiol Ultrasound 2000;41(5):457–60.
7. Vanderperren K, Raes E, Bree HV, et al. Diagnostic imaging of the equine tarsal region using radiography and ultrasonography. Part 2: bony disorders. Vet J 2009;179(2):188–96.
8. McIlwraith CW, Foerner JJ, Davis DM. Osteochondritis dissecans of the tarsocrural joint: results of treatment with arthroscopic surgery. Equine Vet J 1991;23(3):155–62.
9. Laws EG, Richardson DW, Ross MW, et al. Racing performance of standardbreds after conservative and surgical treatment for tarsocrural osteochondrosis. Equine Vet J 1993;25(3):199–202.
10. McIlwraith CW, Nixon A, Wright IM, et al. Diagnostic and Surgical Arthrscopy in the Horse. 3rd ed. 2005 ed. Philadelphia: Elsevier; 2005.
11. van Weeren PR, Barneveld A. The effect of exercise on the distribution and manifestation of osteochondrotic lesions in the Warmblood foal. Equine Vet J Suppl 1999;(31):16–25.
12. Beard WL, Bramlage LR, Schneider RK, et al. Postoperative racing performance in standardbreds and thoroughbreds with osteochondrosis of the tarsocrural joint: 109 cases (1984–90). J Am Vet Med Assoc 1994;204(10):1655–9.
13. van Weeren PR, Sloet van O-O, Barneveld A. The influence of birth weight, rate of weight gain and final achieved height and sex on the development of osteochondrotic lesions in a population of genetically predisposed Warmblood foals. Equine Vet J Suppl 1999;(31):26–30.
14. Barneveld A, van Weeren PR. Conclusions regarding the influence of exercise on the development of the equine musculoskeletal system with special reference to osteochondrosis. Equine Vet J Suppl 1999;(31):112–19.
15. Mirams M, Tatarczuch L, Ahmed YA, et al. Altered gene expression in early osteochondrosis lesions. J Orthop Res 2009;27(4):452–7.
16. Olstad K, Ytrehus B, Ekman S, et al. Epiphyseal cartilage canal blood supply to the tarsus of foals and relationship to osteochondrosis. Equine Vet J 2008;40(1):30–9.
17. Olstad K, Ytrehus B, Ekman S, et al. Epiphyseal cartilage canal blood supply to the metatarsophalangeal joint of foals. Equine Vet J 2009;41(9):865–71.
18. Boero MJ, Kneller SK, Baker GJ, et al. Clinical, radiographic, and scintigraphic findings associated with enthesitis of the lateral collateral ligaments of the tarsocrural joint in standardbred racehorses. Equine Vet J Suppl 1988;(6):53–9.
19. Moll HD, Schumacher J, Wright JC, et al. Evaluation of sodium carboxymethylcellulose for prevention of experimentally induced abdominal adhesions in ponies. Am J Vet Res 1991;52(1):88–91.
20. Laing JA, Caves SF, Rawlinson RJ. Successful treatment of a tarsocrural joint luxation in a pony. Aust Vet J 1992;69(8):200–1.
21. Dik KJ. Ultrasonography fo the equine tarsus. Veterinary Radiology and Ultrasound 1993;34(1):36–43.
22. Raes EV, Vanderperren K, Pille F, et al. Ultrasonographic findings in 100 horses with tarsal region disorders. Vet J 2010;186(2):201–9.
23. Vanderperren K, Raes E, Hoegaerts M, et al. Diagnostic imaging of the equine tarsal region using radiography and

ultrasonography. Part 1: the soft tissues. Vet J 2009;179(2):179–87.

24. Tokateloff N, Carmalt J, Manning S. Trauma resulting in hemarthrosis and long medial collateral ligament desmitis of the tarsocrural joint in a horse. Can Vet J 2011;52(5):519–23.
25. Latorre R, Arencibia A, Gil F, et al. Correlation of magnetic resonance images with anatomic features of the equine tarsus. Am J Vet Res 2006;67(5): 756–61.
26. Blaik MA, Hanson RR, Kincaid SA, et al. Low-field magnetic resonance imaging of the equine tarsus: normal anatomy. Vet Radiol Ultrasound 2000;41(2): 131–41.
27. Smith MR, Wright IM. Arthroscopic treatment of fractures of the lateral malleolus of the tibia: 26 cases. Equine Vet J 2011;43(3):280–7.
28. Tulamo RM, Bramlage LR, Gabel AA. Fractures of the central and third tarsal bones in horses. Journal of the American Veterinary Medical Association 1983;182(11):1234–8.
29. Winberg FG, Pettersson H. Outcome and racing performance after internal fixation of third and central tarsal bone slab fractures in horses. A review of 20 cases. Acta vet Scand 1999;40(2): 173–80.
30. Santschi EM, Adams SB, Fessler JF, et al. Treatment of bacterial tarsal tenosynovitis and osteitis of the sustentaculum tali of the calcaneus in five horses. Equine Vet J 1997;29(3): 244–7.
31. Wright IM. Fractures of the lateral malleolus of the tibia in 16 horses. Equine Vet J 1992;24(6):424–9.
32. Daniel AJ, Judy CE, Rick MC, et al. Comparison of radiography, nuclear scintigraphy, and magnetic resonance imaging for detection of specific conditions of the distal tarsal bones of horses: 20 cases (2006–10). J Am Vet Med Assoc 2012;240(9):1109–14.
33. Stover SM, Hornof WJ, Richardson GL, et al. Bone scintigraphy as an aid in the diagnosis of occult distal tarsal bone trauma in three horses. J Am Vet Med Assoc 1986;188(6):624–8.
34. Lindsay WA, McMartin RB, McClure JR. Management of slab fractures of the third tarsal bone in 5 horses. Equine Vet J 1982;14(1):55–8.
35. Murphey ED, Schneider RK, Adams SB, et al. Long-term outcome of horses with a slab fracture of the central or third tarsal bone treated conservatively: 25 cases (1976–1993). J Am Vet Med Assoc 2000;216(12):1949–54.
36. Welch RD, Auer JA, Watkins JP, et al. Surgical treatment of tarsal sheath effusion associated with an exostosis on the calcaneus of a horse. J Am Vet Med Assoc 1990;196(12):1992–4.
37. Hand DR, Watkins JP, Honnas CM, et al. Osteomyelitis of the sustentaculum tali in horses: 10 cases (1992–1998). J Am Vet Med Assoc 2001;219(3):341–5.
38. Wright IM, Smith MR, Humphrey DJ, et al. Endoscopic surgery in the treatment of contaminated and infected synovial cavities. Equine Vet J 2003;35(6):613–19.
39. Ingle-Fehr JE, Baxter GM. Endoscopy of the calcaneal bursa in horses. Veterinary Surgery 1998;27(6):561–7.
40. Cauvin ERJ, Tapprest J, Munroe GA, et al. Endoscopic examination of the tarsal sheath of the lateral digital flexor tendon in the horse. Equine Veterinary Journal 1999;31(3):219–27.
41. Walmsley EA, Anderson GA, Muurlink MA, et al. Retrospective investigation of prognostic indicators for adult horses with infection of a synovial structure. Aust Vet J 2011;89(6):226–31.
42. Baird DH, Pilsworth RC. Wedge-shaped conformation of the dorsolateral aspect of the third tarsal bone in the Thoroughbred racehorse is associated with development of slab fractures in this site. Equine Vet J 2001;33(6): 617–20.
43. Byam-Cook KL, Singer ER. Is there a relationship between clinical presentation, diagnostic and radiographic findings and outcome in horses with osteoarthritis of the small tarsal joints? Equine Vet J 2009;41(2): 118–23.
44. Murray RC, Dyson SJ, Weekes JS, et al. Scintigraphic evaluation of the distal tarsal region in horses with distal tarsal pain. Vet Radiol Ultrasound 2005;46(2): 171–8.
45. Ehrlich PJ, Dohoo IR, O'Callaghan MW. Results of bone scintigraphy in racing standardbred horses: 64 cases (1992–1994). J Am Vet Med Assoc 1999;215(7):982–91.
46. Ehrlich PJ, Seeherman HJ, O'Callaghan MW, et al. Results of bone scintigraphy in horses used for show jumping, hunting, or eventing: 141 cases (1988–1994). J Am Vet Med Assoc 1998;213(10):1460–7.
47. Branch MV, Murray RC, Dyson SJ, et al. Alteration of distal tarsal subchondral bone thickness pattern in horses with tarsal pain. Equine Vet J 2007;39(2): 101–5.
48. Branch MV, Murray RC, Dyson SJ, et al. Is there a characteristic distal tarsal subchondral bone plate thickness pattern in horses with no history of hindlimb lameness? Equine Vet J 2005;37(5):450–5.
49. Labens R, Mellor DJ, Voute LC. Retrospective study of the effect of intra-articular treatment of osteoarthritis of the distal tarsal joints in 51 horses. Vet Rec 2007;161(18):611–16.
50. Serena A, Schumacher J, Schramme MC, et al. Concentration of methylprednisolone in the centrodistal joint after administration of methylprednisolone acetate in the tarsometatarsal joint. Equine Vet J 2005;37(2):172–4.
51. Sammut EB, Kannegieter NJ. Use of sodium monoiodoacetate to fuse the distal hock joints in horses. Aust Vet J 1995;72(1):25–8.
52. Dowling BA, Dart AJ, Matthews SM. Chemical arthrodesis of the distal tarsal joints using sodium monoiodoacetate in 104 horses. Aust Vet J 2004;82(1–2): 38–42.
53. Bohanon TC, Schneider RK, Weisbrode SE. Fusion of the distal intertarsal and tarsometatarsal joints in the horse using intraarticular sodium monoiodoacetate. Equine Vet J 1991;23(4):289–95.
54. Zubrod CJ, Schneider RK, Hague BA, et al. Comparison of three methods for arthrodesis of the distal intertarsal and tarsometatarsal joints in horses. Vet Surg 2005;34(4):372–82.
55. Carmalt JL, Bell CD, Panizzi L, et al. Alcohol-facilitated ankylosis of the distal intertarsal and tarsometatarsal joints in horses with osteoarthritis. J Am Vet Med Assoc 2012;240(2):199–204.
56. Shoemaker RW, Allen AL, Richardson CE, et al. Use of intra-articular administration of ethyl alcohol for arthrodesis of the tarsometatarsal joint in healthy horses. Am J Vet Res 2006; 67(5):850–7.
57. Wyn-Jones G, May SA. Surgical arthrodesis for the treatment of osteoarthrosis of the proximal intertarsal, distal intertarsal and tarsometatarsal joints in 30 horses: a comparison of four different techniques. Equine Vet J 1986;18(1):59–64.
58. Archer RM, Schneider RK, Lindsay WA, et al. Arthrodesis of the equine distal tarsal joints by perforated stainless steel cylinders. Equine Vet J Suppl 1988;(6): 125–30.
59. Axelsson M, Bjornsdottir S, Eksell P, et al. Risk factors associated with hindlimb lameness and degenerative joint disease in the distal tarsus of Icelandic horses. Equine Vet J 2001; 33(1):84–90.
60. Dyson SJ, Kidd L. Five cases of gastrocnemius tendinitis in the horse. Equine Vet J 1992;24(5):351–6.
61. Wright IM, Minshall GJ. Injuries of the calcaneal insertions of the superficial digital flexor tendon in 19 horses. Equine Vet J 2012;44(2):136–42.
62. Pilsworth RC, Head MJ. A study of ten cases of focal peritarsal infection as a cause of severe lameness in the thoroughbred racehorse: clinical signs, differential diagnosis, treatment and outcome. Equine Vet J 2001;33(4): 366–70.

63. Reeves MJ, Trotter GW, Kainer RA. Anatomical and functional communications between the synovial sacs of the equine stifle joint. Equine Vet J 1991;23(3):215–18.
64. Kane AJ, McIlwraith CW, Park RD, et al. Radiographic changes in Thoroughbred yearlings. Part 2: Associations with racing performance. Equine Vet J 2003;35(4):366–74.
65. Bourzac C, Alexander K, Rossier Y, et al. Comparison of radiography and ultrasonography for the diagnosis of osteochondritis dissecans in the equine femoropatellar joint. Equine Vet J 2009;41(7):685–92.
66. Foland JW, McIlwraith CW, Trotter GW. Arthroscopic surgery for osteochondritis dissecans of the femoropatellar joint of the horse. Equine Vet J 1992;24(6): 419–23.
67. Howard RD, McIlwraith CW, Trotter GW. Arthroscopic surgery for subchondral cystic lesions of the medial femoral condyle in horses: 41 cases (1988–1991). J Am Vet Med Assoc 1995;206(6):842–50.
68. Peroni JF, Stick JA. Evaluation of a cranial arthroscopic approach to the stifle joint for the treatment of femorotibial joint disease in horses: 23 cases (1998–1999). J Am Vet Med Assoc 2002;220(7):1046–52.
69. Wallis TW, Goodrich LR, McIlwraith CW, et al. Arthroscopic injection of corticosteroids into the fibrous tissue of subchondral cystic lesions of the medial femoral condyle in horses: a retrospective study of 52 cases (2001–2006). Equine Vet J 2008;40(5):461–7.
70. Jackson WA, Stick JA, Arnoczky SP, et al. The effect of compacted cancellous bone grafting on the healing of subchondral bone defects of the medial femoral condyle in horses. Vet Surg 2000;29(1):8–16.
71. Vachon AM, McIlwraith CW, Powers BE, et al. Morphologic and biochemical study of sternal cartilage autografts for resurfacing induced osteochondral defects in horses. Am J Vet Res 1992;53:1038–47.
72. Kold SE, Hickman J. An experimental study of the healing process of equine chondral and osteochondral defects. Equine vet J 1986;18:18–24.
73. Dik KJ, Enzerink E, van Weeren PR. Radiographic development of osteochondral abnormalities, in the hock and stifle of Dutch Warmblood foals, from age 1 to 11 months. Equine Vet J Suppl 1999;(31):9–15.
74. Olstad K, Ytrehus B, Ekman S, et al. Epiphyseal cartilage canal blood supply to the distal femur of foals. Equine Vet J 2008;40(5):433–9.
75. Dyson S. Stifle trauma in the event horse. Equine Vet Educ 1994;6(5): 234–40.
76. Dyson S, Wright I, Kold S, et al. Clinical and radiographic features, treatment and outcome in 15 horses with fracture of the medial aspect of the patella. Equine Vet J 1992;24(4):264–8.
77. Gibson KT, McIlwraith CW, Park RD, et al. Production of patellar lesions by medial patellar desmotomy in normal horses. Vet Surg 1989;18(6):466–71.
78. Smith BL, Auer JA, Watkins JP. Surgical repair of tibial tuberosity avulsion fractures in four horses. Vet Surg 1990;19(2):117–21.
79. Wright IM, Montesso F, Kidd LJ. Surgical treatment of fractures of the tibial tuberosity in 6 adult horses. Equine Vet J 1995;27(2):96–102.
80. Hunt RJ, Baxter GM, Zamos DT. Tension-band wiring and lag screw fixation of a transverse, comminuted fracture of a patella in a horse. J Am Vet Med Assoc 1992;200(6):819–20.
81. Marble GP, Sullins KE. Arthroscopic removal of patellar fracture fragments in horses: five cases (1989–1998). J Am Vet Med Assoc 2000;216(11):1799–801.
82. Smith LC, Greet TR, Bathe AP. A lateral approach for screw repair in lag fashion of spiral third metacarpal and metatarsal medial condylar fractures in horses. Vet Surg 2009;38(6):681–8.
83. Eliashar E, Smith RK, Schramme MC, et al. Preoperative bending and twisting of a dynamic compression plate for the repair of tibial tuberosity fracture in the horse. Equine Vet J 2000;32(5):447–8.
84. Hance SR, Bramlage LR, Schneider RK, et al. Retrospective study of 38 cases of femur fractures in horses less than one year of age. Equine Vet J 1992;24(5): 357–63.
85. Dabareiner RM, Sullins KE. Fracture of the caudal medial femoral condyle in a horse. Equine Vet J 1993;25(1):75–7.
86. Walmsley JP. Vertical tears of the cranial horn of the meniscus and its cranial ligament in the equine femorotibial joint: 7 cases and their treatment by arthroscopic surgery. Equine Vet J 1995;27(1):20–5.
87. Walmsley JR, Phillips TJ, Townsend HG. Meniscal tears in horses: an evaluation of clinical signs and arthroscopic treatment of 80 cases. Equine Vet J 2003;35(4):402–6.
88. Barrett MF, Frisbie DD, McIlwraith CW, et al. The arthroscopic and ultrasonographic boundaries of the equine femorotibial joints. Equine Vet J 2012;44(1):57–63.
89. Cohen JM, Richardson DW, McKnight AL, et al. Long-term outcome in 44 horses with stifle lameness after arthroscopic exploration and debridement. Vet Surg 2009;38(4): 543–51.
90. Cauvin ERJ, Munroe GA, Boyd JS, et al. Ultrasonographic examination of the femorotibial articulation in horses: imaging of the cranial and caudal aspects. Equine Vet J 1996;28(4):285–96.
91. Muurlink T, Walmsley J, Young D, et al. A cranial intercondylar arthroscopic approach to the caudal medial femorotibial joint of the horse. Equine Vet J 2009;41(1):5–10.
92. Watts AE, Nixon AJ. Comparison of arthroscopic approaches and accessible anatomic structures during arthroscopy of the caudal pouches of equine femorotibial joints. Vet Surg 2006;35(3):219–26.
93. Anderson DR, Woo SL, Kwan MK, et al. Viscoelastic shear properties of the equine medial meniscus. J Orthop Res 1991;9(4):550–8.
94. Rich FR, Glisson RR. In vitro mechanical properties and failure mode of the equine (pony) cranial cruciate ligament. Vet Surg 1994;23(4):257–65.
95. Prades M, Grant BD, Turner TA, et al. Injuries to the cranial cruciate ligament and associated structures: summary of clinical, radiographic, arthroscopic and pathological findings from 10 horses. Equine Vet J 1989;21(5):354–7.
96. Baker GJ, Moustafa MA, Boero MJ, et al. Caudal cruciate ligament function and injury in the horse. Vet Rec 1987;121(14):319–21.
97. Edwards RB, Nixon AJ. Avulsion of the cranial cruciate ligament insertion in a horse. Equine Vet J 1996;28(4):334–6.
98. Walmsley JP. Fracture of the intercondylar eminence of the tibia treated by arthroscopic internal fixation. Equine Veterinary Journal 1997;29(2): 148–50.
99. Mueller PO, Allen D, Watson E, et al. Arthroscopic removal of a fragment from an intercondylar eminence fracture of the tibia in a two-year-old horse. J Am Vet Med Assoc 1994;204(11): 1793–5.
100. Sanders-Shamis M, Bukowiecki CF, Biller DS. Cruciate and collateral ligament failure in the equine stifle: seven cases (1975–1985). J Am Vet Med Assoc 1988;193(5):573–6.
101. McIlwraith CW, Warren RC. Distal luxation of the patella in a horse. J Am Vet Med Assoc 1982;181(1):67–9.
102. Dyson SJ. Normal ultrasonographic anatomy and injury of the patellar ligaments in the horse. Equine Vet J 2002;34(3):258–64.
103. Cahill JI, Goulden BE, Pearce HG. A review and some observations on stringhalt. N Z Vet J 1985;33(7):101–4.
104. Van Hoogmoed LM, Agnew DW, Whitcomb M, et al. Ultrasonographic and histologic evaluation of medial and middle patellar ligaments in exercised horses following injection with ethanolamine oleate and 2% iodine in

almond oil. Am J Vet Res 2002;63(5): 738–43.

105. Baccarin RY, Martins EA, Hagen SC, et al. Patellar instability following experimental medial patellar desmotomy in horses. Vet Comp Orthop Traumatol 2009;22(1):27–31.

106. Martins EA, Silva LC, Baccarin RY. Ultrasonographic changes of the equine stifle following experimental medial patellar desmotomy. Can Vet J 2006;47(5):471–4.

107. Riley CB, Yovich JV. Fracture of the apex of the patella after medical patellar desmotomy in a horse. Aust Vet J 1991;68(1):37–9.

108. Wright JD, Rose RJ. Fracture of the patella as a possible complication of medial patellar desmotomy. Aust Vet J 1989;66(6):189–90.

109. Bathe AP, O'Hara LK, editors. A retrospective study of the outcome of medial patellar desmotomy in 49 horses. 50th Annual Convention of the American Association of Equine Practitioners; 2004; Denver, Colorado, USA.

110. Tnibar MA. Medial patellar ligament splitting for the treatment of upward fixation of the patella in 7 equids. Vet Surg 2002;31(5):462–7.

111. McIlwraith CW. Osteochondral fragmentation of the distal aspect of the patella in horses. Equine Vet J 1990;22(3):157–63.

Soft tissue injuries: tendinitis and desmitis

20

Carol Gillis

CHAPTER CONTENTS

Introduction

Thirteen to 18% of equine athletes sustain a soft tissue injury sufficiently severe to require a period of rest each year. Horses at greatest risk are those whose work load is increasing rapidly, for example, horses undertaking work at racing speed prior to their first race or dressage horses training to achieve the next training level.

Tendons and ligaments have a slow metabolic rate of activity and require a period of 8–14 months to return to the normal tensile strength range after damage, depending on the severity of the injury. Confinement and rehabilitative exercise needed for optimum healing are expensive and time consuming; therefore an accurate diagnosis of all injuries currently affecting the horse is very important to allow for simultaneous rather than sequential treatment. Tendons and ligaments in varying locations respond to treatment and rehabilitation in a relatively similar fashion therefore if one is confronted with a new or unusual injury, basic treatment principles apply. Although the published prognosis is fair or even poor for many soft tissue injuries, early diagnosis, good client compliance with repeated clinical and ultrasound examinations and a controlled exercise program tailored to the stage of healing of the injured tendon or ligament have improved the prognosis for most injuries. The prognosis for return to full athletic soundness is often good when using these principles, as long as adequate care and time are provided to allow for complete healing.

Superficial digital flexor tendinitis

Recognition

History and presenting complaint

Horses presented for superficial digital flexor (SDF) tendinitis are usually in full athletic use. Affected horses often have a workload that consists primarily of galloping and/or jumping (Fig. 20.1). Most tendon injuries are due to cumulative damage rather than a single event, the exception being a fall or a strike from another limb. Horses often develop clinically apparent pain, swelling and lameness 2–3 days following SDF injury.

Physical examination

Lameness ranges from grade 1 to 3 of 5 and is often transient or intermittent. Lameness often resolves rapidly with the use of ice, rest and anti-iflammatory agents. There will acutely be pain on palpation, heat and swelling at the lesion site. Pain on flexed palapetion is often the sign with longest duration as the lameness resolves. Affected horses frequently exhibit a decrease in performance ability after the initial lameness resolves.[1,2]

Luxation of the SDF tendon from its attachment to the calcaneus often presents as an acute injury during exercise, particularly in polo ponies and eventers. An audible pop may be heard, followed by acute lameness. As luxation usually occurs laterally, the tendon can be seen coursing down the lateral aspect of the tarsus. Within a few

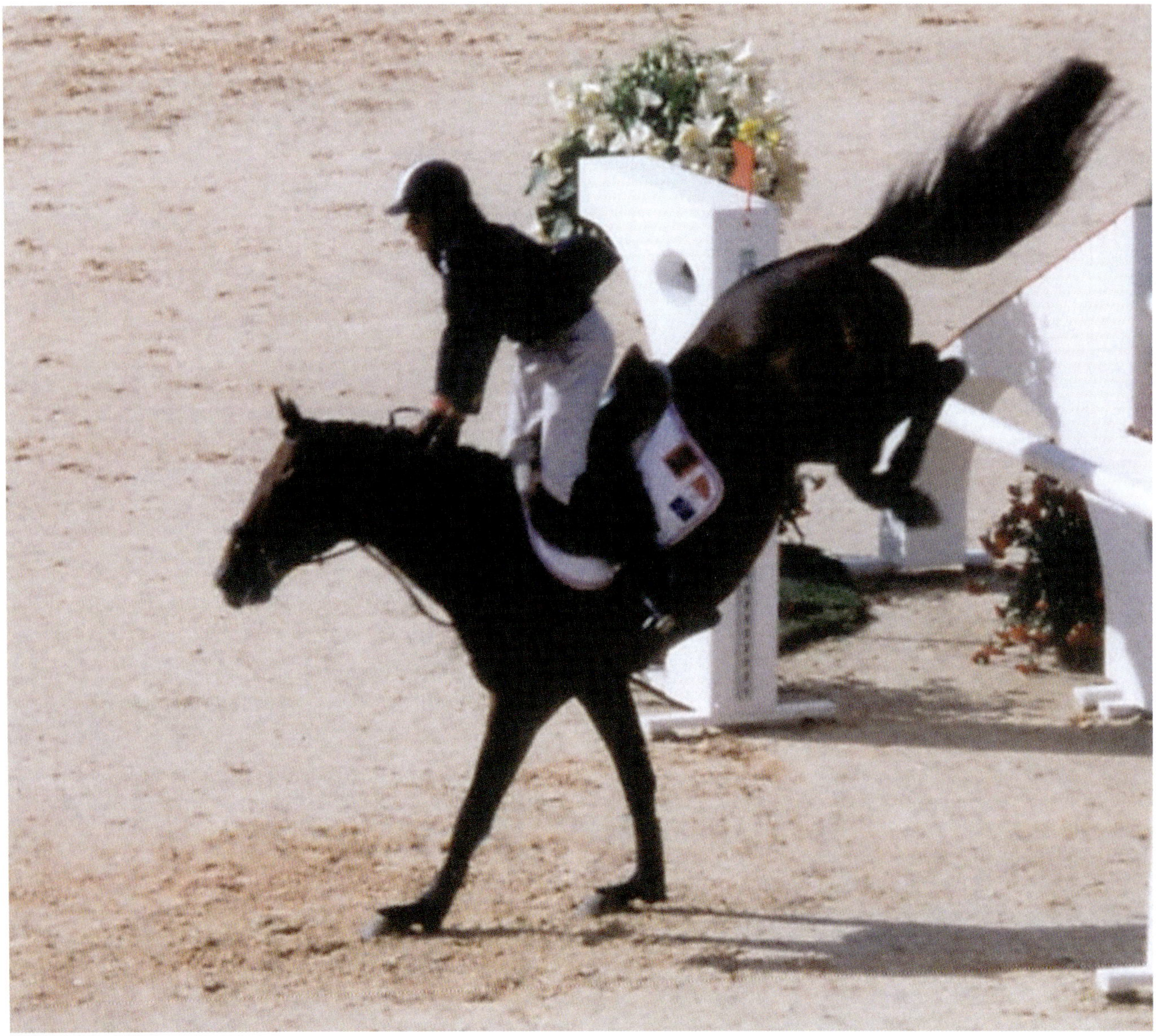

Fig 20.1 Horse competing in the stadium jumping demonstrating extreme stresses on the forelimbs.

days, massive swelling of the limb obscures anatomic details if the injury is not treated aggressively for inflammation.

Differential diagnosis for lesions in the metacarpal/metatarsal region is limited as the SDF tendon is readily palpated and separated from deeper structures. Carpal sheath synovitis may be associated with proximal SDF tendinitis. Digital sheath synovitis may be associated with SDF tendinitis in the fetlock and pastern regions. The manica flexoria portion of the SDF tendon may be damaged deep to the deep digital flexor tendon in conjunction with digital sheath synovitis. Differential diagnosis in the pastern region includes damage to the sesamoidean ligaments or the collateral ligaments of the proximal interphalangeal or distal interphalangeal joints.

Special examination

For SDF branch lesions, a low palmar digital nerve block generally provides analgesia. For SDF lesions in the metacarpal/metatarsal region, a high palmar nerve block resolves the lameness.[3]

Increased size of the affected tendon region combined with loss of echogenicity and normal parallel linear fiber pattern observed with diagnostic ultrasonography provides the definitive diagnosis (Fig. 20.2, Fig. 20.3, Fig. 20.4, Fig. 20.5, Fig. 20.6).[4–10]

Tenoscopy of carpal and digital sheaths provides diagnostic information as well as further treatment options. For example, under arthroscopic guidance debridement of frayed tendon fibers and resection of proliferative synovium and adhesions may be performed.[11,12]

Treatment and prognosis

Therapeutic aims

- to control inflammation and prevent further tendon injury directly, through reducing tendon fiber swelling and influx of inflammatory mediators, or indirectly, through further exercise
- provide adequate tendon support, primarily through shoeing
- provide adequate rest followed by graduated increases in exercise to allow for optimum tendon healing.

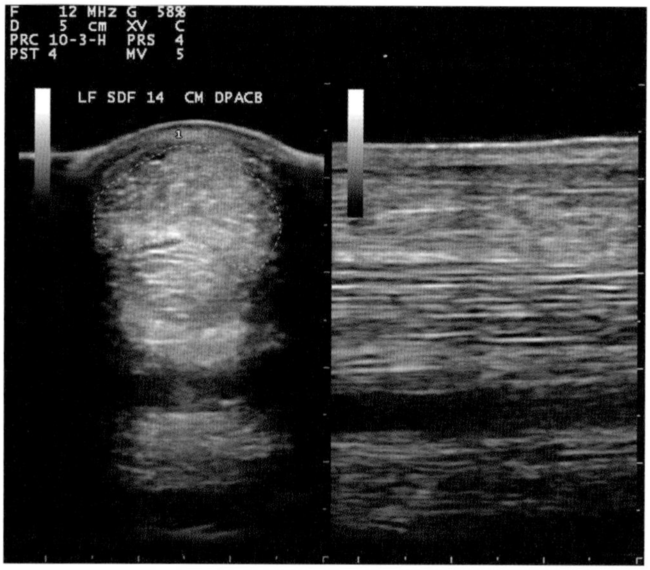

Fig 20.2 Ultrasonographic image of chronic SDF tendinitis in the mid-metacarpal region showing that the SDF tendon is larger than the DDF on the short axis view. The SDF has mixed echogencity with small bright areas of scar (left), and a fair, but not good, fiber pattern on the long axis view (right).

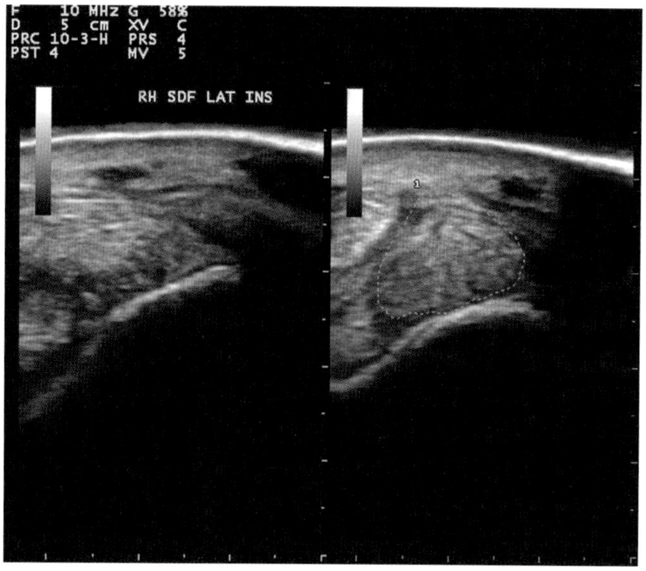

Fig 20.4 Ultrasonographic image of right hind SDF tendinits of the lateral branch at insertion on P1-2. The long axis view (left) shows fair to poor fiber pattern. The short axis view (right) has multiple linear tears within the SDF.

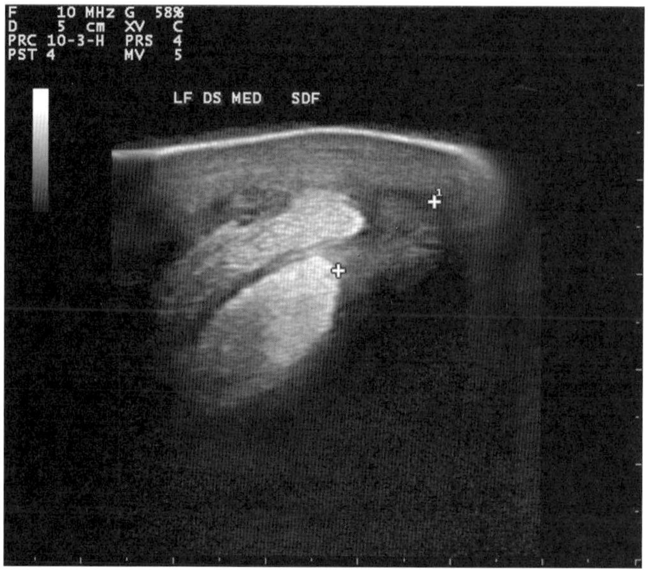

Fig 20.3 Ultrasonographic image of the SDF within the digital sheath which has proliferative synovitis as indicated by the + marks. The palmar border of the SDF has a lesion associated with palmar synovial proliferation.

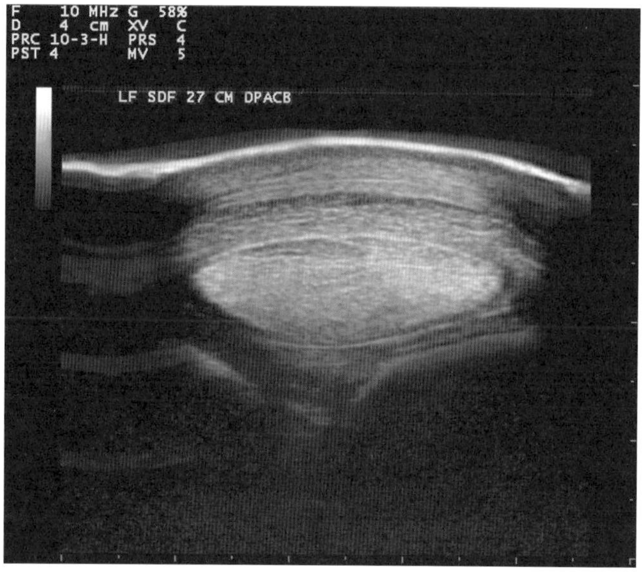

Fig 20.5 Ultrasonographic image of the SDF tendon in the digital sheath in short axis view. The thin echoic line seen encircling the SDF is normal manica flexoria. The thin line dorsal to it is normal digital sheath wall.

Therapy

Initial therapy is directed at controlling excessive inflammation and should include anti-inflammatory therapy such as 1% diclofenac cream applied twice daily to the affected area.

Cold therapy, such as ice for 20 minutes 2–3 times/day for three weeks, is an effective adjunct to reduce inflammation. Treatment with intramuscular polysulfated glycosaminoglycan, 500 mg every four days for seven treatments, has been shown to improve tendon healing.[13]

Foot conformation should be evaluated early in the course of injury. Good caudal heel support should be provided using an egg bar shoe that extends to the level of the heel bulbs unless the horse has sufficient support from his foot shape. Any break in pastern/hoof axis should be corrected at the same time to minimize tension on healing soft tissues.

Although stem cell and platelet rich plasma (PRP) injections are in common use, no contolled study has yet shown that they produce collagen within injured tendon or ligament. A recent paper has shown that mesenchymal stromal cells survivied for approximately 10 days when injected into damaged tendon, and that they did not migrate, indicating little viable activity.[14] Embryonic stem cells were able to survive for 120 days and to migrate indicating that futher research is warranted to determine if embryonic cells might produce

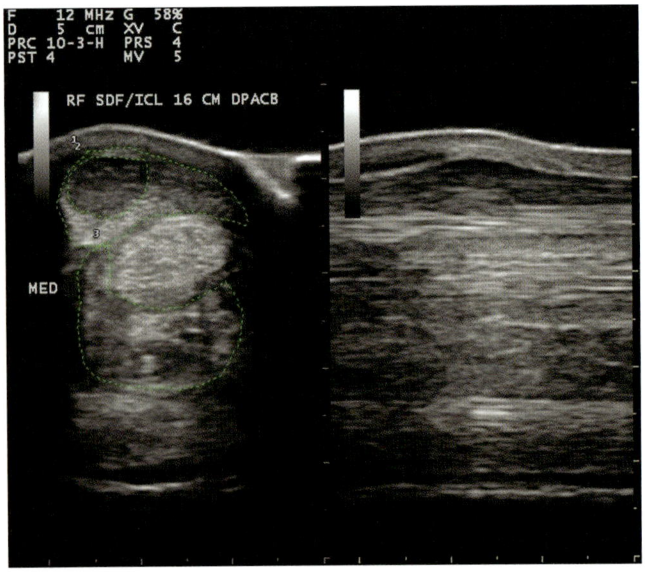

Fig 20.6 Short axcis ultrasonographic image (left) of the SDF tendon with marked swelling and a large core lesion. The AL-DDF has desmitis as seen by enlargement,and mixed echogenicity including scar as well as hypoechoic areas. The long axis view (right) shows loss of normal fiber pattern for the SDF and the AL-DDF.

viable tendon collagen. Another recent paper has shown that insufficient amounts of growth factor are released from platelets using current techniques to induce collagen growth.[15]

Native stem cells present in the patient's injured tendon are capable of producing collagen under appropriate circumstances including controlled exercise, which is the likely reason that horses following a controlled exercise program and whole horse care have as good a prognosis to return to work as those which have received stem cell or PRP injections in addition to controlled exercise. Horses that receive stem cell or PRP injection without adequate time to heal or appropriate rehabilitation have a poor prognosis to return to work without re-injury.

Stall (12′ by 24′) confinement with hand-walking should be initiated following examination. Unless the tendon is so severely damaged that rupture appears likely (rare), hand-walking is an important part of treatment and should not be delayed. If a free or box stall type of mechanical exerciser is available, horses can exercise up through the trot phase on this equipment. Walking times can be moderately increased above hand walking times. All exercise should be under supervision. Aquatic treadmills are also useful for horses when they reach the level of healing equivalent to the trot phase; earlier use may be excessive work for healing soft tissues.[16]

Bandaging is useful to decrease edema in the surrounding tissues. Bandages will not provide significant tendon support. Any concurrent lameness, even slight or chronic, should be treated at the same time.

Following an initial period of stall rest and hand-walking, the SDF tendon should be re-evaluated using physical examination and ultrasonography to assess healing.[17] Increasing exercise should be based upon examination findings rather than time elapsed. The horse should be confined to a space small enough so that it can only walk when not undergoing controlled exercise until healing is sufficient to allow canter work under saddle for one week. Please refer to Tables 20.1–5 for detailed exercise protocols.

Table 20.1 Exercise protocol following the first examination (0–60 days). Horse is confined to a stall or equivalent size paddock (12′ by 24′ maximum)

INJURY	0–30 DAYS	30–60 DAYS
Mild	Hand-walk 15 minutes twice daily	Increase walking time by 5 daily minutes per week
Moderate	Hand-walk 15 minutes twice daily	Increase walking time by 5 daily minutes per 2 weeks
Severe	Hand-walk 10 minutes twice daily	Hand walk 15 minutes twice daily

Table 20.2 Exercise protocol following the second examination (60–120 days). Horse is confined to a stall or equivalent size paddock (12′ by 24′ maximum)

PROGRESS	60–90	90–120 DAYS
Good	Ride at walk 25 minutes daily Increase 5 minutes every 2 weeks	Same protocol
Fair	Same as above	
Poor	Hand-walk 30 minutes twice daily	Ride at a walk for 20 minutes; hand walk for 20 minutes at another time

Table 20.3 Exercise protocol following the third examination (120–180 days). Horse is confined to a stall or equivalent size paddock (12′ by 24′)

PROGRESS	120–150 DAYS	150–180 DAYS
Good	Add a 5 minute trot set every 2 weeks	Add a 5 minute trot set every 2 weeks
Fair	Ride at a walk for 40 minutes daily and hand walk	Add a 5 minute trot set every 2 weeks
Poor	Re-evaluate case to determine cause and discuss further treatment options	

Surgical options

If an anechoic or mostly anechoic core lesion is seen on ultrasonographic examination, ultrasound-guided tendon splitting to decompress the core lesion should be performed as soon as possible, ideally 2–14 days following injury, to prevent further compression injury of the surrounding normal fibers.

If a subcutaneous hematoma is detected, injection of hyaluronic acid between the tendon and the skin should be performed as soon as possible, ideally 2–14 days following injury to attempt to prevent development of adhesions between the subcutaneous tissue and the SDF tendon.

Superior check ligament desmotomy has been shown to improve SDF appearance in the short term; long-term results have been less encouraging. Superior check desmotomy has been associated with significantly increased strains on the SDF tendon and SL.[18] Horses

Table 20.4 Exercise protocol following the fourth examination (180–240 days). Horse can be turned out after riding exercise when it has been cantering five minutes for one week

PROGRESS	180–210 DAYS	210–240 DAYS
Good	Add canter 5 minutes every 2 weeks	Add canter 5 minutes every 2 weeks begin ground pole exercises
Fair	Add trotting 5 minutes every 2 weeks	Add canter 5 minutes every 2 weeks
Poor	Re-evaluate case and discuss further treatment options	

Table 20.5 Exercise protocol following the fifth examination (240–300 days)

PROGRESS	240–270 DAYS	270–300 DAYS
Good	Racing speed work, jumping or other competitive training	Ready for competition
Fair	Add canter 5 minutes every 2 weeks	Full flat work; no racing speed work or jumping
Poor	Re-evaluate case and discuss further treatment options	

treated surgically were 1.2 times more likely to develop recurrent or new injuries after returning to training than horses managed non-surgically. Racehorses that have undergone a superior check ligament desmotomy are 5.5 times as likely to suffer a subsequent suspensory ligament injury as are horses without desmotomy.[19]

Palmar annular ligament (PAL) desmotomy is very helpful in treatment of SDF injuries that extend to the distal metacarpal/ metatarsal region. Resection of the PAL relieves compression of the enlarged SDF and allows for improved tendon gliding. This procedure is most effective when performed soon (within four weeks) after SDF tendon injury. If the procedure is not performed, the proximal portion of the SDF on subsequent ultrasound exams will appear to be healing at a normal rate, while the portion of the SDF just proximal to and at the level of the PAL will heal poorly. Resection is still useful as a treatment for chronic distal SDF tendon injury, although improved healing of the tendon is less dramatic. Although several surgical repair methods have been described for SDF tendon luxation, aggressive medical therapy provides a good long-term outcome without the complications that can occur following surgical attachment/ stabilization at the original site on the calcaneus.

Prognosis

The prognosis is excellent for life and good for return to full athletic use, if aggressive treatment followed by controlled rehabilitation is performed. If the tendon appears 95% healed based on size, echogenicity and fiber pattern on the final ultrasound exam, the horse is at no greater risk of re-injury than of any athletic use injury upon return to full work. A superficial digital flexor tendon that has luxated from its calcaneal attachment also has a good prognosis with aggressive medical treatment for inflammation and a full rehabilitation program.

Etiology and pathophysiology

The SDF tendon, in conjunction with the suspensory ligament, acts to keep the fetlock from extending to the ground when the horse is weight bearing. The SDF actively participates in limb flexion during the swing phase of locomotion through contraction of the SDF muscle.

The SDF tendon has little margin of safety as horses in full work such as galloping or jumping generate forces near to its breaking strength.[20,21] The SDF tendon and the suspensory (interosseous) ligament are the primary load bearing structures in the forelimb[22] and are the soft tissues at greatest risk of injury in the horse that is working at speed. Factors that place excess load on the tendon, such as muscle fatigue which places increasing load on the much smaller, tendinous portion of the muscle/ tendon unit, poor hoof conformation/shoeing or lameness in another limb, place the tendon at increased risk of failure.

Once a few fibers are damaged, strength is reduced and the tendon is predisposed to further fiber rupture with continued work. Hemorrhage at the site of ruptured fibers and associated inflammatory mediator release cause further fiber damage, either through compression by expansion of the hematoma or from the detrimental effects of inflammatory products.

Athletic performance deteriorates in horses with SDF tendinitis due to initial lameness, followed by prolonged tendon weakness during the recovery phase. If excessive exercise is attempted while the tendon is relatively weak, the risk of tendon re-injury is high, leading to a repetitive syndrome of repeated short periods of acute lameness followed by longer periods of inability to perform regular work at a previous or expected level. If the tendon is damaged repeatedly, fibroblast damage occurs (tendinosis), resulting in inability to generate normal repair collagen. At this stage the tendon's ability to heal is compromised.

Prevention

SDF tendinitis prevention consists of:

- increasing work load gradually rather than abruptly. A 5% increase in workload per week is generally a safe guideline
- being attentive to hoof shape and shoeing to avoid a long toe, low heel configuration and to prevent a break in pastern/hoof axis
- early recognition and treatment of other lameness to prevent compensatory tendon overload
- recognition that certain conformational faults, particularly 'back at the knee' conformation, load the SDF additionally and place the horse at increased risk of tendon injury when in full work.
- fifteen minutes of walk warm up prior to faster work in every exercise session will preload the SDF tendon to better withstand the forces applied without injury.

Deep digital flexor tendinitis

Recognition

History and presenting complaint

Forelimb deep digital flexor (DDF) damage occurs most frequently in the pastern region of horses used for athletic pursuits which involve twisting and turning, such as polo, endurance riding in rough terrain or roping. In the foot region of fore- and hindlimbs, DDF tendinitis often occurs in middle-aged horses. It is often concurrent with navicular disease, particularly navicular bursitis. Hindlimb metatarsal region DDF tendinitis is most frequently seen in hunters/jumpers, primarily middle-aged geldings that have had years of work and is often accompanied by tarsal sheath synovitis.

Physical examination

Grade 1–3 out of 5 lameness is observed and is often intermittent or transient. Heat, swelling and pain will be present on palpation of the DDF.

Differential diagnoses depend on location; in the metacarpal/metatarsal region, inferior check ligament(ALDDF or accessory ligament of the deep digital flexor tendon) desmitis is the major differential. Tarsal sheath synovitis may be associated with hindlimb DDF tendinitis. In the pastern the SDF tendon and the sesamoidean ligaments must be included in the differential diagnoses. Digital sheath synovitis is often associated with pastern region DDF tendinitis. In the foot, navicular bursitis, navicular bone changes and other causes of heel pain should be considered as differential diagnoses.

Special examination

Diagnostic nerve blocks will localize the region of the DDF involved and begin the process of elucidating the source(s) of heel pain, if present. Radiographs of the foot will provide information regarding bone and joint involvement. MRI will define both hard and soft tissue injuries and their inter-relationship MRI is providing a large amount of new information that is important in a complete diagnosis but that also needs to be interpreted in light of clinical significance.

Diagnostic ultrasonography will define the presence and extent of DDF damage (Fig. 20.7).[23,24] For a diagnostic examination of the DDF within the hoof, as well as the navicular bursa and the impar ligament, the shoe should be removed and the frog should be pared to provide a level surface for good transducer contact. The foot should be soaked in water overnight to further soften the tissues. The insertion of the DDF on the solar aspect of the distal phalanx, the navicular bursa and the impar ligament can then be evaluated for disease (Fig. 20.8). Ultrasonography will also allow for sequential examinations, which are critical for the accurate assessment of healing stage of injured tendon so that an appropriate treatment and rehabilitation plan can be formulated for each stage of healing.[17]

Treatment and prognosis

Therapeutic aims

As for SDF tendinitis above.

Therapy

For general tendinitis medical treatment, please refer to the section on SDF tendinitis.

DDF tendinitis in the region of the navicular bone is frequently associated with navicular bursitis. If this is the case, therapy should include injection of the navicular bursa with a symptom modulating and preferably a disease modulating agent. Steroids remain the gold standard for anti-inflammatory activity. Hyaluronic acid, IRAP, or polysulfated glycosaminoglycan are also useful. Injection of the coffin joint rarely provides sufficient clinical and ultrasonographic signs of resolution of bursitis, even if the horse responds to coffin joint anesthesia. Reasons include:

- diffusion of local anesthetic across membranes which are not sufficiently permeable to allow diffusion of larger molecules.[25]
- anesthesia of local nerves proximal to the bursa, causing reduction in pain that was not the result of inflammation within the bursa.

Tarsal sheath synovitis may be treated medically in a similar fashion to the digital sheath (see following section. Tenoscopy of the sheath is an effective treatment for chronic/complicated cases with extensive synovial membrane proliferation and/or adhesions.[26]

Prognosis

Prognosis is good for return to athletic use if the tendon alone is involved. Concomitant tarsal sheath synovitis, digital sheath synovitis, and navicular bursitis need to be aggressively managed or they may prove to be the limiting factor(s) in future athletic performance. (Fig. 20.9).

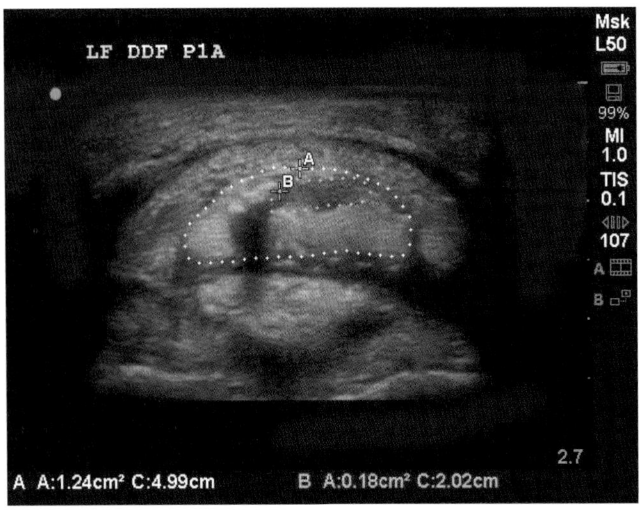

Fig 20.7 Short axis ultrasonographic image of the DDF tendon in the proximal pastern.Cross-sectional area of the DDF tendon is 1.24 cm^2 **(A)**. There is an area of calcification within the DDF that is casting a strong acoutstic shadow (to the left of B); adjacent is a recent hypoechoic core lesion.

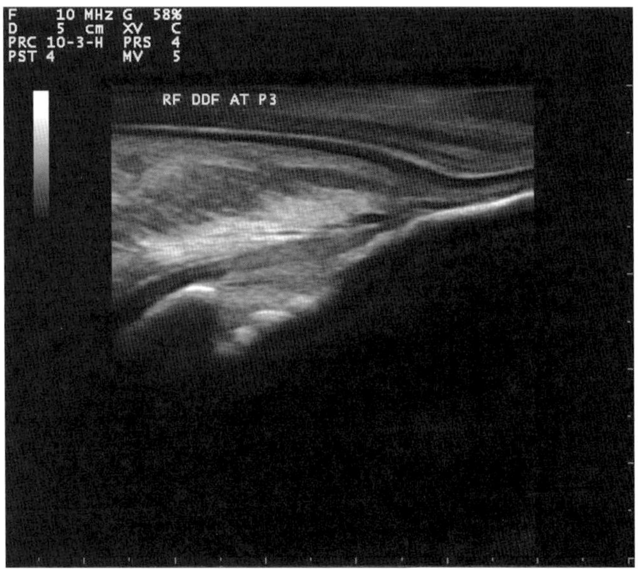

Fig 20.8 Ultrasonographic image showing a transcuneal (imaging across the frog) long axis view. The normal DDF is seen together with the navicular bursa as a hypoechoic line over the bright navicular bone on the lower left of the image. The DDF becomes echoic as it traverses from the navicular bone palmar surface to insert on the solar surface of P3 on the lower right side of the image.

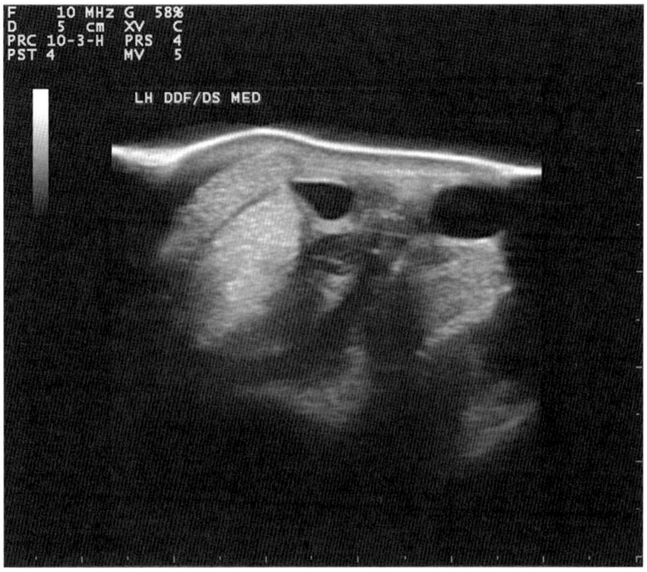

Fig 20.9 Ultrasonographic image of the DDF in the digital sheath. The short axis view shows multiple adhesions to the dorsal surface of the DDF with associated multiple edge tears of the DDF.

Etiology and pathophysiology

The DDF tendon acts to keep the third phalanx/toe of the hoof from overextending and actively participates in flexion of the limb during the swing phase of locomotion through contraction of the DDF muscle. Factors that place excess load on the tendon include the following:

- muscle fatigue, placing increasing load on the much smaller, tendinous portion of the muscle/tendon unit, poor hoof conformation/shoeing, or lameness in another limb
- once a few fibers are damaged, strength is reduced and the tendon is predisposed to further fiber rupture with continued work
- hemorrhage at the site of ruptured fibers and associated inflammatory mediator release cause further fiber damage either through compression by hematoma expansion or the detrimental effects of inflammatory products
- palmar digital neurectomy used to treat heel pain likely leads to atrophy of the deep digital flexor tendon, placing horses at increased risk of DDF injury or rupture after the procedure. Also, following neurectomy horses lose the ability to protect the DDF tendon from over strain or to show clinical signs of DDF damage until they lose control of their ability to place the toe following complete tendon rupture.

Athletic performance deteriorates in horses with DDF tendinitis due to initial lameness, followed by prolonged tendon weakness during the recovery phase. If excessive exercise is attempted while the tendon is relatively weak, the risk of tendon reinjury is high, leading to a repetitive syndrome of repeated short periods of acute lameness followed by longer periods of inability to perform regular work.

Prevention

DDF tendinitis prevention consists of:

- increasing workload gradually rather than abruptly. A 5% increase in workload per week is generally a safe guideline
- being attentive to hoof conformation and shoeing to avoid a long toe, low heel configuration and to prevent a break in pastern/hoof axis
- early recognition and treatment of other lameness to prevent compensatory tendon overload
- recognition that 'heel pain' may be due to excess strain on the DDF and that navicular bursitis may lead to secondary adhesions between the bursa and the DDF, leading to DDF damage.

Accessory ligament of the deep digital flexor tendon desmitis

Recognition

History and presenting complaint

Desmitis of the accessory ligamentof the deep digital flexor tendon (AL-DDFT) is usually observed in horses that are starting into regular work if the condition is developmental, or in middle-aged horses (10–14 years) which have been in regular use, particularly as jumpers.

AL-DDFT desmitis can also occur secondary to moderately severe or severe SDF tendinitis, if the SDF tendon becomes sufficiently enlarged to contact the medial and lateral borders of the AL-DDFT. Adhesions may subsequently develop which cause AL-DDFT inflammation and damage.[27]

Physical examination

Grade 2–3 out of 5 lameness is present and is usually persistent. Heat, swelling and pain are felt on palpation, most often at the accessory ligament-DDFT junction in the palmar/lateral mid-metacarpal region. AL-DDFT desmitis occurs less frequently at the origin of the ligament.

Differential diagnoses include DDF tendinitis and suspensory ligament desmitis. The AL-DDFT is often damaged at the midmetacarpal level, where its fibers join those of the DDF tendon.

Special examination

A high two-point nerve block (lateral and medial palmar nerves) should ablate the lameness and will confirm that the lameness is localized to the metacarpal region.

Diagnostic ultrasonography will reveal AL-DDFT enlargement, loss of echogenicity and deterioration of fiber pattern (Fig. 20.10).[27] AL-DDFT desmitis and associated enlargement of the ligament may cause the DDF tendon to be completely encircled and compressed by the SDF and the AL and may be an additional source of the chronic pain often associated with AL desmitis (Fig. 20.11).

Treatment and prognosis

Therapeutic aims

As above.

Therapy

For general therapy please refer to the section on SDF medical therapy. Following an initial period of stall rest and hand-walking, the AL-DDFT should be re-evaluated using physical examination and ultrasonography to assess healing.[17]

Surgical desmotomy of the AL-DDFT is a final option.[28,29,30] The client must commit to a full 8–10 month healing process. Within four weeks of surgery, granulation tissue will fill the gap between the resected AL-DDFT ends. The AL-DDFT will initially be 2–4 times normal size, then over months of rehabilitation ligament repair will occur, with a functionally lengthened and healed AL-DDFT if surgery and rehabilitation have been successful.[32–35]

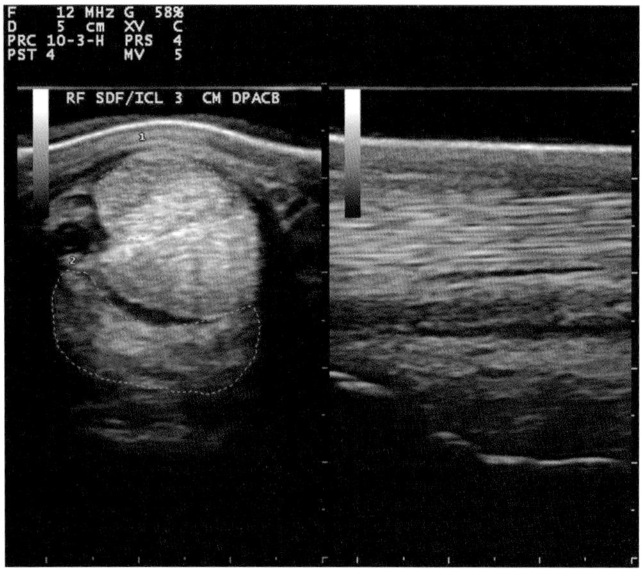

Fig 20.10 Ultrasonographic image of the AL-DDFT (encircled at the bottom of the left image) at its origin on the palmar aspect of the carpus.The short axis view (left) shows a mottled, hypoechoic ligament and the long axis view (right) shows a loss of normal parallel linear fiber pattern.

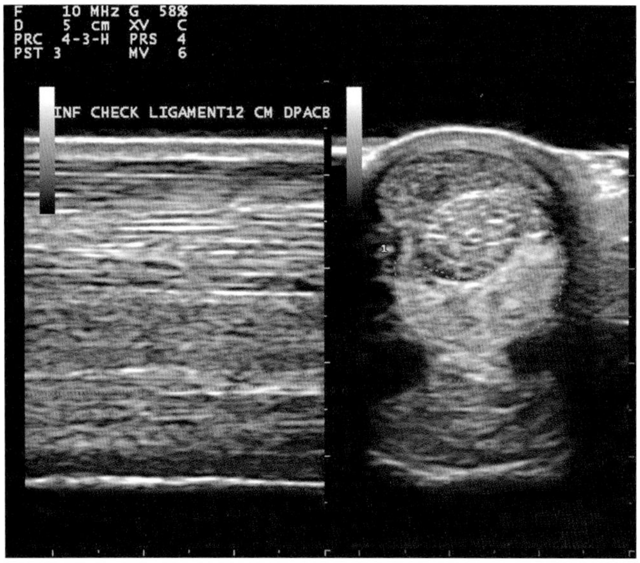

Fig 20.11 Ultrasonographic image of the AL-DDFT (encircled on right image) showing a fair to poor fiber pattern on long axis view (left) and enlargement, multiple small hypoechoic areas and compression of the DDF tendon on the short axis view (right).

AL-DDFT desmotomy in weanlings to correct contracted tendon/club foot syndrome should be followed by a controlled exercise program, minimally by placing the foal (and mare) It is possible for the horse to develop clinical signs of desmitis when the partially healed ligament is subjected to the forces generated by athletic training years later.

Prognosis

Prognosis is fair for return to athletic use. The AL-DDFT causes more long-term lameness than other tendon/ligament injuries.[31,32] Often diagnosis is delayed until AL-DDFT desmitis is chronic and severe, which limits the potential for healing. Horses with AL-DDFT desmitis respond most favorably to a gradual return to work, often with 4–5 days of work per week maximum with rest days in between. Breakdown of adhesions between the AL-DDFT and the SDF tendon may cause transient pain. If the pain, heat and swelling do not respond to 3–4 days of ice, NSAIDs and walking, an ultrasonographic examination is indicated to assess the AL-DDFT for re-injury.

Etiology and pathophysiology

Factors which cause contracted tendons in foals, such as congenital malformation,[33] diet and exercise, contribute to AL-DDFT desmitis, as this ligament is part of the affected DDFT/accessory ligament complex. Chronic overuse of the AL-DDFT due to hyperextension of the limb during athletic work is a second predisposing factor in the older horse, as are changes in biomechanical properties due to the aging process.[34]

Prevention

We are currently unable to detect excess tension on the AL-DDFT prior to the onset of inflammation resulting in pain, heat and swelling.

Prevention of AL-DDFT desmitis hinges primarily on very careful hoof balance, as many horses with AL-DDFT desmitis have had long-term higher than normal heels on the affected limb and lower than normal heels on the opposite limb. Over time this condition tends to become more pronounced.

This condition may have its origins when the patient is a foal, therefore careful attention to hoof trimming in the foal is a primary preventive step. Attempting to lower the high heel substantially often results in acute AL-DDFT pain which may be quite severe. It is preferable to raise low heels on the opposite limb until that foot/pastern axis is balanced and then very gradually lower the high heels.

Suspensory ligament desmitis

Recognition

History and presenting complaint

Suspensory ligament (SL) desmitis is seen most frequently in horses that trot for long periods of time, such as Standardbred racehorses, endurance horses and dressage horses. Pain, heat, swelling and lameness are often noted 1–3 days following hard work or competition. Lameness may resolve quickly following the use of NSAIDs, cold therapy and rest, only to return when the horse is worked vigorously again. Hindlimb SL desmitis is often mistaken for disease of the distal tarsal joints. Treatment of the distal intertarsal and tarsometatarsal joints with steroids may reduce inflammation of the SL temporarily and cause reduction of clinical signs until further SL damage occurs. A frequent complaint with these patients is that they only respond to hock injections over a short period of time.

Physical examination

Grade 1–3 out of 5 lameness is observed and is often intermittent or transient. The SL branches are readily palpated for pain, heat and swelling. The SL origin and body, particularly in the hindlimb, are nestled between MCII-III-IV (MTII-III-IV) and are covered superficially by the flexor tendons, so may only reveal clinical signs on careful deep palpation.

It is helpful to differentiate between hock joint pain and SL damage to compare the horse's response to hindlimb flexion and to deep pressure on the SL body with the heel off the ground but without limb flexion (Fig. 20.12). Rarely, the extensor branches of the SL are injured, resulting in pain, heat and swelling of the affected branch in the dorsolateral or dorsomedial pastern. Differential diagnoses include AL-DDFT damage, metacarpophalangeal joint or collateral ligament injury and tarsal joint disease.

Special examination

Median and ulnar nerve blocks will provide forelimb analgesia with suspensory desmitis.[3,35,36] In the hindlimb, interpretation of nerve blocks is complicated by the potential for anesthesia of the proximal SL and the tarsal sheath when using a high plantar nerve block[37] or, conversely, the possibility of blocking the proximal SL when using a tarsometatarsal joint block.

Radiographic examination of the proximal metatarsus/ metacarpus and the tarsus or carpus respectively will help determine if there is concomitant bone or joint disease. Also, changes in proximal metatarsus/metacarpus bone density on nuclear scintigraphy may indicate abnormalities at the suspensory origin. MRI is a more useful technique to evaluate the relationship between soft tissue and bony changes, particularly in the hindlimb[38] Diagnostic ultrasonography will reveal enlargement of the SL, loss of normal echogenicity and deterioration of fiber pattern.[38–42] To fully examine the origin/proximal SL body in the hindlimb, it is necessary to place the ultrasound probe in a line just below the 'chestnut' and to aim in a plantaromedial dorsolateral direction, otherwise the large proximal portion of MTIV obscures half or more of the SL. Additionally there is muscle mixed with ligament fibers, prominent vascualture, and fat interspersed at the SL origin, causing ultrasonoraphic interpreataion to be more challenging than for the more distal SL body and branches. It is important to evaluate the entire SL from its origins on the palmar carpus/plantar tarsus and proximal MC3/ MT3 to is insertions on the sesamoid bones (Fig. 20.13, Fig. 20.14, Fig. 20.15, Fig. 20.16).

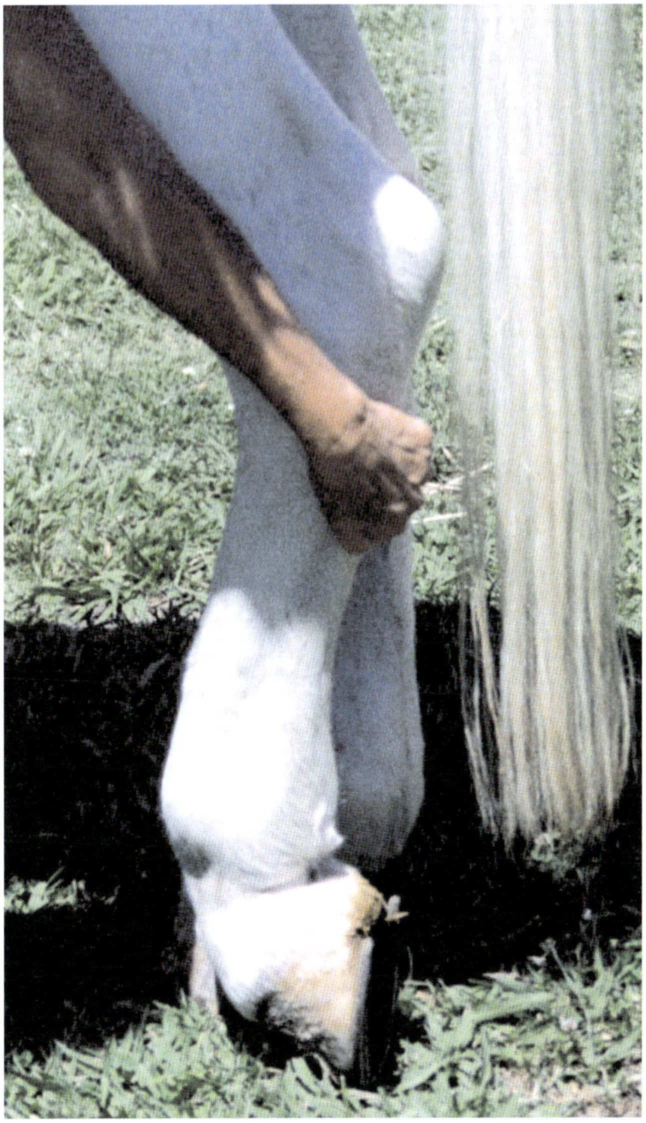

Fig 20.12 Pressure being placed on the proximal hind SL on the medial aspect of the proximal third metatarsal bone.

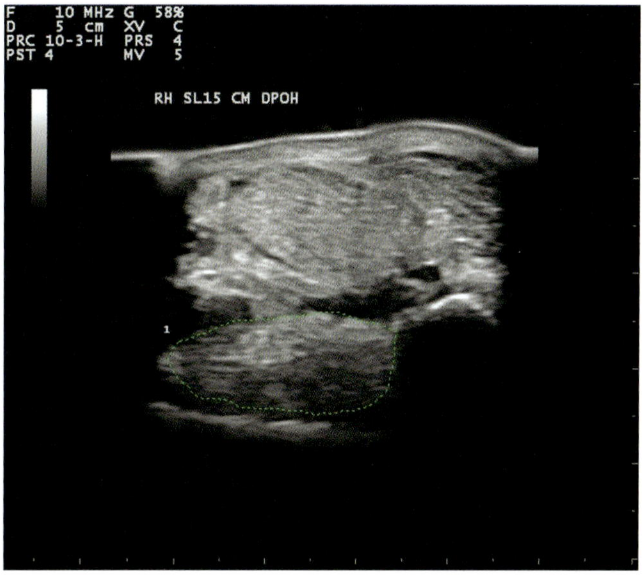

Fig 20.13 Ultrasonographic image of the metatarsal portion of the origin of the SL(encircled) in short axis view. The SL is mottled and hypoechoic and has swollen to fill the metatarsal space.

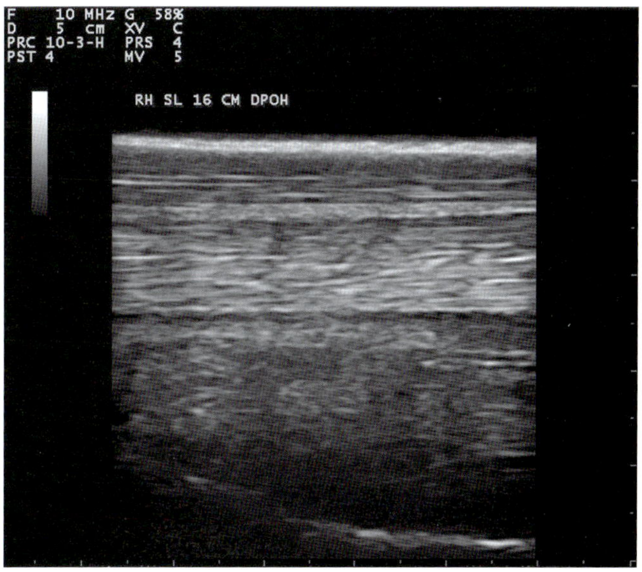

Fig 20.14 Ultrasonographic image of the same SL in Fig 20.13 in long axis view. The SL is bulging in a plantar direction toward the more shallow tendons and has lost its normal parallel linear fiber pattern.

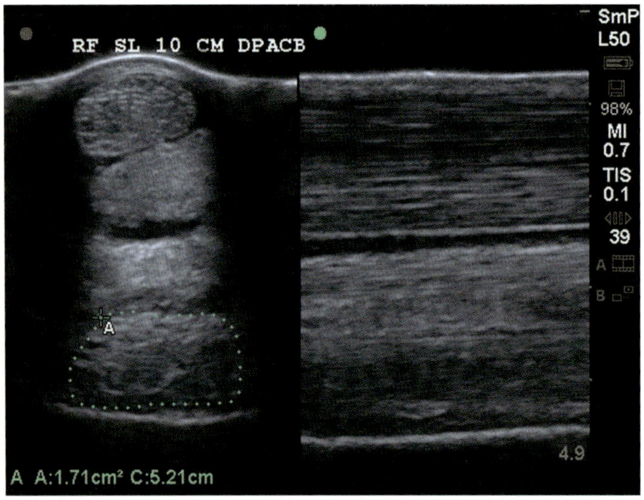

Fig 20.15 Ultrasonographic image of the SL body (encircled). The short axis view (left) shows enlargement and mottled hypoechogencity. The long axis view (right) shows a loss of normal fiber pattern.

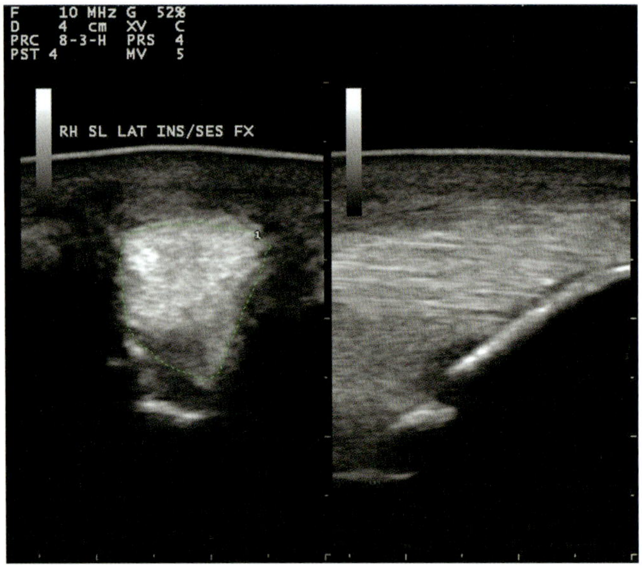

Fig 20.16 Ultrasonographic image of the SL branch at insertion. The short axis view (left) shows acute fiber tearing and discontinuity of the sesamoid. The long axis view (right) shows fiber disruption of the SL and an apical sesamoid fracture (lower left aspect of the hyperechoic line).

Treatment and prognosis

Therapeutic aims

As above.

Therapy

For general therapy please refer to the SDF tendon section (pp 401–3). Because the SL body is confined in a relatively narrow canal between MT2, MT3 and MT4, early resolution of swelling is crucial to prevent further ligament damage and to prevent compression neuropathy of the lateral plantar nerve. Topical NSAID applied twice daily for three weeks and twice daily cold therapy are generally very helpful.

Suspensory ligament injuries respond very favorably to the provision of caudal heel support through the use of an egg bar shoe that extends to the level of the heel bulbs or 1/2″ beyond the heel bulbs for hind SL cases.Hoof/pastern axis should be neutral. Horses which stride up to the front feet with the hind feet can wear bell boots to deter shoe pulling. Many horses tolerate egg bars sufficiently well to wear them through the rehabilitation phase.

Particularly in the first two weeks following injury, splitting with the use of an 18 gauge needle and ultrasound guidance is effective for decompression of lesions in the proximal SL body.

Ultrasonographic examination including evluation of the appearance of the SL relative to MT2-3 and 4 and SL cross-sectional area (CSA) measurement is crucial to monitor SL response to treatment and rest with controlled walking exercise. In the unusual case that does not respond adequately with the necessary reduction in swelling as indicated by decreased CSA, plantar fasciotomy is indicated. Due to SL atrophy following lateral plantar neurectomy[43] and particularly due to reported disastrous sequelae such as SL rupture and/or hind foot laminitis, the author does not recommend neurectomy of the deep branch of the lateral plantar nerve.

Following an initial period of stall rest and hand-walking, the SL should be re-evaluated using physical examination and ultrasonography to assess healing.[17] Increasing exercise should be based upon examination findings rather than time elapsed. The horse should be confined when not undergoing controlled exercise to a space small enough so that it can only walk until healing is sufficient to allow canter work under saddle for one week. Please refer to Table 20.1, Table 20.2, Table 20.3, Table 20.4 and Table 20.5 for detailed exercise protocols.

Prognosis

Prognosis is good for return to athletic use.

Etiology and pathophysiology

See above.

Prevention

The suspensory ligament functions with the SDF tendon to prevent the fetlock from extending to the ground during stance phase. Tendon and ligament respond to appropriate training by increasing in strength.[44] Ensuring that the equine athlete is trained in a stepwise consistent program, gradually building in difficulty, so that muscle fatigue never becomes sufficient to transfer the bulk of the horse's force on to the much smaller tendons and ligaments, is the best prevention for ligament injury. As in human athletes, a history of rapidly increasing work intensity, particularly upon return to work from another injury or as a young horse enters work or a new training situation, is commonly found as a precursor to ligament or tendon injury. Fifteen minutes of walk warm up prior to faster work in every exercise session will preload ligaments and joint capsule as well as joint fluid to better withstand the forces applied without injury.

The second group of athletes which sustain ligament injury are the horses which regularly train using a repetitive protocol; for example, a mature dressage horse which often works 1–2 hours six days per week and which repeats the same maneuvers many times each exercise session. This horse, likely working in a balanced fashion on fore- and hindlimbs, subjects his hind suspensory ligaments to wear and tear injury. Prevention entails cross-training such as hacking on a long rein 1–2 times per week and having a complete rest day, with harder work interspersed between training days. This allows for repair of microdamage to the SL incurred on training days.

Long plantar ligament desmitis (curb)

Recognition

History and presenting complaint

Swelling along the plantar/lateral aspect of the calcaneus to the proximal aspect of MTIV is observed. Long plantar ligament (LPL) desmitis most frequently occurs in Standardbred racehorses and in jumpers. Differential diagnoses include SDF tendinitis and subcutaneous swelling due to trauma.

Physical examination

Grade 1–2 out of 5 lameness is observed and is often transient. Pain, heat and swelling on palpation of the ligament are found.

Special examination

Diagnostic ultrasound will reveal enlargement, loss of echogenicity and deterioration of fiber pattern. The LPL will appear just deep to the SDF in a plantar-dorsal view and should be differentiated from the lateral lobe of the SL origin (Fig. 20.17).

Treatment and prognosis

Therapeutic aims

As above.

Therapy

For general therapy please refer to the SDF tendon section. The LPL is not a weight-bearing tendon so it can be more readily rested by the horse. Generally LPL desmitis healing is sufficiently complete in 4–5 months to allow return to work.

Prognosis

Prognosis is excellent for return to athletic use.

Long digital extensor tendinitis

Recognition

History and presenting complaint

This injury is often seen in horses which jump solid fences such as steeplechase or eventing competitors. The usual presenting complaint is of swelling over the dorsal surface of MTIII and intermittent lameness.

Physical examination

Grade 1–2 out of 5 lameness. Pain, heat and swelling are felt on palpation of the long digital extensor tendon. Damage may extend into the lateral digital extensor tendon as well.

The long digital extensor tendon has a synovial sheath on the dorsum of the tarsus; this may also be involved, filling with hemorrhage, excess synovial fluid, synovial proliferation and adhesions.

Special examination

Diagnostic ultrasound will reveal enlargement of the tendon, loss of echogenicity and deterioration of fiber pattern. Synovitis of the tendon sheath will also be seen, if present, as excess fluid with an increased cell content, synovial proliferation and/or adhesions (Fig. 20.18).

Treatment and prognosis

Therapeutic aims

As above.

Therapy

For general therapy please see the section on SDF tendinitis treatment (pp 401–3).

As extensor tendons are located on the dorsal surface of the bony column of the limb, they do not bear the brunt of the horse's weight as flexor tendons do. This allows the extensor tendons to rest and healing occurs more quickly than in flexors, generally being sufficiently complete in 4–6 months to allow return to work.

The extensor tendon sheath, if affected, should be treated at the time of diagnosis with intrathecal injection of anti-inflammatory medication such as hyaluronic acid.

Extensor tendon injuries are often associated with skin wounds or dermatitis secondary to hitting solid fences. These must be treated aggressively to reduce local inflammation and allow tendon

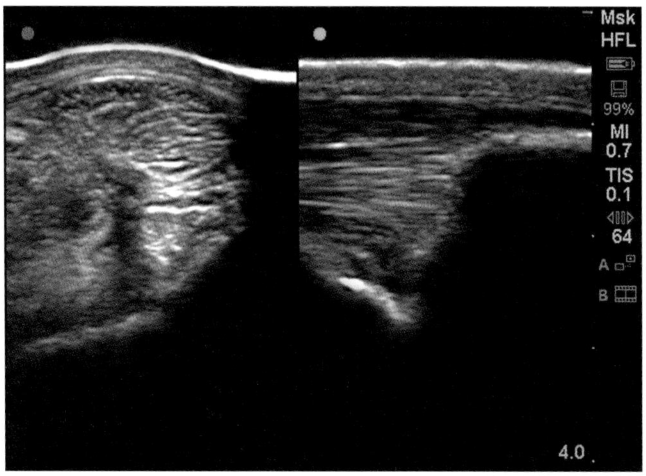

Fig 20.17 Ultrasonographic image of the LPL at insertion on MT4. The short axis view (left) shows the triangular LPL with mottled echogenicity (lower right aspect of image). The long axis view (right) shows LPL mild fiber disruption and scarring.

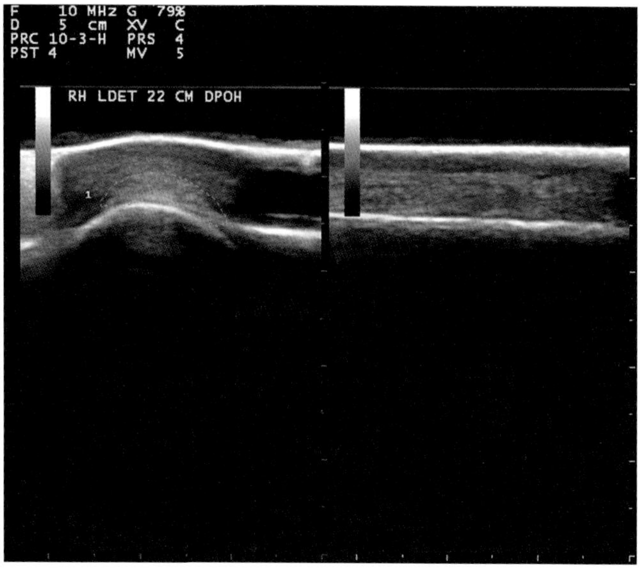

Fig 20.18 Ultrasonographic image of the long digital extensor tendon in the mid-metatarsal region.The short axis view (left) shows hypechogencity. The long axis view (right) shows a loss of normal parallel linear fiber pattern.

healing to progress without adhesion formation between the tendon and the inflamed subcutaneous tissue or the wound if present.

Prognosis

Excellent for return to athletic use.

Prevention

As extensor tendon injuries are often associated with a direct blow to the limb from a fence, the most practical prevention is protective boots for the dorsal surface of MTIII.

Common digital extensor tendinitis

Recognition

History and presenting complaint

See long digital extensor tendinitis (above). Long digital extensor tendinitis, as well as tendon laceration, is far more frequently encountered than common digital extensor tendinitis.[45]

Physical examination

Grade 1–2 out of 5 lameness is observed and is often transient and intermittent. Pain, heat and swelling are felt on palpation. The tendon sheath on the dorsal surface of the carpus may also be warm, swollen and sensitive to palpation.

Special examination

Diagnostic ultrasound will reveal enlargement of the tendon, loss of echogenicity and deterioration of fiber pattern. Synovitis of the tendon sheath will also be seen, if present, as excess, often cellular fluid, synovial proliferation and/or adhesions.

Treatment and prognosis

See long digital extensor tendinitis (above).

Straight sesamoidean ligament desmitis

Recognition

History and presenting complaint

Desmitis of the straight sesamoidean ligament (SSL) is usually seen in horses which twist and turn as part of their sport, such as eventers and cutting horses, or which work on uneven ground, such as endurance horses. This injury also occurs fairly frequently in pasture.

Physical examination

Grade 2–3 out of 5 lameness is observed. Pain, heat and swelling are encountered on palpation of the palmar/plantar aspect of the flexed limb. Differential diagnoses include other sesamoidean ligament injury, collateral ligament damage or pastern joint disease.

Special examination

Nerve blocks at the abaxial sesamoid level will greatly improve or ablate the lameness. Radiographs may reveal bone changes at the site of SSL origin at the base of the sesamoid bones or, more commonly, at the insertion on palmar P2. Diagnostic ultrasound will reveal enlargement, loss of echogenicity and deterioration of fiber pattern. A wedge of muscle tissue located at the SSL insertion on P2 can appear to be a lesion. Placing the limb caudal to the opposite forelimb with the heels touching the ground will compress the muscle, while a true lesion will remain unchanged (Fig. 20.19).

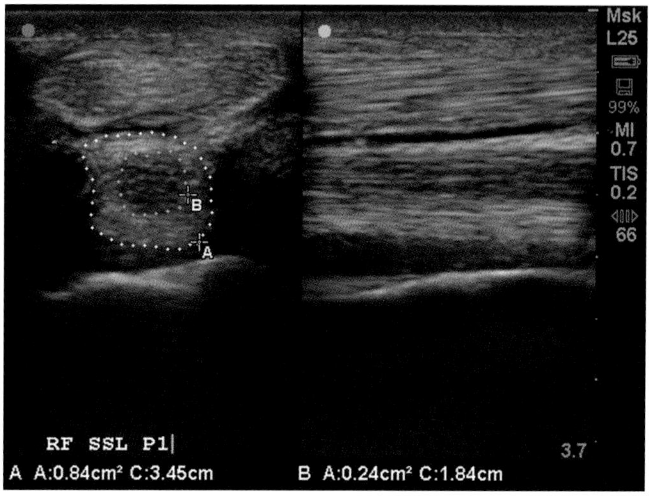

Fig 20.19 Ultrasonographic image of the SSL at mid-palmar P1. The short axis view (left) shows a hypoechoic subacute core lesion. The long axis view (right) shows a marked central loss of normal fiber pattern.

Treatment and prognosis

Therapeutic aims

As above.

Therapy

For general therapy, please refer to the SDF tendon section (pp 401–3).

Caudal heel support through the use of an egg bar shoe to the level of the heel bulbs is very helpful for this injury.

Prognosis

Prognosis is good for return to athletic use.

Etiology and pathophysiology

Torsion of the foot/pastern produces excessive force on the pastern ligaments if:

- the horse is fatigued and muscle contraction is not assisting normally in foot/pastern placement
- the fetlock is sinking excessively during weight-bearing phase due to long toe, low heel foot conformation, muscle fatigue or uneven footing.

Prevention

Balanced shoeing appropriate for the terrain and a well-conditioned horse that does not fatigue excessively during competition are the best prevention.

Oblique sesamoidean ligament desmitis

Recognition

History and presenting complaint

Oblique sesamoidean ligament (OSL) desmitis is usually seen in horses which twist and turn as part of their sport, such as eventers and cutting horses, or which work on uneven ground, such as endurance horses. This injury also occurs fairly frequently in pasture.

Physical examination

Grade 2–3 out of 5 lameness is observed, and is usually persistent. Pain is elicited on palpation of the affected branch from the base of the sesamoid bone to palmar PI.

Differential diagnoses include other sesamoidean ligament injury, collateral ligament damage, or pastern joint disease.

Special examination

Nerve block at the abaxial sesamoid level on the affected side will improve or ablate the lameness. Radiographs may reveal bony changes at the base of the sesamoid or at OSL insertion on palmar (plantar) P1. Diagnostic ultrasound will reveal enlargement, loss of echogenicity and deterioration of fiber pattern (Fig. 20.20).

Treatment and prognosis

See straight sesamoidean ligament (above).

Collateral ligament desmitis of the metacarpophalangeal/ metatarsophalangeal, proximal interphalangeal joints and distal interphalangeal joints

Recognition

History and presenting complaint

This is usually seen in horses which twist and turn as part of their sport, such as eventers and polo ponies.

Physical examination

Grade 2–4 out of 5 lameness is observed. Pain, heat and swelling are palpable on the affected ligament. Palpation is easiest when the distal limb is flexed. Signs of joint inflammation (distended joint and pain on flexion) will be present in acute cases. In chronic cases, osteoarthritis may be present, resulting in reduced flexion and a thickened joint capsule.[46]

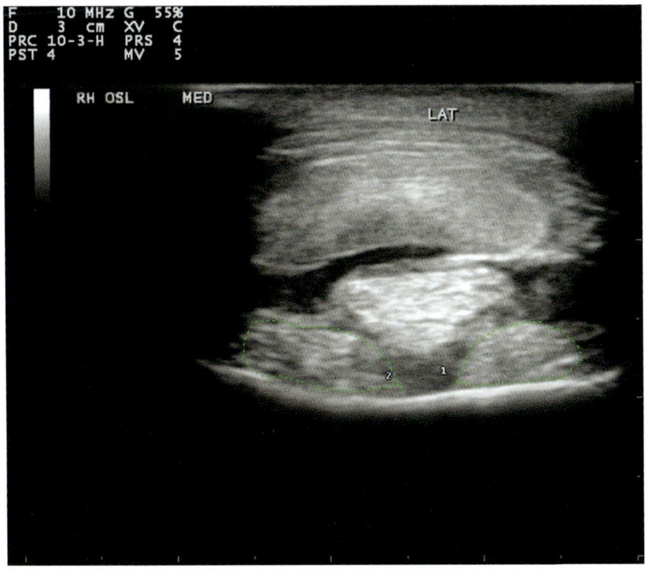

Fig 20.20 Ultrasonographic image of the OSL at mid-plantar P1.The medial branch is enlarged,mottled and hypoechoic in comparison to the lateral branch in this short axis view.

A low four-point nerve block (medial and lateral palmar/ plantar and palmar/plantar metacarpal/metatarsal nerves) greatly improves or ablates the lameness at the level of the fetlock and distal and the abaxial sesamoid block will improve or ablate lameness at the level of the proximal interphalangeal joint. Intra-articular anesthesia generally improves, but does not ablate the lameness.

Special examination

Stress radiographs may reveal medial/lateral joint laxity if damage results in significant ligament laxity. Bony abnormalities at the origin of the collateral ligaments or insertion may be detected. With acute mild to moderate collateral ligament damage radiographs will be within normal limits except for possible joint effusion. Diagnostic ultrasound will reveal ligament enlargement, loss of echogenicity and loss of normal fiber pattern. Associated joints will reveal effusion, synovial proliferation, adhesions and capsule thickening on ultrasonographic examination. The insertion of the collateral ligaments of the distal interphalangeal joint cannot be evaluated using ultrasound because of the interposition of the hoof capsule, however the proximal one-third is readily imaged (Fig. 20.21, Fig. 20.22, Fig. 20.23).

Treatment and prognosis

Therapeutic aims

As above.

Therapy

For general therapy, please refer to the SDF tendon section (pp 401–3).

Shoeing with an extension tapering from flush at the toe to a ½ to 1 inch width beyond the hoof wall at the midquarter of the affected side of the hoof will provide support and make the horse more comfortable, as well as reducing stress on the collateral ligament. Shoeing in this manner may be difficult to maintain if the medial collateral ligament is damaged, as the horse may tend to pull the shoe with the opposite foot. Instead, a shoe with a very wide medial web and narrow, swedged lateral web can be applied. Large bell boots worn at all times are helpful in preventing the shoe from being pulled off by a miss-step. Supportive shoeing should be maintained for 4–6 months. Extensions may be gradually decreased at each shoeing to 1/4 inch as clinical and ultrasonographic signs improve.

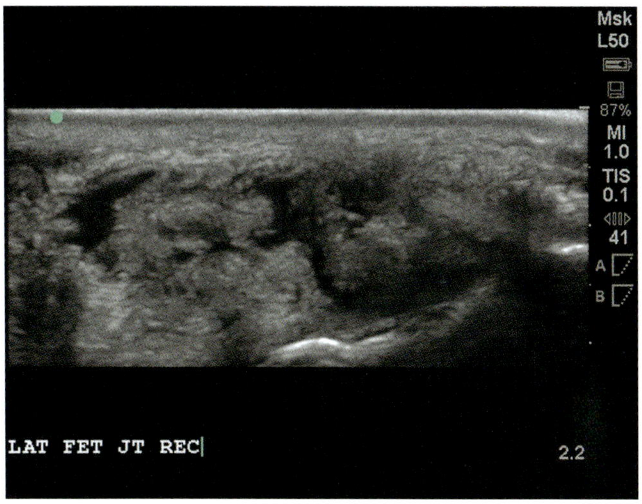

Fig 20.21 Ultrasonographic image of the lateral pouch of the metacarpo-phalangeal joint showing extensive synovial proliferation in response to an injury that also resulted in collateral ligament damage.

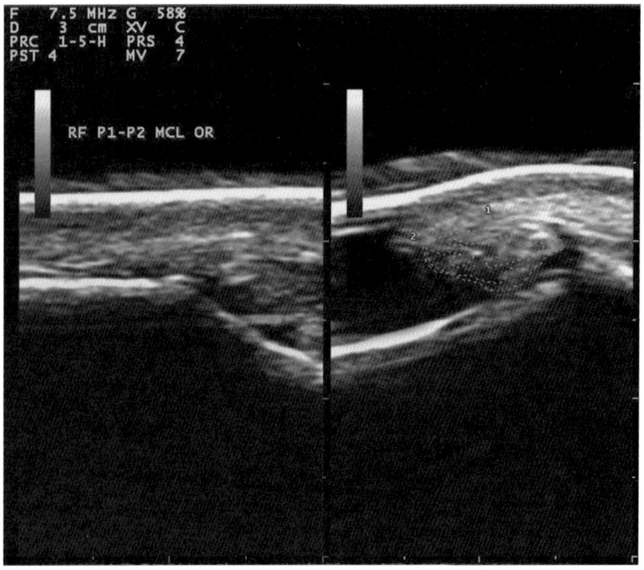

Fig 20.22 Ultrasonographic image of the origin of the proximal interphalangeal joint medial collateral ligament. The long axis view (left) shows loss of normal fiber pattern and periosteal reaction at the origin site on distal P1. The short axis view (right) shows multiple tears in the collateral ligament. There is also joint effusion seen as excessive anechoic fluid.

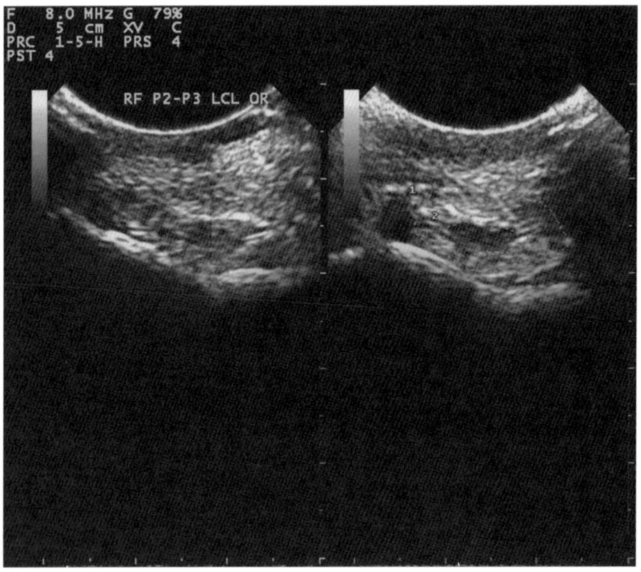

Fig 20.23 Ultrasonographic image of the distal interphalangeal joint lateral collateral ligament origin. The long axis view (left) shows a large defect in fiber alignment. The short axis view (right) shows a central hypoechoic core lesion.

Horses with collateral ligament damage may be lame when turned or circled for up to 90 days following injury. Pain is likely from joint instability as well as ligament trauma. Confinement and regular hand-walking exercise without turns are essential.

Often the joint develops synovitis or capsulitis following this type of injury; treatment of the joint with intra-articular hyaluronic acid or IRAP as well as intramuscular polysulfated glycosaminoglycan (PSGAG) therapy and oral glucosamine and hyaluronicacid, are helpful to relieve joint inflammation. If there has been hemorrhage into the joint, the horse may be in extreme pain and the joint may need to undergo lavage to rid it of inflammatory products. In cases of complete rupture of the collateral ligament(s), surgical repair of the ligament may be necessary.[47,48]

Following an initial period of stall rest and hand-walking, the collateral ligaments should be re-evaluated using physical examination and ultrasonography to assess healing.[17] Increasing exercise should be based upon examination findings rather than time elapsed. The horse should be confined when not undergoing controlled exercise to a space small enough so that it can only walk until healing is sufficient to allow canter work under saddle for 1 week. Please refer to Table 20.1, Table 20.2, Table 20.3, Table 20.4 and Table 20.5 for detailed exercise protocols.

Prognosis

Prognosis is good for return to athletic use. Concomittant joint damage may require long term management to prevent osteoarthritis.

Prevention

Balanced shoeing which provides adequate foot support is an important preventive measure. A well-conditioned horse will withstand the stresses imposed in competition with less chance of injury than a poorly conditioned horse. Fifteen minutes of walk warm up prior to faster work in every exercise session will preload ligaments and joint capsule as well as joint fluid to better withstand the forces applied without injury.

Biceps brachii tendinitis/bicipital bursitis

Recognition

History and presenting complaint

The injury often occurs due to being kicked by another horse or by hitting a solid object such as a fence. Stress injuries are uncommon.

Physical examination

Pain on palpation of the biceps tendon is usually evident. A tendency to stand with the affected limb slightly caudal to the normal one is frequently seen. Pain on extension of the tendon and compression of the bicipital bursa by pulling the limb caudally may also be seen.

Special examination

A radiographic skyline view will reveal concomitant humeral tubercle injury/pathology. Diagnostic ultrasound will reveal tendon enlargement, loss of echogenicity and fiber pattern (Fig. 20.24).[49] Bicipital bursitis is almost always seen concomitantly. Care must be taken on ultrasonographic views to differentiate the bursa from the overlying hypoechoic fibrcartilagenous portion of the biceps tendon that is compressed as it glides over the humeral tubercles. Excess fluid (greater than 3 mm depth) will be seen with effusion. The fluid will be anechoic if there is effusive synovitis present or hypoechoic if it is in the early proliferative phase. Adhesions, if present, may be seen between the bursa and the biceps tendon.

Treatment and prognosis

Therapeutic aims

As above.

Therapy

For general therapy, please see the section on SDF treatment (pp 401–3).

Bicipital bursitis, if present, should be treated as soon as it is recognized. Topical 1% diclofenac cream applied twice daily for two weeks is helpful. Initial treatment should be made with intrathecal hyaluronic acid to prevent adhesion formation and relieve inflammation. The bursa can be readily accessed using a 19 gauge 1½ needle under ultrasound guidance and confirmation of injection into the bursa can be recorded. Often 2–3 injections are required over a period of 4–6 months to resolve the synovitis. As tendon healing progresses, a steroid may be added to hyaluronic acid to increase the anti-inflammatory effect. Physical therapy, such as massage and therapeutic ultrasound to relieve biceps muscle spasm and improve comfort, tends to improve healing.

Prognosis

Chronic biceps tendon/bursa injuries with scar tissue and adhesions respond poorly to treatment, with approximately 25% of such cases returning to athletic use. Early detection of the injury combined with aggressive medical and physical therapy improves the prognosis to 70% return to athletic use.

Etiology and pathophysiology

Direct crushing of the tendon against the humeral tubercles is the most common etiology for biceps brachii damage and concomitant bursitis.This injury is often due to an accident such as hitting a fence or a kick.

Prevention

Careful handling of stallions while breeding mares and avoidance while riding of close proximity to another horse's hindquarters help to prevent accidental injury.

Dorsal spinous ligament and interspinous ligament

Recognition

History and presenting complaint

Horses with injury to one or both ligaments often present with sore or cold backs. They also often resent being saddled or mounted or refuse to jump or to canter. This injury can be seen in any type of equine athlete.[50,51]

Physical examination

Pain on palpation of the affected portion of the dorsal spinous ligament is evident.

Special examination

Radiographs of the dorsal spinous processes may reveal osteoarthrosis, which is likely secondary to chronic ligament injury and subsequent instability. Diagnostic ultrasonography will reveal enlargement, loss of echogenicity and deterioration of the normal fiber pattern of the affected dorsal spinous ligament or interspinous ligament (Fig. 20.25).

Treatment and prognosis

Therapy

For general therapy, please refer to the section on SDF treatment (pp 401–3).

Horses with dorsal spinous or interspinous ligament damage may require 4–6 months of exercise such as ponying or walking and trotting on an exerciser before being worked under saddle.

Prognosis

Prognosis is good for return to athletic use. If dorsal spinous process changes are also present, long term management will be required.

Dorsal sacroiliac ligament (DSIL)

Recognition

History and presenting complaint

Jumpers are particularly susceptible to this injury. Signs may also develop after a fall, either in work or loose in pasture. Horses are usually presented for evaluation of a 'bump' at the croup (sacroiliac region) or changes in gluteal muscle balance.

Physical examination

Intermittent grade 1–3 out of 5 lameness is observed. The tuber sacrale are often uneven when viewed from behind the horse due to concomitant sacroiliac joint subluxation and/or crushing of the tuber sacrum. There is often gluteal wasting of the affected limb. Over time, many horses develop bileratal DSIL injury, likely as a

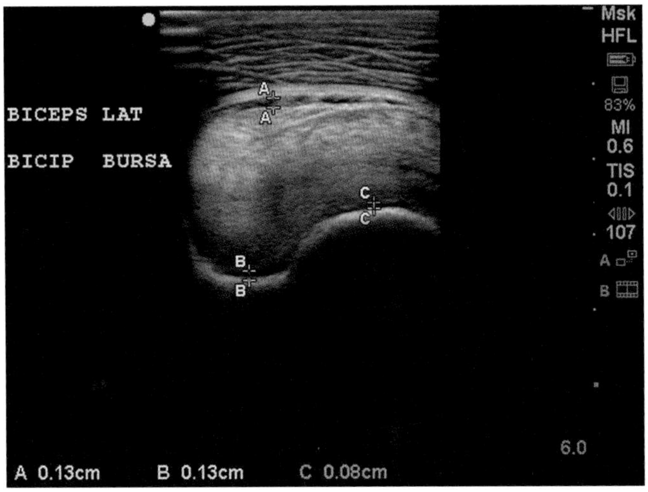

Fig 20.24 Ultrasonographic image of the lateral lobe of the biceps tendon and the bicipital bursa in short axis view. The bursa is within normal limits for fluid depth, however synovial proliferation is seen shallow to the tendon. The biceps tendon is mottled and hypoechoic with three linear tears subsequent to a crush injury.

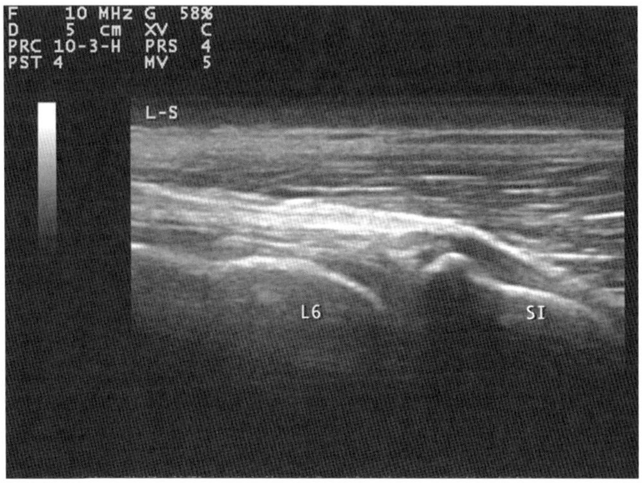

Fig 20.25 Ultrasonographic image of the interspinous ligament in long axis view. There is loss of normal fiber pattern and mild scar. The cranial edge of S1 is reactive, indicating proliferative response to long term inflammation and instability associated with ligament damage.

result of the close attachements of the ligaments to the sacral spine and of the effects of sacroiliac joint subluxation causing uneven loading.

Special examination

Diagnostic ultrasonography will reveal enlargement, loss of echogenicity and deterioration of fiber pattern of the affected ligament(s) (Fig. 20.26). [51]

Treatment and prognosis

For general therapy, please refer to the section on SDF treatment (pp 401–3).

Horses with dorsal spinous ligament damage may require 4–6 months of exercise such as ponying or walking and trotting on an exerciser before being worked under saddle. Following an initial period of stall rest and hand-walking, the DSIL should be re-evaluated using physical examination and ultrasonography to assess healing.[17] Increasing exercise should be based upon examination findings rather than time elapsed. The horse should be confined, when not undergoing controlled exercise, to a space small enough. This is so that it can only walk until healing is sufficient to allow canter work under saddle for one week. Please refer to Tables 20.1–5 for detailed exercise protocols.

Prognosis is good for return to work if rehabilitation is successfully completed and any concomittant issues such assacroiliac joint subluxation and/or lower hind limb pathology are addressed.

Gastrocnemius (achilles) tendinitis

Recognition

History and presenting complaint

Achilles tendon damage is often seen after a fall or after having the hindlimb trapped in a fence or gate.

Physical examination

Persistent grade 2–3 out of 5 lameness is observed. Pain, heat and swelling of the affected portion of the tendon are palpable. The tarsus will be dropped if sufficient damage of the tendon has occurred.

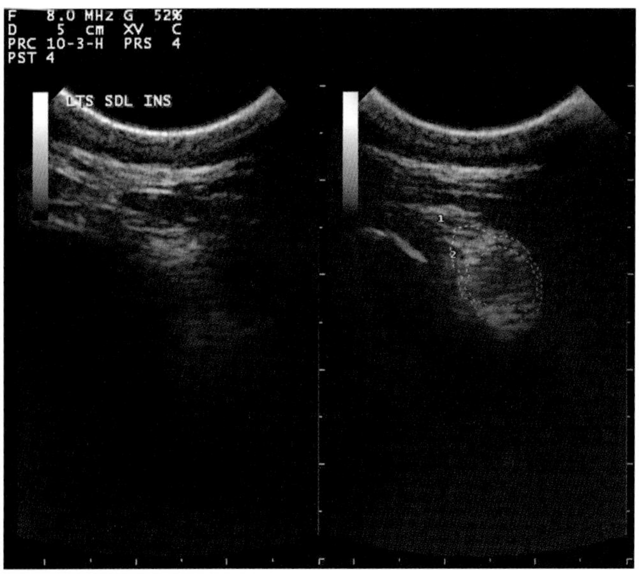

Fig 20.26 Ultrasonographic image of the insertion of the DSIL on the sacrum with the long axis (left) showing a large gap in the fiber pattern and the short axis (right) showing a large hypoechoic core lesion.

Special examination

A tibial nerve block will improve the lameness.[52] Diagnostic ultrasound will reveal enlargement, loss of echogenicity and deterioration of fiber pattern. The tendon is seen proximally as two muscular heads, which join at the musculotendinous junction. Just proximal to the tarsus the gastrocnemius tendon twists from its position superficial to the SDF tendon and becomes deep to it.

Treatment and prognosis

Therapy

Core lesions, if seen, can be decompressed effectively in the acute stage (less than two weeks) using ultrasound guidance.

Prognosis

Prognosis is fair to good for return to athletic use.

Prevention

This is usually an accidental injury.

Digital sheath syndrome

Recognition

The digital sheath is a complex synovial structure[53,54] which surrounds the superficial (SDF) and deep (DDF) flexor tendons from proximal to the fetlock joint distally to midpastern. Normally, the synovium secretes a small amount of fluid which promotes gliding of the flexor tendons around the palmar/plantar aspect of the fetlock joint. With inflammation, the sheath can become greatly distended, reaching to midmetacarpus proximally and/or 'herniating' palmar/planatar to the SDF tendon on the midline.

History and presenting complaint

Generally, digital sheath (DS) synovitis presents as a cumulative wear and tear type of injury which progresses over time. Horses have often been in hard work for a period of time and progress from a non-painful blemish to a syndrome that causes gradually increasing lameness.

Physical examination

Clinical signs of digital sheath synovitis reflect the degree of inflammation, which is divided into three stages. It is not uncommon for athletic horses to present with mild to moderate effusion of the digital sheaths (stage 1 synovitis) of both forelimbs, both hindlimbs or all four limbs. Often, sheath distension decreases following exercise. The distension is fluidly fluctuant on palpation. The patient is sound, non-painful to sheath palpation and negative to fetlock flexion. The lay term often used to describe stage 1 DS synovitis is 'wind-puffs'.

If synovitis progresses from the effusive stage to synovial proliferation (stage 2), clinical signs include mild to moderate lameness. This is often first seen as an attempt by the horse to guard the affected sheath by failing to fully extend the fetlock, manifested as a decreased drop in the fetlock during the stance phase of gait in comparison to the opposite fetlock. The digital sheath will feel firm rather than fluid on palpation and one aspect of the sheath, usually the lateral aspect, will be more distended (Fig. 20.27). The horse will be positive to fetlock flexion, as this maneuver compresses the sheath.

If synovitis progresses to stage 3, synovial proliferation and inflammatory product secretion may cause the patient to be severely lame.[55] The horse will be reluctant to place the heels of the foot on

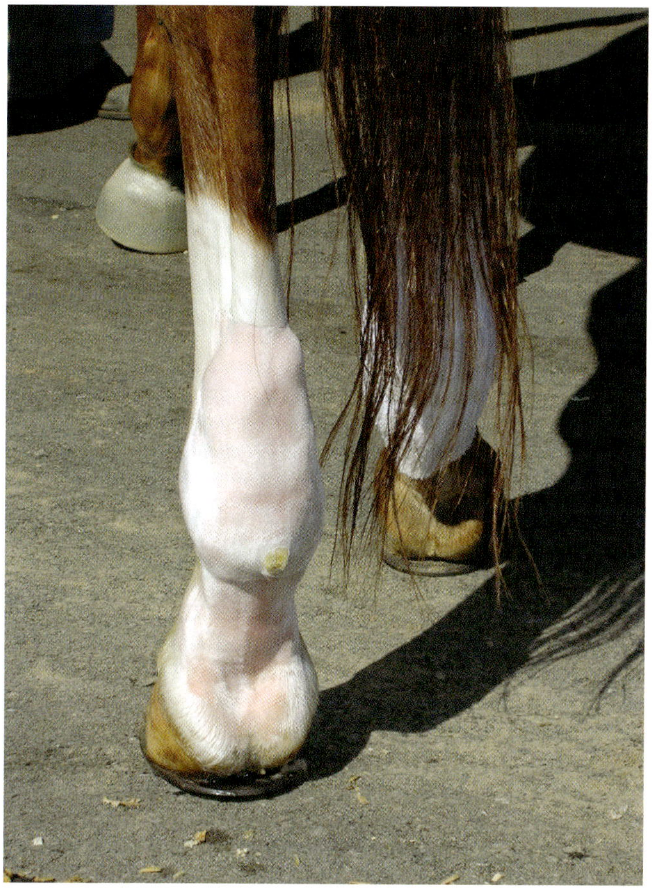

Fig 20.27 Photo of the left hind digital sheath of a horse with stage 2 synovitis.

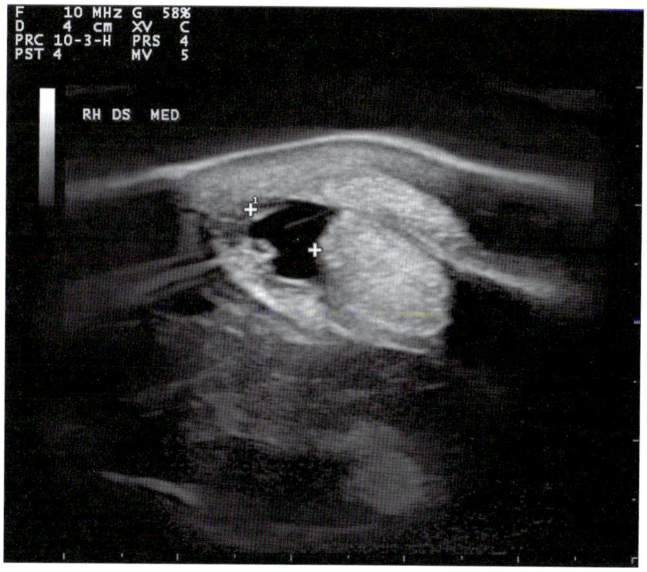

Fig 20.28 Ultrasonographic image of the right hind digital sheath in short axis view showing effusion, synovial proliferation and edge tears of the DDF tendon.

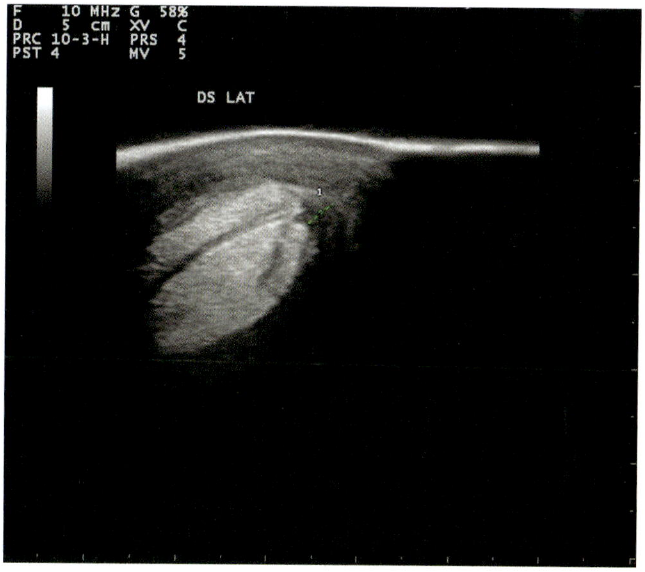

Fig 20.29 Ultrasonographic image of the lateral spect of a digital sheath in short axis view showing a linear tear in the DDF tendon.

the ground and may not tolerate fetlock flexion. The digital sheath will be distended, painful and firm on palpation.

Often, stage 2 and stage 3 digital sheath synovitis are accompanied by damage to either the superficial or deep flexor tendons.[56] This is probably due to the same wear and tear process that caused sheath synovitis. The synovitis advances by prolonged exposure to inflammatory mediators circulating in the sheath, being compressed by synovial proliferation and, finally, due to active pulling on the tendons by adhesions within the sheath. Palmar annular ligament (PAL) desmitis, likely due to chronic stretching of the ligament by the distended digital sheath, may result in a thickened PAL which further compresses the digital sheath, causing a cycle of increasing inßammation, swelling and constriction.

Special examination

A low four-point nerve block will improve/ablate lameness. Ultrasonographic examination of stage 1 synovitis reveals a moderate amount of fluid in the affected sheath(s), with no evidence of synovial proliferation or adhesions.

Ultrasonographic examination of stage 2 synovitis will reveal distension of the sheath with fluid and proliferative synovium. Proliferative tissue may also begin to cover the surfaces of the flexor tendons. Ultrasonographic examination of stage 3 synovitis will reveal extensive synovial proliferation, often covering the surfaces of the flexor tendons, and one or more adhesions between the tendons and the sheath wall (Fig. 20.28). At any stage, but particularly in stages 2 and 3, SDF, DDF or PAL pathology may also be observed (Fig. 20.29).

Treatment and prognosis

Therapeutic aims

Inflammation of the digital sheath should be vigorously treated to reduce excessive synovial proliferation and the onset of restrictive scar formation.

Therapy

Treatment of stage 1 synovitis is medical and may consist of anti-inflammatory medication, cold hosing/icing of the affected limb(s), administration of intramuscular or intrathecal PSGAG or IRAP. Foot balance should be checked and lameness in any other limb that is leading to overload should be recognized and treated.

Treatment of stage 2 synovitisincludes the above plus a series of three injections of first steroid and hyaluronic acid, second hyaluronic acid alone and third steroid and hyaluronic acid spaced 2–3 weeks apart. During this time, the horse is confined and is ridden at a walk or hand walked twice daily.[56] Patients that do not respond promptly and fully to medical treatment require tenoscopy to remove excess proliferative synovial tissue and adhesions. The PAL may be resected[57] tenoscopically at this time to provide relief from compression.

Treatment of stage 3 synovitis requires medical and surgical treatment, as outlined above for stage 2.

Surgical intervention

In cases with thickening and constriction of the annular ligament, some portion of the surgery may be designed to relieve the restrictive effects of this structure. Resection of the PAL[58] will temporarily interrupt the inflammatory cycle but regrowth of the ligament is inevitable and unless the primary problem of synovitis is corrected, the end result will be a progressively more painful sheath that has distended to meet its new dimensions following PAL resection.

Tenoscopic exploration will detect abnormalities of the tendon sheath, superficial digital flexor tendon, deep digital flexor tendon and intersesamoidean ligament Proliferative masses can be removed as well as frayed tendon edges. Adhesions present between the tendons and the tendon sheath are also debrided.[59,60]

Paramount to the success of this procedure is the strict adherence to an aggressive postoperative protocol, including medical therapy as outlined above, for a period of weeks followed by a clinical and ultrasonographic re-evaluation.

Prognosis

Prognosis for stage 1 synovitis is good. As long as the horse is in full athletic use, medical treatment may be required to prevent progression to stage 2 synovitis. Prognosis for stage 2 synovitis is good for full athletic work, if appropriate treatment is performed in a timely manner. Prognosis for stage 3 synovitis is fair for full athletic use. Without treatment, these patients may progress to lameness even at a walk.

Etiology and pathophysiology

Either acute direct trauma or over-extension of the fetlock can cause hemorrhage into the sheath space that initiates a marked inflammatory reaction. Alternatively, repetitive fetlock extension over time results in an ongoing inflammatory process.[22]

Stifle ligament injuries

Recognition

Two groups of horses generally present with stifle joint abnormalities. The first group consists of young horses beginning training. These horses generally have developmental orthopedic disease which becomes apparent when regular exercise is initiated, or intermittent upward fixation of the patella secondary to lack of muscle development. The second group consists of mature horses in full work which sustain (usually) cumulative wear and tear injuries or suffer a traumatic event such as a fall over a fence or directly hitting the stifle.

History and presenting complaint

Stifle ligament injuries generally present with a history of intermittent lameness that is most pronounced 2–3 days after hard exercise. Ligament damage leads to joint laxity; therefore joint effusion is often also noticed, most frequently in the medial femorotibial joint.

Physical examination

Lameness, either unilateral or bilateral, is localized to the stifle(s) by palpation of the joints for effusion and pain, positive response to stifle manipulation and intra-articular anesthesia. Horses which have intermittent upward fixation of the patella are suspect for medial patellar ligament desmitis. These horses are generally not lame or mildly so. They tend to have femoropatellar joint effusion that is mild. Horses with collateral ligament and meniscal injuries are initially Grade II-III/V lame and positive to flexion. There is generally moderate to marked femorotibial joint effusion. As 75% of meniscal injuries are to the medial meniscus and to the medial collateral or meniscotibial ligaments[61], clinical signs will usually be most prominent on the medial aspect of the limb. The examiner should be aware that horses with patellar ligament or collateral ligament injuries, subchondral bone cysts, or severe stifle pathology such as fractures, advanced osteoarthritis and severe cruciate ligament tears may respond partially or not at all to intra-articular anesthesia.[62]

Special examination

Radiography is useful to determine osseous abnormalities associated with ligament injuries, such as osteoarthritis secondary to chronic joint instability or changes at the origins and insertions of the cruciate ligaments. Ultrasonography provides visualization of the collateral, patellar, and meniscal ligaments (Fig. 20.30). The cruciate ligaments can be partially seen on flexed views. The amount of synovial fluid seen in the joints and the amount of fibrin, synovial proliferation and capsule thickening can be detected and measured ultrasonographically (Fig. 20.31). This information can be used on subsequent sequential examinations to assist in determining efficacy of therapy during ligament rehabilitation. Ongoing femorotibial joint effusion, for example, may indicate that arthroscopy is indicated to remove frayed cruciate ligament or meniscal fibers.

Treatment and prognosis

For general therapy, please see the section on SDF tendinitis (pp 401–3).

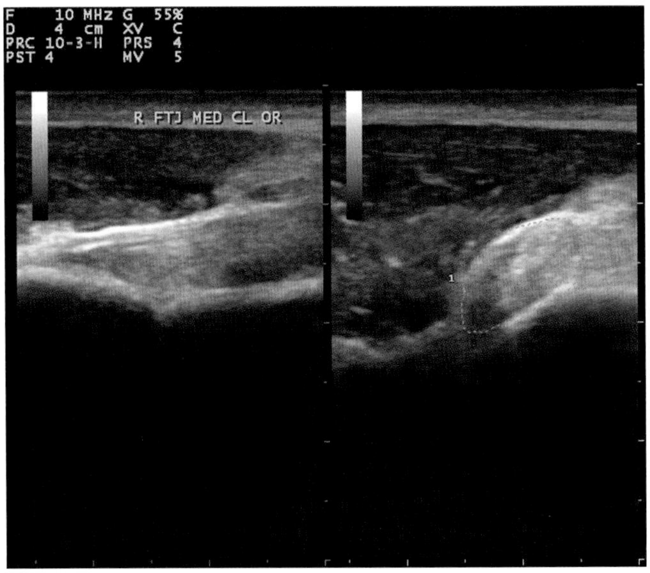

Fig 20.30 Ultrasonographic image of the medial collateral ligament of the femorotibial joint. The long axis (left) image shows disruption of the normal parallel linear fiber pattern. The short axis view (right) shows focal loss of normal echogenicity in the area of the ligament with torn fibers.

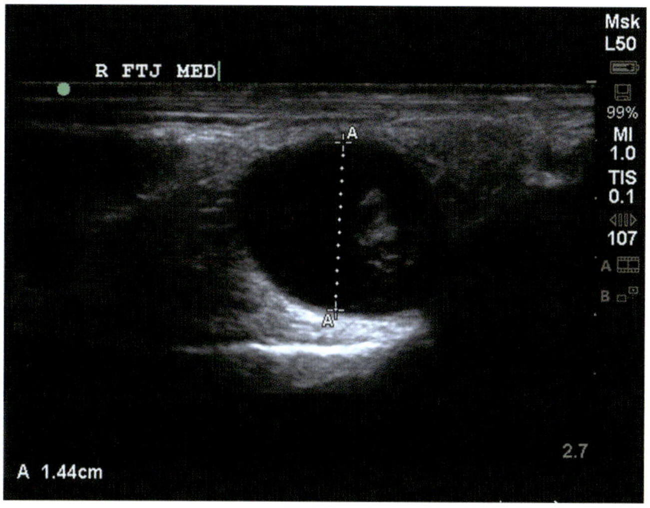

Fig 20.31 Ultrasonographic image of the medial femorotibial joint space. There is effusion as seen by the rounded appearance of the joint and by measurement of 14.4 mm of fluid depth. Echogenic fibrin is also seen within the joint space.

Therapeutic aims

To relieve inflammation and halt further ligament damage by initiating rest and controlled exercise.

Therapy

Stifle ligaments respond to the same rehabilitation protocol as do flexor tendons and require the same time frame to heal. Many horses with intermittent upward fixation of the patella and secondary patellar ligament desmitis have straight hindlimbs and low hind heels with broken back hoof pastern axes. This conformation makes it difficult for the quadriceps muscle to exert effective tension on the medial patellar ligament for its release from the medial femoral trochlea. Raising the heels to align the hoof/pastern axes alleviates or eliminates intermittent upward fixation of the patella and allows healing of the medial patellar ligament through controlled exercise. Horses often present with a combination of ligamentous and primary or secondary joint diesase. The joint injuries if present should be treated with systemic and topical NSAID administration, polysulfated glycosaminoglycan, cold therapy, oral glucosamine and hyaluronic acid, and IRAP as choices to interrupt the inflammatory cycle and promote healing. One or a series of intra-articular injections of anti-inflammatory and disease modulating medications may also be required, generally at three week intervals. Response to treatment is assessed clinically and ultrasonographically.

Prognosis

Although prognosis is reported as fair, this can be improved to good by using an approach that acknowledges both ligamentous and joint injury follwed by appropriate treatment and rehabilitation. As stifle injuries are often accompanied by back and/or lower limb pathology, these issues must also be detected and treated for a successful outcome.

Etiology and pathophysiology

The stifle and associated ligaments are affected strongly by the stay apparatus, which also causes synchronous flexion/extension of the hock. Developmental orthopedic disease frequently affects the femur; abnormal use of the limb due to bone pain may place mensicii and ligaments at increased risk of over load and injury. The medial aspect of the thigh has little musculature in comparison to the lateral aspect; this may contribute to the much higher incidence of medial stifle ligament injury.

The author acknowledges the assistance of Cathy Hebert in preparation of the figures.

References

1. Rapp HJ, Becker M, Heisse K, et al. [Diagnosis and therapy of tendinitis exemplified by the athletic horse]. Sportverletz Sportschaden 1992;6(2):77–88.
2. Meershoek LS, Lanovaz JL, Schamhardt HC, et al. Calculated forelimb flexor tendon forces in horses with experimentally induced superficial digital ßexor tendinitis and the effects of application of heel wedges. Am J Vet Res 2002;63(3):432–7.
3. Keg PR, van der Belt AJ, Merkens HW, et al. The effect of regional nerve blocks on the lameness caused by collagenase induced tendinitis in the midmetacarpal region of the horse: a study using gait analysis, and ultrasonography to determine tendon healing. Zentralbl Veterinarmed A 1992;39(5):349–64.
4. Gibson KT, Burbidge HM, Anderson BH. Tendinitis of the branches of insertion of the superficial digital flexor tendon in horses. Aust Vet J 1997;75(4):253–6.
5. Pickersgill CH, Marr CM, Reid SW. Repeatability of #diagnostic ultrasonography in the assessment of the equine superficial digital flexor tendon. Equine Vet J 2001;33(1):33–7.
6. Reef VB. Superficial digital flexor tendon healing: ultrasonographic evaluation of therapies. Vet Clin North Am Equine Pract 2001;17(1):159–78, vii–viii.
7. van Schie HT, Bakker EM, Jonker AM, et al. Ultrasonographic tissue characterization of equine superficial digital ßexor tendons by means of gray level statistics. Am J Vet Res 2000;61(2):210–9.
8. Micklethwaite L, Wood AK, Sehgal CM, et al. Use of quantitative analysis of sonographic brightness for detection of early healing of tendon injury in horses. Am J Vet Res 2001;62(8):1320–7.
9. Gillis C, Sharkey N, Stover SM, et al. Ultrasonography as a method to determine tendon cross-sectional area. Am J Vet Res 1995;56(10):1270–4.
10. Gillis C, Meagher DM, Cloninger A, et al. Ultrasonographic cross-sectional area and mean echogenicity of the superficial and deep digital flexor tendons in 50 trained thoroughbred racehorses. Am J Vet Res 1995;56(10):1265–9.
11. Cauvin ER, Munroe GA, Boyd JS. Endoscopic examination of the carpal flexor tendon sheath in horses. Equine Vet J 1997;29(6):459–66.
12. Southwood LL, Stashak TS, Kainer RA. Tenoscopic anatomy of the equine carpal flexor synovial sheath. Vet Surg 1998;27(2):15–157.
13. Dow SM, Wilson AM, Goodship AE. Treatment of acute superficial digital flexor tendon injury in horses with polysulphated glycosaminoglycan. Vet Rec 1996;139(17):413–6.
14. Guest DJ, Smith RW, Allen WR. Equine embryonic stem-like cells and mesenchymal stromal cells have different survival rates and migration patterns following their injection into damaged superficial digital flexor tendon. Equine vet J 2010;42(7):636–42.
15. Textor JA, Norris JW, Tablin F. 'Effects of preparation method, shear force, and exposure to collagen on release of growth factors from equine platelet-rich plasma'. Am J Vet Res 2011;72:271–8.
16. Scott R, Nankervis K, Stringer C, et al. The efect of water height on stride frequency,stride length and heart rate during water treadmill exercise.Equine Vet J 2010;42(38):662–4.

17. Gillis C. Ultrasonography for monitoring healing and rehabilitation. Clin Tech in EQ Practice 2007;6(3):174–8.
18. Alexander GR, Gibson KT, Day RE, et al. Effects of superior check desmotomy on flexor tendon and suspensory ligament strain in equine cadaver limbs. Vet Surg 2001;30(6):522–7.
19. Gibson KT, Burbidge HM, Pfeiffer DU. Superficial digital flexor tendinitis in thoroughbred racehorses: outcome following non-surgical treatment and superior check desmotomy. Aust Vet J 1997;75(9):631–5.
20. Dowling BA, Dart AJ, Hodgson DR, et al. Superficial digital ßexor tendinitis in the horse. Equine Vet J 2000;32(5):369–78.
21. Meershoek LS, Schamhardt HC, Roepstorff L, et al. Forelimb tendon loading during jump landings and the influence of fence height. Equine Vet J 2001;33(suppl):6–10.
22. Harrison SM, Whitton RC, Kawcak CE, Stover SM, Pandy MG. Relationship between muscle forces, joint loading and utilization of elastic strain energy in equine locomotion. J Exp Biol 2010;213: 3998–4009.
23. Busoni V, Denoix JM. Ultrasonography of the podotrochlear apparatus in the horse using a transcuneal approach: technique and reference images. Vet Radiol Ultrasound 2001;42(6):534–40.
24 Rabba S, Bolen G, Verwhilghen D. et al. Ultrasonographic findings in horses with foot pain without radiographically detectableosseus abnormalities. Vet Radiol Ultrasound 2011;52(1):95–102.
25. Hoffer MA, Leach DH, Doige CE. The developmental anatomy of the equine navicular bursa and associated structures. Anat Embryol 1989;179(4):355–67.
26. Cauvin ER, Taprest J, Monroe GA, et al. Endoscopic examination of the tarsal sheath of the lateral digital flexor tendon in horses. Equine Vet J 1999;31(3):219–27.
27. Denoix JM, Busoni V. Ultrasonographic anatomy of the accessory ligament of the superficial digital flexor tendon in horses. Equine Vet J 1999;31(3):186–91.
28. Becker CK, Savelberg HH, Buchner HH, et al. Long-term consequences of experimental desmotomy of the accessory ligament of the deep digital flexor tendon in adult horses. Am J Vet Res 1998;59(3):347–51.
29. Todhunter PG, Schumacher J, Finn-Bodner ST. Desmotomy for treatment of chronic desmitis of the accessory ligament of the deep digital flexor tendon in a horse. Can Vet J 1997; 38(10):637–9.
30. White NA 2nd. Ultrasound-guided transection of the accessory ligament of the deep digital flexor muscle (distal check ligament desmotomy) in horses. Vet Surg 1995;24(5):373–8.
31. Buchner HH, Savelberg HH, Becker CK. Load redistribution after desmotomy of the accessory ligament of the deep digital flexor tendon in adult horses. Vet Q 1996;18(suppl 2):S70–74.
32. van den Belt AJ, Becker CK, Dik KJ. Desmitis of the accessory ligament of the deep digital flexor tendon in the horse: clinical and ultrasonographic features. A report of 24 cases. Zentralbl Veterinarmed A 1993;40(7):492–500.
33. Embertson RM. Congenital abnormalities of tendons and ligaments. Vet Clin North Am Equine Pract 1994;10(2):351–64.
34. Becker CK, Savelberg HH, Barneveld A. In vitro mechanical properties of the accessory ligament of the deep digital flexor tendon in horses in relation to age. Equine Vet J 1994;26(6):454–9.
35. Keg PR, Schamhardt HC, van Weeren PR, et al. The effect of the high palmar nerve block and the ulnar nerve block on lameness provoked by a collagenase-induced tendinitis of the lateral branch of the suspensory ligament. Vet Q 1996;18(suppl 2):S103–105.
36. Muylle S, Desmet P, Simoens P, et al. Histological study of the innervation of the suspensory ligament of the forelimb of the horse. Vet Rec 1998;142(22):606–10.
37. Dyson SJ, Romero JM. An investigation of injection techniques for local analgesia of the equine distal tarsus and proximal metatarsus. Equine Vet J 1993;25(1):30–5.
38. Dyson SJ. The suspensory apparatus. In: Dyson SJ, Ross MW, editors. Diagnosis and management of lameness in the horse. 2nd ed. St Louis: Elsevier; 2011. p. 738–60.
39. Gillis CL. Suspensory ligament desmitis and associated fractures.Proc 40th Convention AAEP 2004;40:187–8
40. Dyson SJ, Arthur RM, Palmer SE, et al. Suspensory ligament desmitis. Vet Clin North Am Equine Pract 1995;11(2): 177–215.
41. Dyson S. Proximal suspensory desmitis in the hindlimb: 42 cases. Br Vet J 1994;150(3):279–91.
42. Dyson S. Proximal suspensory desmitis: clinical, ultrasonographic and radiographic features. Equine Vet J 1991;23(1):25–31.
43. Pauwels FE. Neurectomy of the deep branch of the lateral plantar nerve can cause neurogenic atrophy of the muscle fibres in the proximal part of the suspensory ligament (M. interosseous III). Equine Vet J 2009;41(5):508–10.
44. Bukowiecki CF, Bramlage LR, Gabel AA. In vitro strength of the suspensory apparatus in training and resting horses. Vet Surg 1987;16(2):126–30.
45. Belknap JK, Baxter GM, Nickels FA. Extensor tendon lacerations in horses: 50 cases (1982–1988). J Am Vet Med Assoc 1993;203(3):428–31.
46. Simmons EJ, Bertone AL, Weisbrode SE. Instability-induced osteoarthritis in the metacarpophalangeal joint of horses. Am J Vet Res 1999;60(1):7–13.
47. Collard XR, Danse EM, Rombouts JJ. [The syndrome of external ligament sprain in the horse.] Acta Orthop Belg 2000;66(3):229–41.
48. van der Harst MR, Rijkenhuizen AB. The use of a polypropylene mesh for treatment of ruptured collateral ligaments of the equine metatarsophalangeal joint: a report of two cases. Vet Q 2000;22(1):57–60.
49. Crabill MR, Chaffin MK, Schmitz DG. Ultrasonographic morphology of the bicipital tendon and bursa in clinically normal quarter horses. Am J Vet Res 1995;56(1):5–10.
50. Jeffcott LB. Disorders of the thoracolumbar spine of the horse: a survey of 443 cases. Equine Vet J 1980;12(4):197–210.
51. Gillis C. Spinal ligament pathology. Vet Clin North Am Equine Pract 1999;15(1):97–101.
52. Dyson SJ, Kidd L. Five cases of gastrocnemius tendinitis in the horse. Equine Vet J 1992;24(5):351–6.
53. Hago BE, Plummer JM, Vaughan LC. Equine synovial tendon sheaths and bursae: an histological and scanning electron microscopical study. Equine Vet J 1990;22(4):264–72.
54. Hago BE, Vaughan LC, Plummer JM. Equine synovial tendon sheaths and bursae: a transmission electron microscope study. Equine Vet J 1991;23(6):475–8.
55. Dyson SJ, Dik KJ. Miscellaneous conditions of tendons, tendon sheaths, and ligaments. Vet Clin North Am Equine Pract 1995;11(2):315–37.
56. Gaughan EM, Nixon AJ, Krook LP, et al. Effects of sodium hyaluronate on tendon healing and adhesion formation in horses. Am J Vet Res 1991;52(5):764–73.
57. van den Berg MJ, Rijkenhuizen AB, Nemeth F, et al. The fetlock tunnel syndrome: a macroscopic and microscopic study. Vet Q 1995;17(4):138–42.
58. Barr AR, Dyson SJ, Barr FJ, et al. Tendinitis of the deep digital ßexor tendon in the distal metacarpal/ metatarsal region associated with tenosynovitis of the digital sheath in the horse. Equine Vet J 1995;27(5):348–55.
59. Fortier LA, Nixon AJ, Duchorme NG, et al. Tenoscopic examination and proximal annular ligament desmotomy for treatment of equine complex digital sheath tenosynovitis. Vet Surg 1999;28(6):429–35.
60. Dik KJ, Dyson SJ, Vail TB. Aseptic tenosynovitis of the digital flexor tendon sheath, fetlock and pastern annular ligament constriction. Vet Clin North Am Equine Pract 1995;11(2):151–62.
61. Hoegaerts M, Nicaise M, van Bree H, et al. Cross sectional anatomy and comparative ultrasonography of the equine medial femerotibial joint and its related structures. Equine Vet J 2005;37(6):520–9.
62. Walmsley JP. The stifle. In: Dyson SJ, Ross MW, editors. Diagnosis and management of lameness in the horse. 2nd ed. St Louis: Elsevier; 2011. p. 532–49.

Back and pelvis

21

Kevin K. Haussler Leo B. Jeffcott

CHAPTER CONTENTS

Introduction and historical perspectives

Historical reports of back disorders in horses provide few firm facts from the many lengthy accounts in old farriery and veterinary textbooks. In 1876 Lupton remarked that back injuries 'are among the most common and least understood of equine afflictions'.[1] In those days diagnosis was based simply on clinical observation (Fig. 21.1) and the opinions expressed were many and varied. These early writers were often excellent horsemen and were particularly knowledgeable on aspects of conformation. In relation to the incidence of spinal damage, Youatt believed that the short-backed horse showed less tendency to back problems and could be expected to carry more weight and possess greater endurance, but it did not have much potential for speed.[2] The long-backed horse was built for speed but was much more prone to weakness when ridden. Conformationally correct horses should have a gentle ventral curve immediately behind the withers, followed by a straight line to the lumbar region. An increase in this ventral vertebral curvature (i.e. lordosis) would increase the tendency to weakness and strain. Dorsal curvature (kyphosis), however, was considered to be a more severe defect, which seriously impaired usefulness and performance.

Back problems in horses cause a considerable degree of wastage and lost performance in almost all types of athletic horses. However, reports of their incidence are limited to a survey from general practice in the United Kingdom in the 1960s that showed an incidence of only 1% in 6588 horses.[3] This is probably an underestimate and no breakdown of these cases into the specific diagnosis was made, but a later review of 443 horses with back problems did categorize cases further into osseous, soft tissue and miscellaneous disorders.[4] Definitive diagnosis is often difficult due to vague clinical signs and the lack of good diagnostic imaging coupled with pathological reports.[5,6] This has inevitably resulted in widespread controversy engendering many unsubstantiated opinions about the incidence and clinical significance of back problems, which only increase the state of confusion. Much of this controversy has resulted from the general dearth of knowledge of the functional aspects of the equine thoracolumbar spine and scientific studies on the pathogenesis of back problems in horses. It is also clear that many horses perform poorly without an underlying back problem and many other horses perform surprisingly well in spite of one. In recent years there has been an encouraging progression of studies and biomechanical research to improve this situation.[7-12] There is also much more willingness for those involved with traditional methods of clinical medicine to work closely alongside those involved with spinal manipulative therapy and complementary medicine.[13] The purpose of this chapter is to try and combine all these aspects for the benefit and treatment of suspected cases of back pain.

Anatomic and functional considerations

Thoracolumbar vertebral column

Individual vertebrae are connected by an intricate system of ligaments and musculotendinous structures that provide stability while at the same time supporting movement of the vertebral column. The three principal mechanical functions of the vertebral column are:

1. protection of the spinal cord and associated nerve roots (i.e. vertebral arch)
2. providing support for weight bearing and soft tissue attachment (i.e. vertebral body and vertebral processes)
3. maintaining movement for flexibility and locomotion (i.e. articulations, ligaments, and muscles).

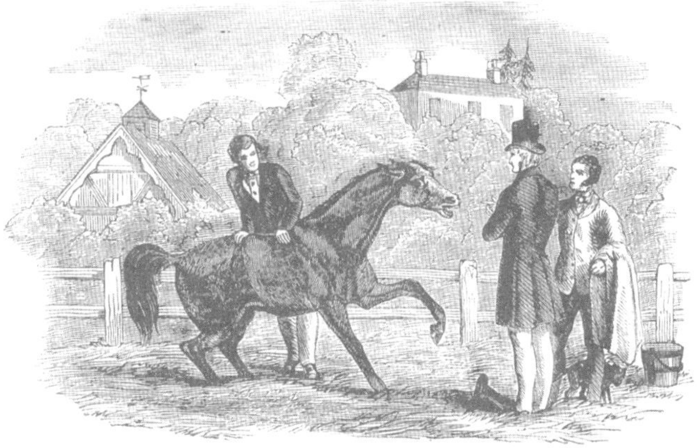

Fig 21.1 A test for rick of the back.[1]

The equine thoracolumbar vertebral region consists of an average of 24 individual vertebrae, based on the typical vertebral formula (C7, T18, L6, S5, Cd15–21).[14] However, variations in the number of vertebrae within the thoracolumbar vertebral region are common and are often compensated by a reduction or increase in the number of vertebrae in an adjacent vertebral region.

Vertebral motion segment

The structural and functional unit of the vertebral column is the vertebral motion segment. A vertebral motion segment consists of two adjoining vertebrae and interposed soft tissue structures (Fig. 21.2). The typical vertebra is characterized by a vertebral body, vertebral arch and vertebral processes that vary in each vertebral region according to structural and functional demands. The vertebral body is a ventral cylindrical structure covered dorsally by the vertebral arch, which includes bilateral pedicles and laminae. Vertebral processes include one spinous process, two transverse processes and two pairs of cranial and caudal articular processes on each vertebra. Mamillary processes are additional vertebral processes found only in the thoracolumbar region that provide added paraspinal muscle attachment sites. Dorsally, the articular processes create bilateral synovial articulations (i.e. zygapophyseal joints) that provide segmental stability and mobility to the vertebral motion segment. Ventrally, the vertebral bodies and intervertebral disks form fibrocartilaginous joints that also provide segmental vertebral stability and mobility. Additional connecting soft tissues include both short and long spinal ligaments and muscles. The vertebrae, vertebral articulations and ligaments are innervated segmentally by sensory branches of the dorsal rami and recurrent meningeal nerves. These nerves mediate nociception and proprioception within the vertebral column.

The vertebral motion segments of the upper cervical region (i.e. occiput-C1–C2) are a highly mobile, specialized joint complex. The cervical vertebrae have rudimentary spinous processes and characteristic transverse foramina for the passage of vertebral vessels. The thoracic vertebrae are characterized by tall spinous processes (highest at T5 or T6), costal articulations and an anticlinal vertebra at T15 or T16. The lumbar vertebrae have long, horizontally flattened transverse processes and intertransverse joints in the caudal region (L4–S1) that are unique to horses. The sacrum is usually made up of five fused segments and has bilateral sacroiliac joints for articulation with the pelvis. The caudal vertebrae are characterized by progressively rudimentary vertebral arches and vertebral processes.

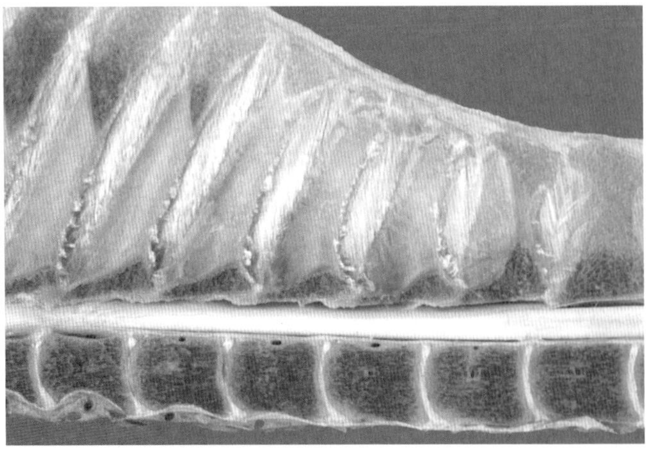

Fig 21.2 Sagittal section of the thoracic vertebral region (T8–T14) demonstrating osseous vertebral structures and supporting spinal ligaments.

Vertebral body and intervertebral disk

The vertebral bodies form the foundation on which the remaining vertebral structures are placed. The cranial vertebral body is convex in shape and the caudal vertebral body is concave (Fig. 21.2). Therefore, most equine intervertebral joints resemble a shallow ball-and-socket configuration, which provides stability without restricting mobility. Vertebral bodies provide support for weight bearing, connective tissue attachment and muscular attachment sites for the diaphragm and psoas muscles in the lumbar vertebral region. The intervertebral disks connect adjacent vertebral bodies and together are classified as fibrocartilaginous articulations. An intervertebral disk consists of an outer annulus fibrosus and central nucleus pulposus. The nucleus pulposus is rudimentary in the thoracolumbar vertebral regions compared to the cervical and caudal vertebral regions (Fig. 21.2). The dorsal and ventral longitudinal ligaments, and the costovertebral ligaments, provide additional reinforcement to the periphery of the intervertebral disk. The intervertebral disk is active in weight bearing, axial shock absorption and maintaining vertebral flexibility. The outer one-third of the intervertebral disk is innervated by both proprioceptive and nociceptive fibers.

Spinous processes

The spinous processes project dorsally from the vertebral arch and vary in size, shape and orientation in different vertebrae and vertebral regions (Fig. 21.3). The spinous processes function as a series of levers for muscle and ligamentous attachment that provide support and movement to the vertebral column. Spinal extension and rotation are produced by contraction of muscles attached to the spinous processes. The supraspinous ligament stabilizes the apex of the spinous processes and aids in resisting excessive spinal flexion. The spinous processes in the cranial thoracic vertebral region are angled caudally and elongated in the region of T2 to T12 to form the withers. The cranial thoracic vertebral region must provide a foundation for stability for and resist forces produced by the head, neck and forelimbs, whereas the caudal thoracic and lumbosacral vertebral region has to resist significant forces associated with the hind limbs and locomotion. The divergent spinous processes of the lumbosacral junction produce a wide interspinous space, compared with the adjacent interspinous spaces.[15-17] The lumbosacral spinous process divergence supports an increased range of motion at the lumbosacral junction without the risk of spinous process impingement.

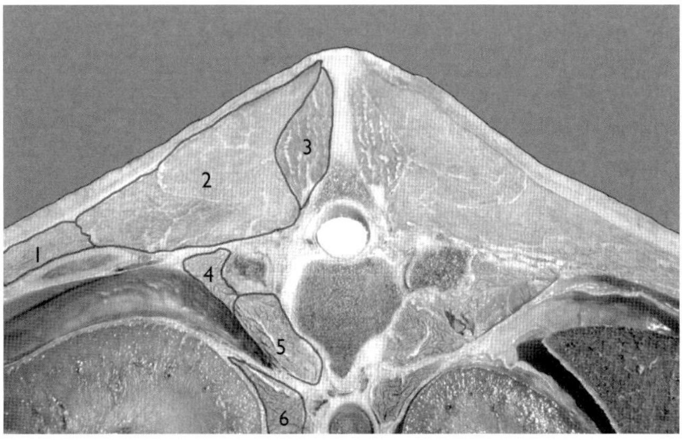

Fig 21.3 Transverse section at the T18 vertebral region. Outline of the muscles represented are: (1) iliocostalis, (2) longissimus, (3) multifidi, (4) psoas major, (5) psoas minor and (6) crus of the diaphragm.

Articular processes

Two pairs of cranial and caudal articular processes arise dorsolaterally from the vertebral arch. An articular surface on the articular processes contributes to the formation of bilateral synovial articulations (i.e. zygapophyseal joints). The articular surfaces in the thoracic vertebral region lie horizontally (i.e. dorsal plane) with the cranial articular surfaces facing dorsally and the caudal articular surfaces facing ventrally. Vertebral motion in the thoracic vertebral region is limited mostly to rotation and lateral bending. The lumbar vertebral region has articular surfaces that predominantly lie vertically (i.e. sagittal plane). Vertebral motion in the lumbosacral vertebral region is limited mostly to dorsoventral flexion. The articular processes function in support and movement of the vertebral arch. The amplitude and direction of segmental vertebral motion are related to the size, shape and orientation of the articular surfaces and functional status of the articulations.[15,16,18] Regional and overall spinal motion is due to the cumulative effects of small amounts of segmental vertebral motion. The zygapophyseal joint capsule has a dense outer fibrous layer, vascular central layer and an inner layer consisting of the synovial membrane. The zygapophyseal joint capsule is richly innervated with sensory nerve fibers from the medial branch of the dorsal rami of several adjacent nerve roots. Proprioception and nociception are two important neurologic functions of the zygapophyseal joints.[19,20] Multilevel spinal innervation of the zygapophyseal articulation produces non-localized pain patterns, which contribute to the difficulty of identifying and localizing back problems.[21]

Transverse processes

The transverse processes provide support and movement to the vertebral column via muscular and ligamentous attachments. Transverse processes are used as lever arms by the deep spinal muscles to maintain posture and to induce rotation and lateral bending.[21] In the thoracic region, the transverse processes contain articular surfaces that contribute to the costotransverse articulations. The lumbar vertebral region has elongated, horizontally flattened transverse processes that provide attachment sites for the large dorsal paraspinal muscles and ventral psoas muscle group. Species of the genus Equus have intertransverse synovial articulations between the transverse processes of the last two or three lumbar vertebrae and at the lumbosacral junction.[15,16] Biomechanically, the intertransverse joints aid in the transfer of propulsive forces from the hindlimbs to the vertebral column and provide resistance to lateral bending and axial rotation of the spine.

Sacroiliac joint

The pelvis articulates with the vertebral column at bilateral sacroiliac articulations, located at the junction between the ventral wing of the ilium and the dorsal wing of the sacrum (Fig. 21.4). Dynamically, the sacroiliac joints aid in locomotion via transfer of hind limb propulsive forces to the vertebral column.[22] The articular surfaces of the sacroiliac joint are nearly flat and closely apposed to support small amounts of gliding movements. The sacroiliac joint is typically L-shaped with the convex border directed caudoventrally. The sacroiliac joint capsule is thin and closely follows the margins of the sacroiliac articular cartilage. The sacroiliac joint is supported by three bilateral sets of strong sacroiliac ligaments that act to support weight of the caudal vertebral column. The dorsal sacroiliac ligaments, consisting of a dorsal and lateral portion, connect the tuber sacrale to the sacrum. The interosseous sacroiliac ligaments are the most robust of the sacroiliac ligaments, spanning

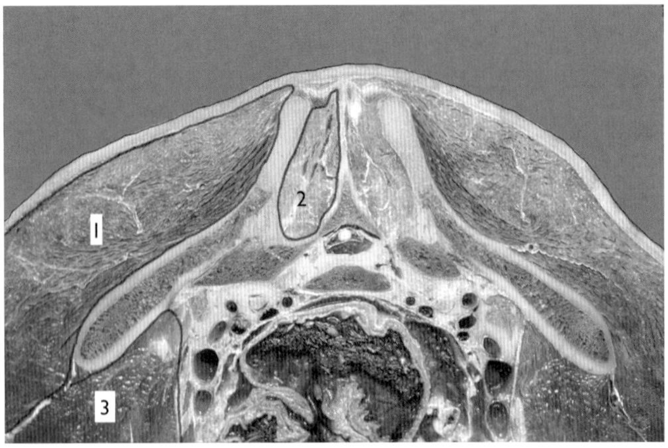

Fig 21.4 Transverse section at the lumbosacral and sacroiliac articulations. Outline of the muscles represented are: (1) gluteus medius, (2) sacrocaudalis dorsalis, (3) iliopsoas (psoas major and iliacus). The tuber sacrale and the interosseous and ventral sacroiliac ligaments are also shown.

the space between the ventral wing of the ilium and the dorsal wing of the sacrum and function as a sling to support the entire mass of the caudal trunk. The ventral sacroiliac ligaments connect the ventral wings of the sacrum to the ilium. The sciatic nerve, cranial gluteal nerve and cranial gluteal artery and vein travel through the greater sciatic foramen, immediately ventromedial to the sacroiliac articulation, which need to be taken in consideration during caudal approaches for injecting the sacroiliac joint.

Spinal ligaments

A series of long and short spinal ligaments contribute to vertebral column stability. Three separate longitudinal spinal ligaments span the length of the vertebral column and provide regional vertebral stability. The nuchal ligament in the cervical vertebral region continues as the supraspinous ligament in the thoracolumbar vertebral region and joins the tips of the spinous processes. The dorsal longitudinal ligament connects the dorsal vertebral bodies within the vertebral canal and acts to reinforce the intervertebral disk (Fig. 21.2). The ventral longitudinal ligament attaches to the ventral vertebral bodies and blends with fibers of the intervertebral disk. The short spinal ligaments interconnect individual vertebral structures and function to protect the spinal cord and to provide segmental vertebral stability. Interspinous ligaments connect adjacent spinous processes. The ligamenta flava span the space between adjacent vertebral laminae and contain a high proportion of elastin. Specialized costovertebral and costotransverse ligaments provide additional stability to the thoracic vertebral region and ribs. The intertransverse ligaments connect adjacent transverse processes in the lumbar vertebral region and limit lateral bending. The intervertebral disk can be considered a specialized connective tissue structure that connects adjacent vertebral bodies.

Intrinsic spinal muscles

Muscles that attach only to the axial skeleton are considered intrinsic spinal muscles. The spinal musculature can be categorized into epaxial or hypaxial muscle groups based on their location relative to the transverse processes of the vertebral column. The epaxial muscles lie dorsal to transverse processes, are segmentally innervated by dorsal branches of spinal nerves and produce spinal extension and lateral bending. Hypaxial muscles lie ventral to transverse processes, are segmentally innervated by ventral branches of spinal nerves and produce spinal flexion and lateral bending. The thoracolumbar fascia is an aponeurosis that serves as an attachment site for many spinal and proximal limb muscles. The thoracolumbar fascia is strong and attaches to the thoracolumbar spinous processes and the cranial edge of the ilial wing. At the lumbosacral junction, the thoracolumbar fascia consolidates along the dorsal midline to form bilateral robust tendons that insert onto the cranial aspect of the tubera sacralia. The largest group of epaxial muscles is organized into three parallel columns. These include (from lateral to medial) the iliocostalis, longissimus and spinalis muscle groups (Fig. 21.3). The iliocostalis muscles are a thin muscle group that attaches to the angle of the ribs and the tips of the lumbar transverse processes. The longissimus muscles are by far the largest and longest group of back muscles. These muscles primarily attach to the dorsal spinous and transverse processes of the thoracolumbar vertebral region and the wing of the ilium and help to support the weight of saddle and rider. The spinalis muscles cover the lateral aspects of spinous processes of the withers and may be compromised by a narrow saddle. The transversospinalis muscle group is the deepest and most medial muscle group (Fig. 21.3) and is largely composed of multifidi muscles in the thoracolumbar vertebral region. The multifidi muscle group is a series of short musculotendinous units that originate from transverse, articular and mamillary processes and insert on adjacent spinous processes. These short muscles span 2–4 vertebrae and are segmentally innervated by dorsal spinal branches.

The epaxial muscles produce spinal extension when activated bilaterally, and lateral bending and rotation when activated unilaterally. Superficial muscle groups usually span one or more vertebral regions, whereas deep spinal muscles usually only span a few vertebrae.[22] The spinal musculature is important for movement, posture and flexibility. The superficial spinal muscles are usually more dynamic and play a role during regional vertebral motion, energy storage and force redistribution during locomotion.[22] Deep, short spinal muscles have more of a static function and are active in segmental stabilization, proprioception and posture.

Extrinsic spinal muscles

Muscles that have attachments on both proximal limbs and the axial skeleton can be considered extrinsic spinal muscles (or shoulder girdle or pelvic girdle limb muscles). The general function of the extrinsic spinal muscles is to induce proximal limb movements required in locomotion or to assist vertebral mobility, depending on whether the vertebral column or limbs are held stationary relative to each other. The shoulder girdle muscles can be categorized into dorsal or ventral muscle groups.[23] The dorsal muscles of the shoulder girdle act to suspend the forelimbs from the neck and trunk. The dorsal shoulder muscles include the brachiocephalicus, omotransversarius, trapezius, rhomboideus, cutaneous trunci and latissimus dorsi. The ventral muscles of the shoulder girdle function in suspending the neck and trunk from the forelimbs. The ventral shoulder muscles include the subclavius, superficial pectoral, deep pectoral and serratus ventralis.

The pelvic girdle muscles are best characterized as cranial-caudal and lateral-medial muscle groups.[23] The cranial muscles of the pelvic girdle function in hind limb protraction and hip flexion. Muscles in this group include the sartorius, iliopsoas, tensor fasciae latae and rectus femoris. The caudal muscles of the pelvic girdle produce hind limb retraction and hip extension. Muscles in this group include the biceps femoris, semitendinosus and semimembranosus. The lateral muscles of the pelvic girdle mostly cause hind limb abduction and include the superficial, middle and deep gluteal muscles. The medial muscles of the pelvic girdle produce hind limb adduction and include the gracilis, pectineus and adductor muscles.

The hypaxial or sublumbar muscles include the psoas minor, psoas major and iliacus. The psoas minor and psoas major originate on the ventral vertebral column (T16 to L6) and insert on the pelvic inlet and lesser trochanter of the femur, respectively. Together, the psoas major and iliacus form the iliopsoas, the largest flexor of the coxofemoral joint (Fig. 21.4). If the hindlimb is stabilized, then the iliopsoas muscle induces flexion of the lumbar spine and pelvic flexion about the sacroiliac articulations.

Diagnostic challenges

Back problems – a syndrome

The general description of a horse having 'back problems' is not particularly useful from either a diagnostic or therapeutic perspective. Affected horses could have differing combinations, severity, chronicity, distribution, and locations of soft tissue, articular, neurologic or even behavioral issues related to chronic pain and discomfort. From this perspective, a horse could also be described as having 'lameness' or 'colic', which signifies that a potential disease process is present but it is does not specify in any way the pathophysiology or affected tissues, which is often a prerequisite for providing a definitive diagnosis and focused treatment.

A proposed approach for describing the vague and sometimes complex clinical features associated with back problems in horses is to define back problems as a syndrome. A syndrome is typically defined as a collection of clinically recognizable features that often occur together and the presence of one of these features should alert the practitioner to the possibility of the presence of other findings. Within a syndrome, the reason that the clinical signs occur together typically has not yet been discovered (i.e., pathophysiology). The majority of musculoskeletal injuries are characterized by signs of acute inflammation, which include heat, swelling, pain, altered function, and in some cases redness. Chronic musculoskeletal injures are also characterized by altered function and chronic pain (i.e., lameness) and swelling most likely due to effusion, fibrosis or osteophytosis. Therefore, the syndrome of acute back problems includes signs of heat, pain and altered function (e.g., stiffness, muscle hypertonicty) and occasional swelling due to the deep location of most spinal structures. All of these signs are clearly observable and measurable with existing objective outcome measures such as infrared thermography, pressure algometry, myotonometry, goniometry or other measures of spinal range of motion. Chronic back problems are characterized by signs of stiffness and chronic pain, which may include behavioral issues in some horses. The presence of any one of these clinical signs within the axial skeleton should then alert the examiner to the possibility of the existence of other related signs of back problems or spinal dysfunction.

Back pain perception

Quantifying the degree of pain in horses and establishing the precise site of pain has always been difficult[24] and horses with back pain are no exception. The situation is further complicated as the major clinical sign recognized by owners in many horses with a back problem is impaired or poor performance and not overt thoracolumbar pain. On the other hand, many horses apparently perform satisfactorily in spite of some low-grade back pain. To add to this confusion, some horses appear to be naturally sensitive or 'thin-skinned' and resent being groomed or palpated along the back. In these patients, both owners and clinicians may interpret an evasive response to innocuous stimuli (i.e., allodynia) as a sign of back pain. Another difficulty in the assessment of back pain involves the condition known as 'cold back' in which there is apparent hypersensitivity over the back with a transient stiffness and extension (lordosis)) of the trunk as the rider gets into the saddle. There are usually no other demonstrable clinical signs, although in severe cases the horse may buck and rear when first mounted and ridden. In some instances the thoracolumbar spine is notable flexed (kyphosis) and the epaxial muscles are severely hypertonic. The initial stiffness from being saddled or mounted usually subsides within a few minutes and thereafter no effect on performance is noted. Whether this condition is actually painful, associated with some previous back pain or illi-fitting saddle or is merely a matter of temperament is unclear.

Many of the difficulties in clinical diagnosis of back problems would be solved if some meaningful criteria for the assessment of pain and an objective system of quantifying it could be established. The origin of primary back pain is irritation of the dorsal nerve roots and the branches of the spinal nerves. The back, like most tissues of the body, is innervated nerve endings that are particularly sensitive to tissue dysfunction (Fig. 21.5). Nociceptive receptors include plexiform and free ending arrangements of unmyelinated nerve fibers. Nociceptive fibers are distributed throughout the skin and subcutaneous tissues, adipose tissues, fasciae and ligaments, periosteum, dura mater, adventitia of blood vessels and fibrous capsules

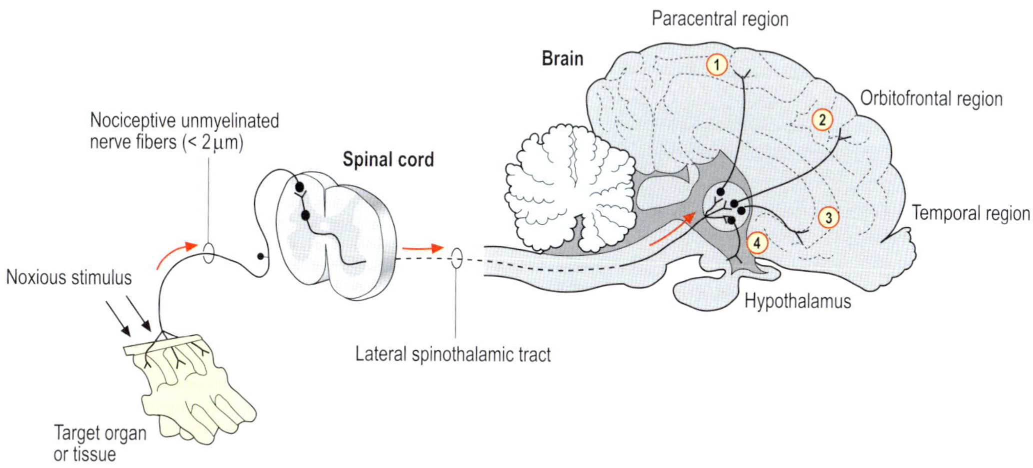

Fig 21.5 Pain pathways associated with the thoracolumbar spine.

of interneural articulations and sacroiliac joints. In normal circumstances this receptor system is relatively inactive but it is activated when chemical, mechanical or other damaging factors are applied to the tissues containing the unmyelinated nerve endings. Primary back pain therefore results from trauma or irritation of these nociceptive receptor nerve endings. Various other pain syndromes are recognized in humans and include secondary, referred and psychosomatic low back pain, but their importance in the horse is unproven as yet.

Another important factor to be considered is the marked variation in response to pain. Even in humans a meaningful measurement of 'pain threshold' is unrealistic as patients can vary in the intensity of their experience of pain from day to day and even at different times during the day. In horses, temperament is considered an important factor in the assessment of both acute and chronic pain. It is suggested that the reduced performance is sometimes due to the horse attempting to guard its back even though the clinical signs of pain have abated some time previously. Some credence has been given to this idea by the induction of back pain in trotting horses and recent research into motor learning and compensatory gait mechanisms.[25] The principal sign of primary induced back pain is not lameness, but stiffness and reduced performance.

Difficulties of palpating the anatomical structures involved

Many of the lesions associated with back problems involve osseous structures of the thoracolumbar spine that are difficult, if not impossible, to palpate effectively (e.g. vertebral bodies, articular and transverse processes). In the thoracolumbar spine it is only possible to palpate the apicess of the dorsal spinous processes. Locating the site of pain within the epaxial muscles is also difficult as typical palpation procedures may precipitate spasm or contraction of the entire longissimus muscle and an overall exaggerated or guarded response. The longissimus muscle runs the entire length of the trunk from its origin at the caudal cervical spine to the insertion on the wing of ilium and sacral spinous processes. The sacroiliac and lumbosacral joints are also virtually impossible to palpate, except partially along their ventral aspects via rectal palpation. The supraspinous ligament and a portion of the dorsal sacroiliac ligaments are readily palpable, but unfortunately other vertebral or pelvic ligaments (e.g. interspinous, ventral sacroiliac, etc.) are not accessible.

Dearth of appropriate pathological studies

There have been no systematic pathological studies on a large series of back cases in horses. There have been a number of studies on congenital deformities[26,27] and reports on diskospondylitis.[28,29] Some investigations on acute and chronic sacroiliac disease have been reported.[30,31] Much has been written about the clinical and surgical treatment of over-riding or impinged dorsal spinous processes (i.e. kissing spines),[32] but very little research has been done on its etiopathogenesis. The widespread use of ultrasonography to diagnose soft tissue injuries of the epaxial structures has dramatically increased the ability to diagnose desmitis within the supraspinous and dorsal sacroiliac ligaments, but no pathological studies have been completed to confirm these clinical findings.[33-35]

Frequency of multiple lesions at multiple sites

Many back problems in horses are associated with chronic or long-standing injuries. It is also common for there to be more than one spinal lesion that contributes to the clinical signs and poor performance. A breakdown of diagnoses of one of the authors' cases (LBJ) from 1992 to 1997 shows a total of 395 diagnoses made from 268 cases presented for examination of the back to a referral clinic (Box 21.1). It is particularly common for cases of over-riding or impinged dorsal spinous processes to be associated with injury of the supraspinous ligament, sacroiliac disease or low-grade hock lameness. Therefore confirmation of such secondary lesions can have important implications for the management and prognosis of horses with primary back problems.

Types of back problems

A serious stumbling block to progress in the diagnosis and treatment of equine back problems is the wide range of opinions that exist. This is true not only within the veterinary profession, but between veterinarians and physical therapists, horse owners and trainers. The lack of authenticated reports and specific studies in this field makes it impossible to set standards for definitive diagnosis and therefore clear guidelines for treatment. The primary clinical sign of back problems in horses is a loss or reduction in performance, whatever the underlying pathogenesis; other clinical signs may be more difficult to precisely define.

Opinions vary as to whether horses genuinely suffer from back problems at all or whether the signs exhibited are referable to damage elsewhere in the skeleton. In our experience genuine back problems do occur, but in a variety of forms (Table 21.1). First, there are those with identifiable lesions in the thoracolumbar spine or epaxial structures (i.e. primary back problems). A second important category are those due to secondary back problems that occur as a result of the pressure or strain exerted from lesions in the appendicular or axial skeleton (i.e. particularly fore- or hind limb lameness). Finally, there is a category of apparent or alleged back problems which, despite popular opinion, have limited anatomic or pathophysiologic evidence to support their occurrence (Table 21.2). This group of 'back problems' forms the basis of much controversy between veterinarians and other professionals (e.g. chiropractors) or non-professionals (e.g. lay practitioners). These difficulties are exacerbated by the fact that many horses suffer low-grade and chronic lesions. Malalignment or displacement of the caudal thoracic or lumbar dorsal spinal processes is reputed to be a common cause of back trouble in horses.[36] One or more spinous summits are said to become laterally displaced (i.e. 'out of place') and these can apparently be replaced by sharp pressure at the appropriate site (i.e. 'put back into place'). From an anatomic point of view this claim is not acceptable; these structures are not moveable like this either in life or at post-mortem. In spite of the tendency for intervertebral disks to degenerate with age in the thoracolumbar spine, they do not appear to cause any clinical signs similar to those seen so commonly in humans and in dogs. Nerve 'pinching' and peripheral nerve lesions are often claimed to be important causes of back problems, but as yet there has been no scientific evidence to substantiate this belief in horses. However, anecdotal necropsy evidence does support the existence of spinal nerve compression at

Box 21.1 Distribution of the general categories of chronic back problems (1992–97)

Total number of horses	268
Primary back problem	268
Secondary back problem	105
Tertiary back problem	32
Total diagnoses	395

Table 21.1 Differential diagnoses to consider for a horse with potential back problems

TYPE OF BACK PROBLEM	GENERAL CATEGORY	SPECIFIC LESION OR PROBLEM
Primary back problem	Soft tissue injury	Longissimus muscle strain Supraspinous ligament sprain or desmitits Dorsal sacroiliac ligament sprain or desmitits Exertional rhabdomyolysis (tying up) Non-specific soft tissue injury
	Osseous injury	Conformational or developmental abnormality Over-riding or impinged dorsal spinous processes Osteoarthritis (e.g. articular processes) Vertebral fracture Spondylosis Diskospondylitis Spinal neoplasia (primary and secondary)
	Neurologic disorders	Equine protozoal myeloencephalitis (EPM) Equine degenerative myeloencephalopathy (EDM) Equine herpesvirus myeloencephalitis (EVH-1) Equine motor neuron disease (EMND)
	Tack associated	Poor saddle fit or excessive pressure
	Idiopathic	No clinical abnormalities detected
Secondary back problem		Hindlimb lameness (e.g. spavin), Forelimb lameness Neck problem (e.g. stenotic myelopathy) Acute sacroiliac injury Chronic sacroiliac disease Pelvic fracture
Presumed back problem		Bad temperament Lack of ability (rider or horse) Lack of fitness Improper tack fit or use Dental problems

Table 21.2 Conditions alleged to cause back problems in horses for which there is currently no definitive scientific evidence

GENERAL CATEGORY	SPECIFIC LESION OR PROBLEM
Vertebral subluxation	Subluxation of thoracolumbar vertebral bodies or articular processes Misalignment of thoracolumbar dorsal spinous processes
Intervertebral disk injury	Intervertebral disk prolapse or herniation
Peripheral neuropathy	Compromise of thoracolumbar spinal nerves at the intervertebral foramen

the lumbosacral junction (i.e., L6 ventral spinal nerve) due to bony proliferation and osteophytosis at the associated intervertebral foramen adjacent to the medial aspect of the L6-S1 intertransverse joints, which would be expected to produce similar clinical signs to 'sciatica' or lumbar spinal nerve compression in humans.

Frequency of spontaneous recovery

Many of the problems causing poor performance in horses are long-standing (i.e. many weeks or months in duration) and there is a tendency for these cases to recover spontaneously. In a survey of cases followed over two years, a 65% recovery rate was reported irrespective of the diagnosis and the treatment or management regime.[5] The prevalence of spontaneous recovery therefore can hamper elucidation of diagnosis and make evaluation of treatment regimes difficult.

Relationship of back pain to lameness

Lameness is not a typical feature of horses suffering primary back problems. However, secondary back pain is often associated with lameness as the underlying condition causing poor performance. Most primary back cases exhibit only low-grade hind limb lameness, which is often bilateral and most commonly associated with hock injury. A study in which back pain was induced using lactic acid injections into the longissimus muscles did not produce any signs of hindlimb lameness.[25] However, in other studies that evaluated naturally-occurring clinical cases of thoracolumbar or sacroiliac pain, the prevalence of limb lameness varied from 35% up to 74–85%.[37–39] Conversely, in horses presented for primary limb lameness, the prevalence of back problems varied between 23–32%.[38,39] Therefore, it appears that a large percentage of horses with back pain have concurrent lameness versus a smaller proportion of horses with lameness also have back pain. The clinical significance of this is that practitioners that focus solely on back problems (e.g., equine chiropractors) are likely not addressing concurrent lameness issues if they are not collaborating with limb lameness specialists. Conversely, practitioners that focus solely on limb lameness without considering the potential adverse effects on spinal function are likely not providing comprehensive treatment of musculoskeletal pain and poor performance.

Causes of sacroiliac joint pain or injury have been postulated to be the result of sacroiliac or lumbosacral osteoarthritis, sacroiliac desmitis or sprain, sacroiliac subluxation or luxation, pelvic stress fractures, complete ilial wing fractures or sacral fractures.[40] Additional differential diagnoses include thrombosis of caudal aorta or iliac arteries, exertional rhabdomyolysis, trochanteric bursitis and impinged dorsal spinous processes in the lumbar vertebral region.[41] Horses with presumed thoracolumbar vertebral problems may also have concurrent chronic sacroiliac joint injuries. In a report on 443 horses with back problems, chronic sacroiliac joint problems were identified in 15%.[4] Clinical signs of lower hind limb lameness may overlap and mimic signs of presumed sacroiliac joint pathology. It is important that a thorough and complete lower limb lameness evaluation is completed prior to or in conjunction with a proximal hind limb or sacroiliac joint work-up.

Diagnostic protocol to assess back problems

A standardized protocol should be used to systematically examine horses with potential back problems (Box 21.2).

Box 21.2 Diagnostic protocol for the evaluation of horses with potential back problems

Case history

- Signalment and use of the horse
- Onset and duration of clinical signs
- Response to treatment, particularly NSAIDs and manipulation
- Temperament and ability to perform
- Assessment of management and training routine
- Evaluation of predisposing factors
- Experience of the rider

Clinical examination

- Visual inspection of conformation, posture and musculoskeletal symmetry
- Gait evaluation: in hand, lunged, ridden, or driven
- Evaluation of concurrent lameness
- Neurologic evaluation
- Postexercise palpation and manipulation
- Soft tissue and osseous palpation
- Regional and segmental joint manipulation
- Rectal palpation
- Examination of tack, particularly saddle fit

Diagnostic imaging

- Radiographic examination – osseous pathology

Standing: lateral view of the thoracolumbar (T2–L4) and sacrocaudal (S2-Cd4) regions

General anesthesia: ventrodorsal view of the lumbosacral (L4–S5) region

- Ultrasonography – articular or spinous processes, supraspinous or sacroiliac ligament desmitis
- Nuclear scintigraphy – active inflammation or bone turnover
- Thermography – back or gluteal muscle injury, altered vasomotor tone
- Linear tomography – sacroiliac joint pathology

Laboratory examination

- Hematology
- Biochemistry: muscle-derived enzymes (AST and CK), before and after exercise test
- Serology: vitamin E and selenium levels, viral isolation
- Cerebrospinal fluid analysis
- Muscle biopsy

Additional diagnostic aids

- Diagnostic injections of interspinous spaces, articular processes or sacroiliac joint
- Electrical muscle stimulation
- Therapeutic trial of NSAIDs – effect on performance
- 'Slap test' for evidence of cervical vertebral stenosis causing hindlimb ataxia

History

The value of obtaining a thorough clinical history cannot be overestimated, as the clinical signs and behavioral changes of thoracolumbar disorders are many and varied.[42] Details dating back to the time when the owner first acquired the horse are extremely helpful in deciding whether or not one is dealing with a genuine back problem. In this regard, information on management, tack and performance should always be sought.

Acute versus chronic onset

The history in acute back injuries is usually straightforward as some traumatic incident will have been noticed. For example, young horses with multiple fractures of the dorsal spinous processes from T2 to T10 often have a history of rearing up and falling over backwards onto the withers. Most acute cases involve soft tissue injuries and strain of the longissimus muscles is particularly common.

Chronic problems are commonly encountered when no obvious initiating incident is recognized. One consistent feature of a long-standing back problem is an alteration in the horse's behavior or temperament. This may be insidious in onset and it may take some time before the owner fully appreciates that the change has taken place (e.g. a normally good-natured horse becomes sour and rather fractious to handle or there may be a loss of enthusiasm to work). There also seems to be a correlation between nervous or temperamental horses and the presence of back problems.

Use of the horse

There also seems to be an association with the type of back injury and the type of work the horse is involved in. Jeffcott reported that the differences in incidence of specific back problems varied quite noticeably according to whether the horse jumped at speed, jumped competitively or was not used for jumping at all.[5] Acute sacroiliac strain or subluxation was more prevalent in horses jumping at speed, whereas impinged or over-riding dorsal spinous processes were most common in showjumpers. The incidence of soft tissue damage was much the same in both of these groups and age was not nearly such an important factor in equine back disorders as it is in humans. Spondylosis appeared more frequently in mares, whereas over-riding dorsal spinous processes was most often seen in short-backed Thoroughbred geldings.

Sacroiliac pain is common in dressage horses and causes impaired performance, usually without lameness. Standardbred harness racing also shows a high incidence of sacroiliac and hindquarters problems but over-riding or impinged spinous processes are rare. Back injuries in reining, barrel racing and rodeo horses are not common but are usually associated with muscle injuries. In endurance horses back problems resulting from long periods of extreme exercise and saddle-induced injuries are common.

Concurrent lameness and loss of performance

Positive clinical signs at exercise may include uni- or bilateral hindlimb lameness, a loss of enthusiasm for work or an inability to stride out at fast paces. Owners will often mention a stiffness in the hindlimb action and a loss of suppleness of the back when ridden, although the action when loose in the paddock appears satisfactory. Jumping with a fixed hollow back is frequently encountered or there may well be a reluctance to jump, particularly combination-type fences. The horse may also lose its fluidity and timing during jumping and become tense, tending to rush over the fences. Signs of head shaking and an increased tendency for tail swishing are other occasional features found in horses with back problems.

Medication and treatment

Since many back problems are chronic in nature, the horse may well have received multiple treatments before your examination. It is therefore important to know what type of medications or therapy have been tried and whether or not they provided any improvement. A clinical trial of phenylbutazone (2 g, p.o., b.i.d. for 4–5 days) is often used to assess the inflammatory component of a back problem. The use of non-steroidal anti-inflammatory drugs (NSAIDs) will often produce an improvement in osseous or articular pathologies although this may be partial and short-lived. A similar clinical trial of methocarbamol (15–44 mg/kg, p.o., s.i.d.) will help some horses with muscle-related back soreness or hypertonicity. Inquiries into the response to rest or changes in activities, such as cross-training, are often helpful in assessing the mechanism of action of the back problem. Some horses, like humans, appear to get burnt out when asked to do repetitive or monotonous disciplines without any changes in routine. Many forms of physiotherapy or spinal manipulative treatment may give temporary improvement, but a lasting success is unlikely without establishing a definitive diagnosis of the back problem.

Management and training ability

It is common for owners to blame poor competitive ability on a problem in the thoracolumbar spine when it is simply due to poor schooling or equitation. It is now well recognized that the most consistent feature in a back problem is a loss of performance, particularly in the ability to jump effectively. Acute soreness in the back muscles is often associated with falling or some other traumatic incident, but a history of obvious pain in the thoracolumbar spine is not always reported, particularly in long-standing cases. Horses with severe back pain may have difficulty in standing to urinate or defecate or there may be a reluctance to lie down or to roll. There may also be resentment to placement of a blanket or to grooming over the loins and hindquarters. In some cases the farrier may note resentment to having a hind limb picked up or difficulty in standing while being shod.

A history of resentment to any weight on the horse's back is sometimes reported with a tendency to collapse behind when ridden. Saddling up may become a problem, particularly when the girth is tightened. The horse may buck when first mounted, although this is usually due to temperament rather than back pain. The owner may also note reluctance to move backwards or reining back when being ridden. Dramatic signs of bucking and rearing are not usually associated with acute back injuries as it is too painful for the horse to fully flex or extend the trunk.

Query into the size and the time spent in stalls, paddocks, or turnout in pasture is indicated for any horse with back problems. In humans, a primary contributing factor for recurrent back problems is bed rest and inactivity.[43] Horses that are stalled for the majority of the day or large portions of the year do not have the opportunity to maintain back flexibility, which may contribute to back stiffness and dysfunction. In addition, horses that are turned out in paddocks with knee-deep mud, large rocks, poor footing or steep hills may aggravate pre-existing back problems.

Rider ability

Equestrian competition involves two athletes – the horse and the rider. There is no question that poor riding can either predispose to a back problem or exacerbate an existing one. Inexperienced or poor riders may blame the poor performance of their horse on a back problem when in fact the blame lies with them. It is also crucial that the saddle used not only fits but is also appropriate for the type of work or competition being undertaken.

Predisposing factors

The conformation and intended use of the horse can have an important bearing on the injury involved. For example, specific spinal malformations (e.g. lordosis and scoliosis) tend to predispose to injury through the inherent weakness of the thoracolumbar spine.[5] These conditions place extra strain on the epaxial muscles of the back that can lead to recurrent soft tissue injuries. The majority of horses do not have severe gross deformities, but conformational defects are common. Horses which are short-backed with restricted flexibility of the spine tend to exhibit more vertebral lesions than the longer backed horses, which have relatively more suppleness and seem to be more prone to muscular or ligamentous strain. Large-framed horses with comparatively weak hindquarters appear to be more susceptible to sacroiliac problems.

Age and gender of the horse are not nearly as important as predisposing factors as they are in humans. The highest incidence of back problems in horses is during middle age, 5–10 years of age,[4] although older horses, like elderly humans, are susceptible to loss of vertebral column flexibility, joint degeneration and loss of muscle strength. Aged horses also have increased healing times and increased chances of having chronic conditions or abnormal musculoskeletal compensations from prior injuries.

Management problems

There are a wide range of management issues that may lead either to a back problem or a suspected one from poor performance. Many of these issues may be due to inexperience or ignorance by the owner and result in inappropriate management, producing signs suggestive of back pain.

Temperament

Horses with an excitable temperament seem to be more prone to back-related problems. This may simply be due to low pain threshold or hypersensitivity, but hyperexcitability often results in excessive tension or spasm of the back muscles. This in turn reduces spinal flexibility and causes impaired impulsion from the hindquarters, which is seen clinically as poor hindlimb action and performance. These horses may become uncontrollable and buck and kick violently rather than settle down to exercise properly. A careful examination is required in these horses to be confident there is no underlying spinal pathology or pathoanatomic explanation for the perceived avoidance behavior suggestive of back pain. In addition to employing diagnostic imaging, a short course of analgesics (e.g. NSAIDs) is useful as some improvement would be expected if any musculoskeletal inflammation or injury exists.

Cold back

The signs of a cold back are usually exhibited when the saddle is put on, the girth tightened or as the rider mounts. The horse will then extend or flex its back and be very stiff as it moves off. In most cases these signs disappear quickly and within a few minutes the horse's performance is satisfactory. There is no doubt that horses with a cold back worry owners a great deal. In our experience, many of these cases are not associated with underlying pathological findings and are therefore thought to be temperamental or behavioral in origin. There are many different ways to manage these horses, including using saddle pads, warming the horse up before saddling (e.g. lungeing) or medicating mares with estrogen.

Mares in season

Owners sometimes report that mares in estrus have associated back pain and poor performance. It is often difficult to substantiate these claims, although some mares do improve during the winter or if medicated with estrus-suppressive drugs (e.g. altrenogest). Rectal palpation and evaluation of abnormal ovarian structures are indicated in any mare with recurrent or refractory back problems.

Schooling and work regime

Failure to keep a horse properly fit for its purpose may lead to fatigue or muscle strain. Horses can be bored with a dull work schedule and become soured or reluctant to work. This can easily be misinterpreted as poor performance related to a back problem.

Dental problems and bitting

General management of the teeth is part of good equine husbandry. Any problem in the mouth, from sharp teeth to an inappropriate bit, can lead to evasion when working. Affected horses often have a raised head carriage, tension or stiffness of the back muscles and poor hindlimb impulsion.

Inspection

Visual inspection is an important initial aspect of examining horses with back problems. General temperament and behavior are evaluated for signs of pain or discomfort. Horses with back problems often have a sudden change in behavior and become easily irritated by previously innocuous stimuli. Pinning the ears, swishing the tail, refusal to move or exaggerated movements away from everyday objects (e.g. curry comb or saddle pad) are signs of changes in behavior.

Evaluation continues with observation of the patient from a distance while turned loose in the stall or paddock while assessing the use and co-ordination of the limbs and trunk. The exam is focused on evaluating the dynamic characteristics of the musculoskeletal system. Owners may report that the head or neck is carried in an abnormal position, the trunk is held rigid or the horse refuses to move or bucks when asked to go forward. The horse should be able to readily raise and lower its head and neck and bend the trunk to either side. Neck injuries can present as the inability to lower the head and neck to graze or, just as common, the consistent inability to raise the head and neck above a certain level. Both instances often have a history of substantial head or neck trauma associated with getting the head or neck trapped in a fence or pulling back or flipping over in the cross-ties. It is important to note the general body conditioning of the horse and to differentiate poor condition (i.e. cachexia) from specific wastage of the longissimus, gluteal and thigh musculature. The presence of any lumps, scars, saddle marks on the back or any undue curvature of the spine must also be noted as they may have some bearing on the underlying condition.

A more detailed examination of the back is best carried out with the horse restrained in stocks (Fig. 21.6). It is important that the horse is not stressed or tense, as this will make assessment of back pain even more difficult. If the horse resents the stocks it is better to carry out the examination in the stable. For in-hand evaluation, the horse should be standing quietly and comfortably with all four limbs on a firm, level surface. The horse is then evaluated for the static characteristics of the musculoskeletal system, which include conformation, posture and muscular and osseous symmetry.

Conformation

Conformation is defined as the static or structural relationship of body segments, whereas postural analysis involves the dynamic or functional assessment within and between body regions. Vertebral column conformation is evaluated with special attention to neck development, height and shape of the withers, length of the trunk relative to the height and osseous pelvic symmetry. Conformationally, it is thought that short-backed horses have a higher incidence of osseous disorders, whereas long-backed horses are more prone to soft tissue injuries.[6]

Posture

The posture is evaluated for head and neck carriage, development and symmetry of the trunk, tail carriage and a preferred or shifting stance. Alterations in trunk posture include lordosis, kyphosis and scoliosis. Abnormal spinal curvatures are often readily visualized and are common primary presenting complaints. Altered spinal posture has both structural and functional etiologies that can

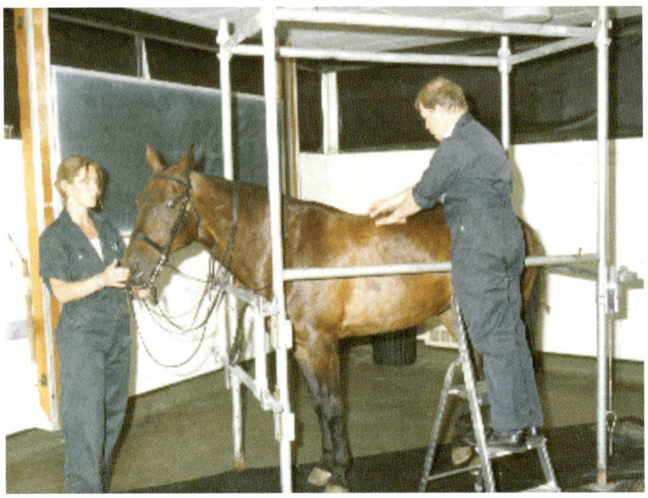

Fig 21.6 Examination of the horse's back while restrained in stocks. The clinician uses a set of steps to facilitate palpation and manipulation of the thoracolumbar spine.

often be differentiated based on history, onset and duration of the condition. Congenital vertebral malformations often produce structural changes in the trunk conformation, whereas developmental injuries produce functional changes in the trunk posture. In adult horses, acute changes in spinal curvatures are often functional adaptations to back pain or muscle imbalances. Correction of the underlying problem often returns the trunk to its original posture. Excessive lordosis is often an age-related change in trunk posture and may be improved with induced trunk elevation (i.e. flexion) and abdominal muscle-strengthening exercises. Horses with sacropelvic injuries will often carry their tail off to one side, lack tail tone or movement or have an abnormal tail set.

Muscular symmetry

The pectoral region, dorsal scapular and wither region, epaxial and gluteal muscles are carefully evaluated for abnormal muscle development and left-to-right asymmetries. This is a crucial part of the examination and needs to be carried out in as objective a fashion as possible. Muscular asymmetries are often due to disuse or neurogenic atrophy.[42] Alterations in the pectoral or pelvic girdle muscles need to be localized to the affected muscles, to aid in the differentiation of a primary lower limb, upper limb or vertebral column dysfunction. Localized or segmental muscle atrophy of the epaxial muscles may be due to vertebral segment dysfunction or a consequence of poor saddle fit. Generalized back muscle atrophy needs to be differentiated from lack of muscle development (i.e. poor conditioning) and disuse atrophy associated with chronic hindlimb lameness. Neurologic diseases that produce local or regional muscle atrophy (e.g. equine protozoal myeloencephalitis) need to be ruled out in horses that present with back problems and gluteal muscle asymmetry. It is unwise to assume that instances of asymmetric hindquarters or a 'hunter's bump' are caused by sacroiliac damage.

Osseous symmetry

The dorsal midline of the back is viewed from above (by standing on a mounting block behind the horse) with the horse standing squarely on all four limbs to see if the back is straight and evenly developed bilaterally. Any lateral curvature of the spine suggests a degree of muscle spasm on one side (i.e. spastic scoliosis). The presence of a 'hunter's bump' may be seen although it is not necessarily associated with overt clinical signs of a back problem. It is associated with a prominence of the tuber sacrale due to atrophy of the longissimus and gluteal muscles (Fig. 21.7). Changes in the height of the tuber sacrale should be assessed relative to the apex of the second sacral spinous process (S2). Visual acuity is high and even slight (<5 mm) deviations can be perceived. Confirmation of pelvic bone asymmetry can also be performed by palpating the main skeletal features (i.e. tuber sacrale, tuber coxae and tuber ischii) while standing directly behind the horse or by getting two assistants to identify the osseous landmarks for left and right comparisons. Guidelines are:

- unilateral gluteal muscle atrophy on one hindquarter without pelvic bone malalignment: suspect hindlimb lameness (hock or stifle) or acetabular damage
- elevation of one tuber sacrale with or without gluteal muscle atrophy: suspect thickening and damage to dorsal sacroiliac ligament or stress fracture of wing of ilium on opposite side (i.e. lowered quarter)
- lowering of tuber sacrale with muscle atrophy and lowering of the ipsilateral tuber coxae: suspect ipsilateral chronic sacroiliac disease or ipsilateral complete ilial wing fracture
- lowering of tuber coxae without lowering of tuber sacrale or tuber ischii: suspect fracture of the tuber coxae
- lowering of tuber ischii without deviation of tuber sacrale or tuber coxae: suspect fracture of tuber ischii.

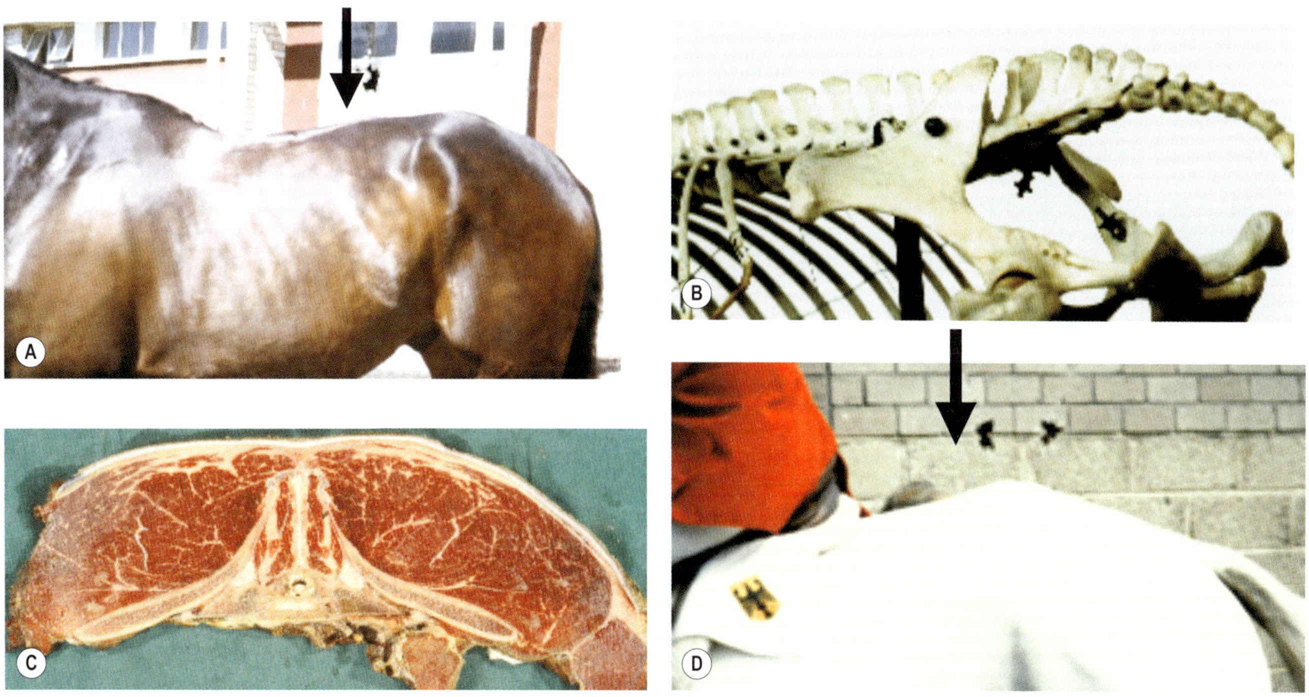

Fig 21.7 Photograph of a hunters' bump and associated muscle wastage in the lumbar and gluteal regions. **(A)** Five-year-old Thoroughbred gelding with prominent lumbar spinous processes. **(B)** Horse's skeleton showing the pelvic and lumbosacral region with the lumbar and sacral spinous processes. **(C)** Transverse section of the quarters showing the wings of ilium and normal musculature of the region. **(D)** Fourteen-year-old showjumper with prominent tuber sacrale and poor muscling of quarters.

Evaluation of tack fit and use

Saddle fit

A frequent cause of back discomfort can be either an inappropriate saddle used or the saddle not fitting properly. Most poorly fitting saddles produce pressure or pinching over the caudal withers region, hence the appearance of white hairs in the midline. Horses change shape, particularly the contour of the back, when they are out of work (i.e. deconditioned) or if they have an increase in bodyweight. Many saddle-fitting techniques provide a static assessment of the fit of the saddle to the shape and contour of the withers and back. Unfortunately, saddles do not come in a wide variety of sizes for individual fit and comfort, like clothes or shoes for humans. Most horses have to conform to only a few different tree widths and saddle types. Ideally, the saddle should fit comfortably and provide as large an area of contact as possible to help to distribute the rider's weight across the withers and back musculature. Computerized pressure pads help to provide both a static and dynamic assessment of saddle fit, pad thickness and placement, rider influences and changes in pressure associated with different gaits.

Assessment of saddle fit begins with checking the tree for straightness, symmetry and intact bars. The panels are evaluated for left-to-right symmetry and any lumps or depressions that might contribute to uneven pressure. The gullet should be 2–3 fingers wide to provide clearance for the dorsal spinous processes and to provide uniform weight distribution on the panels. The best saddles have wide panels that provide maximal weight distribution of the rider over the thoracolumbar epaxial musculature. Deep palpation of the entire fleece surface of the Western saddle should be done to identify any sharp points from nails or loose conchos.

The owner is asked to place only the saddle, without any pads, on the horse's back in the usual position. The analogy of properly fitting shoes (i.e. saddle) and the appropriate socks (i.e. saddle pad) to your feet works well for assessing saddle fit in horses. The chances are that if the shoe does not fit your foot then adding socks will not, in most instances, make the shoe fit any better. Optimally, there should be 2–3 fingers width of dorsal clearance between the pommel at the front of the saddle and the spinous processes of the withers. If there is less clearance, then the additional weight of the rider in the saddle will most likely reduce the space and cause direct contact and dorsal wear of the pommel on the withers. Greater than three fingers width of clearance is indicative of too narrow a tree that will cause increased lateral pressure on the withers. The rider may also feel unstable in the saddle due to an elevated center of gravity relative to the horse.

Most saddles are positioned with the front panels over the caudal border of the scapula. During locomotion, the scapula normally rotates caudally as the forelimb is fully protracted. If the panels are not flared outward slightly to accommodate the scapula, then the scapula cannot rotate caudally during limb protraction. This results in a shortened stride of the forelimbs. This is a common fault of many Western saddles with rigid, non-flared front panels. The contact between the front panel and the caudal scapula should be constant and uniform. An analogy of the desired pressure is the contact felt with your hand as it slides between the seat of the chair and the bottom of your thigh when you are sitting down. Saddles that are too wide will have increased pressure and contact at the dorsal withers, but the bottom of the panel will gape and protrude away from the lateral scapula. Saddles with too narrow a tree will have severe focal pressure on the dorsal scapular cartilage and you will not be able to fit your hand between the saddle and the scapula, even without the weight of the rider in the saddle. A simple correction on most horses is to slide the saddle back 0.5 to 1″ off the dorsal scapula. The seat should remain level to maintain rider comfort and to prevent unnecessary cranial or caudal displacements of the rider.

Saddle pads

The use of extraneous saddle pads or wedges is often a sign of potential saddle fit problems. When it comes to saddle pads, less is often better. The saddle pad should be tented up into the gullet of the saddle so that it provides clearance over the withers and dorsal spinous processes. Unfortunately, gel pads and other specialty pads often do not extend to the ventral edge of the front panel and cause a step defect and concentration of forces at the edge of the pad, which usually occurs directly over the caudal border of the scapula. Properly fitting saddles and pads can be evaluated by the dirt or sweat marks present on the saddle pad. Proper fit is identified by the presence of a symmetric or butterfly-shaped dirt pattern, indicative of uniform panel contact over the dorsum of the withers and back. Asymmetric, clean or dry spots on the saddle pad suggest bridging or uneven saddle contact. Blankets, if not fit properly, can also cause severe wear injuries over the withers.

Restraint devices

Evaluation of proper tack fit and use requires that the horse and rider are evaluated while participating in their specific equestrian activities. Harness racing utilizes a plethora of restraint devices, such as stickers, overchecks and hobbles, that need to be assessed as potential contributors to back problems. Additional tack that needs to be evaluated is the appropriate use and fit of the noseband or cavesson, standing or running martingales, draw reins and the chambon during lungeing exercises. Most of these devices are used to correct altered body positioning or use associated with pain or avoidance, inexperience, inability or the induction of artificial gaits. If horses are sound and have good flexibility and strength, then most of these devices are unnecessary.

Gait evaluation

A careful examination at exercise is an important part of the clinical assessment of a horse with a potential back problem. Gait analysis for back problems focuses on evaluating regional vertebral mobility and pelvic motion symmetry, in addition to the typical lameness assessment. Gait analysis may help to rule out lower limb disorders and rule in vertebral dysfunction although limb lameness has been reported in up to 85% of horses with back problems.[37] Motion asymmetries, restricted vertebral or pelvic mobility, not tracking straight or lack of propulsion are a few characteristics that are evaluated. Tape on the vertebral column midline may help to visualize subtle lateral bending motion asymmetries or scoliosis. Tape on the tuber coxae may help to visualize subtle pelvic motion asymmetries.

Exercise in hand

The horse is first walked and then trotted on a loose rein in hand in a straight line to detect any obvious abnormalities in gait. Many horses with chronic back trouble show a restricted hind limb action with poor hock flexion and a tendency to drag the toes of one or both hind limbs. If there is moderate to severe pain, a wide straddling hind limb gait is usually seen, but in horses with a low-grade problem the action behind will be very close (i.e. plaiting). Next, the horse is turned as short as possible in both directions to induce lateral bending of the trunk. If back pain is present and there is loss of suppleness, turning is often difficult, resulting in rather jerky movements and spasm of the back muscles. On backing there is sometimes an initial reluctance to move, then the head is raised, the back arched more than usual and some spasm of the back muscles occurs. Another sign of discomfort is the dragging of the forelimb toes on moving backwards. Horses with chronic sacroiliac joint injury will often resent being backed up or down a slope. Severe lameness in one or both hind limbs is not usually a feature of a thoracolumbar disorder and diagnostic nerve blocks should be used to differentiate this from a genuine back problem. Mild shifting lameness or simply an unevenness of action of one hind limb is much more commonly seen in horses with back problems. Flexion tests (i.e. spavin test) rarely have any effect on the gait in horses with primary back problems, but are very useful in identifying secondary hock or stifle problems.

Lungeing exercise

A session of 10–15 minutes exercise on the lunge line in a sand ring helps to critically assess a horse's gait. This also provides an opportunity to see any improvement or deterioration in the action as the horse warms up. Horses with stiff backs often show exaggerated contractions or spasms of the longissimus muscles with each stride although this is also seen in horses that are unfit. Horses with restricted hind limb gait often show poor tracking of the hindfeet (i.e. placement of the hindfeet behind the imprint of the ipsilateral forefoot) and a tendency to drag or plait with the hindtoes. The head carriage may be elevated and the horse looks uncomfortable in work. A poor action is usually best seen at the trot. Some horses with back pain will lunge only at a collected canter. Some difficulty is often seen when changing gait (i.e. transitions) along with an inability to lead on the correct leg (i.e. disunited). The action behind appears to lack impulsion and swishing of the tail is often a feature. However, tail swishing is not always indicative of back pain. Placing a surcingle around the thorax and tightening it has also been used to demonstrate acute or active back pain.

Ridden or driven exercise

Evaluation of the response to placing a saddle and being ridden is important for a complete assessment of horses with back problems. Inspection of the tack for proper use and fit is always suggested on initial examination. Saddles and restraint devices should be evaluated for proper fit, padding and positioning on the horse. It is useful to see the horse saddled up and to note if there is any pain or resentment to tightening the girth or when mounting. A horse may have a 'cold back' when mounted, but this does not necessarily imply an underlying spinal problem. The horse should next be ridden in its intended use or discipline by its regular rider, if possible, during a routine training exercise to assess back and limb use at the walk, trot and canter. Showjumpers should also be jumped over the type of fences that usually cause the most challenge (i.e. combination-type fences). For harness racing horses it is of great benefit to have the horse driven so as to assess the performance and trotting or pacing gait at fast exercise.

Post-exercise examination

After allowing the horse to cool down, it should be exercised in hand again to see if there is any change in the action. This is particularly useful in horses with a low-grade exertional myopathy (i.e. mild rhabdomyolysis or tying up) as they show increased stiffness of the hock and hindquarters.

Orthopedic evaluation

The objective of carrying out an orthopedic evaluation of suspected back cases is to be able to rule out or identify concurrent cervical problems and distal limb lameness, and so assist in confirming a primary thoracolumbar or lumbosacral condition.

Cervical conditions

Neck pain or stiffness will often be associated with poor performance, thoracolumbar stiffness and restricted hind limb impulsion. Systematic palpation of the cervical region may pinpoint a painful region. Flexion and lateral bending of the neck, either manually or by offering food or a treat to induce cervical bending, will confirm neck stiffness. Further diagnostic tests, including scintigraphy, radiography and thermography, are indicated to confirm diagnosis of a neck problem.

Forelimb lameness

Gait evaluation in a straight line and on the lunge line should highlight the presence of forelimb lameness. Hoof testers, flexion tests and diagnostic nerve or joint blocks assist in identifying and localizing the site of forelimb lameness.

Hindlimb lameness

Gait evaluation may be more difficult particularly if lameness is mild and bilateral (e.g. hock or stifle). Horses with chronic sacroiliac joint injuries often have compensatory stiffness and pain in the proximal hindlimb.[41] Induced hock flexion (i.e. spavin test) is often negative in horses with back problems.[31] In many cases the use of nuclear scintigraphy will help in identifying areas of increased bone activity that may be the seat of lameness. Hoof testers, flexion tests and diagnostic nerve or joint blocks should confirm that you are not dealing with a primary back problem.

Neurologic evaluation

The majority of horses with back problems do not have concurrent neurologic disorders. If a neurologic disease is suspected, then a thorough neurologic evaluation should be pursued before any further back evaluation or imaging modalities are completed. A neurologic examination is indicated in the evaluation of horses with back problems to rule out traumatic, infectious and toxic etiologies. Postural reactions also help to assess the proprioceptive status (i.e. ataxia), weakness or spasticity, which often occur in spinal cord compromise.[44] Suspect horses are moved in tight circles to evaluate fore and hindfoot placement and backed up to assess willingness, strength and co-ordination of the hind limbs. Walking up and down curbs or over ground poles also helps to assess foot placement. Horses with back pain may drag the hind limbs.[42] Once a neurologic disease has been diagnosed or treated, any residual back problems should be assessed in light of the past or current neurologic signs.

Medical evaluation

Rectal palpation

Rectal palpation is an important diagnostic test in horses with back problems. Soft tissue injuries, osseous pathology and articular instability of the sacropelvic region may not be evident externally, but only palpable internally. It is also possible to rule out urogenital or gastrointestinal causes of back pain (e.g. colic, infection, masses). The psoas major and psoas minor muscles are palpable at the ventral aspect of the lumbar vertebrae. The iliacus and psoas major together form the iliopsoas muscle, which lies along the lateral wall of the pelvic inlet. These hypaxial muscles are evaluated for pain, swelling (i.e. hemorrhage) or asymmetry, and muscle hypertonicity. In horses with vague, upper hind limb lameness, the terminal aorta and iliac arteries also need to be examined for the presence of strong and regular pulses or possible thrombi.

Osseous palpation during rectal examination is useful for evaluating pelvic or sacral fractures, pelvic canal symmetry and lumbosacral or sacroiliac degenerative joint disease. Acute pelvic fractures produce substantial pain and possible crepitus with rocking of the pelvis side-to side. Bony callous or bony asymmetries palpable on the shafts of the ilium or ventral sacrum are indicative of prior fractures. The ventral aspects of the caudal lumbar vertebrae are evaluated for irregular bony proliferation, indicative of spondylosis. The sacroiliac joints lie deep to the bifurcation of the iliac arteries, at the dorsolateral pelvic canal. Some horses with acute sacroiliac joint injuries will strongly resent deep palpation either unilaterally or bilaterally over the sacroiliac joint region. Rectal palpation while walking or during externally induced pelvic motions (e.g. dorsoventrally or laterally) helps to directly assess lumbosacral and sacroiliac joint motion internally. Rectal palpation for chronic sacroiliac joint subluxation is usually unrewarding and not diagnostic unless bony proliferation, excess sacroiliac joint motion or joint crepitus during externally applied movements is identified.[41]

Laboratory analysis

A thorough laboratory diagnostic work-up, when clinically indicated, is important for the appropriate differential diagnosis and rehabilitation of horses with back problems. Two common serum enzymes indicative of skeletal muscle injury or inflammation include creatine kinase (CK) and aspartate aminotransferase (AST). Lactate dehydrogenase (LDH) is not as specific for skeletal muscle injury but the elevation of specific isoenzymes does have diagnostic value.[45] In most instances, these enzymes are not elevated in horses with primary back problems. In suspect horses, a submaximal exercise tolerance test can be performed in a treadmill or after trotting for 10 minutes.[42] Baseline serum samples are taken prior to exercise and compared to four-hour (peak CK) and 24 hour (peak AST) postexercise values. Urinalysis is indicated if exercise-associated muscle damage (i.e. exertional rhabdomyolysis) is suspected in horses with back muscle pain or hypertonicity. The presence of myoglobinuria is indicative of recent or active ongoing muscle injury.[45]

Hematology is indicated in suspected vertebral osteomyelitis and diskospondylitis to evaluate the presence of anemia, hyperproteinemia, hyperfibrinogenemia, leukocytosis or neutrophilia.[44] Cerebrospinal fluid (CSF) analysis and culture is useful if meningitis is also present. Electrolyte imbalances can be found in exhausted endurance horses, especially when coupled with dehydration or poor thermoregulation. To rule out hyperkalemic periodic paralysis (HYPP), serum potassium levels or the submission of whole blood for genetic testing may be indicated in Quarter Horses with muscle fasciculations and weakness.[45] Serum vitamin E (α-tocopherol) and selenium levels are important in the pathogenesis of nutritional myodegeneration (white muscle disease), sporadic exertional rhabdomyolysis and equine degenerative myeloencephalopathy (EDM). In suspect horses, whole-blood analysis of selenium-dependent glutathione peroxidase (GSH-Px) may also be indicated to assess the selenium status.[45]

Viral isolation and PCR techniques on nasopharyngeal swabs or peripheral blood samples are indicated in suspected outbreaks of equine herpesvirus myeloencephalitis (EVH-1).[44] Paired serum titers can reveal elevated or increasing titers in suspect horses. Serology (e.g. titer or Western blot) may also be indicated in horses with a history or clinical presentation suggestive of Lyme disease or equine protozoal myeloencephalitis (EPM). However, due to difficulties in serology interpretation, synovial tissue biopsies and CSF immunoblot analysis are preferred tests. CSF analysis may reveal elevated protein levels, xanthochromia or pleocytosis in cases of EVH-1, polyneuritis equi, EPM and equine motor neuron disease (EMND). CSF creatine kinase may also be elevated in horses infected with EPM or EMND.[44]

Muscle biopsies may be indicated to rule out EMND, polysaccharide storage myopathy (PSSM) and recurrent exertional rhabdomyolysis (RER).[46] Muscle biopsies provide assessment of muscle fibers, neuromuscular junctions, nerve branches, connective tissue and blood vessels.[45] Both light and electron microscopy, combined with histochemistry, are required for the diagnosis and prognostication of muscle disorders. Dietary analysis is indicated in horses with RER and PSSM. High grain diets may need to be replaced with fat supplementation, rice bran and access to high-quality hay.

Physical examination

The focus of the physical examination of the vertebral column is to identify if a back problem exists and to localize the injury to either soft tissue, osseous or neurologic structures. Traditional orthopedic and neurologic evaluations are important adjunctive assessments used to rule out other, more common causes of lameness and neurologic disorders. The spinal examination also helps to determine if the back problem is acute or chronic and if the vertebral dysfunction is segmental and localized or regional and diffuse.

Subjective assessment and grading of back problems

Vertebral dysfunction is most often characterized by localized pain, muscle hypertonicity, reduced joint motion and subsequent functional disability. The challenge, as with any musculoskeletal injury, is to identify the specific musculoskeletal structures affected and quantify the associated disability or altered function. The most common categorization of musculoskeletal injury consists of mild, moderate or severe degrees. Further quantification should include attempts to localize the vertebral levels and potential tissues affected and may involve the use of a 0–10 scale in an attempt to objectively monitor changes in pain, muscle hypertonicity, reduced joint motion or functional disability (Table 21.3). Subjective parameters can then be assigned a numerical value that can be assessed before and after treatment. The progression or regression of the individual parameters can then be recorded over time since most clinical back problems tend to be chronic or recurrent in nature.

Regional joint motion

Joint range of motion can be assessed either regionally via induced vertebral movements or segmentally via mobilization of individual vertebral motion segments. Vertebral range of motion is evaluated to detect whether a particular movement is normal, restricted or hypermobile. Regional causes of vertebral movement restrictions may include Intra-articular pathology (i.e. osteoarthritis), periarticular soft tissue adhesions, musculotendinous contractures or protective muscle spasms.

Table 21.3 Subjective assessment and grading of spinal dysfunction

GRADE	SCALE	PAIN	MUSCLE HYPERTONICITY	JOINT STIFFNESS	OVERALL FUNCTIONAL ABILITY
Absent	0	No clinical evidence of pain	No clinical evidence of muscle hypertonicity	No clinical evidence of joint stiffness	Full functional capability
Mild	1	Mild pain Precipitate with firm pressure only	Mild muscle hypertonicity Precipitate with firm pressure only	Mild joint stiffness No resistance to any induced movement	Mild restriction in ability Able to work at the walk and trot
	2	Localized pain Deep structures affected Soft tissue OR osseous structures Chronic pain condition	Segmental muscle hypertonicity Unilateral muscle hypertonicity One muscle group affected No fasciculations induced with firm palpation	Segmental joint stiffness Unilateral joint stiffness Good overall flexibility Reduced dorsoventral OR lateral bending	Able to perform while ridden Work limited during canter, gallop or jumping Unable to do advanced maneuvers Noticeable dysfunction during certain activities
	3	Occasional, mild reaction to grooming	Hypertonicity varies with applied pressure	Stiffness due to muscular restrictions	Mild incoordination present
Moderate	4	Moderate pain Precipitate with moderate pressure Regional pain	Moderate muscle hypertonicity Precipitate with moderate pressure Regional muscle hypertonicity	Moderate joint stiffness Tolerates some induced movements Regional joint stiffness	Moderate restriction in ability Able to work adequately at the walk. Difficult to perform with rider
	5	Superficial OR deep structures affected Several soft tissue AND osseous structures. Chronic OR acute pain condition	Unilateral OR bilateral muscle hypertonicity Two different muscle groups affected Fasciculations induced with firm palpation	Unilateral OR bilateral joint stiffness Limited flexibility in one *OR* more directions Reduced dorsoventral *AND* unilateral bending	Work limited to walk or trot only Unable to do lateral work or inclines Performs activity with much effort
	6	Consistent, moderate reaction to grooming	Hypertonicity worse with applied pressure	Stiffness due to connective tissue restrictions	Moderate incoordination present
Severe	7	Severe pain Precipitate easily with mild pressure or touch Generalized pain	Severe muscle hypertonicity Precipitate easily with mild pressure or touch Generalized muscle hypertonicity	Severe joint stiffness Resents any induced movements Generalized joint stiffness	Severe restriction in ability Able to stand comfortably Unable to perform with rider
	8	Superficial *AND* deep structures affected Multiple soft tissue *AND* osseous structures. Acute pain condition	Bilateral muscle hypertonicity Multiple muscle groups affected Spontaneous fasciculations present	Bilateral joint stiffness Poor flexibility in multiple directions Reduced dorsoventral *AND* bilateral bending	Work limited to walk only Unable to back up Resents all activities
	9	Consistent, strong avoidance response	Constant, severe muscle spasms	Stiffness due to Intraarticular restrictions	Severe incoordination present
Incapacitated	10	Severe, generalized, unrelenting pain All soft tissue and osseous structures affected	Severe, generalized, constant muscle spasms All muscle groups bilaterally affected	Severe, generalized joint stiffness No flexibility induced in any direction	Unable to perform at any level Unable to stand comfortably

Active range of motion

The diagnostic evaluation of regional active range of motion (AROM) involves using a carrot or other treat to induce flexion, extension and lateral bending of the neck and trunk. The willingness, coordination and amount of vertebral motion are compared bilaterally. Resistance, struggling to grasp the treat and left-to-right range of motion asymmetries are documented. Similar procedures can be used therapeutically as stretching exercises to increase neck or trunk range of motion.

Active lateral bending range of motion

The horse is positioned parallel against the stall wall to stabilize the trunk and pelvis and to provide a surface for the horse to lean against if needed during the active stretches. The positioning also helps to prevent the horse from chasing the treat holder around the stall during the evaluation. The treat is directed towards the elbow and held against the lateral girth region. This motion assesses mid to lower neck flexibility in lateral bending and rotation. Normally, horses should be able to readily touch their nose to the girth and hold the stretch for five seconds. The treat is then advanced along the ribs towards the point of the hip (i.e. tuber coxae). This motion assesses trunk flexibility in lateral bending. Normally, horses should be able to readily touch their nose to the point of the hip and hold the stretch for five seconds. Horses with back pain or stiffness will not be able to reach their nose to their tuber coxae and notable left-to-right asymmetries in range of motion will be seen if a back problem only affects structures on one side of the body. The distance of the nose from the tuber coxae can be measured (e.g. 10″ or able to reach the 15th rib) and changes assessed over time.

Active flexion range of motion

A treat is directed cranially between the forelimbs and towards the front feet. This motion assesses flexion flexibility of the mid to lower neck and withers. The clinician needs to place a hand on the ipsilateral carpus to prevent knee flexion during the range of motion assessment. Normally, horses should be able to readily touch their nose between the front feet and hold the stretch for five seconds. Those with pain or stiffness in the withers or back will not be able to reach their nose to their front feet and will flex one or both of their knees to compensate while reaching for the treat.

Passive range of motion

Passive range of motion (PROM) is assessed by measuring the amount and characteristics of joint motion beyond the active joint ranges of motion. These procedures require muscle relaxation so that passive joint motion can be induced and evaluated. However, there may be a high risk of injury if the excessive forces are applied to the body regions, without protective muscle tone. This is especially true when evaluating joint range of motion while under sedation or anesthesia. Most passive joint range of motions are assessed segmentally in non-sedated horses with more refined and detailed mobilization techniques (see later section).

Active assisted range of motion

Active assisted range of motion (AAROM) or spinal reflexes are often assessed with firm pressure applied to specific body regions that secondarily induce characteristic vertebral column movements. Diagnostically, the induced movements are graded as reduced, normal and exaggerated. Therapeutically, the induced movements are often held for a set period of time to induce stretch of hypertonic muscles and creep relaxation of shortened connective tissue (i.e. fascia or ligaments) or to strengthen weak or unco-ordinated agonist muscles via concentric contractions.

Wither elevation

Firm pressure applied along the ventral midline at the level of the sternum and cranial linea alba will induce elevation of the withers via isometric contraction of the thoracic portion of the serratus ventralis muscle. Pressure is applied with the fingertips or fingernails of one or both hands. Normally, horses will readily elevate the withers and midthoracic vertebrae (T7–T17) approximately 3–4 cm and hold the position for 5–10 seconds. Horses with cranial thoracic pain or stiffness will not be able to elevate the withers and will resent the applied pressure. Caution needs to be applied to horses with girth sensitivity or pain, since they often resent the applied pressure and may kick out with a hind limb. This exercise is often indicated therapeutically to induce relaxation of a hypertonic spinalis muscle associated with poor saddle fit (i.e. too narrow a tree).

Trunk elevation

Firm pressure applied bilaterally along the muscular groove between the biceps femoris and semitendinosus muscles induces elevation of the back via isometric contraction of the rectus abdominis muscle. The muscular groove is located approximately 10 cm (4″) lateral to the base of the tail. Pressure is applied bilaterally with equal pressure from the fingernail of the index fingers or needle caps, if needed. A variation of the technique involves the application of firm manual compression at the sacrocaudal junction but the response is often less consistent or dramatic. Normally, horses should readily elevate the thoracolumbar vertebrae (T12–L5) approximately 10–12 cm. The induced movement should be controlled and co-ordinated and able to be held for 20–30 seconds. Horses with back pain or stiffness will not be able to elevate the trunk and will resent the applied pressure. Other horses may immediately flex their pelvis and slightly hop upwards on the hind limbs or step away from the applied pressure. This exercise is similar to muscular efforts required during collection while performing certain dressage movements. It is often indicated therapeutically to induce relaxation of the thoracic or lumbar longissimus muscle hypertonicity associated with back pain, poor collection and coupling of the lumbosacral region and lack of impulsion from the hind limbs.

Spinal reflexes

Firm pressure applied unilaterally along the length of the longissimus muscles will induce localized contraction of the stimulated back or croup musculature. Light pressure with a needle cap or ballpoint pen is applied either along the long axis of the spine or transversely across the longissimus or middle gluteal muscles. There seems to be some confusion as to the clinical significance of the observed response to the applied stimuli. Some clinicians place significance on exaggerated or rapid movement away from the applied pressure, which is believed to be indicative of muscle pain. However, horses often have differing amounts of skin sensitivity or inconsistent responses to various stimuli, which may not be reliable indicators of back pain.[42] Some clinicians believe that resistance or lack of movement away from the applied pressure is clinically significant and indicative of severe muscle guarding or pain and the horse is unable or unwilling to move its back despite the applied pressure. In the author's opinion, the procedure often appears to be an unnecessary and noxious stimulus for most horses with back pain. Other, less noxious means of assessment are more informative in most horses with back pain. The procedure should be reserved for very stoic horses, where a question exists about the ability to actively lateral bend or flex and extend the trunk.

Blunt pressure applied unilaterally to the epaxial musculature will induce three characteristic and repeatable spinal reflexes. The first portion of the reflex occurs as a stimulus is applied to the saddle region (T10–L3). Normally, the horse will respond with an induced contralateral lateral bending and extension of the trunk away from the applied stimulus. Horses with back pain may have an exaggerated response and will rapidly and dramatically move away from the applied stimuli. Other horses, presumably due to excessive muscle guarding or nervousness, will not move away from the applied stimulus and will resist moving their trunk in the characteristic pattern of contralateral lateral bending and extension. The second portion of the reflex occurs as a stimulus is continued along the cranial croup region (L4–S3). Normally, the horse will respond with an induced extension of the lumbosacral joint. Horses with back pain may have an exaggerated response and will rapidly and dramatically move away from the applied stimulus. Horses with hypertonic or injured iliopsoas muscles would theoretically resent any induced extension of the lumbosacral junction due to secondary stretching of the iliopsoas muscles. The third portion of the reflex occurs as a stimulus is continued along the caudal croup region (S4–tuber ischii) along the muscular groove between the biceps femoris and semitendinosus muscles. Normally, horses will respond with an induced flexion of the lumbosacral joint and ipsilateral lateral bending of the trunk towards the applied stimuli. Horses with back pain may have an exaggerated response to the applied stimuli and will rapidly and dramatically immediately flex the pelvis and step away from the applied pressure. Bilateral application of pressure in the same location will induce flexion of the lumbosacral joint without lateral bending, as described above.

Soft tissue palpation

Any palpation of the musculoskeletal system requires a quiet and co-operative patient. Horses that are moving around and not willing to stand quietly are difficult to assess fully for back problems. The horse's response to being approached and its anticipation of palpation are often used as an indication of potential back pain or hypersensitivity. Many owners will report a change in behavior (i.e. pinned ears, swishing tail) as a horse with back pain anticipates being touched or having the saddle placed on its back. Other complaints include a newly developed sensitivity to being groomed in one particular location on the trunk. The hallmarks of vertebral segment dysfunction include localized pain and abnormal paraspinal muscle tonicity.[47]

Palpation is often a reliable technique used to localize and identify soft tissue and osseous structures for changes in texture, tissue mobility or resistance to pressure.[6,48] The soft tissue layers are evaluated from superficial to deep without simply increasing digital pressure but also shifting attention with discrete palpatory movements. Shapes of structures, transitions between structures and attachment sites may also be palpated.[43] Soft tissue texture and mobility can be compared between the skin, subcutaneous tissues, thoracolumbar fascia and muscle.

Skin and subcutis

Acute back pain and inflammation will produce local areas of palpable heat, whereas chronic back problems can be identified by focal regions of colder temperatures, relative to the surrounding or contralateral tissues. Thermography provides an objective measure of temperature variations within the superficial tissues of horses with back problems. The hair, epidermis, dermis and subcutaneous tissues should be evaluated systematically with detailed palpation and observation for potential contributing factors to back pain or discomfort. The hair coat is evaluated for changes in hair texture or alopecia, which are often indicative of abnormal saddle or blanket wear. Asymmetric dirt or sweat patterns after removal of the saddle pad are also important indicators of poor saddle fit. A common presenting complaint for horses with back problems is localized sensitivity to routine grooming or brushing.

The skin around the withers should be evaluated for evidence of acute injuries associated with poor saddle fit or improper blanket wear, which are characterized by localized hair loss, open skin lesions (saddle galls) and signs of inflammation. Chronic saddle fit or blanket wear lesions are identified by the presence of white hairs and scar tissue over the dorsal or lateral aspects of the withers. In some horses, localized sites of edema or hives may occur after riding with a poor-fitting saddle or pad.[42] The epidermis should be evaluated for scabs, scrapes, lacerations, fly bites (ventral dermatitis), sarcoids and dermatophilus (rain scald), which may be primary causes of back pain or are irritated with saddle or girth placement. The dermis is palpated over the trunk region for eosinophilic granulomas or melanomas. Eosinophilic granulomas may regress spontaneously or enlarge and become ulcerated with continued friction in the saddle region. The subcutaneous tissues are palpated for edema or cellulitis, masses, fat deposits and the mobility of the skin over the underlying loose connective tissue. Chronic scar tissue, adhesions and fibrosis may produce back pain if the affected tissues are restricted or pulled on during locomotion or trunk movements. Blood vessels, nerves and lymph nodes are important structures that reside within the subcutaneous tissues.

Connective tissue palpation

Connective tissue structures, such as the fascia and ligaments, are systematically evaluated for clinical signs of acute or chronic injury.

Fascia

The dense connective tissue that forms the superficial and deep fascia is systematically evaluated for masses, rents, scar tissue and tonicity. The overlying skin and subcutaneous tissues are mobilized by a firm, broad contact. The superficial fascia is assessed for smoothness and uniform tonicity or compliance. The superficial fascia typically forms a superficial covering of muscle bellies, whereas the deep fascia forms folds of connective tissue between muscle bellies and anchors to deeper osseous structures. Severe or deep trauma to the myofascial tissues (e.g. kicks, deep lacerations or abscesses) can produce residual fibrosis that limits adjacent muscular activity and fascial extensibility. The thoracolumbar fascia is the most prominent fascia of the trunk and is particularly evident at the thoracolumbar junction as it blends medially with the supraspinous ligament. In the lumbar region, the thoracolumbar fascia attaches to the cranial aspects of the tuber sacrale and iliac wing, deep to the overlying middle gluteal muscle.

Spinal ligaments

The spinal ligaments are systematically palpated for masses, fiber disruption, fibrosis and signs of desmitis (i.e. swelling or pain). The nuchal ligament forms a broad attachment to the dorsal apexes of the spinous processes of the withers and continues caudally as the supraspinous ligament. The supraspinous bursa lies between the nuchal ligament and the T3–T5 dorsal spinous processes. The supraspinous bursa is not normally palpable, unless distended or possibly infected (i.e. fistulous withers). Firm digital pressure is applied dorsally and laterally to the nuchal and supraspinous ligaments and ligamentous attachments at the dorsal spinous processes. The entire length of the supraspinous ligament is palpated by lateral compression between the index finger and thumb. The induction of spinal flexion will cause the supraspinous ligament to be more prominent and readily palpable.

Pelvic ligaments

Unfortunately, most of the pelvic ligaments are inaccessible due to their location deep to the gluteal musculature or within the acetabular region of the hip. The dorsal portion of the dorsal sacroiliac ligament and the caudal portion of the sacrosciatic ligaments are the only palpable ligaments of the pelvic region. The dorsal sacroiliac ligaments are palpable in the croup region as two large round ligaments that originate on the caudal aspect of the tuber sacrale and converge caudally on the sacral spinous processes. Firm digital pressure is applied dorsally and laterally to the dorsal sacroiliac ligaments, bilaterally and individually, to lateralize any localized pain or swelling, indicative of desmitis. The caudal attachment of the sacrosciatic ligament at the tuber ischii is palpable and should be evaluated for pain and symmetry in tonicity. Horses that consistently carry their tail off to one side or have a history of sacral fractures may have palpable differences in sacrosciatic ligament tonicity. The trochanteric bursa is located between the tendon of the accessory gluteal muscle and the greater trochanter of the femur. Like other bursae, it is not palpable unless inflamed or distended. Trochanteric bursitis often presents as upper hind limb lameness and not as a back problem.

Muscle palpation

The trunk and pelvic musculature is evaluated systematically from superficial to deep with detailed palpation of abnormal muscle tonicity, pain or fasciculations. Muscle palpation is done with light but firm pressure applied by a broad contact with the entire hand, not only the fingertips, which may unduly localize the applied pressure and precipitate a pain response (i.e. false positive). Regional muscle tone and development of the neck, trunk and proximal limb musculature is assessed and compared left to right. Muscles are then individually identified and evaluated for masses, fibrosis, swellings or depressions. Individual muscles and their attachments are assessed unilaterally and then compared bilaterally for tonicity and the response to manual palpation (i.e. sensitivity). Local or regional alterations in temperature or texture are carefully palpated for signs of active inflammation.

Muscle development

Muscle evaluation begins with observation and palpation of the neck, shoulder, pectoral, wither, trunk, gluteal and thigh muscle development and symmetry. Muscle atrophy can be due to partial or complete denervation, disuse, malnutrition or immune-mediated disorders.[45] Obese horses are often difficult to palpate due to poor muscle development and indistinct myofascial borders. Epaxial muscle development is assessed by laying a hand transversely across the longissimus and middle gluteal muscles. Horses with exceptional back muscle development should have a palpable convexity or outward curvature of the muscles along the entire distance from the withers to the croup. Deconditioning or poor flexibility may contribute to epaxial muscles that are palpably flat between the dorsal spinous processes and the ribs laterally. Horses with chronic back problems or poor saddle fit will have a palpable concavity or inward curvature of the epaxial muscles at the withers or along the trunk. Asymmetries in muscle development may be palpable cranial to caudal, medial to lateral or left to right. The thoracic portion of the spinalis muscle is the most commonly affected muscle in the wither region. The longissimus muscle is the most commonly affected trunk muscle. The middle gluteal and the vertebral portions of the biceps femoris, semitendinosus and semimembranosus muscle are common areas to visualize or palpate muscle asymmetries in the pelvic region.

Muscle tonicity

The general muscle tone varies between horses and breeds. Nervous or excited horses will have overall increased muscle tone, whereas stoic, depressed or systemically ill horses will have reduced or sometimes flaccid muscle tone. Arabians tend to carry more muscle tone, whereas most Warmbloods or draft breeds will allow deep palpation of their generally relaxed muscles. Muscle tonicity is an indirect measure of muscle activity or contraction. Electromyography (EMG) provides a direct assessment of muscle activity but it is not readily available in most clinical situations and it is often difficult to perform and interpret.[45]

Muscle tonicity is categorized as hypotonicity, normal tonicity and hypertonicity. Normal epaxial muscles are not contracted in a quietly standing horse, but are relaxed and malleable. Muscle hypotonicity or flaccidity is indicative of neuropathies, such as disuse or denervation atrophy. Muscle hypertonicity is the most commonly palpable abnormality in horses with acute or chronic back problems and can have either neural or myopathic origins.[45] Generalized muscle hypertonicity may affect a small portion of a muscle (i.e. trigger point), an entire muscle belly or a regional group of muscles. Muscle spasms are an acute, severe form of muscle hypertonicity, with substantial pain and loss of muscle function. Detailed palpation and a thorough knowledge of muscular anatomy will help to identify which muscle or muscles are primarily affected, and which adjacent muscles are likely to have secondary guarding due to common biomechanical or neurologic factors. In general, localized muscle hypertonicity is considered an acute or primary back problem whereas regional longissimus muscle hypertonicity is often associated with a chronic hind limb lameness or systemic disease.

Trigger points are characterized as localized bands or foci of muscle contracture and pain within a muscle belly.[49,50] Muscle contractures are not associated with normal neural firing and subsequent depolarization of the muscle membrane.[45] Trigger points occur in consistent and predicable locations, presumably due to alterations in local muscle function caused by changes in posture or biomechanics. In horses with back or pelvic problems, focal hypertonic muscle bands with a lower pain pressure threshold (i.e. increased sensitivity) can often be found in the middle gluteal muscle. The clinical significance of trigger points in the middle gluteal muscle is difficult to determine since they do not always correlate with the presence or severity of lameness or back problems.

Muscle spasms or splinting are characterized as involuntary, pronounced and unremitting muscle contractions in response to severe and unrelenting pain (e.g. colic) or metabolic disturbances (e.g. electrolyte imbalances or exertional rhabdomyolysis). Horses with acute or severe back pain may present with muscle splinting but other underlying medical conditions that may be more life threatening or critical need to be ruled out immediately. Muscle splinting severely restricts the ability to evaluate trunk mobility and the palpation of underlying soft tissue structures. Therefore, medical treatment of the primary problem or the administration of muscle relaxants is often required before a complete evaluation of the vertebral column can be accomplished.

Muscle pain

The assessment of muscle pain is often subjective and is dependent on the evaluator's tactile skills and interpretation of clinical significance. The clinical assessment of acute versus chronic pain is relatively straightforward but determination of the exact etiology and appropriate treatment regime are diagnostically challenging. Acute muscle pain is characterized by heat, firm swelling or edema, substantial hypertonicity and pain and dysfunction of the affected muscle region. Acute muscle pain may be due to direct trauma (e.g. kick or other blunt trauma) or metabolic disorders (i.e. exertional rhabdomyolysis). The thoracic portion of the spinalis muscle is a common site of muscle pain, associated with a poor-fitting saddle (i.e. too narrow a tree). Chronic muscle pain has a more neurogenic basis and is due less to direct inflammatory mediators.

Horses with acute sacroiliac joint injuries may have localized sensitivity to palpation of the gluteal musculature and surrounding soft tissues in the dorsal croup region.[31] Protective muscle spasms may be palpated in the adjacent middle gluteal musculature and the vertebral portions of the biceps femoris, semitendinosus and semimembranosus muscles. A localized region of edema may occasionally be palpated over the lumbosacral junction[40] but this is not a specific finding related to sacroiliac joint injury.

Pressure algometry

In humans, the diagnosis of chronic fatigue syndrome or fibromyalgia is often based on the presence of decreased pain thresholds at a set number of standardized musculoskeletal locations. The clinical syndrome of myofascial pain in horses is common and quite similar to humans. Unfortunately, we often have a poor understanding of the etiopathogenesis and the objective assessment of muscle pain. Pressure algometry of soft tissue structures provides an objective measure of muscle or ligamentous mechanical nociceptive thresholds (i.e. the minimum force that causes discomfort or pain).[51] It utilizes a force gauge and plunger to measure left-to-right asymmetries or identify subnormal values.[50] In horses, normal mechanical nociceptive threshold values for soft tissue landmarks are typically 20–30 pounds/cm^2. Horses with myofascial pain often have mechanical nociceptive threshold values of less than 10 pounds/cm^2.

Guarding of the back is an exaggerated response to typically innocuous stimuli or sudden movements. This abnormal response is commonly seen in nervous horses or those with back pain. Pronounced muscle guarding with movement away from any anticipated contact or placement of the saddle is considered abnormal. Horses should not react adversely to any grooming or superficial or deep muscle palpation[42] although a few sensitive horses may have a mild, temporary avoidance to deep muscle palpation. Any exaggerated attempts to avoid palpation or the presence of prolonged muscle contractions or fasciculations should be considered abnormal. Horses with back pain and muscle soreness may have localized areas of muscle fasciculations depending on the amount and type of pressure applied.

Muscle fasciculation

Muscle fasciculations are usually indicative of profound muscle weakness, electrolyte imbalances, or primary muscle pathology although, muscles may fasciculate at characteristic locations distant to an area of palpation.[42] In humans, this is indicative of referred pain, which is difficult to truly assess in horses due to the lack of verbal feedback. In horses with back or gluteal muscle pain, it is common to find areas of muscle fasciculations in the mid-lumbar longissimus muscles when firm, localized pressure is applied to hypertonic or painful areas (i.e. trigger points) within the middle gluteal muscles. This is an intriguing response since the motor innervation of the reactive lumbar longissimus muscles is provided segmentally by dorsal branches of the spinal nerves of L2–L4 and the middle gluteal muscle is innervated by ventral branches of the spinal nerves that contribute to the cranial gluteal nerve (L6–S2).

Osseous palpation

Osseous palpation involves evaluating osseous structures for pain, morphology, asymmetries and alignment. Individual thoracic, lumbar and sacral spinous processes are palpated for a painful response with firm digital pressure applied to the osseous structures of the dorsal midline.[52] Typical signs of discomfort include tossing the head upwards, extension of the back or withers away from the applied pressure or localized secondary muscle spasms. Algometry (pain pressure thresholds) of osseous landmarks provides an objective measure of bony pain and allows monitoring of the effectiveness of treatment protocols. Normal algometry values for osseous landmarks are higher than soft tissue values and typically exceed 30–40 pounds/cm^2. Horses with bone pain often have osseous algometry values less than 10 pounds/cm^2.

Dorsal spinous processes

The morphology of individual dorsal spinous processes is compared to adjacent spinous processes. It is common to palpate seemingly higher, wider or laterally displaced dorsal spinous processes. However, unless there is also localized pain or muscle hypertonicity adjacent to the affected dorsal process, then the spinous process deviation is probably not clinically significant. Individual spinous process deviation is common, but it is not often associated with spinous process fracture or vertebral malposition (i.e. bone out of place), as is commonly thought. Overlapping or malaligned dorsal spinous processes are often caused by spinous process impingement, developmental asymmetries in the neural arch or isolated dorsal spinous process deviation of unknown etiology.[53,54] Palpably taller or wider dorsal spinous processes occur presumably due to avulsion fractures or osseous proliferation within or at supraspinous ligament insertion sites (i.e. enthesopathies). Radiographs, ultrasonography and scintigraphy are useful modalities to document the cause of palpable differences in dorsal spinous processes.

Tuber sacrale

The tuber sacrale of the pelvis are palpated for height asymmetries and pain response to manual compression. Unilateral or bilateral prominence of the tuber sacrale may be noted, but is not usually clinically significant unless associated with clinical signs of localized pain or inflammation or positive findings on diagnostic imaging (e.g. scintigraphy). In acute sacroiliac injuries, asymmetry in gluteal muscle development is uncommon, unless pronounced osseous pelvic asymmetry is also present. Firm digital pressure applied to the dorsal aspect of the tuber sacrale has been reported to produce a variable and inconsistent pain response.[55] In the author's opinion, dramatic and consistent pain responses have been produced in affected horses with specific provocation tests that are useful to establish a presumptive diagnosis of sacroiliac joint injury or pelvic stress fractures.

The procedure involves simultaneous manual compression of the dorsal aspects of both tuber sacrale, which induces a bending moment on the iliac wing and presumably compresses the sacroiliac articulations (Fig. 21.8). Normally, horses will not have any response or only a mild response to the applied pressure. Mild contraction of the lumbar longissimus muscles and slight extension of the lumbosacral joint is normal for most horses. Acutely affected horses may have a dramatic reaction to this manipulation and will demonstrate severe longissimus muscle contractions and sudden collapse of the hind limbs which is indicative of pelvic injury or sacroiliac joint pain.[42] Practitioners should gradually apply increasing pressure since affected horses may actually collapse in the hind

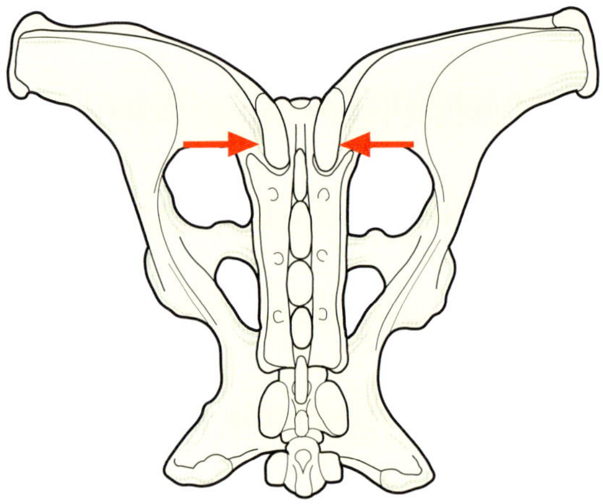

Fig 21.8 Forces applied during a sacroiliac joint provocation test (dorsal view). Firm pressure is applied bilaterally with both hands, compressing the dorsal aspects of the tuber sacrale.

limbs and fall to the ground if excess force is applied to the painful tuber sacrale. This test is not specific for sacroiliac joint pathology, as horses with incomplete or stress fractures of the ilial wing may respond even more dramatically to the applied pressure.

The apex of the second sacral spinous process is a reliable landmark used to evaluate relative tuber sacrale displacement. Normally, the dorsal apices of the tuber sacrale and the second sacral spinous process lie in close apposition and follow the contour of the croup. Using palpation, ultrasound or radiographs, a physical discrepancy in height can often be identified between the dorsal profile of the sacral spinous processes (which should remain constant, unless fractured) and the potentially ventrally or dorsally displaced unilateral or bilateral tuber sacrale. In this manner, either unilateral (i.e. tuber sacrale height asymmetry) or bilateral tuber sacrale displacement (i.e. hunters' or jumpers' bumps) can be diagnosed, depending on whether one or both tuber sacrale are elevated relative to the apices of the sacral spinous processes. Tuber sacrale height asymmetry is evident in sacroiliac joint subluxation (the higher side is affected) and complete ilial wing fractures (the lower side is affected). Bilateral tuber sacrale displacement has an unknown clinical significance and may be present in many high-level competition horses.[40] Theoretically, the hunters' or jumpers' bumps may provide a longer lever arm for the strong longissimus and thoracolumbar fascia to produce extension at the lumbosacral joint, resulting in increased impulsion and range of hindlimb motion with subsequent improved performance.

Pelvis

Lateral compression of the tuber coxae and tuber ischii is indicated in horses with acute pelvic lameness to help rule out complete pelvic fractures. Palpation or auscultation of the dorsal pelvic region during repetitive side-to-side movements also assist in the diagnosis of pelvic crepitus. Normally, the tuber sacrale move in unison during locomotion. A palpable or visible independent movement of the tuber sacrale at a walk or during treadmill locomotion is indicative of sacroiliac joint luxation or a complete pelvic fracture. Horses with acute sacroiliac joint injuries may also resent flexion of the contralateral hind limb. Rectal palpation is also indicated to assess osseous morphology (e.g. displaced fracture fragments or callus) and soft tissue pain or swelling (i.e. hemorrhage) in horses with suspected pelvic fractures.

Segmental vertebral joint motion

A vertebral motion segment is the functional unit of the spine and includes two adjacent vertebrae and the associated soft tissues that bind them together. To utilize palpation in the evaluation of the musculoskeletal system fully, an understanding of how joint motion is assessed is required.[43] Joint motion can be categorized into three zones of movement: physiologic, paraphysiologic and pathologic. The physiologic zone of movement includes both active and passive ranges of motion and is the site where joint mobilization is applied. Moving an articulation from a neutral position first involves evaluating a range of motion that has minimal, uniform resistance. As the articulation is moved toward the end of that range of motion there is a gradual increase in the resistance to movement (i.e. joint end-feel). End range of motion starts when any change in resistance to passive joint manipulation is palpable. Joint end-feel is evaluated by bringing the articulation to tension and applying rhythmic oscillations to the joint to qualify the resistance to movement. The normal joint end-feel is initially soft and resilient and gradually becomes more restrictive as maximal joint range of motion is reached. A pathologic or restrictive end range of motion is palpable earlier in passive joint movement and has an abrupt, restrictive end-feel when compared with normal joint end-feel. The paraphysiologic zone of movement occurs outside the joint's normal elastic barrier and is the site of joint cavitation and manipulation. The anatomic barrier of the joint marks the junction of the paraphysiologic and pathologic zones of movement. The pathologic zone of movement lies outside the limits of normal anatomic joint integrity and is characterized by joint injury (e.g. sprain, subluxation or luxation).

Combining the evaluation of segmental joint range of motion and the presence or absence of pain at the extremes of motion, diagnostic interpretations can be implied.[56] Normal joint motion is painless, suggesting that articular structures are intact and functional. Normal joint mobility that has a painful end range suggests that a minor sprain of the associated articular tissues is present. Painless joint hypomobility suggests that a contracture or adhesion is present. Painful hypomobility suggests an acute strain with secondary muscle guarding. Painless hypermobility may indicate a complete rupture and a painful hypermobility suggests a partial tear of the evaluated structure.

Mobilization

Mobilization is used to evaluate each individual vertebral and pelvic articulation for loss of normal joint motion and overall resistance to induced motion. The goal of palpating joint movement is to evaluate the initiation of motion resistance, the quality of joint motion and end-feel, and the overall joint range of motion (ROM). Similar palpatory findings can be noted in other soft tissues such as skin, connective tissue, muscles or ligaments.[48] Each vertebral segment is evaluated for altered mobilization findings in flexion and extension, right and left lateral bending and right and left rotation. Segmental causes of vertebral movement restrictions include soft tissue (e.g. capsular fibrosis, muscle spasms or contractures) and osseous (e.g. malformations, osteoarthritis, ankylosis) pathologies. Vertebral segments with altered mobilization findings (i.e. joint stiffness) can occur with or without localized muscle hypertonicity and pain. Comparisons of mobilization findings before and after manipulation or stretching exercises are made to evaluate the vertebral motion segment response to treatment.

Wither mobilization

Lateral forces are applied to individual dorsal spinous processes of the withers (T3–T12) to assess lateral bending and rotation of individual thoracic vertebral motion segments. The practitioner stands facing the withers. To stabilize the cranial and caudal vertebral segments, the bases of both hands are applied to the ipsilateral surface of the spinous processes adjacent to the vertebra being evaluated. The index fingers contact the contralateral surface of the dorsal spinous process to be assessed. A compressive force is applied between the index fingers and base of the hands to induce slight rotation of an individual thoracic spinous process. Normally, 3–4 mm of spinous process movement is palpable, without any evidence of pain or muscles spasms in response to the applied force. In horses with wither discomfort due to poor saddle fit, an obvious pain response (e.g. a rapid elevation of the head, depression of the withers) and local muscle hypertonicity will be precipitated with the applied pressure. In chronic forelimb lameness (e.g. laminitis), individual spinous process motion will not be detectable and the entire withers will move as a unit due to presumed chronic fibrosis and muscle guarding.

Trunk lateral bending mobilization

Lateral forces are applied to individual dorsal spinous processes of the trunk (T13–L6) to assess lateral bending and rotation of individual thoracolumbar vertebral motion segments. The practitioner stands facing the trunk. The base of the tail is grasped in the caudal hand, which provides side-to-side motion during the procedure. The base of the cranial hand is positioned against or between the spinous processes of interest. A lateral bending moment (i.e. wiggle) is induced as the cranial hand rhythmically pushes laterally and the caudal hand pulls laterally. The cranial hand is repositioned at the sequential dorsal spinous processes from cranial to caudal in order to assess lateral bending and rotation at individual thoracolumbar vertebral segments. Normally, a slight springy end-feel of joint motion is palpable at each motion segment, without any evidence of pain or muscle spasms in response to the applied force. In horses with back problems, restricted vertebral motion or stiffness is palpable and there is evidence of local pain and muscle spasms in response to the applied pressure. In general, acute or primary back problems produce segmental stiffness, pain and muscle hypertonicity. Chronic or secondary back problems produce regional stiffness, pain and muscle hypertonicity or atrophy.

Rib mobilization

Lateral compressive forces are applied to the individual ribs and costochondral junctions to assess pain and mobility. The base of the hand is positioned over individual ribs as a medial motion is induced, similar to expiration. The hand is repositioned at the sequential ribs and costochondral junctions from cranial to caudal. The amount of rib motion, resentment and secondary muscle spasms are noted during the induced movements. Normally, a slight springy feel is palpable at each rib, without any evidence of pain or muscle spasms. In horses that are girthy, cinchy, or have back problems, restricted rib motion or stiffness is palpable and there is evidence of local pain, resentment and muscle spasms in response to the applied pressure.

Trunk flexion-extension mobilization

While standing on an elevated surface, ventrally directed forces are applied rhythmically over individual dorsal spinous processes to assess flexion and extension of individual thoracolumbar (T13–L6) vertebral motion segments. The palm of one hand is placed over the dorsal aspect of the spinous process of interest. The other hand grasps the wrist and both hands apply a ventral force equally. An extension moment and rebound flexion (i.e. bounce) is induced as the hands rhythmically push ventrally. The hands are repositioned at sequential dorsal spinous processes from cranial to caudal. Normally, a slight springy end-feel of joint motion is palpable at each motion segment, without any evidence of pain or muscle spasms. In horses with back problems, restricted motion or stiffness is palpable and there is evidence of local pain and muscle spasms in response to the applied pressure.

Lumbosacral flexion-extension mobilization

Ventrally directed forces are also applied rhythmically over the tuber coxae to induce extension of the sacroiliac and lumbosacral articulations. The practitioner stands facing the pelvis. The fingers are placed over the dorsal aspect of the tuber coxae to induce the ventral motion. A normal response to the induced movement is fluid vertical motion of the lumbosacral region with 1–2 cm of dorsoventral displacement over the lumbar dorsal spinous processes. Horses with pelvic or lumbar dysfunction will have a noticeable pain response, resent the induced movement or will have protective gluteal or sublumbar muscle spasms that limit the induced movement. The vertically directed force primarily induces movement at the lumbosacral junction, but sacroiliac joint motion and potential injury must also be differentiated with this procedure.

Sacroiliac ligament stress tests

The sacroiliac ligaments are not readily palpable in horses. However, specific forces applied to the pelvic prominences (i.e. tuber sacrale, tuber coxae or tuber ischii) or the sacral apex can provide an indirect method to assess the structural and functional status of the supporting ligaments.

Dorsoventral sacroiliac ligament stress tests

Sacroiliac ligament injury can be identified by rhythmically applying a ventrally directed force over the lumbosacral dorsal spinous processes in an effort to stress the supporting sacroiliac ligaments. This procedure requires the practitioner to get up on an elevated surface (i.e. mounting block) so that the two separately applied forces can be directed vertically over the L6 and S2 dorsal spinous processes, respectively. Horses with sacroiliac ligament injuries would be expected to resent the induced movement over the L6 dorsal spinous process since it specifically stresses the interosseous sacroiliac ligament (i.e. ligamentous sling of the sacropelvic junction). Horses with lumbosacral vertebral joint dysfunction (i.e. localized pain, reduced joint motion and muscle hypertonicity without structural pathology) may also resent this procedure. Rhythmically applied ventrally directed forces over the dorsal spinous processes at the sacrocaudal junction would be expected to specifically stress the dorsal portion of the dorsal sacroiliac ligament. A positive response to this test combined with positive ultrasound findings of desmitis of the dorsal sacroiliac ligament would be highly suggestive of clinically significant dorsal sacroiliac ligament injury.

Lateral sacroiliac ligament stress test

Sacral apex deviation can be assessed by applying simultaneous, but opposite directed, lateral forces to the tuber sacrale and the sacrocaudal junction (Fig. 21.9). Sacroiliac joint or ligament injuries can also be localized by evaluating pain and ligamentous laxity in the sacroiliac joint. These procedures are similar to valgus-varus stress tests used to evaluate the collateral ligaments of the distal limb articulations. Care should be taken not to apply excessive force due to the long lever arm action of the sacral apex on the sacroiliac ligaments, which can unduly stress unstable or partially torn ligaments or aggravate an acutely inflamed sacroiliac joint. The proposed mechanism of action of these tests is to use the base of the tail and sacrum as a handle to apply a lateral (horizontal plane) stress to the sacroiliac joint as the wing of the ilium is stabilized.

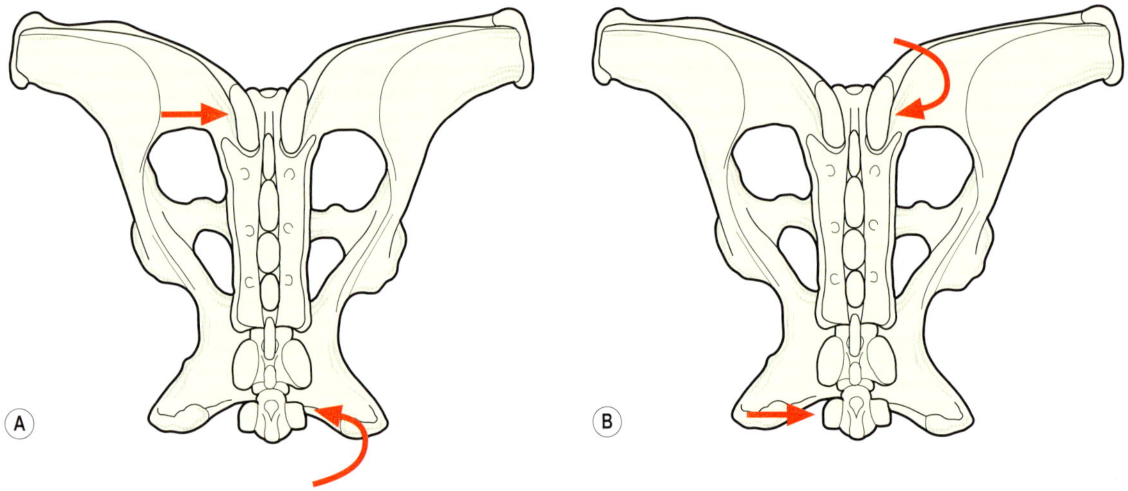

Fig 21.9 Forces applied during a sacroiliac ligament stress test (dorsal view). **(A)** Firm pressure is applied by both hands, pushing with the hand at the ipsilateral tuber sacrale away from the examiner while simultaneously pulling with the hand at the tail head toward the examiner. **(B)** Firm pressure is applied by both hands; pulling with the hand at the contralateral tuber sacrale toward the examiner while simultaneously pushing with the hand at the tail head away from the examiner.

The technique involves two parts. First, the base of the hand closest to the horse's head is placed over the lateral aspect of the tuber sacrale. The hand closest to the tail grasps the base of the tail head (Cd2–3). The sacroiliac joints are then evaluated as firm pressure is simultaneously applied by both hands, pushing with the hand at the tuber sacrale away from the examiner and pulling with the hand at the tail head toward the examiner (Fig. 21.9A). Theoretically, this maneuver produces compression of contralateral and distraction of ipsilateral sacroiliac articular surfaces.

The second portion of the technique involves repeating the procedure and reversing the direction of the applied forces (Fig. 21.9B). The fingers of the hand closest to the horse's head are placed over the contralateral tuber sacrale and the base of the hand closest to the tail is placed against the ipsilateral base of the tail head (Cd2–3). The sacroiliac joints are again evaluated as firm pressure is applied by both hands, pulling with the hand at the tuber sacrale toward the examiner and pushing with the hand at the tail head away from the examiner. Theoretically, the contralateral sacroiliac articular surfaces are distracted and the ipsilateral sacroiliac articular surfaces are compressed. A pain response to the induced movements may be identified either unilaterally or bilaterally, depending on the extent of inflammation or injury present. In general, sacroiliac joint compression would be expected to aggravate osteoarthritic changes, whereas joint distraction would be expected to stress any injured or inflamed sacroiliac ligaments.

Proximal limb evaluation

In horses with back or pelvic problems, the proximal limbs are often affected either primarily or secondarily. Primary thoracic or pelvic girdle muscle or joint dysfunction is often evident as lameness in the affected limb. However, back or pelvic problems can also induce secondary proximal limb dysfunction that needs to be differentiated. Muscular or osseous asymmetry of the shoulder or pelvic regions are often indications of limb dysfunction or lameness. The pectoral region is viewed cranially to assess muscular symmetry. The dorsal scapula and wither region are viewed caudally from an elevated surface to assess bilateral symmetry and muscle development related to proper saddle fit. The croup or gluteal region is also viewed caudally to assess symmetry and muscle development. Horses with pelvic lameness or EPM often have noticeable gluteal muscle atrophy or asymmetry. The tuber sacrale are assessed for osseous asymmetry associated with pelvic fractures, sacroiliac joint subluxation or developmental factors. Changes in the height of the tuber sacrale should be assessed relative to the apex of the second sacral spinous process (S2).

Abnormal tonicity of the thoracic or pelvic girdle muscles is identified by hypotonicity or flaccidity, and hypertonicity associated with local trigger points or regional muscle spasms. The proximal limbs are also evaluated for normal ranges of motion or flexibility. In the forelimb, the scapulothoracic and shoulder joints are evaluated. In the hindlimb, the sacroiliac and coxofemoral joints are assessed. The fore- and hindlimbs are individually examined in protraction, retraction, abduction, adduction and flexion for resistance to the applied movements, joint stiffness or muscle hypertonicity. Horses with back or pelvic problems will resent certain movements, have reduced limb motion and will not actively extend and stretch the limbs. Normally, horses will actively stretch their fore- and hindlimbs when positioned in protraction and retraction. Extension of the hindlimb caudally will apply a stretch to the hindlimb protractor muscles, which include the iliopsoas, rectus femoris and tensor fascia latae. Injury to these muscles will produce resentment to passive stretching of the hindlimb. Iliopsoas muscle injury or hypertonicity can also be confirmed with rectal palpation.

Diagnostic injections

The use of injections of local anesthetics into painful or inflamed musculoskeletal structures is the basis of lameness evaluation. Fortunately, the same principle can be applied to painful soft tissue, articular or osseous structures of the back and pelvis.

Muscle

Injection into areas of perceived muscle pain or reactive acupuncture points helps to assess the contribution of muscle pain to the observed back problem, cause of poor performance, vague gait abnormalities or resentment to placement of the saddle.[42] Before and after comparisons of the muscle response to applied pressure (i.e. pressure algometry) or changes in gait help to confirm the clinical significance of the muscle pain to the primary presenting complaint. In humans, trigger point therapy relies on the use of intramuscular injections of local anesthetic to reduce focal areas of muscle pain and hypertonicity. Similar techniques have been applied in horses with mixed results, which are mostly related to the inability to adequately define and measure muscle pain and dysfunction.

Interspinous spaces

Injections of local anesthetics into narrowed interspinous spaces or areas of interspinous pseudoarthrosis can be used diagnostically and therapeutically to assess the influence of over-riding or impinged spinous processes on back pain. The clinical significance of impinged spinous processes is often difficult to assert based solely on radiographic findings, since impinged spinous processes are often diagnosed in horses without obvious back pain. Firm digital palpation of affected dorsal spinous processes often produces a localized painful response (e.g. cutaneous trunci reflex or active extension of the back). Confirmation of the clinical significance of potential impinged spinous processes can be achieved with injections of local anesthetics. At sites of severe impingement or proliferation, it is often impossible to pass a needle directly on midline into the interspinous space. In this instance, a paramedian approach to the interspinous space provides lateral access to the area of pathology, which reduces the need to advance a needle through a collapsed interspinous space, although bilateral injections of the affected interspinous spaces are required. Nuclear scintigraphy is also an important adjunct in the definitive diagnosis and localization of impinged spinous processes as a contributing cause to back pain. Therapeutically, interspinous injections with anti-inflammatories (i.e. corticosteroids) provide variable effectiveness and durations of pain relief and normal spinal function.

Articular processes

Articular process osteoarthritis is a common pathology and an important contributor to back pain. Like articular limb lameness, intra- or periarticular injections of the articular processes can assist in the localization and treatment of the presumed back pain. Periarticular injections of articular processes in the thoracolumbar spine can be used both diagnostically and therapeutically. Ultrasound guidance is recommended due to the deep location and close proximity to the spinal neurovascular structures that exit the intervertebral foramen.[33] Intra-articular injections of the articular processes are difficult due to the small articulation and sparse joint capsule; therefore periarticular injections are often performed. A 15 cm spinal needle can be used with ultrasound guidance to assess the articular process joint capsule in most horses.

Sacroiliac joint

The ante-mortem diagnosis of sacroiliac osteoarthritis is often frustrating and based on exclusion of other possible causes of hindlimb lameness.[31,57] In humans, periarticular injections of the sacroiliac joint are easy to perform, safe and seemingly effective in controlling pain associated with sacroiliac joint osteoarthritis.[58–60] The deep overlying croup musculature and seemingly inaccessible anatomic location of the sacroiliac joint has limited the clinical application of Intra-articular or periarticular sacroiliac joint injections in horses.[31,57,61] Injection of the general sacroiliac region for diagnostic and therapeutic purposes has been performed, but inappropriate needle placement or the use of too short needles explain why most techniques have had suboptimal diagnostic or therapeutic effects.[40,62,63]

A medial approach to the sacroiliac joint provides the most direct, safe and consistent periarticular injection technique (Fig. 21.10).[64] Periarticular injections are made as close as possible to the caudomedial sacroiliac joint margin due to the high prevalence of degenerative changes affecting the caudomedial sacroiliac joint margin.[54,65] Important neurovascular structures to be avoided include the sciatic nerve and the cranial gluteal nerve, artery and vein that pass through the greater sciatic foramen, directly caudal to the sacroiliac joint.[66] Osseous topographic landmarks used to identify the needle entry site and the direction of needle advancement include the contralateral tuber sacrale and the ipsilateral tuber coxae and greater trochanter of the femur. The midpoint of the distance from the cranial aspect of the tuber coxae and the cranial aspect of the greater trochanter is used as a target for needle advancement. The needle entry site is 2 cm cranial to the contralateral tuber sacrale. The needle entry site and the midpoint of the tuber coxae and greater trochanter are connected with white tape to indicate the direction of needle advancement. A 25 cm, 15 gauge spinal needle is bent slightly in the direction of the bevel of the needle to match the medial curvature of the iliac wing. The needle is inserted with the bevel facing toward the targeted sacroiliac joint and advanced along the medial aspect of the iliac wing until it firmly engages the dorsal surface of the sacral wing, near the medial border of the sacroiliac joint. Poor performance or vague proximal hind limb lameness associated with sacroiliac osteoarthritis can be diagnosed and treated with this reliable and easy-to-use injection technique.[64]

Diagnostic imaging

Radiographic examination

For diagnosing lower limb lameness, radiographs are usually the first imaging modality used. However, due to difficulties associated with radiographing the equine back, other diagnostic imaging modalities may be used initially to localize the presumed inciting cause of back pain or dysfunction.

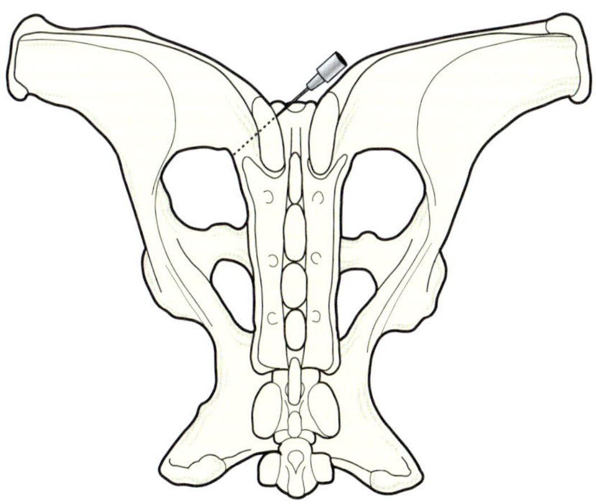

Fig 21.10 Diagram of a medial approach to the sacroiliac joint for diagnostic or therapeutic purposes (dorsal view). The needle is directed from the cranial aspect of the contralateral tuber sacrale toward the caudomedial aspect of the affected sacroiliac joint.

Standing position

It is possible to take good-quality lateral views of the thoracic (T1–T18) and cranial lumbar spine (L1–L4) in the standing position.[67] Using portable equipment, the dorsal apexes of the spinous processes for T2–L3 can usually be visualized. Powerful equipment is necessary for radiographic examination of the horse's vertebral column, because exposures of up to 150 kV and 500 mA may be required in large horses.[68] Exposure values will vary according to the system employed, but a few suggested radiographic techniques are given in Table 21.4.[69]

One of the major problems encountered in radiography of such a thick subject is the inevitable production of secondary radiation. However, there are a number of ways to minimize scatter. The tube can be mounted on an overhead gantry system and linked to a cassette holder on the far side of the horse. The primary beam can then be automatically directed to the center of the cassette and the beam size can be carefully collimated to the size of the film. This system makes it possible to use high-ratio and crosshatch grids with confidence to effectively reduce scatter. The fastest possible system of intensifying screens and film (e.g. rare earth screens) should be employed so that exposures can be kept to a minimum. Most radiographic film cassettes contain lead in the backing, but at exposures over 100 kVp, it is advisable to place an additional lead sheet behind the cassette to absorb backscatter. As the scatter is oriented perpendicular to the ground with a film-focus distance of 150 cm, an air gap exists between the spine and the cassette and this helps to reduce the amount of scatter reaching the film. There is a considerable difference in tissue attenuation between the tips of the spinous processes and the vertebral bodies; thus, at least two radiographs of the same region at different exposures must be taken or some form of beam filtration is necessary. Considerable improvement in radiographic quality can be obtained by filtering (dodging) part of the primary beam to help compensate for the marked variation in thickness of the horse's spine.[68]

The horse should be sedated prior to radiography to reduce the degree of movement and to allow the handler to stand well out of range of the beam. Stocks are also useful to prevent movement. Lead markers placed midline on the horse's back are useful for orientation on the radiographs. The horse must be standing completely square, as the spine rotates to some extent if one leg is non-weight bearing. For the dorsal apexes of the spinous processes, the beam should be centered 5 cm ventral to the dorsal skin surface; for the region of the vertebral bodies, it should be centered 15–20 cm below the dorsum depending on the size of the horse. The beam should normally be horizontal but for visualization of the dorsal articular facets in the cranial lumbar region, it is useful to angle the beam from a ventral to dorsal orientation at an angle of 20–30° to avoid superimposition by the transverse processes. As a grid is being used, the cassette must be tilted accurately at the same angle of 20–30°.[69]

Table 21.4 Suggested radiographic techniques for imaging the thoracolumbar spine

VERTEBRAL STRUCTURES OR REGION (PEAK)	KILOVOLT	MILLIAMPS	GRID
Spinous processes			
Withers (T3–T8)	75	30	No
Midthoracic (T9–T15)	70	55	Yes
Thoracolumbar (T16-L4)	85	80	Yes
Articular processes			
Midthoracic (T9–T15)	100 +	200–300	Yes
Vertebral bodies			
Thoracic (T5–T18)	75	55	Yes
Lumbar (L1–L5)	100 +	200–300	Yes

Under general anesthesia

It is not possible to take radiographs of diagnostic quality of the caudal lumbar (L3–L6) and sacroiliac regions in a standing horse. The horse must be anesthetized and placed on its back in the frog-legged position so that the cassette can be inserted beneath the pelvis for a ventrodorsal view. Even in very large horses (i.e. weighing over 700 kg), exposures above 150 kV are not required, although up to 500 mA have been used on some occasions. To limit scattered radiation, it is necessary to use crossed, high-ratio grids and to put additional lead on the back of the cassette to prevent backscatter.

Normal radiographic anatomy

The thoracolumbar spine of the newborn foal has a more pronounced curvature (i.e. dorsally convex) in the midthoracic region than does the adult horse.[69,70] The dorsal spinous processes appear short in relation to the length of the vertebral bodies, and in the midthoracic region they are blunt ended or spatula shaped, with wide interspinous spaces. The vertebral bodies have well-defined cranial and caudal epiphyses, but all the other ossification centers in the vertebral bodies and neural arch have fused before birth. During the first few months of life the thoracolumbar spine straightens out to some extent. In the mid and caudal region there is some alteration in shape of summits as well as a general lengthening and reduction in size of the interspinous spaces. At about 12 months of age, calcification of separate ossification centers on the summits of the cranial spinous processes occurs, and these persist without fusion into old age (i.e. 15 years or older). The tallest point of the vertebral column is at the withers, usually T4–T6. Areas of periosteal irregularity are frequently seen in the midportion of the thoracic spine, but these are of no clinical significance. The spines beneath the saddle region, T11–T17, are considerably shorter and more upright; the anticlinal vertebra is usually T15. Caudal to this, the spinous processes are increasingly slanted forward and the interspinous spaces are considerably narrowed. The summits are variable in shape, but they have cranially directed, often beak-shaped tips.

In the adult the thoracolumbar spine lies horizontal when the horse stands squarely on a level surface. The ventral portions of the vertebral bodies are clearly visible radiographically as far back as T16, because they form the roof of the thoracic cavity. It is difficult to see the articulations of the ribs and the articular and transverse processes unless oblique views are taken. Behind the diaphragm, the lumbar vertebrae as far back as L3 can be defined, as well as the articular and transverse processes. Closure of the vertebral epiphyses occurs at 3–3.5 years of age. In the region of the midback the width of the interspinous spaces varies and some impingement or Overriding of the spinous summits may occur. This is more often seen in Thoroughbreds than in other breeds and seems to be related to the conformation of the back; it is more common in stocky, short-coupled horses. The reduction or obliteration of the interspinous spaces, chiefly in the region from T13 to T18, is associated with local periosteal reaction and focal areas of radiolucency. The spinous summits sometimes overlap one another and become misshapen presumably because of the continued pressure from the adjacent spines. In one survey of clinically normal horses, 34% showed some degree of spinous process impingement.[70] There are few variations noted in the normal radiographic anatomy apart from the changes associated with impingement or over-riding dorsal spinous processes in the midback region. Other osseous findings (e.g. abnormal spinal curvature, osteoarthritis, vertebral fracture or spondylosis) are incidental or are rarely encountered.[103]

Primary indications for radiography of the pelvis include acute or severe pelvic asymmetries, upper hindlimb lameness and pelvic crepitus or fractures.[71] Ilial wing overlap and the deep anatomic location of the sacroiliac joint make radiographic imaging difficult at best. The radiographic features of chronic sacroiliac joint disease are minimal and include non-specific increases in the joint space and apparent enlargement of the caudomedial aspect of the sacroiliac joint.[31] Linear tomography has also been used to examine the lumbosacral and sacroiliac regions of horses, but limited access to equipment has restricted its clinical usefulness.[72] Positive findings include widening of the sacroiliac joint and irregular joint outlines with osteophyte formation at the caudal aspect of the joint. Osseous changes are common bilaterally, but may be more pronounced on the clinically affected side.[72]

Scintigraphic examination

A useful adjunct to clinical diagnosis in recent years has been the advent of nuclear scintigraphy for horses.[73–76] The technique involves intravenous injection of a radionuclide and detection of 'hotspots' of increased radioactivity in the bone phase by use of a gamma camera. Scintigraphy is helpful in detecting over-riding or impinged spinous processes, vertebrae fractures, osteoarthritis, spondylosis, stress fractures of the wing of ilium and some sacroiliac osteoarthritis. Scintigraphy is particularly valuable in identifying bony lesions at sites not accessible with conventional radiography.

The radiopharmaceutical most commonly used for equine scintigraphy is 99 m technetium-labeled methylene diphosphonate (^{99m}Tc-MDP). A weight-dependent dose between 3 and 6 GBq (100–150 mCi) of ^{99m}Tc-MDP is injected intravenously and images of the bone phase are obtained 2–3 hours later. Due to the initial high renal and bladder radioactivity, vascular phase and soft tissue phase images of the thoracolumbar spine cannot be obtained. Damaged skeletal muscle can be detected by abnormal soft tissue uptake of ^{99m}Tc-MDP during bone-phase imaging, but usually only if the horse has been strenuously exercised before the scintigraphic examination.[77]

For a complete examination, the horse should be imaged from both the left and the right; otherwise some subtle lesions, for example those located at the articular processes, can easily be missed. A high-resolution, low-energy, parallelhole collimator should be used; this gives a geometrical resolution of 4.4 mm at a distance of 5 cm from the collimator face. For the caudal thoracic and lumbar regions, the camera is positioned obliquely at an angle of 50–65° to the horizontal. This allows the distance between the camera and spine to be minimized. Positioning the camera horizontally above the spine results in superimposition of all the vertebral structures. The camera can be oriented perpendicular to the floor for views of the cranial thoracic spine. When the camera is positioned over the lumbar spine, the image quality may be improved by shielding the kidney using a lead sheet.

The images are acquired on the basis of either counts or time. One million counts or more are optimal for maximal resolution of the caudal regions of the equine back and the pelvis. This large number of counts requires several minutes of immobility on the part of the horse, however, and thus generally cannot be achieved without general anesthesia. Movement of the standing horse can be minimized by appropriate sedation and quiet handling of both the horse and camera. Blinders and cotton earplugs for the horse may help. Nuclear medicine software that is able to correct for motion is now available and this compensates for the slight swaying of the horse and respiratory movements.

Normal scintigraphy findings

In normal horses, regions of bone close to the skin surface such as the tuber sacrale and tuber coxae appear 'hotter' (i.e. increased radiopharmaceutical uptake) than adjacent bone structures, as there is less soft tissue attenuation. Other superficial sites that appear slightly 'hot' are the apices of the spinous processes, particularly at the withers. In good-quality images, the individual vertebra can be clearly distinguished. The spinous processes and articulations have a slightly higher uptake, but this should be equal for all joints in the region. On lateral oblique views, each rib is located cranial to its respective vertebra. As an aid to orientation, on left lateral views the 16th rib usually overlies the cranial pole of the right kidney.

Any scintigraphic abnormality appears as increased radiopharmaceutical uptake (a 'hotspot'), whereas areas of diminished uptake are difficult to detect due to poor image resolution. The most common sites for increased uptake are at the apices of the spinous processes, the articular processes or the sacroiliac region.

Nuclear scintigraphy is considered by some authors to be an accurate and diagnostically useful technique for identifying acute and chronic sacroiliac joint injuries.[55] Subjective evaluation or quantitative analysis of bone scans are typically able to identify asymmetric radioisotope uptake over the affected tuber sacrale. However, presumed normal horses, without a history of hindlimb or sacroiliac joint injuries, may also have asymmetric uptake over the tuber sacrale. A dorsal view of the sacrum is considered the most diagnostic image for evaluating and comparing the sacroiliac joints.[55] However, there is usually extensive overlap of uptake in the tuber sacrale and the sacroiliac joints on the dorsal view. Oblique views of the ilial wings are recommended to confirm left-to-right asymmetries in radioisotope uptake and to separate the tuber sacrale dorsally from the sacroiliac joint region ventrally,[78] although oblique views may be difficult to interpret due to inconsistent camera positioning on the left and right sides. The thick overlying gluteal musculature may also attenuate radiopharmaceutical uptake from an affected sacroiliac joint. Stress fractures of the ilial wing may be difficult to differentiate from sacroiliac joint injuries due to the common location and extension of the incomplete fracture line into the sacroiliac joint.[55,79,80]

Ultrasonographic examination

There has been considerable interest in recent years concerning the value of ultrasonography for evaluation of the epaxial structures, particularly the supraspinous and dorsal sacroiliac ligaments.[33,81]

Supraspinous ligament

A 7.5 or 10 mHz linear array transducer is used to examine the supraspinous ligament that runs dorsal to the thoracic and lumbar spinous processes. It is necessary to clip the hair over an area of approximately 20 cm in width extending from the withers to the base of the tail. The ligament has an echogenic, striated appearance similar to tendon. It is thinner and wider in the caudal withers region and becomes narrower and thicker in the lumbar region. It is always thinner as it runs over the spinous processes. The dorsal convex surface of the spinous processes can be clearly seen and impinged or over-riding spinous processes can be identified by visualizing narrowed interspinous spaces. There may also be evidence of false joint formation between impinging spines. The echogenicity of the ligament may vary somewhat and a more clearly defined fibrous pattern seen in the caudal thoracic and lumbar regions. In the withers (T6–T9) it is sometimes possible to see hyperechogenicity that may cast acoustic shadows. These are associated with the secondary centers of ossification on the dorsal tips of the spinous processes. A little caudal to this (T9–T12) it is possible to see hypoechoic areas that may be associated with cartilage metaplasia adjacent to the ligament insertion into the dorsal spinous process. This does not usually have any clinical significance. A high prevalence of ultrasonographic lesions have been reported in ridden, unridden and back pain horses with an increased incidence of lesions localized to the T14-T17 vertebral region.[35] Every horse within this study had at least one site (range 2 to 11) of supraspinous desmitis; however, no significant difference was found between the three groups in the number or location of abnormal images. Therefore, the presence of supraspinous desmitis on ultrasonography cannot always be considered a clinically relevant cause of back pain.

Dorsal sacroiliac ligament

The dorsal portion of the dorsal sacroiliac ligament can be visualized with a 7.5–10 mHz linear array transducer as it runs from the tuber sacrale to the summits of the sacral spinous processes.[82] The sacroiliac region is first viewed on midline in transverse section. The tuber sacrale are seen as hyperechoic convex lines on either side of the sacral spinous processes. The transducer is then moved laterally over the tuber sacrale so that the dorsal portion of the dorsal sacroiliac ligament appears as a crescent-shaped echogenic structure. Longitudinal views of the dorsal sacroiliac ligament are then examined. The ligaments are examined for alterations in echogenicity and fiber orientation, but particularly for any increase in size.

Additional pelvic and vertebral structures

It is possible to examine the dorsal surface of the iliac wing and caudal margin of the sacroiliac articulation to identify dorsal cortex irregularities associated with incomplete and complete ilial wing fractures.[83,84] Denoix has elegantly demonstrated the visualization of the thoracolumbar articular processes, transverse processes, lumbosacral and caudal lumbar intervertebral disk spaces and the sacroiliac joint.[33] The ventral sacroiliac ligament and the ventral joint margins of the sacroiliac joint can also be visualized on transrectal ultrasonography.[81] Ventral periarticular remodeling of the sacroiliac joint has been observed with transrectal ultrasound approaches. Muscle injuries are more difficult to detect ultrasonographically, although in severe cases of muscle strain an increased echogenicity with thickening of the connective tissue septae within the muscle may be identified.

Thermographic examination

Thermography has been used successfully as an aid to diagnose back problems. However, it is important to have the right equipment and to establish normal thermal profile parameters. Even so interpretation of infrared thermography imaging can be difficult. A single thermal study has little or no prognostic value. Von Schweinitz concludes:

> *Thermal imaging reveals important information about the neural outflow of the spine in terms of sympathetic tone. The thermal findings are a compilation of local tissue factors and vasomotor tone requiring care in interpretation. The relevance of disturbed vasomotor tone, especially persistent vasoconstriction, is well established in chronic back pain syndromes in man. Many of these syndromes involve disturbing sensory faults (e.g. allodynia, burning, aching) which can neither be directly communicated by our patients nor readily described by any other current diagnostic test.*[85]

Thermography provides quick, safe and non-invasive assessment of the whole patient. It takes into account a major aspect of homeostasis and prompts one to investigate all other thermally abnormal sites. With current diagnostic technologies, it often provides the only objective evidence confirming cases of equine back disease. Routine use of thermal imaging in equine poor performance syndromes confirms that thoracolumbar and sacral neuromuscular disease is a common condition.[85] Thermography has been used to diagnose muscle strain or inflammation in the sacroiliac and croup regions.[86] Horses with sacroiliac joint injuries are expected to have protective muscle spasms in the adjacent musculature. Palpation of muscle sensitivity has been correlated with abnormal thermographic images in most cases.[86]

Magnetic resonance imaging (MRI) and computed tomography (CT)

These are emerging modalities that have not yet been applied to the problems involving the thoracolumbar spine. However, the detail and quality of both skeletal and soft tissue structures elsewhere in the horse's body mean that once the technological difficulties have been overcome there is great potential for improved diagnostic ability for the thoracolumbar and lumbosacral spine.

Specific pathologic conditions

Clinical signs associated with spinal muscle pathology include atrophy, focal swelling and palpable tenderness of the epaxial muscles. Spinal muscle biopsies help to evaluate suspected back disorders, but are best used with a complete physical examination and imaging procedures. Spinal ligament injuries affect the supraspinous and sacroiliac ligaments. Osseous pathology has been observed at the vertebral processes, intervertebral articulations and sacroiliac joints in horses. Degenerative changes are common in many articular processes, intertransverse, lumbosacral and sacroiliac articulations. Osseous spinal lesions tend to affect multiple vertebral locations.

Vertebral anomalies and deformities

Developmental variations in the morphology of thoracolumbar vertebral bodies, processes and joints in horses are known to occur, but usually result in secondary rather than primary back problems.[14–16,26,53] Congenital abnormalities that affect the normal spinal curvature include scoliosis, lordosis and kyphosis. In newly born foals signs of scoliosis and lordosis are sometimes seen in association with other in utero postural deformities (e.g. limb contractures, bent face and torticollis). These may be severe and necessitate euthanasia or be mild when they show an apparent complete recovery. The condition of kyphosis (i.e. roach-back) is most frequently seen during the period of active growth after weaning although the underlying cause does not appear to be in the vertebral column. The problem may be associated with a progressive straightening of the hind limb conformation during a growth spurt or perhaps be secondary to a stifle or hock problem (e.g. osteochondrosis). The condition of congenital lordosis (i.e. dipped or sway-back) has been associated with hypoplasia of the cranial and caudal intervertebral articular processes in the cranial thoracic region T5–T10.[87] There is overextension of one or more of these articulations leading to the ventral curvature of the midthoracic spine. In older horses acquired lordosis is sometimes seen, particularly in brood mares after a number of pregnancies, but usually no clinical problems are associated with it.

All these vertebral deformities predispose to some weakness of the thoracolumbar spine, leading to poor performance and soft tissue injuries. Diagnosis can be confirmed by radiography revealing abnormal curvature of the vertebral column, principally in the cranial thoracic region (T5–T10) with lordosis, mid- to caudal thoracic region with scoliosis and the cranial lumbar region (L1–L5) with kyphosis.

Soft tissues injuries

Muscle strain

Damage to the epaxial tissues is undoubtedly the most common cause of back injury in the horse.[4] The main action of the longissimus muscle is to extend the back (i.e. to dorsiflex) or, if acting singly, to laterally bend the spine. The primary role of these muscles is to control the stiffness of the back rather than to actively assist locomotor movements. Strain or injury to all or part of the longissimus muscles most frequently occurs during ridden exercise because of a slip, fall or poorly executed jump. It may be caused through fatigue or inadequate fitness. The clinical signs are an acute onset of poor performance often accompanied by a change of temperament. Local swelling and heat of the muscles may occur, particularly in the lumbar region. The back is kept rigid and there is a restriction in the hindlimb gait at exercise, often with a wider than normal hindlimb stance. There may be difficulty in maintaining normal tracking action of the hindlimbs. Disunited canter and frequent breaking of stride are also frequently seen. Stiffness of the hindlimb and back is seen particularly in short turns, but no clear signs of lameness are evident. There is obvious pain on palpation and a marked reduction in flexibility of the thoracolumbar spine. In the acute stages some elevation (i.e. 2–4 times baseline levels) in the plasma levels of muscle-derived enzymes (CK and AST) will be noted after mild exercise. If the sublumbar muscles are involved, pain will be easily elicited on rectal palpation.

Classic signs of exertional myopathy (i.e. rhabdomyolysis) are not difficult to differentiate from muscle strain of the back. However, the atypical low-grade form of exertional myopathy is more difficult to diagnose as it can occur after varying amounts of exercise, but is more commonly seen in horses on a high-protein diet and in highly strung fillies or mares in excellent bodily condition. Diagnosis can usually be confirmed by determination of muscle-derived enzymes after exercise. In exertional myopathy, levels will be increased greater than five times over baseline values.

Polysaccharide storage myopathy (PSSM) has been recently diagnosed from longissimus muscle biopsies in showjumpers, dressage and draft horses.[46] The horses showed typical signs of a soft tissue back injury and biopsies from the longissimus lumborum muscles revealed high glycogen levels with abnormal deposits of amylase-resistant polysaccharide. This study indicates that muscle biopsy may be an important diagnostic aid in some chronic back problem cases.

Ligamentous damage

Clinical conditions affecting the spinal ligaments include mild, moderate or severe sprains. Severe injuries are characterized by complete ligamentous disruption and joint laxity (i.e. joint luxation). A fairly common site of thoracolumbar injury in Thoroughbred gallopers and jumpers is the supraspinous ligament which runs all the way down the middle of the back and is adherent to the summits of the thoracic and lumbar dorsal spinous processes. It is made up of a continuous ligament to which the multiple tendon insertions of the longissimus muscles contribute. The composite structure is subject to strain in the same way as the muscle injuries just described. The clinical signs are essentially similar, but tend to persist for longer and the ultimate prognosis is less favorable. The cranial lumbar region is the most common site of injury. The ligament is often visibly thickened above the spinous summits and pain is easily elicited on palpation. Reduced lateral bending of the thoracolumbar spine is seen in one or both directions. By taking low-exposure radiographs, the soft tissue thickening and some focal radiodensity in the ligament may be seen in long-standing cases. Detached flakes from the spinous summits are also noted on occasion and are associated with periosteal irregularity and sclerosis on the dorsal surfaces of the spinous summits. This may also be seen in the caudal withers' regions, but care must be taken not to confuse elevated periosteum with a vestigial center of ossification on the dorsal tips of the T3–T12 spines. Diagnosis can be assisted by ultrasonographic examination.[33,34] The prognosis for supraspinous ligament strain is usually guarded, largely because of the likelihood of recurrence. Some horses do recover but go on to develop signs of a 'cold back', which is defined as temporary stiffness and a dipped back, without affecting their competitive performance.

Other soft tissue lesions

These include such disorders as skin lesions (e.g. wounds, scars, warbles, pruritic conditions), which may cause secondary signs of back pain. Pressure or chaffing from an ill-fitting saddle, particularly in endurance competitions, may also be observed.

Thoracolumbar osseous pathology

Spinal disorders and sacroiliac joint injuries have been identified as significant causes of chronic poor performance in horses.[4,31,88] In humans, the most common known sources of back pain are related to the intervertebral disks, zygapophyseal joints and sacroiliac articulations.[89] Intervertebral disk disease is uncommon in horses, but significant and widespread degenerative changes of the thoracolumbar zygapophyseal joints and sacroiliac articulations have been reported, even in active racehorses.[54]

Articular pathophysiology

The zygapophyseal joints are synovial articulations that undergo joint capsule pathology and joint degeneration similar to other synovial joints. Articular degeneration usually progresses through three phases of pathology: dysfunction, instability and degeneration. Joint dysfunction is characterized by restricted joint motion, localized pain and inflammation, and abnormal paraspinal muscle hypertonicity. Restricted articular motion stimulates local biochemical alterations and the release of inflammatory products. The inflammatory process can alter the Intra-articular environment and further contribute to joint capsule pathology and periarticular fibrosis. Muscle hypertonicity may restrict joint motion and contribute to adhesion formation. Joint immobilization also produces bone demineralization, capsular adhesions and loss of ligamentous strength. Restoring joint motion can lead to normal joint function, depending on the amount and duration of the immobilization.

Joint motion is essential for the prevention of joint contracture and adhesion formation. Progressive joint immobilization is characterized by initial musculotendinous contractures, followed by capsular and periarticular adhesions and eventual intra-articular adhesions.

Joint degeneration progresses as the dysfunctional joint is unable to distribute normal biomechanical stresses. The instability phase of joint degeneration is characterized by cartilaginous, meniscal, capsular and ligamentous deformation and degeneration. Abnormal joint and paraspinal tissue biomechanics induce additional subchondral bone changes and joint derangement. Reduced or asymmetric motion in one vertebral motion segment may induce compensatory hypermobility in adjacent vertebral segments due to injuries to the joint capsule or ligamentous laxity. The increased joint mobility results in joint instability, joint derangement and secondary muscle hypertonicity. Joint instability also affects the neurologic influences of proprioception and the central neuromotor control of movement and posture. Potential radiographic findings of articular instability may include osteophyte formation or vertebral instability (i.e. listhesis). The spinal degenerative phase is characterized by attempts at stabilization of the degenerative tissues. Chronic joint immobilization can lead to fibrocartilaginous replacement of the joint cavity and eventual ankylosis. Radiographic signs of advanced osteoarthritis and osteophyte formation, spinal ligament ossification and spinal ankylosis can be visualized at this stage.

Articular process degenerative joint disease

As with any synovial articulation, loss of motion or aberrant joint physiology can be a primary source of pain.[21] Jeffcott states that degenerative joint disease of the articular processes (i.e. zygapophyseal joints) is common in older horses, but probably not clinically significant.[90] However, Denoix reports that zygapophyseal joint pathology at the thoracolumbar junction and lumbar vertebral region is one of the most common spinal disorders associated with back pain.[91] In a necropsy survey of 36 Thoroughbred racehorses, severe articular process degenerative changes were reported in 25% of specimens (Fig. 21.11).[54] Articular surface lipping, osteophytes, periarticular erosions, Intra-articular erosions and ankylosis (in order of increasing severity) were noted. Articular surface lipping and periarticular erosions of the articular processes were common at the thoracolumbar junction and cranial lumbar spine. Intra-articular erosions and ankylosis were restricted to the caudal lumbar vertebral segments, where vertebral mobility is normally limited.[92] Additional studies may help to show that the zygapophyseal joints are a clinically significant source of back pain in horses, as has been shown in humans.[89]

Impinged or over-riding spinous process

Spinous process overlap, without any evidence of osseous impingement, has been noted in horses.[54] In humans, isolated spinous

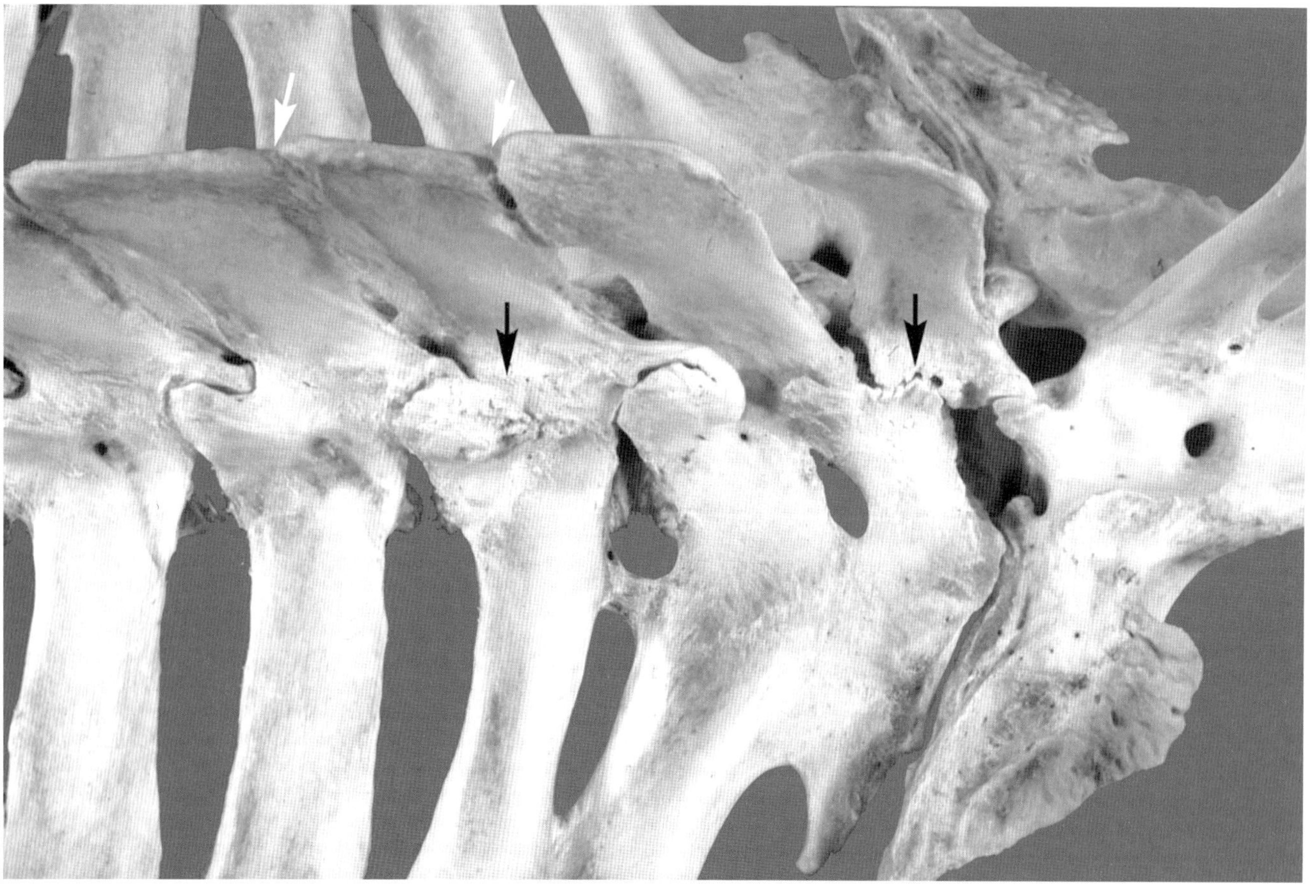

Fig 21.11 Dorsolateral view of the lumbosacral vertebral region (L2–S2) of a four-year-old racing Thoroughbred that fractured the right front sesamoids during a race. Varying degrees of spinous process impingement (white arrows), vertebral lamina stress fractures (black arrows), articular process ankylosis (L4–L6) and bilateral intertransverse joint ankylosis (L5–L6) are present.

process deviation is a common finding and can be related to vertebral rotation (i.e. scoliosis) or developmental asymmetries in the neural arch, but rarely is it associated with spinous process fracture or malposition of the entire vertebra.[93] Impinged or over-riding spinous processes (i.e. kissing spines) are reported to be the most common osseous cause of back pain in horses.[4]

Spinous process impingement in the thoracic spine occurs most commonly between T13 and T18, reportedly related to altered spinous process morphology.[53,94] Thoroughbreds have a higher prevalence of spinous process impingement or overriding compared with other breeds due to misshapen dorsal apices and narrower interspinous spaces.[4,53] Competitive jumping or dressage horses reportedly have a higher prevalence of thoracolumbar spinous process impingement related to ventroflexion or demanding spinal maneuvers.[4] However, dorsoventral vertebral mobility in the caudal thoracic spine has not been reported to differ from other adjacent vertebral regions, therefore increased dorsoventral movement may not fully account for the vertebral distribution of spinous process impingement.[92,94] Additional weight-carrying requirements have also been implicated because this vertebral region is covered by the saddle while being ridden,[37] although thoracolumbar spinous process impingement has been reported in Standardbreds and an extinct equine species, *Equus occidentalis*, which presumably have not had extraneous weight placed on their backs.[95] Aging has not been found to be a factor in the pathogenesis of thoracolumbar spinous process impingement.[4,53,94]

The diagnosis of impinged or over-riding spinous processes is difficult since apparently normal horses often have a high prevalence of osseous changes radiographically.

Vertebral lamina stress fractures

Stress fractures are usually characterized by bone-specific predilection sites, periosteal and endosteal callus, an incomplete fracture line that may progress to complete fracture, tendency to occur bilaterally, a predominance in athletes undergoing strenuous or repetitive activities, and a patient history of periodic, recurrent, low-grade lameness.[80,83,96] In a necropsy sample of Thoroughbred racehorses, 50% (18 of 36) of specimens had incomplete fractures and focal periosteal proliferation of the vertebral lamina, characterized as vertebral stress fractures (see Fig. 21.11).[79] Incomplete fractures of the vertebral lamina occurred consistently at the cranial aspect near the junction of a cranial articular process and the spinous process. Most vertebral stress fractures were continuous with vertical articular clefts of the cranial articular processes, which may provide a site for stress concentration and may contribute to the etiopathogenesis of equine vertebral stress fractures.[97] Thoracolumbar articular process morphology may also contribute to the development of vertebral lamina stress fractures. The articular processes of the caudal thoracic and lumbar portions of the spine (T16–L6) are deeply interlocking and restrict axial rotation.[16,94] Complete articular process fractures in this vertebral region are thought to result from excessive axial rotation.[94] Most specimens had one vertebra affected unilaterally, but several specimens had multiple vertebral lamina stress fractures and some were bilateral. Bilateral complete fractures of the vertebral lamina were noted in one specimen, so that the dorsal L6 vertebral arch and spinous process could be removed.

Spondylosis

Spondylosis is a degenerative disease of the vertebral joints that produces large osteophytes that bridge the ventral vertebral bodies. The exact cause of vertebral body osteophytes is unknown, but biomechanical and biochemical mechanisms have been proposed.[98] Abnormal joint loading produces microtrauma and degeneration of the annulus fibrosis and periarticular tissues. Portions of the annulus fibrosis and ventral longitudinal ligaments become ossified and produce partial bridging of the involved joints. As the osteophytes increase in size, nerve roots may be compressed at the intervertebral foramen or spinal cord compression occurs if the proliferation extends dorsally into the vertebral canal. The cycle of altered joint biomechanics and inflammatory mediators may continue until complete ankylosis and obliteration of the joint occurs. The forming vertebral osteophytes and the ankylosed vertebral bodies are susceptible to fracture due to the reduced ability to absorb or transfer normal locomotor forces through the ossified ligaments and fused vertebral joints. Several vertebral bodies are usually involved, especially in advanced stages.

Vertebral fractures

Spinous process fractures of the withers (T2–T9) are usually due to falling over backwards and landing on the highest point of the back. Conservative care is usually recommended. Proper saddle fit is difficult following fracture due to lateral displacement of the multiple fracture fragments. Spinous process fractures do not typically cause spinal cord compromise.[99]

Vertebral end-plate fractures occur more commonly in foals and are usually related to a fall or significant trauma. Vertebral body compression fractures have been reported in the thoracolumbar vertebral region (T1–T3, T9–T16 and T18–L6) and are frequently due to physical trauma, electric shock or lightning strike.[99–102] Depending on the severity of the vertebral fracture, minimal fracture displacement is usually found. A complete neurologic examination will help to localize the fracture site if spinal cord compromise is present.[103,104] Isolated hind limb paresis or paralysis with normal forelimb function suggests a spinal cord lesion caudal to T2.

Sacral fractures are a common cause of cauda equina injury. Horses that forcefully back into a solid object or fall backwards can fracture the sacrocaudal vertebral region and produce abnormal perineal neurologic signs. Careful palpation may help to localize a site of pain or vertebral asymmetry.

Neurologic diseases

Conditions that are primarily neurologic in origin must always be considered in differential diagnosis of a back problem. However, there are few disorders that can be specifically related to the thoracolumbar vertebral column.

Ataxia

The most common group of conditions are those that cause ataxia and proprioceptive deficits. These conditions include cervical vertebral stenosis (CVS or wobbler disease), equine protozoal myeloencephalitis (EPM), equine degenerative myeloencephalopathy (EDM) and equine herpesvirus 1 vasculitis (EHV-1). Some of the signs in these conditions will be similar to back problems mainly because of ataxia or incoordination resulting in stiffness or splinting of the back muscles. The hind action with varying degrees of proprioceptive deficit will cause stiffness (hypomelia), weakness and toe dragging. Horses with EPM may also exhibit some lameness and neurogenic atrophy of skeletal muscles. Other causes of ataxia that are usually seasonal are associated with ingestion of certain types of grass (e.g. rye grass, Bermuda and Dallis grass). For more information see Chapter 24.

Lower motor neuron diseases

The condition of stringhalt can produce severe and bizarre signs affecting the hindlimbs.[105] However, in milder cases stiffness and exaggerated action of one or both hind limbs may be seen. The specific etiology of this condition is not known, but morphologically it appears to be distal axonopathy.[106] Another long-established but little understood condition is that of 'shivering'. It is assumed to be of neurologic origin, but its etiology is completely unknown. The clinical signs involve muscle fasciculations of the back and hindquarters, particularly if a hindlimb is picked up and fully flexed. The condition rarely affects performance and does not appear to be the cause of a genuine back problem. 'Shivers' may also be confused with polysaccharide storage myopathy (see Chapter 6).

Other neurologic diseases

Lyme disease (borreliosis) may need to be considered in some locations where various species of ticks are present. The infective agent is a spirochete, *Borrelia burgdorferi,* which may cause neurologic signs of lethargy or aggression due to low-grade meningitis. Musculoskeletal pain is usually due to polyarthritis or intermittent lameness. Serological confirmation (i.e. IFA, ELISA and Western blot) is possible and response to treatment with amoxicillin or tetracycline for two weeks may support a diagnosis of Lyme disease.

Sacropelvic pathology

The ante-mortem diagnosis of sacroiliac joint injury in horses is difficult and often based on a diagnosis of exclusion.[55] Based on a review of the literature, osteoarthritis of the sacroiliac joint is the most prevalent disease process affecting horses with sacroiliac joint pain or dysfunction, although its clinical significance remains uncertain.[31,54,65,107] Degenerative changes tend to be bilaterally symmetric and localized to the medial aspect of the sacroiliac joint (Fig. 21.12).

Sacroiliac ligament desmitis has been documented ultrasonographically in the dorsal portion of the dorsal sacroiliac ligament.[34,81,82] A diagnosis of sacroiliac ligament desmitis is based on loss of normal echogenicity on a short-axis view and a decrease in parallel fiber pattern on the long-axis view. Complete sacroiliac ligament disruption is most likely due to substantial trauma, such as flipping over backwards or catastrophic musculoskeletal injuries associated with race training.[54] However, few cases of complete rupture of the sacroiliac ligaments have been reported in the veterinary literature.[54,108]

The pathogenesis of apparent spontaneous or insidious differences in tuber sacrale height needs to be further researched.[31] The presumed diagnosis of sacroiliac joint subluxation based solely on the presence of tuber sacrale height asymmetry is inappropriate.[58] Variable degrees of tuber sacrale height asymmetry occur frequently and may be due to chronic asymmetric muscular or ligamentous

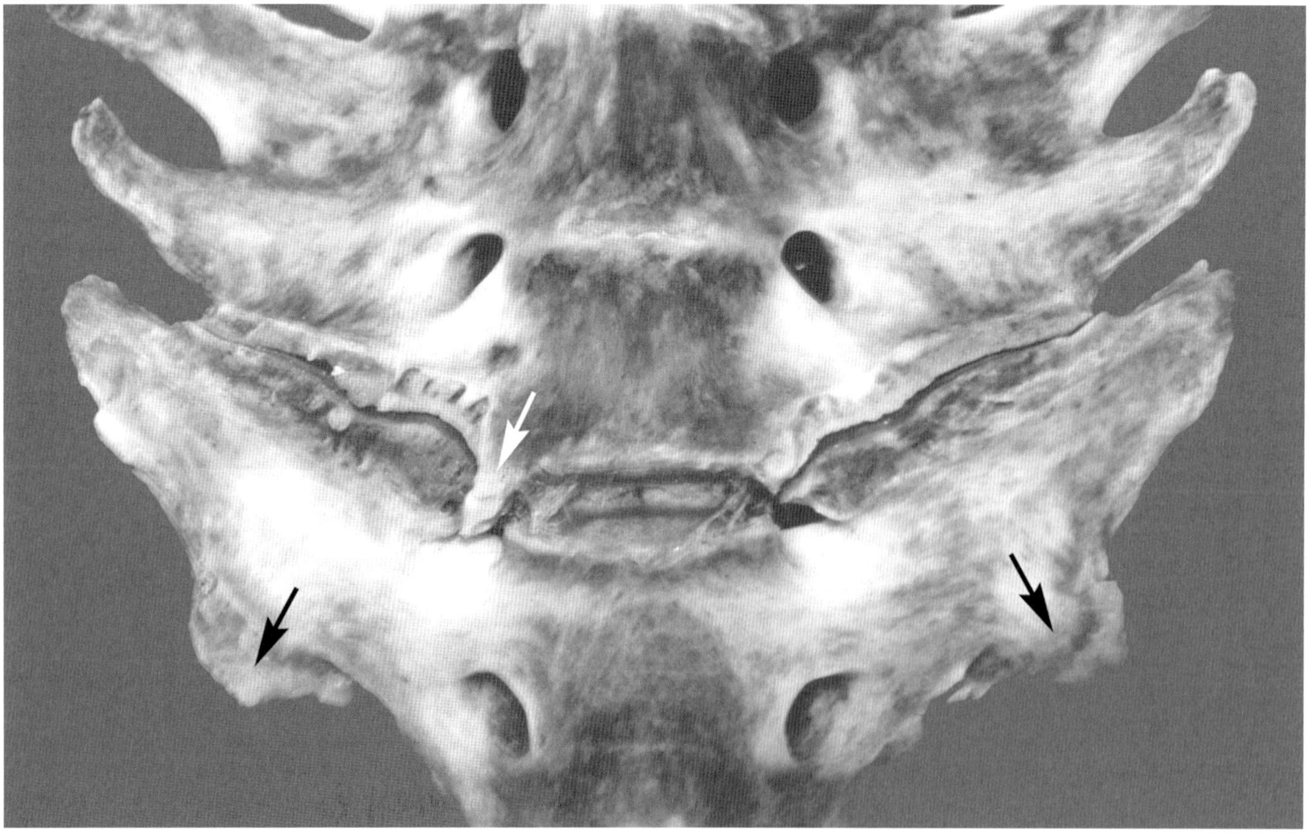

Fig 21.12 Ventral view of the lumbosacral vertebral region (L5–S2) of a 23-year-old Thoroughbred used for dressage. The horse had a clinical history of psoas muscle soreness and chronic pain localized to the lumbosacral junction. Bilateral intertransverse joint ankylosis (L4–L6), a large osteophyte at the right ventral lumbosacral intervertebral foramen (white arrow) and proliferative changes of the sacral articular surface of the sacroiliac joints (black arrows) are present.

forces acting on the malleable osseous pelvis and not direct sacroiliac ligament injury.[109] Horses with chronic sacroiliac problems and presumed sacroiliac joint subluxation have not had identifiable changes in the sacroiliac ligaments at necropsy.[31] In addition, Standardbred trotters with substantial tuber sacrale height asymmetries did not have significant increases in sacroiliac pain compared to horses with lesser degrees of asymmetry.[110] An ante-mortem diagnosis of sacroiliac joint luxation can only be supported if an acute change in tuber sacrale height asymmetry due to substantial trauma has been documented or if sacroiliac joint instability (i.e. crepitus or independent tuber sacrale movement) is evident during physical examination.

Pelvic stress fractures also need to be ruled out in horses with sacroiliac pain or dysfunction.[37] A high prevalence of occult pelvic stress fractures has been reported in Thoroughbred racehorses.[79,80,96,111] Pelvic stress fractures occur in consistent locations on the caudal border of the ilium adjacent to the sacroiliac joint.[78,83,96] The incomplete fracture lines extend into the caudomedial aspect of the sacroiliac joint, which could possibly produce concurrent sacroiliac joint inflammation and degradation. Complete ilial wing fractures (the most common type of pelvic fracture) typically produce a palpably depressed tuber sacrale on the affected side.[80]

Treatment and management

Medical management

The basic principles of medical management are to reduce pain and muscle spasms to permit better healing, followed by a program of rehabilitation and measures to prevent further injury or stress to the back. It is therefore necessary in many cases to use a combination of medications (e.g. NSAIDs, muscle relaxants, corticosteroids, local irritants or analgesics) in addition to physiotherapy or manipulative therapies (Table 21.5).

Non-steroidal anti-inflammatory drugs (NSAIDs)

For acute and severe pain from muscle strain, fractured withers and acute sacroiliac injury, intravenous NSAIDs followed by oral doses are beneficial. Phenylbutazone (1–2 g, p.o., b.i.d.) is still the drug of choice for many equine practitioners. Other NSAIDs include ketoprofen (2.2 mg/kg (1 mL/100 lb), i.v., s.i.d. for up to five days) or naproxen (5–10 mg/kg, p.o., b.i.d. for up to 14 days). If severe muscle spasms are present, then diazepam (0.08 mg/kg, i.v. or p.o.) may also be administered.[112] In mild or chronic cases, oral naproxen once or twice daily (5–10 mg/kg) is recommended. Phenylbutazone in low doses (1 g, p.o., s.i.d.) for mild aches and stiffness can be beneficial, but may mask signs of developing tendinitis or other musculoskeletal injuries with long-term use.[112] In chronic cases with low-grade bone pathology (e.g. over-riding dorsal spinous processes or osteoarthritis), a course of NSAIDs can be useful in conjunction with a progressive exercise program. Exercise should begin with a graduated program of lunging to build up and loosen the back and hindquarter muscles. Once the horse is fairly fit on the lunge line, riding work may begin. At this time oral phenylbutazone (i.e. 4 g/day for four days; 3 g/day for four days; 2 g/day for four days; 1 g/day for four days and 1 g every other day for eight days) can be given as the exercise is gradually increased.

Muscle relaxants

Muscle relaxants such as dantrolene sodium (2 mg/kg, p.o., s.i.d.) and methocarbamol (15–44 mg/kg, p.o., s.i.d.) have been

Table 21.5 Techniques used in the treatment of back problems in horses

CATEGORY	SPECIFIC METHODS
Rest	Stall rest Paddock turnout Restricted or controlled exercise
Management	Replace or reflock saddle Therapeutic saddle pads Change stable and work routine Attempt reschooling or try another training approach Graduated exercise program Assess or modify rider's equitation
Pharmaceuticals	NSAIDs (oral, parenteral or local injection) Corticosteroids (oral or local injection) Muscle relaxants Sclerosing agents (local injection) Sweats or counterirritants Hormonal therapy RVI injections
Surgery	Compound or comminuted fracture of the withers Impinged dorsal spinous processes
Physiotherapy	Heat (hot packs, infrared heat lamp, poultice, short-wave diathermy)
Thermal	Therapeutic ultrasound
Mechanical	Hydrotherapy and swimming
Electrical	Electrical muscle stimulation Magnetic therapy (static and pulsed) Shock-wave therapy
Manual therapy	Osteopathic techniques
Articular techniques	Chiropractic techniques (high velocity, low amplitude)
Soft tissue techniques	Physical therapy techniques (mobilization, soft tissue techniques) Manipulation under general anesthesia (MUA) Massage therapy Stretching exercises
Acupuncture	Dry needle, aquapuncture, low-level laser puncture Moxibustion
Nutraceuticals	Chondroitin sulfate Glucosamine Glycosaminoglycans MSM
Botanicals	Western herbs Chinese herbs
Homeopathy	Arnica montana

advocated for many years, but their effectiveness does not seem to be uniform in all horses.[113] These drugs may not have any specific effects other than reducing muscle tension or spasm in order to allow natural healing to progress. Thiocolchicoside (2–4 mg/100 kg, i.m., twice weekly for four weeks) and repeated injections of methocarbamol (10 mg/kg, i.v.) have also been advocated in Europe.[114]

Corticosteroids

The systemic use of corticosteroids is rarely indicated for primary back problems because of the possible side effects of laminitis, arthropathy and alimentary problems. NSAIDs are usually more effective and are associated with fewer adverse effects. The use of local injections into the interspinous spaces for the diagnosis or treatment of impinged or overriding dorsal spinous processes has been successful.[112] The injection mixture includes methylprednisolone acetate, isoflupredone acetate and serapin with approximately 5 mL injected at each interspinous space of concern. Improvement usually takes 2–6 days and repeated treatment is sometimes necessary. Occasionally, a local infection at the injection site can be a complication, which needs to be treated immediately with antibiotics. Denoix & Dyson recommend local injections of corticosteroids (flumethasone, 0.5–1 mg per injection site with a maximum total dose of 4 mg; dexamethasone 1.5–2.5 mg per injection site, with a maximum total dose of 10 mg; methylprednisolone acetate, 40–60 mg per injection site, with a maximum total dose of 200 mg), sometimes in association with muscle relaxants or serapin.[114] Injections of corticosteroids around the sacroiliac joint region have been used quite extensively, but currently there are no well-designed or controlled trials reported in the literature. Larger doses of corticosteroids (20 mL) mixed with serapin have been advocated for sacroiliac joint injections.[112]

Additional medications

This is another controversial area and one where there is really only anecdotal information on efficacy of a range of different preparations. However, they have been widely used in practice, often in combination with acupuncture or physical therapy.

Serapin

Serapin is an aqueous solution derived from the pitcher plant *(Sarraseniaceae)*, which is said to block selectively the C fibers that carry pain sensation in peripheral nerves. Serapin is used alone or in combination with other drugs (i.e. corticosteroids) and may be used for both soft tissue (muscle and ligament injuries) and osseous problems (e.g. over-riding dorsal spinous processes). Small doses of 1–2 mL of serapin are given at multiple sites.

Sclerosing agents

Again a number of proprietary agents have been used particularly around the sacroiliac joint and in the region of the ventral sacroiliac ligament. Horses are reported to improve their performance, but no scientific reports of their use are available.

Iodine

For chronic muscle soreness, multiple injections of 2% iodine in oil (Hypodermin or McKay's solution, 3–4 mL, i.m., at multiple sites) within the sore muscle (e.g. longissimus and middle gluteal muscles) have been recommended.[112] The injection area is massaged and the horse walked out the next day. Light work can then be resumed. Scientific reports on the beneficial action of iodine on muscle soreness are not currently available.

Hormones

The estrus-suppressing drug altrenogest (0.044 mg/kg (1 mL/110 lb), p.o., s.i.d.) has been useful in some mares that exhibit apparent back pain when they are in estrus. Also in young Thoroughbreds that show signs of 'cold back' the use of estrone sulfate (0.1–0.15 mg/kg, i.m., every two weeks) may be beneficial.

Rubeola virus immunomodulator (RVI)

Some practitioners have promoted RVI injections to assist in the reduction of chronic muscle soreness in some horses. RVI (2 mL, SQ, s.i.d. for six or more days) is an inactivated rubeola virus that is reported to have immunomodulatory effects that reduce chronic myofascial inflammation. However, the exact mechanism of action and extensive clinical reports are not currently available.

Mesotherapy

Mesotherapy is a technique that has been used for more than 30 years in France.[115] It consists of multiple intradermal injections with fine 5 mm needles into the dermatomes corresponding to the site of the lesion. The mechanism of action apparently involves type I and II nerve fibers coming from the skin which have collateral fibers that can inhibit pain transmission in the spinothalamic fasciculus, from deep structures of the same spinal segment to the thalamus and cerebrum.[114]

Mesotherapeutic injections are made using a mixture of local anesthetic solution (7 mL of lidocaine, 140 mg), short-acting corticosteroid (7 ml of dexamethasone, 15 mg), and muscle relaxant (8 ml of thiocolchicoside, 20 mg). The injections are made at the level of the lesion and caudal to it, taking into account the caudal orientation of the segmental nerves. For example, if treating over-riding dorsal spines between T10 and T15, the treated region extends from T10 to L1. Two to three rows of injections are made on each side of the median plane. The horse is restricted to light work on the lunge for three days. Normal training is progressively resumed over five days. A substantial improvement is anticipated within 7–14 days. The expected duration of action varies between three and 12 months.

Surgical management

There are few surgical indications for treatment of back problems except for impinged or over-riding dorsal spinous processes. In young horses that fracture the dorsal spines in the withers (T3–T10) surgery is not necessary unless the fractures are highly comminuted, when it may be necessary to debride the site to prevent infection or osteomyelitis.

Resection of dorsal spinous processes

Surgery for over-riding spinous processes was first reported by Roberts[116] and since then there have been a number of modifications to the technique.[32,117,118] However, the principle is the same, which is to remove the parts of the spinous processes that impinge. We believe that it is absolutely essential to confirm the correct diagnosis and select the most appropriate spines to alleviate the condition. There are many horses that show radiographic findings of over-riding spinous processes that do not exhibit clinical signs of a back problem.[70] Furthermore, many milder cases of over-riding spinous processes will respond to medical and conservative therapy.[53]

A recent paper reported by far the largest series to date and recorded a good response to surgery in those horses that failed to respond to conservative management.[32] The surgical technique involved placing the horse in lateral recumbency. A midline incision is made through the skin, subcutis and supraspinous ligament. The incision extends from one spinous process cranial to those identified for resection to one process caudal to them. The dorsal 4–5 cm of the dorsal spinous processes are dissected free of the supraspinous ligament, the interspinous ligaments and adjacent muscle tissue. Partial resection of the processes is performed with an oscillating saw to a depth that ensures that there is a minimum gap of 5 mm between the remaining bodies of each process resected. The minimum number of processes are resected in each case (e.g. if two processes are affected then one is removed, and if three are affected only the middle one is removed). One centimeter of the dorsal apex of the adjacent spinous process is also removed so that the change from resected to unresected processes is less abrupt. The supraspinous ligament and muscles are sutured and a simple interrupted suture placed between these sutures. The subcutis is sutured using three metric polyglycolic acid sutures and the skin is closed. The wound is protected by a stent bandage sutured over it. In the series, 72% of horses returned to full work and a further 9% improved sufficiently to be used for some athletic work.[32]

Chiropractic

Mechanism of action

Chiropractic evaluation focuses on evaluating and localizing segmental vertebral dysfunction (i.e. chiropractically defined 'subluxation') which is characterized by localized pain, muscle hypertonicity and reduced joint motion.[119] A thorough knowledge of vertebral anatomy, joint physiology and biomechanics is required for proper chiropractic evaluation and treatment. Alterations in articular neurophysiology from mechanical or chemical injuries can affect both Mechano-receptor and nociceptor function via increased joint capsule tension and nerve ending hypersensitivity.[120] Mechanoreceptor stimulation induces reflex paraspinal musculature hypertonicity and altered local and systemic neurologic reflexes. Nociceptor stimulation results in a lowered pain threshold, sustained afferent stimulation (i.e. facilitation), reflex paraspinal musculature hypertonicity and abnormal neurologic reflexes.

The goal of chiropractic treatment is to restore normal joint motion, stimulate neurologic reflexes and to reduce pain and muscle hypertonicity. Multiple theories have been proposed and tested over the years to explain the pathophysiology of vertebral segment dysfunction and its interactions and influences on the neuromusculoskeletal system.[119,121] Chiropractic treatment is thought to affect mechanoreceptors (i.e. Golgi tendon organ and muscle spindles) to induce reflex inhibition of pain and reflex muscle relaxation and to correct abnormal movement patterns.[47,122] Anecdotal evidence and clinical experience suggest that chiropractic is an effective adjunctive modality for the diagnosis and conservative treatment of select musculoskeletal-related disorders in horses.[123,124] However, therapeutic trials of chiropractic manipulations are often used since we currently have limited formal research available about the effectiveness of chiropractic procedures in equine practice.

During treatment, a 'release' or movement of the restricted articulation is often palpable. An audible 'cracking' or 'popping' sound may also be heard during chiropractic treatment as the applied force overcomes the elastic barrier of joint resistance.[125,126] The rapid articular separation produces a cavitation of the synovial fluid.[127] In humans, radiographic studies of synovial articulations after manipulation have shown a radiolucent cavity within the joint space (i.e. vacuum phenomenon) that contains 80% carbon dioxide and lasts for 15–20 minutes. A second attempt to recavitate the joint will be unsuccessful and potentially painful until the Intra-articular gas has been reabsorbed (i.e. refractory period). The static position of the vertebral or sacroiliac joints in humans has been studied before and after manipulation by roentgen stereophotogrammetric analysis, which allows precise measurements of three-dimensional articular movement.[128] Static palpation changes were noted before and after manipulation, but no changes were seen with the roentgen stereophotogrammetric analysis. Therefore, soft tissue responses such as joint capsules, muscles, ligaments, tendons and postural neuromuscular reflex patterns should be the focus of future spinal manipulative studies and not articular malpositioning (i.e. bone out of place).[128]

Indications

The principal indications for equine chiropractic evaluation are back or neck pain, localized or regional joint stiffness, poor performance and an altered gait that is not associated with overt lameness. A thorough diagnostic work-up is required to identify soft tissue and osseous pathology, neurologic disorders or other lameness conditions that may not be responsive to chiropractic care. The primary clinical signs that equine chiropractors look for are localized musculoskeletal pain, muscle hypertonicity and restricted joint motion. This triad of clinical signs can be found in a variety of lower limb disorders, but is most evident in neck or back problems. Chiropractic care can help manage the muscular, articular and neurologic components of select musculoskeletal injuries in performance horses. Musculoskeletal conditions that are chronic or recurring, not readily diagnosed or are not responding to conventional veterinary care may be indicators that chiropractic consultation is needed. Chiropractic care is usually contraindicated in the acute stages of soft tissue injury. However, as the soft tissue injury heals, chiropractic has the potential to help restore normal joint motion, thus limiting the risk for future reinjury.[43] Chiropractic care may provide symptomatic relief in early degenerative joint disease if related to joint hypomobility and subsequent joint degeneration. Chiropractic is usually much more effective in the early clinical stages of disease versus end-stage disease where reparative processes have been exhausted.

Contraindications

Chiropractic is not a 'cure all' for all back problems and is not suggested for treatment of fractures, infections, neoplasia, metabolic disorders or non-mechanically related joint disorders. Acute episodes of sprains or strains, degenerative joint disease or impinged spinous processes are also relative contraindications for chiropractic treatment. All neurologic diseases should be fully worked up to assess the potential risks or benefits of chiropractic treatment. Serious diseases requiring immediate medical or surgical care need to be ruled out and treated by conventional veterinary medicine before routine chiropractic treatment is begun. However, chiropractic care may contribute to the rehabilitation of most postsurgical cases or severe medical conditions by helping in the restoration of normal musculoskeletal function. Chiropractic care cannot reverse severe degenerative processes or overt pathology.

Acupuncture

Mechanism of action

Acupuncture involves the insertion of fine needles into specific predetermined locations (i.e. acupuncture points) to produce therapeutic effects.[129] Acupuncture points are often chosen within the same dermatome as the lesion or condition being treated, as well as local tender or painful sites, points cranial or caudal, proximal or distal to the localized lesion.[130] Additional methods of stimulation include acupressure, aquapuncture, electrostimulation and low-level laser therapy. Theoretically, each acupuncture point, or combination of points, has specific therapeutic actions when stimulated.

The primary benefit of acupuncture for back problems is pain management via opioid (i.e. enkephalin and β-endorphin) and non-opioid (e.g. serotonin) pathways.[130] Pain relief is often immediate, but may have variable durations of effectiveness, depending on the type and severity of musculoskeletal dysfunction. Acute injuries often respond rapidly and require fewer treatment sessions, whereas chronic musculoskeletal conditions may require periodic or long-term treatment. Acupuncture is often the treatment of choice for trigger points, which are localized tight, painful bands of muscle at characteristic locations within large muscle groups, particularly the middle gluteal muscle.

Indications

Clinical studies and experimental reports indicate that acupuncture is a safe and effective modality for specific musculoskeletal conditions if used properly.[129] Disease conditions managed by acupuncture include trauma, osteoarthritis and muscle hypertonicity.[131] Pain is the primary indication for acupuncture in horses with back problems.[132] Acupuncture does not have any known direct effects on reducing joint stiffness, as do manual therapies. Therefore, synergistic effects are often obtained with combined chiropractic and acupuncture treatment that cannot be obtained consistently with either modality by itself. The immediate pre-race use of acupuncture is banned by many racing jurisdictions and athletic organization regulations due to its potential misuse of analgesic properties.

Contraindications

There are few specific contraindications for acupuncture since the majority of medical and surgical conditions have associated indications for acupuncture. Fractures, active infections and bleeding tendencies are relative contraindications. Risks and complications associated with needle placement include infection, puncture of organs or pneumothorax. Solid needles or aquapuncture are often recommended over the thoracolumbar region due to the risk of breaking off a portion of the needle within the epaxial muscles from the action of the thoracolumbar fascia on the needle.

Physical therapy

Mechanism of action

Physical therapy modalities that may have direct application to back problems in horses include devices that apply electrical currents for pain control or neuromuscular rehabilitation; thermal modalities (i.e. superficial and deep heat or cold applications) for influencing inflammatory mediators, collagen extensibility and altering nerve conduction; and mechanical approaches (e.g. massage, vibration, stretching and training exercises) for maximizing musculoskeletal rehabilitation.

Indications

In the absence of trauma or documented pathologic findings, the primary goal of treatment should address restoration of function and prevention of future disability.[43] Management should be systematically and methodically directed toward developing co-ordination and proprioception, flexibility, strength and endurance. The negative effects of immobilization and deconditioning should be minimized with early mobilization and controlled activity. Increased mobility is addressed with joint mobilization and muscle stretching.[133] Altered movement patterns are addressed with co-ordination via proprioceptive retraining, postural re-education, muscle strengthening and endurance training.[43]

The primary indications of physical therapy for back or pelvic problems include localized or generalized pain, joint motion restrictions and altered back muscle tonicity.[134] Pain modulation can be provided by influencing inflammatory mediators, altering pain perception and transmission, and increasing β-endorphin levels. Physical therapy modalities involved in pain control include electrical stimulation (i.e. muscle stimulation, transcutaneous electrical nerve stimulation (TENS)), the application of hot or cold, mechanical vibration and electromagnetic modalities. Soft tissue and articular motion restrictions (i.e. stiffness) can be directly addressed with specific stretching exercises to induce creep and stress relaxation within fibrotic or shortened periarticular soft tissues.[135] With minimal training, horses and their owners can be taught how to do simple but effective passive joint mobilization and active stretching exercises (i.e. carrot stretches) to improve both axial skeleton and limb flexibility.[136] Cryotherapy (i.e. ice packs or ice massage) is indicated in the first 24–48 hours post injury to reduce pain, induce muscle relaxation and reduce inflammation. The application of heat or electrical stimulation can provide increased soft tissue extensibility, reduced inflammation and adhesion formation, and pain control to help facilitate the restoration of normal joint motion.[120]

Abnormal muscle tone can be addressed with modalities that increase or decrease muscle contractility or coactivation and nerve conduction or inhibition. Some of these modalities include hydrotherapy, electrical stimulation and rehabilitative exercises that specifically address issues of reduced flexibility, coordination, strength and endurance. In humans, anti-inflammatories and other drugs can be delivered into superficial soft tissues via electrical currents (i.e. iontophoresis) or via mechanical sound waves (i.e. phonophoresis). However, preliminary equine research indicates that a heavy hair coat, thick skin and deep articular structures may limit the overall effectiveness of these novel drug delivery systems for back problems.

Contraindications

Contraindications for massage include active skin lesions, open wounds, acute inflammation or persistent muscle hypertonicity (i.e. exertional rhabdomyolysis).[137] Contraindications for electrical modalities include active skin lesions, open wounds, pain of unknown origin or pain conditions where masking the pain may be detrimental (e.g. pre-race).[138] Contraindications for superficial or deep heating modalities include acute injury or inflammation, open wounds, recent or potential hemorrhage, neoplasms or impaired sensation.[120] Precautions or contraindications for cryotherapy include open wounds, vascular compromise or peripheral vascular disease due to the induced vasoconstriction produced by the ice.[120]

Future areas of research

In horses with back pain, specific functional pathologies that need to be addressed in addition to initial pain relief include trigger points, hypertonic muscles, weak muscles, abnormal movement patterns and joint dysfunction. Compared to their human counterparts, veterinarians and equine athletes often have a very limited selection of options for the treatment of musculoskeletal disorders. Currently, we do not have objective measurement or rehabilitation tools to specifically assess soft tissue or articular pain, reduced flexibility and joint stiffness, muscle hypertonicity, trigger points or alterations in proprioception or co-ordination associated with musculoskeletal or nerve dysfunction. Normal kinematics of the thoracolumbar spine have been investigated[8,9,11,139,140] but continued work needs to be done to assess segmental vertebral motion and its response to specific and defined articular and soft tissue injuries. Objective measures of spinal stiffness have been investigated[141] but the effects of pain, muscle hypertonicity, articular process osteoarthritis and concurrent lameness have not been explored.

Functional outcome measures assess how well a horse is able to do the job asked of it (e.g. speed, flexibility, coordination, strength and endurance). Quantitative assessments of pain include the use of a 0–10 pain scale, algometry or pain pressure threshold measurements, and mapping areas of pain. A 0–10 visual analog scale or pain scale is easy to use and provides a semi-objective means of following pain, dysfunction, performance or any other musculoskeletal parameter either immediately before and after treatment or over several days or weeks of treatment. Measurements can be compiled independently by both the owner and the veterinarian, with similarities or differences evaluated.

Other areas of musculoskeletal treatment that need further scientific investigation include well-defined, scientifically validated strength and endurance training programs tailored for the unique athletic demands of the various equestrian events. It is hoped that new insights into measuring musculoskeletal dysfunction and the pathophysiology of chronic pain syndromes will assist in assessing the effectiveness of many of the traditional and complementary modalities currently applied to horses with the rationale of reducing morbidity and improving overall performance in our elite equine athletes.

References

1. Lupton. Mayhew's illustrated horse management. London: Allen; 1876.
2. Youatt W. The horse: With a treatise on draught. London: Baldwin and Cardock; 1831.
3. British Equine Veterinary Association. Survey of equine disease. Vet Rec 1965;77:528–38.
4. Jeffcott LB. Disorders of the thoracolumbar spine of the horse – a survey of 443 cases. Equine Vet J 1980;12(4):197–210.
5. Jeffcott LB. Back problems in the horse – a look at past, present and future progress. Equine Vet J 1979;11(3):129–36.
6. Cauvin E. Assessment of back pain in horses. In Practice 1997;19:522–33.
7. Licka T, Peham C. An objective method for evaluating the flexibility of the back of standing horses. Equine Vet J 1998; 30(5):412–15.
8. Pourcelot P, Audigié F, Degueurce C, et al. Kinematics of the equine back: a method to study the thoracolumbar flexion-extension movements at the trot. Vet Res 1998;29:519–25.
9. Audigié F, Pourcelot P, Degueurce C, et al. Kinematics of the equine back: flexion-extension movements in sound trotting horses. Equine Vet J 1999;30(Suppl):210–13.
10. Denoix J-M. Spinal biomechanics and functional anatomy. Vet Clin North Am Eq Pract 1999;15(1):27–60.
11. Licka TF, Peham C, Zohmann E. Treadmill study of the range of back movement at the walk in horses without back pain. Am J Vet Res 2001;62:1173–9.
12. Faber M, Johnston CJ, Schamhardt HC, et al. Basic three-dimensional kinematics of the vertebral column of horses trotting on a treadmill. Am J Vet Res 2001;62:757–64.
13. Haussler KK, Bertram JEA, Gellman K. In-vivo segmental kinematics of the thoracolumbar spinal region in horses and effects of chiropractic manipulations. Am Assoc Eq Pract 1999;45:327–9.
14. Getty R. Sisson and Grossman's the anatomy of the domestic animals. 5th ed. Philadelphia, PA: Saunders; 1975.
15. Stecher RM. Lateral facets and lateral joints in the lumbar spine of the horse: a descriptive and statistical study. Am J Vet Res 1962;23(96):939–47.
16. Townsend HGG, Leach DH. Relationship between intervertebral joint morphology and mobility in the equine thoracolumbar spine. Equine Vet J 1984;16(5):461–5.
17. Denoix J-M. Aspects fonctionnels et approche sémiologique des régions lombo-sacrale et sacro-iliaque chez le cheval. Swiss Vet 1991;8:89–106.
18. Jeffcott LB, Dalin G. Natural rigidity of the horse's backbone. Equine Vet J 1980;12(3):101–8.
19. Giles LGF. Anatomical basis of low back pain. Baltimore, MD: Williams and Wilkins; 1989.
20. Bogduk N, Twomey LT. Clinical anatomy of the lumbar spine, 2nd edn. Melbourne, Australia: Churchill Livingstone; 1991.
21. Cramer GD, Darby SA. Basic and clinical anatomy of the spine, spinal cord and ANS. St Louis, MD: Mosby-Year Book; 1995.
22. Nickel R, Schummer A, Sieferle E, et al. The anatomy of the domestic animals: volume 1. The locomotor system of the domestic mammals. 5th ed. New York: Springer-Verlag; 1986.
23. Budras K-D, Sack WO, Röck S. Anatomy of the horse: an illustrated text. 2nd ed. London: Mosby-Wolfe; 1994.
24. Rutherford KMD. Assessing pain in animals. Animal Welfare 2002;11:31–53.
25. Jeffcott LB, Dalin G, Drevemo S, et al. Effect of induced back pain on gait and performance of trotting horses. Equine Vet J 1982;14(2):129–33.
26. Rooney JR. Congenital equine scoliosis and lordosis. Clin Orthoped Rel Res 1969;62(Jan/Feb):25–30.
27. Lerner DJ. Congenital kyphoscoliosis in a foal. J Am Vet Med Assoc 1978;172(3):274–6.
28. Adams SB, Steckel RR, Blevins WE. Discospondylitis in five horses. J Am Vet Med Assoc 1985;186:270–2.
29. Hillyer MH, Innes JF, Patteson MW, et al. Discospondylitis in the adult horse. Vet Rec 1996;139:519–21.
30. Rooney JR, Delaney FM, Mayo JA. Sacroiliac luxation in the horse. Equine Vet J 1969;1:287–9.
31. Jeffcott LB, Dalin G, Ekman S, et al. Sacroiliac lesions as a cause of chronic poor performance in competitive horses. Equine Vet J 1985;17(2): 111–18.
32. Walmsley JP, Pettersson H, Winberg F, et al. Impingement of the dorsal spinous processes in two hundred and fifteen horses: case selection, surgical technique and results. Equine Vet J 2002;34(1):23–8.
33. Denoix J-M. Ultrasonographic evaluation of back lesions. Vet Clin North Am Eq Pract 1999;15(1): 131–60.
34. Gillis C. Spinal ligament pathology. Vet Clin North Am Eq Pract 1999;15(1): 97–101.
35. Henson FM, Lamas L, Knezevic S, et al. Ultrasonographic evaluation of the supraspinous ligament in a series of ridden and unridden horses and horses with unrelated back pathology. BMC Vet Res 2007;3:3.

36. Herrod-Taylor EE. A technique for manipulation of the spine in horses. Vet Rec 1967;81:437–9.
37. Steckel RR, Kraus-Hansen AE, Fackelman GE, et al. Scintigraphic diagnosis of thoracolumbar spinal disease in horses: a review of 50 cases. Am Assoc Eq Pract 1991;37:583–91.
38. Landman MA, de Blaauw JA, van Weeren PR, et al. Field study of the prevalence of lameness in horses with back problems. Vet Rec 2004;155: 165–8.
39. Dyson S. The interrelationships between back pain and lameness: a diagnostic challenge. Proc Congr Brit Equine Vet Assoc 2005;44:137–8.
40. Marks D. Back pain. In: Robinson NE, editor. Current therapy in equine medicine 4. Philadelphia, PA: Saunders; 1997. p. 6–12.
41. Stashak TS. Adams' lameness in horses. 5th ed. Philadelphia, PA: Lippincott Williams and Wilkins; 2002.
42. Martin BB Jr, Klide AM. Physical examination of horses with back pain. Vet Clin North Am Eq Pract 1999; 15(1):61–70.
43. Liebenson C. Rehabilitation of the spine. Baltimore, MD: Williams and Wilkins; 1996.
44. Cox JH, Murray RC, DeBowes RM. Diseases of the spinal cord. In: Kobluk CN, Ames TR, Geor RJ, editors. The horse: diseases and clinical management. Philadelphia, PA: Saunders; 1995. p. 443–67.
45. Valberg SJ, Hodgson DR. Diseases of muscle. In: Smith BP, editor. Large animal internal medicine. 3rd ed. St. Louis, MO: Mosby; 2002. p. 1266–91.
46. Quiroz-Rothe E, Novales M, Aguilera-Tejero E, et al. Polysaccharide storage myopathy in the M. longissimus lumborum of showjumpers and dressage horses with back pain. Equine Vet J 2002;34(2):171–6.
47. Gatterman MI. Foundations of chiropractic. St Louis, MO: Mosby-Year Book; 1995.
48. Chaitow L. Palpation skills. New York, NY: Churchill Livingstone; 1997.
49. Fischer AA. Pressure algometry over normal muscles: standard values, validity and reproducibility of pressure threshold. Pain 1987;30:115–26.
50. Fischer AA. Application of pressure algometry in manual medicine. Man Med 1990;5:145–50.
51. Tunks E, McCain GA, Hart LE, et al. The reliability of examination for tenderness in patients with myofascial pain, chronic fibromyalgia and controls. J Rheumatol 1995;22:944–52.
52. Dung HC. A simple new method for the quantitation of chronic pain. Am J Acupuncture 1985;13(1):57–62.
53. Jeffcott LB. Radiographic features of the normal equine thoracolumbar spine. Vet Radiol 1979;20:140–7.
54. Haussler KK, Stover SM, Willits NH. Pathology of the lumbosacral spine and pelvis in Thoroughbred racehorses. Am J Vet Res 1999;60(2):143–53.
55. Tucker RL, Schneider RK, Sondhof AH, et al. Bone scintigraphy in the diagnosis of sacroiliac injury in twelve horses. Equine Vet J 1998;30(5):390–5.
56. Kessler RM, Hertling D. Assessment of musculoskeletal disorders. In: Hertling D, Kessler RM, editors. Management of common musculoskeletal disorders: physical therapy principles and methods. 2nd ed. Philadelphia, PA: Lippincott; 1990. p. 68–71.
57. Adams OR. Subluxation of the sacroiliac joint in horses. Am Assoc Eq Pract 1969;15:198–207.
58. Cassidy JD, Townsend HGG. Sacroiliac joint strain as a cause of back and leg pain in man – implications for the horse. Am Assoc Eq Pract 1985;31:317–33.
59. Luukkainen R, Nissila M, Asikainen E, et al. Periarticular corticosteroid treatment of the sacroiliac joint in patients with seronegative spondylarthropathy. Clin Exp Rheumatol 1999;17:88–90.
60. Maugars Y, Mathis C, Berthelot JM, et al. Assessment of the efficacy of sacroiliac corticosteroid injections in spondyloarthropathies: a double-blinded study. Br J Rheumatol 1996;35:767–70.
61. Rooney JR. The horse's back: biomechanics of lameness. Equine Pract 1982;4(2):17–27.
62. Hardy J, Marcoux M. L'Arthrose sacro-iliac chez le cheval Standardbred. Med Vet Quebec 1985;15:185–9.
63. Snyder JR. Selected Intra-articular injections in the horse. Proceedings of the 7th Congress on Equine Medicine and Surgery, Geneva, Switzerland, 2001; 115–23.
64. Engeli E, Haussler KK, Erb HN. A diagnostic injection technique of the sacroiliac joint in horses. 12th Annual ACVS Veterinary Symposium: Equine Proceedings, San Diego, CA, 2002;7.
65. Dalin G, Jeffcott LB. Sacroiliac joint of the horse. 1. Gross morphology. Anat Histol Embryol 1986;15:80–94.
66. Dyce KM, Sack WO, Wensing CJG. Textbook of veterinary anatomy. 2nd ed. Philadelphia, PA: Saunders; 1996.
67. Butler JA, Colles CM, Dyson SJ, et al. The spine. In: Clinical radiology of the horse. Oxford: Blackwell Science; 1993. p. 355–98.
68. Jeffcott LB. Back problems in the horse – a method of clinical examination. Vet Rec 1979;1(Suppl 5):4–15.
69. Weaver MP, Jeffcott LB, Nowak M. Radiology and scintigraphy. Vet Clin North Am Eq Pract 1999;15(1):113–29.
70. Jeffcott LB. Radiographic examination of the equine vertebral column. Vet Radiol Ultrasound 1979;20:135–9.
71. Butler JA, Colles CM, Dyson SJ, et al. The pelvis and femur. In: Clinical radiology of the horse. Oxford: Blackwell Science; 1993. p. 399–421.
72. Jeffcott LB. Radiographic appearance of equine lumbosacral and pelvic abnormalities by linear tomography. Vet Radiol 1983;24(5):201–13.
73. Ueltschi G. Bone and joint imaging with 99mTc labeled phosphates as a new diagnostic aid in veterinary orthopedics. J Am Vet Radiol Soc 1977;18:80–4.
74. Devous M, Twardock A. Techniques and applications of nuclear medicine in the diagnosis of equine lameness. J Am Vet Med Assoc 1984;184:318–25.
75. Lamb CR, Koblik PD. Scintigraphic evaluation of skeletal disease and its application to the horse. Vet Radiol Ultrasound 1988;29:16–27.
76. Steckel RR. The role of scintigraphy in lameness evaluation. Vet Clin No Am Eq Pract 1991;7:207–39.
77. Morris EA, Seeherman HJ, O'Callaghan MW, et al. Scintigraphic identification of skeletal muscle damage in horses 24 hours after strenuous exercise. Equine Vet J 1991;23:347–52.
78. Hornof WJ, Stover SM, Koblik PD, et al. Oblique views of the ilium and the scintigraphic appearance of stress fractures of the ilium. Equine Vet J 1996;28(5):355–8.
79. Haussler KK, Stover SM. Stress fractures of the vertebral lamina and pelvis in Thoroughbred racehorses. Equine Vet J 1998,30(5).374–81.
80. Pilsworth RC, Shepherd MC, Herinckx BMB, et al. Fracture of the wing of the ilium, adjacent to the sacroiliac joint, in Thoroughbred racehorses. Equine Vet J 1994;26(2):94–9.
81. Denoix J-M. Ligament injuries of the axial skeleton in the horse: supraspinal and sacroiliac desmopathies. Dubai International Equine Symposium 1996;273–86.
82. Tomlinson JE, Sage AM, Turner TA, et al. Detailed ultrasonographic mapping of the pelvis in clinically normal horses and ponies. Am J Vet Res 2001;62:1768–75.
83. Shepherd MC, Pilsworth RC. The use of ultrasound in the diagnosis of pelvic fractures. Equine Vet Educ 1994;6(4):223–7.
84. Reef VB. Diagnosis of pelvic fractures in horses using ultrasonography. Vet Radiol Ultrasound 1992;33:121.
85. von Schweinitz DG. Thermographic diagnostics in equine back pain. Vet

Clin North Am Eq Pract 1999;15(1): 161–77.

86. Turner TA. Thermography as an aid in the localization of upper hindlimb lameness. Pferdeheilkunde 1996;12(4): 632–4.
87. Rooney JR, Prickett ME. Congenital lordosis of the horse. Cornell Vet 1967; 57(3):417–28.
88. Wagner PC. Diseases of the spine. In: Mansmann RA, McAllister ES, editors. Equine medicine and surgery. 3rd ed. Santa Barbara, CA: American Veterinary Publications; 1982. p. 1145–58.
89. Bogduk N. The anatomical basis for spinal pain syndromes. J Manip Physiol Ther 1995;18(9):603–5.
90. Jeffcott LB. The horse's back – muscle, soft tissue and skeletal problems. Their diagnosis and management. Dubai International Equine Symposium 1996;337–59.
91. Denoix J-M. Diagnosis of the cause of back pain in horses. In: Lindiven A, editor. 1st Conf Equine Sports Med & Sci. Wageningen Pers, Wageningen, The Netherlands; 1998. p. 97–110.
92. Townsend HGG, Leach DH, Fretz PB. Kinematics of the equine thoracolumbar spine. Equine Vet J 1983;15(2):117–22.
93. van Schaik JPJ, Verbiest H, van Schaik FDJ. Isolated spinous process deviation: a pitfall in the interpretation of AP radiographs of the lumbar spine. Spine 1989;14(9):970–6.
94. Townsend HGG, Leach DH, Doige CE, et al. Relationship between spinal biomechanics and pathological changes in the equine thoracolumbar spine. Equine Vet J 1986;18(2):107–12.
95. Klide AM. Overriding vertebral spinous processes in the extinct horse, *Equus occidentalis*. Am J Vet Res 1989;50(4): 592–3.
96. Stover SM, Ardans AA, Read DH, et al. Patterns of stress fractures associated with complete bone fractures in racehorses. Am Assoc Eq Pract 1993;39:131–2.
97. Haussler KK, Stover SM, Willits NH. Developmental variation in lumbosacropelvic anatomy of Thoroughbred racehorses. Am J Vet Res 1997;58(10):1083–91.
98. Clyne MJ. Pathogenesis of degenerative joint disease. Equine Vet J 1987;19:15–18.
99. Jeffcott LB, Whitwell KE. Fractures of the thoracolumbar spine of the horse. Am Assoc Eq Pract 1976;22:91–102.
100. Wagner PC. Surgical treatment of traumatic disease of the spinal column. In: Auer JA, editor. Equine surgery. Philadelphia, PA: Saunders; 1992. p. 1093–8.
101. Rhoads WS, Cox JH. What is your diagnosis? J Am Vet Med Assoc 1997;210(6):755–6.
102. DeBowes RM, Wagner PC, Gavin PR, et al. Vertebral compression fracture in a foal following electric shock. J Vet Orthop 1981;2(2):14–19.
103. Moyer WA, Rooney JR. Vertebral fracture in a horse. J Am Vet Med Assoc 1971; 159(8):1022–4.
104. Chiapetta JR, Baker JC, Feeney DA. Vertebral fracture, extensor hypertonia of thoracic limbs, and paralysis of pelvic limbs (Schiff-Sherrington syndrome) in an Arabian foal. J Am Vet Med Assoc 1985;186(4):387–8.
105. Huntington PJ, Jeffcott LB, Friend SCE, et al. Australian stringhalt. Epidemiological, clinical and neurological investigations. Equine Vet J 1989;21:266–73.
106. Slocombe RF, Huntington PJ, Friend SCE, et al. Pathological aspects of Australian stringhalt. Equine Vet J 1992;24(3):174–83.
107. Townsend HGG. Pathogenesis of back pain in the horse. Equine Sports Med 1987;6:29–32.
108. Rooney JR. Sacroiliac luxation. Mod Vet Pract 1979;60:45–6.
109. Haussler KK. Anatomy of the thoracolumbar vertebral region. Vet Clin North Am Eq Pract 1999;15(1):13–26.
110. Dalin G, Magnusson L-E, Thafvelin BC. Retrospective study of hindquarter asymmetry in Standardbred Trotters and its correlation with performance. Equine Vet J 1985;17(4):292–6.
111. Shepherd MC, Pilsworth RC, Hopes R, et al. Clinical signs, diagnosis, management and outcome of complete and incomplete fracture to the ilium. Am Assoc Eq Pract 1994;40:177–80.
112. Marks D. Medical management of back pain. Vet Clin North Am Eq Pract 1999; 15(1):179–94.
113. Marks D. Notes on treatment and management on thoracolumbar pain in the horse. Am Assoc Eq Pract 1985;30:353–7.
114. Denoix J-M, Dyson SJ. The thoracolumbar spine. In: Ross M, Dyson S, editors. Diagnosis and management of lameness in the horse. Philadelphia, PA: Saunders; 2003. p. 509–21.
115. Denoix J-M. Personal communication. 2000.
116. Roberts EJ. Resection of thoracic or lumbar spinous processes for the relief of pain responsible for lameness and some other locomotor disorders of horses. Am Assoc Eq Pract 1968;14: 13–29.
117. Jeffcott LB, Hickman J. The treatment of horses with chronic back pain by resecting the summits of the impinging dorsal spinous processes. Equine Vet J 1975;7(3):115–19.
118. Steckel RR, Krasu-Hansen AE, Fackelman GE, et al. Clinical aspects of thoracolumbar spinal disease in horses: a review of 50 cases. Am Assoc Eq Pract 1991;36:583.
119. Leach RA. The chiropractic theories: principles and clinical applications. 3rd ed. Baltimore, MD: Williams and Wilkins; 1994.
120. Cameron MH. Physical agents in rehabilitation. Philadelphia, PA: Saunders; 1999.
121. Haldeman S. Principles and practice of chiropractic, 2nd edn. Norwalk, CT: Appleton and Lange; 1992.
122. Cassidy JD, Lopes AA, Yong-Hing K. The immediate effect of manipulation versus mobilization on pain and range of motion in the cervical spine: a randomized controlled trial. J Manip Physiol Ther 1992;15(9):570–5.
123. Haussler KK. Review of manual therapy techniques in equine practice. J Equine Vet Sci 2009;29:849–69.
124. Haussler KK. Current status of integrative medicine techniques used in equine practice. J Equine Vet Sci 2009; 29:639–41.
125. Brodeur R. The audible release associated with joint manipulation. J Manip Physiol Ther 1995;18(3):155–64.
126. Reggars JW, Pollard HP. Analysis of zygapophyseal joint cracking during chiropractic manipulation. J Manip Physiol Ther 1995;18(2):65–71.
127. Herzog W, Zhang YT, Conway PJW, et al. Cavitation sounds during spinal manipulative treatments. J Manip Physiol Ther 1993;16(8):523–6.
128. Tullberg T, Blomberg S, Branth B, et al. Manipulation does not alter the position of the sacroiliac joint. Spine 1998;23(10):1124–9.
129. Altman S. Small animal acupuncture: scientific basis and clinical applications. In: Schoen AM, Wynn SG, editors. Complementary and alternative veterinary medicine: principles and practice. St Louis, MO: Mosby; 1998. p. 147–67.
130. Fleming P. Equine acupuncture. In: Schoen AM, Wynn SG, editors. Complementary and alternative veterinary medicine: principles and practice. St Louis, MO: Mosby; 1998. p. 169–84.
131. Shmalberg J, Xie H. The clinical application of equine acupuncture. J Equine Vet Sci 2009;29:645–52.
132. Tangjitjaroen W, Shmalberg J, Colahan PT, et al. Equine Acupuncture Research: An Update. J Equine Vet Sci 2009;29: 698–709.
133. Porter M. Stretching for the horse. In: Porter M, editor. The new equine sports therapy. Lexington, KY: The Blood-Horse; 1998. p. 31–42.
134. Porter M. Physical therapy. In: Schoen AM, Wynn SG, editors. Complementary

and alternative veterinary medicine: principles and practice. St Louis, MO: Mosby; 1998. p. 201–12.

135. Frick A. Stretching exercises for horses: are they effective? J Equine Vet Sci 2010;30:50–9.

136. Paulekas R, Haussler KK. Principles and practice of therapeutic exercise for horses. J Equine Vet Sci 2009;29: 870–93.

137. Porter M, Bromiley MW. Massage therapy. In: Schoen AM, Wynn SG, editors. Complementary and alternative veterinary medicine: principles and practice. St Louis, MO: Mosby; 1998. p. 213–16.

138. Bromiley MW. Physical therapy for the equine back. Vet Clin North Am Eq Pract 1999;15(1):223–48.

139. Faber M, Schamhardt HC, van Weeren R, et al. Basic three-dimensional kinematics of the vertebral column of horses walking on a treadmill. Am J Vet Res 2000;61(4):399–406.

140. Haussler KK, Bertram JEA, Gellman K, et al. Segmental in vivo vertebral kinematics at the walk, trot and canter: a preliminary study. Equine Vet J 2001;33:160–4.

141. Haussler KK. Dorsoventral spinal mobility in horses: chiropractic treatment versus control group comparisons. 2nd International Symposium on Rehabilitation and Physical Therapy in Veterinary Medicine, Knoxville, TN, 2002; 207–8.

Repetitive strain injuries of the skeleton in high performance equine athletes

22

Christopher M. Riggs Rob Pilsworth

CHAPTER CONTENTS

Introduction

Bone injuries are common among racehorses. Catastrophic fractures account for over 80% of all racecourse fatalities.[1] Stress fractures lead to significant loss of training days and disease of subchondral bone affects a high proportion of horses, often leading to permanent impairment of joint function and consequent loss of performance and premature retirement.[2] A large body of evidence has accumulated over the last 20 years to demonstrate that the majority of these injuries are the end result of a progressive process associated with fatigue damage of the bone.

The vital nature of bone, including its ability to undergo repair and stimulate an adaptive response to changes in its mechanical environment, are widely documented. Under ideal circumstances, the size and shape of bones will perfectly match ambient conditions of loading and any damage that may be incurred will soon be repaired through the coordinated action of bone cells. The fact that injuries are so common indicates that circumstances are frequently not ideal; we expect too much of the skeleton or, simply, we fail to understand the mechanisms of adaptation and repair, and to modify training regimes to suit their natural response rates.

Increasingly, fatigue-related injuries are referred to in the literature as examples of 'maladaptation', or by some other, equally unfortunate, term. 'Adaptation' suggests a physiological process that confers some advantage, which is, presumably, why it has endured the processes of natural selection. That this process should become a 'disease' in its own right confuses the simple fact that the limits of adaptation or repair are frequently overwhelmed through over-demanding training schedules. It also overlooks that bone undergoes pathological processes, such as infarction, necrosis etc., like any other tissue.

The very fact that many skeletal injuries in high-performing horses are the end result of a progressive process can be viewed as potentially very encouraging. Once we learn to detect damage early enough in the process, we can recommend intervention strategies to allow healing to occur before serious harm is done; many more racing fractures will be prevented and the incidence of joint disease will be greatly reduced. Equally, through understanding the pathophysiological mechanisms of failure that lead to stress fractures, training regimes can be modified to reduce the risks. For instance, the introduction of nuclear scintigraphy to Thoroughbred racehorse practice in the mid 1980s was a great advance in the detection of early bone pathology and led to a significant reduction in the incidence of catastrophic fractures associated with certain common stress fractures.

Clinical signs associated with early fatigue damage of bone are often minimal and can easily be mistaken for other, less significant, injuries. In addition, associated changes in bone structure are often so subtle as to be difficult or impossible to detect by radiography and ultrasonography. The application of specialized techniques, such as nuclear scintigraphy, computed tomography or magnetic resonance imaging, can successfully indicate the presence of or visualize these injuries but these techniques are not suitable as routine screening tools. The application of knowledge from epidemiological studies to the analysis of training and race records, or by performing routine testing for biomarkers in serum or urine, could be used to identify 'at risk individuals'. This would facilitate the selective application of higher level imaging to these animals. However, it is likely that much better outcomes could probably be achieved than at present, simply by using the current routine techniques more effectively. This would require better application of existing knowledge and skills, and a greater awareness of the possibility of fatigue injury and the lesions that could develop from it, in order to encourage owner, trainer and veterinary surgeon to take mild but significant signs seriously. It could also involve active screening of horses known to be at higher risk, e.g. those returning from a period of rest. It would involve education to help veterinary surgeons to recognize the anatomical predilection sites for injuries, and encourage them to routinely use 'specialist' radiographic projections and ultrasonographic views that are most effective at showing up subtle early signs of bone damage and to recognize these signs on images acquired.

In order to achieve the best outcomes for racehorses, clinicians need to have a good understanding of bone physiology and pathology and the reader is encouraged to study Chapter 8 for a review of relevant information. In addition, clinicians must have a working knowledge of the types of lesion that arise, their specific anatomical locations and the subtle radiographic and ultrasonographic features that may be associated with them.

Clinical syndromes associated with repetitive strain injury of bone

Recurrent strain injury of subchondral bone associated with synovial articulations

A growing body of work convincingly demonstrates the progressive nature of many of the injuries associated with joints in Thoroughbred racehorses, which are presumed to arise as a consequence of repetitive, high strains experienced by these tissues while horses train and race. A significant proportion of common, severe racing fractures (e.g. parasagittal fractures of the distal condyles of the third metacarpal bone, frontal slab fractures of the third carpal bone) originate from pre-existing pathology in subchondral bone. In addition, osteochondral chip fractures arise in areas of diseased subchondral bone and degenerative change of hyaline articular cartilage is often preceded by primary disease of underlying subchondral bone.

While pathological changes in subchondral bone have been characterized in numerous studies, there is no unifying hypothesis to explain how they culminate in clinical lesions. We speculate the following may happen: Increased volume fraction of subchondral bone (due to infilling of trabecular spaces with new bone and which may be apparent radiographically as 'sclerosis') in response to higher loads associated with greater exercise, reflects an adaptive response. The resultant structure will be stronger but the more dense bone will be less compliant and, therefore, more prone to injury during impact loading. In the face of a continued cyclical burden, injury may manifest in the form of microdamage and/or osteocyte necrosis. The matrix will become hypermineralized following osteonecrosis, making it more brittle and, therefore, further prone to damage. Disruption of blood supply following more extensive matrix damage exacerbates the rate of osteonecrosis. At some stage (e.g. following a period of reduced loading) a remodeling response to remove damaged or necrotic bone is initiated. This may result in a focal defect in subchondral bone that acts as a stress-riser, which predisposes to fracture. Alternatively, if a relatively large volume of subchondral bone is affected, a void may be created between vital and necrotic tissue during the initial resorptive phase of remodeling. On resumption of loading the superficial, necrotic tissue may collapse into the void, resulting in a depression in the joint surface or may fracture away from the parent bone, leaving a deep ulcer in the joint surface (Fig. 22.1). Longitudinal studies with suitable imaging techniques are required to substantiate this hypothesis.

There are specific anatomical predilection sites in joints for repetitive strain injury in the Thoroughbred racehorse. The reasons why particular animals appear more prone to these injuries than others remain obscure. Attempts to demonstrate material abnormalities of bone, which may predispose to injury, have been unrewarding. Conformational abnormalities or fine variations in neuromuscular control, both of which lead to altered loads on the skeleton, are more likely to be involved. These would affect all limbs symmetrically, and would be consistent with the observed injuries, which are frequently bilateral or quadrilateral. The progressive nature of the disease process results in a continuum of clinical signs and associated findings on diagnostic imaging and the severity of lameness often show poor correlation with extent of structural changes identified.

Subchondral bone disease in the third carpal bone

Recognition

Presentation

Affected horses trot with reduced cranial phase to the stride and often show incomplete flexion of the carpus. The head is held low and does not assume its normal degree of excursion during trotting. This gives a stiff, stilted action with a paddling gait in front and a staccato beat to the trot produced by the short choppy nature of the stepping pattern. There may or may not be effusion of the middle carpal joint. Usually one carpus is slightly more painful than the other giving a very mild observable lameness but instillation of local anesthetic into the middle carpal joint will give immediate marked unilateral lameness in the contralateral limb.

Diagnosis

It is vital that a properly positioned third carpal skyline projection (flexed dorsal 60° proximal-dorsodistal oblique) is included in radiographic examination of the carpus to demonstrate structural changes associated with this syndrome. While easy to accomplish with practice, this projection is often poorly executed and, therefore, significant abnormalities are overlooked. The lesions are most commonly visualized in the radial articular facet of the third carpal bone but can also occur in the intermediate facet. The radiographic appearance of the bone progressively changes as the inter-trabecular spaces are filled with new bone, resulting in an amorphous radiopaque 'haze' as the normal trabeculated pattern of the bone is steadily lost. As the disease advances, focal areas of resorption, often associated with nutrient foraminae, appear within the sclerosis[3] (Fig. 22.2). Fissure fracture of the dorsal cortex may become visible and in advanced cases, sagittal or curvilinear slab fracture lines may be visualized. On scintigraphic examination, moderate increased radiopharmaceutical uptake (IRU) is visualized over the entire outline of the third carpal bone and this will become more intense and focal in the event of fracture (Fig. 22.3).

Management

On first diagnosis of third carpal bone disease in youngsters, the speed, intensity and duration of the horse's training workload should be rapidly reduced to avoid irreversible injury. A period of one month of stable rest will usually result in significant reduction in radiopacity of the third carpal bone. Full training should be heldup until the radiographic appearance of third carpal bone approaches normality. This may take two to three months removed from full speed work, the remainder of which can be walking, trotting and slow canter work, or pasture turnout if available and practical.

Marked sclerosis of the third carpal bone in the older horse often reflects conformational abnormalities rather than inappropriate

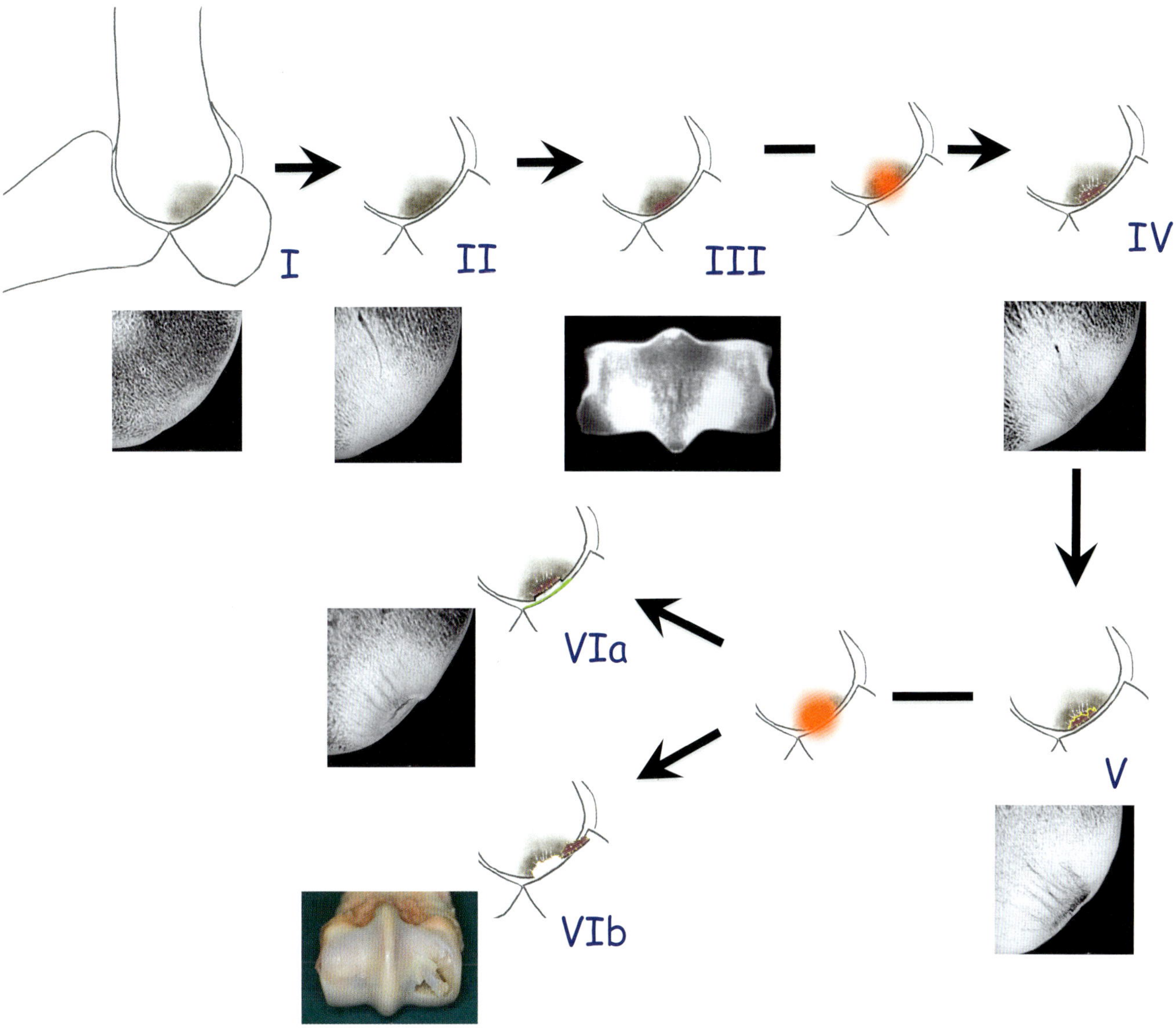

Fig 22.1 Line drawings supported by microradiographs in the parasagittal plane of the palmar quadrant of the medial condyle, computed tomographic slice in the transverse plane and gross image of the palmar articular surface plane of the distal condyles of third metacarpal bones from Thoroughbred racehorses, illustrating hypothetical pathogenesis of subchondral bone disease (Palmar Osteochondral Disease): I – relatively open, porous trabecular structure in a young horse that has undertaken minimal work; II & III – with exercise new bone forms on the trabeculae, progressively filling the vascular spaces and increasing apparent density (volume fraction) of the bone; IV – further exercise (and impact loading of the brittle bone volume) results in death of osteocytes and hypermineralization of bone tissue and early in-growth of new blood vessels; V – recruitment and activation of osteoclasts and focal resorption of damaged bone at the interface between living and dead bone (probably accelerated by a period of low strain – rest). Further intense exercise in the face of the localized porosity leads to either: VIa – collapse of more superficial, dead subchondral bone into the cavity, resulting in a depression at the articular surface, or: VIb – saucer fracture of undermined segment of subchondral bone.

Microradiographs courtesy of Professor Alan Boyde, Barts and The London School of Medicine and Dentistry, Queen Mary University of London.

training strategies, but can also be present when the warning signs in the two year old are ignored, and training is continued. Consequently, these horses are more difficult to manage; long periods of rest from training might result in partial resolution of the sclerosis, but there is a degree of bone change in some horses which appears to be irreversible, irrespective of the length of time off. In some horses, lameness returns as soon as high speed training is resumed, presumably due to abnormal forces as a result of the conformational defect. Corrective shoeing to help balance loads on the limb, particularly with carpal valgus and 'offset' knees, may help. Careful selection of training surface and avoidance of firm ground can help in some cases also.

Subchondral bone disease of the distal condyles of the third metacarpal and third metatarsal bones

Recognition

Presentation

Progressive disease of the bone underlying the articular surface of the mid palmar/plantar aspect of the condyles of the third metacarpal and third metatarsal bones is extremely common in Thoroughbred racehorses.[2,4,5] Originally termed 'traumatic osteonecrosis', it has more recently been referred to as 'palmar osteochondral disease'.[2] Lesions arise at the point of articulation with the basilar half of the proximal sesamoid bones when the joint is at full extension and are presumed to be due to excessive, repetitive stress at these points. A spectrum of pathology is seen, from faint bruising of subchondral bone, visible through the articular cartilage, to deep ulcers associated with saucer-shaped complete, displaced fractures of a 2–3 mm depth of articular cartilage and subchondral bone[5,6] (Fig. 22.4). It is assumed that the different degrees of pathology represent varying stages of the same process. In addition, lameness in which the only related findings are pain localized to the distal condyles of the third metacarpal or metatarsal bone, associated with IRU in the palmar/plantar condyles of these bones is extremely common. It is likely that this is part of the same syndrome.

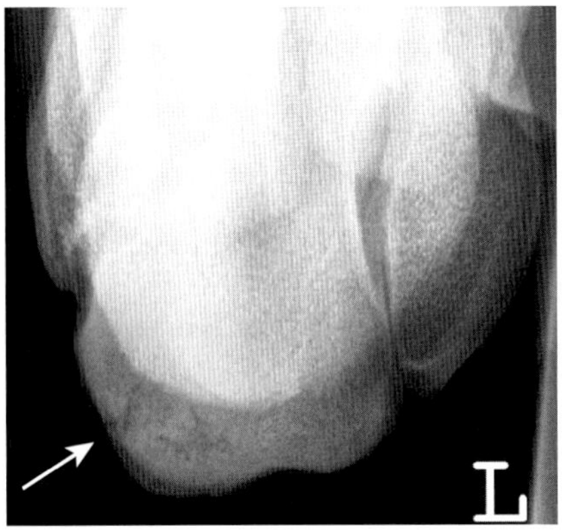

Fig 22.2 Flexed dorsal 60° proximal-dorso distal oblique radiograph of the left third carpal bone. The radial facet has lost it's normal trabecular pattern when compared to the adjacent bones as a result of hyper-mineralization, and lucent areas representing bone necrosis and/or resorption are evident within it. There is a non-displaced irregular sagittal fracture in the center of this area of abnormally 'stiff' bone, extending from the dorsal cortex towards the center of the third carpal bone (white arrow).

Lesions are more common and progress to a greater extent in the medial condyles of the third metacarpal bone and lateral condyle of the third metatarsal bone.[7] However, the clinical condition commonly occurs bilaterally or quadrilaterally and this is reflected in the pattern of gait abnormality seen. Associated lameness is typified by a shortened protraction of each limb at the trot, a low limb flight and a lack of animation or 'bounce' in the gait. Low limb flight and increased pelvic excursion seen with bilateral metatarsal disease often leads to the horse catching its toes, giving a characteristic wear pattern to the feet.

Riders often report that affected horses feel 'wrong' behind and describe that they are not pushing during exercise. These horses also have a characteristic gait at the canter where they will often 'bunny hop' for the first few steps as they break into that gait.

Occasionally a severe bone injury occurs unilaterally causing single leg lameness, although some form of unilateral angular limb deformity almost always accompanies this.

Diagnosis

Early stages of the disease are associated with few clinical signs other than lameness and there is little heat or effusion of the affected

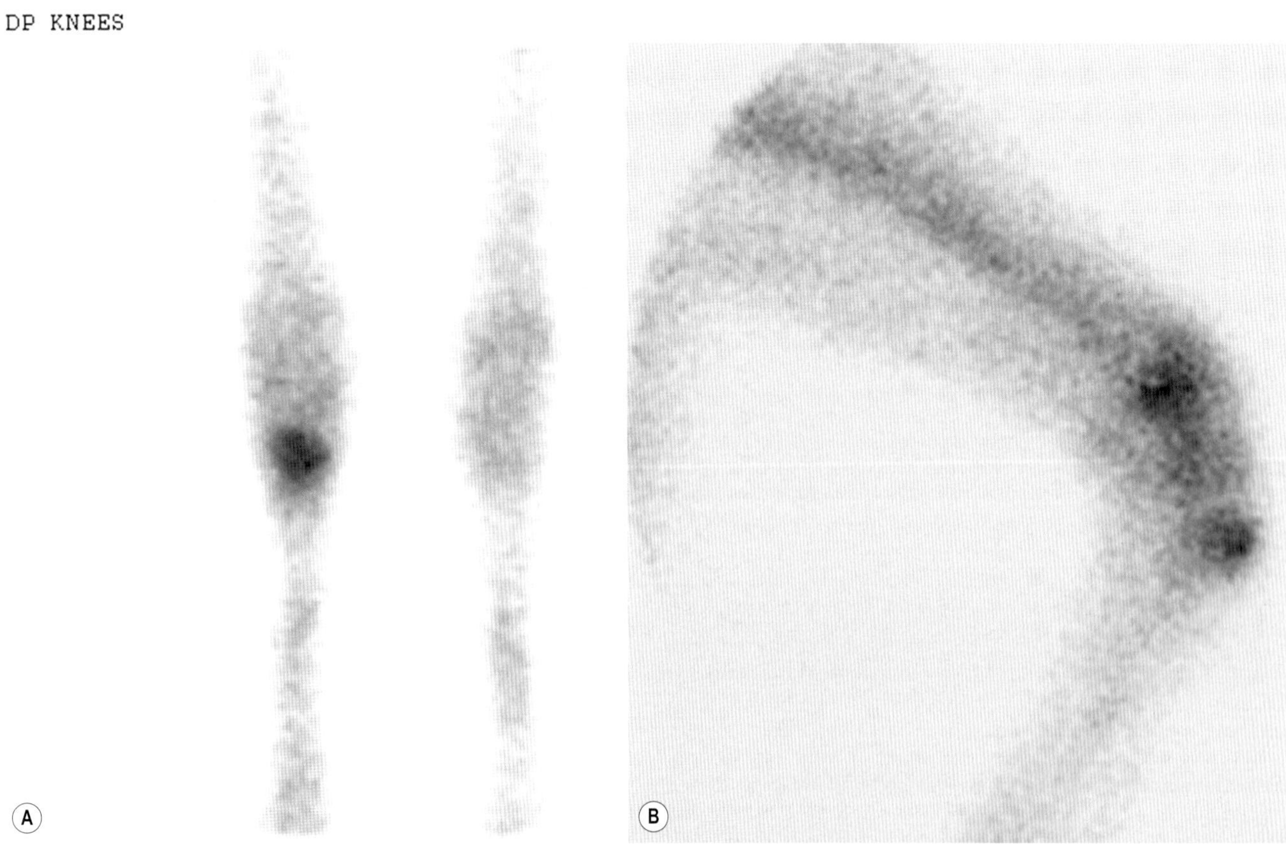

Fig 22.3 **(A)** Dorsal scintigraphic view of the carpi. There is focal intense IRU in the medial aspect of the third carpal bone of the right knee (left image) typical of that seen in fracture in the site of hyper-mineralized bone in the radial facet. **(B)** A flexed lateral view is useful in confirming that this is in C3 and not proximal Mc 3.

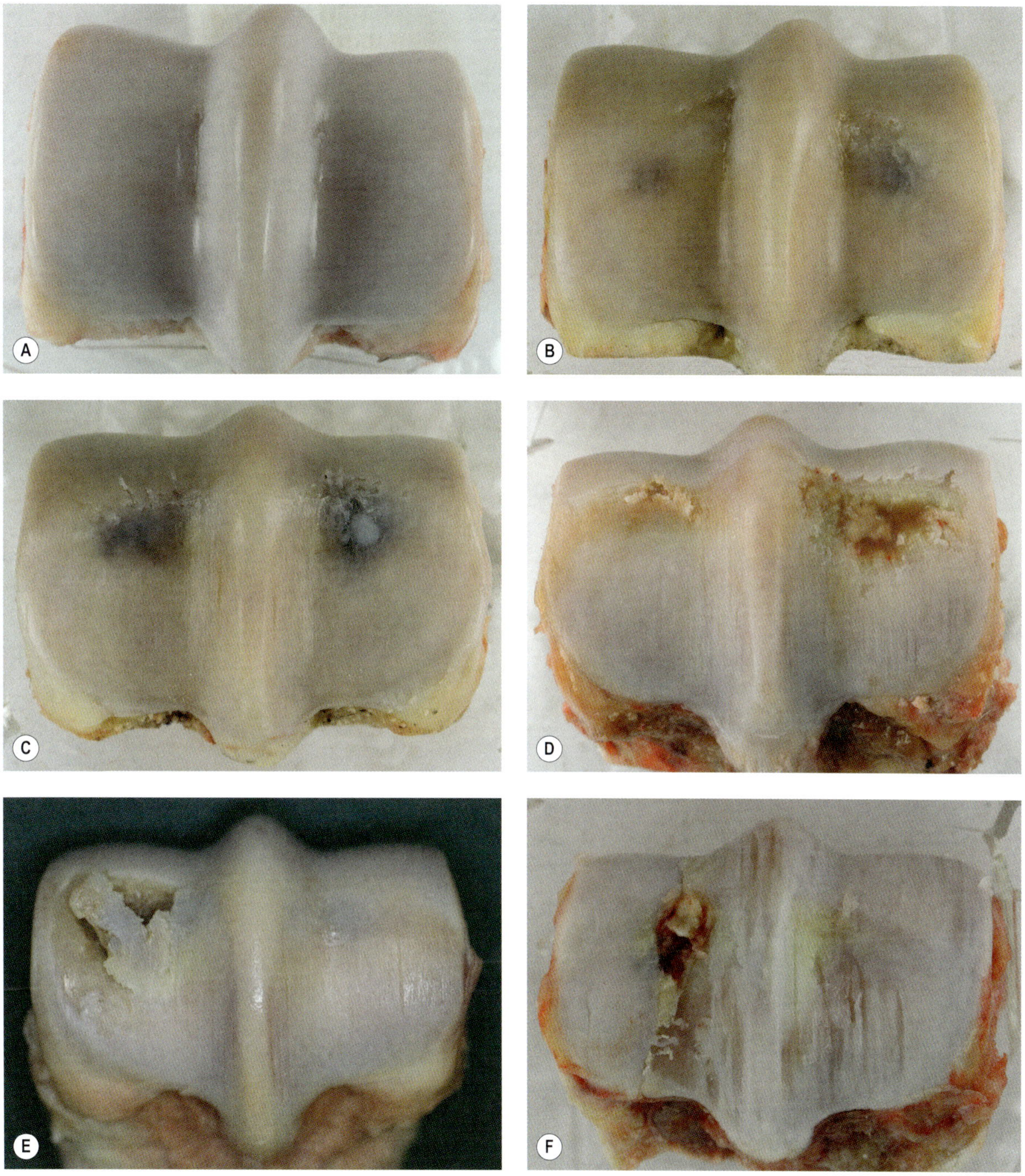

Fig 22.4 Gross images of the palmar aspect of the distal condyles of the third metatarsal (22.4a, b) and third metacarpal (22.4c, d, e, f) bones of Thoroughbred racehorses illustrating a spectrum of pathology associated with osteonecrosis of subchondral bone in the palmar aspect of the condyles. **(A)** Six-year-old gelding; lateral to the right. Normal appearance to subchondral bone in both condyles but faint linear fissures visible in medial and lateral condylar grooves. **(B)** Seven-year-old gelding; lateral to the right. Bruising of subchondral bone visible through intact overlying articular cartilage. Grade I palmar osteochondral disease (POD) lesion medial condyle, Grade II POD, lateral. There is a small linear fissure in the medial condylar groove. **(C)** Seven-year-old gelding, lateral to the right. Grade II POD lateral condyle and Grade I POD medially. There is localized fibrillation of articular cartilage in the region of the transverse ridge in both condyles. There are multiple, marked wear lines in the articular cartilage overlying both condyles and the sagittal ridge. **(D)** Seven-year-old gelding, lateral to the left. Grade III POD medial condyle associated with severe disruption of the articular surface with complete ulceration of articular cartilage and a deep cavity in the underlying subchondral bone, which is filled with fibrin. Focal erosion and tearing of articular cartilage overlying the transverse ridge in the lateral condyle. There are multiple, marked wear lines in the articular cartilage overlying both condyles and the sagittal ridge. **(E)** Five-year-old gelding, lateral to right. Grade III POD medial condyle associated with incomplete saucer fracture of superficial bone and articular cartilage overlying a large defect deeper in the subchondral bone (note that the articular cartilage overlying the fracture fragment is intact). Grade I POD lateral condyle. There are multiple, marked wear lines in the articular cartilage overlying both condyles and the sagittal ridge. **(F)** Four-year-old gelding. Lateral to the left. Complete lateral condylar fracture (one month after surgical repair) associated with a Grade III POD lesion lateral condyle. There are multiple, marked wear lines in the articular cartilage overlying both condyles and the sagittal ridge.

joint. Sometimes a mild pain response on flexion can be elicited. Perineural anesthesia will localize pain to the fetlock region: a four- or six-point block above the fetlock joint will usually give partial or complete resolution of the lameness. Intra-articular anesthesia often improves but does not abolish lameness. Deeper subchondral bone may be partially innervated by nerves leaving the bone at the nutrient foramen. This may explain why some horses, which improve to low 4- or 6- point blocks, are only rendered sound by sub-carpal or sub-tarsal anesthesia.

In horses showing bilateral lameness, very often blocking the medial and lateral palmar metacarpal/tarsal nerves alone, adjacent to the 'button' of the splint (two point block) will abolish most of the pain from the condyles and reveal a marked to moderate degree of lameness in the contralateral limb.

Radiography is unrewarding at early stages of the disease. Attempts to demonstrate sclerosis of subchondral bone in the palmar or plantar aspect of the condyles is hampered by superimposition of other radiopaque structures. Dorsal 45° proximal 45° lateral-plantarodistomedial oblique and the opposite oblique projections[8] provide a relatively unobscured image of a small area of each respective condyle and can demonstrate structural changes associated with increased bone volume fraction in some cases (Fig. 22.5). In more advanced cases of disease that are associated with defects in the subchondral bone plate created by collapse or ulceration of the subchondral bone, crescent shaped radiolucent defects can be identified on lateromedial or flexed dorsopalmar/plantar projections (Fig. 22.6). In these end stages of palmar osteochondral disease the joint surface can collapse or sustain a saucer fracture, leading to severe pathology of articular cartilage (Fig. 22.4). This almost always results in obvious signs of inflammation of the affected joint and is associated with profound lameness.

Scintigraphy

In early stages of the disease, when there are no appreciable radiographic findings, scintigraphy will reveal marked focal IRU in the region of the palmar/plantar condyles (Fig. 22.7). However, this is

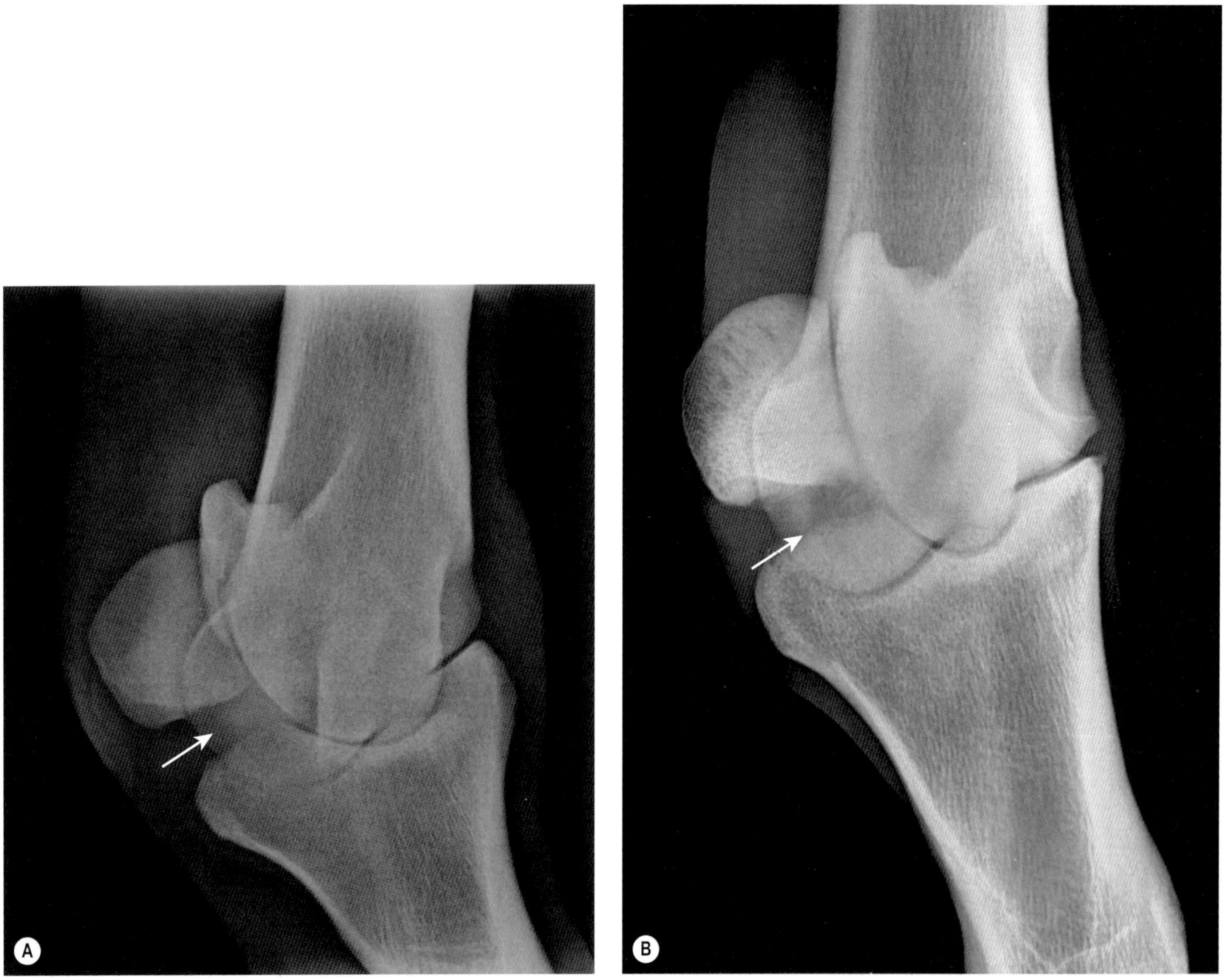

Fig 22.5 **(A)** Dorsal 45°proximal 45° lateral-plantarodistomedial oblique projection of the right hind fetlock. There is a large area of sclerosis (arrow) in the center of the lateral condyle typical of hyper-mineralization in this site as a response to focal repetitive bone stress. **(B)** The same projection in a more advanced case of plantar osteochondral disease, where subchondral bone necrosis has resulted in a focal lucent zone (arrow) in the center of the area of sclerosis.

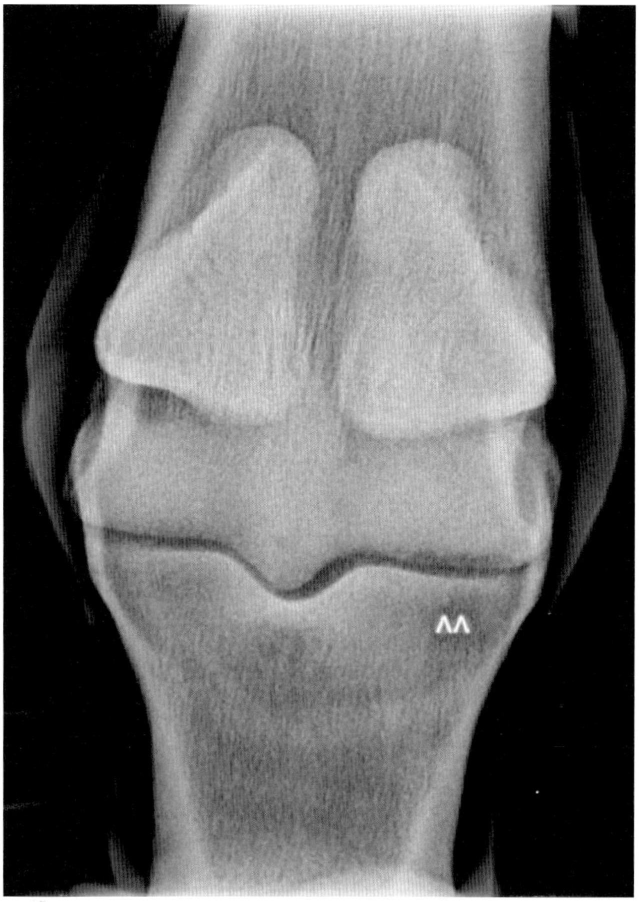

Fig 22.6 Flexed dorsal 125° distal-palmaroproximal oblique projection of the right fore fetlock. There is a broad area of irregular subchondral lucency extending over most of the medial condyle (white arrows), probably representing cartilage loss and subchondral bone resorption. This severity of change carries a poor prognosis for racing soundness.

also seen in horses that show no clinical signs of subchondral bone disease and so must be interpreted in light of clinical findings. The increased radiopharmaceutical uptake is focal and often intense and typically involves the lateral condyle in the hindlimb and the medial condyle in the front limb.[9] On a dorsal or plantar view, IRU in the distal condyles may easily be mistaken as originating from the proximal sesamoid bones because the outline of uptake is similar to the shape of these bones. However, a well-positioned lateral view will differentiate these two regions and confirm the anatomical location of uptake. Flexed lateral views of the hind leg and flexed dorsal views of the front leg aid considerably in identifying the precise location of observed I.R.U. (Fig. 22.7).

MRI Examination

Information obtained from MRI is revolutionizing our knowledge of structural changes in subchondral bone in response to exercise and as a consequence of injury. However, until MRI findings have been correlated fully with pathological studies and longitudinal investigations are performed to document the clinical significance of subtle findings, results from this modality must be interpreted with caution.

New bone formation resulting in increased density (volume fraction) of subchondral bone shows as focal areas of decreased signal on T1 weighted images. However, the area of signal loss often appears to occupy a greater volume of bone than is seen to be affected by *post mortem* studies, suggesting that something in addition to new bone is displacing fat.

There is an urgent need for far more normal racehorses, not showing overt lameness, to undergo MRI examination of the fetlock region in order to map the continuum of normal variation, but this is obviously difficult to justify to individual owners and trainers.

Management

Treatment is difficult and there is no one protocol that results in uniform resolution of lameness. Many different treatment regimes have been used including direct medication of the joint with

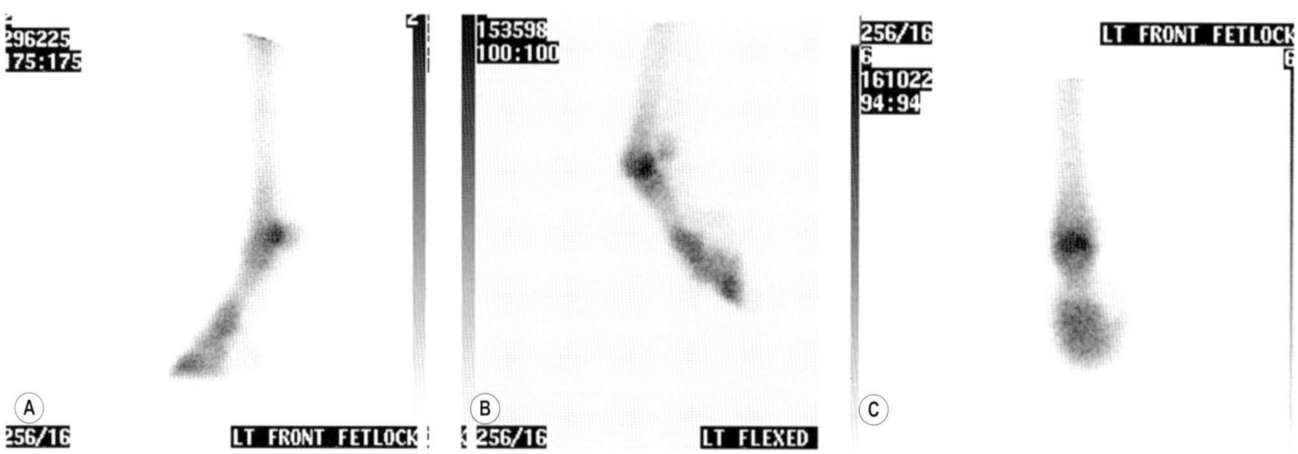

Fig 22.7 **(A)** Lateral view of the left front fetlock. There is intense focal IRU in either the proximal sesamoid bone, the palmar aspect of the condyles, or both. **(B)** The flexed lateral view of the same joint allows this IRU to be definitively located in the palmar condyle only, and likely to represent subchondral bone injury. **(C)** The flexed dorsal view shows that both condyles are affected, but that in this horse, unusually for a front fetlock, the lateral condyle (to the right) shows greater IRU than in the medial one. *(Courtesy of Sue Dyson, Animal Health Trust, Newmarket, U.K.)*

hyaluronan and/or corticosteroids, systemic medication with aspirin and with polysulfated glycosaminoglycans, and rest for varying periods of time.[10] Often the lameness resolves rapidly after a period of rest, but returns when the horse resumes fast galloping exercise, even after prolonged lay off and carefully managed return. Although some horses have been able to perform without further problems following rest, others have not, and predicting which horses may respond favorably is currently not possible. Cases in which radiolucent defects are seen radiographically in the subchondral bone of the palmar or plantar condyle usually remain lame. This does not mean that these horses cannot perform, and many racehorses seem to withstand training despite persistent lameness. However, this is often a performance-limiting problem that determines the level at which the horse can compete.

Limiting the amount of high speed exercise a horse undergoes, with alternate days swimming or using a horse walker or water-walker of some sort seems logical, given that we know the injury is linked epidemiologically to the number of furlongs horses have galloped and raced.[2]

Assuming that the spectrum of pathology identified represents the fact that the disease is progressive in nature and that once fracture or collapse of the articular surface occurs the prognosis deteriorates significantly, it is wise to advise a break from intense training as soon as the condition is diagnosed in two year olds and to allow at least three months of rest. This can consist of free paddock turnout if facilities for this exist.

Appropriate duration of rest is critical. While still unproven, there is circumstantial evidence that resorption is inhibited while the horse remains in work and only activated once the horse rests. There is a danger that return to exercise too quickly may predispose to saucer fracture of the articular surface as the area of diseased subchondral bone is undermined by the remodeling processes at its deeper surface (Fig. 22.1). The authors have experience of clinical cases that fit this model.

When the clinical syndrome first arises in a horse aged three or above, the prognosis appears to be worse than when in two year olds that were allowed to rest. End-stage structural changes are more common in older horses, although these horses may well have been trained through the problem at two years of age, with a low-grade bilateral lameness that was not recognized.

Some horses first show lameness associated with lesions that are usually in the lateral condyles of MtIII or medial condyle of McIII after a race on unsuitably firm ground. They are often described by trainers as 'jarred up'. Although clinical appearance of a jarred-up horse has long been recognized, no precise definition of the syndrome has ever been made. The syndrome may well represent multifocal subchondral bone pain. Affected horses sometimes never regain normal action. The reasons why some horses become progressively lamer while others can race with success and maintain a steady-state lameness are not understood.

A large study into palmar/plantar osteochondral disease (POD) in Thoroughbred racehorses at the Hong Kong Jockey Club (HKJC), which retrospectively correlated *post mortem* findings with clinical and race records revealed some interesting facts around the epidemiology of this example of subchondral bone disease:[11]

- The development of POD lesions was associated with longevity and fast work. In other words, to some extent, it is an occupational hazard of the racehorse and will have greater prevalence in older populations containing horses that have raced longer.
- POD was also associated with the total number of races that horses had taken part in and the total number of gallops in the most recent season.
- There was a decreased risk of POD when a horse had an interval of greater than six weeks out of work in the most recent season prior to euthanasia, which may hint at the possibility of partial healing and resolution in some of these cases.
- What was even more interesting is that for the horses that had the most severe lesions, there were other horses in the cohort group that had raced just as much and performed just as much high-speed exercise, but which had never gone on to develop significant lesions. This suggests some form of inherent variability between horses, either in conformation or the actual constitution of the bone and cartilage, which allows one horse to race on throughout a long career with no problems and yet another horse to end its career with an area of collapsing osteonecrotic bone in the end of the cannon bone. Given the high prevalence of this condition in Thoroughbred racehorses answers to these questions are worthy of further pursuit.

Stress fractures

Stress fractures are most common in horses undergoing a rapid increase in exercise speed and intensity. Consequently, affected animals are usually young, although these injuries will occur in any age class of horse subjected to sudden increases in loading. For this reason, they are also common in horses such as National Hunt racehorses, which have a cyclical training pattern (pasture turnout in the summer followed by intensive race training in the winter) or in horses returning to training after a significant period of lay off.

Many stress fractures present as acute onset lameness, although the changes that lead to the eventual failure of the bone have been taking place over many days or weeks before this. For this reason, it is not uncommon for horses to show subtle gait deficits, or pain on response to palpation of the affected region, for some time preceding the fracture.[12] Stress fractures occur at predilection sites in the skeleton, which makes their diagnosis more straightforward, although the fact that prodromal changes often arise bilaterally can make the use of comparative diagnostic images between contralateral limbs misleading.[8] Even when the pathology is bilateral it will often lead to a unilateral lameness because the lesions develop at different speeds in each limb.[13]

Thoracolumbar spine

Location

Haussler and co-workers first demonstrated that stress fractures in the thoracolumbar spine are relatively common in Thoroughbred racehorses.[14] Although marked changes were often present on routine necropsy, affected horses had not been diagnosed as clinical cases in training, suggesting that the injury often goes undiagnosed. The predilection site is the laminae of the lumbar vertebrae, which show a range of pathology from marginal new bone formation to complete fracture.

Clinical signs and diagnosis

Unilateral thoracolumbar stress fracture can result in ipsilateral hindlimb lameness, but more commonly the horse presents with a gait where hind limb propulsion is lacking. The horse trots with shortened protraction and with the back 'hunched up'. Plaiting of the hind limbs may be observed but this is common with many other causes of hind limb lameness. Clinical examination will often reveal a profound guarding response to palpation of the lumbar spine. However, this is also common in racehorses, particularly those carrying a degree of lameness for other reasons, in which secondary back pain in the longissimus muscles of the lumbar spine is a frequent sequel. Radiography in this site is impractical and the diagnosis is most consistently achieved by scintigraphy of the lumbar spine and pelvis (Fig. 22.8). Ultrasonographic examination of the lumbar facet joints can show the presence of callus as a 'cauliflower' shaped dome of bone obscuring the normally sharp 90° angle of the laminae and lateral facet joints.

Pelvis

Location

Predilection sites in the pelvis include the ilial wing approximately 5–10 cm from the tuber sacrale, the tuber coxa, the ilial shaft and the ischium. While fractures may arise at these locations due to trauma, they also arise in association with pre-existing bone pathology. By far the commonest presentation is that of sagittal plane fracture of the ilial wing. These injuries can vary from a complete displaced comminuted fracture with obvious ventral displacement of the tuber sacrale, to an incomplete stress fracture represented by periosteal new bone on the surface of the pelvis (Fig. 22.9).

Clinical signs and diagnosis

Lameness can vary from mild shortening of protraction of each hindlimb (similar to the appearance of a horse with exertional rhabdomyolysis or ER), through stiffness at the trot and a roached back appearance to non-weight-bearing lameness. Often the tail is held awkwardly and to the side. These horses will show pain, 'guarding', and muscle fasciculation on firm palpation over the fracture site, just as in cases of ER. Sometimes muscle enzymes will also be mildly elevated further confounding the diagnosis.

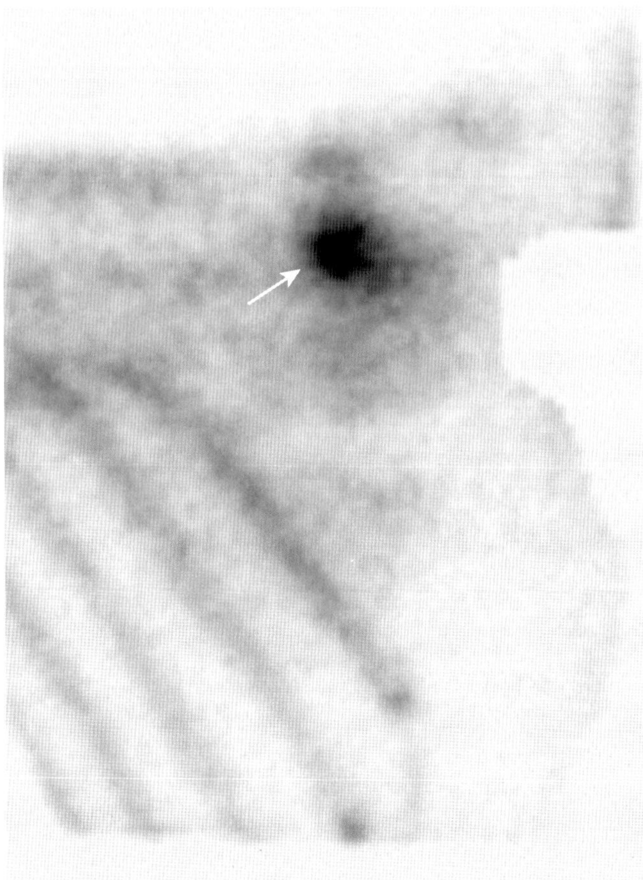

Fig 22.8 Lateral oblique scintigraphic image of the caudal lumbar spine (cranial is to the left). There is marked focal IRU (arrow) in the site of the vertebral articulation of L3/4 in the site typical of vertebral laminar stress fracture.

In cases of unilateral pelvic stress fracture, the lameness can vary from mild to non-weight bearing depending on the exact structure affected and its degree of damage and displacement. Displaced stress fractures of the ilial shaft will present with the most profound lameness, with the horse often unwilling to bear any weight on the limb and hopping on three legs when forced to move. Stress fracture of the ischium is usually associated with swelling on the caudal aspect of the quarter with a central depression. Over time this depression becomes more pronounced and the contour of the back of the thigh changes to a 'stoved in' appearance compared to the other limb. This can be best assessed from the side with the tail held elevated by an assistant. Affected horses are often unwilling to allow the heel of the limb to sink to the ground during weight-bearing, presumably as a consequence of pain associated with load-bearing on the 'hamstring' muscle group. Pain can often be elicited by direct palpation of ischial and ilial wing fractures externally.

Ilial shaft fractures often result in a profound guarding response to palpation of any part of the pelvis and can sometimes be appreciated per rectum either as a swelling associated with haemorrhage along the inner surface of the ilial shaft or as crepitis when the horse is rocked gently from side to side with the hand and arm present within the rectum.

Ultrasonographic examination of the surface of the ilium is quick and easy to carry out[15] and will confirm a variety of changes from periosteal callus to step displacement of the fracture or the presence of comminuted fragments (Fig. 22.10). Ultrasound is also useful for investigating ischial fractures, where a consistent finding is loss of the normally smooth semicircular outline of the ischium.

Scintigraphy is an important adjunct to investigation of pelvic fracture and will often help in planning of convalescence by alerting the clinician to comminution and displacement (Fig. 22.11).

Scapula

Location

Scapula fractures are relatively infrequent accounting for 2% of Thoroughbred and 6% of Quarter Horse racehorse musculoskeletal fatalities in California.[16] Predilection sites have been identified and are frequently identified by periosteal callus on necropsy.[17] The commonest site involves the neck of the scapula. Pathological change is first noted at the level of the distal limit of the scapula spine and involves intracortical resorption associated with periosteal new bone formation. This may eventually progress to transverse fracture at the same location. In some cases, the fracture extends in the frontal plane into the glenoid.

Clinical signs and diagnosis

Although early pathological changes are frequently present at the predilection site in both forelimbs lameness is usually unilateral. Lameness is normally marked (grade 3–4 out of 5) and protraction of the limb at the walk is usually shortened. Horses will often object to forced manipulation of the shoulder, particularly abduction. Diagnostic analgesia is usually not of use and is probably contraindicated because of the risk of propagation and comminution of a fracture during forced locomotion. Scintigraphy is the most sensitive tool for detecting these cases as they characteristically show marked IRU associated with the distal scapula spine and

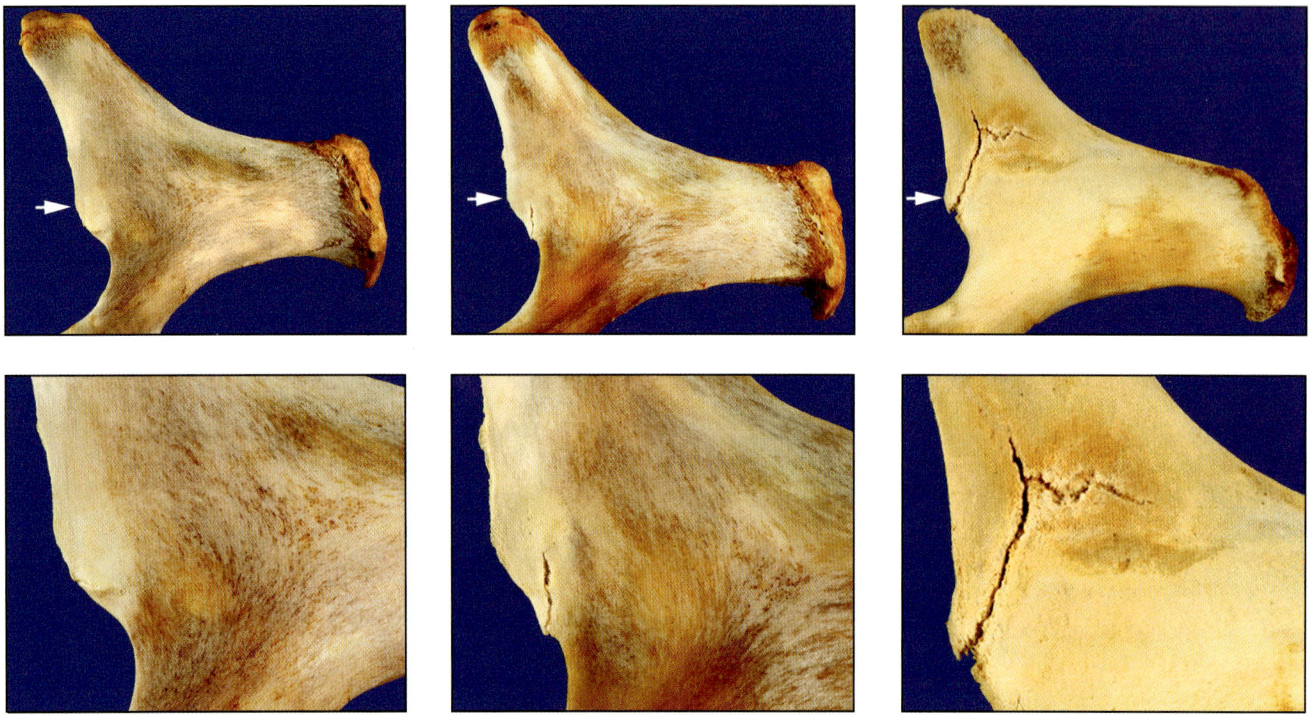

Fig 22.9 Dorsal (top row) and close-up, (bottom row) photographs of the right ilial wing of three horses illustrating mild, moderate and severe examples of stress fracture in the typical predilection site adjacent to the sacroiliac joint 'clamp', the point where maximal bending of the bone 'blade' takes place during propulsion.

*From Haussler K.K. and Stover S.M. (1998) Equine Vet J, **30**, 374-381, courtesy of Sue Stover, University of California, Davis, U.S.A. and the Equine Veterinary Journal.*

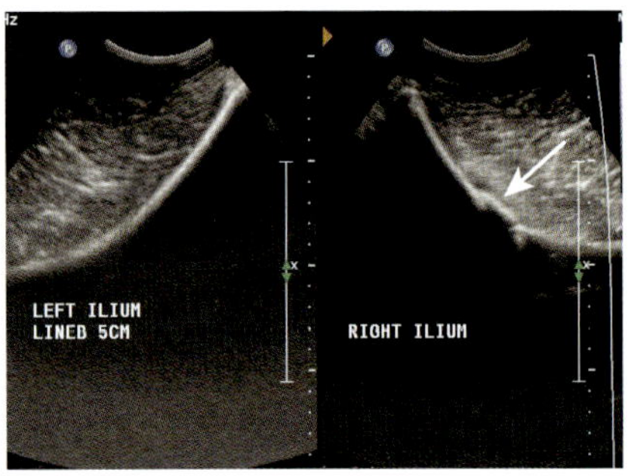

Fig 22.10 Percutaneous ultrasound scan of the right and left ilial wings obtained using a 5 MHz sector scanner. The left ilium shows the normal smooth surface curve extending from tuber sacrale dorsally out towards the tuber coxa laterally (left image). The right ilium (right image) shows two step-defects in the bone surface and irregular periostial callus (arrow) at the site of a slightly displaced complete ilial wing stress fracture.

supraspinous fossa. Radiography is often unhelpful because of the lack of a specific projection to highlight periosteal new bone on the scapula spine. Ultrasound however can be utilized and was useful in one case series in confirming half of the cases.[18] Ultrasonographic findings of use were minimally displaced cortical fracture and irregular periosteal new bone formation at the predilection site on the distal scapula spine. Some cases also showed haematoma formation associated with the stress fracture in the distal scapula supraspinous fossa.

Humerus

Location

Humeral stress fractures are relatively common in racehorses. Predilection sites are:

- the proximocaudal aspect of the humerus, where periosteal new bone is often visualized radiographically, sometimes in association with indistinct incomplete fracture lines and,
- the cranial and caudal cortex of the distal humerus just proximal to the elbow joint.[19]

Return to training after a period of more than eight weeks rest has been documented as a significant risk factor for these injuries.[20] Under these circumstances, fractures may occur even when the horse's exercise is limited to canter only.

Clinical signs and diagnosis

Lameness is usually moderate to marked (grade 3 to grade 5 out of 5) and acute in onset. The horse walks with a significantly shortened cranial phase to the stride and unwillingness to fully flex the proximal limb results in dragging of the toe in some cases. Clinical examination often reveals an unwillingness of the horse to allow forced protraction of the limb with the hand firmly placed on the shoulder joint, although direct palpation of the humerus is often unremarkable. As with other stress fractures, lameness may diminish rapidly within a few days of rest. Scintigraphy has a high sensitivity for detection of humeral stress fracture and, given the catastrophic consequence of complete fracture of this bone, should be carried out in any racehorse showing relevant clinical signs. Marked IRU is usually seen only in the common predilection sites already discussed.

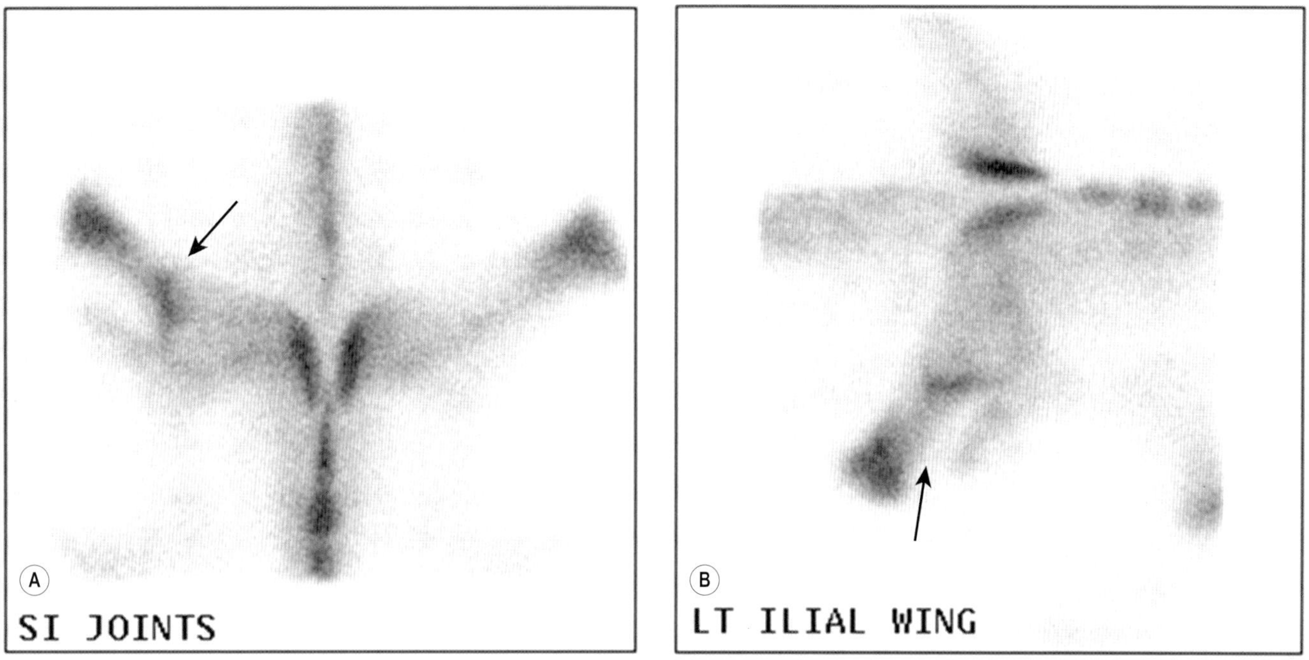

Fig 22.11 (A) Dorsal scintigraphic image of the pelvis (cranial is to the top). There is a focal sagittal 'band' of IRU just lateral to the sacroiliac joint (arrow) and an irregular defect in the ilium caudolateral to this. **(B)** Dorsal 45° lateral oblique view of the left ilium (cranial is to the left). This view confirms that this is a comminuted displaced fracture, with a large fragment (arrow) pulled away from the ilium by the distractive forces of the gluteal muscle mass.

Tibia

Location

Stress fractures commonly occur in the tibia especially in the naïve two year old at one of three predilection sites (Fig. 22.12):

1. the caudolateral cortex, approximately 7–10cm distal to the tibial plateau. This fracture can occur in any age class but is particularly common in two year olds. Radiolucent 'cracks' in the lateral cortex, at 45° to the long-axis of the bone, can sometimes be seen on caudocranial or slightly oblique caudocranial radiographic projections but more often there is abundant, loose, 'fluffy' periosteal new bone present at this site
2. mid-diaphysis. Although fractures at this location can occur in any age class, they are more common in the older horse. They are characterized by endosteal new bone formation and, occasionally, incomplete unicortical fracture lines can be visualized
3. the caudal cortex of the distal tibia, approximately two thirds down the length of the bone. Stress fracture in this site is usually associated with marked sclerosis extending endosteally from the caudal cortex, best visualized on the lateromedial projection. In addition, an indistinct linear fracture line may be visualized on a caudocranial or slightly oblique caudocranial projection.

Clinical signs and diagnosis

These fractures usually present with acute lameness, the degree of which varies with the fracture configuration and site. Lameness will often diminish significantly after a few days of stable rest only to return immediately on cantering exercise. Pain can often be elicited by direct palpation of the predilection sites (distal caudal tibia and proximolateral tibia) or by torsion of the tibia. Forced flexion of the hock will often result in profound unwillingness to bear weight for a few seconds in cases of fracture in the distal caudal cortex. Lesions often develop bilaterally and so affected horses may present with a stiff, short gait behind and, as with pelvic fractures, can closely mimic the typical gait of exertional rhabdomyolosis. Serum muscle enzymes in these cases will usually be normal. Another differentiating factor is that although cases of ER walk with a stiff action, they are not usually lame when forced to trot, whereas bilateral tibial stress fractures still show a markedly abnormal gait.

Diagnosis has been considerably enhanced by scintigraphy. IRU can be surprisingly mild for mid shaft and distal third lesions, but is usually intense in those occurring in the proximo-lateral cortex. Diagnostic analgesia is not helpful, and can even be misleading, in that the pain from mid to distal third cortical fractures can be abolished by tibial and fibular nerve blocks, which then tends to focus attention on the tarsus or below subsequently.

Carpus

Location

Osteochondral chip fractures of the dorsal margins of the carpal bones all arise as a consequence of fatigue damage to associated bone. The more severe example involves the third carpal bone, which usually presents as a frontal slab or, less commonly, sagittal fracture. Almost all horses that develop this injury show prodromal lameness linked to progressive, degenerative change of the subchondral bone at the fracture site.[21] Affected horses frequently have poor carpal conformation and suffer low-grade bilateral lameness leading up to fracture and so the horse may be classed simply as 'shuffly' or a poor mover.

Clinical signs and diagnosis

Fracture results in acute onset, severe, unilateral forelimb lameness with obvious effusion of the carpus, especially if the fracture is displaced. Complete, displaced fractures can be visualized on almost all radiographic projections but incomplete fractures of the

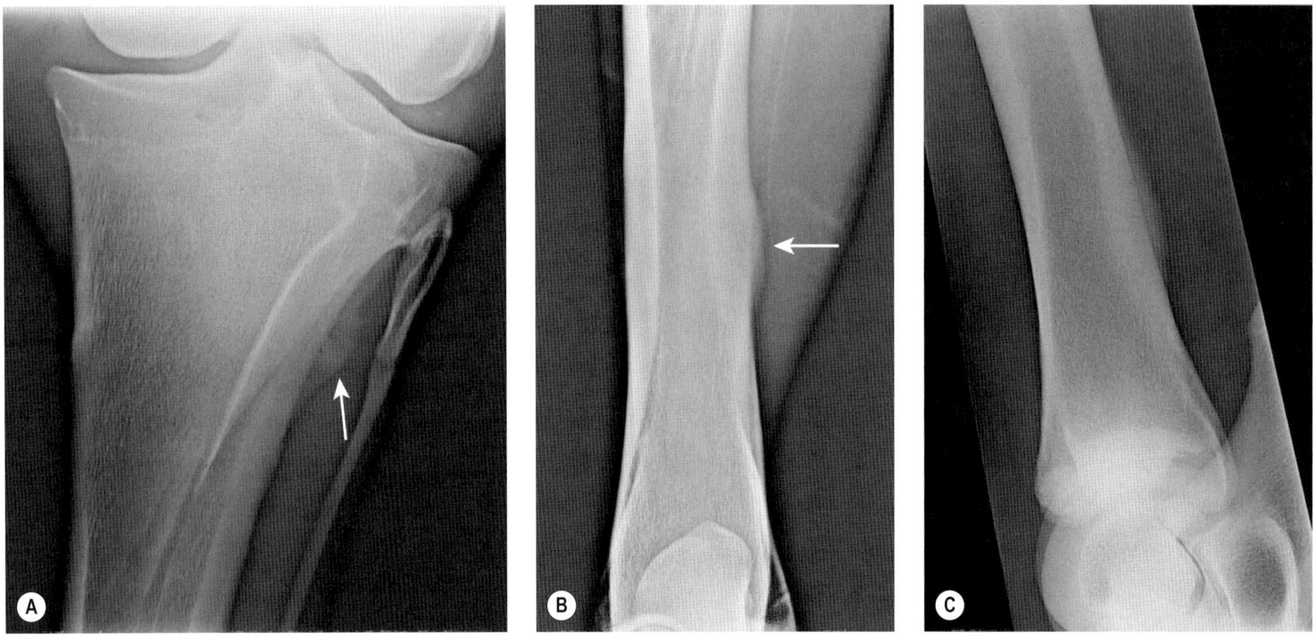

Fig 22.12 The three main areas of focal bone strain (and therefore of the development of stress fracture) in the equine tibia. **(A)** Proximolateral cortex 8–10 cm from the femorotibial joint surface (arrow) : this is the most common site for stress fracture in the naïve two year old, but fractures can also occur here in older horses. (Caudocranial projection of the right tibia, lateral is to the right) **(B)** Mid lateral cortex: stress fractures here are associated with both endosteal and periosteal new bone formation as in this case, and frequently show a fine tangential fracture line in the cortex (arrow). (Caudocranial projection of the right tibia, lateral is to the right.) **(C)** Distal caudal cortex situated approximately 3/4 of the distance between the femorotibial and tarsocrural joints. These stress fractures are best visualized on the lateromedial projection, and are typified by endosteal and periosteal new bone formation. Fracture lines can sometimes be seen in the middle of the zone of sclerosis so produced on the caudocranial projection, or on lesion-oriented oblique projections just medial or lateral to true caudocranial. (Lateromedial projection of the left tibia, caudal is to the right)

Figures 12a and 12b courtesy of Gaynor Minshall, Newmarket Equine Hospital, U.K.

third carpal bone are often only visualized on the flexed dorsal 60° proximal-dorsodistal oblique ('skyline') projection of the third carpal bone. This projection must be taken at an angle of 30 degrees to the horizontal in order to best visualize as much of the radial facet as possible. Associated changes usually include intense sclerosis of the subchondral bone forming the radial facet often with areas of resorption around the nutrient foraminae, in addition to the fracture line (Fig. 22.2).

Third metacarpal bone

Location

Repetitive strain injuries of the third metacarpal bone are most frequently associated with the dorsal or dorsolateral cortex, although stress fractures of the palmar proximal cortex and palmarolateral aspect of the distal diaphysis are increasingly being recognized.[22,23] Occasionally the latter two may culminate in the catastrophic failure of the bone.

Clinical signs and diagnosis

Stress fracture of the dorsal/dorsolateral cortex may occur anywhere along the length of the bone and is usually associated with lameness after a high-speed exercise. Unlike generalized periostitis the pain response to palpation of the shin is usually localized and associated with focal swelling and heat. These fractures typically manifest as unicortical fissures running oblique to the long axis of the bone. They are more common in three-year-old Thoroughbreds. Radiography usually reveals a linear fracture line best visualized either on the lateral and lateral oblique projection or on the dorsopalmar projection, or can be seen by utilizing lesion oriented oblique projections a few degrees dorsomedial and dorsolateral of true dorsopalmar. If fracture lines are not evident, then they may well appear if radiography is repeated in two weeks. Alternatively scintigraphy is a sensitive modality for diagnosis of metacarpal stress fracture where the lesion will appear as a very marked intense focal region of IRU.

Stress fracture of the palmarolateral cortex of the distal metacarpus often present with lameness associated with painful, oedematous swelling over the lateral aspect of the distal metacarpus, which may be confused as cellulitis or bruising from a knock.[23] Early radiographic signs are subtle but the full extent of the fracture is often alarming once it becomes apparent. These fractures occasionally present catastrophically during fast work as complete, transverse fracture through the distal metaphysis.

Fractures of the palmar cortex of the proximal third metacarpal bone are also relatively frequent in association with fatigue injury at that site.[22] Recently pre-fracture change comprising bone marrow oedema like signal has been described from MRI studies in association with lameness, and the later development of obvious radiographic changes.[24]

Parasagittal fractures of the distal condyles of the third metacarpal bone and third metatarsal bones

Location

Condylar fractures frequently originate from pathological defects in the palmar aspect of the distal condyles of the third metacarpal or metatarsal bone. The majority involves linear fissures in the mineralized cartilage and subchondral bone, which arise in either the medial or lateral condylar groove[25] (Fig. 22.4A and Fig. 22.4B). The remainder originates from larger defects in the subchondral bone that are located more centrally within the condyle, associated with palmar osteonecrosis disease lesions (Fig. 22.4F).

Clinical signs and diagnosis

Presentation is always as acute onset lameness immediately during or following exercise. With non-displaced short incomplete fractures, the horse will often finish the exercise without evidence of lameness but become increasingly lame over the following 12 hours. Heat may be present in the joint, but synovial effusion is often absent. With complete non-displaced or complete displaced and comminuted fractures the horse will often pull up during the exercise because of profound lameness. There is normally swelling in the fetlock joint with a painful oedematous plaque along the distolateral aspect of the third metacarpal bone in cases of complete lateral condylar fracture. Medial condylar fractures have a tendency to propagate in a spiral fashion up the bone and are usually associated with a greater degree of lameness. They are more common in hind legs than front legs but both fracture configurations can occur in both legs. In the hind limb, lateral condylar fractures often originate more abaxial to the parasagittal groove than in the front limb and exit the lateral cortex quite distally, therefore producing a relatively small fracture fragment. This can present difficulties for fixation and stabilization.

Diagnosis

Complete displaced fractures are relatively easily diagnosed because of obvious pain on flexion of the fetlock joint, profound swelling of the joint as a result of haemorrhage and the presence of swelling associated with the displacement of fracture fragments. Short incomplete fractures can be difficult to diagnose. Lameness is usually abolished by perineural anesthesia of the palmar and palmar metacarpal nerves at the level of the distal extremity of the splint bone (four point block) but is usually not abolished by intra-articular analgesia of the fetlock joint, although some improvement may occur. Very often these fissures are only visible on the flexed dorsal 125° distal to palmaroproximal oblique projection of the metacarpophalangeal joint and plantar 60° proximal – dorsodistal oblique projection of metatarsophalangeal joint[4,8] Consequently, this projection should be included as routine among all radiographic studies of the racehorse fetlock joint. Even with these projections some short incomplete condylar fractures will show no evidence of their existence on radiography until two to three weeks after occurrence. Therefore, it is advisable that horses with acute onset lameness referable to the fetlock joint of the severity that could include incomplete condylar fracture are not returned to full training until such time has elapsed for any possible lesion to be visualized on repeat radiographs.

Scintigraphy is a sensitive detector of these injuries and can also be used to confirm the presence of a fracture in suspicious cases where radiography is inconclusive.

Magnetic Resonance Imaging (MRI) is sensitive at detecting incomplete fractures early in their course. Incomplete fractures appear as linear features with reduced signal on T1-weighted images and with increased signal on T2-weighted and short tau inversion recovery (STIR) images.[26] In addition, it provides critical, detailed anatomical information that is lacking from scintigraphy. However, details of the clinical relevance of the spectrum of MRI findings still need to be resolved. For instance, in one study in normal horses conducted to document the normal appearance of the fetlock joint on MRI scan, linear features with hypointense signal on T2-weighted images were documented in horses with no history of lameness.[27] Also, the common interpretation that large areas of reduced signal on T1 images of the palmar condyles of the third metacarpal bone are solely due to increased bone volume fraction doesn't always equate with anatomical findings, especially when markedly asymmetric between condyles.

A *post mortem* study on clinical fractures of the distal condyles of the third metacarpal/metatarsal bone, using material from racehorse fatalities from the UK racing authorities, compared MRI findings with those from gross examination of the same bones.[28] This showed good correlation between the presence of fracture and the dorsal extent of increased bone density of the palmar/plantar condyles, as seen on MRI images of the condyles in the sagittal plane. This was present equally in both the fracture limb and the contralateral limb, implying that MRI screening could have been used to detect the horses most at risk of bone failure. Hyperintense signal in the distal condyles on T2-weighted and STIR images are usually thought to be consistent with replacement of fat with other sources of hydrogen ions and is a finding of concern because of the likelihood of impending, radiographically silent osteochondral failure. Studies conducted over the next few years should help to place the changes we see on MRI scan in these cases along a clinical continuum from 'normal' to 'at great risk', which could be a valuable tool in the management of horses at risk of pathology in this region.

Fractures that originate away from the condylar groove are usually associated with ulcerative lesions associated with osteonecrosis of the subchondral bone. Consequently, there is frequently fragmentation of the articular margins and ulceration of articular cartilage on the surface of the proximal sesamoid bone that apposes the site of lesion. This considerably worsens the prognosis for these cases even following surgical fixation.

Proximal sesamoid bones

Association between transverse fracture of the mid body or base of the proximal sesamoid bones and focal lytic defects in the palmar aspect of the bones has been reported.[29] The inference is that tissue in the palmar (tension) cortex is subject to excessive cyclical loading and undergoes fatigue damage and focal resorption, resulting in risk of fracture along the lines of the classic 'stress fracture' model. Currently there is minimal data to support this hypothesis although clinicians should be aware of the possible etiology of these potentially catastrophic injuries. Repeat radiographic studies, focused on the palmar cortex, and/or scintigraphic studies are indicated in suspicious cases.

Sagittal fractures of the first phalanx

Location

Fracture configurations reflect the focal origin and progressive nature of this injury and vary from short fissures to every variant ending in multiple comminuted displaced and even compound fracture of the first phalanx. The fracture always originates in the sagittal groove, most commonly in the dorsal cortex.

This injury was for many years considered one of the few genuinely acute traumatic fractures of the racehorse; the result of one supraphysiological loading incident. This dogma has recently been questioned by the demonstration of prodromal changes in the first phalanx in lame horses on MRI examination, which were not visible on radiography.[30] However, whereas almost all cases of lateral condylar fracture show some prodromal gait abnormality or lameness prior to fracture, sagittal fractures of the first phalanx often occur in horses which have previously shown no observable sign of previous gait change.

Diagnosis

Complete fracture is generally straightforward to diagnose: the horse is non-weight bearing on the limb, the fetlock joint and pastern are swollen, there is profound pain on palpation and flexion of the joint and crepitus can be felt in cases where the fracture is comminuted. Incomplete fissures can present more of a diagnostic challenge, as there is often no swelling in the joint and limited pain on flexion. However, almost all of these horses will show a profound pain response to firm digital pressure on the dorsal midline of the proximal aspect of the first phalanx. Early radiographic findings of subchondral sclerosis, with the suggestion of faint linear sagittal lucency always underestimate the extent of the fracture. Consequently, follow-up studies, two to four weeks after the initial incident, should be routine if surgical fixation is not carried out, to reveal the full extent of fracture.

Conclusions

Research over the past 20 to 30 years has revealed the true aetiology and pathogenesis of the majority of injuries that affect the appendicular skeleton of horses that undertake intense race training. We now know that few fractures or joint injuries are truly spontaneous but, rather, the end result of progressive deterioration of focal areas of the skeleton. We understand that in nearly every case, there is a window of opportunity to modify the horse's training which would arrest the process and allow complete healing to occur. However, we still struggle to identify the changes early enough. On occasion, this is through ignorance or negligence and failure to apply routine techniques to their full effect (e.g. omitting a flexed dorso-palmar projection of the metacarpophalangeal joint during radiographic examination of a racehorse's fetlock.[31] On others it is because the changes are just too subtle to resolve with routine screening tools and more sophisticated imaging techniques, such as scintigraphy or MRI are not available, too expensive or simply inappropriate for use on large numbers of cases. Widespread screening of blood samples for biomarkers that indicate subtle but critical osteochondral pathology have been on the horizon for some time.[32] However, these have not yet attained a sensitivity or specificity to be of great practical value. Epidemiology has helped to identify patterns of management or training that predispose to injury which can be explained by histological studies (e.g. increased risk of fracture on resumption of high-speed exercise after a short period of rest explained by increased porosity of the bone associated with remodeling). Future studies may identity subtle differences in neuromuscular control that mildly but critically alter the pattern of loading on structures in the distal limb that predispose certain individuals to injury.

References

1. Johnson BJ, Ardans A, Stover S, et al. California racehorse post mortem program: a 4-year overview. Proc Am Assoc of Equine Pract 1994;40: 167–9.
2. Barr ED, Pinchbeck GL, Clegg PD, et al. Post mortem evaluation of palmar osteochondral disease (traumatic osteochondrosis) of the metacaro/metatarsophalangeal joint in Thoroughbred racehorses. Equine Vet J 2009;41:366 71.
3. Young A, O'Brien T, Pool R. Exercise related sclerosis in the third carpal bone of the racing Thoroughbred. Proc Am Ass Equine Pract 1988;34:339–46.
4. Hornof W, O'Brien T. Radiographic evaluation of the palmar aspect of the equine metacarpal condyles: a new projection. Vet Radiol 1980;21:161–7.
5. Pool RR. Pathologic manifestations of joint disease in the athletic horse. In: McIlwraith CW, Trotter GW, editors. Joint Disease in the Horse. 1st ed. Philadelphia: WB. Saunders Co; 1996. p. 87–104.
6. Riggs CM. Osteochondral Injury and Joint Disease in the Athletic Horse. Equine Vet Educ 2006;18:100–12.
7. Pinchbeck GL, Clegg PD, Boyde A, et al. Pathological and clinical features associated with palmar osteochondral disease of the metacarpo/metatarsophalangeal joint in Thoroughbred racehorses. Equine Vet J 2012; – *submitted for publication.*
8. Ross MW. Scintigraphic and clinical findings in the Standardbred metatarsophalangeal joint: 114 cases (1993–1995). Equine Vet J 1998;30: 131–8.
9. Trope GD, Anderson GA, Whitton RC. Patterns of scintigraphic uptake in the fetlock joint of Thoroughbred racehorses and the effect of increased radiopharmaceutical uptake in the distal metacarpal/tarsal condyle on performance. Equine Vet J 2011;43: 509–15.
10. Tull TM, Bramlage LR. Racing prognosis after cumulative stress-induced injury of the distal portion of the third metacarpal and third metatarsal bones in Thoroughbred racehorses: 55 cases (2000–9). JAVMA 2011;238:1316–22.
11. Pinchbeck GL, Clegg PD, Boyde A, et al. Horse, training and race-level risk factors for palmar/plantar osteochondral disease in the racing Thoroughbred. Equine Vet J 2012; – *submitted for publication.*
12. Hesse KL, Verheyen KL. Associations between physiotherapy findings and subsequent diagnosis of pelvic or hindlimb fracture in racing Thoroughbreds. Equine Vet J 2010;42: 234–9
13. Johnson BJ, Stover SM, Daft BM, et al. Causes of death in racehorses over a 2 year period. Equine Vet J 1994;26: 327–30.
14. Haussler KK, Stover SM. Stress fractures of the vertebral lamina and pelvis in Thoroughbred racehorses. Equine Vet J 1998;30:374–81.
15. Shepherd MC, Pilsworth RC. The use of ultrasound in the diagnosis of pelvic fractures. Equine Vet Educ 1994;6:223–7.
16. Stover SM, Murray A. The California Postmortem Program: leading the way. Vet Clin North Am Equine Pract 2008;24: 21–36.
17. Vallance SM, Spriet M, Stover SM. Catastrophic scapular fractures in Californian racehorses: pathology, morphometry and bone density. Equine Vet J 2011;43:676–85
18. Vallance SA, Lumsden JM, O'Sullivan CB. Scapular stress fractures in the Thoroughbred racehorse: eight cases(1997–2006). Equine Vet Educ 2009;21:554–9
19. O'Sullivan CB, Lumsden JM. Stress fractures of the tibia and humerus in Thoroughbred racehorses: 99 cases (1992–2000). JAVMA 2003;222:491–8
20. Stover SM, Johnson BJ, Daft BM, et al. An association between complete and incomplete stress fractures of the humerus in racehorses. Equine Vet J 1992;24:260–3.
21. Schneider RK, Bramlage LR, Gabel AA, et al. Equine Incidence, location and classification of 371 third carpal bone fractures in 313 horses. Vet J Suppl 1988;6:33–42.
22. Morgan R, Dyson S. Incomplete longitudinal fractures and fatigue injury of the proximopalmar medial aspect of

the third metacarpal bone in 55 horses. Equine Vet J 2012;44:64–70.

23. O'Sullivan CB, Lumsden JM. Distal third metacarpal bone palmar cortical stress fractures in four Thoroughbred racehorses. Equine Vet Educ 2002;14:70–6.
24. Powell SE, Ramzan PH, Head MJ, et al. Standing magnetic resonance imaging detection of bone marrow oedema-type signal pattern associated with subcarpal pain in 8 racehorses: a prospective study. Equine Vet J. 2010;42:10–7.
25. Riggs CM, Whitehouse GH, Boyde A. Pathology of the distal condyles of the third metacarpal and metatarsal bones of the horse. Equine Vet J 1999;31: 140–8.
26. Murray R, Werpy N. Image interpretation and artifacts. In: Equine MRI, editor. Murray RC: Wiley Blackwel; 2011. p. 101–46.
27. Smith MA, Dyson SD, Murray RC. The appearance of the equine metacarpophalangeal region on high-field vs. standing low-field magnetic resonance imaging. Vet Radiol Ultras 2010;52:61–70.
28. Parkin TD. Epidemiology of racetrack injuries in racehorses. Vet Clin North Am Equine Pract 2008;24(1):1–19.
29. Anthenill LA, Gardner IA, Pool RR, et al. Comparison of macrostructural and microstructural bone features in Thoroughbred racehorses with and without midbody fracture of the proximal sesamoid bone. Am J Vet Res 2010;71:755–65.
30. Ramzan PH, Powell SE. Clinical and imaging features of suspected prodromal fracture of the proximal phalanx in three Thoroughbred racehorses. Equine Vet J 2010;42:164–9.
31. Richard E, Alexander K. Nonconventional radiographic projections in the equine orthopaedic examination. Equine Vet Educ 2007;19:551–9
32. Frisbie DD, McIlwraith CW, Arthur RM, et al. Serum biomarker levels for musculoskeletal disease in two- and three-year-old racing Thoroughbred horses: A prospective study of 130 horses. Equine Vet J 2010; 42:643–51.

Pharmacotherapy of joint and tendon disease

23

Carl A. Kirker-Head   Hillary Feldmann

CHAPTER CONTENTS

Introduction

Pharmacotherapy describes the treatment of disease through the administration of drugs.[1] In the context of this chapter, drugs are chemical substances used to mitigate disease or otherwise enhance physical or mental wellbeing. This chapter excludes discussion of biologics which are also chemical moieties used to treat disease but more generally composed of sugars, proteins, nucleic acids or more complex combinations of these substances, including cells and tissues.[2]

Pharmacotherapeutic drugs are designed to assist the body in the healing process. They are an integral component of the combination therapy that veterinarians frequently prescribe for their patients that also utilizes rest, physical therapy and possibly surgery to ensure proper healing and restoration of function. An effective therapeutic plan is based on careful assessment of patient signalment, the history and duration, location, type, and severity of the injury, as well as the economics.

The common denominator in all equine athletic injuries is inflammation, which is a protective attempt by the organism to remove the injurious stimuli and to initiate the healing process. The cellular mediators and biochemical processes associated with inflammation prompt important beneficial effects such as pain which limits unwanted motion. However, inflammation also prompts deleterious effects, such as ongoing tissue destruction. The goal of pharmacotherapeutic intervention is, therefore, to control the cellular mediators and biochemical processes of inflammation such as to limit their deleterious effects, while attenuating pain, restoring function, and returning the horse to soundness with minimal loss of condition. A sound understanding of the mechanism of action, indications for use, effective dosages, drug interactions, toxicity, and expected results for the available veterinary drugs is essential. The goal of this chapter is to provide information pertaining to drugs used to treat the equine athlete with a joint or tendon disorder. The knowledge gained from this chapter should facilitate the optimum selection and application of the pharmacotherapeutic agents.

Anti-inflammatory drug therapy in horses

Anti-inflammatory medications are commonly administered to horses for the treatment of inflammatory and infectious diseases, and for traumatically- or surgically-induced injuries of the musculoskeletal system. The most commonly used anti-inflammatory drugs include corticosteroids and nonsteroidal anti-inflammatory drugs (NSAIDs), however, other drugs such as polysulfated glycosaminoglycans and hyaluronate are also believed to have anti-inflammatory effects. The NSAIDs are commonly administered systemically for their analgesic and inhibitory effects on inflammation, fever, and edema. Numerous NSAIDs are available with phenylbutazone, (PBZ), flunixin meglumine (FLM), and firocoxib (FCB) being most commonly used. Aspirin (ASP), ketoprofen (KTP), carprofen (CRP), dipyrone (DPN), meclofenamic acid (MFA) and naproxen (NPX) are examples of other NSAIDs used in horses. Although corticosteroids are rarely used systemically to treat musculoskeletal disease in horses, they are commonly administered locally, particularly in joints affected by synovitis and arthritis. Knowledge of the mechanisms of action, pharmacologic properties, pharmacokinetic behavior, and therapeutic and toxic effects of the medications will enable veterinarians to select the optimum anti-inflammatory pharmacotherapeutic regimen for their equine patients.

Nonsteroidal anti-inflammatory drugs

Nonsteroidal anti-inflammatory drugs represent a class of drugs that inhibit one or more of the pathways involved with the synthesis of prostaglandins (PGs) and thromboxanes (TBXs) from arachidonic acid. The principal mechanism of action is through inhibition of the enzyme cyclooxygenase (COX). Prostaglandins, particularly those of the E-series, are involved in synovial inflammation and depletion of proteoglycan from articular cartilage matrix.[3–4] There is substantial evidence to suggest that PGE_2 is the principal PG involved in joint degeneration. Synoviocytes and chondrocytes synthesize PGE_2 in response to exposure to lipopolysaccharide (LPS) and other inflammatory mediators, and increased concentrations of PGE_2 have been reported in the synovial fluid of horses with osteoarthritis.[5–6] Additionally, there is also evidence to suggest that PGs may modulate latent matrix metalloprotease release with resultant cartilage matrix degradation.[7–8]

Classification and mechanism of action

Nonsteroidal anti-inflammatory drugs are classified based upon their chemical structure into carboxylic and enolic acids. A majority of NSAIDs belong to the carboxylic acid group, while fewer are enolic acids. Many texts additionally divide NSAIDs into numerous and often confusing sub-categories based, for example, on their chemical properties, mode of action, or pharmacologic effect.[9] This text will focus instead on their cyclooxygenase enzyme (COX)-1, -2 and -3 selectivity.

Most NSAIDs have a similar mechanism of action as well as physical and chemical properties.[10–11] Nonsteroidal anti-inflammatory drugs inhibit the synthesis of prostaglandins (PGs) and thromboxanes (TBXs) from arachidonic acid by inhibiting COX. Most NSAIDs are also competitive COX antagonists; this mechanism of action of NSAIDs requires the continued presence of the active drug to exert the effect. Aspirin, however, is an irreversible antagonist that deactivates COX by acetylation. Because platelets are nonnucleated and thus do not have the capacity to synthesize new COX, ASP has a profound effect on platelet function.

There are at least two COX isomers, namely the constitutive (COX-1) found throughout the body and the so-called inducible (COX-2) isoforms.[9] The COX-1 isomer is the 'housekeeping' enzyme responsible for basal synthesis of PGs necessary for physiologic functions, including maintenance of vasomotor tone (intestinal mucosal and renal blood flow), prevention of platelet aggregation and adhesion and maintenance of gastric cytoprotection.[9] The COX-2 isomer is responsible for increased eicosanoid synthesis associated with inflammation and is induced by lipopolysaccharide (LPS), cytokines and other inflammatory mediators. However, the 'good' COX-1 versus 'bad' COX-2 dichotomy has proved overly simplistic. COX-2 has been shown to exert its own physiological effects, for instance in regulating renal blood flow[12] and GI mucosal integrity, especially in ulcer healing.[13–14] A third COX isoform, sensitive to acetaminophen and referred to as COX-3, COX 1b or COX-1 variant (because of its similarity to COX-1) has also been identified in some species including the dog.[13] The affinity for the COX isoforms varies among NSAIDs. Some are more potent inhibitors of COX-1, while some are relatively equipotent for their effects on COX-1 and COX-2, and others have a greater selectivity for COX-2. The COX-2/COX-1 ratio is a convention used to reflect the relative selectivity of an NSAID for the COX isomers.[9] Unfortunately, the convention can be confusing to the reader because the numerator/denominator values (COX-2/COX-1) actually reflect the IC_{50} for each isomer. The IC_{50} represents the concentration of a drug that is required for 50% inhibition in vitro.[9b] Hence, an NSAID with a COX-2/COX-1 ratio <1 is preferable in order to maximize the anti-inflammatory effects of the NSAID while minimizing the potential for toxic side effects. With that in mind, an array of COX-2 specific inhibitors, known as coxibs, have been developed and some have been used in horses. Currently, firocoxib (FCB) is the only COX-2 selective drug labeled for use in horses in the United States, while meloxicam (MLX), which is somewhat selective for COX-2, is approved for use in horses in Europe.[15] The concentration of firocoxib required to inhibit 50% of COX-1 activity in horses is reported to be >640 times that required to inhibit 50% of COX-2 activity.[16] Furthermore, concentrations of firocoxib that inhibit 80% and 50% of COX-2 activity in vitro (67 and 30 ng/mL, respectively) are readily achievable in equine plasma following oral administration at the label dose of 0.1 mg/kg.[17] The relative potency of the COX-2 versus COX-1 drugs as analgesics when administered at their approved dose rates has been the subject of debate. However, in a study that compared the efficacy and safety of FCB (0.1 mg/kg, PO, SID) and PBZ (~4.4 mg/kg, PO, SID) paste formulations administered for 12–16 days to 253 horses with chronic arthritis, the proportion of horses clinically improved on day 14 for the FCB group (104/123 [84.6%]) was not significantly different from the proportion for the PBZ group (103/119 [86.6%].[18] In a second study, when FCB was administered as an oral paste (0.1 mg/kg, PO SID) for 14 days to 390 horses afflicted with osteoarthritis, improvement was reported in approximately 80% by day 14.[19] Finally, when oral MLX (0.6 mg/kg) was administered to horses with induced intercarpal joint synovitis, lameness and joint effusion was alleviated compared to placebo-treated joints, as were synovial fluid biomarkers (PGE2, substance P, bradykinin, MMP), and some turnover markers of aggrecan (GAG) and type II collagen (CPII, C2C).[20]

Pharmacokinetics

Absorption

Peak plasma concentrations and the onset of action for NSAIDs after oral administration varies with the timing of administration relative to eating. Mean time to peak plasma concentration for PBZ (4.4 mg/kg PO) in ponies with access to hay was delayed 6 to 12 hours, compared with fasted ponies.[21] Phenylbutazone and other NSAIDs appear to bind to hay and other digesta, thus delaying time to peak plasma concentration. Fermentative digestion of roughage in the large intestine releases the bound drug, which possibly contributes to the propensity of NSAIDs to cause ulcerative disease in the large intestine.[10] The time to reach peak plasma concentration and the elimination half-life can be dramatically prolonged by the timing of administration relative to feeding. This has important clinical implications with regard to the therapeutic efficacy of an orally-administered NSAID as well as with potential problems related to horses in sanctioned competitive events.

There is conflicting data regarding the effects of feeding versus fasting on the absorption of MFA.[9,22] Horses with free access to feed had delayed absorption, decreased maximal plasma concentration, and delayed time to peak concentration, compared with fasted horses, administered FLM. Although it may not be practical, NSAIDs should be administered to horses that have not eaten for at least two hours before, and are withheld from feeding for two hours after, dosing in order to control absorption, time to peak plasma concentration, and elimination half-life.

Metabolism and elimination

Most NSAIDs undergo hepatic metabolism and either renal or biliary excretion. NSAIDs administered to lactating mares are not excreted in milk in concentrations yielding measurable plasma levels in foals. Phenylbutazone undergoes hepatic metabolism to yield oxyphenbutazone, the pharmacologically active metabolite, and γ-hydroxyphenylbutazone, an inactive metabolite. The parent compound and the two metabolites are excreted into the urine, and due to their acidic nature, excretion is more rapid in alkaline than acidic urine.[23–24] Aspirin (acetylsalicylic acid) is rapidly deacetylated to salicylate, the active metabolite of the parent drug. A paucity of data regarding metabolism of MFA exists for horses; it is known that conjugation occurs and between 10–14% is excreted in the urine after oral administration.[11] Although little is known regarding the elimination of FLM, it does not accumulate in the body and approximately 14% is excreted in urine.[11]

Naproxen undergoes hepatic metabolism and along with its principal metabolite, 2-(6-hydroxynaphthyl)propionic acid, are excreted in the urine in high concentrations.[25] Ketoprofen is used clinically as a racemic mixture of the R(−) and S(+) enantiomers with half-lives of 1.1 hours and 1.5 hours, respectively, after IV administration.[26] Ketoprofen accumulates in inflammatory exudates, resulting in substantially prolonged exudate half-lives of 19.7 hours and 22.6 hours for the R(−) and S(+) enatiomers, respectively. Similar to KTP, CRP is used clinically as a racemic mixture of the R(−) and S(+) enantiomers, each with different potencies and pharmacokinetics. There is evidence that the COX inhibitory and anti-inflammatory effects of carprofen are primarily attributable to the S(+) form. However, other evidence suggests that the R(−) enantiomer may be equipotent to the S(+) form as an analgesic and in some other activities such as inhibition of β-glucuronidase release.[27–28] Coincident with decreases in plasma concentrations, CRP accumulates in inflammatory exudates resulting in exudate levels exceeding plasma levels from 2 to 48 hours.[29]

Plasma protein binding

NSAIDs are highly (90 to 99%) bound to plasma proteins, thus, the free active fraction of these drugs is extremely small.[9] Concurrent administration of another highly protein-bound drug (eg, chloramphenicol, rifampin, barbiturates) can cause displacement of the NSAID resulting in an increased free active fraction.[9]

Effect of age on pharmacokinetics

The pharmacokinetics of NSAIDs varies with the age of the horse. The plasma half-life of IV PBZ (4.4 mg.kg) was longer for 8–10 year old adult horses and ponies (5.5 hours) than for three-year-old ponies (3.9 hours)[21]. NSAIDs have substantially different pharmacokinetic profiles in neonatal (<24 hours of age) foals compared with adult horses. In general, neonates have a reduced ability to eliminate NSAIDs, compared with adult horses, after a single IV dose[30–32]. The large volumes of distribution of NSAIDS in neonatal foals may necessitate larger initial doses, however, the relatively long half-lives suggests that the dosing interval should be extended to prevent accumulation of these drugs with resulting potential toxic side effects.

Effect of dose on pharmacokinetics

Unlike most NSAIDS, PBZ can have dose-dependent kinetics, with the half-life increasing from 4 to 8 hours when administered at a dose of 10 mg/kg.[33] This effect is likely due to saturation of hepatic enzymes responsible for PBZ metabolism. Taken together, the effect of dose and age on the pharmacokinetics of PBZ emphasizes the need for caution in the dose and dosing interval when administering this drug to older horses, especially those that are systemically ill or dehydrated.

Tissue kinetics

Phenylbutazone, like many NSAIDs, has dramatically different kinetic values for tissue compared with plasma.[9] The acidic nature and high protein binding of NSAIDs causes them to accumulate at sites of inflammation. For example, the plasma half-life for PBZ is between 4 and 8 hours, whereas the half-life in exudates is approximately 24 hours.[34] Ketoprofen accumulates in inflammatory exudates, and thus the half-lives of the R(−) and S(+) enantiomers are prolonged from 1.1 hours and 1.5 hours to 19.7 hours and 22.6 hours, respectively.[35] Similarly, CRP accumulates in exudates and yields substantially greater concentrations than in plasma between 2–48 hours after administration.[29]

Drug interactions

Concurrent administration of chloramphenicol reduces the clearance and increases the half-life of PBZ, which may accentuate both therapeutic and toxic effects. A single dose (25 mg/kg IV) of chloramphenicol prior to PBZ administration resulted in a significant decrease in the elimination rate, and this effect was accentuated by additional dosing of chloramphenicol.[36] Rifampin induces hepatic biotransformation processes and has been shown to increase the elimination rate of PBZ in horses.[36]

There are anecdotal reports that when PBZ is administered to horses anesthetized with thiobarbiturates increased depth and duration of anesthesia may occur due to competitive plasma protein binding.[37–38] A study evaluating administration of PBZ (8.8 mg/kg IV) nine minutes after thiamylal (11 mg/kg IV) demonstrated no effects of PBZ on thiamylal pharmacokinetic parameters or depth or duration of anesthesia.[39] However, there were changes in PBZ pharmacokinetics, including increased serum concentrations and decreased percentage protein bound PBZ. In another study, administration of PBZ (6.6 mg/kg IV) for four days prior to thiamylal anesthesia did not have a significant effect on recumbency time.[36] Therefore, it seems unlikely that perianesthetic administration of PBZ would alter the intensity or duration of anesthesia. It also seems unlikely that thiamylal administration would have a clinically important effect on the disposition of PBZ.

A study evaluating the pharmacokinetics of steady-state PBZ and single bolus gentamicin administered together revealed that gentamicin pharmacokinetics are altered by concomitant PBZ therapy, however, no effect of gentamicin was found on the pharmacokinetics of PBZ.[40] Gentamicin was administered as a 2.2 mg/kg IV bolus on the fourth day of once daily treatment with PBZ (4.4 mg/kg IV). Phenylbutazone induced a 49% increase in the rate of gentamicin return to the central compartment from peripheral tissues and the half-life and volume of distribution of gentamicin decreased 23% and 26%, respectively. There were no changes in PBZ pharmacokinetics induced by gentamicin. Because PBZ induces changes in the rate and extent of distribution and elimination of gentamicin, caution should be exercised when using this drug combination in horses.

Dosage regimen

The dose, interval, and route of administration for NSAIDs commonly used in horses are given in Table 23.1.[11,22,29,41–47]

Therapeutic uses

NSAIDs are indicated in horses with inflammatory conditions of the musculoskeletal system including tendonitis, myositis, desmitis, laminitis, osteoarthritis, synovitis/tenosynovitis, osteitis/osteomyelitis, septic arthritis, and surgically- or traumatically-

Table 23.1 Recommended dosage regimens for nonsteroidal anti-inflammatory drugs in horses†

DRUG	ROUTE	FORMULATION	DOSE	DURATION	REFERENCES
Acetylsalicylic acid (aspirin)	PO	Tablets, Powder	25–35 mg/kg BID 5–50 mg/kg SID		43 44
Dipyrone	IV, IM	Injectable	5–22 mg/kg 11.1 mg/kg QID		43 11
Firocoxib	PO	Paste	0.1 mg/kg, PO, SID		18
Flunixin meglumine	IV, IM PO	Injectable Granules, Paste	1.1 mg/kg SID-BID 0.25 mg/kg TID 1.1 mg/kg SID-BID	≤5 days	43 43–44 11, 43
Ketoprofen	IV	Injectable	2.2 mg/kg SID		41
Meclofenamic acid	PO	Granules	2.2 mg/kg SID then QOD	5–7 days	11, 22, 43–44
Naproxen	PO	Granules	10 mg/kg BID then SID	≤14 days	11, 43–45
Phenylbutazone	PO IV	Tablets, Powder, Injectable	4.4 mg/kg BID 2.2 mg/kg BID 2.2 mg/kg SID 2.2–4.4 mg/kg SID 4.2 mg/kg SID	1 day 4 days 2 days ≤5 days ≤4 days	11, 22, 43–44 11, 43–44 11
Carprofen	IV PO	Injectable Tablets	0.7 mg/kg SID 0.7 mg/kg SID		29, 46
Eltenac	IV	Injectable	0.5 mg/kg SID	3 days	338
Etodolac	IV	Injectable	23 mg/kg BID		42

PO = per os, IV = intravenous, IM = intramuscular, SID = once daily, BID = twice daily, TID = three times daily, QID = four times daily, QOD = every other day
†Dosages are based on normal horses; may need to adjust dosages if horses are ill, dehydrated, volume depleted, or if administering NSAIDs in combination. Ponies may require lower dosages[10].
Modified from Kallings P: Nonsteroidal Anti-inflammatory Drugs. Vet Clin North Am: Equine Practice 9: 523–541, 1993, with permission from Elsevier.

induced injury. Primary functions include limiting the inflammatory response to injury and concomitantly alleviating associated pain. NSAIDs are similarly administered around the time of surgery to control postoperative pain, fever and prevent excessive edema formation.

Although the mechanism of action is the same, there are apparent differences in the efficacy of different NSAIDs depending upon the type of condition being treated. For example, clinical and experimental data suggest PBZ is more efficacious in providing analgesia for most horses with musculoskeletal disease, whereas FLM is more effective in providing visceral analgesia in horses with colic.[48] These differences in effect may be due to the specificity of certain NSAIDs for different COX isomers or for COX within different tissues. Ketoprofen is reported to be effective in decreasing inflammation and pain associated with musculoskeletal disease and colic.[49–51] Acetylsalicylic acid (ASP) is rarely used as an anti-inflammatory drug in horses because of its extremely short half-life and low potency, however, it is frequently administered to horses with thromboembolic disorders to decrease platelet aggregation.[11,52] Dipyrone is a potent antipyretic agent, but has only mild analgesic properties.[48] Topically administered diclofenac sodium (DLC) is approved in the United States for treatment of horses with osteoarthritis. This formulation provides locally enhanced topical delivery without achieving a clinically important blood concentration of DLC and, when used in the absence of other NSAIDS, alleviates the adverse effects associated with systemically administered NSAIDs.[53]

Other less commonly used NSAIDs include CRP, MFA and NPX. Newer more specific COX-2 inhibitors, such as etodolac, are currently being developed and evaluated in horses.[54–57]

Analgesic effects

NSAIDs appear to mediate their analgesic effect in part by their inhibitory effects on COX, thus preventing or modulating PGE_2 synthesis locally at sites of inflammation.[10] However, because there are several clinically effective NSAIDs that are relatively weak COX inhibitors, anti-inflammatory mechanisms other than inhibition of PG synthesis are believed to be involved. PGE_2 is believed to bind to sensory nerve receptors and promote the discharge of impulses with a consequent increase in pain.[10] Prostaglandin E_2 also sensitizes nerve endings to the effects of numerous physical and chemical stimuli. Overall, PGs amplify peripheral pain by decreasing the nociceptor threshold.[10] Although PGE_2 does not cause pain itself, it can amplify the nocioceptive pathway by affecting the pain-inducing properties of other mediators such as histamine and bradykinin.[10] PGE_2 also seems to affect the body's ability to distinguish between different types of nocioceptive stimuli. There is evidence to suggest that PGs are involved in nocioceptive pathways within the spinal cord, and that NSAIDs have at least some action in inhibiting this cascade. NSAIDs do not exert a direct effect on normal pain perception, but rather reduce hypersensitivity to pain caused by inflammation, and this effect is mediated by a reduction in PGE_2. The analgesic effects of NSAIDS apparently can be dissociated from the anti-inflammatory effects, and require a lower dose. The analgesic effects of NSAIDs are variable depending upon the source of pain and the specific drug. There are limited controlled clinical trials or experimental studies comparing the analgesic effects of commonly used NSAIDs in horses with musculoskeletal disease.

A study evaluating the analgesic effects of PBZ, FLM and CRP administered at the end of various surgical procedures prior to anesthetic recovery, demonstrated that there were no differences in the pain scores or number of horses requiring additional analgesia among the three groups of horses.[58] In horses requiring additional analgesia after surgery, there was a significant difference in the time after surgery that horses required FLM versus PBZ. Horses treated with FLM required additional drug 12.8 ± 4.3 hours after surgery whereas those given PBZ required it at 8.4 ± 4.6 hours after surgery. Horses treated with CRP were intermediate in requiring additional drug 11.7 ± 6.9 hours after surgery. A study evaluating and comparing the inhibition of peripheral pain by FLM and CRP in horses, demonstrated there was no demonstrable analgesic effect for either drug when tested using an external skin-stimulation test for nocioception.[59] However, when the heating element model of nocioception was used, a 1.1 mg/kg IV dose of FLM failed to inhibit peripheral pain whereas a dose of 0.7 mg/kg IV of CRP inhibited the peripheral pain response for approximately 24 hours.[59]

In another study evaluating the analgesic effects of PBZ in horses after arthroscopic surgery, no difference was shown between PBZ-treated and placebo-treated horses regarding plasma βeta-endorphin or catecholamine concentrations.[60] However, horses treated with PBZ had a lower total postoperative pain severity index, which suggests that perioperative treatment with PBZ did exert some analgesic effects.[60] When a series of 9 horses afflicted with navicular disease were administered low (4.4 mg/kg SID or high (8.8 mg/kg SID) dose IV PBZ or saline control in a cross-over design study, clinical lameness scores were significantly decreased at six and 12 hours after PBZ (both low and high dose) treatment, but were significantly decreased at 24 hours only after high dose PBZ treatment. The data suggested that the analgesic effects of both high and low dose IV PBZ is similar, though the duration of analgesia may be longer with high-dose IV PBZ treatment. The authors concluded that there was no benefit to using IV PBZ at dosages higher than 4.4 mg/kg SID, in horses with navicular syndrome, especially considering the toxicities that may result from NSAID-administration.[61]

In another study of the duration of PBZ-mediated analgesic effect, the drug was administered at a dose rate of 4.4 mg/kg IVto eight horses in which lameness was induced using the heart-bar shoe model. Results showed that the PBZ produced profound positive clinical effect on lameness score for six hours after administration of PBZ.[62] In a related study, horses received a single IV treatment of 1) PBZ (4.4 mg/kg bwt), 2) FLM (1.1 mg/kg bwt), or a saline control. Heart rate and lameness score were recorded at rest and every 20 minutes for 5 hours after lameness induction. The horses underwent a standardized exercise test (SET) at four hours at speeds of 2 and 4 m/s on a high-speed treadmill. Results showed that a single-dose IV PBZ or FLM relieved foot pain sufficiently to improve both HR and LS before, during, and after exercise. However, there was no observed difference in efficacy between the two NSAIDs compared to one another. This study also demonstrates that NSAIDs have the ability to 'mask' lameness in the exercising horse, an effect that potentially compromises safety of the horse.[62]

Pretreatment of horses with PBZ prior to carrageenan-induced synovitis was more effective in reducing lameness, joint temperature, synovial fluid volume and synovial fluid PGE_2 concentrations, than pretreatment with KTP.[64] However, KTP administered at the PBZ equimolar dose (3.63 mg/kg) to horses with chronic laminitis reduced chronic hoof pain and lameness to a greater extent that did 2.2 mg/kg PBZ. This effect was still present 24 hours after drug administration.[65] Therefore, it was recommended that a dosage rate of 1.65 times the recommended therapeutic dose of KTP is more potent than PBZ in alleviating chronic hoof pain and lameness in horses.

Anti-inflammatory and chondroprotective effects

Inflammation can lead to pain and edema formation. Inhibition of PG synthesis perioperatively can reduce the inflammatory response secondary to surgery or the primary disease, thus decreasing pain and edema. NSAIDs are commonly administered perioperatively to horses for these reasons. For example, PBZ is often administered for several days after arthroscopic surgery in horses with synovitis secondary to osteochondral chip fractures or osteochondrosis in order to decrease synovitis arising from primary joint disease and from the surgery.

Prostaglandins of the E-series seem to be involved with increased metabolic activity in cartilage, whereas those of the F-series are chondroprotective.[10] Prostaglandin E_2 is responsible for much of the bone resorption associated with osteomyelitis.[10] NSAIDs are therefore useful in acute synovitis and osteomyelitis to decrease PG-mediated synthesis of destructive enzymes and reduce cartilage degradation and bone resorption. However, prolonged administration can accelerate cartilage degeneration. In general, NSAIDs have a suppressive effect on proteoglycan synthesis.[66] In vivo and in vitro studies have investigated the chondroprotective and potentially deleterious effects of NSAIDs, often with contradictory and confusing results. Additionally, the clinical relevance of these effects is not fully known. NSAIDs appear to have a varying ability to inhibit catabolic events in cartilage matrix with several noted differences in their inhibitory effects on the activity of degradative enzymes. Some of the potential beneficial effects of NSAIDs may not result from direct inhibition of these degradative enzymes, but rather suppression of other inflammatory mediators involved in cartilage degeneration.

A study evaluating the effects of orally administered PBZ on proteoglycan synthesis and chrondrocyte inhibition of IL-1β in equine articular cartilage explants revealed that PBZ administration for 14 days caused a significant decrease in proteoglycan synthesis.[67] The investigators concluded that PBZ should be used judiciously in athletic horses with osteoarthritis because prolonged administration could suppress proteoglycan synthesis and potentiate cartilage damage.

Both the R- and S- enantiomers and the racemic mixture of CRP attenuated the increased interleukin (IL)-6 production induced by LPS in equine synoviocytes whereas the S-enantiomer had a similar effect on chondrocytes.[68] Neither enantiomer of the racemic mixture suppressed the LPS-induced IL-1 production in synoviocytes or chondrocytes.

A study evaluating the effect of FLM, tolfenamic acid and both the R- and S-enatiomers of KTP on the response of equine synoviocytes to LPS demonstrated that all four compounds inhibited beta-glucuronidase in a concentration-dependent manner with tolfenamic acid being the most potent.[69] Tolfenamic acid and FLM caused an increased production of IL-6 induced by LPS, but only at their highest concentration (1,000 µmol/l). Flunixin, tolfenamic acid and the S-enantiomer of KTP caused a significant and concentration-dependent increase in IL-1 release. All four drugs caused a marked, concentration-dependent inhibition of PGE_2 synthesis. These findings suggest that by removing the regulator role of PGE_2 on IL-1 synthesis, the long-term use of NSAIDs in horses with arthropathies could potentially enhance cartilage degeneration. In another study evaluating the effect of commonly used NSAIDs on LPS-stimulated equine synovial membrane explants, it was demonstrated that PBZ, FLM, KTP and CRP suppressed PGE_2 production without causing a detrimental effect on viability of function as measured by hyaluronan synthesis.[70]

Effects on bone

With regard to the effect of NSAIDs on bone metabolism, administration of PBZ (4.4 mg/kg PO every 12 hours) for 30 days caused a significant decrease in mineral apposition rate in the tibia and appeared to decrease the healing rate of unicortical bone defects in horses.[71]

Topical administration of NSAIDs

Topical application of 1% DLC liposomal cream to sites of intravenous regional limb perfusion in healthy horses decreased inflammation as judged by visual assessment and ultrasonography. Decreased inflammation may allow extended use of intravenous regional limb perfusion and may result in a reduction in pain in treated horses.[72] In a second study in which induced carpal osteoarthritis was treated with oral PBZ (2g) or topical DLC (7.3g BID), both provided an improvement in lameness when compared with a no treatment control. DLC also induced improved cartilage staining with safranin-O fast green and total articular glycosaminoglycan content when compared with the no treatment control and less cartilage erosion and less radial carpal bone scleorsis when compared with PBZ.[53] Other data have not demonstrated the benefit of using topical diclofenac for induced acute synovitis in horses.[73]

Antipyretic effects

Cytokines such as TNF, IL-1 and IL-6 increase in response to LPS and other inflammatory stimuli and result in the increased production of PGE_2 in the hypothalamus. The net effect of this hypothalamic increase in PGE_2 is to reset the body's thermal set point at a higher temperature, resulting in fever. NSAIDs inhibit endogenous PGE_2, which raises the threshold level of the thermoregulatory center in the hypothalamus[10], thereby preventing or limiting the febrile response. Different NSAIDs seem to have varying antipyretic effects; empirically, DPY seems to be the most effective antipyretic in horses. The antipyretic effects of NSAIDs are observed with doses that inhibit PG synthesis, which is usually much lower than those needed for anti-inflammatory effects.

Antiendotoxic effects

NSAIDs are effective in inhibiting endotoxin-induced prostanoid release, and thus are used to pretreat horses predisposed to develop endotoxemia or to treat horses with suspected endotoxemia to prevent endotoxic shock. Some horse with infectious conditions of the musculoskeletal system such as septic arthritis/tenosynovitis, septic cellulitis, myositis and other potential infectious conditions involving gram-negative bacteria are predisposed to the adverse effects of endotoxemia. Flunixin meglumine reportedly is more effective in ameliorating the cardiovascular effects of endotoxin, whereas PBZ is more selective in blocking the inhibitory effect of endotoxin on gastrointestinal motility.[74] Pretreatment with FLM (0.25 mg/kg IV) decreases the synthesis of TXB-B_2 and 6-ketoprostaglandin $F_{1\alpha}$, the stable metabolites of TXB-A_2 and prostacyclin, respectively, and improves hemodynamic status in experimentally-induced endotoxemia in equids. Flunixin meglumine prevents endotoxin-mediated pregnancy loss in mares during the first 60 days of gestation =if administered in the early stages of endotoxemia (often before clinical signs are present).[75]

Hemostatic and antithrombotic effects

Aspirin and other NSAIDs are sometimes used in horses for treatment or prophylaxis of diseases with a possible thromboembolic component, including thrombophlebitis, intestinal ischemia, and nonstrangulating infarction. Aspirin is recommended because of its irreversible inhibition of platelet COX leading to inhibition of the synthesis of TBX-A_2, which is a pro-aggregatory and vasoconstrictor substance released during blood clotting.[10-11] A single oral dose of ASP (20 mg/kg) prolongs bleeding time and decreases platelet adhesiveness in horses.[76] Aspirin (19 mg/kg) causes complete blockade of serum TXB_2 synthesis for 7 days, 74% inhibition remains at 24 days.[52] This indicates ASP causes complete, irreversible inhibition of platelet COX, and this action probably extends to megakayrocytes in the bone marrow.[52] In vitro studies of equine platelets demonstrate that FLM, PBZ, and NPX also have potent anti-aggregatory properties.[77] Flunixin meglumine and PBZ cause reversible inhibition of platelet COX with serum TXB-B_2 concentrations returning to normal within 48 hours.[52]

Laminitis

Horses with acute gastrointestinal tract disease, other infectious or inflammatory diseases, and horses with severe lameness are predisposed to the development of laminitis. Therefore, NSAIDs are often considered crucial in horses for the prevention and/or treatment of laminitis. Providing analgesia may disrupt the pain-vasoconstriction cycle induced by the release of catecholamines and other vasoconstrictive substances. This may help attenuate the decreased digital blood flow and laminar perfusion characteristics of developmental or acute laminitis. Phenylbutazone is believed by many to be the most effective NSAID for reducing pain associated with laminitis, however, FLM, MFA, and KTP are also effective.[10–11,49] A PBZ equimolar dose of KTP (3.63 mg/kg), which is 1.65 times the recommended therapeutic dose, was more potent than PBZ in alleviating chronic hoof pain and lameness.[49]

The highest observed increase in laminar COX-2 protein concentrations in horses with black walnut extract-induced laminitis was in the developmental phase of the disease before clinical signs became apparent. However, in a carbohydrate- induced model of laminitis, COX-2 activity was only noted during the acute phase.[78] Regardless, NSAIDs given early in the disease's onset may combat COX-2-induced PGE_2 production, be responsible for the expression or activation of matrix metalloproteases (MMPs) which play a central pathophysiologic role in laminar separation in laminitis.[79].

Clinical applications

Clinical and experimental evidence has shown that PBZ be used at 4.4 mg/kg once daily or 2.2 mg/kg once to twice daily for its analgesic and anti-inflammatory properties in musculoskeletal disease.[9] Additionally, clinical experience suggests PBZ also exerts anti-inflammatory effects in reducing surgical wound edema. Clinically, DPY is not a very effective analgesic for musculoskeletal pain and is usually administered IV in horses principally for its antipyretic effects. Aspirin is a poor analgesic, however, its irreversible effect on platelets at low doses makes it potentially useful for horses with pro-thromotic related disease. Meclofenamic acid is apparently most useful for treatment of chronic musculoskeletal pain. In a clinical trial, MFA was shown to improve lameness in 78% of horses with navicular disease, 76% with chronic laminitis, and 61% with osteoarthritis.[80] Another clinical trial comparing seven-day-treatment regimens of MFA (2.2 mg/kg) to PBZ (4.4 mg/kg) in horses with navicular disease and osteoarthritis demonstrated that 60% of those treated with MFA responded favorably compared with 36% treated with PBZ.[11]

Flunixin meglumine is effective and useful in the treatment of lameness in horses, however, because of its comparatively high cost to PBZ, it is usually not the first NSAID administered. In one clinical trial of horses with various musculoskeletal diseases, FLM alleviated clinical signs in 74% of horses.[81] Naproxen is somewhat unique in its relative closeness of the doses required for its analgesic and anti-inflammatory effects. When administered at a dose of 4–8 gm/day for seven days, NPX markedly improved lameness and stride length in horses with experimentally-induced myositis.[82] Naproxen was also reported to be particularly effective in the treatment of inflammatory swelling and lameness.[83] Clinically, 90% of horses with myositis treated with NPX responded favorably within five days. Ketoprofen has been shown to decrease synovial fluid PGE_2 concentrations, joint effusion and lameness in a carrageenan-induced synovitis model in horses.[65] Some veterinarians prefer KTP to FLM or PBZ in the treatment of musculoskeletal inflammation and pain in foals due to its decreased propensity for gastrointestinal ulceration. Carprofen has been shown to decrease inflammatory exudate PGE_2 levels for up to eight hours and ex vivo TXB_2 generation for 15 hours after a single IV dose.[29] Additionally, CRP has been shown to reduce the swelling in an experimental model of soft tissue inflammation in the necks of ponies. Carprofen has also been shown to alleviate cutaneous pain caused by application of a heating element for 24 hours. Carprofen was shown to be equally effective to PBZ and FLM for postoperative analgesia.[58] Ketoprofen and CRP are particularly effective in decreasing inflammation-associated edema and joint effusion in horses.[11,65]

Combination NSAID therapy

Because all NSAIDs have a similar mechanism of action, it was thought that there is no benefit in administering NSAIDs in combination. However, combination NSAID therapy is becoming increasingly common. Although it is true that all NSAIDs inhibit COX, it is currently unknown if there is greater affinity of NSAIDs for COX in some tissues compared with others. Similarly, there may exist a differential affinity for the COX isoforms by the same NSAID. Concurrent administration of FLM (1.1 mg/kg IV) and PBZ (2.2 mg/kg IV) did not alter the disposition or clearance of either drug; therefore, their simultaneous use should not result in increased concentrations of either drug[84]. However, concurrent administration of FLM and PBZ prolongs the pharmacologic effect (TXB-B_2 suppression) and therefore could increase the potential for toxicity.[84] The merits of combining NSAIDs for clinical effect has been studied. Using an adjustable heart-bar shoe to induce lameness, eight healthy horses were administered PBZ (4.4 mg/kg), FLM (1.1 mg/kg), PBZ+FLM (at the same dosages as given individually) or a saline control. Heart rate, used as a measure of pain, was lower in all NSAID-treated horses from 2 h to 10 h post-treatment ($P < 0.05$) and the analgesic effect on lameness score lasted for 12 h post treatment. Lameness score decreased earlier in PBZ and PBZ+FM trials than in FLM trials ($P < 0.05$) but it was concluded that the combination of PBZ+FM was not more effective in alleviationg lameness than either PBZ or FLM alone.[85] In a similar study[86], PBZ paste was administered at a half dose (2.2 mg/kg) PO every 12 hours for five days alone or in combination with FM administered at the full dose 1.1 mg/kg, IV, every 12 hours for five days. Lameness evaluations were performed before and 12 hours after administration of the drugs. Alleviation of lameness was greater after administration of the combination of NSAIDs than after administration of PBZ alone but the combination of NSAIDs did not completely mask lameness. Recognizing that the drug dose rates differed between the two studies, it is difficult to draw conclusions. However, five horses did not improve after either NSAID treatment regimen and one horse administered the combination therapy died of acute necrotizing colitis during the study. Accordingly, consideration should be given to adjusting the dose of each NSAID if administered in combination, and it is imperative to maintain hydration in order to reduce the potential for toxicity.

Adverse effects of NSAIDs

Inhibition of the COX pathway accounts not only for the therapeutic effects of NSAIDs, but also for the potential toxic effects.

Gastrointestinal ulceration and renal papillary necrosis associated with NSAIDs are believed to occur secondarily to decreased PGE_2 synthesis, which is important in maintaining mucosal blood flow and other cytoprotective effects and maintenance of renal medullary blood flow. There may be breed, age, and idiosyncratic differences in the susceptibility to NSAID toxicity. For example, ponies are reportedly more susceptible than horses to the toxic effects of PBZ,[87] and young animals are also believed to be especially sensitive to the adverse effects of NSAIDs.[88–91] Horses that are aged, systemically ill and/or dehydrated also appear to be predisposed to the toxic effects of NSAIDs. In one study, the toxic potential of three commonly used NSAIDs in horses was greatest for PBZ, less for FLM, and least for KTP.[41] Naproxen did not cause clinically apparent toxicity in horses at three times the recommended dose.[25] Although there is not much data, MFA and CRP seem to have minimal toxic effects when used at the recommended dosing regimen.[9,46] Intuitively, COX-2 specific NSAIDs may represent a lower risk for horses and this has been borne out in initial clinical studies. In one, only four of 467 (0.9%) horses that received FCB as prescribed (0.1 mg/kg, PO, q 24 h) had an adverse response.[19] In a second study, only three of 123 horses receiving FCB as prescribed had an adverse effect and none of these could be related to the drug's use.[18]

Gastrointestinal tract effects

Administration of NSAIDs in excessive doses, for prolonged periods, or in the presence of dehydration or volume depletion can lead to a number of serious side effects. Gastrointestinal ulceration (gastric glandular and small and large intestinal mucosa) is a relatively common side effect of NSAID administration in horses. Additionally, horses administered NSAIDs (especially PBZ orally) can develop ulcerations of the oral mucosa as a result of a local irritant effect. Phenylbutazone binds to hay, which delays its absorption. Once the hay reaches the large intestine (cecum and colon), PBZ is released after digestion and fermentation resulting in relatively high concentrations that could have a local effect on the cecal and colonic mucosa. However, this local irritant effect cannot account for all of the toxic effects since similar lesions are noted in horses with parenterally administered NSAIDs.

The gastric ulcerogenic effects of NSAIDs are believed to result at least in part from an NSAID-mediated decrease in mucosal PGE_2, leading to vasoconstriction, hypoxia, and necrosis. Prostaglandins are normally cytoprotective in the gastrointestinal tract. Prostaglandin E_2 and PGI_2 decrease the volume, acidity, and pepsin content of gastric secretions and also stimulate bicarbonate secretion by epithelial cells, produce mucosal vasodilatation, increase mucus production, and stimulate turnover and repair or gastrointestinal epithelial cells.[92] NSAIDs disrupt these normal cytoprotective effects in the gastric mucosal barrier and contribute to the development of gastric glandular mucosal ulceration. Gastrointestinal ulceration is often accompanied by secondary anemia, hypoproteinemia and hypoalbuminemia owing to blood and plasma protein loss. Additionally, horses with NSAID toxicity often demonstrate neutropenia, which has been suggested to be due to suppression of granulopoiesis in the bone marrow, however, this effect is most likely secondary to intestinal inflammation, disruption of the mucosal barrier and subsequent absorption of endotoxin into the circulation. The situation remains confused. In recent studies, PBZ did not decrease gastric or intestinal mucosal PG concentrations in horses 48 hours after administration.[93] There is evidence to suggest that PBZ causes direct injury to the intestinal microvasculature.[93]

In a study focusing on the causation of right dorsal colitis, PBZ treatment (8.8 mg/kg, SID, PO) caused hypoalbuminemia and neutropenia during the first three days of treatment, changes in blood flow in the right dorsal colon (RDC), and alterations in luminal concentrations of volatile fatty acids. The authors proposed these changes to be due to local alterations in the colonic mucosa, including initiation of an inflammatory cascade, recruitment of intestinal immunocytes, dysfunction of the intestinal barrier, and absorption of endotoxin from gram negative bacteria. Intestinal angiogenesis and a subsequent increase in the blood flow in the RDC may have been secondary to complicated mechanisms associated with inflammation that they were unable to elucidate. The authors emphasized that equine veterinarians should be extremely judicious and cautious when making dosing recommendations for phenylbutazone treatment because of the extreme variability in tolerance within horses. Routine hematologic analysis beginning as early as 3– 5 days after initiation of treatment should be performed, and the phenylbutazone dose should be decreased as soon as possible or alternative COX-2 specific NSAIDs should be used.[94]

Juvenile horses are especially predisposed to the ulcerative effects of these drugs on the gastric mucosa, while adult horses are more commonly affected with right dorsal colon ulceration, resulting in abdominal pain, diarrhea, and a protein losing enteropathy.[41] Most reported cases of ulcerative colitis have been in adult horses administered PBZ, however, other NSAIDs can contribute to the development of this disease. The relative ulcerogenic effects of three commonly used NSAIDs in clinically normal adult horses is PBZ > FLM > KTP.[41]

Nonselective COX-1 inhibitors or those with combined COX-1 and COX-2 inhibitory effects are most likely to delay the recovery of ischemic-injured intestinal mucosa.[56] This finding demonstrates that constitutively synthesized PGs are important for mucosal recovery. Etodolac, a potential COX-2 inhibitor in horses, partially inhibited PG synthesis, but had no effect on recovery of ischemic-injured equine jejunal mucosa in vitro, which is in contrast to the FLM, which near-fully inhibited PGs and inhibited mucosal recovery.[56]

Renal toxicity

Papillary necrosis is the major nephrotoxic effect of NSAIDs observed in horses, however, tubular nephritis, can also occur. Renal synthesis of PGs occurs primarily in the medulla.[95] Conditions resulting in renal vasoconstriction (dehydration, volume depletion, shock) induce PG synthesis, and secondary compensatory vasodilatation.[95] Under normal circumstances, vasodilatory PGs play a minor role in maintaining renal blood flow and controlling renal function. However, during certain pathophysiological conditions, vasodilatory PG synthesis is required to maintain adequate renal perfusion and function. Renal medullary ischemia is considered the initiating factor in the development of renal papillary necrosis. This occurs when horses are administered NSAIDs either in excessive doses, for prolonged periods, or concomitant with dehydration or volume depletion.[88–89,96] Without concurrent dehydration, PBZ does not reportedly result in renal papillary necrosis.[89] However, concurrent administration of NSAIDs and aminoglycoside antibiotics can also potentiate the risk of nephrotoxicity.[11] If possible, horses that are dehydrated or volume depleted should have their fluid volume normalized prior to beginning NSAID therapy.

Hemostatic effects

Although NSAIDs impair platelet adhesion and can either lead to or exacerbate bleeding tendencies owing to their inhibition of platelet $TXB\text{-}B_2$ synthesis, these are not frequently observed complications in horses.[48]

Decreased wound healing

Administration of NSAIDs has been reported to contribute to an increased incidence of abdominal incisional complications in horses.[97] Although NSAIDs reportedly have no clinically significant effect on wound healing, their use in horses has been reported to contribute to the development of abdominal incisional complications.[97] Experimentally, the administration of FLM (1.1 mg/kg IV BID) for seven days caused decreased strength in skin, linea alba, and small intestinal enterotomy wounds at seven days in ponies.[98] Another retrospective study reported no association between the administration of NSAIDs and the development of abdominal incisional complications.[99] Clinically, the use of NSAIDs does not appear to affect wound healing.

Thrombophlebitis

Perivascular injection of PBZ causes intense phlebitis and tissue necrosis. Administration of excessive doses of PBZ has been demonstrated to cause degeneration and dilatation of the walls of small veins and microvascular phlebitis, which may contribute to some of the toxic effects on the intestinal mucosa and kidney.[93] Fifty percent of horses administered PBZ develop pulmonary vascular thrombosis observable at necropsy.[100] The clinical significance of these changes is unknown.

Injury predisposition

Because NSAIDs have the propensity to mask pain or otherwise adversely influence metabolism, concern exists that their use, particularly in competition horses, predisposes the patient to unwanted injury. In one series of 161 horses that sustained injury (catastrophic and non-catastrophic) at Kentucky racetracks over the course of one year, average plasma concentrations of FLM and PBZ, as measured by High Pressure Liquid Chromatography, in injured horses were higher than in control horses. However, due to the large number of other variables likely influencing risk of injury (eg, length of race, track condition), further studies must be designed to determine whether higher plasma concentrations of NSAIDs can truly be associated with an increased risk of musculoskeletal injuries.[101]

Corticosteroid therapy

Corticosteroids (CSs) are administered systemically and locally for their anti-inflammatory properties in horses. These drugs are often administered either parenterally or orally for their systemic anti-inflammatory effects or intra-articularly in horses with nonseptic joint disease, again because of their potent anti-inflammatory and associated analgesic properties. Intra-articular injection of CSs into inflamed joints depresses the initial inflammatory events, including capillary dilatation, leukocyte margination and migration, inflammatory cell accumulation, enzyme and inflammatory mediator liberation, and cytokine, prostaglandin and thromboxane synthesis.[102]

Classification and mechanism of action

Glucocorticoids are produced synthetically and are often classified according to their duration of action and route of administration.[103] Corticosteroids commonly administered parenterally in horses with short duration include prednisolone sodium succinate (Solu-Cortef, Pfizer) and methylprednisolone sodium succinate (MPS) (Solu-Medrol, Pfizer). Corticosteroids with intermediate duration include triamcinolone acetonide (Vetalog, Bristol-Myers Squibb Company), and flumethasone (Flucort, Pfizer). Corticosteroids with an intermediate to long duration include betamethasone acetate and betamethasone sodium phosphate (Celestone soluspan, Merch & Co) and methylprenisolone acetate (Depo-Medrol).[104] Long duration CSs include dexamethasone sodium phosphate or dexamethasone in propylene glycol. Parenteral formulations of CSs with rapid onset are usually used in emergency situations such as anaphylaxis and circulatory shock, whereas those with slow onset and long duration are used for synovitis, arthritis or intralesional therapy. Orally administered CS formulations are categorized as rapid onset and short duration (prednisone tablets); rapid onset and short-to-intermediate duration (triamcinolone tablets or powder); and slow onset and long duration (dexamethasone tablets or powder).[103] These formulations are usually used for subacute to chronic inflammatory or allergic conditions.

Corticosteroids are 21-carbon molecules that contain three 6-carbon rings and a 5-carbon ring.[108] Pharmacological activity depends upon the presence of a hydroxyl group at the C-11 location. The corticosteroids available for intra-articular use are 11β-hydroxyl compounds that do not require biotransformation and are generally ester salts prepared as suspensions. The duration of effect appears to be inversely correlated with the water solubility of the corticosteroid and the rate of absorption. Other factors believed to determine the duration of action of intra-articular corticosteroids include the rate of hydrolysis of the drug by enzyme in the synovial cavity as well as the binding affinity of the steroid for the steroid receptors in the target cells of the joint.[105]

The local effect of a CS in the joint is dependent on the rate of hydrolysis within the joint. Methylprednisolone acetate (MPA) is considered a long-acting ester when given IM because of the slow rate of absorption from the site of injection with subsequent hydrolysis in the plasma. However, when injected into a joint, it is rapidly hydrolyzed to the active drug (methylprednisolone, MP) with high local synovial fluid concentrations detectable within two hours postinjection.[106–107] Measurable concentrations of MP were detectable for 5–39 days, whereas MPA was detectable for only 2–6 days postinjection. Although MPA was not detectable systemically after IA injection, it was detectable in the synovial fluid for 24 hours. This resulted in depression of endogenous hydrocortisone for 3–4 days, but the adrenal gland remained responsive to corticotropin.[106]

The biologic potency or activity of CSs is dependent upon many factors, including the total dose administered, the duration of action, duration and frequency of treatment, rate of conversion to biologically active metabolites, crystal size of the suspension and numerous other cell and tissue variables.[105] Corticosteroids exert their effect on cells by binding to plasma membrane and steroid-specific cytosolic receptors of steroid-responsive tissues.[103,108] The CSs apparently passively diffuse into the cytosol of steroid-responsive tissues, bind to cytosolic receptors, which leads to a change in the allosteric nature of the receptor-steroid complex. The activated cytosolic receptors are then translocated to the nucleus where they bind to the steroid response element on nuclear DNA. This results in modulation of gene transcription and mRNA coding for specific proteins that ultimately causes the hormonal effect. Glucocorticoids exert their anti-inflammatory effects via stimulating production of lipocortin, which inhibits the activity of plasma membrane-bound phospholipase A_2 (PLA_2) and thereby inhibits release of arachidonic acid and indirectly the de novo synthesis of inflammatory mediators including PGs, TBXs, LTs, and platelet activating factor. The onset of action at the cellular level is likely immediate, but completion of the necessary steps in this cascade likely takes from a few to several hours, which delays the biologic effect.

Corticosteroids exert their local anti-inflammatory effects by:

- stabilizing lysosomal membranes and the concomitant release of lysosomal enzymes
- decreasing vascular permeability

- inhibiting leukocyte adherence to microvascular endothelium and subsequent diapedesis
- suppressing leukocyte superoxide synthesis
- inhibiting platelet aggregation
- inhibiting PG synthesis by inhibiting the release of arachidonic acid from membrane phospholipids and
- reducing inflammatory effects of the healing process that result in fibrosis.[108]

Importantly, glucocorticoids inhibit the synthesis and release of several soluble mediators including acting on the prostaglandin cascade, and have been shown to inhibit IL-1, the most important mediator of cartilage degradation and tumor necrosis factor (TNFa) at low concentrations.[109–110] Pain relief is attributed to inhibition of PG synthesis, specifically by inhibiting the enzyme phospholipase A2 and COX-2 expression in the arachidonic cascade.[109,111] Glucocorticoid receptors have been identified in neutrophils, lymphocytes, and eosinophils. Corticosteroids typically have greater effects on cellular rather than humoral processes, and on movement rather than function of leukocytes.[105] One of the predominant mechanisms of their anti-inflammatory properties is their inhibitory effect on the migration of neutrophils and macrophages into sites of inflammation. When administered systemically, CSs cause a neutrophillic leukocytosis owing to a prolonged half-life, increased bone marrow synthesis of neutrophils, decreased margination and subsequent egress into sites of inflammation. Corticosteroids also have been shown to exert a dose-dependent effect on neutrophil function, however, this effect occurs to a lesser degree than the effect on leukocyte movement. Higher doses inhibit the release of lysosomal enzymes from neutrophils and neutrophillic phagocytosis is similarly suppressed. There has been poor correlation reported between neutrophil numbers and PGE_2 concentrations in synovial fluid after CS treatment of chronic inflammatory joint disease in people, which suggests a likely alternative source of prostaglandins and/or differential effects of these drugs on cellular function.[112]

Pharmacokinetics

Corticosteroid suspensions generally have a relatively short intra-articular half-life. Considerable variation has been reported for the clearance of corticosteroid suspensions from the synovial cavity after intra-articular administration. Triamcinolone acetate (TCA) has a reported synovial fluid half-life ranging from 1–5 days.[113] The median synovial fluid half-life of MPA and MP in the tarsocrural joint space of normal horses as detected with high performance liquid chromatography was 10.3 and 10.4 hours, respectively.[114] Another study has demonstrated that the active principle of MPA can liberate its active principle in the synovial cavity for up to one month after intra-articular injection.[106]

Therapeutic uses

Joint disease

Although there is appreciable information in the literature regarding the untoward effects of intra-articular corticosteroid therapy, much of this has been shown to be overgeneralizations; there appear to be distinct differences in the effect of steroids on articular cartilage and synovial membrane depending upon the type and dose used. Intra-articular injection of CSs remains a useful treatment for traumatic, degenerative and nonseptic joint disease in the horse. Steroids effectively suppress the pain, heat, and swelling associated with inflammatory joint disease, thus, are effective in treating synovitis and arthritis. Aseptic technique is essential to prevent joint infection.[108]

Several drug formulations are approved for intra-articular administration, such as (1) triamcinolone acetonide (TMA), (2) isoflupredone acetate, (3) betamethasone acetate (BMA), (4) methylprednisolone (MPA), and (5) flumethasone (FMZ).[103]

Experimental and clinical effects of intra-articular corticosteroids

Many in vivo and in vitro experimental and clinical investigations have reported on the therapeutic and deleterious effects of intra-articular corticosteroids in horses.

Methylprednisolone

In vitro studies

Numerous studies have explored the effect of MPS at the cellular and tissue levels. In one, equine articular cartilage explants were treated with MPS at various concentrations ranging from 0.001 to 10 mg/ml for one day and then in fresh medium without MPS.[115] Proteoglycan synthesis was severely depressed by 10 mg/ml MPS for 24 hours in normal cartilage. Cartilage treated with 5 mg/ml had pyknotic chondrocyte nuclei and empty lacunae. MPS concentrations of 1.0 and 0.1 mg/ml depressed proteoglycan synthesis in normal cartilage, however, concentrations recovered within two days after MPS removal from the medium. Concentrations of MPS of 0.01 and 0.001 mg/ml did not have a significant effect on proteoglycan synthesis in normal cartilage explants. MPS concentrations of 1.0 and 0.1 mg/ml alleviated articular cartilage degradation in explants cultured in monocyte-conditioned medium, which suggests that it is possible to identify an intra-articular concentration of CS that will protect articular cartilage from cytokine-induced matrix degradation, but will not have a prolonged or permanent deleterious effect on chondrocyte matrix synthesis.

Equine chondrocytes cultured in monolayer were stimulated with IL-1β and cultured either with or without dexamethasone (DEX) or MPA.[116] The stimulatory effects of IL-1β on matrix metalloprotease 13 (collagenase 3) gene expression in articular chondrocytes was decreased by DEX, and reduced in a dose-dependent manner by MPA. However, in a second in vitro study, neither MPA or TCA counteracted the negative effects of IL-1 on either GAG synthesis or degradation.[117] In another study, the effects of MMP, BMA, and DEX in inhibiting MMP-2 and MMP-9 were assessed using gelatinase and casein degradation assays.[118] Betamethasone had no effect on MMP-2 or -9. Dexamethasone and MPA had no effect on MMP-9, but MMP-2 was significantly inhibited at the highest dose tested for DEX (1 mg/ml) and the higher concentrations of MPA (1.2 and 5 mg/ml). Corticosteroids affect MMP levels in disease by preventing synthesis at the transcriptional level, which has been documented in the horse.[119]

Articular cartilage explants and chondrocyte monolayer cultures obtained from young adult horses were cultured to determine the effect of differing concentrations of MPA on chondrocyte function and viability in vitro.[120] Steady-state levels of type II procollagen mRNA decreased without concomitant decreases in type I procollagen expression as the concentration of MPA in the culture medium increased from 1×10^1 to 1×10^8 pg/ml. Cytotoxicity occurred as MPA concentrations increased to 1×10^8 and 1×10^9 pg/ml. The cartilage specific fibronectin was suppressed in normal and inflamed joints with a single intra-articular injection of 0.1 mg/kg MPA. Collectively, this study demonstrates that MPA suppresses matrix protein markers of chondrocyte differentitation. The investigators speculate that a decreased and altered expression of matrix proteins in chondrocytes likely contributes to corticosteroid-induced cartilage degradation.[120]

An in vitro study evaluating the effect of MPA on proteoglycan and collagen metabolism in cartilage explants from normal equine joints revealed several important findings.[121] Proteoglycans were not lost to the media in response to MPA treatment over a 72-hour period, but there was a decrease in the size of some aggrecan monomers as well as the proteoglycan aggregate. The lowest doses of MPA stimulated protein synthesis, and there was a trend for a similar pattern for proteoglycan and collagen synthesis. A protective effect of MPA against proteoglycan degradation in the explants was observed with higher doses (0.04 to 4.0 mg/ml) as demonstrated by reduced GAG being released into the media. The investigators speculate that MPA may affect post-translational modification of the core protein with the addition of smaller and fewer GAG chains.[121]

Methylprednisolone acetate reduced proteoglycan loss in cartilage explant cultures from the middle carpal joint of horses, however, this effect was not seen at clinically relevant concentrations.[122] MPA caused a dose-dependent inhibition of proteoglycan synthesis at all concentrations tested, however, chondrocyte viability was deleteriously affected only at the 2000 µg/ml dose. In another in vitro study, the deleterious effects of Activated Protein C (APC) on equine cartilage were attenuated by treatment with either MPA, TA or DEX (10–5 M and 10–10 M).[123] Collectively, these results suggest that the therapeutic effect of MPA is not restricted to the anti-inflammatory effects on soft tissues of the joint.

In vivo studies

Intra-articular injection of MPA into the joints of normal horses has shown some regressive effects on articular cartilage.[124–125] However, questions remain regarding the minimal effective dose and the effect this would have in arthritis/synovitis and the effect in joints of exercised horses. Injection of 100 mg of MPA into the middle carpal joint of horses with experimentally-induced osteochondral fragmentation of the distal radial carpal bone did not reduce lameness, but did cause a decrease in synovial fluid PGE_2 concentrations and lowered scores for synovial membrane intimal hyperplasia and vascularity, when compared with polyionic fluid-treated joints.[126] These potential beneficial effects must be weighed against the detrimental findings of articular cartilage erosion and morphologic lesions associated with MPA treatment. The deleterious effects of MPA in this model is in contrast to the favorable effects of TMA on clinical lameness, synovial fluid, synovial membrane and articular cartilage morphologic and biochemical parameters in the same model.[127]

A study of acute synovitis of the radiocarpal and middle carpal joints induced by four injections of LPS (0.5 ng) at two-day intervals in ponies demonstrated that intra-articular injection of MPA (0.1 mg/kg) concomitant with the last dose of LPS two days before euthanasia had substantial effects on proteoglycan, protein and collagen synthesis in harvested cartilage explants.[128] Methylprednisolone alone caused a decrease in proteoglycan synthesis and increased protein and collagen synthesis in cartilage explants. Synovial membrane protein synthesis was also increased by MPA. However, there were no differences in protein or proteoglycan synthesis in explants from horses with synovitis whether or not they were treated with MPA. Acute synovitis appeared to prevent changes induced by intra-articular MPA alone.[128] Thus the effects of intra-articular MPA appear to be different in inflamed versus normal joints.

A study evaluating the effects of LPS-induced acute synovitis and the effects of MPA on transcription of cartilage matrix proteins in ponies demonstrated that articular chondrocytes increase type-II procollagen and aggrecan synthesis in response to synovitis and that MPA alters chondrocyte function in both inflamed and normal joints.[129] In another study, synovial fluid samples were collected weekly from the radiocarpal joints of normal horses and MPA (60 mg) was injected into the radiocarpal joints at two-week intervals beginning on week 3 to quantify synovial fluid volume and keratan sulfate, cartilage aggrecan, C-propeptide and cartilage type II procollagen.[130] Synovial fluid volume was significantly reduced by MPA at weeks 4, 6, 7 and 8, but had returned to pre-teatment values by week 9, which corresponded to two weeks after the last injection of MPA. It is known that CSs suppress synovial membrane hyaluronic acid synthesis in vitro, and this may have contributed to the reduction in synovial fluid volume encountered in normal joints. Keratan sulfate and cartilage aggrecan were significantly increased in the synovial fluid of joints treated with MPA, when compared with non-treated controls. C-propeptide was significantly decreased in synovial fluid of MPA-treated joints. These results suggest that repeated use of intra-articular MPA leads to potentially deleterious inhibition of procollagen II synthesis and increased release of degradation products of proteoglycan aggrecan from articular cartilage. This study also demonstrated that MPA did not influence articular cartilage aggrecan metabolism in the contralateral joint, which is in contrast to remote-site effects of TMA on articular cartilage GAG content.[127]

Betamethasone

Horses were administered either 2.5 mL of BMA (3.9 mg betamethasone sodium phosphate and 12 mg betamethasone acetate per mL) or an equivalent volume of saline intra-articularly 14 and 35 days after experimentally-induced osteochondral fragmentation of the distal radial carpal bone.[131] Some horses were exercised on a high-speed treadmill and others were kept in a box stall, and all horses were evaluated serially and then euthanatized 56 days after fragmentation. The BMA did not cause any histologic, histochemical or biochemical evidence of articular cartilage alterations in horses with or without exercise.[131] The exercised horses also had comparable glycosaminoglycan (GAG) concentrations as the saline-treated control joints. Therefore, the intra-articular injection of BMA in the middle carpal joint did not cause any consistently observable detrimental effects in exercised or non-exercised horses.

Triamcinolone

In vitro studies

In an in vitro study, articular cartilage explants challenged with LPS (100 ng/mL) exhibited a significant decrease in chondral damage when compared with untreated controls implying that treatment with TMA supported chondrocyte morphology in culture and protected chondrocytes from the toxic effects of LPS.[132]

In vivo studies

Intra-articular TMA (12 mg) may also exert chondroprotective effects in the horse in vivo. Using an experimentally induced osteochondral fragmentation model of OA[127] horses treated with TMA were less lame than horses with osteochondral fragments treated with polyionic fluids and horses without osteochondral fragments injected with polyionic fluids. Joints treated with TMA had less synovial membrane inflammatory cell infiltrate, intimal hyperplasia and subintimal fibrosis. Additionally, TMA -treated joints had better articular cartilage morphologic scores and increased hyaluronic acid (HA) concentrations. These findings support a chondroprotective effect of TMA. Despite previous reports of nondetectable CS levels in the contralateral joint of horses,[114] there was an observable beneficial remote-site effect in the non-treated joints of these horses. This remote-site effect of TMA in joints contralateral to the treated joints suggests a possible treatment effect perhaps unrelated to detectable levels of the drug and involving a mechanism of action that may not be pharmacologically mediated.[127]

In another report of the effects of intra-articular TMA (12 mg) on subchondral bone in horses with experimentally-induced osteochondral fragmentation of the distal radial carpal bone, it was demonstrated that treated horses were significantly less lame than non-treated ones.[133] In an in vivo study of 10 healthy horses, repeat intra-articular injections of 12 mg TMA at week intervals (three total) prompted loss of resident and/or newly-synthesized aggrecan and collagen molecules.[134] In the event that TMA does exert a detrimental effect on cartilage in vivo, researchers have considered combination therapy using IGF-1, along with TMA. Using IL-1 conditioned equine articular cartilage explants, TA (1.2 mg/ml), in combination with 500 ng/ml IGF-1 provided an increase in GAG synthesis, a protective response against IL-1-induced degradation, and the least total GAG released into the media. Authors suggested investigation into the effects of this combination therapy on an in vivo model of OA.[135]

When metacarpophalangeal joint synovitis was experimentally induced with lipopolysaccharide (LPS) in 18 horses, TMA (9 mg) reduced lameness, edema, and the concentration of synovial fluid protein. In that study, some horses were also treated with mepivicaine in combination with TMA but the outcome was unchanged. The authors concluded that TMA was a potent analgesic and anti-inflammatory medication for acute synovitis in horses and that simultaneous administration of mepivacaine did not alter the potency or duration of action of TMA.[136]

In a clinical study assessing the outcome of the IA treatment of 51 horses afflicted with OA of the centrodistal and tarsometatarsal joints with either MPA or TMA, horses treated once with MPA or TA, either with or without HA, improved after a median of 56 days. There was no significant difference in outcome between MPA or TMA. There was no significant further improvement in the horses treated twice. In horses in which there was a diffuse increase in the uptake of a radiopharmaceutical by the distal tarsal joints, identified by scintigraphy, the lameness tended to improve ($P = 0.032$), whereas in the horses in which the uptake was focal, it did not. Importantly, at telephone follow-up, only 13 of 34 horses were reported to have had a positive outcome. However, concomitant injury to adjacent structures such as the proximal suspensory was not ruled out and horses with OA of the distal intertarsal and tarsometatarsal joints did better than horses afflicted with proximal intertarsal OA.[137] These findings of observing clinical effectiveness at 56 days are supported by studies using the osteochondral or chip fracture model when effectiveness was still observed at Day 70 when treatments with TA and MPA had been given at Days 14 and 28.[109]

Tendon disease

Many overuse tendinopathies in humans have been treated with intra-or peri-lesional injection of CSs but meta-analysis data shows that while they may help reduce pain in some conditions in the short term (<8 weeks), they have little clinical benefit in the long term.[138] The intra- or peri-lesional use of CSs in equine tendinopathies is now substantially curtailed, not least because we recognize the pathologic process to be degenerative rather than inflammatory.[139–140] Also, the histopathologic appearance of equine tendon injected with CS mimics the histologic features of tendinopathy,[109,141] implying their adverse effect when administered in this manner. The intrathecal injection of CS does however continue in clinical practice,[142] particularly with regard to management of distal limb lameness involving lesions of the DDFT. The clinical outcome is nonetheless guarded for affected horses, many of whom have multiple lesions affecting more than one structure.[140]

Dosage regimen

The formulation and dose of corticosteroid suspensions commonly used for intra-articular administration in horses is given in Table 23.2.

Adverse effects of corticosteroids

Administration of CSs into joints can have both therapeutic and detrimental effects.[108] The detrimental effects include decreased cartilage elasticity and glycosaminoglycan content with progressive cartilage degeneration; formation of calcium deposits on the surface of hyaline cartilage; cartilage thinning and fissure formation; and decreased synovial fluid viscosity and hyaluronic acid content. The predominant adverse effects include 'steroid arthropathy', post-injection flare, septic arthritis, and osseous metaplasia.[108] These deleterious effects have been shown to be both drug- and dose-dependent.

Table 23.2 Corticosteroid suspensions for intra-articular use in horses[102]

CORTICOSTEROID SUSPENSION	TRADE NAME	CONCENTRATION (mg/ml)	DOSE (mg)	POTENCY RELATIVE TO HYDROCORTISONE	RELATIVE DURATION OF ACTION
Betamethasone	Celestone soluspan	6*	3–18	30	M–L
Flumethasone	Flucort	0.5	1.25–2.5	120	M
Isoflupredone acetate	Predef 2X	2	5–20	50	S–M
Methylprednisolone acetate	Depo-Medrol	40	40–120	5	M–L
Triamcinolone acetonide	Vetalog	6	6–18	5	M

*Each ml contains 3 mg betamethasone acetate and 3 mg betamethasone sodium phosphate.
Modified from Caron JP. Principles of treatment of joint disease. In: Auer DE, Stick JA, editors. Equine Surgery. 2nd ed. Philadelphia: W. B. Saunders; 1999. p. 678–696, with permission from Elsevier.

Because of the intense reduction in inflammation and associated pain caused by intra-articular injection of CSs, there is some concern that horses may over-use an injured, 'pain-free' joint, thus accelerating joint degeneration. This concern has been substantiated by at least some studies showing that CSs can have deleterious effects on chondrocyte metabolism. However, the beneficial effects on reducing inflammation and the associated degradative mediators released from inflammatory cells versus the potential direct deleterious effects must be weighed when considering the use of CSs in an inflamed joint. At high concentrations, CSs inhibit proteoglycan synthesis and have a negative influence on the structure of collagen in the articular cartilage.[124,143] However, there is debate over the clinical importance of decreased proteoglycan content, particularly when lower doses of steroids are used. More recently, BMA or TMA injected into the joints of horses with experimentally induced cartilaginous lesions followed by exercise on a treadmill did not cause any exacerbation of cartilage damage beyond that observed in control animals.[131,133] Therefore, it appears that worsening of cartilaginous damage in horses undergoing strenuous exercise may not be as much of a concern as has been reported previously. This is particularly true when using lower doses of CSs, particularly TMA and BMA.

Corticosteroids can lead to steroid arthropathy by delaying fracture healing and reducing synovial inflammation and associated pain, which enables the horse to continue strenuous exercise, thereby exacerbating the degenerative joint disease.[108] Steroid arthropathy is characterized by an accelerated rate of joint damage, radiographic evidence of severe degenerative joint disease, joint enlargement owing to capsular distention and osteophytic new bone growth, decreased range of motion, and crepitation. This condition usually occurs following intra-articular injection of CSs into joints with pre-existing cartilage damage or those not rested appropriately after injection. Recommended doses of CSs injected into a normal joint may not lead to CS-induced arthropathy, even with strenuous exercise. However, injured joints should be allowed to rest following CS injection in order to allow the HA content to return to normal levels. Despite the fact that HA content increases with prolonged CS use, the catabolic effect on cartilage matrix increases the vulnerability of cartilage to traumatic injury. Corticosteroids administered at higher doses or at more frequent intervals than recommended can lead or contribute to steroid arthopathy.

Injection of some CSs can lead to a nonseptic inflammatory response ('steroid flare') characterized by heat, swelling, and pain.[108] This inflammatory response can begin as early as a few hours following injection and may last from a few hours up to several days. The reaction is believed to be in response to the microcrystalline suspension of the CS ester, and occurs in approximately 2% of injected joints.[108] Septic arthritis can occur subsequent to any intra-articular injection secondary to inadvertent contamination of the joint during arthrocentesis.[108] Because CSs suppress the local immune response in the joint following intra-articular injection, the environment is conducive for infection to develop. Inadvertent deposition of long-acting CSs in peri-articular soft tissues can cause idiopathic metaplastic bone formation.[108] This condition does not occur with short-acting steroids, which suggests a reaction to the vehicle in the long-acting formulations. The ossification may take several months to develop, and mechanical interference can occur if the lesions become sufficiently large.

Empirical evidence suggests that higher doses of glucocorticoids can trigger laminitis in the horse and this is the main reason higher doses are not typically recommended. However, no studies have been published that show the dose or dosing regimen that is required to reliably induce laminitis. It's unlikely that glucocorticoids induce laminitis via inflammatory pathways or the expression of MMPs but the potential for glucocorticoids to induce equine laminitis via tissue catabolism, lamellar epithelial apoptosis, insulin resistance (hyperglycemia), GI damage or vasoconstriction, exists.[144] In one study, nine horses were treated intradermally with DEX for 6 consecutive days. A local cooling of the skin resulted, suggesting that DEX may also cause reduced laminar perfusion.[145] However, in one retrospective, uncontrolled study of the clinical use of TMA in 205 mature horses, only 1 (0.5%) developed laminitis in association with TMA therapy, though this horse had been treated previously for laminitis.[146] In a third publication, the author reported that laminitis associated with IA injection of corticosteroids had occurred in 3/2000 (0.15%) cases. The majority of the time TMA was used and the upper total dose ranged 20–45 mg.[147]

The possible existence of a relationship between IA CS therapy and catastrophic injury has been the focus of much interest in recent years. However, direct support of any relationship is largely lacking. In one report on the effects of intra-articular TMA (12 mg) on subchondral bone in horses with experimentally-induced osteochondral fragmentation of the distal radial carpal bone, there were no deleterious effects on the dynamics of bone remodeling and fragility.[133] However, the investigators mentioned their concern that the treated horses, which were less lame, did not have increased subchondral bone formation as expected from their improved weight bearing and increased loading. They speculated that TMA might have caused a slight reduction in the normal subchondral bone remodeling response.[133] In a second study comparing the mechanical effects of intra-articular MPA in horses undergoing short-term treadmill exercise, no effect on subchondral bone or underlying cancellous bone hardness was noted.[148]

Systemic effects of intra-articularly administered corticosteroids

Once intra-articularly administered CSs are absorbed from the synovial cavity, they undergo hepatic biotransformation and renal excretion.[105] Corticosteroids administered intra-articularly are absorbed and can have systemic effects, which has been shown by suppression of the endogenous cortisone levels.[106] Serum concentrations of TMA after injection of 6 mg into three joints of horses peaked 4 hours postinjection and became undetectable by 48 hours postinjection.[149] Only extremely small concentrations of isoflupredone became measurable in serum 24 hours postinjection of 4 mg despite concentrations of both drugs remaining detectable in the synovial fluid of treated joints for up to 10 days after injection.[114] Neither drug was detected in the synovial fluid of the contralateral joint despite detectable quantities in serum. Concentrations of the parent drug or metabolites of both MPA and isoflupredone were detected in urine for 24 and 72 hours, respectively. The study demonstrates the rapid elimination of these two CS preparations from the synovial fluid and serum of horses.

Sodium hyaluronate

Mechanism of action

Hyaluronate (HA) is endogenously synthesized by synoviocytes and chondrocytes. The viscoelasticity of the synovial fluid and the boundary lubrication function of the synovial membrane are directly proportional to the concentration and polymerization of the hyaluronate synthesized and present within the joint.[150–153] Hyaluronate incorporated into the extracellular matrix of articular cartilage forms the nucleus for proteoglycan aggregates within the equine joint.[154] Exogenous HA is thought to supplement the actions of depleted or depolymerized endogenous HA; and modulate the increased synthesis of endogenous HA.[155–164] The half-life of intra-articular HA injected into the normal equine joint is estimated to be 96 hours.[165] The half-life of intra-articular HA injected into the arthritic joints of sheep decreased from 20.8 hours to 11.5 hours.[166] The short half-life suggests that a majority of the exogenous hyaluronate is rapidly cleared from the joint; and that only a portion remains within the joint associated with the synovial tissues influencing the metabolic activity of these cells.[165–167] It is this reduction in half-life that prompts some surgeons to delay the use of IA HA upon completion of routine arthroscopic surgery until some days have passed to allow joint inflammation to subside. That said, other studies show that the concentration of synovial fluid HA measured in joints affected with acute synovitis or acute and chronic arthritis does not differ significantly from the concentrations within normal equine joints; however, joints affected by septic arthritis or with radiographic evidence of osteoarthritis have significantly lower HA concentrations than normal controls.[168–169]

The anti-inflammatory effects of exogenous HA have been demonstrated in numerous in vitro studies. These affects include inhibition of macrophage and granulocyte chemotaxis, inhibition of lymphocyte migration, and reduction of granulocyte and macrophage phagocytosis.[166,170–177] HA is thought to interact with the CD44 cell receptor of neutrophils inhibiting neutrophil-mediated degradation and PGE_2 production; this interaction is concentration and molecular weight dependent.[178] Hyaluronate has an indirect effect upon articular cartilage mediated through the HA binding domain of the proteoglycan molecule at the chondrocyte cell surface.[179] High concentrations of intra-articular HA bind the domain and suppress IL-1β and TNF-α-induced proteoglycan degradation, thus reducing inflammation and inhibiting cartilage degeneration and early osteoarthritis.[180–183] Hyaluronic acid also induces chondrogenesis of equine mesenchymal stem cells (MSCs), setting the stage for tissue engineering applications of MSC in chondral defects, as the natural environment in the joint is favorable for chondrogenic differentiation.[184] A study using partially meniscectomized rabbit stifles demonstrated the ability of high molecular weight HA to inhibit cartilage degeneration and early osteoarthritis in the femoral condyle and tibial plateau of the treated joints.[180,185] Despite research results, clinical reports, and anecdotal success, the exact mechanisms by which HA exerts its beneficial effect upon diseased joints remains speculative.

Indications for use

Joint disease

The use of HA for the treatment of joint disease in the horse was first reported in 1970.[162] Since that time, clinical reports have supported the use of HA for the treatment of equine joint disease. However, a majority of the evaluations are subjective, the criteria for successful treatment are absent, the duration of post-treatment observation is highly variable, and the specific diagnosis for the condition being treated is lacking.[156,158,160,164–165,171–172,186–189]

In vitro studies

With regard to more objective in vitro studies of effect, equine synoviocytes were grown in monolayer culture and stimulated with LPS and simultaneously treated with various concentrations of HA or polysulfated glycosaminoglycan (PSGAG) for 48 hours. The highest concentrations of HA and PSGAG tested inhibited PGE_2 production, prompting the authors to suggest that this anti-inflammatory action may be a mechanism through which these agents exert their anti-arthritic effect.[190] In a second study, proteoglycan release in response to recombinant human IL-1beta (rh-IL-1beta), was measured in equine cartilage explants and fibrocartilage. Hyaluronan (0.2 microgram/mL) significantly reduced rh-IL-1beta-induced proteoglycan release in metacarpal hyaline cartilage ($P < 0.01$), but had no effect or the opposite effect in navicular tissue.[191]

In vivo studies

A more objective report, utilizing a bilateral osteochondral fracture model created with an arthrotomy, concluded that IA HA had a protective effect on the articular cartilage and resulted in reduced lameness. However, both treated and non-treated limbs returned to pre-operative weight-bearing values.[163,187] In a double-blind study using IA hylan, an HA derivative, gait analysis found no beneficial effect in the treatment of acute amphotericin-induced synovitis.[188] When synovial fluid was collected from the tarsometatarsal joint of 25 horses without hindlimb lameness (controls) and 25 lame horses, HA concentration in the synovial fluid as determined by ELISA revealed no significant difference between lame and control horses. Nor was there a correlation between levels of synovial fluid HA and radiographic changes.[192]

Other investigations have evaluated the effect of intravenous HA on carpal joints in exercising horses after arthroscopic surgery and osteochondral fragmentation. The investigators concluded that intravenous HA appears to alleviate signs of lameness by interacting with synoviocytes, and by decreasing the production and release of inflammatory mediators. Treated horses had lower lameness scores, significantly better synovial membrane histologic scores, and significantly lower concentrations of total protein and PGE_2 within the synovial fluid when compared to placebo-treated horses. No significant effects were noted for GAG content, synthetic rate or morphologic score in articular cartilage, or other synovial fluid measurements.[189]

The effects of an oral formulation of hyaluronan gel on joint effusion following arthroscopic surgery of the tarsocrural joint for OCD have also been assessed in yearling Thoroughbreds. Twenty-four horses (27 joints) were treated with 100 mg of HA orally for 30 days post operatively and 24 (30 joints) with a placebo orally for 30 days. The mean 30 day effusion score of the HA treated group was 0.67 while the mean of the 30 day placebo group was 2.05 ($P <$ or $=0.0001$), implying that oral HA reduced joint effusion post operatively.[193]

Tendon lesions

Hyaluronic acid has been shown to improve tendon healing with naturally occurring tendonitis, and was proposed to have prevented scar formation along the damaged tendon tissue.[194] In an experimental study of collagenase-induced tendonitis, peritendinous injections of HA improved tendon healing in areas not associated with a tendon sheath.[195] Intra-thecal injections of HA improved tendon healing as measured by ultrasound, increased the HA content of tendon sheath synovial fluid, and reduced the number of adhesions formed between the tendon and sheath. Histologically, the HA reduced inflammatory cell infiltrate, improved tendon structure, and minimized intra-tendinous hemorrhage.[196] Another study of collagenase-induced tendonitis examined the effect of subcutaneous peri-tendinous HA upon lameness, ultrasonographic healing, biochemical indices, biomechanical strength, and inflammation.[197] The study did not reveal significant benefits of treatment with HA outside the synovial sheath on tendon repair in collagenase-induced tendonitis.[197]

Intrasynovial HA injections have has been used extensively, particularly in combination with corticosteroids, for the clinical management of foot pain. Outcome is unpredictable but treatment can extend the duration of soundness in some horses.[140,198] The direct benefit of injection of HA into the navicular bursa or the digital flexor tendon sheath of horses which have deep digital flexor tendon lesions as part of their pathology is questionable since animals with DDFT lesions generally have a poorer clinical outcome.[140]

Effective dose

Early in vitro work demonstrated that HA with a molecular weight greater than 5×10^2 kDa stimulated the synthesis of HA in a concentration-dependent manner, and that HA preparations with a molecular weight below 5×10^2 kDa had little or no effect except at high concentrations when HA synthesis was depressed.[199] Therefore in vitro, the effect of molecular weight has been clearly demonstrated, but the correlation between molecular weight and clinical effect remains less clearly defined. A comparative study, utilizing five HA products for the treatment of traumatic arthritis, found that horses treated with HA of a molecular weight greater than 2×10^3 kDa were sound significantly longer than those horses treated with HA with a molecular weight less than 2×10^3 kDa.[200] A study utilizing 77 trotters with moderate to severe joint injuries, investigated the comparative effect of HA, PSGAG, and a placebo in a double-blind, randomized design. No difference was detected between treatment groups with regard to prevalence or cumulative incidence of soundness; however, the treatment groups did have reduced lameness scores and significantly better results than the placebo.[201] To add to the controversy, another blinded study looking at the clinical effect of HA in the treatment of 69 Thoroughbreds with carpitis found no therapeutic response or clinically significant difference between HA with molecular weights of 0.13×10^3 kDa and 2.88×10^3 kDa.[202] In an in vitro study assessing the effects of lower and higher molecular weight HA on LPS-challenged fibroblast-like synovial cells, higher molecular weight HA decreased the morphologic change ($P < 0.05$) associated with LPS exposure. Both lower and higher molecular weight HA significantly decreased expression of inflammatory genes (PGE2, IL-6) and catabolic genes (MMP3) and prompted increased expression of anti-inflammatory and anabolic genes. The molecular weight of the HA product did not affect the cell number, the cell viability or the PGE_2, IL-6, or MMP3 production. Taken together, the data supported the pharmacologic benefits of treatment with HA regardless of molecular weight although the higher molecular weight HA provided a cellular protective effect not seen with the lower molecular weight HA.[203]

The molecular weight and manufacturers' dosage recommendations of the currently available HA formulations are given in Table 23.3 and Table 23.4, respectively. The HA formulations currently available for intravenous injection are Legend® (Bayer) in the United States and Hyonate® (Bayer) elsewhere. The manufacturer recommends that Legend®, 40 mg sodium hyaluronate (4 mL) be administered IV once or twice (Hyonate®) or once weekly for a total of three treatments (Legend®). There is substantial inter-individual variability regarding the preferred route of administration of hyaluronate products, whether used alone or in combination with other medications.[204]

Drug interactions

Hyaluronate is frequently combined with CSs for intra-articular treatment of degenerative joint disease in horses. Retrospective studies have shown that intra-articular administration of CSs may suppress effective microbial killing; reducing the immune status within the joints of horses and increase the potential for low numbers of bacteria to establish an infection within the injected joint.[205–208] A prospective study, utilizing intra-articular HA in carpal joints inoculated with *Staphylococcus aureus*, showed no difference in the development of sepsis between HA-injected joints and controls.[209] However, the potential for septic arthritis and the incidence of 'synovial flare' may be increased for combination drug therapy utilizing CSs.[210]

Table 23.3 The average molecular weight of currently available sodium hyaluronate formulations for intra-articular use[102, 339]

TRADE NAME	MANUFACTURER	AVERAGE MOLECULAR WEIGHT IN DALTONS (DA)
Hyalovet	Fort Dodge	$4.0–7.0 \times 10^5$
Hyvisc	Boehringer Ingelheim	2.1×10^6
Synacid	Shering-Plough	$0.15–0.20 \times 10^6$
Hylartin V	Pharmacia & Upjohn	3.5×10^6
HY-50	Bexco Pharma	Not available
Equron	Solvay Animal Health	$1.5–2.0 \times 10^6$
Equiflex	Chesapeake Biological	1×10^6
Legend	Bayer Corporation	3×10^5

Toxicity

No contraindications to HA use are noted on the label, and acute toxicological studies performed in horses demonstrate no evidence for systemic toxicity secondary to acute and chronic overdose.[211] Intra-articular and intravenous HA at one, three, and five times the recommended dose were administered at weekly intervals for a total of nine weeks. Clinical, hematologic, and clinical chemistry parameters remained unchanged. Transient slight to mild post-injection swelling of the joint capsule occurred in horses treated with HA, as well as with the saline control. Neither gross nor histological lesions were noted in either the soft tissues or the articular cartilage of the treated and control joints.[211] The safety of using HA in breeding animals has not been established, and manufacturers caution against its use in these animals.[212]

Polysulfated glycosaminoglycans

Mechanism of action

Polysulafted glycosaminoglycans (PSGAG) are highly sulfated polysaccharides derived from the extract of bovine lung and trachea. The principal glycosaminoglycan present in PSGAG is chondroitin sulfate. PSGAGs are known to inhibit many of the enzymes associated with osteoarthritis and connective tissue degradation. In vitro studies have shown that PSGAGs are capable of inhibiting lysosomal elastase, cathepsins G and B, lysosomal hydrolases, keratin sulfate glycoanhydrolase, serine proteases, neutral metalloproteinase (eg, proteoglycanase, stromelysin, gelatinase, and collagenase), β-glucuronidase, α-glucosidase, β-N-acetylglucosaminidase, and hyaluronidase.[166,213–216] In addition, PSGAGs have been reported

Table 23.4 Manufacturers' recommendations for intra-articular use of sodium hyaluronate in horses[339-345]

TRADE NAME	CONCENTRATION	PACKAGING	RECOMMENDED DOSE
Hyalovet	10 mg/ml	2 ml syringe	20 mg hyaluronate sodium (2 ml) should be administered aseptically in small or medium-sized joints not more than twice weekly for a period not to exceed 4 weeks.
Hyvisc	11 mg/ml	5 ml syringe containing 2 ml dose	22 mg hyaluronate sodium (2 ml) should be administered aseptically in small and medium-sized joints and a double dose or 44 mg hyaluronate sodium (4 mL) in larger joints once weekly for a total of 3 treatments.
Synacid	10 mg/ml	5 ml vial	50 mg of hyaluronate sodium (5 ml) should be given intra-articularly in carpal and fetlock joints. Synacid should be injected under strict aseptic conditions and effusion should be removed prior to injection.
Hylartin V	10 mg/ml	2 ml syringe	20 mg sodium hyaluronate (2 mL) should be administered aseptically in small and medium-sized joints and a double dose or 40 mg hyaluronate sodium (4 mL) in larger joints once weekly for a total of 3 treatments.
Equron	5 mg/ml	2 ml syringe	The dose of Equron in small and medium size joints (fetlock, carpal) is 2 ml (10 mg) administered intra-articularly. In larger joints (hock), the dose is 4 ml (20 mg). Depending on the clinical response and medical judgement of the veterinarian, the treatment may be repeated weekly for a total of 4 treatments.
Legend	10 mg/ml	2 ml vial	20 mg sodium hyaluronate (2 mL) should be administered aseptically in small and medium-sized joints once weekly for a total of 3 treatments.

to inhibit PGE synthesis, influx of leukocytes into inflammatory sites, and the production of superoxide radicals and IL-1 and to have a dose-related effect on fibroblast and tenocyte metabolism resulting in increased production of collagen, noncollagen proteins, and sulfated glycosaminoglycans.[166,217]

Polysulafted glycosaminoglycan has been shown to have a greater affinity for proteoglycans and noncollagenous proteins than for collagen.[214] Fibronectin, which is increased in osteoarthritic cartilage, forms complexes with collagen, which are then stabilized by PSGAG.[214] PSGAGs exert their chondroprotective effect by reducing proteoglycan breakdown, stimulating HA synthesis, and enhancing the production of glycosaminglycan, proteoglycan (glucosamine), and collagen (proline).[217-220]

Joint disease

In vitro studies

In vitro studies on equine cartilage indicate that PSGAG increases collagen and glycosaminoglycan synthesis, and inhibits glycosaminoglycan and collagen degeneration in normal and osteoarthritic articular cartilage explants and cell cultures.[221] However, in vitro work using smaller PSGAG dosages found a dose-dependent inhibition of proteoglycan synthesis, minimal effect on proteoglycan degradation, no effect on proteoglycan monomer size, and no change in monomer aggregation.[222-223] When cultured equine chondrocytes were used to determine the effects of recombinant equine IL-1beta (reIL-1beta) on the expression and activity of inducible nitric oxide synthase (iNOS), their simultaneous exposure to PSGAG significantly reduced iNOS gene expression and media supernatant nitrite concentrations. The authors concluded that the pre-translational regulation of the iNOS gene by PSGAG may contribute to the cartilage-sparing properties of the compound.[224] However, in a related study, PSGAG did not influence COX-2 activity in cultured equine chondrocytes exposed to reIL-1beta.[225] When PSGAG was administered into the joint of horses in which an ostochondral fracture had been purposely created, it had no influence on subchondral bone density, histological appearance or serum bone biomarkers.[226]

In vivo studies

PSGAG is believed to have chondroprotective properties, which make its use preferable when cartilage damage is present in addition to acute synovitis. PSGAGs have been classified as disease modifying osteoarthritis drugs meaning that therapy with this drug is meant to prevent, retard, or reverse the morphologic cartilaginous lesions associated with osteoarthritis.[227]

In vivo work utilizing chemically- and physically-induced models of intercarpal joint osteoarthritis of horses demonstrated less articular fibrillation and erosion, less chondrocyte death, markedly improved safarin-O staining, but no change in the partial or full thickness articular cartilage lesions.[228-229] Investigators concluded:

- that intra-articular PSGAG (250 mg every seven days for five treatments) could markedly decrease the development of osteoarthritis, but was of no benefit in healing cartilage lesions present at the time of initial therapy
- intramuscular PSGAG (500 mg every four days for seven treatments) had an insignificant effect upon physical cartilage defects and only a limited effect upon chemically-induced osteoarthritis as evidenced by a slight degree of improvement in safarin-O staining.[228-229]

Another study investigated the effect of PSGAG, with or without exercise, on the repair of articular cartilage defects and on the development of osteoarthritis in the carpi of ponies. Investigators concluded that PSGAG was effective in ameliorating clinical, radiographic, and scintigraphic signs associated with joint disease, but that repair tissue was more fibrous in the PSGAG treated joints and the synovium of the PSGAG exercised joints had an a greater degree of cellular infiltration.[230–231] When 128 horses with lameness referable to the DIP joint received either three IA injections of PSGAG approximately eight days apart or a single IA injection of MPA, 67% receiving PSGAG had a successful outcome compared with 46% of the group receiving MPA. It should be noted however that a significantly better result was obtained in dressage horses than in jumping horses (eventing and showjumping) and other variables including age, duration of lameness, distribution and degree of lameness were also associated with success of treatment.[232]

In a clinically relevant study, experimentally induced carpal arthritis was treated on study days 14, 21 and 28 with either IA PSGAG (250 mg) and amikacin (125 mg) or HA (20 mg) and amikacin (125 mg). No changes in clinical signs were seen with PSGAG or HA, compared with control horses but histologically, the degree of synovial membrane vascularity and subintimal fibrosis was significantly reduced with PSGAG treatment, compared with controls. Histologically, significantly less fibrillation was seen with hyaluronan treatment, compared with controls.[53] In another study, 12 healthy horses were subject to the monoioidoacetate (MIA) carpitis model, which was allowed to develop for seven days. Horses treated with 500 mg of a PSGAG intramuscularly every four days for seven treatments showed less joint circumference enlargement and lameness and greater carpal flexion compared with controls.[233] PSGAG (Adequan) was the most frequently used disease modifying medication, independent of route of administration) (423/674, 62.8%) in a recent survey.[204] The majority of respondents who used PSGAG chose to administer it IM (643/764 [84.1%]). Most commonly, 78.3% of respondents used it for prophylactic/preventative treatments. It was also used IM by 425/727 (58.5%) in chronic maintenance cases, and by 396/727 (54.5%) in post-operative horses starting back into training. Intramuscular PSGAG was the most common medication selected by respondents for treatment of acute disease in low motion joints (325/727 [44.7%]).

Tendon lesions

Negative charges conferred by sulfate groups cause PSGAG to bind to connective tissues.[213–214,216] In rabbits, radioactively labeled PSGAG is distributed to knee joint articular cartilage, patellar cartilage, meniscus, and intervertebral disk tissue following intramuscular administration.[213–216] The widespread distribution of PSGAG to connective tissue has proven useful in the treatment of tendontis. In rabbits with collagenase-induced tendonitis, treatment with PSGAG resulted in diminished loss of tendon mechanical properties, an increased number of large diameter collagen fibrils, improved organization of repair tissue at the cellular level, and suppression of inflammation.[234] In horses with collagenase-induced tendonitis, those treated with PSGAG had earlier sonographic development of echogenic patterns, a more rapid decrease in core defect size, and less severe lameness, compared with a control group of untreated horses.[235] In a similar study, intralesional PSGAG yielded substantially more organized collagen bundles in the healing superficial digital flexor tendon at 150 days post collagenenase injection than did saline treated controls.[236] In a recent survey, PSGAG was the most common treatment used for a tendon or ligament lesion for 27% (201/727) of respondents[204].

Effective dose

The PSGAGs are most commonly administered by the intramuscular route. Previous work investigating the distribution of radiolabeled PSGAG after IM administration found PSGAG concentrations within the synovial fluid and joint tissues of the carpus consistent with other non-equine studies. No significant difference was found between carpi containing osteochondral fragments and the control joints, suggesting that distribution is not influenced by inflammatory changes. Investigators concluded that intramuscular therapy (500 mg intramuscular every four days) was effective in maintaining anti-inflammatory levels in the joints.[213] Another study, using intramuscular radiolabeled PSGAG in rabbits, demonstrated PSGAG within the superficial digital flexor tendon at concentrations shown to inhibit inflammatory mediators in vitro.[237] Investigators used the label dose for the horse, and concluded that PSGAG may be useful in the treatment of acute tendonitis.[237]

The PSGAG formulations currently available for intra-articular and intramuscular use are Adequan I.A.® (Luitpold) and Adequan I.M.® (Luitpold), respectively. Manufacturer's recommend that Adequan I.A.® (250 mg, 1 mL) be injected aseptically into the affected joint once a week for five weeks; and that Adequan I.M.® (500 mg, 5 mL) be injected aseptically into the muscles of the neck every four days for 28 days or seven treatments. The initial treatment with Adqequan I.M.® at manufacturer's recommended dose and frequency is often followed with one intramuscular dose every 30 days while the horse is in training. Sterile preparation of the injection site accompanied by the use of a single-dose preparation with the addition of 125 mg of amikacin sulfate is standard practice for intra-articular administration of Adequan I.A.®[238]

Drug interactions

The PSGAGs is frequently combined with CSs for IA treatment of degenerative joint disease in horses. Retrospective studies have shown that intra-articular administration of corticosteroids may suppress effective microbial killing; reducing the immune status within the joints of horses and increasing the potential for low numbers of bacteria to establish an infection within the injected joint.[205–208] A prospective study, utilizing IA PSGAG in carpal joints inoculated with *Staphylococcus aureus*, demonstrated significant increase in the potential for sepsis between PSGAG injected joints and controls.[209] Previous in vitro work has shown PSGAG-mediated inhibition of the equine complement activity. Inhibition of the complement cascade within the joint may increase the potential for subinfective doses of bacteria to colonize the synovium resulting in sepsis.[239] Therefore, the potential for septic arthritis and the incidence of 'synovial flare' may be increased with the use of intra-articular PSGAG alone or in combination with CSs.[240]

There is some concern regarding the potential anticoagulant effect of PSGAG which is classified as a heparin analog, and has been known to cause local hematomas and heparin-associated thrombocytopenia in humans.[241] Although it has been suggested that PSGAG not be used in conjunction with other NSAIDs or other anticoagulants; there have been no reports of hemarthrosis, thrombocytopenia, or coagulopathies in horses despite its widespread use both alone and in combination with NSAID administration.[242]

Toxicity

Toxicology studies were conducted in horses: doses as high as 1250 mg PSGAG were administered intra-carpally to six horses once a week for 18 weeks. This dosage is 5.0 times the recommended dosage and 3.6 times the recommended therapeutic regimen. Clinical observations revealed mild, self-limiting swelling and soreness at the injection site in 1.8% of the horses. A dose-related increase in partial thromboplastin time, creatinine, and glucose were noted. Toxicological studies of doses as high as 2500 mg were administered intramuscularly to six horses twice a week for 12 weeks. This dosage is five times the recommended dosage and three times the recommended therapeutic regimen. None of the animals in this study showed any adverse effect on clinical, hemtologic, or clinical chemistry parameters.[240] Studies have not been performed to establish reproductive safety in horses, and manufacturers caution against its use in these animals.

Chondroitin sulfate

Mechanism of action

Chondroitin sulfate (CHS) is the predominant glycosaminoglycan found in adult articular cartilage. CHS is similar to PSGAG in that both contain repeating chains of galactosamine and glucuronic acid disaccharide units, but CHS contains only one sulfate group per dissacharide unit compared with the three or four sulfate groups per disaccharide unit for PSGAG.[243] The presence of sulfate groups is critical to the pharmacology and pharmacokinetic activity of both PSGAG and CHS.[243] Chondroitin sulfate has been classified as a slow-acting, disease-modifying agent (SADMA) and as a slow-acting drug in osteoarthritis (SADOA).[244–246] It has been shown to inhibit degradative enzymes such as leukocyte elastase and N-acetylglycosaminidase in vitro. However, it must be noted that these inhibitory activities refer to intact polymeric CHS molecules, and the efficacy of unsulfated monomeric forms and other degradation products is unknown and untested.[247–248]

Chondroitin sulfate marketed for use as a dietary supplement in horses is usually in combination with glucosamine with or without added vitamins and minerals. The bioavailability of oral CHS remains speculative, and scientific literature provides conflicting results. Absorption of radiolabelled CHS has been reported for man, dogs, and rats; however, less than 15% of the molecules were absorbed as high molecular weight fractions. Investigators concluded that a majority of the CHS was absorbed only after degradation to a smaller molecular weight products and the loss of the sulfate group.[249–252] The absence of absorption of oral CHS has been reported for several studies in humans and rabbits in which a dimethylene blue assay was unable to detect the presence of smaller sulfated glycosaminoglycan molecules.[252–253]

Large intestinal bacteria utilize CHS directly as an energy source; while bacterial sulphatases remove the active sulfate groups from the disaccharide units thus allowing for the appearance of radioactive inorganic sulfate to be present in the body after oral administration of $^{35}SO_4$-labelled CHS.[254] This has led some researchers to conclude that CHS is not absorbed following oral administration, but rather a low molecular weight desulfated degradation product of the disaccharide polymer is absorbed instead. However, absorption of CHS and dermatan sulfate from the gastrointestinal tract has been reported in humans. Treated patients had reduced N-acetylglycosaminidase and granulocyte activity, as well as an increase in HA concentrations.[250] Skeptics would conclude that the existence of a polymer chain and the presence of sulfate groups are necessary for the biologic activity of CHS, therefore any positive clinical response to oral administration of CHS is secondary to the biological activity of its low molecular weight degradation products or from the activity of other substances present in the supplement, such as glucosamine.[255]

Exogenous CHS has been shown in vitro to have no detrimental effects on normal articular cartilage explants.[256] When equine cartilage explants were exposed to LPS in varying concentrations of GLN, CHS or both, the combination of CHS (0.25 mg/ml) and GLN (1 mg/ml) inhibited the synthesis of the mediators of cartilage deterioration.[257] In a second in vitro study using equine articular cartilage incubated with IL-1 conditioned media, there was no detrimental effect of GLN, CHS alone or combined on GAG synthesis nor total GAG content. High doses of GLN + CHS reduced total GAG release into the media.[256] In a 2005 review of the compound, CHS was reported in vitro to increase the synthesis or decrease the turnover of PGs and GAGs.[258] The effects of CHS on the metabolism of type II collagen was also reported to be minimal.[258] CHS was also reported in vitro to inhibit MMP expression and activity and as well as that of aggrecanase in a dose-dependent manner.[258] It has also been shown to increase the concentration and improve the composition (viscosity) of HA which may play a role in its anti-inflammatory effects.[258] In addition, using equine cartilage explants as well as human chondrocyte cultures, CHS has been shown to have the potential to affect the inflammatory cycle via regulation of PGE2 as well as NO production such that both are decreased after CHS administration.[258] Chondroitin sulfate has generally been shown to have a longer duration of action, producing fewer side effects than NSAIDs, while improving the clinical signs associated with OA. In fact, CHS administration may allow for the NSAID dose to be lowered or even discontinued after 6–8 weeks.[259]

Indications for use

Several studies report positive responses to oral CHS therapy for the management of osteoarthritis in the human knee.[260–265] One human study utilizing oral treatment with *Perna canalculus* extract for a period of six months, reported 19 of the 28 rheumatoid and 15 of the 38 osteoarthritis patients felt that they benefited from the oral CHS therapy.[264] Positive results associated with oral CHS therapy have been reported for a rabbit model of osteoarthritis, as well as for a chemically-induced canine synovitis model. Dogs with chemically-induced synovitis pre-treated with CHS combined with glucosamine had reduced soft tissue and bone phase scintigraphic activity as well as reduced lameness scores. However, treatment after the induction of synovitis (without pre-treatment) showed no beneficial effects.[266] When administered in conjunction with glucosamine HCl and N-acetyl-D-glucosamine as an oral supplement to horses for 12 weeks, range of joint motion increased significantly by week eight in the elbow ($P < 0.05$), stifle and hind fetlock ($P < 0.01$). Stride length also increased significantly ($P < 0.05$) with treatment. Swing duration was significantly increased at week 12 ($P < 0.05$), whilst stance duration remained constant, leading to the conclusion that the oral chondroprotective offered symptomatic relief.[267]

Effective dose

A plethora of choices exists regarding oral supplement for the treatment and prevention of joint disease in the horse. Each brand contains varying concentrations of CHS with or without glucosamine (GLN) as key ingredients. These ingredients are then combined with a variety of vitamins, minerals, and frequently a secret compound. The supplements are usually recommended as daily top dressing for feed, and manufacturers provide a measuring device specific to their product. Because these products are classified as dietary supplements and neutraceuticals, the efficacy, safety, and quality assurance programs put forth by the United States Food and Drug Administration do not apply.

Recommendations regarding effective dose, long-term toxicity, drug interaction, and teratogenicity have been largely anecdotal or based on manufacturer's claims.[247,250,252,268–270] One product, Cosequin®, has been clinically and scientifically evaluated. One trial consisted of 25 clinical cases of horses with joint pain treated with oral Cosequin® for a period of six weeks.[271] In this study, lameness, response to flexion, and stride length improved with Cosequin therapy, however, there were no controls. In another study utilizing the Freund's complete adjuvant model of inflammatory joint disease, 12 horses were treated with oral Cosequin® for a total of 36 days.[272] Therapy began 10 days prior to induction of arthritis and continued for 26 days afterward. No benefit was observed for lameness, stride length, carpal circumference, or response to carpal flexion, and synovial fluid protein concentration did not improve.[272] Due to the widespread use and popularity of these products, controlled studies and scientific validation are still needed to address the controversy regarding enteral absorption, pharmacokinetics, toxicity, drug interaction, and clinical efficacy.

Glucosamine

Mechanism of action

Chondrocytes manufacture GLN from glucose as a precursor for the glycosaminoglycan units found within articular cartilage.[273–274] Glucosamine has been classified as a slow-acting, disease-modifying agent, a slow acting drug in osteoarthritis, and as a chondroprotective. When available, GLN becomes the preferred substrate over glucose for chondrocytes synthesis of glycosaminoglycans.

Glucosamine is a small, water-soluble molecule that is absorbed from the small intestine and across biological barriers in the body.[275–276] Glucosamine undergoes gastric dissociation to yield non-ionized glucosamine.[275–276] Glucosamine hydrochloride yields greater quantities of the active non-ionized form of GLN, than glucosamine sulfate. It is the non-ionized form of GLN that directly determines the bioavailability of the GLN compounds.[275–276] Labeling with [^{14}C] label in rats and the use of specific ion-exchange chromatography in dogs and humans, have demonstrated almost complete bioavailability with only 5% fecal loss.[275]

In vitro work has shown a dose-dependent increase in the synthesis of HA, glycosaminoglycan and proteoglycan in response to exogenous GLN.[274,276] Exogenous GLN inhibits superoxide radical generation, lysosomal enzyme production, nitric oxide production, proteoglycan loss, gelatinase activity, and collagenase activity in equine cartilage explants exposed to lipopolysaccharide and recombinant interleukin-1β.[277–278] The anti-inflammatory activity of GLN is achieved through a prostaglandin-independent mechanism, which is thought to contribute to cartilage preservation as well as provide protection against metabolic impairment induced by NSAIDs.[275,279–280] The effects of GLN on articular tissues could also occur via cellular signaling from various other nonarticular tissues.[258]

In vivo studies have demonstrated uniform incorporation of [^{14}C] labeled GLN into newly synthesized proteoglycans located within articular cartilage.[281–282] The anti-inflammatory effect of GLN does not influence or interfere with PG synthesis in rat and dog models, and has been shown to improve experimentally induced morphological damage to articular cartilage.[281–283] In rats, glucosamine counteracts metabolic and morphologic chondrocyte damage produced by intra-articular dexamethasone.[284] A study using human subjects affected with osteoarthritis looked at cartilage biopsies taken before and after four weeks of treatment with either oral glucosamine sulfate or placebo. Glucosamine therapy correlated with reduced use of joint pain analgesics and improved joint function. Electron microscopy performed on biopsy samples taken before treatment confirmed the presence of chronic osteoarthritis. Electron microscopy performed on biopsy samples taken after four weeks of treatment demonstrated evidence for an increase cartilage matrix production and a mild decrease in inflammatory activity, giving the affected cartilage an appearance more similar to healthy cartilage.[270,284]

Indications for use

Oral supplements or nutraceuticals, such as GLN, were initially developed as an alternative to the practical and financial limitations associated with intra-articular and intramuscular HA and PSGAG. Oral GLN administration has been associated with decreased pain and an increased range of motion when compared with placebo in a well-controlled clinical trial in people with osteoarthritis of the knee.[270] Oral GLN has been shown to alleviate the symptoms of chronic arthritis with daily dosing over a 6–8 week period.[285] Publications on the use of GLN in horses are available but meaningful interpretation of the data is often made difficult due to a lack of rigorous scientific method.[286–287] Clinical use is further complicated by inaccurate or misleading manufacturer claims and lack of regulation within the nutraceutical industry. The labeled constituents on GLN and associated nutraceutical products such as chondroitin or combined therapies may also not match the actual constituents. In a study of five GLN, five CHS, and one combination equine products, the actual composition of GLN was 63.6% to 112.2% of the label claim, whereas the concentration for CHS ranged from 22.5% to 155.7%. In addition, the GLN content was 86% of the label claim, and the CHS content was 83.3% of the label claim.[288] In a similar study, the range of measured amounts of product compared to the amount expected in each product based on the label claim was 0–221.2%. Of the 23 products included in that study, 9 (39.1%) contained less GLN than claimed by the manufacturer and 4 (17.4%) less than 30% of the expected amount of GLN.[289]

Effective dose

Two forms of GLN are available for oral administration, glucosamine hydrochloride and glucosamine sulfate. Both disassociate within the stomach, but the hydrochloride salt yields a greater amount of the active, non-ionized glucosamine, which has direct bioavailability. Given the consistency demonstrated for absorption, distribution, and elimination studies in humans, rats, and dogs; the assumption is that a similar effective dose rate of at least 10 grams per day is necessary to treat a 500 kg horse.[255] According to information provided on the product labels of 23 glucosamine containing products, the average recommended daily maintenance dose of GLN was 6302.2 mg (median 5000 mg). Recommendations ranged from 1800 to 12 000 mg GLN per os per day for an average sized mature horse.[289]

Dimethyl sulfoxide

Mechanism of action

Dimethyl sulfoxide (DMSO), a by-product of the lumber industry, was originally used as an industrial solvent. DMSO was first employed as a therapeutic agent in the treatment of interstitial cystitis and arthritis during the early 1960s.[290] Since that time, DMSO has been widely used within the equine industry alone or mixed with corticosteroids to reduce soft tissue swelling, inflammation, and edema secondary to acute trauma.[291–292]

The pharmacological effects of DMSO and its metabolite, dimethyl sulfide, are diverse. DMSO has been shown to possess superoxide dismutase activity. As a result, DMSO can inactivate superoxide radicals; inhibit hydroxyl radical mediated depolymerization of hyaluronan; and suppress PG synthesis by oxygen-derived free radicals.[290,292–295] DMSO is believed to possess analgesic properties secondary to the inhibition of prostaglandins E_2, $F_{2\alpha}$, H_2, and G_2. The analgesic effect of DMSO has been compared to that produced by narcotic analgesics and been found to be efficacious for both acute and chronic musculoskeletal pain.[296]

In addition to its anti-inflammatory effects, DMSO possesses the ability to rapidly and easily penetrate the skin. DMSO serves as a carrier to enhance the penetration of various agents through the skin into underlying synovial, connective, and interstitial tissues.[292,296–297] DMSO has been shown to enhance the penetration of percutaneous steroids three-fold, and the ability of cortisone to locally stabilize lysosomes by 100-fold.[292] In addition, DMSO increases the local anti-arthritic effect of hydrocortisone 10-fold when used as a carrier.[298]

DMSO has an anti-arthritic effect independent of its ability to promote corticosteroid absorption.[299] Topical application of the gel formulation of DMSO decreased the mean synovial white blood cell concentrations in an equine synovitis model.[297] DMSO has been shown to help resolve tissue inflammation through increased blood flow and promote vascular dilation.[292] DMSO causes collagen dissolution, which may help to restore pliability to fibrosed tissues.[292] Topical application of DMSO solution, in rabbits, reduced ankle stiffness in a fracture model of arthritis.[300] Both the anti-inflammatory and anti-arthritic effects of DMSO appear to be more effective when used to treat acute versus chronic inflammatory conditions.[296]

Both DMSO and dimethyl sulfide are extensively and rapidly distributed to all areas of the body after oral, intravenous, and topical administration.[296] The half-life of the parent compound and its metabolite is nine hours.[296] DMSO is primary excreted through the kidney, but secondary elimination through the respiratory tract and bile does occur.[296]

Indications for use

Dimethyl sulfoxide has been used intra-articularly for its anti-inflammatory and free radical scavenging properties in the management of equine inflammatory joint disease.[294–295,297,301–302] Several equine studies reporting the use of DMSO in intra-articular lavage solutions have shown a decrease in total synovial leukocyte counts and a decrease in synovial inflammatory response in DMSO-treated joints without evidence of gross, histological, or histochemical cartilage degradation.[303–305] Juvenile bovine articular cartilage explants repeatedly exposed to a 10% DMSO solution showed a significant time-dependent decrease in the rate of proteoglycan synthesis after 3 or more hours of exposure. Histologically, chondrocyte viability and cartilage matrix water content was decreased.[306] A recent study, evaluating the effect of DMSO on equine articular cartilage metabolism in an explant culture environment, examined proteoglycan synthesis and degradation; lactate metabolism (general indicator of cellular metabolism); and chondrocyte viability after exposure to various concentrations of DMSO for predetermined time intervals.[307] Proteoglycan and lactate metabolism were inhibited in a dose- and time-dependent manner after exposure to DMSO concentrations in excess of 5%. Proteoglycan release and chondrocyte viability were not affected, and the changes in proteoglycan synthesis and lactate metabolism returned to baseline after exposure period. Investigators concluded that DMSO concentrations in excess of 5% suppress equine articular cartilage matrix metabolism by direct inhibition of chondrocyte metabolism without a decrease in chondrocyte number. Thus DMSO induces a state of metabolic dormancy in the chondrocytes, however these effects are reversible and chrondrocyte viability is not affected.[307] In a 2001 study,[70] equine synovial membrane explants exposed to a 10% DMSO solution exhibited a deleterious histomorphologic score and no reduction in the production of PGE2 in response to lipopolysaccharide challenge.

Effective dose

Domoso® (Pfizer Animal Health) is commercially available as a 90% DMSO veterinary gel for topical use. Manufacturer recommendations are for liberal application to skin over affected area 2–3 times per day. The total daily dosage is not to exceed 100 grams, and the duration of therapy is not to exceed 30 days. Domoso® (Pfizer Animal Health) is also available as a 90% veterinary solution. The recommended dose for the solution is 0.25–1.0 grams/kg diluted in saline or 5% dextrose solution at a concentration of not more than 10%. The 10% solution is to be given at a slow rate once daily for three days. The solution can be administered orally through a nasogastric tube at a dose of 1.0 grams/kg diluted in 1 liter of water.

Treatment protocosl for equine septic arthritis include the option of joint lavage with lactated Ringer's solution containing 5% to 40% DMSO. Lavage solutions containing DMSO concentrations in excess of 5% have been shown to have detrimental effects upon articular cartilage matrix metabolism. Until further investigation and pharmacokinetic studies can be performed, the concentration of DMSO contained within intra-articular lavage solutions should not exceed 5%.[307]

The manufacturer cautions against the use of non-medical grade DMSO products, which may contain harmful impurities secondary to the distillation process.[296] Washing of the hands and wearing protective rubber gloves before handling DMSO is strongly recommended in order to avoid transcutaneous penetration of potentially harmful substances.

Drug interactions

Dimethyl sulfoxide possesses anti-cholinesterase activity, and therefore should not be combined or used in conjunction with organophosphates or other cholinesterase inhibitors.[211,296] Death secondary to mercury intoxication has been reported when DMSO was mixed with mercury salts (red blister), and applied topically to the legs of a horse.[296] Caution should be exercised when mixing DMSO with any drug due to enhanced percutaneous absorption and the potential for toxicosis. DMSO potentiates effects of heparin, insulin, corticosteroids, and atropine both topically and systemically.[211,296]

Toxicity

When used at the label dose, DMSO is safe. Local effects such as dermal irritation, exfoliation, erythema, and vesiculation are common even at recommended dosages. Local effects are exacerbated by the use of sweat wraps, blistering agents, heavy bandages, and occlusive dressings. These effects are transient and resolve when therapy is discontinued. When in contact with room air, DMSO will self-dilute to a concentration of 66 to 67% causing an unpleasant garlic smell and taste to which some individuals are highly sensitive.[211,296]

Hemolysis and secondary hemoglobinuria have been reported to occur in horses following rapid intravenous administration of concentrations in excess of 20%. This effect can be prevented by slowing the administration rate and diluting the DMSO with isotonic fluids to a concentration ≤ 10% or by administering the product orally via a nasogastric tube.[296] DMSO is known to be teratogenic and hepatotoxic in laboratory animal species, including rats and rabbits, and been shown to cause intravascular erythrocyte hemolysis and nephritis.[308] DMSO should therefore be used with caution in pregnant mares and individuals suffering from dehydration and renal or liver disease.[240,296]

Pentosan polysulfate

Mechanism of action

Pentosan polysulfate (PPS) is derived from beechwood hemicellulose, and is similar to PSGAG in that it is highly sulfated. Pentosan polysulfate does not possess analgesic activity, but rather works its effect through modification and correction of pathological imbalances associated with osteoarthritis to provide symptomatic relief.[309] Tritiated PPS has been shown to preferentially distribute to the urinary tract after IV administration; the large intestine, liver, and urinary tract after oral administration; and to the articular cartilage and meniscal fibrocartilage after intra-articular administration in rats and rabbits.[310–312] Human studies, using intra-articular administration of tritiated PPS, demonstrated the formation of complexes with the protein components of articular cartilage; while similar rats studies showed localization to cartilage and binding with synoviocytes.[312–313] A new calcium derivative of pentosan polysufate (CAPPS) has been developed that is absorbed more effectively after oral administration than the sodium salt of pentosan polysulfate (NAPPS).[314]

Pentosan polysulfate is a potent inhibitor of human granulocyte elastase, testicular and arterial hyaluronidase, lysosomal chondroitin-4-sulfatase, N-acetylglucosaminidase, cathepsin B_1, and cathepain G.[309,312,315–320] Pentosan polysulfate was able to stimulate the synthesis of proteoglycans by bovine chondrocytes cultured in the presence and absence of IL-1.[321] Pentosan polysulfate in a concentration range of 0.1 to 1.0 μg/ml was able to stimulate the production of HA by cultured synoviocytes obtained from rheumatoid and osteoarthritic joints with maximum stimulation occurring at concentrations of 0.25 μg/ml.[244,322] Pentosan polysulfate at concentrations of 0.1 to 10.0 μg/ml was shown to consistently stimulate proteoglycan synthesis in an in vitro lapine chondrocyte injury model. Synthesis increased to 25% above control level occurred at 1.0 μg/ml after 2–4 days in culture. This concentration is similar to the concentration of achieved in articular cartilage after intramuscular injection of the recommended therapeutic dose; therefore, the in vitro effect could be achieved in vivo.[168,244,322]

An experimental model for joint disease in rabbits demonstrated the ability of oral CAPPS to maintain a ratio of aggrecan to dermatan sulfate similar to normal articular cartilage.[323] A rabbit atrophy model for arthritis showed that PPS given intramuscularly at 10 mg/kg every other day prevented proteoglycan depletion from articular cartilage.[324] An anterior cruciate transection model and a joint atrophy model for canine osteoarthritis demonstrated significant reductions in active stromelysin levels concomitant with increased levels of tissue inhibitor metalloproteinase in the articular cartilage of treated dogs associated with intramuscular PPS given at 2 mg/kg once weekly.[325–326] A sodium iodoacetate-induced model of arthritis reported amelioration of radiographic and histologic indexes of joint degeneration for chickens treated with 1 to 5 μg of PPS.[309] It should be noted that the once weekly for four weeks administration of PPS at dose rates up to 10 mg/kg prompted a dose dependent increase in partial thromboplastin time which, while small, prompted the authors to recommend against activities predisposing to stress or injury within 24 hours of administration. A maximum dose rate of 3 mg/kg was recommended.[327]

Indications for use

Pentosan polysulfate has been found to abrogate the deleterious effects of chronic administration of hydrocortisone when injected simultaneously into the knee joints of rabbits.[328] An owner and clinician-blinded study of 40 dogs with osteoarthritis found significant improvement in stiffness, mobility, and pain on joint manipulation for dogs treated weekly with intramuscular NAPPS at 3 mg/kg for four weeks. The overall responses were measured with a validated scoring system and the effects were evident for a period up to four weeks after the first treatment. NAPPS was evaluated in a randomized prospective study to determine its applicability in the treatment of fragmented coronoid process and osteochondritis dessicans of the elbow compared with conventional surgical management of these disorders in dogs. Dogs treated with intramuscular NAPPS at 3 mg/kg had more rapid improvement of limb function relative to surgically treated dogs as determined by force plate analysis. At nine months, no detectable difference between NAPPS treated and surgically treated dogs was detected. Investigators concluded that NAPPS injections are a valid alternative to surgery for the management of fragmented coronoid process and osteochondritis dessicans in dogs.[329] In an equine in vivo study, osteoarthritis was induced arthroscopically in one middle carpal joint of 18 horses. Nine horses received NAPPS (3 mg/kg, IM) on study days 15, 22, 29, and 36 and the rest received a saline placebo. Articular cartilage fibrillation was substantially reduced by NAPPS treatment, and concentrations of chondroitin sulfate 846 epitope were significantly increased in the synovial fluid of osteoarthritic and non-osteoarthritic joints of horses treated with NAPPS, implying that NAPPS had some beneficial disease-modifying effect.[330]

Bisphosphonates

Bisphosphonates are potent inhibitors of bone resorption. Inhibition of osteoclasts is the main pharmacological action of tiludronate which has seen extensive use in horses for a variety of skeletal ailments. As a consequence, tiludronate slows down bone remodelling and helps in restoring a normal balance between bone resorption and bone formation.[331–332] Tiludronate also has anti-inflammatory properties. It decreases the amount of nitric oxide and cytokines released from activated macrophages, which promotes early inflammation responses. [333] It also inhibits the secretion of cartilage-degrading enzymes induced by IL-1 in the chondrocyte or the synovial cell.[334] An intravenous form of tiludronate (Tildren) has been used in horses at 0.1 mg/kg bwt/day for 10 days for the treatment of navicular disease and bone spavin. Tiludronate's efficacy in treating navicular disease or in improving horses with osteoarthritis of the thoracolumbar vertebral column has been reported.[335–336] In another study, tiludronate was administered as a single IV infusion at a dose of 1 mg/kg for the treatment of bone spavin in 87 horses. Forty-two horses received the tiludronate and they went on to be significantly less lame than placebo treated horses ($P = 0.0318$). The authors concluded that tiludronate treatment has proven to be effective in the treatment of bone spavin in horses in association with a controlled exercise program.[337]

Atropine sulfate

There is anecdotal evidence for the use of atropine in synovial structures of the horse. Atropine is believed to decrease synovial secretions and thus alleviate the gross clinical signs of clinical conditions, such as bog spavin and idiopathic tenosynovitis. Intra-articular and intra-synovial use of atropine alone and in combination with CSs or HA has been reported with the atropine dosages range from 4 mg to 20 mg. The primary indication is distention of synovial structures refractory to drainage and intra-articular treatment with either HA or CSs. There are no anecdotal accounts regarding the use of atropine in osteoarthritis or septic arthritis, and there are

Box 23.1 Abbreviations

ASP = aspirin
BMA = betamethasone
DEX = dexamethasone
CHS = chondroitin sulfate
GAG = glycosaminoglycan
COX = cyclooxygenase
CRP = carprofen
CS = corticosteroids
DLC = diclofenac sodium
DPY = dipyrone
FCB = firocoxib
FLM = flunixin meglumine
FMZ = flumethasone
GLN = glucosamine
HA = hyaluronic acid or hyaluronate or hyaluronan
IA = intra-articular
IL = interleukin
KTP = ketoprofen
LPS = lipopolysaccharide
LT = leukotrienes
MFA = meclofenamic acid
MLX = meloxicam
MMP = matrix metalloprotease
MP = methylprednisolone
MPA = methylprednisolone acetate
MPS = methlprednisolone sodium succinate
MSCs = mesenchymal stem cells
NPX = naproxen
NSAIDs = nonsteroidal anti-inflammatory drug
PBZ = phenylbutazone,
PG = prostaglandin
PPS = pentosan polysulfate
PSGAG = polysulfated glycosaminoglycan
TBX = thromboxane
TCA = triamcinolone acetonide
TNF = tumor necrosis factor

not any clinical or scientific studies to support the use of atropine in the synovial structures of the horse.

The authors and editors gratefully acknowledge the contributions to this chapter by Rustin M. Moore, DVM, PhD, and Honor A. Walesby, DVM, MS, DACVS, both contributors to the previous edition. We also acknowledge the substantial assistance of Corrine D. Nawn in managing the references and tables. Last, but by no means least, we thank our families and friends for tolerating our many absences and oversights during the process of crafting this manuscript.

References

1. Dictionary.com. Retrieved on May 28, 2012. http://dictionary.reference.com/browse/pharmacotherapy
2. US food and Drug Administration. Retrieved on May 28, 2012. http://www.fda.gov/AboutFDA/CentersOffices/OfficeofMedicalProductsandTobacco/CBER/ucm133077.htm.
3. Lippiello L, Yamamoto K, Robinson D, et al. Involvement of prostaglandins from rheumatoid synovium in inhibition of articular cartilage metabolism. Arthritis Rheum 1978;21:909–17.
4. Teitz CC, Chrisman OD. The effect of salicylate and chloroquine on prostaglandin-induced articular damage in the rabbit knee. Clin Orthop Relat Res 1975;108:264–74.
5. Kirker-Head CACV, Agarwal RK, Morris EA, et al. Substance P and PGE2 levels in normal and abnormal equine joint fluids. Am J Vet Res 2000:714–18.
6. May SA, Hooke RE, Peremans KY. Prostaglandin E2 in equine joint disease. In: McIlwraith CW, Trotter GW, editors. Jount Disease in the Horse. Philadelphia: W.B. Saunders; 1996. p. 40.
7. Steinberg JJ, Hubbard JR, Sledge CB. Chondrocyte-mediated breakdown of cartilage. J Rheumatol 1987;14(Spec No):55–8.
8. Mehindate K, al-Daccak R, Aoudjit F, et al. Interleukin-4, transforming growth factor beta 1, and dexamethasone inhibit superantigen-induced prostaglandin E2-dependent collagenase gene expression through their action on cyclooxygenase-2 and cytosolic phospholipase A2. Lab Invest 1996;75:529–38.
9. May SA, Lees P. Nonsteroidal anti-inflammatory drugs. In: McIlwraith CW, Trotter GW, editors. Joint Disease in the Horse. Philadelphia: W. B. Saunders; 1996. p. 223–37.
9b. Sebaugh JL. Guidelines for accurate EC50/IC50 estimation. Pharm Stat 2011;10:128–34.
10. Kallings P. Nonsteroidal anti-inflammatory drugs. Vet Clin North Am Equine Pract 1993;9:523–41.
11. Lees P, Higgins AJ. Clinical pharmacology and therapeutic uses of non-steroidal anti-inflammatory drugs in the horse. Equine Vet J 1985;17:83–96.
12. Berenbaum F. COX-3: fact or fancy? Joint Bone Spine 2004;71:451–3.
13. Hersh EV, Lally ET, Moore PA. Update on cyclooxygenase inhibitors: has a third COX isoform entered the fray? Curr Med Res Opin 2005;21:1217–26.
14. Rodrigues NL, Dore M, Doucet MY. Expression of cyclooxygenase isoforms in ulcerated tissues of the nonglandular portion of the stomach in horses. Am J Vet Res 2010;71:592–6.
15. Davis JL, Marshall JF, Papich MG, et al. The pharmacokinetics and in vitro cyclooxygenase selectivity of deracoxib in horses. J Vet Pharmacol Ther 2011;34:12–16.
16. Kvaternick V, Pollmeier M, Fischer J, et al. Pharmacokinetics and metabolism of orally administered firocoxib, a novel second generation coxib, in horses. J Vet Pharmacol Ther 2007;30:208–17.
17. Letendre LT, Tessman RK, McClure SR, et al. Pharmacokinetics of firocoxib after administration of multiple consecutive daily doses to horses. Am J Vet Res 2008;69:1399–405.
18. Doucet MY, Bertone AL, Hendrickson D, et al. Comparison of efficacy and safety of paste formulations of firocoxib and phenylbutazone in horses with naturally occurring osteoarthritis. J Am Vet Med Assoc 2008;232:91–7.
19. Orsini JA, Ryan WG, Carithers DS, et al. Evaluation of oral administration of firocoxib for the management of musculoskeletal pain and lameness associated with osteoarthritis in horses. Am J Vet Res 2012;73:664–71.
20. de Grauw JC, van de Lest CHA, Brama PAJ, et al. In vivo effects of meloxicam on inflammatory mediators,

MMP activity and cartilage biomarkers in equine joints with acute synovitis. Equine Vet J 2009;41:693–9.
21. Lees P, Maitho TE, Taylor JB. Pharmacokinetics of phenylbutazone in two age groups of ponies: a preliminary study. Vet Rec 1985;116:229–32.
22. Snow DH, Baxter P, Whiting B. The pharmacokinetics of meclofenamic acid in the horse. J Vet Pharmacol Ther 1981;4:147–56.
23. Moss MS, Haywood PE. Persistence of phenylbutazone in horses producing acid urines. Vet Rec 1973;93:124–5.
24. GA M. Disposition of phenylbutazone in the horse. Am Assoc Equine Pract 1974:243–8.
25. T T. Pharmacology review: the nonsteroidal anti-inflammatory drugs I. Phenylbutazone. J Equine Med Surg 1979;6:253–8.
26. Jaussaud P, Bellon C, Besse S, et al. Enantioselective pharmacokinetics of ketoprofen in horses. J Vet Pharmacol Ther 1993;16:373–6.
27. McCormack K, Brune K. Dissociation between the antinociceptive and anti-inflammatory effects of the nonsteroidal anti-inflammatory drugs. A survey of their analgesic efficacy. Drugs 1991;41:533–47.
28. Villanueva M, Heckenberger R, Strobach H, et al. Equipotent inhibition by R(-)-, S(+)- and racemic ibuprofen of human polymorphonuclear cell function in vitro. Br J Clin Pharmacol 1993;35:235–42.
29. Lees P, McKellar Q, May SA, et al. Pharmacodynamics and pharmacokinetics of carprofen in the horse. Equine Vet J 1994;26:203–8.
30. Crisman MV, Wilcke JR, Sams RA. Pharmacokinetics of flunixin meglumine in healthy foals less than twenty-four hours old. Am J Vet Res 1996;57:1759–61.
31. Semrad SD, Sams RA, Ashcraft SM. Pharmacokinetics of and serum thromboxane suppression by flunixin meglumine in healthy foals during the first month of life. Am J Vet Res 1993;54:2083–7.
32. Wilcke JR, Crisman MV, Sams RA, et al. Pharmacokinetics of phenylbutazone in neonatal foals. Am J Vet Res 1993;54:2064–7.
33. Lehmann W, Wintzer HJ, Frey HH. Kinetics of anti-inflammatory drugs in serum and synovia of horses (author's transl). DTW Dtsch Tierarztl Wochenschr 1981;88:218–20.
34. Lees P, Taylor JB, Higgins AJ, et al. Phenylbutazone and oxyphenbutazone distribution into tissue fluids in the horse. J Vet Pharmacol Ther 1986;9:204–12.
35. Higgins AJ, Lees P, Taylor JB, et al. Flunixin meglumine: quantitative determination in and effects on composition of equine inflammatory exudate. Br Vet J 1986;142:163–9.
36. Burrows GE, MacAllister CG, Tripp P, et al. Interactions between chloramphenicol, acepromazine, phenylbutazone, rifampin and thiamylal in the horse. Equine Vet J 1989;21:34–8.
37. McGrath CJ. Drug interactions. In: Short CE, editor. Principles and Practice of Veterinary Anesthesia. Baltimore: Williams & Wilkins; 1987. p. 154–7.
38. Short CE. Principles and Practice of Veterinary Anesthesia. Baltimore: Williams & Wilkins, 1987.
39. Young DB, Ewing PJ, Burrows GE, et al. Effects of phenylbutazone on thiamylal disposition and anaesthesia in ponies. J Vet Pharmacol Ther 1994;17:389–93.
40. Whittem T, Firth EC, Hodge H, et al. Pharmacokinetic interactions between repeated dose phenylbutazone and gentamicin in the horse. J Vet Pharmacol Ther 1996;19:454–9.
41. MacAllister CG, Morgan SJ, Borne AT, et al. Comparison of adverse effects of phenylbutazone, flunixin meglumine, and ketoprofen in horses. J Am Vet Med Assoc 1993;202:71–7.
42. Davis JL, et al. Pharmacokinetics of etodolac in the horse following oral and intravenous administration. J Vet Pharmacol Ther 2007;30:43–8.
43. May SA. Anti-inflammatory agents: Nonsteroidal anti-inflammatory drugs. In: Robinson NE, editor. Current Therapy in Equine Medicine. Philidelphia: WB Saunders; 1992. p. 16–17.
44. Rustin, MM. Principles of therapy: Anti-inflammatory drug therapy in horses. In: Colahan PT, Mayhew IG, Merritt AM, et al, editors. Equine Medicine & Surgery. St. Louis, MO: Mosby, Inc; 1999. p. 155–63.
45. Snow D. Non-steroidal anti-inflammatory agents in the horse. Vet Rec 1981; In Practice:24–31.
46. McKellar QA, Bogan JA, von Fellenberg RL, et al. Pharmacokinetic, biochemical and tolerance studies on carprofen in the horse. Equine Vet J 1991;23:280–4.
47. Hamm D, Turchi P, Johnson JC, et al. Determination of an effective dose of eltenac and its comparison with that of flunixin meglumine in horses after experimentally induced carpitis. Am J Vet Res 1997;58:298–302.
48. Moore RM. Nonsteroidal Anti-Inflammatory Drugs. In: White NA, Moore JN, editors. Current Techniques in Equine Surgery and Lameness. Philideplphia: W. B. Saunders Co.; 1998. p. 25–30.
49. Owens JG, Kamerling SG, Stanton SR, et al. Effects of ketoprofen and phenylbutazone on chronic hoof pain and lameness in the horse. Equine Vet J 1995;27:296–300.
50. Betley MSS, Gregoricka MJ, et al. The analgesic effect of ketoprofen for use in treating equine colic as compared to flunixin meglumine. Equine Pract 1991;13:11–16.
51. Longo E, Autefage A, Bayle R, et al. Efficacy of a non-stroidal anti-inflammatory, ketofen 10%Â® (ketoprofen)in the treatment of colic in horses. J Equine Vet Sci 1992;12:311–15.
52. Lees P, Ewins CP, Taylor JB, et al. Serum thromboxane in the horse and its inhibition by aspirin, phenylbutazone and flunixin. Br Vet J 1987;143:462–76.
53. Frisbie DD, McIlwraith CW, Kawcak CE, et al. Evaluation of topically administered diclofenac liposomal cream for treatment of horses with experimentally induced osteoarthritis. Am J Vet Res 2009;70:210–15.
54. Brideau C, Van Staden C, Chan CC. In vitro effects of cyclooxygenase inhibitors in whole blood of horses, dogs, and cats. Am J Vet Res 2001;62:1755–60.
55. Morton AJYN, Campbell NB, et al. Equine lameness: the role of cyclooxygenase-2. Vet Surg 2002;504–5.
56. Campbell NB, Blikslager AT. The role of cyclooxygenase inhibitors in repair of ischaemic-injured jejunal mucosa in the horse. Equine Vet J Suppl 2000;32: 59–64.
57. Campbell NB, Jones SL, Blikslager AT. The effects of cyclo-oxygenase inhibitors on bile-injured and normal equine colon. Equine Vet J 2002;34:493–8.
58. Johnson CBTP, Young SS, et al. Postoperatie analgesia using phenylbutazone, flunixin or carprofen in horses. Vet Rec 1993;336–8.
59. Schatzmann U, Gugelmann M, Von Cranach J, et al. Pharmacodynamic evaluation of the peripheral pain inhibition by carprofen and flunixin in the horse. Schweiz Arch Tierheilkd 1990;132:497–504.
60. Raekallio M, Taylor PM, Bennett RC. Preliminary investigations of pain and analgesia assessment in horses administered phenylbutazone or placebo after arthroscopic surgery. Vet Surg 1997;26:150–5.
61. Hu HH, MacAllister CG, Payton ME, et al. Evaluation of the analgesic effects of phenylbutazone administered at a high or low dosage in horses with chronic lameness. J Am Vet Med Assoc 2005;226:414–17.
62. Foreman JH, Barange A, Lawrence LM, et al. Effects of single-dose intravenous phenylbutazone on experimentally induced, reversible lameness in the horse. J Vet Pharmacol Ther 2008;31:39–44.
63. Foreman JH, Grubb TL, Inoue OJ, et al. Efficacy of single-dose intravenous phenylbutazone and flunixin meglumine before, during and after exercise in an experimental reversible

model of foot lameness in horses. Equine Vet J 2010;42:601–5.
64. Owens JG, Kamerling SG, Stanton SR, et al. Effects of pretreatment with ketoprofen and phenylbutazone on experimentally induced synovitis in horses. Am J Vet Res 1996;57:866–74.
65. Owens JG, Kamerling SG, Barker SA. Pharmacokinetics of ketoprofen in healthy horses and horses with acute synovitis. J Vet Pharmacol Ther 1995;18:187–95.
66. Hess EV, Herman JH. Cartilage metabolism and anti-inflammatory drugs in osteoarthritis. Am J Med 1986;81:36–43.
67. Beluche LA, Bertone AL, Anderson DE, et al. Effects of oral administration of phenylbutazone to horses on in vitro articular cartilage metabolism. Am J Vet Res 2001;62:1916–21.
68. Armstrong S, Lees P. Effects of carprofen (R and S enantiomers and racemate) on the production of IL-1, IL-6 and TNF-alpha by equine chondrocytes and synoviocytes. J Vet Pharmacol Ther 2002;25:145–53.
69. Landoni MF, Foot R, Frean S, et al. Effects of flunixin, tolfenamic acid, R(-) and S(+) ketoprofen on the response of equine synoviocytes to lipopolysaccharide stimulation. Equine Vet J 1996;28:468–75.
70. Moses VS, Hardy J, Bertone AL, et al. Effects of anti-inflammatory drugs on lipopolysaccharide-challenged and -unchallenged equine synovial explants. Am J Vet Res 2001;62:54–60.
71. Rohde CAD, Bertone AL, et al. Effects of phenylbutazone on bone activity and formation in horses. Am J Vet Res 2000;61:537–43.
72. Levine D, Epsetin K, Neelis D, et al. Effect of topical application of 1% diclofenac sodium liposomal cream on inflammation in healthy horses undergoing intravenous regional limb perfusion with amikacin sulfate. Am J Vet Res 2009;70:1323–5.
73. Schleining JA, McClure SR, Evans RB, et al. Liposome-based diclofenac for the treatment of inflammation in an acute synovitis model in horses. J Vet Pharmacol Ther 2008;31:554–61.
74. King JN, Gerring EL. Antagonism of endotoxin-induced disruption of equine bowel motility by flunixin and phenylbutazone. Equine Vet J Suppl 1989;7:38–42.
75. Daels PF, Stabenfeldt GH, Hughes JP, et al. Effects of flunixin meglumine on endotoxin-induced prostaglandin F2 alpha secretion during early pregnancy in mares. Am J Vet Res 1991;52:276–81.
76. Judson DG, Barton M. Effect of aspirin on haemostasis in the horse. Res Vet Sci 1981;30:241–2.
77. Johnstone IB. Comparative effects of phenylbutazone, naproxen and flunixin meglumine on equine platelet aggregation and platelet factor 3 availability in vitro. Can J Comp Med 1983;47:172–9.
78. Leise BS, Faleiros RR, Watts M, et al. Laminar inflammatory gene expression in the carbohydrate overload model of equine laminitis. Equine Vet J 2011;43:54–61.
79. Blikslager AT, Yin C, Cochran AM, et al. Cyclooxygenase Expression in the Early Stages of Equine Laminitis: A Cytologic Study. J Vet Intern Med 2006;20:1191–6.
80. Conner GH, Riley WF, et al. Arquel (C1-1583) A new non-steroidal anti-inflammatory drug for horses. Am Assoc Equine Pract 1973:81–90.
81. Houdeshell JW, Hennessey PW. A new non-steroidal anti-inflammatory analgesic for horses. J Equine Med Surg 1977:57–63.
82. Kilian JG, Jones EW, Hamm D, et al. The efficacy of equiproxen (naproxen) in a unique equine myositis model. Am Assoc Equine Pract 1974:201–15.
83. Jones EW, Hamm D. Comparative efficacy of phenylbutazone and naproxen in induced equine myositis. J Equine Med Surg 1978:341–7.
84. Semrad SD, Sams RA, Harris ON, et al. Effects of concurrent administration of phenylbutazone and flunixin meglumine on pharmacokinetic variables and in vitro generation of thromboxane B2 in mares. Am J Vet Res 1993;54:1901–5.
85. Foreman JH, Ruemmler R. Phenylbutazone and flunixin meglumine used singly or in combination in experimental lameness in horses. Equine Vet J 2011;43:12–17.
86. Keegan KG, Messer NT, Reed SK, et al. Effectiveness of administration of phenylbutazone alone or concurrent administration of phenylbutazone and flunixin meglumine to alleviate lameness in horses. Am J Vet Res 2008;69:167–73.
87. Snow DH, Douglas TA, Thompson H, et al. Phenylbutazone toxicosis in equidae: a biochemical and pathophysiological study. Am J Vet Res 1981;42:1754–9.
88. Gunson DE. Renal papillary necrosis in horses. J Am Vet Med Assoc 1983;182: 263–6.
89. Gunson DE, Soma LR. Renal papillary necrosis in horses after phenylbutazone and water deprivation. Vet Pathol 1983;20:603–10.
90. Carrick JB, Papich MG, Middleton DM, et al. Clinical and pathological effects of flunixin meglumine administration to neonatal foals. Can J Vet Res 1989;53:195–201.
91. Traub-Dargatz JL, Bertone JJ, Gould DH, et al. Chronic flunixin meglumine therapy in foals. Am J Vet Res 1988;49: 7–12.
92. Conlon PD. Nonsteroidal drugs used in the treatment of inflammation. Vet Clin North Am Small Anim Pract 1988;18: 1115–31.
93. Meschter CL, Maylin GA, Krook L. Vascular pathology in phenylbutazone intoxicated horses. Cornell Vet 1984;74:282–97.
94. McConnico RS, Morgan TW, Williams CC, et al. Pathophysiologic effects of phenylbutazone on the right dorsal colon in horses. Am J Vet Res 2008;69: 1496–505.
95. Kore AM. Toxicology of nonsteroidal anti-inflammatory drugs. Vet Clin North Am Small Anim Pract 1990;20: 419–30.
96. Read WK. Renal medullary crest necrosis associated with phenylbutazone therapy in horses. Vet Pathol 1983;20:662–9.
97. Turner A. Local and systemic factors affecting wound healing. Proc Am Assoc Equine Pract 1978:209–18.
98. Schneiter HL, McClure JR, Cho DY, et al. The effect of flunixin meglumine on early wound healing of abdominal incisions in ponies. Vet Surg 1987:101.
99. Wilson DA, Baker GJ, Boero MJ. Complications of celiotomy incisions in horses. Vet Surg 1995;24:506–14.
100. MacKay RJ, French TW, Nguyen HT, et al. Effects of large doses of phenylbutazone administration to horses. Am J Vet Res 1983;44:774–80.
101. Dirikolu L, Woods WE, Boyles J, et al. Nonsteroidal anti-inflammatory agents and musculoskeletal injuries in Thoroughbred racehorses in Kentucky. J Vet Pharmacol Ther 2009;32:271–9.
102. Caron JP. Principles of treatment of joint disease. In: Auer DE, Stick JA, editors. Equine Surgery. Philidelphia: W.B. Saunders; 1999. p. 678–96.
103. Ferguson DC, Hoenig M. Glucocorticoids, mineralocorticoids, and steroid synthesis inhibitors. In: Adams HR, editor. Veterinary Pharmacology and Therapeutics. Ames, IA: Iowa State University Press; 1995. p. 622–37.
104. GW T, CW M. Joint Disease in the horse. In: Trotter GW, McIlwraith CW, editors. Joint Disease in the Horse. 1st ed. Philadelphia: WB Saunders; 1996.
105. Trotter G. Intra-articular corticosteroids. In: McIlwraith CW, Trotter GW, editors. Joint Disease in the Horse. Philadelphia: W. B. Saunders; 1996. p. 237–56.
106. Autefage A, Alvinerie M, Toutain PL. Synovial fluid and plasma kinetics of methylprednisolone and methylprednisolone acetate in horses following intra-articular administration of methylprednisolone acetate. Equine Vet J 1986;18:193–8.
107. Alvinerie M, Toutain PL. Determination of methylprednisolone and

methylprednisolone acetate in synovial fluid using high-performance liquid chromatography. J Chromatogr 1984;309:385–90.
108. Harkins JD, Carney JM, Tobin T. Clinical use and characteristics of the corticosteroids. Vet Clin North Am Equine Pract 1993;9:543–62.
109. McIlwraith CW. The use of intra-articular corticosteroids in the horse: What is known on a scientific basis? Equine Vet J 2010;42:563–71.
110. Laufer S, Greim C, Bertsche T. An in-vitro screening assay for the detection of inhibitors of proinflammatory cytokine synthesis: a useful tool for the development of new antiarthritic and disease modifying drugs. Osteoarthritis Cartilage 2002;10:961–7.
111. Caron JP. Intra-articular injections for joint disease in horses. Vet Clin North Am Equine Pract 2005;21: 559–73, v.
112. Bombardieri S, Cattani P, Ciabattoni G, et al. The synovial prostaglandin system in chronic inflammatory arthritis: differential effects of steroidal and nonsteroidal anti-inflammatory drugs. Br J Pharmacol 1981;73:893–901.
113. Derendorf H, Mollmann H, Gruner A, et al. Pharmacokinetics and pharmacodynamics of glucocorticoid suspensions after intra-articular administration. Clin Pharmacol Ther 1986;39:313–17.
114. Lillich JD, Bertone AL, Schmall LM, et al. Plasma, urine, and synovial fluid disposition of methylprednisolone acetate and isoflupredone acetate after intra-articular administration in horses. Am J Vet Res 1996;57:187–92.
115. Murphy DJ, Todhunter RJ, Fubini SL, et al. The effects of methylprednisolone on normal and monocyte-conditioned medium-treated articular cartilage from dogs and horses. Vet Surg 2000;29: 546–57.
116. Caron JP, Tardif G, Martel-Pelletier J, et al. Modulation of matrix metalloprotease 13 (collagenase 3) gene expression in equine chondrocytes by interleukin 1 and corticosteroids. Am J Vet Res 1996;57:1631–4.
117. Dechant JE, Baxter GM, Frisbie DD, et al. Effects of dosage titration of methylprednisolone acetate and triamcinolone acetonide on interleukin-1-conditioned equine articular cartilage explants in vitro. Equine Vet J 2003;35: 444–50.
118. Clegg PD, Jones MD, Carter SD. The effect of drugs commonly used in the treatment of equine articular disorders on the activity of equine matrix metalloproteinase-2 and 9. J Vet Pharmacol Ther 1998;21:406–13.
119. Richardson SM, Hoyland JA, Mobasheri R, et al. Mesenchymal stem cells in regenerative medicine: Opportunities and challenges for articular cartilage and intervertebral disc tissue engineering. J Cell Physiol 2010; 222:23–32.
120. Fubini SL, Todhunter RJ, Burton-Wurster N, et al. Corticosteroids alter the differentiated phenotype of articular chondrocytes. J Orthop Res 2001;19:688–95.
121. Todhunter RJ, Fubini SL, Wootton JA, et al. Effect of methylprednisolone acetate on proteoglycan and collagen metabolism of articular cartilage explants. J Rheumatol 1996;23:1207–13.
122. Jolly WT, Whittem T, Jolly AC, et al. The dose-related effects of phenylbutazone and a methylprednisolone acetate formulation (Depo-Medrol) on cultured explants of equine carpal articular cartilage. J Vet Pharmacol Ther 1995;18:429–37.
123. Garvican ER, Vaughan-Thomas A, Redmond C, et al. MMP-mediated collagen breakdown induced by activated protein C in equine cartilage is reduced by corticosteroids. J Orthop Res 2010;28:370–8.
124. Chunekamrai S, Krook LP, Lust G, et al. Changes in articular cartilage after intra-articular injections of methylprednisolone acetate in horses. Am J Vet Res 1989;50:1733–41.
125. Trotter GW, McIlwraith CW, Yovich JV, et al. Effects of intra-articular administration of methylprednisolone acetate on normal equine articular cartilage. Am J Vet Res 1991;52:83–7.
126. Frisbie DD, Kawcak CE, Baxter GM, et al. Effects of 6alpha-methylprednisolone acetate on an equine osteochondral fragment exercise model. Am J Vet Res 1998;59:1619–28.
127. Frisbie DD, Kawcak CE, Trotter GW, et al. Effects of triamcinolone acetonide on an in vivo equine osteochondral fragment exercise model. Equine Vet J 1997;29:349–59.
128. Todhunter RJ, Fubini SL, Vernier-Singer M, et al. Acute synovitis and intra-articular methylprednisolone acetate in ponies. Osteoarthritis Cartilage 1998;6:94–105.
129. MacLeod JN, Fubini SL, Gu DN, et al. Effect of synovitis and corticosteroids on transcription of cartilage matrix proteins. Am J Vet Res 1998;59:1021–6.
130. Robion FC, Doize B, Boure L, et al. Use of synovial fluid markers of cartilage synthesis and turnover to study effects of repeated intra-articular administration of methylprednisolone acetate on articular cartilage in vivo. J Orthop Res 2001;19:250–8.
131. Foland JW, McIlwraith CW, Trotter GW, et al. Effect of betamethasone and exercise on equine carpal joints with osteochondral fragments. Vet Surg 1994;23:369–76.
132. Bolt DM, Ishihara A, Weisbrode SE, et al. Effects of triamcinolone acetonide, sodium hyaluronate, amikacin sulfate, and mepivacaine hydrochloride, alone and in combination, on morphology and matrix composition of lipopolysaccharide-challenged and unchallenged equine articular cartilage explants. Am J Vet Res 2008;69:861–7.
133. Kawcak CE, Norrdin RW, Frisbie DD, et al. Effects of osteochondral fragmentation and intra-articular triamcinolone acetonide treatment on subchondral bone in the equine carpus. Equine Vet J 1998;30:66–71.
134. Céleste C, Ionescu M, Poole AR, et al. Repeated intraarticular injections of triamcinolone acetonide alter cartilage matrix metabolism measured by biomarkers in synovial fluid. J Orthop Res 2005;23:602–10.
135. Sandler EA, Frisbie DD, McIlwraith CW. A dose titration of triamcinolone acetonide on insulin-like growth factor-1 and interleukin-1-conditioned equine cartilage explants. Equine Vet J 2004;36:58–63.
136. Kay AT, Bolt DM, Ishihara A, et al. Anti-inflammatory and analgesic effects of intra-articular injection of triamcinolone acetonide, mepivacaine hydrochloride, or both on lipopolysaccharide-induced lameness in horses. Am J Vet Res 2008;69: 1646–54.
137. Labens R, Mellor D, Voute L. Retrospective study of the effect of intra-articular treatment of osteoarthritis of the distal tarsal joints in 51 horses. Vet Rec 2007;161:611–16.
138. Coombes BK, Bisset L, Vicenzino B. Efficacy and safety of corticosteroid injections and other injections for management of tendinopathy: a systematic review of randomised controlled trials. Lancet 2010;376: 1751–67.
139. Beck S, Blunden T, Dyson S, et al. Are matrix and vascular changes involved in the pathogenesis of deep digital flexor tendon injury in the horse? Vet J 2011;189:289–95.
140. Gutierrez-Nibeyro SD, White Ii NA, Werpy NM. Outcome of medical treatment for horses with foot pain: 56 cases. Equine Vet J 2010;42:680–5.
141. Krook L, Maylin GA. Fractures in Thoroughbred racehorses. Cornell Vet 1988;78(Suppl.):1–133.
142. Wilderjans H, Boussauw B, Madder K, et al. Tenosynovitis of the digital flexor tendon sheath and annular ligament constriction syndrome caused by longitudinal tears in the deep digital flexor tendon: a clinical and surgical report of 17 cases in warmblood horses. Equine Vet J 2003;35:270–5.
143. Oegema Jr TR, Behrens F. Proteoglycan aggregate synthesis in normal and

chronically hydrocortisone-suppressed rabbit articular cartilage. Arch Biochem Biophys 1981;206:277–84.
144. Bailey SR, Elliott J. The corticosteroid laminitis story: 2. Science of if, when and how. Equine Vet J 2007;39:7–11.
145. Cornelisse CJ, Robinson NE, Berney CA, et al. Thermographic study of in vivo modulation of vascular responses to phenylephrine and endothelin-1 by dexamethasone in the horse. Equine Vet J 2006;38:119–26.
146. McCluskey MJ, Kavenagh PB. Clinical use of triamcinolone acetonide in the horse (205 cases) and the incidence of glucocorticoid-induced laminitis associated with its use. Equine Vet Educ 2004;16:86–9.
147. Bathe AP. The corticosteroid laminitis story: 3. The clinician's viewpoint. Equine Vet J 2007;39:12–13.
148. Murray RC, Znaor N, Tanner KE, et al. The effect of intra-articular methylprednisolone acetate and exercise on equine carpal subchondral and cancellous bone microhardness. Equine Vet J 2002;34:306–10.
149. Chen CL, Sailor JA, Collier J, et al. Synovial and serum levels of triamcinolone following intra-articular administration of triamcinolone acetonide in the horse. J Vet Pharmacol Ther 1992;15:240–6.
150. Gibbs DA, Merrill EW, Smith KA, et al. Rheology of hyaluronic acid. Biopolymers 1968;6:777–91.
151. Hamerman D, Rojkind M, Sandson J. Protein bound to hyaluronate: chemical and immunological studies. Fed Proc 1966;25:1040–5.
152. Radin EL, Paul IL. A consolidated concept of joint lubrication. J Bone Joint Surg Am 1972;54:607–13.
153. Swann DA, Radin EL, Nazimiec M, et al. Role of hyaluronic acid in joint lubrication. Ann Rheum Dis 1974;33: 318–26.
154. Freeman MR, Kempsonm GE. Load Carriage. In: Freeman MR, editor. Adult Articular Cartilage. New York: Grune & Stratton; 1972. p. 228–46.
155. Cannon JH. Clinical evaluation of intra-articular sodium hyaluronate in the thoroughbred racehorse. J Equine Vet Sci 1985;5:147–8.
156. Galley R. The use of hyaluronic acid in the racehorse. Am Assoc Equine Pract 1986:657–61.
157. Irwin DH. Sodium hyaluronate in equine traumatic arthritis. J S Afr Vet Assoc 1980;51:231–3.
158. Phillips M. Intra-articular sodium hyaluronate in the horse. Am Assoc Equine Pract 1980:389–94.
159. Roneus B, Lindblad A, Lindholm A, et al. Effects of intraarticular corticosteroid and sodium hyaluronate injections on synovial fluid production and synovial fluid content of sodium hyaluronate and proteoglycans in normal equine joints. Zentralbl Veterinarmed A 1993;40:10–16.
160. Rose RJ. The intra-articular use of sodium hyaluronate for the treatment of osteo-arthrosis in the horse. N Z Vet J 1979;27:5–8.
161. Ruth DT, Swites BJ. Comparison of the effectiveness of intra-articular hyaluronic acid and conventional therapy for the treatment of naturally occurring arthritic conditions in horses. Equine Pract 1985:25–9.
162. Butler J, Rydell NW, Balazs EA. Hyaluronic acid in synovial fluid. VI. Effect of intra-articular injection of hyaluronic acid on the clinical symptoms of arthritis in track horses. Acta Vet Scand 1970;11:139–55.
163. Swanstrom O. Hyaluronate (hyaluronic acid) and its use. Am Assoc Equine Pract 1978:345–8.
164. Vernon G. Clinical successes and failures using new hyaluronic acid-Synacid. Proc Am Assoc Equine Pract 1983:397–402.
165. Fraser JR, Kimpton WG, Pierscionek BK, et al. The kinetics of hyaluronan in normal and acutely inflamed synovial joints: observations with experimental arthritis in sheep. Semin Arthritis Rheum 1993;22:9–17.
166. Gosh P. Osteoarthritis and hyaluronan-palliative or disease modifying treatment? Semin Arthritis Rheum 1993:1–3.
167. Laurent UB, Fraser JR, Engstrom-Laurent A, et al. Catabolism of hyaluronan in the knee joint of the rabbit. Matrix 1992;12:130–6.
168. Saari H, Konttinen YT, Tulamo RM, et al. Concentration and degree of polymerization of hyaluronate in equine synovial fluid. Am J Vet Res 1989;50:2060–3.
169. Tulamo RM, Heiskanen T, Salonen M. Concentration and molecular weight distribution of hyaluronate in synovial fluid from clinically normal horses and horses with diseased joints. Am J Vet Res 1994;55:710–15.
170. Balazs EA, Darzynkiewiez A. The effect of hyaluronic acid on fibroblasts, mononuclear phagocytes and lymphocytes. In: Kulonen E, Pikkarainen JPK, editors. Biology of Fibroblasts. London: Academic Press; 1973. p. 237.
171. Brandt KD. The effect of synovial hyaluronate on the ingestion of monosodium urate crystals by leukocytes. Clin Chim Acta 1974;55: 307–15.
172. Forrester JV, Balazs EA. Inhibition of phagocytosis by high molecular weight hyaluronate. Immunology 1980;40: 435–46.
173. Grecomoro G, Martorana U, Di Marco C. Intra-articular treatment with sodium hyaluronate in gonarthrosis: a controlled clinical trial versus placebo. Pharmatherapeutica 1987;5:137–41.
174. Hakansson L, Hallgren R, Venge P. Effect of hyaluronic acid on phagocytosis of opsonized latex particles. Scand J Immunol 1980;11:649–53.
175. Partsch G, Schwarzer C, Neumuller J, et al. Modulation of the migration and chemotaxis of PMN cells by hyaluronic acid. Z Rheumatol 1989;48:123–8.
176. Pisko EJ, Turner RA, Soderstrom LP, et al. Inhibition of neutrophil phagocytosis and enzyme release by hyaluronic acid. Clin Exp Rheumatol 1983;1:41–4.
177. Treadway WJ, et al. The role of hyaluronic acid flux on modulation of neutrophil function. Arthritis Rheum 1981;24:S94–9.
178. Auer JA, Fackelman GE, Gingerich DA, et al. Effect of hyaluronic acid in naturally occurring and experimentally induced osteoarthritis. Am J Vet Res 1980;41:568–74.
179. McIlwraith CW. Diseases of joints, tendons, ligaments, and related structures. In: Stashak TS, editor. Adams Lameness. Philidelphia: Lippincott Williams & Wilkins; 2002. p. 505–11.
180. Kikuchi T, Yamada H, Shimmei M. Effect of high molecular weight hyaluronan on cartilage degeneration in a rabbit model of osteoarthritis. Osteoarthritis Cartilage 1996;4:99–110.
181. Hilbert BJ, Rowley G, Antonas KN. Hyaluronic acid concentration in synovial fluid from normal and arthritic joints of horses. Aust Vet J 1984;61:22–4.
182. Larsen NE, Lombard KM, Parent EG, et al. Effect of hylan on cartilage and chondrocyte cultures. J Orthop Res 1992;10:23–32.
183. Shimazu A, Jikko A, Iwamoto M, et al. Effects of hyaluronic acid on the release of proteoglycan from the cell matrix in rabbit chondrocyte cultures in the presence and absence of cytokines. Arthritis Rheum 1993;36:247–53.
184. Hegewald AA, Ringe J, Bartel J, et al. Hyaluronic acid and autologous synovial fluid induce chondrogenic differentiation of equine mesenchymal stem cells: a preliminary study. Tissue Cell 2004;36:431–8.
185. Wigren A, Falk J, Wik O. The healing of cartilage injuries under the influence of joint immobilization and repeated hyaluronic acid injections. An experimental study. Acta Orthop Scand 1978;49:121–33.
186. Hilbert BJ, Rowley G, Antonas KN, et al. Changes in the synovia after the intra-articular injection of sodium

hyaluronate into normal horse joints and after arthrotomy and experimental cartilage damage. Aust Vet J 1985;62: 182–4.
187. Gingerich DA, Auer JA, Fackelman GE. Force plate studies on the effect of exogenous hyaluronic acid on joint function in equine arthritis. J Vet Pharmacol Ther 1979;2:291–8.
188. Peloso JG, Stick JA, Caron JP, et al. Effects of hylan on amphotericin-induced carpal lameness in equids. Am J Vet Res 1993;54:1527–34.
189. Kawcak CE, Frisbie DD, Trotter GW, et al. Effects of intravenous administration of sodium hyaluronate on carpal joints in exercising horses after arthroscopic surgery and osteochondral fragmentation. Am J Vet Res 1997;58:1132–40.
190. Frean SP, Lees P. Effects of polysulfated glycosaminoglycan and hyaluronan on prostaglandin E2 production by cultured equine synoviocytes. Am J Vet Res 2000;61:499–505.
191. Frean SP, Gettinby G, May SA, et al. Influence of interleukin-1beta and hyaluronan on proteoglycan release from equine navicular hyaline cartilage and fibrocartilage. J Vet Pharmacol Ther 2000;23:67–72.
192. Taylor SE, Weaver MP, Pitsillides AA, et al. Cartilage oligomeric matrix protein and hyaluronan levels in synovial fluid from horses with osteoarthritis of the tarsometatarsal joint compared to a control population. Equine Vet J 2006;38:502–7.
193. Bergin B, Pierce S, Bramlage L, et al. Oral hyaluronan gel reduces post operative tarsocrural effusion in the yearling Thoroughbred. Equine Vet J 2006;38:375–8.
194. Churchill E. Treating tendonitis with sodium hyaluronate. J Equine Sci 1985;5:217–28.
195. Spurlock GH, Spurlock SL, Parker GA. Evaluation of hylartin-V therapy for induced tendonitis in the horse. J Equine Vet Sci 1989;9:242–6.
196. Gaughan EM, Nixon AJ, Krook LP, et al. Effects of sodium hyaluronate on tendon healing and adhesion formation in horses. Am J Vet Res 1991;52:764–73.
197. Foland JW, Trotter GW, Powers BE, et al. Effect of sodium hyaluronate in collagenase-induced superficial digital flexor tendinitis in horses. Am J Vet Res 1992;53:2371–6.
198. Dabareiner RM, Carter GK, Honnas CM. Injection of corticosteroids, hyaluronate, and amikacin into the navicular bursa in horses with signs of navicular area pain unresponsive to other treatments: 25 cases (1999–2002). J Am Vet Med Assoc 2003;223:1469–74.
199. Smith MM, Ghosh P. The synthesis of hyaluronic acid by human synovial fibroblasts is influenced by the nature of the hyaluronate in the extracellular environment. Rheumatol Int 1987;7: 113–22.
200. Phillips M. Clinical trial comparison of intra-articular sodium hyaluronate products in the horse. Equine Vet Sci 1989;9:39–40.
201. Gaustad G, Larsen S. Comparison of polysulphated glycosaminoglycan and sodium hyaluronate with placebo in treatment of traumatic arthritis in horses. Equine Vet J 1995;27:356–62.
202. Aviad AD, Arthur RM, Brencick VA, et al. Synacid vs hylartin v in equine joint disease. J Equine Vet Sci 1988;8: 112–16.
203. Santangelo KS, Johnson AL, Ruppert AS, et al. Effects of hyaluronan treatment on lipopolysaccharide-challenged fibroblast-like synovial cells. Arthritis Res Ther 2007;9:R1.
204. Ferris DJ, Frisbie DD, McIlwraith CW, et al. Current joint therapy usage in equine practice: A survey of veterinarians 2009. Equine Vet J 2011; 43:530–5.
205. Van Pelt RW. Monarticular idiopathic septic arthritis in horses. J Am Vet Med Assoc 1971;158:1658–73.
206. Schmid FR. Routine drug treatment of septic arthritis. Clin Rheum Dis 1984; 10:293–311.
207. Hackett RP. Intra-articular use of corticosteroids in the horse. J Am Vet Med Assoc 1982;181:292–4.
208. Gustafson SB, McIlwraith CW, Jones RL, et al. Further investigations into the potentiation of infection by intra-articular injection of polysulfated glycosaminoglycan and the effect of filtration and intra-articular injection of amikacin. Am J Vet Res 1989;50: 2018–22.
209. Gustafson SB, McIlwraith CW, Jones RL. Comparison of the effect of polysulfated glycosaminoglycan, corticosteroids, and sodium hyaluronate in the potentiation of a subinfective dose of Staphylococcus aureus in the midcarpal joint of horses. Am J Vet Res 1989;50:2014–17.
210. Arrioja A. Compendium of Veterinary Products. In: Arrioja A, editor. Compendium of Veterinary Products. Canada: North American Compendiums, Ltd; 2001. p. 1665.
211. Arrioja A. Compendium of Veterinary Products. In: Arrioja A, editor. Compendium of Veterinary Products. Canada: North American Compendiums, Ltd; 2001. p. 1346–9.
212. Plumb DC. Hyaluronate sodium. In: Veterinary Drug Handbook. Ames: Iowa University Press; 1999. p. 325–6.
213. Burba DJ, Collier MA, Default LE, et al. In vivo kinetic study on uptake and distribution of intramuscular tritium-labeled polysulfated glycosaminoglycan in equine body fluid compartments and articular cartilage in an osteochondrial defect model. J Equine Vet Sci 1993;13:696–703.
214. Andrews JL, Sutherland J, Ghosh P. Distribution and binding of glycosaminoglycan polysulfate to intervertebral disc, knee joint articular cartilage and meniscus. Arzneimittelforschung 1985;35:144–8.
215. Panse P, Zeiller P, Sensch K. Distribution and excretion of a glycosaminopolysulfate in the rabbit after parenteral application. Arzneimittelforschung 1976;26:2024–9.
216. McIlwraith C, Trotter G. Joint Disease in the Horse. Philadelphia: WB Saunders Co; 1996.
217. Vacha J, Pesakova V, Krajickova J, et al. Effect of glycosaminoglycan polysulphate on the metabolism of cartilage ribonucleic acid. Arzneimittelforschung 1984;34: 607–9.
218. Adam M, Krabcova M, Musilova J, et al. Contribution to the mode of action of glycosaminoglycan-polysulphate (GAGPS) upon human osteoarthrotic cartilage. Biochemical study of the collagen and proteoglycan turnover. Arzneimittelforschung 1980;30:1730–2.
219. Hannan N, Ghosh P, Bellenger C, et al. Systemic administration of glycosaminoglycan polysulphate (arteparon) provides partial protection of articular cartilage from damage produced by meniscectomy in the canine. J Orthop Res 1987;5:47–59.
220. Verbruggen G, Veys EM. Influence of sulphated glycosaminoglycans upon proteoglycan metabolism of the synovial lining cells. Acta Rhumatol Belg 1977;1:75–92.
221. Glade MJ. Polysulfated glycosaminoglycan accelerates net synthesis of collagen and glycosaminoglycans by arthritic equine cartilage tissues and chondrocytes. Am J Vet Res 1990;51:779–85.
222. Caron JP, Eberhart SW, Nachreiner R. Influence of polysulfated glycosaminoglycan on equine articular cartilage in explant culture. Am J Vet Res 1991;52:1622–5.
223. Caron JP, Toppin DS, Block JA. Effect of polysulfated glycosaminoglycan on osteoarthritic equine articular cartilage in explant culture. Am J Vet Res 1993; 54:1116–21.
224. Tung JT, Venta PJ, Caron JP. Inducible nitric oxide expression in equine articular chondrocytes: effects of anti-inflammatory compounds. Osteoarthritis Cartilage 2002;10:5–12.
225. Tung JT, Venta PJ, Eberhart SW, et al. Effects of anti-arthritis preparations on gene expression and enzyme activity of cyclooxygenase-2 in cultured equine chondrocytes. Am J Vet Res 2002;63: 1134–9.

226. Kawcak CE, Frisbie DD, McIlwraith CW. Effects of extracorporeal shock wave therapy and polysulfated glycosaminoglycan treatment on subchondral bone, serum biomarkers, and synovial fluid biomarkers in horses with induced osteoarthritis. Am J Vet Res 2011;72:772–9.
227. McIlwraith C. Intra-articular medication for traumatic joint problems: Do we understand the choices? Comp Cont Educ Pract Vet 1989;11:1287–311.
228. Trotter GW, Yovich JV, McIlwraith CW, et al. Effects of intramuscular polysulfated glycosaminoglycan on chemical and physical defects in equine articular cartilage. Can J Vet Res 1989; 53:224–30.
229. Yovich JV, Trotter GW, McIlwraith CW, et al. Effects of polysulfated glycosaminoglycan on chemical and physical defects in equine articular cartilage. Am J Vet Res 1987;48: 1407–14.
230. Todhunter RJ, Minor RR, Wootton JA, et al. Effects of exercise and polysulfated glycosaminoglycan on repair of articular cartilage defects in the equine carpus. J Orthop Res 1993;11:782–95.
231. Todhunter RJ, Freeman KP, Yeager AE, et al. Effects of exercise and polysulfated glycosaminoglycan on the development of osteoarthritis in equine carpal joints with osteochondral defects. Vet Surg 1993;22:330–42.
232. Kristiansen KK, Kold SE. Multivariable analysis of factors influencing outcome of 2 treatment protocols in 128 cases of horses responding positively to intra-articular analgesia of the distal interphalangeal joint. Equine Vet J 2007;39:150–6.
233. Verde C, Ferrante M, Simpson MI, et al. Efficacy of intramuscular polysulfated glycosaminoglycan in a controlled study of equine carpitis. J Vet Pharmacol Ther 2010;33:357–62.
234. Oryan A. Experimental tendon injury and repair. England: University of Bristol; 1989.
235. Redding W, Booth L, Pool R. Effects of polysulfated glycosaminoglycan on healing of collagenase-induced tendonitis of the equine superficial digital flexor tendon. VCOT 1999;12: 48–56.
236. Moraes JR, Facco GG, Moraes FR, et al. Effects of glycosaminoglycan polysulphate on the organisation of collagen fibres in experimentally induced tendonitis in horses. Vet Rec 2009;165:203–5.
237. Walesby HA, Rosenbusch R, Booth LC, et al. Uptake and distribution of tritium-labeled polysulfated glycosaminoglycan in serum, urine, and superficial digital flexor tendon of rabbits after intramuscular administration. Am J Vet Res 2000;61: 20–3.
238. Nixon AJ. Intra-articular medication. In: Robinson NE, editor. Current Therapy in Equine Medicine. Philidelphia: WB Saunders Co.; 1992. p. 127–31.
239. Rashmir-Raven AM, Coyne CP, Fenwick BW, et al. Inhibition of equine complement activity by polysulfated glycosaminoglycans. Am J Vet Res 1992; 53:87–90.
240. Arrioja A. Compendium of Veterinary Products. Canada: North American Compendiums, Ltd; 2001.
241. Hamm D, Goldman L, Jones E. Polysulfated glycosaminoglycin: A new intra-articular treatment for equine lameness. Vet Med 1984;6:811–16.
242. Plumb DC. Polysulfated glycosaminoglycan. In: Plumb DC, editor. Veterinary Drug Handbook. Iowa: Iowa State University Press; 1999. p. 520–1.
243. Ghosh P, Smith M, Wells C. Second-line agents in osteoarthritis. In: Dixon JS, Furst DE, editors. Second-line Agents in the Treatment of Rheumatic Diseases. New York: Marcel Dekker; 1992. p. 363–427.
244. Ghosh P, Wells C, Smith M, et al. Chondroprotection, myth or reality: an experimental approach. Semin Arthritis Rheum 1990;19:3–9.
245. Avouac B. Slow acting drugs in osteoarthritis: a step towards disease modification. Rev Esp Reumatol 1993; 20:221–2.
246. Lequesne M, Brandt K, Bellamy N, et al. Guidelines for testing slow acting drugs in osteoarthritis. J Rheumatol Suppl 1994;41:65–71; discussion 72–63.
247. Lualdi P. Bioavailability of oral chondroitin sulfate. Rheumatol Int 1993;13:39–43.
248. Baici A, Wagenhauser F. Rheumatol Int 1993;13:41–3.
249. Palmieri L, Conte A, Giovannini L, et al. Metabolic fate of exogenous chondroitin sulfate in the experimental animal. Arzneimittelforschung 1990;40:319–23.
250. Conte A, de Bernardi M, Palmieri L, et al. Metabolic fate of exogenous chondroitin sulfate in man. Arzneimittelforschung 1991;41:768–72.
251. Ronca F, Palmieri L, Panicucci P, et al. Anti-inflammatory activity of chondroitin sulfate. J Osteoarthritis Cartilage 1998;6:14–21.
252. Baici A, Horler D, Moser B, et al. Analysis of glycosaminoglycans in human serum after oral administration of chondroitin sulfate. Rheumatol Int 1992;12:81–8.
253. Yamanashi S, Toyoda H, Furuya N, et al. Metabolic study on chondroitin sulfates in rabbits. Yakugaku Zasshi 1991;111:73–6.
254. Salyers AA, O'Brien M. Cellular location of enzymes involved in chondroitin sulfate breakdown by Bacteroides thetaiotaomicron. J Bacteriol 1980;143:772–80.
255. Wright IM. Oral supplements in the treatment and prevention of joint diseases: a review of their potential application to the horse. Equine Vet Educ 2001;13:135–9.
256. Dechant JE, Baxter GM, Frisbie DD, et al. Effects of glucosamine hydrochloride and chondroitin sulphate, alone and in combination, on normal and interleukin-1 conditioned equine articular cartilage explant metabolism. Equine Vet J 2005;37: 227–31.
257. Orth MW, Peters TL, Hawkins JN. Inhibition of articular cartilage degradation by glucosamine-HCl and chondroitin sulphate. Equine Vet J Suppl 2002:224–9.
258. Trumble. The use of nutraceuticals for osteoarthritis in horses. Vet Clin North Am Equine Pract 2005;21:575–97.
259. Deal CL, Moskowitz RW. Nutraceuticals as therapeutic agents in osteoarthritis. The role of glucosamine, chondroitin sulfate, and collagen hydrolysate. Rheum Dis Clin North Am 1999;25: 379–95.
260. Morreale P, Manopulo R, Galati M, et al. Comparison of the anti-inflammatory efficacy of chondroitin sulfate and diclofenac sodium in patients with knee osteoarthritis. J Rheumatol 1996;23:1385–91.
261. Bourgeois P, Chales G, Dehais J, et al. Efficacy and tolerability of chondroitin sulfate 1200 mg/day vs chondroitin sulfate 3 x 400 mg/day vs placebo. Osteoarthritis Cartilage 1998; 6(Suppl. A):25–30.
262. Bucsi L, Poor G. Efficacy and tolerability of oral chondroitin sulfate as a symptomatic slow-acting drug for osteoarthritis (SYSADOA) in the treatment of knee osteoarthritis. Osteoarthritis Cartilage 1998; 6(Suppl. A):31–6.
263. Uebelhart D, Thonar EJ, Delmas PD, et al. Effects of oral chondroitin sulfate on the progression of knee osteoarthritis: a pilot study. Osteoarthritis Cartilage 1998;6(Suppl. A):39–46.
264. Gibson R, Gibson S, Conway V, et al. Perna canaliculus in the treatment of arthritis. Practitioner 1980;224:955–60.
265. Uebelhart D, Thonar E, Zhang J, et al. Protective effect of exogenous chondroitin 4,6-sulfate in the acute degradation of articular cartilage in the rabbit. J Osteoarthritis Cartilage 1998;6: 6–13.
266. Canapp Jr SO, McLaughlin Jr RM, Hoskinson JJ, et al. Scintigraphic evaluation of dogs with acute synovitis after treatment with glucosamine

hydrochloride and chondroitin sulfate. Am J Vet Res 1999;60:1552–7.
267. Forsyth R, Brigden C, Northrop A. Double blind investigation of the effects of oral supplementation of combined glucosamine hydrochloride (GHCL) and chondroitin sulphate (CS) on stride characteristics of veteran horses. Equine Vet J 2006;Aug:622–5.
268. White G. Is oral supplementation of PSGAG a reliable method of therapy for equine joint disease? J Equine Vet Sci 1989;9:232–3.
269. Muller-Fassbender H, Bach GL, Haase W, et al. Glucosamine sulfate compared to ibuprofen in osteoarthritis of the knee. Osteoarthritis Cartilage 1994;2:61–9.
270. Noack W, Fischer M, Forster KK, et al. Glucosamine sulfate in osteoarthritis of the knee. J Osteoarthritis Cartilage 1994;2:51–9.
271. Hanson R. Oral glycosaminoglycans in treatment of degenerative joint disease in horses. Equine Pract 1996;18:18–22.
272. White G, Jones E, Hamm J. The efficacy of orally administered sulfated glycosaminoglycan in chemically-induced equine synovitis adn degenerative joint disease. J Equine Vet Sci 1994;14:350–3.
273. Roden L. Effect of hexosamines on the synthesis of chondroitin sulphuric acid in vitro. Arkh Kemi 1956;10:345–52.
274. Vidal y Plana RR, Karzel K. Glucosamine: its importance for the metabolism of articular cartilage. 2. Studies on articular cartilage. Fortschritte der Medizin 1980;98:801–6.
275. Setnikar I, Cereda R, Pacini MA, et al. Antireactive properties of glucosamine sulfate. Arzneimittelforschung 1991;41: 157–61.
276. Setnikar I, Pacini MA, Revel L. Antiarthritic effects of glucosamine sulfate studied in animal models. Arzneimittelforschung 1991;41:542–5.
277. Fenton J, Chelebek-Brown K, Peters T. Glucosamino inhibits interleukin-1β and lipopolysaccharide-induced cartilage degeneration in vitro. Vet Surg 1999;28:388–92.
278. Fenton JI, Chlebek-Brown KA, Peters TL, et al. Glucosamine HCl reduces equine articular cartilage degradation in explant culture. Osteoarthritis Cartilage 2000;8: 258–65.
279. Bassleer C, Henrotin Y, Franchimont P. In-vitro evaluation of drugs proposed as chondroprotective agents. Int J Tissue React 1992;14:231–41.
280. Bassleer C, Henrotin Y, Franchimont P. Effects of sodium naproxen on differentiated human chondrocytes cultivated in clusters. Clin Rheumatol 1992;11:60–5.
281. Setnikar I, Giachetti C, Zanolo G. Absorption, distribution and excretion of radioactivity after a single intravenous or oral administration of [14C] glucosamine to the rat. Pharmatherapeutica 1984;3:538–50.
282. Setnikar I, Giacchetti C, Zanolo G. Pharmacokinetics of glucosamine in the dog and in man. Arzneimittelforschung 1986;36:729–35.
283. Eichler J, Noh E. Therapy of deforming arthrosis through the action upon the cartilaginous metabolism. Orthop Prac 1970;9:225–9.
284. Raiss R. Effect of D-glucosamine sulfate on experimentally injured articular cartilage. Comparative morphometry of the ultrastructure of chondrocytes. Fortschritte der Medizin 1985;103: 658–62.
285. Pujalte JM, Llavore EP, Ylescupidez FR. Double-blind clinical evaluation of oral glucosamine sulphate in the basic treatment of osteoarthrosis. Curr Med Res Opin 1980;7:110–14.
286. Pearson W, Lindinger M. Low quality of evidence for glucosamine-based nutraceuticals in equine joint disease: Review of in vivo studies. Equine Vet J 2009;41:706–12.
287. Block JA, Oegema TR, Sandy JD, et al. The effects of oral glucosamine on joint health: is a change in research approach needed? Osteoarthritis Cartilage 2010; 18:5–11.
288. Ramey. An analysis of glucosamine and chondroitin sulfate content in oral joint supplement products. J Eq Vet Sci 2002;22:125–7.
289. Oke S, Aghazadeh-Habashi A, Weese JS, et al. Evaluation of glucosamine levels in commercial equine oral supplements for joints. Equine Vet J 2006;38:93–5.
290. Brayton CF. Dimethyl sulfoxide (DMSO): a review. Cornell Vet 1986;76: 61–90.
291. Koller LD. Clinical application of DMSO by veterinarians in Oregon & Washington. Vet Med Small Anim Clin 1976;71:591–7.
292. Wood DC, Wood J. Pharmacologic and biochemical considerations of dimethyl sulfoxide. Ann N Y Acad Sci 1975;243: 7–19.
293. Fox RB, Fox WK. Dimethyl sulfoxide prevents hydroxyl radical-mediated depolymerization of hyaluronic acid. Ann N Y Acad Sci 1983;411:14–18.
294. Auer DE, Ng JC, Reilly JS, et al. Anti-inflammatory drugs inhibit degradation of equine synovial fluid induced by free radicals. Aust Vet J 1991;68:403–5.
295. Auer DE, Ng JC, Seawright AA. Superoxide production by stimulated equine polymorphonuclear leukocytes inhibition by anti-inflammatory drugs. J Vet Pharmacol Ther 1990;13:59–66.
296. Plumb DC. Dimethyl sulfoxide. In: Plumb DC, editor. Veterinary Drug Handbook. Ames, IA: Iowa State University Press; 1999.
297. Smith G, Bertone AL, Kaeding C, et al. Anti-inflammatory effects of topically applied dimethyl sulfoxide gel on endotoxin-induced synovitis in horses. Am J Vet Res 1998;59:1149–52.
298. Wooley RE, Gilbert JP, Shotts Jr EB. Inhibitory effects of combinations of oxytetracycline, dimethyl sulfoxide, and EDTA-tromethamine on Escherichia coli. Am J Vet Res 1981;42:2010–13.
299. Gorog P, Kovacs IB. Antiarthritic and antithrombotic effects of topically applied dimethyl sulfoxide. Ann N Y Acad Sci 1975;243:91–7.
300. More RC, Kabo JM, Dorey FJ, et al. The effects of dimethyl sulfoxide on posttraumatic limb swelling and joint stiffness. A review and an experimental study in rabbits. Clin Orthop Relat Res 1988;(233):304–10.
301. Honnas CM, Welch RD, Ford TS, et al. Septic arthritis of the distal interphalangeal joint in 12 horses. Vet Surg 1992;21:261–8.
302. Santos L, Tipping PG. Attenuation of adjuvant arthritis in rats by treatment with oxygen radical scavengers. Immunol Cell Biol 1994;72:406–14.
303. Welch RD, DeBowes RM, Liepold HW. Evaluation of the effects of intra-articular injection of dimethylsulfoxide on normal equine articular tissues. Am J Vet Res 1989;50:1180–2.
304. Welch RD, Watkins JP, DeBowes RM, et al. Effects of intra-articular administration of dimethylsulfoxide on chemically induced synovitis in immature horses. Am J Vet Res 1991;52: 934–9.
305. Adair HS, Goble DO, Vanhooser S, et al. Evaluation of use of dimethyl sulfoxide for intra-articular lavage in clinically normal horses. Am J Vet Res 1991;52: 333–6.
306. Palmer JL, Bertone AL. Joint structure, biochemistry and biochemical disequilibrium in synovitis and equine joint disease. Equine Vet J 1994;26: 263–77.
307. Smith CL, MacDonald MH, Tesch AM, et al. In vitro evaluation of the effect of dimethyl sulfoxide on equine articular cartilage matrix metabolism. Vet Surg 2000;29:347–57.
308. Rubin LF. Toxicologic update of dimethyl sulfoxide. Ann N Y Acad Sci 1983;411:6–10.
309. Little C, Ghosh P. Potential use of pentosan polysulfate for the treatment of equine joint disease. In: McIlwraith CW, Trotter GW, editors. Joint Disease in the Horse. Philidelphia: W. B. Saunders; 1996. p. 281–92.
310. Odlind B, Dencker L, Tengblad A. Preferential localization of 3H-pentosanpolysulphate to the urinary

tract in rats. Pharmacol Toxicol 1987;61:162–6.
311. Dencker L, Tengblad A, Odlind B. Preferential localization of 3H-pentosanpolysulfate to the urinary tract in rats. Acta Physiol Scand 1985;124:351–9.
312. Andrews JL, Ghosh P, Lentini A, et al. The interaction of pentosan polysulphate (SP54) with human neutrophil elastase and connective tissue matrix components. Chem Biol Interact 1983;47:157–73.
313. Ghosh P, Hutadilok N. Interactions of pentosan polysulfate with cartilage matrix proteins and synovial fibroblasts derived from patients with osteoarthritis. Osteoarthritis Cartilage 1996;4:43–53.
314. Roberts BJ, Unsworth A, Mian N. Modes of lubrication in human hip joints. Ann Rheum Dis 1982;41:217–24.
315. Baici A, Salgam P, Fehr K, et al. Inhibition of human elastase from polymorphonuclear leucocytes by gold sodium thiomalate and pentosan polysulfate (SP-54). Biochem Pharmacol 1981;30:703–8.
316. Barg WF, Englert ME, Buermann CW, et al. Studies on the effect of pentosan polysulfate on proteoglycan degradation by leukocyte neutral proteases. Biochem Pharmacol 1979;28:2639–43.
317. Kruze D, Fehr K, Menninger H, et al. Effect of antirheumatic drugs on neutral protease from human leukocyte granules. Z Rheumatol 1976;35:337–46.
318. Kruze K, Fehr K, Boni A. Effect of antirheumatic drugs on cathepsin B1 from bovine spleen. Z Rheumatol 1976;35:95–102.
319. Steinmeyer J, Kalbhen DA. Influence of some natural and semisynthetic agents on elastase and cathepsin G from polymorphonuclear granulocytes. Arzneimittelforschung 1991;41:77–80.
320. Aydelotte MB, Kuettner KE. Differences between sub-populations of cultured bovine articular chondrocytes. I. Morphology and cartilage matrix production. Connect Tissue Res 1988;18:205–22.
321. Hutadilok N, Smith M, Cullis-Hill D, et al. Pentosan pentosulphate stimulates hyaluronate and DNA synthesis in synovial fibroblasts and partially reduces the suppressive effect of hydrocortisone on fibroblast metabolism. Curr Ther Res 1988;44:845–60.
322. Burkhardt D, Ghosh P. Laboratory evaluation of glycosaminoglycan polysulphate eseter for chondroprotective activity. Curr Ther Res 1986;40:1034–53.
323. Golding J, Ghosh P. Drugs for osteoarthrosis: 1. The effects of pentosan polysulphate (SP54) on the degradation and loss of proteglycans from articular cartilage in a model of osteoarthrosis induced in the rabbit knee joint by immobilization. Curr Ther Res 1983;32:173–84.
324. Rogachefsky RA, Dean DD, Howell DS, et al. Treatment of canine osteoarthritis with insulin-like growth factor-1 (IGF-1) and sodium pentosan polysulfate. Osteoarthritis Cartilage 1993;1:105–14.
325. Grumbles RM, Howell DS, Howard GA, et al. Cartilage metalloproteases in disuse atrophy. J Rheumatol Suppl 1995;43:146–8.
326. Kongtawelert P, Brooks P, Ghosh P. Pentosan polysulphate (Cartrophen) prevents the hydrocortisone induced loss of hyaluronic acid and proteoglycan from cartilage of rabbit joints as well as normalizes keratin sulphate levels in their serum. J Rheumatol 1989;16:1454–9.
327. Dart. The effect of three different doses of sodium pentosan polysulphate on haematological and haemostatic variables in adult horses. Australian Vet J 2001;79:624–7.
328. Read RA, Cullis-Hill D, Jones MP. Systemic use of pentosan polysulphate in the treatment of osteoarthritis. J Small Anim Pract 1996;37:108–14.
329. Verbruggen G, Veys E, Ghosh P. Pentosan polysulphate treatment in osteoarthritis, serological parameters which could correlate with clinical response. J Osteoarthritis Cartilage 1994;2:60–5.
330. McIlwraith CW, Frisbie DD, Kawcak CE. Evaluation of intramuscularly administered sodium pentosan polysulfate for treatment of experimentally induced osteoarthritis in horses. Am J Vet Res 2012;73:628–33.
331. Ammann P, Rizzoli R, Caverzasio J, et al. Effects of the bisphosphonate tiludronate on bone resorption, calcium balance, and bone mineral density. J Bone Miner Res 1993;8:1491–8.
332. Bonjour JP, Ammann P, Barbier A, et al. Tiludronate: bone pharmacology and safety. Bone 1995;17:473S–7S.
333. Monkkonen J, Simila J, Rogers MJ. Effects of tiludronate and ibandronate on the secretion of proinflammatory cytokines and nitric oxide from macrophages in vitro. Life Sci 1998;62:PL95–102.
334. Emonds-Alt X, Breliere JC, Roncucci R. Effects of 1-hydroxyethylidene-1,1 bisphosphonate and (chloro-4 phenyl) thiomethylene bisphosphonic acid (SR 41319) on the mononuclear cell factor-mediated release of neutral proteinases by articular chondrocytes and synovial cells. Biochem Pharmacol 1985;34:4043–9.
335. Denoix JM, Thibaud D, Riccio B. Tiludronate as a new therapeutic agent in the treatment of navicular disease: a double-blind placebo-controlled clinical trial. Equine Vet J 2003;35:407–13.
336. Coudry V, Thibaud D, Riccio B, et al. Efficacy of tiludronate in the treatment of horses with signs of pain associated with osteoarthritic lesions of the thoracolumbar vertebral column. Am J Vet Res 2007;68:329–37.
337. Gough MR, Thibaud D, Smith RK. Tiludronate infusion in the treatment of bone spavin: a double blind placebo-controlled trial. Equine Vet J 2010;42:381–7.
338. Hamm D, Turchi P, Johnson JC, et al. Determination of an effective dose of eltenac and its comparison with that of flunixin meglumine in horses after experimentaly induced carpitis. Am J Vet Res 1997;58:298–302.
339. Baxter GM. Table 9.2. In: Baxter G, editor. Manual of Equine Lameness. West Sussex, UK: Wiley-Blackwell; 2011. p. 410.
340. Boehringer Ingelheim website. Hyalovet. Available at: http://www.bivetmedica.com/main/by_product/hyalovet.html. Accessed Jul 22, 2013.
341. Boehringer Ingelheim website. Hyvisc. Available at: http://www.bivetmedica.com/main/by_product/hyvisc.html. Accessed Jul 22, 2013.
342. U.S. Food and Drug Administration website. NADA 140-474 Synacid-original approval. Available at: http://www.fda.gov/animalveterinary/products/approvedanimaldrugproducts/foiadrugsummaries/ucm069895.htm. Accessed Jul 22, 2013.
343. Pfizer Animal Health website. Hylartin V. Available at: http://www.hylartinv.com/docs/hylartinv/US_EN_HY_compliance.pdf. Accessed Jul 22, 2013.
344. U.S. Food and Drug Administration website. NADA 139-913 Equron-original approval. Available at: http://www.fda.gov/animalveterinary/products/approvedanimaldrugproducts/foiadrugsummaries/ucm111271.htm. Accessed Jul 22, 2013.
345. Bayer Healthcare LLC Animal Health Division. Legend. Available at: http://bayer.naccvp.com/?m=product_view_basic&id=1040027&u=bayer&p=dvm. Accessed Jul 22, 2013.

Neurologic causes of gait abnormalities in the athletic horse

Elizabeth A. Carr Omar Maher

24

CHAPTER CONTENTS

Introduction

This chapter is not meant to be an exhaustive review of all neurologic disorders, but to focus on neurologic disorders that may result in gait deficits or performance problems in an otherwise healthy horse. There are many neurologic disorders that will not be covered in this chapter simply because the affected individual would generally present with other signs of acute illness. For example, West Nile Virus, Eastern Equine Encephalitis, Equine herpesvirus-1 (EHV-1), Rabies virus infections would all be expected to result in gait deficits in affected horses. However, most of these diseases will also result in other more overt signs of illness including fever, depression and cerebral signs.

West Nile virus myeloencephalitis typically presents with signs of symmetric or asymmetric gait deficits, fever in approximately half of affected horses and cranial nerve deficits in a percentage of cases. Fine muscle fasciculations are often present as well. Eastern equine encephalitis commonly presents with evidence of cerebral involvement with somnolescence or severe depression. Antibody titers in serum or CSF or the finding of viral DNA in CSF are the most accurate diagnostic tests though serology must be interpreted in light of previous vaccination. Lameness is reported to be the most common initial clinical sign in rabies virus infection in horses. Affected horses typically progress to neurologic gait deficits and subsequently develop more profound and diffuse signs including cranial nerve and cerebral dysfunction. Affected horses may be febrile. While vaccination is reported to be efficacious, cases of rabies in vaccinated horses exist.

Equine herpesvirus-1 myeloencephalitis affected horses typically present with hindlimb weakness and ataxia, urinary incontinence and signs of lower motor neuron deficits to the tail, perineal area and caudal region. Clinical deficits usually progress rapidly over hours to days. A history of respiratory signs in the affected horse or herdmates or the introduction of a new horse is often present. Diagnosis of EHV-1 is most commonly made based on the history, clinical signs and the finding of EHV-1 DNA in the CSF. Nasal shedding of EHV-1 has also been considered diagnostic in symptomatic horses though horses may shed EHV-1 without clinical illness during period of stress.

In the last two decades, reports of outbreaks of EHV-1 myeloencephalopathy at performance venues, hospitals and large equestrian farms have increased. Whether this is because of more rapid worldwide distribution of information or truly due to an increase in the incidence is unknown. The spread of EHV-1 at performance venues is a significant concern as mortality rates approach 50% in affected horses and outbreaks result in cancellation of events and significant financial losses to both the event planners and the local economy. Because EHV-1 may be shed asymptomatically and vaccination is not 100% effective in preventing infection vigilance in surveillance and recognition of sick horses is critical in preventing an outbreak. Having precautionary examinations and limiting commingling of animals at show grounds are valuable methods to prevent or detect disease spread. Having a biosecurity plan in place including protocols for quarantine and travel restrictions should an outbreak occur is critical to be able to quickly recognize and limit the spread of disease.

Cervical vertebral malformation

Cervical vertebral malformation-malarticulation (CVM), also referred to as cervical stenotic myelopathy, cervical compressive myelopathy, cervical vertebral stenosis and Wobblers syndrome is one of the most common causes of neurologic gait abnormalities in horses. Clinical symptoms are due to compression of the cervical spinal cord and degeneration of the ascending general proprioceptive pathways and descending upper motor neuron pathways that modulate body and limb position and movement. Clinical signs may be acute in onset or insidious and are often progressive though some owners will report a history of cyclic improvement/deterioration. In some cases, the history is an acute onset after a traumatic event or fall; whether unrecognized neurologic dysfunction precipitated the fall and subsequent deterioration is unknown but often suspected.

Epidemiology and pathogenesis

There are two recognized forms of the disease. Type 1 CVM results in dynamic compression with flexion of the neck and most often occurs in the mid-cervical region (C3-C5). Type I CVM most commonly occurs in young, rapidly growing, male horses. Bony abnormalities are similar to those seen in osteochondrosis and epiphysitis of the appendicular skeleton with cartilage retention and dissecting lesions of the joint surface.[1,2] Type 2 CVM is a static stenosis of the canal most commonly occurring in the caudal neck (C5-T1). Type 2 is reported to occur more commonly in older horses though young horses are also affected. Causes of static compression include cranioventral extension of the dorsal lamina, caudodorsal extension of the caudal vertebral body, hypertrophy of the ligamentum flavum, enlargement of the articular processes of the cervical facets and, less commonly, disc herniation and synovial cyst formation intervertebral disk prolapsed and diskospondylitis in a horse.[3-5]

The underlying etiology of CVM is incompletely understood and is likely multifactorial. Genetics, trauma, high energy diets and micromineral imbalances are all suspect to play a role in the pathogenesis. In addition, similar to humans and other species it is likely that progressive age related degeneration, repetitive movement, instability and trauma may also be factors in the development of this syndrome. Cervical vertebral malformation is most commonly seen in the young, large, rapidly growing, male phenotype with Thoroughbred and Warmblood breeds over-represented.[6,7] While genetics must certainly be a factor in the development of CVM a study breeding CVM-affected horses to CVM-affected horses resulted in an increased incidence of osteochondrosis of the appendicular skeleton without an increased incidence of CVM supporting a similar pathogenesis in these two syndromes.[8] In addition, a study of affected and unaffected Thoroughbreds in Great Britain failed to identify a genetic mode of inheritance.[9]

It is likely that both genetic and environmental factors including diet play a role in the development of CVM. Foals identified as having risk factors for CVM (radiographic changes and or neurologic signs) showed improvement in both radiographic changes and neurologic function when fed a restricted diet and confined to limit exercise. The restricted diet was low in protein and energy with vitamin and mineral composition adjusted for the age and weight of the individual foal.[10] An association between both CVM and osteochondrosis and mineral balance has also been reported.[11,12] Unfortunately because many affected horses are not identified till later in life it is unlikely that dietary modification at that time will affect growth and outcome.

Recognition

Clinical signs

The most common clinical signs of CVM are symmetric ataxia and weakness. Neurologic deficits are due to compression of the long ascending and descending tracks. Hindlimbs are often more severely affected as the tracks that modulate hindlimb movement lie lateral to those that modulate the forelimbs and are more severely compressed. Less commonly, compression at the caudal cervical vertebrae (C6-T1) may result in more severe dysfunction of the forelimbs due to compression of the cervical intumescence. Occasionally, forelimb lameness or neck pain may be present if the spinal roots are involved. Neurologic deficits include, abnormal and irregular foot flight such as hyper or hypometria, circumduction, trunkal sway, knuckling, interfering, spasticity and dragging of the toe. Signs are usually more prominent when horses are asked to circle, back up, go up and down a hill, navigate a curb or obstacle, asked to move with head elevated or blindfolded or when asked to stop suddenly as these movements require greater proprioceptive input and muscle control. Circumduction while circling with bouncing or weakness may be evident when the inside hind is weighted. Horses often exhibit an irregular pace when backing and appear to reach with their hindlimbs while dragging their front limbs. When asked to stop suddenly, many affected animals will sway or stumble due to the loss of coordination. Abnormal wear of the toe of the hoof is often seen as a result of hypometria.

Diagnosis

Diagnostic testing for CVM is generally performed after a presumptive diagnosis is obtained based on historical information, signalment and clinical findings of ataxia and upper motor neuron weakness. Mentation and cranial nerves are generally normal in affected horses unless the horse has fallen and further injured himself. Hematologic and biochemical results are unremarkable and are primarily useful in ruling out other causes of neurologic dysfuction. Cerebral spinal fluid is typically normal though some cases may show xanthochromia or have an elevated protein.

Radiographic evaluation

Screening lateral radiographs of the cervical spinal column are recommended as the first step in the diagnosis of CVM. Radiographs can be taken in the standing, sedated horse. The entire cervical spine can be evaluated taking three images using large cassettes centered over C2, C4 and C6. Standard portable machines are generally not powerful enough to obtain quality cervical films in full size horses however some of the newer portable digital machines appear to be powerful enough to produce acceptable quality images.

Four commonly recognized bony abnormalities may be seen on radiographs including flare of the caudal vertebral epiphysis of the vertebral body, extension of the caudal edge of the dorsal arch of the vertebral body, osteoarthritis of the articular processes and malalignment of adjacent vertebrae (Fig. 24.1).[13] Because these changes can be seen in unaffected horses these findings are supportive but not definitive for a diagnosis of CVM.

In addition to evaluating radiographs for bony changes, narrowing of the canal can be assessed by measuring intra- and intervertebral minimal sagittal diameter ratios (MSDR).[13-15] Minimal sagittal diameter ratios compare the maximum width of the canal within the vertebrae (Intra-) or between vertebrae (inter-) to the maximum width of the body of the cranial cervical vertebrae allowing the assessment of the width of the canal while controlling for magnification effects (Fig. 24.2). It is critical that a true lateral be taken to ensure accuracy. An abnormally low ratio is associated with

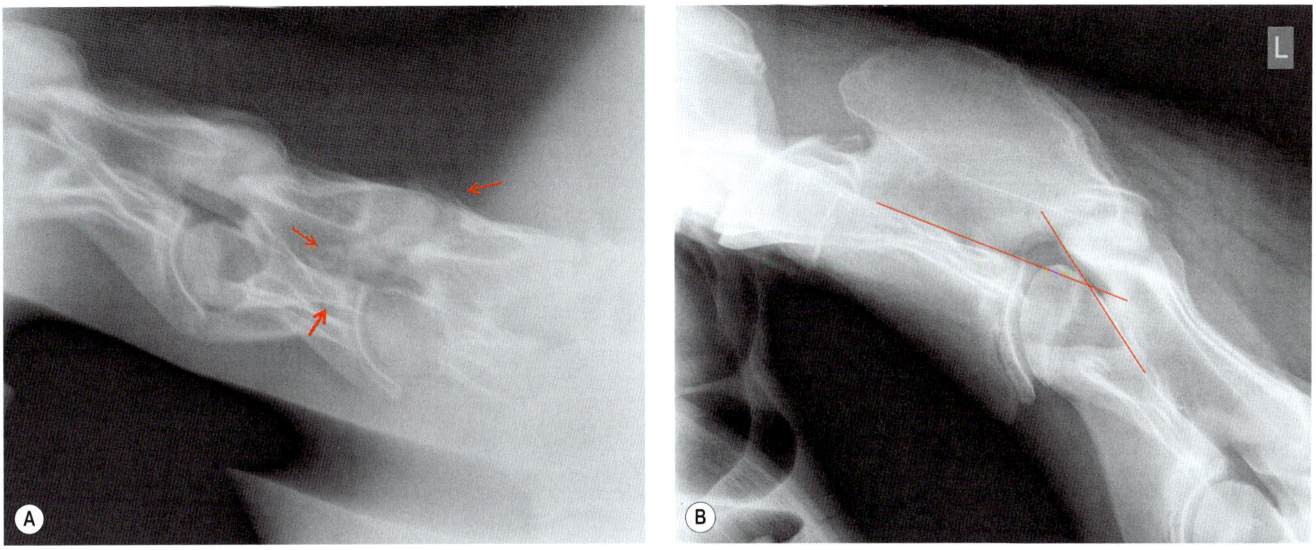

Fig 24.1 **(A)** Lateral survey films illustrating degenerative osteoarthritis of the articular processes at C5-C6 (red arrows) and sclerosis of the associated facet joint. **(B)** Lateral survey films illustrating kyphosis or 'dog nose' appearance at C2-C3 associated with cervical vertebral malformation in a three-year-old Percheron gelding. Post-mortem examination confirmed cervical cord compression at this site.

narrowing of the vertebral canal and suspicious for compression of the spinal cord in this region.

Multiple studies have attempted to predict the likelihood of CVM in suspect cases using scoring systems that utilize bony abnormalities alone or in combination with intra- and inter-MSDRs.[13–18] Papageorges et al concluded that lateral radiographs was not useful in evaluating horses for CVM. In this study only bony abnormalities were scored without determining minimal sagittal diameter ratios. The finding that bony changes alone are not diagnostic for CVM is supported by a recent study determining that cervical facets at C5-C6 and C6-C7 enlarge with age; this enlargement did not correlate with neurologic deficits.[19] Mayhew et al reported on a radiographic scoring system in foals and weanlings that utilized both bony abnormalities and MSDRs. In this study a high score (increased number of abnormalities) was associated with CVM. The authors used the results of this study to determine which individuals were placed on a restricted diet and reported a decrease in both the radiographic scores and neurologic symptoms.[10] The authors noted that certain criteria (angulation and stenosis based on MSDRs) were more accurate in predicting CVM than other criteria. Rush-Moore et al evaluated the accuracy of an intra-vertebral minimal sagittal diameter in predicting CVM in 50 affected and 50 control horse. To be included affected horses had to have histopathologic evidence of CVM at post mortem examination. They concluded that a MSDR cutoff of 0.52 for C_4, C_5 and C_6 and 0.56 for C_7 resulted in the highest sensitivity and specificity. Interestingly, while an abnormal MSDR showed strong correlation in predicting a CVM-affected individual, it was less accurate in predicting the specific site of compression leaving the authors to recommend myelography when planning surgical stabilization. A later study further confirmed the utility of intra- and inter-vertebral minimal sagittal diameters for predicting CVM using a cutoff value of 0.485.[15] Because there is some overlap in MSDR values in affected and unaffected sites a myelogram is strongly recommended to confirm both disease and specific location of compression. To further confuse the interpretation of MSDRs, a recent report showed significant inter and intra-observer variability in measurement of cervical vertebral ratios putting the accuracy of these measurements into question.[18] Given these findings, it is reasonable to conclude that lateral radiographic assessment including measurement of minimum sagittal diameter ratios is useful as a screening tool, but should not be used as the sole diagnostic criteria when evaluating a horse with suspect cervical vertebral malformation.

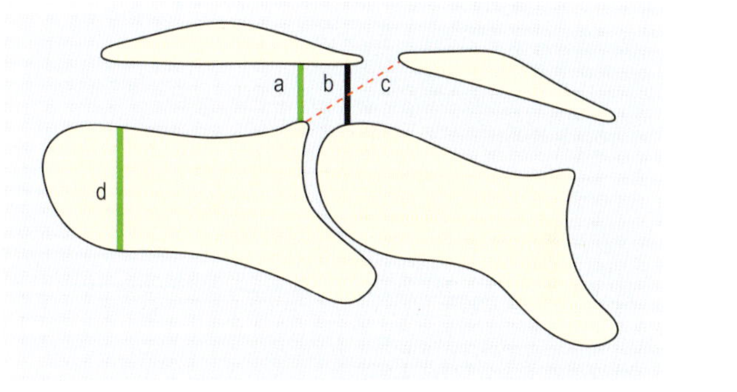

Fig 24.2 Drawing of two vertebra showing the measurements used to determine the intra-vertebral minimal sagital diameter (=a/d) and the inter-vertebral minimal sagital diameter (=b/d or =c/d whichever is smaller). Reprinted from Hahn, C.N., Handel, I., Green, S.L., Bronsvoort, M.B., Mayhew, I.G., (2008) Assessment of the utility of using intra- and intervertebral minimum sagittal diameter ratios in the diagnosis of cervical vertebral malformation in horses, Veterinary Radiology & Ultrasound, 49(1), 1–6.
With permission from John Wiley and Sons.

Myelogram

The gold standard for the diagnosis of CVM has traditionally been the myelogram. A myelogram is performed under general anesthesia though reports exist of myelograms being performed under standing sedation. Iohexol (350 mg iodine/ml), a water-soluble, non-ionic contrast medium has replaced the use of metrizamide as it causes less meningeal irritation and neurotoxicity and is associated with fewer complications.

The technique for performing a myelogram has been well described.[20] Briefly, the horse is placed in lateral recumbency and the poll area clipped and prepped. The land marks for the site are the cranial border of the wings of the atlas on dorsal midline. The poll is flexed and a 3.5 inch 18 gauge needles with a stylet is advanced angled towards the lower incisors. The dura mater must be penetrated and may produce a popping sound when entered. Cerebral spinal fluid will drip from the needle once the trochar is removed. Samples of CSF for additional testing should be collected prior to injection of contrast material. The bevel of the needle is faced caudally and ~40–50 mls of Iohexol injected slowly over a five minute period. The head and neck should be elevated on a wedge platform for five minutes to facilitate flow of contrast down the spinal canal. Radiographic images should be taken in neutral and flexed positions; some clinicians will also take images of the lower spine (C_6-T_1) with extension though this may not be necessary (Fig. 24.3). While extreme flexion and extension may be necessary to achieve a diagnosis it may result in exacerbate of clinical signs and should be performed with caution and only if neutral views are non-diagnostic. Complications include depression, deterioration of neurologic condition, fever, seizures, corneal ulcers, muscle fasciculations, hyperesthesia, stiff neck and meningitis.[20–24] Complications appear to occur less frequently with the use of Iohexol.

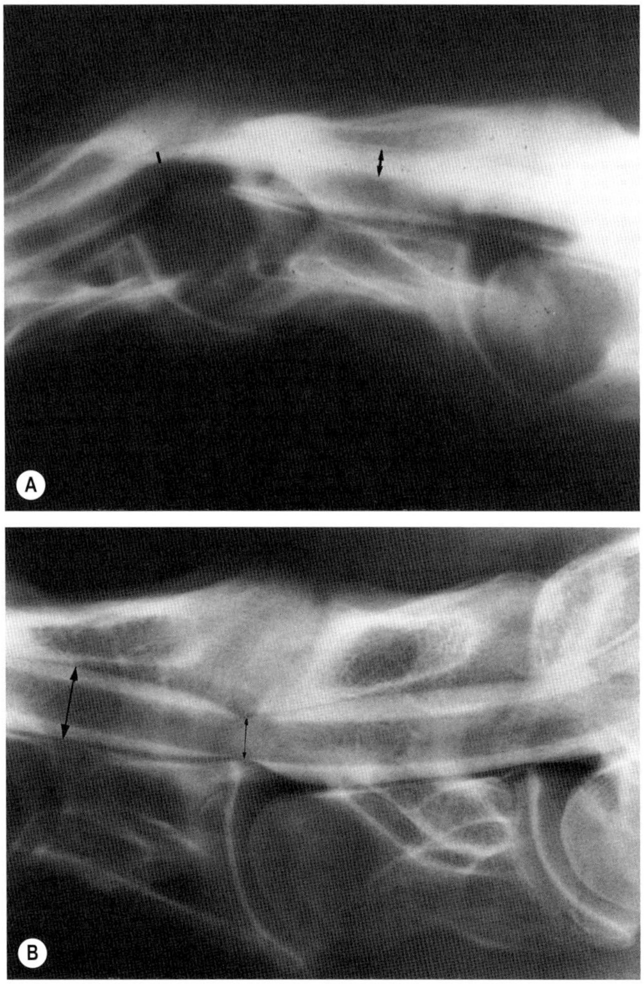

Fig 24.3 (A) Myelographic examination of C4 through C6 with the cervical spine in ventroflexion. Dynamic instability and spinal cord compression are present at C4–C5. The '50% rule' is determined by dividing the dorsal contrast column of the C4–C5 articulation (black line) to the midvertebral, dorsal contrast column caudal to the intervertebral space (double black arrow). **(B)** Myelographic examination of C6–C7 with the cervical spine in neutral position. Static spinal cord compression is demonstrated by obliteration of the dorsal and ventral contrast columns. Percent reduction in dural diameter is determined by comparing the intervertebral space (small black arrow) to the midvertebral site cranial to the intervertebral space (large black arrow). Twenty percent or greater is diagnostic of compression (40% reduction in this case).

Multiple diagnostic criteria have been published. The most common criteria is the finding of a 50% or more height reduction of the minimal dorsal myelographic column (DMC) at the intervertebral site compared to the maximal diameter at the level of the cranial vertebral body. Other reported criteria include the empiric <2 mm DMC and the dural diameter (DD) reduction which is measured by comparing the maximum DD at the cranial vertebral body to the minimum DD at the intervertebral joint. The data behind the development of these criteria is unclear and with one exception, they have not been validated.[25]

A recent report suggests that diagnostic criteria for compression should vary with the vertebral site and neck position (neutral or flexed).[26] The authors conclude that a single diagnostic criteria is not adequate when analyzing a myelographic study. The 50% reduction in the DMC is adequate when evaluating the neutral views of the mid-cervical vertebrae (C_3-C_6) as it has a high specificity (low false-positive rate) but that a more conservative (greater reduction of the DMC) should be used in the flexed view to avoid an increase in false-positive diagnosis. The authors suggest that a cut-off of 50% can be used for a flexed view of C_6-C_7 with a more conservative cut-off (70%) used for this site in a neutral position. Alternatively, a 25% reduction in the DD may be used with either neutral or flexed views at C_6-C_7 with an acceptable sensitivity and specificity.

Treatment and prognosis

Medical treatment

Medical treatment consists primarily of stall rest and anti-inflammatories including NSAIDs and DMSO. Glucocorticoids may be beneficial if an acute exacerbation or injury occurs. Given the underlying pathology medical therapy may temporarily improve clinical signs but is unlikely to resolve the disease. Injection of corticosteroids into the cervical facets may improve clinical signs especially if evidence of neck pain or spinal root compression exists. No data is available on the long term outcome with medical therapy alone. In a multicenter retrospective of long term outcome the majority of severely-affected horses were euthanized or had surgical stabilization; those mildly affected were more likely to be discharged without surgery.[27]

Surgical treatment

Surgical stabilization or decompression is the most effective treatment for CVM.[28–32] Ventral surgical stabilization is recommended for Type 1 CVM when compression is the result of dynamic instability of the intervertebral joint. A stainless steel implant and bone graft are used to fuse the ventral vertebral bodies at the affected joint. Dorsal laminectomy is recommended to immediately decompress the spinal cord when static stenosis is the cause of the neurologic deficits. Removal of the dorsal lamina, ligamentum flavum and joint casule can result in immediate relief. Ventral stabilization can also be beneficial in cases of static stenosis as fusion may result in bony remodeling and atrophy of soft tissue with delayed decompression of the site. Surgical treatment is ideal for animals with acute disease as permanent deficits are more likely with chronic compression. In a retrospective report evaluating surgical treatment of 73 cases using ventral stabilization or dorsal laminectomy neurologic function improved in 77% of horses with 46% returning to athletic performance.[28] Horses with a shorter duration of signs (<1 month) and only one affected site had a better prognosis than those with longer duration and multiple sites of compression. Other studies report similar results with improvement in neurologic function from 44 to 90% and a better prognosis when only one site is affected.[29–32] The risk of surgical complication is relatively high with approximately 10% of horses not surviving to discharge. The successful stabilization of Type 2 CVM using a ventral locking compression plate in a three-month-old foal has also been reported.[33]

Prognosis

The prognosis for for CVM affected horses is fair for life but guarded to poor for performance. Surgical intervention may improve neurologic signs 1 to 2 grades, consequently, mildly affected horses may recovery completely. The prognosis for performance with medical therapy alone is poor.

Equine protozoal myeloencephalitis

Epidemiology and pathogenesis

Equine protozoal myelitis, originally termed segmental myelitis, was first recognized as a cause of neurologic disease in the 1960's.[34] The agent, Sarcocystis neurona, was subsequently cultured from the spinal cord of an affected horse. More recently the protozoal agent Neospora hughesi has been identified in CNS tissue from neurologically affected horses; however it appears to be an infrequent cause of EPM.[35]

Equine protozoal myelitis is recognized in the Western Hemisphere its range corresponding to the range of various opossum species. The opossum is the definitive host of S. neurona and becomes infected after eating muscle containing sarcocysts.[36,37] Sporocysts are passed in the feces of the definitive host and ingested by the intermediate hosts including cats, skunks, armadillos and raccoons.[38–40] Currently, the raccoon is thought to be the most significant intermediate host in North America. After ingestion sporozoits are released and penetrate the gut wall of the intermediate host entering the vascular endothelial cells. Asexual reproduction in the endothelial cell results in release of merozoites into the blood stream. In the natural host, merozoites eventually enter skeletal muscle forming sarcocysts. The life cycle is completed when the opossum eats the dead muscle of the infected intermediate host. Horses are thought to become infected through ingestion of opossum feces containing sporocysts contaminating their feed or environment. The exact route of migration from ingestion to infection of the CNS is unknown but parasitemia has been detected in immunocompromised and one immunocompetent horse.[41,42] The horse is considered a dead end host though mature sarcocysts have been found in the tongue muscle of one horse challenging this assumption.[43]

The pathogenesis of S. neurona in equids is incompletely understood as, despite an apparent high rate of exposure, clinical illness is much less common.[44–48] In a USDA study the average incidence of EPM was 14 cases per 10 000 horses per year.[49] Horses used for competition or racing had a much higher incidence than those used for pleasure or breeding. Certain breeds including Thoroughbreds, Quarter Horses and Standardbreds are over-represented as are young horses, though all breeds and ages can be affected.[50,51] Parasite dose and strain, immune function and physiologic stress (including strenuous exercise) are all thought to play a role in pathogenesis. A common model for inducing EPM is long-distance transport further supporting the role of stress in the pathogenesis of this disease.[52]

Recognition

Clinical signs

Because symptoms vary depending on the location of the organism and subsequent inflammatory response, EPM should be included on almost every differential list for a neurologic horse. Most clinical signs relate to spinal cord and brain stem infection; cerebral disease is uncommon. Slowly progressive onset of asymmetric gait deficits with focal muscle atrophy and/or cranial nerve deficits are the most commonly reported signs though acute onset with rapid progression has been reported.

Diagnosis

Currently there is no perfect test for the diagnosis of EPM as most available immunodiagnostic tests have varying sensitivity and specificity. EPM seroprevalence has been reported to range from 50 to 60% in the United States suggesting that most horses are exposed to S. neurona during their lifetime. Because antibody can move passively across the blood brain barrier (BBB) CSF titers need to be interpreted in light of serum values, the diagnostic test employed and after assessing iatrogenic blood contamination.

The Western Blot (WB) was the first test to be developed and can be performed on both serum and CSF.[53] Because of the high rate of exposure without clinical disease serum testing is useful as a screening test as seronegative horses are unlikely to have EPM. In one study the sensitivity and specificity of the WB was found to be the strongest in neurologic horses.[54] False positive CSF titers may occur due to passive movement of antibody across the BBB, due to iatrogenic blood contamination or due to subclinical infection. A modified Western blot (mWB) was developed to try to decrease false positive results due to cross reaction with other Sarcocystis antigens. Sensitivity and specificity of this mWB was reported to be 100% and 98% by the test developers and 89 and 69% in another study.[55,56] An additional modified Western blot is available that reports the intensity of the staining result as a relative quotient. This modification has not been shown to improve diagnostic value.

More recently an enzyme linked immunosorbent assay (ELISA) was developed against the snSAG-1 protein of S. neurona.[57] An independent study determined the sensitivity and specificity of this test to be poor.[58] In addition, not all S. neurona isolates produce the SAG-1 protein.

A separate research group developed and evaluated a series of ELISA tests against multiple S. neurona surface antigens (sn SAG1-4). The ELISA against the snSAG-2 protein had the highest sensitivity and specificity, 95.5 and 92.9% respectively, using serum and CSF from cases of histopathologically confirmed EPM.[59] A whole organism S.neurona immunofluorescent antibody test (IFAT) is also currently available. In a study comparing the IFAT to the WB and the mWB, the IFAT was reported to have a higher specificity than either WB test.[56,60]

Iatrogenic blood contamination of CSF during collection has been shown to confound results with as little as 11 RBC per microliter causing a false positive CSF Western blot.[61] Evaluation of both serum and CSF as well as performing CSF cytology are recommended when running immunodiagnostic testing for EPM. In addition, because proteins, including antibody, can passively cross the BBB, antibody levels in the CSF can occur in a healthy individual. In theory this passive movement results in CSF antibody levels in proportion to those in the blood, whereas true CNS infection should result in a much higher proportion of specific antibody in the CSF relative to that seen with passive movement from the blood. Consequently, recommendations for interpretation of immunodiagnostic testing of the CSF are to include CSF indices to distinguish intrathecal production from passively acquired antibody in the CSF.[62]

Because there is no ideal diagnostic test for EPM, it is important to establish an accurate list of differentials by considering the signalment, history and progression of neurologic signs, time of year, vaccination history, location and use of the affected animal. Additional diagnostics may include cervical films to rule out cervical vertebral malformation, PCR on CSF to rule out EHV-1 and PCR and/or immunodiagnostic testing of serum and CSF to rule out other infectious diseases such as West Nile Virus or Equine encephalitidies. A diagnosis of EPM is best approached using clinical exam and findings of neurologic signs that are compatible with EPM, ruling out other potential causes of the neurologic symptoms and finally a positive immunodiagnostic test on the CSF.[63]

Treatment, prevention and prognosis

Treatment

Because it is difficult to experimentally reproduce clinical disease in the horse, efficacy of current therapeutics is based on in vitro assays, experimental infections in laboratory animals and clinical trials. There are currently three classes of medications recommended for the treatment of EPM. The first recommended treatment for EPM was a combination of sulfonamides (20 mg/kg) (with or without trimethoprim) and pyrimethamine (1mg/kg).[64] This combination is synergistic blocking protozoal folate synthesis at multiple steps (Beech 1974). In a multicenter field study of clinical cases treated with a combination of pyrimethamine and sulfadiazine (Rebalance, Animal Health Pharmaceuticals, LLC), an overall success rate (defined as an improvement of 1 grade in neurologic deficits or conversion to a negative CSF Western blot) of 53% was reported.[65] Duration of treatment was a minimum of 90 days. Reported side effects in horses receiving the label dose included anemia (22%), leucopenia (19%), neutropenia (5%) and thrombocytopenia (3%). Bone marrow suppression is thought to be due to folate deficiency. In addition, congenital defects in foals born to mares treated with sulfonamides and pyrimethamine during pregnancy have been reported.[66] Horses treated with this combination should be fed good quality green forage (high in folate) to decrease the risk of side effects. Folate supplementation is not thought to be beneficial and may increase the risk of toxicity.[67,68] Though less expensive than other treatment regimes the duration of treatment and risk of side effects may offset the decreased daily cost.

The triazine anticoccidial agent, Ponazuril (Marquis, Bayer Animal Health), was the first FDA approved drug for treatment of EPM. Triazine anticoccidial medications are thought to inhibit the respiratory chain enzymes of the protozoal organism.[69] Recommended oral dosing of Ponazuril is at 5 mg/kg once daily for 28 days. Feeding of two ounces of corn oil immediately prior to dosing has been shown to increase the blood levels by 25%. If neurologic deficits persist, many clinicians will recommend a second 30-day course of therapy. The overall success rate of Ponazuril in the treatment of EPM has been reported to be 62%.[70] Recently another triazine anticoccidial, Diclazuril, has received FDA approval (Protazil, Schering-Plough Animal Health). Currently Diclazuril is marketed as a pelleted oral medication though many clinicians report successful treatment of suspect EPM cases using a compounded intravenous form of Diclazuril. In a multicenter study of clinical cases treated with Protazil the overall success rate was 67% though the percentage dropped to less than half when reviewed by additional experts blinded to the timing of the video exam of enrolled cases.[71]

The thiazolide derivative, Nitazoxanide (Navigator, IDEXX Pharmaceuticals) was approved in 2003 and marketed as the only medication effective in killing S. neurona. Adverse reactions including diarrhea, colic, edema and laminitis were common with this medication leading to recommendations to give one half the recommended dose for five days before starting the full dosing schedule.[72,73] Adverse reactions are common due, in part to Nitazoxanide disturbance of the gastrointestinal flora. Currently Nitazoxanide is no longer on the market. In vitro efficacy of additional thiazolide and thiadiazolide derivatives against S. neurona has been reported.[74] Whether theses derivatives will cause less adverse reactions remains to be determined.

Dosing schedules vary from clinician to clinician and case to case likely due to the lack of data on what constitutes a cure. Recommendations vary from treating until the individual has a negative CSF immunodiagnostic result to treating until 30 days after symptoms stabilize. Most treatment protocols start with a four week treatment followed by re-assessment. A small percentage of cases will have recurrence of clinical EPM. It remains unclear if this constitutes a re-activation of a sub-clinical infection or a new infection.

Additional ancillary treatments include non-steroidal anti-inflammatory medications, DMSO and corticosteroids. Corticosteroids may be beneficial in the acute, severe case but are not recommended for long term use due to their immunosuppressive effects. Vitamin E (20 IU/kg PO daily) has also been recommended as an additional antioxidant. In addition, some clinicians recommend non-specific immunostimulants such as Levamisole and EqStim however, no efficacy data exists.

Prevention

A vaccine was developed against EPM in the mid 1990s. Vaccinated horses may become transiently positive on CSF Western blot making knowledge of vaccination history important when evaluating a suspect case.[75] Efficacy remained unproven and the vaccine is no longer commercially available.

Pretreatment with ponazuril at 5 mg/kg once daily decreased the incidence of clinical EPM in a challenge model.[76] Weekly treatment with 20 mg/kg was also effective in decreasing CSF antibody development in challenged horses. Given the incidence of EPM it is unlikely that prophylactic therapy would be cost effective except in specific circumstances. Current prevention recommendations are primarily targeted on preventing contamination of feeds and environment by S. neurona sporocysts through limiting opossum access to the barn yard and feedstuffs. This can be done by trapping, keeping dogs to discourage opossums from entering the premises and by limiting access to food sources. In particular, keeping equine feedstuffs secure to prevent contamination is strongly recommended.

Prognosis

Approximately two thirds of EPM affected horses will improve at least one grade with treatment regardless of type. A smaller percentage will return to normal. Early recognition and treatment is likely to result in the best outcome.

Neuroaxonal dystrophy and equine degenerative myeloencephalopathy

Epidemiology and pathophysiology

Neuroaxonal dystrophies are a group of degenerative axonopathies recognized in a wide variety of species.[77] Degenerative changes are primarily confined to the central nervous system and may be localized to specific nuclei and tracts or diffuse as seen with Equine Degenerative Myeloencephalopathy (EDM) a severe, diffuse form of neuroaxonal dystophy. Both familial and environmental factors are believed to play a role in the pathophysiology of EDM. Equine degenerative myeloencephalopathy has been recognized in most breeds of horses with reports of familial disease in Appaloosas,[78] Morgans,[79] Standardbreds,[80] Mongolian wild horses,[81] and Quarter Horses.[82,83] Vitamin E deficiency during the rapidly growing stages of life appears to play a role in the development of neuroaxonal dystrophy and EDM particularly in individuals with a familial tendency.[78,80,83,84] In a retrospective case/control study risk factors for EDM include housing on dirt lots, exposure of young foals to insecticides and wood preservatives. Housing in green pasture was found to be protective.[85]

Dietary and serum levels of vitamin E are not always abnormal in affected horses. Serum vitamin E and selenium levels were similar in a retrospective study comparing unaffected to affected horses.[84] In humans, ND has been reported as a result of malabsorption of alpha tocopherol from the gastrointestinal tract.[86] A lack of hepatic vitamin E transfer protein has also been suggested.[87] A deficiency in a metabolic pathway or function of vitamin E cannot be ruled out as some affected individuals appear to have adequate dietary intake of vitamin E. In a study of affected Appaloosa horses, dietary vitamin E was adequate despite low blood vitamin E levels in affected animals.[78] A single serum vitamin E level may not be abnormal as levels can vary in affected animals depending on diet and other unknown factors. In addition, serum vitamin E measurement may not directly correlated with total body levels as <1% is found in the blood.[88] Consequently, serum vitamin E levels are most useful as a screening test for inadequate dietary intake and not definitive evidence of EDM.

Recognition

Clinical signs

Most affected animals develop clinical signs within the first year of life. Bilaterally symmetric ataxia, proprioceptive deficits and weakness are common. Forelimbs may be equally, or less severely affected compared to the hindlimbs. Affected horses may be reported to be 'clumsy' show abnormal placement of limbs, trunkal sway, ataxia, incoordination and/or weakness. Horses may deteriorate over time though the disease appears to be self limiting in the majority of cases. Clinical symptoms are similar to those of cervical vertebral malformation though some differences may be present. Horses affected with EDM often have signs of profound hypometria. Hyporeflexia of the cutaneous trunci may also be reported in cases of EDM; this is not a common finding in CVM-affected horses. EDM-affected horses have normal cranial nerves, no evidence of neurogenic muscle atrophy or loss of skin sensation.

Neuraxonal dystrophy was recently reported in a herd of Quarter Horses. Clinical signs of ataxia, dysmetria, a wide based stance with proprioceptive deficits, an incomplete or sluggish menace and a quiet or obtunded demeanor were reported.[83] Serum and liver vitamin E levels were low in affected animals. Clinical signs did not appear to progress once recognized. Supplementation of vitamin E the following year appeared to decrease the incidence and severity of new cases. Neurodegenerative changes consistent with neuroaxonal dystrophy were found in multiple nuclei of the brain stem and spinal cord as well as axonal loss, demyelinization and astrogliosis in the long tracts of the spinal cord. A common ancestor was present in most affected horses.

Diagnosis

There is no antemortem test for the diagnosis of EDM or neuroaxonal dystrophy. A complete neurologic exam and diagnostic testing including cervical films and CSF tap to rule out other diseases is recommended. A history of confirmed EDM in the blood line of affected horses is strongly supportive of EDM. Early onset (<2 years of age) of symmetric ataxia and weakness coupled with a history of deficient dietary vitamin E or low serum vitamin levels are also strongly suggestive of EDM.

Histopathologic examination of the CNS is necessary for a definitive diagnosis of EDM or neuroaxonal dystrophy of Quarter Horses. Histopathologic abnormalities include neuroaxonal degeneration with spheroid formation within axons, pigment deposition, demyelination and astrogliosis (Fig. 24.4). Histopathologic abnormalities may be localized to specific nuclei or diffuse.[83,89,90]

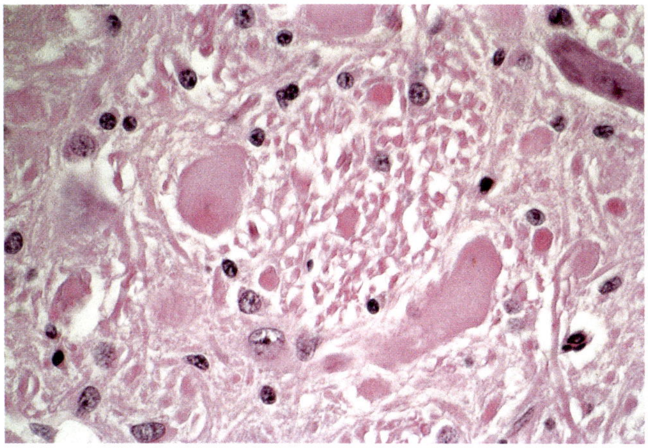

Fig 24.4 Photomicrograph from the brainstem of a six-month-old colt with equine degenerative myeloencephalopathy. Spheroids, representing swollen dystrophic axons, are characteristic of EDM. H&E ×100.

Treatment, prevention and prognosis

Vitamin E supplementation is the cornerstone of treatment of EDM and NAD. Unfortunately, supplementation is unlikely to result in significant improvement of affected animals though reports of improvement in individual horses exist. The vast majority of cases appear to stabilize with or without vitamin E supplementation. Vitamin E supplementation has been shown to decrease the number and severity of new cases on breeding farms.[78–80,89] Prevention is the key to controlling neuroaxonal dystrophies. Preventative measures should be focused on maintaining adequate vitamin E levels in the diet particularly in breeding stock and young horses. Green pasture and fresh, well cured hays are excellent sources of vitamin E. Yearly analysis of hay and concentrates is recommended to determine vitamin E levels and to assess the need for supplementation. In cases with a history of a familial predisposition it is recommended to outcross or avoid breeding suspect horses.

Prognosis

The prognosis for cure in affected horses is poor with most horses stabilizing without improvement. Rare reports of improvement with vitamin E supplementation exist.

Equine motor neuron disease

Epidemiology and pathogenesis

Equine motor neuron disease (EMND) is a diffuse neurodegenerative disorder affecting the somatic, lower motor neurons of horses.[91] The disease occurs sporadically with one or two horses affected on a premise though a report of a large numbers of horses affected in one stable exist.[92] The Quarter Horse breed is over represented and the risk of EMND increases with age with a peak at 16 years followed by a decline.[93] Equine motor neuron disease was first recognized in the Northeastern United States and most cases have been clustered in this region.[94] EMND has been reported across the United States, Canada, Europe, the British Isles, Japan and Brazil.[92,95–98] The exact etiology of EMND is unknown, though a deficiency in dietary vitamin E is thought to play a role. Epidemiologic studies have identified breed, region of residence, housing on dirt paddocks or stabling without access to green pasture, time living on a premises, feeding of pelleted diets and aged, grass hay, and a lack of supplementation for vitamin E and selenium as risk factors.[99,100] Diet and housing alone are not sufficient to cause EMND as many unaffected stable mates are housed and fed similarly to affected individuals. One report of EMND occurring in horses kept on pasture has been published.[101] In a case-control study, controlled for age and breed, plasma vitamin E levels were negatively associated with development of EMND.[93] This association was strengthened by a later case-control report that controlled for season of diagnosis, age, breed and dietary practices. The authors concluded that while plasma vitamin E levels were confounded by age, breed, type of turnout, and type of concentrate fed, plasma vitamin E levels were still negatively associated with EMND when these factors were controlled.[102] Vitamin E is the predominant lipid-soluble antioxidant in mammalian cells. Deficiency of this antioxidant would result in a decreased ability to reduce reactive oxygen species and would make an individual more susceptible to oxidative damage. It is likely that low plasma vitamin E predisposes individuals to EMND but is not the sole cause of this syndrome.

The incidence of EMND appears to have declined in the last two decades. This is likely due to multiple factors including an increase in the nutritional requirement councils recommendation for vitamin E in the equine diet, increased amounts of vitamin E in commercial equine diets, an increased client and veterinary education regarding the risks of vitamin E deficiency and the supplementation of high risk individuals.

Clinical signs are due to degeneration of somatic motor neurons. Histopathologic findings are localized to nuclei of the brain stem and ventral horn of the spinal cord and include chromatolysis, swelling, neurofilamentous accumulations, axonal spheroids and eosinophilic inclusions.[103,104] Secondary lesions resulting from the loss of motor neurons include peripheral nerve degeneration and severe neurogenic muscle atrophy. Muscles units containing a greater percentage of Type 1 fibers are usually more severely affected.[105] These muscle fibers have a higher oxidative activity supporting the conclusion that oxidative stress plays a role in the disease.

A pigment retinopathy has also been reported in the majority of cases examined.[106] Lesions included a reticulated pigment pattern in the tapetal-nontapetal junction extending throughout the fundus in severe cases. Ceroid lipofuscin was deposited in the retinal pigment epithelia. Visual deficits were not reported in affected animals. Retinal photoreceptor membranes contain a large percentage of polyunsaturated fats making them highly sensitive to oxidative damage; pigment accumulation is typical of that seen with lipid peroxidation. These changes are similar to those produced when rats are fed diets lacking antioxidants such as vitamin E.[107] Lipopigment is also seen in the capillary endothelium of the spinal cord in affected horses.[99]

Recognition

Clinical signs

Clinical signs of acute EMND are muscle fasciculatins, almost constant shifting of weight and increased time in recumbency. Affected animals exhibit weight loss and severe muscle atrophy particularly of the appendicular, antigravity muscles including the triceps, gluteals and quadriceps (Fig. 24.5). Affected horses have difficulty standing still for any length of time will frequently shift their weight, tremble and buckle at the knees as they are unable to lock

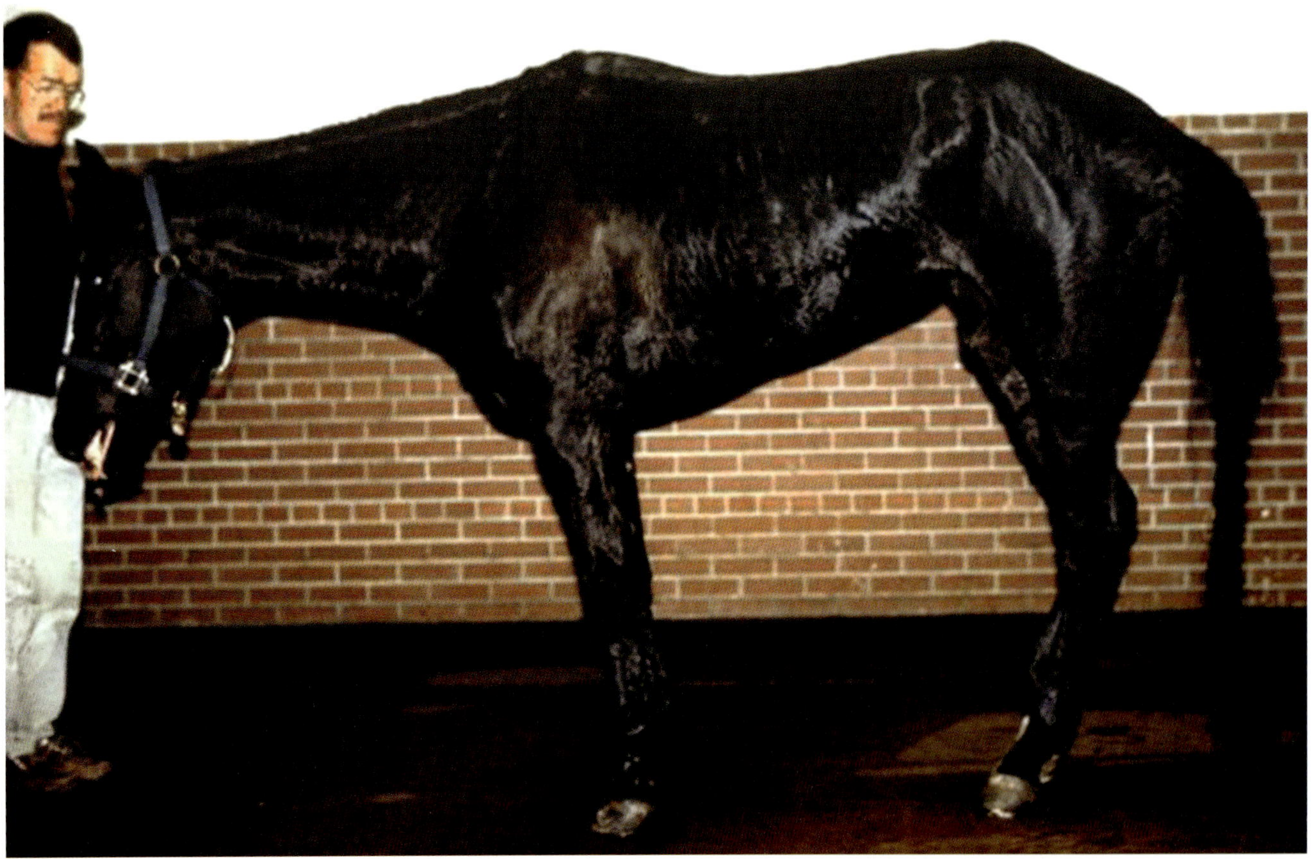

Fig 24.5 Horse with EMND.

and maintain their stay apparatus. When standing, they may adopt a base narrow stance (as if standing on a circus ball) with their head lowered. Elevation of the tail head as a result of atrophy and subsequent contracture of the sacrocaudalis dorsalis medialis muscles may be seen. Appetite is typically normal to excellent. Excessive tartar accumulation (typically black in color) on the canines has been reported. Retinal pigment deposits are noted on ophthalmic exam (Fig. 24.6).

Acutely affected horses often have mild to moderate elevations in creatine kinase (CK) and aspartate aminotransferase (AST). These values often normalize in chronically affected individuals.

Chronic cases may improve or stabilize with or without vitamin E supplementation. In some cases an increase in muscle mass and decrease in fasciculations may occur. These horses may appear normal but often have continued poor performance despite apparent improvement. Other cases may never regain muscle mass with or without improvement in other clinical signs. Individuals may also deteriorate to the point of recumbency requiring humane euthanasia.

Diagnosis

A presumptive diagnosis of EMND can often be made in the acute case based on the characteristic clinical signs. A history of housing on dry lot or stable with little to no pasture and poor quality forage is typical. Mild to moderate elevations in muscle enzymes including serum CK and AST may be seen in acute cases. Needle electromyography (EMG) can be performed in affected horses. Prolonged insertional activity and spontaneous fibrillation potentials and positive sharp waves may be seen. These changes are supportive, but not diagnostic for EMND as they may be seen in other conditions resulting in nerve degeneration or muscle injury.

There are currently two recommended methods for antemortem diagnosis of EMND. Biopsy of the sacrocaudalis dorsalis medialis muscle of the tail head is a relatively simple technique to perform.[105]

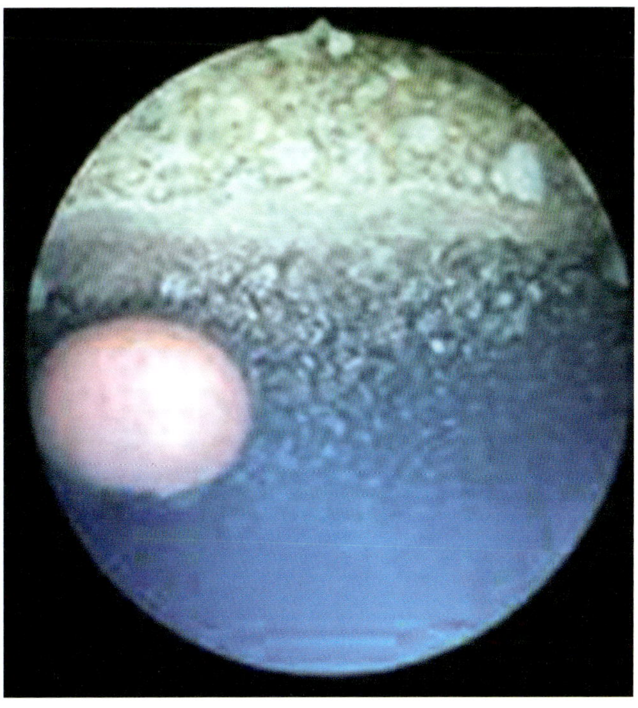

Fig 24.6 Advanced pigment deposition in a horse affected with EMND. Pigment appears as a diffuse yellow-brown accumulation throughout the tapetal zone.

The muscle is located above the tailhead on either side of the dorsal spinous processes of the sacrocoxygeal vertebra (Fig. 24.7). After a surgical prep 2% lidocaine is injected subcutaneously. It is important to avoid injecting lidocaine directly into the muscle belly. A 3–4 cm incision is made cranial to caudal (parallel to the muscle fibers) through the skin and subcutaneous tissue. Two parallel incisions are made into the muscle approximately 1 cm apart. The cranial aspect of the muscle is grasped and the muscle is dissected out. An approximately 1 cm by 2 cm section is ideal. The muscle should be placed in formalin on a wooden tongue depressor to maintain the normal fiber orientation. It is best to contact the laboratory that will be interpreting the muscle biopsy as they may request both formalin and fresh (shipped over night on ice packs) muscle samples to offer the most information in diagnosis. The Neuromuscular Diagnostic Laboratory at the University of Minnesota Equine Center has a very useful web site with directions and photos for obtaining and submitting a muscle biopsy (http://www.cvm.umn.edu/umec/lab/home.html).

An alternative test is to biopsy the spinal accessory nerve as it courses across the neck just deep to the sternocephalicus muscle.[108] Briefly, a 15 cm curvilinear skin incision is made originating at the caudal limit of the linguofacial vein extending along the ventral border of the sternocephalicus muscle. The muscle is isolated using blunt dissection and retracted to expose its dorsomedial surface. The ventral branch of the spinal accessory nerve enters the dorsomedial aspect of the sternocephalicus near the musculotendinous junction. A 5 cm biopsy of the ventral branch is collected and placed on a tongue depressor to retain orientation and placed in Karnovsky fixative. It is recommended that a pathologist familiar with equine neurologic tissue evaluate the biopsy.

The gold standard for diagnosis remains the post mortem examination of the neuromuscular system. Palor of the muscles of the appendicular skeleton may be noted on gross examination. Denervation atrophy particularly of type 1 muscle fibers and oxidative degeneration of the somatic motor neurons with pigment accumulation in the axons, pigmented retinal epithelium and endothelial cells of the spinal cord capillaries is seen. In chronic cases, changes may be subtle and it is recommended that a pathologist with experience in microscopic examination of the equine neuromuscular system perform the examination.

Treatment, prevention and prognosis

The cornerstone of treatment of affected cases is vitamin E supplementation. This can be done by feeding a good quality forage or access to pasture (high in vitamin E) or by supplementation. While the National Research Council recommended daily requirement of vitamin E is approximately 500–1000 U per adult horse per day, the

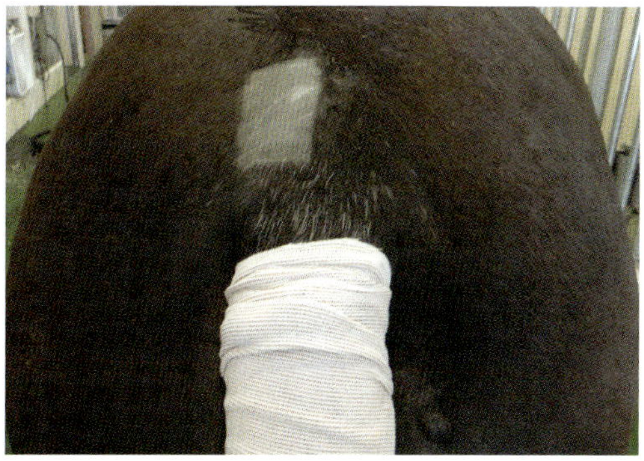

Fig 24.7 Site for biopsy of the sacrocaudalis dorsalis medialis muscle of the tail head.

recommended supplementation in EMND cases is 5000–7000 U vitamin E per day.[99] Supplementation with vitamin E alone is ideal to avoid excessive amounts of other dietary minerals found in combination supplements.

Prognosis

The prognosis for affected horses is poor for return to performance and guarded for life. Acutely affected horses may progress to recumbency necessitating humane euthanasia. In some cases affected horses may stabilize and have improvement in their muscle mass and function with vitamin E supplementation. These horses may appear normal but often have poor performance and may relapse. A third group will stabilize but will fail to regain muscle mass or weight. Chronic cases may develop gait abnormalities due to muscle atrophy and fibrosis. Currently it there is no method other than time, to predict outcome of an individual case.

Shivers

Epidemiology and pathophysiology

Shivers is most commonly seen in draft and Warmblood breeds though reports of shivers in light breeds exist.[109–114] The onset of shivers is variable and reported as early as a year.[109] Shivers is a locomotor-induced movement disorder that is triggered by walking backwards or being asked to raise the hind leg. The exact cause of shivers is unknown. A relationship between shivers and polysaccharide storage myopathy in draft breeds has been postulated however in a prospective study examining Belgium draft horses no association between the two syndromes was found.[115,110] A myopathic cause has been postulated however severity of histopathologic evidence of myopathy does not seem to correlate with severity of shivers. In addition, it is hard to explain why a myopathy would only be apparent when walking backwards with most affected horses having normal forward gaits. Given the breed predispositions, a familial cause is suspected however, infectious, genetic and traumatic hypothesies have all been put forward.[113]

Movement is initiated by the higher centers of the brain including the cerebrum and brain stem. Once initiated cyclic movement, such as walking, is maintained by centers within the spinal cord. Cyclical excitation and inhibition of flexors and extensors of one limb as well as coordination with the other three limbs is controlled by central pattern generators (CPG) located within the cervical and lumbar intumescence. Left to right coordination is maintained by interneurons located in the ventral commissure of the spinal cord. Neurons within these regions maintain the rhythm of a particular gait by excitation and inhibition of various groups of motor neurons. Central pattern generators and commissure interneurons are modulated both by the higher centers as well as sensory input from sensory nerves and muscle spindles within the skeletal muscle. The result is a very highly coordinated interaction between inhibitory and excitatory neurons to maintain the pattern seen in a walk verses a canter or trot. A proposed theory for locomotor-induced movement disorders is a defect in these central pattern generators or interneurons such that this coordination of movement is lost. Such an injury could result in a movement disorder that is apparent at only one gait.[116]

Recognition

Clinical signs

Clinical signs of shivers are characterized by a rapid hyperflexion of the hindlimb with abduction and muscle trembling. The affected animal may hold the limb in flexion for a few seconds to a minute or more before rapidly placing it back on the ground. Shivers is most commonly triggered by walking backwards. Individuals will often exhibit this same rapid flexion and trembling when asked to pick up a hindlimb. Affected animals may be unable to maintain flexion of the limb for any length of time making hoof trimming or shoeing difficult if not impossible. In some cases horses may be reluctant or unable to walk backwards or flex the limb. Clinical signs may be apparent when turned sharply, and occasionally occur in the first few strides of walking forward. Stressful situations such as trailoring may worsen signs. Spastic extension of the tail may be seen in affected individuals especially when asked to back or when the limb is hyperflexed and 'shivering'.[113] Rare reports of forelimb and cranial nerve involvement exist; whether this is the same or a similar syndrome is unknown at this time. Hindlimb weakness is reported in a percentage of affected horses.[110,113] Chronically affected animals may be reluctant to lay down and apparent disuse atrophy of the muscles of the hindquarters may be seen.

Diagnosis

Currently there is no diagnostic test for shivers in horses. The diagnosis is most commonly made based on signalment and clinical signs.

Treatment and prognosis

There is no treatment for shivers syndrome in horses. Clinical signs may improve with rest but will recur with exercise. The prognosis is guarded to poor for performance as affected animals may continue to deteriorate, develop muscle atrophy and weakness limiting their athletic career. Other individuals appear to stabilize and may continue to be useful for several years. Currently there is no method for predicting those horses that will deteriorate and those that will not.

Stringhalt

Epidemiology and pathophysiology

Stringhalt is generally classified into two sub-groups. Plant associated stringhalt is most commonly seen in Australia, but has been reported in North America, Europe, Chile and Japan and likely occurs sporadically in many other countries.[117–121] Outbreaks with multiple horses affected are common in association with ingestion of several related weeds including dandelion (*Taraxacum officinal*), flatweed (*Hypochoeris radicata*) and cheese weed (*Malva parviflora*). The toxic principal is unknown but appears to result in peripheral nerve degeneration. Clinical signs may develop within days of ingestion of the plant. Outbreaks appear to be more common during dry conditions typically during late summer when pastures are less bountiful and horses are forced to eat weeds and other less palatable plants. Reports of horses developing signs after ingestion of the plant in hay exist.[120] Plant associated stringhalt usually affects both hindlimbs though horses may initially develop unilateral signs. Onset may be progressive or sudden.

Sporadic or idiopathic stringhalt typically affects one limb though both limbs can be affected. Idiopathic stringhalt has been reported worldwide. The etiology is unknown, though recent traumatic injury to the distal limb (dorsal tarsus and metatarsus) has been reported in some cases. Whether the underlying cause is adhesion of the extensor tendon or injury to the sensory nerve endings in the muscle or tendon is unknown. The sudden, rapid hyperflexion would suggest dysfunction of the Golgi tendon organ, the stretch receptor in the tendon.

Recognition

Clinical signs

Stringhalt is a locomotor-induced movement disorder or reflex hypertonia characterized by a rapid flexion of the hindlimb during movement. Hyperflexion is towards and under the belly in contrast to shivers where the limb is abducted during flexion. In severe cases the limb will actually hit the underside of the abdomen during the hyperflexion. Symptoms may be seen intermittently or in all gaits. In severe cases the animal may exhibit a hopping gait. Symptoms are exacerbated by excitement or anxiety. In plant associated stringhalt, laryngeal dysfunction with evidence of laryngeal hemiplegia and abnormal vocalization as well as other signs of a more diffuse peripheral neuropathy may be seen.[120,122]

In a descriptive study of a large outbreak of Stringhalt due to plant ingestion, clinical signs in severely affected horses included weight loss and diffuse muscle atrophy despite an increased dietary intake.[120] Multiple horses became recumbent and exhibited hyperextension and increased tonicity of the hind limbs. Behavioral changes were also noted with nine affected individuals showing depression or stupor and one showing aggression.

Pathology

Post-mortem lesions findings in plant associated stringhalt are of the peripheral nerves and muscles.[122] Large, long, myelinated nerves tend to be affected including the deep peroneal, distal tibial, plantar digital, volar and recurrent laryngeal nerves. Histopathologic lesions include demyelination, loss of large myelinated fibers, and Schwann cell proliferation. Wallerian degeneration with swollen vacuolated nerve fibers is present. Muscles innervated by affected nerves showed classic histopathologic changes of denervation atrophy with small angular shrunken myofibers and interspersed hypertrophied pale myofibers. Occasional regenerating myotubes with central nuclei are observed. A multifocal interstitial mono-nuclear-cell infiltrate of the muscle with fibrosis and adipose tissue deposition can be seen in severe cases. Interestingly, atrophy appears to be most severe in the lower limb musculature compared to the upper limb supporting a distal axonopathy. It is unclear why a distal axonopathy results in spastic hyperreflexia. The distal nature of the lesion may result in damage to peripheral sensory receptors such as muscle spindle cells or Golgi tendon organs resulting in an abnormal sensory input and rapid contraction of the muscle.

To the author's knowledge there are no reports on the post-mortem findings in idiopathic stringhalt. Injury and adhesion of the tendon and damage to the myotactic reflex have been postulated as mechanisms for this syndrome.

Diagnosis

Diagnosis is most commonly made based on clinical signs and, in plant associated stringhalt, finding evidence of the associated plants in pasture or hay. Antemortem diagnosis has been reported using histopathologic examination of a peroneal nerve and lateral digital extensor biopsy.[123] This case was initially classified as a spontaneous, idiopathic form, however, it spontaneously resolved after biopsy with no other treatment, an uncommon outcome with idiopathic stringhalt.

Electromyography of affected muscles shows evidence of denervation with increased insertional activity, fibrillation potentials and positive sharp waves.[124,125] These findings are non-specific for denervation and not definitive for stringhalt as other peripheral neuropathies will have similar findings. Interpretation of an EMG requires an experienced clinician. In uncooperative patients, anesthesia may be required to remove the affects of spontaneous movement.

Treatment and prognosis

Medical treatment

In plant associated stringhalt, the most important component of treatment is to prevent ingestion of the plant. Most affected horses will improve over time with reports ranging from days to years for improvement. Even severely affected horses may return to normal though reports of relapses exist.

Treatment with phenytoin a centrally acting anticonvulsant has been recommended to reduce aberrant peripheral nerve activity and excessive muscle contraction.[126] Phenytoin hyperpolarizes the nerve membrane, increases threshold potential and decreases the action potential peak by blockage of Na+ channels and stimulation of the Na+/K+ pump. Its tranquilization effects may also be beneficial as clinical signs are typically worse with excitation. Other tranquilizers (acepromazine) have been recommended to decrease clinical signs in severe cases.

Phenytoin has been reported to be effective in improving clinical signs in affected horses.[120,126] It is recommended to monitor blood levels during treatment as wide variability in absorption exists. Peak plasma concentrations of 5–10 micrograms/ml 1–8 hours after dosing are recommended. A dosing rate of 10–15 mg/kg orally twice daily is usually adequate to reach therapeutic levels. If drug monitoring is not available slowly increasing the dose at 1–2 mg/kg every three days while monitoring for clinical improvement and signs of toxicity is recommended. Because phenytoin is an inducer of the cytochrome P450 system it may increase clearance of drugs metabolized through this route.

Because thiamine deficiency can cause distal axonopathy in humans, it has been suggested for treatment of affected horses. No evidence of a benefit exists.

A recent report on the use of Botox injections to decrease the hypermetric response in stringhalt-affected horses showed a decrease in the number of stringhalt like steps and a decrease in the flexion angle of the hock after repeated injections of Botox into the long and lateral digital extensor.[127]

Surgical treatment

A lateral digital extensor myotenectomy has been reported to have varying success in the treatment of stringhalt. In a case series of 10 horses with idiopathic stringhalt associated with recent injury to the dorsoproximal metatarsus, three of five horses treated surgically had evidence of improvement.[128] Of 13 horses with plant-associated stringhalt treated surgically, 11 horses walked normally after surgery. The two additional case improved but relapsed at a later date and then subsequently improved.[129] Duration of clinical signs prior to surgery ranged from four days to three months. Given that plant-associated stringhalt has been reported to resolve as late as two years after ingestion it is difficult to know if surgical repair is indicated in this type of stringhalt.

Prognosis

The prognosis for idiopathic stringhalt is guarded to poor for performance but excellent for life. Affected animals may not resolve the gait deficit even with medical or surgical therapy. The recent report of the use of Botox may offer a new treatment option for these cases. The prognosis for plant-associated stringhalt is guarded. The majority of horses appear to improve when restricted from ingesting the plant. Resolution of clinical signs may take years.

Severely affected animals may become recumbent and develop severe weight loss making the prognosis for these animals poor.

Laryngeal dysfunction has been reported in association with plant associated stringhalt supporting the assumption of a diffuse peripheral neuropathy. Cerebral signs incuding depression and stupor are reported in some outbreaks.[120] Spontaneous recovery can days to months. In a large outbreak one of the first reported signs associated with recovery was an ability to stretch the hindlimb.[120]

Sweeny

Sweeny is a forelimb gait abnormality that results from instability of the shoulder joint due to injury to the suprascapular nerve. The nerve arises from the 6th and 7th cervical spinal cord segments, it passes between the suprascapularis and subscapularis muscles before coursing around the front of the scapula. Injury is most often reported after a horse collides with another horse, fence or other inanimate object. Injury is thought to result from compression or stretching of the nerve fibers. The subsequent denervation results in atrophy of the supraspinatus and infraspinatus muscles, these muscles are the lateral stabilizers of the joint. As the horse walks, the shoulder bows laterally during the stance phase of the stride. Denervation atrophy is usually apparent by 2–3 weeks post injury however shoulder instability may be seen immediately following injury.

There is some question as to whether injury to the suprascapular nerve alone is sufficient to cause the characteristic atrophy and gait deficits as transection of this nerve in three equids did not result in the typical gait deficits.[130] However, a later study using local anesthesia of the suprascapular nerve resulted in shoulder instability in all subjects.[131] Depending on the severity of the injury, reinervation (from surviving nerve fibers) and muscle re-development may occur months after injury. Maximal recovery is reported to take up to a year.

Recognition

Diagnosis

Diagnosis of Sweeny is made based on gait deficits, presence of atrophy of the surpaspinatus and infraspinatus and a history of trauma to the scapular region.

Treatment and prognosis

Medical treatment

A percentage of horses with injury to the suprascapular nerve will improve with rest over time. In a retrospective study, seven of eight horses had clinical improvement of muscle atrophy, gait and shoulder instability resolving within 3–12 months after injury.[132] The eighth horse was lost to follow up.

Surgical treatment

Scapular notch resection and soft tissue excision is recommended to improve outcome and speed resolution of shoulder instability.[133] Assisted recovery from general anesthesia is recommended because of the shoulder instability and increased risk of fracture of the supraglenoid tubercle. A risk of fracture through the scapular notch exists for six weeks post surgery. Anti-inflammatories are recommended at a tapering dose for one week. Horses should be stall-rested until shoulder instability resolves. Physical therapy and muscle stimulation is recommended to minimize muscle atrophy. Prognosis for return to performance is good.

Headshaking

Epidemiology and pathogenesis

Headshaking is a frustrating, poorly understood syndrome. Headshaking can result from a number of etiologies including trigeminal neuralgia (also known as facial pain syndrome), secondary to aural disease, ear ticks and mites, dental disease, ophthalmic disease, temporomandibular joint disease, upper airway abnormalities, allergic rhinitis, skull fracture or trauma, guttural pouch disease, sinusitis, ethmoid hematoma, ill-fitting tack and behavioral problems.[134–137] Given the list of potential causes it can be a daunting task to evaluate a horse presenting for headshaking. For the purpose of this review, the author will focus on trigeminal neuralgia (also known as facial pain syndrome and, as a subset, photic headshaking). This syndrome is recognized in all breeds and sexes, onset is typically middle age geldings with Warmbloods and Thoroughbreds breeds being over represented.[138] Affected horses shake their head in a characteristic pattern without any obvious external stimuli. Onset is usually sudden and often seasonal beginning in the spring and resolving during the fall or winter months as daylight shortens. Headshaking is often triggered by exercise often leading trainers to feel the horse has a training issue or behavioral problem.

The exact pathogenesis of headshaking syndrome is unknown. A disorder of the trigeminal nerve where sensory stimuli result in an abnormal sensation of discomfort is suspected. In some cases, visual stimuli of the optic nerve (photic headshaking) is thought to result in trigeminal activation due to convergence of the optic and trigeminal nerves. Exercise, sunlight, wind, cold, rain and seasonal changes have all been reported to trigger headshaking. Trigeminal neuralgia in people manifests as sudden facial pain, the exact pathogenesis is unknown trigeminal neuritis, mucosal irritability, allergy and neural hypersensitivity are all suspected.[139] The finding that equine headshaking syndrome appears to be triggered by multiple stimuli supports the idea of enhanced irritability of the trigeminal nerve or optic-trigeminal summation.

Recognition

Clinical signs

Clinical signs of headshaking include sudden, rapid flipping of the nose, avoidance of sunlight, snorting, sneezing, and rubbing of the nose. In some cases, the shaking may be so violent as to make it impossible to safely lead or ride the affected individual. The movement is typically in a dorsal-ventral direction; affected animals flip their nose as if a bee has suddenly gotten up their nostril. Individual cases may rub their nose on the ground, their limbs, or the walls of their stalls, in some cases resulting in self mutilation. Violent repetitive snorting may be seen. Sunlight triggered or photic headshakers may have increased blinking when moved into the sun and seek shade or place their heads in bushes or troughs to avoid sunlight. Exercise triggered cases will show worsening of signs when performing.

Diagnosis

The syndrome of headshaking is generally diagnosed after ruling out all other problems that cause a horse to shake its head. Because of the many etiologies that can result in headshaking examination should include ophthalmologic, otic, endoscopic exam of the upper respiratory tract and guttural pouches, and diagnostic imaging of the skull. Findings are all typically unremarkable in horses with idiopathic headshaking syndrome. After attempting to rule out other etiologies, it is recommended to perform a series of diagnostic steps to best determine effective treatment for idiopathic headshaking. Evaluation of the horse in bright light verses indoors to determine the effects of sunlight (photic head shaking) is recommended. In some cases application of tinted goggles or contacts may improve clinical signs.[136] Application of a nose net or diffuse pressure applied to the skin of the face may improve symptoms in some affected horses.[137,140] Local anesthesia of the rostral portion of the infraorbital nerve at the infraorbital nerve foramen has been shown to temporarily decrease or abolish head shaking in a percentage of cases supporting the theory of trigeminal neuralgia or facial pain syndrome.[141] This technique is relatively simple to perform. The infraorbital foramen can be located by palpation. Approximately 12 mls of mepivicaine is infused at the foramen. Efficacy can be assessed by response to forceps applied to the nares. If analgesia does not decrease headshaking behavior it is recommended to perform local analgesia of the more proximal ethmoidal branch of the trigeminal as it exits the maxillary foramen.[137] This technique is well described.[142] Briefly, a 3 × 4 cm area is clipped and surgically prepared ventral to the zygomatic arch. Mepivacaine (0.5 mls) is injected subcutaneously below the transverse facial artery or between the zygomatic arch and the transverse facial depending on the anatomic variation of the subject. A 7 cm 18 gauge needle is inserted in a rostral direction towards the 6th upper cheek tooth. The stylet is removed and 5 mls of mepivacaine is injected. The effects should be evalulated at 30 minutes, one hour and 90 minutes.

Treatment and prognosis

Medical therapy

The response of horses affected with idiopathic headshaker syndrome to medical therapy is variable. Cyproheptadine (0.3 – 0.6 mg/kg, po BID) is an antihistamine, serotonin antagonist with anticholinergic effects. The mechanism of action for treatment of headshaking in horses is unknown. Cyproheptadine has been reported to be effective for control or improvement of head shaking in approximately two thirds of affected animals.[137,143] Lethargy, depression and anorexia are the most common side effects. It is recommended to treat with cyprohepatadine for at least one week to determine effectiveness.

Carbamazepine is recommended for the treatment of trigeminal neuritis in humans. It has been used for treatment of headshakers alone or combined with cyproheptadine particularly in cases that fail to respond to cyprohepatadine alone.[137] Carbemazepine in combination with cyproheptadine was effective in decreasing signs of headshaking in 8 of 9 treated horses. Melatonin, 12 mg orally in the evening, has been successfully used to treat headshaking in individual cases, no large studies on its effectiveness exist.[136]

Sodium cromoglycated eye drops have been reported to be effective in treating headshakers.[144] Sodium cromoglycate stabilizes mast cell membranes, and inhibits release of histamine. It is used to treat allergic conjunctivitis in humans. In a small case series, two of three cases had resolution of their headshaking with application of sodium cromoglycate to both eyes four times daily. In the third case, clinical symptoms significantly improved. All three horses appeared to have light sensitivity (as evident by increased frequency of blinking when in the bright light) and ocular discharge.

Surgical intervention

Surgical therapy is generally recommended only for cases that fail to respond to medical treatment. Bilateral infraorbital neurectomy was performed in 19 cases a percentage of which had failed to respond to previous medical therapy.[141] Prior to neurectomy the authors recommend that bilateral infraorbital nerve analgesia be performed to determine if neurectomy would be effective. Six horses showed improvement with owners of three horses reporting sustained improvement lasting 3–5 years. Interestingly, one of the three successful cases did not improve after bilateral infraorbital nerve analgesia.

Alternatively, sclerosis of the posterior ethmoidal branch of the trigeminal nerve has been reported to improved clinical signs in all horses with clinical improvement lasting six weeks to nine months.[137] As with neurectomy, posterior ethmoidal nerve analgesia is recommended prior to sclerosis to determine if the procedure will be effective. Sclerosis is performed under general anesthesia. A 20 cm stiletted needles is placed up the infraorbital canal to the level of the maxillary foramen. Positioning is confirmed with fluoroscopy. Once positioned 5 mls of 10% phenol is injected.

Caudal compression of the infraorbital nerve using vascular coils has recently been described.[142,145] Improvement was noted in 35 of 57 horses though recurrence occurred in nine horses. Surgery was repeated in 10 cases with a final success rate of approximately 50%. Approximately two thirds of the cases had post operative complications including self trauma and temporary increase in headshaking.

Successful treatment of headshaking in a horse by coagulation of cystic corpora nigra and behavior modification has been reported.[146] Cystic corpora nigra were obstructing approximately 60% of the pupil. The affected individual exhibited signs when a bridle and blinkers was applied. After surgery the horse continued to respond negatively with headshaking behavior when the blinkers were applied. Behavior modification was successfully used to resolve headshaking completely.

The prognosis for horses with headshaking syndrome is guarded to poor for performance. Unfortunately, while many horses may initially respond to treatment relapse is common.

Temporohyoid osteoarthropathy

Etiology and pathogenesis

Temporohyoid osteoarthropathy (THO) is a disorder characterized by progressive proliferation of the petrous temporal bone and the proximal stylohyoid that eventually results in ankylosis of the temporohyoid (TH) joint. This joint is thought to dampen the movement of the hyoid apparatus as the tongue or larynx move; sudden, forcefull movement of these structures is thought to result in traumatic fracture of the ankylosed joint. There are two major theories regarding the etiology of THO, one theory is that chronic, low-grade otitis media-interna results in local spread of infection to the temporo-hyoid (TH) region. Progressive osteomyelitis results in boney remodeling and eventual ankylosis of the TH joint. The second theory is that THO is a manifestation of progressive degenerative joint disease and osteoarthritis.

There is limited evidence to support both theories. In a study by Blythe et al culture of tympanocentesis aspirates from THO affected horses grew bacteria in 5 of 10 horses.[147,148] Fluid is often present in the middle ear in affected cases.[147–150] Because most affected horses lack a history of ear discomfort or infection it is difficult to know if this fluid is due to otitis media or is a result of fracture and hemorrhage. In a study by Walker et al the majority of horses affected with THO had no evidence of infection at post-mortem examination further supporting the possibility that the fluid is not infectious in origin.[151]

In support of the second theory, THO-affected horses have radiographic and CT evidence of bony remodeling of the TH region.[147–149] In horses with bilateral THO but unilateral neurologic deficits, bony changes are typically more extensive on the affected side. Naylor et al confirmed age related degeneration and bony remodeling of the temporohyoid joint in normal horses.[152] Aged horses had significant anatomic (evaluated by computed tomography) and histopathologic boney and cartilaginous degeneration in the stylohyoid and petrous temporal bones and joint compared to young horses. In some cases ankylosis of the TH joint had occurred without clinical symptoms. The trigger for this degenerative joint disease is unknown though trauma, manipulation of the tongue during biting, dentistry or general chewing may all be factors.

In the early stages, affected horses may be asymptomatic or present with one of two typical complaints. A history of headshaking, behavioral problems particularly when handling the head and overt pain when palpating the ear region is thought to be more common with mild THO.[147] Neurologic signs are thought to result with more severe THO when sudden, rapid movement of the tongue or hyoid apparatus results in fracture, hemorrhage and inflammation in the TH region. Cranial nerve VII and VIII deficits are thought to result from tearing or compression as they pass through the temporal bone and exit the skull.

It is not unusual to find bony changes in unaffected horses or to find bilateral changes in horses with unilateral disease. Currently, there is no formula to predict which horse are at risk for developing a fracture and neurologic signs. In a retrospective study of computed tomography (CT) images of THO-affected horses, the authors concluded that a cumulative width of the TH joint greater than 48 mm was associated with an increased risk of neurologic deficits.[149] Additional data is needed to better predict the risk of clinical disease in affected horses.

Recognition

Clinical signs

The most common clinical signs are an acute onset of unilateral deficits of CN VII and VIII. Occasionally clinical signs will be precipitated while being examined or treated for another problem such as nasogastric intubation or dental examination. About one third of affected horses will present for a corneal ulcer due to unrecognized facial nerve deficits. Because CN VII is motor to the muscle of the eyelid affected horses do not blink adequately resulting in decreased spreading of the tear film and exposure keratitis and corneal ulceration. Diagnosis can be made by identifying poor eyelid tone. It is nearly impossible to fully open the eyelid of a normal horse using one hand but is reasonably easy to perform in horses with CN VII deficits. Decreased lacrimation may also result because the parasympathetic nerve fibers that innervate the lacrimal gland join CN VII as it exits the cranium. An ear droop on the affected side, muzzle deviation towards the normal side and feed may be packed into the cheek and found hanging from the mouth of the affected side. A false menace response may be seen as retraction of the globe (CN 6) will result in partial closure of the eyelids; a careful examination will detect the difference. Complete or partial injury of CN 7 may result in complete or partial paralysis of the ear, eyelid or lip so a careful neurologic exam is necessary to determine deficits. A small percentage of cases will present with bilateral neurologic deficits.

Vestibular signs include a head tilt with the pole titled towards the affected side. Nystagmus with the fast phase towards the normal side may be seen in the acute period but frequently resolves over time. Horses may lean against a wall, drift towards the affected side as they walk or circle compulsively in the direction of the affected side. When blindfolded, affected horses will often dramatically worsen as they rely on vision to overcome vestibular disturbance. A blindfold should only be applied in a safe environment as once blindfolded they can no longer rely on the horizon to stay upright and may fall suddenly to the affected side.

In rare cases deficits of cranial nerves IX and X may occur as these nerves may be compressed or severed if boney proliferation is severe and extensive. Many cases may appear to be painful when chewing or swallowing as well.

In a retrospective study of 33 THO-affected horses a summary of clinical signs included facial nerve deficits (29), vestibulocochlear nerve deficits (23), ataxia (16), corneal ulcer (13), fever (2), convulsive episode (2) and neurologically normal (2).[151]

Diagnosis

The diagnosis of THO is made based on the clinical findings of peripheral facial or vestibular nerve dysfunction coupled with bony remodeling of the temporohyoid region. Because many horses may have degenerative changes of the TH joint without clinical signs, it is difficult to interpret abnormal findings in a normal horse. Currently, guttural pouch endoscopy is the most frequently used diagnostic tool to image the TH region. The proximal stylohyoid bone and TH joint can be imaged as it divides the medial and lateral compartments of the guttural pouches (Fig. 24.8). A baseball bat appearance of the stylohyoid is evidence of bony remodeling and thickening. In some cases there may be evidence of proliferation of the petrous temporal bone though this is less commonly visualized.

Radiographs can also be used to image the TH region. Dorsoventral, lateral and oblique views are recommended. Sedation is necessary as the horses head needs to be low with the pole extended to allow positioning of the film behind the throat latch and the machine above the head. Evidence of bony proliferation of the stylohyoid and temporal bone are evident on the affected side (Fig. 24.9).

Computed tomography has been reported to be very useful in detecting subtle boney changes as well as fractures and fluid in the middle ear. In a recent report, an increase in the width of the TH joint (>48 mm) was associated with an increased risk of neurologic deficits.[149] In the future, computed tomography may be useful to evaluate progression of THO and to determine if prophylactic surgical intervention is indicated.

In suspect cases of otitis media culture of fluid collected from the middle ear via tympanocentesis has been recommended.[147] Because the technique requires general anesthesia and bacterial growth is uncommon it is rarely performed.

Treatment and prognosis

Medical treatment

The goal of medical treatment of THO is to control the inflammation associated with fracture of the ankylosed joint, treat suspect bacterial otitis media and control or prevent secondary complications. A thirty day course of treatment using a broad spectrum antimicrobial is generally recommended if culture results are not available. Nonsteroidals are recommended in the acute stage of the disease and can be tapered and discontinued after 10 to 14 days.[147,148,151] Because medical treatment alone will not resolve the boney remodeling or ankylosis relapse can occur.

Corneal ulceration is a common complication of THO. Treatment of corneal ulcers includes topical antimicrobials, atropine, nonsteroidal antiinflammatories and analgesics. In some cases antifungal medication may be indicated. A conjunctival pedicle graft may be necessary to try to prevent corneal rupture. If eyelid function does not improve enucleation may be necessary as ulceration can be a chronic, recurrent problem. Supplemental tears may help prevent ulceration though frequent treatment is necessary. It is

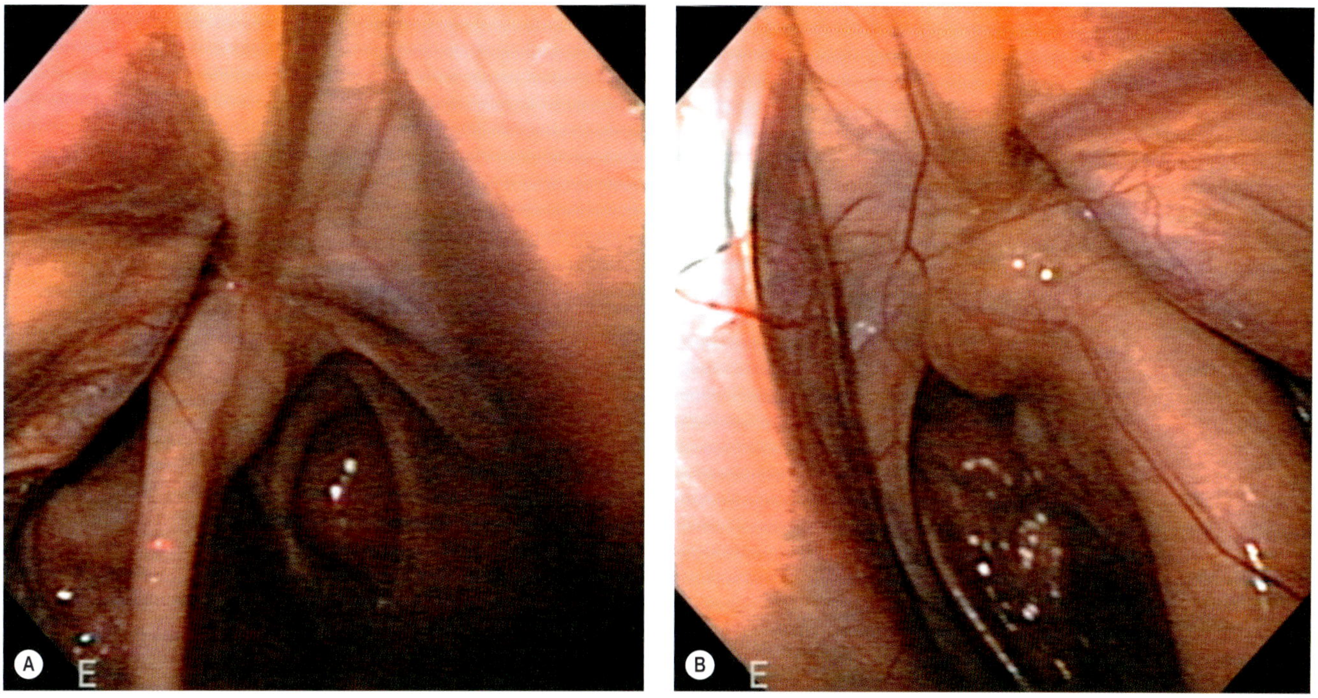

Fig 24.8 Endoscopic imaging of a normal **(A)** and abnormal **(B)** temporohyoid joint and stylohyoid bone in the guttural pouch.

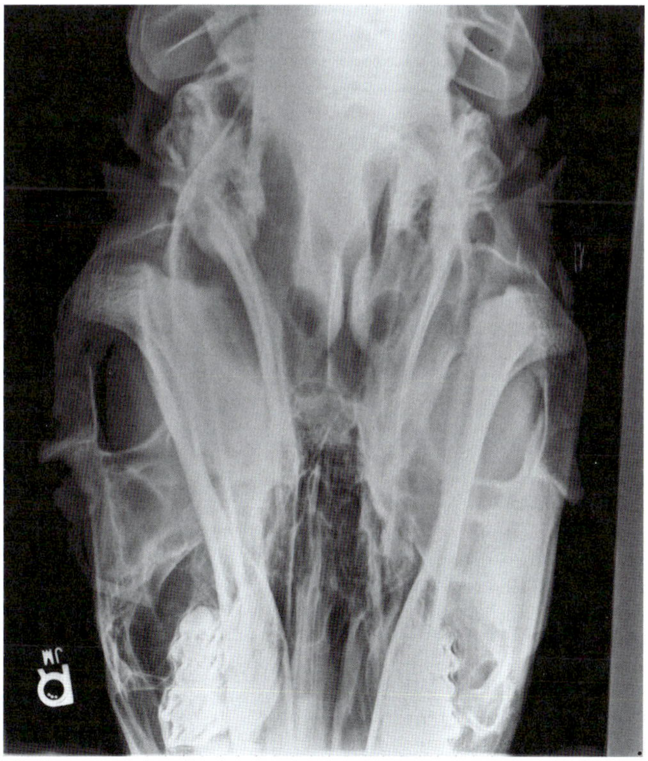

Fig 24.9 Dorsoventral radiograph of a horse with temporohyoid osteopathy of the right temporhyoid joint. Bony remodeling and proliferation are seen in the region of the articulation of the stylohyoid bone and the petrous temporal bone.

important to educate clients of the need for careful daily observation of the eye as early detection of ulceration is important to minimize risk of infection and rupture of the globe.

Surgical treatment

Partial stylohyoidectomy was described to remove the pull of the tongue and larynx on the ankylosed TH joint thereby minimizing the risk of fracture. Post operative complications included laceration of the lingual artery, difficulty masticating hay and dysphagia.[153] A later report described regrowth of the resected portion of the stylohyoid bone as an additional complication in three cases.[150] The authors of this case series described removal of the entire ceratohyoid bone as an alternative procedure. Because complete ceratohyoidectomy results in exposure of two cartilaginous joint surfaces as well as removal of the entire bone and periosteum the risk of boney union is significantly decreased. Risk of vascular laceration from sharp boney edges is also minimized as the bone is disarticulated in its entirety.

Prognosis

The prognosis for life is fair for affected cases. In a retrospective study of 33 THO-affected horses 63% survived long term. Residual neurologic deficits were present in 60% of survivors with facial nerve dysfunction the most commonly reported abnormality. The prognosis for a healthy eye on the affected side is guarded as recurrent ulceration may result in rupture and necessitate enucleation. Because the majority of cases in this retrospective were treated medically theand there is no published data on the success of surgical treatment compared to medical treatment. Clinical impression suggests that surgical treatment has a better long term prognosis. Because surgical removal of part of the hyoid eliminates the pull of the tongue and larynx on the TH joint the risk of recurrence of fracture and clinical symptoms should be minimal.

Vertebral trauma

- The most common sites of vertebral injury in horses vary with the age.
- Diagnosis of vertebral fracture is determined by plain film radiography or nuclear scintigraphy.
- Medical therapy is indicated in ambulatory patients with stable fractures.
- Surgical therapy is indicated in unstable fractures of the cervical or sacral A vertebrae.

Cervical fractures

Traumatic spinal cord injury is a common etiology of spinal ataxia in performance horses, and can be difficult to diagnose. The most common site of traumatic spinal cord injury is dependent on age of the horse.[154] Cervical fractures are more common in foals and result from hyperextension, hyperflexion and luxation. Adult horses are more likely than foals to develop fractures of the caudal thoracic and lumbar spine. Regardless of the site of the fracture, the prognosis is dependent on the severity of the initial injury.

The most common cervical vertebral fracture in foals is axial dens fracture and atlantoaxial subluxation (Fig. 24.10).[155] Atlantoaxial subluxation may result from resisting head restraint (hyperextension) or somersault (hyperflexion) injuries in young horses. Foals with atlantoaxial subluxation will have a stiff, splinted neck and, in some instances, audible crepitation with manipulation of the head. Neurologic gait deficits range from none to marked tetraparesis and ataxia. Foals may have a head tilt, without other signs of vestibular dysfunction, due to mechanical malalignment of the C1–C2 articulation. Radiograph views of the cervical spine reveal widening of the cranial physis of the axis. In foals with neurologic gait deficits, cranioventral luxation of axis usually occurs with increased distance between the spine of the atlas and axis and between the floor of the atlas and the axial dens.

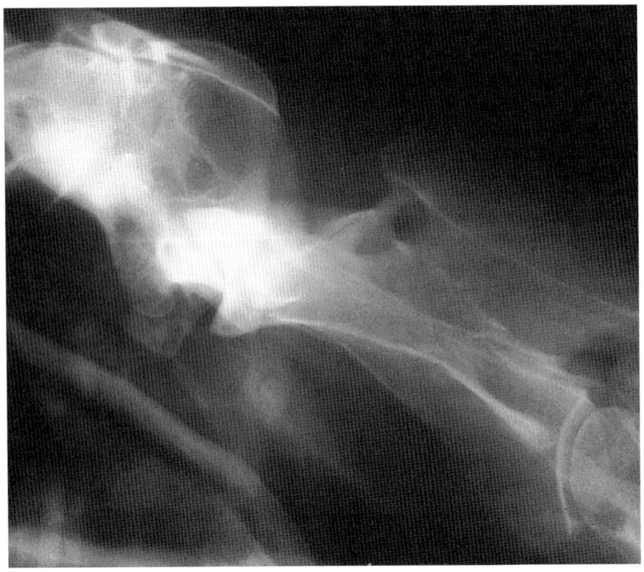

Fig 24.10 Cervical radiograph from a weanling that reared over backward and impacted on the pole. One wing of atlas (C1) is displaced ventrally. The odontoid process (dens) of the axis (C2) is fractured and the entire axis is displaced ventrally. The foal demonstrates grade 2 symmetric ataxia and a mechanical head tilt.

In adult horses, compression fractures of the vertebral body and articular facet fractures are the most common fractures of the cervical vertebrae and occur with head-on collision and falling, rolling injuries in horses (especially jumping and steeple-chasing), respectively (Fig. 24.11).[154] Cervical vertebral fractures are associated with pain, resistance to manipulation and splinting of the neck. Focal sweating, loss of cutaneous sensation and torticollis may be observed if exiting nerve roots are damaged by the fracture. The severity of neurologic gait deficits will range from none to tetraplegia dependent on the degree of vertebral luxation and spinal cord injury.

Thoracic fractures

Thoracic fractures are more common in adult horses than foals and result from falling over a jump or flipping over backwards.[154] The first three thoracic vertebrae are most likely to fracture, followed by T12. Fracture of the thoracolumbar junction is observed in horses that fall and roll down an embankment. Clinical signs in horses with T12 or thoracolumbar fractures include paraparesis and tracking or drifting of the hindlinbs to one side. Dorsal spinous process fractures of T4 to T8 occur in horses that flip over backwards. These fractures are not usually associated with fracture of the vertebral bodies, although neurologic gait deficits may result from contusion of the spinal cord. Sacral fractures occur with dog-sitting incidents and may result in loss of tail function, urinary incontinence, loss of anal tone and fecal retention.

Diagnosis of vertebral fractures can be difficult. Despite the presence of a fracture, overlapping structures and surrounding muscle mass render radiographic projections of the vertebrae difficult to interpret.[156] Vertebral fracture should be investigated in horses that have a history of a traumatic event, pain on palpation, clinical signs of tetra- or paraparesis and/or hyperesthesia or loss of cutaneous sensation. Plain film radiography may identify cervical, sacral and thoracic fractures. Fractures of the lumbar vertebrae are not amenable to radiographic examination due to the soft tissue mass surrounding the vertebral bodies in this region.[154] Nuclear scintigraphy may enable the clinician to identify non-displaced cervical fractures and fractures of the lumbar spine which are inaccessible to radiographic examination. Cerebrospinal fluid is often hemorraghic in horses with CNS trauma. The supernatant will appear

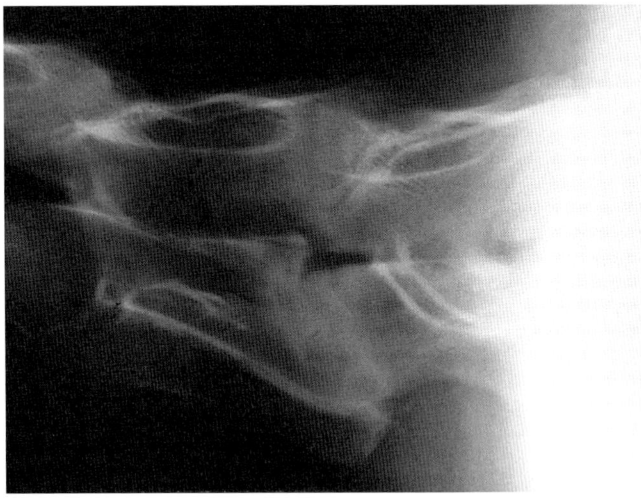

Fig 24.11 Cervical radiograph of C4 through C7 from an adult horse after a head-on collision with a tree. A vertebral body compression fracture is present at C6. The horse was recumbent.

xanthochromic after centrifugation if the hemorrhage is pathologic in origin (as opposed to iatrogenic) (Fig. 24.12).

Treatment and prognosis

Medical therapy

Conservative management, consisting of stall rest and anti-inflammatory therapy, may be rewarding in horses that are ambulatory after vertebral fracture.[156] The therapeutic approach for foals with atlantoaxial subluxation is dependent upon the severity of neurologic deficits and the degree of malalignment and instability of the vertebrae. Stall rest and conservative anti-inflammatory therapy may be successful in foals with relatively stable, non-displaced fractures.

Early medical therapy (less than eight hours after injury) to prevent edema formation consistently produces a more favorable outcome than does late intervention.[156] Glucocorticoids (dexamethasone 0.1–0.2 mg/kg, i.v., q 8–12 h) minimize cerebral edema and secondary injury by prevention of membrane lipoperoxidation and inhibition of arachidonic acid metabolites. Dimethyl sulfoxide (1 g/kg, i.v., s.i.d. to b.i.d.) may prevent or reduce cerebral edema. Rapid administration of the 10% DMSO solution may result in intravascular hemolysis and hemoglobinuria. Mannitol (0.25–1 g/kg, i.v. over 20 minutes as a 20% solution, b.i.d. to t.i.d.) reduces existing CNS edema via hyperosmolar dehydration and may reduce CSF pressure within 30 minutes of administration. Non-steroidal anti-inflammatory drugs have limited ability to reduce CNS edema and inflammation but analgesic properties may relieve malaise and reduce depression. Liberal administration of anti-inflammatory drugs may permit excessive movement by the horse and loss of muscular splinting of the fracture, which may promote displacement of fracture fragments.

Surgical intervention

Surgical intervention is recommended for foals with unstable cervical fractures and severe neurologic gait deficits.[155] Surgical approaches for correction of atlantoaxial subluxation in foals includes compression plating, Steinmann pin fixation, dorsal laminectomy of the caudal atlas and ventral cervical fusion.[154] Partial ostectomy of the dens to correct atlantoaxial subluxation in an adult pony has been reported.[157] Surgical stabilization of vertebral fractures is rarely attempted in adult horses. Successful lag screw fixation of vertebral body fracture and dorsal decompression of a transverse, ventrally displaced sacral fracture have been reported.[158] Surgical intervention has not been reported in horses with thoracic or lumbar vertebral fractures. Dorsal spinous process fractures may require surgical removal if sequestration of bone fragments occurs.

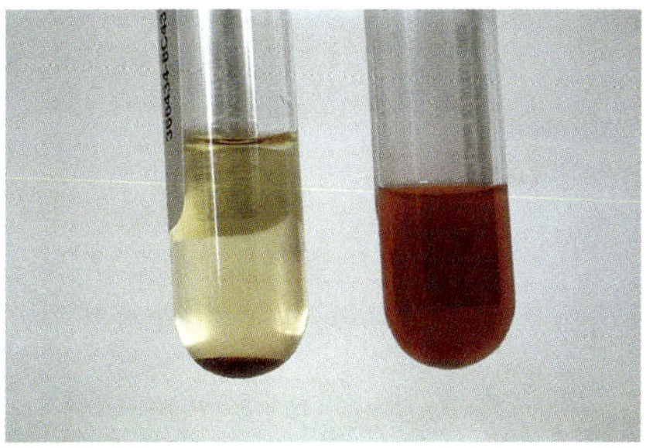

Fig 24.12 Cerebrospinal fluid from a horse with head trauma. CSF appears hemorrhagic prior to centrifugation (right) and xanthochromic (supernatant) with a red cell pellet after centrifugation (left).

Exuberant callus formation may impinge on the spinal cord and produce neurologic gait deficits months after the injury. Therefore, the ultimate usefulness of a horse with traumatic spinal cord damage may not be determined for a prolonged period of time after injury. Nonetheless, response to therapy within the first few days is a good prognostic indicator.

Cervical facet joint injection in the horse

Omar Maher

Degenerative changes and osteochondrosis of the cervical facet (intervertebral synovial) joints are increasingly recognized in horses and are thought to cause a wide array of clinical signs including neck stiffness, non-acceptance of the bit, difficulty with collected gaits, defensive attitudes, poor performance, forelimb lameness, and neurologic proprioceptive deficits.

Medicating these joints in horses has presented a significant challenge. In humans, cervical facet injections are performed using landmark palpation and fluoroscopic guidance. The large muscle mass of the horse's neck prevents accurate palpation of the cervical facet joint, and the size and height of the neck makes using a fluoroscope unpractical, consequently most cervical facet injections are performed using ultrasonographic guidance.

Cervical facet joint injections in horses were first reported in the 1990s and have gained in popularity in the last two decades.[159,160] With advances in diagnostic and ultrasonographic technology, along with the increased awareness of neck pain and cervical pathology in performance horses, cervical facet injections are becoming more and more commonplace in equine veterinary practice.

Anatomy

The most commonly targeted facet joints are those between the third cervical vertebrae and the first thoracic vertebrae. The cervical vertebrae are constituted of a body and an arch. The body presents a head cranially and a fossa caudally. The arch presents transverse processes oriented in a caudo dorsal direction and articular processes. Each cervical vertebra has two cranial and two caudal articular processes (left and right) (Fig. 24.12).

There are three articulation sites between each vertebrae; a symphisis between the vertebral bodies (containing a fibrocartilagenous disk) and two diarthrodial facet joints.

The articular facet joints are formed of the cranial articular processes of the caudal vertebra, and the caudal articular processes of the cranial one (Fig. 24.13). The cranial articular articular processes (of the caudal vertebra) are lateral and ventral to the caudal articular processes (of the cranial vertebra).

Ultrasonographic identification of the transverse processes, the intervertebral foramen and the articular processes forming the facet joints was first described by Berg et al in 2003.[161] The articular processes are the most dorsal contour of the vertebra imaged ultrasonographicallyfrom a lateral approach (Fig. 24.14).

Technique

A careful ultrasonographic evaluation of the cervical spine, using a 5 MHz macroconvex probe perpendicular to the vertebral axis is recommended. Depending on the hair coat, body fat and ultrasound characteristics removal of the hair and application of coupling gel may be necessary to obtain high quality images.

It is important to identify the second vertebra body and the facet joint between the second and third vertebrae and then progress caudally identifying subsequent articulations to the level of the first thoracic vertebrae. Correction fluid (Wite-Out®, Bic USA) or wax crayons can be used to mark the facet joints. These marks should be placed at 90 degree angles from each other such that extension of these lines intersect at the ideal site to image and inject each articulation (typically its cranial aspect). The marks should be placed at a distance from the probe site and intended needle penetration site to delineate the region to be aseptically prepared (Fig. 24.15).

A macroconvex transducer (5 MHz) provides with the most advantages for performing facet injections as it's small footprint allows for easy needle manipulation and its sector shaped beam makes it easier to locate the advancing needle and surrounding structures. However, a convex low frequency transducer, or linear transducer can be used too. Spinal needles are used (3.5 inches, 18 or 20 gauge).

The ultrasound transducer and needle should be manipulated by the same individual. It is helpful to have a second person available to aid in syringe placement and injection once the needle is positioned.

The patient should be adequately sedated to ensure immobility without significant swaying (typically Detomidine at 0.01 mg/kg).

The area to be injected is aseptically prepared and the ultrasound transducer is placed in a sterile glove filled with coupling gel. Alchohol or sterile lubricant should be applied to the sterile field. After obtaining the desired image the needle is advanced from a point approximately 1 cm above the transducer in line with the beam. To visualize the needle it must be advanced in the same plane as the beam (Fig. 24.16). The needle should not be advanced until visualization within the ultrasound image.

It is important that the needle (in its entirety) remains visible within the beam of the ultrasound transducer from insertion through reaching the articular facet joint.

Once the needle is within the joint (Fig. 24.17), the syringe can be connected and medication (maximum volume 3 mls) injected (Fig. 24.18 and Fig. 24.19). Ultrasound visualization should be maintained to ensure that the injection is indeed intra-articular.

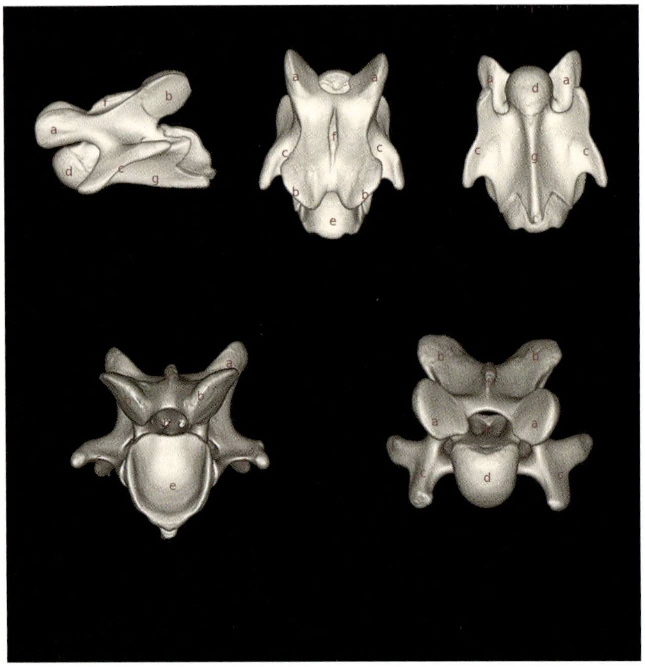

Fig 24.13 a. Cranial articular process b. Caudal articular process c. Transverse process d. Cranial extremity (vertebral head) e. Vertebral fossa f. Spinal process g. Ventral crest h. Spinal canal i. Foramen transversarium j. Intervertebral foramen.

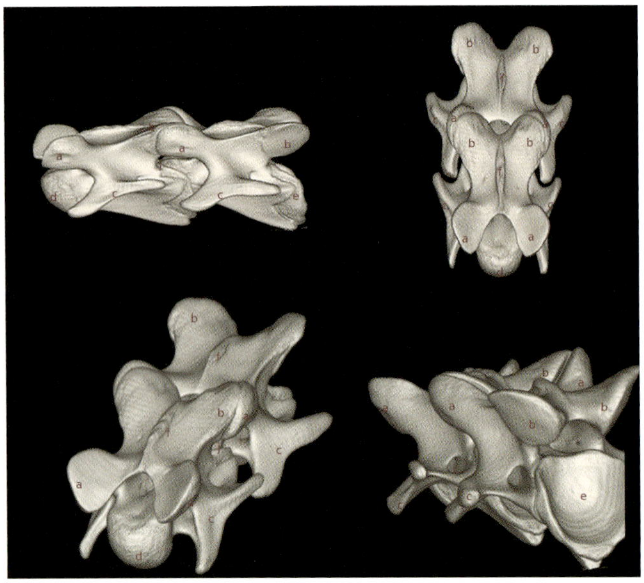

Fig 24.14 a. Cranial articular process b. Caudal articular process c. Transverse process d. Cranial extremity (vertebral head) e. Vertebral fossa f. Spinal process g. Ventral crest h. Spinal canal i. Foramen transversarium j. Intervertebral foramen

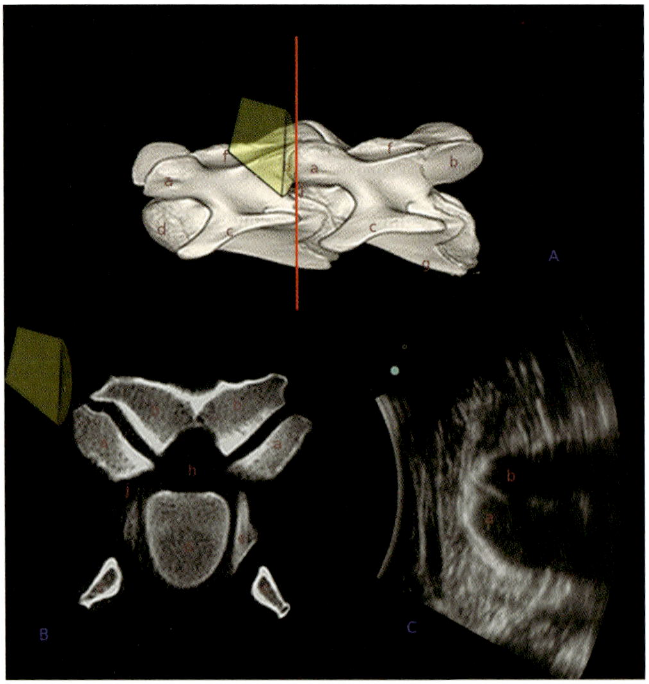

Fig 24.15 The yellow region (A and B) represents the ultrasound beam. C is the representative ultrasound image. **(A)** 3D reconstruction of the cervical spine. The red line represents site at which the cross section is obtained. **(B)** Cross section CT image through the cervical spine. **(C)** Ultrasound image oriented with dorsal towards the top of the picture.

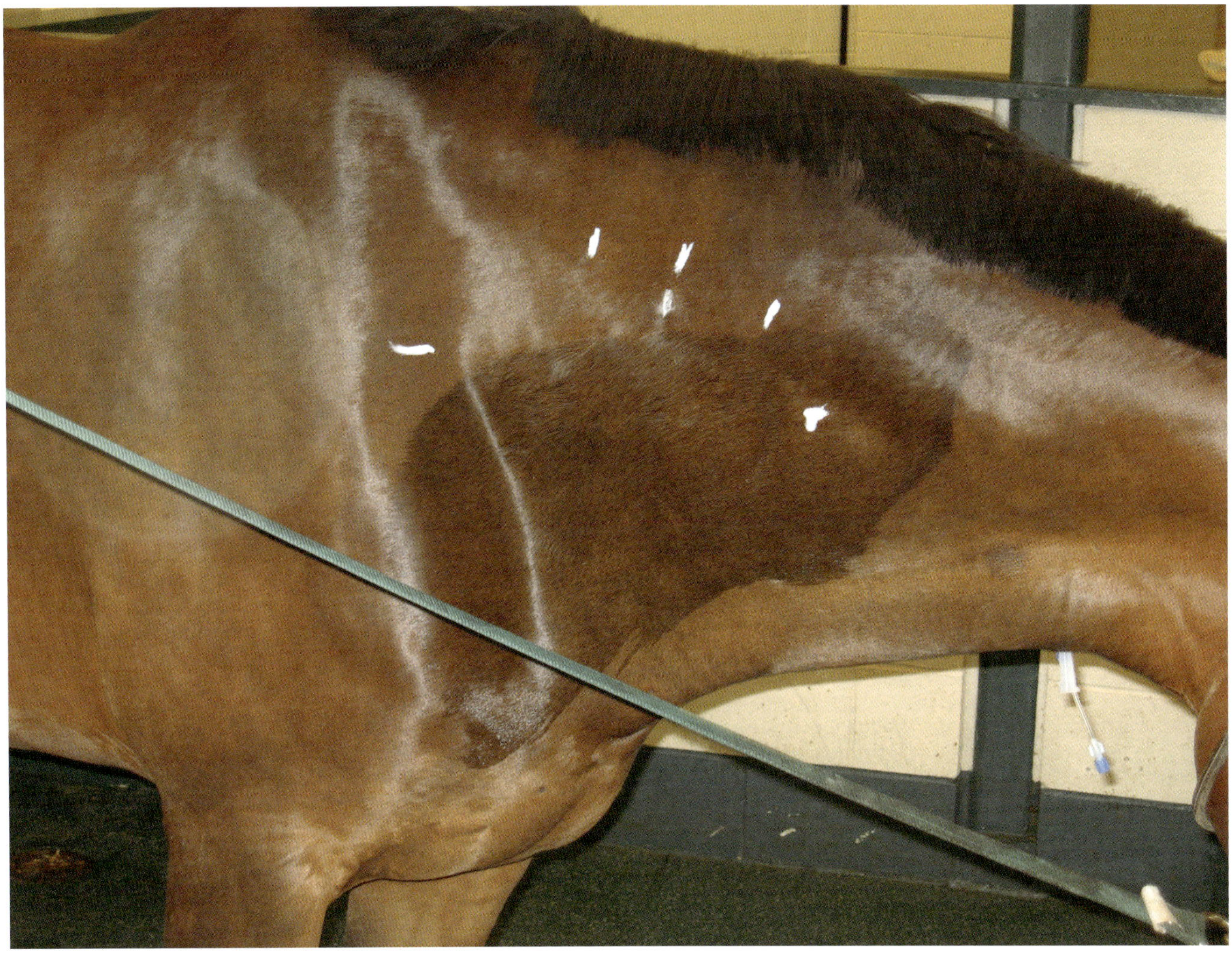

Fig 24.16 Ultrasound of the neck should be performed prior to injection and the injection sites marked with white out (site of ideal probe placement)

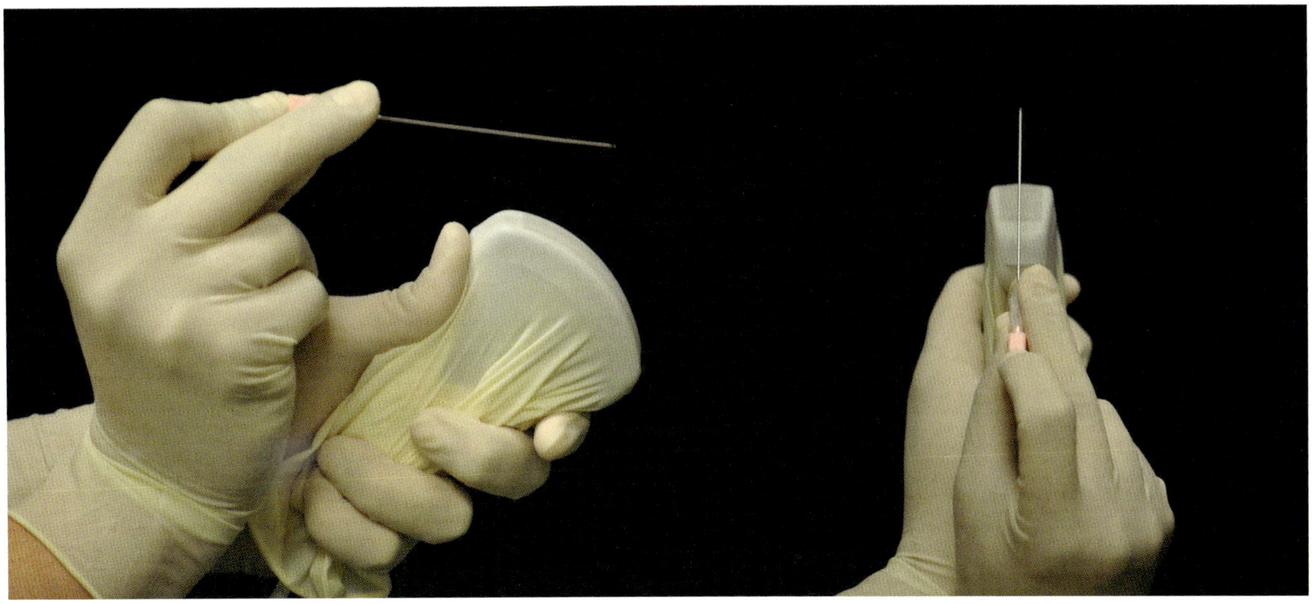

Fig 24.17 Correct orientation of needle with respect to ultrasound probe. The needle is parallel to the ultrasound beam and aligned with the center of the ultrasound beam. The probe should be held transverse with respect to the spinal column.

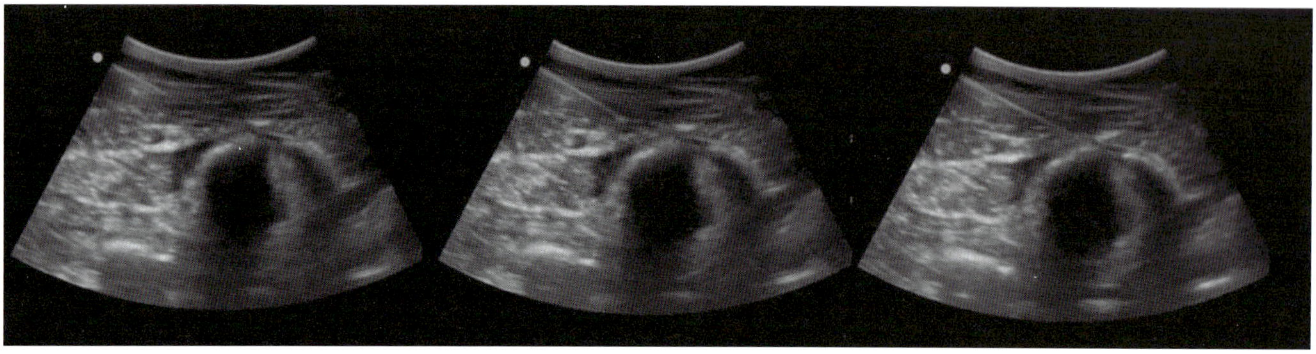

Fig 24.18 Sequence of needle placement with ultrasound guidance. The images are oriented with dorsal towards the left of the picture. The needle should be introduced dorsal to the ultrasound probe and directed ventrally and axially towards the articular facet. Proper placement requires a shallow angle and the needle should be advanced until it goes through the joint capsule (3rd image in the sequence). Once the needle is in place, the stylet can be removed and steroids and antibiotics injected.

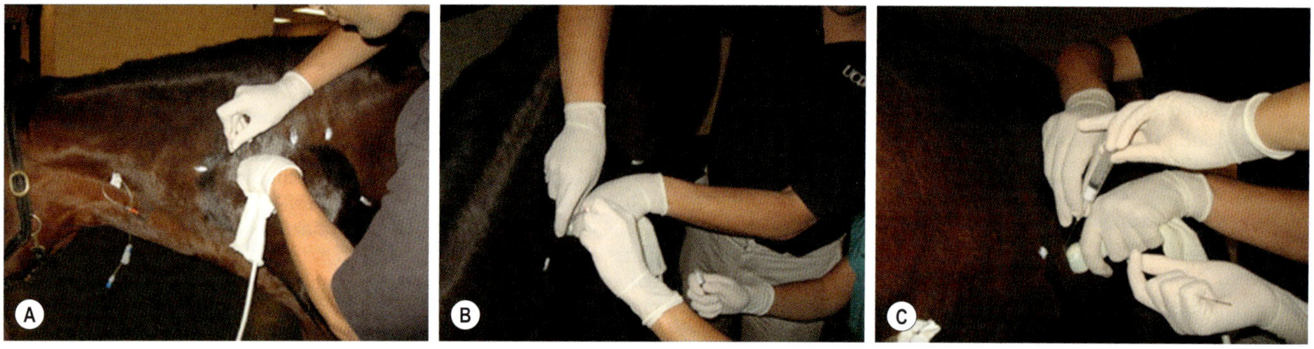

Fig 24.19 **(A)** Proper needle placement requires placement of the needle dorsal to the ultrasound probe in the same plane and parallel to the ultrasound beam. **(B)** The needle is advanced until contact is made with the cranial articular facet within the articular facet joint. **(C)** The stylet is removed once the needle is placed and steroids and antibiotics are injected.

Combinations of corticosteroid (triamcinolone, bethamethasone, methylprednisolone or dexamethasone), hyaluronic acid and an antibiotic (amikacin or gentamicin) are most often injected. The author favors the use of methylprednisolone (40 to 60 mg per joint) for its longer acting effect.

Pitfalls

Inability to visualize the needle usually arises from inappropriate needle placement outside of the ultrasound beam.

If the needle appears to be in the same plan but cannot be visualized, the transducer position may be altered slightly to try and localize the needle. As long as both the facet joint and the needle can be visualized, the needle may be advanced. If this cannot be achieved, it is recommended to remove and redirect the needle. Previous needle tracks will be visible in the tissue as anechoic lines after needle removal and may confuse the inexperienced operator as they resemble the needle.

Results

Accuracy of intra-articular ultrasound guided injection was >72% with inexperienced operators and improved with operator experience.[162]

The duration and degree of improvement after injection depends on the type and severity of clinical signs. In a study by Birmingham et al, 71.2% of horses showed improvement in their clinical signs that lasted from a few weeks to several years.[163]

In the author's experience, for performance issue and neck stiffness, the effect of injections is profound and lasts for 3–18 months. For lameness and neurologic signs, the improvement may last for up to 3–8 months.

References

1. Reed SM, Newbrey J, Norton K, et al. Pathogenesis of cervical vertebral malformation. Amer Assoc Equine Pract 1985;35:37–42.
2. Reed SM, Knight DA, Weisbrode SE, et al. The relationship of cervical vertebral malformation to developmental orthopedic disease. Amer Assoc Equine Pract 1988;34: 139–41.
3. Furr MO, Anver M, Wise M, et al. Intervertebral disk prolapsed and diskospondylitis in a horse. J Amer Vet Med Assoc 1991;198(12):2095–6.
4. Powers BE, Stashak TS, Nixon AJ, et al. Pathology of the vertebral column of horses with cervical static stenosis. Vet Pathol 1986;23:392–99.
5. Yovich JV, Gould DH, Le Couteur RA. Chronic cervical compressive myelopathy in horses: patterns of

astrocytosis in the spinal cord. Aust Vet J 1991;68:334–7.
6. Levine JM, Adam E, MacKay RJ, et al. Confirmed and presumptive cervical vertebral compressive myelopathy in older horses: a retrospective study (1992–2004). J Vet Inter Med 2007;21: 812–19.
7. Levine JM, Scrivani PV, Divers TJ, et al. Multicenter case-control study of signalment, diagnostic features, and outcome associated with cervical vertebral malformation-malarticulation in horses. J Amer Vet Med Assoc 2010; 237:812–22.
8. Wagner PC, Grant BD, Watrous BJ, et al. A study of the heritability of cervical vertebral malformation in horses. Amer Assoc Equine Pract 1985;31:43–50.
9. Falco MJ, Whitwell K, Palmer AC. An investigation into the genetics of 'Wobbler Disease' in Thoroughbred horses in Britain. Equine Vet J 1976;8:165–9.
10. Donawick, WJ, Mayhew IG, Galligan DT, et al. Early diagnosis of Cervical Vertebral Malformation in young Thoroughbred horses and successful treatment with restricted, paced diet and confinement. Amer Assoc Equine Pract 1989;35:525–8.
11. Knight DA, Gabel AA, Reed SM, et al. Correlation of dietary mineral to incidence and severity of metabolic bone disease in Oho and Kentucky. Amer Assoc Equine Pract 1985;31:445
12. Gabel AA, Knight DA, Reed SM. Comparison of incidence and severity of developmental orthopedic disease on 17 farms before and after adjustment of ration. Amer Assoc Equine Pract 1988; 34:163–70.
13. Mayhew IG, Donawick WJ, Green SL, et al. Diagnosis and prediction of cervical vertebral malformation in Thoroughbred foals based on semi-quantitative radiographic indicators. Equine Vet J 1993;25:435–40.
14. Rush Moore B, Reed SM, Biller DS, et al. Assessment of vertebral canal diameter and bony malformations of the cervical part of the spine in horses with cervical stenotic myelopathy. Amer J Vet Res 1994;55:5–13.
15. Hahn CN, Handel I, Green SL, et al. Assessment of the utility of using intra- and intervertebral minimum sagittal diameter ratios in the diagnosis of cervical vertebral malformation in horses. Vet Radiol & Ultrasound 2008;49:1–6.
16. Papageorges M, Gavin PR, Sande RD, et al. Radiographic and myelographic examination of cervical vertebral column in 306 ataxic horses. Vet Rad 1987;28:53–9.
17. Tomizawa N, Nishimura R, Sasaki N, et al. Efficacy of the new radiographic measurement method for cervical vertebral instability in wobbling foals. J Vet Med Sce 1994;56:1119–22.
18. Scrivani PV, Levine JM, Holmes NL, et al. Observer agreement study of cervical-vertebral ratios in horses. Equine Vet J 2011;43:399–403.
19. Down SS, Henson FMD. Radiographic retrospective study of the caudal cervical articular process joints in the older horse. Equine Vet J 2009;41: 518–24.
20. Neuwirth L. Equine Myelography. Compend Cont Ed Pract Vet 1992;14: 72–8.
21. Hubbell JA, Reed SM, Myer CW, et al. Sequela of myelography in the horse. Equine Vet J 1988;20:438–40.
22. Van Biervliet J, Flaminio J, Divers TJ, et al. The febrile response after cervical myelography in the horse: a retrospective analysis and experimental study. ACVIM annual meeting, abstract #35, Minneapolis, MN, 2004.
23. Conrad RL. Metrimazide myelography of the equine cervical spine. Vet Radiol 1984;25:73–7.
24. Nyland HG, Blythe LL, Pool RR, et al. Metrizamide myelography in the horse: clinical, radiographic, and pathologic changes. Amer J Vet Res 1980;4:204–11.
25. Mayhew IG, Green SL. Accuracy of diagnosing CVM from radiographs. British Equine Vet Assoc 2000;39: 74–5.2000
26. Van Biervliet J, Scrivani PV, Divers TJ, et al. Evaluation of decision criteria for detection of spinal cord compression based on cervical myelography in horses: 38 cases (1981–2001). Equine Vet J 2004;36:14–20.
27. Levine JM, Ngheim PP, Levine GJ, et al. Associations of sex, breed, and age with cervical vertebral compressive myelopathy in horses: 811 cases (1974–2007). J Amer Vet Med Assoc 1993;233:1453–8.
28. Rush Moore B, Reed SM, Robertson JT. Surgical treatment of cervical stenotic myelopathy in horses: 73 cases (1983–1992). J Amer Vet Med Assoc 1993;203:108–12.
29. Grant B, Barbee D, Wagner P, et al. Long term results of surgery for equine cervical malformation. Proc Am Assoc Equine Pract 1985;31:75–90.
30. Nixon AJ, Stasak TS. Surgical therapy for spinal cord disease in the horse. Amer Assoc Equine Pract 1985;31:61–74.
31. Nixon AJ, Stashak TS, Ingram JT. Dorsal laminectomy in the horse. III Results in horses with cervical malformation. Vet Surg 1983;12:184–8.
32. Wagner P, Grant B, Bagby G, et al. Evaluation of cervical spinal fusion as a treatment in the equine 'wobbler' syndrome. Vet Surg 1979;8:84–8.
33. Reardon R, Kummer K, Lishcer C. Ventral locking compression plate for treatment of cervical stenotic myelopathy in a 3-month old Warmblood foal. Vet Surg 2009;38: 537–42.
34. Rooney JR, Prickett ME, Delaney FM, et al. Focal myelitis-encephalitis in horses. Cornell Vet 1969;60:494–501.
35. Marsh AE, Barr BC, Madigan J, et al. Neosporosis as a cause of equine protozoal myeloencephalitis. J Amer Vet Med Assoc 1996;209:1907–13.
36. Fenger CK, Granstrom DE, Langemeier JL, et al. Identification of opossums (Didelpis virginiana) as the putative definitive host of Sarcocystis neurona. J Parasitol 1995;81:916–19.
37. Dubey JP, Saville WKA, Lindsay DS, et al. Completion of the life cycle of Sarcocystis neurona. J Parasitol 2000;86:1276–80.
38. Cheadle MA, Yowell CA, Sellon DC, et al. The striped skunk (*Mephitis mephitis*) is an intermediate host for *Sarcocystis neurona*. Int J Parasitol 2001;31:843–9.
39. Dubey JP, Saville WJ, Stanek JF, et al. *Sarcocystis neurona* infections in raccoons (*Procyon lotor*): evidence for natural infections with sarcocysts, transmission of infection to opossums (*Didelphis virginiana*), and experimental induction of neurologic disease in raccoons. Vet Parasitol 2001;100:117–29.
40. Cheadle MA, Tanhauser SM, Dame JB, et al. The nine-banded armadillo (*Dasypus novemcinctus*) is an intermediate host for *Sarcoicystis neurona*. Int J Parasitol 2001;321:330–5.
41. Sellon DC, Knowles DP, Greiner EC, et al. Depletion of natural killer cells does not result in neurologic disease due to Sarcocystis neurona in mice with severe combined immunodeficiency. J Parasitol 2004;90:782–8.
42. Rossano MG, Schott HC, Murphy AJ, et al. Parasitemia in an immunocompetent horse experimentally challenges with Sarcocystis neurona sporocysts. Vet Parasitol 2005:127:3–8.
43. Mullaney T, Murphy A, Kiupel M, et al. Evidence to support horses as natural intermediate hosts for Sarcocystis neurona. Vet Parasitol 2005;133:27–36.
44. Saville WJ, Reed SM, Granstrom DE, et al. Seroprevalence of antibody to Sarcocystis neurona in horses residing in Ohio. J Am Vet Med Assoc 1997;210: 519–24.
45. Bentz BG, Granstrom DE, Stamper S. Seroprevalence of antibodies to Sarcocystis neurona in horses residing in a county of southeastern Pennsylvania. J Am Vet Med Assoc 1997;210:517–18.
46. Blythe LL, Granstrom DE, Hansen DE, et al. Seroprevalence of antibodies to Sarcocystis neurona in horses residing

in Oregon. J Am Vet Med Assoc 1997; 210:525–7.
47. Rossano MG, Kaneene JB, Marteniuk JV, et al. The seroprevalence of antibodies to Sarcocystis neurona in Michigan equids. Prev vet Med 2001;48:113–28.
48. Tillotson K, McCue PM, Grnstrom DE, et al. Seroprevalence of antibodies to Sarcocystis neurona in horses residing in Northern Colorado. J Equine Vet Sci 1999;19:122–6.
49. NAHMS: Equine protozoal myeloencephalitis in the US, Ft. Collins, CO, 2000, USDA: APHIS:VS, CEAH, National animal Health Monitoring System.
50. Fayer R, Mayhew IG, Baird JD, et al. Epidemiology of equine protozoal myeloencephalitis in North America based on histologically confirmed cases. J Vet Intern Med 1990;4:54–7.
51. Boy MG, Galligan DT, Divers TJ. Protozoal encephalomyelitis in horses: 82 cases (1972–1986). J A, Vet Med Assoc 1990;196:632–4.
52. Saville WJ, Stich RW, Reed SM, et al. Utilization of stress in the development of an equine model for equine protozoal myeloencephalitis. Vet Parasitol 2001;95:211–22.
53. Granstrom DE, Dubey JP, Davis SW, et al. Equine Protozoal Myeloencephalitis: Antigen analysis of cultured Sarcocystis neurona merozoites. J Vet Diagn Invest 1993;5:88–90.
54. Daft BM, Barr BB, Gardner IA, et al. Sensitivity and specificity of the western blot testing of cerebralspinal fluid and serum for the diagnosis of equine protozoal myeloencephalitis in horses with and without neurologic abnormalities. J Am Vet Med Assoc 2002;221:1007–13.
55. Rossano MG, Mansfield LS, Kaneene JB, et al. Improvement of wetern blot test specificity for detecting equine serum antibodies to Sarcocystis neurona. J Vet Diagn Invest 2000;12:28–32.
56. Duarte PC, Daft BM, Conrad PA, et al. Comparison of a serum indirect fluorescent antibody test with two Western blot tests for the diagnosis of equine protozoal myeloencephalitis. J Vet Diagn Invest 2003;15:8–13.
57. Ellison SP, Kennedy T, Brown KK. Development of an ELISA to detect antibodies to rSAG1 in horses. Int J Appl Res Vet Med 2003;1:318–27.
58. Johnson AL, Burton AJ, Sweeney RW. Utility of 2 immunological tests for antemortem diagnosis of equine protozoal myeloencephalitis (Sarcocystis neurona infection) in naturally occurring cases. J Vet Intern Med 2010;24:1184–9.
59. Hoane JS, Morrow JK, Saville WJ, et al. Enzyme-linked immunosorbent assays for detection ofequine antibodies specific to Sarcocystis neurona surface antigens. Clin Diagn Lab Immunol 2005;12:1050–6.
60. Duarte PC, Daft BM, Conrad PA, et al. Evaluation and comparison of an indirect fluorescent antibody test for detection of antibodies to Sarcocystis neurona, using serum and cerebrospinal fluid of naturally and experimentally infected, and vaccinated horses. J Parasitol 2004;1:318–27.
61. Miller MM, Sweeney CR, Russell GE, et al. Effects of blood contamination of cerebrospinal fluid on western blot analysis for detection of antibodies against Sarcocystis neurona and on albumin quotient and immunoglobulin G index in horses. J Vet Med Assoc 1999;215:67–71.
62. Furr M, Howe D, Reed S, et al. Antibody coefficients for the diagnosis of equine protozoal myeloencephalitis. J Vet Intern Med 2011;25:138–42.
63. Furr M, MacKay R, Granstrom D, et al. Clinical diagnosis of equine protozoal myeloencephalitis (EPM). J Vet Intern Med 2002;16:618–21.
64. Beech J, et al. Equine Protozoal Myeloencephalitis. Vet Med Small An Clin 1974;69:1562–6.
65. Freedom of Information Summary. Rebalance antiprotozoal oral suspension (sulfadiazine and pyrimethamine. NADA 2004;141–240.
66. Toribio RE, Bain FT, Mrad DR, et al. Congenital defects in newborn foals of mares treted for equine protozoal myeloencephalitis during pregnancy. J Am Vet Med Assoc 1998;212:697–701.
67. Chung MK, Han SS, Roh JK. Synergistic embryotoxicity of combination pyrimethamine and folic acid in rats. Reprod Toxicol 1993;7:463–8.
68. Piercy RJ, Hinchcliff KW, Reed SM. Folate deficiency during treatment with orally administered folic acid, sulphadiazine and pyrimethamine in a horse with suspected equine protozoal myeloencephalitis (EPM). Equine Vet J 2002;34:311–16.
69. Mitchell SM, Zajac AM, Davis WL, et al. the effects of ponazuril on development of apicomplexans in vitro. J eukaryote Microbiol 2005;52:231–5.
70. Furr M, Kennedy T, MacKay R, et al. Efficacy of Ponazuril 15% oral paste as a treatment for equine protozoal myeloencephalitis. Vet Ther 2001;2: 215–22.
71. Freedom of Information Summary. Protazil antiprotozoal pellets. NADA 141–268. 2007
72. McClure S, Palma K. Treatment of equine protozoal myeloencephalitis with nitazoxanide. Equine Vet J 1999;19:639–42.
73. Vatistas N, Fenger C, Palma K, et al. Initial experiences with the use of nitazoxanide in the treatment of equine protozoal encephalitis in Northern California. Equine Pract 1999;21:18–21.
74. Gargala G, Goff LLE, Ballet JJ, et al. In vitro efficacy of nitro- and halogeno-thiazolide/thiadiazolide derivatives against Sarcocystis neurona. Vet Parasit 2009;162:230–5.
75. Witonsky S, Morrow JK, Leger C, et al. Sarcocystis neurona-specific immunoglobin G in the serum and cerebrospinal fluid of horses administered S. neurona vaccine. J Vet Intern Med 2004;18:98–103.
76. Furr M, McKenzie H, Saville WJA, et al. Prophylactic administration of ponazuril reduces clinical signs and delays seroconversion in hores challenged with sarcocystis neurona. J Parasitol 2006;92:637–43.
77. Siso S, Hanzlicek D, Fluehmann G, et al. Neurodegenerative diseases in domestic animals: a comparative review. Vet J 2006;171:20–38.
78. Blythe LL, Hultgren BD, Craig AM, et al. Clinical, viral, and genetic evaluation of equine degenerative myeloencephalopathy in a family of Appaloosas. J Amer Vet Med Assoc 1991;198:1005–13.
79. Beech J, Haskins M. Genetic studies of neuraxonal dystrophy in the Morgan. Amer J Vet Res 1987;48:109–13.
80. Mayhew IG, Brown CM, Stowe HD, et al. Equine degenerative myeloencepalopathy: a vitamin E deficiency that may be familial. J Vet Intern Med 1987;1:45–50.
81. Liu S, Dolensek EP, Adams CR, et al. Myelopathy and vitamin E deficiency in six Mongolian wild horses. J Amer Vet Med Assoc 1983;183:1266–8.
82. Siso I, Ferrer I, Pumarola M. Abnormal synaptic protein expression in two Arabian horses with equine degenerative myeloencephalopathy. Vet J 2003;166: 238–43.
83. Aleman M, Finno CJ, Higgins RJ, et al. Evaluation of epidemiological, clinical, and pathological features of neuroaxonal dystrophy in Quarter Horses. J Amer Vet Med Assoc 2011;239: 823–33.
84. Dill SG, Kallfelz FA, deLaunta A, et al. Serum vitamin E and blood glutathione peroxidase values of horses with degenerative myeloencephalopathy. Amer J Vet Res 1989;50:166–8.
85. Dill SG, Correa MT, Hollis MS, et al. Factors associated with the development of equine degenerative myeloencephalopathy. Amer J Vet Res 1990;51:1300–5.
86. Sokol RJ. Vitamin E and neurologic function in man. Free Radical Biol Med 1989;6:189–207.
87. Sokol RJ, Kayden HJ, Bettis DB, et al. Isolated vitamin E deficiency in the absence of fat malabsorption- familial

and sporadic cases: characterization and investigation of causes. J Lab Clin Med 1988;111:548–59.

88. Horwitt MK, Harvey CC, Dahm CH, et al. Relationship between tocopherol and serum lipid levels for determination of nutritional adequacy. Ann NY Acad Sci 1972;203:223–36.
89. Beech J. Neuroaxonal dystrophy of the accessory cuneate nucleus in horses. Vet Pathol 1984;21:384–93.
90. Blythe LL, Craig AM. Equine degenerative myeloencephalopathy. Part 2 diagnosis and treatment. Compend Cont Educ Pract 1992;14:1633–6.
91. Cummings JF, de Lahunta A, George C, et al. Equine motor neuron disease: a preliminary report. Cornell Vet 1990;80: 357–9.
92. Divers TJ, Mohammed HO, Cummings JF. Equine Motor neuron disease. In Lofstedt J, editor. Vet Clinics N Amer Equine Pract 1997;13:97–105.
93. Mohammed HO, Cummings JF, Divers TJ, et al. Risk factors associated with equine motor neuron disease: a possible model for human MND. Neur 1993;43:966–71.
94. De la Rua-Domenech R, Mohammed HO, Atwill ER, et al. Epidemiologic evidence for clustering of equine motor neuron disease in the Unites States. Amer J Vet Res 1995;56:1433–9.
95. Lofsted J, Ikede BO. Motor neuron disease in a quarter horse from Nova Scotia. Can Vet J 1994;35:507–9.
96. Kuwamura M, Iwaki M, Yamate J, et al. The first case of equine motor neuron disease in Japan. J Vet Med Sci 1994;56: 195–7.
97. Hahn CN, Mayhew IG. Does equine motor neuron disease exist in the United Kingdom? Vet Rec 1993;132:133–4.
98. Landolt G, Feige K, Grest P. Equine motor neuron disease (EMND). A case report. Tierarztl Prax 1997;25:241–3.
99. Divers TJ, Mohammed HO, Cummings JF, et al. Equine motor neuron disease: findings in 28 horses and proposal of a pathophysiologic mechanism for the disease. Equine Vet J 1994;26:409–15.
100. de La Rue-Domenech R, Mohammed HO, Cummings JF, et al. Intrinsic, management, and nutritional factors associated with equine motor neuron disease. J Amer Vet Med Assoc 1997;211:1261–7.
101. McGorum BC, Mayhew IG, Amory H, et al. Horses on pasture may be affected by equine motor neuron disease. Equine Vet J 2006;38:47–51.
102. de La Rue-Domenech R, Mohammed HO, Cummings JF, et al. Association between plasma vitamin E concentration and the risk of equine motor neuron disease. Vet J 1997;154:203–13.
103. Cummings JF, de Lahunta A, Fuhrer GC, et al. Equine motor neuron disease: a preliminary report. Cornell Vet 1990;80:357–9.
104. Cummings JF, de Lahunta A, Summers BA, et al. Eosinophilic cytoplasmic includions in sporadic equine motor neuron disease: an electron microscopic study. Acta Neuropathol 1993;85: 291–7.
105. Valentine BA, de Lahunta A, George C, et al. Acquired equine motor neuron disease. Vet Pathol 1994;31:130–8.
106. Riis RC, Jackson CA, Rebhun WC, et al. Ocular manifestations of equine motor neuron disease. Equine Vet J 1999;31:99–110.
107. Katz ML, Stone WL, Dratz EA. Fluorescent pigment accumulation in retinal pigment epithelium of antioxidant-deficient rats. Invest Ophthalmol vis Sci 1978;17:1049–58.
108. Jackson CA, de Lahunta A, Cummings JF, et al. Spinal accessory nerve biopsy as an ante mortem diagnostic test for equine motor neuron disease. Equine Vet J 1996;28:215–19.
109. Valentine BA, de Lahunta A, Divers TJ, et al. Clinical and pathologic findings in two draft horses with progressive muscle atrophy, neuromuscular weakness, and abnormal gait characteristic of shivers syndrome. J Amer Vet Med Assoc 1999;215: 1661–5.
110. Firshman AM, Baird JD, Valberg SJ. Prevalence and clinical signs of polysaccharide storage myopathy and shivers in Belgian Draft Horses. J Amer Vet Med Assoc 2005;227:1958–64.
111. Hunt LM, Valberg SJ, Steffenhagen K, et al. A retrospective study of myopathies and associated gait abnormalities in 65 Warmblood horses. J Vet Intern Med 2005;19:428–9.
112. Davies PC. Shivering in a Thoroughbred mare. Can Vet J 2000;41:128–9.
113. Baird JD, Firshman AM, Valberg SJ. Shivers (Shivering) in the Horse: A review. Amer Assoc Equine Pract 2006;52:359–64.
114. Andrews fm, Spurgeon TL, Reed SM. Histochemicall changes in skeletal muscles of four male horses with neuromuscular disease. Amer J Vet Res 1986;47:2078–83.
115. Valentine BA, Habacker PL, Patterson JS, et al. Incidence of polysaccharide storage myopathy in draft horse-related breeds: a necropsy study of 37 horses and a mule. J Vet Diagn Invest 2001;13: 63–8.
116. Valberg SJ, Draper A. Movement disorders in horses: Shivers, Stringhalt and other conundrums. In Proceed Amer College Vet Intern Med 2012.
117. Galey FD, Hullinger PJ, McCaskill J. Outbreaks of stringhalt in northern California. Vet Hum Toxicol 1991;33: 176–7.
118. Araya O, Krause A, Solis de Ovando M. Outbreaks of stringhalt in souther Chile. Vet Rec 1998;142:462–3.
119. de Pennington N, Colles C, Dauncey E. Australian stringhalt in the UK. Vet Rec 2011;169:476
120. Domange C, Casteignau A, Collignon G, et al. Longitudinal study of Australian stringhalt cases in France. J Anim Physiol Anim Nutr (Berl) 2010;94:12–20.
121. Takahashi T, Kitamura M, Endo Y, et al. An outbreak of stringhalt resembling Australian stringhalt in Japan. J Equine Sci 2002;13:93–100
122. Slocombe RF, Huntington PJ, Friend SC, et al. Pathological aspects of Australian stringhalt. Equine Vet J 1992;24: 174–83.
123. Armengou L, Anor S, Climent F, et al. Antemortem diagnosis of a distal axonaopathy causing severe stringhalt in a horse. J Vet Intern Med 2010;24: 220–3.
124. Wijnberg ID, Back W, van der Kolk JH. The use of electromyographic examination as a diagnostic tool and phenytoin sodium as treatment in a cse of classic springhalt in a Dutch Warmblood horse. Tijdschr Diergeneeskd 2000;125:743–7.
125. Wijnberg ID, Back W, de Jong M, et al. the role of electromyography in clinical diagnosis of neuromuscular locomotor problems in the horse. Equine Vet J 2004;36:718–22.
126. Huntington PJ, Seneque S, Slocombe RF, et al. Use of phenytoin to treat horses with Australian stringhalt. Aust Vet J 1991;68:221–4.
127. Wijnberg ID, Schrama SE, Elgersma AE, et al. Quantification of surface EMG signals to monitor the effect of Botox treatment in six healthy ponies and two horses with stringhalt: preliminary study. Equine Vet J 2009;41:313–18.
128. Crabhill MR, Honnas CM, Taylor DS, et al. Stringhalt secondary to trauma to the dorsoproximal region of the metatarsus in horses: 10 cases (1986–1991). J amer Vet Med Assoc 1994;205:867–9.
129. Torre F. Clinical diagnosis and results of surgical treatment of 13 cases of acquired bilateral stringhalt (1991–2003). Equine Vet J 2005;37:181–3.
130. Dyson SD. The elbow, brachium and shoulder. In: Ross MW, Dyson SD, editors. Diagnosis and management of lameness in the horse. St Louis: WB Saunders Co; 2003. p. 414.
131. Devin DV, Jann HW, Payton ME. Gait abnormalities caused by selective anesthesia of the suprascapular nerve in horses. Amer J Vet Res 2006;67: 834–6.

132. Dutton DM, Honnas CM, Watkins JP. Nonsurgical treatment of suprascapular nerve injury in horses: 8 cases (1988–1998). J Amer Vet Med Assoc 1999;214:1657–9.
133. Schneider JE, Adams OR, Easley KJ, et al. Scapular notch resection for suprascapular nerve decompression in 12 horses. J Amer Vet Med Assoc 1985;187:1019–20.
134. Cook WR. Headshaking in the horse. Part I. Equine Pract 1979;1:9–17.
135. Cook WR. Headshaking in the horse. Part II. Equine Pract 1979;1:36–9.
136. Madigan JE, Kortz G, Murphy C, et al. Photic headshaking in horses: 7 cases. Equine Vet J 1995;27:306–11.
137. Newton SA, Knottenbelt DC, Eldridge PR. Headshaking in horses: possible aetiopathogenesis suggested by the results of diagnostic tests and several treatment regimes used in 20 cases. Equine Vet J 2000;32:208–16.
138. Madigan JE, Bell SA. Characterisation of headshaking syndrome- 31 cases. Equine vet J 1998;27:28–9.
139. Rappaport ZH, Devor M. Trigeminal neuralgia: the role of self-sustaining discharge in the trigeminal ganglion. Pain 1994;56:127–38.
140. Mills DS, Taylor K. Field study of the efficacy of three types of nose net for the treatment of headshaking in horses. Vet Rec 2003;152:41–4.
141. Mair TS. Assessment of bilateral infra-orbital nerve blockade and bilateral infra-orbital neurectomy in the investigation and treatment of idiopathic headshaking. Equine Vet J 1999;31:262–4.
142. Roberts VL, McKane SA, Williams A, et al. Caudal compression of the infraorbital nerve: A novel surgical technique for treatment of idiopathic headshaking and assessment of its efficacy in 24 horses. Equine Vet J 2009;41:165–70
143. Madigan JE, Bell SA. Owner survey of headshaking in horses. J Amer Vet Med Assoc 2001;219:334–7.
144. Stalin CE, Boydell IP, Pike RE. Treatment of seasonal headshaking in three horses with sodium cromoglycate eye drops. Vet Rec 2008;163:305–6.
145. Roberts VL, Perkins JD, Skarlina E, et al. Caudal anaesthesia of the infraorbital nerve for diagnosis of idiopathic headshaking and caudal compression of the infraorbital nerve for its treatment, in 58 horses. Equine Vet J 2012 (epub).
146. Berger JM, Bell SA, Holmberg BJ, et al. Successful treatment of head shaking by use of infrared diode laser deflation and coagulation of corpora nigra cysts and behavioral modification in a horse. J Amer Vet Med Assoc 2008;233:1610–12.
147. Blythe LL, Watrous BJ, Pearson EG, et al. Otitis media /interna in the horse- A cause of hed shaking and skull fractures. Proc Am Assoc Equine Pract 1990;36:517–22.
148. Blythe LL. Otitis media and interna and temporohyoid osteoarthropathy. Vet Clin North Amer Equine Pract 1997;13:21–42.
149. Hilton H, Puchalski SM, Aleman M. The computed tomographic appearance of equine temporohyoid osteoarthropathy. Vet Radiol Ultrasound 2009;50:151–6.
150. Pease AP, van Biervliet J, Dykes NL, et al. Complications of partial stylohyoidectomy for treatment of temporohyoid osteoarthropathy and an alternative surgical technique in three cases. Equine Vet J 2004;36:546–50.
151. Walker AM, Sellon DC, Cornelisse CJ, et al. Temporohyoid osteoarthropathy in 33 horses (1993–2000). J Vet Intern Med 2002;16:697–703.
152. Naylor RJ, Perkins JD, Allen S, et al. Histopathology and computed tomography of age associated degeneration of the equine temporohyoid joint. Equine Vet J 2010;42:425–30.
153. Blythe LL, Watrous BJ, Schmitz JA, et al. Vestibular syndrome associated with temporohyoid joint fusion and temporal bone fracture in three horses. J Am Vet Med Assoc 1984;185:775–81.
154. Robertson JT, Samii VF. Traumatic disorders of the spinal column. In: Auer JA, Stick JA, editors. Equine surgery. 4th ed. St. Louis: MO Elsevier; 2012. p. 711–20.
155. Nixon AJ, Stashak TS. Laminectomy for relief of atlantoaxial subluxation in four horses. J Am Vet Med Assoc 1988;193(6):677–82.
156. Rush BR. Central nervous system trauma. In: Robinson NE, editor. Current therapy in equine medicine. Philadephia, PA: Saunders; 1997. p. 301–5.
157. Cillan-Garcia E, Taylor SE, Townsend N, et al. Partial ostectomy of the dens to correct atlantoaxial subluxation in a pony. Vet Surg 2011;40:596–600.
158. Collatos C, Allen D, Chambers J, et al. Surgical treatment of sacral fracture in a horse. J Am Vet Med Assoc 1991;198(877):880.
159. Berg LC, Nielsen JV, Thoefner MB, et al. Ultrasonography of the equine cervical region: a descriptive study in eight horses. Equine Vet J 2003;35:647–55.
160. Grisel GB, Grant BD, Rantanen NW. Arthrocentesis of the equine articular facets. Proc Am Ass Equine Practnrs 1996;42:197–8.
161. Mattoon JS, Drost WT, Grguric MR, et al. Technique for equine cervical articular process joint injection. Vet Radiol Ultrasound 2004;45:238–40.
162. Nielsen JV, Berg LC, Thoefnert MB, et al. Accuracy of ultrasound-guided intra-articular injection of cervical facet joints in horses: a cadaveric study. Equine Vet J 2003;35:657–61
163. Birmingham SS, Reed SM, Mattoon JS, et al. Qualitative assessment of corticosteroid cervical articular facet injection in symptomatic horses. Equine Vet Educ 2010;22:77–82.

section 3

Respiratory system

Upper airway function of normal horses during exercise

25

Jon Cheetham Susan J. Holcombe Norm G. Ducharme

CHAPTER CONTENTS

Introduction

The horse is a magnificent athlete that can run in excess of 30 miles per hour. The drive to perform at these high speeds has led to a number of specific adaptations.

At maximal exertion, Thoroughbred and Standardbred racehorses have a maximal oxygen uptake (VO_{2max}) of approximately 160 mL/kg/min which is 40 times the value at rest.[1,2] This increase is far higher than the six to eight fold increase found in endurance trained human athletes and the tenfold increase seen in other mammals.[2,3]

The delivery of oxygen for this uniquely high rate of consumption requires a number of specific cardiovascular and respiratory responses. Resting oxygen consumption (VO_2) in the horse (4.7 mL/kg/min[2,4] is similar to that in other mammals.[5] As the level of exercise increases so does VO_2, and this relationship is linear until maximal oxygen consumption is reached (VO_{2max}) when further increases in speed do not elicit further increases in VO_2 and the extra energy required must be provided by anaerobic pathways.[5,6]

In horses, training can produce a 23% increase in VO_{2max}.[7] To maximize locomotor efficiency, each equine gait has an optimal speed at which oxygen consumption is lowest per distance unit traveled.[8]

In order to accommodate the tremendous oxygen demand of skeletal muscles during such intense exercise, the horse increases its minute ventilation by up to 40 fold. To provide this increase in minute ventilation, tidal volume and respiratory frequency both increase significantly[4,7] (Fig. 25.1). High airflow rates required to meet this ventilatory demand are created principally by diaphragmatic contraction, which produces driving high pressures within the upper airway. As the horse is an obligate nasal breather and rarely breathes orally, the horse's upper airway must quickly prepare for these large changes in airflow and pressures by dilating and becoming more rigid or less compliant. Such accommodation is achieved by the basic structure of the upper airway and synchronous

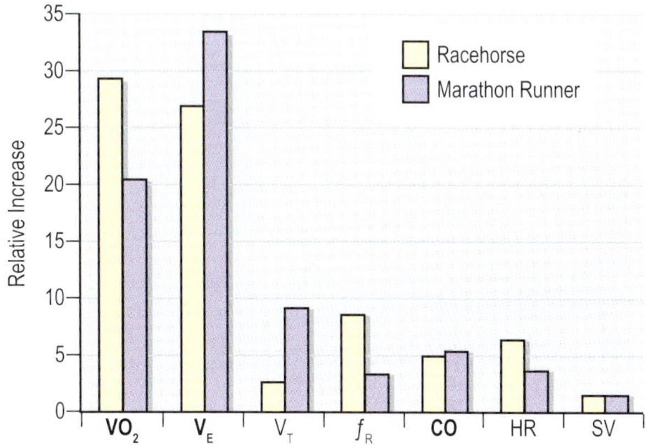

Fig 25.1 Relative increase in cardiorespiratory parameters from rest to exercise for a racehorse and human marathon runner (Body weight 70 kg). Figure shows increases in VO_2, minute volume (V_E), tidal volume (V_T), respiratory frequency (f_R), cardiac output (CO), stroke volume (SV) and heart rate (HR). Parameters in bold are influenced by the unbolded parameters to their right. Human data taken from 129 and 130. Equine data taken from 4 and 7.

and coordinated contraction of upper airway muscles and constriction of capacitance vessels within the mucosa of the upper airway.[9,10]

Obligate nasal breathing

Obligate nasal breathing is a term used to describe a physiological obligation or predisposition to breathe through the nose as opposed to the mouth. It has been suggested that obligate nasal breathing is an adaptation especially useful in prey species, as it allows an animal to feed while preserving their ability to detect predators by scent.[11] To accomplish this, the soft palate is tightly apposed to the base of the larynx, such that there is no communication between the oropharynx and the nasopharynx. Oral breathing does occur in horses, but only in the presence of anatomical abnormalities or disease conditions such as dorsal displacement of the soft palate.[12–14] The horse cannot breathe nor exercise normally in this state.

Basic upper airway mechanics

The equine respiratory system is uniquely adapted to produce a high rate of oxygen delivery to the alveolar surface during sustained high speed exercise.

Moving from the environment to the alveolar surface for gas exchange, the airway consists of the nostrils, nasal cavity, sinuses, guttural pouches nasopharynx, soft palate, larynx, trachea, bronchi, bronchioles and alveoli.

Ventilation

The resting horse is unusual as it has biphasic exhalation and occasionally a biphasic inspiration.[15–18] This flow pattern is lost at exercise or with excitement.[18]

At rest, the horse breathes around its functional residual capacity (FRC) so that inhalation results in a lung volume higher than FRC and exhalation a lung volume lower than FRC. Equine FRC is approximately 25 L.[19]

At walk and trot, respiratory frequency is not related to stride frequency.[15,20] At the canter and gallop, stride frequency and respiratory frequency are synchronized in a 1:1 ratio in fit horses [15,21,22] with the stride lagging approximately 80° behind the respiratory cycle at the canter and 54° at the gallop.[15] The synchronization of gait and respiration, with inhalation when the forelimbs are non-weight bearing and exhalation during the support phase, can offer some mechanical advantage.[21] Despite this, respiratory muscles work harder during exercise.[23,24] In addition, although thoracic expansion occurs at rest, walk, trot and slow canter, at faster speeds there are minimal changes of thoracic circumference with ventilation.[25]

During swallowing or sighing, normal horses may alter this 1:1 ratio.[21] In addition, horses may occasionally take a 'big respiratory cycle' (BRC) with a duration of approximately two strides.[26,27] The incidence of BRCs decreases with training and they can produce improvement in pulmonary gas exchange.[27]

Respiratory minute volume (V_E) in horses is approximately 67 L/min at rest, rising 27 fold to 1800 L/min at exercise.[4] At low speeds (up to 6 m/s), this is mainly due to an increase in respiratory frequency (R_f) which rises from 14 breaths/min to 120 breaths/min.[4,28,29] Above this speed, there is little increase in R_f, as stride and respiratory cycle are linked, and further increases in V_E are due to an increase in tidal volume. Tidal volume (V_T) is approximately 5 L at rest and this increases to 14–18 L at maximal exercise.[4,29,30] Expiration (E) is shorter than inspiration (I) with an E:I ratio of between 0.96 and 0.99.[29,30]

A number of clinical studies have evaluated the airway flows and pressures generated by horses at maximal exercise. Peak inspiratory flow at rest is approximately 3.5 L/s [4] and this rises dramatically at exercise to 65–75 L/s.[4,29–31] Similarly, peak expiratory flow at rest is 5.7 L/s rising to 60–80 L/s at exercise.[4,28–30]

These high flow rates are associated with high tracheal pressures both during inspiration and expiration. Peak inspiratory tracheal pressure has been reported as -18 mmHg to -37 mmHg for clinically normal horses at maximal exercise.[28,32,33] A computational flow model has recently been used to demonstrate that the greatest drops in airway pressure occur at the nostrils and the rostral aspect of the nasopharynx during inhalation.[34,35] This area is susceptible to collapse during inhalation, as it receives only muscular and not bony support. This leads to a reduction in cross-sectional area at this level during inhalation and so the pressure drop. Peak expiratory tracheal pressure has been reported as 6 mmHg to 20 mmHg for clinically normal horses at maximal exercise.[28,29,33] During expiration, airway pressure is greatest over the dorsal surface of the soft palate.[34,35]

High tracheal flow rates and the complex geometry of the upper respiratory tract mean that flow is always in the turbulent range. Tracheal flow in the horse is always turbulent with a Reynolds number (Re) at rest of about 8000.[36] Reynolds number (Re) is a dimensionless number that is the ratio of the inertial force to the viscous force in a fluid:[37]

$$Re = \frac{\rho v L}{\mu}$$

where ρ is the density, v the velocity, and μ is the viscosity of the fluid. L is the diameter of the tube. Turbulent flow occurs at high Reynolds numbers and is characterized by irregular flow with random eddies and vortices. Airflow in tubes such as the trachea becomes turbulent as airflow velocity increases.[38] Flows with Reynolds numbers above 2300 are generally considered turbulent.[37] At maximal exercise, the Reynolds number of inspiratory flow can reach 78000 in vivo.[36] A computational flow model has suggested Re as high as 131000 [34] in the horse at exercising airflows. Under these turbulent conditions, pressure changes in approximate inverse proportion to the fourth power of the radius (Poiseuille's Law). Clinically this is important as small decreases in airway cross-section (for example due to vocal fold collapse) produce profound increases in negative inspiratory pressure which can lead to a cycle of partial collapse, more negative pressure and consequent further collapse.

Resistance to airflow produced by the upper airway during inspiration is approximately twice that during expiration and resistance produced by the nose is approximately twice that at the larynx.[24,39] The nasal passages (26–76%), followed by the larynx (12–30%), produce the greatest resistance to flow within the upper airway.[35]

The peak resistance to airflow is termed impedance. Inspiratory upper airway impedance (Z_I) at exercise in experimental horses is 0.38 to 0.46 mmHg/L/s.[29,30,40] Expiratory impedance is 0.16 to 0.38 mmHg/L/s.[29,40] Adaptive responses to an increase in airway impedance include decreased respiratory frequency, increased driving pressure and increased inspiratory time.[30,33,40] It is important to note that studies measuring airflow and impedance require the use of a nasal mask and this has been shown to affect airway mechanics.[41]

Head position

The position of the horse's head and neck does affect upper airway flow mechanics in exercising horses.[42] Head and neck flexion may cause the airway to be more compliant, because tissues, such as the pharyngeal walls and soft palate, bulge into the airway, or because the nasopharynx shortens with this maneuver. Horses with most types of obstructive upper airway dysfunction show more severe signs of respiratory distress and exercise intolerance while exercising with the head and neck flexed rather than in a neutral or extended position.

Neuromuscular control of upper airway function

During intense exercise, multiple stimuli trigger contraction of upper airway dilating muscles, including chemical stimuli such as hypercapnia and hypoxia, limb movement, central locomotor-linked cortical influences, receptors located in the lower airways, and upper airway sensory receptors.[43–50]

The laryngeal mucosa has an abundant supply of sensory receptors that control a complex pattern of respiratory reflexes that influence the patency of the upper airway and the pattern of breathing.[51] These receptors are mechanoreceptors, chemoreceptors and cold receptors that line the mucous membranes and deeper tissues of the nose, nasopharynx, and larynx.[52–54] The mechanoreceptors can be further divided into pressure (64%), 'drive' (21%) and flow (15%) receptors.[51] The 'drive' receptors are stimulated by the activity of upper airway muscles.[51] These receptors receive afferent innervation from branches of the trigeminal, glossopharyngeal, and vagus nerves.[55,56] Receptors in the nasopharynx are innervated by branches of the glossopharyngeal and trigeminal nerves.[51] These receptors are principally tactile receptors and stimulate the gag response, important in airway protection.

Especially relevant to dilation and stability of the upper airway during exercise are the pressure receptors. Pressure receptors account for 60% of the sensory receptors within the laryngeal mucosa in horses, which is similar to other species.[51,57] These receptors are innervated by the internal branch of the cranial laryngeal nerve which runs through the thyroid notch at the dorsorostral aspect of the thyroid cartilage.[51,52,55,58,59] Through this afferent loop, negative pressure within the upper airway increases the activity of the genioglossus, posterior (dorsal) cricoarytenoid, cricothyroid, nasolabial, sternothyroid and sternohyoid muscles.[59,60] They are stimulated during upper airway obstruction, when large collapsing pressures are produced in the upper airway, and they provide afferent information to the central nervous system, signaling contraction of upper airway muscles to resist dynamic collapse in the upper airway. In horses, negative pressure stimulates increased electromyographic activity in the cricoaryteneoideus dorsalis muscle, the primary laryngeal abductor.[57] During incremental exercise testing the palatinus, palatopharygeus, hyoepiglotticus, sternohyoideus and sternothyroideus, geniohyoideus, and genioglossus muscles all had increasing levels of electromyographic activity as treadmill speed increased, and upper airway pressures became more negative.[61–63]

Topical anesthesia of the luminal surface of the larynx or bilateral superior laryngeal nerve sectioning markedly reduces the response to changes in upper airway pressure and upper airway muscle activity in laboratory species and people.[49,56] In horses, topical anesthesia of the laryngeal mucosa results in increased inspiratory upper airway and nasopharyngeal impedances.[64] The dynamic upper airway obstruction was caused by nasopharyngeal collapse due to decreased skeletal muscle support. Following topical anesthesia of the laryngeal mucosa, horses exhibit dorsal displacement of the soft palate and nasopharyngeal collapse

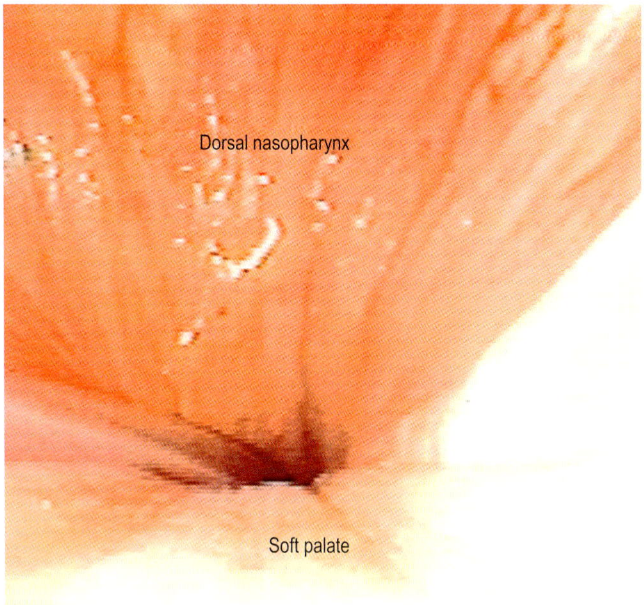

Fig 25.2 Endoscopic image of the nasopharynx while the nares are occluded following topical anesthesia of the laryngeal mucosa. Notice how the nasopharynx collapses, almost forming a sphincter.

during endoscopic examination at rest (Fig. 25.2) and varying degrees of nasopharyngeal collapse during incremental treadmill exercise.[64] These results suggest that local sensory receptors in the upper airway of horses, as has been shown in laboratory species, contribute to upper airway patency and that disrupting the sensory component of the local reflex that controls contraction of upper airway muscles can cause dynamic upper respiratory obstruction in horses.

Nasal occlusion

Because negative pressure induces contraction of upper airway muscles, a nasal occlusion test was developed in horses to challenge the upper airway with more negative pressures during resting videoendoscopic examination, in order to mimic pressure changes that might occur during intense exercise. Peak tracheal inspiratory pressure during nasal occlusion (-24.9 ± 3 cm H_2O) is not significantly different from peak inspiratory pressure while horses exercise at HR_{max} (-25.6 ± 2.7 cm of H_2O), and peak pharyngeal inspiratory pressure is significantly more negative (-28.9 ± 4.9 cm of H_2O) during nasal occlusion than while horses exercise at HR_{max} (-17.5 ± 2.1 cm of H_2O).[65] These data indicate that nasal occlusion in standing horses results in pharyngeal and tracheal inspiratory pressures that equal or exceed those that are generated during exercise at HR_{max}, making it a potentially useful test for evaluating the activity of laryngeal and pharyngeal muscle function. However, anecdotally, horses that exhibit varying degrees of nasopharyngeal collapse at rest frequently have normal airway function during treadmill exercise. As well, horses that readily displace their soft palates at rest frequently displace during treadmill exercise, but the correlation between displacement at rest and during treadmill exercise is not a strong one.

Other sensory receptors within the upper airway include flow and drive receptors. Drive receptors represent 20% of laryngeal sensory receptors in horses.[51,57] These receptors respond to changes in airway deformation, such as collapse, muscle contraction and movement of the laryngeal cartilages.[51] Flow receptors are temperature-sensing receptors.[51] These receptors sense cool air temperatures, which occur as air flow increases. The majority of these receptors are responsive during inspiration, but some (approximately 20%) respond during exhalation, and a small population of the airway sensory receptors is active both during inspiration and expiration.[51]

Muscular anatomy and function of the upper airway

The nose

The horse's nose includes the paired external nares, the nasal cavities, and the paranasal sinuses. The nostril has two compartments: a dorsal blind sac called the nasal diverticulum and the ventral part, which is the true nostril.[66] The alar fold divides the nostril into the dorsal and ventral parts. The nasal cavity is divided in half by the nasal septum and vomer bone. Each nasal cavity has a dorsal and ventral nasal concha, which divide the cavity into dorsal, ventral, middle, and common meatus (Fig. 25.3).[66] The ethmoid turbinates project from the ethmoid bone in the caudal part of the nasal cavity (Fig. 25.4). The nasal valve is the narrowest point in the nasal cavity and, thus, is a major contributor to nasal resistance.[9] This region is caudal to each nostril and immediately rostral to the nasoincisive notch within the dorsal meatus. It is bound medially by the nasal septum, ventrally by the concha, and dorsolaterally by the skin and dorsal conchal fold (Fig. 25.5).[66] Expansion of the nasal valve during exercise occurs by constriction of capacitance vessels and contraction of muscles that pull the skin taught at the dorsal aspect of the notch. The respiratory portion of the nasal cavity has a vascular submucosa, which contains a rich vascular plexus. This plexus

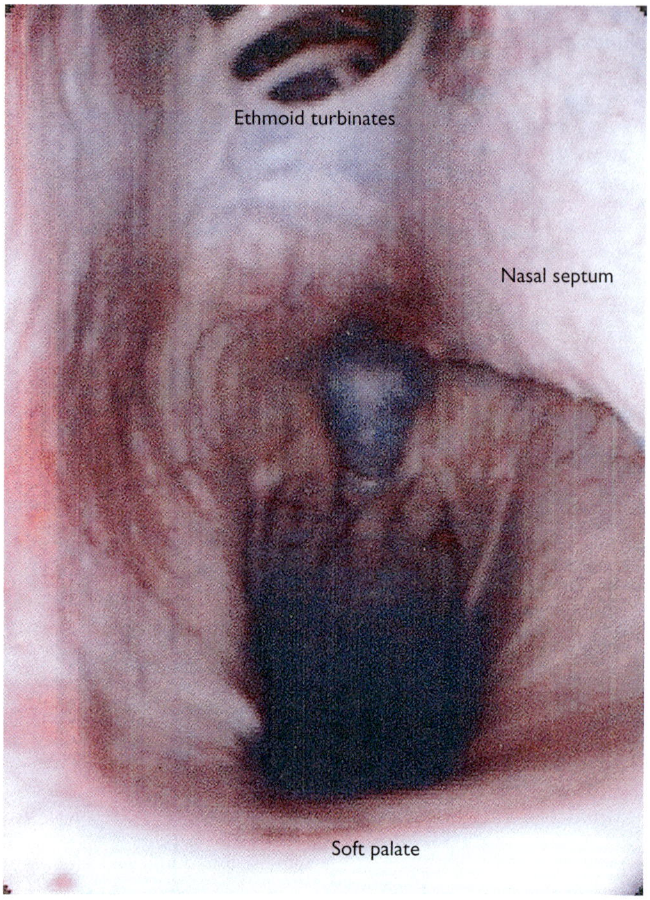

Fig 25.4 Endoscopic image of the ethmoid turbinates and nasopharynx.

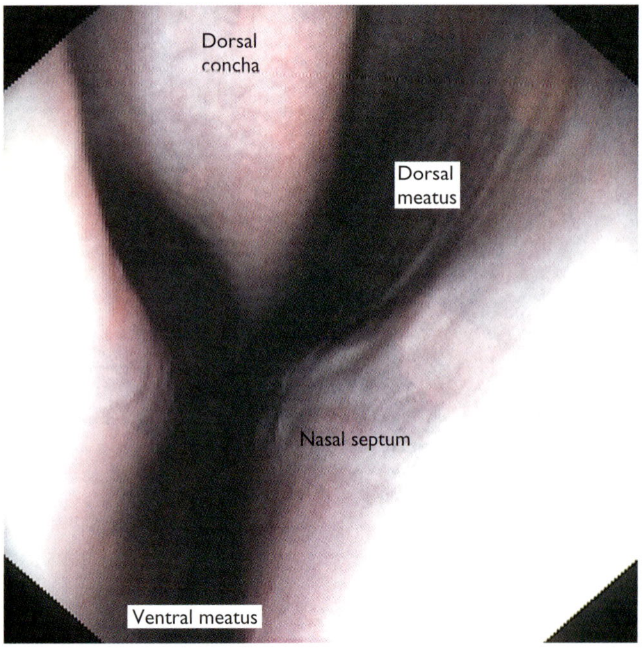

Fig 25.3 Endoscopic image of the concha and turbinates within the nasal passage.

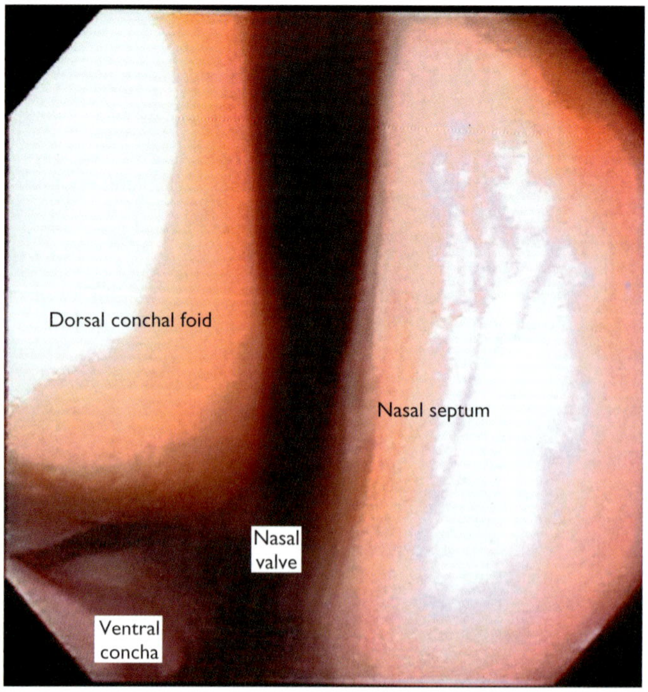

Fig 25.5 Endoscopic image of the nasal valve region.

is concentrated on the ventral portion of the nasal septum and ventral meatus and is important for warming and humidifying air. The capacitance blood vessels in the airways, especially those lining the nasal mucosa, are innervated by sympathetic, parasympathetic, and peptidergic systems that regulate blood flow.[10] This extensive vasculature is responsible for warming and humidifying inspired air. When these vessels are dilated, the sinuses and nasal passages become engorged with blood, resulting in airway narrowing and increased airway resistance. Such nasal congestion is a cause of airway obstruction and poor performance in horses with Horner's syndrome. During exercise, sympathetic stimulation causes vasoconstriction, increasing airway dimensions and decreasing resistance to airflow.[10] The nasal vestibule is lined by fine hairy skin and there is an abrupt change to non-ciliated nasal mucosa over the base of the ventral nasal concha.[18]

In obligate nasal breathers such as the horse, increasing nasal patency during exercise is critical to minimizing work of breathing. At rest, the horse's nostril is shaped like a comma, but as the horse increases its respiratory effort the nostril dilates and becomes circular in shape. Horses can actually decrease their nasal resistance during exercise by increasing nasal volume and flaring their nostrils. Nostril dilation is accomplished by the contraction of four different muscles (Fig. 25.6).[66] Contraction of the lateralis nasi dilates the nostril, rotates the conchal cartilages laterally, and expands the nasal vestibule, which forms the floor of the nasal valve.[66] Other muscles involved in dilatation of the nostrils include the caninus, dilator naris apicales, and levator nasolabialis. These muscles are all innervated by the facial nerve (VII). Contraction of the caninus or dilator naris lateralis muscle helps expand the lateral aspect of the nostrils.[66] Dilator naris apicales is an unpaired muscle that lies between the nostrils and aids in dilatation of the nostrils.[66] Levator nasolabialis dilates the nostrils and also elevates the maxillary lip and commissures.[66] Horses with dysfunction, weakness, or lack of contraction of one or more of these muscles will likely have dynamic nasal obstruction that may limit performance.

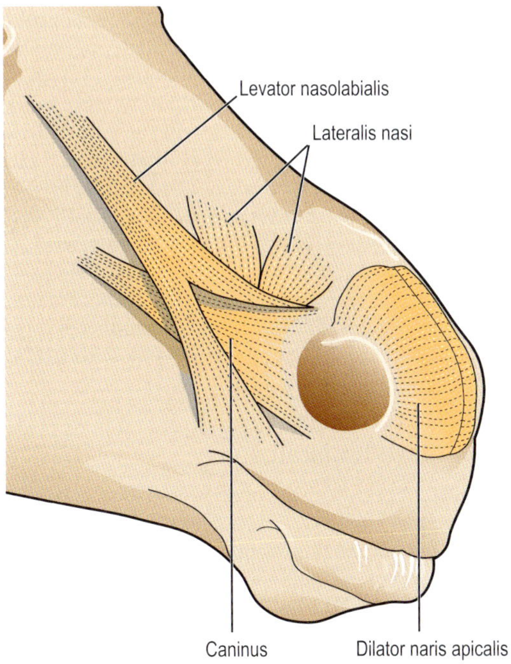

Fig 25.6 Illustration of the dilating muscles of the nares.

The nasopharynx

The nasopharynx is a musculomembranous unit that functions during breathing, deglutition, and vocalization and connects the nasal cavity to the larynx. It is attached to the pterygoid, palatine, and hyoid bone, and to the arytenoid, cricoid, and thyroid cartilages by nasopharyngeal muscles that cause pharyngeal dilation and constriction.[67] The nasopharynx is not directly supported by cartilage or bone, yet contraction of these pharyngeal muscles allows the nasopharynx to withstand large changes in intraluminal pressures that occur during tidal breathing at rest and during exercise. Such activation of these muscle groups is synchronous with breathing and this synchronization is coordinated by multiple stimuli.[46,68] These same muscles are also important during deglutition. This dichotomy of action, contracting the pharyngeal walls during swallowing and dilating the airway during breathing, seems contradictory. But these muscles are uniquely situated to perform both activities, because the pharynx is a conduit for both food and air.

The nasopharynx is lined by pseudostratified columnar ciliated epithelium.[18,69] Elastin fibers are present in the nasopharyngeal submucosa and are more prevalent caudally.[69] The equine nasopharynx at the level of the soft palate has a cross-sectional area of approximately 2430 mm^2.[34] Exhalation results in significant dilation of the nasopharynx to 3920 mm^2 at the same level.[70,71]

Muscles responsible for altering the size and configuration of the nasopharynx, including the muscles that alter the shape and position of the tongue, the muscles that control the position of the hyoid apparatus, a constrictor group of muscles located in the dorsal pharynx, and a group of muscles that regulate the position of the soft palate.

Soft palate

The soft palate completely divides the pharynx into nasal and oral compartments in the horse. Because the horse is an obligate nasal breather, it is critically important that the soft palate remains ventral to the epiglottis, except during swallowing, to allow unimpeded nasal breathing. The soft palate extends caudally from the hard palate to the base of the larynx and consists of the oral mucous membrane, which contains ductile openings of the palatine glands, the palatine glands, the palatine aponeurosis, palatinus and palatopharyngeus muscles, and the nasopharyngeal mucous membrane.[67] The caudal free margin of the soft palate continues dorsally, on either side of the larynx, forming the lateral pillars of the soft palate. These pillars unite dorsally, forming the posterior pillar of the soft palate or the palatopharyngeal arch. The position of the soft palate is determined by the coordinated activity of groups of antagonistic muscles which include the levator veli palatini, tensor veli palatini, palatinus, and palatopharyngeus muscles (Fig. 25.7).[72,73] The *levator veli palatini* muscle attaches to the petrous part of the temporal bone and the lateral lamina of the guttural pouch. It travels along the lateral wall of the nasopharynx and terminates within the soft palate. A branch of the pharyngeal branch of the vagus nerve innervates this muscle.[67] It acts to elevate the soft palate during swallowing and vocalization. The action of the levator veli palatini muscle can be seen during endoscopic examination of the upper airway when the gag reflex is stimulated (Fig. 25.8). A 'sling' forms within the nasopharynx as the nasopharynx contracts into a sphincter.

The *tensor veli palatini* is a flat, fusiform muscle that, like the levator, attaches to the petrous part of the temporal bone, the pterygoid bones, and the lateral lamina of the guttural pouch.[67] Its tendon is reflected around the hamulus of the pterygoid bone, where it is lubricated by a bursa. The tendon then ramifies in the

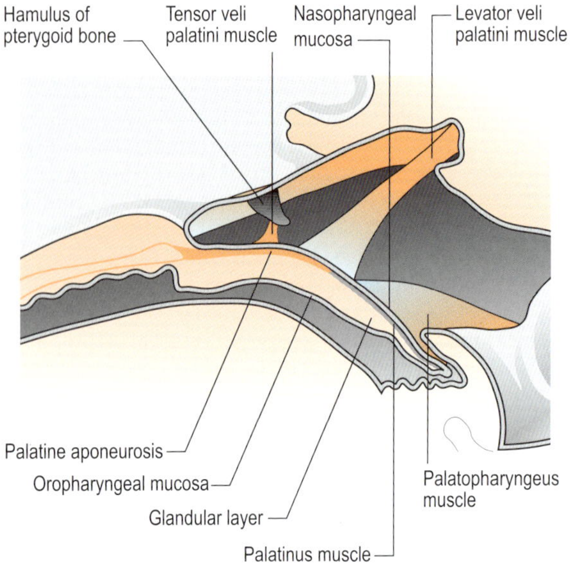

Fig 25.7 Illustration of the muscles of the soft palate.

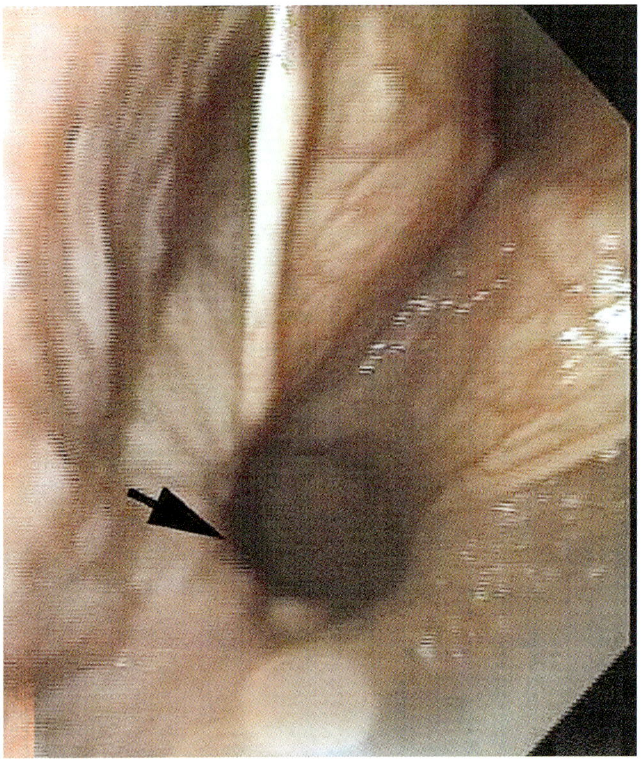

Fig 25.8 Endoscopic image of the nasopharynx during a 'gag' reflex. Notice the 'sling' formed by partial contraction of the levator veli palatini muscles (arrow).

palatine aponeurosis.[67] It receives motor innervation from the mandibular branch of the trigeminal nerve. Contraction of this muscle tenses the palatine aponeurosis and, therefore, the rostral portion of the soft palate, and depresses this portion of the soft palate toward the tongue.[67,72,73] Contraction of the tensor veli palatini muscle also aides in opening the pharyngeal opening of the guttural pouch.[74] Bilateral transection of the tendon of the tensor veli palatini muscle in horses causes instability of the rostral portion of the soft palate resulting in inspiratory obstruction during intense exercise (Fig. 25.9A and B).[75] The rostral portion of the soft palate is more compliant and its action dependent on airway pressures, such that during inspiration the rostral portion of the soft palate billows dorsally in the airway and during expiration, it is depressed toward the tongue by the positive pressure within the airway.[75]

The *palatinus* muscle (uvula retractor muscle) consists of two fusiform muscles that lie on either side of midline of the soft palate, beneath the nasopharyngeal mucosa, extending caudally from the hard palate.[67] The muscles attach to the caudal aspect of the palatine aponeurosis and terminate near the caudal free margin of the soft palate. A small muscle bundle arising from the lateral aspect of each muscle continues a short distance caudodorsally into the palatopharyngeal arch.[67] It receives motor innervation from a branch of the pharyngeal branch of the vagus nerve.[67] Contraction of the palatinus muscle shortens the soft palate.[67,72,73]

The *palatopharyngeus* muscle originates from the palatine aponeurosis and the lateral border of the palatinus muscle.[67] It travels caudally along the lateral wall of the nasopharynx to the pharyngeal raphe, forming part of the superior constrictor muscle group. Contraction of this muscle shortens the soft palate and draws the larynx and esophagus toward the root of the tongue.

Contraction of both the palatinus and palatopharyngeus muscles shortens the soft palate and depresses the caudal portion toward the tongue.[72,73,76] Both the palatinus and palatopharyngeus muscles receive efferent motor innervation from the pharyngeal branch of the vagus nerve.[67] This nerve branches from the parent vagus nerve at the level of the cranial cervical ganglion and courses cranioventrally along the medial wall of the guttural pouch to the dorsal wall of the pharynx where it ramifies in the pharyngeal plexus. Bilateral local anesthesia of the pharyngeal branches of the vagus nerve induced persistent dorsal displacement of the soft palate and dysphasia in horses.[12] Horses can become dysphasic, with or without persistent soft palate dysfunction, following guttural pouch lavage with caustic solutions, guttural pouch empyema, trauma, or mycosis.[77,78] Based on this information, there was convincing evidence to suggest that dysfunction of the neuromuscular group, including the pharyngeal branch of the vagus nerve, palatinus and palatopharyngeus muscles, might be involved in the pathogenesis of intermittent dorsal displacement of the soft palate in exercising horses.

The palatinus muscle is composed of principally type 2A fast twitch fibers (5–25% type 1 and 75–95% type 2A) with darkly staining mitochondria, which suggests that these fibers have increased endurance relative to most skeletal muscle fast-twitch fibers.[79] The palatopharyngeus muscles are also principally composed of type 2A fibers (10–25% type 1 and 75–90% type 2A fibers).[79] Pathological abnormalities are also observed in the palatinus muscle of horses with intermittent DDSP. These abnormalities are consistent with chronic denervation and include fiber type grouping, mild atrophy, moth eaten fibers and target fibers (Fig. 25.10A–D).[79]

Muscles of the hyoid apparatus

The hyoid apparatus in horses consists of an assembly of bony rods, some of which articulate together.[80] Several muscles are attached to this apparatus, and the contraction of theses muscles alters shape and position, which in turn, changes the position and shape of the larynx and nasopharynx.[81,82] The hyoid apparatus consists of the paired stylohyoid, epihyoid, ceratohyoid, thryohyoid bones, and the central basihyoid bone. (Fig. 25.11). The stylohyoid bone articulates with the petrous part of the temporal bone, allowing the

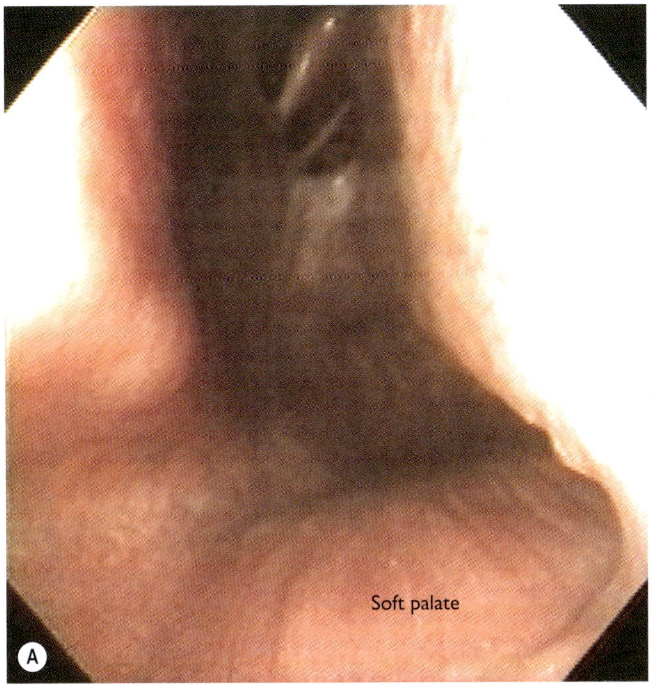

Fig 25.9A Endoscopic image of the nasopharynx during inhalation while the nares are occluded following bilateral tensor veli palatini tenectomy. Notice how the rostral portion of the soft palate billows dorsally into the airway.

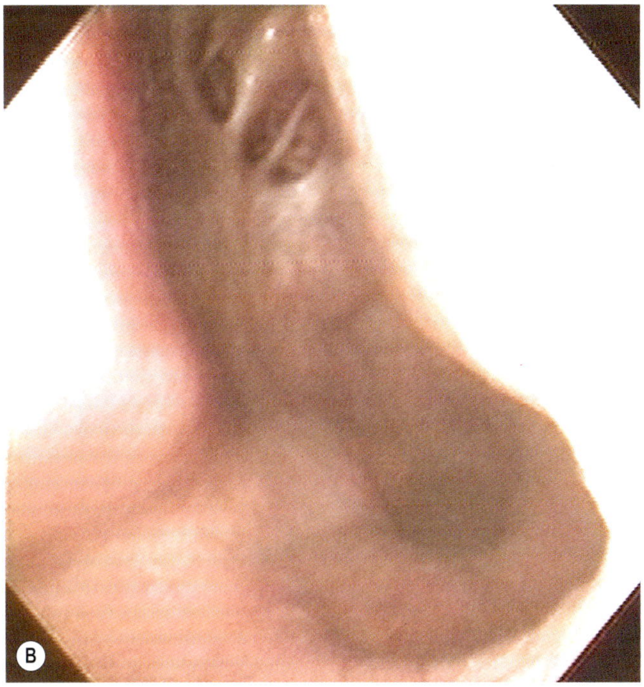

Fig 25.9B Endoscopic image of the nasopharynx during exhalation while the nares are occluded following bilateral tensor veli palatini tenectomy. Notice how the rostral portion of the soft palate billows dorsally into the airway.

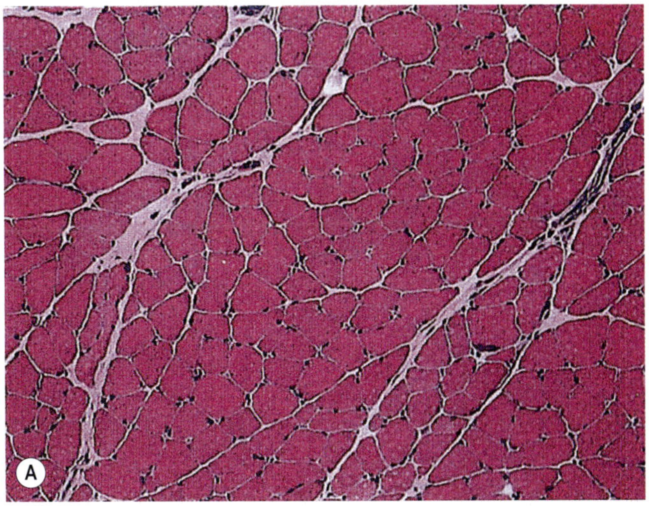

Fig 25.10A H & E stained section of the palatinus muscle from a healthy horse.

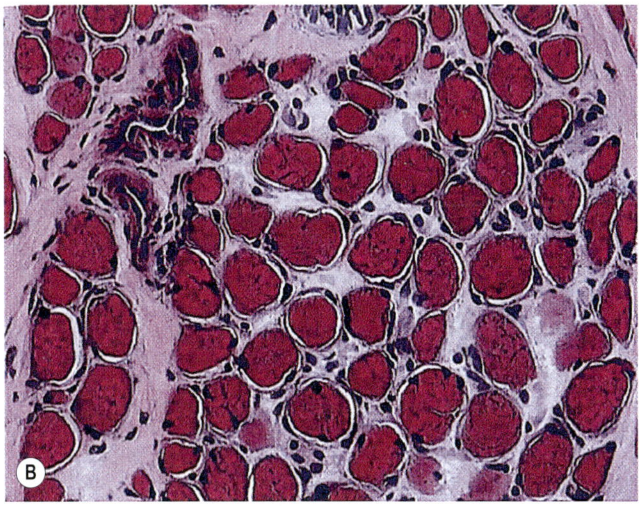

Fig 25.10B H & E stained section of the palatinus muscle from a horse with intermittent dorsal displacement of the soft palate. Notice the increased amount of connective tissue (light pink) and tissue degeneration.

stylohyoid bones to move cranial to caudal, in a pendulous manner. The ceratohyoid bone attaches to the distal end of the stylohyoid bone, and movement at this articulation lengthens the stylohyoid – ceratohyoid unit (Fig. 25.12). The base or root of the tongue is attached to the lingual process of the basihyoid bone. The tongue is located on the floor of the mouth between the rami of the mandible. The base of the tongue is attached to the hyoid apparatus, soft palate, and pharynx.[67] Folds of mucous membrane pass dorsally on either side of the base of the tongue to form the palatoglossal arches, which attach the tongue to the soft palate.[67,51]

The genioglossus, hyoglossus, and styloglossus muscles are extrinsic muscles of the tongue that, in part, control the position and function of the tongue and provide attachments to the hyoid apparatus.[67] The rostral hyoid muscles (hyoglossus, styolglossus, genioglossus and geniohyoideus) are innervated by the hypoglossal nerve and attach to the hyoid apparatus (the hyoglossus to the

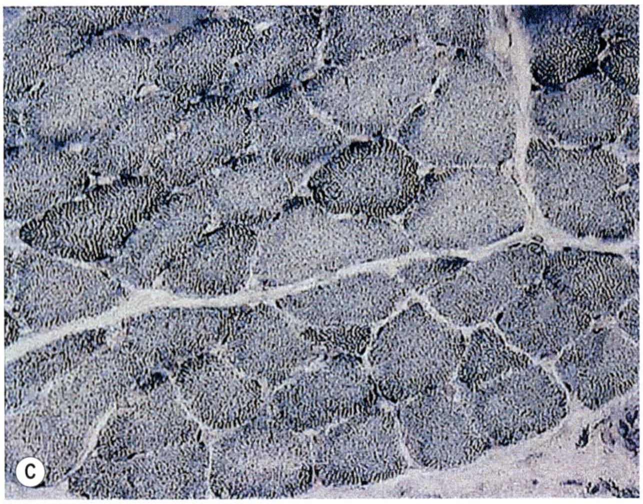

Fig 25.10C NADH stained section of the palatinus muscle from a healthy horse.

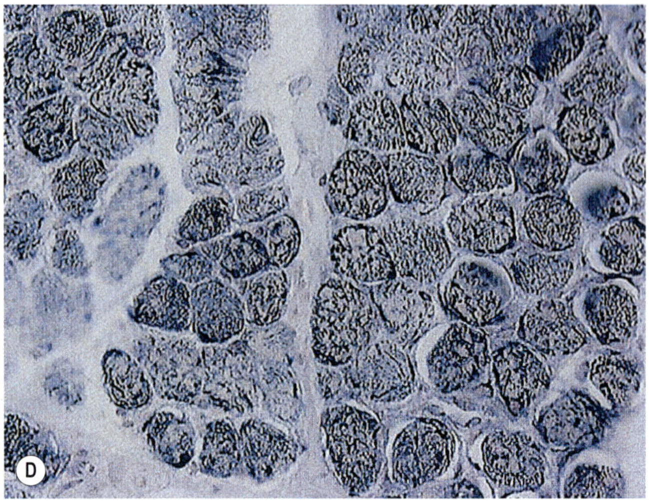

Fig 25.10D NADH stained section of the palatinus muscle from a horse with intermittent dorsal displacement of the soft palate. Notice the moth eaten fibers and areas of increased amounts of connective tissue.

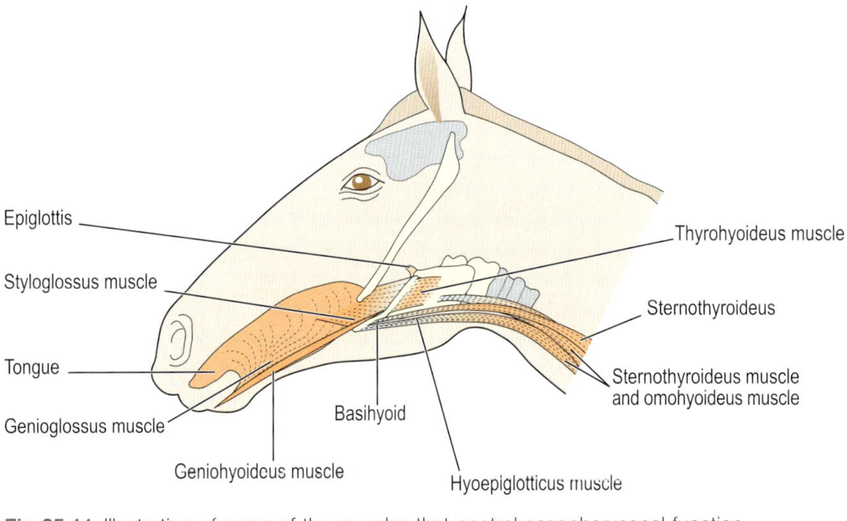

Fig 25.11 Illustration of some of the muscles that control nasopharyngeal function.

basihyoid and thyrohyoid bones, the styloglossus to the stylohyoid bone, the genioglossus to the basihyoid and ceratohyoid bones, and the geniohyoideus to the lingual process of the basihyoid bone) which suspend the larynx from the petrous part of the temporal bone. The hypoglossal nerve also innervates the thyrohyoideus muscle which draws the larynx rostrally and dorsally and the root of the tongue caudally by its attachments to the thyrohyoid and basihyoid bones.[83–85]

The genioglossus is a fan-shaped muscle that lies within and parallel to the median plane of the tongue.[67] The genioglossus muscle originates from the medial surface of the mandible, just caudal to the symphysis and is innervated by the medial branch of the hypoglossal nerve.[67] A large tendon runs throughout the muscle. Muscle fibers radiate rostrally toward the tip of the tongue, dorsally, and distally toward the root of the tongue. The hyoglossus is a flat wide muscle that lies in the lateral portion of the root of the tongue.[67] The hyoglossus originates from the lateral aspect of the basihyoid bone and from portions of the stylohyoid and thyrohyoid bones and is innervated by the lateral branch of the hyopglossal nerve.[67] The styloglossus muscle originates at the distal lateral aspect of the stylohyoid bone and travels the length of the tongue, along its lateral aspect.[67] Near the tip of the tongue the paired muscle meets and ramifies with fibers of intrinsic tongue muscles. Styloglossus contraction retracts the tongue. Contraction of the genioglossus muscle protracts the tongue and pulls the basihyoid bone rostrally. Genioglossus also acts with the hyoglossus muscle to depress and retract the tongue. Hyoglossus and genioglossus activity are synchronous with respiration and activity of these muscles correlates well with increases in pharyngeal airway size during breathing.[81,82,86,87] Hypoxia, hypercapnea, and airway occlusion caused parallel increases in electrical activity of the protrudor and retractor muscle of the tongue, consistently inducing net retraction and depression of the tongue, improved airflow function and enhanced pharyngeal stability.[82,86] Other muscles that attach to the hyoid

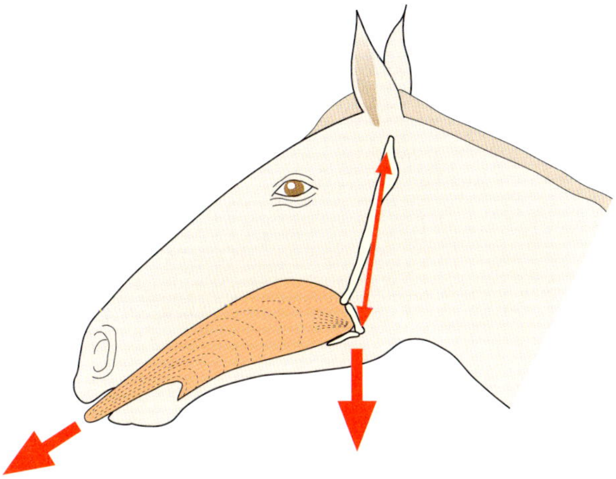

Fig 25.12 Illustration showing the effect of various muscles on hyoid length and position.

apparatus include the geniohyoideus, sternohyoideus and sternothyroideus, omohyoideus, and thyrohyoideus. The geniohyoideus muscle is a fusiform, paired muscle that lies on the ventral surface of the tongue.[88] The geniohyoideus originates from the medial surface of the mandible (near the genioglossus' origin) caudal to the symphysis and inserts on the basihyoid bone and moves the hyoid bone rostrally.[88]

Collectively these muscles that control laryngeal position through their attachment to the hyoid apparatus appear to play an important part in nasopharyngeal stability at exercise. Associations have been shown between laryngeal position and nasopharyngeal stability in horses. Horses with DDSP during treadmill examination have a more ventral basihyoid at rest, although the magnitude of this distance is small.[89] Horses with a more dorsal post-operative basihyoid position are associated with an increased probability of racing following post operatively laryngeal 'tie forward'.[14] The position of the larynx at rest has been shown to be related to the occurrence of Obstructive Sleep Apnea (OSA), a sleep disorder, with major public health consequences affecting 2–4% of adults.[90,91] Changes in laryngeal position are associated with variable airway stability in patients with OSA[92,93] and hyoid bone position is an important predictor of hypoxia reduction with mandibular advancement devices in patients with sleep apnea.[94]

Functionally, bilateral local anesthetic blockade of the distal hypoglossal nerve at the level of the ceratohyoid bone, so disabling the rostral hyoid muscles produces DDSP during high speed exercise.[95] Blockade of the hypoglossal nerve at the level of the guttural pouch produces epiglottic retroversion with inspiratory obstruction.[96]

In a clinical population of horses with DDSP, the frequency of swallowing increases immediately prior to the onset of DDSP.[13] This study suggested that the drive to swallow is diminished in normal horses as they run faster, but that this mechanism can be overridden in horses affected by DDSP. An alternate interpretation is that swallowing directly results in DDSP. The observation of DDSP as an immediate sequel to a swallow[32,97–99] could support either interpretation.

The omohyoideus, sternohyoideus and sternothyroideus muscles are accessory respiratory muscles that insert on the manubrium and extend cranially. The sternothyroideus inserts on the caudal abaxial aspect of the thyroid cartilage, and the sternohyoideus inserts on the basihyoid bone and the lingual process of the hyoid apparatus. Contraction of these muscles results in caudal traction of the hyoid apparatus and larynx, resulting in dilation of the upper airway.[88] These muscles are innervated by branches of the first and second cervical nerves.[88] Both the sternothyroideus and sternohyoideus muscles are sometimes transected as palliative therapy for horses with dorsal displacement of the soft palate, with the goal of reducing caudal retraction at exercise; and if combined with a 'tie-forward' facilitating rostral and dorsal advancement of the larynx. Following myectomy, translaryngeal and tracheal inspiratory pressures and resistance measurements increase, suggesting that these muscles might act to dilate and stabilize the nasopharynx in normal horses.[100] The effects of myectomy on airway mechanics in horses with upper airway obstructive disease is yet unknown. The omohyoideus muscles originates on the subscapular fascia near the shoulder joint and also insert on the on the basihyoid bone and the lingual process of the hyoid apparatus. Contraction of these muscles results in caudal traction of the hyoid apparatus and tongue movement other than retraction.[101] The omohyoideus muscles are innervated by branches of the first and second cervical nerves. The omohyoideus muscles have also been transected for treatment of soft palate displacement in conjunction with the sternohyoideus and sternothyroideus muscles but no experimental data exist to investigate the result of omohyoid transection alone or in conjunction with the sternohyoideus and sternothyroideus muscles in horses during exercise.[102]

The *thyrohyoideus* is a flat rectangular muscle attached to the lateral surface of the thyroid cartilage lamina that inserts on the caudal part of the thyrohyoid bone.[88] It is innervated by the hypoglossal nerve and moves the hyoid bone caudally or the larynx rostrally and dorsally.[88] Bilateral thyrohyoid muscle resection caused intermittent dorsal displacement of the soft palate in exercising horses.[103] This finding formed the basis for the laryngeal 'tie-forward' in which a prosthetic suture is placed to mimic the action of the thyrohyoid muscles.[14,104]

Dorsal pharyngeal constrictors

The action of the dorsal pharyngeal constricting muscles and the stylopharyngeus muscle is responsible for stiffening and dilating the nasopharynx.[105–107] The inferior pharyngeal constrictor (thyropharyngeus muscle), middle pharyngeal constrictor (hyopharyngeus muscle), and superior pharyngeal constrictor (palatopharyngeus and pterygopharyngeus muscles) form the dorsal and caudolateral pharyngeal walls.[105,106] Contraction and shortening of these muscles forms a sphincter, which moves the food bolus caudal into the esophagus during swallowing. During breathing, these muscles have tonic and phasic expiratory activities, that helps to support the nasopharynx.[106,107] The major dilating muscle of the dorsal nasopharynx is the stylopharyngeus muscle.[106] This muscle originates on the axial aspect of the distal portion of the stylohyoid bone and courses rostroventrally to ramify in the wall of the dorsal nasopharynx, by passing between the pterygopharyngeus and palatopharyngeus muscles (Fig. 25.13A and Fig. 25.13B). Contraction of the stylopharyngeus muscles pulls the pharyngeal wall dorsally, to receive the bolus during swallowing.[108] In a similar manner, during breathing, contraction of the stylopharyngeus muscle pulls the nasopharyngeal wall dorsally thereby supporting the dorsal wall of the nasopharynx and preventing dynamic collapse of this area during inspiration.[109] The glossopharyngeal nerve provides motor innervation to the stylopharyngeus muscle.[108] This cranial nerve has mostly sensory fibers, but provides motor innervation to one skeletal muscle, the stylopharygeus muscle. Bilateral glossopharyngeal nerve anesthesia produces stylopharyngeus muscle dysfunction,

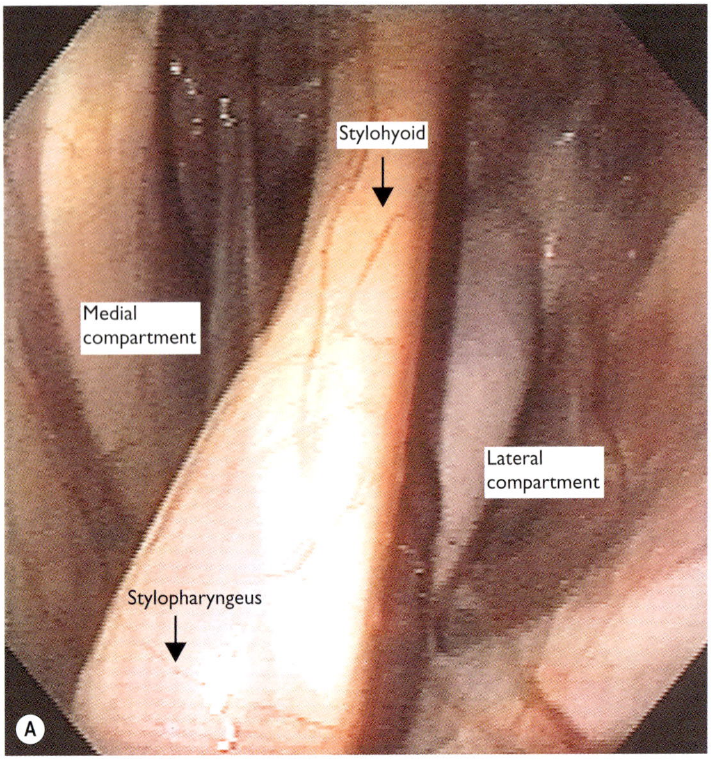

Fig 25.13A Endoscopic image of the origin of the stylopharyngeus muscle on the axial aspect of the stylohyoid bone within the guttural pouch.

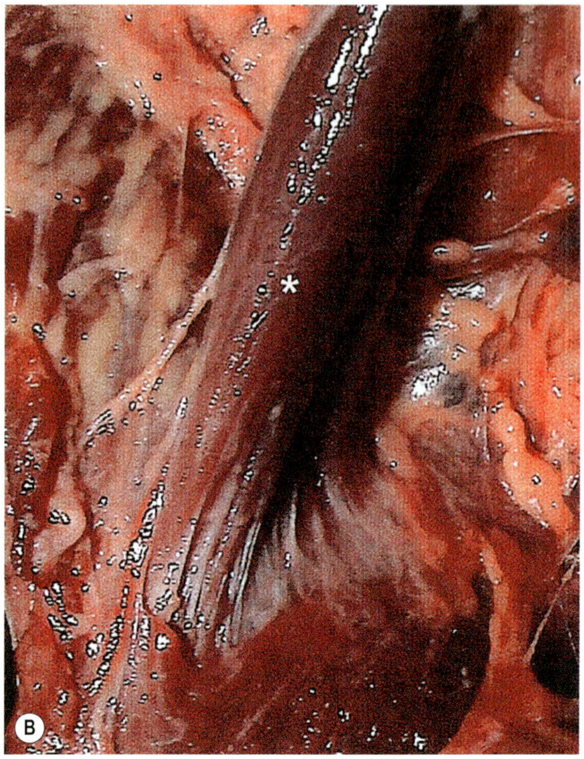

Fig 25.13B Post mortem dissected specimen showing the stylopharyngeus muscle inserting between the pterygopharyngeus and palatopharyngeus muscles.

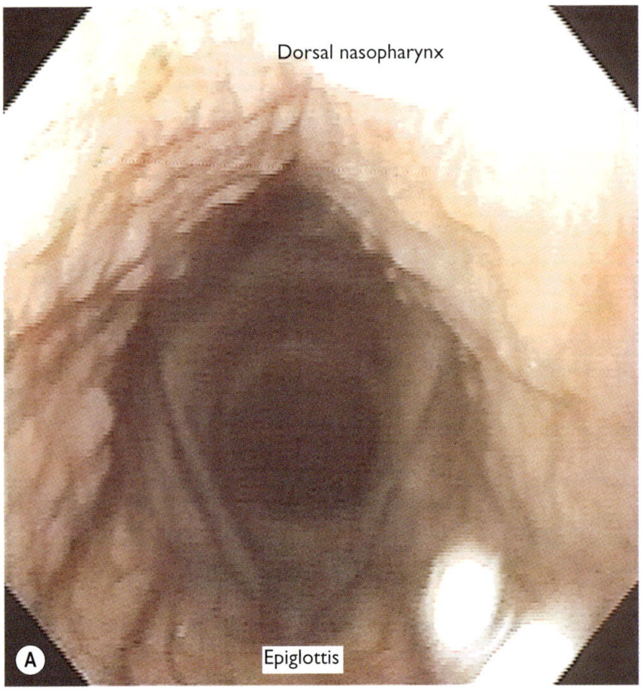

Fig 25.14A Endoscopic image of the nasopharynx following bilateral glossopharyngeal anesthesia with the nares occluded. Notice how the dorsal nasopharynx collapses.

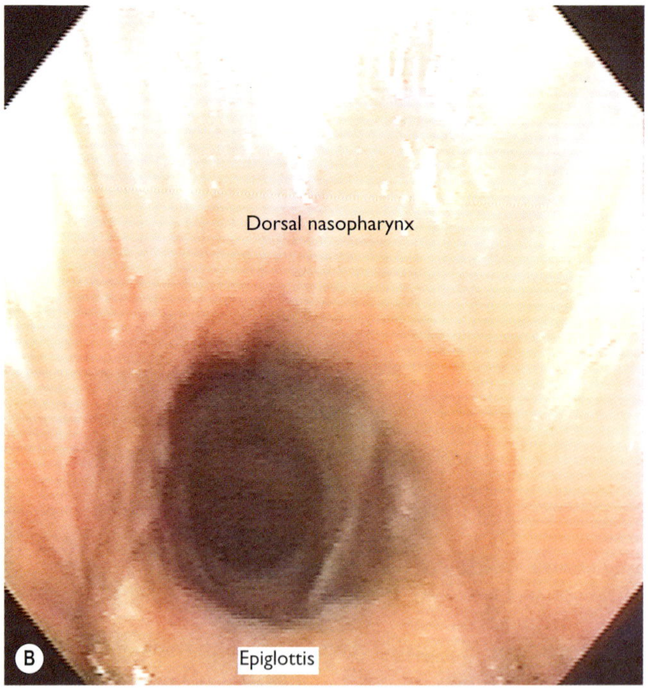

Fig 25.14B Endoscopic image of the nasopharynx following bilateral glossopharyngeal nerve anesthesia during treadmill exercise (12 m/s). Notice how the dorsal nasopharynx collapses, obstructing the view of the corniculate processes.

dorsal pharyngeal collapse both during nasal occlusion and exercise, and airway obstruction in horses (Fig. 25.14A and Fig. 25.14B).[110] Therefore, the stylopharyngeus muscle is an important nasopharyngeal dilating muscle in horses and dysfunction of this muscle may be implicated in clinical cases of dorsal nasopharyngeal collapse.[110]

The larynx

The larynx forms the communicating channel between the pharynx and the trachea and functions during breathing, vocalization, and deglutition. The larynx is composed of cartilage and muscle and is covered with a mucous membrane. The laryngeal cartilages include the cricoid, thyroid, and epiglottic cartilages, which are unpaired, and the arytenoid cartilages, which are paired.[84] The cricoid cartilage is shaped like a signet ring and is positioned rostral to the first tracheal ring and connected to the trachea by the cricotracheal membrane. The thyroid cartilage is the largest of the laryngeal cartilages and is situated just rostral to the cricoid cartilage.[84] The arytenoid cartilages form the dorsal border of the rima glottidis. They are triangular in shape with a dorsal muscular process, which serves as the origin for the cricoarytenoideus dorsalis muscle, a ventral vocal process serving as the attachment of the vocal ligament, and the rostral apex which forms the corniculate process.[84] The arytenoid cartilages are positioned on either side of the cricoid cartilage and are connected to it by the cricoarytenoid articulations. The articulation is a diarthrodial joint that allows the arytenoid cartilage to rotate dorso-laterally during abduction and axially during adduction.[84] The mucous membrane covering the epiglottic cartilage reflects off the lateral border of the epiglottis and blends with the mucous membrane covering the corniculate processes of the arytenoid cartilages, forming the aryepiglottic folds. The mucous membrane covers the vocal ligament, forms the vocal folds, and lines the lateral ventricles, forming the laryngeal saccules (Fig. 25.15). These saccules are 2.5 cm deep with a capacity of 5–6 ml. They extend between the medial surface of the thyroid cartilage and the ventricularis and vocalis muscles. At maximal arytenoid abduction, the cross-sectional area of the *rima glottidis* is approximately 2030 mm^2 which is 7% greater than the cross-sectional area of the trachea.[35] This is more than one order of magnitude greater than the cross-sectional area of the human *rima glottidis* at 126 mm^2.[111] The aryepiglottic fold is a mucous membrane that extends from the lateral aspect of the arytenoid cartilages to the ventrolateral aspect of the epiglottis, where it blends with the subepiglottic mucosa. The ventral aspect of the larynx is lined by epithelium with long cilia.[18]

The intrinsic laryngeal muscles produce changes in caliber of the rima glottidis by abducting and adducting the corniculate processes of the arytenoid cartilages and the vocal folds and hence, altering airway resistance. These actions are accomplished by the contractions of the intrinsic laryngeal muscles. The cricoarytenoideus dorsalis is the principal abductor muscle that widens the laryngeal aperture by abducting the corniculate process of the arytenoid cartilage and tensing the vocal folds. The thyroarytenoideus, arytenoideus transversus, and the cricoarytenoideus lateralis muscles adduct the corniculate processes of the arytenoid cartilages, narrowing the rima glottidis and protecting the lower airway during swallowing.[84,112–116] The cricothyroideus muscle receives efferent motor innervation from the external branch of the superior laryngeal nerve, a branch of the vagus nerve. All other intrinsic laryngeal muscles receive motor innervation from the recurrent laryngeal nerve, which is also a branch of the vagus nerve).[84,112,117,118] The left recurrent laryngeal nerve is the longest motor neuron

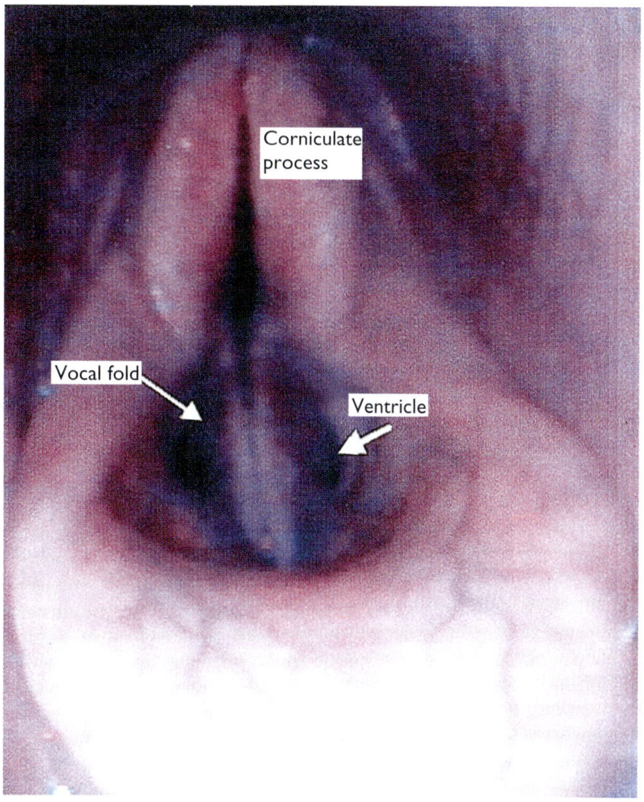

Fig 25.15 Endoscopic image of the larynx during adduction.

in the horse[119–121] with a reported length of between 212 and 250 cm.[118–121] The difference between the left and right RLn can range from 25–30 cm.[118,120,122,123] The RLn provides unilateral motor innervation with no evidence of cross-over motor supply.[118,123] At the caudal boarder of the cricoid cartilage the RLn splits into two branches to innervate the different intrinsic muscles of the larynx.[123]

The epiglottis is principally composed of elastic cartilage and rests on the dorsal surface of the body of the thyroid cartilage and is held there by the thyroepiglottic ligaments. The position of the epiglottis is controlled by the position of the larynx, and hyoid apparatus, and by contraction of the hyoepiglotticus muscle, which is the only muscle that attaches to the epiglottis.[84] The hyoepiglotticus is a bilobed extrinsic laryngeal muscle that originates on the basihyoid bone in horses, and inserts on the ventral body of the epiglottis.[84] In horses, contraction of the hyoepiglotticus muscle pulls the epiglottis toward the basihyoid bone, depressing it against the soft palate, enlarging the airway.[61] The hyoepiglotticus muscle has respiratory-related electromyographic activity in horses that increases with exercise intensity and breathing effort.[61] Furthermore, electrical stimulation of the hyoepiglotticus muscle depresses the epiglottis ventrally against the soft palate, changing the conformation of the epiglottis in some horses (Fig. 25.16A and Fig. 25.16B).[61] The hyoepiglotticus muscle is likely an upper airway dilating muscle, which functions to enlarge the airway, thereby decreasing airway resistance in exercising horses. In addition to dilating the aditus laryngis, contraction of the hyoepiglotticus muscle stabilizes the epiglottis during inspiration, preventing its prolapse through the rima glottidis. Retroversion of the epiglottis is described clinically in exercising horses and can be created experimentally by anesthesia of the hypoglossal nerves.[96,124]

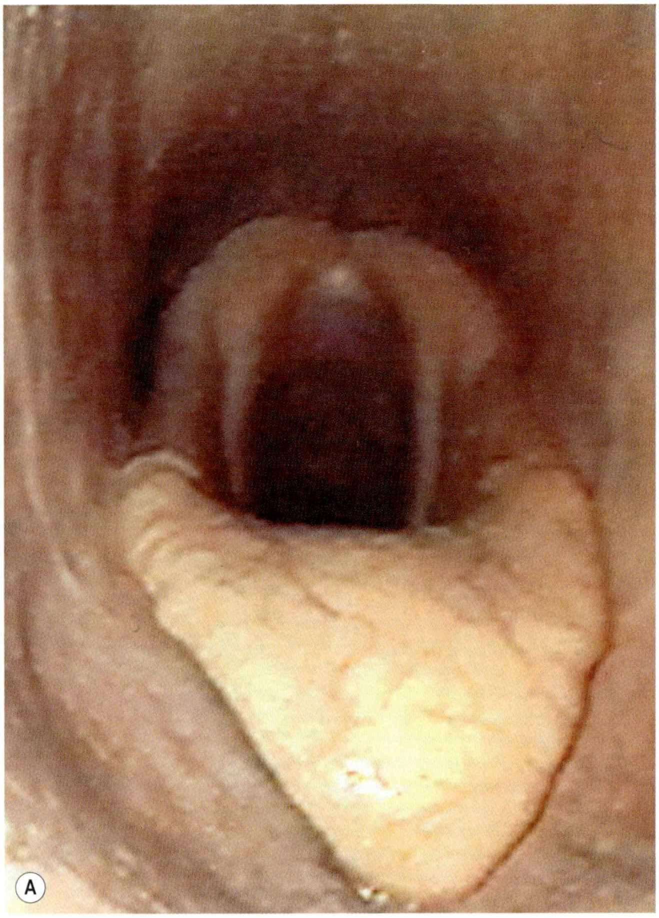

Fig 25.16A Endoscopic image of the larynx.

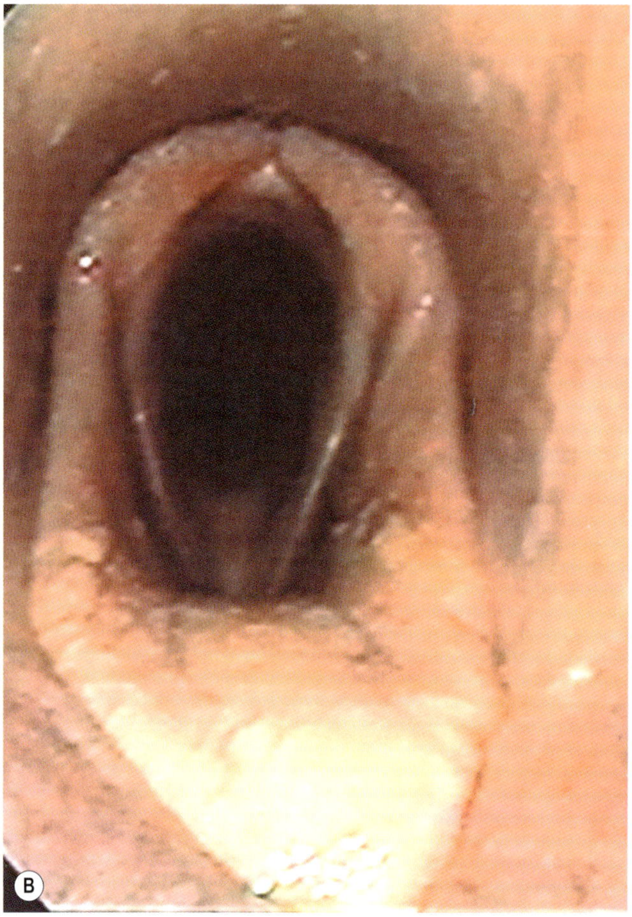

Fig 25.16B Endoscopic image of the same larynx during electrical stimulation of the hyoepiglotticus muscle.

Blockade of these nerves creates hyoepiglotticus dysfunction, and dysfunction of other hyoid muscles including geniohyoideus and genioglossus, and suggests that the clinical problem may be due to paresis of the hyoepiglotticus muscle or other muscles involved in controlling the position of the basihyoid. Active control of epiglottis position by the hyoepiglotticus muscle apparently stabilizes the epiglottis and vigorous recruitment of the muscle activity during inhalation dilates the airway and maintains the nasal breathing route in horses during intense exercise. Conformational changes in the epiglottis that occur during exercise, respiratory stimulation, sedation, or nasal occlusion may not be abnormal, but may be the result of normal activity of the hyoepiglotticus muscle.

Guttural pouches

Physiology

The guttural pouch, or diverticulum of the auditory tube, is unique to the horse and other Perissodactyla. Each pouch has a volume of 300–500 mL and communicates with the nasopharynx through the pharyngeal opening of the auditory tube. The guttural pouch is lined with a thin mucous membrane comprised of pseudostratified, ciliated epithelium interspersed with goblet cells.[125] Mucous glands and lymphatic nodules are found deep to the epithelial layer. Various immunoglobulin isotypes, including IgGa, IgM, and IgA have been detected in the guttural pouch mucosa, submucosa, and lymph nodules, suggesting that the guttural pouch has phylactic ability.[126] Some investigators have suggested that the pouches play a role in cooling the arterial supply to the brain [125] although others have discounted this explanation.[127] After swallowing the nasopharyngeal aperture opens and pressures within the guttural pouches equilibrate with the nasopharynx. Both at rest and during exercise the guttural pouch static pressures are similar to nasopharyngeal pressures, but slightly out of phase with the respiratory cycle.[128]

Anatomy

The openings of the guttural pouches are within the nasopharynx. The floor of the pouches forms the dorsal aspect of the nasopharynx, and the caudal extent of the guttural pouch is at the level of the parotid salivary glands. The guttural pouches are bordered dorsally by the base of the skull and the atlas, ventrally by the nasopharynx and rostral esophagus, medially by the longus capitus muscle, the rectus capitus ventralis muscle and the median septum, and laterally by many blood vessels and muscles, including the digastric muscles. Retropharyngeal lymph nodes can be identified beneath

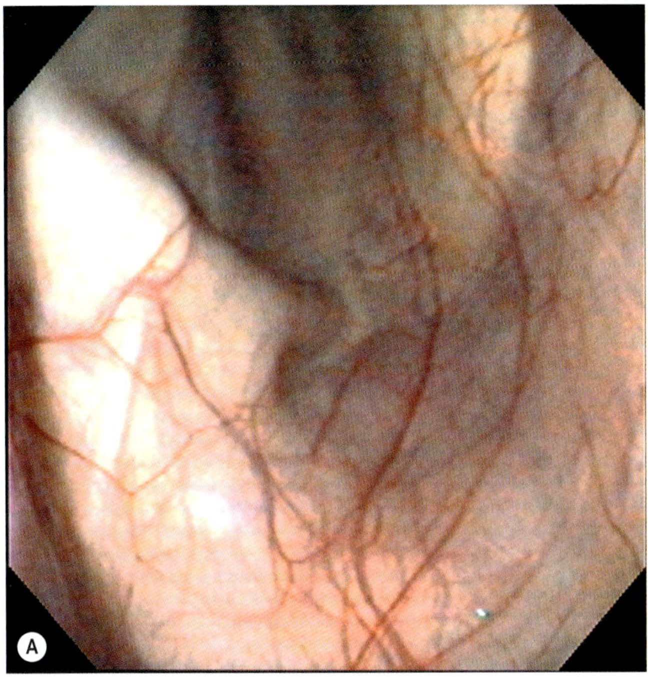

Fig 25.17A Endoscopic image of the ventral medial compartment of the guttural pouch.

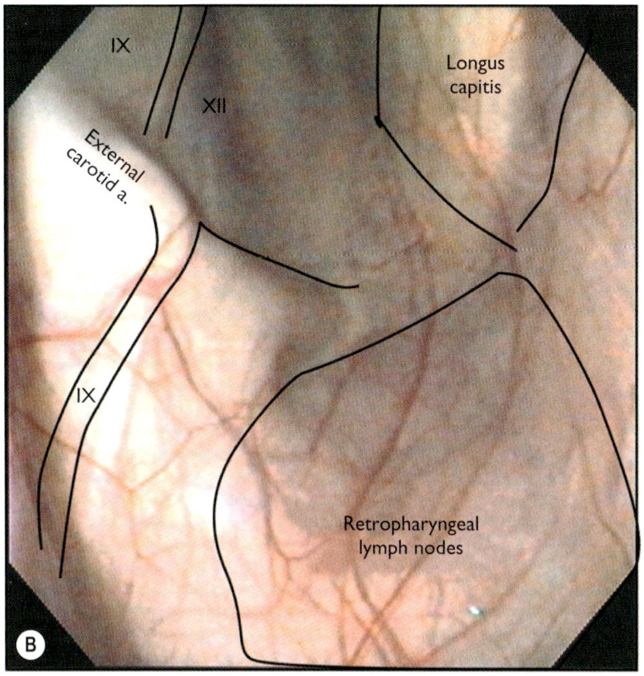

Fig 25.17B Endoscopic image of the ventral medial compartment of the guttural pouch with figure legends. Notice how IX (glossopharyngeal nerve) and XII (hypoglossal nerve) course together, caudal to the external carotid artery. XII dives deep to the external carotid artery, and IX travels across the external carotid artery, rostrally in the guttural pouch. a = artery.

the guttural pouch membrane on the floor of the medial compartment (Fig. 25.17 A and B).

The guttural pouch is divided into medial and lateral compartments by the stylohyoid bone. The caudal portion of the stylohyoid bone articulates with the petrous temporal bone at the base of the skull (Fig. 25.18). Cranial nerves VII (facial) and VIII (vestibulocochlear) exit the cranium near this articulation. The opening from the middle ear into the guttural pouch is with the dorsolateral compartment, near the articulation of the stylohyoid and petrous temporal bones. The medial compartment is approximately twice as large as the lateral compartment and cranial nerves IX (glossopharyngeal), X (vagus), XI (accessory),and XII (hypoglossal), the sympathetic trunk, the cranial cervical ganglion, and the internal carotid artery lie beneath the lining of the medial compartment (Fig. 25.19 A and B and Fig. 25.20 A and B) Cranial nerve X, the sympathetic trunk, and the cranial cervical ganglion are closely associated with the internal carotid artery. The pharyngeal branch of X is given off near the cranial cervical ganglion and can be seen as it runs rostroventrally in the guttural pouch toward the wall of the dorsal pharynx, where it ramifies with the pharyngeal branch of IX in the pharyngeal plexus. The pharyngeal branch of IX can be identified as it runs rostrally across the ventral aspect of the stylohyoid bone (Fig. 25.21). The maxillary artery is a continuation of the external carotid artery, beyond the origin of the superficial temporal artery, and runs dorsally in the lateral compartment of the guttural pouch. The maxillary vein can be seen lateral to and slightly deep to the external carotid artery. A portion of the digastric muscle can be seen along the ventrolateral wall of the lateral compartment (Fig. 25.22 A and B). The levator veli palatini and the tensor veli palatini muscles arise, partially, from the lateral lamina of the auditory tube, and can be seen within the pouch, as they pass rostrally and ventrally along the lateral lamina, the wall of the nasopharynx, to the soft palate. At the most caudal aspect of the guttural pouch, the occipital condyle can be seen.

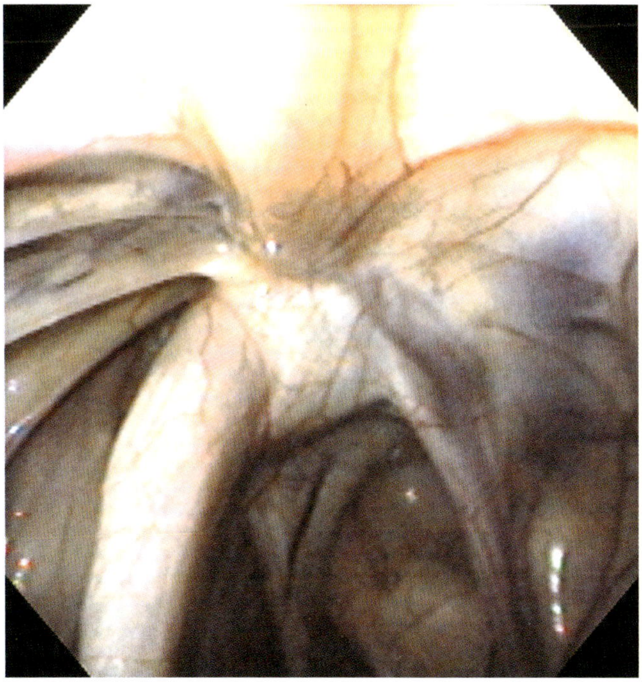

Fig 25.18 Endoscopic image of the dorsal portion of the guttural pouch and stylohyoid/petrous temporal bone articulation.

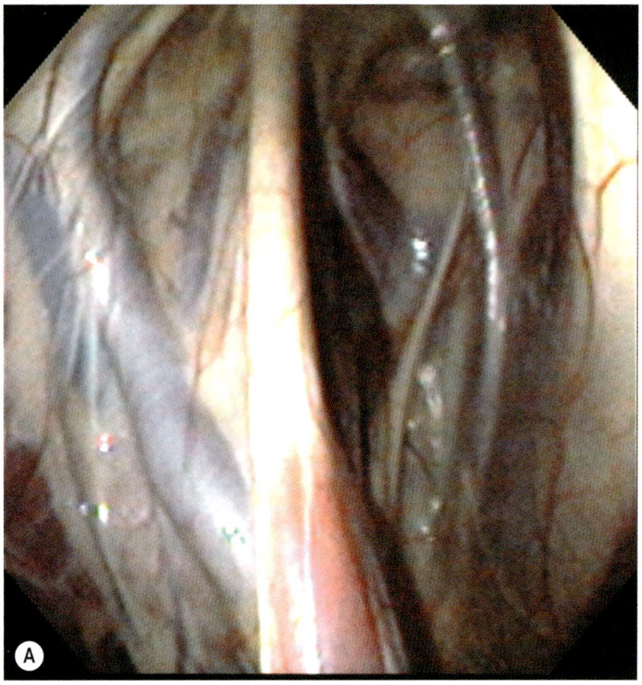

Fig 25.19A Endoscopic image of the medial and lateral compartments of the right guttural pouch. The medial side is to the right of the image.

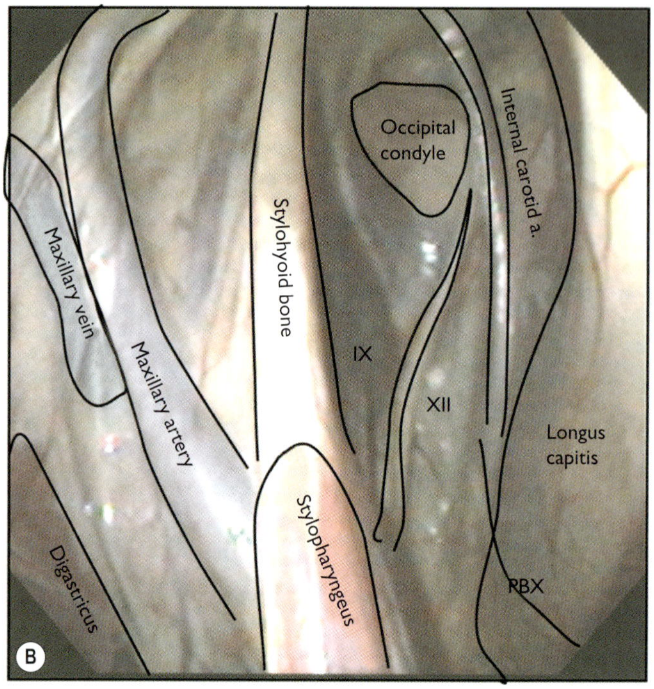

Fig 25.19B Endoscopic image of the medial and lateral compartments of the guttural pouch with figure legends. IX = glossopharyngeal nerve, XII = hypoglossal nerve, PB X = pharyngeal branch of the vagus nerve, a = artery.

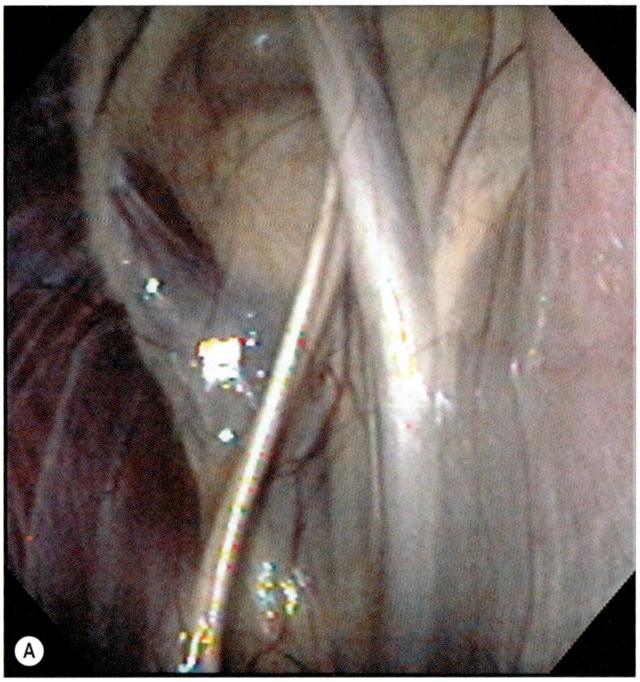

Fig 25.20A Medial compartment of the guttural pouch.

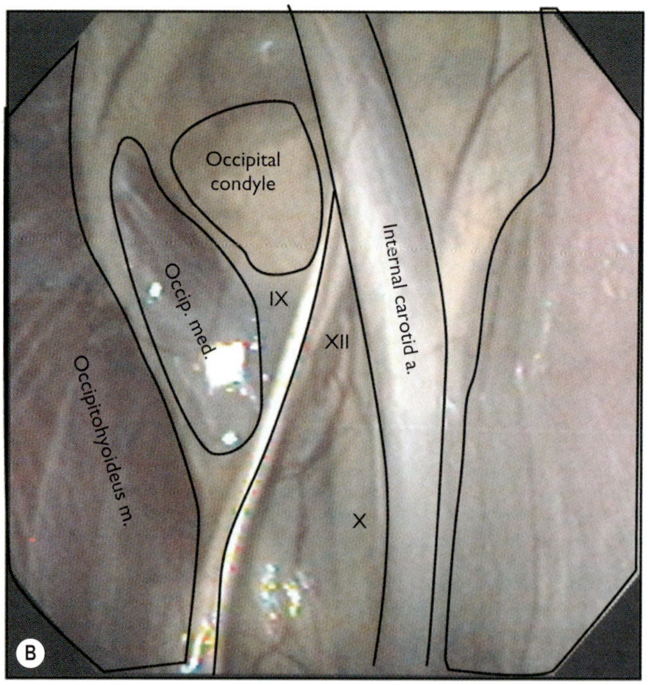

Fig 25.20B Medial compartment of the guttural pouch with figure legends. IX = glossopharyngeal nerve, XII = hypoglossal nerve, X = vagus nerve, a = artery, Occip. Med. = occipitohyoideus, medial belly.

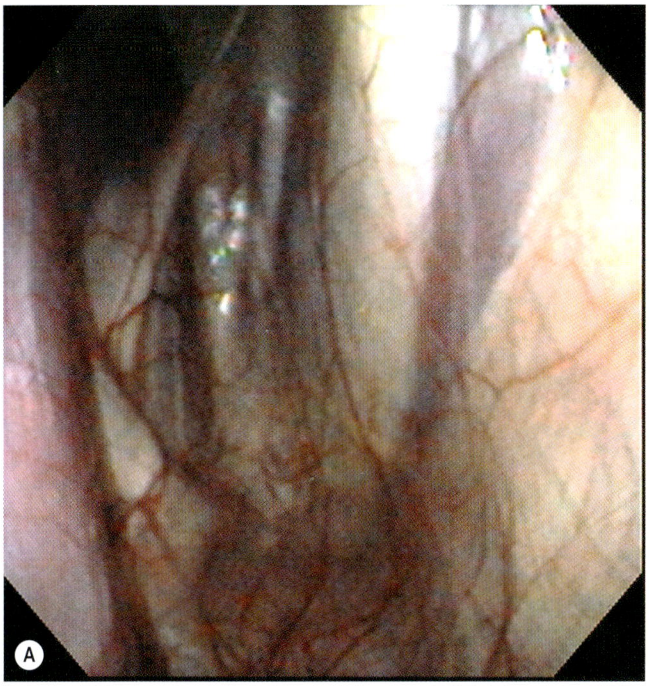

Fig 25.21A Ventral medial compartment of the right guttural pouch. The medial side is to the right of the image.

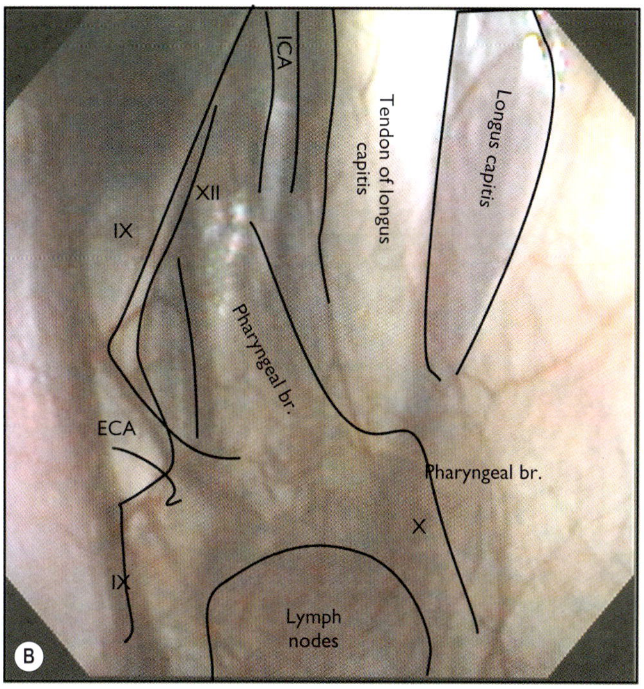

Fig 25.21B Ventral medial compartment of the guttural pouch with figure legends. ICA = internal carotid artery, IX = glossopharyngeal nerve, XII = hypoglossal nerve, ECA = external carotid artery, Pharyngeal br. X = pharyngeal branch of the vagus nerve, Pharyngeal br. IX = pharyngeal branch of the glossopharyngeal nerve.

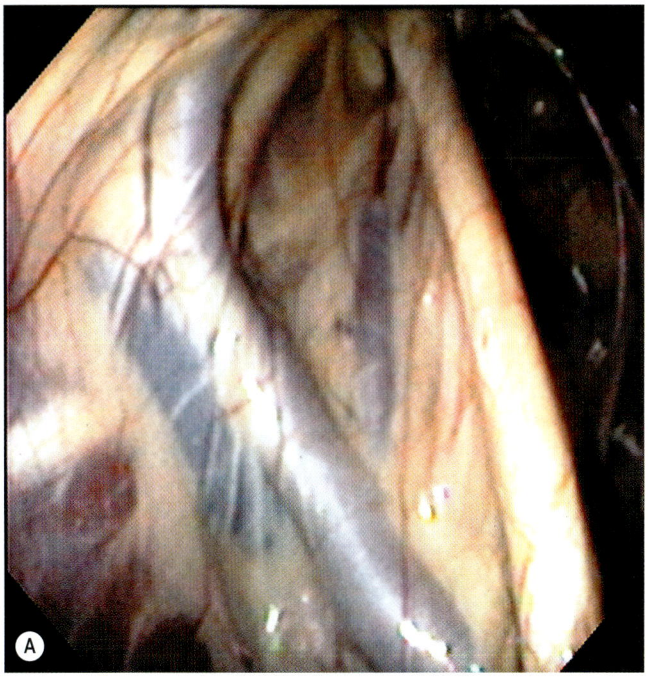

Fig 25.22A Lateral compartment of the right guttural pouch. The medial side is to the right of the image.

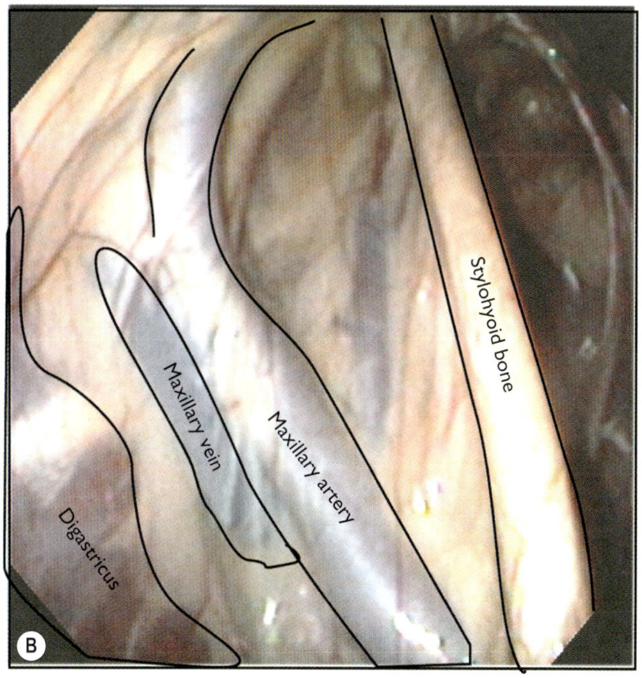

Fig 25.22B Lateral compartment of the guttural pouch with figure legends.

References

1. Morris E. Application of clinical exercise testing for identification of respiratory fitness and disease in the equine athlete. Vet Clin North Am Equine Pract 1991;7(2): 383–401.
2. Weber JM, Dobson GP, Parkhouse WS, et al. Cardiac output and oxygen consumption in exercising Thoroughbred horses. Am J Physiol 1987;253(6 Pt 2):R890–5.
3. Taylor CR, Maloiy GM, Weibel ER, et al. Design of the mammalian respiratory system. III Scaling maximum aerobic capacity to body mass: wild and domestic mammals. Respir Physiol 1981; 44(1):25–37.
4. Butler PJ, Woakes AJ, Smale K, et al. Respiratory and cardiovascular adjustments during exercise of increasing intensity and during recovery in thoroughbred racehorses. J Exp Biol 1993;179:159–80.
5. Seeherman HJ, Taylor CR, Maloiy GM, et al. Design of the mammalian respiratory system. II. Measuring maximum aerobic capacity. Respir Physiol 1981;44(1):11–23.
6. Eaton MD, Evans DL, Hodgson DR, et al. Effect of treadmill incline and speed on metabolic rate during exercise in thoroughbred horses. J Appl Physiol 1995;79(3):951–7.
7. Evans DL, Rose RJ. Cardiovascular and respiratory responses to submaximal exercise training in the thoroughbred horse. Pflugers Arch 1988;411(3): 316–21.
8. Hoyt DF, Taylor CR. Gait and the energetics of locomotion in horses. Nature 1981;292:239–40.
9. Robinson NE, Sorenson PR. Pathophysiology of airway obstruction in horses: a review. J Am Vet Med Assoc 1978;172(3):299–303.
10. Olson LG, Strohl KP. The response of the nasal airway to exercise. Am Rev Respir Dis 1987;135(2):356–9.
11. Negus VE. The Function of the Epiglottis. J Anat 1927;62(Pt 1): 1–8.
12. Holcombe SJ, Derksen FJ, Stick JA, et al. Effect of bilateral blockade of the pharyngeal branch of the vagus nerve on soft palate function in horses. Am J Vet Res 1998;59(4):504–8.
13. Pigott JH, Ducharme NG, Mitchell LM, et al. Incidence of swallowing during exercise in horses with dorsal displacement of the soft palate. Equine Vet J 2010;38(5):393–9.
14. Cheetham J, Pigott JH, Thorson LM, et al. Racing performance following the laryngeal tie-forward procedure: a case-controlled study. Equine Vet J 2008;40(5):501–7.
15. Attenburrow DP. Time relationship between the respiratory cycle and limb cycle in the horse. Equine Vet J 1982;14(1):69–72.
16. Koterba AM, Kosch PC, Beech J, et al. Breathing strategy of the adult horse (*Equus caballus*) at rest. J Appl Physiol 1988;64(1):337–46.
17. McCutcheon FH. The mammalian breathing mechanism. J Cell Physiol 1951;37(3):447–76.
18. Pirie M, Pirie HM, Wright NG. A scanning electron microscopic study of the equine upper respiratory tract. Equine Vet J 1990;22(5):333–7.
19. Lekeux P, Art T. The respiratory system: anatomy, physiology, and adaptations to exercise and training. In: Hodgson DR, Rose RJ, editors. The Athletic Horse: Principles and Practice of Equine Sports Medicine. 1st ed. Philadelphia: W.B. Saunders; 1994. p. 79–127.
20. Young IS, Alexander R, Woakes AJ, et al. The synchronization of ventilation and locomotion in horses (Equus caballus). J Exp Biol 1992;166:19–31.
21. Bramble DM, Carrier DR. Running and breathing in mammals. Science 1983;219(4582):251–6.
22. Ainsworth DM, Eicker SW, Nalevanko ME, et al. The effect of exercise on diaphragmatic activation in horses. Respir Physiol 1996;106(1):35–46.
23. Parks CM, Manohar M. Distribution of blood flow during moderate and strenuous exercise in ponies (Equus caballus). Am J Vet Res 1983;44(10): 1861–6.
24. Gutting SM, Forster HV, Lowry TF, et al. Respiratory muscle recruitment in awake ponies during exercise and CO2 inhalation. Respir Physiol 1991;86(3): 315–32.
25. Marlin DJ, Schrotert RC, Cashman PM, et al. Movements of thoracic and abdominal compartments during ventilation at rest and during exercise. Equine Vet J Suppl 2002;34(34):384–90.
26. Attenburrow DP. Respiratory sounds recorded by radio-stethoscope from normal horses at exercise. Equine Vet J 1978;10(3):176–9.
27. Jolly S, Art T, Lekeux P. Transient respiration locomotion decoupling in galloping Thoroughbreds. Equine Vet J Suppl 1995;18:13–14–17.
28. Ducharme NG, Hackett RP, Ainsworth DM, et al. Repeatability and normal values for measurement of pharyngeal and tracheal pressures in exercising horses. Am J Vet Res 1994;55(3): 368–74.
29. Radcliffe CH, Woodie JB, Hackett RP, et al. A comparison of laryngoplasty and modified partial arytenoidectomy as treatments for laryngeal hemiplegia in exercising horses. Vet Surg 2006; 35(7):643–52.
30. Tetens J, Derksen FJ, Stick JA, et al. Efficacy of prosthetic laryngoplasty with and without bilateral ventriculocordectomy as treatments for laryngeal hemiplegia in horses. Am J Vet Res 1996;57(11):1668–73.
31. Connally BA, Derksen FJ. Tidal breathing flow-volume loop analysis as a test of pulmonary function in exercising horses. Am J Vet Res 1994;55(5):589–94.
32. Rehder RS, Ducharme NG, Hackett RP, et al. Measurement of upper airway pressures in exercising horses with dorsal displacement of the soft palate. Am J Vet Res 1995;56(3): 269–74.
33. Ducharme NG, Hackett RP, Gleed RD, et al. Pulmonary capillary pressure in horses undergoing alteration of pleural pressure by imposition of various upper airway resistive loads. Equine Vet J Suppl 1999;30:27–33.
34. Rakesh V, Datta AK, Ducharme NG, et al. Simulation of turbulent airflow using a CT based upper airway model of a racehorse. J Biomech Eng 2008; 130(031011).
35. Rakesh V, Rakesh NG, Datta AK, et al. Development of equine upper airway fluid mechanics model for Thoroughbred racehorses. Equine Vet J 2008;40(3):272–9.
36. Nielan GJ, Rehder RS, Ducharme NG, et al. Measurement of tracheal static pressure in exercising horses. Vet Surg 1992;21(6):423–8.
37. Reynolds O. An Experimental Investigation of the Circumstances Which Determine Whether the Motion of Water Shall Be Direct or Sinuous, and of the Law of Resistance in Parallel Channels. Philos Trans R Soc Lond 1883;174:935–82.
38. Young DF. Fluid mechanics of arterial stenoses. J Biomech Eng 1979;101: 157–75.
39. Art T, Serteyn D, Lekeux P. Effect of exercise on the partitioning of equine respiratory resistance. Equine Vet J 1988;20(4):268–73.
40. Shappell KK, Derksen FJ, Stick JA, et al. Effects of ventriculectomy, prosthetic laryngoplasty, and exercise on upper airway function in horses with induced left laryngeal hemiplegia. Am J Vet Res 1988;49(10): 1760–5.
41. Holcombe SJ, Beard WL, Hinchcliff KW. Effect of a mask and pneumotachograph on tracheal and nasopharyngeal pressures, respiratory frequency, and ventilation

in horses. Am J Vet Res 1996;57(3): 250–3.

42. Petsche VM, Derksen FJ, Berney CE, et al. Effect of head position on upper airway function in exercising horses. Equine Vet J 1995;18:18–19–22.
43. Krogh A, Lindhard J. The regulation of respiration and circulation during the initial stages of muscular work. J Physiol 1913;47(1–2):112–36.
44. Sullivan J, Fuller D, Fregosi RF. Control of nasal dilator muscle activities during exercise: role of nasopharyngeal afferents. J Appl Physiol 1996;80(5): 1520–7.
45. Van der Touw T, O'Neill N, Amis T, et al. Soft palate muscle activity in response to hypoxic hypercapnia. J Appl Physiol 1994;77(6):2600–5.
46. Bartlett D Jr. Effects of hypercapnia and hypoxia on laryngeal resistance to airflow. Respir Physiol 1979;37(3): 293–302.
47. Van der Touw T, O'Neill N, Brancatisano A, et al. Respiratory-related activity of soft palate muscles: augmentation by negative upper airway pressure. J Appl Physiol 1994;76(1): 424–32.
48. Wheatley JR, Tangel DJ, Mezzanotte WS, et al. Influence of sleep on response to negative airway pressure of tensor palatini muscle and retropalatal airway. J Appl Physiol 1993;75(5): 2117–24.
49. Horner RL, Innes JA, Murphy K, et al. Evidence for reflex upper airway dilator muscle activation by sudden negative airway pressure in man. J Physiol 1991;436:15–29.
50. van Lunteren E, Van de Graaff WB, Parker DM, et al. Nasal and laryngeal reflex responses to negative upper airway pressure. J Appl Physiol 1984;56(3):746–52.
51. Sant'Ambrogio G, Mathew OP, Fisher JT, et al. Laryngeal receptors responding to transmural pressure, airflow and local muscle activity. Respir Physiol 1983; 54(3):317–30.
52. Bartlett D Jr. Respiratory functions of the larynx. Physiol Rev 1989;69(1): 33–57.
53. Sampson S, Eyzaguirre C. Some Functional Characteristics of Mechanoreceptors in the Larynx of the Cat. J Neurophysiol 1964;27:464–80.
54. Mathew OP, Farber JP. Effect of upper airway negative pressure on respiratory timing. Respir Physiol 1983;54(2): 259–68.
55. Mathew OP, Sant'Ambrogio G, Fisher JT, et al. Respiratory afferent activity in the superior laryngeal nerves. Respir Physiol 1984;58(1):41–50.
56. Mathew OP, Sant'Ambrogio G, Fisher JT, et al. Laryngeal pressure receptors. Respir Physiol 1984;57(1):113–22.
57. Mechanoreceptor stimulation in horses. Proceedings of the World Equine Airway Symposium Guelph, ON CANADA; 1998; Aug.
58. Konig HE, Liebich HG. Respiratory system (apparatus respiratorius). In: Konig HE, Liebich HG, editors. Veterinary Anatomy of Domestic Animals. 2nd ed. Stuttgart, Germany: Schattauer GmbH; 2004. p. 343–64.
59. Mathew OP. Upper airway negative-pressure effects on respiratory activity of upper airway muscles. J Appl Physiol 1984;56(2):500–5.
60. Mathew OP, Abu-Osba YK, Thach BT. Influence of upper airway pressure changes on genioglossus muscle respiratory activity. J Appl Physiol 1982;52(2):438–44.
61. Holcombe SJ, Cornelisse CJ, Berney C, et al. Electromyographic activity of the hyoepiglotticus muscle and control of epiglottis position in horses. Am J Vet Res 2002;63(12): 1617–21.
62. Holcombe SJ, Derksen FJ, Robinson NE. Electromyographic activity of the palatinus and palatopharyngeus muscles in exercising horses. Equine Vet J 2007;39(5):451–5.
63. The function of the extrinsic and intrinsic musculature in stabilizing the upper airways. 2nd ed. Edinburgh, Scotland: World Equine Airway Society; 2001.
64. Holcombe SJ, Derksen FJ, Berney C, et al. Effect of topical anesthesia of the laryngeal mucosa on upper airway mechanics in exercising horses. Am J Vet Res 2001;62(11): 1706–10.
65. Holcombe SJ, Derksen FJ, Stick JA, et al. Effect of nasal occlusion on tracheal and pharyngeal pressures in horses. Am J Vet Res 1996;57(9): 1258–60.
66. Sisson S. Equine mycology. In: Getty R, editor. Sisson and Grossman' s The anatomy of the domestic animals, vols. 1 and 2. 5th ed. Philadelphia, USA: W.B. Saunders Company; 1975. p. 377–9.
67. Sisson S. Equine digestive system. In: Getty R, editor. Sisson and Grossman' s The anatomy of the domestic animals, vols. 1 and 2. 5th ed. Philadelphia, USA: W.B. Saunders Company; 1975. p. 454–97.
68. Brouillette RT, Thach BT. A neuromuscular mechanism maintaining extrathoracic airway patency. J Appl Physiol 1979;46(4):772–9.
69. Richardson LE, Wakley GK, Franklin SH. A quantitative study of the equine soft palate using histomorphometry. Vet J 2006;172(1):78–85.
70. Elad D, Liebenthal R, Wenig BL, et al. Analysis of air flow patterns in the human nose. Med Biol Eng Comput 1993;31(6):585–92.
71. Girardin M, Bilgen E, Arbour P. Experimental study of velocity fields in a human nasal fossa by laser anemometry. Ann Otol Rhinol Laryngol 1983;92(3 Pt 1):231–6.
72. Kuehn DP, Folkins JW, Cutting CB. Relationships between muscle activity and velar position. Cleft Palate J 1982;19(1):25–35.
73. Moon JB, Smith AE, Folkins JW, et al. Coordination of velopharyngeal muscle activity during positioning of the soft palate. Cleft Palate Craniofac J 1994; 31(1):45–55.
74. Baptiste K. Functional anatomy observations of the pharyngeal orifice of the equine guttural pouch (auditory tube diverticulum). Vet J 1997;153(3): 311–9.
75. Holcombe SJ, Derksen FJ, Stick JA, et al. Effect of bilateral tenectomy of the tensor veli palatini muscle on soft palate function in horses. Am J Vet Res 1997;58(3):317–21.
76. Trigos I, Ysunza A, Vargas D, et al. The San Venero Roselli pharyngoplasty: an electromyographic study of the palatopharyngeus muscle. Cleft Palate J 1988;25(4):385–8.
77. DeLahunta A. Veterinary neuroanatomy and clinical neurology. Philadelphia: WB Saunders; 1977.
78. Mayhew IG. Large animal neurology: a handbook for veterinary clinicians. Philadelphia: Lea and Febiger; 1989.
79. New thoughts on URT anatomy: Relevancy. Proc. 29th annual surgical forum: American College of Veterinary Surgeons; 2001.
80. Getty R. Equine osteology. In: Getty R, editor. Sisson and Grossman' s The anatomy of the domestic animals, vols. 1 and 2. 5th ed. Philadelphia, USA: W.B. Saunders Company; 1975. p. 336–40.
81. Van de Graaff WB, Gottfried SB, Mitra J, et al. Respiratory function of hyoid muscles and hyoid arch. J Appl Physiol 1984;57(1):197–204.
82. Fregosi RF, Fuller DD. Respiratory-related control of extrinsic tongue muscle activity. Respir Physiol 1997;110(2–3):295–306.
83. Hare WCD. General Respiratory System. In: Getty R, editor. Sisson and Grossman's The Anatomy of the Domestic Animals. 5th ed. Philadelphia, PA: W. B. Saunders Company; 1975. p. 113–44.
84. Sisson S. Equine respiratory system. In: Getty R, editor. Sisson and Grossman's The anatomy of the domestic animals, vols. 1 and 2. 5th ed. Philadelphia, USA: W.B. Saunders Company; 1975. p. 504–11.

85. Ludlow CL. Electrical neuromuscular stimulation in dysphagia: current status. Curr Opin Otolaryngol Head Neck Surg 2010;18(3):159–64.
86. Fuller DD, Williams JS, Janssen PL, et al. Effect of co-activation of tongue protrudor and retractor muscles on tongue movements and pharyngeal airflow mechanics in the rat. J Physiol 1999;519(Pt 2):601–13.
87. Brouillette RT, Thach BT. Control of genioglossus muscle inspiratory activity. J Appl Physiol 1980;49(5): 801–8.
88. Sisson S. Equine myology. In: Getty R, editor. Sisson and Grossman' s The anatomy of the domestic animals, vol. 1 and 2. 5th ed. Philadelphia, USA: W.B. Saunders Company; 1975. p. 386–7.
89. Chalmers HJ, Yeager AE, Ducharme NG. Ultrasonographic assessment of laryngohyoid position as a predictor of dorsal displacement of the soft palate in horses. Vet Radiol Ultrasound 2009; 50(1):91–6.
90. Young T, Palta M, Dempsey J, et al. The occurrence of sleep-disordered breathing among middle-aged adults. N Engl J Med 1993;328(17): 1230–5.
91. Shahar E, Whitney CW, Redline S, et al. Sleep-disordered breathing and cardiovascular disease: cross-sectional results of the Sleep Heart Health Study. Am J Respir Crit Care Med 2001;163(1): 19–25.
92. Riha RL, Brander P, Vennelle M, et al. A cephalometric comparison of patients with the sleep apnea/hypopnea syndrome and their siblings. Sleep 2005;28(3):315–20.
93. Sforza E, Bacon W, Weiss T, et al. Upper airway collapsibility and cephalometric variables in patients with obstructive sleep apnea. Am J Respir Crit Care Med 2000;161(2 Pt 1):347–52.
94. Eveloff SE, Rosenberg CL, Carlisle CC, et al. Efficacy of a Herbst mandibular advancement device in obstructive sleep apnea. Am J Respir Crit Care Med 1994;149(4 Pt 1):905–9.
95. Cheetham J, Pigott JH, Hermanson JW, et al. Role of the hypoglossal nerve in equine nasopharyngeal stability. J Appl Physiol 2009;107(2):471–7.
96. Holcombe SJ, Derksen FJ, Stick JA, et al. Effects of bilateral hypoglossal and glossopharyngeal nerve blocks on epiglottic and soft palate position in exercising horses. Am J Vet Res 1997;58(9):1022–6.
97. Parente EJ, Martin BB, Tulleners EP, et al. Dorsal displacement of the soft palate in 92 horses during high-speed treadmill examination (1993–1998). Vet Surg 2002;31(6):507–12.
98. Lane JG, Bladon B, Little DR, et al. Dynamic obstructions of the equine upper respiratory tract. Part 1: observations during high-speed treadmill endoscopy of 600 Thoroughbred racehorses. Equine Vet J 2006;38(5):393–9.
99. Franklin SH, Naylor JR, Lane JG. Effect of dorsal displacement of the soft palate on ventilation and airflow during high-intensity exercise. Equine Vet J Suppl 2002;34(34): 379–83.
100. Holcombe SJ, Beard WL, Hinchcliff KW, et al. Effect of sternothyrohyoid myectomy on upper airway mechanics in normal horses. J Appl Physiol 1994;77(6):2812–16.
101. Castro HA, Resende LA, Berzin F, et al. Electromyographic analysis of the superior belly of the omohyoid muscle and anterior belly of the digastric muscle in tongue and head movements. J Electromyogr Kinesiol 1999;9(3): 229–32.
102. Zertuche JML, Turner TA, Colahan PT. Strap muscle myectomy for treatment of idiopathic intermittent dorsal displacement of the soft palate in the racing Thoroughbred. Vet Surg 1990;19(1):82.
103. Ducharme NG, Hackett RP, Woodie JB, et al. Investigations into the role of the thyrohyoid muscles in the pathogenesis of dorsal displacement of the soft palate in horses. Equine Vet J 2003;35(3): 258–63.
104. Woodie JB, Ducharme NG, Kanter P, et al. Surgical advancement of the larynx (laryngeal tie-forward) as a treatment for dorsal displacement of the soft palate in horses: a prospective study 2001–2004. Equine Vet J 2005;37(5):418–23.
105. Kuna ST. Effects of pharyngeal muscle activation on airway size and configuration. Am J Respir Crit Care Med 2001;164(7):1236–41.
106. Kuna ST, Vanoye CR. Mechanical effects of pharyngeal constrictor activation on pharyngeal airway function. J Appl Physiol 1999;86(1):411–17.
107. Kuna ST, Smickley JS, Vanoye CR. Respiratory-related pharyngeal constrictor muscle activity in normal human adults. Am J Respir Crit Care Med 1997;155(6):1991–9.
108. Sisson S. Equine digestive system. In: Getty R, editor. Sisson and Grossman' s The anatomy of the domestic animals, vols. 1 and 2. 5th ed. Philadelphia, USA: W.B. Saunders Company; 1975. p. 475.
109. Feroah TR, Forster HV, Pan L, et al. Effect of slow wave and REM sleep on thyropharyngeus and stylopharyngeus activity during induced central apneas. Respir Physiol 2001;124(2):129–40.
110. Tessier C, Holcombe SJ, Derksen FJ, et al. Effects of stylopharyngeus muscle dysfunction on the nasopharynx in exercising horses. Equine Vet J 2004;36(4):318–23.
111. Brancatisano T, Collett PW, Engel LA. Respiratory movements of the vocal cords. J Appl Physiol 1983;54(5): 1269–76.
112. Duncan ID, Griffiths IR. Pathological changes in equine laryngeal muscles and nerves. Proceedings of the nineteenth annual convention of the American Association of Equine Practitioners. December 10th through 12th, 1973. 1974 1974:97–113.
113. Duncan ID, Reifenrath P, Jackson KF, et al. Preferential denervation of the adductor muscles of the equine larynx. II: Nerve pathology. Equine Vet J 1991;23(2):99–103.
114. Anderson LJ, Goulden BE, Munford RE. A study of the weights of some intrinsic laryngeal and palatine muscles in the thoroughbred horse. N Z Vet J 1980; 28(11):222–5.
115. Quinlan T, Goulden BE, Davies AS. Bilateral asymmetry of equine laryngeal muscles. N Z Vet J 1975; 23(7):145–7.
116. Rhee HS, Steel CM, Derksen FJ, et al. Immunohistochemical analysis of laryngeal muscles in normal horses and horses with subclinical recurrent laryngeal neuropathy. J Histochem Cytochem 2009;57(8):787–800.
117. Duncan ID, Griffths IR, McQueen A, et al. The pathology of equine laryngeal hemiplegia. Acta Neuropathol (Berl) 1974;27(4):337–48.
118. Cole CR. Changes in the equine larynx associated with laryngeal hemiplegia. Amer J Vet Res 1946;7:69–77.
119. Hackett MS. The equine nucleus ambiguus: myotopic and neurotopic representations of motor and sensory components of the recurrent laryngeal nerve. 2000.
120. Dixon P, Robinson E, Wade JF, editors. Development and innervation of the larynx. Proceedings of a Workshop on Equine Recurrent Laryngeal Neuropathy, 7–10 September, 2003.; September 7th–10th, 2003; Newmarket, UK: R & W Publications, Ltd.; 2004.
121. Hahn CN, Matiasek K, Dixon PM, et al. Histological and ultrastructural evidence that recurrent laryngeal neuropathy is a bilateral mononeuropathy limited to recurrent laryngeal nerves. Equine Vet J 2008;40(7):666–72.
122. Duncan ID, Griffiths IR, Madrid RE. A light and electron microscopic study of the neuropathy of equine idiopathic laryngeal hemiplegia. Neuropathol Appl Neurobiol 1978;4(6):483–501.
123. Quinlan TJ, Goulden BE, Barnes GR, et al. Innervation of the equine intrinsic laryngeal muscles. N Z Vet J 1982;30(4): 43–5.

124. Parente EJ, Martin BB, Tulleners EP. Epiglottic retroversion as a cause of upper airway obstruction in two horses. Equine Vet J 1998;30(3):270–2.

125. Baptiste KE, Naylor JM, Bailey J, et al. A function for guttural pouches in the horse. Nature 2000;403(6768): 382–3.

126. Manglai D, Wada R, Kurohmaru M, et al. Distribution of immunoglobulin isotypes and subisotypes in equine guttural pouch (auditory tube diverticulum). J Vet Med Sci 2000;62(9):1001–3.

127. Mitchell G, Fuller A, Maloney SK, et al. Guttural pouches, brain temperature and exercise in horses. Biol Lett 2006;2(3):475–7.

128. Rehder RS. Distribution of immunoglobulin isotypes and subisotypes in equine guttural pouch. MS Thesis, Cornell University; 1992.

129. Guyton AC, Hall JE. Chapter 27. Pulmonary Ventilation. In: Guyton AC, Hall JE, editors. Textbook of Medical Physiology. 11th ed. Philadelphia: Elsevier; 2006. p. 471–2–82.

130. Guyton AC, Hall JE. Chapter 84. Sports Physiology. In: Guyton AC, Hall J.E., editors. Textbook of Medical Physiology. 11th ed. Philadelphia: Elsevier; 2006. p. 1055–66.

Abnormalities of the upper airway

26

Norm G. Ducharme   Jon Cheetham

CHAPTER CONTENTS

Introduction

Upper airway obstructive diseases result in resistive breathing (an increase in resistance to passage of air through the upper airways) causing either an abnormal upper respiratory noise, exercise intolerance, or both. Upper airway resistive breathing limits the athletic performance by decreasing minute ventilation, exacerbating exercise-induced hypoxemia, and decreasing maximal oxygen consumption. While some obstructive diseases are static and evident at rest, many obstructive lesions are dynamic and only apparent during exercise. Furthermore, during exercise the coexistence of two or more forms of upper airway obstruction has been reported in 30 to 70% of horses.[1,2] This emphasizes the need for dynamic examination to obtain the full identification of all the upper airway abnormalities in a given horse. A proper assessment including a complete history, signalment, and physical examination, endoscopic examination of the upper airway, both at rest and during treadmill exercise, will establish the etiology of the airway obstruction. In addition to sound analysis, imaging modalities such as radiography, ultrasonography, computed tomography, and nuclear medicine can be valuable in diagnosing performance-limiting lesions of the upper airway.

Redundant alar folds (alar fold collapse)

- The alar fold is formed by a thick fold of skin and mucous membrane extending rostrad from the ventral nasal concha.[3]
- Redundant alar folds are a cause of abnormal respiratory noise. In some horses they are also a cause of exercise intolerance and respiratory noise in performance horses.[4,5] The prevalence has been reported to reach 9.6% in Standardbred racehorses.
- It is seen more commonly in Standardbreds but is also seen in others breeds such as coldblooded trotters and Thoroughbreds.[2,4]
- The diagnosis is made by manually holding the alar folds open during exercise testing, on treadmill exam or securing the alar folds dorsally to document decreased respiratory noise and improved exercise intolerance.[2,4]
- Treatment includes tying the alar folds out of the airway during exercise or alar fold resection.[4]
- Not all horses with alar fold collapse have airway obstruction and therefore improvement in the abnormal noise is not necessarily associated with improvement in performance.

Recognition

History and presenting complaint

Most horses with redundant alar folds make an expiratory fluttering noise during exercise and a smaller percentage might be exercise intolerant. Horses exhibit no clinical signs at rest.[2,4]

Physical examination

No abnormalities are apparent at rest.

Special examination

Other causes of respiratory noise and exercise intolerance should be eliminated by performing an endoscopic examination of the upper airway and evaluating both nasal passages. Confirmation that redundant alar folds are the cause of the airway noise is made by alleviating the abnormal noise by placing a temporary suture through the skin of each nostril, the alar folds, and tying it over the bridge of the nose while the horse exercises (Fig. 26.1).[4] The alar folds can also be held out of the nasal passage manually or with clips.[2] Because dorsal displacement of the soft palate is seen in association with this abnormality, dynamic endoscopic exam during exercise is also indicated.

Laboratory examination

None is indicated.

Diagnostic confirmation

Absence of noise and improved exercise tolerance during exercise with the alar folds secured out of the nasal passage confirms the diagnosis.[2,4] Differential diagnoses for alar fold collapse include obstructive airway diseases that cause exercise intolerance and abnormal respiratory noise during exercise (Table 26.1). Paralysis or paresis of the levator nasolabialis muscle associated with a tight nose band or caveson can allow collapse of the lateral wall of the nostril and could be confused with alar fold paralysis.

Treatment and prognosis

Therapeutic aims

The goal of treatment is to remove or secure the alar folds in an open position during exercise. This can be achieved by suturing the alar folds in an open (i.e. abducted) position during exercise, placement of a nasal insert, or surgically resecting the alar fold. The first two treatments are not permitted in all racing jurisdictions.

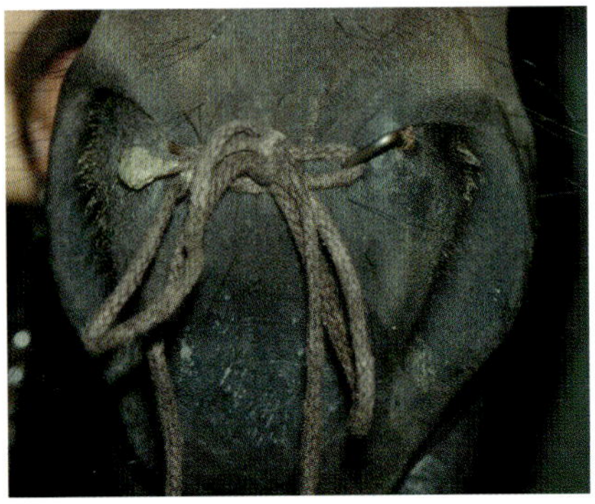

Fig 26.1 The nose of a horse with rings through the alar folds. The string is used to tie the rings together, pulling the alar fold out of the airway.

Therapy

The procedure is most commonly done under general anesthesia in dorsal recumbency or with the horse standing after a bilateral infraorbital nerve block. The alar fold is exposed by retracting or by incising the lateral wall of the nostril. To provide hemostasis in this vascular area, a Glassman intestinal clamp is placed on the dorsal section of the alar fold. Using a blade adjacent to the clamp, the dorsal part of the alar fold is excised, starting immediately caudal to the alar cartilage (Fig. 26.2) and extending caudally along the dorsal limit of the nasal cavity up to the 'V' shape junction of the incisive and nasal bones. At this time a simple continuous pattern uniting the nasal mucosa to the skin at the remnant of the alar fold is done. The Glassman clamp is then placed at the junction of the ventral limit of the alar fold to the ventro-lateral limit of the nasal cavity. A rostral-to-caudal incision completes the alar fold resection.[4] Usually, 1–2 cm of the cartilaginous portion of the ventral nasal concha is excised. The ventral nasal mucosa and the skin of the ventral nasal diverticulum is re-apposed as was done dorsally. If the lateral nasal ala is incised to expose the alar fold, it is closed in two layers.[4]

Prognosis

Reportedly, respiratory tract noise improves in 71% of horses following alar fold resection and 88% of horses race after surgery.[4] Horses with small nares and narrow nasal passages have a poorer prognosis for performance.[2,4] As mentioned earlier, alar fold flutters can result in an abnormal noise not necessarily an airway obstruction.

Prevention

There is generally no known prevention.

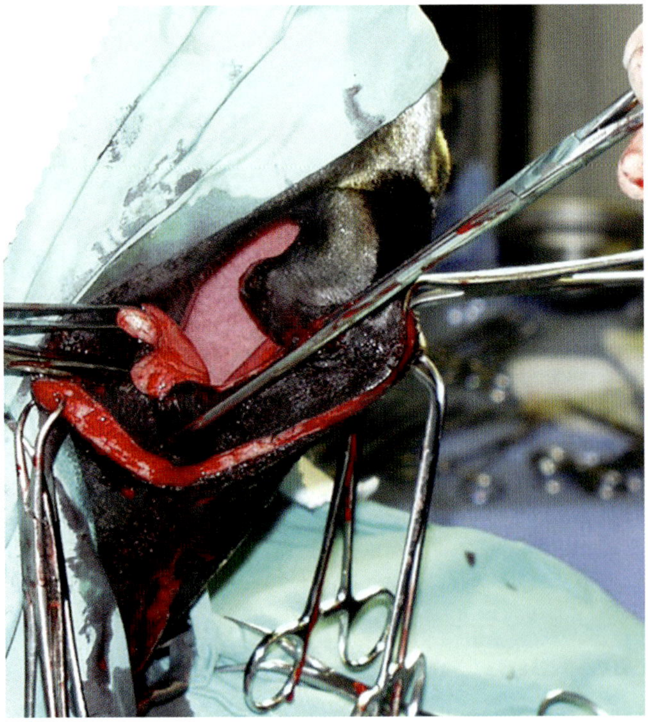

Fig 26.2 Intraoperative view of the left alar fold. The lateral wall of the nostril has been incised and a Glassman forceps is placed on the dorsal aspect of the alar fold.

Table 26.1 Upper airway mechanics measurements and blood gas variables in horses with obstructive upper airway diseases

DISEASE	Pao_2	$Paco_2$	TIP	TEP	Ziu	Zeu	IF	EF	RF	V_T	$\dot{V}_E$
Normal[132]	71.7 (1.6)	54.7 (1.9)	–42.9 (2.8)	9.2 (3.8)	0.53 (0.02)	0.14 (0.06)	80.4 (4.2)	66.6 (4.3)	84 (4)	22.2 (1.6)	1858 (109)
Normal[51]	75 (2.3)	55 (2.3)	–39 (3.3)	12 (1.4)	0.42 (0.05)	0.18 (0.02)	90 (5.2)	91 (4.1)	109 (11.7)	17.1 (1.7)	1690 (130)
Pharyngeal collapse[131]			–40.8 (4.4)	22.0 (6.6)	0.73 (0.02)	0.46 (0.19)	54.2 (4.0)	55.6 (4.1)	76 (4.0)	16.8	1159.4 (94.1)
DDSP[48]			–18.6 (7.6)	36.2 (11.3)	0.41 (0.11)	0.88 (0.38)	44.5 (9.0)	46.7 (10.4)	57 (9.8)	15 (3.31)	875.2 (114.5)
DDSP[51]	64 (3.6)	66 (4.9)	–29 (3.4)	35 (6.7)	0.33 (0.05)	0.66 (0.11)	66 (3.8)	69 (3.4)	98 (8.2)	13.6 (2.5)	1265 (315)
ILH[64]	53	58 (8.3)	–59.4	21.3 (0.47)	1.52	0.49 (9.0)	42.6	42.7 (9)	70		1106.5 (191.5)
Laryngoplasty + ventriculocordectomy[64]	83	39	–45.1 (8.4)		0.82 (0.14)		55.5 (5.0)		77 (20)		1211.5 (95.4)
Arytenoidectomy + ventriculectomy[88]			–40.0 (4.4)		0.81 (0.10)		48.0 (2.0)				1178.5 (38.6)
Epiglottic retroversion[60]			–35.7 (3.80)	13.3 (2.4)					58 (5)		

TIP, tracheal inspiratory pressure (cmH_2O): TEP, tracheal expiratory pressure (cmH_2O); Ziu, inspiratory impedance ($cmH_2O/L/s$); Zeu, expiratory impedance ($cmH_2O/L/s$); IF, peak inspiratory flow (L); EF, peak expiratory flow (L); RF, respiratory frequency (breaths/min); V_T, tidal volume (L); $\dot{V}_E$, minute ventilation (L/min); values in parentheses are standard error of the mean.

Etiology and pathophysiology

Etiology

The etiology of redundant alar folds is unknown, but might involve narrow nasal passages and inappropriate function of the transversus nasi muscles.

Pathophysiology

A thick fold of skin forms the alar fold and mucous membrane extending rostrad from the ventral nasal concha.[3] The space dorsal to the alar fold is the false nostril or diverticulum of the nostril while the true nostril that continues caudally to the nasal passage is ventral to the alar fold. When the nostril is dilated, the alar fold is tensed, obliterating the nasal diverticulum.[4] Excessive alar fold tissue or inappropriate nostril dilation can cause the alar fold to collapse across the nostril, causing airway obstruction and exercise intolerance during inhalation, and a fluttering noise during exhalation.

Epidemiology

Standardbred, Scandinavian coldblooded trotters, and American Saddlebreds might be predisposed to this condition.[2,4]

Mycotic rhinitis

- Rare fungal infection of the nasal cavity.
- Often due to *Aspergillus* spp.
- Diagnosis by endoscopy and laboratory identification of fungus.
- Treatment involves local debridement and topical application of antifungal agent

Recognition

History and presenting complaint

Mycotic rhinitis is rare in horses and occurs most frequently in warm, humid climates. The most common clinical signs include nasal discharge that can be foul smelling, sneezing, and intermittent epistaxis.[4,5,] Horses with nasal granulomas might make an abnormal respiratory noise during exercise and show signs of exercise intolerance. If the fungal infection is invasive and involves the paranasal sinuses, extension to the brain and meninges can occur, resulting in cerebral signs such as depression, dementia, ataxia, and recumbency.

Physical examination

Horses with mycotic rhinitis generally have nasal discharge that is malodorous, and if chronic, they can have alopecia along the ventral aspect of the affected naris.[4,6] If a nasal granuloma is causing airway obstruction, decreased airflow through the affected nostril is detected by holding the hands over each nostril.

Special examination

Endoscopic examination of the affected nasal passage reveals fungal plaques or granulomas affecting the mucocutaneous junction of the nostril, or mucous membrane of the nasal septum and concha.[4,5] Ulceration of the mucosa surrounding the plaque or granuloma can also be seen.[6] If the primary site of infection is the paranasal sinus region, exudate at the nasomaxillary opening within the middle meatus can be evident.

Laboratory examination

Laboratory tests are generally not warranted, but if the infection is chronic, hyperfibrinogenemia might be present.

Diagnostic confirmation

The diagnosis of fungal rhinitis is confirmed by biopsy and culture of the plaque or mass. Fungi that have been reported to cause mycotic rhinitis in horses include *Conidiobolus coronatus, Cryptococcus, Rhinosporidium, Aspergillus fumigatus* and *A. boydii, Coccidioides,* and *Pseudallescheria*.[4–9] The presence of septate hyphae or fungal mycelium on cytological examination is indicative of fungal infection.

Treatment and prognosis

Therapeutic aims

The goal of therapy is to eradicate the fungus from the nasal passage.

Therapy

Surgical debridement of granulomas and lesions followed by topical antifungal lesions have been reported to be effective in the treatment of mycotic rhinitis.[5]For example, *Aspergillus fumigatus* is sensitive to natamycin solution applied topically.[6] Nystatin can be added to the natamycin and used topically or intralesionally.[6] Topical and intralesional injection of amphotericin B and intravenous sodium iodide or oral potassium iodide has been used in the past to treat *Conidiobolus coronatus* infection, but recurrence has been reported.[7] Long-term systemic antifungal therapy has also been effective; oral itraconazole, 3 mg/kg, orally, twice daily, for 3.5–4 months also results in the resolution of *Aspergillus* sp. infection.[8] Alternatively a 1% solution of enilconazole applied topically twice daily for 7 days has been reported to be successful for the treatment of fungal rhinitis.[5]

Prognosis

Mycotic rhinitis due to *Aspergillus* sp. resolves with treatment and recurrence is low.[5,6] *Conidiobolus coronatus* resolves with surgical and medical treatment, but does recur.[7,8] *Cryptococcus* sp. is an invasive fungus that can infect the paranasal sinuses and invade the brain and meninges, and the prognosis is generally poor for resolution.[7,10]

Prevention

No method of prevention is known.

Etiology and pathophysiology

Etiology

Fungi isolated from the nasal cavity of affected horses include *Conidiobolus* spp., *Cryptococcus* spp., *Rhinosporidium, Aspergillus* spp., *Coccidioides,* and *Pseudallescheria.*

Pathophysiology

Inhalation of fungal spores and colonization of the nasal mucosa is the most likely route of infection, resulting in mycotic rhinitis.

Epidemiology

Mycotic rhinitis is rare (reported to represent less than 0.1% of all 21 160 admitted patients to a hospital[5]), but is most commonly seen in hot, humid climates, such as the southeastern USA and tropical areas.

Progressive ethmoid hematoma (PEH)

- Clinical signs include unilateral epistaxis and respiratory stridor.
- Endoscopy of the nasal passage and inspection of the ethmoid region demonstrate ethmoid hematoma.
- The diagnosis is confirmed by histopathology of the mass.
- Most ethmoid hematoma originate at the ethmoid turbinate, but can originate from any of the paranasal sinuses.
- Treatment options include surgical excision, either sharply or with a laser, or chemical ablation.
- Recurrence is approximately 43%.

Recognition

History and presenting complaint

Horses with progressive ethmoid hematoma (PEH) have unilateral or bilateral epistaxis, which can progress to respiratory stridor and variable facial deformity depending on the duration of the condition, and decreased airflow through the affected nostril.[10]

Physical examination

Unilateral nasal obstruction can be diagnosed by holding the hands over each nostril and detecting reduced airflow from the affected nostril. Facial deformity can also be observed as asymmetric convexity of the facial bones, medial and rostral to the orbit.

Special examination

Endoscopic examination of the upper airway, including both nasal passages, is frequently diagnostic for progressive ethmoid hematoma. Ethmoid hematomas originate from the ethmoid turbinate region or paranasal sinuses (Fig. 26.3). The masses are smooth, green to purple in color and can be small and discrete or expansile, invading the entire nasal passage, nasopharynx, or paranasal sinus region.[10,11] If the mass is confined to the maxillary or frontal sinus, sero-sanguineous fluid will be evident at the naso-maxillary opening, yet the mass can be obscured from view.[10,11] Differential diagnoses for progressive ethmoid hematoma include fungal granulomas, neoplasia, and nasal polyps which can be confirmed by biopsy.

Lateral, dorsoventral, and oblique radiographic projections of the paranasal sinus region are taken to define the anatomic limits of the expansile mass (Fig. 26.4).[12] A discrete, round density overlying the ethmoid labyrinth or within the maxillary or frontal sinus is suggestive of progressive ethmoid hematoma.[13] Fluid lines in the sinuses can be present if secondary sinusitis has occurred. Computed tomography is useful to define the extent of the mass prior to surgical excision (Fig. 26.5).[12]

Laboratory examination

Rarely, horses will have evidence of mild, regenerative anemia, though generally blood loss from ethmoid hemotoma is minimal. Depending on the duration, size of the mass, and inflammatory reaction, hyperfibrinogenemia can be present.[13]

Diagnostic confirmation

Differential diagnoses for PEH include neoplasia, fungal granuloma, nasal polyp, sinus cyst or abscess. Definitive diagnosis is made based on the histopathology of the mass. Ethmoid hematoma is a non-neoplastic angiomatous mass covered by respiratory epithelium and fibrous tissue.[11,12] The parenchyma of the mass is composed of blood, fibrous tissue, hemosiderin-laden macrophages, neutrophils and necrotic debris, especially in large, chronic masses, with occasional calcareous deposits.

Treatment and prognosis

Therapeutic aims

The goal of treatment is elimination of the mass. This can be achieved by surgical excision, laser photo ablation, or chemical ablation.[10,11,13,14] Most commonly, PEH is chemically ablated by intralesional injection of formalin.[14,15] In the standing, sedated horse, the mass is injected with 4% formaldehyde or neutral

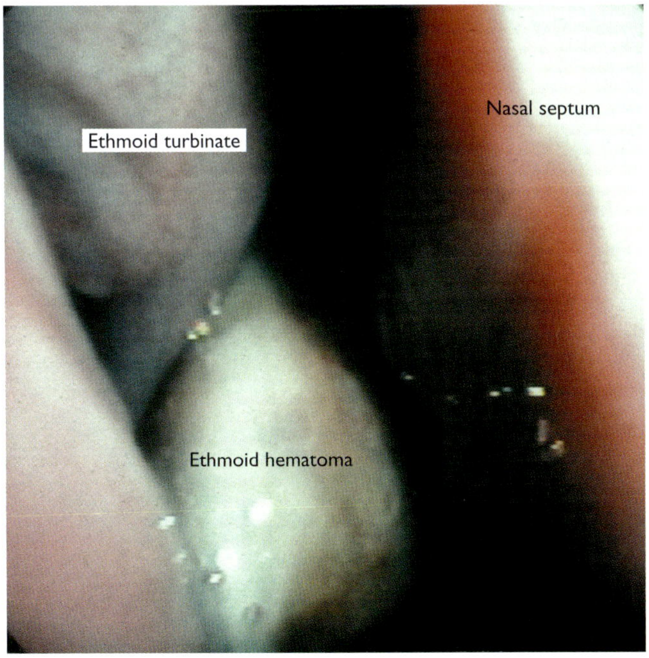

Fig 26.3 Endoscopic image of an ethmoid hematoma.

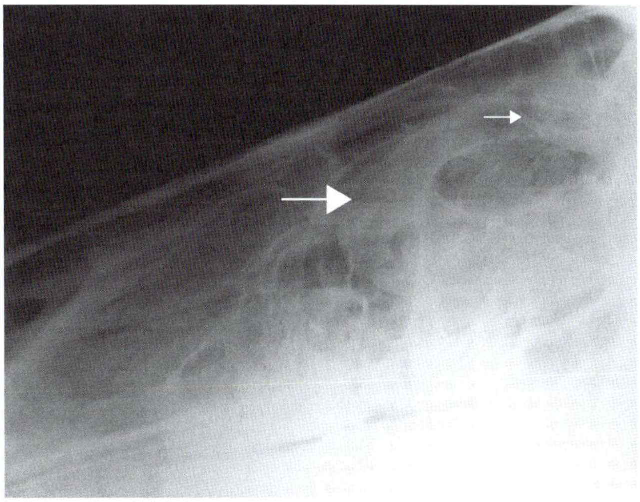

Fig 26.4 Lateral radiograph of the paranasal sinus region of a horse. The large arrow points to the ethmoid hematoma and the small arrow points to the ethmoid turbinates.

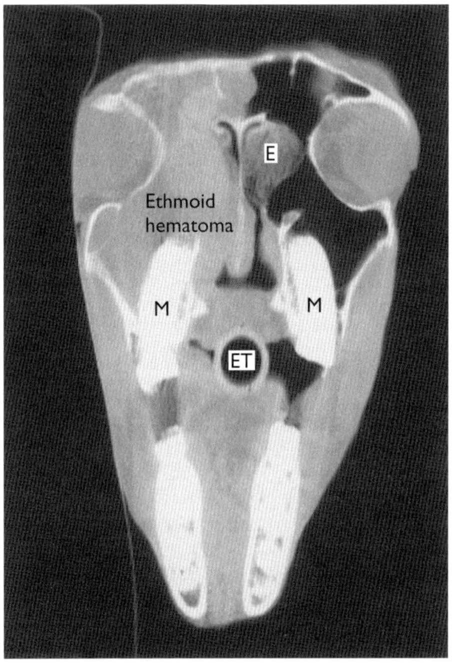

Fig 26.5 Coronal slice of a computed tomographic image of a horse with an ethmoid hematoma. Notice the left sinus region is occupied by the ethmoid hematoma. E = normal ethmoid turbinate; ET = endotracheal tube; M = molars.

buffered 10% formalin until the mass distends using a trans-endoscopic 23-gauge retractable needle (Mill-Rose Laboratories, Inc., Mentor, OH) or through an injection apparatus constructed from polyethylene tubing and a 22- or 25-gauge needle.[13,14] Treatments are repeated every 3–4 weeks until the lesion is obliterated, requiring 1–18 treatments.[15] If the lesion is very large especially if invaded the sinuses surgical excision of progressive ethmoid hematoma is required[10,15–19] Laser excision is rarely indicated.[11] Copious hemorrhage is expected (especially under general anesthesia) and controlled using cold saline and pressure applied with sterile gauze packing.

Complications from surgical excision include severe hemorrhage, chronic sinusitis, surgical site infection, and osteomyelitis of the bone flap.[10] Complications following formalin injection include laminitis, dysphagia, and neurologic disease, if the ethmoid hematoma has eroded through the cribiform plate.[13,14]

Prognosis

Recurrence following surgical excision is 43%, necessitating periodic re-evaluation should the mass recur. Recurrence is slightly higher in horses with bilateral progressive ethmoid hematomas.[10–12,15]

Prevention

There are no known preventive measures.

Etiology and pathophysiology

Etiology

The etiology of PEH is unknown.

Pathophysiology

Progressive ethmoid hematoma is an expanding angiomatous mass originating from the mucosa of the ethmoid conchae or paranasal sinuses. Progressive expansion of the mass occurs due to recurrent hemorrhage and local invasion of tissues. Masses can expand rostroventrally into the nasal passage or nasopharynx, or within the paranasal sinuses.

Epidemiology

Progressive ethmoid hematomas have been reported in horses from 6 months to 20 years old, but are most commonly diagnosed in middle-aged and older horses.[10,16] Thoroughbred horses are overrepresented in case series, though the disease has been reported in many breeds. Bilateral lesions occur 15% of the time.[10,16]

Sinusitis

- The paranasal sinuses include the frontal, maxillary, sphenopalatine, and dorsal and ventral conchal sinuses.
- Sinusitis can be primary or secondary, and is most commonly associated with dental disease, masses, and trauma.
- Clinical signs of sinusitis include nasal discharge and facial swelling.
- Surgical debridement of the sinus is frequently recommended for treatment of primary or secondary sinusitis.

Recognition

History and presenting complaint

Horses with sinusitis frequently have unilateral or bilateral nasal discharge. Sinusitis can be primary if no underlying disease is present or secondary if the sinusitis is due to dental disease or fungal infection.[15] In the latter case the discharge can be foul smelling and is more likely to be bilateral as compared to secondary sinusitis.[15,16] Horses with primary sinusitis frequently have a history of recent upper respiratory tract infection. If the sinusitis is secondary to a cyst or neoplastic mass, facial swelling and deformity of facial bones can be detected as the mass expands within the sinus.[15,16]

Physical examination

Rarely are horses febrile. Facial swelling can be detected and can be painful to palpation.[15,16] Deformity of facial bones overlying the sinus can be evident, especially in chronic cases of expansile masses such as sinus cysts and neoplasia.[15–16]Increased respiratory rate and effort is detected if the airway is obstructed. This occurs when the ventral conchal sinus is affected and compresses the ventral meatus[16] or secondary to intrasinus lesions such as cyst or neoplasia.[15]Airflow obstruction is diagnosed by holding the hands over each nostril and detecting reduced airflow from the affected nostril. Submandibular lymphadenopathy has been reported in 78–83% of affected horses.[16] Epiphora occurs in horses with sinusitis if the nasolacrimal duct is compressed by a mass or swelling in the surrounding tissues.[16] Hair loss can be detected on the horse's face if the epiphora is chronic.

Special examination

Techniques used to diagnose sinusitis include radiography, computed tomography, sinoscopy, endoscopy, and nuclear medicine.[16,17] Generally at least four views of the skull are taken if sinusitis is expected, including the left and right oblique, lateral, and dorsoventral views. The left and right oblique views help to confirm which side of the head is affected. Fluid lines (Fig. 26.6), masses within the sinuses (Fig. 26.7) and periapical tooth root abscessation and abnormal alveolar bone can frequently be detected

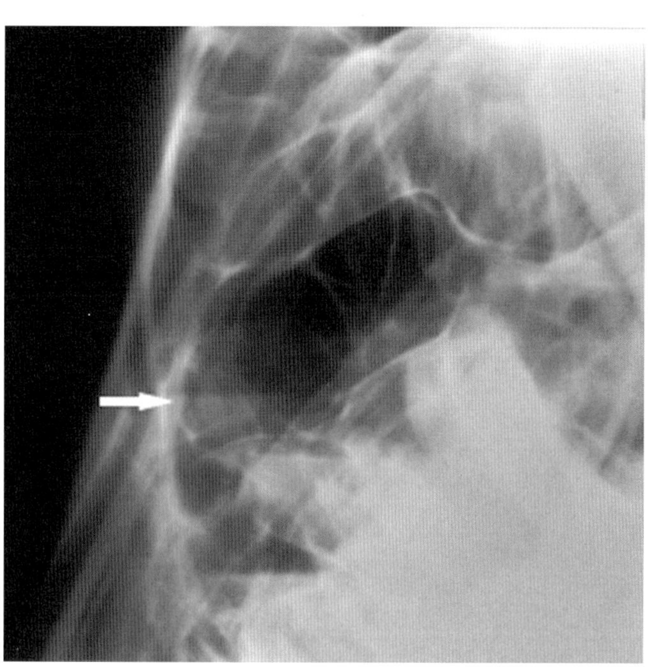

Fig 26.6 Lateral radiograph of the paranasal sinus region of a horse with sinusitis illustrating the fluid line (arrow) within the maxillary sinus.

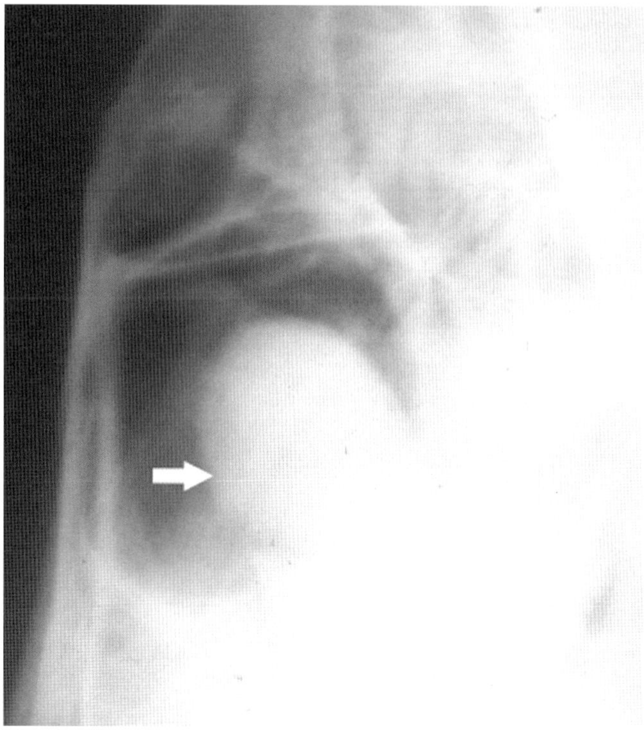

Fig 26.7 Lateral radiograph of the paranasal sinus region of a horse with a mass (arrow) within the maxillary sinus.

radiographically. Computed tomography is performed to localize the lesion more accurately in cases of secondary sinusitis. Sinus cysts, dental disease, neoplasia, ethmoid hematoma, mycotic granulomas, polyps, and epidermal inclusion cysts can cause secondary sinusitis and frequently require surgical removal.[16] The information gained from the computed tomographic scan aids in surgical planning and the surgical approach. Sinoscopy is performed in the sedated, standing horse by inserting a flexible endoscope or arthroscope through a trephine in the frontal, rostral maxillary, or caudal maxillary sinus.[17] Fluid is aspirated from the sinus and submitted for culture and cytology and the sinus can be irrigated to evacuate exudate. The sinuses can be explored and masses or tooth root abscesses identified and biopsied by use of this technique. Endoscopic examination of the nasal passages is useful in cases of sinusitis to confirm that the exudate is coming from the naso-maxillary opening of the middle meatus. The specific origin of the exudate and inciting cause cannot be determined by endoscopy alone. Despite radiography and computed tomography, identifying the affected tooth can at times be difficult. Nuclear medicine is rarely used in cases of sinusitis, but can be used to confirm infected apical tooth root.

Laboratory examination

The results of laboratory tests on blood are generally normal. Fluid aspirates are submitted for culture and sensitivity.

Diagnostic confirmation

The diagnosis of primary sinusitis is made based on a history of previous upper respiratory tract infection, nasal discharge originating from the paranasal sinus region, evidence of fluid within the sinuses on radiographs or computed tomography, and the absence of a secondary cause of the sinusitis.[15–16] Secondary sinusitis is diagnosed based on the presence of an inciting cause of the sinusitis, such as apical tooth root abscess, sinus cyst, neoplastic mass, ethmoid hematoma, mycotic granuloma, polyp, or trauma and facial bone fracture into the sinus.[15–16] Confirmation of the etiology of secondary sinusitis is made by sinoscopy, biopsy, or surgical exploration of the sinuses.

Treatment and prognosis

Therapeutic aims

The goal of therapy is to rid the sinus of infection and remove the inciting cause in cases of secondary sinusitis.

Therapy

The results of culture and sensitivity of fluid aspirated from the sinus dictate the appropriate antimicrobial therapy. Because primary sinusitis frequently is a sequela to upper respiratory tract infection, *Streptococcus* spp. are frequently isolated. Penicillin or trimethoprim sulfonamides are appropriate antibiotics to use in the treatment of primary sinusitis, prior to receipt of culture results. In addition to systemic antibiotics, repeated lavage of the sinus with balanced polyionic solution decreases the exudate and dilutes the organisms and inflammatory mediators within the sinus.[15–16] A chronic irrigation system can be placed following sinus centesis. Sinus centesis can be performed at the cranial or caudal maxillary sinus or frontal sinus. A point 2.5–3 cm dorsal to the facial crest and 3 cm rostral to the medial canthus marks the placement for centesis of the caudal maxillary sinus;[15–16] 2.5–3 cm dorsal to the facial crest and 3 cm caudal to the infraorbital foramen permits access to the cranial maxillary sinus. Centesis of the frontal sinus is performed at a site midway between the medial canthus of the eye and the midline of the head. Following aseptic preparation, a 2–3 mL bleb of local anesthetic is injected subcutaneously. A stab incision is made through the skin and subcutaneous tissue and a 2 mm Steinmann pin in a Jacob's chuck is used to drill a hole into the sinus. Sterile polyethylene tubing is fed through the centesis site and fluid is aspirated using a needle and syringe attached to the tubing. If elected, a chronic irrigation system can be sutured in place. The chronic irrigation system permits irrigation of the sinus with 1–3 liters of solution two to four times daily until exudate is no longer produced.

The goal of treating secondary sinusitis is to treat the primary cause. Depending upon the location, sinus cysts, ethmoid hematomas, neoplasia, polyps, and infected teeth can be approached surgically through a maxillary bone flap or frontal nasal bone flap.[15,18] Standing surgery reduces the amount of the bleeding compared to sinusotomy under general anesthesia. Hemorrhage is controlled during surgery by lavaging the site with cold saline and applying pressure to the bleeding area. Occasionally, but rarely, vessels can be located and ligated. After the mass has been removed, continuous pressure is applied to the area using gauze (within a stockinette) or roll gauze packing placed within the sinus. The end of the packing is exited through a hole in the dorsal or ventral conchal sinus and then out the nose or through a trephine opening in the caudal maxillary sinus. The packing is pulled in 36 to 48 hours.

Prognosis

The prognosis for recovery from primary sinusitis, sinus cysts, trauma, and dental disease is good.[15,19,20] Complications can include chronic drainage from the sinus, recurrence of the cyst if a portion of the cystic lining was left within the sinus, oral nasal fistulas from tooth extraction, incisional infection and sequestration of the bone flap overlying the sinus. Prognosis for most neoplastic masses within the sinus resulting in sinusitis is poor due to the expansile, invasive, and metastatic nature of the tumors.

Prevention

There is no known prevention.

Etiology and pathophysiology

Etiology

Sinusitis can result from a primary infection within the sinus, frequently secondary to an upper respiratory tract infection. Sinusitis can also occur secondary to an apical tooth root abscess, sinus cyst, neoplasia, trauma and fracture of facial bones, ethmoid hematoma, and fungal granuloma.[15,16]

Epidemiology

The prevalence of sinusitis ranges from 0.4 to 1.06%.[20–21]

Nasopharyngeal collapse

- Horses with nasopharyngeal collapse are usually normal at rest.
- The diagnosis of nasopharyngeal collapse is made during exercise (overground or treadmill) endoscopic examination.
- Dorsal nasopharyngeal collapse can be a consequence of excessive thoraco-cervical and atlanto-occipal hyperflexion.
- Dorsal nasopharyngeal collapse can be a manifestation of subclinical guttural pouch tympany and treated by addressing the latter surgically.
- Clinical signs of nasopharyngeal collapse, in young horses or in horses with pharyngitis, can resolve with time.
- Horses with hyperkalemic periodic paralysis are at increased risk for developing nasopharyngeal collapse.

Recognition

History and presenting complaint

Various degrees of nasopharyngeal collapse can cause exercise intolerance and respiratory noise in exercising horses.

Physical examination

This is normal in the resting horse.

Special examination

In affected horses, endoscopic examination of the nasopharynx and larynx at rest is generally normal unless a pharyngitis is present. At rest during nasal occlusion the lateral walls, dorsal aspect of the nasopharynx, or rostral portion of the soft palate can collapse into the airway to an abnormal degree in affected horses, especially horses with hyperkalemic periodic paralysis (HYPP).[22,23] Be aware that sedation and topical application of local anesthetic can create nasopharyngeal collapse. Some horses show signs of nasopharyngeal collapse during resting endoscopic examination, and have normal nasopharyngeal function during exercise.

Dynamic examination is required to confirm the diagnosis (Fig. 26.8). The interpretation of the endoscopic image at exercise is obvious for lateral wall collapse. The interpretation of billowing of the floor of the nasopharynx (i.e rostral nasopharyngeal collapse) as well as the roof of the nasopharynx (i.e dorsal nasopharyngeal collapse) must be made with caution. Normally, the roof of the nasopharynx minimally projects ventrally at the end of expiration due to positive end-expiratory pressure within the guttural pouches resulting in some degree of dorsal pharyngeal collapse at the end of expiration.[24] Dorsal nasopharyngeal collapse has recently been proposed to be artificially created in the dressage horse by the excessive thoraco-cervical and atlanto-occipal hyperflexion (i.e. 'rollkur').[25] Dorsal nasopharyngeal collapse is also reported to be secondary to subclinical tympany of the guttural pouch present only during head flexion.[26] Billowing of the rostral palate can be due to a ventral position of the endoscope in the most rostral aspect of the nasopharynx or caudal aspect of nasal passage during exercise will visually amplify the normal billowing of the rostral palate and cause an inaccurate identification of this condition.

Laboratory examination

None is indicated.

Diagnostic confirmation

The diagnosis is best confirmed by dynamic endoscopic exam during exercise.

Treatment and prognosis

Therapeutic aims

The goal of treatment is to resolve the nasopharyngeal collapse.

Therapy

Horses with nasopharyngeal collapse may be given local or systemic anti-inflammatory agent if upper airway inflammation is present. Horses that are HYPP positive respond to acetazolamide therapy. Horses with dorsal nasopharyngeal collapse may respond to fenestration of the guttural pouches or removal of plica salpingopharyngeal membrane.[26]

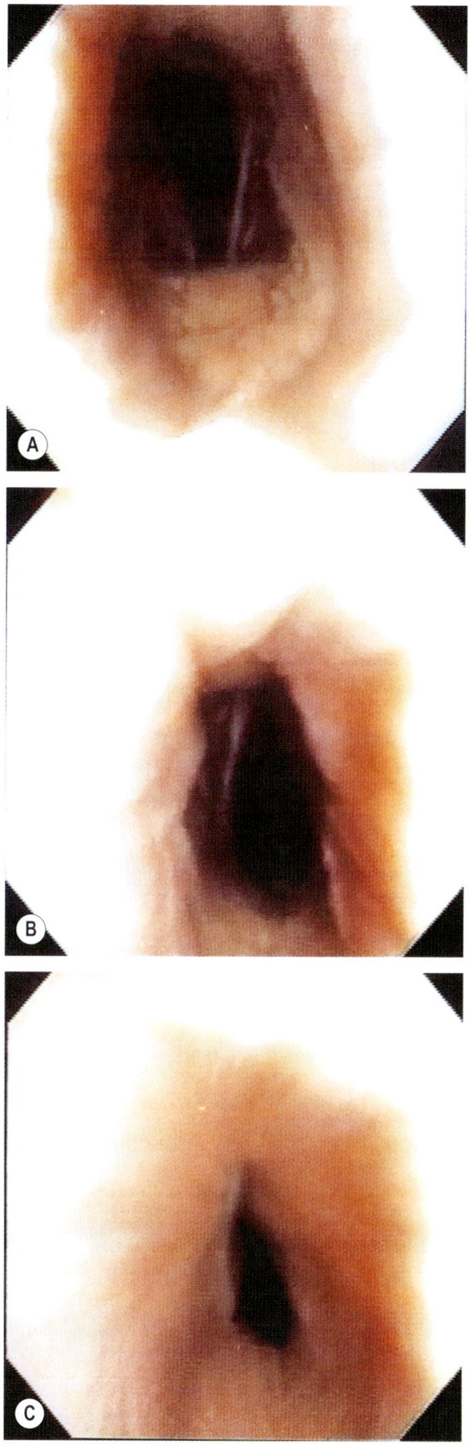

Fig 26.8 Endoscopic images of the nasopharynx of an exercising horse showing progressive nasopharyngeal collapse. Collapse is apparent in the first frame **(A)** and increases with increasing duration of exercise on the treadmill **(B, C)**.

Prognosis

The prognosis is usually unfavorable, especially in horses with underlying disease such as HYPP. The condition resolves in some horses.

Prevention

There is no known prevention.

Etiology and pathophysiology

Etiology

In most cases the etiology of pharyngeal collapse is not known. However in some cases the disease is associated with pharyngitis or HYPP and in foal with muscle disease.

Pathophysiology

Nasopharyngeal collapse can result from some form of exercise-induced guttural pouch tympany or neuromuscular lesion involving the muscles that support the dorsal nasopharynx.[23,26] Horses should be evaluated for neuromuscular or primary muscle disorders, such as equine protozoal neuropathy, selenium and vitamin E deficiency, hyperkalemic periodic paralysis, or upper respiratory inflammatory disease.[22]

Epidemiology

The epidemiology of this condition has not been described. However, this disease is most frequently diagnosed in young racehorses, which can be due to the speed and intensity at which they compete. Nasopharyngeal collapse is also frequently recognized in horses with HYPP, and rather than being a distinct entity, represents a muscle group affected by the disorder.

Retropharyngeal abscesses

Recognition

History and presenting complaint

Horses with retropharyngeal abscessation frequently have palpable swelling in the throat region, nasal discharge, abnormal respiratory noise during exercise, dorsal displacement of the soft palate, and exercise intolerance. If the airway obstruction is severe, horses can show signs of respiratory distress at rest.[27,28] Additional clinical signs include dysphagia, inappetance, and depression.[27]

Physical examination

Palpation of the throat in the area of Viborg's triangle can reveal swelling that can be painful and lead to stridorous upper airway noise. If the horse is dysphagic, feed material and saliva can be seen at the nares. If the horse is in respiratory distress, stridorous breathing and increased respiratory effort might be apparent.

Special examination

Radiography of the throat area reveals soft tissue density in the retropharyngeal region, dorsal to the pharynx and on the floor of the guttural pouch (Fig. 26.9). Compression of the dorsal nasopharynx by the abscessed retropharyngeal lymph node is evident during endoscopic examination of the upper airway (Fig. 26.10). The enlarged lymph node can be best seen within the guttural pouch, on the floor of the medial compartment (Fig. 26.11).

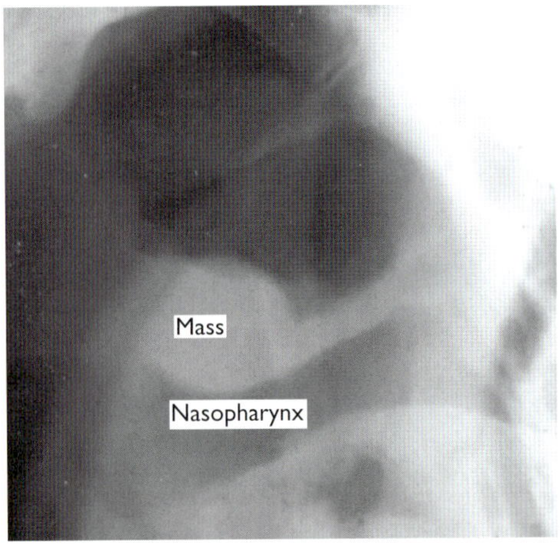

Fig 26.9 Lateral radiograph of the pharyngeal region of a horse with an abscessed retropharyngeal lymph node causing collapse of the dorsal nasopharynx.

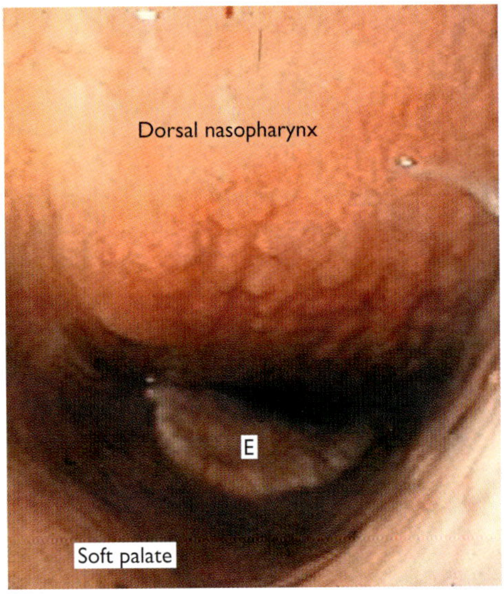

Fig 26.10 Endoscopic image of the nasopharynx of a horse with abscessed retropharyngeal lymph nodes. Notice how the dorsal nasopharynx is collapsed, such that the larynx cannot be seen. E = epiglottis.

Ultrasonographic examination of the throat will show increased soft tissue density containing hyperechoic fluid, or purulent exudates.

Laboratory examination

Results of complete blood count frequently show leukocytosis and neutrophilia with regenerative left shift, and lymphocytosis. Some horses will have hyperfibrinogenemia.

Diagnostic confirmation

The diagnosis is confirmed by aspiration of material from the affected lymph node and real-time PCR or culture of the exudate.[29] Retropharyngeal lymph node abscesses are most frequently caused by *Streptococcus* spp., particularly *Streptococcus equi*. Sequencing of the surface protein (SeM) has been used as an epidemiological tool to identify geographically linked outbreak.[30]

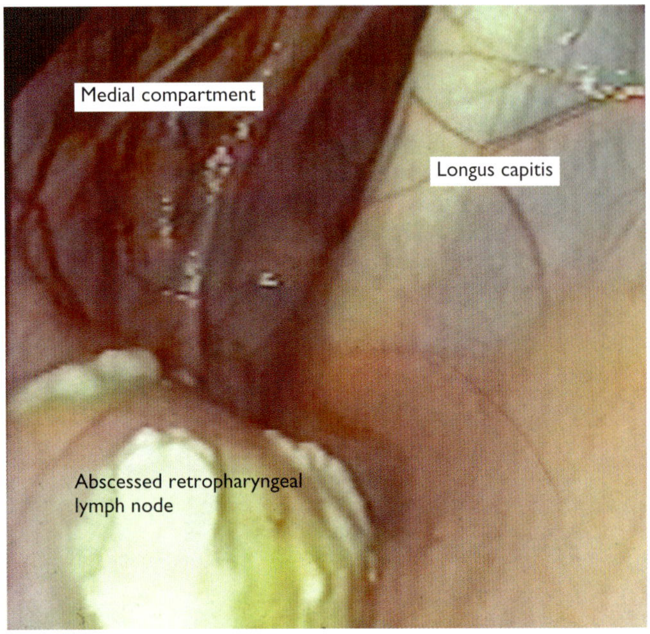

Fig 26.11 Endoscopic image of the medial compartment of the guttural pouch. Notice the abscessed retropharyngeal lymph node.

Treatment and prognosis

Therapeutic aims

The goal of therapy is resolution of the abscess.

Therapy

Emergency tracheotomy

If the horse is in respiratory distress, an emergency tracheotomy is performed in the mid cervical area. After infiltration with local anesthetic and aseptic preparation, a 10–12 cm linear incision is made through the skin, subcutaneous tissue, and cutaneous trunci with a scalpel along the midline. The fascial plane dividing the right and left sternohyoid muscles is sharply incised with a scalpel, Metzenbaum scissors exposing the tracheal rings. A scalpel is inserted through the tracheal ligament parallel to and in between two tracheal rings. Approximately 40% of the ventral aspect of the tracheal ligament is incised and the tracheostomy tube inserted. The tube must be secured such that when the horse moves its head and neck, the tube lumen is not obstructed and the tube is not dislodged from the trachea.

Because most retropharyngeal lymph node abscesses are caused by streptococcal species, penicillin, 22 000–44 000 IU/kg, or sulfamethoxazole-trimethoprim, 15 mg/kg, is administered for 7–10 days. Judicious use of non-steroidal anti-inflammatory medication is appropriate. If the lymph nodes are large, surgical drainage can be required. Following general anesthesia, the horse is positioned in dorsal recumbency. A modified Whitehouse approach is performed on the affected side, exposing the abscessed lymph node. Confirmation of the abscess is made by inserting a needle into the mass and aspirating material from the lymph node that can be submitted for culture and antibiotic sensitivity. A stab incision is then made in the lymph node and the purulent material evacuated.

The incision is left open, to heal by second intention, and the site is lavaged with saline or dilute iodine solution twice daily.

Prognosis

The prognosis for return to normal function within 4–5 months following retropharyngeal lymph node abscess is excellent, or approximately 90%.[27]

Prevention

Decreased exposure to horses infected with *Streptococcus equi* minimizes the occurrence of retropharyngeal lymph node abscess formation. Prophylactic vaccination against *S. equi* can limit lymph node abscess formation, but vaccination is not without risk.

Etiology

Etiology

Most retropharyngeal lymph node abscesses are caused by streptococcal species, principally *S. equi*.

Epidemiology

Retropharyngeal lymph node abscesses are most commonly seen in horses less than 1 year old, and in horses infected with *S. equi*.

Dorsal displacement of the soft palate (DDSP)

Recognition

History and presenting complaint

Horses with intermittent dorsal displacement of the soft palate (DDSP) are exercise intolerant and often make an abnormal expiratory noise during exercise. The displaced soft palate billows dorsally during exhalation as air flows beneath the soft palate (Fig. 26.12). The noise associated with DDSP is a 'gurgling or snoring' noise, and is caused by fluttering of the caudal margin of the soft palate. In approximately 20–30% of horses with DDSP, noise is not heard.[31] The importance of either noise production or exercise intolerance is dependent on the activity of the horse. DDSP in show horses generally affects the horse's performance because of the noise production or coughing, although poor performance is also reported.[32] Horses that perform with the head and neck flexed, such as upper-level dressage horses and Saddlebreds, suffer exercise intolerance with DDSP due to the more negative inspiratory pressure and airway resistance that occurs with head and neck flexion.[33] These horses must be differentiated from horses with collapse of the roof of the nasopharynx, which can also cause a similar abnormal noise and impairment in performance. Dorsal displacement of the soft palate is more common in racehorses, especially 2–4-year-olds.[34,35] The exercise intolerance is often described by trainers and riders or drivers as 'choking down' or 'hitting a wall' because DDSP causes significant expiratory obstruction that limits minute ventilation. Mouth breathing during exhalation is recognized by fluttering of the cheeks as air is diverted underneath the soft palate through the mouth. Occasionally, coughing during exercise is reported in association with the disease; this complaint is more common in sport horses.

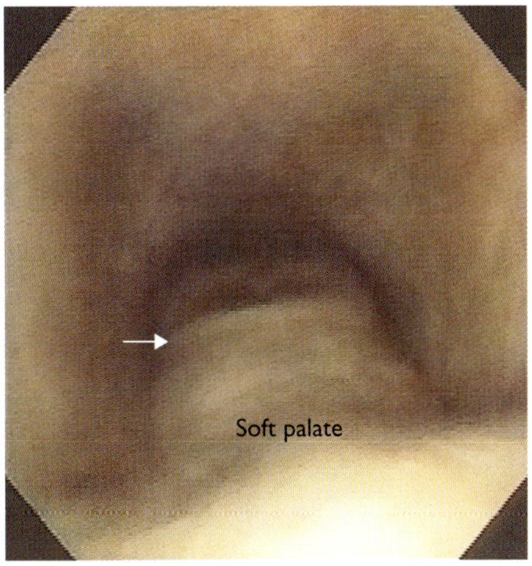

Fig 26.12 Endoscopic image of a horse with dorsal displacement of the soft palate while exercising on a treadmill. Notice how the soft palate billows dorsally in the airway, obstructing the rima glottidis. Arrow, caudal free margin of the soft palate.

Physical examination

Because intermittent DDSP is a dynamic obstructive airway disease that occurs during exercise, most horses are normal at rest. If the soft palate displacement is persistent and associated with dysphagia, feed material can accumulate in the airway, the horse can cough, and have clinical signs of aspiration pneumonia. The primary complaint in these horses is dysphagia and aspiration. This is quite different in horses with intermittent DDSP, where exercise intolerance and respiratory noise are seen.

Some horses with intermittent DDSP have a history of upper respiratory infection. These horses can have nasal discharge, coughing, and enlarged retropharyngeal and submandibular lymph nodes.

Special examination

Intermittent DDSP

Watching and listening to the horse exercise at a racetrack and witnessing the described abnormal noise, open mouth breathing during exhalation and exercise intolerance can be helpful in diagnosing DDSP. The noise is somewhat specific in that it occurs during expiration and has a snoring character, quite different from inspiratory noises associated with laryngeal hemiplegia and other dynamic inspiratory airway abnormalities.

Endoscopic examination of the nasopharynx and larynx at rest in unsedated horses is important to assess nasopharyngeal function and rule in or out other causes of abnormal airway noise and exercise intolerance, such as laryngeal hemiplegia/hemiparesis or epiglottic entrapment. Examination of both guttural pouches can be helpful if dysphagia present. Dorsal displacement of the soft palate is recognized by the dorsal position of the caudal edge of the soft palate obstructing the view of the epiglottis (Fig. 26.12). Occluding the horse's nares for 20–60 seconds, forcing the horse to breathe against the obstruction, can stimulate increased activity in upper airway muscles and induce DDSP. The observation of induced DDSP during nasal occlusion or resting endoscopy is predictive of DDSP at exercise although it is an insensitive test.[36,37] Indeed, the observation of DDSP at rest, coupled with a history of abnormal respiratory noise at exercise, is only correct in approximately half the horses.[36] After withdrawing the endoscope, the caudal edge of the soft palate can be examined for evidence of ulcers (Fig. 26.13), or prior staphylectomy. Ideally a laryngeal forceps is used to elevate the epiglottic cartilage to better examine the caudal edge of the soft palate (Fig. 26.14) and the subepiglottic tissue for ulcers, cysts, granulomas, or swollen aryepiglottic membrane indicative of intermittent aryepiglottic entrapment. During endoscopy, the observations suggestive of DDSP are (1) the ease with which DDSP can be induced by nasal occlusion, (2) more than one swallow is required to correct the DDSP, and (3) ulceration on the caudal edge of the soft palate. Dynamic endoscopic examination of the upper airway is the gold standard to diagnose DDSP.[36,37] Diagnosis is made by observation of DDSP during strenuous exercise or by observation of palatal instability with flaccid epiglottis (presumably both are a reflection of caudal retraction of the larynx). Palatal instability (PI) is interpreted as prodromal to DDSP.[36,37]

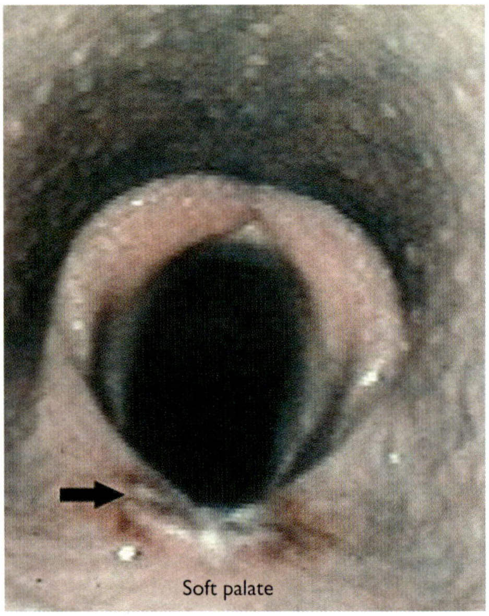

Fig 26.13 Endoscopic image of the nasopharynx of a horse with dorsal displacement of the soft palate. Note the ulcer (arrow) at the caudal free margin of the soft palate.

Persistent DDSP

It is important to evaluate the epiglottis morphology; for instance, subepiglottic masses and epiglottic deformity can result in DDSP. If persistent displacement is present, there are a few techniques that can be used to evaluate the structure and integrity of the epiglottis. Sometimes removing the twitch will relax the horse and allow it to reposition the soft palate appropriately. Sedation can permit replacement of the soft palate.[38] Following application of local anesthetic to the nasopharynx, a laryngeal forceps can be passed in one nostril and used to un-entrap the epiglottis from the soft palate. Evaluation of the epiglottic cartilage and the position of the soft palate can be performed using radiography (Fig. 26.15). Finally, an oral endoscopic examination can be performed on the horse following sedation or general anesthesia and application of a mouth speculum. If the horse is anesthetized, manual palpation of the epiglottic cartilage and soft palate can also be performed.

Diagnostic confirmation

Because horses with intermittent DDSP are generally normal at rest (with clinical signs occurring only during exercise) the diagnosis can be very difficult to confirm. DDSP is best diagnosed by a dynamic endoscopic examination.

Treatment and prognosis

Therapeutic aims

The goal of therapy is to prevent DDSP from occurring. Because the etiology of DDSP is varied, treatment should be directed at the cause.

Therapy

The following discussion should be noted with the concerns expressed in a systemic review[39] recently performed where no treatment could be determined to be superior. This is because most reports in the literature failed to report control or when controls were present, the health status of the control are unknown.[39,40]

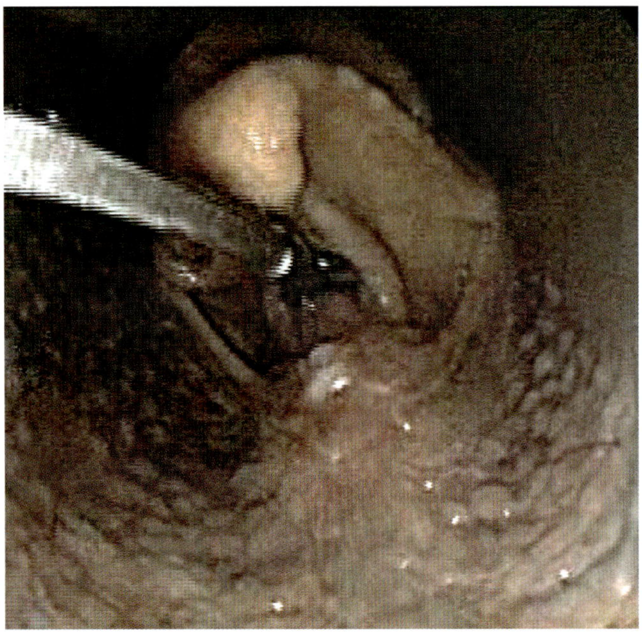

Fig 26.14 Epiglottic cartilage is being lifted with an equine laryngeal forceps, revealing an ulcer on the caudal free edge of the soft palate.

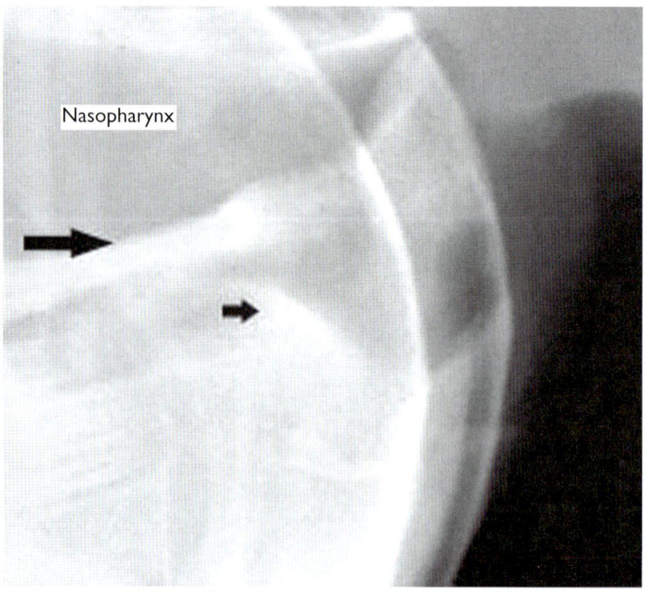

Fig 26.15 Lateral radiograph of the pharyngeal region of a horse with persistent dorsal displacement of the soft palate. Notice the epiglottis (small arrow) positioned ventral to the soft palate (large arrow).

Therapy is directed to the likely cause of the DDSP. Pharyngitis has been associated with DDSP due to inflammation of the nerves and perhaps muscles that stabilize the soft palate.[64] Upper airway inflammation is treated in a plethora of different ways, including systemic administration of corticosteroids (dexamethasone), non-steroidal anti-inflammatory medication, topical anti-inflammatory throat sprays, systemic administration of interferon, and guttural pouch lavage with balanced polyionic solutions with or without dimethyl sulfoxide and corticosteroids. Oral interferon alpha (50–200 IU/day for 10 days to two weeks) is sometimes prescribed. An appropriate treatment regimen for moderate-to-severe nasopharyngeal inflammation, without bacterial infection, might include treatment first with systemic corticosteroids such as prednisolone or dexamethasone and a topical anti-inflammatory throat spray for 2–4 weeks. A common 'throat spray' administered at the rate of 20 cc, orally, every 12 hours consists of: glycerin 250 mL, 250 mL DMSO 90%, nitrofurazone 500 mL, prednisolone 50 mL (25 mg/mL). Horses should be rested (light training without fast speed work) for 10–30 days and the upper airway function re-evaluated periodically.

If there is a structural abnormality, such as epiglottic deformity, entrapment, subepiglottic or soft palate cyst or mass, present then these abnormalities should be addressed. Cysts should be removed either through laser surgery or sharp dissection through a laryngotomy. Granulomas are treated with local anti-inflammatory agents as described above or rarely through resection. Horses with deformed epiglottic cartilage are more difficult to address. In some cases the epiglottic deformity is worsened by partial entrapment by subepiglottic tissues. Those can be released with laser surgery

Whether secondary to an inflammatory process in the upper airways, structural abnormalities and when no structural causes are found, tack modifications such as the use of a bit that keeps the tongue under it (i.e., a 'W' bit, Serena song bit), tongue-ties and the figure-eight noseband are traditional approaches (although unproven) that might be of value in reducing the occurrence of DDSP. There is some circumstantial evidence to support the use of a tongue-tie in the prevention of DDSP or improvement of airway mechanics in exercising horses.[40,41] Finally the use of an external device which positions the larynx in a more forward and dorsal position has been shown to prevent DDSP during treadmill exercise in an experimental model.[42] (Conflict of interest disclosure: one of the authors (N.G.D.) is listed as inventor on a patent owned by both authors' employer, i.e Cornell University).

Many surgical treatments have been reported, including staphylectomy, various bilateral strap muscle resections (sternohyoid, sternothyroid, and omohyoid alone or in combination), epiglottic cartilage augmentation, and various tension or thermal palatoplasty procedures.[43–50] These procedures are performed by some surgeons alone or in various combinations.[49,50] When comparing the results of these surgical treatments to the results of conservative treatment with or without case-control studies, they appear to be little or no advantage to the above procedures.[51–55] Two recent studies looked at the biomechanical/histological results following procedure aims to stiffens the soft palate with laser or injection of sclerosing agent.[56–58] The authors believe that there are two surgical treatments to be considered for treatment of intermittent DDSP: bilateral sternothyroid muscle tenectomy/myotomy transection[46] and laryngeal tie-forward.[58–61]

The goal of the bilateral resection of the tendon of the sternothyroideus (ST) muscles is to prevent caudal retraction of the larynx from the caudal edge of the soft palate.[46] Through a ventral midline incision centered on the cricoid cartilage, the sternothyroideus tendon/muscle is identified and clamped caudal to the cricoid cartilage to avoid damaging the cricothyroid muscles which can lead to vocal cord collapse at exercise.[62] A 2–4 cm section of ST tendon and muscle is resected bilaterally. The incision is left open to heal or can be sutured if desired. Complications are usually minor and include incisional seromas or abscesses requiring appropriate drainage. However, in experimental horses with normal airway function, resection of the sternothyroid and sternohyoid muscles has been observed to result in a less dynamically stable nasopharynx at exercise as measured by an increase in inspiratory tracheal pressure.[63]

Laryngeal tie-forward is based on an experimental model of intermittent DDSP caused by bilateral resection of the thyrohyoideus muscles which was corrected using a suture.[59] This was then shown to be effective in 3 subsequent trials in restoring earnings postoperatively in horses with a clinical diagnosis of DDSP.[58,59,61] Under general anesthesia in dorsal recumbency, a ventral midline incision is made from the base of the lingual process extending 1 cm caudal to the cricoid cartilage. A non-absorbable suture (No. 5 USP) is passed 3–4 times in the caudal edge of the thyroid cartilage over a 1 cm span immediately ventral to the ventral limit of the ST tendon. Both sutures are then passed dorsal to the basihyoid bone with the trailer end of the suture emerging adjacent to the base of the lingual process on the contralateral side while the leading end of the suture emerged adjacent to the base of the lingual process on the ipsilateral side. The procedure is repeated on the contralateral side. The ventral sutures are then tied first advancing the rostral edge of the thyroid cartilage dorsal to the basihyoid bone with an overlap of approximately 1.5 cm. The dorsal sutures are then tied together.

Prognosis

The prognosis following treatment ranged from 53 to 80%.[39, 43–50, 52–55,59–61] These results must be taken with a grain of salt as all outcomes are using some indices of performance as surrogate of success and not actual resolution of the disease. The reported success rate after bilateral tenectomy/myotomy of the sternothyroid muscle is 60%.[45,46] Anecdotally recurrence can occur 3–6 months after surgery. Following laryngeal tie-forward the success rate is 10–20% higher than after bilateral sternothyroid muscle/tendon transection.[59–61]

Etiology and pathophysiology

Etiology

Intermittent DDSP has a multifactorial etiology. Anecdotally physical obstruction (i.e subepiglottic and palatal masses, granulomas, cysts) interferes with the subepiglottic position of the soft palate. Furthermore, epiglottic malformation or chondritis can result in permanent or persistent DDSP.[64]

Damage of the innervation of the soft palate (i.e palatinus and palatopharyngeus muscles),[64] dysfunction of the neuromusculature of the extrinsic laryngeal muscles such as thyrohyoideus muscles,[65] and of the hypoglossal nerves[66] have all, alone, been sufficient to create dorsal displacement of the soft palate.

The innervation of the soft palate is through the pharyngeal branch of the vagus nerve, which with the glossopharyngeal and hypoglossal nerves which course through the guttural pouch and therefore are susceptible to disease processes that specifically affect the lymph node in the floor of the guttural pouches. The pharyngeal branch of the vagus nerve provides motor innervation to the palatinus and palatopharyngeus muscles, two muscles that control the position of the caudal portion of the soft palate. Experimentally desensitizing the pharyngeal branch of the vagus nerve bilaterally causes persistent DDSP at rest with dysphagia.[65] The thyrohyoideus is a flat rectangular muscle attached to the lateral surface of the thyroid cartilage lamina that inserts on the caudal part of the thyrohyoid bone. It is innervated by the hypoglossal nerve and moves the hyoid bone caudally or the larynx rostrally and dorsally. Experimentally bilateral resection of the thyrohyoideus muscles causes intermittent DDSP during exercise in horses.[60] Finally application of local anesthetic around each hypoglossal nerve at the level of the ceratohyoid bone also resulted in DDSP at exercise in experimental horses.[66]

Pathophysiology

Dorsal displacement of the soft palate is an expiratory obstructive syndrome that causes increased expiratory impedance, decreased minute ventilation, hypoxia, and hypercarbia (Table 26.1).[65,67-69] During inhalation, the soft palate is located ventrally (still dorsal to the epiglottis). During exhalation, the soft palate displaces dorsally, thus diverting the flow of air through the oropharynx and mouth. This flow pattern is associated with more negative peak tracheal pressure and increased expiratory impedance.[65,68,69]

Prevention

Preventing DDSP is difficult because the etiology of this disease is unknown. However, timely treatment of upper airway inflammation and appropriate vaccination against upper respiratory tract viruses can decrease the chances of horses developing intermittent DDSP.

Epidemiology

Dorsal displacement of the soft palate (DDSP) is a performance-limiting upper airway condition in horses that was reported to be present in 10–20% of racehorses.[51]

Epiglottic entrapment

- Epiglottic entrapment occurs when redundant aryepiglottic tissue envelops the epiglottis.
- Epiglottic entrapment can be an incidental finding during endoscopic examination of the larynx and not associated with clinical signs.
- The entrapping aryepiglottic tissue can be smooth or edematous and ulcerated.

Recognition

History and presenting complaint

Horses with epiglottic entrapment can have exercise intolerance and make an abnormal respiratory noise during exercise. It must be realized that the performance of some horses with epiglottic entrapment is unaffected[70,71] and therefore treatment may not be needed.

Physical examination

External physical exam is generally normal. On rare occasion, horses with severely ulcerated, swollen entrapping aryepiglottic membrane can be lead to coughing, dysphagia and have signs of aspiration pneumonia.

Special examination

Endoscopic examination reveals that the epiglottis is in its normal position dorsal to the soft palate but is encased in the aryepiglottic membrane so that the normal serrated edge of the epiglottis and its vascular pattern are not visible. The aryepiglottic tissue can be smooth, fitting tightly around the epiglottis, or swollen and ulcerated (Fig. 26.16A, B). The entrapment can also be observed radiographically. If the soft palate is persistently displaced, due to or associated with the entrapment, a laryngeal forceps can be used to either retract the soft palate, or undisplace the soft palate so that the entrapping membrane can be observed. Alternatively an oral exam during general anesthesia will identify the entrapment.

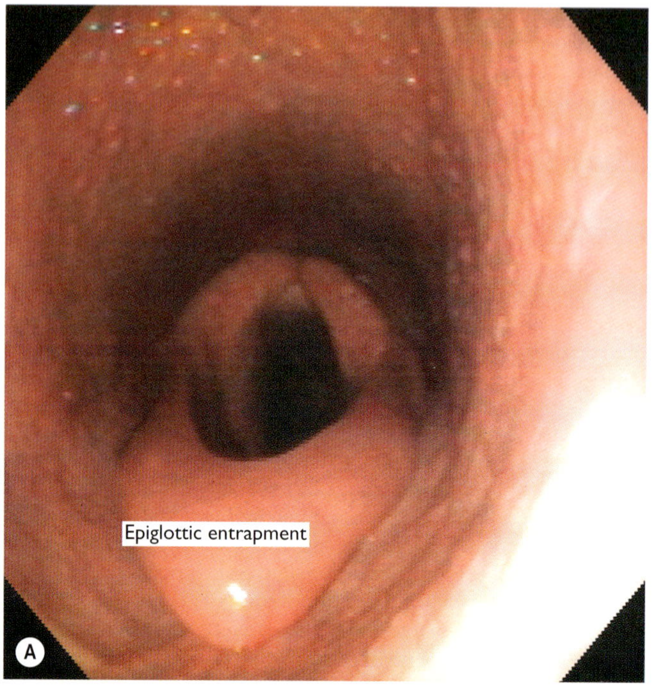

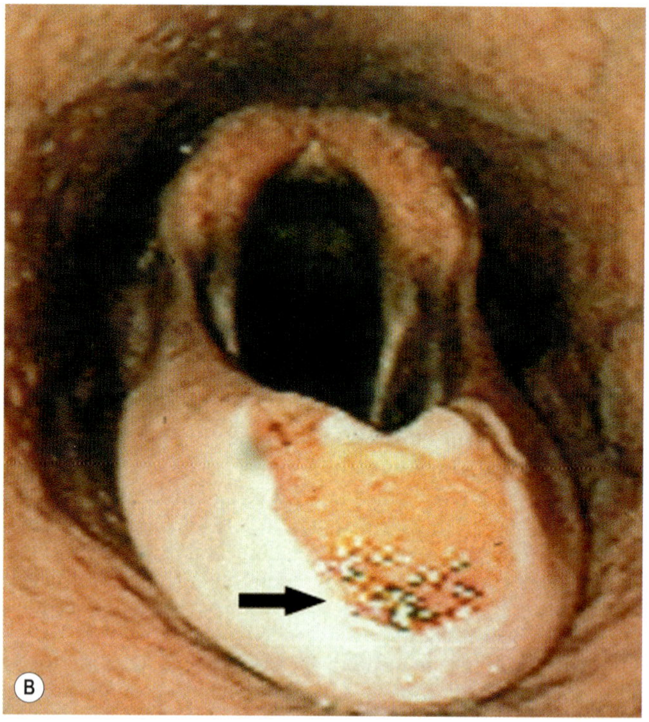

Fig 26.16 **(A)** Endoscopic image of the larynx of a horse with epiglottic entrapment. Note that the epiglottis is encased in the aryepiglottic membrane such that the vascular pattern on the dorsal surface of the epiglottis and the serrated margin of the epiglottis is not visible. **(B)** Endoscopic image of the larynx of a horse with an epiglottic entrapment. Note the ulcerated area (arrow) of the entrapping aryepiglottic tissue.

Occasionally, the epiglottis is entrapped intermittently, during exercise or immediately after swallowing only. In these cases, the diagnosis can be made by dynamic endoscopic examination during exercise.

Laboratory examination

Laboratory examination is normal, but none is usually indicated.

Diagnostic confirmation

Differential diagnoses for epiglottic entrapment include dynamic upper airway lesions that cause exercise intolerance and abnormal respiratory noise during exercise. A definitive diagnosis of epiglottic entrapment is made by static or dynamic endoscopic examination.

Treatment and prognosis

Therapeutic aims

The goal of treatment is to relieve the entrapment. Chronic entrapment can result in epiglottic chondritis and/or deformity.

Therapy

Midline division of the entrapping aryepiglottic membrane can be performed standing by passing a shielded hook bistoury intranasally[72] or by use of a hooked bistoury through the mouth with the horse under general anesthesia (Fig. 26.17).[73,74] It is ill-advised to use an unshielded hooked bistoury transnasally on standing, even on sedated horses, because it exposes the horse to unnecessary morbidity (possibly career ending) such as palatal, esophageal or guttural pouch laceration if the horse swallows or moves. The entrapping membrane can also be divided with the laser.[75] The laser must not come into contact with the epiglottic cartilage, so it is advisable to use a laryngeal forceps or blunt hook to elevate the epiglottic membrane prior to division (Fig. 26.18A,B). The advantage of the laser over the hooked bistoury is that if the aryepiglottic membrane is ulcerated and swollen, the membrane can be resected. Alternatively this resection can be done under general anesthesia through a laryngotomy incision, after everting the epiglottic cartilage in the larynx.[73]

Following midline division of the aryepiglottic membrane, topical and systemic anti-inflammatory therapies are recommended to prevent re-entrapment of the epiglottis. A topical anti-inflammatory solution (throat spray) is applied twice daily using a soft rubber tube (i.e. 12 Fr infant feeding tube) placed in alternating nostrils. In addition, dexamethasone (20 mg, IV, SID for 3 days) and an oral phenylbutazone or flunixin meglumine is recommended for 7–10 days.

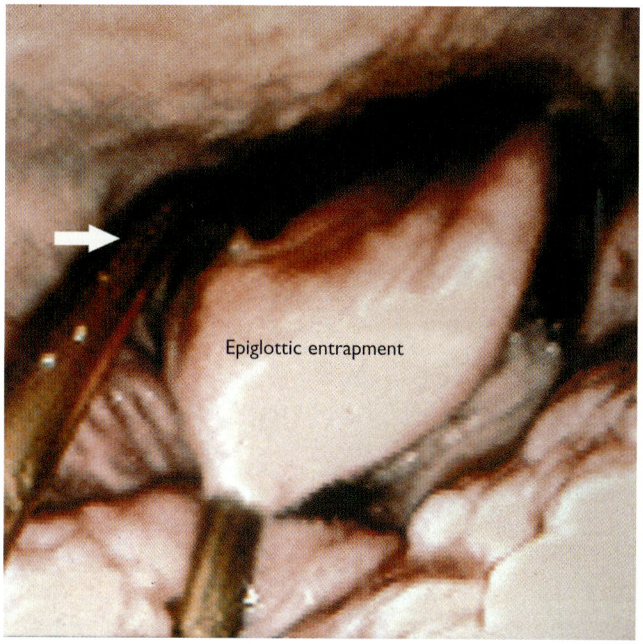

Fig 26.17 Endoscopic image through the oropharynx of a horse where an entrapping aryepiglottic membrane is being excised using a hooked bistoury (arrow) with the horse under general anesthesia.

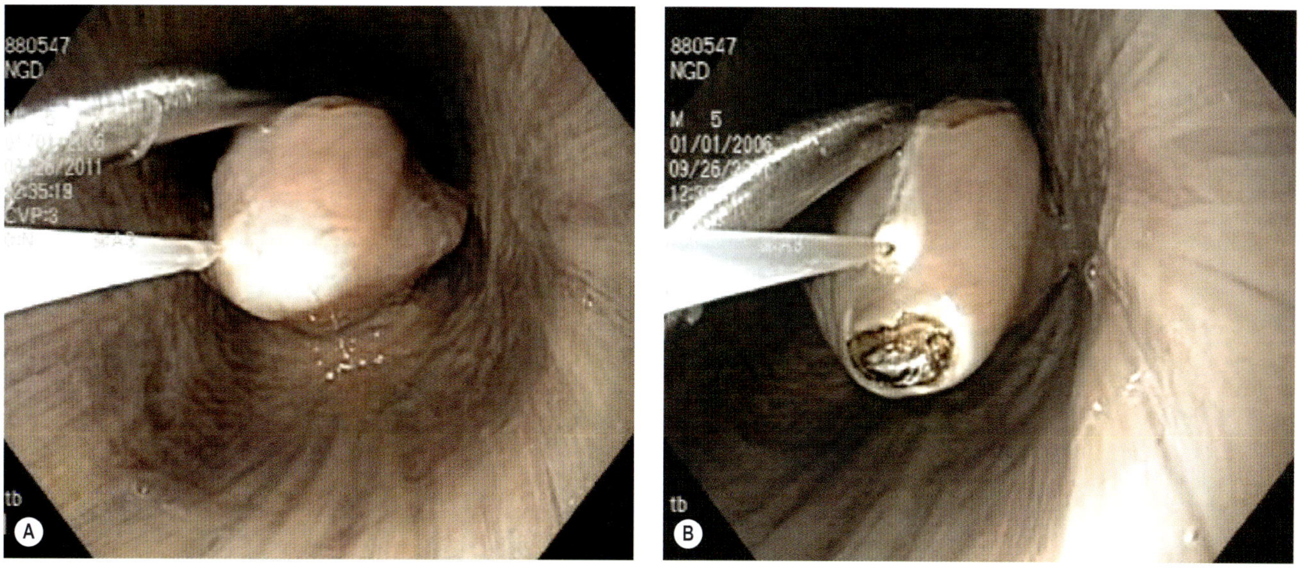

Fig 26.18 (A) Endoscopic image of an epiglottic entrapment being elevated by a blunt laryngeal forceps to protect the epiglottic cartilage from inadvertent contact with the laser. The laser first cut is an horizontal incision to allow the blunt hook to come through the membrane. **(B)** Endoscopic image of the laser-assited midline division of the aryepiglottic membrane.

Prognosis

Seventy-four to 82% of horses have a positive outcome following transoral axial division of the aryepiglottic tissue; 5–10% of horses have recurrence of the entrapment after surgery, and 10–15% of horses develop dorsal displacement of the soft palate following correction of epiglottic entrapment.[72–75]

Prevention

There is no known preventive measure.

Etiology and pathophysiology

Etiology

The etiology is unknown.

Pathophysiology

Aryepiglottic tissue is areolar, mucous membrane that attaches along the ventral margin of the epiglottis and continues between the lateral edges of the epiglottis to the corniculate processes of the arytenoid cartilages. The manner by which the entrapment occurs is unknown, but it can be precipitated by airway inflammation and, specifically, inflammation of the aryepiglottic tissue. It has been suggested that horses with epiglottic hypoplasia, diagnosed by use of endoscopy or radiographic measurement of the thyroepiglottic length, are predisposed to epiglottic entrapment.[73]

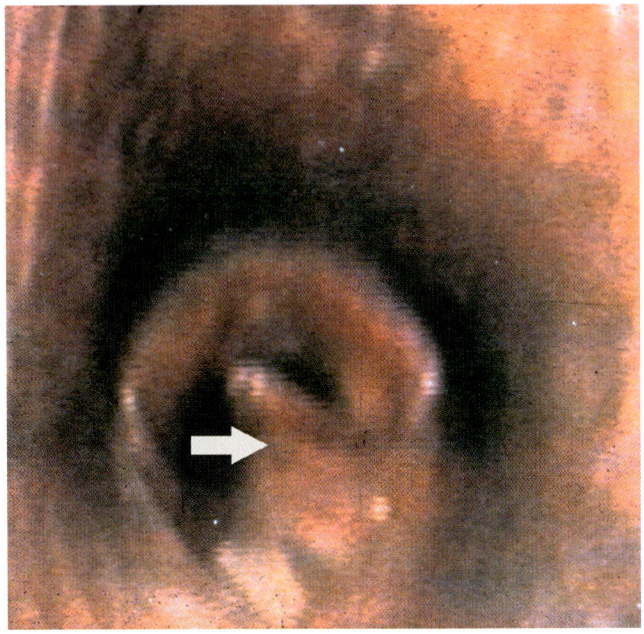

Fig 26.19 Endoscopic image of the larynx of a horse running on a treadmill. Note that the epiglottis (arrow) is retroverted through the rima glottidis, exposing the ventral surface of the epiglottis.

Epidemiology

Between 0.74 and 3% of racehorses have epiglottic entrapment.[70,71,76–79]

Epiglottic retroversion

- Epiglottic retroversion is a rare cause of exercise intolerance and abnormal respiratory noise in horses.
- Epiglottic retroversion is diagnosed during dynamic examination during exercise.
- When the epiglottis retroverts, it prolapses through the rima glottides during inhalation, causing airway obstruction.
- Epiglottic retroversion is probably due to damage to the hyoepiglotticus muscle or the hypoglossal nerve or some of its branches.

Recognition

History and presenting complaint

Epiglottic retroversion is a rare condition that causes abnormal respiratory noise during exercise and exercise intolerance.

Physical examination

The physical examination is normal.

Special examination

Epiglottic retroversion is diagnosed during dynamic endoscopic examination at exercise.[80,81] At rest, the nasopharynx and larynx of affected horses are almost always normal during endoscopic examination. During exercise endoscopy, the epiglottis retroverts such that the ventral surface of the epiglottis faces rostrally (Fig. 26.19). In some horses, the epiglottic retroversion is increased by traction on the lines or reins. Epiglottic retroversion causes dynamic airway obstruction in affected horses (Table 26.1). A rare form of epiglottic retroversion is observed when an exceptionally large subepiglottic cyst is swallowed into the esophagus (see subepiglottic cyst). The horse can then become dyspneic.

Laboratory examination

Laboratory examination is normal, though none is usually indicated.

Diagnostic confirmation

Differential diagnosis of epiglottic retroversion includes those diseases that cause abnormal respiratory noise during inhalation at exercise and can result in exercise intolerance (Table 26.1). The diagnosis of epiglottic retroversion is definitively made during endoscopic examination during exercise.

Treatment and prognosis

Therapeutic aims

The goal of treatment is to stabilize the epiglottis and prevent it from obstructing the airway during inspiration.

Therapy

Little is described in the treatment for epiglottic retroversion. Treatment of two horses is described, with one horse racing successfully after epiglottic augmentation with polytetrafluoroethylene (Teflon), and another horse showing no improvement.[81] The author has performed different fixation (epiglottic 'tie-down') in five cases (four to basihyoid and one to thyroid cartilage) and only one responded to treatment. Currently better results have been obtained using facilitated ankylosis of the thyroepiglottic articulation.

Prognosis

Prognosis is excellent for life, but guarded for athletic endeavors.[80,81]

Special examination

Endoscopic exam at rest allows assessment of the laryngeal anatomy as well as some indication of function by categorizing the degree of arytenoid movement and synchrony (see Table 26.2).[101,102] The diagnosis of RLN with complete paralysis (grade IV) is made by endoscopic examination of the larynx at rest and observation of a midline or paramedian position of the corniculate process without morphological evidence of enlargement or deformation of the cartilage (i.e. arytenoid chondritis). A clinical diagnosis of RLN must not be made solely by observation of motion abnormalities (such as weak, paretic, partially paralyzed, flutter, and/or hesitation) of the arytenoid cartilage at rest. If one suspects laryngeal collapse (arytenoid cartilage collapse [ACC] (Fig. 26.25) or vocal cord collapse [VCC] (Fig. 26.26)), dynamic videoendoscopy (treadmill or overground) is necessary to confirm the diagnosis and identify concomitant obstruction.[1,37,103–105] During exercise, the laryngeal grade can also be classified as grade A, B, or C (Fig. 26.27).[101] Exercise endoscopy allows the precise diagnosis of collapse as well as co-morbid obstruction such that the optimum treatment can be prescribed. For example, horses with partial arytenoid collapse during exercise often have the same or better degree of arytenoid abduction than that obtained after a laryngoplasty. These horses frequently have vocal cord collapse obstructing the ventral aspect of the rima glottidis, with little collapse of the arytenoid cartilage. Therefore ventriculocordectomy might alleviate the obstruction.[106] If a dynamic exam at exercise is not possible, there is a reasonable correlation between laryngeal grade as show in Table 26.2 and laryngeal grade at exercise (Fig. 26.27);[103] horses with a resting laryngeal grade of I or II have a 7% prevalence of laryngeal collapse, while horses with laryngeal grade of III.1, III.2, and III.3 have a prevalence of laryngeal collapse at 44%, 83%, and 100%, respectively.

Another modality less frequently used now that dynamic endoscopy can be done is sound analysis.[31] Frequency analysis of airway sounds during exercise can help quantitate the upper airway sounds of horses such that RLN can be diagnosed during exercise without access to videoendoscopy. RLN is identified by the presence of sound throughout inhalation and exhalation and the presence of three frequency bands centered on 0.3 kHz, 1.6 kHz, and 3.8 kHz are seen during inhalation (Fig. 26.28A, B).[31]

Laryngeal ultrasound is becoming one of the most useful diagnostic modalities in identifying horses with RLN and differentiating them from chondritis. First described in 2006,[99] percutaneous

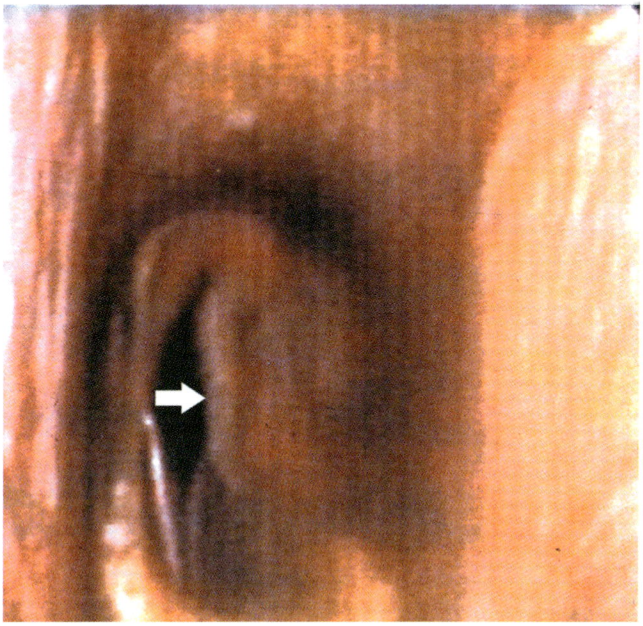

Fig 26.25 Endoscopic image of the larynx of a horse with grade IV idiopathic laryngeal hemiplegia while the horse is running on the treadmill. Notice how the left arytenoid collapses across the rima glottidis (arrow).

Table 26.2 Consensus grading system of laryngeal function performed in the standing unsedated horse[104]

GRADE	DESCRIPTION†	SUB-GRADE
I	All arytenoid cartilage movements are synchronous and symmetrical and full arytenoid cartilage abduction can be achieved and maintained	
II	Arytenoid cartilage movements are asynchronous and/or asymmetrical but full arytenoid cartilage abduction can be achieved and maintained	1. Transient asynchrony, flutter or delayed movements is seen 2. There is asymmetry of the rima glottidis much of the time due to reduced mobility of the affected arytenoid and vocal fold but there are occasions, typically after swallowing or nasal occlusion, when full symmetrical abduction is achieved and maintained
III	Arytenoid cartilage movements are asynchronous and/or asymmetrical but full arytenoid cartilage abduction cannot be achieved and maintained	1. There is asymmetry of the rima glottidis much of the time due to reduced mobility of the arytenoid and vocal fold but there are occasions, typically after swallowing or nasal occlusion, when full symmetrical abduction is achieved but not maintained 2. Obvious arytenoid abductor deficit and arytenoid asymmetry. Full abduction is never achieved 3. Marked but not total arytenoid abductor deficit and asymmetry with little arytenoid movement. Full abduction is never achieved
IV	Complete immobility of the arytenoid cartilage and vocal fold	

†Description generally refers to the left arytenoid cartilage in reference to the right. However, this grading system can apply to the right side (i.e. right grade III.1).)

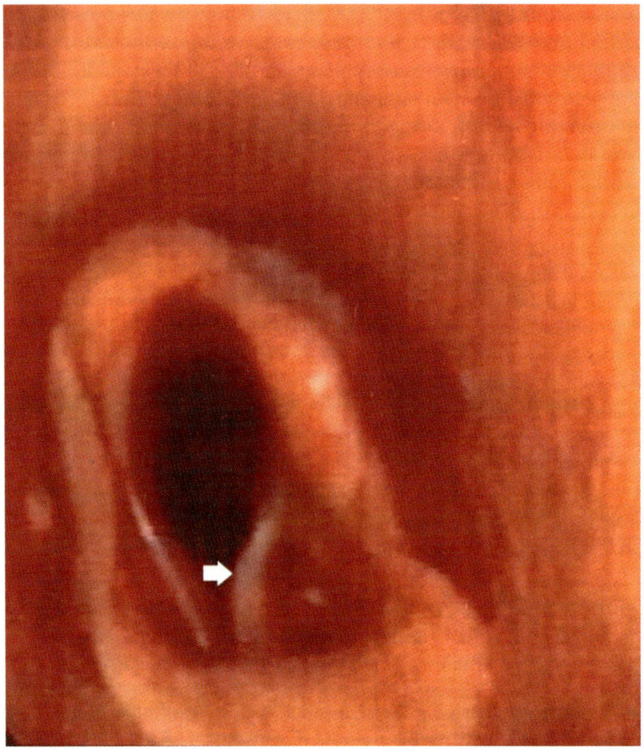

Fig 26.26 Endoscopic image of the larynx of a horse with grade III idiopathic laryngeal hemiplegia and vocal fold collapse. Notice how the left vocal fold collapses across the rima glottidis (arrow) as well as mild collapse of right aryepiglottic fold.

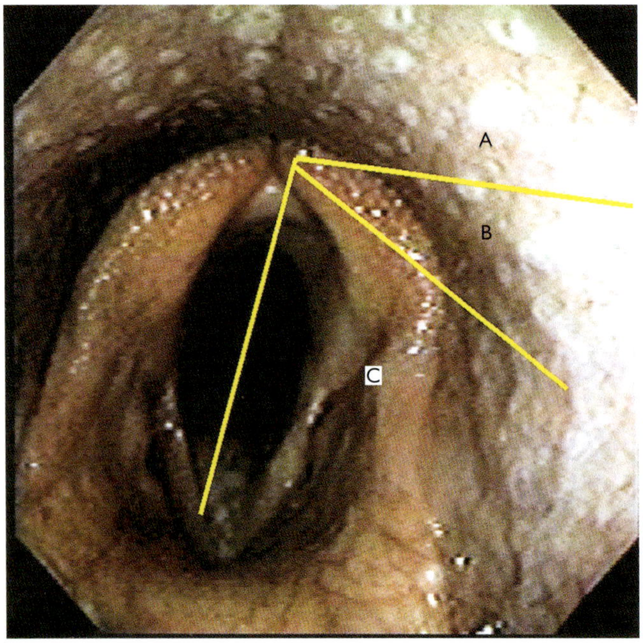

Fig 26.27 Endoscopic image of a larynx showing the position of the corniculate process of the arytenoids cartilage for each grade of laryngeal position. Zone A represents the position (maximal abduction) for grades I and II; Zone B represents the position for grade III (partial abduction); Zone C represents the position for grade IV laryngeal hemiplegia, or complete paralysis with no abduction.

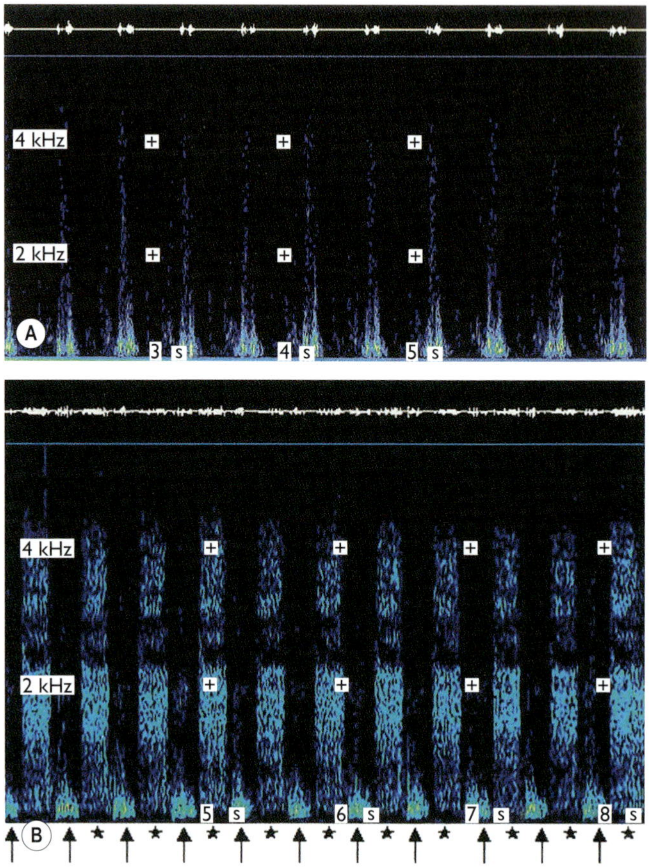

Fig 26.28 **(A)** Spectrogram of respiratory sounds from a horse with normal upper airway function. Time is on the abscissa, frequency on the ordinate. Sound level increases with brightness of the color (black indicates no sound). Inspiration is indicated by a star, expiration by an arrow. The top line of the graph is sound pressure level, a measure of sound intensity. **(B)** Spectrogram of respiratory sounds for a horse with laryngeal hemiplegia. Note the formants of inspiratory noise centered at 0.3, 1.6, and 3.8 kHz.

assessment of the cricoarytenoid lateralis through the caudo-lateral window (Fig. 26.29 A,B) is used as a sentinel for RLN as the adductor muscles are affected earlier and more severely than the abductor muscles.[107] Increase in CAL echogenicity has been shown to correlate with laryngeal collapse at exercise with a sensitivity and specificity of 90 and 98%, respectively.[108]

In sports medicine clinics, airway mechanics can be measured, accurately assessing the degree of laryngeal function and dysfunction.[109,110] In addition, blood gas measurements can help to determine the degree of ventilation compromise caused by laryngeal hemiplegia.[110] Finally electrodiagnostic testing of the thoracolaryngeal reflex latency and velocity has been shown to have no correlation with endoscopic examination and, therefore, is not useful in the assessment of laryngeal function.[111] However preliminary work with nerve conduction velocity suggests that this methodology might be useful in identifying early forms of RLN.[112]

Treatment and prognosis

Therapeutic aims

The goal of therapy is to restore the diameter of the rima glottidis and to prevent dynamic collapse of the vocal cord and arytenoid

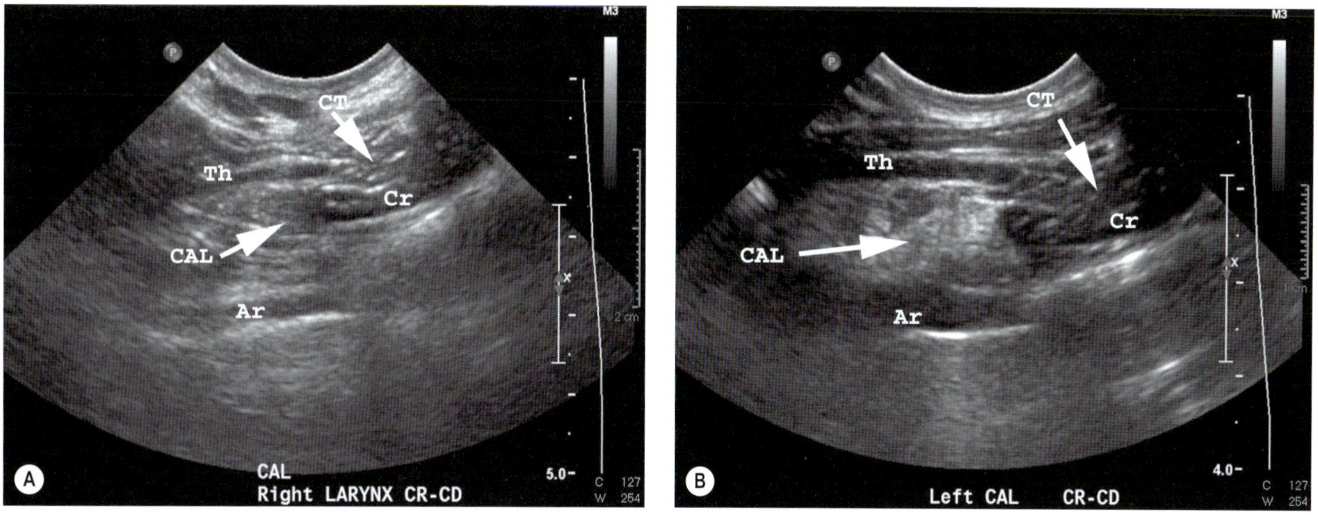

Fig 26.29 Percutaneous ultrasound image showing **(A)** right cricoarytenoid lateralis (CAL) muscle between the thyroid (Th) and arytenoid (Ar) and immediately rostral to the cricoid (Cr) cartilages. Note similar muscle echogenicity between CAL and cricothyroid (CT) muscles. **(B)** Left cricoarytenoid lateralis (CAL) muscle between the thyroid (Th) and arytenoid (Ar) and immediately rostral to cricoid (Cr) cartilages. Note the increased muscle echogenicity compared to right CAL and right and left cricothyroid (CT) muscles.

cartilage during inspiration. The problem resides in the fact that the larynx has both digestive and respiratory functions. The arytenoid cartilage must fully abduct (larynx must be fully dilated) during strenuous exercise and fully adducted (larynx must fully close) during swallowing. Therefore, treatments aimed at permanently increasing the diameter of the rima glottidis tend to interfere with laryngeal adduction during swallowing and protection of the airway.

Therapy

The value of surgical therapy for RLN depends on whether the complaint is exercise intolerance, noise production, or both. Ventriculocordectomy is effective in reducing airway noise and stabilizing the arytenoid cartilage during exercise, but does not improve airway mechanics as well as other surgical procedures.[113] Also, ventriculocordectomy or cordectomy is the surgical treatment of choice for horses with vocal fold collapse as seen in early cases of RLN.[106]

Laryngoprosthesis with unilateral ventriculocordectomy is the current standard surgical treatment for horses with arytenoid collapse at exercise.[114–119] Laryngoplasty reduces the high inspiratory upper airway impedance measured in horses with experimentally induced left laryngeal hemiplegia.[1]

Partial arytenoidectomy[120] is performed in some horses for treatment of RLN but these horses fail to return to their previous level of competition or at the same level as control horses although the return rate into competition can be higher than after laryngoplasty.[121,122] This is probably because, although airway mechanics measurements are improved following partial arytenoidectomy, impedance values are significantly higher than those of horses treated with laryngoplasty or those of normal horses.[115,123] In summary, partial arytenoidectomy is an alternative to laryngoplasty in sport horses and in racehorses where return rate to racing is more important than the level of performance.[124]

The neuromuscular pedicle graft procedure was introduced as a more physiological surgical treatment for RLN and is performed by grafting neuromuscular bundles composed of the first or second cervical nerve and omohyoideus muscle to the atrophied cricoarytenoideus dorsalis muscle or by anastomosing branches of the first cervical nerve to the abductor branch of the left recurrent laryngeal nerve.[124,125] Laryngeal reinnervation returns upper airway mechanics during exercise to normal, but the time required for successful reinnervation is 9–12 months.[125] Therefore, this procedure is generally reserved for yearling racehorses or sport horses.[125] Most recently electrical stimulation of the laryngeal recurrent nerve[126] or the CAD muscle[127] is opening the possibility of early return to function with a more physiological treatment, thus minimizing or eliminating the morbidity of the current treatment.

Prognosis

The clinical results of treatment of laryngeal hemiplegia with collapse of the upper airway (grade III and IV) are highly dependent on the activity of the horse. Horses used for show and jumping have a 90% chance of returning to their same level of function, while the prognosis is worse for racehorses, approximately 60–70%.[116–119,128] Complications of the laryngoplasty include (1) continued exercise intolerance and respiratory noise in 30 to 40% of horses during exercise, (2) chronic coughing due to abduction of the left arytenoid cartilage and the resulting inability of the larynx to protect the trachea from aspiration of ingesta in 20 to 40% of horses, and (3) loosening of the prosthetic suture(s) and loss of an initial degree of abduction in approximately 10% of horses.[116–119,128]

Etiology and pathophysiology

Anatomical considerations

The recurrent laryngeal nerve exits the caudal brainstem as part of the vagus nerve (cranial nerve X) and descends along the trachea dorsal to the common carotid artery with a different course between the left and right recurrent laryngeal nerves. The right recurrent laryngeal nerve leaves the vagus nerve at the level of the second rib turning around the costo-cervical trunk before ascending toward the larynx. The left recurrent laryngeal nerve leaves the vagus nerve as the latter crosses the aortic arch.. Both recurrent laryngeal nerves ascend cranially, ventral to the common carotid artery, to innervate all intrinsic muscles of the larynx except for the cricothyroid muscles, which are innervated by the ipsilateral external branch of the cranial laryngeal nerve.

Pathology

Idiopathic RLN is a peripheral neuropathy characterized by a distal loss of large myelinated fibers (distal axonopathy), is a bilateral mononeuropathy, leading to neurogenic atrophy of the intrinsic laryngeal muscles supplied by the recurrent laryngeal nerve.[95,107,129,130] Histologically, sections of the cricoarytenoideus dorsalis muscle exhibit fiber type grouping intermixed with atrophic fibers, suggestive of denervation and reinnervation.[94,107,129] Interestingly, there is a preferential atrophy of the adductor muscles in some horses so adductor deficit of the left arytenoid cartilage is observed despite normal abductor function in affected horses.[107] In addition, although the disease affects preferentially the left recurrent laryngeal nerve, there are some mild pathological lesions found in the right recurrent laryngeal nerve and associated right intrinsic laryngeal muscles.[130]

There is a significant and reasonable correlation (r = 0.75) between muscle histopathology and clinical disease (as in Table 26.2) or the degree of arytenoid dysfunction.[131] Horses with a clinical laryngeal grade IV RLN have marked pathological lesions. Horses with left-sided RLN can have histopathologic evidence of right-sided lesions without right-sided clinical signs.[131] This subclinical disease and its progression are not well understood. The progression from laryngeal grade I to grade IV is variable. Some horses show no progression in their laryngeal grade and stay at laryngeal grade III for years while others progress over a period of 2–4 months from normal to grade IV.[132,133]

Etiology

The etiology of RLN is unknown. Anatomically, the course of the left recurrent laryngeal nerve around the aorta, combined with the pathological appearance of the nerve, is suggestive of a compressive lesion, and led to the theory that the aortic pulse against the recurrent laryngeal nerve might be involved in the pathological process. Experimentally, constricting sutures were placed around the recurrent laryngeal nerve and a mixed array of abductor and adductor axons were affected along the course of the nerve, which is quite different than what is seen in the clinical disease.[95,134]

Risk factors for RLN include gender, breed, size, and perhaps genetics.[135–138] Male horses are over-represented, as are Thoroughbred and draft horses.[135–137]Horses greater than 16 hands have a higher incidence of RLN and the disease is rarely reported in ponies.[136–138]

Additional causes of ILH included perivascular injections with caustic substances, heart base tumors or other thoracic masses, exposure to organophosphates or lead, thiamine deficiency, and guttural pouch infections, and various neurologic diseases such as equine lower motor neuron disease.

Arytenoid chondritis

- Arytenoid chondritis has three clinical presentations: simple mucosal ulceration, granulation tissue formation (i.e. granulomas), and cartilage deformity.
- The size of the granulomas or of the enlargement of the body of the arytenoid determines the presence and severity of the airway obstruction.
- Clinical signs during exercise mimic those seen in idiopathic RLN.
- Endoscopic examination is diagnostic for arytenoid chondritis.
- Ultrasound exam identifies involvement of the body of the arytenoid cartilage.
- Once the arytenoid cartilage is abscessed and deformed, the treatment is surgical resection by arytenoidectomy.

Recognition

History and presenting complaint

Horses affected only with ulcerative lesions of the mucosa on the axial surface of the corniculate processes of the arytenoid cartilages (Fig. 26.30) are generally asymptomatic at rest and during exercise. These lesions are identified during endoscopic examination for reasons unrelated to abnormal airway function. Horses with granulation tissue originating from the arytenoid cartilage and protruding into the lumen of the rima glottidis (Fig. 26.31A, B) or horses with severe arytenoid cartilage abscessation and deformity (Fig. 26.32) have clinical signs of exercise intolerance and upper respiratory noise very similar to horses with laryngeal hemiplegia. If the abscess within the cartilage is large enough, the arytenoid cartilage can be deformed such that it causes severe obstruction of the rima glottidis.

Physical examination

Palpation of the throat and larynx is usually normal. The larynx has a normal contour and asymmetry of the cricoarytenoideus dorsalis muscles is not detected, as in idiopathic laryngeal hemiplegia. Rarely will there be perilaryngeal swelling associated with infection of the arytenoid cartilage.

Horses with arytenoid chondritis characterized by granulation tissue formation protruding from the arytenoid cartilage, with or without cartilage deformity, can be exercise intolerant and make an abnormal inspiratory noise during exercise. Depending upon the severity of respiratory distress, a tracheostomy can be warranted before further diagnostic evaluation is performed.

Special examination

Endoscopic examination of the larynx is frequently diagnostic for arytenoid chondritis. The morphology of the arytenoid cartilages

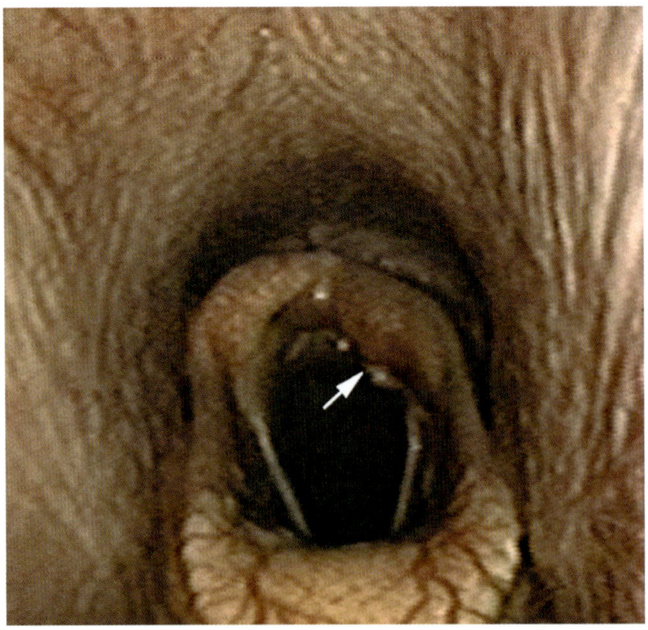

Fig 26.30 Endoscopic image of the larynx of a horse with 'kissing lesions' on the axial aspect of the mucosa covering the corniculate processes of the left arytenoid cartilage (arrow).

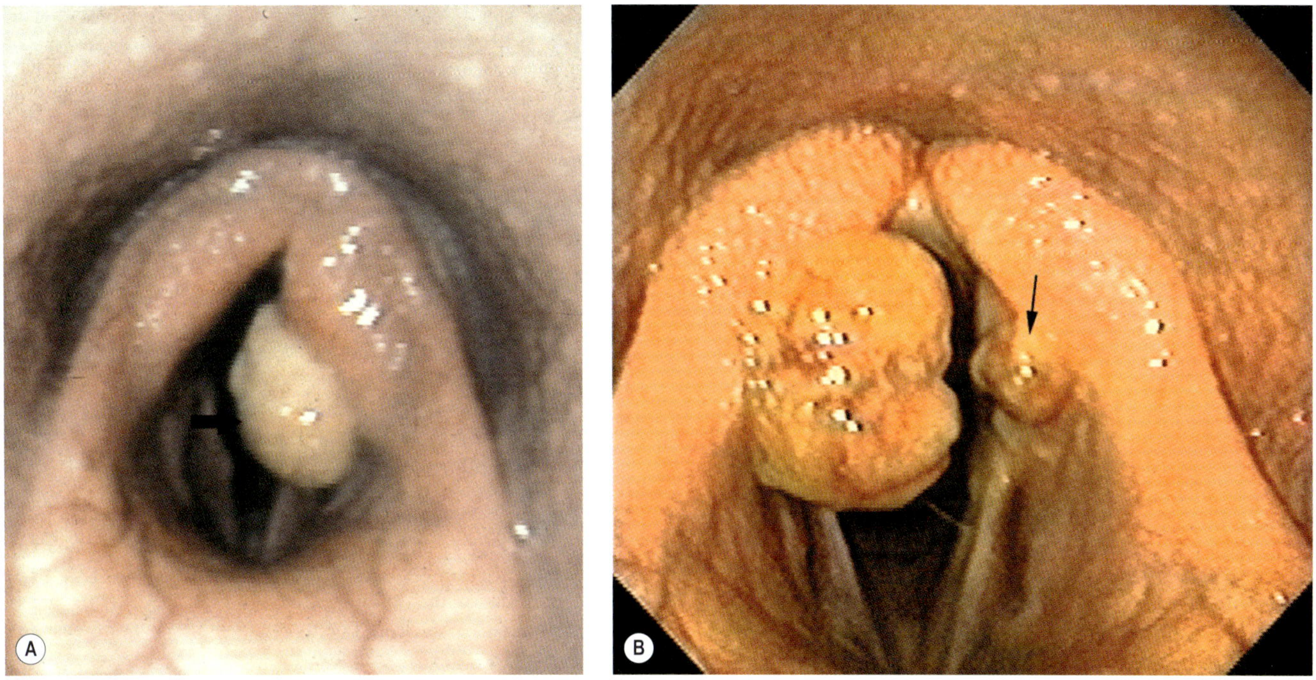

Fig 26.31 Endoscopic image of the larynx of two horse with arytenoid chondritis. **(A)** Note the granulation tissue (arrow) protruding from the left arytenoids. **(B)** A bilateral lesion, where the second smaller lesion (arrow) is thought to secondary to trauma from right granulomas.

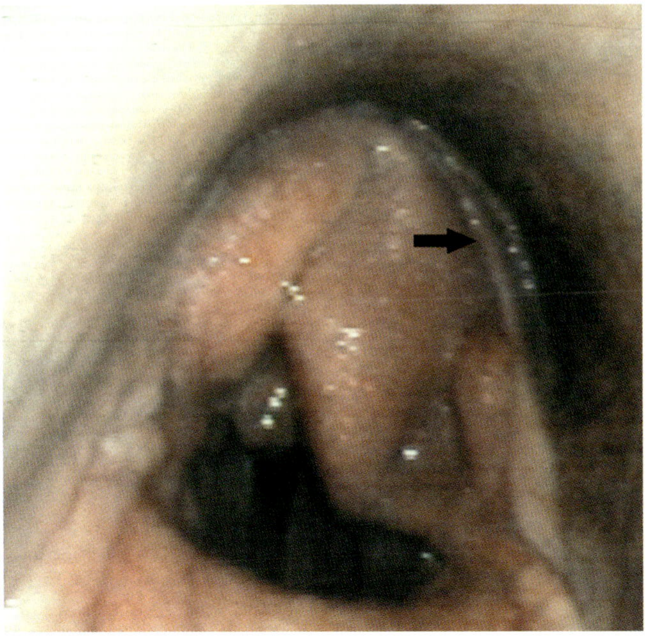

Fig 26.32 Endoscopic image of the larynx of a horse with severe arytenoid chondritis. Note the severely deformed left arytenoid cartilage, with medialization of the corniculate process exposing the palatopharyngeal arch (arrow).

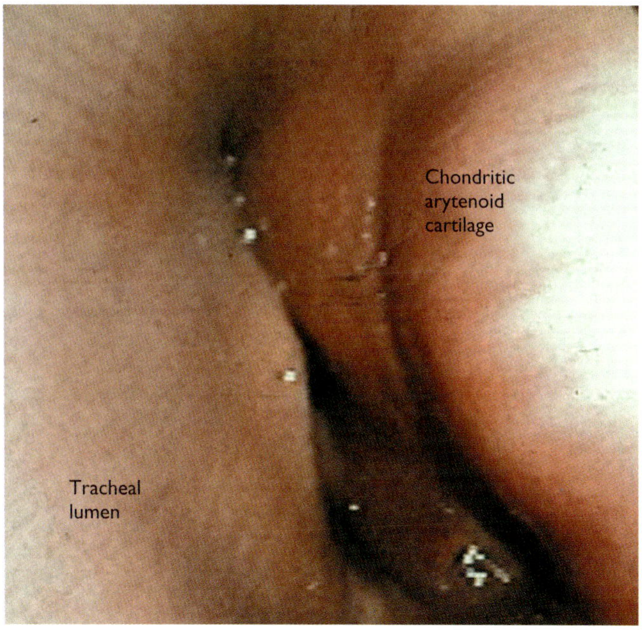

Fig 26.33 Endoscopic image of the lumen of the larynx of a horse with right arytenoid chondritis. Note the abscessed arytenoid cartilage bulging into the laryngeal lumen. The image was taken by passing the endoscope retrograde, through the tracheotomy site.

and the integrity of the overlying mucosa should be evaluated, as well as any purulent exudates draining from the cartilage. In addition, it is important to assess the degree of arytenoid movement. If a tracheostomy has been performed, the endoscope can be passed retrograde through the tracheostomy site to further evaluate the morphology of the arytenoid cartilage (Fig. 26.33).

The most useful technique to identify a lesion extending in the body of the arytenoid is laryngeal ultrasound. Using a caudo-lateral window, an irregular and enlarged body of the arytenoid cartilage (Fig. 26.34) can be detected as well as perilaryngeal abscess if present. In the vast majority of cases the CAL and CAD muscles remain normal in terms of echogenicity (Fig. 26.34). Radiographic and MRI examination can also help to identify enlarged or mineralized arytenoid cartilage but are rarely needed to identify or treat a horse with chondritis.

Treatment and prognosis

Therapeutic aims

If mucosal ulceration of the arytenoid cartilage is the only abnormality and the morphology and function of the arytenoids are normal, the goal of treatment is to reduce the local inflammation and prevent bacterial invasion of the arytenoid cartilage. Systemic and topical anti-inflammatory and antimicrobial therapy form the basis of treatment in these cases. Granulation tissue protruding from the arytenoid cartilage is removed sharply or with a laser, and if no abnormality of the arytenoid cartilage or its function is detected, systemic and topical anti-inflammatory and antimicrobial therapy is prescribed.[139–141] In chronic cases where the arytenoid cartilage is deformed, abscessed, and dysfunctional, the goal of treatment is to restore the diameter of the rima glottidis by surgical removal of the granuloma and the arytenoid cartilage.[142]

Therapy

Ulceration of the mucosa covering the arytenoid cartilage is a subclinical finding that is important because the ulcer can serve as an entrance for bacterial invasion into the arytenoid cartilage, potentially leading to abscessation and deformity of the arytenoids. Treatment consists of local therapy with an anti-inflammatory throat spray applied twice daily. Systemic antibiotics are prescribed for 2–3 weeks (trimethoprim sulfa, 15 mg/kg, p.o. q 12 h) and a nonsteroidal anti-inflammatory drug (phenylbutazone or flunixin meglumine) for 7–10 days.

Protruding buds of granulation tissue with normal arytenoid cartilage abduction are treated with surgical resection of the lesion and medical treatment of the resulting mucosal defect as described above. Endoscopic re-evaluation should be performed to determine if the lesion recurs or the process extends into the arytenoid cartilage, resulting in chondritis and cartilage deformity.

In acute cases of unilateral arytenoid chondritis, medical treatment as described above is initiated. The abscessed cartilage is probed to determine if surgical drainage is possible.[140] To accomplish this, the horse is sedated and, via endoscopy, local anesthetic is liberally applied to the laryngeal mucosa. Under endoscopic control, a No. 15 blade is used to make a stab incision through the skin, muscle, and cricothyroid membrane. A 5 mm trocar is placed through the stab incision and the cricothyroid membrane into the lumen of the larynx. An 18-gauge needle is placed through the mucosal defect into the arytenoid cartilage in the area where the granulation tissue was resected. A curette is used to enlarge the opening, initiating drainage of purulent exudate. Following drainage of the abscess, the lesion can regress completely with return of full cartilage abduction.

In chronic cases of arytenoid chondritis or if following drainage of the abscess, the arytenoid cartilage function failed to return, an arytenoidectomy is performed. Two types of arytenoidectomy can be performed: partial and subtotal arytenoidectomy.[142–144] Partial arytenoidectomy[142,143] includes removal of all portions of the arytenoid cartilage except the muscular process of the arytenoid cartilage. Subtotal arytenoidectomy involves removal of the body of the arytenoid cartilage, leaving the muscular and corniculate processes. Subtotal arytenoidectomy has been shown to yield minimal improvement in airway diameter because the unsupported corniculate process collapses into the rima glottidis during inhalation.[144] However, it best preserves the protective mechanism of the larynx and is associated with less aspiration of feed material. Partial arytenoidectomy provides the best improvement in airway diameter, with a small risk of aspiration of feed material.[143] Following arytenoidectomy, the horses should be fed and watered from the ground to minimize tracheal contamination.

Prognosis

The prognosis for resolution of mucosal ulcers with medical therapy, without the progression to arytenoid chondritis, is excellent. Horses treated with medical therapy for granulation tissue protruding from the arytenoid have a 30% chance of developing arytenoid chondritis. The prognosis for pasture soundness or light riding following arytenoidectomy is very good.[142] In rare cases, tracheal aspiration of feed material occurs at times, resulting in aspiration pneumonia. Bilateral arytenoidectomy has a less favorable prognosis because the potential for aspiration of feed and laryngeal stenosis is increased.[145]

Recent data indicated that in term of resolution of exercise intolerance, the prognosis is good.[121,146]

Etiology and pathophysiology

Etiology

The arytenoid cartilage has two processes: the vocal process where the vocal ligament is attached and the muscular process where the cricoarytenoid dorsalis muscle (the laryngeal abductor muscle) inserts (Fig. 26.35).[3] The comma-shaped corniculate process is attached to the apex of the arytenoid cartilage and forms the dorsal border of the rima glottidis.

Arytenoid chondritis develops following trauma to the mucosa of the arytenoid cartilage and invasion of bacteria into the cartilage. In humans, cattle, and presumably horses, trauma occurs following severe coughing episodes where the arytenoid cartilages contact each other during these marked adduction episodes, creating contact ulcers.[147,148] Other causes include iatrogenic damage to the

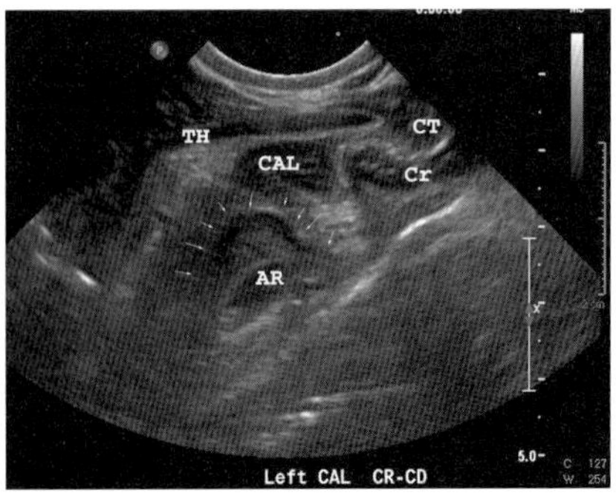

Fig 26.34 Percutaneous ultrasound image using left caudo-lateral window showing enlarged and irregular body of the left arytenoid cartilage. Note that similar to Fig. 26.29A and unlike Fig. 26.29B the cricoarytenoid lateralis (CAL) muscle remains of normal echogenicity. Thyroid cartilage = TH, arytenoid cartilage = AR, cricoid cartilage = Cr, and cricothyroid muscle = CT.

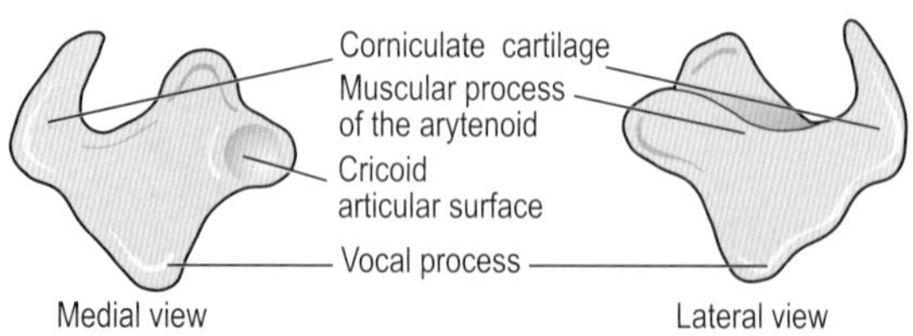

Fig 26.35 Illustration of the anatomy of the arytenoid cartilage.

mucosa of the arytenoid cartilage by coarse feed material, from 'kick back' on dirt tract, or during medical procedures such as nasogastric intubation and endoscopy.[148]

Pathophysiology

Arytenoid chondritis has three clinical presentations affecting one or both arytenoid cartilages: mucosal ulceration, granulation tissue projecting in the lumen of the larynx, and arytenoid cartilage abscessation leading to deformity and dysfunction. Following ulceration of the arytenoid cartilage mucosa, local bacterial invasion of the body of the arytenoid cartilage causes a superficial chondritis resulting in the production of granulation tissues and a fistulous tract. If the infection extends deeper in the body of the cartilage, an abscess can form, and enlargement and deformation of the arytenoid cartilage, and lack of movement results.

The physical presence of the granulation tissue protruding into the rima glottidis causes a static luminal obstruction during both inspiration and expiration. When the cartilage is deformed and immobile, dynamic inspiratory obstruction occurs.

Prevention

Prevention of this syndrome is difficult. Preventing trauma to the arytenoid cartilage by minimizing trauma during nasogastric intubation and endoscopic examination is prudent. Treatment of mucosal ulceration and granulation tissue can prevent further bacterial invasion of the cartilage and more severe chondritis from developing.

There has been one report of an association in Thoroughbred horses of equine lymphocyte antigen A9 and chondritis, suggesting a possible genetic predisposition to this disease.[149]

Rostral displacement of the palatopharyngeal arch (fourth and sixth branchial arch defect, also known as 4-BAD, or cricopharyngeal-laryngeal dysplasia)

- Rostral displacement of the palatopharyngeal arch results most commonly from laryngeal cartilage malformation.
- Rarely are horses affected at rest but they show signs of exercise intolerance and abnormal respiratory noise during exercise.
- Three types of obstruction can be seen with this deformity due to failure of abduction of ipsilateral arytenoid cartilage, DDSP, and collapse of palatopharyngeal arch or its continuation the aryepiglottic fold during inhalation.
- Surgical restoration of the arytenoid cartilage by simple laryngoplasty is usually unsuccessful due to the cartilage deformity, which most commonly involves the thyroid cartilage and the cricothyroid articulation.
- Rostral displacement of the palatopharyngeal arch can also occur secondarily in horses with arytenoid chondritis, due to deformity of the arytenoid cartilage.

Recognition

History and presenting complaint

Horses affected with rostral displacement of the palatopharyngeal arch are usually asymptomatic at rest but this condition can be diagnosed at rest during routine palpation of the larynx or endoscopic examination of the larynx in yearling horses. Clinical signs include poor performance and an inspiratory noise, the severity of which is related to the severity of the congenital malformation. The character of the inspiratory noise resembles that heard in horses with laryngeal hemiplegia except that it is generally less intense and shorter in duration. In a review of 60 cases, 83% of horses made abnormal inspiratory noise, 22% had involuntary aerophagia, 17% had nasal discharge and coughing, and 3% reported tympanic colic.[150]

Physical examination

The most common cause of rostral displacement of the palatopharyngeal arch is congenital malformation of the laryngeal cartilages. The most common abnormality is deformation of the wing(s) of the thyroid cartilage.[150] The larynx should therefore be palpated to detect a gap between the thyroid and cricoid cartilages. In addition it is important to palpate the muscular processes of the arytenoid cartilages because a less prominent or impalpable muscular process suggests arytenoid and/or thyroid cartilage malformation. Paralaryngeal cysts can also be present and cause bulging of the lamina of the thyroid cartilage that can be felt unilaterally or bilaterally around the larynx.

Special examination

The position of the palatopharyngeal arch rostral to the corniculate process of the arytenoid cartilage is pathognomonic for rostral displacement of the palatopharyngeal arch (Fig. 26.36). In a significant proportion of horses affected with rostral displacement of the palatopharyngeal arch, incomplete abduction of one arytenoid cartilage (usually the right) is seen. Dynamic endoscopic examination is performed to assess which airway abnormalities are associated with this malformation.

Radiography of the throat is helpful because horses with rostral displacement of the palatopharyngeal arch frequently have an

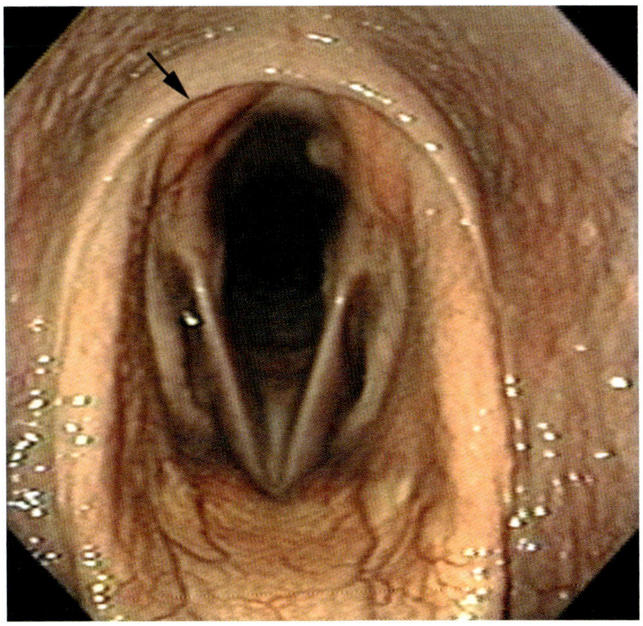

Fig 26.36 Endoscopic image of the larynx of a horse with rostralg displacement of the palatopharyngeal arch. Note how the palatopharyngeal arch (arrow) protrudes over the corniculate processes of the arytenoid cartilages.

anomaly of the cricopharyngeal sphincter, which is seen radiographically as a continuous column of air between the nasopharynx and the esophagus. The presence of redundant tissue dorsal to the corniculate processes of the arytenoid cartilages on radiographs is suggestive of rostral displacement of the palatopharyngeal arch. Laryngeal ultrasound allows the observation of missing cricothyroid articulation. Computer tomography can help identify cartilage malformation such as dorsal border of the thyroid cartilage extending dorsally over the muscular process and also detect paralaryngeal cysts. However MRI exam gives the most detailed evaluation of the abnormal cartilage and muscle such as abnormal cricopharyngeal sphinter and perilaryngeal muscle such as thyrohyoideus.[151]

Diagnostic confirmation

The diagnosis is made by a combination of laryngeal palpation, videoendoscopic examination and imaging of the upper airway.

Treatment and prognosis

Therapeutic aims

The goal of therapy is to restore airway patency during strenuous exercise. It is important to assess which of the possible consequences of 4 BAD contributes to an airway obstruction. DDSP can be treated by laryngeal tie-forward, the redundant palatopharyngeal arch can be resected. If one of the arytenoid cartilages cannot abduct, laryngoplasty used to treat horses with RLN will be ineffective in this instance because the cartilages are malformed; proper resection of a section of the thyroid lamina may be needed to allow abduction of the arytenoid after placement of the laryngoprosthesis. Alternatively a partial arytenoidectomy may need to be performed. If a laryngeal cyst is causing the cartilage malformation, the cyst can be removed.

Therapy

Laryngeal cyts are removed using the lateral laryngeal approach used for laryngoplasty. However, cyst removal does not ensure return of normal abductor function of the arytenoid cartilage. This is because multiple concomitant laryngeal deformations are usually present. Partial arytenoidectomy can be performed in an attempt to maximize the lumen of the airway. Laryngoplasty is generally unsuccessful at abducting the arytenoid cartilage because deformities diminish any abductory movement at the arytenoid cricoid articulation.

Prognosis

The prognosis for athleticism is guarded, and is related to the degree of laryngeal cartilage malformation.

Prevention

Because this congenital malformation is probably heritable, avoiding breeding affected horses will limit occurrence.

Etiology and pathophysiology

Etiology

There is little information on the embryology of horses as it relates to formation of the larynx and nasopharynx.[152] It is, however, well known that the human larynx and its intrinsic musculature, and laryngeal nerves, originate from a combination of the fourth and sixth branchial arches.[153,154] Specifically, the cranial laryngeal nerve originates from the fourth branchial arch and the recurrent laryngeal from the sixth branchial arch. The epiglottic cartilage develops separately as it originates from the hypobranchial eminence.

Abnormalities seen with this congenital disease include absence of cricopharyngeal muscles, deformed thyroid cartilage resulting in an increased space between the thyroid and cricoid cartilage, abnormality of the cricopharyngeus and thyropharyngeus muscles, absence or small muscular process of the arytenoid cartilage, presence of paralaryngeal cyst(s) and associated deformation of laryngeal cartilage.[150,151] Vertical displacement of the lamina of the thyroid cartilage over the muscular process of the arytenoid cartilage can occur, and this deformity prevents arytenoid cartilage abduction. The right side of the larynx is most frequently affected but the deformities can occur bilaterally or on the left side.[150]

Rostral displacement of the palatopharyngeal arch can also be seen unilaterally with arytenoid chondritis or following partial arytenoidectomy. This is thought to be due to the physical loss of the corniculate process of the arytenoid cartilage, caudal to which the palatopharyngeal arch membrane normally sits.

Pathophysiology

Most of the clinical signs associated with rostral displacement of the palatopharyngeal arch are respiratory in origin and are due to obstruction of the rima glottidis. More rarely, associated abnormality of the cricopharyngeal sphincter leads to dysphagia and aerophagia, which can cause tympanic colic in some horses.

Airway obstruction is caused by one or more of the following abnormalities: collapse of one of the arytenoid cartilage, collapse of the palatopharyngeal arch, medial collapse of the aryepiglottic fold and/or DDSP.[150,155–157] Failure of abduction occurs for several reasons including the absence of the muscular process of the arytenoid cartilage, or thyroid cartilage physical obstruction of the arytenoid preventing abduction of the arytenoid cartilage. The absence of the cricothyroid articulation leads to caudal displacement of the arytenoid cartilage instead of abduction.[150] Vertical displacement of the thyroid lamina prevents caudo-lateral displacement of the muscular process of the arytenoid cartilage, a process needed for abduction of the arytenoid cartilage.

When rostral displacement of the palatopharyngeal arch occurs following partial arytenoidectomy, this presentation is unlikely to be of any clinical significance. Decreased performance in horses treated with partial arytenoidectomy can justify dynamic endoscopic examination of the larynx to determine if there is dynamic obstruction of the airway due to unilateral collapse of the palatopharyngeal arch membrane or the remnant of its extension the aryepiglottic membrane.

The digestive dysfunction is rare and caused by regurgitation of esophageal contents back into the nasopharynx due to deficiency in the musculature of the cricopharyngeal sphincter. Regurgitation of feed material back into the nasopharynx and trachea can result in coughing and nasal discharge.[150,] In addition, aerophagia created by the deficient cricopharyngeal sphincter has been reported to result in tympanic colic.[150]

Guttural pouch mycosis

- Associated with a fungal infection usually near or on the internal carotid artery but can extend to the maxillary artery.
- Most commonly recognized by unilateral epistaxis as the lesion erodes in the internal and/or maxillary arteries.
- Medical treatment is risky as horses can die during the next epistaxis episode.

- Simple ligation at the cardiac side does not always prevent continued epistaxis episodes because of retrograde flow from the circle of Willis.
- Embolization of the vessels is needed to prevent retrograde flow.

Recognition

History and presenting complaint

The most common clinical sign of guttural pouch mycosis is severe epistaxis caused by erosion of the internal carotid artery, external carotid artery and/or maxillary artery. Other clinical signs include mucopurulent or hemorrhagic nasal discharge, coughing, dysphagia caused by cranial nerve damage (IX and X), unilateral laryngeal hemiplegia, Horner's syndrome, parotid pain, tongue paresis, and head shaking.[158–161] Endoscopic examination of the nasopharynx can reveal hemorrhage from one or both nasopharyngeal openings.

Physical examination

Physical examination findings vary depending upon the chronicity of the hemorrhage. If the horse has recently bled severely due to erosion of a major artery within the guttural pouch by a mycotic plaque, the horse will show clinical signs of hypovolemic shock, including sweating, tachycardia, weak peripheral pulses, pale mucous membranes, and cold ears and muzzle. Occasionally, if the mycotic plaque forms over cranial nerves, such as branches of the vagus nerve or the sympathetic trunk, the horse can have clinical evidence of dysphagia and aspiration pneumonia or Horner's syndrome.[158–161] Tongue paresis can occur due to hypoglossal nerve involvement.[162]

Special examination

Endoscopic examination of the nasopharynx and guttural pouches is diagnostic for guttural pouch mycosis. Following hemorrhage, a blood clot will protrude from the affected pouch. If the disease is bilateral or the fungus has eroded through the median septum, clots can form at both guttural pouch openings. Inspection of the affected guttural pouch reveals a single fungal plaque or multiple plaques associated with the major arteries of the guttural pouch, including most commonly the internal carotid artery, but also the external carotid artery, and the maxillary artery (Fig. 26.37).[158,161]

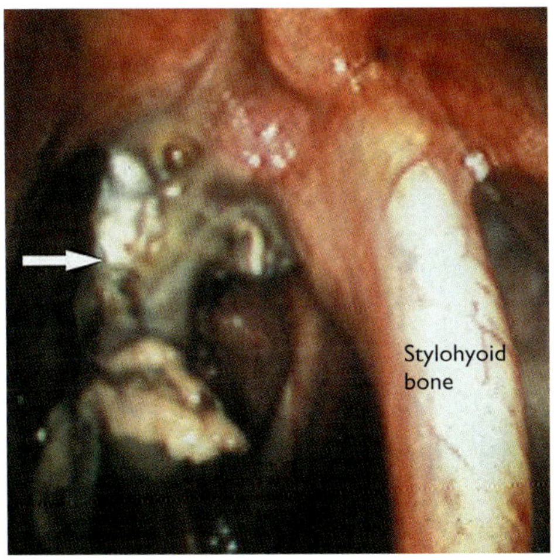

Fig 26.37 Endoscopic image of the guttural pouch of a horse with guttural pouch mycosis. Note the gray-to-black mycotic lesion (arrow).

Laboratory examination

Horses can be anemic if guttural pouch hemorrhage is severe or if multiple bleeding episodes have occurred.

Diagnostic confirmation

Differential diagnosis for guttural pouch mycosis includes other conditions that would result in guttural pouch hemorrhage, the most common being avulsion of the longus capitis muscle from the basisphenoid bone, or trauma.[163] Biopsy and culture of the fungal plaque confirms the diagnosis.

Treatment and prognosis

Therapeutic aims

The goals of treatment are to prevent life-ending hemorrhage and eradicate the fungal infection from the guttural pouch.

Therapy

Medical treatment of guttural pouch mycosis includes topical application of non-irritating antifungal agents that are effective against *Aspergillus* spp., such as itraconazole, micozadole, and enilconazole.[164,165] Medical therapy consists of miconazole 70 mg diluted in 10 mL isotonic saline or in a 400 mg gynecological preparation (must be warmed) administered through a female urinary catheter. The preparation is administered under endoscopic control at the following schedule: Week 1: once a day, Week 2: EOD, and Week 3–4: twice a week. Medical therapy can be justified if hemorrhage has not occurred and the fungal plaques do not involve any blood vessels or if financial constraint prevents surgical options.

If vascular structures are involved, which is most common, the goal of surgical therapy is to occlude the affected arteries.[158,161] Most simply, the internal carotid artery on the affected side can be ligated. This can decrease the hemorrhage, but horses are still at risk for fatal hemorrhage due to collateral circulation through the circle of Willis and the palatine arteries.[161] Alternatively, a combination of internal, external and palatine artery ligation and balloon angioplasty using venous thrombectomy catheters, coil embolization, or nitinol vascular occlusion plugs can be performed.[158,159,161,166,167] These techniques alleviate the possibility of continued hemorrhage through retrograde flow. Following occlusion of the rostral portion of the internal carotid artery, embolization coils/balloon/coils are then placed in the caudal portion of the vessels to prevent normograde blood flow. If the external carotid or maxillary arteries are affected, embolization coil vascular occlusion is performed in the maxillary artery just before the alar foramen, and in the external carotid artery, just after it bifurcates from the linguofacial artery. When obstructing flow into the maxillary artery one should not ligate the palatine artery; instead it should be catheterized so that the obstruction is located at the caudal aspect of the palatine bone; otherwise, blindness can occur due to steal phenomena.[168]

Prognosis

Approximately 50% of horses that bleed severely die from fatal hemorrhage. If appropriate vascular occlusion is successful, the prognosis for life is excellent. Fungal plaques generally resolve without antifungal medication, 30 to 60 days following vascular occlusion. Dysphagia, unilateral laryngeal hemiplegia, and Horner's syndrome can resolve over 6 to 8 months, or can be permanent. Potential complications related to the surgical procedures include unilateral blindness, cerebral ischemia, and recurrent hemorrhage.[158,161,169]

Prevention

There is no known method of prevention.

Etiology and pathophysiology

Etiology

The etiology is unknown, but *Aspergillus* spp. is frequently cultured from the diphtheritic plaques.[165]

Pathophysiology

The fungal plaques grow within the guttural pouch, and if they erode through the walls of the internal, external, or maxillary arteries, life-threatening hemorrhage can ensue.

Epidemiology

There is neither a known geographical predisposition nor age, breed, sex, or occupational predilection for guttural pouch mycosis.

Avulsion of the longus capitis/ rectus capitis ventralis muscles

Recognition

History and presenting complaint

Horses with avulsion or rupture of the longus capitis and rectus capitis ventralis muscles usually have a history of trauma, such as falling over or being tied and pulling free.[163] Occasionally (one case) the trauma can occur as a result of the horse throwing its head and neck overzealously. Affected horses can have bilateral epistaxis, swelling or thickening in the throatlatch area, and can be ataxic or exhibit other signs of neurologic dysfunction.[163]

Physical examination

Horses will often have bilateral epistaxis, may be ataxic or have cranial nerve deficits, and swelling in the area of Viborg's triangle.[163] Affected horses may have signs of vestibular disease (head tilt, falling, ipsilateral weakness, circling), facial nerve injury (palsy of facial muscles, inability to blink, creased lacrimation and keratitis sicca) and cerebral dysfunction (depressed mentation).

Special examination

Endoscopic examination of the nasopharynx reveals collapse of the dorsal nasopharynx due to the hematoma formation within the dorsal and medial tissues of the guttural pouch and blood or blood clots at the nasopharyngeal openings of the guttural pouches. Within the guttural pouch, hemorrhage and hematoma formation are evident along the medial wall (Fig. 26.38). Lateral radiographic projections of the guttural pouch region show soft tissue density within the guttural pouch compression of the dorsal nasopharynx, and avulsion fracture of the basisphenoid bone (Fig. 26.39).

Laboratory examination

Laboratory examination is normal or there is evidence of hemorrhage.

Diagnostic confirmation

Differential diagnosis for avulsion of the longus capitis and rectus capitis ventralis muscles is guttural pouch mycosis. The history of trauma and the appearance of the hematoma within the medial wall of the guttural pouch are diagnostic for this condition.

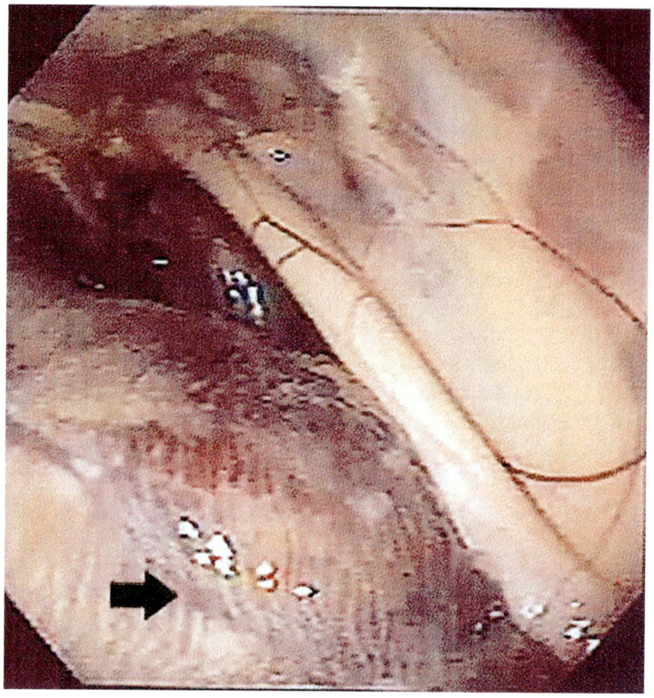

Fig 26.38 Endoscopic image of the guttural pouch of a horse that avulsed the longus capitis and rectus capitis muscles from the basisphenoid and basioccipitus bones at the base of the skull. Note the large hematoma (arrow) within the medial compartment of the guttural pouch.

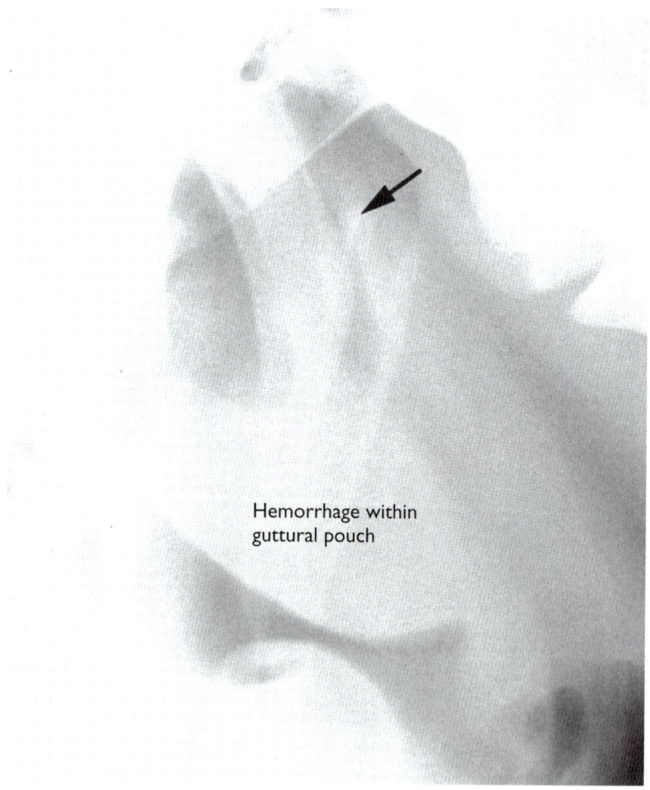

Fig 26.39 Lateral radiograph of the guttural pouch region of a horse that avulsed the longus capitis and rectus capitis muscles from the basisphenoid and basioccipitus bones at the base of the skull. Note the bone fragment (arrow) and the hemorrhage within the guttural pouch.

Treatment and prognosis

Therapeutic aims

The goal of therapy is to provide supportive care if the horse has neurologic signs and confine the horse to minimize the risk of further hemorrhage.

Therapy

Two to three months of stall rest and broad-spectrum antimicrobial therapy are warranted due to the hematoma formation within the guttural pouch.[163] Judicious use of non-steroidal anti-inflammatory therapy for analgesia is recommended. If neurologic signs are severe and the horse is unable to rise, subdural hemorrhage involving the brainstem and cerebral cortex should be suspected and euthanasia is warranted.

Prognosis

The prognosis for return to function is good unless neurologic deficits are severe.[163]

Prevention

There is no known method of prevention.

Etiology and pathophysiology

Etiology

Avulsion of the rectus capitis muscles usually occurs as a result of trauma.

Pathophysiology

Three muscles that flex the head and neck include the large longus capitis muscle and two small muscles, rectus capitis ventralis and rectus capitis lateralis, which course ventrally between the guttural pouches. Simultaneous contraction of these muscles as the horse falls over backwards would lead to avulsion fracture from the basisphenoid and occipital bones, resulting in hemorrhage from the guttural pouch and hematoma formation.

Epidemiology

Horses most commonly affected are young animals early in their training or breaking program. The disease is less common in older horses because they are less likely to fall over backwards or pull back violently when tied.

Temporohyoid osteoarthropathy

- Degenerative disease of unknown cause leading to fusion of the temporohyoid articulation.[169]
- The disease can be unilateral or bilateral.
- Enlargment of the temporohyoid articulation leads to compression of the VII and VIII cranial nerves.[170]
- Clinical signs are associated with deficit of the cranial nerves VII and VIII as well as pain upon movement of the stylohyoid bone by movement of the tongue or pressure on the basihyoid bone.
- Fusion of the temporohyoid articulation can lead to petrous bone fracture and acute death.
- Treatment includes removal of the lever arm action of the stylohyoid bone by removal of the ceratohyoid bone.

Recognition

History and presenting complaint: most horses with temporohyoid osteoarthropathy (THO) have clinical signs suggestive of facial nerve (cranial nerve VII) and/or vestibulocochlear nerve (cranial nerve VIII) deficits. Presenting complaints include facial nerve paralysis and lip droop, head tilt, ataxia or falling, difficulty eating, corneal ulceration/keratitis, nasal discharge, and head shaking/tossing.[170–174]

Physical examination

Physical examination findings include fever, facial and vestibulocochlear nerve deficits, including vestibular signs that can resemble ataxia, pain with manipulation of the jaw or opening the mouth, blepharospasm and corneal ulceration.[170–174]

Special examination

The diagnosis of THO is made based on physical examination findings and endoscopic examination of the guttural pouches. Skull radiographs and computed tomography are sometimes used to help confirm the diagnosis or more fully describe the lesion at the temporohyoid articulation. Osseous proliferation at the proximal aspect of the stylohyoid bone is seen during endoscopic examination of the guttural pouch on the affected side (Fig. 26.40). Dorsoventral radiographic projections of the skull can show enlargement of the temporohyoid region. Computed tomographic scans can show fusion of the temporohyoid joint and osseous proliferation of the proximal portion of the stylohyoid bone. Occasionally, fracture of the stylohyoid or ceratohyoid bones can be seen. Schirmer tear test can be performed to assess tear production from the affected eye, especially if signs of facial neuropathy are present.

CT examination allows the most precise assessment of the condition which will influence or facilitate the surgery by characterizing the plane of the ceratohyoid–stylohyoid articulation, extent of disease on ceratohyoid bone and unilateral or bilateral disease.[175,176]

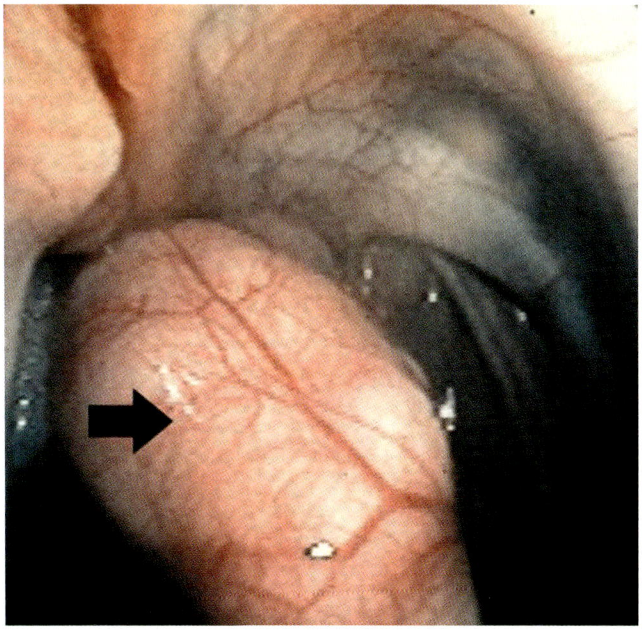

Fig 26.40 Endoscopic image of the articulation of the stylohyoid bone and the petrous portion of the temporal bone in a horse with temporohyoid osteoarthropathy. Note the enlarged region (arrow) of the proximal aspect of the stylohyoid bone.

Laboratory examination

Most frequently, clinical laboratory examination is normal. Leukocytosis, lymphopenia, anemia, and hyperfibrinogenemia can occur.

Diagnostic confirmation

Endoscopic, radiographic, or computed tomographic evidence of temporohyoid fusion or enlargement are diagnostic for temporohyoid osteoarthropathy.

Treatment and prognosis

Therapeutic aims

The goals of therapy include resolution of the vestibular and facial nerve deficits, removing pain associated with swallowing, treatment or prevention of corneal ulceration, and protecting the horse from further trauma resulting from its vestibular disease. Most horses are treated with antibiotics and non-steroidal anti-inflammatory drugs, including trimethoprim sulfa, enrofloxacin, or penicillin and gentamicin for 30 days, and oral phenylbutazone or flunixin meglumine.[171–174] Surgical treatment involves removing the ceratohyoid bone to minimize motion at the temporohyoid articulation.[177] Corneal ulcers are treated with topical medication, and if the eyelid is not functional, a tarsorrhaphy can be performed to protect the cornea until facial neuropathy resolves or improves. Ocular lubricants can be applied to affected eyes several times daily if the cornea is healthy but eyelid function is abnormal.

Prognosis

Following temporohyoid osteoarthropathy, pain is alleviated usually within 24–48 hours: 63% of horses return to athletic activity and most horses return to their intended use, although you may need to maintain the tarsorrhaphy to prevent eye lesions from desiccation. Rehabilitation time can be long, up to 2 years, though many clinical signs will abate within 30 to 60 days.[170,172, 173,174,]

Prevention

There are no known preventive measures.

Etiology and pathophysiology

Etiology

The etiology is unknown.

Pathophysiology

THO is probably the result of primary generative osteoarthritis of the temporohyoid joint associated with age.[169–173] Alternatively, it can be the sequela to otitis media/interna that develops secondary to hematogenous spread of bacteria, ascending infection from the respiratory tract, otitis externa, or extension of guttural pouch empyema.[170,172] The infection and inflammatory reaction of the tympanic bulla, temporohyoid joint, and stylohyoid bone resolves, leaving bony proliferation of the proximal stylohyoid bone and fusion of the temporohyoid joint. Vestibular disease and facial nerve paralysis occur when osseous proliferation impinges on cranial nerves VII (facial) and VIII (vestibulocochlear) or if the petrous temporal bone fractures. The condition is usually unilateral but can be bilateral.

Epidemiology

Temporohyoid osteoarthropathy affects horses of all ages and sex and does not have a geographic predilection.

Tracheal obstructive disease

Primary obstructive tracheal disease in horses is rare, and includes tracheal collapse, fungal granulomas, chondritis, trauma, and foreign bodies. The equine trachea has an oval shape and measures approximately 5 by 7 cm, dorsoventrally to transversely, respectively. It is composed of 48 to 60 incomplete hyaline cartilage rings interspersed by fibroelastic annular ligaments. The dorsal area is made up of fibrous tissue and the trachealis muscle, which is attached to the concave surface of each cartilage ring. The trachealis muscle allows for changes in diameter of the trachea during inhalation and exhalation, while the fibro-elastic annular ligaments permit unimpeded flexion and extension of the head and neck, important in running horses.

Recognition

History and presenting complaint

Horses with primary tracheal obstructive disease are exercise intolerant, make an abnormal respiratory noise during exercise or sometimes at rest, which is characterized as a honking sound, and have bilateral nasal discharge that can be mucopurulent or hemorrhagic.

Physical examination

Physical examination is usually normal. If tracheal trauma has occurred, palpation of the ventral cervical region can reveal a concavity in the area of previous trauma, swelling, or scar tissue. Thickened or abnormal tracheal rings can be palpable in the proximal to middle region of the cervical area if the rings have been traumatized or are chondritic. If the trachea is perforated, subcutaneous emphysema is noted along the neck, withers, and shoulders.

Special examination

Endoscopy, radiography, and ultrasonography can be useful to assess tracheal abnormalities. If the tracheal lesion is caused by a static mass, such as a fungal granuloma, chondritic cartilage, or persistently deformed trachea, endoscopic examination of the trachea at rest will be useful in assessing the tracheal lumen (Fig. 26.41). If dynamic tracheal collapse occurs during exercise, endoscopic examination of the trachea during treadmill exercise is required to diagnose the dynamic collapse.[178] Lateral radiographs of the trachea are useful in assessing extraluminal masses that can cause intraluminal obstruction, as well as the position and extent of the tracheal lesion, if it is cranial to the thoracic inlet. Ultrasonography is also used to evaluate soft tissue densities external to the trachea that can impinge on the tracheal lumen such as abscesses, hematomas, or neoplastic lesions or fracture of the tracheal ring (Fig. 26.42).

Laboratory examination

Complete blood count and serum chemistry values are usually normal.

Diagnostic confirmation

The diagnosis is confirmed based on endoscopic examination of the trachea at rest. Intraluminal masses, such as fungal granulomas, are biopsied and submitted for culture and cytology.[179] Granulomatous tracheitis caused by *Conidiobolus coronatus* can also be confirmed by agar gel immunodiffusion assay performed at the Centers for Disease Control and Prevention, Atlanta, GA.[179] Lesions of the tracheal rings, such as chondritis, are diagnosed based upon endoscopic examination, history of tracheal trauma or injection, and possibly localization of an abscess within the body of the tracheal cartilage. Dynamic tracheal collapse is diagnosed by endoscopic examination of the trachea during exercise if clinical signs are not apparent at rest and endoscopic examination of the upper airway and trachea is normal at rest.

Treatment and prognosis

Therapeutic aims

The goal of treatment is to ameliorate the tracheal obstruction.

Therapy

Discrete intraluminal tracheal masses can be excised by use of transendoscopic laser or sharply through a tracheotomy incision if the mass is within an accessible area of the trachea. Treatment of tracheal trauma includes systemic antimicrobial and non-steroidal anti-inflammatory therapy. Individual tracheal rings that have been traumatically damaged or are chondritic and cause airway obstruction can be resected. Treatment of tracheal collapse is dependent upon the length and accessibility of the trachea involved. Some forms of tracheal collapse can be treated by stenting individual tracheal rings (Fig. 26.43), tracheal prosthesis, or resection and anastomosis of the affected area.[180] Granulomatous tracheitis caused by *Conidiobolus coronatus* was successfully treated by intravenous administration of sodium iodide 20%, 44 mg/kg, once daily for 7 days followed by 1.3 mg/kg organic iodide 4.57%, twice daily for 1 year.[179]

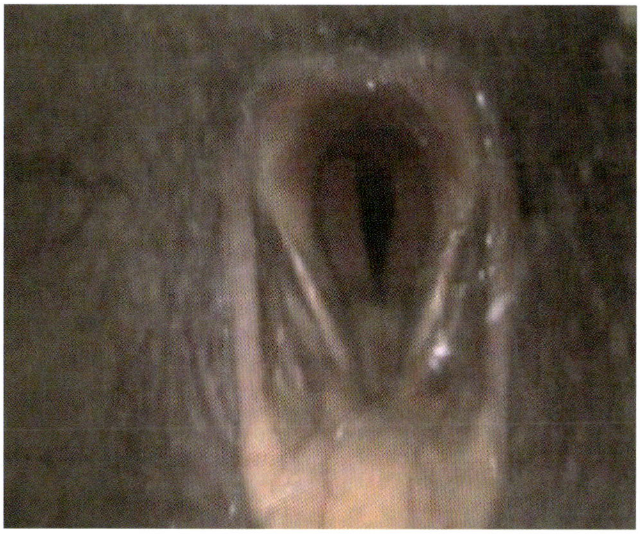

Fig 26.41 Endoscopic image of the lumen of the trachea of a horse with tracheal collapse during exercise.
Courtesy of Dr. Gary Priest, Kentucky.

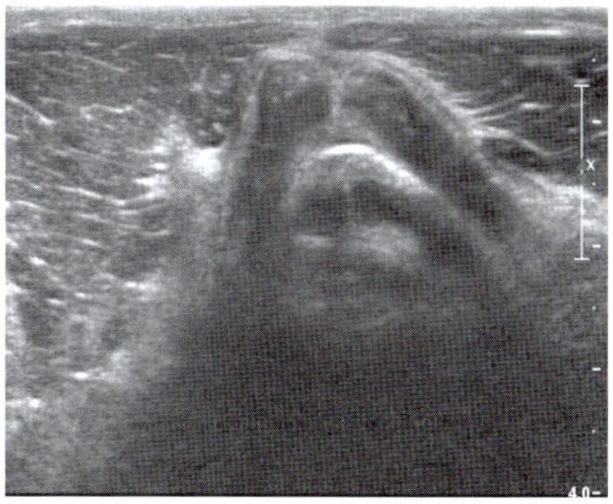

Fig 26.42 Percutaneous ultrasound exam ination of a Thoroughbred filly with an old fracture of the first cervical ring. Note the rounded edge of tracheal cartilage at the side.

Prognosis

Prognosis for removal of discrete intraluminal masses within the trachea and return to function is excellent.

Prevention

There is no known method of prevention of tracheal obstruction.

Etiology and pathophysiology

Etiology

Chondritis of tracheal cartilages can occur following intratracheal injections or transtracheal aspiration, if a tracheal ring is perforated during the injection, trauma, or idiopathically. Alternatively, direct trauma can fracture one or more tracheal rings. Finally, a degenerative process leads to tracheal collapse in miniature horses and ponies.

Pathophysiology

The pathophysiology of tracheal obstruction is based upon the type of obstruction.

Epidemiology

Tracheal obstruction is rare in athletic horses.

With thanks to Susan J. Holcombe, who co-created the original chapter in the first edition.

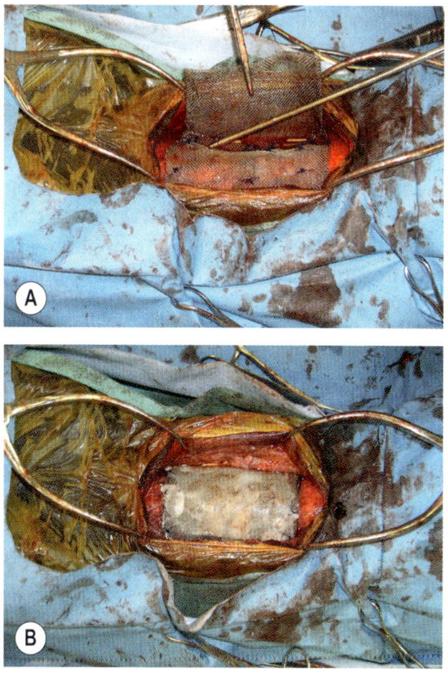

Fig 26.43 Intraoperative view of treatment of a ventral tracheal collapse in a Thoroughbred. **(A)** Tracheal collapse is being repaired by a titanium mesh sutured to the tracheal ring proximal and distal to the collapse area. **(B)** Titanium mesh is then reinforced by PMMA cement to prevent folding of the mesh.

glossopharyngeal nerve blocks on epiglottic and soft palate position in exercising horses. Am J Vet Res 1997;58(9):1022–6.
82. Aitken MR, Parente EJ. Epiglottic abnormalities in mature nonracehorses: 23 cases (1990–2009). J Am Vet Med Assoc 2011;238:1634–8.
83. Hay WP, Baskett A, Abdy MJ. Complete upper airway obstruction and syncope caused by a subepiglottic cyst in a horse. Eq Vet J 1997;97:75–6.
84. Chow TL, Choi CY, Yee-Hing Hui J. Thyroglossal duct cysts in adults treated by ethanol sclerotherapy: a pilot study of a nonsurgical technique. Laryngoscope 2012. doi: 10.1002/lary.23254. [Epub ahead of print]
85. Dougherty SS, Palmer JL. Use of intralesional formalin administration for treatment of a subepiglottic cyst in a horse. J Am Vet Med Assoc 2008;233:463–5.
86. King DS, Tulleners EP, Martin BB, et al. Clinical experience with axial deviation of the aryepiglottic folds in 52 racehorses. Vet Surg 2001;30:151–60.
87. Priest DT, Cheetham J, Regner AL, et al. Dynamic respiratory endoscopy of Standardbred racehorses during qualifying races. Equine Vet J 2012;44(5):529–34.
88. Rakesh V, Ducharme NG, Cheetham J, et al. Implications of different degrees of arytenoid cartilage abduction on equine. Eq Vet J 2008;40:629–35.
89. Hawkins JF, Tulleners EP. Epiglottitis in horses: 20 cases (1988–1993). J Am Vet Med Assoc 1994;205:1577–9.
90. Infernuso T, Watts AE, Ducharme NG. Septic epiglottic chondritis with abscessation in 2 young Thoroughbred racehorses. Can Vet J 2006;47:1007–10.
91. Ortved KF, Cheetham J, Mitchell LM, et al. Successful treatment of persistent dorsal displacement of the soft palate and evaluation of laryngohyoid position in 15 racehorses. Eq Vet J 2010;42(1):23–9.
92. Hahn CN, Matiasek K, Dixon PM, et al. Histological and ultrastructural evidence that recurrent laryngeal neuropathy is a bilateral mononeuropathy limited to recurrent laryngeal nerves. Equine Vet J 2008;40:666–72.
93. Rhee HS, Steel CM, Derksen FJ, et al. Immunohistochemical analysis of laryngeal muscles in normal horses and horses with subclinical recurrent laryngeal neuropathy. J Histochem Cytochem 2009;57:787–800.
94. Duncan ID, Griffith IR. A light and electron microscopic study of the neuropathy of equine idiopathic laryngeal hemiplegia. Acta Neuropathol 1978;4:483–501.
95. Cardiot PJ. Roaring in horses: its pathology and treatment. Swan Sonnenschein 1892;7–78.
96. Witte SHP, Witte TH, Harriss F, et al. Association of owner-reported noise with findings during dynamic respiratory endoscopy in Thoroughbred racehorses. Eq Vet J 2011;43:9–17.
97. Derksen JF, Stick JA, Scott EA, et al. Effects of laryngeal hemiplegia and laryngoplasty on airway flow mechanics in exercising horses. Am J Vet Res 1986;47:16–26.
98. Chalmers HJ, Cheetham J,Yeager AE, et al. Ultrasonography of the equine larynx. Vet Radiol 2006;47(5):476–81.
99. Newton-Clarke MJ, Divers TJ, Valentine BA. Evaluation of the thoraco-laryngeal reflex ('slap test') as an indicator of laryngeal adductor myopathy in the horse. Equine Vet J 1994;26:355–7.
100. Rakestraw PC, Hackett RP, Ducharme NG, et al. Arytenoid cartilage movement in resting and exercising horses. Vet Surg 1991;20:122–7.
101. Anon. Consensus statement on equine laryngeal neuropathy. In: Havermeyer workshop on equine laryngeal neuropathy. Havermeyer monograph series no 11, R& W Publications (Newmarket) Ltd; 2003. p. 93–7.
102. Barakzai SZ, Dixon PM, Correlation of resting and exercising endoscopic findings for horses with dynamic laryngeal collapse and palatal dysfunction. Equine Vet J 2011;43:18–23.
103. Desmaizieres L, Serraud N, Plainfosse B, et al. Dynamic respiratory endoscopy without treadmill in 68 performance Standardbred, Thoroughbred and saddle horses under natural training conditions. Eq Vet J 2009;41:347–52.
104. Pollock PJ, Reardon RJM, Parkin TDH, et al. Dynamic respiratory endoscopy in 67 Thoroughbred racehorses training under normal ridden exercise conditions. Eq Vet J 2009;41:354–360.
105. Taylor SE, Barakzai SZ, Dixon P. Ventriculocordectomy as the sole treatment for recurrent laryngeal neuropathy: long-term results from ninety-two horses. Eq Vet J 2006;35:653–7.
106. Duncan ID, Reifenrath P, Jackson KF, et al. Preferential denervation of the adductor muscles of the equine larynx. II: Nerve pathology. Equine Vet J 1991;23:99–103.
107. Garrett KS, Woodie JB, Embertson RM. Association of treadmill upper airway endoscopic evaluation with results of ultrasonography and resting upper airway endoscopic evaluation. Equine Vet J 2011;43(3):365–71.
108. Tetens J, Derksen JF, Stick JA, et al. Efficacy of prosthetic laryngoplasty with and without bilateral ventriculocordectomy as treatments for laryngeal hemiplegia in horses. Am J Vet Res 1996;57:1668–73.
109. Ducharme NG, Hackett RP, Gleed RD, et al. Measurements of pulmonary capillary pressure in horses undergoing alteration of intrathoracic pressure by imposition of various upper airway resistive loads. Equine Vet J Suppl 1999;30:27–33.
110. Hawe C, Dixon PM, Canhew IG. A study of an electrodiagnostic technique for the evaluation of equine recurrent laryngeal neuropathy. Equine Vet J 2001;33(5):459–65.
111. Cheetham J, Pigott JH, Leal MT, et al. Conduction velocity in horses with normal arytenoid function. Proceedings BEVA, 2008. p. 343.
112. Brown JA, Derksen FD, Stick JA, et al. Ventriculocordectomy reduces respiratory noise in horses with laryngeal hemiplegia. Eq Vet J 2003;35(6):570–4.
113. Shappel KK, Derksen FJ, Stick JA, et al. Effects of ventriculectomy, prosthetic laryngoplasty, and exercise on upper airway function in horses with induced left laryngeal hemiplegia. Am J Vet Res 1988;49:1760–6.
114. Lumsden JM, Derksen FJ, Stick JA, et al. Evaluation of partial arytenoidectomy as a treatment for equine laryngeal hemiplegia. Equine Vet J 1994;24:125–9.
115. Russel AP, Slone DE. Performance analysis after prosthetic laryngoplasty and bilateral ventriculectomy for laryngeal hemiplegia in horses: 70 cases (1986–1991). J Am Vet Med Assoc 1994;204:1235–41.
116. Kidd JA, Slone DE. Treatment of laryngeal hemiplegia in horses by prosthetic laryngoplasty, ventriculectomy and vocal cordectomy. Vet Rec 2002;150:481–4.
117. Strand E, Martin GS, Haynes PF, et al. Career racing performance in Thoroughbreds treated with prosthetic laryngoplasty for laryngeal neuropathy: 52 cases (1981–1989). J Am Vet Med Assoc 2000;217:1689–96.
118. Hawkins JF, Tulleners EP, Ross MW, et al. Laryngoplasty with or without ventriculectomy for treatment of left laryngeal hemiplegia in 230 horses. Vet Surg 1997;26:484–91.
119. White NA, Blackwell RB. Partial arytenoidectomy in the horse. Vet Surg 1980;9:5–12.
120. Witte TH, Mohammed HO, Radcliffe CH, et al. Racing performance after combined prosthetic laryngoplasty and ipsilateral ventriculocordectomy or partial arytenoidectomy: 135 Thoroughbred racehorses competing at less than 2400 m (1997–2007). Eq Vet J 2009;41(1):70–5.
121. Parente E J, Tulleners E P, Southwood LL. Long-term study of partial arytenoidectomy with primary mucosal closure in 76 Thoroughbred racehorses

(1992–2006). Eq Vet J 2008;40(3): 214–18.

122. Radcliffe CH, Woodie JB, Hackett RP et al. A comparison of laryngoplasty and modified partial arytenoidectomy as treatments for laryngeal hemiplegia in exercising horses. Vet Surg 2006; 35(7):643–52.

123. Ducharme NG, Viel L, Partlow GD, et al. Attempts to restore abduction of the paralyzed equine arytenoid cartilage: III. Nerve anastomosis. Can J Vet Res 1989;53:216–23.

124. Fulton IC, Derksen FJ, Stick JA, et al. Treatment of left laryngeal hemiplegia in Standardbreds using a nerve muscle pedicle graft. Am J Vet Res 1991;52: 1461–6.

125. Ducharme NG, Cheetham J, Sanders I, et al. Considerations for pacing of the cricoarytenoid dorsalis muscle by neuroprosthesis in horses. Equine Vet J 2010 42(6):534–40.

126. Cheetham J, Regner A, Jarvis JC, et al. Functional electrical stimulation of intrinsic laryngeal muscles under varying loads in exercising horses. PloS one 2011;6(8):e24258.

127. Dixon PM, McGorum BC, Railton DI, et al. Long-term survey of laryngoplasty and ventriculocordectomy in an older, mixed-breed population of 200 horses. Part 2: Owners' assessment of the value of surgery. Equine Vet J 2003;35(4): 397–401.

128. Duncan ID. The pathophysiology of equine idiopathic laryngeal hemiplegia. Proceedings International Neurology Conference, 1997. p. 108–10.

129. Hahn CN, Matiasek K, Dixon PM, et al. Histological and ultrastructural evidence that recurrent laryngeal neuropathy is a bilateral mononeuropathy limited to recurrent laryngeal nerves. Equine Vet J 2008;40(7):666–72.

130. Collins N, Milne E, Hahn C, et al. Correlation of the Havemeyer endoscopic laryngeal grading system with histopathological changes in equine cricoarytenoideus dorsalis muscles. Ir Vet J 2009;62(5):334–8.

131. Baker GJ. Laryngeal asynchrony in the horses: Definition and significance. In: Snow DH, Persson SHB, Rose RJ, editors. Equine exercise physiology. Cambridge: Granta; 1983. p. 46–50.

132. Dixon PM, McGorum BC, Railton DI, et al. Clinical and endoscopic evidence of progression in 152 cases of equine recurrent neuropathy. Equine Vet J 2002;34(1):29–34.

133. Dyer KR, Duncan ID. The intraneural distribution of myelinated fibres in the equine recurrent laryngeal nerve. Brain 1987;110(Pt 6):1531–43.

134. Ohnesorge B, Deegen E, Miesner K, et al. [Laryngeal hemiplegia in warm blood horses – a study of stallions, mares and their offspring]. Zentralbl Veterinarmed A 1993;40:134–54.

135. Bohanon TC, Beard WL, Robertson JT. Laryngeal hemiplegia in draft horses. A review of 27 cases. Vet Surg 1990;19(6):456–9.

136. Poncet PA, Montavon S. A preliminary report on the possible genetic basis of laryngeal hemiplegia. Equine Vet J 1989;21:137–8.

137. Dupuis MC, Zhang Z, Druet T, et al. Results of a haplotype-based GWAS for recurrent laryngeal neuropathy in the horse. Mamm Genome 2011;22(9–10): 613–20.

138. Kelly G, Lumsden JM, Dunkerly G, et al. Idiopathic mucosal lesions of the arytenoid cartilages of 21 Thoroughbred yearlings: 1997–2001. Equine Vet J 2003;35(3):276–81.

139. Sullins K. Endoscopically guided laser debridement of arytenoid chondritis in standing horses. Abstract 13. In: Proceeding World Equine Airways Society, 2001, CD.

140. Tulleners E, Harrison IW, Raker CW. Management of arytenoid chondropathy and failed laryngoplasty in horses: 75 cases (1979–1985). J Am Vet Med Assoc 1988;192:670–5.

141. White NA, Blackwell RB. Partial arytenoidectomy in the horse. Vet Surg 1980;9:5–12.

142. Lumsden JM, Derksen FJ, Stick JA, et al. Evaluation of partial arytenoidectomy as a treatment for laryngeal hemiplegia. Equine Vet J 1994;26:125–9.

143. Belknap JK, Derksen FJ, Nickels FA, et al. Failure of subtotal arytenoidectomy to improve upper airway flow mechanics in exercising Standardbreds with induced laryngeal hemiplegia. Am J Vet Res 1990;51: 1481–6.

144. Harrison IW, Raker CW. Dorsal glottic stenosis after bilateral arytenoidectomy in two horses. J Am Vet Med Assoc 1988;192:202–4.

145. Parente EJ, Tulleners EP, Southwood LL. Long-term study of partial arytenoidectomy with primary mucosal closure in 76 Thoroughbred racehorses (1992–2006). Equine Vet J 2008;40(3):214–18.

146. Jensen R, Lauerman LH, Braddy PM, et al. Laryngeal contact ulcers in feedlot cattle. Vet Pathol 1980;17:667–71.

147. Smith RL, Perkins, NR, Firth EC, et al. Arytenoid mucosal injury in young Thoroughbred horses – investigation of a proposed aetiology and clinical significance. N Z Vet J 2006;54(4): 173–6.

148. McClure JJ, Koch C, Powell M, et al. Association of arytenoid chondritis with equine lymphocyte antigens but no association with laryngeal hemiplegia, umbilical hernias and cryptorchidism. Anim Genet 1988;19:427–33.

149. Lane GF. Fourth branchial arch defects in Thoroughbred horses: 60 cases. In: Proceeding of the World Equine Airways Symposium, Edinburgh, Scotland, 2001.

150. Garrett KS, Woodie JB, Embertson RM, et al. Diagnosis of laryngeal dysplasia in five horses using magnetic resonance imaging and ultrasonography. Equine Vet J 2009;41(8):766–71.

151. Baxter GM, Allen D, Farrel RL. Paralaryngeal accessory bronchial cyst as a cause of laryngeal hemiplegia in a horse. Equine Vet J 1992;24: 67–9.

152. Wilson RG, Sutton RH, Groenendyk S. Rostral displacement of palatopharyngeal arch in a Thoroughbred yearling. Aust Vet J 1986;63:99–100.

153. Zaw-Tun HA, Burdi AR. Reexamination of the origin and early development of the human larynx. Acta Anat (Basel) 1985;122:163–84.

154. Hast MH. Early development of the human laryngeal muscles. Ann Otol Rhino Laryngol 1972;81:524–30.

155. Goulden BE, Anderson LJ, Davies AS, et al. Rostral displacement of the palatopharyngeal arch: a case report. Equine Vet J 1976;8:95–8.

156. Blikslager AT, Tate LP, Tudor R. Transendoscopic laser treatment of rostral displacement of the palatopharyngeal arch in four horses. J Clin Laser Med Surg 1999;17:49–52.

157. Lepage OM, Piccot-Crézollet C. Transarterial coil embolisation in 31 horses (1999–2002) with guttural pouch mycosis: a 2-year follow-up. Equine Vet J 2005;37(5):430–4.

158. Leveille R, Hardy J, Robertson JT, et al. Transarterial coil embolization of the internal and external carotid and maxillary arteries for prevention of hemorrhage from guttural pouch mycosis in horses. Vet Surg 2000;29(5): 389–97.

159. Greet TRC. Outcome of treatment in 35 cases of guttural pouch mycosis. Equine Vet J 1987;19(5):483–7.

160. Freeman DE, Ross MW, Dona wick WJ, et al. Occlusion of the external carotid and maxillary arteries in the horse to prevent hemorrhage from guttural pouch mycosis. Vet Surg 1989;18(1): 39–47.

161. Kipper A, Frees K. Hypoglossal neuritis with associated lingual hemiplegia secondary to guttural pouch mycosis. Vet Pathol 1993;30(6):547–56.

162. Sweeney CR, Freeman DE, Sweeney RW, et al. Hemorrhage into the guttural pouch (auditory tube diverticulum) associated with rupture of the longus capitis muscle in three horses. J Am Vet Med Assoc 1993;202(7): 1129–31.

163. Ludwig A, Gatineau S, Reynaud MC, et al. Fungal isolation and identification in 21 cases of guttural pouch mycosis in horses (1998–2002). Vet J 2005;169(3):457–61.
164. Davis EW, Legendre AM. Successful treatment of guttural pouch mycosis with itraconazole and topical enilconazole in a horse. J Vet Intern Med 1994;8(4):304–5.
165. Delfs KC, Hawkins JF, Hogan DF. Treatment of acute epistaxis secondary to guttural pouch mycosis with transarterial nitinol vascular occlusion plugs in three equids. J Am Vet Med Assoc 2009;235(2):189–93.
166. Benredouane K, Lepage O. Trans-arterial coil embolization of the internal carotid artery in standing horses. Vet Surg 2012;41(3):404–9.
167. Freeman DE, Ross MW, Dona wick WJ. 'Steal phenomenon' proposed as the cause of blindness after arterial occlusion for treatment of guttural pouch mycosis in horses. J Am Vet Med Assoc 1990;197(7):811–12.
168. Naylor RJ, Perkins JD, Allen S, et al. Histopathology and computed tomography of age-associated degeneration of the equine temporohyoid joint. Equine Vet J 2010;42(5):425–30.
169. Power HT, Watrous BJ, de Lahunta A. Facial and vestibulocochlear nerve disease in six horses. J Am Vet Med Assoc 1983;183:1076–80.
170. Blythe LL, Watrous BJ, Shire MH. Prophylactic partial stylohyoidostectomy for horses with osteoarthropathy of the temporohyoid joint. J Equine Vet Sci 1994;14:32–7.
171. Blythe LL. Otitis media and interna and temporohyoid osteoarthropathy. Vet Clin North Am Equine Pract 1997;13:21–42.
172. Divers TJ, Ducharme NG, de Lahunta A, et al. Temporohyoid osteoarthropathy. Clin Tech Equine Pract 2006;5:17–23.
173. Walker AM, Sellon DC, Cornellisse CJ, et al. Temporohyoid osteoarthropathy in horses: 33 cases (1993–2000). J Vet Intern Med 2002;16(6):697–703.
174. Hilton H, Puchalski SM, Aleman M. The computed tomographic appearance of equine temporohyoid osteoarthropathy. Vet Radiol Ultrasound 2009;50(2):151–6.
175. Pownder S, Scrivani PV, Bezuidenhout A, et al. Computed tomography of temporal bone fractures and temporal region anatomy in horses. J Vet Intern Med 2010;24(2):398–406.
176. Pease AP, van Biervliet J, Dykes NL, et al. Complication of partial stylohyoidectomy for treatment of temporohyoid osteoarthropathy and an alternative surgical technique in three cases. Equine Vet J 2004;36:546–50.
177. Tetens J, Hubert JD, Eddy AL, et al. Dynamic tracheal collapse as a cause of exercise intolerance in a Thoroughbred. J Am Vet Med Assoc 2000;216(5):722–4.
178. Steiger RR, Williams MA. Granulomatous tracheitis caused by *Conidiobolus coronatus* in a horse. J Vet Intern Med 2000;14(3):311–14.
179. Tate LP, Koch DB, Sembrat RF, et al. Tracheal reconstruction by resection and end-to-end anastomosis in the horse. J Am Vet Med Assoc 1981;178(3):253–8.

Lower airway function: response to exercise and training

27

Tatiana Art Warwick Bayly

CHAPTER CONTENTS

Introduction

The major function of the lung is to ensure gas exchange, i.e. the transport of oxygen (O_2) from the ambient air into the blood and of carbon dioxide (CO_2) in the reverse direction. Secondarily, airways play also a role in immune defense, as well as in cleaning, warming and humidifying the inspired air.

During maximal exercise, O_2 consumption (VO_2) and CO_2 output (VCO_2) of the horses can increase to more than 30 times the values at rest. Consequently, the physiologic and biochemical systems involved in the oxygen consumption chain are subjected to dramatic adjustments in order to meet these metabolic requirements.

In most species, the healthy respiratory system is able to ensure adequate ventilation, as evidenced by PaO_2 and $PaCO_2$ values that differ minimally from those at rest, during exercise of any intensity. This is not the situation with horses which develop hypoxemia at relatively low exercise intensities (i.e. 60% VO_{2max}) and hypercapnia at high exercise intensity. [1] Given the numerous and substantial respiratory adjustments that occur in this species during exercise, this impairment of gas exchange can be at first glance surprising. Nevertheless, some anatomic and physiologic peculiarities of this species combined with the huge metabolic demands at the level of the working muscles can explain this relative inability of the lung to maintain adequate gas exchange during heavy exercise.

From a clinical point of view, the importance of a healthy respiratory system in the performance horse is highlighted by several retrospective studies of racing horses or endurance horses with exercise intolerance. All these papers reported a major impact of lower airway disease on exercise capability.[2-4]

This chapter reviews equine respiratory physiology and focuses on the exercise-induced changes in respiratory function.

General overview: structure and function of the lower respiratory airway

Airway

Air is delivered into the deep part of the lung through conducting airways that carry ambient air from the nose to the alveoli during inspiration. Airflow is reversed during expiration. Gas exchange occurs at the level of the alveolar duct and the alveoli, which are lined by an extensive capillary network. The intrathoracic trachea, the bronchi and the bronchioles constitute the lower airway. The trachea is divided into right and left mainstem bronchi that enter the hilum of each lung. Each bronchus in turn divides into lobar, segmental and sub-segmental bronchi which end in bronchioles. The terminal bronchioles are poorly developed respiratory bronchioles, or open directly into alveolar ducts. Epithelium of the tracheobronchial tree is tall columnar pseudostratified interspersed with ciliated cells as well serous and mucus-producing goblet cells.[5] Short ciliated cells and non-ciliated (Clara) cells constitute the epithelium of the bronchioles. Lastly, alveoli are mainly covered by type I pneumocytes, with type II pneumocytes producing surfactant (Fig. 27.1). The latter is essential to maintain the stability of alveoli, especially at low lung volumes.

The epithelium in the large airway is covered by a double mucus layer, this system forming the mucociliary escalator which is an efficient system to clear the airway from the airborne particles deposited by impaction in the deep part of the lung (Fig. 27.1).

Immune cells, including lymphocytes, macrophages, mast cells and, in some inflammatory or infectious conditions, eosinophils and neutrophils, are distributed throughout the lower respiratory tract in the epithelium lining fluid.

Lung

Unlike the lung in most other animals, the horse lung is not divided into distinct lobes. There are fibrous connecting septa comprising an intricate mesh of interconnecting elastic and collagenous tissue fibers[6] that divide the lung into lobules. This separation limits the collateral ventilation between lung regions – the ventilation of adjacent lobules through other pathways than the bronchial tree such as anastomosing bronchioles – but increases pulmonary interdependence (the mechanical interaction between adjacent regions) which enhances synchronization of ventilation of the different regions of the lung.

Because the collateral pathways have a rather high resistance to airflow, they are probably of limited usefulness whatever the respiratory frequency.[6] On the other hand, the interdependence between adjacent lung areas can induce abnormal stresses on some lobules. Indeed, with increased airflow resistance, decreased compliance, or both, the tissues are stretched and compressed by the surrounding lung parts.[7] It has been suggested that exercise-induced pulmonary hemorrhage could be a consequence of this pulmonary overstretching.[8]

Blood supply

The lung is perfused with arterial blood from the pulmonary and bronchial circulations.

The *pulmonary circulation* receives the total cardiac output from the right heart. At rest, it is a low-pressure low-resistance system. The branches of the pulmonary artery carry mixed venous blood to the lung, accompany the bronchi, and form rich capillary plexuses on the walls of the alveoli. The blood is arterialized at this level and returns to the left atrium via the pulmonary veins. The primary function of pulmonary circulation is consequently gas exchange. Other roles are the filtration of emboli or thrombi and the release or the removal of bioactive chemical substances.

Blood flow distribution is mainly influenced by gravity and shows consequently a vertical gradient according to the relative magnitude of pulmonary arterial, venous and alveolar pressures in humans.[9] The ventral regions in the lungs of humans receive more perfusion per unit lung volume than the dorsal regions, and blood flow in the lung can be divided into three or four zones (Fig. 27.2).

It has been long thought that the same was true for horses, but recent work indicates that at rest gravity is a minor factor in determining blood flow distribution, despite the large hydrostatic gradient imposed by the height of the lung. Blood flow is preferentially distributed in the dorsal regions of the lung (thus opposite to gravity),[10] a phenomenon which is exacerbated by exercise.[12] The exercise-induced changes of blood distribution are described later in the text.

There is a large heterogeneity of blood distribution within the same isogravitational plane, showing that pulmonary blood flow depends on factors other than the pressure gradient between pulmonary arteries and veins, such as the vessel's length and resistance in a given area.[11]

The *bronchial circulation* is a high pressure system. It comes from a single vessel, branching from the aorta and receiving, at rest, 2% of the cardiac output. It subsequently divides into a right and left bronchial artery at the hilar region of the lung. It provides nutritional blood flow to the lymphatic, vascular and airway components as well as to the pleura. Bronchial circulation seems to play a role in warming and humidifying the inspired air, as suggested by the increase of its blood flow during exercise.[13] Bronchial circulation could be involved in local inflammatory processes, as suggested by its proliferation occurring in horses with lesions of exercise-induced pulmonary hemorrhage (EIPH).[14]

When pulmonary perfusion is locally impaired, the bronchial circulation can proliferate and at the level of the terminal bronchioles, pulmonary and bronchial circulations can anastomose. Most of these anastomoses occur between capillaries and veins rather than with arteries.[15] They maintain some blood flow throughout the lung, thus contributing partly to gas exchange. Such proliferations also can occur during pulmonary inflammation. Because they are extensive in the dorso-caudal regions of the lungs, which are the sections that sometimes bleed during exercise, this neovascularisation has been related to the occurrence of EIPH.[14]

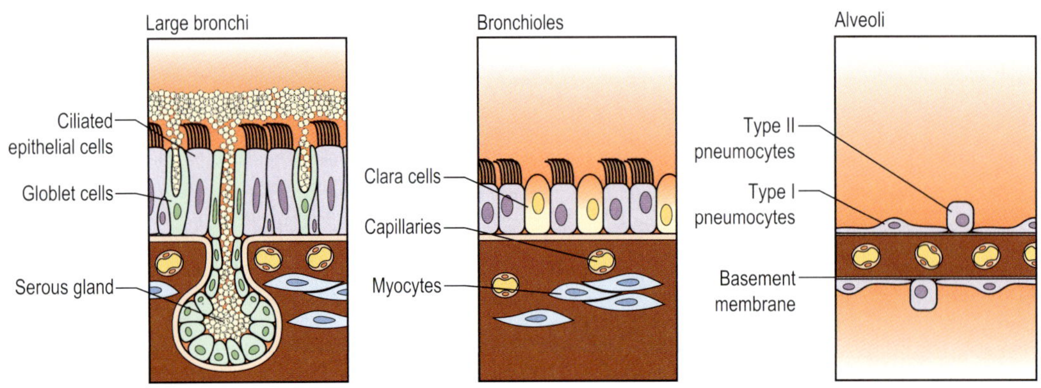

Fig 27.1 Epithelium composition of different parts of the lower airway. Large bronchi: columnar pseudo-stratified epithelium interspersed with ciliated cells and serous and mucus-producing goblet cells; two mucus layers, a deep serous and a superficial mucus. Bronchioles: ciliated cells and non-ciliated (Clara) cells. Alveoli: type I pneumocytes, with spare type II pneumocytes.

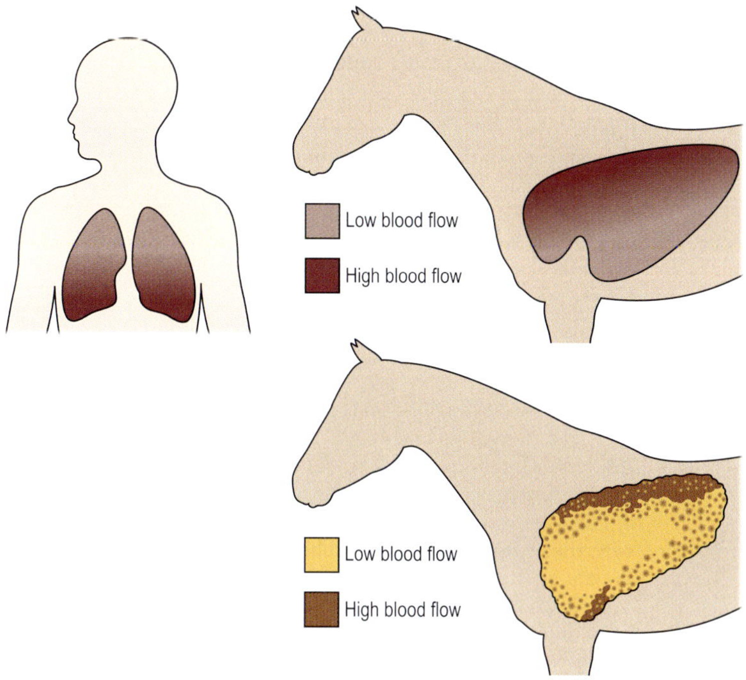

Fig 27.2 Pulmonary blood distribution in resting man (left) and in horse at rest (right) and after exercise (bottom). In the first species, gravity is the main determinant of lung blood perfusion, which results in a vertical perfusion gradient. In horses, for still unclear reasons, blood is preferentially distributed in the dorsal parts, resulting in a caudo-dorsal gradient. Exercise still exacerbates this phenomenon, as assessed by the post-exercise scintigraphic image (bottom).
Courtesy of Dominique Votion.

Thoracic cavity and respiratory muscles

The thorax provides rather rigid protection for the intrathoracic organs. The diaphragm, which separates the thorax from the abdomen, and the external intercostal muscles are the main inspiratory muscles. In horses, the serratus ventralis has an important role in assisting the inspiratory effort of the diaphragm, both at rest[16] and during exercise.[17] The mechanical equilibrium of the equine respiratory system (including thorax, lung parenchyma and muscles) lies at the midpoint of the tidal volume, contrary to other species in which the equilibrium point occurs at functional residual capacity. Consequently, in horses, both inspiration and expiration have a physiological biphasic pattern, with an initial passive and a second active component for each phase[18] (Fig. 27.3).

The intercostal muscles are activated in the second part of inspiration (for the external ones) and expiration (for the internal ones).[16] The transversalis muscle is the principal expiratory muscle. Lastly, the abdominal muscles (external and oblique abdominis, transverse and rectus abdominis, transverse thoracics) participate also to the active phase of expiration. When they contract, they increase the abdominal pressure, forcing the relaxed diaphragm forward and reducing the thoracic volume. However, during exercise, the biphasic shape of the respiratory airflow is no longer visible because of the very high respiratory frequency (Fig. 27.3).

The activity of the respiratory muscles can be assessed either directly by electromyographic measurement or indirectly, by assessment of the respiratory muscle perfusion. Electromyographic studies of respiratory muscle recruitment have been performed in healthy horses at rest,[1,16] and during exercise.[19] Electrical activation of the diaphragm, as well as its mechanical output, increases linearly with exercise intensity.[19] Ventilatory muscle perfusion has been studied in ponies as an indicator of muscle activity.[17,20] The ventilatory muscles receive 10% of the cardiac output at rest and 15% during maximal exercise.

During exercise, despite the activation of the external intercostal muscles (which should move the ribs forward and outwards), the thoracic circumference decreases slightly.[21] This is probably related to the large negative pressures occurring in the thorax when the diaphragm contracts. The role of external intercostal muscle contraction consequently could be a stiffening of the thoracic structure to help to resist its physical deformation, rather than a genuine increase of the thoracic volume. Also, during exercise the abdominal circumference does not change either, which leads to the conclusion that in this circumstance the increase in tidal volume is due to an elongation of the thoracoabdominal segment.[22]

A study was recently performed to assess the effect of girth tension on respiration and performance ability in horses during supramaximal exercise. Although there was a decrease of the time to fatigue associated with high girth tensions, this was not due to alteration of respiratory mechanics or troubles in gas exchange. The authors suggested that this loss in performance could be related to inspiratory muscles working at suboptimal lengths due to thoracic compression or compression of musculature around the chest.[23]

Autonomic innervation

The smooth muscles of the vessels and the bronchioles are innervated by sympathetic, parasympathetic and non-adrenergic non-cholinergic nervous systems. In the healthy horse, the lack of changes in pulmonary resistance after β-adrenergic stimulation or muscarinic blockade[24] reflect that there is no smooth muscle tone in the bronchi of healthy horses at rest.

A modest autonomic innervation, with both adrenergic and cholinergic components, is found in the muscular vessels of the pulmonary circulation but its role remains unclear.

Physiological adjustments to exercise

While at rest, VO_2 is approximately 4.5 ml/kg/min, and VCO_2 4.0 ml/kg/min, when the horse runs at increasing intensity, its VO_2 increases linearly up to a plateau called VO_{2max} (at a speed of approximately 10 m/sec). The value of VO_{2max} can be as high as 175 ml/kg/min in fit Thoroughbred or Standardbred racehorses (although higher values have been recorded), which means that resting values are increased by 30-fold during intense exercise

The main factors involved in gas exchange are:

- ventilation (i.e. how air gets to the alveoli)
- perfusion (i.e. removal of gas from the lungs by the blood)
- ventilation–perfusion ratio (i.e. how matching of air and blood distribution in the lung influences the gas exchange)
- diffusion (i.e. how gas gets across the air–blood barrier)
- gas transport (i.e. how gases are moved from lungs to the tissues)
- mechanics of breathing (i.e. how the lungs are moved) and
- control of breathing (i.e. how gas exchange is adjusted to the metabolic demand).

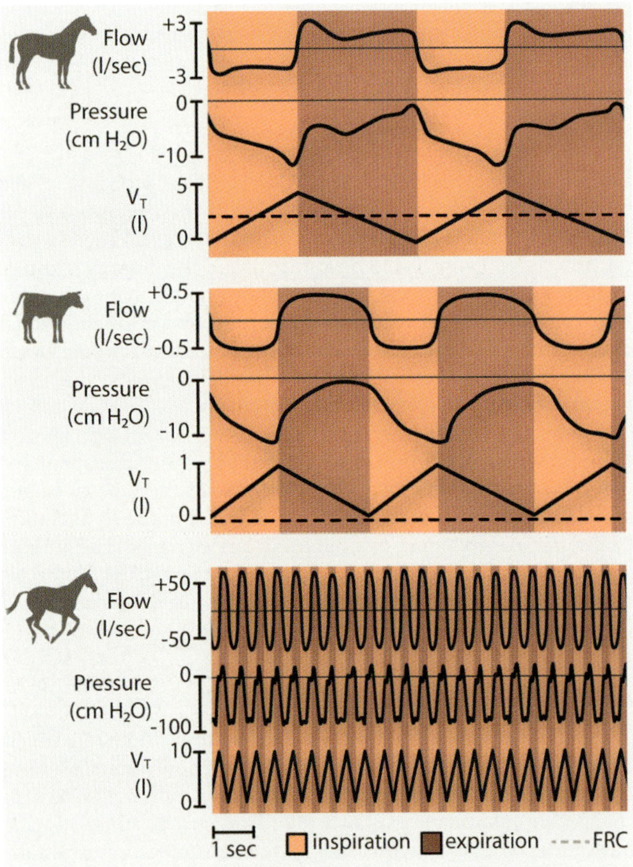

Fig 27.3 Respiratory airflow, esophageal pressure and tidal volume in the horse and the calf. Note that the calf breathes above the functional residual capacity (dashed line), which is the pulmonary volume when the elastic structures are in equilibrium, and has an active inspiration and a passive expiration. On the opposite, the horse at rest breathes around its functional residual capacity, having passive and active phases during both inspiration and expiration and consequently a biphasic shape of the airflow. During exercise (here at gallop at 10 m/sec), however, the airflow curves are monophasic and dome shaped.

Ventilation

Ventilatory data and respiratory strategy

At rest, horses breathe at a frequency of 12–15 breaths/min with a tidal volume of 5–6 L, which means that the expired minute volume is around 60–80 L/min. At the end of expiration, the horse lungs still contain a volume of air of about 20 L (the functional residual capacity). This provides a reserve of air allowing gas exchange to be continuous between each breath, and contributes to airway patency which decreases the work of breathing of the next inhalation.

Exercise imposes a potent stress on the ventilatory pump: as speed increases, expired minute ventilation (the product of tidal volume and breathing frequency) increases almost linearly: while it averages 80 L/min at rest, it can reach values in the vicinity of 2000 L/min during heavy exercise.[25,26] *At the walk and trot*, respiratory and step frequencies are generally independent, although studies have reported that they can be coupled at a trot. However, this coupling is neither constant nor compulsory[27,28] but when it occurs, it seems that the 'abdominal piston' acts in synergy with the respiratory pump[28] probably reducing the oxygen cost of breathing.

Once the *horse gallops*, there is an obligatory linkage between stride and respiratory rates.[22,27,29] Step and respiratory frequencies averaging 110 to 130/min and tidal volume between 12 and 15 L are reported in fast galloping horses.[25,30]

The mechanisms underlying the coupling, as well as its physiological significance, are not yet well understood but it is probably due to a mechanical linkage: the visceral piston, the flexion of the back and the loading of the thorax by the forelimbs probably play an important mechanical role in facilitating breathing.[29] During protraction of the forelimbs, the rib cage is pulled forwards and outwards, the visceral content stays backwards because of inertia, favoring inhalation (Fig. 27.4). During weight-bearing, the rib cage

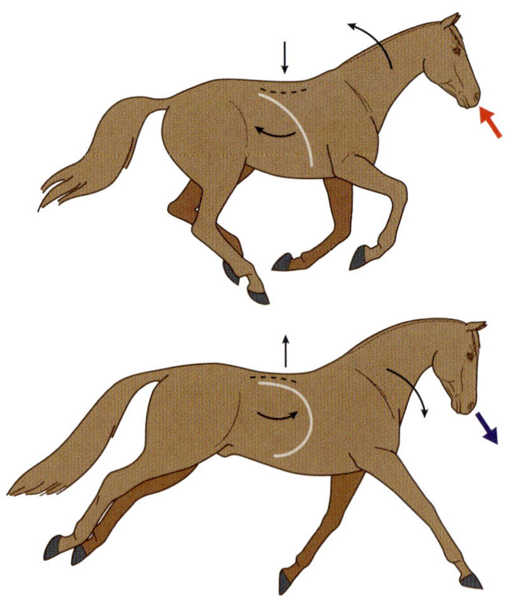

Fig 27.4 Coupling of breathing and locomotion in the galloping horse. (Top) inspiration: protraction of the forelimb, caudal displacement of the visceral piston, lumbo-sacral extension and cervical movement which pulls the rib cage forwards and outwards; (Bottom) expiration: weight-bearing, cranial displacement of the visceral piston, lumbo-sacral flexion, downward movement of the neck.

absorbs forces and is compressed, and the visceral content moves forwards, favoring exhalation (Fig. 27.4).

Experimental evidence shows that in galloping horses it is the back flexion rather than the visceral piston mechanism that assists breathing.[22] The mechanism obviously gives a mechanical advantage to respiration. These conclusions have nevertheless been challenged by work showing no evidence that the diaphragmatic electrical activity or mechanical output was 'spared' as horses ran at progressively increasing intensity such that total diaphragmatic electrical activity and mechanical output were proportional to exercise hyperpnea and independent of the existence of a coupling between gait and respiration.[19]

On the other hand, in Standardbred horses trotting at 10 m/sec on a 6% slope, tidal volume of about 18 L and respiratory frequency of approximately 90 breaths/min have been reported.[31] This breathing strategy is different from that observed in Thoroughbred horses at similar exercise intensities (Table 27.1). However, despite this lack of locomotion/respiration coupling, Standardbred horses do not reach higher expired minute ventilation than do Thoroughbreds, and they are similarly hypoxemic and hypercapnic.[31,32]

A recent work examining the expired minute volume during the first minutes after exercise in Thoroughbred horses after maximal exercise showed that there is a noticeable hyperventilation, similar to the end-exercise level of ventilation (with a sharp increase in VT and a lower f_b) showing that horses can reach their prodigiously high ventilation even when there is no locomotor–respiration coupling.[33]

Moreover, coupling is not always the rule, even in healthy horses. For example, horses galloping either on the track or on the treadmill, can sporadically show 'big respiratory cycles' which continue for two or three strides.[34,35] An extreme value of 29.7 L tidal volume has been observed in a horse decoupling the 1:1 step/respiratory frequency ratio for a 2:1 ratio.[36]

Table 27.1 Ventilatory and arterial gas tension values in trotting and galloping horses. Despite a different combination of respiratory frequency and tidal volume, both are hypoxemic and hypercapnic at high intensity of exercise. At 10m/sec, Standardbreds were running with a slope of 6% and Thoroughbred with a slope of 4°

VALUES	GAIT	REST	4 m/sec	10 m/sec
VT(L)	Trot	5.8	9.4	19.8
	Gallop	4.8	6.4	13.2
f_b(b/min)	Trot	16	79	92
	Gallop	14	91	121
Ve (L/min)	Trot	93	737	1812
	Gallop	78	564	1585
SF (r/min)	Trot	–	94	123
	Gallop	–	121	123
PaO_2 (mmHg)	Trot	110.5	102.3	75.4
	Gallop	92.4	99.0	69.8
$PaCO_2$ (mmHg)	Trot	44.9	42.9	50.6
	Gallop	46.5	43.1	49.2

VT: tidal volume; f_b: breathing frequency, Ve: expired minute volume; SF: stroke frequency; PaO_2 & $PaCO_2$: arterial partial pressure in O_2 and CO_2.

Lastly, breathing pattern during exercise can be altered by respiratory troubles. Qualitative and quantitative assessments of respiratory airflow, pattern of breathing and tidal breathing flow-volume loops at rest and during exercise can, in some cases, help to diagnose clinical and subclinical obstructive respiratory diseases.[37]

Partitioning of the respiratory volumes

Only a portion of the volume of inspired air reaches the area of the lung where gas exchange takes place: this is the *alveolar ventilation*. The remaining portion, i.e. two-thirds of the minute ventilation at rest, ventilates regions of lung where no gas exchange occurs. This is the physiological *dead space ventilation*. It includes the conducting airways (anatomical dead space) and the alveoli which are ventilated but not – or only poorly – perfused (alveolar dead space). The dead space to tidal volume ratio (VD/VT) averages 50–60% in the resting horse,[38] a percentage twice as high as that reported in humans and dogs.

Exercise-induced changes in alveolar ventilation and VD/VT in horses depend on the type of exercise performed.[30,39-41] During mild-to-moderate exercise, the dead space volume does not change significantly,[39] but because minute ventilation increases, VD/VT decreases (40%) and alveolar ventilation is improved.

If the exercise is prolonged at a constant rate, the dead space ventilation increases due to an increase in respiratory frequency and in VD/VT.[39,40] This adaptation probably reflects the thermoregulatory role of the respiratory system.[41]

Lastly, during intense effort, VD/VT decreases from about 60% to 20%,[40] with the physiological dead space reduced from 3.5 L at rest to 2.5 L.

Ventilation distribution

The *distribution of ventilation* is not uniform in the lung, even in healthy horses. Two factors can explain this phenomenon. The main one is that the intrapleural pressure changes are not uniform all over the thoracic cage.[42] A second reason is the existence of inequalities in regional small airways resistance and/or alveoli compliance: inhaled air preferentially enters the areas of the lungs with low resistive airways and highly compliant alveoli (Fig. 27.5).

The resulting ventilatory asynchronism is moderate in healthy horses at rest, and does not have significant effects on gas exchange at low respiratory frequencies. On the contrary, in horses with significant asynchronism (e.g. subclinical obstruction of small airways), this phenomenon can significantly impair gas exchange (Fig. 27.5) especially during exercise, with high respiratory frequency. The lobules which have a long time for filling do not fill adequately before expiration begins and might even 'rebreath' the expired air from other regions. Consequently ventilation/perfusion mismatching and hypoxemia result, possibly leading to exercise intolerance.

Perfusion and vascular adjustments

Blood flow distribution

As already mentioned, blood flow is preferentially distributed to the dorsal regions of the lung[11] (Fig. 27.2) and this pattern is exacerbated during exercise.[12] The greatest perfusion redistribution occurs during moderate exercise intensity, with little further change when intensity further increases. Moreover, there is a considerable heterogeneity in each isogravitational plane,[11] which obviously is in disagreement with the gravitational model for distribution of

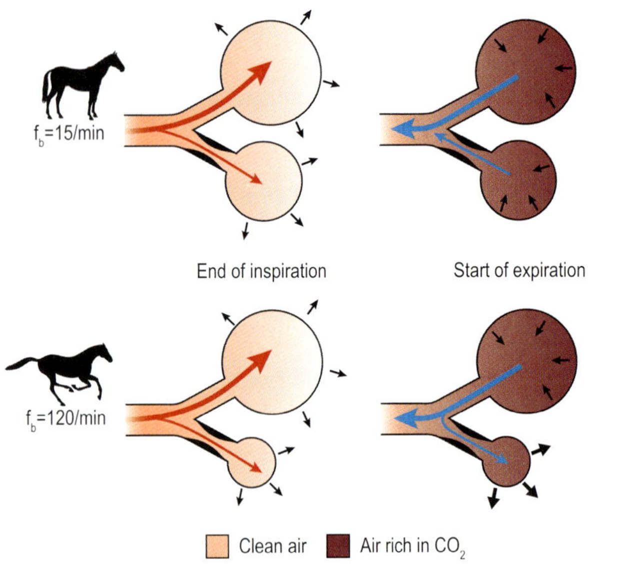

Fig 27.5 Representation of two bronchioles with different resistance to airflow which induces an inhomogeneity of ventilation. This phenomenon leads to ventilatory asynchronism, which means that some alveoli start to expire when other are still inhaling, and to impairment of gas exchange because expired air is inhaled by the alveoli having a sub-obstructed bronchiole. This is especially true during exercise when breathing frequency (f_b) is high.

pulmonary blood flow. More than 70% of variation of pulmonary blood flow at rest and during exercise is determined by a fixed spatial pattern that is most likely related to the structural anatomy of the pulmonary vascular tree. Accordingly, despite a redistribution of pulmonary blood flow, heterogeneity of perfusion remains during effort.[12] Furosemide, which is frequently used for its putative preventive effect on pulmonary hemorrhage in susceptible horses, slightly attenuates this blood redistribution, but does not influence flow heterogeneity.[43] The remaining 30% variation of blood distribution can be attributable to modulation of vascular diameter or other factors, which remain to be elucidated. It must be pointed out that perfusion heterogeneity is greater in horses suffering from recurrent airway obstruction than in healthy horses.[44]

Vascular diameter is modulated by smooth muscles that respond to vasoactive compounds. A wide range of mediators can modulate vascular smooth muscle tone, and among these epinephrine, norepinephrine, dopamine, prostaglandin and endothelin,[45] which is notably potent, are vasoconstrictors, and isoproterenol, bradykinin, histamine, nitric oxide and acetylcholine produce vasodilatation.

Lung volume also plays a role in pulmonary blood flow by passively modulating vascular resistance. A distinction must be made between extra-alveolar vessels and alveolar vessels (thin-walled capillaries which perfuse alveoli). The cross-section of extra-alveolar capillaries is dependent on the pressure changes in the interstitial tissues rather than in the alveoli, while the opposite is true for the intra-alveolar capillaries. Consequently, vascular resistance varies with degree of lung inflation, as shown in Figure 27.6.

During intense exercise, *pulmonary blood flow* increases approximately 10-fold.[46] The pulmonary right-to-left shunt fraction of cardiac output is approximately 1% at rest and 0.4% during heavy exercise.[47] At the same time, mean *pulmonary arterial pressure* rises about 3-fold, from 28 mmHg at rest to about 85 mmHg at a fast gallop, with maximal reported values of 100 mmHg.[47–49] This increase in pulmonary artery pressure is associated with large increases in pulmonary capillary, wedge and venous pressures.[50]

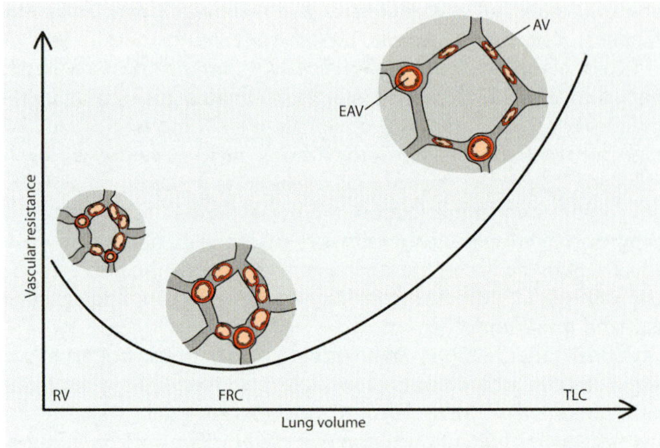

Fig 27.6 The lung volume passively influences the vascular resistance. (1) At residual lung volume (RV), the extra-alveolar vessels (EAV; not gas exchanging) are narrowed, while the alveolar vessels (AV; gas exchanging) are distended. The resistance is increased because of the narrowing of EAV. (2) At functional residual capacity (FRC), the vascular resistance is the lowest, both kinds of vessels being distended. (3) At total lung capacity (TLC), the EAV are distended and the AV become elliptic because of the tension on the alveolar septa. This increases the resistance of the AV and the vascular resistance is consequently increased.

This marked pulmonary *hypertension* is a unique feature of exertion in horses and ponies and might be due, in part, to the high left atrial pressure which is necessary for rapid ventricular filling at maximal heart rates.

This elevation in pulmonary vascular pressure is nowadays largely thought as being one of the major factors responsible for the occurrence of pulmonary hemorrhage during strenuous exercise. While some authors did not find a relationship between pulmonary vascular pressure and occurrence of blood into the airways after exercise,[50] others identified a pressure threshold of 90 mmHg above which hemorrhage occurred in the lungs of horses running on a treadmill.[51]

Pulmonary vascular resistance

Pulmonary vascular resistance (PVR) in horses is low. It is estimated by dividing the pressure gradient between arterial and capillary pressures (the latter being more easily measurable than the left atrial pressure, by use of the arterial occlusion technique) by the cardiac output. Some experiments have suggested that the precapillary sphincters are responsible for the greater part of the PVR.[52] The post-capillary resistance (venous capillaries) is, conversely, very low. This physiological adjustment could offer protection against a large increase in pressure at the level of the capillaries[52] and consequently against pulmonary hemorrhage and the development of pulmonary edema.

With moderate exercise, there is an approximate two-fold decrease in pulmonary vascular resistance (from 0.14 to 0.06 mmHg/ml/min.kg).[53] Dilatation (increase of the cross-sectional area) and recruitment of the vascular bed whereby previously non-perfused or minimally perfused vessels become functional,[54] are probably the major factors contributing to the decrease in vascular resistance. With further increase of exercise intensity, resistance does not change further, despite the increase in cardiac output.

The decrease in vascular resistance occurs despite the existence of several factors that should increase it: compression of the extra-alveolar lung vessels during forced expiration (decrease in lung volume) or alveolar vessels during forced inspiration (lung distended)[9] (Fig. 27.6), increase in circulatory volume and in greater viscosity of blood related to the exercise-induced rise in packed cell volume. An in vitro study has suggested that blood viscosity is not a major factor contributing to vascular resistance in horses,[55] which differs from humans where each increase of 1% in the packed cell volume induces an increase of 4% in the pulmonary vascular resistance.[56] Nevertheless, splenectomized exercising ponies had a lower increase in pulmonary arterial pressure when compared with normal ones.[57]

The great increase in pulmonary arterial pressure together with the exercise-related hypoxemia has led to the suggestion that, in exercising horses, there could be an accumulation of interstitial water and occurrence of an interstitial edema which impairs gas diffusion. In human beings and pigs, this phenomenon exists, leading to worsening of the ventilation/perfusion ratio.[58] However, there is no accumulation of interstitial water in exercising horses[54] which is compatible with the preservation of ventilation/perfusion ratio.[47] Why hypertension and an increase in the rate of *fluid filtration* across the capillary walls of the lung do not result in pulmonary edema can be explained by the fact that in horses, as in other species, the lymphatic system has a substantial capacity to drain the pulmonary interstitial space.[54,56] Moreover, the 'pumping' action associated with the large and frequent pressure changes in the equine thoracic cage during exercise could contribute to the efficiency of the lymphatic drainage.[59]

Ventilation/perfusion ratio

Gas exchange ultimately depends on the matching of pulmonary ventilation and perfusion. It is efficient in lung regions where the ratio is 0.8 to 1.0–1.2, which is the case for most regions. However, there can be regions that are excessively perfused, as indicated by a ventilation/perfusion ratio <0.8, or excessively ventilated, ventilation/perfusion ratio >1.2.[60,61]

In horses, the ventilation/perfusion ratio is not influenced by gravity, being uniform from the top to the bottom of the lung, suggesting that in this species the gradient in lung ventilation is appropriately matched by the gradient in lung perfusion.[10,60,61]

During exercise, there is only a slight mismatch of ventilation to perfusion ratio in horses.[32,47,62] The mismatch accounts for 25%[47] to 40%[32] of the increase in the alveolar–arterial pressure difference in O_2 which averages 4 mmHg at rest, and can reach values as high as 30 mmHg during exercise.[32] This physiological adaptation contrasts with what is observed in humans and pigs, where the ventilation/perfusion ratio is non-uniform at rest, and a true mismatching occurs during exercise.[58] The mechanism of this exercise-induced ventilation/perfusion inequality in horses remains to be understood.

In horses suffering from airway disease, exercise will induce a ventilation/perfusion mismatching, by impairing either ventilation or perfusion, or both. As mentioned before, the collateral ventilation in the horse has little ability to compensate for the occlusion of small airways.[6] The resulting ventilatory asynchronism leads to hypoxemia and sometimes hypercapnia. Studies have also shown that gas exchange impairment during exercise can also result from inappropriate perfusion redistribution in horses with recurrent airway obstruction (heaves).[44]

Gas exchange

Development of hypoxemia/hypercapnia

In resting healthy horses, arterial partial pressure in oxygen (PaO_2) is 85–100 mmHg and that of carbon dioxide ($PaCO_2$) is 40–45 mmHg.

Arterial hypoxemia and hemoglobin desaturation occur when exercise intensity exceeds 60% of VO_{2max}.[1,63] Arterial oxygen tension can be as low as 60 mmHg and carbon dioxide tension as high as 58 mmHg during intense exercise. Theoretically, hypoxemia can be primarily related to one of the following factors:

- right-to-left vascular shunts
- ventilation/perfusion mismatching
- diffusion impairment
- alveolar hypoventilation.

The post-pulmonary shunts between bronchial and pulmonary circulation can theoretically be partly responsible for the exercise-induced hypoxemia. However, with a shunt of 1%, which is a reasonable approximation, the arterial O_2 partial pressure should be reduced by 5 mmHg, which is less than the actual decrease observed during exercise.[47] According to different studies, the V/Q mismatch accounts for 25%[47] to 40%[32] of the increase in the alveolar–arterial pressure difference in O_2, the remaining 60% to 75% of the widening of $(A-a)O_2$ gradient is related to alveolar-capillary diffusion impairment and to alveolar hypoventilation.

Diffusion

During heavy exercise, different and opposite factors can influence the diffusion capacity. On the one hand, several factors should improve diffusion. Firstly, a mixed venous O_2 pressure as low as 16 mmHg has been reported during a fast gallop.[63] Although the alveolar O_2 pressure decreases, the increase in the pressure gradient between capillary blood and alveolar air should improve O_2 extraction and diffusion. Secondly, the increased blood flow recruits alveoli that are not perfused at rest, and therefore, increases the functional vascular exchange surface. Thirdly, the increase of hemoglobin concentration related to splenic contraction promotes O_2 diffusion by increasing the number of binding sites (hemoglobin concentration) available.

But, on the other hand, despite the 50–60% increase in the volume of the pulmonary vasculature (due to the recruitment and enlargement of the capillary bed), the 8-fold increase in cardiac output leads to a dramatic shortening of the capillary transit time and consequently to a decrease of the time for O_2 equilibration, and thus, diffusion impairment[54] (Fig. 27.7).

However, other species have also a very short transit time during exercise (0.29 sec in the dog, 0.35 sec in the pony and 0.5 sec in

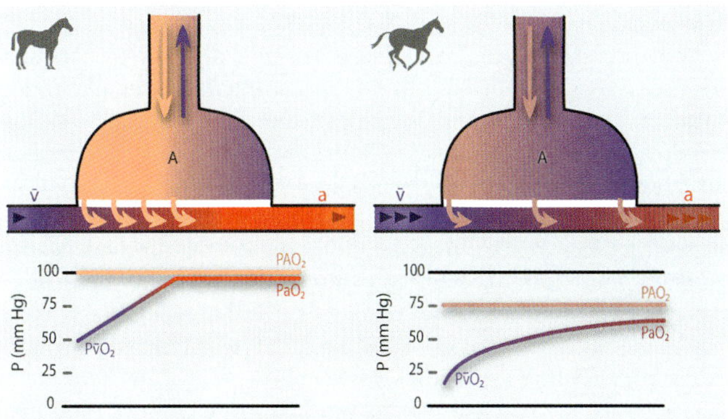

Fig 27.7 Monoalveolar model showing gas exchange at rest (left) and during exercise (right). Arterial hypoxemia probably occurs for several reasons and, among these, the increase of cardiac output reducing the capillary transit time which impairs gas diffusion, a relative hypoventilation (decrease of PAO_2), and the fact that the partial pressure in O_2 in the mixed venous blood is dramatically low. a = arterial; v = mixed venous; A = alveolar.

man) but none of them demonstrate diffusion limitation during exercise.[64] Therefore, it can be hypothesized that these species are able to compensate for their short capillary transit time with other physiological adaptations, which are either lacking or inadequate in the horse.

Alveolar hypoventilation

Lastly *alveolar hypoventilation* can also play a role in the occurrence of hypoxemia during exercise as demonstrated by the narrowing of the high alveolar–arterial gradient in O_2 when a helium–oxygen mixture is substituted for air.[65] Indeed, helium–oxygen mixtures, being less dense than normal air, permit greater alveolar ventilation during intense exercise.

Blood gas transport

The *oxygen content of blood* is mainly determined by the hemoglobin concentration and its degree of saturation with O_2. At rest, when hemoglobin is nearly fully saturated (97%) with O_2, and assuming a hemoglobin concentration of 14 g/L, 100 ml of blood carries about 20 ml of O_2, including the 0.3 ml of O_2 dissolved per 100 ml of plasma.

The saturation of hemoglobin depends on the arterial O_2 partial pressure which, in turn, depends on the amount of O_2 dissolved in the plasma. Above an O_2 partial pressure of approximately 70 mmHg, the oxyhemoglobin curve is essentially flat and any increase in O_2 partial pressure will add little O_2 to hemoglobin because the hemoglobin is nearly saturated and only a few (3–5%) of the binding sites are still available. Below an O_2 partial pressure of 70 mmHg, the oxyhemoglobin curve has a sharply decreasing slope. At the partial pressure encountered in the tissues (about 40 mmHg), blood releases about 25% of its O_2 to the tissues. During exercise, the tissue partial pressure of O_2 is further reduced and more O_2 will be released. Arterial O_2 partial pressure in blood returning from all tissues averages 16 mmHg during heavy exercise. It can consequently be assumed that O_2 tension at the level of the exercising muscle is still lower and this increases the driving pressure for O_2 diffusion at this level. Lastly, increases in blood temperature, in $[H^+]$ (ie a decline in pH), in partial pressure of CO_2 and in intracellular concentration of certain organic phosphates (2,3 DPG) induce a right shift of the curve,[66] promoting a higher O_2 release in the metabolizing tissues (Fig. 27.8), especially during intense exercise, but also pushing the point at which the steep downward slope begins to the right. This means that reduction in arterial saturation of hemoglobin begins at a higher PO_2.

The increase in the packed cell volume and the consequent increase in hemoglobin due to splenic contraction is an adaptation to exercise specific to the horse (and the dog), providing almost 50–60% more binding sites for O_2 during exercise.[67] This represents an adjustment which partly compensates for the fall in arterial O_2 partial pressure and hemoglobin desaturation. It has been hypothesized that too great an increase in packed cell volume can be disadvantageous from a hemodynamic point of view, because it increases the blood viscosity.[68] However, this theory has been invalidated by an in vitro study showing that viscosity is not a major factor contributing to vascular resistance.[55]

Carbon dioxide results from metabolic processes, and, once produced, it diffuses from the cells into the capillary blood. At high intensities of exercise, i.e. above VO_{2max}, the large muscular mass produces an extraordinary amount of CO_2 and the lung seems unable to completely eliminate it. The development of a relative CO_2 retention in horses during intense exercise is unique among mammals.[63] Human athletes develop a compensatory hyperventilation during heavy exercise to ensure high alveolar O_2 partial pressure, which in turn provokes a decrease in the arterial partial pressure of CO_2 to about 30 mmHg.[69] Obviously, in exercising horses, there is a lack of truly compensatory hyperventilation and this contributes to the development of exercise-induced hypercapnia as well as hypoxemia.[63] The partial pressures of O_2 and CO_2 along the oxygen line are summarized in Figure 27.9.

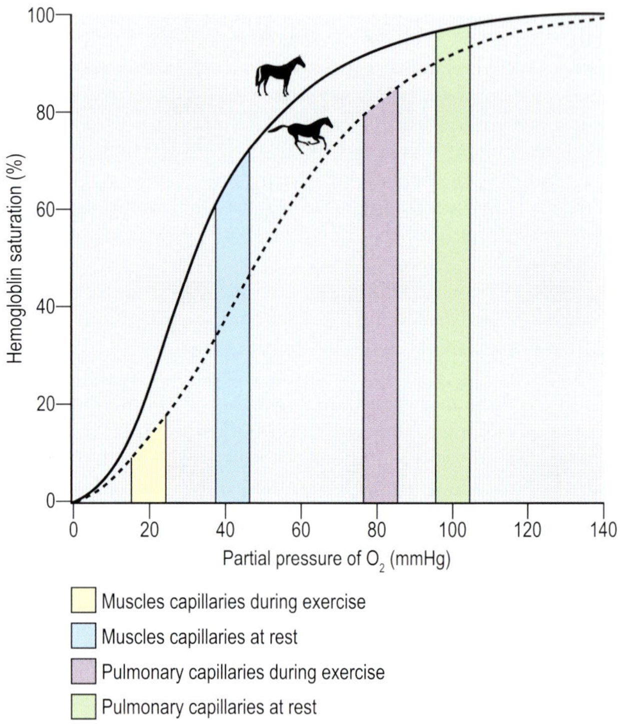

Fig 27.8 Oxyhemoglobin dissociation curve at rest (solid line) and during exercise (dashed line). During exercise, there is a right shift related to the decrease in pH and the increase in blood temperature and PCO_2. This shift facilitates the release of O_2 at the level of the tissue, especially at the level of the muscles during exercise.

Mechanics of breathing

Volume changes in the respiratory apparatus imply that work is being performed on the respiratory system, mainly expanding or compressing the gas in the lungs, and displacing it in and out of the airways. The driving forces exerted by the respiratory muscles are opposed mainly by static forces (elastic, gravitational and surface) and flow resistive forces (viscous and turbulent resistance of the gases and viscous resistance of the tissues). Inertial forces, negligible at rest, are also of importance in running horses.[70]

The study of the relationship between the pressures exerted on the respiratory system and the changes in volume and airflow that result from these pressure changes is the basis of the mechanics of breathing (Fig. 27.10).

The maximal pleural pressure change is the difference between peak inspiratory and peak expiratory pleural pressures ($DPpl_{max}$), and is approximately 0.5 kPa at rest. Once exercise starts, the $DPpl_{max}$ increases, and in Thoroughbred horses during maximal exercise, becomes as high as 8.5 kPa or 80 cmH_2O[25] (Table 27.2). At this intensity of exercise, respiratory frequency is about 120/min, which means that the time for inspiration or expiration is approximately 250 msec.[25]

The *total pulmonary resistance* quantifies the ease with which air flows through the airways. It is influenced by different and opposed

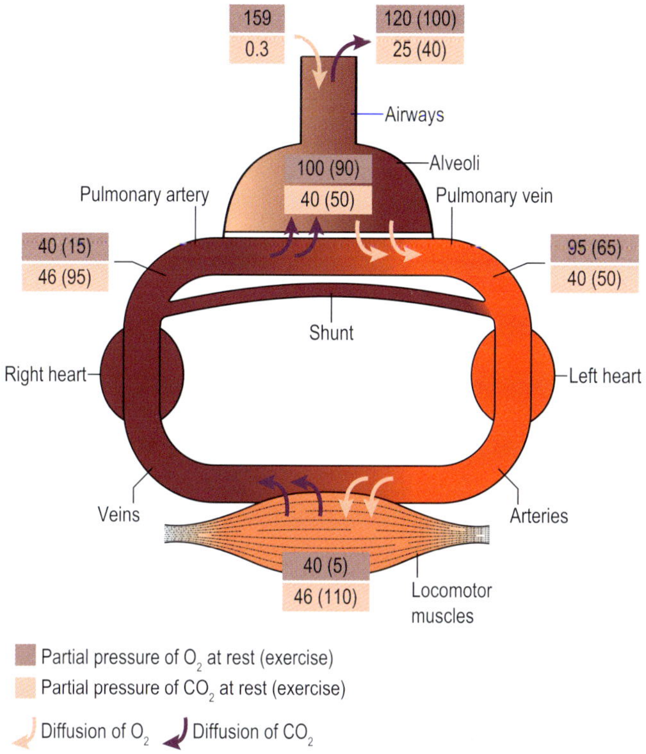

Fig 27.9 Partial pressure of O_2 and CO_2 (given in mmHg) at different levels of the oxygen line at rest and during exercise.

Table 27.2 Mechanics of breathing in horses at exercise

VALUES	REST	4 m/sec	10 m/sec
Tidal volume (L)	4.8	6.4	13.2
Respiratory frequency (r/min)	14	91	121
Expired minute volume (L/min)	78	564	1585
Peak inspiratory flow (L/sec)	5.1	27.6	63.9
Peak expiratory flow (L/sec)	5.1	30.5	78.8
Maximal pressure changes (kPa)	0.043	2.37	8.23
Total pulmonary resistance (kPa/L/sec)	0.021	0.029	0.058
Work of breathing (J/L)	0.41	2.41	6.22

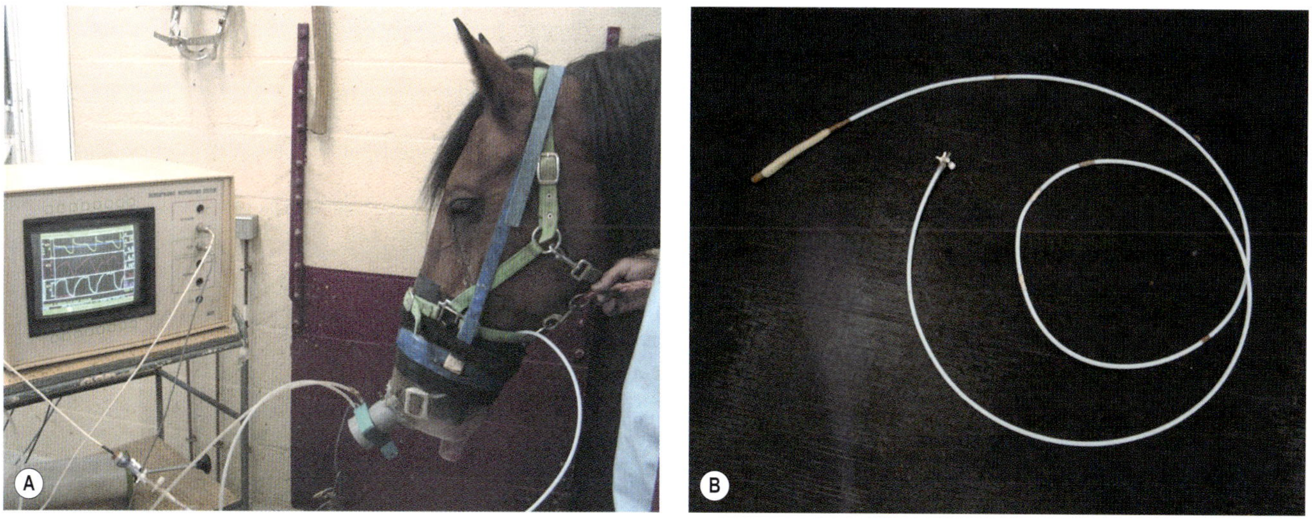

Fig 27.10 Measurement of the mechanics of breathing: **(A)** airflow is measured with a pneumotachograph, simultaneously with the measurement of the pleural (esophageal) pressure (**(B)** esophageal balloon). Tidal volume is obtained by integration of airflow over time, and resistance to airflow and pulmonary compliance are computed.

factors: physiological ones which tend to decrease the resistance (mainly through enlargement of the cross-sectional area of some parts of the airways) and physical ones which tend to increase it (friction, turbulence, inhomogeneous distribution of the resistance along airways and alveoli, and airway cross-sectional area changes induced by compressive transmural pressures). The importance of the cross-sectional area of the airway is highlighted by the the relationship between airway radius and resistance (resistance is proportional to the inverse of the radius raised to the fourth power) such that when the radius of the airway is reduced to one-half (i.e. reduced by a factor of two), the resistance is increased by 16-fold (2^4).

The importance of friction and turbulence has been demonstrated by experiments where trotting horses breathed a helium–oxygen mixture. Being less dense than air and therefore minimizing turbulence and friction, heliox induced a 50% decrease in the total pulmonary resistance and mechanical work of breathing,[71] and as a consequence, an increase in breathing frequency and alveolar and expired minute ventilation.[65,71]

During quiet breathing, 50% of the total pulmonary resistance results from the nasal passages, 30% from the remaining upper airways and 20% from the intrathoracic airways.[72] The resistance of the lower airway is much lesser than that of the upper airway because the sum of the cross-sectional areas of the bronchioles is much greater than the cross-sectional area of the trachea, and because the airflow is laminar in these regions while it is more turbulent in the trachea.

The importance of the relative contribution of the nasal cavities is not specific to horses but this species, in contrast to others, cannot switch from nasal to oro-nasal breathing. Strenuous exercise induces a substantial two-fold increase in the respiratory resistance but it does not significantly modify the relative contribution of each part of the respiratory tract to the total pulmonary resistance.[25,72]

Studies of the inspiratory and expiratory components of the respiratory resistance values in trotting horses have shown that, during inspiration, the extra-thoracic airway accounts for more than 90% of the total pulmonary resistance while, during expiration, the intra-thoracic airway is responsible for more than 50% of the pulmonary resistance (Fig. 27.11).[72] This observation could be explained by dynamic partial collapse of intrathoracic airways during exercise when the pressure surrounding the airways exceeds the pressure within the lumen. When a horse inhales, sub-atmospheric pressures in the extra-thoracic airways can be as low as -5 kPa while the pressure in the surrounding tissues remains atmospheric. During expiration, the intra-thoracic pressure becomes greater than the pressure prevailing inside some of the intra-thoracic airways. When exposed to compressive pressures, these structures tend to collapse, consequently increasing their resistance to airflow.[73] This phenomenon can be expected to be dramatically worsened in horses with partial airway obstruction, a condition that is accompanied by substantial transmural pressure increases during exercise.[73–75]

The *dynamic compliance* (C_{dyn}) gives an estimate of the elastic properties of the lung. The lung has an inherent elasticity due to the tissue elasticity provided by a network of elastin and collagen fibers and the surface tension forces. The latter is lowered by the pulmonary surfactant, a complex material composed of 80% lipids and 20% proteins. At rest, C_{dyn} is approximately equal to 23 L/kPa. Because of (1) technical problems associated with the determination of dynamic compliance during hyperventilation in large animals, and (2) the magnitude of the pressure necessary for flow acceleration, the value of compliance measured during exercise can become negative.[70] Bayly and Slocombe,[76] calculated the dynamic compliance of horses running at 10 m/sec, taking the inertial pressure into account. They concluded that during exercise, C_{dyn} is 25% of its pre-exercise value. However, whether this decrease is the genuine reflection of changes in elastic properties of the horse's lung, or due to an increase in respiratory asynchronism,[75] or related to other technical problems, is not yet elucidated.

Assessment of the *mechanical work of breathing* is based on the measurement of the area of the pressure–volume loops. Although it is well known that the total work of breathing is underestimated by this method, it gives a good estimation of the dynamic components of the work of breathing. It has been shown that the work per respiratory cycle, the work per liter of air ventilated and the work per minute are dramatically increased during exercise.[77] For example, the power output (i.e. the work of breathing per minute) is increased 475 times when the horse gallops.[25]

The relationship between the mechanical work of breathing per minute and the minute volume in running horses is curvilinear with an upwards concavity. The curve is of ever-increasing slope, implying that the mechanical cost of breathing for any additional units of air ventilated becomes greater with any increase in ventilation.[25,77] These observations strongly suggest that the work of breathing could be a limiting or at least a constraining factor to further increases in ventilation during strenuous exercise. Furthermore, in order to evaluate the relative respiratory muscle O_2 uptake compared with total O_2 uptake, the ratio of the *mechanical work of breathing*/O_2 *uptake* has been calculated in galloping horses. This ratio increases exponentially with the minute volume indicating that during exercise, the respiratory muscles O_2 uptake reaches a substantial percentage of the O_2 uptake.[25] This suggests that in horses as in humans,[78] there is a so-called 'critical level of ventilation' above which any further increase in O_2 uptake would be entirely consumed by the respiratory muscles.

Control of breathing

In healthy horses at rest, blood gases and chemical composition of the blood remain steady. The matching of the metabolic needs and the alveolar ventilation is under the control of a central controller

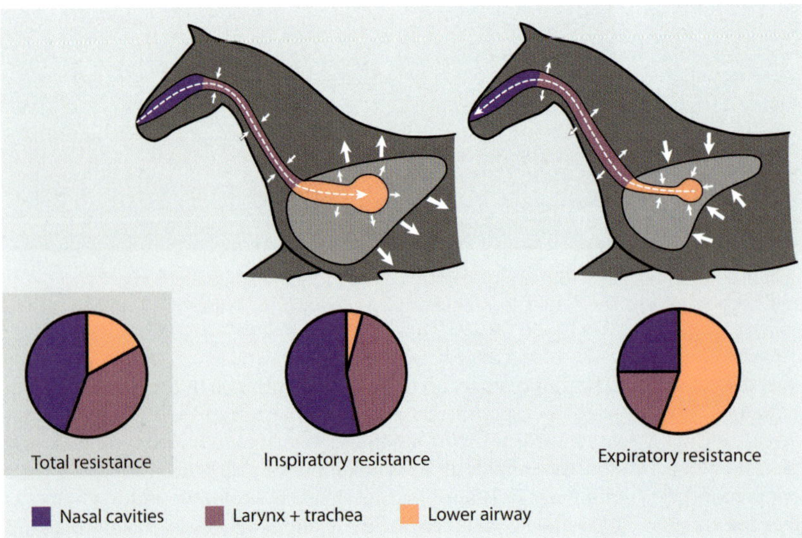

Fig 27.11 Relative contribution of the different parts of the respiratory system to the total pulmonary resistance during exercise. At exercise, the upper airway contributes about 95% to the total resistance during inspiration, while during expiration, lower airway contributes to more than half of the resistance. This is explained by the dynamic changes occurring in the cross-sectional area of the airway related to compressive transmural pressure during inspiration (upper airways) and during expiration (lower airways). Nasal cavities are supported by bones and therefore are much less subject to changes in airway diameter related to intraluminal pressure changes.

located in the pons and in the medulla. Its activity is modulated by a variety of neural inputs coming from peripheral and central receptors, and it regulates, via motor neurons, the ventilatory muscles according to the received information. Higher conscious centers can also modify the pattern of breathing.

Changes in arterial partial pressure of CO_2 and/or pH, detected by both peripheral and central chemoreceptors, are more potent regulators of ventilation than changes in arterial O_2 partial pressure, which are detected by peripheral chemoreceptors only.

The *peripheral chemoreceptors* are located in the carotid bodies at the bifurcation of the common carotid arteries and in the aortic bodies, near the aortic arch. They send afferent impulses to the control center via the vagus and the glosso-pharyngeal nerves. Their activity is enhanced by hypercapnia, hypoxemia and acidosis, but also by hyperthermia and decreased blood pressure. While their response to CO_2 and pH is quite linear, their response to changes in arterial O_2 partial pressure is non-linear and they show enhanced activity only when arterial O_2 partial pressure is below 60 mmHg. The stimulation of these chemoreceptors via hypoxemic challenge increases the inspiratory muscles' activation with little changes in abdominal expiratory muscle activity.[79]

The *central chemoreceptor* tissue is located near the ventral aspect of the medulla. It lies in the intracerebral interstitial fluid and, apparently, responds to changes in the interstitial tissue fluid pH. The latter is induced either by changes in arterial partial pressure of CO_2, giving a fast response (because CO_2 diffuses freely through the blood–brain barrier) or by a change in blood pH, giving a delayed response (because the barrier is relatively impermeable to H^+). Therefore an acute increase of H^+ concentration is at first detected by the peripheral receptors.

The *pulmonary stretch receptors* are nerves ending in the tracheal and bronchial smooth muscles. Their activity is enhanced by the enlargement of airway cross-section: for example, when the lung volume increases, and results in an inhibition of further inspiratory activity. The stretch receptors could be responsible for the adjustment of the pattern of breathing to minimize the energetic cost of breathing. They could also prevent a lung overstretching when the ventilatory demand is high, such as during heavy exercise.

The question of how the ventilatory rate is controlled during exercise is one of the major unresolved issues in respiratory physiology. The controversy mainly comes from the origin of the stimulus that can provide a rapid and adequate adjustment of alveolar ventilation that perfectly meets the metabolic demand. In the human, there are several theories proposing either neural stimuli, or humoral stimuli, or a combination of both.[80] Obviously, because horses do not adopt a compensatory hyperventilation as human do, human respiratory physiology cannot be transposed to horses.

Different research protocols suggested that, in horses, the mechanism of control of breathing seems to be related to the exercise intensity.

During *short-term moderate exercise*, arterial blood gases and chemical composition do not change: the ventilation rate increases in parallel with the metabolic rate. However, gas tensions are far too stable to account for the increase in ventilation on the basis of the simple negative feedback system existing at rest. Although there is a considerable conviction that gas tensions (especially partial pressure of CO_2 and associated H^+ concentration) are involved in the control of ventilation during exercise as well, how they are involved remains enigmatic. It is likely that other drives such as mechanoreflexes originating from motion of the working limbs, changes in cardiac output, thermoregulation, and cortical and psychological factors are involved in the control of ventilation.[81]

During more *intense exercise*, and once the horse reaches 60% of its VO_{2max}, a decrease in arterial O_2 partial pressure and pH is observed. At a higher intensity, there is an increase in arterial partial pressure of CO_2. Despite the fact that these chemical regulators are supposed to strongly stimulate ventilation, the stimuli appear to be insufficient to maintain arterial blood gas homeostasis, which is obviously specific to the equine species.

So, in contrast with other species, the horse does not adopt a compensatory hyperventilation.[47,63] The reason for this hypercapnic hypoventilation remains unclear and numerous hypotheses have been put forward.

Locomotion–respiration coupling has been suggested as a major constraint to the increase in ventilation. Although there is no doubt that respiratory frequency is totally related to step frequency in galloping horses, several experimental observations rule out the coupling as a reason for hypoventilation: (1) Standardbred horses, racing at a trot (a gait where a coupling can exist but is not compulsory), also demonstrate hypoxemia and hypercapnia[32,46](see Table 27.1); (2) the magnitude of hypercapnia is poorly related to the respiratory frequency;[63] (3) the respiratory frequency of the pony – and all other mammals – is also tightly coupled with its step frequency and, nevertheless, it adopts a compensatory hyperventilation and becomes hypocapnic during heavy exercise.[64]

In horses running at 10m/sec a slight increase in ventilation is observed when the CO_2 concentration in the inhaled air is increased from 0 to 3%. But a further increase in inhaled CO_2 up to 6% does not induce any further changes in ventilation, despite the fact that the horses are not at their maximal ventilation capacity,[82] suggesting a *lower sensitivity of the chemoreceptors*.

The compensatory hyperventilation which would be required for the homeostasis of arterial O_2 partial pressure should theoretically be ensured by either:

1. a tidal volume of about 23 L, which together with a respiratory frequency of about 120 breaths/min, implies mean respiratory airflow of more than 100 L/sec, or
2. a coupling 2:1 between respiratory frequency and step frequency, which implies that the respiratory frequency should reach values of about 240 breaths/min.[63]

In terms of *respiratory muscle energetics and force–velocity characteristics*, such a level of ventilation would probably be impossible to reach. In such a situation, energy demand of the respiratory muscles becomes so substantial that the energy supply can be insufficient to satisfy this demand.

Respiratory muscle exhaustion occurs in man after high-intensity short-term exercise as well as during prolonged exercise. This results in a progressive increase in diaphragmatic excitation–contraction decoupling.[83] Although it has been shown that exhaustion during high-intensity short-term exercise is associated with a sudden decrease in expired minute volume and O_2 uptake,[40,84] the occurrence of muscle fatigue as a cause of these observations remains to be demonstrated.

Lastly, during *prolonged heavy, but not maximal, exercise*, the impairment of gas exchange (especially hypercapnia) seems to be progressively compensated after several minutes of exercise.[63,85] This suggests that horses, like humans, could experience a 'second wind' phenomenon related to changes in diaphragmatic function.[86]

To summarize, the fact that the increase in ventilation becomes limited during heavy exercise in horses can be explained by several factors. *Firstly*, during strenuous exercise, the horse could reach a 'critical level of ventilation' above which any further increase in O_2 uptake would be entirely consumed by the respiratory muscles. The advantage of not increasing ventilation further during strenuous exercise can be that extra-flow resistive and elastic work is avoided and that there is a reduction in the O_2 uptake of ventilatory muscles, consequently reducing their energy demand. In terms of performance, hypoxemia and hypercapnia could be less disadvantageous than reaching the critical level of ventilation. *Secondly*, this negative feedback mechanism could protect the ventilatory muscles against exhaustion. *Thirdly*, pulmonary overstretching, i.e. high lung volume, has been shown to increase the fragility of alveolar and vessel walls.[87] By limiting the increase in lung volume, the horse could minimize the risk of tissue rupture, possibly leading to severe exercise-induced pulmonary hemorrhage.

Physiological measurements during exercise

Assessment of lung function and evaluation of the ventilatory response to exercise requires airway instrumentation. Since these measurements alter the breathing pattern and ventilation, and are usually performed in laboratory conditions, they might not reflect the genuine ventilation during physical activities.

Therefore, research has focused during the last decade on non-invasive systems, which can be portable, for unobtrusive and cooperation-independent monitoring of ventilation in exercising horses.

Accurate measurement of ventilation of exercising horses is challenging for numerous technical problems related to the size and anatomy of these animals as well as to their specific breathing physiology. First of all, wearing a mask increases the anatomical dead space and induces re-breathing of CO_2. The mask also increases respiratory resistance, inducing some artifactual adaptations of the breathing strategy, including generally lower respiratory frequency, higher lung volume, and locomotion/respiration decoupling.[88,89] Another problem is the time response of the devices used for the metabolic measurements when they are based on a breath-by-breath approach. Indeed, with respiratory frequency as high as 120 r/min, the time response of the gas (O_2 and CO_2) analyzers is too long and results in a phase lag between the ventilatory and gas signals.[90] Last, but not least, measurements must be done during spontaneous breathing as horses are non-cooperative subjects.

Pulmonary function tests usable in exercising horses include measurements of lung volumes, of pulmonary mechanics, and tests of gas exchange such as arterial blood gas tensions and oxygen consumption measurements.

Ventilation

Measurement of ventilation requires a face mask and a flow measuring system. The face mask must be very light, but rigid and solid, the dead space must be limited to avoid CO_2 rebreathing, but compression of the nares and soft tissues must be avoided. It must be airtight. Several systems are available for breath-by-breath measurement of the airflow and volume: Fleisch, Lilly or ultrasonic pneumotachometers, inductance plethysmography (Fig. 27.12). However, most of these techniques are not applicable during exercise. Indeed, the devices to measure airflow must have a limited weight, have a wide range of measurement and an appropriate frequency response (respiratory airflow can be as high as 100 L/sec and frequency as high as 120 breaths/min); they must be protected against moisture and, above all, they should not add extraresistance to breathing. Ultrasonic pneumotachometers meet these requirements but they are sensitive to presence of water and can, in this case, have severe baseline drift of the volume measurement (i.e. a progressive change in the measured volume, when in fact there is no change).

Pulmonary mechanics

To evaluate the respiratory effort necessary to generate given airflow and ventilation, recording of pleural pressure changes, generally done via the recording of esophageal pressure changes,[42] must be performed simultaneously with the measurement of respiratory airflow and volume. The impulse oscillometry system is also a non-invasive method of measuring the mechanics of breathing, but it is impossible to use this method on running horses.[91]

The maximal changes in pleural pressure, the total pulmonary resistance and the pulmonary dynamic compliance can be determined. These measurements give a quantification of the degree of airflow obstruction of the airway and of the elastic properties of the lung. Other methods such as the forced oscillation technique, tidal breathing flow–volume loops or forced expiration techniques are also useful but have not been used during exercise.

Arterial blood gases

Arterial blood gas analysis helps to investigate pulmonary function as it quantifies the lung's ability to oxygenate and remove CO_2 from the blood. It therefore gives an estimate of the overall capacity of the lung to ensure adequate gas exchange. While at-rest sampling can be done through the puncture of a superficial artery, the sampling of arterial blood gas during exercise requires the catheterization of a superficial artery, the most commonly used being the transverse facial artery (Fig. 27.13).

To obtain reliable data, it is essential to simultaneously measure blood temperature at the site of sampling, especially during exercise, when this temperature can change rapidly with the increase of the metabolism (Fig. 27.14). As previously mentioned horses develop hypoxemia at an exercise intensity of about 60% VO_{2max} and hypercapnia during maximal exercise. The phenomenon is still

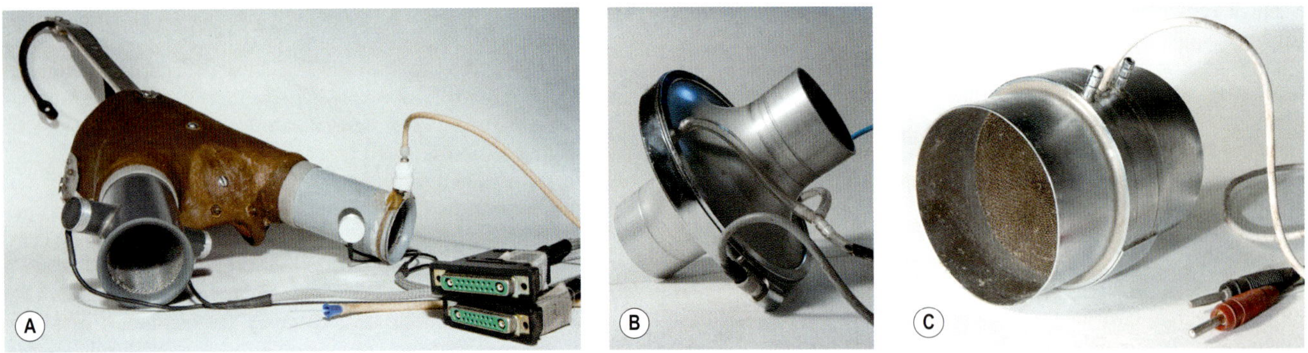

Fig 27.12 Different systems facilitating measurement of airflow in horses: **(A)** ultrasonic pneumotachographs, **(B)** Lilly head, **(C)** Fleisch head No. 5. The first system allows measurements in horses during high-intensity exercise (flow range ± 100 L/sec); the second one is usable at rest only; and the third one in ponies at moderate exercise (flow range ± 35 L/sec).

exacerbated in well-trained horses, because their muscular oxidative capacity is dramatically improved. As a consequence, the O_2 removal at the peripheral level is so high that PvO_2 of 16 mmHg or less can be sometime observed. This venous blood deoxygenation, combined with a further increase of the cardiac output – also related to training – and a lack of improvement of the pulmonary function explain why trained horses show more severe hypoxemia and hypercapnia than untrained subjects.[92]

On the other hand, lower respiratory tract problems can also interfere with the gas exchange (namely by decreasing the quality of the alveolar ventilation or by perturbing the V/Q ratio) and induce exercise hypoxemia.[93] The lack of norms of PaO_2 and $PaCO_2$ during exercise, combined with the possible interference of training and/or illness, makes this measurement rather difficult to interpret for clinical purpose.

Oxygen consumption

The measurement of VO_2 and VCO_2 necessitates the simultaneous recording of the ventilation and the concentration of O_2 and CO_2 in the expired gases. So, the system described above to measure ventilation must be combined with a system of gas analysis (e.g. mass spectrometer) or expired gas collection. The latter method requires a system with expiratory valves which are likely to increase the resistance of the mask and to severely interfere with the physiological adjustment. Alternatively, open-flow systems can be used but they do not give any information on the ventilation.

One of the biggest concerns of these methods used in a laboratory is the fact that they do not reflect the exercise performed in field conditions. Some portable systems, available for the human athlete, have been adapted for horses. However, because of the horse's high level of ventilation with high peak airflows and respiratory frequency, these systems are technically difficult to adapt and can be unreliable in extreme exercise conditions (Fig. 27.15).[90,94]

Response of the respiratory function to training

Training rapidly and significantly improves maximal oxygen consumption.[26,92] The cardiovascular mechanisms underlying the improvement in O_2 uptake with training have been thoroughly studied, but the accompanying ventilatory changes have been less investigated. However, some information is now available.

The increase in VO_{2max} related to training, and the consequent improvement of performance, i.e. speed or resistance, is not accompanied by an improvement of the exercise-induced alterations in blood gas tensions during maximal exercise[46,49] and, on the contrary, hypoxemia and hypercapnia are more pronounced after a training period.[84,95] A possible explanation of this observation is that training induces a substantial increase in stroke volume and cardiac output, and probably reduces the pulmonary capillary transit time, hence worsening the degree of exercise-induced arterial hypoxemia. Moreover, because aerobic capacity of the muscles is improved, their oxygen consumption and carbon dioxide production are increased with, as a consequence, a worsening of the blood gases relative to the pre-training values.

The marked increase in the O_2 uptake induced by training is not accompanied by an equivalent increase in the expired minute volume. In Thoroughbred horses, the ventilatory rate during a maximal exercise test up to fatigue remains unchanged after a period of training (Fig. 27.16).[26,92,95] This leads to a significant decrease of the ventilatory equivalent for O_2 (minute volume to O_2 uptake ratio), occurring even in the early stages of training.[26] In equine athletes, the decrease in the ventilatory equivalent for O_2 after training is associated with an improvement in the alveolar O_2 extraction. However, in contrast to humans, the reason for this improvement is not a change in the pattern of breathing but more probably an increase in the affinity of hemoglobin for O_2.

The lack of ventilatory improvement with training suggests that pulmonary function could be a limiting factor to performance in the well-trained horse (Fig. 27.16).

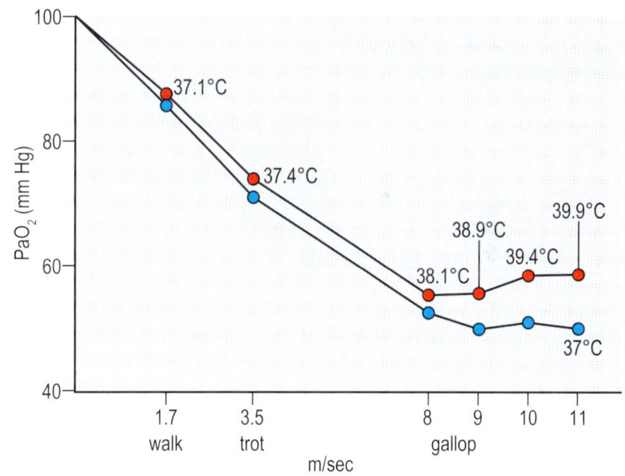

Fig 27.14 Curve of the changes in partial pressure of arterial oxygen during an exercise of increasing intensity, showing the importance of correcting the data for blood temperature, especially at high exercise intensity, in order to avoid underestimation of the results. Blue circles: data without temperature correction (37°C).

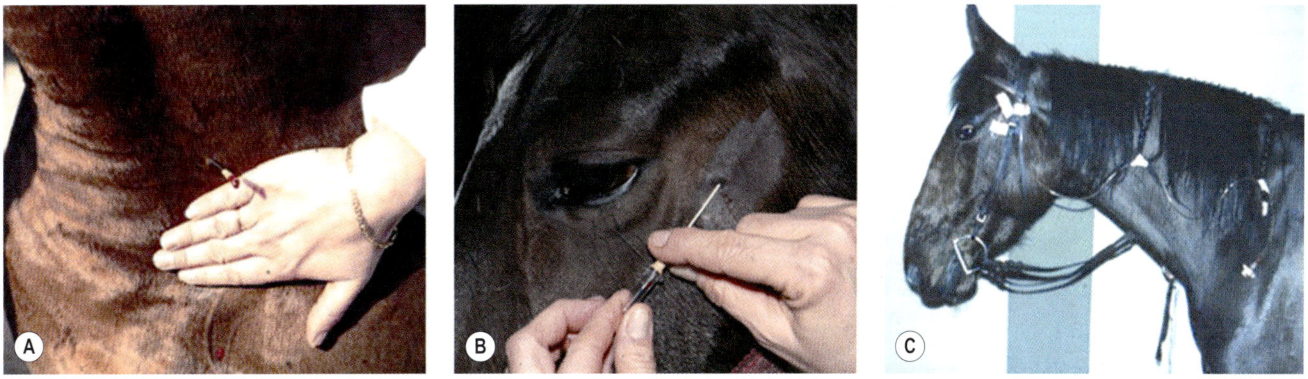

Fig 27.13 Arterial blood can be sampled at rest by puncture of the carotid artery **(A)**. The sampling during exercise necessitates the catheterization of a superficial artery (often the facial artery) (**B** and **C**). Moreover, the arterial blood temperature must be simultaneously measured for data correction.

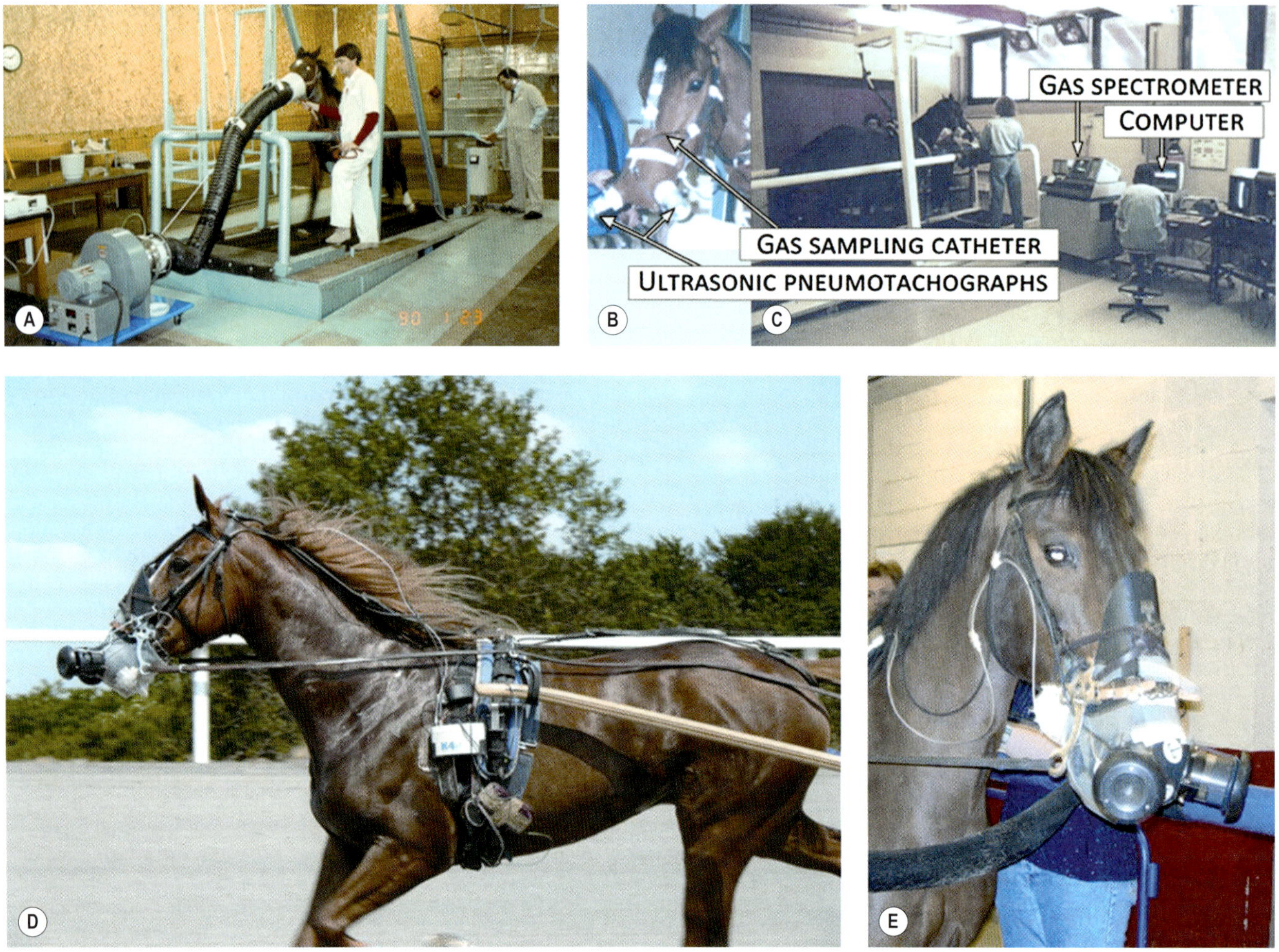

Fig 27.15 Different methods used to measure VO_2 during exercise in horses. Top left: open-flow system; top right: ultrasonic pneumotachographs and gas spectrometer, with the advantage of giving breath-by-breath data; bottom: portable system.

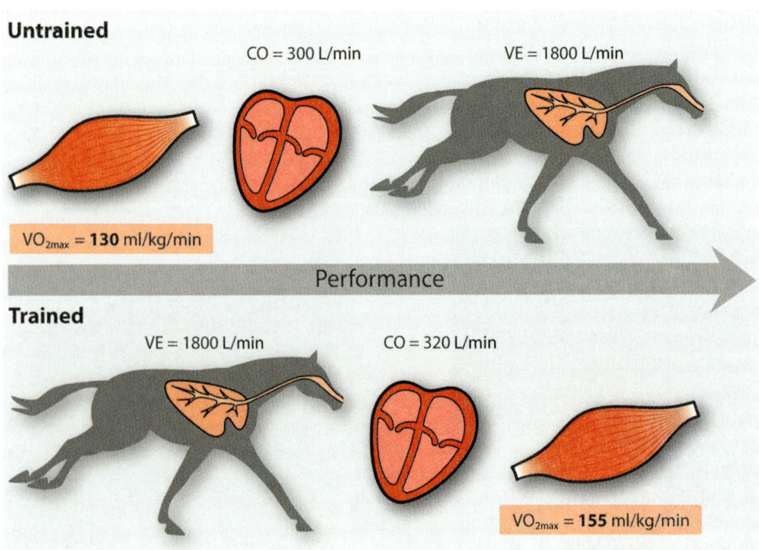

Fig 27.16 Training improves the different steps and systems of the oxygen line, but not the pulmonary function. The latter is redundant in the untrained horse, but becomes the limiting factor of performance in the trained horse.

After a 3 week period of detraining, most of the training-modified ventilatory parameters, i.e. O_2 uptake and ventilatory equivalent for O_2 during a standardized exercise, return to their pre-training level.[26] This indicates that, while the metabolic adaptations occur rapidly when the intensity of training is sufficient, they are nevertheless transient and highly reversible.

Conclusion

The lack of training-induced improvement of the pulmonary function, combined with the high frequency of respiratory problems in athletic horses, means that the respiratory system is the major system limiting performance in sound horses. This explains why the respiratory problems are the second leading cause of retirement of sports and racehorses, and highlight the fact that special attention should be paid to this system when examining horses suffering from exercise intolerance.

With thanks to Dorothy M. Ainsworth, who created the original chapter in the first edition.

References

1. Bayly WM, Grant BD, Breeze RG. The effects of maximal exercise on acid-base balance and arterial blood gas tension in thoroughbred horses. In: Snow DH, Persson SGB, Rose RJ, editors. Equine exercise physiology. Cambridge: Granta Editions; 1983. p. 400–7.
2. van Erck E, Jakesova V, Lekeux P, et al. Field evaluation of poor performance in Standardbred trotters. Pferdeheilkunde 2006;5:625–31.
3. Richard E, Fortier G, Pitel PH, et al. Subclinical diseases affecting performance in Standardbred trotters: diagnostic methods and predictive parameters. Vet J 2010;184(3):282–9.
4. Fraipont A, van Erck E, Ramery E, et al. Subclinical diseases underlying poor performance in endurance horses: diagnostic methods and predictive tests. Vet Rec 2011;169(6):154.
5. Pirie M, Pirie HM, Cranston S, et al. An ultrastructural study of the equine lower respiratory tract. Equine Vet J 1990;22:338–42.
6. Robinson NE, Sorenson PR. Collateral flow resistance and time constant in dog and horse lungs. J Appl Physiol 1978;44:63–8.
7. Mead J, Takishima T, Leith D. Stress distribution in lungs: a model of pulmonary elasticity. J Appl Physiol 1970;28:596–608.
8. Robinson NE. Functional abnormalities caused by upper airway obstruction and heaves: their relationship to the etiology of epistaxis. Vet Clin North Am: Large Anim Practice 1979;1:17–34.
9. Fishman AP. Pulmonary circulation. In: Fishman AP, editor. Handbook Of physiology, Section 3, The respiratory system, vol 1. Bethesda: Circulation and non respiratory functions, American Physiological Society, MD; 1985. p. 93–166.
10. Amis TC, Pascoe JR, Hornof W. Topographic distribution of pulmonary ventilation and perfusion in the horse. Am J Vet Res 1984;45:1597–601.
11. Hlastala MP, Bernard SL, Erickson HH, et al. Pulmonary blood flow distribution in standing horses is not dominated by gravity. J Appl Physiol 1996;81:1051–61.
12. Bernard SL, Glenny RW, Erickson HH, et al. Minimal redistribution of pulmonary blood flow with exercise in racehorses. J Appl Physiol 1996;81:1062–70.
13. Manohar M, Duren SE, Sikkes B, et al. Bronchial circulation during prolonged exercise in ponies. Am J Vet Res 1992;53:925–9.
14. O'Callaghan MW, Pascoe JR, Tyler WS, et al. Exercise-induced pulmonary haemorrhage in the horse: results of a detailed clinical, post mortem and imaging study. IV. Changes in the bronchial circulation demonstrated by C.T. scanning and microradiography. Equine Vet J 1987;19:405–10.
15. McLaughlin RF Jr. Bronchial artery distribution in various mammals and in humans. Am Rev Respir Dis 1983;128:S57–8.
16. Hall LW, Aziz HA, Groenendyk J, et al. Electromyography of some respiratory muscles in the horse. Res Vet Sci 1991;50:328–33.
17. Manohar M. Respiratory muscle perfusion during strenuous exercise. In: Persson SGB, Lindholm A, Jeffcott LB, editors. Equine exercise physiology 3. Davis, California: ICEEP Publications; 1991. p. 1–8.
18. Koterba AM, Kosch PC, Beech J, et al. Breathing strategy of the adult horse (*Equus caballus*) at rest. J Appl Physiol 1988;64:337–46.
19. Ainsworth DM, Eicker SW, Nalevanko ME, et al. The effect of exercise on diaphragmatic activation in horses. Respir Physiol 1996;106:35–46.
20. Manohar M. Inspiratory and expiratory muscle perfusion in maximally exercised ponies. J Appl Physiol 1990;68:544–8.
21. Marlin DJ, Schrotert RC, Cashman PM, et al. Movements of thoracic and abdominal compartments during ventilation at rest and during exercise. Equine Vet J Suppl 2002;34:384–90.
22. Young IS, Alexander R, Woakes AJ, et al. The synchronization of ventilation and locomotion in horses (*Equus caballus*). J Exp Biol 1992;166:19–31.
23. Bowers J, Slocombe RF, Sides RH, et al. Interaction of saddle girth construction and tension on respiratory mechanics and gas exchange during supramaximal treadmill exercise in horses. Aust Vet J 2005;83(1–2):62–7.
24. Bayly WM, Slocombe RF, Schott HC 2nd, et al. Effects of inhalation of albuterol sulphate, ipratropium bromide and frusemide on breathing mechanics and gas exchange in healthy exercising horses. Equine Vet J 2001;33:302–10.
25. Art T, Anderson L, Woakes AJ, et al. Mechanics of breathing during strenuous exercise in thoroughbred horses. Respir Physiol 1990;82:279–94.
26. Art T, Lekeux P. Training-induced modifications in cardiorespiratory and ventilatory measurements in thoroughbred horses. Equine Vet J 1993;25:532–6.
27. Attenburrow DP. Respiration and locomotion. In: Snow DH, Persson SGB, Rose RJ, editors. Equine exercise physiology. Cambridge: Granta Editions; 1983. p. 17–22.
28. Art T, Desmecht D, Amory H, et al. Synchronization of locomotion and respiration in trotting ponies. J Vet Med A 1990;37:95–103.
29. Bramble DM, Carrier DR. Running and breathing in mammals. Science 1983;219:251–6.
30. Bayly WM, Schulz DA, Hodgson DR, et al. Ventilatory response to exercise in horses with exercise-induced hypoxemia. In: Gillespie JR, Robinson NE, editors. Equine exercise physiology 2. Davis, California: ICEEP Publications; 1987. p. 172–82.
31. Art T, Lekeux P. Ventilatory and arterial blood gas tension adjustments to strenuous exercise in Standardbreds. Am J Vet Res 1995;56:1332–7.
32. Nyman G, Björk M, Funkquist P, et al. Ventilation-perfusion relationships during graded exercise in the Standardbred trotter. Equine Vet J Suppl 1995;18:63–9.
33. Padilla DJ, McDonough P, Kindig CA, et al. Ventilatory dynamics and control of blood gases after maximal exercise in the thoroughbred horse. J Appl Physiol 2004;96:2187–93.

34. Jolly S, Art T, Lekeux P. Transient respiration locomotion decoupling in galloping Thoroughbreds. Equine Vet J 1995;(Suppl. 18):S13–17.
35. Curtis RA, Kusano K, Evans DL. Observations on respiratory flow strategies during and after intense treadmill exercise to fatigue in Thoroughbred racehorses. Equine Vet J Suppl 2006;36:567–72.
36. Gillespie JR, Landgren GL, Leith DE. 1:2 ratio of breathing to stride frequencies in a galloping horse breathing 6% CO_2. In: Persson SGB, Lindholm A, Jeffcott LB, editors. Equine exercise physiology 3. Davis, California: ICEEP Publications; 1991. p. 66–70.
37. Art T, Lekeux P. Respiratory airflow patterns in ponies at rest and during exercise. Can J Vet Res 1988;52:299–303.
38. Gallivan GJ, McDonell WN, Forrest JB. Comparative ventilation and gas exchange in the horse and the cow. Res Vet Sci 1989;46:331–6.
39. Pelletier N, Blais D, Vrins A, et al Effect of sub-maximal exercise and training on dead space ventilation in the horse. In: Gillespie JR, Robinson NE, editors. Equine exercise physiology 2. Davis, California: ICEEP Publications; 1987. p. 225–34.
40. Rose RJ, Evans DL. Cardiovascular and respiratory function in the athletic horse. In: Gillespie JR, Robinson NE, editors. Equine exercise physiology 2. Davis, California: ICEEP Publications; 1987. p. 1–2.
41. Hopkins SR, Bayly WM, Slocombe RF, et al. Effect of prolonged heavy exercise on pulmonary gas exchange in horses. J Appl Physiol 1998;84:1723–30.
42. Derksen FJ, Robinson NE. Esophageal and intrapleural pressures in the healthy conscious pony. Am J Vet Res 1980;41:1756–61.
43. Erickson HH, Bernard SL, Glenny RW, et al. Effect of furosemide on pulmonary blood flow distribution in resting and exercising horses. J Appl Physiol 1999;86:2034–43.
44. Harmegnies NF, Duvivier DH, Vandenput SN, et al. Exercise-induced pulmonary perfusion redistribution in horses. Equine Vet J suppl 2002;34:478–84.
45. Benamou AE, Marlin DJ, Callingham BC, et al. Spasmogenic action of endothelin-1 on isolated equine pulmonary artery and bronchus. Equine Vet J 2003;35:190–6.
46. Thornton JR, Essén-Gustavsson B, Lindholm A. Effects of training and detraining on oxygen uptake, cardiac output, blood gas tensions, pH and lactate concentrations during and after exercise in the horse. In: Snow DH, Persson SGB, Rose RJ, editors. Equine exercise physiology. Cambridge: Granta Editions; 1983. p. 470–86.
47. Wagner PD, Gillespie JR, Landgren GL, et al. Mechanism of exercise-induced hypoxemia in horses. J Appl Physiol 1989;66:1227–33.
48. Erickson BK, Erickson HH, Coffman JR. Pulmonary artery, aortic and oesophageal pressure changes during high intensity treadmill exercise in the horse: a possible relation to exercise-induced pulmonary haemorrhage. Equine Vet J Suppl 1990;9:47–52.
49. Manohar M. Pulmonary artery wedge pressure increases with high-intensity exercise in horses. Am J Vet Res 1993;54:142–6.
50. Manohar M, Goetz TE. Pulmonary vascular pressures of exercising Thoroughbred horses with and without endoscopic evidence of EIPH. J Appl Physiol 1996;81:1589–93.
51. Langsetmo I, Meyer MR, Erickson HH. Relationship of pulmonary arterial pressure to pulmonary haemorrhage in exercising horses. Equine Vet J 2000;32:379–84.
52. Sinha AK, Gleed RD, Hakim TS, et al. Pulmonary capillary pressure during exercise in horses. J Appl Physiol 1996;80:1792–8.
53. Manohar M, Goetz TE. Pulmonary vascular resistance of horses decreases with moderate exercise and remains unchanged as workload is increased to maximal exercise. Equine Vet J 1999;30(Suppl):S117–21.
54. Wilkins PA, Gleed RD, Krivitski NM, et al. Extravascular lung water in the exercising horse. J Appl Physiol 2001;91:2442–50.
55. Fedde MR, Wood SC. Rheological characteristics of horse blood: significance during exercise. Respir Physiol 1993;94:323–5.
56. Taylor AE, Rehder K, Hyatt RE, et al. Clinical respiratory physiology. Philadelphia: WB Saunders Company; 1989.
57. Davis JL, Manohar M. Effect of splenectomy on exercise-induced pulmonary and systemic hypertension in ponies. Am J Vet Res 1988;49:1169–72.
58. Schaffartzik W, Poole DC, Derion T, et al. VA/Q distribution during heavy exercise and recovery in humans: implications for pulmonary edema. J Appl Physiol 1992;72:1657–67.
59. Vengust M, Staempfli H, Viel L, et al. Transvascular fluid flux from the pulmonary vasculature at rest and during exercise in horses. J Physiol 2006; 570:397–405.
60. Hedenstierna G, Nyman G, Kvart C, et al. Ventilation-perfusion relationships in the standing horse: an inert gas elimination study. Equine Vet J 1987;19:514–9.
61. Votion D, Vandenput S, Duvivier H, et al. Analysis of equine scintigraphical lung images. Vet J 1997;153:49–61.
62. Seaman J, Erickson BK, Kubo K, et al. Exercise induced ventilation/perfusion inequality in the horse. Equine Vet J 1995;27:104–9.
63. Bayly WM, Hodgson DR, Schulz DA, et al. Exercise-induced hypercapnia in the horse. J Appl Physiol 1989;67: 1958–66.
64. Parks CM, Manohar M. Blood-gas tensions and acid-base status in ponies during treadmill exercise. Am J Vet Res 1984;45:15–19.
65. Erickson BK, Seaman J, Kubo K, et al. Mechanism of reduction in alveolar-arterial PO_2 difference by helium breathing in the exercising horse. J Appl Physiol 1994;76:2794–801.
66. Fenger CK, McKeever KH, Hinchcliff KW, et al. Determinants of oxygen delivery and hemoglobin saturation during incremental exercise in horses. Am J Vet Res 2000;61:1325–32.
67. Persson SGB. On blood volume and working capacity in horses. Acta Vet Scand 1967;19:9–189.
68. Boucher JH, Ferguson EW, Wilhelmsem CL, et al. Erythrocyte alterations during endurance exercise in horses. J Appl Physiol 1981;51:131–4.
69. Wasserman K, Whipp BJ. Exercise physiology in health and disease. Am Rev Respir Dis 1975;122:219–49.
70. Art T, Lekeux P, Gustin P, et al. Inertance of the respiratory system in ponies. J Appl Physiol 1989;67:534–40.
71. Art T, Desmecht D, Amory H, et al. Heliox-induced changes in the breathing mechanics of ponies during exercise. In: Persson SGB, Lindholm A, Jeffcott LB, editors. Equine exercise physiology 3. Davis, California: ICEEP Publications; 1991. p. 47–53.
72. Art T, Serteyn D, Lekeux P. Effect of exercise on the partitioning of equine respiratory resistance. Equine Vet J 1988;20:268–73.
73. Art T, Lekeux P. Mechanical properties of the isolated equine trachea. Res Vet Sci 1991;51:55–60.
74. Rehder RS, Ducharme NG, Hackett RP, et al. Measurement of upper airway pressures in exercising horses with dorsal displacement of the soft palate. Am J Vet Res 1995;56:269–74.
75. Art T, Duvivier DH, Votion D, et al. Does an acute COPD crisis modify the cardiorespiratory and ventilatory adjustments to exercise in horses? J Appl Physiol 1998;84:845–52.
76. Bayly WM, Slocombe RF. Airflow mechanics in models of equine obstructive airway disease under conditions simulating exercise. Res Vet Sci 1997;62:205–11.
77. Art T, Lekeux P. Work of breathing in exercising ponies. Res Vet Sci 1989;46:49–53.
78. Bye PTP, Farkas GA, Roussos C. Respiratory factors limiting exercise. Annu Rev Physiol 1983;45:439–51.

79. Ainsworth DM, Ducharme NG, Hackett RP, et al. Regulation of respiratory muscle activities during chemoreceptor stimulation in the adult horse (*Equus caballus*). Am J Vet Res 1995;56:366 73.

80. Forster HV, Pan LG. Exercise hyperpnea. Ist characteristics and control. In: Crystal RG, West JB, editors. The lung: scientific foundations, vol. 2. New York: Raven Press; 1991. p. 1553–64.

81. Wasserman K, Whipp BJ, Casaburi R. Respiratory control during exercise. In: Fishman AP, editors. Handbook of physiology, Section 3, The respiratory system, vol. 2. part 2, Control of breathing. Bethesda, MD: American Physiological Society; 1986. p. 595–619.

82. Landgren GL, Gillespie JR, Leith DE. No ventilatory response to CO_2 in thoroughbreds galloping at 14 $m.s^{-1}$. In: Persson SGB, Lindholm A, Jeffcott LB, editors. Equine exercise physiology 3. Davis, California: ICEEP Publications; 1991. p. 59–65.

83. Roussos C, Macklem PT. Inspiratory muscle fatigue. In: Fishman AP, Fisher AB, editors. Handbook of physiology, Section 3. The respiratory system, vol. 3, part 2, Mechanics of breathing. Bethesda, MD: American Physiological Society; 1986. p. 511–27.

84. Art T, Lekeux P. Booster vaccination in thoroughbred horses with oily adjuvanted inactived vaccine against influenza and rhinopneumonia. Effect on cardio-respiratory and metabolic adjustments to strenuous exercise and intense training. J Vet Med A 1993;40:481–91.

85. Hodgson DR, Rose RJ, Kelso TB, et al. Respiratory and metabolic responses in the horse during moderate and heavy exercise. Pflügers Arch 1990;417:73–8.

86. Scharf SM, Bark H, Heimer D, et al. 'Second wind' during inspiratory loading. Med Sci Sports Exerc 1984;16:87–91.

87. Fu X, Costello ML, Tsukimoto K, et al. High lung volume increases stress failure in pulmonary capillaries. J Appl Physiol 1992;73:123–33.

88. Bayly WM, Schulz DA, Hodgson DR, et al. Ventilatory responses of the horse to exercise: effect of gas collection systems. J Appl Physiol 1987;63:1210–17.

89. Holcombe SJ, Beard WL Hinchcliff KW. Effect of mask and pneumotachograph on tracheal and nasopharyngeal pressures, respiratory frequency and ventilation in horses. Am J Vet Res 1996;57:250–3.

90. Art T, Duvivier DH, van Erck E. Validation of a portable equine metabolic measurement system. Equine Vet J suppl 2006;36:557–61.

91. van Erck E, Votion D, Art T. Qualitative and quantitative evaluation of equine respiratory mechanics by impulse oscillometry. Equine Vet J 2006;38:52–8.

92. Christley RM, Hodgson DR, Evans DL Rose RJ. Effects of training on the development of exercise-induced arterial hypoxemia in horse. Am J Vet Res 1997;58:653–7.

93. Sanchez A, Couëtil LL, Ward MP, et al. Effect of airway disease on blood gas exchange in racehorses. J Vet Intern Med 2005;19:87–92.

94. Ramseyer A, Sides R, Slinker B, et al. Evaluation of a mask for breath-by-breath respirometry during exercise in horses. Equine Vet J Suppl 2010;42:240–5.

95. Roberts CA, Marlin DJ, Lekeux P. The effects of training on ventilation and blood gases in exercising thoroughbreds. Equine Vet J Suppl 1999;30:57–61.

Inflammatory diseases of the lower airway of athletic horses

28

Laurent L. Couetil

CHAPTER CONTENTS

Introduction

Respiratory and musculoskeletal diseases are the two most common causes of training interruption and poor performance in athletic horses.[1-5] Inflammatory airway disease (IAD) is a chronic respiratory syndrome affecting horses of any age, gender or breed that is characterized clinically by excess tracheobronchial mucus, cough and decreased performance.[13] The negative impact of IAD on performance has been documented both in racehorses and sport horses.[2,6-8] The prevalence of IAD as determined by excess tracheal mucus is high both in racehorses (13–22%),[7,9,10] sports horses (31%)[8] and pleasure horses (20%).[11] Recurrent airway obstruction (RAO) or heaves is another common chronic respiratory disease presenting similarities with IAD. But heaves only affects mature-to-older horses and is characterized by more severe clinical signs and exercise intolerance that may abate at times; nonetheless, horses are affected for life.

Inflammatory airway disease (IAD, small airway disease, small airway inflammatory disease, lower airway disease, bronchiolitis)

- IAD is associated with poor performance, cough and increased respiratory secretions.
- Young athletic horses are commonly affected with IAD.
- Airway endoscopy, bronchoalveolar lavage fluid cytology and exercise testing are valuable diagnostic tools for IAD.
- Horses with IAD exhibit various degrees of airflow obstruction and airway hyperresponsiveness.
- Etiology of IAD appears to be multifactorial, with environmental dusts playing an important role.
- Therapy is aimed at decreasing environmental dusts and controlling airway inflammation.
- Aerosol therapy with corticosteroids and bronchodilators is effective

Recognition

History and presenting complaint

Inflammatory airway disease (IAD) is a respiratory syndrome characterized by mild lower airway inflammation and excess mucus that is commonly encountered in young athletic horses and recognized as a separate entity from recurrent airway obstruction (RAO).[12,13] In the majority of cases, RAO and IAD may be differentiated based on clinical grounds (Table 28.1). It is likely that both conditions represent a continuum of respiratory diseases where mild-to-moderate airway inflammation is represented by horses with IAD and where some horses might progress to severe inflammation and develop RAO. However, there is currently no evidence suggesting which IAD phenotype or risk factors predispose a horse with IAD to develop RAO. In addition, the majority of horses with IAD recover fully after proper therapy. It is also worth noting that IAD is common worldwide, whereas RAO is virtually absent in countries like Australia and South Africa despite reports of high prevalence of IAD.

Horses with IAD typically have a history of cough, increased respiratory secretions and decreased performance or delayed recovery after exercise.[14-16] Foals and older horses can also suffer from IAD.[17-19] In these cases, the diagnosis is often reached by ruling out infectious causes and other non-infectious respiratory diseases, such as RAO. The possibility of IAD should be considered in horses with cough and tracheobronchial mucopurulent exudate that do not respond, or relapse, after antimicrobial therapy. In such cases, further diagnostic tests should be pursued, in particular bronchoalveolar lavage.

Table 28.1 Comparison between recurrent airway obstruction (RAO) and inflammatory airway disease (IAD) in horses

		RAO	IAD
Signalment	Age	>6 years	>1 year
	Activity level	+/++	++/+++
Clinical signs	Duration	Months to years Recurrent	1–6 months Not recurrent
	Cough	Chronic intermittent	38% of cases
	Exudate in airways	Mucopurulent (++/+++)	Mucoid to mucopurulent (+/++)
	Lung sounds	Breath sounds (++/+++), wheezes, crackles	Normal
	Increased respiratory efforts	++/+++	0/++
	Exercise intolerance	++/+++	+/++
Etiology		Allergy to molds	Multifactorial
Pathophysiology	Lower airway obstruction	++/+++	0/+
	BALF cytology	Neutrophilia (>25%)	Neutrophilia (5–20%) Eosinophilia (>1%) Mastocytosis (>2%)
	Airway hyperresponsiveness	+/+++	+/+++
Histopathology	Bronchiolitis	++/+++	+/++

Low/mild: +, medium/moderate: ++; high/severe: +++.

Duration of clinical signs of IAD is seven to nine weeks on average with a range between 4 and 22 weeks, which is longer than most infectious respiratory diseases.[15,20,21] In a study involving 170 Thoroughbred horses in training over a two-year period, it was estimated that horses had some degree of IAD during a third of their time spent in training and each affected horse had an average of two episodes of IAD during the study.[15] IAD is more common in yearlings and two-year-old racehorses with the incidence and prevalence decreasing significantly between the ages of two to four years.[21–23] Horses of any breed can be affected including Quarter Horse, Warmblood, Appaloosa, Thoroughbred cross and American Saddlebred.[9,15,16,18,24,25]

The most common complaints reported by owners of athletic horses, other than racehorses, with IAD are chronic cough, exercise intolerance, poor willingness to perform and prolonged recovery after exercise.[8,16] These horses can be involved in a variety of activities such as barrel racing, show-jumping, three-day event, dressage, or pleasure riding. In some cases, owners report a history of respiratory disease affecting several horses in the barn and all horses recovered except for the one with IAD, which continues to cough intermittently.

There is a strong association between poor performance and IAD, as defined by increased amount of tracheal mucus, both in racehorses and sports horses.[7–9] Detection of more than a few blobs of mucus in the trachea after a race is associated with poor performance in both Standardbreds and Thoroughbreds. More pronounced accumulation of mucus that forms a continuous stream in the trachea has been associated with poor performance in horses competing in dressage and show-jumping.

Physical examination

The most common clinical signs associated with IAD are increased respiratory secretions, cough, and decreased performance.[8,11,14,21,26] Pharyngeal lymphoid hyperplasia is positively correlated with tracheal mucus accumulation in racehorses but not in performance or pleasure horses.[7,8,11] This difference is likely due to the fact that racehorses tend to be younger and pharyngeal lymphoid hyperplasia is most pronounced yearlings and two-year-old horses and then it decreases rapidly with increasing age. Estimation of the quantity of mucus present in the trachea by endoscopy reveals that horses free of respiratory disease have either no mucus or a few isolated flecks and horses with IAD have large blobs of mucus up to a continuous stream of variable width (score 0 or 1, Fig. 28.1).[8,19,23] The prevalence of tracheal exudate increases after strenuous exercise[27] although this finding is not consistent.[28] The amount of tracheal mucus in performance and pleasure horses can be positively, but weakly, correlated with age or not associated with age.[19,29]

Cough is only present in 38 % of horses with IAD; however, 85% of coughing horses have IAD.[15,30] Daily observation of racehorses in training showed that coughing is not noted 62% of the time during which they have IAD and that there is a strong associations between coughing, the amount of mucus present in the upper airways, and pharyngeal lymphoid hyperplasia.[15,22,30] Also, a strong association exists between coughing, isolation of bacteria, and the degree of inflammation in tracheal wash fluid.[23,30] Nevertheless, bacteriological examination of tracheal wash samples reveals that 35–58% of horses with IAD do not contain significant amounts of bacteria. On the other hand, there is a strong association between presence of cough and BAL neutrophilia.[31]

Other clinical signs of respiratory disease such as nasal discharge and fever do not appear to be associated with IAD,[15,21] although one study found a 4.5-fold increased odds of nasal discharge in horses with IAD.[32] Interestingly, the prevalence of nasal discharge is low in racehorses (4% of cases), except in yearlings (>30%).[21] Thoracic auscultation is usually normal; however, some horses with IAD can exhibit increased breath sounds or wheezes. Horses with severe IAD might have a slightly increased respiratory rate and abdominal contraction on expiration. For the most part, IAD is subclinical and can be undetected unless coughing is present or tracheal exudate is detected by endoscopy.[18]

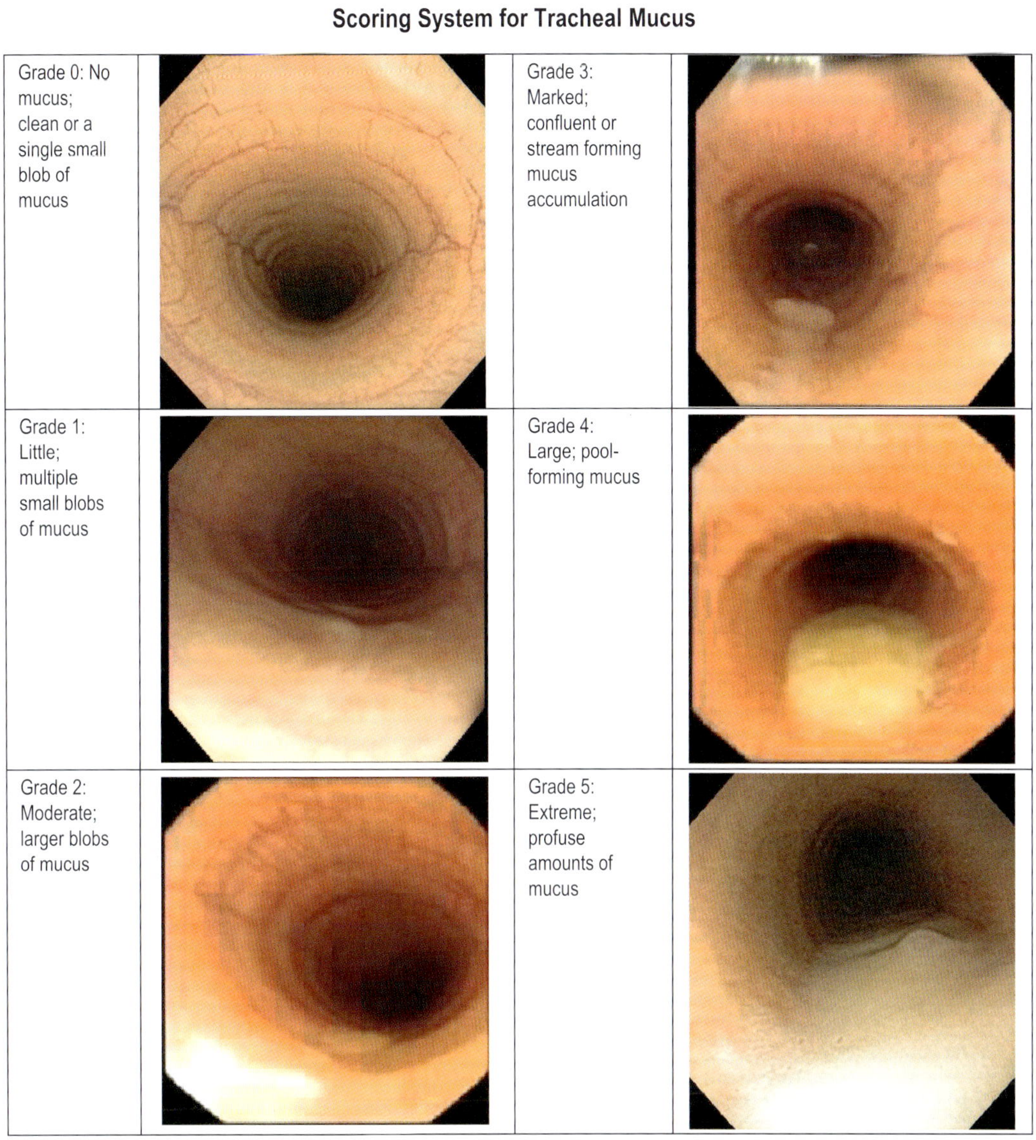

Fig 28.1 Increased mucopurulent secretions visualized by endoscopy of the trachea in a horse with inflammatory airway disease.
Modified from Gerber V, Straub R, Marti E et al. Endoscopic scoring of mucus quantity and quality: observer and horse variance and relationship to inflammation, mucus viscoelasticity and volume, Equine Vet J *2004,36: 576–582 with permission from the* Equine Veterinary Journal.

Special examination

Endoscopic examination of the respiratory tract is a simple, well tolerated by most horses and a valuable diagnostic tool for IAD. Horses with normal respiratory tract have at most a few flecks of mucus visible in the trachea by endoscopy.[29,33] Increased mucopurulent exudate in the tracheobronchial tree is detected in the majority of horses with IAD but tracheal exudate is non-specific and is also present in the majority of pulmonary diseases other than IAD.[33] A semi-quantitative mucus scoring system using a scale between 0 and 5 has been developed and validated for use in the horse (Fig. 28.1).[19,34] This scale is useful to grade severity of IAD since a positive association has been found between tracheal mucus score, BAL neutrophilia and poor performance.[8,19,35] Tracheal septum thickness increases with age but is not greater in IAD as compared to healthy horses.[19,36]

Cytologic examination of respiratory secretions collected from the tracheobronchial tree is important when trying to confirm a diagnosis of pulmonary disease. Tracheal secretions can be collected by direct aspiration or wash of tracheal lumen via transcutaneous catheterization or through an endoscope.[37-39] Normal tracheal fluid cytology usually contains neutrophils representing less than 20% of total nucleated cells.[40,41] Several studies have shown an association between tracheal neutrophilia (>20%), coughing and IAD.[21,30,42,43] A relationship between tracheal mucus accumulation and neutrophilia was found by some investigators but not by others.[43,44] However, cytological examination of tracheal mucus in horses free of respiratory disease is highly variable, with neutrophil percentages ranging between 3 and 83% of total nucleated cells[45,46] and it correlates poorly with pulmonary histopathology.[45,47] Furthermore, mucus score but, not the proportion of neutrophils in tracheal wash, correlates with performance in racehorses as well as in sports horses.[8,35] Therefore, the preponderance of evidence suggests that neutrophil accumulation in tracheal lumen represents a physiological response to contamination of the respiratory tract by inhaled particulates or bacteria in otherwise healthy horses. In some cases, contamination can overwhelm local defense mechanisms (mucociliary clearance, immune response) and result in clinical signs such as cough and excess mucus accumulation.

In contrast, neutrophils represent a small proportion of total nucleated cells present in BAL fluid with most studies reporting neutrophils as <5% of cells in healthy horses (Table 28.2). Furthermore, BAL cytology reportedly correlates well with histopathology of the lungs[48] and does not correlate with tracheal wash cytology.[46,49] A BAL can be easily performed in field conditions using either a flexible endoscope (≥2 meters long) or an equine BAL catheter at least 2.5 meters long and 10 mm diameter with inflatable cuff at the end (Bivona, Gary, IN; Cook, Bloomington; IN, Jorgensen Laboratories, Loveland, CO). The technique has been described in detail previously.[50,51] It is important to always use the same technique during a BAL because the volume of fluid used as well as the number of boluses administered have a significant effect on cell count and differential (see Table 28.2). Fluid samples should be processed within 1–2 hours or stored at 4 °C if sample shipping to the laboratory is to be delayed. Normal BAL fluid should appear slightly turbid with a layer of white foam on the surface (surfactant). Between 50 and 90% of the volume infused is expected to be retrieved.

Measurement of lung function can be done in a variety of ways including assessment of gas exchanges, determination of lung volumes (spirometry), and evaluation of the movement of air in and out the respiratory tract (lung mechanics). Racehorses with IAD exhibit more pronounced exercise-induced hypoxemia than healthy controls during standardized run to fatigue on a high-speed treadmill (Fig. 28.2).[52–54] Both groups of horses had comparable $PaCO_2$, suggesting that impaired gas exchanges were likely a result of ventilation–perfusion mismatching and not hypoventilation. Spirometry is useful in severe obstructive diseases such as RAO but not in milder diseases like IAD. On the contrary, lung mechanics allows quantification of the degree of airflow obstruction present in horses' airways. Airflow obstruction is the basic mechanism responsible, at least in part, for some of the manifestation of IAD such as exercise intolerance and cough. The advantage of lung mechanics is quantification of airflow obstruction, which is often subclinical in horses with IAD. Measurement of the degree of airway obstruction allows the clinician to determine the severity of the disease process and provides objective means of assessing response to therapy. The disadvantage is that sophisticated equipment and a sound understanding of respiratory physiology are required. Therefore, tests of lung mechanics are currently used mainly in the research arena and in some referral clinics. However, one commercially available test (Open Pleth™, Ambulatory Monitoring, Inc., Ardsley, NY) allows lung function testing in the field, in particular measurement of airway responsiveness.[55,56]

There are four main methods used in the horse to evaluate lung mechanics:

1. measurement of pleural pressure changes in relation to airflow at the nose during normal (tidal) breathing or 'conventional lung mechanics',
2. measurement of airflow during forceful exhalation or 'forced expiration',
3. evaluation of the pressure–flow relationship while an oscillating source of flow is applied to the respiratory system during tidal breathing ('forced or impulse oscillometry'),
4. measurement of thoracic and abdominal volume changes by plethysmography in relation to airflow at the nose during tidal breathing ('flowmetrics').

Conventional lung mechanics has been the first test of lung mechanics adapted to the horse[57] and is still commonly used in research.[58–60] However, this test has not been used extensively in clinical settings because it does not permit detection of airway obstruction until it is severe and clinical signs are then evident.[18,61] Recently, some researchers showed that the addition of dead space to the respiratory system increases CO_2 rebreathing and ventilation which is accompanied by a significant rise in lung resistance in horses with IAD as compared to healthy controls.[62] Forced expiration (FE) can be performed in standing, sedated horses.[63] As in people, FE is a sensitive test of airflow obstruction where a reduction in forced expiratory flow during late FE (i.e. $FEF_{95\%}$) is an early indicator of mild airway obstruction such as in IAD (Fig. 28.3).[18] Forced or impulse oscillometry techniques have the advantage of being non-invasive and have been used both in research and clinical cases. Horses with IAD often show frequency dependence of resistance with higher values obtained at the lower frequencies (<10 Hz) suggestive of heterogeneous airway obstruction.[64,65] Finally, flowmetrics or inductance plethysmography (Open Pleth™, Ambulatory Monitoring, Inc., Ardsley, NY, Fig. 28.4) is non-invasive, portable in the field and shows satisfactory correlation with standard lung mechanics.[56,66]

Another means of detecting airway obstruction is by testing airway reactivity in response to inhaled irritant such as histamine. Exaggerated airway narrowing in response to an irritant is called airway hyperresponsiveness. Airway reactivity can be quantified using the four tests of lung mechanics described above.[63,66–68] Airway hyperresponsiveness is a prominent feature of IAD in horses with increased BALF eosinophil and mast cell counts.[31,65,68,69] The sensitivity of forced oscillometry and flowmetrics is enhanced when used to detect airway hyperresponsiveness. This increased bronchoconstriction in response to inhaled irritants plays an important role in the pathogenesis of the cough and presumably exercise intolerance.

Laboratory examination

Hematology and serum biochemistry of horses with IAD are usually within normal limits.

Cytologic specimens of BALF are prepared by centrifugation and processed with Wright's stain. Total cell count in healthy horses is usually less than 400 cells/μl (Table 28.2). Differential cell counts should be determined by examination of at least 200 cells per slide and preferably 500 cells. Cytological analysis of BAL fluid allows recognition of 3 main types of inflammatory profiles in IAD (Table 28.2).[50] The most commonly encountered profile is characterized by an increased total nucleated cell count with mild neutrophilia (5–20 % cells), lymphocytosis, and monocytosis (Fig. 28.5A).[14,16,18,31] Two other cytological profiles characterized by increased percentages of mast cells (>2%, Fig. 28.5B) and eosinophils (>1%, Fig. 28.5C) are also observed in some horses with IAD.[31,69,70] Some horses can also present with a combination of BALF abnormalities such as elevated neutrophils and mast cells, mast cells and eosinophils or all three cell types.[71,72] In contrast, BAL of horses with RAO shows moderate-to-severe neutrophilia (>20% cells), lymphopenia, and decreased alveolar macrophages.[18,73,74] Cytology of BALF collected from horses with RAO in clinical remission can be normal if there has been sufficient time free of exposure to inciting allergens.[75] Some RAO cases can be in clinical remission but still exhibit some degree of pulmonary neutrophilia and, therefore, can be difficult to differentiate from IAD. One way to discriminate RAO from

Table 28.2 Bronchoalveolar lavage (BAL) fluid cytology in control horses and in horses with inflammatory airway disease (IAD) and technique used to perform BAL

BAL TECHNIQUE	HORSES' TYPE/ NUMBER	LEUKOCYTES (cells/μL)	ALVEOLAR MACROPH. %	LYMPHOCYTES %	NEUTROPHILS %	EOSINOPHILS %	MAST CELLS %	REFERENCE
Control horses								
5 × 50 mL saline-syringe-endoscope	training (no racing) / 40	133.5 ± 8.2	56.9 ± 1.9	38.2 ± 1.8	4.1 ± 0.5	0.3 ± 0.2	0.4 ± 0.2	Clarck CK, 1995
50 mL saline-pump-endoscope	pasture / 9	782.2 ± 272.0	54.3 ± 16.4	28.8 ± 16.2	14.4 ± 10.1	0.4 ± 1.0	2.0 ± 1.1	Sweeney CR, 1992
300 mL saline-pump-endoscope	pasture / 8	175.9 ± 110.7	49.5 ± 13.0	40.4 ± 14.6	2.5 ± 1.5	0.1 ± 0.4	7.4 ± 2.7	Sweeney CR, 1992
3 × 100 mL saline-pump-endoscope	pasture / 6	378.3 ± 141.3	59.2 ± 7.4	33.0 ± 8.1	1.2 ± 1.2	0.2 ± 0.4	6.5 ± 2.1	Sweeney CR, 1992
4 × 60 mL saline-syringe-tube	racing / 11		65 ± 6.2	28 ± 5.8	7 ± 3.3	0 ± 0	0.2 ± 0.3	Forgarty U, 1991
1 × 250 mL saline-pump-endoscope	racing / 12	530 ± 170	60.1 ± 4.8	36.7 ± 5.4	2.2 ± 1.4	0.03 ± 0.1	0.4 ± 0.4	Hare JE, 1994
300 mL LRS-BAL tube	racing / 6	153.2 ± 17.1	64.8 ± 4.6	28.3 ± 2.9	3.8 ± 0.3	1.2 ± 0.8	0.3 ± 0.3	Rush B, 1995
2 × 250 mL saline-pump-endoscope	racing / 6	360 (260–540)	67.7 (61–78.8)	31.5 (19–35)	0.4 (0.2–1.4)	0.3 (0–1)	1(0–2.8)	Hare JE, 1998
1 × 250 mL saline-pump-endoscope	racing / 10	445 ± 142	68.8 ± 8.8	22.9 ± 7.4	3.8 ± 5.5	2.0 ± 1.0	1.5 ± 0.3	Couëtil L, 1999
1 × 120 ml saline-syringe-BAL tube	racing / 14	517 ± 229	50.2 ± 10.4	26.2 ± 6.5	15.1 ± 2.8	0	2.1 ± 1.4	Courouce-Malblanc A, 2002
1 × 250 mL saline-pump-endoscope	racing / 10	436 (326–536)	65.0 (63.0–76.7)	25.0 (15.0–29.2)	2.0 (1.0–4.0)			Sanchez A, 2005
3 × 83 ml saline-syringe-BAL tube	racing / 20		73.5 (64.0–79.5)	19.0 (13.8–25.3)	5.5 (3.8–7.0)	0.0 (0.0–0.0)	1.0 (0.0–1.0)	Richard EA, 2012
1 × 300 ml saline-syringe-endoscope	Racing/19		63.0 [49-90]	32.0 [6-47]	2.0 [1-4]	0.0 [0-1]	1.0 [0-1]	Nolen-Walston R, 2013

Continued

Table 28.2 Continued

BAL TECHNIQUE	HORSES' TYPE/ NUMBER	LEUKOCYTES (cells/μL)	ALVEOLAR MACROPH. %	LYMPHOCYTES %	NEUTROPHILS %	EOSINOPHILS %	MAST CELLS %	REFERENCE
IAD horses								
4 × 60 mL saline-syringe-tube	racing / 65		54 ± 15.2	23 ± 11.4	13 ± 12*	0.1 ± 0.3	0.3 ± 0.7	Forgarty U, 1991
1 × 250 mL saline-pump-endoscope	racing / 12	590 ± 290	56 ± 13	37 ± 16	4.1 ± 3.5	0.2 ± 0.2	3.1 ± 1.0*	Hare JE, 1994
300 mL LRS-BAL tube	racing / 32	366.0 ± 16.8	48.4 ± 1.9*	36.0 ± 1.9*	10.4 ± 1.1*	3.8 ± 1.5	1.8 ± 1.5	Rush B, 1995
2 × 250 mL saline-pump-endoscope	racing / 5	650 (320–1100)	58.6 (40.6–62.4)	25.8 (22.6–31.4)	0.8 (0–1.8)	11.8 (6.4–26.4)*	1.4(0.4–2.4)	Hare JE, 1998
1 × 250 mL saline-pump-endoscope	racing / 13	582 ± 122	54.8 ± 10.8*	33.6 ± 10.7	12.0 ± 7.7*	0.4 ± 1.4	1.4 ± 0.4	Couëtil L, 1999
1 × 120 ml saline-syringe-BAL tube	racing / 7	729 ± 229*	22.6 ± 9.9*	21.3 ± 6.6	34.0 ± 15.3*	0	2.9 ± 2.7	Courouce-Malblanc, 2002
1 × 250 mL saline-pump-endoscope	racing / 25	491 (394–634)	54.0 (44.0–58.0)*	37.0 (30.8–48.5)*	5.0 (3.0–13.0)			Sanchez A, 2005
3 × 83 ml saline-syringe-BAL tube	racing / 22		57.0 (51.5–66.3)*	20.0 (12.3–29.3)	14.5 (8.0–18.0)*	0.0 (0.0–0.8)	2.0 (1.0–3.0)*	Richard EA, 2012
1 × 300 ml saline-syringe-endoscope	Racing/40		54.5 [18-80]	36.5 [14-67]	2.0 [0-4]	**3.5 [0-12]***	**3.0 [0-10]***	Nolen-Walston R, 2013
1 × 300 ml saline-syringe-endoscope	Racing/17		55.0 [43-80]	36.0 [14-51]	**6 [5-15]***	0.0 [0-0]	1.0 [0-1]	Nolen-Walston R, 2013

Data expressed as mean ± SD or median (1st quartile – 3rd quartile).
*Significantly different from controls ($P < 0.05$).

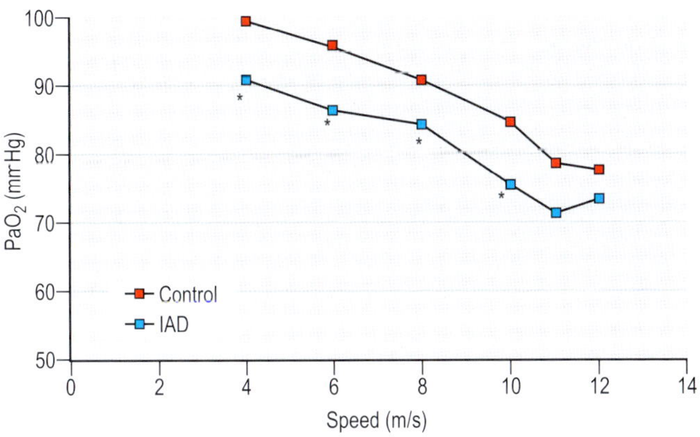

Fig 28.2 Partial pressure of oxygen in arterial blood of racehorses subjected to a standardized treadmill test. *values are significantly different from control horses ($P < 0.05$).

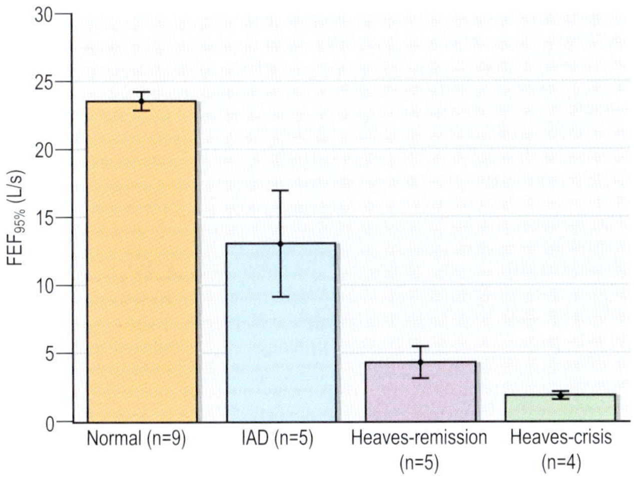

Fig 28.3 Forced expiratory flow at 95% of exhaled vital capacity ($FEF_{95\%}$) measured during forced expiration in healthy horses and horses with inflammatory airway disease, and recurrent airway obstruction during disease remission and exacerbation (crisis).

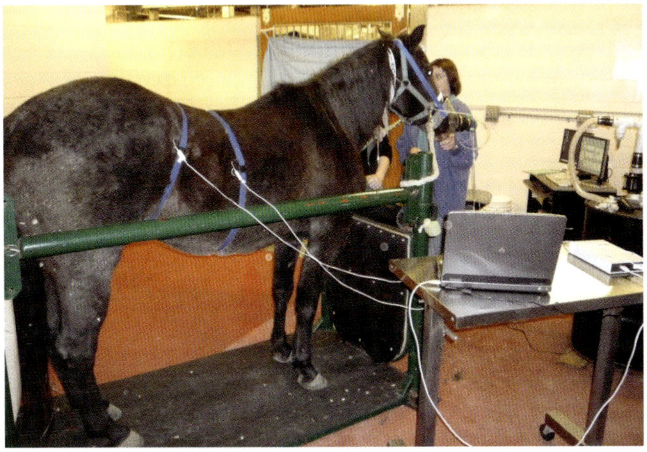

Fig 28.4 Measurement of lung function by inductance plethysmography (Open Pleth™, Ambulatory Monitoring, Inc., Ardsley, NY). Airflow is measured at the nose using a Fleisch pneumotachograph fitted on a facemask. Change in abdominal and thoracic volumes are measured by sinusoid wires placed within elastic bands around the flanks and mid-thorax.

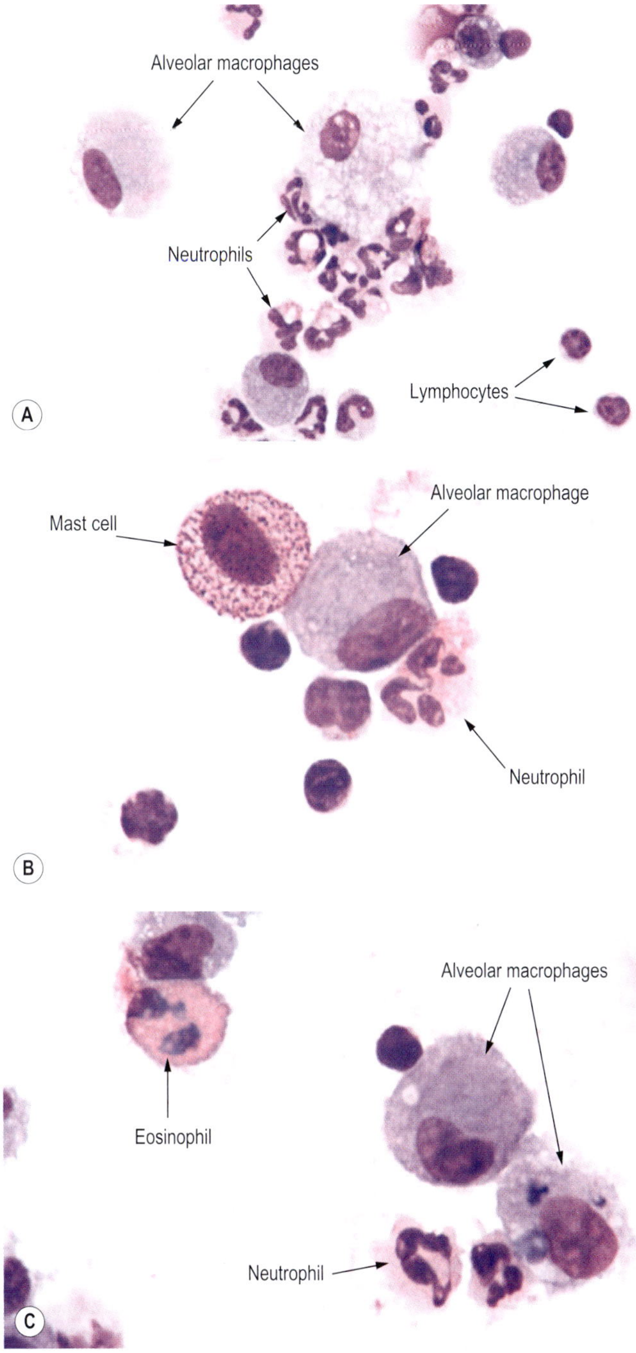

Fig 28.5 Bronchoalveolar lavage fluid cytology in horses with IAD characterized by increased percentage of neutrophils **(A)**, mast cells **(B)**, and eosinophils **(C)**. ×100

IAD is by performing a hay challenge and monitoring clinical signs of respiratory disease, which should develop within a few hours to a few days in RAO-affected horses.[59,76] Horses with IAD exposed to moldy hay exhibit a worsening of coughing and pulmonary neutrophilia; however, they do not develop increased respiratory effort or nostrils flaring like RAO-affected horses do. Although practical, this challenge might not be feasible in client-owned horses and in such situations, pulmonary function testing is indicated.

Tracheal secretions can be collected by direct wash of tracheal lumen with sterile saline via a catheter introduced through the endoscope's working channel or by percutaneous transtracheal aspiration. If microbiologic culture of the fluid is being pursued, tracheal wash (TW) should be performed using a sterile, multiple lumen guarded catheter (double or triple lumen) introduced through the endoscope working channel or via percutaneous catheterization of the trachea in mid-cervical region using a sterile technique. The latter technique requires sedation, whereas the former one can be conducted using only simple restraint such as application of a nose twitch. An abundant commensal flora inhabits nasal passages and nasopharynx (e.g. *Streptococcus zooepidemicus*). Therefore, TW via the instrument channel of the endoscope without a multiple lumen guarded catheter will result in contamination of the sample and will be inappropriate for microbiologic culture and render any such results uninterpretable.[77] Furthermore, coughing during the procedure increases the chances of oropharyngeal contamination of the sample.

A smear of the TW sample should be made as soon as possible after collection. Total nucleated cell count in healthy horses is usually less than 500 cells/μL with few to no red blood cells.[11,78] Differential count should be determined based on 200–300 consecutive cells. Cells in TW are more difficult to identify and count than in BAL because they often are more degenerate and are trapped in abundant mucus strands. Normal TW fluid should contain a majority of macrophages (30–70%), low numbers of epithelial cells (higher if collected with catheter through the endoscope), <20% neutrophils, <10% lymphocytes, <1% eosinophils and very few mast cells (<0.2%).[11,49,77,78] Importantly, several studies have documented the fact that there is no correlation between TW and BAL cytology, indicating that one is not a substitute for the other.[49,79] Tracheal wash is the sample of choice when suspecting an infectious etiology and BAL is preferred otherwise because of the high correlation with lung lesions (as determined by histopathology).

Horses that cough during training more than 4 times in a 10-min period are more likely to have >20% neutrophils in TW, large numbers of bacteria (>10^3 cfu/mL) and intracellular bacteria.[40] The likelihood of isolating bacteria from tracheal wash samples collected from racehorses in training is strongly associated with the TW inflammation and mucus accumulation, in particular in young horses.[15,23,30] But there is no apparent association between TW neutrophilia and mucus in older racehorses.[44] Isolation of more than 10^3 colony-forming units of pathogenic *Streptococcus* spp. is also strongly associated with coughing.[30] Therefore, tracheal inflammation and high bacterial counts are common in racehorses but only excess tracheal mucus is associated with decreased performance, not TW neutrophilia.[7]

Necropsy examination

Histopathological examination of the lungs can be conducted ante-mortem by collecting tissue samples using transcutaneous lung biopsy needles and endobronchial biopsies forceps via the endoscope, or at post-mortem examination. Horses with IAD present similar histopathology findings as horses with RAO but with less severe and chronic changes.[48] Typical morphological findings include peribronchiolitis, bronchiolitis, bronchiolar epithelial hyperplasia, goblet cell metaplasia, luminal mucus, and in some cases alveolitis.[80,81] Severity of histopathologic changes assessed by a scoring system appears to be negatively correlated to various indices of respiratory and cardiovascular function in horses with IAD.[80] Consequently, as pulmonary lesions become more severe, horses become more exercise intolerant. However, histopathology findings obtained from transcutaneous lung biopsies or endobronchial biopsies are highly variable and the potential diagnostic benefit should be weighed against the potential risks associated with transthoracic biopsy such as hemorrhage and pneumothorax.

Diagnostic confirmation

In horses presenting with clinical signs including cough, increased respiratory secretions, and poor performance, detailed history, physical examination, and diagnostic tests should help eliminate differential diagnoses (Fig. 28.5B). Using a validated questionnaire administered to clients is useful to identify horses with heaves;[82] however, the same questionnaire has been unable to differentiate IAD from healthy horses.[16] Horses with IAD are not febrile and presence of a fever suggests infectious respiratory diseases such as viral diseases, bronchopneumonia, pleuropneumonia, or pulmonary abscess. Hematology findings can be helpful to confirm a suspicion of respiratory infection; however, they are often nonspecific. Leukocytosis with neutrophilia is commonly found with bacterial respiratory infections and during the acute phase of a bacterial infection, increased numbers of immature neutrophils ('left shift') may be observed. Neutrophilia can also accompany non-infectious inflammatory diseases (such as caused by toxins), neoplasia, and mycotic and parasitic infections. Hematologic changes during the early phase of a viral respiratory infection, such as influenza, are often characterized by normocytic, normochromic anemia, lymphopenia or lymphocytosis, and sometimes neutropenia.[83,84] Neutrophilia can follow within a week of initial clinical signs, particularly in cases of secondary bacterial infection. Monocytosis can develop during the recovery phase of a viral infection.

Coughing is often chronic, intermittent (>3 weeks) in horses with IAD. Main differential diagnoses are mild cases of heaves (RAO), and parasitic pneumonitis (Fig. 28.6). Horses with RAO typically display exercise intolerance and increased respiratory efforts during periods of disease exacerbation; however, these signs can be subtle during periods of disease remission. In those cases, pulmonary function testing or more simply, moldy hay challenge, will help reaching a definitive diagnosis. Neutrophilia is commonly observed in BAL fluid from horses with RAO and IAD.[14,73,85] The neutrophilia is usually more pronounced (>20%) with RAO than IAD; however, there is significant overlap between diseases.[16,18,86] Eosinophilic inflammation can be associated with IAD, parasitic pneumonitis (*Parascaris equorum, Dictyocaulus arnfieldi*),[87] hypersensitivity pneumonitis, fungal pneumonia, and cutaneous habronemiasis.[70,88,89] Clinical signs of parasitic pneumonitis are non-specific. Fecal flotation (Baermann technique) is often not diagnostic of *P. equorum* infection because migration through the lungs occurs during the pre-patent period.[90] *D. arnfieldi* follows a complete cycle in donkeys, mules, and asses; however, the infection is usually not patent in horses. Therefore, the Baermann fecal flotation is not useful either. *P. equorum* pneumonitis is more commonly detected in foals less than 6 month of age. *D. arnfieldi* usually occurs in horses in contact with infected donkeys and rarely by ingesting larvae excreted by infected horses.[91] A presumptive diagnosis can be reached when respiratory secretions reveal eosinophilic inflammation with sometimes evidence of parasite eggs or larvae, exposure to donkeys exists, and anthelmintic therapy results in clinical improvement.[90] Increased numbers of metachromatic cells (mast cells, basophils) are common in horses with IAD but have not been associated with other types of respiratory disease.[70,92]

Treatment and prognosis

Therapeutic aims

Treatment of IAD should combine environmental changes and medical therapy. The goals of medical therapy are to control airway

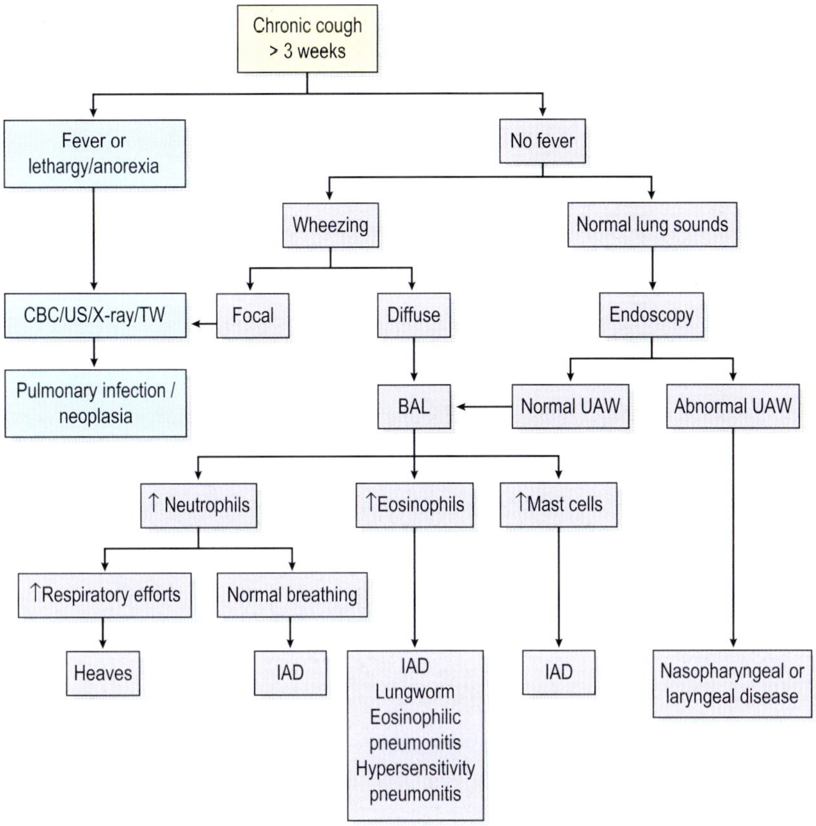

Fig 28.6 Diagnostic approach in horses with chronic cough (>3 weeks). BAL: bronchoalveolar lavage, CBC: complete blood count, IAD: inflammatory airway diseases, UAW: upper airway, U/S: ultrasound, X-ray: radiographs.

inflammation and relieve airflow obstruction using mainly corticosteroids and bronchodilators or antimicrobials when infection is suspected. There are few peer-reviewed clinical trials published, especially concerning aerosol therapy. Therefore, most of the drugs and dosages recommended are based on studies performed on horses with RAO; however, good clinical response of IAD has been observed using those guidelines (Table 28.3). Both systemic and aerosolized drugs are effective; however, the potential for adverse effects and prolonged elimination times is greater with systemic administration. The advantages of aerosol therapy are ease of administration and safety. The disadvantages are cost of delivery of devices and drugs (metered-dose inhalers). Non-steroidal anti-inflammatory and anti-histamine drugs are ineffective for the treatment of IAD.

Therapy

Environmental changes

Inhaled dust particles play an important role in the pathophysiology of IAD and treatment of IAD should always include recommendation to decrease environmental irritants to airways. Several measures help reduce exposure of the horse's airways to respirable particles and are discussed in details in the section on RAO.

Medical therapy

Antibiotics. A large proportion of racehorses suspected of respiratory disease because of poor performance, cough, or nasal discharge are treated with antimicrobials usually without supportive evidence of bacterial infection.[93,94] However, there is currently no controlled study reporting the efficacy of antimicrobials in the treatment of IAD. Available data show no association between response to treatment and the type of antimicrobial used, duration of treatment or time elapsed between repeated examinations.[93] Only 50% of racehorses diagnosed with IAD based on excess tracheal mucus respond favorably to a single course of antibiotic therapy.[93] Therefore, there is currently no evidence-based data supporting the use of antimicrobials in horses with IAD.

Corticosteroids. Two clinical trials have been reported concerning the use of inhaled corticosteroids for IAD and only one in the peer-reviewed literature.[71,95] In a randomized cross-over study, seven horses diagnosed with IAD based on criteria provided in a consensus statement [13] were treated for two weeks with inhaled fluticasone (3000 μg, q 12 h) using an equine aerosol delivery device (AeroHippus™, Trudell Medical International, London, Ontario, Canada, Fig. 28.7) or with intramuscular dexamethasone (0.05 mg/kg q 24 h).[71] After two weeks of therapy, the only significant change detected was a relative decrease in BALF lymphocytes and none of the other BALF cell types were affected by treatment. A second study used a randomized, controlled cross-over design with 8 horses diagnosed with IAD based on elevated tracheal mucus and neutrophil percentages (>20%) and horses were treated for two weeks with either inhaled fluticasone (1000 μg q 12 h), ipratropium bromide (250 μg q 12 h), a combination of the two drugs or a placebo (four horses per treatment group) using a different type of aerosol delivery device (Equine Haler™, Equine HealthCare ApS, Denmark, Fig. 28.7).[95] Results showed that two weeks of inhaled fluticasone with or without ipratropium significantly decreased tracheal neutrophilia (−18.5% and −22%, respectively) as compared to ipratropium alone (−7.9%) or placebo (+14.2%) and most of the improvement occurred during the first week. Since tracheal cytology does not necessarily reflect severity of lesions in lungs, results from this study

Table 28.3 Therapeutic aerosols used for the treatment of inflammatory airway disease (IAD) and recurrent airway obstruction (RAO)*

DRUG	TRADE NAME (LABORATORY)	DOSE DELIVERED PER ACTUATION	NUMBER OF DOSES PER CANISTER	DEVICE	DOSE	DURATION OF ACTION
Bronchodilators						
Albuterol	Torpex (Boehringer & 3M)	120 μg	200	3M ED	1–2 μg/kg†	1 hour
	Combivent (Boehringer)	120 μg (+ 21 μg ipratropium)	200	AeroMask	2–3 μg/kg	1 hour
	Proventil (Schering)	120 μg	200	AeroHippus/ Equine Haler	1 μg/kg	1 hour
Ipratropium bromide	Atrovent (Boehringer)	18 μg	200	AeroMask	0.5–1 μg/kg	4–6 hours
	Atrovent (Boehringer)	0.02 % solution for nebulization	2.5 ml vial	Ultrasonic nebilizer	2–3 μg/kg	4–6 hours
	Combivent (Boehringer)	21 μg (+ 120 μg albuterol)	200			
Fenoterol	Only in Canada			AeroMask	2–4 μg/kg	
Pirbuterol	Maxair inhaler (3M)	200 μg	300	3M ED	1–2 μg/kg	1 hour
Salmeterol	Serevent (Glaxo Wellcome)	25 μg	120 (13 g canister)	3M ED	0.5–1 μg	6–8 hours
Corticosteroids						
Beclomethasone*	Beclovent (Glaxo Wellcome)	42 μg	200 (16.8 g canister)	3M ED AeroMask	1–3 μg/kg, q 12 hours 7–9 μg/kg, q 12 hours	
Fluticasone*	Flovent (Glaxo Wellcome)	220 μg 125 μg	120 (13 g canister)	AeroMask Equine Haler	2–4 μg/kg, q 12 hours 6–12 μg/kg, q 12 hours	
Other						
Sodium cromoglycate	Generic	0.02 % solution for nebulization	2 mL vials	Jet nebulizer Ultrasonic nebulizer	200 mg, q 12 hours 80 mg, q 24 hours	

3M ED: aerosol delivery device for equine developed by 3M Animal Care Products (no longer commercially available), AeroMask: aerosol delivery device for equine developed by Trudell Medical International.
*Dosages reported in this table were taken from studies using CFC propellant. Current aerosols are packaged with HFA propellant that require lower dosages for a given effect when using certain types of corticosteroids (e.g. beclomethasone, see discussion about aerosol therapy for further explanation)
†Approved for use in horses at a dose of 360–720 μg per horse no more than four times per day.

should be interpreted with caution and large field trials are needed before evidence-based recommendations can be made.

Clinical experience suggests that a combination of environmental measures aimed at decreasing dust exposure coupled with inhalation therapy using the same drugs effective against RAO is also beneficial for IAD (Table 28.3). As a general rule, the low end of the dose range recommended for RAO seems appropriate for IAD cases. Currently available aerosol delivery devices used to administer drugs packaged in metered-dose inhalers (MDI) provide similar clinical efficacy (AeroHippus™ and Equine Haler™, Fig. 28.7).[96] Improved clinical signs, decreased airway hyperresponsiveness, and reduced pulmonary inflammation are usually detectable within two weeks of therapy.

Bronchodilators. Bronchodilators are indicated to relax airway smooth muscle and relieve airflow obstruction. Two main classes of inhaled bronchodilators have been used in the horse: beta$_2$-agonists (e.g. albuterol, clenbuterol) and anticholinergic drugs. Horses with IAD have a mild degree of airway obstruction that could be secondary to airway inflammation or bronchospasm.[62,65,97]

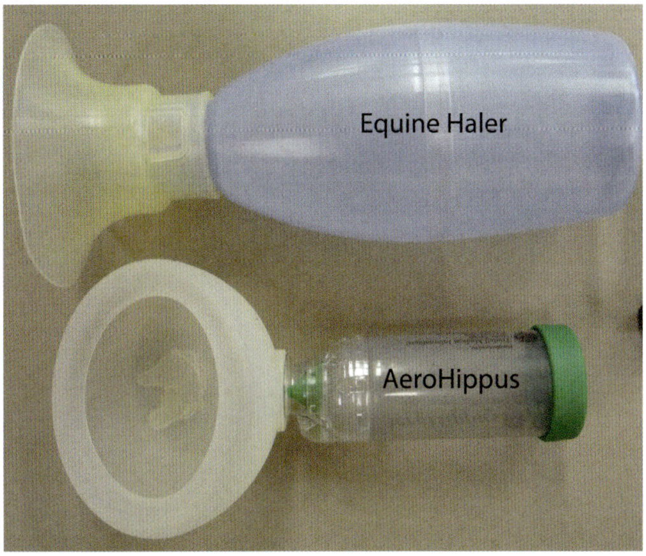

Fig 28.7 Aerosol delivery devices for drugs packaged in metered-dose inhaler (AeroHippus™, Trudell Medical International, London, Ontario, Canada; Equine Haler™, Jørgen Kruuse A/S, Marslev, Denmark).

Another common cause of airway obstruction is bronchial hyperresponsiveness which is particularly evident in horses with IAD associated with increased concentrations of eosinophils or mast cells in BAL lavage fluid.[31,98]

Bronchodilators should not be used as the sole therapy for a prolonged period of time because they do not suppress airway inflammation. However, evidence from ex-vivo and in-vivo studies suggest that clenbuterol (0.8 μg/kg PO or IV, q 12 h) has mild anti-inflammatory properties and reduces airway responsiveness to an irritant challenge in healthy, IAD- and RAO-affected horses.[99–103] The bronchoprotective effect of clenbuterol decreases after 2 weeks of therapy due to tachyphylaxis.[99] In general, bronchodilators should be administered prior to inhalation therapy with corticosteroids to optimize lung deposition of corticosteroids.[104]

Other therapies

Sodium cromoglycate (cromolyn) improves clinical signs and decreases bronchial hyperresponsiveness when administered to horses with IAD characterized by a high mast cell count in BAL fluid (Table 28.3).[70] However, it is ineffective for the treatment of IAD with other inflammatory profiles.

Oral administration of low-dose (50–150 U q 24 h) interferon alpha (IFNα) for five days reduces neutrophil, macrophage, lymphocyte, and total nucleated cell counts in the BALF of racehorses with IAD as well as cough for at least two weeks.[105,106] There is a parallel reduction in concentrations of immunoglobulins and inflammatory mediators in BALF, suggesting plasma exudation as a result of airway inflammation.[107] Higher doses of IFNα (450 U) appear to be less effective. Endoscopic scores based on respiratory exudate, cough, and pharyngeal lymphoid hyperplasia were significantly reduced after one week of therapy but were not different from placebo at two weeks. Mast cell and eosinophil counts did not change after IFNα therapy. Until the pathophysiology of IAD is established, pulmonary anti-inflammatory effects of IFNα could be attributed to antiviral activity or immunomodulatory properties.[107]

Non-specific immunostimulants such as *Propionibacterium acnes* are recommended as an adjunct treatment for a variety of chronic respiratory diseases and as prophylactic agents for stress-associated (e.g. long-distance transport, weaning) respiratory diseases.[108,109] However, the efficacy of such therapy has not been demonstrated conclusively for IAD.

Prognosis

Horses with IAD have a good prognosis for return to previous level of performance. In some cases the disease can recur but in the majority of cases implementation of environmental changes combined with medical therapy results in long-lasting resolution of the clinical signs.

Etiology and pathophysiology

Etiology

Putative causes of IAD include bacteria, viruses, and inhaled environmental pollutants with a modulatory role played by factors such as the horse's immune response and genetic make-up (Fig. 28.8).

The likelihood of isolating bacteria from tracheal wash samples collected from racehorses in training is strongly associated with the cytological degree of inflammation.[15,23,30] Isolation of more than 10^3 colony-forming units/mL of pathogenic *Streptococcus* spp. is strongly associated with coughing.[30] Bacterial species most frequently isolated from tracheal wash are *Streptococcus* spp., *Pasteurella/Actinobacillus* spp., and *Bordetella* spp. *Mycoplasma* organisms, in particular *M. equirhinis*, have been isolated in some horses with IAD.[21] The marked increase in the risk of coughing in horses with high numbers of bacteria in tracheal secretions, the common isolation of bacteria with potential to cause pulmonary disease, and the association between IAD and detection of intracellular bacteria in tracheal secretions argue for a causative role of bacteria in the pathogenesis of IAD. However, results from uncontrolled studies suggest that only 50–69% of racehorses diagnosed with IAD respond favorably to a single course of antibiotic therapy (7–10 days).[93,110]

Several factors suggest that bacteria can be present in the trachea because of contamination during sampling or transient colonization of the proximal airways. First, no bacteria are cultured in 22 to 54% of horses with IAD.[21,23,111] Second, the trachea is not a sterile environment and potentially pathogenic bacteria can be isolated by tracheal wash in 8–25% of healthy horses with isolation of non-pathogenic organisms in as many as 75% of those horses.[112,113] Third, the presence of bacteria in the airways can result from decreased mucociliary clearance and not from primary infection. Fourth, successful treatment of IAD with oral interferon-alpha or inhaled glucocorticoids suggests that infectious agents are not causative agents but rather opportunistic invaders of the tracheobronchial tree.[50,92,95,105]

Contrary to a common belief, respiratory viruses do not appear to play an important role in IAD. Several reports have shown either a low incidence or no evidence of viral infections in horses with IAD based on serology or virus isolation aimed at detecting equine herpesvirus, influenza virus, adenovirus, and rhinoviruses.[15,21,27,30] More recently, detection of viruses by PCR in respiratory samples from athletic horses revealed that equine herpesvirus 2 was identified in a greater proportion of tracheal fluid from horses with IAD or poor performance (33%) than controls (11%).[114] Such association was not found in BAL fluid despite the fact that epithelial cell alterations were significantly associated with equine herpesvirus 2 and 5 only in BAL fluid. These findings raise questions on the significance of PCR detection of herpesviruses in respiratory secretions because it could be due to latent infection or low pathogenicity of otherwise ubiquitous infectious agents.[114,115]

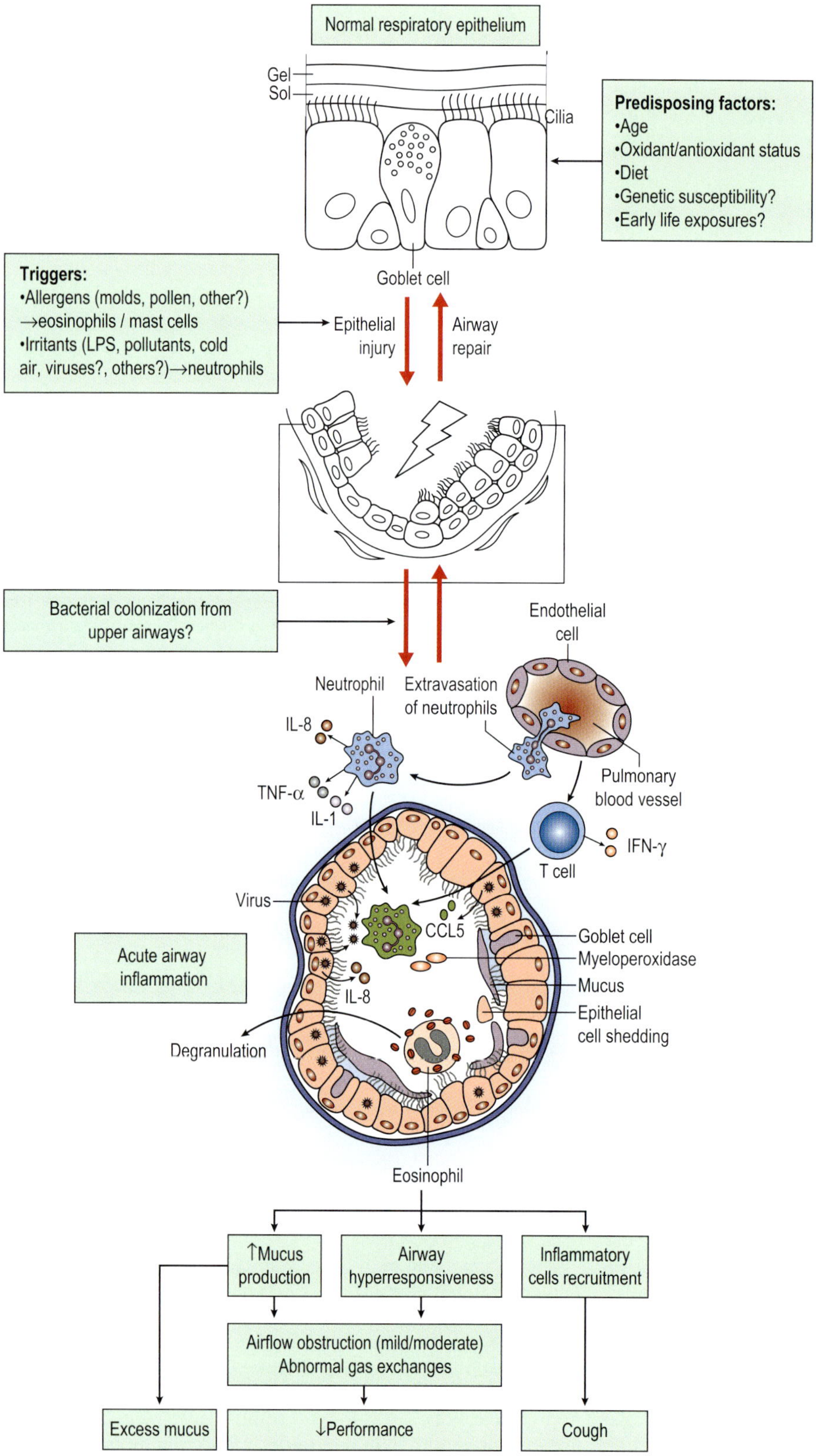

Fig 28.8 Pathophysiology of inflammatory airway disease.

The role of exposure to dust in the pathogenesis of IAD is suggested by several studies. Healthy yearlings fed hay demonstrate a significant increase in BAL fluid neutrophil count and percentage, and a higher airway inflammation score when housed in a stable than when kept on pasture[116] while others have found that these changes occur with housing combined with exercise training but not just stabling.[117] Natural exposure of healthy horses to moldy hay or controlled exposure to organic molds and endotoxins to levels encountered during natural exposure result in BAL fluid neutrophilia[74,118,119] and airway hyperresponsiveness.[120] Also, horses in training kept on straw bedding experience episodes of IAD that last longer than in horses bedded on paper.[15] These findings are consistent with data showing that conventional horse management consisting of indoor housing with straw bedding and feeding of hay result in much larger dust exposure levels than housing of horses on wood shavings and pelleted feed or keeping them on pasture.[121,122] Some horses with IAD demonstrate increased eosinophil or metachromatic cell counts in BAL fluid, suggesting hypersensitivity response of the lower airways to inhaled allergens.[14,19,69,70,92]

Atmospheric oxidants such as ozone have the potential to cause lower airway inflammation in horses, but levels encountered during natural exposure are unlikely to induce IAD in otherwise healthy animals.[123] Nevertheless, horses exercising strenuously while exposed to ozone levels comparable to atmospheric concentrations develop histologic evidence of airway damage and horses with IAD have elevated indices of oxidant injury[124] in BAL fluid, suggesting that oxidant injury could play a role in the pathophysiology if IAD.[123,125]

Several additional factors encountered in athletic horses can contribute to the pathogenesis of IAD. Horses exercising in cold weather (−5 °C) have a mild relative increased proportion of neutrophils in BALF.[126] Transportation of horses over long distances can induce airway inflammation and colonization of the tracheobronchial tree by bacteria.[127,128] Strenuous exercise results in colonization of the lower airways by large numbers of bacteria (10- to 100-fold compared to pre-exercise levels) suggesting that tracheal inflammation post-exercise is expected, in particular influx of neutrophils.[129] However, the duration of this inflammatory response is currently unknown. Both heaves in horses and asthma in people have a significant heritable component.[130–132] Therefore, airway response to environmental challenges is likely modulated by certain genes and study of linkage between respiratory diseases such as heaves and IAD and those genes will help identify animals at risk and design better ways of treating and preventing respiratory diseases.

Pathophysiology

(See Figure 28.8.) The effect of IAD on performance is dependent on the severity of the disease and the intensity of exercise. Pulmonary gas exchanges are the limiting factor to performance in fit horses exercising strenuously as illustrated by the marked exercise-induced arterial hypoxemia and hypercapnia developed by healthy racehorses.[133,134] During strenuous exercise, horses exercise at or above maximum aerobic capacity (VO_{2max}). In this situation, a relatively mild degree of IAD can significantly impair gas exchanges and result in decreased performance.[26,53,54] IAD is not likely to cause exercise intolerance in a horse exercising at less than 50% of VO_{2max} until the disease causes marked airflow obstruction or frequent coughing. Therefore, the clinician needs to select diagnostic tools and interpret test results based on the horse's fitness level and type of activity.

Mechanisms responsible for decreased performance in horses with IAD are mainly speculative at this point in time. A study of Standardbred racehorses performing submaximal exercise test on a treadmill found that horses with IAD exhibited increased pulmonary artery pressure and red cell volume (RCV/kg BW) in comparison to healthy controls.[81] These findings suggested a compensatory response to exercise-induced hypoxemia[135,136] even though significant differences in PaO_2 between IAD and control horses were not found. The elevated pulmonary artery pressure was thought to result from increased vascular resistance. Elevation in RCV/kg BW or packed cell volume has been shown to correlate with increase in pulmonary blood pressure and vascular resistance.[137,138] Also, horses with more severe airway disease such as heaves have significantly elevated pulmonary artery pressure.[139,140] Peripheral airway obstruction can be detected in horses with IAD using sensitive methods such as forced expiration, forced oscillatory mechanics or rebreathing maneuvers (Fig. 28.3).[18,62,64,65,68] Several studies have shown that racehorses with IAD exhibit more pronounced exercise-induced hypoxemia than healthy controls during standardized run to fatigue on a treadmill (Fig. 28.2).[52–54] Exercise-induced hypoxemia is a physiologic phenomenon in horses[133] and the degree of arterial hypoxemia is more pronounced as the level of training increases.[141] Therefore, assessment of the significance of exercise-induced hypoxemia is dependent on control data matched for horses' age and fitness level.

Poor performance can result from a variety of causes such as lameness, exertional rhabdomyolysis, and cardiac and neurologic diseases. More importantly, it is common to diagnose several problems in the same horse.[142] In a retrospective study of 275 horses evaluated because of a complaint of poor performance, Morris and Seeherman reported that 84% of cases were diagnosed with a combination of problems involving one or more body system.[142] These findings underscore the importance of performing a comprehensive evaluation of poorly performing horses.

The mechanism responsible for the influx of neutrophils, mast cells or eosinophils in airways of horses with IAD is still unclear, with some studies showing an association between IAD and Th2-type cytokines[71,126] while others did not.[143]

Prevention

The risk of IAD is significantly lower in older horses, suggesting that development of an appropriate immune response can protect horses from IAD.[22,32,42] Even though viral diseases do not appear to play a major role in IAD, proper vaccination against respiratory pathogens before the introduction of young horses into the stable is recommended.

Air quality, in particular low dust and other irritants levels, is an important part of preventive measures (see discussion of environmental changes in RAO section). For example, horses bedded on wood shavings are exposed to significantly less respirable dust than when bedded on straw and feeding haylage instead of hay results in an even more dramatic decline in exposure.[144] Similarly, soaking hay results in a significant reduction in respirable dust exposure.[145] Horses kept in well-ventilated stalls and bedded on shredded paper are 4 times less likely to develop IAD than horses housed in closed stalls and bedded on straw.[15] Also, a study showed that young healthy horses fed hay while being maintained on pasture for a three-month period did not exhibit signs of respiratory disease; however, they developed pulmonary neutrophilic inflammation within a month of being housed inside a barn on the same diet and bedded on straw.[116] Another study found that adult horses free of respiratory disease initially and exposed to incremental amount of dust for two weeks at a time showed an increased percentage of neutrophils in BAL fluid and an increase in airway responsiveness to histamine challenge (Fig. 28.9A and Fig. 28.9B).[120] These studies suggest that exposure of horses to dust levels commonly encountered in standard housing systems is sufficient to cause airway inflammation and pulmonary dysfunction in otherwise healthy horses.

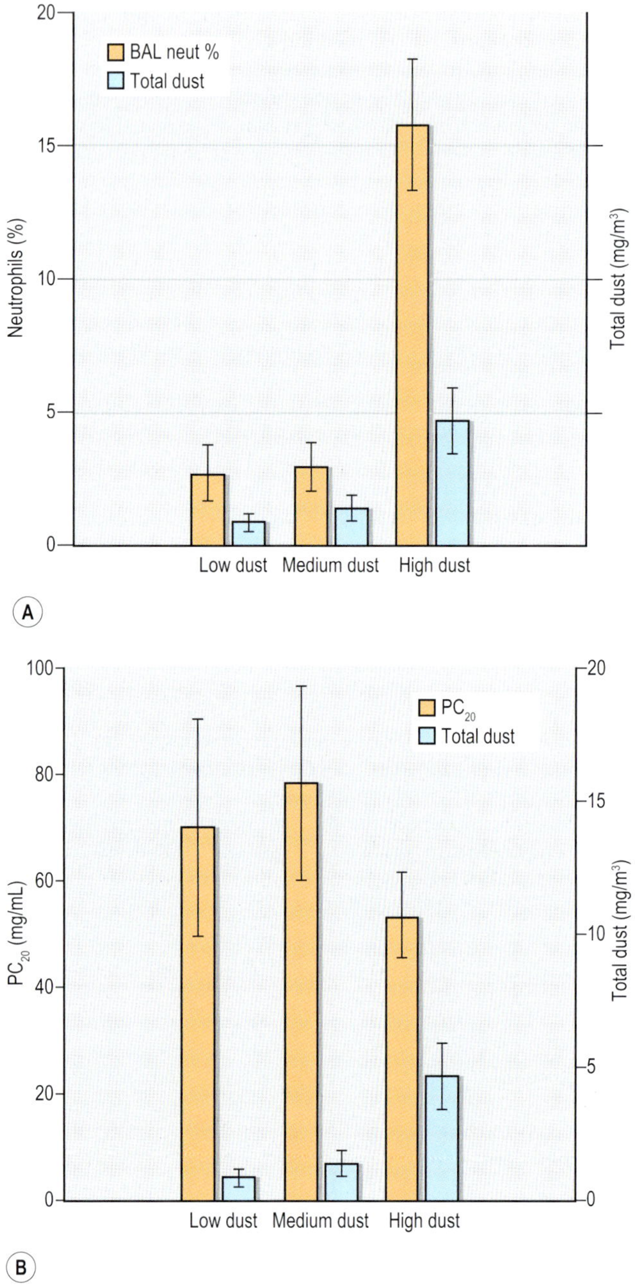

Fig 28.9 Effect of dust exposure on **(A)** bronchoalveolar lavage fluid cytology and **(B)** airway responsiveness to histamine challenge. Low dust: horse in stall fed pellets and bedded on wood shavings. Medium dust: horse in stall fed pellets and bedded on straw. High dust: horse in stall fed moldy hay and bedded on straw. Total dust was measured in the breathing zone of the horse. PC_{20}: provocative concentration of histamine required to decrease $FEV_{1.5}$ by 20%.

Epidemiology

The prevalence of IAD in racehorses varies between 11 % and 65 % depending on the diagnostic criteria used (endoscopy or cytology), the training stable where horses are housed, the age of the horse (highest prevalence in young) and the timing of examination (highest prevalence post-exercise).[7,9,21,23,44] Prevalence of IAD is also high in sports and pleasure horses (20–66%).[8,11,16,19] Monthly fluctuation in the incidence of IAD based on inflammation score in Thoroughbreds in training may vary between 0 and 45%.[15] Age appears to be a significant factor with yearlings and two-year-old horses being significantly more likely to be affected by IAD than older horses.[15,22,32,42]

Recurrent airway obstruction (RAO, SPAOPD, heaves, chronic obstructive pulmonary disease, broken wind)

- RAO is associated with exercise intolerance, increased tracheobronchial exudate, mild-to-severely increased respiratory efforts, and occasionally cough.
- Mature and older horses housed in stables for extended periods and fed hay are commonly affected.
- Horses suffering from summer pasture-associated RAO are clinically indistinguishable from RAO except that they develop clinical signs while at pasture during the summer.
- Bronchoalveolar lavage fluid cytology and response to bronchodilators are valuable diagnostic tools for RAO.
- Horses with RAO exhibit severe airflow obstruction and airway hyperresponsiveness.
- RAO appears to be hypersensitivity to inhaled organic molds with an additional role played by inhaled endotoxins.
- Therapy is aimed at decreasing environmental allergens, decreasing airway inflammation with glucocorticoids, and relieving airway obstruction with bronchodilators.

Recognition

History and presenting complaint

Recurrent airway obstruction (RAO) or heaves is an allergic disease characterized by cough, accumulations of mucopurulent secretions in the tracheobronchial tree, abnormal breath sounds, increased respiratory efforts, and exercise intolerance.[146] Coughing and nasal discharge are frequently reported in horses with RAO (84% and 54%, respectively); however, they are non-specific signs of respiratory disease.[20] Similarly, presence of tracheal exudate is very common (96%) yet it is also found in a variety of pulmonary diseases. Exercise intolerance is usually marked but highly dependent on the level of exertion required of the horse as well as disease severity. Frequent bouts of coughing might be the main perceived cause of exercise intolerance. Horses with RAO exhibiting mild respiratory signs at rest can only show abnormally increased respiratory efforts for a given exercise intensity or prolonged recovery post-exercise. Because of a lack of objective data on 'normal' cardiopulmonary variables during exercise and recovery period in healthy horses, most of the assessment concerning exercise intolerance is based on the owner's or the trainer's perception.[8]

Clinical signs of RAO usually resolve within a few days after placing the horse at pasture (removing it from a stable or barn environment) or improving the air quality of the environment by reducing organic dusts and increasing ventilation in the stall. Conversely, susceptible horses housed indoors and exposed to moldy hay develop clinical signs within a few hours to a few days.[59,67] Summer pasture-associated RAO is clinically indistinguishable from RAO except that historical findings reveal disease flare-ups while horses are kept at pasture during summer months and clinical improvement during winter or after horses are housed indoors.[85,147]

Physical examination

Horses with RAO can present with a wide spectrum of clinical signs depending on disease severity. Horses with mild RAO exhibit little to no clinical signs of respiratory disease except for poor performance and can be difficult to differentiate from horses with IAD (Table 28.1). At the other end of the spectrum, horses with severe RAO show exercise intolerance associated with markedly increased respiratory efforts manifested by nostril flaring, head and neck extension, pronounced abdominal muscle contraction during expiration (heaving), and exaggerated rib excursion during inspiration (Fig. 28.10). Over time, horses develop hypertrophy of the external abdominal oblique muscles resulting in the characteristic 'heave line'. Respiratory rate is quite variable but is usually elevated. These clinical signs result from small airway obstruction secondary to airway inflammation, bronchospasm, mucus plugging of airways, and thickening of the airway wall.

Bilateral mucoid to mucopurulent nasal discharge can be present. A deep cough might be heard intermittently or in bouts of paroxysmal coughing. Thoracic auscultation often reveals increased breath sounds bilaterally, an extended area of auscultation, and abnormal breath sounds including crackles and expiratory wheezes. Horses' thick chest wall render auscultation an insensitive indicator of pulmonary disease with abnormal findings obtained in less than 50% of horses with RAO.[20]

Special examination

Horses with normal respiratory tracts have either no or just a few flecks of mucus visible upon endoscopic examination of the airways.[29,33] The presence of increased amounts of respiratory secretions in the tracheobronchial tree is found in the majority of RAO horses; however, it is also common in horses with IAD and infectious pulmonary diseases.[8,9,27,33] Horses with severe pulmonary disease, including heaves, often exhibit marked airway erythema and bronchial edema illustrated by blunting of the carina and 'bumpiness' of the airway surface (Fig. 28.11). But carina septum thickness markedly overlaps between RAO and healthy horses and is not correlated with tracheal mucus or BAL neutrophilia.[19,36]

Collection of respiratory secretions using TW or BAL techniques is important for diagnostic purposes and monitoring response to therapy. Sedation of the horse prior to BAL collection is mandatory and is sometimes needed for TW. Administration of alpha2-agonist sedatives (xylazine, detomidine, romifidine) to horses with RAO results in significant decrease in respiratory rate, minute ventilation, and variable effects on R_L and lung C_{dyn}.[148–150] PaO_2 in affected horses is either maintained or only mildly decreased after administration of sedatives. Similar effects of sedatives on lung function are reported in healthy horses. Therefore, administration of sedatives to horses with RAO prior to diagnostic procedures is considered safe. The volume of fluid retrieved during BAL procedure is often decreased in RAO horses due to small airway collapse as fluid is aspirated back. However, as long as the volume of fluid infused is sufficient (250–500 mL) there is no significant difference in absolute or differential cell counts between aliquots retrieved sequentially.[151] Therefore, interpretation of BALF cytology in horses with RAO has diagnostic value even if the procedure only yielded a small amount of fluid.

Thoracic radiographs might be useful to rule out pulmonary diseases other than RAO. However, interpretation of radiographs is considered insensitive because radiographic findings correlate poorly with severity of lesions as detected by histopathology of the lungs and interpretation of images is highly variable between examiners.[152] Also, no radiographic findings are specific for a particular inflammatory lung disease, which renders chest radiography of limited value for the diagnosis of RAO.

Pulmonary function tests allow quantification of lung dysfunction using various techniques (see discussion in 'IAD/special examination'). During episodes of disease exacerbation pulmonary changes translate into functional changes such as increased maximal changes in transpulmonary pressure (ΔP_{plmax}), pulmonary resistance (R_L) and decreased dynamic lung compliance (C_{dyn}).[97] However, these measurements are not sensitive and test results usually become abnormal only when horses display obvious clinical signs of heaves. These tests are still useful in clinical practice to evaluate reversibility of airway obstruction after bronchodilation or to assess response to therapy because clinical signs alone are poor predictors of lung function; i.e. a significant degree of airway obstruction may still be present after the course of therapy even though clinical signs have

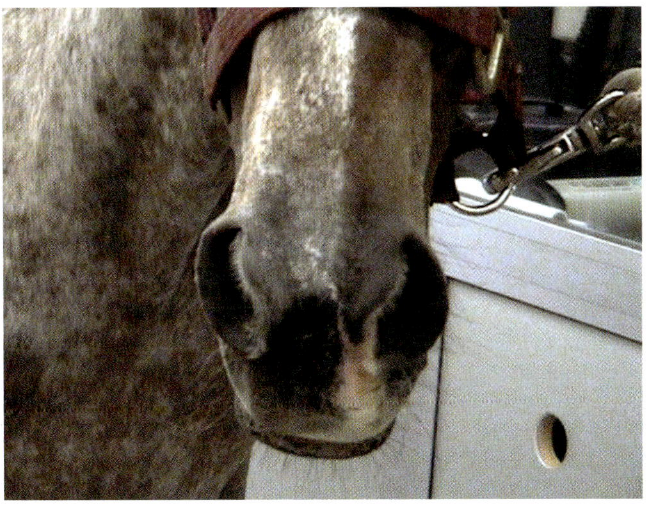

Fig 28.10 Nostril flaring in a horse with recurrent airway obstruction.

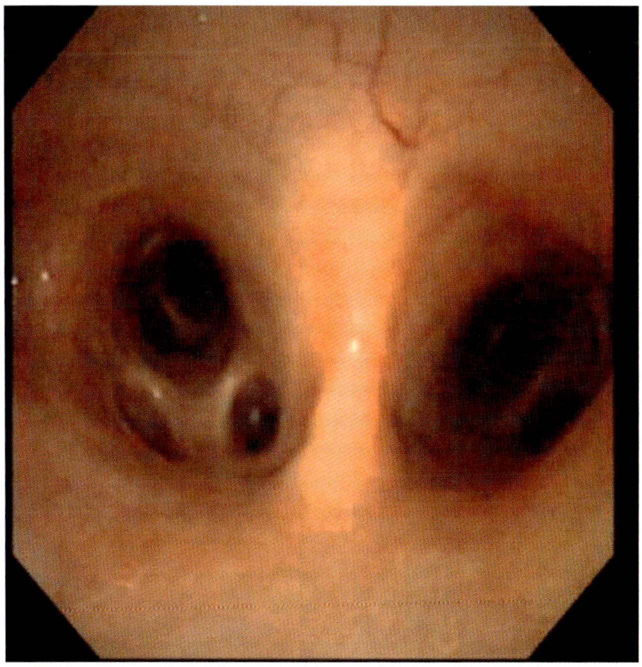

Fig 28.11 Endoscopic view of the carina in a horse with recurrent airway obstruction showing rounded bifurcation between left and right mainstem bronchi consistent with mucosal edema.

resolved.[153] Another non-invasive method that is well suited for field-testing combines the use of respiratory inductance plethysmography and pneumotachography during normal breathing at rest.[66] Airflow measured at the nostril opening by a pneumotachograph is compared to flow signal derived from bands placed around chest and abdomen. In the presence of airway obstruction, gas compression within the airways can result in asynchrony between thoracic and abdominal contractions. Several indices derived from this lung function test correlate with conventional lung mechanics (ΔP_{plmax}, R_L) and allow quantification of airway obstruction in horses with RAO as well as response to bronchodilators or histamine challenge.[55,66]

A unique feature of horses with airway obstruction (RAO, IAD) is their increased airway narrowing in response to challenge with irritants such histamine or methacholine (hyperresponsiveness).[63,66–68,154–158] In general, the greater the airway obstruction, the more pronounced the bronchoconstriction for a given concentration of irritant. Bronchoprovocation can be a useful method for the detection of mild-to-moderate RAO in horses that do not display overt clinical signs.

In addition to alteration in lung mechanics, RAO horses exhibit abnormal gas exchanges at rest during periods of disease exacerbation, leading to hypoxemia and sometimes hypercapnia.[159,160] These blood gas abnormalities are mainly the result of ventilation–perfusion mismatch and increased dead-space ventilation.[139] Horses with mild clinical signs usually have normal blood gases. During exercise, the degree of exercise-induced hypoxemia and hypercapnia is markedly worse in RAO horses in crisis compared to remission.[161] Deterioration in gas exchanges appears to be mainly due to further deterioration in the ventilation–perfusion relationship.

Few studies have examined the relationship between lung histopathology, clinical signs, and lung function in horses with chronic airway disease. Significant correlation between percutaneous lung biopsy scores and clinical signs ($r = 0.58$) has been reported in RAO horses[162] and between mucus score in lung biopsies and clinical signs ($r = 0.78$) in horses with summer pasture-associated RAO.[163]

Laboratory examination

Hemogram and serum biochemistry are usually within the normal range,[73] although some horses with acute severe RAO have mild hyperfibrinogenemia.

Cytologic examination of TW or BAL fluid is useful to reach a final diagnosis. TW fluid obtained from horses with RAO usually reveals a marked increase in neutrophil percentages (>50%, range, 7–96%).[33,38,47,113] Neutrophils are non-degenerate and even if bacteria are isolated in some cases, they do not play a role in the pathogenesis of the disease. Increased amounts of mucus containing casts of inspissated mucus originating from the bronchioles (Curschmann's spirals) are often present in long-standing cases. In the BALF of healthy horses, lymphocytes and alveolar macrophages predominate and neutrophils represent <10% of the total nucleated cell count.[74,74,163,164] A marked absolute and relative neutrophilia (>20%) is usually observed in RAO horses.[73,74,74,163] The range of neutrophil percentages is wide (10–98%) but no significant differences exists between BALF cytology collected from different regions of the lung.[164]

Necropsy examination

The classic histopathologic lesion in horses with RAO is bronchiolitis characterized by peribronchiolar lymphoplasmacytic, neutrophilic, and sometime eosinophilic cell infiltration, bronchiolar goblet cell metaplasia, epithelial and smooth muscle hyperplasia, and accumulation of mucopurulent exudate in the bronchioles' lumen.[162,165–167] Similar changes are also frequently detected in the large airways.[168] Other lesions reported in severely affected horses are peribronchiolar fibrosis and epithelial metaplasia. Emphysema is sometimes present in RAO horses and both centrilobular and panlobular forms have been reported.[169–171] Lungs of affected horses tend to remain over-inflated at post-mortem examination because of air trapping secondary to airway obstruction and not emphysema. In general, there is a good correlation between the degree and extent of histopathological changes and clinical severity.[165,166,168] However, lesions are usually extensive but multifocal in nature, making interpretation based on small size samples (e.g. percutaneous lung biopsy) hazardous.[166]

Ultrastructural changes are characterized by loss of ciliated cells in the larger airways and replacement by a hyperplastic epithelium.[168] Examination of terminal airways and alveoli shows degenerative changes affecting non-ciliated bronchiolar epithelial cells (Clara cells). Suggesting that Clara cells can be the target for antigens and inflammatory mediators during the disease process.[166]

Diagnostic confirmation

Horses presenting an abnormal increase in respiratory efforts should be examined to rule out upper versus lower airway causes (Fig. 28.12). Upper airway obstruction may be associated with loud abnormal respiratory sounds (stridor). Lower airway diseases are often associated with abnormal breath sounds upon thoracic auscultation. Typically, upper airway obstruction results in increased inspiratory efforts, whereas intrathoracic airway obstruction is associated with increased expiratory efforts. Fixed obstructions result in sounds, respiratory efforts, and respiratory times that are comparable during inspiration and expiration. Variable (dynamic) obstructions are characterized by a marked difference between inspiratory and expiratory sounds and time. Endoscopic examination should be performed rapidly in order to localize the disease process.

Decreased lung sounds in the ventral thorax are usually indicative of pleural effusion or diaphragmatic hernia. Decreased lung sounds dorsally associated with increased resonance upon percussion of the thorax is consistent with pneumothorax. Diagnosis may be confirmed by ultrasonography of the thoracic cavity. Presence of abnormal lung sounds (crackles, wheezes) in horses with fever and respiratory distress suggests infectious pulmonary disease (such as bronchopneumonia, pulmonary abscess, interstitial pneumonia, necrotizing pneumonia).[172–174]

A horse with labored breathing, normal rectal temperature, and abnormal lung sounds should be treated with a fast-acting bronchodilator, such as aerosolized albuterol or intravenous administration of *N*-butylscopolammonium bromide to assess the role of bronchoconstriction (Fig. 28.12). Improvement in clinical signs, in particular decrease in respiratory rate, strongly suggests RAO. Lack of improvement can be associated with restrictive pulmonary diseases such as pleural effusion, pulmonary edema, interstitial pneumonia, pulmonary fibrosis, silicosis, or a mediastinal mass,[175,176] loss of lung elastic recoil caused by bronchiectasis or emphysema,[177] or non-respiratory diseases such as heart failure. Thoracic radiography and cardiac ultrasonography are indicated to characterize the disease process and evaluate the severity of the lesion.

Horses in respiratory distress with no abnormal respiratory sounds should be further evaluated (Fig. 28.12). Horses with synchronous diaphragmatic flutter present with pronounced abdominal contractions that might be mistaken for increased respiratory effort. However, in this case spasmodic contractions of the flank are synchronous with the first heart sound and are independent of the normal respiratory cycle.[178] A markedly elevated rectal temperature may be associated with conditions causing hyperthermia (e.g. exercise, hot environment) or fever and contribute to respiratory distress. Hematology is valuable to detect anemia and diseases resulting

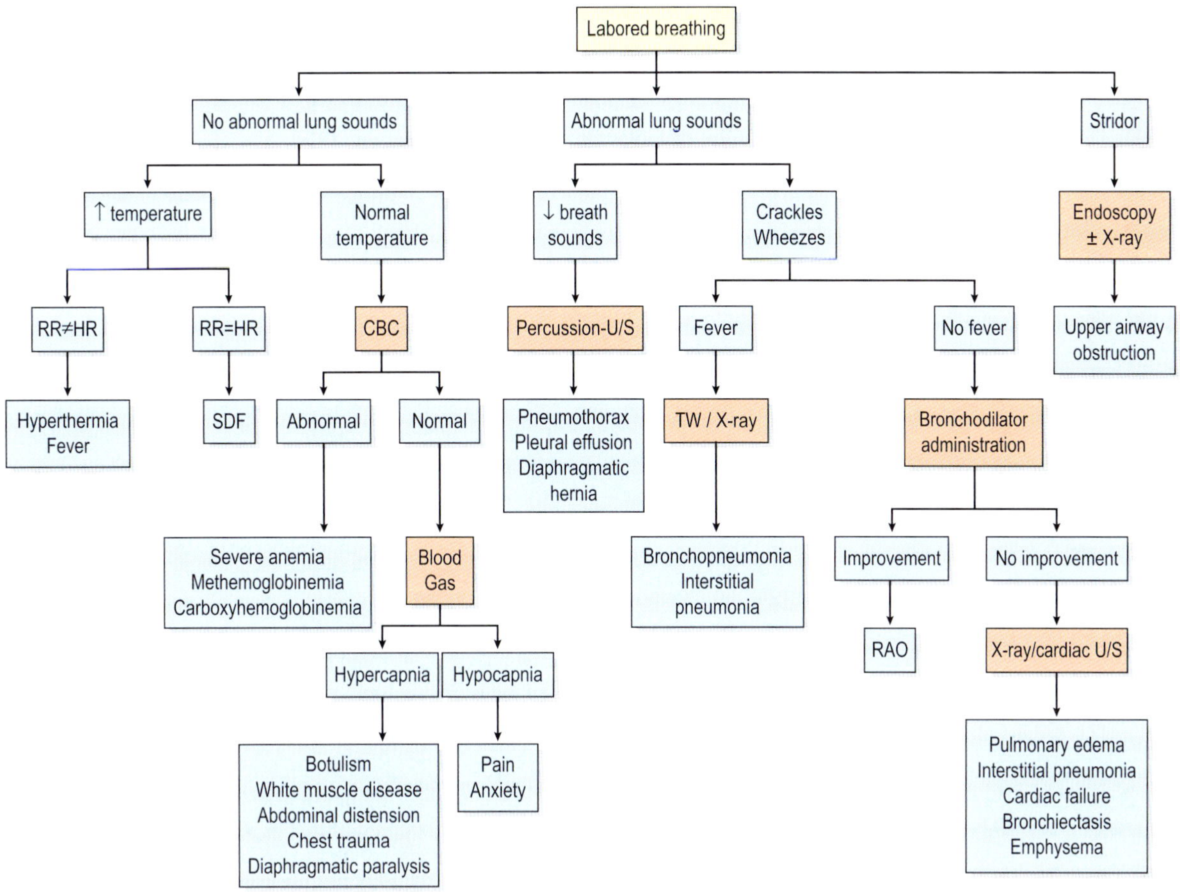

Fig 28.12 Diagnostic approach in horses with labored breathing. CBC: complete blood count, RR: respiratory rate, HR: heart rate, RAO: recurrent airway obstruction, SDF: synchronous diaphragmatic flutter, TW: tracheal wash, U/S: ultrasound, X-ray: radiographs.

in decreased oxygen-carrying capacity of the blood (methemoglobinemia, carboxyhemoglobinemia). Only severe anemia resulting in packed cell volume <8–10% causes labored breathing at rest. Anemia does not cause hypoxemia but a decrease in the delivery of oxygen to tissues (i.e. tissue hypoxia). Therefore, anemic horses have a normal PaO_2 and hyperventilation results from acidification of cerebrospinal fluid secondary to increased anaerobic metabolism. An arterial blood gas sample is indicated in horses with normal hematologic findings. Hypercapnia can be associated with conditions impairing respiratory muscle function (e.g. botulism, nutritional muscular dystrophy, diaphragmatic paralysis) or chest wall movement (e.g. abdominal distension, chest trauma). Hypocapnia indicates hyperventilation and can be in response to painful conditions (e.g. colic) or to anxiety.

Treatment and prognosis

Therapeutic aims

The goals of therapy are to control airway inflammation and relieve airflow obstruction with emphasis on environmental changes.[59,179] Medical therapy is useful to control clinical signs in severely affected animals and when improvement in environmental management is limited. The main classes of drugs recommended for RAO are corticosteroids to treat airway inflammation and bronchodilators to relax airway smooth muscle. Improvement of mucociliary clearance can also help reduce airway obstruction.

It is important to keep in mind that the type of activities the horse is performing as well as the initial complaint from the owner should be taken into consideration before therapy is recommended. For example, a RAO-affected horse used for show-jumping that started exhibiting decreased performance and coughing while being maintained in a low-dust environment should benefit from medical therapy. However, a brood-mare exhibiting an acute RAO crisis two weeks after being housed in the barn for the winter might only need simple environmental control measures (e.g. changing bedding and feed) to be implemented in order to resolve clinical signs even though lung function and BALF cytology can take weeks to improve.

Therapy

Environmental changes

Several measures can reduce exposure of the horse's airways to respirable particles and are discussed in details in the section on RAO prevention. Placing RAO horses in crisis into a low-dust environment composed of wood shavings bedding and pelleted diet results in significant improvement in lung function within three days, even if environmental changes only take place in the affected horse's stall.[180] Horses become free of clinical signs within 1–2 weeks in optimal indoor housing or outside on pasture.[67,181] Some horses might only improve partially after being placed on pasture, especially chronic long-standing cases. Medical therapy will help most of those cases to become free of clinical disease (remission) at which point medication can be discontinued. Subsequently, horses can remain free of clinical disease for extended periods given that they are kept in a low-dust environment.[75] Because of the nature of the disease, susceptible horses can experience another bout of the disease when exposed to allergens.

Horses with summer pasture-associated RAO are affected while at pasture in response to inhaled plant allergens such as pollen and mold spores.[182] In those cases, removal from pasture and confinement to low-dust indoor environment is recommended; however, medical therapy is often needed to provide clinical resolution.[85,183] The management of affected horses may be complicated by the fact that some animals suffer both from classic RAO and summer pasture-associated RAO.[183]

Systemic medical therapy

The cost of systemic therapy is usually less than that of aerosol therapy because of the need to purchase a delivery device (i.e. face mask, inhaler) for aerosol administration. However, systemic therapy with corticosteroids or bronchodilators can have adverse effects.

Corticosteroids

Corticosteroids are potent inflammation inhibitors with demonstrated efficacy for the treatment of heaves. Triamcinolone acetonide is a potent long-acting corticosteroid that can improve lung function for 2–4 weeks after administration of a single dose (0.09 mg/kg, IM) to RAO horses maintained on straw bedding and fed hay.[184] Neutrophil percentage in BALF can also be significantly decreased within two weeks of treatment. Depending on the dose of triamcinolone used, endogenous cortisol production can be suppressed for 2–4 weeks but adrenal gland response to ACTH administration is maintained.[184]

Dexamethasone (0.1 mg/kg, IV, q 24 h) induces a marked improvement in clinical signs and lung function of RAO horses as early as two hours after administration with peak effect at 4–6 hours.[60,185] These beneficial effects persist for at least a week after treatment is discontinued. A reduction in BALF neutrophilia is evident within 3–10 days of therapy.[186,187] Oral bioavailability of dexamethasone is approximately 60% and it is decreased by concomitant feeding.[185] Otherwise, efficacy is similar between oral (0.164 mg/kg in fed horses or 0.082 mg/kg in fasted horses) and intravenous (0.1 mg/kg) administration of dexamethasone.[185] Dexamethasone results in marked adrenal suppression of endogenous cortisol production starting two hours after administration and persisting approximately three days after treatment ends; however, adrenal gland response to exogenous ACTH is maintained.[188,189] Treatment of RAO horses with dexamethasone 21-isonicotinate suspension (0.04 mg/kg, IM, q 72 h) reduces airway obstruction three days after treatment initiation with a maximum effect obtained after seven days.[190] However, the same product administered once as a depot formulation does not result in appreciable improvement within a 10-day period.[191]

Oral administration of prednisone is poorly effective in RAO.[179,180,190] The reason for this lack of efficacy is related to the poor oral absorption of the drug either in tablet or liquid forms.[192] Conversely, both liquid and tablet forms of prednisolone are well absorbed in the horse with a bioavailability of 56 and 65%, respectively.[192] Nevertheless, a dose of prednisolone (1 mg/kg) equipotent to dexamethasone (0.1 mg/kg) will result in slightly lower treatment efficacy.[193]

Bronchodilators

Bronchodilators are indicated to relax airway smooth muscle and relieve airflow obstruction, but they should not be used alone because, with the exception of clenbuterol, they have no anti-inflammatory properties.[101] In addition, prolonged use of certain type of bronchodilators (e.g. beta$_2$-agonists) as solo medication induces airway receptor downregulation and renders the drug less effective after two weeks of therapy.[99,194] This phenomenon is prevented by combined use of beta$_2$-agonists and corticosteroids.

The three classes of drugs available as systemic bronchodilators are anticholinergics, beta$_2$-agonists, and methylxanthines. Atropine (0.01–0.02 mg/kg, IV) is an anticholinergic drug that has been used systemically in horses with heaves and shown to provide rapid and marked improvement in lung function (mean reduction in ΔP_{plmax} of 68–83%) and clinical signs.[195–197] Effects occur within 10 minutes of administration, peak around 30 minutes and last a maximum of 1–2 h. Potentially serious side effects such as ileus and abdominal pain usually develop when higher dosages are used (22–88 mg)[198] but are rare with low-dose atropine (≤ 0.02 mg/kg) unless administration is repeated. *N*-butylscopolammonium bromide (Buscopan®, Boehringer Ingelheim Vetmedica, St. Joseph, MO) is a safer anticholinergic drug that resulted in a marked improvement in lung function within 2–5 minutes of administration (0.3 mg/kg IV, mean reduction in ΔP_{plmax} of 53%).[199]

Clenbuterol hydrochloride syrup (Ventipulmin®, Boehringer Ingelheim Vetmedica, St. Joseph, MO) is approved for the treatment of heaves in horses in the United States. Injectable and oral formulations have been available in other countries for many years. Treatment should be titrated to effect starting with a low dose (0.8 µg/kg, q 12 h) and increasing by 0.8 µg/kg every 3–5 days until improvement is noted or a maximum dose of 3.2 has been reached.[200] It should be recognized that some horses do not respond to treatment even at the highest dose. Clenbuterol therapy also enhances airway mucociliary clearance by increasing ciliary beat frequency.[201] Mild side effects such as sweating, muscle tremors, and excitement occur in less than 9% of horses treated with oral clenbuterol.[200] More concerning side effects are cardiovascular remodeling detected by echocardiographic examination performed immediately after exercise and decreased aerobic capacity in healthy horses treated with medium doses of clenbuterol (2.4 µg/kg, per os q 12 h) for eight weeks.[202,203]

Administration of the beta-adrenergic drug isoproterenol (0.1–0.2 mg/kg, IV) to RAO horses results in clinical and lung function improvement within 15 minutes; however, results are variable between animals and heart rate more than doubles because of stimulation of cardiac beta$_1$-receptors.[195] Terbutaline, a beta$_2$-receptor agonist, is not absorbed orally but intravenous (0.01 mg/kg) and aerosol (0.02 mg/kg) administration improve lung function of RAO horses for up to six hours with marked adverse reactions are such as CNS stimulation, sweating, and trembling likely to occur with the IV route.[196,204]

Methylxanthine and derivatives can be beneficial in horses with heaves; however, plasma levels necessary for bronchodilation vary widely between horses and the range between effective and toxic concentrations is narrow.[205,206] Aminophylline (5–12 mg/kg IV) and theophylline (5–10 mg/kg, per os) administered every 12 hours improve lung function and clinical signs in up to 50% of RAO-affected horses.[195,207] Common side effects are hyperesthesia, hyperexcitability, and muscle tremors. Pentoxifylline (36 mg/kg, per os q 12 h for 14 days) administered to RAO-affected horses results in significant improvement in lung function and is not associated with adverse effects.[208]

Enhancement of mucociliary clearance

Mucociliary clearance may be enhanced by stimulation of the ciliary apparatus or by decreasing mucus viscoelasticity, but the latter appears to be the most important factor.[209] Different types of drugs can enhance clearance of respiratory secretions, including mucolytics (e.g. acetylcysteine, dembrexine hydrochloride) and drugs capable of improving mucociliary transport (e.g. clenbuterol).

Other treatments

Furosemide (1 mg/kg IV or aerosol) also results in significant improvement in the lung mechanics of RAO horses but not in arterial blood gases.[210] Antihistamine drugs are commonly used to treat RAO horses in the field, but they appear to have limited usefulness and no controlled study has proved their efficacy.

A technique of overhydration consisting in the intravenous administration of 30–40 L of isotonic saline solution over a 3–4 hour period has been advocated[211,212] but the method is not without risks including pulmonary edema, electrolyte abnormalities and death and a controlled study showed no benefit for the treatment of heaves.[213]

Aerosol therapy

Administration of therapeutic substances via inhalation has the advantage of delivering high concentration of the drug directly into the lungs while minimizing the amount absorbed systemically and, therefore, reducing the risk of adverse effects. In addition, systemic side effects and drug residue are decreased. Clinical response to aerosol medications is a function of the dose deposited in the airways, which is dependent on the delivery device, the particle size characteristics of the inhaled aerosol, the pattern of breathing, and airway disease.[214]

Airway narrowing increases aerosol deposition in central airways and results in poor deposition in peripheral airways.[214] In horses with RAO, aerosol deposition after administration of inhaled albuterol (360 µg) results in rapid (5 minutes) improvement in peripheral airway deposition.[104] Therefore, corticosteroid therapy for the treatment of RAO should be preceded by bronchodilation in order to maximize anti-inflammatory effectiveness.

Therapeutic aerosols can be produced by nebulizing a solution or administrating aerosols prepackaged in pressurized metered-dose inhalers (pMDI). Several types of device improve delivery of aerosol to the horse's lung such as facemask, nosepiece, and extension tubing (spacer or holding chamber). The fraction of drug deposited into the lungs varies between 0.3 and 7% for nebulizers and 6.1 and 31% for pMDI delivery devices (6.1%, AeroMask™, Fig. 28.13, 8.2%, Equine Haler™, Fig. 28.7, 18.2%, AeroHippus™, Fig. 28.7, 23.3% 3M Equine device).[215–218] The type of propellant used in pMDI is an important factor affecting lung deposition. Until recently, most propellants used were chlorofluorocarbons (CFC) but by the end of 2008 they have been replaced by hydrofluoroalkanes (HFA). Consequently, some of the drugs have been reformulated as solution with HFA instead of suspension (e.g. flunisolide, beclomethasone), resulting in a significantly reduced MMAD and improved lung deposition.[219] As a result, dose recommendation for beclomethasone HFA in people with asthma are approximately half of the dose with beclomethasone CFC. This improvement in lung deposition has not been observed for drugs that remained as suspension in HFA such as fluticasone or triamcinolone. The problem is that most equine studies published used pMDI with CFC except for one study with albuterol HFA.[220] In this context, lung deposition reported for AeroHippus (18.2%) was achieved using beclomethasone HFA while percentage of lung deposition using AeroMask and Equine Haler were obtained with fenoterol CFC and fluticasone HFA, respectively.

Corticosteroids

(See Table 28.3.) At least five different inhaled corticosteroids are available to treat inflammatory lung diseases in humans: beclomethasone dipropionate, budesonide, flunisolide, fluticasone propionate, and triamcinolone acetonide. A common test of potency for inhaled corticosteroids called the McKenzie skin blanching test allows relative ranking of the compounds from least to most potent (relative to dexamethasone potency = 1): flunisolide = triamcinolone acetonide (330) < beclomethasone dipropionate (600) < budesonide (980) < fluticasone propionate (1200).[221] At the time of this writing, only clinical trials with beclomethasone and fluticasone have been reported in the horse.

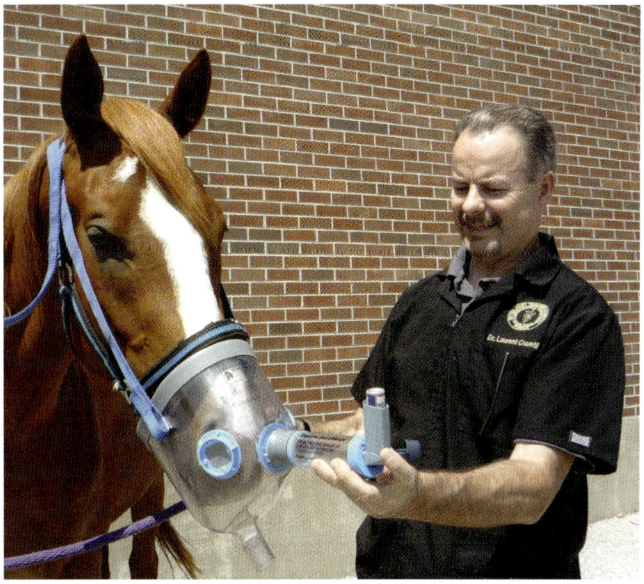

Fig 28.13 Aerosol delivery device for metered-dose inhaler or nebulization (Equine Aeromask™, Trudell Medical International, London, Ontario, Canada).

Clinical trials in horses with RAO indicate that beclomethasone dipropionate at a dose of 1000 µg twice a day administered with the 3M Equine device results in similar clinical and lung function improvement as 3750 µg twice a day administered with the AeroMask™.[222,223] An almost four-fold reduction in dose with the 3M device is consistent with the fact than lung deposition is approximately four times higher (23.3/6.1 = 3.8) with it than with the AeroMask. Therapeutic effects are measurable within 24 hours of administration. Administration of a low-dose of beclomethasone dipropionate (500 µg twice a day) to horses with heaves results in similar efficacy as highdose (>1500 µg twice a day) but with less adrenal suppression.[222] However, the 3M Equine device is no longer on the market. Also, these studies were conducted using CFC as propellant for beclomethasone dipropionate. Only HFA-propelled beclomethasone is currently available as pMDI. Because aerosolized particles of beclomethasone generated with HFA propellant have a lower MMAD, we can estimate that the dose needed to achieve the same effect in RAO-affected horses would be approximately half of the dose needed with CFC-propelled beclomethasone. Therefore, treatment of RAO with a dose equipotent to 3750 µg twice a day administered with the AeroMask™ would be ~ 1875 µg of beclomethasone HFA (3750/2 = 1875) twice a day using the same mask system or ~1250 µg of beclomethasone HFA (3750/3 = 1250) twice a day using an AeroHippus™. Similarly, lung deposition of beclomethasone HFA administered with the Equine Haler would be expected to double in comparison to CFC formulation (8.2 × 2 = 16.4%). Consequently, a dose equipotent to 3750 µg twice a day administered with the AeroMask™ would be ~ 1400 µg of beclomethasone HFA (3750 × 6.1/16.4 ~ 1400) twice a day. Future clinical trials would be required to determine if these estimated dosages can be confirmed.

Fluticasone propionate has been used successfully for the treatment of heaves in horses using 2000 µg twice daily (AeroMask).[224,225] A higher dose of fluticasone (6000 µg) is required to obtained a significant improvement in clinical signs and lung function in a shorter period of time (third day of therapy) using an Equine Haler.[226] Administration of fluticasone (3000 µg) prior to exposure to moldy hay can effectively prevent clinical disease and deterioration in lung function.[226] Treatment of horses with inhaled fluticasone (AeroMask) using 3000 µg twice a day results in adrenal suppression; however, no adrenal suppression is detectable with 2000 µg twice a day.[224,227] Fluticasone propionate is formulated as a suspension both in CFC- and HFA-propelled pMDI. Therefore, lung deposition in horses would be expected to be similar regardless of the type of propellant used as demonstrated in humans.[219]

Comparison of drug efficacies in the treatment of RAO suggest that fluticasone is approximately twice as potent as beclomethasone but currently available pMDI contain beclomethasone HFA that requires approximately twice less drug to achieve the same effect. Therefore, beclomethasone and fluticasone pMDI should be considered equipotent with currently available formulations.

Bronchodilators

The main classes of inhaled bronchodilators used in the horse are beta$_2$-agonists and anticholinergics (Table 28.3). Bronchodilators should not be used as sole therapy for a prolonged period of time because they do not suppress airway inflammation (except for clenbuterol, see IAD therapy) and lose efficacy after two weeks.[101,99]

Beta$_2$-agonists induce airway smooth muscle relaxation regardless of bronchoconstriction mechanism and also inhibit mast cell degranulation.[228] Albuterol, pirbuterol, and fenoterol are short-acting bronchodilators (one hour) with rapid onset of action (five minutes).[229–231] Some horses benefit from the effects of albuterol for up to seven hours.[232] Salmeterol and formoterol are long-acting beta$_2$-agonists (6–8 hours) suitable for twice daily dosing but with slow onset of action (15 minutes).[233] Salmeterol is currently not available as a standalone aerosol medication because of its association with an increased risk of severe asthma exacerbations and asthma-related death in people.

Ipratropium bromide is an anticholinergic drug chemically derived from atropine but devoid of side effects when administered by inhalation. Nebulization of 2 µg/kg causes bronchodilation for approximately six hours with a maximum effect obtained one hour after administration.[234] The effects of anticholinergic drugs on airway smooth muscle are additive to beta$_2$-agonists.[228]

Prognosis

A follow-up survey involving 51 RAO-affected horses revealed that the median survival time after diagnosis was eight years and that 87% of horses would be expected to survive three years after being diagnosed with RAO.[235] Seventy-nine percent of respondents had recurring episodes of heaves and 21% believed that the condition resolved. And while 21% of diagnosed horses were retired, 74% were still used in various athletic activities. These findings are good considering that >77% of horses were still fed hay and housed indoors for at least part of the day.[235] Some investigators found horses diagnosed with more severe disease to be more likely to die within 2–4 years or be euthanized, but others did not.[162,235,236]

Etiology and pathophysiology

Etiology

RAO is associated with exposure to high levels of organic molds particularly abundant in moldy hay and poorly ventilated stables.[237] Susceptible horses are allergic to inhaled spores, and exposure to an environment rich in molds triggers clinical signs within a few hours to a few days.[59,67] Clinical signs usually resolve within days of horses being removed from the dusty environment. Numerous studies have documented that traditional horse's management exposes them to high dust levels originating mainly from bedding and feed.[121,122,238–241] In addition, horses are exposed to higher levels of dust around the nose (breathing zone) than in the stable because of their feeding behavior.[122] As water content of hay at baling increases, mold growth rises to reach a maximum for hay baled at 35–50 % moisture.[242] Approximately 70 species of fungi and actinomycetes have been identified and among them thermophilic molds such as *Aspergillus fumigatus, Faenia rectivirgula* and *Thermoactinomyces vulgaris* are commonly present.[242] These spores have a small diameter (MMAD <5 µm), allowing them to be inhaled in peripheral airways (respirable particles) where they may trigger an inflammatory reaction.[119,243] Furthermore, BALF neutrophilia increases in a dose-dependent fashion as the quantity of inhaled dust rises.[244]

Horses are also exposed to higher endotoxin levels in stables than on pasture and that can potentiate the inflammatory response to inhaled molds.[121,245] Inhalation challenge using hay dust fractions suggests that endotoxin and other substances (e.g. β-glucans) exert a synergistic effect with molds for neutrophil recruitment to the lungs of RAO-affected horses.[246,247] Studies in humans and other species indicate that timing and dose of inhaled endotoxins also play a modulatory role in the induction of airway inflammation as early exposure during childhood may prevent later development of asthma in people but exposure later in life exacerbates airway inflammation and clinical signs.[248]

There is a strong genetic predisposition to RAO in particular bloodlines of Warmblood and Lipizzaner horses.[130,249] Two regions on equine chromosomes 13 and 15 have been associated to RAO and several candidate genes and protein products have been identified.[250,251] These findings strongly suggest that, as in human asthma, genetic susceptibility is an important factor contributing to the development of heaves.

Pathophysiology

RAO causes of exercise intolerance; however, few studies have attempted to understand the mechanisms responsible for this impaired performance. Horses with severe clinical signs are markedly hypoxemic and sometimes hypercapnic at rest, but blood gas values are not different from healthy controls during periods of disease remission.[59,197,252] Pronounced ventilation–perfusion mismatching is mainly responsible for these gas exchange abnormalities.[139,253,254] During submaximal exercise, gas exchanges worsen and these abnormalities are associated with decreased expired minute ventilation and increased work of breathing.[161] These changes likely increase oxygen consumption by respiratory and cardiac muscles and reduce the amount of oxygen available for exercising muscles, resulting in exercise intolerance.[161] This phenomenon has been demonstrated in humans where respiratory muscles consume 10–15% of maximum oxygen consumption in trained athletes and up to 50% in COPD patients.[255]

The cascade of event leading to pulmonary dysfunction starts shortly after susceptible horses are exposed to allergens. Circulating neutrophils are recruited to the lungs within four hours of an allergen challenge and are detectable in BALF in five hours.[119,256] The production of numerous inflammatory mediators is upregulated in respiratory secretions or blood of RAO horses after allergen challenge; however, the complex relationships between effector cells, inflammatory mediators, and clinical signs are still unclear.[251,257,258] The majority of studies suggest a predominant Th2-type lymphocyte response but other studies implicate a Th1 or Th17 bias as in human asthma.[146]

Epidemiology

RAO is an occupational disease of horses housed indoors and fed hay. It is more commonly diagnosed in parts of the world where summers are frequently humid (e.g. northern Europe, northeast of the United States) than in areas with warm and dry climate (e.g. Australia) with prevalence between 11 and 17% reported in Great Britain.[259,260] Conversely, summer pasture-associated RAO is commonly diagnosed in hot and humid climates (e.g. southern United States) where horses spend most of the time on pasture and the highest prevalence of the disease is observed between July and September.[147] Nevertheless, the condition is also diagnosed in areas where RAO is traditionally believed to be more prevalent and some horses can suffer from both conditions.[183,260] A strong genetic predisposition to RAO has been identified in some breeds such as Warmblood and Lippizan.[249]

Horses with RAO tend to be mature (>4 years) to old animals and an increased predilection in certain breeds such as Thoroughbred, American Trotter, Morgan and Arab has been reported by some but not others.[20,147,236,260] Duration of the disease varies from months to years, with periods of disease exacerbation (crisis) alternating with periods of clinical remission of variable duration. Hence, clinical signs are recurrent but the disease is permanent.[12]

Prevention

Inhaled dust particulates play a central role in the pathophysiology of RAO and management of the disease should always include recommendation to decrease environmental exposure. Small respirable particulates tend to be deposited in the lower airways where they can exert their pro-inflammatory effects. Among respirable dust particles, mold spores from hay and straw, including *Aspergillus fumigatus*, *Faenia rectivirgula* (previously called *Micropolyspora faeni*) and *Thermoactinomyces vulgaris*, have been directly implicated.[122,243,261] Two main approaches help reduce exposure of the horse's airways to respirable particles. The first approach is to use feedstuff and bedding that generate low dust levels with emphasis placed on low-dust feed (e.g. wood shavings, cardboard, haylage, soaking hay, grain with molasses).[144,145,241] The second approach is to increase removal of airborne particles and noxious gases by improving ventilation in the building.[262,263]

The ideal environment for horses with RAO is pasture because exposure to dust and endotoxin is significantly less than in stalls, regardless of feed and bedding quality.[121,239,245] If for practical reasons the horse cannot be kept on pasture at all times, ventilation in the barn and stall, the type of bedding, feedstuff, and general management should be scrutinized in order to minimize allergen exposure. However, owners need to realize that RAO horses kept on pasture but exposed to organic dust for just a few hours, such as when bringing horses indoors to be fed or during periods of inclement weather, may be sufficient to recruit inflammatory cells to the lungs, resulting in recurrence of clinical signs.[119,154]

Horses with summer pasture-associated RAO are generally affected between June and September when they spend more than half of each day on pasture.[147] Consequently, the recommended environment for these horses during the summer is low-dust indoor housing.[85,183]

The activity in the barn also affects dust exposure, with peak levels during the day, especially at the time of feeding and cleaning of the stalls, when dust levels can increase by more than 10-fold.[239] Therefore, dust-generating tasks such as cleaning stalls and sweeping floors should be performed when RAO-susceptible horses are outside the barn. Grooming also generates airborne dust particles and should be done outside or using a vacuum cleaner system.

References

1. Wilsher S, Allen WR, Wood JL. Factors associated with failure of Thoroughbred horses to train and race. Equine Vet J 2006;38:113–18.
2. Fraipont A, Van EE, Ramery E, et al. Subclinical diseases underlying poor performance in endurance horses: diagnostic methods and predictive tests. Vet Rec 2011;169:154.
3. Knight PK, Evans DL. Clinical abnormalities detected in post-race examinations of poorly performing Standardbreds. Aust Vet J 2000;78: 344–6.
4. Martin BB Jr, Reef VB, Parente EJ, et al. Causes of poor performance of horses during training, racing, or showing: 348 cases (1992–1996). J Am Vet Med Assoc 2000;216:554–8.
5. Perkins NR, Reid SWJ, Morris RS. Profiling the New Zealand Thoroughbred racing industry. 2. Conditions interfering with training and racing. New Zealand Vet J 2004;53: 69–76.
6. MacNamara B, Bauer S, Iafe J. Endoscopic evaluation of exercise-induced pulmonary hemorrhage and chronic obstructive pulmonary disease in association with poor performance in racing Standardbreds. J Am Vet Med Assoc 1990;196:443–5.
7. Holcombe SJ, Robinson NE, Derksen FJ, et al. Effect of tracheal mucus and tracheal cytology on racing performance in Thoroughbred racehorses. Equine Vet J 2006;38:300–4.
8. Widmer A, Doherr MG, Tessier C, et al. Association of increased tracheal mucus accumulation with poor willingness to perform in show-jumpers and dressage horses. Vet J 2009;182:430–5.
9. MacNamara B, Bauer S, Iafe J. Endoscopic evaluation of exercise-induced pulmonary hemorrhage and chronic obstructive pulmonary disease in association with poor performance in racing Standardbreds. J Am Vet Med Assoc 1990;196:443–5.
10. Allen KJ, Tremaine WH, Franklin SH. Prevalence of inflammatory airway disease in national hunt horses referred for investigation of poor athletic performance. Equine Vet J Suppl 2006;36:529–34.
11. Robinson NE, Karmaus W, Holcombe SJ, et al. Airway inflammation in Michigan pleasure horses: prevalence and risk factors. Equine Vet J 2006;38: 293–9.
12. Robinson N. International workshop on equine chronic airway disease. Equine Vet J 2001;33:5–19.
13. Couetil LL, Hoffman AM, Hodgson J, et al. Inflammatory airway disease of horses. J Vet Intern Med 2007;21: 356–61.
14. Rush Moore B, Krakowka S, Robertson JT, et al. Cytologic evaluation of

bronchoalveolar lavage fluid obtained from Standardbred racehorses with inflammatory airway disease. Am J Vet Res 1995;56:562–7.
15. Burrell M, Wood J, Whitwell K, et al. Respiratory disease in Thoroughbred horses in training: the relationships between disease and viruses, bacteria and environment. Vet Rec 1996;139: 308–13.
16. Wasko AJ, Barkema HW, Nicol J, et al. Evaluation of a risk-screening questionnaire to detect equine lung inflammation: results of a large field study. Equine Vet J 2011;43:145–52.
17. Sellon D. Investigating outbreaks of respiratory disease in older foals. Proceedings of the Am Assoc Equine Pract, 2001, 447–55.
18. Couetil L, Rosenthal F, DeNicola D, et al. Clinical signs, evaluation of bronchoalveolar lavage fluid, and assessment of pulmonary function in horses with inflammatory respiratory disease. Am J Vet Res 2001;62:538–46.
19. Koblinger K, Nicol J, McDonald K, et al. Endoscopic assessment of airway inflammation in horses. J Vet Intern Med 2011;25:1118–26.
20. Dixon P, Railton D, McGorum B. Equine pulmonary disease: a case control study of 300 referred cases. Part 2: Details of animals and of historical and clinical findings. Equine Vet J 1995;27:422–7.
21. Wood JL, Newton JR, Chanter N, et al. Inflammatory airway disease, nasal discharge and respiratory infections in young British racehorses. Equine Vet J 2005;37:236–42.
22. Christley RM, Hodgson DR, Rose RJ, et al. Coughing in Thoroughbred racehorses: risk factors and tracheal endoscopic and cytological findings. Vet Rec 2001;148:99–104.
23. Chapman P, Green C, Main J, et al. Retrospective study of the relationships between age, inflammation and the isolation of bacteria from the lower respiratory tract of Thoroughbred horses. Vet Rec 2000;146:91–5.
24. Vrins A, Doucet M, Nunez-Ochoa L. A retrospective study of bronchoalveolar lavage cytology in horses with clinical findings of small airway disease. J Vet Med A 1991;38:472–9.
25. Bracher V, von Fellenberg R, Winder CN, et al. An investigation of the incidence of chronic obstructive pulmonary disease (COPD) in random populations of Swiss horses. Equine Vet J 1991;23:136–41.
26. Couetil LL, DeNicola DB. Blood gas, plasma lactate and bronchoalveolar lavage cytology analyzes in racehorses with respiratory disease. Equine Vet J Suppl 1999;30:77–82.
27. Burrell MH. Endoscopic and virologic observations on respiratory disease in a group of young Thoroughbred horses in training. Equine Vet J 1985;17:99–103.
28. Gerber V. Mucus in equine lower airway disease. Proceedings of the World Equine Airway Symposium. 2001.
29. Gerber V, Robinson N, Luethi E, et al. Comparison of airway inflammation and mucus between younger versus older stabled clinically healthy horses. Proceedings of the World Equine Airway Symposium. 2001.
30. Christley RM, Hodgson DR, Rose RJ, et al. A case-control study of respiratory disease in Thoroughbred racehorses in Sydney, Australia. Equine Vet J 2001;33:256–64.
31. Bedenice D, Mazan MR, Hoffman AM. Association between cough and cytology of bronchoalveolar lavage fluid and pulmonary function in horses diagnosed with inflammatory airway disease. J Vet Intern Med 2008;22: 1022–8.
32. Wood JL, Newton JR, Chanter N, et al. Association between respiratory disease and bacterial and viral infections in British racehorses. J Clin Microbiol 2005;43:120–6.
33. Dixon PM, Railton DI, McGorum BC. Equine pulmonary disease: a case control study of 300 referred cases. Part 3: Ancillary diagnostic findings. Equine Vet J 1995;27:428–35.
34. Gerber V, Straub R, Marti E, et al. Endoscopic scoring of mucus quantity and quality: observer and horse variance and relationship to inflammation, mucus viscoelasticity and volume. Equine Vet J 2004;36:576–82.
35. Holcombe SJ, Robinson NE, Derksen FJ, et al. Effect of tracheal mucus and tracheal cytology on racing performance in Thoroughbred racehorses. Equine Vet J 2006;38:300–4.
36. Koch C, Straub R, Ramseyer A, et al. Endoscopic scoring of the tracheal septum in horses and its clinical relevance for the evaluation of lower airway health in horses. Equine Vet J 2007;39:107–12.
37. Beech J. Tracheobronchial aspirates. In: Beech J, editor. Equine respiratory disorders. Philadelphia: Lea & Febiger; 1991. p. 41–53.
38. Mair T, Stokes C, Bourne F. Cellular content of secretions obtained by lavage from different levels of the equine respiratory tract. Equine Vet J 1987;19:458–62.
39. Christley RM, Hodgson DR, Rose RJ, et al. Comparison of bacteriology and cytology of tracheal fluid samples collected by percutaneous transtracheal aspiration or via an endoscope using a plugged, guarded catheter. Equine Vet J 1999;31:197–202.
40. Christley RM, Hodgson DR, Rose RJ, et al. A case-control study of respiratory disease in Thoroughbred racehorses in Sydney, Australia. Equine Vet J 2001;33: 256–64.
41. Malikides N, Hughes KJ, Hodgson JL. Comparison of tracheal aspirates before and after high-speed treadmill exercise in racehorses. Aust Vet J 2007;85: 414–19.
42. Chapman P, Green C, Main J, et al. Retrospective study of the relationships between age, inflammation and the isolation of bacteria from the lower respiratory tract of Thoroughbred horses. Vet Rec 2000;146:91–5.
43. Robinson NE, Karmaus W, Holcombe SJ, et al. Airway inflammation in Michigan pleasure horses: prevalence and risk factors. Equine Vet J 2006;38: 293–9.
44. Cardwell JM, Wood JL, Smith KC, et al. Descriptive results from a longitudinal study of airway inflammation in British National Hunt racehorses. Equine Vet J 2011;43:750–5.
45. Larson V, Busch R. Equine tracheobronchial lavage: comparison of lavage cytology and pulmonary histopathologic findings. Am J Vet Res 1985;46:144–6.
46. Derksen F, Brown C, Sonea B. Comparison of transtracheal aspirate and bronchoalveolar lavage cytology in 50 horses. Equine Vet J 1989;21:23–6.
47. Winder N, Gruenig G, Hermann M, et al. Comparison of respiratory secretions cytology and pulmonary histology in horses. J Vet Med A 1989;36:32–8.
48. Viel L. Structural-functional correlations of the lung in horses with small airway disease. Thesis, 1983. University of Guelph, Canada.
49. Malikides N, Hughes KJ, Hodgson DR, et al. Comparison of tracheal aspirates and bronchoalveolar lavage in racehorses. 2. Evaluation of the diagnostic significance of neutrophil percentage. Aust Vet J 2003;81:685–7.
50. Rush Moore B. Lower respiratory tract disease. Vet Clin North Am Equine Pract 1996;12:457–72.
51. Hoffman AM. Bronchoalveolar lavage technique and cytological diagnosis of small airway inflammatory disease. Equine Vet Edu 1999;11:330–6.
52. Couetil L, DeNicola D. Blood gas, plasma lactate, and bronchoalveolar lavage cytology analyzes in racehorses with respiratory disease. Equine Vet J 1999;30:77–82.
53. Sanchez A, Couetil LL, Ward MP, et al. Effect of airway disease on blood gas exchange in racehorses. J Vet Intern Med 2005;19:87–92.
54. Courouce-Malblanc A, Pronost S, Fortier G, et al. Physiological measurements and upper and lower respiratory tract evaluation in French Standardbred Trotters during a standardised exercise

test on the treadmill. Equine Vet J Suppl 2002;34:402–7.

55. Hoffman AM, Oura TJ, Riedelberger KJ, et al. Plethysmographic comparison of breathing pattern in heaves (recurrent airway obstruction) versus experimental bronchoconstriction or hyperpnea in horses. J Vet Intern Med 2007;21:184–92.
56. Nolen-Walston RD, Kuehn H, Boston RC, et al. Reproducibility of airway responsiveness in horses using flowmetric plethysmography and histamine bronchoprovocation. J Vet Intern Med 2009;23:631–5.
57. Gillespie J, Tyler W, Eberly V. Pulmonary ventilation and resistance in emphysematous and control horses. J Appl Physiol 1966;21:416–22.
58. Derksen F, Robinson N, Slocombe R, et al. Pulmonary function tests in standing ponies: reproducibility and effect of vagal blockade. Am J Vet Res 1982;43:598–602.
59. Tesarowski DB, Viel L, McDonell WN. Pulmonary function measurements during repeated environmental challenge of horses with recurrent airway obstruction (heaves). Am J Vet Res 1996;57:1214–19.
60. Rush B, Raub E, Rhoads W, et al. Pulmonary function in horses with recurrent airway obstruction after aerosol and parenteral administration of beclomethasone dipropionate and dexamethasone, respectively. Am J Vet Res 1998;59:1039–43.
61. Petsche V, Derksen F, Robinson N. Tidal breathing flow-volume loops in horses with recurrent airway obstruction (heaves). Am J Vet Res 1994;55:885–91.
62. Pirrone F, Albertini M, Clement MG, et al. Respiratory mechanics in Standardbred horses with sub-clinical inflammatory airway disease and poor athletic performance. Vet J 2007;173:144–50.
63. Couetil L, Rosenthal F, Simpson C. Forced expiration: a test for airflow obstruction in horses. J Appl Physiol 2000;88:1870–9.
64. Hoffman A, Mazan M. Programme of lung function testing horses suspected with small airway disease. Equine Vet Educ 1999;11:322–8.
65. Richard EA, Fortier GD, Denoix JM, et al. Influence of subclinical inflammatory airway disease on equine respiratory function evaluated by impulse oscillometry. Equine Vet J 2009;41:384–9.
66. Hoffman A, Kuehn H, Riedelberger K, et al. Flowmetric comparison of respiratory inductance plethysmography and pneumotachography in horses. J Appl Physiol 2001;91:2767–75.
67. Derksen FJ, Robinson NE, Armstrong PJ, et al. Airway reactivity in ponies with recurrent airway obstruction (heaves). J Appl Physiol 1985;58:598–604.
68. Hoffman A, Mazan M, Ellenberg S. Association between bronchoalveolar lavage cytologic features and airway reactivity in horses with a history of exercise intolerance. Am J Vet Res 1998;59:176–81.
69. Hare J, Viel L. Pulmonary eosinophilia associated with increased airway responsiveness in young racing horses. J Vet Intern Med 1998;12:163–70.
70. Hare JE, Viel L, O'Byrne PM, et al. Effect of sodium cromoglycate on light racehorses with elevated metachromatic cell numbers on bronchoalveolar lavage and reduced exercise tolerance. J Vet Pharmacol Therap 1994;17:237–44.
71. Beekman L, Tohver T, Dardari R, et al. Evaluation of suitable reference genes for gene expression studies in bronchoalveolar lavage cells from horses with inflammatory airway disease. BMC Mol Biol. 2011;12:5.
72. Hughes KJ, Nicolson L, Da CN, et al. Evaluation of cytokine mRNA expression in bronchoalveolar lavage cells from horses with inflammatory airway disease. Vet Immunol Immunopathol 2011;140:82–9.
73. Derksen F, Scott J, Miller D, et al. Bronchoalveolar lavage in ponies with recurrent airway obstruction (heaves). Am Rev Respir Dis 1985;132:1066–70.
74. Tremblay G, Ferland C, Lapointe J-M, et al. Effect of stabling on bronchoalveolar cells obtained from normal and COPD horses. Equine Vet J 1993;25:194–7.
75. Miskovic M, Couetil LL, Thompson CA. Lung function and airway cytologic profiles in horses with recurrent airway obstruction maintained in low-dust environments. J Vet Intern Med 2007;21:1060–6.
76. Dixon P, Railton D, McGorum B. Equine pulmonary disease: a case control study of 300 referred cases. Part 1: Examination, techniques, diagnostic criteria and diagnoses. Equine Vet J 1995;27:416–21.
77. Christley RM, Hodgson DR, Rose RJ, et al. Comparison of bacteriology and cytology of tracheal fluid samples collected by percutaneous transtracheal aspiration or via an endoscope using a plugged, guarded catheter. Equine Vet J 1999;31:197–202.
78. Mair TS, Stokes CR, Bourne FJ. Cellular content of secretions obtained by lavage from different levels of the equine respiratory tract. Equine Vet J 1987;19:458–62.
79. Derksen FJ, Brown CM, Sonea I, et al. Comparison of transtracheal aspirate and bronchoalveolar lavage cytology in 50 horses with chronic lung disease. Equine Vet J 1989;21:23–6.
80. Persson S, Lindberg R. Lung biopsy pathology and exercise tolerance in horses with chronic bronchiolitis. ICEEP Proceedings 1991;3:457–64.
81. Nyman G, Bjork M, Funkquist P. Gas exchange during exercise in Standardbred trotters with mild bronchiolitis. Equine Vet J 1999;30(Suppl.):96–101.
82. Laumen E, Doherr MC, Gerber V. Relationship of horse owner assessed respiratory signs index to characteristics of recurrent airway obstruction in two Warmblood families. Equine Vet J 2010;42:142–8.
83. Wilson W. Equine influenza. Vet Clin North Am Equine Pract 1993;9:257–82.
84. Kastner S, Haines D, Archer J, et al. Investigations on the ability of clenbuterol hydrochloride to reduce clinical signs and inflammation associated with equine influenza A infection. Equine Vet J 1999;31:160–8.
85. Seahorn T, Beadle R. Summer pasture-associated obstructive pulmonary disease in horses: 21 cases. J Am Vet Med Assoc 1993;202:779–82.
86. Costa LR, Eades SC, Venugopal CS, et al. Plasma and pulmonary fluid endothelin in horses with seasonal recurrent airway obstruction. J Vet Intern Med 2009;23:1239–46.
87. Burks B. Parasitic pneumonitis. Compend Contin Educ Pract Vet 1998;20:378–82.
88. Hermann M, Gruning G, Bracher V, et al. Eosinophile granulozyten im tracheobronchialsekret von pferden: anhaltspunkt fur eine parasitare lungenerkrankung? Schweiz Arch Tierheilk 1988;130:19–28.
89. Darien B. Eosinophilic pneumonitis in foals and horses. Compend Contin Educ Pract Vet 1994;16:1210–12.
90. Beech J, Sweeney C. Infections caused by bacteria, mycoplasmas, parasites, and fungi. In: Beech J, editor. Equine respiratory disorders. Malvern: Lea & Febiger; 1991. p. 181–207.
91. Lyons E, Tolliver S, Drudge J, et al. Parasites in lungs of dead equids in Kentucky: emphasis on *Dictyocaulus arnfieldi*. Am J Vet Res 1985;46:924–7.
92. Viel L. Small airway disease as a vanguard for chronic obstructive pulmonary disease. Vet Clin North Am: Equine Pract 1997;13:549–60.
93. Ramzan PH, Parkin TD, Shepherd MC. Lower respiratory tract disease in Thoroughbred racehorses: analysis of endoscopic data from a UK training yard. Equine Vet J 2008;40:7–13.
94. Weese JS, Sabino C. Scrutiny of antimicrobial use in racing horses with allergic small airway inflammatory disease. Can Vet J 2005;46:438–9.
95. Spendlove PJ, Hodgson JL, Hodgson DR. Prevention and control of lower

airway inflammation in horses. 08/051, 1–61. Kingston, Rural Industries Research and Development Corporation; 2008.

96. Bertin FR, Ivester KM, Couetil LL. Comparative efficacy of inhaled albuterol between two hand-held delivery devices in horses with recurrent airway obstruction. Equine Vet J 2011;43:393–8.
97. Couetil LL, Rosenthal FS, DeNicola DB, et al. Clinical signs, evaluation of bronchoalveolar lavage fluid, and assessment of pulmonary function in horses with inflammatory respiratory disease. Am J Vet Res 2001;62:538–46.
98. Hare JE, Viel L. Pulmonary eosinophilia associated with increased airway responsiveness in young racing horses. J Vet Intern Med 1998;12:163–70.
99. Read JR, Boston RC, Abraham G, et al. Effect of prolonged administration of clenbuterol on airway reactivity and sweating in horses with inflammatory airway disease. Am J Vet Res 2012;73: 140–5.
100. Laan TT, Bull S, van Nieuwstadt RA, et al. The effect of aerosolized and intravenously administered clenbuterol and aerosolized fluticasone propionate on horses challenged with *Aspergillus fumigatus* antigen. Vet Res Commun 2006;30:623–35.
101. Laan TT, Bull S, Pirie RS, et al. The anti-inflammatory effects of IV administered clenbuterol in horses with recurrent airway obstruction. Vet J 2006;171:429–37.
102. Laan TT, Bull S, Pirie RS, et al. Evaluation of cytokine production by equine alveolar macrophages exposed to lipopolysaccharide, *Aspergillus fumigatus*, and a suspension of hay dust. Am J Vet Res 2005;66:1584–9.
103. van den Hoven R, Duvigneau JC, Hartl RT, et al. The expression of messenger RNA for tumor necrosis factor-α, interleukins 1β, 6, 8, and 10, tissue growth factor-β, and interferon-γ in bronchoalveolar lavage fluid cells from horses challenged with lipopolysaccharide and treated with clenbuterol. J Equine Vet Sci 2004;24:29–36.
104. Rush B, Hoskinson J, Davis E, et al. Pulmonary distribution of aerosolized technetium Tc 99m pentetate after administration of a single dose of aerosolized albuterol sulfate in horses with recurrent airway obstruction. Am J Vet Res 1999;60:764–9.
105. Rush Moore B, Krakowka S, Cummins J. Changes in airway inflammatory cell populations in Standardbred racehorses after interferon administration. Vet Immunol Immunopathol 1996;49:347.
106. Moore I, Horney B, Day K, et al. Treatment of inflammatory airway disease in young standardbreds with interferon alpha. Can Vet J 2004;45: 594–601.
107. Rush Moore B, Krakowka S, McVey D, et al. Inflammatory markers in bronchoalveolar lavage fluid of Standardbred racehorses with inflammatory airway disease: response to interferon-alpha. Equine Vet J 1997;29:142–7.
108. Evans D, Rollins J, Huff G, et al. Inactivated *Propionobacterium acnes* (Immunoregulin) as adjunct to conventional therapy in the treatment of equine respiratory diseases. Equine Pract 1988;10:17–21.
109. Klimczak C. Immunostimulant quickly aids weanling equine respiratory disease complex (ERDC) cases. Equine Vet Sci 1992;12:68–9.
110. Fogarty U, Buckley T. Bronchoalveolar lavage findings in horses with exercise intolerance. Equine Vet J 1991;23: 434–7.
111. Wood J, Burrell M, Roberts C, et al. Streptococci and *Pasteurella* spp. associated with disease of the equine lower respiratory tract. Equine Vet J 1993;25:314–18.
112. Sweeney C, Beech J, Roby K. Bacterial isolates from tracheobronchial aspirates of healthy horses. Am J Vet Res 1985;46:2562.
113. Nuytten J, Muylle E, Oyaert W, et al. Cytology, bacteriology and phagocytic capacity of tracheo-bronchial aspirates in healthy horses and horses with chronic obstructive pulmonary disease (COPD). Zentralbl Veterinarmed A 1983;30:114–20.
114. Fortier G, Van EE, Fortier C, et al. Herpesviruses in respiratory liquids of horses: putative implication in airway inflammation and association with cytological features. Vet Microbiol 2009;139:34–41.
115. Dunowska M, Howe L, Hanlon D, et al. Kinetics of Equid herpesvirus type 2 infections in a group of Thoroughbred foals. Vet Microbiol 2011;152:176–80.
116. Holcombe S, Jackson C, Gerber V, et al. Stabling is associated with airway inflammation in young Arabian horses. Equine Vet J 2001;33:244–9.
117. Michelotto PV Jr, Muehlmann LA, Zanatta AL, et al. Platelet-activating factor and evidence of oxidative stress in the bronchoalveolar fluid of Thoroughbred colts during race training. J Vet Intern Med 2010;24: 414–19.
118. Pirie R, Dixon P, Collie D. Pulmonary and systemic effects of inhaled endotoxin in control and heaves horses. Equine Vet J 2001;33:311–18.
119. McGorum B, Dixon P, Halliwell R. Responses of horses affected with chronic obstructive pulmonary disease to inhalation challenges with mould antigens. Equine Vet J 1993;25:261–7.
120. Couetil L, Hunt M, Rosenthal F. Effects of dust and endotoxin exposures on lung function and airway cytology of horses. Lunn, DP and Wade, JF. Equine immunology [No. 4], 86. Newmarket, UK, R & W Publications. Havemeyer Foundation Monograph Series; 2001.
121. McGorum B, Ellison J, Cullen R. Total and respirable airborne dust endotoxin concentrations in three equine management systems. Equine Vet J 1998;30:430–4.
122. Woods P, Robinson N, Swanson M, et al. Airborne dust and aeroallergen concentration in a horse stable under two different management systems. Equine Vet J 1993;25:208–13.
123. Mills P, Roberts C, Smith N. Effects of ozone and airway inflammation on glutathione status and iron homeostasis in the lungs of horses. Am J Vet Res 1996;57:1359–63.
124. Davis M, Foster W. Inhalation toxicology in the equine respiratory tract. In: Lekeux P, editor. Equine respiratory diseases. Ithaca, NY: International Veterinary Information Services (www.ivis.org); 2002.
125. Tyler W, Jones J, Birks E. Effects of ozone on exercising horses: a preliminary report. ICEEP Proceedings 1991;3:490–502.
126. Davis MS, Williams CC, Meinkoth JH, et al. Influx of neutrophils and persistence of cytokine expression in airways of horses after performing exercise while breathing cold air. Am J Vet Res 2007;68:185–9.
127. Hobo S, Oikawa M-A, Kuwano A, et al. Effect of transportation on the composition of bronchoalveolar lavage fluid obtained from horses. Am J Vet Res 1997;58:531–4.
128. Raidal S, Bailey G, Love D. Effect of transportation on lower respiratory tract contamination and peripheral blood neutrophil function. Aust Vet J 1997;75:433–8.
129. Raidal S, Love D, Bailey G. Effect of a single bout of high intensity exercise on lower respiratory tract contamination in the horse. Aust Vet J 1997;75:293–5.
130. Marti E, Gerber H, Essich G, et al. The genetic basis of equine allergic disease. 1: Chronic hypersensitivity bronchitis. Equine Vet J 1991;23:457–60.
131. Morrison J. Asthma and COPD genetics and genomics: an overview. In: Hansel T, Barnes P, editors. New drugs for asthma, allergy and COPD. New York: Karger; 2001. p. 358–60.
132. Gerber V, Baleri D, Klukowska-Rotzler J, et al. Mixed inheritance of equine recurrent airway obstruction. J Vet Intern Med 2009;23:626–30.
133. Wagner P, Gillespie J, Landgren G, et al. Mechanism of exercise-induced hypoxemia in horses. J Appl Physiol 1989;66:1227–33.

134. Art T, Lekeux P. Ventilatory and arterial blood gas tension adjustments to strenuous exercise in standardbreds. Am J Vet Res 1995;56:1332–7.
135. Persson S. On blood volume and working capacity in horses. Studies of methodology and physiological and pathological variations. Acta Vet Scand 1967, Suppl 19.9:189.
136. Persson S. Evaluation of exercise tolerance and fitness in the performance horse. In: Snow D, Persson S, Rose R, editors. Equine exercise physiology. Cambridge: Granta Editions; 1983. p. 441–57.
137. Funkquist P, Nyman G, Persson S. Hemodynamic responses to exercise in trotters with red cell hypervolemia and exercise induced pulmonary hemorrhage. Proceedings of the 10th International Conference of Racing Analysts and Veterinarians 1994, 165–7.
138. Davis J, Manohar M. Effect of splenectomy on exercise-induced pulmonary and systemic hypertension in ponies. Am J Vet Res 1988;49: 1169–72.
139. Nyman G, Lindberg R, Weckner D, et al. Pulmonary gas exchange correlated to clinical signs and lung pathology in horses with chronic bronchiolitis. Equine Vet J 1991;23:253–60.
140. Eberly V, Tyler W, Gillespie J. Cardiovascular parameters in emphysematous and control horses. J Appl Physiol 1966;21:883–9.
141. Christley RM, Hodgson DR, Evans DL, et al. Effects of training on the development of exercise-induced arterial hypoxemia in horses. Am J Vet Res 1997;58:653–7.
142. Morris EA, Seeherman HJ. Clinical evaluation of poor performance in the racehorse: the results of 275 evaluations. Equine Vet J 1991;23: 169–74.
143. Riihimaki M, Raine A, Elfman L, et al. Markers of respiratory inflammation in horses in relation to seasonal changes in air quality in a conventional racing stable. Can J Vet Res 2008;72:432–9.
144. Clements JM, Pirie RS. Respirable dust concentrations in equine stables. Part 1: validation of equipment and effect of various management systems. Res Vet Sci 2007;83:256–62.
145. Clements JM, Pirie RS. Respirable dust concentrations in equine stables. Part 2: the benefits of soaking hay and optimising the environment in a neighbouring stable. Res Vet Sci 2007;83:263–8.
146. Leclere M, Lavoie-Lamoureux A, Lavoie JP. Heaves, an asthma-like disease of horses. Respirology 2011;16:1027–46.
147. Seahorn T, Groves M, Harrington K, et al. Chronic obstructive pulmonary disease in horses in Louisiana. J Am Vet Med Assoc 1996;208:248–51.
148. Broadstone R, Gray P, Robinson N, et al. Effects of xylazine on airway function in ponies with recurrent airway obstruction. Am J Vet Res 1992;53: 1813–17.
149. Lavoie J, Phan S, Blais D. Effects of a combination of detomidine and butorphanol on respiratory function in horses with or without chronic obstructive pulmonary disease. Am J Vet Res 1996;57:705–9.
150. Reitemeyer H, Klein H-J, Deegen E. The effect of sedatives on lung function in horses. Acta Vet Scand 1986;82:111–20.
151. Pickles K, Pirie R, Rhind S, et al. Cytological analysis of equine bronchoalveolar lavage fluid. Part 1: comparison of sequential and pooled aliquots. Equine Vet J 2002;34:288–91.
152. Wisner E, O'brien T, Lakritz J, et al. Radiographic and microscopic correlation of diffuse interstitial and bronchointerstitial pulmonary patterns in the caudodorsal lung of adult Thoroughbred horses in race training. Equine Vet J 1993;25:293–8.
153. Robinson N, Olszewski M, Boehler D, et al. Relationship between clinical signs and lung function in horses with recurrent airway obstruction (heaves) during a bronchodilator trial. Equine Vet J 2000;32:393–400.
154. Fairbairn S, Lees P, Page C, et al. Duration of antigen-induced hyperresponsiveness in horses with allergic respiratory disease and possible links with early airway obstruction. J Vet Pharmacol Therap 1993;16:469–76.
155. Armstrong P, Derksen F, Slocombe R, et al. Airway responses to aerosolized methacholine and citric acid in ponies with recurrent airway obstruction (heaves). Am Rev Respir Dis 1986;133: 357–61.
156. Doucet M, Vrins A, Ford-Hutchinson A. Histamine inhalation challenge in normal horses and in horses with small airway disease. Can J Vet Res 1991;55: 285–93.
157. Klein H-J, Deegen E. Histamine inhalation provocation test: method to identify nonspecific airway reactivity in equids. Am J Vet Res 1986;47: 1796–800.
158. Mazan M, Hoffman A, Manjerovic N. Comparison of forced oscillation with the conventional method for histamine bronchoprovocation testing in horses. Am J Vet Res 1999;60:174–80.
159. Willoughby R, McDonnell W. Pulmonary function testing in horses. Vet Clin North Am Large Anim Pract 1979;1:171–97.
160. Gillespie J, Tyler W. Chronic alveolar emphysema in the horse. Adv Vet Sci Comp Med 1969;13:99.
161. Art T, Duvivier D, Votion D, et al. Does an acute COPD crisis modify the cardiorespiratory and ventilatory adjustments to exercise in horses? J Appl Physiol 1998;84:845–52.
162. Naylor J, Clark E, Clayton H. Chronic obstructive pulmonary disease: usefulness of clinical signs, bronchoalveolar lavage, and lung biopsy as diagnostic and prognostic aids. Can Vet J 1992;33:591–8.
163. Rodrigues Costa L, Seahorn T, Moore R, et al. Correlation of clinical score, intrapleural pressure, cytologic findings of bronchoalveolar fluid, and histopathologic lesions of pulmonary tissue in horses with summer pasture-associated obstructive pulmonary disease. Am J Vet Res 2000;61:167–73.
164. McGorum B, Dixon P, Halliwell R, et al. Comparison of cellular and molecular components of bronchoalveolar lavage fluid harvested from different segments of the equine lung. Res Vet Science 1993;55:57–9.
165. Thurlbeck W, Lowell F. Heaves in horses. Am Rev Respir Dis 1964;89: 82–8.
166. Kaup F, Drommer W, Damsch S, et al. Ultrastructural findings in horses with chronic obstructive pulmonary disease (COPD) II: pathomorphological changes of the terminal airways and the alveolar region. Equine Vet J 1990;22:349–55.
167. Herszberg B, Ramos-Barbon D, Tamaoka M, et al. Heaves, an asthma-like equine disease, involves airway smooth muscle remodeling. J Allergy Clin Immunol 2006;118:382–8.
168. Kaup F, Drommer W, Deegen E. Ultrastructural findings in horses with chronic obstructive pulmonary disease (COPD) I: alterations of the larger conducting airways. Equine Vet J 1990;22:343–8.
169. Breeze R. Heaves. Vet Clin North Am Large Anim Pract 1979;1:219–30.
170. Foley F, Lowell F. Equine centrilobular emphysema. Am Rev Respir Dis 1966;93:17–21.
171. Port C, Ketels K, Coffin D, et al. A comparison study of experimental and spontaneous emphysema. J Toxicol Environ Health 1977;2:589–604.
172. Carr E, Carlson G, Wilson W, et al. Acute hemorrhagic pulmonary infarction and necrotizing pneumonia in horses: 21 cases (1967–1993). J Am Vet Med Assoc 1997;210:1774–8.
173. Hoffman A, Viel L, Prescott J, et al. Association of microbiologic flora with clinical signs, endoscopic, and pulmonary cytologic findings in foals with distal respiratory tract infections. Am J Vet Res 1993;54:1615–22.
174. Wong DM, Belgrave RL, Williams KJ, et al. Multinodular pulmonary fibrosis in five horses. J Am Vet Med Assoc 2008;232:898–905.
175. Bell SA, Drew CP, Wilson WD, et al. Idiopathic chronic eosinophilic

pneumonia in 7 horses. J Vet Intern Med 2008;22:648–53.

176. Pusterla N, Pesavento PA, Smith P, et al. Idiopathic granulomatous pneumonia in seven horses. Vet Rec 2003;153: 653–5.

177. Lavoie JP, Dalle S, Breton L, et al. Bronchiectasis in three adult horses with heaves. J Vet Intern Med 2004;18: 757–60.

178. Mansmann R, Carlson G, White N. Synchronous diaphragmatic flutter in horses. J Am Vet Med Assoc 1974;165: 265–70.

179. Couetil LL, Chilcoat CD, DeNicola DB, et al. Randomized, controlled study of inhaled fluticasone propionate, oral administration of prednisone, and environmental management of horses with recurrent airway obstruction. Am J Vet Res 2005;66:1665–74.

180. Jackson C, Berney C, Jefcoat A, et al. Environment and prednisone interactions in the treatment of recurrent airway obstruction (heaves). Equine Vet J 2000;32:432–8.

181. Thomson J, McPherson E. Effect of environmental control on pulmonary function of horses affected with chronic obstructive pulmonary disease. Equine Vet J 1984;16:35–8.

182. Costa LR, Johnson JR, Baur ME, et al. Temporal clinical exacerbation of summer pasture-associated recurrent airway obstruction and relationship with climate and aeroallergens in horses. Am J Vet Res 2006;67:1635–42.

183. Mair T. Obstructive pulmonary disease in 18 horses at summer pasture. Vet Rec 1996;138:89–91.

184. Lapointe J-M, Lavoie J-P, Vrins AA. Effects of triamcinolone acetonide on pulmonary function and bronchoalveolar lavage cytologic features in horses with chronic obstructive pulmonary disease. Am J Vet Res 1993;54:1310–16.

185. Cornelisse CJ, Robinson NE, Berney CE, et al. Efficacy of oral and intravenous dexamethasone in horses with recurrent airway obstruction. Equine Vet J 2004;36:426–30.

186. Rush B, Flaminio J, Matson C, et al. Cytologic evaluation of bronchoalveolar lavage fluid from horses with recurrent airway obstruction after aerosol and parenteral administration of beclomethasone dipropionate and dexamethasone, respectively. Am J Vet Res 1998;59:1033–8.

187. Robinson NE, Jackson C, Jefcoat A, et al. Efficacy of three corticosteroids for the treatment of heaves. Equine Vet J 2002;34:17–22.

188. Rush B, Worster A, Flaminio M, et al. Alteration in adrenocortical function in horses with recurrent airway obstruction after aerosol and parenteral administration of beclomethasone dipropionate and dexamethasone, respectively. Am J Vet Res 1998;59: 1044–7.

189. Toutain PL, Brandon RA, de Pomyers H. Dexamethasone and prednisolone in the horse: pharmacokinetics and action on the adrenal gland. Am J Vet Res 1984;45:1750–6.

190. Robinson N, Jackson C, Jefcoat A, et al. Efficacy of three corticosteroids for the treatment of recurrent airway obstruction (heaves). Equine Vet J 2002;34:17–22.

191. Couetil LL, Art T, de MB, et al. Effect of beclomethasone dipropionate and dexamethasone isonicotinate on lung function, bronchoalveolar lavage fluid cytology, and transcription factor expression in airways of horses with recurrent airway obstruction. J Vet Intern Med 2006;20:399–406.

192. Peroni D, Stanley S, Kollias-Baker C, et al. Prednisone per os is likely to have limited efficacy in horses. Equine Vet J 2002;34:283–7.

193. Courouce-Malblanc A, Fortier G, Pronost S, et al. Comparison of prednisolone and dexamethasone effects in the presence of environmental control in heaves-affected horses. Vet J 2008;175:227–33.

194. Abraham G, Brodde OE, Ungemach FR. Regulation of equine lymphocyte beta-adrenoceptors under the influence of clenbuterol and dexamethasone. Equine Vet J 2002;34:587–93.

195. Pearson E, Riebold T. Comparison of bronchodilators in alleviating clinical signs in horses with chronic obstructive pulmonary disease. J Am Vet Med Assoc 1989;194:1287–91.

196. Murphy J, McPherson E, Dixon P. Chronic obstructive pulmonary disease (COPD): Effects of bronchodilator drugs on normal and affected horses. Equine Vet J 1980;12:10–14.

197. Broadstone R, Scott J, Derksen F, et al. Effects of atropine in ponies with recurrent airway obstruction. J Appl Physiol 1988;65:2720–5.

198. Ducharme N, Fubini S. Gastrointestinal complications associated with the use of atropine in horses. J Am Vet Med Assoc 1983;182:229–31.

199. Hammer J, Perez-Moreno C, Miskovic M, et al. Effects of N-butyl scopolammonium bromide on lung function and clinical signs of horses with recurrent airway obstruction. The 27th Symposium of the Veterinary Comparative Respiratory Society. 2009.

200. Erichsen D, Aviad A, Schultz R, et al. Clinical efficacy and safety of clenbuterol HCl when administered to effect in horses with chronic obstructive pulmonary disease (COPD). Equine Vet J 1994;26:331–6.

201. Turgut K, Sasse H. Influence of clenbuterol on mucociliary transport in horses with chronic obstructive pulmonary disease. Vet Rec 1989;12:526–30.

202. Sleeper M, Kearns C, McKeever K. Chronic clenbuterol administration negatively alters cardiac function. Med Sci Sports Exerc 2001;34:643–50.

203. Beekley MD, Ideus JM, Brechue WF, et al. Chronic clenbuterol administration alters myosin heavy chain composition in standardbred mares. Vet J 2003;165:234–9.

204. Torneke M, Ingvast-Larsson J, Johansson J, et al. Pharmacokinetics and pharmacodynamics of terbutaline in healthy horses. Am J Vet Res 2000;61:761–5.

205. McKiernan B, Koritz G, Scott J, et al. Plasma theophylline concentration and lung function in ponies with recurrent obstructive lung disease. Equine Vet J 1990;22:194–7.

206. Ayres J, Pearson E, Riebold T, et al. Theophylline and dyphylline pharmacokinetics in the horse. Am J Vet Res 1985;46:2500–6.

207. Nuytten J, Deprez P, Picavet T, et al. Euphillin treatment of horses suffering from COPD. Vlaams Diergeneeskundig Tijdschift 1988;57:271–7.

208. Leguillette R, Deseveaux C, Lavoie J. Effects of pentoxifyline on pulmonary function and results of cytological examination of bronchoalveolar lavage fluid in horses with recurrent airway obstruction. Am J Vet Res 2002;63: 459–63.

209. Gerber V, Gehr P, Straub R, et al. Microscopic investigation of mucus qualities, mucus transport velocity and ciliary beat frequency on horse tracheal epithelium. Respir Physiol 1997;107: 67–74.

210. Broadstone R, Robinson N, Gray P, et al. Effect of furosemide on ponies with recurrent airway obstruction. Pulm Pharmacol 1991;4:203–8.

211. Deegen E. Neure methoden der behandlung chronisch hustender pferde. Prakt Tierarzt 1982;63:55–7.

212. Bosler K. Langzeiterfolg der NaCl-hyperinfusions-therapie beim pferd mit chronisch obstruktiver bronchitis. Pferdeheilkunde 1986;2:197–200.

213. Jean D, Vrins A, Lavoie JP. Respiratory and metabolic effects of massive administration of isotonic saline solution in heaves-affected and control horses. Equine Vet J 2004;36:628–33.

214. Dolovich M. Lung dose, distribution, and clinical response to therapeutic aerosols. Aerosol Sci Technol 1993;18:230–40.

215. Viel L, Tesarowski DB. Radioaerosol deposition in equids. 1994, 93–4.

216. Votion D, Ghafir Y, Munsters K, et al. Aerosol deposition in equine lungs following ultrasonic nebulisation versus

jet aerosol delivery system. Equine Vet J 1997;29:388–93.
217. Funch-Nielsen H, Roberts C, Weekes J, et al. Evaluation of a new spacer device for delivery of drugs into the equine respiratory tract. WEAS-CRS Symposium 2001;56.
218. Geor R, Johnston G. Deposition of radiolabelled aerosols within the equine respiratory tract. 1993.
219. Zeidler M, Corren J. Hydrofluoroalkane formulations of inhaled corticosteroids for the treatment of asthma. Treat Respir Med 2004;3:35–44.
220. Derksen FJ, Olszewski MA, Robinson NE, et al. Aerosolized albuterol sulfate used as a bronchodilator in horses with recurrent airway obstruction. Am J Vet Res 1999;60:689–93.
221. Kelly H. Comparison of inhaled corticosteroids. Ann Pharmacother 1998;32:220–32.
222. Rush B, Raub E, Thomsen M, et al. Pulmonary function and adrenal gland suppression with incremental doses of aerosolized beclomethasone dipropionate in horses with recurrent airway obstruction. J Am Vet Med Assoc 2000;217:359–64.
223. Ammann VJ, Vrins AA, Lavoie J-P. Effects of inhaled beclomethasone dipropionate on respiratory function in horses with chronic obstructive pulmonary disease (COPD). Equine Vet J 1998;30:152–7.
224. Viel L, Celly C, Staempfli H, et al. Therapeutic efficacy of inhaled fluticasone propionate in horses with chronic obstructive pulmonary disease. Proceedings Am Assoc Equine Pract 1999, 306–7.
225. Giguere S, Viel L, Lee E, et al. Cytokine induction in pulmonary airways of horses with heaves and effect of therapy with inhaled fluticasone propionate. Vet Immunol Immunopathol 2002;85:147–58.
226. Robinson NE, Berney C, Behan A, et al. Fluticasone propionate aerosol is more effective for prevention than treatment of recurrent airway obstruction. J Vet Intern Med 2009;23:1247–53.
227. Laan T. Serum cortisol concentrations in response to fluticasone propionate inhalation therapy in horses. Proceedings of the WEAS and VCRS Symposium 2001, 25.
228. Barnes P. Current therapy for asthma. In: Hansel T, Barnes P, editors. New drugs for asthma, allergy and COPD. New York: Karger; 2001. p. 6–10.
229. Derksen F, Olszewski M, Robinson N, et al. Aerosolized albuterol sulfate used as a bronchodilator in horses with recurrent airway obstruction. Am J Vet Res 1999;60:689–93.
230. Derksen F, Olszewski M, Robinson N, et al. Use of a hand-held, metered-dose aerosol delivery device to administer pirbuterol acetate to horses with heaves. Equine Vet J 1996;28:306–10.
231. Tesarowski D, Viel L, McDonnell W, et al. The rapid and effective administration of a beta2-agonist to horses with heaves using a compact inhalation device and metered-dose inhalers. Can Vet J 1994;35:170–3.
232. Derksen F, Robinson N, Olszewski M, et al. Clinical studies with Torpex (aerosol albuterol sulfate): Duration of effect. Technical research review, 3–4. Boehringer Ingelheim Vetmedica; 2002.
233. Hendrikson S, Rush B. Efficacy of saltpeter xinafoate in horses with recurrent airway obstruction. J Am Vet Med Assoc 2001;218:1961–5.
234. Robinson N, Derksen F, Berney C, et al. The airway response of horses with recurrent airway obstruction (heaves) to aerosol administration of ipratropium bromide. Equine Vet J 1993;25:299–303.
235. Aviza G, Ainsworth D, Eicker S, et al. Outcome of horses diagnosed with and treated for heaves. Equine Vet Educ 2001;3:318–20.
236. Couetil LL, Ward MP. Analysis of risk factors for recurrent airway obstruction in North American horses: 1,444 cases (1990–1999). J Am Vet Med Assoc 2003;223:1645–50.
237. McPherson E, Lawson G, Murphy J, et al. Chronic obstructive pulmonary disease (COPD): factors influencing the occurence. Equine Vet J 1979;11:167–71.
238. Clarke A. A review of environmental and host factors in relation to equine respiratory disease. Equine Vet J 1987;19:435–41.
239. Crichlow E, Yoshida K, Wallace K. Dust levels in a riding stable. Equine Vet J 1980;12:185–8.
240. Vandenput S, Duvivier D, Votion D, et al. Environmental control to maintain stabled COPD horses in clinical remission: effects on pulmonary function. Equine Vet J 1998;30:93–6.
241. Kirschvink N, Di Silvestro F, Sbai I, et al. The use of cardboard bedding material as part of an environmental control regime for heaves-affected horses: in vitro assessment of airborne dust and aeroallergen concentration and in vivo effects on lung function. Vet J 2002;163:319–25.
242. Clarke A, Madelin T. Technique for assessing respiratory health hazards from hay and other source materials. Equine Vet J 1987;19:442–7.
243. Derksen F, Robinson N, Scott J, et al. Aerosolized *Micropolyspora faeni* antigen as a cause of pulmonary dysfunction in ponies with recurrent airway obstruction (heaves). Am J Vet Res 1988;49:933–8.
244. Pirie R, Collie D, Dixon P, et al. Evaluation of nebulised hay dust suspensions (HDS) for the diagnosis and investigation of heaves. 2: Effects of inhaled HDS on control and heaves horses. Equine Vet J 2002;34:337–42.
245. Berndt A, Derksen FJ, Edward NE. Endotoxin concentrations within the breathing zone of horses are higher in stables than on pasture. Vet J 2010;183:54–7.
246. Pirie R, Dixon P, McGorum B. Evaluation of nebulised hay dust suspension (HDS) for the diagnosis and investigation of heaves. 3: Effect of fractionation of HDS. Equine Vet J 2002;34:343–7.
247. Pirie RS, Dixon PM, McGorum BC. Endotoxin contamination contributes to the pulmonary inflammatory and functional response to *Aspergillus fumigatus* extract inhalation in heaves horses. Clin Exp Allergy 2003;33:1289–96.
248. Doreswamy V, Peden DB. Modulation of asthma by endotoxin. Clin Exp Allergy 2011;41:9–19.
249. Ramseyer A, Gaillard C, Burger D, et al. Effects of genetic and environmental factors on chronic lower airway disease in horses. J Vet Intern Med 2007;21:149–56.
250. Swinburne JE, Bogle H, Klukowska-Rotzler J, et al. A whole-genome scan for recurrent airway obstruction in Warmblood sport horses indicates two positional candidate regions. Mamm Genome 2009;20:504–15.
251. Racine J, Gerber V, Miskovic FM, et al. Comparison of genomic and proteomic data in recurrent airway obstruction affected horses using ingenuity pathway analysis(R). BMC Vet Res 2011;7:48.
252. McPherson E, Lawson G, Murphy J, et al. Chronic obstructive pulmonary disease (COPD): Identification of affected horses. Equine Vet J 1978;10:47–53.
253. Littlejohn A, Bowles F. Studies on the pathophysiology of chronic obstructive pulmonary disease in the horse: VI. The alveolar dead space. Onderstepoort J Vet Res 1982;49:71–2.
254. Votion D, Ghafir Y, Vandenput S, et al. Analysis of scintigraphical lung images before and after treatment of horses suffering from chronic pulmonary disease. Vet Rec 1999;144:232–6.
255. Aliverti A, Macklem P. How and why exercise is impaired in COPD. Respiration 2001;68:229–39.
256. Fairbairn S, Page C, Lees P, et al. Early neutrophil but not eosinophil or platelet recruitment to the lungs of allergic horses following antigen exposure. Clin Exp Allergy 1993;23:821–8.
257. Ramery E, Closset R, Bureau F, et al. Relevance of using a human microarray to study gene expression in heaves-affected horses. Vet J 2008;177:216–21.

258. Venugopal CS, Mendes LC, Peiro JR, et al. Transcriptional changes associated with recurrent airway obstruction in affected and unaffected horses. Am J Vet Res 2010;71:476–82.
259. Robinson N, Derksen F, Olszewski M, et al. The pathogenesis of chronic obstructive pulmonary disease of horses. Br Vet J 1996;152:283–306.
260. Hotchkiss JW, Reid SW, Christley RM. A survey of horse owners in Great Britain regarding horses in their care. Part 2: Risk factors for recurrent airway obstruction. Equine Vet J 2007;39: 301–8.
261. Pirie RS, Collie DD, Dixon PM, et al. Evaluation of nebulised hay dust suspensions (HDS) for the diagnosis and investigation of heaves. 2: Effects of inhaled HDS on control and heaves horses. Equine Vet J 2002;34: 337–42.
262. Webster A, Clarke A, Madelin T, et al. Air hygiene in stables 1: Effects of stable design, ventilation and management on the concentration of respirable dust. Equine Vet J 1987;19:448–53.
263. Walinder R, Riihimaki M, Bohlin S, et al. Installation of mechanical ventilation in a horse stable: effects on air quality and human and equine airways. Environ Health Prev Med 2011;16:264–72.

Exercise-induced pulmonary hemorrhage (EIPH)

29

Kenneth W. Hinchcliff

CHAPTER CONTENTS

Introduction

- Exercise-induced pulmonary hemorrhage is a common disorder of athletic horses, among which it occurs worldwide.
- EIPH is a cause of poor performance and infrequently manifests as epistaxis during or after exercise. It rarely causes death.
- Diagnosis is based on demonstration of blood in the airways after exercise either by tracheobronchoscopy or examination of fluid obtained by tracheal aspiration or bronchoalveolar lavage.
- Furosemide is commonly used to treat EIPH and is efficacious in reducing both severity and frequency of bleeding – efficacy of other medications has not been demonstrated under field conditions.
- EIPH is likely caused by rupture of pulmonary capillaries with subsequent development of pulmonary inflammation, fibrosis and angiogenesis contributing to continued hemorrhage during exercise.

Exercise-induced pulmonary hemorrhage

Recognition

History and presenting complaint

Poor athletic performance or epistaxis is the most common presenting complaint for horses with exercise-induced pulmonary hemorrhage (EIPH). While poor performance can be attributable to any of a large number of causes, epistaxis associated with exercise is almost always attributable to pulmonary hemorrhage (EIPH).

Epistaxis due to EIPH occurs during or shortly after racing, is usually bilateral and resolves within hours of the end of the race. Epistaxis is discussed further under 'Clinical Signs'.

Failure of racehorses to perform to the expected standard (poor performance) is often attributed to EIPH likely because many horses with poor performance have cytologic evidence of EIPH on microscopic examination of tracheobronchial aspirates or bronchoalveolar lavage fluid or have blood evident on endoscopic examination of the tracheobronchial tree.[1,2] A relationship between finishing position and incidence of EIPH, diagnosed by bronchoscopic examination, was not detected in a number of studies of relatively small numbers of horses or a non-random selection of horses.[3,4,5] In contrast, a prospective observational study with strict entrance criteria and which included examination of over 700 horses, approximately 50% of all horses racing during the period of the study, demonstrated that exercise-induced pulmonary hemorrhage is a cause of poor performance in Thoroughbred racehorses.[6] Horses with EIPH of grade 1 or less (on a scale of 0–4)[7] were 4.0 times more likely to win, 1.8 times more likely to finish in the top three positions, 3.0 times more likely to earn above the 90th percentile of earnings than horses with EIPH of grade 2 or greater.[6] Horses with EIPH of grade 2 or greater finished significantly further behind the winner than did horses with less severe hemorrhage or no evidence of hemorrhage. These findings are consistent with a study of 452 Thoroughbred horses examined after racing in Hong Kong which demonstrated that those finishing in the first three positions had less severe EIPH than did horses finishing in lower positions.[8] Of horses finishing in the first three places, 43.9% had evidence of EIPH on tracheobronchoscopic examination after racing, whereas 55.9% of horses finishing in 4th to 14th place had evidence of EIPH. Exercise-induced pulmonary hemorrhage is an important cause of reduced athletic performance in Thoroughbred racehorses because of its high frequency and the magnitude of its association with impaired performance.

Results of studies in Standardbred racehorses indicate either a lack of effect of EIPH on performance or an association between EIPH and superior performance. There was not a relationship between presence of EIPH and finishing position in 29 Standardbred racehorses with intermittent EIPH examined on at least two occasions,[9] nor in 92 Standardbred racehorses examined on one occasion.[10] However, of 965 Standardbred racehorses examined after racing, those finishing first or second were 1.4 times more likely (95% CI 0.9–2.2) to have evidence of EIPH on tracheobronchoscopic examination than were horses that finished in 7th or 8th position.[11] The relationship between EIPH and performance in

Standardbred horses is unclear, largely because of the lack of appropriately designed large-scale studies. An association between EIPH and athletic performance has not been demonstrated for other breeds.

Exercise-induced pulmonary hemorrhage is infrequently associated with sudden death during racing or training. Of 143 horses subject to detailed post-mortem examination after death during racing or training, 50 died with severe pulmonary hemorrhage (the presumed cause of death).[12]

Physical examination

Apart from epistaxis in a small proportion of EIPH-affected horses, there are few abnormalities detectable on routine physical examination of horses with EIPH.[13] Rectal temperature and heart and breathing rates are elevated as a consequence of exercise in horses examined soon after exercise, but values of these variables in horses with EIPH at rest are not noticeably different to horses with no evidence of EIPH.[14] Affected horses might swallow more frequently during recovery from exercise than do unaffected horses, probably as a result of blood in the larynx and pharynx.[15] Coughing is common in horses recovering from strenuous exercise and horses with EIPH are reported to have a hacking cough, although this observation is not very specific.[3] After recovery from exercise, horses with EIPH are no more likely to cough than are unaffected horses.[16] Other clinical signs related to respiratory abnormalities are uncommon in horses with EIPH. Respiratory distress is rare in horses with EIPH and when present indicates severe hemorrhage or other serious lung disease such as pneumonia, pneumothorax or rupture of a pulmonary abscess. Lung sounds are abnormal in a small number of EIPH-affected horses and when present are characterized by increased intensity of normal breath sounds during rebreathing examination.[14] Tracheal rales can be present in horses with EIPH but are also heard in unaffected horses.[15]

Epistaxis associated with exercise is almost always attributable to pulmonary hemorrhage. The severity of epistaxis ranges from flecks or a small amount of blood at one nostril present after the horse lowers its head at the end of exercise to profuse hemorrhage from both nostrils occurring during exercise (Fig. 29.1). Epistaxis occurs in a small proportion racehorses.[3,6,15,17–21] The prevalence of epistaxis in racehorses varies between 0.1 and 9.0%, with the frequency depending on the breed, age and sex of horses selected for study, the type of racing, and the timing and frequency of observation of horses after racing (See 'Epidemiology'). Epistaxis occurs in 0.13% of Thoroughbred racehorses in Japan,[18] 5.9% of Thoroughbreds in Hong Kong,[8] 0.8% of Thoroughbreds in California,[3] 9.0% of Thoroughbreds in Pennsylvania,[4] 0.8% of Thoroughbreds in Australia,[6] and 3.5% of Quarter Horses in the USA.[20]

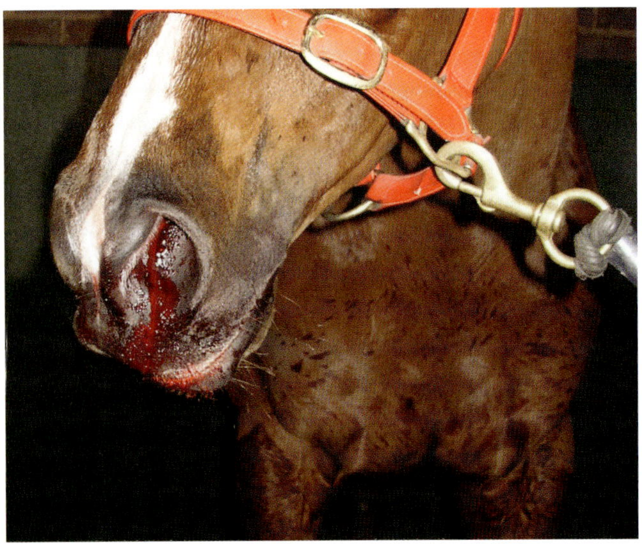

Fig 29.1 Thoroughbred horse with epistaxis that occurred during and after racing.

The recurrence rate after one episode of epistaxis in Thoroughbred horses is approximately 13.5% despite affected horses not being permitted to race for one month after the initial episode of epistaxis.[18] For this reason most racing jurisdictions do not permit horses with epistaxis to race for a period of weeks to months after the initial instance, with more prolonged enforced rest after a subsequent episode of epistaxis and retirement from racing after a third bout. This high rate of recurrence suggests that the inciting pulmonary lesions have not healed.

There are not clinically important abnormalities in routinely measured hematologic, blood gas and blood biochemical tests in resting horses with EIPH.[13]

Diagnostic tests

There are a variety of techniques available for determining the presence and severity of EIPH, including direct visualization of the airways through a flexible endoscope or examination of bronchial lavage fluid or tracheal aspirates for evidence of hemorrhage. The utility of these diagnostic tests varies and choice of examination technique depends on the time between the horse racing and the examination and the desired sensitivity of the test. For instance, tracheobronchoscopic examination is most appropriate if a horse is examined within 1–2 hours of exercise, whereas examination of airway washings is most appropriate if the examination is days to a week after strenuous exercise. Radiography, pulmonary scintigraphic examination and lung function tests are useful in eliminating other respiratory diseases as a cause of poor performance, but are minimally useful in confirming a diagnosis of EIPH or in determining the severity of hemorrhage.

Tracheobronchoscopy

Observation of blood in the trachea or large bronchi of horses 30–120 minutes after racing or strenuous exercise provides a definitive diagnosis of EIPH. The amount of blood in the large airways varies from a few small specks on the airway walls to blood covering most of the luminal surface of the trachea and extending into the larynx, nasopharynx and nasal cavities (Fig. 29.2).[7] If there is a strong suspicion of EIPH and blood is not present on a single examination conducted soon after exercise, the examination should be repeated in 60–90 minutes. Some horses with EIPH do not have blood present in the rostral airways immediately after exercise, but do so when examined 1–2 hours later. Blood is detectable by tracheobronchoscopic examination for 1–3 days with some horses having blood detectable for up to seven days.

Tracheobronchoscopic examination is performed using a 1–1.5 m flexible endoscope. Endoscopes of 1 m length allow visualization of the rostral trachea to the level of the thoracic inlet, but do not permit direct examination of the caudal trachea and large bronchi. Use of an endoscope of at least 1.5 m length is recommended to allow direct examination of all the large airways. The examination is performed with the horse restrained while the endoscope is passed through the ventral meatus into the nasopharynx. Most horses will tolerate passage of an endoscope into the caudal trachea with minimal restraint such as application of a nose twitch. Some horses require administration of sedatives or tranquilizers.

Administration of tranquilizers will alter pharyngeal and laryngeal function and might impair assessment of abnormalities of the upper airway. The nasopharynx and larynx are then examined for the presence of blood or other abnormalities and the endoscope is passed through the larynx into the cranial trachea. The trachea is examined as the endoscope is passed caudally so that the carina and cranial aspects of the left and right bronchi are visualized.

Bronchoscopic examination can be used to estimate the severity of EIPH through use of a grading system.[3,7–9,22] A validated grading system has a scale of 4 levels (Fig. 29.2):[7]

- **Grade 0** = no blood detected in the pharynx, larynx, trachea, or mainstem bronchi
- **Grade 1** = presence of 1 or more flecks of blood or 2 or fewer short (less than one-quarter the length of the trachea) narrow (<10% of the tracheal surface area) streams of blood in the trachea or mainstem bronchi visible from the tracheal bifurcation
- **Grade 2** = 1 long stream of blood (greater than half the length of the trachea) or more than 2 short streams of blood occupying less than a third of the tracheal circumference
- **Grade 3** = multiple, distinct streams of blood covering more than a third of the tracheal circumference, with no blood pooling at the thoracic inlet
- **Grade 4** = multiple, coalescing streams of blood covering more than 90% of the tracheal surface with blood pooling at the thoracic inlet.

There is a high concordance amongst trained observers using this grading system (weighted kappa of 0.75 to 0.80) with fewer than 0.5% of observations differing by two or more grades.[7] It is assumed that a higher score represents more severe hemorrhage, but while the repeatability of this scoring system has been established, the relationship between the amount of blood in the large airways and the actual amount of hemorrhage has not been established.

Examination of airway secretions or lavage fluid

The presence of red cells or macrophages containing either effete red cells or the breakdown products of hemoglobin (hemosiderophages) in tracheal or bronchoalveolar lavage fluid provides evidence of EIPH (Fig. 29.3). Detection of red cells or hemosiderophages in tracheal aspirates or bronchoalveolar lavage fluid is believed to be both sensitive and specific in the diagnosis of EIPH.[1,23] Examination of airway fluids indicates the presence of EIPH in a greater proportion of horses than does tracheobronchoscopic examination after strenuous exercise or racing. The greater sensitivity of examination of airway fluid is likely attributable to the ability of this examination to detect the presence of small amounts of blood

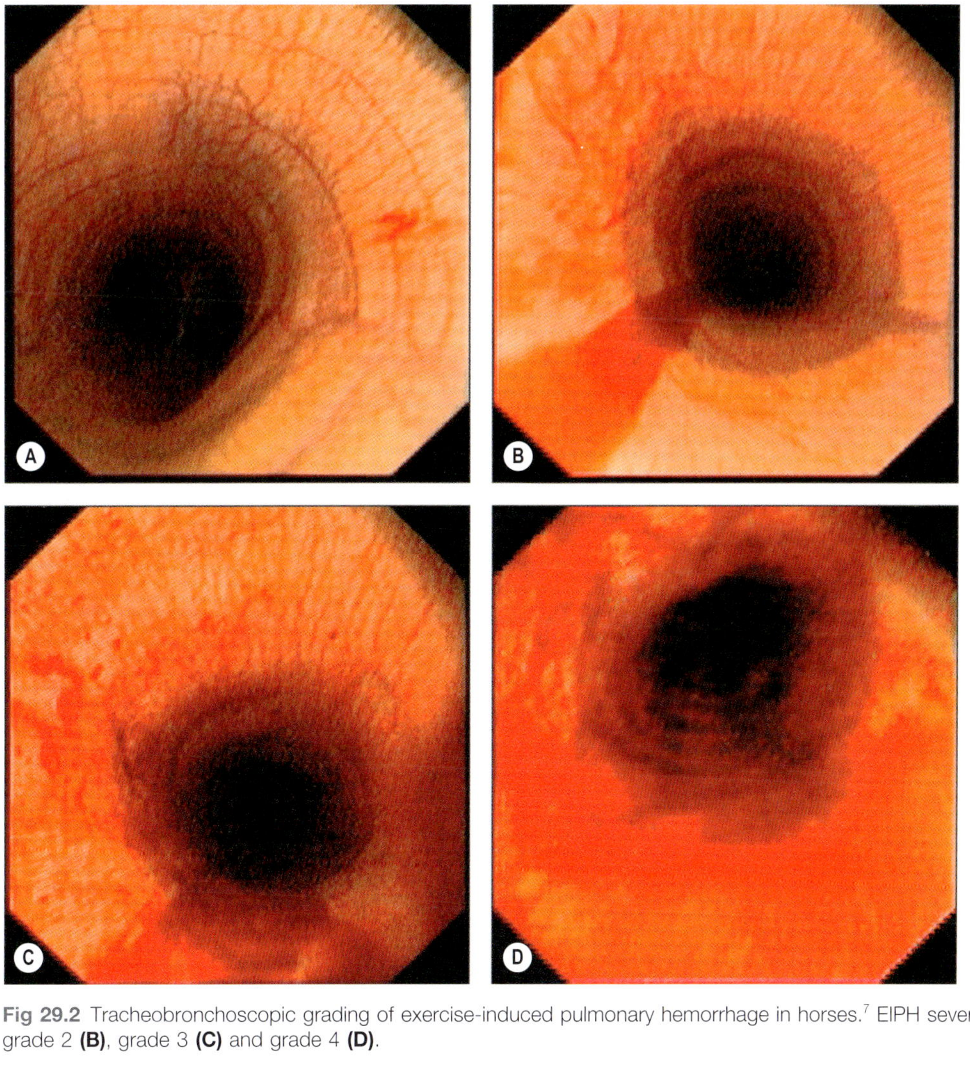

Fig 29.2 Tracheobronchoscopic grading of exercise-induced pulmonary hemorrhage in horses.[7] EIPH severity is depicted as grade 1 **(A)**, grade 2 **(B)**, grade 3 **(C)** and grade 4 **(D)**.

or its residual products and the longevity of these products in the airways. While endoscopic examination detects blood in occasional horses up to seven days after an episode of EIPH, cellular evidence of pulmonary hemorrhage persists for weeks after a single episode.[1,23–26] Red blood cells and macrophages containing red cells are present in bronchoalveolar lavage fluid or tracheal aspirates for at least one week after strenuous exercise or instillation of autologous blood into airways and hemosiderophages are present for at least 21 days and possibly longer.[1,23–26]

Red cell numbers in bronchoalveolar lavage fluid are used as a means of detecting EIPH, a quantitative indicator of severity of EIPH and for monitoring efficacy of treatments.[25,27–30] However, identification of hemosiderophages or red blood cells in tracheal aspirates, or hemosiderophages in bronchoalveolar lavage fluid, does not provide a reliable measure of the severity of pulmonary haemorrhage in a model using intrapulmonary administration of blood.[24] The assumptions underlying the use of this technique are that it is a more sensitive indicator of EIPH than tracheobronchoscopic examination of airways, and that the red blood cell count in lavage fluid is proportional to the severity of haemorrhage. While it is very probable that detection of red blood cells in bronchoalveolar lavage fluid is a more sensitive indicator of EIPH than tracheobronchoscopic examination,[31] the usefulness of red cell counts in bronchoalveolar lavage fluid as an indicator of severity of haemorrhage is less clear given that an unknown area, although presumably small, of the lung is examined by lavage and there is a risk that this area of lung might not be representative of the lung as a whole, similar to the situation of examination of bronchoalveolar lavage fluid of horses with pneumonia.[32,33] However, other methods of determining severity of EIPH, including pulmonary scintigraphy and pulmonary function tests,[34,35] have to date proved unable to detect or quantify hemorrhage, leaving measurement of red cell count in bronchoalveolar lavage fluid as a viable but perhaps less than optimal method of quantification.

Tracheal aspirates may be obtained any time after exercise by either aspiration during tracheobronchoscopic examination or aspiration through a percutaneous intratracheal needle. Aspirates obtained through an endoscope might not be sterile, depending on the collection technique. Bronchoalveolar lavage fluid can be obtained through either an endoscope wedged in the distal airway or through a cuffed tube inserted blindly into a distal airway. Collection of fluid through an endoscope has the advantage of permitting examination of the distal airways and selection of the area of lung to be lavaged. However, it does require the use of an endoscope that is longer (2 m) than those readily available in most equine practices. Use of a commercial bronchoalveolar lavage catheter does not require use of an endoscope and can be readily performed in field situations.

For both endoscopic and lavage tube collection of bronchoalveolar lavage fluid the horse is restrained and sedated (xylazine 0.5–1.0 mg/kg iv, detomidine 20–40 micrograms/kg IV). Some clinicians administer butorphanol (0.02–0.5 mg/kg IV) or local anesthetic (lidocaine, 20 mL of a 2% solution diluted with saline to a total volume of 100 mL and administered into the trachea) to suppress coughing. Application of a nose twitch may be necessary in some horses. The endoscope or lavage tube is passed into the trachea and then advanced caudally until it wedges in the distal airway. The cuff of the lavage tube is then inflated and a quantity of fluid (150–300 mL) of isotonic fluid (phosphate buffered 0.9% sodium chloride or similar) rapidly injected. After allowing the horse several breaths, the fluid is aspirated with the first 20 mL being discarded. Blind passage of the lavage tube usually results in its lodging in the dorsocaudal lung region.[36]

Radiography

Thoracic radiography is of limited sensitivity in detecting horses with EIPH. Radiographs can demonstrate the presence of densities in the caudodorsal lung fields of some horses (Fig. 29.4),[37–39] but many affected horses have minimal to undetectable radiographic abnormalities and unaffected horses can have marked abnormalities. The severity of radiographically apparent pulmonary abnormalities was not significantly different between horses with EIPH and control horses.[13] Examination of thoracic radiographs of horses with EIPH can be useful in ruling out the presence of another disease process, such as a pulmonary abscess, contributing to the horse's pulmonary hemorrhage or poor athletic performance, but are not sensitive for the detection of EIPH.

Pulmonary scintigraphy

Scintigraphic examination of lungs has the potential to detect horses with EIPH, but to date technical limitations have precluded its routine use for this purpose.[35,40]

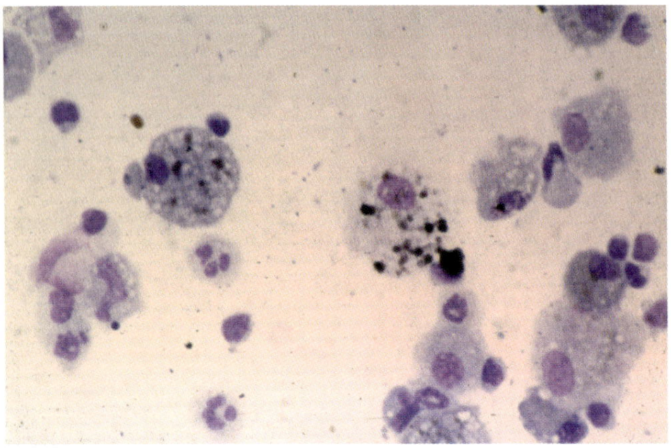

Fig 29.3 Hemosiderophages in bronchoalveolar lavage fluid of Standardbred racehorse.

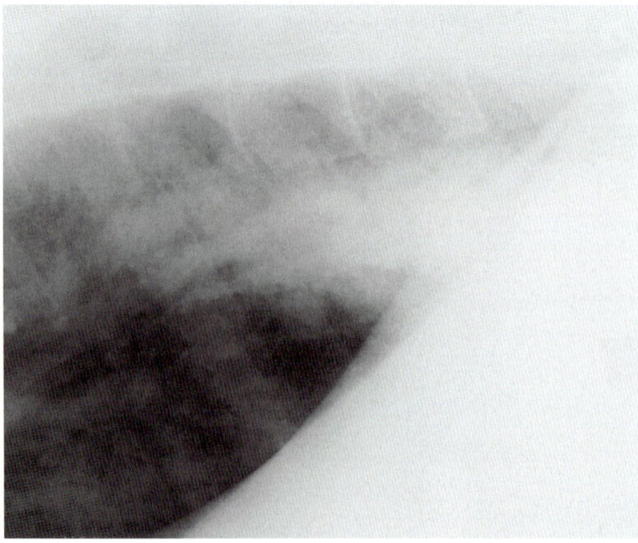

Fig 29.4 Thoracic radiograph of a five-year-old Thoroughbred racehorse. Radiographic signs of EIPH are evident as the wedge-shaped density in the dorsocaudal lung fields.

Exercise testing

During incremental exercise on a treadmill, horses with EIPH have more severe exercise-induced arterial hypoxemia, hypercapnia and higher blood lactate concentrations than do control horses[41] although this is not a consistent finding.[42] These changes indicate abnormalities in gas exchange in horses with EIPH but are not sufficiently large; nor do they have sufficient sensitivity to be useful clinically. Blood gas tensions in resting horses with EIPH are within the normal ranges.

Necropsy examination

Exercise-induced pulmonary hemorrhage is a rare cause of death of racehorses. Necropsy examination of affected horses is usually incidental to examination for another cause of death. Pertinent abnormalities in horses with EIPH are restricted to the respiratory tract. Grossly, horses examined within hours of strenuous exercise, such as horses necropsied because of catastrophic musculoskeletal injuries incurred during racing, can have severe petechiation in the caudodorsal lung fields (Fig. 29.5). Horses with chronic disease have blue/gray or blue/brown discoloration of the visceral pleural surfaces of the caudodorsal lung fields that is often sharply demarcated, especially on the diaphragmatic surface (Fig. 29.6).[43] The discoloration affects both lungs equally with 30–50% of the lung fields being discolored in severe cases.[43] Affected areas do not collapse to the same extent as unaffected areas and, in the deflated lung, have a spleen-like consistency.[43] On cut surface, the discolored areas of lung are predominantly contiguous with the dorsal pleural surface and extent ventrally into the lung parenchyma. Areas of affected lung may be separated by normal lung. There is proliferation of bronchial vessels, predominantly arteries and arterioles, in affected areas.[44] Histologically, affected areas exhibit bronchiolitis, hemosiderophages in the alveolor lumen and interstitial spaces, and fibrosis of interlobular septa, pleural and around vessels and bronchioles.[45]

Diagnostic confirmation

There are a variety of causes of epistaxis, pulmonary hemorrhage or both in horses,[46] although most are not associated solely with exercise (Table 29.1). Presence of EIPH is most immediately confirmed by tracheobronchoscopic examination of the horse after strenuous exercise. Detection of red blood cells or hemosiderophages in

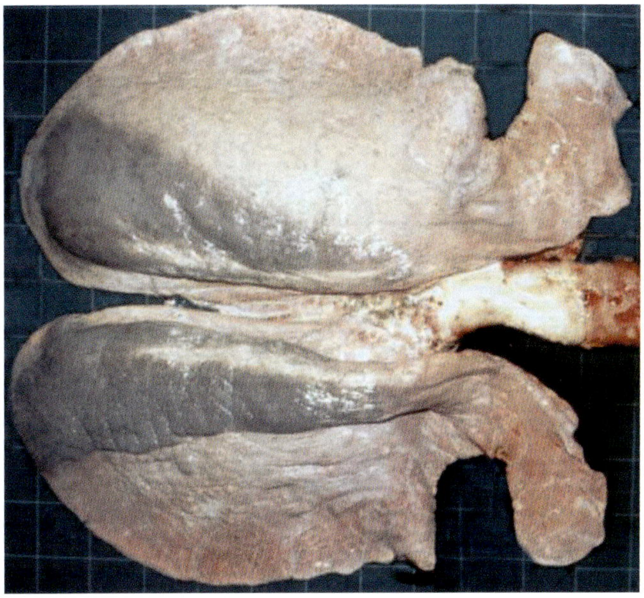

Fig 29.6 Lungs of a Thoroughbred racehorse with exercise-induced pulmonary hemorrhage. The lesions are restricted to the caudodorsal lung fields and produce a blue-gray discoloration of the visceral pleural surface.

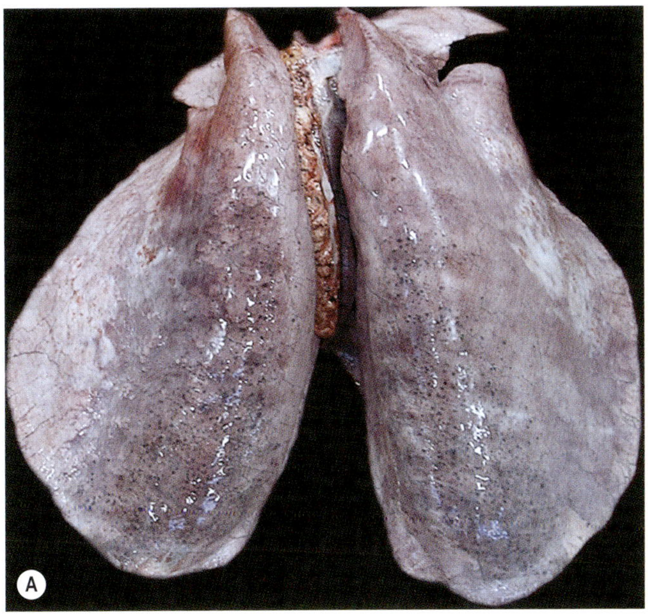

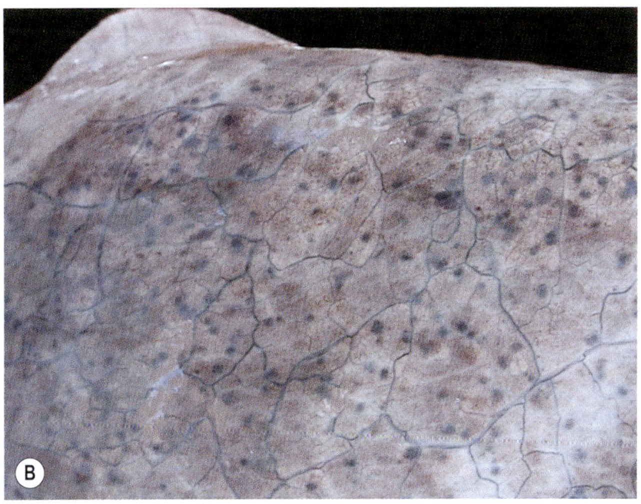

Fig 29.5 **(A)** Lungs of a Thoroughbred racehorse euthanized immediately after racing because of a catastrophic musculoskeletal injury. Lesions of acute EIPH are evident in dorsocaudal lung fields. **(B)** Closer view of lungs in A demonstrating focal nature of hemorrhage.
Courtesy Professor R. F. Slocombe.

Table 29.1 Causes of epistaxis in horses

DISEASE	EPIDEMIOLOGY	CLINICAL SIGNS AND DIAGNOSIS	TREATMENT AND CONTROL
Epistaxis with hemorrhage into trachea or bronchi			
Exercise-induced pulmonary hemorrhage	Horses after strenuous exercise. Most common in Thoroughbred and Standardbred racehorses	Epistaxis is a rare but very specific sign of EIPH. Only occurs after exercise. Endoscopic examination of the airways is diagnostic	Administration of furosemide. Rest – often enforced by regulations of the racing jurisdiction
Trauma	Sporadic. Associated with trauma to head, neck, or chest	Physical examination reveals site and nature of the trauma. Can require endoscopic examination of upper airways	Symptomatic treatment
Pneumonia	Recent shipping or respiratory disease. Can occur as outbreaks though usually individual animals	Fever, tachypnea, abnormal lung sounds, leukocytosis, radiography demonstrates lung lesions. Cytologic and microbiologic examination of tracheal aspirate	Antimicrobials, NSAIDs, oxygen. Control by vaccination and prevention of respiratory disease
Lung abscess	Sporadic. Hemorrhage can occur after exercise	Sometimes no premonitory signs. Fever, depression, anorexia, cough. Hemogram demonstrates leukocytosis. Hyperfibrinogenemia. Ultrasonography or radiography demonstrates lesion. Tracheal aspirates	Antibiotics
Intrabronchial foreign body	Sporadic	Cough, hemoptysis, fever. Endoscopy or radiography reveals foreign body	Removal of foreign body – often not readily achieved
Pulmonary neoplasia	Sporadic. Often older horse, but not always. Hemangiosarcoma	Cough, hemoptysis. Demonstrate mass on ultrasonographic or radiographic examination	None
Epistaxis without hemorrhage into trachea or bronchi			
Guttural pouch mycosis	Sporadic. Acute-onset epistaxis	Severe, life-threatening epistaxis. Tachycardia, anemia, hemorrhagic shock	Surgical ligation or occlusion of arteries
Ethmoidal hematoma	Sporadic	Epistaxis not associated with exercise. Usually unilateral	Surgery or injection of mass with formaldehyde
Thrombocytopenia	Sporadic	Epistaxis, mild, intermittent. Petechiation and ecchymotic hemorrhages. Thrombocytopenia	Glucocorticoids or other immunosuppressive medications
Neoplasia	Sporadic	Neoplasia of upper airways	None
Trauma	Sporadic	Injury to head or pharynx	Symptomatic
Sinusitis	Sporadic	Endoscopic or radiographic examination of sinus	Drainage. Antimicrobials

NSAIDs – non-steroidal anti-inflammatory drugs.

Modified from Radostits et al. Veterinary Medicine. A textbook of the diseases of cattle, horses, sheep, goats and pigs. 10th edition W.B. Saunders. London.

tracheal aspirates or bronchoalveolar lavage fluid is also indicative of EIPH. The finding of hemorrhage in the airways of a horse soon after exercise allows a strong presumptive diagnosis of EIPH.

Treatment and prognosis

Therapeutic aims

The aims of treatment are to reduce the severity of hemorrhage and minimize the adverse sequelae to hemorrhage. Sequelae to hemorrhage include airway and interstitial inflammation and fibrosis.

Treatment

Therapy for EIPH is controversial in that a wide variety of treatments are used but only one, furosemide, has demonstrated efficacy under conditions of racing (Table 29.2).[47,48] There is evidence, based on studies of small numbers of horses running on a treadmill, of efficacy for a small number of other substances but care should be taken in extrapolating results of these studies to horses in the field. Conversely, failure to detect a beneficial effect of a compound or substance during testing using a small number of horses might be related to the low statistical power of the study rather than lack of efficacy.[49,50]

Table 29.2 Pharmacotherapeutic and management interventions used in an attempt to prevent exercise-induced pulmonary hemorrhage in horses

PUTATIVE MECHANISM AND CONTRIBUTING FACTOR	INTERVENTION	EVIDENCE OF EFFICACY
High pulmonary capillary pressure		
High cardiac output	Furosemide Dehydration Other diuretics	Evidence of efficacy of furosemide in control of EIPH
Insufficient pulmonary vasodilation	Antihypertensive agents: Guanabenz Clonidine	No studies to investigate efficacy or effect on PAP
	Enalapril	No effect on PAP during intense exercise
	Nitric oxide donors/analogues: Nitroglycerin Nitroprusside L-arginine	NG reduces PAP of standing horses. No evidence of effect on PAP during exercise No blockade by L-NAME does not affect PAP during intense exercise
	Phosphodiesterase inhibitors: Sildenafil (Viagra) Aminophylline	No effects on PAP or EIPH
Increased blood viscosity (reduced red cell defomability, echinocytosis)	Pentoxifylline	No effect on PAP during intense exercise. Effect on EIPH not reported
Low alveolar pressure – increased upper airway resistance		
Upper airway abnormalities (increased inspiratory resistance)	Surgical correction of obstruction	No demonstrated efficacy on EIPH
Resistance at nares	Nasal dilator strips (FLAIR)	Decreases red cell count in bronchoalveolar lavage fluid collected after intense exercise
Low alveolar pressure – intrathoracic obstruction		
Bronchoconstriction	Bronchodilatory drugs: Clenbuterol Albuterol Ipratropium Pyrroglycolate	No demonstrated efficacy on EIPH, except for ipratropium in two horses. Clenbuterol does not affect PAP
Lower airway inflammation	Anti-inflammatory drugs: Corticosteroids Cromolyn sodium	No demonstrated efficacy of corticosteroids in preventing EIPH. Cromolyn sodium has demonstrated lack of efficacy
	Low allergenic stall bedding (paper)	No efficacy in reducing EIPH
Interstitial inflammation and bronchial angiogenesis		
Progressive lung injury	Rest	No demonstrated efficacy in reducing EIPH
	Corticosteroids	No demonstrated efficacy in reducing EIPH
Coagulopathy or platelet dysfunction		
Excessive fibrinolysis	Aminocaproic acid	Inhibits fibrinolysis. No demonstrated efficacy in preventing EIPH
	Estrogens	Rationale unclear. No demonstrated efficacy in preventing EIPH
Increased platelet aggregation	Aspirin	Inhibits platelet aggregation. No demonstrated effect in preventing EIPH
Capillary fragility	Hesperidin-citrus bioflavonoids, carbazochrome	No detectable effect on EIPH

PAP = pulmonary artery pressure, EIPH = exercise-induced pulmonary hemorrhage.

Therapy of EIPH is usually a combination of attempts to reduce the severity of subsequent hemorrhage and efforts to minimize the effect of recent hemorrhage and is problematic for a number of reasons. Firstly, the pathogenesis of EIPH has not been determined although the available evidence supports a role for stress failure of pulmonary capillaries secondary to exercise-induced pulmonary hypertension (see below). Secondly, there is a lack of information using large numbers of horses under field conditions that demonstrates an effect of any medication or management practice (with the exception of bedding and pre-race administration of furosemide) on EIPH.[47,51] There are numerous studies of small numbers of horses (<~40) under experimental conditions but these studies often lacked the statistical power to detect treatment effects and, furthermore, the relevance of studies conducted on a treadmill to horses racing competitively is questionable. Treatments for EIPH are usually intended to address a specific aspect of the pathogenesis of the disease and will be discussed in that context.

Prevention of stress failure of the pulmonary capillaries

Stress failure of pulmonary capillaries, and subsequent hemorrhage, is believed to occur as a result of the high transmural pressures in pulmonary capillaries that develop in the lungs of horses during strenuous exercise. There is therefore interest in reducing the pressure difference across the pulmonary capillary membrane in an effort to reduce EIPH. Theoretically, this can be achieved by reducing the pressure within the capillary or increasing (making less negative) the pressure within the intrathoracic airways and alveolus.

Reducing pulmonary capillary pressure

Furosemide administration as prophylaxis of EIPH is permitted in a number of racing jurisdictions worldwide (see Fig. 29.7) although its use in some jurisdictions is being reconsidered with a view to restricting use of the medication.[52] Furosemide use on race day is currently permitted in Argentina, Brazil, Canada, Chile, Peru, Saudi Arabia, United States of America, and Venezuela (this is not an exhaustive list).[53] Within the United States and Canada, almost all Thoroughbred, Standardbred and Quarter Horse racing jurisdictions permit administration of furosemide before racing, although this situation is changing rapidly. Approximately 85% of all Thoroughbred racehorses in the United States and Canada receive furosemide at some stage of their career and, on average, 75% of horses in a race receive furosemide.[54] Although accurate numbers are not available, it appears that a smaller proportion of Standardbred and Quarter Horse racehorses receive furosemide before racing. Furosemide is administered to 22–32% of Standardbred racehorses and 19% of racing Quarter Horses in two racing jurisdictions.[55–57]

Furosemide is efficacious for the treatment of EIPH in Thoroughbred racehorses.[47] One hundred and sixty-seven Thoroughbred racehorses competing in races as part of a double-blind, randomized, cross-over field trial were 3.3 to 4.4 times more likely to develop EIPH ≥1 when administered saline than when administered furosemide (1 mg/kg IV). Furthermore, horses were 7 to 11 times more likely to have severe EIPH (≥2) when administered saline rather than furosemide.[47] However, other field studies of large numbers of horses do not demonstrate an effect of furosemide on the prevalence of EIPH.[5,58] Studies of Thoroughbred horses running on a treadmill provide evidence that furosemide reduces the severity of EIPH.[29,59] The weight of evidence clearly indicates that furosemide is efficacious in the reduction of severity and frequency of EIPH in Thoroughbred racehorses.

The mechanism by which furosemide could reduce the severity of EIPH is unknown although it is speculated that furosemide, by attenuating the exercise-induced increase in pulmonary artery and pulmonary capillary pressure of horses, reduces the frequency or severity of pulmonary capillary rupture.[60–62]

Furosemide is associated with superior performance in both Thoroughbred and Standardbred racehorses.[54,55] Thoroughbred horses treated with furosemide were 1.4 times as likely to win the race, earned more money and had a standardized 6 furlong race time 0.56 to 1.09 seconds less than untreated horses.[54] Similarly, furosemide reduced one mile race times of Standardbred pacers by 0.31 to 0.74 seconds.[55]

Antihypertensive agents used in control of systemic (not pulmonary artery) hypertension in humans have been used in an effort to prevent EIPH in horses. Drugs including guanabenz and clonidine have been administered to horses to prevent EIPH, but the efficacy of these drugs in preventing EIPH or reducing pulmonary capillary pressure of exercising horses has not been demonstrated. Enalapril is effective in inhibiting angiotensin converting enzyme (ACE) activity in horses, but does not affect pulmonary artery pressure of exercising horses.[63] Similarly, the efficacy of enalapril,

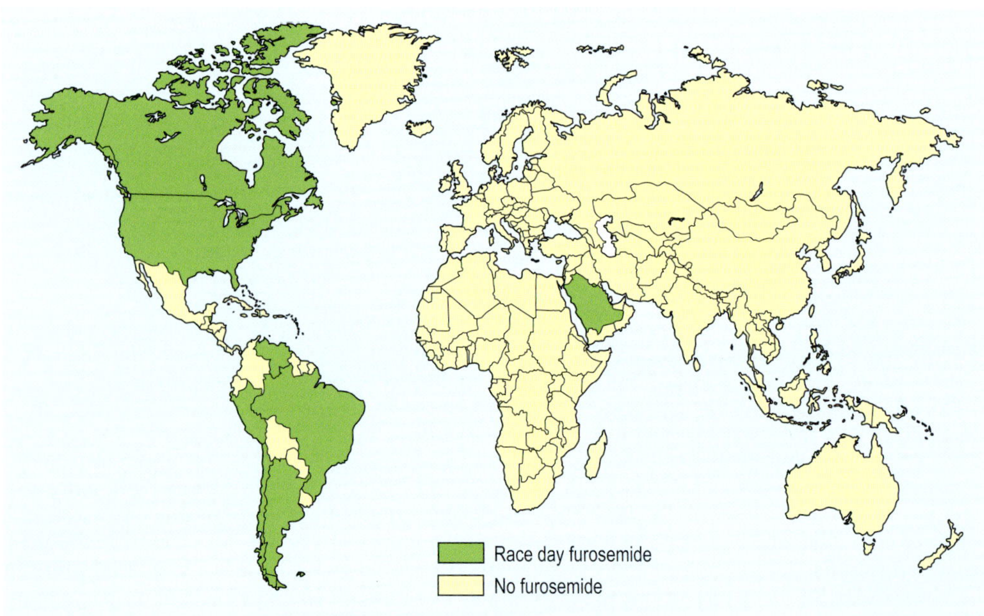

Fig 29.7 Map depicting racing jurisdictions that permit administration of furosemide on the day of racing in 2011.

or other ACE inhibitors, in preventing EIPH has not been demonstrated.

Nitric oxide is a potent vasodilator in many vascular beds. Administration of nitroglycerin (a nitric oxide donor) reduces pulmonary artery pressure of standing horses, but does not affect pulmonary artery pressure of horses during intense exercise.[64] L-arginine is a nitric oxide donor with no demonstrated efficacy in reducing pulmonary capillary pressure or EIPH in horses. The effect of L-NAME, an inhibitor of nitric oxide synthetase, on pulmonary artery pressure during maximal exercise is controversial, with either no effect or a decrease in pulmonary artery pressure reported.[65,66] Interestingly, L-NAME administration caused an increase in severity of EIPH.[65] Sildenafil, a phosphodiesterase inhibitor that accentuates the effect of nitric oxide and is used in the treatment of erectile dysfunction in men, has been administered to horses in an apparent attempt to reduce EIPH.[67] However, sildenafil was not effective in preventing EIPH or reducing pulmonary capillary pressure in horses running on a treadmill.[67] There is a patent for use of a novel type V phosphodiesterase (E4021) in treatment of EIPH but this product was not commercially available in 2012.[68]

An increase in pulmonary capillary pressure secondary to altered rheostatic properties of blood during exercise has been suggested as a possible contributing factor for EIPH.[69] Furosemide increases blood viscosity whereas pentoxifylline increases red blood cell deformability and may attenuate the increase in blood viscosity that occurs during exercise.[70–72] However, pentoxifylline does not affect pulmonary capillary pressure of exercising horses and did not affect the prevalence of EIPH in a small experimental study.[73]

Increasing alveolar inspiratory pressure

Airway obstruction, either intrathoracic or extrathoracic, increases airway resistance and results in a more negative intrathoracic (pleural) pressure during inspiration to maintain tidal volume and alveolar ventilation. Causes of extrathoracic airway obstruction include laryngeal hemiplegia and other abnormalities of the upper airway (see Chapter 27), whereas intrathoracic obstruction is usually a result of bronchoconstriction and inflammatory airway disease. Horses with partial extrathoracic inspiratory obstruction or bronchoconstriction and airway inflammation associated with recurrent airway obstructive disease (heaves) have pleural (and hence alveolar) pressures that are lower (more negative) than those in unaffected horses or in horses after effective treatment.

Partial inspiratory obstruction, such as produced by laryngeal hemiplegia, exacerbates the exercise-induced decrease in intrapleural pressures with a consequent increase in transmural capillary pressures (Fig. 29.8).[74–76] These changes may exacerbate the severity of EIPH although an association between upper airway obstructive disease and EIPH has not been demonstrated. Surgical correction of airway obstruction is expected to resolve the more negative intrapleural pressure but its effect on EIPH is unknown.

The role of the nares in contributing to upper airway resistance, and hence lowering inspiratory intrapleural pressure during intense exercise, has attracted the attention of some investigators (Fig. 29.9). Application of nasal dilator bands (FLAIR® strips) reduces nasal resistance by dilating the nasal valve,[77] and reduces red cell count of bronchoalveolar lavage fluid collected from horses after intense exercise on a treadmill[29,59,78] and during racing.[78]

The role of small airway inflammation and bronchoconstriction in the pathogenesis of EIPH is unclear. However, horses with EIPH are often treated with drugs intended to decrease lower airway inflammation and relieve bronchoconstriction. Beta-adrenergic bronchodilatory drugs such as clenbuterol and albuterol are effective in inducing bronchodilation in horses with

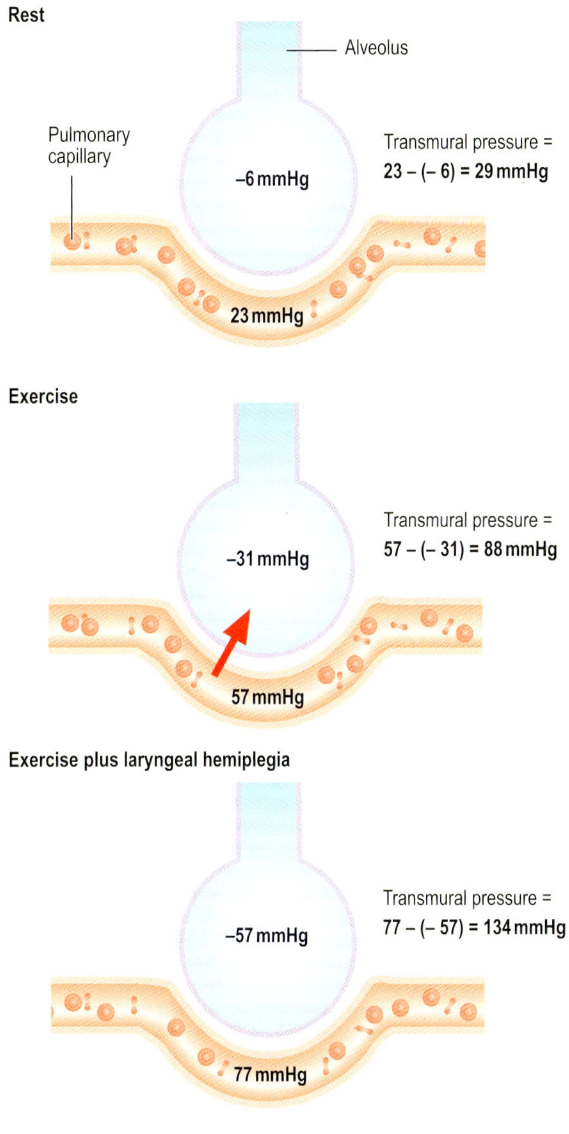

Fig 29.8 Schematic representation of determinants of transmural pressure in a horse at rest, during intense exercise, and during intense exercise with left laryngeal hemiplegia. Data are from Ducharme et al (1999).

bronchoconstriction, but their efficacy in preventing EIPH is either unknown or, in very small studies, is not evident. Clenbuterol does not alter the hemodynamic responses of horses to exertion or attenuate exercise-induced arterial hypoxemia in normal horses.[79,80] Ipratropium, a parasympatholytic drug administered by inhalation, showed promise in a very small study (two horses) of preventing EIPH.[81] Corticosteroids, including dexamethasone, fluticasone and beclomethasone administered by inhalation, parenterally or enterally, reduce airway inflammation and obstruction, but have no demonstrated efficacy in preventing EIPH. Cromolyn sodium (sodium cromoglycate) has no efficacy in preventing EIPH.[82]

Water vapor treatment (inhalation of water-saturated air) has been proposed as a treatment for EIPH because of its putative effect

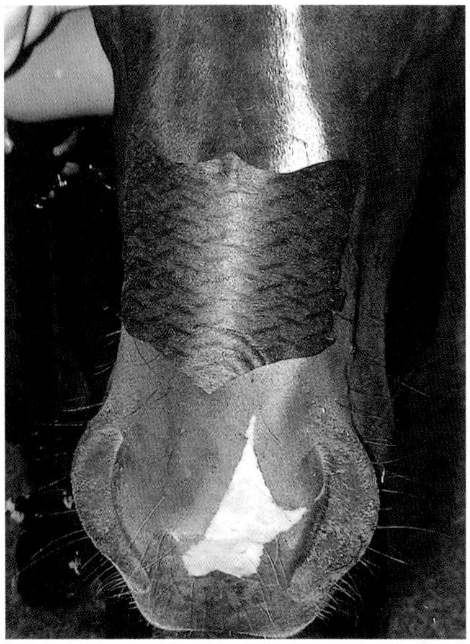

Fig 29.9 Horse wearing a nasal support.
FLAIR® Equine Nasal Strip, with kind permission of Flair, LLC. Photograph courtesy of Dr. S. Holcombe.

on small airway disease. However, water vapor treatment has no effect on EIPH.[83]

The use of bedding of low allergenic potential (shredded paper) to prevent EIPH has no apparent effect on the prevalence of EIPH.[51] While it is suggested that the severity of EIPH could be reduced by preventing or minimizing small airway disease, studies to demonstrate such an effect have not been reported. However, optimizing the air quality in barns and stables and preventing infectious respiratory disease appear sensible precautions.

Interstitial inflammation and bronchial angiogenesis

Hemorrhage into interstitial tissues induces inflammation with subsequent development of fibrosis and bronchial artery angiogenesis.[44,84] The role of these changes in perpetuating EIPH in horses is unclear, but likely is of some importance. Treatments to reduce inflammation and promote healing with minimal fibrosis have been proposed. Rest is an obvious recommendation and many racing jurisdictions have rules regarding enforced rest for horses with epistaxis. While the recommendation for rest is intuitive, there is no information that rest reduces the severity or incidence of EIPH in horses with prior evidence of this disorder.

Similarly, corticosteroids are often administered, either by inhalation, enterally or parenterally, in an attempt to reduce pulmonary inflammation and minimize fibrosis. Again, the efficacy of this intervention in preventing or minimizing severity of EIPH has not been documented.

Excessive bleeding

Coagulopathy and fibrinolysis

Exercise induces substantial changes in blood coagulation and fibrinolysis.[85] However, these is no evidence that horses with EIPH have defective coagulation or increased fibrinolysis,[86] and there is evidence that affected horses might have increased coagulability, although this finding requires verification.[87] Regardless, aminocaproic acid, a potent inhibitor of fibrin degradation, has been administered to horses to prevent EIPH. The efficacy of aminocaproic acid in preventing EIPH has not been demonstrated in either of two studies examining horses running on a treadmill.[49,88] Both studies used small numbers of horses (6–8) and had high variability in red cell count in bronchoalveolar lavage fluid resulting in low statistical power to detect an effect of the medication. Similarly, estrogens are given to horses with the expectation of improving hemostasis although effect of estrogens on coagulation in any species is unclear. There is no evidence that estrogens prevent EIPH in horses.[88]

Vitamin K is administered to horses with EIPH presumably with the expectation that it will decrease coagulation times. However, as EIPH is not associated with prolonged bleeding times, it is unlikely that this intervention will affect the prevalence or severity of EIPH.

Platelet function. Aspirin inhibits platelet aggregation in horses and increases bleeding time.[89] Seemingly paradoxically, aspirin is sometimes administered to horses with EIPH because of concerns that increased platelet aggregation contributes to EIPH.[90] There is no evidence that aspirin either exacerbates or prevents EIPH.

Capillary integrity. Capillary fragility increases the risk of hemorrhage in many species. Various bioflavonoids have been suggested to increase capillary integrity and prevent bleeding. However, hesperidin and citrus bioflavonoids have no efficacy in prevention of EIPH in horses.[91] Similarly, vitamin C is administered to horses with EIPH without scientific evidence of any beneficial effect.

Carbazochrome salicylate (Kentucky Red) is a putative 'capillary stabilizer' administered to horses to reduce EIPH.[50] Carbazochrome, in combination with furosemide, did not reduce red cell count in bronchoalveolar lavage fluid of six Standardbreds running on a treadmill.[50]

Miscellaneous. Concentrated equine serum has been administered intratracheally and intravenously and is reported to reduce the severity of EIPH in horses running on a treadmill.[92] There are no reports of its use in field conditions. Herbal products are often recommended for treatment of EIPH. Yunnan Paiyao and Single Immortal do not prevent EIPH in horses running on a treadmill.[93]

Overview of treatment

Selection of therapy for horses with EIPH is problematic. Furosemide is clearly efficacious but its use on race day is limited or prohibited in many racing jurisdictions. Given that most horses have some degree of pulmonary hemorrhage during most bouts of intense exercise, the decision must be made not only as to the type of treatment and its timing but also which horses to treat. Moreover, the apparent progressive nature of the disease with continued work highlights the importance of early and effective prophylaxis and emphasizes the need for studies of factors, such as air quality and respiratory infections, in inciting the disorder.

Rest is an obvious recommendation for horses with EIPH, but the hemorrhage is likely to recur when the horse is next strenuously exercised. The duration of rest and the optimal exercise program to return horses to racing after EIPH is unknown, although some jurisdictions require exercise no more intense than trotting for two months. Firm recommendations cannot be made on duration of rest because of a lack of objective information.

Although a role for lower airway disease (either infectious or allergic) in the genesis of EIPH has not been demonstrated, control of infectious diseases and minimization of non-infectious lower airway inflammation appears prudent.

Prognosis

The prognosis for racing for horses with clinically significant EIPH is guarded because of the progressive nature of the disease. Horses that have experienced severe EIPH on one occasion are likely to do so again regardless of treatment. However, the risk of horses experiencing a repeated bout of severe hemorrhage and the effect of EIPH on career longevity are unknown.

Pathophysiology and etiology

The likely proximate cause of EIPH is rupture of alveolar capillary membranes with subsequent extravasation of blood into interstitial and alveolar spaces.[94] The source of blood in such instances is the pulmonary circulation. Bleeding from bronchial circulation during exercise has been suggested based on histologic evidence of bronchial angiogenesis in horses that have experienced previous episodes of EIPH.[95] Whether there is a contribution of the bronchial circulation to EIPH has not been determined. Regardless of the contribution of bronchial circulation to blood in the airways, the likely initial lesion is in capillaries associated with the pulmonary circulation. Hemorrhage into the interstitial space and alveoli, with subsequent rostral movement of blood in the airways, results in blood in the trachea and bronchi and, infrequently, epistaxis.

Rupture of alveolar capillaries occurs secondary to an exercise-induced increase in transmural pressure (pressure difference between the inside of the capillary and the alveolar lumen (Fig. 29.8)). If the transmural stress exceeds the tensile strength of the capillary wall, the capillary ruptures.[96] The proximate cause of alveolar capillary rupture is the high transmural pressure generated by positive intracapillary pressures (largely attributable to capillary blood pressure) and the lower intra-alveolar pressure (generated by the negative pleural pressures associated with inspiration). During exercise, the absolute magnitudes of both pulmonary capillary pressure and alveolar pressure increase, with a consequent increase in transmural pressure[76,96] (Fig. 29.8). Strenuous exercise is associated with marked increases in pulmonary artery pressure in horses.[27,61,97] Values for mean pulmonary arterial pressure at rest of 20–25 mmHg increase to greater than 90 mmHg during intense exercise because of the large cardiac output achieved by exercising horses. Although pulmonary capillary pressure cannot be measured directly, it can be estimated from pulmonary artery wedge pressures. Different techniques for estimating pulmonary capillary pressure produce varying values, but invariably exercise induces a marked increase in pulmonary capillary pressure.[76,98,99] Combined with the increase in pulmonary capillary pressure is a marked decrease (more negative) in pleural, and therefore alveolar, pressures during exercise. Pleural pressures of normal horses during inspiration decrease from approximately −0.7 kPa (−5.3 mmHg) at rest to as low as −8.5 kPa (64 mmHg) during strenuous exercise.[100] Together, the increases in pulmonary capillary pressure and decrease (more negative) in intrapleural (alveolar) pressure contribute to a marked increase in stress in the alveolar wall. Although the alveolar wall and pulmonary capillary of horses are stronger than those of other species, rupture may occur because the wall stress in the alveolus exceeds the mechanical strength of the capillary.[101]

Other theories of the pathogenesis of EIPH include (Table 29.3): small airway disease, upper airway obstruction, hemostatic abnormalities, changes in blood viscosity and erythrocyte shape, intrathoracic sheer forces associated with gait, and bronchial artery angiogenesis.[95,102] It is likely that the pathogenesis of EIPH involves several processes, including pulmonary hypertension, lower alveolar pressure and changes in lung structure, that summate to induce stress failure of pulmonary capillaries.

Obstruction of either the upper or lower airways has been proposed as a cause of EIPH.[103] Inspiratory airway obstruction results in more negative intrapleural, and therefore alveolar, pressures. This effect is exacerbated by exercise with the result that alveolar transmural pressure is greater in horses with airway obstruction (see Fig. 29.8).[74] The higher transmural pressure in such horses could increase the severity of EIPH, although this has not been demonstrated. Moreover, while inspiratory airway obstruction could predispose to EIPH, the prevalence of this condition is much less than that of EIPH, indicating that it is not the sole factor inducing EIPH in most horses.

Table 29.3 Potential factors inducing or contributing to the severity of exercise-induced pulmonary hemorrhage

Pulmonary capillary hypertension
Rheologic properties of blood
Negative intrapleural (alveolar) pressures
Extrathoracic airway obstruction (e.g. laryngeal hemiplegia)
Intrathoracic airway obstruction (e.g. bronchoconstriction)
Small airway inflammatory disease
• viral or bacterial infections
• allergy
• air pollution (dust, ozone)
Coagulopathy
• abnormal platelet function
• capillary fragility
Bronchial neovascularization
Veno-occlusive remodeling
Pulmonary fibrosis and altered compliance
Locomotory forces
• foot strike
• abdominal piston

There is debate over the role of inflammation in causing or exacerbating EIPH. Horses with moderate-to-severe EIPH have histologic evidence of inflammation of the small airways,[45,104] and there is a clear association between presence of EIPH and inflammatory changes in bronchoalveolar or tracheal aspirate fluid.[23,105,106] Instillation of autologous blood into the airways induces a marked inflammatory response in normal horses,[26,107] although others have not detected inflammation and fibrosis subsequent to installation of autologous blood into the airways of horses.[108] Regardless of whether blood causes pulmonary inflammation, mild pulmonary inflammation increases the severity of EIPH in an experimental model of the disorder,[109] providing support for a role for inflammation in the disorder. Small airway inflammation and bronchoconstriction have the potential to produce intrathoracic airway obstruction and, therefore, a more negative alveolar pressure. Given that small airway disease is common in horses, there is the potential for an important effect of factors such as viral infections, air pollution and allergic airway disease to contribute to the initiation or propagation of EIPH. However, these associations remain unproved.

Exercise is accompanied by marked changes in blood flow characteristics attributable to an increase in hematocrit and decrease in red cell deformability.[69,110] These changes cause an increase in microvascular shear stress and thus could, conceivably, contribute to capillary rupture.[110] However, there is at present no direct evidence that indicates that this is an important feature of EIPH.

The characteristic location of lesions of EIPH in the caudodorsal lung fields has led to the proposal that hemorrhage is a result of tissue damage occurring when waves of stress, generated by forelimb foot strike, are focused and amplified into by the narrowing cross-sectional area of the caudal lung lobes.[111] According to the theory, the locomotory impact of the forelimbs results in transmission of forces through the scapula to the body wall, from where they pass into the lungs and caudally and dorsally. As the wave of pressure passes into the narrower caudodorsal regions of the lungs it generates progressively greater shearing forces which disrupt tissue and cause EIPH.[102] However, studies of intrapleural pressures have not demonstrated the presence of a systemic pressure wave passing through the lung and do not provide support for this hypothesis.[112]

Horses with EIPH have been suspected of having defects in either hemostasis or fibrinolysis. However, while exercise induces substantial changes in blood coagulation and fibrinolysis,[85] these is no evidence that horses with EIPH have defective coagulation or increased fibrinolysis.[86,87]

There is interest in the heritability or a potential genetic basis for susceptibility to EIPH and while initial studies are suggestive of such a phenomenon, there is no clear evidence of a genetic basis for the disorder.[113,114]

Regardless of the cause, rupture of pulmonary capillaries and subsequent hemorrhage into airways and interstitium causes inflammation of both airways and interstitium with subsequent development of fibrosis and alteration of tissue compliance especially in the caudodorsal lung fields (Fig. 29.10). Heterogeneity of compliance within the lungs, and particularly at the junction of normal and diseased tissue, results in development of abnormal shear stress with subsequent tissue damage. These changes are exacerbated by inflammation and obstruction of small airways with resulting uneven inflation of the lungs. Additionally, there is veno-occulsive remodeling of intralobular veins, collocated with hemosiderosis, fibrosis and hypertrophy of pleural vessels, which is postulated to lead to regional congestion and hemorrhage.[115,116] The structural abnormalities, combined with pulmonary hypertension and the large intrathoracic forces associated with respiration during strenuous exercise, cause repetitive damage at the boundary of normal and diseased tissue with further hemorrhage and inflammation. The process, once started, is lifelong and continues for as long as the horse continues to perform strenuous exercise.[95]

Epidemiology

Exercise-induced pulmonary hemorrhage is characteristically a disorder of horses that run at high speed, such as Thoroughbred or Standardbred racehorses. The disease is uncommon in endurance horses and rare in draft horses. As a general rule, the more intense the exercise or higher the speed attained, the greater the proportion of horses with EIPH.

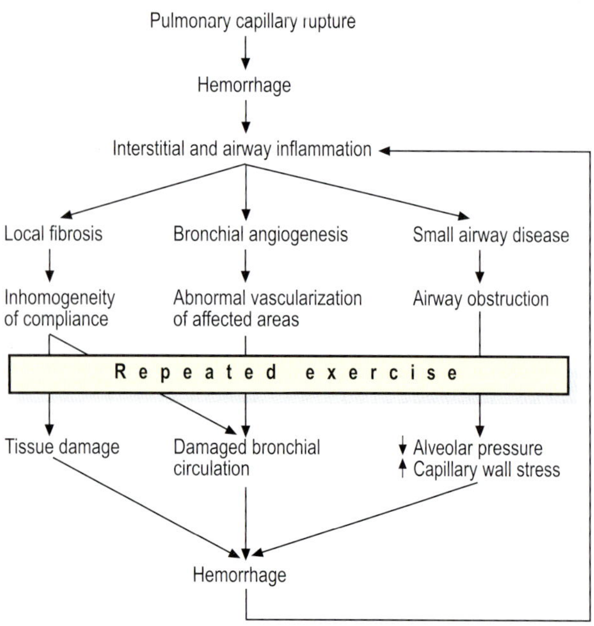

Fig 29.10 Proposed pathogenesis of EIPH.

The prevalence of EIPH varies with the method used to detect it and the frequency with which horses are examined. Almost all Thoroughbred racehorses in active training have hemosiderophages in bronchoalveolar lavage fluid, indicating that all have some degree of EIPH.[1] The prevalence of EIPH decreases when diagnosis is based on endoscopic examination of horses after exercise or racing.

Exercise-induced pulmonary hemorrhage is very common in Thoroughbred racehorses with estimates of prevalence, based on a single endoscopic examination of the trachea and bronchi, of 43 to 75%.[3,4,6,8,47] The prevalence increases with the frequency of examination with over 80% of horses having evidence of EIPH on at least one occasion after examination after each of two or three consecutive races.[47,58] The prevalence of EIPH in Standardbred racehorses is assumed to be lower, with 26–34% of horses reported to have blood in the trachea after racing.[10,117] However, these studies were based on a single examination and one[117] only reported as positive those horses with blood covering more than one-half of the tracheobronchial tree. When examined after each of three races, 87% of Standardbred racehorses have evidence of EIPH on at least one occasion,[9] suggesting that EIPH is as common in Standardbred racehorses as it is in Thoroughbred racehorses.

Exercise-induced pulmonary hemorrhage occurs in approximately 62% of racing Quarter Horses, and has been observed in Quarter Horses used for barrel racing.[20] The disorder occurs in racing Appaloosa horses.[19] Approximately 11% of polo ponies are affected with EIPH.[118] EIPH is rare in draft horses.[119]

Age, or increasing duration of racing career, is reported in some studies as an important risk factor for EIPH with the prevalence of the disorder being higher in older horses.[3,4,8] These studies did not control for the effect of number of lifetime starts and some examined relatively small numbers of horses. A large, prospective study of Thoroughbred racehorses did not identify age, independent of the number of lifetime starts, as being significantly ($P = 0.35$) associated with risk of EIPH.[120] The number of lifetime starts was significantly associated with risk of EIPH ≥ 1.[120] There is no consistent effect of sex on prevalence of EIPH.[3,4,8,120]

Among Thoroughbred racehorses the prevalence of EIPH increases with increasing speed with the prevalence of EIPH in one small study being greater in Thoroughbreds after racing than after breezing (galloping).[4] Lesions of EIPH are not detected in young Thoroughbred racehorses that have not trained at speeds above 7 m per second.[104]

Ambient temperature might be related to risk of EIPH in Standardbred and Thoroughbred racehorses. Standardbred horses racing at colder temperatures, have an increased risk of EIPH as do Thoroughbred.[9,120] The effect is relatively weak and the clinical importance of these risk factors is unclear. There is not a relationship between air quality and risk of EIPH in Thoroughbreds racing in Australia.[120]

Risk factors for epistaxis are not identical to risk factors for EIPH. Epistaxis is more common in horses with longer racing careers, with horses 4–5 years of age or older being 2.7–6.4 times as likely to have epistaxis compared to two-year-old horses or horses with no previous racing.[4,8,15,18,21,121,122] Female Thoroughbreds are 1.4 times as likely as stallions to have epistaxis in Japan although this effect was not detected in the United Kingdom.[18,121] Epistaxis is more common after races <1600 m than in longer races.[18] However, horses in steeplechase or hurdle races, which are typically longer than 2000 m, are at greater risk of epistaxis than are horses in flat races.[15,18,21,121] Horses racing over hurdles are 2.6 times more likely to have epistaxis if the going is 'firm' rather than 'good'.[121]

References

1. McKane SA, Canfield PJ, Rose RJ. Equine bronchoalveolar lavage cytology: survey of thoroughbred racehorses in training. Aust Vet J 1993;70:401–4.
2. Martin Jr BB, Beech J, Parente EJ. Cytologic examination of specimens obtained by means of tracheal washes performed before and after high-speed treadmill exercise in horses with a history of poor performance. J Am Vet Med Assoc 1999;214:673–7.
3. Pascoe JR, Ferraro GL, Cannon JH, et al. Exercise-induced pulmonary hemorrhage in racing thoroughbreds: a preliminary study. Am J Vet Res 1981;42:703–7.
4. Raphel CF, Soma LR. Exercise-induced pulmonary hemorrhage in Thoroughbreds after racing and breezing. Am J Vet Res 1982;43:1123–7.
5. Birks EK, Shuler KM, Soma LR, et al. EIPH: postrace endoscopic evaluation of Standardbreds and Thoroughbreds. Equine Vet J Suppl 2002:375–8.
6. Hinchcliff KW, Jackson MA, Morley PS, et al. Association between exercise-induced pulmonary hemorrhage and performance in Thoroughbred racehorses. J Am Vet Med Assoc 2005;227:768–74.
7. Hinchcliff KW, Jackson MA, Brown JA, et al. Tracheobronchoscopic assessment of exercise-induced pulmonary hemorrhage in horses. Am J Vet Res 2005;66:596–8.
8. Mason DK, Collins EA, Watkins KL. Exercise-induced pulmonary haemorrhage in horses. In: Snow DH, Persson SG, Rose RJ, editors. Equine Exercise Physiology. Cambridge: Granta; 1983. p. 57–63.
9. Lapointe JM, Vrins A, McCarvill E. A survey of exercise-induced pulmonary haemorrhage in Quebec standardbred racehorses. Equine Vet J 1994;26:482–5.
10. Speirs VC. Pulmonary haemorrhage in standardbred horses after racing. Aus Vet J 1982;59:38.
11. Rohrbach BW. Exercise-induced pulmonary hemorrhage, chronic obstructive pulmonary disease, and racing performance. J Am Vet Med Assoc 1990;196:1563–4.
12. Lyle CH. Sudden death in racing Thoroughbred horses: an international multicentre study of post mortem findings. Equine Vet J 2011;43:324.
13. Doucet MY. Clinical, radiographic, endoscopic, bronchoalveolar lavage and lung biopsy findings in horses with exercise-induced pulmonary hemorrhage. Can Vet J 2002;43:195.
14. O'Callaghan MW, Pascoe JR, Tyler WS, et al. Exercise-induced pulmonary haemorrhage in the horse: results of a detailed clinical, post mortem and imaging study. I. Clinical profile of horses. Equine Vet J 1987;19:384–8.
15. Cook WR. Epistaxis in the racehorse. Equine Vet J 1974;6:45.
16. Christley RM. Coughing in thoroughbred racehorses: risk factors and tracheal endoscopic and cytological findings. Vet Rec 2001;148:99.
17. Raphel CF. Endoscopic findings in the upper respiratory tract of 479 horses. J Am Vet Med Assoc 1982;181:470–3.
18. Takahashi T, Hiraga A, Ohmura H, et al. Frequency of and risk factors for epistaxis associated with exercise-induced pulmonary hemorrhage in horses: 251,609 race starts (1992–1997). J Am Vet Med Assoc 2001;218:1462–4.
19. Hillidge CJ, Whitlock TW. Sex variation in the prevalence of exercise-induced pulmonary haemorrhage in racing quarter horses. Res Vet Sci 1986;40:406–7.
20. Hillidge CJ, Lane TJ, Johnson EL, et al. Preliminary investigations of exercise-induced pulmonary hemorrhage in racing Quarter Horses. J Equine Vet Sci 1984;4:21–3.
21. Pfaff G. The incidence of epistaxis in racehorses in South Africa. J S Afr Vet Med Assoc 1976;47:215–18.
22. Pascoe JR, McCabe AE, Franti CE, et al. Efficacy of furosemide in the treatment of exercise-induced pulmonary hemorrhage in Thoroughbred racehorses. Am J Vet Res 1985;46:2000–3.
23. Fogarty U, Buckley T. Bronchoalveolar lavage findings in horses with exercise intolerance. Equine Vet J 1991;23:434–7.
24. Step DL. Cytologic and endoscopic findings after intrapulmonary blood inoculation in horses. J Equine Vet Sci 1991;11:340.
25. Meyer TS. Quantification of exercise-induced pulmonary haemorrhage with bronchoalveolar lavage. Equine Vet J 1998;30:284.
26. McKane SA, Slocombe RF. Sequential changes in bronchoalveolar cytology after autologous blood inoculation. Equine Vet J Suppl 1999;30:126–30.
27. Langsetmo I, Meyer MR, Erickson HH. Relationship of pulmonary arterial pressure to pulmonary haemorrhage in exercising horses. Equine Vet J 2000;32:379–84.
28. Kindig CA, McDonough P, Finley MR, et al. NO inhalation reduces pulmonary arterial pressure but not hemorrhage in maximally exercising horses. J Appl Physiol 2001;91:2674–8.
29. Geor RJ, Ommundson L, Fenton G, et al. Effects of an external nasal strip and frusemide on pulmonary haemorrhage in Thoroughbreds following high-intensity exercise. Equine Vet J 2001;33:577–84.
30. Richard EA. Laboratory findings in respiratory fluids of the poorly-performing horse. Vet J 2010;185:115.
31. Lester G, Clark C, Rice B, et al. Effect of timing and route of administration of furosemide on pulmonary hemorrhage and pulmonary arterial pressure in exercising thoroughbred racehorses. Am J Vet Res 1999;60:22–8.
32. Rossier Y. Bronchoalveolar lavage fluid cytologic findings in horses with pneumonia or pleuropneumonia. J Am Vet Med Assoc 1991;198:1001.
33. Hinchcliff KW. Counting red cells – is it the answer to EIPH? Equine Vet J 2000;32:362–3.
34. Aguilera-Tejero E, Pascoe JR, Smith BL, et al. Evaluation of a technique for detection of pulmonary hemorrhage in horses, using carbon monoxide uptake. Am J Vet Res 1994;55:1032–6.
35. Votion DM, Roberts CA, Marlin DJ, et al. Feasibility of scintigraphy in exercise-induced pulmonary haemorrhage detection and quantification: preliminary studies. Equine Vet J Suppl 1999;30:137–42.
36. McKane SA. Radiographic determination of the location of a blindly passed bronchoalveolar lavage catheter. Equine Vet Educ 1993;5:329.
37. O'Callaghan MW, Pascoe JR, O'Brien TR, et al. Exercise-induced pulmonary haemorrhage in the horse: results of a detailed clinical, post mortem and imaging study. VI. Radiological/pathological correlations. Equine Vet J 1987;19:419–22.
38. O'Callaghan MW. Radiographic changes in the lungs of horses with exercise-induced epistaxis. New Zealand Vet J 1982;30:117.
39. Pascoe JR. Radiographic aspects of exercise-induced pulmonary hemorrhage in racing horses. Vet Radiol Ultrasound 1983;24:85.
40. O'Callaghan MW, Hornof WJ, Fisher PE, et al. Exercise-induced pulmonary haemorrhage in the horses: results of a detailed clinical, post mortem and imaging study. VII. Ventilation/perfusion scintigraphy in horses with EIPH. Equine Vet J 1987;19:423–7.
41. Couetil LL, Denicola DB. Blood gas, plasma lactate and bronchoalveolar lavage cytology analyzes in racehorses with respiratory disease. Equine Vet J Suppl 1999;30:77–82.
42. Davidson EJ. Exercising blood gas analysis, dynamic upper respiratory tract obstruction, and postexercising bronchoalveolar lavage cytology – a comparative study in poor performing horses. J Equine Vet Sci 2011;31:475.

43. O'Callaghan MW, Pascoe JR, Tyler WS, et al. Exercise-induced pulmonary haemorrhage in the horse: results of a detailed clinical, post mortem and imaging study. II. Gross lung pathology. Equine Vet J 1987;19:389–93.
44. O'Callaghan MW, Pascoe JR, Tyler WS, et al. Exercise-induced pulmonary haemorrhage in the horse: results of a detailed clinical, post mortem and imaging study. III. Subgross findings in lungs subjected to latex perfusions of the bronchial and pulmonary arteries. Equine Vet J 1987;19:394–404.
45. O'Callaghan MW, Pascoe JR, Tyler WS, et al. Exercise-induced pulmonary haemorrhage in the horse: results of a detailed clinical, post mortem and imaging study. V. Microscopic observations. Equine Vet J 1987;19:411–18.
46. Barakzai SZ. Epistaxis in the horse. Equine Vet Educ 2004;16:207.
47. Hinchcliff KW. Efficacy of furosemide for prevention of exercise-induced pulmonary hemorrhage in Thoroughbred racehorses. J Am Vet Med Assoc 2009;235:76.
48. Williamson KK, Davis MS. Evidence-based respiratory medicine in horses. Vet Clin North Am 2007;23:215–27.
49. Buchholz BM. Effects of intravenous aminocaproic acid on exercise-induced pulmonary haemorrhage (EIPH). Equine Vet J 2010;42:256.
50. Perez Moreno CI. Effect of furosemide and furosemide–carbazochrome combination on exercise-induced pulmonary hemorrhage in Standardbred racehorses. Can Vet J 2009;50:821.
51. Mason DK, Collins EA, Watkins KL. Effect of bedding on the incidence of exercise induced pulmonary haemorrhage in racehorses in Hong Kong. Vet Rec 1984;115:268–9.
52. Furosemide (Lasix) Banned: Horse Bleeding Drug Not Allowed By American Graded Stakes Committee Huffington Post, 2011. (Accessed March 6, 2012, at http://www.huffingtonpost.com/2011/08/13/furosemide-banned-horse_n_926184.html.)
53. International agreement on breeding, racing and wagering. International Federation of Horseracing Authorities. (Accessed March 6, 2012, at http://www.horseracingintfed.com/resources/2011_choose_eng.pdf.)
54. Gross DK, Morley PS, Hinchcliff KW, et al. Effect of furosemide on performance of Thoroughbreds racing in the United States and Canada. J Am Vet Med Assoc 1999;215:670–5.
55. Soma LR, Birks EK, Uboh CE, et al. The effects of frusemide on racing times of Standardbred pacers. Equine Vet J 2000;32:334–40.
56. Soma LR, Uboh CE, Nann L, et al. Prerace venous blood acid–base values in standardbred horses. Equine Vet J 1996;28:390–6.
57. Sime D, Engen R, Miller-Graber P. Frequency and use of medications in horses racing in Prairie Meadows. Iowa State Uni Vet 1994:54.
58. Sweeney CR, Soma LR, Maxson AD, et al. Effects of furosemide on the racing times of Thoroughbreds. Am J Vet Res 1990;51:772–8.
59. Kindig CA, McDonough P, Fenton G, et al. Efficacy of nasal strip and furosemide in mitigating EIPH in Thoroughbred horses. J Appl Physiol 2001;91:1396–400.
60. Manohar M. Furosemide attenuates the exercise-induced increase in pulmonary artery wedge pressure in horses. Am J Vet Res 1993;54:952–8.
61. Manohar M, Hutchens E, Coney E. Pulmonary haemodynamics in the exercising horse and their relationship to exercise-induced pulmonary haemorrhage. Br Vet J 1993;149:419–28.
62. Gleed FD, Ducharme NG, Hackett RP, et al. Effects of frusemide on pulmonary capillary pressure in horses exercising on a treadmill. Equine Vet J Suppl 1999;30:102–6.
63. Muir 3rd WW, Sams RA, Hubbell JA, et al. Effects of enalaprilat on cardiorespiratory, hemodynamic, and hematologic variables in exercising horses. Am J Vet Res 2001;62:1008–13.
64. Manohar M, Goetz TE. Pulmonary vascular pressures of strenuously exercising Thoroughbreds during intravenous infusion of nitroglycerin. Am J Vet Res 1999;60:1436–40.
65. Kindig CA. Dissociation of exercise-induced pulmonary hemorrhage and pulmonary artery pressure via nitric oxide synthase inhibition. J Equine Vet Sci 2000;20:715.
66. Manohar M. L-NAME does not affect exercise-induced pulmonary hypertension in Thoroughbred horses. J Appl Physiol 1998;84:1902.
67. Colahan PT. The effect of sildenafil citrate administration on selected physiological parameters of exercising Thoroughbred horses. Equine Vet J 2010;42:606.
68. Perry BJ. Inventor Use of type V phosphodiesterase inhibitors in the treatment of exercise induced pulmonary hemorrhage in the equine. USA Patent 8,217,049 B2, July 10, 2012.
69. Fedde MR, Erickson HH. Increase in blood viscosity in the sprinting horse: can it account for the high pulmonary arterial pressure? Equine Vet J 1998;30:329–34.
70. Weiss DJ, Geor RJ, Burger K. Effects of pentoxifylline on hemorheologic alterations induced by incremental treadmill exercise in thoroughbreds. Am J Vet Res 1996;57:1364–8.
71. Weiss DJ, Geor RJ, Burger K. Effects of furosemide on hemorheologic alterations induced by incremental treadmill exercise in thoroughbreds. Am J Vet Res 1996;57:891–5.
72. Weiss DJ, Evanson OA, Geor RJ. The effects of furosemide and pentoxifylline on the flow properties of equine erythrocytes: in vitro studies. Vet Res Commun 1994;18:373–81.
73. Manohar M, Goetz TE, Rothenbaum P, et al. Intravenous pentoxifylline does not affect the exercise-induced pulmonary arterial, capillary or venous hypertension in Thoroughbred horses. J Vet Pharmacol Ther 2000;23:317–22.
74. Hackett RP, Ducharme NG, Ainsworth DM, et al. Effects of extrathoracic airway obstruction on intrathoracic pressure and pulmonary artery pressure in exercising horses. Am J Vet Res 1999;60:485–94.
75. Jackson JA, Ducharme NG, Hackett RP, et al. Effects of airway obstruction on transmural pulmonary artery pressure in exercising horses. Am J Vet Res 1997;58:897–903.
76. Ducharme NG. Pulmonary capillary pressure in horses undergoing alteration of pleural pressure by imposition of various upper airway resistive loads. Equine Vet J 1999;31:27.
77. Holcombe SJ. Effect of commercially available nasal strips on airway resistance in exercising horses. Am J Vet Res 2002;63:1101.
78. Valdez SC, Nieto JE, Spier SJ, et al. Effect of an external nasal dilator strip on cytologic characteristics of bronchoalveolar lavage fluid in Thoroughbred racehorses. J Am Vet Med Assoc 2004;224:558–61.
79. Slocombe RF. Respiratory mechanics of horses during stepwise treadmill exercise tests, and the effect of clenbuterol pretreatment on them. Aus Vet J 1992;69:221.
80. Manohar M, Goetz TE, Rothenbaum P, et al. Clenbuterol administration does not attenuate the exercise-induced pulmonary arterial, capillary or venous hypertension in strenuously exercising Thoroughbred horses. Equine Vet J 2000;32:546–50.
81. Sweeney CR, Soma LR, Bucan CA, et al. Exercise-induced pulmonary hemorrhage in exercising Thoroughbreds: preliminary results with pre-exercise medication. Cornell Vet 1984;74:263–8.
82. Hillidge CJ. Failure of inhaled disodium cromoglycate aerosol to prevent exercise-induced pulmonary hemorrhage in racing Quarter Horses. J Vet Pharmacol Ther 1987;10:257.

83. Sweeney CR, Hall J, Fisher JR, et al. Efficacy of water vapor-saturated air in the treatment of exercise-induced pulmonary hemorrhage in Thoroughbred racehorses. Am J Vet Res 1988;49:1705–7.
84. McKane SA, Slocombe RF. Alveolar fibrosis and changes in equine lung morphometry in response to intrapulmonary blood. Equine Vet J Suppl 2002:451–8.
85. McKeever KH. Changes in coagulation and fibrinolysis in horses during exercise. Am J Vet Res 1990;51:1335.
86. Johnstone IB, Viel L, Crane S, et al. Hemostatic studies in racing standardbred horses with exercise-induced pulmonary hemorrhage. Hemostatic parameters at rest and after moderate exercise. Can J Vet Res 1991;55:101–6.
87. Giordano A, Meazza C, Salvadori M, et al. Thromboelastometric profiles of horses affected by exercise-induced pulmonary hemorrhages. Vet Med Int 2010;2010.
88. Epp TS. Effects of conjugated oestrogens and aminocaproic acid upon exercise-induced pulmonary haemorrhage (EIPH). Comp Exerc Physiol 2008;5:95.
89. Kopp KJ. Template bleeding time and thromboxane generation in the horse: effects of three non-steroidal anti-inflammatory drugs. Equine Vet J 1985;17:322.
90. Mahony C, Rantanen NW, DeMichael JA, et al. Spontaneous echocardiographic contrast in the thoroughbred: high prevalence in racehorses and a characteristic abnormality in bleeders. Equine Vet J 1992;24:129–33.
91. Sweeney CR, Soma LR. Exercise-induced pulmonary hemorrhage in thoroughbred horses: response to furosemide or hesperidin-citrus bioflavonoids. J Am Vet Med Assoc 1984;185:195–7.
92. Epp TS. The effectiveness of immunotherapy in treating exercise-induced pulmonary hemorrhage. J Equine Vet Sci 2009;29:527.
93. Epp TS. The effect of herbal supplementation on the severity of exercise-induced pulmonary haemorrhage. Equine Comp Exerc Physiol 2005;2:17.
94. West JB, Mathieu-Costello O, Jones JH, et al. Stress failure of pulmonary capillaries in racehorses with exercise-induced pulmonary hemorrhage. J Appl Physiol 1993;75:1097–109.
95. Pascoe JR. Exercise-induced pulmonary hemorhage: a unifying concept. In: Proceedings American Association of Equine Practitioners; 1996. p. 220–6.
96. West JB, Mathieu-Costello O. Stress failure of pulmonary capillaries as a mechanism for exercise induced pulmonary haemorrhage in the horse. Equine Vet J 1994;26:441–7.
97. Birks EK, Mathieu-Costello O, Fu Z, et al. Very high pressures are required to cause stress failure of pulmonary capillaries in thoroughbred racehorses. J Appl Physiol 1997;82:1584–92.
98. Manohar M. Pulmonary artery wedge pressure increases with high-intensity exercise in horses. Am J Vet Res 1993;54:142.
99. Sinha AK. Pulmonary capillary pressure during exercise in horses. J Appl Physiol 1996;80:1792.
100. Art T. Mechanics of breathing during strenuous exercise in Thoroughbred horses. Respir Physiol 1990;82:279.
101. Birks EK, Mathieu-Costello O, Fu Z, et al. Comparative aspects of the strength of pulmonary capillaries in rabbit, dog, and horse. Respir Physiol 1994;97:235–46.
102. Schroter RC, Leeming A, Denny E, et al. Modelling impact-initiated wave transmission through lung parenchyma in relation to the aetiology of exercise-induced pulmonary haemorrhage. Equine Vet J Suppl 1999;30:34–8.
103. Cook WR. Hypotheses on exercise-induced pulmonary hemorrhage in horses. J Am Vet Med Assoc 1988;193:8–10.
104. Oikawa M. Exercise-induced haemorrhagic lesions in the dorsocaudal extremities of the caudal lobes of the lungs of young thoroughbred horses. J Comp Pathol 1999;121:339–47.
105. Newton JR, Wood JL. Evidence of an association between inflammatory airway disease and EIPH in young Thoroughbreds during training. Equine Vet J Suppl 2002:417–24.
106. Michelotto PV. Pulmonary inflammation due to exercise-induced pulmonary haemorrhage in Thoroughbred colts during race training. Vet J 2011;190:e3–6.
107. Ainsworth DM. Effects of in vitro exposure to autologous blood and serum on expression of interleukin-8, interleukin-1β, and chemokine (CXC motif) ligand 2 in equine primary bronchial epithelial cell cultures. Am J Vet Res 2012;73:296.
108. Williams KJ. Repeated blood instillation into the airway of the horse does not cause pulmonary fibrosis. Equine Vet J 2011;43:354.
109. McKane SA. Experimental mild pulmonary inflammation promotes the development of exercise-induced pulmonary haemorrhage. Equine Vet J 2010;42:235.
110. Weiss DJ, Smith 2nd CM. Haemorrheological alterations associated with competitive racing activity in horses: implications for exercise-induced pulmonary haemorrhage (EIPH). Equine Vet J 1998;30:7–12.
111. Schroter RC, Marlin DJ, Denny E. Exercise-induced pulmonary haemorrhage (EIPH) in horses results from locomotory impact induced trauma – a novel, unifying concept. Equine Vet J 1998;30:186–92.
112. Jones JH. Heterogeneity of intrapleural pressures during exercise. Equine Vet J 2002;34:391.
113. Weideman H, Schoeman SJ, Jordaan GF. A genetic analysis of epistaxis as associated with EIPH in the Southern African Thoroughbred. S Afr J Anim Sci 2004;34:265–73.
114. Weideman H, Schoeman SJ, Jordaan GF. The inheritance of liability to epistaxis in the southern African Thoroughbred. J S Afr Vet Assoc 2004;75:158–62.
115. Williams KJ. Regional pulmonary veno-occlusion: a newly identified lesion of equine exercise-induced pulmonary hemorrhage. Vet Pathol 2008;45:316.
116. Derksen FJ. Regional distribution of collagen and haemosiderin in the lungs of horses with exercise-induced pulmonary haemorrhage. Equine Vet J 2009;41:586.
117. MacNamara B, Bauer S, Iafe J. Endoscopic evaluation of exercise-induced pulmonary hemorrhage and chronic obstructive pulmonary disease in association with poor performance in racing Standardbreds. J Am Vet Med Assoc 1990;196:443–5.
118. Voynick BT, Sweeney CR. Exercise induced pulmonary hemorrhage in polo and racing horses. J Am Vet Med Assoc 1986;188:301–2.
119. Brackenhoff JE, Holcombe SJ, Hauptman JG, et al. The prevalence of laryngeal disease in a large population of competition draft horses. Vet Surg 2006;35:579–83.
120. Hinchcliff KW. Risk factors for exercise-induced pulmonary haemorrhage in Thoroughbred racehorses. Equine Vet J 2010;42:228.
121. Newton JR, Rogers K, Marlin DJ, et al. Risk factors for epistaxis on British racecourses: evidence for locomotory impact-induced trauma contributing to the aetiology of exercise-induced pulmonary haemorrhage. Equine Vet J 2005;37:402–11.
122. Weideman H, Schoeman SJ, Jordaan GF, et al. Epistaxis related to exercise-induced pulmonary haemorrhage in south African Thoroughbreds. J S Afr Vet Assoc 2003;74:127–31.

Viral respiratory disease in athletic horses

30

Paul S. Morley   Nicola Pusterla

CHAPTER CONTENTS

Importance of viral respiratory infections in athletic horses

Viral respiratory infections are one of the most common health problems in horses throughout the world. These infections are self-limiting and associated disease is not life-threatening, except in extreme cases. However, athletic horses generally have an increased risk of becoming infected and disease associated with these infections has greater consequences for both the horse and owner/trainer because of the effect of disease on athletic capacity and ability to compete successfully.

How big is the problem?

Infectious respiratory disease (IRD) is one of the most common reasons that athletic horses are removed from scheduled training and performances.[1-3] Interestingly, it has been suggested that IRD is also a more frequent cause of performance disability among human athletes than all other diseases combined.[4-7] Even mild respiratory disease can affect equine athletes such they are not able to attain peak performance. Most clinical occurrences of acute IRD in horses are primarily if not solely attributable to viral respiratory infections.[8] While bacteria and mycoplasma can be primary pathogens, bacteria can be more important in exacerbating clinical disease after a primary viral insult. Major exceptions would be disease caused by *Streptococcus equi* subsp *equi* and *Rhodoccus equi*, although the latter is only a clinically important problem in foals.

The importance of respiratory disease among athletic horses is generally well recognized in the equine industries. In 1997 the United States Department of Agriculture (USDA) performed a survey to identify concerns that were of highest priority to the horse industry in the United States.[9] This needs assessment survey showed that problems in horses related to the respiratory system were the third most important health problem reported by all survey respondents (n = 2599), respiratory disease was the top health concern for respondents which used horses primarily for racing, and a majority of respondents considered respiratory disease agents, collectively (e.g., influenza virus, herpesvirus, etc.), to be their highest concern among infectious diseases.[9] A survey of 1200 equine practitioners in the United States found that veterinarians considered viral respiratory disease second only to colic in importance among medical problems of horses.[10] In addition to affecting the success of individual athletic performances, outbreaks of acute infectious respiratory disease can disrupt entire athletic competitions with important economic consequences. For example, dramatic outbreaks have been seen when novel strains of influenza virus are introduced into naïve populations (Fig. 30.1). The worldwide importance of viral IRD is further substantiated by the classification of equine influenza, equine rhinopneumonitis (herpesvirus), and equine viral arteritis as List B diseases for equids by

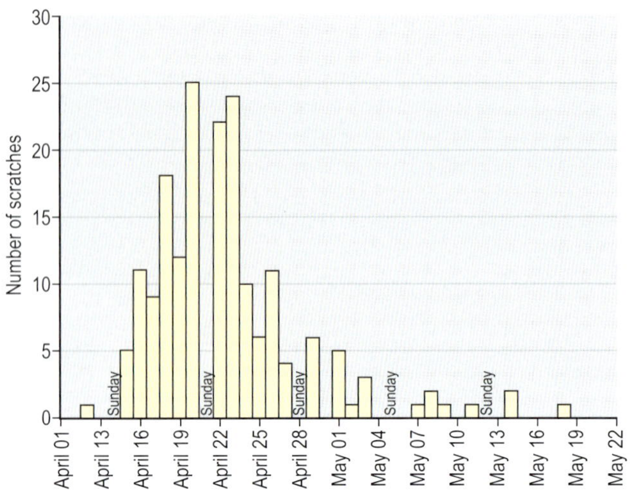

Fig 30.1 Scratches among 600 horses stabled at a racetrack during an influenza epidemic in April 1963. Similar epidemics were observed throughout North America following introduction of influenza A/equine/Miami/63 (H3N8). Note the lower rate of scratches observed after the epidemic during May.
Scholtens and Steele, 1964, Public Health Reports. *Adapted with permission.*

the Office International des Epizooties (OIE) because they are considered to have important effects on international trade of animals and animal products.

Why do equine athletes have an increased risk of viral infections?

Firstly, equine athletes are typically young and often do not have the fully developed immunity to infectious agents that is acquired through repeated exposure to agents that commonly affect horses. Secondly, athletic horses are often congregated in large groups at training and performance facilities which increases the probability of introduction and exposure to novel contagious pathogens. Thirdly, intensive management of equine athletes at training facilities increases the probability of exposure through management practices such as the shared use of tack and other equipment, as well as through increased exposure via respiratory aerosols and contaminated surfaces. Fourthly, environmental conditions encountered by equine athletes can impair non-specific clearance mechanisms through respiratory exposure to noxious chemicals (e.g. ammonia), dust, fungi, and molds. Drying and irritation of mucous membranes caused by airflow across their surfaces have been proposed as factors affecting non-specific immunity in human athletes,[11] and also might impact the health of equine athletes. In addition, racehorses are known to inhale significant quantities of small dirt particles when racing on dirt surfaces. These respiratory irritants can exacerbate non-infectious respiratory problems such as recurrent airway obstruction (heaves), which in turn are strongly believed to be a predisposing factor in viral respiratory infections in humans.[12–13] This is supported by the observation that the amount of airborne particulate matter in stabling environments significantly affects airway inflammation during EHV1 infection.[14,15] Infected horses stabled in barns with adequate ventilation and lower air particulate counts have less lower airway inflammation when compared with infected horses stabled in less suitable environments.

The frequency of IRD among equine and human athletes can also be impacted by important effects that exercise has on immune function. Physical stresses related to athletic activity have been repeatedly shown to be associated with transient changes of in vitro and in vivo measures of systemic and local immune function. This includes changes in catecholamine and cortisol release, neuropeptide hormone release, cytokine release and activity, secretion of mucosal antibody, and the functional activity of blood and pulmonary leukocytes.[16–23] These documented changes provide a basis for the 'open window' model proposed to describe cumulative effects of exercise on the immune system in humans.[16,24,25] According to this theoretical model, moderate exercise stimulates immune function during the event and for a short time after. In contrast, heavy exertion is related to an initial stimulation followed by a longer lasting (i.e. hours) depression in cell-mediated immune function. It is proposed that during this 'open window' of immune depression athletes have an increased risk of becoming infected with a variety of pathogens. Since elite athletes often train intensively on a daily basis, the cumulative time that they are at increased risk of infection is considerable.[16,25,26] In an effort to summarize the relationship between exercise and infectious disease, it has been proposed that the apparent relationship between intensity of exercise and its predisposing effect on the risk of upper respiratory tract infections in humans fits a J-shaped curve.[16,25] This model suggests that the risk of IRD in athletes is attenuated by moderate physical activity, but is exacerbated by chronic, intensive athletic activity. While similar research in horses is not as comprehensive, the limited work that is available suggests that similar effects can be found in horses.[27–37]

This relationship between exercise and immune function is obviously not simple, and is likely modulated by several other factors such as likelihood of exposure to novel pathogens, lack of adequate rest, mental stress, transport, inappropriate nutrition or weight loss, and concurrent infectious or non-infectious disease. This is probably one of the reasons that studies directly evaluating the relationship between exercise and the occurrence of infectious disease in humans have met with equivocal results, even though the effects on various markers of immune function have been repeatedly and convincingly demonstrated.[38] Unfortunately, almost no information is available directly examining the effects of athletic activity on the risk of IRD occurrences in horses.

How common is infectious respiratory disease in horses?

While IRD is very common among all horses there are few comprehensive estimates of the frequency of disease. There are two published estimates of IRD incidence in equine athletes that were obtained through prospective monitoring of racehorse populations.[2,39] A study performed at a single Canadian racetrack where investigators monitored disease occurrence during two race seasons estimated that the incidence of undifferentiated IRD was about 49 IRD cases per 1000 horse-months.[39] A prospective study of a cohort of Thoroughbred horses in Australia estimated the incidence of reported coughing and nasal discharge (infectious or non-infectious) to be approximately 1.8 cases per 1000 horse-months.[2] It is not clear if the difference in observers explains some of the difference between these estimates (reported by research investigators versus owner reported), or if the intensive nature of horse stabling at North American racetracks compared to more extensive management of racehorses elsewhere is partially responsible for differences between these two estimates. The absence of influenza virus as a disease agent in Australia at the time of the study could have also affected these estimates. The largest population-based study estimating the frequency of undifferentiated IRD occurrence among horses was conducted by the USDA as part of the NAHMS Equine '98 study.[40]

While the population for this study of owner-reported disease specifically excluded horses stabled at racetracks, it did include race horses that were stabled at other facilities. However, it should be noted that this data includes respiratory disease occurrences from horses of all ages, including those less than one year old. An estimated 1.5 percent (SE = 0.2) of horses per quarter developed IRD during this study, and the rate of reported IRD among racehorses housed off-track was nearly three times greater than the average for all horses (4.3 percent of horses per quarter, SE = 1.9). The occurrence of IRD was reported to vary by season, and disease incidence was greatest in the spring (March through May, 2.6 percent of horses, SE = 0.6), and least common during the winter (December through February, 0.8 percent of horses, SE = 0.2). In a smaller, but similar longitudinal study, data regarding the occurrence of disease was collected from randomly selected horse operations in Michigan, and the estimated incidence of undifferentiated respiratory disease was 33 cases per 1000 horse-years.[41]

Recognizing infectious respiratory disease

Clinical signs

Horses with IRD generally develop similar clinical signs regardless of which primary or secondary agents are causing clinical disease.[8] Disease is most frequently typified by the occurrence of mucopurulent nasal discharge and sometimes coughing. In a three-year study of respiratory disease at a Canadian racetrack, regardless of etiology, 80–95% of affected horses developed mucopurulent nasal discharge, while the occurrence of coughing was less common and more variable (30–75% coughed depending upon the etiology; Fig. 30.2).[8] In two more recent surveillance studies enrolling randomly selected horses with acute onset of upper respiratory tract infections, fever, coughing and nasal discharge varying from serous to mucopurulent were amongst the most common reported clinical signs.[42,43] Increased serous nasal discharge may be noted prior to becoming more mucoid. Paroxysmal coughing in a majority of affected animals may be suggestive of influenza virus infection, but this is not always predominant during influenza outbreaks, especially if clinical disease is mild. Fever (rectal temperature >38.5°C or 101.5°F) is less commonly noted in affected animals (10–30%).[8] Abscessation and dramatic enlargement of submandibular lymph nodes can sometimes allow differentiation of animals infected with *Streptococcus equi* subsp. *equi*, but not all infected animals develop this pathognomonic sign.[8,43] Many horses infected with viral respiratory agents remain asymptomatic, especially if they are older and are more immune. Others might only show vague signs such as lethargy, decreased appetite, and sub-optimal performance. Evaluation of horses with mild signs and sub-optimal performance can reveal evidence of lower respiratory tract infections (visible airway inflammation, inflammatory cytology, recovery of bacterial agents such as *S. zooepidemicus* subsp *zooepidemicus*). It is not clear if viral agents play a major role in less acute lower respiratory disease. However, seroconversion to equine herpesvirus was found to be associated with occurrences of less severe lower airway inflammatory disease, in addition to the isolation of *S. zooepidemicus* subsp. *equi* and *S. pneumoniae*.[44]

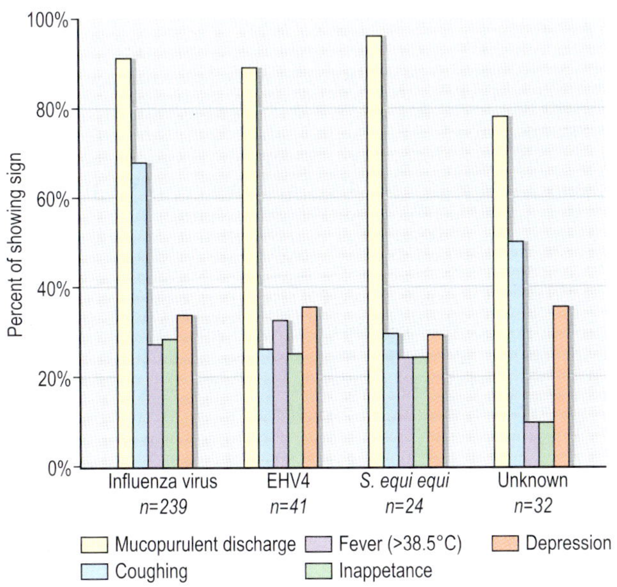

Fig 30.2 Clinical signs in racehorses diagnosed with IRD during a three-year study in Canada.

While most acute viral respiratory infections have been thought to primarily or solely affect the upper respiratory tract, the lower respiratory tract can also be affected during acute viral respiratory infections.[45] Ultrasound examinations showed that horses either experimentally and naturally infected with influenza virus can develop substantial areas of pulmonary consolidation and peripheral (pleural and subpleural) irregularities.[45] However, it is not clear if these lesions are principally caused by viral damage, or if this is a result of viral–bacterial co-infection. The bacterial flora of the upper respiratory tract change dramatically after viral infections, and this is principally characterized by proliferation of beta-hemolytic streptococci (Fig. 30.3; PS Morley, KW Hinchcliff, RD Slemons, DK Gross, unpublished data).[46] However, it is not clear whether this change is simply a result of viral mucosal damage and solely coincidental with clinical disease, or whether this change contributes significantly to clinical disease in horses with IRD. Pneumonia is a well-recognized sequela to severe viral respiratory infections in humans, and has also been reported after introduction of novel influenza viruses to naïve equine populations.[28,47–50] However, this is an infrequently recognized complication of most viral respiratory infections in horses. Interestingly, the significant pulmonary consolidation that was seen after severe experimental influenza virus infections resolved uneventfully without any treatment, even in horses that continued to exercise after infection.[45] There are few published results from objective investigations of clinical parameters in horses with viral IRD. Horses infected with influenza virus have been shown to have increased resting respiratory rates and heart rates which coincided with the occurrence of fever.[45] Pulmonary auscultation of horses experimentally and naturally infected with influenza virus often develop abnormal lung sounds, which was most frequently characterized as wheezing (DK Gross, PS Morley, K Hinchcliff, RD Slemons, unpublished data).[45,51,52]

Other systemic disease signs are sometimes reported in association with viral respiratory infections. These signs are perhaps most commonly recognized in association with equine herpesvirus type 1 (EHV1) infection; abortion and neurologic disease are well recognized in association with EHV1 infections. While essentially all EHV1 infections are thought to originate in the respiratory tract, signs of respiratory disease are not always evident before abortion or the onset of neurologic disease. While equine arteritis virus is considered an infrequent cause of respiratory disease, it has also been associated with edema of the head, legs, prepuce and abdomen, and abortion. Other systemic signs including myocarditis, rhabdomyolysis, and purpura hemorrhagica, have been reported as possible sequela of influenza virus infections. A recent study determined

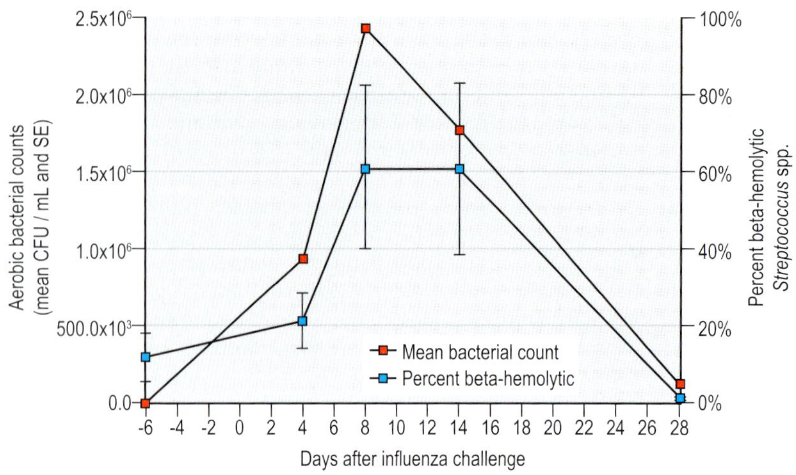

Fig 30.3 Bacteria recovered from aerobic culture of transtracheal wash fluid following influenza challenge in naïve horses.

cardiac troponin I concentrations in ponies experimentally challenged with equine influenza virus (A/eq/Kentucky/91).[53] The study demonstrated no evidence of severe myocardial necrosis secondary to equine influenza virus challenge with 10^8 EID_{50}, but transient increase in cardiac troponin I suggested that mild myocardial injury occurred. This is consistent with the fact that influenza virus is strongly epitheliotropic and that viremia is not a recognized feature of influenza virus infections.[50] While myocarditis has by recognized in humans in association with viral infections, this condition is more likely to be identified in association with Parvo B19, enteroviruses, adenoviruses, or cytomegalovirus, and is very rarely found in association with influenza virus infections.[54] It seems likely that myocardial damage or purpura hemorrhagica found in association with IRD would result from disseminated streptococcal infection in horses rather than viral respiratory infections.

Laboratory diagnosis

Viral IRD is often diagnosed based solely upon clinical evaluation and history. However, clinical signs associated with one virus cannot be used to reliably distinguish IRD caused by other pathogens. This is important because establishing an etiologic diagnosis can be very important for targeting disease prevention efforts early in some disease outbreaks. Viral agents have been clearly shown to vary in their clinical importance as well as in their infectious and contagious nature. However, efforts to control IRD in horses can be hampered because it can be difficult to quickly establish an etiological diagnosis for IRD.

Hematology

Routine hematologic analysis should routinely be performed in horses with respiratory signs in order to distinguish between an infectious and a non-infectious process. It must be emphasized that the timing of blood sampling and carefully standardized laboratory techniques are essential if interpretation of leukocyte patterns, in relation to viral infections, is to be useful as a diagnostic aid. It is also necessary to be aware of the various physiological (age, breed, diurnal variation, exercise) and pathological (stress) states which can influence the total and differential leukocyte count in the horse.[55] Ideally, horses with acute disease processes should be sampled during the first 24 hours of the febrile phase and because the leukocyte response is transient, sequential sampling of individual horses is necessary to detect all changes. The most consistent findings in horses with viral infectious disease of the respiratory tract are initial lymphopenia, mild normocytic, normochromic anemia and occasional mild thrombocytopenia.[45,56,57] A decrease in neutrophils and monocytes also occurs, but the absolute values of both cell types remain within normal limits. The blood work rapidly normalizes within a few days and often a transient mild monocytosis and relative lymphocytosis can be observed following the acute onset. It is not uncommon for horses with viral respiratory tract infection to develop a mild increase in fibrinogen post-exposure as a reflection of inflammation.

Serology

Viral infection is most often confirmed in horses using serology, which may be the most sensitive method available. However, even when isolation and epidemiologic data point to a single etiology for outbreaks of respiratory disease, serologic investigations found that only 72% of horses with disease thought to be caused by influenza virus infection seroconverted to this virus during epidemics, and only 36% of horses with disease thought to be caused by EHV4 seroconverted to herpesvirus.[8,39] By far the most commonly recognized viral agents associated with respiratory disease in horses are influenza and EHV4. However, diagnostic laboratories do not routinely test for other types of viral infections. In addition, regardless of the etiology, most serological tests require evaluation of multiple blood samples; the first must be obtained soon after infection and at least two or more weeks later. It might not be logistically possible to obtain samples at these times or it might not be practically relevant or important to veterinarians or owners.

Virus isolation

Virus isolation is a very specific method for diagnosis of viral infection, but culture techniques need a week or more for completion and require specialized laboratory equipment and skills. Early identification and sampling of affected horses is critical for virus isolation as horses shed viruses for only a short period after infection. Isolation techniques have also been found to be quite insensitive as a diagnostic test during several field investigations.[8,39,58] Because it can take weeks to obtain results, data from serology or virus isolation is often not very useful for enacting measures to control respiratory disease. As such, it would be useful to have simple tests available for rapid diagnoses of virus infections at the onset of epidemics so that control measures could be instituted.

Rapid diagnostic tests

In recent years rapid detection assays have been developed in research laboratories for identification of several viral agents (e.g., antigen capture ELISA, PCR), but most of these tests are not widely available for use in disease prevention efforts. Rapid antigen detection kits for influenza virus are, however, commercially available throughout the world. While it would be useful to have rapid tests available for other equine respiratory pathogens, influenza virus probably causes a majority of IRD cases among athletic horse populations (where it is present in the world; Fig. 30.4), and it is one of the most contagious pathogens which increases the importance of early intervention efforts. Most of these rapid influenza detection assays are based upon using monoclonal or polyclonal antibodies to detect highly conserved viral antigens. Most of these commercial assays can be completed in about 15–30 minutes and several have been proved to be useful for detection of influenza virus in horses.[59–63] Because they have been standardized and are sold in kits, they are more useful for a broad variety of diagnostic applications than are isolation techniques. While these tests are rapid and extremely useful, they have limitations. Optimal timing of sampling is important for antigen detection assays just as it is for virus isolation. Evaluation of nasal secretions collected from horses naturally infected with influenza virus suggests that only about one-third of clinically affected horses would be positive using the Directigen® assay (Becton Dickinson Microbiology Systems, Cockeysville, Maryland), which has been the most widely used assay in horses.[59] Other rapid influenza tests might be more sensitive, but they might also be less specific, which can be very important when these tests are used as part of stringent disease control programs.[55,56] It is important to note that more sensitive influenza detection assays have been shown to detect viral antigen in horses recently vaccinated with modified-live intranasal products, as well as from non-vaccinated horses that were in-contact with vaccinated horses.[62] This can be particularly important to consider if both vaccination and rapid detection assays are being used in disease prevention efforts during outbreaks.

Despite intensive investigative efforts, veterinarians frequently diagnose clinical IRD respiratory disease without identifying a primary etiologic agent. Potential pathogens were not identified from about 25% of IRD outbreaks investigated in England over a six-year period.[63] Investigators in Kentucky were unable to determine the etiology of 34% (14/41) of IRD outbreaks investigated over a five-year period.[64] Among 168 respiratory disease occurrences investigated during 1979, pathogens were identified for 44%.[65] Investigators in Canada were not able to identify an etiology for 14% (32/277) of IRD cases identified during a two-year longitudinal study of respiratory disease among racehorses (Fig. 30.4).[66] A recent voluntary surveillance study on 761 equids from the United States with clinical signs of acute onset of respiratory tract infection determined that 26.4% of index cases tested PCR positive for one or more of four selected common respiratory pathogens (equine herpesvirus-1/-4, equine influenza virus, *Streptococcus equi* subsp. *equi*).[43] The highest detection rate was for EHV4, followed by equine influenza virus, *Streptococcus equi* subsp. *equi* and EHV1. The lack of etiological diagnosis for some IRD cases observed in these investigations is at least partially attributable to concentrating diagnostic efforts on identifying infection with agents that most frequently cause disease. It is likely that more comprehensive diagnostic efforts would identify agents in affected animals that tend to cause either less dramatic outbreaks or sporadic rather than epidemic disease (e.g. gammaherpesviruses or equine rhinitis virus).

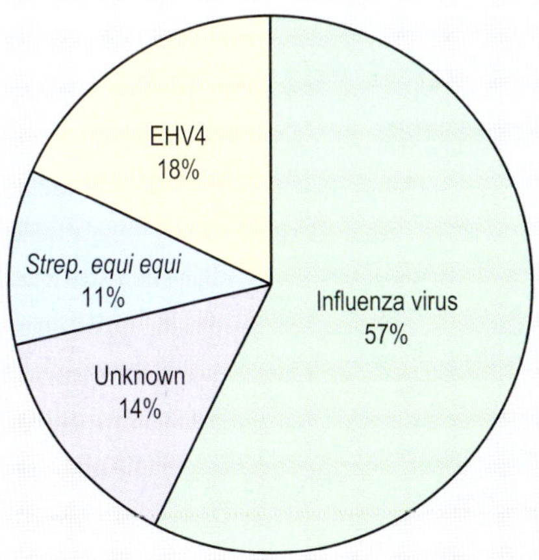

Fig 30.4 Etiology of IRD identified in a two-year longitudinal study at a Thoroughbred racetrack in Canada (n = 277).

The most obvious change in the laboratory diagnosis of viral respiratory pathogens has been the appearance and increasing importance of nucleic acid (NA) amplification-based techniques, primarily the polymerase chain reaction (PCR), at the expense of traditional methods of clinical microbiology.[67] The PCR has become an increasingly important tool in microbial diagnosis in recent years, mainly because of its rapidity, high sensitivity and high specificity. These superior characteristics have propelled the field of PCR-based molecular diagnostics into the arena of applied diagnostics for infectious agents. Because the number of published and offered PCR assays is steadily rising, there is a need for critical evaluation, comparison of performance, and eventually also standardization of methods to enable equine practitioners to select the optimal methodology. The sample of choice for the molecular detection of viruses associated with IRD is nasal secretions, which are generally collected from the nasal passages and/or the nasopharynx using rayon- or Dacron-tipped swabs. The use of viral transport medium for the transportation of nasal swabs is not needed for PCR detection, since nucleic acid-based assays do not rely on viability of the target pathogen. In order to increase the detection yield of viral respiratory pathogens, many molecular diagnostic laboratories offer panel testing for several viruses associated with infectious respiratory tract diseases. Collectively, PCR assays testing for the presence of equine influenza virus, EHV1 and EHV4 have shown increased sensitivity compared to antigen-capture ELISAs, conventional culture systems or both. Another advantage of molecular assays is their ability to detect non-viable virus, a situation which can occur when nasal or nasopharyngeal samples are frozen or not adequately stored and/or shipped to a diagnostic laboratory. Further, novel PCR platforms allow quantitation of DNA or RNA content in a given sample. This is of interest in order to assess the kinetics of viral shedding, to determine the infectious nature of a clinically or subclinically infected horse and the response to treatment.

In a recent study of 369 horses that were present at two major horse shows and two major Thoroughbred, newly arrived horses were sampled to identify subclinical and clinical shedding of EIV, EHV1 and EHV4.[68] Nasal swabs obtained from horses were tested using qPCR. On arrival at the four events the overall prevalence of EHV1 shedding was 3.3%, EHV4 shedding was detected in 1.1% of horses, and EIV shedding was found in 0.8%. In all instances EHV1 was detected at very low levels, and detection of EHV1 and EHV4 in nasal swab samples was not associated with clinical disease. EIV was detected only in horses sampled at a Thoroughbred sale and was associated with an outbreak of clinical respiratory disease but EHV1 and EHV4 shedding were not associated with respiratory disease. Horses under two years of age had a significantly greater risk of shedding EHV1 compared to older horses.

Ancillary diagnostic procedures

Although rarely utilized in most horses with viral IRD, information obtained from radiography, ultrasonography, and endoscopy may be useful for evaluating the extent and nature of guttural pouch and lower respiratory tract involvement. However, there is little published literature regarding findings of these ancillary diagnostics when applied in horses infected with various viral respiratory agents. Horses have been shown to developed marked consolidation after experimental infection with influenza virus which resolved without treatment or complication.[45] Similar findings have also been observed by these investigators in naturally infected horses. Endoscopic examination of these experimentally infected horses showed mild erythema and inflammation of the pharynx and airways, with increased amounts of mucoid respiratory secretions. Transtracheal wash fluid collected from horses infected with influenza virus was found to have increased cellularity and marked neutrophilia when compared with pre-infection values.[45] These changes were most severe for a week after infection, but changes could be detected for much longer. Intracellular bacteria were noted in about 25% of horses for up to 14 days after infection

Treatment and prognosis for viral respiratory disease in horses

Almost all viral respiratory infections are self-limiting and the primary therapeutic aim is to provide supportive care. Care should be taken to ensure that affected horses have access to clean water and adequate quantities of palatable feed as infected horses have been shown to lose weight and body condition.[45] Providing stabling in areas with minimal dust and ammonia exposure tends to lessen airway irritation and decrease the likelihood of secondary bronchitis and pharyngitis which can limit athletic performance.

Rest

It is often recommended that athletic horses with typical IRD be rested for an extended period after illness, sometimes for several weeks. This is intended to reduce the risk of serious complication such as pneumonia, pleuritis, and exercise limiting reactive airway disease. However, there are no published reports documenting the efficacy of this practice. One investigation specifically investigated whether moderate exercise exacerbated clinical disease in horses experimentally infected with influenza virus.[45] This study found that all of the horses developed pneumonia after infection and that there was an exacerbated loss of body condition and mild differences in resting heart and respiratory rates among exercised horses. However, all of the horses fully recovered without treatment according to parameters investigated, regardless of whether they were rested. It should be noted, however, that this study evaluated a small number of horses and did not specifically evaluate performance parameters that might be important for equine athletes.

Antibacterial and antiviral agents

Horses with uncomplicated viral respiratory infections will likely recover without drug therapy; use of anti-inflammatory drugs and other non-specific treatments may reduce fever and make affected animals more comfortable, but it is not clear whether they alter the course of disease. Severely affected horses might benefit from antimicrobial therapy as the bacterial flora of the respiratory tract changes dramatically during viral infections (PS Morley, KW Hinchcliff, RD Slemons, and DK Gross, unpublished data).[8] Bacteria can be recovered from the lower airways of horses that exhibit signs of primary viral IRD,[44,69,70] but it should be noted that there are no published studies evaluating the ability of antimicrobial (antibacterial) drugs to alter the course of IRD in horses with primary viral infections. Even horses with documented pulmonary consolidation and pneumonia secondary to experimental influenza infections were shown to recover uneventfully without the use of antimicrobial drugs.[45] Most horses affected by viral IRD show marked clinical improvement within a week of the onset of disease. Ongoing respiratory disease may reflect complications related to more severe pulmonary involvement, and these horses should be evaluated using ancillary diagnostics including pulmonary ultrasound and cytology and culture of transtracheal wash fluids.

Specific antiviral therapies for equine influenza virus and equine herpesvirus have been evaluated in equine and mouse models. However, none are licensed in the United States for this use in horses. In addition, considering the self-limiting nature of viral IRD, cost alone would preclude their use in most horses, regardless of safety or efficacy. In addition, use of antiviral drugs in humans is known to select for resistant strains. Amantadine and rimantadine have been used in humans infected with influenza virus, and both have demonstrated in vitro activity against equine influenza virus.[51,63] Oral administration of rimantadine has been evaluated in a small number of horses and administration of 30 mg/kg, PO, q 12 h for four days was associated with amelioration of clinical signs.[51] However, given the self-limiting nature of untreated influenza virus infections in horses, this therapy is of questionable value. Absorption of amantadine administered orally is inconsistent and effective plasma concentrations cannot be reliably attained.[71] In addition, while IV administration yielded more reproducible plasma concentrations, horses have a relatively small therapeutic margin and treatment can result in seizures.[71] Use of this drug is therefore not recommended. There are a variety of reports regarding evaluation of antiviral compounds against equine herpesvirus in in vitro and mouse models, but only limited published report of use in horses.[72–78] Respiratory disease associated with equine herpesviruses is generally mild and self-limiting, but use of these drugs in horses with other clinical disease syndromes (e.g., neurologic disease) or valuable pregnant mares could be warranted in some circumstances to reduce spread of infection amongst horses or prophylactically to attenuate the severity of disease in infected or exposed horses.

Prevention of viral respiratory disease in horses

The basic features of infectious disease control programs for horse populations are similar, regardless of the type of disease or the agent that is being targeted. Specific practices employed need to be tailored to the population of horses, the facilities involved, and the diseases of greatest concern.[79,80] Consider the following basic requirements and features for effective disease prevention programs:

- Understand the mode of transmission and important biological aspects for infectious diseases of interest.
- Identify management or host factors that facilitate transmission (considering the previous item in this outline)
- Categorize animals according to risk of having or acquiring the disease of interest or infecting others. Prioritize prevention and control efforts according to those risk categories:

- Appropriate categorization may be accomplished based upon known risk factors or history (e.g., age, history of travel, vaccination status, etc.)
- This categorization can be facilitated by use of diagnostic procedures when appropriate (e.g., serology to help in characterizing immunity to an agent and therefore susceptibility to infection or disease).
- Grouping horses according to these risk categories will facilitate management and decrease the risk of transmission to animals in other risk categories. However, it is possible to manage individual horses appropriately according to their disease risk category assuming that adequate rigor is employed.
- Prepare contingency plans for changes in disease risk when IRD is detected in the population. This can include the need to move horses to facilitate management, or to restrict movement and access to control disease transmission.

- Monitor for evidence of disease in the population. As the adage goes, 'you cannot manage what is not measured.' Viral respiratory agents can be extremely contagious, and large portions of susceptible populations can be affected when they are introduced. Early intervention can decrease the impact of these outbreaks, but this requires active monitoring of the population and swift action when disease is detected. Employment of rapid diagnostic tests to assist in identifying viral etiologic agents is useful in providing timely, measured responses that are appropriate for the degree of contagiousness of the different agents and the significance of associated disease.
- Employ prophylactic measures that have a reasonable expectation of efficacy and are appropriate for the degree of risk aversion and the budget of the facility (e.g., vaccination, hygiene practices such as hand washing, barrier nursing precautions, foot baths, etc.):
  - Ordering available prophylactic measures based upon cost and degree of efficacy will assist in determining which should be applied first, and which should only be considered if the degree of risk aversion is high.
  - These practices might vary depending upon the risk category of the animals.
  - Decisions to employ prophylactic measures often must be made far in advance of identifying IRD if they are to be of maximal benefit. For example, appropriate immunological priming is critical for vaccination to be of maximal benefit. This often requires a series of vaccinations given over several weeks.
  - Avoid wasting time, money, and effort employing prophylactic measures that do not have reasonable expectation of efficacy. More treatments are not necessarily better! Try to use only vaccines that have demonstrated efficacy. Employing non-efficacious treatments also creates a false sense of security for owners and managers, as well as increasing the likelihood that that they will be dissatisfied with previous veterinary advice.
- Do not forget or underestimate the importance of optimizing the overall health and well-being of horses when designing disease prevention programs. Minimize stress when possible. Optimize nutrition, and provide clean, fresh water ad libitum. Maximize cleanliness, hygiene, air quality, and comfort in stabling environments. Avoid treatments and management practices that unnecessarily increase the risk of infection.

Preventing transmission

The most important aspect of preventing IRD is to minimize the likelihood of adequate direct or indirect contact that allows exposure to agents that is adequate to establish infection. As testament to this statement, it is possible to identify large, isolated horse populations in the United States and Canada that are naïve to influenza virus despite the fact that this agent is frequently recognized and considered endemic in those countries. These populations have minimal protective immunity and are highly susceptible to disease, which is a major reason that they are frequently used for experimental research on IRD.[45,81,82] These populations remain disease free because of their closed nature and the minimal likelihood of exposure to influenza virus. Given the ubiquitous nature of some IRD agents (e.g., EHV1 and EHV4), it is harder to prevent all exposure, but frequent high-risk contact increases the risk of introducing highly contagious and highly pathogenic strains. Studies of IRD in racehorses have shown that horses with higher concentrations of serum antibody to influenza virus have decreased risk of disease during EHV4 epidemics, and horses with higher EVH4 concentrations have lower risk of disease during influenza epidemics.[8] This suggests that horses with increased risk of exposure to one respiratory virus likely have an increased risk of exposure to all respiratory viruses. This emphasizes the importance of non-specific control measures such as stringent biosecurity measures.

Indirect transmission

Direct contact among horses is obviously important for transmission of infectious respiratory agents, but the importance of indirect contact must not be overlooked. Viral IRD agents vary in their contagiousness via respiratory aerosols, and this mode of transmission seems most important in propagation of influenza epidemics. In addition, indirect transmission via contaminated surfaces and fomites can play a critical role in introduction of respiratory agents.[83–85] In many instances outbreaks in susceptible populations occur as result of indirect transmission, and epidemics can certainly be exacerbated by this route. During a longitudinal study of respiratory disease it was noted that grooms would often wipe the face and body of affected horses with a rag, and then repeat the same procedure on unaffected horses using the same grooming tool.[39] Tattooing of young horses using the same instrument was thought to be associated with spread of infection in another outbreak.[39] Contaminated trailers, tack, watering facilities and equipment, and even clothing of handlers have also been implicated in introduction of respiratory agents.

Barrier nursing precautions and personal hygiene

An important concept related to care of patients with contagious diseases is the use of barrier nursing precautions. Barrier nursing precautions (e.g., gloves and water-impervious gowns) can be used whenever working with high-risk patients to prevent strike-through and to minimize the potential for cross-contamination between patients. Barrier gowns are assigned for use with specific animals so that clothing most likely to be contaminated essentially stays with the patient. Disposable gloves, and separate coveralls or inexpensive disposable plastic barrier gowns (PolyWear gowns, #GEB-4250; PolyConversions Inc., Rantoul, IL 61866) could be assigned for use with specific animals. Rubber boots and disinfectant footbaths can also be used to reduce the risk of footwear serving to traffic infectious agents between stalls. In addition, limiting the number of people contacting high-risk patients and assigning specific people to care for animals in different risk categories will also reduce the risk of transmission.

Personal hygiene and cleanliness is indisputably an important cornerstone of infection control. All personnel contacting animals should be required to wear clean, appropriate attire at all times. Contaminated hands are perhaps the most frequent route of indirect nosocomial transmission in all species.[86] Frequent hand washing should be required particularly before and after handling affected animals. Alcohol-based hand sanitizing gels are available for use when it is not possible to wash hands. These hand sanitizing gels have equal efficacy to full surgical scrub when properly applied, but gross contamination of dirt and biological material must be removed by hand washing. We often illustrate the common-sense importance of hand hygiene as a disease control measure with students by asking them to look closely at their hands and to consider whether they would appreciate a physician with similar cleanliness performing an examination or an invasive procedure on them.

Cleaning and disinfection

Effective cleaning and disinfection are critical for breaking transmission cycles for viral and bacterial agents in horse populations. Stalls should be cleaned and thoroughly disinfected between all horses, especially when they have been used to house high-risk animals. Particular attention should be paid to disinfecting feeders, watering equipment, and surfaces frequently contacted by hands. Cleaning tools should not be used for animals in different risk categories unless they have been appropriately cleaned and disinfected. Bedding and feces should be removed from stalls between horses to facilitate more thorough cleaning. Dumpsters, wheelbarrows, and cleaning tools should be visibly marked for easy identification, and different sets should be assigned for use with a specific risk group. Several reviews are available regarding disinfection recommendations for livestock facilities.[87–89] Applying copious amounts of disinfectant to dirty surfaces is not effective for decontamination. Disinfectants are quickly inactivated in the presence of even small amounts of dirt and organic debris and can only be truly relied upon when applied to clean surfaces. Physical disruption is generally required to adequately remove gross contamination and surface films to ensure adequate disinfection. High-pressure washing can be an efficient method for cleaning large areas but it is also possible to further disseminate surface contaminants as they may be aerosolized in the cleaning process. Some disinfectants such as phenolics and peroxygen compound are more effective in the presence of organic material, but they are also more likely to cause irritation with skin contact in horses or personnel. Bleach, chlorhexidine, and quaternary ammonium-based products are less irritating, but are easily inactivated. Mist application of a peroxygen compound has been described as a means of inactivating airborne viruses as opposed to relying upon surface disinfection.[90] Mist application can also be an effective means for applying peroxygen disinfectants to surfaces in large buildings.[91] However, this should only be performed with appropriate personal protection equipment for personnel and also should only be used with products that are less irritating and toxic for humans and animals.

Housing and facility design

Design of animal facilities is a critical consideration for optimal performance of disease prevention programs. Stalls and buildings should be constructed to minimize the potential for direct and indirect contact between horses. In addition, it is extremely useful to have areas that can be separated to quarantine newly introduced animals, as well as provide separation between horses in different risk categories. Care should be given to ensure that animals can receive adequate care in these different areas, preferably without trafficking animals or equipment through the environment of horses in different risk categories. At a minimum, consideration should be given to separating high-risk animals from other animals with an empty stall. Cleanable surfaces should be maintained throughout practice environments whereever possible. Concrete floors are preferable to dirt, particularly for housing animals shedding contagious pathogens, as it is impossible to completely disinfect the latter. Rubber stall mats are usually quite porous, and it is very difficult to maintain effective seals at edges. This has been shown to be important in outbreaks documented in several veterinary teaching hospitals. Sealing or painting exposed wood and other porous surfaces greatly increases the ease of cleaning. However, it is important to consider quality of products and maintenance of painted surfaces when selecting sealants, as chipped and peeling paint provide a niche for bacterial contamination that is difficult clean. Attention must also be paid to controlling wildlife (e.g. mice and birds) and insect vectors, although these are usually not considered important as a means of transmitting viral respiratory disease among horses.

Management of disease control efforts

Perhaps one of the greatest obstacles to implementing a comprehensive infection control program for all horses at large facilities is obtaining cooperation from all of the owners, managers, and veterinarians. In many training or performance facilities, athletic horses are congregated in large groups with different people responsible for care of each different group. Generally, owners only want to pay for care of their own animals and thus procedures and costs for a comprehensive control program would need to be agreed upon and shared. Even if most owners and managers wish to employ such a program, like a chain with a single weak link, it only takes one hold-out employing less optimal biosecurity practices to allow introduction of a highly contagious agent, thus placing all horses at the facility at risk. In these situations it is useful to develop a cooperative agreement among all users of a facility, and empower a single individual to direct or oversee disease control efforts. This person could also oversee surveillance efforts so that there is uniform rigor in detection and management of sick horses. This would also facilitate prompt intervention which may help decrease the severity of outbreaks when they occur. This proactive approach has been very useful for control of infectious diseases of all types among horses hospitalized at Colorado State University, U.C. Davis, and other large referral centers.

Vaccination

Vaccines can play an important role in decreasing susceptibility to infectious agents, but their use should not replace other control efforts. The efficacy of specific influenza vaccines has been well demonstrated.[27,81,92,93] but other vaccines have limited efficacy.[94,95] or published information from properly designed efficacy studies is not available. Data regarding protection provided by herpesvirus vaccines is even more equivocal[8,95–99] Equine arteritis virus is the only other respiratory virus for which there are commercial vaccines, but their use can be restricted because of importation restrictions on seropositive stallions. Development of efficacious vaccines for respiratory viruses is complicated by the apparent shortduration of immunity which follows even natural exposure, and the genetic variability and rapid genetic mutation in some viruses. While most manufacturers recommend annual boosters on vaccine labels, many equine experts recommend vaccination at much shorter intervals (e.g. every three months or less).[49] A vaccine that must be boosted every three months or more frequently is obviously performing sub-optimally; managers and veterinarians should view this as strong evidence of the imperfect protection provided by some commercial vaccines. One of the challenges that manufacturers of equine vaccines have faced is the strong aversion among owners and managers for any overtly detectable local or systemic response to vaccination. The primary concern should be whether vaccines can be used safely to evoke a protective immune response, i.e., the risk of acceptable local or systemic reaction is worth the benefit of protective immunity. Unfortunately, many managers would prefer to pay for and employ ineffective vaccines at frequent intervals rather than have any observable response to vaccination. Veterinarians have been known to be no longer employed by owners or trainers when vaccinations have resulted in local swelling at injection sites. This would seem to be an incredibly short sighted and inadvisable approach to selection of vaccines. Consider that vaccines are commonly used for children when they are known to cause local (swelling, pain, induration) as well as systemic responses (fever, malaise, inappetance) as long as use provides the benefit of protective immunity.

Etiology of viral respiratory disease in horses

The most important viral agents associated with respiratory disease in athletic horses are influenza virus, EHV4, EHV1, and equine arteritis virus (EAV). Influenza virus and EHV4 are the viral agents most commonly identified in association with respiratory disease (Fig. 30.4). Herpesvirus type 1 is important because of its ubiquitous nature as well as the significance of non-respiratory clinical disease that is less commonly seen in association with infection (neurologic disease and abortion). Disease associated with EAV is much less common than infection, and this agent is more important because of associated reproductive losses. Other viral agents have been isolated from horses with IRD, including equine adenovirus, equine rhinitis virus and gammaherpesviruses. While infection with these agents may be associated with the occurrence of clinical disease, particularly sporadic cases, there is very little controlled evidence documenting the significance of these agents in relation to other more common agents.

Influenza virus

Characteristics

Influenza virus is a pleomorphic orthomyxovirus with a segmented double-stranded RNA genome. The segmented RNA genome predisposes this virus to genetic reassortment and mutation which promotes rapid viral evolution. There are three types of influenza virus (types A, B, and C) that are differentiated by their highly conserved internal proteins (matrix protein and nucleoprotein); horses are only infected by some Type A influenza viruses. The more variable surface glycoproteins, hemaglutinin and neuraminidase, contain the major antigenic determinants and are used to characterize subtypes of influenza virus (e.g. H3N8). RNA viruses are more prone to genetic variation, which likely influences important variability identified in antigenically dominant surface epitopes. Three distinct subtypes of influenza virus have been isolated from horses since 1956. These are represented by the following prototype strains: influenza A/equine/Prague/56 (H7N7) which is sometimes referred to as A1 equine influenza, influenza A/equine/Miami/63 (H3N8) which is sometimes referred to as A2 equine influenza, and influenza A/equine/Jilin/89 (H3N8). Only strains that evolved from the Miami/63 isolate are currently circulating in horse populations, but this virus has evolved into genetically and antigenically distinguishable clusters:[100–102] a so-called 'Eurasion' lineage, and an 'American' lineage. The 'American' lineage viruses can be further differentiated into three evolutionary strains.[103] Contrary to geo-specific strain names, 'American' lineage viruses are commonly isolated from horses in Europe and Asia, and a 'Eurasian' lineage virus was isolated from horses in Canada in 1991.[103] Tracking antigenic variation among strains of influenza virus is important because natural exposure and vaccination tend to promote strain-specific immunity. For example, while serum antibody concentrations tend to correlate well with immunity, antibody concentrations have been shown to be more strongly correlated with protection when animals were challenged with influenza virus from homologous lineage compared to when they were challenged with virus from a heterologous lineage.[104]

While some investigators have hypothesized that strains of H7N7 influenza may still circulate and that it is important to continue inclusion in vaccines, this strain of virus appears to no longer circulate as the last two reported isolations of this virus subtype occurred in Maylasia in 1977[105] and in India in 1987.[106] In 1989 a novel strain of H3N8 influenza virus emerged in horses in China and was thought to have been directly transmitted from birds,[28,107] but this strain also appears to have failed to be sustained in equine populations.[108]

Distribution

Equine influenza virus affects horses throughout the world, with only a few exceptions. Some member countries report to the OIE that they are free from disease,[50] but the rigor of scientific evidence to support this status varies considerably. Rigorous investigations in countries such as New Zealand has never found evidence of infection in resident horses, and there are some countries such as Singapore, Japan, South Africa and Australia that have previously had infected horses, but which have apparently eliminated the virus through rigorous control efforts.[50,109]

Transmission and pathogenesis

Influenza virus is spread via aerosols, as well as by direct and indirect contact with infected horses and contaminated surfaces. As an enveloped virus, influenza virus is not particularly hardy in the environment, but epidemics have been known to result from contact with people and fomites that have been moved from one operation to another. The incubation period is 24 to 48 hours, and clinical disease is highly variable. Virus can only be recovered from horses for about 10 days after infection at most, but viral antigen has been recovered from respiratory secretions only for as long as 21 days post-infection.[110] Influenza virus infects epithelial cells throughout the respiratory tract. Cell death and damage to mucociliary apparatus results in airway irritation and accumulation of cellular debris and respiratory secretions. Disease may be enhanced by proliferation of respiratory bacteria and secondary bacterial infections of respiratory tissues (Fig. 30.3). Disease is self-limiting in most cases.

Epidemiology and risk factors

Influenza virus is capable of being spread throughout large geographic areas and even continents when novel viruses are introduced to naïve horse populations.[84,85,106,107,111] For example, a study of sanctioned Thoroughbred and Standardbred race meetings in the United States after introduction of a novel virus in 1963 found that the outbreaks had been detected in 78% of respondent racetracks (49/63), and the virus spread throughout the United States and Canada during a six-month period (Fig. 30.5).[84] This spread of disease highlights the importance of disease control in athletic horses which tend to be the most mobile sector of equine populations in most countries. Introduction of horses that travel from one horse population to another has been repeatedly shown to be the major inciting incident for influenza epidemics. As horses do not become persistently infected with influenza virus, animals with acute infections are critical for the introduction of virus into susceptible populations. Unfortunately horses can be infected and shed influenza virus while remaining asymptomatic, or at least only mildly affected. Considering this, some disease control programs have employed the use of rapid antigen detection tests as a screening tool for newly introduced horses.[112] Assuming that the prevalence of infection among these horses would generally be very low, the negative predictive value for this test would be quite high, and regulatory officials could be quite certain that test-negative animals were truly uninfected. However, the positive predictive value would be unavoidably very low, and positive tests would frequently be false-positive in these testing conditions.[62] However, this testing is fairly innocuous and very rapid, and the consequences of introducing influenza virus can be very significant. Some inaccuracy in testing is unavoidable and as such, this low positive predictive value may be acceptable if the managers are highly risk averse.

Just as frequent contact between populations increases the risk of introduction, frequent direct and indirect contact among horses within a population increases the risk of infection during influenza outbreaks. Care must be taken to reduce inadvertent contact, and to consider all horses in a population as being significant in the control of disease. Longitudinal studies in Canada showed exercise ponies had much greater risk of disease during influenza epidemics which was probably attributable to their frequent contact with other horses.[113] In addition, there was less concern about their health than there was for racehorses, which ironically increased the risk for all horses in the population.

Factors related to specific immunity against influenza virus are also very important in determining a horse's risk of disease. Several studies have repeatedly shown that serum antibody concentrations strongly correlate with the risk of disease, and even small increases can be associated with a dramatic decrease in disease risk. For example, horses with high antibody concentrations were shown during a series of influenza epidemics to have 2–6 times lower odds of disease compared to those with low antibody concentrations, and about 10–40 times lower odds of disease compared to those that were seronegative.[113] In a recent nation-wide cross-sectional study conducted by the USDA, only about one-third of all horses tested had high antibody concentrations to influenza virus; about one-third were seronegative and one-third had low antibody concentrations. Age is also associated with the risk of influenza infection, which probably is a surrogate marker of the probability of previous exposure to disease agents. This is supported by studies documenting a relationship between age and increasing antibody concentrations.[40] This age-associated disease risk is particularly important for athletic horses given the predominance of young horses in these populations.

The strength and repeatability of the association between age and measures of previous exposure demonstrate their importance as predictors of disease risk. As such, these factors can be used as important factors in categorizing horses for future disease risk, and help in targeting control measures on horses in the highest risk categories. Serum antibody concentrations could be measured as horses enter populations and more rigorous biosecurity precautions could be employed with those horses having low antibody concentrations. This information could also be used to specifically target vaccination protocols. Information collected from longitudinal studies in Canada suggested that 25% IRD associated with influenza virus would have been prevented during epidemics if all horses had high serum antibody concentrations prior to exposure.[111] While efficacious killed virus vaccines administered intramuscularly invoke protection by stimulating humoral immunity it is important to note that a new modified-live intranasal vaccine has been shown to be efficacious without stimulating increases in serum antibody concentrations.[81] If vaccines are to be used in prevention efforts, it is critical to only use products with reasonable expectation of efficacy.[81,92,93] as several equine influenza vaccines that are available commercially have been shown to perform sub-optimally.[94,95]

Equine herpesvirus

Characteristics

Herpesviruses are subdivided into three subfamilies based upon genetic structure: alpha, beta, and gamma. There are five

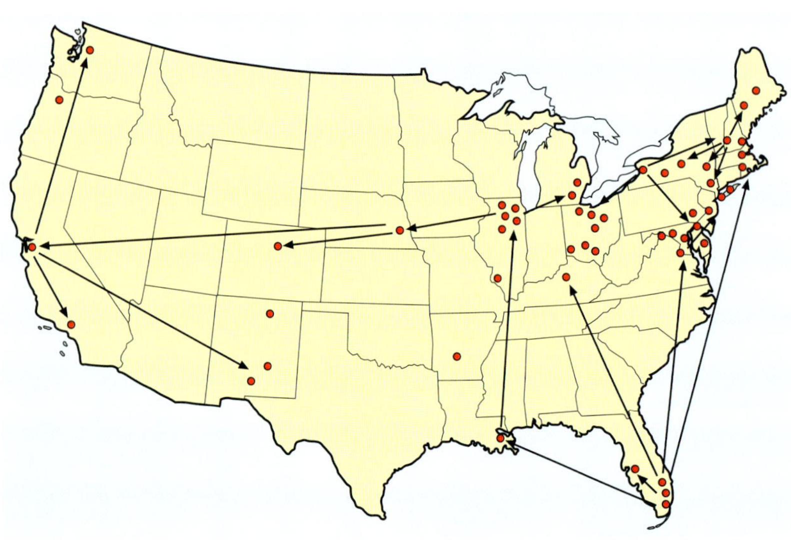

Fig 30.5 Spread of influenza A/equine/Miami/63 (H3N8) at racetracks in the six-month period following introduction in 1963. Dots indicate racetracks with influenza outbreaks, arrows represent movement of horses thought to be associated with transmission.
Scholtens and Steele, 1964, Public Health Reports. *Reprinted with permission.*

herpesviruses known to infect horses, four of which have been shown to infect tissues of the respiratory tract.[114] EHV4 is an alphaherpesvirus that is thought to be a frequent cause of respiratory disease in horses.[43] EHV1 is also an alphaherpesvirus, and while infections typically originate in the respiratory tract, it is more commonly associated with other severe systemic illness (neurologic disease and abortion) and less commonly with respiratory disease. EHV2 and EHV5 are slow-growing gammaherpesviruses that have been recovered from numerous tissues of healthy and clinically diseased horses. Their role and importance in the occurrence of clinical IRD has not been fully elucidated. All of these viruses are known to cause latent infections: that is, infection results in the viral genome being retained in host cells for long periods without transcription or translation. In practical terms, this essentially means that horses are infected for life, and that viral infections can recrudesce repeatedly throughout an animal's life. This recrudescence can result in clinical disease or be unapparent. Recent investigations suggest that essentially all foals are infected with EHV1, EHV4, EHV2, and EHV5 at very young ages.[115,116] Viruses that are homologous to EHV1, EHV2, and EHV3 have been isolated from donkeys and have been designated asinine herpesviruses (AHV3, AHV2, and AHV1, respectively). Herpesviruses are enveloped and are relatively sensitive to a variety of disinfectants and environmental conditions.

EHV4 and EHV1 were once considered the same virus (EHV1) and older descriptions of associated disease can therefore confuse readers that are not aware of the timing of this differentiation. Classically described herpesvirus rhinopneumonitis is now believed to be most commonly associated with EHV4 infections. There is extensive genetic and structural homology between these viruses especially for antigenically dominant surface glycoproteins.[114] This gives rise to apparent cross-reactivity in immunity, especially in horses that have been exposed to both viruses on multiple occasions. As such, serology is often performed against one virus or the other, and the results are assumed to reflect antibody that will react with both viruses. This cross-reactivity is also of interest relative to vaccination.

EHV2 and EHV5 were also considered the same virus until recently. The association between infections with these viruses and the occurrence of clinical IRD is less well established. EVH2 and EHV5 have been recovered from horses with non-specific signs of IRD, but they are also commonly recovered from unaffected horses. In more objective studies, virus was more likely to be recovered from foals and horses with clinical respiratory disease compared to asymptomatic animals.[117-119] As methods designed to emphasize recovery of EHV2 and EHV5 have not been included in recent large-scale epidemiologic studies, it seems likely that they cause some disease currently classified as having an unknown etiology (Fig. 30.4). EHV2 and EHV5 genetically resemble Epstein–Barr virus of humans, which is also a gammaherpesvirus.[66] There appears to be significant variability among EHV5 isolates,[120] which may affect the likelihood that horses can be reinfected, as well as the ability to diagnose and investigate EHV5 using serology or PCR. These viruses appear to be as ubiquitous as EHV1 and EHV4, and limited studies suggest that foals are infected early in life.[116]

Distribution

EHV1 and EHV4 have been studied extensively and all available data suggests that the viruses are ubiquitous in all horse populations throughout the world. Information about the distribution of disease as recorded on the OIE website suggests that IRD associated with herpesvirus is not present among horses in some countries. However despite the importance of these viruses and the OIE List B status of equine rhinopneumonitis, this undoubtedly is an example of regulatory under-reporting and lack of investigative rigor. Although not extensively studied, EHV2 and EHV5 infections have been identified in horses in North America, Europe, Australia, and New Zealand, suggesting that these viruses have worldwide distribution.

Transmission and pathogenesis

It is believed that all EHV1 and EHV4 infections originate in the respiratory tract, and result in the virus genome being inserted as an episome in host cell nuclei. New infections and recrudescence both result in lymphocyte-associated viremia which allows virus to spread to tissues at distant sites. Viremia is more commonly detected with EHV1. EHV1 and EHV4 are believed to become latent in lymph nodes associated with the respiratory tract, and although not considered neurotropic, viral genome has also been identified in trigeminal ganglia. Strains vary in their tendency to cause disease, and specific strains of EHV1 are more likely to cause neurologic disease or abortion. The most intriguing recent discovery may be the apparent association of a single nucleotide polymorphism (SNP) in the DNA polymerase (DNA_{pol}) gene and the occurrence of EHM.[121,122] Retrospective analyzes of panels of isolates from over 100 EHV1outbreaks (either involving EHM or with no reported neurologic signs) suggested that that variability of a single amino acid of the DNA polymerase (DNA_{pol}) was associated with increased risk of EHM occurring in at least one horse during the outbreaks. The mechanism underlying CNS endothelial infection is unknown, as are the risk factors that determine its occurrence. While viral factors are certain to be important, such as the DNA_{pol} SNP described below, host and environmental factors also have a critical role.[8,12] Unlike neurologic disease associated with herpesvirus in cattle, humans and pigs, herpesvirus myeloencephalitis in horses is not believed to be commonly associated with direct infection of neurologic tissues.[114] Abortion is thought to result from both placental and neonatal infections. Little is know about transmission and pathogenesis associated with EHV2 and EHV5. Viral infections can be detected in essentially all foals,[116] and virus has been isolated from peripheral blood leukocytes, suggesting that viremia and latency are similar to that of EHV1 and EHV4.

Epidemiology and risk factors

Repeated EHV1 and EHV4 infections are common among horses of all ages, which is also probably true for EHV2 and EHV5. Respiratory disease associated with EHV4 has also been documented to occur repeatedly in young horses. Compared to influenza virus, EHV4 is a much more common cause of IRD in horses under one year, and a less common cause of large IRD outbreaks among horses under two years old. Younger racehorses have been shown to have an increased risk of IRD during outbreaks associated with EHV4. The frequency of disease associated with EHV2 and EHV5 has not been well described, but these agents may also be associated with sporadic disease or small outbreaks. Recrudescence is always a potential source of virus given the ubiquitous nature of equine herpesviruses, and this may be a common cause of sporadic IRD. However, epidemiologic data also suggests that novel disease-causing strains of EHV1 and EHV4 can be introduced into populations resulting in outbreaks of respiratory disease, neurologic disease, or abortion, suggesting that horizontal transmission is an important source of EHV1 and EHV4 during epidemics. These viruses can be transmitted by aerosols, but epidemiologic data regarding patterns of disease during outbreaks suggest that direct transmission, and indirect transmission via fomites and contaminated surfaces, are more important methods of transmitting virus during outbreaks. Horses that frequently come into contact with other horses have been shown to have increased risk of IRD associated with EHV4.[8]

Because of the cell-associated nature of herpesvirus infections, it has been suggested that cell-mediated immunity is far more important than humoral immunity in protecting horses from disease. As such, the use of killed-virus vaccines and the relationship between serum antibody and protective immunity has been questioned. Cell-mediated immunity is undoubtedly important for protecting horses. However, field investigations have shown that higher serum antibody titers are associated with decreased IRD risk in association with EHV4 infections.[8,58] It is not clear if humoral immunity was protective or whether it was simply a marker of horses with stronger CMI against these agents. It was also shown that horses with high influenza virus antibody titers had lower risk of disease during an EHV4 outbreak, supporting the idea that antibody titers may to some degree be simple markers of previous exposure, and not entirely direct indicators of immunity.

Equine arteritis virus

Characteristics

Equine arteritis virus (EAV) is the prototype virus of the recently established genus *Arterivirus*. It is an enveloped RNA virus and is therefore relatively sensitive to drying and common disinfectants. While some variability has been demonstrated in the viral genome, there is only one recognized serotype. EAV has a limited host range and is only known to infect equids. Infections are far more common than is the occurrence of respiratory disease and EAV is primarily a concern because of associated reproductive disease. EAV is particularly problematic to the equine industries because of its ability to establish a carrier state in intact stallions. These carrier animals are important for introducing and maintaining the virus in equine populations, as well as because of their impact on trade of horses and semen. Infection is apparently more common among some breeds, especially Standardbred and Warm Blood horses. There is evidence for a correlation between variation in the genotype of horses and phenotypic differences in terms of the extent of viral replication, presence and severity of clinical signs and cytokine gene expression caused by exposure to EAV.[123,124]

Distribution

EAV is thought to have a worldwide distribution, even though outbreaks are reported only occasionally. However, despite having OIE List B status, many countries report that they have never recognized this agent or disease.[50] Again, this is likely attributable to underreporting and lack of investigative rigor. There has been an apparent decrease in the number of reported outbreaks which may be attributable to increased availability of diagnostic testing as well as increased awareness throughout the world regarding disease impact and effective disease control measures. Recent broad-based investigation of EAV infection in the United States found that about 2% of unvaccinated horses were seropositive, and another investigation based on selective sampling in the United Kingdom found that 2% or less of unvaccinated horses were seropositive.[125,126]

Transmission and pathogenesis

EAV is shed via the respiratory tract by acutely infected horses, in the semen of carrier stallions, as well in amniotic fluid, placenta, and fetuses of aborted mares. Less important sources of virus include blood, feces, and urine of acutely infected animals. Infections in carrier stallions are inapparent even though virus is shed in their semen for their entire life, or until they are castrated. EAV infections do not apparently affect fertility of stallions. Asymptomatic infections are common, and stallions may become long-term carriers of the virus even without showing signs of disease. The incubation period in clinically affected animals is about 3–7 days. Clinical disease can be indistinguishable from that caused by other IRD agents, but affected horses may also develop swelling and edema that is most commonly noted in the legs, scrotum, sheath, or udder, as well as abortion in pregnant mares. Modified live and killed virus vaccines are commercially available. Control recommendations for EAV from the American Horse Council include the use of modified live vaccines,[127] and the killed virus vaccine is used in Great Britain and Ireland.[128] It should be noted that vaccination decreases the risk of disease, but does not prevent infection.[128]

Epidemiology and risk factors

Perhaps the most dominant factor affecting spread and maintenance of EAV in populations is the presence of persistently infected stallions that shed virus in semen. Further, while outbreaks of clinical disease are sometimes reported, most infections result in very mild or no clinical signs. This allows opportunity for further spread of virus without the presence of identifiable disease that might trigger enactment of more rigorous control strategies. Seroprevalence has been repeatedly shown to vary among breeds, and is highest among Standardbred horses, which may be attributable to the number of persistently infected stallions. In a broad-based cross-sectional study performed by the USDA, the seroprevalence among adult non-vaccinated Standardbreds was about 24%, compared to 4.5% among Thoroughbreds, 3.6% among Warmbloods, and about 1% among other horses.[125] Horses from operations used primarily for breeding or for boarding and training were more likely to be seropositive compared to other operations.[125] Various countries have enacted control strategies centered on identifying persistently infected stallions, reducing the likelihood of exposure to acutely infected horses, and use of vaccines to decrease the risk of disease and decrease the risk of stallions becoming persistently infected.

Other respiratory viruses

Several other viruses have been recovered from the respiratory tract of horses showing signs of IRD, as well as from clinically normal horses. The role that these viruses play in the occurrence of respiratory disease in horses is not clear. While it is interesting that these viruses can be recovered from horses with clinical IRD, these data would be more convincing if evidence of infection were found more commonly in disease cases compared to non-cases in the same populations. A brief description of two of these agents follows.

Equine rhinitis virus

Horses are commonly infected with equine rhinitis-A virus and equine rhinitis-B virus (formerly classified as equine rhinovirus types 1 and 2, respectively). Seroprevalence has been shown to approach 100% in young and adult horses. Limited experimental challenge studies indicate that this agent can cause IRD under some conditions. Horses commonly shed virus in nasal secretions and in urine. Studies evaluating the distribution of this agent have not been performed in many countries, but infections have been documented in North America, Australia, New Zealand, United Kingdom and Europe, suggesting a worldwide distribution.

Equine adenovirus

Equine adenovirus type 1 has been isolated from horses throughout the world, and seroprevalence can approach 100% in mature horses. In most horses infection is not believed to cause clinical disease, or it is very mild. However, adenovirus infections cause significant disease in Arabian foals with primary, severe combined immunodeficiency disease (PSCID). A limited study of experimental challenge in two immunocompetent foals showed that infection can result in pathologic changes under certain conditions.

References

1. Bailey CJ, Rose RJ, Reid SW, et al. Wastage in the Australian Thoroughbred racing industry: a survey of Sydney trainers. Aust Vet J 1997;75(1):64–6.
2. Bailey CJ, Reid SW, Hodgson DR, et al. Impact of injuries and disease on a cohort of two- and three-year-old Thoroughbreds in training. Vet Rec 1999;145(17):487–93.
3. Hernandez J, Hawkins DL. Training failure among yearling horses. Am J Vet Res 2001;62(9):1418–22.
4. Ryan AJ, Dalyrmple W, Dull B, et al. Round table: Upper respiratory infections in sports. Phys Sports Med 1975;3:29–42.
5. Hanley DF. Medical care of the US Olympic Team. JAMA 1976;236(2): 147–8.
6. Weidner TG. Literature review: upper respiratory illness and sport and exercise. Int J Sports Med 1994;15(1): 1–9.
7. Weidner TG, Anderson BN, Kaminsky LA, et al. Effect of a rhinovirus-caused upper respiratory illness on pulmonary function test and exercise responses. Med Sci Sports Exer 1997;29:604–9.
8. Morley PS. The epidemiology of infectious upper respiratory tract disease in horses. Ph.D. dissertation, University of Saskatchewan; 1995.
9. NAHMS. NAHMS Equine '98: Needs Assessment Survey Results. #N207.597. [Web Page]. 1997; Available at http://www.aphis.usda.gov/vs/ceah/cahm/Equine/eq98na.pdf. (Accessed 11 April 2003).
10. Traub-Dargatz JL, Salman MD, Voss JL. Medical problems of adult horses, as ranked by equine practitioners. J Am Vet Med Assoc 1991;198(10):1745–7.
11. Peters EM, Bateman ED. Ultramarathon running and upper respiratory tract infections. S Afr Med J 1983;64:582–4.
12. Weigl JA, Puppe W, Schmitt HJ. The incidence of influenza-associated hospitalizations in children in Germany. Epidemiol Infect 2002;129(3):525–33.
13. Zimmerman RK, Middleton DB, Smith NJ. Vaccines for persons at high risk due to medical conditions, occupation, environment, or lifestyle, 2003. J Fam Pract 2003;52(Suppl. 1):S22–35.
14. Clarke AF, Madelin TM, Allpress RG. The relationship of air hygiene in stables to lower airway disease and pharyngeal lymphoid hyperplasia in 2 groups of Thoroughbred horses. Equine Vet J 1987;19(6):524–30.
15. Clarke AF, Madelin TM, Allpress RG. The relationship of air hygiene in stables to lower airway disease during an outbreak of equid herpesvirus-1 infection. In: Equine Infectious Diseases V: Proceedings of the Fifth International Conference on Equine Infectious Diseases. Lexington, Kentucky: University Press of Kentucky; 1988. p. 268–71.
16. Nieman DC. Special feature for the Olympics: effects of exercise on the immune system: exercise effects on systemic immunity. Immunol Cell Biol 2000;78(5):496–501.
17. Gleeson M, Pyne DB. Exercise effects on mucosal immunity. Immunol Cell Biol 2000;78(5):536–44.
18. Gleeson M, Pyne DB. Special feature for the Olympics: effects of exercise on the immune system: exercise effects on mucosal immunity. Immunol Cell Biol 2000;78(5):536–44.
19. Woods JA, Lu Q, Ceddia MA, et al. Exercise-induced modulation of macrophage function. Immunol Cell Biol 2000;78(5):545–53.
20. Woods J, Lu Q, Ceddia MA, et al. Special feature for the Olympics: effects of exercise on the immune system: exercise-induced modulation of macrophage function. Immunol Cell Biol 2000;78(5):545–53.
21. Jonsdottir IH, Hoffmann P. The Significance of intensity and duration of exercise on natural immunity in rats. Med Sci Sports Exerc 2000;32(11): 1908–12.
22. Jonsdottir IH. Exercise immunology: neuroendocrine regulation of Nk-cells. Int J Sports Med 2000;21:S20–3.
23. Jonsdottir IH. Special feature for the Olympics: effects of exercise on the immune system: neuropeptides and their interaction with exercise and immune function. Immunol Cell Biol 2000;78(5):562–70.
24. Pedersen BK, Ullum H. Nk cell response to physical activity – possible mechanisms of action. Med Sci Sports Exerc 1994;26(2):140–6.
25. Nieman DC. Is infection risk linked to exercise workload? Med Sci Sports Exerc 2000;32(7):S406–11.
26. Pedersen BK, Bruunsgaard H. How physical exercise influences the establishment of infections. Sports Med 1995;19(6):393–400.
27. Lunn DP, Hussey S, Sebring R, et al. Safety, efficacy and immunogenicity of a modified-live equine influenza virus vaccine in ponies after induction of exercise-induced immunosuppression. J Am Vet Med Assoc 2001;218(6):900–6.
28. Guo Y, Wang M, Kawaoka Y, et al. Characterization of a new avian-like influenza A virus from horses in China. Virology 1992;188(1):245–55.
29. Guo Y, Wang M, Zheng GS, et al. Seroepidemiological and molecular evidence for the presence of two H3N8 equine influenza viruses in China in 1993–94. J Gen Virol 1995;76:2009–14.
30. Horohov DW, Keadle TL, Pourciau SS, et al. Mechanism of exercise-induced augmentation of lymphokine activated killer (LAK) cell activity in the horse. Vet Immunol Immunopathol 1996;53(3–4):221–33.
31. Horohov DW, Dimock A, Guirnalda P, et al. Effect of exercise on the immune response of young and old horses. Am J Vet Res 1999;60(5):643–7.
32. Kurcz EV, Lawrence LM, Kelley KW, et al. The effect of intense exercise on the cell-mediated immune response of Horses. J Equine Vet Sci 1988;8: 237–9.
33. Keadle TL, Pourciau SS, Melrose PA, et al. Acute exercise stress modulates immune function in unfit horses. J Equine Vet Sci 1993;13:226–31.
34. Wong CW, Smith SE, Thong YH, et al. Effects of exercise stress on various immune functions in horses. Am J Vet Res 1992;53:1414–17.
35. Rose RJ. Hematological changes associated with endurance exercise. Vet Rec 1982;110(8):175–7.
36. Snow DH, Ricketts SW, Mason DK. Hematological response to racing and training exercise in Thoroughbred horses, with particular reference to the leukocyte response. Equine Vet J 1983;15(2):149–54.
37. Rose RJ, Hodgson DR. Hematological and plasma biochemical parameters in endurance horses during training. Equine Vet J 1982;14(2):144–8.
38. Shephard RJ. Special feature for the Olympics: effects of exercise on the immune system: overview of the epidemiology of exercise immunology. Immunol Cell Biol 2000;78(5):485–95.

39. Morley PS, Townsend HG, Bogdan JR, et al. Descriptive epidemiologic study of disease associated with influenza virus infections during three epidemics in horses. J Am Vet Med Assoc 2000;216(4):535–44.
40. NAHMS. Infectious Upper Respiratory Disease in U.S. Horses: Disease Frequency. #N342.1001 [Web Page]. 2001; Available at http://www.aphis.usda.gov/vs/ceah/cahm/Equine/iurd98.pdf. (Accessed 11 April 2003).
41. Kaneene JB, Saffell M, Fedewa DJ, et al. The Michigan equine monitoring system. 1. Design, implementation and population estimates. Prev Vet Med 1997;29(4):263–75.
42. Diaz-Mendez A, Viel L, Hewson J, et al. Surveillance of equine respiratory viruses in Ontario. Can J Vet Res 2010;74(4):271–8.
43. Pusterla N, Kass PH, Mapes S, et al. Surveillance programme for important equine infectious respiratory pathogens in the USA. Vet Rec 2011;169(1):12.
44. Burrell MH, Wood JL, Whitwell KE, et al. Respiratory disease in Thoroughbred horses in training: the relationships between disease and viruses, bacteria and environment. Vet Rec 1996;139(13):308–13.
45. Gross DK, Hinchcliff KW, French PS, et al. Effect of moderate exercise on the severity of clinical signs associated with influenza virus infection in horses. Equine Vet J 1998;30(6):489–97.
46. Morley PS, Townsend HG, Bogdan J, et al. Infectious upper respiratory tract disease caused by influenza virus in horses stabled at a racetrack. Proceedings of the Annual Convention of the American Association of Equine Practitioners. 1995. p. 174–5.
47. Marois P, Pavilanis V, Boudreault A, et al. An outbreak of Type A2 influenza among horses. Can J Comp Med 1963;27:257–60.
48. McQueen JL. Review of influenza in animals: Equine. CDC Zoonoses Surveillance. Spec Rep: Anim Influenza 1965;Report #5:6–13.
49. Aiello SE, editor. The Merck Veterinary Manual – Equine Influenza [Web Page]. Available at http://www.merckvetmanual.com/mvm/index.jsp?cfile=htm/bc/121304.htm&word=equine%2cinfluenza. (Accessed 11 April 2003).
50. Handistatus II [Web Page]. Available at http://www.oie.int/hs2/report.asp?lang=en. (Accessed 11 April 2003).
51. Rees WA, Harkins JD, Lu M, et al. Pharmacokinetics and therapeutic efficacy of rimantadine in horses experimentally infected with influenza virus A2. Am J Vet Res 1999;60:888–94.
52. Mumford JA, Hannant D. Equine influenza. Virus Infections of Equines. New York: Elsevier; 1996. p. 285–94.
53. Durando MM, Birks EK, Hussey SB, et al. Cardiac troponin I concentrations in ponies challenged with equine influenza virus. J Vet Intern Med 2011;25(2):339–44.
54. Maisch B, Ristic AD, Portig I, et al. Human viral cardiomyopathy. Front Biosci 2003;8:S39–67.
55. Rose RJ, Allen JR. Hematologic responses to exercise and training. Vet Clin North Am Equine Pract 1985;1(3):461–76.
56. Gerber H. Clinical features, sequelae and epidemiology of equine influenza. In: Bryans JT, editor. Equine Infectious Diseases IV: Proceedings of the Second International Conference on Equine Infectious Diseases, Paris, France. Basel: Karger; 1970. p. 63–80.
57. Newton JR, Mumford JA. Equine influenza. In: Coetzer JA, Tustin RC, editors. Infectious Diseases of Livestock. Oxford: Oxford University Press; 2005. p. 766–74.
58. Mumford EL, Traub-Dargatz JL, Salman MD, et al. Monitoring and detection of acute viral respiratory tract disease in horses. J Am Vet Med Assoc 1998; 213(3):385–90.
59. Morley PS, Bogdan JR, Townsend HG, et al. Evaluation of Directigen Flu A assay for detection of influenza antigen in nasal secretions of horses. Equine Vet J 1995;27(2):131–4.
60. Chambers TM, Shortridge KF, Li PH, et al. Rapid diagnosis of equine influenza by the Directigen FLU-A enzyme immunoassay. Vet Rec 1994;135(12):275–9.
61. Townsend HGG, Moore SL, Bogdan JR, et al. Evaluation of an optical immunoassay for the diagnosis of equine influenza. Salman MD, Morley PS, Ruch-Gallie R, editors Proceedings of the 9th Symposium of the International Society for Veterinary Epidemiology and Economics. International Society for Veterinary Epidemiology and Economics, 2000: Abstract number 508.
62. Adam EN, Morley PS, Chmielewski KE, et al. Detection of cold-adapted vaccine-strain influenza virus using two commercial assays. Equine Vet J 2002; 34(4):400–4.
63. Powell DG, Burrows R, Spooner PR, et al. A study of infectious respiratory disease among horses in Great Britain, 1971–1976. In: Bryans JT, editor. Equine Infectious Diseases IV: Proceedings of the Fourth International Conference on Equine Infectious Diseases. Princeton, NJ: Veterinary Publications, Inc.; 1978. p. 451–9.
64. Ostlund EN, Powell D, Bryans JT. Equine Herpesvirus 1: A Review. Proceedings of the 36th Annual Convention of the American Association of Equine Practioners. 1991. p. 387–95.
65. Burrows R, Goodridge D, Denyer M, et al. Equine influenza infections in Great Britain, 1979. Vet Rec 1982;110: 494–7.
66. Browning GF, Agius CT. Equine herpesvirus 2 and 5 infections. In: Studdert MJ, editor. Virus Infections of Equines. New York: Elsevier; 1996. p. 47–62.
67. Pusterla N, Leutenegger CM. Molecular diagnostics in large animals. In: Smith BP, editor. Large Animal Internal Medicine. St. Louis: Mosby Elsevier; 2009. p. 436–50.
68. Carlson JK, Traub-Dargatz JL, Lunn DP, et al. Equine viral respiratory pathogen surveillance at horse shows and sales. Equine Vet J [submitted 2012].
69. Wood JL, Burrell MH, Roberts CA, et al. Streptococci and *Pasteurella* spp. associated with disease of the equine lower respiratory tract. Equine Vet J 1993;25(4):314–18.
70. Ward CL, Wood JL, Houghton SB, et al. *Actinobacillus* and *Pasteurella* species isolated from horses with lower airway disease. Vet Rec 1998;143(10):277–9.
71. Rees WA, Harkins JD, Woods WE, et al. Amantadine and equine influenza: pharmacology, pharmacokinetics and neurological effects in the horse. Equine Vet J 1997;29(2):104–10.
72. Gibson JS, Slater JD, Field HJ. The activity of (S)-1-[(3-hydroxy-2-phosphonyl methoxy) propyl] cytosine (HPMPC) against equine herpesvirus-1 (EHV-1) in cell cultures, mice and horses. Antivir Res 1992;19(3):219–32.
73. Henninger RW, Reed SM, Saville WJ, et al. Outbreak of neurologic disease caused by equine herpesvirus-1 at a university equestrian center. J Vet Intern Med 2007;21(1):157–65.
74. Garré B, Shebany K, Gryspeerdt A, et al. Pharmacokinetics of acyclovir after intravenous infusion of acyclovir and after oral administration of acyclovir and its prodrug valacyclovir in healthy adult horses. Antimicrob Agents Chemother 2007;51(12):4308–14.
75. Maxwell LK, Bentz BG, Bourne DW, et al. Pharmacokinetics of valacyclovir in the adult horse. J Vet Pharmacol Ther 2008;31(4):312–20.
76. Garré B, Gryspeerdt A, Croubels S, et al. Evaluation of orally administered valacyclovir in experimentally EHV1-infected ponies. Vet Microbiol 2009; 135(3–4):214–21.
77. Garré B, Baert K, Nauwynck H, et al. Multiple oral dosing of valacyclovir in horses and ponies. J Vet Pharmacol Ther 2009;32(3):207–12.
78. Tsujimura K, Yamada M, Nagata S, et al. Pharmacokinetics of penciclovir after oral administration of its prodrug famciclovir to horses. J Vet Med Sci 2010;72(3):357–61.

79. Morley PS. Biosecurity of veterinary practices. Vet Clin North Am Food Anim Pract 2002;18(1):133–55, vii.
80. Traub-Dargatz JL, Morley PS, Dargatz DA, et al. Infection control strategies in horses for the new millennium. Proceedings of the 46th Annual Convention of the American Association of Equine Practitioners. 2000. p. 36–41.
81. Townsend HG, Penner SJ, Watts TC, et al. Efficacy of a cold-adapted, intranasal, equine influenza vaccine: challenge trials. Equine Vet J 2001; 33(7):637–43.
82. Kastner SB, Haines DM, Archer J, et al. Investigations on the ability of clenbuterol hydrochloride to reduce clinical signs and inflammation associated with equine influenza A infection. Equine Vet J 1999;31(2): 160–8.
83. Kitchen RH, Kehler WH, Henthorne JC. The 1963 Equine influenza epizootic. J Am Vet Med Assoc 1963;143:1108–10.
84. Scholtens RG, Steele JH, Dowdle WR, et al. United States epizootic of equine influenza, 1963. Public Health Rep 1964;79(5):393–402.
85. Guthrie AJ, Stevens KB, Bosman PP. The circumstances surrounding the outbreak and spread of equine influenza in South Africa. Rev Sci Tech 1999;18(1):179–85.
86. Larson EL. APIC guideline for handwashing and hand antisepsis in health care settings. Am J Infect Control 1995;23(4):251–69.
87. Fotheringham VJ. Disinfection of livestock production premises. Rev Sci Tech 1995;14(1):191–205.
88. Ford WB. Disinfection procedures for personnel and vehicles entering and leaving contaminated premises. Rev Sci Tech 1995;14(2):393–401.
89. Dwyer RM. Disinfecting equine facilities. Rev Sci Tech 1995;14(2): 403–18.
90. Antec International Ltd. Animal health: equine menu [Web Page]. Available at http://www.antecint.co.uk/main/equine.htm. (Accessed 11 April 2003).
91. Patterson G, Morley PS, Blehm KD, et al. Efficacy of directed misting application of a peroxygen disinfectant for environmental decontamination of a veterinary hospital. J Am Vet Med Assoc 2005;227:597–602.
92. Mumford JA, Jessett D, Dunleavy U, et al. Antigenicity and immunogenicity of experimental equine influenza ISCOM vaccines. Vaccine 1994;12(9): 857–63.
93. Mumford JA, Wilson H, Hannant D, et al. Antigenicity and immunogenicity of equine influenza vaccines containing a Carbomer adjuvant. Epidemiol Infect 1994;112(2):421–37.
94. Morley PS, Townsend HG, Bogdan JR, et al. Efficacy of a commercial vaccine for preventing disease caused by influenza virus infection in horses. J Am Vet Med Assoc 1999;215(1):61–6.
95. Mumford EL, Traub-Dargatz JL, Carman J, et al. Occurrence of infectious upper respiratory tract disease and response to vaccination in horses on six sentinel premises in northern Colorado. Equine Vet J 2003;35(1):72–7.
96. Ellis JA, Bogdan JR, Kanara EW, et al. Cellular and antibody responses to equine herpesviruses 1 and 4 following vaccination of horses with modified-live and inactivated viruses. J Am Vet Med Assoc 1995;206(6):823–32.
97. Gerber JD, Marron AE, Bass EP, et al. Effect of age and pregnancy on the antibody and cell-mediated immune responses of horses to equine herpesvirus 1. Can J Comp Med 1977;41(4):471–8.
98. Goodman LB, Wagner B, Flaminio MJ, et al. Comparison of the efficacy of inactivated combination and modified-live virus vaccines against challenge infection with neuropathogenic equine herpesvirus type 1 (EHV-1). Vaccine 2006;24(17):3636–45.
99. Goehring LS, Wagner B, Bigbie R, et al. Control of EHV-1 viremia and nasal shedding by commercial vaccines.Vaccine 2010;28(32):5203–11.
100. Banks J, Speidel EC, McCauley JW, et al. Phylogenetic analysis of H7 haemagglutinin subtype influenza A viruses. Arch Virol 2000;145(5): 1047–58.
101. Lai AC, Chambers TM, Holland RE Jr, et al. Diverged evolution of recent equine-2 influenza (H3N8) viruses in the Western Hemisphere. Arch Virol 2001;146(6):1063–74.
102. Daly JM, Lai AC, Binns MM, et al. Antigenic and genetic evolution of equine H3n8 influenza A viruses. J Gen Virology 1996;77:661–71.
103. Lewis NS, Daly JM, Russell CA, et al. Antigenic and genetic evolution of equine influenza A (H3N8) virus from 1968 to 2007. J Virol 2011;85(23):12742–9.
104. Yates P, Mumford JA. Equine influenza vaccine efficacy: the significance of antigenic variation. Vet Microbiol 2000;74(1–2):173–7.
105. Loke CT. Outbreak of equine influenza in Malaysia and Singapore. Singapore Vet J 1981;5:53–4.
106. Singh G. A note on the concurrent isolation, from horses and ponies, of influenza A/EQ 1 and A/EQ 2 viruses from an epidemic of equine influenza in India. Comp Immunol Microbiol Infect Dis 1995;18:73–4.
107. Webster RG, Guo Y. New influenza virus in horses. Nature 1991;351:527.
108. Mumford J, Wood J. WHO/OIE meeting: consultation on newly emerging strains of equine influenza. 18–19 May 1992, Animal Health Trust, Newmarket, Suffolk, UK. Vaccine 1993;11:1172–5.
109. Watson J, Halpin K, Selleck P, et al. Isolation and characterisation of an H3N8 equine influenza virus in Australia, 2007. Aust Vet J 2011; 89(Suppl. 1):35–7.
110. Sutton GA, Viel L, Carman PS, et al. Study of the duration and distribution of equine influenza virus subtype 2 (H3N8) antigens in experimentally infected ponies in vivo. Can J Vet Res 1997;61(2):113–20.
111. Webster RG, Kawaoka Y, Guo Y. Equine influenza in China. Foreign Anim Dis Rep 1991;19:3.
112. Powell DG, Watkins KL, Li PH, et al. Outbreak of equine influenza among horses in Hong Kong during 1992. Vet Rec 1995;136(21):531–6.
113. Morley PS, Townsend HG, Bogdan JR, et al. Risk factors for disease associated with influenza virus infections during three epidemics in horses. J Am Vet Med Assoc 2000;216(4):545–50.
114. Crabb BC, Studert MJ. Equine rhinopneumonitis and equine abortion (Equine herpesviruses 4 and 1). In: Studdert MJ, editor. Virus Infections of Equines. New York: Elsevier; 1996. p. 11–38.
115. Gilkerson J, Jorm LR, Love DN, et al. Epidemiological investigation of equid herpesvirus-4 (EHV-4) excretion assessed by nasal swabs taken from Thoroughbred foals. Vet Microbiol 1994;39(3–4):275--83.
116. Dunowska M, Wilks CR, Studdert MJ, et al. Equine respiratory viruses in foals in New Zealand. New Zealand Vet J 2002;50(4):140–7.
117. Murray MJ, Eichorn ES, Dubovi EJ, et al. Equine herpesvirus type 2: prevalence and seroepidemiology in foals. Equine Vet J 1996;28(6):432–6.
118. Borchers K, Wolfinger U, Goltz M, et al. Distribution and relevance of equine herpesvirus type 2 (EHV–2) infections. Arch Virol 1997;142(5):917–28.
119. Dunowska M, Wilks CR, Studdert MJ, et al. Viruses associated with outbreaks of equine respiratory disease in New Zealand. New Zealand Vet J 2002;50(4): 132–9.
120. Dunowska M, Holloway SA, Wilks CR, et al. Genomic variability of equine herpesvirus-5. Arch Virol 2000;145(7): 1359–71.
121. Nugent J, Birch-Machin I, Smith KC, et al. Analysis of equid herpesvirus 1 strain variation reveals a point mutation of the DNA polymerase strongly associated with neuropathogenic versus nonneuropathogenic disease outbreaks. J Virol 2006;80:4047–60.

122. Perkins GA, Goodman LB, Tsujimura K, et al. Investigation of the prevalence of neurologic equine herpes virus type 1 (EHV-1) in a 23-year retrospective analysis (1984–2007). Vet Microbiol 2009;139:375–8.

123. Go YY, Cook RF, Fulgêncio JQ, et al. Assessment of correlation between in vitro CD3+ T cell susceptibility to EAV infection and clinical outcome following experimental infection. Vet Microbiol 2012;157(1-2):220–5.

124. Go YY, Bailey E, Cook DG, et al. Genome-wide association study among four horse breeds identifies a common haplotype associated with in vitro CD3+ T cell susceptibility/resistance to equine arteritis virus infection. J Virol 2011;85(24):13174–84.

125. NAHMS. Equine Viral Arteritis (EVA) and the U.S. Horse Industry. #N312.0501. [Web Page]. 2000; Available at http://www.aphis.usda.gov/vs/ceah/cahm/Equine/eq98eva.pdf. (Accessed 11 April 2003).

126. Newton JR, Wood JL, Castillo-Olivares FJ, et al. Serological surveillance of equine viral arteritis in the United Kingdom since the outbreak in 1993. Vet Rec 1999;145(18):511–16.

127. Equine Viral Arteritis Protocol [Web Page]. 2000; Available at http://www.horsecouncil.org/health/evaproto.html. (Accessed 11 April 2003).

128. De Vries AAF, Rottier PJM, Glaser AL, et al. Equine viral arteritis. In: Studdert MJ, editor. Virus Infections in Equines. Elsevier, Amsterdam; 1996. p. 171–200.

section 4

Cardiovascular system

Heart and vessels: function during exercise and training adaptations

31

David C. Poole Howard H. Erickson

CHAPTER CONTENTS

Introduction

The horse is often considered one of, if not the, premier athletic mammalian species. However, depending upon the criterion used, there are other distinct (and sometimes surprising) contenders for that title. For example, as seen in Figure 31.1, compared with the Thoroughbred racehorse (40 miles/h, 65 km/h), the cheetah can achieve speeds in excess of 70 miles/h (120 km/h) and several species of antelope, as well as the blackbuck, gnu, and ostrich, are all faster than the horse (fastest human 27–28 miles/h, ~44 km/h). The fastest horses ever clocked are Quarter Horses, which reach speeds of 50–55 miles/h (~85 km/h).[1] Because body length determines the distance that individual muscles shorten, it might be more appropriate to judge athletic ability in terms of speed relative to body length.[2] From this perspective, the Merriam kangaroo rat is superlative, achieving 110 body lengths per second, which is three times faster than the cheetah (32 length/s) and an order of magnitude faster than the horse (~10 length/s).

Within humans, the aerobic capacity or maximal oxygen uptake ($\dot{V}O_{2max}$) is considered an excellent (though by no means the sole) indicator of performance for running events over 1 minute in duration. Across the spectrum of terrestrial mammalian species, aerobic capacity increases over five orders of magnitude as a function of body size from approximately 0.001 L/min in the 2 g Etruscan shrew (world's smallest mammal) to in excess of 80 L/min in the elite Thoroughbred racehorse. Whereas it is possible that a large rapidly walking elephant may have a higher total $\dot{V}O_2$, this remains to be demonstrated. When aerobic capacity is expressed relative to body mass, the diminutive Etruscan shrew ($\dot{V}O_{2max}$ ~400 mL O_2/kg/min)[2,3] reigns supreme, as this measure of performance decreases systematically with increasing body mass. Amongst the larger animals, the pronghorn antelope ($\dot{V}O_{2max}$ ~300 mL O_2/kg/min)[4] and the horse ($\dot{V}O_{2max}$ > 200 mL O_2/kg/min)[2,5] are outstanding and each can consume more O_2 in toto and per unit body mass than any other mammal of their respective sizes.

This chapter addresses the structural and functional capacities of the cardiovascular system that permit the horse to achieve such prodigious O_2 flows and athletic performances. As we shall see, a large, high-capacity heart is requisite. Whereas animals such as the shrew and pronghorn antelope have evolved in accordance with the laws of nature, the horse has been subjected to several thousand years of selective breeding (Fig. 31.2)[6a] based upon athletic performance. As detailed below, this practice has produced a disproportionate increase in the horse's heart size and pumping capacity (cardiac output, $\dot{Q}$) compared to lung capacity; the consequence of this is a structural and functional failure of the respiratory system during maximal exercise.

The purpose of this chapter is to present those features of the equine heart and cardiovascular system that facilitate this animal's extraordinary performance. Those mechanisms underlying

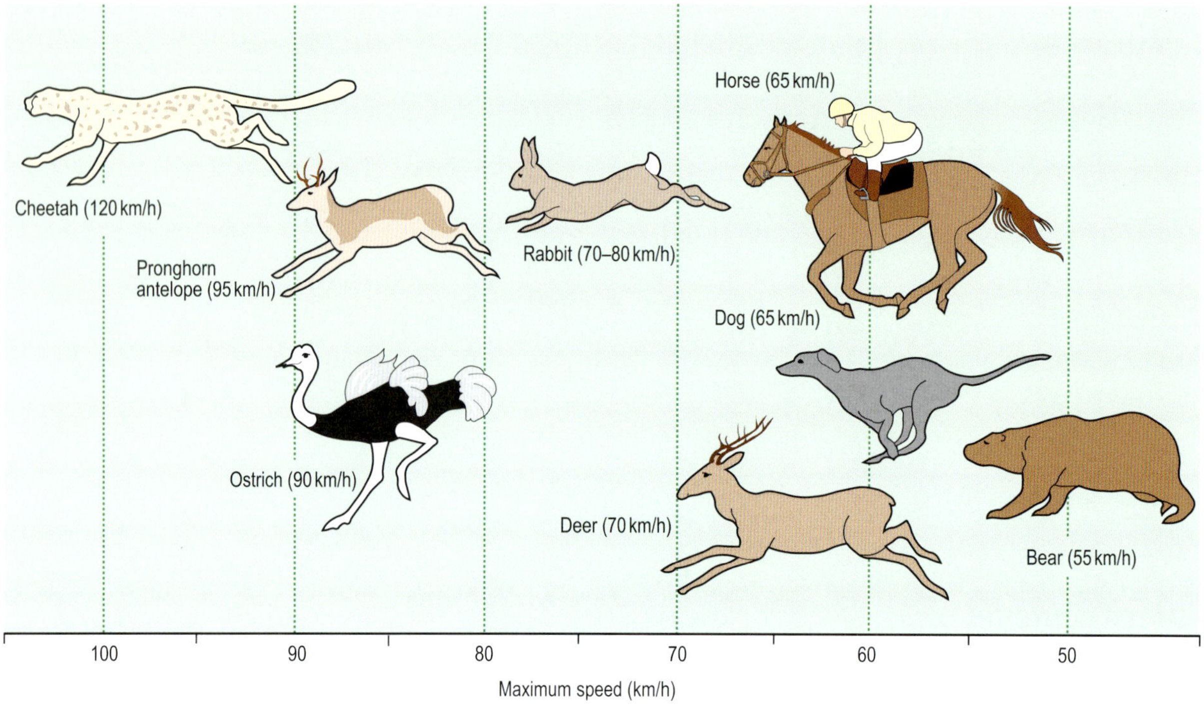

Fig 31.1 Approximate maximum speeds for a variety of terrestrial mammalian species and the ostrich. Please note that the Quarter Horse has been clocked close to 90 km/h (55 miles/h)[1] whereas maximal speeds for the Thoroughbred as seen in this figure with rider are somewhat lower. For converting to other commonly used units: 10 km/h = 6.2 miles/h or 2.8 m/s.

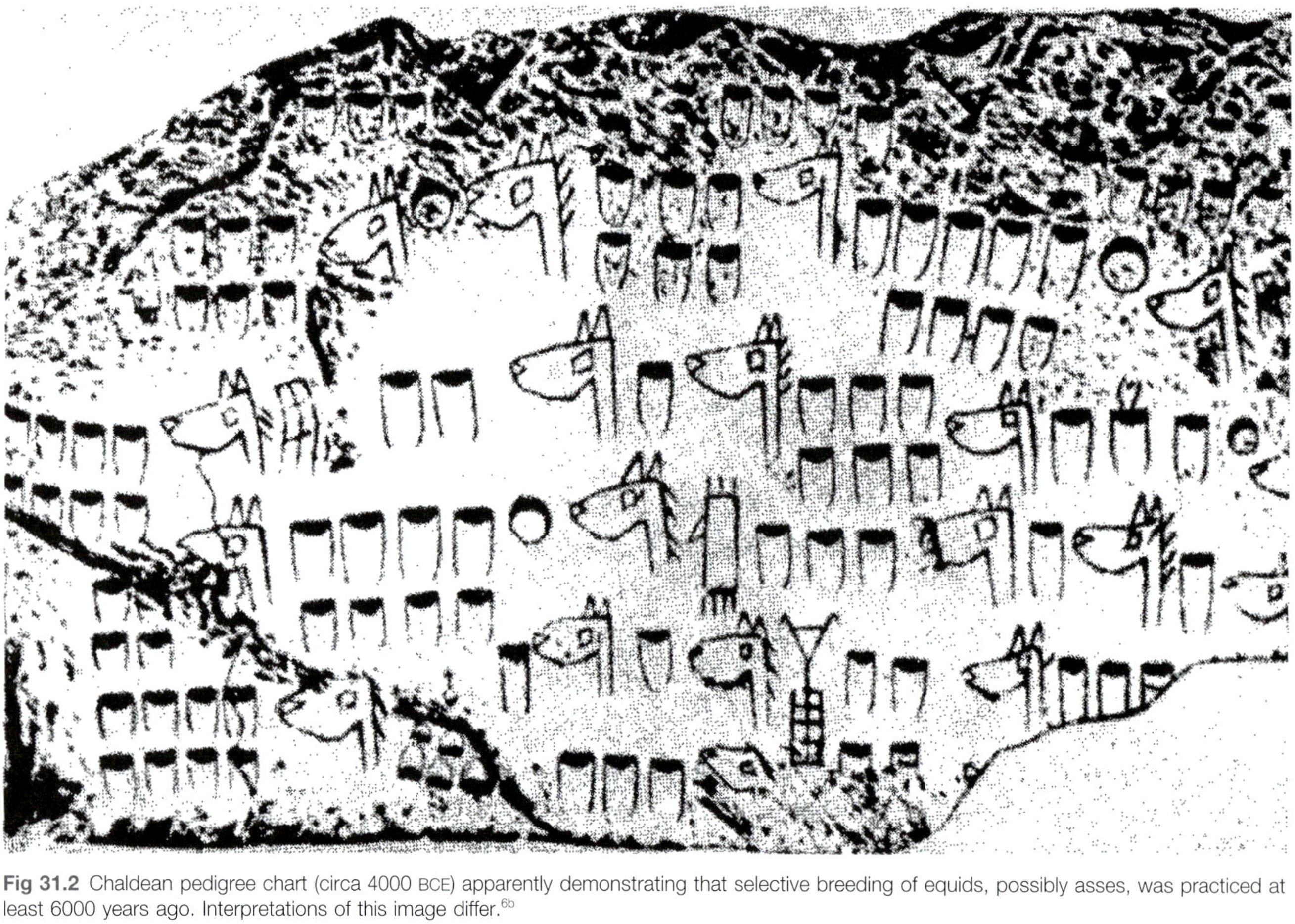

Fig 31.2 Chaldean pedigree chart (circa 4000 BCE) apparently demonstrating that selective breeding of equids, possibly asses, was practiced at least 6000 years ago. Interpretations of this image differ.[6b]

Reproduced with kind permission from Lyons & Petrucelli[6a] and the World Health Organization, Geneva.

respiratory system failure will be discussed as they relate intimately to the cardiovascular system. Particular attention will be afforded to the plasticity of the equine cardiovascular system to exercise training and, although such changes are important, compared with the magnitude of inherited inter-animal variations, they are relatively modest. Throughout this chapter and contingent upon available data, reference will be made to several other species, including the human, dog, ox, and camel, as a basis for comparison (Fig. 31.3).[7]

Role of the heart and cardiovascular system in setting aerobic capacity $\dot{V}O_{2max}$

The energetic capability of skeletal muscle is so high that it far surpasses the capacity of the respiratory and cardiovascular systems to deliver O_2. In Thoroughbreds, skeletal muscle comprises over 50% of body mass[8] and aerobic capacity ($\dot{V}O_{2max}$) (at least of Standardbreds) increases as a function of fat-free mass.[9] Moreover, under many conditions $\dot{V}O_{2max}$ is considered to be O_2 supply-limited because the mitochondrial oxidative enzyme capacity for utilizing O_2 exceeds that of the cardiorespiratory systems to deliver O_2. In support of this notion, there is strong evidence that increasing muscle O_2 delivery during intense exercise will elevate $\dot{V}O_{2max}$. Specifically:

- Breathing high O_2 mixtures elevates arterial O_2 content and $\dot{V}O_{2max}$ in horses[10] and humans.[11]
- With respect to equine $\dot{V}O_{2max}$, there is recent evidence that horses run to maximal speeds on an incline (6°) exhibit higher cardiac output ($\dot{Q}$) (Fig. 31.4) and $\dot{V}O_{2max}$ values than on the flat. This increased $\dot{Q}$ and $\dot{V}O_{2max}$ results from an elevated stroke volume[12] and may relate to greater hindlimb muscle recruitment, greater swings in intrapleural pressures (higher tidal volume) aiding heart function, and/or increased hydrostatic pressures improving muscle blood flow.
- Pericardectomy elevates stroke volume, cardiac output and $\dot{V}O_{2max}$ in dogs[13] and pigs.[14]
- Restricting the exercising muscle mass in humans to 2–3 kg (knee extensors) rather than the 15–20 kg recruited during running or cycling elevates mass specific $\dot{V}O_{2max}$ substantially.[15,16]
- Blood doping (reinfusion of autologous red cells) elevates $\dot{V}O_{2max}$ in humans.[17]

Several steps in the pathway of O_2 from the atmosphere to its site of utilization within muscle mitochondria may limit the achievable $\dot{V}O_{2max}$.[18,19] These include O_2 diffusion across the blood-gas barrier in the lungs, conductive transport of O_2 in the blood $\dot{Q}$, and O_2 concentration (CaO_2), and diffusion of O_2 from the skeletal muscle capillary into the myocyte. The coordinated function of respiratory, cardiovascular, and muscular systems provides for rapid changes in O_2 flux from lungs to mitochondria (Fig. 31.5) and in most species, including the horse, human, and dog, the strongest determinant of $\dot{V}O_{2max}$ is the capacity of the cardiovascular system to transport O_2 (i.e. $\dot{Q}O_2$, Fig. 31.6). However, during maximal exercise in the horse other steps in the O_2 pathway assume greater importance for limiting $\dot{V}O_{2max}$ than in other species, in large part because of the disproportionality between the cardiovascular and respiratory systems. For example, O_2 loading in the lung is impaired and arterial hypoxemia becomes manifested (see *'Cardiovascular physiology and responses to exercise'* below). In addition, the ability to offload O_2 in the muscle capillary is constrained by the finite O_2-diffusing capacity of skeletal muscle which is determined by the capillary bed and blood flow within those capillaries. Figure 31.7 integrates the conductive and

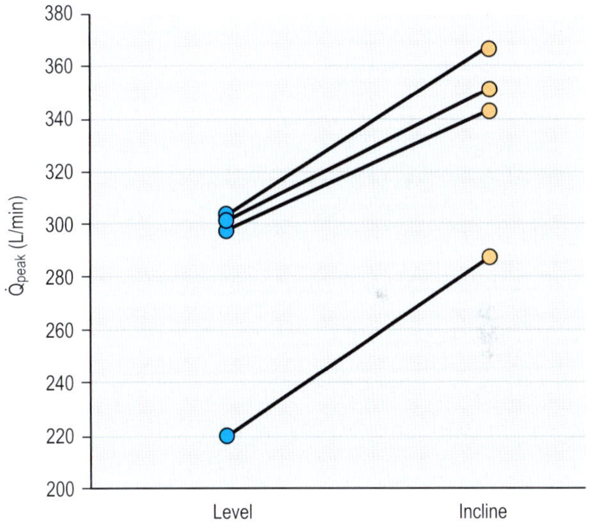

Fig 31.4 Running on an incline (6°) significantly increases cardiac output at maximal exercise ($\dot{Q}_{peak}$) and also elevates $\dot{V}O_{2max}$.
Reprinted from McDonough P, Kindig CA, Hildreth T, et al. Effect of body incline on cardiac performance. Equine Vet J Suppl 2002; 34:506-509, with permission of the Equine Veterinary Journal.

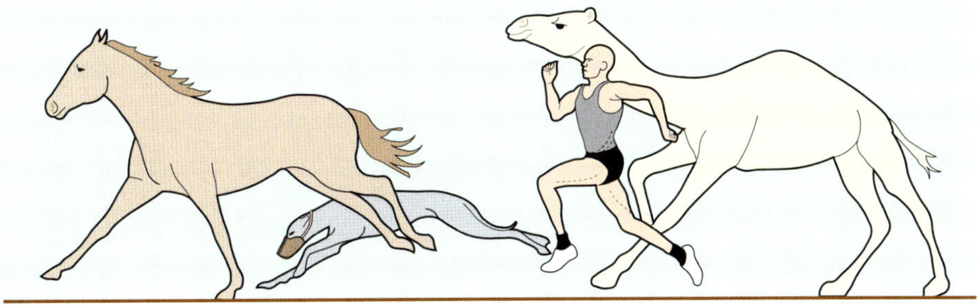

Fig 31.3 Relative maximum speed in m/s of the four main athletic species. For converting to other commonly used units: 10 m/s = 36 km/h or 22 miles/h.
Adapted from Derman KD, Noakes TD. Comparative aspects of exercise physiology. In: Hodgson DR, Rose RJ, eds. The athletic horse. Philadelphia: WB Saunders; 1994; 15, with permission from Elsevier.

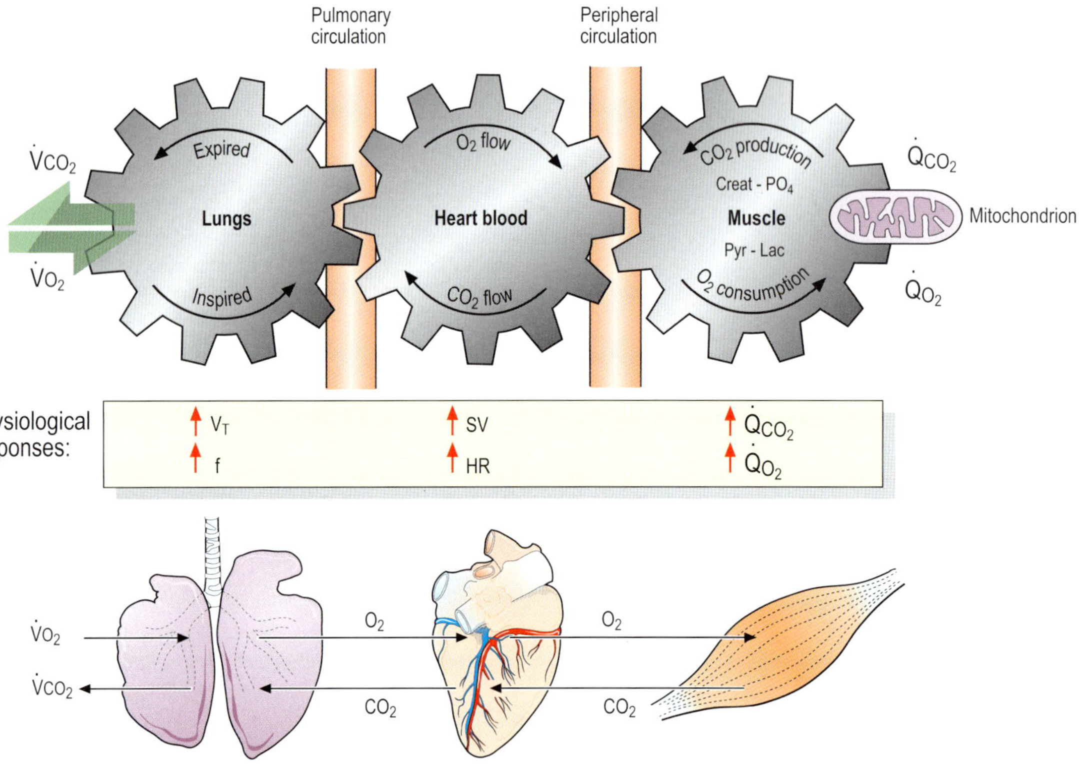

Fig 31.5 Illustration of the pathway for oxygen (O_2) from the atmosphere to its site of utilization within muscle mitochondria. The cogs demonstrate that the respiratory (lungs), cardiovascular (heart and blood vessels), and muscle systems must increase O_2 flux in a tightly coordinated fashion for effective delivery of adequate O_2 to facilitate muscular performance. $\dot{Q}O_2$, mitochondrial O_2 delivery/utilization; $\dot{V}O_2$, oxygen uptake; $\dot{V}CO_2$, CO_2 output, SV, stroke volume; HR, heart rate; V_T, tidal volume; f, breathing frequency; CO_2, carbon dioxide; Creat-PO_4, creatine phosphate; Pyr, pyruvate; Lac, lactate; $\dot{Q}CO_2$, mitochondrial carbon dioxide production.

Reprinted from Wasserman K, Hansen JE, Sue DY, et al. Principles of exercise testing and interpretation, 2nd edn. Philadelphia: Lea & Febiger; 1987, with permission from John Wiley and Sons, © 1988 Wiley Periodicals, Inc.

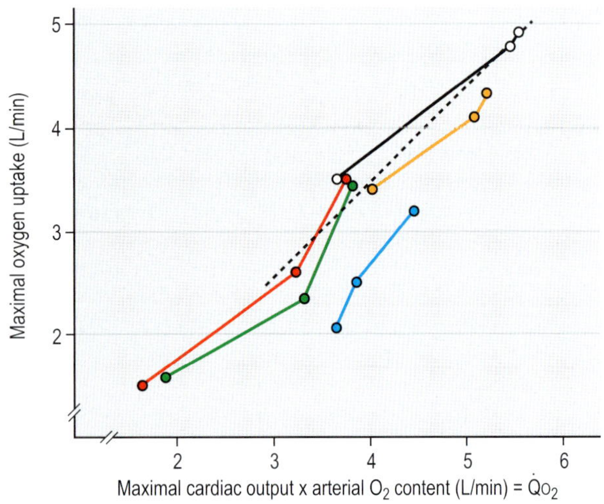

Fig 31.6 Relationship between increased O_2 delivery ($\dot{Q}O_2$) and maximal oxygen uptake ($\dot{V}O_2$) after bedrest and exercise training in five humans.

Reprinted from Saltin B, Blomqvist G, Mitchell JH, et al. Response to exercise after bed rest and after training. Circulation 1968; 38 (suppl VII):1-78, with permission of Wolters Kluwer Health.

diffusive elements of O_2 transport to demonstrate how the horse achieves its very high $\dot{V}O_{2max}$.

Conductive O_2 transport (lungs to muscle)

Given that high rates of O_2 delivery ($\dot{Q}O_2$) are of paramount importance for achieving this high $\dot{V}O_{2max}$, it is instructive to break down the components of $\dot{Q}O_2$:

$$O_2 \text{ delivery} = \text{cardiac output} \times \text{arterial } O_2 \text{ content}$$

$$\dot{Q}O_2 = \dot{Q} \times CaO_2$$

$$\dot{Q} = HR \times SV$$

Therefore:

$$CaO_2 = ([Hb] \times 1.34 \times \%Sat) + {\sim}0.3\ \text{mL}/100\ \text{mL dissolved } O_2$$

$$\dot{Q}O_2 = (HR \times SV \times [Hb] \times 1.34 \times \%Sat) + {\sim}0.3\ \text{mL}/100\ \text{mL}$$

$$\dot{Q}O_2 = \text{Heart rate} \times \text{stroke volume} \times \text{hemoglobin concentration} \times O_2 - \text{binding capacity of Hb} \times \%\text{ of } O_2 \text{ binding sites filled}$$

In the horse during maximal exercise, SV is determined principally by heart size and HR may approach 240 beats/min in young adults, which is unusually high for such a large animal (though it does decrease with advancing age and other factors[20]). Circulating hemoglobin concentration ([Hb]) increases nearly twofold above rest as red blood cells are released from the large muscular spleen in response to increased sympathetic activity. Table 31.1

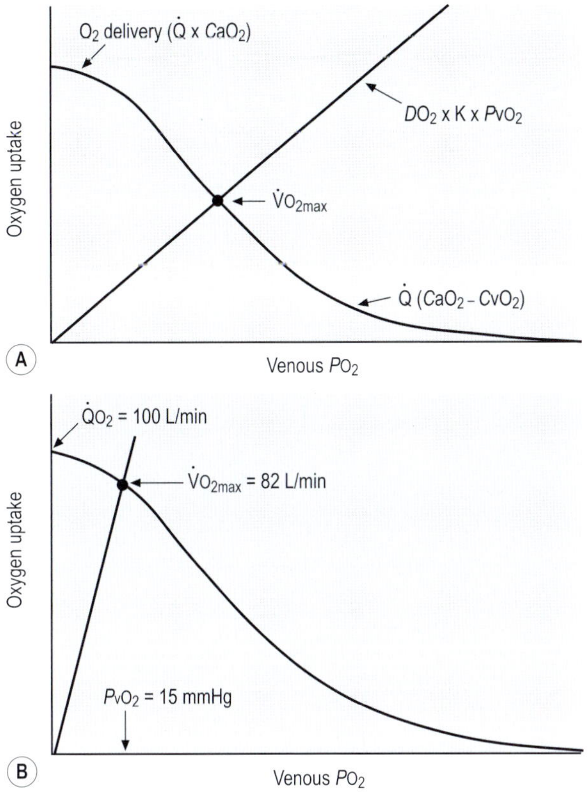

Fig 31.7 Determination of maximal O_2 uptake ($\dot{V}O_{2max}$) by conductive ($\dot{Q}O_2$) and diffusive movement of O_2 by the cardiovascular and muscle microcirculatory systems ('Wagner' diagram[18]). The curved line denotes mass balance according to the Fick principle and the straight line from the origin represents Fick's law of diffusion. DO_2 is effective diffusing capacity and K is a constant that relates venous PO_2 to mean capillary PO_2. PvO_2, CaO_2, and CvO_2 are the partial pressure of venous O_2 and the concentrations of O_2 in arterial and venous blood, respectively. $\dot{V}O_{2max}$ occurs at the intersection of the two relationships. **(A)** is a general schematic whereas **(B)** presents actual values for a very fit Thoroughbred at maximal exercise. Understanding the conductive and diffusive determinants of $\dot{V}O_{2max}$ is essential for interpreting the structural and functional mechanisms that increase $\dot{V}O_{2max}$ with exercise training . See pp. 670 and 671 for additional details.
Wagner PD, Hoppeler H, Saltin B. Determinants of maximal oxygen uptake. In: Crystal RG, West JB, Barnes PJ, et al, eds. The lung: scientific foundations, 2nd edn. New York: Lippincott-Raven; 1997; 2033-2041.

demonstrates that the size of the heart and spleen is relatively larger in the horse than in either the ox or man. Relative heart size in the athletic dog (i.e., greyhound[24–26]) approaches that found in the horse, but the horse is unusual in that the spleen is so large. Note that in the horse, the proportion of skeletal muscle is very high (close to 50%) and the lungs are relatively small (particularly with respect to heart size, see *'Cardiovascular physiology and responses to exercise'* below). A comparison between actual heart size and $\dot{V}O_{2max}$ in the athletic horse and human is shown in Figure 31.8.

Diffusive O_2 transport within muscle

$\dot{V}O_{2max}$ is the product of $\dot{Q}_{max}$ and the extraction of O_2 primarily by the muscles as described by the Fick equation:

$$\dot{V}O_{2max} = \dot{Q}_{max} \times (CaO_2 - CvO_2)$$

where CaO_2 and CvO_2 denote arterial and mixed venous O_2 contents. Figure 31.7 demonstrates that the effective muscle diffusing

Table 31.1 Relative comparison of the mass of organs key to the loading and transport of O_2 as a % of body mass

	HORSE	DOG	OX	MAN
Spleen	up to 1.1	0.3	0.2	0.3
Heart	0.7–2.0	0.8	0.4	0.5
Lungs	**0.9–1.5**	**0.9**	**0.7**	**1.4**

Data from Webb and Weaver[23] and Haun.[31] Note 'Dog' excludes greyhounds.

capacity (estimated by the slope of the line projecting from the origin) determines the level to which CvO_2 will fall at maximal exercise (i.e. extraction) and also the $\dot{V}O_{2max}$. The section *'Cardiovascular physiology and responses to exercise'* details the determinants of muscle O_2 diffusing capacity.

This chapter deals primarily with horses in their athletic prime and considers their maximal capacities irrespective of age per se. In this respect, horses increase their cardiovascular (Fig. 31.9) and muscle oxidative enzyme (Table 31.2) capacities substantially during their first 3 years. Thus, 3- to 4-year-old horses have larger hearts,[27,29] and a lower HR[27] (larger stroke volume) at a given running speed, as well as a reduced blood lactate response to submaximal running speeds (Fig. 31.10).[27] The mechanistic bases for these last two alterations, as they relate to increased heart size and vascular adaptations which improve muscle O_2 delivery and exchange, are encompassed within the training section of this chapter (*'Exercise training'*).

Anatomy of the cardiovascular system

Heart size

The size of the heart is a key determinant of maximum stroke volume, cardiac output, and hence aerobic capacity and exercise performance (Figs 31-11-31.14). This relationship has been documented in humans by examination of the electrocardiogram (ECG), ultrasound, radiographs, and post-mortem examination of heart size. For example, Paavo Nurmi, multiple Olympic champion distance runner, reportedly had a heart mass nearly three times larger than predicted for his body size. At post-mortem, the heart of the seven-time Boston Marathon winner, Clarence DeMar, who died of a non-myocardial cancer, was substantially larger than normal and his coronary arteries were threefold larger than found in his non-athletic counterparts.[31]

In horses, heart mass approximates 0.9–1% of body mass, which is greater than that for other non-athletic species (Fig. 31.14) and may exceed 1.1% of body mass in trained horses, possibly reaching ~2% in elite horses.[23,26] Amongst different horse breeds, racing horses have proportionally larger hearts (Fig. 31.14) and Table 31.3 lists some famous horses and their heart masses. The heaviest horse heart actually weighed was that of Sham at 18 lb (8.2 kg), who was consistently runner-up to Secretariat. Secretariat was a Triple Crown winner and holds the track record at Belmont Park (2 min 24.4 s for 1.5 miles on turf). Tragically, Secretariat's heart was never weighed. However, the same pathologist, Dr Thomas Swerczek, who weighed Sham's heart estimated that Secretariat's heart weighed 22 lb (10 kg) and he considered it to be in perfect condition.[31] If

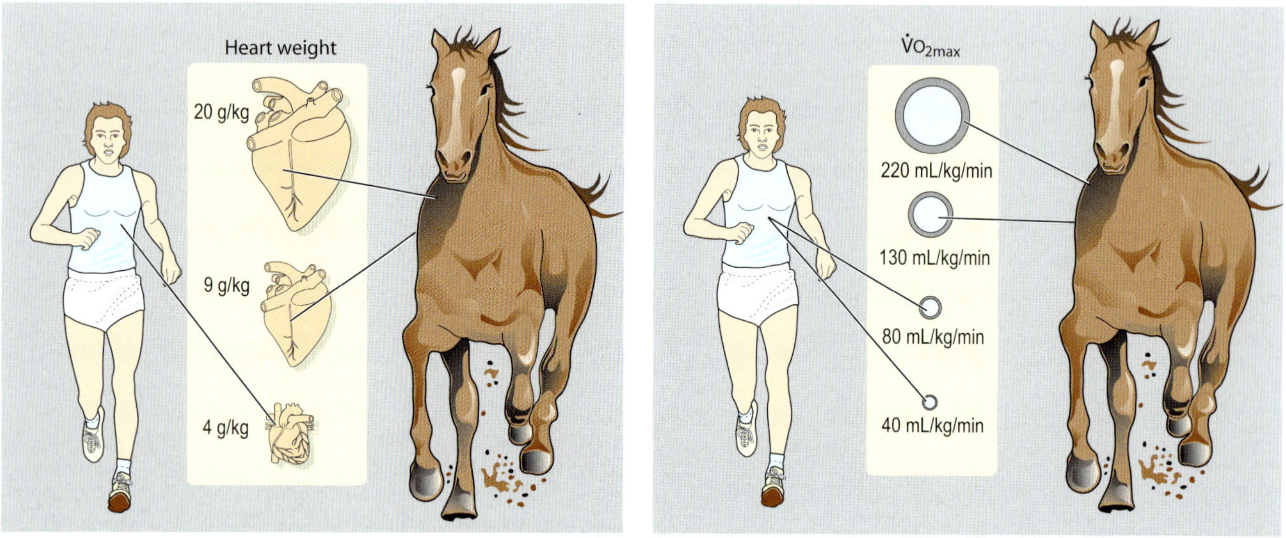

Fig 31.8 Comparison of heart size (per kg body mass) and $\dot{V}O_{2max}$ ranges within healthy human and equine populations. Note that exercise training increases heart size and mass and also $\dot{V}O_{2max}$ (see Table 31.7 for references).

Table 31.2 Relative citrate synthase (CS, carbohydrate metabolism), 3-hydroxy-acyl CoA dehydrogenase (HAD, fat metabolism) and lactate dehydrogenase (LDH, lactate→pyruvate interconversion) activities in the middle gluteal muscle of Thoroughbreds and Standardbreds of different ages

		ENZYME ACTIVITIES (SCALED TO 1 AT AGE 1 FOR MARES (M, FILLY) AND STALLIONS (S, COLT))					
		Thoroughbreds			Standardbreds		
Age	Sex	CS	HAD	LDH	CS	HAD	LDH
1	M	1	1	1	1	1	1
1	S	1	1	1	1	1	1
2	M	1.4	1.1	1.2	1.2	1.1	1
2	S	1.3	1.2	0.8	1.4	1.1	0.9
3	M	2.1	1.6	0.9	1.9	1.1	0.7
3	S	1.8	1.7	0.9	1.8	1.43	0.68
4–6	M	2.2	1.6	0.8	1.9	1.1	0.9
4–6	S	2.1	2.1	0.8	2.3	1.5	0.8
Age		XXX	XXX	XX	XXX	NS	XXX
Sex		NS	NS	NS	NS	NS	NS

Significance over the four age groups: XX, $P < 0.01$; XXX, $P < 0.001$.
(Based upon data from Snow and Valberg.[28])

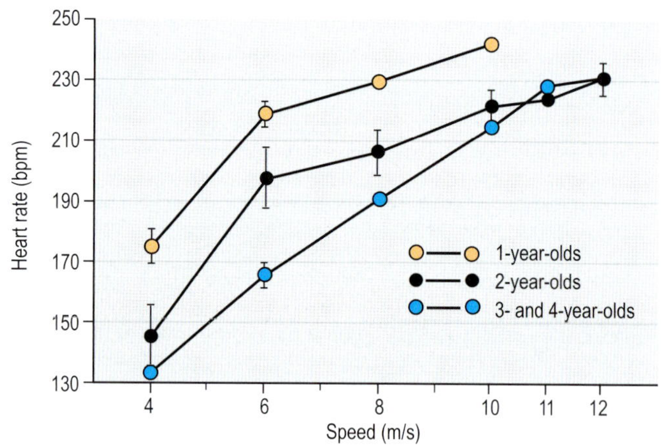

Fig 31.9 Reduction in heart rate response to running as a function of age which reflects increased heart size and stroke volume at 2–4 years of age in comparison with 1 year old.

Reprinted from Rose RJ, Hendrikson DK, Knight PK. Clinical exercise testing in the normal thoroughbred race horse. Aust Vet J 1990; 67:345-348, © 2008, John Wiley and Sons.

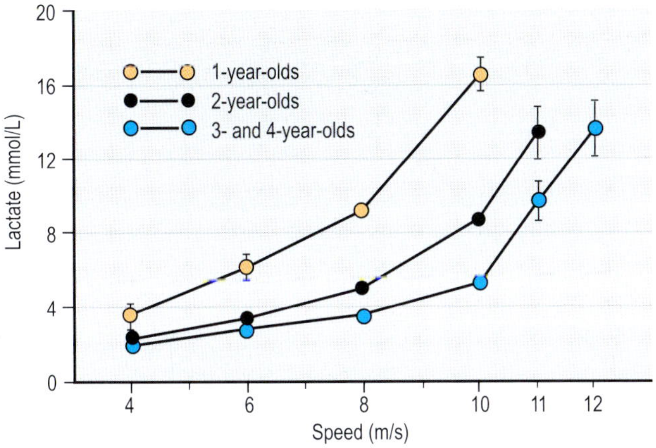

Fig 31.10 Decreased blood lactate response to submaximal running speeds for horses aged from 1 to 3 and 4 years.
Reprinted from Rose RJ, Hendrikson DK, Knight PK. Clinical exercise testing in the normal thoroughbred race horse. Aust Vet J 1990; 67:345-348, © 2008, John Wiley and Sons.

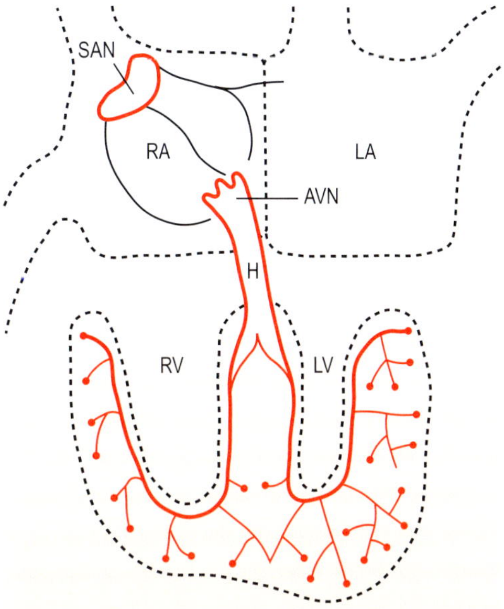

Fig 31.12 Conduction system of the equine heart which is composed of specialized cardiac muscle fibers rather than nerves. Note the extensive arborization of the Purkinje fibres across the ventricular walls that is characteristic of the horse heart and which results in effective depolarization from multiple points. SAN, sinoatrial node; RA, right atrium; LA, left atrium; AVN, atrioventricular node; H, bundle of His; RV, right ventricle; LV, left ventricle.
Courtesy of R. Hamlin.

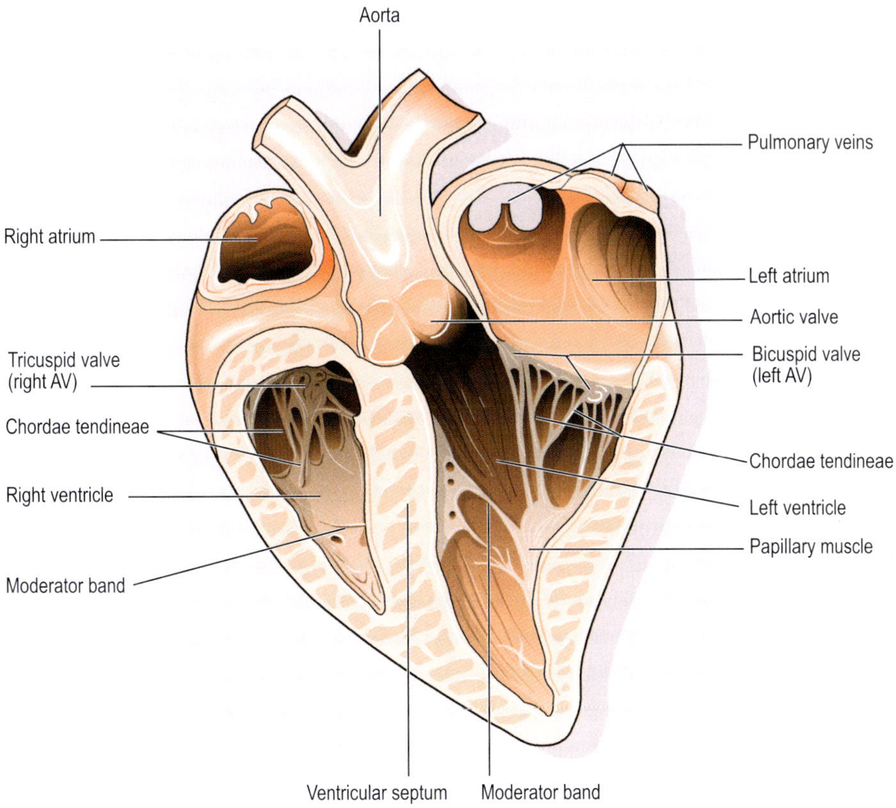

Fig 31.11 Cross-section of the equine heart showing principal anatomic structures. AV, atrioventricular valve (see Fig. 31.12).

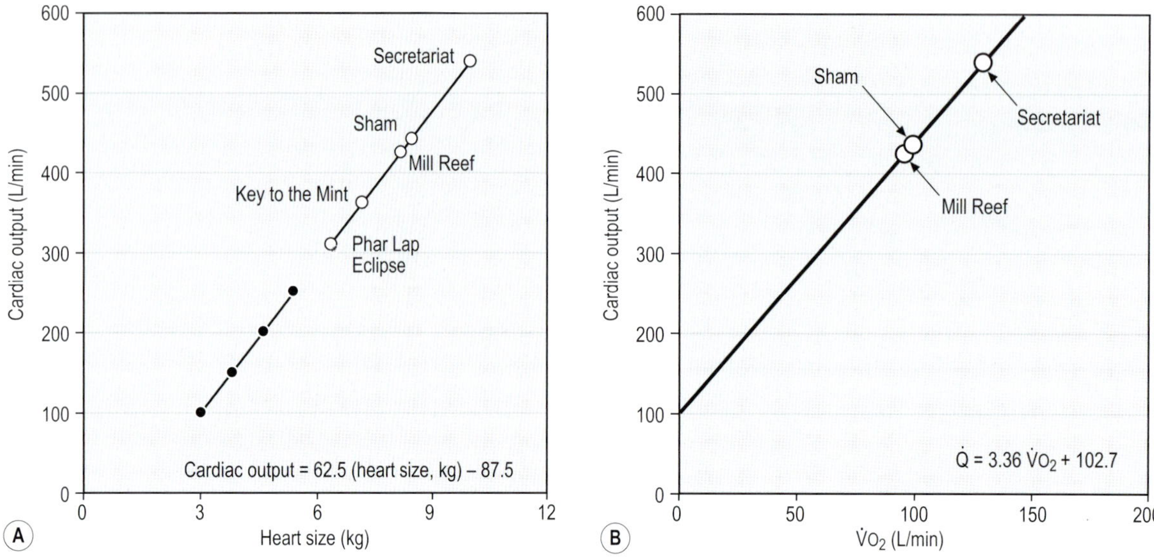

Fig 31.13 Relationship between heart size and cardiac output ($\dot{Q}$) **(A)** and $\dot{V}O_2$ and cardiac output at maximum exercise **(B)**. **(A)** The solid symbols are determined from the data of Evans and Rose (1988);[30] the hollow symbols are determined from that relationship and the measured or estimated (Secretariat) heart masses published for each named horse.[31] **(B)** An arterial–venous O_2 difference of 22.8 mL/100 mL of blood is assumed to estimate $\dot{V}O_{2max}$ values for Secretariat and Sham. The echocardiographic data of Young et al.[5] are consistent with this relationship. Note Secretariat's extraordinary $\dot{Q}$ (~ 540 L/min) and $\dot{V}O_{2max}$ (over 120 L/min, which would be 240 mL O_2/kg/min at 500 kg body mass).

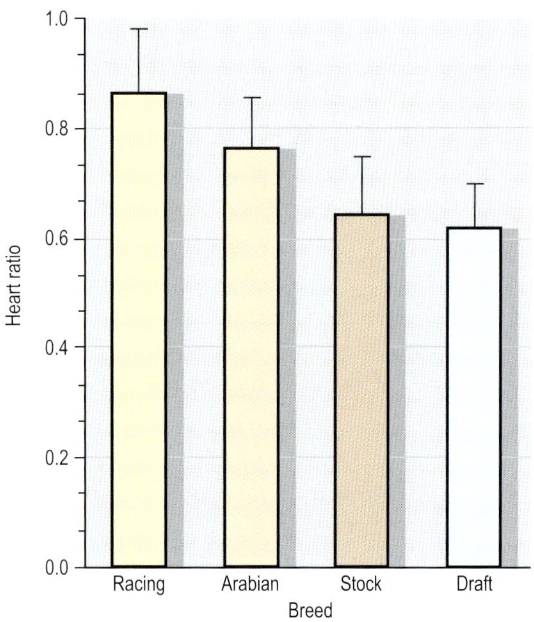

Fig 31.14 Heart ratio (heart mass as a percentage of body mass) with standard deviations for racing, Arabian, stock, and draft horses. Note that, after training, heart ratio may reach 1.1% or higher (~2% in exceptional horses i.e., Sham and Secretariat).[23,26]

Reprinted from Kline H, Foreman JH. Heart and spleen weights as a function of breed and somatotype. Equine Exerc Physiol 1991; 3:17-21, with permission from Wageningen Academic Publishers.

that mass is correct, Figure 31.13A predicts that Secretariat may have achieved a cardiac output in excess of 500 L/min and Figure 31.13B a $\dot{V}O_{2max}$ over 120 L/min! To place heart size in visual perspective, Figure 31.15 compares Key to the Mint's 15.8 lb (7.2 kg) heart to that of an unexceptional stallion.

Given the crucial importance of heart size in setting athletic potential, there has been great interest in establishing a convenient and accurate non-invasive method of estimating this variable in horses. The mean/average duration of the QRS complex (in ECG leads I, II, and III, Fig. 31.16) has been shown to correlate with heart mass at autopsy and also racing performance.[32] Thus, larger hearts have a wider QRS complex and the so-called 'heart score' measured in milliseconds has been related to heart mass and subsequently predicted stroke volume and cardiac output, as shown in Table 31.4 and Table 31.5. It should be noted, however, that other studies have not been able to confirm the relationship between heart score and heart mass.[33-37] Based upon the inheritance of heart scores in racehorses,[38] there is currently great interest in identifying the gene, located on the X-chromosome, that codes for heart mass.[31] Echocardiographic and cardiac ultrasound techniques have demonstrated that a significant relationship exists between left ventricular mass and $\dot{V}O_{2max}$ in Thoroughbred racehorses.[5] Moreover, positive relationships among left ventricular size, systolic function, and race performance are emerging.[39,40] These latter findings offer some hope that non-invasive evaluation methods may prove valuable in helping to select for athletic potential.

An important feature of the equine heart that may contribute to exercise-induced pulmonary hypertension concerns the disparity in size of the right and left atrioventricular (AV) valves. Specifically, at Kansas State University, Professors M. Roger Fedde and Howard H. Erickson (unpublished findings) have determined that the cross-sectional area of the left AV valve is only 63% that of the right AV valve (i.e. 38.1 vs 60.8 cm^2). As the smaller cross-sectional area will substantially elevate resistance to blood flow, this is expected to raise left atrial, pulmonary venous, pulmonary capillary, and, ultimately, pulmonary arterial pressures.

Spleen

As shown above, O_2 delivery depends not only upon cardiac output ($\dot{Q}$) but also upon arterial O_2 content (CaO_2), and the equine spleen

Table 31.3. Heart mass and heart scores of famous racehorses

NAME OF HORSE (COLOR, SEX, YEAR BORN)	HEART MASS lb	HEART MASS kg	HEART SCORE (ms)
Secretariat (ch.s. 1970)	22	10	
Sham[a] (ch.s. 1970)	18	8.2	
Mill Reef[a] (b.s. 1968)	16.9	7.7	
Key to the Mint (b.s. 1969)	15.8	7.2	157
Easy Goer (ch.s. 1986)	15	6.8	
Althea (ch.m. 1981)	15	6.8	
Eclipse (ch.s. 1764)	14	6.4	
Phar Lap (ch.g. 1926)	14	6.4	
Star Kingdom (ch.s. 1946)	14	6.4	
Tulloch (b.s. 1954)	13.5	6.2	136
Killaloe (b.m. 1970)	12.9	5.9	
Northern Dancer (b.s. 1961)			150
Soviet Problem (ch.m. 1990)			150
Moscow Ballet (b.s. 1982)			147
The Last Red (ch.m. 1993-twin)			140
Desert Secret (b.s. 1990)			140
Hyperion (ch.s. 1930)			133
Vo Rouge (b.g. 1983)			130

[a]Some pathologic enlargement (may add 2–3 lb to heart mass).
(Reprinted from Haun M, 1997, The X factor – what it is and how to find it, with kind permission from Flying Island LLC.)
b, bay; ch, chestnut; g, gelding; m, mare; s, stallion.

Table 31.4 Relationship derived between heart mass and heart score

HEART SCORE (ms)	HEART MASS lb	HEART MASS kg
100	6.6	3.0
110	7.4	3.4
120	10.1	4.6
130	11.9	5.4
140	13.6	6.2
150	15.4	7.0
160	17.2	7.8

(Reprinted from Haun M, 1997, The X factor – what it is and how to find it, with kind permission from Flying Island LLC.)

Table 31.5 Relationships derived among heart score, heart mass, and stroke volume and cardiac output at maximal exercise

HEART SCORE (ms)	HEART MASS (kg)	STROKE VOLUME (L)[a]	CARDIAC OUTPUT (L/min AT MAX EXERCISE)[b]
100	3.0	0.5	100
110	3.8	0.75	150
120	4.6	1.0	200
130	5.4	1.25	250

[a]Estimated by Steel (unpublished data 1977).
[b]Assuming a heart rate of 200 beats/min.

is of paramount importance for setting the horse's high exercising blood hemoglobin concentration ([Hb]) and thus CaO_2. Splenic contraction may dump 12 L or more of red cells into the circulation, thereby doubling the number of circulating red blood cells.[41–44] In keeping with the importance of $\dot{Q}O_2$ in determining racing performance, splenectomy reduces $\dot{V}O_{2max}$ by over 30% in the Thoroughbred.[43] Splenic reserve is correlated with spleen mass and total blood volume but not body mass per se.[36,41,44] Racing horses have a significantly greater splenic mass than non-racing breeds, i.e. Arabian, stock, draft[32] (Fig. 31.17). There is some evidence that erythropoietin treatment increases $\dot{V}O_{2max}$ via elevated circulating hemoglobin concentration in Standardbred horses.[45] However whether this is efficacious for the racing Thoroughbred who may already be at a hematocrit approaching 70% remains to be determined.

Systemic circulation and microcirculation

In the Thoroughbred, total blood volume approximates 10% of body mass[46,47] and of this approximately 50 L of blood, 75% resides in the systemic circulation, of which 60% is in the highly distensible venous system and only 15% in the arteries. Depending upon the activity undertaken (e.g. digestion, thermal stress, exercise), the cardiovascular system must redistribute $\dot{Q}$ amongst the appropriate organs. Physical exercise produces the most profound physiological stress to the horse and, as shown in Figure 31.18, the percentage of $\dot{Q}$ that perfuses the splanchnic region and kidneys is reduced from ~50% at rest to only 5% at maximal exercise. By contrast, exercising skeletal muscle may receive 80–90% of $\dot{Q}$ compared with only 10–20% at rest. Such flexible and precise control over blood flow distribution demands a network of powerful muscular arterioles that provide the principal resistance to flow in the systemic circulation and which can dilate or constrict rapidly in response to the vasoactive effects of muscle metabolites, prostacyclins, and nitric oxide (dilation), or sympathetic stimulation, angiotensin, and endothelin (constriction). From rest to maximal exercise, skeletal muscle blood flow may increase over 60–70-fold. Although the perfusion pressure does increase substantially, elevated muscle vascular conductance (dilation) constitutes the primary mechanism by which the increased muscle blood flow ($\dot{Q}m$) is achieved, and this response is detailed in the section *'Cardiovascular physiology and responses to exercise'* below. Following a systematic series of bifurcations through several orders of progressively narrower arterioles, the

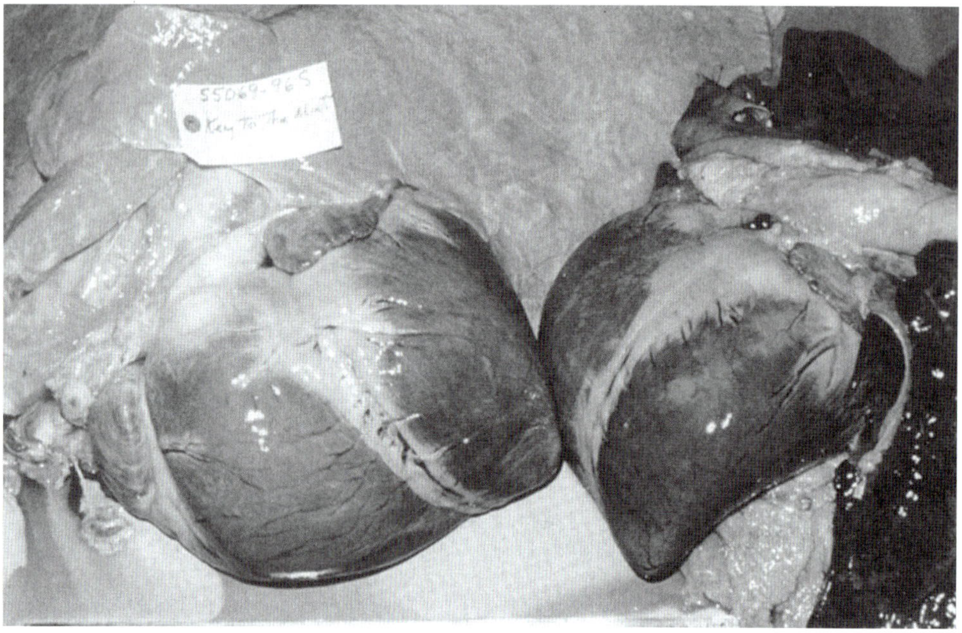

Fig 31.15 Comparison of Key to the Mint's heart on the left (15.8 lb (7.2 kg), heart score 157) with that of an unremarkable stallion on the right (12 lb (5.5 kg)).

Reprinted from Haun M, 1997, The X factor – what it is and how to find it, with kind permission from Flying Island LLC, and Dr Thomas Swerczek.

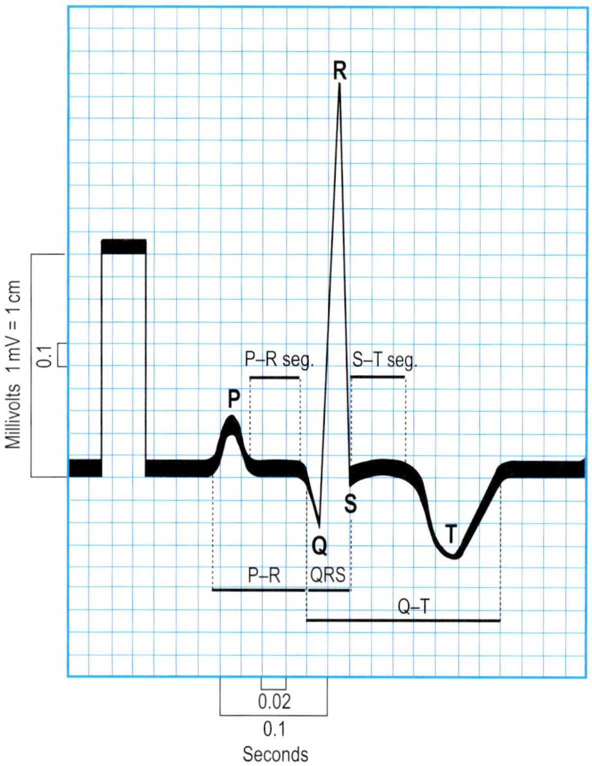

Fig 31.16 The heart score is calculated from the width of the QRS complex (in milliseconds) on the electrocardiogram shown here. In general, the larger the heart, the wider the QRS complex and the greater the heart score. See text for further details.

Reprinted from Haun M, 1997, The X factor – what it is and how to find it, with kind permission from Flying Island LLC.

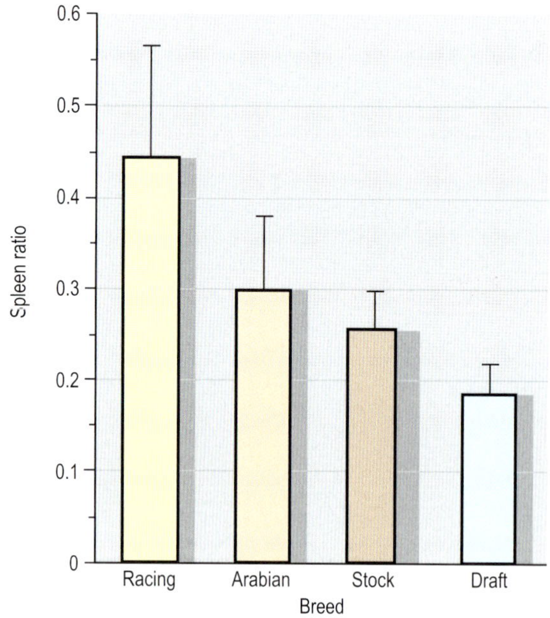

Fig 31.17 Spleen ratio (spleen mass as a percentage of body mass) with standard deviations for racing, Arabian, stock, and draft horses. Note that absolute ratio reflects post-mortem mass when spleens are largely depleted of red cells.

Reprinted from Kline H, Foreman JH. Heart and spleen weights as a function of breed and somatotype. Equine Exerc Physiol 1991; 3:17-21, with permission from Wageningen Academic Publishers.

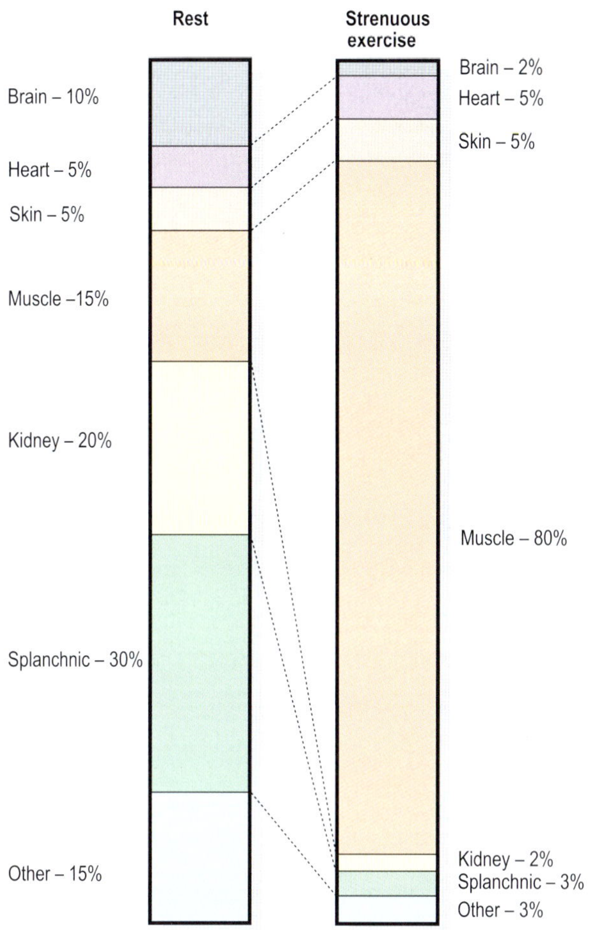

Fig 31.18 Distribution of cardiac output ($\dot{Q}$) at rest and during maximal exercise. In the highly trained, very fit Thoroughbred, it is possible that skeletal muscle blood flow may reach as much as 90% of cardiac output.

Values from Erickson et al.[48]

vascular tree ramifies into a series of capillaries which form the principal site for blood-tissue exchange (Fig. 31.19). The capillary wall is devoid of smooth muscle and presents a barrier typically less than 1 µm thick between the capillary blood and the myocyte sarcolemma. The density, volume, and surface area of the skeletal muscle capillary bed are correlated closely with oxidative capacity and thus muscle fiber type.[51,52] In equine muscle (transverse section across fibers), there may be between 400 and 800 capillaries per square millimeter with a mean diameter of 4–6 µm,[49,53] and these contain over 80% of the intramuscular blood volume. As we shall see in the section *'Cardiovascular physiology and responses to exercise'* below, the capillary volume is crucial for setting red blood cell transit time in the capillary and facilitating O_2 offloading during exercise (or loading in the pulmonary capillary).

Pulmonary circulation and microcirculation

At rest, the pulmonary circulation holds about 20% of total blood volume (mostly in larger compliant vessels rather than the capillaries) which decreases at exercise onset. Because the pulmonary circulation has to accept the whole output of the right ventricle, it is a low-pressure, high-conductance system with arteries and arterioles that are far less muscular than seen for the systemic circulation. Approximately half of the pulmonary vascular resistance is precapillary and the capillaries themselves constitute an important site of resistance, particularly at high lung volumes and when alveolar pressure is positive during breathhold or forced exhalation.

The pulmonary vasomotor tone can be influenced by a variety of neural and humoral factors. Specifically, pulmonary arteries have both sympathetic and parasympathetic innervation and respond to serotonin, epinephrine (adrenaline), norepinephrine (noradrenaline), isoproterenol, acetylcholine, angiotensin II, leukotrienes, prostacyclins, histamine, thromboxane, bradykinin, and arachidonic acid. However, as seen in Figure 31.20, the horse has relatively little pulmonary vascular smooth muscle compared with cattle and pigs.[54] Thus, the horse exhibits only a weak vasoconstrictive response which is most evident in the low susceptibility of the horse to pulmonary hypoxic vasoconstriction but which causes a profound pulmonary hypertension in cattle and pigs at altitude. During exercise, the elevated pulmonary arterial pressures induce recruitment and distension of the vascular bed, which reduces vascular resistance, elevates vascular conductance, and increases pulmonary capillary volume (Fig. 31.21). Despite this elevated conductance, pulmonary vascular pressures do become extraordinarily high during maximal exercise (see *'Cardiovascular physiology and responses to exercise'* below).

The pulmonary capillaries form a dense plexus around each alveolus and, unlike their systemic counterparts, are not embedded within a supporting tissue matrix and thus are subject to collapse at positive alveolar pressures, particularly when perfusion pressure is low. In the horse, these vessels are about 6–7 µm in diameter[56] (which is narrower than found in dog or rabbit lungs) and have a total wall thickness (capillary endothelium, basement membrane, alveolar epithelium) which averages only 0.9 µm (Fig. 31.22). Consequently, even at relatively low transmural pressures (positive luminal plus negative alveolar), these vessels bulge into the alveolar space and may rupture during exercise (exercise-induced pulmonary hemorrhage). Pulmonary capillary blood volume constitutes only a very small fraction of that present in the pulmonary circulation, which confers the advantage of maximizing blood-gas spatial contact but has the consequence of limiting red blood cell transit time in the capillary. Pulmonary capillary blood volume in the horse is 60–80% greater than that of a steer of the same mass.[57]

In healthy animals as for humans, active vasomotor control is traditionally thought to play a relatively minor role (compared with the effects of hydrostatic pressure gradients, lung volume, and alveolar pressure) in setting the distribution of blood flow within the pulmonary circulation.[53] However, more recent investigations have demonstrated that there is a gravity-independent distribution of $\dot{Q}$ toward the dorsal aspect of the equine lung (Fig. 31.23).[58] This effect may be explained by a regionally dependent arteriolar reponsiveness. For example, arterioles in the upper lung regions exhibit a pronounced vasodilation to methacholine (an endothelium-dependent vasodilator) whereas those at the bottom do not.[59]

Cardiovascular physiology and responses to exercise

Cardiac output

Cardiac output ($\dot{Q}$) is defined as the volume of blood ejected from the right or left ventricle and is usually expressed per minute. As illustrated in Table 31.6, cardiac output is the most important means of increasing muscle O_2 delivery during exercise and is the principal determinant of $\dot{V}O_{2max}$, which can vary from 90 to 220 mL/kg/min[5,60] or possibly even higher (Secretariat). Very fit Thoroughbreds have had $\dot{Q}$ values measured in excess of 350 L/min and, as

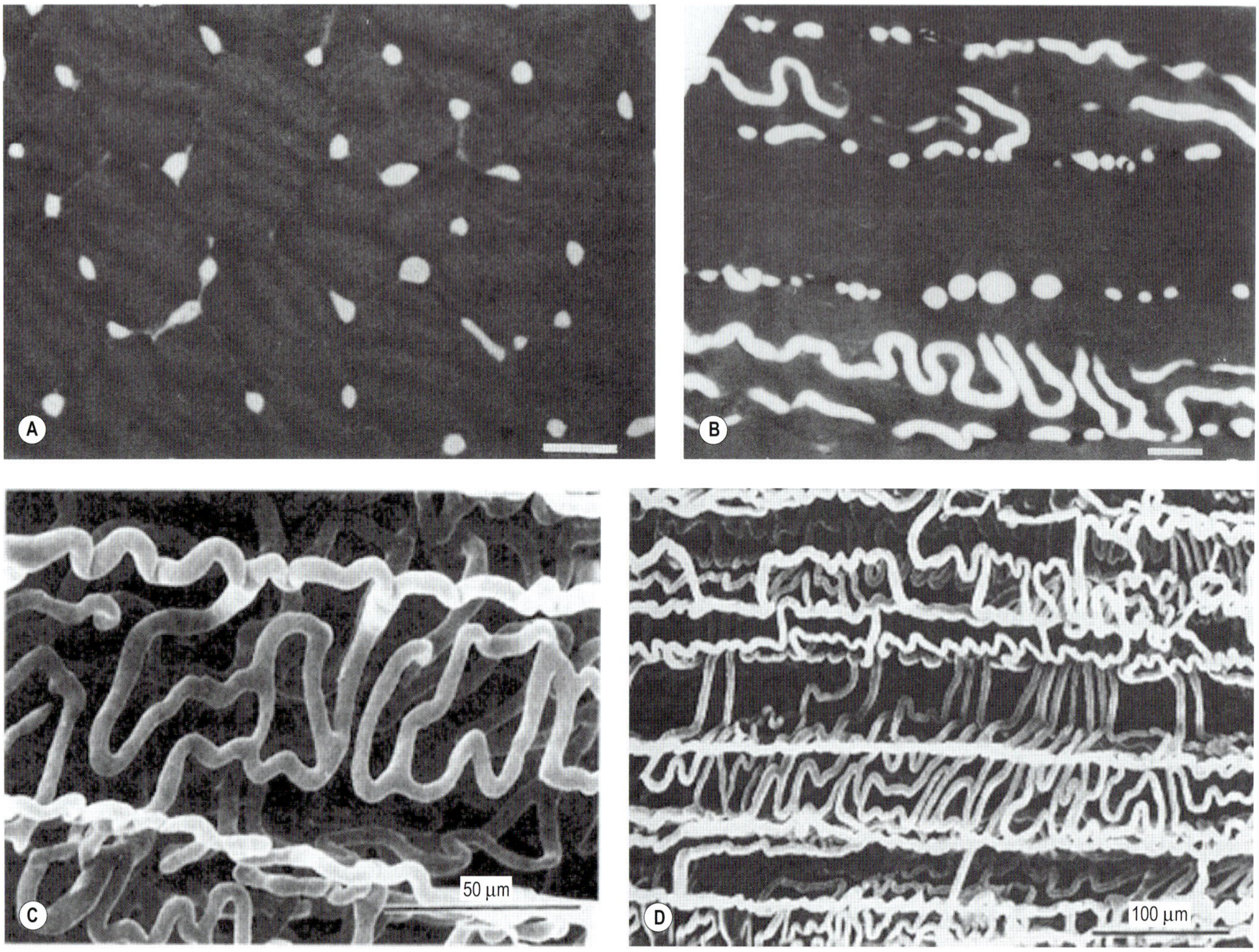

Fig 31.19 The capillary bed of skeletal muscle possesses a complex three-dimensional geometry with extensive branching and capillaries that become extremely tortuous at short muscle sarcomere lengths forming a convoluted network around the fibers. **(A, B)** Light micrographs of pony vastus medialis muscle perfusion-fixed at 1.90 μm sarcomere length and cut transverse **(A)** and longitudinal **(B)** to the fiber longitudinal axis. Capillaries have been flushed clear of red cells and appear white surrounding the perimeter of the individual muscle fibers **(A)**. **A, B** scale bar = 25 μm. **(C, D)** Corrosion casts (muscle fibers have been corroded away) of the mouse soleus muscle that demonstrates superbly the three-dimensional geometry of the muscle capillary bed.

(A) and (B) Reprinted from Mathieu-Costello O, Hoppeler H, Weibel ER. Capillary tortuosity in skeletal muscles of mammals depends on muscle contraction. J Appl Physiol 1989; 66:1436-1442, with permission from The American Physiological Society. (C) and (D) Ishikawa H, Sawada H, Yamada E. Surface and internal morphology of skeletal muscle. In: Peachy LD, Adrian RH, Geiger SR, eds. Handbook of physiology. Section 10: skeletal muscle; 1983; 1-22, reprinted with permission of the American Physiological Society.

mentioned above, based upon estimated heart size, it is likely that superlative athletes have achieved $\dot{Q}$ values between 400 and 540 L/min (Fig. 31.13A and B, Fig. 31.14). During submaximal exercise, $\dot{Q}$ (and body O_2 delivery, $\dot{Q}O_2$) increase linearly with running speed and also $\dot{V}O_2$.[61–63] Increased $\dot{Q}$ in combination with the splenic-induced polycythemia may elevate $\dot{Q}O_2$ over 20-fold in a very fit Thoroughbred racehorse from rest to maximal exercise. Increases in $\dot{Q}$ are driven most powerfully by heart rate, with a smaller contribution from elevated stroke volume (Table 31.6).

Heart rate

At exercise onset, heart rate increases rapidly from approximately 30 beats/min at rest to approximately 110 beats/min via parasympathetic withdrawal, with the consequence that at low running speeds heart rate may elicit an early overshoot (Fig. 31.24).[30,64,65] At faster speeds, further heart rate elevations are achieved less rapidly and are driven by the sympathetic nervous system and circulating catecholamines. Maximum heart rate varies between 204 and 241 beats/min and, as mentioned above, a reduction with age has been described recently in horses.[20,66] In human populations a decrease of 1 beat/min/year has been well established.[67,68] However, among horses other factors likely contribute more to their variance in maximum HR.[20,66] Maximum heart rate is not considered to be an important measure of fitness and, as seen in the section *'Exercise training'* below, does not change with training. The speed or velocity a horse can achieve or sustain at a submaximal heart rate of 140, 170, or 200 beats/min (i.e. V_{140}, V_{170}, and V_{200}) provides information about stroke volume and cardiovascular capacity and pertains directly to fitness and racing potential.[60] Both heart rate[30,64] and $\dot{V}O_2$[69] increase faster after a warm-up, although as cardiac output does not appear to limit $\dot{V}O_2$ kinetics at exercise onset,[70,71] the two are probably not linked mechanistically. There is a linear relationship between heart rate and running speed and between $\%HR_{max}$ and $\%\ \dot{V}O_{2max}$ (Figs. 31.25 and 31.26).[60,72–74] However, at a constant running speed in the heavy intensity domain, heart rate may continue to rise and this is accompanied by rising ventilation, $\dot{V}O_2$, and $\dot{Q}$.[75] This 'slow component' of the cardiorespiratory response is driven by elevated metabolic requirements within the exercising muscles,[76] a progressive fall in blood volume, and also thermoregulatory responses to the rising body temperature.

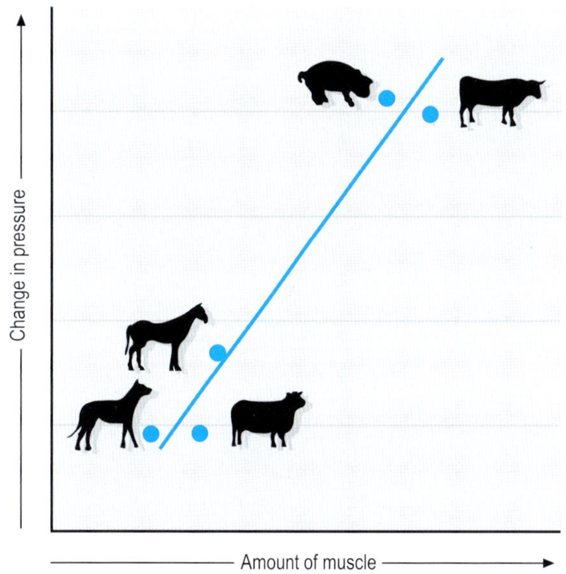

Fig 31.20 Species variation in the muscle thickness in the walls of small pulmonary arteries and the change in pulmonary arterial pressure evidenced during hypoxic exposure. Note that the horse has far less muscle (and thus change in pulmonary arterial pressure) than the cow and the pig when exposed to hypoxia.

Reprinted from Robinson NE. Respiratory function. In: Cunningham JG, ed. Textbook of veterinary physiology, 3rd edn. London: WB Saunders; 2002; 481, with permission from Elsevier.

Stroke volume

Stroke volume refers to the volume of blood ejected per beat from the left or right ventricle and increases from approximately 1000 mL (2–2.5 mL/kg) at rest up to 1700 mL (3–4 mL/kg) or higher at maximal exercise (Table 31.6).[12,60,61,63,73] If a maximum heart rate of 225 beats/min is assumed for Secretariat, his stroke volume would have been well in excess of 2000 mL/beat. Typically, stroke volume increases sharply at exercise onset up to around 40% $\dot{V}O_{2max}$ consequent to increased blood volume, venous return, and filling pressures according to the Frank–Starling mechanism.[30,77] What is particularly remarkable is that ventricular filling (and thus stroke volume) does not appear to be compromised at maximal exercise despite heart rates of 4 beats/s.

Arterial O_2 content (CaO_2) and O_2 delivery ($\dot{Q} \times CaO_2 = \dot{Q}O_2$)

As described in the first section of this chapter, arterial O_2 content, CaO_2, is determined principally by blood hemoglobin

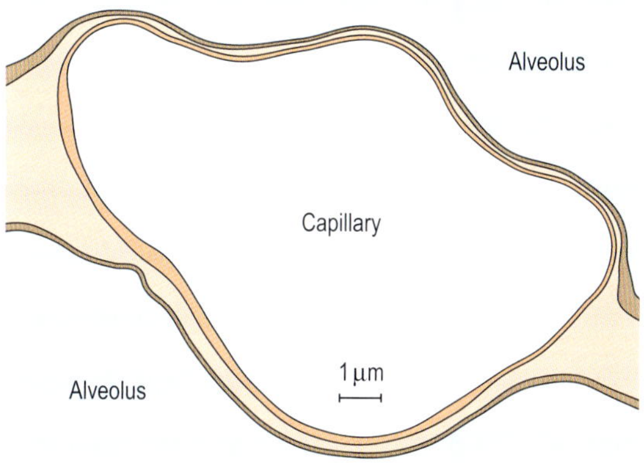

Fig 31.22 Pulmonary capillary interposed between two alveoli. Note the exquisitely thin blood-gas barrier.

Reprinted from Birks EK, Mathieu-Costello O, Fu Z, et al. Comparative aspects of the strength of pulmonary capillaries in rabbit, dog, and horse. Respir Physiol 1994; 97:235-246, with permission from Elsevier.

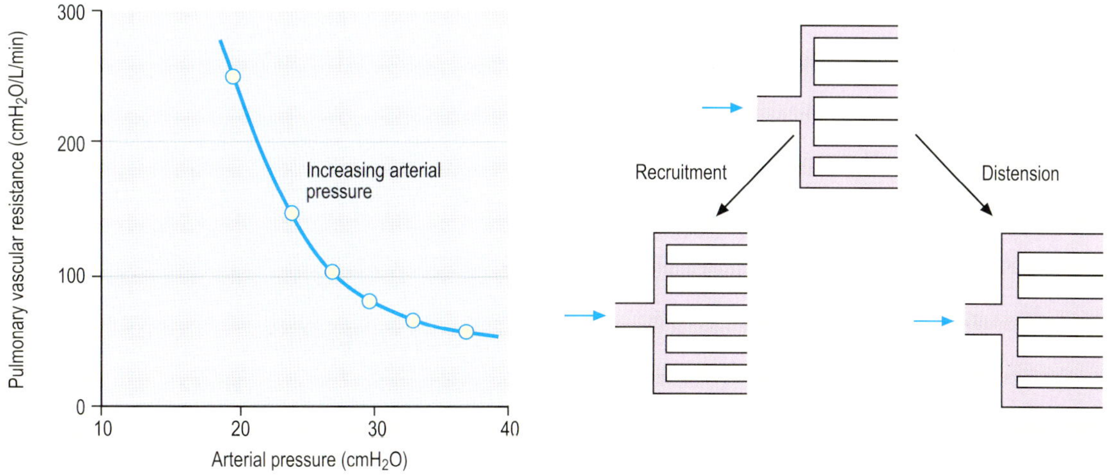

Fig 31.21 Elevated pulmonary arterial pressure reduces pulmonary vascular resistance because it forces a recruitment of previously non-perfused vessels and distends those vessels recruited.

Revised from West.[55]

Table 31.6 Cardiovascular responses to maximal exercise in a 500 kg horse

VARIABLE	REST	EXERCISE	EXERCISE/REST RATIO
Heart rate (beats/min)	30	210–250	7–8
Cardiac output (L/min)	30	240–>450	8–13
Stroke volume (mL)	1000	>1700	1.7
Systolic/diastolic arterial Blood pressure (mmHg)	130/80	230/110	1.6
Pulse pressure (mmHg)	50	120+	3–4
Pulmonary artery pressure (mmHg)	20–30	90–140	3–4
Hemoglobin concentration (g/dL)	13	17–24	1.3–1.6
O_2 uptake (mL/min/kg) (L/min)	2–4 1.0–2.0	160–>220 80–>110	40–110 40–110
a – vO_2 difference (mL/100 mL)	5	20–25	4–5

(Data from Erickson and Poole.[48])

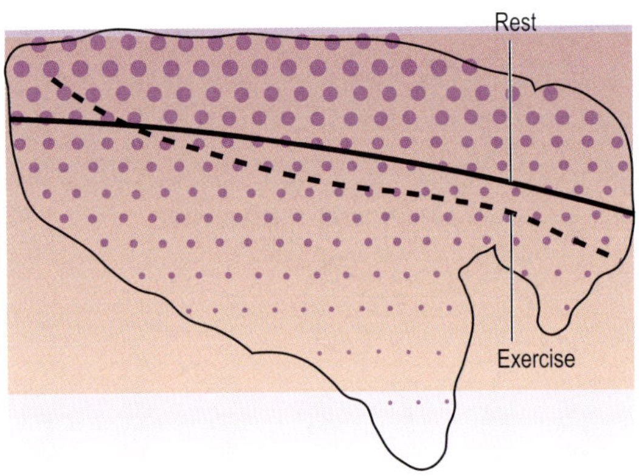

Fig 31.23 Distribution of pulmonary blood flow in the lung at rest. The shading indicates relative blood flow (the darker the area, the greater the blood flow) and the solid and broken lines indicate relative dorsal–caudal blood flow at rest and during exercise, respectively. Note that pulmonary blood flow is not regulated by gravity, as once thought.

Reprinted from Robinson NE. Respiratory function. In: Cunningham JG, ed. Textbook of veterinary physiology, 4th edn. London: WB Saunders; 2007; p. 580, with permission from Elsevier.

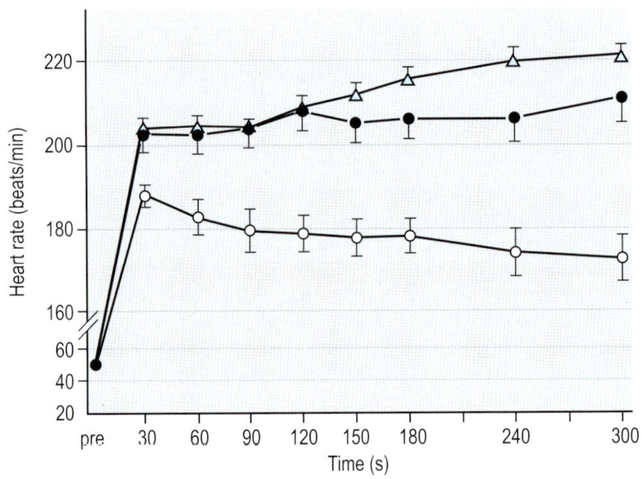

Fig 31.24 Heart rate response following the onset of exercise at 50% (hollow circles), 75% (solid circles), and 100% (triangles) $\dot{V}O_{2max}$ in Standardbred racehorses. Note the pronounced early overshoot at 50% $\dot{V}O_{2max}$.

Springer and the Journal of Comparative Physiology B: Biochemical, Systemic, and Environmental Physiology, 157, (6); 791-799, 1988, Dynamics of cardiorespiratory function in standardbred horses during constant load exercise, Evans DL, Rose RJ. With kind permission from Springer Science and Business Media.

concentration (which sets the O_2-carrying capacity) and the % saturation of those hemoglobin-binding sites with O_2. At rest, arterial hemoglobin concentration is 12–14 g/100 mL, whereas at maximal exercise the spleen has expelled sufficient red blood cells to increase this up to 21–24 g/100 mL. This corresponds to a packed cell volume increase from 35% at rest to 70% at maximal exercise. Thus, at maximal exercise, if hemoglobin was 100% saturated with O_2, each 100 mL of blood would hold between 27 and 31 mL O_2. However, as discussed below, arterial O_2 saturation falls from around 95% at rest to below 85% at maximal exercise,[10] and this will decrease CaO_2 to 23–26 mL/100 mL. Even considering this effect, with a $\dot{Q}$ of 400 L/min, the Thoroughbred can deliver a prodigious 100 L O_2/min to the body during maximal exercise.

Determinants of O_2 loading

Pulmonary circulation

The rapid increase in pulmonary blood flow at exercise onset in concert with the polycythemic hyperviscosity[41,78–80] elevates pulmonary vascular pressures (Fig. 31.27) and forces recruitment of non-flowing vessels and distension of flowing vessels (Fig. 31.21). This behavior elevates pulmonary vascular conductance several-fold but does not prevent mean pulmonary arterial pressure from

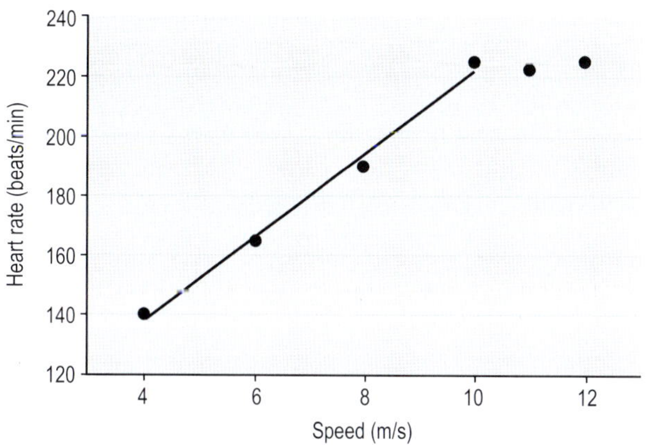

Fig 31.25 Relationship between running speed and heart rate from 4 m/s to maximal speed (12 m/s) in a race-fit Thoroughbred racehorse.

Reprinted from Evans DL. The cardiovascular system: anatomy, physiology, and adaptations to exercise and training. In: Hodgson DR, Rose RJ, eds. The athletic horse. Philadelphia: WB Saunders; 1994; 129-144, with permission from Elsevier.

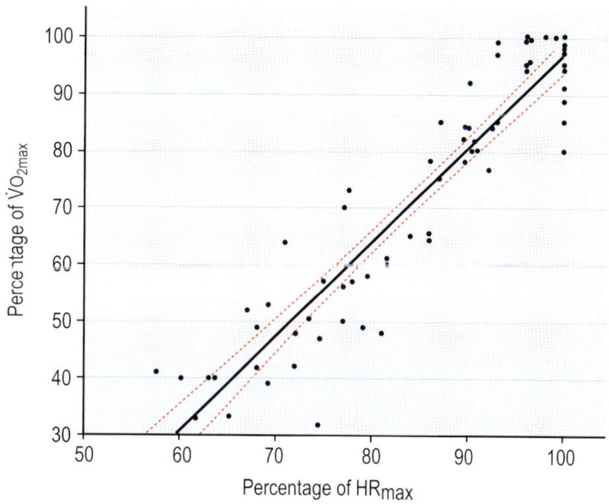

Fig 31.26 Relationship between % maximum heart rate and % $\dot{V}O_{2max}$ in horses of varying fitness levels.

Reprinted from Evans DL, Rose RJ. Maximal oxygen consumption in race horses: changes with training state and prediction from submaximal indices of cardiorespiratory function. In: Gillespie JR, Robinson NE, eds. Equine exercise physiology 2. Equine Vet J, 20(4); 241-242, with permission from the Equine Veterinary Journal.

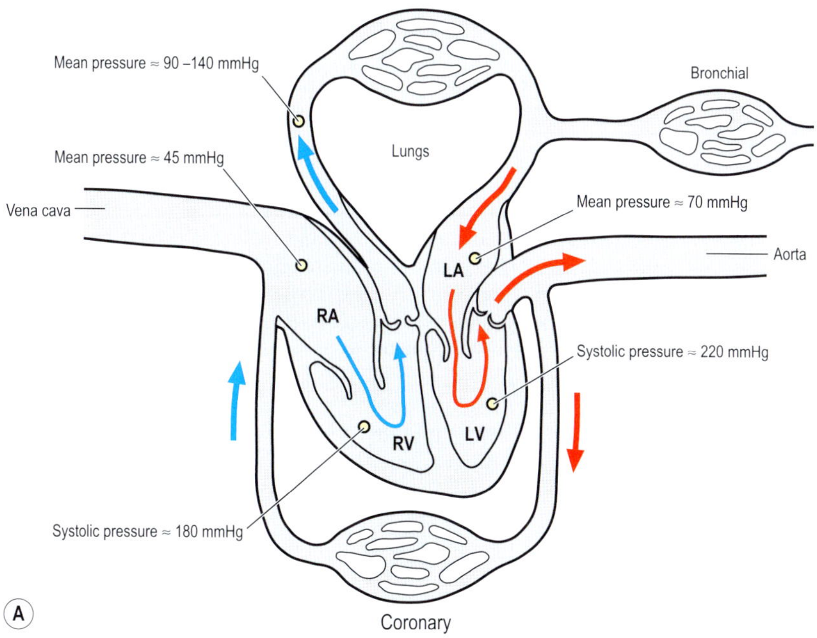

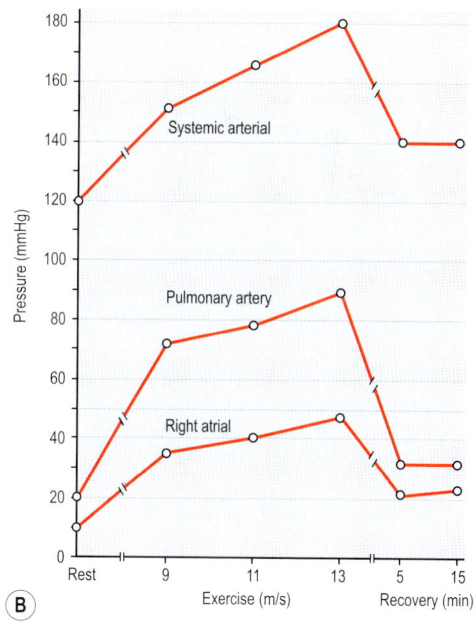

Fig 31.27 **(A)** Pressures within the pulmonary and systemic circulations during maximal exercise. **(B)** Mean systemic and pulmonary arterial and right atrial pressures at rest and during exercise and recovery.

Courtesy of S.C. Olsen.

exceeding 120 mmHg in fit horses.[70,81-85] The consequences of this hypertension include exercise-induced pulmonary hemorrhage (EIPH) and are detailed below. Splenectomy (reduced blood viscosity),[43,80] diuretic therapy (furosemide),[85-89] and nitric oxide (vasodilator)[84] are all effective modalities for reducing maximal pulmonary arterial pressures during exercise. However, splenectomy reduces $\dot{Q}O_2$ and thus negatively impacts both $\dot{V}O_{2max}$ and performance.[43] As mentioned in the section, *'Anatomy of the cardiovascular system'*, in contrast to conventional wisdom, it has now been established that gravity is not the sole or even the primary regulator of the regional distribution of blood flow within the equine lung. Elegant fluorescent microsphere studies by Bernard, Hlastala, Erickson, and colleagues have determined that pulmonary $\dot{Q}$ is preferentially distributed toward the dorsal aspect of the lung at rest and during exercise (Fig. 31.23)[58,90] likely due to a regional variation in sensitivity to endothelium-induced vasodilation.[59]

Exercise-induced arterial hypoxemia

As demonstrated in Figure 31.28, blood leaving the horse's lung during maximal exercise is profoundly hypoxemic.[10,91] Several mechanisms impair O_2 loading in the pulmonary capillary. These are described below in order of importance.

Alveolar–capillary O_2 diffusion limitation (~70% of alveolar-to-capillary O_2 pressure gradient)

During maximal exercise the horse develops a significant alveolar-to-capillary O_2 pressure (P) gradient.[91] Unlike in other species such as man, in whom alveolar hyperventilation drives arterial $P\text{CO}_2$ below resting and in which alveolar $P\text{O}_2$ becomes elevated during intense exercise, in the horse alveolar $P\text{O}_2$ may fall and consequently the increased alveolar-to-capillary O_2 pressure gradient results from the reduced arterial $P\text{O}_2$. The primary reason for the elevated alveolar-to-capillary O_2 pressure gradient and arterial hypoxemia relates to the prodigious values of $\dot{Q}$ achieved. The average transit time for a red blood cell (RBC) within the pulmonary capillary is determined by the ratio between pulmonary capillary blood volume and $\dot{Q}$. In the horse at rest, pulmonary capillary volume is some 1.8-fold that of an equivalently sized steer[57] and RBCs probably spend 0.75–1 s within the capillary, which is thought to be three to four times longer than necessary for equilibration with the alveolar O_2 (Fig. 31.28). However, during maximal exercise, when $\dot{Q}$ may increase from rest by up to 13-fold, capillary volume does so by only a small fraction of this. Consequently, red cell capillary transit time will decrease. Morphometric estimation of mean exercising red cell transit time places it at 0.3–0.5 s.[57,92] This is probably a gross overestimate of that present in very fit racehorses that can achieve $\dot{Q}$ values around 400 L/min and it is pertinent that, even if this were the mean transit time, there would exist a substantial population of red cells with considerably shorter transit times. Because of the sigmoid shape of the O_2 dissociation curve, it is not possible for those cells with longer

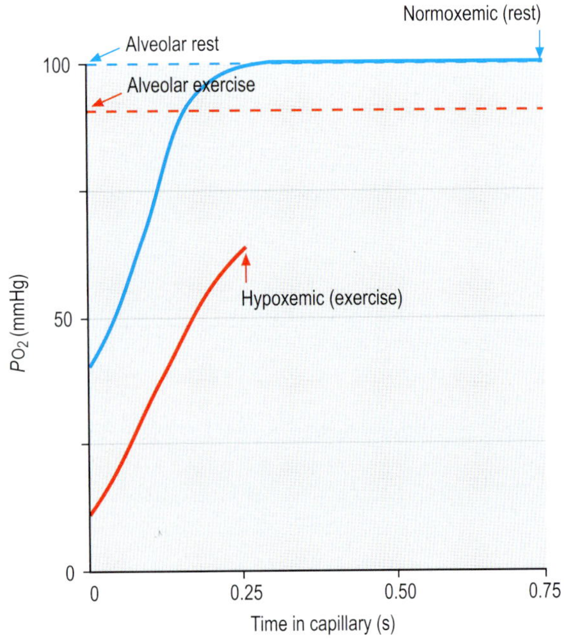

Fig 31.28 Partial pressure of O_2 ($P\text{O}_2$) in the red blood cell as a function of pulmonary capillary transit time at rest and during exercise. Note the reduction in alveolar $P\text{O}_2$ during exercise (alveolar hypoventilation) and the profound decrease in red cell $P\text{O}_2$ as it enters and leaves the capillary during maximal exercise.

transit times to compensate for those that do not equilibrate with the alveolar gas. The consequence of this mixing of hypoxemic with normoxemic blood in the pulmonary veins will be arterial hypoxemia. In addition, the rightward shift of the O_2 dissociation curve consequent to elevated blood temperatures, arterial hypercapnia, and acidosis will reduce the hemoglobin-O_2 affinity and further exacerbate alveolar–capillary disequilibrium.

Alveolar hypoventilation

As mentioned above, at maximal exercise the horse's arterial $P\text{CO}_2$ may exceed 65 mmHg.[10,79,81,93] Calculated from the alveolar gas equation, this will cause alveolar $P\text{O}_2$ to fall from approximately 100 mmHg at rest to approximately 90 mmHg at maximal exercise (Fig. 31.28). The opinion that this hypoventilation results somehow from the constraints of locomotory–respiratory coupling (LRC, locking breathing and stride frequencies, which was considered necessary to achieve exercising tidal volumes >14 L/breath) has been undermined by the observation that tidal volumes may actually increase further (as well as minute ventilation itself) during recovery from the gallop.[94]

Mild ventilation-to-perfusion ($\dot{V}_A/\dot{Q}$) mismatch

During exercise, the horse develops a small but significant degree of $\dot{V}_A/\dot{Q}$ mismatch. However, this is not thought to contribute in a quantitatively important fashion to the exercise-induced arterial hypoxemia.[91,95] The percentage of $\dot{Q}$ that does not come into contact with alveolar gas (i.e. shunt) is trivially small (≤1%).

Exercise-induced pulmonary hemorrhage

Exercise-induced pulmonary hemorrhage (EIPH) is characterized by rupture of the blood-gas barrier and the presence of blood in the alveolar space and airways. In extreme cases, frank epistaxis may occur. EIPH is prevalent in Thoroughbreds, Standardbreds, and also Quarter Horses during sprint racing, where repeated endoscopic examination indicates an incidence approaching 95%.[96–101] Importantly, it isn't just sprint or severe intensity exercise that causes EIPH. Epp and colleagues[102] at Kansas State University found significant EIPH in horses after trotting for ~25 minutes. Microspheres (10–15 μm) injected into the jugular vein have identified the pulmonary rather than the bronchial (systemic) vasculature as the site of EIPH[82] and elegant electron microscopy studies have captured red cells actually erupting from breaks in the fragile blood-gas barrier (Fig. 31.29).[103,104]

EIPH isn't simply an acute condition but leads to extensive destruction and remodeling of lung structure. Specifically, postmortem examination of lungs from racing Thoroughbreds evidence interstitial fibrosis, pleural/interlobular septal thickness and elevated venous wall thickness and veno-occlusive remodeling particularly within the dorsocaudal lobe.[105,106] Whereas free blood within the alveolar/airway spaces does promote inflammation[107] such inflammation in-and-of itself is not thought to be responsible for the fibrosis/accumulation of interstitial collagen that characterizes the racehorse towards the end of its career.[108]

EIPH must ultimately arise from high positive intraluminal pressures coupled with very negative alveolar pressures which summate across the blood-gas barrier causing failure (Fig. 31.29).[81,109,110] However, the etiology of EIPH is complex and numerous mechanisms have been implicated.[101] These include:

- Alveolar pressure fluctuations which may be exacerbated by upper airway obstruction (inspiratory nasal collapse;[111] laryngeal hemiplegia[112]).

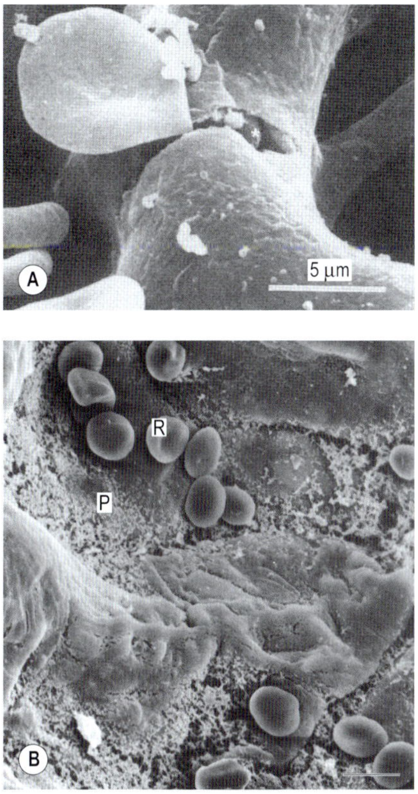

Fig 31.29 Rupture of the pulmonary capillaries. **(A)** Red blood cell emerging from a split in the blood-gas barrier into the alveolar space. **(B)** Exercise-induced pulmonary hemorrhage in the alveolar space of a pony lung. R, red blood cell; P, proteinaceous material. Scale bar = 5 μm.

*(A) Reprinted from Fu Z, Costello ML, Tsukimoto K, et al. High lung volume increases stress failure in pulmonary capillaries. J Appl Physiol 1992; 73(1):123-133, with permission from the American Physiological Society. **(B)** Reprinted from Erickson HH, McAvoy JL, Westfall JA. Exercise-induced changes in the lung of Shetland ponies: ultrastructure and morphometry. J Submicrosc Cytol Pathol 1997; 29:65-72, reprinted with kind permission.*

- Pulmonary hypertension consequent to high $\dot{Q}$ values (>120 mmHg mean pulmonary artery pressure[81,82,87,110]), exercise-induced hyperviscosity,[78,113] and possibly arteriolar vasoconstriction.[79,83,84] In this regard, Thoroughbred horses have higher pulmonary vascular pressures than Standardbred horses and this has been linked to the greater incidence/severity of EIPH in the former.[114] Importantly, RV internal dimensions are greater in horses suffering from more extreme EIPH supporting the connection between elevated vascular pressures and RV remodeling in athletic horses.[115] Repeated bouts of venous hypertension are known to produce regional vein wall remodeling and collagen accumulation as well as venous occlusion[106] and these may be distributed in regions of high blood flow.[116a]
- Redistribution of blood within the lung.[90]
- Mechanical stresses of respiration and locomotion.[116b]

Additional factors that may contribute to elevated pulmonary arterial pressures include flow limitation induced by the relatively small cross-sectional area of the atrioventricular (AV) valves,[101] possible regurgitation through the AV valves consequent to high ventricular pressures, and also a left ventricular relaxation rate that may be too slow to allow rapid filling at lower left atrial pressures.[101,117,118] With regard to valvular regurgitation, Young and Wood[119] performed cardiac auscultation on 111 Thoroughbreds aged 2–5 years old and reported that the incidence of mitral and tricuspid regurgitation was 7% and 13%, respectively. After training, this increased significantly to 22% (mitral) and 26% (tricuspid).

Following the observation that pulmonary artery pressures and capillary transmural pressures reach extraordinarily high levels in the exercising horse and that there are threshold pulmonary arterial and capillary pressures above which the integrity of the blood-gas barrier is disrupted,[110,120] EIPH research and therapeutic interventions have focused on reducing these pressures.[101] Diuretic treatment with furosemide, which lowers pulmonary vascular pressures, has the greatest proven track record in this regard.[85,87,121–123] However, this therapy also improves performance by decreasing body mass[124] and may also mask the presence of other illicit drugs. Nasal passage support with the FLAIR nasal strip also reduces EIPH to a similar extent by reducing alveolar pressure swings and the transmural pressure gradient, which lowers the work of breathing.[85,111,122,125] Other treatment strategies involving Chinese herbal remedies,[126] antifibrolytic treatment with aminocaproic acid,[127] sildenafil citrate (Viagra)[128] or endothelin-1A antagonism[129] have not proven efficacious.

Pulmonary inflammation increases the opportunity for developing EIPH during intense exercise[107] and immunomodulation with concentrated equine serum reduces the severity of EIPH possibly through a reduction in parenchymal/airway inflammation and damage.[130] This is consistent with the observation that severe EIPH is associated with elevated IL-6 levels.[131]. Experiments using furosemide,[85] nitric oxide inhalation,[84] inhibition of nitric oxide synthase[79,83] and inclined running[132] have demonstrated that interventions which lower peak pulmonary artery pressure may not necessarily induce a corresponding reduction in EIPH.[101] Thus, regulation of the distribution of pulmonary $\dot{Q}$ and vascular conductance may be crucial for limiting EIPH and continues to be an active and important avenue of research. Intriguing recent observations that race distances, speed, age, track hardness and air quality could not be linked to EIPH development, but that ambient temperatures below 20°C could,[133] merit future scientific consideration.

Systemic circulation

Cardiovascular control must subserve two crucial and sometimes conflicting demands: namely, muscle $\dot{Q}$ must achieve a level commensurate with O_2 and substrate requirements (up to 100-fold resting) whilst maintaining systemic mean arterial pressure (MAP) within acceptable limits. Excessive vasodilation lowers MAP and compromises blood flow to critical organs such as the brain. By contrast, excessive MAP impairs vascular integrity, elevates vascular fluid exudation, and causes tissue damage.

MAP is the product of $\dot{Q}$ and total peripheral resistance (TPR). TPR is determined principally by the aggregate cross-sectional area of all recruited arterioles and also blood viscosity. Figure 31.30 details many of the factors controlling vascular smooth muscle, and thus vascular conductance, within skeletal muscle. Even at maximal exercise, there is a profound sympathetic vasoconstrictor tone within skeletal muscle[135] and blood pressure regulation depends upon the interaction of central nervous system reflexes emanating from the brain (central command) and those within the working muscle.[136–140] MAP rises from 110–138 mmHg at rest to as high as 200 mmHg during maximal exercise (Table 31.6, Fig. 31.27).[60,62,79,83,141,142] In addition to MAP, systolic left ventricular and right atrial pressures increase substantially[60,63,73,82] and myocardial contractility (peak derivative of left ventricular pressure, LV$dp/dt$) rises progressively with running speed.[60]

From rest to exercise, skeletal muscle arterial and arteriolar vasodilation allows TPR to fall precipitously, which facilitates enormous $\dot{Q}$ values with a relatively modest rise in MAP. Specifically, if $\dot{Q}$ increases from 30 (rest) to 450 (maximal exercise) L/min for a corresponding increase in MAP from 120 to 180 mmHg, TPR must fall by 90% (i.e., 4 to 0.4 mmHg/L/min). The control of skeletal muscle vasomotor tone involves a complex array of mechanical (muscle pump, shear stress, myogenic), humoral (vasoactive metabolites, catecholamines) and neural (sympathetic, anteriograde and retrograde conducted vasodilation) mechanisms (Fig. 31.30). Recent findings from Kindig and colleagues[79,83,84] indicate a major role for nitric oxide in increasing systemic and vascular conductances during intense running (Fig. 31.31). There have been several excellent recent reviews on the regulation of muscle vascular conductance[138–140,143] and it is apparent that the precise mechanisms which mediate the rapid increase of muscle $\dot{Q}$ and $\dot{Q}O_2$ at exercise onset remain to be resolved.[144] The matching between $\dot{Q}O_2$ and $\dot{V}O_2$ during exercise is so precise that it has inspired the suggestion that the system behaves as though there is an O_2 sensor located within the muscle or its vascular bed.[140] However, if present, such a sensor remains elusive.

During exercise, muscle $\dot{Q}$ ($\dot{Q}m$) is distributed heterogeneously among and within muscles depending on their recruitment, oxidative capacity, fiber type, and $\dot{V}O_2$ demands.[139] Thus, in the exercising horse, $\dot{Q}$ in heavily recruited, highly oxidative red muscles in the

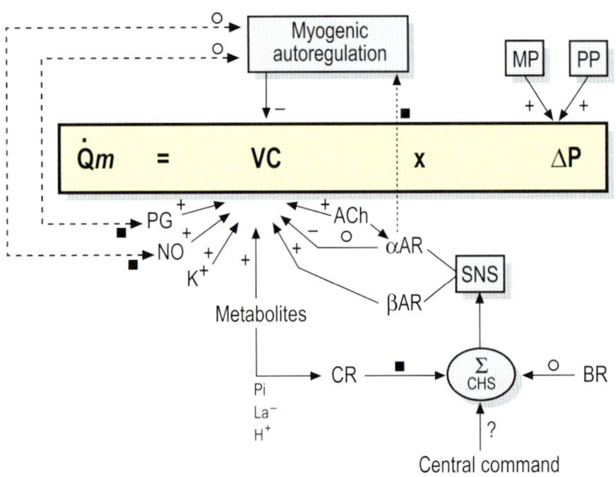

Fig 31.30 Muscle blood flow ($\dot{Q}m$) is regulated by the interaction of multiple mechanical (top row) and non-mechanical (bottom) factors which act directly on vascular smooth muscle to either reduce (–) or increase (+) limb vascular conductance (VC). $\dot{Q}m$ will also increase if the pressure gradient (DP) across the capillary bed is enhanced by the muscle pump (MP) following muscle contraction or elevated perfusion pressure (PP). In addition, VC may be changed by the action of the sympathetic nervous system (SNS) after integration of opposing reflex inputs arising from the baroreflexes (BR) and chemoreflexes (CR) and also from higher centers within the brain. There are also other factors that may potentiate (solid squares) or constrain (hollow circles) the effect of other regulatory agents (dotted lines). The net blood flow response to exercise is the result of all of these factors. PG, prostaglandins; NO, nitric oxide; K^+, potassium ion; Pi, inorganic phosphate; La^-, lactate ion; βAR, beta-adrenergic receptor; αAR, alpha-adrenergic receptor; ACh, acetylcholine; H^+, hydrogenion. *Reprinted from Shoemaker JK, Hughson RL. Adaptation of blood flow during the rest to work transition in humans. Med Sci Sports Exerc 1999; 31:1019-1026, with permission from Wolter Kluwer Health.*

limbs and respiratory system may achieve peak values of 1–3 L/min/kg.[53,145–147] Specifically, Armstrong and colleagues[53] measured vastus intermedius $\dot{Q}m$ at 1.5 L/min/kg in Standardbred horses running at $\dot{V}O_{2max}$ (134 mL/kg/min; $\dot{Q}$ 288 L/min). Within the thigh muscles sampled, the vastus intermedius had the highest citrate synthase activity (mitochondrial volume density, 9%) and myoglobin concentration, and exhibited the greatest $\dot{Q}m$. Indeed, across the several muscles/muscle portions sampled there was a strong correlation ($r = 0.947$) between citrate synthase activity and $\dot{Q}m$ at $\dot{V}O_{2max}$.

The respiratory muscles, and in particular the diaphragm, are extremely oxidative and during near-maximal exercise diaphragm $\dot{Q}m$ may exceed 2.5 L/min/kg.[145,146] Vasodilation and inspiratory resistance studies have revealed that, even at $\dot{V}O_{2max}$, the diaphragm retains a considerable vasodilator reserve. Specifically, prodigious diaphragm $\dot{Q}m$ values close to 4 L/kg/min are feasible.[145–148] It is quite possible that exceptional athletes or individuals with laryngeal hemiplegia exhibit substantially higher diaphragm blood flows than their less fit but healthy counterparts and that the respiratory muscles 'steal' $\dot{Q}m$ from the exercising limb muscles,[149] thereby compromising running performance.

The heart, in keeping with its great energetic demands, rich vascularity, and mitochondrial content,[150] sustains an extraordinarily high blood flow during exercise. Specifically, in Standardbreds run at $\dot{V}O_{2max}$, left and right ventricular and septal blood flows increase from their pre-exercise value (0.4–0.6 L/kg/min) up to 2.6–2.9 L/kg/min.[53,151] Atrial blood flows are somewhat lower at rest (0.3 L/kg/min) and at $\dot{V}O_{2max}$ (1.3–1.4 L/kg/min). One remarkable feature of the equine heart is that there is little or no gradation of blood flow across the myocardial wall. This is surprising given the high compressive forces to which the subendocardial vessels are subjected as systolic pressures greatly exceed 200 mmHg. There is also evidence that the myocardium retains a substantial vasodilator reserve during maximal exertion, at least in ponies.[152]

Muscle blood flow ($\dot{Q}m$) and O_2 delivery ($\dot{Q}O_2m$) across the rest–exercise transition

The close matching between $\dot{Q}O_2m$ and $\dot{V}O_2$, leading to O_2 extractions ≥90%, presents a strong case for $\dot{Q}O_2m$ being controlled ultimately by muscle metabolism.[16,138,140,153–156] In contrast, $\dot{Q}O_2m$ increases within the first one or two contractions at exercise onset and this time course is generally accepted to be far faster than that of $\dot{V}O_2$;[154] it is thus too rapid to be explained by metabolic feedback.[156] However, recent evidence suggests that, contrary to previous notions,[158] endothelial smooth muscle can relax sufficiently fast in response to increased flow and acetylcholine[159] and that this does indeed occur.[160–162] It is also considered that the muscle pump, which substantially reduces venular pressure, is key to increasing the pressure differential across the muscle vascular bed and augmenting flow almost instantaneously (Fig. 31.32).[157,162,140,163] Another component of increased vascular conductance is conducted vasodilation, initiated within the capillaries adjacent to active muscle fibers, which causes vasodilation upstream within the arteriolar bed.[143,164] Kindig and colleagues[70,71] have demonstrated recently that inhibition of nitric oxide formation using L-NAME actually speeds the rate of $\dot{V}O_2$ increase at exercise onset in Thoroughbreds (Fig. 31.33) as does prior warm-up (or priming) running particularly at higher intensities.[165–167] Thus, despite any L-NAME-induced $\dot{Q}O_2$ reduction,[79,168,169] relief of nitric oxide-mediated mitochondrial inhibition[70,71] allows a more rapid $\dot{V}O_2$ increase. This provides the most compelling evidence to date that muscle O_2 delivery does not limit the energetic ($\dot{V}O_2$ kinetics) response to exercise.

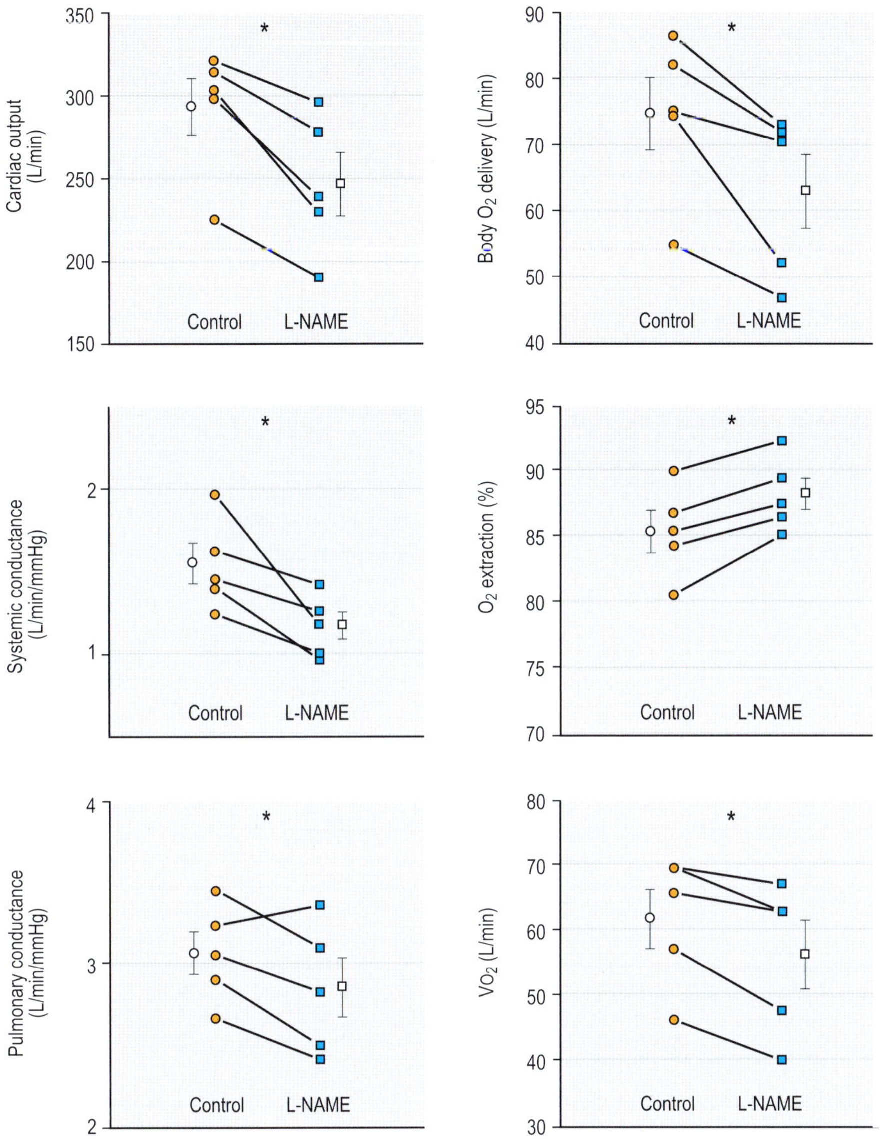

Fig 31.31 Effect of inhibition of nitric oxide production by L-NAME (nitric oxide synthase inhibitor, N^G-L-nitro-arginine methyl ester) on cardiovascular responses, O_2 delivery ($\dot{Q}O_2$), O_2 extraction and O_2 uptake ($\dot{V}O_2$) at maximum exercise. Solid symbols denote individual horses, hollow symbols are mean ± standard error. The L-NAME condition significantly (*$P < 0.05$) reduced all variables in addition to the maximum speed attained.

Reprinted from Kindig CA, Quackenbush D, Gallatin LL, et al. Cardiorespiratory impact of nitric oxide synthase inhibition in the exercising horse. Respir Physiol 2000; 120:151-166, with permission from Elsevier.

Determinants of O_2 exchange within skeletal muscle: the microcirculation

In skeletal muscle, O_2 diffuses down its pressure gradient from the capillary towards the mitochondria at a rate ($\dot{V}O_2$) that is determined by the O_2 pressure (PO_2) difference between capillary and mitochondria and the tissue-diffusing capacity for O_2 (D) according to Fick's law ($\dot{V}O_2 = D[PO_2 \text{ cap} - PO_2 \text{ mito}]$). The enduring dogma that there is a large PO_2 gradient from the myocyte sarcolemma to the most distant mitochondrion is at odds with the more recent observation that intramyocyte PO_2 during exercise is low (1–3 mmHg) and without appreciable transverse or longitudinal variation (Fig. 31.34).[170] This is important because it means that the greatest fall in PO_2 occurs in very close proximity (1–2 μm) to the RBC even in the presence of potentially long diffusion distances (>40 μm) to the mitochondrion. Intramyocyte O_2 transport is thought to be facilitated by myoglobin, particularly within fibers in which oxidative enzyme activity is high. In addition, the mitochondrial system comprises a catenated network that may, in and of itself, enhance O_2 and high-energy phosphate transport.[171,172]

From the above, the inescapable conclusion is that the size (surface area) and geometry (luminal diameter, tortuosity, branching) of the muscle capillary network combined with the flux and distribution of RBCs within that network are of paramount importance for gas exchange. Within skeletal muscle, capillary surface area is regulated as a function of fiber mitochondrial volume,[51] which itself is indicative of maximal O_2 demand (Fig. 31.35). Within the major limb muscles there are 700–800 km of capillary length per kg which supply 40–50 mL of mitochondria.[49,53] The capillaries form a dense, interconnecting network of vessels, which average 4–6 μm in diameter (equine RBCs are 5.5 μm in diameter), that becomes extremely tortuous at short muscle sarcomere lengths.[49] By contrast, at long sarcomere lengths (>2.8 μm), the capillaries become straight and highly aligned with the muscle fibers. As the capillaries stretch, their luminal diameter is reduced and this increases their resistance to RBC passage.[173,174]

Observation of capillary RBC flux and distribution during muscle contractions presents a formidable challenge to scientists. It is only very recently that events within muscle capillaries have been observed across the rest–contractions transition. At rest in rat spinotrapezius

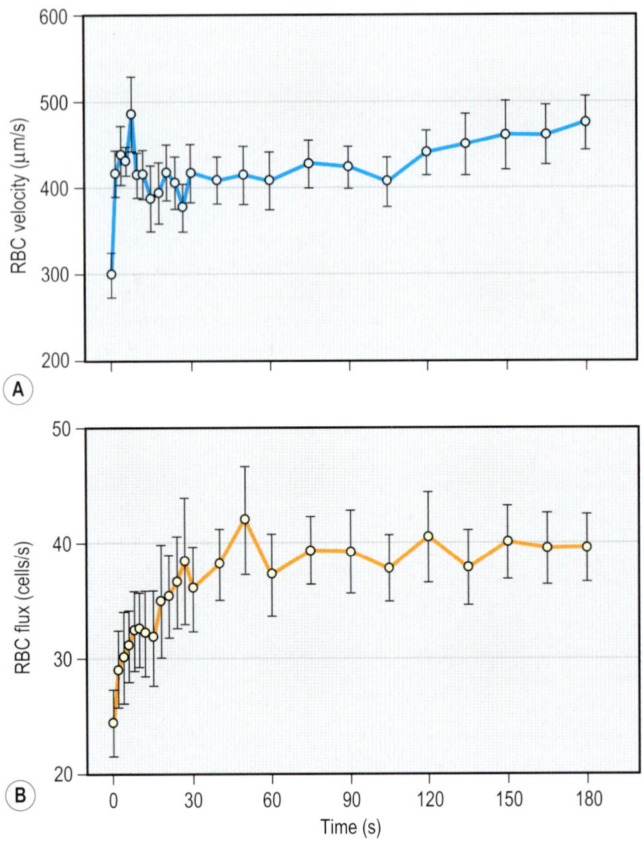

Fig 31.32 Within the capillary bed of skeletal muscle, red blood cell (RBC) velocity **(A)** and flux **(B)** increase within the first few contractions at the start of exercise.

Reprinted from Kindig CA, Richardson TE, Poole DC. Skeletal muscle capillary hemodynamics from rest to contractions: implications for oxygen transfer. J Appl Physiol 2002; 92:2513-2520, with permission from The American Physiological Society.

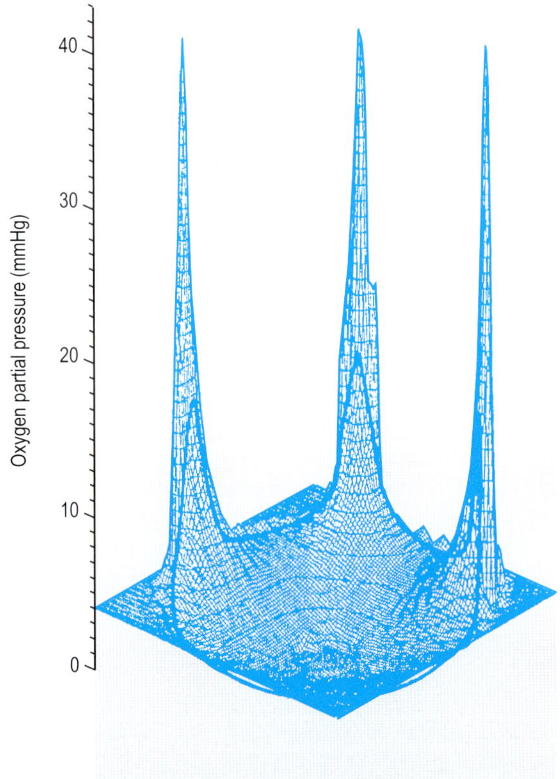

Fig 31.34 Three-dimensional reconstruction of the O_2 partial pressure (PO_2) profile within the muscle capillary and the contracting myocyte. Sarcolemma is indicated by thick line. Notice that the principal drop in PO_2 occurs in close proximity (within 1 µm) to the capillary spikes and that the intramyocyte PO_2 profile is remarkably flat without appreciable PO_2 gradients. This suggests that, at least in red muscle fibers containing myoglobin, even relatively large intracellular O_2 diffusion distances to the mitochondria are of little consequence.

Redrawn from Honig CR, Gayeski TEJ, Groebe K. Myoglobin and oxygen gradients. In: Crystal RG, West JB, Weibel ER, et al, eds. The lung: scientific foundations. New York: Raven; 1997; 1925-1933.

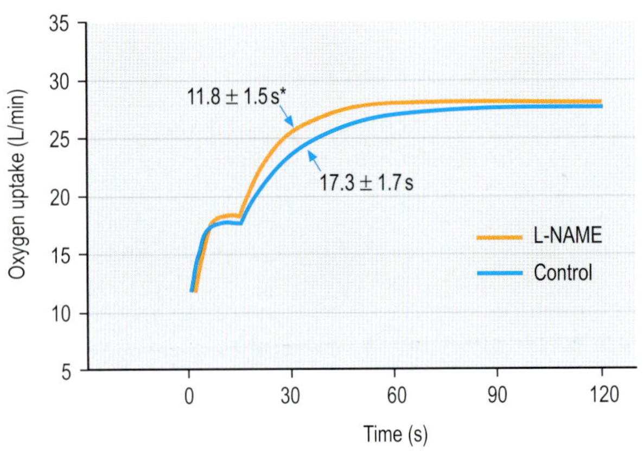

Fig 31.33 Inhibition of nitric oxide production by L-NAME (nitric oxide synthase inhibitor, N^G-L-nitro-arginine methyl ester) significantly speeds the O_2 uptake ($\dot{V}O_2$) response at the onset of moderate speed running (7 m/s).

Reprinted from Kindig CA, McDonough P, Erickson HH, et al. Nitric oxide synthase inhibition speeds oxygen uptake kinetics in horses during moderate domain running. Resp Physiol Neurobiol 2002; 132:169-178, with permission from Elsevier.

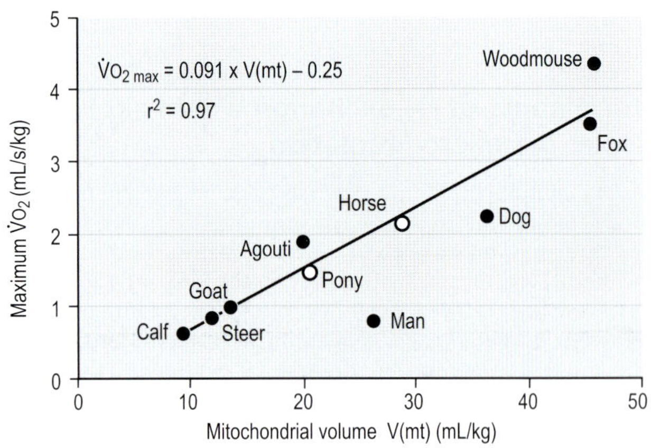

Fig 31.35 There is a close relationship between whole body mitochondrial content and $\dot{V}O_{2max}$ across a wide range of mammalian species. This supports the notion that $\dot{V}O_{2max}$ increases in proportion to the structural capacity for muscle to utilize O_2. V(mt), mitochondrial volume.

Redrawn from Wagner PD, Hoppeler H, Saltin B. Determinants of maximal oxygen uptake. In: Crystal RG, West JB, Barnes PJ, et al, eds. The lung: scientific foundations, 2nd edn. New York: Lippincott-Raven; 1997; 2033-2041.

muscle, approximately 80% of capillaries support RBC flow[174] at a velocity of approximately 250 µm/s and a capillary tube hematocrit that averages only 25–50% of systemic values.[172] The instantaneous muscle O_2-diffusing capacity is thought to be determined by the number of RBCs in the capillary lying adjacent to the muscle fiber.[175] Consequently, the total length of capillaries adjacent to a muscle fiber in combination with their hematocrit (i.e. number of RBCs per unit length of capillary) will set the potential for O_2 flux. As muscle begins rhythmic contractions and blood flow increases, capillary RBC velocity and flux are elevated rapidly (Fig. 31.32) and hematocrit increases towards systemic values.[162] If we extrapolate what is known from microscopic observations in contracting rodent muscle to the exercising horse using equine capillary morphometric[49] and blood flow[53] data, from rest to maximal exercise capillary hematocrit is predicted to increase from approximately 10% up to approximately 60% and mean RBC capillary transit time decreases to about 1–2 s (which is substantially longer than seen in the pulmonary capillaries). This presents a remarkable scenario. Specifically, during maximal exercise, if the systemic polycythemia is expressed at the microcirculatory level (as suggested from rodent studies), the sixfold increase in capillary hematocrit will facilitate rapid blood-to-muscle O_2 exchange. Moreover, as capillary RBC transit time is not thought to become limiting for O_2 offloading until values less than 0.3–0.5 s are reached, the mean transit time of 1–2 s in horse muscle is so long that there likely exists only a small proportion of capillaries where O_2 offloading is limited. These considerations help explain how the horse achieves such excellent O_2 extractions (up to 85–90%) at very high cardiac outputs.

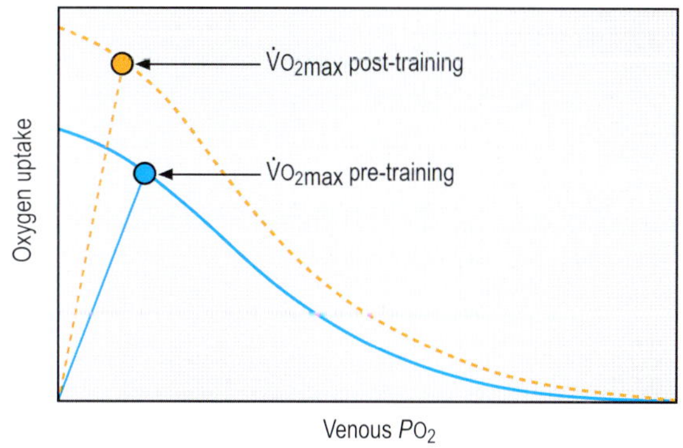

Fig 31.36 The Wagner diagram demonstrates that exercise training increases $\dot{V}O_{2max}$ by elevating both conductive (curved line, due to increased stroke volume) and diffusive (straight line, due principally to increased muscle capillarity and events within the capillaries) O_2 transport. Note that even a modest reduction in venous PO_2 (5–10%)[182] after training requires a substantial increase (~30%) in muscle O_2-diffusing capacity. Moreover, if training solely increased convective O_2 delivery and there was no augmentation of muscle-diffusing capacity, venous PO_2 would rise after training. This has not been observed. For additional information see legend to Figure 31.7 and Table 31.7.

Exercise training

Regular physical exercise or exercise training produces a coordinated pattern of structural and functional adaptations within the cardiovascular and muscular systems. The first three main sections of this chapter dealt with the anatomy and physiology of these systems and their responses to acute exercise (i.e. a single bout). This section details the remarkable plasticity of the cardiovascular and muscular systems in response to training and focuses primarily on those adaptations which elevate $\dot{V}O_{2max}$ and running performance. For our purposes the training mode considered is running either on the track, pasture or the motor-driven treadmill. So far, water training[176] has not proven effective in driving many of the cardiovascular/muscular adaptations considered herein. There exists a substantial literature on this topic in other species such as the human, dog, and rat,[52,138,156,177] and this section will avoid an exhaustive overview. Rather it will focus on understanding the mechanistic bases for the elevated training-induced $\dot{V}O_{2max}$ that occurs in both young and old horses.[66]

Historically, $\dot{Q}$ and $\dot{Q}O_2$ have been considered the principal, if not the sole, determinants of $\dot{V}O_{2max}$ and its increase with training. However, the insightful modeling and novel experiments of Professor Peter D. Wagner at the University of California at San Diego[18] and others[178–181] have established that $\dot{V}O_{2max}$ and training-induced increases thereof are the result of a coordinated sequence of adaptations that increases the capacity for conductive and diffusive movement of O_2 from the atmosphere to its site of utilization within muscle mitochondria. The 'Wagner' diagram combines these conductive and diffusive elements (as seen in Fig. 31.7), and it is instructive to use this diagram to understand how training increases $\dot{V}O_{2max}$ (Fig. 31.36). The relationship seen in Figure 31.36 presents the increased $\dot{V}O_{2max}$ as an elevated cardiovascular O_2 delivery ($\dot{Q}O_2$) concomitant with an elevated fractional O_2 extraction (increased CaO_2 – CvO_2) that reduces muscle effluent and mixed-venous PO_2. Typically, training-induced increases in fractional O_2 extraction and reduction of venous PO_2 are relatively modest, and this observation has led to the erroneous belief that adaptations to training within muscle that increase O_2-diffusing capacity (e.g. increased muscle capillarity and associated capillary hemodynamics) are of no, or at least, lesser importance than those cardiovascular changes that elevate $\dot{Q}O_2$. Nothing could be further from the truth. Notice from Figure 31.36 that simply increasing $\dot{Q}O_2$ at the same diffusing capacity (i.e. slope of line from the origin to $\dot{V}O_{2max}$) will *decrease* O_2 extraction and *elevate* venous PO_2. That this response is not seen after training is the result of adaptations within the capillary bed (Table 31.7) that substantially increase muscle O_2-diffusing capacity.[51,156,183] Table 31.7 lists the primary adaptations to training that produce the response evident in Figure 31.36.

Training usually increases $\dot{V}O_{2max}$ between 10 and 25% and, as in other species,[52,138,156,177] the % improvement in the horse is dependent upon initial fitness, with fitter individuals having less room for adaptation. In addition to an increased muscle O_2-diffusing capacity, the higher post-training $\dot{V}O_{2max}$ is driven by an elevated $\dot{Q}$ (and $\dot{Q}O_2$) consequent to increased SV. At maximal exercise neither heart rate nor MAP changes appreciably with training and hence the elevated $\dot{Q}$ must be countered by a precisely matched fall in total peripheral resistance.[138]

Mechanistic bases for training-induced stroke volume (SV) increase

After training, ventricular mass and volume are increased.[29,184] Training elevates blood/plasma volume and subsequently end-diastolic volume, and this stretches the myocardial fibers and increases both the force and velocity of contraction. This adaptation occurs in the absence of any substantial changes in myocardial contractility per se[138,185,186] and, as MAP is unchanged by training, it cannot be caused by modulation of cardiac afterload. Training expands plasma volume[182,187] and this may elevate ventricular preload by increasing central venous pressure. However, experiments in humans have not demonstrated that expanding plasma volume consistently increases central venous pressure and SV.[138] What is certain is that removal of the pericardium does increase SV

Table 31.7 Principal cardiovascular effects of exercise training in the horse at maximal exercise.

VARIABLE	% INCREASE	REFERENCE(S)
$\dot{V}O_{2max}$	10–25	74,182,192–195
Mean arterial pressure (at max)	NC	
Total peripheral resistance	Decreased	
Conductive O_2 transport (at max)		
Heart weight	10+	23,29
LV mass	33	29,184
LV internal diameter	7	184
Cardiac output, max	10+	
Stroke volume, max	10+	73
Plasma volume	19–30	182,187,196
Central venous pressure	?	
Pericardial hypertrophy	Yes?	
Systemic [hemoglobin]/hematocrit	NC or decreased	182
Arterial O_2 content	NC or decreased	
Red cell mass	15	182
Heart rate (max)	NC	66,192,197
Muscle O_2 diffusing capacity		
Arterial – venous O_2 extraction, max	5	182
Capillarity		
Capillary density	13–36	195,198,199
Capillary-fiber ratio	70	195,200
Myoglobin	?	
Oxidative enzymes	up to 100	193,198,199,201–203,204
Mitochondrial volume	75–200	195,205
Capillary hematocrit	Increased?	
Capillary RBC transit time	?	
Velocity – submaximal heart rates/blood lactate concentrations		
V200	NC or increased	206
V140	Increased	207
V_{La4}	Up to 31	199,208
La_9	–51	208
Run time to fatigue (90–100% $\dot{V}O_{2max}$)		
Time	140	195

NC, no change; ?, unknown.
$\dot{V}O_{2max}$, maximal O_2 uptake; V200, V140, running velocity at a heart rate of 200 and 140 beats/min, respectively; V_{La4}, running velocity that induces a lactic acidosis of 4 mmol/L; La_9, blood lactate concentration at a running velocity of 9 m/s.

and maximal $\dot{Q}$ in the absence of altered preload.[13,14] Indeed, in dogs and pigs removing the pericardial constraint to myocardial expansion produces an increased maximal $\dot{Q}$ similar to that found after weeks or months of training.[13,14] There is evidence that volume overload chronically stretches the pericardial sac[188] and decreases its stiffness[189] such that after training a much smaller rise in cardiac filling pressure is needed to increase SV[138] and a greater SV can be achieved. To date, there is no available evidence that pericardectomies have been performed as an ergogenic aid in racing horses. It is pertinent that training-induced increases in heart size may promote valvular (mitral and tricuspid) insufficiencies and regurgitation which will act to limit the improvement in cardiac output.[107,190] However, neither regurgitation or murmurs in racing Thoroughbreds have been associated with poor performance per se.[191] It appears that any impediment to maximal $\dot{Q}$ generation resulting from such conditions is outweighed by the genetic or training-induced large SV that may have contributed to these defects in the first place.

Mechanistic bases for increased muscle vascular conductance and O_2-diffusing capacity (and increased $Ca_{O_2} - Cv_{O_2}$) after training

Arterial O_2 content (Ca_{O_2}) is not elevated by training (although small increases in arterial P_{O_2} during submaximal exercise may be found);[207] hence any increased $Ca_{O_2} - Cv_{O_2}$ must result from a decreased Cv_{O_2}. This decreased Cv_{O_2} does not arise from a greater vasoconstriction in other organs or inactive muscle vascular beds, but rather from a preferential redistribution of the training-induced $\dot{Q}$ increase towards the active muscles[138,139,209] and a greater total and fractional extraction of O_2 within those muscles.

Exercise training induces a rapid and profound growth of arterioles and capillaries within skeletal muscle[52,210–213] and increases the sensitivity of cardiac[214] and skeletal muscle[215,216] arterioles to vasoactive mediators such as prostaglandins, catecholamines, and nitric oxide. Moreover, training increases the availability of nitric oxide in the myocardium by upregulating endothelial nitric oxide synthase, which is the enzyme responsible for much of the nitric oxide production within the arterial tree.[217] It is quite probable that this latter adaptation occurs also in skeletal muscle. Exercise training increases $\dot{Q}$ capacity in muscles composed of both slow- and fast-twitch fibers provided they are recruited during exercise.[218] The distribution of $\dot{Q}$ within and among muscles is altered after training, which may be important for improving the matching of O_2 delivery ($\dot{Q}_{O_2}$) to O_2 utilization ($\dot{V}_{O_2}$).[139,172] After training, capillary length and surface area per fiber volume, as well as capillary surface-to-fiber surface contact, is increased in proportion to the elevated muscle oxidative enzyme capacity.[51,52,156,211,219] Such capillary proliferation increases the capillary surface area available for O_2 exchange and, by increasing capillary volume, may prevent or at least constrain any reduction in capillary RBC transit time that would otherwise result from the elevated muscle $\dot{Q}$. It is pertinent that the effect of training on capillary RBC transit time will depend on the precise proportionality between increased $\dot{Q}$ and elevated capillary volume. Moreover, the effect of training on capillary hematocrit (a key determinant of blood–muscle O_2 movement) is not at present known. What is certain is that muscle O_2-diffusing capacity increases dramatically with training to facilitate a substantially increased total blood–muscle O_2 flux (Fig. 31.36).

Conclusions

Both the cardiovascular and muscular systems evidence great plasticity. During maximal exercise after training, improved cardiac function elevates total $\dot{Q}$ and muscle $\dot{Q}$ (and $\dot{Q}_{O_2}$) Synchronized muscle vascular and intramyocyte oxidative enzyme proliferation permits trained muscle to accept this increased $\dot{Q}$, elevate O_2 exchange, and facilitate a greater O_2 utilization at maximal exercise (increased $\dot{V}_{O_{2max}}$). At submaximal running speeds, exercise training speeds $\dot{V}_{O_2}$ kinetics,[26,156] thereby tightening metabolic control which reduces glycolysis and glycogen utilization,[52,150,177] and elevates stroke volume, thereby lowering heart rate. This in turn may actually reduce the $\dot{V}_{O_2}$ cost of running at submaximal speeds.[156] The training response may be augmented by hypoxia and is modulated by running speed, frequency, and duration. In contrast to humans, training-induced adaptations may be maintained, at least in young Thoroughbred horses, for at least 10 weeks provided that they are permitted spontaneous (pasture) activity.[220]

References

1. Pratt GW. Clocking the fastest horses on earth. Quarter Racing J 1991;4:36–40.
2. Jones JH, Lindstedt SL. Limits to maximal performance. Ann Rev Physiol 1993;55:547–69.
3. Weibel ER. The pathway for oxygen: structure and function in the mammalian respiratory system. London: Harvard University Press; 1984. p. 399–404.
4. Lindstedt SL, Hokanson JF, Wells DJ, et al. Running energetics in the pronghorn antelope. Nature 1991;353: 748–50.
5. Young LE, Marlin DJ, Deaton C, et al. Heart size estimated by echocardiography correlates with maximal oxygen uptake. Equine Vet J Suppl 2002;34:467–71.
6a. Lyons AS, Petrucelli RJ. Medicine: an illustrated history. New York: Harry N Abrams; 1987. p. 603.
6b. Jochle, W. Chaldean Pedigree Chart, indicating selective breeding of horses circa 4000 BC: Something is wrong. J Eq Vet Sci 2005;25(1):6–7.
7. Derman KD, Noakes TD. Comparative aspects of exercise physiology. In: Hodgson DR, Rose RJ, editors. The athletic horse. Philadelphia: WB Saunders; 1994. p. 15.
8. Gunn HM. Muscle, bone and fat proportions and muscle distribution of Thoroughbreds and other horses. In: Gillespie JR, Robinson NE, editors. Equine exercise physiology 2. Davis, CA: ICEEP; 1987. p. 253–64.
9. Kearns CF, McKeever KH, John-Adler H, et al. Relationship between body composition, blood volume and maximal oxygen uptake. Equine Vet J Suppl 2002;34:485–90.
10. Wagner PD, Erickson BK, Seaman J, et al. Effects of altered F_{IO_2} on maximum $\dot{V}_{O_2}$ in the horse. Respir Physiol 1996;105:123–34.
11. Knight DR, Schaffartzik W, Poole DC, et al. Effects of hyperoxia on maximal leg O_2 supply and utilization in men. J Appl Physiol 1993;75:2586–94.
12. McDonough P, Kindig CA, Hildreth T, et al. Effect of body incline on cardiac performance. Equine Vet J Suppl 2002;34:506–9.
13. Stray-Gundersen J, Musch TI, Haidet GC, et al. The effect of pericardiectomy on maximal oxygen consumption and maximal cardiac output in untrained dogs. Circ Res 1986;58:523–30.
14. Hammond HK, White FC, Bhargava V, et al. Heart size and maximal cardiac output are limited by the pericardium. Am J Physiol 1992;263:H1675–1681.
15. Andersen P, Saltin B. Maximal perfusion of skeletal muscle in man. J Physiol 1985;366:233–49.
16. Richardson RS, Poole DC, Knight DR, et al. High muscle blood flow in man: is maximal O_2 extraction compromised? J Appl Physiol 1993;75:1911–16.
17. Gledhill N. Blood doping and related issues: a brief review. Med Sci Sports Exerc 1982;14:183–9.
18. Wagner PD, Hoppeler H, Saltin B. Determinants of maximal oxygen uptake. In: Crystal RG, West JB, Barnes PJ, et al, editors. The lung: scientific foundations. 2nd ed. New York: Lippincott-Raven; 1997. p. 2033–41.
19. Hoppeler H, Weibel ER. Limits for oxygen and substrate transport in mammals. J Exp Biol 1998;201: 1051–64.
20. Vincen TL, Newton JR, Deaton CM, et al. Retrospective study of predictive variables for maximal heart rate (HRmax) in horses undergoing strenuous treadmill exercise. Equine Vet J Suppl 2006;36:146–52.
21. Wasserman K, Hansen JE, Sue DY, et al. Principles of exercise testing and interpretation. 2nd ed. Philadelphia: Lea & Febiger; 1994.
22. Saltin B, Blomqvist G, Mitchell JH, et al. Response to exercise after bed rest and after training. Circulation 1968; 38(suppl VII):1–78.

23. Webb AI, Weaver BMQ. Body composition of the horse. Equine Vet J 1979;11:39–47.
24. Staaden RV. The exercise physiology of the racing greyhound. Doctoral thesis, School of Veterinary Studies, Murdoch University, Perth, Western Australia, 1984. p. 1–273.
25. Staaden RV. Exercise and training. In: Bloomberg MS, Dee JF, Taylor RA, editors. Canine sports medicine and surgery. London: Saunders, 1998. p. 357–63.
26. Poole DC, Erickson HH. Highly athletic terrestrial mammals: horses and dogs. Comp Physiol 2011;1:1–37.
27. Rose RJ, Hendrikson DK, Knight PK. Clinical exercise testing in the normal Thoroughbred racehorse. Aust Vet J 1990;67:345–8.
28. Snow DH, Valberg SJ. Muscle anatomy, physiology, and adaptations to exercise. In: Hodgson DR, Rose RJ, editors. The athletic horse. Philadelphia: WB Saunders; 1994. p. 145–79.
29. Kubo K, Senta T, Sugimoto O. Relationship between training and heart in the Thoroughbred racehorse. Exp Rep Equine Health Lab 1974;11:87–93.
30. Evans DL, Rose RJ. Cardiovascular and respiratory responses to exercise in Thoroughbred horses. J Exp Biol 1988; 134:397–408.
31. Haun M. The X factor. What it is and how to find it. Neenah, WI: Russell Meerdink; 1997.
32. Kline H, Foreman JH. Heart and spleen weights as a function of breed and somatotype. Equine Exerc Physiol 1991;3:17–21.
33. Gross DR, Muir WM, Pipers FS, et al. Reevaluation of the equine heart score. South West Vet 1974;27: 231–3.
34. Leadon DP, Cunningham EP, Mahon GA, et al. Heart score and performance ability in the United Kingdom. Equine Vet J 1982;14:89–90.
35. Leadon DP, McAllister H, Mullins E, et al. Electrocardiographic and echocardiographic measurements and their relationships in Thoroughbred yearlings to subsequent performance. In: Persson SGB, Lindholm A, Jeffcot LB, editors. Equine exercise physiology 3. CA: ICEEP; 1991. p. 22–9.
36. Hanson CM, Kline KH, Foreman JH. Measurements of heart scores and heart weights in horses of two different morphic types. Comp Biochem Physiol 1993;108A:175–8.
37. Sampson SN, Tucker RL, Bayly WM. Relationship between $\dot{V}O_{2max}$, heart score and echocardiographic measurements obtained at rest and immediately following maximal exercise in Thoroughbred horses. Equine Vet J Suppl 1999;30:190–4.
38. Steel JD, Beilharz RG, Stewart GA, et al. The inheritance of heart score in racehorses. Aust Vet J 1977;53:306–9.
39. Young LE. Equine athletes, the equine athlete's heart and racing success. Exp Physiol 2003;88:659–63.
40. Young LE, Rogers K, Wood JL. Left ventricular size and systolic function in Thoroughbred racehorses and their relationships to race performance. J Appl Physiol 2005, in press.
41. Persson SGB, Ekman L, Lydin G, et al. Circulatory effects of splenectomy in the horse. II. Effect on plasma volume and total and circulating red-cell volume. Zentralbl Veterinarmed A 1973;20: 456–68.
42. Moore J. Nature's supercharger. Equus 1994;198:30–4.
43. Wagner PD, Erickson BK, Kubo K, et al. Maximum oxygen transport and utilisation before and after splenectomy. Equine Vet J Suppl 1995;18:82–5.
44. Persson SGB, Bergsten G. Circulatory effects of splenectomy in the horse. IV. Effect on blood flow and blood lactate at rest and during exercise. Zentralbl Veterinarmed A 1975;22:801–7.
45. McKeever KH, Agans JM, Geiser S, et al. Low dose exogenous erythropoietin elicits an ergogenic effect in standardbred horses. Equine Vet J Suppl 2006;36:233–8.
46. Persson SGB. On blood volume and working capacity. Acta Vet Scand Suppl 1967;19:1–189.
47. Altman PL, Dittmer DS. Biology data book, vol. 2, 2nd ed. Bethesda, MD: FASEB; 1974. p. 1847.
48. Erickson HH, Poole DC. Exercise physiology. In: Reece WO, editor. Dukes physiology of domestic animals. 12th ed. Ithaca: Cornell University Press; 2004. p. 360.
49. Mathieu-Costello O, Hoppeler H, Weibel ER. Capillary tortuosity in skeletal muscles of mammals depends on muscle contraction. J Appl Physiol 1989;66:1436–42.
50. Ishikawa H, Sawada H, Yamada E. Surface and internal morphology of skeletal muscle. In: Peachy LD, Adrian RH, Geiger SR, editors. Handbook of physiology. Section 10: skeletal muscle. Bethesda, MD: American Physiological Society; 1983. p. 1–22.
51. Poole DC, Mathieu-Costello O. Relationship between fiber capillarization and mitochondrial volume density in control and trained rat soleus and plantaris muscles. Microcirculation 1996;3:175–86.
52. Saltin B, Gollnick PD. Skeletal muscle adaptability: significance for metabolism and performance. In: Peachy LD, Adrian RH, Geiger SR, editors. Handbook of physiology. Section 10: skeletal muscle. Bethesda, MD: American Physiological Society; 1983. p. 555–631.
53. Armstrong RB, Essén-Gustavsson B, Hoppeler H, et al. O_2 delivery at $\dot{V}O_{2max}$ and oxidative capacity in muscles of standardbred horses. J Appl Physiol 1992;73:2274–82.
54. Robinson NE. Respiratory function. In: Cunningham JG, editor. Textbook of veterinary physiology. 3rd ed. London: WB Saunders; 2002. p. 481.
55. West JB. Respiratory physiology. 4th ed. Baltimore: Williams & Wilkins; 1995. p. 36–7.
56. Birks EK, Mathieu-Costello O, Fu Z, et al. Comparative aspects of the strength of pulmonary capillaries in rabbit, dog, and horse. Respir Physiol 1994;97:235–46.
57. Constantinopol M, Jones JH, Weibel ER, et al. Oxygen transport during exercise in large mammals. II. Oxygen uptake by the pulmonary gas exchanger. J Appl Physiol 1989;67:871–8.
58. Hlastala MP, Bernard SL, Erickson HH, et al. Pulmonary blood flow distribution in standing horses is not dominated by gravity. J Appl Physiol 1996;81:1051–61.
59. Pelletier N, Robinson NE, Kaiser L, et al. Regional differences in endothelial function in horse lungs: possible role in blood flow distribution? J Appl Physiol 1998;85:537–42.
60. Evans DL. The cardiovascular system: anatomy, physiology, and adaptations to exercise and training. In: Hodgson DR, Rose RJ, editors. The athletic horse. Philadelphia: WB Saunders; 1994. p. 129–44.
61. Bayly WM, Gabel AA, Barr SA. Cardiovascular effects of submaximal aerobic training on a treadmill in Standardbred horses using a standardized exercise test. Am J Vet Res 1983;44:544–53.
62. Parks CM, Manohar M. Distribution of blood flow during moderate and strenuous exercise in ponies (*Equus caballus*). Am J Vet Res 1983;44: 1861–6.
63. Thomas DP, Fregin GF, Gerber NH, et al. Effects of training on cardiorespiratory function in the horse. Am J Physiol 1983;245:R160–5.
64. Evans DL, Rose RJ. Dynamics of cardiorespiratory function in standardbred horses during constant load exercise. J Comp Physiol [B] 1988;157:791–9.
65. Hamlin RL, Klepinger WL, Gilpin KW, et al. Autonomic control of heart rate in the horse. Am J Physiol 1972;222:976–8.
66. Betros CL, McKeever KH, Kearns CF, et al. Effects of aging and training on maximal heart rate and $\dot{V}O_{2max}$. Equine Vet J Suppl 2002;34:100–5.

67. Astrand P-O, Rodahl K. Textbook of work physiology. 3rd ed. New York: McGraw-Hill; 1986.
68. Brooks GA, Fahey TD, White TP. Exercise physiology: human bioenergetics and its applications. 2nd ed. London: Mayfield; 1996.
69. Rose RJ, Evans DL. Cardiovascular and respiratory function in the athletic horse. In: Gillespie JR, Robinson NE, editors. Equine exercise physiology 2. Davis, CA: ICEEP; 1987. p. 1–24.
70. Kindig CA, McDonough P, Erickson HH, et al. Effect of l-NAME on oxygen uptake kinetics during heavy intensity exercise in the horse. J Appl Physiol 2001;91:891–6.
71. Kindig CA, McDonough P, Erickson HH, et al. Nitric oxide synthase inhibition speeds oxygen uptake kinetics in horses during moderate domain running. Resp Physiol Neurobiol 2002;132:169–78.
72. Lindholm A, Saltin B. The physiological and biochemical response of standardbred horses to exercise of varying speed and duration. Acta Vet Scand 1974;15:310–24.
73. Thomas DP, Fregin GF. Cardiorespiratory and metabolic responses to treadmill exercise in the horse. J Appl Physiol 1981;50:864–8.
74. Evans DL, Rose RJ. Maximal oxygen consumption in racehorses: changes with training state and prediction from submaximal indices of cardiorespiratory function. In: Gillespie JR, Robinson NE, editors. Equine exercise physiology 2. Davis, CA: ICEEP; 1987. p. 52–67.
75. Thomas DP, Fregin GF. Cardiorespiratory drift during exercise in the horse. Equine Vet J Suppl 1990;9:61–5.
76. Langsetmo I, Weigle GE, Fedde MR, et al. $\dot{V}O_2$ kinetics in the horse at moderate and heavy exercise. J Appl Physiol 1997;83:1235–41.
77. Stephenson RB. Cardiovascular physiology. In: Cunningham JG, editor. Textbook of veterinary physiology. 3rd ed. New York: WB Saunders; 2002. p. 109–219.
78. Fedde MR, Erickson HH. Increase in blood viscosity in the sprinting horse: can it account for the high pulmonary arterial pressure? Equine Vet J 1998;30:329–34.
79. Kindig CA, Quackenbush D, Gallatin LL, et al. Cardiorespiratory impact of nitric oxide synthase inhibition in the exercising horse. Respir Physiol 2000;120:151–66.
80. Davis JL, Manohar M. Effect of splenectomy on exercise-induced pulmonary and systemic hypertension in ponies. Am J Vet Res 1988;49: 1169–72.
81. Erickson BK, Erickson HH, Coffman JR. Pulmonary artery, aortic and oesophageal pressure changes during high-intensity treadmill exercise in the horse: a possible relation to exercise induced pulmonary haemorrhage. Equine Vet J Suppl 1990;9:47–52.
82. Jones JH, Smith BL, Tyler WS, et al. Why do horses bleed? Source and cause of exercise-induced pulmonary hemorrhage in horses. In: Clarke AF, editor. Proceedings of the International Exercise Induced Pulmonary Hemorrhage Conference. Guelph: Equine Research Center; 1993. p. 23–4.
83. Kindig CA, Erickson HH, Poole DC. Dissociation of exercise-induced pulmonary hemorrhage and pulmonary artery pressure via nitric oxide synthase inhibition. J Equine Vet Sci 2000;20: 715–21.
84. Kindig CA, McDonough P, Finley MR, et al. Nitric oxide inhalation reduces pulmonary hypertension but not hemorrhage in maximally exercising horses. J Appl Physiol 2001;91:2674–80.
85. Kindig CA, McDonough P, Fenton G, et al. Efficacy of nasal strip and furosemide in mitigating exercise-induced pulmonary hemorrhage in Thoroughbred horses. J Appl Physiol 2001;91:1396–400.
86. Hopper MK, Pieschl RL, Pelletier NG, et al. Cardiopulmonary effects of acute blood volume alteration prior to exercise. In: Persson SGB, Lindholm A, Jeffcot LB, editors. Equine exercise physiology 3. Davis, CA: ICEEP; 1991. 3. p. 9–16.
87. Olsen SC, Coyne CP, Lowe BS, et al. Influence of furosemide on hemodynamic responses during exercise in horses. Am J Vet Res 1992;53:742–7.
88. Hinchcliff KW, McKeever KH. Frusemide. Equine Vet J Suppl 1995;18:256–8.
89. Langsetmo I, Weigle GE, Erickson HH, et al. Influence of frusemide on dynamic cardiac variables during exercise. Equine Vet J Suppl 1999;30: 170–3.
90. Bernard SL, Glenny RW, Erickson HH, et al. Minimal redistribution of pulmonary blood flow with exercise in racehorses. J Appl Physiol 1996;81: 1062–70.
91. Wagner PD, Gillespie JR, Landgren GL, et al. Mechanism of exercise-induced hypoxemia in horses. J Appl Physiol 1989;66:1227–33.
92. Karas RH, Taylor CR, Jones JH, et al. Adaptive variation in the mammalian respiratory system in relation to energetic demand. VII. Flow of oxygen across the pulmonary gas exchanger. Respir Physiol 1987,69:101–15.
93. McDonough P, Kindig CA, Erickson HH, et al. Mechanistic basis for the gas exchange threshold in the Thoroughbred horse. J Appl Physiol 2002;92:1499–505.
94. Padilla DJ, McDonough P, Kindig CA, et al. Ventilatory dynamics and control of blood gases after maximal exercise in the Thoroughbred horse. J Appl Physiol 2004;96:2187–93.
95. Seaman J, Erickson BK, Kubo K, et al. Exercise induced ventilation/perfusion inequality in the horse. Equine Vet J 1995;27:104–9.
96. Burrell MH. Endoscopic and virologic observations on respiratory disease in a group of young Thoroughbred horses in training. Equine Vet J 1985;17:99–103.
97. Hillidge CJ, Lane TJ, Johnson EL. Preliminary investigations of EIPH in racing Quarter Horses. J Equine Vet Sci 1984;4:21–3.
98. Lapointe JM, Vrins A, McCarvill E. A survey of exercise-induced pulmonary haemorrhage in Quebec Standardbred racehorses. Equine Vet J 1994;26: 482–5.
99. Mason DK, Collins EA, Watkins KL. Respiratory system. In: Snow DH, Persson SGB, Rose RJ, editors. Equine exercise physiology. Cambridge: Granta; 1983. p. 57–63.
100. Raphel CF, Soma LR. Exercise-induced pulmonary hemorrhage in Thoroughbreds after racing and breezing. Am J Vet Res 1982;43:1123–7.
101. Erickson HH, Poole DC. Exercise-induced pulmonary hemorrhage. In: Lekeux P, editor. Equine respiratory diseases. Ithaca: International Veterinary Information Services; 2002. p. B0320.0102.
102. Epp TS, McDonough P, Padilla DJ, et al. Exercise-induced pulmonary haemorrhage during submaximal exercise. Equine Vet J Suppl 2006;36: 502–7.
103. Fu Z, Costello ML, Tsukimoto K, et al. High lung volume increases stress failure in pulmonary capillaries. J Appl Physiol 1992;73:123–33.
104. Erickson HH, McAvoy JL, Westfall JA. Exercise-induced changes in the lung of Shetland ponies: ultrastructure and morphometry. J Submicrosc Cytol Pathol 1997;29:65–72.
105. Williams KJ, Derksen FJ, de Feijter-Rupp H, et al. Regional pulmonary veno-occlusion: a newly identified lesion of equine exercise-induced pulmonary hemorrhage. Vet Pathol 2008;45:316–26.
106. Derksen FJ, Williams KJ, Pannirselvam RR, et al. Regional distribution of collagen and haemosiderin in the lungs of horses with exercise-induced pulmonary haemorrhage. Equine Vet J 2009;41:586–91.
107. McKane SA, Slocombe RF. Experimental mild pulmonary inflammation promotes the development of exercise-induced pulmonary haemorrhage. Equine Vet J 2010;42(Suppl 38):235–9.

108. Williams KJ, Derksen FJ, Defeijter-Rupp HL, et al. Repeated blood instillation into the airway of the horse does not cause pulmonary fibrosis. Equine Vet J 2011;43:354–8.
109. West JB, Mathieu-Costello O, Jones JH, et al. Stress failure of pulmonary capillaries in racehorses with exercise-induced pulmonary hemorrhage. J Appl Physiol 1993;75:1097–109.
110. West JB, Mathieu-Costello O. Structure, strength, failure, and remodeling of the pulmonary blood-gas barrier. Annu Rev Physiol 1999;61:543–72.
111. Poole DC, Kindig CA, Fenton G, et al. Effects of external nasal support on pulmonary gas exchange and EIPH in the horse. J Equine Vet Sci 2000;20: 579–85.
112. Cook WR, Williams RM, Kirker-Head CA, et al. Upper airway obstruction (partial asphyxia) as the possible cause of exercise-induced pulmonary hemorrhage in the horse: an hypothesis. Equine Vet Sci 1988;8:11–26.
113. Fedde MR, Wood SC. Rheological characteristics of horse blood: significance during exercise. Respir Physiol 1993,94.323–35.
114. Hackett RP, Ducharme NG, Gleed RD, et al. Do Thoroughbred and Standardbred horses have similar increases in pulmonary vascular pressures during exertion? Can J Vet Res 2003;67:291–6.
115. Young LE, Helwegen MM, Rogers K, et al. Associations between exercise-induced pulmonary haemorrhage, right ventricular dimensions and atrioventricular valve regurgitation in conditioned national hunt racehorses. Equine Vet J Suppl 2006;36:193–7.
116a. Williams KJ, Robinson NE, Defeijter-Rupp H, et al. Distribution of venous remodeling in exercise-induced pulmonary hemorrhage of horses follows reported blood flow distribution in the equine lung. J Appl Physiol 2013;114:869–78.
116b. Schroter RC, Marlin DJ, Denny E. Exercise-induced pulmonary haemorrhage (EIPH) in horses results from locomotory impact induced trauma – a novel, unifying concept. Equine Vet J 1998;30:186–92.
117. Manohar M, Hutchens E, Coney E. Pulmonary hemodynamics in the exercising horse and their relationship to exercise-induced pulmonary hemorrhage. Br Vet J 1993;149:419–28.
118. Erickson HH. A review of exercise-induced pulmonary hemorrhage and new concepts for prevention. Proc Am Assoc Equine Practs 2000;46:193–6.
119. Young LE, Wood JLN. Effect of age and training on murmurs of atrioventricular valvular regurgitation in young Thoroughbreds. Equine Vet J 2000;32: 195–9.
120. Langsetmo I, Fedde MR, Meyer TS, et al. Relationship of pulmonary arterial pressure to pulmonary haemorrhage in exercising horses. Equine Vet J 2000;32: 379–84.
121. Erickson HH, Hildreth TS, Poole DC, et al. Management of exercise-induced pulmonary hemorrhage in non-racing performance horses. Comp Cont Educ Pract Vet 2001;23:1090–3.
122. Geor RJ, Ommundson L, Fenton G, et al. Effects of an external nasal strip and furosemide on pulmonary hemorrhage in Thoroughbreds following high-intensity exercise. Equine Vet J 2001;33:577–84.
123. Hinchcliff KW, Morley PS, Guthrie AJ. Efficacy of furosemide for prevention of exercise-induced pulmonary hemorrhage in Thoroughbred racehorses. J Am Vet Med Assoc 2009;1(235):76–82.
124. Zawadzkas XA, Sides RH, Bayly WM. Is improved high speed performance following frusemide administration due to diuresis-induced weight loss or reduced severity of exercise-induced pulmonary haemorrhage? Equine Vet J Suppl 2006;36:291–3.
125. Holcombe SJ, Cornelisse CJ, Derksen FJ, et al. The effect of FLAIR nasal strips on upper airway mechanics in exercising horses. Am J Vet Res 2002;63:1101–5.
126. Epp TS, McDonough P, Padilla DJ, et al. The effect of herbal supplementation on the severity of exercise-induced pulmonary hemorrhage. Equine Comp Exerc Physiol 2005;2:17–25.
127. Buchholz BM, Murdock A, Bayly WM, et al. Effects of intravenous aminocaproic acid on exercise-induced pulmonary haemorrhage (EIPH). Equine Vet J 2010;42(Suppl 38):256–60.
128. Colahan PT, Jackson CA, Rice B, et al. The effect of sildenafil citrate administration on selected physiological parameters of exercising Thoroughbred horses. Equine Vet J 2010;42(Suppl 38):606–12.
129. Padilla DJ, Epp TS, McDonough P, et al. Effects of a specific endothelin-1A antagonist on exercise-induced pulmonary haemorrhage (EIPH) in Thoroughbred horses. Equine Vet J Suppl 2006;36:198–203.
130. Epp TS, McDonough P, Behnke BJ, et al. The effects of concentrated equine serum on exercise-induced pulmonary hemorrhage in Thoroughbred horses. Equine Comp Exerc Physiol 2006;2: 17–25.
131. Saulez MN, Godfroid J, Bosman A, et al. Cytokine mRNA expressions after racing at a high altitude and at sea level in horses with exercise-induced pulmonary hemorrhage. Am J Vet Res 2010;71: 447–53.
132. Kindig CA, Ramsel C, McDonough P, et al. Inclined running increases pulmonary haemorrhage in the Thoroughbred horse. Equine Vet J 2003;35:581–5.
133. Hinchcliff KW, Morley PS, Jackson MA, et al. Risk factors for exercise-induced pulmonary haemorrhage in Thoroughbred racehorses. Equine Vet J 2010;42(Suppl 38):228–34.
134. Shoemaker JK, Hughson RL. Adaptation of blood flow during the rest to work transition in humans. Med Sci Sports Exerc 1999;31:1019–26.
135. Rowell LB, Saltin B, Kiens B, et al. Is peak quadriceps blood flow in humans even higher during exercise with hypoxemia? Am J Physiol 1986;251: H1038–44.
136. Mitchell JH, Kaufman MP, Iwamoto GA. The pressor reflex: its cardiovascular effects, afferent mechanisms, and central pathways. Annu Rev Physiol 1983;45: 229–42.
137. Rowell LB, O'Leary DS. Reflex control of the circulation during exercise: chemoreflexes and mechanoreflexes. J Appl Physiol 1990;69:407–18.
138. Rowell LB. Human cardiovascular control. Oxford: Oxford University Press; 1993. p. 255–88.
139. Laughlin MH, McAllister RM, Delp MD. Heterogeneity of blood flow in skeletal muscle. In: Crystal RG, West JB, Weibel ER, et al, editors. The lung: scientific foundations. New York: Raven; 1997. p. 1945–55.
140. Duling BR, Dora K. Control of striated muscle blood flow. In: Crystal RG, West JB, Weibel ER, et al, editors. The lung: scientific foundations. New York: Raven; 1997. p. 1935–43.
141. Bergsten G. Blood pressure, cardiac output and blood gas tension in the horse at rest and during exercise. Acta Vet Scand Suppl 1974;48:1–88.
142. Hornicke H, von Engelhardt W, Ehrlein HJ. Effect of exercise on systemic blood pressure and heart rate in horses. Pflugers Arch 1977;372:95–9.
143. Segal SS. Integration of blood flow control to skeletal muscle: key role of feed arteries. Acta Physiol Scand 2000;168:511–18.
144. Hughson RL, Tschakovsky ME, Houston ME. Regulation of oxygen consumption at the onset of exercise. Exer Sport Sci Rev 2001;29:129–33.
145. Manohar M. Vasodilator reserve in respiratory muscles during maximal exertion in ponies. J Appl Physiol 1986;60:1571–7.
146. Manohar M. Costal vs. crural diaphragmatic blood flow during submaximal and near-maximal exercise in ponies. J Appl Physiol 1988;65: 1514–19.
147. Manohar M. Inspiratory and expiratory muscle perfusion in maximally exercised ponies. J Appl Physiol 1990;68:544–8.

148. Manohar M. Blood flow in respiratory muscles during maximal exertion in ponies with laryngeal hemiplegia. J Appl Physiol 1987;62:229–37.
149. Harms CA, Wetter TJ, McClaran SR, et al. Effects of respiratory muscle work on cardiac output and its distribution during maximal exercise. J Appl Physiol 1998;85:609–18.
150. Poole DC, Mathieu-Costello O. Analysis of capillary geometry in rat sub-epicardium and sub-endocardium. Am J Physiol 1990;259:H204–10.
151. Manohar M, Goetz TE, Hutchens E, et al. Atrial and ventricular myocardial blood flows in horses at rest and during exercise. Am J Vet Res 1994;55:1464–9.
152. Manohar M. Transmural coronary vasodilator reserve and flow distribution during maximal exercise in normal and splenectomized ponies. J Physiol 1987;387:425–40.
153. Knight DR, Poole DC, Schaffartzik W, et al. Relationship between body and leg $\dot{V}O_2$ during maximal cycle ergometry. J Appl Physiol 1992;73:1114–21.
154. Poole DC, Gaesser GA, Hogan MC, et al. Pulmonary and leg $\dot{V}O_2$ during submaximal exercise: implications for muscular efficiency. J Appl Physiol 1992;72:805–10.
155. Laughlin MH, Korthuis RJ, Duncker DJ, et al. Control of blood flow to cardiac and skeletal muscle during exercise. In: Rowell LB, Shepherd JT, editors. Handbook of physiology. New York: Oxford University Press; 1996. p. 705–69.
156. Poole DC. Influence of exercise training on skeletal muscle oxygen delivery and utilization. In: Crystal RG, West JB, Weibel ER, et al, editors. The lung: scientific foundations. New York: Raven; 1997. p. 1957–67.
157. Delp MD. Control of skeletal muscle perfusion at the onset of dynamic exercise. Med Sci Sports Exerc 1999;31:1011–18.
158. Wunsch SA, Muller-Delp J, Delp MD. Time course of vasodilatory responses in skeletal muscle arterioles: role in hyperemia at onset of exercise. Am J Physiol 2000;279:H1715–23.
159. Behnke BJ, Delp MD. Aging blunts the dynamics of vasodilation in isolated skeletal muscle resistance vessels. J Appl Physiol 2010;108:14–20.
160. Tschakovsky ME, Sheriff DD. Immediate exercise hyperemia: contributions of the muscle pump vs. rapid vasodilation. J Appl Physiol 2004;97:739–47.
161. Clifford PS, Tschakovsky ME. Rapid vascular responses to muscle contraction. Exerc Sport Sci Rev 2008;36:25–9.
162. Kindig CA, Richardson TE, Poole DC. Skeletal muscle capillary hemodynamics from rest to contractions: implications for oxygen transfer. J Appl Physiol 2002;92:2513–20.
163. Sheriff DD, Hakeman AL. Role of speed vs. grade in relation to muscle pump function at locomotion onset. J Appl Physiol 2001;91:269–76.
164. Berg BR, Cohen KD, Sarelius IH. Direct coupling between blood flow and metabolism at the capillary level in striated muscle. Am J Physiol 1997;272:H2693–700.
165. Geor RJ, McCutcheon LJ, Hinchcliff KW. Effects of warm-up intensity on kinetics of oxygen consumption and carbon dioxide production during high-intensity exercise in horses. Am J Vet Res 2000;61:638–45.
166. Mukai K, Hiraga A, Eto D, et al. Effects of warm-up intensity on oxygen transport during supramaximal exercise in horses. Am J Vet Res 2008;69:690–6.
167. Mukai K, Hiraga A, Takahashi T, et al. Effects of three warm-up regimens of equal distance on $\dot{V}O_2$ kinetics during supramaximal exercise in Thoroughbred horses. Equine Vet J 2010;42(Suppl 38):33–9.
168. Musch TI, McAllister RM, Symons JD, et al. Effects of nitric oxide synthase inhibition on vascular conductance during high speed treadmill exercise in rats. Exp Physiol 2001;86:749–57.
169. Shen W, Xu X, Ochoa M, et al. Role of nitric oxide in the regulation of oxygen consumption in conscious dogs. Circ Res 1994;75:1086–95.
170. Honig CR, Gayeski TEJ, Groebe K. Myoglobin and oxygen gradients. In: Crystal RG, West JB, Weibel ER, et al, editors. The lung: scientific foundations. New York: Raven; 1997. p. 1925–33.
171. Wagner PD. Determinants of maximal oxygen transport and utilization. Ann Rev Physiol 1996;58:21–50.
172. Poole DC, Musch TI. Pulmonary and peripheral gas exchange during exercise. In: Roca J, Rodriguez-Roisin R, Wagner PD, editors. Pulmonary and peripheral gas exchange in health and disease. New York: Marcel Dekker; 2000. p. 469–523.
173. Poole DC, Mathieu-Costello O. Capillary and fiber geometry in rat diaphragm perfusion fixed in situ at different sarcomere lengths. J Appl Physiol 1992;73:151–9.
174. Poole DC, Musch TI, Kindig CA. In vivo microvascular structural and functional consequences of muscle length changes. Am J Physiol 1997;272:H2107–14.
175. Federspiel WJ, Popel AS. A theoretical analysis of the effect of the particulate nature of blood on oxygen release in capillaries. Microvasc Res 1986;32:164–89.
176. Borgia LA, Valberg SJ, Essen-Gustavsson B. Differences in the metabolic properties of gluteus medius and superficial digital flexor muscles and the effect of water treadmill training in the horse. Equine Vet J 2010;42(Suppl 38):665–70.
177. Holloszy JO, Coyle EF. Adaptations of skeletal muscle to endurance exercise and their metabolic consequences. J Appl Physiol 1984;56:831–8.
178. Weibel ER. Understanding the limitation of O_2 supply through comparative physiology. Respir Physiol 1999;118:85–93.
179. Hogan MC, Bebout DE, Wagner PD, et al. Maximal O_2 uptake of in situ dog muscle during acute hypoxemia with constant perfusion. J Appl Physiol 1990;69:570–6.
180. Roca J, Hogan MC, Story D, et al. Evidence for tissue diffusion limitation of $\dot{V}O_{2max}$ in normal humans. J Appl Physiol 1989;67:291–9.
181. Bebout DE, Hogan MC, Hempleman SC, et al. Effects of training and immobilization on $\dot{V}O_2$ and DO_2 in dog gastrocnemius muscle in situ. J Appl Physiol 1993;74:1697–703.
182. Knight PK, Sinha AK, Rose RJ. Effects of training intensity on maximum oxygen uptake. In: Persson SGB, Jeffcott LB, editors. Equine exercise physiology 3. Davis, CA: ICEEP; 1991. p. 77–82.
183. Roca J, Agusti AG, Alonso A, et al. Effects of training on muscle O_2 transport at $\dot{V}O_{2max}$. J Appl Physiol 1992;73:1067–76.
184. Young LE. Cardiac responses to training in 2-year-old Thoroughbreds: an echocardiographic study. Equine Vet J Suppl 1999;30:195–8.
185. Scheuer J, Tipton CM. Cardiovascular adaptations to physical training. Annu Rev Physiol 1977;39:221–5.
186. Schiable TF, Scheuer J. Cardiac adaptations to chronic exercise. Prog Cardiovasc Dis 1985;27:297–324.
187. McKeever KH, Schurg WA, Jarrett SH, et al. Exercise training induced hypervolemia in the horse. Med Sci Sports Exerc 1987;19:21–7.
188. Freeman GL, LeWinter MM. Pericardial adaptations during chronic cardiac dilation in dogs. Circ Res 1984;54:294–300.
189. Lee M-C, LeWinter MM, Freeman G, et al. Biaxial mechanical properties of the pericardium in normal and volume overload dogs. Am J Physiol 1985;249:H222–30.
190. Lightfoot G, Jose-Cunilleras E, Rogers K, et al. An echocardiographic and auscultation study of right heart responses to training in young national hunt Thoroughbred horses. Equine Vet J Suppl 2006;36:153–8.

191. Young LE, Rogers K, Wood JL. Heart murmurs and valvular regurgitation in Thoroughbred racehorses: epidemiology and associations with athletic performance. J Vet Intern Med 2008;22:418–26.
192. Evans DL, Rose RJ. Cardiovascular and respiratory responses to submaximal exercise training in the Thoroughbred horse. Pflugers Arch 1988;411:316–21.
193. Eaton MD, Hodgson DR, Evans DL, et al. Effects of low- and moderate-intensity training on metabolic responses to exercise in Thoroughbreds. Equine Vet J Suppl 1999;30:521–7.
194. Katz LM, Bayly WM, Roeder MJ, et al. Effects of training on oxygen consumption of ponies. Am J Vet Res 2000;61:986–91.
195. Tyler CM, Golland LC, Evans DL, et al. Skeletal muscle adaptations to prolonged training, overtraining and detraining in horses. Pflugers Arch 1998;436:391–7.
196. McKeever KH, Scali R, Geiser S, et al. Plasma aldosterone concentration and renal sodium excretion are altered during the first days of training. Equine Vet J Suppl 2002;34:524–31.
197. Foreman JH, Bayly WM, Grant BD, et al. Standardized exercise test and daily heart rate responses of Thoroughbreds undergoing conventional race training and detraining. Am J Vet Res 1990;51: 914–20.
198. Essén-Gustavsson B, McMiken D, Karlstrom K, et al. Muscular adaptation of horses during intensive training and detraining. Equine Vet J 1989;21:27–33.
199. Serrano AL, Quiroz-Rothe E, Rivero J-LL. Early and long-term changes of equine skeletal muscle in response to endurance training and detraining. Pflugers Arch 2000;441:263–74.
200. Rivero JL, Ruz MC, Serrano AL, et al. Effects of a 3 month endurance training programme on skeletal muscle histochemistry in Andalusian, Arabian and Anglo-Arabian horses. Equine Vet J 1995;27:51–9.
201. Essén-Gustavsson B, Lindholm A. Muscle fiber characteristics of active and inactive Standardbred horses. Equine Vet J 1985;17:434–8.
202. Guy PS, Snow DH. The effect of training and detraining on muscle composition in the horse. J Physiol (Lond) 1977;269:33–51.
203. Hodgson DR, Rose RJ, Dimauro J, et al. Effects of training on muscle composition in horses. Am J Vet Res 1986;47:12–15.
204. Lovell DK, Rose RJ. Changes in skeletal muscle composition in response to interval and high intensity training. In: Persson SGB, Lindholm A, Jeffcot LB, editors. Equine exercise physiology 3. Davis, CA: ICEEP; 1991. p. 215–22.
205. Straub R, Dettwiler M, Hoppeler H, et al. The use of morphometry and enzyme activity measurements in skeletal muscles for the assessment of the working capacity of horses. In: Snow DH, Persson SGB, Rose RJ, editors. Equine exercise physiology. Cambridge: Granta; 1983. p. 193–9.
206. Courouce CA, Chretien M, Valette JP. Physiological variables measured under field conditions according to age and state of training in French trotters. Equine Vet J 2002;34:91–7.
207. Sexton WL, Erickson HH, Coffman JR. Cardiopulmonary and metabolic responses to exercise in the Quarter Horse: effects of training. In: Gillespie JR, Robinson NE, editors. Equine exercise physiology 2. Davis, CA: ICEEP; 1987. p. 77–91.
208. Evans DL, Rainger JR, Hodgson DR, et al. The effects of intensity and duration of training on blood lactate concentrations during and after exercise. Equine Vet J Suppl 1995;18:422–5.
209. Saltin B, Rowell LB. Functional adaptations to physical activity and inactivity. Fed Proc 1980;39:1506–13.
210. Hudlicka O, Brown M, Egginton S. Angiogenesis in skeletal and cardiac muscle. Physiol Rev 1992;72:369–417.
211. Poole DC, Mathieu-Costello O, West JB. Capillary tortuosity in rat soleus muscle is not affected by endurance training. Am J Physiol 1989;256:H1110–16.
212. Hansen-Smith F, Egginton S, Hudlicka O. Growth of arterioles in chronically stimulated adult rat skeletal muscle. Microcirculation 1998;5:49–59.
213. Suzuki J, Kobayashi T, Uruma T, et al. Time-course changes in arteriolar and venular portions of capillary in young treadmill-trained rats. Acta Physiol Scand 2001;171:77–86.
214. Griffin KL, Woodman CR, Price EM, et al. Endothelium-mediated relaxation of porcine collateral-dependent arterioles is improved by exercise training. Circulation 2001;104: 1393–8.
215. Lash JM. Exercise training enhances adrenergic constriction and dilation in the rat spinotrapezius muscle. J Appl Physiol 1998;85:168–74.
216. Koller A, Huang A, Sun D, et al. Exercise training augments flow-dependent dilation in rat skeletal muscle arterioles. Role of endothelial nitric oxide and prostaglandins. Circ Res 1995;76: 544–50.
217. Laughlin MH, Pollock JS, Amann JF, et al. Training induces nonuniform increases in eNOS content along the coronary arterial tree. J Appl Physiol 2001;90:501–10.
218. Laughlin MH, Ripperger J. Vascular transport capacity of hindlimb muscles of exercise-trained rats. J Appl Physiol 1987;62:438–43.
219. Rietbroek NJ, Dingboom EG, Schuurman SO, et al. Effect of exercise on development of capillary supply and oxidative capacity in skeletal muscle of horses. Am J Vet Res 2007;68:1226–31.
220. Mukai K, Ohmura H, Hiraga A, et al. Effect of detraining on cardiorespiratory variables in young Thoroughbred horses. Equine Vet J Suppl 2006;36: 210–13.

Diseases of the heart and vessels

32

Lesley E. Young Gunther van Loon

CHAPTER CONTENTS

Introduction

Cardiac murmurs and arrhythmias are detected commonly in performance horses, creating problems for veterinarians who must then determine their significance.[1–4] This chapter will address the diseases and abnormalities affecting the heart and vessels of the athletic horse:

- abnormalities of cardiac rhythm
- cardiac murmurs
- diseases of the myocardium and pericardium
- diseases of the vessels.

When performance horses are presented with a cardiac arrhythmia, or murmur, an accurate history and a thorough physical examination are often all that is required to determine the relevance of the abnormality. As determination of the significance of cardiac abnormalities detected by auscultation forms the largest part of performance horse cardiology, this chapter will first address the general approach to equine cardiology cases, including the technique of cardiac auscultation. During discussion of specific cardiovascular abnormalities, emphasis will be placed on diagnosis, the physical signs used to assess severity and prognosis, and the most useful ancillary aids for determining the significance of cardiovascular dysfunction in performance horses.

General approach to equine cardiology

Overall approach

The horse is equipped with enormous cardiac reserve (Chapter 31) and as a result, evaluation of the equine cardiovascular system at rest provides limited information relevant to function during intense exercise. Only when increased demand is placed on the heart during exercise will the effect of more subtle cardiac or vascular lesions become obvious. It is clearly important not to lose sight of the plethora of other reasons that cause horses to fail to perform to owner expectations.[5] As has been emphasized elsewhere in this book, the probability of heart disease is low on the list of causes of poor performance, compared to orthopedic or respiratory disease. Clearly field, or treadmill, exercise tests provide the optimal environment to assess cardiac function in equine athletes, but it is often impractical or inappropriate to evaluate the heart at the limits of its reserve. As a result, the clinician must rely on clinical history to provide a subjective assessment of exercise tolerance and physical examination to assess the hemodynamic effect of any lesions present. In many cases, resting and exercising electrocardiography and echocardiography provide the additional information needed to determine a diagnosis and prognosis.

Clinical history

The importance of obtaining a thorough case history cannot be over-emphasized in considering the importance of cardiac murmurs or dysrhythmias in horses. It will usually be obvious if a horse is in overt heart failure, but this is not a frequent diagnosis in performance horses. It is much more common to discover a cardiac murmur or dysrhythmia in an apparently normal horse during a pre-purchase examination, when the horse is presented with a history of poor performance, or when a horse is examined because of illness. As a result, the clinician must rely on clinical history to provide a subjective assessment of exercise tolerance and physical examination to assess the hemodynamic effect of any lesions present.

Cardiac auscultation

Despite advances in technology, cardiac auscultation remains the most important technique for the diagnosis of cardiac disease in horses. It is important to develop a systematic, logical approach to cardiac auscultation for it to yield maximum information. The suggestion that equine clinicians find interpretation of auscultation findings difficult only serves to emphasize the importance of developing the necessary skills to perform this very important technique with confidence.[6]

Findings from cardiac auscultation must always be used in combination with performance history, patient details and the remainder of the clinical examination to evaluate the significance of any suspected cardiovascular abnormalities.

Technique

Rules

- Always auscultate both sides of the chest.
- Always palpate for an apex beat on both sides of the chest. (See Fig. 32.1.)
- Always listen for at least 30 seconds to calculate the horse's heart rate and establish the normality of its cardiac rhythm before worrying about the presence or absence of cardiac murmurs.
- Always maintain a standard systematic approach for listening to the whole cardiac cycle at each valve area.

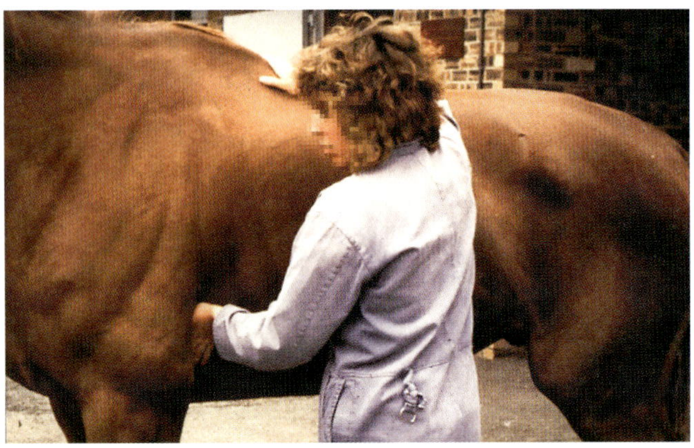

Fig 32.1 Palpation of the cardiac apex beat. The apex beat provides an excellent starting point for auscultation on the left hemithorax.

Location of valve areas

Classically, landmarks for localization of cardiac valve areas have been described with reference to rib spaces and anatomical landmarks.[7] The mental effort of remembering the landmarks, coupled with marked breed variation in thoracic conformation, makes this approach difficult to put into practice. It also encourages the clinician to remove the stethoscope from the horse's chest, to examine each valve individually, potentially leaving wide areas of the cardiac auscultation area unexamined. An alternative approach is suggested.

Left hemithorax

Palpation of the left apex beat (Fig. 32.1) provides an easy landmark for the mitral valve auscultation area. The apex beat should be palpated with the flat of the left hand. The stethoscope is then placed exactly over the apex beat. The point of maximal intensity (PMI) of sounds associated with the mitral valve is usually in this area. In this region the first heart sound, S_1, caused by various vibrations at the onset of ventricular systole, should be loud. The third sound, S_3, associated with the end of rapid early ventricular filling, might also be audible. It is important to appreciate that the normal diastolic sounds S_3 and S_4 are not always clearly audible in every horse. Once positioned at the apex beat, the examiner should initially concentrate only on cardiac rate and rhythm for at least 30 seconds, so that the heart rate and underlying rhythm are established before the examiner is distracted by the absence or presence of any cardiac murmurs. Then the examiner should concentrate specifically on both diastole and systole for a number of complete heart cycles, before the stethoscope is then moved slowly and deliberately in radiating directions around the mitral valve area while maintaining contact with the chest wall, until S_1 is no longer clearly audible.

The remaining valve areas on the left are then accessed by gradually moving the stethoscope in a cranial direction from the mitral valve area. Once more, the stethoscope remains in contact with the chest wall at all times. As the stethoscope is advanced slightly dorsal and cranial, the relative loudness of S_1 and S_2 is reversed, and S_2 is accentuated relative to S_1. As this occurs, the stethoscope is positioned at the point of maximal intensity of the semilunar valves. The first, more caudal and dorsal, valve encountered is the aortic valve. Once in the outflow and aortic and pulmonic valve areas, the clinician must again specifically listen for adventitious sounds in both systole and diastole, before performing the same radial scan of the area as for the mitral valve. S_2 will be loudest over the pulmonary valve, which is situated more cranial and slightly ventral to the area in which S_2 first becomes accentuated. Occasionally an audible splitting of S_2 can be heard in the area of the pulmonic valve. Usually the sound is split due to earlier closure of the aortic valve compared to the pulmonic valve, but the situation can also be reversed in horses.[8] The fourth heart sound, S_4, composed of vibrations arising from active atrial contraction, is usually heard best in the area cranial and dorsal to the apex beat.

Right hemithorax

It should also become standard to palpate for an apex beat on the right hemithorax. The vibrations are often palpable in narrow-chested athletic horses. If an apex beat is detected, it represents an excellent starting point for thoracic auscultation. The auscultation area is more cranial on the right, and forward placement of the forelimb is necessary in many horses (Fig. 32.2). The only valve sounds reliably heard in this area are associated with the tricuspid valve. After once more concentrating specifically on systole and diastole, a similar radiating survey, with the stethoscope in contact with the chest wall, should be performed around the point of maximal intensity of the heart sounds on the right side. Many clinicians find auscultation of the right side unrewarding, because the heart sounds are usually quieter here and there is more variation between horses. When difficulties arise, it is usually because the stethoscope is not positioned sufficiently cranial, the horse is excessively fat, or the horse's leg is insufficiently protracted.

Abnormalities of cardiac rhythm

General principles

- Dysrhythmias occur commonly in athletic horses[9] and the majority, with the notable exception of atrial fibrillation (AF) and atrial flutter (AFL), usually do not affect performance.
- In horses, use of limb leads for recording ECG traces is ill-advised. Wires and crocodile clips attached to their limbs are poorly tolerated and subject to a large amount of movement artifact. In addition, the pattern of depolarization of the equine ventricle precludes using multiple leads for assessment of cardiac size and mean electrical axis.[10–12]
- The base-apexlead system or modifications of it are used exclusively for rhythm diagnosis in equine medicine (Fig. 32.3). This lead system produces large complexes, which are easy to identify.[13] Recording of multiple leads can be useful to identify buried P waves or slight alterations in QRS morphology (such as caused by fusion beats) (Fig. 32.4).
- Diagnosis of arrhythmias has been greatly enhanced by improvements in technology that allow ECG recordings to be taken readily in resting and exercising horses (Figs 32.5 and 32.6). Digital ECGs, based on laptop and android technology are now readily affordable for equine veterinarians (Figs 32.4 and 32.5). Increased availability and practicability of this equipment means that disorders of cardiac rhythm are diagnosed more frequently in horses at rest and during exercise.

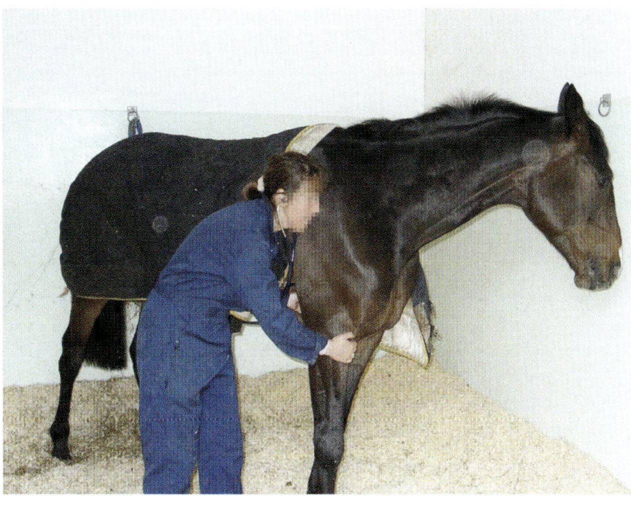

Fig 32.2 Auscultation of the heart from the right hemithorax is best achieved when the right forelimb is pulled forward.

Cardiac disease is a rare primary cause of poor performance in the equine athlete, but on the rare occasion that performance is affected by cardiac disease, dysrhythmia is the commonest underlying cause.[5] Paradoxically, alterations in cardiac rhythm are common in athletic horses because of their normal high parasympathetic drive,[14] so the equine clinician is faced with a wide variety of normal rhythms in resting horses. Bradydysrhythmias (slow rhythms) are normal findings in athletic horses, as are sinus and atrioventricular block.[9,15] Despite this, on rare occasions, all of these normal rhythms can also result from cardiac disease, when the dysrhythmia causes serious decrements to performance and presents important risks to the rider and horse.[16] Conversely, obvious arrhythmia such as atrial fibrillation might have no obvious effect on the performance of horses engaged in activities that are not aerobically challenging (dressage or show jumping). In contrast, if all of the cardiac reserve must be used, the effect of the same dysrhythmia on performance is devastating (racing, three-day eventing).[17–19] Finally, cardiac rhythm disturbances often occur as a result of disease in other body systems or metabolic disturbances.[20,21] In such cases, the arrhythmia is unlikely to be associated with primary heart disease.

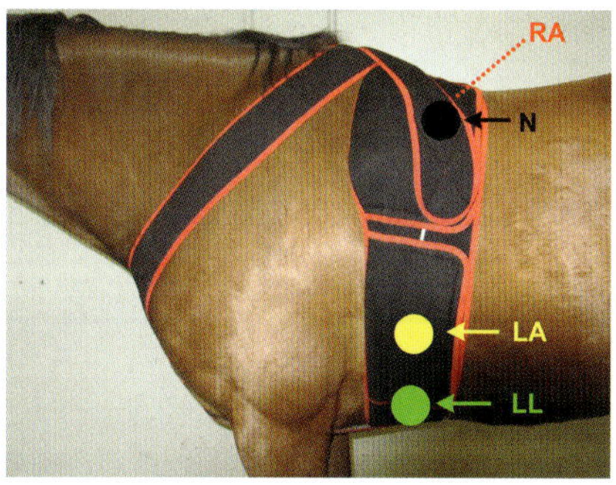

Fig 32.3 Photograph showing placement of four electrodes suitable for recording an electrocardiogram at rest (ambulatory or 24-hour ECG) or during lunging exercise. High-quality adhesive electrodes must always be used. This lead configuration to be used here is a modified base-apex system. When the ECG recorder is equipped with four leads, as in most cases, its leads will usually be labeled and color coded according to the Einthoven system: right arm (red), left arm (yellow), left leg (green) and earth (black), although these color conventions can vary depending on the country of origin. Right arm and neutral are placed right and left to the withers, respectively. Left leg is placed on the left ventral thorax. By putting the left arm electrode 15 to 20 cm dorsal to the left leg electrode, this lead (lead III) is useful at rest to identify buried P waves or small changes in QRS morphology (e.g. fusion beats) (see Fig. 32.4). During exercise however, abundant artifacts occur on this lead. To record a true, base-apex lead, the positive or left arm (LA) electrode should be positioned at the cardiac apex, and the right arm (RA) negative electrode, two-thirds of the way down the jugular groove on the right. The third, left leg and fourth (earth) electrode, if present are then placed in remote positions away from the heart. The standard base-apex ECG can then be recorded from lead 1 of an Einthoven ECG recorder. This lead configuration will give maximum deflections for both atrial and ventricular waveforms, but is completely unsuitable for prolonged monitoring, or exercising recordings. The vertical modification shown will still produce large 'QRS' deflections, but the atrial deflection ('P' wave) will be slightly lower in amplitude than that of a true base-apex configuration.

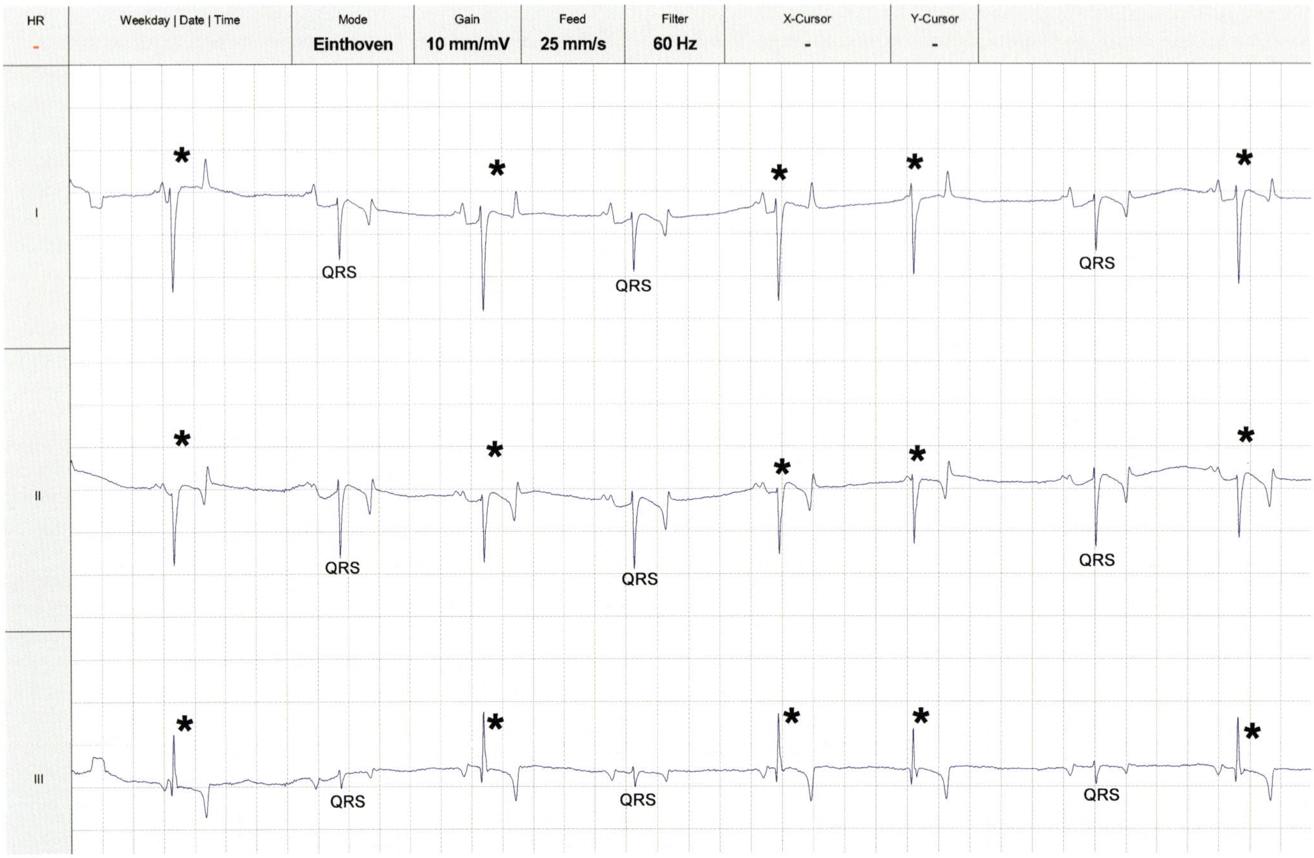

Fig 32.4 Multiple lead recording is useful as it facilitates identification of buried P waves (e.g. P wave buried in previous T wave) and small alterations in QRS morphology. This picture shows a three lead recording in a horse with ventricular premature beats with electrodes placed as shown in Fig. 32.3. Normal QRS complexes are indicated (QRS). The abnormal morphology (asterisks) of certain ventricular premature beats could be missed on lead I and II but is very obvious on lead III, which is recording the potential difference between the lowermost left arm and left leg electrodes.

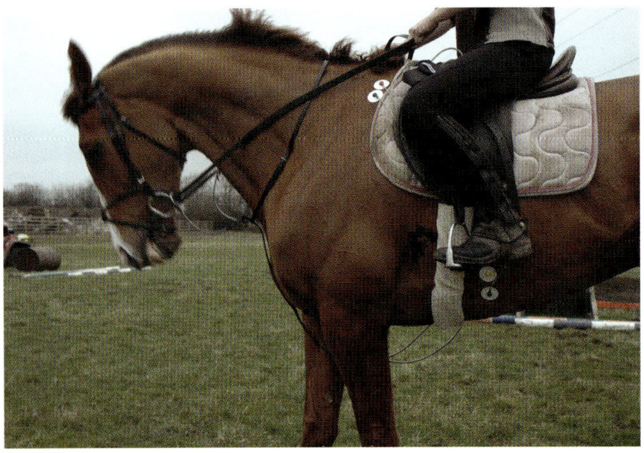

Fig 32.5 Placement of four silver/silver chloride adhesive electrodes suitable for recording an electrocardiogram during ridden exercise. To record an exercising electrocardiogram from a horse, often only a single vector is used. The electrodes are positioned slightly different as depicted in Fig. 32.3, so that they remain visible to the rider and/or examiner. As a result they can be reattached easily, should they become dislodged and are unlikely to be affected by saddle or girth slipping backwards during fast exercise. Depending on the rider's leg/stirrup length, the vertical position of the lower electrodes might need to be positioned more ventral. The recording device is visible, attached to the front 'D' ring of the saddle, where it usually causes minimal disruption and rider discomfort.

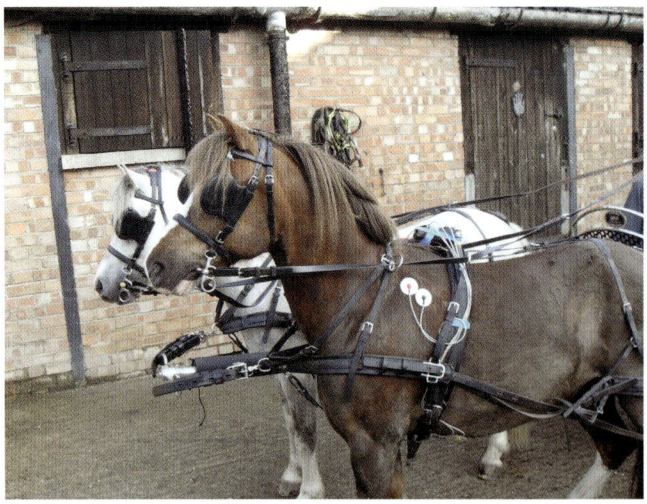

Fig 32.6 For harness racing and carriage horses the electrodes are positioned similarly away from moving harness straps. Use of a surcingle with a breast plate facilitates recording and exercising ECG from horses on the lunge. To gain maximum information from exercising ECG, it is imperative that exercise of appropriate type is used and that its intensity meets or preferably exceeds the subject's usual activities.

The main hemodynamic effect of abnormalities of cardiac rhythm is to change cardiac output. These alterations can result from effects on heart rate or stroke volume. In some cases, especially when the abnormal rhythm is fast, arrhythmia begets further arrhythmia as myocardial oxygen demand increases and coronary perfusion declines in the face of reduced diastolic blood pressure. It remains an important general rule that treatment of arrhythmia is only indicated when the abnormal rhythm has, or is likely to have, an important effect on cardiac function, or when treatment is likely to resolve the arrhythmogenic mechanism (e.g. correction of acid–base and electrolyte imbalances).

Atrial fibrillation (AF) and atrial flutter (AFL)

- Re-entrant rhythm disorders are usually characterized by an irregularly irregular rhythm (Figs 32.7–32.12).
- Both abnormal rhythms can occasionally self-correct within hours to days of becoming established (Fig. 32.10).
- AF is the commonest cardiovascular cause of poor performance in racehorses and those engaged in other aerobically challenging sports (eventing, hunting) but also

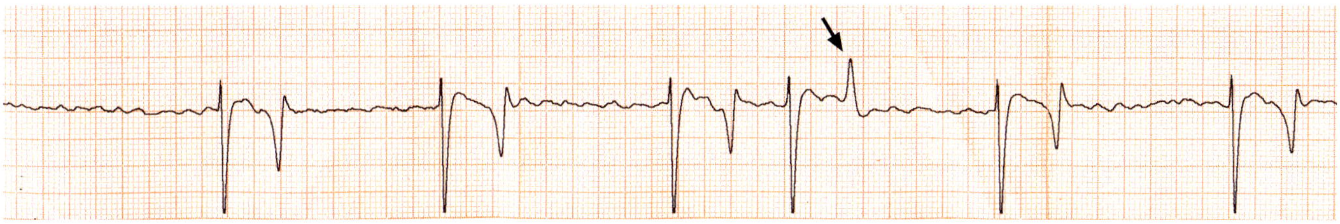

Fig 32.7 Electrocardiogram (base-apex configuration) of a horse with atrial fibrillation. The typical characteristics include an irregularly irregular rhythm, absence of P waves, coarse baseline irregularity called fibrillation ('f') waves and 'QRS' complexes of normal width and morphology. Note that for short RR intervals the T wave has opposite polarity to the QRS complexes that follow longer diastolic intervals; the same phenomenon occurs in ECGs recorded during exercise compared to at rest. In the same horse, even in the same ECG trace, coarse and fine fibrillation waves can be present, representing the chaotic nature of the underlying electrical activation of the atria.

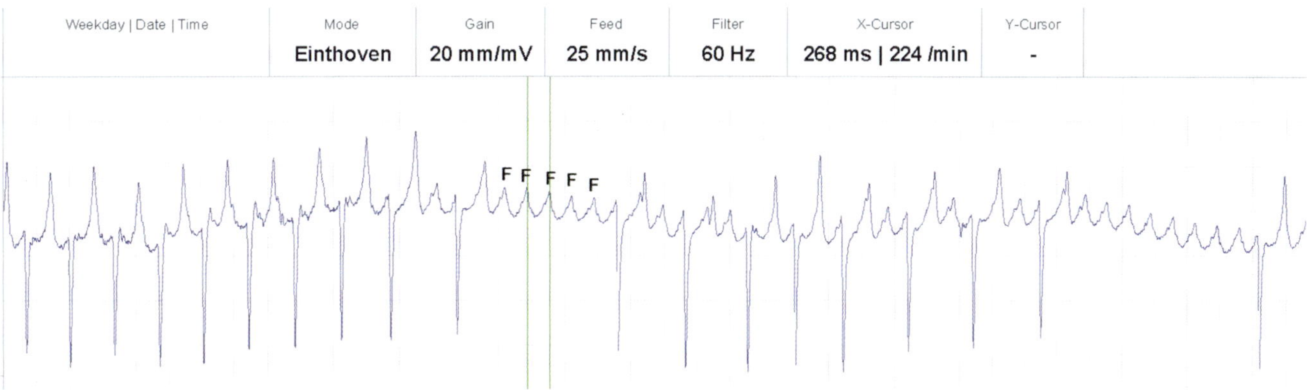

Fig 32.8A Base-apex ECG obtained from a five-year-old trotter with a 14-day history of reduced athletic performance. The ECG shows atrial flutter with a cycle length of 268 ms (rate 224 per minute).

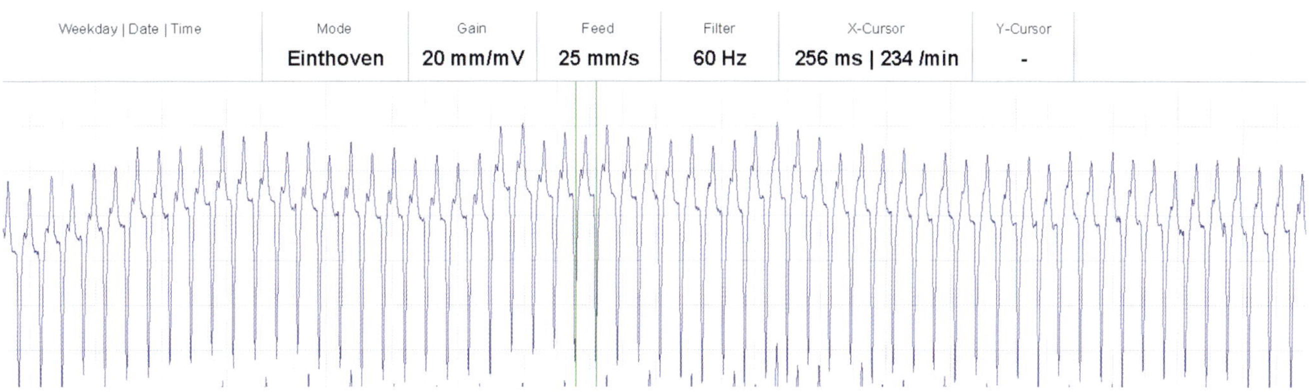

Fig 32.8B During exercise and during periods of excitement 1:1, 1:2 and 1:3 atrioventricular conduction of the flutter waves occurred and the horse's heart rate rhythm sounded regular by auscultation. This ECG recording was obtained during and immediately after pulling up from trot on the lunge. 1:1 conduction of F waves as parasympathetic tone is withdrawn results in an excessively high heart rate for the work being undertaken, but the horse's cardiac rhythm is now completely regular. The horse was subsequently converted by transvenous electrical cardioversion at the first 125 J shock, whereupon he returned to his previous level of exercise.

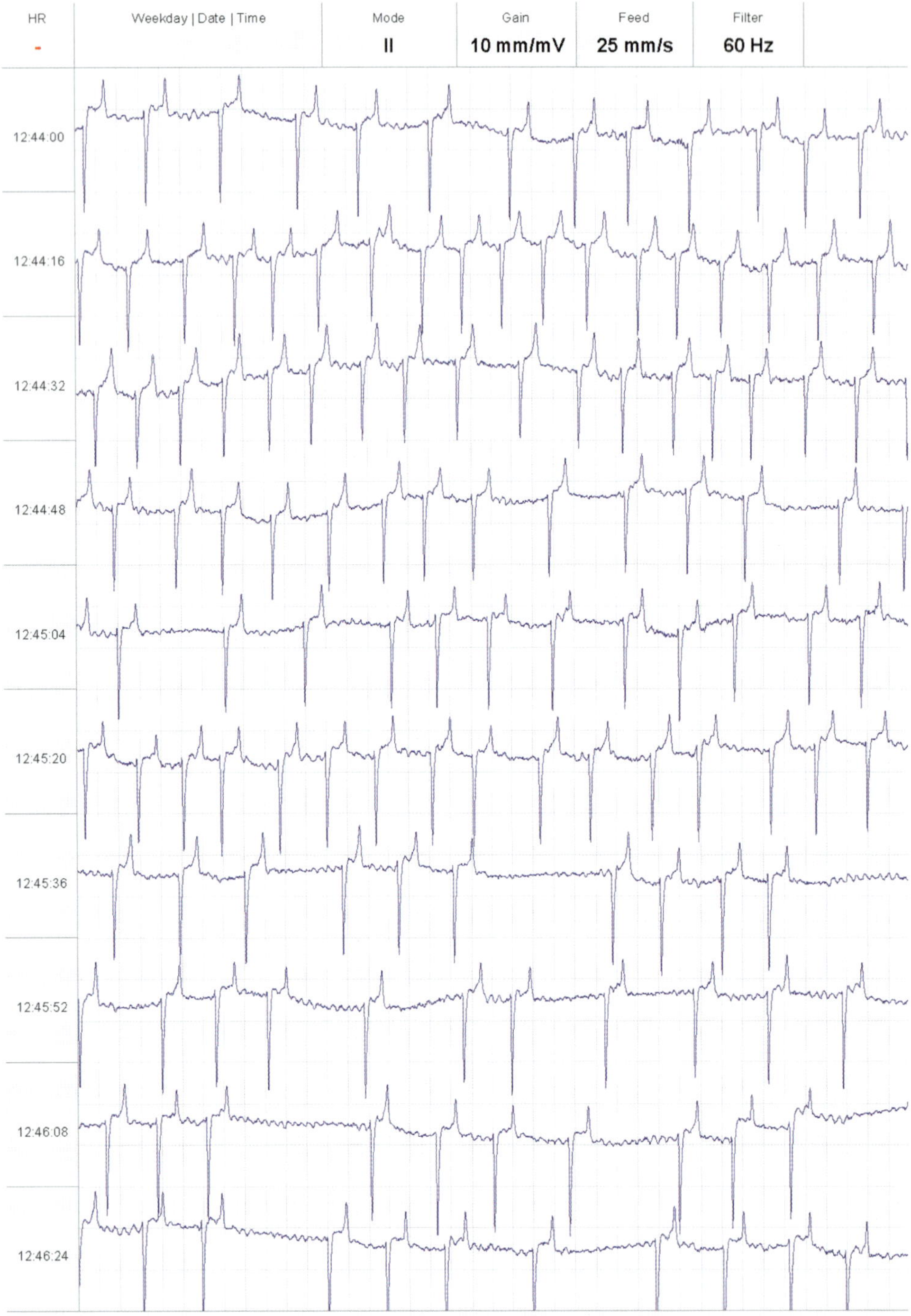

Fig 32.9 Summary of a continuous ECG recording from a five-year-old trotter horse. The summary clearly demonstrates the irregular irregularity of atrial fibrillation that would become obvious with prolonged monitoring by auscultation. Notice that during periods of rapid conduction, the rhythm can seem almost regular, and during periods of slow conduction, it might be mistaken for sinus arrhythmia and 2° AV block. As a result, AF can easily be missed if a cursory examination by auscultation is performed.

jumping or dressage horses might present with loss of performance.

- It can be an incidental finding in horses performing in less aerobically challenging disciplines.
- AF can be associated with severe cardiac disease (Figs 32.13 and 32.14), or occur in the absence of any significant cardiac dysfunction.
- Its presence leads to excessively high ventricular rates during exercise, increased prevalence of ventricular premature beats, ventricular tachycardia and occasionally R-on-T phenomenon (Fig. 32.11). These features will predispose affected horses to exercise-associated collapse and sudden death (Fig. 32.12).
- Treatment depends on whether underlying cardiac disease is present (Fig. 32.14A and B).

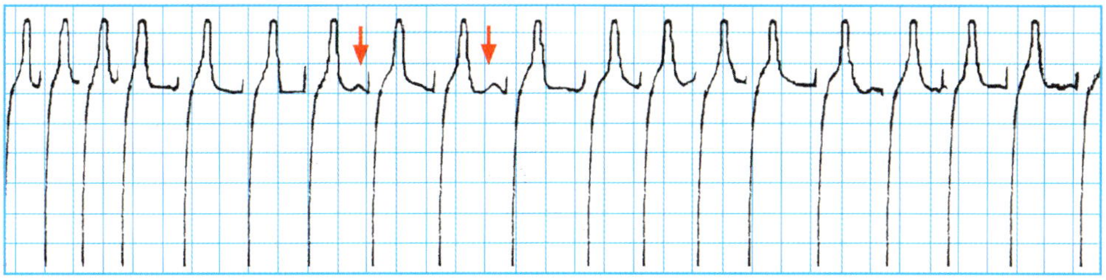

Fig 32.10 Base-apex ECG taken from a seven-year-old Thoroughbred mare, 20 minutes after dramatically fading during fast work. Heart rate is still elevated (average rate 140 bpm) and the rhythm is irregularly irregular. The 'QRS' complex width and morphology is normal and 'P' waves are not visible.

There are positive baseline undulations between the 7th and 8th and 9th and 10th beat that could be mistaken for 'P' waves. Closer inspection reveals them to be too close to the 'QRS' complex that follows and more characteristic 'f' waves are visible in the long diastolic interval before the final 'QRS complex. This trace illustrates the high heart rate maintained by horses affected with paroxysmal atrial fibrillation.

The horse spontaneously converted to normal sinus rhythm within 5 hours of the abnormal rhythm becoming established.

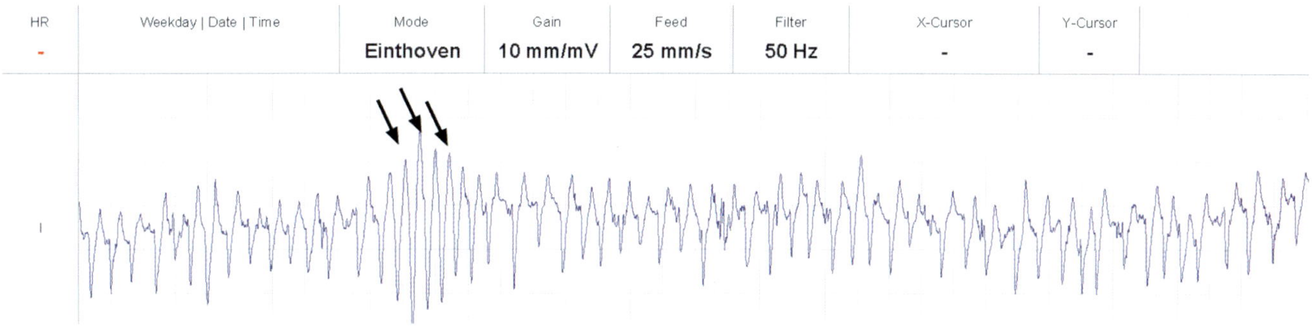

Fig 32.11 Horses with AF show a high prevalence of ventricular premature beats, ventricular tachycardia and even R-on-T phenomenon during sudden stress or exercise. During (only) lunge exercise, this horse with lone AF showed short runs of ventricular tachycardia with R-on-T morphology and a heart rate up to 388 bpm (arrows). Sinus rhythm was successfully restored by transvenous delivery of a 200 J biphasic shock and the horse returned to his previous level of exercise.

- Prognosis for successful treatment and return to previous athletic function in the absence of cardiac disease is good, but treatment failure and recurrence of the arrhythmia are also possible.

Recognition

History

Atrial fibrillation (AF) and atrial flutter (AFL) can occur in horses with no other evidence of cardiac disease, or these can be precipitated by atrial dilation secondary to underlying heart disease, most commonly long-standing mitral regurgitation[17] (Figs 32.13 and 32.14). When AF occurs in isolation, it is often larger breed horses that are affected. Affected animals usually present with a history of poor performance. The more demanding the sports discipline, the more likely clinical signs are to occur. The lack of an atrial contribution to ventricular filling, which is especially important during exercise when the time available for early diastolic filling is reduced, is coupled with a very high ventricular response rate to the atrial arrhythmia. Both these factors combine to reduce the length of diastole and contribute to inadequate ventricular filling. This results in a deleterious effect on forward cardiac output and aerobic capacity in affected horses. The disproportionately high ventricular rate during AF is the result of an increased sympathetic tone that allows a high number of atrial impulses to be conducted to the ventricles. Instantaneous heart rates of over 300 bpm are often found (Fig. 32.11). At such high rates, ventricular filling is even more reduced, further decreasing cardiac output during exercise. In some horses, AF is associated with epistaxis.[18,22]

If AF develops suddenly, during fast work, there is an acute decrease in cardiac output, and affected horses can pull up suddenly, sometimes with ataxia and distress. Immediate thoracic auscultation reveals a rapid chaotic rhythm. Obvious performance decrements are not invariably the case, however, as affected horses can appear to work normally at lower intensity. The rhythm, once initiated, can be sustained, but short-lived paroxysmal AF also occurs during exercise (Fig. 32.10).[23] Paroxysmal AF resolves in the minutes, hours or days following exercise and can be difficult to detect. As a result, AF is a possible cause for fading during racing or competition when horses are subsequently presented in normal sinus rhythm.[24] AF can also develop in association with deranged electrolyte and fluid balance in endurance horses after endurance events. In such cases, the rhythm usually resolves spontaneously with rehydration and restitution of electrolyte balance.

Clinical signs of atrial flutter are similar as for AF, although maximal heart rates during exercise equalize rapidly to the atrial flutter rate with withdrawal of parasympathetic tone; although the peak heart rates will be ultimately lower compared with that of horses affected by AF, the condition is usually still performance limiting (Fig. 32.8B).

Physical examination

Auscultation findings in cases of AF will depend on the underlying cause. The irregularly irregular rhythm will be common to

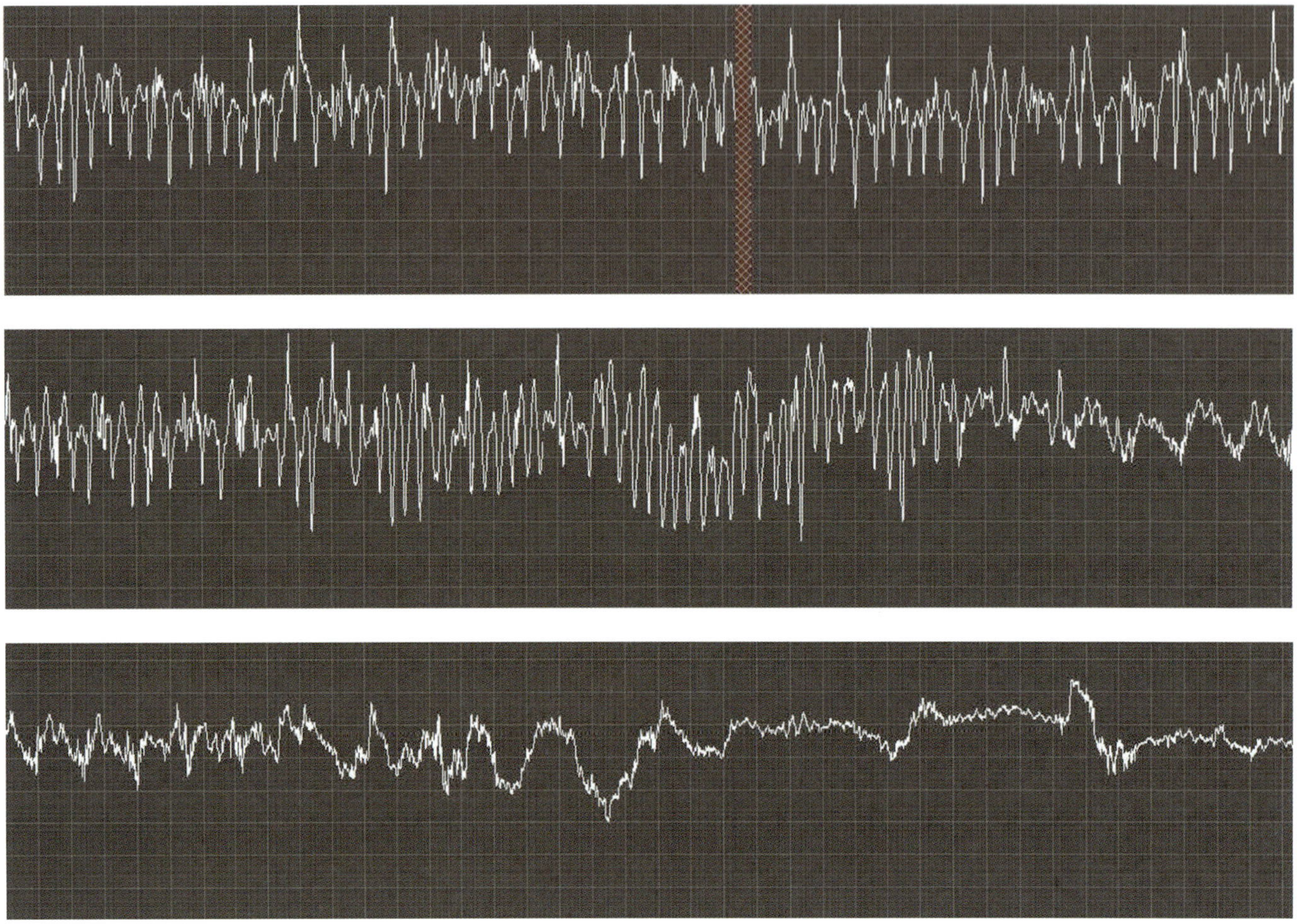

Fig 32.12 Continuous sequence of ECG recorded during ridden exercise from a nine-year-old three-day event horse, who had been diagnosed with atrial fibrillation after pulling up unexpectedly during the cross country phase of an event, three weeks earlier. The horse performed a short bout of trot and light canter at an excessively high average heart rate (252 bpm), before runs of wide complex beats, probably ventricular in origin became evident (first trace). Over the next 90 seconds (second and third traces), the rhythm degenerated to ventricular tachycardia, fibrillation followed by asystole. During the same period, the horse appeared to stagger and whinnied. The rider was told to dismount, whereupon the horse fell, lost consciousness and died. Subsequent post mortem examination, including full histologic examination of the heart, was unremarkable.

ECG courtesy of the Dr KJ Blissett, Royal (Dick) School of Veterinary Studies Edinburgh.

all cases of sustained AF, but in horses with AF secondary to atrial dilation from cardiac disease, there will also be an elevated heart rate, characteristic cardiac murmurs and physical signs of heart failure. Careful auscultation of these cases will reveal the underlying cause such as mitral regurgitation or ventricular septal defect. Horses with AF but no significant underlying heart disease, usually have a normal resting heart rate. Vagal tone at the atrioventricular node will cause waxing and waning of the cardiac rhythm that can appear deceptively similar to second-degree atrioventricular block.[25] This feature can be confusing, but the two rhythms can always be differentiated with patient auscultation because an unexpected early beat will be always be detected (Fig. 32.9).

Because of the absence of pre-systolic closure of the atrioventricular valves, the intensity of the first heart sound is usually increased. Other findings include a complete absence of the fourth heart sound (associated with atrial contraction), often coupled with increased intensity of the third sound. During very long diastolic intervals, over-filling of the atria results in backward filling of the jugular veins. Other clinical signs will be evident if the abnormal rhythm is associated with heart failure.

The less common variant, atrial flutter, occasionally presents with a more regular and rapid rhythm when a constant ratio of flutter waves are blocked at the AV node. (Fig. 32.8B). The regular rapid atrial activity provoked by the flutter waves is occasionally audible if there are long diastolic intervals.

Special examination

Electrocardiography will reveal an irregularly irregular rhythm with a complete absence of P waves and normal QRS morphology. Cardiac rate will depend on the presence or absence of associated cardiac disease and atrioventricular conduction. Fibrillation waves are visible on the surface ECG and often change between coarse and fine fibrillation waves in the same horse (Fig. 32.7).

When atrial flutter is present, P-like, often bifid, undulations at a rate of 170–250 per minute cycle continuously (Fig. 32.8A). Horses with atrial flutter have a regular or irregular ventricular rhythm depending on atrioventricular conduction and prevailing autonomic tone. At elevated heart rates, ventricular rhythm is regular because of a 1 : 1, 2 : 1, 3 : 1 atrioventricular conduction. RR intervals will be a constant multiple of the atrial flutter cycle length (Fig. 32.8B).

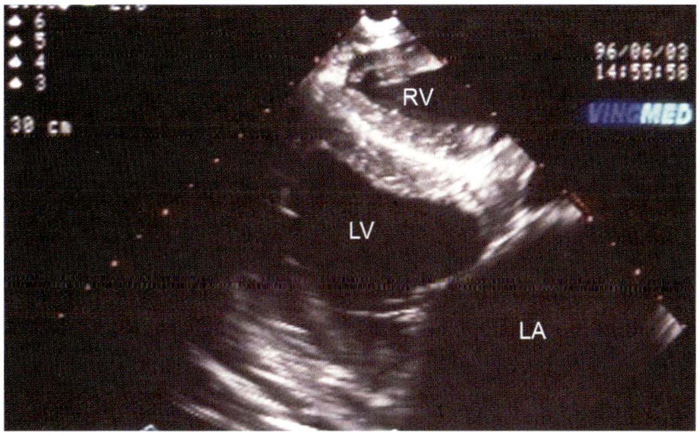

Fig 32.13 Two-dimensional echocardiograph from a three-year-old colt in training with a season-long history of poor performance, believed by the trainer to be due to chronic foot lameness. When the colt developed a cough, veterinary examination revealed a fast irregular heart rhythm and a grade 5/6 murmur suggestive of mitral valve regurgitation. The image is taken from the right hemithorax and shows massive left atrial enlargement from long-standing severe mitral regurgitation. Although the colt had no physical signs of heart failure, treatment was not attempted and the horse was euthanized. (LA = left atrium, LV = left ventricle, RV = right ventricle).

In both AF and atrial flutter, echocardiography is important to determine the presence or absence of cardiac lesions and assess chamber size, when important cardiac disease cannot be ruled out from the physical examination and clinical history (Figs 32.13 and 33.14A and B). An exercising ECG should be performed if the owners decide against any treatment, even if the rhythm is an incidental finding and the horse's performance is believed to be unaffected. This procedure will ascertain whether the horse is able to perform its duties comfortably within its reduced cardiac reserve and will confirm that withdrawal of parasympathetic tone during exercise does not result in accelerated conduction of wavelets, excessive tachycardia, or other malignant cardiac rhythms (Fig. 32.11) that could increase the horse's risk of exercise-related injury, or predispose it to collapse and sudden death (Fig. 32.12).

Laboratory tests

Paroxysmal and sustained AF can be associated with alterations in electrolyte status. Plasma or serum concentrations of cardiac troponin I (cTnI), markers of myocardial injury and inflammation, are rarely elevated in cases of AF, unless the condition is associated with toxic damage to the heart, or end-stage valvular of congenital heart disease. Mild elevations are often recorded in the first 24–48 hours after the rhythm becomes established but the significance of this elevation is unknown and could also be the result of mild exercise-associated elevations in cTnI.[26]

Treatment and prognosis

The therapeutic aims vary depending on the circumstances and cause of AF. When the horse is expected to perform and there is no evidence of underlying heart disease, therapy aims to convert AF to normal sinus rhythm and to prevent its recurrence. However, if AF is not associated with poor performance, provided underlying heart disease can be ruled out and the horse's heart rate and rhythm appear to be acceptable during the horse's normal activities, treatment might not be necessary. Nevertheless, recent clinical evidence that this rhythm can degenerate in some individuals during exercise means that horses affected with sustained AF could still be at a

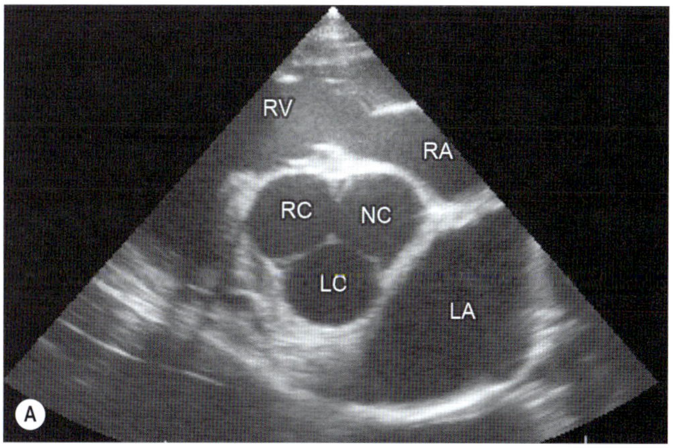

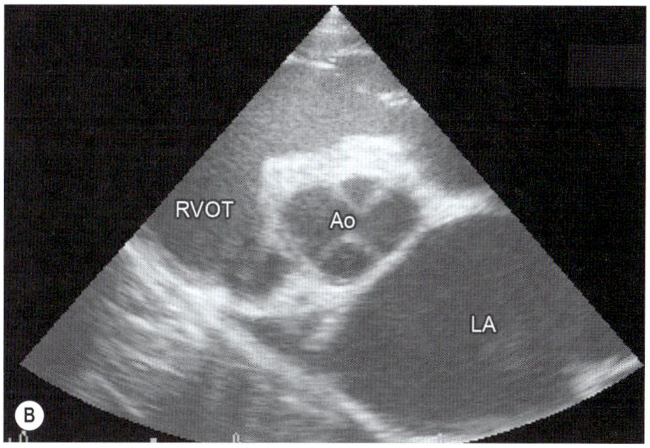

Fig 32.14 **(A)** Two-dimensional echocardiograph from an eight-year-old Thoroughbred racehorse with atrial fibrillation associated with a sudden decrease in race performance. Image is derived from the right hemithorax with the transducer positioned to obtain a short-axis view of the atrium and aorta. Comparison of the relative width of the left atrium with respect to the aortic root provides useful reference for determination of left atrial enlargement, regardless of horse size. Normal horses have a left atrial to aortic root ratio of <1.2 : 1. Although there was a grade 2/6 murmur of mitral regurgitation, left atrial : aortic width ratio was within normal limits. The horse converted to normal sinus rhythm after administration of 45 g of quinidine per os. (LC = left coronary cusp of aortic valve; NC = non-coronary, RC = right coronary cusp, LA = left atrium, RV = right ventricle, RA = right atrium.)

(B) Two-year-old Thoroughbred flat racing filly with atrial fibrillation that presented with lethargy and poor exercise tolerance. Image is derived from the right hemithorax with the transducer positioned to obtain a short-axis view of the atrium and aorta. Visual inspection of the same image as Fig. 32.14A shows the greatly increased left atrial : aortic width ratio (2.9 : 1). The difference is accentuated as low output cardiac failure has reduced left ventricular stroke volume and blood pressure and concurrently aortic diameter has also reduced. The filly was treated using digoxin to control cardiac rate, diuretics to reduce congestion, an angiotensin-converting enzyme inhibitor (enalapril) to reduce cardiac afterload and a calcium sensitizing agent and phosphodiesterase inhibitor (pimobendan) to enhance myocardial contractility and further reduce afterload. Quinidine treatment is not appropriate when atrial fibrillation occurs secondary to left atrial enlargement. (Ao = aorta, RVOT = right ventricular outflow tract, LA = left atrium.)

tangibly increased risk of collapse and sudden death during exercise than their peers. When AF coexists with heart failure, the abnormal rhythm should not be specifically treated. Treatment goals in this instance include control of ventricular response rate, reduction of volume overload by diuretics and angiotension-converting enzyme inhibitors, and cardiac afterload reduction by vasodilation.[27,28]

Before therapy is contemplated, any underlying fluid, electrolyte or acid–base abnormalities should be corrected. When horses become dehydrated, or develop abnormalities of acid–base and electrolyte abnormalities, as might occur during three-day events or endurance competitions, restoration of fluid and electrolyte balance alone is likely to be sufficient for normal sinus rhythm to restore itself in case of recent-onset AF.

Successful cardioversion can be achieved by pharmacological treatment or by electrical cardioversion. The most commonly used pharmacological treatment consists of oral quinidine sulfate, a class 1A antiarrhythmic.[29,30] Intravenous administration of quinidine gluconate has been described,[31] but this preparation, though more convenient, is less effective when the arrhythmia is long-standing.[30,32] In many countries, the intravenous preparation of quinidine gluconate is not available and production of quinidine sulfate has been discontinued. As a result quinidine must now be imported and as difficulty in obtaining quinidine sulfate increases, there has been a drive to investigate alternative treatments of equine AF. As a result of these efforts, the most promising new technique appears to be direct current transvenous electrical cardioversion (TVEC) under general anesthesia. This method is efficacious and it appears to have the least side effects and a high success rate for conversion of AF in many horses.[33–35]

Treatment of atrial flutter is similar to that of AF, but it can generally be expected to have a higher success rate because the arrhythmia is more organized and therefore amenable to conversion. Overdrive intra-atrial pacing has also been used successfully to treat refractory atrial flutter in one horse.[36]

Treatment of atrial fibrillation with quinidine sulfate

Horses should not be treated for the first 72–96 hours after development of AF, as a proportion will spontaneously return to normal sinus rhythm. Treatment should be contemplated if there is no evidence of cardiac failure, if there is compromise of athletic ability or if exercise results in accelerated conduction, excessive tachycardia or other malignant cardiac rhythms.

Regime

Traditionally the administration of a test dose of quinidine sulfate (10 mg/kg per os) was given to check for idiosyncratic reactions before commencing treatment. However, this is not necessary and treatment is begun with 20 mg/kg quinidine sulfate administered via nasogastric tube (10 g per 500 kg horse). This dosage is repeated every two hours until sinus rhythm is restored, signs of intoxication develop, or a maximum total dose of 60–80 g (120 mg/kg) is achieved. Individual differences in quinidine resorption and elimination are considerable.[37] Especially when mild signs of intoxication develop, the two-hour interval can be prolonged between two and six hours to avoid more severe intoxication. The longer quinidine can be kept at therapeutic level, the higher the statistical chance for conversion to sinus rhythm. Treatment must be performed in a quiet area with immediate IV access available. A continuous telemetric ECG should be available to monitor heart rate and rhythm throughout the treatment. Horses receiving quinidine should not be moved, as quinidine causes hypotension, through alpha receptor blockade.[38]

Signs of intoxication include urticaria, diarrhea, anorexia, weakness, ataxia and tachycardia.[18,30] Nasal edema with stertorous breathing and depression are commonly observed after only a few doses. A relationship has been demonstrated between high plasma quinidine concentrations, ataxia and respiratory tract stridor, but not between plasma quinidine concentrations and tachycardia, diarrhea or colic.[30] Conversion to normal sinus rhythm is less likely when there are signs of quinidine intoxication.[30] Laminitis has also been reported after quinidine treatment, but this adverse effect appears to be rare. Sudden death can also occur and is most likely the result of a malignant ventricular rhythm (Fig. 32.15). In common with all class 1A antiarrhythmic drugs, quinidine has proarrhythmic properties.[39] By lengthening the myocardial cell refractory period, quinidine increases the risk of severe ventricular rhythm disturbances.[38] Because the drug increases AV nodal conduction, it has the potential to produce rapid supraventricular, as well as ventricular tachycardia.[38] ECG should be monitored throughout the treatment and QRS and QT interval measured before each treatment. Although a 25% increase in QRS duration is reported as being clinically important,[30] exact measurement is often difficult during AF due to superposition of f-waves. In addition, increased atrioventricular conduction during treatment can result in QRS broadening due to use-dependent sodium channel blockade and aberrant conduction. Therefore it is easy to confuse supraventricular tachycardia with ventricular tachycardia (Fig. 32.16A), although management is very different. Tachycardia is often encountered, most commonly due to supraventricular tachycardia (SVT). Low dose of alpha2-adrenergic agonist administration, provided significant signs of hypotension are absent, can depress atrioventricular nodal conduction sufficiently to immediately abolish supraventricular tachycardia and reduce QRS duration (Fig. 32.16B). Further emergency treatment includes intravenous administration of bicarbonate at 1 mEq/kg body weight to increase protein binding of quinidine and therefore decrease the concentration of unbound drug, which is the biologically active form. Supraventricular tachycardia can be treated by the intravenous administration of 0.002 mg/kg digoxin IV, or if unsuccessful, 0.03 mg/kg propranolol IV[30] to slow AV nodal conduction. Digoxin, however, has a slow onset of action and concurrent use of quinidine and digoxin might increase toxicity of both quinidine and digoxin because of competitive protein binding. Propranolol should be administered with caution as it can enhance hypotension and negative inotropism. Life-threatening ventricular tachycardia can be treated with magnesium sulfate IV (4 mg/kg every two minutes up to 50 mg/kg) followed by lidocaine IV (0.25 to 0.5 mg/kg every five minutes up to 2–4 mg/kg).

In many horses, cardioversion is a progressive event related to the cumulative quinidine dose. Intra-atrial electrograms show that the initial fibrillation 'rate' is usually between 300 and 450 depolarizations per minute. Due to quinidine, fibrillation becomes more organized and fibrillation rate decreases, thereby producing fibrillation waves that start to appear as flutter waves or P' waves. Close to conversion, atrial rate can drop towards 170 to 100 per minute, while 2 : 1 conduction results in a ventricular rate between 50 and 85 bpm. Occasionally, the ECG can resemble sinus rhythm while in fact a fibrillation wave is still buried in each preceding QRS or T wave (Fig. 32.17). This means that AF is still present. Termination of treatment at this stage can result in gradual return of fine fibrillation waves as quinidine concentrations in plasma decline. This should not be regarded as early recurrence of AF.

Horses that fail to revert to sinus rhythm after administration of 120 mg/kg quinidine, or that develop unacceptable adverse effects during cumulative dosing, sometimes respond to a second series of 20 mg/kg treatments after waiting 24-hours without further drug administration. Indeed some horses convert to normal sinus rhythm up to 24 hours after the final dose of quinidine has been administered without any additional drugs being administered.

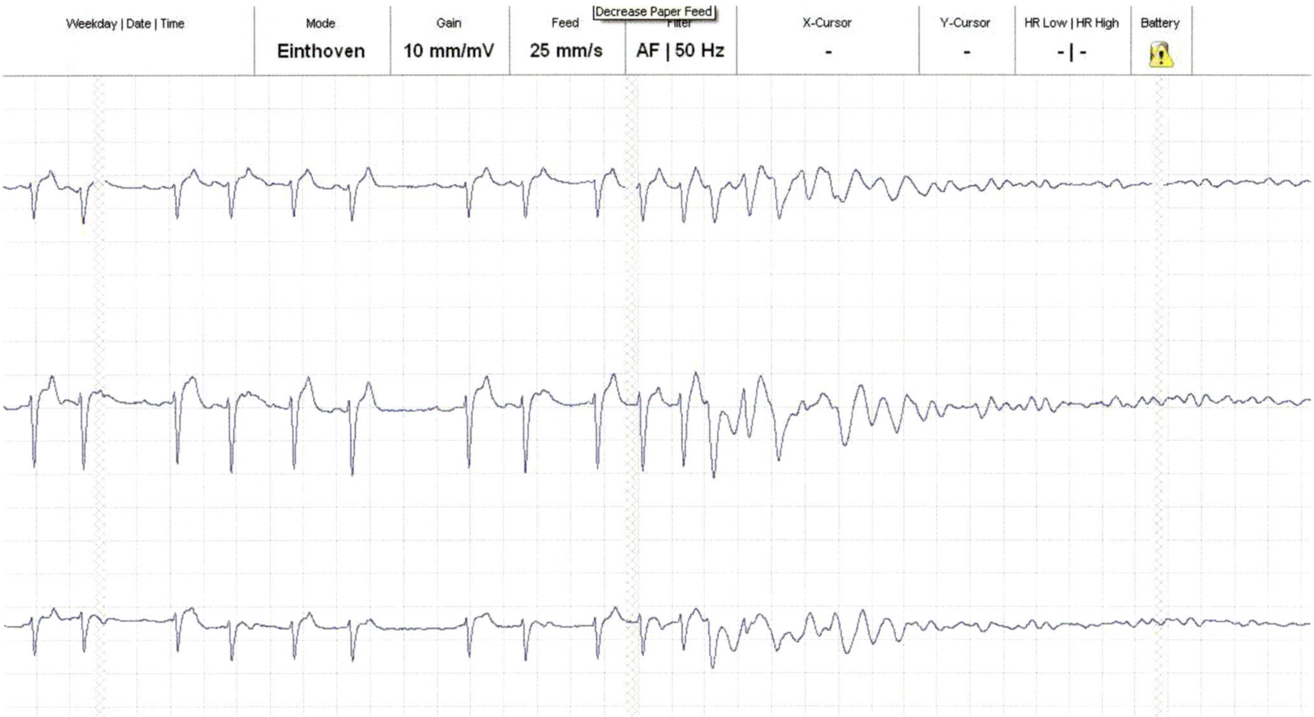

Figure 32.15 Sudden cardiac death in a horse approximately 12 hours after a cumulative dose of 50 g of quinidine sulfate had been administered in four divided doses for the treatment of sustained lone atrial fibrillation. Although sinus rhythm had not been restored, treatment was abandoned due to development of increasing gastrointestinal side effects, including gaseous distension and colic. The horse died suddenly at an average heart rate of 60 bpm some time after resolution of his gastrointestinal side effects. The ECG shows that one abnormal ventricular complex triggered ventricular fibrillation and asystole within a period of 4–5 seconds.
ECG courtesy of Dr John Keen, Royal (Dick) School of Veterinary Studies, University of Edinburgh.

Such delayed conversion could be explained by slower quinidine elimination in some individuals, whereby the prolonged duration of a therapeutic quinidine level increases the statistical likelihood for cardioversion. The potential severity of quinidine's side effects, have led to modifications of the traditional cumulative two-hourly regime and an alternative regime has been suggested.[30] If a horse fails to respond to the initial two-hourly treatments, when signs of toxicity develop, or when the maximum dose of quinidine has been reached, quinidine administration is continued at six-hourly intervals. These workers also recommend that digoxin (0.01 mg/kg) be given orally every 12 hours until sinus rhythm is restored. From a theoretical point of view, digoxin tends to stabilize AF by increasing the number of wavelets circulating in the atria and decreasing their wavelength.[40] However, digoxin has beneficial vagotonic effects on the atrioventricular node and is used therapeutically in humans and dogs to reduce the ventricular response to stable AF. It is therefore possible that a horse given digoxin might be better able to tolerate quinidine at its therapeutic levels without the development of tachycardia, thereby increasing the probability of conversion. The use of digoxin in the treatment of AF remains somewhat controversial.

Other pharmacological treatments for atrial fibrillation

The class 1C antiarrhythmic flecainide is more efficacious than quinidine in returning human patients to sinus rhythm after sustained[41] and paroxysmal AF[42] and its use has been investigated in horses.[43] Initial reports suggested that flecainide at 0.2 mg/kg/min IV over 10 minutes was effective in returning horses to normal sinus rhythm after AF was induced by rapid atrial pacing.[44] However, use in horses with naturally occurring AF, but also in recent-onset experimental AF (G. van Loon, unpublished results), was associated with potentially dangerous wide-QRS tachycardia and risk for sudden death[45] (Fig. 32.18). The class 3 agent amiodarone showed moderate efficacy (50%) in equine AF but its use was associated with adverse effects such as diarrhea and temporary hind limb weakness, especially when administered for longer than 48 hours.[46,47] Because of its low bioavailability, amiodarone should be administered intravenously.[48] Median half-lives of amiodarone and desethylamiodarone were 24.1 and 58.6 hours, respectively.[48] In some countries, the cost of this product might be prohibitive.

Other drugs such as propafenone (class 1C) and sotalol (class III), both with beta-adrenergic blocking activity, have been sporadically used in horses. No data on pharmacokinetics, adverse effects and pro-arrhythmic properties of these drugs in horses have been reported to date. Cibenzoline treatment in two horses with AF did not restore sinus rhythm and was associated with severe ventricular pro-arrhythmia.[49]

Transvenous electrical cardioversion of atrial fibrillation

Direct current electrical cardioversion of tachyarrhythmias is a well-known and very effective technique for treatment of human tachyarrhythmias and can be applied via a transthoracic, transvenous or a combined approach. The adult horses' size makes transthoracic cardioversion of AF very difficult. However, transvenous electrical cardioversion (TVEC) of AF has proven to be very effective with success rates of 90 to 98%.[33,35] The technique also seems to be well suited for conversion of chronic AF cases or horses that failed to convert on quinidine.[33,35] In a study of 72 treatments, treatment outcome was not predicted by AF duration as 71 horses converted.[35] Although mild increases in cTnI are occasionally observed, increases have been judged to be clinically unimportant.[50] As electrical cardioversion is painful, it always necessitates general anesthesia,

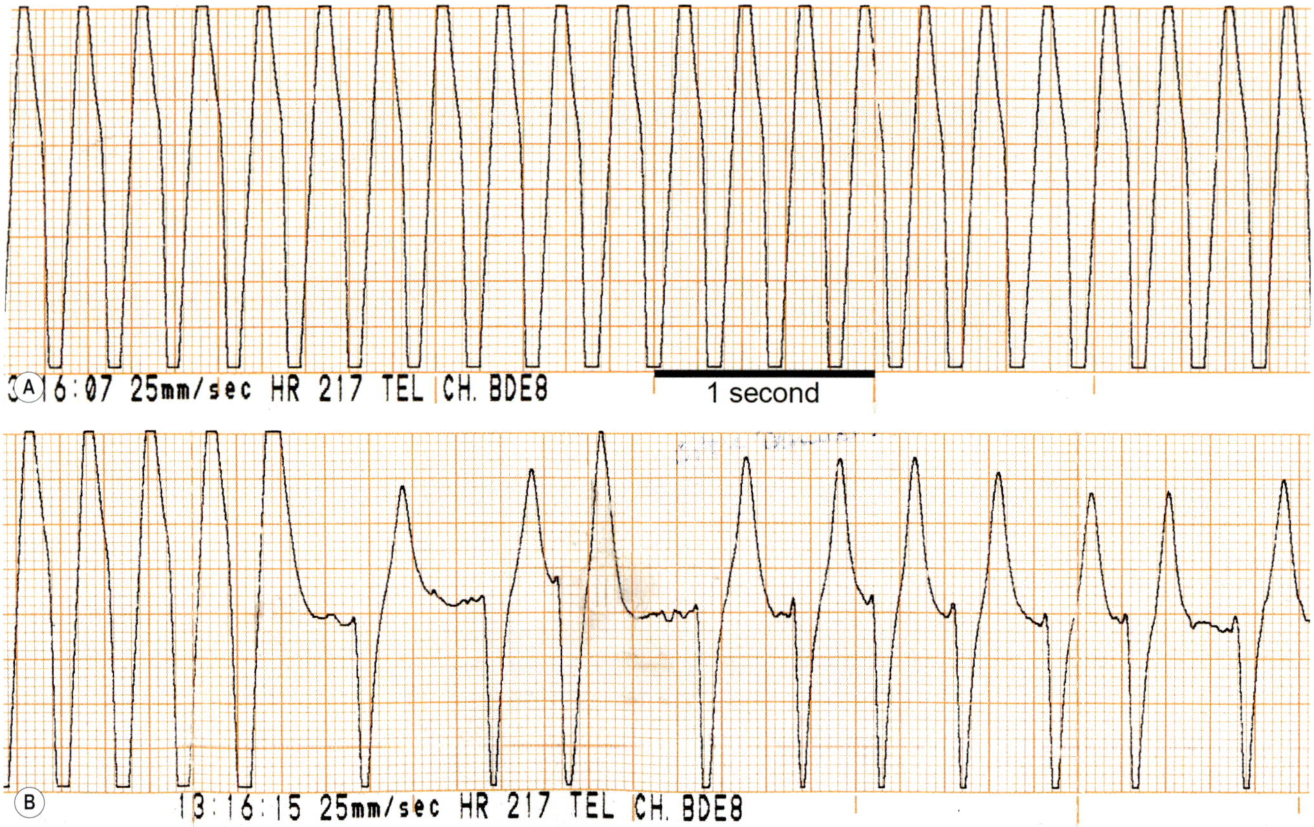

Fig 32.16 (A) Sustained supraventricular tachycardia at 217 bpm per minute developed suddenly in this horse with lone atrial fibrillation, 20 minutes after the second 22 mg/kg dose of quinidine sulfate. Note the broadening of the QRS complexes.

(B) ECG trace of the same horse as in Fig. 32.16A, 10 seconds after IV administration of 5 μg/kg detomidine. Note the sudden slowing of atrioventricular conduction and immediate shortening of the QRS complexes.

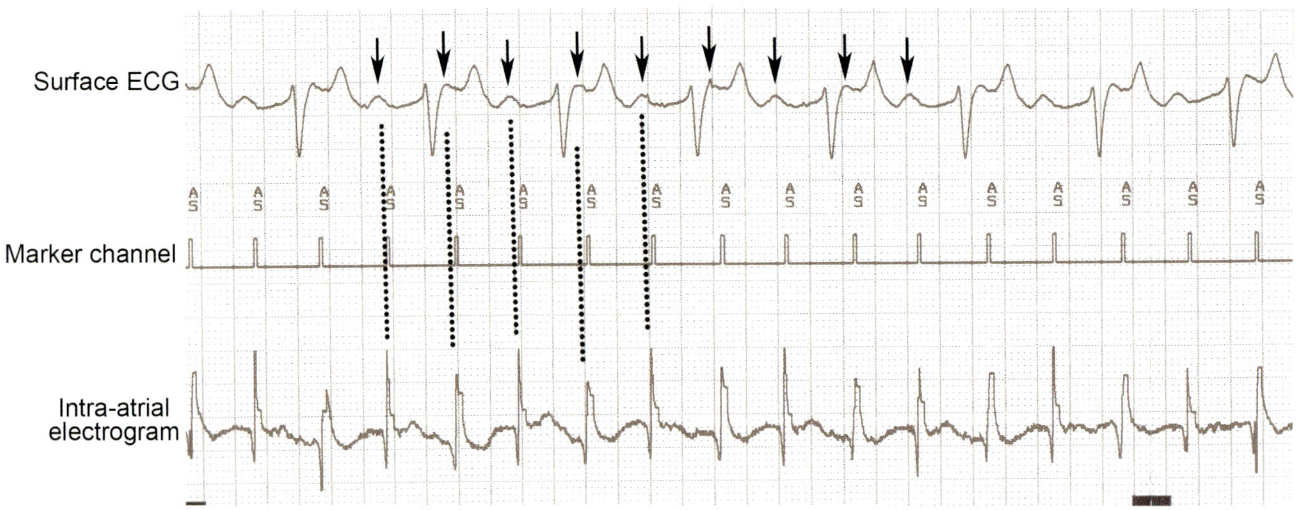

Fig 32.17 Quinidine slows the rate of atrial fibrillation, often resulting in a flutter-like situation before cardioversion occurs. In this horse with lone AF, the surface ECG is regular and mimics sinus rhythm. Close inspection. However, shows that f waves are buried in the QT interval. This is confirmed by a simultaneous recording of an intra-atrial electrogram: RR interval is 840 ms while atrial fibrillation cycle length (ff interval) is 420 ms. The horses has not converted at this stage. Cessation of treatment can result in a gradual acceleration of atrial fibrillation rate as quinidine levels drop. This should not be misinterpreted as early recurrence of AF.

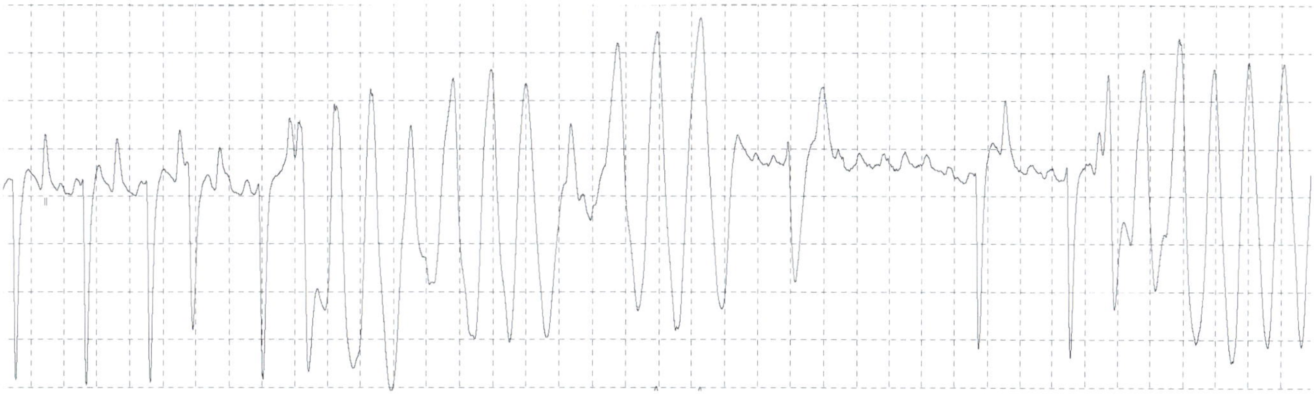

Fig 32.18 Polymorphic wide-QRS tachycardia develops in a horse with lone atrial fibrillation during intravenous treatment with flecainide. Action of the drug is rate dependent and results in QRS widening at increased ventricular rates (due to increased atrioventricular conduction). Administration of an alpha2-adrenergic agonist slowed ventricular rate immediately and terminated wide-QRS tachycardia. The horse did not convert but was subsequently converted with quinidine sulfate and returned to competition.

which carries independent risks for morbidity and death.[51] Despite the presence of AF, cardiovascular function was well maintained during anesthesia and was not affected by shock application. Cardiac index and stroke index increased and SAP decreased after cardioversion.[52]

The cardioversion procedure starts with insertion of two cardioversion catheters via the jugular vein in the standing horse. These catheters possess a large surface area electrode at the tip for shock delivery. Under ultrasound guidance, one catheter needs to be positioned in the right atrium while the second catheter is maneuvered 10–20 cm into the left pulmonary artery (Fig. 32.19). Both right and left parasternal images are useful for exact catheter localization. A pressure trace recording from the catheter gives additional insight into the position of the catheter top. On occasion, shock delivery can result in temporary asystole and, consequently. The use of an additional right ventricular temporary pacing catheter is also advised (Fig. 32.20A and B).[53] When all catheters are in place, general anesthesia is induced. Catheter position is then confirmed by ultrasound and the catheters repositioned, as necessary. Radiography has also been used to check catheter and electrode location during anesthesia.[54] The right ventricular pacing catheter is first connected to a temporary pacing unit. Both cardioversion catheters and a surface ECG are then connected to the defibrillator, which is operated in synchronous mode. This detects the R wave of the ECG and will automatically deliver the shock timed exactly on the R wave after the button of the defibrillator is pressed (Fig. 32.21). Correct detection of the R wave is vital as shock delivery on a T wave almost inevitably results in fatal ventricular fibrillation. When the defibrillator wrongly identifies the T wave as an R wave, position of the surface electrodes must be changed. Biphasic, rather than monophasic, shocks should be used because they are most effective. Incremental shocks are applied, starting at 125 to 360 J, with attempts being made to minimize total energy delivered. Most horses convert between 125 and 250 J, with an impedance of 30 to 50 ohms (Fig. 32.21).[33,35] If cardioversion is not achieved, shock delivery after administration of an antiarrhythmic drug, such as amiodarone, occasionally promotes successful electrical cardioversion (G. van Loon, unpublished data). Also if there is a high frequency of atrial premature beats immediately after cardioversion, antiarrhythmic drugs can reduce the risk for immediate recurrence of AF (IRAF). After restoration of sinus rhythm, catheters are gently withdrawn and the horse is allowed to recover.

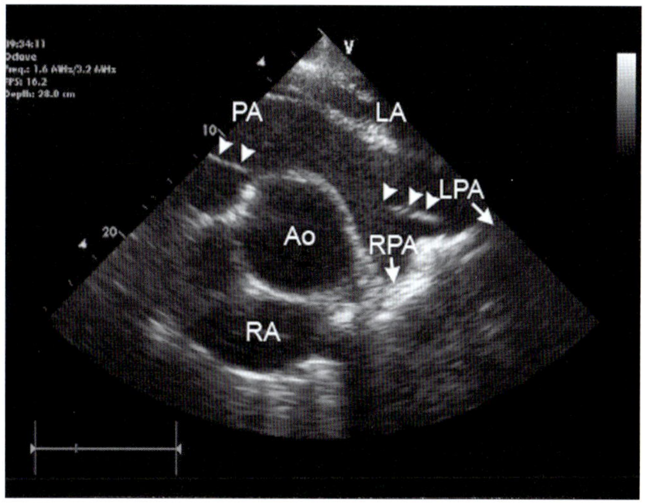

Fig 32.19 Image taken from the left hemithorax, optimized for visualization of the pulmonary artery (dorsal angulation, right on screen is caudodorsal). The cardioversion catheter (arrowheads) is positioned in the pulmonary artery (PA) and enters the left branch of the pulmonary artery (LPA) (RPA = right pulmonary artery; Ao = aorta; RA = right atrium; LA = left atrium).

Aftercare

Following successful conversion to normal sinus rhythm, aftercare is similar irrespective of the method used to achieve it.

A high burden of atrial premature depolarizations and especially the presence of runs of atrial tachycardia on a 24-hour ECG monitoring one week after cardioversion have been associated with an increased risk for AF recurrence (G. van Loon, unpublished data). In these circumstances, treatment with anti-inflammatory, antiarrhythmic drugs, or both coupled with prolonged rest (2–4 months) have been suggested in an attempt to reduce the risk of the AF recurring. Anecdotal data suggest that oral sotalol administration could have some role in reducing atrial ectopy and, consequently, the likelihood of recurrence but the dosage used remains empirical and the risk of this therapy has not been studied. Unfortunately, there are no data available to assess critically the benefit

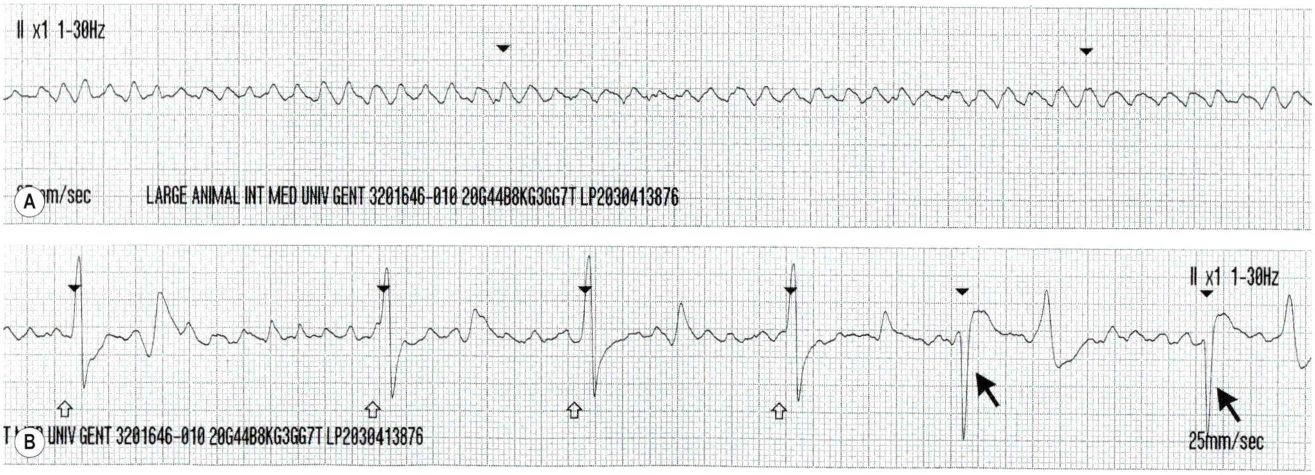

Fig 32.20 **(A)** Immediately following transvenous delivery of a 200 J biphasic shock, this 610 kg Warmblood develops temporary atrioventricular block that results in temporary asystole. Note that atrial fibrillation is still present but no ventricular depolarization occurs.
(B) Continuation of the ECG trace from Fig. 32.20A: right ventricular pacing (open arrows) is started and immediately restores ventricular function. Cardiac pacing is continued until the patient's own ventricular depolarizations start to reappear (black arrows). Note the difference in QRS morphology between the paced and normal ventricular depolarizations. In this horse, subsequent 250 J shock delivery restored sinus rhythm.

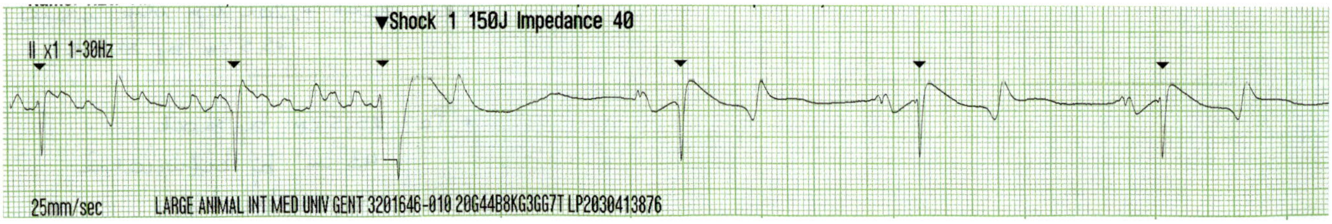

Fig 32.21 Transvenous electrical cardioversion, using one 150 J biphasic shock, instantaneously restores sinus rhythm in this 590 kg Warmblood horse with lone atrial fibrillation with suspected duration of 3.5 months. The horse was rested for six weeks, after which it returned to high-level showjumping. Note that the defibrillator correctly detects all R waves, as indicated by the black arrowheads. The defibrillator is operated in synchronous mode, which means that the shock is automatically delivered on the R wave. One should carefully position surface electrodes so that no T waves are detected as shock delivery on the T wave will almost invariably lead to ventricular fibrillation and death.

of these various treatment and management strategies for horses following successful conversion to normal sinus rhythm. As a result, in commercial practice when there are considerable financial pressures for horses to perform, coupled with a short competitive season, only after a horse reverts repeatedly to AF would such measures be contemplated.

AF results in progressive electrical and contractile remodeling of the atrial myocardium. Reverse remodeling after successful conversion depends on the chronicity of the arrhythmia. Experimental studies showed that after one week of AF, reverse remodeling was complete within 1–2 days, while AF of 4–6 months duration took longer (3–4 weeks) to fully return to normal baseline values.[55–58] A resting period that allows full recovery is optimal but not always possible due to financial and time constrains. Therefore, even when AF has been long-standing, horses are often rested for about a week and then gradually return to fast training over 3–4 weeks. Owners/trainers are advised to monitor cardiac rhythm regularly by palpation of the apex beat (Fig. 32.1), especially before and after fast work and if the horse ever performs below expectation.

Prognosis

Horses with long-standing AF (>4 months) are thought to be less likely to convert to normal sinus rhythm and more likely to revert to fibrillation after treatment than horses with more recent onset of the arrhythmia.[17,30] The success rate for conversion from lone AF to normal sinus rhythm using quinidine varies between 82 and 87%[18,30] in racehorses but is lower in Warmbloods. The lower success rate in Warmbloods is probably related to their larger size (more stable AF due to the larger atrial size) and the fact that they are more frequently presented with chronic AF compared to racehorses. Transvenous electrical cardioversion has a success rate of 90–98% and is known to be more effective in chronic cases compared to quinidine.[35] Therefore, transvenous electrical cardioversion can still be efficacious in horses that fail to convert with quinidine. When treatment of AF is successful, horses can return to their previous exercise tolerance. In a series of 70 horses treated for AF, AF recurrence rate at 4 months was 22% and at 1 year 35% (racehorses) to 40% (G. van Loon, unpublished data). In some horses, recurrence of paroxysmal or sustained AF is a problem, although some owners and trainers become aware of the trigger factors and learn to manage them accordingly. In such cases, and before treatment is attempted, it is important to establish that the rhythm is present in isolation and has not occurred secondary to atrial enlargement and heart failure (Figs 32.13 and 33.14A and B). In other cases when frequent recurrence or poor tolerance of treatment occur, an alternative career can sometimes be found for the horse. The rider must, however, appreciate that some individuals with AF have excessively high ventricular rates increased prevalence of ventricular arrhythmias and even R-on-T phenomenon during low-level exercise,[59] (Fig. 32.11). As a consequence, such horses can be at an increased risk of collapse or sudden death during exercise compared to their age-matched peers (Fig. 32.12). When AF exists with signs of heart failure, prognosis for return to athletic activity is hopeless.

Etiology and pathophysiology

AF is a re-entrant rhythm disturbance. The arrhythmia is initiated by ectopic foci (atrial premature depolarizations), which act as a trigger. The mechanism that was widely held to underlie the arrhythmia was that of multiple wavelets, a model that hypothesized that large numbers of wavelets moved randomly through the atria.[60] Recently, evidence from complex electrophysiological mapping studies in man have suggested the wavefronts often originate from uninterrupted periodic activity of ectopic foci in myocardial sleeves in the pulmonary veins.[61] Maintenance of the arrhythmia is enhanced by large atrial size and by short refractoriness and differences in electrophysiological characteristics between anatomical sites in the atria and between the left and right atria themselves. The large mass of tissue allows cells to repolarize before the initial wavefront has died out. As a result, waves of excitation continuously circle around the atria and provide a self-sustaining source of electrical activity independent of the sinus node. Once AF is initiated, electrical remodeling occurs rapidly (within hours to days), leading to a shortening of the atrial refractory period and thereby promoting perpetuation of AF.[55–58] When the arrhythmia has persisted for 3–5 days the remodeling is sufficient to prevent the arrhythmia from terminating spontaneously. Both atrial flutter and AF occur in the horse. The difference reflects the number of wavelets circulating around the atria. Multiple, chaotic wavelets are present during AF while one rotating depolarization wave at a fixed anatomical path (macro-reentry) is present during atrial flutter (Fig. 32.8A and B). This explains the more rapid (300–500 per minute) and chaotic atrial electrical activity in AF producing fine and coarse f waves often found in the same animal, on the same ECG trace. In contrast the wavelets in atrial flutter are more organized, slower and less frequent (170–250 per minute), often resulting in a bifid morphology that can closely resemble P′ waves.[36]

The risk of re-entry becoming established is increased with changes in autonomic tone.[62] Both parasympathetic and sympathetic stimulation increase the inhomogeneity of refractoriness within the atria, by changing the refractory period of the myocytes.[63] Most commonly in horses these changes occur during fast exercise or recovery, but they can also be invoked by use of vagotonic drugs such as alpha-adrenoreceptor agonists (xylazine, romifidine and detomidine) and opiates (butorphanol). Paroxysmal and sustained AF can also follow sedation, anesthesia,[64] and occasionally occur after disease in other body systems.[65,66]

AF results in a decreased stroke volume due to the loss of the atrial contribution to filling. This loss of atrial contractile function is caused by both the chaotic electrical activation and by contractile remodeling. After initiation of AF, atrial contractile dysfunction develops within days to weeks.[55–58] The atria contribute up to 15–20% to ventricular filling, but in most horses at rest the loss of the atrial contraction has little effect on cardiac output.[65] However during exercise when the heart rate is high and the time available for ventricular filling is reduced, the atrial contribution to filling becomes important. More importantly, AF is associated with disproportionally high ventricular rates during exercise. Indeed, at rest, the naturally high vagal tone increases the blocking function of the atrioventricular node, thereby decreasing the number of atrial depolarizations conducted to the ventricles. Increased sympathetic tone due to stress or exercise abolishes this vagal predomination and the atrioventricular node suddenly starts to conduct a higher proportion of the atrial impulses, occasionally resulting in excessively high ventricular rates (250 to over 400 bpm during exercise) (Fig. 32.11). Because of these mechanisms, horses with AF have reduced performance only during strenuous exercise, unless there is some other underlying cardiac disease that has precipitated the dysrhythmia. AF always affects performance in racehorses, hunters and event horses, but occasionally show jumping and dressage horses can also show some reduction in their athletic prowess, even though the cardiovascular demands of their normal exercise is much lower.

In addition, many horses with AF present abnormal (broadened) QRS complexes and even short runs of R-on-T rhythms during exercise (Fig. 32.11) (G. van Loon, unpublished data). Whether these represent ventricular ectopy or aberrant conduction of supraventricular impulses is not known (such as bundle branch block). During runs of accelerated conduction and supraventricular tachycardia, instantaneous heart rates of up to 450 bpm occur not infrequently.

Experimental studies in healthy horses with AF induced by pacing has suggested that extensive electromechanical remodeling of the atrial muscle cells, shortened refractoriness and loss of contractile dysfunction both promote AF perpetuation and probably help to explain why sinus rhythm is more difficult to recapture in many horses when the condition is chronic.[55–58] Presence of atrial fibrosis is another important factor that influences AF stability and recurrence rate. In the series of cases examined by Else and Holmes,[67] 36/45 affected horses had gross lesions affecting the atria, including dilation, thinning and fibrosis. The left atrium was more commonly affected than the right. Eighty percent of affected horses had lesions affecting the cardiac valves, most commonly the mitral valve, confirming clinical evidence that left atrial enlargement and mitral valve disease are important in the pathogenesis of sustained AF in horses. Atrial fibrosis did not develop after prolonged experimental AF, suggesting that fibrosis is probably a cause rather than a consequence of AF (G. van Loon, unpublished data).

Immediately after restoration of sinus rhythm, electrical and contractile remodeling can be detected by electrophysiological studies and cardiac ultrasound.[55–58,68] Reverse remodeling then occurs within days when acute AF is present (e.g. AF of one week duration) or weeks when AF is chronic (eg. 4–6 months duration).[55–58]

Epidemiology

This dysrhythmia is the commonest cardiovascular cause of poor performance in horses. The prevalence of acute AF in racehorses varies between 0.02 and 0.05% of race starts.[23,69] When large numbers of horses from a mixed population were examined, the prevalence of AF varied between 0.5 and 2.4%[67] and increased with age, an observation that probably explains the difference between these groups. Else and Holmes also observed that draught and heavy horses were over-represented in their affected horses. The prevalence of the sustained form of AF is lower in smaller Thoroughbreds, but it appears to have a similar prevalence in Standardbred horses.[17] It is likely that paroxysmal AF occurs more commonly than is recognized in horses of all types, because only when performance is obviously affected, will the rhythm be noticed,[23] a situation that is similar in people.[70] Standardbreds, young horses, and males predominated in a group of 67 horses studied by Reef and colleagues,[17] but it is likely that these data reflect the bias of sex, breed and age in athletic horses, rather than relate to prevalence of AF in the horse population per se. In the same study the majority of horses affected with AF had no clinical evidence of other cardiac disease (56.7%).

Supraventricular premature depolarizations

- Supraventricular premature beats arise from tissue at or above the level of the atrioventricular node. They usually originate in the atria and occur not infrequently in athletic horses.
- Their importance and underlying etiology are not well understood, although increased excitability of atrial tissue is associated with atrial stretch in severe cardiac disease (Figs 32.13 and 32.14B).
- They can also be associated with primary myocardial damage (myocarditis), systemic disease and electrolyte and acid–base derangement.
- Electrocardiographic examination is required for a definitive diagnosis.
- Electrocardiographic monitoring during appropriate exercise will be required to assess the effects of changes in autonomic tone and to determine the effect, if any, of the arrhythmia on performance.
- Five or more consecutive atrial premature beats constitute atrial tachycardia.
- Frequent atrial ectopy increases the risk for development of atrial fibrillation, or more rarely atrial flutter.

Recognition

History

Supraventricular premature beats are usually detected incidentally during cardiac auscultation or palpation of arterial pulses in otherwise normal horses. Occasional isolated supraventricular premature beats at rest, during exercise or recovery were frequently found in healthy Thoroughbreds, jumping and dressage horses.[71–73] Most premature beats occurred at low heart rates and their total number was low. Supraventricular premature beats can also be detected in association with myocardial inflammation or, more commonly, severe cardiac disease that has resulted in atrial dilation, e.g. atrioventricular valve disease, large ventricular septal defect. Supraventricular arrhythmia can also accompany systemic disease or any condition that modifies autonomic tone and alters electrolyte and acid–base status.

Physical examination

Isolated cardiac contractions are noted to follow too early in an otherwise normal rhythm during cardiac auscultation, or pulse palpation. The first heart sound of the premature beat usually has a normal or decreased intensity. During supraventricular tachycardia, a fast regular rhythm might be noted by auscultation.

Special examination

A definitive diagnosis and the origin of all ectopic complexes must be determined by electrocardiography (Figs 32.22 and 32.23A). Premature P′ waves appear on the ECG and might be abnormal or normal in morphology (depending on the site of origin) (Fig. 32.23A). Occasionally the premature P′ wave will be buried in the preceding T wave and can be difficult to locate (Fig. 32.22). Depending on the prematurity, the P′ is followed (Fig. 32.22) (close to normal PQ interval) or not followed (Fig. 32.23) by a QRS complex that has a normal morphology and duration. Usually, the supraventricular premature depolarization resets the 'clock' of the sinus node, resulting in a non-compensatory pause, although one should be aware that this is not invariably the case. On rare occasions the supraventricular ectopic beat arises at the atrioventricular node, resulting in a premature QRS complex with normal morphology without a preceding P wave.

In horses with isolated atrial premature beats without underlying disease, an electrocardiogram during appropriate ridden exercise will be required to assess the effect of exertion upon the arrhythmia and to evaluate its effect on athletic performance (Fig. 32.23A–C)

Other tests

In all cases of persistent supraventricular ectopic activity in horses, thorough evaluation of electrolyte status and assessment of other body systems should precede expensive specialized cardiac examinations.

Laboratory analysis of blood samples for concentrations of cardiac troponin I can be useful to assess active myocardial necrosis and inflammation.

Echocardiography is also used to rule out cardiac chamber enlargement, major structural lesions and abnormal wall motion suggestive of previous myocardial damage. In the majority of cases the results of all these examinations are unremarkable, or equivocal.

Treatment and prognosis

Therapeutic aim

It is a general rule that an arrhythmia should always be considered in the context of the horse's concurrent disease. Treatment of an atrial rhythm disturbance is only warranted when there is obvious decrement to cardiac function as a result of the abnormal rhythm, or if the rhythm is likely to degenerate into a more sinister life-threatening arrhythmia, a situation that is unlikely for most atrial dysrhythmias. In selected cases, antiarrhythmic therapy can be used for suppression of an ectopic focus when trying to prevent initiation or recurrence of atrial fibrillation.

As isolated atrial premature beats are not infrequently encountered in performance horses, they present a dilemma to the veterinarian. Usually specific anti-arrhythmic treatment is not indicated, as the premature beats are too infrequent to significantly affect cardiac output at rest. Clearly in these animals it is important to establish what happens to heart rhythm during exercise. In many cases when sinus rate exceeds the firing rate of the single ectopic focus, there is overdrive suppression of the ectopic focus and cardiac rhythm is normal (Fig. 32.23A–C). However, it is important to be aware of the fact that atrial premature beats can easily be obscured by ventricular complexes and artifacts during exercise and the automated analysis software of digital ECG recorders will often fail to detect them when heart rate exceeds 180 bpm, even if a low detection limit of 10% or less is used.

Therapy

It has been suggested that atrial arrhythmias due to confirmed or suspected non-infectious myocardial disease can respond to treatment with anti-inflammatory agents (dexamethasone 0.02–0.2 mg/kg) and rest. However the efficacy of this treatment is not proven and a period of rest alone (2–3 months) can also result in resolution of the arrhythmia. We have also used oral prednisolone therapy in some cases. This treatment's efficacy is not proven either, but seems to be well tolerated. Our usual regimen for a 500-kg horse is 500 mg prednisolone, orally, once daily for 4–7 days, 250 mg prednisolone daily for 4–7 days, and then 100 mg prednisolone daily for 4–7 days. Anecdotal data suggest that oral sotalol can be efficacious in suppression of ectopy. However, to date, the administered

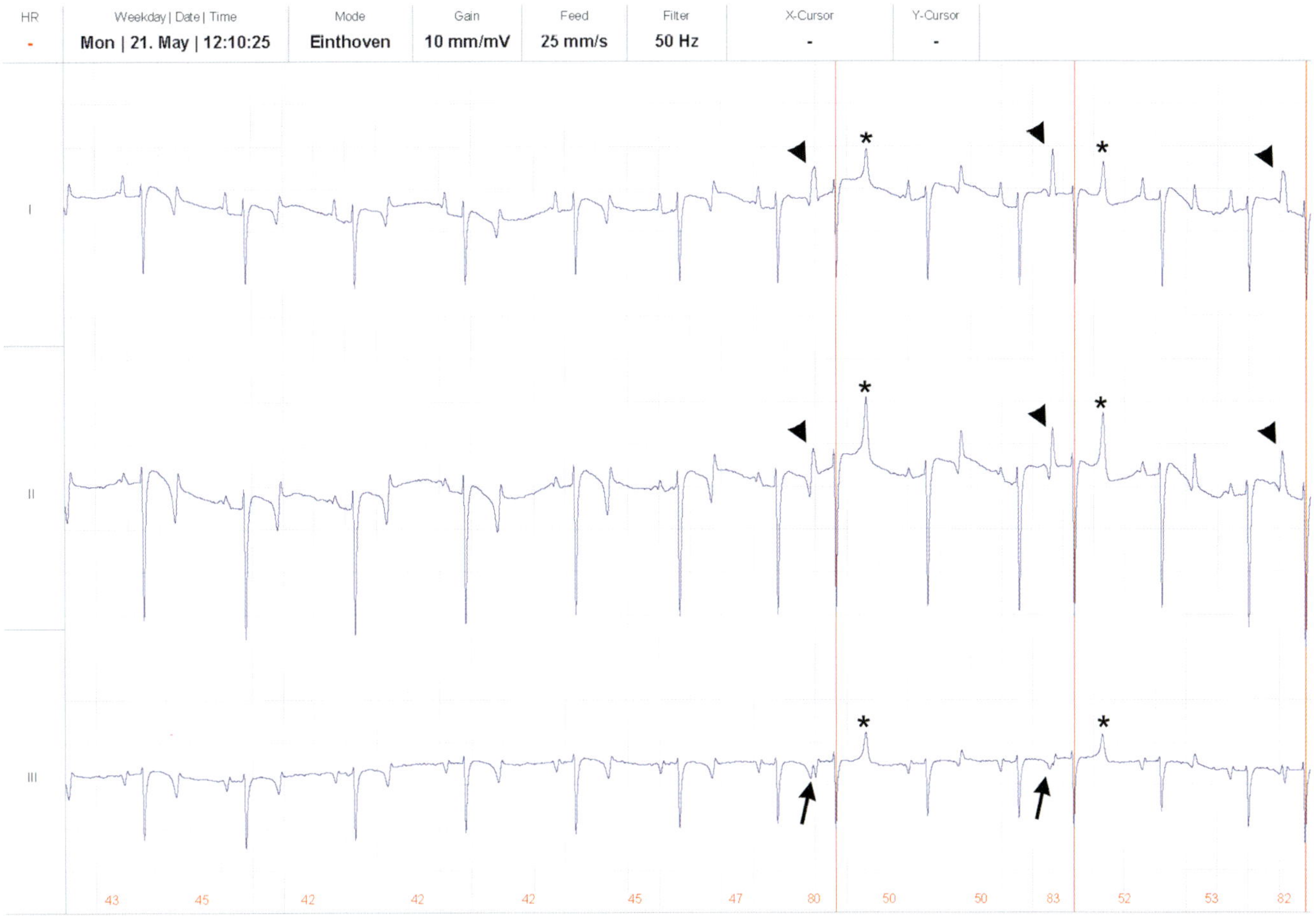

Fig 32.22 Atrial premature beats in five-year-old Warmblood. The cardiac rhythm is broken by QRS complexes of normal morphology and width, that appear too early as indicated by red markers. Their origin is not immediately obvious, as discrete associated ectopic P' waves (arrows) are difficult to discern because of their close proximity to the preceding T wave. Closer inspection of those T waves (arrowheads) reveals them to be subtly different from the sinus T waves, suggesting that they also contain a P' wave. The P'R interval that precedes the ectopic beat is normal. Note that in this horse the T wave following the atrial premature beat (asterisk) is opposite to the QRS complex and therefore also different from the sinus T waves because of the short RR interval that results in altered repolarization (see also Fig. 32.7). Electrodes are positioned as described in Fig. 32.3.

dose is empirical and there are no data available on pharmacokinetics or safety.

Prognosis

The prognosis for horses with atrial prematurity in absence of cardiac disease is good. In these horses, the arrhythmia is only rarely associated with poor performance and although there is a theoretical increased risk of atrial fibrillation developing in affected horses, this complication is predominantly seen in large horses with a high burden of ectopy. Usually the horses remain in full work and competition, the arrhythmia either resolve, or is evident at each subsequent examination. When the arrhythmia is associated with laboratory or echocardiographic evidence of myocarditis or atrial enlargement and fibrosis, the prognosis is more guarded, although a percentage of affected animals will return to athletic performance following rest, steroid therapy, or the combination. When supraventricular arrhythmia is associated with severe cardiac disease, the prognosis is poor and the likelihood of atrial fibrillation developing is high.

Etiology and pathophysiology

Specific information regarding the etiology of supraventricular ectopic beats in horses is lacking, but based on data from other species, the condition is associated with cardiac disease resulting in atrial dilation, stretch and hypoxia. In absence of specific cardiac pathology, electrolyte abnormalities alter atrial myocyte automaticity and coupled with alterations in autonomic balance, promote ectopic activity and dysrhythmias in other species. In horses, it has been suggested that the ectopic foci come from areas of local ischemia in the atria that provide the physiological substrate for increased automaticity as the myocytes become hypoxic and die. Indeed areas of diffuse and focal fibrosis are common in the equine myocardium at post mortem examination.[74,75] The precise etiology of the lesions is unknown, but the hypothesis that they are important in the pathogenesis of atrial arrhythmia is supported by a case report[76] which identified areas of myocytolysis and replacement with fibrous tissue in the atrial myocardium of a Quarter Horse with multiple atrial dysrhythmias.

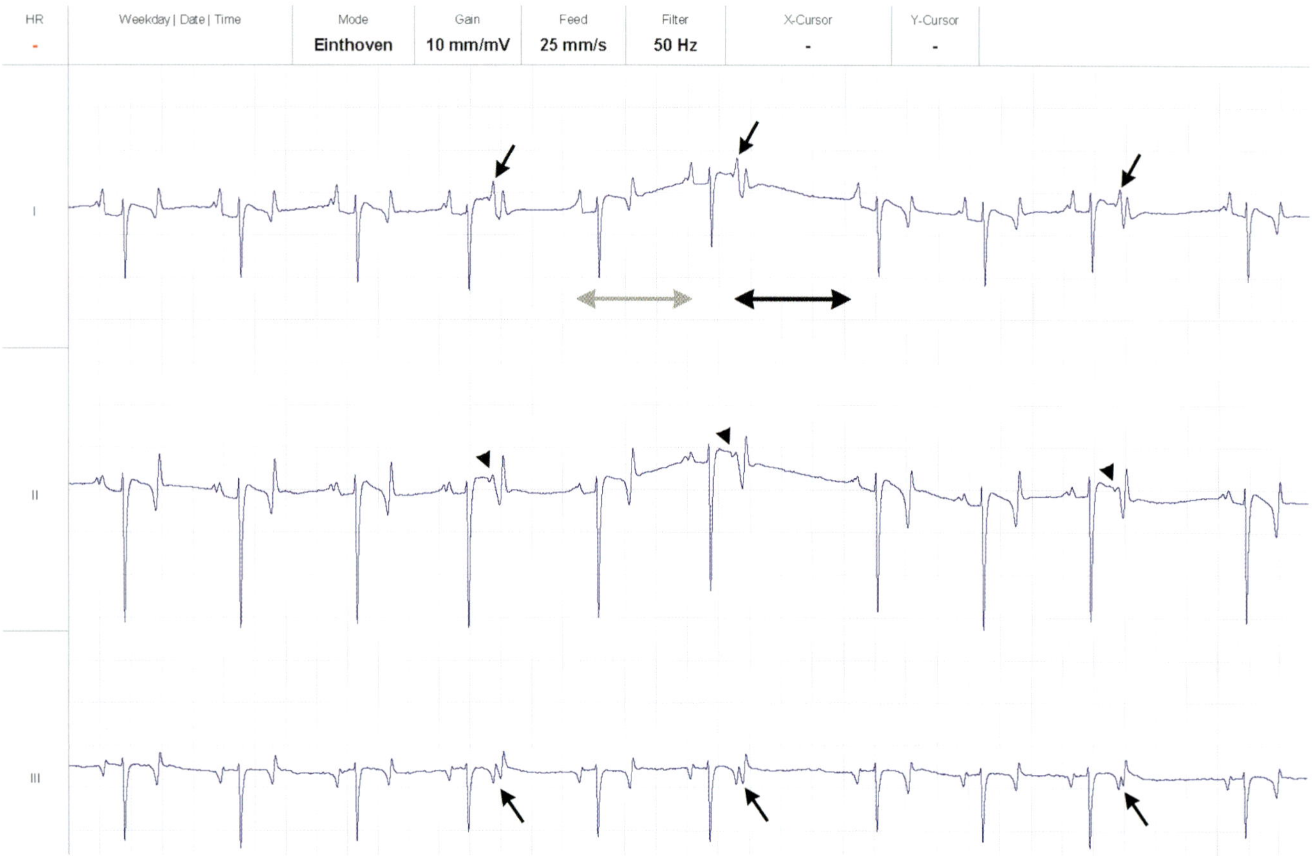

Fig 32.23A Atrial premature beats in a five-year-old trotter with normal performance, detected during routine clinical examination. Note that three premature P' waves (arrows) are partially buried in the preceding T wave, which makes them more difficult to spot, especially on the second lead (arrowheads). Because P' appears during the T wave, the atrioventricular node and ventricle are still refractory: there is no conduction to the ventricle and therefore no QRS complex. The distance from P' to the next normal P (black horizontal arrow) is approximately the same as the normal PP interval (grey horizontal arrow). As a result, and seemingly contradictory, the RR interval for this premature arrhythmia is prolonged, not shortened. Electrodes are positioned as described in Fig. 32.3.

Ventricular premature depolarizations

- Ventricular premature beats arise from tissue below the level of the atrioventricular junction, i.e. the ventricular myocardium (Figs 32-4-32.6).
- Five or more consecutive ventricular premature beats constitute ventricular tachycardia, a rapid and potentially life-threatening rhythm that can lead to ventricular fibrillation and death.
- If five or more consecutive ventricular premature beats occur (a rate that is similar, but just slightly faster, than the prevailing sinus rate), the rhythm is more correctly described as an accelerated ventricular rhythm.
- The importance and underlying etiology of ventricular premature beats in horses are not well understood, although in common with other species, increased excitability of equine ventricular myocardium is associated with ventricular dilation and myocardial hypoxia, inflammation or necrosis.
- In horses ventricular premature beats are most often associated with disease of other body systems, electrolyte and acid–base derangement, toxicoses or aortic regurgitation.[20]
- Ventricular premature beats occur commonly in the early cardiac slowing period after maximal and near-maximal exercise in athletic horses when their presence rarely indicates cardiac disease (Fig. 32.26).
- Because of the possibility of life-threatening ventricular tachycardia developing during exercise, horses with ventricular premature beats at rest should be retired from ridden work until thorough systemic and cardiovascular examinations can be performed.

Recognition

History

Ventricular premature beats are usually detected incidentally during cardiac auscultation or palpation of arterial pulses in otherwise normal horses. Ventricular premature beats at rest, during exercise or recovery were frequently found in healthy Thoroughbreds and dressage horses but their total number was low.[73,77] They can be detected in association with severe cardiac disease that has resulted in ventricular dilation, e.g. aortic valve disease, myocardial inflammation, e.g. myocarditis or toxicosis, or during disruption of the normal intracardiac conduction system, e.g. intra-interventricular septal rupture of an aortic root aneurysm.[78] Ventricular arrhythmia can also accompany systemic disease[21] or extreme exertion,[79] and any other conditions that modify autonomic tone, induce hypoxia and alter electrolyte and acid–base status.[20]

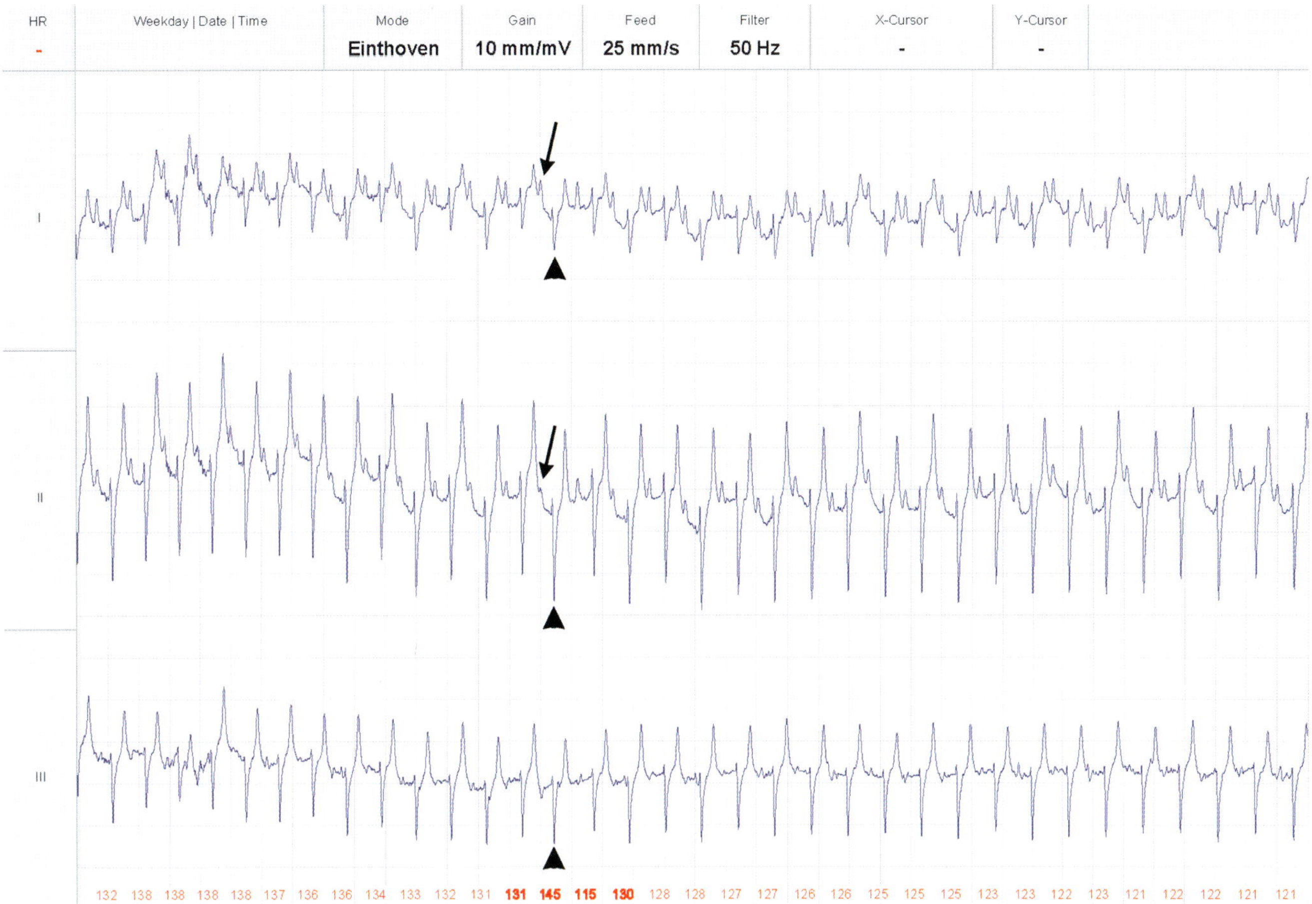

Fig 32.23B Same horse as in Fig. 32.23A. On mild exercise the ectopic focus was predominantly overridden, with only a rare atrial premature beat at this heart rate of 130 bpm, as shown in this figure. P waves can still be identified. On one occasion, a shortened RR interval with normal QRS morphology appears (arrowhead). Close inspection reveals a premature P wave (arrows), partially buried in the preceding T wave. Therefore the premature beat is atrial in origin.

Isolated and multiple ventricular ectopic beats are commonly detected in horses during the immediate early slowing period after maximal exercise.[80,81] They rarely seem to be associated with primary cardiac disease and probably should not be over-interpreted when they appear only at this time. In race-fit Standardbreds, isolated ventricular premature beats and short episodes of polymorphic ventricular tachycardia occurred in 11.6% and 15.9% of the cases and were often associated with sudden cardiac slowing after exercise.[80] The reason for ectopy might be that during exercise the increase in catecholamines counteracts the harmful effects of acidosis and hyperkalaemia and vice versa. After cessation of exercise, potassium levels drop while catecholamine concentrations remain high, making the heart more vulnerable for arrhythmias.[82] If ventricular ectopic beats occur at a high frequency during work, the situation is quite different and an underlying cause should be sought and treated if possible. In the meantime the horse should probably be retired from ridden work because the risk of ventricular fibrillation is a significant danger to both horse and rider.

In general, when considering ventricular ectopic beats in horses, *'judge them according to the company they keep'.*

Physical examination

Ventricular premature beats are usually detected incidentally during cardiac auscultation or palpation of arterial pulses, when they can be difficult to distinguish from supraventricular premature beats. Depending on their proximity to the previous conducted beat, they can be associated with a louder first heart sound or a palpable pulse deficit. Isolated cardiac contractions are noted to follow too early in an otherwise normal rhythm and are usually followed by an obvious compensatory pause that might help to distinguish them from atrial premature contractions.

During sustained ventricular tachycardia, a fast (usually in excess of 100 bpm) regular rhythm will be noted by auscultation. At very high rates, aortic valve opening can not occur for every ventricular depolarization, rendering the heart sounds and the rhythm irregular at auscultation. Horses with sustained ventricular tachycardia (e.g. 150 bpm or more) eventually develop biventricular heart failure and will often develop jugular pulsations, ventral edema and even ascites within 1–3 days.

Special examination

A definitive diagnosis and the origin of the ectopic complexes can be determined by electrocardiography. When the complexes are ventricular in origin, one or more premature complexes with a (sometimes slightly) abnormal QRS morphology will break the regular cardiac rhythm. Although QRS morphology can vary, these complexes are always dissociated from normal sinus activity. The sinus node continues to fire at its normal rate, since the atria are

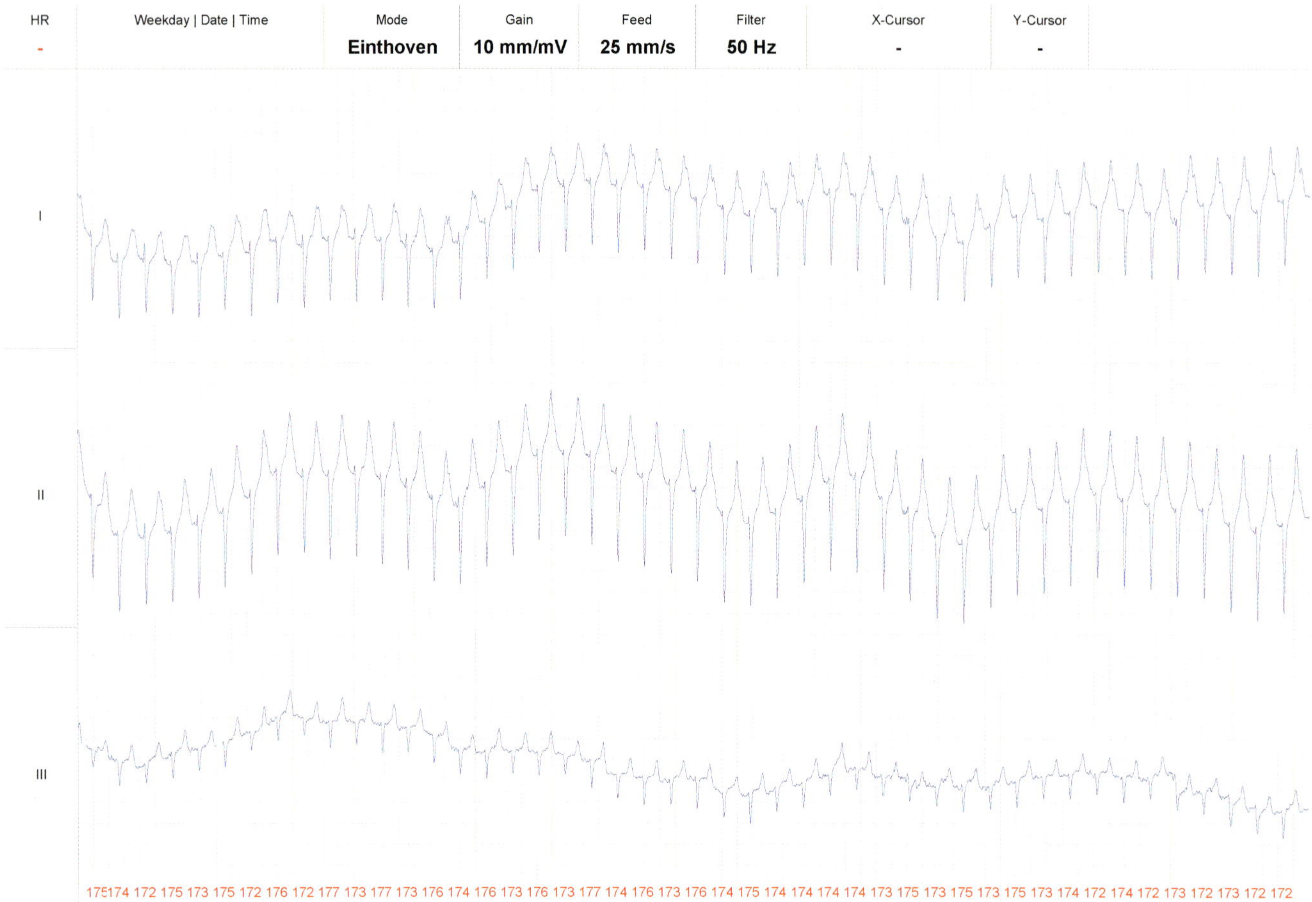

Fig 32.23C Same horse as in Fig. 32.23A and Fig. 32.23B. At higher heart rates (HR = 176) the P wave becomes increasingly difficult to discern, as it is now buried in the preceding T wave, but the RR interval is absolutely regular. There is thus no evidence that the atrial arrhythmia present should be affecting performance in this individual. Cardiac troponin I was normal. The condition was not treated and the horse continued to race successfully.

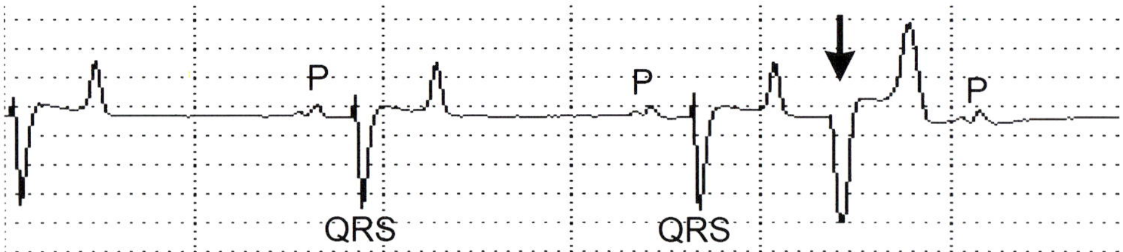

Fig 32.24A Base-apex ECG obtained from a nine-year-old Thoroughbred racehorse with an arrhythmia at rest. A wide bizarre complex occurs after the third sinus beat (arrow). The bizarre shape of the premature QRS complex suggests a ventricular origin and this is confirmed by the presence of the dissociated sinus P wave that follows at the normal sinus rate. Atrioventricular (AV) dissociation is another hallmark of ventricular prematurity. The sinus P wave follows as normal, but is not conducted to the ventricles, as they remain refractory due to the premature beat. In cases like this it is important to determine the effect of exercise on the ectopic focus and cardiac rhythm. In this case treadmill exercise was used.

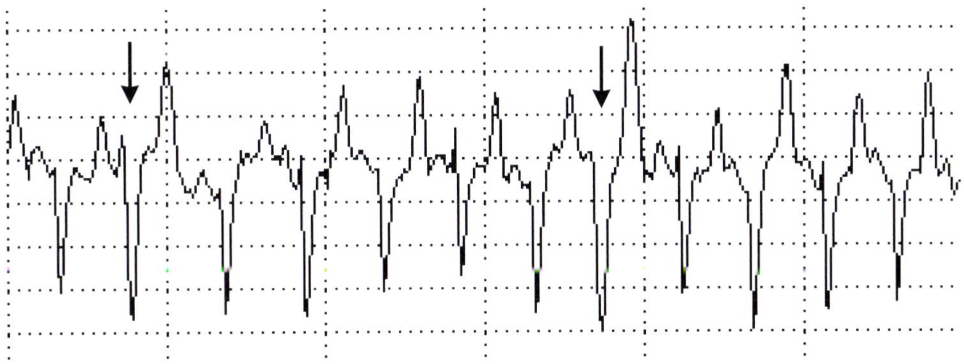

Fig 32.24B Base-apex ECG from the same horse during trot. Note the increased sinus rate (heart rate 120). Two premature beats occur (arrows), which have a slightly different conformation and are slightly wider, suggesting a ventricular origin. There is still AV dissociation, but as sinus rate has increased the P wave is just visible at the start of the QRS complex of the premature beat.

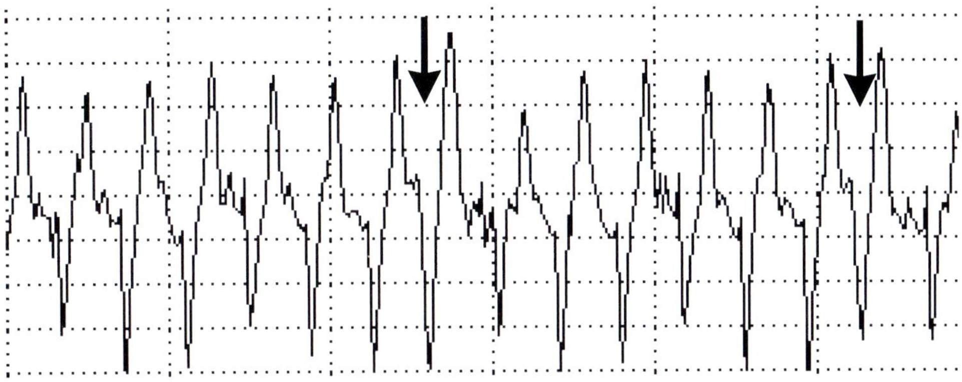

Fig 32.24C As in Figs 32.24A and B, the ventricular prematurity continues (arrows) during hack canter at 10 m/s.

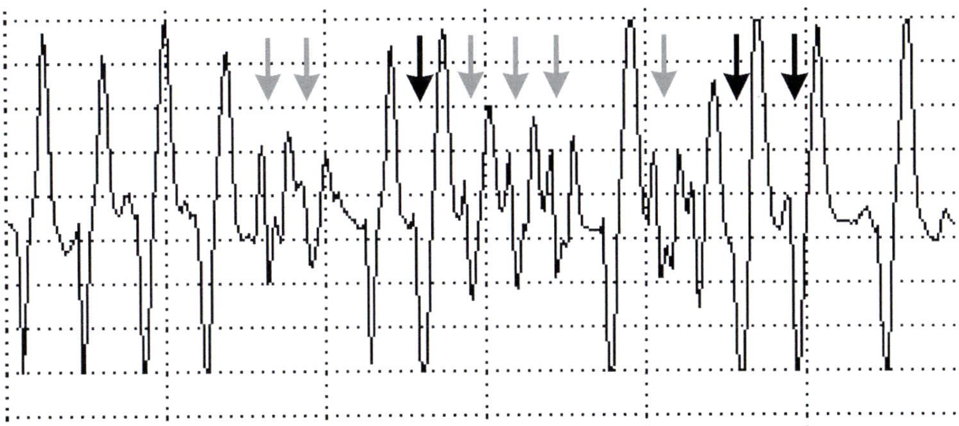

Fig 32.24D Base-apex ECG from the horse in Fig. 32.24A–C 30 seconds after exercise to fatigue. Although ectopic beats are common in the early recovery period after exercise in athletic horses (see Fig. 32.25), this horse suffered multiple sustained runs of ventricular prematurity. Note that ventricular premature beats of different morphology (black and gray arrows) are present, suggesting that ectopy occurs at different sites in the ventricular myocardium. This horse was rested for three months and repeat exercise testing showed the ectopic focus to have resolved. The horse returned to full competition.

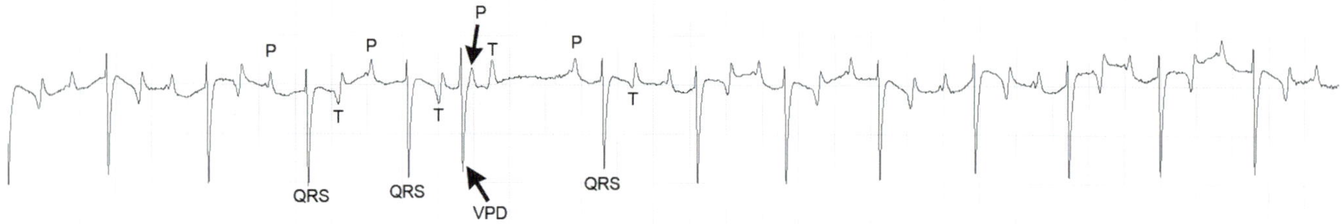

Fig 32.25 Junctional ventricular ectopic beats in a horse presented with poor performance.

The normal rhythm is broken by a ventricular premature depolarization (VPD) with a morphology that is only slightly different from the normal sinus beats (QRS). Within the QT interval of the VPD a P wave can be identified (P wave indicated by arrow) because the normal sinus rhythm is not interrupted. The P wave does not result in a QRS complex as the ventricle is still refractory. This atrioventricular dissociation is a hallmark of ventricular prematurity. Although the complex is not noticeably wider than the sinus beats, it is still ventricular in origin. Its configuration suggests that it originates from the atrioventricular junctional, or His-Purkinje system and has been conducted using (part of) the normal conduction pathways. Note that the T wave preceding the VPD is exactly the same as the other sinus T waves, so that an ectopic P' wave could not have been hidden within it (compare with Fig. 32.22).

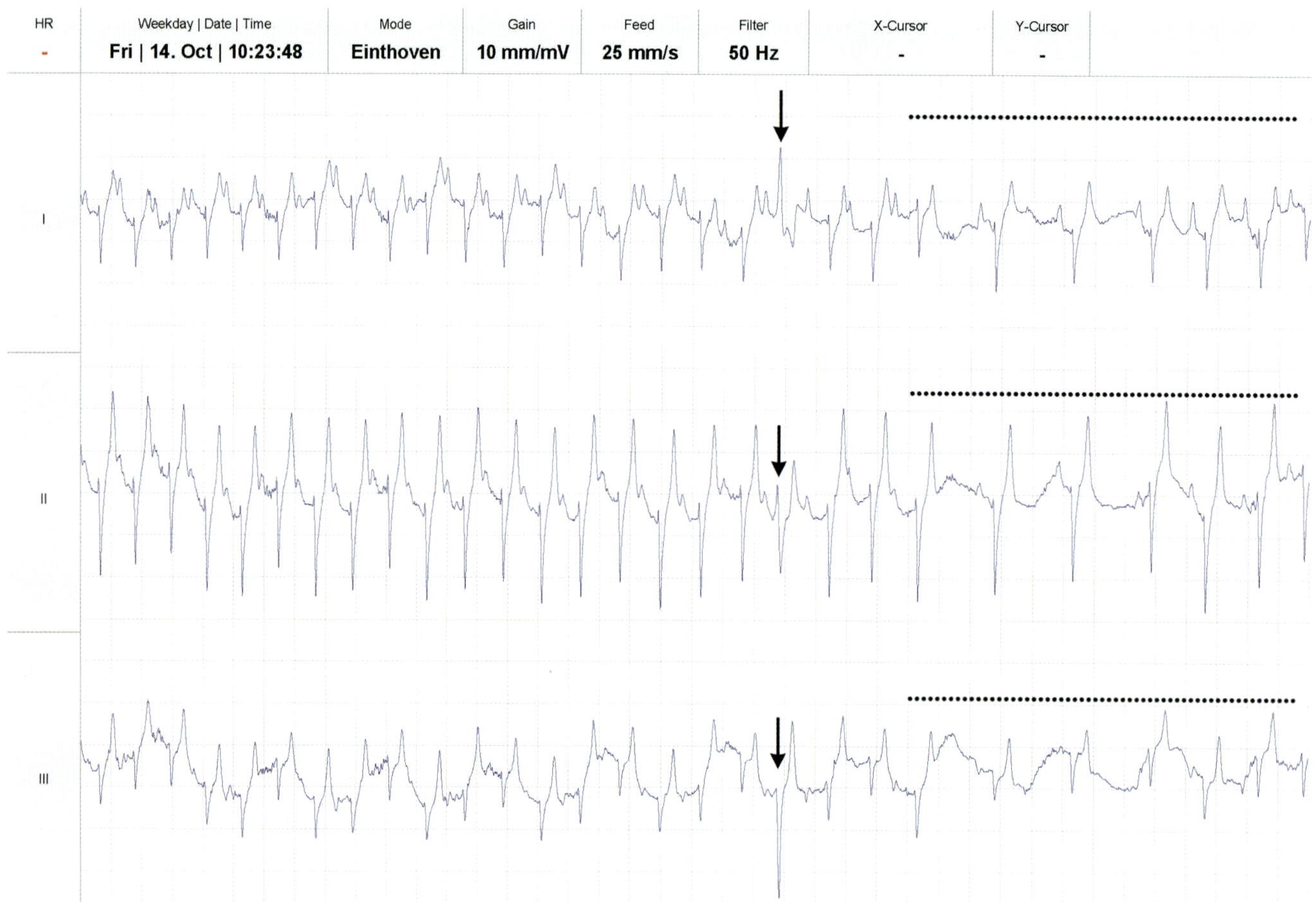

Fig 32.26 The difficulty of interpretation of post exercise ventricular ectopy is illustrated by the trace obtained from a horse during recovery from work at home. The horse worked only at 3/4 pace. This rhythm shows a ventricular ectopic beat. In this case the abnormal complex is not unduly wider than the normal sinus beats. This finding is not uncommon in horses. A definite diagnosis of a ventricular origin is possible however: the complex has a different morphology, a shortened PQ interval and is followed by a compensatory pause. At the end of the ECG (dotted line) sinus arrhythmia is present, characterized by normal P–QRS relation and morphology and gradual change in sinus rate. This recording was taken from an eight-year-old National Hunt horse, highly rated in the National Hunt racehorses in the UK. The trace was recorded two weeks after the horse had won a race and one week before finishing second in another race. The ECG was taken during normal work at home on a 'slow' day. There was no history of poor performance. The horse lost his place in the second race after jumping badly. There was no evidence of cardiorespiratory or other systemic disease in this individual.

electrically isolated from the ventricles and the site of ectopic activity (Figs 32.24A and 32.25). Therefore, the ventricular premature beat will usually be followed by a noticeable compensatory pause. If the premature beat originates in the ventricular myocardium, remote from the normal His-Purkinje system, it will have a wide and bizarre configuration (Figs 32.24A and 32.26). In contrast, if it arises from close to the atrioventricular junctional tissue or the His-Purkinje system, the QRS complex can differ only slightly from the normal sinus beats (Fig. 32.25). In this case, the premature impulse is still largely conducted through the ventricle using part of the normal conduction pathways and therefore it is only slightly altered in shape and might be normal in duration. A ventricular premature beat that occurs at (almost) the same time as the normal QRS can result in a 'fusion beat' with a bizarre morphology that is a mixture of the normal and abnormal QRS. At high heart rates, there is a physiologic shortening of the QRS complex, such that the QRS duration of ventricular premature beats or ventricular tachycardia at high rates will often not exceed the reference values reported in the equine literature.

Presence of multiple abnormal QRS morphologies indicates multiple ectopic foci and more severe cardiac or underlying disease.

Other tests

In all cases of persistent ventricular ectopic activity in horses, thorough evaluation of electrolyte status and assessment of other body systems should precede expensive specialized cardiac examinations. Although diseases such as Lyme disease, babesiosis, leptospirosis, influenza and atypical myopathy,[83,84] can be associated with ventricular arrhythmia in some individuals, their precise effects on the equine heart remain poorly understood.

Laboratory determination of plasma or serum concentrations of cardiac troponin I might be useful to assess active myocardial inflammation and necrosis. In rare cases where intoxication with cardiac glycosides is considered, determination of plasma digoxin concentrations can be useful. One should be aware that digoxin levels due to plant poisoning (e.g. oleander) can be at or below therapeutic level as only a small proportion of the numerous cardiac glycosides from the plant is captured by the assay.[85]

Echocardiography is also used to rule out cardiac chamber enlargement, structural abnormalities and abnormal wall motion suggestive of myocardial damage. The results of all these examinations can be unremarkable or equivocal.

Treatment and prognosis

Therapeutic aim

The therapeutic aims are to treat the underlying disease process, restore normal electrolyte and acid–base status, return the heart to normal sinus rhythm if the ventricular rhythm disturbance is life threatening, and abolish abnormal ventricular automaticity.

Therapy

It is a general rule that an arrhythmia should always be considered in the context of the horse's concurrent disease. Premature depolarizations are usually associated with hypoxia, myocardial disease, electrolyte and metabolic disturbances, elevated sympathetic tone, fever and toxemia. Therefore the first therapeutic aim is to treat any of the predisposing disorders rather than the arrhythmia per se.

Treatment of a ventricular rhythm disturbance with antiarrhythmic agents is only warranted when there is obvious decrement to cardiac function as a result of the abnormal rhythm, or if the rhythm is likely to degenerate into a more sinister life-threatening arrhythmia (ventricular fibrillation). This scenario is most likely to occur during general anesthesia, the postoperative period, or during generalized sickness. The class 1B, fast sodium channel blocker lidocaine is generally accepted to be the drug of choice for treatment and management of ventricular arrhythmia in this context.[59] In unresponsive cases, IV administration of magnesium sulfate and other drugs such as quinidine gluconate, amiodarone, procainamide, propafenone and phenytoin have been suggested. Intracardiac (biventricular) electrical cardioversion has been applied successfully in one case of drug-refractory ventricular tachycardia (G. van Loon, unpublished data).

Specific anti-arrhythmic treatment for ventricular ectopic beats in performance horses is usually not indicated, as they are too infrequent to significantly affect cardiac output at rest. However ventricular ectopic beats can be the only abnormal finding in horses presented for poor or loss of performance when their significance is much more perplexing. In most cases the ectopic beats do not occur with sufficient frequency during exercise to significantly compromise cardiac output (Fig. 32.24A–D), yet despite extensive investigations, no other cause of poor performance can be established. It seems possible that increased ventricular automaticity reflects myocardial cellular damage or is a marker of subtle damage to other elements of the oxygen transfer chain that, in themselves, are responsible for reduced aerobic capacity and performance limitation. The precise nature of the insult and its etiology are unknown and further studies of affected horses are clearly required. However, clinical experience and anecdotal evidence suggest that a clinical syndrome of poor performance associated with ventricular ectopy and reduced heart rate recovery following fast exercise exists in Thoroughbred racehorses in the UK. Usually biochemical markers of myocardial damage (cardiac troponin I) are not significantly elevated at the time horses are presented. There is usually no specific indication to treat the arrhythmia, so treatment is usually empirical and includes rest with, or without, steroid therapy (see therapy of supraventricular premature beats).

Prognosis

The prognosis for ventricular prematurity and ventricular dysrhythmia is dependent upon the severity of the underlying disease. When the arrhythmia is associated with laboratory or echocardiographic evidence of myocarditis, the prognosis is guarded or poor. The time course or likelihood of resolution of ventricular ectopy in otherwise asymptomatic horses presenting with poor performance is impossible to predict, although a percentage of such horses do return to their previous athletic performance following protracted rest, steroid therapy or both.

Ventricular ectopic beats that occur only in recovery from fast exercise are not usually regarded as having any clinical significance, but they could be of importance in the etiology of sudden cardiac death (Fig. 32.26).[86]

Etiology and pathophysiology

Specific information regarding the etiology of ventricular ectopic beats in horses is lacking, but based on data from other species, increased automaticity of ventricular myocytes is associated with cardiac disease resulting in ventricular dilation, stretch and hypoxia. In the absence of primary cardiac pathology, electrolyte abnormalities, hypoxia, toxins and alterations in acid–base status can provide the physiological substrates for increased myocyte and pacemaker irritability and invoke re-entry.[87]

It has been suggested that isolated ventricular ectopic beats emanate from ischemic foci that provide the physiological substrates for increased ventricular automaticity during myocyte death. There is circumstantial evidence to support this hypothesis, as areas of focal fibrosis are common in the equine myocardium at post mortem examination.[74,75,88] The precise etiology of these lesions is unknown, although small coronary artery occlusion by arterial atherosclerosis has been proposed as a possible underlying cause.[88,89] There is a significant association between the occurrence of proximal aortic *Strongylus vulgaris* lesions and the presence of focal ischemic lesions in the myocardium.[88] They hypothesized that this association was not the result of direct larval damage to the heart but was caused by microembolization from the parasitic lesions in the proximal aorta that caused myocardial obstructive arteriosclerosis. The role of myocardial cell death and ischemia in the etiology of ventricular rhythm disturbances in horses is supported by case reports. Areas of myocytolysis and replacement fibrosis were identified in the ventricular myocardium of horses after fatal ventricular dysrhythmias.[90,91]

Ventricular premature beats and even short runs of ventricular tachycardia are often found in healthy horses immediately after maximal exercise. These dysrhythmias might suddenly deteriorate in ventricular fibrillation which is a fatal condition. The importance of arrhythmias in sudden death in horses is difficult to establish as an ECG recording at the time of death is usually not available. When pulmonary edema, congestion and/or hemorrhage are the only finding, fatal arrhythmia is the most probable etiology because sudden lack of cardiac activity causes a sudden and massive increase in left atrial pressure. Cardiac failure was suspected as the cause of death in 25–56% of racecourse fatalities in a recent multicenter post mortem study.[92]

Bradydysrhythmias

- These include sinus bradycardia and arrest (see Fig. 32.28), second- and third-degree atrioventricular (AV) block (see Fig. 32.29).
- All these rhythms, except third-degree atrioventricular block, are also normal findings in athletic horses, reflecting high resting parasympathetic tone.
- When clinically important, they are characterized by an inappropriately low heart rate and blunted chronotropic responses to exercise, or sympathomimetic agents (atropine)
- Third-degree AV block is rarely diagnosed in athletic horses, but when present it always affects performance and carries a guarded prognosis.

Recognition

History

The usual presenting signs for horses with significant bradydysrhythmias include syncope, ataxia, exercise intolerance and collapse.

Significant cardiac disease can usually be ruled out in horses with a very low resting heart rate or marked arrhythmia at rest, if excitement or exercise restore rate and rhythm to normal.

It is common for a marked arrhythmia to be noticed within a minute of cardiac slowing after fast exercise in athletic horses. This arrhythmia is a normal manifestation of increasing parasympathetic influence and usually occurs when heart rate falls from 150 to 60 bpm. When electrocardiographic examination is performed, the dysrhythmia is usually a marked sinus arrhythmia and it is thus described as transient post-exercise sinus arrhythmia (see Fig. 32.30). The arrhythmia is usually short-lived, but can cause alarm for an inexperienced examiner. Post-exercise sinus arrhythmia is another normal arrhythmia, found commonly in athletic horses, that does not indicate cardiac dysfunction.

Physical examination

In horses affected with significant bradydysrhythmia, auscultation usually reveals an inappropriately slow resting heart rate that can be regular. Resting heart rate can be less than 20 bpm.

Occasionally horses present with evidence of unexplained trauma when collapse occurs at night, or is not observed.

During severe second-degree AV block, one or more isolated fourth (atrial) heart sounds, S_4, will be audible during the long diastolic pauses. In sinus block, S_4 will be absent and the diastolic pauses silent. In third-degree AV block, S_4 can be audible in a regular fast rhythm underlying the predominant slow ventricular rhythm. In third-degree AV block pronounced waves, 'cannon a waves', that travel rapidly all the way up the jugular vein are also obvious. Increased atrial pressure causes the augmented waves as the atria contract against the closed tricuspid valve. Horses with profound bradycardia often keep their head low and lifting the head can sometimes elicit collapse. Collapse usually last for seconds (to minutes), after which the horse immediately stands up.

Special tests

Electrocardiography will provide a definitive diagnosis (Figs 32.27–33.30). For third-degree atrioventricular block P waves generally occur at increased rate (50–95 per minute) but have no relation to the slower ventricular rate. QRS complexes have a normal (atrioventricular nodal or His bundle origin) or abnormal (ventricular myocardial origin) morphology and duration and occur at regular or irregular intervals. Ideally, 24-hour ambulatory ECG monitoring (Holter) should be employed for a definitive diagnosis in cases of collapse. Affected cases often have blunted chronotropic responses to both exercise and parasympatholytic agents, but these tests are frequently difficult to interpret.

Plasma concentrations of cardiac troponin I are useful to detect active myocardial damage. Development of congestive heart failure often results in mildly increased plasma activity of gamma-glutamyl transferase.

Treatment and prognosis

Therapeutic aims

Aims are restore normal sinus rhythm, normal heart rate at rest and to normalize heart rate response to exercise.

Therapy

Clinically important sinus bradycardia is found most commonly in elderly performance horses. Occasionally horses affected with profound second-degree AV block and sinus bradycardia respond favorably to daily oral administration of β_2-adrenoreceptor agonist drugs, e.g. clenbuterol.

Third-degree AV block is very rare in horses, and is rarely amenable to medical treatment. In most species with third-degree AV block, permanent and transvenous pacing is required for permanent relief of clinical signs. A standardized technique for temporary pacing[93] and dual chamber pacemaker implantation has been described[94] and successfully applied in clinical cases.[16,95] The technique has also been used successfully to allow horses to return to competition.[16,95] Successful pacing for more than 10 years has been achieved in horses (G. van Loon, unpublished results)

On rare occasions, third-degree AV block can be transient and normal sinus activity can resume after variable periods of time elapse. It seems likely that in these cases, a reversible inflammatory process causes transient complete block at the AV junction. Based on this unproven hypothesis, use of corticosteroid drugs is sometimes recommended for these individuals.[31]

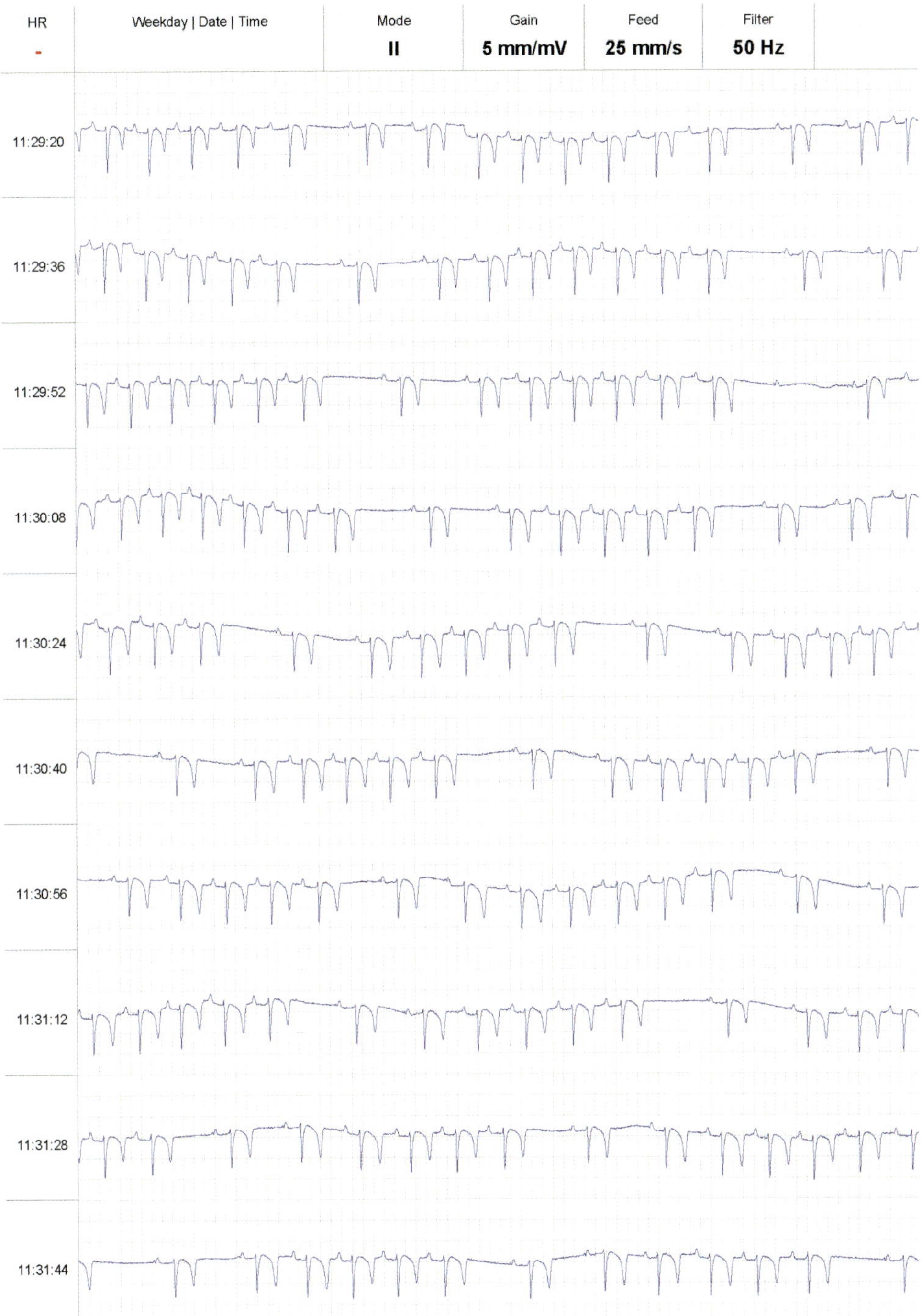

Fig 32.27A Sustained base-apex ECG recording at rest from a two-year-old colt presented for poor performance. Atrial fibrillation was suspected during cardiac auscultation. The summary trace shows that the arrhythmia is caused by apparent variations in sinus firing rate (sinus arrhythmia) and second-degree atrioventricular block. Close inspection of the trace reveals that P waves precede each QRS complexes.

Prognosis

In all cases of symptomatic bradyarrhythmia, the prognosis is guarded to poor. In some horses the condition can be transient and reversible and these horses return to their previous levels of activity. Transvenous pacing carries a fair prognosis for return to certain athletic performance, but as in all species, the technique can be associated with complications.[96] One should be aware that fully pacemaker-dependent horses cannot achieve heart rates higher than 180 bpm due to the technical specifications of the device. Furthermore, ventricular contractile function during ventricular pacing is lower than when the rhythm originates from above the atrioventricular node. Consequently, ventricular pacemaker-dependent horses are unlikely to be able to compete successfully in aerobically demanding sports.

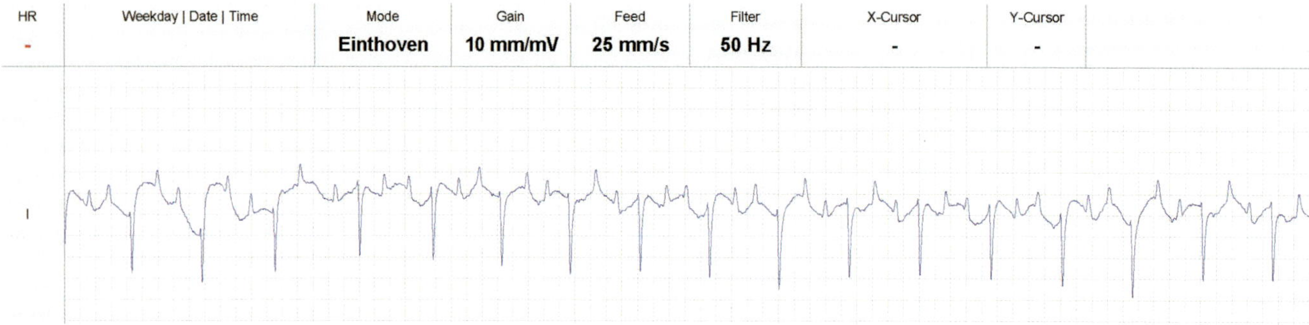

Fig 32.27B Same horse as in Fig. 32.27A. Excitement or exercise rapidly restored the rhythm to normal. Heart rate and rhythm during fast exercise were also normal. Treadmill exercise testing revealed the colt to have dynamic airflow obstruction caused by dorsal displacement of the soft palate.

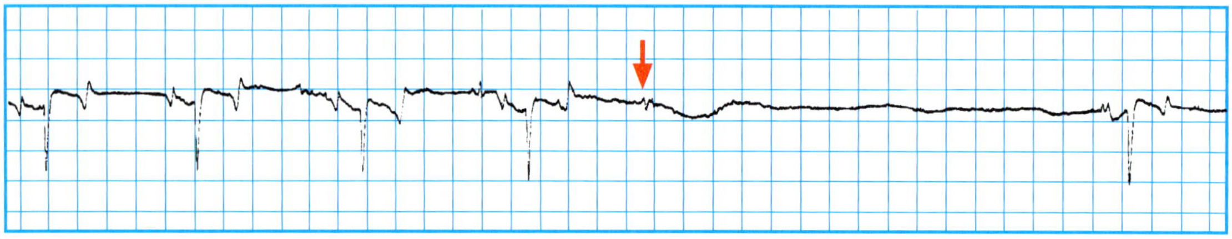

Fig 32.28 Sinus arrest and second-degree block in a 14-year-old endurance horse. One non-conducted 'P' wave (red arrow) is visible during the long pause followed by complete sinus arrest. There is a total absence of ventricular escape activity. The clinical history that follows is fairly typical. The horse initially presented with traumatic uveitis. Two weeks later she was found with a severely swollen carpus and damage to buckets in the loose box. One week later the horse was observed to collapse by her owner. 24-hour Holter monitoring showed maximum pauses of 10 seconds, but as is frustratingly common in these cases, no collapse occurred during the monitoring period. The horse responded to oral clenbuterol therapy and after a period of six months rest, returned to ridden work. The response to treatment in older animals can be less impressive, possibly because the underlying lesion is advanced disease of the conduction tissues.

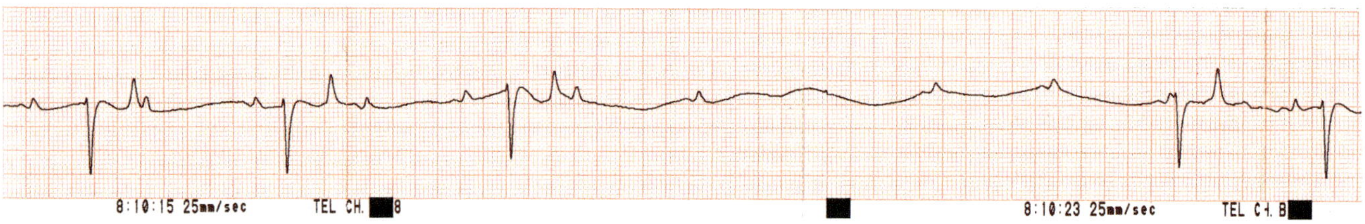

Fig 32.29 Third-degree atrioventricular block in a 15-year-old Grand Prix dressage horse. There is complete atrioventricular dissociation because of third-degree AV block. PQ interval is highly variable because they have no relation; the fourth QRS complex occurs simultaneously with a P wave. Bifid 'P' waves occur at a rapid rate because of associated hypotension. In this case the QRS morphologies are similar but their rate is slow and rhythm is irregular. They are junctional ventricular escape complexes. The gelding presented acutely after multiple episodes of collapse in a single day. The referring veterinarian administered antibiotics and corticosteroids and referred the horse for pacemaker implantation. At presentation, third-degree atrioventricular block was present but ventricular escape rhythm was sufficiently high to prevent collapse. Within 48 hours he reverted to normal sinus rhythm. No pacemaker was implanted. The gelding was closely monitored and returned to dressage after six months. He was retired 2.5 years later because of chronic tendinitis.

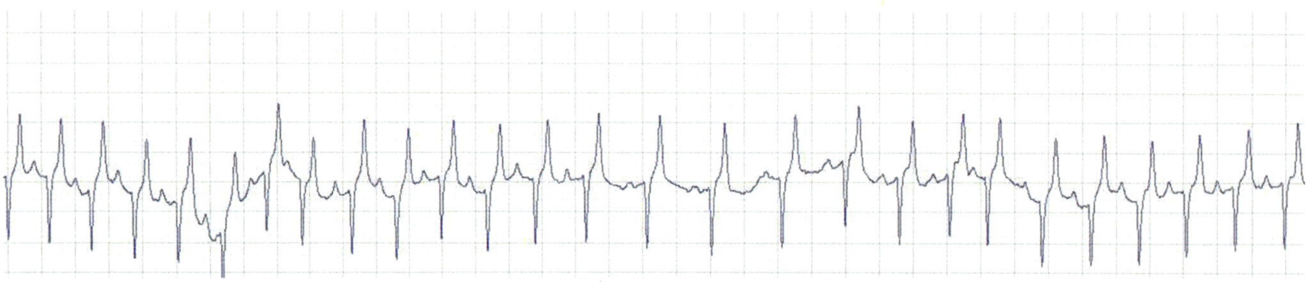

Fig 32.30 Electrocardiographic recording taken from a Thoroughbred racehorse, 20 seconds after completion of exercise to fatigue. There is some baseline interference as the horse is walking and blowing heavily. The rhythm is noticeably irregular but the relation between P waves and QRS complexes is correct. The PP intervals, and also RR intervals, show a progressive increase and decrease (accordion-like variation). The trace illustrates transient post-exercise sinus arrhythmia, which is a common finding in athletic horses following exercise.

Etiology and pathology

In the resting horse most bradydysrhythmias are of no clinical significance, as within limits, cardiac output is maintained by increased stroke volume. The trained horse has an increased resting stroke volume and therefore the resting heart rate is usually low. During exercise however, there is an increased requirement for muscle perfusion, systemic vascular resistance falls and cardiac output must increase in order to maintain arterial blood pressure. As increasing heart rate is the major cause of the increased cardiac output, if low heart rate is maintained during exercise, cardiac output will be inadequate and performance will be limited. Although second-degree AV block is the commonest manifestation of high vagal tone in horses, other bizarre sinus arrhythmias, including sinus block, can occasionally be encountered in normal individuals (Fig. 32.27). Normal heart rate responses to exercise and excitement rule out significant pathology in these individuals.

Pathological sinus, second- and third-degree AV block indicates total or partial block in conduction in the sinus, atria, or AV node. This clearly results from cardiac lesions, thought to be associated with transient or permanent inflammation or degeneration and fibrosis of the intracardiac conduction system.

Epidemiology

Profound sinus bradycardia, pathological second- and third-degree AV block occur only rarely in athletic horses, being much more common in aged animals. Sporadically the condition can be seen in younger horses and is more likely to be transient where it is believed to be associated with inflammation of the conduction system and/or myocardium.

Cardiac murmurs

General principles

This section will cover the basic approach to heart murmurs in athletic horses, their diagnosis, prognosis and assessment of their significance.

A number of murmurs occur in normal horses that are not associated with underlying cardiac disease. These murmurs have been variously called, functional, physiological, innocent or flow murmurs. These murmurs are common in athletic horses of all breeds.

Murmurs associated with mitral and tricuspid valve regurgitation are also commonly detected in performance horses (Table 32.1).[1,2,97]

Although there is no doubt that severe regurgitation, secondary atrial fibrillation and cardiac failure cause performance decrements,[98,99] recent data showed that compensated aortic, mitral and tricuspid valve regurgitation had no negative associations with performance in flat or jump racehorses in the UK.[1,100]

Recent data have shown that atrioventricular (AV) valve regurgitation increases after six months race training in Thoroughbreds[3] and in Standardbred trotters.[101] It seems likely that the eccentric cardiac hypertrophy and increased blood volume that accompany athletic training[102] result in secondary stretch of the valve annulus and increased regurgitation.

Endocarditis is a rare condition causing valvular regurgitation and cardiac murmurs. Blood-borne bacteria colonize the valves (usually mitral and aortic) and the resulting inflammation and deformation leads to chronic regurgitation. *Pasteurella*, *Actinobacillus* and *Streptococcus* species are most likely to be causative in horses,[103] although other agents have also been reported.[104–106] Prognosis is poor, even if the horse survives the early acute phase and bacterial cure is achieved; there can be sufficient damage to the cardiac valves to preclude return to previous performance, or cause death from heart failure.[107]

Physiological murmurs

Systolic ejection murmurs

Systolic ejection murmurs are commonly heard over the pulmonary and aortic valves in normal horses. Usually the murmur is early–mid systolic, crescendo–decrescendo in character, and variable in intensity. Usually these murmurs are heard best over the left hemithorax, cranial over the heart base when S_2 becomes accentuated. Submaximal exercise often increases the intensity of these murmurs. In some horses, and in foals, it can be difficult to separate a functional ejection murmur from a murmur of mitral regurgitation, but an ejection murmur, unlike the murmur of mitral regurgitation, should end before S_2 in the resting horse. Ejection murmurs

Table 32.1 Prevalence of cardiac murmurs by auscultation in two-year-old Thoroughbreds in training

	% OF POPULATION AFFECTED		
MURMUR	YOUNG & WOOD[3]	KRIZ ET AL.[1]	PATTESON & CRIPPS[2]
Mitral regurgitation	21	3.8	1.2
Tricuspid regurgitation	25.5	27.4	4.7
Aortic regurgitation	2	0.5	0
Diastolic flow	65	33	44
Systolic ejection	34	57.4	55
No murmurs	11	18.9	24.7

Note: Patteson and Cripps defined mitral and tricuspid valve regurgitation as pansystolic murmurs only. As it is now generally accepted that murmurs of mitral and tricuspid valve prolapse may not extend throughout systole, this may explain the difference in prevalences of atrioventricular valve regurgitation. Patteson and Cripps also noted a much higher prevalence of systolic murmurs on the left and right hemithorax, suggesting that some early systolic murmurs of mitral and tricuspid valve prolapse were classified as systolic ejection murmurs.

will disappear at maximal heart rates, but the amount of exercise needed to achieve this varies according to the fitness of the horse. Ejection murmurs are equally prevalent in other conditions that provoke high sympathetic tone, e.g. colic, anemia, sepsis, pain or fever, whereupon their duration can be longer. A major feature of all physiological murmurs is their variability with changes in heart rate and or excitement.

Functional diastolic murmurs: diastolic filling murmurs

Most physiological filling murmurs occur either, in early diastole (before S_3), or are pre-systolic (after S_4, but before S_1). The *pre-systolic* murmurs are associated with vibrations in the atria, and are usually low pitched and rumbling. The murmur can be heard on either side of the chest. The *early diastolic murmurs*, closely following S_2, are soft and blowing and are believed to be associated with rapid ventricular filling. They usually end at S_3 and are heard from the left and right hemithorax. An early diastolic musical murmur is not infrequently heard in conditioned horses. This murmur is very variable, and is usually heard best from the mitral or tricuspid valve area. The murmur follows S_2 by a short interval and ends abruptly at S_3. It is commonly known as a *'two-year-old squeak'*, although it is present in athletic horses of all ages. Diastolic murmurs are also very variable, depending on heart rate and excitement.

Murmurs associated with cardiac dysfunction

Tricuspid regurgitation

See Figure 32.31.

Recognition

History

This is usually detected incidentally during cardiac auscultation. Tricuspid regurgitation is unlikely to be a primary cause of poor performance or heart failure.

A murmur of tricuspid regurgitation is often detected in horses presenting with heart failure due to mitral valve insufficiency. Severe pulmonary hypertension results in secondary dilation of the right ventricle and tricuspid annulus and causes tricuspid valve regurgitation.

Physical examination

The murmur of tricuspid regurgitation (TR) is a systolic murmur heard over the right side of the thorax. It is usually soft and band shaped and extends throughout systole and can incorporate S_1 and S_2. Occasionally tricuspid regurgitation is crescendo in character and might not occupy all of systole; in this case it is usually described as 'tricuspid valve prolapse'.

Special examination

Color flow Doppler echocardiography will confirm the presence of tricuspid regurgitation. Use of pulsed or continuous wave Doppler techniques allows an estimate of pulmonary artery systolic pressure to be obtained from the modified Bernoulli equation.[108] Two-dimensional and M-mode echocardiography allows cardiac chamber size to be visually assessed. The non-symmetric shape of the right ventricle and atrium mean that it is very difficult to obtain repeatable and meaningful measurements of chamber size[109,110] and it is probably advisable to visually appraise the two chambers relative to the left ventricle. The tricuspid valve of affected horses invariably appears morphologically normal, but can prolapse into the right atrium during systole (Fig. 32.32).

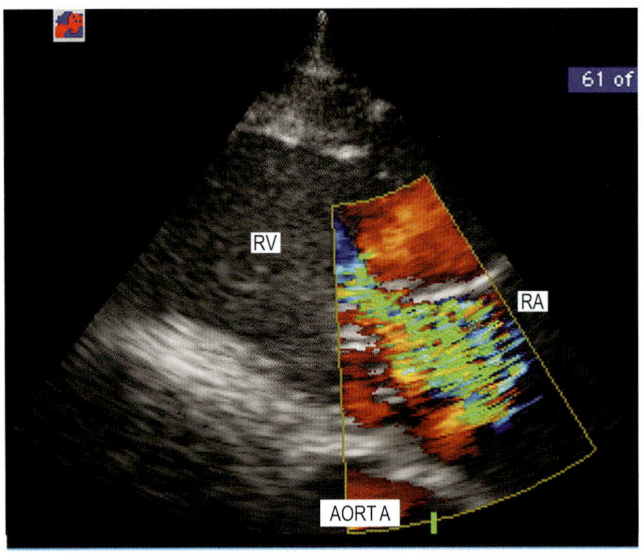

Fig 32.31 Color flow Doppler study of tricuspid valve regurgitation in an eight-year-old racehorse. A grade 4/6 systolic murmur on the right hemithorax was detected incidentally at a veterinary examination. The horse was a successful handicap steeplechaser with no history of poor race performance. A green jet of blood can be seen entering the right atrium through the closed tricuspid valve. (RA = right atrium, RV = right ventricle).

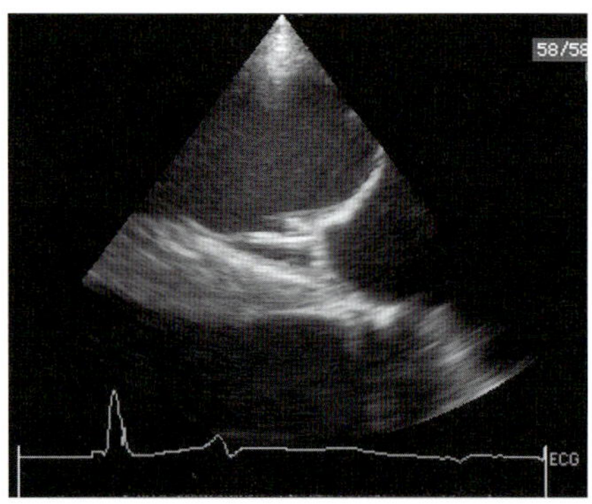

Fig 32.32 Two-dimensional image of the tricuspid valve of the horse shown in Fig. 32.31. Abnormal systolic valve motion was visible in real time. The anterior valve leaflet buckled backwards into the right atrium during systole. However, there is no structural valve abnormality. Abnormal systolic movement is the most frequently encountered echocardiographic feature of tricuspid valve dysfunction in performance horses. Unfortunately due to their geometry, right atrial and ventricular echocardiographic measurements are not very repeatable in horses, making assessment of volume overload of the right heart very difficult. It is rare to see convincing evidence of right heart enlargement due to primary tricuspid valve dysfunction in performance horses.

Treatment and prognosis

Treatment

There is no specific treatment available.

Prognosis

Echocardiographic follow-up of an increasing number of horses affected with tricuspid valve regurgitation indicates that the valve dysfunction rarely progresses to cause clinical signs of heart disease. The condition does not seem to predispose to rupture of chordae tendinae, nor readily result in congestive heart failure. There is also no evidence that compensated tricuspid valve regurgitation, in isolation, causes performance-related problems.[100]

Although all tricuspid regurgitation is not physiological, the condition is certainly very widespread (Table 32.1) and, in horses without evidence of valve lesions, the condition carries an excellent prognosis. Although theoretically right atrial enlargement as a result of severe tricuspid regurgitation should increase the risk of development of atrial fibrillation, this rarely appears to be the case. It is important to note that AF is common in large athletic horses, a group in which the prevalence of audible tricuspid regurgitation is high (Table 32.2). This apparent association does not necessarily mean that the two conditions are causative: indeed, clinical experience suggests this is unlikely.

Etiology and pathophysiology

Tricuspid valve regurgitation is the commonest valve insufficiency in athletic horses.[1–4,100,111,112] Tricuspid regurgitation is also increased after athletic training,[3,101,111,113,114] suggesting that training-induced eccentric hypertrophy is important in the pathogenesis of the condition. Also in elite female athletes, tricuspid regurgitation was more common than in sedentary women.[115] Fibrous thickening and distortion of tricuspid valve leaflets and chordae tendinae have been reported.[74,75] Haemorrhagic lesions were also reported on the right ventricular first-order chordae and their presence led the authors to speculate that these lesions might be precursors to chordae rupture. However, the prevalence of tricuspid valve lesions in the post mortem study was much lower than the prevalence of murmurs of tricuspid valve regurgitation and regurgitation detected by Doppler techniques in athletic horses (Tables 32.1–32.3), supporting the growing suspicion that in many athletic horses, tricuspid regurgitation is physiological, rather than caused directly by valve disease.

Secondary dilation of the tricuspid valve annulus resulting in tricuspid regurgitation also occurs during severe pulmonary hypertension.[67] Increased pressure in the pulmonary circulation increases afterload on the right heart and stimulates eccentric and concentric right ventricular hypertrophy. Deformation of the tricuspid valve apparatus then results in tricuspid valve regurgitation. Pulmonary hypertension is associated most commonly with left-sided cardiac failure and more rarely with pulmonary thromboembolic and hypoxic pulmonary diseases.

Epidemiology

Our work[100] shows that isolated TR is the most commonly encountered murmur in National Hunt horses, occurring in almost 50% of mature horses at full race fitness (Table 32.2). The prevalence is less in flat-racing Thoroughbreds and Standardbred trotters based on these data and those of others.[1,2,97,101]

Mitral regurgitation

See Figures 32.33 and 32.34.

Table 32.2 Prevalence of cardiac murmurs by auscultation and color flow Doppler echocardiography in older race-fit National Hunt steeplechase horses

	% PREVALENCE BY AUSCULTATION		% PREVALENCE BY DOPPLER
REGURGITATON	PATTESON & CRIPPS[2]	YOUNG & WOOD[4]	YOUNG & WOOD[4]
Mitral	5.6	22	58
Tricuspid	16.4	47	88
Aortic	2.2	4	62

Table 32.3 Prevalence of murmurs and regurgitation by color flow Doppler echocardiography at the aortic, mitral and tricuspid valves in 50 two-year-old Thoroughbreds before and after six months' race training[3]

	% PREVALENCE BEFORE TRAINING		% PREVALENCE AFTER TRAINING	
REGURGITATION	AUSCULTATION	DOPPLER	AUSCULTATION	DOPPLER
Mitral	7.3	25	21	35
Tricuspid	12.7	57	25.5	66
Aortic	0	18	2	44

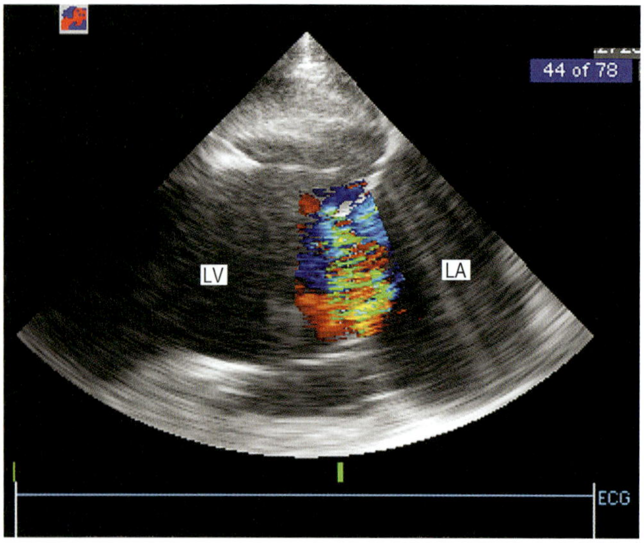

Fig 32.33 Color flow Doppler image showing moderate-to-severe mitral valve regurgitation in a six-year-old Thoroughbred racehorse. The horse had a grade 5/6 murmur over the apex beat area of the left hemithorax. A grade 3/6 murmur of tricuspid regurgitation was also audible at the right hemithorax. The murmurs were detected incidentally during epidemiological studies on the horse's training yard. Despite the moderate-to-severe regurgitation present over two years of the study, the horse had won races and been moderately successful as a handicap steeplechaser (LA = left atrium; LV = left ventricle).

Recognition

History

Mitral regurgitation (MR) is usually detected incidentally during cardiac auscultation.

The murmur of mitral regurgitation is often detected in horses that present in heart failure, as severe mitral valve insufficiency is the most common cause of the heart failure syndrome in horses.[116]

Physical examination

The murmur of mitral regurgitation is loudest on the left hemithorax, in the area of the apex beat. It can radiate forwards towards the heart base, which can cause confusion, if there is a coexistent functional ejection murmur. In common with tricuspid regurgitation, the murmur is usually band shaped and pansystolic. It should not vary with exercise. If mitral regurgitation is severe, resulting in the retrograde flow of large quantities of blood into the left atrium, S_3 will be more pronounced.

Occasionally mitral regurgitation is crescendo in character and can be musical or vibrant. In this case the murmur might not occupy all of systole. The presence and intensity of the murmur can also be variable or disappear with exercise. When the murmur has these characteristics it is usually classified as 'mitral valve prolapse'.

Rupture of a major mitral chord (Fig. 32.35) or severe long-standing mitral regurgitation, usually results in acute left-sided heart failure and a plethora of associated signs:

- Pulmonary edema and increased respiratory rate (Fig. 32.35).
- Increased heart rate.
- Rapid acute onset cardiac cachexia (Fig. 32.36).
- Poor peripheral pulses (Fig. 32.37) and cold extremities.

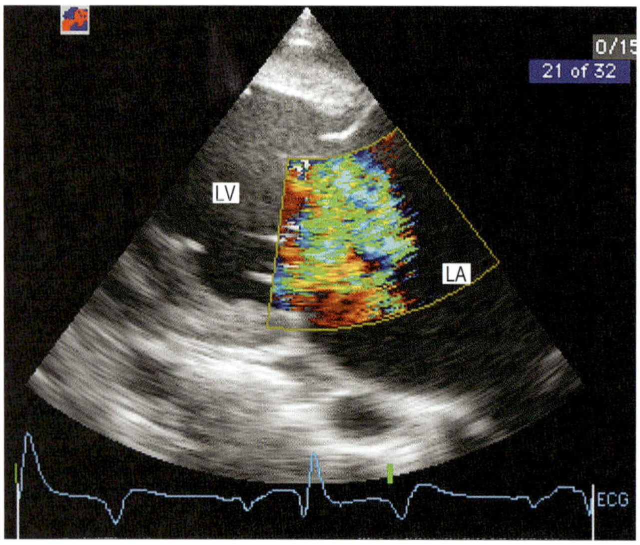

Fig 32.34 Color flow Doppler study showing severe mitral regurgitation in a two-year-old filly in training. There is a large green/blue regurgitant jet entering a grossly dilated left atrium. The filly presented with recurrent pyrexia due to repeated bouts of respiratory infection. A grade 5/6 left-sided cardiac murmur and elevated heart rate (58 bpm) were noted on auscultation. Despite being in left-side heart failure, poor performance was not noted by the trainer, as the filly had only just begun canter work. As in this case, coughing usually arises due to secondary bacterial infection, rather than primarily from the interstitial and alveolar edema present concurrently (LA = left atrium; LV = left ventricle).

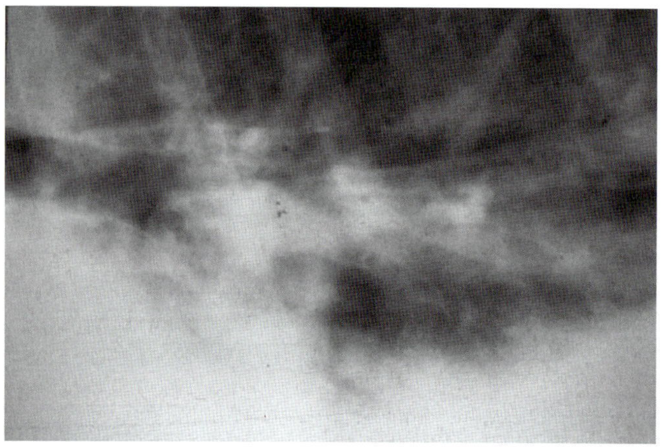

Fig 32.35 Thoracic radiograph from a horse with acute rupture of a major mitral chordae tendinae. There is an alveolar and interstitial pattern most marked in the cardiophrenic angle in this lateral radiograph. Coughing is not a feature usually noted with pulmonary edema in horses, unless there is secondary bacterial infection, which occurs not infrequently. Alveolar and interstitial edema occurs as a consequence of marked elevations in left atrial pressure, from left-sided heart failure. Thoracic auscultation is frequently disappointing in these patients even though pulmonary edema is known to be present. The increased respiratory rate that always accompanies severe alveolar edema is the most reliable method for detecting pulmonary congestion in horses. Occasionally white (occasionally blood-tinged) frothy edema fluid can appear at the nostrils.

- While the murmur associated with such catastrophic valve dysfunction might be expected to be very loud, this is not invariably the case. The murmur is usually associated with a precordial thrill, and will invariably radiate over very large areas of the chest wall.

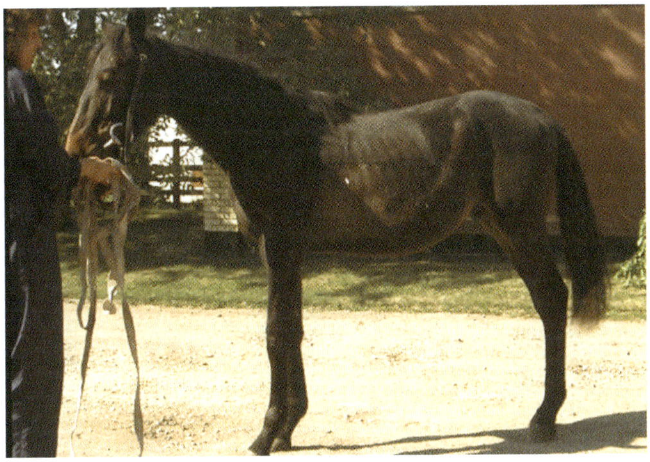

Fig 32.36 Yearling Thoroughbred colt with severe mitral valve regurgitation and atrial fibrillation. Cardiac cachexia or loss of lean body mass is an inevitable consequence of heart failure and occurs in the absence of obvious inappetence. It is often dramatic in onset, occurring within a very short time of cardiac decompensation. It is usually most obvious in the highly muscled areas, e.g. the hindquarters in mature conditioned horses or, as in this case, in the neck and shoulder of young stock.

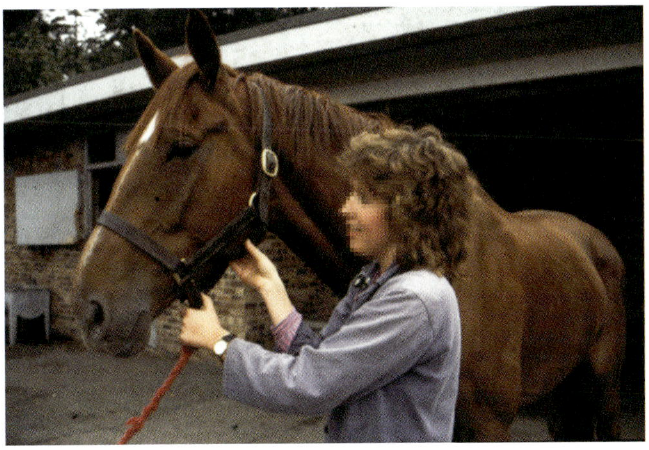

Fig 32.37 Palpation of a peripheral pulse provides a 'window' to the heart's function as a pump. It can also provide a clue to the severity of valve lesions that are picked up on auscultation. The facial artery provides a convenient site for examination. If a patient is in heart failure, heart rate will be elevated above the normal expected value for the animal's type and fitness. These patients usually sustain their heart rates between 55 and 80 bpm dependent on type and severity of disease. Pulse quality reflects the difference between the systolic and diastolic blood pressure. The difference between the two, rather than the magnitude of either, is detected when the pulse is palpated. To obtain an estimate of mean arterial pressure, the amount of digital pressure needed to occlude the pulse can be assessed. Pulse quality can also reflect the severity or type of underlying cardiac disease. A characteristically bounding pulse (i.e. a wide difference between systolic and diastolic pressure) can be indicative of marked aortic insufficiency in older horses, or extracardiac left-to-right shunts in foals.

- Severe left atrial enlargement (Figs 32.13 and 32.14B), not uncommonly results in the development of atrial fibrillation (Fig. 32.7).
- Although heart failure almost always results from primary mitral valve dysfunction, horses not infrequently present with biventricular failure, the signs of which include:
  - peripheral edema (Figs 32.38 and 33.39)
  - jugular engorgement
  - a loud right-sided murmur of tricuspid regurgitation develops (Fig. 32.31).

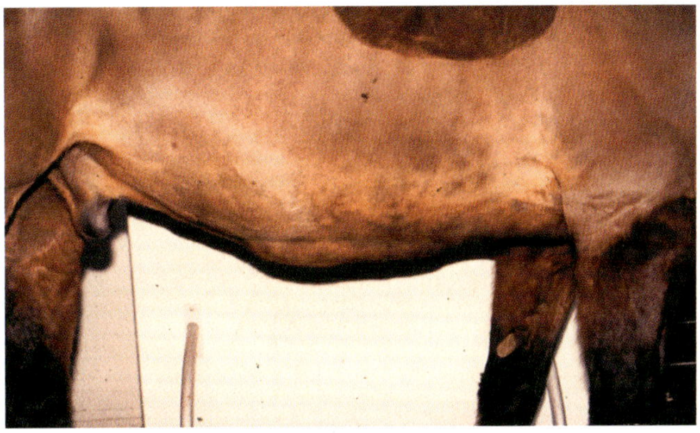

Fig 32.38 Dependent edema in a nine-year-old hunt horse, two weeks after rupture of a mitral chordae tendineae. A plaque of pitting edema is visible in the most dependent area of the ventral abdomen. Occasionally the sheath and brisket are also involved. Although the underlying cause of heart failure in this case was left sided, as is typical, after a variable period of time, if the condition is left untreated, increased pulmonary vascular pressures cause secondary failure of the right ventricle, resulting in systemic venous congestion.

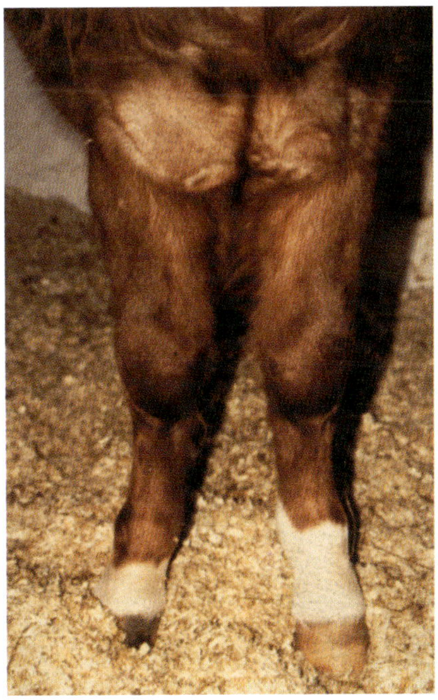

Fig 32.39 Edema of the lower limbs occurs commonly in horses, but is rarely associated with cardiac disease. This six-year-old riding pony has end-stage heart failure from a large ventricular septal defect. He has edema of his brisket and the antebrachium, but minimal swelling of his lower limbs.

Special examination

Color flow Doppler echocardiography will confirm the presence of mitral regurgitation (Figs 32.33, 32.34, and 32.40). Use of continuous wave Doppler will allow an estimate of transmitral pressure gradient to be obtained and thence assessment of left ventricular systolic function to be made, provided it is possible to obtain parallel alignment with the regurgitant flow. Two-dimensional and M-mode echocardiography are used to evaluate cardiac chamber size and left ventricular wall motion. In severe mitral regurgitation, there is dilation and septal hypermotility as the volume-overloaded left ventricle ejects into the low-pressure left atrium. The left atrium will be dilated, as evidenced by an increase in the ratio of the aortic diameter to that of the left atrium (Fig. 32.14A, B). There can be evidence of pulmonary hypertension and dilation of the main pulmonary artery, best assessed by comparison with the diameter of the aorta.

In mild disease, cardiac dimensions will remain within normal range and often the valve appears morphologically normal. Valve thickening or noticeably abnormal valve motion can be observed in more severe cases. Occasionally a flail valve leaflet can be visible after mitral chordae rupture has occurred.

In horses with mild–moderate mitral regurgitation and without evidence of heart failure, electrocardiographic examination during appropriate exercise is recommended to assess heart rate response to exercise. This is especially important when the cardiac murmur is implicated in poor performance or is detected at a pre-purchase examination.

When there is overt heart failure, thoracic radiography is useful to confirm the presence of the alveolar-interstitial infiltrate characteristic of pulmonary edema.

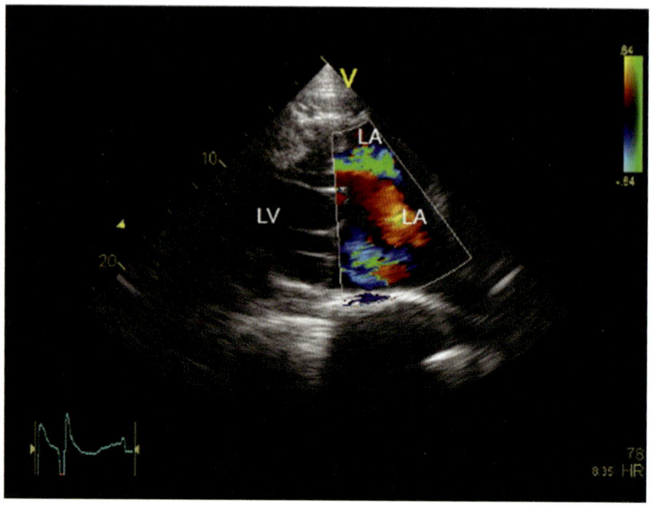

Fig 32.40 Color flow Doppler echocardiograph obtained from the left hemithorax of a nine-year-old Thoroughbred racehorse. The image shows two discrete regurgitant jets entering the left atrium through the closed mitral valve in systole. The horse had a grade 2-3/6 murmur of mitral valve regurgitation. It not uncommon to visualize more than one regurgitant jet in horses with mitral valve dysfunction. In this case, the jets were small, traveled at high velocity and occupied only a small area of the left atrium. Left atrial and ventricular size was normal.

Treatment and prognosis

Treatment

There is no specific treatment for valve regurgitation and in horses with compensated valve dysfunction, no treatment is indicated. When signs of heart failure become evident (Figs 32.13 and 32.14B) therapy focuses upon control of heart rate (digoxin), reduction of volume overload (diuretics) and reduction of cardiac afterload (angiotensin-converting enzyme inhibitors). Once signs of heart failure are present, the horse must be immediately retired from ridden exercise. Aggressive treatment is expensive and palliative only; it will not return the horse to its previous athletic performance. In view of the hopeless prognosis, many owners request immediate euthanasia for their horses and, as a result, treatment is rarely performed.

Prognosis

Mitral valve disease of sufficient severity to cause cardiac failure will have a detrimental effect on athletic performance and a very poor prognosis. The prognosis for isolated compensated mitral regurgitation remains much less certain. This is because overall the condition is less common than tricuspid valve regurgitation and, although there has been some long term follow-up of horses with mild-to-moderately loud mitral valve murmurs, mitral valve disease remains the commonest cause of congestive heart failure in horses. Despite this, the general consensus amongst most cardiologists is that, like tricuspid valve dysfunction, provided valve lesions do not accompany the regurgitation and there is no significant adverse left atrial remodeling, prognosis is generally good.

Most investigators agree that isolated, compensated MR (Fig. 32.40) should not affect athletic performance. There is now epidemiological evidence to support this view because the condition had no effect on the athletic performance of a large group of Thoroughbred racehorses in the UK.[100] It is therefore reasonable to conclude that the condition will have little or no effect on the performance of horses engaged in less aerobically challenging disciplines, unless the associated secondary cardiac remodeling results in the development of atrial fibrillation.

Of all murmurs detected, isolated MR is most problematic when detected during pre-purchase examinations. Because of the relative paucity of high-quality follow-up information on affected horses, there is no definitive solution and ultimately the prospective rider/owner/trainer must make up his or her own mind regarding the suitability of the horse using an informed guess about likelihood of progression. Most investigators are confident that a horse with low-grade MR and a normal resting heart rate is safe to ride, and that its performance is likely to remain unaffected for as long sinus rhythm is maintained and full compensation continues. Auscultation is useful to monitor the progression of regurgitation over long periods, but in a one-off physical examination, the veterinarian knows nothing about the appearance of the valves, the extent of cardiac remodeling, or the previous and subsequent rate that dysfunction developed. Invariably, when a moderately loud murmur is detected at a pre-purchase or insurance examination, it is usually advisable to refer the horse for specialist echocardiographic and electrocardiographic examinations. In the majority of performance horses, it is unlikely that the murmur has arisen as a result of serious progressive valve lesions, but this can never be guaranteed in the absence of these more detailed examinations. In some cases, commercial pressures dictate that the veterinarian informs the prospective client of the existence of the murmur and is then forced to make an educated assessment of its likely impact. In these cases, when heart rate and work history are normal and the murmur is equal to or less than grade 3/6 in intensity, it is fairly unlikely that the murmur will be rapidly progressive. Referral to a specialist center for cardiac ultrasound examination is the best approach whenever any doubt exists regarding the origin or importance of a murmur detected during pre-purchase or insurance examination. It is important to note that murmurs of mitral valve regurgitation are rare in young Thoroughbreds, though the prevalence of murmurs increases in older horses[100] (Table 32.1).

The variable systolic murmurs of mitral valve prolapse are generally considered to carry a good prognosis. In other species, notably dogs and humans, mitral valve prolapse is a precursor of progressive mucinous valvular degeneration and severe mitral valve regurgitation. Similar data are not available for horses, but current opinion suggests that isolated mitral prolapse rarely progresses to cause significant cardiac disease during the career or lifetime of most performance horses.

Etiology and pathophysiology

During mitral insufficiency, blood is ejected retrograde into the left atrium. For the most part the regurgitant fraction is small and the condition remains well compensated. Only when regurgitant fraction is large, or increases through progressive valve dysfunction, will forward cardiac output be compromised and volume and pressure overload of the left atrium begin. As a progressively greater proportion of the left ventricular output is ejected into the low-pressure left atrium, progressive dilation of both chambers occurs and stretching of the fibrous annulus further exacerbates mitral valve incompetence. Reduction in arterial blood pressure as forward cardiac output decreases causes activation of neurohumeral reflexes that further accelerate the vicious cycle of the heart failure syndrome, a syndrome that is always fatal. Signs of congestive heart failure develop when horses with severe mitral valve disease survive low-output left-sided failure for even a short period of time. Increased left atrial pressure causes pulmonary venous congestion and increased afterload to the right ventricle. Subsequently, there is pressure overload of the right ventricle and dilation of the tricuspid valve annulus, such that progressive tricuspid regurgitation develops. Meanwhile low-output failure of the left ventricle and pulmonary edema compromise coronary perfusion and oxygenation and worsen the mechanical function of both ventricles.

The recently observed variability of mild mitral valve murmurs with changes in sympathetic tone and exercise, can be explained because the mitral valve is an apparatus composed of leaflets, chordae and papillary muscles, and not simply an inert fibrous structure. Changes in the loading conditions of the heart and papillary muscles and alterations in myocardial function with changing neurohumoral drive probably change leaflet coaptation, thus preventing, reducing or increasing the regurgitation present at the valve.

The mitral valve was the valve most likely to be affected by gross post mortem changes.[74,75] Microscopic changes included variable fibrosis and infiltration of the superficial valve layers (atrialis and spongiosa) with histiocytes, lymphocytes and fibroblasts.[74,75] Occasionally the deeper (fibrosa and ventricularis) layer of the valve were involved and their involvement usually resulted in deformation of the valve cusps. The precise etiology of valvular damage was not established, but the absence of polymorphonucleated cells, except in two animals, lead these authors to speculate that an infectious cause was unlikely in the majority of cases. Their speculation is supported by clinical evidence suggesting that bacterial endocarditis occurs only rarely in horses.[103] Rupture of a first-order mitral chordae has been repeatedly reported in association with severe mitral regurgitation and heart failure in horses,[117-119] but the precise etiology of the damage to the chordae is yet to be fully explored or explained.

Epidemiology

Recent data shows that the prevalence of MR in racing Thoroughbreds varies between 3.8 and 21% (Tables 32.1 and 32.2). As there is convincing evidence that athletic training increases the prevalence of atrioventricular valve regurgitation (mitral and tricuspid) in Thoroughbreds, this relationship might in part explain the difference in prevalence of AV valve regurgitation found by different investigators (Table 32.3). The effect of age on prevalence of AV valve regurgitation has yet to be established, although from ongoing epidemiological studies, the prevalence of AV valve murmurs assessed by color flow Doppler and auscultation in Thoroughbred racehorses and Standardbreds increased with advancing age and time in training.[100,101,114] The prevalence of gross mitral valve lesions also increased with age in a large post mortem study.[74,75]

Ventricular septal defect

See Figures 32.41-32.43.

- The ventricular septal defect is the most commonly occurring congenital heart defect in horses. Experience suggests that although the defect can be found in all breeds, it seems especially common in Arabians, Standardbreds and small pony breeds (Welsh, Section A, and Shetland ponies).

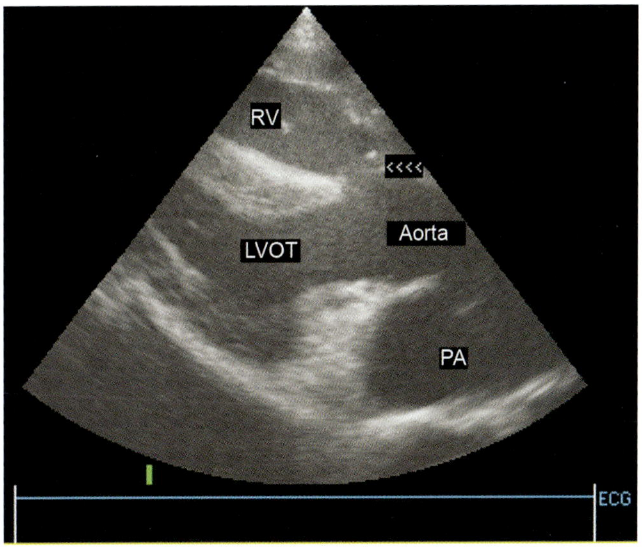

Fig 32.41 Two-dimensional echocardiograph from the right hemithorax of a yearling Thoroughbred with a grade 5/6 pansystolic murmur with point of maximal intensity on the right side. There is a moderately large ventricular septal defect (labeled <<<<) at the top of the interventricular septum. This image has been optimized to visualize the septal defect so that the right pulmonary artery (RPA) is transected obliquely, rather than in true short axis. Failure to attain standard images of intra- and extracardiac structures can lead to errors in measurements of chamber and vessel size and great caution must be applied when interpreting non-standard views. Despite this, the PA does appear to be dilated when compared to the aorta, seen here in oblique long axis. This observation was repeatable in other 2D images that were optimized for the vessels. This observation suggests that there is significant pulmonary over-perfusion, a finding supported by an increased right ventricular stroke volume as estimated by pulsed Doppler echocardiography. Although the filly is compensating for the defect, the defect size and the resultant large left-to-right shunt fraction suggests that she is unlikely to be successful in flat racing. Smaller restrictive defects, despite being associated with a loud murmur, are often compatible with a successful athletic career at the highest levels (RV = right ventricle, LVOT = left ventricular outflow tract, PA = right pulmonary artery).

- The condition is not restricted to foals. Because of the large cardiac reserve of the horse, big lesions are often detected before athletic training commences at insurance or pre-purchase examinations. Indeed this is probably the most frequently encountered clinical presentation.
- The defect can also be associated with other more complex congenital abnormalities (Figs 32.42 and 32.49), but these cases are rare.

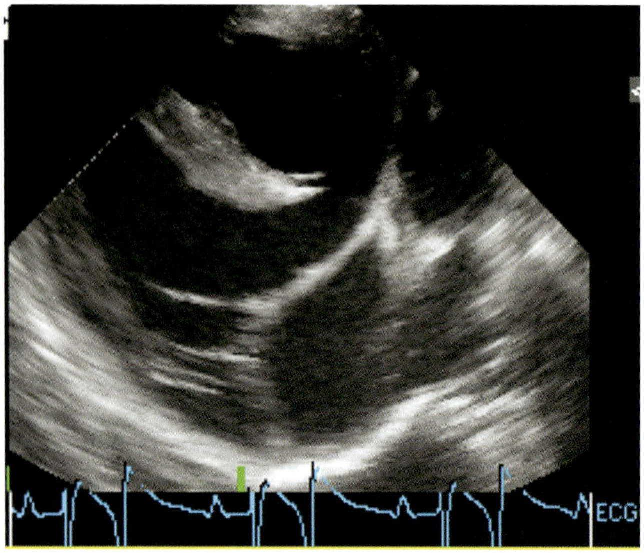

Fig 32.42 Large ventricular septal defect in an 18-month-old Thoroughbred colt, examined after failing an veterinary examination for insurance because of a loud heart murmur. The large septal defect was found in association with other complex congenital abnormalities, including dextroposition of the aorta, right ventricular hypertrophy and subvalvular pulmonic stenosis,. These abnormalities are collectively known as *tetralogy of Fallot.* Despite such severe congenital abnormalities, the colt was fully grown and had no history suggestive of cardiac disease.

- Ventricular septal defects can cause secondary aortic valve insufficiency.

Recognition

History

Usually loud cardiac murmurs are detected during a pre-purchase or insurance examination of a horse without clinical signs. However when the ventricular septal defect is large, the horse/pony might present in biventricular heart failure, although this presentation occurs only very rarely.

Presenting signs

The murmur of a membranous ventricular septal defect is loudest cranial on the right side of the chest. It is usually coarse and band shaped and is often associated with a precordial thrill. This murmur is caused by blood shunting across the defect, from the left ventricle to the right. Most ventricular septal defects occur in the membranous septum, close to the aortic valve (Fig. 32.41). The resultant high-velocity jet of blood then impinges on the right ventricular free wall and swirls ventrally towards the pulmonary artery (Fig. 32.43). The vibrations caused by this flow pattern result in the characteristic cranial and ventral radiation of the right-sided murmur. The murmur can be audible as far ventral as the sternum.

Though much less common, defects can also occur in the muscular part of the interventricular septum (Fig. 32.44) or in the area of the pulmonary outflow. The former still result in a right-sided cardiac murmur, but the pattern of radiation of the murmur differs. In contrast, defects which open into the pulmonary outflow tract result in a murmur whose point of maximal intensity is cranial and ventral on the left hemithorax at the level of the pulmonary valve.

Another discrete murmur is often also heard in association with large septal defects in horses. It is best heard over the heart base on the left hemithorax. This murmur is not always simply referred from the right side. This is also an ejection murmur component, with a PMI over the pulmonary valve area. This is known as a murmur of

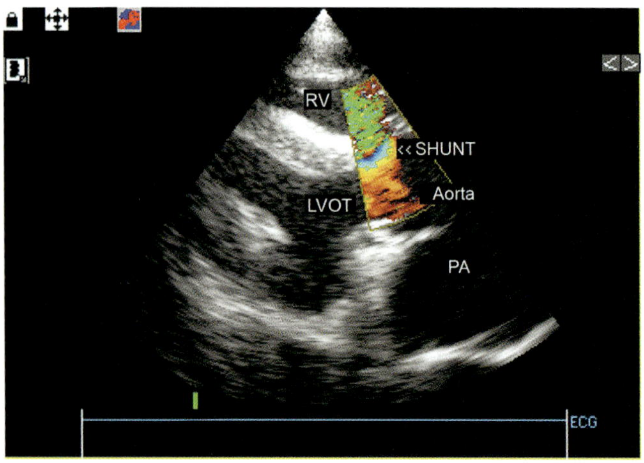

Fig 32.43 Color flow Doppler study obtained from the filly in Fig. 32.41 The color flow study demonstrates left-to-right flow of blood through the defect during systole. The shunted blood travels through the defect and swirls ventrally and cranially towards the pulmonary valve, giving rise to the characteristic ventral and cranial radiation of the murmurs associated with membranous septal defects (RV = right ventricle, LVOT = left ventricular outflow tract, RPA = right pulmonary artery).

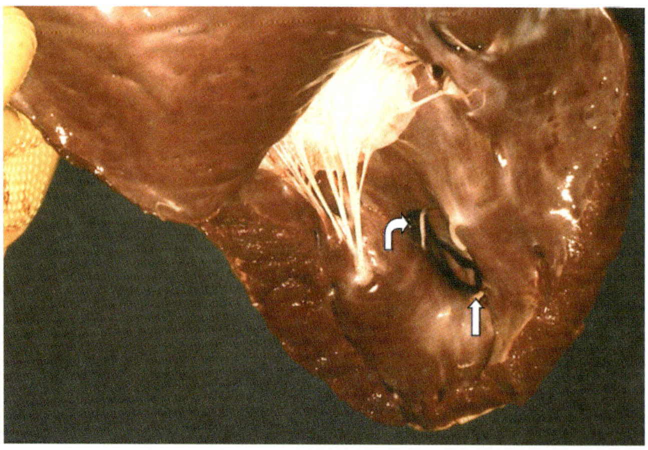

Fig 32.44 Post mortem specimen showing a large muscular ventricular septal defect in a two-year-old Arabian filly. A widely radiating grade 5/6 murmur was detected from her right hemithorax at a pre-purchase examination. There was no medical history consistent with cardiac disease and the filly appeared to have normal exercise tolerance relative to her peer group. As her prognosis for useful athletic performance and sale was hopeless and her congenital cardiac defect rendered her unsuitable for breeding, her owners elected for her euthanasia.

relative pulmonary stenosis. It arises as a result of augmented flow of blood through a normal pulmonary valve.

A further secondary finding, associated with a large defect and shunt fraction, is an increased intensity of S_3 that results from augmented filling of the left ventricle in diastole. When the defect is large, the resultant left atrial and ventricular enlargement eventually results in left heart failure and the plethora of associated clinical signs.

Special tests

Two-dimensional and M-mode echocardiography is necessary to evaluate the size of the defect. The loudness of the primary murmur is not helpful in assessing the clinical importance of this condition, since loud murmurs are often associated with small defects that are restrictive to blood flow. It has been suggested that defects less than 2.5 cm in diameter in an adult horse are compatible with normal athletic performance and are unlikely to result in heart failure.[120] Since ponies and small horses are often affected, a more universally applicable method is to use Doppler echocardiography to measure peak flow across the defect, or to compare stroke volume from the right and left ventricle. Reef and colleagues[120] suggested that velocity across the defect that exceeded 4 m/s was likely to be associated with a restrictive defect. When using these methods, it is crucial to ensure that the continuous wave ultrasound beam is aligned parallel to the shunt flow and that other reasons for right ventricular or pulmonary artery hypertension are absent. If adequate alignment is not achieved, blood flow velocity will be significantly underestimated and the defect's significance overestimated. Left atrial size and pulmonary artery dilation can also be assessed using two-dimensional methods and these measurements are also helpful in determining a prognosis for life and performance. On occasion, the typically positioned, inlet, membranous septal defect can interfere with support of the closely apposed aortic valve, resulting in aortic valve regurgitation, causing further volume overload of the left heart and potentially impacting on overall prognosis.

While auscultation findings and clinical signs are helpful in assessing size of a defect and its clinical impact, only two-dimensional and Doppler echocardiography are ultimately able to provide information about the severity of volume overload, a quantitative assessment of defect size, the presence of additional congenital anomalies and the degree of involvement of adjacent valves.

Treatment and prognosis

Treatment

No surgical or medical treatment for ventricular septal defects is currently available for horses. Due to the position of the membranous defect, close to the aortic valve, application of a transvenous occlusion device is hampered. Only if heart failure develops is treatment warranted and should include drugs to control heart rate (digoxin), diuretics to reduce volume overload and angiotensin-converting enzyme inhibitors for reduction of cardiac afterload.

Prognosis

The prognosis for small defects that restrict transeptal blood flow and that are found incidentally in performance horses is generally good. Certainly absence of a separate murmur of relative pulmonary stenosis and loud S_3 sounds indicate that the volume of abnormal blood flow through the defect is small and that the defect is likely to be restrictive. Such defects rarely progress to cause clinical problems. Progression of disease, even with moderately large defects, can be slow, affected horses often compensating well into adulthood. As with all cases of heart disease, echocardiographic examination of an affected horse allows the size of lesion and its hemodynamic impact to be determined. Whether an animal is suitable for athletic duties will depend upon the size of the defect and the degree of volume overload, the involvement of other valves and the type of work to be performed.

When detected at pre-purchase examination all septal defects undoubtedly constitute unsoundness, but the horse may still be able to perform a useful job, when the defects are small and restrictive to blood flow. The integrity and function of the aortic valve should always be assessed, even when defects are small and restrictive.

Etiology and pathophysiology

The condition occurs as a result of anomalous development of any of the components of the interventricular septum, most commonly the dorsal membranous portion that forms part of the fibrous skeleton of the heart. Although the precise genetics and mechanisms of inheritance of the condition in horses are unknown, affected animals should probably not be used for breeding.

Restrictive defects that result in a small shunt are usually well tolerated and have minimal hemodynamic impact. When defects are large, left-sided heart failure develops due to volume overload of the left atrium. The right ventricle tends to be relatively spared, because the pulmonary valve is open when the bulk of the shunt volume is propelled by the left ventricle across the defect and it passes directly into the pulmonary artery. Pulmonary over-circulation occurs and marked dilation of the pulmonary artery can result in pulmonary artery rupture. As a result horses with evidence of pulmonary over-circulation should not be used for ridden work.

Epidemiology

In the series of 27 cases described by Reef,[120] Standardbreds and Arabians were over-represented compared to the hospital population and Thoroughbreds were under-represented. European experience suggests that the condition occurs sporadically in Thoroughbreds and Warmblood horses, but that Welsh section A ponies have a disproportionately high prevalence of the condition.

Aortic insufficiency

See Figure 32.45.

Recognition

History

Usually a diastolic cardiac murmur is detected incidentally. Occasionally horses can have a history of ataxia during exercise or die suddenly, usually during exercise. Aortic regurgitation can be found in association with congestive heart failure, atrial fibrillation and mitral valve regurgitation.

Presenting signs

Aortic insufficiency (AI) occurs commonly in older horses. The murmur is diastolic, usually decrescendo, and has a PMI at the aortic valve, although it will often radiate widely towards the apex. Because the aorta is a midline structure, as the disease progresses, the murmur often becomes audible over the right hemithorax. It is thus the only murmur that can be routinely osculated from both sides of the thorax. The murmur often has a musical quality and can appear to 'buzz' or 'whoo'. The musical quality is believed to arise as the regurgitant jet hits the anterior leaflet of the mitral valve, or due to resonance and vibration of the aortic root, or interventricular septum.

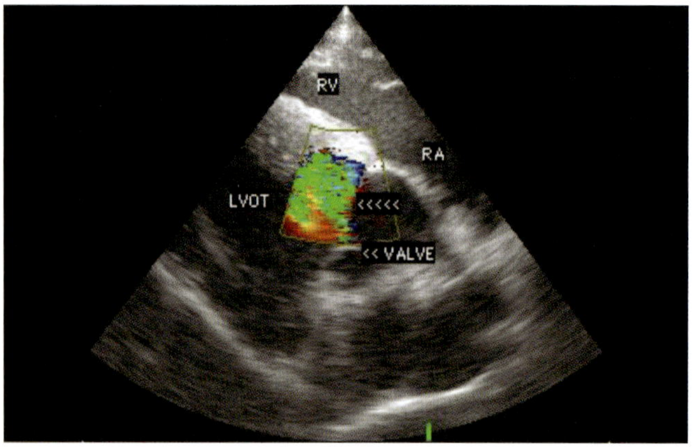

Fig 32.45 Color flow Doppler study of aortic valve regurgitation in a 16-year-old Grand Prix dressage horse.

The image shows a green jet of blood travelling from the center of the aortic valve towards the interventricular septum. The two-dimensional image showed valve leaflet thickening typical of nodular degeneration in the older horse. The was no evidence of exercise-induced arrhythmias and left ventricular dimensions were still within normal limits. The horse is subject to regular echocardiographic and electrocardiographic examinations as aortic valve degeneration is progressive. Currently he is able to remain in full competition, as he has no significant left ventricular dilation and his risk of developing exercise-induced cardiac arrhythmias was not increased above that of his peers. This was confirmed by a normal ECG taken from him during appropriate ridden exercise (RA = right atrium, LVOT = left ventricular outflow tract, RV = right ventricle).

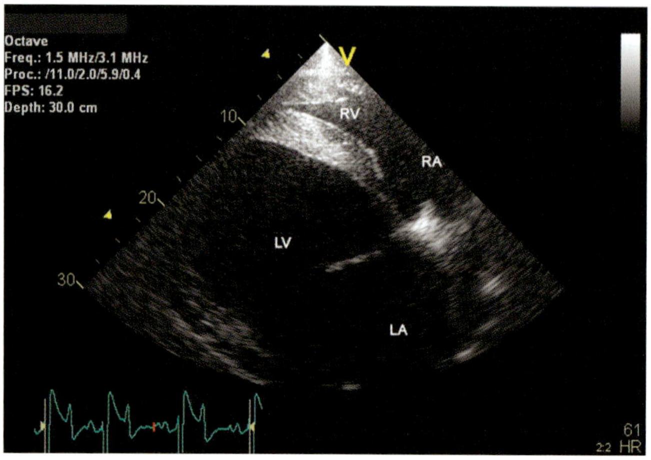

Fig 32.46 Two-dimensional echocardiograph from the right hemithorax from an 11-year-old riding horse with a grade 5/6 murmur of aortic regurgitation. Note the rounded bloated appearance of the dilated left ventricle. Dilation results in increased afterload to the left ventricle and increases both myocardial work and oxygen demand. Coronary perfusion is simultaneously reduced as diastolic aortic pressure falls. Stretch and hypoxia increase the likelihood of ventricular dysrhythmia and there is increasing risk of exercise-induced dysrhythmias and sudden death. Severe volume overload also causes dilation of the mitral valve annulus, resulting in secondary development of mitral regurgitation that can ultimately result in left-sided heart failure. (LA = left atrium, LV = left ventricle, RA = right atrium, RV = right ventricle).

When severe, the condition can result in noticeably bounding arterial pulses (Fig. 32.37). This occurs because there is a rapid run off of aortic pressure in diastole, as blood leaks backwards into the low-pressure chamber of the relaxed left ventricle.

When the regurgitant fraction is large, there is volume overload of the left ventricle (Fig. 32.46). There is also dilation of the mitral valve annulus and, in consequence, secondary mitral regurgitation can occur. Thus when a systolic murmur of MR is heard, in conjunction with the diastolic murmur of AI, prognosis is much more guarded.

Special examination

Color flow Doppler echocardiography will confirm the presence of aortic regurgitation (Fig. 32.45). Pulsed or continuous wave Doppler techniques allow estimates of right and left ventricular stroke volume and regurgitant fraction to be made. Two-dimensional and M-mode echocardiography are used to evaluate cardiac chamber size and left ventricular wall motion. In severe aortic regurgitation, there is left ventricular dilation (Fig. 32.46) and secondary mitral regurgitation.

Careful examination of the aortic valve using two-dimensional and color flow Doppler techniques can demonstrate the underlying cause of the valve dysfunction. Typical findings include valve leaflet prolapse (Fig. 32.47) and nodular degeneration, thickening of the valve leaflets, or evidence of a small ventricular septal defect. There is often diastolic fluttering of the anterior mitral valve leaflet visualized by two-dimensional or M-mode echocardiography.[121] In severe volume overload and secondary mitral regurgitation, premature closure of the mitral valve and septal hyperkinesis can also be a feature.[122]

In horses with mild–moderate aortic valve regurgitation and without evidence of heart failure, electrocardiographic examination during appropriate exercise is mandatory to ensure that there is an absence of exercise-induced ventricular dysrhythmias (Fig. 32.48).

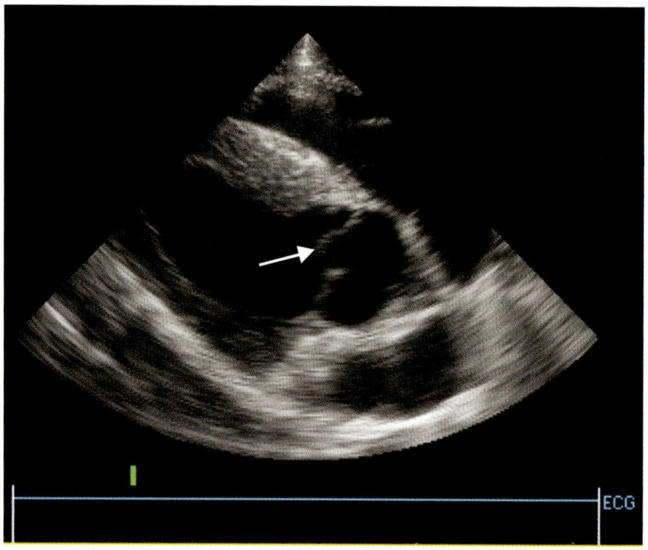

Fig 32.47 Two-dimensional echocardiograph from a nine-year-old National Hunt racehorse with a grade 3/6 murmur of aortic regurgitation. The image has been optimized to show the aortic valve (center). The non-coronary leaflet (arrow) has prolapsed into the left ventricular outflow tract. There is a bright echogenic nodule at the coaptation point of the valve, the usual site of nodular degeneration in older horses.

Treatment and prognosis

Treatment

There is no specific treatment for aortic valve regurgitation available and, in horses with compensated valve dysfunction, none is

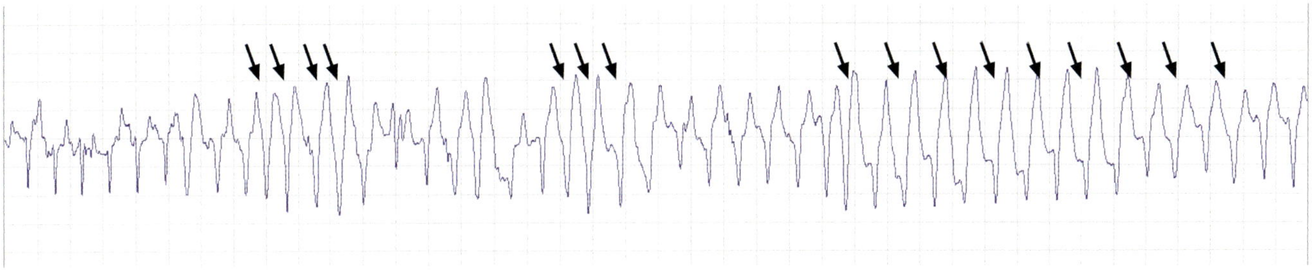

Fig 32.48 ECG obtained during fast canter exercise in a 17-year-old Thoroughbred with grade 5/6 aortic valve regurgitation. The horse had an internal left ventricular diameter in diastole of 17.0 cm and the owners had continued to use their horse for ridden work, despite veterinary advice that he should be retired 18 months earlier. Note the development of multiform ventricular tachycardia (arrows), a trigger for ventricular fibrillation and exercise-associated sudden cardiac death.

indicated. When signs of left ventricular volume overload become evident (Fig. 32.46), or signs of heart failure are present, the horse must be immediately retired from ridden exercise. Palliative therapy focuses upon control of heart rate (digoxin), reduction of volume overload (diuretics) and reduction of cardiac afterload (angiotensin-converting enzyme inhibitors). On the rare occasion that valve dysfunction is caused by endocarditis, targeted antibiotic therapy will be required.

Prognosis

Most commonly the condition arises due to normal progressive aging changes to the valve leaflets and when the murmur is detected in older horses the prognosis for life and performance is generally good. In such cases performance problems are rarely reported and the ultimate cause of death or euthanasia in these horses is usually, but not invariably, non-cardiac.[123] In older horses, the condition usually progresses slowly and they are usually able to continue their normal activities, provided they are monitored regularly by echocardiography and electrocardiography.

Aortic insufficiency also occurs sporadically in younger horses when the only abnormalities on echocardiography include leaflet prolapse, dilatation of the aortic root and/or premature degenerative changes (thickening or nodular degeneration). In these horses the condition might progress to heart failure during the course of the horse's athletic career. In some cases progression is very slow and the horse's career might not be noticeably compromised, but progression of regurgitation and volume overload is impossible to predict in individuals, so all affected cases must be carefully monitored. As a result when the murmur is encountered during a pre-purchase examination, although each horse must be considered individually, as a general rule this murmur should be viewed with extreme caution.

When a systolic murmur of MR is heard in conjunction with a loud diastolic murmur of AI, or there is hyperkinesis of peripheral pulses, it is likely that there is a large regurgitant fraction and that MR has developed secondary to severe left ventricular volume overload. As a result prognosis is extremely guarded and the horse must immediately be retired from ridden duties.

Etiology and pathophysiology

Usually the condition arises due to fibrous and nodular degeneration of the valve leaflets, a change that appears to be age-related.[74,75] When a loud murmur of AI is detected in a horse under 15 years of age, there has been premature progression of aortic valve disease and a complicating reason, other than normal aging processes, is implicated. Vegetative endocarditis, though very rare, can affect both aortic and mitral valves in horses,[103] and prognosis for performance and survival is poor. More commonly premature regurgitation is caused by prolapse of the non-coronary cusp of the aortic valve (Fig. 32.47).[120] Congenital malformations, including fenestrations of the aortic valve, also occur sporadically.[124]

When the regurgitant fraction is large, there is volume overload of the left ventricle (Fig. 32.46) and dilation of the mitral valve annulus, resulting in mitral regurgitation. The severely dilated ventricle also becomes prone to exercise-induced ventricular dysrhythmias. This increased susceptibility occurs due to increased cardiac work and myocardial oxygen demand caused by increased cardiac preload and the augmented afterload of cardiac dilation. These factors are coupled with reduced diastolic blood pressure and thence coronary perfusion pressure. The risk of dysrhythmia is heightened when myocardial oxygen demand increases and diastole shortens during exercise. As a result, affected horses should be monitored regularly by echocardiography and exercising electrocardiography as long as they remain in ridden work (Fig. 32.48).

Epidemiology

In a population of 1159 horses comprising many retired animals, the presence of a diastolic murmur of aortic insufficiency was significantly associated with age.[125] The murmur is only infrequently detected in racehorses (Tables 32.1 and 32.2), but the prevalence is greater in older National Hunt Thoroughbreds than those engaged in flat racing (Tables 32.1 and 32.2).[100]

Complex congenital lesions

A wide variety of complex cardiac abnormalities have been reported in foals.[126–135] They are, however, uncommon[136] and often result in early signs of heart failure and cyanosis. Complex developmental abnormalities have a higher incidence in Arabian foals, but they can occur in all breeds, occasionally presenting at adulthood or adolescence[137] (Fig. 32.49). Complex congenital lesions are not compatible with athletic performance, but depending upon the amount of intracardiac shunting and venous admixture, can carry a surprisingly good prognosis for short to medium-term survival.

Diseases of the myocardium

- Diseases of the myocardium are poorly understood in horses.
- They are characterized by loss of performance, arrhythmias at rest and during exercise and/or ventricular contractile dysfunction (Fig. 32.50).

- Serum or plasma concentration of cardiac troponin I will be elevated in severe acute cases of myocardial inflammation and necrosis.
- Dilated cardiomyopathy occurs rarely in athletic horses and has been associated with nutritional deficiencies in young horses and cattle.

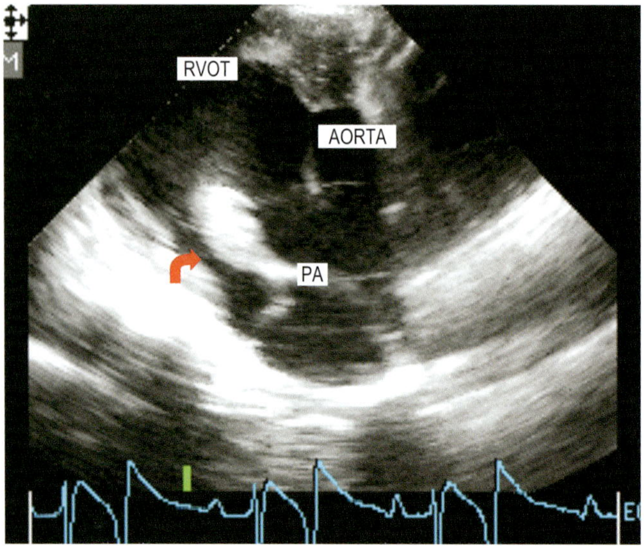

Fig 32.49 Two-dimensional echocardiograph from the right hemithorax of an 18-month-old Thoroughbred with tetralogy of Fallot. This is a cranial short-axis view of the right ventricular outflow tract (RVOT). The outflow tract connects directly with a dilated aorta and a pulmonary artery (PA). Subvalvular pulmonic stenosis is severe (red arrow).

- Occasionally toxic damage to myocytes occurs when a cardiotoxin is accidentally introduced into equine feed. The ionophores lasalocid, salinomycin and monensin have caused a number of such outbreaks throughout the world.[138–147]
- Horses that survive ingestion of cardiotoxins usually develop a dilated hypocontractile ventricle that mimics dilated cardiomyopathy.
- Ingestion of cardiac glycoside-containing plants, such as foxglove, oleander and adonis, can result in cardiac arrhythmias, hemodynamic collapse and sudden death.[85] In these cases measurement of serum digoxin concentrations is helpful for diagnosis.
- Dilated cardiomyopathy as occurs in other species has not been convincingly identified in horses, but there have been recent reports of arrhythmogenic right ventricular cardiomyopathy.[148]

Recognition

History

Myocarditis has been linked to poor performance syndromes occurring in individuals, or in outbreaks in racing stables. Myocarditis can be the underlying cause of atrial and ventricular dysrhythmia in athletic horses. In the acute phases of toxic damage to the myocardium, one or more horses can die suddenly from fatal ventricular dysrhythmia.

Physical examination

In many mildly affected cases, the horse is normal on physical examination at rest. A cardiac rhythm disturbance might be present during auscultation, or during palpation of the apex beat or peripheral pulse. If cardiac function is severely compromised,

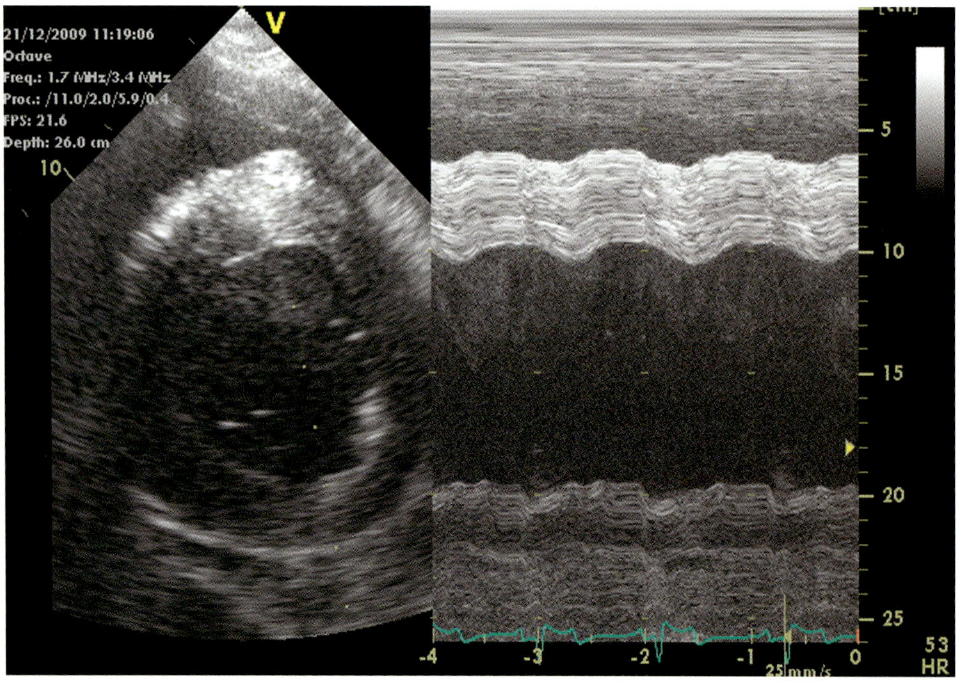

Fig 32.50 M-mode shows severe left ventricular contractile dysfunction in a horse due to intoxication with the ionophore lasalocid. Left ventricular fractional shortening is 14%. The horse died one day after the image was taken.

the horse will present with signs of biventricular heart failure (see mitral regurgitation) with jugular pulsation and ventral edema.

Special examination

A definitive diagnosis of the origin of the ectopic complexes (atrial or ventricular) will be determined by electrocardiography (see supraventricular and ventricular premature beats). In cases of poor performance, an ECG during appropriate exercise is advisable. Glycoside or ionophore intoxication can be associated with atrial standstill, second-degree atrioventricular block, and polymorphic ventricular premature beats, ventricular tachycardia and ventricular fibrillation.

In acute cases, measurement of serum cardiac troponin I can sometimes provide a definitive diagnosis of active myocardial inflammation and necrosis. However, normal troponin I values do not rule out myocardial damage, as lesions can be too small to result in a measurable troponin increase in the circulation. Furthermore, when horses present with suspected myocardial dysfunction, it is possible that active myocardial damage is no longer present as the acute insult to the heart or any causative agent is no longer present. The importance of infectious organisms or toxic agents in equine myocardial disease is poorly documented and therefore, additional tests to find the exact etiology in suspected cases of myocardial disease are rarely performed. Nevertheless, *Streptococcus* spp., *Salmonella*, *Clostridium*, *Borrelia burgdorferi*, piroplasmosis, influenza, herpes virus, infectious anemia and *Strongylus vulgaris*, have all been associated with myocardial disease and require further investigation. In selected cases, samples should be analyzed to diagnose vitamin E or selenium deficiency, or to confirm intoxication (ionophores, cantharidin, glycosides). In the case of glycoside intoxication, e.g. by oleander ingestion, serum or plasma levels for digoxin are often sufficiently diagnostic. However, in such cases, the assay will often show only very low levels of digoxin even if intoxication is present because digoxin is only one of the numerous glycosides that are contained in this family of plants.[85] Although atypical myopathy can be associated with cardiac damage (long QT and abnormal wall motion)[84] overt signs of skeletal muscle damage predominate in this disease.

Resting echocardiography is also useful to assess the cardiac chambers and systolic function. Horses with glycoside intoxication often present increased inotropy in the initial stage while ionophore-intoxicated animals show reduction in systolic function (Fig. 32.50). Abnormal wall motion suggestive of localized myocardial damage can be present, or there can be extensive areas of fibrosis and calcification of the myocardium and endocardium. Two-dimensional speckle tracking and tissue Doppler imaging have proven to be useful in the detection of myocardial dysfunction in horses with ionophore intoxication and atypical myopathy.[84,147] In many cases, echocardiographic examination is unremarkable or equivocal, especially in horses with vague signs of poor performance or lone dysrhythmias.

It has also been suggested that post-exercise echocardiography can be a more sensitive method to detect mild ischemic damage to the myocardium in horses.[149,150] M-mode echocardiography is used within 60 seconds of exercise to fatigue in an attempt to mimic the stress echocardiography that is carried out during exercise in people to detect subclinical disease.[151] Unfortunately it is not practical to perform the examination during steady-state exercise in horses and the technique appears to have a very high coefficient of variation in normal horses.[152] Despite this limitation, the method's advocates claim that the technique has been useful in horses undergoing performance evaluation on the treadmill.[150]

Treatment and prognosis

Therapeutic aim

Treat underlying disease process and any life-threatening dysrhythmia. Remove access to toxin. Improve nutritional status.

Therapy

In all suspected outbreaks, or in individual animals, thorough evaluation of previous medical history, bacteriological or serological examination, toxicological analyzes and assessment of nutritional status of affected horses and their in-contacts should be undertaken.

In most cases of extensive myocardial damage or necrosis, treatment is ineffectual once clinical signs are apparent. Therapy is therefore aimed at control of clinical signs and amelioration of cardiac failure with use of appropriate antiarrhythmic drugs to treat life-threatening rhythm disturbances. Affected horses should always be completely rested to reduce myocardial oxygen demand.

In less severely affected cases with signs of poor performance or lone dysrhythmia, rest and steroid therapy have been advocated (see supraventricular premature beats). When biochemical markers of myocardial damage are elevated at diagnosis, their levels can be used to monitor progress.

Prognosis

The prognosis for myocardial disease is dependent upon the severity of the underlying damage to the myocardium. In general the prognosis for return to athletic function is very guarded, if there is echocardiographic evidence of reduced systolic function or marked chamber dilation. The prognosis for survival is also poor.

When myocarditis is suspected in horses presenting with poor performance and arrhythmia, and when there are no echocardiographic or biochemical abnormalities, prognosis is fair. A percentage of affected horses will return to their previous athletic performance following rest and/or steroid therapy. In the absence of a definitive test to diagnose myocarditis in horses, unfortunately it is questionable whether true myocardial inflammation was ever present in many of these cases. Myocardial biopsy is an invasive, high-risk procedure, and as a result it seems unlikely that our understanding of this condition will improve in the foreseeable future.

Etiology and pathophysiology

In man, the usual underlying cause of myocardial damage is ischemia resulting from coronary artery occlusion, usually arteriosclerosis. A similar etiology can underlie the condition in horses as areas of focal fibrosis are common in the equine myocardium at post mortem examination.[74,75,88] There is a relationship between proximal aortic *Strongylus vulgaris* lesions and the presence of focal ischaemic lesions in the myocardium and hypothesized that microembolization from parasitic lesions in the proximal aorta, produced obstructive arteriosclerotic lesions in myocardial arterioles.[88] In most horses, the areas of fibrosis are focal and do not penetrate the whole thickness of the ventricular myocardium,[74,75,88] but it is possible that during cell ischemia and death, before fibrosis occurs, these areas act as foci for arhythmogenesis. In more severely affected horses, there can be sufficient damage to wide areas of myocardium to provoke extensive remodeling and lasting damage to cardiac function. Unfortunately in most post mortem studies the fibrotic lesions cannot be correlated to clinical signs before death and in many cases the lesions appear inactive. In addition, improved anthelmintic management of equidae has resulted in a marked reduction in the incidence of thrombo-ischemic lesions associated with large strongyle infestations. Although the precise etiology was uncertain, a number of authors have found post mortem evidence of acute myocarditis in horses presenting with severe ventricular dysrhythmia and poor performance.[89,91,153,154]

Ionophores, such as monensin,[155,156] lasalocid[146,147] and salinomycin,[145] and cantharidin, cardiac glycosides and rattlesnake poison[157] cause direct damage to myocytes resulting in cell death, replacement fibrosis, arrhythmia and/or loss of systolic function.

In the poor performance syndrome in racing yards, the cardiac signs are often observed some time after an outbreak of infectious respiratory disease, but despite extensive serological and bacteriological investigations, in most cases, a causative agent cannot be identified. More research is needed in this area. In humans, viruses are believed to be associated with dilated cardiomyopathy[158] and during influenza virus epidemics there is unexpected high mortality of humans due to cardiovascular diseases.[159] The precise mechanism of viral damage to the myocardium is not fully understood, but can involve procoagulant effects.[159] It is possible that similar sporadic cases of virus-associated or post-viral myocarditis occur in the equine population, but at the moment this is entirely speculative. There is, however, evidence that equine viruses including equine viral arteritis, equine herpesvirus-1 and African horse sickness virus, replicate in epicardial or myocardial blood vessels in natural and experimental disease,[160–162] and myocarditis has been reported in horses infected with influenza virus.[163,164]

Idiopathic dilated cardiomyopathy in dogs and humans results from various genetic mutations of the proteins involved in cardiac contraction. There is reduced contractile function and ultimately cell death and fibrous remodeling that result in a dilated poorly contractile ventricle and symptoms of heart failure and dysrhythmia. There have been clinical and anecdotal reports of a similar syndrome in horses, based on the post mortem, or echocardiographic diagnosis of a large dilated heart. However it is important to appreciate that myocardial failure and dilation accompanies all types of heart failure in endstages, so that echocardiographic evidence of dilated poorly contractile ventricle is not diagnostic of dilated cardiomyopathy.

Epidemiology

No epidemiological information is currently available, as myocarditis is too poorly understood in horses.

Diseases of the pericardium

See Figure 32.51.

Recognition

History

Affected horses can present with general signs of malaise or evidence of heart failure including weakness and collapse.[165]

Presenting signs

In horses affected with bacterial pericarditis, there will be associated signs of infection and sepsis. Cardiovascular signs depend upon the volume of pericardial fluid. In cardiac tamponade (large effusion compressing the right atrium), jugular distension, subcutaneous edema, ascites, pleural effusion and abdominal enlargement will be evident. Peripheral pulse quality is poor and heart rate is increased. There can by muffling of the heart sounds with the presence of pericardial friction rubs in some cases.[165,166]

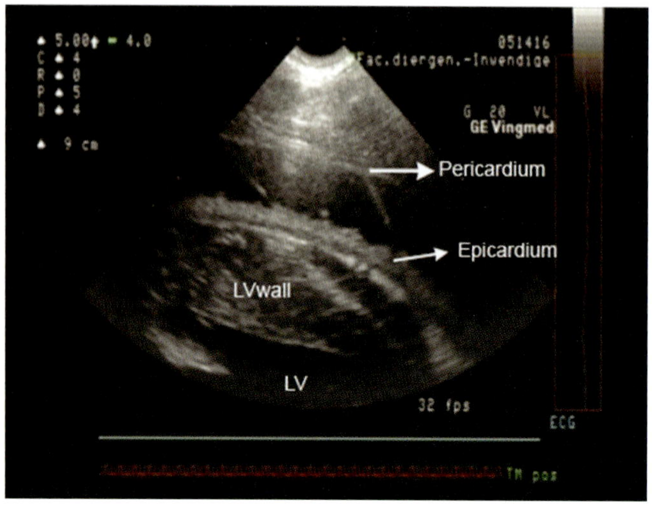

Fig 32.51 Six-year-old endurance horse with fever and jugular distention shows fluid in the pericardial space. A fibrin layer is present on the epicardium and fibrin strands are visible between epicardium and pericardium. The horse returned to endurance competition six months after repeated pericardial lavages and eight weeks' antibiotic treatment (LVwall = left ventricular wall, LV = left ventricle).

Special tests

Two-dimensional echocardiography will identify fluid in the pericardial space. There can be obvious compression of the right cardiac structures, depending upon the volume of effusate present (Fig. 32.51).

Electrocardiography will reveal sinus tachycardia, but the QRS amplitude will be less than usual. Electrical alternans, as occurs in other species, is rare in horses.[165,166]

Hematology, bacteriology and analysis and culture of pericardial fluid are valuable in determining etiology and treatment in cases of septic pericarditis.

Therapeutic aims

Aims are to release pressure on the right heart chambers and restore normal cardiac filling and to achieve bacteriological cure in cases of septic pericarditis.

Treatment and prognosis

Treatment

Aggressive pericardial drainage and lavage have been recommended for effusions associated with cardiac compromise.[165] Additional antibiotic therapy as indicated by culture and sensitivity will also be indicated in bacterial pericarditis. In cases of non-septic idiopathic pericarditis, corticosteroids are recommended.[165,166] Surgical pericardectomy was also attempted as a treatment for restrictive pericarditis in a horse, but the results were disappointing and the condition recurred.[167]

Prognosis

In a series of 18 cases,[165] all 14 of the horses treated successfully returned to their previous athletic performance. Only one treated horse died in the series of 10 cases of idiopathic pericarditis,[166] suggesting that with aggressive treatment prognosis is good. In contrast to other species, there are few reports of effusion returning repeatedly after drainage. If effusion results from sepsis, or trauma, the prognosis is more guarded and will depend upon the nature of the effusion and the response to antimicrobial agents.

Etiology and pathophysiology

In the series of 18 cases,[165] pericarditis was defined as idiopathic in six horses. A bacterial cause was identified in five horses and the remaining horses had non-septic pericarditis associated with bacterial (five horses) and viral respiratory disease (two horses). Laboratory analysis of pericardial fluid samples from 10 cases of idiopathic pericarditis classified six cases as aseptic serofibrinous, three cases as eosinophilic, and one case as histiocytic.[166]

The hemodynamic effect of pericardial effusion depends upon the volume of effusion and the amount of compression of the thin-walled right atrium. Increased pericardial pressure impedes ventricular filling and increases end diastolic pressure. Reduced stroke volume of the right heart causes reduction in arterial blood pressure and activates the renin–angiotensin system, resulting in massive retention of Na and water. Backward failure of the right ventricle rapidly occurs, resulting in jugular distension and abdominal, pleural and subcutaneous fluid accumulation. Low-output failure simultaneously results in weakness and exercise intolerance.

Epidemiology

Isolated cases of pericarditis occur only rarely in athletic horses and no specific epidemiological information is available. In the spring of 2001 in central Kentucky, outbreaks of pericarditis and uveitis were recognized in grazing yearlings.[168] The outbreaks occurred concurrently with mare reproductive loss syndrome on breeding establishments. The syndrome was only detected in horses at grass and, as a result, athletic animals were not affected.[169] The precise etiology of the syndrome remains uncertain at this time. Mare reproductive loss syndrome is associated with ingestion of eastern tent caterpillars.[170]

Diseases of the vessels

General

Three general syndromes of large vessel disease are recognized in performance horses. These are:

- sudden death or acute heart failure due to large vessel rupture/dissection
- acute or recurrent colic due to arteritis and thrombosis of the cranial mesenteric arteries
- renal arteries and a vague history of increasingly poor performance and hind limb lameness with aortoiliacofemoral thrombosis.

Aortic and great vessel rupture

Recognition

History and presenting signs

Horses present with sudden death or sudden-onset pallor, tachycardia and weakness usually during exercise. Subacute cases can also present with ventricular dysrhythmia, usually ventricular tachycardia.[78] Rapid weak pulses with pulse deficits are usually obvious.

In cases of dissection of a sinus of Valsalva aneurysm (Figs 32.52 and 32.53) there is often extreme distress and profuse sweating during the dissection phase. Affected horses are not uncommonly presented for colic. If the aneurysm eventually dissects through the septum and ruptures into the right heart (Fig. 32.52), a coarse continuous cardiac murmur suddenly develops that is usually associated with a pre-cordial thrill. If the fistula is large and the shunt flow through it substantial, the horse might present acutely with all of the physical signs of acute congestive heart failure. If the shunt fraction is small, the condition can present incidentally when a new continuous cardiac murmur is detected in an otherwise asymptomatic animal.

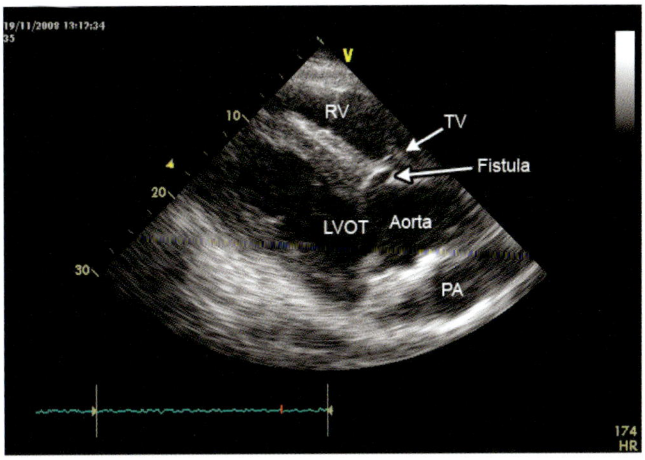

Fig 32.52A Right parasternal long-axis view of the left ventricular outflow tract of an 18-year-old three-day eventer obtained two weeks after she was presented for acute colic. At presentation, rectal examination was unremarkable, but the mare was sweaty and uncomfortable with a rapid regular heart rate, but no cardiac murmurs. Her heart rate remained elevated after analgesics and non-steroidal anti-inflammatory drugs were administered and ECG examination revealed a monomorphic ventricular tachycardia. Within 24 hours of hospitalization, a continuous grade 5/6 murmur with point of maximal intensity on the right hemithorax became audible, the mare's heart rate fell, normal sinus rhythm resumed and she no longer required analgesia. The ultrasound image shows that a fistula is now present between her right coronary sinus and her right ventricle, exiting in the typical position underneath the tricuspid valve. (LVOT = left ventricular outflow tract, PA = xxxx. RV = right ventricle, TV = tricuspid valve).

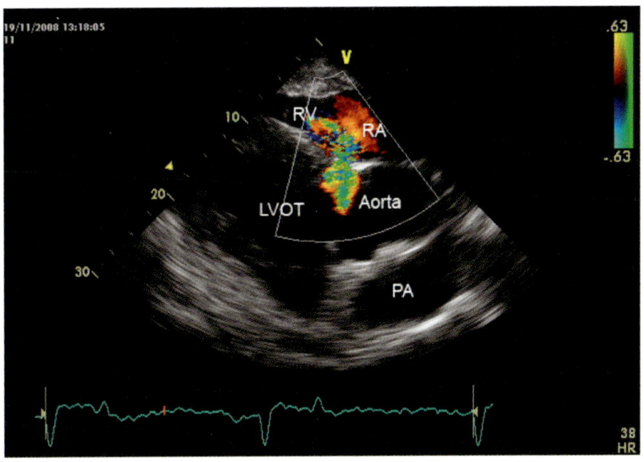

Fig 32.52B Color flow Doppler image of high-velocity flow between the aorta and right ventricle in the same mare. Because aortic pressure exceeds right ventricular pressure throughout the cardiac cycle, continuous flow of blood through the fistula results in a characteristic, continuous coarse, crescendo–decrescendo murmur. This murmur cannot be present at first presentation, because the dissecting aneurysm has not yet exited the interventricular septum. (LVOT = left ventricular outflow tract, PA = xxxx, RA = right atrium, RV = right ventricle).

In a recent study on sudden death in 268 racing Thoroughbreds, 24 horses had extrapulmonary vascular rupture of which only two had aortic rupture.[92] Hemothorax occurred in two other cases (origin unidentified) and hemoabdomen in 17 cases (rupture of external iliac artery, internal spermatic artery, mesenteric vessels, posterior vena cava, vaginal artery or an unidentified vessel).

A unique form of aortic rupture, and probably genetic disorder, is seen in Friesian horses.[171,172] The aorta ruptures close to the ligamentum arteriosum in transverse direction (often 3.5 to 6.5 cm in size) (Figs 32.54 and 32.55). Although hemothorax can result, many horses develop one or two pseudoaneurysms that rupture into the pulmonary artery. As such, an aortopulmonary fistula is formed which can be detected by echocardiography. Due to the large communication between systemic and pulmonary circulation, pulmonary vascular pressures suddenly equilibrate with systemic blood pressure. Different clinical presentations result. Sudden death at rest or during exercise occurs due to aneurysm rupture and hemothorax. Aortopulmonary fistulation more often leads to exercise intolerance, colic signs, persistent sinus tachycardia, coughing, leading to cardiac failure and death. Affected horses can survive for hours or days. Occasionally, horses with an aortopulmonary fistula, following initial signs of colic, and sinus tachycardia, jugular pulsation and edema, are able to stabilize and survive for weeks or months before eventually developing right cardiac failure. An important differential clinical sign of aortopulmonary fistulation in Friesian horses is the presence of a strong bounding pulsation in the carotid artery. Due to the equalization of aortic and pulmonary pressures only a soft systolic and early-to-mid diastolic murmur are usually present, dorsal to the aortic valve area. Clinical signs are not always definitive and the diagnosis must be confirmed

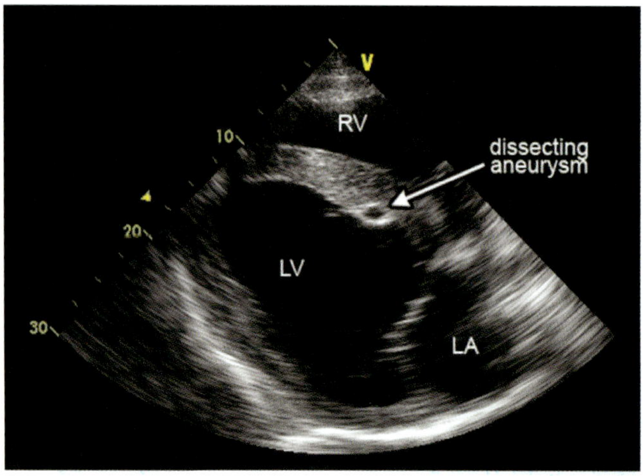

Fig 32.53A More rarely, the aneurysm can dissect ventrally under the septal endocardium on the left ventricular side.

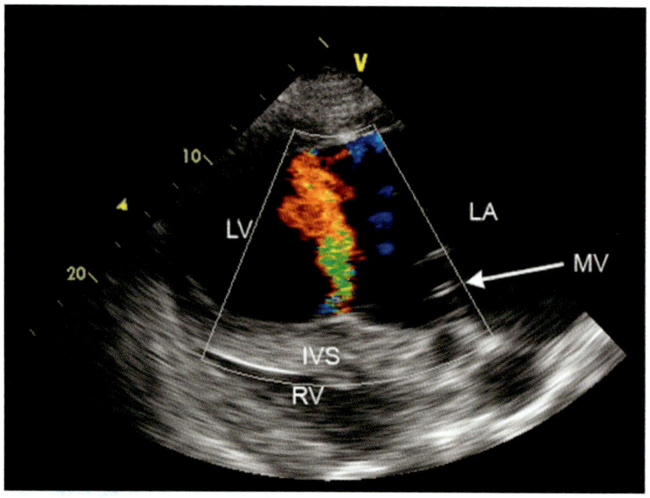

Fig 32.53B In this case, the aneurysm dissected until it eventually exited into the left ventricle, The horse presented with a diastolic murmur at his left hemithorax. This is because during systole aortic and LV pressures are the same, so flow through the fistula can only occur in diastole.

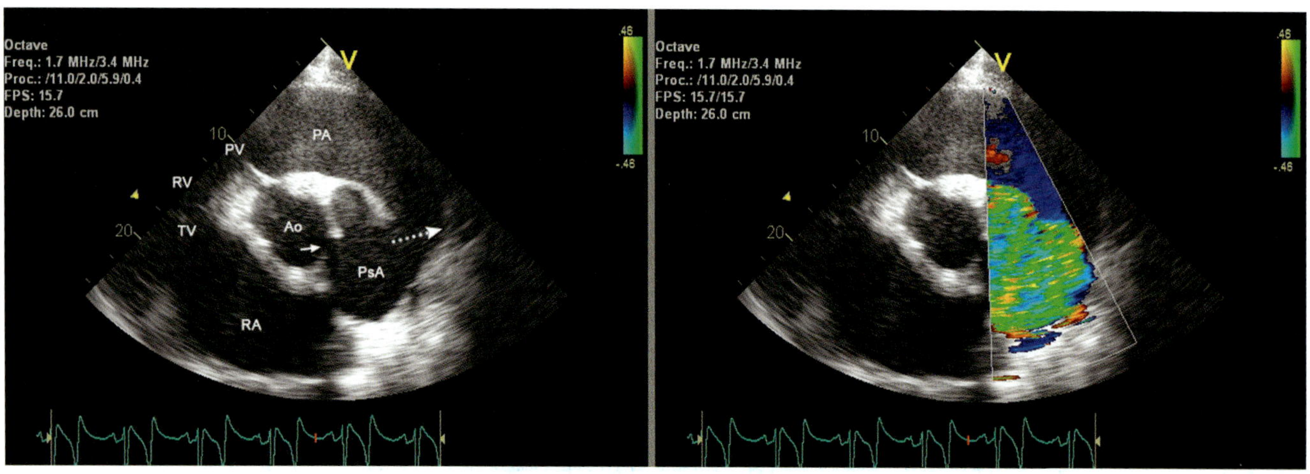

Fig 32.54 Two-dimensional (left) and color flow (right) image, taken pre-mortem from the left hemithorax of a four-year-old Friesian gelding, presented for exercise intolerance, ventral edema and loss of appetite. Right on screen is caudodorsal. The aorta (Ao) has ruptured (arrow) into a pseudoaneurysm (PsA), which in turn is connected (dotted arrow) to the pulmonary artery (PA), forming an aortopulmonary fistulation. A massive amount of turbulent blood flow is seen leaving the aorta and entering the pseudoaneurysm and pulmonary artery. Pressure and partial oxygen tension measurements during cardiac catheterization confirmed the diagnosis. Due to the grave prognosis and severity of his clinical signs, the horse was euthanized.

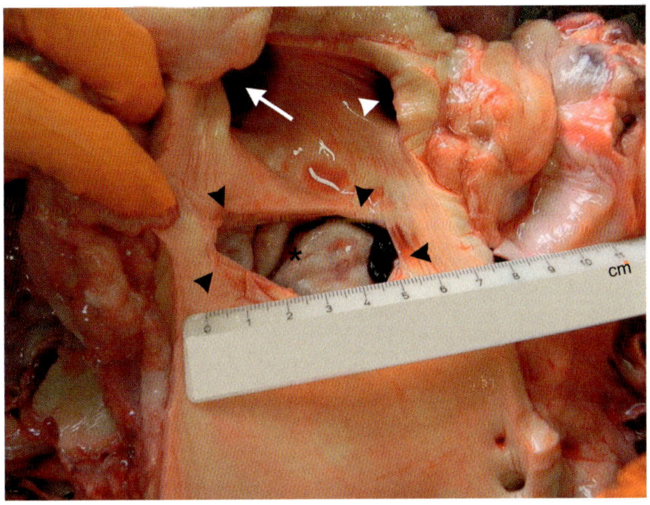

Fig 32.55 Post mortem specimen of the same horse as in Fig. 32.54, diagnosed with an aortopulmonary fistula. A 5 cm transverse rupture (arrowheads) of the aorta was present and through a pseudoaneurysm (*) it connected to the pulmonary artery, forming an aortopulmonary fistula. The white arrow indicates the aortic valves and the white arrowhead points to the brachiocephalic trunk.

by ultrasound. In 10/10 cases of aortopulmonary fistulation ultrasonography clearly identified the lesion in all cases (G. van Loon, unpublished results). The fistulous tract with pseudoaneurysm is best visualized from left parasternal oblique images (Fig. 32.54). Cardiac catheterization will confirm the presence of severe pulmonary hypertension with diastolic, systolic and mean pressures around 40–50, 90–140 and 60–90 mmHg, respectively. Blood gas analysis of blood samples taken during catheterization will demonstrate a significant increase in partial pressure of oxygen and Hb saturation in samples obtained from the right ventricle compared to the distal (right) pulmonary artery. The latter will approach results from arterial blood samples.

Treatment and prognosis

Treatment

There is no specific treatment.

Large vessel rupture into the thorax, lung or abdomen is invariably fatal. The time taken for the horse to succumb depends on the size and nature (artery or vein, systemic or pulmonary) of the vessel involved.

For dissecting sinus of Valsalva aneurysms, antiarrhythmic drugs can be needed to control the associated ventricular rhythm disturbance and analgesic/anti-inflammatory drugs are also indicated to control pain. Response to antiarrhythmic therapy is variable and will depend upon the extent of damage to the conduction tissues. Horses that survive the acute phase of dissection generally improve clinically and arrhythmia subsides when aneurysmal rupture occurs, usually into the right ventricle (Fig. 32.52A and B), but occasionally into the left ventricle (Fig. 32.53A and B), right atrium, or even more rarely, the pericardial space.[78,173] Transcatheter occlusion of an aortocardiac fistula and an aortopulmonary fistula have been attempted.[173,174]

Prognosis

Large vessel rupture

The prognosis for large vessel rupture is hopeless.

Sinus of Valsalva aneurysm

Death can occur acutely or very soon after dissection due to fatal ventricular arrhythmia.

When dissection is followed by rupture into the right heart, the horse can present subacutely with a sudden-onset continuous heart murmur, ventricular dysrhythmia, and/or acute distress. Prognosis for subacute cases depends on the site and size of the aortic rupture.

Etiology and pathogenesis

Rupture of the aorta, at the level of the sinus of Valsalva, aortic arch, or the main pulmonary artery and its branches can occur.[92,175-177] When a large vessel ruptures into the thoracic cavity, death is immediate through rapid hypovolemic shock. Aortic aneurysms are reported most frequently at or around the right coronary sinus up to the brachiocephalic trunk.[178-181] It seems likely that an aneurysmal weakness at the site of vessel rupture also underlies sudden death and rupture is most likely during strenuous exercise when arterial and pulmonary vascular pressure increases. These sites are also commonly affected with lesions associated with *Strongylus vulgaris* migration[88] and parasitic damage to arteries has been postulated to underlie great vessel rupture in horses. In subacute cases rupture of the aneurysm usually occurs at the level of the right coronary artery from whence it dissects into the interventricular septum,[78] pulmonary artery,[182] or the right heart.[183] When the aneurysm dissects through the interventricular septum, there is widespread damage of the cardiac conduction system, resulting in the characteristic ventricular rhythm disturbances. Occasionally volume overload leads to right heart failure after rupture of the aneurysm into the right ventricle.[183]

Pulmonary artery aneurysm and vessel rupture can be associated with severe pulmonary hypertension in left heart failure.

Epidemiology

Large vessel rupture and sinus of Valsalva aneurysmal dissection tend to occur most frequently, but not exclusively, in older performance horses. The former is usually associated with strenuous exercise. Rupture occurs due to systemic hypertension during exercise. However, the age factor not only plays a role in exercise-related cases of arterial wall rupture.[184,185] Therefore, one might consider that age-associated alterations in arterial wall stiffness might occur in horses, as in man.[186]

Aortoiliacofemoral thrombosis

Recognition

Presenting signs

Clinical signs vary from mild hind limb stiffness that reduces performance to more severe unilateral or bilateral hind limb lameness induced by strenuous exercise. Fairly commonly, increasingly poor performance is often noted before the onset of more dramatic clinical signs. The affected limb can feel cooler after fast exercise. Affected horses can also become distressed and unpredictable and sweat profusely immediately following very strenuous work. There can be reduced saphenous venous refill time in the affected limb after exercise and the affected limb can feel cooler. In long-standing cases there can be unilateral hind limb muscle atrophy.[187,188]

Special tests

Aortoiliacfemoral thrombosis can be diagnosed by careful rectal palpation revealing vessel occlusion/aneurysm at the bifurcation of the caudal aorta. Two-dimensional ultrasonography is the most practical method to make a definitive diagnosis,[189] although Doppler and nuclear scintigraphic methods[190] have also been used. In athletic horses, the thrombus is usually only partially occlusive at presentation and flow limitation occurs initially at maximal exercise. As the thrombus increases in size, flow limitation occurs with progressively less strenuous activity.

Therapeutic aims

The aim is to relive signs of hind limb ischemia by restoring limb blood flow. Strategies include preventing further thrombus formation, encouraging thrombolysis, providing analgesia and allowing a collateral circulation to develop.

Treatment and prognosis

Treatment

Specific treatments with various anticoagulant agents[191] and surgical removal of thrombus have been described. None have been critically assessed and recovery will always depend upon the development of collateral circulation and prevention of further clot formation. In athletic horses, daily administration of aspirin is often recommended, but its efficacy is unknown.[187] Monthly administration of ivermectin coupled with twice daily administration of phenylbutazone has also been suggested, but the efficacy of this regimen is also difficult to assess as improvements in clinical signs can result from development of collateral circulation alone.[192]

Prognosis

The prognosis for return to previous levels of athletic performance after aortoiliacofemoral thrombosis is poor.

Etiology and pathophysiology

Characteristically organized lesions are found at the aortic quadrifurcation and extend into the distal portions of the femoral and internal iliac arteries. The lesions can be partially or completely occlusive and consist of well-organized and well-vascularized fibrous tissue, occasionally containing hemorrhagic or degenerate areas. Proximal to the organized masses, thrombi are often present.[188] The pathogenesis of the lesions remains unclear. *Strongylus vulgaris* larval damage has been implicated, but actual larvae or inflammatory cells are not usually present in the lesions[188] and the larvae rarely migrate to such caudal arterial locations.[193] In addition, the disease is most frequently reported in athletic animals with a good standard of management. Others have suggested that condition can be similar to arteriosclerosis obliterans in humans when intimal damage, expression of inflammatory mediators, thrombus formation and fibrosis result in progressive vessel occlusion.[188] It has been proposed that equine iliac arteries can be predisposed to damage because of vessel branching that results in turbulent flow at a location that is already predisposed to damage because of large forces of locomotion and tight fascial attachments to surrounding tissues.[192]

Epidemiology

The condition has been documented in horses of all ages and sexes, but clinical signs are more frequently reported in male performance horses.[188] It is possible this observation reflects the higher proportion of males engaged in strenuous activity rather than a true sex difference in prevalence of arterial damage. The average age of horses in a series of 15 cases was 5.2 years.[188]

Jugular vein thrombosis

Recognition

History

Often associated with prolonged intravenous catheterization following surgical procedures. Horses with endotoxemia and septicemia are at increased risk.[194] Venous thrombosis and thrombophlebitis also occur with repeated jugular venipuncture, particularly when the drugs being administered are irritant, or intravenous injection technique is poor.

Presenting signs

When one vein is affected there might be no obvious clinical signs except localized firmness and cording of the vessel. When both vessels are affected, there will be proximal engorgement of vessels coupled with subcutaneous and local edema. Head and laryngeal swelling can occur in extreme cases. Head swelling is always exacerbated when the head is lowered, e.g. during grazing. When a long length of vein is occluded by thrombus, there can be bacterial colonization resulting in pyrexia, depression, neck stiffness, heat and pain. Inadvertent perivascular deposition of irritant drugs such as phenylbutazone, guiafenesin, thiopentone and hypertonic solutions also results in heat, swelling and localized pain. If sufficiently severe, the initial chemical irritation can be followed by a marked inflammatory response, tissue necrosis and skin sloughing.

Special examination

Two-dimensional ultrasound examination is useful to assess the extent of the thrombus, or check jugular vein patency in cases of severe perivascular inflammation and swelling. An echodense cavitating thrombus is usually present within the jugular vein. The appearance of brightly echogenic areas within the thrombus suggests that gas-forming bacteria are present and that aggressive treatment will be required. Hematological and biochemical investigation usually demonstrates leukocytosis, neutrophilia and hyperfibrinogenemia.

Treatment and prognosis

Therapeutic aims

Therapy is focused upon the need to discourage further thrombus formation and control and prevention of infection, thus reducing the chances of septic embolization and systemic complications. In mild or unilateral cases treatment cannot be required as spontaneous recanalization occurs in many affected horses.

Therapy

Prolonged systemic antibiotic therapy will be required when bacterial infection is present. All intravenous catheters must be removed and further venipuncture cease. Surgical excision and removal of the affected vein can be required when the lesion is extensive and infected.[195–197] Concurrent administration of non-steroidal anti-inflammatory drugs, hot packing and massage can also provide analgesia and relief during the acute phase.

When inadvertent perivascular injection of a known irritant has occurred, the drug should be diluted by instilling large volumes (at least 1 L) of isotonic electrolyte solution around the site. Local anesthetic agents (without epinephrine) can be added to the diluent solution to provide analgesia.

Prognosis

In most cases prognosis is good and normal jugular filling returns after recanalization occurs. If there is infection and septic embolization, prognosis is more guarded. If early aggressive treatment is not performed after perivascular injection of a known irritant, there can be extensive necrosis and sloughing of neck skin that ultimately requires reconstructive surgery. Occasionally there can be damage to the recurrent laryngeal nerves, carotid artery, ventral neck muscles and the vago-sympathetic trunk.

Etiology and pathogenesis

Localized or diffuse vascular endothelial damage exposes endothelial collagen and promotes platelet and fibrin adhesion and thrombus formation. When the thrombus is occlusive there is increased venous pressure resulting in swelling and edema in dependent areas. When thrombus or thrombophlebitis is complicated by sepsis there will pyrexia and the possibility of septic emboli causing disease in other body systems. Horses with a hypercoagulable state, or with endotoxemia and sepsis, are at a higher risk of thrombosis and thrombophlebitis.[194] Although the jugular vein is most commonly affected, thrombosis of other systemic veins has also been reported.[198]

Epidemiology

Jugular thrombosis and thrombophlebitis occur sporadically in performance horse and are usually iatrogenic, associated with administration of drugs or intravenous catheterization.

Immune-mediated vasculitis

Recognition

History

Immune-mediated vasculitis is associated with previous and ongoing infections including *Streptococcus equi* (strangles), equine viral arteritis, ehrlichiosis, equine infectious anemia and equine influenza. Occasionally the syndrome occurs after other systemic diseases including neoplasia and colitis.[199] As a result the condition is rare in athletic horses.

Presenting signs

Immune-mediated vasculitis usually results in cutaneous lesions (crusting, ulceration), edema, erythema, pyrexia, reluctance to move, depression and inappetance.

Treatment and prognosis

Treatment depends upon the underlying cause, although corticosteroids are recommended in the absence of active infection. Prognosis depends on the underlying cause, speed of recognition of clinical signs and patient response to early aggressive treatment.

References

1. Kriz NG, Hodgson DR, Rose RJ. Prevalence and clinical importance of heart murmurs in racehorses. J Am Vet Med Assoc 2000;216(9):1441–5.
2. Patteson MW, Cripps PJ. A survey of cardiac auscultatory findings in horses. Equine Vet J 1993;25(5):409–15.
3. Young LE, Wood JL. Effect of age and training on murmurs of atrioventricular valvular regurgitation in young Thoroughbreds. Equine Vet J 2000; 32(3):195–9.
4. Young LE, Wood JLN. Effect of age and training on Thoroughbred valvular competence. Proceedings of the 19th Annual Veterinary Medical Forum 2001:347–8.
5. Martin BB Jr, Reef VB, Parente EJ, et al. Causes of poor performance of horses during training, racing, or showing: 348 cases (1992–1996). J Am Vet Med Assoc 2000;216(4):554–8.
6. Naylor JM, Yadernuk LM, Pharr JW, et al. An assessment of the ability of diplomates, practitioners, and students to describe and interpret recordings of heart murmurs and arrhythmia. J Vet Intern Med 2001;15(6):507–15.
7. Patterson DF, Detweiler DK, Glendenning SA. Heart sounds and murmurs of the normal horse. Ann N Y Acad Sci 1965;127(1):242–305.
8. Welker FH, Muir WW. An investigation of the second heart sound in the normal horse. Equine Vet J 1990;22(6):403–7.
9. Scheffer CW, Robben JH, Sloet van Oldruitenborgh-Oosterbaan MM. Continuous monitoring of ECG in horses at rest and during exercise. Vet Rec 1995;137(15):371–4.
10. Hall MC, Steel JD, Stewart GA. Cardiac monitoring during exercise tests in the horse. 2. Heart rate responses to exercise. Aust Vet J 1976;52(1):1–5.
11. Holmes JR. Equine electrocardiography – Some practical hints on technique. Equine Vet J 1984;16(5):477–9.
12. Physick-Sheard PW, Hendren CM. Heart score: Physiological basis and confounding variables. Cambridge: Burlington Press Ltd; 1998.
13. Patteson MW. Equine cardiology. Oxford: Blackwell Science; 1996.
14. Hamlin RL, Klepinger WL, Gilpin KW, et al. Autonomic control of heart rate in the horse. Am J Physiol 1972;222(4): 976–8.
15. Raekallio M. Long term ECG recording with Holter monitoring in clinically healthy horses. Acta Vet Scand 1992;33(1):71–5.
16. Reef VB, Clark ES, Oliver JA, et al. Implantation of a permanent transvenous pacing catheter in a horse with complete heart block and syncope. J Am Vet Med Assoc 1986;189(4):449–52.
17. Reef VB, Levitan CW, Spencer PA. Factors affecting prognosis and conversion in equine atrial fibrillation. J Vet Intern Med 1988;2(1):1–6.
18. Deem DA, Fregin GF. Atrial fibrillation in horses: a review of 106 clinical cases, with consideration of prevalence, clinical signs, and prognosis. J Am Vet Med Assoc 1982;180(3):261–5.
19. Bonagura JD. Equine heart disease. An overview. Vet Clin North Am Equine Pract 1985;1(2):267–74.
20. Reimer JM, Reef VB, Sweeney RW. Ventricular arrhythmias in horses: 21 cases (1984–1989). J Am Vet Med Assoc 1992;201(8):1237–1243.
21. Cornick JL, Seahorn TL. Cardiac arrhythmias identified in horses with duodenitis/proximal jejunitis: six cases (1985–1988). J Am Vet Med Assoc 1990;197(8):1054–9.
22. Fregin GF, Deem DA. Epistaxis in horses with atrial fibrillation. Proceedings of the Annual Convention of the American Association of Equine Practitioners 1980;26(Nov):431–3.
23. Holmes JR, Henigan M, Williams RB, et al. Paroxysmal atrial fibrillation in racehorses. Equine Vet J 1986;18(1): 37–42.
24. Rose RJ, Davis PE. Paroxysmal atrial fibrillation in a racehorse. Aust Vet J 1977;53(11):545–9.
25. Gelzer AR, Moise NS, Vaidya D, et al. Temporal organization of atrial activity and irregular ventricular rhythm during spontaneous atrial fibrillation: an in vivo study in the horse. J Cardiovasc Electrophysiol 2000;11(7):773–84.

26. Nostell K, Haggstrom J. Resting concentrations of cardiac troponin I in fit horses and effect of racing. J Vet Cardiol 2008;10(2):105–9.
27. Packer M. How should physicians view heart-failure – the philosophical and physiological evolution of 3 conceptual models of the disease. Am J Cardiol 1993;71(9):C3–11.
28. Smith TW, Braunwald E, Kelly RA. The management of heart failure. In: Braunwald E, editor. Heart disease: a textbook of cardiovascular medicine. Philadelphia: W.B. Saunders; 1992.
29. McGuirk SM, Muir WW. Diagnosis and treatment of cardiac arrhythmias. Vet Clin North Am Equine Pract 1985;1(2):353–70.
30. Reef VB, Reimer JM, Spencer PA. Treatment of atrial fibrillation in horses: new perspectives. J Vet Intern Med 1995;9(2):57–67.
31. Muir WW, Reed SM, McGuirk SM. Treatment of atrial fibrillation in horses by intravenous administration of quinidine. J Am Vet Med Assoc 1990;197(12):1607–10.
32. Marr CM. Treatment of arrhythmias and cardiac failure. In: Robinson NE, editor. Current therapy in equine medicine. Philadelphia: W.B. Saunders Company; 1997. p. 250–9.
33. De Clercq D, van Loon G, Schauvliege S, et al. Transvenous electrical cardioversion of atrial fibrillation in six horses using custom made cardioversion catheters. Vet J 2008;177:198–204.
34. McGurrin MKJ, Physick-Sheard PW, Kenney DG, et al. transvenous electrical cardioversion in equine atrial fibrillation: technique and successful treatment of 3 horses. J Vet Intern Med 2003;17(5):715–18.
35. McGurrin MKJ, Physick-Sheard PW, Kenney DG. Transvenous electrical cardioversion of equine atrial fibrillation: patient factors and clinical results in 72 treatment episodes. J Vet Intern Med 2008;22(3):609–15.
36. van Loon G, Jordaens L, Muylle E, et al. Intracardiac overdrive pacing as a treatment of atrial flutter in a horse. Vet Rec 1998;142(12):301–3.
37. McGuirk SM, Muir WW, Sams RA. Pharmacokinetic analysis of intravenously and orally administered quinidine in horses. Am J Vet Res 1981;42(6):938–42.
38. Opie LH. Drugs for the heart. 4th ed. Philadelphia: WB Saunders Company; 1995.
39. Fagbemi SO, Chi L, Lucchesi BR. Antifibrillatory and profibrillatory actions of selected class I antiarrhythmic agents. J Cardiovasc Pharmacol 1993;21(5):709–19.
40. Wang J, Bourne GW, Wang Z, et al. Comparative mechanisms of antiarrhythmic drug action in experimental atrial fibrillation. Importance of use-dependent effects on refractoriness. Circulation 1993;88(3):1030–44.
41. Miller MR, McNamara RL, Segal JB, et al. Efficacy of agents for pharmacologic conversion of atrial fibrillation and subsequent maintenance of sinus rhythm – a meta-analysis of clinical trials. J Fam Pract 2000;49(11):1033–46.
42. Naccarelli GV, Dorian P, Hohnloser SH, et al. Prospective comparison of flecainide verses quinidine for the treatment of paroxysmal atrial fibrillation flutter. Am J Cardiol 1996;77(3):A53–9.
43. Ohmura H, Hiraga A, Aida H, et al. Determination of oral dosage and pharmacokinetic analysis of flecainide in horses. J Vet Med Sci 2001;63(5):511–14.
44. Ohmura H, Nukada T, Mizuno Y, et al. Safe and efficacious dosage of flecainide acetate for treating equine atrial fibrillation. J Vet Med Sci 2000;62(7):711–15.
45. van Loon G, Blissitt KJ, Keen JA, et al. Use of intravenous flecainide in horses with naturally-occuring atrial fibrillation. Equine Vet J 2004;36(7):609–15.
46. De Clercq D, van Loon G, Baert K, et al. Effects of an adapted intravenous amiodarone treatment protocol in horses with atrial fibrillation. Equine Vet J 2007;39(4):344–9.
47. De Clercq D, van Loon G, Baert K, et al. Intravenous amiodarone treatment in horses with chronic atrial fibrillation. Vet J 2006;172:129–34.
48. De Clercq D, Baert K, Croubels S, et al. Evaluation of the pharmacokinetics and bioavailability of intravenously and orally administered amiodarone in horses. Am J Vet Res 2006;67(3):448–54.
49. van Loon G. Methods of treatment and new management techniques in horses with atrial fibrillation. Paper presented at Veterinary Cardiovascular Society, 2003. Loughborough, UK.
50. Jesty SA, Kraus M, Gelzer A, et al. Effect of transvenous electrical cardioversion on plasma cardiac troponin I concentrations in horses with atrial fibrillation. J Vet Intern Med 2009;23(5):1103–7.
51. Johnston GM, Eastment JK, Wood JLN, et al. The confidential enquiry into perioperative equine fatalities (CEPEF): mortality results of Phases 1 and 2. Vet Anaesth Analg 2002;29(4):159–70.
52. Schauvliege S, van Loon G, De Clercq D, et al. Cardiovascular responses to transvenous electrical cardioversion of atrial fibrillation in anaesthetized horses. Vet Anaesth Analg 2009;36(4):341–51.
53. van Loon G, De Clercq D, Tavernier R, et al. Transient complete atrioventricular block following transvenous electrical cardioversion of atrial fibrillation in a horse. Vet J 2005;170(1):124–7.
54. Preiss EE, Kenney DG, McGurrin MKJ, et al. Influence of electrode position on cardioversion energy requirements during transvenous electrical cardioversion in horses. Am J Vet Res 2011;72(9):1193–203.
55. De Clercq D, van Loon G, Tavernier R, et al. Atrial and ventricular electrical and contractile remodeling and reverse remodeling owing to short-term pacing-induced atrial fibrillation in horses. J Vet Intern Med 2008;22(6):1353–9.
56. De Clercq D, van Loon G, Tavernier R, et al. What happens after induction and termination of chronic atrial fibrillation in horses? In: Association Vétérinaire Equine Française (AVEF). France: Deauville; 2009. p. 204–5.
57. van Loon G, Duytschaever M, Tavernier R, et al. An equine model of chronic atrial fibrillation: methodology. Vet J 2002;164(2):142–50.
58. van Loon G. Atrial fibrillation in equines: prevalence, symptoms and pathophysiology. Paper presented at: Veterinary Cardiovascular Society, 2003. Loughborough, UK.
59. Verheyen T, Decloedt A, Van Der Vekens N, et al. Ventricular response during lunging exercise in horses with lone atrial fibrillation. Equine Vet J 2012;45(3):309–14.
60. Moore EN, Spear JF. Electrophysiological studies on atrial fibrillation. Heart Vessels Suppl 1987;2:32–9.
61. Nattel S. New ideas about atrial fibrillation 50 years on. Nature 2002;415(6868):219–26.
62. Coumel P. Management of atrial fibrillation. Isr J Med Sci 1996;32(10):871–2.
63. Coumel P, Thomas O, Leenhardt A. Drug therapy for prevention of atrial fibrillation. Am J Cardiol 1996;77(3):A3–9.
64. Muir WW, McGuirk SM. Hemodynamics before and after conversion of atrial fibrillation to normal sinus rhythm in horses. J Am Vet Med Assoc 1984;184(8):965–70.
65. Collatos C, Clark ES, Reef VB, et al. Septicemia, atrial-fibrillation, cardiomegaly, left atrial mass, and *Rhodococcus equi* septic osteoarthritis in a foal. J Am Vet Med Assoc 1990;197(8):1039–42.
66. Gelberg HB, Smetzer DL, Foreman JH. Pulmonary hypertension as a cause of atrial fibrillation in young horses: four cases (1980–1989). J Am Vet Med Assoc 1991;198(4):679–82.

67. Else RW, Holmes JR. Pathological changes in atrial fibrillation in the horse. Equine Vet J 1971;3(1):56–64.
68. Schwarzwald CC, Schober KE, Bonagura JD. Echocardiographic evidence of left atrial mechanical dysfunction after conversion of atrial fibrillation to sinus rhythm in 5 horses. J Vet Intern Med 2007;21(4):820–7.
69. Ohmura H, Hiraga A, Takahashi T, et al. Risk factors for atrial fibrillation during racing in slow-finishing horses. J Am Vet Med Assoc 2003;223(1):84–8.
70. Petch MC. Atrial fibrillation: bad news for man and horse? Equine Vet J 1986;18(1):3–4.
71. Buhl R. Valvular regurgitations in the horse: the importance of an exercise ECG. Vet J 2010;183(2):117–18.
72. Barbesgaard L, Buhl R, Meldgaard C. Prevalence of exercise-associated arrhythmias in normal performing dressage horses. Equine Vet J 2010;42: 202–7.
73. Ryan N, Marr CM, McGladdery AJ. Survey of cardiac arrhythmias during submaximal and maximal exercise in Thoroughbred racehorses. Equine Vet J 2005;37(3):265–8.
74. Else RW, Holmes JR. Cardiac pathology in the horse. 1. Gross pathology. Equine Vet J 1972;4(1):1–8.
75. Else RW, Holmes JR. Cardiac pathology in the horse. 2. Microscopic pathology. Equine Vet J 1972;4(2):57–62.
76. Button C, Scrutchfield WL, Clark RG, et al. Multiple atrial dysrhythmias in a horse. J Am Vet Med Assoc 1980;177(8): 714–19.
77. Buhl R, Meldgaard C, Barbesgaard L. Cardiac arrhythmias in clinically healthy showjumping horses. Equine Vet J 2010;42:196–201.
78. Marr CM, Reef VB, Brazil TJ, et al. Aorto-cardiac fistulas in seven horses. Vet Radiol Ultrasound 1998;39(1): 22–31.
79. Leroux AJ, Schott HC, Hines MT. Ventricular tachycardia associated with exhaustive exercise in a horse. J Am Vet Med Assoc 1995;207(3):335–7.
80. Physick-Sheard PW, McGurrin MKJ. Ventricular arrhythmias during race recovery in Standardbred Racehorses and associations with autonomic activity. J Vet Intern Med 2010;24(5): 1158–66.
81. Jose-Cunilleras E, Young LE, Newton JR, et al. Cardiac arrhythmias during and after treadmill exercise in poorly performing Thoroughbred racehorses. Equine Vet J Suppl 2006:163–70.
82. Paterson DJ. Antiarrhythmic mechanisms during exercise. J Appl Physiol 1996;80(6):1853–62.
83. Diana A, Guglielmini C, Candini D, et al. Cardiac arrhythmias associated with piroplasmosis in the horse: A case report. Vet J 2007;174(1):193–5.
84. Verheyen T, Decloedt A, De Clercq D, et al. Cardiac changes in horses with atypical myopathy. J Vet Intern Med 2012;26(4):1019–26.
85. Durie I, van Loon G, De Clercq D, et al. Nerium oleander intoxication in horses: 3 cases. Paper presented at: 47th British Equine Veterinary Association Congress; April 10–14, 2008, Liverpool, UK.
86. Lyle CH, Blissitt KJ, Kennedy RN, et al. Risk factors for race-associated sudden death in Thoroughbred racehorses in the UK (2000–2007). Equine Vet J 2012;44(4):459–65.
87. Opie LH. Electricity out of control: ventricular arrhythmias. New York: Lippincott Raven; 1998.
88. Cranley JJ, McCullagh KG. Ischaemic myocardial fibrosis and aortic strongylosis in the horse. Equine Vet J 1981;13(1):35–42.
89. Kiryu K, Machida N, Kashida Y, et al. Pathologic and electrocardiographic findings in sudden cardiac death in racehorses. J Vet Med Sci 1999;61(8): 921–8.
90. Traub-Dargatz JL, Schlipf JW Jr, Boon J, et al. Ventricular tachycardia and myocardial dysfunction in a horse. J Am Vet Med Assoc 1994;205(11): 1569–73.
91. Machida N, Nakamura T, Kiryu K, et al. Cardiopathological observation on a case of persistent ventricular tachycardia in a pony mare. J Vet Med Sci 1992;54(6):1213–16.
92. Lyle CH, Uzal FA, McGorum BC, et al. Sudden death in racing Thoroughbred horses: an international multicentre study of post mortem findings. Equine Vet J 2011;43(3):324–31.
93. van Loon G, Laevens H, Deprez P. Temporary transvenous atrial pacing in horses: threshold determination. Equine Vet J 2001;33(3):290–5.
94. van Loon G, Fonteyne W, Rottiers H, et al. Dual chamber pacemaker implantation via the cephalic vein in healthy equids. J Vet Intern Med 2001;15(6):564–71.
95. van Loon G, Fonteyne W, Rottiers H, et al. Implantation of a dual-chamber, rate-adaptive pacemaker in a horse with suspected sick sinus syndrome. Vet Rec 2002;151(20):541–5.
96. Hamir AN, Reef VB. Complications of a permanent transvenous pacing catheter in a horse. J Comp Pathol 1989;101(3): 317–26.
97. Zucca E, Ferrucci F, Stancari G, et al. The Prevalence of cardiac murmurs among standardbred racehorses presented with poor performance. J Vet Med Sci 2010;72(6):781–5.
98. Reef VB. Heart murmurs in horses: determining their significance with echocardiography. Equine Vet J Suppl 1995;(19):71–80.
99. Reef VB, Bain FT, Spencer PA. Severe mitral regurgitation in horses: clinical, echocardiographic and pathological findings. Equine Vet J 1998;30(1): 18–27.
100. Young LE, Rogers K, Wood JLN. Heart murmurs and valvular regurgitation in Thoroughbred racehorses: epidemiology and associations with athletic performance. J Vet Intern Med 2008;22(2):418–26.
101. Buhl R, Ersboll AK, Eriksen L, et al. Use of color Doppler echocardiography to assess the development of valvular regurgitation in Standardbred trotters. J Am Vet Med Assoc 2005;227(10): 1630–5.
102. Young LE. Cardiac responses to training in 2-year-old Thoroughbreds: an echocardiographic study. Equine Vet J Suppl 1999;30:195–8.
103. Maxson AD, Reef VB. Bacterial endocarditis in horses: ten cases (1984–1995). Equine Vet J 1997;29(5): 394–9.
104. Buergelt CD, Cooley AJ, Hines SA, et al. Endocarditis in six horses. Vet Pathol 1985;22(4):333–7.
105. Ewart S, Brown C, Derksen F, et al. *Serratia marcescens* endocarditis in a horse. J Am Vet Med Assoc 1992;200(7): 961–3.
106. McCormick BS, Peet RL, Downes K. *Erysipelothrix rhusiopathiae* vegetative endocarditis in a horse. Aust Vet J 1985;62(11):392.
107. Dedrick P, Reef VB, Sweeney RW, et al. Treatment of bacterial endocarditis in a horse. J Am Vet Med Assoc 1988;193(3): 339–42.
108. Long KJ. Doppler echocardiography – clinical applications. Equine Vet Educ 1993;5:161–6.
109. Long KJ. Echocardiographic studies of valvular and ventricular function in horses [PhD]. Edinburgh: University of Edinburgh, United Kingdom; 1993.
110. Helwegen MM, Young LE, Rogers K, et al. Measurements of right ventricular internal dimensions and their relationships to severity of tricuspid valve regurgitation in national hunt Thoroughbreds. Equine Vet J Suppl 2006;36:171–7.
111. Buhl R, Ersboll AK, Eriksen L, et al. Changes over time in echocardiographic measurements in young Standardbred racehorses undergoing training and racing and association with racing performance. J Am Vet Med Assoc 2005;226(11):1881–7.
112. Zucca E, Ferrucci F, Stancari G, et al. Evaluation of cardiac Troponin I serum concentration in standardbred horses

before and after strenuous exercise on treadmill. Ippologia 2010;21(4):3–9.
113. Lightfoot G, Jose-Cunilleras E, Rogers K, et al. An echocardiographic and auscultation study of right heart responses to training in young National Hunt Thoroughbred horses. Equine Vet J 2006;38(S36):153–8.
114. Buhl R, Ersboll AK. Echocardiographic evaluation of changes in left ventricular size and valvular regurgitation associated with physical training during and after maturity in Standardbred trotters. J Am Vet Med Assoc 2012;240(2):205–12.
115. Pollak SJ, McMillan SA, Knopff WD, et al. Cardiac evaluation of women distance runners by echocardiographic color Doppler flow mapping. J Am Coll Cardiol 1988;11(1):89–93.
116. Davis JL, Gardner SY, Schwabenton B, et al. Congestive heart failure in horses: 14 cases (1984–2001). J Am Vet Med Assoc 2002;220(10):1512–15.
117. Holmes JR, Miller PJ. Three cases of ruptured mitral valve chordae in the horse. Equine Vet J 1984;16(2):125–35.
118. Reef VB. Mitral valvular insufficiency associated with ruptured chordae tendineae in three foals. J Am Vet Med Assoc 1987;191(3):329–31.
119. Marr CM, Love S, Pirie HM, et al. Confirmation by Doppler echocardiography of valvular regurgitation in a horse with a ruptured chorda tendinea of the mitral valve. Vet Rec 1990;127(15):376–9.
120. Reef VB. Evaluation of ventricular septal defects in horses using two-dimensional and Doppler echocardiography. Equine Vet J Suppl 1995;(19):86–95.
121. Reef VB, Spencer P. Echocardiographic evaluation of equine aortic insufficiency. Am J Vet Res 1987;48(6):904–9.
122. Bonagura JD, Pipers FS. Echocardiographic features of aortic valve endocarditis in a dog, a cow, and a horse. J Am Vet Med Assoc 1983;182(6):595–9.
123. Stevens KB, Marr CM, Horn JNR, et al. Effect of left-sided valvular regurgitation on mortality and causes of death among a population of middle-aged and older horses. Vet Rec 2009;164(1):6–10.
124. Taylor SE, Else RW, Keen JA. Congenital aortic valve dysplasia in a Clydesdale foal. Equine Vet Educ 2007;19(9):463–8.
125. Horn JNR. Sympathetic nervous control of cardiac function and its role in equine heart disease [PhD]. London: University of London, United Kingdom; 2002.
126. Reppas GP, Canfield PJ, Hartley WJ, et al. Multiple congenital cardiac anomalies and idiopathic thoracic aortitis in a horse. Vet Rec 1996;138(1):14–16.
127. Bayly WM, Reed SM, Leathers CW, et al. Multiple congenital heart anomalies in five Arabian foals. J Am Vet Med Assoc 1982;181(7):684–9.
128. Zamora CS, Vitums A, Nyrop KA, et al. Atresia of the right atrioventricular orifice with complete transposition of the great arteries in a horse. Anat Histol Embryol 1989;18(2):177–82.
129. Vitums A, Bayly WM. Pulmonary atresia with dextroposition of the aorta and ventricular septal defect in three Arabian foals. Vet Pathol 1982;19(2):160–8.
130. Vitums A, Grant BD, Stone EC, et al. Transposition of the aorta and atresia of the pulmonary trunk in a horse. Cornell Vet 1973;63(1):41–57.
131. Critchley KL. An interventricular septal defect, pulmonary stenosis and bicuspid pulmonary valve in a Welsh pony foal. Equine Vet J 1976;8(4):176–8.
132. Muylle E, De Roose P, Oyaert W, et al. An interventricular septal defect and a tricuspid valve insufficiency in a trotter mare. Equine Vet J 1974;6(4):174–6.
133. Prickett ME, Reeves JT, Zent WW. Tetralogy of fallot in a Thoroughbred foal. J Am Vet Med Assoc 1973;162(7):552–5.
134. Gumbrell RC. Atresia of the tricuspid valve in a foal. N Z Vet J 1970;18(11):253–6.
135. De Clercq D, van Loon G, Deprez P. Truncus arteriosus persistens in an Arabian foal. Vlaams Diergeneesk Tijdschr 2007;76(1):49–54.
136. Crowe MW, Swerczek TW. Equine congenital defects. Am J Vet Res 1985;46(2):353–8.
137. van Loon G, Deprez P. Echographic diagnosis of complex congenital cardiac anomalies in two adult horses. Vlaams Diergeneesk Tijdschr 1998;67(5):288–92.
138. Bezerra PS, Driemeier D, Loretti AP, et al. Monensin poisoning in Brazilian horses. Vet Hum Toxicol 1999;41(6):383–5.
139. Bila CG, Perreira CL, Gruys E. Accidental monensin toxicosis in horses in Mozambique. J S Afr Vet Assoc 2001;72(3):163–4.
140. Doonan GR, Brown CM, Mullaney TP, et al. Monensin poisoning in horses – an international incident. Can Vet J 1989;30(2):165–9.
141. Hughes KJ, Hoffmann KL, Hodgson DR. Long-term assessment of horses and ponies post exposure to monensin sodium in commercial feed. Equine Vet J 2009;41(1):47–52.
142. Muylle E, Vandenhende C, Oyaert W, et al. Delayed monensin sodium toxicity in horses. Equine Vet J 1981;13(2):107–8.
143. Nuytten J, Bruynooghe D, Muylle E, et al. Accidental monensin intoxication in horses – acute and subacute symptoms. Vlaams Diergeneesk Tijdschr 1981;50(4):242–9.
144. Sarcey G, Lorgne G. Equine intoxications by polyether antibiotics. Pratique Veterinaire Equine 1993;23:45–50.
145. Guthrie AJ, Killeen VM, Mulders MS, et al. Use of the cardiopulmonary flow index to evaluate cardiac function in Thoroughbred horses. J S Afr Vet Assoc 1991;62(2):43–7.
146. Decloedt A, Verheyen T, De Clercq D, et al. Acute and long-term cardiomyopathy and delayed neurotoxicity after accidental lasalocid poisoning in horses. J Vet Intern Med 2012;26(4):1005–11.
147. Decloedt A, Verheyen T, Sys S, et al. Tissue Doppler imaging and 2-dimensional speckle tracking of left ventricular function in horses exposed to lasalocid. J Vet Intern Med 2012;26(5):1209–16.
148. Freel KM, Morrison LR, Thompson H, et al. Arrhythmogenic right ventricular cardiomyopathy as a cause of unexpected cardiac death in two horses. Vet Rec 2010;166(23):718–21.
149. Reef VB. Stress echocardiography and its role in performance assessment. Vet Clin North Am Equine Pract 2001;17(1):179–89.
150. Reef VB. Electrocardiography and echocardiography in the exercising horse. In: Robinson NE, editor. Current therapy in equine medicine. Philadelphia: W.B. Saunders Company; 1997. p. 234–9.
151. Feigenbaum H. Evolution of stress-testing. Circulation 1992;85(3):1217–18.
152. Durando MM, Reef VB, Birks EK. Right ventricular pressure dynamics: relationship to stress echocardiography. Equine Vet J Suppl 2002;34:472–7.
153. Fisher EW, Pirie HM, Andrew H. Clinical-pathological correlation of an equine cardiac arrhythmia. Vet Rec 1970;86(17):499–502.
154. Schwarzwald CC, Hardy J, Buccellato M. High cardiac troponin I serum concentration in a horse with multiform ventricular tachycardia and myocardial necrosis. J Vet Intern Med 2003;17(3):364–8.
155. Blomme EAG, La Perle KMD, Wilkins PA, et al. Ionophore toxicity in horses. Equine Vet Educ 1999;11(3):153–8.
156. Matsuoka T, Novilla MN, Thomson TD, et al. Review of monensin toxicosis in horses. J Equine Vet Sci 1996;16(1):8–15.
157. Dickinson CE, TraubDargatz JL, Dargatz DA, et al. Rattlesnake venom poisoning in horses: 32 cases (1973–1993). J Am

Vet Med Assoc 1996;208(11):1866–1871.
158. Opie LH. Heart failure and neurohumoral responses. New York: Lippincott Raven; 1998.
159. Visseren FLJ, Bouwman JJM, Bouter KP, et al. Procoagulant activity of endothelial cells after infection with respiratory viruses. Thromb Haemost 2000;84(2):319–24.
160. Del Piero F. Equine viral arteritis. Vet Pathol 2000;37(4):287–96.
161. Brown CC, Meyer RF, Grubman MJ. Presence of African horse sickness virus in equine tissues, as determined by in situ hybridization. Vet Pathol 1994;31(6):689–94.
162. Machida N, Taniguchi T, Nakamura T, et al. Cardio-histopathological observations on aborted equine fetuses infected with equid herpesvirus 1 (EHV-1). J Comp Pathol 1997;116(4):379–85.
163. Powell DG. Equine infectious respiratory disease. Vet Rec 1995;96:30–4.
164. Wilson WD. Equine influenza. Vet Clin North Am Equine Pract 1993;9(2):257–82.
165. Worth LT, Reef VB. Pericarditis in horses: 18 cases (1986–1995). J Am Vet Med Assoc 1998;212(2):248–53.
166. Freestone JF, Thomas WP, Carlson GP, et al. Idiopathic effusive pericarditis with tamponade in the horse. Equine Vet J 1987;19(1):38–42.
167. Hardy J, Robertson JT, Reed SM. Constrictive pericarditis in a mare – attempted treatment by partial pericardiectomy. Equine Vet J 1992;24(2):151–4.
168. Seahorn JL, Slovis NM, Reimer JM, et al. Case-control study of factors associated with fibrinous pericarditis among horses in central Kentucky during spring 2001. J Am Vet Med Assoc 2003;223(6):832–8.
169. Dwyer RM, Garber L, Traub-Dargatz J, et al. An epidemiological investigation of mare reproductive loss syndrome: breaking ground on a new disease. Society for Veterinary Epidemiology and Preventive Medicine, Vicenary Proceedings 2002:44–7.
170. Webb BA, Barney WE, Dahlman DL, et al. Eastern tent caterpillars (*Malacosoma americanum*) cause mare reproductive loss syndrome. J Insect Physiol 2004;50(2–3):185–93.
171. van Loon G, De Clercq D, de Bruijn CM, et al. Clinical findings and diagnosis of aortopulmonary fistula in 4 Friesian horses. Paper presented at 49th British Equine Veterinary Association congress; September 8–11, 2010, Birmingham, UK.
172. van Loon G, De clercq D, de Bruijn CM, et al. Aortic rupture and aortopulmonary fistulation: increased prevalence in Friesian horses and importance of early ante-mortem diagnosis. Paper presented at: 39ième Congrès de l'Association Vétérinaires Equines Française; 2–4 December 2011, Lyon, France.
173. Javsicas LH, Giguere S, Maisenbacher HW, et al. Percutaneous transcatheter closure of an aorto-cardiac fistula in a Thoroughbred stallion using an Amplatzer occluder device. J Vet Intern Med 2010;24(4):994–8.
174. van Loon G, Verheyen T, Decloedt A, et al. Use of a transcatheter occlusion device in a 9-year old Friesian gelding with aortopulmonary fistula. Paper presented at: 44th European Veterinary Conference Voorjaarsdagen; April 27–29, 2011, Amsterdam, The Netherlands.
175. Platt H. Sudden and unexpected deaths in horses – a review of 69 cases. Br Vet J 1982;138(5):417–29.
176. Gelberg HB, Zachary JF, Everitt JI, et al. Sudden-death in training and racing Thoroughbred horses. J Am Vet Med Assoc 1985;187(12):1354–6.
177. Brown CM, Kaneene JB, Taylor RF. Sudden and unexpected death in horses and ponies – an analysis of 200 cases. Equine Vet J 1988;20(2):99–103.
178. Sleeper MM, Durando MM, Miller M, et al. Aortic root disease in four horses. J Am Vet Med Assoc 2001;219(4):491–6.
179. Derksen FJ, Reed SM, Hall CC. Aneurysm of the aortic-arch and bicarotid trunk in a horse. J Am Vet Med Assoc 1981;179(7):692–4.
180. Reef VB, Klumpp S, Maxson AD, et al. Echocardiographic detection of an intact aneurysm in a horse. J Am Vet Med Assoc 1990;197(6):752–5.
181. Shirai W, Momotani E, Sato T, et al. Dissecting aortic aneurysm in a horse. J Comp Pathol 1999;120(3):307–11.
182. Holmes JR, Rezakhani A, Else RW. Rupture of a dissecting aortic aneurysm into the left pulmonary artery in a horse. Equine Vet J 1973;5(2):65–70.
183. Roby KA, Reef VB, Shaw DP, et al. Rupture of an aortic sinus aneurysm in a 15-year-old broodmare. J Am Vet Med Assoc 1986;189(3):305–8.
184. Arnold CE, Payne M, Thompson JA, et al. Periparturient, hemorrhage in mares: 73 cases (1998–2005). J Am Vet Med Assoc 2008;232(9):1345–51.
185. Frederick J, Giguere S, Butterworth K, et al. Severe phenylephrine-associated hemorrhage in five aged horses. J Am Vet Med Assoc 2010;237(7):830–4.
186. van Loon G, De Witte M, Rossel N, et al. Measurement of arterial diameter distension to assess arterial wall stiffness in horses: preliminary results Paper presented at 5th Congress of the European College of Equine Internal Medicine; February 2–4, 2012, Edinburgh, UK.
187. Dyson SJ, Worth LT. Aortailiacofemoral thrombosis. Philadelphia: W. B. Saunders Company; 1997.
188. Maxie MG, Physick-sheard PW Aortic-iliac thrombosis in horses. Vet Pathol 1985;22(3):238–49.
189. Reef VB, Roby KAW, Richardson DW, et al. Use of ultrasonography for the detection of aortic-iliac thrombosis in horses. J Am Vet Med Assoc 1987;190(3):286–8.
190. Boswell JC, Marr CM, Cauvin ER, et al. The use of scintigraphy in the diagnosis of aortic-iliac thrombosis in a horse. Equine Vet J 1999;31(6):537–41.
191. Branscom BL. Treatment of arterial thrombosis in a horse with sodium gluconate. J Am Vet Med Assoc 1968;152(11):1643–6.
192. Harris PA. Musculoskeletal system. In: Reed SM, Bayly WM, editors. Equine internal medicine. Philadelphia: W. B. Saunders Company; 1998. p. 371–426.
193. Morgan SJ, Stromberg PC, Storts RW, et al. Histology and morphometry of *Strongylus vulgaris*-mediated equine mesenteric arteritis. J Comp Pathol 1991;104(1):89–99.
194. Lankveld DPK, Ensink JM, van Dijk P, et al. Factors influencing the occurrence of thrombophlebitis after post-surgical long-term intravenous catheterization of colic horses: a study of 38 cases. J Vet Med A Physiol Pathol Clin Med 2001;48(9):545–52.
195. Rijkenhuizen AB, van Swieten HA. Reconstruction of the jugular vein in horses with post thrombophlebitis stenosis using saphenous vein graft. Equine Vet J 1998;30(3):236–9.
196. Wiemer P, Ugahary F. Surgical treatment of complete thrombosis of the jugular vein in a horse with a synthetic vascular graft. Tijdschr Diergeneeskd 1998;123(2):40–4.
197. Ben Chehida N, Bellagha A, Bardi K. Treatment of thromobophlebitis in a horse using a polytetrafluoroethylene (PTFE) prosthesis. Pratique Veterinaire Equine 1994;26:169–73.
198. Brianceau P, Divers TJ. Acute thrombosis of limb arteries in horses with sepsis: five cases (1988–1998). Equine Vet J 2001;33(1):105–9.
199. Morris DD. Cutaneous vasculitis in horses – 19 cases (1978–1985). J Am Vet Med Assoc 1987;191(4):460–4.

section 5

Metabolism and nutrition

Metabolic responses to exercise and training

33

Dominique Votion

CHAPTER CONTENTS

Introduction

A sustained supply of energy within skeletal muscle is fundamental to physical activity. Muscle contraction and relaxation are dependent on the hydrolysis of high-energy phosphate bonds. Adenosine-5′-triphosphate (ATP) is the primary energy currency; ATP contains three phosphate groups, two of which can be utilized in energy-requiring processes. This chapter reviews the whole-body and muscular metabolic responses to exercise and also describes the effects of training adaptation on these processes.

Physiological response to exercise

Overview

Integration of various body systems

The physiological response to exercise is a coordinated event that involves integration of various body systems to sustain ATP turnover at the level of working muscles. Several hormones act on the lungs, heart, spleen, vasculature and muscles to increase metabolic rate. Physiological adaptations to exercise increase blood flow and oxygen delivery to muscles while maintaining thermal homeostasis. In addition, the supply of energy substrates to muscle is increased via the mobilization of reserves in the liver and in adipose tissue, in addition to catabolic processes within muscle (Fig. 33.1).

The overall response to exercise is regulated by several hormones released into circulation. The initial response to exercise is primarily controlled by epinephrine and norepinephrine, two catecholamines synthesized and released by the adrenal medulla of the adrenal glands in response to the exercise-induced stress. Norepinephrine is also a neuromodulator of the peripheral sympathetic nervous system where it is released from synaptic vesicles. Among other effects, catecholamines stimulate the cardiovascular and respiratory systems, and induce splenic contraction. They contribute to the redistribution of blood flow to working muscles and promote catabolic processes to provide energy. The increase in catecholamine concentrations occurs at the onset of exercise and is proportional to exercise intensity. In horses during maximal effort, the responses are several-fold greater than in humans.[1–3] Mobilization of fuel for muscular work is also under the dependence of hormones such as glucagon that acts on the liver to induce glycogenolysis and gluconeogenesis. Glucocorticoids, in particular cortisol, also play a role in enhancing substrate availability.

High aerobic capacity (expressed as the maximal rate of oxygen consumption [VO_{2max}]) underpins the athletic power of horses.[4,5] On a mass specific basis, racehorses typically have values for VO_{2max} at least double those of elite human athletes (>200 mL.min^{-1}.kg^{-1} [6] versus 80 mL.min^{-1}.kg^{-1} [7]). The up to 50-fold increase in oxygen consumption from rest to maximal exercise is facilitated by adjustments in cardiopulmonary function, including a large increase in oxygen extraction from blood perfusing the muscles and increases in pulmonary blood flow and ventilation. During high-intensity exercise, respiratory rate increases 10-fold and the tidal volume three-fold; consequently, the minute ventilation may reach 1500 L/min with peak expiratory airflow as high as 90 L/s.[8,9] During exercise, cardiac output may increase 10-fold (versus 6-fold in human athletes) whereas the heart rate may exceed 230 beats/min[8,10,11] (versus 170–190 beats/min in trained men[12]). Also, in response to the sympathetic stimulation of exercise, the oxygen-carrying capacity of the blood is enhanced by the release into circulation of red blood cells (RBCs) stored in the spleen with total circulating RBCs increasing by as much as 50%.[13] The muscle vascular bed accommodates such an increase in blood flow via capillary dilatation mediated by the autonomic nervous system and locally produced vasoactive substances. At VO_{2max}, skeletal muscle

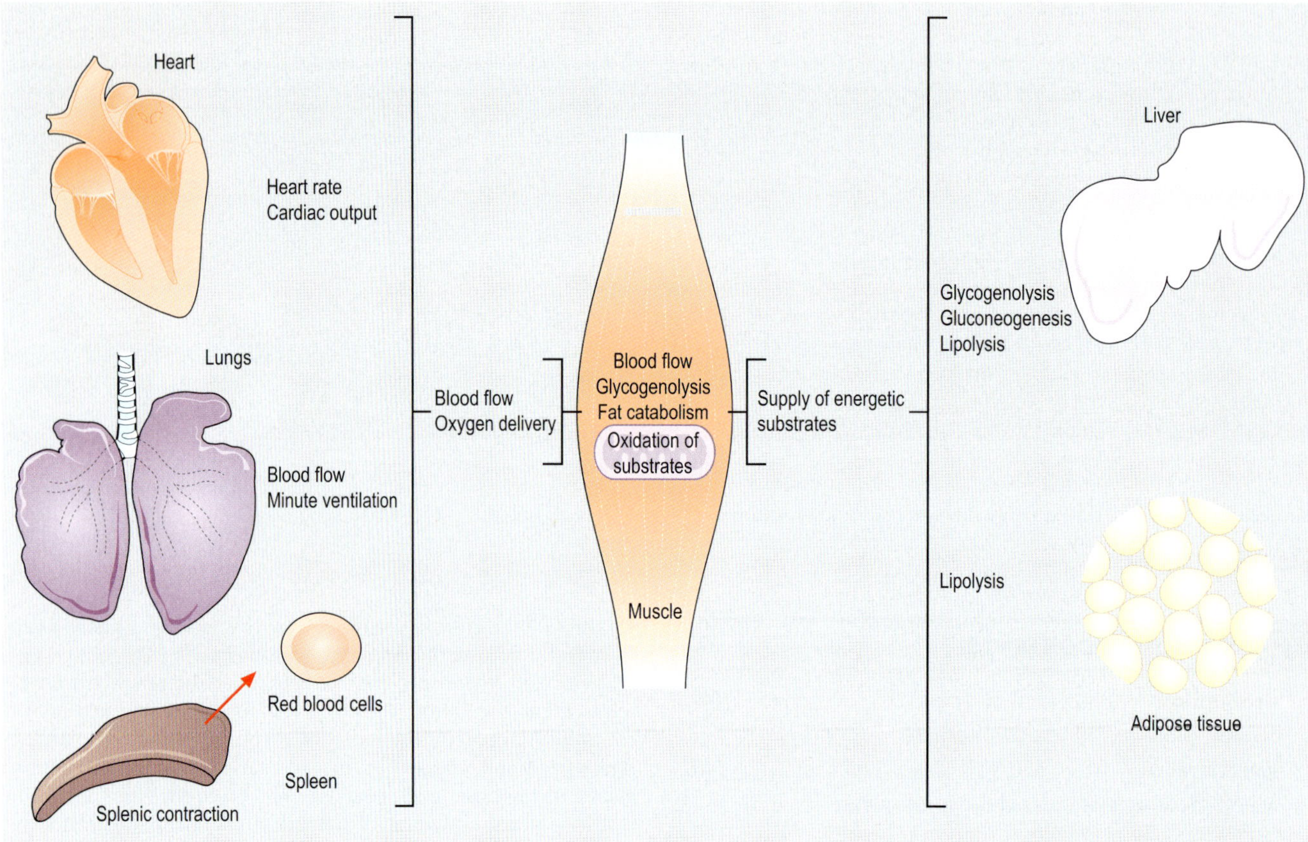

Fig 33.1 Catecholamines and other hormones exert effects on the spleen, circulatory and respiratory systems to increase the oxygen delivery to the muscle and substrate availability. Exercise stimulates (1) liver glycogenolysis and gluconeogenesis to supply glucose to the myofiber, and (2) lipolysis to release fatty acids from adipose tissue and/or liver stores. At the muscle level, vasodilatation occurs and muscle glycogen, triglycerides and if necessary proteins are used to produce ATP. Free fatty acids and pyruvate (i.e. the end product of glycolysis and amino acid catabolism) may be oxidized by the mitochondria in muscle to produce ATP.

receives about 80% of total cardiac output[14] while, at the same time, there is an increase in blood flow to the skin to facilitate heat loss.[15] Oxygen delivery to skeletal muscle is thought to be the primary limiting factor in $\dot{V}O_{2max}$[5] as muscle mitochondrial oxidative capacity far exceeds the ability of the respiratory and cardiovascular systems to deliver oxygen.[16] Mitochondrial oxidative capacity appears to be fixed among species including the horse, with average values of ~5 mL $O_2.min^{-1}.mL^{-1}$ of mitochondrial volume.[17–19] According to the theory of symmorphosis, therefore, improved muscle oxidative capacity with training would only result from increased muscle mitochondrial density.[20] However, recent investigations have demonstrated functional plasticity of mitochondria and thus have challenged an exclusively quantitative effect of training on mitochondrial oxidative capacity.[21,22]

Sources of metabolic fuel

The hydrolysis of ATP supports the cross-bridge cycle as well as the activity of ion pumps and channels participating in excitation–contraction coupling, in particular, the sarcoplasmic reticulum calcium ATPase pump. As local ATP reserves can only sustain contraction for a few seconds, the synthesis of ATP from other substrates is of primary importance to sustained muscular activity. The first source of energy for muscle contraction is phosphocreatine (PCr), which has a high-energy phosphate bond similar to that of ATP. Hydrolysis of PCr enables transfer of the phosphate group to ADP in order to reconstitute ATP. The mitochondrial isoform of the creatine kinase enzyme produces phosphocreatine in the mitochondrion, whereas the myofibrillar isoform catalyzes ATP reformation in the sarcoplasm. The amount of phosphocreatine stored is very small and is rapidly depleted, supporting ATP production for a few seconds only. Other sources of energy are therefore needed for resynthesis of ATP and PCr; the primary sources are glycogen and triglycerides stored in muscle and blood-derived glucose and free fatty acids.

Equine skeletal muscle, especially fast twitch fibers, contains high glycogen stores. Expressed on dry weight basis, the glycogen concentration varies from 300 to 650 μmol/g dry weight depending on the muscle, training status and diet.[23,24] The content of triglycerides in equine skeletal muscle has been found to be highly variable (from 7 to 128 μmol/g dry weight in the middle gluteal muscle.[25] Proteins (amino acids) also may contribute to the energy supply, particularly during prolonged low-intensity exercise such as endurance races.[26]

Fatty acids released from triglycerides stored in adipose tissue, myocytes or very low density lipoproteins (VLDL) are a major energy source. Horses differ from other athletic animals in that there is an increase in the circulating triglycerides during exercise.[27] Triglycerides are released from the liver as very low density lipoproteins;[27] the increase during exercise may reflect enhanced synthesis in response to increased delivery of non-esterified fatty acids (NEFA) to the liver. Lipoprotein lipase located on the outer side of the endothelial membranes in muscle capillaries will release fatty acids from circulating VLDL-triglycerides for oxidation in muscles. NEFA released from the hydrolysis of triglycerides in adipose tissue are transported in blood bound to serum albumin and enter myocytes via specific fatty acid transporter proteins. The glycerol from hydrolyzed triglycerides is converted to glycerol-3-phosphate and enters the glycolytic pathway.[28,29] In the liver, glycerol is a gluconeogenic substrate, as are lactate and alanine (Fig. 33.2).

Epinephrine, glucagon and cortisol are key hormones involved in the mobilization of stored energy substrates during exercise. The increase in epinephrine concentration, for example, is thought to augment the hepatic output of glucose and also increases glycogenolysis and glycolysis in muscle.

The release of nutrients from the gastrointestinal tract depends on pre-exercise feeding regimens (e.g. glucose absorbed after digestion of a pre-exercise grain meal may be utilized during exercise). In general, equine diets are rich in carbohydrates (e.g. hemicellulose) that are not degraded by pancreatic amylase, but rather are subjected to bacterial fermentation in the cecum and colon. Short-chain (or volatile) fatty acids, mainly acetate, propionate and butyrate, are produced by this process. At rest, acetate may provide approximately 30% of the energy utilized by the hindlimb[30] while propionate is used mainly for gluconeogenesis.[31,32] The direct contribution of these substrates to energy use during exercise is not known.

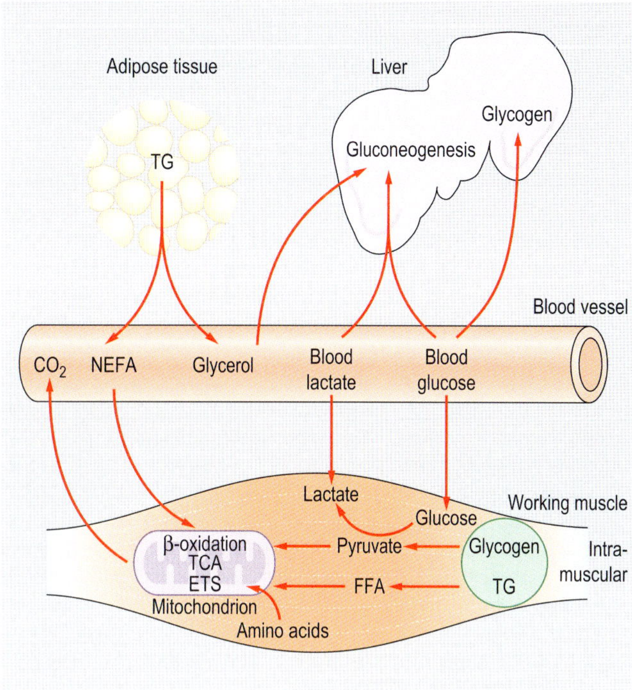

Fig 33.2 During exercise, energy stores in muscle, liver and adipose tissue are mobilized by the action of catecholamines and other hormones. Non-esterified fatty acids (NEFA) are released from triglycerides (TG) in adipose tissue and transported by circulation to the working muscles. Muscle glycogen is the body's main store of carbohydrates, but additional glucose from liver glycogen and gluconeogenesis is provided via circulation. So, sources of energy for muscle contraction are intramuscular glycogen and triglycerides, as well as blood-borne glucose and NEFA fatty acids and amino acids. These substrates are transformed (by intermediary metabolism) into their reducing equivalents (NADH + H^+ or $FADH_2$), which may be further oxidized by the mitochondrion to generate ATP in the presence of oxygen.

Major pathways for energy transduction

Ultimately, the metabolism of the above-mentioned energy substrates generates reduced nicotinamide adenine dinucleotide (NADH + H^+) or reduced flavine adenine dinucleotide ($FADH_2$) that are further oxidized by the mitochondrion to generate ATP. The main muscle energy metabolic pathways are illustrated in Figure 33.3. The preferential use of an energetic substrate is dependent on its availability, the activity of oxidative enzymes, oxygen availability, and mitochondrial density. Also, the sources of energy for aerobic and anaerobic metabolism as well as the relative contribution of

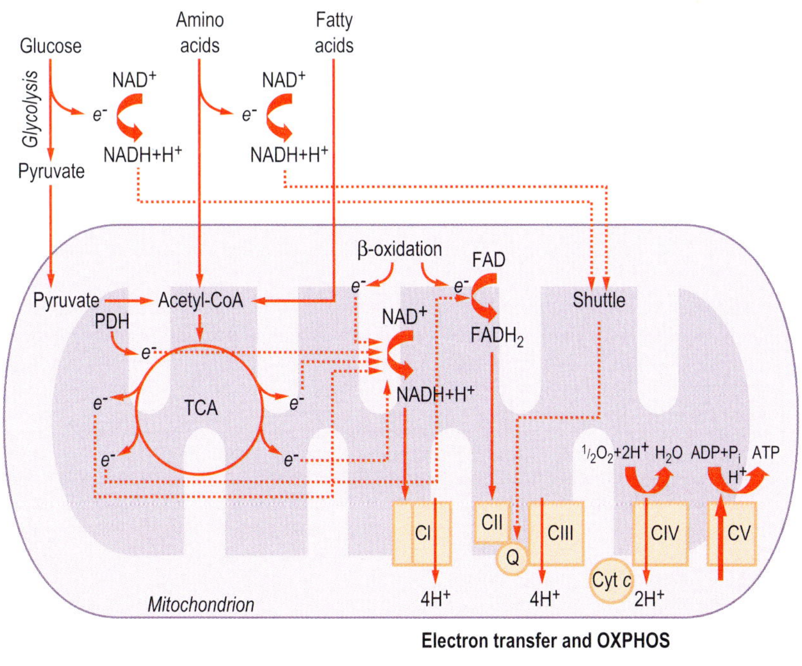

Fig 33.3 Catabolism of proteins, fats, and carbohydrates yields acetyl-CoA that enters the tricarboxylic acid (TCA) cycle. Electrons removed at the different steps are carried by reduced nicotinamide adenine dinucleotide (NADH + H^+) or reduced flavine adenine dinucleotide ($FADH_2$) to be channeled into the electron transfer system, providing the energy for ATP synthesis by oxidative phosphorylation (OXPHOS). A specific shuttle operates in skeletal muscle to move NADH from the cytosol to the mitochondrial matrix.

Abbreviations: PDH = pyruvate dehydrogenase complex; Cyt *c* = cytochrome *c*; Q = coenzyme Q; CI, CII, CIII, CIV, and CV = complexes I, II, III, IV and V, respectively.

both pathways depend on the intensity, type and duration of the exercise. Nutrition and training are also important determinants of the relative contributions of different substrates to energy transduction (for a review, see Reference 33).

Glycolysis

Two pathways are available to extract energy from glycogen or glucose in muscle: *anaerobic* and *aerobic* glycolysis. Glucose 6-phosphate derived from blood glucose or from mobilized stored intracellular glycogen is the first substrate in the glycolytic pathway. Blood glucose crosses the plasma membrane of the muscle cells through specific glucose carriers (GLUTs); glucose transporter 4 (GLUT-4) is the major isoform in the skeletal muscle.[34] The translocation of GLUT-4 to the cell surface is a major rate-limiting step in glucose utilization; translocation occurs in response to insulin as well as muscle contraction.[35] Once in the cytoplasm, glucose is phosphorylated by hexokinase into glucose 6-phosphate. Glycogenolysis releases glucose 1-phosphate molecules from glycogen that are subsequently converted into glucose 6-phosphate. The key regulatory enzyme of glycolysis is phosphofructokinase, which converts fructose 6-phosphate to fructose 1,6-diphosphate. This enzyme is considered to be an *indicator of the anaerobic metabolism* because its activity is regulated by the ATP/ADP ratio; when this ratio decreases, the activity of phosphofructokinase increases, thus resulting in a greater production of pyruvate.

Under anaerobic conditions, the pyruvate produced in the cytoplasm is converted to lactate by lactate dehydrogenase (LDH), utilizing electrons from NADH + H^+. In anaerobic glycolysis, one glucose molecule produces a net gain of two ATP molecules but the conversion of glucose to pyruvate also yields NADH + H^+. Indeed, when the NADH/NAD^+ ratio increases, glycolysis switches to the anaerobic mode and pyruvate is reduced to lactate. This decreases the NADH/NAD^+ ratio and restores NAD^+, which allows glycolysis to continue at the maximum rate. This process occurs in the cytoplasm and is only moderately efficient in terms of energy production but is efficient with respect to speed (Table 33.1).

Under aerobic conditions, pyruvate is transported into the mitochondrion and undergoes oxidative decarboxylation to form acetyl-CoA, which enters the citric acid cycle (also named tricarboxylic acid cycle (TCA) or Krebs cycle). The irreversible conversion of pyruvate to acetyl-CoA is catalyzed by the pyruvate dehydrogenase (PDH) complex. Aerobic glycolysis is much more efficient in terms of energy yield than the anaerobic process but not in terms of kinetics. Aerobic and anaerobic metabolism are connected, with lactate generation serving to reoxidize NADH + H^+ and thus maintaining the cytosolic NAD^+ pool needed for continued glycolysis and generation of pyruvate.

β-Oxidation of free fatty acids

β-Oxidation of fatty acids occurs within the mitochondrial matrix. Sarcoplasmic short and medium-chain fatty acids (chain lengths up to 12 carbons) can freely enter the mitochondrial matrix. In contrast, long-chain fatty acids must be transported into the mitochondria by the carnitine shuttle, which is a rate-limiting step.[29]

Table 33.1 Total ATP yield from major pathways for ATP regeneration

MOLECULE	PROCESS	DIRECT ENERGETIC PRODUCTS	END PRODUCTS	FINAL ATP[1]
Phosphocreatine	*Hydrolysis*	ATP		1
		Total per phosphocreatine	Creatine	1
Glucose	*Anaerobic glycolysis*			
	Glycolysis to lactate	2 NADH (cytosolic) + 2 ATP		3[2] + 2
		Total per glucose	Lactate	5
	Aerobic glycolysis			
	Glycolysis to pyruvate[3]	2 NADH (cytosolic) + 2 ATP		3[2] + 2
	Pyruvate to acetyl-CoA	2 NADH (mitochondrial)		5
	TCA	6 NADH (mitochondrial)		15
		+ 2 $FADH_2$ + 2 ATP (or 2GTP)	CO_2, H_2O	+ 3[4] + 2
		Total per glucose		30
Fatty Acids	*Oxidation*			
	β-Oxidation of palmitate[5]	7 NADH + 7 $FADH_2$		28
	Acetyl-CoA in TCA[6]	24 NADH + 8 $FADH_2$ + 8 ATP		80
		Total per palmitate	CO_2, H_2O	108
ADP + phosphocreatine	*Creatine kinase reaction*	ATP		
		Total	Creatine	1
2 ADP	*Adenylate kinase pathway*	ATP		
		Total	AMP	1

[1]These calculations assume that mitochondrial oxidative phosphorylation produces 1.5 ATP per $FADH_2$ oxidized and 2.5 ATP per NADH oxidized.
[2]In the muscle, cytosolic NADH are delivered to ubiquinone of the ETS by the glycerol 3-phosphate shuttle and thus, the reducing equivalents from NADH are directed to Complex III and not Complex I, providing only 1.5 ATP molecules per pair of electrons rather than 2.5 ATP molecules when this pair of electron passes from Complex I to O_2.
[3]2 molecules of pyruvate are produced per glucose molecule.
[4]$FADH_2$ passes its electrons into the ETS at the level of Complex II and generates 1.5 molecules of ATP.
[5]Palmitate (C16:0) is one of the major individual acids in the fatty acids of adipose tissue in horses.[231]
[6]8 molecules of acetyl-CoA are produced per palmitate.

β-Oxidation involves the sequential removal of 2-carbon segments in the form of acetyl-CoA[29] and production of shortened acyl-CoA, with concurrent reduction of one FAD and one NAD^+. The electrons carried by NADH + H^+ and $FADH_2$ immediately enter the electron transfer system (ETS) of the oxidative phosphorylation (OXPHOS) system, whereas acetyl-CoA enters the TCA cycle (Fig. 33.3).[29,36]

Degradation of amino acids

Tissue proteins can be degraded to provide fuel and a net protein degradation may occur during prolonged exercise.[26] There is no large energetic storage form (like glycogen for glucose or triglycerides for fatty acids) for amino acids; thus amino acids used for energy are provided by structural and functional proteins. When necessary, these proteins are degraded into amino acids that are transported via the blood to other tissues. Some of the amino acids are oxidized as fuel (where their metabolites enter the TCA cycle), whereas the rest provide substrates for gluconeogenesis in the liver and possibly for acid–base regulation.

Tricarboxylic acid cycle

The major pathways for oxidative metabolism of glucose, fatty acids and amino acids converge in the TCA cycle. In this mitochondrial process, several oxidation steps culminate in the formation of oxaloacetate that can be used to repeat the cycle. The oxidants used are NAD^+, FAD and guanosine 5′-diphosphate (GDP) or ADP. For each acetyl-CoA that undergoes the whole process, three $NADH^+ + H^+$, one $FADH_2$, and one ATP (or one guanosine 5′-triphosphate (GTP) that is energetically equivalent) are generated. NADH and $FADH_2$ are reoxidized by the mitochondrial ETS to provide ATP (Fig. 33.3).

The electron transfer system

Under aerobic conditions, glycolysis, *β*-oxidation of free fatty acids and the TCA cycle generate reducing equivalents (i.e. NADH + H^+ and $FADH_2$) which are oxidized in mitochondria owing to the ETS localized in the inner mitochondrial membrane. The ETS is made of five complexes and two mobile carriers named ubiquinone (also called coenzyme Q, or simply Q) and cytochrome *c* (Fig. 33.4). From I to IV, complexes are named NADH dehydrogenase (or NADH:ubiquinone oxidoreductase), succinate dehydrogenase (or succinate-coenzyme Q reductase or succinate-ubiquinone oxidoreductase), coenzyme Q:cytochrome *c* – oxidoreductase (or cytochrome bc_1 complex or ubiquinone:cytochrome *c* oxidoreductase) and cytochrome *c* oxidase (frequently abbreviated as COX). Mitochondrial NADH transfers its electrons to Complex I whereas cytosolic NADH requires a specific shuttle (i.e. the glycerol 3-phosphate shuttle in the skeletal muscle and brain versus the malate-aspartate shuttle which operates in liver, kidney and heart mitochondria) to pass its electrons to Q. $FADH_2$ transfers its electrons into the ETS at the level of Complex II. There is also an entry at the level of Q for electrons transferred at the first step in the *β*-oxidation of fatty acyl-CoA by the electron transferring flavoprotein (ETF) (Fig. 33.5). The mitochondrial ETS reduces oxygen to water and generates the electrochemical gradient of protons used by ATP synthase (i.e. Complex V) to phosphorylate ADP and produce ATP. The oxygen consumed by the ETS must be constantly provided to mitochondria from the blood (transferred via myoglobin). OXPHOS is highly efficient in producing ATP and thus mitochondria have a central role in ATP replenishment (Table 33.1).

Other pathways

Consumption of ATP during exercise results in the accumulation of ADP. During intense exercise, in addition to the ATP regeneration via the enzyme creatine kinase (that catalyzes the replenishment of ATP using the phosphocreatine as a source of phosphoryl groups), muscle can temporarily generate ATP using the adenylate kinase pathway. This fully reversible reaction catalyzes the generation of one ATP and one adenosine monophosphate (AMP) using two ADP molecules. The AMP molecule can then be deaminated to inosine monophosphate (IMP) within the purine nucleotide cycle, with concurrent production of ammonia. The accumulation of IMP closely mirrors the loss of ATP.[37] This reaction cascade eventually leads to loss of adenine nucleotides and myofibrillar fatigue.

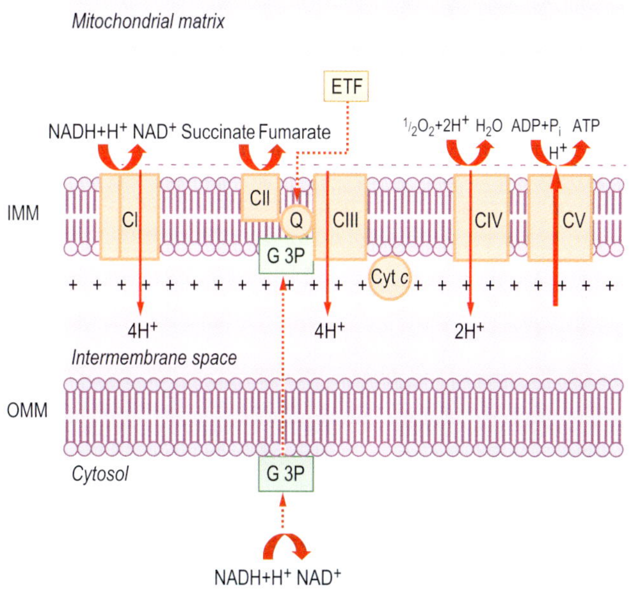

Fig 33.4 Cytosol and mitochondrial matrix are separated by two membranes, i.e. the outer and inner mitochondrial membranes separated by an intermembrane space. Electrons from donors (i.e. NADH and $FADH_2$) pass through a series of carriers arranged asymmetrically in the inner membrane of the mitochondria. In this chemiosmotic model, the electron transport from coenzymes to oxygen is accompanied by proton transfer (owing to proton pumps at the level of CI, CIII and, CIV) across the membrane, producing an electrochemical gradient across the inner mitochondrial membrane: the membrane is negatively charged at its inner surface and positively charged at its outer (i.e. intermembrane) space. The inner mitochondrial membrane is impermeable to protons that can re-enter the matrix only through proton specific channels at the level of complex V. ATP synthesis relies on the maintenance of this proton gradient.
Abbreviations: IMM = inner mitochondrial membrane; OMM = outer mitochondrial membrane; Q = ubiquinone or coenzyme Q; Cyt *c* = cytochrome *c*; CI, CII, CIII, CIV, and CV = complexes I, II, III, IV and V, respectively; G 3P = glycerol 3-phosphate shuttle; ETF = electron-transferring flavoprotein.

Methods of assessing metabolic response to exercise and training

Assessment of the metabolic responses to exercise may guide conditioning programs that target the optimization of athletic performance. This goal raises the question of the physiological determinants of performance and requires understanding of whether specific responses represent physiological or pathophysiological events. For example, oxidative stress during exercise is a physiological event, whereas inappropriate antioxidant capacity may result in muscle homeostasis disturbances, fatigue and injury.[38–40]

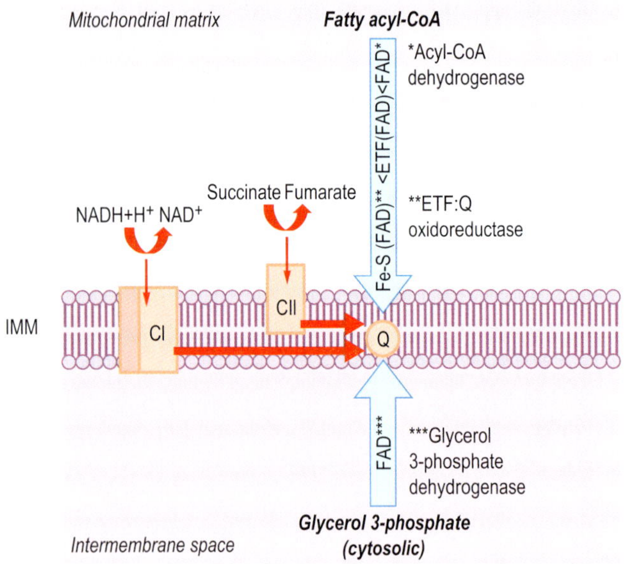

Fig 33.5 Electrons from reduced nicotinamide adenine dinucleotide (NADH + H^+), succinate, fatty acyl-CoA and glycerol 3-phosphate converge to ubiquinone (coenzyme Q). The term respiratory chain or electron transfer chain for the mitochondrial electron transfer system is a misnomer since the system is not arranged as a chain but rather is a non-linear system with a convergence of electron flow at the Q-junction.

Abbreviations: IMM = inner mitochondrial membrane; Q = coenzyme Q; CI = Complex I; CII = Complex II.

Several exercise testing methodologies enable evaluation of the state of physical conditioning and therefore an indication as to whether the horse is fit for the intended activity.[22,41–48] They may be used repeatedly to adjust the degree of exercise load during the conditioning program.[45] Indeed, it is well documented that training induces biochemical adaptations that moderate exercise-induced muscle damage.[49–51] The monitoring of specific biomarkers also may facilitate avoidance of overexertion and training-associated injuries,[52,53] while standardized assessment of the metabolic response to exercise can aid in the investigation of poor performance.[54–56]

Methods for laboratory (treadmill) and field exercise testing are covered in Chapters 2 and Chapter 3. In brief, treadmill testing offers several advantages, including the ability to control the environmental and exercise conditions, use sophisticated equipment for physiological monitoring, and easily obtain blood samples from the horse during running. However, physiologic and metabolic responses to treadmill exercise may not mirror exercise over ground.[57,58] In contrast, field testing offers environmental conditions closer those of competition but is more difficult to standardize and in general allows for a more limited range of measurements when compared to treadmill tests. Nonetheless, the advent of newer methodologies and equipment[22,48,55,56,59–62] has increased the clinical usefulness of field exercise testing.

Samples and measurements to study the effects of exercise

The metabolic responses to exercise may be studied at different levels: (1) at the whole-body level, for example by measuring oxygen consumption or by analyzing blood, substrates, enzyme activities or the end products of energetic metabolism (e.g. lactate); or (2) across the organ at the cellular level (e.g. muscle biopsy) or at the molecular level (e.g. study of the proteome, transcriptome or metabolome).

Whole-body level measurements

Non-invasive techniques to study metabolic rate include *direct calorimetry* that is based on the law of conservation of energy (energy may neither be created nor destroyed). Direct calorimetry requires the animal to be placed in a calorimeter chamber for the measurement and is not feasible for exercise studies. However, given the link between the amount of heat released during metabolism and the amount of oxygen consumed, measurement of oxygen consumption (i.e. *indirect calorimetry*) is a feasible means for estimation of metabolic rate and ATP turnover in horses during exercise.

Indirect calorimetry can be used to estimate whole-body rates of carbohydrate and lipid utilization during submaximal exercise, while isotopic tracer techniques enable quantification of the turnover of specific metabolic substrates such as glucose.[63–68] Using stoichiometric equations for the combustion of carbohydrate and fat, values for the respiratory exchange ratio (R, the ratio of carbon dioxide produced to oxygen consumed) can be used to estimate the relative contribution of these substrates to energy expenditure during submaximal exercise.[65] These calculations assume that measures of gas exchange at the level of the lung accurately reflect the actual metabolic gas exchange at the cellular level. In addition, it is assumed that protein makes a negligible contribution to energy metabolism. This approach is invalid at high work intensities wherein a portion of expired CO_2 is derived from the bicarbonate buffer system (the buffering of lactic acid) and values for R may be greater than 1.0. So, this technique enables the quantification of aerobic energy release (i.e. whole-body aerobic production of ATP) from the combustion of carbohydrates and fats.

Several studies in horses have employed an infusion of a stable isotopically labeled tracer of glucose in order to calculate rates of glucose production (mainly hepatic glucose production) and utilization (mainly muscle glucose uptake) in horses during submaximal exercise.[63–69] In contrast with measurement of blood glucose concentrations, this technique allows assessment of the dynamics of glucose turnover during exercise or after feeding.[68,69] From concurrent calculations of whole-body rates of carbohydrate oxidation and the rate of plasma glucose disappearance, it is also possible to estimate the contribution by blood glucose and muscle glycogen (plus lactate) to total carbohydrate utilization.[65] The main assumption is that the rate of glucose disappearance is equal to the actual oxidation rate of glucose derived from the blood, although it is possible that some glucose is used for glycogen resynthesis during low-to-moderate-intensity exercise. This technique is expensive due to the price of stable-isotope labeled substrates and the instrumentation required for measurement of isotopic enrichment.[70,71]

Recently, the hyperglycemic clamp technique has been used to estimate glucose utilization in horses during exercise.[72] In this non-isotopic method,[73] the plasma glucose concentration is acutely raised to a fixed concentration by injection of glucose and then maintained at a hyperglycemic plateau by use of a variable rate glucose infusion. Because the plasma glucose concentration is held constant, the glucose infusion rate is an index of glucose disposal.[74] By maintaining the fixed hyperglycemic plateau for about 2 h, it is assumed that endogenous hepatic glucose production is suppressed and (with appropriate corrections for glucose loss via the glucose space and urine) and that the rate of glucose disposal is equal to the glucose infusion rate.[72] However, the induced hyperglycemia may affect muscle metabolism by favoring the use of glucose rather than fat.

Aerobic capacity, measured as maximum oxygen uptake (VO_{2max}), correlates with running speed over 2000 m in Thoroughbreds.[44] The measurement of VO_{2max} is also useful because thereafter it is possible to express workloads as a percentage of VO_{2max}.[75] Comparison of studies performed among sport centers is feasible since the type of exercise protocols used to determine VO_{2max} does not markedly influence the results.[76]

In horses, methods to quantify anaerobic energy metabolism are the measurement of maximal accumulated oxygen deficit ('MAOD', calculated from the difference of calculated O_2 demand and maximum oxygen uptake[77]) and blood lactate measurement. These methods lack accuracy due to the fact that anaerobic ATP production is an intracellular process. The peak blood lactate concentration is often used as a measure of anaerobic release during exercise but this does not take into account the energy release from stored ATP and phosphocreatine. In addition, blood lactate does not quantify muscle lactate concentration. However, it may be used to indicate increased glycolytic activity within exercising skeletal muscle[78] as lactate and hydrogen ions (end products of anaerobic glycolysis) are released from muscle into the circulation. Indeed, the initial rise in blood lactate does not necessarily mean hypoxia in muscle cell; rather it is an indication that the rate of pyruvate delivery to the mitochondria has exceeded the ability of the organelle to oxidize pyruvate, leading to accelerated generation of lactic acid. Therefore, lactate accumulation is intimately linked to the oxidative capacity of muscle fibers.

Lactate threshold (V_{La4}, i.e. velocity at 4 mmol/L of blood lactate) and the velocity (running speed) at a heart rate of 200 bpm (V_{200}) are frequently used in the evaluation of fitness and state of training. These indices are easy to measure, can be determined both on a track and a treadmill and do not require any expensive equipment. Metabolically, lactate threshold represents the maximal work intensity at which ATP is produced aerobically, i.e. there exists a steady-state situation in blood lactate concentration, wherein lactate is released (mainly from muscles) into circulation at the same rate as it is used by other tissues. Based on studies in humans, it has been shown that blood lactate concentration starts to increase exponentially around a concentration of 4 mmol/L. Similarly, in horses lactate threshold is expressed as the speed of the treadmill or the speed of the horse on a track at which blood lactate reaches 4 mmol/L (see Fig. 33.6).

The analysis of blood lactate is complex since equine RBCs behave differently from that of other athletic species,[79] functioning as lactate sink. Up to 50% of blood lactate can be found in RBCs[80,81]

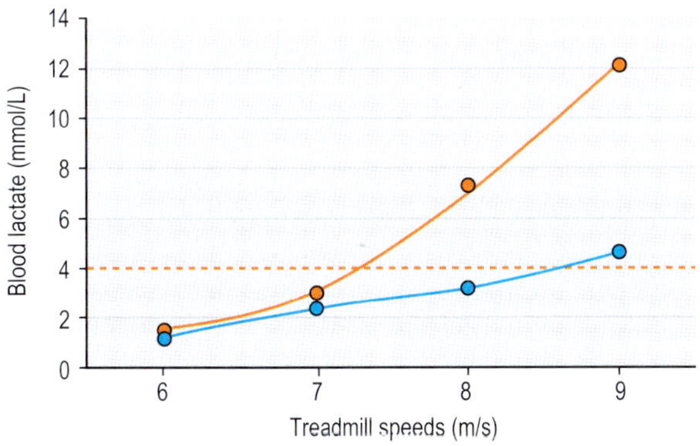

Fig 33.6 Blood lactate response to submaximal treadmill exercise depends on the aerobic capacity of the horse. In untrained horses (red circles) two-minute steps at speeds indicated on the x-axis induce a rapid increase in blood lactate concentration, while the higher aerobic capacity of trained horses (blue circles) allows energy transduction without accumulation of lactic acid.

versus only 20% in human athletes.[82] There is a close correlation between whole-blood and plasma lactate concentrations[80,83] but the uptake of lactate into RBCs varies interindividually[81,84,85] according to activity of monocarboxylate transporters (MCT) that facilitate the transport of lactate across membranes in RBCs but also from the muscles into plasma.[86] On the basis of lactate transport activity in RBCs, horses can be divided into two populations of unequal size: the large majority with high transport activity versus the other one with low lactate transport activity in their RBCs.[85,87] Low lactate transport activity in the Standardbred is inherited as an autosomal recessive trait.[87] Horses with high lactate transport activity have higher RBC lactate concentration after submaximal and maximal exercise[81,88] and have been shown to be better performers.[89] It is hypothesized that the influx of lactate from plasma into RBC sustains the gradient between muscle cell and plasma, thereby facilitating lactate efflux from muscle.[80,90] Further studies are needed to demonstrate a correlation between lactate transport activity and performance.[91]

Blood samples are easy to collect and many research studies have been directed at finding the best markers of performance and athletic ability. It is worth noting that several factors may influence the results obtained in laboratory analysis. Sources of variation include the laboratory that may use different methodologies for the measurement of the same biochemical parameters. At animal level, breed, age and sex are significant sources of variation in blood variables.[92]

Two other major factors influencing the results of blood analyzes are the site of collection and methods of sample handling. The sample collection site (e.g. jugular vein, carotid artery, systemic artery) can have important effects on the results. From a metabolic viewpoint, the most relevant samples would be those taken from veins coming directly from exercising muscles, especially if combined with arterial samples. These samples would allow for measurement of oxygen extraction, the consumption of various fuels, and the efflux of catabolic products. However, for practical reasons samples are most often taken from the jugular vein, which represents mixed venous blood. For some metabolites, the concentrations in jugular venous blood are similar to those in arterial blood, while others such as glucose, ketones and lactate differ.[93,94] It should, however, be kept in mind that the concentration of any substance in blood is a sum of its release into and its disappearance from the blood and does not provide information about the rate of these events. Blood lactate measurement is a good example of the importance for standardization in sampling, given the differences in arterial and venous lactate concentrations[93] as well as the inter-individual variation in RBC lactate transport activity that induces different kinetics in blood lactate metabolism.

The choice of anticoagulants for determination of specific biochemical parameters in plasma is also crucial. Heparin is the anticoagulant of choice for most chemical determination requiring plasma; however, it must be excluded for specific measurements such as myeloperoxidase (MPO) enzyme activity (ethylenediamineteraacetic acid [EDTA] should be used).[95,96] On the other hand, EDTA is a chelating agent which interferes with several chemical determinations. Fluoride/oxalate halts glycolysis by the RBC and thus is the best choice for blood glucose determination.

In field testing, analysis of sample may be delayed and appropriate storage of samples is required. Collection of serum necessitates clotting before centrifugation. Plasma separation from the RBC must be done soon after sampling to avoid in vitro hemolysis of RBC and/or changes in substrates or metabolites due to RBC activity. For delayed analysis, serum and plasma can be frozen on dry ice on site and then stored in an ultra-low temperature freezer. Repeated freezing and thawing alters some analytes and thus samples to be used in several assays or analyzed in more than one laboratory should be aliquoted into 1–2 mL volumes.

Exercise and training induce alterations in enzyme activities related to energy metabolism.[97] For example, the activities of plasma malate (MDH) and lactate dehydrogenase (LDH) change with training and reflect alterations in oxidative capacity and lipid mobilization. As previously mentioned, fatty acids with a chain length longer than 12 carbons must be transported into the mitochondria by the carnitine shuttle in which their acyl group is transiently attached to the hydroxyl group of carnitine to form fatty acyl-carnitine.[98] Determination of plasma acyl-carnitine and fatty acid profiles might be of interest to better understand fatty acids metabolism in the exercising horse[99] but will require the establishment of reference ranges.

In the future, proteomic and metabolomic approaches may provide new insight into the metabolic responses to exercise and training. While the genome is a steady entity, its proteomes may differ according to the cell and to specific post-translational modifications that are critical to define function. In equine exercise physiology, proteomics is in its early infancy but one preliminary study has provided evidence that a proteomic approach may be useful for assessment of training level as well as detection of subclinical exercise-related conditions.[100] In this study, prolonged physical exercise was demonstrated to affect plasma proteins involved in pathways related to inflammation, coagulation, immune modulation, oxidant/antioxidant activity, and cellular damage. Metabolomic profiling also may provide new insights about the responses of specific metabolic pathways.[101]

Metabolic evaluation at the organ level

Metabolic changes in muscle are primarily determined by analysis of muscle samples taken by the percutaneous needle biopsy technique that was introduced to equine research by Lindholm and Piehl[102] as well as by Snow and Guy.[103] Biochemical, histochemical, immunohistochemical, and morphological studies performed on muscle biopsy samples have provided most of our knowledge about muscle energetic.[33] Biopsy samples are usually taken from the middle gluteal muscle at a defined depth (e.g. 2, 4 or 6 cm) and at a specific location. Standardization of the site of the muscle biopsy is imperative because equine skeletal muscles have a heterogeneous distribution of muscle fiber types within the muscle.[104–106]

The glycolytic capacity of muscle fibers may be evaluated using stains for enzymes of the glycolytic pathway, whereas pre- and post-exercise muscle biopsy may be used to estimate glycogen utilization and to follow the recovery of glycogen stores, e.g. by use of histological stains.[107–111] Immunofluorescent and immunohistochemical stains are useful to locate GLUT-4 in intracellular storage pools and in their active position within the sarcolemma.[112] Assessment of the concentrations of triglycerides, glycogen, glucose 6-phosphate, pyruvate, lactate and adenine nucleotides may provide further information regarding the metabolic state of muscle at the time of biopsy. However, these local measures are 'static' in the same way as blood samples, and do not allow quantitative assessment of the actual rate of substrate use.

In horses, muscle oxidative capacity has been classically evaluated by the activity of mitochondrial enzymes such as succinate dehydrogenase, by examining the capillary supply of muscles and/or by determining the mitochondrial volume density.[19,43,102,113–116] These techniques have contributed to the characterization of the metabolic properties of diverse muscles[105] in different types of horses,[102,104,117,118] to study effects of growth on muscle characteristics,[119] to describe muscle response to exercise and/or training,[49,120–123] to improve conditioning programs (for a review, see Reference 47), and define athletic potential.[124,125] These measurements have also highlighted the possible contribution of muscle oxidative capacity to maximal metabolic rate in mammals.[18,19]

Determination of oxidative capacity based on histological methods does not provide information on the integrative nature of mitochondrial function. Among others, the coupling of phosphorylation to oxygen consumption, transport of metabolites into the mitochondrial membrane, activity of dehydrogenases and the structural integrity of the mitochondria are key determinants of aerobic energy production. Quantitative determination of single marker enzymes or mitochondrial volume density does not take into account this fundamental concept of integrated function and assume that mitochondrial markers define oxidative capacity. Only one study has reported direct measurement of respiratory capacity, specifically by use of a Clark electrode on mitochondria isolated from equine muscle samples collected by percutaneous needle biopsy.[126]

High-resolution respirometry (HRR) is an advanced technology that enables the monitoring of mitochondrial respiration in small samples of permeabilized muscle fibers.[127] This in situ approach allows the analysis of integrated mitochondrial function by controlling metabolic pathways. Under controlled experimental conditions, the functional capacities of mitochondria are determined by feeding various substrates, uncouplers and inhibitors into the ETS. Mitochondrial function is screened at different steps of the OXPHOS system and may be analyzed to define the various modes of mitochondrial respiratory control[127] (Fig. 33.7). Standardized protocols to determine OXPHOS capacity and respiratory control patterns with HRR in horse skeletal muscle have been validated.[22,128] The technique is minimally invasive since the protocol may be performed using microbiopsies collected with a 14G biopsy needle (about 20 mg of tissue is sampled by puncture). Given that fiber-type distribution is not homogeneous within the muscle,[105,106] an accurate standardization of the sampling site and depth is required. The triceps brachii muscle has been selected as the reference muscle in equine studies because of its mixed composition of type I (slow-twitch) and type II (fast-twitch) fibers.[105] Conveniently, the triceps brachii is safer to access for the investigator than the propulsive muscles of the hindlimb. In addition to this important advantage, the hindlimb muscles include a greater proportion (up to 90% in thoroughbred horses) of type II fibers,[105] thus rendering them less useful for screening. Muscle specimens remain viable for up to 4 days when kept in a specific medium and under controlled temperature;[22] thus, this methodology may be applicable for the evaluation of horses in field settings.[128]

Proteomic, metabolomic and transcriptomic approaches offer great potential for the investigation of metabolic adaptations at the muscle cellular level, as demonstrated by recent studies in horses.[129–132]

Metabolic responses and mechanisms

Metabolic responses to exercise and the underlying mechanisms depend on several parameters such as the type and duration of the exercise (for a review, see Reference 33). The level of training[47] and warm-up[133,134] are also important determinants of the relative contributions of different metabolic pathways to energy transduction. Other key elements in the metabolic response to exercise include hydration status, hormonal status and nutrition, as well as ambient temperature, humidity and the degree of acclimatization. Other factors that are beyond the 'simple' physiological explanation such as motivation might also be unsuspected components of metabolic response to exercise and in particular to the poorly understood mechanisms of fatigue.

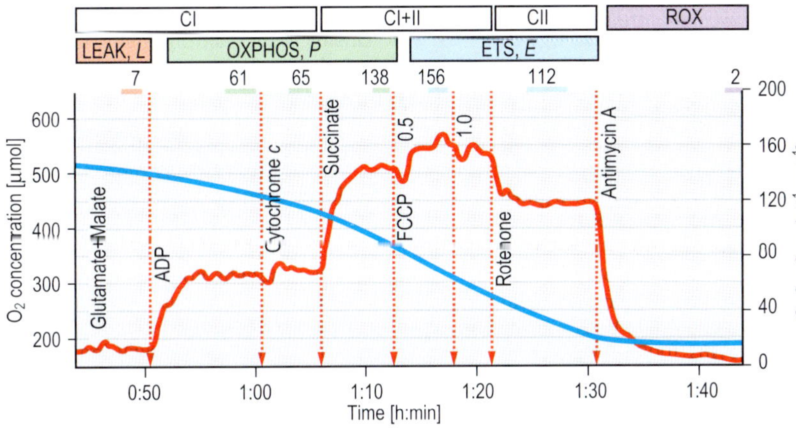

Fig 33.7 Respirometric protocol with permeabilized fibers from horse skeletal muscle (triceps brachii). The oxidative phosphorylation (OXPHOS) and electron transfer system (ETS) capacities per unit of muscle mass are determined by the sequential addition of different substrate combinations that furnish electrons upstream of the Q-junction. In this study, electron flow through Complex I (CI) is supported by the NADH-linked substrates glutamate+malate in the presence of ADP. ADP-stimulated respiration with various substrate combinations represents OXPHOS capacity (State *P*). The addition of cytochrome *c* allows assessment of the integrity of the outer mitochondrial membrane. Injury of the outer mitochondrial membrane will lead to loss of cytochrome *c* from the mitochondria, and in this experiment it would have led to significant stimulation of respiration following addition of exogenous cytochrome *c* to the respiration medium. At the next step, convergent electron flow through Complexes I and II (CI+II) is obtained by adding succinate (in the mitochondria; succinate is formed in the TCA cycle and is a substrate of Complex II (CII), feeding electrons into the Q-junction through flavin adenine dinucleotide [$FADH_2$]). By stepwise addition of the uncoupler FCCP (induces the dissipation of the electrochemical proton gradient; thus, electron flow is no longer coupled to OXPHOS), the ETS capacity (*E*), with convergent electron flow through CI+II is obtained. Electron input into the Q-junction through CII alone was subsequently induced by inhibition of CI by rotenone. Finally, residual oxygen consumption (ROX) is obtained by addition of antimycin A to block electron transfer through Complex III (CIII).

Oxygen concentration (μmol; blue line) and muscle mass-specific oxygen flux (pmol $O_2.s^{-1}.mg^{-1}$ wet weight; red line). Marked sections correspond to steady-state fluxes at different coupling states (*L, P and E*) and substrate states. Numbers on top of traces are tissue mass-specific fluxes at various metabolic states (pmol $O_2.s^{-1}.mg^{-1}$).

Adapted from Votion et al. 2012.[22]

Responses in metabolite concentrations in plasma

During exercise, hormonal changes facilitate the mobilization of metabolic fuels such as NEFA and glucose into circulation. NEFA is released from adipose tissue together with glycerol but, of these two, glycerol is a more reliable indicator of lipolysis.[135,136] Muscle tissue, which accounts for more than 40% of the bodyweight of horses, is the main user of NEFA and thus even small changes in the oxidation of fatty acids in the muscle will greatly influence the concentration of NEFA in plasma. On the other hand, the concentration of glycerol is not influenced by changes in muscle metabolism as it is mainly utilized by the liver. This is demonstrated by studies in which NEFA and glycerol concentrations have been measured in tests where the intensity of exercise varies. The results show that NEFA concentration decreases significantly during intense exercise, while glycerol concentration increases steadily.[27,136,137]

Changes in blood glucose concentration depend on the type of exercise. Plasma glucose concentration tends to decrease during prolonged exercise (>3 h), but during short, intense exercise both decreases and increases have been recorded[108,136,138–140] depending on exercise intensity and training and feeding status of the horse. The regulation of blood glucose during exercise is complex, but changes in prevailing hormone concentrations are important. The exercise-associated increase in hepatic glucose output is mainly mediated via a decrease in the insulin : glucagon ratio, whereas the rate of uptake and utilization in exercising muscle is restrained by increases in circulating epinephrine.[64]

Lactate is the end product of anaerobic metabolism and lactate concentrations in blood increase during high-intensity exercise. Lactate concentrations after different types of competitions and exercise tests are shown in Table 33.2. Usually, the highest lactate concentrations are seen 2–10 min after exercise. In equine blood, a significant amount of lactate may be in RBC; uptake is rapid and depends on the activity of MCT on the RBC membrane,[81] as previously described.

As a result of ATP degradation during high-intensity exercise, breakdown products of purine nucleotides such as ammonia, hypoxanthine, uric acid and allantoin appear in blood.[37,89,141,142] In horses, the predominant end products of purine catabolism are uric acid and allantoin. The time to peak concentration varies individually and peak concentrations are reached as late as 30 min after exercise.[142,143] Marked accumulation of uric acid, allantoin and ammonia is seen mainly after intense exercise and the breakdown of adenine nucleotides is probably triggered by accumulation of ADP and the decrease in muscle pH.[37,143,144] In horses, the threshold value for accumulation of these breakdown products is a muscle pH of 6.8, which represents a lactate concentration of 80 mmol/kg dry weight in muscle and about 12 mmol/L in blood.[37,142] It has been suggested that the peak concentration of uric acid or ammonia is useful as an indicator of ATP degradation in muscles.[143]

Changes in muscle

At rest, when energy transduction is fully aerobic, muscle may use volatile fatty acids, lipids and carbohydrates. Equine diets are usually low in lipids and plasma NEFA concentration is also low at rest. Thus, during periods of inactivity the utilization of lipids for energy may be limited by their low concentration, and the main energy sources are acetate and glucose.[30]

For most types of exercise muscle glycogen is utilized. Glycogen utilization increases with increasing work intensity; during interval

Table 33.2 Maximal lactate concentrations after exercise (values are means ± standard error of the mean)

	DISTANCE/TIME	BLOOD LACTATE (mmol/L)	PLASMA LACTATE (mmol/L)	REFERENCES
Endurance races	80–100 km	1.6 ± 0.1	0.50 ± 0.2	178, 232, 233
Standardbred races (trotting)	2100 m	21.6 ± 0.9	24.5 ± 0.7	80, 201
Standardbred races (pacing)	1760–2160 m		20.9 ± 4.1	234
Thoroughbred races	1100–3800 m	29.6 ± 4.7	33 ± 1.9	37, 233, 235–237
Three-day event, cross-country	6200 m		19.1 ± 4.2	233, 238
Showjumping			9.0 ± 0.9	239
Donkey after exercise			10 ± 1.4	240

work, its use is more pronounced during the first work bouts.[11,107,145] Glycogen is stored as macro- and proglycogen molecules which are two distinct populations of glycogen particles. These populations contribute differently to the release of glucose molecules according to the intensity of exercise. During an endurance race, macroglycogen is utilized to a greater extent than proglycogen.[26] During intense exercise both pro- and macroglycogen contribute equally to glycogenolysis.[146]

During low-intensity submaximal exercise, muscle triglycerides, blood glucose and free fatty acids (released from adipose tissue and/or liver stores) are the main sources of energy for oxidative fibers.[109] With prolonged low-intensity exercise, the uptake of free fatty acids by muscle increases substantially, gradually becoming the major source of energy.[109] As exercise continues, further motor units are recruited, including finally those of glycolytic fibers.[109,110] Catabolism of protein and amino acid metabolism may also contribute to provision of energy during this type of endurance exercise.[26]

In horses performing high-intensity maximal exercise, motor units of glycolytic fibers are rapidly recruited in addition to those of oxidative fibers: anaerobic glycolysis is the main source of energy and large amounts of lactate are produced, leading to acidosis.[143,145,147] Accumulation of lactate correlates with the amount of glycogen utilized but depends also on the oxidative capacity of muscle (i.e. horses with muscles containing a high proportion of fibers with low oxidative capacity have higher lactate concentrations in their muscles after high-intensity exercise[148]) and activity of the muscle lactate transporters,[149] which are highly influenced by training.[116] Muscle lactate concentrations up to 200 mmol/kg dry weight have been measured in equine muscle.[37,150] Muscle can temporarily generate ATP using breakdown of phosphocreatine but this source of energy is rapidly depleted.[89,143,147,151] However, its resynthesis post exercise is very rapid and, thus, results of its quantization within muscle are greatly influenced by the time of sampling at recovery. In situations of high energy demand (i.e. when ATP consumption exceeds the capacity for ADP rephosphorylation), ADP molecules accumulate and activate the muscle adenylate kinase pathway with the subsequent production of ATP and AMP molecules. AMP-activated protein kinases initiate cascades of phosphorylation events and stimulate the expression of genes involved in ATP production, while reducing that of genes involved in ATP consumption. AMP is further deaminated to IMP and the accumulation of this molecule closely mirrors the loss of ATP.[37] Thus, high lactate, ammonia and IMP levels and low ATP levels are seen in muscle after intense exercise, especially in fast-glycolytic fibers.[144,151,152]

To sustain muscle contraction beyond the first few minutes of exercise, horses rely heavily on glycogen, which is the obligate substrate to sustain anaerobic ATP production.[11] The importance of muscle glycogen reserves as an anaerobic energetic fuel to prevent fatigue during high-speed exercise has been highlighted in studies that manipulated muscle glycogen stores after strenuous exercise.[153,154] For instance, substantial depletion of muscle glycogen stores in horses before exercise is associated with decreased anaerobic capacity, during a subsequent high-speed exercise test.[153,154] Replenishment of muscle glycogen stores by glucose infusion after glycogen-depleting exercise restores anaerobic capacity, evident as restoration of the MAOD and run time to fatigue during high-speed exercise.[154]

Evidence of the role of muscle glycogen as a major energy substrate during submaximal exercise was clearly demonstrated by combined use of isotopic tracer and indirect calorimetry methods. Intramuscular carbohydrates (primarily glycogen) account for about 50% of the total energy expenditure during submaximal exercise performed at 30% of maximum oxygen uptake during the early phase of the exercise (0–30 min). However, as the exercise duration increases, glycogen utilization counts for only 20% of the total energy expenditure, with a concomitant increase in lipid utilization at 60–90 min of exercise.[64] Conversely, with increased work intensity (from 30 to 60% of maximum O_2 uptake), there is an increase in the rates of both muscle glucose uptake and muscle glycogen breakdown, with concomitant decrease in lipid oxidation (Fig. 33.8). Indeed, the increase in energy expenditure associated with increased workload was met almost entirely by an increase in muscle glycogen utilization, which was 60% of the total energy expenditure[64] (see Fig. 33.8).

Changes in the concentration of triglycerides in muscle fibers with exercise are difficult to interpret because of large inter-individual variation, both in triglycerides content and amount of triglycerides utilized.[25,148] Furthermore, muscle are made of different fibers types with different triglyceride contents, i.e. lipids are mainly stored in type I (oxidative) fibers.[109] Endurance-type exercise induces a decrease in muscle triglyceride content;[109,155] a decrease also has been observed after maximal exercise.[148]

Although the majority of studies have examined exercise-induced alterations in metabolic fuel content, recent work has provided data on changes in the muscle transcriptome. By examining global mRNA expression in the gluteus medius muscle of Thoroughbred racehorses before, immediately after, and 4 h post exercise it was demonstrated that genes involved in the stress response, metabolism and intracellular signaling are temporally expressed following exercise.[130] Also, expression of mitochondrial genes may be induced by exercise.[132]

A few studies have evaluated the effects of exercise on muscle mitochondrial function in horses.[126,128] Gollnick et al.[126] reported a transitory depression in respiratory capacity in middle gluteal muscle after high-intensity exercise. More recently, the HRR method was used to measure mitochondrial respiratory function in triceps brachii and middle gluteal muscle of endurance horses following training.[128] Changes appeared to be muscle group specific and were highly variable among horses that successfully completed a 2-star endurance ride. In some horses, OXPHOS and ETS capacities were markedly decreased while in others, mitochondrial capacities were significantly increased. There was a significant negative correlation between the percentage decrease in mitochondrial respiration and the exercise-associated increase in serum creatine kinase (CK) activity. The highest oxygen fluxes were observed in muscle from horses with the lowest serum CK activities.[128] Overall, the changes in mitochondrial respiratory function after training were consistent with increased fatty acid oxidation and decreased aerobic glycolysis,[128] appropriate adaptations in the face of increased energy demand.[21,156,157]

Effects of warm-up

The purpose of a warm-up is to enhance the transition from rest to exercise and thereby gain the dual benefits of enhanced performance and reduced risk of injury by a gradual increase in exercise intensity. An active warm-up increases body and muscle temperature by about 1 °C as a result of the heat generated during muscular activity. Warm-up improves tissue oxygenation, because epinephrine and norepinephrine released during warm-up increase respiratory rate, tidal volume and heart rate, cause the spleen to contract and release stored RBC into the circulation, and increase blood flow to skeletal muscles. Catecholamines also activate glycogenolysis and lipolysis and thus increase the supply of energy fuels to the muscle, while elevated temperature decreases the activation energy of metabolic reactions. A higher temperature also increases elasticity of muscles, tendons and ligaments, which may reduce the risk of injury and allow for full range of motion in the joints.

A brief period (5–10 min) of warm-up exercise, completed 5 min before the start of treadmill exercise at 115–120% of VO_{2max}, results in a significant acceleration in VO_{2max} kinetics, i.e. the rate of rise in VO_2 after exercise onset.[133,134] This change in oxygen uptake kinetics enhances the ability of muscle to work aerobically and reduces lactate accumulation during high-intensity exercise.[133,134,158,159] Both a low- and a high-intensity warm-up resulted in a significant increase in the run time to fatigue during intense treadmill exercise when compared to exercise undertaken without prior warm-up[158] (Fig. 33.9) and the comparison of different warm-up regimens indicates that high-intensity warm-up accelerates VO_2 kinetics and reduces reliance on net anaerobic power compared with low-intensity warm-up at the onset of the subsequent sprint.[160]

The ideal duration and intensity of warm-up exercise is not known and likely depends on the nature of the subsequent exercise task and the prevailing ambient conditions. On the one hand, if the warm-up period is too brief to allow time for the rise in body temperature the desired effect is not gained, whereas if exercise intensity during warm-up is too high significant lactate accumulation will be present at the onset of performance exercise. Even a low-intensity warm-up (e.g. 5 min of trotting exercise) is beneficial in terms of an enhancement in aerobic energy metabolism during subsequent galloping exercise.[133,134,159] The benefits of warm-up are likely diminished if the rest period between warm-up and performance is extended so that the horse cools down.

Mechanisms of fatigue

In horses performing high-intensity maximal exercise anaerobic glycolysis is the main source of energy.[77,78,143] In muscle, high lactate, ammonia and IMP concentrations and low ATP are observed after fatiguing exercise, especially in glycolytic fibers.[24,67,109] Excessive production of lactic acid is believed to alter metabolism of the muscle cells[161] and induce sarcoplasmic reticulum dysfunction.[162,163] For

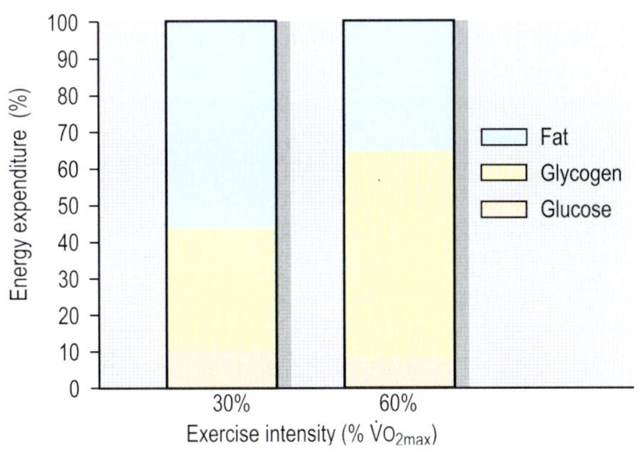

Fig 33.8 The estimated relative contributions of lipid, plasma glucose and muscle glycogen to energy expenditure in horses during exercise at approximately 30% and 60% of maximum aerobic capacity ($\dot{V}O_{2max}$). When compared to exercise at 30% $\dot{V}O_{2max}$, there is increased reliance on muscle glycogen (and a decreased energy contribution from fat) for energy transduction during exercise at 60% $\dot{V}O_{2max}$.

Adapted and reprinted from Geor RJ, Hinchcliff KW, Sams RA. Beta-adrenergic blockade augments glucose utilization in horses during graded exercise. J Appl Physiol 2000;89(3):1086-98, with permission from The American Physiological Society.

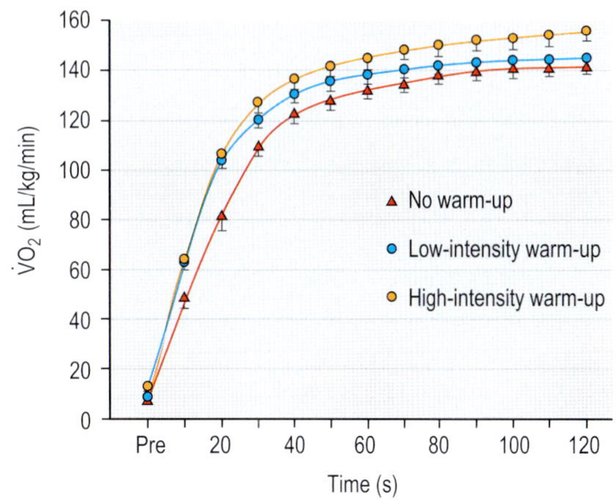

Fig 33.9 Effects of a low- and high-intensity warm-up on oxygen consumption (VO_2) in six horses during 2 min of intense exercise (~115% of maximum aerobic capacity). Note the acceleration in the rate of rise in VO_2 when exercise was preceded by a warm-up.

Adapted and reprinted from Geor RJ, McCutcheon LJ, Hinchcliff KJ. Effects of warm-up intensity on kinetics of oxygen consumption and carbon dioxide production during high-intensity exercise in horses. Am J Vet Res 2000;61(6): 638-45, with permission from the American Veterinary Medical Association. http://avmajournals.avma.org/loi/ajvr.

example, low muscle pH (values as low as 6.5–6.3 have been measured) following intense, fatiguing exercise[164] inhibits phosphofructokinase, thus decreasing the efficiency of the anaerobic glycolysis. The glycolytic enzymes are in close proximity to the sarcoplasmic reticulum calcium transport system.[165] Impaired glycolytic flux and selective depletion of muscle glycogen associated with the sarcoplasmic reticulum may impair excitation–contraction coupling and calcium flux, further contributing to fatigue.[166,167] On the other hand, products of AMP deamination stimulate glycolytic enzymes. The means to prevent intramuscular acidosis include buffers, the most important of which are proteins, the bicarbonate system, phosphate and carnosine.[161,168] Although buffering capacity of equine muscle is higher than in other species, it is still not enough to prevent acidosis. The second mechanism for regulation of cell pH is the transport of protons out of the cell.[169,170] Only the acid form, lactic acid, is able to diffuse through cell membranes; both protons and lactate anions require a transporter for transmembrane movement. In skeletal muscle, there are two carriers that may facilitate the efflux of protons: the Na^+/H^+ exchange protein and monocarboxylate transporters.[169,170] During Na^+/H^+ exchange, one Na^+ is transported into the cell and simultaneously one H^+ is carried out from the cell. There are no studies on the activity of Na^+/H^+ exchange in equine muscle, but in human muscle this carrier plays a minor role and monocarboxylate transporters (MCT), which simultaneously transport one proton together with one lactate anion, are responsible for most proton efflux.[169,170] Several isoforms of MCTs have been characterized, but only MCT1 and MCT4 have been found in equine skeletal muscle.[86] In human athletes, MCT1, which is the main lactate carrier in oxidative muscles, is upregulated by exercise. On the other hand, the content of MCT4, which is the dominant isoform in glycolytic fibers, increases only with high-intensity training.[171,172] In human subjects, the endurance training-associated decrease in muscle lactate accumulation during exercise is associated with an increase in skeletal muscle MCT content,[149] demonstrating the importance of MCTs for the regulation of intramuscular pH (Fig. 33.10). In Norwegian-Swedish Coldblooded Trotters, expression of MCT1 differed among fiber types and was related to the oxidative capacity of the fibers, which is increased with training.[116]

During high-intensity exercise, acidification may be the main reason for fatigue but a reduction in energy stores and accumulation of P_i, ADP, AMP and further degradation products as well as, elevated muscle temperature[37,107,135,173–175] may be other contributing factors. In particular, fatigue is thought to be related to the depletion of muscle glycogen stores, especially in oxidative fibers.[111,153,154,173] Depletion of sources of energy in these fibers will induce progressive recruitment of glycolytic fibers and further lactate production. Indeed, to sustain muscle contraction beyond the first few minutes of exercise, horses rely heavily on glycogen, which is the obligate substrate to sustain anaerobic ATP production.[11] Thus, the metabolic response to such exercise is highly influenced by the muscle fiber composition and by the oxidative and glycolytic capacities of the muscle fibers. Those properties are most probably responsible for the different resistance to fatigue observed between horses.[148] Capillary supply of muscles, and especially of glycolytic fibers, is of importance for aerobic capacity and exercise tolerance in Standardbred trotters.[115]

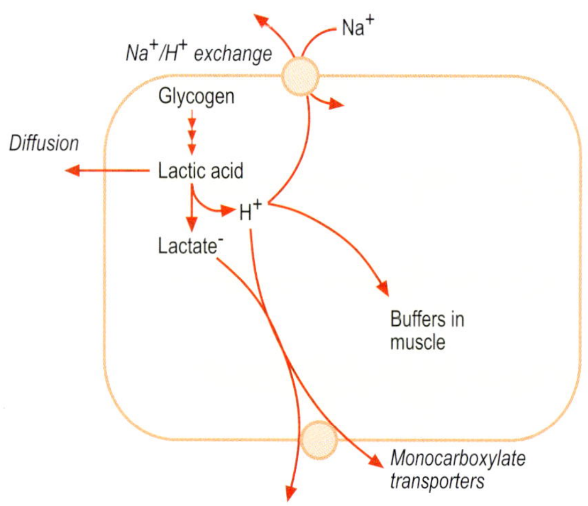

Fig 33.10 Lactic acid formed via anaerobic glycolysis is almost completely dissociated into a lactate anion and a proton. The means to prevent acidification of the cell include different buffer systems and transport of hydrogen ions out from the muscle cell. Most hydrogen ions are transported by the monocarboxylate transporter (MCT) with Na^+/H^+ exchange playing a minor role.

In prolonged low-to-moderate-intensity (submaximal) exercise, lipids are the predominant source of energy. During endurance exercise, there is usually no marked accumulation of lactic acid[108,109,176–178] and, therefore, acidification may not be a major cause of fatigue. From a metabolic viewpoint, the major contributing factor to the development of fatigue is a shortage of fuel, especially depletion of glycogen stores,[109] as demonstrated by a correlation between the extent of glycogen depletion and the duration of exercise.[179] Indeed, after an endurance rides, depletion of glycogen is seen and, in some horses, muscle biopsy samples may be completely devoid of glycogen.[108,177] Glycogen depletion in oxidative fibers[180] contributes to fatigue[145] because acetyl-CoA produced by free fatty acid oxidation needs oxaloacetate to enter the Krebs cycle and proceed to sufficient ATP synthesis through oxidative phosphorylation. Low blood glucose concentration also may contribute as it limits the glucose availability to the central nervous system. In addition, central fatigue may be due to increased formation of serotonin in the central nervous system.[181] During endurance exercise, factors not related to substrate supply also may be more important in the development of fatigue; these include dehydration, electrolyte and acidbase disturbances, and hyperthermia.

Metabolism during recovery from exercise

Lactate removal

After cessation of exercise, the rate of oxygen consumption remains elevated[182] and blood lactate concentration continues to increase, with peak concentrations attained 2–10 min post exercise. During exercise the main tissues that use lactate are the liver, which converts lactate back to glucose, and the heart, in which lactate is used directly for energy. There also may be some utilization of lactate by oxidative muscle fibers. However, during recovery the major consumer of lactate is, due to its large mass, skeletal muscle with oxidation of lactate by all fiber types.[183]

The rate of lactate removal from blood depends on the metabolic state. At rest the need for energy is low, but even light exercise increases the oxygen consumption of muscles and thereby the oxidation of lactic acid.[183–185] Following high-speed treadmill exercise, the half-life of lactate is decreased by 50% in horses that exercise lightly in comparison to those that remain stationary.[185] The rate of lactate disappearance is independent of concentration, which implies that the rate-limiting step in the process is saturable[185] (Fig. 33.11).

Glycogen synthesis

Because glycogen is a limiting fuel for contracting muscle for both high- and low-to-moderate-intensity exercise, the capacity to maximize muscle glycogen replenishment after exercise is an important factor for optimizing performance in horses competing on successive days or on several occasions during the same day.[180] However, in horses, recovery of glycogen is typically slow. During the first 24 h practically no repletion occurs and complete resynthesis of muscle glycogen stores requires 48–72 h after intense exercise that results in a greater than 60–70% reduction in muscle glycogen concentrations.[180,186–188] Intravenous glucose administration (6 g/kg bodyweight over 12 h) hastened glycogen stores replenishment after strenuous exercise[154] but a high starch diet did not enhance muscle glycogen resynthesis within the first 24 h after exercise.[189] A 30% increase in muscle glycogen concentrations in horses fed starch-rich meals was observed only 72 h after exercise compared with horses fed conventional diet.[186] Mechanisms underlying the slow glycogen replenishment after exercise in horses are not known, but may include limited ability of the small intestine to digest starch, slower activity of the muscle glycogen synthase enzyme and lower recruitment of GLUT-4 at the plasma membrane compared with values reported in humans and rodents.[186,190] For instance, glycogen synthase activity increased twofold after glycogen-depleting exercise in horses, whereas a 5- to 10-fold increase was reported in humans under similar condition.[186] Furthermore, in contrast with other species, GLUT-4 protein content is unchanged or only mildly increased immediately after exercise,[186,191] and intravenous glucose infusion after exercise enhanced muscle glycogen synthesis but attenuated the increase in GLUT-4 protein content.[191] A lack of post-exercise enhancement in insulin sensitivity in skeletal muscle also may contribute to slow glycogen resynthesis.[192–195]

The two forms of glycogen (i.e. the proglycogen and macroglycogen) have a different rate of resynthesis. The fraction most depleted during exercise (i.e. macroglycogen)[146] had no resynthesis during the first hour of recovery but then had the highest rate of resynthesis during the remainder of the first 24 h period. The rate of muscle glycogen resynthesis thereafter was slower and did not differ between the two forms of glycogen up to 72 h.[187] Another possible factor for low glycogen resynthesis may be a shortage of fuel during recovery. Skeletal muscle has to maintain its normal functions and only the available substrate (glucose) in excess of these demands is available for the resynthesis of glycogen. After exercise, catecholamine concentrations decrease within minutes and, consequently, lipolysis slows and the plasma concentration of NEFA decreases to a very low level.[137] Therefore, the predominant substrate available for muscle will be glucose (Fig. 33.12).

Because of the slow rate of glycogen synthesis (up to three days), the interval between exercise bouts may be inadequate for complete or partial restoration of muscle glycogen stores, which may contribute to a decline in performance during subsequent exercise in the horse.[196]

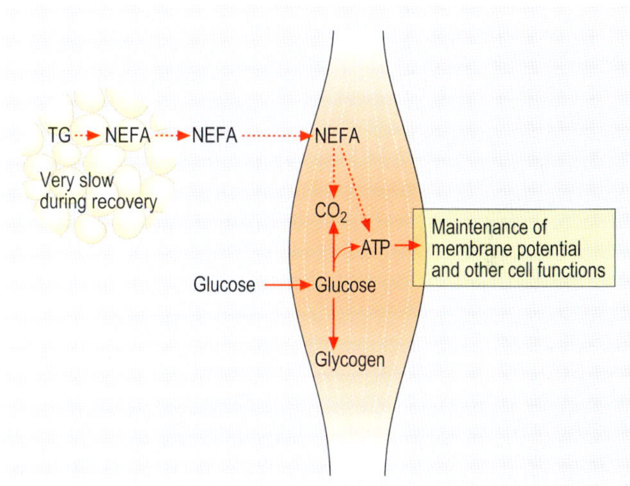

Fig 33.12 During recovery the rate of lipolysis decreases, leading to low concentrations of fatty acids (NEFA) in plasma. Therefore, the predominant substrate for muscle metabolism is blood glucose. The use of glucose in the maintenance of cell functions will affect the availability of glucose for the resynthesis of glycogen.

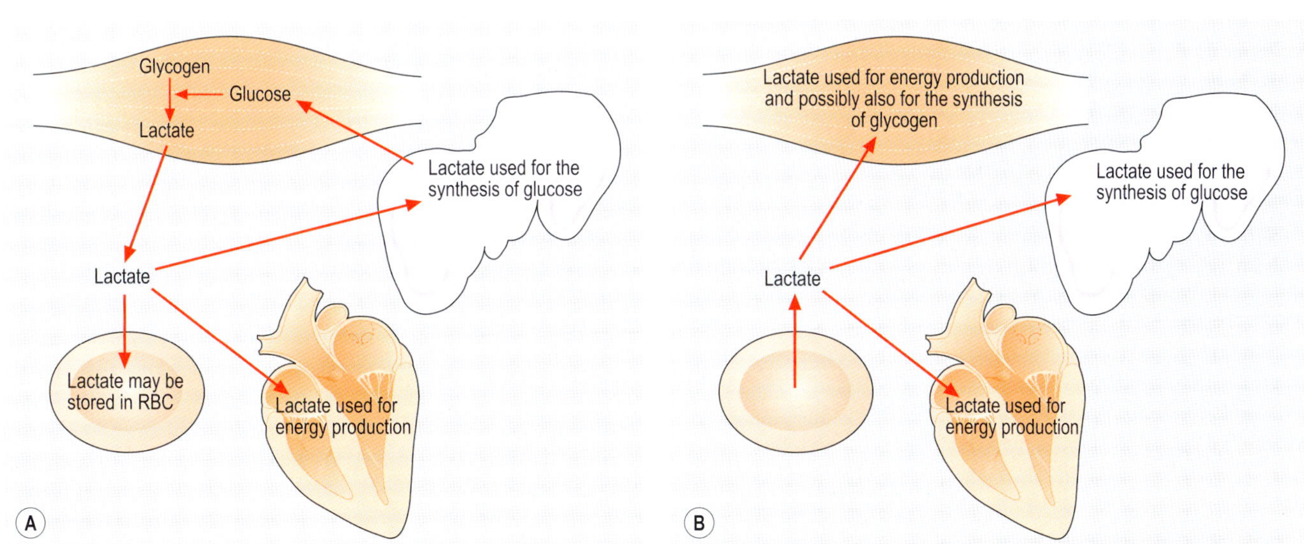

Fig 33.11 During exercise **(A)** lactate is formed in the working muscles and the flow of lactate is from muscle cells into blood plasma and further into tissues such as heart and liver that may use lactate for energy or glucose production. In horses, a substantial proportion of lactate produced in muscle may also be taken up by red blood cells (RBC). During recovery **(B)** the direction of lactate flow is reversed, i.e. from RBC to plasma, and the main user of lactic acid is skeletal muscle. Light exercise during the recovery period that increases muscle energy requirements will also increase the rate of lactate disappearance.

Physiological response to training

Overview

Horses are used for diverse and often highly specialized disciplines that require specific training programs.[47] Conditioning exercises or any repetitive activities induce changes in muscle structure and function that will increase the overall capacity of the muscle to respond to the energy demand associated with exercise. Ultimately, training increases oxidative capacity as measured at the whole-body and muscle levels. The extent of the whole-body adaptations to training, quantified as increases in VO_{2max}, depends on the intensity and duration of training as well as the pre-training status. This effect of training on VO_{2max} results mainly from the remarkable plasticity of the cardiovascular and muscular systems. At the muscle level, oxidative capacity increases as a result of several morphological and functional adaptations including increased mitochondrial density[51,197] in accordance to the concept of symmorphosis.[20] However, measurement of oxygen consumption at the level of the mitochondria by HRR[22,128] suggests that higher oxidative capacity with training in muscle is not due to an exclusively quantitative effect (i.e. increased mitochondrial volume density) but also to changes in functional properties of the ETS.[22]

Metabolic responses and mechanisms

Responses in metabolite concentrations in plasma

The rate of lactate production is intimately linked to the oxidative capacity of the muscle cells. Thus, training that increases the muscle oxidative capacity may reduce lactate concentrations in blood. Effluxes of lactate from the muscle and to the RBC are also primary determinants of blood lactate concentrations. Training has been shown to increase RBC lactate transport activity in reindeer and sled dogs, but not in horses.[79] On the other hand, training increases the number of MCT proteins on the sarcolemma that regulate the efflux of lactate from muscle, thus favoring an increase in blood lactate concentrations. This lactate may be taken up by tissues that oxidize lactate, such as the liver, but also inactive muscles. Lactate clearance is increased by training,[198,199] such that trained horses have significantly lower blood lactate concentrations during exercise[200,201] and are able to run faster before attainment of the lactate threshold when compared to untrained animals.[148] However, at the point of fatigue, plasma lactate is increased with training because of enhanced ability to remove lactate from muscle.[175]

Changes in muscle

Skeletal muscle undergoes major adaptations in response to conditioning. Specific training has the ability to change significantly the fiber type composition, metabolic properties, fiber size and/or capillarization within the skeletal muscle.[121,202–204] For example, endurance-trained horses show some enlargement of oxidative fibers (hypertrophy) and an increased number of capillaries surrounding them in their locomotory muscles.[121] Also, long-term endurance training modifies the fiber type composition with an increase in high-oxidative fibers and a decrease in fast-glycolytic fibers.[205,206] Studies have also demonstrated an increase in muscle glycogen stores in the early phase and, later on, in triglyceride content after endurance training.[207]

Generally speaking, training results in significant changes in muscle composition towards more oxidative fibers,[116,208,209] even in Thoroughbreds,[210–214] while additional high-intensity training programs have the potential to increase anaerobic capacity.[215,216] In addition to a fiber type transition that results in increased oxidative capacity, there is increased ability of muscle to metabolize fat after training. This adaptation occurs due to an increase in enzymes involved in β-oxidation as well as the increase in activity of TCA cycle enzymes.[50,217] Also, increased mitochondrial volume density contributes to the increased muscle oxidative capacity.[19,197] Increases in muscle mitochondrial volume of up to 70% have been observed after training in previously untrained horses.[197]

Training improves glucose availability to muscle owing to increased muscle concentration of glycogen stores,[215,218,219] increased muscle GLUT-4 content[220] and insulin sensitivity,[194,195] and a better perfusion of the muscle fibers owing to the development of capillary network.[221,222] Because of increased oxidative capacity, less glycogen is used and respiratory exchange ratio decreases during both high-[223] and moderate-intensity[67] exercise. Some studies report that exercise post training resulted in a nearly identical reduction in muscle glycogen concentrations while the concentration at rest (i.e. before exercise) was higher after conditioning.[23,215,219]

Overall, therefore, training results in increased aerobic (oxidative) and anaerobic capacity. These changes are accompanied by a significant increase in run time to fatigue during sprinting. It is worth noting that increases in anaerobic capacity may not be reflected in blood lactate concentrations measured during intense, exhaustive exercise or during recovery from such exercise.[215] Indeed, the effects of training on blood lactate concentrations after such maximal effort are controversial as some studies show no differences[200,215] while others show significantly higher lactate concentrations after training.[136,201] As previously mentioned, this finding may be related to increased expression and activity of the MCTs in muscle. Another factor that could modify blood lactate concentrations after training is an increase in muscle buffering capacity. Studies in horses have reported both an increase[175,224,225] and no change in muscle buffering capacity with training.[215]

In trained Standardbred horses, proteomics also confirms training-induced structural changes towards a higher oxidative capacity, an increased capacity to take up long-chain fatty acids, and to store energy in the form of glycogen.[129] In Thoroughbred racehorses, transcriptomic approaches have identified changes in the expression of functional groups of genes related to metabolism, oxidative phosphorylation and muscle structure.[131]

In addition to an increase in mitochondrial biogenesis, training induces an increase in mitochondrial performance, e.g. aerobic ATP production by OXPHOS.[128] In a longitudinal study, the effects of training (two 10-week periods) on quantitative and qualitative changes in muscle mitochondrial respiration were determined by HRR in the triceps brachii and gluteus medius muscles of endurance horses.[128] Training effects were more pronounced in the triceps brachii than in the gluteus medius. A greater training-induced increase in the oxidative capacity of the triceps brachii versus a locomotor muscle (i.e. semimembranosus) has previously been documented.[49] Analysis of respirometric parameters indicated not only quantitative but also sequential qualitative functional changes. Specifically, OXPHOS capacity supported by NADH-linked substrates (i.e. electron entry at the level of Complex I) was significantly increased after the first session of training (in both muscles) whereas OXPHOS capacity at the level of Complex II (i.e. where succinate is oxidized with reduction of FAD into $FADH_2$ and subsequent electron flow) was only increased after the second training period and only in the triceps brachii. This preliminary study demonstrated that the sampling of the triceps brachii is useful for the evaluation of changes in mitochondrial respiratory function in endurance horses during training. Mitochondrial respiratory capacity is affected by training and body condition score; the maximum tissue-mass-specific OXPHOS and ETS capacities increased 1.7-fold as a function of these two parameters (Fig. 33.13).

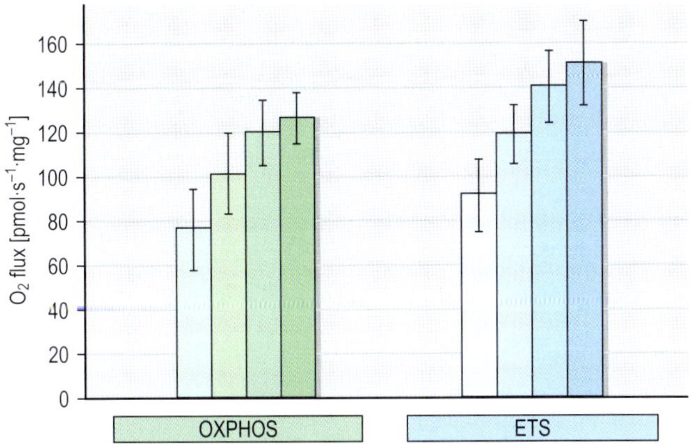

Fig 33.13 Maximal oxidative phosphorylation (OXPHOS) and electron transfer system (ETS) capacities (pmol.s^{-1}.mg^{-1} wet weight) with Complexes I and II (CI+II) substrates supply as a function of physical fitness level. From light green or blue to dark green or blue: overweight-untrained (N = 3) → untrained with optimal body condition score (BCS; N = 8) → trained with optimal BCS (N = 16) → competitive with optimal BCS (N = 5); N: number of horses.
Adapted from Votion et al. 2012.[22]

Training intensity and duration

Significant training effects are apparent even when the intensity of training exercise is low or moderate, but these changes mainly reflect an increase in aerobic capacity and reactions related to aerobic metabolism. Decreases in the rate of glycogenolysis, increases in oxidative enzymes and increases in oxygen extraction by tissues are evident after as little as 2 weeks of training,[226,227] sometimes even before any measurable changes in indices of muscle oxidative capacity can be detected.[223] In general, most of the training-induced increase in aerobic capacity occurs during the initial 6-week period of training.[228] However, further increments in VO_{2max} occur if a training stimulus is maintained.[228] The study by Hinchcliff et al.,[215] however, clearly shows that high-intensity training is necessary for improvements in anaerobic capacity. It is possible that intense exercise is also necessary for maximum improvements in aerobic capacity because adaptive changes in aerobic processes appear to require hypoxia as an inducer of gene activity, e.g. the induction of erythropoiesis, capillary growth and the synthesis of glycolytic enzymes appear to be regulated by hypoxia.[229]

Detraining

Most of the changes in metabolism require synthesis of new proteins and thus require days or weeks to develop; these adaptations also persist for several weeks after the cessation of regular physical activity (detraining).[221,230] In general, adaptive training responses in skeletal muscle persist for 5–6 weeks after the cessation of regular physical activity.[50,207] Similarly, there is minimal change in maximum oxygen uptake after 2–4 months of detraining.[228,230] However, in a study by Butler et al.[230] lactate accumulation during intense exercise was higher after a 15-week period of detraining, indicating a decrease in aerobic capacity. The fiber type changes during detraining occur in reverse order to the changes during training.[50,207]

With thanks to A. Reeta Pösö, Seppo Hyyppä and Raymond J. Geor, who created the original chapter in the first edition.

References

1. Nagata S, et al. Plasma adrenocorticotropin, cortisol and catecholamines response to various exercises. Equine Vet J Suppl 1999;30: 570–4.
2. Kokkonen UM, et al. Exercise-induced changes in atrial peptides in relation to neuroendocrine responses and fluid balance in the horse. J Vet Med A Physiol Pathol Clin Med 2002;49(3): 144–50.
3. Snow DH, et al. Effects of high-intensity exercise on plasma catecholamines in the thoroughbred horse. Equine Vet J 1992;24(6):462–7.
4. Taylor CR, et al. Design of the mammalian respiratory system. III Scaling maximum aerobic capacity to body mass: wild and domestic mammals. Respir Physiol 1981;44(1): 25–37.
5. Poole D. Current concepts of oxygen transport during exercise. Equine Comp Exerc Physiol 2004;1(1): 5–22.
6. Young L, et al. Heart size estimated by echocardiography correlates with maximal oxygen uptake. Equine Vet J Suppl 2002;34:467–71.
7. Saltin B, Astrand P-O. Maximal oxygen uptake in athletes. J Appl Physiol 1967;23:353–8.
8. Evans D, Rose R. Cardiovascular and respiratory responses in Thoroughbred horses during treadmill exercise. J Exp Biol 1988;134:397–408.
9. Art T, Lekeux P. Ventilatory and arterial blood gas tension adjustments to strenuous exercise in Standardbreds. Am J Vet Res 1995;56(10):1332–7.
10. Asheim A, et al. Heart rates and blood lactate concentrations of Standardbred horses during training and racing. J Am Vet Med Assoc 1970;157(3):304–12.
11. Lindholm A, Saltin B. The physiological and biochemical response of Standardbred horses to exercise of varying speed and duration. Acta Vet Scand 1974;15(3):310–24.
12. McArdle WD, Foglia GF, Patti AV. Telemetered cardiac response to selected running events. J Appl Physiol 1967;23(4):566–70.
13. Thomas DP, Fregin GF. Cardiorespiratory and metabolic responses to treadmill exercise in the horse. J Appl Physiol 1981;50(4):864–8.
14. Armstrong RB, et al. O_2 delivery at VO_{2max} and oxidative capacity in muscles of Standardbred horses. J Appl Physiol 1992;73(6):2274–82.
15. Hodgson DR, et al. Dissipation of metabolic heat in the horse during exercise. J Appl Physiol 1993;74(3): 1161–70.
16. Weibel ER, et al. Design of the mammalian respiratory system. IX. Functional and structural limits for oxygen flow. Respir Physiol 1981;44(1):151–64.
17. Hoppeler H, Lindstedt SL. Malleability of skeletal muscle in overcoming limitations: structural elements. J Exp Biol 1985;115:355–64.
18. Weibel ER, et al. Allometric scaling of maximal metabolic rate in mammals: muscle aerobic capacity as determinant factor. Respir Physiol Neurobiol 2004;140(2):115–32.
19. Kayar SR, et al. Total muscle mitochondrial volume in relation to aerobic capacity of horses and steers. Pflugers Archiv 1989;413(4): 343–7.
20. Weibel ER, Taylor CR, Hoppeler H. The concept of symmorphosis: a testable

hypothesis of structure–function relationship. Proc Natl Acad Sci U S A 1991;88(22):10357–61.
21. Pesta D, et al. Similar qualitative and quantitative changes of mitochondrial respiration following strength and endurance training in normoxia and hypoxia in sedentary humans. Am J Physiol Regul Integr Comp Physiol 2011;301(4):R1078–87.
22. Votion DM, et al. Physical fitness and mitochondrial respiratory capacity in horse skeletal muscle. PLoS One 2012;7(4):e34890.
23. Guy PS, Snow DH. The effect of training and detraining on muscle composition in the horse. J Physiol 1977;269(1):33–51.
24. Snow DH, et al. Glycogen repletion following different diets. In: Gillespie JR, Robinson NE, editors. Equine exercicse physiology 2. Davis, CA: ICEEP; 1987. p. 701–10.
25. Hyyppa S, Saastamoinen M, Reeta Poso A. Effect of a post exercise fat-supplemented diet on muscle glycogen repletion. Equine Vet J Suppl 1999;30:493–8.
26. Essén-Gustavsson B, Jensen-Waern M. Effect of an endurance race on muscle amino acids, pro- and macroglycogen and triglycerides. Equine Vet J Suppl 2002;(34):209–13.
27. Pösö AR, et al. Exercise-induced transient hyperlipidemia in the racehorse. Zentralbl Veterinarmed A 1989;36(8):603–11.
28. Guyton AC, Hall JE. Metabolism of carbohydrates, and formation of adenosine triphosphate. In: Guyton AC, Hall JE, editors. Textbook of medical physiology. Philadelphia: Elsevier Saunders; 2006. p. 829–39.
29. Nelson DL, Cox MM. Fatty acid catabolism. In: Lehninger AL, editor. Principles of biochemistry. 4th ed. New York: WH Freeman and Company; 2005. p. 631–55.
30. Pethick DW, et al. Nutrient utilisation by the hindlimb of thoroughbred horses at rest. Equine Vet J 1993;25(1): 41–4.
31. Ford EJ, Simmons HA. Gluconeogenesis from caecal propionate in the horse. Br J Nutr 1985;53(1):55–60.
32. Simmons HA, Ford EJ. Gluconeogenesis from propionate produced in the colon of the horse. Br Vet J 1991;147(4): 340–5.
33. Votion DM, et al. Muscle energetics in exercising horses. Equine Comp Exerc Physiol 2007;4(3/4):105–18.
34. Hayashi T, Wojtaszewski JF, Goodyear LJ. Exercise regulation of glucose transport in skeletal muscle. Am J Physiol 1997;273(6 Pt 1):E1039–51.
35. Holloszy JO, Constable SH, Young DA. Activation of glucose transport in muscle by exercise. Diabetes Metab Rev 1986;1(4):409–23.
36. Guyton AC, Hall JE. Lipid metabolism. In: Guyton AC, Hall JE, editors. Textbook of medical physiology. Philadelphia: Elsevier Saunders; 2006. p. 383–401.
37. Sewell DA, Harris RC. Adenine nucleotide degradation in the thoroughbred horse with increasing exercise duration. Eur J Appl Physiol Occup Physiol 1992;65(3):271–7.
38. Kinnunen S, et al. Exercise-induced oxidative stress and muscle stress protein responses in trotters. Eur J Appl Physiol 2005;93(4):496–501.
39. Kinnunen S, et al. Oxygen radical absorbance capacity (ORAC) and exercise-induced oxidative stress in trotters. Eur J Appl Physiol 2005; 95(5–6):550–6.
40. Kinnunen S, et al. alpha-Lipoic acid modulates thiol antioxidant defenses and attenuates exercise-induced oxidative stress in Standardbred trotters. Free Radic Res 2009;43(8):697–705.
41. Courouce A, et al. Comparison of exercise tests in French trotters under training track, racetrack and treadmill conditions. Equine Vet J Suppl 1999;30: 528–32.
42. Erck EV, et al. Evaluation of oxygen consumption during field exercise tests in Standardbred trotters. Equine Comp Exerc Physiol 2007;4(1):43–9.
43. Escribano BM, et al. Utility of the discriminant analysis to categorize untrained Spanish Pure Bred horses on the basis of biochemical and muscle variables before and after a standardized exercise test. Res Vet Sci 2011;91(3): e144–8.
44. Harkins JD, Beadle RE, Kamerling SG. The correlation of running ability and physiological variables in thoroughbred racehorses. Equine Vet J 1993;25(1):53–60.
45. Lindner A, et al. Effect of different blood-guided conditioning programmes on skeletal muscle ultrastructure and histochemistry of sport horses. J Anim Physiol Anim Nutr (Berl) 2012.
46. Noel de Burlin A, et al. Routine standardized tests to assess fitness in endurance horses. PVE 1994;26(1): 25–30.
47. Rivero JL. A scientific background for skeletal muscle conditioning in equine practice. J Vet Med A Physiol Pathol Clin Med 2007;54(6):321–32.
48. Vermeulen AD, Evans DL. Measurements of fitness in thoroughbred racehorses using field studies of heart rate and velocity with a global positioning system. Equine Vet J Suppl 2006;(36):113–7.
49. Kim JS, et al. Exercise training increases oxidative capacity and attenuates exercise-induced ultrastructural damage in skeletal muscle of aged horses. J Appl Physiol 2005;98(1):334–42.
50. Serrano AL, Quiroz-Rothe E, Rivero JL. Early and long-term changes of equine skeletal muscle in response to endurance training and detraining. Pflugers Archiv 2000;441(2–3):263–74.
51. Tyler CM, et al. Skeletal muscle adaptations to prolonged training, overtraining and detraining in horses. Pflugers Archiv 1998;436(3):391–7.
52. Franck T, et al. Specific immuno-extraction followed by enzymatic detection (SIEFED) of myeloperoxidase and mitochondrial complex I in muscular microbiopsies: preliminary results in endurance horses. Equine Vet J 2010;42(Suppl. 38):296–302.
53. Serteyn D, et al. Effect of a 120 km endurance race on plasma and muscular neutrophil elastase and myeloperoxidase concentrations in horses. Equine Vet J 2010;42(Suppl. 38): 275–9.
54. Barrey E, et al. Gene expression profiling in blood cells of endurance horses completing competition or disqualified due to metabolic disorder. Equine Vet J Suppl 2006;(36):43–9.
55. Evans DL. Physiology of equine performance and associated tests of function. Equine Vet J 2007;39(4): 373–83.
56. Fraipont A, et al. Subclinical diseases underlying poor performance in endurance horses: diagnostic methods and predictive tests. Vet Rec 2011; 169(6):154.
57. de Moffarts B, et al. Effect of exercise on blood oxidant/antioxidant markers in Standardbred horses: comparison between treadmill and race track tests. Equine Vet J Suppl 2006;(36):254–7.
58. Nostell K, et al. The physiological responses to simulated race tests on a track and on a treadmill in Standardbred trotters. Equine Vet J Suppl 2006;(36):123–7.
59. Art T, et al. Validation of a portable equine metabolic measurement system. Equine Vet J Suppl 2006;(36):557–61.
60. Butudom P, et al. Validation and comparison of two methods of measuring lactate in equine plasma. Equine Vet J Suppl 2010;(38):155–60.
61. Votion DM, et al. New perspective for field measurement of cardiorespiratory parameters in exercising horses. Pferdeheilkunde 2006;22(5):619–24.
62. Guhl A, Lindner A, von Wittke P. Reproducibility of the blood lactate-running speed curve in horses under field conditions. Am J Vet Res 1996;57(7):1059–62.
63. Treiber KH, et al. Single-injection glucose kinetics with compartmental modelling during rest and low-intensity exercise in horses. Equine Vet J Suppl 2010;(38):361–9.

64. Geor RJ, Hinchcliff KW, Sams RA. beta-adrenergic blockade augments glucose utilization in horses during graded exercise. J Appl Physiol 2000;89(3):1086–98.
65. Geor RJ, et al. Epinephrine inhibits exogenous glucose utilization in exercising horses. J Appl Physiol 2000;88(5):1777–90.
66. Geor RJ, Hinchcliff KW, Sams RA. Glucose infusion attenuates endogenous glucose production and enhances glucose use of horses during exercise. J Appl Physiol 2000;88(5):1765–76.
67. Geor RJ, et al. Training-induced alterations in glucose metabolism during moderate-intensity exercise. Equine Vet J Suppl 2002;(34):22–8.
68. Jose-Cunilleras E, et al. Glycemic index of a meal fed before exercise alters substrate use and glucose flux in exercising horses. J Appl Physiol 2002;92(1):117–28.
69. Jose-Cunilleras E, et al. Ingestion of starch-rich meals after exercise increases glucose kinetics but fails to enhance muscle glycogen replenishment in horses. Vet J 2006;171(3):468–77.
70. Klein HJ, et al. Metabolism of naturally occurring [13C]glucose given orally to horses. Am J Vet Res 1988;49(8):1259–62.
71. Schulze E, et al. Glucose entry rate in dairy cattle as determined by stable isotope 13C-labelled glucose at different stages of reproduction. Comp Biochem Physiol B 1991;100(1):167–71.
72. Rijnen KE, van der Kolk JH. Determination of reference range values indicative of glucose metabolism and insulin resistance by use of glucose clamp techniques in horses and ponies. Am J Vet Res 2003;64(10):1260–4.
73. DeFronzo RA, Tobin JD, Andres R. Glucose clamp technique: a method for quantifying insulin secretion and resistance. Am J Physiol 1979;237(3):E214–23.
74. Kemmink A, Westermann CM, van der Kolk JH. Assessment of glucose disposal with the hyperglycaemic clamp technique during low intensity exercise in Warmblood horses. Equine Vet J Suppl 2010;(38):147–51.
75. Evans DL, Rose RJ. Maximum oxygen uptake in racehorses: changes with training state and prediction from submaximal cardiorespiratory measurements. In: Gillespie JR, Robinson NE, editors. Equine exercise physiology 2. Davis: ICEEP Publications; 1987. p. 52–67.
76. Rose RJ, et al. Kinetics of VO_2 and VCO_2 in the horse and comparison of five methods for determination of maximum oxygen uptake. Equine Vet J Suppl 1990;(9):39–42.
77. Eaton MD, et al. Maximal accumulated oxygen deficit in thoroughbred horses. J Appl Physiol 1995;78(4):1564–8.
78. Gauvreau GM, et al. The relationship between respiratory exchange ratio, plasma lactate and muscle lactate concentrations in exercising horses using a valved gas collection system. Can J Vet Res 1996;60(3):161–71.
79. Vaihkonen LK, et al. Lactate-transport activity in RBCs of trained and untrained individuals from four racing species. Am J Physiol Regul Integr Comp Physiol 2001;281(1):R19–24.
80. Pösö AR, Lampinen KJ, Räsänen LA. Distribution of lactate between red blood cells and plasma after exercise. Equine Vet J Suppl 1995;18:231–4.
81. Vaihkonen LK, Hyyppä S, Pösö AR. Factors affecting accumulation of lactate in red blood cells. Equine Vet J Suppl 1999;30:443–7.
82. Juel C, et al. Lactate and potassium fluxes from human skeletal muscle during and after intense, dynamic, knee extensor exercise. Acta Physiol Scand 1990;140(2):147–59.
83. Persson SGB, et al. Plasma, red cell and whole blood lactate concentrations during prolonged treadmill exercise at VLA4. Equine Vet J Suppl 1995;18:104–7.
84. Rainger JE, et al. Distribution of lactate in plasma and erythrocytes during and after exercise in horses. Br Vet J 1995;151(3):299–310.
85. Vaihkonen LK, Poso AR. Interindividual variation in total and carrier-mediated lactate influx into red blood cells. Am J Physiol 1998;274(4 Pt 2):R1025–30.
86. Koho NM, Hyyppa S, Poso AR. Monocarboxylate transporters (MCT) as lactate carriers in equine muscle and red blood cells. Equine Vet J Suppl 2006;(36):354–8.
87. Vaihkonen LK, Ojala M, Poso AR. Age-related changes and inheritance of lactate transport activity in red blood cells. Equine Vet J Suppl 2002;(34):568–72.
88. Koho NM, Vaihkonen LK, Poso AR. Lactate transport in red blood cells by monocarboxylate transporters. Equine Vet J Suppl 2002;(34):555–9.
89. Rasanen LA, Lampinen KJ, Pösö AR. Responses of blood and plasma lactate and plasma purine concentrations to maximal exercise and their relation to performance in Standardbred trotters. Am J Vet Res 1995;56(12):1651–6.
90. Juel C, et al. Human skeletal muscle and erythrocyte proteins involved in acid–base homeostasis: adaptations to chronic hypoxia. J Physiol 2003;548(Pt 2):639–48.
91. Mykkanen AK, et al. Expression of lactate transporters MCT1, MCT2 and CD147 in the red blood cells of three horse breeds: Finnhorse, Standardbred and Thoroughbred. Equine Vet J Suppl 2010;(38):161–6.
92. Persson SG. Heart rate and blood lactate responses to submaximal treadmill exercise in the normally performing Standardbred trotter – age and sex variations and predictability from the total red blood cell volume. Zentralbl Veterinarmed A 1997;44(3):125–32.
93. Harris P, Snow DH. The effects of high intensity exercise on the plasma concentration of lactate, potassium and other electrolytes. Equine Vet J 1988;20(2):109–13.
94. Russell MA, Rodiek AV, Lawrence LM. Effects of exercise, training, and sampling location on selected plasma free amino acids in horses. Can J Anim Sci 1986;66:827–31.
95. Franck T, et al. Development of an enzyme-linked immunosorbent assay for specific equine neutrophil myeloperoxidase measurement in blood. J Vet Diagn Invest 2005;17(5):412–9.
96. de la Rebiere G, et al. Effects of unfractionated and fractionated heparins on myeloperoxidase activity and interactions with endothelial cells: possible effects on the pathophysiology of equine laminitis. Vet J 2008;178(1):62–9.
97. Li G, Lee P, Mori N, et al. Long term intensive exercise training leads to a higher plasma malate/lactate dehydrogenase (M/L) ratio and increased level of lipid mobilization in horses. Vet Res Commun 2012;36(2):1439–55.
98. Nelson DL, Cox MM. Fatty acid catabolism. In: Lehninger AL, editor. Principles of biochemistry. 4th ed. New York: WH Freeman and Company; 2005. p. 631–55.
99. Westermann CM, et al. Plasma acylcarnitine and fatty acid profiles during exercise and training in Standardbreds. Am J Vet Res 2008;69(11):1469–75.
100. Scoppetta F, et al. Plasma protein changes in horse after prolonged physical exercise: a proteomic study. J Proteomics 2012.
101. Lewis GD, et al. Metabolic signatures of exercise in human plasma. Sci Transl Med 2010;2(33):33ra37.
102. Lindholm A, Piehl K. Fibre composition, enzyme activity and concentrations of metabolites and electrolytes in muscles of Standardbred horses. Acta Vet Scand 1974;15:287–309.
103. Snow DH, Guy PS. Percutaneous needle muscle biopsy in the horse. Equine Vet J 1976;8:150–5.

104. Sewell DA, Harris RC, Marlin DJ. Skeletal muscle characteristics in 2-year-old race-trained thoroughbred horses. Comp Biochem Physiol Comp Physiol 1994;108(1):87–96.
105. van den Hoven R, et al. Variation of fiber types in the triceps brachii, longissimus dorsi, gluteus medius, and biceps femoris of horses. Am J Vet Res 1985;46:939–41.
106. Kline KH, Bechtel PJ. Changes in the metabolic profile of the equine gluteus medius as a function of sampling depth. Comp Biochem Physiol A Comp Physiol 1988;91(4):815–9.
107. Gottlieb M. Muscle glycogen depletion patterns during draught work in Standardbred horses. Equine Vet J 1989;21(2):110–5.
108. Snow DH, Baxter P, Rose RJ. Muscle fibre composition and glycogen depletion in horses competing in an endurance ride. Vet Rec 1981;108(17):374–8.
109. Essén-Gustavsson B, Karlstrom K, Lindholm A. Fibre types, enzyme activities and substrate utilisation in skeletal muscles of horses competing in endurance rides. Equine Vet J 1984;16(3):197–202.
110. Lindholm A, Bjerneld H, Saltin B. Glycogen depletion pattern in muscle fibres of trotting horses. Acta Physiol Scand 1974;90(2):475–84.
111. Valberg S. Glycogen depletion patterns in the muscle of Standardbred trotters after exercise of varying intensities and durations. Equine Vet J 1986;18(6):479–84.
112. Annandale EJ, et al. Insulin sensitivity and skeletal muscle glucose transport in horses with equine polysaccharide storage myopathy. Neuromuscul Disord 2004;14(10):666–74.
113. Quiroz-Rothe E, Rivero JL. Coordinated expression of myosin heavy chains, metabolic enzymes, and morphological features of porcine skeletal muscle fiber types. Microsc Res Tech 2004;65(1–2):43–61.
114. Snow DH, Guy PS. Muscle fibre type composition of a number of limb muscles in different types of horse. Res Vet Sci 1980;28:137–44.
115. Karlstrom K, et al. Capillary supply in relation to muscle metabolic profile and cardiocirculatory parameters. In: Third International Conference on Equine Exercise Physiology. Uppsala, Sweden: ICEEP Publications; 1991.
116. Revold T, et al. Effects of training on equine muscle fibres and monocarboxylate transporters in young Coldblooded Trotters. Equine Vet J Suppl 2010;(38):289–95.
117. Rivero JL, et al. Skeletal muscle histochemistry in male and female Andalusian and Arabian horses of different ages. Res Vet Sci 1993;54(2):160–9.
118. Gunn HM. Differences in the histochemical properties of skeletal muscles of different breeds of horses and dogs. J Anat 1978;127(Pt 3):615–34.
119. Kim JS, et al. Age-related changes in metabolic properties of equine skeletal muscle associated with muscle plasticity. Vet J 2005;169(3):397–403.
120. Rivero JL, et al. Effects of intensity and duration of exercise on muscular responses to training of thoroughbred racehorses. J Appl Physiol 2007;102(5):1871–82.
121. Rivero JL, et al. Effects of a 3 month endurance training programme on skeletal muscle histochemistry in Andalusian, Arabian and Anglo-Arabian horses. Equine Vet J 1995;27(1):51–9.
122. Rivero JL. Muscle biopsy as a tool for assessing muscular adaptation to training in horses. Am J Vet Res 1996;57(10):1412–6.
123. Rivero JL, et al. Coordinated changes of kinematics and muscle fibre properties with prolonged endurance training. Equine Vet J Suppl 2001;33:104–8.
124. Rivero JL, Serrano AL, Henckel P. Activities of selected aerobic and anaerobic enzymes in the gluteus medius muscle of endurance horses with different performance records. Vet Rec 1995;137(8):187–92.
125. Rivero JL, Henckel P. Muscle biopsy index for discriminating between endurance horses with different performance records. Res Vet Sci 1996;61(1):49–54.
126. Gollnick PD, et al. The effect of high-intensity exercise on the respiratory capacity of skeletal muscle. Pflugers Arch 1990;415:407–13.
127. Gnaiger E. Capacity of oxidative phosphorylation in human skeletal muscle: new perspectives of mitochondrial physiology. Int J Biochem Cell Biol 2009;41(10):1837–45.
128. Votion DM, et al. Alterations in mitochondrial respiratory function in response to endurance training and endurance racing. Equine Vet J 2010;42(Suppl. 38):268–74.
129. Bouwman FG, et al. Differential expression of equine muscle biopsy proteins during normal training and intensified training in young Standardbred horses using proteomics technology. Comp Biochem Physiol D Genomics Proteomics 2010;5(1):55–64.
130. McGivney BA, et al. Transcriptional adaptations following exercise in thoroughbred horse skeletal muscle highlights molecular mechanisms that lead to muscle hypertrophy. BMC Genomics 2009;10:638.
131. McGivney BA, et al. Characterization of the equine skeletal muscle transcriptome identifies novel functional responses to exercise training. BMC Genomics 2010;11:398.
132. Nam GH, et al. Identification of ORF sequences and exercise-induced expression change in thoroughbred horse OXCT1 gene. Gene 2012;496(1):45–8.
133. Geor RJ, McCutcheon LJ, Hinchcliff KW. Effects of warm-up intensity on kinetics of oxygen consumption and carbon dioxide production during high-intensity exercise in horses. Am J Vet Res 2000;61(6):638–45.
134. Tyler CM, Hodgson DR, Rose RJ. Effect of a warm-up on energy supply during high intensity exercise in horses. Equine Vet J 1996;28(2):117–20.
135. Havel RJ, et al. Turnover rate and oxidation of different free fatty acids in man during exercise. J Appl Physiol 1964;19:613–18.
136. Snow DH, Mackenzie G. Some metabolic effects of maximal exercise in the horse and adaptations with training. Equine Vet J 1977;9(3):134–40.
137. Hyyppa S, Rasanen LA, Poso AR. Resynthesis of glycogen in skeletal muscle from Standardbred trotters after repeated bouts of exercise. Am J Vet Res 1997;58(2):162–6.
138. Pösö R, Hyyppä S. Metabolic and hormonal changes after exercise in relation to muscle glycogen concentrations. Equine Vet J Suppl 1999;30:332–6.
139. Rose RJ, Purdue RA, Hensley W. Plasma biochemistry alterations in horses during an endurance ride. Equine Vet J 1977;9(3):122–6.
140. Pösö AR, Soveri T, Oksanen HE. The effect of exercise on blood parameters in Standardbred and Finnish-bred horses. Acta Vet Scand 1983;24(2):170–84.
141. Schuback K, Essen-Gustavsson B, Persson SG. Incremental treadmill exercise until onset of fatigue and its relationship to metabolic response and locomotion pattern. Equine Vet J Suppl 1999;30:337–41.
142. Rasanen LA, et al. Accumulation of uric acid in plasma after repeated bouts of exercise in the horse. Comp Biochem Physiol B Biochem Mol Biol 1996;114(2):139–44.
143. Harris RC, et al. Muscle ATP loss and lactate accumulation at different work intensities in the exercising Thoroughbred horse. Eur J Appl Physiol Occup Physiol 1991;62(4):235–44.
144. Essén-Gustavsson B, Valberg SJ. Blood and muscle ammonia concentrations in horses during treadmill work and after racing. In: Gillespie JR, Robinson NE, editors. Equine exercise

physiology 2. Davis: ICEEP Publications; 1987. p. 456–63.
145. Valberg S, et al. Blood chemistry and skeletal muscle metabolic responses during and after different speeds and durations of trotting. Equine Vet J Suppl 1989;21(2):91–5.
146. Brojer J, et al. Pro- and macroglycogenolysis in skeletal muscle during maximal treadmill exercise. Equine Vet J Suppl 2002;(34):205–8.
147. Schuback K, Essen-Gustavsson B. Muscle anaerobic response to a maximal treadmill exercise test in Standardbred trotters. Equine Vet J 1998;30(6): 504–10.
148. Valberg S, et al. Energy metabolism in relation to skeletal muscle fibre properties during treadmill exercise. Equine Vet J 1985;17(6):439–44.
149. Green H, et al. Increases in muscle MCT are associated with reductions in muscle lactate after a single exercise session in humans. Am J Physiol Endocrinol Metab 2002;282(1):E154–60.
150. Valberg SJ, et al. Skeletal muscle metabolic response to exercise in horses with 'tying-up' due to polysaccharide storage myopathy. Equine Vet J 1999;31(1):43–7.
151. Essén-Gustavsson B, Roneus N, Poso AR. Metabolic response in skeletal muscle fibres of Standardbred trotters after racing. Comp Biochem Physiol B Biochem Mol Biol 1997;117(3):431–6.
152. Gottlieb M, et al. Cardio-respiratory and muscle metabolic responses to draught work on a treadmill in Standardbred horses. In: Gillespie JR, Robinson NE, editors. Cardio-respiratory and muscle metabolic responses to draught work on a treadmill in Standardbred horses. Davis: ICEEP Publications; 1987. p. 384–92.
153. Lacombe V, et al. Exercise that induces substantial muscle glycogen depletion impairs subsequent anaerobic capacity. Equine Vet J Suppl 1999;30:293–7.
154. Lacombe VA, et al. Muscle glycogen depletion and subsequent replenishment affect anaerobic capacity of horses. J Appl Physiol 2001;91(4): 1782–90.
155. Pagan JD, et al. The effect of dietary energy source on exercise performance in Standardbred horses. In: Gillespie JR, Robinson NE, editors. Equine exercise physiology 2. Davis: ICEEP Publications; 1987. p. 686–700.
156. Benard G, et al. Mitochondrial bioenergetics and structural network organization. J Cell Sci 2007;120(Pt 5): 838–48.
157. Benard G, Rossignol R. Ultrastructure of the mitochondrion and its bearing on function and bioenergetics. Antioxid Redox Signal 2008;10(8):1313–42.
158. McCutcheon LJ, Geor RJ, Hinchcliff KW. Effects of prior exercise on muscle metabolism during sprint exercise in horses. J Appl Physiol 1999;87(5): 1914–22.
159. Mukai K, et al. Effects of warm-up intensity on oxygen transport during supramaximal exercise in horses. Am J Vet Res 2008;69(5):690–6.
160. Mukai K, et al. Effects of three warm-up regimens of equal distance on VO_2 kinetics during supramaximal exercise in Thoroughbred horses. Equine Vet J Suppl 2010;(38):33–9.
161. Hyyppa S, Poso AR. Fluid, electrolyte, and acid–base responses to exercise in racehorses. Vet Clin North Am Equine Pract 1998;14(1):121–36.
162. Byrd SK, et al. Altered sarcoplasmic reticulum function after high-intensity exercise. J Appl Physiol 1989;67(5): 2072–7.
163. Wilson JA, et al. Sarcoplasmic reticulum responses to repeated sprints are affected by conditioning of horses. J Anim Sci 1998;76(12):3065–71.
164. Harris RC, et al. Effect of freeze-drying on measurements of pH in biopsy samples of the middle gluteal muscle of the horse: comparison of muscle pH to the pyruvate and lactate content. Equine Vet J 1989;21(1):45–7.
165. Xu KY, Becker LC. Ultrastructural localization of glycolytic enzymes on sarcoplasmic reticulum vesticles. J Histochem Cytochem 1998;46(4): 419–27.
166. Xu KY, Zweier JL, Becker LC. Functional coupling between glycolysis and sarcoplasmic reticulum Ca^{2+} transport. Circ Res 1995;77(1):88–97.
167. Lees SJ, Williams JH. Skeletal muscle sarcoplasmic reticulum glycogen status influences Ca^{2+} uptake supported by endogenously synthesized ATP. Am J Physiol Cell Physiol 2004;286(1): C97–104.
168. Harris RC, Dunnett M, Snow DH. Muscle carnosine content is unchanged during maximal intermittent exercise. In: Persson SGB, Lindholm A, Jeffcott LB, editors. Equine exercise physiology 3. Davis: ICEEP Publications; 1991. p. 257–61.
169. Juel C. Lactate–proton cotransport in skeletal muscle. Physiol Rev 1997;77(2): 321–58.
170. Juel C. Muscle pH regulation: role of training. Acta Physiol Scand 1998; 162(3):359–66.
171. Pilegaard H, et al. Effect of high-intensity exercise training on lactate/H^+ transport capacity in human skeletal muscle. Am J Physiol 1999;276(2 Pt 1): E255–61.
172. Dubouchaud H, et al. Endurance training, expression, and physiology of LDH, MCT1, and MCT4 in human skeletal muscle. Am J Physiol Endocrinol Metab 2000;278(4):E571–9.
173. Essén-Gustavsson B, Gottlieb-Vedi M, Lindholm A. Muscle adenine nucleotide degradation during submaximal treadmill exercise to fatigue. Equine Vet J Suppl 1999;30:298–302.
174. Snow DH, Harris RC, Gash SP. Metabolic response of equine muscle to intermittent maximal exercise. J Appl Physiol 1985;58(5):1689–97.
175. McGowan CM, et al. Effects of prolonged training, overtraining and detraining on skeletal muscle metabolites and enzymes. Equine Vet J Suppl 2002(34):257–63.
176. Castejon F, et al. Uric acid responses to endurance racing and relationships with performance, plasma biochemistry and metabolic alterations. Equine Vet J Suppl 2006(36):70–3.
177. Snow DH, et al. Alterations in blood, sweat, urine and muscle composition during prolonged exercise in the horse. Veterinary Record 1982;110(16):377–84.
178. Lucke JN, Hall GN. Further studies on the metabolic effects of long distance riding: Golden Horseshoe Ride 1979. Equine Vet J 1980;12(4):189–92.
179. Hodgson DR, Rose RJ, Allen JR. Muscle glycogen depletion and repletion patterns in horses performing various distances of endurance exercise. In: Snow DH, Persson SGB, Rose RJ, editors. Equine exercise physiology. Cambridge: Granta Editions; 1983. p. 229–36.
180. Jensen-Waern M, et al. The effects of an endurance ride on metabolism and neutrophil function. Equine Vet J Suppl 1999;30:605–9.
181. Farris JW, et al. Effect of tryptophan and of glucose on exercise capacity of horses. J Appl Physiol 1998;85(3):807–16.
182. Langsetmo I, Poole DC. $V(O_2)$ recovery kinetics in the horse following moderate, heavy, and severe exercise. J Appl Physiol 1999;86(4):1170–7.
183. Lovell DK, Rose RJ. Effects of post exercise activity on recovery from maximal exercise. Equine Vet J Suppl 2010;27(18):188–99.
184. Hubbell JA, et al. Cardiorespiratory and metabolic effects of walking, standing, and standing with a splint during the recuperative period from maximal exercise in horses. Am J Vet Res 1997;58(9):1003–9.
185. Marlin DJ, et al. Influence of post-exercise activity on rates of muscle and blood lactate disappearance in the Thoroughbred horse. In: Gillespie JR, Robinson NE, editors. Equine exercise physiology 2. Davis: ICEEP Publications; 1987. p. 321–31.
186. Lacombe VA, et al. Effects of feeding meals with various soluble-carbohydrate

content on muscle glycogen synthesis after exercise in horses. Am J Vet Res 2004;65(7):916–23.

187. Brojer J, et al. Synthesis of proglycogen and macroglycogen in skeletal muscle of Standardbred trotters after intermittent exercise. Equine Vet J Suppl 2006(36):335–9.
188. Snow DH, Harris RC. Effects of daily exercise on muscle glycogen in the Thoroughbred racehorse. In: Persson SGB, Lindholm A, Jeffcott LB, editors. Equine exercise physiology 3. Davis: ICEEP Publications; 1990. p. 299–304.
189. Jose-Cunilleras E, et al. Expression of equine glucose transporter type 4 in skeletal muscle after glycogen-depleting exercise. Am J Vet Res 2005;66(3):379–85.
190. Lacombe VA, et al. Effects of dietary glycaemic response after exercise on blood concentrations of substrates used indirectly for muscle glycogenesis. Equine Vet J Suppl 2006(36):585–9.
191. Lacombe VA, Hinchcliff KW, Devor ST. Effects of exercise and glucose administration on content of insulin-sensitive glucose transporter in equine skeletal muscle. Am J Vet Res 2003;64(12):1500–6.
192. Geor RJ, et al. Route of carbohydrate administration affects early post exercise muscle glycogen storage in horses. Equine Vet J Suppl 2006(36):590–5.
193. McCutcheon LJ, et al. Effects of prior exercise on components of insulin signalling in equine skeletal muscle. Equine Vet J Suppl 2006(36):330–4.
194. Pratt SE, Geor RJ, McCutcheon LJ. Effects of dietary energy source and physical conditioning on insulin sensitivity and glucose tolerance in Standardbred horses. Equine Vet J Suppl 2006(36):579–84.
195. Stewart-Hunt L, Geor RJ, McCutcheon LJ. Effects of short-term training on insulin sensitivity and skeletal muscle glucose metabolism in Standardbred horses. Equine Vet J Suppl 2006(36):226–32.
196. Lacombe VA, Hinchcliff KW, Taylor LE. Interactions of substrate availability, exercise performance, and nutrition with muscle glycogen metabolism in horses. J Am Vet Med Assoc 2003;223(11):1576–85.
197. Straub R, et al. The use of morphometry and enzyme activity measurements in skeletal muscles for the assessment of the working capacity of horses. In: Snow DH, Persson SGB, Rose RJ, editors. Equine exercise physiology. Cambridge: Granta Editions; 1983. p. 193–9.
198. Donovan CM, Brooks GA. Endurance training affects lactate clearance, not lactate production. Am J Physiol 1983;244(1):E83–92.
199. Phillips SM, et al. Increased clearance of lactate after short-term training in men. J Appl Physiol 1995;79(6):1862–9.
200. Rainger JE, et al. Blood lactate disappearance after maximal exercise in trained and detrained horses. Res Vet Sci 1994;57(3):325–31.
201. Roneus N, et al. Plasma lactate response to submaximal and maximal exercise tests with training, and its relationship to performance and muscle characteristics in Standardbred trotters. Equine Vet J 1994;26(2):117–21.
202. Snow DH, Guy PS. The effect of training and detraining on several enzymes in horse skeletal muscle. Arch Int Physiol Biochim 1979;87(1):87–93.
203. Cutmore CM, Snow DH, Newsholme EA. Activities of key enzymes of aerobic and anaerobic metabolism in middle gluteal muscle from trained and untrained horses. Equine Vet J 1985;17(5):354–6.
204. Snow DH, Valberg SJ. Muscle anatomy, physiology, and adaptations to exercise and training. In: Hodgson DR, Rose RJ, editors. The athletic horse: principles and practice of equine sports medicine. Philadelphia. WB Saunders Company; 1994. p. 145–79.
205. Rivero JL, Serrano AL. Skeletal myosin heavy chain composition and carriage training. Equine Vet J Suppl 1999;30:318–23.
206. Gottlieb M, et al. Effects of a draft-loaded interval-training program on skeletal muscle in the horse. J Appl Physiol 1989;67(2):570–7.
207. Serrano AL, Rivero JL. Myosin heavy chain profile of equine gluteus medius muscle following prolonged draught-exercise training and detraining. J Muscle Res Cell Motil 2000;21(3):235–45.
208. Roneus M, et al. Skeletal muscle characteristics in young trained and untrained Standardbred trotters. Equine Vet J 1992;24(4):292–4.
209. Essén-Gustavsson B, Lindholm A. Muscle fibre characteristics of active and inactive Standardbred horses. Equine Vet J 1985;17(6):434–8.
210. Yamano S, et al. Effect of growth and training on muscle adaptation in Thoroughbred horses. Am J Vet Res 2002;63(10):1408–12.
211. Hodgson DR, et al. Effects of training on muscle composition in horses. Am J Vet Res 1986;47(1):12–5.
212. Miyata H, et al. Muscle adaptation of Thoroughbred racehorses trained on a flat or sloped track. Am J Vet Res 1999;60(12):1536–9.
213. Lindholm A, et al. Muscle histochemistry and biochemistry of Thoroughbred horses during growth and training. In: Snow DH, Persson SGB, Rose RJ, editors. Equine exercise physiology. Cambridge: Granta Editions; 1983. p. 211–17.
214. Ronéus M, Essén-Gustavsson B. A field study of circulatory response and muscle characteristics in young Thoroughbreds. In: Gillespie JR, Robinson NE, editors. Equine exercise physiology 2. Davis: ICEEP Publications; 1987. p. 376–83.
215. Hinchcliff KW, et al. High intensity exercise conditioning increases accumulated oxygen deficit of horses. Equine Vet J 2002;34(1):9–16.
216. Eto D, et al. Effect of high intensity training on anaerobic capacity of middle gluteal muscle in Thoroughbred horses. Res Vet Sci 2004;76(2):139–44.
217. Mole PA, Oscai LB, Holloszy JO. Adaptation of muscle to exercise. Increase in levels of palmityl Coa synthetase, carnitine palmityltransferase, and palmityl Coa dehydrogenase, and in the capacity to oxidize fatty acids. J Clin Invest 1971;50(11):2323–30.
218. Gansen S, et al. Effects of conditioning horses with lactate-guided exercise on muscle glycogen content. Equine Vet J Suppl 1999;30:329–31.
219. Foreman JH, et al. Muscle responses of thoroughbreds to conventional race training and detraining. Am J Vet Res 1990;51(6):909–13.
220. McCutcheon LJ, Geor RJ, Hinchcliff KW. Changes in skeletal muscle GLUT4 content and muscle membrane glucose transport following 6 weeks of exercise training. Equine Vet J Suppl 2002(34):199–204.
221. Essén-Gustavsson B, et al. Muscular adaptation of horses during intensive training and detraining. Equine Vet J 1989;21(1):27–33.
222. Hoppeler H. [Morphology of human skeletal muscle and its adaptability to different training conditions]. Sportverletz Sportschaden 1987;1(2):71–5.
223. Geor RJ, McCutcheon LJ, Shen H. Muscular and metabolic responses to moderate-intensity short-term training. Equine Vet J Suppl 1999;30:311–17.
224. Fox G, et al. Skeletal muscle buffer capacity changes in Standardbred horses: effects of growth and training. In: Gillespie JR, Robinson NE, editors. Equine exercise physiology 2. Davis: ICEEP Publications; 1987. p. 341–7.
225. Sinha AK, Ray SP, Rose RJ. Effect of training intensity and detraining on adaptations in different skeletal muscles. In: Persson SGB, Lindholm A, Jeffcott LB, editors. Equine exercise physiology 3. Davis: ICEEP Publications; 1991. p. 223–30.
226. Eaton MD, et al. Effects of low- and moderate-intensity training on metabolic responses to exercise in thoroughbreds. Equine Vet J Suppl 1999;30:521–7.

227. Knight PK, Sinha AK, Rose RJ. Effects of training intensity on maximum oxygen uptake. In: Persson SGB, Lindholm A, Jeffcott LB, editors. Equine exercise physiology 3. Davis: ICEEP Publications; 1991. p. 77–82.
228. Tyler CM, et al. Changes in maximum oxygen uptake during prolonged training, overtraining, and detraining in horses. J Appl Physiol 1996;81(5):2244–9.
229. Boutilier RG, St-Pierre J. Surviving hypoxia without really dying. Comp Biochem Physiol A Mol Integr Physiol 2000;126(4):481–90.
230. Butler PJ, et al. The effect of cessation of training on cardiorespiratory variables during exercise. In: Persson SGB, Lindholm A, Jeffcott LB, editors. Equine exercise physiology 3. Davis: ICEEP Publications; 1991. p. 71–6.
231. Robb J, et al. Chemical composition and energy value of the body, fatty acid composition of adipose tissue, and liver and kidney size in the horse. Anim Prod 1972;14(01):25–34.
232. Dybdal NO, et al. Alterations in plasma corticosteroids, insulin and selected metabolites in horses used in endurance rides. Equine Vet J 1980;12(3):137–40.
233. Desmecht D, et al. Relationship of plasma lactate production to cortisol release following completion of different types of sporting events in horses. Vet Res Commun 1996;20(4):371–9.
234. Evans DL, Priddle TL, Davie AJ. Plasma lactate and uric acid responses to racing in pacing Standardbreds and relationships with performance. Equine Vet J Suppl 2002(34): 131–4.
235. Harris P, Snow DH. The effects of high intensity exercise on the plasma concentration of lactate, potassium and other electrolytes. Equine Vet J 1988;20(2):109–13.
236. Keenan DM. Changes of blood metabolites in horses after racing, with particular reference to uric acid. Aust Vet J 1979;55:54–7.
237. Kelso TB, et al. Bicarbonate administration and muscle metabolism during high-intensity exercise. In: Gillespie JR, Robinson NE, editors. Equine exercise physiology 2. Davis: ICEEP Publications; 1987. p. 438–47.
238. White SL, et al. Heart rate response and plasma lactate concentrations of horses competing in the speed and endurance phase of 3-day combined training events. Equine Vet J Suppl 1995(20):52–6.
239. Art T, et al. Effect of show jumping on heart rate, blood lactate and other plasma biochemical values. Equine Vet J Suppl 1990(9):78–82.
240. Mueller PJ, et al. Effect of increasing work rate on metabolic responses of the donkey (*Equus asinus*). J Appl Physiol 1994;77(3):1431–8.

Endocrine function during exercise and response to training

34

Johannes H. van der Kolk

CHAPTER CONTENTS

Introduction

Exercise is a stress situation that challenges homeostasis for which the body must find a new dynamic equilibrium. This dynamic process requires, among other things, adaptive responses of the hormonal systems.[1] For instance, the neuroendocrine reflex arch is characterized mainly by the activation of the hypothalamic-pituitary-adrenocortical (HPA) axis, whereas the autonomic branch consists of the activation of the hypothalamic–sympathetic–adrenomedullary axis. Interestingly, both the neuroendocrine and the autonomic efferent arcs of the generalized stress response converge on the adrenal glands, albeit on different timescales and with different final endpoints: the autonomic response occurs rapidly, triggered by sympathetic neural outputs that stimulate the secretion of adrenomedullary catecholamines (like adrenaline), and the neuroendocrine response occurs on a slower timescale, triggered by hypothalamic–pituitary hormone output and resulting in adrenocortical glucocorticoid secretion.[2,3] This response, in turn, stimulates other endocrine glands to secrete hormones that potentiate fuel mobilization and regulate water and electrolyte concentrations. As duration of exercise increases, nutrient and ion (electrolyte) concentrations also influence hormonal responses.[4] The study of exercise-associated hormonal alterations is of growing interest because of the implications for adaptation, performance, welfare and health. Interpretation of results, however, is difficult because of the numerous factors that affect plasma hormone concentrations. Changes in plasma volume and/or hormone clearance rate, as well as the influence of timing and method of blood sampling and analysis must be considered when evaluating endocrine responses to exercise. Other factors that must be considered are the design of exercise protocols, and various characteristics of the horses studied.[4]

Physical activity plays an important role in tissue anabolism, growth and development, but the mechanisms that link patterns of exercise with tissue anabolism are not completely understood. One of the unique features of exercise is that it leads to a simultaneous increase of antagonistic mediators. For instance, on the one hand, exercise stimulates anabolic components of the growth hormone (GH)-insulin-like growth factor-I (IGF-I) axis, but, on the other hand, exercise is also associated with an increase in catabolic pro-inflammatory cytokines. This emphasizes the importance of optimal adaptation to exercise. The very fine balance between the anabolic and inflammatory/catabolic response to exercise will determine the effectiveness of exercise training and the health consequences of exercise.[5] The effectiveness of physical training depends on the training load and on the individual ability to tolerate it, and an imbalance between the overall strain experienced during exercise and the athlete's tolerance of such effort may induce overreaching/overtraining syndrome[5,6] or undertraining.[5] In addition, the stress of exercise might inhibit the gonadal function especially concerning the female human athlete that many authors describe as the so-called 'exercise-related female reproductive dysfunction'.[1] In comparison, moderate exercise (six days/week) in mares suppressed peak LH concentrations, decreased the number of follicles sized 6–20 mm, and lengthened the interovulatory interval,[7] whereas repeated strenuous exercise in stallions induced negative influences on semen quality.[8]

Growth hormone

Major actions of growth hormone

Phylogenetically, GH is an ancestral hormone that has been identified in the pituitary of primitive vertebrates.[9] In addition, signal transducers and activators of transcription (STAT) 5, a principal intracellular mediator of GH signaling, exhibits a very high degree of homology between invertebrate and prevertebrate species, reflecting the ancient nature of the GH/STAT signaling system.[10] Intriguingly, it also appears that insulin-like peptides, such as IGF-I and proinsulin, are much older than both the pancreas and insulin.[11] In line with this phylogenetic hierarchy, GH, together with prolactin and human placental lactogen, stimulates β-cell proliferation, insulin gene expression, and insulin biosynthesis and secretion.[12]

GH may be viewed as the primary anabolic hormone during stress and fasting. During fasting, GH contributes to the switch from carbohydrate utilization to lipolysis and lipid oxidation.[13] GH exerts anabolic effects directly as well as indirectly by stimulation of hepatic IGF-I production. When subjects are well nourished, the GH-induced stimulation of IGF-I and insulin are important for anabolic processes. The most prominent metabolic effect of GH is a marked increase in lipolysis and concurrent FFA concentrations. GH is a counter-regulatory hormone that antagonizes the hepatic and peripheral effects of insulin on glucose metabolism via mechanisms involving the concomitant increase in FFA flux and uptake. The ability of GH to induce insulin resistance (IR) is significant for the defense against hypoglycemia, for the development of 'stress' diabetes during fasting and inflammatory illness, and perhaps for the 'dawn' phenomenon (the increase in insulin requirements in the early morning hours).[13]

Regulation of GH secretion

GH is a protein hormone secreted by the anterior pituitary gland in a pulsatile fashion under the regulation of two hypothalamic peptides: GH-releasing hormone (GHRH) stimulates GH synthesis and secretion while somatostatin inhibits GH release. Whereas GHRH is required for the initiation of GH pulses, the amplitude of GH pulses is modulated by somatostatin, resulting in a pattern of volleys of GH-secretory pulses with intervening periods of relative secretory quiescence. The amplitude and frequency of GH-secretory pulses are regulated by a complex array of external and internal stimuli[14,15] with exercise and sleep being robust physiological stimulators of GH secretion.[16,17] As a protein hormone, GH is rather species specific, is not lipophylic, and binds to a specific cell membrane receptor.

In the normal human population, a gradual and progressive fall in spontaneous GH (and associated IGF-I) secretion occurs with increasing age; this age-associated decrease in GH secretion is termed 'the somatopause'. It remains to be determined whether this fall in GH secretion is an important physiological safety event of the normal aging process by preventing relative GH excess, or whether it marks the development of GH deficiency which would benefit from GH replacement.[16] In comparison, chronic recombinant equine GH administration (up to 12.5 mg/d SC for 43 days) did not affect body weight or muscle mass dimensions in geriatric horses.[18]

Effects of exercise and training on secretion and circulating GH concentrations

The development of computerized algorithms to quantify episodic GH release has offered new insights into the pathophysiological regulation of GH secretion in humans[19,20] and horses.[20b] So-called pulse detection algorithms and deconvolution analysis were developed to aid in the unraveling of GH release dynamics. A pulse detection program[19] was designed to describe concentration peaks in a data series. However, it does not provide information on the two events that together determine the concentration peak: namely, hormonal secretion and clearance. Deconvolution analysis will render a quantitative description of GH secretory and clearance dynamics for the number, amplitude, duration, and temporal locations of all significant underlying secretory bursts and the half-life of endogenous GH disappearance.[21] In order to use deconvolution analysis with sufficient accuracy, it is of importance to fulfill the following criteria necessary to obtain a valid GH concentration curve:[22]

1. a sensitive GH assay with a known precision of low, middle, and high hormone concentrations
2. a long enough sampling period during which pulses can be detected
3. optimally, the sample frequency should be approximately 0.25 times the hormone half-life.

In order to meet the last criterion, the disappearance half-life of the hormone should be known.[21] Mean endogenous and exogenous

GH half-life in yearling Standardbred geldings has been estimated at 18 and 26 min, respectively, associated with a mean endogenous basal secretion of 0.012 ± 0.014 μg/L/min.[23]

There is some evidence in horses that a single bout of exercise causes an increase in plasma GH concentration[24,25,26,27,28] although the majority of these studies used heterologous GH assays. In a report based on a homologous GH assay, maximal treadmill exercise (comprising 2 min intervals at 30, 50, and 70% VO_{2max} then to fatigue at 100% VO_{2max}) in Standardbred geldings increased plasma GH transiently from 0.51 ± 0.076 to 8.43 ± 3.36 μg/L with normal secretion restored within 24 h.[27]

In contrast, nocturnal GH pulsatility was not affected by 18 weeks of moderate-intensity training in young Standardbreds preceded by 4 weeks of acclimatization to exercise, as determined by deconvolution analysis.[29] On the other hand, overtraining in young Standardbreds following 24 weeks of moderate-intensity training was associated with an increase in concentration peak number (3.6 versus 2.0), a smaller peak secretion pattern with a prolonged GH half-life (15.2 versus 7.3 min), and an increased irregularity of nocturnal GH pulsatility pattern (as reflected by approximate entropy 0.89 versus 0.49) compared to control horses. As mentioned before, the amplitude of GH pulses is modulated by somatostatin resulting in a pattern of volleys of GH-secretory pulses with intervening periods of relative secretory quiescence. The observed absence of relative secretory quiescence suggests (relative) somatostatin deficiency. Four weeks of detraining did not lead to full recovery of the nocturnal GH pulsatility pattern (see Fig. 34.1). However, as basal GH secretion was not affected[20b] the presence of absolute GH deficiency is unlikely in overtrained horses. The fact that GH administration did not change aerobic capacity in young Standardbreds in exercise training also does not support the presence of absolute GH deficiency.[30a]

In horses at rest, mean IGF-I concentration was 34.2 ± 13.6 nmol/L. In post-race samples (Thoroughbreds and Standardbreds mixed without specified racing conditions), IGF-I mean concentration was 24.5 ± 13.1 nmol/L, indicating that exercise does not affect plasma IGF-I concentration.[30b]

Actions of growth hormone during exercise

Based on computerized algorithms it has been shown that there is a linear relationship between the magnitude of the acute increase in GH release and exercise intensity in human athletes.[31] GH and its primary downstream mediator, IGF-I, play a critical role in formation, maintenance, and regeneration of skeletal muscles[31,32,33,34] although it is not anabolic toward the contractile (i.e. myofibrillar) muscle tissue in healthy humans.[35] However, it remains to be clarified whether skeletal muscle hypertrophy after exercise is stimulated primarily by endocrine or paracrine/autocrine IGF-I.[32]

Glucose tolerance

The maintenance of normal blood glucose concentrations at rest and during exercise is critical and depends on the coordination and integration of several physiological systems, including the sympathetic nervous system and the endocrine system.[36] Besides being the most important energy substrate for the central nervous system, glucose has a very important role in providing energy for muscular contraction. In horses, muscle glycogen, and to a lesser extent plasma glucose, are utilized in substantial amounts during low-, moderate- and high-intensity exercise because of stimulation of hepatic glycogenolysis, due to sympathoadrenergic mechanisms operating directly via hepatic sympathetic innervation or indirectly via circulating adrenaline[37,38] (see also Chapter 33). Although carbohydrate availability to skeletal muscle affects maximal exercise performance in humans, this relationship is not very well described in horses.[39]

Glucose utilization and production are regulated in part by insulin.[40] Glucose tolerance has been long studied in the equine species.[41] During an oral glucose tolerance test (OGTT), the normal response to the absorption of the carbohydrate load is both to suppress hepatic glucose output and to enhance glucose uptake in muscle and liver. This requires a prompt increase in insulin secretion as well as adequate hepatic and muscle sensitivity to insulin. In particular, impaired fasting glycemia (or failure of plasma glucose concentration to decrease in response to fasting) is associated with decreased peripheral insulin sensitivity (IS), most importantly at the level of skeletal muscle (being the main site of glucose disposal). In human medicine, neither impaired glucose tolerance nor impaired fasting glycemia are considered clinical entities in their own right; rather they are risk factors for diabetes mellitus and represent metabolic states intermediate between normal glucose homeostasis and diabetic hyperglycemia.[40] It is worth stressing that impaired glucose tolerance and impaired fasting glycemia are not interchangeable and that they represent metabolically distinct abnormalities with a different prevalence in humans.[42a,42b,43]

Impaired fasting glycemia has also been associated with decreased peripheral IS in the equine species (5.9 ± 1.4 in PPID and 4.9 ± 0.3 mmol/L in controls).[44] The OGTT reflects the efficiency of the body to dispose of glucose after an oral glucose load. Thus, the OGTT provides useful information about glucose tolerance, but not insulin sensitivity/resistance per se.[43]

Insulin

Major actions of insulin

Insulin is a peptide hormone essential for appropriate tissue development, growth, and maintenance of whole-body glucose homeostasis by regulating carbohydrate, lipid and protein metabolism.[45] It suppresses hepatic glucose and triglyceride production, inhibits adipose tissue lipolysis and whole-body and muscle proteolysis, and stimulates glucose uptake in muscle.[45] These effects of insulin serve to promote the synthesis of carbohydrate, fat and protein; therefore, insulin is considered to be an anabolic hormone.[46] As a protein hormone, insulin is rather species specific, is not lipophylic, and binds to a specific cell membrane receptor (see Fig. 34.2).

Regulation of insulin secretion

Insulin is secreted by the β-cells of the pancreatic islets of Langerhans predominantly in response to increased circulating levels of glucose and amino acids.[46,47] The early insulin response in horses was similar to that reported in other species, both during an IV glucose challenge[49] and a standardized exercise test.[50]

Effects of exercise and training on secretion and circulating insulin concentrations

A decline in plasma insulin is important for the rise in glucose production during exercise in a variety of species. In horses, as in humans and other species, there is suppression of insulin secretion during exercise. This suppression appears to have a threshold of 50% of VO_{2max}.[51] β-blockade (propranolol at 0.22 mg/kg BW IV) lowered the exercise-associated plasma insulin levels during

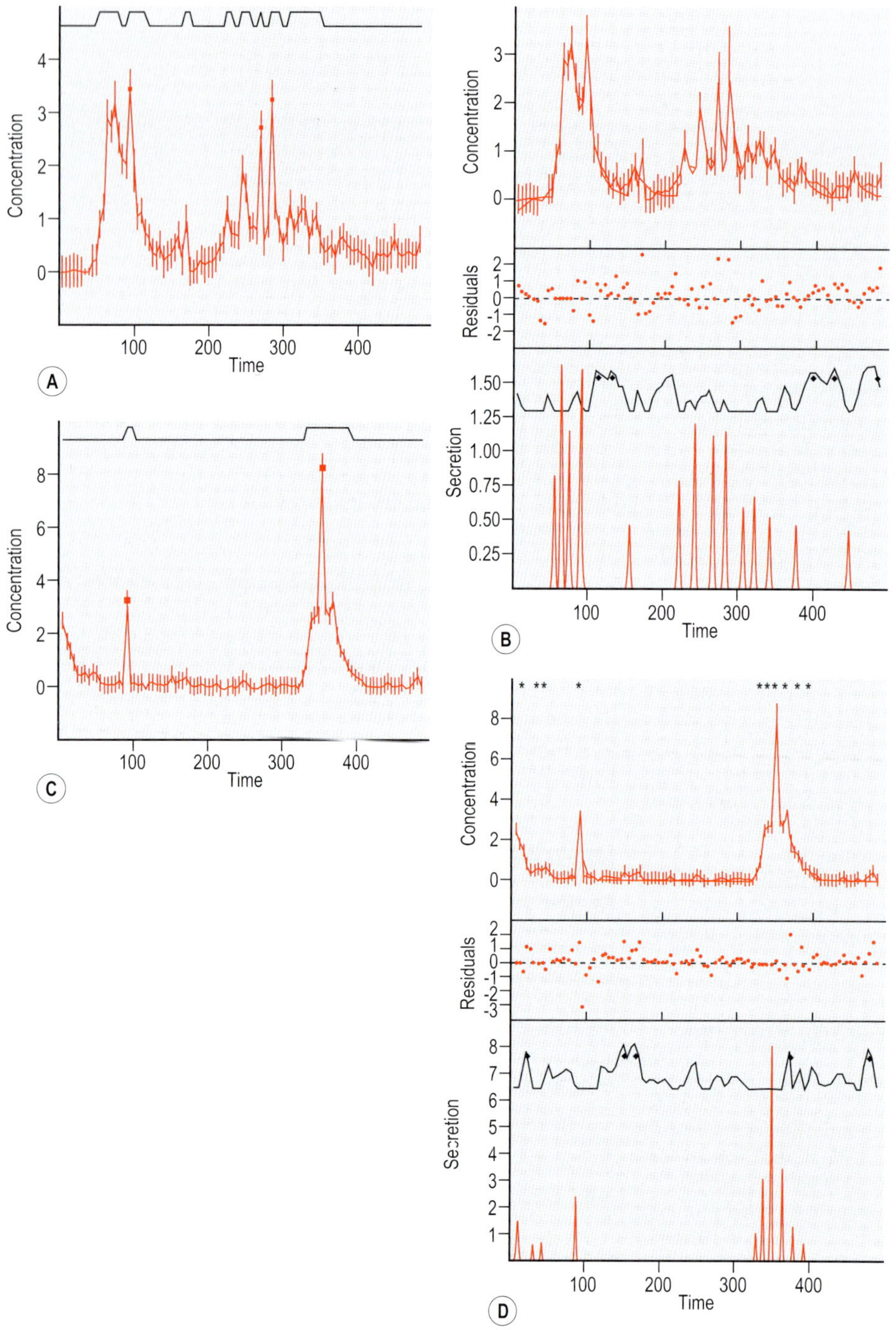

Fig 34.1 Growth hormone data series (based on plasma samples taken at 5-min intervals for eight hours from 22:00 until 06:00) analyzed with a pulse detection program called Cluster 8 as a discrete peak-detection method not based on deconvolution analysis: **(A)** Analysis revealed eight peaks, seven nadirs and three probable outliers as shown by the black line in upper part of graph. A pulse analysis algorithm based on deconvolution analysis called Autodecon was used to provide crucial information about secretion-event burst mass, elimination half-lives, and basal secretion. **(B)** The upper panel shows the growth hormone concentration curve and the lower panel the calculated growth hormone secretion curve depicted as bursts for an overtrained horse four weeks after detraining. In comparison, results with Cluster 8 **(C)** and Autodecon **(D)** in a control horse four weeks after detraining. Cluster 8 revealed two peaks, two nadirs, and two probable outliers in the control horse (y-axis, GH concentration in μg/L; x-axis, time in minutes).

Pulse_XP, Pulse Analysis Software, University of Virginia, Charlottesville, VA, USA.

consecutive 30-min bouts of low and moderate exercise in mixed-breed, conditioned horses compared to no change over time without treatment.[38] In other reports, plasma insulin concentrations decreased by 35% following an incremental exercise test in untrained Standardbred mares[52] and in horses competing in a 160 km endurance ride.[53] Although decreased blood glucose concentrations did not occur in all horses following an 80 km endurance ride, insulin concentrations also fell in all horses examined associated with increased plasma concentrations of both adrenaline and noradrenaline post ride.[54] However, rather than studying the

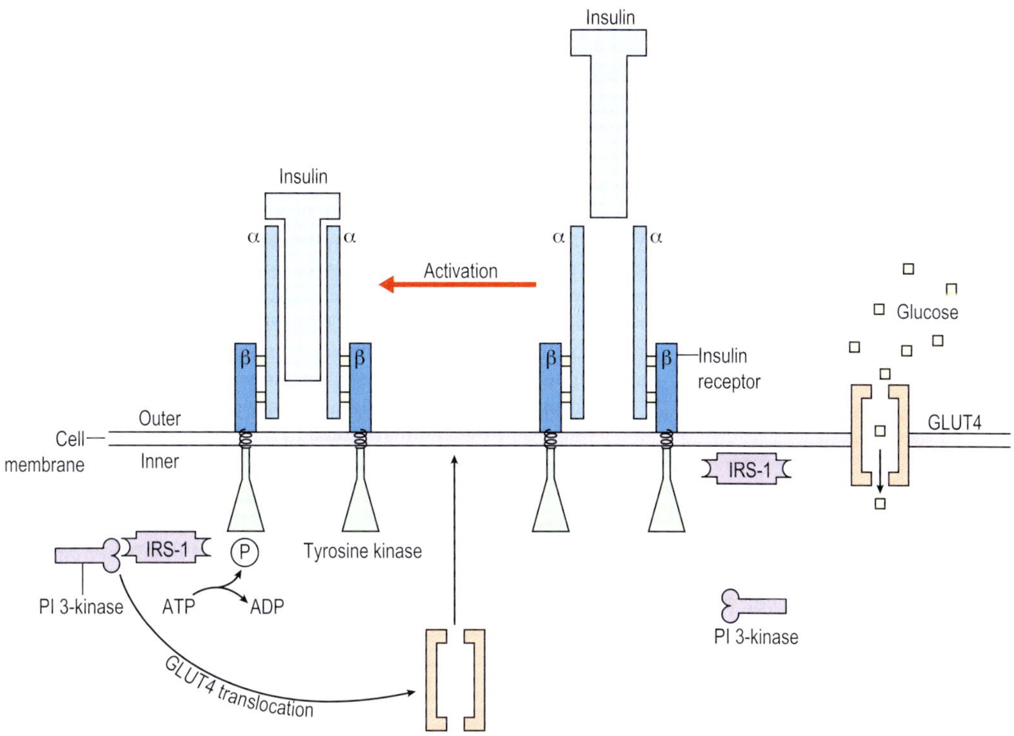

Fig 34.2 Insulin binding to its receptor activates a tyrosine kinase that initiates a cascade of signaling events, the initial step being the tyrosine phosphorylation of insulin receptor substrate 1 (IRS-1). The activation of phosphatidylinositiol 3-kinase (PI 3-kinase) ultimately leads to the translocation of GLUT4.

relationship between exercise or training and plasma insulin concentration it is more appropriate to assess effects on IS itself.

Actions during exercise and training

During prolonged exercise, increased demand for glucose by contracting muscle is in part met by an increase in glucose transport into muscle via glucose transporter-4 (GLUT4) proteins.[55] Both insulin and muscle contraction increase the translocation of GLUT4 from intracellular sites to the plasma membrane (see Fig. 34.2) and transverse tubules, albeit by activation of different signaling pathways. This perhaps explains why in humans with IR, an acute bout of exercise but not insulin results in increased muscle glucose uptake.[55,56] Furthermore, muscle contractions not only stimulate muscle glucose uptake independent of insulin but also increase IS. The contraction signaling pathway does not increase insulin receptor kinase or PI 3-kinase activity. However, the possibility that two distinct GLUT4 pools may be targeted, one by insulin and the other by contractions, cannot be excluded.[57] Unlike insulin-stimulated glucose transport, in which permeability is reversed rapidly upon removal of the insulin, the increase in membrane permeability following contractile activity can persist for many hours in human athletes.[56]

Similarly to other species, the equine GLUT4 cDNA encodes 509 amino acids. The calculated molecular weight of the resulting protein is 54.8 kDa.[39] In equine skeletal muscle, GLUT4 is expressed in a fiber type selective manner predominantly expressed in the cytosol of fast-type 2B as shown in vastus lateralis fibers of Warmblood horses.[58] GLUT4 translocation in semitendinosus muscle of Shetland ponies is insulin-dependent as has been described in other species,[59] although active cell-surface GLUT4 protein content might not have been assessed optimally in this study, possibly explaining the reported poor responsiveness to insulin.[60]

The effects of exercise training on skeletal muscle GLUT4 content are similar to those found in other mammals and man. Prolonged, submaximal exercise[61,62] and short periods of strenuous training[39,63] increased skeletal muscle GLUT4 protein and mRNA content in horses, but single bouts of intense exercise had no significant effect on equine skeletal muscle GLUT4 protein[61,64] and mRNA expression.[65]

Insulin resistance selectively decreased active basal cell-surface GLUT4 in equine semimembranosus muscle, without altering total GLUT4 content and further enhancement of cell-surface GLUTs after in vitro insulin stimulation. The observed lack of substantial increase in insulin-stimulated GLUT4 translocation in healthy insulin-sensitive horses may be the result of the insulin-dependent signaling pathways regulating GLUTs already being at near maximal physiologic limits for the species.[60] In addition, a single bout of moderate-intensity exercise in Standardbred horses increased the glucose disposal under hyperinsulinemic conditions (5.6 ± 1.1 versus 3.3 ± 0.9 mg/kg BW/min in controls) without enhanced non-insulin-mediated glucose uptake post-exercise[66] perhaps suggesting that the insulin-stimulated glucose transport by far exceeds the increase in membrane permeability following contractile activity.

Insulin sensitivity and resistance

Insulin has concentration-dependent saturable actions to increase whole-body glucose disposal. The maximal effect of insulin defines 'insulin responsiveness', whereas the insulin concentration required for a half-maximal response defines 'insulin sensitivity'.[42a] IS is the reciprocal of IR.[40] IR is associated with defective signal

are mediated by specific receptors (e.g. androgen receptors (AR) and glucocorticoid receptors (GR)) located in the cytosol of target cells that regulate the transcription of deoxyribonucleic acid.[96,97,98] The identification of steroid receptors on the membrane of cells provides a new viewpoint for understanding the biological effects of steroid hormones.[96,99] Similar to basal testosterone secretion, there does appear to be a loading threshold before acute exercise-induced changes in androgen receptor content may occur.[100,101] The specificity of the AR and GR responses to exercise and training is likely to support the biological effects at target tissue, by activating those signaling processes that contribute to the long-term steroid actions (i.e. gene transcription).[99]

Testosterone

Testosterone, a primary anabolic hormone (anabolic steroid), increases protein synthesis and decreases protein degradation.[100] In males, the steroid sex hormone testosterone is produced by Leydig cells, situated in the testicular interstitium. The Leydig cells produce testosterone in response to hormonal stimulation by the pituitary gonadotropin luteinizing hormone (LH).[102] Interestingly, it has been shown in rats that testosterone secretion is also regulated by a direct inhibitory neural connection between the brain and testes independently of the pituitary. This neurocircuitry is activated via β-receptors in the paraventricular nucleus of the hypothalamus.[103,104,105,106,107]

Effects of exercise and training on secretion and circulating testosterone concentrations

It has been reported that plasma testosterone concentrations were not significantly different between young Standardbreds with a tentative diagnosis of maladaptation to training (based on an abnormal weight loss during their first months of training only) and controls.[108] On the other hand, no controlled studies on horses yet exist to show whether anabolic steroids improve physical performance in comparison with that of similarly trained control horses, and at least three studies demonstrate that anabolic steroids offer no beneficial effect on exercise performance.[109,110,111,112]

Actions during exercise/training

Although anabolic steroid treatment increased the rate of muscle glycogen repletion after exercise,[111] it also caused delayed closure of epiphyseal growth plates in Standardbreds advocating against use of anabolic steroids in equine medicine.[113] Recent studies in untrained men have indicated that physiological increases in hormones (GH, IGF-I, cortisol, and testosterone) do not necessarily enhance protein metabolism, muscle growth or strength.[114,115,116,117] As a consequence, it appears that anabolic hormones may have a permissive (i.e. need to be present) rather than primary effect on improving muscle form and function in human subjects during physical conditioning.

The hypothalamic–pituitary–adrenocortical axis and cortisol

Major actions of cortisol

The primary role of cortisol (a primary catabolic hormone) as a glucocorticoid is to stimulate gluconeogenesis and glycogenolysis via glycogen, protein and lipid metabolism and through its permissive actions on other hormones (e.g. catecholamines and glucagon).[99] Although glucocorticoids increase lipolysis via an increase in hormone-sensitive lipase expression in adipose tissue, they clearly have antilipolytic effects regarding adipocytes. In rats, it has been show that glucocorticoids have both lipolytic and antilipolytic effects within adipocytes, depending on the dose and duration of exposure, although the mechanism by which these metabolic effects occur are still unclear.[118]

Regulation of cortisol secretion

Cortisol production is situated in the adrenal cortex (see Fig. 34.3). The production of cortisol by the adrenal gland is induced by ACTH. The first 25 amino acids of ACTH are rigorously conserved between species.[119] At rest and during some perturbations, AVP is the immediate stimulus for ACTH release. Even ACTH micropulses, previously thought to occur spontaneously, appear to be regulated by AVP in horses. Cortisol had a significant negative feedback effect on

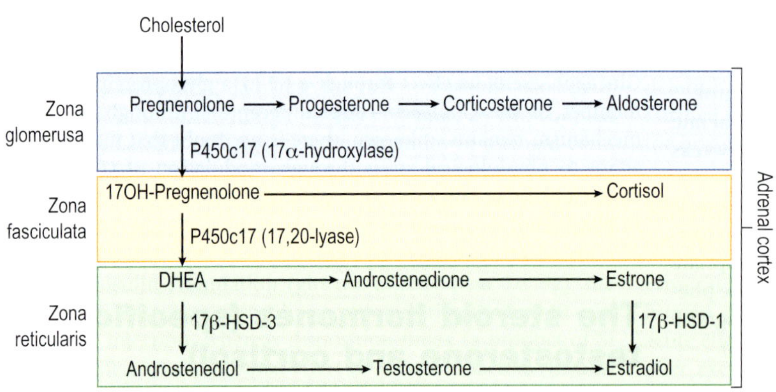

Fig 34.3 Cortisol synthesis occurs in the adrenal cortex. Qualitative regulation, which determines the type of steroid produced in a cell, is principally at the level of P450c17 (CYP17). In the absence of P450c17 in the zona glomerulosa of the adrenal gland, C21 deoxy steroids are produced, leading to the synthesis of the mineralocorticoid aldosterone. In the presence of the 17α-hydroxylase but not the 17,20-lyase activity of P450c17 in the zona fasciculata, C21, 17-hydroxy steroids are produced, leading to the glucocorticoid cortisol. When both the 17α-hydroxylase and 17,20-lyase activities of P450c17 are present in the zona reticularis, the androgen precursor DHEA is produced (see also Miller[187]).

basal ACTH secretion by equine anterior pituitary cells in vitro at 30 min after the start of cortisol perfusion. Also in vitro, cortisol can differentially affect the response of the pituitary gland to CRH and arginine vasopressin (AVP). The significant inhibitory effect of cortisol on stimulated ACTH secretion was more apparent when CRH was the secretagogue than when AVP was the secretagogue.[120] On the other hand, CRH secretion and pituitary responsiveness to CRH rise when cortisol falls, suggesting that a major role for CRH is to fix the cortisol setpoint.[121] However, the ACTH pulse frequency was unchanged, raising the possibility that glucocorticoids may have a greater effect on pulse amplitude than on pulse frequency.[122] Furthermore, a circadian cortisol rhythm exists also in horses and this rhythm can be obliterated by the minor perturbation of removing the horse from its accustomed environment. By contrast, the rhythm occurs in trained Standardbreds, suggesting either that they have adapted to their environment, thereby allowing an endogenous rhythm to emerge, or that the rhythm is entrained by their daily routine. These observations highlight the difficulties in determining the cortisol status of a horse, since measurements will be affected by time of day, the occurrence of short-term fluctuations, and how accustomed the horse is to its environment.[123]

Effects of exercise and training on secretion and circulating cortisol concentrations

There is robust evidence in horses that a single or repeated bout of exercise causes an increase in plasma cortisol[123,124,125,126,127,128,129] with the exception of old Standardbred mares,[130] whereas younger horses show higher concentrations after exercise than older horses.[127] Maximum ACTH concentrations were recorded at the end of exercise in Hanoverian horses trained for 20 weeks when they had to canter for 20 min at 450 m/min at 3% inclination, and maximum cortisol concentrations were recorded 20–30 min later.[129] Plasma ACTH and cortisol concentrations increased as function of the intensity and duration of exercise, with rapid increases during cantering.[129,131] In contrast, the plasma ACTH response during exercise was more sensitive to the intensity of exercise than that of cortisol in Thoroughbreds undergoing an incremental exercise test with the plasma cortisol response associated with the duration of exercise.[128] Post-exercise cortisol concentrations have been reported to decline faster toward resting values after training.[132] In contrast, no difference in the post-exercise concentrations was found between trained and untrained horses even after 20 weeks of training.[129]

The use of measurements of basal cortisol concentrations in resting horses are of no use in the diagnosis of over-training syndrome in Standardbred horses.[133] Moreover, adrenocortical insufficiency is not evident in overtrained Standardbreds.[133,134] Interestingly, stimulation of cortisol production by an IV bolus injection of 250 μg of ACTH resulted in lower net plasma cortisol concentrations at 30 min after exercise in 24 weeks, trained (57.0 ± 3.2 ng/mL) horses than in untrained (73.9 ± 3.0 ng/mL) Hanoverian geldings. There was also a significant difference in the net increase of plasma cortisol concentrations between trained and untrained horses following a standardized exercise treadmill test with values in trained horses being lower. As there was no overlap between the highest value in net plasma cortisol concentrations of trained horses and the respective lowest value in the group of untrained horses at 30 min after exercise, discrimination between trained horses (receiving additional endurance training) and horses that are only trained for dressage and jumping is possible.[129]

The cortisol net response (the mean value of two samples taken before exercise subtracted from exercise value) to a standardized exercise test (carried out four times) was highly repeatable (r = 0.75) within individuals, nicely illustrating an individual response.[129] In addition, plasma cortisol concentration also increased (by 79%) following cross-country jumping,[135] swimming,[136] and in horses competing in a 56 km,[137] 80 km[54] or 160 km endurance rides.[52] Overall, the degree of exercise-induced hypercortisolemia was related to both the intensity and the duration of exercise for various sporting events, but the endurance ride induced the most and show-jumping the least serious post-exercise changes in plasma cortisol concentration.[137,138] Significant elevations in jugular cortisol (1.6 times) and AVP (4.9 times) concentrations were observed as compared with pre-exercise values in contrast with jugular CRH concentrations immediately after a single bout of light-intensity exercise in trained Standardbreds. Similarly, there was an immediate and dramatic rise in ACTH and AVP secretion during exercise which peaked during galloping with 24-fold for ACTH and 52-fold for AVP in pituitary venous effluent compared to peripheral jugular concentrations.

Acute exercise caused a transient increase in ACTH secretion, which occurs synchronously with an increase in AVP secretion. CRF does not appear to play a major role in mediating the initial ACTH response to exercise.[139] Furthermore, competition induced a significant increase in cortisol and ACTH responses in both jumping and dressage horses. This effect was more apparent in dressage horses. When horses were most experienced (not specified), cortisol and ACTH responses were much lower. Jumping horses displayed higher baseline cortisol concentrations, whereas dressage horses showed lower baseline cortisol concentrations. Both showjumping and dressage horses showed lower basal ACTH plasma concentrations compared to control horses.[140] Plasma cortisol concentrations were not affected by moderate-intensity training on a high-speed treadmill during 20 weeks in Hanoverian geldings,[129] 24 weeks in Standardbred geldings[29] or 34 weeks in Standardbreds.[133]

In addition, it has been shown that a 56 km endurance ride triggers a large increase (6 times) in the adrenal secretion rate of cortisol, which is not accurately reflected by the more limited increase (2–3 times) in plasma cortisol concentration and as a consequence the actual measurement of plasma cortisol clearance is needed for accurate assessment of adrenal gland function during exercise.[137]

Actions of cortisol during exercise

Testosterone is a primary anabolic hormone, whereas cortisol is a primary catabolic hormone regarding protein metabolism. The net result might be an increase, decrease or maintenance in muscle fiber and whole muscle size, especially with resistance training.[141,142,143,144] The force-generating capacity of muscle is related to its cross-sectional area, so it is generally agreed that testosterone and cortisol contribute to the expression of human performance by regulating longer-term (i.e. weeks to months) changes in skeletal muscle size.[99,145] In addition, these steroids also induce neural modifications.[99] In animals, the most recognized effect of testosterone and cortisol lies in the remodeling of skeletal muscle protein, leading to rapidly modulating Ca^{2+} influx and Na^+-K^+pump activity, especially in type II muscle fibers.[146,147,148] It is also clear that the effects of steroid hormones are dose dependent. However, the exact contribution of these steroid hormones to the training process remains unclear because most studies have not taken accurate measurements of muscle size (e.g. muscle fiber cross-sectional area) and neural activity (e.g. electromyography as by Wijnberg[149]).

The dual steroid response

The steroid hormones (specifically testosterone and cortisol) are recognized as important mediators for improving the morphological (e.g. muscle size) and/or functional (e.g. strength, power) qualities of the neuromuscular system. To date, little research has addressed the concept of dual steroid effects, namely the short-term effects of testosterone and cortisol on the neuromuscular system and the dose-response training role of these hormones with the second tier being a possible moderator of human movement during exercise.[99]

The dual steroid response has been well described in horses in two acute studies only. In stallions, plasma testosterone (1.5–2.8 times) and cortisol (1.4 times) increased significantly following repeated strenuous exercise (around the anaerobic threshold of plasma lactate) on a high-speed treadmill.[8] Comparable effects were found in Standardbred geldings following a maximal exercise test. Maximal exercise disrupted basal plasma concentration of testosterone for 26–32 h post-exercise, thereby reflecting the minimum recovery period required before evaluation of the resting concentrations of various hormones in horses undergoing strenuous exercise.[27]

Of interest, a recent human study addressed the prospect of prescribing training based on individual hormonal response patterns.[150] The prescription of resistance exercise and training programs based on individual hormonal data is a novel area for further research in horses.

β-endorphin

The proopiomelanocortin (POMC) gene was most likely derived from an ancestral opioid-coding gene following the 1R chordate genome duplication event. During the radiation of the jawless fish, the POMC organization plan emerged multiple melanocortin sequences (α-MSH/ACTH and β-MSH) and a C-terminally extended opioid sequence (β-endorphin). POMC is synthesized in the pituitary gland and in neurons of the hypothalamus, where an array of post-translational processing mechanisms, such as endoproteolytic cleavage and N-acetylation, generate distinct sets of end products in these tissues.[119]

Acute maximal graded exercise on a high-speed treadmill elevated plasma β-endorphin concentration in unfit Standardbred mares.[130] However, there was a large variation in the β-endorphin response of horses that underwent a standardized strenuous treadmill exercise test. The increase in β-endorphin was correlated significantly and inversely with the treadmill velocity at which maximal oxygen uptake was reached. It was also significantly and directly correlated with the heart rate during recovery, the increase in plasma lactate concentration and the change in blood pH, indicating that the exercise-induced increase in β-endorphin concentration was smaller in horses with a higher aerobic capacity.[126] In addition, a critical exercise threshold exists for β-endorphin concentration in horses, which is 60% VO_{2max} or less and is related to exercise intensity and duration. Even under conditions of controlled exercise there may be considerable differences in β-endorphin concentrations between horses. This makes the value of comparing horses on the basis of their β-endorphin concentration questionable.[151] Furthermore, total concentration of β-endorphin in Standardbred geldings was not significantly different after 34 weeks of moderate-intensity training on a high-speed treadmill.[133]

Adrenaline

Major actions of adrenaline

The term 'adrenergic' originates from 'adrenaline' and describes hormones or drugs whose effects are similar to those of epinephrine. Adrenergic stress is mediated by stimulation of adrenergic receptors and activation of post-receptor pathways.[152] Adrenaline (or *epinephrine*) is the prototypical stress hormone and is the most effective endogenous agonist at the β_2-receptor. Its stimulation of all α- and β-adrenergic receptors elicits short-term systolic hypertension, hyperglycemia, lipolysis, and insulin resistance. In the longer term, however, epinephrine prevents hypertension during stress and improves glucose tolerance.[151]

Regulation of adrenaline secretion

Adrenaline release from the adrenal medulla increases during exercise via the autonomic efferent arcs, but at a given absolute work intensity the magnitude of this response is less pronounced in endurance trained versus sedentary humans most likely due to a lower sympathetic stimulation of the adrenal medulla. However, when trained and untrained subjects are compared at identical relative workloads as well as in response to numerous non-exercise stimuli, endurance trained athletes have a higher adrenaline secretory capacity compared to sedentary individuals. This indicates development of a so-called 'sports adrenal medulla' as a result of a long-term adaptation to physical training. Such an adaptation is parallel to adaptations taking place in other tissues like skeletal muscle and the heart and can be advantageous in relation to exercise performance in the competing athlete.[154]

Effects of exercise and training on secretion and circulating adrenaline concentrations

A few reports have documented plasma catecholamine concentrations in horses undergoing high-intensity exercise.[128,155,156,157,158] In Thoroughbreds in training, plasma catecholamines measured 5 min after competition exercise were increased 6-7 fold, while cortisol was increased only by 25%.[155] Plasma noradrenaline and adrenaline responses during exercise were sensitive to the intensity of exercise in Thoroughbreds undergoing an incremental exercise test with maximal catecholamine concentrations occurring at the point of fatigue.[128] Adrenaline and noradrenaline concentrations were similar over all speeds,[128] although in one study there was a tendency for the increase in noradrenaline to be greater than that of adrenaline at lower speeds.[156] In addition, 5 min after a maximal speed race of 1200 m in Thoroughbreds, both plasma adrenaline and noradrenaline concentrations increased by 1.5 and 1.7 times, respectively with the increment of adrenaline being greater in high-performance as compared to low-performance horses (77 versus 44%). Similarly, erythrocyte membrane β-adrenergic receptors and dissociation constant (^{3}H-dihydroalprenolol binding to erythrocyte membranes) decreased 5 min after racing as compared to basal values (1.9 and 2.1 times, respectively) possibly mediated by catecholamines.[158] It has been shown that β-adrenergic stimulation (via intravenous administration of epinephrine) directly inhibited glucose uptake into equine skeletal muscle during moderate-intensity exercise.[37]

Actions of adrenaline during exercise

Exercise-associated changes in plasma adrenaline and noradrenaline in horses were much greater than recorded in man and emphasize the importance of catecholamines in mediating the physiological response of the horse to exercise.[156]

Thyroid hormones

There are two thyroid lobes located dorsolaterally of the trachea in the equine species. The thyroid gland is unique in that it has a follicular structure and is the only tissue of the body which is able to accumulate iodine in large quantities and incorporate it into hormones. Thyroid hormone exists in three forms: 3,5,3′,5′-tetraiodothyronine (T_4), 3,5,3′-triiodothyronine (T_3), and 3,3′5′-triiodothyronine (reverse T_3). The two biologically most active iodothyronines secreted by the thyroid gland are thyroxine (T_4) and triiodothyronine (T_3). Reverse T_3 (rT_3), which is formed by target cells, is biologically inactive.[159] Like rT_3, the bound fractions of T_4 and T_3 are biologically inactive. Once released into the circulation, $0.20 \pm 0.21\%$ of T_3 and $0.058 \pm 0.040\%$ of T_4 are free or unbound.[160] Monodeiodination to form reverse T_3 provides a mechanism to attenuate the overall metabolic effects of thyroid hormones even prior to any change in serum concentrations.[159] Thyroxine-binding globulin (TBG) and thyroxine-binding prealbumin (TBPA) exist in the horse, with TBPA mobility anodal to albumin on electrophoresis.[161]

Major actions of thyroid hormones

Thyroid hormone nuclear receptors (TRs) mediate the biological activities of T_3 via transcriptional regulation. Traditionally, T_4 and T_3 were the only thyroid hormones considered to have metabolic effects. However, T_3 as well as 3,5-diiodothyronine (T_2), have important effects on mitochondrial energetic, lipoprotein metabolism and on the cytoskeleton.[162,163,164] Modulation of the basal proton leak in mitochondria accounts for heat production caused by iodothyronines and a substantial component of cellular oxygen consumption. Thyroid hormones also act on the mitochondrial genome via imported isoforms of nuclear TRs to affect several mitochondrial transcription factors.[163] In addition, thyroid hormones increase Na^+-K^+-ATPase activity in skeletal muscle.[165]

Regulation of thyroid hormone secretion

Thyrotropin or thyroid-stimulating hormone (TSH) from the pituitary gland increases the biosynthesis and secretion of thyroid hormones. T_3 probably is more active physiologically than T_4.[159] In addition to their negative feedback effect on the stimulatory hormones thyrotropin-releasing hormone (TRH) and TSH, thyroid hormones also regulate their receptors in various physiological and pathological conditions. Upregulation and downregulation of the thyroid receptors fine-tune the biological effects exerted by the thyroid hormones. Interestingly, the deiodinase enzyme system is another intrinsic regulator of thyroid physiology that adjusts the availability of thyroid hormones to the tissues, which is essential for normal growth and development.[166]

The sympathoadrenal system, including the sympathetic nervous system and the adrenal medulla, interacts with thyroid hormones at various levels. Both systems are evolutionarily old and regulate independent functions, playing probably independent roles in poikilothermic species. With the advent of homeothermy, thyroid hormones acquired a new role, which is to stimulate thermogenic mechanisms and synergize with the sympathoadrenal system to produce heat and maintain body temperature. An important part of this function is mediated through coordinated and, most of the time, synergistic interactions with the sympathoadrenal system. Catecholamines, in turn, activate thyroid hormones in a tissue-specific manner, most notably in brown adipose tissue. Such interactions are important in cold adaptation and in states needing high-energy output. Emerging results suggest the possibility that disrupted interactions between the two systems contribute to metabolic variability.[167]

Effects of exercise and training on secretion and circulating thyroid hormone concentrations

Most investigations of thyroid gland function in exercising horses have measured circulating concentrations of total T_4, free T_4, total T_3, and free T_3. Short bouts of high-intensity exercise tend to produce transient increases in T_4 and T_3 in horses, although findings have been inconsistent.[158,168,169] Five minutes after a maximal speed race of 1200 m, T_3 (by 46%) but not T_4 concentrations increased in Thoroughbreds under conventional race training.[158] In show jumpers, there also is an inconsistent picture regarding plasma iodothyronine concentrations following jumping sessions.[170]

Regarding a single bout of exercise, it should be realized that after a single injection of thyroid hormones into mammals, physiological alterations (e.g. changes in oxygen consumption rates) are detectable after a lag period of ~48 hours.[164] Circulating concentrations of total and free iodothyronines in horses decrease in response to endurance exercise (without a progressive increase in rT_3) indicating that circulating thyroid hormones are either more rapidly utilized or degraded. Serum iodothyronine concentrations were also unchanged from the start to finish of a 60 km endurance simulation ride on a treadmill, with the exception of a decrease by 32% in T_3 concentration. After 12 hours of recovery, total T_4, free T_4 and T_3 were all lower than pre-exercise values. Serum concentrations of all iodothyronines had returned to pre-exercise values by 24 hours of recovery.[171]

Early work by Irvine[172] documented increased thyroid hormone production and utilization during training similar to findings regarding T_3 concentrations in Thoroughbreds in training.[173] During training, resting concentrations of T_4 below the lower end of the reference range are commonly found[173] and this observation might suggest a hormonal status similar to that of euthyroid sick syndrome (ESS), with suppression of T_3 and elevation of rT_3 plasma levels. In young Standardbreds suspected of maladaptation (based on an abnormal weight loss during their first months of training only), a significantly lower plasma T_4 concentration was found compared to controls.[108] Low-intensity training had no detectable effect on the concentration of the Na^+, K^+-pumps in Shetland ponies.[174]

Actions of thyroid hormones during exercise

The stress of chronic exercise induces certain changes to the thyroid axis. Peripheral thyroid hormone metabolism suppression is observed, and the result is a hormonal status similar to that of euthyroid sick syndrome (ESS), with suppression of T_3 and elevation of rT_3 plasma levels. One mechanism proposed involves exercise-activated pathways participating in the pathogenesis of ESS. This is realized through norepinephrine's activation of NF-κB resulting in inactivation of T_3-dependent 5′-deiodinase gene expression and enzyme activity. Thus, ESS is generated in the periphery.[2]

Adipocyte hormones

Catecholamines, natriuretic peptides, and insulin are considered to be the major regulators of lipolysis in humans. However, autocrine/paracrine factors such as metabolites and prostaglandins may also participate in its regulation.[175] Although once thought to be a mere storage depot of excess energy, it is now apparent that adipose tissue is an endocrine organ that plays a prominent role in the regulation of energy metabolism. For example, leptin is a satiety hormone secreted by adipose tissue. In addition to leptin, other proteins like tumor necrosis factor (TNF)-α, interleukin-6 (IL-6), resistin, visfatin, acylation stimulation protein, and adiponectin have been identified as adipose-secreted proteins that are collectively referred to as adipocytokines.[176] Adipocytokines signal a variety of metabolic functions, including satiety, lipid mobilization and utilization, and modulate insulin-mediated glucose disposal. Their secretion is modulated by energy flux, i.e., carbohydrate and lipid availability.[177] Of the various adipocytokines, decreased adiponectin appears to show the strongest relationship with IR and obesity in humans. Although exercise is a common recommendation for the management of IR, when body weight is maintained there appears to be little effect of exercise on the secretion of adiponectin and leptin. As adipocytokines and exercise (muscle contraction) act via the same (AMPK activation) pathway in regards to alterations in insulin action, modulation of adipocytokine concentrations may not be necessary for exercise-induced improvements in IS,[176] whereas in man, weight loss does appear to regulate adipocytokines in a manner that may enhance insulin action.[176,178,179]

In accordance with the above findings, plasma concentrations of ghrelin, leptin, and adiponectin were unchanged following an incremental exercise test in untrained Standardbred mares.[52] Of interest, leptin's effects are largely absent in the obese hyperleptinemic state, probably due to leptin resistance or tolerance.[180] Changes in the expression of tissue-specific adiponectin receptor isoforms in skeletal muscle, rather than circulating total adiponectin levels, may be of physiological importance.[181]

Fluid-regulating hormones

Plasma volume expansion usually occurs with acute endurance exercise and endurance training both in humans and in animals. In most cases, the increase in plasma volume is associated with lower hematocrit without red cell mass change or an actual reduction in red cell mass, causing relative or true anemia, respectively. The combination of exercise and heat acclimation (which produces also hypervolemia, but at a lesser degree than exercise) enhances hypervolemia induced by exercise training alone. The onset of the phenomenon is extremely rapid: hypervolemia is observed within minutes or hours of the cessation of exercise. Fluid-regulating hormones (aldosterone from the adrenal zona glomerulosa, arginine vasopressin (AVP) synthesized in the hypothalamus and released from the posterior lobe of the pituitary gland and atrial natriuretic peptide (ANP) from the cardiac atrium) in conjunction with an elevation in plasma protein content promote hypervolemia. Hypervolemia can improve performance by inducing better muscle perfusion, and by increasing stroke volume and maximal cardiac output. By increasing skin blood flow, plasma volume expansion also enhances thermoregulatory responses to exercise. This leads to the important concept of optimal plasma volume and hematocrit, and performance.[182]

It has been stated that the long-lasting post-exercise increase in plasma atrial peptides in horses after a graded submaximal exercise test on a treadmill is most probably explained by elevated central blood volume and that the role of vasoactive hormones is small.[183] In accord, elevated blood osmolality triggered synchronous central AVP and ACTH secretion, without altering pituitary venous CRH. The source of pituitary venous AVP was presumably the magnocellular/neurohypophysial pathway, which is thought to respond primarily to changes in blood osmolality and pressure.[121]

A 3-day exercise training period caused substantial elevations in both pre-exercise (967%) and post-exercise (+3013%) plasma aldosterone concentrations, suggesting that mechanisms affecting tubular conservation of electrolytes contribute to the early response to training.[184] Furthermore, linear correlations were found between treadmill exercise intensity (and duration) and plasma renin activity (PRA) and plasma aldosterone concentration.[185] In contrast, exercise on a treadmill up a 6 degree grade for 20 min at a speed calculated to require a power equivalent to 80% of VO_{2max} did not reveal significant differences between arterial or mixed venous ANP concentration at rest or during exercise.[186] It should be realized that corrections should be made for plasma volume shifts when examining the endocrine responses to exercise. On the other hand, uncorrected hormonal values better represent what target tissue is actually exposed to.

Conclusions

Exercise is a stress situation that challenges homeostasis, requiring, among other things, adaptive responses of the hormonal systems. It cannot be excluded that endocrine changes following exercise may take more time and as a consequence repeated bouts of exercise might be indicated for the assessment of the performance level in horses. In the equine species, both the GH–IGF I axis and the relationship between IS and peripheral glucose disposal are most likely to be adversely affected by long-term exercise given their derailment following overtraining.

References

1. Mastorakos G, Pavlatou M, Diamanti-Kandarakis E, et al. Exercise and the stress system. Hormones (Athens) 2005;4:73–89.
2. Mastorakos G, Pavlatou M. Exercise as a stress model and the interplay between the hypothalamus-pituitary-adrenal and the hypothalamus-pituitary-thyroid axes. Horm Metab Res 2005;37:577–84.
3. Tasker JG, Herman JP. Mechanisms of rapid glucocorticoid feedback inhibition of the hypothalamic-pituitary-adrenal axis. Stress 2011;14:398–406.
4. Bunt JC. Hormonal alterations due to exercise. Sports Med 1986;3:331–45.
5. Nemet D, Eliakim A. Growth hormone-insulin-like growth factor-1 and inflammatory response to a single exercise bout in children and adolescents. Med Sport Sci 2010;55:141–55.
6. Urhausen A, Gabriel H, Kindermann W. Blood hormones as markers of training stress and overtraining. Sports Med 1996;20:251–76.
7. Kelley DE, Gibbons JR, Smith R, et al. Exercise affects both ovarian follicular dynamics and hormone concentrations in mares. Theriogenology 2011;76:615–22.
8. Janett F, Burkhardt C, Burger D, et al. Influence of repeated treadmill exercise on quality and freezability of stallion semen. Theriogenology 2006;65:1737–49.
9. Kawauchi H, Sower SA. The dawn and evolution of hormones in the adenohypophysis. Gen Comp Endocrinol 2006;148:3–14.
10. Schindler C, Levy DE, Decker T. JAK-STAT signaling: from interferons to cytokines. J Biol Chem 2007;282:20059–63.
11. Hernández-Sánchez C, Mansilla A, de la Rosa EJ, et al. Proinsulin in development:

new roles for an ancient prohormone. Diabetologia 2006;49:1142–50.

12. Nielsen JH, Galsgaard ED, Møldrup A, et al. Regulation of beta-cell mass by hormones and growth factors. Diabetes Suppl 2001;1:S25–9.
13. Møller N, Jørgensen JO. Effects of growth hormone on glucose, lipid, and protein metabolism in human subjects. Endocr Rev 2009;30:152–77.
14. Hartman ML, Veldhuis JD, Thorner MO. Normal control of growth hormone secretion. Horm Res 1993;40:37–47.
15. McMahon CD, Radcliff RP, Lookingland KJ, et al. Neuroregulation of growth hormone secretion in domestic animals. Domest Anim Endocrinol 2001;20:65–87.
16. Savine R, Sönksen PH. Is the somatopause an indication for growth hormone replacement? J Endocrinol Invest Suppl 1999;22:142–9.
17. Widdowson WM, Healy ML, Sönksen PH, et al. The physiology of growth hormone and sport. Growth Horm IGF Res 2009;19:308–19.
18. Malinowski K, Christensen RA, Konopka A, et al. Feed intake, body weight, body condition score, musculation, and immunocompetence in aged mares given equine somatotropin. J Anim Sci 1997;75: 755–60.
19. Merriam GR, Wachter KW. Algorithms for the study of episodic hormone secretion. Am J Physiol 1982;243:E310–18.
20. Veldhuis JD, Carlson ML, Johnson ML. The pituitary gland secretes in bursts: appraising the nature of glandular secretory impulses by simultaneous multiple-parameter deconvolution of plasma hormone concentrations. Proc Natl Acad Sci U S A 1987;84: 7686–90.

20b. de Graaf-Roelfsema E, Veldhuis PP, Keizer HA, et al. Overtrained horses alter their resting pulsatile growth hormone secretion. Am J Physiol Regul Integr Comp Physiol 2009;297:R403–11.

21. Johnson ML, Veldhuis JD. Evolution of deconvolution analysis as a hormone pulse detection method. Methods Neurosci 1995;28:1–24.
22. Johnson ML. Pulse_XP User's Guide, version 1.0. Charlottesville, Virginia, USA: University of Virginia; 2004.
23. de Graaf-Roelfsema E, Veldhuis PP, van Dam KG, et al. Assessment of endogenous growth hormone pulsatility in gelded yearling horses using deconvolution analysis. Vet Q 2011;31:63–71.
24. Thompson DL Jr, Rahmanian MS, DePew CL, et al. Growth hormone in mares and stallions: pulsatile secretion, response to growth hormone-releasing hormone, and effects of exercise, sexual stimulation, and pharmacological agents. J Anim Sci 1992;70:1201–7.
25. Thompson DL Jr, DePew CL, Ortiz A, et al. Growth hormone and prolactin concentrations in plasma of horses: sex differences and the effects of acute exercise and administration of growth hormone-releasing hormone. J Anim Sci 1994;72:2911–18.
26. Sticker LS, Thompson DL Jr, Bunting LD, et al. Feed deprivation of mares: plasma metabolite and hormonal concentrations and responses to exercise. J Anim Sci 1995;73: 3696–704.
27. Golland LC, Evans DL, Stone GM, et al. Maximal exercise transiently disrupts hormonal secretory patterns in standardbred geldings. Equine Vet J Suppl 1999a;30:581–5.
28. Cartmill JA, Thompson DL Jr, Storer WA, et al. Endocrine responses in mares and geldings with high body condition scores grouped by high vs. low resting leptin concentrations. J Anim Sci 2003;81(9):2311–21.
29. de Graaf-Roelfsema E, van Ginneken ME, van Breda E, et al. The effect of long-term exercise on glucose metabolism and peripheral insulin sensitivity in Standardbred horses. Equine Vet J Suppl 2006;36:221–5.

30a. Gerard MP, Hodgson DR, Lambeth RR, et al. Effects of somatotropin and training on indices of exercise capacity in Standardbreds. Equine Vet J Suppl 2002;34:496–501.

30b. Popot MA, Bobin S, Bonnaire Y, et al. IGF -I plasma concentrations in non-treated horses and horses administered with methionyl equine somatotropin. Res Vet Sci 2001;71:167–73.

31. Wideman L, Weltman JY, Hartman ML, et al. Growth hormone release during acute and chronic aerobic and resistance exercise: recent findings. Sports Med 2002;32:987–1004.
32. Borer KT. The effects of exercise on growth. Sports Med 1995;20:375–97.
33. Frystyk J. Exercise and the growth hormone-insulin-like growth factor axis. Med Sci Sports Exerc 2010;42: 58–66.
34. Nindl BC, Pierce JR. Insulin-like growth factor I as a biomarker of health, fitness, and training status. Med Sci Sports Exerc 2010;42:39–49.
35. West DW, Phillips SM. Anabolic processes in human skeletal muscle: restoring the identities of growth hormone and testosterone. Phys Sportsmed 2010;38:97–104.
36. Suh SH, Paik IY, Jacobs K. Regulation of blood glucose homeostasis during prolonged exercise. Mol Cells 2007;23:272–9.
37. Geor RJ, Hinchcliff KW, McCutcheon LJ, et al. Epinephrine inhibits exogenous glucose utilization in exercising horses. J Appl Physiol 2000a;88:1777–90.
38. Geor RJ, Hinchcliff KW, Sams RA. Beta-adrenergic blockade augments glucose utilization in horses during graded exercise. J Appl Physiol 2000;89:1086–98.
39. Jose-Cunilleras E, Hayes KA, Toribio RE, et al. Expression of equine glucose transporter type 4 in skeletal muscle after glycogen-depleting exercise. Am J Vet Res 2005;66:379–85.
40. Kahn CR. Insulin resistance, insulin insensitivity, and insulin unresponsiveness: a necessary distinction. Metabolism Suppl 1978;2:1893–902.
41. Link RP. Glucose tolerance in horses. J Am Vet Med Assoc 1940;97:261–2.

42a. Unwin N, Shaw J, Zimmet P, et al. Impaired glucose tolerance and impaired fasting glycaemia: the current status on definition and intervention. Diabet Med 2002;19:708–23.

42b. Hanley AJ, Williams K, Gonzalez C, et al. San Antonio Heart Study; Mexico City Diabetes Study; Insulin Resistance Atherosclerosis Study. Prediction of type 2 diabetes using simple measures of insulin resistance: combined results from the San Antonio Heart Study, the Mexico City Diabetes Study, and the Insulin Resistance Atherosclerosis Study. Diabetes 2003;52:463–9.

43. Muniyappa R, Lee S, Chen H, et al. Current approaches for assessing insulin sensitivity and resistance in vivo: advantages, limitations, and appropriate usage. Am J Physiol Endocrinol Metab 2008;294:E15–26.
44. Klinkhamer K, Menheere PP, van der Kolk JH. Basal glucose metabolism and peripheral insulin sensitivity in equine pituitary pars intermedia dysfunction. Vet Q 2011;31:19–28.
45. Chakraborty C. Biochemical and molecular basis of insulin resistance. Curr Protein Pept Sci 2006;7:113–1121.
46. Magkos F, Wang X, Mittendorfer B. Metabolic actions of insulin in men and women. Nutrition 2010;26: 686–93.
47. Dimitriadis G, Mitron P, Lambadiari V, et al. Insulin effects in muscle and adipose tissue. Diabetes Res Clin Pract Suppl 2011;1:S52–9.
48. Sticker LS, Thompson DL Jr, Gentry LR. Pituitary hormone and insulin responses to infusion of amino acids and N-methyl-D,L-aspartate in horses. J Anim Sci 2001;79:735–44.
49. Giraudet A, Hinchcliff KW, Kobn CW, et al. Early insulin response to intravenous glucose tolerance test in horses. Am J Vet Res 1994;55: 379–81.

50. Jager MM, de Graaf-Roelfsema E, van Breda E, et al. Changes in plasma glucose and insulin concentrations during standardised exercise tests and during experimentally induced early overtraining in Standardbreds. Proceedings 7th International Conference on Equine Exercise Physiology. August 26–31, Fontainebleau, France. Abstract 154, 2006.
51. McKeeever KH. The endocrine system and the challenge of exercise. Vet Clin North Am Equine 2002;18: 321–53.
52. Gordon ME, McKeever KH, Betros CL, et al. Exercise-induced alterations in plasma concentrations of ghrelin, adiponectin, leptin, glucose, insulin, and cortisol in horses. Vet J 2007;173:532–40.
53. Dybdal NO, Gribble D, Madigan JE, et al. Alterations in plasma corticosteroids, insulin and selected metabolites in horses used in endurance rides. Equine Vet J 1980;12:137–40.
54. Snow DH, Rose RJ. Hormonal changes associated with long distance exercise. Equine Vet J 1981;13:195–7.
55. Ivy JL. The insulin-like effect of muscle contraction. Exerc Sport Sci Rev 1987;15:29–51.
56. Goodyear LJ, Kahn BB. Exercise, glucose transport, and insulin sensitivity. Annu Rev Med 1998;49:235–61.
57. Cortright RN, Dohm GL. Mechanisms by which insulin and muscle contraction stimulate glucose transport. Can J Appl Physiol 1997;22:519–30.
58. van Dam KG, van Breda E, Schaart G, et al. Investigation of the expression and localization of glucose transporter 4 and fatty acid translocase/CD36 in equine skeletal muscle. Am J Vet Res 2004;65:951–6.
59. Duehlmeier R, Hacker A, Widdel-Bigdely A, et al. Insulin stimulates GLUT4 translocation in the semitendinosus muscle of Shetland ponies. Vet J 2010;184:176–81.
60. Waller AP, Burns TA, Mudge MC, et al. Insulin resistance selectively alters cell-surface glucose transporters but not their total protein expression in equine skeletal muscle. J Vet Intern Med 2011;25:315–21.
61. McCutcheon LJ, Geor RJ, Hinchcliff KW. Changes in skeletal muscle GLUT4 content and muscle membrane glucose transport following 6 weeks of exercise training. Equine Vet J Suppl 2002;34:199–204.
62. Stewart-Hunt L, Geor RJ, McCutcheon LJ. Effects of short-term training on insulin sensitivity and skeletal muscle glucose metabolism in standardbred horses. Equine Vet J Suppl 2006;36:226–32.
63. Lacombe VA, Hinchcliff KW, Devor ST. Effects of exercise and glucose administration on content of insulin-sensitive glucose transporter in equine skeletal muscle. Am J Vet Res 2003;64:1500–6.
64. Pratt SE, Geor RJ, Spriet LL, et al. Time course of insulin sensitivity and skeletal muscle glycogen synthase activity after a single bout of exercise in horses. J Appl Physiol 2007;103:1063–9.
65. Nout YS, Hinchcliff KW, Jose-Cunilleras E, et al. Effect of moderate exercise immediately followed by induced hyperglycemia on gene expression and content of the glucose transporter-4 protein in skeletal muscles of horses. Am J Vet Res 2003;64:1401–8.
66. Geor RJ, Stewart-Hunt L, McCutcheon LJ. Effects of prior exercise on insulin-mediated and noninsulin-mediated glucose uptake in horses during a hyperglycaemic clamp. Equine Vet J Suppl 2010;38:129–34.
67. Kim B, Feldman EL. Insulin resistance in the nervous system. Trends Endocrinol Metab 2012;23(3): 133–41.
68. DeFronzo RA, Tobin JD, Andres R. Glucose clamp technique: a method for quantifying insulin secretion and resistance. Am J Physiol 1979;237:E214–23.
69. Wallace TM, Matthews DR. The assessment of insulin resistance in man. Diabet Med 2002;19:527–34.
70. Ayala JE, Bracy DP, McGuinness OP, et al. Considerations in the design of hyperinsulinemic-euglycemic clamps in the conscious mouse. Diabetes 2006;55:390–7.
71. Powell DM, Reedy SE, Sessions DR, et al. Effect of short-term exercise training on insulin sensitivity in obese and lean mares. Equine Vet J Suppl 2002;34:81–4.
72. Rijnen KEPM, van der Kolk JH. Determination of reference range values indicative of glucose metabolism and insulin resistance by use of glucose clamp techniques in horses and ponies. Am J Vet Res 2003;64:1260–4.
73. Sessions DR, Reedy SE, Vick MM, et al. Development of a model for inducing transient insulin resistance in the mare: preliminary implications regarding the estrous cycle. J Anim Sci 2004;82:2321–8.
74. Pratt SE, Geor RJ, McCutcheon LJ. Repeatability of 2 methods for assessment of insulin sensitivity and glucose dynamics in horses. J Vet Intern Med 2005;19:883–8.
75. Geor RJ. Metabolic predispositions to laminitis in horses and ponies: obesity, insulin resistance and metabolic syndromes. J Equine Vet Sci 2008;28:753–9.
76. Tiley HA, Geor RJ, McCutcheon LJ. Effects of dexamethasone on glucose dynamics and insulin sensitivity in healthy horses. Am J Vet Res 2007;68:753–9.
77. Yang YJ, Youn JH, Bergman RN. Modified protocols improve insulin sensitivity estimation using the minimal model. Am J Physiol 1987;253(6 Pt 1):E595–602.
78. Hoffman RM, Boston RC, Stefanovski D, et al. Obesity and diet affect glucose dynamics and insulin sensitivity in Thoroughbred geldings. J Anim Sci 2003;81:2333–42.
79. Eiler H, Frank N, Andrews FM, et al. Physiologic assessment of blood glucose homeostasis via combined intravenous glucose and insulin testing in horses. Am J Vet Res 2005;66:1598–604.
80. Chen H, Sullivan G, Quon MJ. Assessing the predictive accuracy of QUICKI as a surrogate index for insulin sensitivity using a calibration model. Diabetes 2005;54:1914–25.
81. Bergman RN, Finegood DT, Ader M. Assessment of insulin sensitivity in vivo. Endocr Rev 1985;6:45–86.
82. Kronfeld DS, Treiber KH, Geor RJ. Comparison of nonspecific indications and quantitative methods for the assessment of insulin resistance in horses and ponies. J Am Vet Med Assoc 2005;226:712–19.
83. Firshman AM, Valberg SJ. Factors affecting clinical assessment of insulin sensitivity in horses. Equine Vet J 2007;39:567–75.
84. Bergman RN, Ider YZ, Bowden CR, et al. Quantitative estimation of insulin sensitivity. Am J Physiol 1979;236:E667–77.
85. Funk R, Wooldridge A, Stewart A, et al. Seasonal changes in the combined glucose-insulin tolerance test in normal aged horses. J Vt Intern Med2012;26(4):1035–41.
86. Borghouts LB, Keizer HA. Exercise and insulin sensitivity: a review. Int J Sports Med 2000;21:1–12.
87. Koopman R, Manders RJ, Zorenc AH, et al. A single session of resistance exercise enhances insulin sensitivity for at least 24 h in healthy men. Eur J Appl Physiol 2005;94:180–7.
88. Carter RA, McCutcheon LJ, Valle E, et al. Effects of exercise training on adiposity, insulin sensitivity, and plasma hormone and lipid concentrations in overweight or obese, insulin-resistant horses. Am J Vet Res 2010;71:314–21.
89. Treiber KH, Hess TM, Kronfeld DS, et al. Glucose dynamics during exercise: dietary energy sources affect minimal model parameters in trained Arabian geldings during endurance exercise. Equine Vet J Suppl 2006;36:631–6.

90. Freestone JF, Beadle R, Shoemaker K, et al. Improved insulin sensitivity in hyperinsulinaemic ponies through physical conditioning and controlled feed intake. Equine Vet J 1992;24:187–90.
91. Henriksen EJ. Invited review: Effects of acute exercise and exercise training on insulin resistance. J Appl Physiol 2002;93:788–96.
92. de Graaf-Roelfsema E, Keizer HA, van Breda E, et al. The effect of overtraining and subsequent detraining on glucose metabolism and peripheral insulin sensitivity in Standardbred horses. Am J Vet Res 2012;73(9):1386–93.
93. Ramnanan CJ, Edgerton DS, Kraft G, et al. Physiologic action of glucagon on liver glucose metabolism. Diabetes Obes Metab Suppl 2011;1:118–25.
94. Hall GM, Adrian TE, Bloom SR, et al. Changes in circulating gut hormones in the horse during long distance exercise. Equine Vet J 1982;14:209–12.
95. Taborsky GJ Jr, Mundinger TO. Minireview: the role of the autonomic nervous system in mediating the glucagon response to hypoglycemia. Endocrinology 2012;153:1055–62.
96. Falkenstein E, Tillmann HC, Christ M, et al. Multiple actions of steroid hormones – a focus on rapid, nongenomic effects. Pharmacol Rev 2000;52:513–56.
97. Lavoie C. Glucagon receptors: effect of exercise and fasting. Can J Appl Physiol 2005;30:313–27.
98. Falkenstein E, Tillmann HC, Christ M, et al. Multiple actions of steroid hormones – a focus on rapid, nongenomic effects. Pharmacol Rev 2000;52:513–56.
99. Makara GB, Haller J. Non-genomic effects of glucocorticoids in the neural system. Evidence, mechanisms and implications. Prog Neurobiol 2001;65:367–90.
100. Heinlein CA, Chang C. The roles of androgen receptors and androgen-binding proteins in nongenomic androgen actions. Mol Endocrinol 2002;16:2181–7.
101. Crewther BT, Cook C, Cardinale M, et al. Two emerging concepts for elite athletes: the short-term effects of testosterone and cortisol on the neuromuscular system and the dose-response training role of these endogenous hormones. Sports Med 2011;41:103–23.
102. Matsakas A, Nikolaidis MG, Kokalas N, et al. Effect of voluntary exercise on the expression of IGF-I and androgen receptor in three rat skeletal muscles and on serum IGF-I and testosterone levels. Int J Sports Med 2004;25:502–8.
103. Vingren JL, Koziris LP, Gordon SE, et al. Chronic alcohol intake, resistance training, and muscle androgen receptor content. Med Sci Sports Exerc 2005;37:1842–8.
104. Haider SG. Cell biology of Leydig cells in the testis. Int Rev Cytol 2004;233:181–241.
105. James P, Rivier C, Lee S. Presence of corticotrophin-releasing factor and/or tyrosine hydroxylase in cells of a neural brain-testicular pathway that are labelled by a transganglionic tracer. J Neuroendocrinol 2008;20:173–81.
106. Selvage DJ, Rivier C. Importance of the paraventricular nucleus of the hypothalamus as a component of a neural pathway between the brain and the testes that modulates testosterone secretion independently of the pituitary. Endocrinology 2003;144:594–8.
107. Selvage DJ, Lee SY, Parsons LH, et al. A hypothalamic-testicular neural pathway is influenced by brain catecholamines, but not testicular blood flow. Endocrinology 2004;145:1750–9.
108. Leleu C, Haentjens F. Morphological, haemato-biochemical and endocrine changes in young Standardbreds with 'maladaptation' to early training. Equine Vet J Suppl 2010;38:171–8.
109. Snow DH, Munro CD, Nimmo MA. Effects of nandrolone phenylpropionate in the horse: (2) general effects in animals undergoing training. Equine Vet J 1982;14:224–8.
110. Thornton JR, Dowsett KF, Mann R, et al. Influence of anabolic steroids on the response to training of 2 year old horses. In: Persson SGB, Lindhom A, Jeffcott LB, editors. Equine Exercise Physiology 3. Davis, CA, USA: ICEEP Publications; 1991. p. 503–8.
111. Hyyppä S, Räsänen LA, Persson SG, et al. Exercise performance indices in normal and anabolic steroid treated trotters. Equine Vet J Suppl 1995;18: 443–7.
112. Hyyppä S. Effects of nandrolone treatment on recovery in horses after strenuous physical exercise. J Vet Med A Physiol Pathol Clin Med 2001;48: 343–52.
113. Koskinen E, Katila T. Effect of 19-norandrostenololylaurate on serum testosterone concentration, libido, and closure of distal radial growth plate in colts. Acta Vet Scand 1997;38:59–67.
114. West DW, Kujbida GW, Moore DR, et al. Resistance exercise-induced increases in putative anabolic hormones do not enhance muscle protein synthesis or intracellular signalling in young men. J Physiol 2009;587(Pt 21):5239–47.
115. West DW, Burd NA, Tang JE, et al. Elevations in ostensibly anabolic hormones with resistance exercise enhance neither training-induced muscle hypertrophy nor strength of the elbow flexors. J Appl Physiol 2010;108:60–7.
116. Buresh R, Berg K, French J. The effect of resistive exercise rest interval on hormonal response, strength, and hypertrophy with training. J Strength Cond Res 2009;23:62–71.
117. Wilkinson SB, Tarnopolsky MA, Grant EJ, et al. Hypertrophy with unilateral resistance exercise occurs without increases in endogenous anabolic hormone concentration. Eur J Appl Physiol 2006;98:546–55.
118. Peckett AJ, Wright DC, Riddell MC. The effects of glucocorticoids on adipose tissue lipid metabolism. Metabolism 2011;60:1500–10.
119. Dores RM, Baron AJ. Evolution of POMC: origin, phylogeny, posttranslational processing, and the melanocortins. Ann N Y Acad Sci 2011;1220:34–48.
120. Evans MJ, Marshall AG, Kitson NE, et al. Factors affecting ACTH release from perifused equine anterior pituitary cells. J Endocrinol 1993;137:391–401.
121. Alexander SL, Irvine CH, Donald RA. Dynamics of the regulation of the hypothalamo-pituitary-adrenal (HPA) axis determined using a nonsurgical method for collecting pituitary venous blood from horses. Front Neuroendocrinol 1996;17:1–50.
122. Livesey JH, Donald RA, Irvine CHG, et al. The effects of cortisol, vasopressin (AVP), and corticotropin-releasing factor administration on pulsatile adrenocorticotropin, α-melanocyte-stimulating hormone, and AVP secretion in the pituitary venous effluent of the horse. Endocrinology 1988;123:713–20.
123. Irvine CH, Alexander SL. Factors affecting the circadian rhythm in plasma cortisol concentrations in the horse. Domest Anim Endocrinol 1994;11:227–38.
124. Wilson DW, Kingery S, Snow DH. The effect of training on adrenocortical function in Thoroughbred racehorses. In: Persson SGB, Lindholm A, Jeffcott LB, editors. Equine Exercise Physiology 3; Davis, USA: ICEEP Publications; 1991. p. 482–9;
125. Keadle TL, Pouciau SS, Melrose PA. Acute exercise stress modulates equine immune function. J Equine Vet Sci 1993;13:226–31.
126. Art T, Franchimont P, Lekeux P. Plasma beta-endorphin response of thoroughbred horses to maximal exercise. Vet Rec 1994;135:499–503.
127. Horohov DW, Dimock A, Guirnalda P, et al. Effect of exercise on the immune response of young and old horses. Am J Vet Res 1999;60:643–7.
128. Nagata S, Takeda F, Kurosawa M, et al. Plasma adrenocorticotropin, cortisol and catecholamines response to various exercises. Equine Vet J Suppl 1999;30:570–4.

129. Marc M, Parvizi N, Ellendorff F, et al. Plasma cortisol and ACTH concentrations in the warmblood horse in response to a standardized treadmill exercise test as physiological markers for evaluation of training status. J Anim Sci 2000;78:1936–46.
130. Malinowski K, Shock EJ, Rochelle P, et al. Plasma beta-endorphin, cortisol and immune responses to acute exercise are altered by age and exercise training in horses. Equine Vet J Suppl 2006;36:267–73.
131. Rose RJ, Hodgson DR, Sampson D, et al. Changes in plasma biochemistry in horses competing in a 160 km endurance ride. Aust Vet J 1983;60:101–5.
132. Church DB, Evans DL, Lewis DR, et al. The effect of exercise on plasma adrenocorticotrophin, cortisol and insulin in the horse and adaptation with training. In: Gillespie JR, Robinson NE, editors. Equine Exercise Physiology 2. Davis, CA, USA: ICEEP Publications; 1987. p. 506–15.
133. Golland LC, Evans DL, Stone GM, et al. Plasma cortisol and beta-endorphin concentrations in trained and over-trained standardbred racehorses. Pflugers Arch 1999b;439:11–17.
134. de Graaf-Roelfsema E, Keizer HA, van Breda E, et al. The influences of overtraining on the hypothalamo-pituitary-adrenocortical axis in Standardbred horses. Conference on equine sports medicine and science (CESMAS) Utrecht, the Netherlands, July 9–13, 2008. p. 159–61.
135. Linden A, Art T, Amory H, et al. Comparison of the adrenocortical response to both pharmacological and physiological stresses in sport horses. Zentralbl Veterinarmed A 1990;37:601–4.
136. Garcia MC, Beech J. Endocrinologic, hematologic, and heart rate changes in swimming horses. Am J Vet Res 1986;47:2004–6.
137. Lassourd V, Gayrard V, Laroute V, et al. Cortisol disposition and production rate in horses during rest and exercise. Am J Physiol 1996;271:R25–33.
138. Desmecht D, Linden A, Amory H, et al. Relationship of plasma lactate production to cortisol release following completion of different types of sporting events in horses. Vet Res Commun 1996;20:371–9.
139. Alexander SL, Irvine CH, Ellis MJ, et al. The effect of acute exercise on the secretion of corticotropin-releasing factor, arginine vasopressin, and adrenocorticotropin as measured in pituitary venous blood from the horse. Endocrinology 1991;128: 65–72.
140. Cayado P, Muñoz-Escassi B, Domínguez C, et al. Hormone response to training and competition in athletic horses. Equine Vet J Suppl 2006;36:274–8.
141. Salehian B, Kejriwal K. Glucocorticoid-induced muscle atrophy: mechanisms and therapeutic strategies. Endocr Pract 1999;5:277–81.
142. Herbst KL, Bhasin S. Testosterone action on skeletal muscle. Curr Opin Clin Nutr Metab Care 2004;7:271–7.
143. Viru A, Viru M. Cortisol – essential adaptation hormone in exercise. Int J Sports Med 2004;25:461–4.
144. Crewther B, Keogh J, Cronin J, et al. Possible stimuli for strength and power adaptation: acute hormonal responses. Sports Med 2006;36:215–38.
145. Bruce SA, Phillips SK, Woledge RC. Interpreting the relation between force and cross-sectional area in human muscle. Med Sci Sports Exerc 1997;29:677–83.
146. Krotkiewski M, Kral JG, Karlsson J. Effects of castration and testosterone substitution on body composition and muscle metabolism in rats. Acta Physiol Scand 1980;109:233–7.
147. Hyyppä S, Karvonen U, Räsänen LA, et al. Androgen receptors and skeletal muscle composition in trotters treated with nandrolone laureate. Zentralbl Veterinarmed A 1997;44: 481–91.
148. Ustünel I, Akkoyunlu G, Demir R. The effect of testosterone on gastrocnemius muscle fibres in growing and adult male and female rats: a histochemical, morphometric and ultrastructural study. Anat Histol Embryol 2003;32:70–9.
149. Wijnberg ID, van Dam KG, Graaf-Roelfsema E, et al. (Over)training effects on quantitative electromyography and muscle enzyme activities in standardbred horses. J Appl Physiol 2008;105:1746–53.
150. Beaven CM, Cook CJ, Gill ND. Significant strength gains observed in rugby players after specific resistance exercise protocols based on individual salivary testosterone responses. J Strength Cond Res 2008;22:419–25.
151. Mehl ML, Schott HC 2nd, Sarkar DK, et al. Effects of exercise intensity and duration on plasma beta-endorphin concentrations in horses. Am J Vet Res 2000;61:969–73.
152. Dünser MW, Hasibeder WR. Sympathetic overstimulation during critical illness: adverse effects of adrenergic stress. J Intensive Care Med 2009;24:293–316.
153. Ziegler MG, Elayan H, Milic M, et al. Epinephrine and the metabolic syndrome. Review. Curr Hypertens Rep 2012;14:1–7.
154. Kjaer M. Adrenal medulla and exercise training. Eur J Appl Physiol Occup Physiol 1998;77:195–9.
155. Martínez R, Godoy A, Naretto E, et al. Neuroendocrine changes produced by competition stress on the Thoroughbred race horse. Comp Biochem Physiol A Comp Physiol 1988;91:599–602.
156. Snow DH, Harris RC, MacDonald IA, et al. Effects of high-intensity exercise on plasma catecholamines in the thoroughbred horse. Equine Vet J 1992;24:462–7.
157. Valberg S, Häggendal J, Lindholm A. Blood chemistry and skeletal muscle metabolic responses to exercise in horses with recurrent exertional rhabdomyolysis. Equine Vet J 1993;25:17–22.
158. González O, González E, Sánchez C, et al. Effect of exercise on erythrocyte beta-adrenergic receptors and plasma concentrations of catecholamines and thyroid hormones in Thoroughbred horses. Equine Vet J 1998;30:72–8.
159. Pineda MH, Dooley MP. McDonald's Veterinary Endocrinology and Reproduction. 5th ed. Ames, Iowa: Iowa State Press; 2003.
160. Messer NT, Johnson PJ, Refsal KR, et al. Effect of food deprivation on baseline iodothyronine and cortisol concentrations in healthy, adult horses. Am J Vet Res 1995;56:116–21.
161. Larsson M, Pettersson T, Carlstrom A. Thyroid hormone binding in serum of 15 vertebrate species: isolation of thyroxine-binding globulin and prealbumin analogs. Gen Comp Endocrinol 1985;58:360–75.
162. Cioffi F, Lanni A, Goglia F. Thyroid hormones, mitochondrial bioenergetics and lipid handling. Curr Opin Endocrinol Diabetes Obes 2010;17:402–7.
163 Cheng SY, Leonard JL, Davis PJ. Molecular aspects of thyroid hormone actions. Endocr Rev 2010;31:139–70.
164. Weitzel JM, Iwen KA. Coordination of mitochondrial biogenesis by thyroid hormone. Mol Cell Endocrinol 2011;342:1–7.
165. Clausen T. Na^+-K^+ pump regulation and skeletal muscle contractility. Physiol Rev 2003;83:1269–324.
166. Tarım Ö. Thyroid hormones and growth in health and disease. J Clin Res Pediatr Endocrinol 2011;3:51–5.
167. Silva JE, Bianco SD. Thyroid-adrenergic interactions: physiological and clinical implications. Thyroid 2008;18:157–65.
168. Powell D, Lawrence LM, Brewster-Barnes T, et al. The effect of diet composition and feeding state on the response to exercise in feed-restricted horses. Equine Vet J Suppl 1999;30:514–18.
169. Greene HM, Cogger EA, Miltenberger TL, et al. Metabolic and osmoregulatory function at low and high (3800 m) altitude. Equine Vet J Suppl 2002;34:545–50.

170. Cravana C, Medica P, Prestopino M, et al. Effects of competitive and noncompetitive showjumping on total and free iodothyronines, β-endorphin, ACTH and cortisol levels of horses. Equine Vet J Suppl 2010;38:179–84.

171. Graves EA, Schott HC 2nd, Marteniuk JV, et al. Thyroid hormone responses to endurance exercise. Equine Vet J Suppl 2006;36:32–6.

172. Irvine CH. Thyroxine secretion rate in the horse in various physiological states. J Endocrinol 1967;39:313–20.

173. Bayly WM, Andrea R, Smith B, et al. Thyroid hormone concentrations in racing Thoroughbreds. Pferdeheilkunde 1996;12:534–8.

174. Suwannachot P, Verkleij CB, Kocsis S, et al. Prolonged food restriction and mild exercise in Shetland ponies: effects on weight gain, thyroid hormone concentrations and muscle $Na^{(+)}$,$K^{(+)}$-ATPase. J Endocrinol 2000;167:321–9.

175. Kolditz CI, Langin D. Adipose tissue lipolysis. Curr Opin Clin Nutr Metab Care 2010;13:377–81.

176. Berggren JR, Hulver MW, Houmard JA. Fat as an endocrine organ: influence of exercise. J Appl Physiol 2005;99: 757–64.

177. Havel PJ. Update on adipocyte hormones: regulation of energy balance and carbohydrate/lipid metabolism. Diabetes Suppl 2004;1:S143–51.

178. Hulver MW, Houmard JA. Plasma leptin and exercise: recent findings. Sports Med 2003;33:473–82.

179. Bouassida A, Chamari K, Zaouali M, et al. Review on leptin and adiponectin responses and adaptations to acute and chronic exercise. Br J Sports Med 2010;44:620–30.

180. Mantzoros CS, Magkos F, Brinkoetter M, et al. Leptin in human physiology and pathophysiology. Am J Physiol Endocrinol Metab 2011;301: E567–84.

181. Vu V, Riddell MC, Sweeney G. Circulating adiponectin and adiponectin receptor expression in skeletal muscle: effects of exercise. Diabetes Metab Res Rev 2007;23:600–11.

182. Fellmann N. Hormonal and plasma volume alterations following endurance exercise. A brief review. Sports Med 1992;13:37–49.

183. Kokkonen UM, Pösö AR, Hyyppä S, et al. Exercise-induced changes in atrial peptides in relation to neuroendocrine responses and fluid balance in the horse. J Vet Med A Physiol Pathol Clin Med 2002;49:144–50.

184. McKeever KH, Scali R, Geiser S, et al. Plasma aldosterone concentration and renal sodium excretion are altered during the first days of training. Equine Vet J Suppl 2002;34:524-31.

185. McKeever KH, Hinchcliff KW, Schmall LM, et al. Plasma renin activity and aldosterone and vasopressin concentrations during incremental treadmill exercise in horses. Am J Vet Res 1992a;53:1290-3.

186. McKeever KH, Hinchcliff KW, Cooley JL, et al. Arterial-venous difference in atrial natriuretic peptide concentration during exercise in horses. Am J Vet Res 1992;53:2174–7.

187. Miller WL. Androgen synthesis in adrenarche. Rev Endocr Metab Disord 2009;10:3–17.

Endocrine and metabolic disorders of the equine athlete

35

Catherine M. McGowan   Raymond J. Geor

CHAPTER CONTENTS

Introduction

Unlike their sedentary or aged counterparts, endocrine and metabolic disorders of the athletic horse are relatively rare. However, when horses are excessively exercised without the appropriate acclimation or conditioning, or when horses are chronically overtrained, marked metabolic and endocrine derangements can occur. This chapter describes two metabolic/endocrine conditions of athletic horses: the exhausted horse and overtraining syndromes. Synchronous diaphragmatic flutter, which can occur in exhausted horses, is described elsewhere in this book (Chapter 40).

Exhausted horse syndrome

- This is a multisystemic condition due to the combined effects of dehydration, hypovolemia, acid–base and electrolyte disturbances, energy substrate depletion, and hyperthermia.
- Clinical signs include depression, lack of impulsion and shortened stride, muscle fasciculations and soreness, increased capillary and jugular refill times, hyperthermia, delayed recovery of heart rate, and reduced or absent borborygmi.
- Treatment focuses on correction of fluid and electrolyte deficits and aggressive cooling of the overheated horse.
- Despite extensive supportive care, severely affected horses may die.

Recognition

History and presenting complaint

The exhausted horse syndrome is a term used to describe a multisystem disorder that can develop in horses participating in athletic activity over an extended period (e.g. three-day events, endurance racing, and other long-distance rides), particularly when exercise is performed in hot ambient conditions.[1–3] The clinical presentation is variable and dependent upon the severity and speed of onset of fatigue as well as the individual horse's tolerance to physiological strain. In general, clinical signs are reflective of dehydration, electrolyte and acid–base disturbances, depletion of energy reserves, hyperthermia and muscle pain.[2,3]

Physical examination

Initially, there are subtle signs of fatigue with mild alterations in mental state (alertness and attitude) and inconsistencies in gait that may be due to muscle soreness. Clinical evidence of exhaustion becomes more pronounced if exercise is continued; muscles start to show localized hardening and pain on palpation, the gait becomes stiff and stilted, and muscle spasms and cramps may occur, as may synchronous diaphragmatic flutter (SDF).[2,3] Severely affected horses are often unwilling to continue to exercise, are depressed and are unwilling to eat or drink. They may show incoordination (ataxia), become recumbent, and show other neurologic signs such as head pressing and seizures.

Temperature, heart and respiratory rates are elevated and after cessation of exercise show a delayed return to resting values. Although the heart and respiratory rates of an exhausted and a non-exhausted horse may be similar immediately following exercise, these rates return to normal (heart rate <60 bpm, respiratory rate <25 breaths/min) within 10 to 20 minutes of exercise cessation in the non-exhausted horse but not in the exhausted one. Rectal temperature may be 42 °C or higher. However, measured rectal temperature may be lower than true body temperature if the horse has diminished anal sphincter tone. Respiratory rate is elevated in an attempt to increase respiratory heat loss; heart rate is elevated to maintain cardiac output. Auscultation of the heart may reveal cardiac irregularities, capillary refill time is increased and both pulse pressure and jugular distensibility are decreased.

Dehydration is expressed clinically as decreased skin turgor, sunken eyes, dry mucous membranes, firm, dry feces and decreased urine output. Mild signs of dehydration usually become apparent at a body water deficit of 4–5%. Subjectively, the sweating response may appear inappropriate relative to the level of hyperthermia (e.g. a patchy appearance or, in severe cases, a hot and dry coat). Despite significant dehydration, affected horses often are not interested in water or feed. Intestinal stasis commonly occurs with decreased or absent borborygmi, poor anal tone and, occasionally, colic.[2,3]

In severely affected horses, a number of serious complications may develop immediately or over the following 1–4 days. These complications include exertional rhabdomyolysis, renal failure secondary to muscle necrosis and myoglobinuria, hepatic dysfunction, gastrointestinal dysfunction, laminitis and central nervous system disorders. Despite intensive supportive care, the horse may die.

Laboratory examination

In an exhausted horse, early clinicopathologic findings include increased packed cell volume (PCV) and plasma protein concentration due to dehydration, normo- or slight hyponatremia, hypokalemia, hypocalcemia (ionized), hypochloremia, and azotemia.[1–3] The PCV of endurance horses eliminated from races due to metabolic problems may be as high as 55–65%, while plasma protein concentration may exceed 10 g/dl (typical reference range, 5.9 to 7.5 g/dl). As a result of muscle exertion or damage, increases in muscle enzyme activity (e.g. creatine kinase, CK; and aspartate amino transferase, AST) and plasma phosphorus concentration may be evident. Plasma creatinine values may be elevated, suggesting a reduction in glomerular filtration rate because of dehydration. Urine samples appear dark due to myoglobinuria, hematuria, proteinuria and glycosuria.[4,5] Serum electrolyte concentrations may be decreased (especially, K^+, Cl^-, Ca^{2+} and Mg^{2+}). Metabolic alkalosis is the most common acid–base disturbance although metabolic acidosis may develop in horses with profound hypovolaemia and circulatory shock.[6] Metabolic alkalosis along with hypocalcemia and hypokalemia contribute to the development of SDF. Profound neutropenia with a left shift is sometimes observed within 24 h of the onset of exhaustion.[3]

It should be noted that laboratory evidence of muscle damage as well as disturbances in electrolyte and acid–base balance also may be present in horses that successfully complete endurance races. Conversely, some exhausted horses may not show substantial alterations in clinicopathological variables at the time of diagnosis. During endurance races, muscle enzyme activities and serum creatinine concentration increase as a function of distance covered and in one study were not useful for the early diagnosis of metabolic stress.[7]

Necropsy examination

Necropsy findings include skeletal and myocardial muscle damage, gastrointestinal ulceration, renal necrosis and sometimes renal infarction as well as laminitis.[8]

Diagnosis

Diagnosis is based on history, clinical signs and laboratory findings. Although diagnosis is straightforward in severe cases, early recognition of the exhausted horse is difficult due to the subtlety of clinical signs and lack of objective clinical and/or clinicopathological diagnostic criteria. Careful observation during rest stops is essential to identify horses at risk of severe exhaustion. A lack of interest in feed or water in the face of dehydration indicates the need for aggressive intervention, including elimination from the race and prompt initiation of fluid therapy.

Treatment and prognosis

Therapeutic aims

Cooling the overheated horse and fluid therapy to replace fluid and electrolyte losses and to assist in restoration of circulating blood volume are essential components of therapy.

Therapy

Exercise must cease to minimize further damage and a horse with marked hyperthermia (rectal temperature 41°C or greater) should be cooled down as quickly as possible. Repeated application of cool or cold water by sponges or by hosing down and ventilation via a natural breeze or a fan will enhance heat loss via convection and evaporation. Ice-water enemas can be effective in a severely compromised patient. Cooling should continue until the body temperature is reduced to nearly normal (<39°C).

For mildly affected horses, rest together with cooling out and access to water, salt and feed may be sufficient. However, fluid therapy is required if the horse does not drink or eat within 15–30 minutes. In severe cases, fluid therapy should be started immediately. Under most circumstances, it is better to treat a horse in the field and not to attempt a trailer ride until it has been rehydrated. Oral fluid therapy may be considered in mildly affected horses that have adequate gut sounds and no evidence of colic. Oral fluid administration offers the advantages of speed and convenience and can be used if the horse has normal gut sounds. Between 4–8 L of fluid can be given via nasogastric tube every 30–60 min until the horse shows signs of improvement. Oral administration can be started immediately after exercise, because consumption of 10–15 L of cool (~16°C) water within 3–5 min of completing exercise is not harmful.[9,10] Isotonic solutions containing sodium, potassium, calcium, chloride and glucose are often well tolerated and fairly rapidly absorbed. Commercial electrolyte powders should be those formulated for horses. For example, electrolyte formulations designed for use in calves with diarrhea usually contain bicarbonate, lactate or citrate. Therefore, these preparations are not the best choice for the treatment of horses with exercise-induced dehydration because of their alkalinizing effects. The oral administration of hypertonic solutions should also be avoided because they may cause a transient reduction in plasma volume due to movement of water into the bowel lumen.[9,11] Oral administration should be halted if any discomfort or gastric reflux becomes apparent.

Many exhausted horses are severely dehydrated (fluid deficits in the range of 30 to 60 L) and/or have evidence of compromised gut function (absent gut sounds, gastric reflux), thus necessitating use of the intravenous (i.v.) route. The rate of fluid administration will depend on the extent of hypovolemia and dehydration. In general, a 14-gauge jugular catheter is adequate for delivery of i.v. fluids; however, a larger-bore catheter (10- or 12-gauge) and/or the insertion of a second catheter may be indicated in severely affected horses to facilitate a rapid rate of fluid administration during the first hour of therapy. The initial rate of fluid administration should be in the range of 15 to 20 ml/kg/h (7.5 to 10 L/h for a 500 kg horse). The subsequent rate of fluid administration should be based on ongoing clinical assessment. Some horses will require as much as 60–80 L of fluid over a 6–12 h period, while others will show marked clinical improvement after receiving 20–25 L (e.g. restoration of gut sounds, initiation of eating and drinking) and may not require further i.v. fluid therapy. Preferred fluids are isotonic or only slightly hypertonic solutions containing sodium, potassium, chloride, calcium and glucose (e.g. Normosol-R or Ringer's solution with 5% glucose). An alternative is 0.9% saline with glucose and potassium added: 1–3 g of potassium chloride/L and 5 to 10 g of glucose/L. The added glucose will also assist in the replacement of energy deficits. In horses with SDF, a 23% calcium borogluconate solution (100 to 300 ml) should be administered by slow i.v. infusion. Calcium should be added to the fluids of horses with evidence of hypocalcemia (ionized calcium <1.25 mmol/L); correction of hypocalcemia may help to improve gastrointestinal motility.

Lactated Ringer's solution (LRS) is not the ideal fluid choice because exhausted horses often have metabolic alkalosis; however, the volume of administered fluid rather than its composition is of primary importance for correction of hypovolemia and cardiovascular compromise, i.e. LRS should be used if it is the only sterile i.v. fluid available.

The use of hypertonic solutions (e.g. 1–2 L of a 7.5% NaCl solution) for resuscitation of severely dehydrated, hypovolemic horses is controversial due to concern that the administration of a hyperosmotic solution will exacerbate intracellular dehydration. In one study of endurance horses disqualified from a race for metabolic conditions, the administration of 2 L 7.2% NaCl in combination with 5 L of LRS solution resulted in greater decreases in PCV, total plasma protein, and albumin concentration and earlier onset of urine production when compared to treatment with LRS alone.[12] It was concluded that the i.v. administration of hypertonic solutions appears to be safe in the treatment of dehydrated endurance horses but this treatment must always be accompanied by the administration of isotonic fluids for correction of fluid deficits.[12]

The administration of non-steroidal anti-inflammatory drugs (NSAIDs) and phenothiazine agents such as acepromazine should be avoided during the initial phase of treatment of the exhausted horse. Renal perfusion during hypovolemia is in part dependent on the local production and action of prostaglandins I_2 and E_2. As such, the administration of NSAIDs that block prostaglandin synthesis may compromise renal blood flow in dehydrated or hypovolemic horses and increase risk for NSAID toxicity. The administration of acepromazine may potentiate hypotension in exhausted horses due to its peripheral vasodilatory effects. Treatment with NSAIDs – flunixin meglumine (0.5–1.0 mg/kg), phenylbutazone (2.2–4.4 mg/kg) or ketoprofen (0.5–1.0 mg/kg) – for control of pain and inflammation can be initiated once the horse has received sufficient fluids to induce diuresis. The lower end of the recommended dosage range should initially be used.

A thorough physical examination, including evaluation for gastric reflux, palpation per rectum, and abdominal ultrasonography, should be performed in horses with colic. Ileus appears to be primary cause of colic pain in exhausted horses and the colic often resolves with fluid therapy and an improvement in intestinal motility. Pain should be managed with xylazine (0.33 to 0.55 mg/kg i.v.), butorphanol (0.01 to 0.02 mg/kg i.v.), or a combination of the two. Surgical lesions (e.g. small intestinal volvulus) have been reported in endurance horses after racing;[3] repeated examinations are therefore imperative for horses that show persistent colic in the face of medical treatment.

Close clinical monitoring is indicated during and after initial treatment for exhaustion, including the frequency and volume of urination, serum BUN, creatinine and electrolyte concentrations, gastrointestinal function (gastric reflux, gut sounds, fecal characteristics), and clinical signs of laminitis (foot pain, increased digital pulse amplitude and hoof wall temperature). Intravenous fluid therapy should be continued in horses with evidence of compromised renal function (i.e. persistent azotemia and/or oliguria). Treatment with furosemide (loading dose of 0.15 mg/kg i.v., followed by a constant-rate infusion [CRI] of 0.12 mg/kg bwt per hour) should be considered if ongoing fluid therapy fails to induce an increase in urine production. In hypoproteinemic horses (e.g. secondary to diarrhea or renal disease), colloids and/or plasma may be necessary to limit development of pulmonary or peripheral edema. The initiation of laminitis prophylactic treatments (e.g. digital cryotherapy, aspirin 15 mg/kg per os every 24 or 48 hours) should be considered although the efficacy of these measures for prevention of laminitis in exhausted horses is not known.

Some clinicians advocate the administration of broad-spectrum antibiotics (e.g. a combination of procaine penicillin and gentamicin) and anti-endotoxin medications (e.g. polymyxin B, 3000 iu/kg, i.v., every 12 hours) to counter sepsis and/or endotoxemia, particularly for exhausted horses with profound leukopenia.

Prognosis

Prognosis is good for mildly and moderately affected horses; these horses generally respond to conservative treatment and can be returned to training after 1–2 weeks of rest. The prognosis for more severely affected horses is guarded; some exhausted develop serious sequelae that lead to death or necessitate euthanasia.

Etiology and pathophysiology

Exhaustion occurs when the horse is required to exercise beyond its physiological limit, with the combined effects of dehydration, hypovolemia, electrolyte loss, acid–base disturbances, energy substrate depletion, and hyperthermia contributing to the pathophysiology of exhaustion and its sequelae (Fig. 35.1). Risk of exhaustion is greatest when horses compete under conditions of high heat and humidity, especially in under-conditioned animals or those not properly acclimated to exercise in hot ambient conditions. Lameness also may contribute to the development of exhaustion by altering a horse's gait, leading to increased use of certain muscle groups and earlier onset of fatigue. Depletion of energy stores in endurance horses, especially during 100 km or longer rides,[13] may contribute to the onset of exhaustion.

Dehydration and a decrease in effective circulating volume occur as a result of sweat fluid losses (and the failure to replenish at least some of these losses during performance). Physical exercise leads to considerable heat production, because only 20 to 25% of the energy utilized in muscles is converted to mechanical energy.

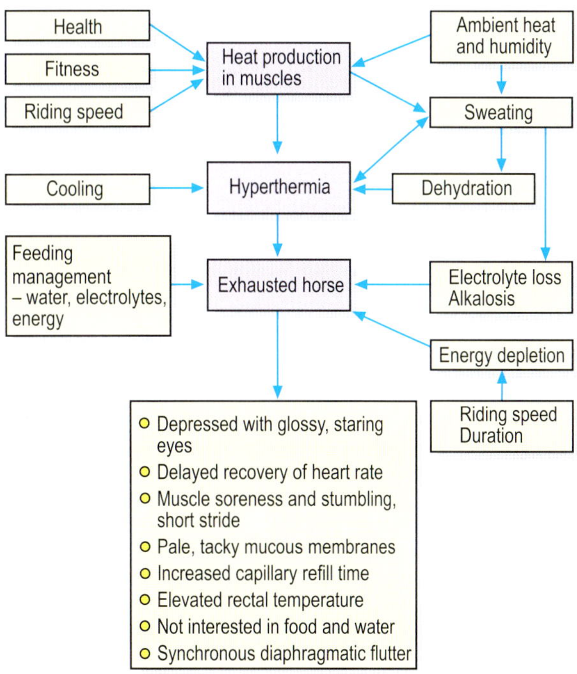

Fig 35.1 Both internal and external factors contribute to dehydration, electrolyte loss , energy substrate depletion and excessive hyperthermia, which, if untreated, may lead to the exhausted horse syndrome.

Evaporation of sweat is the most efficient means of heat loss during exercise and may be the only means of heat dissipation in a hot environment. The amount of sweat produced depends on the horse's size and fitness, on work intensity and the environmental conditions. Under cool climatic conditions, horses may sweat 5 to 8 L/h but in hot weather sweat production may amount to 10 to 15 L/h when activity levels are maintained at a high rate (e.g. 15 km/h). During endurance competitions, horses routinely lose 4 to 7% of their bodyweight but in hot conditions, net water loss may be about 40 L or close to 10% of bodyweight.[14] Respective values during the endurance phase of a three-day event range from 2% to 4% of bodyweight under normal conditions[15] and in hot conditions deficits greater than 9% of bodyweight have been reported.[16] During sweating, water is mainly lost from the extracellular fluid and the consequent decreases in blood and plasma volumes[1,11,17] can reduce perfusion in skeletal muscle and in other vital organs. Inadequate tissue perfusion leads to inefficient oxygen and substrate transport, and hampers thermoregulation. If severe, this cardiovascular compromise may contribute to impaired renal and intestinal function.

Sweating-induced dehydration is always accompanied by electrolyte loss. Equine sweat is isotonic or slightly hypertonic relative to plasma and contains high concentrations of sodium, potassium and chloride and also some calcium and magnesium.[10,18] Abundant sweating will incur significant ion deficits; these will lead to alterations in skeletal muscle ion content, increasing the potential for muscular dysfunction and contributing directly to fatigue.[18]

The most consistent acid–base alteration associated with endurance exercise in a hot environment is metabolic alkalosis.[6] Endurance horses exercise at moderate work intensities at a fairly constant speed between 10 and 20 km/h and rely almost totally on aerobic energy metabolism, with minimal accumulation of lactate in blood. Typical plasma lactate concentrations during such exercise are 1.0 to 3.3 mmol/L.[18] The degree of metabolic alkalosis is dependent on the severity of hypochloremia and hypokalemia. Hypochloremia is associated with an increase in plasma bicarbonate because in the kidney when chloride concentration is low, bicarbonate (HCO_3^-) is resorbed. As plasma sodium concentration tends to decrease due to loss in sweat, the kidney conserves sodium at the expense of potassium and hydrogen ions, which also contributes to the alkalosis.[1,14] Potassium, magnesium, and calcium depletion associated with metabolic alkalosis may alter membrane potential and neuromuscular transmission, contributing to gastrointestinal stasis, cardiac arrhythmias and muscle cramps and spasms including SDF.[14]

The situation differs during the endurance phase of a three-day event and the marathon phase in combined driving, during which anaerobic metabolism significantly contributes to energy transduction, plasma lactate concentrations are very high (up to 38.5 to 40.2 mmol/L),[6,19,20] and horses may develop metabolic acidosis. After exercise, the acidosis is resolved through oxidation of lactate during a 30-min to 2-h period. Thereafter, metabolic alkalosis prevails.

During exercise, there is redistribution of blood flow, with a decrease in flow to the intestinal tract and other visceral organs (e.g. kidneys) and concomitant increases in blood flow to the locomotor muscles to meet metabolic demands and to the skin for heat dissipation. With severe exercise-associated dehydration and hypovolemia, there likely is a further reduction in blood flow to visceral organs and eventually to working muscle and the skin, resulting in impairment to the efficiency of sweating and evaporative cooling. Heat dissipation is markedly compromised when dehydration is severe (>10% of bodyweight). If exercise is continued, the thermoregulatory system will be overwhelmed and this will lead to an excessive elevation of body temperature (hyperthermia). Ultimately this may cause life-threatening heat stroke, with damage to the central nervous system. Heat stroke is more often observed in three-day horses and combined driving horses that do fast anaerobic work at a high rate of heat production, but it may also occur in endurance horses.

Epidemiology

Published data on the epidemiology and risk factors for exhausted horse syndrome are not available. Anecdotally, the syndrome is most often seen in association with long-distance riding, but may also be seen in horses competing in the endurance phase of a three-day event or in the marathon phase of combined driving, in which horses perform moderate- and high-intensity exercise for a period of 1–2 hours, depending on the level of competition. As ambient temperature and humidity and the duration of exercise increase, the incidence of exhausted horse syndrome appears to rise. For example, in 160 km endurance rides, up to 40-50% of the horses may retire from the competition or be eliminated at veterinary checks.

Endurance horses are typically eliminated for one of three reasons: lameness; metabolic problems (including exhaustion, colic, SDF, and myopathy); or for other reasons, including overtime (failure to reach a veterinary gate by a certain time point) and a rider option to withdraw. In a retrospective study of veterinary records for 3493 endurance horse competition starts during 2007 in the United States, the overall elimination proportion was 18.9% (660/3493).[21] Lameness was listed as the reason for elimination for 312 horses, and metabolic causes were listed for 147 horses. A number of examination variables assessed prior to or during the ride were associated with elimination, including HR, cardiac recovery index, and abnormal gastrointestinal sounds.[21] Examination of 4326 endurance horse starts for FEI sanctioned events in nine countries demonstrated a higher rate of elimination (54%); lameness and metabolic reasons accounted for, respectively, 69.2% and 23.5% of all eliminations (see Chapter 52). Specific reasons for metabolic elimination of endurance horses are not well documented; however, dehydration and poor HR recovery, colic, myopathy or SDF were listed as the primary reason for metabolic elimination of horses competing in the Tevis Cup race.[22]

Prevention

Thorough physical conditioning (fitness), the absence of underlying lameness problems, acclimatization to competition exercise in the prevailing ambient conditions, and close clinical monitoring during events can help to prevent development of exhaustion in horses competing in endurance-type events. Although a high level of fitness should lower risk of developing metabolic problems, even fit horses may be ridden beyond their performance limits by inexperienced riders. Accordingly, the rider must develop an awareness of the early signs of fatigue (e.g. subtle changes in gait) and, when these signs are recognized, be prepared to stop exercise before exhaustion (Fig. 35.2).

Provision of an adequate period of recovery after transportation will help to ensure correction of travel-associated dehydration and muscle fatigue. During transport, a horse typically experiences substantial loss of weight (approximately 3 kg/h of transport) and will become dehydrated. The horse therefore requires sufficient time to recover from a long trailer ride such that hydration state and electrolyte balance are normal at the start of the event. Athletic horses do not regulate their salt intake according to need, at least not when offered salt from salt blocks.[23] It is therefore recommended to include salt and other electrolyte supplements in the ration.

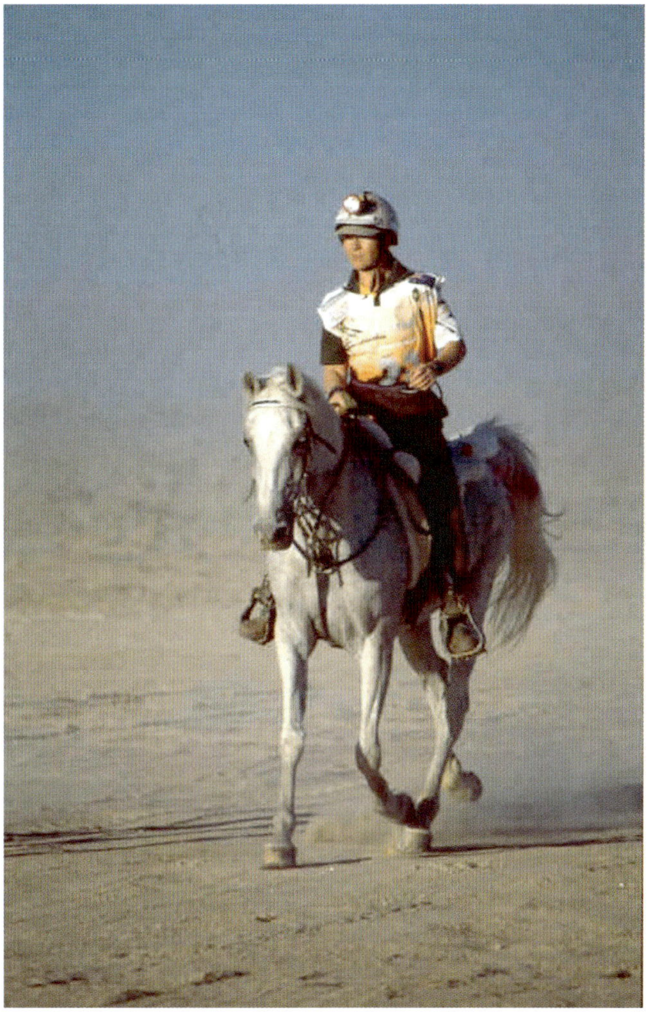

Fig 35.2 Endurance ride is a competition to test the speed and endurance ability of a horse. But equally important is the horsemanship of the rider so that he understands the physiology of the horse and can take care of him during a competition. Horse and rider approaching the first veterinary check point in good condition during the World Endurance Championship 1998 in the United Arab Emirates.

Photo by S. Hyyppä.

Electrolyte loading by feeding supplemental electrolytes for several days prior to competition is not effective because the kidneys readily excrete excess electrolytes within a few hours of administration. Nevertheless, electrolytes administered in the few hours immediately before a prolonged exercise competition may be of benefit if adequate water is also ingested (see Chapter 37).[9]

During the endurance ride, it is critical to give the horse a chance to drink as often as possible. Ideally, horses should be taught to drink electrolyte solutions because plain water, although better than nothing at all, is inadequate. Water intake without electrolyte replacement exacerbates dilution of sodium in the extracellular fluid such that the osmotic thirst stimulus is mitigated. An isotonic, polyionic electrolyte solution that replaces some of the electrolyte deficit is therefore more beneficial. Frequent sponging of the horse with cool water will assist in evaporative heat loss and cool the horse. However, riders should keep in mind that especially during warm and hot climatic conditions, even when a horse is a good drinker, it is impossible to compensate for all the losses during the ride. It is therefore important to monitor the horse very carefully and adjust the speed accordingly or retire from the ride if necessary.

In the endurance phase of a three-day event and in the marathon phase of combined driving, the sequence of the competitions does not allow for proper rehydration because the 10-minute rest occurs towards the end of the ride. It is unlikely that fluid consumed at this point will be absorbed in time to significantly assist rehydration and thus improve performance. On the contrary, if a large volume of fluid is given, the extra weight that the horse must carry could limit performance during the last part of the competition. Therefore, in hot weather, the best strategy is to use the rest periods to effectively cool the horse.

During the recovery period, the fullest restoration of fluid losses can be achieved by the inclusion of salts in the ration and by allowing free access to both isotonic electrolyte solution and water. Achieving complete replenishment of fluid and electrolytes is important because in the case of multiday rides, horses may fail to replenish bodyweight losses overnight and may enter the next day's competition with some degree of dehydration. A bodyweight deficit of 2% or more is thought to impair performance on the following day.[17]

Good veterinary supervision is vital to prevent horses from being overrridden by excessively ambitious riders. At vet gates, horses must be carefully monitored when deciding whether they are 'fit to continue'. Attending veterinarians should also be well prepared to handle any metabolic disorders and other problems that may occur. The availability of point-of-care blood analysis devices facilitates early recognition and treatment of clinicopathologic abnormalities.

Overtraining syndrome

- Overtraining syndrome is a syndrome of chronic fatigue and poor performance due to an imbalance between training and recovery.
- Overtraining syndrome should be suspected in horses with sustained decreased performance in association with one or more physiological, endocrine or psychological (behavioral) signs.
- Overtraining syndrome should not be diagnosed unless the poor performance remains after two weeks rest. Horses that recover during this period are said to have been overreached.
- Physiological signs in horses may include a decrease in bodyweight, elevated heart rates during exercise, lower plasma cortisol response to exercise, elevated muscle enzymes or gamma glutamyl transferase concentrations.
- Behavioral signs are a consistent and early marker of overtraining syndrome in longitudinal studies in horses.

Racehorse trainers have long used the terms 'overtraining', 'staleness' or 'sourness' to describe a syndrome of poor performance, failure to recover from exercise, and prolonged fatigue, but it has only been relatively recently that longitudinal studies in horses have shown that overtraining is a real and reproducible syndrome. Overtraining syndrome is a significant cause of poor athletic performance in horses, as it is in humans, although overtraining syndrome must be distinguished from overreaching, which may have some of the signs of overtraining syndrome including a reduction in performance. While overreaching is an acute maladaptation to an increased training load, taking only a short time for recovery (an average of two weeks), overtraining syndrome is a chronic condition that may require many weeks or months for a full recovery[24,25] or in some cases can be career ending.[26] (See Fig. 35.3.)

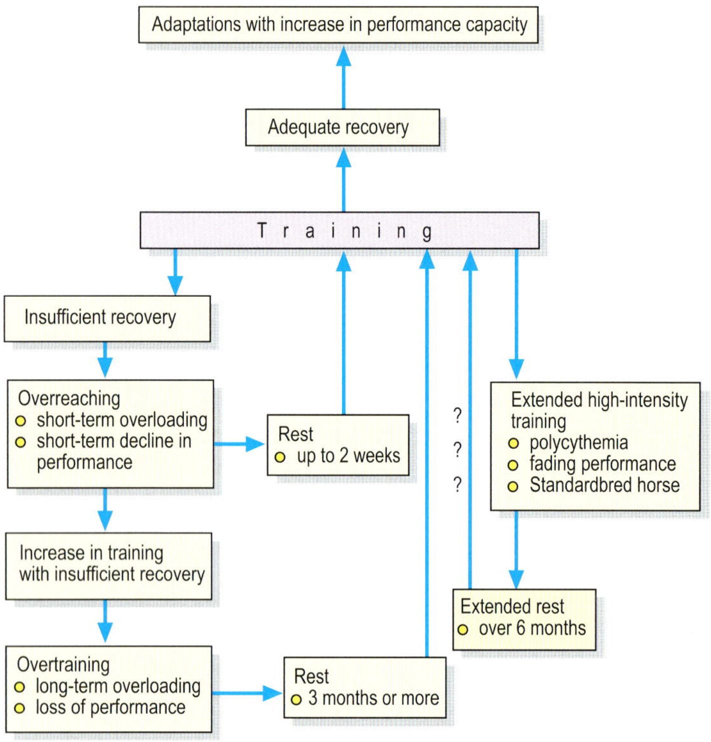

Fig 35.3 A balanced training program leads to adaptation and increase in performance capacity while an overly strenuous training load, with insufficient recovery between training sessions, may cause loss of performance. In Standardbred trotters, training-induced red cell hypervolemia may signal the end of a successful racing career.

Recognition

History and presenting complaint

Overtraining is a syndrome of poor performance and prolonged fatigue that does not resolve for weeks or months. By definition signs should persist after two or more weeks rest or reduced activity.[24,25] The main presenting complaint is evidence of sustained decreased performance, despite the maintenance of or an increase in training effort which cannot be explained by any discrete pathology. In addition there may be one or more physiological or psychological (behavioral) signs.[27–29]

Physical examination

Physical examination is usually unremarkable unless secondary or concurrent disease syndromes are present. No single physiological marker is able to identify the syndrome; however, many horses may display accompanying physiological, endocrine or behavioral signs as listed in Table 35.1.

Table 35.1 Signs of overtraining in horses which may accompany poor performance

Physiological signs
Decrease in bodyweight[27,30]
Elevated heart rates during exercise[27]
Elevated muscle enzymes[27,31]
Elevated gamma glutamyl transferase[31,32]
Subtle changes on hemogram/leukogram occurrence of illnesses[31]
Endocrine signs
Lower plasma cortisol response at rest or in response to exercise[33]
Altered overnight growth hormone pulsatile release[29]
Behavioral signs
Decreased interaction with other horses[34]
Unwillingness to train[27,28,35]
Sour/cranky/nervous behavior[27–29,36,37]

Bodyweight and heart rate

A decrease in bodyweight was found in longitudinal models of overtraining syndrome in Standardbred horses trained on the track or treadmill.[27,30] The decrease was small and only represented 10–15 kg bodyweight or around 3% of bodyweight on average and therefore required accurate electronic horse scales for diagnosis.

The decreased bodyweight is most likely to be linked to decreased muscle glycogen stores rather than altered feed intake. The training volumes required to induce overtraining may have interfered with complete glycogen resynthesis[38] as a decrease resting glycogen has been measured prior to training without alteration of the glycogen utilization.[39] Muscle glycogen increases muscle weight by increasing muscle water content.[40] Further, overtrained horses showed no alteration to feed intake or roughage concentrate ratio[31] or a greater severity of gastric ulceration[41] than control horses.

Overtrained horses have a significant decrease in the velocity at a heart rate of 200 beats per minute (V200), compared to control horses.[27,37]

Hematological findings

Leukograms have long been used as an indicator of stress in horses. Typically, a 'stress leukogram' consists of an elevated total leukocyte count, with a neutrophilia, lymphocytopenia and eosinopenia. Longitudinal studies have not shown typical stress leukograms in overtrained horses during the overtraining period.[31] However, both control and overtrained horses increased their neutrophil: lymphocyte ratio with training (relative percentages from 59 : 41–66 : 33 over 32 weeks). Overtrained horses showed a reduction in eosinophils to below normal range (reference range >0.1 × 10^9/L),[31] and individual horses that had clinical signs of illness showed an absolute eosinopenia. Thus, eosinopenia should not be ignored as an indicator of training stress.[32]

Red cell hypervolemia has been associated with chronic, naturally occurring overtraining syndrome in Swedish Standardbred Trotters, affecting mostly stallions.[26,36] See also Chapter 44. While this has not been seen in experimental models of overtraining in horses, these more acute experimental models may not be directly comparable to the situation in the field.[27,29,31,35]

Decreases in packed cell volume (PCV) or hematocrit have been frequently reported in horses with viral respiratory tract disease which may accompany overtraining. However, the actual decrease in red cell indices merely indicates the presence of disease and not a reduction in oxygen-carrying capacity.[42] The reduced PCV has been postulated to be due to reduced resting sympathetic activity and relatively more splenic sequestration of erythrocytes.[43]

Clinicopathological findings

Elevated serum activity of the muscle enzymes CK and AST may be present in overtrained horses in the absence of metabolic muscle disease as an indicator of cumulative subclinical muscle damage.[27,31] Increases in CK and AST are only mild to moderate (CK 523–1119 U/L, AST 647–4612 U/L).[31] Serial monitoring of serum biochemistry at a 2–4 week interval is often carried out during an equine training period, in which case AST is the better indicator of subclinical muscle damage due to its longer half-life (Fig. 35.4). While elevated AST may support a diagnosis of overtraining syndrome, it is not specific for the syndrome, but a similar increase in muscle enzymes has been seen in overreached rugby players and overtrained athletes.[44–45]

Gamma glutamyl transferase (GGT) is a liver enzyme that appears to be induced with training. Although the mechanism for induction is unclear, it may involve increased glycogen depletion and repletion during intense training (pers. comm. A. Lindholm). In Standardbred horses undergoing prolonged training and overtraining, prolonged training resulted in a linear increase in GGT with this

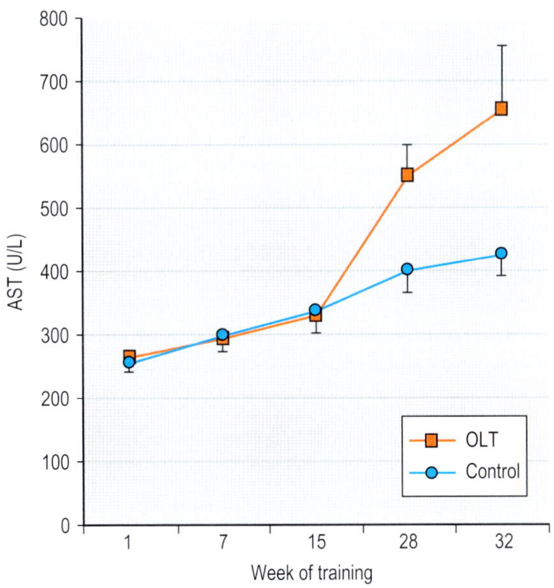

Fig 35.4 Changes in aspartate amino transferase (AST) through a 32-week training period. All horses completed the same training until week 16 where the Overload Training (OLT) group completed increasing intensity, frequency and duration of training until a performance decrement was observed (overtraining confirmed in week 34 after two weeks of rest) and Control group which continued a steadily increasing training program over the same period.[31]

increase being greater in overtrained horses.[31] GGT increased from a mean value of 14 U/L prior to training (after four months detraining) to a mean of 51 U/L in the control, and 70 U/L in overtrained horses after 32 weeks of training.[31] This increase in GGT in overtrained horses has also been described in some horses with poor performance where very high values of 100 U/L or more were detected and further – those horses with high GGT values showed a markedly reduced incidence of increased GGT following reduction in training intensity in subsequent years.[46,47]

Endocrine signs

A variety of endocrinological perturbations have been seen in overtrained horses, although neuroendocrine changes are less consistent in overtrained horses than humans and some changes are complex to measure in the clinical situation.

A reduced cortisol response to adrenocorticotropic hormone (ACTH) administration has been observed with overtraining syndrome and poor performance in Standardbreds, especially those horses with red cell hypervolemia[37] and certainly some racehorses may eventually develop adrenocortical exhaustion with prolonged training stress. However, again, this tends to be only seen in chronic field overtraining and has not occurred in experimental studies[33] where no reduction in cortisol response to administration of ACTH has been observed in overtrained compared to control horses.[33]

A decrease in the cortisol concentration has been measured after a maximal exercise test in acutely overtrained Standardbred pacers trained on the track[27] or treadmill.[33] The mean peak cortisol concentrations after intense treadmill exercise were 320 nmol/L before overtraining, and had decreased to 245 nmol/L when horses were overtrained.[33] However, as performance was also reduced in each instance, the cortisol measured most likely simply reflected the reduced overall work effort during the exercise period rather than a physiological variation associated with the syndrome.

Increased irregularity of nocturnal growth hormone (GH) pulsatility pattern indicative of a loss of coordinated control of GH regulation has been measured in overtrained Standardbreds.[29] This alteration in resting pulsatile growth hormone secretion is likely to represent an overall loss of coordination of the hypothalamic–growth hormone–insulin-like growth factor-1 axis. Monitoring the pattern of spontaneous GH secretion is labor-intensive and difficult, so further work to validate challenge tests using growth hormone releasing hormone to measure maximal GH secretory response or serum concentrations of IGF-1 and IGF-2 and their binding proteins as proxies of GH status is warranted.

Behavioral signs

In human athletes, profiles of mood state (POMS) are still considered one of the most sensitive indicators of overtraining.[48] Similarly in all the major studies on overtraining in horses, behavioral changes were observed[27–29,36,37] In the majority of studies, the main behavioral sign was irritability and an unwillingness to complete training. However, in one study, behavioral changes were described as manifest in a variety of ways, including in a not wanting to get on or off the treadmill, tossing their head while exercising, barging, pushing very hard against the front or back straps of the treadmill and sudden stopping when galloping on the treadmill.[31] A more recent study examined POMS using three assessments of behavior.[34] Horses were observed during treadmill training and using video surveillance in their stalls and during a standardized 'novel horse test'. Overtrained horses showed altered gait on the treadmill and reduced response to the novel horse test – both reduced interaction with the horse and reduced exploration of the arena and reduced response to the novel horse leaving.[34]

Diagnostic confirmation

A diagnosis of overtraining is dependent on the finding of a performance decrement accompanied by one or more physiological, endocrine or behavioral signs as mentioned above. It is important to have a thorough veterinary poor performance investigation to rule out clinical or subclinical disease which may have contributed to the development of overtraining, arisen secondary to overtraining or may be the primary problem. Overtraining due to subclinical disease versus disease secondary to overtraining may not be clearly distinguishable and deciding which the predominant problem is may not be simple. For example gastric ulceration or mild muscle pain may create stress to precipitate overtraining in a horse, but equally may arise as a result of overtraining. In all cases though, serial monitoring of hematology and biochemistry and good record keeping provide more information than samples taken after poor performance has developed. This will assist detection of subclinical disease and cumulative damage from training, which can be an early indicator of overtraining.

A diagnosis of overtraining cannot be reached until the decrement in performance has been shown to persist after two weeks of reduced training load. Any horses suspected of overtraining should immediately be taken out of training and given field rest or light exercise for two weeks.

If the horse was overreached, its performance should have improved during the two weeks, while if poor performance persists without evidence of or following resolution of clinical or subclinical disease, a diagnosis of overtraining is confirmed.

Treatment and prognosis

Therapeutic aims

The principal aims in treatment of overtraining are to maximize recovery time and reduce associated stresses. Overtraining will often result when additional stresses are added to an athlete's program.[49] Such stresses should be identified and eliminated and can include a monotonous training routine or social stresses. A horse in training is exposed to the stresses of intensive housing, absence of foraging, inability to exercise for most of the day and loss of its natural herd structure, all of which may contribute to external stresses in horses.[50] In addition, transport stress, and subclinical or low-grade disease, gastric ulceration, respiratory disease or lameness might occur, adding additional stresses that could precipitate overtraining syndrome. Sometimes the stresses may be inapparent, but a new trainer or environment can improve the performance.

As part of maximizing recovery, consideration should be made as to the intensity of the training program as more intense training is more likely to result in overtraining.[28] Further, consideration to the type of exercise and routine should be made. A horse that only exercises in the same direction on the track may respond to a more varied training routine which could include underwater treadmill/horse walker, flat work, or even small jumps or pole work. Quieter athletes may respond to hacking exercise.

Prognosis

The prognosis for return to athletic performance is guarded to poor if chronic overtraining is induced. In studies of overtraining in horses, performance improves with rest but had not returned to normal three months[30] and three years[26] after diagnosis. However, more acute overtraining and overreaching may respond in two weeks to three months.[27,34] This highlights the importance of monitoring, recognition and appropriate treatment before overtraining becomes chronic.

Etiology and pathophysiology

In elite human athletes, overload training techniques are commonly employed to optimize performance at the time of competition. This involves progressively increasing training loads followed by appropriate periods of reduced training or tapering prior to competition.[44,51] Such techniques are closely monitored by trainers and sports psychologists to ensure the athlete does not develop signs of overreaching or overtraining. Overtraining arises from an imbalance between training and recovery where the training stimulus is too great or the recovery too short, resulting in a syndrome of fatigue and poor performance usually accompanied by altered POMS and one or more other signs.[24,25,28,48,49]

While it was originally theorized that the principle of overload training was based on a positive period of physiological adaptation (or supercompensation) during the recovery phase, this has been shown to be less important than the reduction of accumulated fatigue associated with training.[51] The tapering period is more important to reduce the negative physical and psychological factors associated with training.[51] When overload training and tapering are poorly managed, overreaching manifest as a performance decrement can result.[44,48,49] If this is allowed to continue unchecked for a long period, overtraining syndrome can result.

The precipitating factor in overtraining is unaccounted for or new stresses in an athlete's life and can include emotional stress and anxiety as well as physical stress.[52] Sources of physical stress are not only limited to training but also include environmental temperature, altitude, improper nutrition and a monotonous routine.[52,53] Increases in the training volume and/or intensity can contribute to overtraining syndrome.[53]

The accumulation of these physical and psychological stresses without appropriate recovery periods can result is a state of prolonged fatigue, characterized by decreased or stagnant performance despite continued training which may be accompanied by dysfunction of a range of physiological and endocrine systems and altered mood states.[24,25,28,48,49] However, while these manifestations of overtraining syndrome are now better recognized, the pathophysiological mechanisms underlying the condition are still poorly understood. Overtraining syndrome may be the result of a chronic, systemic inflammatory response to exercise, principally due to repeated trauma or microtrauma to muscles, joints and connective tissues.[54,55] This supports the earlier work by Kibler et al.[45] who defined overtraining syndrome as a series of physiological, biomechanical and anatomical stresses that eventually cause either a relative, or an absolute, force overload on the musculotendinous unit. The theory of microtrauma is also supported by studies in human and equine athletes reporting elevated muscle enzymes in athletes with overtraining syndrome.[27,31,32,44,56] Such cytokines may be responsible for central actions resulting in 'sickness' type behavior patterns encouraging rest and recovery and altering endocrine and other physiological functions.[49,55] Systemic cytokine stimulation may also be responsible for some of the changes in immune function shown in overtrained athletes[49,57] with decreased IFN gamma function detected in fatigued athletes.[58] Overtraining syndrome has several parallels with chronic fatigue syndrome and clinical depression, in particular persistent fatigue, mood state disturbances, and muscle soreness.[59]

Epidemiology

Young horses at the beginning of their training are especially susceptible to overreaching when too much is attempted too soon. It may, however, also occur in well-trained horses if training is dramatically increased or the workout routine altered. Overtraining is primarily related to a sustained high training load, such as that undertaken by Standardbred and Thoroughbred racehorses. Both overreaching and overtraining are of importance in horses due to the potential frequency of overreaching as a result of short time frames and costs involved in getting a horse to the racetrack. This may be more likely where a horse has suffered an injury and has lost time in training as a result.

Prevention

Prevention of overtraining is important and one method of ensuring adequate recovery is tapering. A three-week cycle of linear reduction in training load while maintaining an equivalent training volume was shown to enhance performance in Standardbred racehorses compared to control horses that continued their usual program.[60] A new exercise program should begin slowly, with increases in intensity or duration of a workout schedule being accomplished gradually. As a general rule, to minimize the risk of overrreaching, horses should not perform the same type of strenuous conditioning exercise on consecutive days.

Increase in training load should be moderate, so that the horse has time to respond to the present load before any new requirement is imposed. Monotonous training should be avoided. After strenuous exercise, recovery is essential to allow time for training gains to take place and to permit further heavy work. Even when the training load is increased, the program for light exercise days should not be increased.

No two horses will react in the same to an equivalent exercise regimen. Each horse should therefore be monitored daily by measurement of resting heart rate and rectal temperature, by palpation of legs and muscles for swelling and soreness, by assessment of gait for any irregularities and by observance for any change in attitude or appetite. If any irregularities are noted, training volume should be reduced or a short rest period given. Adequate nutrition must be maintained.

With thanks to Seppo Hyyppa and A. Reeta Poso, who created the original chapter in the first edition.

References

1. Carlson GP. Thermoregulation, fluid and electrolyte balance. In: Snow DH, Persson SGB, Rose RJ, editors. Equine Exercise Physiology. Cambridge, UK: Granta Editions; 1983. p. 291–309.
2. Foreman JH. The exhausted horse syndrome. Vet Clin North Am Equine Pract 1998;14:205–19.
3. Whiting J. The exhausted horse. In: Robinson NE, Sprayberry K, editors. Current Therapy in Equine Medicine. 6th ed. Philadelphia, PA: W.B. Saunders Co.; 2009. p. 926–9.
4. Chapman DI, Haywood PE, Lloyd P. Occurrence of glucosuria in horses after strenuous exercise. Equine vet J 1981;13:259–60.
5. Schott HC II, Hodgson DR, Bayly WM. Haematuria, pigmenturia and proteinuria in exercising horses. Equine vet J 1995;27:67–72.
6. Kingston JK, Bayly WM. Effect of exercise on acid–base status of horses. Vet Clin North Am Equine Pract 1998;14:61–73.
7. Trigo P, Castejon F, Riber C, et al. Use of biochemical parameters to predict metabolic elimination in endurance rides. Equine vet J 2010;42(Suppl. 38): 142–6.
8. Sloet van Oldruitenborgh-Oosterbaan MM. The treatment of the exhausted horse under field conditions. Equine Pract 1994;16:27–33.
9. Sosa Leon LA. Treatment of exercise-induced dehydration. Vet Clin North Am Equine Pract 1998;14:159–73.
10. Geor RJ, McCutcheon LJ. Thermoregulatory adaptations associated with training and heat acclimation. Vet Clin North Am Equine Pract 1998;14:97–120.
11. Schott HC II, Hinchcliff KW. Treatments affecting fluid and electrolyte status during exercise. Vet Clin North Am Equine Pract 1998;14:175–204.
12. Fielding CL, Magdesian KG. A comparison of hypertonic (7.2%) and isotonic (0.9%) saline for fluid resuscitation in horses: a randomized, double-blinded, clinical trial. J Vet Intern Med 2011;25:1138–43.
13. Essen-Gustavsson B, Karlström K, Lindholm A. Fiber types, enzyme activities and substrate utilisation in skeletal muscle of horses competing in endurance rides. Equine vet J 1984;16:197–202.
14. Flaminio MJBF, Rush BR. Fluid and electrolyte balance in endurance horses. Vet Clin Equine Pract 1998;14:147–58.
15. White SL. Fluid, electrolyte, and acid–base balance in three-day, combined-training horses. Vet Clin North Am Equine Pract 1998;14:137–45.
16. Andrews FM, Ralston SL, Sommerdahl CS, et al. Weight, water, and cation losses in horses competing in three-day event. J Am Vet Med Assoc 1994;205:721–4.
17. Hyyppä S, Saastamoinen M, Pösö AR. Restoration of water and electrolyte balance in horses after repeated exercise in hot and humid conditions. Equine vet J 1996;22(Suppl):108–12.
18. Schott HC II, Hichcliff KW. Fluids, electrolytes, and bicarbonate. Vet Clin North Am Equine Pract 1993;9:577–604.
19. Marlin DJ, Harris PA, Schroter RC, et al. Physiological, metabolic and biochemical responses of horses competing in the speed and endurance phase of a CCI**** 3-day-event. Equine vet J 1995;20(Suppl):37–46.
20. White SL, Williamson LH, Maykuth PL, et al. Heart rate response and plasma lactate concentrations of horses competing in the cross-country phase of combined training events. Equine vet J 1995;20(Suppl):47–51.
21. Fielding CL, Meier CA, Balch OK, et al. Risk factors for elimination of endurance horses from competition. J Am Vet Med Assoc 2011;239:493–8.
22. Fielding CL, Magdesian KG, Rhodes DM, et al. Clinical and biochemical abnormalities in endurance horses eliminated from competition for medical complications and requiring emergency medical treatment: 30 cases (2005–2006). J Vet Emerg Vet Crit Care 2009;19:473–8.
23. Jansson A, Rytthammar A, Lindberg JE, et al. Voluntary salt (NaCl) intake in Standardbred horses. Pferdeheilkunde 1996;12:443–5.
24. Kuipers H, Keizer HA. Overtraining in elite athletes: review and directions for the future. Sports Med 1988;6:79–92.
25. Halson SL, Jeukendrup AE. Does overtraining exist? An analysis of overreaching and overtraining research. Sports Med 2004;34:967–81.
26. Persson SG, Osterberg I. Racing performance in red blood cell hypervolaemic standardbred trotters. Equine vet J Suppl 1999;30:617–20.
27. Hamlin MJ, Shearman JP, Hopkins WG. Changes in physiological parameters in overtrained Standardbred racehorses. Equine vet J 2002;34:383–8.
28. McGowan CM, Whitworth DJ. Overtraining syndrome in horses. Comp Exerc Physiol 2008;5:57–65.
29. De Graaf-Roelfsema E, Veldhuis PP, Keizer HA, et al. Overtrained horses alter their resting pulsatile growth hormone secretion. Am J Physiol Regul Integr Comp Physiol 2009;297: R403–11.
30. Tyler CM, Golland LC, Evans DL, et al. Changes in maximum oxygen uptake during prolonged training, overtraining and detraining in horses. J Appl Physiol 1996;81:2244–9.
31. Tyler-McGowan CM, Golland LC, Evans DL, et al. Haematological and

biochemical responses to training and overtraining. Equine vet J 1999;30(Suppl):621–5.

32. McGowan C. Clinical pathology in the racing horse: the role of clinical pathology in assessing fitness and performance in the racehorse. Vet Clin North Am Equine Pract 2008;24:405–21
33. Golland LC, Evans DL, Stone GM, et al. Plasma cortisol and β-endorphin concentrations in trained and over-trained Standardbred racehorses. Pflugers Arch 1999;439:11–17.
34. De Graaf-Roelfsema E. Endocrinological ad behavioural adaptations to experimentally induced physical stress in horses. Dissertation, Utrecht University, Faculty of Veterinary Medicine; 2007. p. 168–8.
35. Bruin G, Kuipers H, Keizer HA, et al. Adaptation and overtraining in horses subjected to increasing training loads. J Appl Physiol 1994;76:1908–13.
36. Persson SGB. On blood volume and working capacity of horses. Acta Vet Scand 1967;19(Suppl):1–189.
37. Persson SGB, Larsson M, Lindholm A. Effects of training on adrenal-cortical function and red-cell volume in trotters. Zentrabl Veterinarmed A 1980;27:261–8.
38. Bröjer J, Holm S, Jonasson R, et al. Synthesis of proglycogen and macroglycogen in skeletal muscle of standardbred trotters after intermittent exercise. Equine vet J 2006;36(Suppl): 335–9.
39. McGowan CM, Golland LC, Evans DL, et al. Effects of prolonged training, overtraining and detraining on skeletal muscle metabolites and enzymes. Equine vet J 2002;34:257–63.
40. Olsson KE, Saltin B. Variation in total body water with muscle glycogen changes in man. Acta Physiol Scand 1970;80:11–18.
41. De Graaf-Roelfsema E, Keizer HA, Wijnberg ID, et al. The incidence and severity of gastric ulceration does not increase in overtrained Standardbred horses. Equine vet J 2010;38(Suppl):58–61.
42. Carlson GP. Haematology and body fluids in the equine athlete: a review. In: Gillespie JR, Robinson NE, editors. Equine Exercise Physiology 2. Davis, California: ICEPP Publications; 1987. p. 393–425.
43. Rose RJ, Allen JR. Hematologic responses to exercise and training. Vet Clin North Am Equine Pract 1985;1:461–76.
44. Coutts A, Reaburn P, Piva TJ, et al. Changes in selected biochemical, muscular strength, power, and endurance measures during deliberate overreaching and tapering in rugby league players. Int J Sports Med 2007;28:116–24.
45. Kibler WB, Chandler TJ, Stracener ES. Musculoskeletal adaptations and injuries due to overtraining. In: Holloszy JD, editor. American College of Sports Medicine Series: Exercise and Sport Sciences Reviews, Vol. 20. Baltimore: Williams and Wilkins; 1992. p. 99–126.
46. Snow DH, Gash SP, Rice D. Field observations on selenium status, whole blood glutathione peroxidise and plasma gamma-glamyl transferase activities in Thoroughbred racehorses. In: Gillespie JR, Robinson NE, editors. Equine Exercise Physiology 2. Davis, California: ICEPP Publications; 1987. p. 494–505.
47. Snow DH, Harris P. Enzymes as markers of physical fitness and training of racing horses. Adv Clin Enzymol 1988;6: 251–8
48. Urhausen A, Kindermann W. Diagnosis of overtraining: what tools do we have? Sports Med 2002;32:95–102.
49. MacKinnon LT. Special feature for the Olympics: effects of exercise on the immune system: overtraining effects on immunity and performance in athletes. Immunol Cell Biol 2000;78:502–9.
50. Henderson AJ. Don't fence me in: managing psychological well being for elite performance horses. J Appl Anim Welf Sci 2007;10:309–29.
51. Mujika I, Padilla S. Scientific bases for precompetition tapering strategies. Med Sci Sports Exerc 2003;35:1182–7.
52. Costill DL. Peaking for performance. In: Inside Running. Indiananapolis: Benchmark Press; 1986. p. 123–34.
53. Hooper SL, MacKinnon LT, Howard A, et al. Markers for monitoring overtraining and recovery. Med Sci Sports Exerc 1995;27:106–12.
54. Smith LL. Cytokine hypothesis of overtraining: a physiological adaptation to excessive stress? Med Sci Sports Exerc 2000;32:317–31.
55. Smith LL. Tissue trauma: the underlying cause of overtraining syndrome? J Strength Cond Res 2004;18:185–93.
56. Fry AC, Kraemer WJ, van Borselen F, et al. Performance decrements with high-intensity resistance exercise overtraining. Med Sci Sports Exerc 1994;26:1165–73.
57. Mackinnon LT, Hooper SL, Jones S, et al. Hormonal, immunological, and hematological responses to intensified training in elite swimmers. Med Sci Sports Exerc 1997;29:1637–45.
58. Clancy RL, Gleeson M, Cox A, et al. Reversal in fatigued athletes of a defect in interferon gamma secretion after administration of *Lactobacillus acidophilus*. Br J Sports Med 2006;40:351–4.
59. Shephard RJ. Chronic fatigue syndrome: an update. Sports Med 2001;31:167–94.
60. Shearman JP, Hamlin MJ, Hopkins WG. Effect of tapered normal and interval training on performance of Standardbred pacers. Equine vet J 2002;34:395–9.

Nutrition for the equine athlete: nutrient requirements and key principles in ration design

36

Patricia A. Harris Raymond J. Geor

CHAPTER CONTENTS

Introduction

Although nutritional management (i.e. diet composition, feeding management) will not improve the intrinsic ability of a horse, a sound nutritional program enables the horse to train and compete to its athletic potential. Poor or inappropriate nutrition, on the other hand, may impose limits on the animal's ability to perform. Appropriate nutritional management goes beyond the provision of a ration that meets basic nutrient and energy requirements (for maintenance of bodyweight, etc.) to consider how the type and amount of nutrients provided can help optimize individual performance, maintain health and help reduce the risk of disease. For any athletic horse, the primary goals of nutritional management therefore should include:

- provision of substrates for maintenance of bodyweight and replenishment of energy reserves in working muscle and other tissues
- promotion of tissue adaptation, growth and repair
- promotion of general health and well-being
- application of competition feeding strategies appropriate to the athletic task.

This chapter provides an overview of the nutrient requirements of athletic horses and also discusses key aspects to consider in the development of an appropriate ration. Given the large array of equestrian disciplines and circumstances, it is not feasible to make specific feeding recommendations (i.e. diet recipes). Also beyond the scope of this chapter is discussion on nutrition during growth (i.e. from gestation to adulthood), which is clearly fundamental to the development of a horse that is athletically sound.

What nutrients does an athletic horse need?

As for all animals, athletic horses require an adequate and balanced intake of energy, protein, vitamins, minerals (macro and micro) and water in order to support health and activity. The background details to why and how these nutritional components are digested, utilized and stored can be found elsewhere;[1,2] the focus of this chapter is to place this information into the context of feeding management for the athletic horse. A summary of the nutrients required and some specific comments with respect to the exercising horse are given in Table 36.1.

Building a ration for an individual horse

The feeding program for an individual animal will depend on many factors including temperament, level of training and competition, age, owner/rider preference, housing and feedstuffs available. Nonetheless, in designing a ration, the first thing to consider is the energy requirement and how this will be provided.

Which units and requirements to use?

Globally, several different feeding systems (e.g. NRC, INRA, GEH) and units (e.g. digestible vs. net energy) are used for the description of energy and nutrient requirements.[3,4] Requirements can be expressed as a function of actual bodyweight or on the basis of metabolic bodyweight (typically $BW^{0.75}$) and also quantified on either an *'as fed'* (actual feed weight that includes water content) or *'dry matter'* (the weight of feed after removal of moisture) basis. Most concentrate feeds such as cereal grains, cubes, pellets, etc., contain around 10% moisture with a dry matter content therefore of ~88–92%, whilst the water content of preserved forage typically

Table 36.1 Guide to the nutrient requirements for a 500-kg athletic horse as well as typical nutrient concentrations in some common feedstuffs ('As fed basis' unless otherwise stated). Due to marked variations due to cultivar, processing, etc., these data only represent the average nutrient content of feedstuffs. Requirements need to be adapted to the individual circumstances

NUTRIENT	REQUIREMENTS BASED ON NRC 2007 (VALUES IN PARENTHESIS REPRESENT THE AUTHORS' CURRENT RECOMMENDATIONS)	HIGH SOURCE	MODERATE SOURCE	LOW SOURCE	COMMENTS
Energy – Is not a nutrient per se Units MJ or Mcal I Mcal = 4.184 MJ	DE: Based on one of 4 levels of exercise: 20–34.5 Mcal (Base on NRC but adapt to the individual)	Vegetable oils ~35 MJ/Kg as fed	Oats ~10–12 MJ/kg Barley ~13 MJ/kg Corn ~14 MJ/kg Mature grass hays ~6–12 MJ/kg	Wheat straw ~6 MJ/kg Rice hulls ~2 MJ/kg	*Essential to all cellular functions.* Important to consider source of energy as well as quantity. Base intake on previous diet or NRC and then adapt to the individual. Need to continue to monitor (body condition, behavior, etc.) as requirements will change with environmental conditions, availability of grass during any turnout, nature of the forage, body condition, etc.
Protein – Expressed as crude protein (CP) or digestible protein (DP varies from ~40 to 80% CP)	699–1004 g (750–1500 g)	Oil seed meals ~22% sunflower seeds whole ~45% soyabean meal	Alfalfa hay ~15–20%	Grass hays ~8% Grains variable and influenced by growing conditions ~6–12%	*Maintaining building and repairing body tissues.* Too little and too much protein may be detrimental to performance. Especially with higher amounts need to ensure adequate water intake and good stable hygiene
Amino acids e.g. Lysine: an essential amino acid which must be provided by the diet as cannot be made by the horse	30–43 g (30–50: allow up to 0.1 g/kg BW in hard/intensive work). Threonine possibly 80% of the lysine level	Soyabean meal ~28 g/kg lysine ~20 g/kg threonine ~6 g/kg methionine	Linseed ~12 g/kg lysine ~11 g/kg threonine ~4 g/kg methionine	Cereals ~2–3 g/kg lysine Grass /cereal hay <2 g/kg lysine	*Protein quality*. i.e. Amino acid profile may be more important than total protein intake. Lysine is thought to be the first limiting amino acid in typical horse rations and if the lysine requirement is met, unless synthetic amino acids are used to supplement the diet, then it is believed the requirement for other amino acids will most likely be met. Requirements for the other amino acids have not been established for the horse
Fats/fatty acids *There may be a need for certain fatty acids such as linoleic acid but actual amount required*	(Up to 1 ml/kg BW without additional nutritional advice but around 5–10% of the diet may be advantageous for some performance animals)	Vegetable oils ~99%. Corn oil/soy oil more commonly used. *Possible advantage of including some*	Whole oil seeds ~20% Rice brans ~25%	Grains ~1–3% Hays ~2% Beans ~1%	*Concentrated starch free source of energy.* Add gradually, consider the vitamin (esp. vit E) and mineral balance of the final diet. Only use fresh non-rancid oils. Fatty acid profile may be important but not known for the

	amount is controversial and needs to be adapted to the individual and take into account core ration – especially for endurance horses	can be high from ~20–50 g/kg			but for those in harder work higher levels may be required. Authors' current general advice is to provide reasonable levels in the core daily diet and then provide during / immediate post competition ~1/3 of estimated losses but this needs to be adapted to individual circumstances. Continue with a fortified diet post exercise
Potassium – K Mineral Electrolyte	28.5–53 g: NB may be higher if undergoing prolonged endurance work (minimum of 35 + at least 0.5 g/L sweat)	Sugar beet molasses – variable ~10–35 g/kg KCl ~ 14 g/28 g or ounce	Forages ~15–25 g/kg – in hay	Grains <5 g/kg	*Major intracellular cation essential for normal cellular function including heart and muscle.* Potential risk of a reduced or even deficient intake when on low forage intakes, especially if the forage fed is haylage/silage
Chloride – Cl Mineral Electrolyte	47–93 g (40 + ~3 g/L sweat)	Salt ~17 g Cl /28 g or ounce	Sugar beet mollases ~10 g Cl/kg DM	Cereals ~<1 g/kg DM salt ~0.6 g Cl/kg	*Closely interrelated to sodium plus osmotic pressure*
Calcium – Ca Mineral Electrolyte	30–40 g (45 g + 0.2 g/kg sweat loss)	Limestone flour (~40% Ca – 400 g/kg)	Legumes e.g. alfalfa ~1.2% Sugar beet pulp ~0.6% (DM basis)	Cereals ~0.15% some very low less than 1 g/kg	*Bone formation, nerve and muscle function, blood clotting, etc.* May need to provide higher amounts when first go into training and and during 'lay off' periods
Phosphorus – P Mineral Electrolyte	18–29 g (25–30+ in proportion with the Ca intake)	Dicalcium phosphate ~23% Ca and 18% P	NB high content in most cereal brans (~11 g/kg) but due to high phytate level limited bioavailability estimated ~2 g/kg Legume hays ~2 g/kg	Cereals (0.3–0.6% P) NB still high relative to Ca content	*Bone formation, energy metabolism, essential component of cell membranes.* Ratio of Ca: P may be as important as total amount – aim for a ratio of Ca : P between 1.5 and 2.1. Potentially need to provide higher amounts when first go into training (e.g. 35 g/500 kg horse)

Continued

Table 36.1 Continued

NUTRIENT	REQUIREMENTS BASED ON NRC 2007 (VALUES IN PARENTHESIS REPRESENT THE AUTHORS' CURRENT RECOMMENDATIONS)	HIGH SOURCE	MODERATE SOURCE	LOW SOURCE	COMMENTS
Magnesium – Mg Mineral Electrolyte	9–5 – 15 g (15 g + 0.125 g/kg sweat loss)	Rice brans ~0.9% Wheat bran ~0.55% Canola seeds ~0.55%	Sugar beet molasses ~0 23% Oil seeds ~0.3%	Timothy mature hay ~0.08% Oats ~0.8%	*Bone, muscle contraction, metabolism.* Claims for behavior-modifying effect when fed in moderately increased amounts have not been confirmed but large amounts given iv will be sedative. Availability from synthetic sources will be highly variable – i.e. low from MgO and higher from sources such as magnesium aspartate
Copper – Cu Micromineral	100–125 mg (125–175 mg)	Synthetic sources Molasses can be ~50 mg/kg	Legume hays ~10–16 mg/kg Some cereals may have ~10 mg/kg	Many cereals and hays <4 mg/kg	*Cofactor for many enzymes associated with energy metabolism collagen and elastin synthesis – bone formation, immunity.* Copper to Zn ratio in the diet may be important – current advice is to try to maintain around 3.5–4.5 : 1. Authors' advice is not >33% of the intake comes from chelated sources
Zinc – Zn Micromineral	400–500 mg (500–700 mg)	Synthetic sources Inorganic sources	Synthetic sources Chelates and bioplexes Full-fat soya ~50 mg/kg	Legume hays and cereals ~20–25 mg/kg	*Component of many metalloenzymes involved in protein and carbohydrate metabolism, important to several hormones including insulin, immunity.* Authors' advice is not >33% of the intake comes from chelated sources
Manganese – Mn Micromineral	400–500 mg (500–700 mg)	Synthetic sources	Legume hays ~30–60 mg/kg Oats can be high 35 mg/kg or low	Grass hays Corn ~5 mg/kg Barley intermediate	*Cartilage (formation chondroitin sulfate) Metabolism* Authors' advice is not >33% of the intake comes from chelated sources
Iron – Fe Micromineral	400–500 mg (500–625 mg)	Inorganic supplements Oaten chaff ~350 mg/kg	Legume hays 140–210 mg/kg Cereals <100 mg/kg		*Incorporated into hemoglobin, myoglobin, certain enzymes; oxygen transfer; metabolism.*

4% cobalt				low ~0.05 mg/kg	
Selenium – Se Micromineral	1–1.25 mg (2–3 mg)	Synthetic sources Certain selenium accumulating plants	Selenium yeast	Cereals and hays – but variable some plant species can have very high levels. Cereals <0.2 mg/kg	*Part of the cellular antioxidant defeness.* Toxicity can occur. Recommended not more that 1 mg/100 kg BW, i.e. <5 mg/500 kg horse
Iodine – I Micro-mineral	3.5–4.4 mg (2–3 mg)	Seaweed meal Iodized salt Potassium iodate	Legume hay ~0.15 mg/kg	Cereals usually <0.1 mg/kg	*Essential component of thyroid hormones.* Very difficult to assess iodine levels from organic materials. Seaweeds contain very variable and sometimes high levels of iodine
Vitamin A – fat soluble Main source is β-carotene from green herbage. Toxicity is unlikely to result from high intakes of β-carotene as the horse is thought able to reduce the conversion of β-carotene to vitamin A	22 500 iu (50 000 iu as mix Vit A and β carotene)	Leafy green plants Vitamin A equivalents ~200 000 iu/kg but will vary with plant maturity, season, etc. Cod liver oil ~200 000 iu/20 ml Different synthetic sources may have different availabilities	Yellow maize ~2000 iu/kg Legume hays early stage 50 000 iu/kg	'Aged' preserved forages – rapid loss in cured hays Oats <500 iu/kg Barley <1000 iu/kg	*Normal growth, vision, maintenance of skin and epithelial tissue, support for infection resistance.* Requirements for exercising horses in the literature vary between ~45 and 200 iu/kg BW – the authors' currently recommenc a more optimal intake level of 100 iu/kg BW
Vitamin D A hormone Fat soluble Synthesized in skin under exposure to sunlight	3300 iu (5000 iu)	Action of sunlight on the skin Synthetic sources Cod liver oil ~2000 iu/20 ml	Sun-cured forages Alfalfa hay ~1500 iu/kg	Little or none in cereals & preserved aged forages	*Normal bone growth. Believed involvement in Ca metabolism may not be as great under normal conditions as in other species.* Currently levels between 5 and 13 iu/kg BW suggested for exercising animals. The authors' recommend around 10 iu/kg BW. Higher levels may be required for stabled animals and young animals entering training; BUT toxicity possible. Recent research into Vit D in other species suggests has a much broader role in immunity, metabolism, etc.

Continued

Table 36.1 Continued

NUTRIENT	REQUIREMENTS BASED ON NRC 2007 (VALUES IN PARENTHESIS REPRESENT THE AUTHORS' CURRENT RECOMMENDATIONS)	HIGH SOURCE	MODERATE SOURCE	LOW SOURCE	COMMENTS
Vitamin E Fat soluble 1 mg ~ 1 iu	800–1000 iu (1500–2500 iu – plus 1–2 iu/ml of additional oil)	Synthetic or natural concentrated tocopherols. Supplementation most beneficial if given orally daily	Oils of some grain seeds e.g. wheat germ 2.1 mg/20 ml Green forage 100–450 iu/kg	Cereals <30 iu/kg Alfalfa hay 10–30 iu/kg Haylage and hay levels may be very low	*Antioxidant, normal muscle metabolism, promotes immune function.* Higher intakes may be advantageous re the oxidative stress and immunity challenges associated with exercise. Levels in the literature typically vary from 1.5 to 5 mg/kg BW but as high as 11 mg have been suggested. The authors' recommend from 3 to 5 mg/kg BW depending on work load plus 1–2 iu/ml additional oil depending on the oil and the background level of Vit E in the oil. Recommend other than for specific clinical reasons not >10 iu/kg BW
Vitamin K Fat soluble Synthesized by intestinal bacteria and sourced from good-quality hay and pasture	Unknown	Synthetic sources Some suggestion that certain synthetic sources (e.g. injectable menadione) may have increased toxicity	Most forages and hays are thought to be adequate sources		*Blood clotting/bonemetabolism.* Typically thought not to be required in the diet as synthesized in hind gut. Whether additional Vit K is required on top of a forage-based diet has not been proven but some recent work suggests that it may not be as bioavailable from forage as previously thought and supplementation may be of value for young growing /exercising animals
Thiamine Vitamin B_1 Water soluble S	30–62.5 mg (60–65 mg)	Brewers' and bakers' yeast contain 150–160 mg/kg. Yeast is a good source of thiamine as well as other B	Cereal by-products 10–15 mg/kg if contain the scutellum and germ which s rich in thiamine	Legume hays ~3 mg/kg Cereals ~5 mg/kg Hays 0.2–4.5 mg/kg DM	*Growth, energy production, nerve function.* In the literature 0.07–0.13 mg/kg BW/day have been suggested. Potential for increased requirements in animals with reduced appetite or reduced forage intake depending on the core ration

		kg dried yeast	Wheat bran ~0.4 mg/kg		Suggested that 2–3 mg/100 kg BW/day required to maintain healthy hooves and 3–5 mg/100 kg BW to improve hoof quality or for those with hoof problems. NB not all hoof problems respond to biotin supplementation. Response may take up to 9 months or more to have an effect, if at all
Folic acid	Unknown	Brewers' yeast (10–15 mg/kg) Synthesized by bacteria in the GIT	Wheat bran 0.8–1.8 mg/kg Alfalfa meal dehydrated ~1.6 mg/kg Rice bran ~1.6 mg/kg	Cereal grains variable ~0.1–0.6 mg/kg	*Associated with vitamin B_{12} and blood cell production.* Increased erythropoiesis during training may increase requirements of folate to support the cell turnover. Serum concentrations may be reduced in hard working/stabled animals. Intakes of 0.012–0.043 mg/kg BW suggested in the literature
Vitamin C Ascorbic acid Water soluble Synthesized in the liver	(5 g – respiratory support)	Manufactured within body – absorption from synthetic sources not always good and individually variable	Pasture contains variable amounts		*Formation of cartilage and bone, antioxidant, Immune system and wound healing.* Additional vitamin C may be of value in certain conditions, e.g., infections, 'stress' especially respiratory challenge. Levels of 30–40 mg/kg BW have been recommended in such instances. The authors' currently recommend ~1 g/100 kg BW for exercising or stabled animals (of a stable bioavailable form). Advise that vitamin C supplementation should not be stopped abruptly

Adapted from Harris PA (2013) Nutrition in Equine Veterinary Nursing Manual Coumbe K (ed) with kind permission from John Wiley & Sons Ltd.[88]

ranges between 10 and 50%. It is important to be aware of these differences – a single system should be chosen and consistently applied when evaluating or developing an equine ration.

Calculation of energy requirements

In the UK and USA energy requirements for athletic horses are most commonly expressed as megacalories (Mcal – USA) or megajoules (MJ – UK) of digestible energy (DE), where 1 Mcal = 4.184 MJ. Energy requirements are the sum of maintenance requirements plus an allowance for the work being undertaken and will depend not only on work duration and intensity but also the environmental conditions, terrain, weight of the rider and tack, ability of the rider, and fitness of the horse, etc.[3] Two primary approaches can be used to estimate energy requirements:[3,4]

- *Categorization of workload:* The *NRC Nutrient Requirements for Horses* uses the work categories of light, moderate, heavy and very heavy exercise to estimate DE requirements (e.g. NRC 2007). For *light work* (e.g. horses at the start of a training program), the DE requirements in Mcal/day are stated as (0.0333 × BW) × 1.20, whereas for *very heavy work* (e.g. all racing animals and elite three-day event horses) the requirements are given as (0.0363 × BW) × 1.9. These estimates do not take into account different training and exercise workloads for different animals and disciplines.[5] Nonetheless, surveys of racehorse trainers have indicated that these estimates compare favorably with feeding practices.[6–8]
- *Individual estimate of workload:* A second approach is to base requirements on some measure of the *individual work load,* usually running speed e.g. DE (kJ per kilogram of horse, rider and tack) = $4.184 \times \{[e^{(3.02 + 0.0065Y)} - 13.92] \times 0.06\}/0.57$ where Y is running speed (meters per minute) and 0.57 accounts for the efficiency of utilization of DE.[9] This method also does not take into account fitness, jumping efforts, environmental conditions, etc.

An alternative approach is to base DE requirements on the horse's *current diet,* bearing in mind that laboratory analysis of feed samples are needed for reasonably accurate assessment of DE content. Regardless of the method used, it is important to realize that these estimates only provide a starting point for ration development; regular assessment of body weight and condition will inform the need for adjustments in DE provision. Underfeeding of DE in relation to workload, etc., will result in weight loss, lethargy and poor performance, while horses provided too much DE will gain weight and may become hyperactive.[3,10]

The relationship between body fatness, fat free mass (FFM) and running performance has not been studied in great detail in the horse. Ultrasound-measured depth of subcutaneous fat over the rump was used to estimate percentage body fat and FFM, and then examine the relationship of these variables with maximum aerobic capacity (VO_{2max}) and running performance.[11–13] Both sprint and endurance performance were inversely correlated with estimated body fat in these studies; however, it should be recognized that measurement of rump fat depth has not been fully validated for estimation of body fat and FFM in the horse.[14] The concept of optimal BW has been proposed for racehorses; Lim[15] reported that race performance was negatively affected by deviations >1.5% from optimal BW, with performance less affected by the horse being overweight as compared to being underweight. The amount of energy needed for athletic activity is directly related to the weight being moved (horse, rider and tack) as well as the speed of running, the incline, jump efforts, etc.[16] Therefore, a change in total weight will affect the energy cost of locomotion. The addition of a 10% load to horses exercising on a horizontal treadmill increased oxygen consumption by 15%,[17] the administration of furosemide resulted in decreased anaerobic energy expenditure during brief high-intensity work at least in part due to an acute BW reduction.[18]

For endurance-type events (e.g. endurance racing, three-day event), being 'thin' (i.e. body condition score, BCS ≤ 3/9) might be a disadvantage because of lower energy reserves (and potentially lower muscle mass) when compared to a higher BCS. Over-conditioning (BCS ≥ 6/9) also could adversely affect performance due to the insulating effects (and potential impairment to heat dissipation) of excess subcutaneous adipose tissue. For most athletic activities, therefore, a BCS of 4–5 should be targeted and monitored regularly, with DE intake adjusted as needed. The authors recommend use of the Henneke BCS system[19] as modified by Kohnke.[20]

Sources of dietary energy

Energy is supplied to the horse via the diet but fundamentally energy is not a nutrient. The chemical energy or gross energy contained within feeds needs to be converted into a form of energy that the cells can use for mechanical work or movement (useable or net energy, NE). The feedstuffs commonly provided to the horse can be divided into forages, cereals (and their by-products), vegetable oils, primary protein sources, vitamin/mineral supplements and other additives. 'Sweet feeds/concentrates' are commercially manufactured mixtures of these core feedstuffs (but do not typically include forage although recently fiber mixes have entered the feed market and combine specific fiber components, including chopped preserved forage, with the added nutrition of a concentrate feed). Different feeds contain varying amounts of the four potential sources of dietary energy:

- *hydrolysable carbohydrates,* e.g. simple sugars and starch
- *fermentable fibers,* a component of dietary fiber, e.g., cellulose, pectins, hemicelluloses
- *oils/fats*
- *protein* (note, however, that protein should not be included in the ration as an energy source).

Figure 36.1 is a schematic that depicts how energy is provided to the horse by the three principal dietary sources. The efficiency conversion of these energy sources into useable or NE varies considerably.[3,21] In general, cereals provide more NE than hay, and hay provides more than twice the NE of straw. Vegetable oils contain proportionally more energy than cereals (~2.5 times as much DE as maize/corn and three times as much as oats). The art and science of feeding the performance horse depends to a large extent on the relative proportions of the energy sources provided to the horse and the feedstuffs used. Different athletic disciplines will require different strategies, e.g. the provision of a high-fiber, roughage-based diet may be advantageous to an endurance horse as it is likely to provide an ongoing supply of energy during a race. Additionally, this type of ration is thought to increase the size of the fluid and electrolyte reservoir in the hindgut (which may help offset sweat fluid losses during exercise). However, excess gut fill may be energetically disadvantageous during high-intensity, short-duration exercise. Nonetheless, forage provision should be the starting point in designing any ration for an athletic horse.

Forage

As non-ruminant herbivores, horses are well adapted to eating high-fiber feedstuffs that undergo microbial fermentation primarily within the caecum and colon with production of short-chain or volatile fatty acids (SCFA). The SCFA propionic acid is an important precursor for gluconeogenesis, acetate is important in the production and storage of long-chain fatty acids, while butyrate is a primary energy source for the hindgut mucosa.[22,23] The inclusion of some long-stem forage in the diet is thought to be important for maintenance of hindgut function and health, and also may reduce risk of gastric ulceration and abnormal behaviors.[24] The continual fermentation and absorption of SCFA (predominately acetate and propionate) *also* means that fiber can provide ongoing energy during prolonged exercise.

Most equine feedstuffs contain some fiber but forage is the primary source. For most horses, the daily forage intake will be based around fresh or dried/preserved 'grass'. Preserved forages should be as free as possible of contaminants such as molds. Hay that is baled at high moisture content is likely to heat and become heavily contaminated with molds that can exacerbate chronic airway diseases such as recurrent airway obstruction and inflammatory airway disease. In areas with high rainfall during the growing and haymaking season (e.g. the UK), the feeding of ensiled hay or 'haylage' is increasingly practiced. Haylage can be a suitable alternative to hay providing that it is stored correctly and fed in sufficient quantity to ensure adequate fiber intake. One concern with especially large bale haylage is the potential for clostridial growth and production of botulinum toxin.[25] Haylage, unlike properly made silage, can still have a high WSC content (average 21% in a recent UK survey – Briars, personal communication 2013) and nutritionally very variable. Haylage should be examined carefully for the presence of mold and other contaminants before feeding, and sealed haylage bales should be fed within a few days of opening. Recently, there has been increased use of small hay-bale steamers that significantly reduce the fungal spore count of the hay.[26] Comments on the main types of preserved forage are provided in Table 36.2.

Although several factors can affect the nutrient value of conserved forages, the most important is the stage of maturity at the time of harvest (Fig. 36.2). The energy content, digestibility and palatability of forage all decrease with increasing maturity. Therefore, forages harvested at an early stage of plant maturity should be fed to working horses to maximize nutritional value and intake of the offered quantities. This will also help reduce the amount of fecal bulk and therefore gut fill. An exception to this recommendation is the feeding of a very high-quality alfalfa, which may not contain adequate fiber (specifically, acid detergent fiber [ADF]) to support hindgut function. Figure 36.3 illustrates how the energy content of the forage affects the relative proportions of forage and energy concentrates required to meet the energy needs of an athletic horse.

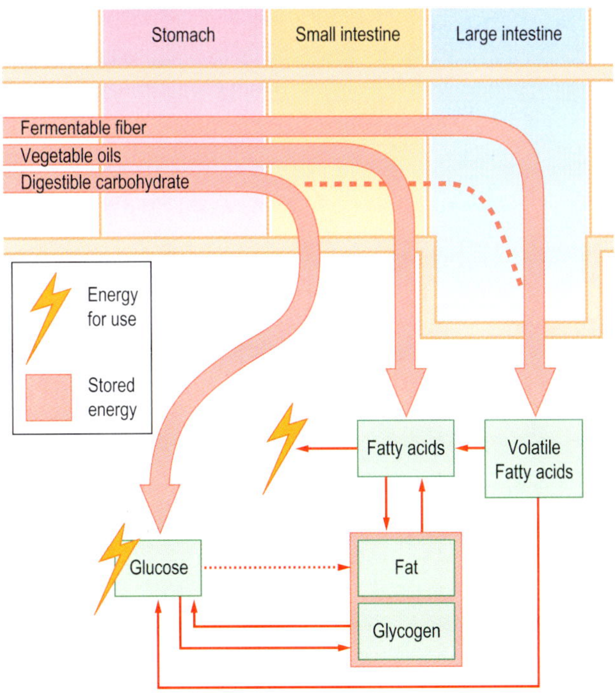

Fig 36.1 Schematic of the absorption and processing of the three main dietary energy sources in the horse.
Reproduced with kind permission from Mars HorseCare (UK) Ltd.

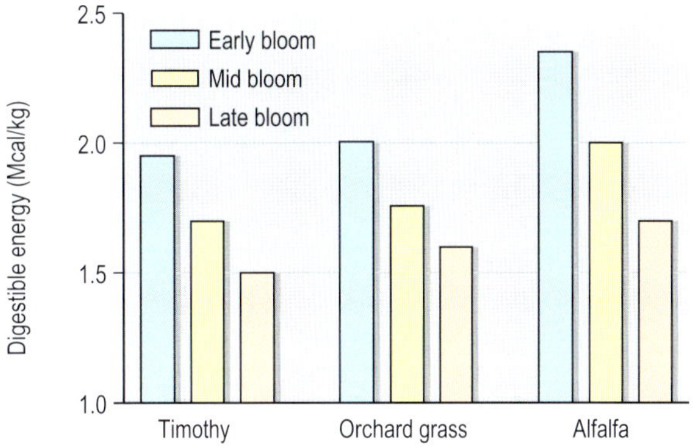

Fig 36.2 The effects of maturity at the time of harvest on estimated digestible energy content of timothy, orchard grass and alfalfa hay.

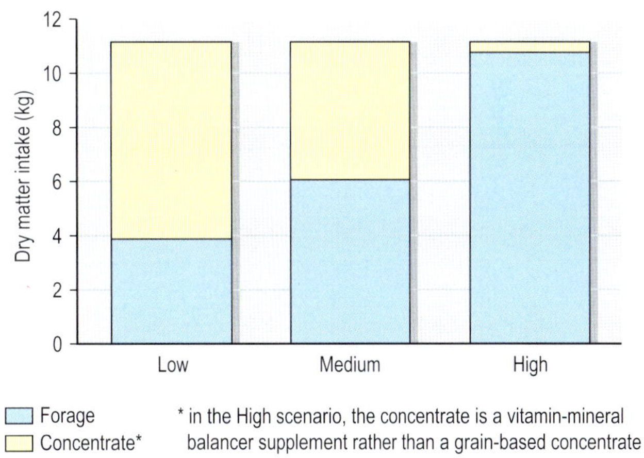

Fig 36.3 The effects of forage energy content on the proportions of hay and a grain-based energy concentrate required to meet the energy requirements of a 500-kg horse with daily digestible energy (DE) needs of approximately 30 Mcal/day. This example assumes a daily dry matter (DM) intake of 11.5 kg (~2.2% of bodyweight) and the use of hay with either **Low** (DE 1.5 Mcal/kg DM), **Medium** (DE 2.0 Mcal/kg DM) or **High** (DE 2.5 MCal/kg DM) energy content. The energy concentrate feed contains ~3.3 Mcal DE/kg DM. In order to achieve the 30 Mcal DE/day intake, the proportions of hay and concentrate in the diet will be: **Low** (4 kg hay and 7.5 kg concentrate, or a ratio of 35 : 65); **Medium** (6.25 kg of hay and 5.25 kg of concentrate, or a ratio of 54 : 46); and **High** (11.5 kg of the forage and a vitamin-mineral forage balancer). Alternatively, it would be possible to meet the energy requirements with a lower DM intake if fed the High hay (e.g. 7.5 kg forage and 3.3 kg concentrate). Note that the Low energy forage scenario results in a forage intake that is below the recommended target minimum of 6.25 kg (1.25% BW/day). Additionally, depending on the composition of the concentrate feed, starch intake is likely to be considerably higher than 2 g/kg BW/day.

Table 36.2 A guide to the main types of forage available and their nutrient content. Please note that this is only a general guide as forages vary between countries and even from field to field

	GENERAL COMMENTS	PROTEIN/ENERGY	MINERALS	SOME COMMENTS SPECIFIC TO ATHLETIC HORSE
Meadow hay 10–15% Moisture	Typically from permanent pastures with a range of grass species (plus often herbs and other plants). Resulting in plants at different stages of maturity when cut – so can be referred to as 'soft' hay. Note: due to different growing conditions late harvested hay from one region may have higher nutrient value than an early cut from another region	Provide higher protein (typically 8–12% DM) and digestible energy levels (typically around 2–2.5 MCal/kg DM: 8–11 MJ/kg DM) than most seed hays. Lysine values vary but can be up to 4.5% of the CP values	The Na content will be low in all forages & Na and Cl supplementation will typically be required for performance horses on forage-based diets. Cu, Zn and Se contents can be low in hays. Ca/P vary	Energy and nutritive value will vary mainly due to fiber content and fiber quality. Younger less mature hays tend to be more digestible and suitable for the exercising animal – but the reduced fiber content may be an issue if low levels of forage are fed
Seed hay 10–15% Moisture	Produced from specially seeded leys, usually 1–3 years old, and contains predominantly one or two grass species (often rye grass or timothy)	Typically, seed hay has lower energy (for example around 1.5–2 Mcal: 7–9 MJ/kg DM) and protein levels (around 4–8% DM) and a lower digestibility than meadow hay	The mineral levels in seed hay also tend to be lower than for meadow hay, although this will depend on the soil upon which the hay was grown	For all hays the hygienic quality (dust, molds, etc.) is important. Soaking or more recently steaming hays may improve hygiene status
Legume hay 10–15% Moisture	Alfalfa is perhaps the most commonly fed legume hay today. It can have multiple harvests and can be found as a pure hay or in a mix with other grass types or for example barn dried and packaged in a short chopped form in plastic-covered bales	Due to nitrogen-fixing properties, higher protein levels than seed or meadow hay often CP >20%. Starch content variable but can be high	Calcium content will be higher in legume hays	For endurance horses often recommended to choose hay with a low-to-moderate protein content (i.e. grass hay) rather than a legume hay because of the concerns regarding high protein intake. If a grass alfalfa hay is used currently recommend that alfalfa is < 30% of the mix
Silages Recommended that the DM should be greater than 35% and preferably in excess of 40%	Unstable weather conditions at harvest have resulted in an exponential increase in the use of forage preservation by ensiling. The extent of fermentation is influenced by the moisture content, resulting in less fermentation with increasing DM content. *Less commonly fed to horses than haylage*		Mineral content will depend on the original grass type	Very important that the pH/DM/organic acids/ammonia content. etc., suggests good silage quality and that the silage is appropriate for horses, e.g. horses may find very low pH material unpalatable and silage with a pH of less than 4.5 may be rejected by some horses. Effect of some fermentation products in the horses not fully appreciated. Note: Vitamin D_2 is not made during the ensiling process and Vit E will be destroyed

Continued

Table 36.2 Continued

	GENERAL COMMENTS	PROTEIN/ENERGY	MINERALS	SOME COMMENTS SPECIFIC TO ATHLETIC HORSE
Haylages 25–45% Moisture (but lower moistures measured in some so-called haylages fed to horse)	A hybrid of hay and silage, haylage is grown and cut similarly to hay, but baled before it is dry, generally when there is about 35–40% of the moisture remaining. To prevent mould spoilage, it is then bagged or wrapped to exclude air. Haylage has less fermentation products (including lactic acid) and a higher pH vs silage (with its lower DM content). This means that it will have reduced aerobic stability after opening of the bales	The nutritive value of haylage normally is higher than hay. Will vary however in a similar way to hay depending on the time of harvest, e.g. CP 80 to 130 g/kg DM from the same sward. WSC content can be relatively high, as often little fermentation. Actual level depends on the original grass content and can be similar to that found in hays	Mineral content will depend on the original grass type	Increased palatability can increase intake rate – which may result in weight gain or less time spent on foraging activities. Nutritional value and quality of haylage can be very variable. Low potassium as well as low-fiber intakes can result when replaced wt for wt for hay. Vitamin E levels can be very low

Adapted from Harris PA (2013) Nutrition in Equine Veterinary Nursing Manual Coumbe K (ed) with kind permission from John Wiley & Sons Ltd.[88]

Accounting for pasture forage intake

Many competition horses, including racehorses, spend part of the day out at pasture. Currently it is not practically feasible to determine the nutrient contribution of pasture to a mixed diet and only rough estimates can be made. Grass intake of ponies can approach 5% of BW (as DM) when they have 24 h access, with up to 1% BW consumed within 3 h of turnout.[27,28] Grass intake by horses, however, is perhaps lower at ~2–2.5% BW/day on a DM basis.[29,30] As a guide the contribution of pasture to the daily DM intake can be estimated by subtracting the amount of supplemental feeds/forage provided from a given daily DM intake level (e.g. 4% of BW for ponies out at grass for >16–18 h/day; 2–3% BW for horses). The alternate approach is to estimate intake as a function of time at pasture – for horses 0.4% BW as DM per 3 h of turnout up to a maximum of 1% BW when turned out during the day and stabled at night. Higher values (at least double) can perhaps be used for ponies. Intake from pasture can perhaps be ignored, especially in horses if only minimal turnout time is provided (i.e. ≤1 h/day) given the likely increase in energy expenditure associated with this activity.

Cereals and cereal by-products

Cereals vary in their nutrient content, especially fiber and starch (see Table 36.3). Overall, however, all cereals contain substantially greater quantities of sugar and starch than more fibrous feeds such as hay. The horse has a limited capacity to hydrolyze starch in the small intestine and any starch that is not digested there will be rapidly fermented in the hindgut with potential adverse clinical consequences.[10,31,32] Pre-cecal starch digestibility varies with the type of grain and the nature of any mechanical or thermal processing. For example, whereas oat starch (at up to 2–3 g/kg BW per meal) has a pre-cecal digestibility greater than 80%, approximately 35% of an equivalent dose of cornstarch reaches the caecum undigested.[33] Heat treatments such as micronization, extrusion and steam flaking significantly improve the pre-cecal starch digestibility of barley and corn.[10,22] Accordingly, meal size, starch/sugar content, and the grain type and level of processing will affect both the glycemic and insulinemic response to the diet as well as the potential for undigested substrate to be delivered to the hindgut.[33,34] In addition, there are potential adverse effects of large amounts of starch and sugar on gastric mucosal health.[35]

In general, the nutrient profiles of cereal by-products such as wheat bran, rice bran and maize (corn) feed flour vary depending on the production process. Crude protein, crude fat and fiber are typically higher when compared to the parent cereal grain, whereas starch content is usually lower. Cereal by-products often have an imbalanced Ca:P ratio, high phytate content, and low lysine levels, all of which must be taken into consideration in feed formulation.

Highly digestible fibers

Readily fermentable fiber sources such as sugar beet pulp and soya hulls can be used to replace some of the cereal grains in a ration.[36–38] When compared to more traditional fiber sources like hay, these 'super fibers' contain lower indigestible/non-fermentable material (e.g. lignin) and higher amounts of non-starch polysaccharides, pectins and gums that can be extensively degraded within a timeframe that such a feedstuff would be resident in the gastrointestinal tract.[39] This translates to a higher energy yield[36,40] than their gross nutrient specification would suggest. These fiber sources may

Table 36.3 Comments on the most common cereals fed to horses, including typical nutrient content on a DM basis. Note that nutrient content will vary considerably according to the variety as well as conditions during growth, harvesting and processing

FEEDSTUFF CONTENT	TYPICAL FEED FORMS	GOOD POINTS	POTENTIAL POINTS TO CONSIDER
Cereals	Most are palatable to horses and well digested – typically fed whole or more commonly processed. Included primarily as a source of energy, which is present mainly as starch. Rice is high in starch content, and is followed in descending order by maize, wheat, barley and oats. Starch consists of polymers of glucose, and the starch grains of different cereals vary in chemical structure (ratio of amylose to amylopectin) and size, which can significantly alter their digestibility in the small intestine. Glucose availability tends to be higher with the amylopectin type of starch. Fiber content increases from rice to maize, then wheat, triticale, dehulled oats, barley and finally oats. The nature of the fiber also varies significantly. Protein content tends to be highest for triticale, and decreases progressively for wheat, dehulled oats, oats, barley, rice and maize; the protein quality is higher in oats, barley and rice (3.7–4.2% lysine of CP) than in wheat and maize (3.0–3.1% lysine of CP). Oats and maize are relatively high in fat content (4–5.5%) and contain ~ twice the amount present in wheat and rice. Controversy over the relative effects of the different cereals on the behavior and activity level of individual animals. Some have suggested that behavior is influenced by the total energy/starch intake or glycemic response.		Generally low in lysine and methionine. Calcium generally low – unbalanced ratio of Ca:P as P relatively high. Sodium levels generally low (~0.2 g Na / kg DM). Trace element intake often low in unfortified high-cereal-containing rations. Contain up to 1% phytates, which make the phosphorus less available and bind calcium, even though the phytates may be broken down in the hindgut the released minerals cannot be absorbed from there. Rancidity and spoilage rate increases with processing
Oats DM 88% CF 100 Oil 40 CP 110 Starch 470 Ca 0.8 P 3.5	Whole most common, bruised, rolled and crushed possible. 'Naked' or 'dehulled' without husks – lower fiber, higher starch and oil content plus higher protein content and quality. 'Clipped' or racehorse oats have part of the fibrous hull removed and therefore increase the relative starch-to-fiber ratio.	Higher fiber than many cereals in relation to its starch content – oat starch well digested in small intestine, if not fed in excess, making it a more 'safe' cereal with respect to hindgut disturbances. Lowish energy content. Sugar ~1.5%	No proven advantage of processing unless horse has poor dentition. Lowest energy content of most commonly fed grains – increases the bulk needed for intensively exercising horses to meet energy. High variability in nutrient content. Processing tends to reduce storage life
Corn/Maize DM ~87% CF 20 Oil 40 CP 90 Starch 700 Ca 0.2 P 3.0	Flaking, steaming, micronising improves small intestinal starch digestion	Energy-dense cereal more than twice the energy per unit volume of oats although the difference is only 20% on a dry matter basis *Should feed on a weight not volume basis.* Less waste heat of fermentation, so potentially more helpful in hot conditions. Fair source of Vit. A unless aged. Sugar ~1% DM basis	Lowest CP of commonly fed cereals (~8–10% DM). Cracked corn commonly fed in USA but unprocessed corn is not well digested in the small intestine, with an increased risk of excess starch reaching the hindgut. Corn is prone to mold infestation and production of mycotoxins. Adding mollases may substantially increase intake rate
Barley DM ~86% CF 50 Oil 20 CP 120 Starch 530 Ca <1 P 4.0	Generally fed rolled, crimped or soaked in an attempt to improve palatability (by opening up the closely attached hull). However, cooking (steam/micronizing) is required to significantly increase SI digestibility	Higher level of energy than oats but lower than corn. Lower oil content, so less risk of rancidity after processing. Like oats, has a hull. Sugar ~3.5%	Whole barley is harder and less palatable than oats. Contains hordenine. Increased risk of weevil infestation
Wheat DM ~85% CF 25 Oil 18 CP 120 Starch 660 Ca 0.5 P 3.5	Cracked or coarsely ground – often dusty and must be introduced gradually. Can be steam flaked	Small grain – higher energy content on a weight basis (than corn and nearly 2½ times as much as oats on a volume basis). Naked grain has ~66% starch and 5.5% sugar on a DM basis. Low fiber (~2.5% DM)	Often more expensive. Hard grain needs to be chewed thoroughly otherwise increased risk of undigested starch reaching the hindgut. If feed more than 20% as finely ground wheat may form a glutinous mass with increased risk of gastric colic. Typically less palatable than corn and oats

Adapted from Harris PA (2013) Nutrition in Equine Veterinary Nursing Manual Coumbe K (ed) with kind permission from John Wiley & Sons Ltd.[88]

augment the size of the large intestinal fluid and electrolyte reservoir, which may represent as much as 8–10% of bodyweight and 10–20% of total body Na, K and Cl.[41,42] Fiber composition of the diet also may affect total body water and core temperature during endurance-type exercise.[43]

Oils

Vegetable oil is a rich source of energy – 450 ml of oil (~420 g) provides about 3.3 Mcal (~14 MJ) of DE, or about 3× as much DE as an equivalent quantity of oats and 2× that of corn. As such, the addition of vegetable oil to the ration can allow DE requirements to be met by a reduced amount of feed. Other potential advantages may include decreased heat production, calmer demeanor, and improved athletic performance.[3,32] Although animal fat (tallow or lard) has been fed to horses, palatability and digestibility are inferior when compared to vegetable oils and their use is not recommended. Therefore, most commercial oil-supplemented feeds for horses contain a vegetable oil such as soy, corn or canola. Other oils that may be used in equine rations include peanut, safflower, coconut, linseed or flaxseed. Vegetable oils are highly palatable,[44] although there can be slight variation in acceptance, depending on oil type, how the oil is introduced, method of processing, and horse variability.

Other sources of oil that are used commonly in horse rations include stabilized rice bran (18–22% fat), flaxseed meal (40% fat) and copra meal (8–9% fat). Rice bran (as a powder or an extruded pellet) is well accepted by horses, and has been fed at a rate of 0.5 to 2.5 kg per day to mature horses, providing 90 to 500 g oil per day. Rice bran is rich in phosphorus and has an inverted Ca/P ratio; many commercial rice bran products contain added calcium (e.g. calcium carbonate) to correct this imbalance. Alternatively, a mineral supplement can be added to the ration to ensure an appropriate Ca/P ratio (at least 1:1) in rations containing rice bran.

The ideal amount and type of dietary fat for horses has not been determined, although Kronfeld et al.[45] estimated daily endogenous loss of 0.22 g fat/kg BW and the NRC (2007)[1] recommends a dietary minimum for linoleic acid of 0.5% DM. Minimal information is available regarding the effects of fatty acid chain length or degree of saturation on metabolism and health in horses. The NRC (2007)[1] notes that: '*the data from studies in which horses were fed diets enriched with omega – 3(n-3) fatty acids (linseed, flaxseed or fish oils) have demonstrated modulation of inflammatory mediator synthesis by cells harvested from blood peritoneal fluid or respiratory secretions. However, physiological importance of these findings is unclear*.'

Any supplemental oil should be introduced slowly (over 14–21 days) to avoid intestinal disturbances as the capacity to hydrolyze lipids appears to need time to adapt. However, the equine pancreas has high lipase activity,[46] which might explain why horses are able to digest and utilize up to 20% or more of the diet as oil when fully adapted.[45] Commercially, the level of fat or oil added to a concentrate is often limited by manufacturing constraints (e.g. poor pellet quality when large amounts of oil are included in pelleted feeds; greasy appearance of concentrate mixes). Therefore, oil-supplemented concentrates designed for performance horses usually contain between 5 and 14% oil (as fed), providing between 8 and 30% of the DE. However, as these concentrates are fed with forage, the amount of oil on a total diet basis is much lower (3%–8% oil, or 4 to 15% of the DE from oil assuming a 50% concentrate, 50% forage diet).

Mean apparent fat digestibilities of 55% for forages, 81% for mixed diets with added oil, and 95–100% for added oil have been reported.[45] In a recent meta-analysis of the effects of supplementary oil (15.5 to 217.5 g/kg DM) on protein and fiber digestibility in the horse,[47] it was suggested that whilst added oil can decrease ADF digestibility this effect is unlikely to have any practical relevance. In mature horses and ponies, absorption of calcium, phosphorus and magnesium appears to be largely unaffected by moderate amounts of additional oil[48] but in growing animals it is recommended to ensure that the diet provides more than the minimal requirement for these minerals.

Many horse owners and trainers add vegetable oil to existing rations. A suggested upper limit of oil supplementation is 1 ml/kg BW/day. For reference, one standard measuring cup contains 250 ml (8 fluid ounces) of oil (~225 g) and provides approximately 1.8 Mcal (7.6 MJ) of DE. For a 500-kg horse in moderate work (daily DE needs of 26 Mcal) the inclusion of 500 ml oil/day will provide about 14% of the DE requirement. The DE of one cup of oil is roughly equivalent to that provided in ~0.6 kg oats or rice bran and ~0.5 kg corn. There should be a gradual introduction to oil feeding to avoid digestive disturbances (loose and oily feces). Initially, ¼ cup of oil/day can be added to the ration. Over a 2–3 week period, the amount of added oil can be increased to ~2 cups/day, divided into at least 2–3 feedings.

One concern with the addition of vegetable oils (or rice bran) to an existing diet is the potential for nutrient imbalances. Unlike other high-energy sources such as cereals, oil does not provide any additional protein, vitamins (vitamin E content can be variable) or minerals; ensuring nutrient balance of the overall ration is therefore very important. Commercial energy concentrates with added oil are fortified to maintain appropriate nutrient-to-calorie ratios, and are designed to complement the forage source. On the other hand, the on-farm addition of a substantial amount of oil (e.g. 400–500 ml per day) to an existing ration may result in an unbalanced diet. Consultation with a nutritionist is recommended in these situations and especially if more than 1 ml/kg BW/day is being added. Supplementation with vitamin E (1–1.5 iu/ml added oil) is recommended for prophylaxis against oxidant stress when oil is directly added to the ration.

Amounts of forage and concentrate feed in the ration

Forage

The DE requirement of an athletic horse can be more than twofold greater when compared to a horse at maintenance, although the exact amount will be affected by several factors, including training load and individual horse variation. The use of grass, legume or cereal (usually oaten) hays (or other forms of preserved forages made from these species) often depends on availability and personal preference. Legume hays such as alfalfa usually have higher DE, protein and mineral (particularly calcium) content when compared to the grass species. These differences will influence the type and quantity of energy concentrate that may be required to be fed with hay. However, even within a plant species, the nutrient composition of preserved forage can vary greatly depending on growing conditions, plant maturity and harvesting methods. Thus, proximate analysis (including crude protein, neutral detergent fiber, and macrominerals) should be performed whenever possible to best guide ration balancing and the selection of an appropriate energy concentrate.

For the majority of horses, forage should comprise at least 50% of the diet (DM basis). Endurance horses typically would be fed 75% or more of their daily DM intake as forage/pasture.[49] This means feeding at least 1.5–2.0 kg forage DM per 100 kg BW. For horses in only moderate work (i.e. only a 30–50% increase in DE requirements over maintenance) or those with a nervous temperament, forage may constitute the majority of the ration. Less mature hays that have higher digestibility and DE content than more mature hays should be considered, especially for horses with high DE requirements, i.e. elite-level performance horses (see Table 36.2).

Is there a maximum or minimum forage intake?

For horses with high DE needs, forage alone will not meet the requirement, e.g. a 500-kg, three-day eventing horse requires ~60 MJ NE on the day of the cross-country discipline.[3] About 22 kg (or ~4.5% BW on a DM basis) of timothy hay would be needed to meet this requirement. Whereas ponies may achieve this level of DM intake when allowed to feed ad libitum,[50] the daily DM intake of performance horses is ~2.0–2.7% BW – and may be lower due to other constraints on feeding activity, e.g. time spent in other activities on the day of competition. The relatively low-energy content of many forages coupled with physical limitations to the amount that can be ingested are two key reasons why the ration of most high-performance horses includes alternative sources of energy. An additional concern is that 'filling' a horse with forage reduces appetite for other feeds (e.g. cereal grains) and therefore reduces daily energy intake.

However, perhaps the main reason that most trainers are reluctant to feed high forage-based diets is that for every kg of dry hay, around 2.5–3.5 kg of water may be consumed; this will add to the weight of the horse and may adversely affect athletic performance. Therefore, many trainers believe that forage should be restricted to reduce gut fill and BW in high-performance horses. There is some evidence that a short-term reduction in forage intake is beneficial in horses undertaking high-intensity exercise. When compared to ad libitum hay consumption, restricting hay intake to ~1% BW for a three-day period before a treadmill exercise test (2 min at 115% VO_{2max}) resulted in a 2% BW decrease and a reduction in anaerobic energy expenditure during exercise, as evidenced by reduced oxygen deficit and plasma lactate concentrations. The reduction in BW was attributed to a decrease in bowel ballast (gut fill).[51] However, the practical implications of these findings are uncertain given that many racehorses routinely do not consume more than 1% BW per day as forage. In fact, the actual feeding value or quality of the forage can have as much of an effect on gut fill and water turnover as the amount of forage being fed. Therefore, high-performance horses should be fed high-quality forage to minimize the impact on gut fill. Low-fiber diets may predispose horses to behavioral problems as well as gastrointestinal dysfunction (e.g. gastric ulcers, colic). Recent work has suggested that a ration of just high-quality haylage may be suitable for trotting horses.[52]

The amount of forage in the ration should be calculated on a DM basis rather than an as-fed basis due to the low fiber content of some very immature hays, especially alfalfa, and haylages/silages. To ensure gastrointestinal and behavioral health, the authors recommend that forage (grass and preserved forages) is provided at a minimum of 15 g DM per kg BW/day, even for horses with high energy requirements (in which case young, less mature high-energy content forages should be used). The absolute minimal level for animals undergoing restriction for weight loss purposes is 10 g DM per kg BW/day and a target minimum for elite-level athletic horses is 12.5 g DM per kg BW/day (1.25% of BW/day).

Concentrate or complementary feeds (including oil)

The next step in formulating a ration is to determine the combination of alternative energy sources required to be fed along with forage so that daily energy and nutrient requirements can be met. In most situations, these calculations are not based on actual nutrient analysis of forages and feeds; instead, book data or information provided by a feed manufacturer is used to estimate the relative quantities of different feeds needed to meet requirements. Figure 36.4 compares the sources of DE in a traditional racehorse diet (forage plus grain) and a diet in which an oil and fiber energy concentrate is fed.

Some epidemiological studies have identified the level of grain feeding as a risk factor for colic, e.g. odds ratios of 4.8 and 6.3 (relative to no episode of colic) have been reported for horses fed, respectively, 2.5 kg/day and more than 5.0 kg/day of concentrate.[53,54] Similarly, recent (within the previous two weeks) changes in the type or amount of grain or concentrate fed, or feeding more

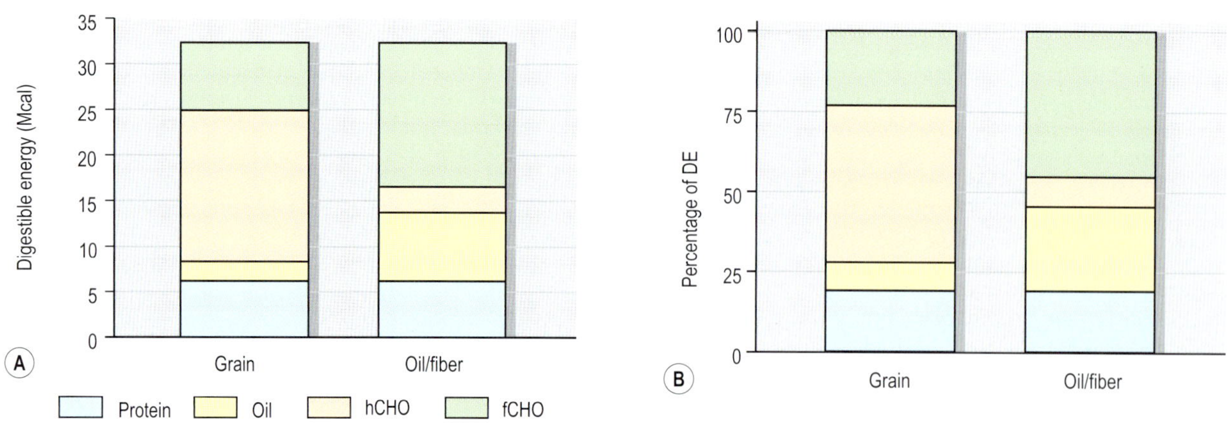

Fig. 36.4 Graphical representation of the sources of energy in a traditional grain and hay diet (**Grain**) and a contemporary oil and fiber energy concentrate and hay diet (**Oil/fiber**) fed to a 500-kg racehorse requiring approximately 32 Mcal of digestible energy (DE) per day. Both diets include 6.25 kg of mid-bloom timothy hay and, on a total diet basis, provide 12% crude protein. For Grain, the horse is fed ~7 kg of an energy concentrate composed of oats (57%), cracked corn (37%) and sugar cane molasses (6%). The same quantity of energy concentrate is fed in Oil/fiber (~13% fat), the primary ingredients of which are beet pulp, rice bran, soy hulls and vegetable oil. **(A)** Estimates of the absolute DE provided by protein, oil, hydrolyzable carbohydrate (hCHO; starch and sugar), and fiber carbohydrates (fCHO) in the respective diets. **(B)** The percentage contribution of the four energy sources to the total DE intake. Note the dramatic reduction in hCHO intake in the Oil/fiber when compared to the Grain diet.

than 2.7 kg of oats per day have been associated with increased risk of an episode of colic.[55] In Standardbred horses in training that were fed a forage:concentrate diet with a starch intake of 0.54 g per kg BW/day, there was evidence of reduced microbial stability of fecal flora as well as an increase in members of the *Streptococcus bovis/equis* complex and other lactate-producing species when compared to the feeding of a forage-only diet.[56]

These data raise the question, 'What is a safe level of starch (and simple sugar) feeding?' Although there is no clear answer to this question, the authors recommend ≤2 g/kg BW starch (and simple sugar) per meal and, more preferably, ≤1 g/kg BW per meal and ≤2 g/kg BW/day. Practically, these targets are very difficult to achieve, especially in Thoroughbred racehorses under typical management conditions. As oats are ~40% starch and corn ~60% starch (as-fed basis), the above recommendations would mean that a 500-kg horse should be fed only 1.25 kg oats or 0.8 kg corn per meal, with no more than two meals per day! The compromise is to adhere to the recommendation related to the size of individual concentrate meals (and therefore the amount of starch provided per meal) but allow for a higher total daily intake of starch with the higher intake achieved by feeding more than 2 meals per day rather than by an increase in the size of morning and evening feedings. Alternatively, larger meals (~2 kg for a 500-kg horse) can be fed if a lower starch (25%) feed with highly digestible fibers and oil is provided. Use of these alternative energy sources facilitates a reduction in the level of starch feeding without compromising the caloric density of the ration. Whilst there does not appear to be a minimal starch requirement for athletic horses, anecdotally trainers report reduced performance if the intake is too restricted.

Balancing the ration for protein and amino acids

After selection of the forage and concentrate feed, the resultant ration needs to be assessed for the quantity and quality of protein. The dietary protein requirement is a function of amino acid needs, the amino acid composition of the dietary protein, and the digestibility of the protein. Horses have negligible ability to utilize non-protein nitrogen, which means that nitrogen requirements must be provided in the form of protein or amino acids. Furthermore, it is thought that intact amino acids are not absorbed to any significant extent from the large intestine. Therefore, the horse's essential amino acid requirements must be met from protein sources that are digested in the small intestine.

There is still controversy in both the human and equine fields with respect to the role of protein as an energy source during (or after) exercise and to what extent exercise increases protein requirements. High protein diets may be undesirable in horses because of the effects of excess dietary protein on heat production, acid–base balance, water requirements and, potentially, respiratory health.[57–60] In one study, for example, horses consuming 1741 g CP per day (>3 g/kg BW) excreted more urea in sweat and had higher plasma urea when compared to horses consuming 836 g CP per day.[57] It has been estimated that a change in dietary CP content from 10% to 15% would increase water requirement by approximately 5% because of an obligate increase in urine production for clearance of endogenous urea loads.[58,60] Moreover, the higher urinary urea load could adversely affect the respiratory health of confined horses because urea is converted to ammonia, a known respiratory irritant. One recommendation is to restrict digestible protein intake to 2 g/kg BW/day or ~3–4 g CP (depending on the feedstuff) per kg BW/day, especially for endurance horses.[49] It is worth noting that the NRC (2007)[1] reduced its recommendation for CP requirements for horses in hard work from 2.5–2.6 g/kg BW/day to ~2 g/kg BW/day. Note that the maintenance recommendation is 1.1–1.45 g CP/kg BW/day.[1]

Athletic horses in training likely require a protein intake that exceeds the maintenance requirement in order to accommodate muscular development, the need for muscle repair post-exercise, and to replenish the nitrogen lost in sweat (~20 g/kg sweat loss[1]). The most recent NRC recommendation is 1.4 to 2.0 g CP/kg BW/day depending on workload and sweat loss.[1] However, given:

1. the uncertainty regarding the assumptions made by the NRC (e.g. digestibility of dietary protein taken as 79%, whereas the digestibility of many feeds and forages may be lower than this – *personal observations*)
2. variability of the amino acid composition of horse feeds
3. the difficulty in assessing sweat nitrogen losses.

The authors recommend that unless the quality of the protein is known, most high-performance horses should be fed at least 2 g CP/kg BW/day. For horses in very intense work, up to 3 g CP/kg BW/day may be advisable (providing stable hygiene is good and water intake is not restricted). Further work in this area is needed.

The quality of the protein fed is likely important, especially for horses in hard work as well as young horses in training that are still growing. The NRC (2007)[1] suggests a maintenance lysine intake of 4.3% of the protein requirement. The authors currently recommend around 0.08–0.1 g lysine/kg BW/day for the intensively working horse. As threonine has been proposed to be the second limiting amino acid for growth, the threonine content of the diet of competition/actively exercising horses should also be considered. Based on the recommendation to feed threonine at 80% of the lysine requirement, the authors recommend 0.64–0.8 g threonine/kg BW/day. The amount of supplemental lysine needed in the ration will depend on lysine contents of the hay, pasture and other feed components (see Table 36.2, Table 36.3 and Table 36.4).

Typical feeds used to provide additional protein are peas, beans, linseed and soyabeans. Peas, for example, typically contain ~15–18 g lysine/kg DM and 8–10 g threonine/kg DM. Full-fat soya beans are ~40% protein (as fed) with high levels of essential amino acids (lysine ~24 g/kg DM). The lysine content of 'defatted' soyabean meal can be even higher (~36 g lysine/kg DM). There are a number of other considerations when using these ingredients, e.g. the potential presence of anti-nutritive factors and the need to account for the energy provided by these ingredients and therefore adjust the quantity of other ration components.

Other nutrients

Minerals

Based on their daily requirements, minerals are usually classified as macrominerals (e.g. calcium, phosphorus, sodium, potassium, and chloride) or trace elements (e.g. selenium, iron, zinc, and copper). These nutrients are important in a large array of body functions (Table 36.1).[1,61] Several minerals and trace elements, such as magnesium, iron, zinc and copper, act as enzyme activators in glycolysis and oxidative phosphorylation. Minerals (electrolytes) are also critical to nerve and muscle function.

Once the ration has been balanced with respect to the protein and amino acid intake, an assessment as to how closely the ration matches mineral, trace element and vitamin requirements needs to be made (see Table 36.1).[1] Obvious deficiencies can be addressed through the use of specific supplements or more generic commercial balancers: e.g. balancers targeted at cereal-based or forage-based rations. Requirements may need to take into account the age of the animal and its prior exercise history. For example, additional Ca and P may be required to support the remodeling of bone associated with exercise in young racehorses;[5] additional Ca and P also may be indicated during recovery after intense exercise and during periods of inactivity.[5] It is therefore difficult to be prescriptive. It is rare that any ration will exactly meet all requirements and intake will often exceed the recommended intake for one or more of the trace elements. In most cases, however, intake levels will not exceed stated upper limits[1] but it is possible that the excess intake or imbalanced ratio may result in a short- or long-term adverse effect on the health, behavior or performance of the horse. Table 36.1 presents some practical upper limits for some nutrients. A nutritionist should be consulted if there is concern regarding excessive intake of one or more nutrients or in regards to a nutritionally unbalanced ration.

Table 36.4 Comments on the most common protein sources fed to horses, including typical nutrient content on a DM basis. Note that nutrient content will vary considerably according to the variety as well as conditions during growth, harvesting and processing

FEEDSTUFF CONTENT	TYPICAL FEED FORMS	GOOD POINTS	POTENTIAL POINTS TO CONSIDER
Peas DM ~87% CF 60 Oil 18 CP 240 Starch 400–500 Ca 1 P 5	Micronized, flaked, split	Good protein source with a reasonable amino acid profile (lysine ~15–18 g/kg DM: threonine 8–10 g/kg DM). Sugars ~55 g/kg DM	Certain varieties, including those fed in the UK contain trypsin inhibitors and other anti-nutritive factors and therefore must be cooked before feeding. Other varieties from other countries may contain far lower amounts and therefore can be fed whole or more commonly rolled or flaked
Beans – Winter DM ~85–90% CF 83 Oil 14 CP 280 Starch 400 Ca 1 P 9	Often cracked, crushed or coarsely ground or rolled following micronization, but can be fed whole. Cooked or micronized for certain varieties such as winter horse beans, and field beans where potentially toxic factors are present. Field bean is the main variety grown in the UK. Not normally fed in large quantities	High in energy and protein with a reasonable lysine content, especially the field beans ~15 g/kg. They are suited to horses in hard work or breeding/growing animals but soyabean has a better amino acid profile. Rich in phosphorus but poor in calcium and manganese (~8 mg/kg DM)	Bean protein is not believed to be as well digested in the small intestine as other protein sources, especially if uncooked. Most varieties of beans are best cooked before feeding as they contain low levels of a trypsin (the enzyme that breaks peptides into amino acids) inhibitor and other anti-nutritive factors. They are normally micronized or cooked and split open. Field beans, for example, also contain tannins which can have adverse effects; again, appropriate cooking processes are needed to reduce such anti-nutritive factors
Soya beans Meal dehulled: – DM ~90% CF 34 Oil 15 CP 470 Starch 34 Ca 3 P 8	Soya is commonly fed to horses with the oil removed (soya meal ~1% oil); as full-fat soya which contains 18–19% oil and can be used as a meal or more commonly micronized as a flake	Good source of protein. Full-fat soya ~40% protein as-fed with high levels of essential amino acids (dehulled meal around 36 g lysine/kg DM – full-fat soya ~24 g/kg DM). Low starch around 1–3% DM and 8–10% DM sugar	Needs to be appropriately cooked or micronized before feeding to reduce the protease inhibitors, anti-coagulant factors, allergenic and goitrogenic factors. Meal is not always very palatable and may need to be gradually added to the diet, anti-nutritive factors should be significantly reduced in meal production. Micronized or extruded full-fat soyabean flakes have enhanced palatability and digestion and improved stability.

Table 36.4 Continued

FEEDSTUFF CONTENT	TYPICAL FEED FORMS	GOOD POINTS	POTENTIAL POINTS TO CONSIDER
Linseed meal DM ~89% CF 100 Oil 80 CP 350 Starch 50 Ca 4.5 P 8.5	Small, oval, flat, shiny, dark brown seeds. Linseed meal or cake, where the seeds are cooked and most of the oil extracted and then compressed together into small rectangles, or linseed oil (bought ready prepared) can be used. Newer forms of processed linseed now on the market designed to be fed without additional cooking	Linseed contains good protein levels (26%) and a very high oil level (39%). Mechanically expelled meal has a higher protein of around 35%, with a much lower oil content (~4–8%), with a high linolenic acid level and is still thought to have beneficial effects on coat condition. Linseed meal contains a mucilage (30–200 g/kg) that may help maintain softer droppings without any irritation compared to bran	Contains an enzyme which it is thought can release hydrocyanide from the glycoside compounds contained within the seed, especially after soaking unless cooked – therefore seeds tend to be boiled until they spilt open, making a gruel, tea or jelly (dependent on the amount of water added). The cake or meal making process will inactivate the enzyme but may not destroy all the anti-nutritive factors, so amount fed should still be limited. Solvent extracted meal contains low levels of oil (<2%), so less effect on coat condition. Lower lysine content than soyabean meal or other high protein sources such as canola and only around 50–60% of the amount of other essential amino acids

Adapted from Harris PA (2013) Nutrition in Equine Veterinary Nursing Manual Coumbe K (ed) with kind permission from John Wiley & Sons Ltd.[88]

Limited information is available with respect to the effects of regular exercise on trace mineral requirements. As sweat contains a small amount of iron and other trace minerals (e.g. zinc), there may be a slightly increased requirement with exercise.

Iron

During training the apparent absorption of iron is increased and this appears to compensate for any exercise-associated increase in iron turnover.[62] Dietary supplementation has failed to produce changes in hemoglobin or hematocrit and there is the potential for excessive doses of iron to result in hepatopathy if the iron-binding capacity is exceeded.[63] Practically, common horse feedstuffs provide iron well in excess of requirements and iron deficiency anemia is rare in the horse. Iron supplementation is therefore not justified other than for horses with anemia due to external blood loss. The NRC 2007 maintenance requirement for iron is 40 mg/kg of diet (DM basis) or approximately 0.8 mg/kg BW/day (400 mg/day for a 500-kg horse); the recommendation for horses in hard work is 1 mg/kg BW. The authors' more optimal recommendation for hard-working animals is up to 1.25 mg/kg BW/day. Forages usually contain >100 mg Fe/kg DM and most grains >50 mg/kg DM. Thus, even a diet of 6.25 kg DM of hay and 6.25 kg of an unfortified grain-concentrate for a 500-kg horse would provide >900 mg Fe.

Selenium

Selenium is a functional component of a number of selenoproteins and Se-dependent enzymes, including the intracellular enzymes glutathione peroxidase and thioredoxin reductase. Selenium, in concert with vitamin E, is important in the defense of cells against oxidant stress, and Se deficiency is associated with vitamin E/Se responsive nutritional myodegeneration. Selenium is also essential for the development of acquired immunity. There is wide geographical variation in the Se content of feeds and forages (including the presence of Se-accumulating plants in some locations) but in general horse feedstuffs have a low Se content and dietary fortification is commonly required.[64] Whether or not regular physical activity increases the Se requirement is disputed.[64,65] The NRC (2007)[1] recommendation for a 500-kg horse in hard work is 1.25 mg Se/day (vs 1 mg/day for maintenance) due to the role of Se as an antioxidant, immune function, etc., whereas the authors currently recommend ~0.25 mg/100 kg BW for maintenance and up to ~0.4–0.6 mg/100 kg BW (2–3 mg/500 kg/day) for heavily exercising horses due to its important roles. However, the total diet should provide not more than 1 mg Se/100 kg BW/day. The relative merits of organic vs inorganic sources of Se are also controversial but, based on the available data, it can be concluded that both types are suitable for equine diets.

Chelated/organic sources

Studies in other species have demonstrated higher digestibility and retention of organic vs inorganic source trace elements; however, findings in the horse are equivocal.[65] The authors personally recommend that, when included in the diet of horses, chelated trace elements comprise no more than 33% of the total requirement.

Dietary cation-anion balance (DCAB)

Rations with a DCAB <100 mEq/kg DM can be acidogenic and, in theory, will promote the demineralization of bone as well as increased renal Ca loss.[66,67] Cereal grains have a low DCAB (<100 mEq/kg DM), which may be a concern for young, growing and exercising animals. However, there is evidence of adaptation to low-DCAB diets.[68] In addition, the roughage to concentrate ratio and type of roughage strongly influences the effect of diet on acid–base balance.[69] Feeding even currently recommended levels of salt to exercising horses may cause a mild metabolic acidosis unless there is an adequate intake of roughage.[70]

Vitamins

The classification of vitamins is based on their relative solubility: fat-soluble vitamins (A, D, E and K) are more soluble in organic solvents, whereas the B vitamins and vitamin C are more soluble in water. Most vitamins participate in processes related to muscle contraction and energy expenditure. Vitamins of the B complex group (e.g. thiamine, riboflavin, vitamin B_6, niacin, biotin and pantothenic acid) act as cofactors for enzymes regulating glycolysis, citric acid cycle, oxidative phosphorylation, β-oxidation of fatty acids, and amino acid catabolism. Folic acid and vitamin B_{12} are needed for heme synthesis. The antioxidant vitamins (mainly vitamins C and E) participate in a buffer system against free radicals. B-complex vitamins are synthesized by intestinal microorganisms, and are normally also present in adequate amounts in feeds commonly fed to horses (except vitamin B_{12}).[71,72] These two sources are normally considered to be adequate to meet the B-vitamin requirements of adult horses. However, it is possible that changes in the ration, introduction of intense exercise and other stressful conditions may change the microflora and result in inadequate B-vitamin synthesis.[72] There is in fact very limited information regarding the vitamin requirements of horses and even fewer data concerning the effects of habitual exercise on these requirements or the effects on performance of reduced or increased intakes.[73]

Antioxidant vitamins E and C

In recent years, there has been considerable interest regarding the role of vitamins C and E (and other antioxidant nutrients such as β-carotene and lipoic acid) in the mitigation of oxidative stress and lipid peroxidation in horses during exertion. Vitamins E (α-tocopherol) and C, along with glutathione, are important non-enzymatic antioxidants. Vitamin E acts as a non-specific chain-breaking type of antioxidant that prevents the propagation of lipid peroxidation, particularly in membranes and plasma lipoproteins. Vitamin C is located in the aqueous phase of cells where it scavenges free radicals and recycles vitamin E to its active form. Vitamin E also plays an important role in the maintenance of immune function. Exercise causes a dramatic increase in oxidative metabolism and, therefore, the production of reactive oxygen species (ROS). During prolonged and/or strenuous exercise, the extent of ROS production may overwhelm antioxidant systems such that the susceptibility of cells and tissues to damage by ROS (lipid peroxidation) is enhanced, particularly in animals with inadequate endogenous stores of the antioxidant nutrients. For example, in a recent study a higher concentration of thiobarbituric acid reactive substances (indicator of oxidative stress) before an endurance race was associated with a reduced likelihood of completing the race.[74] This finding supported previous work suggesting that horses with low antioxidant reserves may be more prone to lipid peroxidation from ROS during endurance exercise.[75] It is not known whether additional antioxidant supplementation prior to or during the race may be advantageous; however, it has been suggested that under certain circumstances high doses of antioxidants may be detrimental by impeding physiological adaptations to exercise training.[76] Moreover, in other species there is increasing evidence that vitamin E can have an antioxidant, neutral or even pro-oxidant effect depending on the level of intake. The pro-oxidant effect may occur in conditions of high oxidative stress, particularly when there is low availability of co-antioxidants such as vitamin C or the appropriate mixture of the different forms of vitamin E forms is not present.[77] The balance of antioxidants, therefore, may be as, if not more, important than the amount of an individual antioxidant.

For vitamin E, the NRC (2007)[1] requirement is set at 1–2 mg/kg BW depending on workload. This level of dietary inclusion is considerably lower than other recommendations for athletic horses in hard work, with as much as 4 mg/kg BW recommended by some authors.[73] In support of this higher recommendation, Saastamoinen and Juusela[78] reported that 3–5 mg/kg BW was required to maintain or increase serum vitamin E concentrations in horses in training during winter. Siciliano et al.[79] demonstrated a decrease in plasma and muscle α-tocopherol concentrations in working horses fed a diet supplemented with 80 iu α-tocopherol per kg DM, whereas plasma concentrations were maintained when horses were supplemented with 300 iu/kg DM. Similarly, plasma concentrations of α-tocopherol were significantly higher in hard-working polo ponies fed a diet providing 300% of the current NRC recommendation for vitamin E (240 iu/kg vs 80 iu/kg diet).[80]

Further research is needed to better define the vitamin E requirements for different classes of athletic horse. In the meantime, it is recommended that athletic horses be fed a diet providing at least 2 mg/kg BW and preferably 3 mg/kg BW. Intensely working horses (e.g. race and endurance horses) may benefit from higher levels of vitamin E (4–5 mg/kg BW or around 200–250 iu/kg DM). Most equine feedstuffs contain less that 50 iu/kg DM. Therefore, supplemental vitamin E must be added to horse rations to meet requirements. Supplementation appears to be most beneficial if given daily to maintain a constant level of vitamin E in serum, liver and muscles.[81] Vitamin E supplementation is often used in horses with a history of exertional rhabdomyolysis. Although it is important to ensure that the diet of these horses contains adequate vitamin E, the authors caution that such supplementation will not necessarily protect against exercise-induced muscle damage.[82]

Horses have no dietary vitamin C requirement because they have L-gluconolactone oxidase, the enzyme required for the synthesis of vitamin C (ascorbic acid) from glucose. However, the demand for ascorbic acid may be increased by regular exercise because it is thought to spare tissue vitamin E by reducing the tocopheroxyl radical and restoring the radical scavenging activity of vitamin E.[83] Ascorbic acid is thought to be the primary antioxidant to neutrophil-derived oxidants in recurrent airway obstruction (RAO)[84] and chronic airway inflammation in RAO-affected horses results in reduced levels of ascorbic acid in the plasma and epithelial lining fluid (ELF).[85] ELF ascorbic acid concentration can be elevated in RAO-affected horses by appropriate dietary supplementation[85] and specific dietary antioxidant supplementation has also been demonstrated to decrease endoscopic inflammation scores in RAO-affected horses.[86]

Water

The 1989 NRC guidelines[87] recommend 2–4 L water per kg of DM intake while the 2007 NRC[1] notes that average maintenance intakes are ~5 L/100 kg BW/day when horses are fed 1.5 kg DM/100 kg BW (i.e. 25 L for a 500-kg horse receiving 7.5 kg DM/day). However, diet, ambient conditions, level of activity and inter-horse variability will all modify the water requirement. Related to diet, it has been estimated that ~3.5 L water is required per kg feed for horses on an all-hay diet, with ~2.4 L per kg on a hay-grain diet. Sweat fluid losses also must be accounted for in estimating water needs. For a 500-kg horse undergoing moderate exercise for one hour (sweat loss of 5 L), being fed in total 10 kg DM (7.5 kg forage and 2.5 kg sweet feed) and being maintained at an ambient temperature of 20°C, the water requirement using these guidelines would be between ~25 and 45 L of water. Water intake by horses living in warm climates (>25–30°C daytime temperature) may be increased by 15–30%, whereas heavy work in warm-to-hot ambient conditions may increase water requirement by as much as 200–300% due to large sweat fluid losses. From a practical viewpoint, however, horses should have clean drinking water available at all times.

References

1. Anon. Nutrient Requirements of Horses. 6th revised ed. Washington, DC: National Research Council, The National Academies Press; 2007.
2. Geor RJ. Endocrine and metabolic physiology. In: Geor RJ, Harris PA, Coenen MC, editors. Equine Applied and Clinical Nutrition. London: Saunders Elsevier; 2013. p. 33–63.
3. Harris PA. Energy requirements of the exercising horse. Ann Rev Nutr 1997;17:185–210.
4. Ellis AD. Energy systems and requirements. In: Geor RJ, Harris PA, Coenen MC, editors. Equine Applied and Clinical Nutrition. London: Saunders Elsevier; 2013. p. 96–112.
5. Nielsen BD. Practical considerations for feeding racehorses. In: Geor RJ, Harris PA, Coenen MC, editors. Equine Applied and Clinical Nutrition. London: Saunders Elsevier; 2013. p. 261–71.
6. Gallagher K, Leech J, Stowe H. Protein, energy and dry matter consumption by racing Thoroughbreds: A field survey. J Equine Vet Sci 1992;12:43–8.
7. Gallagher K, Leech J, Stowe H. Protein, energy and dry matter consumption by racing Standardbreds: A field survey. J Equine Vet Sci 1992;12:382–6.
8. Southwood L, Evans DL, Bryden WL, et al. Nutrient intake of horses in Thoroughbred and Standardbred stables. Aust Vet J 1993;70:164–8.
9. Pagan JD, Hintz HF. Equine energetics II. Energy expenditure in horses during submaximal exercise. J Anim Sci 1986;63:822–30.
10. Kronfeld DS, Harris PA. Equine grain associated disorders. Comp Cont Educ Pract Vet 2003;25:974–83.
11. Kearns C, McKeever, KH, Kumagai, K, et al. Fat-free mass is related to one-mile race performance in elite standardbred horses. Vet J 2002;163:260–6.
12. Kearns C, McKeever KH, John-Alder H, et al. Relationship between body composition, blood volume and maximal oxygen uptake. Equine Vet J 2002;(Suppl. 34):S485–90.
13. Lawrence L, Jackson SJ, Kline K, et al. Observations on body weight and condition of horses in a 150-mile endurance ride. J Equine Vet Sc 1992;12:320–4.
14. Dugdale AH, Curtis GC, Cripps P, et al. Effect of dietary restriction on body condition, composition and welfare of overweight and obese pony mares. Equine Vet J 2010;42:600–10.
15. Lim AS. Body weight and performance in racehorses. In: Proceedings of the 4th International Conference on Control of the Use of Drugs in Racehorses, Melbourne, Australia; 1988. p. 93–4.
16. Jones JH, Carlson G. Estimation of metabolic energy cost and heat production during a 3-day-event. Equine Vet J 1995;(Suppl. 20):S23–31.
17. Garlinghouse S, Burrill MJ. Relationship of body condition score to completion rate during 160 km endurance races. Equine Vet J 1999;(Suppl. 30):S591–5.
18. Hinchcliff KW. Effects of furosemide on athletic performance and exercise-induced pulmonary haemorrhage in horses. J Am Vet Med Assoc 1999;215:630–5.
19. Henneke D, Potter G, Kreider J, et al. Relationship between condition score, physical measurements and body fat percentage in mares. Equine Vet J 1983;15:371–2.
20. Kohnke J. Feeding and nutrition: the making of a champion. Australia: Birubi Pacific; 1992. p. 163–6.
21. Martin Rosset W, Vermorel M, Doreau M, et al. The French horse feed evaluation systems and recommended allowances for energy and protein. Livestock Prod Sci 1994;40:37–56.
22. Moore-Colyer MJS, Hyslop JJ, Longland AC, et al. Intra-cecal fermentation parameters in ponies fed botanically diverse fiber-based diets. Anim Feed Sci Tech 2000;84:183–97.
23. Guilloteau P, Martin L, Eeckhaut V, et al. From the gut to the peripheral tissues: the multiple effects of butyrate. Nutr Res Rev 2010;23:366–84.
24. Hothersall B, Nicol CJ. Effects of diet on behaviour – normal and abnormal. In: Geor RJ, Harris PA, Coenen MC, editors. Equine Applied and Clinical Nutrition. London: Saunders Elsevier; 2013. p. 443–54.
25. Whitlock RH. Feed additives and contaminants. Vet Clin North Am Equine Pract 1990;6:467–78.
26. Moore-Colyer MJS, Fillery BG. The effect of three different treatments on the respirable particle content, total viable count and mould concentrations in hay for horses. In: Saastamoinen M, Fradinho MJ, Santos AS, et al, editors. Forages and Grazing in Horse Nutrition. EAAP Publication No. 132, 2012. p. 101–7.
27. Longland AC, Ince J, Harris PA. Estimation of pasture intake by ponies from liveweight change during six weeks at pasture. J Equine Vet Sci 2011;31:275–6.
28. Longland AC, Barfoot C, Harris PA. The effect of wearing a grazing muzzle vs. not wearing a grazing muzzle on pasture dry matter intake by ponies. J Equine Vet Sci 2011;31:282–3.
29. Edouard N, Fleurance G, Dumont B, et al. Does sward height affect feeding patch choice and voluntary intake in horses? Appl Anim Behav Sci 2009;119: 219–28.
30. Cuddeford D. Factors affecting feed intake. In: Geor RJ, Harris PA, Coenen MC, editors. Equine Applied and Clinical Nutrition. London: Saunders Elsevier; 2013. p.64–79.
31. Milinovich GJ, Burrell PC, Pollitt CC, et al. Microbial ecology of the equine hindgut during oligofructose-induced laminitis. ISME J 2008;2: 1089–100.
32. Geor RJ, Harris PA. Laminitis. In: Geor RJ, Harris PA, Coenen MC, editors. Equine Applied and Clinical Nutrition. London: Saunders Elsevier; 2013. p. 469–86.
33. Kienzle E, Pohlenz J, Radicke S. Morphology of starch digestion in the horse. J Vet Med A 1997;44:207–21.
34. Harris PA, Geor RJ. Primer on dietary carbohydrates and the utility of the glycemic index in equine nutrition. Vet Clin North Am Equine Pract 2009;25:23–38.
35. Luthersson N, Nielsen KH, Harris PA, et al. Risk factors associated with equine gastric ulceration syndrome in 201 horses in Denmark. Equine Vet J 2009;41: 625–30.
36. Longland AC, Moore-Colyer M, Hyslop JJ, et al. Comparison of the in sacco degradation of the non-starch polysaccharide and neutral detergent fiber fractions of four sources of dietary fiber by ponies. Proceedings 15th Equine

Nutrition and Physiology Symposium, College Station, Texas; 1997. p. 120–121.

37. Crandell KG, Pagan JD, Harris PA, et al. A comparison of grain, oil and beet pulp as energy sources for the exercised horse. Equine Vet J 1999;(Suppl. 30):S485–9.
38. Palmgren-Karlsson C, Jansson A, Essen-Gustavsson B, et al. Effect of molassed sugar beet pulp on nutrient utilisation and metabolic parameters during exercise. Equine Vet J 2002;(Suppl. 34):S44–9.
39. Moore-Colyer M, Longland AC. The effect of plain sugar beet pulp on in vitro gas production and the in vivo apparent digestibility of hay when offered to ponies. In: 17th Conference of the Equine Nutrition and Physiology Society, Lexington, Kentucky; 2001. p. 145–7.
40. Lindberg J, Palmgren-Karlsson C. Effect of replacing oats with sugar beet pulp and maize oil on nutrient utilisation in horses. Equine Vet J 2001;33:585–90.
41. Meyer H, Coenen M. Influence of exercise on the water and electrolyte content of the alimentary tract. In: 11th Conference of the Equine Nutrition and Physiology Symposium; 1989. p. 3–7.
42. Warren L, Lawrence LM, Roberts A, et al. The effect of dietary fiber on gastrointestinal fluid volume and the response to dehydration and exercise. In: 17th Conference of the Equine Nutrition and Physiology Society, Lexington, Kentucky; 2001. p. 148–9.
43. Spooner HS, Nielsen BD, Harris, PA, et al. Hydration status of horses during endurance exercise as affected by dietary fiber type. In: Proceedings of the 20th Equine Science Symposium, Baltimore, Maryland; 2007. p. 24–25.
44. Holland JL Kronfeld DS, Rich GA, et al. Acceptance of fat and lecithin containing diets by horses. Appl Animal Behav Sci 1998;56:91–6.
45. Kronfeld DS, Holland JL, Rich V, et al. Fat digestibility in *Equus caballus* follows increasing first order kinetics. J Anim Sci 2004;82:1773–80.
46. Lorenzo-Figueras M, Morisset SM, Morisset J, et al. Digestive enzyme concentrations and activities in healthy pancreatic tissue of horses. Am J Vet Res 2007;68:1070–2.
47. Sales J, Homolka P. A meta-analysis of the effects of supplemental dietary fat on protein and fibre digestibility in the horse. Livestock Sci 2011;136:55–63.
48. Meyer H, Flothow C, Radicke S. Preileal digestibility of coconut fat and soybean oil in horses and their influence on metabolites of microbial origin of the proximal digestive tract. Arch Anim Nutr 1997;50:63–74.
49. Harris PA. Feeding management of elite endurance horses. Vet Clin North Am Equine Pract 2009;25:137–54.
50. Dugdale AH, Curtis GC, Cripps P, et al. Effects of season and body condition on appetite, body mass and body composition in ad libitum fed pony mares. The Vet J 2011;190:329–37.
51. Rice O, Geor R Harris PA, et al. Effects of restricted hay intake on body weight and metabolic responses to high intensity exercise in Thoroughbred horses. In: 17th Conference of Equine Nutrition and Physiology Society, Lexington, Kentucky; 2001. p. 273–9.
52. Essén-Gustavsson B, Connysson M, Jansson A. Effects of crude protein intake from forage-only diets on muscle amino acids and glycogen levels in horses during training. Equine Vet J 2010;42(Suppl. 38):S341–6.
53. Durham AE. Intestinal disease. In: Geor RJ, Harris PA, Coenen MC, editors. Equine Applied and Clinical Nutrition. London: Saunders Elsevier; 2013. p. 568–81.
54. Tinker M, White NA, Lessard P, et al. Prospective study of equine colic risk factors. Equine Vet J 1997;29: 454–8.
55. Hudson J, Cohen ND, Gibbs PG, et al. Feeding practices associated with colic in horses. J Am Vet Med Assoc 2001;219:1419–25.
56. Willing B, Vörös A, Roos S, et al. Changes in faecal bacteria associated with concentrate and forage-only diets fed to horses in training. Equine Vet J 2009;41:908–14.
57. Miller-Graber P, Lawrence LM, Foreman J, et al. Effect of dietary protein level on nitrogen metabolites in exercised Quarter horses. In: Persson S, Lindholm A, Jeffcott LB, editors. Equine Exercise Physiology 3. Davis, CA: ICEEP Publications; 1991. p. 305–14.
58. Kronfeld DS. Dietary fat affects heat production and other variables of equine performance, under hot and humid conditions. Equine Vet J 1996;(Suppl. 22):S24–34.
59. Graham-Thiers PM, Kronfeld DS, Kline KA, et al. Dietary protein restriction and fat supplementation diminish the acidogenic effect of exercise during repeated sprints in horses. J Nutr 2001;131:1959–64.
60. Kronfeld D. Body fluids and exercise: Influences of nutrition and feeding management. J Equine Vet Sci 2001;21:417–28.
61. Coenen MC. Macro and trace elements in equine nutrition. In: Geor RJ, Harris PA, Coenen MC, editors. Equine Applied and Clinical Nutrition. London: Saunders Elsevier; 2013. p. 190–228.
62. Inoue Y, Matsui A, Asai Y, et al. Effect of exercise on iron metabolism in horses. Biol Trace Elem Res 2005;107: 33–42.
63. Jackson SG. Trace minerals for the performance horse: known biochemical roles and estimates of requirements. Irish Vet J 1997;50:668–74.
64. Dunnett CE, Dunnett M. Organic selenium and the exercising horse. In: Saastamoien MT, Martin-Rosset W, editors. Nutrition of the Exercising Horse. EAAP Publication No. 125. Wageningen Academic Publishers; 2008. p. 255–66.
65. Vervuert I. Major mineral and trace element requirements and functions in exercising animals. In: Saastamoien MT, Martin-Rosset W, editors. Nutrition of the Exercising Horse. EAAP Publication No. 125. Wageningen Academic Publishers; 2008. p.207–18.
66. Baker LA, Topliff DA, Stoecker B. The comparison of two forms of sodium and potassium and chloride versus sulfur in the dietary cation-anion difference equation: Effects on acid-base status and mineral balance in sedentary horses. J Equine Vet Sci 1998;18: 389–95.
67. Baker LA, Topliff DA, Freeman DW, et al. Effect of dietary cation-anion balance in mineral balance in anaerobically exercised and sedentary horses. J Equine Vet Sci 1993;13:557–61.
68. Cooper SR, Topliff DR, Freeman DW, et al. Effect of dietary cation-anion difference on mineral balance serum osteocalcin concentration and growth in weanling horses. J Equine Vet Sci 2000;20:39–44.
69. Kienzle E, Sturmer K, Ranz D, et al. A high roughage/concetrate ratio decreases the effect of ammonium chloride on acid-base balance in horses. J Nutr 2006;136:2048S–9S.
70. Romanowski K, Hacke S, Vernunft A, et al. Effects of different doses of oral sodium chloride on acid-base and mineral balance of exercised horses fed a hay-based diet. Proceedings of the 15th ESVCN Congress; 2011. p. 83.
71. Caroll FD, Goss H, Howell CE. The synthesis of B vitamins in the horse. J Anim Sci 1949;8:290–9.
72. Linerode PA. Studies on the synthesis and absorption of B-complex vitamins in the horse. Proceedings of the 13th Annual Convention of the American Association of Equine Practitioners; 1967. p. 283–314.
73. Saastamoinen MT, Harris PA. Vitamin requirements and supplementation in exercising horses. In: Saastamoien MT, Martin-Rosset W, editors. Nutrition of the Exercising Horse. EAAP Publication No: 125. Wageningen Academic Publishers; 2008. p. 233–55.
74. Holbrook TC, McFarlance D, Schott HC. Neuroendocrine and non-neuroendocrine markers of inflammation associated with performance in endurance horses. Equine Vet J 2010;(Suppl. 38):S123–8.
75. Hargreaves B, Kronfeld DS, Waldron JN, et al. Antioxidant status and muscle cell

leakage during endurance exercise. Equine Vet J 2002;(Suppl. 34):S116–21.
76. Neubauer O, Reichhold S, Nics L, et al. Antioxidant response to an acute ultra-endurance exercise: impact on DNA stability and indications of an increased need for nutritive antioxidants in the early recovery phase. Br J Nutr 2010;104:1129–38.
77. Nieman DC, Henson DA, Mcanulty SR, et al. Vitamin E and immunity after the Kona Triathlon world championship. Med Sci Sports Exerc 2010;36: 1328–35.
78. Saastamoinen MT, Juusela J. Serum vitamin concentration of horses on different vitamin E supplementation levels. Acta Agric Scand Sect A Anim Sci 1993;43:52–5.
79. Siciliano P, Parker AL, Lawrence LM. Effect of dietary vitamin E supplementation on the integrity of skeletal muscle in exercised horses. J Anim Sci 1997;75:1553–60.
80. Hoffman R, Morgan KL, Phillips A, et al. Dietary vitamin E and ascorbic acid influence nutritional status of exercising polo ponies. In: 17th Conference of the Equine Nutrition and Physiology Society, Lexington, Kentucky; 2001. p. 129–30.
81. Roneus BO, Hakkarainen RV, Lindholm A, et al. Vitamin E requirements of adult Standardbred horses evaluated by tissue depletion and repletion. Equine Vet. J. 1986;18:50–8.
82. Harris PA. Feeding and management advice for tying up/azoturia/Monday Morning disease/equine rhabdomyolysis syndrome. In: Harris PA, Mair TS, Slater JD, et al, editors. Equine Nutrition for All. Proceedings of the1st BEVA & WALTHAM Nutrition Symposia, Harrogate, UK; 2005. p.113–18.
83. Packer L. Oxidants, antioxidant nutrients and the athlete. J Sports Sci 1997;15:353–63.
84. Deaton CM, Marlin DJ, Smith NC, et al. Antioxidant and inflammatory responses of healthy horses and horses affected by recurrent airway obstruction to inhaled ozone. Equine Vet J 2005;37: 243–9.
85. Deaton CM, Marlin DJ, Smith NC, et al. Antioxidant supplementation in horses affected by recurrent airway obstruction. J Nutr 2004;134:2065S–7S.
86. Kirschvink N, Fievez L, Bougnet A, et al. Effect of nutritional antioxidant supplementation on systemic and pulmonary antioxidant status, airway inflammation and lung function in heaves-affected horses. Equine Vet J 2002;34:705–12.
87. Anon. Nutrient Requirements of Horses. 5th revised ed. Washington, DC: National Research Council, The National Academies Press; 1989.
88. Harris PA. Nutrition. In: Coumbe K, editor. Equine Veterinary Nursing Manual. Wiley-Blackwell; 2013. p. 97–120.

37 Nutrition for the equine athlete: above and beyond nutrients alone

Raymond J. Geor Patricia A. Harris

CHAPTER CONTENTS

Introduction

As described in Chapter 36, the main considerations in ration formulation are:

1. provision of adequate fiber (roughage) to maintain normal gut and digestive function (and to support the horse's natural chewing behavior and thereby reduce the risk of certain behavioral disturbances)
2. targeting of an overall energy density that will allow energy requirements to be met at typical fed intakes
3. provision of the optimal amounts and balance of other essential nutrients (i.e., protein/amino acids, minerals, trace elements and vitamins)
4. use of only the highest hygienic quality feedstuffs that have been stored appropriately.

In addition to these basic principles, there are a number of other topics related to the nutritional management of the athletic horse during training and competition that warrant discussion, including:

- the timing of feeding before exercise, i.e. when and what should be fed before bouts of heavy exercise
- electrolyte supplementation, i.e. what quantity and type of electrolytes should be given, and when
- the effect of diet and post-exercise feeding strategy on muscle glycogen content
- what nutritional adjustments are indicated for the management of specific problems that commonly occur in athletic horses, e.g. gastric ulcer syndrome, equine rhabdomyolysis syndrome
- the potential benefits of oil (fat)-supplemented rations
- whether there is any rationale for the addition of 'specialized supplements' to the ration of an athletic horse.

Time of feeding before exercise

The timing and composition of meals consumed before exercise may impact health and performance via effects on fluid balance, blood flow distribution, metabolism and perhaps also mechanical discomfort associated with gut fill. A full stomach may restrict the space available for lung expansion during exercise although there are no published data to support or refute this contention. Pre-exercise feeding also might alter the distribution of blood flow, with potentially adverse effects on blood flow to the respiratory and locomotor muscles. However, one study in horses during moderate exercise demonstrated no adverse effect of a pre-exercise meal on blood flow distribution when compared to the control treatment.[1] Presumably the exercise-associated increases in heart rate and cardiac output were sufficient to meet the competing demands for blood flow to the splanchnic bed as well as the respiratory and locomotor muscles. Whether the same is true in regards to feeding before high-intensity exercise in horses is not known.

Several studies have examined the effects of the timing and composition of a meal consumed before exercise on metabolic responses in horses.[2–5] Most notably, the hyperglycemia and insulinemia associated with the digestion and absorption of starch-rich (grain) meals affects the mix of substrates utilized during a bout of exercise. Insulin is a potent inhibitor of lipolysis and fatty acid oxidation in skeletal muscle, and also promotes glucose uptake into muscle via recruitment of the transporter protein GLUT4 to the sarcolemma. Thus, hyperinsulinemia at exercise onset will suppress FFA availability and lipid oxidation and increase reliance on carbohydrate stores (including plasma glucose) for energy transduction. Accordingly, several equine studies have demonstrated that a grain meal (1–3 kg of oats, corn or a mixture of the two) consumed 3 hours or less before exercise results in hyperglycemia, hyperinsulinemia (Fig. 37.1) and decreased plasma FFA concentration at the start of exercise, and a subsequent marked decrease in plasma glucose concentration during the initial period of exercise.[2–5] Jose-Cunilleras and colleagues[6] utilized isotopic tracer methods and indirect calorimetry to determine the effects of hay (alfalfa cubes; ~3 kg) and starch (cracked corn; 1.7 kg) feeding on glucose flux and substrate oxidation during exercise. The alfalfa cubes were consumed between 2 and 3 hours before exercise, while the cracked corn was ingested 90 min pre-exercise. Feeding corn before exercise resulted in increased utilization of blood-borne glucose and whole-body carbohydrate oxidation when compared to a meal of alfalfa or not feeding (Fig. 37.2). In another study in which smaller amounts of forage and cereals were fed (~1 kg each) 1.5–2 h before a simulated trotting race (2600 m on a 2.5% incline at around 90% of VO_{2max}), no differences in blood glucose and insulin values were found between the pre-exercise samples and resting pre-prandial samples.[7]

The effects of pre-exercise grain feeding on endurance exercise performance in horses per se have not been reported. In humans, carbohydrate ingestion during exercise unequivocally improves performance during prolonged (more than 2 hours) moderate-intensity (>50–60% of VO_{2max}) exercise, presumably by maintaining glucose supply in skeletal muscle at a time when glycogen stores are depleted. On the other hand, the performance effects of pre-exercise glucose feedings in human athletes are more equivocal. For horses performing prolonged (endurance) exercise, the acceleration in carbohydrate oxidation (and suppression of fat oxidation) associated with pre-exercise grain feeding might impair performance as a result of carbohydrate depletion. The impact of feeding during endurance rides may be more complex as in these circumstances exercise-associated alterations in hormones (e.g., increased catecholamines, decreased insulin) may counterbalance the effect of any hormonal changes induced by feeding. One study in horses looked at the effect of feeding a grass meal based pellet with or without either 50% glucose or fructose before and during a simulated 30 km endurance ride.[8] Plasma glucose concentrations were elevated during the simulated endurance exercise after glucose feeding, but no counter-regulation by insulin occurred. Plasma insulin, FFA and lactate levels showed exercise-related changes but dietary treatment did not affect these results.

As demonstrated in the study by Jose-Cunilleras et al.,[6] together with the results of earlier studies by Pagan and Harris,[5] forage meals (<2 kg) consumed 2–3 hours before exercise have minimal effect on substrate availability and oxidation during sustained exertion. However, free choice consumption of hay in the 12–24 hour period before exercise may adversely affect performance because of an increase in body weight (gut fill), especially in horses not adapted to such a ration or when hays with a reduced digestibility are fed. Large meals (hay or grain or a combination) consumed near the start of exercise will also result in a decrease in plasma volume as a result of fluid shifts into the gastrointestinal tract.[5] Such reductions in plasma volume could compromise cardiovascular function during exercise. There is some evidence that a short-term reduction in forage intake may be beneficial in horses undertaking high-intensity exercise – although this may depend on the pre-reduction intake; e.g. when compared to ad libitum hay consumption, restricting hay intake to ~1% of bodyweight for a three-day period before a treadmill exercise test (2 min at 115% VO_{2max}) resulted in a 2% decrease in body weight and a reduction in anaerobic energy expenditure during exercise, as evidenced by reduced oxygen deficit

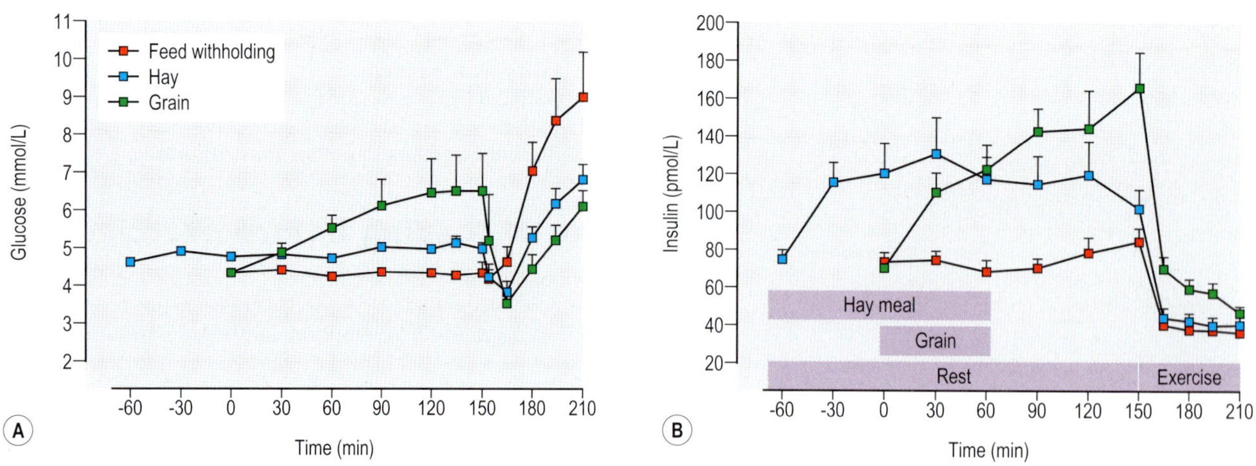

Fig 37.1 Plasma glucose **(A)** and serum insulin **(B)** concentrations at rest and during 60 min of exercise at 50% of maximum oxygen uptake in horses that were fasted for 18 hours (feed withholding) or fed alfalfa cubes (Hay) or cracked corn (Grain) 2–3 h before exercise. The hay and grain meals were approximately iscaloric. Grain feeding was associated with hyperglycemia and hyperinsulinemia before exercise (compared to feed withholding and Hay), and lower glucose concentrations but higher utilization of blood-borne glucose during exercise when compared to feed withholding.

Reprinted from Jose-Cunilleras E, Hinchcliff KW, Sams RA, et al. Glycemic index of a meal fed before exercise alters substrate use and glucose flux in exercising horses. J Appl Physiol 2002;92:117–28, with permission from The American Physiological Society.

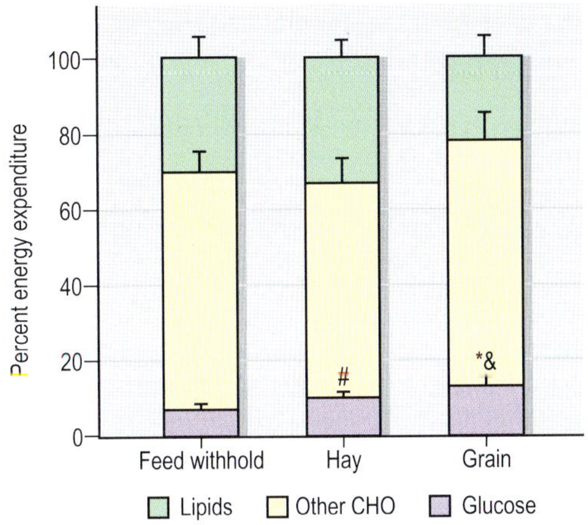

Fig 37.2 Effects of pre-exercise feeding on the partitioning of energy expenditure from different substrate sources (blood glucose, other carbohydrate [CHO; muscle glycogen and lactate], or lipids) in horses during the 5–30 min period of exercise at 50% of maximum oxygen uptake. Horses were either fasted (18 h of feed withholding), or fed alfalfa cubes (Hay) or cracked corn (Grain) 2–3 h before exercise. Grain feeding resulted in a significant ($P < 0.05$) increase in the caloric contribution from utilization of glucose when compared to the fast (*) and hay feeding (&) trials. The utilization of blood-borne glucose also was higher in the hay feeding (#) when compared to the feed withholding trial.

Reprinted from Jose-Cunilleras E, Hinchcliff KW, Sams RA, et al. Glycemic index of a meal fed before exercise alters substrate use and glucose flux in exercising horses. J Appl Physiol 2002;92:117–28, with permission from The American Physiological Society.

and plasma lactate concentrations. The reduction in body weight was attributed to a reduction in gut fill.[9]

In summary, small forage meals consumed 2–3 hours before exercise are likely to have minimal effect on substrate metabolism during exertion. However, meals containing hydrolyzable carbohydrate (starch and sugar) >1g/kg BW consumed within 3 hours of the start of exercise accelerate carbohydrate utilization and decrease free fatty acid availability and lipid oxidation. Although the performance effects of these feeding practices are not known, this suppression in lipid oxidation may be detrimental during endurance exercise (e.g. endurance races; speed and endurance test of a three-day event). Practical recommendations therefore include:

- Limit the size of pre-exercise grain or complementary feed meals (<1 kg/500-kg horse) and ideally do not feed this type of feed within 2–3 hours of the event. Feed <1 g/kg BW of starch and sugar in the pre-exercise meal
- Provide 1–2 kg forage (500-kg horse) (e.g. in a double hay net/haylage net) 2–3 hours pre-exercise to promote slow chewing and salivation without excessive gut fill
- Do not bed on straw or wood shavings during the period of feed withholding before exercise. The consumption of bedding materials (e.g. straw, wood shavings) may increase under conditions of forage restriction.[10] This intake of bedding material might increase the risk of colic in some horses. There also is a potential increased risk of colic when horses are provided access to a new bedding source at a competition
- The inclusion of alfalfa in the pre-exercise forage meal should be considered as some studies have suggested that alfalfa feeding may be beneficial with respect to prevention of exercise-associated gastric ulceration.[11]
- Avoid feed changes. A recent change in hay or forage feeding (as well as grain or concentrate feeding) is associated with increased risk for an episode of colic (the period of highest risk is 2 weeks post change).[12,13] Clinical experience suggests that changing from one batch to another of the same forage type carries less risk of colic when compared to a change from preserved to fresh forage or from a forage-only diet to a mixed forage-concentrate diet. Ideally, *any changes in the diet should be done gradually.*
- A slight reduction in training effort linked with maintenance of an appropriate diet should help to ensure that muscle and liver glycogen stores are as close to optimal as possible prior to the undertaking of competition exercise (see below). It has been suggested that the feeding of a high glycemic meal the night before competition may facilitate the 'topping-up' of liver glycogen stores; this strategy should only be applied in horses adapted to grain.

Electrolyte supplementation

Whether or not electrolyte supplementation has a beneficial effect on health and performance, especially during prolonged exercise, is a controversial topic in equine nutrition (see Harris and Schott[14] and also Chapter 40 and Chapter 52). Electrolyte supplementation of athletic horses is a common practice and it is generally held that at least partial replacement of sweat ion losses is needed for avoidance of fluid, electrolyte and acid–base disturbances that may adversely affect health and performance. No adverse effects were detected in eventing horses that received no or 'inadequate' amounts of additional sodium chloride supplementation.[15] As well, some elite endurance horses are apparently not provided electrolyte supplementation during rides up to 120 km in distance. Nonetheless, a study of French endurance horses suggested that in such circumstances renal mechanisms were not able to compensate for electrolyte losses during the ride.[16] The authors of this study concluded that their findings supported 'the benefit of electrolyte supply during rides'.[16] Furthermore, when horses were exercised at 30% VO_{2max} 1 hour after the administration of 3 L of an electrolyte solution, the radiolabeled sodium in the solution appeared in the sweat by 10 min of exercise and the duration of exercise to voluntary fatigue was increased by 33 ± 10%.[17] These findings provide a rationale for electrolyte supplementation, particularly during long endurance rides, although questions regarding the timing, amount and composition of supplementation require additional research. The following comments are particularly relevant to electrolyte supplementation of endurance horses but the principles also can be applied to horses used in other activities that elicit substantial sweat fluid loss:

- The amount of sweat produced depends on environmental conditions, nature of the work performed (which also depends on the rider's ability and terrain) and the animal's fitness.[18]
- Under mild ambient conditions, horses (~500 kg BW) may lose 5–7 liters of sweat per hour of steady trotting and cantering.[19,20] However, under conditions of high heat and humidity, sweat rates may approach 10–12 liters per hour.[19,21]
- In addition, to the large amounts of water that can be lost in sweat by horses performing several hours of endurance exercise, equine sweat contains 110–130 mmol Na^+ (2.5–3.0 g/L), 120–140 mmol Cl^- (4.3–5.0 g/L), and 30–40 mmol K^+ (1.2–1.6 g/L) per liter.[19,20]

- In theory, intake of water and electrolytes via (1) the oral administration of hypertonic electrolyte slurries followed by voluntary drinking or (2) by initially offering salt water followed by plain water, should limit dehydration and enhance recovery, but supporting data are lacking. Similarly, the effects of electrolyte supplementation on performance are not well established. There are potential risks associated with repeated electrolyte administration, especially by hypertonic pastes (e.g. increased risk of gastric ulceration) and if supplied to dehydrated animals (potential for further dehydration due to initial influx of fluid into the gastrointestinal tract).
- Using a typically applied factorial approach to electrolyte replenishment that is based on body weight loss and estimated sweat electrolyte content appears to overestimate the daily requirements of horses, especially those that lose large quantities of sweat fluid. Basing salt requirements according to energy expenditure also overestimates sodium requirements and depending on the core diet may influence acid–base status.[22]
- A forage-based diet should provide adequate potassium, and for most animals also adequate calcium and magnesium; therefore the main concern should be for salt replenishment during training (note that low-forage, high-cereal rations may not provide sufficient calcium or potassium).
- Salt should be introduced or removed from a feed gradually.
- For many horses in light work, access to a salt block or free salt is likely to be sufficient. When a commercial feed or a vitamin-mineral supplement is being fed, the block should be pure salt rather than a salt-mineral type (blocks formulated for other species should not be used). However, some horses may not consume adequate salt when a salt block is the sole source. Accordingly, loose salt should be provided to horses in moderate/hard work (either added to feed or provided in a separate vessel).
- During competitions, a conservative starting point for supplementation is to add 1.2 g Na per kg of sweat loss to the ration, i.e. over and above maintenance requirements. This supplemented amount represents ~30–40% of estimated losses.
- The optimal level of salt supplementation likely varies between horses, and will depend on many factors during a competition including environmental conditions and the fitness of the horse.
- During endurance competitions, additional potassium chloride supplementation is often provided (in a 3 : 1 ratio of NaCl : KCl) although there is some dispute whether such potassium provision should occur during loops undertaken at high intensities.
- Provide supplementary electrolytes during the 24 h post-race period – the inclusion of potassium in this supplement is recommended.

The timing of electrolyte supplementation pre-exercise is also controversial. The thirst response peaks around 2–3 hours after the administration of hypertonic electrolyte slurries, with urinary excretion continuing for up to 6 hours post-administration. The aforementioned study in which radiolabeled electrolytes were administered orally demonstrated the appearance of Na and K in the plasma within 10 min of administration, with peak values at 20–40 min and a more rapid clearance of K than Na from plasma.[17] The authors recommend that any electrolytes should be administered at around 2 hours pre-exercise but only in animals that are fully hydrated. Fresh, clean drinking water must be available to the horse when electrolyte pastes/slurries are administered.

Dietary manipulation of muscle glycogen content

Muscle glycogen and exercise performance

The increased demand for energy (adenosine triphosphate, ATP) to sustain muscle contraction during exercise is matched by the increased utilization of energy substrates. The primary fuel sources within muscle are ATP, phosphocreatine (PCr), glycogen and triglycerides (TG), while the primary extramuscular fuel sources are blood-borne glucose (from hepatic glycogen and gluconeogenesis) and NEFA (from adipose TG stores). There are three immediately available energy sources in skeletal muscle: ATP, PCr and adenylate kinase (myokinase). These phosphagens have very low capacity with respect to providing fuel for contraction, and energy from glycolytic and oxidative metabolism is needed to sustain all but very brief (<20–30 s) periods of exercise.[23] Muscle glycogen is the primary energy source for anaerobic glycolysis and oxidative phosphorylation during intense exercise in horses, and also is an important fuel during prolonged, lower-intensity exercise. Indeed, experimental studies have suggested that most of the energy for exercise at intensities above 50% VO_{2max} is derived from carbohydrates (muscle glycogen, blood glucose, and lactate).[24]

The chemical energy required for muscle contraction is ultimately provided in the diet. Therefore, inasmuch as diet can influence the storage of glycogen and TG in muscle, there is an obvious relationship between dietary intake and skeletal muscle exercise metabolism. Studies in human athletes have unequivocally demonstrated that a high carbohydrate (CHO) and low fat diet will result in higher muscle glycogen concentration when compared to a more conventional, lower CHO diet.[25] Furthermore, there is a direct relationship between initial muscle glycogen stores and performance during moderate-intensity (50–80% of VO_{2max}) endurance exercise in humans.[26] Thus, for human athletes, dietary strategies that boost muscle glycogen stores enhance exercise performance. Conversely, a low CHO and high fat diet impairs endurance exercise performance, in part due to lower initial muscle glycogen concentrations.

The depletion of muscle glycogen reserves is also likely to contribute to fatigue and poor performance in high-intensity as well as endurance exercise in horses. Depletion of muscle glycogen stores has been associated with fatigue in horses during endurance racing,[27] and the time to exhaustion in horses running at 6–7 mph was decreased by 35% when pre-exercise muscle glycogen content was 70% lower than in control horses.[28] Anaerobic work capacity in horses during a sprint treadmill exercise test was decreased by approximately 28% when muscle glycogen content was 60–70% lower relative to a control treatment.[29] Taken together, there is a rationale for feeding and training strategies that optimizes muscle glycogen content in preparation for competition exercise.

Post-exercise muscle glycogen synthesis

Post-exercise replenishment of muscle glycogen is two- to threefold fold slower in horses than in man and other mammals.[30] During the first 24 hours post-exercise, very little repletion occurs under conventional feeding conditions and full recovery after exhausting exercise may take up to 3 days. As a result, hoses that are exercised frequently (on a single day or on consecutive days) may have low muscle glycogen stores at the start of subsequent exercise bouts, which may impair physical performance.

In humans, muscle glycogen synthesis following glycogen-depleting exercise follows two phases.[31] Initially, there is a period of rapid synthesis that functions independent of external factors such as insulin and last about 30–60 minutes. Exercise-induced translocation of glucose transport protein-4 (GLUT4) to the sarcolemmal membrane, with increased permeability of the muscle membrane to glucose, is a key determinant of this rapid phase of glycogen resynthesis. The second phase of resynthesis is slower and lasts several hours. Systemic glucose availability, insulin stimulation of glucose uptake into muscle, and the activity of glycogen synthase (GS; the 'rate-limiting' enzyme in glycogen synthesis) interact to control the rate of glycogen synthesis during this phase (Fig. 37.3).[31] Another important component of this slower phase is a post-exercise enhancement in skeletal muscle insulin sensitivity to glucose transport, an effect that persists for as long as glycogen stores remain below resting concentrations.[32]

Several factors may account for the comparatively slow rate of muscle glycogen resynthesis in horses.[30] In humans, an up to six-fold increase in muscle GS activity has been observed after glycogen-depleting exercise and GS activity is further increased in response to carbohydrate feedings or IV insulin administration.[33] Skeletal muscle GS activity in horses is much lower when compared to humans,[34,35] only increases to a modest extent following exercise that depletes glycogen by 40–50%,[34] and no further increase in post-exercise GS activity is observed in response to hyperinsulinemia[35] or following starch-rich meals.[36] Additionally, a post-exercise enhancement in insulin-stimulated glucose disposal (insulin sensitivity) does not occur in horses.[35] Taken together, these observations suggest that glucose transport into muscle and the activity of GS restrain glycogen resynthesis in horse skeletal muscle and, at least in part, may explain why nutritional strategies that emphasize hyperinsulinemia and increased glucose availability provide only a modest enhancement in the rate of muscle glycogen resynthesis.

Diet and muscle glycogen storage

The relatively low (with respect to horses) glycogen content of human muscle (~300 mmol/kg dry muscle [dm]) can be doubled by a combination of exercise and diet. Originally this 'glycogen loading' involved a 2–3 day depletion phase of hard training on a low carbohydrate diet followed by a 2–3 day loading phase of high carbohydrate intake with a tapering of exercise. It now is evident that the combination of exercise taper and high daily CHO intake (~7–10g/kg BW/day) will increase muscle glycogen storage.[37] This level of starch and sugar feeding is difficult to achieve in horses and not recommended given the recognized associations between high dietary starch and risk of gastric ulcer syndrome, intestinal disturbances, etc.

Several different feeding strategies for enhancement of the post-exercise rate of muscle glycogen synthesis have been evaluated in horses, with a primary focus on carbohydrate feedings (glucose, glucose polymers or starch-rich meals) largely because these approaches have proven successful in human athletes.[30] The primary conclusion from this work is that feeding (or administering) glucose or starch in amounts comparable to that used with success in humans does not substantially (if at all) alter muscle glycogen recovery in horses. For example, oral administration of a glucose polymer (3 g/kg BW) within 60 min of the completion of glycogen-depleting exercise[38] or 1 g glucose/kg BW given at 0, 2 and 4 h post-exercise[34] did not enhance or alter the rate of muscle glycogen resynthesis in Standardbred horses (Fig. 37.4). Provision of a 80% grain (corn, oats and barley mix):20% hay diet modestly increased glycogen recovery over a 72-h period when compared to hay only or 50:50 grain:hay diets.[36] Feeding two meals of cracked corn at 0 and 4 h after glycogen-depleting exercise (2.2 kg corn/meal, total digestible energy intake of ~15 Mcal) enhanced systemic glucose supply (threefold increase in whole body glucose kinetics) but minimally enhanced muscle glycogen replenishment at 24 h post-exercise when compared to feed withholding or isocaloric feedings of hay (grass and alfalfa hay mix) (Fig. 37.5).[39] In contrast, intravenous administration of glucose (6 g/kg BW over 12 hours,[40,41] or about 0.5 g/kg BW/h) was demonstrated to increase muscle glycogen recovery by 24 h post-exercise.

Alternative strategies for the enhancement of muscle glycogen recovery in horses have been examined, including the addition of amino acids to glucose feedings, short-chain (volatile) fatty acid supplementation, and provision of a hypotonic electrolyte solution. Studies in humans have shown that the addition of protein hydrolysates or certain amino acids to carbohydrate/glucose feedings can enhance insulinemic response and glycogen replenishment when compared to carbohydrate alone.[42] Leucine is an insulin secretagogue and, in rodent studies, has been demonstrated to increase muscle glucose uptake; both mechanisms may promote muscle glycogenesis when leucine is fed along with glucose. It should be

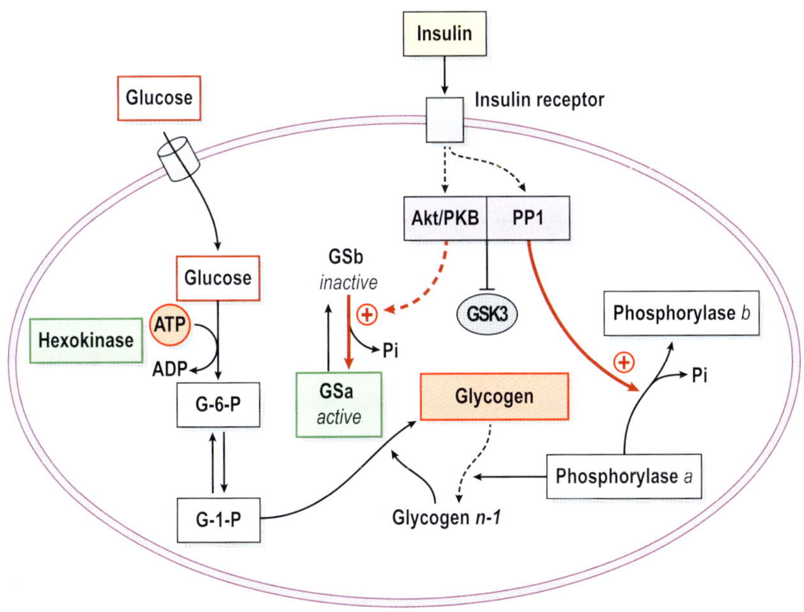

Fig 37.3 Simplified schematic of the biochemical pathways for the synthesis of glycogen in skeletal muscle under conditions of increased circulating glucose and insulin. Glucose entering the cell is phosphorylated to form glucose-6-phosphate (G-6-P) in a reaction catalyzed by hexokinase. Glycogen synthase (GS) catalyzes the addition of glucosyl units to the glycogen polymer. GS is regulated by the concentrations of glycogen (autoregulation) and G-6-P, as well as insulin. Stimulation of GS by insulin involves activation of Akt (protein kinase B, PKB) that, in turn, leads to deactivation of glycogen synthase kinase 3 (GSK3). Deactivation of GSK3 enables conversion of GS from its inactive (GSb) to active form (GSa). Protein phosphatase 1 (PP1) also glycogen synthetic activity via dephosphorylation reactions that activate GS and deactivate glycogen phosphorylase.

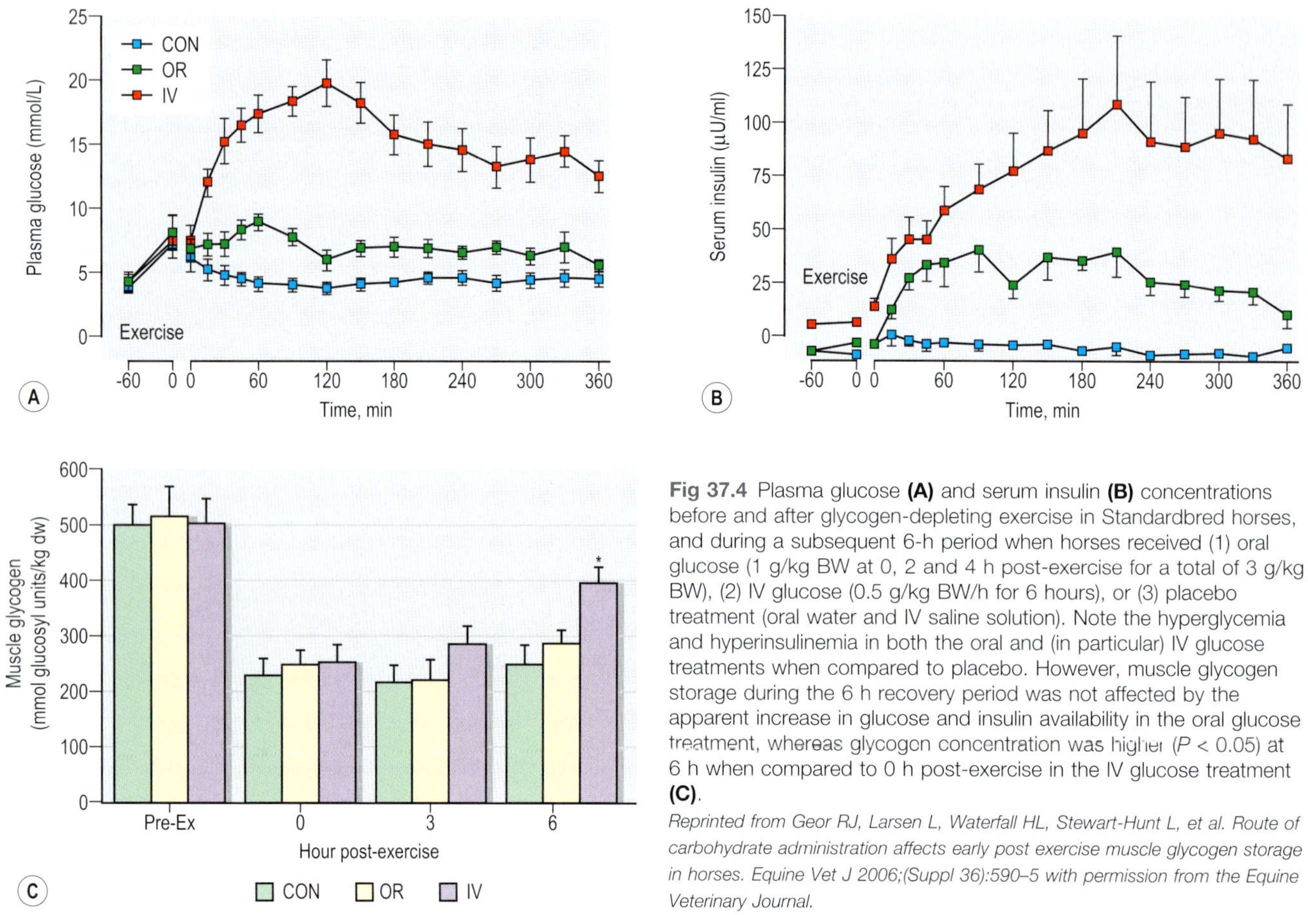

Fig 37.4 Plasma glucose **(A)** and serum insulin **(B)** concentrations before and after glycogen-depleting exercise in Standardbred horses, and during a subsequent 6-h period when horses received (1) oral glucose (1 g/kg BW at 0, 2 and 4 h post-exercise for a total of 3 g/kg BW), (2) IV glucose (0.5 g/kg BW/h for 6 hours), or (3) placebo treatment (oral water and IV saline solution). Note the hyperglycemia and hyperinsulinemia in both the oral and (in particular) IV glucose treatments when compared to placebo. However, muscle glycogen storage during the 6 h recovery period was not affected by the apparent increase in glucose and insulin availability in the oral glucose treatment, whereas glycogen concentration was higher ($P < 0.05$) at 6 h when compared to 0 h post-exercise in the IV glucose treatment **(C)**.

Reprinted from Geor RJ, Larsen L, Waterfall HL, Stewart-Hunt L, et al. Route of carbohydrate administration affects early post exercise muscle glycogen storage in horses. Equine Vet J 2006;(Suppl 36):590–5 with permission from the Equine Veterinary Journal.

noted that protein or amino acid supplementation does not augment muscle glycogenesis in humans when larger amounts of carbohydrate are consumed during recovery (~1.2 g CHO/kg BW/h) which is considered the optimal dosage for enhancement of glycogen resynthesis.[43]

In horses, the addition of 0.1 g/kg BW[44] or 0.3 g/kg BW[45] leucine to a glucose dose was shown to substantially increase post-exercise plasma insulin responses when compared to glucose alone. However, the administration of leucine (0.1 g/kg BW at 0 and 4 h post-exercise) in concert with glucose (1.0 g/kg BW at 0, and 4 h post-exercise) did not alter post-exercise glycogen replenishment in Standardbred horses.[46] Whereas amino acid supplementation may not enhance early post-exercise glycogen recovery, recent work has suggested that protein nutrition can affect muscle glycogen content. Specifically, the muscle glycogen concentration of Standardbred trotters fed a forage-only diet with 16.6% crude protein (CP) was higher (~630 mmol/kg DM) when compared to a forage diet providing 12.5% CP (~550 mmol/kg DM), and there also was a trend for faster post-exercise glycogen recovery in horses fed the higher protein diet.[47] However, the 16.6% CP hay also had greater NSC content and this difference may have contributed to the higher muscle glycogen concentration in this treatment.

Low availability of lipid metabolites during the post-exercise recovery period may limit muscle glycogenesis by redirecting glucose away from glycogen synthesis to support immediate energy needs through the tricarboxylic acid (TCA) cycle,[48] i.e. available glucose is partitioned to oxidation rather than storage. Therefore, post-exercise feeding strategies that directly or indirectly (e.g. via production of volatile fatty acids by microbial fermentation) increase the availability of alternative substrates for the TCA cycle (such as acetate) could support glycogen synthesis. The ingestion of a glucose/acetate solution increased glycogen replenishment and GS activity in rats after exercise when compared to glucose alone.[49] In horses, Waller et al.[50] reported that the administration of a sodium acetate–electrolyte solution (containing 500 g sodium acetate, 250 ml acetic acid, 32 g KCl, and 300 g glucose in 8 L of water) modestly enhanced the early rate (measured at 4 h) of muscle glycogen synthesis in horses after glycogen-depleting exercise. The authors suggested that the administered acetate was rapidly taken up by skeletal muscle, converted to acetyl-CoA and acetylcarnitine and, in turn, metabolized to CO_2 and water via the TCA cycle.[50] Synthesis of ATP by this mechanism would allow the partitioning of glucose into storage (glycogenesis) rather oxidative pathways. The acetate–acetic acid mixture, however, appeared to depress appetite and may have elicited intestinal discomfort,[50] and such a treatment cannot be recommended for use in the field pending further investigations of different acetate formulations.

There has been interest in the effects of higher oil diets on muscle glycogen storage and replenishment rate in horses. Although early studies suggested that fat/oil supplementation was associated with higher 'resting' muscle glycogen concentrations,[51] more recent studies have reported no effect of oil supplementation on muscle glycogen stores.[52,53] One study in horses reported that the ingestion of a diet containing 50 g oil/kg DM intake rapeseed oil reduced the rate of post-exercise glycogen repletion. This effect, however, was not apparent when horses were adapted for 3 weeks to a diet containing 50 g oil/kg DM intake.[53] McCue et al.[54] reported that the administration of 217 ml of either corn or triheptanoin (a triglyceride containing fatty acid moieties with a chain length of seven carbons) 120 min before exercise did not influence post-exercise glycogen repletion.

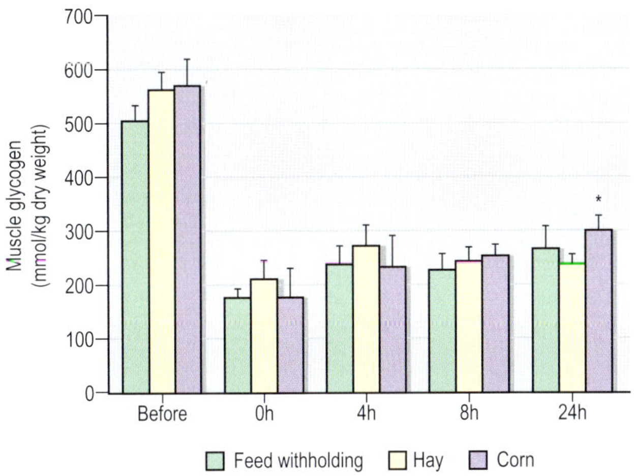

Fig 37.5 Muscle glycogen concentrations (mean ± SEM) before and 0, 4, 8 and 24 h after a glycogen-depleting exercise protocol in seven horses. In a randomized, crossover design horses were either not fed for 8 h, fed half of the daily energy requirements (~15 Mcal digestible energy [DE]) as hay, or fed an isocaloric amount of corn 15 min and 4 h after exercise. Grain feeding resulted in moderate hyperglycemia and hyperinsulinemia and threefold higher glucose kinetics when compared to feed withholding; however, these differences were not associated with enhancement in the rate of muscle glycogen resynthesis (* indicates that muscle glycogen concentration in corn-fed horses is higher [$P = 0.04$] at 24 h vs 0 h).

Reprinted from Jose-Cunilleras E, Hinchcliff KW, Lacombe VA, et al. Ingestion of starch-rich meals after exercise increases glucose kinetics but fails to enhance muscle glycogen replenishment in horses. Vet J 2006;171:468–77 with permission from Elsevier.

There is evidence that dehydration affects glycogen synthesis in muscle and liver. Within these tissues, glycogen is stored in a hydrated form associated with about 3 g water and 0.5 mmol K^+ per gram of glycogen, and adequate intracellular water and K^+ are required for glycogen synthesis. Indeed, studies in rodents have shown that cell shrinkage, as occurs with dehydration, impairs glycogen synthesis in skeletal muscle while cell swelling has the opposite effect.[55] It is therefore possible that exercise-associated dehydration is one factor that constrains the post-exercise rate of muscle glycogen resynthesis in horses. To test this hypothesis, Waller et al.[56] evaluated the effects of a hypotonic (~210 mOsmol/kg) electrolyte solution (12 g Na, 24 g Cl, 9 g K, 1 g Ca and Mg in 8 liters of water) on whole-body and muscle hydration state plus glycogen synthesis in horses after glycogen-depleting exercise. When compared to the control trial, the electrolyte treatment resulted in quicker restoration of hydration, evidenced by faster recovery of plasma protein concentration, maintenance of plasma osmolality and greater muscle intracellular fluid volume. Additionally, the electrolyte treatment enhanced the rate of muscle glycogen resynthesis; at 4 h and 24 h of recovery, muscle glycogen was significantly higher than in the control treatment. Total water intake, including the 8 liters given via nasogastric intubation, was higher in the electrolyte treatment; at 24 h of recovery total water consumption in the electrolyte and control treatments was, respectively, 49.5 ± 4.2 and 34.8 ± 2.2 liters.[56] Rehydration via administration of electrolyte solutions (and ensuring that horses have free access to fresh, palatable water) therefore may be important in the context of muscle glycogen recovery.

In summary, nutritional interventions with proven efficacy for enhancement of muscle glycogen recovery in humans and other species are not effective in horses, likely reflecting differences in physiology – in particular lower insulin sensitivity in horses vs other mammals. Very high starch diets (e.g. grain at 70–80% of the as-fed ration) have been shown to modestly increase the rate of muscle glycogen resynthesis, but even then 48 hours or more are needed for complete replenishment and the risks of intestinal disturbances associated with high starch diets may outweigh any benefit with respect to muscle glycogen recovery. The composition of post-exercise meals should largely mirror the current base ration, with forage the first feedstuff offered after exercise.

The interval between hard exercise events is likely the most important consideration with respect to the optimization of muscle glycogen stores. A 1600 m Thoroughbred race may result in substantial (~30–40%) decrease in muscle glycogen concentration but horses competing in such races are not likely to perform another hard training session or race for a few days, by which time muscle glycogen will have returned to baseline values. It is recognized that for other athletic disciplines (e.g. show jumpers competing multiple times per day, Standardbred racehorses running more than one heat in a single day, or three-day eventers performing the stadium jumping test the day following the cross-country test) muscle glycogen replenishment will be incomplete due to the short interval between exercise bouts.

Feeding management for horses at risk for specific conditions

Equine gastric ulcer syndrome (EGUS)

The horse is a basal acid producer, meaning that it secretes acid into the stomach continuously. The saliva produced by normal grazing behavior helps to buffer this gastric acid. In addition, living under natural conditions encourages the horse to move freely and may promote more efficient gastric emptying when compared to horses kept in confinement housing. Arguably, the modern management of athletic horses, including meal feeding, low fiber/high concentrate diets and intensive training programs, may result in a poorly buffered, acidic gastric environment that contributes to high prevalence of gastric ulcers in performance horses. As discussed in detail elsewhere in this book (Chapter 47), the prevalence and severity of ulceration has been correlated with the intensity of training that the horse undergoes. Additional contributing factors associated with gastric lesions include high concentrate (starch and sugar-based) diets, low hay diets, forage type, meal feeding, and feed deprivation.[57]

Exceeding 2 g/kg BW of starch intake per day (or >1 g/kg starch in a single meal) was associated with a twofold increase in the likelihood for gastric sqamous lesions (grade 2 or higher ulcer scores) in Danish horses.[58] In this same study, the risk of significant gastric squamous ulcers was increased (4.5-fold) when straw was the only forage provided. In contrast, there is some evidence that the feeding of alfalfa hay reduces the severity of ulcer scores in horses undergoing exercise training. Differences in buffering capacity (protein and calcium contents) between straw and alfalfa may account for this apparent effect of forage type on gastric ulceration. The length of time between forage feeding is another consideration; Luthersson et al.[58] observed that greater than 6 hours between forage meals increased the likelihood of non-glandular ulcers. These authors also reported that horses without access to water in their paddock were more likely to have clinically significant gastric ulcers (ulcer score ≥ 2/4).

The primary dietary recommendations for management of gastric ulcer disease are to limit the amount of starch-rich feeds and increase the quantity of forage, with inclusion of some alfalfa. Specific recommendations to help reduce the risk of EGUS include:

- feeding a ration with not less than 1.5% on a DM basis of BW as forage (i.e. 7.5 kg dry matter [DM] for a 500-kg horse) and preferably 2% or more. When restricted forage intakes are required (i.e. during weight loss regimens), appropriate measures need to be instigated to maximize the time the horses spend chewing and foraging
- including some alfalfa hay. Although the optimal amount is not known, for horses with a propensity for EGUS the inclusion of about one-quarter of the hay ration as alfalfa is recommended
- limiting daily starch intake to no more than 2 g/kg BW/day and restricting the starch content of individual meals to no more than 1g/kg BW. These goals are difficult to achieve in racehorses that are traditionally provided grain-rich (e.g. >6–7 kg/day) rations that far exceed the recommended level of daily starch intake. Nonetheless, it is possible to substantially decrease starch intake by these animals by providing a higher quantity of forage together with a higher oil and fiber feed that has been formulated for the performance horse
- providing pasture turnout. It should be recognized, however, that gastric ulcers may develop and/or persist in pasture-managed animals especially if they are still being fed high levels of starch and sugar-rich feeds and/or are in hard work
- providing access to water at all times, including when at pasture
- wherever possible, avoiding stressful situations such as long-distance travel, changes in living environment, and long periods of confinement where the horse cannot freely move around. Horses should be provided access to forage during transportation and immediately on arrival.

Note that dietary and management changes alone will rarely result in resolution of gastric lesions. Medical therapy (see Chapter 47) should be instituted to facilitate ulcer healing; longer-term medical therapy may be needed in some cases.

What about the use of supplements?

A number of studies have examined the potential for specific cocktails of ingredients to positively influence gastric ulcer healing or prevent ulcer development. A specific pectin–lecithin complex, however, did not prevent development of squamous mucosal lesions induced by intermittent feed deprivation.[59] The feeding of a product derived from sea buckthorn berries and pulp to stall confined horses had no apparent efficacy for the treatment or prevention of naturally occurring squamous mucosal ulcers; however, glandular mucosa ulcer scores were significantly lower in the treated animals after feed deprivation.[60] Another product containing a mixture of bentonite, psyllium, dicalcium phosphate, soybean hydrolysate, marsh mallow, orange peel, dandelion, rosemary, mint, dried grass meal, lecithin and yeast was reported to have a beneficial effect on ulcer healing but the study design did not include a non-treated control group.[61]

Equine rhabdomyolysis syndrome

Based on current knowledge, the authors divide horses affected by the equine rhabdomyolysis syndrome (ERS) into two groups (see also Chapter 7):

1. Those in which the primary underlying susceptibility is intrinsic to the muscle; often referred to as *chronic*.
   - Currently two main subgroups are recognized within this category. One involves a disorder in muscle contractility or excitation–contraction coupling and is often referred to as recurrent exertional rhabdomyolysis (RER), and the other is associated with increased muscle glycogen content (polysaccharide storage myopathy [PSSM]).
   - In both RER and PSSM, a lack of routine daily exercise and a diet high in starch are common predisposing factors for an episode.
2. Those in which *an intrinsic muscle defect does not appear to be present* (or, is as yet unrecognized): sometimes referred to as *sporadic*. Dietary and other management factors are also thought to contribute to this form of rhabdomyolysis, including:
   - exercising after a period of (relative) over-feeding and under-exercising
   - electrolyte imbalances (dietary or individual animal in origin)
   - provision of low fiber, high non-structural carbohydrate (NSC) rations.

For all horses with ERS, forage should be the basis of their ration. Other management practices to consider include (see also Harris and Rivero[62]):

- not turning the horse out onto 'lush' fast-growing pastures, especially pastures with a high fructan, high starch (e.g. high clover/legume cover) or water-soluble carbohydrate content, but providing prolonged daily periods out in a sparse paddock can often be beneficial
- providing regular daily exercise including the opportunity for free (unstructured) physical activity – some horses appear to be more 'stressed' when exercised alone while others appear more relaxed in this situation – it is important to choose the exercise format that appears to cause minimum 'stress'
- using more digestible fiber sources such as soya hulls and unmolassed sugar beet pulp if additional energy is required over and above forage. These are often most easily provided by use of a commercial feed containing these ingredients
- utilizing supplementary oil as a concentrated energy source rather than cereal grains – either by the addition of high oil feedstuffs such as rice bran (ensure correct overall calcium: phosphorus balance of the diet) or the addition of vegetable oil, e.g. corn oil, sunflower or soya oil. Any supplemental oil should be introduced slowly – over 2–3 weeks depending on the amount to be added (see below)
- ensuring that the diet provides a sufficient intake of electrolytes (appropriate use of the urinary fractional electrolyte excretion test may aid in the assessment of the adequacy of electrolyte intake)
- ensuring adequate dietary vitamin E and selenium intake (see below).

For horses with RER or PSSM, there should be a significant reduction in NSC intake and increased use of oil and fibers as energy sources. With respect to PSSM, the diet should be devoid of grain (starch) and sugar such that, on a total diet basis, less than 15% of DE is supplied by NSC. There is some controversy with respect to the amount of supplemental oil required for management of PSSM.[63] 'Easy keeper' horses PSSM that are only in light work will maintain condition on a diet that is predominantly medium-quality hay (supplied at approximately 1.5% of BW as DM), with a small quantity of oil (e.g. 0.5 to 1 kg rice bran per day or ½ to 1 cup of oil) and a vitamin-mineral supplement. For horses with PSSM, forage should have low starch and sugar content – the authors recommend <12% NSC on a DM basis – to minimize post-feeding glycemic and insulinemic responses.[64] Lush pasture and legume hays (alfalfa) should be avoided because these forages can supply a substantial quantity of sugar/starch. Possible options for meeting the energy needs of affected horses in harder training include the provision of larger quantities of rice bran (e.g. 1–2 kg/day), a combination of hay pellets and vegetable oil (up to 1 ml per kg BW/day), or a 'fat and fiber' energy concentrate. The latter utilize a combination of vegetable oils (oils and/or rice bran) and highly fermentable fibers (sugar beet pulp and/or soya hulls). Some of these feeds provide less than 15% of DE from NSC and up to 20% of DE as fat.

A typical racehorse with RER is consuming greater than 30 Mcal of DE per day, with much of the energy supplied by starch. Indeed, it is not uncommon for racehorses to consume 7–10 kg/day of a grain-concentrate, and this level of starch intake appears to contribute to an increased frequency of tying-up episodes.[63,65] Therefore, as with PSSM, a lower starch, higher fat and fermentable fiber diet is indicated in the management of horses with RER. One recommendation for racehorses in intense work is a diet that provides no more than 20% of DE from starch/sugars, with a minimum of 20% DE from fat. Practically, providing a low/restricted starch commercial feed or not feeding more than ~2.5 kg/day of cereal-based feed (for a 500-kg horse) is a reasonable starting point although the level of starch/sugar that can be tolerated appears to be individual in nature.

Vitamin E and/or selenium deficiency may be *permissive* to the development of ERS in some circumstances and therefore it is important to take into account factors such as local geography that may contribute to low selenium or vitamin E in forages and feedstuffs. The potential for ERS to be associated with a vitamin E/selenium deficiency is unlikely when the daily intakes of vitamin E and selenium are, respectively, 3–5 iu/kg BW and 0.003–0.006 mg/kg BW. An additional 1–1.5 iu vitamin E should be provided per ml of supplemental oil.

These dietary interventions are not a panacea for the prevention of PSSM and RER. As discussed in Chapter 7, a number of other management changes are needed for the successful management of horses with chronic rhabdomyolysis. For example, along with strict dietary control, daily exercise is critical to the successful management of horses with PSSM, while strategies for reduction of stress and excitability are important in the management of RER-susceptible horses.

Effects of oil-supplemented diets in athletic horses

Metabolic responses to exercise

The inclusion of vegetable oil in diets for athletic horses is now widespread. Oil supplementation in horses is characterized by an increase in plasma phospholipids and cholesterol and a decrease in plasma TGs.[66,67] Changes in the activities of lipoprotein lipase and the enzymes of β-oxidation also suggest that horses adapted to a oil-supplemented diet have increased capacity for the uptake and oxidation of fatty acids in muscle. Indeed, some studies have shown lower respiratory exchange ratio in oil-adapted horses during low- and moderate-intensity exercise.[68,69] Pagan et al.[68] also reported a decrease in glucose flux during low intensity in horses adapted to a diet providing 29% of DE from corn oil. Thus, oil supplementation enhances lipid oxidation and spares the use of endogenous CHO (plasma glucose, muscle glycogen) during moderate exercise (Fig. 37.6). Theoretically, such a glycogen-sparing effect could improve exercise performance; however, the actual effects of oil supplementation on endurance exercise performance under competition conditions still remain to be proven scientifically.

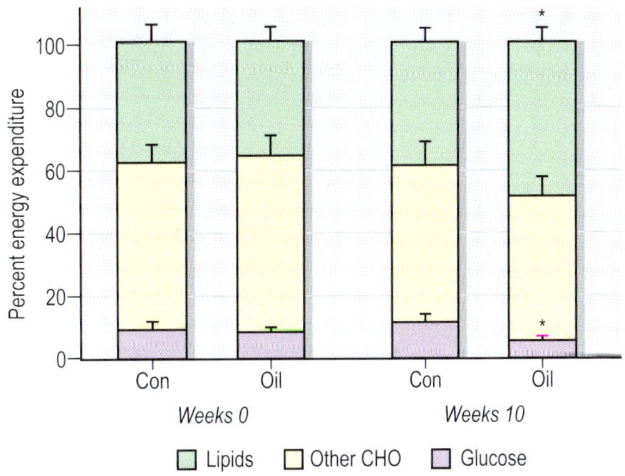

Fig 37.6 Relative contributions of energy from different substrate sources (blood glucose, other carbohydrate [CHO; muscle glycogen and lactate], or lipids) during 90 min of exercise at ~35% of maximal oxygen uptake in horses before (Week 0) and after (Week 10) adaptation to a control [Con] diet (hay and sweet feed) or an oil-supplemented diet (Oil). The total amount of digestible energy supplied by oil in the Con and Oil diets was 7% and 29%, respectively. Adaptation to the oil-supplemented diet resulted in a decrease in the rate of carbohydrate utilization and an increase in the rate of lipid oxidation.

Reprinted from Pagan JD, Geor RJ, Harris PA, et al. Effects of fat adaptation on glucose kinetics and substrate oxidation during low intensity exercise. Equine Vet J 2002;(Suppl 34):33–38, with permission from the Equine Veterinary Journal.

The length of time required for metabolic adaptation to dietary oil is also a somewhat contentious issue. Some nutritionists believe that a minimum of 10–12 weeks is required for full adaptation.[70] However, metabolic adaptations to oil supplementation have been observed as early as 3–5 weeks after the start of supplementation.[66,68] Thus, whereas a 2–3 month period may be required for complete adaptation to an oil-supplemented diet, some of the metabolic responses are evident much earlier. In one study, the metabolic responses to oil supplementation were abolished within 5 weeks of withdrawal of the oil-supplemented diet.[66] The putative benefits of oil-supplemented diets in horses are therefore dependent on continued use of such rations.

Athletic performance

Lay articles on equine nutrition and feed company marketing literature commonly state that higher oil diets enhance athletic performance. There may be benefits associated with oil substitution for starch and sugar due to improved behavior, reduced thermal load, etc. (see below), but the effects of oil supplementation on actual exercise performance are equivocal, especially in regards to high-intensity exercise. Harkins et al.[71] reported improved racetrack performance in Thoroughbreds fed a fat-supplemented diet, while Eaton et al.[72] reported that a fat-supplemented diet resulted in a small but statistically significant increase in run time to fatigue and maximal accumulated oxygen deficit (MAOD) in horses undertaking treadmill exercise at an intensity equivalent to 120% of VO_{2max}. In other studies, providing more than 12–15% of DE as fat was associated with faster times during repeated sprints[73–75] and greater total work effort during cutting events.[76] Feeding trotting horses 250 g and 500 g of oil/day vs the control diet resulted in decreases in exercise-associated elevations of heart and respiratory rates, body temperature, PCV and blood lactate.[77] In contrast, a number of studies have reported no change in exercise performance when horses received similar amounts of supplemental fats or oils.[78–80] Differences between study findings may be attributed to variation in experimental design, level of oil supplementation, etc., coupled with the difficulty in assessing performance per se. The mechanism(s) of any effect of fat/oil supplementation on exercise performance is not known, although muscle glycogen-sparing, improved power-to-weight ratio resulting from reduced DM intake and bowl ballast, and a reduction in acidemia and metabolic heat generated during exercise have been proposed.[81]

Thermal load

It has been proposed that the feeding of fat/oil-enriched diets reduces the thermal burden of exercise.[81] Kronfeld[81] employed a theoretical model to compare estimated heat production in horses provided rations with different proportions of fermentable CHO, hydrolysable CHO (starch/sugars) and fat. It was concluded that a hay, oat and corn oil ration (45:45:10% of intake, respectively) would result in ~2% less heat produced during moderate-to-heavy exercise and an ~5% reduction in total daily heat load compared to a diet of hay and oats (50:50). Although this calculated reduction in total heat load is small, it might be enough to benefit horses living and competing in hot and/or humid environments. The practical implications of these theoretical calculations have not been determined.

Behavior

An increase in dietary oil (and concurrent decrease in NSC) may positively impact performance in some athletic disciplines (e.g. dressage) via effects on behavior. Anecdotally, horses owners have reported that horses are more tractable when provided diets with added fat/oil. In support of these observations, spontaneous activity and reactivity to pressure, loud noise and visual stimuli were reduced in horses fed a diet containing 10% soy lecithin and corn oil,[82] while horses in dressage training had lower resting cortisol concentrations and a reduction in the intensity of their responses to a startle reaction test when fed a diet with 11% DM fat compared to an isocaloric diet with higher starch.[83]

Free fatty acid (FFA) profile

The profile of FFA contained within an oil-supplemented diet may also be important as it will influence the FFA profile of stored triglycerides and, therefore, the FFA mobilized with exercise. FFA constitute a broad spectrum of molecules, from the so-called short to long fatty acids, which may have different rates of diffusion into cells, thereby affecting their rate of utilization with exercise. No studies have been undertaken in the horse to examine specifically the utilization of the different FFAs during exercise. Medium-chain triglycerides (MCTs) have been evaluated as a potential ergogenic aid in humans because, when compared to longer-chain fats, they are more rapidly digested and absorbed directly into systemic circulation rather than transported to the liver as a component of chylomicrons. Furthermore, MCTs do not require the acetyl transferase system for transport across the inner mitochondrial membrane. Orally supplied MCTs, however, do not lead to a sparing of muscle glycogen use during moderate-to-intense exercise in humans and their effect on performance is questionable.[84] Limited work in horses also has not demonstrated an effect of MCT supplementation on performance.[85]

Putative ergogenic supplements

One of the tenets of a sound nutritional management is to feed the horse as an individual, and the feeding of supplements are a potential means by which the diet can be tailored. A supplement enables specific individual conditions (e.g. a horse with a nervous temperament or poor hooves) or environmental risks (e.g. the effect of housing on lung health; the impact of travel on the immune system) to be taken into account. Supplementation in such circumstances may work to counteract the imbalance between nutrient supply and demand and help to restore 'normality'. In other situations supplementation may help to provide additional boost or support to enable enhanced performance. It is this last category that tends to provoke the most controversy because horsemen often feed a variety of supplements in an attempt to enhance a horse's performance. Depending on the nature of the supplement and the sport, such supplementation may be within or contrary to the rules of that discipline. Equally as relevant and controversial are the safety and efficacy of these so-called ergogenic supplements. The term *ergogenic* means 'work generating';[86] thus, an ergogenic supplement is one that enhances work performance (e.g. an increase in speed, endurance or strength). Possible ways that ergogenic supplements may improve performance could include (Fig. 37.7):[87]

- psychological effects
- improved coordination or recruitment of muscle fibers
- provision of a supplementary fuel source or the feeding of a feed with a higher energy content
- increased levels of available stored energy
- improved efficiency of conversion of the chemical energy of the feed, or stored energy, to mechanical energy for work
- improved ATP/ADP homeostasis in contracting muscle fibers
- decreased substrate depletion
- decreased end-product accumulation including improved intracellular acid–base regulation.

Innate athletic ability can be modified by various factors, in particular training but also nutrition. In the human sports medicine field, there has been a shift in the rationale for the type of nutritional support given to elite athletes from being primarily focused on recovery between training sessions to a focus on ways that nutrition can 'help promote the adaptations that take place in tissues in response to the training stimulus.'[88] There is very little published work on these aspects in the horse; indeed, in general there has been very little work on putative ergogenic supplements for horses. This does not necessarily imply a lack of efficacy but rather a lack of evidence of efficacy. The following discussion is restricted to some of the supplements that have been evaluated in the horse; a discussion on herbs, spices, pre- and probiotics as well as chondroprotective compounds is outside the scope of this chapter.

Creatine

Creatine (methylguanidine-acetic acid) is a compound derived from amino acids that is stored primarily in skeletal muscle at typical concentrations of 100–150 mmol/kg dry weight (dw) of muscle. About 60–65% of this creatine is phosphorylated. Creatine phosphate provides a rapid but brief source of phosphate for the resynthesis of ATP during intense exercise, and therefore helps to maintain normal ATP/ADP homeostasis. A large number of studies have evaluated the performance effects of creatine supplementation in humans. Although the results have varied between studies and sporting event,[89–92] the general view is that creatine supplementation enhances performance involving repeated sprints, probably related to an increase in the rate of creatine phosphate resynthesis

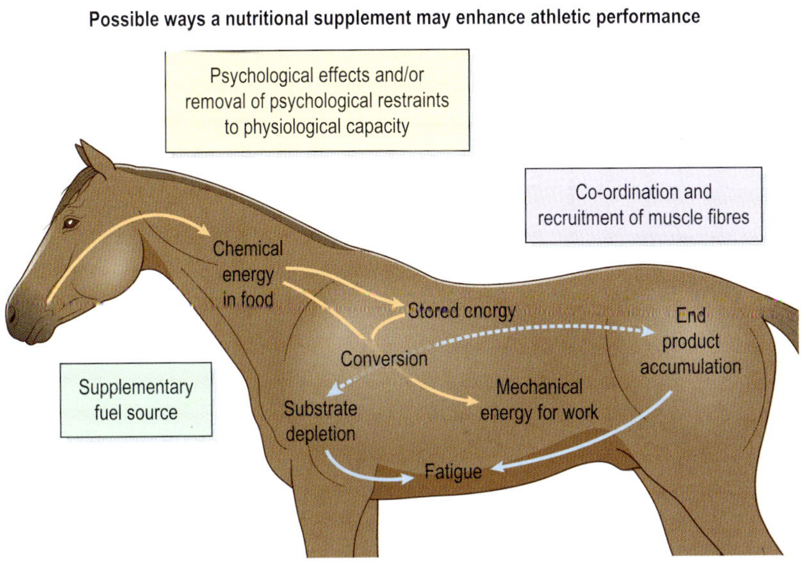

Fig 37.7 Schematic indicating possible mechanisms by which a nutritional supplement may have an ergogenic (performance-enhancing) effect. The supplement may boost performance via central mechanisms (e.g. psychological effects) or by peripheral effects on metabolism or muscle function (e.g. decrease end-product accumulation in muscle; increase substrate supply; decrease substrate depletion; enhance the efficiency of conversion of chemical into mechanical energy).
Figure with permission from copyright holder, Mars Horsecare UK Ltd.

during recovery between bouts of exercise. However, oral creatine supplementation is not considered ergogenic for single-bout or first-bout sprints, or for prolonged submaximal exercise. The evidence is inconclusive for effects on muscle strength, although creatine supplements are widely used by body builders and weight lifters. Several potential mechanisms may account for an ergogenic effect of creatine supplementation, including direct effects in skeletal muscle (increased muscle glycogen and phosphocreatine, faster phosphocreatine resynthesis, and enhanced muscle buffering capacity) or indirectly through increased training volume.[89]

Studies in man have demonstrated that a daily creatine dose of 20–25 g (~250 mg/kg BW/day), divided into four doses, results in increased muscle creatine concentrations, with an apparent upper threshold of 150–160 mmol/kg dw. About 20% of the increased muscle creatine content is stored as creatine phosphate, and saturation occurs 2–3 days after the start of supplementation.[93] The increase in muscle creatine content is greatest in those subjects with a low initial concentration. Lower daily doses of 3 g/day (~40–44 mg/kg BW) will achieve a slower loading over 14–28 days, and elevated muscle creatine stores can be maintained by continued daily supplementation of 2–3 g creatine.[94] Creatine is transported into muscle against a high concentration gradient, via saturable transport processes that are stimulated by exercise[94] and by insulin.[95]

In horses, Sewell and Harris[96] demonstrated that, in contrast to man and dog, creatine is poorly absorbed. The intragastric administration of 50 mg Cr per kg BW resulted in an increase in plasma creatine concentration from 40 to 100 fmol/L after 4–6 hours. By comparison, the same dose in humans results in plasma concentrations of 800–1000 fmol/L.[93] Furthermore, the administration of creatine at 150 mg/kg per day (divided into three doses) for 13 days had no effect on muscle creatine content.[96] In a randomized, crossover design, Schuback et al.[97] fed Standardbred trotters 25 g creatine monohydrate twice daily (total daily dose of ~100–120 mg/kg BW) for 14 days. Before and after the period of supplementation, horses completed an incremental treadmill exercise test until exhaustion. There was no significant effect of supplementation on plasma or muscle creatine concentrations, nor an effect on treadmill run time and the muscle metabolic response to exercise.[97] A more recent study found no changes in ultrasound measurements of cross-sectional area of the longissimus dorsi muscle when 75 g of creatine monohydrate was fed to Arabian horses for 90 days during aerobic training.[98]

Thus, creatine supplementation in the horse at dosages shown to be effective in man has failed to result in an increase in muscle creatine content. Without a change in muscle creatine content, creatine supplementation is unlikely to exert an ergogenic effect in horses. The reason for the apparent low bioavailability of orally administered creatine in horses has not been determined. It is possible that, as an herbivorous animal, the horse's gastrointestinal tract is not adapted to the absorption of creatine.

L-carnitine

L-carnitine is a component of the enzymes carnitine-palmityltransferase I, carnitine- palmityltransferase II, and carnitine-acylcarnitine translocase that are involved in the transport of long-chain fatty acids across the inner mitochondrial membrane.[99] As such, long-chain fatty acid oxidation is carnitine dependent and, therefore, it has been proposed that increased availability of L-carnitine by supplementary ingestion might upregulate the capacity to transport fatty acids into the mitochondria and increase fatty acid oxidation.[86] This augmentation in fat oxidation could be of benefit during endurance exercise. Another role of carnitine is to act as a 'sink' for acetyl-CoA units produced during high-intensity exercise. The conversion of acetyl-CoA to acetyl-carnitine maintains CoA availability and decreases the ratio of acetyl-CoA : CoA. As such, an increase in carnitine availability could enhance substrate flux through the citric acid cycle and increase the activity of pyruvate dehydrogenase, which is otherwise inhibited by high levels of acetyl-CoA. These mechanisms would serve to increase oxidative metabolism of glucose, decrease lactate production, and perhaps enhance performance during exercise tasks that might be limited by excess hydrogen ion and lactate accumulation.[86]

However, the weight of evidence from human studies indicates that oral carnitine supplementation has no effect on muscle carnitine concentration. In addition, there is no evidence that muscle carnitine content limits fat oxidation other than in patients with inborn errors in metabolism that result in inadequate muscle carnitine. This is also likely to be the case in horses, as the carnitine content of equine skeletal muscle is 2–3-fold higher when compared to human muscle.[100] Supplementation studies in humans have failed to demonstrate an effect of carnitine on measures of fat oxidation or muscle metabolism during exercise.[86,99]

Studies in humans[101] and in horses[102,103] have demonstrated that the oral bioavailability of L-carnitine is poor. In horses, large oral doses of L-carnitine (10–60 g) are required to effect an approximate doubling in plasma carnitine concentration.[102] Importantly, supplementation at these levels for 58 days had no effect on muscle carnitine content. In a subsequent study, intravenous doses of 10 g L-carnitine were administered daily for 26 days.[103] These infusions resulted in peak plasma carnitine concentrations 30-fold higher when compared to pre-injection values, and concentrations remained threefold higher after 6 hours. Yet, there was no change in muscle carnitine content. Thus, from the available data there is no compelling evidence that muscle carnitine content is enhanced as a result of oral or IV L-carnitine supplementation.

Although the weight of evidence suggests that L-carnitine is unlikely to be ergogenic in horses, one study has provided evidence that supplementation during conditioning may augment training-associated skeletal muscle adaptations.[104] In a small group of 2-year-old Standardbred horses subjected to a 10-week conditioning program, supplementation with L-carnitine (10 g/day per os) was associated with significant increases in the percentage of type IIA muscle fibers and the intensity of periodic acid Schiff staining (an indicator of intrafiber glycogen content) when compared to untreated control horses.[104] The mechanism of these effects is unclear and somewhat perplexing given that previous studies have failed to demonstrate a change in muscle carnitine content in horses receiving an identical carnitine dosage. Further studies are required to determine the performance implications of these apparent carnitine-induced muscular adaptations.

Amino acids

Amino acid or 'refined' protein supplements are often touted for their ability to 'build' muscle mass. Although there has been limited work in horses on this subject, the results of a few studies have provided evidence that amino acid supplementation may support greater muscle development (e.g. in old horses[105]).

The branched-chain amino acids (BCAA; leucine, isoleucine, valine) have been suggested to enhance endurance performance by modifying factors that contribute to central fatigue.[106,107] In addition, it has been proposed that BCAA supplementation during exercise may provide carbon intermediates for the citric acid cycle at a time when endogenous carbohydrate reserves are depleted, thereby delaying the onset of fatigue.[86] The 'central fatigue' hypothesis proposes that increased brain serotonin contributes to fatigue development during prolonged moderate-intensity exercise.[107] The increase in brain serotonin synthesis occurs as a result of increased transport of free (unbound) tryptophan transfer across the blood–brain barrier. Key to this increase in tryptophan uptake is an increase in the plasma ratio of free tryptophan to BCAA.[107] This ratio may increase for two reasons. First, as blood free fatty acid (FFA) concentration rises during exercise, the FFAs compete with tryptophan for binding sites on albumin, and the FFAs displace some of the tryptophan molecules from albumin; therefore, free tryptophan concentration increases. Second, an increase in the oxidation of BCAA in muscle results in a decrease in blood BCAA concentration. As BCAA and tryptophan compete for carrier-mediated entry into the central nervous system, an increase in the free tryptophan to BCAA ratio leads to increased tryptophan transport. Therefore, it has been theorized that BCAA supplementation could reduce the exercise-induced increase in brain tryptophan uptake and thus delay fatigue.[107] Interestingly, when horses were infused with tryptophan (100 mg/kg, IV) during submaximal exercise, run time to fatigue was decreased by ~15% relative to the placebo treatment, providing evidence that an increase in circulating tryptophan adversely affects endurance performance in horses.[108] In another study where tryptophan was administered before exercise, there was neither a positive nor a negative effect on exercise performance, nor any effect on metabolic responses to exercise.[109] The oral ingestion of a tryptophan solution that markedly increased plasma free tryptophan concentration and estimated brain tryptophan uptake also had no effect on time to exhaustion in exercising humans.[110] Furthermore, in this and other studies, the ingestion of large quantities of BCAA also had no effect on endurance performance.[86,110] These data cast some doubt on the 'central fatigue' hypothesis and suggest that BCAA supplementation is not ergogenic during dynamic exercise in humans.

BCAA supplements are marketed for use in horses, but there are no published data regarding the effects of BCAA supplementation on exercise performance per se. Glade[111] reported that BCAA supplementation mitigated the increase in blood lactate during exercise. However, the exercise test involved treadmill walking and the applicability of these results to equine athletic activities is questionable. Other studies have failed to demonstrate a beneficial effect of BCAA supplementation in horses. The administration of a mixture of L-leucine (9 g), isoleucine (4.5 g), and L-valine (9 g) to Standardbreds 1 hour before training had no measurable effect on energy metabolism during intense exercise.[112] Similarly, there was no change in plasma biochemical variables during and after exercise in horses fed BCAA three times per week for 5 weeks.[113]

Several studies in humans have demonstrated that increased amino acid availability early in the post-exercise period modifies protein metabolism in skeletal muscle.[114–117] Specifically, hyperaminoacidemia resulting from ingestion or intravenous infusion of amino acids increases post-exercise muscle protein synthetic rate and prevents the exercise-induced increase in protein degradation. Thus, post-exercise amino acid or protein supplementation may promote anabolism in skeletal muscle during conditioning. Matsui et al.[118] used radiolabeled phenylalanine to investigate amino acid metabolism in horse muscle after strenuous exercise and reported that the IV administration of a mixture of 10 amino acids reduced protein breakdown and increased protein synthesis in the hindlimb. In another study, the oral administration of a mixture of 18 amino acids to horses after high-intensity exercise increased the intramuscular pool of amino acids and decreased the 4-h post-exercise expression of ubiquitin mRNA in muscle, raising the possibility that supplementation altered the rate of muscle proteolysis.[119] More research is needed before recommendations can be made regarding post-exercise amino acid supplementation in horses.

Carnosine

Physicochemical buffers that include organic and inorganic phosphates, amino acids, and proteins, and dipeptides of histidine and β-alanine comprise the primary defense against an increase in intracellular hydrogen ion concentration.[120] The primary intracellular buffer in muscle is carnosine (β-alanyl-L-histidine) and recent studies in humans have shown strong associations between increased muscle carnosine and high-intensity exercise performance.[120] Carnosine also is the primary intracellular buffer in equine muscle, accounting 30% or more of the physicochemical buffering in type II fibers where it is found in highest concentrations.[121] Although its importance to intracellular acid–base regulation is evident, the physiology governing its synthesis and metabolism remain to be elucidated. In humans, several studies have demonstrated that muscle carnosine increases by 60–80% with 4–10 weeks of β-alanine supplementation, the increase occurring equally in all muscle fiber types.[122] When administered at doses greater than 10 mg/kg body mass, β-alanine supplementation in humans is associated with symptoms of paresthesia, a form of neuropathic pain although potentially this can be avoided through the use of sustained release tablets where the rate of absorption into plasma is controlled.[122] Supplementation of Thoroughbred horses with 100 mg/kg BW oral β-alanine and 12.5 mg/kg BW L-histidine for 30 days significantly increased the carnosine content of type IIa and IIb muscle fibers in some but not all horses, with no change in the carnosine content of type I fibers.[123] Although naturally found in low levels in horse diets (carnosine is a component of pantothenic acid/coenzyme-A in plants) there also may be bacterial synthesis of carnosine via propionate. Further studies in horses are needed to evaluate the effects of β-alanine and L-histidine supplementation on exercise performance.

With thanks to Seppo Hyyppä and A. Reeta Pösö, who created the original chapter in the first edition.

References

1. Duren SE, Manohar M, Sikkes S, et al. Influence of feeding and exercise on the distribution of intestinal and muscle blood flow in ponies. Pferdeheilkunde 1992;9:24 (abstract).
2. Lawrence LM, Soderholm LV, Roberts AM, et al. Feeding status affects glucose metabolism in exercising horses. J Nutr 1993;123:2151–7.
3. Lawrence LM, Hintz HF, Soderholm LV, et al. Effect of time of feeding on metabolic response to exercise. Equine Vet J 1995;(Suppl. 18):392–5.
4. Stull C, Rodiek A. Effects of post prandial interval and feed type on substrate availability during exercise. Equine Vet J 1995;(Suppl. 18):362–6.
5. Pagan JD, Harris PA. The effects of timing and amount of forage and grain on exercise response in Thoroughbred horses. Equine Vet J 1999;(Suppl. 30): 451–7.
6. Jose-Cunilleras E, Hinchcliff KW, Sams RA, et al. Glycemic index of a meal fed before exercise alters substrate use and glucose flux in exercising horses. J Appl Physiol 2002;92:117–28.
7. Palmgren Karlsson C, Jansson A, Essén-Gustavsson B, et al. Effect of molassed sugar beet pulp on nutrient utilisation and metabolic parameters during exercise. Equine Vet J 2002;(Suppl. 34):44–9.
8. Vervuert I, Coenen M, Bichman M. Comparison of the effects of fructose and glucose supplementation on metabolic responses in resting and exercising horses. J Vet Med A Physiol Pathol Clin Med 2004;51:171–7.
9. Rice O, Geor R, Harris P, et al. Effects of restricted hay intake on body weight and metabolic responses to high-intensity exercise in Thoroughbred horses. In: Proceedings of the 17th Meeting of the Equine Nutritional and Physiology Society, 2001. p. 273–9.
10. Curtis GC, Barfoot CF, Dugdale AHA, et al. Voluntary ingestion of wood shavings by obese horses under dietary restriction. Br J Nutr 2011;106:S178–82.
11. Nadeau JA, Andrews FM, Mathew AG, et al. Evaluation of diet as a cause of gastric ulcers in horses. Am J Vet Res 2000;61:784–90.
12. Archer DC, Proudman CJ. Epidemiological clues to preventing colic. Vet J 2006;172:29–39.
13. Hudson JM, Cohen ND, Gibbs PG, et al. Feeding practices associated with colic in horses. J Am Vet Med Assoc 2001;219:1419–25.
14. Harris PA, Schott HC II. Nutritional management of elite endurance horses. In: Geor RJ, Harris PA, Coenen M, editors. Equine Applied and Clinical Nutrition. Saunders Elsevier; 2013. p. 272–88.
15. Brunner J, Wichert B, Burger D, et al. A survey on the feeding of eventing horses during competition. J Anim Physiol Anim Nutr (Berl) 2012;96:878–84.
16. Robert C, Goachet A-G, Fraipont A, et al. Hydration and electrolyte balance in horses during an endurance season. Equine Vet J 2010;42(Suppl 38):98–104.
17. Lindinger MI, Ecker GL. Gastric emptying, intestinal absorption of electrolytes and exercise performance in electrolyte-supplemented horses. Exp Physiol 2013;98:193–206.
18. Ecker GL, Lindinger MI. Effects of terrain, speed, temperature and distance on water and ion losses. Equine Vet J 1995;(Suppl. 18):298–305.
19. McCutcheon LJ, Geor RJ, Hare MJ, et al. Sweating rate and sweat composition during exercise and recovery in ambient heat and humidity. Equine Vet J 1995;(Suppl. 18):153–7.
20. Kingston JK, Geor RJ, McCutcheon LJ. Rate and composition of sweat fluid losses are unaltered by hypohydration during prolonged exercise in horses. J Apply Physiol 1997;83:1133–43.
21. Carlson GP. Thermoregulation and fluid balance in the exercising horse. In: Snow DH, Persson SGB, Rose RJ, editors. Equine Exercise Physiology. Cambridge: Granta Editions; 1983. p. 291–309.
22. Zeyner A, Schwarzer U, Fürll M. Effects of an oral sodium chloride load at different levels on acid-base balance and renal mineral excretion in horses. Proceedings of the 9th Congress of the European Society of Veterinary Clinical Nutrition, Grugliasco, Italy, 2005. p. 124 (abstract).
23. Brooks GA. Bioenergetics of exercising humans. Compr Physiol 2012;2: 537–62.
24. Geor RJ, Hinchcliff KW, Sams RA, et al. Beta-adrenergic blockade augments glucose utilization in horses during graded exercise. J Appl Physiol 2000; 89:1086–98.
25. Spriet LL, Peters SJ. Influence of diet on the metabolic response to exercise. Proc Nutr Soc 1998;57:25–33.
26. Bergström J, Hermansen L, Hultman E, et al. Diet, muscle glycogen and physical performance. Acta Physiol Scand 1967;71:140–50.
27. Snow DH, Baxter P, Rose RJ. Muscle fibre composition and glycogen depletion in horses competing in an endurance ride. Vet Rec 1981;108: 374–8.
28. Topliff DR, Potter GD, Kreider JL. Diet manipulation, muscle glycogen metabolism and anaerobic work performance in the equine. In: Proceedings of the 9th Equine Nutrition and Physiology Symposium. Champaign, IL: American Society of Animal Science; 1985. p. 224–9.
29. Lacombe VA, Hinchcliff KW, Geor RJ, et al. Muscle glycogen depletion and subsequent replenishment affect anaerobic capacity of horses. J Appl Physiol 2001;91:1782–90.
30. Waller AP, Lindinger MI. Nutritional aspects of post exercise skeletal muscle glycogen synthesis in horses: a comparative review. Equine Vet J 2010;42:274–81.
31. Jentjens R, Jeukendrup A. Determinants of post-exercise glycogen storage during short-term recovery. Sports Med 2003; 33:117–44.
32. Cartee GD, Young DA, Sleeper M, et al. Prolonged increase in insulin-stimulated glucose transport in muscle after exercise. Am J Physiol Endocrin Metab 1989;256:E494–E499.
33. Bergstrom J, Hultman E, Roch-Norlund AE. Muscle glycogen synthetase in normal subjects. Basal values, effect of glycogen depletion by exercise and a carbohydrate-rich diet following exercise. Scand J Clin Lab Invest 1972;29:231–6.
34. Geor RJ, Larsen L, Waterfall HL, et al. Route of carbohydrate administration affects early post exercise muscle glycogen storage in horses. Equine Vet J 2006;(Suppl. 36):590–5.
35. Pratt SE, Geor RJ, Spriet LL, et al. Time course of insulin sensitivity and skeletal muscle glycogen synthase activity after a

single bout of exercise in horses. J Appl Physiol 2007;103:1063–9.
36. Lacombe VA, Hinchcliff KW, Kohn CW, et al. Effects of feeding meals with various soluble carbohydrate content on muscle glycogen synthesis after exercise in horses. Am J Vet Res 2004;65:916–23.
37. Burke LM, Hawley JA, Wong SH, et al. Carbohydrates for training and competition. J Sports Sci 2011;29(Suppl. 1):S17–27.
38. Davie AJ, Evans DL, Hodgson DR, et al. The effects of an oral glucose polymer on muscle glycogen resynthesis in standardbred horses. J Nutr 1994; 124(12 Suppl):2740S–1S.
39. Jose-Cunilleras E, Hinchcliff KW, Lacombe VA, et al. Ingestion of starch-rich meals after exercise increases glucose kinetics but fails to enhance muscle glycogen replenishment in horses. Vet J 2006;171:468–77.
40. Davie AJ, Evans DL, Hodgson DR. Effects of intravenous dextrose infusion on muscle glycogen resynthesis after intense exercise. Equine Vet J 1995;(Suppl. 18):195–8.
41. Lacombe VA, Hinchcliff KW, Geor RJ, et al. Muscle glycogen depletion and subsequent replenishment affect anaerobic capacity of horses. J Appl Physiol 2001;91:1782–90.
42. Ivy JL, Goforth HW, Damon BM, et al. Early postexercise muscle glycogen recovery is enhanced with a carbohydrate-protein supplement. J Appl Physiol 2002;93:1337–44.
43. Jentjens R, Van Loon LJ, Mann CH, et al. Addition of protein and amino acids to carbohydrates does not enhance postexercise muscle glycogen synthesis. J Appl Physiol 2001;91: 839–46.
44. Pösö AR, Hyyppä S. Metabolic and hormonal changes after exercise in relation to muscle glycogen concentrations. Equine Vet J 1999;(Suppl. 30):332–6.
45. Urschel KL, Geor RJ, Waterfall HL, et al. Effects of leucine or whey protein addition to an oral glucose solution on serum insulin, plasma glucose and plasma amino acid responses in horses at rest and following exercise. Equine Vet J 2010;42(Suppl. 38):347–54.
46. Bröjer JT, Nostell K, Essen-Gustavsson B, et al. Effects of repeated post-exercise supplementation with glucose and leucine on post-exercise glycogen storage and insulin response in horses. Am J Vet Res 2012;73:867–74.
47. Essén-Gustavsson B, Connysson M, Jansson A. Effects of crude protein intake from forage-only diets on muscle amino acids and glycogen levels in horses during training. Equine Vet J 2010;42(Suppl. 38):341–6.
48. Hyyppä S, Räsänen LA, Pösö AR. Resynthesis of glycogen in skeletal muscle from standardbred trotters after repeated bouts of exercise. Am J Vet Res 2007;58:162–6.
49. Fushimi T, Tayama K, Fukaya M, et al. The efficacy of acetic acid for glycogen repletion in rat skeletal muscle after exercise. Int J Sports Med 2002;23: 218–22.
50. Waller AP, Geor RJ, Spriet LL, et al. Oral acetate supplementation after prolonged moderate intensity exercise enhances early muscle glycogen resynthesis in horses. Exp Physiol 2009;94:888–989.
51. Meyers MC, Potter GD, Evans JW, et al. Physiologic and metabolic responses of exercising horses to added dietary fat. J Eq Vet Sci 1989;9:218–23.
52. Eaton MD, Hodgson DR, Evans DL. Effect of a diet containing supplementary fat on the capacity for high-intensity exercise. Equine Vet J 1995;(Suppl. 18):353–6.
53. Hyyppä S, Saastamoinen M, Pösö AR. Effect of a post-exercise fat supplemented diet on muscle glycogen repletion. Equine Vet J 1999;(Suppl. 30):493–8.
54. McCue ME, Valberg SJ, Pagan JD, et al. Effect of triheptanoin on muscle metabolism during submaximal exercise in horses. Am J Vet Res 2009;70: 1043–52.
55. Low AY, Rennie MJ, Taylor PM. Modulation of glycogen synthesis in rat skeletal muscle by changes in cell volume. J Physiol 1996;495:299–303.
56. Waller AP, Heigenhauser GJF, Geor RJ, et al. Fluid and electrolyte supplementation after prolonged moderate-intensity exercise enhances muscle glycogen resynthesis in horses. J Appl Physiol 2009;106:91–100.
57. Jonsson H, Egenvall A. Prevalence of gastric ulceration in Swedish Standardbreds in race training. Equine Vet J 2006;38:209–13.
58. Luthersson N, Nielsen KH, Harris PA, et al. Risk factors associated with equine gastric ulceration syndrome (EGUS) in 201 horses in Denmark. Equine Vet J 2009;41:625–30.
59. Murray MJ, Grady TC. The effect of a pectin-lecithin complex on prevention of gastric mucodal lesions induced by feed deprivation in ponies. Equine Vet J 2002;34:195–8.
60. Huff NK, Auer AD, Garza F Jr, et al. Effect of sea buckthorn berries and pulp in a liquid emulsion on gastric ulcer scores and gastric juice pH in horses. J Vet Int Med 2012;26:1186–91.
61. Berger S, Schmidt C, van den Hoven R. The effect of AcidProtect on ulcer healing in standardbred horses in active training. Pferdeheilkunde 2011;27:26–30.
62. Harris PA, Rivero JLL. Exercise-associated muscle disorders. In: Geor RJ, Harris PA, Coenen M, editors. Equine Applied and Clinical Nutrition. Saunders Elsevier; 2013. p. 521–35.
63. McKenzie E, Valberg SJ, Pagan JD. Nutritional management of exertional rhabdomyolysis. In: Robinson N, editor. Current Therapy in Equine Medicine 5. Philadelphia: W.B. Saunders; 2003. p. 727–34.
64. Borgia L, Valberg S, McCue M, et al. Glycaemic and insulinaemic responses to feeding hay with different non-structural carbohydrate content in control and polysaccharide myopathy-affected horses. J Anim Physiol Anim Nutr (Berl) 2011;95:798–807.
65. McKenzie E, Valberg SJ, Godden SM, et al. Effects of dietary starch, fat, and bicarbonate on exercise responses and serum creatine kinase activity in equine recurrent exertional rhabdomyolysis. J Vet Int Med 2003;17:693–701.
66. Orme CE, Harris RC, Marlin DJ, et al. Metabolic adaptation to a fat-supplemented diet by the Thoroughbred horse. Br J Nutr 1997;78:443–58.
67. Geelen SN, Sloet van Oldruitenborgh-Oosterbaan MM, Beynen AC. Dietary fat supplementation and equine plasma lipid metabolism. Equine Vet J 1999;(Suppl. 30):475–8.
68. Pagan JD, Geor RJ, Harris PA, et al. Effects of fat adaptation on glucose kinetics and substrate oxidation during low intensity exercise. Equine Vet J 2002;(Suppl. 34):33–8.
69. Dunnett CE, Marlin DJ, Harris RC. Effect of dietary lipid on response to exercise: relationship to metabolic adaptation. Equine Vet J 2002;(Suppl. 34):75–80.
70. Harris PA, Kronfeld DS. Influence of dietary energy source on health and performance. In: Robinson NE, editor. Current Therapy in Equine Medicine 5. Philadelphia: WB Saunders Co; 2003. p. 698–704.
71. Harkins JD, Morris GS, Tulley RT, et al. Effect of added dietary fat on racing performance in Thoroughbred horses. J Equine Vet Sci 1992;12:123–9.
72. Eaton MD, Hodgson DR, Evans DL, et al. Effect of a diet containing supplementary fat on the capacity for high intensity exercise. Equine Vet J 1995;(Suppl. 18):353–6.
73. Scott BD, Potter GD, Greene LW, et al. Efficacy of a fat-supplemented diet on muscle glycogen concentrations in exercising Thoroughbred horses maintained in varying body conditions. J Equine Vet Sci 1992;12:105–9.
74. Oldham SL, Potter GD, Evans JW, et al. Storage and mobilization of muscle glycogen in exercising horses fed a fat-supplemented diet. J Equine Vet Sci 1990;10:353–9.
75. Meyers MC, Potter GD, Evans JW, et al. Physiologic and metabolic response of

exercising horses to added dietary fat. J Equine Vet Sci 1989;9:218–23.
76. Webb SP, Potter GD, Evans JW. Physiologic and metabolic response of race and cutting horses to added dietary fat. Proc 10th Equine Nutr Physiol Soc Symp, Fort Collins, CO, 1987. p. 115.
77. Mattos F, Araújo KV, Leite GG, et al. Uso de óleo na dieta de equinos submetidos ao exercício. Rev Bras Zootecnia 2006;35:1373–80.
78. Topliff D, Potter GD, Dutson TR, et al. Diet manipulation and muscle glycogen in the equine. In: Proceedings of the 8th Equine Nutrition and Physiology Symposium, 1983, p. 224–9.
79. Pagan JD, Essen-Gustavsson B, Lindholm A, et al. The effect of dietary energy source on exercise performance in Standardbred horses. In: Gillespie JR, Robinson NE, editors. Equine Exercise Physiology 2. Davis, CA: ICEEP Publications; 1987. p. 686–700.
80. Essen-Gustavsson B, Blomstrand E, Karlstrom K, et al. Influence of diet on substrate metabolism during exercise. In: Persson SGB, Lindholm A, Jeffcott LB, editors. Equine Exercise Physiology 3. Stockholm, Sweden: ICEEP Publications; 1991. p. 288–98.
81. Kronfeld DS. Dietary fat affects heat production and other variables of equine performance, under hot and humid conditions. Equine Vet J 1996;(Suppl. 22):24–34.
82. Holland JL, Kronfeld DS, Meacham TN. Behavior of horses is affected by soy lecithin and corn oil in the diet. J Anim Sci 1996;74:1252–5.
83. Redondo AJ, Carranza J, Trigo P. Fat diet reduces stress and intensity of startle reaction in horses. Appl Anim Behav Sci 2009;118:69–75.
84. Jeukendrup AE, Aldred S. Fat supplementation, health, and endurance performance. Nutrition 2004;20:678–88.
85. Warren LK, Vineyard KR. Fat and fatty acids. In: Geor RJ, Harris PA, Coenen M, editors. Equine Applied and Clinical Nutrition. Saunders Elsevier; 2013. p. 135–55.
86. Wagenmakers A. Nutritional supplements: effects on exercise performance and metabolism. In: Lamb D, Murray R, editors. Perspectives in Exercise Science and Sports Medicine. The Metabolic Basis of Performance in Exercise and Sport. Carmel, IN: Cooper Publishing; 1999. p. 207–60.
87. Harris P, Harris RC. Nutritional ergogenic aids in the horse: uses and abuses. In: Pagan J, Geor RJ, editors. Advances in Equine Nutrition II. Nottingham: Nottingham Press; 2001. p. 491–507.
88. Maughan RJ, Shirreffs SM. Nutrition for sports performance: issues and opportunities. Proc Nutr Soc 2012;71:112–19.
89. Hespel P, Derave W. Ergogenic effects of creatine in sports and rehabilitation. Subcell Biochem 2007;46:245–59.
90. Glaister M, Lockey RA, Abraham CS, et al. Creatine supplementation and multiple sprint running performance. J Strength Cond Res 2006;20:273–7.
91. Izquierdo M, Ibanez J, Gonzalez-Badillo JJ, et al. Effects of creatine supplementation on muscle power, endurance and sprint performance. Med Sci Sports Exerc 2002;34:332–43.
92. Van Loon LJ, Oosterlaar AM, Hartgens F, et al. Effects of creatine loading and prolonged creatine supplementation on body composition, fuel selection, sprint and endurance performance in humans. Clin Sci (Lond) 2003;104:153–62.
93. Hultman E, Soderlund K, Timmons JA, et al. Muscle creatine loading in men. J Appl Physiol 1996;81:232–7.
94. Harris R, Soderlund K, Hultman E. Elevation of creatine in resting and exercised muscle in normal subjects by creatine supplementation. Clin Sci (Lond) 1992;83:367–74.
95. Green A, Simpson EJ, Littlewood JJ, et al. Carbohydrate ingestion augments creatine retention during creatine feeding in man. Acta Physiol Scand 1996;158:195–202.
96. Sewell D, Harris RC. Effect of creatine supplementation in the Thoroughbred horse. Equine Vet J 1995;(Suppl. 18):239–42.
97. Schuback K, Essen-Gustavsson B, Persson SGB. Effect of creatine supplementation on muscle metabolic response to a maximal treadmill exercise test in Standardbred horses. Equine Vet J 2000;32:533–40.
98. D'Angelis FH, Ferraz GC, Boleli IC, et al. Aerobic training, but not creatine supplementation, alters the gluteus medius muscle. J Anim Sci 2005;83:588–94.
99. Brass E. Supplemental carnitine and exercise. Am J Clin Nutr 2000;(Suppl. 77):618S–23S.
100. Forster C, Harris RC, Snow DH. Total carnitine content of the middle gluteal muscle of Thoroughbred horses: normal values, variability and effect of acute exercise. Equine Vet J 1992;24:52–7.
101. Ceretelli P, Marconi C. L-carnitine supplementation in humans: the effects on physical performance. Int J Sports Med 1990;11:1–14.
102. Forster C, Harris RC, Snow DH. The effect of oral L-carnitine supplementation on the muscle and plasma concentration in the Thoroughbred horse. Comp Biochem Physiol A 1988;91:827–35.
103. Harris R, Forster CV, Snow DH. Plasma carnitine concentration and uptake into muscle with oral and intravenous administration. Equine Vet J 1995;(Suppl. 18):382–7.
104. Rivero J, Sporleder HP, Quiroz-Rothe E, et al. Oral L-carnitine combined with training promote changes in skeletal muscle. Equine Vet J 2002;(Suppl. 34):269–74.
105. Graham-Thiers PM, Kronfeld DS. Amino acid supplementation improves muscle mass in aged and young horses. J Anim Sci 2005;83:2783–8.
106. Blomstrand E, Hasseman P, Ek S, et al. Influence of ingesting a solution of branched-chain amino acids on perceived exertion during exercise. Acta Physiol Scand 1997;159:41–9.
107. Davis J. Carbohydrates, branched-chain amino acids and endurance: the central fatigue hypothesis. Int J Sports Med 1995;(Suppl. 5):S29–38.
108. Farris J, Hinchcliff KW, McKeever KH, et al. Effect of tryptophan and of glucose on exercise capacity of horses. J Appl Physiol 1998;85:807–16.
109. Vervuert I, Coenen M, Watermulder E. Metabolic responses to oral tryptophan supplementation before exercise in horses. J Anim Physiol Anim Nutr (Berl) 2005;89:140–5.
110. Van Hall G, Raaymakers JSH, Saris WHM, et al. Ingestion of branched-chain amino acids and tryptophan during sustained exertion: failure to affect performance. J Physiol 1995;486:789–94.
111. Glade M. Effects of specific amino acid supplementation on lactic acid production by horses exercised on a treadmill. In: 11th Conference of the Equine Nutrition and Physiology Symposium, 1989. p. 244–8.
112. Stefanon B, Bettini P, Guggia P. Administration of branched-chain amino acids to Standardbred horses in training. J Equine Vet Sci 2000;20:115–19.
113. Casini L, Gatta L, Magni B, et al. Effect of prolonged branched-chain amino acid supplementation on metabolic response to anaerobic exercise in Standardbreds. J Equine Vet Sci 2000;20:120–3.
114. Rennie M, Tipton KD. Protein and amino acid metabolism during and after exercise and the effects of nutrition. Ann Rev Nutr 2000;20:457–83.
115. Tipton K, Ferrando AA, Phillips SM, et al. Postexercise net protein synthesis in human muscle from orally administered amino acids. Am J Physiol 1999;276:E628–34.
116. Tipton K, Rasmussen BB, Miller SL, et al. Timing of amino acid-carbohydrate ingestion alters anabolic

response of muscle to resistance exercise. Am J Physiol 2001;281: E197–206.

117. Volpi E, Ferrando AA, Yeckel CW, et al. Exogenous amino acids stimulate net muscle protein synthesis in the elderly. J Clin Invest 1998;101:2000–7.

118. Matsui A, Ohmura H, Asai Y, et al. Effect of amino acid and glucose administration following exercise on the turnover of muscle protein in the hindlimb femoral region of thoroughbreds. Equine Vet J 2006;(Suppl. 36):611–16.

119. van den Hoven R, Bauer A, Hackl S, et al. A preliminary study on the changes in some potential markers of muscle-cell degradation in sub-maximally exercised horses supplemented with a protein and amino acid mixture. J Anim Physiol Anim Nutr (Berl) 2011;95:664–75.

120. Derave W, Everaert I, Beeckman S, et al. Muscle carnosine metabolism and beta-alanine supplementation in relation to exercise and recovery. Sports Med 2010;40:247–63.

121. Sewell DA, Harris RC, Marlin DJ, et al. Estimation of the carnosine content of different fibre types in the middle gluteal muscle of the thoroughbred horse. J Physiol 1992;455:447–53.

122. Stellingwerff T, Decombaz J, Harris RC, et al. Optimizing human in vivo dosing and delivery of beta-alanine supplements for muscle carnosine synthesis. Amino Acids 2012;43:57–65.

123. Dunnett M, Harris RC. Influence of oral beta-alanine and L-histidine supplementation on the carnosine content of the gluteus medius. Equine Vet J 1999;(Suppl. 30):499–504.

section 6

Fluids and electrolytes

Body fluids and electrolytes: responses to exercise and training

38

Eduard Jose-Cunilleras Kenneth Harrington McKeever

CHAPTER CONTENTS

Introduction

The exercising horse produces a tremendous amount of metabolic heat. This byproduct of the transduction of potential energy into kinetic energy can raise core body temperature in the horse from 37°C at rest to temperatures exceeding 42°C in a matter of minutes.[1-6] Normal cellular function, however, requires active and efficient ways to keep core body temperature within narrow limits. To do this a horse must move heat produced in the muscles to the periphery.[1-6] Other mammalian species, like the rabbit and dog, have an enhanced countercurrent brain blood-flow mechanism that couples with panting to provide for cooling of the brain while permissively allowing heat storage in the rest of the body and a rise in body temperature.[7,8] Similarly, horses have a singular anatomical feature involved in brain cooling; their internal carotid arteries are in close contact with the air-filled guttural pouches and it is suggested that blood reaching the brain has a lower temperature compared to mixed venous blood given this unique arrangement (see Chapter 41).[9,10] Horses and humans are the only species that cool primarily through the evaporation of sweat.[1,5,7,8] Sweating can produce tremendous fluid and electrolyte losses that, if uncompensated for, can lead to cardiovascular and thermoregulatory instability. These fluid deficits and their effects are even more pronounced during endurance exercise and exercise performed during periods of high environmental temperature and humidity.[1-3,5-7] Work focused on preventing thermal injuries in horses has documented findings similar to those published in the human sports medicine literature: namely, that strategies aimed at maintenance of fluid and electrolyte balance prevent dehydration and provide thermoregulatory and cardiovascular stability.[1-8,11-14] Data demonstrate that optimal fluid and electrolyte balance delays the onset of fatigue. The present chapter reviews the current literature on the effects of exercise and training adaptations on fluid balance and renal function in horses.

Body fluid compartments

Like all animals, the body of the horse is primarily composed of water and electrolytes. Those solutions are compartmentalized within and outside the cells. This combination of intracellular and extracellular water is referred to as the total body water (TBW). The TBW accounts for 50–70% of bodyweight, or 250–350 kg of the bodyweight of a typical 500 kg horse.[1,2,11] TBW can be measured using various indicator dilution techniques, stable isotope techniques, and bioelectric impedance technologies.[1,2,11] Each of these techniques has advantages and disadvantages, with the use of stable isotope infusion being one of the most accurate but technically demanding and bioelectric impedance technology the least reliable.

The TBW is divided by cell membranes into two primary fluid compartments, the intracellular fluid compartment (ICF) and the extracellular fluid compartment (ECF).[1,2,8,11] Approximately two-thirds of the TBW (~200 L) is contained within the cells of the body, leaving one-third of the water in the ECF space (~100 L) (Fig. 38.1). According to Carlson,[2] the latter is further compartmentalized into fluid contained within the vascular space, the interstitial fluid space, the lymphatics, and transcellular fluids. This last category includes the fluid content of the gastrointestinal tract, which represents a large reservoir of fluid.[2]

The vascular space or total blood volume is filled with a mixture of fluid and cells, the latter primarily red blood cells, but also including white blood cells and platelets. Thus, the total blood volume (BV) is the combination of the plasma volume (PV) and the red cell volume (RCV) or stated as a formula:[2] BV = PV + RCV. Blood volume varies from breed to breed, with age, body composition, hydration status, and training status.[2,15] Across breeds, studies have reported total blood volumes ranging from 61 mL/kg in draft horses to 137 mL/kg in racehorses.[1,2,11] In the average 450 kg horse, total BV would be about 36 L, PV ~20 L and RCV around 16 L.[1,2,11]

The eloquent work of Persson[15] and many others[2,16–18] has shown that there is a strong relationship between red blood cell volume and aerobic performance in the horse. Oxygen uptake and delivery is dependent on both optimal volume to insure cardiac filling pressure and an optimal number of red blood cells to carry oxygen. Much focus has been placed on the need to have red blood cells to carry oxygen to the working muscles. However, while RCV and PV are usually looked at independently, they are interdependent in the optimization of blood flow during exercise. Blood flow can be affected by changes in viscosity; thus, too many red blood cells and not enough plasma can cause a substantial change in viscosity, as well as other factors related to resistance to flow. The values for BV, PV, and RCV in the literature also vary with the differing methodologies used in different laboratories to measure and/or calculate total blood volume.[2,15–18] For the most part, studies of equine blood volume have not used direct measurement of BV. Instead, they have generally used dye or indicator dilution techniques to measure PV and then calculated BV using the measured PV and hematocrit (HCT):[2,15–18]

$$BV = \left(\frac{PV}{100 - HCT}\right) \times 100$$

The measurement of PV using dye or indicator dilution techniques requires the use of an indicator that stays within the vascular compartment for a long enough time to reach full steady-state distribution without substantial removal through the metabolism of the dye by the tissues.[2,17] Ideally, this requires an indicator that binds to a large molecule that does not readily leave the vascular compartment. Two substances commonly used to measure PV in the horse are indocyanine green (IC-green or cardiac green) dye and Evans Blue dye.[2] While IC-green dye has been used to measure plasma volume in the horse, one must caution that because it is rapidly cleared from the vascular compartment, it is better suited for the repeated injections required for the measurement of cardiac output. The rather short half-life of IC dye means it can be cleared before reaching full distribution, affecting the accuracy and repeatability of PV measurements in the horse. Evans Blue dye binds to albumin and, thus, has a relatively long half-life and stays for the most part in the vascular compartment.[2,15,17] However, one must caution that albumin can shift out of the vascular compartment if there is an increase in hydrostatic pressure induced by manipulations such as exercise or epinephrine infusion. Thus, the measurement of PV using the Evans Blue dye dilution technique requires that a horse be standing relatively quietly and unperturbed by exercise or pharmacological manipulations for the 15- to 20-min mixing period between collection of a blank plasma sample and injection of the dye and the collection of a postinjection blood sample.[17] Anything that disturbs the steady state of the cardiovascular system affects distribution of the dye; therefore, one should view with extreme caution published studies reporting PV, BV, and RCV values calculated using a postinjection sample obtained after exercise as the readings can be skewed in two ways:[15] first, decreases in PV due to water shifts out of the vascular compartment caused by increases in hydrostatic pressure that would give artificially high concentration of the dye and, second, errors caused by the loss of dye from the vascular compartment due to extrusion of albumin out of the bloodstream by the same increases in hydrostatic pressure.[3,19–22] Plasma volume can decrease 15–20% after only three 1-min steps of an incremental exercise test;[19] therefore, errors in the measurement of plasma volume due to non-steady-state sampling would also affect the calculation of BV and RCV using the above formula.

Another factor that must be considered in the calculation of total BV in the horse is the splenic reserve volume. The horse is somewhat unique compared to most other mammalian species in that the spleen is a very capacious and capricious organ, storing between 6 and 12 L of red-cell-rich blood at rest.[2,15,20,22] Splenic blood typically has a hematocrit of ~65–75%.[2,15,20,22] Thus, studies of total BV become somewhat problematic because measurement of the total circulating BV requires an accounting for the splenic reserve volume, a measurement that requires mobilization of the splenic red cell reserve. Most studies to date have utilized exercise or infusion of epinephrine or an α-adrenergic agonist drug to cause splenic contraction, with a blood sample obtained for the measurement of hematocrit after the accommodation and the mixing of the extra volume of blood. Complete mixing takes only 1–2 min; however, in many studies, the hematocrit used to calculate BV and RCV was taken at the end of or after an incremental exercise test.[15,18] While this is an accepted way to cause splenic contraction and a viable

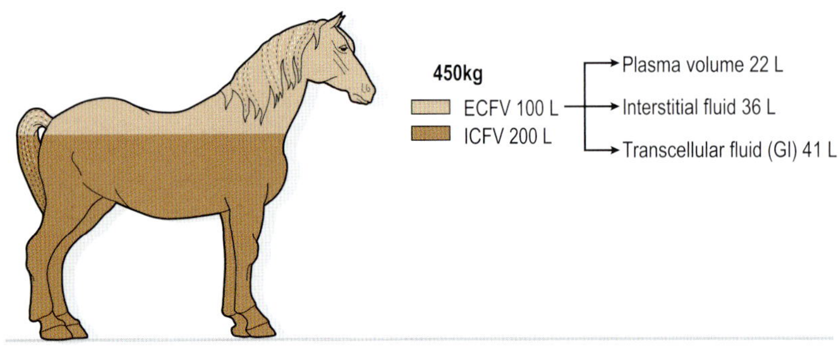

Fig 38.1 Estimated body fluids compartments in a 450 kg horse.

way to *estimate* the contribution of the splenic reserve to the total circulating blood volume, the resulting hematocrit values are skewed upward by the dynamic fluid shifts caused by the changes in flow and hydrostatic pressure induced by the exercise or pharmaceutical manipulation. Therefore, the hematocrit used to calculate total BV would reflect both the contribution of splenic reserve mobilization and reductions in plasma volume and would be an overestimation of total blood volume. This is essentially an offset error and, because acute reductions in PV caused by exercise-induced fluid shifts are linked to exercise intensity,[3,19–21] the fluid shifts that lead to this overestimation only become a problem if a study's experimental design uses different exercise intensities to measure the hematocrits used in comparisons between treatment groups or comparisons made before and after training. For example, if one calculates BV using a hematocrit obtained at the 10 m/s step of a treadmill test it will yield a different result than the value calculated using the hematocrit collected at the 11 or 12 m/s step of an incremental treadmill test.

As mentioned above, the absolute value for resting plasma volume can be determined using Evans Blue dye. However, measurement of PV during exercise and any resulting decreases are problematic because of mixing time, the requirement for steady-state conditions, and the potential for overwhelming the vascular space with dye through repeated injections. Percent changes in PV can be measured using changes in protein concentration.[19] However, because some protein leaves the vascular compartment, this method tends to underestimate the reduction in PV.[19] To get around these methodological problems, studies of human athletes[23–25] have utilized changes in hematocrit to calculate percent changes in PV (Box 38.1,). Absolute volume changes in liters are then calculated using the previously measured absolute resting PV determined using Evans Blue dye.[23–25] The calculation of percentage change in PV using hematocrit is feasible because red blood cells do not leave the vascular compartment like protein molecules and any change in their concentration must be due to changes in plasma volume.[23–25] In humans, the calculation is simple and involves the use of a pre-exercise hematocrit (HCTb) and hematocrits measured during or after exercise (HCTa).[23–25] For example, if the hematocrit measured before exercise (HCTb) was 43 and the hematocrit measured in a blood sample obtained after 10 min of exercise was 45, then the change in plasma volume is – 7.9%. Thus, one can see that a relatively small change in hematocrit represents a much larger change in plasma volume.

However, it is important to note that the use of this formula requires that there is no addition of red blood cells to the central circulation or change in the size of the cells.[23–25] The latter has been shown to not be a problem if exercise duration is less than 120 min.[25] The former makes the use of this formula problematic for those doing horse research because the spleen adds RBCs to the central circulation. Fortunately, McKeever et al. have developed a correction factor obtained after comparing sequential blood samples taken from splenectomized and intact horses.[19] These studies demonstrated that the spleen contracts very rapidly with both the extruded volume and cells accommodated and mixed with the central circulation within the first 1 to 1.5 min of exercise.[19] Changes in hematocrit from the point of full mixing onward paralleled each other in both groups of horses. Thus, the changes in hematocrit from that point on were due to decreases in plasma volume caused by fluid shifts and loss of water from the vascular compartment.[19] More importantly, the difference between the pre-exercise and the 2-min values for hematocrit in the intact horses represented an offset due to splenic reserve mobilization that could be used as a correction factor.[19]

The example in Box 38.2 demonstrates how to use hematocrit in the horse to calculate percent changes in PV. For example, if a horse had a resting hematocrit (HCTb) of 35 and the hematocrit measured at 2 min of exercise (HCT_{raw}) was 55 then the difference between the two would be the calculated correction factor ($HCT_{corrected}$) to be used to correct all the hematocrits measured after the 2-min point of exercise onward. Thus, in the example in Box 38.2, if the uncorrected hematocrit obtained at 15 min of exercise was 58 (HCT), then the value for HCTa to be used in the formula would be obtained by subtracting the correction factor from the uncorrected hematocrit.

More recently, multifrequency-bioelectrical impedance analysis (MF-BIA) has been applied to estimate fluid volumes and their fluctuations in adult horses. This technique offers the advantage of providing immediate results and is non-invasive. Indicator dilution methods have been used to estimate total body water (TBW), extracellular fluid volume (ECFV), intracellular fluid volume (ICFV) by difference of these two, and plasma volume (PV). Specifically, deuterium oxide has been used to estimate TBW in adult horses,[26–28] bromide and sodium thiocyanate have been used to determine ECFV,[27,29,30] and plasma and blood volume have been estimated by

Box 38.1 Example: Calculation of the percent change in plasma volume using uncorrected hematocrit as in humans

$$\%\Delta PV = \left(\frac{100}{100-HCTb}\right)\times\left[100\times\frac{(HCTb-HCTa)}{HCTa}\right]$$

$$\%\Delta PV = \left(\frac{100}{100-43}\right)\times\left[100\times\frac{(43-45)}{45}\right]$$

$$\%\Delta PV = \left(\frac{100}{57}\right)\times\left[100\times\frac{(-2)}{45}\right]$$

$$\%\Delta PV = (1.8)\times[-4.4]$$

$$\%\Delta PV = -7.9$$

Box 38.2 Example: Calculation of the percentage change in plasma volume using corrected hematocrit in horses

$HCTb = 35$

$HCT_{raw} = 58$

$HCT_{2min} = 55$

$HCTa = HCT_{raw} - HCT_{correction}\ [HCT_{2min} - HCT_b = 58 - (55 - 35) = 58 - 20 = 38$

$$\%\Delta PV = \left(\frac{100}{100-HCTb}\right)\times\left[100\times\frac{(HCTb-HCTa)}{HCTa}\right]$$

$$\%\Delta PV = \left(\frac{100}{100-35}\right)\times\left[100\times\frac{(35-38)}{38}\right]$$

$$\%\Delta PV = \left(\frac{100}{65}\right)\times\left[100\times\frac{(-3)}{38}\right]$$

$$\%\Delta PV = (1.54)\times[-7.89]$$

$$\%\Delta PV = -12.15$$

McKeever, Hinchcliff et al. 1993[17]

use of Evans blue dye.[17,27] However, indicator dilution methods are not clinically applicable in situations of rapidly changing fluid balance because they require time to reach steady state, prolonged equilibration periods, and specialized laboratory equipment, and as such they are not practical for everyday clinical use.[31] In studies recently performed in adult horses at rest, after prolonged exercise and after experimentally induced fluid shifts, MF-BIA appears to be a useful technique to estimate changes in TBW and ECFV, but not as reliable to estimate ICFV.[31,32]

Plasma osmolality and the concentration of key electrolytes

Normal cellular function is vitally linked to maintenance of fluid, electrolyte and acid–base balance within a narrow range.[2,3,25,33–35] Thus, the composition of both the plasma within the vascular compartment and the fluid within the intracellular fluid space is tightly controlled.[2,3,25,33–35] Key to maintenance of the internal environment is a regulation of overall plasma osmotic concentration or osmolality as well as the concentration of key electrolytes such as sodium, potassium, chloride.[2,3,25,33–35] Sodium is the major cation contributing to osmolality and is the major cation in the extracellular fluid space.[2,3,25,33–35] Potassium on the other hand is the primary cation found within the cells.[2,3,25,33–35] Other important cations include calcium and magnesium, both primarily intracellular ions.[2,3,25,33–35] When considering exercise, it is the calcium found within the muscle in the tubular sarcoplasmic reticulum that is important.[2,3,25,33–35] This calcium plays a vital role in the process of excitation contraction coupling. Magnesium found within the cells is an important cofactor in many of the reactions involved in various metabolic pathways.[2,3,25,33–35] Major anions include chloride, bicarbonate, and the phosphates.[2,3,25,33–35] Normal values for resting concentrations of the major electrolytes found in plasma, interstitial fluid, intracellular fluid and sweat can be found in Table 38.1. All of the electrolytes contribute to the osmotic concentration of the body fluids, a variable that is tightly regulated to prevent cell dehydration or cell swelling.

The osmotic concentration or osmolality of the plasma is essentially the same as that of the rest of the interstitial fluids.[36,37] Normal plasma osmolality in the horse and most other mammals averages 290 mOsm/L.[2] Plasma osmolality is the total number of dissolved particles in solution, independent of the elemental species making up that solution.[36] Plasma osmolality reflects the osmolality of both the extracellular fluid space and the intracellular fluid space[36] and is important for two reasons. First, large molecules in solution exert osmotic force across semipermeable membranes such as capillaries and cell membranes. Thus, plasma osmolality is a measure of the total 'osmotic pull' or osmotic force that is exerted by the sum of freely moving particles in solution exerting an effect on water in surrounding tissues.[36,37] Because water tends to move down a concentration gradient from an area of low concentration to an area of high concentration, an increase or decrease in plasma osmolality has the capacity to dramatically alter normal cellular function by causing fluid shifts into and out of the cells, shifts that can decrease cell function.[36,37] Second, a change in osmolality reflects expansion or contraction of the extracellular fluid compartment.[36,37] Optimal cardiovascular function is highly dependent on fluid volume status and mechanisms associated with the maintenance of plasma osmolality and extracellular fluid volume serve as one of the first lines of defense in the regulation of cardiac filling volume and pressure and ultimately mean arterial pressure and the ability to perfuse the tissues.[20,36,37] During exercise the horse can lose tremendous volumes of isotonic to slightly hypertonic sweat, presenting a serious challenge for maintaining the volume and the composition of the body fluids.[1,2,20] Dramatic changes can compromise cellular function.[37] It can also compromise cardiovascular stability through a reduction in venous return and cardiac output. Therefore, it is vitally important that the body regulates plasma osmolality within very narrow limits.[37] Defense of osmolality is vitally intertwined with the defense of extracellular fluid volume, plasma volume, and cardiac filling pressure.[20,37] Thus, defending plasma osmolality involves an integrative response of multiple systems, including the cardiovascular, neural, endocrine, and renal systems.[6,12,20,36–39] Changes in plasma osmolality are sensed by specialized cells within the supraoptic and paraventricular nuclei of the hypothalamus.[20,36–38] These osmoreceptors are very sensitive and changes in plasma osmolality as small as 2 mOsm/L can evoke a change in the synthesis and secretion of the hormone arginine vasopressin (antidiuretic hormone) by the posterior pituitary.[38] Changes in circulating vasopressin concentration occur rapidly and can cause dramatic alterations in renal handling of water within minutes, thus correcting volume deficits and swings in the concentration of osmotically active substances through losses of plasma water or electrolytes in the sweat.[38,39] Vasopressin also

Table 38.1 Electrolyte composition (mEq/L) of plasma, interstitial fluid, intracellular fluid (muscle), and sweat

ELECTROLYTE	PLASMA	INTERSTITIAL FLUID	SKELETAL MUSCLE CELL	SWEAT
Cations				
Na^+	140	143	10	120 (range 115–150)
K^+	4	4.1	142	35 (range 25–50)
Ca^{2+} (ionized)	2.5	2.4	4	10 (range 3–20)
Mg^{2+} (ionized)	1.1	1.1	34	5
Anions				
Cl^-	100	113	4	150 (range 140–190)
HCO_3^-	25	28	12	
$H_2PO_4^-$, HPO_4^{2-}	2	2	40	
Lactate$^-$	≈1			
Protein	14	0	50	
Other	7	7	84	

stimulates thirst and drinking, which ultimately affects water balance and osmolality.[38]

Plasma concentration versus plasma content

When considering the effects of acute exercise on changes in key electrolytes one must distinguish between changes in the concentration versus changes in the total content of those electrolytes.[25,40] By definition, the concentration of a substance is the amount of solute in a given volume of solvent. Content, on the other hand, is the total amount of that solute in the fluid compartment or body depending on the focus of analysis. For example, normal plasma concentration sodium is 140 mEq/L or, put another way, there are 140 mEq of sodium per liter of plasma. Plasma content of sodium would be obtained by multiplying the concentration of sodium by the plasma volume:[25,40]

$$\frac{140\ \text{mEq}}{\text{Liter}} \times \frac{26\ \text{Liters}}{1} = 3640\ \text{mEq}$$

Calculation of changes in the content of key electrolytes and other substances allows one to determine if changes in the concentration of a substance is the result of addition or loss of the substance or just due to changes in plasma water.[25,40] When viewed on a whole-body level, changes in content allow one to make calculations giving insight into how concentrations of tightly regulated plasma constituents are affected through routes of intake or loss that affect whole-body balance of said constituent.[25,40] Acutely, calculation of relative or percent changes in the content of plasma volume and the plasma constituents gives one insight into the dynamic changes that occur in response to the challenge of exertion.[25,40] To that end, human exercise physiologists for years have used key formulae to calculate percentage changes in plasma volume and percentage changes in the content of various plasma constituents during exercise (Box 38.3).[23–25] If one knows the resting plasma volume, then once one calculates the percentage change in the content of a plasma constituent, one can calculate the total amount of that substance lost during exercise from the vascular compartment.[25,40] On a practical level, calculation of changes in the content of various plasma constituents can give insight into their disposition. An example of this would be an examination of sodium and chloride losses during short-term versus endurance exercise. Plasma sodium and chloride concentrations are held within very narrow limits. During short-term exercise, plasma sodium and chloride concentrations undergo minimal changes.[40] However, the plasma content of sodium and presumably chloride decreases, suggesting the fluid shifts that occur during short-term exercise involve an isotonic shift of fluid.[40] During longer-term exertion there can be minimal changes in plasma sodium concentration but content can change dramatically.[25,40] With chloride there is a dramatic disproportional decrease both in the plasma concentration and content due to large amounts lost in the sweat.[25,40] Measuring total content lost gives a more complete picture of how much supplementation must occur to replenish exercise-related losses. When one looks at changes in plasma potassium concentration and content one sees a different picture. Both the concentration and content of potassium go up during high-intensity exercise. When one looks at the change in content one can see that the change in concentration is due to both the loss of plasma water and the addition of potassium to the plasma when it leaks out of the contracting muscle cells.

Box 38.3 Example: Calculation of percent change in the content of a plasma constituent using corrected hematocrit[40]

HCTb = Resting hematocrit

HCTa = Corrected hematocrit

Cnb = Resting concentration

Cna = Post-concentration

Co = Content of solute

$$\%\Delta Co = \frac{Cna - [HCTa\,(100 - HCTb) \times (Cnb)]/HCTb\,(100 - HCTa)}{HCTa\,(100 - HCTb) \times (Cnb)/HCTb\,(100 - HCTa)} \times 100$$

Effects of acute exercise on fluid and electrolyte balance

Hypothetically, fluid and electrolytes can shift from the intracellular space to the extracellular space as well as between each of the compartments through active, passive, and facilitative mechanisms.[6–8,13,20,21,25,41,42] This dynamic exchange of fluid and electrolytes between compartments moves nutrients and waste products, provides fluid and electrolytes for the production of sweat and allows the horse to defend the internal environment of the cells.[6–8,13,20,21,25,41,42] To maintain cellular homeostasis the horse must regulate blood volume, blood pressure, and the osmotic composition of the intracellular and extracellular fluid compartments. Acute fluid and electrolyte shifts have differing functional significance related to the timing of the response during exercise. Early shifts appear more related to a system-wide redistribution of blood and fluid from capacitance vessels and the interstitial space so as to increase venous return and augment cardiac output.[6–8] Later responses provide fluid and electrolytes for the production of sweat and thermoregulation[6,13,19,25] Finally, decreases and depletion of fluid stores lead to dehydration, thermoregulatory, and cardiovascular instability and fatigue. [6,13,19,25] This latter challenge stimulates an expansion of plasma volume and the contents of the various electrolytes, a beneficial adaptive response known as a training-induced hypervolemia. [6,13,19,25]

Intercompartmental fluid shifts at the onset of exercise

Senay[43] demonstrated, in humans, that in the first seconds at the onset of exercise, there is a rapid net movement of protein and fluid from the interstitial space and lymphatics into the vascular compartment.[43] This inward flux of protein and water causes a transient, short-lived increase in plasma volume, an intercompartmental shift of body fluids that couples with a redistribution of blood from the venous capacitance side of the vascular system to the arterial side to provide adequate venous return to maintain cardiac filling pressure.[6–8,43] This important redistribution of blood and fluid from the capacitance side of the vascular system is important because of the need for extra venous return at a time when there is rapid vasodilation in the working muscles.[6–8,43–45] Similar phenomena have been demonstrated in dogs and probably also occur in horses.[44,45] Studies have demonstrated a shift in the albumin-to-globulin ratio in the horse consistent with an inward flux of fluid from the interstitial space.[46] At rest albumin is the primary protein found in the vascular space and globulin represents the most prevalent protein found in the lymphatics.[46] This dramatic change in albumin-to-globulin ratio suggests that the horse experiences a similar influx in fluid at the onset of exercise as described in humans.[43,46] Plasma is also added to the central circulation upon mobilization of the splenic reserve.[15,19] Splenic blood is rich in red blood cells, with a hematocrit between 65 and 75%.[15,19] However, this also means that there is an addition of plasma to the central circulation. Splenic blood volume averages range from 8 to 12 L; thus, there is an addition of a 1.6 to 3.6 L plasma to the central circulation in addition to the volume added by intercompartmental fluid shifts.[15,19] This extra volume of plasma serves a role in cardiovascular control and it also increases circulating protein that provides extra buffering capacity to the central circulation.[15,19]

Plasma volume decreases rapidly after this initial intercompartmental redistribution of water and electrolytes.[6,19,21,25,41,42,47] These secondary fluid shifts are caused by significant increases in mean arterial pressure and consequentially capillary hydrostatic pressure that cause water, electrolytes, and a small amount of protein to be extruded from the vascular compartment.[6,25] Studies of horses[19,20,22] performing moderate incremental exercise have demonstrated that this decrease in plasma volume is rapid and intensity dependent with a 15 to 20% decrease observed after only four 1-min steps of an incremental exercise test (Fig. 38.2). This movement of water and salts bathes the interstitial space, where it can be taken up into the working muscles, used to form sweat, or returned to the vascular compartment.[19,20,22] In recent studies of Standardbred horses performing high-intensity track exercise, a decrease by 27%, 16% and 2% in plasma volume, ECFV and TBW, respectively, was detected within minutes of recovery from exercise.[48] Similarly, in horses performing prolonged submaximal exercise on the treadmill, a decrease of 10%, 10% and 4% in plasma volume, ECFV and TBW, respectively, was detected at the time of recovery.[49]

In mammals there is a dynamic flux of fluid into and out of the vascular compartment that is governed by Starling forces (Fig. 38.3).[2,6–8,13] Net filtration and reabsorption across a vascular bed is the sum of forces affecting the movement of fluid and osmotically active substances in both the arterial and venous capillaries.[2,6–8,13] These forces include the capillary and interstitial hydrostatic pressures and the capillary and interstitial oncotic pressures. On the arterial side of the resting capillary bed, hydrostatic pressure and interstitial oncotic pressure outweigh interstitial pressure and intravascular oncotic pressure.[2,6–8,13] This favors a net movement of fluid out of the vascular compartment. However, resting venous oncotic forces outweigh the other forces and favor a movement of fluid back into the vascular space.[2,6–8,13] Some fluid is not returned via the influx into the venous capillaries and is returned through the lymphatic system.[2,6–8,13] During exercise, the balance of Starling forces is greatly affected by a larger increase in arterial hydrostatic pressure.[2,6–8,13] At the arteriole level this amounts to a ~20 mmHg increase in hydrostatic pressure enhancing the net force of fluid

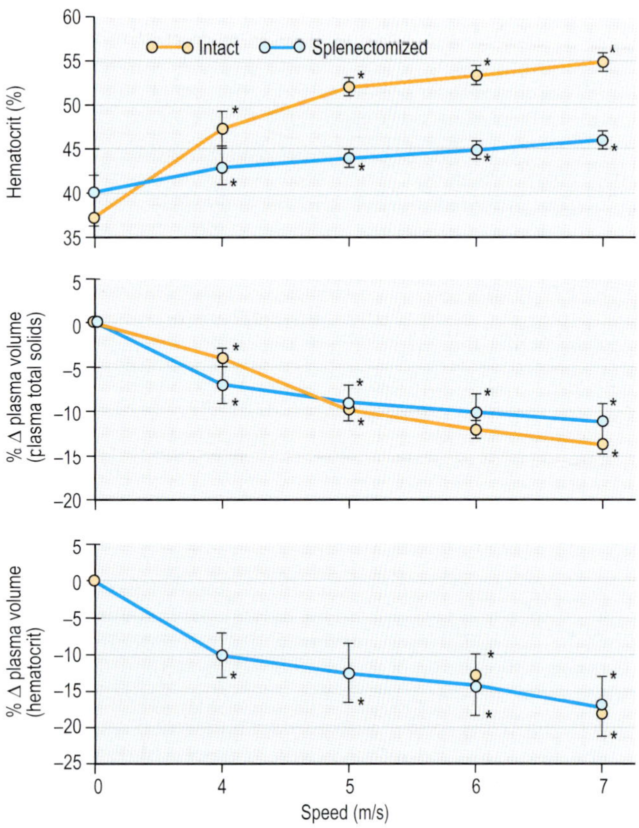

Fig 38.2 Percentage change in plasma volume during incremental exercise. Values are means ± SE for hematocrit, percentage change in plasma volume calculated using total solids (i.e. protein) and percentage changes in plasma volume calculated using corrected hematocrit.

McKeever KH, Hinchcliff KW, Reed SM, et al. Role of decreased plasma volume in hematocrit alterations during incremental treadmill exercise in horses, Am J Physiol 1993;265(2 Pt 2):R404–8, with permission from the American Physiological Society.

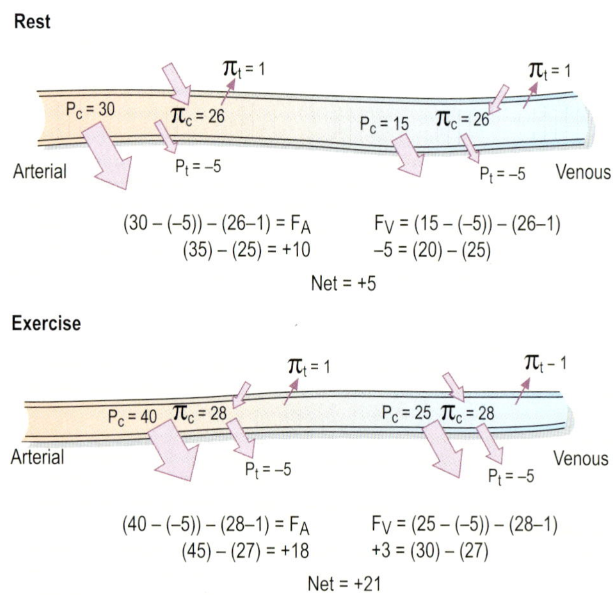

Fig 38.3 Starling forces affecting the movement of fluid in and out of the vascular compartment. Rest: at rest, the balance of forces on the arterial side of the capillary bed is positive (+10), favoring an outward movement of fluid. On the venous side of the capillary bed the balance of forces is negative (–5), favoring the inward movement of fluid. However, the net difference between the arterial and venous sides of the capillary beds is positive (+5) and thus not all the fluid is returned to the bloodstream. The excess must be returned via the lymphatic system. Exercise: during exercise, hydrostatic pressure increases in both sides of the capillary bed enhancing the movement of fluid outward into the interstitial space for transport and for sweat production. Thus, during exercise, lymphatics play an important role in returning fluid not lost as sweat.

outward.[2,6–8,13] On the venous side of the capillary beds, hydrostatic pressure is also elevated with a tendency for a net positive outward force. This means that more fluid is shifted into the interstitial space when compared to rest. This extra dynamic outward flux of fluid has a functional significance and is beneficial as it can either be excreted as sweat or returned to the vascular compartment via the lymphatics. The net result is a decrease in plasma volume and a dynamic flux of fluid that provides for removal of metabolic waste products and for removal of heat produced during exercise.[2,19,22] The key here is that the decrease in plasma volume seen at the onset of exercise[2,19,22] is dynamic and intensity dependent (Fig. 38.4) and occurs before the onset of sweat losses.[19,22] However, plasma volume decreases seen after these initial fluid shifts are the result of reductions in total body water caused by sweating.[1,2]

Fluid and electrolyte losses associated with longer acute exercise

Exercise continued beyond a few seconds causes pronounced hemodynamic changes and, because of sweat production, fluid and electrolyte losses.[1,2,6] Evaporative cooling via sweating is by far the most efficient way to remove a large amount of heat from the body.[1,2,4–6,50] But this ability to maintain body temperature comes at a cost to the cardiovascular system. First, a portion of blood flow that could be used to supply the working muscles is redistributed to the skin to transport heat from the core to the surface.[5–8] At moderately heavy work intensities limited circulating blood volume and cardiac output cause transient alterations in cardiac filling volume and mean arterial pressure that are sensed, respectively, by the cardiopulmonary baroreceptors (volume receptors) and by the high pressure baroreceptors.[5–8] Optimal perfusion of working muscles requires that the cardiovascular system keeps mean arterial pressure within narrow limits.[5–8] However, there is an upward change in the set point during exercise that removes the check on the system that would tend to limit an increase in cardiac output. Rowell[7,8] has suggested that a feedforward mechanism allows blood pressure to increase during exercise via integrated responses of the above mentioned two layers of defense.[7,8] Control of mean arterial pressure during increasing exercise intensity necessitates shunting of blood away from non-obligate tissues.[6–8,44,45] These non-obligate tissues include the splanchnic and renal vascular beds.[6–8,44,45,51,52] The changes in vascular tone are so pronounced that they are facilitated by both nervous system and endocrine effector signals.[6–8,51,52] Interestingly, these neural and endocrine factors (catecholamines, plasma renin activity, vasopressin, etc.) influencing vascular tone in the splanchnic and renal vascular beds increase at intensities above 50–60% $\dot{V}O_{2max}$[6–8,38,42,51,53–55] in most cases prior to any substantial loss of sweat. These adjustments in cardiovascular function and renal blood flow thus appear to be a response to the 'stress of exercise' itself rather than fluid and electrolyte imbalance.[51] As exercise progresses, acute fluid shifts from the vascular compartment to the interstitial space provide water for sweat production.[6–8] Sweat loss causes a net reduction in total body water and a decrease in plasma volume that, if not replaced by water intake, eventually results in decreased venous return and cardiac filling pressure.[6–8] The horse has evolved to have a large reservoir of fluid in its digestive tract.[6] This is not an inconsequential amount as the horse can utilize fluid from the large colon as well as fluid contained in its cecum. Thus, in the wild the horse does not need to stop to drink while running from a predator. There are limits to these fluid reserves and the horse produces a huge volume of hypertonic sweat that eventually can lead to a compromised vascular volume. The cardiopulmonary volume receptors sense the drop in cardiac filling pressure and volume. To keep cardiac output constant the resultant fluid-loss-induced decrease in stroke volume must be countered by an increase in heart rate.[6–8] This tachycardiac adjustment to progressive fluid loss is referred to as cardiovascular drift.[6–8] More dramatic reductions in flow to non-obligate tissues can occur if increased heart rate cannot compensate for the decrease in cardiac filling pressure. Sweat-induced reductions in total body water initially come at the expense of plasma volume; however, as exercise progresses water loss causes a progressive cellular dehydration.[1,2,4–6,11,50,55] The resultant cellular fluid deficit eventually leads to decreased cell function, fatigue, and a failure to thermoregulate properly.[56,57] Other problems can be caused by significant simultaneous electrolyte losses.[2,4,5,50,55–57] Along with heavy sweat production comes loss of electrolytes, which stimulates a variety of endocrine responses that function to correct the concentration of these vital substances.[6] Human sweat is hypotonic: that is, the concentration of sodium is less than that found in the plasma.[2] While prolonged exercise can result in severe electrolyte disturbances, recent research has shown that they are much less frequent in humans compared to those seen in horses.[2,6,55–57] Equine sweat, on the other hand, is hypertonic and excessive sweat loss can rapidly result in severe problems related to both the hypovolemia and to the resulting electrolyte imbalance.[2,50] Several papers have documented that severe electrolyte loss can lead to weakness, muscle cramps, acid–base imbalance, and decreased performance.[2,5,6,55–57] Interestingly, trained humans appear to start sweating earlier and in greater amounts than untrained individuals exercising at similar relative work intensities.[6,34,58] Trained human athletes also appear to have a more hypotonic sweat[13,58] that results from aldosterone's action on the sweat glands.[20,22,34,35,58] Studies have not yet demonstrated similar training-induced adaptations in the neuroendocrine control of sweating and fluid balance in horses.

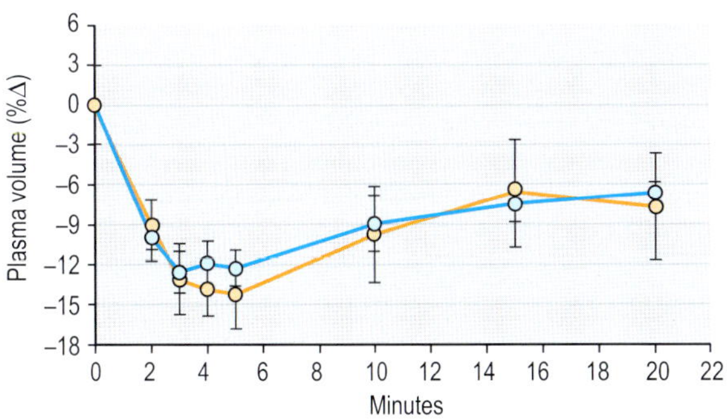

Fig 38.4 Changes in plasma volume with steady-state exercise. Initial drop in plasma volume (0–3 min) due to fluid shifts, secondary changes due to fluid loses.

McKeever KH, Hinchcliff KW, Reed SM, et al. Role of decreased plasma volume in hematocrit alterations during incremental treadmill exercise in horses, Am J Physiol 1993;265(2 Pt 2):R404–8, with permission from the American Physiological Society.

Sweat losses and the combined effects of exercise and environment

The transduction of potential energy into kinetic energy is a rather inefficient process, with only 20–30% of potential energy effectively utilized for work.[5] The rest is heat that must be liberated from the body.[5] In general, the greater the exercise intensity of the event, the greater the heat load generated and the greater the need for heat dissipation.[5] Even under mild ambient conditions, the exercising horse is presented with a significant thermoregulatory challenge that requires an integrated response to transport heat from the core to be transferred to the environment.[5] The major method for the transfer of heat from the body involves sweating and evaporative cooling.[5] Evaporative cooling is several times more effective than other routes of heat exchange. Because evaporative cooling is so essential, the horse appears to have evolved with several species specific adaptations that enhance the ability to move fluid from the vascular compartment to the sweat glands and ultimately to the exterior as sweat.[5] First, as previously mentioned, increases in hydrostatic pressure during exercise enhance fluid shifts from the vascular compartment to the interstitial space, increasing the availability of fluid for sweat production.[5,6,20,22] Second, the sweat gland of the horse is very simple compared to the well-organized sweat glands seen in humans.[5,50] Therefore, sweat excretion is a less complex process. Additionally, the equine sweat gland, unlike the human sweat gland, is not responsive to aldosterone and thus it cannot conserve sodium.[50] Put simply, the equine sweat gland almost acts like a funnel to allow a slightly hypertonic solution of electrolytes to move from the interstitial space to the surface. Teleologically, producing a hypertonic sweat may be beneficial as the solvent drag would tend to facilitate the movement of a greater amount of water outward. The extra salt in the sweat, as well as the protein lather in, also alters the evaporation point of the sweat, possibly enhancing evaporative cooling. Functionally, this is significant as the horse has a less favorable surface area to volume ratio when compared to humans. The downside to these adaptations is the potential for large fluid and electrolyte deficits.

Recent studies have reported that during submaximal exercise, under conditions of high heat and humidity, sweat losses in horses can exceed rates of 12 L per hour.[5,50,55,59–66] This large volume of sweat results in proportional decreases in body weight, total body water, and plasma volume. This, in turn, can compromise venous return, cardiac filling pressure, cardiac output, and the ability to thermoregulate. Thermoregulatory stability requires a large cardiac output and peripheral blood flow to carry heat from the core of the body to blood vessels in the skin.[5] At the same time, the heart must pump blood to the working muscles, to the brain, and to other 'obligate' tissues that cannot suffer from reduced perfusion. To maintain cardiac output during intense exercise, baroreflexes cause selective vasoconstriction and blood flow redistribution.[6–8] This reduces blood flow to non-obligate tissue beds like the viscera and kidneys and allows for increased blood flow to the working muscles[7,8] (see Chapter 31, Fig. 31.18). As core heat accumulates, various feedback mechanisms cause blood flow to increase to the skin to enhance the transport of heat from deep in the core of the body to the surface.[5] If exercise proceeds for a long enough time, sweat loss leads to progressive dehydration and loss of plasma water from the bloodstream. Dehydration causes a decrease in circulating blood volume and cardiac stroke volume. A horse can keep going despite this reduction in vascular fluid volume; however, to maintain cardiac output, heart rate must increase ('cardiovascular drift').[5–8] When dehydration cannot be compensated for by cardiovascular adjustments, body temperature rises and is soon followed by decreased performance and fatigue. Maintaining cardiac output and mean arterial pressure (MAP) is vital to keeping perfusion pressure at the level needed to distribute flow to the working muscles, skin, and other obligate tissues. Thus, at the onset of exercise both mean arterial blood pressure and skin blood flow are defended.[5–8,20] However, as a horse becomes dehydrated MAP is defended preferentially at expense of skin blood flow and thermoregulation, adding to the resulting increase in body temperature.[5–8,20] Several laboratories have observed that, even under cool conditions, endurance exercise performed in the field or on a treadmill laboratory will cause a substantial rise in core temperature, a substantial amount of sweat production, and a dramatic loss of total body water.[1,2,5,50,55,59–66] In field trials, it has been documented that even with the combination of proper hydration, adequate sweating, and maximal rates of evaporative cooling, a horse's body temperature can reach 105–106 °F (40.5–41 °C) during endurance rides performed under moderate climatic conditions.[1,2,5,50,55,59–66] Under hot humid conditions, evaporative cooling becomes ineffective because sweat will not evaporate. The resulting hyperthermia can cause fatigue, cramps, heat stroke, and other thermal injuries.[1,4,6] Thus, in a hot and humid environment, even a well-hydrated horse can encounter potential life-threatening situations in a relatively short time. However, most of these injuries can be prevented with proper feeding, adequate watering, and advanced planning of exercise training sessions and athletic events.

Almost all studies reporting sweat electrolyte concentrations in horses during exercise demonstrate that the horse loses a large amount of key electrolytes.[1,2,5,50,55,59–66] The range of sweat electrolyte concentrations varies, with older studies suggesting tremendous sodium and chloride losses.[2] The magnitude of electrolyte loss reported in some studies is questionable and most likely is a function of the methodologies utilized. Older studies relied on sweat scrapings and other sampling techniques that overestimate actual losses. Several newer studies have utilized more refined methods adapted from human research, preventing the errors due to evaporation of water or addition of salt from areas already contaminated by prior sweating.[59–61] Nevertheless, more recent studies still demonstrate that equine sweat is slightly hypertonic relative to plasma and that without replacement there are substantial electrolyte deficits in horses competing in endurance activities. While sodium and chloride are the primary electrolytes lost in equine sweat, other key electrolytes like magnesium and calcium are lost.[50] Most important is a disproportional loss of chloride ions that can potentially lead to a serious metabolic alkalosis.[11,50] The loss of sodium can become an even greater problem during recovery if a horse drinks too much water.[11] As with human marathon runners, some endurance horses can develop a hyponatremia that, if untreated, can lead to collapse and death.[57] Thus, provision of water as well as electrolyte supplements, is warranted after endurance activities accompanied by large fluid and electrolyte losses.

Thirst, drinking, and electrolyte intake

Hormonal changes stimulate thirst and drinking and it is well recognized that the horse has a finely tuned regulatory system to maintain fluid and electrolyte balance.[1,2,6,20] Mechanistically, thirst can be stimulated by increases in circulating concentrations of angiotensin, arginine vasopressin (AVP), and by changes in the concentration of calcium and other electrolytes in the cerebrospinal fluid.[6,33–35,37,67–70] These systems are modulated by changes in osmolality sensed by the paraventricular and supraoptic nuclei of the hypothalamus.[6,33–35,37,67–70] Thus, a small increase in plasma osmolality will result in the release of AVP by the posterior pituitary.[6,33–35,37,67–70] These drives for thirst and drinking are finely tuned for the resting horse; however, it has been documented that strenuous, high-intensity, exercise can paradoxically suppress thirst and the central drive for drinking behavior in humans, dogs, and more recently horses.[6,33–35,37,67–70] Mechanistically, it appears that early in exercise there is a suppression of AVP release associated with the role the cardiopulmonary baroreceptors play in the accommodation of fluid shifts and the mobilization of the splenic reserve.[20,71]

Comparative studies of dogs, humans, and other species have also shown that there is a general suppression of the drive for drinking, as well as additional suppression of thirst and drinking during exercise when cold hypotonic water passes by nerves in the mouth and throat.[6,33–35,37,67–70] This suppression of drinking behavior may be a protective mechanism – an ingrained defensive behavior that prevents an individual from stopping for water while on the run from a predator. Horse owners and veterinarians monitoring endurance events have reported a similar suppression of drinking in horses.[6,11,12] In many cases, endurance horses will not drink at the end of a race and some clinicians have reported that this suppression of thirst and drinking behavior can last for several hours after exercise.[1,2,12] Unfortunately, this is the time when rehydration should be taking place. In some cases, it is the horse with the most severe fluid and electrolyte deficit that is the one that will not drink right away or is the one that will consume a volume that is not sufficient to replace the amount of water lost during competition.[12] Some researchers have speculated that there is a threshold where severe dehydration itself accentuates this paradoxical suppression of drinking.[34,37,67–70] Interestingly, recent research demonstrated that endurance horses could be taught to drink warm water with electrolytes during competition without a resulting suppression of thirst and drinking.[72–76] An equine athlete can usually recover from moderate acute exercise-induced fluid and electrolyte losses. And, in most cases, fluid and electrolyte losses following acute exercise can be compensated for through the provision of adequate water, a normal diet, and a salt and mineral supplement.[12,77] However, some scenarios can potentially cause problems for competing animals.[12,77] One scenario might result from larger-than-normal fluid and electrolyte losses resulting from exercise in hot or hot and humid conditions. In this case, fluid losses may need to be replaced rapidly to avoid thermal injuries.[12] Competition following long periods of trailering to an event with limited amount of water supplied for drinking while in transit presents another scenario for problems.[12] In this case, a horse owner should provide access to water prior to competition.[12] If the distance to the event is long, one should consider providing opportunities for drinking at rest stops along the way.[12] Another situation that can result in severe dehydration can occur when there is limited recovery time between phases during three-day competitions or other multiple event competitive formats.[12] Logistics of these events may prevent an animal from drinking enough water or prevent a horse from getting adequate electrolytes via dietary replacement.[12] Clinicians monitoring the status of competing horses should insure that all animals have had an ample opportunity to recover between days, phases, or heats of a competition.[12] The amount of water consumed by a horse varies with the individual, diet, climate, and amount of exercise.[12,76] The National Research Council guidelines for feeding horses recommend 2–4 L of water per kilogram of dry matter feed intake.[12,77] This amount can increase 15–20% for horses in warm environments.[12,76] For example, a recent paper reported that non-exercised horses in Arizona consumed between 30 and 40 L of water in the hot months of June and July.[16] Water intake may increase 300% or more with prolonged exercise and some studies have documented that an active horse can consume 100 liters of water per day under some conditions.[1,2,50,72]

Renal function during exercise

Alterations in renal blood flow and renal function vary with both the duration and the intensity of exercise.[6,51,78,79] In general, exercise affects both renal blood flow and the delivery of water and electrolytes to the kidney and it affects mechanisms associated with the tubular reabsorption of water and electrolytes.[6,51] Acute and chronic renal responses to exercise are part of an integrative defense of blood volume, blood pressure, and osmolality.[6,51] Zambraski[51] suggests that the alterations in renal function are both a response to the stress of exercise alone and also to perturbations in fluid and electrolyte balance (Fig. 38.5). Acute demands of exercise result in a decrease in renal blood flow, sparing cardiac output so as to allow the cardiovascular system to meet the increased circulatory demand associated with exertion.[51] Post-exertional changes in renal function, on the other hand, are part of a long-term mechanism to restore lost water and electrolytes.[6,51] The kidneys also function as major effector organs in the adaptive expansion of plasma volume and electrolyte content balance referred to as the hypervolemic response to exercise training.[6,51]

Effects of exercise on renal blood flow

During submaximal exercise absolute renal blood flow (RBF) is not reduced in humans or horses.[51,80] However, it has been documented that low-intensity exercise results in a reduction of renal blood flow as a percentage of cardiac output.[51,80] For example, Hinchcliff et al.[80] reported that renal blood flow averaged 15 mL/kg/min and did not change during exercise. However, because cardiac output increased, RBF did decrease as a percentage of cardiac output, dropping from 23% at rest to 6% during exercise.[80] High-intensity exercise, on the other hand, causes substantial reductions in absolute renal blood flow in swine, horses and humans, but not in normal dogs.[6,51,81,82] Renal vasoconstriction appears to occur when work intensities exceed a threshold of 50–60% of $\dot{V}O_{2max}$[6,51] a point coincident with detectable increases in renal nerve activity, circulating catecholamines, and plasma renin activity.[6,51–53]

Schott and co-workers[81] were the first to demonstrate that high-intensity exertion causes a reduction both in absolute RBF and relative RBF (i.e. RBF expressed as a percentage of cardiac output) in the horse. Absolute RBF decreased from 9.0 L/min to 2.4 L/min when horses were exercised at a speed shown to produce an oxygen

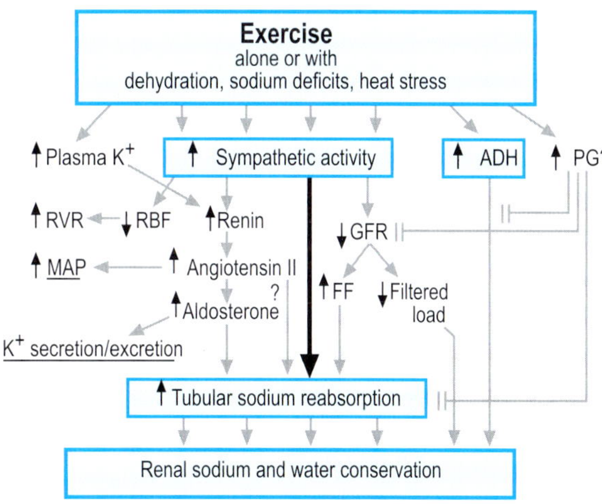

Fig 38.5 Renal response to high-intensity exercise. FF, filtration fraction; GFR, glomerular filtration rate; MAP, mean arterial pressure; PG, prostaglandins; RBF, renal blood flow; RVR, renal vascular resistance.

Reprinted from Zambraski EJ. Renal regulation of fluid homeostasis during exercise. In: Gisolfi CV, Lamb DR, editors. Perspectives in exercise science and sports medicine, vol 3. Fluid homeostasis during exercise, 1990, p. 245-280, with kind permission of Cooper Publishing Group, Traverse City, MI, USA.

uptake that was 100% of $\dot{V}O_{2max}$.[81] Amazingly, RBF decreased as a percentage of cardiac output from 22% at rest down to 0.09% during maximal exercise.[81] This reduction in RBF resulted in a substantial drop in glomerular filtration rate and subsequently a drop in urine flow, and the excretion of solute-free water and various electrolytes. Interestingly, a follow-up study demonstrated that phenylbutazone and furosemide did not appear to alter the renal response to high-intensity exercise.[82]

Effect of exercise on glomerular filtration rate, filtration fraction

Blood flowing through the renal artery is filtered through millions of glomeruli in the kidney.[51] The glomerulus is part of the nephron, the basic structural unit of the kidney.[51] It is a complex structure made up of the afferent artery, Bowman's capsule, and the efferent artery.[51] Algebraically, glomerular filtration rate is representative of the sum of the action of all the nephrons, and is autoregulated over a wide range of kidney blood flow. As with RBF, the effects of exercise on glomerular filtration rate (GFR) in the horse varies with the intensity of the exercise.[80-82] GFR has been shown to increase or decrease during submaximal exercise depending on hydration status.[51] In studies where the subjects were hyperhydrated, GFR did not change during submaximal exertion.[51] However, when individuals were euhydrated or hypohydrated, changes in GFR were intensity and/or duration dependent, changing the most when individuals performed high-intensity exercise.[51] Interestingly, while RBF can be dramatically reduced during exercise, studies of humans show that decreases in GFR do not necessarily parallel the decreases in RBF.[51] Thus, glomerular filtration is somewhat protected in the face of exercise-induced reductions in RBF with a resultant increase in filtration fraction (i.e. the ratio GFR/RBF).[51] Zambraski[51] has suggested some possible mechanisms to explain the exercise-induced increase in filtration fraction (FF) observed in humans and other species. First, maintenance of glomerular hydrostatic pressure and preservation of GFR through greater constriction of the efferent arteriole relative to the afferent arteriole.[51] However, data from comparative species are lacking or have not fully supported this hypothesis. A second hypothesis for exercise-induced increases in FF postulated that changes in glomerular capillary Kf simultaneous to decreases in glomerular capillary hydrostatic pressure would 'assist in maintaining GFR'.[51] While not directly tested, this mechanism fits teleologically with data from human and animal studies documenting exercise-induced increases in substances that affect Kf, such as vasopressin, the prostaglandins, and angiotensin II.[51] The effects of exercise on GFR and FF appear to be similar in the exercising horse and in exercising humans. Hinchcliff and co-workers[80] reported that, as in humans, there appear to be no alterations in GFR or FF during standing control or submaximal (50–60% $\dot{V}O_{2max}$) exercise in horses. In that study, creatinine clearance (GFR) ranged between 2.0 and 2.5 mL/min/kg and FF averaged 23%.[80] High-intensity exercise, on the other hand, produces a significant decrease in GFR and a significant increase in FF in the horse.[81] Schott and co-workers[81] demonstrated that GFR decreased 73% from a mean of 1.9 mL/kg/min to 0.5 mL/kg/min during exercise performed at an intensity shown to produce $\dot{V}O_{2max}$. As with humans, horses performing high-intensity exercise had significant increases in FF from 16% at rest to 23.2% following running.[81] While drugs like furosemide and phenylbutazone affect renal blood flow, they do not appear to alter GFR and FF in the horse during submaximal or maximal exercise.[82] These observations were interpreted to suggest that the renal prostaglandins play a minimal role in mediating changes in GFR and RBF in the horse during exercise.[82]

Renal tubular function and excretion during exercise

In simple terms, the kidneys filter the blood at the glomerulus and then selectively reabsorb or secrete essential and non-essential substances in the tubules[6,51] (Fig 38.6). Normal fluid and electrolyte homeostasis requires the kidneys to eliminate excess water and electrolytes or, if there is a deficit, to reabsorb those vital components of the blood[6,51] (Fig 38.7). Alterations in GFR and/or tubular handling of water and solutes ultimately affects the volume of urine produced and the rate volume of essential electrolytes excreted over a given period of time.[6,51] Studies of humans, dogs, and horses have demonstrated that changes in tubular handling of water and solutes varies with work intensity.[6,51] These changes appear to be secondary to alterations in renal blood flow, GFR, and the filtered load of a given substance.[6,51] We are aware of only a few studies of the effects of exertion on renal tubular function. One study (Fig. 38.8) examined the effects of 1 h of submaximal exercise on endocrine changes and renal tubular function[83] and the others examined the effects of high-intensity exercise on renal function during and after exercise.[81] During submaximal exercise, performed at an intensity below 60% of $\dot{V}O_{2max}$, urine flow increases in humans and horses.[51,78,80] However, in horses, while low-intensity exercise resulted in a significant 45% increase in urine production, the total volume of extra water lost (~6 mL/min) was reported to be small compared with the increased volume lost as sweat.[81] McKeever et al.[83] reported that the increase in urine flow was due to an exercise-induced increase in osmotic clearance induced primarily by a natriuresis and a kaliuresis.[83] The increase in sodium excretion appeared to be mediated by a concomitant increase in plasma atrial natriuretic peptide (ANP).[83] Even so, the total amount of sodium lost via renal excretion was minimal. The authors suggested that, during exercise, ANP (a potent vasodilator) functioned primarily to facilitate decreased vascular resistance in the working muscles[83] so as to accommodate increased atrial pressure caused by exercise-induced increases in venous return. The relatively small but significant increase in sodium excretion observed in horses and humans during the early part of a bout of endurance exercise appeared to be a minor secondary response to the potent cardiovascular action of this hormone.[83] Interestingly, the authors of that same study demonstrated that there was a significant kaliuresis as well as the aforementioned natriuresis and suggested that the increase in potassium excretion was due primarily to a rise in plasma aldosterone concentration.[83] The increase in plasma K^+ concentration seen in submaximally exercised horses coincided with an increase in plasma aldosterone concentration.[83] The authors speculated that because there were limited decreases in plasma Na^+ concentration, the increases in aldosterone release may have been primarily in response to the rise in plasma K^+ concentration.[83] This phenomenon has been demonstrated by other researchers, who have shown that the most potent stimulus for aldosterone secretion is an increase in circulating potassium.[83] Functionally, this prevents excessive increases in plasma K^+ concentration, which can alter electrophysiological gradients in the muscles and other tissues.[83] Several studies have documented that excessive increases in plasma K^+ concentration appear to be one of many factors contributing to the onset of muscle fatigue.[6,83] Thus, the reported increase in plasma aldosterone release and the kaliuretic action of ANP may function to limit an excessive rise in plasma K^+ concentration during lower-intensity exercise.[83] The increase in plasma K^+ concentration is due to its efflux from active skeletal muscle during high-intensity exercise, which is only partially offset by uptake by non-contracting muscle and by kaliuresis.[84]

Another major problem associated with exercise in the horse is an excessive and disproportional loss of chloride via the sweat.[83]

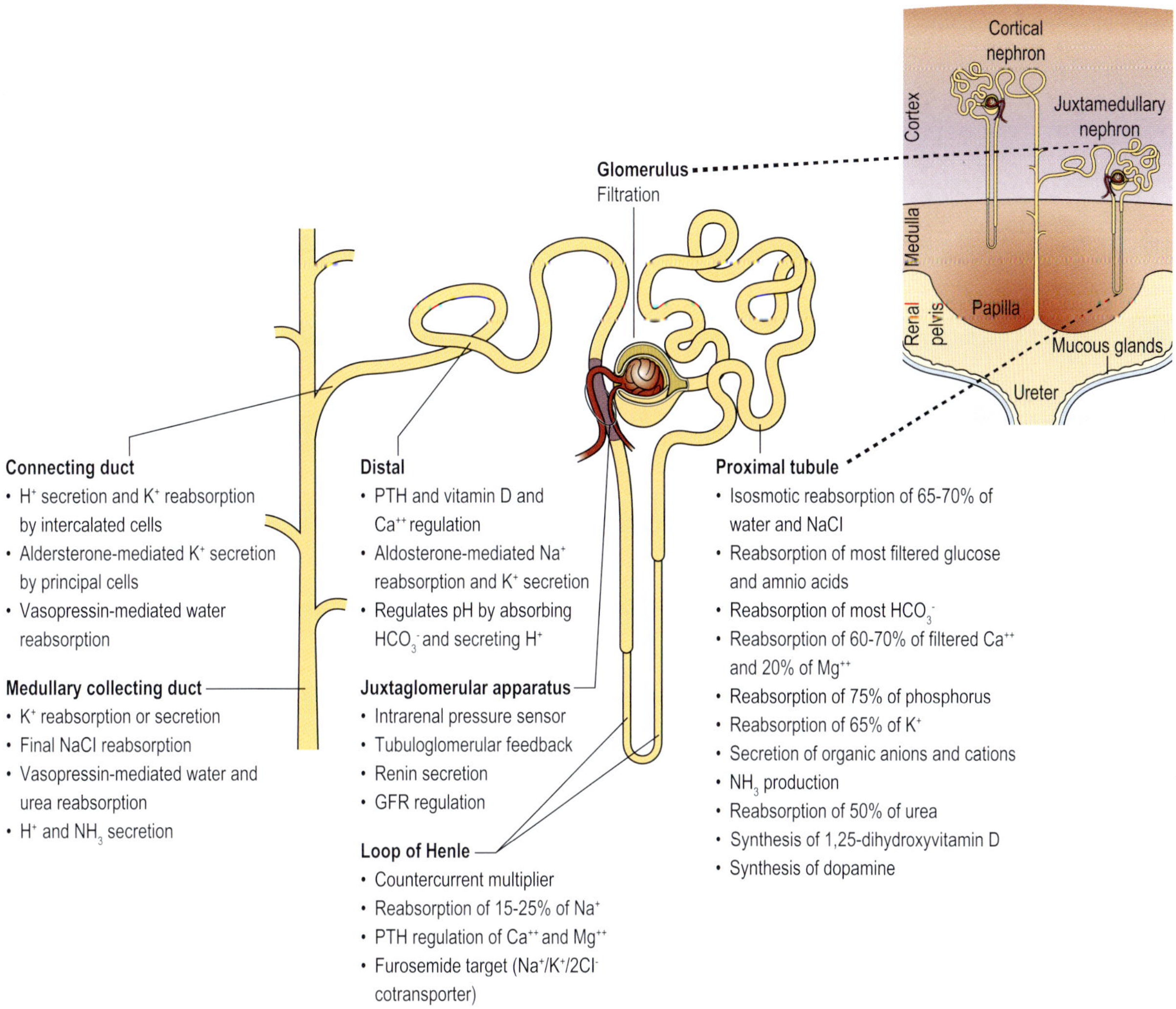

Fig 38.6 Structure and function of the nephron.
Courtesy of Toribio R, The Ohio State University, Columbus, OH; with permission. Essentials of equine renal and urinary tract physiology. Vet Clinics North Am Equine Pract 2007;23:533–561.

McKeever et al[83] demonstrated that renal chloride losses decrease when plasma chloride concentrations fall. Similar reductions in chloride excretion are also seen in exercising humans.[6,51] As Na^+ and K^+ excretion increased in submaximally exercised horses, the authors suggested that mechanisms affecting the conservation of those electrolytes could not have been responsible for the increase in Cl^- reabsorption.[83] Interestingly, the same horses became alkalotic during the hour-long bout of exercise.[83] Thus, the authors suggested that, based on other reports,[51,83] renal mechanisms affecting reabsorption of Cl^- and secretion of HCO_3^- by the antiporter in the apical membrane of the intercalated cell of the cortical collecting duct may have led to conservation of chloride.[51] Lastly, solute-free water clearance does not appear to be altered by submaximal exercise in the horse despite significant increases in plasma osmolality and plasma vasopressin concentrations.[83] Similar observations have been made in exercising humans.[51] This paradox has several possible explanations. First, a decrease in renal blood flow potentially could decrease the filtered load of solute-free water available for reabsorption by the action of AVP on the collecting ducts.[51] This explanation would not be supported by the observation that submaximal exercise does not affect absolute RBF or GFR.[6,58,80] It may, however, be possible that the extrarenal functions of vasopressin are more important during exercise and actions on the kidneys are overridden. Such functions may include vasopressin's role in vasoconstriction of vascular beds in non-obligate tissues, its role in central mechanisms that stimulate thirst and drinking, and its action on the gut.[6,35,85,86] In the gut, vasopressin appears to act on the epithelium of the large intestine, enhancing the uptake of sodium and water.[85] This protective effect would aid in the limitation of exercise-related fluid deficits more than potential reductions in free water clearance.

High-intensity exercise appears to have effects that are dramatically different from submaximal exertion. Sodium excretion is dramatically reduced during high-intensity exercise in horses, pigs, and humans.[6,51,80] Inconsistent changes in sodium excretion have been observed in the exercising dog.[51] Several mechanisms could be responsible for the decrease in sodium excretion, including: (i) a decrease in filtered load of sodium; (ii) activation of the renin–angiotensin cascade; (iii) elevation of plasma aldosterone concentration; and (iv) direct neurogenic control.[51] In the first instance, a change in filtered load sodium would mean that less solute would be presented to the tubules for reabsorption. This would require a reduction in GFR; as this does not change in humans, pigs, or horses,[6,51,80] it does not appear to be a viable mechanism for the

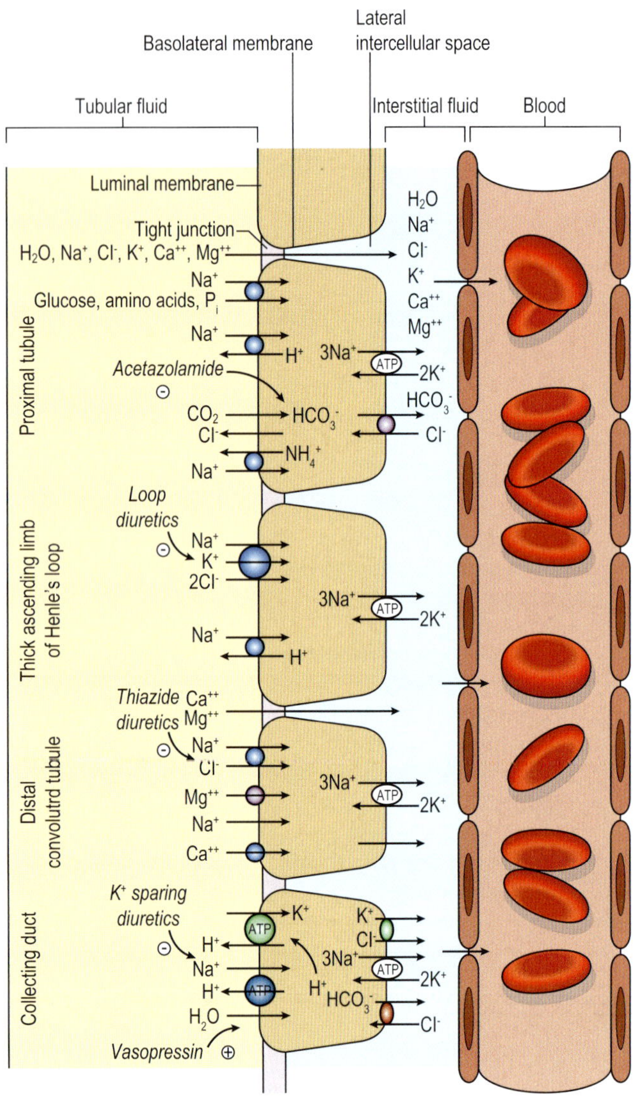

Fig 38.7 A schematic depicting sites of solute, electrolyte and acid–base regulation by the renal tubular cells.

Courtesy of Toribio R, The Ohio State University, Columbus, OH; with permission. Essentials of equine renal and urinary tract physiology. Vet Clinics North Am Equine Pract 2007;23:533–561.

decrease in sodium excretion. More recent information has been published that shows that the decrease in sodium excretion is not blocked by pharmacological blockade of the renin–angiotensin cascade.[51] Aldosterone concentration increases in the horse without a change in sodium excretion.[83] In other species, the observation that sodium excretion rapidly returns to baseline after exercise suggested that aldosterone was not the mediator of the antinatriuresis seen during exercise.[51] The speed of the recovery has been further interpreted to suggest a neural mechanism. This theory is consistent with a reported intensity-dependent increase in renal sympathetic nerve activity during exercise.[51] Zambraski[51] and others have suggested that, based on all the current evidence, the mechanism behind exercise-induced increases in sodium reabsorption is primarily direct neurogenic control.

Schott et al.[81,82] reported that urine flow almost stopped during supramaximal exercise and was still below pre-exercise levels in the period immediately after exercise. High-intensity exercise also caused a decrease in urine osmolality and osmotic excretion.[81,82] Interestingly, one would have predicted a significant reduction in electrolyte excretion; however, there were only non-significant reductions in the bulk excretion of K^+ and Cl^- during exercise and no change in Na^+ excretion, despite a reduction in urine flow.[81] This response contrasts with changes observed in other species.[51] One explanation for this aberrational finding may be the design of the experiment. In the experiment, exercise was performed during part of one of the 15-min collection periods.[81] Data for the entire 15-min collection period were pooled and included a post-exercise period characterized by diuresis, natriuresis, and kaliuresis (see below). These post-exercise changes may have offset any exercise-induced decreases in electrolyte excretion that should have occurred with a reduction in RBF and urine flow.

High-intensity exercise appears to also affect urinary pH, an observation of interest to racing chemists.[87] Gerken et al.[87] reported that high-intensity exercise caused a transient reduction in urine pH that lasted for up to 60 min of recovery. The authors suggested that the more acidic urine may affect the results of the battery of tests used to detect foreign substances.[87] More interestingly, they suggested that alkalinizing agents like sodium bicarbonate may alter post-exertion pH, thus further complicating drug detection efforts.

Post-exercise changes in renal function

While the studies of Schott et al.[81,82] did not document a change in tubular function, the authors did report a substantial post-exercise increase in urine flow. Data were consistent with a diuresis, kaliuresis, and natriuresis.[81,82] Excretion rates for these substances returned to baseline by 30 min of recovery. The authors suggested that the increase in sodium and potassium excretion was most likely due to an increase in atrial natriuretic peptide, which had been shown to increase during exercise in the horse.[81] Long term, the adaptations to exercise training involves reduction in 24 h urine output and an expansion of plasma volume with a concomitant increase in the content of sodium in the vascular compartment.[16,88]

Adaptive response to repeated exercise (training)

Training-induced hypervolemia

Repeated exercise or training usually evokes an adaptive response that better prepares the horse's various physiological systems for subsequent bouts of acute exertion.[6,13,16,58,89] Disturbances in fluid and electrolyte balance require a two-phase response, with the early phase resulting in the replenishment of acute fluid and electrolyte losses and a secondary or adaptive phase that results in an enhanced ability to cope with future systemic disturbances.[6,13,16,58] This 'hypervolemic' response to training is an adaptive response that involves a beneficial increase in blood volume due to an increase in plasma volume.[58] The training-induced hypervolemia is beneficial because it enhances both cardiovascular and thermoregulatory stability during the challenge of acute exercise.[58,90] The increase in total body water provides extra fluid that insures cardiovascular stability by providing the extra volume needed to maintain venous return and thus cardiac output.[6,58] Thermoregulatory benefits are two-fold, including an increase in the ability to increase skin blood flow to enhance transport of heat from the core to the surface and an increase in the amount of fluid available for sweat production and evaporative cooling.[58] Functional evidence for the latter benefit can be seen in studies of humans that have demonstrated that trained individuals have an earlier onset to sweating and produce more

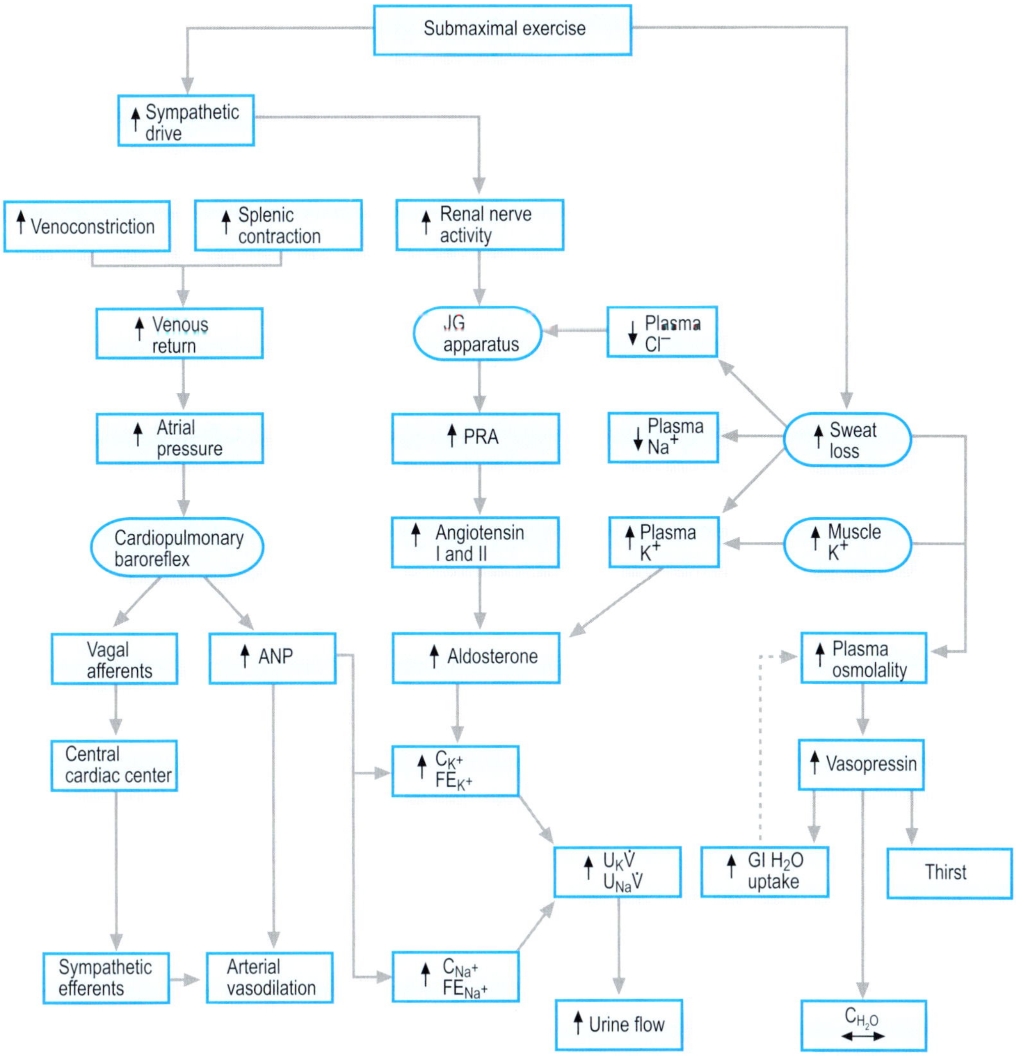

Fig 38.8 Renal, cardiovascular, and endocrine response to low-intensity exercise in the horse. ANP, atrial natriuretic peptide; C_{K^+}, potassium clearance; C_{Na^+}, sodium clearance; C_{H_2O}, water clearance, FE_{K^+}, fractional excretion of potassium; FE_{Na^+}, fractional excretion of sodium; GI, gastrointestinal, JG, juxtaglomerular (apparatus); PRA, plasma renin activity; $U_K\dot{V}$, potassium excretion; $U_{Na}\dot{V}$, sodium excretion.
McKeever KH, Hinchcliff KW, Schmall LM, et al. Renal tubular function in horses during submaximal exercise. Am J Physiol - Regulatory, Integrative and Comparative Physiology 1991;261(3 Pt 2):R553–60, with permission from the American Physiological Society.

sweat compared to untrained individuals exercising at the same relative submaximal work intensity.[58] It is likely that there are similar training-induced changes in cardiovascular function and thermoregulation in the horse.[90] Mechanistically, the retention of water and electrolytes that leads to a training-induced hypervolemia reflects the effort of multiple systems to defend volume, plasma osmolality, and blood pressure.[6,13,16,20,58] Comparative studies have demonstrated that approximately 60% of the mechanism behind the hypervolemic response is related to stimuli associated with the demands of thermoregulation.[58] The remaining 40% of the response appears to be related to mechanisms directly associated with exertion.[58] These mechanisms counter acute fluid and electrolyte losses by stimulating the intake of water and by reducing renal losses of water and electrolytes (Fig. 38.9).

Interestingly, rats, humans, dogs, and horses all expand their plasma volume in response to exercise training.[16,58,91] However, there are profound species differences in the mechanism behind the hypervolemic response to exercise training. Dogs expand their total body water through drinking; in fact, water is consumed at a greater rate than an observed training-induced natriuresis and diuresis.[91] Cooling in dogs involves a large loss of respiratory water and saliva, which results in acute increases in plasma tonicity and osmolality.[91] Thus, dogs must either drink to take in water to dilute the hyperosmotic hypertonic plasma or they must use renal mechanisms to excrete the excess electrolytes sensed in the plasma.[91] Humans and horses, on the other hand, lose a large amount of electrolytes in their sweat; therefore, there is a drive to replenish fluid and electrolytes to defend both volume and tonicity.[16,58,88] In horses and humans, drinking during and immediately after exercise at best only slows or partially counters the development of a fluid deficit, but does not counter any electrolyte deficit.[16,58,88] Studies of horses and humans are mixed as to the role of water and electrolyte intake in the long-term response to exercise training.[16,58,88] Humans use both an increase in thirst and drinking and renal mechanisms to increase

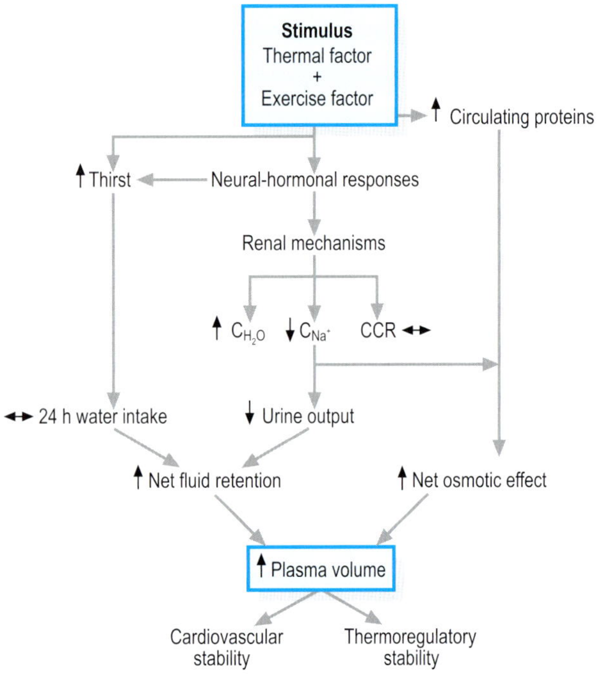

Fig 38.9 Suggested mechanisms for the exercise training-induced hypervolemia seen in horses. CCR, creatinine clearance.

Adapted from Convertino. Reprinted from Convertino, V., 1991, Blood volume: its adaptation to endurance training, Medicine & Science in Sports & Exercise, 23(12), with permission from Wolters Kluwer Health.

net fluid retention.[58] Drinking in humans, however, does not account for all of the net water retention, with most of the actual expansion of total body water coming through renal mechanisms.[58] One recent study of the horse reported that water intake increased with training; however, the authors did not measure renal losses or conduct a balance study that would determine if the amount ingested contributed to an expansion of plasma volume.[6] Other studies have shown that exercise training does not alter water intake in the horse.[6,88] Instead, they reported that the horse appears to rely on renal mechanisms and an overall reduction in urine water loss[16,88] to retain the sodium and water needed to expand plasma and blood volume.

In both humans and horses, this decrease in urine output seen with training is due to alterations in postglomerular mechanisms rather than a change in filtration rate.[16,58,88] These renal adjustments are an adaptive or training response rather than a countermeasure to the perturbations of acute exercise. In humans an aldosterone-mediated retention of sodium and water seems to cause a net retention of water.[92–94] Until recently, the mechanism behind the hypervolemic response was not as clear in the horse. An early study did not demonstrate any change in renal mechanisms affecting the retention of sodium and water, and instead suggested that urea rather than sodium may be the solute responsible for the renal retention of water that leads to a training-induced expansion of plasma volume in the horse.[16] However, the authors paradoxically demonstrated that there was a highly significant increase in plasma sodium content that paralleled the increase in plasma volume.[16] Interestingly, this net increase in retained sodium and water occurred despite increased losses via sweating.[16] As the rate of sodium intake was held constant, the only other routes for a training-induced retention of sodium would have been either a more efficient uptake of electrolytes and water from the gut and/or a net retention by the kidneys early in the first days of training, as seen in humans, where most of the response occurs in the first days of training. To solve this mystery, a more recent paper[88] focused on the first days of training and demonstrated dramatic reductions in urine output and excretion of sodium during the first days of training. Thus, like humans, the horse appears to undergo a similar aldosterone-mediated retention of sodium and water by the kidneys.[88] However, it was also found that renal retention of sodium and water did not fully counter losses seen in the sweat during the first days of training and the authors suggested that an enhanced aldosterone-mediated uptake of sodium and water from the large intestine may also contribute to the retention of electrolytes and water.[88] This makes sense because the horse's large intestine serves as a fluid reservoir. Such an additional response in the horse may be a warranted species-specific adaptation in response to the relatively larger electrolyte deficits associated with the production of hypertonic sweat. Enhanced intestinal uptake of sodium and water is supported by other published studies[95] demonstrating that aldosterone may enhance the transport of electrolytes and water from the digestive tract of the horse.

Concurrent with the aforementioned retention of water, sodium, and other vital electrolytes (which keeps the retained fluid isotonic), is an increase in the plasma protein content.[16,58,88] This increase in protein functions to keep the plasma iso-oncotic; thus, holding water within the vascular space. Human studies suggest that the early increase in plasma protein content comes about from inward shifts of protein from the lymphatics and interstitial space, and later from an overall net increase in plasma protein synthesis.[58] The hypervolemic response to training in the horse also appears to involve an increase in the content of plasma protein, most likely through a net increase in synthesis.[16,88] One aspect of the effect of training yet to be studied in the horse is whether there are alterations in the cardiopulmonary baroreceptors that allow for the retention of the extravascular volume. Human studies have shown that training results in a downregulation of the ANP and neuroendocrine response to exercise, quite possibly to accommodate the hypervolemia associated with exercise training.[58]Future research should determine if downregulation of these important control mechanisms also occurs in horses.

It is important to note that short-term horizontal studies of humans, dogs, and horses have demonstrated that the increase in plasma volume occurs early in training and is followed by a subsequent slow increase in red blood cell volume (Fig. 38.10).[96] Thus, early in training, if one only looks at hematocrit, there is a false impression of a 'sports anemia'.[96] Interestingly, in humans there appears to be an overshoot in the expansion of plasma volume.[96] As red cell volume slowly increases, the early increases in plasma volume appear to level off and even decrease.[96] Thus, after weeks and months of training there is a greater blood volume, with both plasma and red cell volume remaining greater than pretraining levels,[96] most likely at a level that optimizes both blood viscosity and oxygen-carrying capacity.[97]

A syndrome of red cell hypervolemia has been reported in Scandinavian Standardbred trotters associated with overtraining or poor performance.[15,98–102] These reports were based on cross-sectional studies of normal and poor performance horses, where an excess of red blood cells was observed associated with limited performance or overtraining.[15,98–102] However, a direct cause and effect has not been reported in horses or any other species.[103] In addition, longitudinal studies of overtraining in horses, using controls and objective measurements to show the existence of overtraining, convincingly demonstrate that there were no differences in red cell volume between overtrained and normal horses.[104]

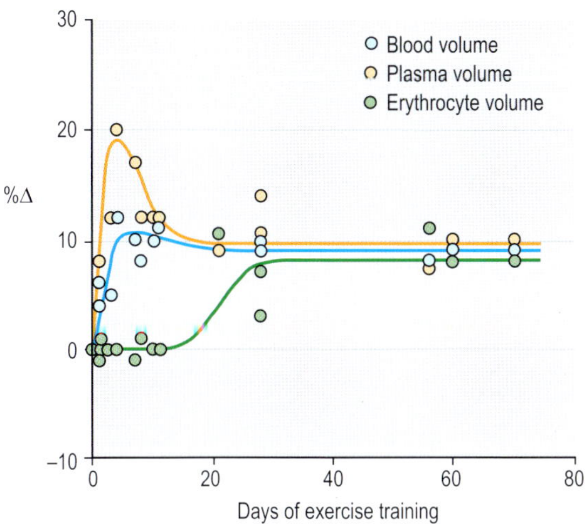

Fig 38.10 Estimated time course of relative (%) changes in blood volume (blue line), plasma volume (orange line), and erythrocyte volume (green line) during exercise. Each point represents the average change reported in a group of (human) subjects from one investigation. Data were extracted from 18 investigations in which all three vascular volumes were reported.

Reprinted from Sawka M,Convertino V, Eichner E, et al. 2000, Blood volume: importance and adaptations to exercise training, environmental stresses, and trauma/sickness, 32(2), Medicine & Science in Sports & Exercise, with permission from Wolters Kluwer Health.[96]

Effects of aging on the acute and chronic response to exercise

A limited number of data have been reported comparing the thermoregulatory responses of older and younger men and women during exercise in the heat.[105,106] It has been concluded that age influences thermoregulatory function during exercise.[105] Suggested reasons for this age-related decline in the ability to thermoregulate properly during exercise in humans include lower cardiovascular capacity due to the age-related decrease in cardiac output, alterations in mechanisms associated with the control of skin blood flow, and a possible state of hypohydration in the elderly.[105] While there are an abundance of papers that have examined thermoregulation in young horses, few studies have addressed the effects of age on the thermoregulatory response to exercise in the horse.[107,108] McKeever and co-workers[107,108] exercised young and old horses at the same submaximal absolute work intensity of 1625 watts until they reached a core body temperature of 40°C. Older horses reached a core temperature of 40°C in almost half the time required by the younger mares.[107,108] The heart rates of the older mares were also substantially higher than the heart rates of the younger mares at 40°C.[107,108] Interestingly, both groups had similar heart rates and core temperatures by 10 min after exercise.[107,108] Even with the more rapid heart rate, older horses were still unable to dissipate the heat generated from exercise as quickly as younger mares, therefore leading to a faster increase in core temperature after the onset of exercise. Age-related changes in fluid and electrolyte balance and cardiovascular function may contribute to the impaired thermoregulatory capacity. Older humans commonly have lower total body water, plasma volume and reserves of fluid for sweating.[105] In the above-mentioned studies of aged horses the changes in markers of fluid status suggested that acute fluid shifts were of a similar magnitude when compared to younger animals. However, a subsequent study[109] demonstrated that older horses had a substantially lower pre-exercise plasma volume compared to younger animals. A lower plasma volume could result in lower venous return, stroke volume, and cardiac output and a compromise of thermoregulatory stability.

Summary

Exercise places large demands on the cardiovascular system, and is further complicated by environmental factors. Performance is limited in many respects by fluid and electrolyte stores and the ability to maintain cardiovascular and thermoregulatory stability in the face of severe sweat losses. Studies of the exercising horse have been primarily descriptive and/or associative with only a limited number seeking to identify physiological mechanisms associated with the control of fluid and electrolyte balance. More mechanistic studies are needed to fully understand the integration of the cardiovascular, endocrine and renal systems in the defense of plasma osmolality, blood volume, and blood pressure.

References

1. Carlson G. Thermoregulation, fluid and electrolyte balance. In: Snow DH, Persson SGB, Rose RJ, editors. Proc. International Conference. Equine exercise physiology. Oxford UK: Granta Ed.; 1982. p. 291–309.
2. Carlson GP. Hematology and body fluids in the equine athlete: a review. In: Gillespie JR, Robinson NE, editors. Proc. 2nd International Conference. Equine exercise physiology. Davis, CA: ICEEP; 1987. p. 393–425.
3. Greenleaf JE, Morimoto T. Mechanisms controlling fluid ingestion: thirst and drinking. In: Buskirk ER, Puhl SM, editors. Body fluid balance: exercise and sport. New York: CRC; 1996. p. 3–17.
4. Geor RJ, McCutcheon LJ. Thermoregulatory adaptations associated with training and heat acclimation. Vet Clin North Am Equine Pract 1998;14(1):97–120.
5. McConaghy FF. Thermoregulation. In: Hodgson DR, Rose RJ, editors. The athletic horse: principles and practice of equine sports medicine. Philadelphia: WB Saunders; 1994. p. 181–204.
6. McKeever KH. Fluid balance and renal function in exercising horses. Vet Clin North Am Equine Pract 1998;14:23–44.
7. Rowell LB. Human cardiovascular control. New York: Oxford University Press; 1993. p. 441–79.
8. Rowell LB. Cardiovascular adjustments to thermal stress. Handbook of physiology, The cardiovascular system. Peripheral circulation and organ blood flow. Bethesda, MD: American Physiological Society; 1983. p. 967–1023.
9. Baptiste KE, Naylor JM, Bailey J, et al. A function for guttural pouches in the horse. Nature 2000;403(6768): 382–3.
10. McConaghy FF, Hales JR, Rose RJ, et al. Selective brain cooling in the horse during exercise and environmental heat stress. J Appl Physiol 1995;79(6): 1849–54.
11. Schott HC 2nd, Hinchcliff KW. Fluids, electrolytes, and bicarbonate. Vet Clin North Am Equine Pract 1993;9(3): 577–604.
12. McKeever KH. Electrolyte and water balance in the exercising horse. Nutrition manual for veterinarians. St Louis: AAEP and Purina Mills; 1997. p. 79–86.
13. Convertino VA. Fluid shifts and hydration state: effects of long-term

exercise. Can J Sport Sci 1987;12(Suppl. 1):136S–9S.
14. Eichner E. Other medical considerations in prolonged exercise. Perspectives in exercise science and sports medicine, vol. 1, Prolonged exercise. Indianapolis: Benchmark; 1988. p. 415–22.
15. Persson SGB. On blood volume and working capacity. Acta Vet Scand 1967;(Suppl. 19):1–189.
16. McKeever KH, Schurg WA, Jarrett SH, et al. Exercise training-induced hypervolemia in the horse. Med Sci Sports Exerc 1987;19(1):21–7.
17. McKeever KH, Schurg WA, Convertino VA. A modified Evans blue dye method for the measurement of plasma volumen in the horse. J Equine Vet Sci 1988;8:208–12.
18. Rose RJ, Hodgson DR. Hematology and biochemistry. In: Hodgson DR, Rose RJ, editors. The athletic horse: principles and practice of equine sports medicine. Philadelphia: WB Saunders; 1994. p. 63–78.
19. McKeever KH, Hinchcliff KW, Reed SM, et al. Role of decreased plasma volume in hematocrit alterations during incremental treadmill exercise in horses. Am J Physiol 1993;265(2 Pt 2):R404–8.
20. McKeever KH, Hinchcliff KW. Neuroendocrine control of blood volume, blood pressure, and cardiovascular functions in horses. Equine Vet J Suppl 1995;18:77–81.
21. Nose H, Mack GW, Shi XR, et al. Shift in body fluid compartments after dehydration in humans. J Appl Physiol 1988;65(1):318–24.
22. McKeever KH, Hinchcliff KW, Reed SM, et al. Splenectomy alters blood pressure response to incremental treadmill exercise in horses. Am J Physiol 1993;265(2 Pt 2):R409–13.
23. Dill DB, Costill DL. Calculation of percentage changes in volumes of blood, plasma, and red cells in dehydration. J Appl Physiol 1974;37(2):247–8.
24. Van Beaumont W, Greenleaf JE, Juhos L. Disproportional changes in hematocrit, plasma volume, and proteins during exercise and bed rest. J Appl Physiol 1972;33(1):55–61.
25. Harrison MH. Effects on thermal stress and exercise on blood volume in humans. Physiol Rev 1985;65(1):149–209.
26. Fielding CL, Magdesian KG, Elliott DA, et al. Use of multifrequency bioelectrical impedance analysis for estimation of total body water and extracellular and intracellular fluid volumes in horses. Am J Vet Res 2004;65(3):320–6.
27. Forro M, Cieslar S, Ecker GL, et al. Total body water and ECFV measured using bioelectrical impedance analysis and indicator dilution in horses. J Appl Physiol 2000;89(2):663–71.
28. Andrews FM, Nadeau JA, Saabye L, et al. Measurement of total body water content in horses, using deuterium oxide dilution. Am J Vet Res 1997; 58(10):1060–4.
29. Fielding CL, Magdesian KG, Elliott DA, et al. Pharmacokinetics and clinical utility of sodium bromide (NaBr) as an estimator of extracellular fluid volume in horses. J Vet Intern Med 2003;17(2):213–17.
30. Carlson GP, Harrold D, Rumbaugh GE. Volume dilution of sodium thiocyanate as a measure of extracellular fluid volume in the horse. Am J Vet Res 1979;40(4):587–9.
31. Fielding CL, Magdesian KG, Carlson GP, et al. Estimation of acute fluid shifts using bioelectrical impedance analysis in horses. J Vet Intern Med 2007;21(1): 176–83.
32. McKeen G, Lindinger MI. Prediction of hydration status using multi-frequency bioelectrical impedance analysis during exercise and recovery in horses. Equine Comp Exerc Physiol 2004;1(3):199–209.
33. Nadel ER, Mack GW, Takamata A. Thermoregulation, exercise and thirst: interrelationships in humans. In: Gisolfi CV, Lamb DR, Nadel ER, editors. Perspectives in exercise science and sport medicine, vol. 6. Exercise, heat and thermoregulation. Carmel, IN: Brown & Benchmark; 1993. p. 225–56.
34. Wade CE, Freund BJ, Claybaugh JR. Fluid and electrolyte homeostasis during and following exercise: hormonal and non-hormonal factors. In: Claybaugh JR, Wade CE, editors. Hormonal regulation of fluids and electrolytes. New York: Plenum; 1989. p. 1–44.
35. McKeever KH. The endocrine system and the challenge of exercise. Vet Clin North Am Equine Pract 2002:321–53.
36. Johnson PJ. Physiology of body fluids in the horse. Vet Clin North Am Equine Pract 1998:1–22.
37. Szlyk-Modrow PC, Francesconi RP, Hubbard RW. Integrated control of body fluids. In: Buskirk ER, Puhl SM, editors. Body fluid balance: exercise and sport. New York: CRC; 1996. p. 117–36.
38. Wade CE, Freund BJ. Hormonal control of blood volume during and following exercise. In: Gisolfi CV, Lamb DR, editors. Perspectives in exercise science and sports medicine, vol. 3. Fluid homeostasis during exercise. Carmel, IN: Benchmark; 1990. p. 207–45.
39. Convertino VA, Keil LC, Bernauer EM, et al. Plasma volume, osmolality, vasopressin, and renin activity during graded exercise in man. J Appl Physiol 1981;50(1):123–8.
40. McKeever KH, Hinchcliff KW, Reed SM, et al. Plasma constituents during incremental treadmill exercise in intact and splenectomised horses. Equine Vet J 1993;25(3):233–6.
41. Freund BJ, Claybaugh JR, Dice MS, et al. Hormonal and vascular fluid responses to maximal exercise in trained and untrained males. J Appl Physiol 1987;63(2):669–75.
42. Freund BJ, Shizuru EM, Hashiro GM, et al. Hormonal, electrolyte, and renal responses to exercise are intensity dependent. J Appl Physiol 1991;70(2):900–6.
43. Senay LC Jr. Early response of plasma contents on exposure of working men to heat. J Appl Physiol 1978;44(2): 166–70.
44. Delgado R, Sanders TM, Bloor CM. Renal blood flow distribution during steady-state exercise and exhaustion in conscious dogs. J Appl Physiol 1975;39(3):475–8.
45. Musch TI, Friedman DB, Pitetti KH, et al. Regional distribution of blood flow of dogs during graded dynamic exercise. J Appl Physiol 1987;63(6):2269–77.
46. Coyne CP, Carlson GP, Spensley MS, et al. Preliminary investigation of alterations in blood viscosity, cellular composition, and electrophoresis plasma protein fraction profile after competitive racing activity in Thoroughbred horses. Am J Vet Res 1990;51(12):1956–63.
47. Convertino VA, Keil LC, Greenleaf JE. Plasma volume, renin, and vasopressin responses to graded exercise after training. J Appl Physiol 1983;54(2): 508–14.
48. Waller A, Lindinger MI. Time course and magnitude of fluid and electrolyte shifts during recovery from high-intensity exercise in Standardbred racehorses. Equine Comp Exerc Physiol 2005;2(2):77–87.
49. Lindinger MI, McKeen G, Ecker GL. Time course and magnitude of changes in total body water, extracellular fluid volume, intracellular fluid volume and plasma volume during submaximal exercise and recovery in horses. Equine Comp Exerc Physiol 2004;1(2):131–9.
50. McCutcheon LJ, Geor RJ. Sweating. Fluid and ion losses and replacement. Vet Clin North Am Equine Pract 1998; 14(1):75–95.
51. Zambraski EJ. Renal regulation of fluid homeostasis during exercise. In: Gisolfi CV, Lamb DR, editors. Perspectives in exercise science and sports medicine, vol. 3. Fluid homeostasis during exercise. Carmel, IN: Benckmark; 1990. p. 245–80.
52. Zambraski EJ, Tucker MS, Lakas CS, et al. Mechanism of renin release in exercising dog. Am J Physiol 1984; 246(1 Pt 1):E71–6.

53. Jimenez M, Hinchcliff KW, Farris JW. Catecholamine and cortisol responses of horses to incremental exertion. Vet Res Commun 1998;22(2):107–18.
54. McKeever KH, Hinchcliff KW, Schmall LM, et al. Plasma renin activity and aldosterone and vasopressin concentrations during incremental treadmill exercise in horses. Am J Vet Res 1992;53(8):1290–3.
55. Lindinger M, ECKER GL. Ion and water losses from body fluids during a 163 km endurance ride. Equine Vet J 1995;27(S18):314–22.
56. Sawka MN, Pandolf KB. Effects of body water loss on physiologic function and exercise performance. In: Gisolfi CV, Lamb DR, editors. Perspectives in exercise science and sports medicine, vol. 3. Fluid homeostasis during exercise. Carmel, IN: Benchmark; 1990. 1–38.
57. Sejersted OM. Electrolyte imbalance in body fluids as a mechanism of fatigue during exercise. In: Lamb DR, Gisolfi CV, editors. Perspectives in exercise science and sports medicine, vol. 5. Energy metabolism in exercise and sport. Dubuque, IA: Brown & Benchmark; 1992. p. 149–206.
58. Convertino VA. Blood volume: its adaptation to endurance training. Med Sci Sports Exerc 1991;23(12):1338–48.
59. Geor RJ, McCutcheon LJ, Lindinger MI. Adaptations to daily exercise in hot and humid ambient conditions in trained Thoroughbred horses. Equine Vet J Suppl 1996;22(22):63–8.
60. Geor RJ, McCutcheon LJ. Hydration effects on physiological strain of horses during exercise-heat stress. J Appl Physiol 1998;84(6):2042–51.
61. Kingston JK, McCutcheon LJ, Geor RJ. Comparison of three methods for estimation of exercise-related ion losses in sweat of horses. Am J Vet Res 1999;60(10):1248–54.
62. Kingston JK, Geor RJ, McCutcheon LJ. Rate and composition of sweat fluid losses are unaltered by hypohydration during prolonged exercise in horses. J Appl Physiol 1997;83(4):1133–43.
63. McCutcheon LJ, Geor RJ. Influence of training on sweating responses during submaximal exercise in horses. J Appl Physiol 2000;89(6):2463–71.
64. McCutcheon LJ, Geor RJ, Ecker GL, et al. Equine sweating responses to submaximal exercise during 21 days of heat acclimation. J Appl Physiol 1999;87(5):1843–51.
65. McCutcheon L, Geor R. Sweat fluid and ion losses in horses during training and competition in cool vs. hot ambient conditions: implications for ion supplementation. Equine Vet J 1996;28(S22):54–62.
66. McCutcheon LJ, Geor RJ, Hare MJ, et al. Sweating rate and sweat composition during exercise and recovery in ambient heat and humidity. Equine Vet J Suppl 1995;20(20):153–7.
67. Hubbard RW, Szlyk PC. Solute model or cellular energy model? Practical and theoretical aspects of thirst during exercise. In: Marriott BM, editor. Fluid replacement and heat stress. Washington, DC: National Academy Press; 1994. p. 16–193.
68. Hubbard RW, Szlyk PC, Armstrong LE. Influence of thirst and fluid palatability on fluid ingestion during exercise. In: Gisolfi CV, Lamb DR, editors. Perspectives in exercise science and sports medicine, vol. 3. Fluid homeostasis during exercise. Carmel, IN: Benchmark; 1990. 39–86.
69. Thrasher TN, Nistal-Herrera JF, Keil LC, Ramsay DJ. Satiety and inhibition of vasopressin secretion after drinking in dehydrated dogs. Am J Physiol 1981;240(4):E394–401.
70. Greenleaf JE. Environmental issues that influence intake of replacement beverages. In: Marriott BM, editor. Fluid replacement and heat stress. Washington DC: National Academy Press; 1994. p. 194–214.
71. McKeever KH, Hinchcliff KW, Cooley JL. Acute volume load during exercise in horses: atrial natriuretic peptide, vasopressin, and hemodynamics. Med Sci Sports Exerc 1991;23:S104.
72. Sosa Leon LA. Treatment of exercise-induced dehydration. Vet Clin North Am Equine Pract 1998:159–73.
73. Sosa Leon LA, Hodgson DR, Carlson GP, et al. Effects of concentrated electrolytes administered via a paste on fluid, electrolyte, and acid base balance in horses. Am J Vet Res 1998;59(7):898–903.
74. Sosa Leon LA, Hodgson DR, Rose RJ. Gastric emptying of oral rehydration solutions at rest and after exercise in horses. Res Vet Sci 1997;63(2):183–7.
75. Sosa Leon LA, Davie AJ, Hodgson DR, et al. The effects of tonicity, glucose concentration and temperature of an oral rehydration solution on its absorption and elimination. Equine Vet J Suppl 1995;20(20):140–6.
76. Butudom P, Schott HC 2nd, Davis MW, et al. Drinking salt water enhances rehydration in horses dehydrated by frusemide administration and endurance exercise. Equine Vet J Suppl 2002;34(34):513–18.
77. Lawrence L. Nutrition and the athletic horse. In: Hodgson DR, Rose RJ, editors. The athletic horse: principles and practice of equine sports medicine. Philadelphia: WB Saunders; 1994. p. 205–30.
78. Kachadorian WA, Johnson RE. Renal responses to various rates of exercise. J Appl Physiol 1970;28(6):748–52.
79. Grimby G. Renal clearances at rest and during physical exercise after injection of bacterial pyrogen. J Appl Physiol 1965;20:137–41.
80. Hinchcliff KW, McKeever KH, Schmall LM, et al. Renal and systemic hemodynamic responses to sustained submaximal exertion in horses. Am J Physiol 1990;258(5 Pt 2):R1177–83.
81. Schott HC, Hodgson DR, Bayly WM, et al. Renal responses to high intensity exercise. In: Persson SGB, Lindholm A, Jeffcott LB, editors. Proc. 3rd International Conference. Equine exercise physiology. Davis, CA: ICEEP; 1991. p. 361–7.
82. Schott HC, Ragle CA, Bayly WM. Effects of phenylbutazone and frusemide on urinary excretory responses to high intensity exercise. Equine Vet J Suppl 1995;18:426–31.
83. McKeever KH, Hinchcliff KW, Schmall LM, et al. Renal tubular function in horses during submaximal exercise. Am J Physiol 1991;261(3 Pt 2):R553–60.
84. Schott HC 2nd, Bohart GV, Eberhart SW. Potassium and lactate uptake by noncontracting tissue during strenuous exercise. Equine Vet J Suppl 2002;34(34):532–8.
85. Bridges RJ, Rummel W. Vasopressin-stimulated Na transport in rat colon descendens. In: Skadhauge E, Heintze K, editors. Intestinal absorption and secretion. Boston, MA: MTP; 1984. p. 265–72.
86. Gisolfi CV, Summers RW, Schedl HP. Intestinal absorption of fluids during rest and exercise. In: Gisolfi CV, Lamb DR, editors. Perspectives in exercise science and sports medicine, vol. 3. Fluid homeostasis during exercise. Carmel, IN: Benchmark; 1990. p. 129–80.
87. Gerken DF, Sams RA, McKeever KH, et al. Urinary pH effects on the renal clearance of lidocaine and phenylbutazone in exercising horses. Toxicologist 1991;11:96.
88. McKeever KH, Scali R, Geiser S, et al. Plasma aldosterone concentration and renal sodium excretion are altered during the first days of training. Equine Vet J Suppl 2002;34(34):524–31.
89. Lindinger MI, McCutcheon LJ, Ecker GL, et al. Heat acclimation improves regulation of plasma volume and plasma Na(+) content during exercise in horses. J Appl Physiol 2000;88(3):1006–13.
90. Kearns CF, McKeever KH, John-Alder H, et al. Relationship between body composition, blood volume and maximal oxygen uptake. Equine Vet J Suppl 2002;34(34):485–90.
91. McKeever KH, Schurg WA, Convertino VA. Exercise training-induced hypervolemia in greyhounds: role of

water intake and renal mechanisms. Am J Physiol 1985;248(4 Pt 2):R422–5.
92. Costill DL, Branum G, Fink W, et al. Exercise-induced sodium conservation changes in plasma renin and aldosterone. Med Sci Sport Exerc 1976;8:209–13.
93. Kirby CR, Convertino VA. Plasma aldosterone and sweat sodium concentrations after exercise and heat acclimation. J Appl Physiol 1986;61(3):967–70.
94. Luetkemeier MJ, Flowers KM, Lamb DR. Spironolactone administration and training-induced hypervolemia. Int J Sports Med 1994;15(6):295–300.
95. Jansson A, Lindholm A, Dahlborn K. Effects of acute intravenous aldosterone administration on Na(+), K(+), and water excretion in the horse. J Appl Physiol 2002;92(1):135–41.
96. Sawka MN, Convertino VA, Eichner ER. Blood volume: importance and adaptations to exercise training, environmental stresses, and trauma/sickness. Med Sci Sports Exerc 2000;32:332–48.
97. Birchard GF. Optimal hematocrit: theory, regulation, and implications. Amer Zool 1997;37:65–72.
98. Persson SG, Larsson M, Lindholm A. Effects of training on adreno-cortical function and red-cell volume in trotters. Zentralbl Veterinarmed A 1980;27(4):261–8.
99. Persson SG, Osterberg I. Racing performance in red blood cell hypervolaemic standardbred trotters. Equine Vet J Suppl 1999;30:617–20.
100. Funkquist P, Wagner PD, Hedenstierna G, et al. Ventilation-perfusion relationships during exercise in standardbred trotters with red cell hypervolaemia. Equine Vet J Suppl 1999;30:107–13.
101. Funkquist P, Nyman G, Persson SG. Haemodynamic response to exercise in Standardbred trotters with red cell hypervolaemia. Equine Vet J 2000;32(5):426–31.
102. Funkquist P, Sandhagen B, Persson SG, et al. Effects of phlebotomy on haemodynamic characteristics during exercise in standardbred trotters with red cell hypervolaemia. Equine Vet J 2001;33(4):417–24.
103. McKeever KH. Overtraining syndrome in standardbred horses: new insights into the role of red blood cell hypervolaemia. Vet J 2003;165(3):190–2.
104. Golland LC, Evans DL, McGowan CM, et al. The effects of overtraining on blood volumes in standardbred racehorses. Vet J 2003;165(3):228–33.
105. Kenney WL. Body fluid and temperature regulation as a function of age. In: Lamb DR, Gisolfi CV, Nadel ER, editors. Perspectives in exercise and sports medicine, vol. 8. Exercise in older adults. Carmel, IN: Cooper; 1995. p. 305–52.
106. Armstrong CG, Kenney WL. Effects of age and acclimation on responses to passive heat exposure. J Appl Physiol 1993;75(5):2162–7.
107. McKeever KH. Exercise physiology of the older horse. Vet Clin North Am Equine Pract 2002:469–90.
108. McKeever KH, Eaton TL, Geiser S. Thermoregulation in old and young horses during exercise. Med Sci Sports Exerc 2000;32:S156.
109. McKeever KH, Kearns CF. Aging-induced alterations in plasma volume in horses. Med Sci Sports Exerc 2001;33:S257.

Acid-base physiology at rest, during exercise and in response to training

39

Michael I. Lindinger

CHAPTER CONTENTS

Introduction

The purposes of this chapter are to provide an overview of acid-base state in athletic horses at rest, and to introduce acid-base assessment in clinically normal horses at rest and performing exercise of different intensities and durations. The physicochemical approach to acid-base assessment will be explained and used to exemplify the origins of acid-base disturbances during exercise. Also, the impact of diet, alkalinizing agents, furosemide (frusemide, Lasix) and selected clinical conditions on acid-base status will be briefly explored. A brief discussion on the topic of acidosis and skeletal muscle fatigue is provided to address some of the myths and confusion surrounding lactate, H^+ and muscle fatigue.

Why is it important to understand acid-base balance? Acid-base balance represents the integrated sum of many simultaneously acting physiological processes on physical and chemical state of body fluids. These processes include cellular respiration, ventilation at the lungs, renal function, hepatic function, and cellular (primarily skeletal muscle) ion transport processes. An understanding of acid-base state allows the practitioner to better understand the state of the horse at any point of time, how it got there, and to develop effective approaches for normalizing acid-base state when it had been pathophysiologically disturbed. This is important because 'clinically normal' acid-base state is tolerated within relatively wide physiological limits. We often read that plasma and intracellular pH are maintained within narrow limits; however, this contention is not supported by the research literature in any animal so far studied, including horses. In clinically normal humans and horses, plasma pH may vary from 7.0 to 7.6, although the norm lies close to 7.4. The large range of change in pH represents a 4-fold change in $[H^+]$, specifically 25 to 100 nEq/L, with normal plasma $[H^+]$ of 40 nmol/L. While this range of plasma $[H^+]$ can be tolerated, it is true that such changes are eventually accompanied by the activation of mechanisms that return $[H^+]$ back towards 40 nEq/L. Within skeletal muscle, pH at rest is about 7.0 ($[H^+]$ = 100 nEq/L) but with very high-intensity exercise muscle pH may approach 6.0 ($[H^+]$ = 1000 nEq/L). These are much wider ranges than generally appreciated. Also, they are tolerated, albeit briefly, and normal.

Let us start by considering what is meant by acid-base balance. In traditional terms acid-base balance refers to the balance between pH, PCO_2 and $[HCO_3^-]$ in physiological solution. While it is true that pH, representing the acidity or alkalinity of the fluid, is directly related to the PCO_2 and $[HCO_3^-]$, it is not true that changes in $[HCO_3^-]$ determine pH. The reason for this, as detailed below, is that it is not physically possible to change $[HCO_3^-]$ with simultaneously changing either the PCO_2, or the concentration of one or more of the ions in solution. Therefore, similar to pH, $[HCO_3^-]$ is dependent on the PCO_2 and the concentrations of all of the ions in solution. From this it follows that all of the ions in solution contribute to the acid-base state. Therefore acid-base state represents the physicochemical balance between PCO_2 and all ions in solution, including many large molecules such as albumin, lactate and intracellular proteins.

Acid-base balance in resting horses

The past 20 years has seen considerable interest in the acid-base state of racehorses at rest. This is in large part due to the practice of horsemen administering alkalinization agents to horses for the purpose of enhancing race performance, i.e. delaying onset of muscle fatigue.[1] The reader is referred to the following papers for discussion of ergogenic effects of alkalinizing agents.[2] Because of the potential of alkalinizing agents to enhance race performance, regulations have been put in place by all major racing jurisdictions. Most jurisdictions use a threshold for total CO_2 (TCO_2) of either 36 or 37 mmol/L for horses that have not been given furosemide; the corresponding $[HCO_3^-]$ thresholds are 34 and 35 mmol/L. Furosemide administration produces a dehydration with attendant changes in plasma ion concentrations, which typically raises TCO_2 by ~1.5 mmol/L. Therefore in racing jurisdictions that allow furosemide administration the TCO_2 testing threshold can be as high as 39 mmol/L. Racing jurisdictions also contend that all horses having a TCO_2 at or above the threshold have been given an alkalinizing agent for the purposes of enhancing exercise performance. Horsemen caring for horses that have been tested at or above the threshold are generally heavily penalized. There is scientific evidence both for and against the use of TCO_2 / $[HCO_3^-]$ testing thresholds, and this has led to considerable debate and legal wrangling. Two main points arise from objective review of the acid-base literature as it pertains to resting horses:

1. Acid-base state and TCO_2 are more variable and of a wider range than admitted by racing jurisdictions; a review of the literature shows a large range of natural variability in Standardbred racehorses (Table 39.1).
2. Many factors can contribute to elevated TCO_2 in horses that have not been administered alkalinizing agents. From these peer-reviewed studies it can be concluded that plasma $[HCO_3^-]$ and TCO_2 have a wide range of 'normal' values within racing populations of Standardbred and Thoroughbred horses.

Table 39.1 Acid-base state of race horses in non-race situations

Auer et al. 1993:[3] TCO_2 27–33[1]; 192 horses in stable; Australia
Auer et al. 1993:[3] TCO_2 27–36; 61 horses on raceday, *after* bicarbonate testing implemented; Australia
Kallings, Bondesson and Houghton 1994:[4] TCO_2 31.4 – 35.2; 6 trotters, Sweden
Short 1992:[5] $[HCO_3^-]$ 27–37; 205 trotters and pacers; New Zealand; 'data from a large group of horses under race-day conditions in which there is reasonable assurance that no bicarbonate was given.'
Short 1992:[6] $[HCO_3^-]$ 25–33; 95 racehorses; Australia
Soma et al. 1996:[7] $[HCO_3^-]$ 24.6–33.6; 30 racehorses, Pocono Downs, non-race day
Soma et al. 1996:[7] $[HCO_3^-]$ 28.1–34.6; 30 racehorses, Meadows, non-race day
Frey et al. 1995:[8] $[HCO_3^-]$ 33–36, mean = 34.5; 12 racehorses in controlled research trial; USA. Therefore TCO_2 in 2 of these 12 horses would be between 37 and 38
Waller and Lindinger 2005:[9] TCO_2 of 30–39, mean 35; 13 Standardbred racehorses on training days at rest, prior to exercise and after morning feeding
Nostell et al. 2006:[10] $TCO_2 = 33.2 \pm 1.8$ (mean ± SE; n = 5)
Cohen et al. 2006:[11] TCO_2 = 31; range 24–37.5; 2,439 Thoroughbred racehorses in California
Waller et al. 2010:[12] TCO_2 of 33.1 ± 2.9 mmol/L; range 25.66–42.9; 211 horses in race training

Overview of acid-base balance

Moderate to high intensity muscular exercise results in acidification of muscles and blood. The acidification primarily results from the generation of protons (H^+) within contracting skeletal muscle. The protons are of the product of biochemical and physicochemical reactions associated with increased rates of anaerobic energy production that result in intracellular lactate accumulation, intracellular K^+ depletion and increased CO_2 production.[13] The resultant large and rapid efflux of acid equivalents from contracting muscle produces the systemic metabolic acidosis associated with moderate to high intensity exercise.

In the exercising horse, whole-body acid-base balance is dependent on the integrated responses of the muscular, respiratory, vascular, hepatic, cutaneous and renal systems. The muscular system, in addition to providing the locomotory force requirement for activity, generates considerable amounts of acid equivalents, resulting in acidification of the intracellular and extracellular fluid compartments. Non-contracting skeletal muscle also provides the largest tissue mass within the body for the removal of lactate and acid equivalents during high intensity exercise and the initial recovery period. The respiratory system plays a key role in eliminating acid equivalents as CO_2 at the lung in addition to extracting the oxygen needed to fuel aerobic cellular metabolism. The vascular system plays an integral role in the transport and distribution of acid and base equivalents throughout the body – this system provides for the 'buffering' of the acid-base disturbance by distributing acid equivalents from acid-generation sites (contracting skeletal muscle) to other sites (non-contracting skeletal muscle and other tissues).[13] Within the vascular system itself, bicarbonate, plasma proteins and hemoglobin within red blood cells are also involved in the transport and temporary storage (buffering) of acid equivalents. The hepatic system is a major tissue mass involved in the removal of lactate from the vascular system, thereby removing acid equivalents from the circulation. The cutaneous system is heavily involved in the production and secretion of sweat to the surface of the skin during and immediately following moderate to high intensity exercise. Sweat contains large amounts of Na^+, K^+ and Cl^- and different rates of excretion of each ion affects acid-base state of blood leaving the skin.[14] The kidneys are capable of excreting H^+ and lactate at greatly elevated rates during recovery from high intensity exercise, aiding in the process of recovery from the acidosis of exercise.

Each of the systems described above is capable of modifying the water, electrolyte and acid-base composition of the extracellular (blood plasma, lymph, interstitial fluids) and intracellular fluid compartments. Therefore it must be appreciated that the acid-base status of the blood depends greatly on where and when the blood is sampled. Blood draining intensely contracting skeletal muscle has very high concentrations of H^+, lactate, K^+ and CO_2 while blood that drains relatively inactive tissues (jugular venous blood for example) has markedly lower concentrations of these metabolites and ions; arterial blood is intermediate in composition. Also, the magnitude of change is proportional to the intensity and duration of exercise, and the concentrations of these and other substances change with time of exercise and recovery.

Why is acid-base balance important? A detailed analysis of acid-base balance can provide a complete biochemical and physicochemical description of the state of the organism, or of individual organs and tissues within the body. Furthermore, severe acid-base disturbances are often associated with high intensity exercise, prolonged duration exercise and with many pathologies. Therefore an understanding of the origins of acid-base disturbance is of interest to both basic and clinical physiologists. Within the context of the present chapter, exercise physiologists remain keenly interested in acid-base balance because of a close association between acidification and muscle fatigue.[13] The content of this chapter is primarily directed to moderate to high intensity exercise because exercise at these intensities produces a significant acid-base disturbance, while exercise at low intensities does not (unless markedly prolonged with underlying dehydration and metabolic abnormalities). For detailed reviews of skeletal muscle acid-base balance during exercise the reader is referred to Hultman and Sahlin[15] and Lindinger and Heigenhauser.[13] Treatments of plasma acid-base status have been provided by Constable,[16,17] Johnson et al.[18] and Lindinger and Heigenhauser.[13] There are also a number of brief reviews on the effects of exercise on acid-base status in horses.[16,17,19,20] There are also a number of clinical primers on assessing and treating acid-base disturbances.[17,21–23]

Acidosis and skeletal muscle fatigue

There is no question that high intensity muscle contraction results in intracellular acidification[13,39,40] that generates an extracellular, systemic acidosis in the whole organism that can be very pronounced and long lasting.[9] It is also clear that intracellular acidosis and fatigue are associative during high intensity exercise, with mounting evidence that increased $[H^+]$ reduces the calcium sensitivity of the contractile proteins.[41] Furthermore, acidosis imposed prior to the period of high intensity exercise results in an earlier onset and more pronounced skeletal muscle fatigue.[42–44] Intracellular acidosis may, however, only exert these effects during high intensity muscle contraction. Recent evidence has shown that the contributions of intracellular acidosis to fatigue process have yet to be fully understood (Table 39.2). Westerblad and colleagues[33] have suggested that increased intracellular concentrations of inorganic phosphate may be a more important contributor to muscle fatigue

Table 39.2 Effects of increased intramuscular $[H^+]$ and functional consequence(s) in muscle

Decreased glycogenolytic (phosphorylase) activity[24,25] → decreased anaerobic ATP production → ATP supply is limited → fatigue
Decreased glycolytic (phosphofructokinase) activity[24,26,27] → decreased anaerobic ATP production → ATP supply is limited → fatigue
Decreased pyruvate dehydrogenase activity[24] → decreased aerobic ATP production → ATP supply is limited → fatigue
Decreased sarcolemmal and SR Ca^{2+}-ATPase activity[28–30] → elevated cytosolic $[Ca^{2+}]$ → decreased myosin ATPase activity[29] → decreased rate of actin-myosin cross-bridge cycling → slowed rate of muscular contraction → fatigue
Increased $[H^+]$ increases the [diprotonated inorganic phosphate] → Inhibition of actin-myosin cross-bridge interaction resulted[31–33]
Inhibition of Ca^{2+} binding to troponin C,[29,34,35] resulting in decreased number of actin-myosin cross-bridges formed → decreased strength of force production → fatigue
Increased acetyl-CoA, indicative of increased intramuscular triacylglycerol hydrolysis[24] → increased citric acid cycle dehydrogenase activities → stimulate aerobic metabolism
Decreased lactate efflux from muscle cells[36] → prolongation of intracellular acidification by retaining a strong acid anion
Increased intracellular $[H^+]$ → improved membrane excitability[37,38]

than the increase in $[H^+]$. Pedersen et al.[37,38] have shown that intracellular acidosis can contribute to sustaining muscle function during contractile activity by improving membrane excitability, an effect that appears to involve alterations of sarcolemmal chloride conductivity.[45,46]

Skeletal muscle fatigue is also associated with an increased interstitial $[K^+]$ as a result of rapid rates of K^+ loss through sarcolemmal K^+ channels during the recovery phase of action potentials.[47,48] This increase in interstitial $[K^+]$ results in a marked depolarization of the sarcolemma and decreased contractile force.[48,49] In contrast to the dogma that we have long been taught, the loss in both sarcolemmal excitability and tetanic force resulting from elevated interstitial $[K^+]$ (8–12 mEq/L) was actually **reversed** when intracellular acidosis (either 20 mmol/L lactic acid or increased CO_2) was imposed.[37,50,51] While these muscles were only stimulated to perform one contraction every 10 min, this allowed a separation between the fatigue associated with repetitive contraction versus that associated with sarcolemmal depolarization and intracellular acidification.

As summarized by Fitts[52] and Allen,[40] increased $[H^+]$ does contribute to decreased force production *during* high intensity muscle contraction (see Fig. 39.1), and there is reasonably good evidence that these effects occur at the level of: (i) impaired Ca^{2+} binding to troponin C, which therefore impairs the ability of actin to form cross-bridges with myosin; (ii) slowing SR Ca^{2+}-ATPase activity; (iii) increasing the leak of Ca^{2+} from the SR; (iv) and at key sites of biochemical control within glycogenolysis (decreased glycogen phosphorylase *a* activity) and glycolysis (decreased phosphofructokinase activity. The latter study also demonstrated an increased reliance on fat metabolism to meet the energy demands of contracting muscle during exercise in humans made acidotic by ingestion of 0.3 g/kg ammonium chloride.[24]

It may be concluded that intracellular acidosis may have two main effects that, when taken together, are of long-term benefit for muscle function and survival (prevention of destruction resulting from overuse). First, acidification restores the sarcolemmal excitability and contractility resulting from elevated interstitial $[K^+]$, and the former is very important for cells maintaining the composition of their intracellular environment within physiological limits. Second, the muscle retains the ability to contract while the force and rate of contraction and rates of glycogenolysis / glycolysis are slowed as a result of the acidosis. This in turn slows the demand for energy and the production of acid equivalents, while allowing the animal to continue to move if need be.

Assessment of acid-base balance and factors that affect acid-base regulation

In traditional terms, many of us remember being taught that acid-base balance is represented by the relationships among PCO_2, pH and the HCO_3^- in blood plasma. While this is true, using only these three variables provides for only a very limited understanding of the factors that contribute to acid-base imbalances. The approach taken within this chapter is to use a comprehensive, physicochemical approach to identify the causes or origins of acid-base disturbances during exercise, and to discuss how the disturbance is resolved during recovery from exercise.[13] Several key papers have used this approach in horses.[9,12,53–58]

While the traditional variables of acid-base – PCO_2, pH and the HCO_3^- – are useful in identifying whether an acid-base disturbance is metabolic or respiratory in nature, they are insufficient to identify the physicochemical origins of the acid-base disturbance. It is nonetheless important for the student of acid-base physiology to be familiar with the concepts presented using the traditional approach, and to be able to use these concepts as an important foundation on which to apply the physicochemical approach. This chapter will emphasize the use of the physicochemical approach as this method provides for a detailed physiological and clinical assessment of acid-base disturbances. It is worth pointing out that the traditional approaches to assessing acid-base status are not incorrect, but rather they were a simplification introduced in the 1960s to make use of readily available and relatively simple measurements of PCO_2 and pH. Technology developed from the 1970s onwards has simplified the measurements of the other important acid-base variables in blood plasma and skeletal muscle, allowing us to take a more comprehensive approach.

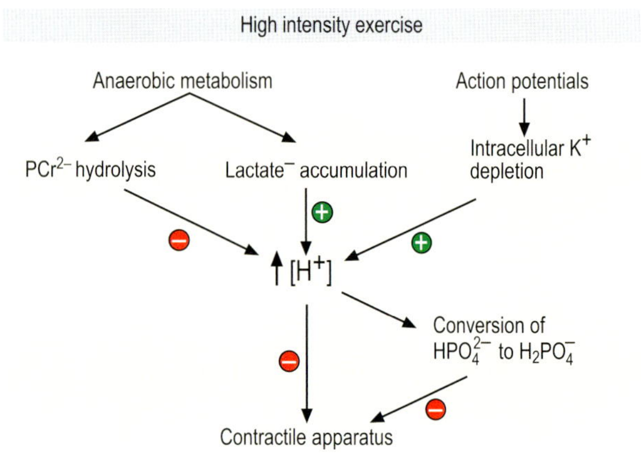

Fig 39.1 Overview of events contributing to the intracellular acidosis and fatigue of skeletal muscle during high intensity exercise. A – indicates a decrease in accumulation of function, while a + indicates a positive contribution to the increase in $[H^+]$.

The physicochemical approach presented here was detailed by Peter Stewart.[59–62] The foundation for this approach lies on the work of van Slyke and co-workers,[63,64] and builds on the work of many others including Hastings, Dill, Henderson and Siggaard-Anderson.[13]

Physicochemical characteristics refer to those properties and reactions that are physical and chemical in nature; they proceed in the absence of enzymes and life and occur as a result of the physical and chemical properties of the solvent and solute molecules. Also, biochemical reactions, those catalyzed by enzymes, may alter the physicochemical properties of a solution. However, for the purposes of discussing acid-base balance, biochemical reactions may be considered distinct from physicochemical reactions. The main physicochemical reactions are detailed below.

The advantages and disadvantages of the physicochemical approach are listed in Table 39.3. The development and widespread use of ion selective electrodes and combination blood gas–electrolyte analyzers has greatly simplified the process of obtaining the necessary measurements with the accuracy needed to perform detailed assessments of acid-base balance.[13] The advantages of this approach lie in the ability to quantitatively determine the physical and chemical origins of acid-base disturbances. This is therefore a very powerful approach and an important step towards understanding acid-base physiology and pathophysiology. This approach provides an essential foundation for the effective treatment of pathological acid-base disorders.

Physicochemical determinants of acid-base balance

Prior to detailing the physicochemical reactions that increase $[H^+]$ within contracting skeletal muscle, it is necessary to provide an introduction to the physicochemical system of acid-base

Table 39.3 Disadvantages and advantages of the physicochemical approach

Disadvantages
• requires accurate measurement of many variables including plasma PCO_2, $[Na^+]$, $[K^+]$, $[Cl^-]$, $[lactate^-]$, [plasma protein] and in muscle additionally $[A_{tot}]$ • requires advanced calculator or computer to perform calculations • requires consideration of physical chemistry, biochemistry and physiology – it is truly an integrative approach
Advantages
• provides for detailed analysis of why changes in $[H^+]$ and $[HCO_3^-]$ occurred, giving insight into the pathophysiology of any type of acid-base disorder • allows for the determination of the individual independent variables, i.e. $[Na^+]$, $[lactate^-]$, [plasma protein] …, that is the origin of the acid-base disturbance • identification of the origins of the acid-base disturbance allows one to determine the physiological or biochemical mechanism(s) responsible for the alteration(s) in independent variables • knowledge of the physicochemical origins and physiological/biochemical mechanism(s) behind the acid-base disturbance allows for the development and administration of effective treatment strategies for correcting the acid-base disturbance with minimal untoward side effects

balance. This approach is founded on three underlying physical premises:

1. A dissociated proton molecule (H^+) is only in physical existence for a fleeting instance of time, approximately 10^{-5} second. The proton is highly reactive, associating briefly with negative charges on proteins, ^-OH molecules, HCO_3^- molecules and amino acids to name a few. The proton is therefore very unlike inorganic electrolytes such as Na^+, K^+ and Cl^- that are relatively unreactive.
2. Protons are a main constituent of water, the most prevalent molecule within the body. Water thus provides an almost limitless source of H^+ for biochemical and physicochemical reactions. Protons are part of the solvent that comprises the milieu of the body. It is because of its ability to so rapidly dissociate and re-associate H^+ and ^-OH that water is the 'universal' solute.
3. Because of these physical attributes of protons and water, it is physically impossible to add protons to a physiological solution without adding water. Take hydrochloric acid (HCl) as an example. HCl exists only in aqueous form and is characterized by a very high concentration of Cl^- and H^+ in solution. The H^+ is an integral part of the aqueous system. It will be described below that it is the strong acid anion Cl^- that makes this solution so acidic. The strong acid anion Cl^- can be neutralized by the addition of an equivalent amount of the strong base cation Na^+ to the solution, but without an accompanying acid anion such as Cl^-, HCO_3^-, of $H_2PO_4^-$. Thus NaOH would be added – the strong anions Cl^- and Na^+ remain fully dissociated in solution while there occurs a rapid reaction between H^+ and ^-OH that decreases $[H^+]$. The resultant solution is saline at neutral pH.

The physicochemical approach to acid-base balance recognizes that there are three groups of independent variables that determine the concentrations of the traditional acid-base variables pH and $[HCO_3^-]$. The three groups of independent variables are: (1) the strong ion difference (SID), which represents the sum (charge considered) if the strong acid anions and strong base cations; (2) the total weak acid concentration (A_{tot}), which represents the sum (charge considered) of the weak acids and bases; and (3) the carbon dioxide (CO_2) concentration, which is usually measured and used as the partial pressure of CO_2 (PCO_2).

Strong ions and strong ion difference

The terms strong acid anion and strong base cation were introduced in the preceding section and they will be defined here. The term 'strong' refers to the fact that the ion will be fully, or nearly so, dissociated in aqueous solutions (Fig. 39.2). Most of the inorganic ions are 'strong' and hence nearly fully dissociated within the body fluids (Table 39.4). Some organic ions are also strong, such as lactate$^-$ (acid dissociation constant of 3.9) and phosphocreatine^{2-} (PCr^{2-}; acid dissociation constant of 4.5). Anions possess negative charge while cations possess positive charge. An anion is an acid by definition because the addition of that strong anion, in the absence of an accompanying strong base, will result in acidification of the solution. Using the example of HCl above, the addition of HCl to plasma will result in acidification. Similarly, the addition of HLactate will also result in acidification. In contrast, the addition of the strong base Na^+ in the absence of accompanying strong anion (as $NaHCO_3^-$) will result in alkalinization. The values for the key variables used in the physicochemical assessment of acid-base balance, for resting horses, are provided in Table 39.5.

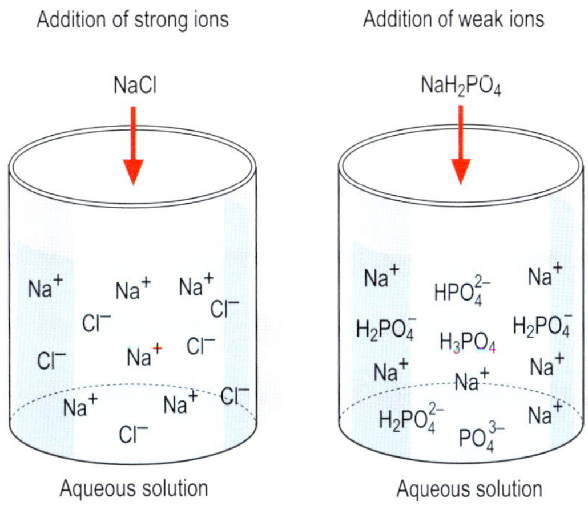

Fig 39.2 Representation of strong ions and weak ions in an aqueous solution. The addition of NaCl to an aqueous solution results in the complete dissociation into the strong ions Na^+ and Cl^-. In contrast, the addition of sodium phosphate results in the complete dissociation of all of the sodium into Na^+, but the phosphate is capable of reacting with H^+ in solution to form the following weak ions: H_3PO_4, $H_2PO_4^-$, HPO_4^{2-} and PO_4^{3-}.

Table 39.4 A summary of acid-base terminology

The following definitions are placed in order of functional similarities, as opposed to alphabetical order.

Base: any cation in biological fluids[65]

Buffer base: base equivalent to the sum of buffer anion concentrations (including $[HCO_3^-]$) in mEq/L[65]

base excess / deficit: represents the accumulation of non-volatile base / acid in the blood (excludes plasma $[HCO_3^-]$ and blood hemoglobin concentration)[66]

Alkali (alkaline) reserve: the proton buffering ability of plasma bicarbonate when bases or non-volatile acids are added to or taken from the body fluid[65]

$[A_{tot}]$: a physicochemical term that defines the *total* concentration of weak anions in solution[60–62]

[SID]: a physicochemical assessment term that refers to the sum of all strong base cations minus the sum of all strong acid anions[60–62]

$$[SID] = \Sigma[\text{strong base cations}] - \Sigma[\text{strong acid anions}]$$

Strong ion: that ions that are fully, or nearly so, dissociated in physiological solutions. In general, if the dissociation constant is ≤ 4.5, then the molecule is considered to be a strong anion; if the dissociation constant is greater than 9, then the molecule is considered to be a strong cation.

Anion gap: a traditional term that is defined as:

$$\text{anion gap} = ([Na^+] + [K^+]) - ([Cl^-] + [HCO_3^-])$$

Strong ion gap: a term coined by Constable et al.[23] as an alternate way of determining the concentration of unmeasured strong ions in plasma:

$$\text{strong ion gap} = 2.24 \times \text{total [protein] (g/dl)} / (1 + 10^{(6.65-pH)}) - AG$$

(where AG is anion gap).

Unmeasured anions: unmeasured anions contribute to the anion gap, strong ion difference and strong ion gap. The unmeasured anions include both strong (SO_4^{2-}, some amino acids, pyruvate) and weak (inorganic phosphate, carbonate, carbamates, some amino acids) anions. The negative charges on plasma protein contribute to the anion gap, strong ion difference and strong ion gap, but this is usually a 'measured' anion.

Table 39.5 Physiologically important acid-base variables, and their concentrations, in arterial plasma and skeletal muscle of horses at rest

VARIABLES	PLASMA		SKELETAL MUSCLE	
Dependent variables	**'normal' value**	**normal range**	**'normal' value**	**normal range**
$[H^+]$ nEq/L	40	33–45	100	71–126
pH	7.40	7.35–7.48	7.0[a,b]	6.90–7.15[a,b]
$[HCO_3^-]$ mEq/L	28	22–34	10[a]	8–12[a]
Independent variables				
PCO_2 mmHg	40	35–45		
[total CO_2] mmol/L	30	23–36	10[a]	8–12[a]
[SID] mEq/L	40	37–43	110[c]	60–130[c]
Strong ions				
$[Na^+]$ mEq/L	140	132–146	15	8–30
$[K^+]$ mEq/L	3.7	2.7–4.7	140	110–165
$[Ca^{2+}]$ mEq/L	2.5	2–3	0.4	0.2–1.0
$[Mg^{2+}]$ mEq/L	1.0	0.5–2.0	5	3–7
$[Cl^-]$ mEq/L	105	99–109	10	5–25
$[lactate^-]$ mEq/L	1.0	0.5–1.5	1.5	1.0–2.0
$[PCr^{2-}]$ mEq/L	na	na	15	12–18
$[SO_4^{2-}]$ mEq/L	0.5	0.3–0.7	–	–
Weak ions				
$[A_{tot}]$ mEq/L	12	11–13	140	120–170
[plasma protein] g/dl	5.5	5.0–6.0	na	na
[albumin] g/dl			na	na
[globulins] g/dl			na	na
$[HPO_4^{2-}] + [H_2PO_4^-]$ mmol/L	2.7	2.0–3.5	8	7–9
carnosine mmol/L	na	na	6[b]	3–9[b]
Protein histidine concentration mmol/L	–	–	46[b]	30–60[b]

na = not applicable.
[a]Sahlin et al.[67] – human muscle.
[b]Hultman and Sahlin[15] – human muscle.
[c]Lindinger.[13,68]

The concentrations of strong acid anions and strong base cations within a fluid compartment are summed, with consideration of the charge, to yield the strong ion difference, or [SID].

Within plasma and the extracellular fluid compartment, the [SID] may be calculated as:

$$[SID]\,(mEq/L) = ([Na^+]+[K^+]+[Mg^{2+}]+[Ca^{2+}]) - ([Cl^-]+[lactate^-]+[SO_4^{2-}])$$

Note that it is the free or ionized concentrations of the divalent ions that must be used, and not the total concentration; considerable amounts of the divalent ions are bound to plasma proteins or to each other. The concentrations measured using ion selective electrodes are that of the free or ionized or dissociated ion in the aqueous portion of the solution (i.e. mEq/L of plasma water), so long as the instrument does not use a calculation to modify the 'concentration' to total (not free) concentration or mEq/L of plasma. Thus, while these divalent ions are 'strong', the interactions with charged moieties on protein molecules removes some of the ion from solution. In practice, the free concentrations of the divalent cations and anions are approximately equivalent and can be ignored, leaving:

$$[SID]_{plasma}\,(mEq/L) = ([Na^+]+[K^+]) - ([Cl^-]+[lactate^-])$$

In some treatments of acid-base balance using the physicochemical approach, [lactate$^-$] is also ignored. However [lactate$^-$] cannot be ignored in the exercising and recovering animal.

Within skeletal muscle, PCr^{2-} and Mg^{2+} must be used within the equation because their free concentrations are large and change substantially during exercise:

$$[SID]_{muscle}\ (mEq/L) = ([Na^+]+[K^+]+[Mg^{2+}]) - ([Cl^-]+[lactate^-]+[PCr^{2-}])$$

The strong ions are important determinants of the concentrations of $[H^+]$ and $[HCO_3^-]$ because they directly affect the associated state of H_2O, and thereby determine the concentrations of H^+ and ^-OH.

A decrease in the SID (without concurrent change in PCO_2 or A_{tot}), due to either a decrease in strong cation concentration OR an increase in strong anion concentration will increase $[H^+]$ and decrease $[HCO_3^-]$ – an acidification occurs. Conversely, an increase in SID has an alkalinizing effect and decreases $[H^+]$ and increases $[HCO_3^-]$.

Weak acids and bases, and $[A_{tot}]$

The term 'weak' refers to those anion acids and cation bases that are not fully dissociated in solution. Thus when sodium phosphate (Na_2HPO_4) is added to an aqueous solution, two Na^+ are added and fully dissociates and a weak anion HPO_4^{2-} is added. In contrast to Na^+, the HPO_4^{2-} cannot achieve full dissociation due to reactions of the molecule with H^+ within the solution. Thus the HPO_4^{2-} is also partially and instantaneously transformed into H_3PO_4, $H_2PO_4^-$ and PO_4^{3-} (Fig. 39.2). This physical attribute of phosphate is what makes phosphates, and many other weak acid anions such as bicarbonate and albumin, good proton 'buffers'. The predominant weak acid anion in plasma and ECF is albumin, while the predominant weak acid anions within skeletal muscle cells are the histidine residues on proteins.

The main weak acids and bases within the extracellular fluid compartment are albumin, globulin, phosphate and bicarbonate. Bicarbonate, however, is part of the CO_2 system and thus is not used in the calculation, or estimation, of $[A_{tot}]$. As for the strong ions, the weak ions also directly affect the concentrations of H^+ and HCO_3^- in solution. Within skeletal muscle it is primarily the histidine moieties on proteins that contribute to $[A_{tot}]$, with creatine, Pi, ATP and other molecules also contributing.[68] While it is theoretically possible to measure the concentration of weak acids and bases in both extracellular and intracellular fluid compartments, this tends to be prohibitive and appears not to be necessary to be able to effectively estimate acid-base state. Rather, an effective $[A_{tot}]$ and apparent dissociation constant K'a have been determined in equine plasma and rat skeletal muscle (Table 39.6). A value for $[A_{tot}]$ has not been determined in equine or human skeletal muscle. Muscle $[A_{tot}]$ is equivalent to the non-bicarbonate proton buffering capacity of adult rat plantaris muscle,[68–70] and is similar to that of human vastus lateralis.[15,71,72] When rat plantaris values for $[A_{tot}]$ and K'a were applied to human muscle, reasonably good data were generated.[68] Equine muscle, compared to human muscle, has a much greater non-bicarbonate proton buffering capacity: 43 mEq.kg dry muscle^{-1}.pH^{-1} in trained humans, vs 58 and 93 mEq.kg^{-1}.pH^{-1} in untrained and trained equine skeletal muscle.[73] Assuming proportionality with rat hindlimb skeletal muscle (buffer capacity of ~40 mEq.kg^{-1}.pH^{-1} = $[A_{tot}]$ of ~140 mmol/L[68]), this translates to an $[A_{tot}]$ of ~315 mmol/L in trained equine muscle.

The carbon dioxide system

The concentration of CO_2 is the third independent variable of acid-base balance. Carbon dioxide is effectively a strong acid, and because it is a major end-product of cellular respiration is often referred to as a respiratory acid. Also, the primary means for eliminating excess CO_2 from the body is through the respiratory system.[13,18]

Carbon dioxide is a strong acid by virtue of its ability to combine with water to increase the concentration of H^+ while at the same time increasing the weak acid $[HCO_3^-]$. This reaction effectively acidifies the solution to which CO_2 has been added. The majority (about 95%) of the total CO_2 within the body is in the form of HCO_3^-, with much smaller amounts of H_2CO_3, CO_3^{2-}, dissolved CO_2 ($CO_{2(d)}$) and some that is bound to amino groups on protein to form carbamino compounds. The chemical reactions involved in the hydration and dehydration of CO_2 are:

$$CO_2 + H_2O \rightleftharpoons H_2CO_3 \rightleftharpoons H^+ + HCO_3^- \rightleftharpoons 2H^+ + CO_3^{2-}$$

Table 39.6 Values of the constants used within the acid-base equations

PARAMETER	CONSTANT	REFERENCE
K_A – plasma	2.11 or 2.12 × 10^{-7} Eq/L	Constable 1997;[17] Staempfli et al. 1999[74]
	1.74 × 10^{-7} Eq/L	Waller et al. 2010[12]
K_A – resting muscle	1.64 × 10^{-7} Eq/L	Lindinger 1995[68]
K_A – exercised muscle	1.98 × 10^{-7} Eq/L	Lindinger 1995[68]
K_3	6.0 × 10^{-11} Eq/L	Stewart 1983[62]
K_C	2.46 × 10^{-11} (Eq/L)^2/mmHg	Stewart 1983[62]
K'_w	4.4 × 10^{-14} (Eq/L)^2	Stewart 1983[62]

Solving equations to determine acid-base balance

With this background, the following five mass action equations and one equation expressing electrical neutrality of solutions describe the physicochemical characteristics of any aqueous, physiological solution:[60–62]

Water dissociation:

$$K'_w = [H^+]\cdot[^-OH]$$

Weak electrolyte system:

$$K_A \cdot [HA] = [H^+]\cdot[A^-]$$
$$[A_{tot}] = [HA] + [A^-]$$

Carbon dioxide system:

$$K_c \cdot PCO_2 = [H^+]\cdot[HCO_3^-]$$
$$K_3 \cdot [HCO_3^-] = [H^+]\cdot[CO_3^{2-}]$$

Electrical neutrality:

$$[SID] + [H^+] - [HCO_3^-] - [A^-] - [CO_3^{2-}] - [^-OH] = 0$$

It is noteworthy that $[H^+]$ appears in each of these equations and its dependence on the concentrations of strong and weak acids/base and CO_2 is evident. These six equations can be combined into a single equation that may then be solved for $[H^+]$ when the three independent variables and the constants are known:

$$[H^+]^4 + \{K_A = [SID]\}[H^+]^3 = \{K_A([SID]-[A_{tot}]) - (K_C pCO_2 + K'_w)\}$$
$$[H^+]^2 - \{K_A(K_C pCO_2 + K'_w) + K_3 K_C pCO_2\}$$
$$[H^+] - K_A K_3 K_C pCO_2 = 0$$

Contracting skeletal muscle: proton generating and removing reactions

When considering the acid-base changes that occur in blood during exercise, it is important to have an understanding of the changes that occur within skeletal muscle because that tissue forms 40–60% of the mass of the horse.[75] Contracting skeletal muscle generates the disturbance[76,77] and non-contracting cells are capable of ameliorating the disturbance.[78,79] The role of non-contracting muscle may be small to negligible in horses performing moderate to high intensity exercise because most skeletal muscles are used for locomotion and maintenance of posture. That is in contrast to bipedal humans where many activities require leg muscles and leave many other muscles relatively inactive. This section will thus focus on the time course and magnitude of changes that occur within contracting skeletal muscle, primarily gluteus medius, during moderate to high intensity exercise.

Exercise is a consequence of muscular contraction, and muscular contraction results in an increase in cellular energy demand compared to the resting state. The increased energy demand is due to activation of myosin ATPase needed for release of actin-myosin cross-bridge interaction, increased activity of sarcoplasmic reticulum Ca^{2+}-ATPase activity resulting from increased cytosolic $[Ca^{2+}]$ and increased rates of Na,K-ATPase activity needed to maintain transmembrane Na^+ and K^+ gradients and repolarization of the muscle membrane potential.

The acid-base changes that occur within contracting skeletal muscle and in blood during exercise are the results of the biochemical (metabolic) and physicochemical reactions that occur within contracting muscle cells.[13] The onset of muscular contraction sets into motion a series of biochemical events that result in stimulation and inhibition of numerous metabolic pathways. Those pathways within the aerobic energy systems are relatively slow to increase, while those of the anaerobic pathways (ATP utilization, phosphocreatine degradation, glycolysis) increase rapidly. Thus the onset of exercise (rest to work transition) may be associated with muscular acidification for reasons described below. Similarly, transitions from low to high work rates, as well as exercise at moderate to high intensities, result in increased rates of anaerobic metabolism. Full activation of aerobic pathways may be achieved within minutes of the onset of exercise, but until this is achieved anaerobic pathways continue to supply ATP. Activation of aerobic metabolism results in increased mitochondrial respiration with CO_2 production – while this CO_2 is acidic, its rate of production and removal from the cell can easily be matched by CO_2 elimination rates at the lung. Therefore aerobic CO_2 production can be ignored in most discussions of the acid-base changes of exercise.

Muscle characteristics and acid-base

Skeletal muscle is composed of different fiber types, some of which produce acid equivalents at high rates (the anerobic, fast twitch, glycolytic fibers) while others do not (the aerobic, slow twitch, oxidative fibers). Fiber types continue to be classified on the basis of their twitch characteristics, oxidative / glycolytic capacities and on their myosin heavy chain composition.[80] The acid-base changes that occur reflect the fiber type composition of the contracting muscles, and may reflect breed differences and type of activity performed. This is tempered by the high degree of variability in muscle fiber type proportions in most horse breeds.[81,82]

Within individual muscle groups, such as the well-studied gluteus medius of equids, skeletal muscle fibers of different composition are in close proximity and form integrated functional units that are selectively recruited by appropriate motor units depending on the locomotory requirements of the animal.[83] Muscle fibers with high oxidative capacity that have low glycoytic capacity, slow contractile properties with low myosin ATPase activity, are fatigue resistant and primarily function in the maintenance of posture (Table 39.7). These slow twitch oxidative fibers have the ability to oxidize all the pyruvate generated from glycolysis and, during exercise, they have the ability to take up and oxidize lactate released into the interstitium from nearby glycolytic muscle fibers – the intramuscular lactate shuttle.[84] At the other extreme, fibers of high glycolytic capacity with low oxidative capacity have fast contractile properties with high myosin ATPase activity. These fibers function to generate power at high rates for high intensity sprinting, jumping and pulling activities. The majority of the acid-base disturbance that occurs during high intensity exercise is generated within the fast twitch glycolytic

Table 39.7 Skeletal muscle fiber types in horses and relationship to acid-base balance

	FIBER TYPE		
	SO – TYPE I	FOG – TYPE IIA	FG – TYPE IIB
% of total fibers[1,2]	15	45	40
Total H^+ buffer capacity[1]	88	98	130
Carnosine H^+ buffer capacity[1]	18	58	60
Carnosine % of total[1]	20	29	45
Carnosine content[1]	54 ± 15	85 ± 15	180 ± 15
Glycogen phosphorylase activity[2]	122 ± 20	71 ± 20	172 ± 20
Citrate synthase activity[2]	168 ± 15	167 ± 15	37 ± 15
Glycogen content[3]	+	++	++

[1,2]Averaged data from Sewell et al.[94] (n = 20 2–3-year-old racing Thoroughbreds); Sewell et al.[87] (n = 50 2–3-year-old racing Thoroughbreds).
[1]Data from Sewell et al.[94]
[2]Data from Sewell et al.[87]
[3]Data from Quiroz-Rothe and Rivero.[96]

(type IIB or type IID/X) that are endowed with a high glycogen content, high activities of glycogen phosphorylase and lactate dehydrogenase, and a high content of carnosine[85] to buffer metabolically generated H^+.[86] These fibers also fatigue rapidly due to the loss of membrane excitability, as well as their high rate of intracellular acidification[70] that effectively downregulate muscle fiber function at multiple membrane and intracellular sites.[48,52]

It is noteworthy that Quarter Horses and Thoroughbreds, the two fastest horse breeds, have the lowest proportion of slow oxidative (type I) fibers and high proportions of both fast twitch oxidative glycolytic (type IIA) and fast twitch glycolytic (type IIB) fibers. These fast twitch fibers are also known to have high activities for glycogen phosphorylase,[87] catalyzing the initial reaction in glycogenolysis, and lactate dehydrogenase[88–90] for converting pyruvate to lactate. Indeed, in racing Thoroughbreds and Standardbreds there is a high degree of correlation between type IIB fiber proportion and lactate accumulation:[90] fiber type specific lactate content 6 min AFTER the end of 1200–2700 m races was greater in gluteus medius type IIB fibers (97.3 ± 2.1) than in type I (82.6 ± 3.8 μmol/kg dry muscle; n = 8), with type IIA fibers intermediate (93.6 ± 2.1). This is consistent with observations that type IIB fiber proportion is positively correlated with elevated plasma [$lactate^-$] during submaximal and maximal exercise in Standardbred trotters.[90–92] Of interest and importance to muscle acid-base regulation is the observation that in type I fibers [$lactate^-$] was only 15 mEq/kg dry muscle (equivalent to about 3 mEq/L) less than in type IIB fibers. This supports the idea that lactate produced in type IIB fibers diffuses out of these fibers into the interstitium where the lactate can be taken up by oxidative fibers[84,92,93] to be used as a fuel source both during and following exercise.

The fast-twitch fibers are also endowed with an important physicochemical feature that aids in the regulation of intracellular acid-base balance. There is an increasing content of the histidine dipeptide, carnosine, with increasing glycolytic capacity. Carnosine has a pK_a ~6.9 and, as such, is an effective H^+ buffer and contributes substantively to the non-bicarbonate H^+ buffer capacity of muscle, particularly in fast twitch glycolytic fibers.[85,94] Indeed, if the contribution of carnosine to non-bicarbonate buffering is removed, then each of the different fiber types have similar non-bicarbonate H^+ buffering capacities; thus carnosine confers all of the fiber type difference in non-bicarbonate H^+ buffering capacity.[87,94] Quarter Horses have a higher carnosine content (39.2 ± 1.8 mmol/kg wet muscle; n = 6) compared to Thoroughbreds (31.3 ± 2.9 mmol/kg wet muscle; n = 6) and Standardbreds (27.6 mmol/kg wet muscle; n = 5).[95] The high H^+ buffering capacity of glycolytic fibers is important given the high rates of metabolic H^+ production resulting from ATP hydrolysis, glycogenolysis and glycolysis (described above). Without the ability to buffer this rapidly produced H^+ during exercise, cellular [H^+] would rapidly increase to concentrations inhibitory for actin-myosin cross-bridge cycling and for many metabolic reactions.[29,52] Buffering of H^+ within the cells in which it is produced also reduces the extent of extracellular acidification that occurs. Cessation of activity and resynthesis of ATP and glycogen results in a lowering of intracellular [H^+] and a decrease in the quantity of H^+ buffered by histidine groups within the cell.

Physicochemical origins of [H^+] changes in skeletal muscle during exercise

Increased flux through numerous biochemical pathways results in altered cytosolic concentrations of muscle metabolites and redox state that have been associated with changes in muscle acid-base state. Because the relationships between biochemistry and acid-base state are associative (not cause and effect) we will focus on considering how physicochemical changes occurring within the intracellular compartment of contracting muscle contribute to the acid-base changes of exercise. There is involvement of each of the three independent physicochemical variables; however, the changes in the concentrations of strong ions predominates, as will be exemplified below. The physicochemical descriptions complement the biochemical descriptions provided above, and as exemplified in the descriptions that follow.

Muscle [SID] during exercise

The time course and magnitude of changes in muscle [SID], and of the factors contributing to it, have not been well studied in horses. This is due in large part to the fact that muscle biopsies cannot truly be taken during exercise – the exercise must be stopped and the horse restrained in order to safely obtain a useful piece of muscle. Also, most studies have taken post-exercise muscle biopsies between 2 and 20 min after cessation of exercise, during which time there are substantial changes in organic and inorganic strong ions. Accordingly, studies that measured muscle [K^+] showed no change[97] or a small increase[98] after brief periods of high intensity exercise and this may be attributed to rapid recovery processes. The limited equine data will be used with what is known from human experiments to profile the changes occurring within muscle during exercise and recovery. The focus will be on high intensity exercise because the changes are more pronounced and hence somewhat easier to follow. Changes with moderate intensity exercise are attenuated compared to those occurring with high intensity exercise.[99–101] Muscle acid-base responses to low intensity exercise have not been specifically studied and, indeed, changes in metabolites that affect acid-base state are minimal.[102,103] With prolonged, endurance exercise it is expected that the major players would be [SID] changes resulting from net K^+ loss, with Na^+ and Cl^- gain, water loss or gain[104] and changes in [A_{tot}] primarily resulting from changes in intracellular water content.[68,70]

The main variables changing within muscle during exercise that affect [SID] are [PCr^{2-}], [$lactate^-$], [K^+][68] and water content.[97,105] The osmotic shift of water from plasma and non-contracting tissues into contracting muscle at the onset of exercise is very large and rapid and can be attributed to the accumulation of osmolytes such as creatine, inorganic phosphate and $lactate^-$.[106] This fluid shift produces a large decrease in plasma volume (see below) and the 10% increase in intracellular volume at the end of two minutes of high intensity exercise in horses[105] effectively dilutes intracellular metabolites and electrolytes and reduces [A_{tot}]. It is the actual concentrations of these variables that determine the acid-base state of the cell at any given point in time.

When working from metabolite or electrolyte data expressed in mmol/kg dry muscle or mmol/kg wet muscle it is necessary to convert to units of mmol/L or mEq/L of intracellular water. The water content of resting, non-exercised skeletal muscle is 0.75 L/kg wet muscle[107] and increases by about 10% with high intensity exercise;[105] resting muscle thus has a wet:dry weight ratio of ~4 which increases to ~4.5 with high intensity exercise. Therefore, a resting PCr^{2-} content of 85 mmol/kg dry muscle equates to 21 mmol/kg wet muscle (85/4) and 28 mmol/L (21/0.75) or 56 mEq/L. The doubling from 28 mmol/L to 56 mEq/L recognizes the divalent negative charge on PCr^{2-}.

With the onset of exercise, the initial few seconds of contraction results in the rapid hydrolysis of PCr^{2-} to regenerate ATP being used by myosin-, Ca^{2+} and Na,K-ATPases. The hydrolysis of PCr^{2-} effectively removes a strong acid anion from solution, which increases intracellular [SID] and has an alkalinizing effect (Fig. 39.3). The alkalizing effect resulting from PCr^{2-} hydrolysis is short-lived. With high intensity exercise, the high rates of H^+ and lactate$^-$ (a strong acid anion that decreases [SID]) production rapidly acidifies the intracellular environment. Concurrent increases in [lactate$^-$][100,108] and decreases in [K^+][98,109] effectively decrease [SID] which accounts for the majority of intracellular acidification during high intensity exercise.[13,70] As may be expected, the accumulation of muscle lactate$^-$ contributes substantially to the exercise-induced acidosis because lactate$^-$ is a strong acid anion that increases [H^+]. Intracellular lactate$^-$ concentrations greater than 60 mEq/L (234 mmol/kg dry weight) have been reported in the gluteus medius of trained Standardbreds after trotting 1600 m at a high speed of 11 m/s.[110,111] With lower intensity exercise PCr^{2-} is resynthesized during the subsequent period of steady state exercise, thus contributing to decreases in [SID] and increased intracellular acidification.

The physicochemical factors contributing to intracellular acidification will now be examined in more detail. Thoroughbreds exercising at high intensity hydrolyzed 32% of PCr^{2-} in 40 s (600 m sprint; Gollnick et al.,[108]) and 42% after 5 min at 100% of peak VO_2.[101] In these studies muscle biopsies were obtained within 60s of stopping exercise and thus the amount of post exercise PCr^{2-} resynthesis was low at the time of muscle sampling. In resting equine muscle, [PCr^{2-}] of 21 mmol/kg wet muscle[100,107,108] equates to 56 mEqv/L (21 mmol/kg wet muscle / 0.75 L/kg intracellular water). Thus, after 40 s of sprinting, muscle [PCr^{2-}] was reduced by 34 mEq/L, which effectively raises [SID] by 34 mEq/L; by virtue of this increase in [SID] it is evident that PCr^{2-} hydrolysis has an alkalinizing effect. This effect, however, is completely offset by the accumulation of lactate$^-$, with muscle [lactate$^-$] reaching 45 mEq/L.[108] Very similar results for PCr^{2-} degradation were reported by Lindholm and Saltin[100] in five racing Standardbreds completing 2100 m in 178 s; however, these trained racehorses experienced considerably less muscle lactate$^-$ accumulation (~20 mEq/L), a likely training adaptation.

Combining the effects of changes in [PCr^{2-}] and [lactate$^-$] decreases [SID] by 11 mEq/L,which has a net acidifying effect. This effect alone, however, only accounts for about 50% of the observed decrease in muscle intracellular pH from 7.01 to 6.86;[108] this is equivalent to an increase in [H^+] from 98 to 138 nEq/l. The other contributor to the decrease in [SID] is the rapid and pronounced decrease in [K^+] during high intensity exercise. In the gluteus medius of Standardbreds at rest, intracellular [K^+] is 122 ± 7 mEq/L (92 ± 5 mEq/kg wet wt, with water content of 75%[107]). There are no reports of equine muscle [K^+] *during* exercise[97,98,107] and, on the basis of the large increases in plasma [K^+] and sweat K^+ losses[14,112] seen during exercise in horses,[113] it is expected that horses experience similar rates and magnitudes of muscle K^+ loss as do humans. In humans, 30 s of high intensity exercise decreased muscle [K^+] by 20 mEq/L and, with increases in muscle [Na^+] and [Cl^-] balancing each other, the decrease in [SID] is thus approximately 20 + 11 = 31 mEq/L. Based on titrimetric studies conducted on rat fast twitch skeletal muscle the 31 mEq/L decrease in [SID] is sufficient to account for about 3/4 of the increase in [H^+].[68] In summary, using this example of muscle after 40 s of high intensity exercise, the decrease in [SID] can account fully for the increase in [H^+]. Coincidently, the decrease in [SID] approximates the increase in [lactate$^-$], and the decrease in [PCr^{2-}] was similar to the decrease in [K^+]. Further study is needed to determine if this relationship holds during high intensity exercise, but if it does it means that decreases in [SID] during high intensity exercise may be estimated from the increase in [lactate$^-$] alone. Changes in muscle [SID] account for the majority of the change in muscle [H^+] (Fig. 39.4).

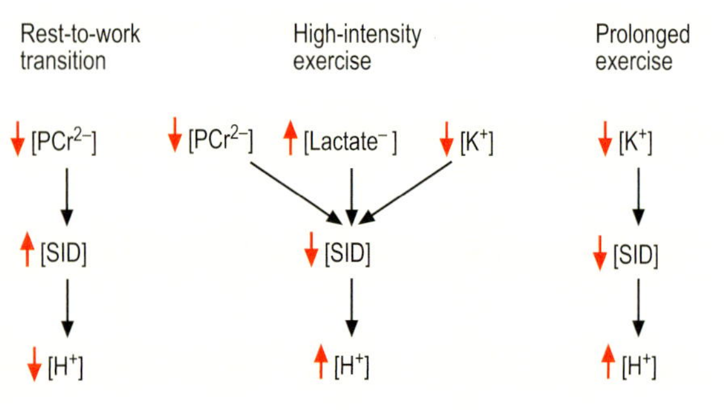

Fig 39.3 Factors that affect muscle [SID], and the impact on muscle [H^+], during exercise.

Muscle [A_{tot}] during exercise

Exercise affects the intracellular protein portion of [A_{tot}] (which has units of concentration) primarily through changes in cell volume or intracellular water content.[105] These volume changes are pronounced during the first several minutes of exercise[114] and also much later during prolonged exercise resulting in intracellular dehydration.[115] The impact of cell volume changes on skeletal muscle [A_{tot}] and acid-base state has not been studied; however, it appears that the total capacity to buffer protons may not be appreciably affected because the content of carnosine remains constant.[116]

With high intensity exercise a number of the minor variables contribute to changes in [A_{tot}], including an increase in [creatine] resulting from PCr^{2-} hydrolysis, a decrease in [ATP] and an increase in [Pi]. The increases in [creatine] result from PCr^{2-} hydrolysis, while increases in Pi are due to ATP hydrolysis, increases in glycolytic phosphates, and decreases in ATP.[68,69] Taken together, the increases in [creatine] and [Pi] account for all of the increase in [A_{tot}] during high intensity contractions in rat skeletal muscle. The production of H^+ with increase in [H^+] does not affect [A_{tot}], but does decrease [A^-] and increase [HA] as H^+ is buffered by this non-bicarbonate buffer system. Because the concentrations of the constituents comprising [A_{tot}] changes during exercise, the K_A also changes. The increases in [A_{tot}] and K_A accounted for 19% and 7%, respectively, of the increase in [H^+] during 5 min of high intensity exercise in rat muscle;[68,69] these have yet to be determined in equine muscle.

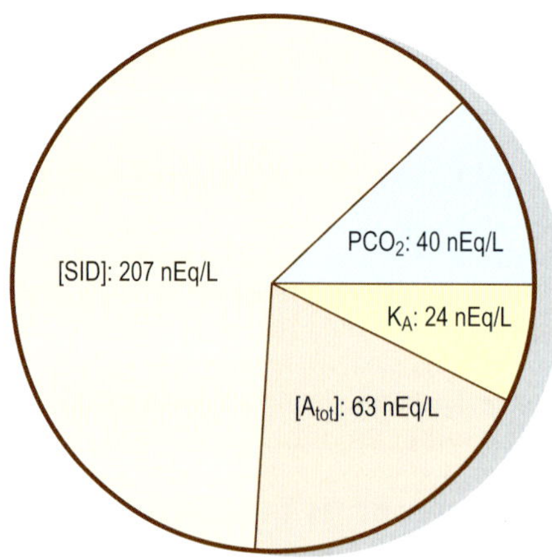

Fig 39.4 Effects of changes in independent physicochemical variables on muscle [H^+] after high intensity exercise. The example provided is a brief period of very high intensity exercise resulting in a decrease in muscle pH from 7.00 to 6.48, equal to an increase in [H^+] from 100 to 334 nEq/L.

Data taken from Lindinger.[13,68]

Muscle CO_2 during exercise

During high intensity exercise CO_2 is produced primarily as a result of H^+ buffering by HCO_3^-, with a minor although increasing amount from tricarboxylic acid (TCA) cycle activity. Within the TCA cycle, the dehydrogenation of oxalosuccinate to α-ketoglutarate and of α-ketoglutarate to succinyl CoA produces one molecule of CO_2 for each carbon entering the cycle.

Muscle $[H^+]$ responds in near linear manner to increases in intracellular PCO_2, with a 90 mmHg increase in PCO_2 (40–130 mmHg) increasing $[H^+]$ from 100 to 140 nEq/L.[68] Therefore, increases in CO_2 contribute relatively little to contraction-induced changes in intracellular $[H^+]$, compared to the relatively large effect of CO_2 on plasma $[H^+]$ (Fig. 39.4). The contribution of CO_2 to the intracellular acid-base of exercise can only be estimated using venous plasma PCO_2 in blood draining intensely contracting muscles; this estimate assumes that intracellular muscle PCO_2 is similar to muscle venous PCO_2.[117] This is reasonable given that CO_2 is highly diffusible and that there is substantial carbonic anhydrase within the interstitium, cells and on the sarcolemma to catalyze the conversion of HCO_3^- to CO_2. It is likely that the majority of the increase in PCO_2 results from the reaction of metabolically and physicochemically produced H^+ with HCO_3^- to produce CO_2 and water.

Draught exercise

While the responses described above are typical of racing horses, very similar responses appear to occur in horses pulling heavy loads. As occurs with racing, increasing exercise intensity results in increasing recruitment of fast motor units and fast glycolytic fiber types. Standardbreds performing incremental draught loading exercise while trotting slowly (4.8 m/s) showed a similar muscle metabolic profile[118] to that seen during racing.[108] Indeed, after 10–12 min of incremental draught loading, muscle $[PCr^{2-}]$ decreased by 15 mEq/L and $[lactate^-]$ increased by 20 mEq/L, with one horse achieving a muscle $[lactate^-]$ of 57 mEq/L.[118] This study is noteworthy in that the muscle biopsies were obtained 10 s after cessation of the exercise.

Changes in plasma acid-base state during exercise and recovery

As noted previously, the acid-base disturbance within the plasma during exercise is generated within contracting skeletal muscle. It must therefore be appreciated that the venous plasma draining contracting muscles display the greatest and most rapid changes in metabolite, electrolyte and gas concentrations compared to mixed venous or arterial plasma. The changes in mixed venous plasma will be greater than those in arterial plasma, and those in arterial plasma will be greater than those seen in venous plasma draining non-contracting tissues (i.e. jugular vein).[119–121] Therefore, difference in blood sampling site is an important consideration when evaluating the acid-base and electrolyte profile of exercised horses. In laboratory conditions, acid-base determinations are best performed on arterial and on venous plasma draining contracting skeletal muscle. While blood samples have been collected from the iliac vein in resting horses,[122] the technique does not yet appear to have been applied to exercising horses. The only real difference in acid-base composition between mixed venous and arterial plasma is due to CO_2 loss at the lung but this, together with associated measures of PO_2, provides valuable information on the respiratory system during exercise and recovery.[18] When an acid-base assessment is performed on jugular venous plasma (as it often must be due to ethical or field considerations) then it must be kept in mind that a less severe and somewhat erroneous picture of whole body acid-base status will be the result.

As with muscle, it must also be appreciated that the rapid loss of water and some electrolytes from the plasma compartment with the onset of exercise is among the factors that produces changes in measured concentrations of electrolytes, metabolites protein and red cells (hematocrit or packed cell volume – PCV).[114,123] Indeed, about 50% of the increase in plasma $[K^+]$, all of the increase in [plasma protein] and 50% of the increase in PCV is due to loss of water from the plasma compartment. The remainder of the increase in plasma $[K^+]$ is due to net loss of K^+ from contracting skeletal muscle and the remaining increase in PCV is due to splenic contraction resulting in discharge of red cells into the circulation.

Assessment of acid-base status in the blood is performed on constituents measured within the plasma compartment. Therefore concentrations of metabolites measured on samples of lysed whole blood cannot be used because the concentrations of these substances within red cells differs from that measured in plasma. The differences between plasma and red cell intracellular concentrations diminish within the syringe after blood sampling.[124] It is therefore important to separate red cells from plasma immediately after sampling the blood from exercising horses so that the plasma sample is as close to a true reflection of what was in the plasma of the horse at the exact time of blood sampling. As noted above, the PCO_2 at different blood sampling sites varies considerably and is an important consideration when determining whole-animal acid-base status, and some of this can be due to marked temperature differences. Determination of the actual pH, PCO_2 and PO_2 (as opposed to that measured by an instrument at 37°C), and hence $[HCO_3^-]$, requires a non-linear correction of the blood gas and pH values to the temperature within each blood sampling site.[125,126] Increases in temperature result in increases in PCO_2, PO_2 and $[H^+]$ (decreased pH).

As in contracting muscle, the main changes that affect plasma [SID] during moderate to high intensity exercise are increases in $[K^+]$, $[lactate^-]$[113] and $[Na^+]$ but not $[Cl^-]$[120,121] due to the greater rate of loss of water (than of Na^+) from plasma into contracting muscle. Examples of these types of exercise include incremental exercise to fatigue, maximal intensity sprints, and constant rate submaximal exercise tests.

The arterial PCO_2 responses to exercise are highly dependent on running velocity and, during incremental exercise tests, on the duration of time spent at each running velocity. Arterial PCO_2 remains unchanged during low to mild intensity exercise. During incremental exercise to fatigue, arterial PCO_2 decreased slightly but mixed venous PCO_2 increased markedly from 50 mmHg at rest to 80–95 mmHg at the highest work load corresponding to 100% VO_{2peak}.[120] In Fenger et al.'s study[120] running velocity was increased in small increments (0.5 to 1 m/s) and each velocity sustained for 90s to achieve near steady state of cardiovascular and respiratory responses.[127,128] When velocity was consistently increased at 0.5 m/s increments with 4 min at each speed, increasing exercise duration was associated with a marked and progressive hypocapnia[126] indicative of increasing alveolar ventilation.[129] In contrast, when velocity is increased in large (2 m/s) increments with only 1 min at each speed[130,131] or when single high intensity (running at >10 m/s) exercise bouts are performed the increase in PCO_2 is similar to that achieved during high intensity sprint exercise.[53,131,132] In horses sprinting at 115% of peak VO_2 arterial PCO_2 increased from 42 mmHg at the walk to 48 and 59 mmHg at 45 and 75 s of the sprint, comparable to the 58 mmHg PCO_2 seen with rapid, non-steady state incremental exercise test.[131] From these and other similar results it can be concluded that sprinting or rapid increases in exercise intensity result in elevations in arterial PCO_2 indicating that the respiratory system cannot keep the pace of metabolic and physicochemical CO_2 production. However, if sufficient time (90s) is allowed at each running velocity the respiratory system is capable keeping or exceeding the rate of CO_2 production.

Incremental steady state exercise

Let us now conduct an acid-base evaluation during the incremental 'steady state' exercise test of Fenger et al.[120] The reason for choosing this type of a test is because it is a very good design for the controlled, clinical assessment of respiratory and metabolic systems during and following exercise. Although the $[A_{tot}]$ data are incomplete, this particular study provides a reasonably good assessment of acid-base state using arterial plasma.

In arterial plasma, the dependent variable $[H^+]$ increased by 21 nEq/L at maximal exercise, while $[HCO_3^-]$ decreased from 32.8 to 16.2 mEq/L (Table 39.8). The independent variable [SID] remained unchanged (36.8 at rest and 35.5 mEq/L at maximal exercise) and thus had no effect on the changes in $[H^+]$ or $[HCO_3^-]$. Arterial PCO_2 decreased from 44 at rest to 35.5 mmHg at maximal exercise; this reduction appeared to be due to an increase in alveolar ventilation during the progressive exercise test and effectively reduced the mixed venous PCO_2 of 83 mmHg to below resting values. By solving for $[H^+]$ with this decrease in PCO_2, but holding [SID] and $[A_{tot}]$ constant at resting values, the decrease in PCO_2 alone (independent of any other changes) contributed to a 7.7 nEq/L decrease in $[H^+]$, indicative of considerable sensitivity of $[H^+]$ to changes in PCO_2. Because this decrease in PCO_2 caused a decrease in $[H^+]$, it means that increases in either or both of $[A_{tot}]$ and [SID] had to contribute to the increased $[H^+]$ (acidosis). The numerical (though not statistically significant) 1.3 mEq/L decrease in [SID] only accounts for 5.3 nEq/L of the 21 nEq/L increase in $[H^+]$. Therefore, the increase in $[A_{tot}]$ accounts for the difference between measured change in $[H^+]$ and the decrease in $[H^+]$ due to decreased PCO_2 as well as the difference between change in measured $[H^+]$ and the increase in $[H^+]$ due to the increase in $[A_{tot}]$ (Table 39.8). It may appear unusual that [SID] was unchanged at maximal exercise, compared to rest, so we will examine this in more detail. As expected, the main contributor to a decrease in [SID] during exercise is an increase in $[lactate^-]$, and indeed lactate increased to 17 mEq/L at maximal exercise; the 16 mEq/L increase in $[lactate^-]$ thus contributed to a 16 mEq/L decrease in [SID]. This effect of increased $[lactate^-]$ (from 1 to 17 mEq/L), however, was offset by a simultaneous 11 mEq/L increase in $[Na^+]$ and a 3 mEq/L increase in $[K^+]$ with no change in $[Cl^-]$.

The important points about arterial acid-base balance during this type of exercise are that the increases in plasma total weak acids (primarily albumin) and inorganic phosphate are the primary contributors to the acidosis. While the 16 mEq/L increase in the strong acid anion $[lactate^-]$ did have a pronounced acidifying effect (the increase in $[lactate^-]$ alone effectively increased $[H^+]$ by ~55 nEq/L) this effect is offset by the increases in plasma strong base cations $[Na^+]$ and $[K^+]$. The increase in $[Na^+]$ results from the net movement of a low $[Na^+]$ plasma filtrate into skeletal muscle while the increase in $[K^+]$ arises from net K^+ loss by contracting skeletal muscle.[106,109] Finally, within mixed venous plasma the increases in $[A_{tot}]$ and PCO_2 both contribute substantially to the acidosis, and this PCO_2 effect is abolished upon transit of the blood through the lungs.

High intensity sprint exercise

The second example to be illustrated is using high intensity sprint exercise. We will specifically examine the second and ninth sprints of a series of 9 sprints performed by trained Arabian horses, as described by Kronfeld and colleagues.[53] Each sprint lasted for 60 s, with a 4 min active recovery between sprints. After a warm up, the first sprint was performed at 7 m/s (6% incline) and the remaining 8 sprints at 10 m/s. Another noteworthy feature of this study is that jugular venous plasma was used, and this raises some points of interest that will be addressed as we work through the data.

At the end of sprint 2, as in Fenger's et al's[120] study, there was only a small 1 mEq/L decrease in [SID] that theoretically contributed 1 nEq/L to the 5 nEq/L increase in $[H^+]$ (Table 39.9). In the Table, this is reported as −0.6 nEq/L because this more accurately represents the mean of the individual calculations for eight horses. The point is that changes in [SID] are small and do not play a major role in acid-base balance during this type of exercise. While a 4.3 mEq/L increase in plasma $[lactate^-]$ contributed to an acidifying effect, this was offset by increases in plasma $[Na^+]$ (1.7 mEq/L) and $[K^+]$ (1.4 mEq/L). As the number of sequential sprints increased, plasma $[lactate^-]$ continued to increase to 9.5 mEq/L at the end of sprint 9; this now offset the increases in $[Na^+]$ and $[K^+]$ resulting in a 3.6 mEq/L decrease in [SID] that could alone account for all of the increase (3.8 nEq/L) increase in $[H^+]$.

PCO_2 peaked at the end of the sprint 2, then progressively decreased to below resting by the end of sprint 6. This indicates

Table 39.8 Contributions to increases in arterial plasma dependent variables $[H^+]$ and $[HCO_3^-]$ by each of the independent variables [SID], PCO_2 and $[A_{tot}]$ during incremental 'steady state' exercise in horses, using data from Fenger et al[120]

VARIABLE	RESTING	MAXIMAL EXERCISE	CHANGE FROM REST	CONTRIBUTION TO CHANGE IN $[H^+]$ (nEq/L)
$[H^+]$ nEq/L (pH)	33 (7.47)	54 (7.26)	+21	–
$[HCO_3^-]$ mEq/L	32.8	16.2	−16.6	–
[SID] mEq/L	36.8	35.5	−1.3	+5.3
PCO_2 mmHg	44.0	35.5	8.5	−7.7
$[A_{tot}]$ mmol/L	Not given	Not given		+23.4*

*Calculated as $[H^+]$ change from rest[21] – ([SID] and PCO_2 effects)

Table 39.9 Contributions to increases in jugular venous plasma dependent variables [H$^+$] and [HCO_3^-] by each of the independent variables [SID], PCO_2 and [A_{tot}] at the end of the 2nd and 9th sprints in horses, using data from Kronfeld et al[53]

VARIABLE	REST	2nd SPRINT	CHANGE FROM REST	CONTRIBUTION TO CHANGE IN [H$^+$] (nEq/L)
[H$^+$] nEq/L	38.7	43.7	5.0	–
[SID]	48.6	47.6	−1.0	−0.6
PCO_2	51.6	57.5	+5.9	4.1
[A_{tot}]	18.5	19.5	+1.0	1.5
VARIABLE	**REST**	**9th SPRINT**	**CHANGE FROM REST**	**CONTRIBUTION TO CHANGE IN [H$^+$] (nEq/L)**
[H$^+$] nEq/L	38.7	42.1	+3.8	–
[SID]	48.6	45	−3.6	+4.4
PCO_2	51.6	48.2	−3.4	−2.4
[A_{tot}]	18.5	20	+1.5	+2.0

both a lowering of glycolytic metabolism and resultant decrease in metabolic H$^+$ production[101,133] that reduces the generation of PCO_2 (from H$^+$ combining with HCO_3^-) and an improvement in alveolar ventilation as the exercise progresses. Nonetheless, the decrease in PCO_2 to below resting values contributed to alkalinizing effect equivalent to reducing [H$^+$] by 2.4 nEq/L. A further small increase in [A_{tot}] also contributed to an acidifying affect that offset most of the alkalinizing effect of lowered PCO_2.

In summary, comparing the results of sprints 2 and 9 we see a marked difference in the origins of the acid-base disturbance. The primary acidifying influence at the end of sprint 2 was the increase in PCO_2, whereas at the end of sprint 9 PCO_2 had decreased and contributed to an alkalinizing effect. This is an important regulatory aspect, for this later alkalinizing effect of lowered PCO_2 markedly reduced the acidifying effects of decreased [SID] (which account for 2/3 of the acidification) and increased [A_{tot}] (1/3 of the acidification at the end of sprint 9). In sprint 2, there was negligible effect of [SID]; however, as [lactate$^-$] continued to increase in plasma with repeated sprints, a progressively decreasing [SID] played an increasing role in systemic acidification. In classical acid-base physiology one may refer to this acidosis at the end of sprint 2 as a primary respiratory acidosis that progresses to a primary metabolic acidosis with respiratory compensation by the end of sprint 9.

It should be noted that repeated sprints result in a sequential lowering of $PaCO_2$ with each successive sprint[53,132] that is attributed to a significant increase in alveolar ventilation and not to increased breathing frequency which is tightly coupled to stride frequency.[129,132] After five sprints, an increasing arterial hypocapnia is observed with each successive sprint.[53] In a similar vein, when a low intensity exercise warm-up precedes a bout of high intensity exercise, there is an increase in VCO_2 during the first minute of exercise compared to when no warm-up precedes the high intensity exercise.[134,135] Rather than evoking an increase in alveolar ventilation to explain this result, however, these authors suggested that the warm-up resulted in increased tissue CO_2 storage that then reduced the amount of CO_2 during the subsequent bout of high intensity exercise – this also does not preclude an increase in alveolar ventilation after a warm-up. Furthermore, since the increase in VCO_2 occurred within seconds of starting the high intensity exercise,[134] it is unlikely that the rapidity of the augmented VCO_2 response could be explained by a reduced ability to store CO_2. It can be concluded that the augmented VCO_2 during high intensity exercise after warm-up is due primarily to increased alveolar ventilation, similar to that seen with high intensity steady state exercise. In further support, during heavy exercise (4.5 m/s at a 10% grade = 60% of peak VO_2) of 30 min duration, a progressive decrease in $PaCO_2$ was primarily due to a progressive increase in alveolar ventilation secondary to increases in both respiratory frequency and tidal volume.[136]

Steady state submaximal exercise

This section exemplifies the changes and contributions seen during steady state, submaximal exercise in well-trained horses. A time point of 15 min into exercise was selected because this is well past the rapid changes that occur with the onset of exercise and was at least 10 min prior to the onset of fatigue at this intensity with this group of horses (Lindinger MI, Geor RJ, McCutcheon LJ, Ecker GL, unpublished). One of the most noteworthy features of submaximal steady state exercise in trained horses is the alkalosis that occurs during the steady state period (Table 39.10). Plasma pH rose in both arterial (carotid artery) and mixed venous (pulmonary artery). In arterial plasma, the alkalosis was completely due to the decrease in $PaCO_2$, since there was negligible change in [SID] (2 mEq/L increase in [lactate$^-$] balanced by 1 mEq/L decrease in [Cl$^-$] and 1.3 mEq/L increase in [K$^+$]) and a 1.3 mEq/L increase in [A_{tot}] had an acidifying effect. The decrease in arterial plasma [HCO_3^-] is a hallmark of 'metabolic acidosis' in the clinical acid-base sense and, indeed that is what one would expect to see with exercise. Importantly, however, this decrease is primarily due to the increase in total weak acid concentration (primarily plasma proteins) and secondarily to the decrease in $PaCO_2$ (despite the marked 14.4 mmHg decrease). It must be emphasized that such modest increases in [K$^+$] and [lactate$^-$] with the alveolar hyperventilation are features of well-trained horses.

In mixed venous plasma, there was a small decrease in $PmvCO_2$' indicating that the influence of alveolar hypoventilation persisted within the peripheral circulation and that the rates of metabolic H$^+$ production were low; metabolism was primarily aerobic, as evidenced by the low plasma [lactate$^-$] of 3.25 mEq/L. The sole contributor to an acidifying effect was the increase in [PP] resulting

Table 39.10 Contribution to increases in arterial and mixed venous dependent variables $[H^+]$ and $[HCO_3^-]$ by each of the independent variables [SID], PCO_2 and $[A_{tot}]$ at 15 min of steady state exercise prior to onset of fatigue

VARIABLE	RESTING	EXERCISE	CHANGE FROM REST	CONTRIBUTION TO CHANGE IN $[H^+]$	CONTRIBUTION TO CHANGE IN $[HCO_3^-]$
Arterial plasma					
$[H^+]$ nEq/L (pH)	37 (7.43)	26 (7.58)	−10	–	–
$[HCO_3^-]$ mEq/L	28.3	26.3	−2.0	–	–
[SID] mEq/L	39.9	39.6	−0.3	+0.4	−0.3
PCO_2 mmHg	42.7	28.3	14.4	−12.0	−0.6
$[A_{tot}]$ mmol/L	13.5	14.8	+1.3	+1.4	−1.0
Mixed venous plasma					
$[H^+]$ nEq/L (pH)	43 (7.37)	38 (7.42)	−5	–	–
$[HCO_3^-]$ mEq/L	28.4	31.0	+2.6	–	–
[SID] mEq/L	39.9	43.8	+3.9	−4.8	+3.7
PCO_2 mmHg	49.2	48.1	−1.1	−0.9	0.0
$[A_{tot}]$ mmol/L	13.6	14.9	+1.3	+1.6	−1.0

Data represent averages obtained from four trained Standardbreds, from Lindinger MI, Geor RJ, McCutcheon LJ, Ecker GL (unpublished).

from the fluid shift into contracting muscle. The 4 mEq/L increase in [SID] thus accounted for all of the alkalinizing effect. Plasma [SID] increased due to a 2 mEq/L increase in $[Na^+]$, a 1.4 mEq/L increase in $[K^+]$ and a 2 mEq/L decrease in $[Cl^-]$ that offset the 1.9 mEq/L rise in $[\text{lactate}^-]$. Mixed venous plasma $[HCO_3^-]$ increased during steady state exercise, in contrast with what was seen in arterial plasma and what would also be seen in jugular venous plasma. Again, this is solely due to the increase in [SID], as the increase in $[A_{tot}]$ had the effect of reducing $[HCO_3^-]$ by 1 mEq/L.

It is evident from this analysis, using relatively small changes in both dependent and independent acid-base variables, that $[H^+]$ has similar sensitivities to physiological changes in the independent variables; however, $[HCO_3^-]$ is much more sensitive to changes in [SID] and $[A_{tot}]$ than to changes in PCO_2.

Endurance exercise

Low speed endurance exercise, such as draught horses pulling loads for 8 hours per day for 5 consecutive days produces no significant acid-base disturbances. When the speed of endurance exercise is increased, with ensuing sweat losses of water and electrolytes occurring at elevated rates, then a slowly progressing metabolic alkalosis develops.[137–139] It is important to point out that when the hydration status of the horses is maintained, through the use of effective strategies of electrolyte supplementation, this alkalosis does not develop.

The metabolic alkalosis associated with dehydration during endurance rides, or indeed during prolonged transport of the horse, is a direct result of sweating. Equine sweat has a tonicity similar to that of plasma[14] in contrast to the very dilute sweat produced by humans. The reasons for the high tonicity of equine sweat is that the equine sweat gland does not appear to have the ability to resorb ions from within the lumen of the sweat glands. Rather, some ions, such as K^+ and Cl^-, appear to be secreted for their concentrations in sweat are much greater than in plasma and extracellular fluid.[14] Although the electrolyte composition of equine sweat changes over time, in general sweat $[Na^+]$ ranges from 65 to 170, $[K^+]$ ranges from 25 to 55 and charge balance is made up by $[Cl^-]$ in the range 100–180 mEq/L (McCutcheon et al. 1995). The total amount of electrolyte loss during a 100 mile endurance ride can be excess of 1 mole for Na^+ and Cl^-, representing substantial depletion of body stores,[115] so it is instructive to determine the origins of the electrolyte losses. Because the tonicity and $[Na^+]$ of equine plasma and sweat are similar, there is little if any change in plasma osmolality and $[Na^+]$ during prolonged endurance exercise.[103,115,140] Additionally, when plasma $[K^+]$ is measured, after allowing sufficient time after exercise has stopped for re-equilibration of plasma and muscle K^+ pools, there is little change in plasma $[K^+]$ and clearly the K^+ losses are not borne by the extracellular compartment. Therefore, the K^+ appearing in the sweat originates largely from cells, and likely contracting muscle cells that are known to lose K^+ during the period of exercise.[104] It is important to recall that the bulk of the body's Na^+ and Cl^- stores are extracellular, and it is Cl^- that balances the positive charge on Na^+ and K^+ lost in sweat. Therefore, sweat $[Cl^-] = [Na^+] + [K^+]$. Because the extracellular losses of Cl^- exceeds those of Na^+ by a factor ranging between 1.3 and 1.8, extracellular and plasma $[Cl^-]$ must decrease, and indeed does by 10 to 15 mEq/L as measured in numerous studies.[103,115,137,140] It is this large decrease in plasma $[Cl^-]$ that is responsible for the alkalosis, for this results in a large increase in plasma [SID].

A detailed assessment of acid-base status in horses during the time course of an endurance ride has not yet been performed. Using the principles of acid-base assessment provided above, an extreme case of plasma $[Cl^-]$ depletion (−15 mEq/L[139]) will be used to exemplify the effect of acid-base status:

$$[SID] = ([Na^+] + [K^+]) - ([Cl^-] + [\text{lactate}^-])$$

Before endurance exercise:

$$38\ \text{mEq/L} = (135+4)-(100+1)$$

After endurance exercise:

$$53\ \text{mEq/L} = (135+4)-(85+1)$$

The increase in [SID] alone has a large alkalinizing effect and can be calculated to decrease plasma [H^+] from 36.6 to 23.9 nEq/L (pH increase from 7.436 to 7.622), with [HCO_3^-] increasing from 26.9 to 41.2 mEq/L. The fact that such large changes do not occur is primarily attributed to the simultaneous increase in plasma [A_{tot}] resulting from the loss of extracellular water, which raises plasma [proteins] ([PP]). An increase in [PP] from 60 to 75 g/L, typical of endurance rides, increases [A_{tot}] from 13 to 16.25 mmol/L and this change alone (independent of change in [SID] or PCO_2) has the effect of raising [H^+] from 36.6 to 40.5 nEq/L. The combined effect of increased [A_{tot}] and decreased [SID] results in an [H^+] of 25.6 nEq/L (pH 7.591) and [HCO_3^-] of 38.4 mEq/L. There is negligible change in PCO_2 during endurance exercise, and the small changes that occur can be neglected for the purposes of assessing acid-base status. Therefore, the acidification resulting from the increase in plasma [A_{tot}] only partially offsets the alkalinization caused by the increase in [SID], resulting in the observed alkalosis.

It is very important to note that, in the dehydrated horse, there is little change in plasma [Na^+] and osmolality. Horses can lose 30 liters or more of fluid as sweat with minimal alteration of plasma osmolality and [Na^+]. This is solely because sweat osmolality and [Na^+] differs little from that of sweat. To complicate the interpretation, the decrease in plasma [Cl^-] is seemingly inconsistent with dehydration. The key hematological variables for diagnosis of dehydration in the horse are a decrease in plasma [Cl^-] coupled with increases in [PP] and PCV.

Simulated racing: Standardbred racehorses

Recovery from race-intensity exercise was studied in a group of nine Standardbred racehorses fitted with catheters in the jugular vein for repeated blood sampling.[9] The detailed acid-base analysis is provided in the paper, so will not be replicated here as with the previous examples. Horses warmed up with 1 mile of walking followed by 2.5 miles of jogging at submaximal intensity. This was followed by 45 min of rest at the stall. The second phase of exercise comprised a warm-up of 1 mile walking, 1 mile jogging, then 1 mile at race speed. The first recovery blood sample was taken 60 s after completion of this fast mile. Plasma [H^+] increased from 39.1 ± 1.0 nEq/L at rest to 44.8 ± 2.7 nEq/L at 1 min of recovery. A decreased [SID] due to a [$lactate^-$] of 16 ± 3 mEq/L was the primary contributor to the increased [H^+] immediately at the end of exercise. Plasma [$lactate^-$] was highest at 1 min of recovery, reflecting a high rate of cellular $lactate^-$ clearance in the immediate post-exercise period. Plasma [Na^+] and [K^+] were increased by 6.5 ± 0.7 and 1.14 ± 0.06 mEq/L, respectively, at 1 min of recovery. The increased plasma [Atot], due to increased plasma [protein] resulting from extra- to intracellular fluid shift, was a minor contributor to the acidosis. A decreased PCO_2 at 1 min of recovery, due to the pronounced hyperventilation, had a slight alkalinizing effect. Acid-base state recovered with a half time of 15–20 min, with full recovery from race-intensity exercise requiring 90–120 min.

Other types of exercise

It is worth noting some interesting features of acid-base balance reported in the literature in horses performing different types of activities ranging from draught work to show jumping. Show jumping competition resulted in a decrease in jugular venous PCO_2, once again illustrating the degree of alveolar ventilation and an ability of lowered PCO_2 to offset the acidifying effects due to increases in [A_{tot}].[141] In these horses [SID] increased by 2 mEq/L, which also had an alkalinizing effect; a 2 mEq/L decrease in [Cl^-] and 3 mEq/L increase in [Na^+] more than offset the 3.8 mEq/L increase in [$lactate^-$].

The second day of three-day eventing consists of a steeplechase, a roads and tracks phase and a cross country phase with each separated by a rest / cool down period. Rose and colleagues[142,143] assessed the acid-base changes occurring within jugular venous blood during this period. Similar to the other forms of exercise described above, plasma [H^+] decreased from 42 to 37 nEq/L at the end of the roads and tracks phase, and was subsequently 41 nEq/L at the end of the cross country phase. The main reasons for the decrease in [H^+] at the end of roads and tracks was a 6 mmHg decrease in PCO_2 with a 2.3 mEq/L increase in [SID]. The increase in [SID] resulted from increases in [Na^+] and [K^+] and decreases in [Cl^-] that offset the 1.5 mEq/L increase in [$lactate^-$]. Together, the combined effects of lowered PCO_2 and increased [SID] more than offset the acidifying effects of the 1.2 mmol/L increase in [A_{tot}], producing the mild alkalosis. At the end of the cross country, plasma [$lactate^-$] had risen to 8.2 mEq/L, negating the effects of increased [Na^+] and lowered [Cl^-] and leaving [SID] at resting values (40 mEq/L). The sole contributor to an acidifying effect was thus the 3 mmol/L increase in [A_{tot}] (resulting from dehydration [57%] and exercise-induced fluid shift [43%]) and this was completely offset by a further decrease in PCO_2 to 31.5 mmHg, resulting in a normal [H^+] (41.3 nEq/L). As expected, the combined effects of increased [A_{tot}] and reduced PCO_2 lowered [HCO_3^-] from 28 mEq/L at rest and at the end of roads and tracks to 18 mEq/L at the end of the cross country. Within 30 min of the cross country, both [H^+] and [HCO_3^-] had normalized to pre-exercise values despite an elevated [A_{tot}] (at this point due solely to dehydration) whose acidifying effects were offset by a continued depression of PCO_2.

Polo consists of periods of low to moderate activity interspersed with brief periods of burst activity while carrying the rider. The total duration of activity for individual horses ranges from 1 to 2 hours, allowing time for dehydration to occur as a result of sweating (see endurance exercise section below). Polo exercise results in a modest acidosis of metabolic origin that lasts during the period of activity.[144] The mild to modest acidosis has its sole origins in the decrease in [SID] associated with mild lactate accumulation, as there tends to be little to no change in plasma [protein] and PCO_2 is decreased.[145] After cessation of exercise, a mild alkalosis may develop, concomitant with decreased plasma [Cl^-] resulting from sweat losses (see endurance exercise section on page 868).

Clinical notes

In a clinical vein, the nature of the generation of the acid-base disturbance, and its subsequent regulation during and following the period of exercise, results in its eventual amelioration over a period of minutes to hours depending on the intensity and duration. Very high intensity exercise is capable of lowering arterial plasma pH to 7.1.[113] Therefore caution may be required with repeated sprints of very high intensity due to the cumulative effects of increasing [$lactate^-$] and [PP] that may be capable of decreasing arterial pH below 7.1. It must the understood that the severity of the mixed venous acidosis would be measurably greater than the arterial acidosis. At somewhat lower intensity, horses are capable of several repeated sprints without incurring a severe acid-base disturbance.[53] The final caution pertains to dehydration that results from

skeletal muscle glycogen, and ensuing decrements in exercise performance, during moderate-to-high intensity prolonged exercise (eventing and endurance). In theory, exogenous carbohydrate is converted to glucose, which is taken up by contracting skeletal muscle to be used by glycolysis, and reducing the need for sustained rates of glycogenolysis. This has not been shown by experimental research one way or the other, and effects on acid-base balance also have not been studied. The results in the field have been very mixed, with several instances of poor performance related to the use of inappropriate loading strategies. It appears that in most instances riders administer insufficient carbohydrate to elicit a performance-enhancing effect, but sufficient amounts to downregulate uptake and oxidation of free fatty acids by contracting muscle. This appears to result in an increased reliance on carbohydrate metabolism and has resulted in high rates of liver glycogen depletion, as evidenced by hypoglycemia (Lindinger MI, McKeen G, Ecker GL, unpublished results).

Dietary fat

The effects of dietary fat on performance and acid-base balance have received more attention than starch and protein. In resting horses, substituting some of the starch energy with fat (soybean oil) resulted in a mild acidifying effect on plasma, with increased PCO_2 with no significant effect on renal base excretion.[176] The increase in urine base Graham-Thiers et al.[173] found no effect of dietary fat (0 vs 10%) on acid-base balance at rest and during repeated sprint exercise, although there was evidence for an increased reliance of fat as an energy source. In contrast, an earlier study of repeated sprint exercise reported that horses on a 10% fat diet showed an increased plasma acidosis with increased [lactate$^-$][177] and decreased PCO_2 and [SID] than horses on the control diet.[178] Peak effects of the high fat diet required between 6 and 11 weeks of feeding. When horses were on a high fat (10%) diet for a relatively short duration of 4 weeks, there was a tendency for the high fat diet to increase plasma [lactate$^-$] during exercise.[179] This was associated with faster gallop speeds during the third and fourth repeated gallops that Duren et al.[179] attributed to an increased activation of glycolysis and glycogenolysis[180] with associated increases in power output with repeated sprint exercise. It appears that, with high intensity exercise, horses must be maintained on a high fat diet for at least 6 weeks and that the chronic high fat diet results in an increased reliance on glycolysis to produce the ATP needed to generate the high power outputs. The effects of a high fat diet on acid-base balance during high intensity exercise appear to be minor. The effects of dietary fat on acid-base balance during prolonged low and moderate intensity exercise do not appear to have been studied.

Selected clinically relevant issues for seemingly 'normal' horses

Age

Aguilera-Tejero et al.[181] provided a detailed comparison of plasma acid-base status in young (less than 9 years) and old (greater than 19 years). The only differences were a reduced (by 1.5 mmHg) arterial PCO_2 that resulted in a lower pH (7.428 vs 7.404) and this was associated with a lower PO_2 (90 vs 102 mmHg); there were no differences in measured weak and strong ion concentrations. A similar effect of age on arterial PCO_2 has previously been reported.[182] Aguilera-Tejero et al.[181] suggested that the apparent hypoxemia in older horses results in an increased ventilation that would thereby reduce arterial PCO_2.

Idiopathic laryngeal hemiplegia

A number of racehorses, both Thoroughbred and Standardbred, may perform poorly[186] due, in part, to a syndrome known as idiopathic laryngeal hemiplegia (ILH). ILH is a peripheral neuropathy characterized by dysfunction of the left recurrent laryngeal nerve innervating most of the left laryngeal muscles.[185] Between 35%[183] and 50% of large breed horses have some degree of laryngeal synchrony and asymmetry at rest.

Impaired regulation of acid-base balance occurs during exercise in horses having grade 4 or 5 laryngeal function,[184,185] where grade 5 is complete hemiplegia. The primary manifestation during a standard exercise test to fatigue is a marked elevation in arterial PCO_2 (grade 4, 69 mmHg; grade 5, 75 mmHg) compared to grade 1 (normal laryngeal function, 58 mmHg) that is associated with a reduced arterial PO_2 (by 8 mmHg) and increased (by 5–6 mEq/L) plasma [lactate$^-$].[185,186] Surgical correction of ILH improved but did not fully achieve a normal acid-base profile.[184,187]

Small airway inflammation and exercise-induced pulmonary hemorrhage (EIPH) also commonly occur in racehorses, leading to decrements in performance.[188] Poorly performing horses with these respiratory diseases manifested a pronounced and sustained hypocapnia with lower arterial PO_2, [HCO_3^-] and pH and higher blood [lactate$^-$] during recovery from high intensity exercise. The more pronounced increase in [lactate$^-$] is consistent with impaired blood oxygenation at the lungs, resulting in a greater reliance on anaerobic mechanisms to produce energy during high intensity exercise. The author's conclusion that the hypocapnia was due to the lactic acidosis[188] cannot be supported. While the hypocapnia itself would blunt the arterial chemoreceptor drive to ventilate, this may be offset by the increased [H^+]. The hypocapnia can be explained in terms of alveolar hyperventilation, which would facilitate rapid release of CO_2 at the lungs while maintaining compromised the ability to extract oxygen.

Administration of alkalinizing substances and other purported ergogenic aids

Alkalinizing substances

There is an extensive literature on the administration of bicarbonate salts and other alkalinizing agents in both horses and humans, and the interested reader is referred to the following reviews.[2,13,189,190] There is also consistent evidence that the administration of alkalinizing agents will result in enhanced performance with exercise at moderate to high intensities, and that this is due to increased rates of strong acid (i.e. lactate$^-$) removal from contracting muscle. This section will focus on the physicochemical aspects of inducing and correcting the acid-base disturbance resulting from the administration of bicarbonate-, citrate- and phosphate-containing compounds.

At the outset it must be explained that the administration of HCO_3^- does not in and of itself result in an increase in plasma [HCO_3^-]. When sodium bicarbonate, or baking soda, is dissolved in water all of the Na^+ completely dissociates from HCO_3^- by virtue of Na^+ being a strong ion; by definition strong ions are completely dissociated in solution. The HCO_3^- in solution readily participates in physicochemical reactions with H^+, CO_2 and H_2O as described above. In this simple solution consisting of water and added baking soda, the [HCO_3^-] will be determined by the [Na^+] and by the PCO_2. Since this solution will come into equilibrium with the CO_2 in the air, the resulting PCO_2 will be very low once equilibrium is achieved. The addition of carbonic anhydrase to this solution would greatly increase the speed of the reactions establishing equilibrium.

When a freshly mixed baking soda solution is administered nasogastrically into the stomach of a horse, which is an acidic environment, acid within the stomach and upper intestinal tract reacts rapidly with the HCO_3^- in solution. The HCO_3^- that was in solution rapidly dissipates, producing CO_2 and H_2O:

$$HCO_3^- + H^+ \rightarrow CO_2 + H_2O$$

The CO_2 readily diffuses into the blood where most is transformed by the action of carbonic anhydrase to HCO_3^-, transported to the lungs, reconverted to CO_2 and eliminated in expired air. The ingested water and Na^+ are absorbed within the small intestine, resulting in increased plasma water content and $[Na^+]$ – the excess is ultimately removed from the body through normal renal processes. Since the ingested HCO_3^- becomes part of the open CO_2 system, which is in a dynamic equilibrium with inspired air and the tissues, PCO_2 is rapidly normalized through ventilation.[146] Therefore the only changes remaining within the plasma (and extracellular) compartment are increased $[Na^+]$ and decreased concentrations of other plasma ions, both strong and weak. Notably, the concentrations of the predominant weak acid, protein, and strong acid Cl^- are decreased, resulting in decreased $[A_{tot}]$ and $[Cl^-]$. Both the decrease in $[Cl^-]$ and the increase in $[Na^+]$ contribute to a increase in [SID]. Both the increase in [SID] and the decrease in $[A_{tot}]$ contribute to increased $[HCO_3^-]$, decreased $[H^+]$ while PCO_2 remains unchanged.[146]

Because of the nature of these physicochemical reactions, it does not matter which cation salts of bicarbonate are dissolved in water and administered to the horse – all will result in a very similar extracellular alkalosis, at least initially. If calcium salts are used, these are slowly absorbed and the onset of the alkalosis will be slow. If a sufficient amount of calcium is used to induce an alkalosis, it is likely that this would be toxic. Potassium bicarbonate has also been used. Potassium, in contrast to Na^+, does not remain in the extracellular compartment but is rapidly taken up by the tissues, reducing the extent of the extracellular alkalosis presumably at the expense of alkalinizing the intracellular compartment.[146]

Time course

The administration of an alkalinizing agent results in a lowering of plasma and extracellular $[H^+]$, with a concurrent increase in $[HCO_3^-]$, with peak effects appearing to depend on the volume of water administered with the dose. When 1 L of water was administered with $NaHCO_3$ doses of 0.4 g/kg body mass, peak effects occurred 2–4 h after administration.[191] In contrast, when 2–4 L of water was used to administer doses ranging from 0.25 to 1.5 g/kg, peak effects occurred only 6–8 hours after administration.[192–195] Similar time courses occurred with a range of alkalinizing agents (sodium citrate, sodium acetate, sodium lactate, sodium acetate) administered at a dose of 0.5 g/kg in 2 L of water.[196]

As noted above, the administration of an alkalinizing agent with 4 L of water should result in a transient increase in plasma volume. The time course of PV change has not been studied, although it is known that any early changes in PV that would occur are corrected 6 h after administration.[197] Therefore, after this 6 h period the sole cause for the acid-base disturbance is the increase in extracellular $[Na^+]$ (or other administered cation).

Mechanism for enhanced lactate efflux

The rate of lactate$^-$ transport into muscle is facilitated by the monocarboxylate transporter (MCT1), whereas efflux of lactate$^-$ from muscle is facilitated by MCT4[158,198,199] and is dependent on the chemical gradient and driving force for H^+ and lactate$^-$.[199] Extracellular [lactate$^-$] is very low compared to muscle [lactate$^-$] in horses performing moderate-to-high intensity exercise,[200,201] providing a high driving force for lactate$^-$ diffusion out of contracting muscle cells. Similarly, extracellular $[H^+]$ is low compared to intramuscular $[H^+]$ and this is increased for a prolonged duration (up to 16 h) after administration of alkalinizing agents.[196] This combination of chemical changes results in an enhanced rate of removal of lactate$^-$ from contracting muscle during high intensity exercise, producing a higher plasma [lactate$^-$] and lower muscle [lactate$^-$] at the end of exercise.[201] In order to be able to detect these changes the dose administered may be important: Greenhaff et al.[201] used a $NaHCO_3$ dose of 0.6 mg/kg, while when a dose of 0.4 mg/kg was used no differences in muscle and blood lactate were found.[200]

Creatine supplementation

The practice of creatine supplementation is used in humans to improve performance associated with short-term high intensity exercise.[202] Attempts to replicate similar effects in horses with a dose of 25 g creatine monohydrate twice daily have shown no effect on performance, metabolism and related acid-base variables.[203]

Furosemide

Furosemide also known as frusemide or Lasix, is a loop diuretic that is extensively used to treat racehorses exhibiting symptoms of exercise-induced pulmonary hemorrhage (EIPH) in some racing jurisdictions.[204,205] There is evidence that furosemide administration improves racing performance[206,207] despite the pronounced diuresis with loss of water and electrolytes.[208,209] In addition, administration of the drug appears to result in a pronounced shift in fluid from the extracellular to the intracellular compartment[210] that, in part, contributes to the increase in plasma $[A_{tot}]$, which has a mild acidifying effect. The mechanism by which furosemide induces a long-lasting mild alkalosis is through reductions in plasma $[Cl^-]$ due to marked increases in renal Cl^- excretion without concomitant increases in renal strong cation excretion[56,208,211] and movement of plasma Cl^- into red blood cells. Because furosemide results in a pronounced loss of water, Na^+ and titratable acid from (primarily) the extracellular fluid compartment, this results in increased plasma $[Na^+]$ (by 8 mEq/L) and decreased plasma $[Cl^-]$ (by 8 mEq/L) between 5 and 10 h after administration of 1 mg/kg im.[208] In this study, it appears that plasma [SID] increased by 13 mEq/L 8 h after administration. Carlson and Jones[56] reported a 7 mEq/L increase in plasma [SID] 4 h after administering 1 mg/kg furosemide. This large increase in [SID] fully explains the increase in pH (7.383 to 7.445) and increase in $[HCO_3^-]$ (3 mEq/L) in arterial plasma.[56] The effect of increased [SID] alone would have been greater; however, the concomitant increase in [PP], and hence $[A_{tot}]$, due to the extracellular dehydration, results in an acidifying effect. Arterial and mixed venous PCO_2 remains unchanged in resting horses.[56] During high intensity treadmill running exercise (4 h after 0.5 or 1 mg/kg furosemide administration), the elevations in arterial and mixed venous pH and $[HCO_3^-]$ were maintained in furosemide-treated horses through to the last minute of maximal exercise; furosemide did not appear to result in increased lactate accumulation within blood.[56,212]

In many ways, the alkalosis resulting from furosemide administration qualitatively resembles that resulting from administration of $NaHCO_3$ and related alkalinizing agents. The main feature in common that produces the increased plasma pH and [HCO_3^-] is the pronounced decrease in plasma [Cl^-]. The main differences are elevations in [PP] and [Na^+] with furosemide, while these variables remain largely unchanged with alkalinizing agents. The alkalosis resulting from even high-dose furosemide (1 mg/kg) is relatively mild compared to the moderate alkalosis resulting from high-dose $NaHCO_3$ (>0.5 mg/kg), although the effects appear to be similar in duration.

References

1. Williams RB. Sodium bicarbonate loading and the rules of racing. Br Vet J 1995;151(5):473–5.
2. Matson LG, Tran ZV. Effects of sodium bicarbonate ingestion on anaerobic performance: a meta-analytic review. Int J Sport Nutr 1993;3(1):2–28.
3. Auer DE, Skelton KV, Tay S, et al. Detection of bicarbonate administration (milkshake) in Standardbred horses. Aust Vet J 1993;70:336–40.
4. Kallings P, Bondesson U, Houghton E, editors. Effects of Sodium Bicarbonate on Total Carbon Dioxide in Blood and Plasma Lactate in the Horse. Newmarket, UK: R&W Publications; 1994.
5. Short CR, editor. Control of Administration of Sodium Bicarbonate and Other Alkalis: the New Zealand Experience. Newmarket, UK: R&W Publications; 1992.
6. Short CR, editor. The Detection and Performance Effects of Sodium Bicarbonate Administration in the Racehorse. Newmarket, UK: R&W Publications; 1992.
7. Soma LR, Uboh CE, Nann L, et al. Prerace venous blood acid-base values in standardbred horses. Equine Vet J 1996;28(5):390–6.
8. Frey LP, Kline KH, Foreman JH. Effects of prerace exercise, frusemide, sex and ambient temperature on blood sodium, bicarbonate and pH values in standardbred horses. Equine Vet J 1995;27(3):170–3.
9. Waller A, Lindinger MI. Physicochemical analysis of acid-base status during recovery from high intensity exercise in Standardbred racehorses. Equine Comp Exerc Physiol 2005;2:119–27.
10. Nostell K, Funkquist P, Nyman G, et al. The physiological responses to simulated race tests on a track and on a treadmill in standardbred trotters. Equine Vet J Suppl 2006;36:123–7.
11. Cohen ND, Stanley SD, Arthur RM, et al. Factors influencing pre-race serum concentration of total carbon dioxide in Thoroughbred horses racing in California. Equine Vet J 2006;38(6):543–8.
12. Waller AP, Pearson W, Lindinger MI. Factors contributing to plasma TCO_2 and acid-base state in Ontario Standardbred racehorses. Equine Vet J 2010;42(Suppl. 38):592–600.
13. Lindinger MI, Heigenhauser GJF. Effects of gas exchange on acid-base balance. Compr Physiol 2012;2:1–52.
14. McCutcheon LJ, Geor RJ, Hare MJ, et al. Sweating rate and sweat composition during exercise and recovery in ambient heat and humidity. Equine Vet J Suppl 1995;20:153–7.
15. Hultman E, Sahlin K. Acid-base balance during exercise. Exerc Sport Sci Rev 1980;8:41–128.
16. Constable PD. The physicochemical approach for evaluating acid-base balance in exercising horses. Equine Vet J Suppl 1999;30:636–8.
17. Constable PD. A simplified strong ion model for acid-base equilibria: application to horse plasma. J Appl Physiol 1997;83(1):297–311.
18. Johnson R, Heigenhauser G, Hsia C, et al. Determinants of gas exchange and acid-base balance during exercise. Handbook of Physiology. Section 12. Exercise Regulation and Integration of Multiple Systems. New York: Oxford University Press; 1996. p. 515–84.
19. Hyyppa S, Poso AR. Fluid, electrolyte, and acid-base responses to exercise in racehorses. Vet Clin North Am Equine Pract 1998;14(1):121–36.
20. Kingston JK, Bayly WM. Effect of exercise on acid-base status of horses. Vet Clin North Am Equine Pract 1998;14(1):61–73.
21. Whitehair KJ, Haskins SC, Whitehair JG, et al. Clinical applications of quantitative acid-base chemistry. J Vet Intern Med 1995;9(1):1–11.
22. Johnson PJ. Electrolyte and acid-base disturbances in the horse. Vet Clin North Am Equine Pract 1995;11(3):491–514.
23. Constable PD, Hinchcliff KW, Muir WW 3rd. Comparison of anion gap and strong ion gap as predictors of unmeasured strong ion concentration in plasma and serum from horses. Am J Vet Res 1998;59(7):881–7.
24. Hollidge-Horvat MG, Parolin ML, Wong D, et al. Effect of induced metabolic acidosis on human skeletal muscle metabolism during exercise. Am J Physiol 1999;277(4 Pt 1):E647–58.
25. Chasiotis D, Hultman E, Sahlin K. Acidotic depression of cyclic AMP accumulation and phosphorylase b to a transformation in skeletal muscle of man. J Physiol 1983;335:197–204.
26. Gevers W, Dowdle E. The effect of pH on glycolysis in vitro. Clin Sci 1963;25:343–9.
27. Trivedi B, Danforth WH. Effect of pH on the kinetics of frog muscle phosphofructokinase. J Biol Chem 1966;241(17):4110–12.
28. Nakamaru Y, Schwartz A. The influence of hydrogen ion concentration on calcium binding and release by skeletal muscle sarcoplasmic reticulum. J Gen Physiol 1972;59(1):22–32.
29. Fabiato A, Fabiato F. Effects of pH on the myofilaments and the sarcoplasmic reticulum of skinned cells from cardiac and skeletal muscles. J Physiol 1978;276:233–55.
30. Fitts RH, Courtright JB, Kim DH, et al. Muscle fatigue with prolonged exercise: contractile and biochemical alterations. Am J Physiol 1982;242(1):C65–73.
31. Cooke R, Pate E. The effects of ADP and phosphate on the contraction of muscle fibers. Biophys J 1985;48(5):789–98.
32. Wilkie DR. Muscular fatigue: effects of hydrogen ions and inorganic phosphate. Fed Proc 1986;45(13):2921–3.
33. Westerblad H, Allen DG, Lannergren J. Muscle fatigue: lactic acid or inorganic phosphate the major cause? News Physiol Sci 2002;17:17–21.
34. Williams GJ, Collins S, Muir JR, et al. Observations on the interaction of calcium and hydrogen ions on ATP hydrolysis by the contractile elements of cardiac muscle. Recent Adv Stud Cardiac Struct Metab 1975;5:273–80.
35. Donaldson SK, Hermansen L, Bolles L. Differential, direct effects of H^+ on Ca^{2+}-activated force of skinned fibers from the soleus, cardiac and adductor magnus muscles of rabbits. Pflugers Arch 1978;376(1):55–65.
36. Mainwood GW, Worsley-Brown P. The effects of extracellular pH and buffer concentration on the efflux of lactate from frog sartorius muscle. J Physiol 1975;250(1):1–22.
37. Pedersen TH, Nielsen OB, Lamb GD, et al. Intracellular acidosis enhances the excitability of working muscle. Science 2004;305(5687):1144–7.
38. Pedersen TH, de Paoli F, Nielsen OB. Increased excitability of acidified skeletal muscle: role of chloride conductance. J Gen Physiol 2005;125(2):237–46.
39. Furusawa K, Kerridge PM. The hydrogen ion concentration of the muscles of the cat. J Physiol 1927;63(1):33–41.
40. Allen DG, Lamb GD, Westerblad H. Skeletal muscle fatigue: cellular mechanisms. Physiol Rev 2008;88(1):287–332.
41. Chin ER, Allen DG. The contribution of pH-dependent mechanisms to fatigue at

different intensities in mammalian single muscle fibres. J Physiol 1998;512(Pt 3):831–40.
42. Jones NL, Sutton JR, Taylor R, et al. Effect of pH on cardiorespiratory and metabolic responses to exercise. J Appl Physiol 1977;43(6):959–64.
43. Ehrsam RE, Heigenhauser GJ, Jones NL. Effect of respiratory acidosis on metabolism in exercise. J Appl Physiol 1982;53(1):63–9.
44. Spriet LL, Matsos CG, Peters SJ, et al. Effects of acidosis on rat muscle metabolism and performance during heavy exercise. Am J Physiol 1985;248(3 Pt 1):C337–47.
45. de Paoli FV, Ortenblad N, Pedersen TH, et al. Lactate per se improves the excitability of depolarized rat skeletal muscle by reducing the Cl^- conductance. J Physiol 2010;588(Pt 23):4785–94.
46. Bandschapp O, Soule CL, Iaizzo PA. Lactic acid restores skeletal muscle force in an in-vitro fatigue model: are voltage-gated chloride channels involved? Am J Physiol Cell Physiol 2012.
47. Sejersted OM, Sjogaard G. Dynamics and consequences of potassium shifts in skeletal muscle and heart during exercise. Physiol Rev 2000;80(4): 1411–81.
48. Cairns SP, Lindinger MI. Do multiple ionic interactions contribute to skeletal muscle fatigue? J Physiol 2008;586(17): 4039–54.
49. McKenna MJ, Bangsbo J, Renaud JM. Muscle K^+, Na^+, and Cl disturbances and Na^+-K^+ pump inactivation: implications for fatigue. J Appl Physiol 2008;104(1):288–95.
50. Nielsen OB, de Paoli F, Overgaard K. Protective effects of lactic acid on force production in rat skeletal muscle. J Physiol 2001;536(Pt 1):161–6.
51. Kristensen M, Albertsen J, Rentsch M, et al. Lactate and force production in skeletal muscle. J Physiol 2005;562(Pt 2):521–6.
52. Fitts RH. Cellular mechanisms of muscle fatigue. Physiol Rev 1994;74(1):49–94.
53. Kronfeld DS, Ferrante PL, Taylor LE, et al. Partition of plasma hydrogen ion concentration changes during repeated sprints. Equine Vet J Suppl 1999;30:380–3.
54. Graham-Thiers PM, Kronfeld DS, Kline KA. Dietary protein influences acid-base responses to repeated sprints. Equine Vet J Suppl 1999;30:463–7.
55. Forster HV, Murphy CL, Brice AG, et al. Plasma $[H^+]$ regulation and whole blood $[CO_2]$ in exercising ponies. J Appl Physiol 1990;68(1):309–15.
56. Carlson GP, Jones JH. Effects of frusemide on electrolyte and acid-base balance during exercise. Equine Vet J Suppl 1999;30:370–4.
57. Bayly WM, Kingston JK, Brown JA, et al. Changes in arterial, mixed venous and intraerythrocytic concentrations of ions in supramaximally exercising horses. Equine Vet J Suppl 2006;36:294–7.
58. Viu J, Jose-Cunilleras E, Armengou L, et al. Acid-base imbalances during a 120 km endurance race compared by traditional and simplified strong ion difference methods. Equine Vet J 2010;42(Suppl. 38):76–82.
59. Stewart CP, Frazer SC. Magnesium. Adv Clin Chem 1963;6:29–65.
60. Stewart PA. Independent and dependent variables of acid-base control. Respir Physiol 1978;33(1):9–26.
61. Stewart P. How to Understand Acid-Base: A Quantitative Acid-Base Primer for Biology and Medicine. New York: Elsevier/North-Holland; 1981.
62. Stewart PA. Modern quantitative acid-base chemistry. Can J Physiol Pharmacol 1983;61(12):1444–61.
63. Van Slyke D, Wu H, McLean F. Studies of gas and electrolyte equilibria in the blood. V. Factors controlling the electrolyte and water distribution in the blood. J Biol Chem 1923;56: 767–849.
64. van Slyke D, Hastings A, Hiller A, et al. Studies of gas and electrolyte equilibria in blood. XIV. The amounts of alkali bound by serum albumin and globulin. J Biol Chem 1928;79:769–80.
65. Singer RB, Hastings AB. An improved clinical method for the estimation of disturbances of the acid-base balance of human blood. Medicine (Baltimore) 1948;27(2):223–42.
66. Siggaard-Andersen O. The Acid-Base Status of the Blood. Copenhagen: Munksgaard; 1974.
67. Sahlin K, Alvestrand A, Brandt R, et al. Intracellular pH and bicarbonate concentration in human muscle during recovery from exercise. J Appl Physiol 1978;45(3):474–80.
68. Lindinger MI. Origins of $[H^+]$ changes in exercising skeletal muscle. Can J Appl Physiol 1995;20(3):357–68.
69. Lindinger MI, Heigenhauser GJF. Acid Base Systems in Skeletal Muscle and Their Response to Exercise. Champaign, IL: Human Kinetics; 1990. p. 341–57.
70. Lindinger MI, Heigenhauser GJF. The roles of ion fluxes in skeletal muscle fatigue. Can J Physiol Pharmacol 1991;69(2):246–53.
71. Mannion AF, Jakeman PM, Willan PL. Skeletal muscle buffer value, fibre type distribution and high intensity exercise performance in man. Exp Physiol 1995;80(1):89–101.
72. Mannion AF, Jakeman PM, Willan PL. Determination of human skeletal muscle buffer value by homogenate technique: methods of measurement. J Appl Physiol 1993;75(3):1412–18.
73. McCutcheon LJ, Kelso TB, Bertocci LA, et al. Buffering and aerobic capacity in equine muscle: variation and effect of training. Equine Exercise Physiology 1987. p. 348–58.
74. Stampfli HR, Misiaszek S, Lumsden JH, et al. Weak acid-concentration Atot and dissociation constant Ka of plasma proteins in racehorses. Equine Vet J Suppl 1999,30.438–42.
75. Gunn HM. Muscle, bone and fat proportions and muscle distribution of Thoroughbreds and other horses. Equine Exercise Physiology 1987;2:253–64.
76. Kowalchuk JM, Heigenhauser GJ, Lindinger MI, et al. Factors influencing hydrogen ion concentration in muscle after intense exercise. J Appl Physiol 1988;65(5):2080–9.
77. Lindinger MI, Heigenhauser GJ, McKelvie RS, et al. Blood ion regulation during repeated maximal exercise and recovery in humans. Am J Physiol 1992;262(1 Pt 2):R126–36.
78. Lindinger MI, Heigenhauser GJ, McKelvie RS, et al. Role of nonworking muscle on blood metabolites and ions with intense intermittent exercise. Am J Physiol 1990;258(6 Pt 2):R1486–94.
79. Kowalchuk JM, Heigenhauser GJ, Lindinger MI, et al. Role of lungs and inactive muscle in acid-base control after maximal exercise. J Appl Physiol 1988;65(5):2090–6.
80. Rivero JL, Serrano AL, Barrey E, et al. Analysis of myosin heavy chains at the protein level in horse skeletal muscle. J Muscle Res Cell Motil 1999;20(2):211–21.
81. Weijs W, Dingboom E, van Ginkel F. Experimental analysis of error sources in fibre type counts of biopsies in horses. Eur J Morphol 2002;40(3):145–52.
82. Revold T, Ihler CF, Karlstrom K, et al. Muscle characteristics in young Norwegian-Swedish Coldblooded Trotters and associations with breeding index, body size and early training. Equine Vet J 2011;43(6):701–7.
83. Eto D, Yamano S, Hiraga A, et al. Recruitment pattern of muscle fibre type during flat and sloped treadmill running in thoroughbred horses. Equine Vet J Suppl 2006;36:349–53.
84. Brooks GA. Lactate shuttles in nature. Biochem Soc Trans 2002;30(2): 258–64.
85. Harris RC, Wise JA, Price KA, et al. Determinants of muscle carnosine content. Amino Acids 2012.
86. Harris RC, Marlin DJ, Dunnett M, et al. Muscle buffering capacity and dipeptide content in the thoroughbred horse, greyhound dog and man. Comp

Biochem Physiol A Comp Physiol 1990;97(2):249–51.

87. Sewell DA, Harris RC, Marlin DJ. Skeletal muscle characteristics in 2 year-old race-trained thoroughbred horses. Comp Biochem Physiol Comp Physiol 1994;108(1):87–96.

88. Valberg S. Glycogen depletion patterns in the muscle of standardbred trotters after exercise of varying intensities and durations. Equine Vet J 1986;18(6):479–84.

89. Rivero JL, Serrano AL, Henckel P. Activities of selected aerobic and anaerobic enzymes in the gluteus medius muscle of endurance horses with different performance records. Vet Rec 1995;137(8):187–92.

90. Valberg S, Essén-Gustavsson B. Metabolic response to racing determined in pools of type I, IIA and IIB fibres. In: Gillespie JR, Robinson NE, editors. Equine Exercise Physiology 2. Davis, CA: ICEEP Publications; 1987. p. 290–310.

91. Roneus M, Persson SG, Essen-Gustavsson B, et al. Skeletal muscle characteristics in red blood cell normovolaemic and hypervolaemic standardbred racehorses. Equine Vet J 1994;26(4):319–22.

92. Valberg S, Essen-Gustavsson B, Lindholm A, et al. Energy metabolism in relation to skeletal muscle fibre properties during treadmill exercise. Equine Vet J 1985;17(6):439–44.

93. Essen B, Haggmark T. Lactate concentration in type I and II muscle fibres during muscular contraction in man. Acta Physiol Scand 1975;95(3):344–6.

94. Sewell DA, Harris RC, Marlin DJ, et al. Estimation of the carnosine content of different fibre types in the middle gluteal muscle of the thoroughbred horse. J Physiol 1992;455:447–53.

95. Bump KD, Lawrence LM, Moser LR. Effect of breed type on muscle carnosine. Proc 11th Eq Nutr Physiol Symp 1989:252–6.

96. Quiroz-Rothe E, Rivero JL. Co-ordinated expression of contractile and non-contractile features of control equine muscle fibre types characterised by immunostaining of myosin heavy chains. Histochem Cell Biol 2001;116(4):299–312.

97. Wilson JA, Kronfeld DS, Gay LS, et al. Sarcoplasmic reticulum responses to repeated sprints are affected by conditioning of horses. J Anim Sci 1998;76(12):3065–71.

98. Gottlieb-Vedi M, Dahlborn K, Jansson A, et al. Elemental composition of muscle at rest and potassium levels in muscle, plasma and sweat of horses exercising at 20 degrees C and 35 degrees C. Equine Vet J Suppl 1996;22:35–41.

99. Valberg S, Gustavsson BE, Lindholm A, et al. Blood chemistry and skeletal muscle metabolic responses during and after different speeds and durations of trotting. Equine Vet J 1989;21(2):91–5.

100. Lindholm A, Saltin B. The physiological and biochemical response of standardbred horses to exercise of varying speed and duration. Acta Vet Scand 1974;15(3):310–24.

101. Chen J, Gollnick PD. Effect of exercise on hexokinase distribution and mitochondrial respiration in skeletal muscle. Pflugers Arch 1994;427(3–4):257–63.

102. Essen-Gustavsson B, Karlstrom K, Lindholm A. Fibre types, enzyme activities and substrate utilisation in skeletal muscles of horses competing in endurance rides. Equine Vet J 1984;16(3):197–202.

103. Snow DH, Kerr MG, Nimmo MA, et al. Alterations in blood, sweat, urine and muscle composition during prolonged exercise in the horse. Vet Rec 1982;110(16):377–84.

104. Lindinger MI, Sjogaard G. Potassium regulation during exercise and recovery. Sports Med 1991;11(6):382–401.

105. Harris RC, Marlin DJ, Snow DH. Metabolic response to maximal exercise of 800 and 2,000 m in the thoroughbred horse. J Appl Physiol 1987;63(1):12–19.

106. Lindinger MI, Spriet LL, Hultman E, et al. Plasma volume and ion regulation during exercise after low- and high-carbohydrate diets. Am J Physiol 1994;266(6 Pt 2):R1896–906.

107. Lindholm A, Piehl K. Fibre composition, enzyme activity and concentrations of metabolites and electrolytes in muscles of standardbred horses. Acta Vet Scand 1974;15(3):287–309.

108. Gollnick PD, Bertocci LA, Kelso TB, et al. The effect of high-intensity exercise on the respiratory capacity of skeletal muscle. Pflugers Arch 1990;415(4):407–13.

109. Lindinger MI, McKelvie RS, Heigenhauser GJ. K^+ and Lac^- distribution in humans during and after high-intensity exercise: role in muscle fatigue attenuation? J Appl Physiol 1995;78(3):765–77.

110. Essen-Gustavsson B, Roneus N, Poso AR. Metabolic response in skeletal muscle fibres of standardbred trotters after racing. Comp Biochem Physiol B Biochem Mol Biol 1997;117(3):431–6.

111. Roneus N, Essen-Gustavsson B. Skeletal muscle characteristics and metabolic response to exercise in young standardbreds. Am J Vet Res 1997;58(2):167–70.

112. McCutcheon LJ, Geor RJ. Sweat fluid and ion losses in horses during training and competition in cool vs. hot ambient conditions: implications for ion supplementation. Equine Vet J Suppl 1996;22:54–62.

113. Harris P, Snow DH. Plasma potassium and lactate concentrations in thoroughbred horses during exercise of varying intensity. Equine Vet J 1992;24(3):220–5.

114. Lindinger MI, Geor RJ, Ecker GL, et al. Plasma volume and ions during exercise in cool, dry; hot, dry; and hot, humid conditions. Equine Vet J Suppl 1995;20:133–9.

115. Ecker GL, Lindinger MI. Water and ion losses during the cross-country phase of eventing. Equine Vet J Suppl 1995;20:111–19.

116. Harris RC, Dunnett M, Snow DH. Muscle carnosine content is unchanged during maximal intermittent exercise. Equine Exercise Physiology 1991;3:257–61.

117. Hogg RJ, Pucacco LR, Carter NW, et al. In situ PC_2 in the renal cortex, liver, muscle, and brain of the New Zealand white rabbit. Am J Physiol 1984;247(3 Pt 2):F491–8.

118. Gottlieb M, Essen-Gustavsson B, Skoglund-Wallberg H. Blood and muscle metabolic responses to draught work of varying intensity and duration in horses. Res Vet Sci 1989;47(1):102–9.

119. Taylor R, Jones NL. The reduction by training of CO_2 output during exercise. Eur J Cardiol 1979;9(1):53–62.

120. Fenger CK, McKeever KH, Hinchcliff KW, et al. Determinants of oxygen delivery and hemoglobin saturation during incremental exercise in horses. Am J Vet Res 2000;61(10):1325–32.

121. Harris P, Snow DH. The effects of high intensity exercise on the plasma concentration of lactate, potassium and other electrolytes. Equine Vet J 1988;20(2):109–13.

122. Pethick DW, Rose RJ, Bryden WL, et al. Nutrient utilisation by the hindlimb of thoroughbred horses at rest. Equine Vet J 1993;25(1):41–4.

123. Lindinger MI, McCutcheon LJ, Ecker GL, et al. Heat acclimation improves regulation of plasma volume and plasma Na(+) content during exercise in horses. J Appl Physiol 2000;88(3):1006–13.

124. Vaihkonen LK, Hyyppa S, Reeta Poso A. Factors affecting accumulation of lactate in red blood cells. Equine Vet J Suppl 1999;30:443–7.

125. Fedde MR. Blood gas analyzes on equine blood: required correction factors [see comment]. Equine Vet J 1991;23(6):410–12.

126. Taylor LE, Kronfeld DS, Ferrante PL, et al. Blood-gas measurements adjusted

for temperature at three sites during incremental exercise in the horse. J Appl Physiol 1998;85(3):1030–6.

127. Evans DL, Rose RJ. Cardiovascular and respiratory responses in Thoroughbred horses during treadmill exercise. J Exp Biol 1988;134:397–408.

128. Evans DL, Rose RJ. Cardiovascular and respiratory responses to submaximal exercise training in the thoroughbred horse. Pflugers Arch 1988;411(3): 316–21.

129. Bayly WM, Hodgson DR, Schulz DA, et al. Exercise-induced hypercapnia in the horse. J Appl Physiol 1989;67(5):1958–66.

130. Roberts CA, Marlin DJ, Lekeux P. The effects of training on ventilation and blood gases in exercising thoroughbreds. Equine Vet J Suppl 1999;30:57–61.

131. Christley RM, Evans DL, Hodgson DR, et al. Blood gas changes during incremental and sprint exercise. Equine Vet J Suppl 1999;30:24–6.

132. Manohar M, Goetz TE, Hassan AS. Effect of prior high-intensity exercise on exercise-induced arterial hypoxemia in Thoroughbred horses. J Appl Physiol 2001;90(6):2371–7.

133. Spriet LL, Lindinger MI, McKelvie RS, et al. Muscle glycogenolysis and H^+ concentration during maximal intermittent cycling. J Appl Physiol 1989;66(1):8–13.

134. Geor RJ, McCutcheon LJ, Hinchcliff KW. Effects of warm-up intensity on kinetics of oxygen consumption and carbon dioxide production during high-intensity exercise in horses. Am J Vet Res 2000;61(6):638–45.

135. Tyler CM, Hodgson DR, Rose RJ. Effect of a warm-up on energy supply during high intensity exercise in horses. Equine Vet J 1996;28(2):117–20.

136. Hopkins SR, Bayly WM, Slocombe RF, et al. Effect of prolonged heavy exercise on pulmonary gas exchange in horses. J Appl Physiol 1998;84(5):1723–30.

137. Fluid and electrolyte alteration in endurance trained horses. 1975.

138. Gillespie JR, Kauffman A, Steere J, et al. Arterial blood gases and pH during long distance running in the horse. Proc 1st Int Symp Equine Hematology 1975:450–68.

139. Rose RJ, Ilkiw JE, Martin IC. Blood-gas, acid-base and haematological values in horses during an endurance ride. Equine Vet J 1979;11(1):56–9.

140. Rose RJ, Arnold KS, Church S, et al. Plasma and sweat electrolyte concentrations in the horse during long distance exercise. Equine Vet J 1980;12(1):19–22.

141. Aguilera-Tejero E, Estepa JC, Lopez I, et al. Quantitative analysis of acid-base balance in show jumpers before and after exercise. Res Vet Sci 2000;68(2): 103–8.

142. Rose RJ, Ilkiw JE, Arnold KS, et al. Plasma biochemistry in the horse during 3-day event competition. Equine Vet J 1980;12(3):132–6.

143. Rose RJ, Ilkiw JE, Sampson D, et al. Changes in blood gas, acid-base and metabolic parameters in horses during three-day event competition. Res Vet Sci 1980;28(3):393–5.

144. Craig L, Hintz HF, Soderholm LV, et al. Changes in blood constituents accompanying exercise in polo horses. Cornell Vet 1985;75(2):297–302.

145. Ferraz GC, Soares OA, Foz NS, et al. The workload and plasma ion concentration in a training match session of high-goal (elite) polo ponies. Equine Vet J 2010;42(Suppl. 38):191–5.

146. Lindinger MI, Franklin TW, Lands LC, et al. Role of skeletal muscle in plasma ion and acid-base regulation after $NaHCO_3$ and $KHCO_3$ loading in humans. Am J Physiol 1999;276(1 Pt 2):R32–43.

147. Geor RJ, McCutcheon LJ, Shen H. Muscular and metabolic responses to moderate-intensity short-term training. Equine Vet J Suppl 1999;30:311–17.

148. Serrano AL, Quiroz-Rothe E, Rivero JL. Early and long-term changes of equine skeletal muscle in response to endurance training and detraining. Pflugers Arch 2000;441(2–3):263–74.

149. Putman CT, Jones NL, Hultman E, et al. Effects of short-term submaximal training in humans on muscle metabolism in exercise. Am J Physiol 1998;275(1 Pt 1):E132–9.

150. Romijn JA, Coyle EF, Sidossis LS, et al. Regulation of endogenous fat and carbohydrate metabolism in relation to exercise intensity and duration. Am J Physiol 1993;265(3 Pt 1):E380–91.

151. Art T, Lekeux P. Training-induced modifications in cardiorespiratory and ventilatory measurements in thoroughbred horses. Equine Vet J 1993;25(6):532–6.

152. Rose RJ, Allen JR, Hodgson DR, et al. Responses to submaximal treadmill exercise and training in the horse: changes in haematology, arterial blood gas and acid base measurements, plasma biochemical values and heart rate. Vet Rec 1983;113(26–27):612–18.

153. Sewell DA, Harris RC, Dunnett M. Carnosine accounts for most of the variation in physicochemical buffering in equine muscle. Equine Exercise Physiology 1991;3:276–80.

154. Sahlin K, Henriksson J. Buffer capacity and lactate accumulation in skeletal muscle of trained and untrained men. Acta Physiol Scand 1984;122(3):331–9.

155. Marlin DJ, Harris RC, Gash SP, et al. Carnosine content of the middle gluteal muscle in thoroughbred horses with relation to age, sex and training. Comp Biochem Physiol A Comp Physiol 1989;93(3):629–32.

156. Hinchcliff KW, Lauderdale MA, Dutson J, et al. High intensity exercise conditioning increases accumulated oxygen deficit of horses. Equine Vet J 2002;34(1):9–16.

157. Roberts AD, Billeter R, Howald H. Anaerobic muscle enzyme changes after interval training. Int J Sports Med 1982;3(1):18–21.

158. Bonen A. The expression of lactate transporters (MCT1 and MCT4) in heart and muscle. Eur J Appl Physiol 2001;86(1):6–11.

159. Greene HM, Wickler SJ, Anderson TP, et al. High-altitude effects on respiratory gases, acid-base balance and pulmonary artery pressures in equids. Equine Vet J Suppl 1999;30:71–6.

160. Greene HM, Hurson MJ, Wickler SJ. Haematological and respiratory gas changes in horses and mules exercised at altitude (3800 m). Equine Vet J Suppl 2006;36:551–6.

161. Foreman JH, Waldsmith JK, Lalum RB. Environmental stress and 3-day eventing: effects of altitude. Equine Vet J Suppl 1999;30:394–7.

162. Waller A, Armstrong S, Smithurst KJ, et al. Effects of diet, feeding and daily variation on acid-base balance in horses. Equine Comp Exerc Physiol 2004;1:153–65.

163. Baker LA, Topliff DR, Freeman DW. The comparison of two forms of sodium and potassium, and chloride versus sulfur in the dietary cation-anion difference equation: effects on acid-base status and mineral balance in sedentary horses. J Equine Vet Sci 1998;18:389–96.

164. Waller A, Smithurst KJ, Ecker GL, et al. Daily variation in plasma electrolyte and acid–base status in fasted horses over a 25 h period of rest. Equine Comp Exerc Physiol 2006;3:29–36.

165. Waller A, Smithurst KJ, Ecker GL, et al. Cyclical plasma electrolyte and acid–base responses to meal feeding in horses over a 24-h period. Equine Comp Exerc Physiol 2005;2: 159–69.

166. Baker LA, Topliff DR, Freeman DW. Effect of dietary cation-anion balance on acid-base status in horses. J Equine Vet Sci 1992;12:160–3.

167. Topliff DR, Kennerly MA, Freeman DW, et al. Changes in urinary and serum calcium and chloride concentrations in exercising horses fed varying cation-anion balances. Proc 11th Equine Nutr Physiol Symp 1989;1–4.

168. Baker LA, Wall DL, Topliff DR. Effect of dietary cation-anion balance on mineral balance in anaerobically exercised and

sedentary horses. J Equine Vet Sci 1993;13:557–61.
169. Cooper SR, Kline KH, Foreman JH, et al. Effects of dietary cation-anion balance on pH, electrolytes, and lactate in standardbred horses. J Equine Vet Sci 1998;189:662–6.
170. The effect of dietary cation-anion balance on acid-base balance and blood parameters in anaerobically exercised horses. 1993.
171. van den Hoven R, Bauer A, Hackl S, et al. A preliminary study on the changes in some potential markers of muscle-cell degradation in sub-maximally exercised horses supplemented with a protein and amino acid mixture. J Anim Physiol Anim Nutr (Berl) 2011;95(5): 664–75.
172. Connysson M, Muhonen S, Lindberg JE, et al. Effects on exercise response, fluid and acid-base balance of protein intake from forage-only diets in standardbred horses. Equine Vet J Suppl 2006;36:648–53.
173. Graham-Thiers PM, Kronfeld DS, Kline KA, et al. Dietary protein restriction and fat supplementation diminish the acidogenic effect of exercise during repeated sprints in horses. J Nutr 2001;131(7):1959–64.
174. Mueller RK, Topliff DR, Freeman DW, et al. Effect of varying DCAD on the acid-base status of mature sedentary horses with varying starch source and level of intake. Animal Science Research Report 1999:189–93.
175. Southwood LL, Evans DL, Hodgson DR, et al. The effect of roughage source on exercise performance and metabolism in thoroughbred horses. Cornell Vet 1993;83(3):243–55.
176. Zeyner A, Kirbach H, Furll M. Effects of substituting starch with fat on the acid-base and mineral status of female horses. Equine Vet J Suppl 2002;34:85–91.
177. Lactate and glucose responses to exercise in the horse are affected by training and dietary fat. 1993.
178. Acid-base responses to exercise in horses trained on a diet containing added fat. 1993.
179. Duren SE, Pagan JD, Harris PA, et al. Time of feeding and fat supplementation affect plasma concentrations of insulin and metabolites during exercise. Equine Vet J Suppl 1999;30:479–84.
180. Storage and mobilization of muscle glycogen in exercising horses fed a fat-supplemented diet. 1990.
181. Aguilera-Tejero E, Estepa JC, Lopez I, et al. Arterial blood gases and acid-base balance in healthy young and aged horses. Equine Vet J 1998;30(4):352–4.
182. Grandy JL, Steffey EP, Miller M. Arterial blood PO_2 and PCO_2 in horses during early halothane-oxygen anaesthesia. Equine Vet J 1987;19(4):314–18.
183. Brakenhoff JE, Holcombe SJ, Hauptman JG, et al. The prevalence of laryngeal disease in a large population of competition draft horses. Vet Surg 2006;35(6):579–83.
184. Tate LP, Corbett WT, Bishop BJ, et al. Blood gas tensions, acid-base status, heart rates, and venous profiles in exercising horses with laryngeal hemiplegia before and after corrective surgery. Vet Surg 1993;22(3): 177–83.
185. Christley RM, Hodgson DR, Evans DL, et al. Cardiorespiratory responses to exercise in horses with different grades of idiopathic laryngeal hemiplegia. Equine Vet J 1997;29(1):6–10.
186. King CM, Evans DL, Rose RJ. Cardiorespiratory and metabolic responses to exercise in horses with various abnormalities of the upper respiratory tract. Equine Vet J 1994;26(3):220–5.
187. Bayly WM, Grant BD, Modransky PD. Arterial blood gas tensions during exercise in a horse with laryngeal hemiplegia, before and after corrective surgery. Res Vet Sci 1984;36(2): 256–8.
188. Couetil LL, Denicola DB. Blood gas, plasma lactate and bronchoalveolar lavage cytology analyzes in racehorses with respiratory disease. Equine Vet J Suppl 1999;30:77–82.
189. Schott HC 2nd, Hinchcliff KW. Fluids, electrolytes, and bicarbonate. Vet Clin North Am Equine Pract 1993;9(3):577–604.
190. Carr AJ, Hopkins WG, Gore CJ. Effects of acute alkalosis and acidosis on performance: a meta-analysis. Sports Med 2011;41(10):801–14.
191. Harkins JD, Kamerling SG. Effects of induced alkalosis on performance in thoroughbreds during a 1,600-m race. Equine Vet J 1992;24(2):94–8.
192. Greenhaff PL, Snow DH, Harris RC, et al. Bicarbonate loading in the thoroughbred: dose, method of administration and acid-base changes. Equine Vet J Suppl 1990;9:83–5.
193. Kline KH, Foreman JH, Hanson MS, et al. Changes in blood gases and electrolytes of horses given varying doses of sodium bicarbonate. J Equine Vet Sci 1995;15:487–91.
194. Lloyd DR, Rose RJ. Effects of sodium bicarbonate on fluid, electrolyte and acid-base balance in racehorses. Br Vet J 1995;151(5):523–45.
195. Rivas LJ, Hinchcliff KW, Kohn CW, et al. Effect of sodium bicarbonate administration on blood constituents of horses. Am J Vet Res 1997;58(6):658–63.
196. Effects of several alkalinising agents on acid base balance in horses. 1996.
197. Hanson CM, Kline KH, Foreman JH, et al. The effects of sodium bicarbonate administered nasogastrically on plasma volume, electrolytes and blood gases in resting quarter horses. J Equine Vet Sci 1993;10:593–5.
198. Kitaoka Y, Masuda H, Mukai K, et al. Effect of training and detraining on monocarboxylate transporter (MCT) 1 and MCT4 in Thoroughbred horses. Exp Physiol 2011;96(3):348–55.
199. Juel C. Current aspects of lactate exchange: lactate/H^+ transport in human skeletal muscle. Eur J Appl Physiol 2001;86(1):12–16.
200. Kelso TB, Hodgson DR, Visscher AR, et al. Some properties of different skeletal muscle fiber types: comparison of reference bases. J Appl Physiol 1987;62(4):1436–41.
201. Greenhaff PL, Harris RC, Snow DH, et al. The influence of metabolic alkalosis upon exercise metabolism in the thoroughbred horse. Eur J Appl Physiol Occup Physiol 1991;63(2):129–34.
202. Casey A, Greenhaff PL. Does dietary creatine supplementation play a role in skeletal muscle metabolism and performance? Am J Clin Nutr 2000;72(2 Suppl):607S–17S.
203. Schuback K, Essen-Gustavsson B, Persson SG. Effect of creatine supplementation on muscle metabolic response to a maximal treadmill exercise test in Standardbred horses. Equine Vet J 2000;32(6):533–40.
204. Hinchcliff KW, Morley PS, Guthrie A. Use of furosemide for exercise-induced pulmonary hemorrhage in racehorses. J Am Vet Med Assoc 2011;239(11): 1407.
205. Hinchcliff KW, Morley PS, Guthrie AJ. Efficacy of furosemide for prevention of exercise-induced pulmonary hemorrhage in Thoroughbred racehorses. J Am Vet Med Assoc 2009;235(1):76–82.
206. Soma LR, Birks EK, Uboh CE, et al. The effects of frusemide on racing times of Standardbred pacers. Equine Vet J 2000;32(4):334–40.
207. Zawadzkas XA, Sides RH, Bayly WM. Is improved high speed performance following frusemide administration due to diuresis-induced weight loss or reduced severity of exercise-induced pulmonary haemorrhage? Equine Vet J Suppl 2006;36:291–3.
208. Freestone JF, Carlson GP, Harrold DR, et al. Influence of furosemide treatment on fluid and electrolyte balance in

horses. Am J Vet Res 1988;49(11):1899–902.

209. Bosken JM, Tobin T, Mundy GD, et al. Effect of furosemide on urine specific gravity and osmolality in thoroughbred racehorses. Vet Ther 2003;4(3):292–8.

210. Forro M, Lindinger MI. Frusemide results in an extracellular to intracellular fluid shift in horses. Equine Vet J Suppl 2006;36: 245–53.

211. Schott HC 2nd, Hinchcliff KW. Treatments affecting fluid and electrolyte status during exercise. Vet Clin North Am Equine Pract 1998;14(1):175–204.

212. Hinchcliff KW, McKeever KH. Frusemide and weight carriage alter the acid:base responses of horses to incremental and to brief intense exertion. Equine Vet J Suppl 1999;30:375–9.

Abnormalities of body fluids and electrolytes in athletic horses

40

Eduard Jose-Cunilleras

CHAPTER CONTENTS

Introduction

The cardiovascular system delivers oxygen and nutrients to all tissues. During exercise the cardiovascular system is also involved in transferring the heat load generated in working skeletal muscles to the skin. Heat is lost by convection (transfer between media of different temperatures), conduction (direct transfer between surfaces in contact), radiation (energy absorbed or emitted at the body surface) and evaporation (conversion of a liquid to vapor and consequent cooling effect at the surface at which the change of state occurs). In equine athletes the most important route of heat transfer during exercise is the evaporation of sweat[1] accounting for approximately two-thirds of heat dissipation. Therefore, sweating is an essential mechanism to avoid hyperthermia during exercise. Equine sweat is an isotonic to slightly hypertonic fluid with electrolyte concentrations equal or higher than that of plasma. Consequently, horses performing athletic events of several hours' duration, in which thermal balance is maintained by evaporation of sweat, will lose considerable amounts of water and electrolytes. When fluid and electrolyte deficits are not partially or totally replaced during and/or after exercise horses may develop clinical signs of dehydration and exhaustion. Clinical disorders associated with fluid, electrolyte and acid-base imbalances are most commonly observed in horses competing in different modalities of endurance rides and three-day events.

Fluid and electrolyte balance is not only important from a medical perspective but also because it relates to exercise performance. The reduction in plasma volume associated with dehydration can impair the ability to maintain adequate perfusion to the working skeletal muscle, potentially leading to fatigue, and to the skin, which may lead to excessive hyperthermia and fatigue. The relationship between hydration status and/or fluid and electrolyte supplementation and exercise performance has not been formally investigated in horses. It has been established that horses dehydrated prior to exercise will have compromised thermoregulatory function, and fluid and/or electrolyte supplementation during and immediately after exercise will hasten recovery. However, the effects of dehydration prior to exercise or fluid/electrolyte supplementation upon direct measurements of athletic performance in endurance exercise have not been formally addressed. In human athletes it is well established that exercise performance, assessed as an increase in time to exhaustion at a given exercise intensity, or as a decrease in time to complete a given distance, is enhanced by ingestion of electrolyte-containing solutions during exercise.[2]

Understanding of some concepts related to fluid composition is necessary for discussion of fluid and electrolyte disturbances, as well as disorders of acid-base balance. Concentrations of electrolytes in plasma or fluids are commonly reported in a variety of forms: weight per volume (mg/dL, g/L or %), or number of mols, osmols or equivalents per volume (mmol/L, mOsm/kg or mEq/L). One mol of any substance is the molecular weight of the substance in grams (Na^+ 23 g/mol, K^+ 39.1 g/mol, Cl^- 35.5 g/mol, Ca^{2+} 40.1 g/mol, Mg^{2+} 24.3 g/mol). Electrolytes in body fluids combine based on their charge, the number of positively charged particles (cations) and negatively charged particles (anions) is always equal, and it is often useful to express electrolyte concentrations as mEq/L. One equivalent is defined as the number of mols times its valence or number of ionic charges (valence is 1 for Na^+, K^+ and Cl^-, and 2 for Ca^{2+} and Mg^{2+}). Osmolality refers to the number of dissociated particles per kg of solvent (e.g. water) and osmolarity refers to the number of dissociated particles per liter of solvent. Those particles in solution that cannot freely diffuse across cellular membranes will exert an osmotic effect, and are referred to as effective osmols. The effective osmolality of a solution is referred to as tonicity. Isotonic fluids are those with a concentration of osmotically active particles similar to that of plasma (osmolality of equine plasma is 270–300 mOsm/kg). Hypotonic and hypertonic fluids are those with an osmolality much lower or much higher than 300 mOsm/kg, respectively. Acid-base balance physiology and its regulation is further discussed in greater detail in Chapter 39. Suffice here to say that plasma pH is determined by strong ion difference (SID), non-volatile weak buffers (A_{tot}) and partial pressure of CO_2 (pCO_2). Measured strong ion difference (SID_m) is usually calculated as $SID_m = (Na + K) - (Cl + lactate)$, in other words, the difference between cations and anions. An increased SID (due to hypochloremia or hypernatremia) will result in metabolic alkalosis, whereas decreases in SID (due to hyponatremia or hyperlactacidemia) will result in metabolic acidosis. Non-volatile weak buffers (A_{tot}) are those weak acids that are not fully dissociated in blood and have a smaller impact on acid-base balance, mainly albumin, globulins and phosphate. An increased A_{tot} (due to dehydration and increased plasma proteins) will result in mild metabolic acidosis, whereas decreases in A_{tot} (due to protein loss and/or hemodilution) will induce mild metabolic alkalosis. Finally, decreased partial pressure of CO_2 (due to hyperventilation) will result in respiratory alkalosis, and increased pCO_2 (due to hypoventilation) will result in respiratory acidosis.

Exercise-associated dehydration/ exhaustion

- Most commonly seen in horses competing in endurance events (e.g. endurance races, competitive trail rides and three-day eventing).
- Exhaustion is due to the compound effects of heat accumulation, alterations in electrolyte, fluid and acid-base, and substrate depletion.
- Therapeutic strategy: stop exercise, cool the horse, and provide access to water and hay in mild cases. In more severe cases administration of oral electrolyte solutions via nasogastric tube and/or intravenous fluids is a must.
- Prevention: acclimatization to environment in the case of extreme heat, humidity, or altitude. Administer electrolytes and offer water to horses during endurance exercise. Avoid competitive endurance exercise with unfit or otherwise unsuitable horses (e.g. overweight Quarter Horses). Provide supplementary electrolytes in the diet to compensate for electrolyte losses in sweating.

Recognition

History and presenting complaint

Exercise-induced dehydration/exhaustion is most commonly recognized as a condition that requires medical intervention in horses exercising for protracted periods in hot environments. It is most commonly observed in horses competing in endurance rides and less frequently in horses undertaking three-day events or combined training competitions. The presenting complaint is severe depression, and lack of thirst and appetite despite apparent dehydration.

Physical examination

Clinical signs observed in horses suffering exercise-induced dehydration/exhaustion include depression, anorexia, lack of thirst despite persistent dehydration, persistently elevated rectal temperature, heart rate and respiratory rate.[3,4] Other clinical signs related to dehydration and poor cardiovascular function include dryness of mucous membranes (gums, conjunctiva), delayed capillary refill time, decreased pulse pressure, and persistent skin-fold test. Dry feces, minimal urine production, poor gastrointestinal motility, poor anal tone, ileus, and colic may also be observed. Other less common signs associated with dehydration and exhaustion include cardiac arrhythmia, muscle cramps, and/or synchronous diaphragmatic flutter.

The severity of dehydration can be subjectively assessed based on the clinical signs observed (Table 40.1). Dehydration below 5% is not detectable clinically, whereas acute dehydration above 10–12% is considered incompatible with life.

In endurance competitions, horses are evaluated at regular intervals in an attempt to assure that only those capable of safely continuing to exercise remain in the competition. At each mandatory rest period ('vet gates'), fitness to continue is assessed based on examination of general appearance, attitude, gait, pulse and respiratory rates, and evaluation of dehydration, capillary refill time, color of mucous membranes, and gastrointestinal motility. The cardiac recovery index is performed routinely in some countries during the veterinary examination at a mandatory stop. The cardiac recovery index involves taking a resting heart rate, the horse is then trotted 30 m (33 yards) out and back and the heart rate is taken again 1 minute after starting the trot out. Generally, if the resting heart rate is low (50 bpm or less), and the heart rate taken after trotting is equal or lower than the resting heart rate, the horse is considered fit to continue.[5,6] Close examination of horses at the mandatory stop and use of the cardiac recovery index may help to identify those horses with significant dehydration/exhaustion, as it has been suggested in a recent study of a 160-km endurance ride in Western Australia.[7]

Laboratory examination

Routine hematology reveals alterations related to dehydration and stress, which include increased plasma total protein, packed cell volume, red blood cell count, and hemoglobin; and the total white blood cell count and differential generally show neutrophilia and lymphopenia.[8–10]

Plasma electrolyte concentrations in dehydrated/exhausted horses are variable. Moderate hypochloremia is most commonly observed after endurance exercise in exhausted and non-affected horses. However, the degree of dehydration and hypochloremia, with consequent metabolic alkalosis due to increased strong ion difference (SID), is generally more pronounced in affected horses. Although the characteristic acid-base abnormality is hypochloremic metabolic alkalosis, it is also reported that the fastest horses in an endurance race may develop mild metabolic acidosis due to lactate production,[9,11] which probably results in a mixed acid-base disorder with concurrent lactic acidosis and hypochloremic metabolic

Table 40.1 Clinical signs observed depending on severity of dehydration

	% OF BODY WEIGHT	VOLUME DEFICIT (L) IN 450 kg HORSE	CLINICAL SIGNS
Mild	5–6	≈20–30	Tacky mucous membranes, decreased skin turgor
Moderate	7–9	≈30–40	Dry mucous membranes, depression, sunken eyes
Severe	>9	>40	Cold extremities, recumbency, moribund

acidosis. In a recent study of a 120-km endurance race, most horses had complex acid-base imbalances characterized by mild strong ion alkalosis (due to hypochloremia attenuated by hyperlactacidemia), non-volatile buffer acidosis and compensatory mild respiratory acidosis.[12] Other abnormalities can include hypokalemia, hypocalcemia, hypomagnesemia and hypo- or hypernatremia. Substantial decreases in total body electrolyte content due to sweating will be poorly reflected by changes in plasma electrolyte concentrations, because fluid and electrolyte losses are isotonic and of similar composition to plasma. Plasma electrolyte concentrations observed in horses performing endurance rides and three-day events are shown in Table 40.2 and Table 40.3.

Plasma glucose concentrations in dehydrated/exhausted horses are quite variable. Hyperglycemia can occur in exhausted horses and those with heat-stroke due to high concentrations of stress hormones, such as the catecholamines and cortisol. Hypoglycemia can also occur during protracted exercise because of depletion of liver glycogen, which will lead to fatigue and altered mentation due to lack of glucose availability to neurons.

Dehydration and possibly renal disease may be apparent by elevation in blood urea nitrogen and creatinine concentrations in horses performing protracted exercise. If urine can be obtained, it may be highly concentrated due to severe dehydration, or may be poorly concentrated despite severe dehydration in cases of ischemic renal tubular damage. The use of urinary specific gravity, urinary to plasma creatinine ratios and fractional excretion ratios of electrolytes in the diagnosis and management of acute renal failure is discussed below under the heading *'Acute renal failure'*.

Table 40.2 Plasma electrolyte concentrations (from jugular venous blood unless specified otherwise) observed in horses competing in endurance rides (average ± SD, except Lindinger 1995,[12,17] Schott 2006[100] and Viu 2010[12] average ± SE)

	BEFORE RIDE	32–50 km	80–120 km	160 km	REFERENCE
Na^+ mEq/L	138.6 ± 0.5	136.4 ± 1.0	133.7 ± 1.8	–	Rose 1980[101]
	139.6 ± 2.5	–	138.5 ± 2.6	136.6 ± 4	Carlson 1974[102]
	139.1 ± 2.5	–	134.9 ± 3.0	–	Carlson 1976[103]
	139.7 ± 0.4	137.7 ± 1.2	141.8 ± 2.6	138.6 ± 0.5	Lindinger 1995[17]
	136.5 ± 1.4	–	–	130.4 ± 3.9	Schott 2006[100]
	137 ± 0.3	137 ± 0.6	134 ± 1.0	–	Viu 2010[12]
K^+ mEq/L	3.8 ± 0.1	3.4 ± 0.1	3.2 ± 0.2	–	Rose 1980[101]
	3.6 ± 1.8	–	3.5 ± 0.6	3.2 ± 0.5	Carlson 1974[102]
	3.6 ± 0.4	–	2.7 ± 0.3	–	Carlson 1976[103]
	3.6 ± 0.04	2.8 ± 0.11	2.7 ± 0.08	3.2 ± 0.27	Lindinger 1995[17]
	4.0 ± 0.4	–	–	3.4 ± 0.7	Schott 2006[100]
	3.5 ± 0.1	3.1 ± 0.1	3.1 ± 0.1	–	Viu 2010[12]
Cl^- mEq/L	99.8 ± 0.8	90.1 ± 1.1	84.5 ± 1.2	–	Rose 1980[101]
	101.1 ± 2.4	–	93.3 ± 4.3	93.9 ± 6.8	Carlson 1974[102]
	101.1 ± 2.4	–	90.8 ± 4.8	–	Carlson 1976[103]
	104.8 ± 0.6	100.9 ± 1.1	105.2 ± 1.6	101.6 ± 3.0	Lindinger 1995[17]
	97.4 ± 1.7	–	–	89.2 ± 4.9	Schott 2006[100]
	102 ± 0.4	99 ± 0.1	96 ± 1.3	–	Viu 2010[12]
iCa^{2+} mmol/L	1.8 ± 0.01	1.6 ± 0.05	1.6 ± 0.03	1.6 ± 0.03	Lindinger 1995[17]
	1.6 ± 0.01	–	1.4 ± 0.01	–	Aguilera-Tejero 2001[104]
	1.6 ± 0.04	–	–	1.37 ± 0.08	Schott 2006[100]
	1.6 ± 0.01	1.5 ± 0.03	1.5 ± 0.03	–	Viu 2010[12]
tCa^{2+} mmol/L	3.1 ± 0.2	–	2.6 ± 0.2	2.7 ± 0.2	Carlson 1974[102]
	3.1 ± 0.2	–	2.9 ± 0.4	–	Carlson 1976[103]
	3.2 ± 0.1	–	–	3.1 ± 0.1	Schott 2006[100]
tMg^{2+} mmol/L	0.78 ± 0.04	–	0.70 ± 0.08	0.74 ± 0.12	Carlson 1974[102]
	0.80 ± 0.08	–	0.86 ± 0.20	–	Carlson 1976[103]
HCO_3^- mEq/L	25.4 ± 1.7	26.5 ± 3	25.8 ± 4.2	–	Rose 1979[9]
	24.4 ± 0.4	26.4 ± 1	25.3 ± 1.4	–	Rose 1980[101]
	29.5 ± 2.4	–	32.7 ± 2.3	–	Carlson 1976[103]
	29.9 ± 1.6	–	–	31.4 ± 3.7	Schott 2006[100]
	29 ± 0.3	32 ± 0.7	30 ± 0.6	–	Viu 2010[12]
Total protein g/L	65 ± 7	76 ± 7	89 ± 11	–	Rose 1979[101]
	67 ± 3	–	72 ± 6	67 ± 4	Carlson 1974[102]
	70 ± 4	–	–	79 ± 7	Carlson 1976[103]
	66 ± 2	73 ± 1	72 ± 2	69 ± 3	Lindinger 1995[17]
	73 ± 4	–	–	74 ± 5	Schott 2006[100]
	66 ± 1	74 ± 1	75 ± 1	–	Viu 2010[12]

iCa^{2+}, ionized calcium; tCa^{2+} total calcium; tMg^{2+} total magnesium.

Table 40.3 Plasma electrolytes concentrations observed in horses competing in three-day event competitions (average ± SD, except Ecker 1995[20] average ± SE)

	BEFORE RIDE	END PHASE B	END PHASE C	END PHASE D	REFERENCE
Na^+ mEq/L	139.0 ± 1.6	143.5 ± 2.7	141.5 ± 1.6	143.7 ± 2.9	Williamson 1996[105]
	137.6 ± 4.1	–	–	143.5 ± 7.3	Andrews 1995[19]
	139 ± 2	–	–	142 ± 2	Marlin 1995[21]
	135 ± 1.2	–	–	134 ± 2.3	Hinchcliff 1995[106]
	140.2 ± 0.3	–	144.0 ± 0.5	–	Ecker 1995[20]
K^+ mEq/L	3.5 ± 0.5	5.2±0.7	4.2 ± 0.5	4.5 ± 0.7	Williamson 1996[105]
	3.6 ± 0.3	–	–	4.2 ± 0.3	Andrews 1995[19]
	3.6 ± 0.4	–	–	3.8 ± 0.3	Marlin 1995[21]
	4.0 ± 0.3	–	–	3.9 ± 0.2	Hinchcliff 1995[106]
	3.7 ± 0.1	–	3.7 ± 0.1	–	Ecker 1995[20]
Cl^- mEq/L	104.5 ± 1.2	104.4 ± 1.7	102.3 ± 1.7	102.4 ± 2.8	Williamson 1996[105]
	103 ± 5.3	–	–	97.7 ± 5.5	Andrews 1995[19]
	99 ± 2	–	–	96 ± 1	Marlin 1995[21]
	101 ± 1.9	–	–	97 ± 1.8	Hinchcliff 1995[106]
	102.2 ± 0.6	–	102.7 ± 0.5	–	Ecker 1995[20]
tCa^{2+} mmol/L	3.1 ± 0.1	3.0 ± 0.1	3.0 ± 0.1	3.1 ± 0.2	Williamson 1996[105]
	3.2 ± 0.2	–	–	3.3 ± 0.2	Andrews 1995[19]
	3.0 ± 0.1	–	–	3.0 ± 0.2	Marlin 1995[21]
	3.0 ± 0.1	–	–	2.9 ± 0.1	Hinchcliff 1995[106]
iCa^{2+} mmol/L	1.7 ± 0.07	1.5 ± 0.07	1.5 ± 0.07	1.4 ± 0.1	Williamson 1996[105]
	1.7 ± 0.1	–	–	1.4 ± 0.1	Andrews 1995[19]
	1.9 ± 0.05	–	–	1.6 ± 0.1	Hinchcliff 1995[106]
	1.6 ± 0.02	–	1.2 ± 0.05	–	Ecker 1995[20]
tMg^{2+} mmol/L	0.75 ± 0.05	–	–	0.72 ± 0.08	Marlin 1995[21]
HCO_3^- mmol/L	29.5 ± 0.7	–	–	23.7 ± 3.1	Hinchcliff 1995[106]
pH	7.37 ± 0.02	7.30 ± 0.06	7.42 ± 0.03	7.30 ± 0.09	Williamson 1996[105]
	7.40 ± 0.02	–	–	7.31 ± 0.1	Andrews 1995[19]
	7.41 ± 0.03	–	–	7.38 ± 0.05	Hinchcliff 1995[106]
Total protein g/L	66.6 ± 5.6	75.9 ± 4.1	69.8 ± 4.0	77.6 ± 5.0	Williamson 1996[105]
	65 ± 4	–	–	77 ± 5	Andrews 1995[19]
	65.7 ± 2.6	–	–	74.9 ± 3.0	Marlin 1995[21]
	61.8 ± 2.6	–	–	71.8 ± 3.3	Hinchcliff 1995[106]
	75.2 ± 1.3	–	79 ± 1.3	–	Ecker 1995[20]

iCa^{2+}, ionized calcium; tCa^{2+} total calcium; tMg^{2+} total magnesium.

Plasma concentrations of creatine kinase (CK) and aspartate aminotransferase (AST or GOT) may be elevated as a consequence of recent muscular activity, and in case of exertional rhabdomyolysis these enzymes are elevated 20–100-fold or more.

Treatment and prognosis

Prognosis varies from favorable to very grave depending upon severity of clinical signs, promptness of medical therapy, and potential complications. Exercise-induced dehydration and exhaustion is responsive to medical therapy if fluid therapy is aggressive. Unfortunately, loss of horses competing in endurance events still occurs, and the importance of close veterinary supervision and diligent therapeutic intervention cannot be overemphasized.

Immediate care should include stopping exercise and, if possible, moving the horse into the shade. If available, fans should be placed close to the horse to promote cooling. The horse should be cooled by repeated rinsing/bathing with abundant volume of cold water over the entire body. In studies performed under field and laboratory conditions, repeated application of cold water over the entire body surface decreases rectal temperature more quickly than no bathing or bathing with water at ambient temperature.[13,14] These treatments do not cause muscle cramps or myopathies. Wet sheets or towels left in place over the horse's neck or trunk should be avoided, unless cold water is sprayed repeatedly because wet towels will only serve to provide unneeded insulation in a heat-compromised patient.[3]

The choice of oral versus intravenous fluid administration or a combination of both should be based mostly on severity of the clinical signs, but cost and manpower may be other considerations. Oral fluid therapy may be considered in mildly affected horses that may not drink sufficiently on their own. It is generally recommended to administer isotonic electrolyte solutions at a rate of 6–8 liters every 30–60 minutes via nasogastric tube. Contraindications for oral fluid therapy are nasogastric reflux and signs of colic. If the patient's clinical condition does not improve within the following

2–4 hours, intravenous fluids should be administered as soon as possible. Table 40.4 lists some recipes for homemade isotonic solutions.

A balanced polyionic solution that is approximately isotonic is recommended. To that effect, Carlson[4] described the following formula, which is similar in composition to electrolytes lost in sweat and is close to isotonic:

Mix 1 level tablespoon of table salt (16.6 g NaCl) and 1 level tablespoon of Lite salt (16.9 g of 50:50 mixture of NaCl:KCl) in 4 L (~1 gallon) of water (Na^+ 107 mEq/L, K^+ 28 mEq/L and Cl^- 135 mEq/L, 270 mOsm/L).[4]

The effect of tonicity, glucose supplementation and temperature of oral electrolyte solutions is discussed below under the heading *'Rehydration after exercise'*.

Intravenous fluid therapy

Intravenous fluids are classified as crystalloids or colloids. Crystalloid fluids are solutions containing electrolyte and non-electrolyte solutes capable of distributing among the body compartments. Colloid fluids contain large-molecular-weight particles, which do not normally pass through capillary membranes, and some smaller more diffusible particles. Colloid fluids include dextrans, glucose polymer mixtures of low (dextran 40) or high-molecular-weight (dextran 70 and dextran 75), gelatins, modified bovine collagens (oxypolygelatin), and hydroxyethyl starch preparations (hetastarch and pentastarch). Colloid fluids are indicated in those patients suffering increased capillary permeability and hypoproteinemia. Exhausted and dehydrated athletic horses will not generally require colloid fluids. Therefore, the following discusses the administration of crystalloid fluids that are used commonly in field situations for treatment of athletic horses.

The ionic composition, pH and osmolality of commonly used crystalloid fluids are presented in Table 40.5. The composition of polyionic fluids resembles that of extracellular fluid. Note that Ringer's solution and 0.9% saline solution have a relative excess of sodium, and especially chloride, when compared to extracellular fluid concentrations. Exhausted/dehydrated horses generally have

Table 40.4 Composition and tonicity of homemade recipes for electrolyte solutions for nasogastric administration

	1 LITER	1 GALLON (3.8 LITERS)	ELECTROLYTE COMPOSITION (mEq/L)	TONICITY
0.45% NaCl	4.5 g (0.16 oz)	17 g (0.6 oz, 1 tbsp)	Na^+ 77 and Cl^- 77	hypotonic
0.9% NaCl	9 g (0.32 oz)	34 g (1.2 oz, 2 tbsp)	Na^+ 154 and Cl^- 154	isotonic
Dr Carlson's formula[4]	–	1 tbsp table salt + 1 tbsp Lite salt in 4 liters	Na^+ 107 , K^+ 28 and Cl^- 135	isotonic
Dr Smith's formula[107]	–	1 part $CaCO_3$ (ground limestone) + 3 parts Lite salt; 2 oz per gallon	Na^+ 96, K^+ 75, Cl^- 154, Ca^{2+} 75 and HCO_3^- 25	slightly hypertonic
Dr Monreal's formula[108]	6 g NaCl + 3 g KCl	23 g (0.8 oz) NaCl + 11.5 g KCl (0.4 oz) per gallon	Na^+ 103, K^+ 40, Cl^- 143	isotonic

Note: Lite salt: mixture of KCl:NaCl at 50:50, Morton Lite salt mixture, Morton International, Rohm and Haas, Philadelphia, PA, USA; tsp, teaspoon (5 mL); tbsp, tablespoon (15 mL), oz, ounce (28.35 g), 1 US gallon = 3.8 L.

Table 40.5 Electrolyte composition of selected common sterile intravenous fluids

	Na^+ (mEq/L)	K^+ (mEq/L)	Cl^- (mEq/L)	Ca^{2+} (mEq/L)	Mg^{2+} (mEq/L)	Buffer‡ (mEq/L)	pH	mOsm/L	SID
0.9% NaCl	154	0	154	0	0	0	5.0	308	0
Dextrose 2.5% in 0.45% NaCl	77	0	77	0	0	0	4.5	280	0
Ringer's solution[a]	147	4	156	4	0	0	5.5	310	0
Lactated Ringer's sol.[b]	130	4	109	3	0	28 (L)	6.5	274	28
Plasma-Lyte A[c] and Normosol-R[d]	140	5	98	0	3	27 (A)	7.4	294	50

‡Buffers used: lactate (L), acetate (A).
[a]Ringer's injection, Abbott Laboratories, Abbott Park, IL, USA.
[b]Lactated Ringer's injection, Abbott Laboratories, Abbott Park, IL, USA.
[c]Plasma-Lyte A, Baxter Healthcare Corp, Deerfield, IL, USA.
[d]Normosol-R, Abbott Laboratories, Abbott Park, IL, USA.

Recognition

History and presenting complaint

Horses afflicted with acute renal failure (ARF) will generally have a history of participating in an athletic event that induced moderate or severe dehydration and frequently concomitant NSAID administration. The presenting complaint may be oliguria (decreased urine production), although urine production may be variable.

Physical examination

Acute renal failure is generally suspected in horses showing marked depression, anorexia, and a lack of urine production within the first 6–12 h of initiation of fluid therapy. Alternatively, affected horses are unable to concentrate urine despite clinical signs of dehydration. However, clinical signs observed are most often those related to the inciting condition.

Renal ultrasonography may be of use in diagnosing acute renal failure. Nephrolithiasis and congenital renal disorders may be ruled out by renal ultrasonography. Ultrasonographic findings described in horses with ARF include perirenal edema, loss of detail of the corticomedullary junction, or dilation of the renal pelvis.[86]

Laboratory examination

Plasma biochemical measurements of horses with acute renal failure will demonstrate increases in plasma urea nitrogen (also referred as BUN) and creatinine concentrations (i.e. azotemia). However, azotemia is only indicative of decreased glomerular filtration and may be solely a consequence of dehydration (prerenal ARF). Determination of the specific gravity of the urine by refractometry is one of the few readily available tests in the field to determine presence of ARF in horses. In cases of oliguria due solely to dehydration, urine specific gravity is usually above 1.025; however, in cases of intrinsic ARF it is generally below 1.020. These cut-off values will only be valid when performed in urine collected before initiation of fluid therapy or administration of diuretics (e.g. furosemide) or α_2-agonist sedatives (e.g. xylazine).

Hyponatremia and hypochloremia are fairly common in horses with renal failure due to increased loss of sodium and chloride in urine because of decreased renal tubular reabsorptive function. Hypocalcemia and hypophosphatemia are often found in horses with acute renal failure.

Urinalysis and urine sediment evaluation

Urine can be collected as a midstream catch during voiding or via urethral catheterization. It is recommended to obtain a urine sample for urinalysis assessment whenever renal failure is suspected in athletic horses.

Horse urine is normally alkaline (pH 7 to 9). However, aciduria may develop as a consequence of exercise-induced fluid and electrolyte losses. In an attempt to maintain plasma volume in the face of dehydration, renal tubular reabsorption of sodium is maximal and sodium is reabsorbed in exchange for potassium. When potassium depletion occurs due to continued losses in sweat, sodium continues to be reabsorbed in the renal tubules in exchange for hydrogen ions. This results in paradoxic aciduria, which describes a state of alkalosis in which the kidneys do not compensate by urinary elimination of an alkaline urine but rather maintain sodium reabsorption at the expense of elimination of inappropriately acidic urine.

Reagent strip analysis is useful to obtain an estimate of pH and the presence or absence of blood, protein, glucose, ketone bodies, and bilirubin. A positive result for blood indicates presence of red blood cells, hemoglobin, or myoglobin. To distinguish between these pigments one can examine the urine sediment for presence of red blood cells, examine plasma to assess if it appears hemolytic (pink or red tinge in normally light yellow plasma) and measure the activities of creatine kinase (CK, normal 145–380 units/L) and aspartate aminotransferase (AST, normal 220–600 units/L) as indicators of rhabdomyolysis and thus the potential for myoglobinuria. A false-positive result for urine protein is common in alkaline urine, and the presence of protein in urine is better assessed with other more specific biochemical assays. Proteinuria and hematuria may transiently follow exercise.[87] Proteinuria is a characteristic finding in glomerulonephritis due to filtration of albumin and other proteins into the urine. A urine protein to urine creatinine ratio above 2:1 is indicative of clinically significant proteinuria in a patient. Glucose should not be detected in normal equine urine and glucosuria may be observed in cases of acute renal failure. Ketones are rarely detected in equine urine, even in cases of catabolic states. Bilirubinuria may be observed in cases of hemolysis and liver disease; however, other plasma biochemical data (total and conjugated bilirubin, bile acids, alkaline phosphatase, aspartate aminotransferase, γ-glutamyl transferase and sorbitol dehydrogenase) may be more useful in assessing liver disease.

Sediment examination of equine urine is a simple and very useful technique to evaluate presence and magnitude of renal tubular disease and to determine presence or not of infectious or inflammatory disorders. However, sediment examination should be performed within 1 h of collection, because casts are unstable in alkaline urine. A normal horse urine sediment should not contain casts, fewer than five red blood cells and fewer than ten white blood cells should be seen per high power field. Briefly, a urine sediment examination is performed by centrifugation of a 6–10 mL urine sample at 1000 rpm for 5 min. The supernatant is discarded and the sediment is resuspended in a couple of drops of sediment staining solution and transferred to a glass slide with a coverslip on top. The sediment is examined first at low power to evaluate for casts (long cylindrical molds of protein and cells shed from the renal tubules; Fig. 40.4). The presence of casts is indicative of renal tubular necrosis. Increased numbers of red blood cells can result from inflammation, infection, and neoplasia, and it is transiently observed after exercise.

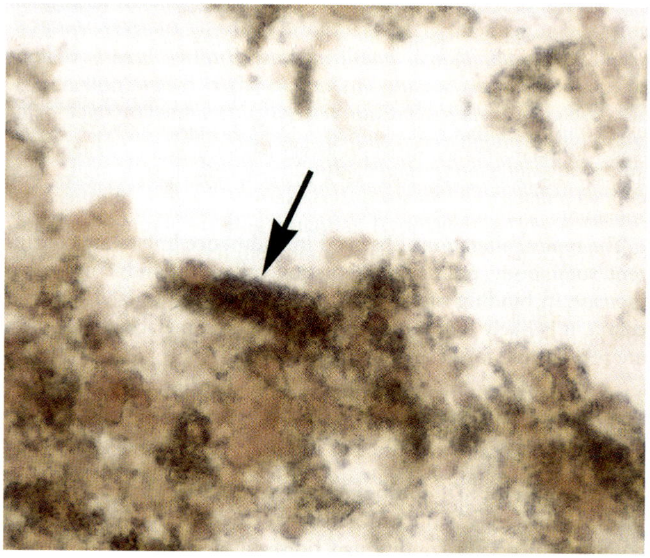

Fig 40.4 Microscopic evaluation of urine sediment from a horse with acute renal failure. Note the presence of granular casts, one of them in the center of the image (arrow) (x42).

Renal tubular function is assessed by clearance rates of electrolytes. However, the clearance rate of a substance in urine requires volumetric urine collection, which is not practical in clinical settings. Fractional creatinine clearance values, more commonly referred to as fractional excretion ratios, allow a similar assessment of renal tubular function by comparing the clearance of an electrolyte to creatinine clearance. Fractional excretion ratios are calculated after measurement of electrolytes in plasma and urine, and obviate the need for volumetric urine collection. Fractional excretion ratio of substance X (i.e. Na^+) is calculated as:

$$\frac{Cl_X}{Cl_{Cr}} = \left(\frac{\text{Urine [X]}}{\text{Plasma [X]}} \Big/ \frac{\text{Urine [Cr]}}{\text{Plasma [Cr]}} \right) \times 100$$

Normal fractional clearance values are less than 1% for sodium, less than 1.6% for chloride, 20–60% for potassium, less than 1% for phosphorus and 2–6% for calcium.[66] However, the results of these calculations must be interpreted taking into consideration fluid therapy and dietary intake. Fractional clearances of potassium, calcium, and phosphorus will vary greatly depending upon dietary intake. Potassium intake is generally adequate and excessive amounts are readily excreted in the urine. The kidneys also play an important role in calcium and phosphorus homeostasis and urinary loss of these electrolytes varies with dietary intake.

Once fluid therapy has been initiated, urine specific gravity and fractional excretion ratios will not be useful because the results are altered by fluid diuresis. However, urine sediment microscopic evaluation will still be useful in assessing ongoing renal damage.

Treatment and prognosis

Therapy for acute renal failure is aimed at removing the primary cause and restoring normal fluid balance by correcting dehydration and electrolyte and acid-base disorders. The prognosis will depend upon the initiating cause and the severity of renal damage. In those cases due to hypoperfusion or ischemia, the prognosis is favorable when the condition is treated promptly. In cases where fluid replacement has been delayed and/or the kidneys suffer multiple simultaneous insults from different nephrotoxins, as in a dehydrated horse that is 'tying-up' (rhabdomyolysis) and is given phenylbutazone, the prognosis is guarded to poor.

Fluid therapy

Regardless of the cause of acute renal failure, initial therapy should include replacement of fluid deficits (preferably by intravenous administration) and correction of any electrolyte or acid-base abnormalities. After these have been corrected, one should attempt to monitor urinary output. Other than subjective assessment of frequency and volume of urination, monitoring of bodyweight will be useful in assessing excessive fluid retention in cases of oliguric renal failure. As described under the heading 'exercise-associated dehydration/exhaustion', the fluid of choice in horses after prolonged endurance-type exercise is Ringer's solution, although other balanced polyionic solutions also are suitable.

Adjunctive medications

When urine output remains reduced after replacement of fluid deficits over the first 6–12 h, administration of drugs that increase renal blood flow, glomerular filtration and urinary flow may be indicated.

Diuretics

Furosemide is a loop diuretic; it blocks the $Na^+/K^+/2Cl^-$ cotransporter in the ascending limb of the loop of Henle, which promotes natriuresis and diuresis. The aim of furosemide administration is to turn oliguric renal failure into non-oliguric renal failure, which facilitates the management of fluid and electrolyte status. The efficacy of furosemide in treating horses with acute renal failure is not documented. In human patients with ARF, administration of furosemide does not affect the long-term outcome. The use of furosemide is contraindicated in horses with suspected urinary tract obstruction or rupture.

Mannitol is an osmotic diuretic that increases intravascular osmolality, causing an increase in intravascular volume and, as a consequence, it increases renal blood flow and glomerular filtration rate. These osmotic effects cause an increase in urinary output and may be effective in the treatment of ARF characterized by tubular obstruction and swelling of the tubular cells.[88]

Renal vasodilators

Dopamine activates dopaminergic receptors present in the renal cortex and induces increased renal blood flow and urine output when infused at 5 μg/kg/ min, without significant alteration in arterial blood pressure and heart rate. However, some horses develop dysrhythmias with dopamine infusion.[89] Fenoldopam is a selective, α_1-dopaminergic agonist that, in animal models and humans, increases renal blood flow, glomerular filtration rate, and urinary output without unwanted side effects.[90,91] The effect of fenoldopam on renal hemodynamics in horses is unknown.

Prevention

Acute renal failure in athletic horses will be prevented using those strategies that minimize the risk of development of clinically significant dehydration that may compromise renal perfusion. Avoidance of commonly used nephrotoxic drugs is of the utmost importance in horses that show clinical signs of dehydration/ exhaustion. If administration of an NSAID is considered necessary, it is advisable to delay administration until fluid and electrolyte deficits have been at least partially corrected by administration of oral and/or intravenous fluids.

Etiology and pathophysiology

Acute renal failure in the horse results from toxic causes or from ischemic or hemodynamic causes.[88,92] Causes of nephrotoxic acute renal failure include aminoglycoside antibiotics (neomycin being the most nephrotoxic), non-steroidal anti-inflammatory drugs, vitamin K_3, myoglobin, vitamin D, heavy metals, mycotoxins, and acorns.

Aminoglycoside antibiotics (gentamicin, amikacin, neomycin, streptomycin, kanamycin, and tobramycin) are toxic to the tubular epithelial cells. These antibiotics are reabsorbed from the urine and accumulate in tubular epithelial cells, which causes disruption of the cellular metabolism resulting in tubular swelling and sloughing.[93]

Phenylbutazone and other NSAIDs exert their analgesic and anti-inflammatory effects by inhibition of cyclo-oxygenase, an enzyme responsible for prostaglandin and thromboxane synthesis. However, NSAIDs inhibit also the synthesis of local protective vasodilator prostaglandins in the kidney, thereby reducing blood flow to the renal medulla and inducing renal papillary necrosis.[94,95] Acute renal failure is more likely when NSAIDs are administered in abnormally high doses or when administered to hypovolemic or dehydrated horses. Ketoprofen may be less nephrotoxic when compared to other NSAIDs.[95]

Vitamin K_3 (menadione sodium bisulfite) had been a common cause of acute renal failure in the USA before its withdrawal from the market. The development of ARF appears to be an idiosyncratic reaction.[96]

Acute tubular necrosis may occur in cases of moderate or severe myoglobinuria or hemoglobinuria.[88,92] The pathogenesis for this condition is not completely understood; hemoglobin or myoglobin casts present within the renal tubules may result in ischemic injury, and these pigments also reduce renal blood flow by direct vasoconstrictor effects. In addition, myoglobin deposited in the renal tubules appears to induce oxidative damage of components of tubular cell membranes.[97]

Dehydration and decreased renal blood flow may cause acute renal damage due to hypoxic damage of tubular epithelial cells. Tubular epithelial cells are more susceptible to hypoxia because these cells are involved in solute reabsorption, which demands a high metabolic rate and high demand for oxygen. However, due to unique physiologic and anatomic features of the kidneys, only about 10–20% of the total renal blood flow reaches the medullary portion of the kidney. The low medullary blood flow is required to provide a functional countercurrent mechanism; however, it also renders the medulla relatively hypoxic and more susceptible to ischemic injury.

Epidemiology

Incidence of acute renal failure in the general horse population and specifically in athletic horses is not well documented. The more common causes of acute renal failure are described to be ischemic renal tubular damage due to renal hypoperfusion or NSAIDs (most commonly phenylbutazone and flunixin meglumine), and gentamicin nephrotoxicity.

References

1. Hodgson D, McCutcheon L, Byrd S, et al. Dissipation of Metabolic Heat in the Horse during Exercise. J Appl Physiol 1993;74:1161–70.
2. Coyle EF, Hamilton M. Fluid replacement during exercise: effects on physiological homeostasis and performance. In: Gisolfi CV, Lamb DR, editor. Perspectives in Exercise Science and Sports Medicine, vol. 3. Fluid homeostasis during exercise. Carmel, IN: Benchmarck Press Inc; 1990. p. 281–308.
3. Foreman JH. The Exhausted Horse Syndrome. Vet Clin North Am Equine Pract 1998;14:205–19.
4. Carlson GP. The exhausted horse syndrome. In: Robinson NE, editor. Current Therapy in Equine Medicine. WB Saunders; 1987. p. 482–5.
5. Ridgway K. Inride Veterinary Examination, Postride Examination, and Judging of Best Condition. Proc 37th Annu Conv Am Assoc Equine Pract 1992:826.
6. Robert C, Benamou-Smith A, Leclerc JL. Use of the Recovery Check in Long-distance Endurance Rides. Equine Vet J 2002;34:106–11.
7. Barnes A, Kingston J, Beetson S, et al. Endurance Veterinarians Detect Physiologically Compromised Horses in a 160 km Ride. Equine Vet J 2010;42:6–11.
8. Carlson GP, Ocen PO, Harrold D. Clinicopathologic Alterations in Normal and Exhausted Endurance Horses. Theriogenology 1976;6:93–104.
9. Rose R, Ilkiw J, Martin I. Blood-Gas, Acid-Base and Haematological Values in Horses during an Endurance Ride. Equine Vet J 1979;11:56–9.
10. Snow DH, Kerr MG, Nimmo MA, et al. Alterations in Blood, Sweat, Urine and Muscle Composition during Prolonged Exercise in the Horse. Vet Rec 1982;110:377–84.
11. Lucke J, Hall G. A Biochemical Study of the Arab Horse Society's Marathon Race. Vet Rec 1980;107:523.
12. Viu J, Jose-Cunilleras E, Armengou L, et al. Acid-Base Imbalances during a 120 km Endurance Race Compared by Traditional and Simplified Strong Ion Difference Methods. Equine Vet J 2010;42:76–82.
13. Kohn CW, Hinchcliff KW, McKeever KH. Evaluation of Washing with Cold Water to Facilitate Heat Dissipation in Horses Exercised in Hot, Humid Conditions. Am J Vet Res 1999;60:299–305.
14. Williamson L, White S, Maykuth P, et al. Comparison between Two Post Exercise Cooling Methods. Equine Vet J 1995;27:337–40.
15. Schott HC 2nd, McGlade KS, Molander HA, et al. Body Weight, Fluid, Electrolyte, and Hormonal Changes in Horses Competing in 50- and 100-Mile Endurance Rides. Am J Vet Res 1997;58:303–9.
16. Ecker GL, Lindinger M. Effects of Terrain, Speed, Temperature and Distance on Water and Ion Losses. Equine Vet J 1995;27:298–305.
17. Lindinger M, Ecker GL. Ion and Water Losses from Body Fluids during a 163 km Endurance Ride. Equine Vet J 1995;27:314–22.
18. Andrews F, Ralston S, Sommardahl C, et al. Weight, Water, and Cation Losses in Horses Competing in a Three-Day Event. J Am Vet Med Assoc 1994;205:721–4.
19. Andrews F, Ralston SL, Williamson LH, et al. Weight Loss, Water Loss and Cation Balance during the Endurance Test of a 3-day Event. Equine Vet J 1995;27:294–7.
20. Ecker G, Lindinger M. Water and Ion Losses during the Cross-Country Phase of Eventing. Equine Vet J 1995;(Suppl. 20):S119.
21. Marlin DJ, Harris PA, Schroter RC, et al. Physiological, Metabolic and Biochemical Responses of Horses Competing in the Speed and Endurance Phase of a CCI*****3-Day-Event. Equine Vet J Suppl 1995;(20):37–46.
22. McCutcheon LJ, Geor RJ. Sweating. Fluid and Ion Losses and Replacement. Vet Clin North Am Equine Pract 1998;14:75–95.
23. Fielding CL, Magdesian KG. A Comparison of Hypertonic (7.2%) and Isotonic (0.9%) Saline for Fluid Resuscitation in Horses: A Randomized, Double-Blinded, Clinical Trial. J Vet Intern Med 2011;25:1138–43.
24. Hew-Butler T, Almond C, Ayus JC, et al. Consensus Statement of the 1st International Exercise-Associated Hyponatremia Consensus Development Conference, Cape Town, South Africa 2005. Clin J Sport Med 2005;15:208.
25. Greenleaf J, Castle B. Exercise Temperature Regulation in Man during Hypohydration and Hyperhydration. J Appl Physiol 1971;30:847–53.
26. Geor RJ, McCutcheon LJ. Hydration Effects on Physiological Strain of Horses during Exercise-Heat Stress. J Appl Physiol 1998;84:2042–51.
27. Sosa Leon LA, Davie A, Hodgson D, et al. Effects of Oral Fluid on Cardiorespiratory and Metabolic Responses to Prolonged Exercise. Equine Vet J 1995;27:274–8.
28. Sosa Leon L, Hodgson D, Evans D, et al. Effects of Hyperhydration on Cardiorespiratory and Metabolic Responses to Exercise in Horses during a Simulated 2nd Day of the 3-Day-Event. Pferdeheilkunde 1996;12:459–62.
29. Sosa Leon L, Hodgson DR, Evans DL, et al. Hyperhydration Prior to Moderate-Intensity Exercise Causes Arterial Hypoxaemia. Equine Vet J Suppl 2002;(34):425–9.
30. Marlin D, Scott C, Mills P, et al. Effects of Administration of Water versus an Isotonic Oral Rehydration Solution

(ORS) at Rest and Changes during Exercise and Recovery. Vet J 1998;155:69–78.
31. Freund B, Montain S, Young A, et al. Glycerol Hyperhydration: Hormonal, Renal, and Vascular Fluid Responses. J Appl Physiol 1995;79:2069–77.
32. Schott HC 2nd, Patterson K, Eberhart S. Glycerol Hyperhydration in Resting Horses. Vet J 2001;161:194–204.
33. Schott HC 2nd, Dusterdieck KF, Eberhart SW, et al. Effects of Electrolyte and Glycerol Supplementation on Recovery from Endurance Exercise. Equine Vet J Suppl 1999;30:384–93.
34. Dusterdieck KF, Schott HC 2nd, Eberhart SW, et al. Electrolyte and Glycerol Supplementation Improve Water Intake by Horses Performing a Simulated 60 km Endurance Ride. Equine Vet J Suppl 1999;30:418–24.
35. Coenen M, Meyer H, Steinbrenner B. Effects of NaCl Supplementation before Exercise on Metabolism of Water and Electrolytes. Equine Vet J 1995;27:270–3.
36. Nyman S, Jansson A, Dahlborn K, et al. Strategies for Voluntary Rehydration in Horses during Endurance Exercise. Equine Vet J 1996;28:99–106.
37. Butudom P, Schott HC 2nd, Davis MW, et al. Drinking Salt Water Enhances Rehydration in Horses Dehydrated by Frusemide Administration and Endurance Exercise. Equine Vet J Suppl 2002;34:513–18.
38. Ralston S, Larson K. The Effect of Oral Electrolyte Supplementation during a 96 Kilometer Endurance Race for Horses. J Equine Vet Sci 1989;9:13–19.
39. Costill D, Saltin B. Factors Limiting Gastric Emptying during Rest and Exercise. J Appl Physiol 1974;37:679–83.
40. Coyle EF, Montain SJ. Benefits of Fluid Replacement with Carbohydrate during Exercise. Med Sci Sports Exerc 1992;24:S324–30.
41. Marlin D, Scott C, Mills P, et al. Rehydration Following Exercise: Effects of Administration of Water versus an Isotonic Oral Rehydration Solution (ORS). Vet J 1998;156:41–9.
42. Monreal L, Garzon N, Espada Y, et al. Electrolyte vs. Glucose-Electrolyte Isotonic Solutions for Oral Rehydration Therapy in Horses. Equine Vet J 1999;31:425–9.
43. Sosa Leon LA, Davie AJ, Hodgson DR, et al. The Effects of Tonicity, Glucose Concentration and Temperature of an Oral Rehydration Solution on its Absorption and Elimination. Equine Vet J Suppl 1995;(20):140–6.
44. Gisolfi C, Summers R, Schedl H, et al. Intestinal Water Absorption from Select Carbohydrate Solutions in Humans. J Appl Physiol (Bethesda, Md.: 1985) 1992;73:2142.
45. Lacombe VA, Hinchcliff KW, Taylor LE. Interactions of Substrate Availability, Exercise Performance, and Nutrition with Muscle Glycogen Metabolism in Horses. J Am Vet Med Assoc 2003;223:1576–85.
46. Bergstrom J, Hermansen L, Hultman E, et al. Diet, Muscle Glycogen and Physical Performance. Acta Physiol Scand 1967;71:140–50.
47. Lacombe VA, Hinchcliff KW, Geor RJ, et al. Muscle Glycogen Depletion and Subsequent Replenishment Affect Anaerobic Capacity of Horses. J Appl Physiol 2001;91:1782–90.
48. Waller A, Heigenhauser GJ, Lindinger MI. Electrolyte Supplementation after Prolonged Moderate-Intensity Exercise Results in Decreased Plasma [TCO_2] in Standardbreds. Equine Comp Exerc Physiol 2007;4:149–58.
49. Hyyppa S, Saastamoinen M, Poso AR. Restoration of Water and Electrolyte Balance in Horses after Repeated Exercise in Hot and Humid Conditions. Equine Vet J Suppl 1996;(22):108–12.
50. Schott HC, Axiak SM, Woody KA, et al. Effect of Oral Administration of Electrolyte Pastes on Rehydration of Horses. Am J Vet Res 2002;63:19–27.
51. Sosa Leon LA, Hodgson DR, Carlson GP, et al. Effects of Concentrated Electrolytes Administered via a Paste on Fluid, Electrolyte, and Acid Base Balance in Horses. Am J Vet Res 1998;59:898–903.
52. Holbrook TC, Simmons RD, Payton ME, et al. Effect of Repeated Oral Administration of Hypertonic Electrolyte Solution on Equine Gastric Mucosa. Equine Vet J 2005;37:501–4.
53. Carlson G. Thermoregulation, fluid and electrolyte balance. In: Snow DH, Persson SGB, Rose RJ, editors. Proc 1st Intl Conf Equine Exercise Physiology. Oxford UK: Granta Ed; 1982. p. 291–309.
54. Argenzio RA. Functions of the Equine Large Intestine and Their Interrelationship in Disease. Cornell Vet 1975;65:303–30.
55. Meyer H. Influence of Feed Intake and Composition, Feed and Water Restriction, and Exercise on Gastrointestinal Fill in Horses, Part 1. Equine Pract 1996;18(7):29.
56. Meyer H. Influence of Feed Intake and Composition, Feed and Water Restriction, and Exercise on Gastrointestinal Fill in Horses, Part 2. Equine Pract 1996;18 (9):20–3.
57. Webb A, Weaver BMQ. Body Composition of the Horse. Equine Vet J 1979;11:39–47.
58. Warren LK, Lawrence LM, Brewster-Barnes T, et al. The Effect of Dietary Fibre on Hydration Status after Dehydration with Frusemide. Equine Vet J Suppl 1999;30:508–13.
59. Meyer H, Coenen M. Influence of Exercise on the Water and Electrolyte Content of the Alimentary Tract. Proc 11th Equine Nutrition and Physiology Symposium. 1989:3–7.
60. Jansson A, Dahlborn K. Effects of Feeding Frequency and Voluntary Salt Intake on Fluid and Electrolyte Regulation in Athletic Horses. J Appl Physiol 1999;86:1610.
61. Houpt KA, Northrup N, Wheatley T, et al. Thirst and Salt Appetite in Horses Treated with Furosemide. J Appl Physiol 1991;71:2380–6.
62. McCutcheon L, Geor R. Sweat Fluid and Ion Losses in Horses during Training and Competition in Cool vs. Hot Ambient Conditions: Implications for Ion Supplementation. Equine Vet J 1996;28:54–62.
63. Robert C, Goachet AG, Fraipont A, et al. Hydration and Electrolyte Balance in Horses during an Endurance Season. Equine Vet J 2010;42:98–104.
64. Naylor JR, Bayly WM, Gollnick PD, et al. Effects of Dehydration on Thermoregulatory Responses of Horses during Low-Intensity Exercise. J Appl Physiol 1993;75:994–1001.
65. Naylor J, Bayly WM, Schott H, et al. Equine Plasma and Blood Volumes Decrease with Dehydration but Subsequently Increase with Exercise. J Appl Physiol 1993;75:1002–8.
66. Schott HC 2nd, Hinchcliff KW. Treatments Affecting Fluid and Electrolyte Status during Exercise. Vet Clin North Am Equine Pract 1998;14:175–204.
67. Kingston JK, McCutcheon LJ, Geor RJ. Comparison of Three Methods for Estimation of Exercise-Related Ion Losses in Sweat of Horses. Am J Vet Res 1999;60:1248–54.
68. Pickar JG, Spier SJ, Snyder JR, et al. Altered Ionic Permeability in Skeletal Muscle from Horses with Hyperkalemic Periodic Paralysis. Am J Physiol – Cell Physiol 1991;260:C926–C933.
69. Gottlieb-Vedi M, Dahlborn K, Jansson A, et al. Elemental Composition of Muscle at Rest and Potassium Levels in Muscle, Plasma and Sweat of Horses Exercising at 20 Degrees C and 35 Degrees C. Equine Vet J Suppl 1996;(22):35–41.
70. Johnson PJ, Goetz TE, Foreman JH, et al. Effect of Whole-Body Potassium Depletion on Plasma, Erythrocyte, and Middle Gluteal Muscle Potassium Concentration of Healthy, Adult Horses. Am J Vet Res 1991;52:1676–83.
71. Wilson JA, Kronfeld DS, Gay LS, et al. Sarcoplasmic Reticulum Responses to

Repeated Sprints are Affected by Conditioning of Horses. J Anim Sci 1998;76:3065–71.
72. Rose BD, Post TW. Clinical Physiology of Acid-Base and Electrolyte Disorders, New York: McGraw-Hill Professional; 2001. p. 371.
73. Burger D, Dollinger S. Raisons d'élimination, Etat De Santé Et Carrière Sportive Des Chevaux Dans Les Raids d'endurance en Europe et dans Les Pays Arabes: Approche Statistique. Prat Vet Equine 1998;30:91–7.
74. Nagy A, Murray JK, Dyson S. Elimination from Elite Endurance Rides in Nine Countries: A Preliminary Study. Equine Vet J 2010;42(Suppl. 38): S637–43.
75. Leroux AJ, Schott HC 2nd, Hines MT. Ventricular Tachycardia Associated with Exhaustive Exercise in a Horse. J Am Vet Med Assoc 1995;207:335–7.
76. Holbrook TC, Birks EK, Sleeper MM, et al. Endurance Exercise is Associated with Increased Plasma Cardiac Troponin I in Horses. Equine Vet J Suppl 2006;(36):27–31.
77. van Eps AW. Therapeutic Hypothermia (Cryotherapy) to Prevent and Treat Acute Laminitis. Vet Clin North Am Equine Pract 2010;26:125–33.
78. Fielding CL, Magdesian KG, Rhodes DM, et al. Clinical and Biochemical Abnormalities in Endurance Horses Eliminated from Competition for Medical Complications and Requiring Emergency Medical Treatment: 30 Cases (2005–2006). J Vet Emerg Crit Care 2009;19:473–8.
79. Balch O. AERC Ride Related Horse Deaths. AERC Research Summit 2009;2012: http://www.aerc.org/ENOct09Research.asp.
80. Mansmann RA, Carlson GP, White NA 2nd, et al. Synchronous Diaphragmatic Flutter in Horses. J Am Vet Med Assoc 1974;165:265–70.
81. Freestone JF, Carlson GP, Harrold DR, et al. Furosemide and Sodium Bicarbonate-Induced Alkalosis in the Horse and Response to Oral KCl or NaCl Therapy. Am J Vet Res 1989;50:1334–9.
82. Oetzel GR. Meta-Analysis of Nutritional Risk Factors for Milk Fever in Dairy Cattle. J Dairy Sci 1991;74:3900–12.
83. McKenzie EC, Valberg SJ, Godden SM, et al. Plasma and Urine Electrolyte and Mineral Concentrations in Thoroughbred Horses with Recurrent Exertional Rhabdomyolysis after Consumption of Diets Varying in Cation-Anion Balance. Am J Vet Res 2002;63:1053–60.
84. Carlson G. Medical Problems Associated with Protracted Heat and Work Stress in Horses. Compend Contin Educ Pract Vet 1985;7:s550.
85. Coffman J, Amend J, Garner H, et al. A Conceptual Approach to Pathophysiologic Evaluation of Neuromuscular Disorders in the Horse. J Equine Med Surg 1978;2:90.
86. Divers T, Yeager AE. The Value of Ultrasonographic Examination in the Diagnosis and Management of Renal Diseases in Horses. Equine Vet Educ 1995;7:334–41.
87. Schott HC 2nd, Hodgson D, Bayly W. Haematuria, Pigmenturia and Proteinuria in Exercising Horses. Equine Vet J 1995;27:67–72.
88. Bayly WM. Acute renal failure. In: Reed SM, Bayly WM, Sellon DC, editors. Equine Internal Medicine. 3rd ed. WB Saunders Co; 2009. p. 1176–82.
89. Trim CM, Moore JN, Clark ES. Effects of Dopamine Infusion in Conscious Horses. Equine Vet J 1989;Suppl 7: 124–8.
90. Singer I, Epstein M. Potential of Dopamine A-1 Agonists in the Management of Acute Renal Failure. Am J Kidney Dis 1998;31:743–55.
91. Wood AJJ, Murphy MB, Murray C, et al. Fenoldopam – a Selective Peripheral Dopamine-Receptor Agonist for the Treatment of Severe Hypertension. N Engl J Med 2001;345:1548–57.
92. Divers T, Whitlock R, Byars T, et al. Acute Renal Failure in Six Horses Resulting from Haemodynamic Causes. Equine Vet J 1987;19: 178–84.
93. Humes HD, Weinberg JM, Knauss TC. Clinical and Pathophysiologic Aspects of Aminoglycoside Nephrotoxicity. Am J Kidney Dis 1982;2:5–29.
94. Gunson D. Renal Papillary Necrosis in Horses. J Am Vet Med Assoc 1983;182:263–6.
95. MacAllister CG, Morgan SJ, Borne AT, et al. Comparison of Adverse Effects of Phenylbutazone, Flunixin Meglumine, and Ketoprofen in Horses. J Am Vet Med Assoc 1993;202:71–7.
96. Rebhun WC, Tennant BC, Dill SG, et al. Vitamin K_3-Induced Renal Toxicosis in the Horse. J Am Vet Med Assoc 1984;184:1237–9.
97. Moore KP, Holt SG, Patel RP, et al. A Causative Role for Redox Cycling of Myoglobin and its Inhibition by Alkalinization in the Pathogenesis and Treatment of Rhabdomyolysis-Induced Renal Failure. J Biol Chem 1998;273:31731–7.
98. Pitts RF. Physiology of the Kidney and Body Fluids. 2nd ed. Chicago: Year Book Medical Publishers; 1968. p. 169.
99. Leaf A, Cotran R. Renal Pathophysiology. New York: Oxford University Press; 1976. p. 116.
100. Schott HC 2nd, Marlin DJ, Geor RJ, et al. Changes in Selected Physiological and Laboratory Measurements in Elite Horses Competing in a 160 km Endurance Ride. Equine Vet J Suppl 2006;(36):37–42.
101. Rose RJ, Arnold KS, Church S, et al. Plasma and Sweat Electrolyte Concentrations in the Horse during Long Distance Exercise. Equine Vet J 1980;12:19–22.
102. Carlson GP, Mansmann RA. Serum Electrolyte and Plasma Protein Alterations in Horses used in Endurance Rides. J Am Vet Med Assoc 1974;165:262–4.
103. Carlson GP, Ocen PO, Harrold D. Clinico Pathologic Alterations in Normal and Exhausted Endurance Horses. Theriogenology 1976;6: 93–104.
104. Aguilera-Tejero E, Estepa JC, Lopez I, et al. Plasma Ionized Calcium and Parathyroid Hormone Concentrations in Horses After Endurance Rides. J Am Vet Med Assoc 2001;219:488–90.
105. Williamson LH, Andrews FM, Maykuth PL, et al. Biochemical Changes in Three-Day-Event Horses at the Beginning, Middle and End of Phase C and After Phase D. Equine Vet J Suppl 1996;(22):92–8.
106. Hinchcliff KW, Kohn CW, Geor R, et al. Acid:Base and Serum Biochemistry Changes in Horses Competing at a Modified 1 Star 3-Day-Event. Equine Vet J Suppl 1995:105–10.
107. Smith C. Electrolyte Imbalances and Metabolic Disturbances in Endurance Horses. Compend Contin Educ Pract Vet 1985;7:s575–85.
108. Monreal L, Navarro M, Armengou L, et al. Enteral Fluid Therapy in 108 Horses with Large Colon Impactions and Dorsal Displacements. Vet Rec 2010;166:259–63.
109. Ott EA, Chairman & Subcommittee on Horse Nutrition. Nutrient Requirements of Horses. 5th ed. Washington, DC: National Research Council, National Academy Press; 1989.
110. Meyer H. Nutrition of the equine athlete. In: Gillespie JR, Robinson NE, editors. Equine Exercise Physiology 2. Davis, CA: ICEEP Publications; 1987. p. 673.
111. Flaminio MJ, Rush BR. Fluid and Electrolyte Balance in Endurance Horses. Vet Clin North Am Equine Pract 1998;14:147–58.
112. Schott HC 2nd, Hinchcliff KW. Fluids, Electrolytes, and Bicarbonate. Vet Clin North Am Equine Pract 1993;9:577–604.
113. Frazier DL. Synchronous Diaphragmatic Flutter. Proc 37th Ann Conv Am Assoc Equine Pract 1991:833.

41 Thermoregulation and exercise-associated heat illnesses

L. Jill McCutcheon Raymond J. Geor

CHAPTER CONTENTS

Introduction

Body heat is produced by metabolism and is also gained from the environment. In homeotherms, internal temperature is normally maintained within a narrow range (37–40 °C) by integrated neurophysiologic mechanisms that balance heat production and heat loss. Thermoregulation is the process by which the internal temperature is regulated to maintain body temperature within this thermoneutral zone. For example, during heat exposure or exercise, when heat gain occurs, the thermoregulatory system will provoke mechanisms for heat loss such that the rise in internal (or core) body temperature is mitigated. It is the most important regulation system in homeothermic animals.[1,2]

In horses, as in humans and other mammalian species, an excessive elevation in body temperature limits performance capacity. Therefore, a thorough understanding of thermoregulation and means for enhancement of these mechanisms is crucial to management of the athletic horse. The fact that horses often train and compete in hot weather, ambient conditions that substantially increase the risk of thermal injury, further underscores the importance of such understanding.

Heat production and dissipation

Core body temperature is a dynamic equilibrium between factors that add or remove heat. This balance is maintained by integration of mechanisms that vary the body's rate of heat production, alter the transfer of heat to the periphery (e.g. skin), and regulate evaporative cooling. The hypothalamus contains the central coordinating center for the various processes of thermoregulation. Specialized heat- and cold-sensitive neurons within the preoptic and anterior nuclei of the hypothalamus act as a thermostat to initiate thermoregulatory adjustments to deviations from normal body temperature. Input from thermal receptors in the skin (as well as the abdominal viscera, large veins, and spinal cord) provide information to the hypothalamus. This input, compared and integrated with detected changes in the temperature of blood perfusing the anterior hypothalamus, forms the basis for the initiation of thermoregulatory adjustments.[3,4]

The greatest disequilibrium in heat balance occurs during exercise. Conversion of chemical energy (i.e. stored substrates) to mechanical energy (e.g. muscular contraction) is inefficient, with approximately 70–80% of the total chemical energy released as heat rather than physical work.[4–6] As such, the rate of metabolic heat production increases markedly with the onset of exercise and is accompanied by increases in muscle and core body temperatures. The increase in core temperature provokes activation of heat dissipatory mechanisms such that increases in body temperature are mitigated. However, whether balance between heat gain and heat loss can be re-established will depend on the duration and intensity of exercise and the efficiency of heat dissipation. The latter is primarily influenced by ambient conditions but also modified by hydration state and by physiological adaptations (e.g. conditioning, heat acclimatization) in heat dissipatory mechanisms.[4,7,8]

Heat production

For living organisms, biologic work is either external, which includes moving the body or other objects through muscular contraction, or internal work that would include all other forms of biologic work, such as smooth muscle contraction, synthesis of molecules and compounds, or active transport within cells. With the exception of periods of growth, ultimately all this work is transformed into heat that is either stored or liberated. Energy expenditure by the body can therefore be expressed by the following equation:

$$\text{Total energy} = \frac{\text{internal heat production} + \text{external work}}{\text{expenditure performed} + \text{energy stored}}$$

The body has a basal level of energy expenditure or basal metabolic rate (BMR) that is lowest when environmental temperature range is within a thermoneutral zone. This BMR minimizes energy expenditure required to maintain normal body temperature. The BMR is altered by numerous factors, both internal and within the environment, which increase or decrease energy expenditure. Metabolic rate is normally lowered during sleep and increases with any form of work or stress. Perturbations of BMR such as exercise, fever, catecholamine release, feed consumption (thermic effect of feed), or dealing with a cold environment can therefore affect heat balance. In mammals, there have been extensive investigations of the relationship between bodyweight and heat production,[5,9] which have demonstrated that resting heat production is proportional to body mass to the power of 0.75 in adults but not in growing animals. There are, however, differences between species and it could be expected that within a species such as the horse with extensive variation in size and weight based on breed, lighter breeds may have a significantly lower resting heat production when compared to heavier breeds.[10]

Heat production in horses is influenced by dietary factors, including the quantity and quality of feed and water intake. Replacing hay in the diet with grains has been demonstrated to decrease heat production,[11] with a further reduction in heat production possible with fat supplementation.[12] When exposed to hot or cold environments, water restriction and dehydration can also reduce heat production.

During exercise, the workload or speed is the main determinant of the rate of heat production. Other factors such as the weight of rider and tack, and the nature of the terrain and footing will also contribute to the overall workload.[13,14] Heat production during exercise can be estimated from oxygen consumption data:

$$\text{Metabolic heat} = \dot{V}O_2(\text{liters per min}) \times k \times \text{exercise duration (min)}$$

where $\dot{V}O_2$ = oxygen consumption and k = amount of heat liberated per liter of oxygen consumed. Values for k range from 4.7 kcal to 5.1 kcal depending on the substrate oxidized (lowest value for pure fat oxidation, highest value for pure carbohydrate oxidation).[9]

Metabolic rate in horses is 40- to 60-fold higher during exercise at maximum oxygen uptake ($\dot{V}O_{2max}$) when compared to the resting state. For a 500 kg horse with a $\dot{V}O_{2max}$ of 80 L/min, this equates to metabolic heat production in excess of 400 kcal/min (~1.3 MJ/min) of exercise. Production of this quantity of heat without any ability for heat dissipation would result in an increase in body temperature of approximately 1 °C per minute during exercise. Although the rate of metabolic heat production is lower during endurance exercise, the overall heat load is substantially higher because of the longer work duration. For example, it has been estimated that the metabolic heat production of an endurance horse running at 8 m/s is about 150–200 kcal/min; if no heat was dissipated, this heat load would result in an increase in core temperature of approximately 21 °C per hour. These hypothetical measurements emphasize that effective heat-loss mechanisms are crucial and serve to further underline the additional impact severe ambient conditions will impose on the horse's ability to lose heat to the surrounding environment.

In contrast to most other large domestic species in which skeletal muscle comprises 30–40% of total bodyweight, half the total bodyweight of the Thoroughbred is working muscle. This higher percentage of bodyweight from muscle contributes to the horse's higher mass-specific $\dot{V}O_2$ when compared to other athletic species, including man. Furthermore, a running horse uses a greater proportion of its body mass for locomotion than does a human performing running or leg cycling exercise. Thus, the mass-specific heat load for the exercising horse is as much as two- to three-fold higher compared to that of exercising humans. Despite a substantially higher rate of heat production in the horse, the ratio of surface area to body mass is approximately 50% less than that of humans (man = 1 : 35–40 m²/kg; horse = 1 : 90–100 m²/kg).[13,14] As a result, the horse has a significantly smaller surface area over which to dissipate a relatively larger metabolic heat load and, at any given workload, must dissipate approximately four times more heat per unit of body surface area during exercise than human athletes. The disadvantage posed by a smaller surface area to body mass ratio can be partially offset by higher rates of cutaneous and respiratory heat loss. However, it is apparent that exercise is a considerable thermoregulatory challenge to the horse, with prolonged exercise representing one of the most demanding situations.

Mechanisms of heat transfer

Conductive, convective, radiative, and evaporative heat loss are the four basic mechanisms for heat transfer. Heat loss by *conduction* involves direct transfer of heat through a liquid, solid, or gas from one molecule to another. Although most of the body heat is transferred to the periphery by the circulation, a small amount moves by conduction directly through the deep tissues to the cooler surface. Heat loss by conduction then occurs by the warming of air molecules and cooler surfaces in contact with the skin. The rate of conductive heat loss is directly proportional to the temperature gradient between the skin and surrounding surfaces, and inversely proportional to the thickness of the hair coat. Heat loss by conduction from the surfaces of the head, neck and distal limbs is more effective due to a higher surface area to mass ratio in these regions when compared to proximal limbs, thorax and abdomen.

Convection represents the transfer of heat between two media, such as the skin surface and surrounding air. The effectiveness of heat loss by convection depends on how rapidly the air near the body is exchanged once it is warmed. Conductive heat loss is most effective when the warm air surrounding the body is continually replaced by cooler air, as occurs as a running horse moves through the air and/or wind speed is moderate to high. On the other hand, the trapping of air within a long hair coat will impede convective heat transfer to the environment. Convective heat transfer also occurs in the respiratory tract, the rate of which is dependent on pulmonary ventilation and the temperature difference between inspired and expired air.

Radiative heat transfer occurs when waves of electromagnetic radiation are emitted or absorbed at the skin surface. As body temperature is normally higher than the environment, there is a net loss of radiative heat energy at the skin surface. However, in hot ambient conditions, when the temperature of objects in the environment exceeds skin temperature, radiant heat energy is absorbed from the surroundings. Under these conditions, the only avenue for heat loss is evaporative cooling. A gain of radiant heat energy also occurs via direct (or reflected) sunlight. It has been suggested that solar radiation can contribute up to 15% of the heat gain in horses during exercise in sunny conditions.[15]

For the horse, the most important mechanism for heat loss is *evaporative* cooling including the evaporation of sweat from skin surfaces and water from the respiratory tract. The efficacy of this mechanism is dependent upon the extent of the vapor pressure gradient between body surface and environment. Calculations of the estimated heat loss are based on the latent heat of vaporization of water (from a liquid to a vapor – 598 kcal [2501 kJ] for each gram of water at 0°C).[16] After accounting for possible variations in the thermodynamic properties of sweat when compared to water, it is estimated that the evaporation of 1 L of sweat from the skin surface will dissipate approximately 580 cal (2428 kJ or 2.4 MJ) of body heat.[17] The quantity of heat (~2.4 MJ) dissipated in association with the evaporation of 1 L of sweat in thermoneutral conditions is approximately equivalent to the heat generated by 2 min of high-intensity exercise or 6 min of moderate-intensity exercise. In optimum conditions (i.e. when relative humidity is low) the evaporation of sweat is a very efficient mechanism of heat loss and can account for as much as 65% of total heat loss during exercise. However, several environmental factors will influence the efficacy of evaporative heat loss. These include ambient temperature and relative humidity, the extent of the vapor pressure gradient between the skin surface, and the rate of air movement.[18–20] At high ambient humidity, the vapor pressure gradient between the body surface and the environment narrows, thereby constraining evaporative cooling and increasing the rate of heat storage.

The extensive surface area of the respiratory tract also provides a mechanism for heat dissipation. This process relies upon the difference in vapor pressure between the inspired air and that of the epithelial surface of the respiratory tract. The external nares of the horse contribute considerable surface area for heat exchange. Similarly, the extensive surface area of the upper respiratory tract, including the internal nares and nasal turbinates provide an environment in which air entering the nasal passages contacts the highly vascularized epithelium of the upper respiratory tract. Horses, like humans, lack a carotid rete, a vascular heat exchanger that can serve to cool blood shortly before it enters the brain. However, horses have a unique anatomical arrangement by which their internal carotid arteries are enveloped by a pair of air-filled guttural pouches. Studies by Baptiste et al[21] suggest exercising horses utilize these guttural pouches to cool blood en route to the brain. It is surmised that this heat loss from the upper respiratory tract contributes to selective brain cooling, whereby the temperature of blood reaching the brain is lower when compared with that measured in mixed venous (pulmonary artery) blood or within skeletal muscle.[22] The extent of selective brain cooling in the horse is questionable as not all studies to date have reported a lower hypothalamic vs carotid artery temperature during and following exercise.[23]

Heat loss from the respiratory tract is dependent upon relative humidity and minute ventilation. Under cool, dry conditions, the extent of heat loss via this mechanism is estimated to be between 15 and 25% of total heat loss. In hot, humid conditions, when cutaneous evaporative cooling is compromised, respiratory heat loss may account for a relatively higher proportion of total heat loss and therefore represent 25% or more of total heat loss. While elevations in the respiratory rate increase the proportion of heat loss from the respiratory tract in these conditions, mechanical limitations imposed during exercise (e.g. the coupling of stride to respiration during canter and gallop) may ultimately limit heat loss from the respiratory tract.

Mechanisms of sweat formation

In only a limited number of species, including some bovidae, primates and equidae, is the sweat gland primarily a thermoregulatory organ.[11,24] In the horse, sweat glands are present in both haired and relatively hairless skin with regional variation in the density of glands that is not dependent on the presence of a haircoat. Structurally, the gland is similar to that of many other domestic species, consisting of a fundus and a duct connecting the fundus with the skin surface. Throughout most of its length, the duct lining is composed of two layers, with a single layer of keratinocytes lining the duct at the skin surface. Located within the dermis, the fundus is lined by an inner layer of secretory epithelium interspersed with myoepithelial cells and surrounded by a fenestrated sheath of fibrocytes that encloses a layer of connective tissue.[25] Although sweating appears to be under sympathetic nervous control, there is no evidence of direct sympathetic innervation of the sweat gland. Rather, sweating appears to occur via humoral stimulation of β_2-adrenergic receptors on sweat glands. As a result, sweating can be initiated by epinephrine (adrenaline) release in advance of any stimulus related to an increase in core temperature. However, Scott et al[26] reported peak sweating rates in standing horses in response to infusion of epinephrine (adrenaline) were significantly lower than rates previously measured by these investigators during exercise, which supported the concept of a dual control of sweating that integrates hormonal and neural input.

As most studies to date have investigated sweating rate and composition in Thoroughbred horses, the degree to which sweating rate and composition varies between breeds is unknown. To date, it appears that the basic composition of sweat is similar between breeds. Spooner et al[27] noted that sweat sodium concentration measured in Arabian horses performing endurance exercise was lower than values for sweat sodium measured in previous studies but this have been a reflection of the low sodium diet imposed for this study. Equine sweat, unlike that of humans, is isotonic to slightly hypertonic relative to plasma.[18,22,28] Equine sweat is also unique in having a high protein content, a consequence of the presence of latherin. This surface-active, non-glycosylated protein significantly reduces water surface tension, aiding the translocation of sweat fluid through the haired coat to facilitate rapid evaporation.[29] Sweat ion concentrations are largely a reflection of sweating rate and therefore are subject to alteration based on environmental conditions and exercise intensity (Table 41.1). Although there is some variation in sweat ion composition of equine sweat, individual differences in sweat composition do not appear to be as extensive in horses when compared to human athletes. Epinephrine (adrenaline) infusion will produce a more dilute sweat and may account for the less concentrated sweat produced during high-intensity exercise when compared to low-intensity exercise.[18,22,30]

During exercise, an increase in body temperature as a result of metabolic heat production is the primary stimulus for sweating. Normally, sweating is initiated at a specific core temperature and continues in proportion to the increase in core temperature.[31] demonstrated that increases in sweating rate at three different exercise intensities (40%, 65%, and 90% of $\dot{V}O_{2max}$) were closely related to elevations in carotid artery blood temperature (Fig. 41.1). Rate of rise in body temperature and the concentration of circulating

Table 41.1 Sweating rate, ion concentrations, and osmolality at two exercise intensities and three different ambient conditions after 10 minutes of exercise

VARIABLE	CD HIGH	CD LOW	HD LOW	HH LOW
Sodium (mmol/L)	124.0 ± 6.7	116.7 ± 6.1	133.6 ± 2.3	130.6 ± 1.7
Potassium (mmol/L)	25.8 ± 2.1	32.6 ± 1.4	41.5 ± 1.1	28.1 ± 0.9
Chloride (mmol/L)	142.0 ± 5.6	144.3 ± 4.3	155.8 ± 3.2	149.5 ± 2.9
Osmolality (mOsm/kg)	313 ± 18	303 ± 6	339 ± 6	327 ± 5
Sweating rate (mL/m²/min)	40.4 ± 3.7	21.1 ± 5.2	32.8 ± 5.1	27.0 ± 6.2

CD = cool, dry (room temperature [T] = 20°C, relative humidity [RH] = 45–55%); HD = hot, dry (T = 32–34°C, RH = 45–55%); HH = hot, humid (T = 32–34°C, RH = 80–85%); High = exercise at 90% of maximum oxygen consumption ($\dot{V}O_{2max}$); low = exercise at 50% of $\dot{V}O_{2max}$.
Data from McCutcheon LJ, Geor RJ, Hare MJ, et al. Sweat composition: comparison of collection of methods and effects of exercise intensity. Equine Vet J Suppl 1995;18:279–84. McCutcheon LJ, Geor RJ, Hare MJ, et al. Sweating rate and sweat composition during exercise and recovery in ambient heat and humidity. Equine Vet J Suppl 1995;20:153–7. (Refs 18, 132).

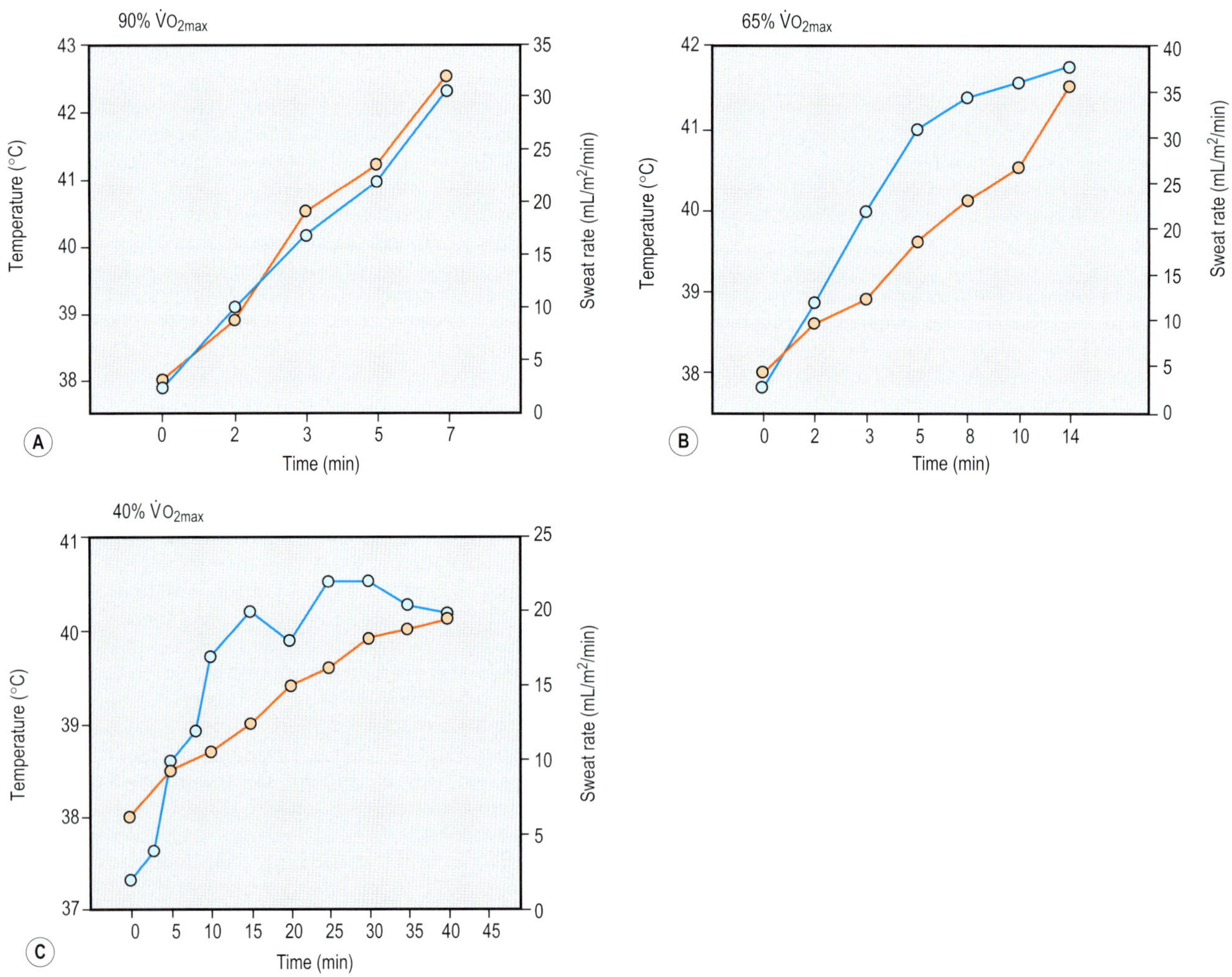

Fig 41.1 Carotid artery temperature (blue circles) and sweat rate (red circles) in horses exercising at **(A)** 90%, **(B)** 65%, and **(C)** 40% of maximal O_2 uptake ($\dot{V}O_{2max}$). Ambient temperature was 21–23.5°C.
Adapted from Hodgson DR, McCutcheon LJ, Byrd SK, et al. Dissipation of metabolic heat in the horse during exercise. J Appl Physiol 1993;74(3):1161–70, with permission from the American Physiological Society.[31]

catecholamines associated with different exercise intensities could also contribute to the determination of sweating rate.

Thermoregulation during exercise

During exercise, metabolic heat from working muscles must be transferred to the skin surface to be lost to the environment. Peripheral thermoreceptors in skin, spinal cord, skeletal muscle, abdomen, and hypothalamus detect changes in thermal load and produce a proportional output that is integrated in the hypothalamus to allow adequate thermoregulatory effector activity, particularly by the circulatory system and sweat glands. The primary physiologic mechanisms driving heat loss are an increase in the proportion of cardiac output directed toward the cutaneous circulation and an increase in the rate of sweat secretion. The increase in cardiac output and blood flow to contracting muscles enables a substantial increase in convective heat transfer away from the muscle. The circulation carries the heat to the body core, resulting in an increase in core temperature. Increasing core temperature and, to a lesser extent, increasing skin temperature provides the afferent signal for reflex increases in skin blood flow and sweating, thereby facilitating heat transfer to the skin surface and its dissipation to the environment.

Skin blood flow is substantially increased by the opening of capillary beds that are normally bypassed by arteriovenous anastamoses that connect arteries directly to veins. The increase in blood flow through the vascular beds of the skin allows heat to be lost to the environment via convection and direct radiation of heat from the skin surface. The efficacy of transfer of heat by convection and radiation varies according to the rate of air movement across the skin (wind speed) and the gradient of skin temperature to environmental temperature. Increased skin blood flow also provides the latent heat for vaporization of sweat and as well as the fluid required for sweat production. The attempt to maximize blood flow for increased activity and thermoregulation is also reflected in decreased splanchnic and adipose tissue blood flow.[32] Greater oxygen demand increases respiratory rate and respiratory blood flow and both activities will enhance the extent of evaporative cooling by the respiratory system.

Sweating rates of ~20 to 55 mL/m^2/min have been measured on the necks and backs of horses exercising on a treadmill in a laboratory.[31,33–35] Assuming a body surface area of 4.5 to 5.0 m^2 for a 500 kg horse, these sweating rates correspond to fluid losses of 6–15 L per hour. This estimate of hourly sweat fluid loss is in agreement with sweat rates calculated on the basis of the decrease in body mass during prolonged exercise under field conditions.[36] When expressed in terms of sweating rate per unit area of skin, these sweating rates are two- to three-fold greater than those reported for human subjects.

At any given point in time during exercise, core body temperature reflects the balance between heat production and dissipation. Soon after the onset of exercise, the rate of heat production greatly exceeds the rate of heat dissipation such that there is a rapid increase in muscle temperature.[37] During short-term, high-intensity exercise (e.g. racing), the rate of heat production will exceed the rate of heat loss throughout exercise and body temperature will continue to increase until the cessation of exercise. In this circumstance, a large proportion of the metabolic heat load will be dissipated during the recovery period. Conversely, during more prolonged low- to moderate-intensity exercise in temperate ambient conditions, activation of heat dissipatory mechanisms progressively attenuates the rate of rise of body temperature. Eventually, the rate of heat loss increases sufficiently to balance metabolic heat production, allowing a near steady-state core temperature to be achieved.[37]

Effects of environmental heat load on exercise responses

Not surprisingly, the thermal response to exercise is affected by the ambient conditions. As environmental temperature increases, the thermal gradient between the skin and the environment is reduced, and sensible heat loss (i.e. convective and radiative heat transfer) is impaired. When ambient temperature exceeds skin temperature (>35–36°C), the gradient for heat transfer is reversed and the body gains heat from the environment. If humidity is low, a decrease in sensible heat loss can be offset by an increase in sweating rate and evaporative cooling. As humidity rises, the gradient between skin and ambient dew point is reduced and evaporative heat loss is also impaired. The decrease in sweat evaporation is manifested by excessive wetting of the skin surface and drippage of sweat from the body. Sweat that drips from the body only removes 5% to 10% of the heat that can be dissipated by evaporation of sweat. Therefore, during exercise under conditions of high ambient heat and humidity, the rate of heat dissipation may be inadequate to prevent the progressive rise in body temperature. The impact of the environment on the rate of rise of core body temperature in exercising horses is depicted in Figure 41.2. The rate of heat storage when exercising in hot, humid conditions may be more than twice the rate occurring during exercise at the same intensity in cool, dry conditions.[20,38–40] Increased demands for respiratory heat loss are reflected by an increase in respiratory rate and during and after exercise. Kohn and Hinchcliff[41] reported a 20% to 25% increase in the respiratory rate of horses during speed and endurance tests in hot when compared to cool conditions. In laboratory experiments, an approximately two-fold increase in post-exercise respiratory rate has been observed in horses under hot, humid when compared to cool, dry environmental conditions.[20,38] When ponies were exposed to heat (41°C dry bulb temperature), there were three-fold increases in respiratory rate and blood flow to tissues of the upper respiratory tract,[42] reflecting the role of the respiratory system in heat dissipation. Similarly,

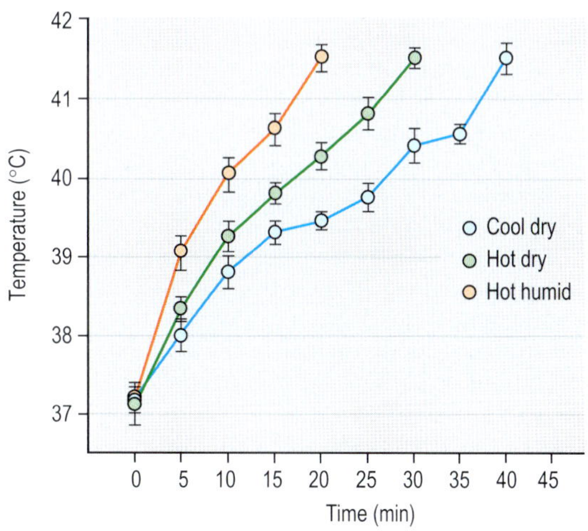

Fig 41.2 Time course of rise in pulmonary artery blood temperature (T_{pa}) during exercise at 50% of maximal O_2 uptake in cool, dry (room temperature [T] = 20°C; relative humidity [RH] = 45–55%), hot dry (T = 32–34°C, RH = 45–55%), and hot, humid (T = 32–34°C, RH = 80–85%) ambient conditions. Exercise was discontinued when T_{pa} reached 41.5°C.
Adapted from Geor RJ, McCutcheon LJ, Ecker GL, et al. Thermal and cardiorespiratory responses of horses to submaximal exercise under hot and humid conditions. Equine Vet J 1995;(Supp. 2):S125–32, with permission from the Equine Veterinary Journal.[20]

during moderate-intensity (~30% $\dot{V}O_{2max}$) exercise respiratory rate was five-fold greater in hot than in thermoneutral conditions.[32]

An important consequence of the impairment to heat dissipation during exercise in the heat is a decrease in the time to attainment of a critical upper limit in core body temperature. In humans, it is clearly established that time to exhaustion in trained subjects during exercise in the heat is inversely related to the initial level of body temperature and directly related to the rate of heat storage.[43] That the lowering of core temperature prior to the start of exercise[44] or cooling the body during the period of exercise[45] will delay attainment of the critically high body temperature and extend exercise duration is further evidence for the relationship between body temperature and exercise performance.

Several factors may contribute to a decrease in performance when exercise is undertaken in hot versus cool conditions. These include the effects of hyperthermia on brain and muscle function, and compromise of cardiovascular and respiratory function. There appears to be a critical body temperature above which mammals will not continue to exercise voluntarily, likely a protective mechanism to protect the human or animal from reaching tissue temperatures that harm cell function.[40] Thus, a more rapid attainment in critical body temperature will translate to a reduction in exercise duration.[46] In trained humans exercising over a range of work intensities in the heat, voluntary fatigue occurs at a core (esophageal) temperature of 39.7–40.0 °C.[43,47–49] Elevations in core body temperature (either through passive heat exposure or exercise) also increase serotonergic (5-hydroxytryptamine; 5-HT) and dopaminergic pathway activity. There is evidence that both pathways contribute to the vasodilatory component of thermoregulatory control and to the release of neuroendocrine hormones that can contribute to the behavioral (motivational) response to exercise. Intrinsic differences in these pathways have been proposed as one mechanism contributing to differences in heat tolerance between individuals. For example, differences in receptor density or neurotransmitter release to a given stimulus could produce variations in the thermoregulatory or behavioral responses to a given thermal load.[50] Furthermore, following heat acclimation procedures that enhance thermoregulatory mechanisms and reduce the rate of heat storage during exercise, the core temperature at the onset of fatigue is unchanged.[48,51] Measurements of central blood (pulmonary artery) temperature in horses during heavy exercise have demonstrated that fatigue occurs as blood temperature approaches 42.5–43 °C;[31,52] muscle temperature may reach 44–45 °C during such high-intensity exercise. Hypothalamic blood temperature, on the other hand, is approximately 1 °C lower than central blood temperature in horses during heavy exercise in moderate ambient conditions.[22] The difference between the temperatures in these two regions provides evidence for the existence of a mechanism for selective brain cooling in the horse. Particularly during exercise in the heat, the onset of fatigue at some critical upper limit in brain temperature may represent a mechanism to avoid heat stroke.

Human studies, dating back to the work of Asmussen and Boje,[53] have indicated that a moderately elevated, but steady-state core body temperature is advantageous to muscle function and to the dissociation of oxygen from red blood cells within muscle tissue. The increase in muscle temperature acts on glycolytic and glycogenolytic enzymes, altering flux rate through these pathways.[54,55] This Q_{10} effect is accentuated during exercise in the heat. However, at high muscle temperature (>46 °C) deleterious structural and functional alterations in skeletal muscle proteins can be induced.[56] These proteins play essential roles in mitochondrial respiration, regulation of calcium by the sarcoplasmic reticulum and the subsequent interactions of myosin and actin, and control of electrolyte movement across the sarcolemma.[43,57] As a consequence, substantial detrimental alterations to skeletal muscle metabolism may occur with elevation of muscle temperature to this critical range.

During exercise heat stress, circulatory adjustments must be regulated to maintain adequate blood flow to contracting muscle and to the thermoregulatory tissues, particularly the skin and the upper respiratory tract.[17,58] Given a finite cardiac output, the increased demands for blood flow to these thermoregulatory tissues may compromise blood flow to skeletal muscle, thereby limiting oxygen delivery and, possibly, exercise duration. Studies in ponies have provided data on the effects of environmental heat load (41 °C dry bulb) on the redistribution of cardiac output during exercise.[31] Blood flow to the fore- and hindlimbs during moderate- (~30% $\dot{V}O_{2max}$) and high-intensity (~65% $\dot{V}O_{2max}$) exercise was reduced by as much as 25–30% when compared to similar exercise in thermoneutral conditions. This reduction in muscle blood flow during exercise heat stress is likely to restrict performance and contribute to an early onset of fatigue.

A reduction in maximal aerobic power is another potential reason for decreased physical performance during exercise in the heat. A reduction in peak oxygen uptake has been demonstrated in human subjects exercising in the heat.[59–61] When non-heat acclimatized horses performed an incremental treadmill exercise test in hot, humid conditions (temperature 30 °C, relative humidity 75%), peak expired minute ventilation, oxygen uptake and oxygen pulse were significantly lower and plasma lactate concentrations higher when compared to exercise in temperate conditions (15 °C, 55% relative humidity).[62] Although the mechanism of the reduction in peak oxygen uptake in horses exercising in heat and humidity has not been determined, it is possible that alterations in breathing strategy that favor heat loss from the upper respiratory tract (dead space ventilation) and compromise of skeletal muscle blood flow result in decreased oxygen uptake and delivery. Regardless of mechanism, such a reduction in peak oxygen uptake is likely to impair performance relative to exercise performed in temperate conditions.

Physiologic factors affecting thermoregulatory capacity

The term 'exercise heat tolerance' refers to an ability to withstand high internal and external heat loads during exercise. In humans it is well recognized that high aerobic fitness and a period of acclimatization in the heat improves both physiological and psychological responses to the challenge of exercise in the heat.[63] Adaptations in heat dissipatory mechanisms improve cardiovascular stability, decrease the rate of heat storage, and increase the duration of exercise before volitional fatigue. However, highly trained athletes are also able to tolerate higher levels of hyperthermia when compared to untrained individuals: that is, volitional fatigue occurs at a higher core temperature.[64] Conversely, regardless of training or heat acclimatization, dehydration decreases exercise heat tolerance, as evidenced by an increase in the rate of heat storage and the development of volitional fatigue at a lower level of hyperthermia. There is now evidence that these physiological factors also modify the thermoregulatory capacity of horses. Specifically, conditioning and heat acclimatization improve tolerance to exercise in the heat, whereas dehydration adversely affects heat dissipation in horses during exercise.

Other factors that can influence thermoregulation in exercising horses include coat color and the density of the hair coat. Coat color will affect the quantity of solar heat absorbed, while a long hair coat will limit evaporative heat loss. Breed-associated physiological traits have also been implicated in thermal tolerance and the extent of seasonal adaptation to environmental temperature.[10,65–67]

Conditioning

Physical training in a cool environment is broadly accepted to improve exercise heat tolerance. The extent to which heat dissipatory effector mechanisms are stimulated and the duration of that stimulus will determine the effectiveness of training in improving exercise-heat tolerance. Detectable changes in heat tolerance are evident in human athletes after 1–2 weeks of training but are much more substantial if regular training is sustained for 8–12 weeks.[68–70] In human subjects, the stimulus must be sufficient to elevate core temperature by approximately 1.5 to 2.0 °C for a minimum of 30 min/day.[68,70,71]

At a given percent of maximal oxygen uptake ($\dot{V}O_{2max}$), trained athletes have a higher metabolic rate and, hence, greater heat production at any given relative exercise intensity. Despite this higher metabolic rate, the trained individual is able to maintain a similar core temperature when compared to the untrained subject, indicating an enhanced ability to dissipate heat. Improved cutaneous blood flow and whole-body sweating have been measured in trained individuals and are the main contributions to more effective heat dissipation in human subjects.[72] However, highly trained human athletes have been shown to have less extensive sweat fluid losses during exercise[73,74] and there is evidence for similar sweating economy in horses following training.[75] Specifically, eights weeks of moderate intensity treadmill conditioning resulted in a 1.6-fold increase in sweating sensitivity and an approximately 0.7 °C decrease in sweating threshold in horses during exercise in hot, dry conditions (temperature 32–34 °C, relative humidity 45–55%). Despite higher sweating rates for a given core temperature during exercise, decreases in recovery sweating rates resulted in an overall reduction in sweat fluid losses (Fig. 41.3).[75]

Enhancement in sweating economy as a result of training may assist in minimizing demands placed on the circulatory system by reducing the extent of dehydration associated with fluid losses.

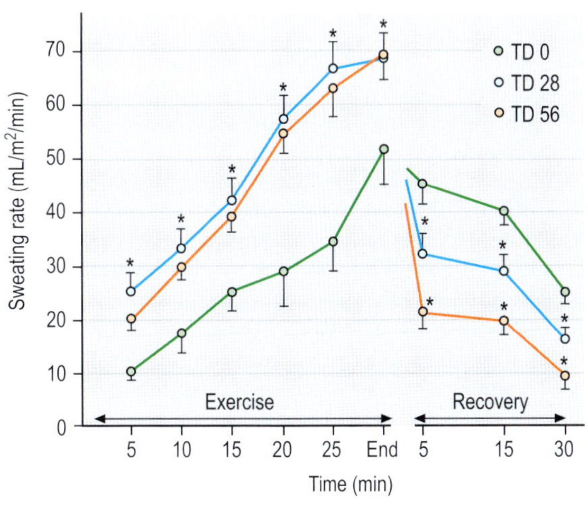

Fig 41.3 Mean sweating rate for five horses averaged for 5 min intervals during an exercise test in hot, dry conditions (32–34°C and 45–55% relative humidity) at 50% of maximal O_2 uptake ($\dot{V}O_{2max}$) on training days (TD) 0, 28, and 56 of an eight-week training regimen. *Significantly different from TD0 ($P < 0.05$).

Data from McCutcheon LJ and Geor RJ. Influence of training on sweating responses during submaximal exercise in horses. J Appl Physiol 2000;89:2463–71.[75]

Alterations in sweat composition following training in horses appear to reflect changes in the rate of sweat production rather than a modification of the sweat gland itself.[35,75] Similarly, a recent study comparing untrained and trained human subjects exercising in hot conditions reported that sweat sodium was affected by sweating rate and the expanding mismatch between sodium secretion and reabsorption with increasing sweating rate but was unaffected by training state.[76] Even a short period of training in cool conditions can provide a significant improvement in heat dissipation in a hot environment. When unfit horses completed 10 consecutive days of conditioning in a cool dry environment (19–21 °C, relative humidity 45–55%), lower pulmonary, rectal and muscle temperature were evident during the latter portion of a standardized submaximal exercise test in hot conditions (temperature 32–34 °C, relative humidity 45–55%). Whereas sweating rates during exercise did not differ from those measured in a similar test conducted prior to the 10-day period of conditioning, a more rapid rate of decline in sweating rate during recovery resulted in an overall reduction in sweat fluid losses.[77]

Improvements to cardiovascular function are one of the hallmarks of training. The increase in plasma volume, stroke volume and cardiac output all contribute to increased cardiac stability during exercise and, in particular, a lower heart rate at the same work output.[78] Expanded plasma volume in the trained athlete also improves thermoregulatory capacity by reducing the extent to which cutaneous blood flow is compromised. Increased resting plasma volume reduces the risk of a fall in cardiac output during exercise in the face of the decline in plasma volume associated with sweat fluid losses. In studies of human subjects, Roberts et al[79] observed earlier onset of cutaneous vasodilation in trained individuals. Similarly, work by Fritzsche and Coyle[72] demonstrated that cutaneous blood flow was higher in trained than in untrained individuals at the same relative work load despite similar core (esophageal) body temperatures. Conversely, when trained human subjects were subjected to 10% hypohydration prior to exercise in hot conditions, thresholds for sweating and for cutaneous vasodilation were increased, reversing the improvements in these heat dissipatory mechanisms to levels measured prior to training.[80] In the horse, as in human subjects, enhanced capacity for heat dissipation is, in part, a reflection of an expansion of blood volume[81] and likely a higher proportion of blood flow directed to the skin surface.

The time course of decay in training-induced thermoregulatory adaptations after the onset of detraining has not been determined in horses. In humans there is a strong association between aerobic fitness and exercise-heat tolerance, and the decline in thermoregulatory function with detraining tends to parallel the reduction in aerobic fitness.[64,68]

Heat acclimatization

The term 'acclimatization' is used to describe adaptive changes that occur when a subject undertakes repeated, prolonged exposure to severe environmental conditions (*acclimation* refers to the adaptations produced in controlled laboratory conditions). In the context of the present discussion, hot conditions are normally considered those that will induce the greatest thermoregulatory challenge for horses. As indicated previously, exercise training in a cool environment improves physiological responses when horses exercise in hot conditions. The adaptive responses to training and acclimatization are qualitatively the same. However, the more profound thermal stimulus used during acclimatization will result in thermoregulatory adaptations of a greater magnitude.[81,82] Furthermore, factors that modify the environment in which acclimatization is undertaken will influence the extent of alterations. These differences are apparent in the higher rate of sweat production during exercise when acclimatization occurs in hot, dry versus hot, humid conditions.[83]

Human studies have demonstrated that the process of heat acclimation begins within a few (3–5) days of regular exposure to and exercise in the heat, with most adaptations complete within a 14-day period.[48,51,68,70,82] The most notable changes are an increase in plasma volume, a decrease in heart rate and core temperature during exercise, an increase in sweating rate and initiation of sweating at a lower body temperature, and redistribution of cardiac output such that there is an increase in blood flow to capillary beds of the skin.[84] In general, the cardiovascular adaptations are complete during the first week of acclimation, whereas alterations in sweating responses require 10–14 days of repeated heat exposure.[81,82] Heat acclimation also may result in an improved efficiency of biochemical energy transformation in contracting muscles, thereby attenuating heat production in the acclimated versus unacclimated state.[38] With heat acclimation comes an increase in heat shock protein expression and an enhancement of thermotolerance at the cellular level. These proteins respond to numerous stressors, including reduced energy availability and increased temperature, upregulating signaling pathways of critical cytoprotective mechanisms.[85–87]

In horses, there is evidence that regular exercise in the heat results in physiological adaptations that are consistent with thermal acclimation. Marlin and coworkers[52] subjected five horses to 15 consecutive days of treadmill exercise in 30°C and 85% relative humidity. Training consisted of a combination of low-, medium- and high-intensity exercise, with a total duration of exercise-heat exposure of 80 min per day. Before and after acclimation, horses undertook a treadmill exercise test designed to simulate the speed and endurance test of a three-day event at 30°C and 85% relative humidity. Following acclimation, four of the five horses were able to complete a significantly greater amount of phase D in the exercise test (pre: 6.3 ± 0.3 min; post: 7.3 ± 0.3 min; target time = 8 min), suggesting an improvement in heat tolerance. Resting body temperatures (rectal, pulmonary artery, tail skin) were lower after acclimation, whereas plasma volume was unchanged.[52]

In another study, six conditioned horses were exposed for 4 h to heat and humidity (temperature 33–35°C, relative humidity 80–85%) for 21 days.[88–91] One hour of low- and moderate-intensity treadmill exercise (30–60% $\dot{V}O_{2max}$) was completed during daily heat exposure. At regular intervals during the 21-day period, horses undertook a standardized submaximal (50% $\dot{V}O_{2max}$) exercise test in the same environmental conditions. In addition, before and after 18 days of acclimation, the horses performed the same exercise test in hot, dry conditions (relative humidity 45–50%). Exercise duration was defined as the time taken for attainment of a pulmonary artery blood temperature of 41.5°C. Similar to the findings of Marlin et al,[52] there were significant decreases in resting body temperatures after 5–7 days of heat acclimation. However, in contrast to Marlin's findings, there was a 7–10% increase in plasma volume during the first week of heat acclimation. Thereafter, plasma volume tended to decrease and was not different from preacclimation values at the end of the experimental period.[90] There was a 25% increase in exercise duration when comparing trials performed in the hot, dry conditions before and after acclimation (Fig. 41.4). However, heat acclimation did not increase exercise duration in the hot, humid environment,[89] further emphasizing the biophysical limitations to heat dissipation in such conditions ('uncompensable heat stress').

Sweating rates greatly exceeded evaporative capacity throughout the 21-day period of humid heat exposure, as evidenced by profuse drippage of sweat from the body. In contrast to the findings of some studies in human subjects, whole-body sweat loss was attenuated with repeated heat exposure. Although sweating rates were slightly higher during exercise after acclimation, a more rapid abatement of sweating during the recovery period after exercise resulted in a significant reduction in overall sweat losses (Table 41.2). Similarly, calculated sweat ion losses were 26% lower after acclimation, for the most part a result of a 10% decrease in mean sweat sodium concentration. The more rapid decline in sweating rate during recovery may represent an adaptive mechanism for conservation of water and ions. An increase in respiratory heat loss as a result of humid heat acclimation, evidenced by an increase in post-exercise respiratory rate, may have partially offset the decrease in cutaneous heat loss during the recovery period.[88,89]

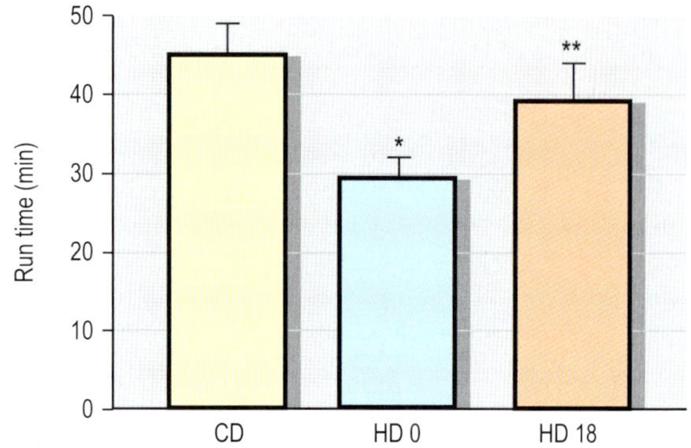

Fig 41.4 Mean ± SE exercise duration during a standardized exercise test (SET) at 50% maximal O_2 uptake ($\dot{V}O_{2max}$) in cool dry (CD) and hot dry conditions before (HD 0) and after 18 days of heat acclimation (HD 18). *Significantly different from CD and HD 18; **significantly different from HD 0 ($P < 0.05$).
Data from Geor RJ, McCutcheon LJ, Ecker GL, et al. Heat storage in horses during submaximal exercise before and after humid heat acclimation. J Appl Physiol 2000;89:2283–93.

In summary, horses undergo a number of physiological adaptations to repeated cycles of exercise heat stress that are consistent with a heat acclimation response. These adaptations are evident after 7–14 days and appear to confer a modest improvement in tolerance for exercise in the heat, although, similar to observations in human subjects,[51] this improvement is largely negated when exercise is performed in uncompensable heat stress conditions (high heat and humidity).

The physiologic adaptations associated with acclimatization to heat will diminish in the absence of the thermoregulatory stimulus. In human subjects, the rate of decay is reported to vary from one to several weeks.[82,83,92,93] In physically fit individuals, there is a slower rate of decay of the thermoregulatory adaptations, emphasizing the importance of exercise training in augmenting the benefits of heat acclimatization.[88,94] The time course of the decay in thermoregulatory adaptations in horses has not been reported.

Hydration state

Prolonged exercise, particularly when it is performed in hot and humid ambient conditions, can result in large fluid deficits that limit thermoregulatory and cardiovascular function. Studies in humans have demonstrated that dehydration of as little as 2–3% of body weight can impair heat transfer from the body core to the periphery, decrease sweating sensitivity (the increase in sweating rate per unit increase in core temperature), and increase the rate of rise in core body temperature during exertion.[95–97] Furthermore,

Table 41.2 Run time, pre-exercise body mass and change in body mass on days 0, 3, 7, 14 and 21 of heat acclimation

	RUN TIME (min)	BODY MASS (kg)	TOTAL SWEAT FLUID LOSS ASSOCIATED WITH SET (L)	SWEAT LOSS DURING EXERCISE (mL)	% OF TOTAL LOSS (EXERCISE)	SWEAT LOSS DURING RECOVERY (mL)	% OF TOTAL LOSS (RECOVERY)
Day 0	19.09 ± 1.41	454.1 ± 11.7	11.67 ± 1.23	3844 ± 380	33.8 ± 2	7413 ± 953	66.2 ± 2
Day 3	20.92 ± 1.98	452.0 ± 12.0	12.00 ± 0.86	4179 ± 645	38.0 ± 4	6452 ± 818	62.1 ± 4
Day 7	19.59 ± 1.70	449.5 ± 11.5	11.50 ± 0.99	4324 ± 756	39.8 ± 3	5772 ± 875	59.8 ± 3
Day 14	20.42 ± 1.78	449.7 ± 10.1	10.08 ± 1.31	4451 ± 577	41.7 ± 3*	5323 ± 444	58.0 ± 3*
Day 21	19.61 ± 1.86	445.7 ± 8.7	8.67 ± 0.71*	4452 ± 490	50.7 ± 3*	4193 ± 435*	49.1 ± 3*

Values are mean ± SE for six horses. Run time represents duration of exercise at 50% $\dot{V}O_{2max}$ to attainment of a pulmonary artery temperature of 41.5°C. Total sweat fluid loss includes exercise and one hour of recovery. Exercise includes exercise at 50% $\dot{V}O_{2max}$ only. Recovery includes 1 hour of recovery only.
SET = standardized exercise test. *Significantly different from *Day 0*, P < 0.05.
(Data from McCutcheon LJ, Geor RJ, Ecker GL, et al. Equine sweating responses to submaximal exercise during 21 days of heat acclimation. J Appl Physiol 1999; 87:1843–51.[91])

dehydration decreases exercise heat tolerance such that fatigue occurs at a lower core temperature when compared to exercise undertaken in the euhydrated state.[98,99] In horses during 40 min of exercise eliciting 40% $\dot{V}O_{2max}$, pre-exercise dehydration (4% of body weight) induced by water withholding or furosemide administration decreased cardiac output and increased pulmonary artery blood and middle gluteal muscle temperatures (by approximately 1°C) when compared to the euhydrated state. Peak sweating rates during exercise were not affected by hydration state.[100] The authors concluded that the dehydration-induced impairment of thermoregulation was primarily due to a decreased transfer of heat from core to periphery.

The effects of dehydration on thermoregulatory function in horses are magnified during exercise in the heat. During 90 min of treadmill running at 50% $\dot{V}O_{2max}$ under hot ambient conditions (room temperature 33–35°C; relative humidity 50–55%), progressive dehydration equivalent to 6–8% of body weight was associated with decreases in stroke volume, cardiac output and sweating rate, and higher blood, muscle and rectal temperatures when compared to trials in which hydration state was maintained by the administration of oral fluid equivalent to approximately 85% of the incurred sweat fluid losses.[39] In summary, pre-exercise dehydration or the progressive dehydration incurred as a result of sweat fluid losses during prolonged exercise will impair thermoregulation in horses. This impairment of thermoregulation will be reflected by a more rapid rise in body temperature. Such an exacerbation of hyperthermia would be expected to reduce exercise capacity due to earlier attainment of a critical upper limit in core and brain temperatures.

Old age

Almost all the studies that have addressed thermoregulatory responses to exercise in horses have used young subjects.[13,20,31,52,75] As a result, there are very limited data on the effects of age on thermoregulatory function during activity in older horses. McKeever and coworkers[101] demonstrated that older horses had higher heart rates and attained a core body temperature of 40°C in approximately 50% less time than younger mares when both groups were required to work at the same absolute work output (1625 watts). Despite their inability to dissipate heat load at a similar rate during exercise when compared to the younger mares, the older horses had similar heart rates and core temperatures 10 min post exercise.[101,102]

In human studies, older subjects have been shown to have lower total body water and plasma volume and, as a result, will have a smaller fluid volume that is available to produce sweat.[103,104] There is some suggestion that older subjects are chronically hypohydrated and that these age-related alterations in fluid and electrolyte status will add to an age-related reduction in thermoregulatory capacity. However, based on the limited data available regarding older horses, it appears that the fluid shifts during exercise are of similar magnitude in aged and young horses.[101,102]

The sweating rate in older horses has been determined to be higher when working at the same absolute work intensity as younger mares. However, it would appear that this increased sweating rate did not improve the ability of the older horses to dissipate heat when compared to their younger counterparts. This could suggest that higher sweating rates occurred in the presence of lower skin blood flow in older versus younger horses.[101] An apparent decline in maximal heart rate and stroke volume measured in older horses may contribute to this reduced heat dissipatory capacity.[105,106] While skin blood flow measurements were not undertaken in these studies, impaired cutaneous blood flow has been demonstrated in older human subjects in response to exercise.[104] The mechanism for this age-related change in skin blood flow has not been determined. Chronic hypohydration and a concomitant decrease in plasma volume have been suggested as a contributing factor for differences in thermoregulatory capacity in older versus young human subjects.[103,104] In one study by McKeever and coworkers,[101] pre-exercise plasma volume was lower in old when compared to younger mares. These investigators have speculated that the relative hypovolemia imposed by a lower absolute plasma volume could impair the thermoregulatory responses of older horses.[102,107] A recent study, comparing highly trained older (51–63 years) human subjects with groups of younger moderately and highly trained individuals reported that body temperature during exercise in the heat was not different in older athletes and differences in cardiovascular and evaporative heat loss responses were consistent with an age-related diminishment in maximal aerobic capacity.[108] To date, no studies have assessed thermoregulatory responses in highly trained older horses.

Recommendations for preparation for exercise or competition in hot conditions

Although it is not possible to eliminate the effects of adverse effects of environmental conditions on exercise performance, there is evidence from human and animal (including equine) studies that a thorough exercise training program together with a subsequent period of acclimatization will mitigate the impact of the environment. Careful planning is needed for horses transported from a temperate to a hot, humid climate, and then required to train and compete in the hot environment. These horses should attain a high level of event-specific fitness before the trip, and be given adequate time for acclimatization to exercise in the hotter conditions. The hair coat should be clipped to facilitate cutaneous heat loss.[109] For the 1996 Olympic Games in Atlanta, Georgia, the International Equestrian Federation recommended that horses arrive approximately three weeks in advance of the events. This recommendation was based on research studies[52,88–91] that demonstrated physiological adaptations consistent with heat acclimatization after 14 consecutive days of exercise conditioning in heat and humidity. Minimal training was recommended in the first week, to allow horses to recover from the effects of prolonged transportation. There should not be the expectation of conducting the major portion of a horse's conditioning during this period. More recently, the equestrian events of the 2008 Olympic Games were again held in a hot environment (August 8–24, 2008 in Hong Kong, China). Building on previous recommendations, careful preparations were undertaken to ensure horses would not become heat stressed while competing in these hot, humid conditions (mean temperature 31.6 °C, relative humidity 77%). Weather data gathered in 2006 and 2007 and a test event held in August 2007 provided the basis for recommendations regarding optimum time of day, length of events and placement of cooling stations and allowed the events to be carried out safely. Despite the high ambient temperature, the use of cooling fans and application of chilled water within 10 minutes of completion of the cross country course provided effective cooling measures for horses competing in this event.[110] However, careful preparation of horses prior to training and competition in hot conditions is essential. Initially, only light exercise should be undertaken during the heat of the day, with harder workouts performed during cooler periods, e.g. early morning. Subsequently, there should be a gradual increase in the duration and intensity of exercise performed in the heat. It is important that some exercise be performed at the intensity required of the horse during competition. Careful clinical monitoring is required to assess successful adaptation to the environment. Collection of detailed clinical data should begin 1–2 weeks before travel to the hotter climate. These data will provide baseline information against which to compare clinical responses during initial days of training in the hot conditions. In addition, evaluation of this information will provide an objective assessment of how well the horse is adapting to the hot environment. Water and feed intake should be measured on a daily basis. Heart rate, respiratory rate, and rectal temperature should be recorded before and after training sessions. The intensity of work efforts can be estimated by use of a heart rate monitor. Daily weighing is useful for estimation of the extent of fluid losses associated with travel and training.

Assuming similarity in the duration and intensity of exercise bouts undertaken in both cool and hot ambient conditions, the exercise-induced increase in rectal temperature will serve as an indicator of the added thermal burden associated with the hotter conditions. The monitoring of post-exercise rectal temperature is critical to early detection of heat exhaustion and other heat illnesses. As there is a lag in the rise in rectal temperature, particularly after heavy exercise in hot and humid conditions, it is important to continue to monitor rectal temperature during the first 5 to 10 min after exercise. A rectal temperature that exceeds 42 °C (108 °F) indicates the need for immediate and vigorous cooling. Hyperthermia of this magnitude also may signal the need for a reduction in the intensity or duration of exercise in the hot ambient conditions. There may be an increase in resting respiratory rate following the transition from cool to hot ambient conditions. This increase reflects the thermoregulatory role of the respiratory system. Similarly, the post-exercise respiratory rate is typically 30–40% higher following exercise in hot ambient conditions than in cool to moderate environments. In very hot and humid conditions (ambient temperature of 33–35 °C, relative humidity 60–75%), particularly when the horse is not cooled by the application of cold water, the respiratory rate may remain increased (up to 80–100 breaths/min) for 20–30 min after exercise. Persistence of tachypnea after the horse is placed in a cooler environment or is vigorously cooled may indicate that body temperature is still markedly elevated.

Maintenance of fluid and electrolyte balance is important for successful adaptation to a hot environment. Indeed, studies in humans have demonstrated that any thermoregulatory benefits derived from heat acclimation are overwhelmed by the elevated heat stress imposed by hypohydration.[82,99] The first concern is the fluid deficit resulting from the period of transport to the new location. Even when access to food and water is maintained during travel, horses typically incur a substantial loss of weight (approximately 3 kg/h of transport). Fluid losses will be higher during road transport in hot weather. As many horses drink poorly during the initial days in a new environment, this dehydration may persist for 3–4 days after arrival. Oral or intravenous fluid support is often provided to recently transported horses in an attempt to hasten correction of fluid balance. Dehydration of as little as 2–3% of body weight not only impairs thermoregulation and exercise performance but also prevents the expansion in plasma volume that typically occurs during the early phases of heat acclimatization. Thus, it is imperative that dehydration is corrected before commencement of training in the heat.

Given the increased fluid losses associated with a period of exercise training in a hot climate, an increase in daily water consumption is to be anticipated. A 30–50% increase in 24-h water consumption was observed in horses undergoing heat acclimation; this change occurred within 10 days of the start of heat exposure and largely reflected an increase in water consumption in the 1-h period after exercise.[88]

Electrolyte or salt supplementation is recommended for horses training and competing in hot climates (see Chapter 40). Fat supplementation has been advocated as a means for reducing thermal stress in horses exercising in hot climates. A high-fat diet (8–10% on a total diet basis) may reduce the heat generated by colonic fermentation when compared to a more traditional diet that is higher in roughage.[12] In addition, lower roughage intake may decrease 'bowel ballast', which may be beneficial during high-intensity exercise. However, the actual effects of these dietary manipulations on thermal load in exercising horses have not been quantified. A limited number of studies have demonstrated that fat supplementation has no effect on fluid and electrolyte balance in horses performing daily exercise in hot conditions (mean daily temperature of 29.2 °C).[111,112]

Regardless of the level of training and acclimatization to hot conditions, it should be recognized that it is possible to overwhelm the thermoregulatory capacity of horses with a high level of physical conditioning when exercise is prolonged and/or there are adverse environmental conditions that will impair heat dissipatory mechanisms. Under such conditions, seeking shade at stops to reduce solar heating, using fans to improve convective cooling, and frequent, copious application of cool water will reduce the rate at which heat is stored. The extent of fluid losses can also be ameliorated if horses are trained to drink fluids at rest stops during competition. Close monitoring of horses exercising under hot conditions is essential to ensure early recognition of hyperthermia which, left unattended, can progress to the development of heat exhaustion and heat stroke.

Diseases caused by inadequate thermoregulation

In human medicine, several terms are used to describe syndromes associated with environmental heat exposure or exercise-induced hyperthermia; these include heat stress, heat exhaustion and heat stroke. Heat stress is defined as 'perceived discomfort and physiological strain associated with exposure to a hot environment, especially during physical work', whereas heat illness, exhaustion and stroke refer to mild-to-severe illness arising from exposure to high environmental temperatures or strenuous physical exercise and the resulting inability to maintain normal body temperature.[113–116]

As discussed above, heat stress can occur when horses are exercised in warm ambient conditions, wherein physiological strain is evidenced by a more rapid rise in core body temperature, more severe exercise-induced dehydration, and higher heart and respiratory rates during recovery when compared to similar exercise in cool or moderate environments. The horse's prodigious capacity for sweating comes at a cost; high rates of sweat fluid loss can result in moderate to severe dehydration and electrolyte abnormalities that predispose to development of muscle cramping, rhabdomyolysis and synchronous diaphragmatic flutter (SDF). Furthermore, dehydration can impair heat dissipation and contribute to the progression from heat stress to heat exhaustion or heat stroke.

Anhidrosis ('dry coat')

- Anhidrosis is defined as an inability to sweat effectively in response to suitable stimuli such as heat or exercise.
- It occurs almostexclusively in horses living in hot or hot and humid climates.
- The mechanism of anhidrosis is not fully understood, but involves gradual failure of sweat gland secretory mechanisms following downregulation of sweat gland β_2-receptors.[117]
- Clinical signs include patchy and inadequate sweating, marked hyperthermia in response to exercise, and delayed recovery of rectal temperature, heart rate and respiratory rate after exercise. Horses with long-standing anhidrosis may exhibit dry and flaky skin with alopecia.
- Exercise during cooler periods of the day, housing the horse in an air-conditioned stall, or relocation to a more temperate climate are possible preventive strategies.

Recognition

History and presenting complaint

Affected horses often present with a history of poor or decreased exercise performance or exercise intolerance. On occasion, a dermatologic abnormality is the initial presenting complaint. An absent or inappropriate sweating response is often not detected by owners and trainers. Instead, they report poor exercise performance, labored breathing after exercise, and deterioration of the hair coat. The condition is normally more evident during hotter summer months.

Physical examination

Affected horses develop the problem in the summer months and usually recommence sweating in the winter. The primary clinical signs of anhidrosis reflect inadequate cutaneous evaporative heat loss, and include failure to sweat, tachypnea at rest, elevated rectal temperature, and a delayed post-exercise recovery in rectal temperature and respiratory rate. Tachypnea (>60–80 breaths per min) with marked nostril flare can persist for 60 or more minutes after exercise. Affected horses may seek shade or attempt to cool themselves with water (e.g. stand in water troughs), particularly during the heat of the day.

The degree of anhidrosis is variable, ranging from partial sweat production to complete absence of sweating. Body areas that may retain the ability to sweat include under the mane, the saddle and halter regions, and the axillary, inguinal and perineal regions. Sweat gland density is highest in these regions, and these areas appear to the last affected prior to onset of complete anhidrosis. Dermatologic abnormalities in horses with long-standing anhidrosis include a dry, sparse hair coat with excessive scaling and alopecia, particularly of the face, neck and shoulders.

Diagnosis

The diagnosis of anhidrosis is predominantly based on history and repeated demonstration of inadequate sweating in response to adequate thermogenic stimuli. Semiquantitative data on sweating response may be obtained by intradermal skin testing using injection of a specific β_2-agonist such as terbutaline or salbutamol.[118] Serial dilutions (10^{-3} to 10^{-8} [w/v]) of the β_2-agonist and a control saline solution are injected into shaved areas over the neck. Normal horses sweat in response to all dilutions, usually within 15–20 min of injection. Horses with partial anhidrosis sweat only in response to the highest β_2-agonist concentration, whereas horses with more severe anhidrosis may be refractory to all concentrations. Histological examination of skin sections may be unrewarding, although ultrastructural changes in the sweat glands and surrounding tissues may be evident. These changes include thickening of the basal lamina and connective tissues, and a marked reduction in the number of secretory cell vesicles. The lumen of sweat gland ducts may be obstructed with cellular debris, and luminal microvilli are often absent.

Anhidrosis should be differentiated from respiratory diseases that result in an increase in respiratory rate.

Treatment and prognosis

Therapy

Given the paucity of knowledge as to the underlying mechanisms for the altered pattern and intensity of sweating, no effective treatment has been determined. However, the risk of heat stress and heat stroke can be mitigated by a combination of environmental and management strategies. The only recognized effective treatment is to remove affected horses to a cooler environment, either physically (i.e. move to a more temperate climate) or by the use of air conditioning or other means of assisted cooling. Some change in exercise routine is required. Heavy training and competition during the summer months should be discouraged. On the other hand, anhidrotic horses that are rested during the summer may train and compete successfully during the cooler winter months. Anecdotally, affected horses resume a more normal sweating response as night-time temperatures begin to decline. For horses maintained in exercise training during the summer, workouts should be conducted during cooler periods of the day (e.g. early morning) and horses should be cooled aggressively after exercise (e.g. the liberal and repeated application and removal of cool water over the entire body).

A variety of nutritional supplements have been advocated in the treatment of anhidrosis, but objective data on the efficacy of these products is not available. Anecdotally, some veterinarians and trainers have reported that horses with a history of anhidrosis that are treated with electrolyte supplements (especially sodium and potassium) before the onset of hot weather and during the summer months do not develop further episodes of anhidrosis. As tyrosine is thought to be important for the resensitization of β_2-receptors, supplementation with this amino acid has been recommended for horses with anhidrosis. Similarly, some veterinarians have claimed success when affected horses are supplemented with vitamin E (1000–3000 U/day) or iodinated casein (10–15 g/day for 4–8 days).

Prognosis

There is anecdotal evidence that most affected horses respond favorably to a change in environment and begin to sweat normally after a few days to weeks. A complete return to normal sweating function may take 3–4 months in some horses. There are no published reports on the long-term follow-up of horses with anhidrosis. However, it is genererally believed that horses with a history of anhidrosis will become anhidrotic when again exposed to hot, humid conditions.

Etiology and pathophysiology

The pathophysiological mechanisms underlying anhidrosis are not known. Various factors have been suggested, including electrolyte imbalances, hypothyroidism, sweat gland exhaustion, plugging or blocking of the sweat gland ducts to the surface, failure of secretory function, and a downregulation of glandular sensitivity. The most plausible cause is altered sweat gland receptor function. Recent evidence implicates overstimulation of sweat gland β_2-receptors and purinoreceptors results in diminished function via desensitization or downregulation of the receptors that may eventuate as an irreversible degeneration in sweat gland function.[119] Even apparently normally sweating horses have reduced sensitivity to intradermal epinephrine (adrenaline) in a hot and humid environment.[120] That many anhidrotic horses once again achieve adequate sweat production upon removal to a cooler climate emphasizes the importance of environmental conditions to the development of clinical disease. One hypothesis is that increased circulating epinephrine (adrenaline) concentrations result in overstimulation of the sweat glands. Beadle et al.[121] reported higher resting epinephrine (adrenaline) concentrations in anhidrotic horses compared with control horses in the same hot and humid climate. However, other studies[120,122] did not detect a difference in epinephrine (adrenaline) concentrations between control and anhidrotic horses. Water channel proteins, known as aquaporins have a role in passage of water across plasma membranes. Aquaporin-5 (AQP-5) has been found to be expressed in apical plasma membrane epithelial cells in mouse, rat, human and equine sweat glands. Although the exact role of this protein has not been elucidated, lack of sweat gland function in AQP-5 knockout mice suggests these channel proteins have a role in sweat secretion. Level of expression of AQP-5 is reported to be reduced in severely anhidrotic horses, suggesting a role for water channel protein impairment in this disorder.[123]

For the equine athlete, the loss of an adequate sweating response translates into a reduction in the efficacy of heat loss through evaporation and an early and excessive increase in core temperature in response to moderate exercise. Exercise intolerance and poor performance can be attributed to hyperthermia. Increased respiratory rate, both at rest and after exercise, reflects an attempt to dissipate heat via the respiratory tract.

Epidemiology

Anhidrosis is almost exclusive to horses living in hot or hot and humid climates.[124] It is estimated that as much as 20% of the population of athletic horses exercising in hot humid climates experience some degree of anhidrosis. However, more severe signs of anhidrosis are recognized in a smaller percentage of horses.[125] Anecdotally the disease was attributed to acclimization stress in horses bred and raised in cooler climates and transported to a warm and humid climate for training or competition and a in recent study of horses in Florida a survey indicated greater susceptibility in horses originating from the western or midwestern regions of the United States.[126] Sneddon et al (2008)[127] noted seasonal adaptations in skin thickness and sweat gland volume differed between breeds, being most pronounced in Thoroughbreds. These morphological differences and their use in highly athletic activities may contribute to a higher prevalence of anhidrosis in this breed.

Prevention

There is no proven strategy for the prevention of anhidrosis in horses kept in hot and humid climates. However, further episodes of anhidrosis may be prevented by relocation to a cooler climate. When physical removal from the hot climate is not possible, exercise and environmental management can prevent excessive hyperthermia and minimize the risk of heat stress or stroke.

Heat exhaustion/heat stroke

- Heat illnesses can result from exposure to high environmental temperature (non-exertional heat stroke) or, more commonly, from strenuous exercise (exertional heat stroke) undertaken in hot and/or humid ambient conditions.
- Heat exhaustion is a mild-to-moderate illness characterized by hyperthermia, tachypnea, dehydration, and fatigue. A more severe exhaustion syndrome attributed to the combined effects of hyperthermia, fluid and electrolyte deficits, and substrate depletion occurs in horses undertaking endurance exercise.
- Heat stroke is a severe illness in which there is thermoregulatory failure and development of multi-organ dysfunction, including encephalopathy.
- Clinical features common to heat exhaustion and heat stroke include hyperthermia, tachypnea with panting, tachycardia, evidence of dehydration, and fatigue. Other signs may include reduced sweat production with dry hot skin, synchronous diaphragmatic flutter (SDF), muscle cramps, and colic. With heat stroke, these signs are accompanied by neurologic abnormalities including weakness, ataxia progressing to collapse, convulsions, coma, and death.
- Exhausted horses that have sustained large sweat fluid losses may develop a 'postexhaustion syndrome' characterized by

renal failure, laminitis, hepatic failure, myonecrosis and a high mortality rate.
- Therapy includes rapid assisted cooling, intravenous fluids for correction of dehydration and electrolyte and acid–base abnormalities, and judicious use of anti-inflammatory drugs.

Recognition

History and presenting complaint

Heat exhaustion and heat stroke can occur in any environmental condition but are more likely to occur in a hot and humid environment. These conditions should be viewed as a continuum; a state of heat stress can progress rapidly to heat exhaustion or heat stroke. Most often, heat stroke is recognized in association with exercise, particularly when undertaken in hot and humid ambient conditions. Affected horses may have a history of anhidrosis or prior episodes of heat exhaustion. Less commonly, heat stroke may develop in horses confined in closed trailers or buildings during hot weather. Affected horses may present with complaints of fatigue, depression, weakness, stilted gait, respiratory distress, and neurologic abnormalities including seizures.

Physical examination

The clinical signs of heat exhaustion reflect the deleterious effects of hyperthermia, dehydration, hypovolemia, and electrolyte disturbances on the function of many body systems. Hyperthermia (rectal temperature >41–42 °C), elevated heart rate (>60–80 bpm), rapid, shallow respirations (>80–100 breaths/min), dehydration, and evidence of fatigue are often present. Horses that have completed prolonged exercise in hot weather (e.g. an endurance race) are often dehydrated and hypovolemic. Therefore, skin elasticity may be decreased, capillary and jugular refill time delayed, and mucous membranes tacky or dry. Cardiac auscultation or electrocardiographic examination may indicate a tachyarrhythmia. Horses may be unwilling to drink despite moderate to severe dehydration. While fatigued, these horses do not necessarily appear depressed, although they might exhibit a slightly stiff gait and possibly lameness in association with muscle cramping or soreness. High metabolic heat load is often reflected in a delayed post-exercise recovery of heart and respiratory rates (more than 20–30 min) and excessive sweating. Rectal temperature may continue to rise during the 5–10 min period immediately following the cessation of exercise. Decreased anal tone, muscle cramping and SDF may be evident.

By definition, both hyperthermia and central nervous system dysfunction must be present for a diagnosis of heat stroke. Signs of heat stress or exhaustion are accompanied by evidence of brain dysfunction, including a weak, staggering gait, depression or poor mentation, convulsions and coma. There may be excessive sweating with a uniformly wet hair coat or, especially in dehydrated animals, a hot dry skin with dilated cutaneous vasculature.

A number of serious complications can develop in horses with heat exhaustion or stroke. In horses undertaking prolonged exercise that results in exhaustion, glycogen depletion, and marked fluid and electrolyte deficits, such as endurance rides of 50–150 miles, a 'postexhaustion syndrome' characterized by multi-organ dysfunction or failure may develop. These horses may develop laminitis, colic, renal and/or hepatic failure, or myonecrosis in the 1–3-day period after the strenuous exercise. Similarly, horses that recover from the acute phases of heat stroke may develop a syndrome of multi-organ dysfunction characterized by renal and hepatic failure, laminitis, pulmonary edema and respiratory distress, and disseminated intravascular coagulation.

Diagnosis

A number of clinicopathologic abnormalities may be present in horses with heat exhaustion or stroke. Respiratory alkalosis due to hyperventilation is usually present. Metabolic alkalosis or acidosis (lactic acid accumulation) may be present depending on the nature of the exercise performed. There is an increased PCV, Hb, red cell count, and TPP and elevated creatine kinase and aspartate aminotransferase activity and decreased serum electrolytes (P, Cl, Ca [total and ionized], Mg, and possibly Na). A stress neutrophilia and lymphopenia with possible degenerative left shift and leukopenia in face of impending diarrhea may be evident. Severe dehydration and the possible onset of renal disease may be reflected in elevated blood urea nitrogen and creatinine. Urinalysis may reveal high specific gravity (with dehydration and normal renal function) or low specific gravity when renal disease is present with or without evidence of protein or blood in urine. A clotting profile may indicate disseminated intravascular coagulation (thrombocytopenia, increased fibrin degradation products, and prolonged prothrombin time).

Treatment and prognosis

Therapy

Horses exhibiting signs of heat stroke require immediate and aggressive use of cooling techniques and intravenous fluid administration. The horse should be removed from direct sunlight to minimize further radiative heat gain. Unnecessary tack should be removed and the horse left unblanketed.[128] If available, the horse should be positioned in front of high-output fans to increase convective heat loss. Cold water should be applied to the head, neck and body; this will increase the temperature gradient between the skin and the environment, and therefore increase conductive heat loss. The applied water must be quickly removed by use of a skin scrapper with subsequent application of further cool water to maintain this gradient. Misting fans are sometimes available at competitions held during the summer months; these also assist heat dissipation. Internal cooling techniques, such as the intragastric or rectal administration of cold water, may be attempted. However, the latter obviates use of the rectum for monitoring the temperature response to therapy. Assisted cooling should be continued until rectal temperature is less than 39 °C.

Large-volume intravenous fluid replacement is indicated. Normal saline (0.9% NaCl) is the fluid of choice in cases of metabolic alkalosis, but any balanced polyionic solution (e.g. lactated Ringer's solution) is suitable in the face of hypovolemia and dehydration. As much as 60–80 L of fluid may be required over a 6–12-h period in severely dehydrated horses. Subsequent fluid therapy should be guided by clinical assessment and the results of serum biochemical analysis. Supplemental calcium may be required in horses with SDF. Oral fluid therapy may be considered, providing the horse has normal gut sounds and no clinical evidence of colic or gastric reflux. Further details on the correction of exercise-induced dehydration and electrolyte disturbances are presented in Chapter 40.

The role of antipyretic and anti-inflammatory agents (e.g. nonsteroidal anti-inflammatory drugs [NSAIDs]) in the management of heat stroke is unknown. Animal studies have demonstrated that the correction of hyperthermia after the onset of heat stroke may not prevent inflammation, coagulation, and progression to multi-organ dysfunction. On the other hand, treatment with glucocorticoids and immunomodulators such as interleukin-1 (IL-1) receptor antagonists improves survival in animals with heat stroke.[120] Other studies have shown that salicylates and NSAIDs enhance cellular protection against heat stress via induction of the transcription and translation of heat-shock proteins.[129] Accordingly, there may be rationale for the judicious use of NSAIDs (e.g. flunixin meglumine, 1.0 mg/kg) and glucocorticoids (e.g. methylprednisolone sodium succinate, 2–4 mg/kg i.v.) in horses with heat stroke. NSAIDs should also be administered if the horse has pain associated with colic, exertional rhabdomyolysis, or laminitis.

Rest is paramount and therefore it is advisable to transport the horse back to a stabling area once the condition has been stabilized to avoid the requirement for further exercise. Close clinical monitoring is required for a 3–5-day period after an episode of heat exhaustion or heat stroke. This should include clinical assessment of attitude, appetite, hydration status, gastrointestinal function and digital pulses. Serial measurements of serum biochemistries should also be performed. These evaluations will guide further therapy.

Prognosis

There are no reports of long-term follow-up of horses that have suffered an episode of heat stroke. Clinical experience has indicated that the prognosis for heat stroke is variable, depending on severity. The recovery of central nervous system function during cooling is a favorable prognostic sign. On the other hand, persistence of neurologic abnormalities and/or the development of complications such as pulmonary edema, laminitis, renal or hepatic failure and disseminated intravascular coagulation indicate a much poorer prognosis.

Etiology and pathophysiology

A complex interplay of physiological alterations that accompany hyperthermia, including circulatory failure, hypoxia, increased metabolic demand, and inflammatory and coagulation responses, result in the development of heat stroke and the associated progressive multi-organ dysfunction.[113] Heat stress induces thermoregulatory, heat shock and acute-phase responses. Thermoregulatory failure, altered expression of heat-shock proteins and an excessive acute-phase response individually or collectively contribute to the development of heat stroke. Studies in animal models have demonstrated increased production of nitrogen or reactive oxygen species with splanchnic hypoperfusion, the result of the diversion of blood flow to the cutaneous circulation and away from the gut.[113]

Subsequent mucosal injury and hyperpermeability allows the escape of endotoxin into circulation, further stimulating the acute-phase response and the production of pyrogenic cytokines and nitric oxide, both of which can further interfere with thermoregulatory mechanisms. The production of these cytokines and nitric oxide can therefore precipitate hyperthermia, hypotension, and heat stroke (Fig. 41.5).

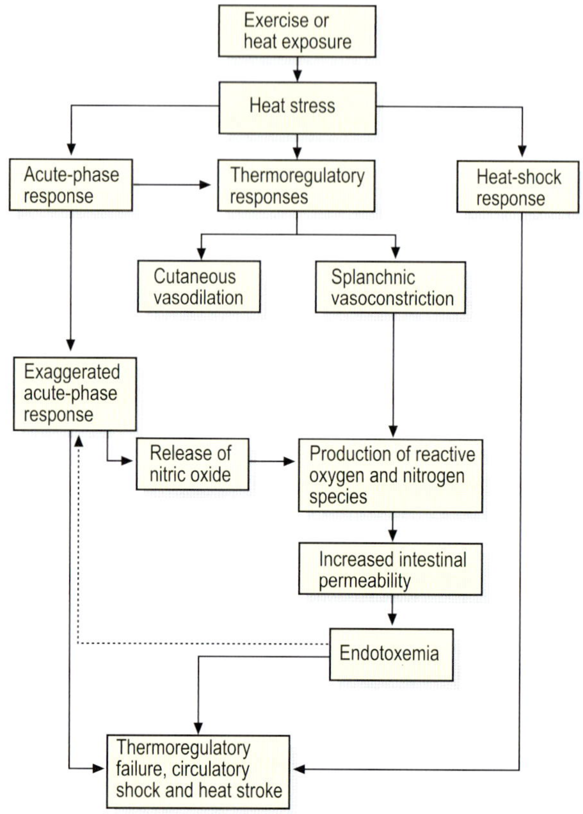

Fig 41.5 Proposed sequence of events in the development of heat stroke in mammals. Heat stress induces thermoregulatory, acute-phase, and heat-shock responses. The redistribution of cardiac output to accommodate cutaneous heat loss results in splanchnic hypoperfusion and ischemia and the increased production of reactive oxygen and nitrogen species. These mediators may induce intestinal mucosal injury and an increase in permeability that allows the entry of endotoxin into circulation. Endotoxin enhances the acute-phase response, leading to production of pyrogenic cytokines and nitric oxide. These mediators can disrupt thermoregulation and precipitate heat stroke. Solid arrows indicate pathways for which there is experimental evidence; broken arrows indicate putative pathways. *From Bouchama A, Knochel JP. Heat stroke. N Engl J Med 2002;346:1978–88. © 2002 Massachusetts Medical Society. Reprinted with permission from Massachusetts Medical Society.*[113]

In addition to the leakage of endotoxin from the intestine, hyperthermia can also lead to the release of IL-1 and IL-6 proteins from muscle. The release of these proteins may result in upregulation of cell-surface adhesion molecules, and shedding of soluble cell-surface adhesion molecules as well as activation of coagulation and inhibition of fibrinolysis. Direct cytotoxic effects to cells and the inflammatory and coagulation responses result in endothelial injury and microthrombosis.[113,116]

A critical thermal maximum beyond which lethal injury occurs has been determined in several mammalian species.[130] In humans, critical thermal maximum is a core body temperature of 41.6°C to 42°C for 45 min to 8 h. The critical core temperature for horses has not been determined. However, exercise-associated elevation in muscle temperature above 43°C (109.4°F) results in alterations in muscle mitochondria and sarcoplasmic reticulum in horses.[131] As previously discussed, the onset of volitional fatigue in humans occurs at a core (esophageal or rectal) temperature of approximately 40°C, whereas studies in horses indicate that voluntary exhaustion does not occur until core or rectal temperatures of 42°C or greater. It is possible that horses have higher heat tolerance when compared to humans. Alternatively, the thermal limit to exercise may be very similar to that associated with the induction of heat stroke,[40] further emphasizing the need for the close monitoring of horses exercising in warm conditions.

Epidemiology

Epidemiological data on risk factors for heat stroke in horses are not available. However, poor physical conditioning, lack of heat acclimatization, prolonged exercise in hot and humid ambient conditions, dehydration, long hair coat, and obesity are factors that may increase the risk of exertional heat stroke. Horses with a history of anhidrosis are obviously at higher risk for heat stroke. In addition, the heavily muscled breeds (e.g. Warmbloods) may be at higher risk because of a low body mass to surface area ratio.

Prevention

One of the most important criteria for the prevention of heat stress is ensuring that horses have undertaken a training program that is adequate for the level of exercise or competition that will be demanded of them. However, it should be recognized that it is possible to overwhelm the thermoregulatory capacity of horses with a high level of physical conditioning when exercise is prolonged and/or there are adverse environmental conditions that will impair heat dissipatory mechanisms. Under such conditions, seeking shade at stops to reduce solar heating, using fans to improve convective cooling, and frequent, copious application of chilled water will reduce the rate at which heat is stored.

As stated previously, an adequate training program will substantially improve thermoregulatory efficiency during exercise. When there is a requirement to compete in severe (i.e. hot) environmental conditions, then acclimatization to hot conditions will further enhance the horse's ability to thermoregulate. Under such conditions greater attention needs to be paid to ensuring that there are an adequate number of stops during which cooling can take place. The extent of fluid losses can be ameliorated if horses are trained to drink fluids at rest stops during competition. Early recognition of hyperthermia and heat exhaustion with aggressive medical intervention will prevent development of heat stroke.

References

1. Gordon MS, Bartholomew GA, Grinnell AD, et al. Body temperature and energy metabolism. In: Gordon MS, Bartholomew GA, Grinnell AD, et al, editors. Animal physiology. 4th ed. New York: MacMillan; 1982. p. 333.
2. Hales JRS, Hubbard RW, Gaffin SL. Limitation of heat tolerance. In: Blatteis C, Fregly M, editors. Handbook of physiology: environmental physiology. Bethesda, MD: American Physiological Society; 1996. p. 285.
3. Armstrong LE, Boulant JA. Neuroendocrine influences on temperature regulation in hot environments. In: Kraemer WJ, Rogol AD, editors. The endocrine system in sports and exercise. Malden: Blackwell; 2006. p. 466.
4. Wendt D, van Loon LJC, van Marken Lichtenbelt WD. Thermoregulation during exercise in the heat. Sports Med 2007;37:669–82.
5. Brody S. Bioenergetics and growth. New York: Reinhold; 1945.
6. Brooks G. Bioenergetics of exercising humans. Compr Physiol 2012;2: 537–62.
7. Armstrong LE, Maresh CM. Effects of training, environment, and host factors on the sweating response to exercise. Int J Sports Med Suppl 1998;19:S103–5.
8. Lorenzo S, Halliwill JR, Sawka MN, et al. Heat acclimation improves exercise performance. J Appl Physiol 2010;109:1140–7.
9. Kleiber M. The fire of life: an introduction to animal energetics. New York: John Wiley; 1961.
10. Castanheira M, Rezende S, Louvandini H, et al. Multivariate analysis for characteristics of heat tolerance in horses in Brazil. Trop Anim Health Prod 2010;185–91.
11. Lovatt Evans C. Physiological mechanisms that underlie sweating in the horse. Br Vet J 1966;122:117–23.
12. Kronfeld D. Dietary fat affects heat production and other variables of equine performance under hot and humid conditions. Equine Vet J 1996;(Suppl. 22):S24–34.
13. Hodgson DR, Davis RE, McConaghy FF. Thermoregulation in the horse in response to exercise. Br Vet J 1994;150:219–35.
14. Jones JH, Carlson GP. Estimation of metabolic energy costs and heat production during a 3-day event. Equine Vet J 1995;(Suppl. 20):S23–30.
15. Guthrie AJ, Lund RJ. Thermoregulation: base mechanisms and hyperthermia. In: Hinchcliff KW, editor. Veterinary clinics of North America: equine practice; fluids and electrolytes in athletic horses. Philadelphia: WB Saunders; 1998;14(1). p. 45–59.
16. Ingram DL, Mount LE. Man and animals in hot environments. Berlin: Springer-Verlag; 1975.
17. Rowell LB. Human circulation: regulation during physical stress. New York: Oxford University Press; 1986. p. 363–407.
18. McCutcheon LJ, Geor RJ, Hare MJ, et al. Sweating rate and sweat composition during exercise and recovery in ambient heat and humidity. Equine Vet J 1995;(Suppl. 20):S153–7.
19. Monteith JL. Specification of the environment for thermal physiology. In: Monteith JL, Mount LE, editors. Heat loss from animals and man. London: Butterworths; 1973. p. 1–35.
20. Geor RJ, McCutcheon LJ, Ecker GL, et al. Thermal and cardiorespiratory responses of horses to submaximal exercise under hot and humid conditions. Equine Vet J Suppl 1995;20:125–32.
21. Baptiste KW, Naylor JM, Bailey J, et al. A function for guttural pouches in the horse. Nature 2000;403:382–3.
22. McConaghy FF, Hales JRS, Rose RJ, et al. Selective brain cooling in the horses during exercise and environmental heat stress. J Appl Physiol 1995;79:1849–54.
23. Mitchell G, Fuller A, Laloney SK, et al. Guttural pouches, brain temperature and exercise in horses. Biol Lett 2006;2:475–7.
24. Jenkinson D McE. Thermoregulatory function. In: Thody AJ, Friedman PS, editors. Scientific basis of dermatology. Edinburgh: Churchill Livingstone; 1986. p. 89–95.
25. Jenkinson DE, Elder HY, Bovell DL. Equine sweating and anhidrosis. Part 1 – equine sweating. Vet Dermatol 2006;17:361–92.
26. Scott CM, Marlin DJ, Schroter RC. Quantification of the response of equine apocrine sweat glands to beta2-adrenergic stimulation. Equine Vet J 2001;33:605–12.
27. Spooner HS, Nielsen BD, Schott HC, et al. Sweat composition in Arabian horses performing endurance exercise on forage-based, low Na rations. Equine Vet J Suppl 2010;38:382–6.
28. McCutcheon LJ, Geor RJ. Sweat fluid and ion losses during training and competition in cool vs. hot conditions: implications for ion supplementation. Equine Vet J 1996;(Suppl. 22): S54–62.
29. Kennedy MW. Latherin and other biocompatible surfactant proteins. Biochem Soc Trans 2011;39:1017–22.
30. Carlson GP, Ocen PO. Composition of equine sweat following exercise in high environmental temperatures and in response to intravenous epinephrine administration. J Equine Med Surg 1979;3:27–32.
31. Hodgson DR, McCutcheon LJ, Byrd SK, et al. Dissipation of metabolic heat in the horse during exercise. J Appl Physiol 1993;74:1161–70.
32. McConaghy FF, Hodgson DR, Hales JR, et al. Thermoregulatory-induced compromise of muscle blood flow in ponies during intense exercise in the heat: a contributor to the onset of fatigue? Equine Vet J Suppl 2002;34:491–5.
33. Kingston JK, Geor RJ, McCutcheon LJ. Rate and composition of sweat fluid losses are unaltered by hypohydration

during prolonged exercise in horses. J Appl Physiol 1997;83: 1133–43.
34. McCutcheon LJ, Geor RJ. Sweating: fluid and ion losses and replacement. In: Hinchcliff KW, editor. Veterinary clinics of North America: equine practice; fluids and electrolytes in athletic horses. Philadelphia: WB Saunders; 1998;14. p. 75–95.
35. McConaghy FF, Hodgson DR, Evans DL, et al. Effects of two types of training on sweat composition. Equine Vet J 1995;(Suppl. 18):S285–8.
36. Carlson GP. Thermoregulation, fluid and electrolyte balance. In: Snow DH, Persson GB, Rose RJ, editors. Equine exercise physiology. Cambridge: Granta Editions; 1983. p. 291–309.
37. Nadel ER. Temperature regulation and prolonged exercise. In: Gisolfi CV, Lamb DR, Nadel ER, editors. Perspectives in exercise science and sports medicine. Exercise, heat, and thermoregulation. Dubuque, IA: Brown; 1988. p. 125–46.
38. Geor RJ, McCutcheon LJ. Thermoregulatory adaptations associated with training and heat acclimation. In: Hinchcliff KW, editor. Veterinary clinics of North America: equine practice; fluids and electrolytes in athletic horses. Philadelphia: WB Saunders; 1998;14. p. 97–120.
39. Geor R, McCutcheon LJ. Hydration effects on physiological strain of horses during exercise-heat stress. J Appl Physiol 1998;84:2042–51.
40. Lindinger ML. Exercise in the heat: thermoregulatory limitations to performance in humans and horses. Can J Appl Physiol 1999;24:135–46.
41. Kohn CW, Hinchcliff KW. Physiological responses to the endurance test of a 3-day event during hot and cool weather. Equine Vet J 1995;(Suppl. 20): S31–6.
42. McConaghy FF, Hodgson DR, Rose RJ, et al. Redistribution of cardiac output in response to heat exposure in the pony. Equine Vet J 1996;(Suppl. 22):S42–6.
43. Gonzalez-Alonzo J, Teller C, Andersen SL, et al. Influence of body temperature on the development of fatigue during prolonged exercise in the heat. J Appl Physiol 1999;86:1032–9.
44. Lee DT, Haymes EM. Exercise duration and thermoregulatory responses after whole body precooling. J Appl Physiol 1995;79:1971–6.
45. MacDougall JD, Reddan WG, Layton CR, et al. Effects of metabolic hyperthermia on performance during prolonged heavy exercise. J Appl Physiol 1974;36:538–44.
46. Nielsen B, Nybo L. Cerebral changes during exercise in the heat. Sports Med 2003;33:1–11.
47. Gonzalez-Alonso J, Mora-Rodriguez R, Below PR, et al. Dehydration markedly impairs cardiovascular function in hyperthermic endurance athletes during exercise. J Appl Physiol 1997;82:1229–36.
48. Nielsen B, Hales JRS, Strange S, et al. Human circulatory and thermoregulatory adaptations with heat acclimation and exercise in a hot, dry environment. J Physiol (Lond) 1993;460:467–85.
49. Nielsen B, Savard G, Richter EA, et al. Muscle blood flow and muscle metabolism during exercise and heat stress. J Appl Physiol 1990;69:1040–6.
50. Bridge MW, Weller AS, Rayson M, et al. Responses to exercise in the heat related to measures of hypothalamic serotonergic and dopaminergic function. Eur J Appl Physiol 2003;89:451–9.
51. Nielsen B, Strange S, Christensen N, et al. Acute and adaptive responses to exercise in a warm, humid environment. Pflug Arch 1997;434:49–56.
52. Marlin DJ, Scott CM, Schroter RC, et al. Physiological responses of horses to a treadmill simulated speed and endurance test in high heat and humidity before and after humid heat acclimation. Equine Vet J 1999;31: 31–42.
53. Asmussen E, Boje O. Body temperature and work capacity. Acta Physiol Scand 1945;10:1–22.
54. Kozlowski S, Brzezinska Z, Kruk B, et al. Exercise hyperthermia as a factor limiting physical performance: temperature effect on muscle metabolism. J Appl Physiol 1985;59:766–73.
55. Young AJ. Energy substrate utilization during exercise in extreme environments. Exer Sports Sci Rev 1990;18:65–117.
56. Brooks GA, Hittelman KJ, Faulkner JA, et al. Temperature, skeletal muscle mitochondrial functions, and oxygen debt. Am J Physiol 1971;220:1053–9.
57. Willis WT, Jackman MR. Mitochondrial function during heavy exercise. Med Sci Sports Exerc 1994;26:1347–54.
58. Crandall CG, Gonzalez-Alonso J. Cardiovascular function in the heat-stressed human. Acta Physiol 2010;199:407–23.
59. Galloway SD, Maughan RJ. Effects of ambient temperature on the capacity to perform prolonged cycle exercise in man. Med Sci Sports Exerc 1997;29:1240–9.
60. Febbraio MA. Temperature, muscle metabolism and performance. In: Lamb DR, Murray R, editors. Perspectives in exercise science and sports medicine. Carmel, IN: Cooper Publishing; 1999. p. 315–54.
61. Nybo L, Jensen T, Nielsen B, et al. Effects of marked hyperthermia with and without dehydration on VO_2 kinetics during intense exercise. J Appl Physiol 2001;90:1057–64.
62. Art T, Leukeux P. Respiratory adjustments in unacclimatised horses exercised under hot, humid conditions. Equine Vet J 1995;(Suppl. 18):S289–93.
63. Aoyagi Y, McLellan TM, Shephard RJ. Effects of 6 versus 12 days of heat acclimation on heat tolerance in lightly exercising men wearing protective clothing. Eur J Appl Physiol 1995;71:187–96.
64. Cheung SS, McLellan TM. Heat acclimation, aerobic fitness, and hydration effects on tolerance during uncompensable heat stress. J Appl Physiol 1998;84:1721–39.
65. Anufriev Ai, Yadrikhinishii VF, Isaev AP. Body temperature changes in purebred and hybrid Yakut horses under the conditions of Yakutia. Dokl Biol Sci 2009;427:358–61.
66. Arnold W, Ruf T, Kuntz R. Seasonal adjustment of energy budget in a large wild mammal, the Przewlski horse (*Equus ferus przewalskii*) II. Energy Expenditure. J Experimental Biol 2006;209:4566–73.
67. Brinkmann L, Gerken M, Riek A. Adaptation strategies to seasonal changes in environmental conditions of a domesticated horse breed, the Shetland pony (*Equus ferus caballus*). J Exp Biol 2012;215:1061–8.
68. Armstrong LE, Pandolf KB. Physical training, cardiorespiratory fitness and exercise heat tolerance. In: Pandolf KB, Sawka MN, Gonzalez RR, editors. Human performance physiology and environmental medicine at terrestrial extremes. Indianapolis, IN: Benchmark; 1988. p. 199–226.
69. Gisolfi GV. Work-heat tolerance derived from interval training. J Appl Physiol 1973;35:349–54.
70. Gisolfi GV. Influence of acclimatization and training on heat tolerance and physical endurance. In: Hales JRS, Richards DAB, editors. Heat stress: physical exertion and environment. Amsterdam: Elsevier Science; 1987. p. 355–66.
71. Gisolfi GV, Cohen JS. Relationships among training, heat acclimation, and heat tolerance in men and women: the controversy revisited. Med Sci Sports 1979;11:56–9.
72. Fritzsche RG, Coyle EF. Cutaneous blood flow during exercise is higher in endurance-trained humans. J Appl Physiol 2000;88:738–44.
73. Araki T, Matsushita K Umeno K, et al. Effect of physical training on exercise-induced sweating in women. J Appl Physiol 1981;51:1526–32.

74. Yamauchi M, Matsumoto T, Ohwatari N, et al. Sweating economy by graded control in well-trained athletes. Eur J Physiol 1997;433:675–8.
75. McCutcheon LJ, Geor RJ. Influence of training on sweating responses during submaximal exercise in horses. J Appl Physiol 2000;89:2463–71.
76. Hamouti N, Del Coso J, Ortega JF, et al. Sweat sodium concentration during exercise in the heat in aerobically trained and untrained humans. Eur J Appl Physiol 2011;111:2873–81.
77. McCutcheon LJ, Geor RJ. Effects of short-term training on thermoregulatory and sweat responses during exercise in hot conditions. Equine Vet J Suppl 2010;38:135–41.
78. Convertino VA. Blood volume: its adaptation to endurance training. Med Sci Sports Exerc 1991;23: 1338–51.
79. Roberts MF, Wenger CG, Stolwijk JAJ, et al. Cutaneous blood flow and sweating changes following exercise training and heat acclimation. J Appl Physiol 1977;43:133–7.
80. Ikegawa S, Kamijo Y, Okazaki K, et al. Effects of hypohydration on thermoregulation during exercise before and after 5-day aerobic training in a warm environment in young men. J Appl Physiol 2011;110:972–80.
81. Armstrong LE, Maresch CM. The induction and decay of heat acclimation in trained athletes. Sports Med 1991;12:302–12.
82. Wenger CB. Human heat acclimatization. In: Pandolf KB, Sawka MN, Gonzalez RR, editors. Human performance physiology and environmental medicine at terrestrial extremes. Indianapolis, IN: Benchmark; 1988. p. 153–97.
83. Nadel EF, Pandolf KB, Roberts MF, et al. Mechanisms of thermal acclimation to exercise and heat. J Appl Physiol 1974;37:512–20.
84. Lorenzo S, Minson CT. Heat acclimation improves cutaneous vascular function and sweating in trained cyclists. J Appl Physiol 2010;109:1736–43.
85. Horowitz M. From molecular and cellular to integrative heat defense during exposure to chronic heat. Comp Biochem Physiol 2002 part A;131:475–83.
86. Kregel KC. Heat shock proteins: modifying factors in physiological heat stress responses and acquired thermotolerance. J Appl Physiol 2002;92:2177–86.
87. Schneider EM, Niess AM, Lorenz I, et al. Inducible Hsp70 expression analysis after heat and physical exercise. Transcriptional, protein expression, and subcellular localization. Ann NY Acad Sci 2002;973:8–12.
88. Geor RJ, McCutcheon LJ, Lindinger MI. Adaptations to daily exercise in hot and humid ambient conditions in trained thoroughbred horses. Equine Vet J 1996;(Suppl. 22):S63–9.
89. Geor RJ, McCutcheon LJ, Ecker GL, et al. Heat storage in horses during submaximal exercise before and after humid heat acclimation. J Appl Physiol 2000;89:2283–93.
90. Lindinger MI, McCutcheon LJ, Ecker GL, et al. Heat acclimation improves regulation of plasma volume and plasma Na(+) content during exercise in horses. J Appl Physiol 2000;88:1006–13.
91. McCutcheon LJ, Geor RJ, Ecker GL, et al. Equine sweating responses to submaximal exercise during 21 days of heat acclimation. J Appl Physiol 1999;87:1843–51.
92. Daanen HA, Jonkman AG, Layden JD, et al. Optimising the acquisition and retention of heat acclimation. Int J Sports Med 2011;32:822–8.
93. Weller AS, Linnane DM, Jonkman AG, et al. Quantification of the decay and re-induction of heat acclimation in dry-heat following 12 and 26 days without exposure to heat stress. Eur J Appl Physiol 2007;102:57–66.
94. Garrett AT, Rehrer NJ, Patterson MJ. Induction and decay of short-term heat acclimation in moderately and highly trained athletes. Sports Med 2011;41:757–71.
95. Montain SJ, Smith SA, Mattot RP, et al. Hypohydration effects on skeletal muscle performance and metabolism: a 31P-MRS study. J Appl Physiol 1998;84:1889–94.
96. Montain SJ, Coyle EF. Influence of graded dehydration on hyperthermia and cardiovascular drift during exercise. J Appl Physiol 1992;73:1340–50.
97. Montain SJ, Latzka WA, Sawka MN. Control of thermoregulatory sweating is altered by hydration level and exercise intensity. J Appl Physiol 1995;79:1434–9.
98. Sawka MN. Body fluid responses and hypohydration during exercise heat stress. In: Pandof KB, Sawka MN, Gonzalaz RR, editors. Human performance physiology and environmental medicine at terrestrial extremes. Indianapolis, IN: Benchmark; 1988. p. 227–66.
99. Sawka MN, Toner MM, Francesconi RP, et al. Hypohydration and exercise: effects of heat acclimation, gender and environment. J Appl Physiol 1983;55:1147–53.
100. Naylor JR, Bayly WM, Gollnick PD, et al. Effects of dehydration on thermoregulatory responses of horses during low intensity exercise. J Appl Physiol 1993;75:994–1001.
101. McKeever KH, Eaton TL, Geiser S, et al. Thermoregulation in old and young horses during exercise. Med Sci Sport Exerc 2000;32:S156.
102. McKeever KH. Exercise physiology in older horses. In: MacLeay JM, editor. Veterinary clinics of North America: equine practice; geriatrics. Philadelphia: WB Saunders; 2002. p. 469–90.
103. Armstrong CG, Kenney WL. Effects of aging and acclimation on responses to passive heat exposure. J Appl Physiol 1993;75:2162–7.
104. Kenney WL. Body fluid and temperature regulation as a function of age. In: Lamb DR, Gisolfi CV, Nade ER, editors. Perspectives in exercise and sports medicine, vol. 8, exercise in older adults. Carmel, IN: Cooper Publishing; 1995. p. 305–52.
105. McKeever KH, Kearns CF. Aging-induced alterations in plasma volume in horses. Med Sci Sport Exerc 2001;33:S257.
106. Betros CL, McKeever KH, Kearns CF, et al. Effects of aging and training on maximal heart rate and VO_{2max}. Equine Vet J 2002;(Suppl. 34):S100–5.
107. McKeever KH, Eaton TL, Geiser S, et al. Age related decreases in thermoregulation and cardiovascular function in horses. Eq Vet J Suppl 2010;38:220–227.
108. Best S, Caillaud C, Thompson M. The effect of ageing and fitness on thermoregulatory response to high-intensity exercise. Scand J Med Sci Sports 2012;22(4):29–37.
109. Morgan K, Funquist P, Nyman G. The effect of coat clipping on thermoregulation during intense exercise in trotters. Equine Vet J 2002;(Suppl. 34):S564–7.
110. Jeffcott L, Leung WM, Riggs C. Managing the effects of the weather on the Equestrian Events of the 2008 Beijing Olympic Games. Vet J 2009;182:412–29.
111. Hower MA, Potter GD, Greene LW, et al. Plasma aldosterone and electrolyte concentrations in exercising Thoroughbred horses fed two diets in summer and winter. J Equine Vet Sci 1995;15:445–9.
112. Hoyt JK, Potter GD, Greene LW, et al. Electrolyte balance in exercising horses fed a control and a fat-supplemented diet. J Equine Vet Sci 1995;15:429–33.
113. Bouchama A, Knochel JP. Heat stroke. N Engl J Med 2002;346:1978–88.
114. Coris EE, Ramirez AM, Van Durme DJ. Heat illness in athletes. The dangerous combination of heat, humidity and exercise. Sports Med 2004;34: 9–16.
115. Jardine DS. Heat illness and heat stroke. Pediatr Rev 2007;28:248–58.

116. Yeo TP. Heat stroke. A comprehensive review. AACN Clin Issues 2004;15:280–93.
117. Jenkinson DE, Elder HY, Bovell DL. Equine sweating and anhidrosis. Part 2 – anhidrosis. Vet Dermatol 2007;18:2–11.
118. MacKay RJ. Quantitative intradermal terbutaline sweat test in horses. Eq Vet J 2008;40:518–20.
119. Wilson DCS, Corbett AD, Steel C, et al. A preliminary study of the short circuit current (I_{SC}) responses of sweat gland cells from normal and anhidrotic horses to purinergic and adrenergic agonists. Vet Dermatol 2007;18:152–60.
120. Lovatt Evans C, Smith DFG, Ross KA, et al. Physiological factors in the condition of 'dry coat' in horses. Vet Rec 1957;69:1–15.
121. Beadle RE, Norwood GL, Brencick VA. Summertime plasma catecholamine concentrations in healthy and anhidrotic horses in Louisiana. Am J Vet Res 1982;43:1446–8.
122. Marlin DJ, Schroter RC, Scott CM, et al. Sweating and skin temperature responses of normal and anhidrotic horses to intravenous adrenaline. Equine Vet J Suppl 1999;30: 362–9.
123. Bovell DL, Lindsay SL, Corbett AD, et al. Immunolocalization of aquaporin-5 expression in sweat gland cells from normal and anhidrotic horses. Vet Dermatol 2006;17:17–23.
124. Hubert JD, Beadle RE, Norwood G. Equine anhidrosis. Vet Clin North Am Equine Pract 2002;18:355–69.
125. Warner AE, Mayhew IG. Equine anhidrosis: a survey of affected horses in Florida. J Am Vet Med Assoc 1982;180:627–30.
126. Johnson EB, MacKay RJ, Hernandez JA. An epidemiologic study of anhidrosis in horses in Florida. J Am Vet Med Assoc 2010;236:1091–7.
127. Sneddon JC, Ritruechai P, Staats de Yanes G, et al. Seasonal influences on quantitative changes in sweat-associated anatomy in native and thoroughbred horses. Vet Dermatol 2008;19:163–73.
128. Foreman JH, Benson GJ, Foreman MH. Effects of a pre-moistened multilayered breathable fabric in promoting heat loss during recovery after exercise in hot conditions. Equine Vet J Suppl 2006;36:303–7.
129. Polla BS, Bachelet M, Elia G, et al. Stress proteins in inflammation. Ann N Y Acad Sci 1998;851:75–85.
130. Bynum GD, Pandolf KB, Schuette WH, et al. Induced hyperthermia in sedated humans and the concept of critical hyperthermia. Am J Physiol 1978;235:R228–36.
131. Byrd SK, McCutcheon LJ, Hodgson DR, et al. Altered sarcoplasmic reticulum function after high intensity exercise. J Appl Physiol 1989;76:2072–7.
132. McCutcheon LJ, Geor RJ, Hare MJ, et al. Sweat composition: comparison of collection methods and effects of exercise intensity. Equine Vet J Suppl 1995;18:279–84.

section 7

Hematology and immunology

Hematology and serum biochemistry of the equine athlete

42

Erica C. McKenzie

CHAPTER CONTENTS

Introduction

The circulation of blood and its many components to and from the major organs, including the exercising musculature, represents one of the most critical aspects of exercise physiology. Since evaluation of the hemogram and serum or plasma biochemistry analyzes can provide insights into oxygen transport, organ function, and fluid, electrolyte and acid–base balance, it is not surprising that such tests currently rank among the most frequent diagnostic techniques employed during investigation of suboptimal performance or disease in equine athletes.[1,2] Although these methods provide a broad assessment of possible inflammation or dysfunction of various organ systems, training and exercise both can influence multiple hematologic and biochemistry variables in healthy horses. Therefore a comprehensive understanding of expected changes in response to these stimuli is essential for accurate interpretation of laboratory analyzes. In addition, among other factors, sample collection and processing can substantially impact analysis results; thus, exemplary sample collection, handling and processing techniques should always be employed.[3]

Methods

Blood for hematologic analysis should be collected from the jugular or cephalic vein atraumatically to minimize hemolysis or activation of platelets and clotting factors.[3] Blood should be obtained into an EDTA tube, which is subsequently inverted gently multiple times, with inspection for clumping or clotting. In horses in which an accurate platelet count is desirable, an additional sample should be collected using sodium citrate as the anticoagulant rather than EDTA, to prevent platelet clumping and subsequent pseudothrombocytopenia. Since even relatively brief delays in processing can result in deterioration of equine leukocyte morphology, samples to be transported for analysis should be accompanied by a thin blood smear prepared at the time of collection.[3]

The use of automated cytometers in clinical practice has expanded rapidly in the last few years and has greatly improved the convenience of performing on-site hematologic analysis.[3] However, microscopic examination of a stained blood film should always accompany automated analysis to verify the accuracy of reported leukocyte, red cell and platelet counts, and to ensure an accurate differential cell count and description of cellular morphology is obtained.[3] This is particularly critical for diseased patients in which abnormal cell counts and distributions are considered likely or in which abnormalities of cell morphology might be present.[3] In addition a spun hematocrit should be performed, and plasma or serum total protein values obtained by refractometry should be interpreted with caution in patients in which hyperlipemia is possible since falsely high values may be obtained.[3] The spun hematocrit represents one of the most accurate and reproducible methods of determining blood erythrocyte concentrations in horses, providing the EDTA tube into which the blood sample is obtained is appropriately filled to avoid osmotic shrinkage of the cells, the blood sample is appropriately mixed before filling the microhematocrit tubes, and the microhematocrit tube is appropriately centrifuged and correctly interpreted.[3]

Quantitative biochemical analyzes can be performed on serum or plasma, depending on the preference of the analyzing laboratory or the specific equipment to be used for in-clinic analyzes.[3] Plasma may be preferable in emergency situations to facilitate more timely results. Heparinized plasma should be used for biochemical analyzes rather than EDTA-preserved plasma to avoid erroneous results, particularly for concentration of specific electrolytes such as calcium (which might be below artifactually low) and potassium (which might be artifactually high). Whole blood samples should be centrifuged within 30 minutes followed by separation of serum or plasma to reduce changes associated with ongoing red cell metabolism. Samples specifically designated for plasma lactate analysis can be collected into sodium fluoride tubes and chilled if lactate concentrations will not be obtained from gas analysis of heparinized whole blood.[3] Blood intended for chemistry analyzes, which will include measurement of serum glucose concentrations, can be preserved with appropriate quality by collection into serum separator tubes or for samples intended only for measurement of glucose concentration, tubes containing sodium fluoride or a similar inhibitor of glycolysis.[4] However, changes in multiple blood chemistry variables should be expected even in separated samples if they are stored at room temperature for 24 hours or more.[5] Therefore, if prolonged delays in sample analysis are anticipated, refrigeration of samples at 4 °C is appropriate prior to biochemical or hematological analyzes, after preparation of an accompanying slide to preserve original cell morphology.[3,4] Samples for venous or arterial blood gas analysis should be collected into evacuated glass tubes, or into a 1 or 3 mL glass or quality plastic syringe containing minimal retained heparin volume, and which is capped immediately after the sample is obtained.[3] The use of plastic heparinized vacutainer tubes results in substantial increases in the oxygen content of equine blood samples, accompanied by lesser alterations in carbon dioxide content, and should therefore be avoided.[6] Arterial blood is the ideal sample to determine blood oxygenation status and cardiorespiratory function, though venous blood gas analysis can provide convenient information regarding metabolic disorders and electrolyte status. The transverse facial artery provides the most convenient site for arterial blood sampling in the standing adult horse. Analysis of both venous and arterial samples should be performed as rapidly as possible after collection.

A variety of factors must be taken into account when evaluating the results of common laboratory analyzes, particularly so for the complete blood count.[7] These factors include the horse's age and breed, the stage of the daily routine in relationship to the timing of blood collection, and the horse's demeanor at the time of blood collection.[7] Differences generated by these various factors are described in more detail below, but are usually mild to moderate in degree, and unlikely to result in values outside of appropriate reference limits. However, these factors are particularly relevant when repeated analyzes are performed within the same individual, and therefore attention should be paid to the timing of blood sampling in relationship to the daily routine when serial sampling is expected.[8] Conditioning of horses stimulates a variety of changes, including endocrine alterations directed at increasing plasma volume and defending tonicity, which may result in changes in hematologic and biochemical variables over time in training individuals, or in differences in results obtained from fit versus unfit individuals.[9] Plasma volume expansion likely peaks within eight weeks of submaximal training in the horse, and is likely more pronounced in younger horses.[10] Reference intervals for a variety of equine breeds and activity groups are outlined in Appendices 1 and 2.

Consumption of a relatively large meal (4–5 kg) of forage or concentrate can also elicit substantial changes in plasma volume associated with increased saliva production and extracellular fluid shifts associated with digestion (Fig. 42.1).[11,12] Packed cell volume (PCV) has been reported to increase as much as 16% from pre-feeding values, peaking one to five hours after feeding.[11,13] Comparable but more transient increases in plasma total protein concentration may occur, in addition to transient mild increases in serum sodium and decreases in serum potassium concentrations. These phenomena reflect a decline in plasma volume with feed ingestion and the effects of subsequent aldosterone release.[12,13] Changes are reported to be more pronounced in horses receiving intermittent large meals compared to horses eating more frequent meals.[11,12] However, a study of feed ingestion and voluntary sodium intake in conditioned athletic horses did not identify significant differences in PCV or plasma aldosterone concentrations when horses were fed two times compared to six times per day, though minor transient increases in plasma protein concentration and plasma osmolality were observed after horses consumed a large meal.[14] It was concluded in this study that voluntary sodium intake had the most significant impact on fluid and electrolyte regulation in conditioned horses, and that feeding frequency had minimal influence. It is possible that the differences between the findings of these studies reflect the superior capacity of conditioned individuals to preserve plasma volume in the face of challenges such as exercise and feeding.[14] However, even in conditioned individuals participating in a twice-daily feeding schedule, it remains prudent to obtain samples for hemogram analysis prior to a meal or several hours after a meal to reduce the possible effects of feed ingestion on subsequent results.

Excitability or apprehension at the time of blood sampling can result in catecholamine-mediated splenic contraction, producing substantial increases in PCV.[15] Increases in leukocyte and platelet numbers can also occur since these blood components are also sequestered in the spleen. Obtaining a blood sample quickly and calmly within 30 seconds of encountering the horse will help circumvent catecholamine-related effects. Therefore if blood collection is anticipated as part of the assessment of a performance horse, it best precedes more extensive physical examination procedures in nervous horses in particular.[16] In addition, recent exercise can increase PCV and peripheral leukocyte counts, and can alter the neutrophil : lymphocyte ratio.[8,17–20] Hence, where possible, blood samples are likely best collected in the morning prior to exercise. Similarly, transport and tranquilization can also affect complete

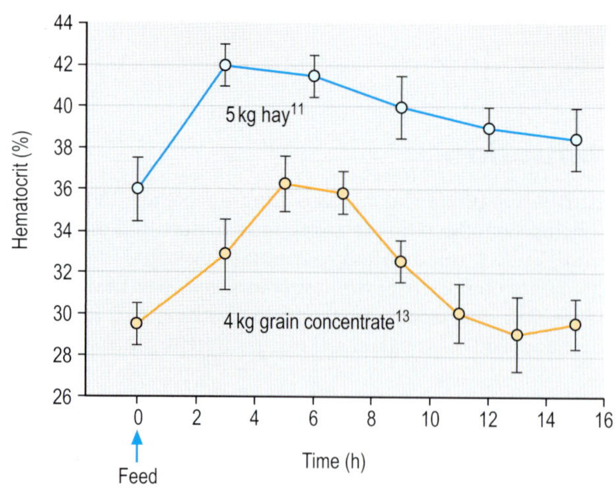

Fig 42.1 The effect of a single feeding of 5 kg of hay[11] or 4 kg of grain concentrate[13] on the hematocrit.

blood count results and therefore sample collection should be temporally distant from such events.

Finally, the clinician should ensure that results are interpreted in light of individual reference limits specific to the laboratory or equipment involved in the analyzes, and that reference limits are in comparable units for all provided results. Where possible, reference limits relevant to the age, breed and conditioning of the horse being examined should also be taken into account (Appendices 1 and 2).

Hematology: structure and function

Erythrocytes and gas exchange

Erythrocytes are anucleate cells which primarily function to transport oxygen to the tissues, carbon dioxide to the lungs, and to buffer hydrogen ions in the blood, all largely as a result of their substantial hemoglobin content. On average, there are approximately 9×10^6 mature erythrocytes per microliter of equine blood, with a circulating life span of approximately 150 days.[3] In comparison to some of the other domestic species, horses do not usually have circulating reticulocytes (immature erythrocytes with stainable cytoplasmic RNA) even during regenerative anemia states; however, some hematology analyzers will report low concentrations of reticulocytes in equine blood.[3] A common measure of erythrocyte mass applied in the horse is the hematocrit (frequently used synonymously with PCV), which represents the percentage of the blood volume filled with erythrocytes.[3] This value can be calculated from the mean cell volume (MCV) and erythrocyte concentration, in which case it is often referred to as hematocrit or calculated hematocrit, or else it can be determined from measurement of a centrifuged microhematocrit tube, in which case it is often referred to as the packed cell volume (PCV) or spun hematocrit. Hematocrit values usually reliably reflect blood hemoglobin and erythrocyte concentrations in the horse, though it should be recognized that blood hemoglobin concentration represents the most direct measure of the blood's capacity to carry oxygen.[3]

Though plasma contains a small amount of dissolved oxygen (3 mL per liter of blood) this is inadequate to meet normal tissue oxygen demands, let alone the dramatically enhanced oxygen demands associated with exercise. Hence oxygen transport in the blood is achieved primarily via the reversible combination of hemoglobin and oxygen molecules within erythrocytes, which increases the oxygen-carrying capacity of the blood to above 200 mL per liter.[21] The high pressure of oxygen (~100 mmHg) within the alveolar air of the lung facilitates rapid diffusion of oxygen into the less well oxygenated pulmonary capillary blood (PO_2 ~40 mmHg) and subsequently into the erythrocytes, where it saturates the four oxygen-binding sites of each hemoglobin molecule. The relationship between the partial pressure of oxygen in the blood and the oxygen saturation of hemoglobin is represented by the oxygen–hemoglobin dissociation curve (Fig. 42.2).[22] The affinity of hemoglobin for oxygen progressively increases as successive oxygen molecules bind, reflected by the steep aspect of the sigmoidal curve. However, at oxygen pressures exceeding 50 to 60 mmHg, the curve flattens, representing a plateau in oxygen saturation that occurs in spite of an increasing partial pressure of oxygen in the blood.[21] The characteristics of this system promote the release of oxygen molecules to the tissues when PO_2 is low, such as in the peripheral tissue capillaries, while oxygen saturation of the blood can be maintained at the pulmonary capillary level even if alveolar oxygen pressure declines to some degree. Directional shifts in the oxygen–hemoglobin dissociation curve can occur and represent changes in the affinity of hemoglobin for oxygen. A rightward shift in the curve reflects a decreased affinity of hemoglobin for oxygen, and is elicited by increases in body temperature, plasma hydrogen ion concentration, plasma CO_2 partial pressure, and the concentration of 2,3-bisphosphoglycerate in the erythrocytes.[3,21] These changes enhance the dissociation of oxygen from hemoglobin and therefore facilitate the subsequent distribution of oxygen to the tissues. Many of these changes are provoked by exercise, consequently causing a rightward shift in the oxygen–hemoglobin dissociation curve and enhancing the delivery of oxygen to contracting muscle tissue.

Carbon dioxide is transported in the blood as dissolved CO_2 (~5%), bicarbonate ions (~70–90%), and carbamate bound to hemoglobin and plasma proteins (~5–10%).[21] However, it should be recognized that the proportions of these various states is very dynamic, and that the contributions of each likely change substantially during exercise activity.[23] Carbon dioxide transport is coupled closely with oxygen transport to the benefit of both systems, as demonstrated in Figure 42.3. Carbon dioxide produced by the tissues diffuses into the tissue capillaries and subsequently the erythrocytes, facilitating the release of oxygen molecules from hemoglobin to the tissues. Within the erythrocytes, CO_2 is converted to

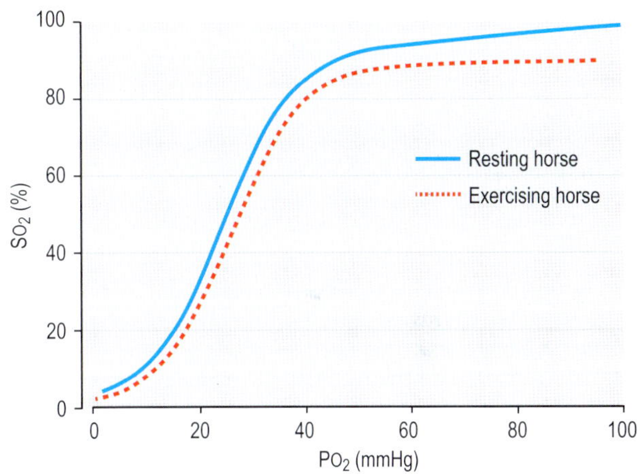

Fig 42.2 The oxygen–hemoglobin dissociation curve in resting (solid line) and heavily exercising (dashed line) horses. PO_2, partial pressure of oxygen; SO_2, percentage saturation of hemoglobin.[22]

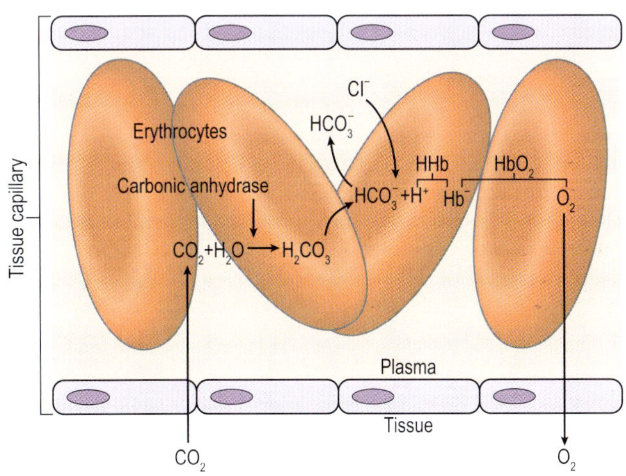

Fig 42.3 Carbon dioxide and oxygen exchange at the level of the systemic tissue capillary. Hb = hemoglobin, HHb = protonated hemoglobin.[21]

bicarbonate ions and protons in a process greatly facilitated by the high carbonic anhydrase activity within red cells, and accommodated by a shift of chloride ions into the red cells in exchange for bicarbonate. The greater affinity of reduced hemoglobin for protons compared to oxyhemoglobin facilitates this process and enables transport of a large proportion of the carbon dioxide load from the tissues to the lungs in the form of plasma bicarbonate, though the contribution of dissolved CO_2 to gas exchange also increases substantially during exercise.[23] Reversal of the carbonic anhydrase reaction when erythrocytes return to the pulmonary capillary drives the off-loading of CO_2 into the alveolar air to be expired.[3,21]

Leukocytes

Leukocytes represent a major fraction of the complete blood count encompassing neutrophils, eosinophils, basophils, monocytes, and lymphocytes. Leukocytes have considerably shorter circulating times than erythrocytes, sometimes mere hours, and therefore their presence in the peripheral blood reflects their transit from their site of production to their site of function or destruction. Although total white blood cell count (WBC) is a commonly assessed value on the routine complete blood count, it is of limited use without specific differential counts to help identify the specific cell types altered in number by processes such as exercise or disease. Similarly to erythrocytes, leukocytes may be sequestered in the spleen, and can also marginalize in capillary beds, and therefore their presence in the peripheral blood may be substantially affected by recent activities altering the horse's cortisol and catecholamine profile, including excitement and exercise.[3,19]

Platelets

Platelets represent fragments of the cytoplasm of late-stage megakaryocyte cells shed into circulation from the bone marrow. Platelets circulate for between five to ten days in the peripheral blood if they are not sequestered or consumed. Their major purpose is to repair vascular damage and to prevent persistent bleeding, although they are also recognized to have increasingly more complex roles in the body, including in wound healing and inflammation.[3] Similarly to erythrocytes and leukocytes, platelets are also subject to splenic sequestration and might therefore increase in number in the peripheral blood in response to exercise or excitement-induced splenic contraction.[3]

Evaluation of the resting hemogram as a predictor of performance potential has long been a source of interest in equine sports medicine.[7,16,24,25] Particular emphasis has been placed on evaluation of the red cell indices, including PCV, red blood cell count and blood hemoglobin concentration, since these specific variables are critical to athletic function. However, attempts to link one or more of these variables in resting horses to athletic performance have met with mixed results.[16,18,25] Though some studies have reported lower values for these variables in poor-performing compared to well-performing horses, the degree of difference between these groups is relatively small, making it challenging to attribute clinical significance to results in the individual animal.[26] This phenomenon is demonstrated in Figures 42.4 and 42.5, in which significant but small differences in hematocrit and hemoglobin concentrations were reported between normal (control) and intermediate and poor performing Standardbred trotters at rest and after an exercise test.[26] In addition, given the dynamic and variable nature of the equine hemogram, and the complicated multifactorial nature of oxygen transport in exercising horses, a reliable link between specific features of the resting hemogram and subsequent performance is unlikely to

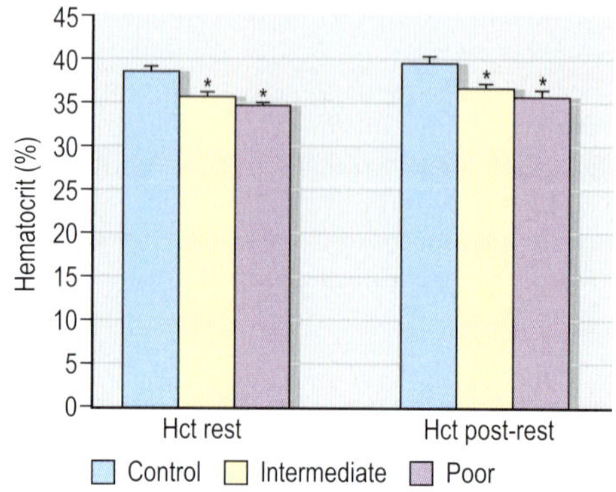

Fig 42.4 Differences in hematocrit (%) at rest and after a 1275 m sand racetrack test in Standardbred trotters reported to have normal (control), intermediate and poor performance, respectively.
Data from Richard et al.[26]

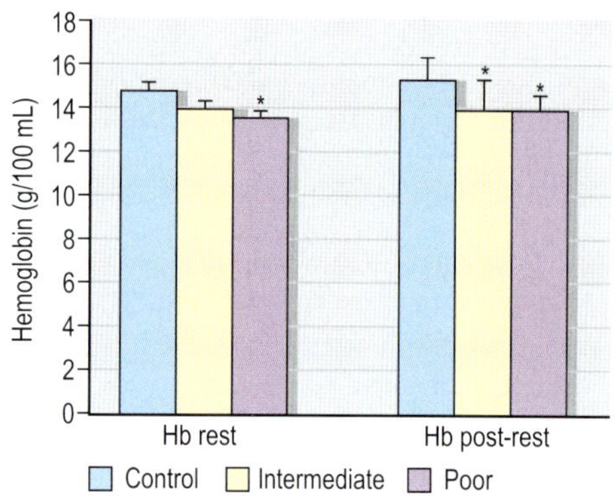

Fig 42.5 Differences in blood hemoglobin concentration (g/100 mL) at rest and after a 1275 m sand racetrack test in Standardbred trotters reported to have normal (control), intermediate and poor performance respectively.
Data from Richard et al.[26]

be firmly established.[16] However, values outside of appropriate reference limits, or changes over time in a specific individual, should be evaluated carefully if suboptimal performance is a complaint.

Hematologic responses to exercise

Changes in the hemogram, particularly the hematocrit, evoked by exercise are expected to correlate to the intensity and duration of the exercise stimulus (Fig. 42.6).[16,19,27–32] However, even light to moderate exercise may create substantial alterations to the hemogram, particularly if exercise is prolonged in duration or associated with significant apprehension or excitement.[15,18] Changes that may arise with moderate exercise include a mild increase in PCV and plasma protein, reflecting a combination of the effects of splenic contraction and exercise-induced fluid shifts. Prolonged endurance exercise is associated with substantial fluid losses, contributing to an increase in packed cell volume of 8 to 10% or more, with concurrent mild increases in serum or plasma total protein concentration.[33] More pronounced alterations in these variables may occur in horses completing these distances at higher speeds, less fit horses, or in horses encountering metabolic failure.[18,33,34]

Intense exercise stimulates more dramatic changes in the hemogram, accommodating the delivery of more than 80 liters of oxygen per minute to the tissues of the elite Thoroughbred racehorse during

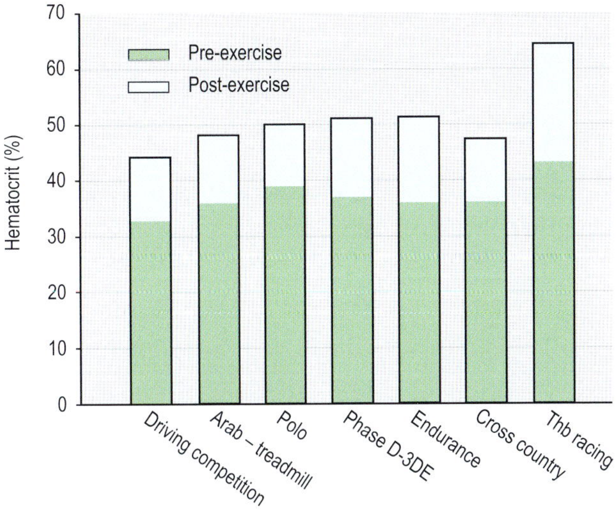

Fig 42.6 The effect of different types of exercise on the hematocrit including the cross-country phase of driving trail competition,[27] low-intensity treadmill exercise,[32] during a polo match,[31] phase D of a three-day event,[30] an 80-km endurance ride,[29] the cross-country phase of a three-day event,[28] and Thoroughbred racing.[19]

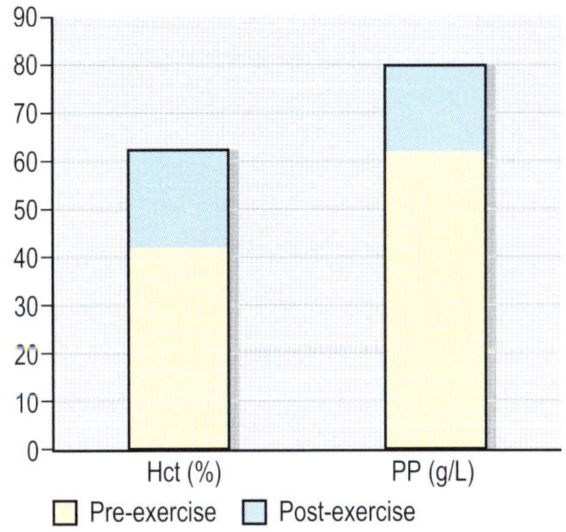

Fig 42.7 Hematocrit (Hct) and plasma protein concentration (PP) in Thoroughbred horses at rest and after completion of a 1600 m race.[39]

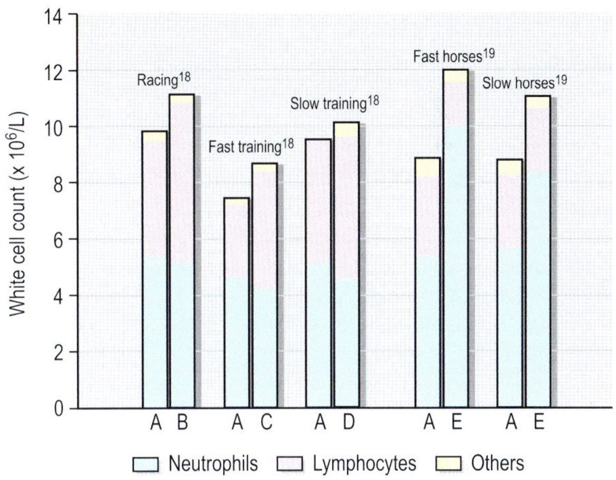

Fig 42.8 The effect of different types of exercise on peripheral leukocyte numbers. Data from Rose[18] and Snow, et al.[19] **(A)** resting; **(B)** immediately after racing; **(C)** immediately after fast training (11–12 m/s); **(D)** immediately after slow training (13 m/s); **(E)**, immediately after a 160-km endurance ride.

maximal activity.[35] The horse is to some degree unique among many species in that at the onset of exercise, catecholamine-mediated contraction of the spleen can result in a veritable doubling of the PCV to as much as 70%, with concurrent increases in red cell count and hemoglobin concentrations.[35] However, breed specificity exists, and Thoroughbred horses have considerably higher peak hematocrit values than other athletic breeds such as the Arabian horse.[36] Differences in hemogram values related to age and training also exist, with increases in hemoglobin and hematocrit expected with age and increased training experience. Gender differences in these variables appear to be insignificant.[8,24,37]

The increase in PCV, red cell count and hemoglobin and plasma protein concentrations that occur at the commencement of both submaximal and intense exercise efforts contribute to substantial increases in blood viscosity in horses (Fig. 42.7).[28,38,39] Increases in blood viscosity during exercise may be further exacerbated by reduced erythrocyte deformability, and external factors such as furosemide administration.[40] Increased blood viscosity can impair oxygen delivery to the exercising tissues and is likely one of the phenomena contributing to the routine development of arterial hypoxemia in conditioned horses.[41] A syndrome of red cell hypervolemia and its subsequent effects on variables including blood viscosity has been extensively investigated in Standardbred trotters, and possible associations of this syndrome with exercise-induced pulmonary hemorrhage, poor performance, and overtraining syndrome have been reported.[42] However, red cell hypervolemia syndrome has not been definitively identified in other breeds or groups, and currently its significance in the general athletic horse population is controversial.[43] Nonetheless, exercise equal to or exceeding 60% of maximal oxygen uptake has been recorded as producing intravascular hemolysis and transient hematuria, pigmenturia and proteinuria in exercising horses, illuminating the stresses that even submaximal exercise can place on multiple body systems of the healthy horse, and particularly on the red cells.[44]

The impact of exercise on the leukogram of equine athletes is less consistent than for the red cell indices (Fig. 42.8). Both endurance exercise and intense trotting and galloping exercise may result in leukocytosis characterized by an increased neutrophil : lymphocyte ratio, with absolute neutrophilia persisting for approximately one to six hours.[20,45–47] Exhaustive high-intensity exercise may promote an increased leukocyte count in horses that persists for 24 hours, and changes to the leukogram have been documented to occur on consecutive days of exercise.[45,46] Neutrophilia, when present, likely reflects demargination of cells from the vascular endothelium and also potentially the release of leukocytes from the bone marrow, but does not necessarily correlate with increases in blood cortisol concentration.[17,47]

Hematologic responses to training

Training activity in horses stimulates increases in resting red blood cell count, PCV and hemoglobin concentration to accommodate the periodic demand for increased oxygen delivery to exercising muscle tissue.[8,16,37,48] This phenomenon is most pronounced in young horses newly encountering the training stimulus, though less profound alterations to the hemogram over time also occur in previously conditioned horses returning to training after a period of rest.[8,49] Substantial changes in the hemogram are also more likely to occur with faster-paced race training compared to submaximal or endurance training.[10,49] However, the extensive changes in plasma volume that can occur in response to training can confound accurate assessment of changes in the total erythrocyte mass.[10]

Nonetheless, values that fall outside appropriate reference limits for the horse's age, breed and state of training are most likely to carry clinical significance during evaluation of horses with poor performance.

Neither submaximal nor intense exercise training have been reported to significantly alter the leukogram of horses, beyond those changes previously described occurring in proximity to exercise bouts.[20,45–47] However, a mild increase in the neutrophil : lymphocyte ratio was identified in horses training intensively over 32 weeks, with concurrent eosinopenia identified in a group of horses defined as overtrained, indicating that eosinopenia can reflect inappropriately heavy training stress.[48]

Plasma or serum biochemistry overview

Plasma or serum biochemistry analysis encompasses assessment of several organ systems relevant to the athletic horse, including the renal, hepatic and muscular systems.[3] Hence biochemical analyzes can provide valuable indications of specific disease issues in athletic horses with suboptimal performance. However, similarly to the hemogram, specific biochemical variables can be influenced by exercise and training, and therefore evaluation of biochemistry results from athletic horses must be undertaken with care to avoid erroneous interpretation. Routine serum biochemical analyzes often include measurements of plasma protein fractions (total protein, albumin, and total globulin), indicators of renal function (urea nitrogen and creatinine concentrations), and enzyme activities associated with the muscular and hepatic systems (including creatine kinase [CK], aspartate transaminase, gamma-glutamyltransferase, and sorbitol dehydrogenase).[3] Additional variables may include measurement of bilirubin (total concentration and conjugated and unconjugated fractions), triglycerides, electrolyte concentrations (sodium, potassium, and chloride) and mineral concentrations (phosphorus, total calcium, and magnesium). The clinician should be intimately familiar with each variable of the routine chemistry profile in regard to origin and significance, and the specific vulnerability of each variable to artifactual changes as a result of sample handling or hemolysis. In addition, knowledge of the release or production characteristics of specific enzymes is important to ensure appropriate timing of sample collection in relationship to exercise or specific disease processes.

Changes in plasma or serum biochemistry associated with exercise

Plasma proteins

Exercise prompts a complicated redistribution of fluid and electrolytes within the body compartments, resulting in a rapid decline in plasma volume following the onset of exercise, proportional to the intensity and duration of effort.[50] This decline in plasma volume commonly elicits transient increases in circulating total protein and albumin concentrations during maximal exercise efforts, which usually persist for less than an hour. Prolonged exercise is associated with further plasma volume decline as a result of fluid loss via sweating and other processes.[50] Hence more significant and sustained increases in plasma protein concentration can be observed during or immediately after prolonged exercise activity, with the greatest increases evident in more severely dehydrated horses.[33,51]

Liver-derived enzymes

Currently, the most commonly evaluated hepatic enzymes in horses include sorbitol dehydrogenase (SDH), glutamate dehydrogenase (GLDH), gamma-glutamyl transferase (GGT), aspartate transaminase (AST) and alkaline phosphatase (ALP).[3] Lactate dehydrogenase activity is often reported in routine biochemical profiles, but unless isoenzyme analysis is performed, the highly non-specific nature of this enzyme precludes accurate interpretation regarding its origin.[3] The serum or plasma activities of SDH, GLDH and GGT reliably reflect liver-related anomalies in the horse due to a high degree of tissue specificity.[3] Plasma ALP activity tends to be an insensitive marker of cholestasis in horses, and increases can also reflect osteoblastic activity in bone, especially in younger animals.[3] Increases in serum AST activity which are not accompanied by alterations of any other hepatic enzyme are most likely to reflect muscular origin in a non-hemolyzed sample.[3] Although liver enzyme activities are relatively sensitive indicators of hepatic injury, they are poor indicators of liver function, which can be investigated by assessment of other relevant biochemistry variables (urea nitrogen, bilirubin, glucose, albumin) and from measurement of serum bile acid concentrations, plasma ammonia and blood coagulation times.

Single episodes of exercise have minimal impact on the serum or plasma activities of liver-derived enzymes in the horse, though increases in GGT activity have been reported during endurance exercise.[52]

Muscle-derived enzymes

The health and function of the muscular system of athletic horses is routinely assessed via measurement of serum or plasma activity of CK and AST. Plasma lactate dehydrogenase activity can also reflect muscle injury but is not tissue specific, which limits its application unless isoenzyme analysis is performed.[3] Increases in plasma or serum CK activity provide the most sensitive and specific indication of recent skeletal muscle injury in the horse, though due to a brief half-life, samples for measurement of CK activity are best collected within four to six hours after exercise, training, or the suspected muscular insult. In comparison, AST activity can remain persistently increased for days after a muscular insult, though it should always be interpreted in conjunction with CK and the other liver enzymes to account for its lesser tissue specificity.[3]

Maximal exercise in horses commonly induces mild to moderate increases in CK and AST activity, of usually less than 400 U/L in magnitude.[53,54] More substantial increases are induced by prolonged endurance exercise, and serum CK commonly increases several thousand units per liter or more in apparently healthy endurance horses after racing.[33,34,55] A comparison of the impact of endurance exercise and racing exercise on serum CK activity is displayed in Figure 42.9. Considerably more dramatic increases in serum CK activity can be observed in individual horses participating in either endurance or high-intensity exercise, but should be considered highly suggestive of subclinical or clinical muscular pathology associated with an exertional rhabdomyolysis disorder.[56,57]

Electrolytes and minerals

Changes in specific electrolyte and mineral concentrations with exercise are most likely to occur during high-intensity or prolonged submaximal exercise. High-intensity exercise in horses induces mild to marked hyperkalemia (plasma potassium concentrations can reach 8–10 mEq/L), mild to marked increases in plasma sodium concentration (~10–20 mEq/L increase) and decreased arterial bicarbonate concentrations.[58] These changes reflect the combined

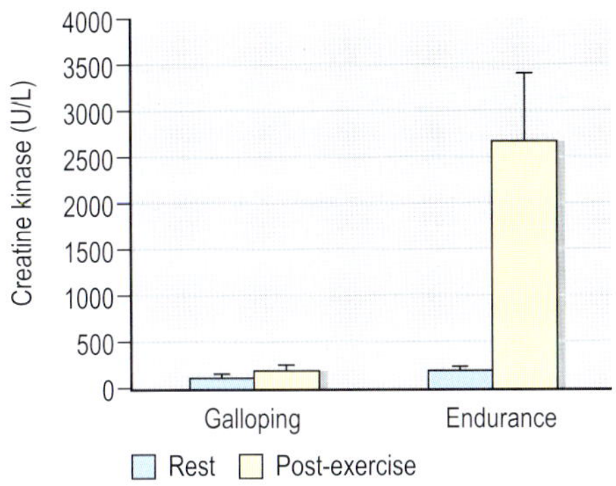

Fig 42.9 Serum CK activity at rest, and in Thoroughbred horses after a 1200 m race (galloping)[39] and in Arabian horses after a 120 km race (endurance).[55]

effects of plasma volume contraction and metabolic and respiratory acidosis, which can become profound enough to cause plasma pH to fall below 7.0 during maximal exercise. However, these changes are transient and generally resolve within 60 to 90 minutes after exercise ceases, during which time transient hypokalemia may be observed.[58]

Prolonged strenuous and submaximal exercise can also elicit substantial changes in the electrolyte profile as a result of the loss of sodium, chloride, potassium, calcium and other electrolytes and minerals into sweat, particularly in hot and humid ambient conditions.[59] Due to concurrent plasma volume loss and the variable concentration of the different ions in sweat relative to plasma, sustained exercise most frequently provokes hypochloremic metabolic alkalosis with normal to mildly decreased plasma sodium and potassium concentrations.[59] These changes can be more pronounced in endurance horses encountering metabolic compromise during racing.[34,51,57]

Changes in plasma or serum biochemistry associated with training

In general, training has a limited impact on resting biochemical values in athletic horses. The most notable phenomenon is a progressive increase in serum or plasma GGT activity in racehorses in training.[48] Increases in serum bilirubin have also been reported in training horses.[8,48] The significance of these changes is unclear, though attempts have been made to link increases in GGT activity with overtraining or poor-performance syndromes.[48,60] Usually GGT increases in training horses are not accompanied by other evidence of hepatic disease, and the cause of this phenomenon remains unknown. Similar phenomena have occasionally been reported in elite human athletes.

Training tends to attenuate serum CK and AST alterations over time, although this is dependent on the intensity and frequency of training.[61] In one study, strenuous training of Standardbred horses resulted in a several hundred unit/liter increase in serum AST over time.[48] In another study of mature Thoroughbreds, serum CK activity measured 12 hours after exercise was higher in horses that were trained only once or twice per week compared to horses being exercised three times per week.[62] In general, in horses adapting appropriately to training stresses, serum CK or AST activity after exercise should remain within reference limits or increases should not exceed more than a few hundred units per liter. Increases can be more prominent in younger horses that have had less exposure to training stress.

Conclusion

Hematology and plasma or serum biochemistry analyzes represent convenient tools for assessing the health of the performance horse. Currently they cannot be reliably used to predict performance potential or to determine maladaptation to training. In addition, the clinician must be aware of the multitude of factors relevant to the athletic horse that can impact many specific variables of these analyzes.

With thanks to Janene K. Kingston, who created the original chapter in the first edition.

References

1. McGowan C. Clinical pathology in the racing horse: the role of clinical pathology in assessing fitness and performance in the racehorse. Vet Clin North Am Equine Pract 2008;24: 405–21.
2. Fraipont A, Van Erck E, Ramery E, et al. Subclinical diseases underlying poor performance in endurance horses: diagnostic methods and predictive tests. Vet Rec 2011;169:154.
3. Stockham SL, Scott MA. Fundamentals of Veterinary Clinical Pathology. 2nd ed. Ames, IA: Blackwell Publishing; 2008.
4. Bush VJ, Janu MR, Bathur F, et al. Comparison of BD Vacutainer SST Plus Tubes with BD SST II Plus Tubes for common analytes. Clin Chim Acta 2001;306:139–43.
5. Rendle DI, Heller J, Hughes KJ, et al. Stability of common biochemistry analytes in equine blood stored at room temperature. Equine Vet J 2009;41:428–32.
6. Noël PG, Couëtil L, Constable PD. Effects of collecting blood into plastic heparinised vacutainer tubes and storage conditions on blood gas analysis values in horses. Equine Vet J Suppl 2010;42:91–7.
7. Carlson GP. Haematology and body fluids in the equine athlete: a review. In: Gillespie JR, Robinson NE, editors. Equine Exercise Physiology 2. Davis, CA: ICEEP Publications; 1987. p. 393–425.
8. Allen BV, Powell DG. Effects of training and time of day of blood sampling on the variation of some common haematological parameters in normal Thoroughbred racehorses. In: Snow DH, Persson SGB, Rose RJ, editors. Equine Exercise Physiology. Cambridge, UK: Granta Editions; 1983. p. 328–53.
9. McKeever KH, Schurg WA, Jarrett SH, et al. Exercise training-induced hypervolemia in the horse. Med Sci Sports Exerc 1987;19:21–7.
10. Golland LC, Evans DL, McGowan CM, et al. The effects of overtraining on blood volumes in Standardbred racehorses. Vet J 2003;165:228–33.
11. Kerr MG, Snow DH. Alterations in haematocrit, plasma proteins and electrolytes in horses following the feeding of hay. Vet Rec 1982;110:538–40.
12. Clarke LL, Argenzio RA, Roberts MC. Effect of meal feeding on plasma volume

and urinary electrolyte clearance in ponies. Am J Vet Res 1990;51:571–76.
13. Clarke LL, Ganjam VK, Fichtenbaum B, et al. Effect of feeding on renin-angiotensin-aldosterone system of the horse. Am J Physiol 1988;254:R524–30.
14. Jansson A, Dahlborn K. Effects of feeding frequency and voluntary salt intake on fluid and electrolyte regulation in athletic horses. J Appl Physiol 1999;86:1610–16.
15. Revington M. Haematology of the racing Thoroughbred in Australia 1: reference values and the effect of excitement. Equine Vet J 1983;15:141–4.
16. Bayly WM. The interpretation of clinicopathologic data from the equine athlete. Vet Clin North Am Equine Pract 1987;3:631–47.
17. Rossdale PD, Burguez PN, Cash RS. Changes in blood neutrophil/lymphocyte ratio related to adrenocortical function in the horse. Equine Vet J 1982;14:293–8.
18. Rose RJ. Haematological changes associated with endurance exercise. Vet Rec 1982;110:175–7.
19. Snow DH, Ricketts SW, Mason DK. Haematological response to racing and training exercise in Thoroughbred horses, with particular reference to the leukocyte response. Equine Vet J 1983;15:149–54.
20. Art T, Franck T, Gangl M, et al. Plasma concentrations of myeloperoxidase in endurance and 3-day event horses after a competition. Equine Vet J Suppl 2006;36:298–302.
21. West JB. Gas transport by the blood. In: Respiratory Physiology: The Essentials. 8th ed. Baltimore, MD: Lippincott, Williams & Wilkins; 2008. p. 75–93.
22. Lekeux P. Pulmonary function in healthy, exercising and diseased animals. Ghent, Belgium: V. D. T. Publications; 1993.
23. Geers C, Gros G. Carbon dioxide transport and carbonic anhydrase in blood and muscle. Physiol Rev 2000;80:681–715.
24. Allen BV. Comparison of the haemogram between three-year-old Thoroughbred stayers and sprinters. Vet Rec 1986;118:555–6.
25. Revington M. Haematology of the racing Thoroughbred in Australia 2: haematological values compared to performance. Equine Vet J 1983;15: 145–8.
26. Richard EA, Fortier GD, Pitel PH, et al. Sub-clinical diseases affecting performance in Standardbred trotters: diagnostic methods and predictive parameters. Vet J 2010;184:282–9.
27. Snow DH. Haematological, biochemical and physiological changes in horses and ponies during the cross country stage of driving trial competitions. Vet Rec 1990;126:233–9.
28. Sommardahl CS, Andrews FM, Saxton AM, et al. Alterations in blood viscosity in horses competing in cross country jumping. Am J Vet Res 1994;55:389–94.
29. Snow DH, Kerr MG, Nimmo MA, et al. Alterations in blood, sweat, urine and muscle composition during prolonged exercise in the horse. Vet Rec 1982;110:377–84.
30. Andrews FM, Geiser DR, White SL, et al. Haematological and biochemical changes in horses competing in a 3-star horse trial and 3-day-event. Equine Vet J Suppl 1995;40:57–63.
31. Craig L, Hintz HF, Soderholm LV, et al. Changes in blood constituents accompanying exercise in polo horses. Cornell Vet 1985;75:297–302.
32. Rubio D, Riber C, Santisteban R, et al. Hematologic alterations as an index of exercise tolerance in different breeds of horses. Equine Athlete 1994;7:10–12.
33. Schott HC 2nd, Marlin DJ, Geor RJ, et al. Changes in selected physiological and laboratory measurements in elite horses competing in a 160 km endurance ride. Equine Vet J Suppl 2006;36:37–42.
34. Muñoz A, Riber C, Trigo P, et al. Muscle damage, hydration, electrolyte balance and vasopressin concentrations in successful and exhausted endurance horses. Pol J Vet Sci 2010;13:373–9.
35. Poole DC, Erickson HE. Cardiovascular function and oxygen transport: responses to exercise and training. In: Hinchchcliff KW, Geor RJ, Kaneps AJ, editors. Equine Exercise Physiology – The Science of Exercise in the Athletic Horse. Philadelphia, PA: Elsevier Limited; 2008. p. 212–45.
36. Prince A, Geor R, Harris P, et al. Comparison of the metabolic responses of trained Arabians and Thoroughbreds during high- and low-intensity exercise. Equine Vet J Suppl 2002;34:95–9.
37. Seeherman HJ, Morris EA. Comparison of yearling, two-year-old and adult Thoroughbreds using a standardised exercise test. Equine Vet J 1991;23:175–84.
38. Geor RJ, Weiss DJ, Smith CM 2nd. Hemorheologic alterations induced by incremental treadmill exercise in Thoroughbreds. Am J Vet Res 1994;55:854–61.
39. Snow DH, Mason DK, Ricketts SW, et al. Post-race blood biochemistry in Thoroughbreds. In: Snow DH, Persson SGB, Rose RJ, editors. Equine Exercise Physiology. Cambridge, UK: Granta Editions; 1983. p. 389–99.
40. Weiss DJ, Geor RJ, Burger K. Effects of furosemide on hemorheologic alterations induced by incremental treadmill exercise in Thoroughbreds. Am J Vet Res 1996;57:891–5.
41. Caillaud C, Connes P, Bouix D, et al. Does haemorheology explain the paradox of hypoxemia during exercise in elite athletes or Thoroughbred horses? Clin Hemorheol Microcirc 2002;26:175–81.
42. Funkquist P, Wagner PD, Hedenstierna G, et al. Ventilation-perfusion relationships during exercise in Standardbred trotters with red cell hypervolaemia. Equine Vet J Suppl 1999;30:107–13.
43. Rivero JL, van Breda E, Rogers CW, et al. Unexplained underperformance syndrome in sport horses: classification, potential causes and recognition. Equine Vet J 2008;40:611–18.
44. Schott HC 2nd, Hodgson DR, Bayly WM. Haematuria, pigmenturia and proteinuria in exercising horses. Equine Vet J 1995;27:67–72.
45. Korhonen PA, Lilius EM, Hyyppä S, et al. Production of reactive oxygen species in neutrophils after repeated bouts of exercise in Standardbred trotters. J Vet Med A Physiol Pathol Clin Med 2000;47:565–73.
46. Donovan DC, Jackson CA, Colahan PT, et al. Assessment of exercise-induced alterations in neutrophil function in horses. Am J Vet Res 2007;68:1198–204.
47. Cywińska A, Wyszyńska Z, Górecka R, et al. The effect of the 162 km endurance ride on equine peripheral blood neutrophil and lymphocyte functions. Pol J Vet Sci 2010;13:279–85.
48. Tyler-McGowan CM, Golland LC, Evans DL, et al. Haematological and biochemical responses to training and overtraining. Equine Vet J Suppl 1999;30:621–5.
49. Ohmura H, Hiraga A, Matsui A, et al. Physiological responses of young Thoroughbreds during their first year of race training. Equine Vet J Suppl 2002;34:140–6.
50. McKeever KH. Body fluids and electrolytes. In: Hinchchcliff KW, Geor RJ, Kaneps AJ, editors. Equine Exercise Physiology – The Science of Exercise in the Athletic Horse. Philadelphia, PA: Elsevier Limited; 2008. p. 328–49.
51. Fielding CL, Magdesian KG, Rhodes DM, et al. Clinical and biochemical abnormalities in endurance horses eliminated from competition for medical complications and requiring emergency medical treatment: 30 cases (2005–2006). J Vet Emerg Crit Care (San Antonio) 2009;19:473–8.
52. Rose RJ, Hodgson DR, Sampson D, et al. Changes in plasma biochemistry in horses competing in a 160 km endurance ride. Aust Vet J 1983;60:101–5.
53. Judson GJ, Frauenfelder HC, Mooney GJ. Biochemical changes in Thoroughbred racehorses following submaximal and maximal exercise. In: Snow DH, Persson SGB, Rose RJ, editors. Equine Exercise Physiology. Cambridge, UK: Granta Editions; 1983. p. 408–15.
54. Harris PA, Marlin DJ, Gray J. Plasma aspartate aminotransferase and creatine

kinase activities in Thoroughbred racehorses in relation to age, sex, exercise and training. Vet J 1998;155:295–304.
55. Serteyn D, Sandersen C, Lejeune JP, et al. Effect of a 120 km endurance race on plasma and muscular neutrophil elastase and myeloperoxidase concentrations in horses. Equine Vet J Suppl 2010;42:275–9.
56. Martin BB Jr, Reef VB, Parente EJ, et al. Causes of poor performance of horses during training, racing, or showing: 348 cases (1992–1996). J Am Vet Med Assoc 2000;216:554–8.
57. Barnes A, Kingston J, Beetson S, et al. Endurance veterinarians detect physiologically compromised horses in a 160 km ride. Equine Vet J Suppl 2010;42:6–11.
58. Bayly WM, Kingston JK, Brown JA, et al. Changes in arterial, mixed venous and intraerythrocytic concentrations of ions in supramaximally exercising horses. Equine Vet J Suppl 2006;36:294–7.
59. Flaminio MJ, Rush BR. Fluid and electrolyte balance in endurance horses. Vet Clin North Am Equine Pract 1998;14:147–58.
60. Leleu C, Haentjens F. Morphological, haemato-biochemical and endocrine changes in young Standardbreds with 'maladaptation' to early training. Equine Vet J Suppl 2010;42:171–8.
61. Siciliano PD, Lawrence LM, Danielsen K, et al. Effect of conditioning and exercise type on serum creatine kinase and aspartate aminotransferase activity. Equine Vet J 1995;27:243–7.
62. Lindner A, Signorini R, Brero L, et al. Effect of conditioning horses with short intervals at high speed on biochemical variables in blood. Equine Vet J Suppl 2006;36:88–92.

Biochemical abnormalities of athletic horses

43

Erica C. McKenzie

CHAPTER CONTENTS

Introduction

Clinical pathology, including serum or plasma biochemical analyzes, plays a pivotal role in the assessment of athletic horses with suspected poor performance or other disorders.[1] Given the finely tuned nature of the performance athlete, it is not surprising that even relatively minor clinicopathologic anomalies might reflect processes capable of substantially reducing the potential for athletic success. However, since both training and exercise can also influence a variety of serum biochemistry variables in a somewhat predictable manner, the clinician must be familiar with expected biochemistry changes in the equine athlete to more accurately determine when disease might be present.[1] In general, values that fall outside appropriate reference limits, or that are substantially different from previous measurements in the same individual, or which are accompanied by additional indications of disease, are likely to carry the greatest clinical significance. Obviously a wide array of disease situations can promote abnormal serum or plasma biochemistry results in horses, hence in this chapter, emphasis will be placed on serum or plasma biochemistry changes that hold particular relevance for the performance horse.[2]

Methods of sample collection for biochemical analyzes are described in the preceding chapter, and as previously noted, exemplary sample handling techniques are essential to avoid errors of interpretation.[2] Blood samples should be centrifuged within 30–60 minutes after collection, and the separated serum or plasma ideally stored at 4°C until the time of analysis. Where in-clinic analyzes are routinely performed, the equipment should be properly maintained by frequent assessment and calibration. The staff performing the analyzes should be adequately trained in all relevant procedures, and participation in external quality control programs is necessary to ensure consistent provision of accurate results.[3] Professional laboratory services provide a convenient and reliable means of biochemical analysis in non-urgent situations, provided samples are appropriately prepared, stored and transported as described in the preceding chapter. Prior communication with the receiving laboratory will often elicit valuable information regarding sample collection and submission, further reducing the potential for preparation or handling errors to affect the quality of the obtained results.[2,3]

Clinical chemistry as an indicator of disease

Plasma proteins

Currently over 1000 different plasma proteins have been characterized; however, only a minute fraction are individually measured on a routine basis in equine plasma.[3] Specific proteins that can be useful indicators of systemic inflammation or disease are broadly categorized into three groups; positive acute phase proteins, negative acute phase proteins, and delayed response proteins.[4] Positive acute phase proteins are those which increase in concentration in response to an inflammatory process, and include fibrinogen, serum amyloid A (SAA), ferritin, and haptoglobin. Negative acute phase proteins, such as albumin and transferrin, decrease in concentration when inflammation is present, usually due to loss from the body or vascular space, or reduced production, respectively. Delayed response proteins are those which increase in concentration one to three weeks after the onset of inflammation, and include the various immunoglobulin fractions (immunoglobulins A, G, M, and E) and the complement proteins.[3,4]

Dysproteinemia is characterized by abnormal concentrations of total protein, albumin or globulin in the serum or plasma. It should be recognized that plasma total protein and serum total protein differ quantitatively due to the absence of fibrinogen in the latter, and that 'globulin' represents the cumulative total of *all* plasma proteins excluding albumin.[3] Serum protein electrophoresis (SPE) can be used to more accurately qualify dysproteinemia situations by separating out protein fractions based on their migration characteristics through a medium to which an electrical field is applied. Typically, equine total serum protein will separate into a large albumin fraction, representing approximately 50% of the serum protein content, with the remaining fractions comprising the alpha 1-globulins, alpha 2-globulins, beta 1-globulins, beta 2-globulins and gamma-globulins (Fig. 43.1).[3-5] Alterations in SPE morphology associated with a variety of pathologic conditions have been described in horses.[4,5] In general, however, this procedure has limited diagnostic value and should be utilized in conjunction with additional diagnostics appropriately tailored to the clinical signs or disease process of concern.[3]

Simple quantitative measurement of total protein and albumin concentrations in performance horses can provide useful information regarding infectious or parasitic disease. Hypoproteinemia resulting from low blood albumin concentrations most frequently reflects some form of gastrointestinal disease in horses. Given that many performance horse populations are composed of young, potentially immunosuppressed horses exposed to variable extremes of management and crowding, gastrointestinal parasitism should be considered among the likely possible causes of hypoalbuminemia in young horses, particularly if history or inspection suggests they are dwelling in suboptimal management situations.[6] In addition, protein losing enteropathy associated with *Lawsonia intracellularis* infection is most prevalent in weanling Thoroughbred and Standardbred horses destined for performance careers, potentially also reflecting the intensive management of some performance horse operations.[7,8] *Lawsonia* infection in horses is characterized by moderate to profound hypoproteinemia which is variably associated with additional anomalies including ventral edema, diarrhea, fever, neutrophilia, hyperfibrinogenemia and serum electrolyte disturbances.[7,8] Other potential causes of hypoproteinemia that are possibly relevant to the performance horse include administration

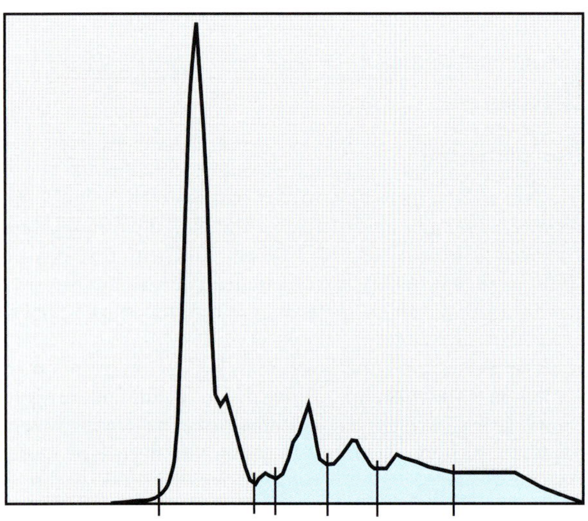

Fraction	Rel %	g/L
1	5.0	1.10
2	26.1	5.74
3	20.6	4.53
4	24.9	5.48
5	23.5	5.17

Total g/L 22.0

Fig 43.1 Serum protein electrophoresis trace from a healthy horse.[5]

of non-steroidal anti-inflammatory drugs, sand ingestion, severe gastric ulceration, and infectious disease situations including pleuropneumonia, which occurs with a greater prevalence in racing Thoroughbred horses compared to other equine populations.[9-11]

Given the nature of the diseases that can cause protein loss in horses, evaluation of the hypoproteinemic performance horse should likely include thorough physical examination, fecal analysis for the presence of parasite ova and complete blood count analysis to identify any additional indicators of inflammation or infection including hyperfibrinogenemia, neutrophilia, and anemia. Additional diagnostic procedures should then be selected based on detailed anamnesis and the results of the physical examination and initial diagnostic tests, and may include thoracic and abdominal ultrasonography, tracheal wash procedures, gastric endoscopy, and abdominocentesis.[12] If *Lawsonia intracellularis* infection is suspected, blood and fecal samples should be submitted for serologic assays (immunofluorescence or immunoperoxidase monolayer assay) and polymerase chain reaction analysis, respectively.[7]

Plasma fibrinogen represents a very commonly measured acute phase protein (APP) in equine populations.[4] Fibrinogen can be accurately measured from fresh whole blood samples collected into EDTA or sodium citrate anticoagulants, but should not be measured in heparinized blood; hence, care should be taken when collecting samples for fibrinogen analysis via indwelling venous catheters to avoid heparin contamination.[3] Fibrinogen is considered a positive moderate APP partly because of its slow response dynamics, taking days to weeks to peak and return to normal plasma concentrations.[4] The combination of this behavior with a fairly wide reference interval in healthy horses makes fibrinogen a fairly insensitive indicator of inflammation in the horse.[4]

Serum amyloid A (SAA) currently represents the most sensitive and only major positive APP analyzed with frequency in horses.[4] This protein is normally present in the serum of healthy horses at undetectable to low concentrations, and production of SAA by the hepatocytes increases rapidly in response to a variety of inflammatory and disease situations. Extra-hepatic isoforms of SAA also exist and can be measured locally at their sites of production (for example, measurement of SAA3 can be performed in joint fluid).[4] Several methods of assay for SAA exist, including ELISA, latex agglutination and immunoturbidimetric techniques. Reference intervals also vary with the most broad reference limits currently in use suggesting values of between 0 to 20 mg/mL to be appropriate in healthy horses.[4] Concentrations of SAA increase rapidly and substantially in 24 hours in response to inflammation or infectious conditions, including viral and bacterial respiratory infections, colic, surgery and experimentally induced septic arthritis.[4,13] Rapid methods of quantifying equine SAA have been reported from Europe where measurement of SAA as a screening assessment in poor-performing horses or for determining fitness to return to training after an illness is anecdotally reported. However, further research to conclusively define the utility of this assay for such purposes is required.[4,13,14]

Nonetheless, the application of SAA measurement in athletic horse populations appears to be currently expanding. In a study of 20 endurance horses participating in 120 or 160 kilometer distance endurance races, all horses with a pre-competition SAA concentration exceeding 1000 ng/mL (1.0 mg/L) failed to complete their event, with 9 of these 12 horses subsequently removed from competition due to the occurrence of lameness conditions.[15] However, plasma SAA concentrations after competition were found to be equally elevated in successful and eliminated horses, and remained below 20 mg/mL in all but one horse (Fig. 43.2).[15] Similar elevations in SAA were reported in another study of endurance horses competing in races of 120 or 160 km; however, serum haptoglobin

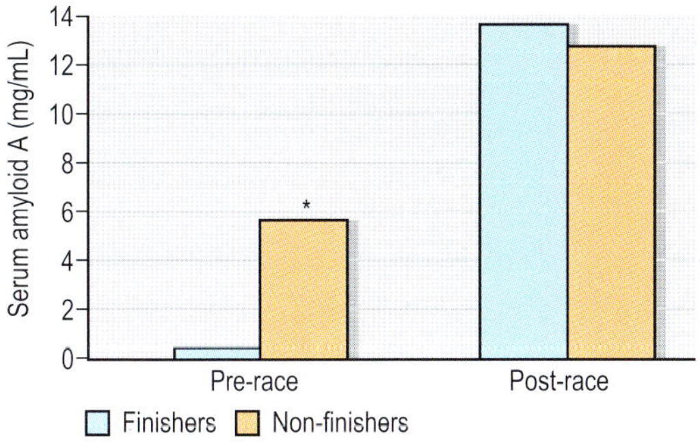

Fig 43.2 Serum amyloid A concentrations in endurance horses prior to and after completing (finishers) or failing to complete (non-finishers) endurance races of 120 km or 160 km in length.[15]

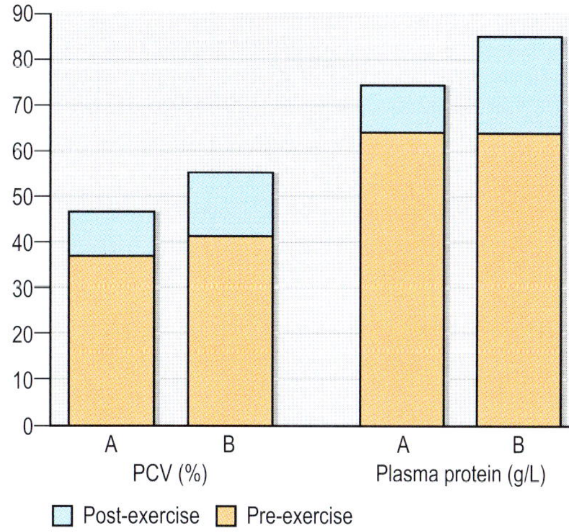

Fig 43.3 Pre- and post-exercise PCV (%) and plasma protein concentrations (g/L) in endurance horses; (A) after successfully completing a 91 km endurance race or (B) after elimination from a 91 km race due to exhaustion, dehydration or lack of heart rate recovery.[26]

and C-reactive protein concentrations in the same horses were unchanged.[16] Additionally, serum concentrations of SAA, haptoglobin, and C-reactive protein were not observed to increase significantly in endurance horses completing limited distance events (34 and 60 km).[16] Collectively, these findings indicate that long-distance endurance exercise increases SAA concentrations in horses, though values usually remain within current broad reference limits. Further investigation is therefore indicated to define appropriate reference limits for SAA concentrations in healthy athletic horses, and to elucidate the discriminatory power of SAA measurement in various equine performance activities.

At the onset of exercise, inter-compartmental fluid shifts promote rapid and transient increases in plasma protein and albumin concentrations in healthy horses.[17] More pronounced and persistent changes are noted in horses undertaking endurance exercise, in which fluid shifts are compounded by progressive and substantial fluid losses over time, related to sweat losses which can exceed 10 L/h in a warm environment.[18] Metabolic derangement associated with perturbations of fluid and electrolyte balance is one of the most common causes of elimination of horses from endurance competition.[19–21] Increases in plasma protein concentration and hematocrit commonly occur in endurance horses, and to a large degree will reflect the immensity of body water losses.[22–24] Therefore monitoring changes in hematocrit and plasma protein, in addition to other clinical and laboratory variables, constitutes one valuable method of potentially identifying horses at risk of metabolic derangement during or after endurance competitions. Previous reports have identified higher plasma protein, hematocrit or both in horses that are eliminated from endurance racing or which require treatment for metabolic derangements.[23–25] Supporting this finding, a large-scale study of endurance horses competing in races of 72 to 169 km in length found both PCV and plasma protein concentration to provide good prediction ability for metabolic elimination.[21] Plasma protein concentrations had greater sensitivity and specificity for this purpose than PCV, perhaps reflecting the confounding impact of splenic contraction on PCV. Ultimately the authors concluded that PCV values exceeding 52% and plasma protein concentrations exceeding 82 g/L were associated with the development of metabolic alterations in competing horses.[21] Similar values have been reported in other studies of endurance horses competing in similar distance races, with higher PCV and plasma protein values reported in horses developing metabolic derangements during or after racing (Fig. 43.3).[25,26] Hence, where possible, assessment of PCV and plasma protein concentrations should be incorporated into the assessment of individual endurance horses considered at risk of metabolic derangement during competition.

Muscle enzyme activities

Due to the relatively high prevalence of exertional rhabdomyolysis disorders in various equine athletic performance groups, including Thoroughbreds, Warmbloods, Quarter Horses and related breeds, measurement of muscle enzyme activity should be routinely included in the assessment of poor-performing horses.[27,28] Muscle damage in the horse is currently most accurately reflected by an increase in serum or plasma creatine kinase (CK) activity, which peaks within 4 to 6 hours after muscle injury has occurred. However, due to its brief half-life (approximately 2 hours), serum CK activity declines rapidly if the injury is transient in nature.[3] Aspartate transaminase (AST) activity peaks approximately 12–24 hours after muscle or liver injury in the horse but has a longer half-life of approximately seven to eight days.[3] Therefore, interpretation of serum CK activity, combined with assessment of AST and additional liver enzyme activities (sorbitol dehydrogenase, gamma-glutamyl transferase) can accurately distinguish the source of enzyme derangements and can be a valuable means of delineating acute and chronic muscle disease in performance horses (Fig. 43.4).[5] Although lactate dehydrogenase activity is often measured in serum biochemical panels, it has a low degree of tissue specificity without isoenzyme measurement.[3] In horses, the LDH-5 isoenzyme is derived largely from muscle and liver tissue, and therefore increases can be interpreted similar to increases in AST activity if this specific isoenzyme fraction is analyzed.[3]

Generally, brief maximal exercise efforts provoke minimal derangement in serum CK and AST activity in healthy horses, with increases rarely exceeding several hundred units per liter.[28–30] Submaximal training efforts usually do not alter muscle enzyme values in healthy individuals; however, endurance competition commonly results in a several thousand units per liter increase in serum CK activity in apparently healthy horses.[15,16,21–23,31,32] Exertional rhabdomyolysis disorders of the performance horse, including recurrent exertional rhabdomyolysis (RER) and polysaccharide storage myopathy (PSSM), are described in detail in other chapters of this text. However, it should be recognized that serum enzyme elevations can be extremely variable in horses affected with these disorders, and increases can range from between several thousand to hundreds of thousands of units per liter in affected individuals.[27,28,33] Hence it

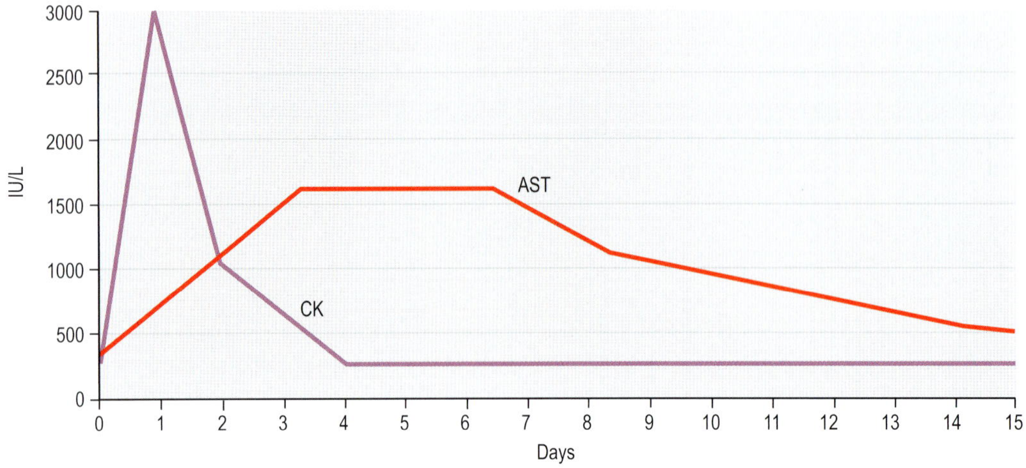

Fig 43.4 Schematic diagram depicting serum AST and CK activities following a single mild episode of exertional rhabdomyolysis.[5]

can be challenging, particularly in unfit individuals exposed to an inappropriate level of exertion, to determine whether increases in muscle enzyme activity after exercise reflect a transient, sporadic phenomenon or are truly attributable to an underlying muscular disorder. Muscle disease should be considered when there are persistent increases in activity of serum muscle enzymes at rest; significant repeated increases in muscle enzyme activity after exercise or increases that seem disproportionate for the level of exertion occurring prior to measurement, and whenever there are accompanying clinical signs of muscular discomfort such as stiffness, myoglobinuria, inappropriate sweating and tachycardia.[28] However, it should also be recognized that occasional individuals with exertional rhabdomyolysis disorders can have dramatic elevations in muscle enzyme activity without obvious clinical abnormalities.[22,23,27] This phenomenon is of particular concern in endurance horses due to the prolonged nature of their competition and the possibility of continued exercise in the face of significant, but clinically occult rhabdomyolysis.[22,23]

Although specific diagnostic techniques including muscle biopsy and genetic testing are frequently indicated in the evaluation of horses with possible exertional rhabdomyolysis disorders, an exercise test represents a simple initial method for assessing an individual horse's muscular response to exercise.[28] Serum for CK and AST analysis can be obtained prior to performing 10 to 15 minutes of trotting exercise, during which time the horse is examined for any signs of stiffness or sweating which may prompt premature termination of the test. Horses that display greater than a 2- to 4-fold increase in serum CK activity from analysis of a second blood sample obtained four hours after the exercise task are likely to have underlying muscle disease.[23,28] It should also be borne in mind that serum CK activity in horses with exertional rhabdomyolysis disorders can be strongly influenced by exercise and dietary regime.[34,35] More pronounced elevations in serum CK activity might occur in horses that have been stall rested for 48 hours or longer prior to testing, and in horses consuming diets with a high starch content. Likewise, changes in muscle enzyme activity may be minimal in spite of underlying muscle disease if horses have recently received consecutive days of exercise or have been consuming a low-starch diet (Fig. 43.5).[34] Hence failure to demonstrate an increase in serum creatine kinase after an exercise response test does not preclude the diagnosis of an exertional rhabdomyolysis disorder, also because intermittent increases in muscle enzyme activity can occur in affected horses. Therefore in those individuals in which the history, clinical signs or other clinicopathologic findings suggest the possibility of a muscular disorder, further diagnostics appropriate for assessment of muscular disorders should be pursued even if an exercise response test is inconclusive.[28] Additional diagnostic procedures might include genetic tests, skeletal muscle biopsy, and calculation of urinary fractional excretion ratios to assess dietary electrolyte and mineral requirements, depending on the breed of the horse and the characteristics of the suspected disorder.[28]

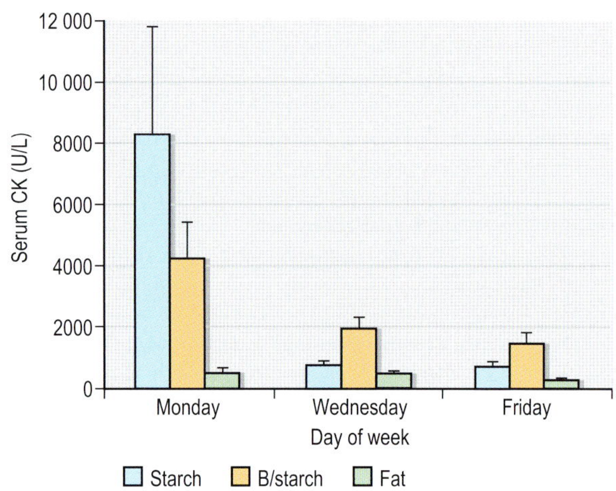

Fig 43.5 Post-exercise serum CK activity in five Thoroughbred horses with recurrent exertional rhabdomyolysis consuming diets high in starch (starch or bicarbonate/starch) or fat and exercising five days per week (Monday to Friday) after two days of stall rest on Saturday and Sunday.[34]

Measurement of serum CK isoenzyme fractions has been used extensively in human medicine to differentiate skeletal muscle injury from cardiac muscle injury, delineated by increases in the skeletal muscle isoform (MM CK) and cardiac muscle isoform (MB CK) of CK, respectively.[36] However, in horses, MB CK activity is greatest in splenic and intestinal tissue, and present only in small amounts in myocardial tissue, preventing it from being a useful indicator of cardiac damage in this species.[37] Hence, CK isoform analysis has limited application in horses, and cardiac damage in this species is currently best determined through measurement of plasma cardiac troponin concentrations.[38]

Cardiac troponin I

Cardiac troponin I (cTnI) is a myocardial polypeptide which can be accurately measured in equine plasma as a sensitive biomarker for myocardial injury.[38] Significantly elevated cTnI concentrations have been recorded in a variety of clinical disorders in adult horses, including colic, renal failure and septicemia, as well as primary cardiac disorders.[38,39] Values do not correlate with the etiology or pathogenesis of myocardial disease, but represent a useful method for quantifying and monitoring myocardial damage.[38] Suggested reference limits for cTnI have been established in athletic Thoroughbred, Standardbred and Warmblood populations, and in horses with monensin-induced cardiac disease, but are potentially assay dependent.[38,40–43] Most healthy horses have low plasma cTnI values in the absence of cardiac disease, regardless of whether they are sedentary or involved in regular athletic training.[38,40] Brief intense racing exercise can provoke mild elevations in some individuals that might persist for more than 14 hours.[41] In a large study of horses participating in endurance races of 80 and 160 km in distance, substantial cTnI elevations (exceeding 0.1 ng/mL) were observed in up to 27% of horses in some events.[44] Plasma cTnI concentrations after racing were comparable between the two distances studied and no association between plasma cTnI concentration and metabolic elimination was identified. One horse with a cTnI value of 0.94 ng/mL developed paroxysmal atrial fibrillation during competition; however, the importance of this finding is unclear, and athletic horses with lone chronic atrial fibrillation rarely display cTnI increases.[44,45] However, substantial elevations in cTnI, particularly those unassociated with exercise, should prompt appropriate cardiac evaluation to determine the possible cause of cardiac damage.

Liver enzymes

Hepatic disease in horses is suggested by leakage of hepatocellular enzymes into the serum, including sorbitol dehydrogenase, glutamate dehydrogenase, and lactate dehydrogenase (isoenzyme 5) and by increased production and release into circulation of the cholestatic enzymes (alkaline phosphatase and gamma-glutamyl transferase).[2] Since these enzymes vary substantially in regard to their origin, half-lives, and stability, they should not be assessed singly and in isolation, but as part of a complete serum or plasma biochemistry analysis. It should also be remembered that hepatic enzyme measurements infer limited information regarding hepatic function, which must be assessed via evaluation of non-specific (serum or plasma urea nitrogen, glucose and bilirubin concentrations) and specific (serum bile acid concentration) indicators of hepatic function.

Performance horses are prone to the same wide variety of hepatic diseases as sedentary horses, which are thoroughly described in current veterinary internal medicine texts. However, one peculiarity of the performance horse is the common and idiopathic increase in serum GGT activity that is frequently observed in horses in athletic training.[46,47] Progressive mild to moderate elevations in GGT have been reported in apparently healthy horses during athletic training, and correlation exists between GGT activity and training intensity.[46,47] In a study of young Standardbred horses participating in a 32-week training schedule, those horses exposed to training efforts of higher intensity and frequency from 16 weeks onwards displayed GGT values approximately 20 U/L higher than less strenuously trained horses by the end of the experiment (Fig. 43.6).[47] Another study of maladaption to training in Standardbred trotters also demonstrated mildly higher GGT activity in Standardbred trotters, in conjunction with weight loss, higher white cell counts and lower red cell counts than similarly trained horses classified as

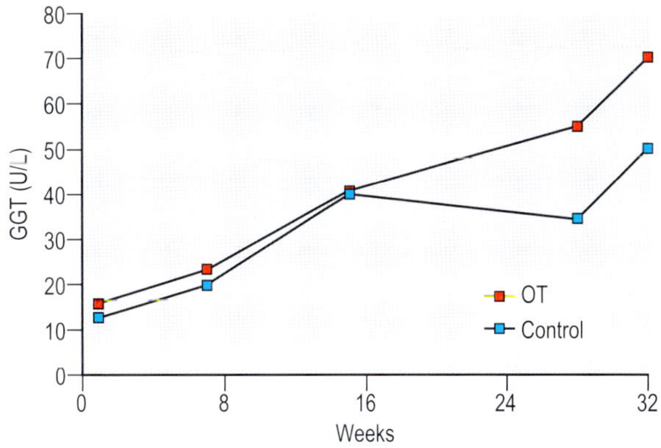

Fig 43.6 Changes in serum GGT activity measured during 32 weeks of training in Standardbred horses participating in a normal training protocol (control) or an overtraining protocol (OT), the latter commencing after 15 weeks of training.[47]

adapting well to the training stress.[48] However, beyond reflecting training intensity, the significance of increased plasma GGT activity in training horses is unclear, and the relatively small differences in values between healthy and training maladapted horses make it challenging to define a specific plasma activity at which excessive training stress is likely. One anecdotal report indicated that poor performance was perceived in Thoroughbred racehorses with plasma GGT activity equal to or exceeding 100 U/L.[46] Although the significance of increased plasma GGT activity in training racehorses is unclear, maladaptation to training might be suspected in athletic horses with plasma GGT activity approaching 100 U/L that also display weight loss, reduced performance despite continued training, and behavioral and appetite disturbances among other clinical anomalies.[46–48] Serum GGT should return to within reference limits if training intensity is decreased or training stopped.[2,46] Reduced hepatic function or other evidence of hepatic pathology has not been noted in athletic horses with mildly elevated plasma GGT activity, though mild elevations in serum bilirubin have been concurrently reported.[2,47] However, horses with substantial increases in serum GGT or additional biochemical or clinical findings suggestive of hepatic disease should be thoroughly evaluated for hepatic dysfunction via serum bile acid measurement, hepatic ultrasound examination, and where indicated, hepatic biopsy.

Renal variables and urinary fractional excretion

Measurement of plasma or serum creatinine and urea nitrogen concentrations can provide useful information about hydration status and renal function in athletic horses. Where possible, these values are often best interpreted in conjunction with concurrent urine specific gravity to assist delineation of pre-renal from renal azotemia.[3] Performance horses are vulnerable to the same renal diseases as the general population, withstanding perhaps a greater likelihood of kidney injury from repeated exposure to non-steroidal anti-inflammatory drugs. Renal dysfunction is suggested by increased plasma or serum creatinine and urea nitrogen concentrations, in conjunction with isosthenuria (urine specific gravity of 1.008–1.014) or suboptimal urine concentration (urine specific gravity < 1.020).[49] Severe chronic renal disease is usually accompanied by overt clinical signs including polyuria and polydipsia, weight loss, poor hair coat quality, lethargy and poor athletic performance.

Since creatinine is released from the musculature on a remarkably constant basis for excretion via the kidneys it provides a convenient method for determining urinary electrolyte and mineral excretion rates in horses with normal renal function.[3,50] Calculation of urinary fractional excretion rates of specific electrolytes and minerals can be useful for investigating specific nutritional imbalances, and have also been used to monitor electrolyte balance in athletic horses during training and in horses predisposed to exertional rhabdomyolysis.[33,49,51,52] Concurrent blood and urine samples (within 1 to 72 hours of each other) should be obtained from a non-sedated horse, and creatinine concentration and the concentrations of the specific electrolytes and minerals to be assessed subsequently measured in both samples. Percentage urinary fractional excretion (%FE) of each electrolyte or mineral (X) can then be calculated using the equation:

$$\mathrm{FE\%}\,(\mathrm{X}) = \frac{[\mathrm{Cr}]\,\mathrm{serum}}{[\mathrm{Cr}]\,\mathrm{urine}} \times \frac{[\mathrm{X}]\,\mathrm{urine}}{[\mathrm{X}]\,\mathrm{serum}} \times 100$$

where [X] is the concentration of the specific electrolyte or mineral in the urine and serum, and [Cr] is the concentration of creatinine in the urine and serum.[3,49]

Fractional excretion rates are most commonly calculated for sodium, potassium, chloride, magnesium, calcium, and phosphate. Confidence intervals (95%) for urine FE values based on non-centrifuged and acidified urine samples (to completely incorporate urine mineral content) have been reported (Table 43.1).[51] Sodium, chloride, potassium, magnesium and calcium FE% values below reference limits are suggestive of conservation of those specific substances and possible inadequate dietary intake.[33,49] Values of phosphate that exceed reference limits are suggestive of inadequate calcium intake or of a calcium : phosphorus ratio imbalance. High sodium excretion can be observed in horses with acute renal tubular dysfunction or in horses receiving excessive dietary sodium supplementation.[49]

Urinary fractional excretion values can vary considerably between individuals consuming similar diets, between methods of urine collection and as a result of common activities including eating and exercise.[51,53] Abnormal values are therefore most likely to be significant if they are repeatable on consecutive days from samples obtained at the same stage of the daily routine, preferably prior to exercise activity or feeding.[51]

Assessment of plasma creatinine concentration in conjunction with other biochemical variables has been examined as an indicator of metabolic derangement in endurance horses.[22,24,26] Mild to moderate increases in plasma creatinine concentration commonly occur in endurance horses and tend to correlate with other indicators of hydration status including hematocrit and plasma protein. Significantly higher increases in creatinine, plasma protein and packed cell volume have been reported in endurance horses encountering metabolic failure during competition, though this is not necessarily a consistent finding, and the influence of speed and distance on these variables during endurance competition is also inconsistent.[22,24,26,54]

Table 43.1[51]

VARIABLE	% FRACTIONAL EXCRETION
Sodium	0.1–0.55%
Potassium	18.0–51.5%
Chloride	0.1–1.4%
Calcium	6.0–15.0%
Phosphate	0–5.0%
Magnesium	7.8–22.5%

Serum and plasma electrolytes and minerals

As described in the preceding chapter, maximal exercise in healthy horses can induce significant transient hyperkalemia and mild to moderate hypernatremia, reflecting plasma volume alterations and ion flux from exercising muscle tissue. These changes normally resolve rapidly after exercise ceases. Prolonged strenuous or submaximal exercise can create more persistent alterations in serum or plasma electrolyte and mineral concentrations, largely related to the loss of large volumes of water, electrolytes and minerals in sweat, and potentially also to alterations in urinary electrolyte excretion during exercise.[52,53,55]

The most common electrolyte abnormality that occurs with prolonged sweat loss is hypochloremia, reflecting the considerably greater concentration of chloride in equine sweat relative to equine plasma.[55] Other changes documented in endurance horses include complicated acid-base disturbances that often ultimately result in a dominant metabolic alkalosis, and variable hyponatremia, hypokalemia, and ionized hypocalcemia.[22,23,55–57] Severe derangements may result in cardiac arrhythmias, synchronous diaphragmatic flutter, ileus and other disorders.[23,58] Some studies have identified more profound hypochloremia and other electrolyte derangements in endurance horses encountering metabolic problems during competition than in horses that complete events successfully, though the exact role of these specific imbalances in eliciting the clinical signs of concern is not always clear.[23–26]

Conclusion

Serum or plasma biochemistry analysis is a convenient and useful tool that can help to determine the presence of various pathologic conditions in performance horses, including inflammatory conditions of various organ systems, and potentially maladapation to training stress. It achieves its greatest value when combined with careful anamnesis, a thorough physical examination, and additional appropriate diagnostic procedures. The line between physiologic and pathologic changes however is frequently indistinct, and familiarity with expected changes induced by exercise and training will help to determine when further investigations are warranted.

With thanks to Sidney A. Ricketts, who created the original chapter in the first edition.

References

1. McGowan C. Clinical pathology in the racing horse: the role of clinical pathology in assessing fitness and performance in the racehorse. Vet Clin North Am Equine Pract 2008;24:405–21.
2. Carlson GP. Clinical chemistry tests. In: Smith BP, editor. Large Animal Internal Medicine. 4th ed. St Louis, MO: Mosby Elsevier; 2009. p. 375–97.
3. Stockham SL, Scott MA. Fundamentals of Veterinary Clinical Pathology. 2nd ed. Ames, IA: Blackwell Publishing; 2008.
4. Crisman MV, Scarratt WK, Zimmerman KL. Blood proteins and inflammation in

the horse. Vet Clin North Am Equine Pract 2008;24:285–97.
5. Ricketts SW. Hematologic and biochemical abnormalities in athletic horses. In: Hinchcliff KW, Kaneps AJ, Geor RJ, editors. Equine Sports Medicine and Surgery. St Louis, MO: Elsevier Limited; 2004. p. 949–66.
6. Peregrine AS, McEwen B, Bienzle D, et al. Larval cyathostominosis in horses in Ontario: an emerging disease? Can Vet J 2006;47:80–2.
7. Frazer ML. *Lawsonia intracellularis* infection in horses: 2005–2007. J Vet Intern Med 2008;22:1243–8.
8. McGurrin MK, Vengust M, Arroyo LG, et al. An outbreak of *Lawsonia intracellularis* infection in a Standardbred herd in Ontario. Can Vet J 2007;48:927–30.
9. Reed SK, Messer NT, Tessman RK, et al. Effects of phenylbutazone alone or in combination with flunixin meglumine on blood protein concentrations in horses. Am J Vet Res 2006;67:398–402.
10. Roy MA, Vrins A, Beauchamp G, et al. Prevalence of ulcers of the squamous gastric mucosa in Standardbred horses. J Vet Intern Med 2005;19:744–50.
11. Austin SM, Foreman JH, Hungerford LL. Case-control study of risk factors for development of pleuropneumonia in horses. J Am Vet Med Assoc 1995;207:325–8.
12. Sanchez LC. Diseases associated with malabsorption and maldigestion In: Reed SM, Bayly WM, Sellon DC, editors. Equine Internal Medicine. 3rd ed. St. Louis, MO: Saunders Elsevier; 2010. p. 850–6.
13. Jacobsen S, Kjelgaard-Hansen M, Hagbard Petersen H, et al. Evaluation of a commercially available human serum amyloid A (SAA) turbidometric immunoassay for determination of equine SAA concentrations. Vet J 2006;172:315–19.
14. Petersen HH, Nielsen JP, Heegaard PMH. Application of acute phase protein measurements in veterinary clinical chemistry. Vet Res 2004;35:163–87.
15. Cywinska A, Gorecka R, Szarska E, et al. Serum amyloid A level as a potential indicator of the status of endurance horses. Equine Vet J Suppl 2010;42: 23–7.
16. Cywińska A, Szarska E, Górecka R, et al. Acute phase protein concentrations after limited distance and long distance endurance rides in horses. Res Vet Sci 2012;93:1402–6.
17. McKeever KH. Body fluids and electrolytes. In: Hinchchcliff KW, Geor RJ, Kaneps AJ, editors. Equine Exercise Physiology – The Science of Exercise in the Athletic Horse. Philadelphia, PA: Elsevier Limited; 2008. p. 328–49.
18. Geor RJ, McCutcheon LJ. Thermoregulatory adaptations associated with training and heat acclimation. Vet Clin North Am Equine Pract 1998;14:97–120.
19. Nagy A, Murray JK, Dyson S. Elimination from elite endurance rides in nine countries: a preliminary study. Equine Vet J 2010;42:637–43.
20. Fielding CL, Meier CA, Balch OK, et al. Risk factors for the elimination of endurance horses from competition. J Am Vet Med Assoc 2011;239:493–8.
21. Trigo P, Castejon F, Riber C, et al. Use of biochemical parameters to predict metabolic elimination in endurance rides. Equine Vet J Suppl 2010;42:142–6.
22. Schott HC 2nd, Marlin DJ, Geor RJ, et al. Changes in selected physiological and laboratory measurements in elite horses competing in a 160 km endurance ride. Equine Vet J Suppl 2006;36:37–42.
23. Barnes A, Kingston J, Beetson S, et al. Endurance veterinarians detect physiologically compromised horses in a 160 km ride. Equine Vet J Suppl 2010;42:6–11.
24. Muñoz A, Riber C, Trigo P, et al. Muscle damage, hydration, electrolyte balance and vasopressin concentrations in successful and exhausted endurance horses. Pol J Vet Sci 2010;13:373–9.
25. Fielding CL, Magdesian KG, Rhodes DM, et al. Clinical and biochemical abnormalities in endurance horses eliminated from competition for medical complications and requiring emergency medical treatment: 30 cases (2005–2006). J Vet Emerg Crit Care (San Antonio) 2009;19:473–8.
26. Muñoz A, Riber C, Trigo P, et al. Dehydration, electrolyte imbalances and renin-angiotensin-aldosterone-vasopressin axis in successful and unsuccessful endurance horses. Equine Vet J Suppl 2010;42:83–90.
27. Martin BB Jr, Reef VB, Parente EJ, et al. Causes of poor performance of horses during training, racing, or showing: 348 cases (1992–1996). J Am Vet Med Assoc 2000;216:554–8.
28. MacLeay JM. Disorders of the musculoskeletal system. In: Reed SM, Bayly WM, Sellon DC, editors. Equine Internal Medicine. 3rd ed. St. Louis, MO: Saunders Elsevier; 2010. p. 488–544.
29. Harris PA, Marlin DJ, Gray J. Plasma aspartate aminotransferase and creatine kinase activities in Thoroughbred racehorses in relation to age, sex, exercise and training. Vet J 1998;155:295–304.
30. Snow DH, Mason DK, Ricketts SW, et al. Post-race blood biochemistry in Thoroughbreds. In: Snow DH, Persson SGB, Rose RJ, editors. Equine Exercise Physiology. Cambridge, UK: Granta Editions; 1983. p. 389–99.
31. Rose RJ, Allen JR, Hodgson DR, et al. Responses to submaximal treadmill exercise and training in the horse: changes in haematology, arterial blood gas and acid base measurements, plasma biochemical values and heart rate. Vet Rec 1983;113:612–18.
32. Serteyn D, Sandersen C, Lejeune JP et al. Effect of a 120 km endurance race on plasma and muscular neutrophil elastase and myeloperoxidase concentrations in horses. Equine Vet J Suppl 2010;42:275–9.
33. McKenzie EC, Valberg SJ, Pagan JD. Nutritional management of exertional rhabdomyolysis. In: Robinson NE, editor. Current Therapy in Equine Medicine. 5th ed. St Louis, MO: Saunders; 2003. p. 727–34.
34. McKenzie EC, Valberg SJ, Godden SM, et al. Effect of dietary starch, fat, and bicarbonate content on exercise responses and serum creatine kinase activity in equine recurrent exertional rhabdomyolysis. J Vet Intern Med 2003;17:693–701.
35. Firshman AM, Valberg SJ, Bender JB, et al. Epidemiologic characteristics and management of polysaccharide storage myopathy in Quarter Horses. Am J Vet Res 2003;64:1319–27.
36. Lewandrowski K. Point-of-care testing for cardiac markers in acute coronary syndromes and heart failure. Clin Lab Med 2009;29:561–71.
37. Argiroudis SA, Kent JE, Blackmore DJ. Observations on the isoenzymes of creatine kinase in equine serum and tissues. Equine Vet J 1982;14:317–21.
38. Serra M, Papakonstantinou S, Adamcova M, et al. Veterinary and toxicological applications for the detection of cardiac injury using cardiac troponin. Vet J 2010;185:50–7.
39. Schwarzwald CC, Hardy J, Buccellato M. High cardiac troponin I serum concentration in a horse with multiform ventricular tachycardia and myocardial necrosis. J Vet Intern Med 2003;17:364–8.
40. Phillips W, Giguère S, Franklin RP, et al. Cardiac troponin I in pastured and race-training Thoroughbred horses. J Vet Intern Med 2003;17:597–9.
41. Nostell K, Häggström J. Resting concentrations of cardiac troponin I in fit horses and effect of racing. J Vet Cardiol 2008;10:105–9.
42. Begg LM, Hoffmann KL, Begg AP. Serum and plasma cardiac troponin I concentrations in clinically normal Thoroughbreds in training in Australia. Aust Vet J 2006;84:336–7.
43. Kraus MS, Jesty SA, Gelzer AR, et al. Measurement of plasma cardiac troponin I concentration by use of a point-of-care analyzer in clinically normal horses and horses with experimentally induced

cardiac disease. Am J Vet Res 2010;71:55–9.
44. Holbrook TC, Birks EK, Sleeper MM, et al. Endurance exercise is associated with increased plasma cardiac troponin I in horses. Equine Vet J Suppl 2006;36:27–31.
45. Jesty SA, Kraus MS, Gelzer AR, et al. Effect of transvenous electrical cardioversion on plasma cardiac troponin I concentrations in horses with atrial fibrillation. J Vet Intern Med 2009;23:1103–7.
46. Snow DH, Gash SP, Rice D. Field observations on selenium status, whole blood glutathione peroxidase and plasma gamma-glutamyl transferase activities in Thoroughbred racehorses. In: Gillespie JR, Robinson NE, editors. Equine Exercise Physiology 2. Davis, CA: ICEEP Publications; 1987. p. 494–505.
47. Tyler-McGowan CM, Golland LC, Evans DL, et al. Haematological and biochemical responses to training and overtraining. Equine Vet J Suppl 1999;30:621–5.
48. Leleu C, Haentjens F. Morphological, haemato-biochemical and endocrine changes in young Standardbreds with 'maladaptation' to early training. Equine Vet J Suppl 2010;42:171–8.
49. Savage CJ. Urinary clinical pathologic findings and glomerular filtration rate in the horse. Vet Clin North Am Equine Pract 2008;24:387–404.
50. Harris PA, Gray J. The use of the urinary fractional electrolyte excretion test to assess electrolyte status in the horse. Equine Vet Educ 1992;4:162–6.
51. McKenzie EC, Valberg SJ, Godden SM, et al. Comparison of volumetric urine collection versus single sample urine collection in horses consuming diets varying in cation-anion balance. Am J Vet Res 2003;64:284–91.
52. Robert C, Goachet AG, Fraipont A, et al. Hydration and electrolyte balance in horses during an endurance season. Equine Vet J Suppl 2010;42: 98–104.
53. McKeever KH, Hinchcliff KW, Schmall LM, et al. Renal tubular function in horses during submaximal exercise. Am J Physiol 1991;261:R553–60.
54. Barton MH, Williamson L, Jacks S, et al. Body weight, hematologic findings, and serum and plasma biochemical findings of horses competing in a 48-, 83-, or 159-km endurance ride under similar terrain and weather conditions. Am J Vet Res 2003;64:746–53.
55. Flaminio MJ, Rush BR. Fluid and electrolyte balance in endurance horses. Vet Clin North Am Equine Pract 1998;14:147–58.
56. Viu J, Jose-Cunilleras E, Armengou L, et al. Acid-base imbalances during a 120 km endurance race compared by traditional and simplified strong ion difference methods. Equine Vet J 2010;42:76–82.
57. Rose RJ, Ilkiw JE, Martin IC. Blood-gas, acid-base and haematological values in horses during an endurance ride. Equine Vet J 1979;11:56–9.
58. Foreman JH. The exhausted horse syndrome. Vet Clin North Am Equine Pract 1998;14:205–19.

Abnormalities of the erythron

44

Colin C. Schwarzwald

CHAPTER CONTENTS

Anemia

Adequate oxygen delivery to the tissues is critical for life and is of upmost importance during extreme athletic performance. As hemoglobin is the major determinant of the arterial oxygen content (CaO_2), a normal hemoglobin concentration is one of the prerequisites for normal performance.[1] There is evidence for a strong positive relationship between blood volume, red blood cell volume, and aerobic capacity in humans, dogs, and horses.[2,3] Conversely, a decrease in total red blood cell volume will negatively affect aerobic capacity and performance in athletes.

Anemia is defined as a decrease in red cell mass leading to a reduction in measured erythrocyte concentration, hemoglobin concentration, and hematocrit below the reference interval.[4,5] Anemia is functionally characterized by a reduced oxygen-carrying capacity of the blood.[6–8] Several compensatory mechanisms serve to increase tissue oxygenation in the presence of anemia.[4,5,9] One of the initial adaptations to anemia is an increase in 2,3-biphosphoglycerate (2,3-BPG; formerly called 2,3-diphosphoglycerate, 2,3-DPG) content of the red blood cells. It is probably caused by a change in intracellular pH, and leads to a decreased oxygen affinity of hemoglobin; oxygen is therefore more readily released to the tissue. Blood viscosity is markedly decreased at lower erythrocyte concentrations,[10] while tissue hypoxia activates mechanisms of local blood flow regulation and causes peripheral vessels to dilate.[11] This results in a dramatic fall in peripheral vascular resistance, a baroreceptor-mediated sympathetic activation, an increase in cardiac output, and improvement in oxygen delivery to the tissues.[4,5,9,12] Individual changes in vascular tone result in redistribution of blood from non-vital areas (skin, intestine) to highly oxygen-dependent tissues (heart, brain, muscles). Finally, diminished oxygen supply to the kidneys leads to increased synthesis of erythropoietin, which accelerates erythropoiesis in the bone marrow and elicits a regenerative response to anemia.[5]

These mechanisms can, at least partially, compensate for the decreased hemoglobin concentration and attenuate the decrease in oxygen delivery to tissues. Even severe anemia is therefore relatively well tolerated at rest, as long as it meets the following criteria:

- It does not occur acutely.
- It is not associated with acute hemolysis or blood loss.
- There is no loss of blood volume.
- No other disease processes or conditions (such as infection, fever, severe injury, exercise, agitation, or advanced pregnancy) are present which increase oxygen demand.

Free hemoglobin in solution, as present in intravascular hemolysis, exerts strong vasoconstrictor effects due to binding of nitric oxide,[13] and has an increased affinity for oxygen due to a loss of 2,3-BPG.[14] The resulting decline of effective oxygen delivery and release in the tissue contributes to the pathophysiologic effects of hemolytic anemia. When tissue oxygen demand is increased, or when anemia becomes severe enough to exceed the compensatory capacity of the organism, the degree of oxygen extraction from the blood cannot be increased, and the oxygen uptake by the tissue decreases as the oxygen supply decreases (supply dependent oxygen uptake; Fig. 44.1). The resulting anaerobic metabolism leads to accumulation of lactate and metabolic acidosis.[6,7,15] Ultimately, tissue hypoxia and limited metabolic capacity of the affected tissue can lead to tissue damage and organ failure.[5,16]

Diagnosis of anemia

Recognition

Clinical signs

Decreased oxygen-carrying capacity of the blood and related compensating mechanisms are responsible for most of the clinical signs associated with anemia. The severity and rate of development of anemia determine the efficacy of physiologic compensatory mechanisms. Patients with chronic anemia tolerate a much lower red blood cell mass than do patients with rapidly developing acute anemia.

Subtle anemia is difficult to detect and has mild clinical effects. Total red cell volume and hemoglobin concentration are correlated with the exercise capacity of a horse.[17-19] During exercise, tissue demand for oxygen is increased. Small decrements in red cell mass lower the level of exercise intensity at which tissue hypoxia occurs, and therefore result in reduced exercise capacity.[9]

More severe anemia is characterized by depression, weakness, tachypnea, tachycardia, hyperkinetic pulses, and pale or icteric mucous membranes. Systolic, functional heart murmurs are frequently associated with anemia. Hemoglobinuria or bilirubinuria can be seen in horses with hemolytic anemia. Cardiac arrhythmias may indicate myocardial hypoxia. Abdominal pain and signs of functional intestinal ileus are likely related to splanchnic ischemia, which can lead to sloughing of the intestinal mucosa, endotoxemia, and bacteremia.[15,16]

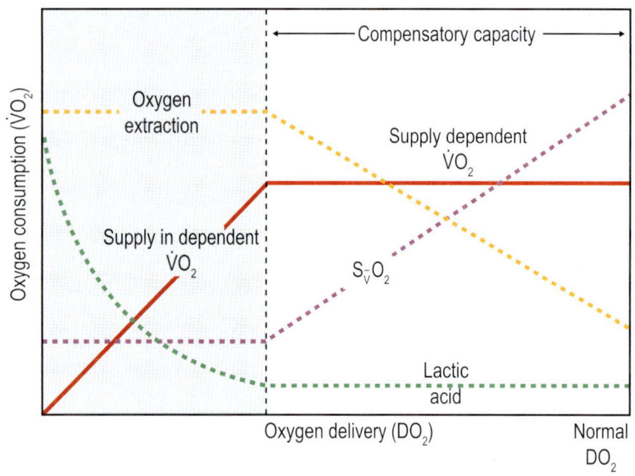

Fig 44.1 Schematic diagram showing the interrelationship between oxygen delivery (DO_2), oxygen consumption ($\dot{V}O_2$), and oxygen extraction in the systemic circulation. DO_2 can decline either because of a decrease in cardiac output or a decrease in arterial oxygen concentration, which largely depends on hemoglobin concentration and % saturation of hemoglobin with oxygen. As DO_2 decreases, a compensatory increase in oxygen extraction in the tissue allows maintaining the $\dot{V}O_2$ at a constant level (red line). Consequently, the mixed-venous oxygen saturation ($S_{\bar{v}}O_2$) decreases, the arterio-venous oxygen difference widens, and the oxygen extraction ratio increases. Once the compensatory capacity is exceeded (shaded area), the level of maximal oxygen extraction is reached and the $\dot{V}O_2$ becomes supply dependent, hence decreases parallel to the DO_2. Anaerobic metabolism in the tissues then leads to accumulation of lactic acid and metabolic acidosis. Venous (mixed venous) oxygen saturation, blood pH, and blood lactate concentration are clinically useful for assessment of oxygen delivery and oxygen extraction in the tissues.

Hematology

Anemia is diagnosed when hematocrit, hemoglobin concentration, and erythrocyte concentration on a complete blood count (CBC) are below the reference range for the respective breed. The clinical definition of anemia can be problematic, as hydration status and splenic contraction due to exercise, excitement, or stress can also influence the hematologic values. Changes in hematocrit and hemoglobin concentration might therefore not reflect the true change in oxygen-carrying capacity of the blood.[4,20]

The traditional approach to determine the etiology and pathogenesis of anemia is to establish whether the anemia is regenerative or non-regenerative.[21] In horses, assessment of a regenerative response is difficult based on a routine hemogram, because reticulocyte maturation is mostly completed in the bone marrow and release of reticulocytes into the blood is minimal compared to other species, even in response to severe anemia.[20,22,23] However, horses under severe erythropoietic stress may release reticulocytes with unique characteristics into the circulation, which may be detected using sensitive modern hematology analyzers.[24] Reticulocytes and nucleated red blood cells can be found in cases with severe hemolysis.[25]

Young erythrocytes are usually larger than normal erythrocytes. Therefore, a regenerative response in most species is characterized by release of macrocytes into the bloodstream, independent of reticulocytosis.[21,22] Macrocytosis and anisocytosis may therefore be used as indicators of regeneration in the peripheral blood of horses.[21,24] It can be detected by determination of erythrocyte indices (mean corpuscular volume and red blood cell distribution width), red blood cell cytograms and volume distribution histograms, or blood smear evaluation.[21]

The mean corpuscular volume (MCV) is not very sensitive for detection of abnormal or variable sizes of erythrocytes. Large numbers of macrocytes are necessary to increase the MCV above the normal range.[21,22,26,27] Macrocytosis is more pronounced in hemolytic anemia than in anemia due to acute blood loss.[28,29] The mixture of pre-existing normocytes and newly produced macrocytes during the recovery period in regenerative anemias leads to anisocytosis.[30] The red blood cell distribution width (RDW) is an index of anisocytosis and is calculated by many automated hematology systems as coefficient of variation of the erythrocyte volume distribution.[22,27] Significant increases in MCV and RDW are detectable 14 to 20 days after onset of anemia and can persist for several weeks [22,27] Although the RDW might be somewhat more sensitive than the MCV in detecting a regenerative response in horses, its increase is not a consistent indicator of regeneration, and it does not occur in mildly anemic horses.[22] Therefore, absence of these two findings does not exclude regenerative anemia.

Red blood cell (RBC) cytograms, RBC volume distribution curves, and hemoglobin concentration histograms are more sensitive in detecting changes in erythrocyte size or hemoglobin content, and allow earlier detection of abnormal erythrocyte subpopulations than the routine erythrocyte indices (MCV, RDW).[21,22 26,27,31] Most modern automated hematology analyzers will report this information on request (Fig. 44.2).

Single hematologic measurements may be difficult to assess. Series of samples can reveal the severity of anemia and the presence

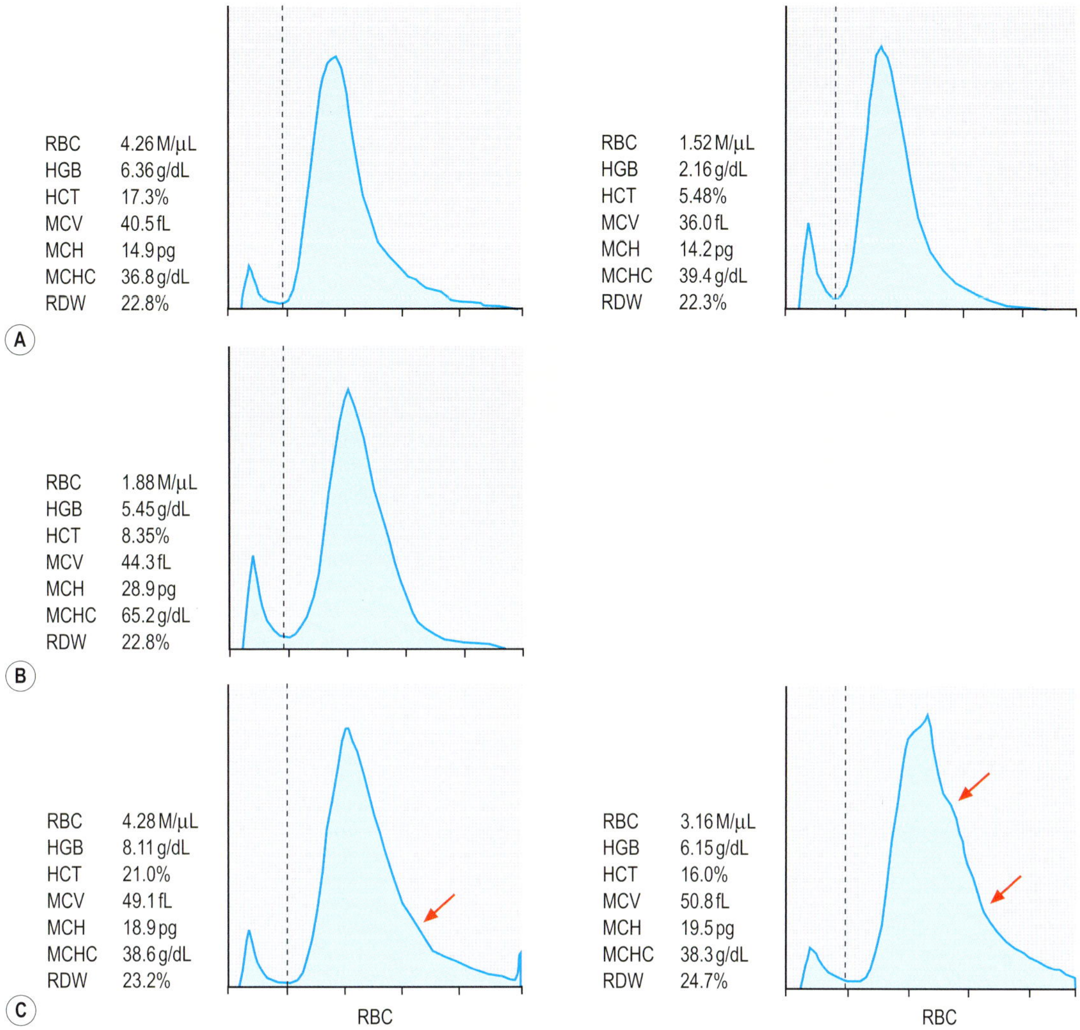

Fig 44.2 Red blood cell indices and erythrocyte volume histograms. **(A)** Pure red cell aplasia associated with administration of rhEPO. The RBC indices and erythrocyte volume histograms of two examinations 80 days apart indicate lack of regenerative response despite decreasing hematocrit (PCV). **(B)** Heinz body hemolytic anemia due to maple leaf toxicity. RBC indices and erythrocate volume histograms four days after onset of the clinical signs do not indicate regeneration. **(C)** Erythrocyte volume histogram of the same horse two days (left) and eight days (right) later. Widening of the right tail of the histograms (arrows) indicate increased numbers of macrocytes consistent with a regenerative response. Note that the MCV and RDW are increasing over time, but do not exceed the upper limit of the normal range. (Normal ranges: MCV 43–55 fL; RDW 19.8–25.4%).

of a regenerative response. The nadir of the hematocrit is reached around 2–7 days after acute blood loss and as late as 13–22 days after onset of hemolysis.[22,23,27–29] Reported daily increases in hematocrit following hematocrit nadir in regenerative anemias in horses vary between 0.32 and 0.67%, and are slower than reported in other species.[22,23] The rate of erythrocyte and hemoglobin production after hemolysis is higher than after acute blood loss, probably because iron and protein is not lost from the body and is readily available for erythropoiesis.[20,27,29,30]

Concurrent measurements of total plasma protein concentration may also be useful for determination of the type of anemia. Regenerative anemia, associated with a low, increasing plasma protein concentration, is consistent with blood loss, whereas a normal protein concentration more likely indicates hemolysis.[20]

The mean cellular hemoblogin concentration can be calculated as: MCHC = [Hb] (g/dL) / PCV (%) × 100, where [Hb] is the whole blood hemoglobin concentration and PCV is the packed cell volume. Normal MCHC varies little and equals 32–38 g/dL.[32] Intravascular hemolysis causes the PCV to decrease while [Hb] remains unchanged, leading to an increased MCHC. Conversely, iron deficiency anemia causes a decrease in MCHC.

Although not routinely used in horses, haptoglobin may be helpful to screen for and monitor intravascular hemolytic anemia. Haptoglobin is an acute-phase protein that is synthesized in the liver.[33] It binds free hemoglobin in the plasma and forms a hemoglobin–haptoglobin complex, which is then quickly removed by the reticuloendothelial system, allowing the recycling of iron and globin. A decrease in haptoglobin concentrations is therefore consistent with intravascular hemolysis.[34–37] Conversely, in extravascular hemolysis, hemoglobin is not released in the circulation and haptoglobin concentrations remain normal. Haptoglobin concentration in healthy horses may differ depending on breed, age, and laboratory assay (see Table 44.4). Furthermore, haptoglobin concentrations increase in the presence of inflammatory diseases, which may limit its diagnostic value for detection of intravascular hemolysis in some patients.

Blood smears

Blood smear evaluation is an easy and very important procedure in diagnosing anemia. Autoagglutination, alterations in erythrocyte morphology, presence of blood parasites, or the brown color of methemoglobin cannot be accurately detected by automated hematology analyzers.[21,38]

The physiologic property of equine erythrocytes to aggregate and form rouleaux on the peripheral blood smear (Fig. 44.3) requires special consideration and should be distinguished from pathologic autoagglutination. The latter leads to formation of irregularly shaped erythrocyte clusters of different sizes, whereas rouleaux formation leads to a more orderly association with the erythrocytes lining up in rows. Mixing of the blood with normal saline (in a ratio of 1 part blood to 4 parts saline) will break up rouleaux, but not agglutinated erythrocytes.[20,39,40]

Wedge smears of EDTA-anticoagulated whole blood can be made using two clean glass slides. The smears are then air dried and stained with Romanowsky-type stains (Wright, Giemsa, Diff-Quick).[38] New methylene blue stain can be used to detect Heinz bodies. Normal equine erythrocytes are approximately 5.4 µm in diameter. Changes in erythrocyte morphology may be useful to determine the underlying mechanism of anemia.[38] Table 44.1 summarizes common findings in blood smears of anemic horses.

Bone marrow evaluation

Bone marrow evaluation is the most accurate method for assessment of a regenerative response in horses. It is indicated in cases for which the hemogram does not adequately provide evidence of normal bone marrow function.[21,30,41] Bone marrow aspirate cytology allows evaluation of individual cellular morphology and the use of special stains and procedures, but might not reflect true cellularity

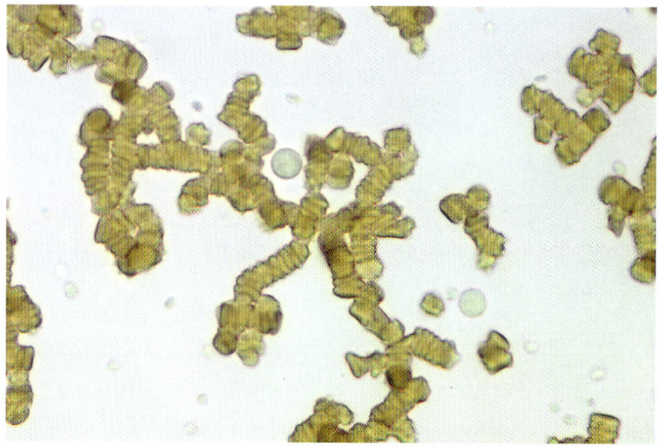

Fig 44.3 Normal rouleaux formation of equine erythrocytes.

Table 44.1 Common findings on peripheral blood smears in anemic horses[20,21,38]

FINDING	DESCRIPTION / APPEARANCE	CAUSE
Rouleaux formation	Erythrocytes lining up in rows, very prominent in equine blood	Normal
Howell–Jolly bodies	Round, basophilic inclusion bodies, found near the periphery of the erythrocytes	DNA remnants, found in 0.1% of normal erythrocytes; more often with severe (regenerative) anemia
Heinz bodies	Pale-pink (Romanowsky stain) or dark-blue (new methylene blue stain) round protrusions of the erythrocyte membrane or bodies within the cell	Denaturated aggregates of hemoglobin due to oxidative damage (maple leaf, onion, or phenothiazine toxicity)
Eccentrocytes ('hemighosts')	Erythrocytes with small peripheral cytoplasmatic clearing	Alterations in the erythrocyte membrane and condensation of hemoglobin in the remainder of the cell due to severe oxidative damage (maple leaf toxicity)
Schistocytes (erythrocyte fragments)	Small, irregularly shaped erythrocyte fragments with two to four angular or pointed projections	Endothelial damage and alterations in the microcirculation, associated with DIC, neoplasia, or inflammation of very vascular organs (liver, spleen, lung, kidney, bone marrow, placenta)
Autoagglutination	Irregularly shaped erythrocyte clusters of different sizes	Immune-mediated hemolytic anemia, adverse effect of unfractioned heparin, occasionally incidental finding as a result of anti-erythrocyte IgM antibodies present in normal animals
Echinocytes	Uniformly spaced, pointed membrane projections	Crenation artifact, electrolyte depletion
Macrocytosis	Large erythrocytes	Regenerative anemia, prolonged storage of blood
Microcytosis	Small erythrocytes	Iron deficiency, chronic blood loss
Spherocytes	Small round erythrocytes with lack of central pallor (difficult to detect in horses)	Result from partial removal of red cell membrane by macrophages secondary to antibody or complement attachment (immune-mediated) or oxidative damage (maple leaf toxicity)
Parasites	Teardrop-shaped inclusions with two or four ('maltese cross') organisms per cell	*Babesia caballi* or *Theileria equi*

of the bone marrow and might be affected by hemodilution. Core biopsy examination is indicated if repeated aspirates are of marginal cellularity, if hypoplasia, aplasia, inflammation, necrosis, or myelofibrosis is suspected, or when megakaryocyte numbers should be determined.[42] In some cases only a combination of both techniques provides the desired information. Both procedures are easy to perform on the standing sedated horse and carry small risk of complications. Standard techniques for bone marrow collection, sample preparation, and staining have been described.[42–45]

For aspirates, a 13 to 15 gauge two-inch needle with stylet is recommended. For core biopsies, a larger needle (11 to 13 gauge) should be used (Fig. 44.4). Several types of bone marrow collection needles are commercially available. An alternative biopsy technique using an electric drilling machine has been described.[46] Possible sites for bone marrow sampling in horses are the cranial sternum, tuber coxae, and the dorsal third of the ribs where hematopoietic activity is maintained throughout life. The sternum is most frequently used. The sampling is performed in the ventral midline on an imaginary line between the two elbows. The site is clipped, aseptically prepared, and 5 to 10 mL of a local anesthetic is injected into the subcutis down to the periosteum. A stab incision is then made at the sampling site and the bone marrow needle with stylet is inserted through the skin to the sternum. To take a bone marrow aspirate, the needle is then advanced approximately 1 to 1.5 centimeters with a rotational movement using firm pressure. The stylet is removed, a 10 mL syringe is attached, and aspiration is performed. The risk of extensive contamination of the sample with peripheral blood can be reduced by forceful, rapid aspiration. The suction should be released when blood becomes evident in the syringe. The marrow specimen should be processed immediately to avoid coagulation and to preserve cellular morphology. The sample is transferred through the needle to several glass slides and direct smears are made before the sample clots. Alternatively, bone marrow aspirates can be transferred onto a Petri dish containing 0.5 to 1 mL 2% to 3% EDTA or a citrate-phosphate-dextrose solution for anticoagulation. The marrow particles adhere to the Petri dish and can be easily detected as small, granular, gray particles, even when some blood contamination is present. They are selected and transferred to glass slides using a Pasteur pipette. Bone marrow squash preparations are made using a second slide. The slides are then air-dried. Multiple smears (4 to 10, depending on volume of material obtained) should be submitted for routine stains and for additional special stains.

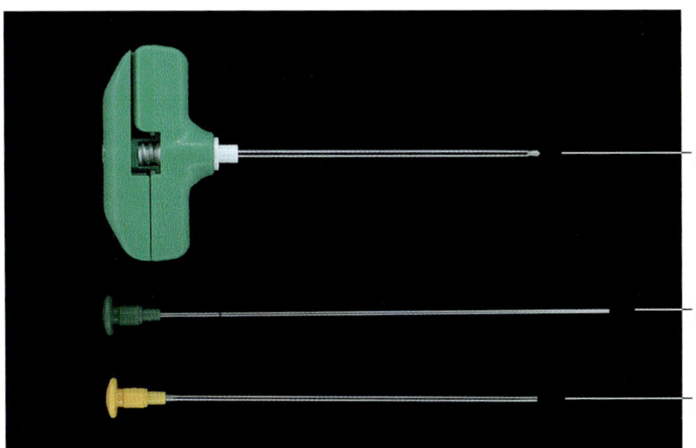

Fig 44.4 Bone marrow sampling device: **(A)** needle with stylet, **(B)** probe, **(C)** extraction cannula (optional use). TrapSystem™ bone marrow biopsy/aspiration needle.
With kind permission of Inomed Ltd.

To obtain a core biopsy, the needle is inserted through the skin and the cortex of the sternum as described above. After removing the stylet, the needle is advanced with a rotating motion an additional 1 to 2 centimeters into the bone marrow cavity. The needle is then withdrawn rapidly from the sternum, and the biopsy specimen is removed retrograde from the lumen of the needle with a probe or with the stylet. Some needles offer alternative techniques or require particular handling and the manufacturer's instructions should be followed carefully. Core biopsy samples are fixed in 10% neutral buffered formalin. Before placing in formalin, the specimen can be gently rolled across a glass slide to obtain impression smears for cytologic examination.

Common problems encountered when performing these procedures are failure to obtain a bone marrow aspirate or biopsy, and excessive blood contamination of aspirate specimens. In this case, multiple attempts at slightly different sites should be made to obtain diagnostically interpretable samples. Complications of bone marrow aspiration or biopsy are rare. Iatrogenic infections can be avoided by sterile technique. Excessive bleeding in patients with coagulation disorders, pneumothorax, hemothorax, and cardiac laceration may occur. The risk can be minimized by sedation of the horse, proper restraint, use of a needle guard and careful monitoring the needle length during the procedure. Bone marrow collection from the ribs contains similar risks, as the needle can slip off the bone and enter the thoracic cavity. Bone marrow sampling at the tuber coxae appears safer for examiner and horse, and may be associated with fewer complications. However, it is difficult to obtain bone marrow samples from the tuber coxae of older horses.

Cytologic examination of bone marrow aspirates or histologic examination of bone marrow biopsies should be assessed together with a complete blood count and differential taken on the same day and, if available, with results from previous CBCs and bone marrow evaluations.[21,42,45] Accurate interpretation of bone marrow samples requires training and considerable expertise. Routine bone marrow aspirate cytology is performed using Romanowsky-type stains (Wright, Giemsa, Diff-Quick). These stains allow assessment of particle cellularity; megakaryocyte numbers and maturity; erythroid and myeloid development, maturation, and morphology; and the presence of lymphoid cells, macrophages, stromal cells, and unusual cell populations.[45] Normocellular bone marrow particles contain 50% fat and 50% cells (Table 44.2). Hypocellularity is consistent with decreased hematopoiesis, whereas hypercellularity suggests hematopoietic response, infiltrative disease, or neoplasia.[45] Normocellular bone marrow with normal-appearing erythroid cells and increased iron deposits in the marrow is seen in anemia of inflammatory disease.[21,47] Erythroid hyperplasia, accompanied by a lack of hemosiderin in macrophages, is seen in iron deficiency.[21] Aplastic anemia (aplastic pancytopenia) is characterized by peripheral pancytopenia and bone marrow panhypoplasia. The bone marrow space is replaced by adipose tissue.[48] Infiltration and replacement of the bone marrow by inflammatory cells, neoplastic cells, or fibrous tissue (myelofibrosis) is referred to as myelophthisis. The marrow usually appears normocellular or hypercellular.[48] Myelodysplasia is characterized by morphologic abnormalities in hemic cells. Excessive blast cell content of the bone marrow is indicative for leukemia.[21] Severe suppression of only the erythroid cell line is called pure red cell aplasia.[48]

Although subjective microscopic evaluation is a valuable and important method, it is often inadequate to assess regenerative response to anemia. Differential cell counts should be determined to increase the accuracy of quantification of myeloid and erythroid cells.[41] The myeloid-to-erythroid ratio (M:E ratio) is commonly used to assess the erythroid compartment. The ratio is determined by counting 200 to 500 cells and dividing the number of cells of

Table 44.2 Normal and abnormal bone marrow findings used for assessment of anemia in horses

FINDING (STAINING METHOD)	NORMAL	REGENERATIVE RESPONSE	HYPOPROLIFERATIVE BONE MARROW
Cellularity	50% fat, 50% cells	>50% cells, dense cellular aggregates	<50% cells, mainly fat
M:E ratio	0.5–1.5	<0.5	>1.5
PRBCs (Romanowsky)	<2/HPF	>5/HPF	
Reticulocytes (new methylene blue)	0.5–1% of erythroid cells	>3–5% of erythroid cells	
Stainable iron (Prussian blue)	Many or all erythroblasts contain one to many hemosiderin granules	Normal in blood loss anemia ⇑ in hemolytic anemia	⇓ or absent in iron deficiency anemia Normal or ⇑ in anemia of inflammatory disease

PRBC = polychromatophilic erythrocytes ; HPF = high power field (100x oil immersion); M:E ratio = myeloid-to-erythroid ratio.

the myeloid series by the number of cells of the erythroid series. The normal M:E ratio in horses is between 0.5 and 1.5. A regenerative response leads to a decrease in M:E ratio, whereas a hypoproliferative anemia is characterized by an increased M:E ratio.[41,49–51] The regenerative response after acute loss of 25% of blood volume (20 mL/kg) leads to an expansion of the erythroid compartment within the first three days, and the peak erythroid response is reached after nine days, corresponding with the lowest M:E ratio. The regenerative response in horses is prolonged and may be detected for more than one month.[41] Coexisting changes in the myeloid compartment can also influence the M:E ratio and should be taken into consideration. Leukocytosis with left shift, as detected on complete blood count, results from augmented granulopoiesis. In this instance an activation of the myeloid series increasing the M:E ratio is to be expected.

In addition to the M:E ratio, determination of the number of young erythrocytes in bone marrow is useful to assess erythropoietic activity.[52] Anucleate erythrocytes in Romanowsky-stained smears are referred to as polychromatophilic erythrocytes (PRBC). In new methylene blue-stained smears, these cells appear as reticulocytes.[45] The presence of more than 5 PRBCs per high power field (100× oil immersion) and more than 3% reticulocytes (up to 66%) in relation to the total red blood cells confirm a regenerative response.[20,41,52–54]

Prussian blue stain allows semiquantitation of iron storage in the bone marrow. Normal bone marrow particles contain a moderate to large amount of erythroblasts with hemosiderin granula.[50] The amount of stainable iron is decreased in horses with chronic blood loss and iron deficiency.[51] Normoblasts and macrophages containing iron-rich granules (siderocytes, sideromonocytes) can be seen in horses with hemolytic anemia.[55,56] Anemia of inflammatory (chronic) disease leads to increased iron storage,[47,50] whereas iron deficiency anemia leads to decreased iron storage in bone marrow.[57,58]

Serum biochemistry

Determination of the serum bilirubin concentration can be useful in diagnosis of anemia. Bilirubin is a breakdown product of hemoglobin metabolism. Horses frequently develop mild increases in serum unconjugated (indirect, prehepatic) bilirubin concentrations (up to 6–8 mg/dL [103–137 μmol/L]) as a result of anorexia. Larger increases of unconjugated bilirubin concentrations in anemic horses support the diagnosis of hemolysis. The degree of elevation depends on the rate of red cell destruction and the capacity of the liver to conjugate and excrete the newly formed bilirubin.[59] Monitoring of the serum creatinine and serum urea nitrogen concentrations is critical in horses with hemolytic anemia, as hemoglobinuria and bilirubinuria can lead to acute tubular nephrosis (pigment nephropathy). Hypovolemia associated with acute blood loss is characterized by prerenal azotemia. Furthermore, moderate non-regenerative anemia can occur secondary to chronic renal failure.[59,60] Serum activities of sorbitol dehydrogenase (SDH), other liver-derived enzymes, and bile acid concentrations can be increased with severe acute anemia due to hypoxic or ischemic liver damage or increased iron storage and iron overload with severe hemolytic anemia.[59,61] Increased cardiac troponin I serum concentrations can indicate hypoxic myocardial damage.

Urinalysis

Hemoglobinuria and bilirubinuria are common features associated with severe intravascular hemolysis, potentially leading to acute tubular nephrosis. Monitoring of renal function in cases with hemolytic anemia includes repeated analyzes of urine samples.[59]

Blood gas analysis and lactate

Blood gas analysis and measurement of blood or plasma lactate concentration can be useful for assessment of tissue oxygenation in horses with severe anemia. Metabolic acidosis, increased anion gap, and elevated blood or plasma lactate concentration (i.e., >4 mmol/L) is consistent with tissue hypoxia or ischemia. A low venous or (preferably) mixed venous oxygen partial pressure ($p_vO_2 < 25–30$ mmHg) in association with normal pulmonary function and adequate arterial oxygenation ($p_aO_2 > 90$ mmHg) indicates increased oxygen extraction from the blood secondary to inadequate oxygen delivery (see Fig. 44.1).[4,7,62,63] However, the clinical application of these measurements to assess the severity of anemia, tissue oxygenation, and the need of blood transfusions in horses with anemia has not been well established and requires further investigation.

Assessment of minerals, trace elements, and vitamins

Iron

Iron exists in several anatomically, chemically, and functionally distinct compartments in the organism.[64,65] The functional pool contains approximately 70% of the total body iron. It consists of hemoglobin, myoglobin, and several iron-containing or iron-dependent enzymes. Iron is stored primarily in bone marrow, spleen, and liver, either in a soluble form (ferritin), or as insoluble, aggregated deposits (hemosiderin). Plasma transferrin is the major iron transport protein.

The iron content of several of these compartments can be determined to assess a patient's iron metabolism. Hemoglobin, the largest iron compartment of the body, is most commonly measured and routinely included in complete blood counts. However, hemoglobin is probably the least sensitive variable for detection of iron deficiencies. Overt anemia occurs only in late stages of severe iron deficiency.[64,65] Serum iron, ferritin, iron-binding capacity, and evaluation of the iron content of bone marrow are more accurate indicators of the iron status (Table 44.3 and Table 44.4).[57,58,64,65] Total serum iron concentration is low with chronic iron deficiency, but it is also decreased in inflammatory disease, hypoproteinemia, and renal disease.[66] Serum ferritin concentration correlates well with body iron stores and is a sensitive indicator of iron deficiency.[66,67] It is also an acute-phase reactant protein and can increase secondary to inflammation or liver disease, leading to an overestimation of total body iron content. Serum ferritin should therefore be assessed together with a complete blood count and plasma fibrinogen concentration.[68] Plasma transferrin is indirectly measured after complete saturation with iron, with the resulting iron content referred to as total iron-binding capacity (TIBC). The TIBC is typically increased in iron deficiency states, but decreased with acute-phase reactions and inflammatory disease. The amount of stainable iron in bone marrow samples correlates well with iron stores[69] and is a

Table 44.3 Variables used for assessment of iron status in horses[57,58,64,65,68,70]

	INCREASED	DECREASED
Serum iron	Hemolytic anemia Refractory anemia Iron overload Liver disease	Iron deficiency Acute-phase reactions Chronic inflammation Hypoproteinemia Renal disease Stress response (transport)
Serum ferritin	Iron overload Hemolysis Acute-phase reactions Inflammation Liver disease Some neoplasia	Iron deficiency
Total iron-binding capacity	Iron deficiency	Acute-phase reactions Chronic inflammation Hypoproteinemia Renal disease
Haptoglobin	Acute-phase reactions	Intravascular hemolysis
Bone marrow stainable iron	Acute-phase reactions Inflammation	Iron deficiency

Table 44.4 Normal values for the evaluation of the iron status in horses

VALUE	(n) BREED	NORMAL VALUES*	REFERENCE
Serum iron (μg/dL)	n.d.	111 ± 11	71
	(14) Arabian	129 ± 29	72
	(33) Quarter Horse	154 ± 34	72
	(18) Thoroughbred	109 ± 12	72
	(28) n.d.	124 ± 36.9	66
	(23) Standardbred	147 ± 36.8	73
Serum ferritin (ng/mL)	(28) n.d.	152 ± 54.6	67
	(23) Standardbred	88.4 ± 31.8	73
TIBC (μg/dL)	n.d.	330 ± 32	71
	(14) Arabian	189 ± 17	72
	(33) Quarter Horse	337 ± 49	72
	(18) Thoroughbred	297 ± 47	72
	(28) n.d.	343 ± 56.0	66
Transferrin saturation (%)	(14) Arabian	68.3	72
	(33) Quarter Horse	45.7	72
	(18) Thoroughbred	36.7	72
Haptoglobin (g/L)	(97) Thoroughbred/Arabian	2.19 ± 1.54	74
	(15) Standardbred	2.02 ± 0.4	34
	(6) Thoroughbred	0.98 ± 0.16	75
	(17) Thoroughbred	1.11 ± 0.70	33

n.d. = not determined. *Normal values expressed as mean ± SD, where applicable.

sensitive indicator for evaluation of the iron metabolism (see above). The amount of marrow stainable iron is decreased with iron deficiency, and increased with inflammatory disease.

Copper

Copper deficiency might be commonly overdiagnosed in horses because of inappropriately high reference ranges available for horses. Normal serum copper concentrations in healthy horses probably vary between 0.5 and 1.5 mg/L (8–24 μmol/L).[76–79] Concentrate ration feeding and copper supplementation increase the serum copper concentrations to 1–1.7 mg/L (17–26.6 μmol/L).[80] Serum copper concentrations lower than 0.7 mg/L (11.5 μmol/L) can indicate copper deficiency.[81]

Liver copper concentration and plasma ceruloplasmin activity can be used in addition to serum copper concentration to assess copper status of an animal.[77,81,82] Normal copper concentrations in liver tissue vary between 3.2 and 11 mg/kg (51–176 μmol/kg) fresh weight.[81,83,84] Mean plasma ceruloplasmin activity in mature Standardbreds has been determined to be 39.1 ± 0.5 IU/L (mean ± s.d.),[78] and serum ceruloplasmin concentration in adult horses varies between 4.07 ± 0.41 and 6.06 ± 0.74 mg/mL.[85] Acute-phase reactions can increase copper metabolism and cause the plasma copper concentration and ceruloplasmin activity to rise.[76,82,85] Complete blood count and plasma fibrinogen concentration should therefore be assessed together with serum copper concentrations to detect falsely elevated values.

Folic acid and vitamin B_{12} (cobalamin)

Data on normal folate and vitamin B_{12} serum concentrations for horses are limited, and comparison between different studies is complicated by differences in feeding and management regimen. Serum folate concentrations in non-supplemented stabled horses and intensively training Thoroughbreds and Standardbreds (range: 1.5–15.1 ng/mL) are generally lower than in pastured horses (range: 6.4–21.7 ng/mL) or in racehorses receiving dietary folate supplements (range: 2.0–21.1 ng/mL).[86–89] Similar differences were found for red cell folate concentrations, with racehorses in training having lower values (35–372 ng/mL) compared to stabled horses (70–630 ng/mL) or horses on pasture (123–986 ng/mL).[89] Measurement of red cell folate concentration could be more accurate for the assessment of the folate metabolism of horses.[89,90] Serum vitamin B_{12} concentrations in non-supplemented horses vary between 1.25 and 5.4 μg/L.[88,89] Vitamin B_{12} levels do not seem to be significantly affected by feeding and exercise.

Measurements of serum or red cell folate concentrations and vitamin B_{12} levels might be indicated in horses with macrocytic or normocytic anemia, leukopenia, and hypoplastic bone marrow. However, interpretation of the results can be difficult, as specific cut-off values for determination of vitamin deficiency have not been established.

Specific causes of anemia

Anemia is caused by hemorrhage (blood loss anemia), red blood cell destruction (hemolytic anemia), or lack of erythrocyte production (hypoproliferative anemia).[20,21] Blood loss anemias and hemolytic anemias are referred to as regenerative anemias, whereas hypoproliferative anemias are non-regenerative (see Table 44.5).

Table 44.5 Causes of anemia in athletic horses

REGENERATIVE ANEMIA		
BLOOD LOSS ANEMIA	**HEMOLYTIC ANEMIA**	**NON-REGENERATIVE (HYPOPROLIFERATIVE) ANEMIA**
Acute • Trauma • Surgery • Guttural pouch mycosis • Severe exercise-induced pulmonary hemorrhage • Internal abdominal or thoracic bleeding • Coagulation disorders **Chronic** • Gastrointestinal (ulceration, neoplasia, parasites) • Respiratory (ethmoidal hematoma, guttural pouch mycosis, pulmonary hemorrhage) • Urogenital • Coagulation disorders	**Infectious** • Equine infectious anemia (EIA) • Piroplasmosis (*Babesia caballi, Theileria equi*) • Anaplasmosis (*Anaplasma phagocytophilum*) **Immune-mediated hemolytic anemia (IMHA)** • Secondary IMHA (clostridial or streptococcal infection, penicillin, lymphoma, purpura hemorrhagica) • Autoimmune hemolytic anemia • Transfusion incompatibility **Oxidative injury (Heinz body anemia and methemoglobinemia)** • Maple leaf toxicity • Onion/garlic poisoning • Phenothiazine poisoning **Others** • Exercise-induced intravascular hemolysis • Terminal liver failure • Snake bite • Intravenous administration of concentrated dimethyl sulfoxide (DMSO) or hypotonic solutions	**Anemia of inflammatory (chronic) disease** • Chronic infection • Chronic inflammation • Severe trauma • Neoplasia **Nutritional deficiencies** • Iron deficiency (chronic hemorrhage, rarely nutritional) • Folate deficiency **Immune-mediated hypoproliferative anemia** • Pure red cell aplasia caused by treatment with erythropoiesis-stimulating agents • Immune-mediated hemolytic anemia affecting erythroid precursors **Infectious** • Equine infectious anemia **Others** • Chronic organ dysfunction • Aplastic anemia • Myelophthisic disorders • Myelodysplastic syndromes

Acute blood loss anemia

- External or internal bleeding can lead to decreased circulatory volume and hypovolemic shock.
- External bleeding is usually obvious, whereas internal bleeding can be difficult to diagnose.
- Anemia and hypoproteinemia usually become evident within 12 to 24 hours after onset of acute hemorrhage.
- Treatment consists of controlling the hemorrhage and reversing hypovolemia, rather than increasing the hemoglobin content of the blood.
- Whole blood transfusion should only be considered after assessment of appropriate transfusion triggers and after weighing benefits against potential risks.
- The prognosis is favorable for controlled hemorrhage, and guarded for uncontrolled hemorrhage.

Acute hemorrhage is defined as major external or internal hemorrhage that occurs within a few minutes to several hours. Severe acute blood loss results in acutely reduced blood volume, cardiovascular collapse, hypovolemic shock, and death.[15,16,91,92]

Recognition

History and presenting complaint

A history of recent trauma or surgery might be obtained. Overt bleeding is a common, but not invariate presenting sign. Exercise intolerance, weakness, depression, anorexia, colic, and dyspnea can be present.[93]

Physical examination

Clinical signs principally reflect the loss of blood volume rather than the loss of hemoglobin.[91] They vary depending on the underlying cause and rapidity, severity (volume), and duration of blood loss. Depression, weakness, tachycardia, tachypnea, pale mucous membranes, weak peripheral pulses, dehydration, and cold extremities are signs of hypovolemia and hypovolemic shock. Occasionally, anxiety and agitation occur. Death due to cardiovascular collapse can occur within 30 minutes with severe acute hemorrhage.[93–95]

Hemothorax is generally associated with dyspnea,[95] whereas hemoperitoneum commonly present with signs of abdominal pain.[93,96–99] Colic can also arise from malperfusion of the intestine and tissue ischemia resulting from compensatory cardiovascular mechanisms.[94]

Special examination

Endoscopic examination of the upper airways and guttural pouches is indicated to determine the cause of severe epistaxis. Rectal examination, ultrasonographic examination of the abdominal and thoracic cavity, followed by abdominocentesis or thoracocentesis, should be performed if internal hemorrhage is suspected.[93,94,100]

Laboratory examination

Initially, hematocrit and erythrocyte count are normal due to the simultaneous loss of blood cells and plasma. Splenic contraction can initially increase the hematocrit in horses with acute blood loss. The hematocrit is therefore not an accurate indicator of the severity of blood loss, especially in early stages of hemorrhage.[91,95,100] The severity of blood loss must therefore be estimated from clinical signs or, if possible, from measurement of the volume of blood loss. Blood volume is restored by shifting water from the interstitial fluid compartment to the intravascular compartment and by gastrointestinal and renal reabsorption of fluid. Anemia and hypoproteinemia usually become evident within 12 to 24 hours after acute hemorrhage, indicating blood loss anemia.[20,28,91,100] The plasma protein concentration usually begins to increase within 2 to 3 days and reaches normal values within 5 to 7 days, unless there is ongoing blood loss.[91,100] Three to seven days after acute blood loss, regenerative response can be detected by sequential measurements of the hematocrit.[23,27,28,91]

Internal hemorrhage is more difficult to detect based on measurements of hematocrit and plasma protein concentration, because up to two-thirds of the erythrocytes and most of the plasma proteins are recycled. The hematocrit can therefore increase more rapidly and the plasma protein concentration can be normal or only slightly decreased.[31,33,100]

The diagnostic work-up should include a platelet count and coagulation profile if the etiology of the hemorrhage is not obvious.[94] Bone marrow evaluation is rarely indicated, unless inadequate regenerative response to blood loss anemia is suspected. Erythroid hyperplasia and decreased M:E ratio usually become apparent within the first 3 to 5 days after hemorrhage.[91,95] The increase in red cell production reflects the severity of the anemia. However, concomitant iron deficiency, chronic renal disease, inflammation, bone marrow disorders, or blood transfusions can decrease the erythrocyte response.[91]

Diagnostic confirmation

Usually ongoing blood loss or signs of recent hemorrhage are evident on physical examination. However, hematologic examination, abdominal ultrasonography, abdominocentesis, and thoracocentesis might be required to detect internal bleeding.

Treatment and prognosis

Therapeutic aims

Initial treatment is aimed at controlling the hemorrhage and reversing the hypovolemic shock rather than increasing the hemoglobin concentration in the blood.[4,91,100] If blood pressure, circulatory volume, cardiac output, and tissue perfusion are adequate, tissue oxygenation will usually be maintained even in severely anemic horses.[62,100]

Therapy

External hemorrhage can usually be controlled by external pressure or surgical ligation of large vessels. Control of internal hemorrhage can often not be achieved effectively and surgical intervention is rarely practical.[95,100]

Reduction of stress, placement in a quiet environment, and moderate fluid therapy are essential points of treatment of uncontrolled bleeding. The circulatory volume should be restored by rapid administration of crystalloid solutions, hypertonic saline, colloid solutions, or equine plasma (Table 44.6).[92,94,100] Hypertonic saline[101–103] and colloid solutions[104–108] allow rapid resuscitation with smaller volumes of fluids, but subsequent administration of crystalloid solutions is required. A plasma protein concentration of less than 4.0 g/dL or a colloid osmotic pressure of less than 10 mmHg indicate the need for colloid solutions or equine plasma. Colloid solutions are readily available and usually well tolerated, but can exert anticoagulatory effects at high doses or after repeated administration.[109] Therefore, restrictive use of colloid solutions is advised in cases of acute hemorrhage. Alternatively, fresh frozen plasma can be used.[94,110]

Excessive volume replacement in the setting of uncontrolled hemorrhage can exacerbate the bleeding tendency and increase blood loss, due to the increased blood pressure and cardiac output.[94,96] Restrictive and carefully titrated volume replacement is therefore preferred, but only after initial volume losses have been restored to ensure adequate circulatory volume, cardiac output, blood pressure (i.e., mean arterial pressure >70 mmHg), and peripheral perfusion.[111,112] Sedation with acepromazine (0.02–0.055 mg/kg IV or IM) reduces stress and leads to peripheral vasodilation and drop in blood pressure, which potentially reduces severity of hemorrhage and permits clot formation. However, acepromazine can exacerbate shock and cause acute collapse. Pain control might be necessary, particularly in cases with internal hemorrhage. Flunixin meglumine (0.5 to 1.0 mg/kg IV) and butorphanol tartrate (0.02 to 0.1 mg/kg IV) are commonly used. If more analgesia is required, a multimodal approach using combinations of non-steroidal anti-inflammatory drugs, opioids, alpha-2 agonists, acepromazine, lidocaine, or ketamine should be considered.[113]

Several pharmacologic agents have been recommended to treat acute hemorrhage, although clinical efficacy has not been proven in horses. The antifibrinolytic agents aminocaproic acid and tranexamic acid have been used with the intention to stabilize fibrin clots and stop further hemorrhage (Table 44.7).[93,94,100,114,115] Intravenous administration of 10% buffered formalin might help to control bleeding,[94,116,117] although no effect on hemostatic variables can be detected in healthy horses and the mechanism of action remains unknown.[118] Naloxone hydrochloride, an opiate antagonist with dopaminergic activity, can reverse the effects of endogenous opioids on cardiovascular dynamics and attenuate cardiovascular responses associated with acute hemorrhage,[94,100] but can potentially result in increased pain perception.[93]

Following initial volume replacement and stabilization, the patient should be reassessed for the necessity of whole blood transfusion. The decision for transfusion should be based on clinical and clinicopathologic assessment. Transfusion is indicated if:

- the hematocrit rapidly falls below 15% and continues to decrease
- the hematocrit is below 10%
- there is severe, uncontrolled bleeding
- the quantitated blood loss is more than 30% of the total blood volume
- the tissue oxygen demand increases due to fever or agitation
- gastrointestinal signs (colic, diarrhea) indicate possible intestinal hypoxia
- cardiac arrhythmia and increased cardiac troponin I serum concentrations indicate myocardial hypoxia
- tachycardia, tachypnea, depression and weakness persist after initial restoration of the circulatory volume.[63,95,100,119]

Table 44.6 Therapies for intravenous volume restoration and increase of oxygen-carrying capacity of the blood[94,95,100,101]

TREATMENT	DOSAGE RECOMMENDATIONS	COMMENTS
Isotonic crystalloid solutions	3 times estimated volume of blood loss at a rate of 40–80 mL/kg/h	Shock dose
Hypertonic saline (7.2%)	4–6 mL/kg over 10–15 min	Followed by 40 mL/kg of an isotonic solution within 2 hours
Hetastarch 6% Pentastarch 10%	10 (–20) mL/kg	Colloid solutions Caution: might exert anticoagulatory effects. Use cautiously with acute hemorrhage
Equine fresh frozen plasma	12–16 mL/kg (initial rate: 0.1 mL/kg for 10 minutes, monitor for adverse reactions)	Estimate: 7 L plasma (PP 70 g/L) raises plasma protein concentration by 10 g/L in a 500-kg horse
Whole blood	12–16 mL/kg or 20–40% of estimated blood loss at a rate of 20 mL/kg per h (initial rate: 0.1 mL/kg for 10 minutes, monitor for adverse reactions)	May need to repeat due to destruction of transfused red blood cells. Caution: should only be considered after assessment of transfusion triggers and weighing benefits against potential risks. Estimate: 1 L blood (PCV 40%) raises PCV by 1% in a 500-kg horse

Table 44.7 Commonly used dosages for anecdotal treatment of acute hemorrhage in horses[93,94,100,114–117]

TREATMENT	DOSAGE RECOMMENDATIONS	COMMENTS
Aminocaproic acid	Bolus: 20–80 mg/kg IV, diluted in 1 liter 0.9% saline, over 30–60 min. Infusion: 52.5 mg/kg IV over 15 min, followed by 0.25 mg/kg/min CRI IV	Antifibrinolytic agents. Can be redosed as needed Tranexamic acid is approximately 8 times as potent as aminocaproic acid. Contraindications: thromboembolic disease, DIC
Tranexamic acid	5–25 mg/kg IV q12h	
Naloxone hydrochloride	0.01–0.02 mg/kg IV	Opioid antagonist
10% buffered formalin	0.02–0.08 mL/kg IV, diluted in 1 liter 0.9% saline	Efficacy and mechanism of action unknown

The use of blood gas measurements and oxygen extraction ratios (O_2ER) as transfusion triggers have not been well established in horses. However, a low venous oxygen partial pressure ($pO_2 < 25–30$mmHg) with normal pulmonary function, the presence of metabolic acidosis, and increased blood lactate concentrations (>4 mmol/L) indicate inadequate tissue oxygenation and the need of blood transfusion.[4,7,62,63,120]

If available, cross-match testing should precede transfusion. Alternatively, blood can be transfused without cross-matching, if the donor (preferably a gelding or stallion) and the recipient have not received prior transfusions.[94,95,119] Adult horses can donate safely 10 to 16 mL/kg (5 to 8 L for a 500-kg horse) whole blood without fluid replacement, and up to 25 mL/kg (12.5 L for a 500-kg horse) whole blood when the withdrawn volume is replaced with isotonic solutions.

Transfusion of whole blood is critical in the management of acute hemorrhage, but per se may be associated with adverse outcome.[121] The decision to transfuse must therefore weigh the potential benefits and harms. Adverse effects of administration of whole blood include immediate and delayed transfusion reactions and suppression of the normal bone marrow response to anemia.[110,119,122,123] Therefore, whole blood transfusion should only be considered after thorough clinical and clinicopathologic assessment and consideration of all available variables that may serve as transfusion triggers (see above). Blood transfusions are only temporarily effective, and further transfusions may be required, when the transfused erythrocytes are degraded or removed from the circulation.[94,95]

Prognosis

Generally, the prognosis for anemias caused by acute hemorrhage is good, provided that the hemorrhage can be controlled and appropriate treatment is initiated in a timely fasion.[91] The erythrocyte variables usually return to prehemorrhage levels within 8 to 14 weeks after acute hemorrhage.[28,91] The prognosis for internal, uncontrolled bleeding is usually guarded, with survival rates between 39 and 74% reported for hemoperitoneum.[93,97–99]

Etiology and pathophysiology

Acute blood loss anemia occurs with severe hemorrhage due to trauma or surgery. Infectious, neoplastic, or parasitic lesions can cause erosion of vessel walls. Severe epistaxis can occur due to trauma or guttural pouch mycosis, and less commonly due to pulmonary hemorrhage or nasal neoplasia.[95,100] Occasionally, internal hemorrhage can occur into the abdominal or thoracic cavity. It is caused by trauma, vascular abnormalities, neoplasia, abscesses, amyloidosis, parasite damage, or postoperative complications, and originates from large vessels, liver, spleen, kidneys, intestine, reproductive tract, or lungs. However, the underlying cause is often not identified.[92–94,96–100] Rarely, coagulation disorders (e.g., warfarin intoxication, thrombocytopenia, disseminated intravascular coagulation, hemophilia) lead to significant acute hemorrhage.[100]

While the decreased oxygen-carrying capacity of the blood and the increased cardiac output are the main pathophysiologic effects in other types of anemia (see above), decreased circulatory blood volume, hypotension, decreased cardiac output, and hypovolemic shock are the primary sequelae in severe hemorrhagic anemia.[4,91,100] The total blood volume equals approximately 8% of body weight (40 L in a 500-kg horse). A small amount of acute blood loss is well tolerated, while a loss of larger volume may lead to overt clinical signs. Acute blood loss of more than 30% of total blood volume (13 L/500 kg) results in hypovolemic shock, whereas loss of 50% or more (20 L/500 kg) leads to death if untreated.[91,100]

Chronic blood loss anemia

- Chronic blood loss is uncommon in horses.
- Diagnosis is made by identification of the source of bleeding and exclusion of other causes of anemia.
- Differential diagnoses of chronic blood loss anemia are anemia of inflammatory disease, iron deficiency anemia, and low-grade hemolysis.

Recognition

Pale mucous membranes and clinical signs associated with the underlying disease may be noted. Physiologic adaptation to the gradually developing anemia usually masks overt signs of anemia until the hematocrit is less than 15%. The anemia is typically regenerative, unless chronic blood loss results in iron deficiency and depletion of the iron stores (see below). Plasma protein concentration is usually normal, although in some cases hypoproteinemia (e.g., because of intestinal blood and protein loss) or hyperproteinemia (e.g., because of hyperglobulinemia and chronic immunologic stimulation) can be present.

Diagnostic confirmation

Diagnosis is based on characterization of the anemia, identification of a source of chronic blood loss, and exclusion of other causes for anemia. Diagnostic procedures may include complete blood count, bone marrow aspirate, coagulation profile, gastroscopy, fecal occult blood test, fecal parasite egg count, abdominocentesis, endoscopy of upper and lower airways, bronchoalveolar lavage, urinalysis and Coggins test for equine infectious anemia. Differential diagnoses for anemia of chronic blood loss are anemia of inflammatory disease, iron deficiency anemia, and low-grade hemolysis.

Treatment and prognosis

Treatment of the underlying cause is the cornerstone in management of chronic blood loss. Treatment of the anemia is rarely indicated, although horses with secondary iron deficiency anemia may benefit from oral supplementation with ferrous sulfate.

The prognosis depends on the underlying disease.

Etiology and pathophysiology

Chronic blood loss may result from bleeding gastrointestinal ulcers, parasites, gastrointestinal neoplasia, exercise-induced pulmonary hemorrhage, ethmoid hematoma, guttural pouch mycosis, or urogenital hemorrhage. Coagulopathies should always be considered.[95,100,124] Chronic blood loss can lead to iron depletion and iron deficiency anemia.

Equine infectious anemia (EIA)

- Equine infectious anemia is a viral disease characterized by development of persistent subclinical infections with possible recrudescence of disease. Chronic carriers remain infectious.
- Transmission occurs most commonly via insect vectors.
- Anemia occurs because of immune-mediated intravascular and extravascular hemolysis and bone marrow suppression.
- Depression, peripheral edema, weight loss, and recurrent episodes of fever are typical clinical signs of EIA. Laboratory abnormalities include anemia and thrombocytopenia.
- The diagnosis is based on serologic testing with agar gel immunodiffusion (Coggins) or ELISA tests. Infected horses

remain carriers for life and, with very few exceptions, yield a positive serological test result.
- EIA occurs worldwide and is a reportable disease. Prevention and regulatory measures are important for control of the disease.
- No effective treatment is available.

The equine infectious anemia virus (EIAV) is a retrovirus of the Lentivirinae subfamily. [125] Infected animals remain life-long carriers and a potential source of infection for other animals. Performance of chronically infected horses is impaired, despite lack of clinical signs of disease.[126] Equine infectious anemia occurs in all parts of the world and has important implications on horse trading as well as national and international equestrian sports. Equine infectious anemia is a reportable disease (World Organization for Animal Health [OIE] listed disease).[127]

Recognition

History and presenting complaint

Horses with acute EIA typically present with lethargy, anorexia, and fever.[125,128] Only a small percentage of EIAV-infected horses develop a severe, fatal form, while most horses only show mild clinical signs of disease and remain undetected. The subacute to chronic stage is characterized by recurrent episodes of fever, lethargy, peripheral edema, and weight loss. Periodic exacerbation of clinical disease may be associated with environmental stressors, transportation, strenuous exercise, concomitant diseases, or corticosteroid therapy.

Physical examination

The acute form is characterized by high fever, lethargy, petechial hemorrhages, pale or icteric mucous membranes, and occasionally death within days. Horses with subacute to chronic EIA show additional signs of lymphadenopathy, edema, and weight loss. Recurrent fever is typical. Neurologic signs have been reported.[125]

Laboratory examination

Thrombocytopenia, marked anemia and hyperbilirubinemia are seen during active febrile episodes. Chronic carriers show low normal erythrocyte indices or occasionally mild to moderate anemia. Persistent non-specific hypergammaglobulinemia may indicate low-grade chronic infection.[128,129]

Serologic testing for EIA should be performed in all horses with anemia if the etiology is not evident. Horses usually seroconvert within 14 to 45 days after infection.[125,130] The most widely accepted diagnostic test is the Coggins test, an agar gel immunodiffusion procedure, which is sensitive and specific for antibodies against EIA core protein antigens.[125,128,131] Highly sensitive enzyme-linked immunosorbent assays are also available.[125,128,131]

Necropsy examination

Necropsy findings vary with the stage of the disease process. During active disease, splenomegaly, hepatomegaly, lymphadenopathy, hemorrhages, and edema are common findings. Histopathologic findings include lymphoid necrosis and perivascular lymphocytic infiltrates of most organs and widespread hemosiderosis, especially in the liver.[125,128]

Diagnostic confirmation

The diagnosis of EIA is based on a positive Coggins test or ELISA. Virus isolation or PCR is usually not necessary.[131] Infected horses remain carriers for life and, with very few exceptions, yield a positive serological test result.[131]

Treatment and prognosis

Therapeutic aims

No effective treatment is available to eliminate the infection.

Therapy

Clinical recovery can be achieved with rest and supportive treatment.

Prognosis

The prognosis is unfavorable. Most horses spontaneously recover from the initial viremic episode, but latent infection persists, and recrudescence of clinical signs is common. Most horses become inapparent carriers with time, and few horses progress to a debilitating form of the disease.[125]

Etiology and pathophysiology

Equine infectious anemia virus infects and replicates primarily in tissue macrophages and integrates into the host genome.[125,132,133] Transmission of the disease requires a vector allowing blood transfer from an infected to a susceptible horse. Interrupted feeding of large hematophagous insects (Tabanidae; horseflies, deerflies, stable flies) is the principal mechanism of disease transmission.[129,134] Iatrogenic, transplacental, transmammary, and venereal transmission by asymptomatic carriers can occur as well.[125,128,135] The incubation period is 1 to 3 weeks, but can be as long as three months.[125,131]

Infection of a naive host leads to acute EIA and causes an immune response that finally leads to a remission of clinical sings and latent infection. Anemia is primarily caused by complement-mediated intravascular and extravascular hemolysis secondary to virus-antibody attachment to erythrocytes.[125,129] Direct bone marrow suppression and sequestration of iron in the reticuloendothelial system further contributes to anemia.[136,137] Recurrence of the disease is associated with recrudescence of viremia, with production of antigenetically novel virus strains that temporarily escape the host's immune system.[125,128] The severity of clinical signs decreases with each viremic episode and the host mounts an immune response against all common variants of EIAV, leading to the chronic subclinical carrier stage,[125] which can be a source of infection of other animals.[125,135]

Epidemiology

Equine infectious anemia occurs worldwide with variable prevalence. The potential of chronic inapparent carriers to serve as a source of infectious virus is of epidemiologic importance and emphasizes the need for rigorous disease control measures. Disease information, including current disease outbreak and distribution maps and detailed country disease incidence, is available online.[138]

Prevention

Equine infectious anemia is a reportable disease. Depending on local procedures and regulations, Coggins test or ELISA are required for traveling across state or country borders, change of ownership, and participation in exhibitions, sales markets, and equestrian sports events. Testing of horses before introduction into a new population is generally recommended, particularly in regions with a high prevalence of disease. Tests should be performed following a quarantine of 60–90 days' duration after potential exposure to EIAV.

The OIE Terrestrial Animal Health Code (2011)[139] lists the following recommendations for the importation of equines: Veterinary authorities of importing countries should require the presentation of an international veterinary certificate attesting that:

- the animals showed no clinical sign of EIA on the day of shipment and during the 48 hours prior to shipment; and
- no case of EIA has been associated with any premises where the animals were kept during the three months prior to shipment; and
- the animals were subjected to a diagnostic test for EIA with negative results on blood samples collected during the 30 days (if imported on a permanent basis) or 90 days (if imported on a temporary basis) prior to shipment.

Control measures are usually aimed at elimination of inapparent carriers, although the regulations for Coggins-positive horses may vary. Under certain circumstances, keeping affected horses in isolation is permitted. Insect control and strict prevention of iatrogenic transmission is required.[125,128,130,134] All horses that were within 200 yards of a confirmed EIA-positive horse should be considered exposed. They should be held under quarantine and tested at 30- to 60-day intervals until all positive horses have been removed from the population and all horses have been tested negative 60 days after the last positive result.[125]

Equine piroplasmosis (babesiosis, theileriosis)

- Equine piroplasmosis is a tick-borne protozoal disease characterized by hemolytic anemia, fever, peripheral edema, and weight loss.
- Development of immunity leads to a chronic carrier state, characterized by chronic anemia and poor performance.
- *Theileria equi* is considered more pathogenic than *Babesia caballi*.
- The diagnosis is based on direct detection of intraerythrocytic parasites (blood smears or polymerase chain reaction) or indirect serologic tests.
- Treatment is aimed towards resolution of the clinical sings. Infections with *T. equi* are difficult to eliminate with the currently available drugs.
- The worldwide distribution of the disease is related to the presence of the tick vectors.
- Equine piroplasmosis is a reportable disease. Regulatory measures aim at prevention of introduction of infectious organisms into equine piroplasm-free areas.

Piroplasmosis is a tick-borne disease of horses, caused by the intraerythrocytic protozoa *Babesia caballi* and *Theileria equi* (formerly *Babesia equi*). Potential tick vectors are present in many disease-free countries and would allow the disease to become endemic once introduced into the native horse population by carrier animals. Equine piroplasmosis is an OIE-listed disease.[127] Import regulations of various countries restrict entering of horses that have been tested positive for *B. caballi* or *T. equi*. The disease has therefore important implications in the international equestrian sports and trade of horses.[140–143]

Recognition

History and presenting complaint

Clinical cases are more frequently caused by *T. equi*, while *B. caballi* seems to be less pathogenic and infection tends to be milder or inapparent.[140,144] Acute forms usually present with depression, anorexia, fever, and peripheral edema. Subacute cases show similar signs, accompanied by weight loss, and occasionally colic and diarrhea. The fever can be intermittent. In chronic cases, unspecific clinical signs including poor performance, mild inappetence, and weight loss are the major complaints. Inapparent carriers do not show obvious clinical signs but may have compromised athletic performance compared with uninfected horses.[143]

Physical examination

Acute and subacute piroplasmosis is characterized by high fever, tachycardia, tachypnea, peripheral edema, swelling of the eyelids, and hemoglobinuria.[140,143,144] The mucous membranes appear from congested to pale pink to pale yellow or bright yellow. Untreated cases become severely anemic and weak. Physical examination in chronic cases is often unremarkable or reveals unspecific signs of chronic inappetence, poor performance, and weight loss.

Laboratory examination

Hemolytic anemia, neutropenia, lymphopenia, and thrombocytopenia are common in acute infections.[145] Varying degrees of hemoglobinuria are observed in acute and subacute cases.[140] Laboratory abnormalities may be minimal in chronic cases and in inapparent carriers, and marked hyperbilirubinemia may the only abnormality found in these horses.

Direct detection of the parasites during the acute phase of the infection can be achieved by examination of Giemsa-stained blood smears (Fig. 44.5).[140,142,145–147] In carrier animals and in most cases of *B. caballi* infection, parasitemia is very low and detection on routine blood smears is usually not possible.[143,144] Polymerase chain reaction (PCR) has been shown to be highly specific and sensitive for diagnosis of piroplasmosis in horses and is useful for detection of carrier animals.[143,146,147]

Several serologic tests are available for diagnosis of piroplasmosis in horses.[142,144,146] Antibody titers become detectable between 2 and 20 days after infection, depending on the type of assay used. The complement fixation test (CFT) used to be the official standard test for qualifying horses for international import/export. However, the CFT is characterized by low sensitivity and specificity and is not able to detect latent infections.[142,146,148] Therefore, it has now been replaced by the indirect fluorescent antibody test (IFAT) and the competitive enzyme-linked immunosorbent assay (cELISA) as the prescribed tests for international horse trading.[143,147] Antibody titers remain positive during the latent phase of infection.[142,143,146,148]

Necropsy examination

Gross pathological findings include generalized pallor or icterus, subcutaneous and subserosal edema, emaciation, hepato- and splenomegaly, enlarged kidneys, ascites, hydrothorax, pericardial effusion, pulmonary edema, and lymphadenopathy.

Diagnostic confirmation

The detection of intraerythrocytic parasites or positive direct or indirect tests in an animal with clinical signs of piroplasmosis is diagnostic.

Treatment and prognosis

Therapeutic aims

The first goal of treatment is resolution of the clinical signs. The second goal is elimination of the parasites from affected horses. Clinical recovery is usually achieved, but infections with *T. equi* are difficult to eliminate with the currently available drugs and horses usually remain carriers, probably for life.[141,142,144]

Therapy

Imidocarb is the drug of choice for treatment of piroplasmosis. For *B. caballi*, two doses of 2.2 mg/kg IM at a 24-hour interval are

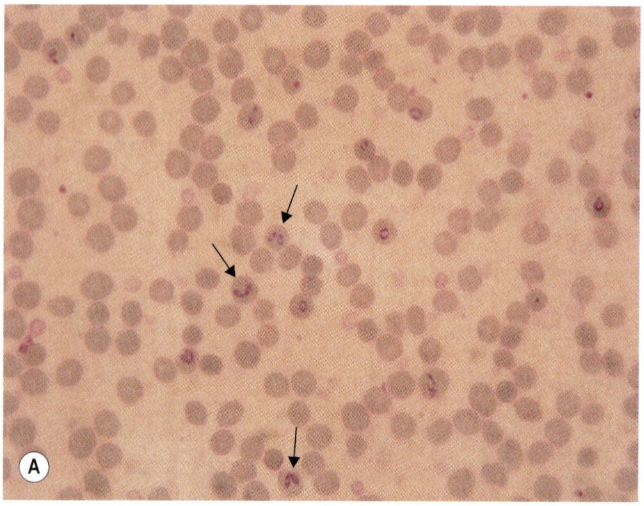

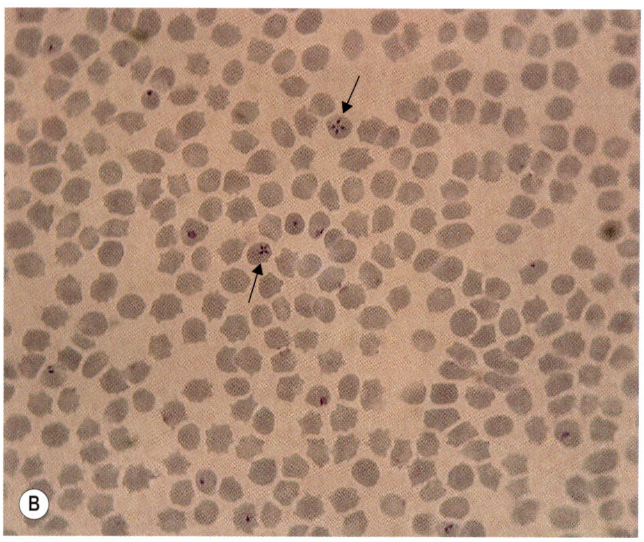

Fig 44.5 Blood smears of horses with piroplasmosis: **(A)** *B. caballi* is characterized by large paired intraerythrocytic merozoites (arrows) forming an acute angle. **(B)** *T. equi* is characterized by four smaller merozoites forming a 'Maltese cross' (arrows).

Courtesy of Dr Heinz Sager, Institute of Parasitology, University of Bern, Switzerland.

recommended, although higher doses might be necessary to clear infection and eliminate transmission risk.[149,150] *T. equi* should be treated with four doses of 4 mg/kg IM at a 72-hour interval.[140,143,144,151] The risk of cholinergic adverse reactions (salivation, sweating, heavy breathing, restlessness, abdominal pain, GI hypermotility) may be reduced by administering half this dose initially, followed by the remainder of the dose 1–2 hours later, and combining the drug with butylscopolamine (0.1–0.2 mg/kg IV) and metamizole (dipyrone, 20–40 mg/kg IV). Combined treatment with buparvaquone (4 mg/kg IV) and imidocarb (4 mg/kg IM) has been suggested for elimination of *T. equi*.[152,153]

Administration of polyionic electrolyte solutions is indicated to prevent or treat acute renal failure due to pigmenturia. Blood transfusions are only indicated if signs of tissue hypoxia are present in cases with severe anemia.[63]

Prognosis

Early treatment is effective even without completely eliminating the etiologic agent. Chronic carriers are resistant to new infections.

Etiology and pathophysiology

During the life cycle of *B. caballi* and *T. equi*, ticks (*Dermacentor*, *Hyalomma*, and *Rhipicephalus* spp.) serve as vectors for transmission of the disease between host animals.[143,144,154] The incubation period varies from 5 to 30 days.[140,143,144,152] The protozoa usually infect 0.1–1% (*B. caballi*) and 1–7% (*T. equi*) of erythrocytes, respectively, thereby causing intravascular hemolysis.[143,145] Development of immunity without expression of clinical signs is common in endemic areas.[140,154] Acute infections are followed by a chronic carrier state that leads to persistent anemia and can result in decreased performance in racehorses.[154]

Epidemiology

Piroplasmosis occurs most commonly in subtropic and tropic regions in South and Central America, Africa, Asia, the Middle East, and Eastern and Southern Europe. It is however not strictly confined to these areas. The United States, Canada, Australia, Japan, England, and Ireland are considered non-endemic areas, although epidemic foci and introduction of the disease by imported horses have been reported.[142,144,155] The worldwide distribution is related to the presence of tick vectors.[140,144] Disease information, including current disease outbreak and distribution maps and detailed country disease incidence, is available online.[138]

Prevention

Currently, effective vaccines for equine piroplasmosis are not available. Control of equine piroplasmosis largely relies on drug therapy, tick-vector control, and restrictions in the movement of infected animals.[143] It is important to prevent introduction of both infected horses and ticks into equine piroplasm-free areas.[143,155]

The OIE Terrestrial Animal Health Code (2011)[139] lists the following recommendations: For the importation of equines, veterinary authorities of importing countries should require the presentation of an international veterinary certificate attesting that the animals:

- showed no clinical sign of equine piroplasmosis on the day of shipment;
- were subjected to diagnostic tests for equine piroplasmosis (*T. equi* and *B. caballi*) with negative results during the 30 days prior to shipment;
- were maintained free from ticks, by preventive treatment when necessary, during the 30 days prior to shipment.

Depending on local regulations, temporary import of competition horses that have been tested positive for piroplasmosis might be permitted, if the horses are accompanied by a passport and an international veterinary certificate attesting that the animals showed no clinical sign of equine piroplasmosis on the day of shipment, were treated against ticks within the seven days prior to shipment, are kept in an area where necessary precautions are taken to control ticks, and are regularly examined for the presence of ticks under the direct supervision of the veterinary authority.[139]

Immune-mediated hemolytic anemia

- True autoimmune hemolytic anemia is uncommon in horses. Secondary IMHA has been reported secondary to infections,

administration of certain drugs, and neoplasia, or in association with other immunologic diseases.
- Immune-mediated erythrocyte destruction leads to intravascular or extravascular hemolysis.
- The primary disease often predominates the clinical picture.
- Typical laboratory findings are autoagglutination of the blood and the presence of spherocytes. Coombs' test and direct immunofluorescence flow cytometry tests can confirm the diagnosis.
- Therapy consists of elimination of the primary cause, administration of corticosteroids, and supportive treatment.
- The prognosis depends on the underlying disease.

Recognition

History and presenting complaint

Lethargy, depression, weight loss, anorexia, and tachypnea are frequent presenting complaints. A history of recent drug administration or infectious disease may be obtained.

Physical examination

Hemolysis can be acute and severe or chronic and insidious.[129] Clinical signs depend on the severity of the anemia, the rate of erythrocyte destruction, and the underlying disease process. Often, the clinical signs of the primary disease predominate the clinical picture. Lethargy, depression, pyrexia, tachycardia, tachypnea, icterus, and hemoglobinuria are found. Pallor of the mucous membranes can occur but is not a consistent finding.[124,129]

Special examination

Ultrasonographic examination of abscesses and local swellings (myositis, cellulitis) can be useful to detect clostridial infections (gas and fluid accumulation). Rectal examination and ultrasonographic examination of abdominal and thoracic cavity should be performed to detect possible neoplasia. Splenomegaly is occasionally found and is likely caused by splenic hypertrophy or an underlying disease (neoplasia).

Laboratory examination

Complete blood count and bone marrow analysis reveal signs for regenerative anemia within days after onset of hemolysis.[40] Serial measurements of hematocrit are helpful to detect ongoing hemolysis or regenerative response. Occasionally, the immune reaction also affects red blood cell precursors in the bone marrow, leading to non-regenerative anemia.[39,40] The presence of spherocytes is highly suggestive for immune-mediated hemolytic anemia.[39] Autoagglutination of red blood cells (Fig. 44.6) is a consistent finding in immune-mediated hemolytic anemia and should be distinguished from normal rouleaux formation (see above).[25,39,40] Moderate neutrophilic leukocytosis is a common feature[156] and, occasionally, immune-mediated hemolytic anemia is associated with thrombocytopenia.[25,157,158] Red discoloration of the plasma after centrifugation indicates hemoglobinemia. The plasma protein concentration is typically normal. Hyperbilirubinemia can be present.[124]

The direct antiglobulin test (Coombs' test) using multivalent, species-specific reagent detects IgM (cold agglutinin) and IgG (warm agglutinin) anti-erythrocyte antibodies as well as complement protein C3 on the erythrocyte surface.[40] Although the specificity of the Coombs' test is very high, its sensitivity is low and a negative test does not rule out immune hemolytic anemia.[39] Previous corticosteroid treatment might lead to false-negative test results.[156] Direct immunofluorescence flow cytometry has been used for

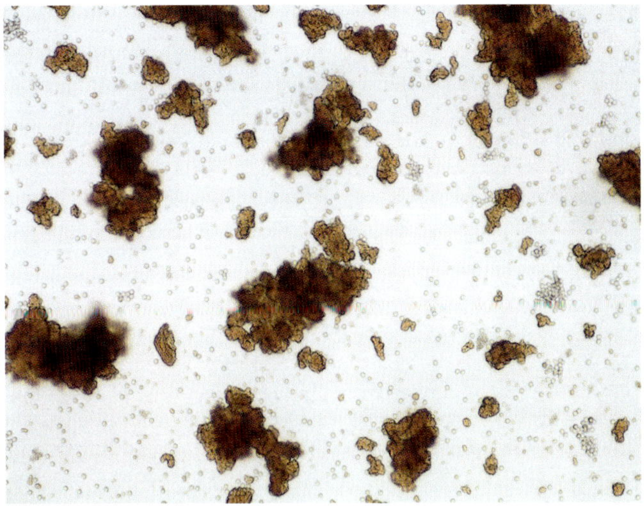

Fig 44.6 Autoagglutination of erythrocytes in a horse with immune-mediated hemolytic anemia secondary to clostridial myositis.

diagnosis of immune-mediated hemolytic anemia in horses.[159,160] This method allows the detection, differentiation, and quantification of cell-bound IgG, IgM, and IgA antibodies. The sensitivity of the test is thought to be very high, whereas its specificity is somewhat lower than in the Coombs' test, occasionally leading to false-positive results.

Agar gel immunodiffusion for EIA (Coggins) should be submitted in all cases of hemolytic anemia. If the horse is living in or was imported from an area in which piroplasmosis is endemic, appropriate further diagnostic should be performed (see above). Tests for anti-penicillin IgG antibodies can be performed when penicillin-associated hemolytic anemia is suspected.[161–163] Clostridial infection (myositis or cellulitis) can be diagnosed by fine needle aspirate, cytologic examination, Gram stains, and bacterial culture. Cytologic evaluation of abdominal or pleural fluid is recommended in cases with detectable effusion. Fine needle aspiration of mass lesions is indicated to diagnose neoplasia.

Necropsy examination

Generalized pallor or icterus is present on post-mortem examination. Lesions of primary disease can be found predominantly. Hemosiderosis of liver and kidneys, bone marrow erythroid hyperplasia, and extramedullary hematopoiesis are present.[56]

Diagnostic confirmation

Immune-mediated hemolytic anemia is confirmed by ruling out other causes of hemolytic anemia, detection of autoagglutination of red blood cells, positive Coombs' test, positive flow cytometry test, and response to treatment with corticosteroids.

Treatment and prognosis

Therapeutic aims

Treatment of the underlying disease, suppression of the abnormal immune response, and supportive care are the basic principles for successful treatment of immune-mediated hemolytic anemia. Monitoring and support of renal function is important. If signs of tissue hypoxia and organ dysfunction are present, blood transfusions should be considered.[63]

Therapy

The treatment depends on the severity and the primary cause of the anemia. Previously administered drugs should be discontinued. If antibiotic treatment is necessary, the class of the antimicrobial agent should be altered. Treatment with isotonic crystalloid solutions is crucial to avoid pigment nephropathy and acute renal failure in cases with severe hemolysis and hemoglobinuria.

Corticosteroids stabilize cell membranes, decrease the antibody production, decrease the affinity of the antibodies to the red blood cells, and decrease the rate of RBC destruction by macrophages of the reticuloendothelial system.[25,39,164] An initial daily dose of 0.05–0.1 mg/kg of dexamethasone IM or IV usually leads to a clinical and hematological response within 5–6 days. Alternatively, prednisolone can be administered orally at an initial dose of 1–1.5 mg/kg once daily. The dose should then be gradually reduced and continued for the total duration of 3 to 6 weeks, depending on the clinical response. Prior to initiation of corticosteroid treatment, possible infectious causes of immune hemolytic anemia should be precluded. In these cases, corticosteroids should be used with caution, as immune suppression can lead to exacerbation of the disease.[156]

Cytotoxic drugs including cyclophosphamide can be considered for severe therapy-resistant cases.[164] There is one report of treatment of a horse with cyclophosphamide and azathioprine.[56] Other therapies occasionally used in humans and dogs, including splenectomy, administration of intravenous immunoglobulins, and plasmapheresis, have not been well established in horses.[39]

Clostridial myositis or cellulitis requires surgical debridement of necrotic tissue, analgesia, fluid therapy, and correction of electrolyte and acid–base disturbances.[165] Although penicillin is commonly recommended as antimicrobial agent of choice, experimental data suggest that treatment with oxytetracycline and metronidazole are more effective in decreasing toxin production and increasing overall survival rate.[166–168]

If signs of tissue hypoxia and organ dysfunction indicate the need to increase the oxygen-carrying capacity of the blood, the use of whole blood transfusions or packed red cells should be considered (see 'Acute blood loss anemia').[63] However, transfusion of blood or erythrocyte concentrates can have limited benefits, as transfused cells are rapidly removed from the circulation and put additional workload on the reticuloendothelial system. Compatible donors often are not available and cross-matching is usually positive.

Prognosis

The response to corticosteroid treatment is usually good in horses.[39] However, recurrence of the anemia after cessation of the treatment is possible, especially when the primary disease process is still present. The prognosis is best for patients with penicillin-associated anemia and primary idiopathic autoimmune hemolytic anemia. The prognosis for patients with neoplastic disease is usually poor.[39,156,169] Repeated monitoring of the hematologic indices is recommended for 6 to 12 months after cessation of treatment.

Etiology and pathophysiology

Immune-mediated hemolytic anemia is caused by antibodies directed against erythrocyte membrane proteins or membrane-bound antigens. Initiating factors are thought to be alterations of the erythrocyte membrane, alterations in immune regulation, or stimulation by other antigens, leading to a production of cross-reacting antibodies.[39,40] Erythrocyte destruction is the result of complement-mediated intravascular hemolysis or, more commonly, phagocytosis of antibody-coated erythrocytes by the macrophages of the reticuloendothelial system in liver and spleen (extravascular hemolysis).[39,40] Occasionally, autoantibodies are also directed against bone marrow erythroid precursors, thereby interfering with erythropoiesis and leading to acquired pure red cell aplasia.[39,40] In patients in which no demonstrable underlying disease is present, the anemia is referred to as primary idiopathic autoimmune hemolytic anemia.[25,169] More commonly, immune-mediated hemolytic anemia occurs in association with other disease processes (secondary immune-mediated hemolytic anemia). A variety of causes has been described in association with immune-mediated hemolytic anemia in horses.

Immune-mediated hemolytic anemia secondary to clostridial myositis or cellulitis is not uncommon in horses.[165,170,171] Autoagglutination can occur without clinically detectable hemolysis. Clostridial myositis or cellulitis is most commonly caused iatrogenically as a result of intramuscular injections of non-antibiotic drugs (flunixin meglumine, ivermectin, antihistamines, B-complex vitamins, prostaglandins, dipyrone, phenylbutazone).[165,171] Although *Clostridium perfringens* alpha toxin has a direct hemolytic effect resulting from massive acute destruction of the red cell membranes,[165,171,172] clinical and laboratory findings (delayed-onset hemolysis, autoagglutination) suggest an immune-mediated cause of the anemia.[171] The pathomechanism could be related to bacterial synthesis of neuraminidase and subsequent enzyme-mediated exposure of a membrane-bound antigen (Thomsen-Friedenreich cryptantigen).[165,173] However, the contribution of this mechanism to the hemolytic process is unknown.

Immune-mediated hemolytic anemia is a rare complication after administration of penicillin[161–163,174] and possibly trimethoprim-sulfamethoxazole[175] in horses. Presumably the drugs act as haptens. They bind to erythrocyte membrane proteins and plasma proteins and induce production of anti-penicillin IgG antibodies. Binding of the antibodies to the erythrocyte-bound penicillin leads predominantly to extravascular hemolysis and to a lesser extent to complement-mediated intravascular hemolysis.[161,163] In part, the anemia might also result from pooling of red blood cells in the microcirculation or in the spleen, which would explain the rapid rise in hematocrit seen in some horses after cessation of penicillin treatment and initiation of corticosteroid treatment.[162]

Lymphosarcoma and other neoplasms are commonly associated with anemia of chronic disease and blood loss anemia. Occasionally, immune-mediated hemolytic anemia (and thrombocytopenia) is found.[25,157,176]

Other primary disorders which can be associated with immune-mediated hemolytic anemia are purpura hemorrhagica and systemic lupus erythematosus, inflammatory bowel disease, and chronic bacterial infections or abscesses.[25,177,178] Etiology and pathogenesis of equine infectious anemia and piroplasmosis were described above.

Prevention

Administration of drugs that are known to cause immune-mediated hemolytic anemia and intramuscular injection of irritating drugs (e.g., flunixin meglumine, ivermectin) that could cause clostridial myositis or cellulitis should be avoided.

Heinz body hemolytic anemia

- Heinz body anemia results from toxic effects of maple leaves, wild onions, phenothiazines, or methylene blue.
- Oxidative damage to erythrocytes leads to hemolytic anemia characterized by the presence of Heinz bodies and eccentrocytes on the blood smear.

- Maple leaf toxicity also leads to methemoglobinemia and brown discoloration of mucous membranes, urine, and blood.
- Prognosis with rapid developing severe anemia is poor.

Recognition

History and presenting complaint

Clinical signs vary depending on type and amount of toxin, time since exposure, and occurrence of complicating factors like pigment nephropathy and acute renal failure. Horses usually present with weakness, depression, anorexia, exercise intolerance, and signs of hematuria. Colic, ataxia, or acute death can occur.[129,179–181]

Physical examination

Tachycardia, tachypnea and icterus are common findings. Brown discoloration of the mucous membranes, blood, and urine indicate methemoglobinuria, commonly found with maple leaf toxicity (Fig. 44.7 and Fig. 44.8).[129,179,181]

Laboratory examination

Moderate to severe anemia, hyperbilirubinemia, hemoglobinemia, and hemoglobinuria are present. Heinz bodies and eccentrocytes can be detected on blood smears (Fig. 44.9).[129,179] Measured blood methemoglobin concentration is increased in cases with maple leaf toxicity and can exceed 50% of total cellular hemoglobin concentration (normal methemoglobin fraction is less than 2% of total hemoglobin).[129,181] Serum biochemistry and urinalysis should be performed to monitor liver and kidney function. Blood gas analysis and serum lactate measurements may be used to assess severity and metabolic consequences of the anemia.

Diagnostic confirmation

Clinical diagnosis is established based on history, clinical signs, specific laboratory findings, negative Coombs' test, and exclusion of other causes of anemia.

Treatment and prognosis

Treatment consists of removal of the source of the toxin, administration of activated charcoal via nasogastric tube to decrease toxin absorption, intravenous fluid therapy to support renal function, and administration of high doses of vitamin C (30 mg/kg IV twice daily) as an antioxidant agent.[179,182,183] Whole blood transfusion might be necessary as indicated by transfusion triggers including indices of tissue hypoxia and organ dysfunction (see 'Acute blood loss anemia').[63]

The prognosis depends on the amount of the ingested toxin, occurrence of complicating factors, and the response to treatment. With rapidly progressive severe anemia, the prognosis is poor. The mortality rate with maple leaf toxicity is 60 to 65%.[179,181]

Etiology and pathophysiology

Heinz body hemolytic anemia results from acute oxidative damage to the erythrocytes, caused by ingestion of maple leaves (red maple, *Acer rubrum*, and potentially sugar maple, *A. saccharum*, and silver maple, *A. saccharinum*), onions and garlic (*Allium* spp.), or certain drugs including phenothiazines or methylene blue.[36,129,179,180,184]

Oxidative denaturation and aggregation of hemoglobin results in development of typical Heinz body inclusions, increased osmotic fragility of the erythrocytes, and enhanced cell clearance by mononuclear phagocytes, leading to intravascular and extravascular hemolysis. Maple leaf toxicity is also associated with formation of methemoglobin, which is incapable of carrying oxygen to the tissue.[129,179]

Exercise-induced intravascular hemolysis

- Exercise-induced intravascular hemolysis is seen after exercise of various intensity.
- It results from increased erythrocyte fragility that is likely of multifactorial etiology.
- It can reflect a normal physiologic response to exercise and is unlikely to cause clinically relevant anemia.
- No abnormal clinical signs are noticed and diagnosis usually requires measurement of free plasma hemoglobin and detection of pigmenturia.
- Dietary supplementation of vitamin E and selenium may be beneficial to reduce exercise-related oxidative damage to the erythrocytes.

Exercise-induced intravascular hemolysis is a condition recognized in horses after endurance rides, races, and treadmill exercise of various intensity.[34,35,37,185] The hemolysis is mild and transient and might reflect a normal physiologic response to exercise rather than a pathologic condition.[186]

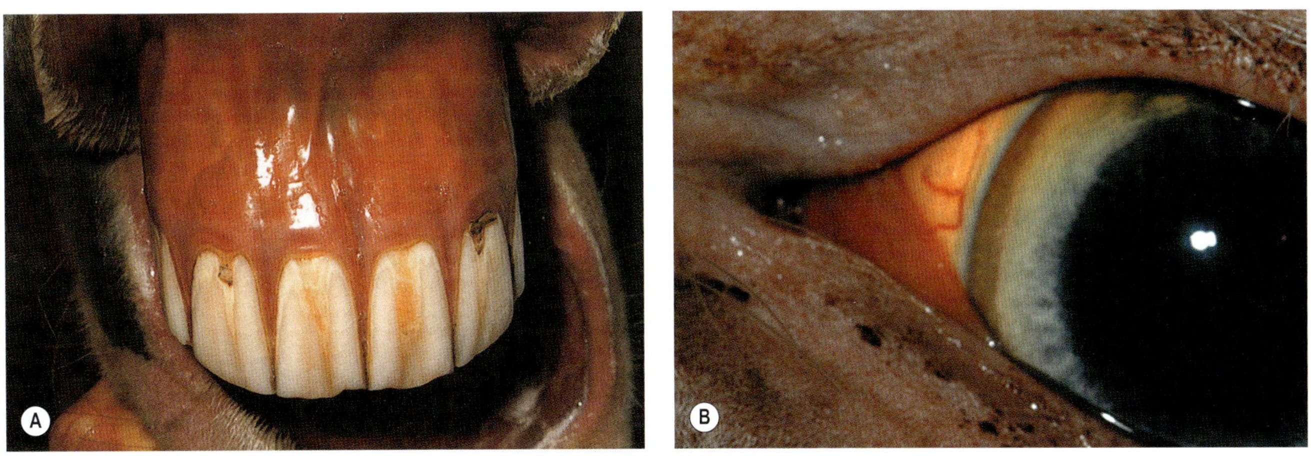

Fig 44.7 Brown discoloration of mucous membranes **(A)** and conjunctivae **(B)** indicate severe methemoglobinemia associated with red maple leaf toxicity. The methemoglobin fraction in this horse was 44.3% of the total hemoglobin.

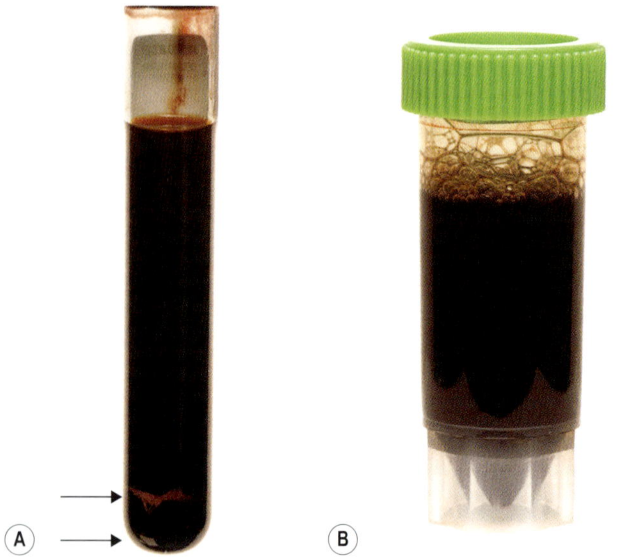

Fig 44.8 **(A)** Blood sample of the same horse (Fig. 44.7) after complete sedimentation of the erythrocytes (arrows). Severe hemolysis and methemoglobinemia leads to a dark red-brown discoloration of the plasma. **(B)** Dark brown urine is consistent with hemoglobinuria and methemoglobinuria.

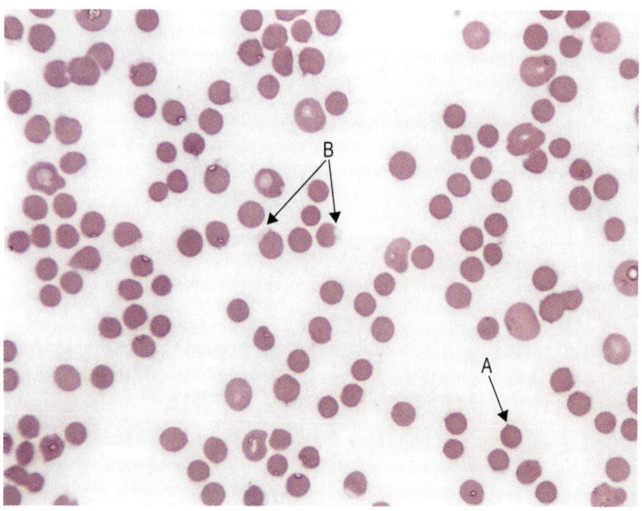

Fig 44.9 Heinz bodies (A) and eccentrocytes (B) in a blood smear of a horse with hemolytic anemia due to red maple leaf toxicity.

Recognition

History and presenting complaint

Usually, no clinical signs are noticed. Because of the mild and transient nature of pigmenturia, the dilutional effects resulting from increased urine flow after exercise, and the dark yellow to amber color of normal urine, gross pigmenturia is unlikely to be observed following exercise of healthy horses.[185] Gross discoloration of post-exercise urine samples is therefore indicative of a pathologic process and warrants further examination for muscular or urinary tract disease.[185]

Physical examination

Physical examination does not reveal any abnormal clinical signs. Gross pigmenturia is usually not noticeable.

Laboratory examination

Intravascular hemolysis is characterized by an increase of free plasma hemoglobin accompanied by a decrease in serum haptoglobin concentrations and occurrence of transient pigmenturia.[34,35,37,185] Total bilirubin concentrations in athletic horses are slightly increased on the day after a sports event, likely as a result of mild hemolysis.[34]

Diagnostic confirmation

Confirmation of exercise-induced hemolysis requires analysis of blood and urine samples for presence of free hemoglobin. However, a thorough diagnostic evaluation may not be necessary unless hemolysis and pigmenturia are severe and persistent or other abnormal clinical signs are evident.

Treatment and prognosis

Therapeutic aims

No specific therapy is necessary.

Prognosis

Exercise-induced hemolysis is generally mild and does not seem to negatively affect general health or performance in athletic horses.

Etiology and pathophysiology

Exercise-induced intravascular hemolysis can result from increased fragility of erythrocytes because of frequent accumulation in the spleen, strong shear forces associated with hemoconcentration and increased blood flow, oxidative stress, and anaerobic exercise leading to decrease in blood pH, increase in partial pressure of carbon dioxide, and increase in blood lactate concentration.[37,75,185–188] The decrease in haptoglobin concentrations observed after exercise is consistent with intravascular hemolysis, since the role of this protein is to bind the free hemoglobin in the plasma in order to form a complex, which is then quickly removed by the reticuloendothelial system, allowing the recycling of iron and globin.[34]

The magnitude of changes is related to intensity and duration of exercise. The fact that intravascular hemolysis has been reported after treadmill exercise of moderate intensity suggests that common training sessions in racehorses could also cause intravascular hemolysis.[35,37,185] However, the clinical consequences of repeated episodes of exercise-induced hemolysis in horses are not well known. Considering that hemolysis is mild and transient, it is unlikely to exceed the rate of red cell production in healthy athletic horses and may simply rejuvenate the circulating erythrocytes.[186] Although pigmenturia might increase urinary iron losses, iron deficiency anemia related to exercise-induced hemolysis has not been documented in horses. The results of a study in Thoroughbred horses indicate that three weeks of exercise of moderate to high intensity induces hemolysis and decreases serum iron concentration, total iron-binding capacity, and transferrin saturation, but leads to an increase in apparent iron absorption that compensates for the adverse effect of exercise on iron status.[35] The reduction of the available iron pool was slight and did not induce iron deficiency anemia.

Epidemiology

In one study, exercise-induced intravascular hemolysis after strenuous treadmill exercise exceeding the aerobic–anaerobic threshold appeared to be limited to mares, while stallions were not affected.[37] However, exercise-induced hemolysis has also been detected in male horses and in mixed populations.[34,35,187,189]

Prevention

The suggested role of oxidative stress in the pathogenesis of exercise-induced hemolysis implies that dietary supplementation of vitamin E and selenium might be beneficial to reduce the severity of erythrocyte destruction.[190–192] (See Chapter 36 and Chapter 37 for more on nutrient requirements.) Furthermore, adequate training protocols might increase antioxidant defenses and thereby reduce oxidative damage to erythrocytes.[190,193–196]

Anemia of inflammatory disease (AID)

- Non-regenerative anemia secondary to inflammatory or chronic disease is the most common type of anemia in horses.
- It is characterized by moderate anemia associated with normal or decreased serum iron concentration and total iron-binding capacity, and normal or increased serum ferritin and bone marrow iron stores.
- The pathogenesis is multifactorial, including sequestration of iron, decreased erythrocyte survival, and decreased bone marrow response to anemia.
- Treatment is directed against the primary disease process.
- The prognosis depends on the underlying problem.

Anemia of inflammatory disease (AID) is a mild to moderate, non-regenerative anemia, associated with inflammatory disease, chronic infections, traumatic conditions, and neoplastic disorders.[47] It is also commonly referred to as anemia of chronic disease, although the syndrome can include anemias associated with diseases that are not chronic.[47,197] Anemia of inflammatory disease is considered the most common type of anemia in veterinary medicine, but it is usually a secondary finding of little clinical significance.[47]

Recognition

History and presenting complaint

The presenting complaints usually result from the primary underlying disease. Often, a history of poor performance, chronic weight loss, long-lasting disease processes, and infectious conditions might be obtained.

Physical examination

Signs of the primary disorder usually predominate the clinical picture. Weight loss and fever are often present. Because of the mild to moderate character of the anemia, pale mucous membranes are not consistently found.

Laboratory examination

Laboratory findings include slightly to moderately decreased PCV and erythrocyte counts, and a low-normal or decreased MCV. Neutrophilic leukocytosis, monocytosis, and increased plasma fibrinogen and globulin concentrations usually indicate chronic inflammation.[198] Serum iron concentration and TIBC are normal or decreased, whereas serum ferritin and bone marrow stainable iron are normal or increased.[57,197] Bone marrow evaluation reveals increased stainable iron deposits with a nearly normal cellular pattern (Fig. 44.10).[47]

Diagnostic confirmation

The presence of (often chronic) inflammatory or neoplastic disease associated with mild to moderate non-regenerative anemia is highly suggestive for AID. Diagnostic confirmation of AID can be achieved by evaluation of the body iron status.[47]

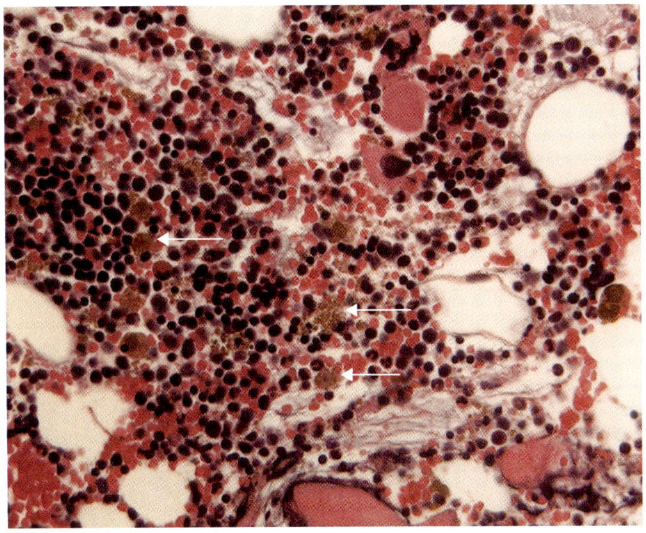

Fig 44.10 Sternal bone marrow biopsy of a horse with anemia of inflammatory disease. Using conventional staining, increased hemosiderin deposits appear as brown aggregates (arrows). The cellular pattern is normal (hematoxylin-eosin staining).

Treatment and prognosis

Therapeutic aims

Treatment is directed against the primary disease process. The anemia is rarely severe enough to require specific treatment.

Therapy

Supplementation of iron is not useful, as the body is not iron deficient.

Prognosis

The prognosis depends on the primary disease. The anemia usually resolves within weeks or months after resolution of the primary disease.

Etiology and pathophysiology

The conditions leading to AID are inflammatory diseases, chronic infections, traumatic injuries, or neoplastic disorders. The anemia usually develops slowly to reach a plateau after the first one or two months of illness, but initial changes in hematocrit and hemoglobin concentration can occur after 3–10 days. There is no correlation between the duration of the disease and the severity of the anemia.[47]

The pathogenesis of AID is multifactorial, including sequestration of iron into storage forms in liver and bone marrow, decreased erythrocyte survival, and decreased bone marrow response to anemia.[47,197]

Increased sequestration of iron in macrophages and decreased absorption of iron from the intestinal tract is part of the acute-phase reaction, mediated by inflammatory mediators (e.g., interleukin-1, tumor necrosis factor alpha). This is considered part of a non-specific antibacterial immune response, reducing the availability of iron for bacterial growth.

Increased erythrocyte destruction can be a major factor in the early stage of AID, presumably due to alterations in the red cell membrane, binding of IgG, and activation of the macrophages leading to a more efficient clearing of senescent and IgG-coated red blood cells from the circulation. Finally, decreased erythropoiesis results from blunted erythropoietin release in response to anemia, diminished bone marrow response to erythropoietin, and limited availability of iron.

Some chronic diseases and organ dysfunctions (chronic renal disease, hepatic disease, endocrine disease, and gastrointestinal disease) are associated with anemia that differs from AID in regards to pathophysiologic mechanism and iron metabolism.[197,198] However, no difference exists regarding treatment and prognosis of this type of anemia.

Iron deficiency anemia

- Iron deficiency anemia is rare in adult horses. It usually occurs secondary to chronic blood loss.
- The primary disease might predominate the clinical picture.
- Iron deficiency anemia is characterized by microcytic non-regenerative anemia with low serum iron and serum ferritin concentrations, low bone marrow iron stores, and normal or increased iron-binding capacity.
- Treatment consists of elimination of the underlying disease process and iron supplementation.
- The prognosis depends on the primary cause of iron deficiency.
- Prevention should focus on potential causes of iron deficiency rather than daily supplementation of iron.

Recognition

History and presenting complaint

Clinical signs vary depending on cause and severity of the anemia and the presence of other concomitant disorders.[57] Poor performance, depression, weakness, and weight loss are common, but unspecific features of iron deficiency anemia.[57]

Physical examination

Physical examination usually reveals signs of mild to moderate anemia. Pale mucous membranes, diarrhea, hematuria, hematochezia, melena, and epistaxis can be found in affected horses.[57] The primary disease may predominate the clinical picture.

Special examination

Gastroscopy, fecal parasite egg counts, fecal occult blood test, urinalysis, and bronchoalveolar lavage may be performed in order to identify the underlying process leading to chronic blood loss and iron deficiency (see below).

Laboratory examination

Anemia due to chronic blood loss is initially macrocytic and regenerative. Only after weeks or months, in very late stages of severe iron depletion, microcytic non-regenerative anemia develops.[57,58] The RDW can be increased because of presence of microcytes together with normocytic cells. Hypochromasia is rarely apparent in horses with iron deficiency anemia.[57] Hypoproteinemia is often associated when substantial recent or ongoing blood loss is present.[57]

Evaluation of the body iron status typically reveals low serum iron concentrations and increased TIBC. Serum ferritin concentration correlates directly with body iron stores and is usually low in iron deficiency anemia.[57,58,64,65] Bone marrow evaluation is the most sensitive method for detection of iron deficiency, prior to development of microcytic anemia.[57,58,199] Typically, erythroid hyperplasia and ineffective erythropoiesis with asynchrony and shift to later rubricytes are found. Reduced erythropoiesis is apparent at later stages. Stainable iron in the bone marrow is minimal or absent.

Diagnostic confirmation

Primary differential diagnosis in cases with mild to moderate non-regenerative anemia is anemia of inflammatory disease. Diagnostic confirmation of iron deficiency anemia can be achieved by evaluation of the body iron status (see Table 44.8).

Treatment and prognosis

Therapeutic aims

Treatment should be directed towards elimination of the underlying process that causes the chronic blood loss.

Therapy

Besides treatment of the primary disease process, iron supplementation is recommended. Oral supplementation of iron compounds is safe and can be achieved by administration of commercially available hematinics containing ferrous sulfate, copper, and various B vitamins.[65] Parenteral iron dextran preparations should not be used due to severe tissue irritation (thrombophlebitis, myositis), possible related anaphylaxis, and fatal reactions.[57,65]

Prognosis

The prognosis largely depends on the underlying disease causing the iron deficiency.

Several months can be required to replenish body iron stores and to normalize hematocrit and red cell indices.

Table 44.8 Differentiation between anemia of inflammatory disease and iron deficiency anemia[47,57,58]

	IRON DEFICIENCY ANEMIA	ANEMIA OF INFLAMMATORY DISEASE
MCV	⇓	Normal or ⇓
RDW	Normal or ⇑	Normal
Serum iron	⇓	⇓ or normal
Serum ferritin	⇓	Normal or ⇑
Total iron-binding capacity	Normal or ⇑	⇓ or normal
Bone marrow stainable iron	⇓ or absent	Normal or ⇑

Etiology and pathophysiology

Iron deficiency anemia is rare in adult horses.[20,57,58,66] It usually occurs secondary to chronic blood loss due to gastrointestinal ulcers, parasites, neoplasia, and urinary or pulmonary hemorrhage. Dietary causes are rare. Unless the anemia is severe, clinical signs of iron deficiency are more likely the result of the underlying disease and the impaired function of iron-containing enzymes rather than the reduction of the oxygen-carrying capacity of the blood.[70]

Prevention

The administration of hematinics (iron- and B vitamin-containing compounds) to horses is common practice, although efficacy of these treatments to enhance performance has not been proven.[58,65,70,200] Recommendations suggest that the iron requirements vary between 500 and 1200 mg/day for a 500-kg horse, depending on work intensity.[200] Although exact iron requirements for athletic horses in training are not known, the usual dietary sources are considered adequate to maintain a sufficient supply of iron for hemoglobin synthesis and function of iron-dependent enzymes.[64,65,200,201] Prevention should therefore focus on potentially underlying disease processes rather than iron supplementation.

Other nutritional deficiency anemias

Deficiencies of copper, folic acid, vitamin B_{12} (cobalamin), and cobalt can potentially lead to hypoproliferative anemia in humans and animals. However, reports on anemias due to nutritional deficiencies are often based on response to supplementation or treatment rather than demonstration of deficiency of a defined nutrient.[199] The true incidence of this type of anemias is therefore often unknown. Copper, folic acid, and cobalamin are common ingredients of modern horse feed and hematinic preparations which are used empirically in horses.[65]

Copper

Copper, as part of a copper-containing plasma protein (ceruloplasmin), plays an important role for transmembranous iron transport and transfer of iron from ferritin (ferrous form) to transferrin (ferric form).[57,64] Although not well defined, daily copper requirements are estimated to be 131 to 187 mg/day for a 500-kg horse.[82,200] Copper deficiency can lead to impaired iron metabolism and accumulation of iron stores with signs of functional iron deficiency. There is evidence of a relationship between developmental orthopedic disease and dietary copper intake in foals.[82,84] However, adult horses are usually not affected by copper deficiency.

Folic acid, vitamin B_{12}, and cobalt

Folic acid and vitamin B_{12} (cobalamin) belong to the group of water-soluble vitamins (B vitamins). Interactive reactions of folic acid and vitamin B_{12} are involved in DNA synthesis and amino acid metabolism. These two vitamins are therefore essential for cell division and proliferation, especially in rapidly dividing cells such as the hematopoietic cells and the gastrointestinal endothelium.[90,202]

Requirements for vitamin B_{12} and folic acid are likely met by microbial synthesis within the large intestine of horses. Intake of folic acid is further provided by oral dietary intake.[65,84,202–204] Cobalt is essential for vitamin B_{12} synthesis.

Macrocytic or normocytic normochromic non-regenerative anemia caused by folate or vitamin B_{12} deficiency occurs in humans and ruminants. Although cases of poor performance and anemia have occasionally been associated with folate deficiency,[88] it seems to occur rarely in horses.[21,84,199,202] Horses also appear to be unaffected by vitamin B_{12} and cobalt deficiency.[84,203] However, serum folate concentrations in stabled, intensively training Thoroughbred and Standardbred horses are generally lower than in pastured horses,[86–89] and additional dietary folic acid may be indicated for some horses in training.

Administration of sulfadiazine and pyrimethamine to treat equine protozoal myeloencephalitis requires special consideration regarding folate metabolism. Both drugs sequentially limit folate synthesis, by inhibition of protozoal enzymes and competition with para-aminobenzoic acid, which is a precursor of folic acid.[90] Mammals are less sensitive to these effects, but intestinal uptake of folic acid can be inhibited. A rapid and significant reduction of serum folate concentrations occurs after administration of sulfadiazine and pyrimethamine to horses.[86]

Anemia, leukopenia, glossitis, oral ulcerations, and bone marrow hypoplasia has been reported in a horse during long-term treatment with orally administered folic acid, sulphadiazine, and pyrimethamine.[90] Experimental evidence from other species suggests that concomitant oral administration of folic acid and pyrimethamine can result in decline, rather than an increase, in plasma folate concentrations. This paradoxical effect is likely due to competition of the orally administered inactive form with endogenous folates for intestinal absorption and interruption of the enterohepatic circulation of folic acid.[90,205] Monitoring of serum or erythrocyte folate concentrations and hemograms might therefore be indicated in horses treated with sulfadiazine and pyrimethamine. However, against common recommendations, the use of folic acid as a dietary supplement with sulfadiazine/pyrimethamine treatment may be contraindicated.

Pure red cell aplasia caused by treatment with erythropoiesis-stimulating agents

- Erythropoiesis-stimulating agents (ESA) such as recombinant human erythropoietin (rhEPO) and erythropoietin analogues are sometimes used in horses with the intention to enhance athletic performance.
- This form of doping is dangerous and can lead to severe pure red cell aplasia.
- The proposed underlying pathophysiologic mechanism is the production of anti-erythropoietin antibodies that cross-react with endogenous erythropoietin and thereby suppress erythropoiesis.
- Diagnosis is based on exclusion of other causes for hypoproliferative anemia, bone marrow examination, and a history of ESA administration.
- The prognosis is guarded.
- Administration of ESA to horses is not recommended.

Erythropoiesis-stimulating agents (ESA) are commonly used to treat human patients, dogs, and cats with chronic renal failure or other chronic or neoplastic disease.[206–208] Although ESA are not routinely used for therapeutic purposes in horses, they have been administered to equine athletes as performance-enhancing agents, in order to increase the total red cell mass and oxygen-carrying capacity of the blood.[209,210] However, this form of doping is dangerous. Similar to dogs, cats, and some people,[206,207,211,212] multiple administrations of ESA to horses can cause erythroid hypoplasia and severe non-regenerative anemia.[213–215]

Recognition

History and presenting complaint

The horses usually present with a history of poor performance, depression, anorexia, and weight loss.[213] Detailed information about previous administration of ESA is sometimes not readily available from trainers or owners.

Physical examination

Poor body condition, lethargy, weakness, tachycardia, tachypnea, and pale mucous membranes are found in cases of severe anemia. Cardiac arrhythmia may indicate hypoxic myocardial damage. Earlier in the course of the disease, the anemia can be less profound and the clinical signs may be mild. Due to the slow development, the chronicity of the anemia, and effective compensating mechanisms (see above), most horses can tolerate even severe anemia.

Laboratory examination

Laboratory evaluation usually reveals profound anemia without any signs of regenerative response. The severity of the anemia varies between individual horses and depends on the time since administration of the drug.[214] The PCV decreases continuously and can reach values as low as 5%.[215] White blood cell counts, leukocyte differential, and platelet counts are usually within normal limits. Mild elevations of liver enzyme activities and cardiac troponin I serum concentrations may occur, most likely due to tissue hypoxia secondary to severe anemia.[214] Measurements of serum urea nitrogen, serum creatinine concentration, and urinalysis should be performed to rule out primary kidney disease and chronic renal failure.

Coombs' test and Coggins test are negative. Evaluation of the serum iron concentration, percent saturation of transferrin, ferritin concentration and total iron-binding capacity indicate adequate iron supply and precludes iron deficiency anemia.[213] Bone marrow evaluation typically reveals generalized hypocellularity with markedly decreased numbers or complete absence of erythroid precursors and increased M:E ratio (Fig. 44.11). The myeloid series appears normal and the number of megakaryocytes is adequate. There is no evidence for a myelophthisic process. The findings are consistent with erythroid hypoplasia or pure red cell aplasia.[213,214]

Clonogenic assays can be performed to determine whether the serum of affected horses contains substances inhibiting erythroid development. Positive results suggest presence of anti-erythropoietin antibodies.[213] However, established methods for specific detection of anti-erythropoietin antibodies in horses are not routinely available.

Measurements of endogenous serum erythropoietin concentrations in affected horses are known to be inconsistent and results vary considerably between different assays, possibly due to interference by anti-erythropoietin antibodies.[214] In recent years, methods for detection of rhEPO and erythropoietin analogues in equine plasma have been described with regard to doping control in athletic horses.[216–221] However, measurements of serum concentrations of ESA are of limited value for the diagnosis of ESA-associated anemia. Clearance of ESA from plasma in horses is rapid, which often precludes the possibility of detection of ESA at the time of onset of clinical signs of severe anemia.[222,223]

Necropsy examination

The bone marrow found on necropsy has a markedly pale appearance, due to the lack of erythropoiesis (Fig. 44.12). Histopathology shows generalized hypocellularity with severe erythroid hypoplasia, normal myeloid series, and adequate numbers of megakaryocytes. There is no evidence of myelophthisic disease. Evidence for hypoxic damage of kidneys, liver, myocardium, and other organs may be present.

Diagnostic confirmation

Exclusion of other causes for non-regenerative anemia, together with a history of ESA administration, strongly suggest ESA-associated anemia.

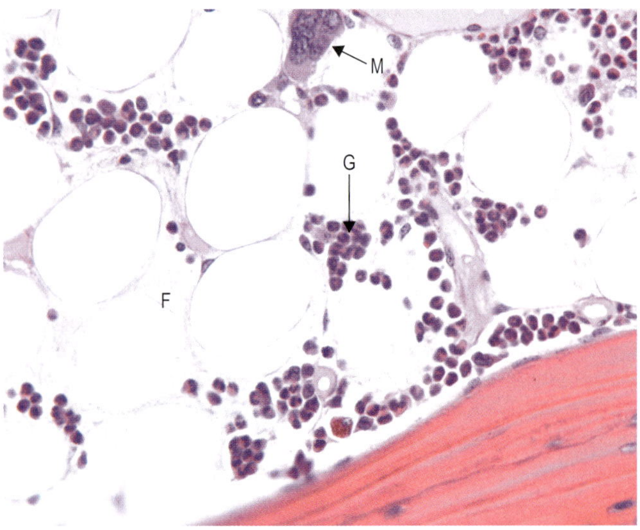

Fig 44.11 Histologic preparation of a bone marrow biopsy taken from the sternum of a horse with rhEPO-induced pure red cell aplasia (PCV 5%). The bone marrow appears hypocellular. Cells of the granulocytic series (G), megakaryocytes (M), and fat (F), but no cells of the erythroid series are present.

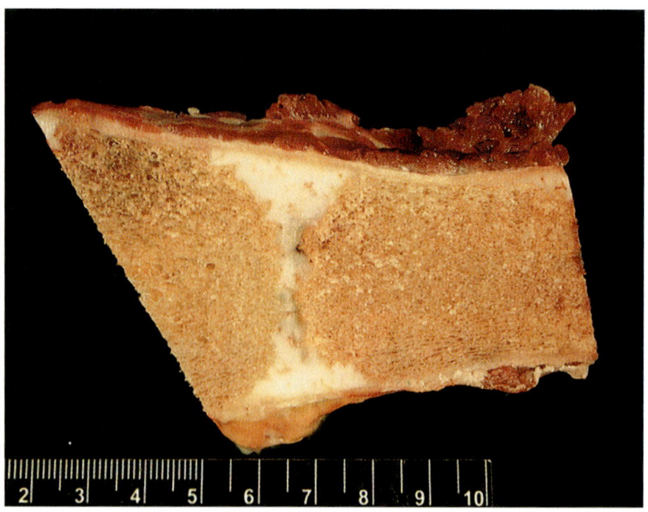

Fig 44.12 Diaphyseal bone marrow of the tibia in a horse with rhEPO-induced pure red cell aplasia. The yellow-fatty appearance of the marrow indicates absence of hematopoietic tissue. Although this would be expected for diaphyseal marrow in normal horses, there should be a hematopoietic response given this horse's severe anemia (PCV 5%).

Treatment and prognosis

Therapeutic aims

The initial goal of treatment is to provide adequate oxygen-carrying capacity to avoid hypoxic organ damage, organ failure, and death. The second therapeutic aim is suppression of the immune response against erythropoietin.

Therapy

If still ongoing, administration of ESA should be discontinued immediately. Blood transfusions should be performed when the PCV is below 10% or if signs of severe tissue hypoxia are present (see the section 'Acute blood loss anemia').[63] Experience has shown that even large volumes of blood transfusions are not able to increase the PCV significantly and persistently, although clinical signs might improve.[214]

Dexamethasone or prednisolone have been used to attempt to suppress the hypothesized immune response that is causing the anemia.[90,214] The dose should be adjusted according to clinical response and considering possible adverse effects. The efficacy of corticosteroid treatment is unknown. In addition to corticosteroids, treatment with immunoglobulins, plasmapheresis, cyclophosphamide, cyclosporine, and other immunosuppressive drugs has been described in humans.[207,211,224–226] Recently, hematide, a synthetic, peptide-based erythropoietin receptor agonist with no homology to native erythropoietin, has been shown to be effective in the treatment of human patients with pure red cell aplasia caused by anti-erythropoietin antibodies.[227]

Prognosis

ESA-induced anemia can be reversible in some cases after cessation of treatment and decline in circulating anti-erythropoietin antibodies.[90,206,212] However, the overall prognosis in horses is guarded. Potential recovery may take several months or years,[207,211] and death due to chronic hypoxia and organ failure is possible if the anemia remains untreated.

Etiology and pathophysiology

The anemia is most likely the result of production of anti-erythropoietin antibodies that cross-react with endogenous erythropoietin and inhibit its effect on bone marrow erythroid precursors.[206,207,211,213,214] Twenty to thirty percent of cats and dogs treated with rhEPO develop anti-rhEPO antibodies.[206,212] The incidence of ESA-induced pure red cell aplasia in horses is unknown, but susceptibility for this adverse reaction and severity of the anemia seem to vary considerably between individual horses.[214] Development of anemia is probably dose independent, but can require repeated exposure to the antigen.[213] Although not well described in horses, all commercially available erythropoietin analogues could have the potential to cause pure red cell aplasia as they do in people.[208] Factors associated with composition of the different preparations, storage, and handling might also influence the incidence of adverse effects.[208,225] Due to the long half-life of equine erythrocytes, the development of the anemia is slow and clinical signs of anemia can occur with a delay of 2–6 months after administration of the drug and onset of the adverse reaction.[213,214,228] The clinical signs result directly from a reduced oxygen-carrying capacity of the blood, related compensatory mechanisms, and ensuing organ dysfunction.

Prevention

Administration of ESA to horses should be strictly avoided.

Other causes of hypoproliferative anemia

Other very rare types of hypoproliferative anemia in horses are anemia secondary to organ dysfunction, aplastic anemia, myelophthisic disorders, and myelodysplastic syndromes.

Mild to moderate hypoproliferative anemia can occur in association with chronic renal failure, liver disease, gastrointestinal disease, or chronic endocrine disorders, which suppress hematopoiesis independent of alterations in iron metabolism that characterize anemia of inflammatory disease.[198]

Aplastic anemia is characterized by pancytopenia in peripheral blood, bone marrow panhypoplasia with fatty replacement, and the absence of primary disease processes infiltrating the bone marrow or suppressing hematopoiesis.[48,229] Clinical signs include hemorrhagic diathesis due to severe thrombocytopenia, increased susceptibility to infections due to neutropenia, and non-regenerative anemia.[230] The cause usually remains undetermined.[231–233] An association with administration of phenylbutazone has been suspected in some cases, but has not been conclusively proven.[234] The underlying pathophysiologic mechanism of aplastic anemia could be immune-mediated in most cases.[229,233] Infectious agents, drugs, and toxins might also be responsible for development of aplastic anemia.[48]

Myelophthisis is characterized by normo- or hypercellular bone marrow and replacement of normal hematopoietic cells by neoplastic cells[235] or proliferating fibroblasts (myelofibrosis).[236]

Myelodysplastic syndromes are a heterogenous group of disorders characterized by peripheral cytopenias and normocellular or hypercellular bone marrow with abnormal morphology.[229,237] Refractory, severe anemia is usually accompanied by leukopenia and thrombocytopenia in variable degrees.

Anemia associated with administration of heparin

A distinct type of apparent anemia in horses cannot be categorized in the classical groups of regenerative and non-regenerative anemias. Anticoagulatory treatment with unfractioned heparin (sodium or calcium heparin) has been reported to decrease hematocrit, hemoglobin concentration, and erythrocyte concentration by as much as 50%.[238–241] This adverse effect of heparin is unique to horses. It is associated with erythrocyte agglutination and is thought to occur secondary to sequestration of the red cell agglutinates in the microcirculation, potentially leading to impairment of microvascular blood flow. The effect is reversible and resolves within three to four days after discontinuation of heparin therapy. Similar adverse effects are not encountered with use of low-molecular-weight heparin.[242,243]

Increase in red cell mass

Erythrocytosis

Erythrocytosis is defined as an increase in peripheral erythrocyte concentration, hemoglobin concentration, and hematocrit above the reference interval.[32,244] Erythrocytosis can be classified based on pathogenesis (Fig. 44.13).

Recognition

History and presenting complaint

In horses with relative erythrocytosis, the underlying condition usually predominates the clinical picture. Horses with absolute erythrocytosis can exhibit signs of depression, decreased appetite, weight loss, poor performance, weakness, and syncope.[245–253] Other

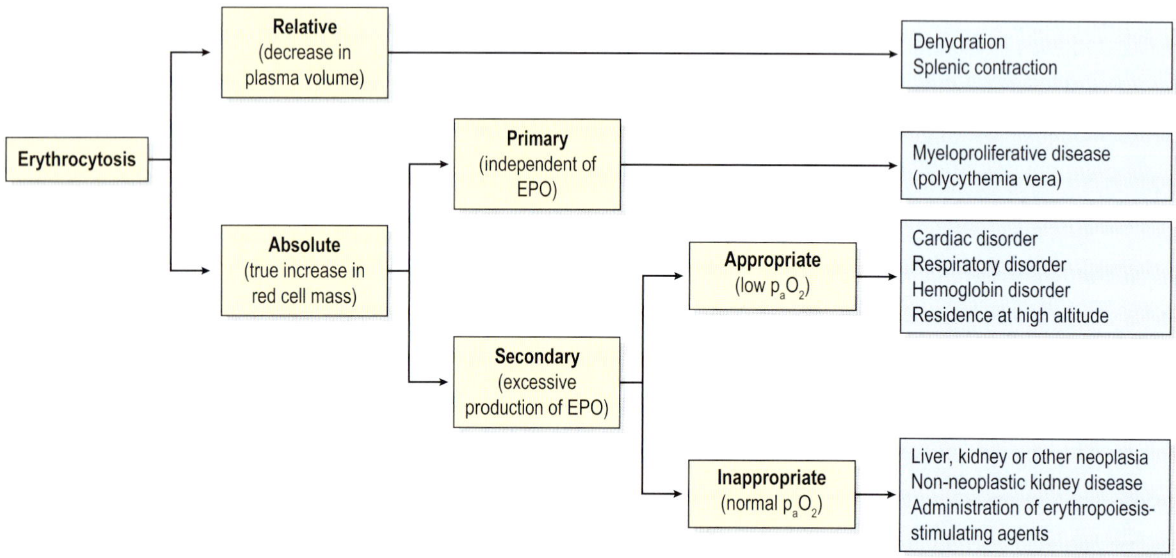

Fig 44.13 Classification of erythrocytosis.

signs may be observed depending on the underlying condition. A history of administration of erythropoiesis-stimulating agents may be obtained.

Physical examination

Relative erythrocytosis due to hemoconcentration usually goes along with clinical signs of dehydration including slow capillary refill time, dry mucous membranes, prolonged skin tenting, and often tachycardia. Furthermore, signs of the underlying condition are present.

Clinical signs associated with persistent absolute erythrocytosis may include muddy red, brick red, or cyanotic mucous membranes, prolonged capillary refill time, tachycardia, tachypnea, lethargy, neurologic disturbances (ataxia, weakness, seizures, blindness, behavioral changes), and increased bleeding tendency or thrombosis.[32,245–254] Other clinical signs may result from concurrent disorders, including cardiovascular disease, respiratory disease, kidney disease, liver disease, or neoplasia.

Laboratory examination

Hematologic examination shows increases in hematocrit, hemoglobin concentration, and red blood cell count. In horses with relative erythrocytosis, the hematocrit rarely exceeds 60–65%. Conversely, untreated absolute erythrocytosis is usually characterized by a hematocrit higher than 60%.[245–253]

Relative erythrocytosis caused by hemoconcentration is often accompanied by an increase in total plasma protein concentration, unless the underlying condition causes concurrent protein loss. Serum biochemistry and urinalysis reveal azotemia and hypersthenuria. In cases of absolute erythrocytosis, plasma volume and plasma protein concentration often remain normal. Azotemia is absent and urinalysis is unremarkable, unless the erythrocytosis is associated with kidney disease. Liver enzymes might be elevated because of underlying liver disease or because of hypoxic liver damage resulting from severe erythrocytosis. Hypercalcemia might indicate presence of renal or neoplastic disease.[251] Hypoglycemia may be observed because of enhanced glucose utilization by the increased number of red blood cells in vivo or in vitro.

Measurement of plasma erythropoietin (EPO) concentration and arterial blood gas analysis serve to differentiate primary (decreased to normal EPO, normal arterial oxygenation), secondary appropriate (high EPO, arterial hypoxemia), and secondary inappropriate (high EPO, normal arterial oxygenation) erythrocytosis (Fig. 44.13). Blood gas analysis can further reveal metabolic acidosis resulting from impaired oxygenation of the peripheral tissues. In this case, blood or plasma lactate concentrations are increased.

Although hemoglobinopathies have not been described in horses, they should be considered in cases of unexplained secondary erythrocytosis. Note that with hemoglobinopathies, the partial pressure of oxygen in the arterial blood (p_aO_2) would be normal, whereas the arterial oxygen content (c_aO_2) would be decreased. The work-up includes testing for abnormal hemoglobin[255] and calculation of the hemoglobin dissociation curve and P_{50} value (i.e., the partial pressure of oxygen at which the saturation of hemoglobin with oxygen is 50%).[253,256]

Special examination

Further diagnostics are required to diagnose pathologic conditions that cause absolute erythrocytosis. These can include echocardiography (including agitated saline contrast studies) and possibly angiography or cardiac catheterization, airway endoscopy, tracheal and/or bronchoalveolar fluid analysis, thoracic radiography, rectal examination, thoracic and abdominal ultrasonography, thoracocentesis or abdominocentesis, and needle biopsy of liver, kidney, spleen, or unidentified mass lesions. Bone marrow aspirate and/or biopsy can be obtained for evaluation of erythroid and myeloid cell lines and detection of unusual cell populations. Typically, histopathologic examination of a bone marrow biopsy will show erythroid hyperplasia with a low myeloid : erythroid ratio.

Necropsy examination

Post-mortem examination of horses with relative or absolute erythrocytosis will primarily show abnormalities related to the primary underlying disease or alterations caused by hypoxic organ damage. Erythroid hyperplasia with a low myeloid : erythroid ratio will be present in the bone marrow.

Diagnostic confirmation

Complete resolution of erythrocytosis after appropriate fluid therapy and treatment of the underlying condition is indicative for relative erythrocytosis. Confirmation of absolute erythrocytosis requires measurement of total red cell mass.[245] However, persistently high hematocrit, hemoglobin concentration, and erythrocyte concentration that are resistant to aggressive fluid therapy usually confirm the presence of absolute erythrocytosis in clinical practice.

Treatment and prognosis

Therapeutic aims

The first therapeutic aim is to increase oxygen delivery to the peripheral tissues in order to improve organ function and minimize hypoxic organ damage. This is achieved by increasing the circulating plasma volume (in case of relative erythrocytosis) or by reduction of circulating red cell mass (in case of absolute erythrocytosis) to improve rheological characteristics of the blood. Generally, the hematocrit should be maintained well below 60%.[245]

The second therapeutic aim is the correction or alleviation of the underlying disease processes that may be causing relative or absolute erythrocytosis.

Therapy

Treatment of relative erythrocytosis consists of correction of the underlying problem and intravenous fluid therapy to replace fluid deficits and ongoing losses and to provide maintenance requirements.

Absolute erythrocytosis does not respond well to intravenous fluid therapy and hematocrit will often remain elevated despite aggressive treatment. Periodic phlebotomy (e.g., every 5–7 days) and removal of several liters (e.g., 10–15 mL/kg/week) of blood with subsequent equal volume of crystalloid fluid replacement may be required to maintain hematocrit at an acceptable level, but may induce iron deficiency over time.[32,245,246] Therapeutic erythrocytapheresis with removal of red blood cells and reinfusion of the plasma into the patient's circulation may be more effective compared to traditional phlebotomy, but has not been described in horses to date.[257,258]

Chemotherapy may aid in suppression of bone marrow red cell production. Hydroxyurea has been used in one case,[245] but true efficacy of chemotherapy for treatment of erythrocytosis in horses is unknown.

Whenever possible, long-term treatment of secondary erythrocytosis should be directed towards the underlying cause.

Prognosis

Relative erythrocytosis can usually be corrected with adequate fluid therapy, normalization of oral fluid uptake, and reduction of excessive fluid losses by treating the underlying disease. Most horses with absolute primary or secondary erythrocytosis have a guarded to poor prognosis.[32]

Etiology and pathophysiology

Classification of erythrocytosis is shown in Figure 44.13. Relative erythrocytosis is most common in horses and is associated with hemoconcentration (because of excessive fluid losses and/or reduction in fluid uptake) or splenic contraction.[32,244] The latter is caused by exercise, excitement, stress, or exogenous administration of adrenergic agents and can result in an increase of hematocrit by as much as 50% of resting values.[32,259,260]

Primary erythrocytosis (polycythemia vera) is a rare chronic, myeloproliferative disorder characterized by expansion of erythroid precursors independent of erythropoietin.[32,244–246] It may be accompanied by thrombocytosis and leukocytosis. Secondary erythrocytosis develops from excessive production of erythropoietin in response to systemic hypoxia (physiologically appropriate response) or unrelated to systemic hypoxia (inappropriate response).[32,244]

Appropriate secondary erythrocytosis aims at increasing the oxygen-carrying capacity of the blood to improve tissue oxygenation in the presence of severe systemic hypoxia (i.e., $p_aO_2 < 60$ mmHg) that triggers erythropoietin release from the kidneys. Tissue hypoxia can result from congenital cardiac defects associated with right-to-left shunting of blood, chronic severe pulmonary disease, hemoglobin disorders that affect oxygen transport, or residence at high altitude.[247,261,262] Cyanotic heart disease is usually detected in foals, but survival to adult age is possible.[261] Most chronic pulmonary diseases do not cause severe enough hypoxemia to induce secondary erythrocytosis. Hemoglobin disorders have not been described in horses and true secondary erythrocytosis in horses at high altitude is poorly documented.[32,263,264]

Inappropriate secondary erythrocytosis results from excess production of erythropoietin caused by hepatic or renal neoplasia, other neoplasia, non-neoplastic renal disease, or administration of erythropoiesis-stimulating drugs.[248–252]

Most of the clinical manifestations of erythrocytosis are related to increased blood viscosity. In fact, blood viscosity rises steeply as the hematocrit increase above normal values. In turn, hyperviscosity slows blood flow, distends small vessels and capillaries, increases the risk of thrombosis and rupture of these vessels, and reduces tissue oxygen delivery.[1,32,244] Vascular changes, including dilated and tortuous retinal vessels and occasionally retinal hemorrhage, can be visualized on ophthalmologic examination.[244] Prolonged, persistent erythrocytosis can result in hypertension, tissue hypoxia, thrombosis, and hemorrhage.[32]

Red cell hypervolemia in Swedish Standardbred trotters

- Red cell hypervolemia has been described in Standardbred trotters in Sweden, but there are no published data suggesting a widespread incidence of this condition in horses worldwide.
- Affected racehorses gradually deteriorate in performance after a long, often successful racing career. They show no specific findings upon clinical examination.
- Early studies suggested that red cell hypervolemia is caused by overtraining and results in a loss of performance.
- However, it has been shown that overtraining does not result in red cell hypervolemia in horses, and that red cell hypervolemia is not a mechanism for the loss of performance in overtrained Standardbred horses.
- Diagnosis is based on an increased red cell volume compared to normal horses of corresponding age and sex.
- The pathophysiology and the clinical relevance of the condition are largely unresolved.

Horses with red cell hypervolemia have a significantly increased red cell volume and higher maximal hematocrit after exercise in comparison to normal horses of corresponding age and sex.[17,265] Red cell hypervolemia has been reported to occur in Standardbred trotters in Sweden that are presented with a complaint of impaired performance capacity.[17,266,267] Red cell hypervolemia has been diagnosed in Standardbred trotters both with American and French origin.

Early studies on overtraining in horses largely focused on red cell hypervolemia that, hypothetically, was limiting performance.[17,265,268,269] However, this seems paradoxical, since there is evidence for a strong positive relationship between blood volume, red blood cell volume, and aerobic capacity in horses.[2,270] Furthermore, increased production of red blood cells has not been observed as a cause or a sequel of overtraining syndrome in other athletic species. Lastly, reports on red cell hypervolemia are mostly based on cross-sectional studies of clinically normal horses and horses with red cell hypervolemia within a regional population of Standardbred trotters in Scandinavia, but there are no published data suggesting a widespread incidence of this condition in horses worldwide.[270,271]

Prospective, horizontal studies on overtraining in horses convincingly demonstrate that there are no differences between normal and overtrained horses in regards to total red cell mass, suggesting that red cell hypervolemia is not a mechanism for the loss of performance in overtrained Standardbred horses.[272–275]

Recognition

History and presenting complaint

The condition is mainly found in stallions or geldings at an age between 3 and 9 years (average around 6 years) that have recently experienced a gradual decline in performance.[268] Generally, affected horses have initially been very successful on the race tracks in comparison to the average population. In order for the horse to remain competitive, the trainers often train these horses very hard with a lot of high-speed interval training.

Many of these horses also have a history of epistaxis in association with intense exercise.[267,269,276] Furthermore, behavioral changes including excitement and anxiety associated with racing or training, muscle tremor, tachycardia, excessive pulling during the race, sweating, and sometimes loose feces are reported.

Physical examination

Generally, horses diagnosed with red cell hypervolemia show no specific findings upon physical examination. In some cases, the condition is reported to be associated with other clinical disorders such as small airway disease.[276–278]

Special examination

Screening test

One screening method to determine if a horse suffers from red cell hypervolemia is to measure the maximal hematocrit after exercise. This can be done at the race track. The horse should be exercised at a heart rate exceeding 200 bpm to induce maximum emptying of the splenic red cell reservoir and the blood sample for measurement of hematocrit should be collected within 1 min after the end of exercise.[17,267,279] If the horse's post-exercise hematocrit is more than 2 standard deviations above the expected average of healthy horses, the horse should be suspected to have red cell hypervolemia.

Calculation of total red cell volume

If the above screening test suggests red cell hypervolemia, the total red cell volume and total blood volume should be determined in order to confirm the diagnosis. This is done using the Evans blue dye dilution technique to measure plasma volume, and determination of the maximal hematocrit after exercise, which then allows calculation of the total blood volume and red cell volume (Table 44.9).[17,279]

Standardized exercise testing

Standardized submaximal incremental stepwise exercise tests on an inclined treadmill can be conducted on horses suspected of having red cell hypervolemia.[17,267] Heart rate and blood lactate concentration are measured at the end of each speed step and V_{La4} and V_{200} are calculated.

Red cell hypervolemic horses have an abnormally high heart rate in relation to their red cell volume during submaximal exercise.[17,267] However, V_{200} does not seem to differ between red cell hypervolemic and normal horses during submaximal exercise.[280,281] Red cell hypervolemic horses do have a tendency to have lower blood lactate concentrations immediately post-exercise in comparison to normal horses.[282]

During exercise, red cell hypervolemic horses have higher pulmonary artery pressures (PAP), pulmonary vascular resistance, and systemic arterial pressures (SAP) compared to normal trotters.[276]

Furthermore, affected horses have a more pronounced hypoxemia during exercise in comparison to normal horses.[278] This has been attributed to an increase in ventilation-perfusion (V/Q) mismatch, which is likely caused by a mild interstitial pulmonary edema that occurs as a result of an increased fluid transudation secondary to the pulmonary hypertension[283,284] (see Fig. 44.14).

Endoscopy

Endoscopy of the respiratory tract and bronchoalveolar lavage performed within 90 min after the submaximal exercise test often suggests exercise-induced pulmonary hemorrhage (EIPH).[269] In fact, Standardbred trotters with red cell hypervolemia seem to have a higher incidence (92%) of EIPH in comparison to normal Standardbred trotters (23–45%), possibly related to increased blood viscosity and stress failure of the capillary endothelial layers[267,269,283] (S. Adehed and P. Funkquist, unpublished data).

Table 44.9 Reference values (mean ± SD) for body weight (BWT), packed cell volume (PCV), total red cell volume (RCV/BWT), total blood volume (TBV/BWT), and plasma volume (PV/BWT) relative to BWT and in different age and sex groups in normally performing Standardbred trotters after exercise

AGE	SEX	N	BWT	PCV	RCV/BWT	TBV/BWT	PV/BWT
(years)			(kg)	(L/L)	(mL/kg)	(mL/kg)	(mL/kg)
2		30	416 ± 38	0.510 ± 0.035	52.2 ± 6.8	102.1 ± 7.6	49.9 ± 3.1
3		45	437 ± 40	0.560 ± 0.032	66.3 ± 8.6	118.0 ± 10.0	51.7 ± 3.4
≥4	Fillies	45	429 ± 42	0.571 ± 0.030	68.5 ± 8.3	119.6 ± 10.4	51.2 ± 4.3
	Geldings	44	455 ± 39	0.574 ± 0.021	74.4 ± 6.5	129.4 ± 8.4	55.0 ± 3.3
	Colts	41	451 ± 46	0.597 ± 0.026	79.6 ± 7.3	133.4 ± 9.2	53.7 ± 4.2
All	Horses	205	439 ± 43	0.566 ± 0.039	69.1 ± 11.3	121.5 ± 13.6	52.4 ± 4.1

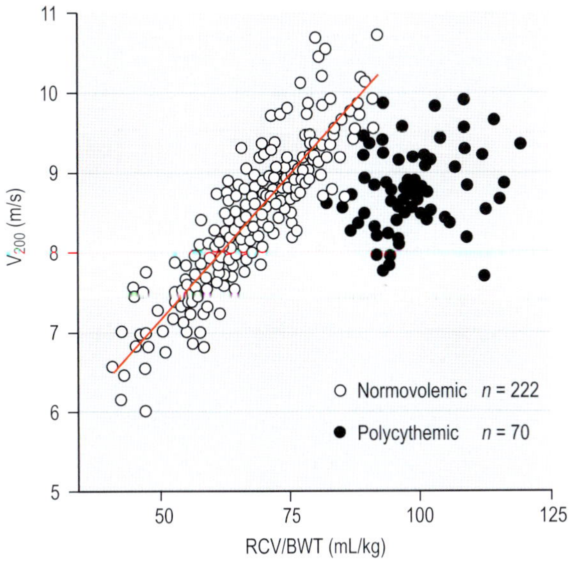

Fig 44.14 The relationship between speed at a heart rate of 200 bpm (V_{200}) and the total red cell volume in relation to body weight (RCV/BWT) in normal horses (○; n = 222) and horses with red cell hypervolemia (●; n = 70).

Muscle biopsy

Histochemical analysis of muscle biopsies of horses with red cell hypervolemia showed that the muscle fiber composition and fiber area do not differ from normal horses.[285,286] However, horses with red cell hypervolemia had a higher percentage of type IIB fibers with a high oxidative capacity and expressed less of the isoform of myosin heavy chain MHC IIX in comparison to well-trained normal horses.[285,287] Horses with red cell hypervolemia also had a lower capillary supply in muscles compared to well-trained normal horses.[281]

Laboratory examination

Blood viscosity is higher in red cell hypervolemic horses than in normal horses (P. Funkquist, unpublished data: 6.67 ± 0.37 mPa × s, range 6.27–7.19, at maximal exercise to fatigue).

Red cell hypervolemic horses also appear to suffer from an adrenocortical dysfunction, characterized by decreased resting plasma cortisol concentrations and a decreased response to exogenous ACTH.[266]

Necropsy examination

Generally, horses with red cell hypervolemia are not euthanized. Therefore, little is known regarding specific findings on necropsy.

Diagnostic confirmation

Measurement of maximal hematocrit after exercise and determination of the total blood volume and total red cell volume are used to diagnose this condition. Differential diagnoses that need to be precluded include other disorders that cause an increase in red cell mass (see previous section and Fig. 44.13).

Treatment and prognosis

Therapeutic aims

When absolute or relative erythrocytosis can be attributed to a specific underlying disease (Fig. 44.13), the therapeutic guidelines discussed in the previous section should be followed. However, for horses that fit the clinical picture of red cell hypervolemia as discussed in this section, the therapeutic approach is less clear. Generally, it has been suggested that treatment should be aimed towards diminishing potential stress factors and reducing the intensity of training. However, the pathophysiology of this condition is incompletely understood. Since there is convincing evidence that red cell hypervolemia is not a cause for the loss of performance in Standardbred horses, it is unclear if and how this condition should be treated.

Therapy

Alterations in training regimes

Horses with red cell hypervolemia often have a history of very intense interval training at high speed, suggesting increased stress and possible overtraining. Therefore, it has been recommended that horses with red cell hypervolemia rest completely for a period of 3–6 months, after which training at a lower intensity should be commenced and the frequency and intensity of racing should be reduced. Furthermore, it was suggested to move these horses from the busy large training camps to smaller and quieter stables. However, because a number of prospective studies did not allow to prove a causative relationship between overtraining and red cell hypervolemia in horses,[272–275] these recommendations may be useful to address clinical signs related to overtraining, but they may not be effective to reduce total red cell mass in affected horses.

Phlebotomy

Repeated phlebotomy decreases the maximal hematocrit and the maximal hemoglobin concentration in horses with red cell hypervolemia.[269] Furthermore, blood viscosity, pulmonary artery pressures, pulmonary vascular resistance, and severity of EIPH are lower after phlebotomy. However, it has been shown that reversal of the red cell hypervolemia does not increase performance. Rather, the treadmill run time to fatigue is shorter and oxygen delivery as well as maximum oxygen uptake is decreased after phlebotomy,[269] suggesting that the loss of performance is not due to the red cell hypervolemia.

Castration

The prevalence of red cell hypervolemia is higher in stallions compared to mares. Stallions have been shown to have a larger red cell volume and total blood volume in relation to body weight in comparison to both mares and geldings, probably due to the erythropoietic effect of testosterone.[17] Thus, one therapeutic method that has been suggested to decrease erythropoiesis in stallions is castration. However, there are no studies regarding the effect of castration on the red cell volume that supports castration as a treatment for horses with this condition.

Prognosis

Although a slight improvement can be seen after a longer period of rest and alterations in training regimes, horses with red cell hypervolemia rarely reach their previous racing capacity.[268] However, this might not be related to the persistence of red cell hypervolemia, since red cell hypervolemia is not a mechanism for the loss of performance.

Etiology and pathophysiology

The exact cause of the development of red cell hypervolemia in Swedish Standardbred trotters is still unclear. It has been suggested that these horses suffer from a chronic stress syndrome.[266] However, it has been demonstrated that overtraining does not result in red cell hypervolemia in horses.[272-275]

Unfortunately, none of the cross-sectional studies suggesting the existence of red cell hypervolemia and its association with overtraining syndrome attempted to measure plasma erythropoietin concentration or give some mechanistic insight into why erythropoiesis would be disrupted by the stress of training.[270] Also, the potential use of erythropoiesis-stimulating agents has not been convincingly precluded in these studies.

Horses with loss of performance and concurrent red cell hypervolemia have a history of superior racing performance.[268] However, the loss of performance was not shown to occur at the same time as red cell hypervolemia developed. It is therefore possible, that the red cell hypervolemia in those horses was inherent and was indeed a factor associated with their superior performance.[273]

Prevention

As the pathophysiology of red cell hypervolemia is unclear, it is difficult to give any recommendations for prevention of this condition. Considering that it could well be an inherent characteristic of very successful racehorses, the condition might not be prevented at all. Under any circumstances, excessive training should be avoided in horses with declining performance. Instead, appropriate diagnostic measures should be undertaken in an attempt to identify all possible factors that may result in poor performance.

With thanks to Katarina Schuback, who co-created the original chapter in the first edition.

References

1. Muir WW, Wellman ML. Hemoglobin solutions and tissue oxygenation. J Vet Intern Med 2003;17:127–35.
2. McKeever KH, Hinchcliff KW. Neuroendocrine control of blood volume, blood pressure and cardiovascular function in horses. Equine Vet J 1995;27(S18):77–81.
3. Convertino VA. Blood volume: its adaptation to endurance training. Med Sci Sports Exerc 1991;23:1338–48.
4. Marino PL. Anemia and red blood cell transfusions in the ICU. In: Marino PL, editor. The ICU book. 3rd ed. Philadelphia: Lippincott Williams & Wilkins; 2007. p. 659–80.
5. Aird B. Clinical and hematologic manifestations of anemia. In: Feldman BF, Zinkl JG, Jain NC, editors. Schalm's veterinary hematology. 5th ed. Philadelphia: Lippincott, Williams & Wilkins; 2000. p. 140–2.
6. Mellema M. Cardiac output, wedge pressure, and oxygen delivery. Vet Clin North Am Small Anim Pract 2001;31:1175–205.
7. Marino PL. Oxygen and carbon dioxide transport. In: Marino PL, editor. The ICU book. 3rd ed. Philadelphia: Lippincott Williams & Wilkins; 2007. p. 21–38.
8. Guyton AC, Hall JE. Transport of oxygen and carbon dioxide in the blood and body fluids. In: Guyton AC, Hall JE, editors. Textbook of medical physiology. 10th ed. Philadelphia: W. B. Saunders Company; 2000. p. 463–73.
9. Guyton AC, Hall JE. Red blood cells, anemia, and polycythemia. In: Guyton AC, Hall JE, editors. Textbook of medical physiology. 10th ed. Philadelphia: W. B. Saunders Company; 2000. p. 382–91.
10. Guyton AC, Hall JE. Overview of the circulation: Medical physics of pressure, flow, and resistance. In: Guyton AC, Hall JE, editors. Textbook of medical physiology. 10th ed. Philadelphia: W. B. Saunders Company; 2000. p. 144–51.
11. Guyton AC, Hall JE. Local control of blood flow by the tissues; and humoral regulation. In: Guyton AC, Hall JE, editors. Textbook of medical physiology. 10th ed. Philadelphia: W. B. Saunders Company; 2000. p. 175–83.
12. Guyton AC, Hall JE. Cardiac output, venous return, and their regulation. In: Guyton AC, Hall JE, editors. Textbook of medical physiology. 10th ed. Philadelphia: W. B. Saunders Company; 2000. p. 210–22.
13. Meyer R. Current topics in fluid therapy: Oxyglobin. In: Gleed RD, Ludders JW, editors. Recent advances in veterinary anesthesia and analgesia: Companion animals. Ithaca, NY: International Veterinary Information Service (www.ivis.org); 2001:Document No. A1407.0501.
14. Rentko VT, Sharpe TA. Red blood cell substitutes. In: Feldman BF, Zinkl JG, Jain NC, editors. Schalm's veterinary hematology. 5th ed. Philadelphia: Lippincott, Williams & Wilkins; 2000. p. 874–8.
15. Moore KE, Murtaugh RJ. Pathophysiologic characteristics of hypovolemic shock. Vet Clin North Am Small Anim Pract 2001;31:1115–28.
16. Kumar A, Parrillo JE. Shock: Classification, pathophysiology, and approach to management. In: Parrillo JE, Dellinger RP, editors. Critical care medicine: Principles of diagnosis and management in the adult. 2nd ed. St. Louis: Mosby; 2001. p. 371–420.
17. Persson S. On blood volume and working capacity in horses: Studies of methodology and physiological and pathological variations. Acta Vet Scand 1967;Suppl 19:1–189.
18. Persson SGB. Blood volume, state of training and working capacity of racehorses. Equine Vet J 1968;1:52–62.
19. Persson SG. Heart rate and blood lactate responses to submaximal treadmill exercise in the normally performing standardbred trotter – age and sex variations and predictability from the total red blood cell volume. J Vet Med A 1997;44:125–32.
20. Lassen ED, Swardson CJ. Hematology and hemostasis in the horse: normal functions and common abnormalities. Vet Clin North Am Equine Pract 1995;11:351–89.
21. Tvedten H, Weiss DJ. Classification and laboratory evaluation of anemia. In: Feldman BF, Zinkl JG, Jain NC, editors. Schalm's veterinary hematology. 5th ed. Philadelphia: Lippincott, Williams & Wilkins; 2000. p. 143–50.
22. Radin MJ, Eubank MC, Weiser MG. Electronic measurement of erythrocyte volume and volume heterogeneity in horses during erythrocyte regeneration associated with experimental anemias. Vet Pathol 1986;23:656–60.
23. Smith JE, Agar NS. Studies on erythrocyte metabolism following acute blood loss in the horse. Equine Vet J 1976;8:34–7.
24. Cooper C, Sears W, Bienzle D. Reticulocyte changes after experimental anemia and erythropoietin treatment of horses. J Appl Physiol 2005;99:915–21.
25. Mair TS, Taylor FG, Hillyer MH. Autoimmune haemolytic anaemia in eight horses. Vet Rec 1990;126:51–3.
26. Weiser MG. Erythrocyte volume distribution analysis in healthy dogs, cats, horses, and dairy cows. Am J Vet Res 1982;43:163–6.
27. Easley JR. Erythrogram and red cell distribution width of Equidae with experimentally induced anemia. Am J Vet Res 1985;46:2378–84.
28. Lumsden JH, Valli VE, McSherry BJ, et al. The kinetics of hematopoiesis in the light horse II. The hematological response to hemorrhagic anemia. Can J Comp Med 1975;39:324–31.
29. Lumsden HJ, Valli VE, McSherry BJ, et al. The kinetics of hematopoiesis in the light horse III. The hematological response to hemolytic anemia. Can J Comp Med 1975;39:332–9.

30. Fernandez FR, Grindem CB. Reticulocyte response. In: Feldman BF, Zinkl JG, Jain NC, editors. Schalm's veterinary hematology. 5th ed. Philadelphia: Lippincott, Williams & Wilkins; 2000. p. 110–16.
31. Weiser G, Kohn C, Vachon A. Erythrocyte volume distribution analysis and hematologic changes in two horses with immune-mediated hemolytic anemia. Vet Pathol 1983;20:424–33.
32. Sellon DC, Wise LN. Disorders of the hematopoietic system. In: Reed SM, Bayly WM, Sellon DC, editors. Equine internal medicine. 3rd ed. St. Louis: Saunders Elsevier; 2010. p. 730–76.
33. Pollock PJ, Prendergast M, Schumacher J, et al. Effects of surgery on the acute phase response in clinically normal and diseased horses. Vet Rec 2005;156:538–42.
34. Pellegrini Masini A, Tedeschi D, Baragli P, et al. Exercise-induced intravascular haemolysis in standardbred horses. Comp Clin Path 2003;12:45–8.
35. Inoue Y, Matsui A, Asai Y, et al. Effect of exercise on iron metabolism in horses. Biol Trace Elem Res 2005;107:33–42.
36. Pearson W, Boermans HJ, Bettger WJ, et al. Association of maximum voluntary dietary intake of freeze-dried garlic with Heinz body anemia in horses. Am J Vet Res 2005;66:457–65.
37. Cywinska A, Szarska E, Kowalska A, et al. Gender differences in exercised-induced intravascular haemolysis during race training in thoroughbred horses. Res Vet Sci 2011;90:133–7.
38. Latimer KS, Rakich PM. Peripheral blood smears. In: Cowell RL, Tyler RD, editors. Diagnostic cytology and hematology of the horse. 2nd ed. St. Louis: Mosby; 2002. p. 200–16.
39. Barker RN. Anemia associated with immune response. In: Feldman BF, Zinkl JG, Jain NC, editors. Schalm's veterinary hematology. 5th ed. Philadelphia: Lippincott, Williams & Wilkins; 2000. p. 169–77.
40. Day MJ. Immune-mediated hemolytic anemia. In: Feldman BF, Zinkl JG, Jain NC, editors. Schalm's veterinary hematology. 5th ed. Philadelphia: Lippincott, Williams & Wilkins; 2000. p. 799–806.
41. Malikides N, Kessell A, Hodgson JL, et al. Bone marrow response to large volume blood collection in the horse. Res Vet Sci 1999;67:285–93.
42. Freeman KP. Bone marrow evaluation. In: Feldman BF, Zinkl JG, Jain NC, editors. Schalm's veterinary hematology. 5th ed. Philadelphia: Lippincott, Williams & Wilkins; 2000. p. 29–32.
43. Russell KE, Sellon DC, Grindem CB. Bone marrow in horses: Indications, sample handling, and complications. Comp Cont Educ Pract Vet 1994;16:1359–65.
44. Taylor FGR, Hillyer MH. Blood disorders. In: Taylor FGR, Hillyer MH, editors. Diagnostic techniques in equine medicine. 1st ed. London: W. B. Saunders; 1997. p. 137–58.
45. Latimer KS, Andreasen CB. Bone marrow. In: Cowell RL, Tyler RD, editors. Diagnostic cytology and hematology of the horse. 2nd ed. St. Louis. Mosby, 2002. p. 217–26.
46. Steiger R, Geyer H, Provencher A, et al. Equine bone core biopsy: Evaluation of collection sites using a new electric drilling machine. Equine Pract 1999;21:14–21.
47. Waner T, Harrus S. Anemia of inflammatory disease. In: Feldman BF, Zinkl JG, Jain NC, editors. Schalm's veterinary hematology. 5th ed. Philadelphia: Lippincott, Williams & Wilkins; 2000. p. 205–9.
48. Weiss DJ. Aplastic anemia. In: Feldman BF, Zinkl JG, Jain NC, editors. Schalm's veterinary hematology. 5th ed. Philadelphia: Lippincott, Williams & Wilkins; 2000. p. 212–15.
49. Tschudi P, Archer RK, Gerber H. The cells of equine blood and their development. Equine Vet J 1975;7:141–7.
50. Franken P, Wensing T, Schotman AJH. The bone marrow of the horse. 1. The techniques of sampling and examination and values of normal warmblooded horses. J Vet Med A 1982;29:16–22.
51. Franken P, Wensing T, Schotman AJH. The bone marrow of the horse. 2. Warmblooded horses with anemia. J Vet Med A 1982;29:23–7.
52. Schalm OW. Bone marrow erythroid cytology in anemias of the horse. In: First International Symposium on Equine Hematology. Michigan State University; 1975. p. 17–25.
53. Schalm OW. Equine hematology: Part IV – Erythroid marrow cytology in response to anemia. Equine Pract 1980;2:35–40.
54. Tablin F, Weiss L. Equine bone marrow: a quantitative analysis of erythroid maturation. Anat Rec 1985;213:202–6.
55. Tschudi P, Archer RK, Gerber H. Cytochemical staining of equine blood and bone marrow cells. Equine Vet J 1977;9:205–7.
56. Messer NT, Arnold K. Immune-mediated hemolytic anemia in a horse. J Am Vet Med Assoc 1991;198:1415–16.
57. Harvey JW. Microcytic anemias. In: Feldman BF, Zinkl JG, Jain NC, editors. Schalm's veterinary hematology. 5th ed. Philadelphia: Lippincott, Williams & Wilkins; 2000. p. 200–4.
58. Carlson GP. A survey of the iron status of thoroughbred horses in race training. In: Proceedings of the10th Annual ACVIM Forum. San Diego; 1992. p. 448–9.
59. Carlson GP. Clinical chemistry tests. In: Smith BP, editor. Large animal internal medicine. 3rd ed. St. Louis: Mosby; 2002. p. 389–412.
60. Schott II HC, Van Metre DC, Divers TJ. Diseases of the renal system. In: Smith BP, editor. Large animal internal medicine. 3rd ed. St. Louis: Mosby; 2002. p. 824–72.
61. Pearson EG. Diseases of the hepatobiliary system. In: Smith BP, editor. Large animal internal medicine. 3rd ed. St. Louis: Mosby; 2002. p. 790–823.
62. Klein HG, Higgins MJ. Use of blood components in the intensive care unit. In: Parrillo JE, Dellinger RP, editors. Critical care medicine: Principles of diagnosis and management in the adult. 2nd ed. St. Louis: Mosby; 2001. p. 1416–38.
63. Divers TJ. Liver failure and hemolytic anemia. In: Orsini JA, Divers TJ, editors. Equine emergencies: Treatment and procedures. 3rd ed. St. Louis: Saunders Elsevier; 2008. p. 237–58.
64. Andrews GA, Smith JE. Iron metabolism. In: Feldman BF, Zinkl JG, Jain NC, editors. Schalm's veterinary hematology. 5th ed. Philadelphia: Lippincott, Williams & Wilkins; 2000. p. 129–34.
65. Geor RJ, Weiss DJ. Drugs affecting the hematologic system of the performance horse. Vet Clin North Am Equine Pract 1993;9:649–67.
66. Smith JE, Cipriano JE, DeBowes R, et al. Iron deficiency and pseudo-iron deficiency in hospitalized horses. J Am Vet Med Assoc 1986;188:285–7.
67. Smith JE, Moore K, Cipriano JE, et al. Serum ferritin as a measure of stored iron in horses. J Nutr 1984;114: 677–81.
68. Smith JE, Cipriano JE. Inflammation-induced changes in serum iron analytes and ceruloplasmin of Shetland ponies. Vet Pathol 1987;24:354–6.
69. Franken P, Wensing T, Schotman AJ. The concentration of iron in the liver, spleen and plasma, and the amount of iron in bone marrow of horses. J Vet Med A 1981;28:381–9.
70. Mills PC, Marlin DJ. Plasma iron in elite horses at rest and after transport. Vet Rec 1996;139:215–17.
71. Kaneko JJ, Harvey JW, Bruss ML. Blood analyte reference values in large animals. In: Kaneko JJ, Harvey JW, Bruss ML, editors. Clinical biochemistry of domestic animals. 5th ed. San Diego: Academic Press; 1997. p. 890–4.
72. Osbaldiston GW, Griffith PR. Serum iron levels in normal and anemic horses. Can Vet J 1972;13:105–8.

73. Kohn CW, Jacobs RM, Knight D, et al. Microcytosis, hypoferremia, hypoferritemia, and hypertransferrinemia in standardbred foals from birth to 4 months of age. Am J Vet Res 1990;51:1198–205.
74. Taira T, Fujinaga T, Okumura M, et al. Equine haptoglobin: isolation, characterization, and the effects of ageing, delivery and inflammation on its serum concentration. J Vet Med Sci 1992;54:435–42.
75. Hanzawa K, Hiraga A, Yoshida Y, et al. Effects of exercise on plasma haptoglobin composition in control and splenectomized thoroughbred horses. J Equine Sci 2002;13:89–92.
76. Suttle N, Small J, Jones D. Overestimation of copper deficiency in horses? Vet Rec 1995;136:131.
77. Auer DE, Ng JC, Seawright AA. Assessment of copper and zinc status of farm horses and training thoroughbreds in south-east Queensland. Aust Vet J 1988;65:317–20.
78. Cymbaluk NF, Bristol FM, Christensen DA. Influence of age and breed of equid on plasma copper and zinc concentrations. Am J Vet Res 1986;47:192–5.
79. Stubley D, Campbell C, Dant C, et al. Copper and zinc levels in the blood of thoroughbreds in training in the United Kingdom. Equine Vet J 1983;15:253–6.
80. Mee JF, McLaughlin J. 'Normal' blood copper levels in horses. Vet Rec 1995;136:275.
81. Suttle NF, Small JN, Collins EA, et al. Serum and hepatic copper concentrations used to define normal, marginal and deficient copper status in horses. Equine Vet J 1996;28:497–9.
82. Pearce SG, Grace ND, Firth EC, et al. Effect of copper supplementation on the copper status of pasture-fed young Thoroughbreds. Equine Vet J 1998;30:204–10.
83. Pearce SG, Firth EC, Grace ND, et al. Liver biopsy techniques for adult horses and neonatal foals to assess copper status. Aust Vet J 1997;75:194–8.
84. Radostits OM, Gay CC, Blood DC, et al. Diseases caused by nutritional deficiencies. In: Radostits OM, Gay CC, Blood DC, Hinchcliff KW, editors. Veterinary medicine: A textbook of the diseases of cattle, sheep, pigs, goats and horses. London: W. B. Saunders; 2000. p. 1477–560.
85. Okumura M, Fujinaga T, Yamashita K, et al. Isolation, characterization, and quantitative analysis of ceruloplasmin from horses. Am J Vet Res 1991;52:1979–85.
86. Colahan PT, Bailey JE, Johnson M, et al. Effect of sulfadiazine and pyrimethamine on selected physiologic and performance parameters in athletically conditioned thoroughbred horses during an incremental exercise stress test. Vet Ther 2002;3:49–63.
87. Allen BV. Serum folate levels in horses, with particular reference to the English thoroughbred. Vet Rec 1978;103:257–9.
88. Seckington IM, Huntsman RG, Jenkins GC. The serum folic acid levels of grass-fed and stabled horses. Vet Rec 1967;81:158–61.
89. Roberts MC. Serum and red cell folate and serum vitamin B_{12} levels in horses. Aust Vet J 1983;60:106–11.
90. Piercy RJ, Hinchcliff KW, Reed SM. Folate deficiency during treatment with orally administered folic acid, sulphadiazine and pyrimethamine in a horse with suspected equine protozoal myeloencephalitis (EPM). Equine Vet J 2002;34:311–16.
91. Aird B. Acute blood loss anemia. In: Feldman BF, Zinkl JG, Jain NC, editors. Schalm's veterinary hematology. 5th ed. Philadelphia: Lippincott, Williams & Wilkins; 2000. p. 151–3.
92. Moore RM. Pathophysiology of circulatory shock. In: Colahan PT, Merritt AM, Moore JN, Mayhew IGJ, editors. Equine medicine and surgery. 5th ed. St. Louis: Mosby; 1999. p. 210–18.
93. Jeffrey SC. Managing hemoperitoneum in horses. Equine Pract 1996;91:850–6.
94. Edens LM. Abdominal hemorrhage. In: Robinson NE, editor. Current therapy in equine medicine 4. Philadelphia: W. B. Saunders; 1997. p. 211–14.
95. Morris DD. Diseases associated with blood loss or hemostatic dysfunction. In: Smith BP, editor. Large animal internal medicine. 3rd ed. St. Louis: Mosby; 2002. p. 1039–48.
96. McCarthy PF, Hooper RN, Carter GK, et al. Postparturient hemorrhage in the mare: Managing ruptured arteries of the broad ligament. Equine Pract 1994;89: 147–52.
97. Pusterla N, Fecteau ME, Madigan JE, et al. Acute hemoperitoneum in horses: A review of 19 cases (1992–2003). J Vet Intern Med 2005;19:344–7.
98. Dechant JE, Nieto JE, Le Jeune SS. Hemoperitoneum in horses: 67 cases (1989–2004). J Am Vet Med Assoc 2006;229:253–8.
99. Conwell RC, Hillyer MH, Mair TS, et al. Haemoperitoneum in horses: A retrospective review of 54 cases. Vet Rec 2010;167:514–18.
100. Collatos C. Blood loss anemia. In: Robinson NE, editor. Current therapy in equine medicine 4. Philadelphia: W. B. Saunders; 1997. p. 276–7.
101. Muir 3rd WW. Small volume resuscitation using hypertonic saline. Cornell Vet 1990;80:7–12.
102. Schmall LM, Muir WW, Robertson JT. Haemodynamic effects of small volume hypertonic saline in experimentally induced haemorrhagic shock. Equine Vet J 1990;22:273–7.
103. Schmall LM, Muir WW, Robertson JT. Haematological, serum electrolyte and blood gas effects of small volume hypertonic saline in experimentally induced haemorrhagic shock. Equine Vet J 1990;22:278–83.
104. Hermann M, Bretscher R, Thiebaud G, et al. [Preliminary experiences with the treatment of shock in horses with a plasma expander from a starch base]. Schweiz Arch Tierheilkd 1990;132:5–12.
105. Jones PA, Bain FT, Byars TD, et al. Effect of hydroxyethyl starch infusion on colloid oncotic pressure in hypoproteinemic horses. J Am Vet Med Assoc 2001;218:1130–5.
106. Jones PA, Tomasic M, Gentry PA. Oncotic, hemodilutional, and hemostatic effects of isotonic saline and hydroxyethyl starch solutions in clinically normal ponies. Am J Vet Res 1997;58:541–8.
107. Rudloff E, Kirby R. The critical need for colloids: Administering colloids effectively. Comp Cont Educ Pract Vet 1997;20:27–43.
108. Rudloff E, Kirby R. The critical need for colloids: Selecting the right colloid. Comp Cont Educ Pract Vet 1997;19:811–25.
109. Hughes D, Boag A. Fluid therapy with macromolecular plasma volume expanders. In: DiBartola SP, editor. Fluid, electrolyte, and acid-base disorders in small animal practice. 4th ed. St. Louis: Elsevier Saunders; 2012. p. 647–64.
110. Hohenhaus AE. Blood Transfusion and blood substitutes. In: DiBartola SP, editor. Fluid, electrolyte, and acid-base disorders in small animal practice. 4th ed. St. Louis: Elsevier Saunders; 2012. p. 585–604.
111. Capone AC, Safar P, Stezoski W, et al. Improved outcome with fluid restriction in treatment of uncontrolled hemorrhagic shock. J Am Coll Surg 1995;180:49–56.
112. Stern SA. Low-volume fluid resuscitation for presumed hemorrhagic shock: helpful or harmful? Curr Opin Crit Care 2001;7:422–30.
113. Lerche P, Muir WW. Perioperative pain management. In: Muir WW, Hubbell JAE, editors. Equine anesthesia: Monitoring and emergency therapy. St. Louis: Saunders Elsevier; 2009. p. 369–80.
114. Ross J, Dallap BL, Dolente BA, et al. Pharmacokinetics and pharmacodynamics of ε-aminocaproic acid in horses. Am J Vet Res 2007;68:1016–21.

115. Heidmann P, Tornquist SJ, Qu A, et al. Laboratory measures of hemostasis and fibrinolysis after intravenous administration of epsilon-aminocaproic acid in clinically normal horses and ponies. Am J Vet Res 2005;66:313–18.
116. Roberts SJ. The effects of various intravenous injections on the horse. Am J Vet Res 1943;4:226–39.
117. Jones W. IV formalin to control hemorrhage. J Equine Vet Sci 1998;18:581.
118. Taylor EL, Sellon DC, Wardrop KJ, et al. Effects of intravenous administration of formaldehyde on platelet and coagulation variables in healthy horses. Am J Vet Res 2000;61:1191–6.
119. Collatos C. Blood and blood component treatment. In: Robinson NE, editor. Current therapy in equine medicine 4. Philadelphia: W. B. Saunders; 1997. p. 290–2.
120. Magdesian KG, Fielding CL, Rhodes DM, et al. Changes in central venous pressure and blood lactate concentration in response to acute blood loss in horses. J Am Vet Med Assoc 2006;229:1458–62.
121. Theusinger OM, Spahn DR, Ganter MT. Transfusion in trauma: why and how should we change our current practice? Curr Opin Anaesthesiol 2009;22:305–12.
122. Hurcombe SD, Mudge MC, Hinchcliff KW. Clinical and clinicopathologic variables in adult horses receiving blood transfusions: 31 cases (1999–2005). J Am Vet Med Assoc 2007;231:267–74.
123. Hart KA. Pathogenesis, management and prevention of blood transfusion reactions in horses. Equine Vet Educ 2011;23:343–5.
124. Morris DD. Review of anemia in horses, Part II: Pathophysiologic mechanisms, specific diseases and treatment. Equine Pract 1989;11:34–46.
125. Mealey RH. Equine infectious anemia. In: Sellon DC, Long MT, editors. Equine infectious diseases. St. Louis: Saunders Elsevier; 2007. p. 213–19.
126. Coggins L, Auchnie JA. Control of equine infectious anemia in horses in Hong Kong. J Am Vet Med Assoc 1977;170:1299–301.
127. World Organization for Animal Health (OIE). OIE listed diseases. Paris: 2012. http://www.oie.int/animal-health-in-the-world/oie-listed-diseases-2012/.
128. Carlson GP. Equine infectious anemia. In: Smith BP, editor. Large animal internal medicine. 3rd ed. St. Louis: Mosby; 2002. p. 1056–8.
129. Sellon DC. Hemolytic anemia. In: Robinson NE, editor. Current therapy in equine medicine 4. Philadelphia: W. B. Saunders; 1997. p. 278–82.
130. Sellon DC. Coggins positive: An owner's nightmare. In: Proceedings of the 14th ACVIM Forum. St. Antonio; 1996. p. 413–15.
131. World Organization for Animal Health (OIE). Equine infectious anaemia. In: World Organization for Animal Health (OIE), editor. Manual of diagnostic tests and vaccines for terrestrial animals. Paris; 2011. http://www.oie.int/fileadmin/Home/eng/Health_standards/tahm/2.05.06_EIA.pdf.
132. Sellon DC, Perry ST, Coggins L, et al. Wild-type equine infectious anemia virus replicates in vivo predominantly in tissue macrophages, not in peripheral blood monocytes. J Virol 1992;66:5906–13.
133. Swardson CJ, Lichtenstein DL, Wang S, et al. Infection of bone marrow macrophages by equine infectious anemia virus. Am J Vet Res 1997;58:1402–7.
134. Issel CJ, Foil LD. Studies on equine infectious anemia virus transmission by insects. J Am Vet Med Assoc 1984;184:293–7.
135. Tashjian RJ. Transmission and clinical evaluation of an equine infectious anemia herd and their offspring over a 13-year period. J Am Vet Med Assoc 1984;184:282–8.
136. McGuire TC, Henson JB, Quist SE. Impaired bone marrow response in equine infectious anemia. Am J Vet Res 1969;30:2099–104.
137. Swardson CJ, Kociba GJ, Perryman LE. Effects of equine infectious anemia virus on hematopoietic progenitors in vitro. Am J Vet Res 1992;53:1176–9.
138. World Organization for Animal Health (OIE). World Animal Health Information Database (WAHID). Paris: 2012. http://web.oie.int/wahis/public.php?page=home.
139. World Organization for Animal Health (OIE). Terrestrial Animal Health Code. Paris: 2011. http://www.oie.int/en/international-standard-setting/terrestrial-code/access-online/.
140. De Waal DT. Equine piroplasmosis: A review. Br Vet J 1992;148:6–14.
141. Knowles Jr D. Equine babesiosis (piroplasmosis): A problem in the international movement of horses. Br Vet J 1996;152:123–6.
142. Bruning A. Equine piroplasmosis: an update on diagnosis, treatment and prevention. Br Vet J 1996;152:139–51.
143. Rothschild CM, Knowles DP. Equine Piroplasmosis. In: Sellon DC, Long MT, editors. Equine infectious diseases. St. Louis: Saunders Elsevier; 2007. p. 465–73.
144. Friedhoff KT, Soule C. An account on equine babesioses. Rev Sci Tech 1996;15:1191–201.
145. Gaunt SD. Hemolytic anemias caused by blood Rickettsial agents and protozoa. In: Feldman BF, Zinkl JG, Jain NC, editors. Schalm's veterinary hematology. 5th ed. Philadelphia: Lippincott, Williams & Wilkins; 2000. p. 154–62.
146. Böse R, Jorgensen WK, Dalgliesh RJ, et al. Current state and future trends in the diagnosis of babesiosis. Vet Parasitol 1995;57:61–74.
147. World Organization for Animal Health (OIE). Equine proplasmosis. In: World Organization for Animal Health (OIE), editor. Manual of diagnostic tests and vaccines for terrestrial animals. Paris: 2011. http://www.oie.int/fileadmin/Home/eng/Health_standards/tahm/2.05.08_EQUINE_PIROPLASMOSIS.pdf.
148. Böse R, Peymann B. Diagnosis of *Babesia caballi* infections in horses by enzyme-linked immunosorbent assay (ELISA) and western blot. Int J Parasitol 1994;24:341–6.
149. Schwint ON, Ueti MW, Palmer GH, et al. Imidocarb dipropionate clears persistent *Babesia caballi* infection with elimination of transmission potential. Antimicrob Agents Chemother 2009;53:4327–32.
150. Butler CM, Nijhof AM, van der Kolk JH, et al. Repeated high dose imidocarb dipropionate treatment did not eliminate *Babesia caballi* from naturally infected horses as determined by PCR-reverse line blot hybridization. Vet Parasitol 2008;151:320–2.
151. Belloli C, Crescenzo G, Lai O, et al. Pharmacokinetics of imidocarb dipropionate in horses after intramuscular administration. Equine Vet J 2002;34:625–9.
152. Zaugg JL. Babesiosis. In: Smith BP, editor. Large animal internal medicine. 3rd ed. St. Louis: Mosby; 2002. p. 1051–5.
153. Zaugg JL, Lane VM. Efficacy of buparvaquone as a therapeutic and clearing agent of *Babesia equi* of European origin in horses. Am J Vet Res 1992;53:1396–9.
154. Homer MJ, Aguilar-Delfin I, Telford SR, et al. Babesiosis. Clin Microbiol Rev 2000;13:451–69.
155. Short MA, Clark CK, Harvey JW, et al. Outbreak of equine piroplasmosis in Florida. J Am Vet Med Assoc 2012;240:588–95.
156. Carlson GP. Autoimmune hemolytic anemia. In: Smith BP, editor. Large animal internal medicine. 3rd ed. St. Louis: Mosby; 2002. p. 1058–9.
157. Reef VB, Dyson SS, Beech J. Lymphosarcoma and associated immune-mediated hemolytic anemia and thrombocytopenia in horses. J Am Vet Med Assoc 1984;184:313–17.
158. Lubas G, Ciattini F, Gavazza A. Immune-mediated thrombocytopenia

and hemolytic anemia (Evans' syndrome) in a horse. Equine Pract 1997;19:27–32.

159. Davis EG, Wilkerson MJ, Rush BR. Flow cytometry: Clinical applications in equine medicine. J Vet Intern Med 2002;16:404–10.
160. Wilkerson MJ, Davis E, Shuman W, et al. Isotype-specific antibodies in horses and dogs with immune-mediated hemolytic anemia. J Vet Intern Med 2000;14:190–6.
161. McConnico RS, Roberts MC, Tompkins M. Penicillin-induced immune-mediated hemolytic anemia in a horse. J Am Vet Med Assoc 1992;201:1402–3.
162. Step DL, Blue JT, Dill SG. Penicillin-induced hemolytic anemia and acute hepatic failure following treatment of tetanus in a horse. Cornell Vet 1991;81:13–18.
163. Blue JT, Dinsmore RP, Anderson KL. Immune-mediated hemolytic anemia induced by penicillin in horses. Cornell Vet 1987;77:263–76.
164. Tizard IR. Drugs and other agents that affect the immune system. In: Tizard IR, editor. Veterinary immunology – An introduction. 6th ed. Philadelphia: W.B. Saunders; 2000. p. 426–33.
165. Jeanes LV, Magdesian KG, Madigan JE, et al. Clostridial myositis in horses. Comp Cont Educ Pract Vet 2001;23:577–87.
166. Stevens DL, Maier KA, Laine BM, et al. Comparison of clindamycin, rifampin, tetracycline, metronidazole, and penicillin for efficacy in prevention of experimental gas gangrene due to *Clostridium perfringens*. J Infect Dis 1987;155:220–8.
167. Stevens DL, Maier KA, Mitten JE. Effect of antibiotics on toxin production and viability of *Clostridium perfringens*. Antimicrob Agents Chemother 1987;31:213–18.
168. Stewart AJ. Clostridial myositis and collapse in a standardbred filly. Vet Clin North Am Equine Pract 2006;22:127–43.
169. Beck DJ. A case of primary autoimmune haemolytic anaemia in a pony. Equine Vet J 1990;22:292–4.
170. Weiss DJ, Moritz A. Equine immune-mediated hemolytic anemia associated with *Clostridium perfringens* infection. Vet Clin Path 2003;32:22–6.
171. Reef VB. *Clostridium perfringens* cellulitis and immune-mediated hemolytic anemia in a horse. J Am Vet Med Assoc 1983;182:251–4.
172. Hübl W, Mostbeck B, Hartleb H, et al. Investigation of the pathogenesis of massive hemolysis in a case of *Clostridium perfringens* septicemia. Ann Hematol 1993;67:145–7.
173. Batge B, Filejski W, Kurowski V, et al. Clostridial sepsis with massive intravascular hemolysis: rapid diagnosis and successful treatment. Intensive Care Med 1992;18:488–90.
174. Robbins RL, Wallace SS, Brunner CJ, et al. Immune-mediated hemolytic disease after penicillin therapy in a horse. Equine Vet J 1993;25:462–5.
175. Thomas HL, Livesey MA. Immune-mediated hemolytic anemia associated with trimethoprim-sulphamethoxazole administration in a horse. Can Vet J 1998;39:171–3.
176. Ogilvie GK. Paraneoplastic syndromes. Vet Clin North Am Equine Pract 1998;14:439–49.
177. Geor RJ, Clark EG, Haines DM, et al. Systemic lupus erythematosus in a filly. J Am Vet Med Assoc 1990;197:1489–92.
178. Collins JD. Autoimmune haemolytic anemia in the horse. In: First International Symposium on Equine Hematology. Michigan State University; 1975. p. 342–8.
179. Corriher CA, Parviainen AKJ, Gibbons DS, et al. Equine red maple leaf toxicosis. Comp Cont Educ Pract Vet 1999;21:74–80.
180. Carlson GP. Heinz body hemolytic anemia. In: Smith BP, editor. Large animal internal medicine. 3rd ed. St. Louis: Mosby; 2002. p. 1059–61.
181. Alward A, Corriher CA, Barton MH, et al. Red maple (*Acer rubrum*) leaf toxicosis in horses: A retrospective study of 32 cases. J Vet Int Med 2006;20: 1197–201.
182. McConnico RS, Brownie CF. The use of ascorbic acid in the treatment of 2 cases of red maple (*Acer rubrum*) – poisoned horses. Cornell Vet 1992;82:293–300.
183. Loscher W, Jaeschke G, Keller H. Pharmacokinetics of ascorbic acid in horses. Equine Vet J 1984;16:59–65.
184. Boyer JD, Breeden DC, Brown DL. Isolation, identification, and characterization of compounds from *Acer rubrum* capable of oxidizing equine erythrocytes. Am J Vet Res 2002;63:604–10.
185. Schott HC, Hodgson DR, Bayly WM. Haematuria, pigmenturia and proteinuria in exercising horses. Equine Vet J 1995;27:67–72.
186. Hanzawa K, Watanabe S. Changes in osmotic fragility of erythrocytes during exercise in athletic horses. J Equine Sci 2000;11:51–61.
187. Hanzawa K, Kubo K, Kal M, et al. Effects of exercise on erythrocytes in normal and splenectomised Thoroughbred horses. Equine Vet J 1995;27:439–42.
188. Matsuki N, Tamura S, Ono K, et al. Exercise-induced phospholipid degradation in the equine skeletal muscle and erythrocytes. J Vet Med Sci 1991;53:1001–7.
189. Mills P, Smith N, Casas I, et al. Effects of exercise intensity and environmental stress on indices of oxidative stress and iron homeostasis during exercise in the horse. Eur J Appl Physiol Occup Physiol 1996;74:60–6.
190. Avellini L, Chiaradia E, Gaiti A. Effect of exercise training, selenium and vitamin E on some free radical scavengers in horses (*Equus caballus*). Comp Biochem Physiol B Biochem Mol Biol 1999;123: 147–54.
191. Ono K, Inui K, Hasegawa T, et al. The changes of antioxidative enzyme activities in equine erythrocytes following exercise. Jpn J Vet Sci 1990;52:759–65.
192. Motta S, Letellier C, Ropert M, et al. Protecting effect of vitamin E supplementation on submaximal exercise-induced oxidative stress in sedentary dogs as assessed by erythrocyte membrane fluidity and paraoxonase-1 activity. Vet J 2009;181:288–95.
193. Sentürk ÜK, Gündüz F, Kuru O, et al. Exercise-induced oxidative stress leads hemolysis in sedentary but not trained humans. J Appl Physiol 2005;99:1434–41.
194. Janiak M, Suska M, Dudzińska W, et al. Blood glutathione status and activity of glutathione-metabolizing antioxidant enzymes in erythrocytes of young trotters in basic training. J Anim Physiol Anim Nutr 2010;94:137–45.
195. Piccione G, Giannetto C, Marafioti S, et al. Training-induced modifications of circadian rhythmicity of peroxidative parameters in horses. J Anim Physiol Anim Nutr 2011. doi: 10.1111/j.1439-0396.2011.01209.x.
196. de Moffarts B, Kirschvink N, Art T, et al. Impact of training and exercise intensity on blood antioxidant markers in healthy Standardbred horses. Equine Comp Exerc Physiol 2004;1:211–20.
197. Means RT Jr, Krantz SB. Progress in understanding the pathogenesis of the anemia of chronic disease. Blood 1992;80:1639–47.
198. Carlson GP. Depression anemia. In: Smith BP, editor. Large animal internal medicine. 3rd ed. St. Louis: Mosby; 2002. p. 1063–5.
199. Watson ADJ, Canfield PJ. Nutritional deficiency anemias. In: Feldman BF, Zinkl JG, Jain NC, editors. Schalm's veterinary hematology. 5th ed. Philadelphia: Lippincott, Williams & Wilkins; 2000. p. 190–5.
200. Jackson SG. Trace minerals for the performance horse: Known biochemical

roles and estimates of requirements. Irish Vet J 1997;50:668–74.
201. Pearson EG, Andreasen CB. Effect of oral administration of excessive iron in adult ponies. J Am Vet Med Assoc 2001;218:400–4.
202. Rucker RB, Morris JG. The vitamins. In: Kaneko JJ, Harvey JW, Bruss ML, editors. Clinical biochemistry of domestic animals. 5th ed. San Diego: Academic Press; 1997. p. 703–39.
203. Alexander F, Davies ME. Studies on vitamin B_{12} in the horse. Br Vet J 1969;125:169–76.
204. Salminen K. Cobalt metabolism in horse. Serum level and biosynthesis of vitamin B_{12}. Acta Vet Scand 1975;16:84–94.
205. Toribio RE, Bain FT, Mrad DR, et al. Congenital defects in newborn foals of mares treated for equine protozoal myeloencephalitis during pregnancy. J Am Vet Med Assoc 1998;212:697–701.
206. Cowgill LD, James KM, Levy JK, et al. Use of recombinant human erythropoietin for management of anemia in dogs and cats with renal failure. J Am Vet Med Assoc 1998;212:521–8.
207. Casadevall N, Nataf J, Viron B, et al. Pure red-cell aplasia and antierythropoietin antibodies in patients treated with recombinant erythropoietin. N Engl J Med 2002;346:469–75.
208. Pollock C, Johnson DW, Hörl WH, et al. Pure red cell aplasia induced by erythropoiesis-stimulating agents. Clin J Am Soc Nephrol 2008;3:193–9.
209. Barragry T. Drugs, doping and current sporting problems: 1. Irish Vet J 2000;53:312–19.
210. Kearns CF, Lenhart JA, McKeever KH. Cross reactivity between human erythropoietin antibody and horse erythropoietin. Electrophoresis 2000;21:1454–7.
211. Casadevall N. Antibodies against rHuEPO: Native and recombinant. Nephrol Dial Transplant 2002;17(Suppl. 5):42–7.
212. Giger U. Erythropoietin and its clinical use. Comp Cont Educ Pract Vet 1992;14:25–34.
213. Piercy RJ, Swardson CJ, Hinchcliff KW. Erythroid hypoplasia and anemia following administration of recombinant human erythropoietin to two horses. J Am Vet Med Assoc 1998;212:244–7.
214. Woods PR, Campbell G, Cowell RL. Nonregenerative anaemia associated with administration of recombinant human erythropoietin to a Thoroughbred racehorse. Equine Vet J 1997;29:326–8.
215. Schwarzwald CC, Hinchcliff KW. Recombinant human erythropoietin as a cause of non-regenerative anemia in a stable of racing Thoroughbreds. In: Proceedings of the 50th Annual Convention of the American Association of Equine Practitioners. Denver, CO, 2004.
216. Lasne F, Popot M-A, Variet-Marie E, et al. Detection of recombinant epoetin and darbepoetin alpha after subcutaneous administration in the horse. J Anal Toxicol 2005;29:835–7.
217. Chang Y, Maylin GM, Matsumoto G, et al. Screen and confirmation of PEG-epoetin β in equine plasma. Drug Test Anal 2011;3:68–73.
218. Yu N, Ho E, Wan T, et al. Doping control analysis of recombinant human erythropoietin, darbepoetin alfa and methoxy polyethylene glycol-epoetin beta in equine plasma by nano-liquid chromatography-tandem mass spectrometry. Anal Bioanal Chem 2010;396:2513–21.
219. Guan F, Uboh CE, Soma LR, et al. Confirmatory analysis of continuous erythropoietin receptor activator and erythropoietin analogues in equine plasma by LC-MS for coping control. Anal Chem 2010;82:9074–81.
220. Guan F, Uboh CE, Soma LR, et al. LC-MS/MS method for confirmation of recombinant human erythropoietin and darbepoetin α in equine plasma. Anal Chem 2007;79:4627–35.
221. Guan F, Uboh CE, Soma LR, et al. Differentiation and identification of recombinant human erythropoietin and darbepoetin alfa in equine plasma by LC-MS/MS for doping control. Anal Chem 2008;80:3811–17.
222. Souillard A, Audran M, Bressolle F, et al. Pharmacokinetics and haematological parameters of recombinant human erythropoietin after subcutaneous administrations in horses. Biopharm Drug Dispos 1996;17:805–15.
223. Jaussaud P, Audran M, Gareau RL, et al. Kinetics and haematological effects of erythropoietin in horses. Vet Res 1994;25:568–73.
224. Sawada K, Fujishima N, Hirokawa M. Acquired pure red cell aplasia: Updated review of treatment. Br J Haematol 2008;142:505–14.
225. Summers S, Holdsworth S, Sharples E. The (re)challenging question of erythropoiesis-stimulating agents inducing pure red cell aplasia. Nephrol Dial Transplant 2008;23:3053–5.
226. Macdougall IC. Epoetin-induced pure red cell aplasia: Diagnosis and treatment. Curr Opin Nephrol Hypertens 2007;16:585–8.
227. Macdougall IC, Rossert J, Casadevall N, et al. A peptide-based erythropoietin-receptor agonist for pure red-cell aplasia. N Engl J Med 2009;361:1848–55.
228. Lappin TRJ, Maxwell AP. Recombinant human erythropoietin and the anaemic horse: Flogging a dead horse? Equine Vet J 1997;29:255–6.
229. Young NS, Maciejewski J. The pathophysiology of acquired aplastic anemia. N Engl J Med 1997;336:1365–72.
230. Morris DD. Aplastic anemia. In: Smith BP, editor. Large animal internal medicine. 3rd ed. St. Louis: Mosby; 2002. p. 1065–6.
231. Ward MV, Mountan PC, Dodds WJ. Severe idiopathic refractory anemia and leukopenia in a horse. Calif Vet 1980;12:19–22.
232. Berggren PC. Aplastic anemia in a horse. J Am Vet Med Assoc 1981;179:1400–2.
233. Lavoie JP, Morris DD, Zinkl JG, et al. Pancytopenia caused by bone marrow aplasia in a horse. J Am Vet Med Assoc 1987;191:1462–4.
234. Dunavant ML. Clinical evidence of phenylbutazone induced hypoplastic anemia. In: First International Symposium on Equine Hematology. Michigan State University; 1975. p. 383–5.
235. Lester GD, Alleman AR, Raskin RE, et al. Pancytopenia secondary to lymphoid leukemia in three horses. J Vet Int Med 1993;7:360–3.
236. Angel KL, Spano JS, Schumacher J, et al. Myelophthisic pancytopenia in a pony mare. J Am Vet Med Assoc 1991;198:1039–42.
237. Durando MM, Alleman AR, Harvey JW. Myelodysplastic syndrome in a quarter horse gelding. Equine Vet J 1994;26:83–5.
238. Moore JN, Mahaffey EA, Zboran M. Heparin-induced agglutination of erythrocytes in horses. Am J Vet Res 1987;48:68–71.
239. Mahaffey EA, Moore JN. Erythrocyte agglutination associated with heparin treatment in three horses. J Am Vet Med Assoc 1986;189:1478–80.
240. Gerhards H. Low dose calcium heparin in horses: Plasma heparin concentrations, effects on red blood cell mass and on coagulation variables. Equine Vet J 1991;23:37–43.
241. Duncan SG, Meyers KM, Reed SM. Reduction of the red blood cell mass of horses: Toxic effect of heparin anticoagulant therapy. Am J Vet Res 1983;44:2271–6.
242. Feige K, Schwarzwald CC, Bombeli T. Comparison of unfractioned and low molecular weight heparin for prophylaxis of coagulopathies in 52

horses with colic: A randomised double-blind clinical trial. Equine Vet J 2003;35:506–13.

243. Monreal L, Villatoro AJ, Monreal M, et al. Comparison of the effects of low-molecular-weight and unfractioned heparin in horses. Am J Vet Res 1995;56:1281–5.
244. Randolph JF, Peterson ME, Stokol T. Erythrocytosis and polycythemia. In: Weiss DJ, Wardrop KJ, editors. Schalm's veterinary hematology. 6th ed. Ames, Iowa: Wiley-Blackwell; 2010. p. 162–6.
245. McFarlane D, Sellon DC, Parker B. Primary erythrocytosis in a 2-year-old Arabian gelding. J Vet Intern Med 1998;12:384–8.
246. Steiger R, Feige K. [Case report: Polycythemia in a horse]. Schweiz Arch Tierheilkd 1995;137:306–11.
247. Belli CB, Baccarin RY, Ida KK, et al. Appropriate secondary absolute erythrocytosis in a horse. Vet Rec 2011;169:609.
248. Roby KA, Beech J, Bloom JC, et al. Hepatocellular carcinoma associated with erythrocytosis and hypoglycemia in a yearling filly. J Am Vet Med Assoc 1990;196:465–7.
249. Lennox TJ, Wilson JH, Hayden DW, et al. Hepatoblastoma with erythrocytosis in a young female horse. J Am Vet Med Assoc 2000;216:718–21, 685.
250. Axon JE, Russell CM, Begg AP, et al. Erythrocytosis and pleural effusion associated with a hepatoblastoma in a Thoroughbred yearling. Aust Vet J 2008;86:329–33.
251. Cook G, Divers TJ, Rowland PH. Hypercalcaemia and erythrocytosis in a mare associated with a metastatic carcinoma. Equine Vet J 1995;27:316–18.
252. Koch TG, Wen X, Bienzle D. Lymphoma, erythrocytosis, and tumor erythropoietin gene expression in a horse. J Vet Int Med 2006;20:1251–5.
253. Beech J, Bloom JC, Hodge TG. Erythrocytosis in a horse. J Am Vet Med Assoc 1984;184:986–9.
254. McMichael M, Smith SA, McConachie EL, et al. In-vitro hypocoagulability on whole blood thromboelastometry associated with in-vivo expansion of red cell mass in an equine model. Blood Coagul Fibrinolysis 2011;22:424–30.
255. Bain BJ. Haemoglobinopathy diagnosis: Algorithms, lessons and pitfalls. Blood Rev 2011;25:205–13.
256. Cambier C, Di Passio N, Clerbaux T, et al. Blood-oxygen binding in healthy Standardbred horses. Vet J 2005;169:251–6.
257. Vecchio S, Leonardo P, Musuraca V, et al. A comparison of the results obtained with traditional phlebotomy and with therapeutic erythrocytapheresis in patients with erythrocytosis. Blood Transfus 2007;5:20–3.
258. Zarkovic M, Kwaan HC. Correction of hyperviscosity by apheresis. Semin Thromb Hemost 2003;29:535–42.
259. Archer RK, Clabby J. The effect of excitation and exertion on the circulating blood of horses. Vet Rec 1965;77:689–90.
260. Torton M, Schalm O. Influence of the equine spleen on rapid changes in the concentration of erythrocytes in peripheral blood. Am J Vet Res 1964;25:500.
261. Bonagura JD, Reef VB, Schwarzwald CC. Cardiovascular diseases. In: Reed SM, Bayly WM, Sellon DC, editors. Equine internal medicine. 3rd ed. St. Louis: Saunders Elsevier; 2010. p. 372–487.
262. Bayly WM, Reed SM, Leathers CW, et al. Multiple congenital heart anomalies in five Arabian foals. J Am Vet Med Assoc 1982;181:684–9.
263. Wickler SJ, Anderson TP. Hematological changes and athletic performance in horses in response to high altitude (3,800 m). Am J Physiol Regul Integr Comp Physiol 2000;279:R1176–81.
264. Greene HM, Hurson MJ, Wickler SJ. Haematological and respiratory gas changes in horses and mules exercised at altitude (3800 m). Equine Vet J 2006;38:551–6.
265. Persson SG, Funkquist P, Nyman G. Total blood volume in the normally performing Standardbred trotter: age and sex variations. J Vet Med A 1996;43:57–64.
266. Persson SG, Larsson M, Lindholm A. Effects of training on adreno-cortical function and red-cell volume in trotters. J Vet Med A 1980;27:261–8.
267. Persson SGB. Evaluation of exercise tolerance and fitness in the performance horse. In: Snow DH, Persson SGB, Rose RJ, editors. Equine exercise physiology 1. Cambridge: Granta Publications; 1983. p. 441–57.
268. Persson SG, Osterberg I. Racing performance in red blood cell hypervolaemic standardbred trotters. Equine Vet J 1999;Suppl 30:617–20.
269. Funkquist P, Sandhagen B, Persson SG, et al. Effects of phlebotomy on haemodynamic characteristics during exercise in standardbred trotters with red cell hypervolaemia. Equine Vet J 2001;33:417–24.
270. McKeever KH. Overtraining syndrome in Standardbred horses: New insights into the role of red blood cell hypervolaemia. Vet J 2003;165: 190–2.
271. Rivero JLL, Van Breda E, Rogers CW, et al. Unexplained underperformance syndrome in sport horses: Classification, potential causes and recognition. Equine Vet J 2008;40:611–18.
272. Bruin G, Kuipers H, Keizer HA, et al. Adaptation and overtraining in horses subjected to increasing training loads. J Appl Physiol 1994;76:1908–13.
273. Golland LC, Evans DL, McGowan CM, et al. The effects of overtraining on blood volumes in Standardbred racehorses. Vet J 2003;165:228–33.
274. Hamlin MJ, Shearman JP, Hopkins WG. Changes in physiological parameters in overtrained Standardbred racehorses. Equine Vet J 2002;34:383–8.
275. Tyler-McGowan CM, Golland LC, Evans DL, et al. Haematological and biochemical responses to training and overtraining. Equine Vet J 1999;31:621–5.
276. Funkquist P, Nyman G, Persson SGB. Haemodynamic response to exercise in trotters with red cell hypervolaemia and exercise induced pulmonary haemorrhage. In: Proceedings of the 10th International Conference of Racing Analysts and Veterinarians. Newmarket; 1994. p. 165–7.
277. Persson SGB. Lung biopsy pathology and exercise intolerance in horses with chronic bronchiolitis. In: Persson SGB, Lindholm A, Jeffcott LB, editors. Equine exercise physiology 3. Davis, CA: ICEEP Publications; 1991. p. 457–64.
278. Funkquist P, Wagner PD, Hedenstierna G, et al. Ventilation-perfusion relationships during exercise in standardbred trotters with red cell hypervolaemia. Equine Vet J Suppl 1999;30:107–13.
279. Persson SGB. Practical aspects of blood volume measurement. Procedure for determination of total red cell volume (CV) in the horse. In: Proceedings of the International Conference on Equine Sports Medicine. 1986. p. 51.
280. Pösö AR, Essen-Gustavsson B, Persson SG. Metabolic response to standardised exercise test in standardbred trotters with red cell hypervolaemia. Equine Vet J 1993;25:527–31.
281. Karlström K, Essén-Gustavsson B, Persson SGB. Capillaries of muscle in red cell hypervolaemic versus normovolaemic Standardbred horses. Equine Vet J 1995;Suppl 18:228–30.
282. Persson SGB. Blood volume in relation to exercise tolerance in trotters. J S Afr Vet Assoc 1974;45:293–9.
283. West JB, Mathieu-Costello O, Jones JH, et al. Stress failure of pulmonary capillaries in racehorses with exercise-induced pulmonary hemorrhage. J Appl Physiol 1993;75:1097–109.
284. Birks EK, Mathieu-Costello O, Fu Z, et al. Very high pressures are required to cause stress failure of pulmonary

capillaries in thoroughbred racehorses. J Appl Physiol 1997;82:1584–92.

285. Roneus M, Persson SG, Essen-Gustavsson B, et al. Skeletal muscle characteristics in red blood cell normovolaemic and hypervolaemic standardbred racehorses. Equine Vet J 1994;26:319–22.

286. Funkquist P, Essen-Gustavsson B, Nyman G. Muscle characteristics in Standardbred trotters with red cell hypervolemia and pronounced hypertension during exercise. In: Proceedings of the Association of Equine Sports Medicine. San Antonio; 1997. p. 31–4.

287. Karlstrom K, Essen-Gustavsson B. Myosin heavy chain-based fibre types in red cell hyper- and normovolaemic Standardbred trotters. Equine Vet J Suppl 2002:279–82.

Exercise and immunity in horses

45

Tatiana Art

CHAPTER CONTENTS

Introduction

Living organisms are continuously exposed to infectious agents such as viruses, bacteria and other pathogens. Without an immune system, animals would soon die from disease caused by these infectious agents. The immune system includes all the mechanisms available to protect the body against disease caused by these agents and neoplastic cells. The immune system is extremely adaptable and can generate a great diversity of cells and molecules able to recognize and eliminate a large variety of potential pathogens. From a functional point of view, two sub-divisions can be considered: the innate (or non-specific) immunity that confers basal resistance to illness, immediately functional at birth and the first-line defense; and the adaptive (or acquired) immunity, which generates specific reactions, with immunological memory, against each potential biological invader.

Innate immunity includes anatomical barriers (skin, mucous membranes, bronchial epithelial cells) and physiological reaction (fever, pH variation), as well as humoral and chemical transmitters such as interferons, lysozyme, inflammatory proteins, cytokines, complement and others. Lastly, it includes specialized cells such as phagocytes (neutrophils, monocytes and macrophages), killer cells, called natural killers or NK, and lymphokine-activated killers or LAK. The innate inflammatory response is orchestrated by cytokines. These small signaling proteins secreted by numerous – immune and other – cells ensure intercellular communication. They bind to specific receptors and induce a response in the target cells, modulating cell function by modifying its gene expression. Cytokines can have pro-inflammatory effects (e.g. IL-6, IL-8, IL-12, TNF-α) or anti-inflammatory effects (IL-10). Others have antiviral effects (INF type 1) or play a regulating role of the adaptive immunity (IL-4, IL-7, IL-23).

Acquired immunity is mediated by humoral and cellular components. Specialized cells are effector T cells such as cytotoxic T lymphocytes that have both antigen specificity and immunological memory. T helper cells regulate the adaptative response by producing cytokines. Lymphocytes B and T secrete a broad panel of substances including compounds such as antibodies and cytokines.

Antigen-presenting cells (APCs) represent the link between both immune systems. They are efficient at internalizing antigens, either by phagocytosis or endocytosis: they then display fragments of foreign antigen bound with a class II major histocompatibility complex (MHC) located on their membrane. The T cell recognizes and interacts with the antigen-class II MHC molecule complex on the membrane of the antigen-presenting cell. An additional co-stimulatory signal is then produced by the antigen-presenting cell, leading to activation of the T cell. Dendritic cells have the broadest range of antigen presentation, and are probably the most important APC.

Exercise is recognized as one of the most potent physiological stresses that a healthy organism might experience. The question of knowing if this stress is compatible with health and whether it influences immunity is still poorly elucidated in humans and horses.

The relationship between exercise, immune function and infectious or inflammatory diseases remains poorly resolved.[1–4] The difficulty of assessing this relationship is due to numerous factors, among which the complexity of the immune function, the variability of the exercise considered (which varies by equestrian discipline, intensity and duration), the population studied (sedentary, athletic, young, mature, trained or untrained), what function or what cells have been analyzed to assess the immunity, the timing of sampling used (during exercise, just after, or 1, 24 or 48 hours after); and the difficulty of dissociating the effect of the effort from other effects (psychological stresses, environment). Last but not least, it is difficult to determine the genuine clinical significance of the changes observed in some parameters of the immunity.

Assessment of immunity

The relationship beteween immunity and exercise is evaluated through either epidemiological studies or experimental biocellular or biomolecular studies.

Epidemiological studies help to assess the effect of physical activity on a given population but do not bring any mechanistic information.

Experimental studies focus on one isolated component of the immune function and help to understand some mechanisms. Nevertheless, it is often difficult to assess the clinical relevance of these findings as they might not reflect the overall immune status.

The general principle of the experimental studies related to immunity is the sampling of biological fluids, leukocytes, or both, to evaluate:

- some cellular components: quantitative evaluation and proportion of each type of leukocyte (cells counting, identification by flow cytometry)
- some functional parameters of the phagocytic cells: phagocytic capacity, oxidative burst, functional immune capacity of neutrophils by evaluating capacity of adherence, chemotaxis, ingestion and digestion of foreign substances; cytotoxicity
- lymphoproliferation after non-specific (mitogens) or specific (antigens) stimulation of lymphocytes
- cells response after stimulations that mimic an attack by a pathogen
- dosage of immunoglobulins.

Recent discoveries in molecular biology have opened new prospects for studying the non-specific response of the first-line defender cells when microorganisms invade the organism. Among these findings, are pattern recognition receptors (PRR) such as Toll-like receptors (TLRs) and NOD-like receptors (NLRs) that seem to play a key role in the defense against microbes.[5,6] These receptors are activated after recognizing specific pathogen-associated molecular pattern (PAMP) or damage-associated molecular pattern (DAMP). When these receptors bind and recognize their specific ligand, they induce a cascade of events leading to the activation of transcription factors, resulting in production of chemokine/cytokine, upregulation of cell adhesion molecules, phagocytic cellular infiltration, and finally clearance of the microorganisms.

The study of TLRs activation by specific ligands is being investigated in equids.[7–10] For example, TLR4 is located in the cellular membrane and is involved in the recognition of several bacterial signals. The TLR4 cascade is activated by the classical addition of bacterial endotoxins (lipopolysaccharide or LPS) on cultured peripheral blood mononucleated cells (PBMC) or pulmonary alveolar macrophages (PAM) and results in the production of pro-inflammatory cytokines such IL-1α, IL-6 and TNF-α. These tests, overall, evaluate the response of the phagocytic cells in front of a bacterial attack.

In young racehorses in training, respiratory problems are frequently related to viral diseases (EHV4, influenza) which induces acute respiratory disease with temporary incapacity to work, and that can 'prepare the ground' for secondary infectious and/or inflammatory complications.[11] It is therefore of paramount importance to examine the capacity of the immune system to protect against disease caused by these viruses. Polyinosinic-polycytidylic acid (poly I:C) has a structure similar to the double strand of RNA contained in some viruses and, consequently, is a tool used in research to evaluate the immune response against viral attack. It is a stimulant of the Toll-like receptor type 3 (TLR3), an intracellular receptor included in the endosome membrane and which is involved in the recognition of viral DNA/RNA. It is expressed in lymphocytes T cells, dendritic cells and phagocytes. The recognition of its ligand will mainly result in the production of INFβ. Experimental induction of the TLR3 pathway can be obtained by adding poly I:C (which has a structure similar to the viral RNA) on cultured PBMC, or PAM or bronchial epithelial cells (Fig. 45.1).

Current research is aimed at studying the response of PBMC, PAM and bronchial epithelial cells to specific stimulation of TLR with synthetic ligands. The cells are put in a culture medium and stimulated by LPS (specific of TLR4), poly I:C (specific of TLR3), and other specific ligands for the different TLRs (Table 45.1). The cytokines in the supernatant are then analyzed (when ELISA homologous for the horses is available) and the white cells are recovered for extraction of RNA and transcriptomic study (when ELISA are not available). These methods have shown a probable decrease of resistance to virus 24 hours after an exercise to fatigue in Thoroughbred horses.[10]

Epidemiologic data

Epidemiological studies carried out in man have led to the following observations:

- Moderate regular physical activity confers a protection against chronic inflammatory diseases (cardiac, type 2 diabetes,

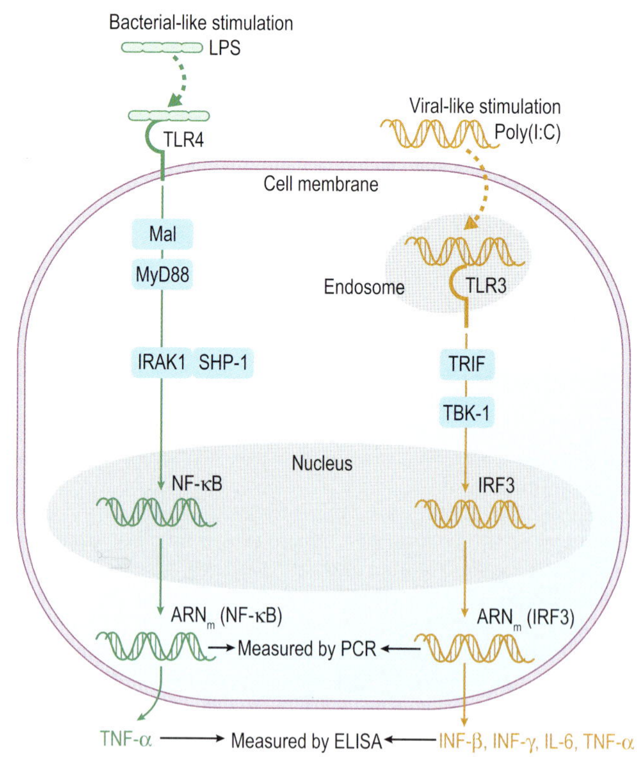

Fig 45.1 The specific stimulation of pattern recognition receptors such as Toll-like receptors is a method used to assess innate immune response. The bond between the receptor and its specific ligand (generally a synthetic ligand is used in experimental conditions) induces a cascade of intracellular events leading to a modification (up- or downregulation) of gene expression, which can be assessed by RT-PCR, and/or by a change in cytokine secretions, which can be measured by ELISA, when equine kits are available.

chronic obstructive pulmonary disease) and reinforces the resistance of the subjects to the infectious viral and bacterial diseases. This is especially true in the elderly.[3,4]

- Intense physical activity, and particularly a competition, induces an increased (+150%) susceptibility to upper airway respiratory diseases, just after the exercise. Moreover, intense exercise seems to reactivate latent infections.[3,12,13] (see Fig. 45.2).
- The susceptibility to infections of the upper airway is greater in 'overtrained' subjects.[12]
- There is a much higher prevalence of asthma and bronchitis in human athletes, especially in marathon runners, than in the sedentary population. Air quality and characteristics (chemical, biological and physical) as well as high level of ventilation are thought to be favoring factors.[4]

In horses, epidemiological studies have also shown an increased susceptibility to infectious disease in young racehorses, despite appropriate vaccination.[11]

Table 45.1 Toll-like receptors and some of their specific experimental ligands

TLR	LIGANDS
TLR-1&2 (heterodimer)	Peptidoglycan, lipoproteins, zymosan
TLR-1&6 (heterodimer)	Peptidoglycan, lipoproteins, zymosan
TLR-3	dsRNA
TLR-4 (dimer)	LPS (Gram-), lipoteichoic acid (Gram+)
TLR-5	Flagellin
TLR7	ssRNA
TLR-8	G-rich oligonucleotide
TLR-9	Unmethylated CPG DNA

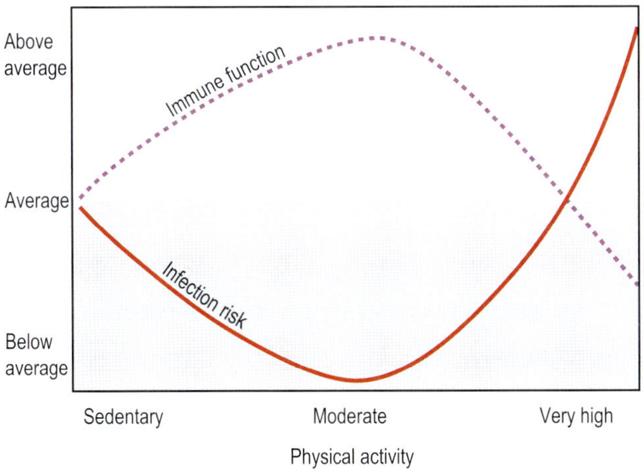

Fig 45.2 Relationship between the level of physical activity and the risk for infectious diseases in man. Moderate and regular exercise is associated with a decreased risk for infection, while inactivity or high-level activity is accompanied by an increased risk. These observation led to the 'inverted J hypothesis' proposed by Woods et al.[3]

Another characteristics of racehorses regularly trained and involved in competition is the fact that they frequently suffer from chronic inflammation of the airway, a syndrome commonly known as inflammatory airway disease (IAD).[14] The primum novens and the mechanisms of occurrence of IAD remain poorly defined to date. Most probably, the problem is related to an inappropriate response of the innate immune system. Dysregulation of immunity in IAD could be due either to an uncontrolled chronic inflammation or, on the contrary, a subdued inflammatory response, favoring the occurrence of secondary microbial and fungal infections. The fact that some scientists propose to treat IAD by anti-inflammatory drug administration while others recommend to control it by giving stimulants of immunity gives an idea of the extent of the lack of knowledge on this syndrome (Fig. 45.3).

Experimental data

There is a great discrepancy in the results and sometimes contradictions in the conclusions of research into immunity and exercise in horses, a result of the diversity of the methodologies used.

Effect of exercise

In humans, several changes occur *at the beginning of the effort*: increase in the number of circulating neutrophils, lymphocytes and monocytes, in NK and LAK, a burst of pro-inflammatory cytokines (TNF-α, MIP-1, IL-1β, IL-6, IL-8, IL-12, granulocytes/macrophages colony stimulating factor, i.e. GMC-SF) but also an increase of anti-inflammatory cytokines (IL-6, IL-10, IL-1ra), and an increase in concentration of an inflammatory protein (CRP).[4,15] Equine phagocytes sampled during exercise have an increased phagocytic capacity.[2,16]

Many changes also occur during the period after exercise. Exercise at 60%, or less, of VO_{2max} appears to have only moderate effects on innate immunity,[17] while exhausting exercise has an immunosuppressor effect during the recovery period. This decrease of immunity, called by the physiologist the 'Open Window Period' continues, depending on the protocols, from 3 to 72 hours after the exercise[4] (Fig. 45.4).

During the Open Window Period, the observed changes are namely:[15]

- a reduction in the phagocytic capacity and oxidative burst of the neutrophils
- a loss of the capacity of the macrophages to present the antigens to the lymphocytes (under-expression of the MHCII)
- a lack of activation of the macrophages stimulated with LPS, during six hours
- a lymphopenia with reduction of the T cells
- a reduction in the cytotoxic activity of the NK (however exacerbated during the effort) to half of the resting capacity, two hours after the effort
- a reduction in the TLR 1,2 and 4 on the monocytes
- a decrease in nasal and salivary IgA concentration.

It should be emphasized that most of these immunosuppressor effects reduce the resistance to infections for a short period, but also reduce the acute inflammatory reactions which could result from an intense exercise (e.g. at the muscular and osteoarticular levels). This decrease of immunity (reactivity) could therefore have a physiological justification and could finally result in a net beneficial effect.

Most of the studies in the horse are focused on the innate immunity response and, more particularly, on its blood cellular component (neutrophils, monocytes, NK, LAK).[17-20] The functionality of

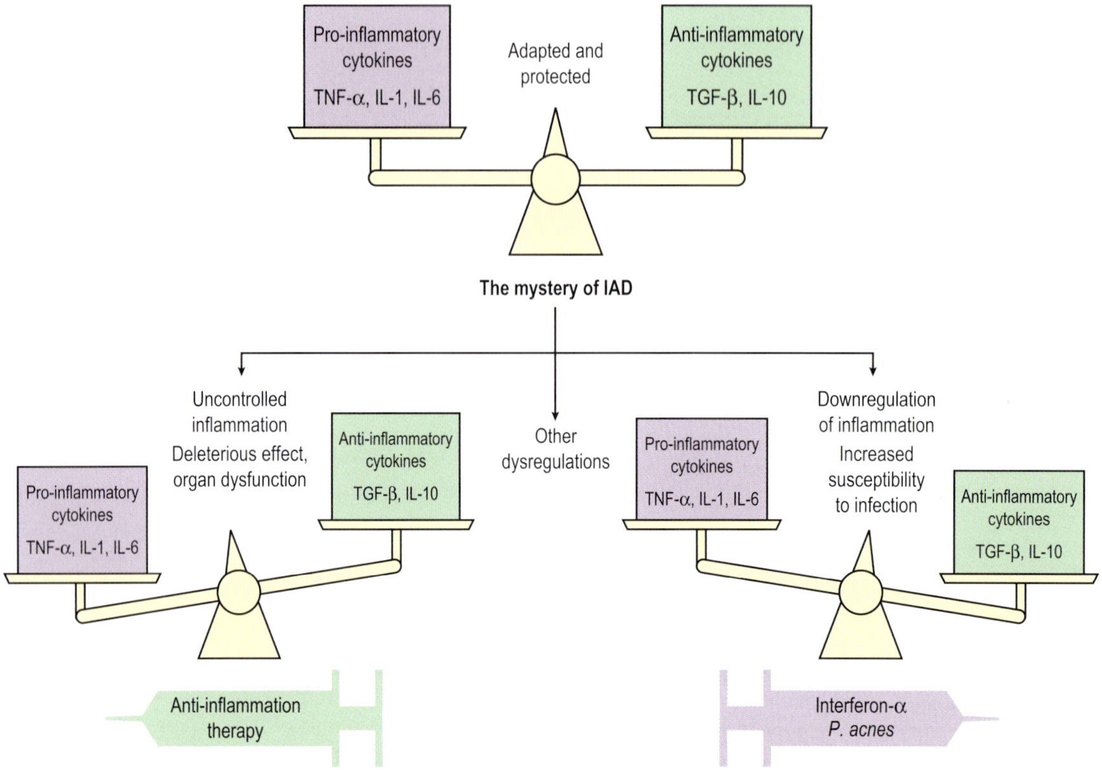

Fig 45.3 Inflammation regulation is the results of pro and anti-inflammatory cytokine secretion. It must be controlled and balanced to be efficient and to result in the elimination of the pathogen. IAD is probably related to an inappropriate response of the innate immune system: either an uncontrolled chronic inflammation or, on the contrary, a too low inflammatory response, favoring the occurrence of secondary microbial and fungal infections. The fact that some scientists propose to treat the IAD by anti-inflammatory drugs administration while others recommend to control it by giving stimulants of immunity gives an idea of the extent of the lack of knowledge on this syndrome.

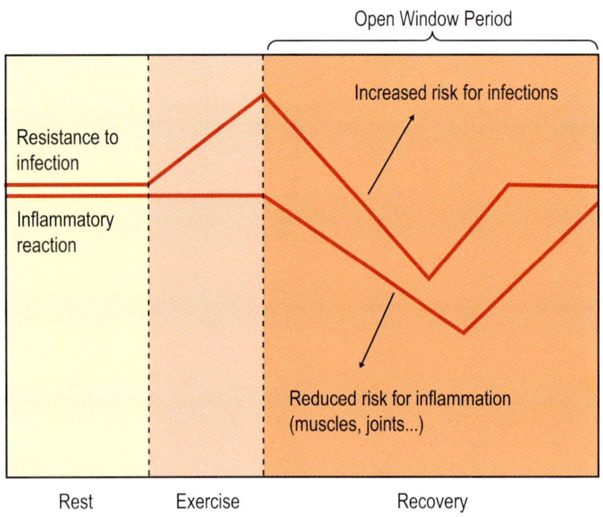

Fig 45.4 Inflammatory reaction and resistance to infection, before, during and after an intense exercise in man. The recovery period is associated with an immunodepression called the 'Open Window Period'.[4] There is an increased risk for infection but also a down-regulation of inflammation, suggesting that this phenomenon could finally result in a positive balance for the individual.

the innate response is evaluated through in vitro studies of the phagocytic and/or oxidative capacities of the macrophages and neutrophils, and on the cytotoxicity of the NK[1,2] (Table 45.2).

Studies of adaptive immunity are less frequent and related to lymphocyte proliferation after specific or non-specific stimulation, and the dosage of cytokines, as well as to the production of antibody.[9,19,21]

The observations reported in the horses are rather similar to those observed in humans: namely

- an intense – or prolonged – effort is associated with an early neutrophil burst (and leukocytes in general); secretion of pro-inflammatory cytokines during exercise and augmentation of LAK activity[22–24]
- a later impairment of the innate immunity during the recovery period.[10,16,25,26,27,28]

Mechanisms involved in these changes

Hormonal secretions

Modulation of innate immunity during exercise is dependent on the hormonal millieu.[29] Epinephrine and norepinephrine, cortisol, growth hormone, prolactin, leptin and β-endorphins increase during exercise[30–32] and could be partially responsible for the observed modifications in immunity[33,34] (Fig. 45.5).

For example, catecholamines could be responsible for the leukocytosis observed during exercise and the functional depression of the lymphocytes, but they could also induce the demargination of

Table 45.2 Some immune changes with intense exercise

CELL OR FUNCTION	CELL NUMBER	FUNCTION	REFERENCES
Leukocytes	↑	↑	27
Neutrophils (same observation in endurance)	↑	Phagocytosis/chemotaxis/O_2 burst ↓	20,27 (28)
Lymphocytes	↑	Proliferation ↓ or =	16,21,24–26
LAK cells	–	↑ activity, later ↓	19
Alveolar macrophages	= or ↓	Phagocytic activity ↓ (3 days after) Respiratory burst = or ↓ Response to stimulation of TLR3 ↓ (24 h after)	26,40 10

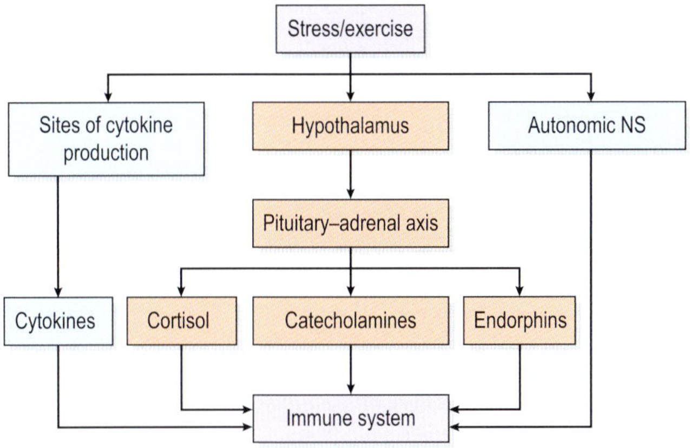

Fig 45.5 The stimulation of the hypothalamic–pituitary–adrenal axis is probably the most important factor modulating immunity during exercise. However, other factors also probably play a non-negligible role, such as the stimulation of the autonomic system, or the secretion of pro- or anti-inflammatory cytokines.

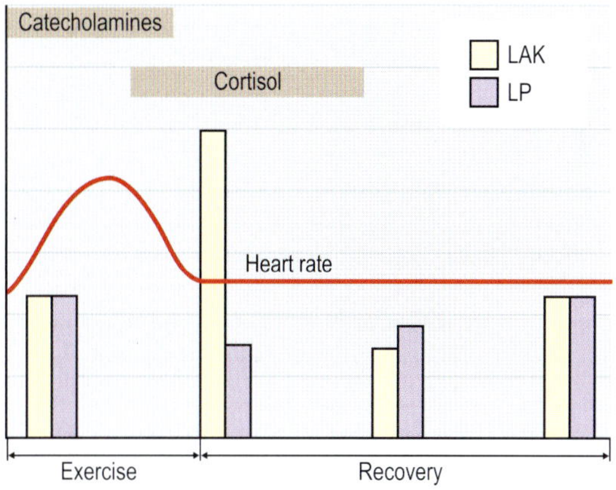

Fig 45.6 Equine exercise–immunology model.[2] Exercise is associated with the early production of catecholamines and an increase in heart rate. Cortisol production occurs later and is intensity dependent. Lymphokine-activated killer (LAK) cell activity and the lymphoproliferative (LP) response to mitogens are at a baseline level prior to exercise. Upon completion of exercise, LAK activity increases, with a concomitant decrease in the LP response. Later in the recovery period, both LAK and LP responses are suppressed, although eventually they will return to baseline levels.

the neutrophils and, consequently, increase their phagocytic capacity during exercise. The cortisol, which increases later, could be the main factor responsible for the immunosuppression that occurs after exercise[33] (Fig. 45.6). However, horses are more resistant to corticoids than other species: immune suppression by corticosteroïds can be absent or require higher doses and prolonged exposure to occur.[2,35]

Cytokine IL-6 and other factors

Recently, IL-6 has also been involved in the immunodepression induced by exercise. Skeletal muscle acts as an endocrine organ, secreting mediators that have the ability to reduce or enhance systemic inflammation. In man, during exercise, the muscle is the primary source of IL-6: both muscular genic expression and circulating IL-6 are strongly increased.[36] The physiological importance of this increase in IL-6 is still subject to discussion. Although having pro-inflammatory effects, it could have, in the case of exercise, anti-inflammatory effects for several reasons: it could be the signal responsible for the rise in the cortisol concentrations (by increasing ACTH but also by direct stimulation on the adrenal gland), for the secretion of two anti-inflammatory cytokines (IL-10 and IL-1ra) and for the reduction of secretion of TNF-α. The anti-inflammatory effect of this usually pro-inflammatory cytokine is called the 'IL-6 paradox'.[4]

Other hypothetical and/or experimentally assessed factors are:

- decrease of plasma glutamine, an amino acid essential for the function of some leukocytes
- exercise-induced endotoxemia. During efforts of high intensity or long duration, endotoxemia is observed in humans and horses. It is probably from the gastrointestinal tract and related to a change in the permeability of the intestinal barrier, perhaps secondary to splanchnic hypoperfusion. The endotoxin can have deleterious effects through stimulation of release of endogenous mediators by the mononucleated cells. This exercise-induced endotoxemia is therefore proposed by some scientists as a factor modulating innate immunity in athletes[34]
- inhalation of cold air could also influence the pulmonary innate immunity, but the theory is not confirmed by experimental data in humans. In horses, breathing cold air during exercise increases the secretion of pro-inflammatory cytokines in the BAL (IL-1, IL6; IL-8 and TNF-α) for 24 to 48 hours after exercise.[37]

Effect of training

Modification of innate immunity in response to exercise is transitory and, generally, a return to the basal level is observed 72 hours after exercise (at the latest). After this period, it is not possible to discriminate an athlete from a sedentary subject, as regards their innate immunity. So, suprisingly, and in contradiction with the epidemiologic data, in humans there is no measurable effect of training. This is in opposition to the clinical observation that chronic inflammatory problems are less frequent in the active person than in the sedentary person. This effect appears to be a consequence of the reduction in the adipose tissue in active individuals. Adipocytes and macrophages located in fatty tissue secrete pro-inflammatory cytokines and leptin. For this reason, fat is regarded as a neuroendocrine organ favoring the development of chronic inflammation[4] and its disappearance with regular physical activity probably explains the anti-inflammatory effect of moderate activity in man. In horses, there is also a positive correlation between obesity and the blood level of pro-inflammatory cytokine (TNF-α).[38]

Effect of overtraining

When human athletes overtrain there is no more functional recovery of innate immunity during periods of rest, probably because there is an overlap of the immunosuppressed periods (Open Window Period) induced by intense exercise. The strategy exposes the athletes to a significant risk of disease.[12] There is no information about the effect of overtraining on the immunity in horses.

Modulation of the adaptations of the innate immunity by nutritional strategies

Nutritional strategies (glutamine, vitamin C, indomethacin, carbohydrates [HCO]) are proposed to attenuate the post-effort immunosuppression in humans. For example, providing HCO during the exercise reduces the increase in plasma concentration catecholamines and cortisol and, consequently, reduces the disturbances in immunity.[39]

Innate immunity and inflammation

The term *inflammation* is used to describe the biological environment produced by activated macrophages, including the presence of cytokines, chemokines and other proteins that are involved in the innate immunity response. The inflammatory response can be acute as in transitory physical injury or infection, and generally in this case, it is favorable for the organisms. But it can also be of low grade and chronic, as in long-term infections, autoimmune diseases or chronic inflammation. In this case, inflammation is deleterious for the organisms and is associated with innate immunity dysregulation[4] (Fig. 45.7). As previously mentioned, the anti-inflammatory effect of exercise in man has been suggested to result from several factors, including activation of the hypothalamic–pituitary–adrenal axis, resulting in glucocorticoid suppression of immune response; reduction of adipose tissues; reduction of the macrophage accumulation in the adipose tissue; and secretion of IL-6 by the exercising muscles.[29] Currently, it is not known whether the same mechanisms exists in horses. Nevertheless, when considering the epidemiology of diseases in racehorses, training seems to favor occurrence of inflammatory processes rather than to prevent it.[14] This could be because in horses athletes are very young and exercise rarely at moderate intensity but generally at very high intensity. This point remains to be better understood.

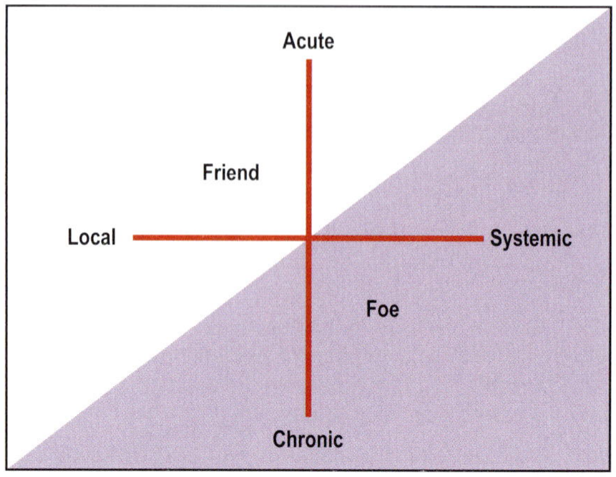

Fig 45.7 Friend or foe? The inflammatory response can be acute as in transitory physical injury or infection, and generally, in this case, it is favorable for the organism and helps to eliminate the infectious agent. But it might be also low grade and chronic, as in long-term infections, autoimmune diseases or chronic inflammation. In this case, inflammation is deleterious for the organism and is associated with innate immunity dysregulation.

Effects of exercise on the innate immunity in the respiratory system

Up to now, most of the studies related to the modifications of immunity with exercise in the horse have been focused on the actors of innate immunity in the blood, while there are few scientific papers available on the effect of the effort on pulmonary defenses in this species.[18]

In humans, studies are focused on the IgA in saliva and at the level of upper airway mucosal membranes, probably because respiratory infections in athletes are frequently observed at this level,[13] and because tracheal washes or broncho-alveolar lavages (BAL) are not routinely performed in humans.

Alveolar macrophages are the main phagocytes located in the lower airway. They play a key role in the non-specific immunity of the lung, particularly as the first-line antiviral defense. They also play a central role in the initiation and the regulation of the inflammatory pulmonary response to external aggressions. Other cells also take part in the non-specific defense at the pulmonary level: these are the neutrophils, the lymphocytes specialized cells (the natural killer), and the epithelial cells.

The effort does not induce any change in the cellular composition of BAL fluid but induces a depression of alveolar macrophage function up to 3 days after an intense exercise.[26,40] On the other hand, at the end of the period of training, there is an increase in the number of cells in the BAL and particularly of the neutrophils, suggesting the occurrence of a pulmonary inflammation. The post-effort phagocytic capacity of the macrophages is reduced with training, but , by contrast, their oxidative burst is increased after the effort before and after training.[40]

An interesting finding is also the possible role of the exercise-induced pulmonary hemorrhage. Observation of erythrocytes around macrophages in BAL fluid in some horses suggests impairment of the phagocytic capacity of the alveolar macrophages due to the presence of the red cells in the lung. This is possibly due to spatial occupation of the receptors and reduction in the oxidative capacity after phagocytosis of erythrocytes.[40] This observation suggests that (1) from a experimental point of view, it is necessary to lyse the red cells contained in the BAL before testing the phagocytic capacity; and, (2) on the other hand, that it could have a genuine clinical consequence in the racehorses, which are known to regularly suffer from pulmonary hemorrhages.

Recently, studies realized on TLR3 and TLR4 response to specific stimulation demonstrated a possible decrease in viral resistance at the level of the BAL leukocytes 24 hours after a strenuous exercise in Thoroughbreds.[10]

Conclusions

Our knowledge on the effect of exercise on immunity is still incomplete, especially in the horses. This lack of informations is related to the difficulty of assessing the response of the immune system and to standardize the experimental conditions. There are numerous factors that influence the results and conclusions of the scientific works: the type of cells and the function studied, the cytokine examined, the kind of exercise performed, the time of sampling, the level of training, the age of the athlete and other factors. Moreover, it is up to now difficult to assess the genuine clinical importance of experimental findings.

Information from human medicine suggest that (i) exercise is associated to an hypereactivity of the immune system during the effort, followed by (ii) a hyporeactivity (immunosuppression) in the hours, or even days, after the effort, (iii) that the chronic repetition of light to moderate exercise could be useful to improve immunity and decrease the inflammatory reactions and (iv) that overtraining induces immunosuppression. The results of the studies performed in horses show the same trends. However, the direct transposition of the conclusions of human studies to horses might be hazardous given the differences between the species. For example, field observations show that, while human athletes frequently suffer from upper airway diseases, horses, on the contrary, suffer frequently from lower airway disease and that moderate exercise in man decreases the risk of inflammation while the opposite is observed in horses. The presence of erythrocytes in the airway related to exercise-induced pulmonary hemorrhage in horses might play a role in the efficiency of pulmonary macrophages function. Furthermore, the horse seems to be less sensitive to increases in serum cortisol concentration than other species, adipose tissue is of very low importance in this species and we do not know whether the working muscles secrete IL-6 during exercise. Further work is therefore necessary to improve our understanding of the effect of exercise and training on the innate immunity and inflammation in this species.

References

1. Hines MT, Schott HC, Bayly WM, et al. Exercise and immunity: a review with emphasis on the horse. J Vet Intern Med 1996;10:280–9.
2. Horohov DW. Immunological response to exercise and training. In: Hinchcliff KW, Kaneps AJ, Geor RJ, editors. Equine Sports Medicine and Training. Edinburgh: Saunders; 2004. p. 1000–10.
3. Woods JA, Davis JM, Smith JA, et al. Exercise and cellular innate immune function. Med Sci Sports Exerc 1999;31:57–66.
4. Woods JA, Vieira VJ, Keylock KT. Exercise, Inflammation and innate immunity. Immunol Allergy Clin North Am 2009;29:381–93.
5. Takeda K, Kaisho T, Akira S. Toll-like receptors. Annu Rev Immunol 2003;21:335–76.
6. Akira S, Uematsu S, Takeuchi O. Pathogen recognition and innate immunity. Cell 2006;124:783–801.
7. Figueiredo MD, Vandenplas ML, Hurley DJ, et al. Differential induction of MyD88- and TRIF-dependent pathways in equine monocytes by Toll-like receptor agonists. Vet Immunol Immunopathol 2009;127:125–34.
8. Kwon S, Vandenplas ML, Figueiredo MD, et al. Differential induction of Toll-like receptor gene expression in equine monocytes activated by Toll-like receptor ligands or TNF-alpha. Vet Immunol Immunopathol 2010;138:213–17.
9. Wattrang E, Palm AK, Wagner B. Cytokine production and proliferation upon in vitro oligodeoxyribonucleotide stimulation of equine peripheral blood mononuclear cells. Vet Immunol Immunopathol 2012;146:113–24.
10. Mignot CC, Pirottin D, Farnir F, et al. Effect of strenuous exercise and ex vivo TLR3 and TLR4 stimulation on inflammatory gene expression in equine pulmonary leukocytes. Vet Immunol Immunopathol 2012;47:127–35.
11. Wood JL, Newton JR, Chanter N, et al. Association between respiratory disease and bacterial and viral infections in British racehorses. J Clin Microbiol 2005;43:120–6.
12. MacKinnon LT. Special feature for the Olympics: effects of exercise on the immune system: overtraining effects on immunity and performance in athletes. Immunol Cell Biol 2000;78:502–9.
13. Nieman DC. Exercise, upper respiratory tract infection, and the immune system. Med Sci Sport Exer 1994;26:128–39.
14. Richard EA, Fortier GD, Pitel PH, et al. Sub-clinical diseases affecting performance in Standardbred trotters: diagnostic methods and predictive parameters. Vet J 2010;184:282–9.
15. Romeo J, Wärnberg J, Pozo T, Marcos A. Physical activity, immunity and infection. Proc Nutr Soc 2010;69:390–9.
16. Nesse LL, Johansen GI, Blom AK. Effects of racing on lymphocyte proliferation in horses. Am J Vet Res 2002;63:528–30.
17. Escribano BM, Castejon FM, Vivo R, et al. Nonspecific immune response of peripheral blood neutrophils in two horse breeds (Anglo-Arabian and Spanish-Arabian): response to exercise. Comp Immunol Microbiol Infect Dis 2005;28:145–54.
18. Ainsworth DM, Appleton JA, Eicker SW, et al. The effect of strenuous exercise on mRNA concentrations of interleukin-12, interferon-gamma and interleukin-4 in equine pulmonary and peripheral blood mononuclear cells. Vet Immunol Immunopathol 2003;91:61–71.
19. Horohov DW, Dimock A, Guirnalda P, et al. Effect of exercise on the immune response of young and old horses. Am J Vet Res 1999;6:643–7.
20. Raidal SL, Love DN, Bailey GD, et al. Effect of single bouts of moderate and high intensity exercise and training on equine peripheral blood neutrophil function. Res Vet Sci 2000a;68:141–6.
21. Folsom RW, Littlefield-Chabaud MA, French DD, et al. Exercise alters the immune response to equine influenza virus and increases susceptibility to infection. Equine Vet J 2001;33:664–9.
22. Horohov DW, Keadle TL, Pourciau SS, et al. Mechanism of exercise-induced augmentation of lymphokine activated killer (LAK) cell activity in the horse. Vet Immunol Immunopathol 1996;53: 221–33.
23. Jensen-Waern M, Lindberg A, Johannisson A, et al. The effect of an endurance ride on metabolism and neutrophil function. Equine Vet J Suppl 1999;30:605–9.
24. Keadle TL, Pourciau SS, Melrose PA, et al. Acute exercise stress modulates immune function in unfit horses. J Equine Vet Sci 1993;13:4–9.
25. Kurcz EV, Lawrence LM, Kelley KW, et al. The effect of intense exercise on the cell-mediated immune response of horses. Equine Nutr Physiol Soc 1988;8:237–9.
26. Wong CW, Thompson HL, Thong YH, et al. Effect of strenuous exercise stress on chemiluminescence response of equine alveolar macrophages. Equine Vet J 1990;22:33–5.

27. Wong CW, Smith SE, Thong YH, et al. Effects of exercise stress on various immune functions in horses. Am J Vet Res 1992;53:1414–17.
28. Robson P, Alston T, Myburgh K. Prolonged suppression of the innate immunity system in the horse following a 80km endurance race. Equine Vet J 2003;35:133–7.
29. Webster JI, Tonelli L, Sternberg EM. Neuroendocrine regulation of immunity. Annu Rev Immunol 2002;20:125–63.
30. Nagata S, Takeda F, Kurosawa M, et al. Plasma adrenocorticotropin, cortisol and catecholamines response to various exercises. Equine Vet J Suppl 1999;30:570–4.
31. Lassourd V, Gayrard V, Laroute V, et al. Cortisol disposition and production rate in horses during rest and exercise. Am J Physiol 1996;271:R25–33.
32. Art T, Franchimont P, Lekeux P. Plasma beta-endorphin response of thoroughbred horses to maximal exercise. Vet Rec 1994;135:499–503.
33. Dohms JE, Metz A. Stress – mechanisms of immunosuppression. Vet Immunol Immunop 1991;30:89–109.
34. Griffin T, Frank J. Stress and immunity: a unifying concept. Vet Immunol Immunopathol 1989;20:263–312.
35. Magnuson NS, McGuire TC, Banks KL, et al. In vitro and in vivo effects of corticosteroids on peripheral blood lymphocytes from ponies. Am J Vet Res 1978;39:393–8.
36. Malm C. Exercise-induced muscle damage and inflammation: fact or fiction? Acta Physiol Scand 2001;171:233–9.
37. Davis MS, Williams CC, Meinkoth JH, et al. Influx of neutrophils and persistence of cytokine expression in airways of horses after performing exercise while breathing cold air. Am J Vet Res 2007;68:185–9.
38. Suagee JK, Corl BA, Crisman MV, et al. Relationships between body condition score and plasma inflammatory cytokines, insulin, and lipids in a mixed population of light-breed horses. J Vet Intern Med 2013;27(1):157–63.
39. Gleeson M, Lancaster GI, Bishop NC. Nutritional strategies to minimise exercise-induced immunosuppression in athletes. Can J Appl Physiol 2001;26(Suppl):S23–35.
40. Raidal SL, Love DN, Bailey GD, et al. The effect of high intensity exercise on the functional capacity of equine pulmonary alveolar macrophages and BAL-derived lymphocytes. Res Vet Sci 2000;68: 249–53.

section 8

Gastrointestinal system

Effects of exercise on gastrointestinal function

46

Mireia Lorenzo-Figueras Alfred M. Merritt

CHAPTER CONTENTS

Introduction

Based upon the design of its gastrointestinal tract (GIT) alone, the horse would be an unlikely animal for humans to choose as their athletic alter ego. The very large cecum and folded large colon, normally filled with ingesta, must certainly not be the easiest of structures to move around. Likewise, the anatomical arrangement and complexity of function of these fermentation vats could, theoretically at least, set the system up for any number of exercise-induced abnormalities. When left to their own devices in the wild, herbivores, whether they be the forestomach fermenters or the hindgut fermenters which include the equidae, spend the large majority of their day quietly grazing or resting.[1] Instances of movement faster than a walk are usually brief and in response to attack by a predator or a rival.

'Domesticated' horses, on the other hand, are often subject to many situations that result in a greater percentage of their level of daily activity being much more vigorous than just walking and standing around grazing. In human medicine, *physical activity* is defined as any bodily movement produced by skeletal muscles that results in energy expenditure, whereas *exercise* is a subset of physical activity that is planned, structured and repetitive with a final objective of maintenance or improvement of physical fitness.[2] While hard data concerning the effect of any form of exertion on the equine GIT, whether it be physical activity or exercise, are scarce, we have some results showing that even the anticipation of an upcoming training session on a treadmill, such as turning on the treadmill motor, will evoke an increase in intra-abdominal pressure, reflecting tensing of the abdominal muscles.[3] One outstanding effect this pressure increase, and that associated with subsequent trotting or galloping, has on the stomach, for example, will be discussed later in this chapter. The point is that the intra-abdominal pressure response could have far-reaching effects on abdominal viscera, and that the character of the response could vary depending upon the type and duration of the exertion. Galloping may have a different effect than trotting, while trotting may have a different effect than pacing. Jumping may have entirely unique consequences. Effects could include distortion and/or displacement of viscera, redirection of blood flow, and release of various regulatory peptides.

A study of human subjects that were 'encouraged to perform at near-maximal effort' indicated that runners have more complaints of gastroesophageal reflux (GERD) than do cyclists.[4] Could this be because, in the bent over position in which they ride, cyclists create less abdominal muscle press than do runners? Or is it because, as one report has suggested, the physical displacement of the abdominal viscera associated with the 'pounding of the pavement' results in an irritation that produces symptoms – the so-called 'cecal slap syndrome'?[5] Or, could it be a question of experimental methodology, since two subsequent studies found that subjects asked to perform at up to 90% VO_{2max} on a stationary bicycle experienced gastroesophageal reflux that was exercise-intensity dependent?[6,7] Then, another study found that GERD symptoms and reflux were even more prevalent in weight lifters than either runners or cyclists.[8]

that is, type, duration and intensity of exercise all need to be considered from the standpoint of potentially differential effects on the gut.

Finally, considering all of the things humans ask horses to do in the form of exertion, are some forms more stressful than others? In general, existent data indicate a direct relationship between plasma ACTH and cortisol concentrations and intensity and duration of exercise, respectively, in horses.[9–11] But in one study, for instance, galloping caused no significant increase in pituitary venous blood corticotropin-releasing factor (CRF), although ACTH concentration did increase significantly.[12] These issues must also be factored in with respect to the potential impact on the GIT.

This chapter considers the effects of exercise on:

- digestion
- absorption
- secretion
- motility
- maintenance of mucosal barrier integrity
- liver specific functions.

These functions are directly influenced by blood flow status, and activity within the enteric nervous system (ENS), which may be strictly intrinsic or may be modified by input from the central nervous system (CNS). With respect to horses, some special species-relevant aspects of these functions deserve note.

Digestion

Some fermentation of soluble carbohydrate occurs within the stomach, with subsequent production of lactic and volatile fatty acids (VFAs).[13] Whether and to what extent these products are absorbed across the gastric wall and into the bloodstream is not known, although a large proportion should be in the non-ionized, diffusable form, given the acidic environment and they may have some ulcerogenic effects on the non-glandular (squamous) mucosa.[14] Pancreatic secretion, on the other hand, while being large in volume, is relatively low in amylase and protease activity.[15] The usual complement of small intestinal (brush border) disaccharide enzymes is present in horses, but small intestinal proteolytic enzymes have not been measured.[16] From a comparative perspective, the one thing that makes horses unique with respect to other domestic species is the degree of cecal and colonic digestion of dietary fiber; up to 35% of daily caloric needs may be derived from the volatile fatty acids produced from the fermentation of dietary fiber.[17]

Absorption

As indicated above, one of the most unique aspects of equine gut function is the fermentation of carbohydrates at both ends of the tract. While we still know little about where and how the products of gastric fermentation are absorbed, we do know that absorption of VFAs produced in the cecum and colon requires mucosal Na^+/H^+ exchange.[18] A mole of water follows each mole of VFA to be absorbed. Furthermore, aldosterone plays an important role in determining the amount of Na, and the water that follows it, that is resorbed by the lower parts of the colon. It follows that disruption of any of the mechanisms involved in support of normal mucosal function, because of an exercise-related event for example, could have major consequences on water and electrolyte balance, and nutrition. In addition, under conditions where the cecum and colons are presented with a large amount of fermentable carbohydrate over a short period of time, the production rate of the VFAs may initially outstrip absorption and, through the osmotic gradient created, pull water from plasma into the colonic lumen.[19]

Secretion

Gastric acid secretion occurs in the horse even under fasting conditions.[20] The important role played by acid in gastric squamous mucosal ulcerogenesis has been demonstrated, especially as related to the high incidence of this form of gastric ulcer disease in horses under intensive training conditions.[3,21–23] This association probably provides one of the clearest representations to date of how exertion can affect the equine GIT (see below). At least when the stomach is empty, small intestinal contents, made up primarily of pancreatic juice, periodically reflux into the stomach, providing some buffering of the acid present.[24] Effects of exercise, if any, on this process still need to be investigated. Finally, the horse undoubtedly possesses all the intestinal secretory mechanisms that have been described in other species, but to what degree needs to be defined. What must be remembered is that, in contrast to humans and animals with relatively simple colons, a hypersecretion of strictly small intestinal origin in the horse would not manifest as diarrhea because of the ability, from a water balance perspective, of the ceco-colon to compensate for that malfunction.[25] Thus, diarrhea in adult horses is indicative of a large bowel dysfunction, which could include hypersecretion at this level.

Motility

As an extension of the human experience,[26] horse trainers often try to schedule the training sessions for a time when they think the horse has a relatively empty stomach. Humans in general do not feel that they can perform maximally on a 'full stomach.' It has been shown that pedaling exercise slows gastric emptying rate in humans, although more runners than cyclists complain of GI problems.[4,27–29] Effects of exercise on gastric motility and emptying function in horses are not known as they may have important implications regarding squamous mucosal ulcerogenesis, among other things. As in other species, the proximal stomach relaxes in response to active ingestion (receptive relaxation), and the degree of this relaxation is directly related to the amount of feed ingested.[30] A more sustained, but less profound, post-ingestion proximal relaxation (accommodation) then occurs, along with peristaltic-like contractions that begin in the middle of the gastric body and traverse through the antrum and promote emptying of gastric contents into the duodenum. The presence of those contents within the duodenum will, in turn, have modulatory effects on the rate of gastric emptying, the degree of which will depend upon their specific composition.[31] This complex regulatory process could be affected by exertion. As indicated earlier, intragastric fermentation of ingested soluble carbohydrates occurs to a considerable degree in horses and this implies gas production as a result.[13] It follows that this gas must also be moved aborally into the duodenum, since horses do not normally eructate. Likewise, the large amount of gas that is generated from hindgut fermentation must be moved aborally, along with the contents, to be expelled via the anus. Thus, any condition that could adversely reduce the delivery of gas and/or contents, such as an exercise-induced dysmotility, could result in notable abdominal discomfort and/or diarrhea.

Maintenance of mucosal barrier integrity

Normal gut function is dependent upon a reasonably intact barrier between luminal contents and the submucosa.[32–34] Maintenance of barrier integrity is dependent upon numerous factors that include blood flow, mucosal cell turnover rate and immunological tolerance to luminal antigens. Methods for experimentally evaluating the 'leakiness' of GI mucosa are discussed below. From the few in vivo and in vitro studies done to date, it appears that horses probably will not differ fundamentally from other species with respect to regional mucosal barrier characteristics, although this needs much more investigation.[35–40]

Liver specific functions

Irrespective of species, normal liver function is critical to good health, and this is highly dependent upon adequate blood supply from both arterial and portal venous sources. Blood supply is emphasized here because it is probably the aspect of liver function most prone to modification by exercise. From a species-specific perspective, it should also be kept in mind that certain detoxifying and conjugative functions of the equine liver might be prone to modulation by fasting and fever, as is the case for endogenously generated bilirubin.[41]

Available methodologies to document the effects of exercise on the equine gastrointestinal system

Methods that have been used in horses

Transit markers

Gastrointestinal transit time can be measured by the use of indigestible, non-absorbable markers. The rate of passage is normally expressed as mean retention time (amount of marker excreted at a certain time after administration of the marker), cumulative excretion or % recovery rate. Comparison of rate of digesta passage during rest and light to moderate exercise has been evaluated in horses and donkeys. Some of the markers used in these studies were cobalt-EDTA, for liquid phase, chromium-mordanted fiber, for solid phase, and ruthenium-phenanthroline and ytterbium chloride, for particulates passage.[42–44] A recent review of the subject found that published values for mean retention time (MRT) for digesta passage through the equine GIT ranged from 18 to 60 hours, depending upon many factors, including type of food and marker used, with most of the variability most likely occurring within the large intestine.[45]

Non-absorbable markers, such as phenol red in man,[27,46,47] and horse,[48] and polyethylene glycol in dog,[49] have been used to measure the effect of different levels of exercise on gastric emptying (GE) of liquid meals. After ingestion of a labeled meal, gastric contents are aspirated through a nasogastric tube or recovered by drainage through a gastric cannula. The amount of marker remaining in the stomach after exercise will depend on the rate of GE of the labeled meal. Sosa et al. reported that GE of a single dose of isotonic fluid administered after intense exercise (70% VO_{2max}) in the horse did not differ from rest, which suggests that GE is not a limitation for rehydration. However, as discussed by the authors of this study, the results were highly variable, suggesting high measurement error due to the technique.[48]

Apparent digestibility of diet

Apparent digestibility is calculated as the difference between specific components of the diet and those found in feces, expressed as percent utilization. Changes in efficiency of dietary fiber utilization in response to exercise may reflect changes in the passage rate of digesta, the activity or population of microbes within the gut, or mucosal integrity.[50] The effect of exercise on digestibility has been studied in horses with inconsistent results.

Pearson and Merritt studied the effect of a 14-km walk in donkeys, and neither GI transit nor the digestibility of hay was affected.[42] On the other hand, Pagan et al. showed that 8 km of trotting and galloping by a group of Thoroughbreds resulted in a small, but significant decrease in dry matter digestibility, whereas transit rates of both a forage diet and a forage/grain diet were increased at 24 hours after the exercise.[43] Orton et al. studied the effect of 12-km daily trotting in yearling horses and recorded an increase in apparent digestibility of dry matter transit rate of particulates, but decreased transit rate of the fluid phase[44] (Fig. 46.1). Similarly, Goachet et al. saw an increased apparent digestibility in Arabian horses after endurance training (Table 46.1)[51]. As Goachet et al. point out,

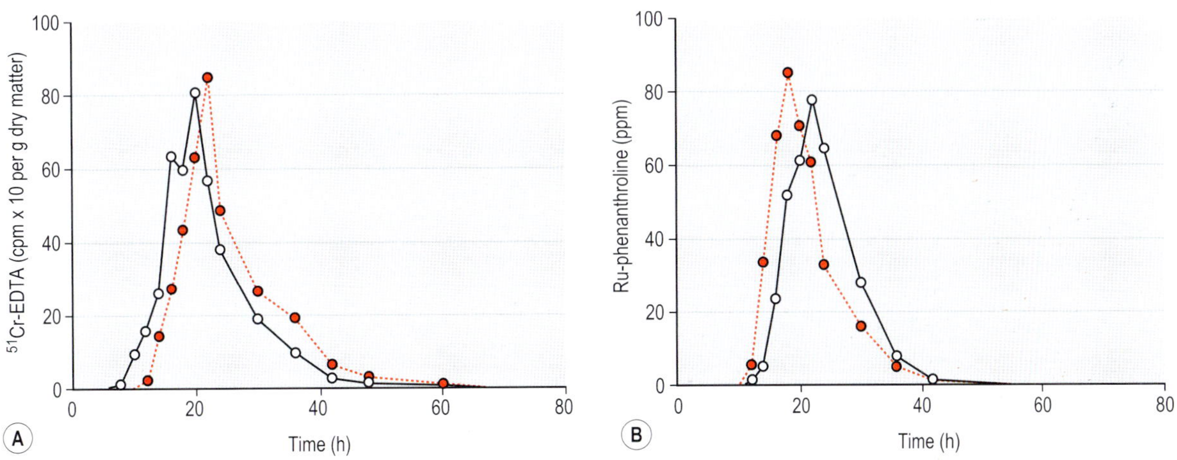

Fig 46.1 Effect of exercise on rate of passage of fluid **(A)** and particulate **(B)** digesta. **(A)** Concentration of ^{51}Cr-EDTA in the feces of exercised (broken red line) and non-exercised (solid black line) yearling horses. Four animals per group. **(B)** Concentration of ruthenium (Ru)-phenanthroline in the feces of exercised (broken red line) and non-exercised (solid black line) yearling horses. Four animals per group. Exercise: 12 km trotting at 12 km/h. Transit of the fluid phase marker **(A)** was delayed in exercised horses, whereas transit of the particulate phase marker **(B)** was accelerated. These results are supported by Pagan et al,[32] who observed that fecal excretion of the particulate marker ytterbium was accelerated in Thoroughbreds trotted and galloped for 8 km/day.

Reprinted from Orton RK, Hume ID, Leng RA. Effects of exercise and level of dietary protein on digestive function in horses. Equine Vet J 1985;17:386-390, with permission from the Equine Veterinary Journal.

experimental conditions, particularly exercise regimen during measurements, may explain these contradictions as they can cause misconception between short-term effects of exercise and long-term adaptations through physical activity. Clearly, many more studies need to be done on this subject.

Table 46.1 Digestibility measurements performed in Arabian horses at the control level (P01) and after conditioning periods corresponding to incremental endurance racing levels at 60 and 90 km. During the measurement periods, feed intake and diet composition were similar

N = 7	P01	P60	P90	s.e.	P VALUE
bwt (kg)	442[a]	434[a,b]	430[b]	3	0.03
BCS	3.4[a]	3.2[a]	2.7[b]	0.06	<0.0001
DMd (%)	57.7[a]	60.5[a,b]	64.4[b]	1.1	0.008
OMd (%)	52.4[a]	55.3[a,b]	59.7[b]	1.4	0.010
NDFd (%)	36.2[a]	39.7[a]	43.8[b]	1.8	0.031

Means in rows with different superscripts are significantly different ($P < 0.05$). bwt, Bodyweight; BCS, body condition score; DMd, dry matter total tract apparent digestibility; OMd, organic matter total tract apparent digestibility; NDFd, neutral detergent fiber total tract apparent digestibility. Adapted from Goachet A-G, Varloud M, Philippeau C et al. Long-term effects of endurance training on total tract apparent digestibility, total mean retention time and faecal microbial ecosystem in competing Arabian horses. Eq Vet J 2010; 42, Suppl 38:387-392, with permission from John Wiley and Sons.

Barostat

The electronic barostat has been extensively used to document gastrointestinal motility in many species, including horses.[3,52–54] Unlike other methods, this system is more useful for recording changes in smooth muscle tone than active, phasic contractions. The principle of the barostat is to maintain a constant pressure within a plastic bag of infinite compliance, positioned within the lumen of the segment to be studied. When the internal pressure of the organ increases for any reason (e.g. contraction, increased mural tone), the barostat aspirates air from the bag to maintain the intra-bag pressure constant. Conversely, when the internal pressure decreases, air is injected into the bag. Therefore, as the bag follows the movement of the visceral walls, changes in bag volume are an indirect measurement of changes in tone of the organ[55] (Fig. 46.2).

In other instances, changes in bag volume reflect changes in external pressure exerted over the organ containing the bag. As we mentioned earlier, we observed such changes in the proximal stomach of horses under a training session and related them to increased intra-abdominal pressure caused by tensing of the abdominal muscles during exercise.[3] Interestingly, we also observed relaxation of the proximal stomach in some horses soon after exercise (*data not published*). What effect this might have on gastric emptying, for instance, could provide some useful information concerning optimal timing of feeding with respect to a given exercise schedule.

Blood flow measurement

Adequate local perfusion is necessary for normal gut tissue activity, which requires oxygen and nutrients supplied by peripheral blood. Exercise leads to blood flow diversion from the gastrointestinal tract

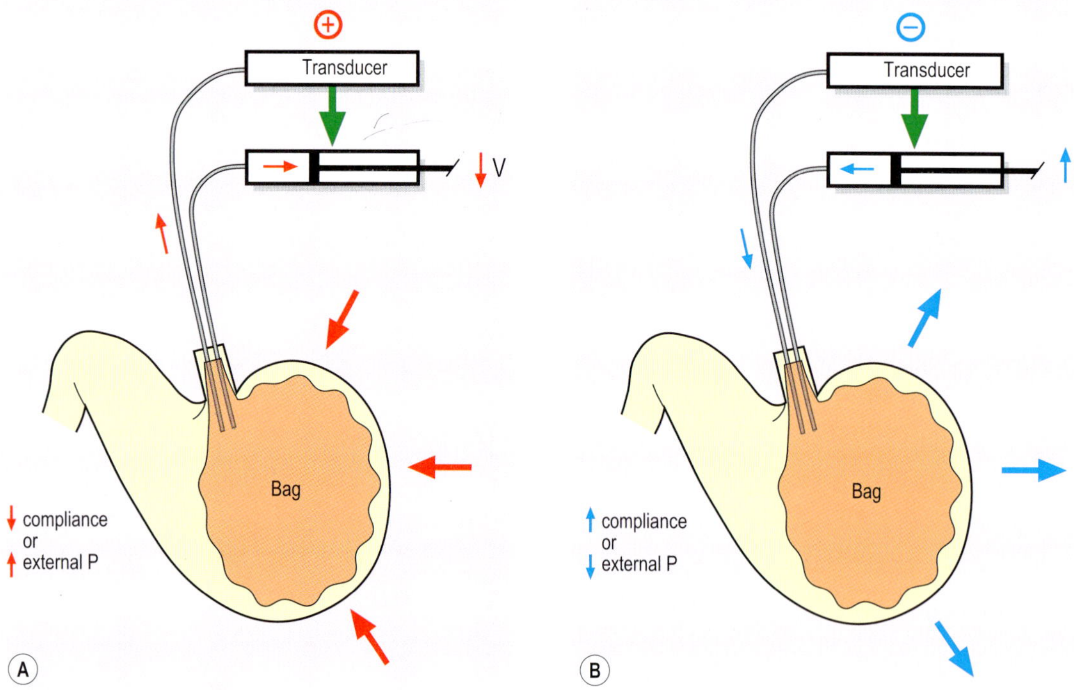

Fig 46.2 Motility of the stomach can be indirectly measured by an electronic barostat. The barostat maintains a constant pressure (P) within an intragastric bag. **(A)** When the stomach relaxes or the gastric wall becomes more compliant, the system injects air into the bag. **(B)** Conversely, when the stomach contracts or the gastric wall becomes less compliant, air is aspirated from the bag. Changes in bag volume (V) can also reflect changes in pressure exerted extraluminally upon the stomach. The same method could be applied to study motility at any site of the intestine.

to the working skeletal muscles and the skin.[56] Decreased perfusion or ischemic damage may result in impairment of normal function of the gastrointestinal tissues, including mechanisms of mucosal protection, membrane secretory and absorptive functions, and motility.

The effect of short-term exercise on blood flow of abdominal organs has been measured in the horse, using radionuclide-labeled microspheres.[57] Once injected into the general circulation, the distribution of microspheres is proportional to the blood flow during its first transit through the circulation.[58,59] In the above-mentioned study by Manohar et al. significant vasoconstriction occurred in all gastrointestinal tract tissues during short-term exercise, which caused blood flow to be diverted away from these vascular beds.[57]

Additionally, hepatic blood flow can be quantified by IV infusion of a marker, such as, bromsulphalein (BSP). As BSP is highly extracted by the liver, hepatic clearance of BSP is mainly dependent on liver blood flow. Decreases in blood clearance of BSP in horses have been attributed to exercise-induced splanchnic vasoconstriction, leading to decreased portal vein blood flow.[60]

Continuous pH monitoring

Continuous pH monitoring of the GIT luminal contents with a self-referencing pH electrode may be useful for tracking the effects of exercise on digestive function. The stomach and distal small colon are accessible without special preparation; other parts of the tract would need to be surgically cannulated. Continuous recording of pH changes within the proximal portion of the stomach has indicated that exposure of the non-glandular (squamous) mucosa to hydrochloric acid is increased during periods when forage ingestion is reduced and during exercise.[3,61]

(See Fig. 46.3.) To date, there is nothing in the literature that describes pH changes within the small colon in response to exercise. Such data have the potential to provide information about the effect of exercise on mucosal secretion, net electrolyte flux and fermentation activity within the large intestine.

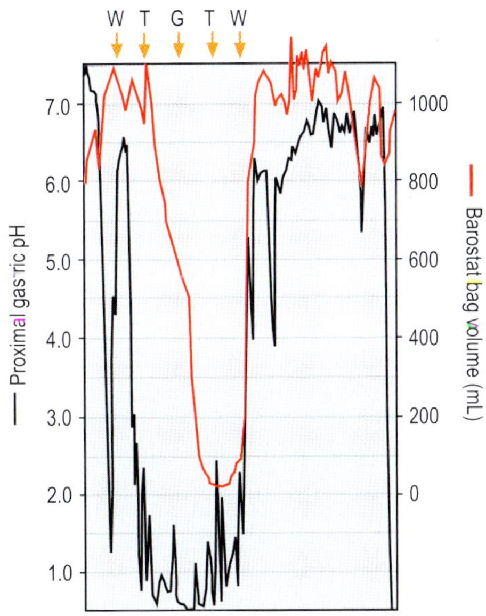

Fig 46.3 Composite of continuous pH and intragastric barostat bag volume monitoring in two different horses, respectively, during exercise. **In red**: changes in intragastric pressure were indirectly measured by changes in volume of a bag placed within the proximal stomach, with its internal pressure constantly controlled at 6 mmHg by an electronic barostat. The decrease in volume indicates increased pressure >6 mmHg on the bag. **In black:** intragastric pH was measured by a self-referencing pH electrode positioned 2 cm below the entrance of the stomach. Both patterns are characteristic responses to exercise (W = walk; T = trot; G = gallop).

Measurement of GI regulatory peptides and steroids

Modification of gastrointestinal regulatory peptides and steroids in response to exercise may either result in, or reflect changes in, gastrointestinal function. Some of these substances have been measured in horses under different exercise regimens, varying in type, intensity and duration.

Exercise stimulates adrenal secretion and activity of the sympathetic autonomic nervous system. This stimulation is reflected in increased plasma levels of ACTH, catecholamines, cortisol and β-endorphins, which are used as indices of physical stress.[9–11,62–64] As the horse's fitness improves, these hormonal responses to exercise diminish.[65] Variations in plasma cortisol are more sensitive to duration of exercise, whereas ACTH and catecholamine levels are more closely correlated with exercise intensity.[9,11,66] The effect of variations of stress hormone levels upon equine gastrointestinal function is still unknown. In other species, cortisol can have a deleterious effect on mucosal immune function and epithelial permeability,[67] whereas catecholamines have the potential to delay gastric emptying, prolong transit time,[68,69] and decrease perfusion of the gastric mucosa.[70]

Gastrin is a major regulatory peptide of acid secretion, the plasma concentration of which was increased after prolonged exercise in the horse in one study,[71] but not in another.[72] In a third study, gastrin concentration did not increase after short, sprint exercise, but was higher postprandially in trained horses, compared to non-trained horses.[73] Whether this has any significant effect on the pH of gastric contents remains to be determined. Plasma concentrations of inhibitors of gastric acid secretion, such as somatostatin in man[74] and vasoactive intestinal polypeptide (VIP) in man[75] and horse,[71] may increase with exercise. Additionally, somatostatin may favor colonic electrolyte transport and inhibit nutrient absorption.[76]

Potential exercise-induced changes in fluid absorption and secretion within the gut may reflect changes in expression of some regulatory hormones, and vice versa. Exercise increases plasma levels of secretagogues, such as VIP and glucagon, in the horse,[71] and secretin, gastric inhibitory polypeptide and prostaglandins in man.[74,77,78] On the other hand, atrial natriuretic peptide and aldosterone, which favor sodium absorption, also increase during prolonged exercise in horses.[63,79]

Agents such as corticotropin-factor (CRF), motilin,[80] neuropeptide Y[81] and prostaglandins[78] can affect motility and are released during endurance-type exercise in man and the same could be expected in horses.[10] For instance, activation of CRF signaling pathways mediates both the inhibition of upper gastrointestinal (GI) and the stimulation of lower GI motor function through interaction with different CRF receptor subtypes.[82] The effect of exercise on GI motility can, therefore, be indirectly studied by measuring endogenous expression of hormones that control the motility.

Finally, alterations of peptide expression may result from a decrease in GIT blood flow, leading to decreased hepatic and renal clearance.[56] VIP[71] and arginine vasopressin[12] in horses, and endothelin-1[83] and angiotensin II[84] in other species, are released during exercise and act as vasoconstrictors. The resulting decrease in blood flow may affect function and regulation of the GIT;

for instance, mucosal integrity is compromised by splanchnic ischemia.[85]

Methods that could potentially be useful in horses, based upon experience in other species

Gastric motility and emptying

In contrast to the phenol red technique mentioned above, barium contrast radiography[86] and scintigraphy[87] have the advantage of non-invasiveness, and have been previously applied to equine studies. An additional advantage of the latter technique is the differentiation between solid and liquid-phase emptying. Also, installation of acetominophen solution into the stomach followed by tracking of its appearance into the blood through sequential sampling is a reasonable relatively non-invasive measurement of emptying rate of *liquid* contents from the equine stomach.[87]

Breath tests employing stable isotopically labeled *solid meal* tracers are potentially very useful, since they are non-invasive, non-radioactive and easy to perform (Fig. 46.4). As it empties the stomach, the ^{13}C-enriched marker is readily absorbed in the proximal intestine and metabolized to CO_2. Thus, breath $^{13}CO_2$ enrichment reflects the rate of GE of the labeled meal. The effect of exercise on GE of carbohydrate meals marked with ^{13}C acetate has been studied in humans.[88,89] The ^{13}C-octanoate breath test has been validated in the horse[90] and its use in exertional studies is promising.

Imaging of the stomach by ultrasound has shown that strenuous exercise disrupts gastric motility in man, although the examination was done right after, rather than during, the active exertion.[91] Another available technique in humans is electrogastrography (EGG), which consists of measuring gastric myoelectrical activity by electrodes positioned on the surface of the epigastrium.[92] Although both techniques as applied to the stomach are unsuitable in the horse for anatomical reasons, they could be potentially used to measure cecal motility percutaneously – also known as electrocecography[93] – during the recovery period after exercise.

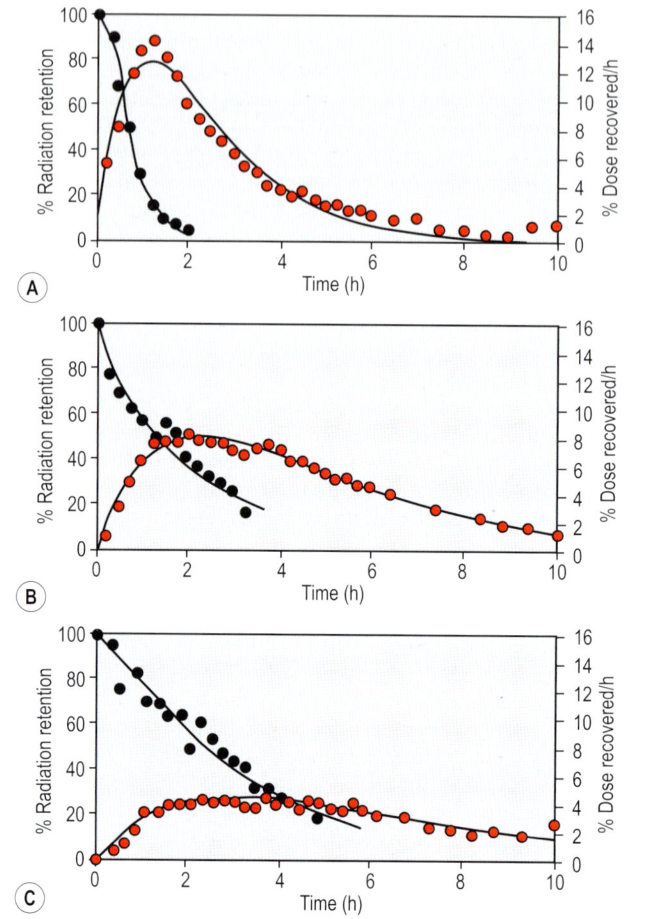

Fig 46.4 Results of simultaneous ^{13}C-octanoic acid breath test and gastric radioscintigraphy in three typical cases. **(A)** Rapid gastric emptying rate (T1/2 = 0.73 h). **(B)** Normal gastric emptying curve (T1/2 = 1.34 h). **(C)** Slow gastric emptying pattern (T1/2 = 2.62 h). Scintigraphic data • on the left y-axis and breath test data on the right y-axis are plotted against time. The continuous lines represent a modeled fit.

Reprinted with permission from Sutton DG, Bahr A, Preston T, et al. Validation of the 13C-octanoic acid breath test for measurement of equine gastric emptying rate of solids using radioscintigraphy. Equine Vet J 2003;35:27–33, with permission from the Equine Veterinary Journal.

Gastric secretion

Collection of gastric contents from cannulated dogs has allowed constant measurement of acid and pepsin during exercise.[49] This method could be useful in determining changes in acid secretion and other gastric components in cannulated horses; however, it would require that the animal be fasted. Alternatively, Varloud et al. have described a method of collecting gastric contents from conscious horses via nasogastric tube but, again, potential effects of the intubation have to be considered.[94]

Gastric blood flow

Air tonometry measures changes in luminal intragastric P_{CO_2} and seems to be more reliable indicator of gastric ischemia than measuring splanchnic blood flow. Detection of ischemia is based on the difference between arterial P_{CO_2} and intragastric P_{CO_2}, which better reflects mucosal balance between needed and supplied levels of O_2.[95] It would be interesting to apply this technique to the horse.

Intestinal transit and motility

In humans, mouth-to-cecum transit time has been measured by the H_2 *breath test* during exercise.[96,97] For this test, lactulose, a non-absorbable disaccharide, is added to the meal. Breath H_2 starts rising when lactulose reaches the cecum and is degraded by bacterial fermentation. Although fermenting bacteria are also present in the equine stomach and small intestine, the cecum and the large colon are the primary sites of microbial fermentation.[18] However, not all horses exhale excess hydrogen after ingestion of lactulose, so this technique may not be reliable.[98] Lactose, another disaccharide, has been used as a marker for H_2 breath test,[98] since adult horses appeared to be lactose intolerant.[99] Yet, the presence of brush border lactase in the small intestine of adult horses has been recently reported,[16] and also excludes the usefulness of this sugar to measure oro-cecal transit time (OCTT). However, the lactose ^{13}C ureide breath test (LUBT) has recently been validated as a measurement of OCTT in horses.[100] The labeled lactose ureide reaches the cecum intact, where it is hydrolyzed by bacteria, producing ^{13}C-labeled CO_2. In contrast to the H_2 breath test, LUBT seems to be a repeatable and more reliable method, especially for the horse.

Transcutaneous ultrasonography has recently been used to non-invasively record intestinal motility in horses. Accordingly, Williams et al. found that large intestinal motility in stabled horses was significantly reduced when compared to pastured horses,[101] and this procedure could be similarly applied after various forms of more strenuous exercise (Fig. 46.5).

Motor activity of the intestinal tract can be studied by several invasive techniques. For example, *electrodes* implanted on the serosa of the gut can detect surface potentials or voltages generated by the gastrointestinal muscle. These electrodes measure two different patterns of electrical potentials: *slow waves*, which reflect basal electric rhythm, and *action potentials*, which correlate with contractions. By implantation of bipolar electrodes in dogs, slow wave patterns and the migrating motor complex (MMC) of the proximal jejunum have been studied in relation to exercise of different intensities.[102] This technique has certainly been successfully applied to horses,[103–105] but not, as yet, to evaluate the effects of exercise.

Strain gauge transducers have also been secured onto the serosa of the GI segment to be studied; they measure mechanical instead of myoelectrical activity. They detect unidirectional, isometric muscle contractions and monitor the stress/tension applied by these muscle contractions on them. Colonic MMCs have been evaluated during long-distance exercise in dogs using this method.[106] As with the serosally applied electrodes, this technique has been used successfully in horses but never in association with exercise.[107,108]

Manometers and transducers are used to measure changes in intraluminal pressure, which are interpreted as contractions that generate them. This technique has been used to study changes in the small intestinal MMC in dogs during exercise.[49] In contrast to the other methods previously mentioned, this one does not need surgical implantation so long as the GIT section of interest is accessible by either mouth or anus.

Mucosal permeability and absorption

Intestinal permeability can be assessed non-invasively in vivo by *orally administered markers*. These markers are cleared unaltered by renal excretion, wherein their concentrations in urine can be quantified over a specified post-feeding time period to determine the amount absorbed. Appearance, or not, of these markers in the urine will depend on the integrity of the intestinal mucosa since they are not absorbed through intact mucosa.[109]

Polyethylene glycol (PEG) polymers of different molecular weights have been widely used for assessment of permeability. This marker is also used to determine net water absorption, which is calculated directly by changes in PEG concentration within the gut contents.[110] PEGs of high molecular weights have also been used as markers of gastrointestinal transit time in the horse.[111] PEG is not, however, an ideal marker for these kinds of studies, since its purported size can be somewhat variable, and too large a dose can induce an osmotic hypersecretion.[112]

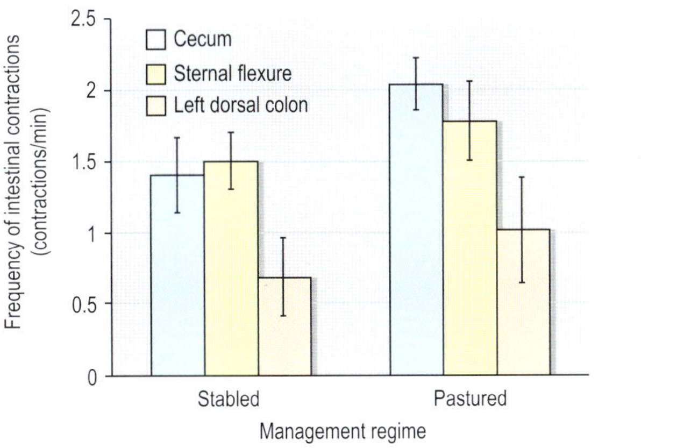

Fig 46.5 Mean ± s.d. frequency of intestinal contractions assessed by ultrasonography in the cecum, sternal flexure and left dorsal colon for horses when stabled (n = 13) and pastured (n = 7).
Reprinted with permission from Williams S, Tucker CA, Green MJ, et al. Investigation of the effect of pasture and stable management on large intestinal motility in the horse, measured using transcutaneous ultrasonography. Equine Vet J 2011;43(supp39):93–97, with permission from John Wiley and Sons.

Sugars are also commonly used as probes to evaluate intestinal integrity. Disaccharides, such as lactulose and sucrose, and monosaccharides, such as L-rhamnose, D-xylose, 3-O-D-methyl M-glucose and mannitol are used to assess both transcellular and paracellular transport capacity across the intestinal mucosa. Their natural transport across the epithelium may be impaired by cellular damage, whereas compromise of the mucosa barrier (e.g. ulceration, ischemia) may facilitate their passive movement into the bloodstream. Sugars have been used in humans to study the effect of running and cycling on intestinal transport.[113,114] Agents such as these are preferable over PEG because of their uniformity of respective size, making them better discriminators at specific sites of GIT permeability. However, in a recent study in horses that measured sucrose translocation as an indicator of gastric ulceration, it was found that it was much less invasive and more reliable to measure plasma rather than urinary appearance in this species.[115]

Finally, *isotopic tracers* like ^{51}Cr-labeled ethylenediaminetetraacetic acid (^{51}Cr-EDTA) and ^{99m}Tc-diethylenetriaminopentaacetate (^{99m}Tc-DTPA) can be added to drinks and used to measure unidirectional flux, from the intestinal lumen to the vascular compartment. Although the activity of these tracers in blood is readily measured, their radioactive character is a clear disadvantage, largely limiting application to a laboratory setting.[95]

Exercise and gastrointestinal function: what is known in other species that is pertinent to horses

Gastric motility and emptying

Different GI symptoms occur in as many as 30 to 50% of human participants in endurance events.[28,116,117] Lower GI symptoms, which include diarrhea, rectal incontinence, urge to defecate, rectal bleeding and abdominal cramps, are more common than upper GI symptoms, such as gastroesophageal reflux, nausea, vomiting and stomach pain. A direct effect of exercise on GI motility has been hypothesized to explain many of these disorders. Because of this high prevalence and the severity of some of the symptoms, many experiments have focused on the study of gastrointestinal motor function and transit. In the horse, exercise does not seem to directly result in signs of GI disturbance, but this observation should not exclude the possibility of GI alterations in response to the high demand imposed on the horse's body. Dehydration, musculoskeletal or metabolic disorders may mask mild GI tract dysfunction during long, intense exercise.

During moderate exercise (less than 75% VO_{2max}), gastric emptying in man occurs at a rate similar or slightly greater than that during rest; however, more intense exercise appears to inhibit it.[27,118] In equine events where oral supplementation with electrolyte and carbohydrate solutions may be important to compensate a deficit of water, electrolytes and carbohydrates, the rate of gastric emptying may limit the availability of administered fluids.[119] Solutions with higher carbohydrate concentration seem to delay gastric emptying in humans,[47] although increasingly larger volumes leave the stomach at faster rates.[46,120] Pyloric closure and reduced antral contractions, observed by ultrasound after exercise, may be in part responsible for the delay in gastric emptying in humans.[91] In contrast, as mentioned above, one study in horses found that gastric emptying of an isotonic fluid preparation was not affected by exercise, but this is only one study in 4 horses.[48]

Intestinal motility and transit

In humans, inactivity has often been considered a cause of constipation; conversely, physical activity seems to promote colonic transit. Soffer et al. found that bicycle exercise could convert the motor-fed pattern of the small intestine into an migrating motor complex (MMC), and that this effect was intensity related, although there was no effect on oro-cecal transit time.[97] In contrast, Moses et al.[121,122] observed that moderate and intense treadmill exercise delayed small intestinal transit in humans and van Nieuwenhoven et al.[29] documented increased oro-cecal transit time. Yet, Dainese et al.[123] found that mild physical activity enhanced intestinal gas propulsion and Strid et al. documented an acceleration of small bowel but not colonic transit during 'heavy' exercise.[124] In a study performed in fed dogs, moderate treadmill exercise decreased jejunal myoelectric activity only when exercise was prolonged beyond 30 minutes, and this inhibitory effect continued during recovery.[102] Furthermore, prolonged exercise induced MMCs characteristic of the interdigestive motor pattern in the jejunum of fed dogs,[102] whereas it can interrupt MMCs in the stomach and duodenum of fasted dogs.[49] Therefore, exercise can alter motor activity, which may explain some of the GI symptoms associated with exercise in humans.

Increased stool frequency and diarrhea induced by strenuous exercise in humans has been attributed to accelerated colonic transit time, or alternatively, to changes in absorption/secretion by the intestinal epithelium.[116] Acute graded bicycle exercise decreases colonic phasic motor activity in an intensity-dependent way. This may facilitate transit by offering less resistance to colonic flow. After the end of exercise, propagated activity is increased, and this also may enhance colonic propulsion.[125] In fasted dogs, exercise decreases the frequency of colonic MMCs, and stimulates non-migrating colonic contractile activity within 3 hours after ingestion of a meal. Exercise also stimulates defecation, giant migrating contractions and mass movements in the colon, in both fasted and postprandial states.[106]

As mentioned, release of catecholamines and β-endorphins into the bloodstream, and stimulation of the sympathetic nervous system occur in the horse and in other species in response to exercise. This effect correlates with intensity of exercise and diminishes with continued training.[62–65] Each of the components of this stress response affects gastrointestinal motor function. Inhibition of gastric emptying and stimulation of colonic motor function are the characteristic pattern in response to different stressors. Central corticotropin-releasing factor (CRF) seems to be a main component in the induction of this stress-related motor response. Activation of CRF signaling pathways mediates both the inhibition of upper gastrointestinal (GI) and the stimulation of lower GI motor function through interaction with different CRF receptor subtypes.[82] In some studies, CRF modulation of autonomic nervous system activity was found to be independent of activation of pituitary-adrenal hormone release.[126] Alexander et al. measured plasma concentrations of CRF and adrenocorticotropin (ACTH) in the horse during and after acute intense exercise; ACTH was elevated, whereas CRF concentrations were not different from resting values.[12] However, as suggested above, central rather than peripherally circulating CRF may be responsible for the gastrointestinal motor changes[82,126] and could be involved in the exercise-induced changes in GI transit documented in horses.[43,44]

Gastrointestinal blood supply

Numerous studies in humans have documented a significant reduction in splanchnic blood flow during exercise of varying intensities, with gut barrier dysfunction, activation of the intestinal inflammatory response and mild hepatic damage being the most outstanding consequences,[127] although these effects have not been universally documented.[128,129] Reduced splanchnic blood flow during high-intensity exercise may also play a role in slowing the rate of gastric emptying. Manohar et al. reported a significant reduction in splanchnic blood flow during moderate exercise in the horse[57] (Fig. 46.6). Likewise, acute exercise decreased the clearance of BSP from the blood in an intensity-dependent manner in horses as a result of decreased splanchnic blood flow[60] (Fig. 46.7). Splanchnic vasoconstriction in the horse may be induced by epinephrine and norepinephrine,[7] or by release of hormones such as arginine vasopressin and VIP.[12,71] Endothelin, another potent vasoconstrictor released by endothelial cells, increases with exercise in humans[130] and horses.[131] Its effect should be further investigated in horses, especially in view of a recent study that demonstrated a significant association between plasma endothelin-like immunoreactivity and pathogenesis of certain GIT disorders.[132]

Reduced blood flow during exercise also disrupts intestinal absorption. Carrier-mediated glucose uptake decreased with intense cycling in humans.[133] This decrease in absorptive capacity may be a consequence of impaired blood flow and insufficient energetic supply for glucose active transport, which relies on ATPase activity, and could (1) prevent adequate plasma volume restitution, or (2) increase osmotic pressure within the gut, which could result in diarrhea or loose stools.[56,134] On the other hand, one hour of exercise on a treadmill at 71% VO_{2max} did not affect glucose, D-xylose, water, sodium, chloride and bicarbonate intestinal uptake in humans.[135] In the horse, impaired glucose absorption could lead to its accumulation within the intestinal lumen, creating an osmotic load and/or an increase in the substrate available for bacterial digestion within the large intestine, but it is unlikely that this would have any significant detrimental effects on the animal.

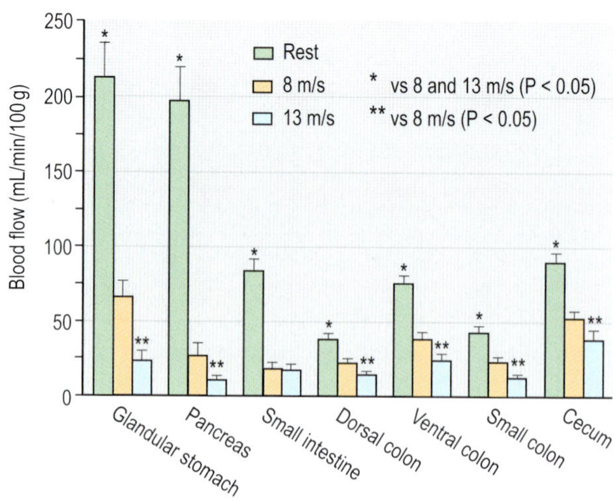

Fig 46.6 Blood flow to pancreas and various gastrointestinal tract tissues in standing (rest) and exercised horses (n = nine horses). *Reprinted with permission from Manohar M, Goetz TE, Saupe B, et al. Thyroid, renal, and splanchnic circulation in horses at rest and during short term exercise. Am J Vet Res 1995;56:1356–1361, with permission from the American Journal of Veterinary Research, http://avmajournals.avma.org/loi/ajvr*

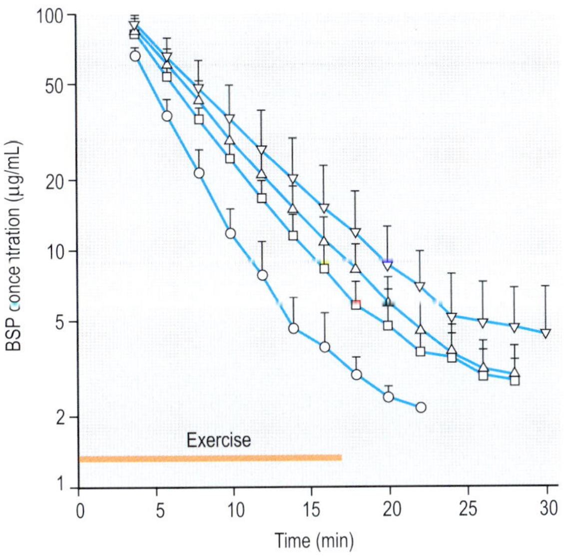

Fig 46.7 Mean (± SD) plasma concentrations of bromsulphalein (BSP) for eight horses exercising on a treadmill at four intensities. Bromsulphalein (5 mg/kg of bodyweight) was administered intravenously during a 45- to 60-second period. Symbols: ○ = resting; □ = 40% VO_{2max}; △ = 60% VO_{2max}; ▽ = 80% VO_{2max}.

Reprinted with permission from Dyke TM, Sams RA, Hinchcliff KW. Intensity-dependent effects of acute submaximal exercise on the pharmacokinetics of bromsulphalein in horses. Am J Vet Res 1998;59:1481–1487, with permission from the American Journal of Veterinary Research, http://avmajournals.avma.org/loi/ajvr

Mechanical factors

Mechanical bouncing of the body during exercise or compression of the viscera by abdominal muscles may also affect gastrointestinal motility, since GI symptoms in humans occur more frequently during running than cycling events. Some cases of post-running volvulus have been reported in humans.[134] Although light exercise has often been used as a way to facilitate passage of gas and promote transit in the large intestine of sick horses, strenuous exercise may promote excessive visceral movement. This, especially if combined with GIT dysmotility, could potentially promote intestinal displacement. The amount of colonic filling could have an influence on this bouncing effect.

Increased concentrations of prostaglandins and VIP, released by rubbing of the intestinal mucosa and distension,[134] may shift intestinal absorption into secretion. Upregulated expression of these agents in the horse, especially within the distal large intestine, could theoretically result in diarrhea.

Mucosal barrier integrity

Fecal occult blood has been documented repeatedly in endurance athletes, but its etiology is still unknown. Yet, the stomach is the most frequent site of running-associated hemorrhage in humans, possibly due to ischemic damage or trauma from the diaphragm.[116,117] Bleeding may reflect pronounced tissue damage. Inadequate perfusion to the intestinal epithelium can compromise the protective barrier function. Compromised barrier function might also facilitate bacterial and endotoxin translocation and initiate a local immune response. Subsequent production and release of inflammatory mediators would exacerbate this whole process.[127,128,136] Reduced mesenteric blood flow may also generate O_2 free radicals which can also contribute to tissue damage.[136,137] For example, running by some human subjects at 80% VO_{2max} increased small intestinal permeability of lactulose compared with rest and running at 40 and 60% VO_{2max}. Since lactulose crosses the epithelium only paracellularly, its increased transport is a strong indication of breakdown of the small intestinal barrier.[138] To date, no studies have been done to *directly* investigate the effect of exercise on the integrity of the mucosal barrier in horses.

Clinical implications of exercise-associated changes in gastrointestinal function

As has already been suggested, the anatomically and physiologically complex ceco-colon of horses could, in particular, predispose them to GIT disturbances during athletic training and competition. Undoubtedly a major confounding factor in this consideration is the feeding program, especially abrupt changes in diet composition or feeding routine. In fact, with respect to incidence of colic, the majority of the recent epidemiological studies more strongly indicate change in feeding program than type or duration of athletic activity as a high risk factor.[139–143] Concerning the effect of exercise, Cohen et al. reported that primary use of the horse was not significantly associated with colic, although they then remarked that horses with colic were significantly more likely than control horses to have had a change in activity level during the two-week period prior to examination.[140] Likewise, Tinker et al. found that horses used for eventing or training had a significantly higher incidence rate of colic when compared to mature horses that were sedentary.[142] This is not to say that the origin of the problem in all these cases was large intestinal (there was no information on site in the report) but, because of that organ's complexity, it must be considered as a highly likely origin nonetheless.

Anatomical considerations

From an anatomical standpoint, the fact that a large section of mid-colon floats freely within the abdominal cavity makes it prone to various forms of displacement that can result in serious colic. Whether any of these conditions may result from, for example, a combination of physical characteristics of the contents therein (e.g. collected sand; the gas : ingesta ratio) and type of exercise the horse is asked to perform remains to be established.

Physiological considerations

From a physiological standpoint, at least three areas deserve attention in future research on the effects of exercise on GIT function in horses. The first concerns factors that determine daily net water movement across the gut mucosa, between lumen and plasma. It is a common practice to withhold food hours before an event to decrease gut fill, and consequently, body weight. However, eating before or during a competition may have beneficial effects, as observed in human endurance athletes.[144] Ingestion of food may attenuate the reduction in blood flow induced by moderate to severe exercise.[145] Accordingly, blood flow to the digestive tract during exercise seems to be higher in fed than fasted ponies.[58] Fed horses may start with elevated blood flow of the GI tract, so that the impact of exercise on blood distribution is not so marked. Ingestion of food is accompanied by saliva production, and gastric and pancreatic secretion. Forage stimulates more water ingestion and digestive secretions than concentrate meals.[146] Factors which determine daily net water flux across ceco-colonic mucosa are complex and are characterized by regional compartmentalization.[147,148] Such factors include timing and composition of ingested food which impact directly on fermentative activity, water and electrolyte status of the horse, and efficacy of gastrointestinal motility. For instance, Clarke et al. have shown that during early postprandial stages of a large meal of balanced ration pellets, the VFA production from its fermentation within the colons may outstrip the subsequent VFA absorption, resulting in a large flux of water into the colonic lumen from the plasma space.[19] This can deplete plasma volume to a point where renin–angiotensin and aldosterone are released to promote plasma water conservation, the degree of which may be great enough to result in significant rebound dehydration of distal colonic contents.[19,149] (Fig.46.8) Combine a strenuous training session on top of this, and you have the makings of a serious impaction. In contrast, when that same meal was split into small volumes and given over 12 hours, mass movement of plasma water into the colons did not occur.[19]

Second, the effect of exercise on increasing GI mucosal permeability in humans has been discussed earlier in the chapter. Brouns and Becker mention cramps, diarrhea (sometimes bloody) and urge to defecate as symptoms associated with exhausting endurance events.[144] And, in the study by Ashton et al., a majority of subjects reported 'chills and nausea' sometime within the 24 hours following the strenuous exercise they had endured.[136] Both these studies suggest that exercise-related endotoxemia could account for the symptoms reported. It is safe to assume that there is, at any given time, a much greater load of endotoxin within the equine cecocolonic lumen than in that of humans.[150] Detrimental effects of endotoxemia in horse are well-recognized and include leucopenia, hypotension, and intestinal dysmotility and hypersecretion.[150,151] Clearly, if athletic activities consistently caused signs indicative of endotoxemia in a large number of horses, the beast would not be used for the many things humans ask of it. However, it would still be important to know if exercise, especially if strenuous, does cause a degree of endotoxemia that could be clinically important.[32,34] This suggestion is further supported by the observation that physical stress enhances colonic epithelial permeability in rats via peripheral release of CRF.[152] Accordingly, Baker et al.[153] reported in 1988 that a group of racing-fit horses had significantly higher serum anti-LPS concentrations than a similar group of horses that were not trained, suggesting that increased intestinal permeability could have occurred as a result of their repeated exertion. Barton et al. and Donovan et al. reported a similar phenomenon occurring in horses during endurance racing and after high-speed treadmill exercise, respectively.[154–155] More studies following up on these important observations need to be done.

Third, the transient defecation of non-formed, sometimes quite watery feces from some horses when they are subjected to a training session or race environment is a well-recognized phenomenon. It is usually of little consequence to the horse, but can be very bothersome to owners and trainers, especially when it occurs during a public display. Commonly, it is attributed to 'nerves', which could be one reasonable explanation. Nonetheless, this is an exercise-related event and it would be interesting to know its functional basis because it might be controllable. Probably the first place to look would be the small colon, where final desiccation of colonic contents takes place resulting in the formation of the fecal balls. This process involves a coordinated interaction between mechanisms that control motility and net transmucosal water flux; this is undoubtedly closely monitored by the enteric nervous system, much of which we still need to learn about with respect to equine small colon function. What we do know is that at least some of the water absorption is determined by a Na^+/K^+-ATPase pump, the functional status of which is under the control of aldosterone.[37] It seems unlikely, however, that the transient, exercise-related loose feces problem would be due to a downregulation of this system. More likely possibilities would be either a small colon dysmotility that allows more rapid passage of contents through the organ, the upregulation of a secretagogue such as CRF, VIP, or some combination thereof.

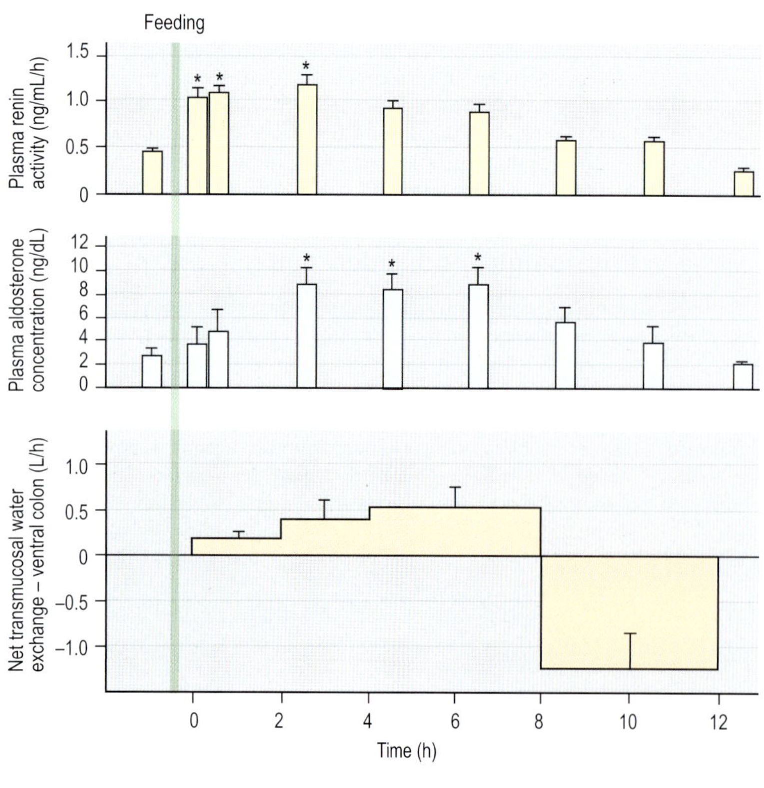

Fig 46.8 Postprandial activation of the renin–angiotensin–aldosterone system superimposed on net fluid transport in pony ventral colon. Rapid accumulation of bacterially produced volatile fatty acids within the colon after ingestion of a single large meal results in net flux of water from the plasma compartment into the colonic lumen. In response to this plasma volume depletion, renin–angiotensin and aldosterone are released to promote water absorption from the luminal compartment back into the vascular system. Addition of strenuous exercise during this period could exacerbate dehydration of colonic contents, and therefore, increase the risk of colonic impaction. (*Significantly [$P < 0.05$] greater than preceding value.)

Reprinted with permission from White NA. The Equine Acute Abdomen. 1990;25–35, with permission from Teton New Media.

References

1. Houpt KA. Biological rhythms and behavior. In: Houpt KA, editor. Domestic animal behavior for veterinarians and animal scientists. 3rd ed. Ames: Iowa State University Press; 1998. p. 95–8.
2. Casperson CJ, Powell KE, Christenson GM. Physical activity, exercise, and physical fitness: definitions and distinctions for health-related research. Publ Health Rep 1985;100:126–31.
3. Lorenzo-Figueras M, Merritt AM. Effects of exercise on gastric volume and pH in the proximal portion of the stomach of horses. Am J Vet Res 2002;63:1481–7.
4. Clark CS, Kraus BB, Sinclair J, et al. Gastroesophageal reflux induced by exercise in healthy volunteers. JAMA 1989;261:3599–601.
5. Porter AM. Case report: marathon running and the caecal slap syndrome. Br J Sports Med 1982;16:178.
6. Soffer EE, Merchant RK, Duethman G, et al. Effect of graded exercise on esophageal motility and gastroesophageal reflux in trained athletes. Dig Dis Sci 1993;38:220–4.
7. Soffer EE, Wilson J, Duethman G, et al. Effect of graded exercise on esophageal motility and gastroesophageal reflux in nontrained subjects. Dig Dis Sci 1994;39:193–8.
8. Collings K L., Pratt FP, Rodriguez-Stanley S, et al. Esophageal reflux in conditioned runners, cyclists, and weightlifters. Med Sci Sports Exerc 2003;35:730–5.
9. Nagata S, Takeda F, Kurosawa M, et al. Plasma adrenocorticotropin, cortisol and catecholamines response to various exercises. Equine Vet J 1999;(Suppl. 30):570–4.
10. de Graaf-Roelfsema E, Keizer HA, van Breda E, et al. Hormonal responses to acute exercise, training and overtraining. A review with emphasis on the horse. Vet Q 2007;29:82–101.
11. Jiminez M, Hinchcliff KW, Farris JW, et al. Catecholamine and cortisol responses of horses to incremental exertion. Vet Res Comm 1998;22:107–18.
12. Alexander SL, Irvine CH, Ellis MJ, et al. The effect of acute exercise on the secretion of corticotropin-releasing factor, arginine vasopressin, and adrenocorticotropin as measured in pituitary venous blood from the horse. Endocrinology 1991;128:65–72.
13. Argenzio RA, Southworth M, Stevens CE. Sites of organic acid production and absorption in the equine gastrointestinal tract. Am J Physiol 1974;226:1043–50.
14. Andrews FM, Buchanan BR, Smith SH, et al. In vitro effects of hydrochloric acid and various concentrations of acetic, propionic, butyric, or valeric acids on bioelectric properties of equine gastric squamous mucosa. Am J Vet Res 2006;67:1873–82.
15. Alexander F, Hickson JCD. The salivary and pancreatic secretion of the horse. In: Phillipson AT, editor. Physiology of digestion and metabolism in the ruminant. Newcastle upon Tyne: Oriel; 1970. p. 375–89.
16. Dyer J, Fernandez-Castano Merediz E, Salmon KS, et al. Molecular characterisation of carbohydrate digestion and absorption in equine small intestine. Equine Vet J 2002;34:349–58.
17. Begaut M. Occurrence, absorption and metabolism of short chain fatty acids in the digestive tract of mammals. Comp Biochem Physiol 1987;86B:439–72.
18. Argenzio RA, Southworth M, Lowe JE, et al. Interrelationship of Na, HCO_3, and volatile fatty acid transport by equine large intestine. Am J Physiol 1977;233:E469–78.
19. Clarke LL, Roberts MC, Argenzio RA. Feeding and digestive problems in horses. Physiologic responses to a concentrated meal. Vet Clin North Am Equine Pract 1990;6:433–50.
20. Campbell-Thompson ML, Merritt AM. Basal and histamine-stimulated gastric secretion in young horses. Am J Physiol 1990;259:R1259–66.
21. Birschneider H, Blikslager AT, Roberts MC. Role of duodenal reflux in nonglandular gastric ulcer disease of the mature horse. Equine Vet J 1999;(Suppl. 29):24–9.
22. Widenhouse TV, Lester GD, Merritt AM. Effect of hydrochloric acid, pepsin, or taurocholate on bioelectrical properties of gastric squamous mucosa of horses. Am J Vet Res 2002;63:744–9.
23. Andrews FM, Sifferman RL, Bernard W, et al. Efficacy of omeprazole paste in the treatment and prevention of gastric ulcers in horses. Equine Vet J 1999;(Suppl. 29):81–6.
24. Kitchen DL, Burrow JA, Hartless CS, et al. Effect of pyloric blockade and infusion of histamine or pentagastrin on gastric secretion in horses. Am J Vet Res 2000;61:1133–9.
25. Merritt AM, Cimprich RE, Beech J. Granulomatous enteritis in nine horses. J Am Vet Med Assoc 1976;169:603–9.
26. Parmelee-Peters K, Moeller JL. Gastroesophageal reflux in athletes. Curr Sports Med Rep 2004;3:107–11.
27. Leiper JB, Broad NP, Maughan RJ. Effect of intermittent high-intensity exercise on gastric emptying in man. Med Sci Sports Exerc 2001;33:1270–8.
28. Simons SM, Kennedy RG. Gastrointestinal problems in runners. Curr Sports Med Rep 2004;3:112–16.
29. van Nieuwenhoven MA, Brouns F, Brummer RM. Gastrointestinal profile of symptomatic athletes at rest and during physical exercise. Eur J Appl Physiol 2004;91:429–34.
30. Lorenzo-Figueras M, Jones G, Merritt AM. Effects of various diets on gastric tone in the proximal portion of the stomach of horses. Am J Vet Res 2002;63:1275–8.
31. Mayer EA. The physiology of gastric storage and emptying. In: Johnson LR, editor. Physiology of the gastrointestinal tract. 3rd ed. New York: Raven; 1994. p. 929–76.
32. Soderholm JD, Perdue MH. Stress and gastrointestinal tract. II. Stress and intestinal barrier function. Am J Physiol 2001;280:G7–13.
33. Sanderson IR. Nutritional factors and immune functions of gut epithelium. Proc Nutr Soc 2001;60:443–7.
34. Lyte M, Vulchanova L, Brown DR. Stress at the mucosal surface: catecholamines and mucosa-bacteria interactions. Cell Tissue Res 2011;343:23–32.
35. Campbell NB, Blikslager AT. The role of cyclooxygenase inhibitors in repair of ischaemic-injured jejunal mucosa in the horse. Equine Vet J 2000;(Suppl. 32):59–64.
36. Campbell NB, Jones SL, Blikslager AT. The effects of cyclo-oxygenase inhibitors on bile-injured and normal equine colon. Equine Vet J 2002;34:493–8.
37. Clarke LL, Roberts MC, Grubb BR, et al. Short-term effect of aldosterone on Na-Cl transport across equine colon. Am J Physiol 1992;262:R939–46.
38. Freeman DE. In vitro concentrative accumulation of D+xylose by jejunum from horses and rabbits. Am J Vet Res 1993;54:965–9.
39. Rotting AK, Freeman DE, Eurell JAC, et al. Effects of acetylcysteine and migration of resident eosinophils in an in vitro model of mucosal injury and restitution in equine right dorsal colon. Am J Vet Res 2003;64:1205–12.
40. Marshall JF, Blikslager AT. The effect of nonsteroidal anti-inflammatory drugs on the equine intestine. Eq Vet J 2011;43(Suppl. 39):140–4.
41. Engleking LR, Anwer MS. Liver and biliary tract. In: Anderson NV, editor. Veterinary gastroenterology. 2nd ed. Philadelphia: Lea & Febiger; 1992. p. 211–74.
42. Pearson RA, Merritt JB. Intake, digestion and gastrointestinal transit time in resting donkeys and ponies and exercised donkeys given ad libitum hay and straw diets. Equine Vet J 1991;23:339–43.
43. Orton RK, Hume ID, Leng RA. Effects of exercise and level of dietary protein on

digestive function in horses. Equine Vet J 1985;17:386–90.
44. Pagan JD, Harris P, Brewster-Barnes T, et al. Exercise affects digestibility and rate of passage of all-forage and mixed diets in thoroughbred horses. J Nutr 1998;128(Suppl):2704S–7S.
45. Van Weyenberg S, Sales J, Janssens GPJ. Passage rate of digesta through the equine gastrointestinal tract: a review. Livestock Sci 2006;99:3–12.
46. Mitchell JB, Voss KW. The influence of volume on gastric emptying and fluid balance during prolonged exercise. Med Sci Sports Exerc 1991;23:314–19.
47. Owen MD, Kregel KC, Wall PT, et al. Effects of ingesting carbohydrate beverages during exercise in the heat. Med Sci Sports Exerc 1986;18:568–75.
48. Sosa León LA, Hogdson DR, Rose RJ. Gastric emptying of oral rehydration solutions at rest and after exercise in horses. Res Vet Sci 1997;63:183–7.
49. Kondo T, Naruse S, Hayakawa T, et al. Effect of exercise on gastroduodenal functions in untrained dogs. Int J Sports Med 1994;15:186–91.
50. Drogoul C, de Fombelle A, Julliand V. Feeding and microbial disorders in horses: 2: Effect of three hay:grain ratios on digesta passage rate and digestibility in ponies. JEVS 2001;21:487–91.
51. Goachet A-G, Varloud M, Philippeau C, et al. Long-term effects of endurance training on total tract apparent digestibility, total mean retention time and faecal microbial ecosystem in competing Arabian horses. Equine Vet J 2010;42(Suppl. 38):387–92.
52. Azpiroz F, Malagelada JR. Physiological variations in canine gastric tone measured by an electronic barostat. Am J Physiol 1985;248:G229–37.
53. Desai KM, Sessa WC, Vane JR. Involvement of nitric oxide in the reflex relaxation of the stomach to accommodate food or fluid. Nature 1991;351:477–9.
54. Vu MK, Straathof JW, v d Schaar PJ, et al. Motor and sensory function of the proximal stomach in reflux disease and after laparoscopic Nissen fundoplication. Am J Gastroenterol 1999;94:1481–9.
55. Whitehead W, Delvaux M. Standardization of barostat procedures for testing smooth muscle tone and sensory thresholds in the gastrointestinal tract. Dig Dis Sci 1997;42:223–41.
56. Brouns F, Saris WH, Rehrer NJ. Abdominal complaints and gastrointestinal function during long-lasting exercise. Int J Sports Med 1987;8:175–89.
57. Manohar M, Goetz TE, Saupe B, et al. Thyroid, renal, and splanchnic circulation in horses at rest and during short term exercise. Am J Vet Res 1995;56:1356–61.
58. Reddy VK, Kammula RG, Randolph A, et al. Regional blood flow to the stomach and small intestine in ponies. Am J Vet Res 1977;38:2047–8.
59. Neutze JM, Wyler F, Rudolph AM. Use of radioactive microspheres to assess distribution of cardiac output in rabbits. Am J Physiol 1968;215:486–95.
60. Dyke TM, Sams RA, Hinchcliff KW. Intensity-dependent effects of acute submaximal exercise on the pharmacokinetics of bromsulphalein in horses. Am J Vet Res 1998;59:1481–7.
61. Husted L, Sanchez LC, Baptiste KE, et al. Effect of a feed/fast protocol on pH in the proximal equine stomach. Equine Vet J 2009;41:658–62.
62. Golland LC, Evans DL, Stone GM, et al. Maximal exercise transiently disrupts hormonal secretory patterns in standardbred geldings. Equine Vet J Suppl 1999;30:581–5.
63. Kokkonen UM, Poso AR, Hyyppa S, et al. Exercise induced changes in atrial peptides in relation to neuroendocrine responses and fluid balance in the horse. J Vet Med A Physiol Pathol Clin Med 2002;49:144–50.
64. Mehl ML, Sarkar DK, Schott HC 2nd, et al. Equine plasma beta-endorphin concentrations are affected by exercise intensity and time of day. Equine Vet J Suppl 1999;30:567–9.
65. McCarthy RN, Jeffcott LB, Funder JW, et al. Plasma beta-endorphin and adrenocorticotrophin in young horses in training. Aust Vet J 1991;68:359–61.
66. Desmecht D, Linden A, Amory H, et al. Relationship of plasma lactate production to cortisol release following completion of different types of sporting events in horses. Vet Res Commun 1996;20:371–9.
67. Soderholm JD, Perdue MH. Stress and gastrointestinal tract. II. Stress and intestinal barrier function. Am J Physiol Gastrointest Liver Physiol 2001;280:G7–13.
68. Oshi M, Tominaga K, Tanaka F, et al. Effect of chronic stress on gastric emptying and plasma ghrelin levels in rats. Life Sci 2008;82:862–8.
69. Rees MR, Clark RA, Holdsworth CD, et al. The effect of beta-adrenoreceptor agonists and antagonists on gastric emptying in man. Br J Clin Pharmacol 1980;10:551–4.
70. Holzer P, Livingston EH, Paul HG. Neural, metabolic, physical, and endothelial factors in the regulation of the gastric circulation. In: Johnson LR, editor. Physiology of the gastrointestinal tract. 3rd ed. New York: Raven; 1994. p. 1311–29.
71. Hall GM, Adrian TE, Bloom SR, et al. Changes in circulating gut hormones in the horse during long distance exercise. Equine Vet J 1982;14:209–12.
72. Sandin A, Girma K, Sjoholm B, et al. Effects of differently composed feeds and physical stress on plasma gastrin concentration in horses. Acta Vet Scand 1998;39:265–72.
73. Furr M, Taylor L, Kronfeld D. The effects of exercise training on serum gastrin responses in the horse. Cornell Vet 1994;84:41–5.
74. Hilsted J, Galbo H, Sonne B, et al. Gastroenteropancreatic hormonal changes during exercise. Am J Physiol 1980;239:G136–40.
75. MacLaren DP, Raine NM, O'Connor AM, et al. Human gastrin and vasoactive intestinal polypeptide responses to endurance running in relation to training status and fluid ingested. Clin Sci (Lond) 1995;89:137–43.
76. Walsh JH. Gastrointestinal hormones. In: Johnson LR, editor. Physiology of the gastrointestinal tract. 3rd ed. New York: Raven; 1994. p. 1–128.
77. Hurley RS, Bossetti BM, O'Dorisio TM, et al. The effect of exercise training on body weight and peptide hormone patterns in normal weight college-age men. J Sports Med Phys Fitness 1991;31:52–6.
78. Demers LM, Harrison TS, Halbert DR, et al. Effect of prolonged exercise on plasma prostaglandin levels. Prostaglandins Med 1981;6:413–18.
79. Schott HC 2nd, McGlade KS, Molander HA, et al. Body weight, fluid, electrolyte, and hormonal changes in horses competing in 50- and 100-mile endurance rides. Am J Vet Res 1997;58:303–9.
80. Sullivan SN, Champion MC, Cristophides ND, et al. Gastrointestinal regulatory responses in long -distance runners. Phys Sportsmed 1984;12:78–82.
81. Saelsen L, Andersen HB, Bratholm P, et al. Radioimmunoassay of plasma neuropeptide Y using HPLC for separation of related peptides and fragments. Scand J Clin Lab Invest 1994;54:207–14.
82. Stengel A, Taché Y. Neuroendocrine control of the gut during stress: corticotropin-releasing factor signaling pathways in the spotlight. Ann Rev Physiol 2009;71:219–39.
83. Maeda S, Miyauchi T, Waku T, et al. Plasma endothelin-1 level in athletes after exercise in a hot environment: exercise-induced dehydration contributes to increases in plasma endothelin-1. Life Sci 1996;58:1259–68.
84. Stebbins CL, Symons JD. Role of angiotensin II in hemodynamic responses to dynamic exercise in miniswine. J Appl Physiol 1995;78:185–90.

85. Strid H, Simren M. The effects of physical activity on the gastrointestinal tract. Internat Sport Med J 2005;6:151–61.
86. Ross MW, Donawick WJ, Sellers AF, et al. Normal motility of the cecum and right ventral colon in ponies. Am J Vet Res 1986;47:1756–62.
87. Lohmann KL, Roussel AJ, Cohen ND, et al. Comparison of nuclear scintigraphy and acetaminophen absorption as a means of studying gastric emptying in horses. Am J Vet Res 2000;61:310–15.
88. Mudambo KS, Leese GP, Rennie MJ. Gastric emptying in soldiers during and after fi eld exercise in the heat measured with the [13C]acetate breath test method. Eur J Appl Physiol Occup Physiol 1997;75:109–14.
89. van Nieuwenhoven MA, Wagenmakers AJ, Senden JM, et al. Performance of the [13C]-acetate gastric emptying breath test during physical exercise. Eur J Clin Invest 1999;29:922–8.
90. Sutton DG, Bahr A, Preston T, et al. Validation of the 13C-octanoic acid breath test for measurement of equine gastric emptying rate of solids using radioscintigraphy. Equine Vet J 2003;35:27–33.
91. Brown BP, Ketelaar MA, Schulze-Delrieu K, et al. Strenuous exercise decreases motility and cross-sectional area of human gastric antrum. A study using ultrasound. Dig Dis Sci 1994;39: 940–5.
92. Koch KL, Stern RM. Functional disorders of the stomach. Semin Gastrointest Dis 1996;7:185–95.
93. Koening JB, Martin CEW, Nycamp SG, et al. Use of multichannel electrointestinography for noninvasive assessment of myoelectrical activity in the cecum and large colon of horses. Am J Vet Res 2008;69:709–15.
94. Varloud M, Fonty G, Roussel A, et al. Postprandial kinetics of some biotic and abiotic characteristics of the gastric ecosystem of horses fed a pelleted concentrate meal. J Anim Sci 2007;85:2508–16.
95. Otte JA, Oostveen E, Geelkerken RH, et al. Exercise induces gastric ischemia in healthy volunteers: a tonometry study. J Appl Physiol 2001;91:866–71.
96. Kayaleh RA, Meshkinpour H, Avinashi A, et al. Effect of exercise on mouth-to-cecum transit in trained athletes: a case against the role of runners' abdominal bouncing. J Sports Med Phys Fitness 1996;36:271–4.
97. Soffer EE, Summers RW, Gisolfi C. Effect of exercise on intestinal motility and transit in trained athletes. Am J Physiol 1991;260:G698–702.
98. Murphy D, Reid SW, Love S. Breath hydrogen measurement in ponies: a preliminary study. Res Vet Sci 1998;65:47–51.
99. Roberts MC. Carbohydrate digestion and absorption studies in the horse. Res Vet Sci 1975;18:64–9.
100. Sutton DG, Preston T, Love S. Application of the lactose 13C-ureide breath test for measurement of equine orocaecal transit time. Equine Vet J 2011;43(Suppl. 39):49–55.
101. Williams S, Tucker CA, Green MJ, et al. Investigation of the effect of pasture and stable management on large intestinal motility in the horse, measured using transcutaneous ultrasonography. Equine Vet J 2011;43 (Suppl. 39):93–7.
102. Kenney MJ, Flatt A, Summers RW, et al. Changes in jejunal myoelectrical activity during exercise in fed untrained dogs. Am J Physiol 1988;254:G741–7.
103. Merritt AM, Campbell-Thompson ML, Lowrey S. Effect of xylazine treatment on equine proximal gastrointestinal tract myoelectrical activity. Am J Vet Res 1989;50:945–9.
104. Lester GD, Merritt AM, Neuwirth L, et al. Myoelectric activity of the ileum, cecum, and right ventral colon, and cecal emptying of radiolabeled markers in clinically normal ponies. Am J Vet Res 1998;59:313–19.
105. Roussel AJ, Hooper RN, Cohen ND, et al. Prokinetic effects of erythromycin on the ileum, cecum, and pelvic flexure of horses during the postoperative period. Am J Vet Res 2000;61:420–4.
106. Dapoigny M, Sarna SK. Effects of physical exercise on colonic motor activity. Am J Physiol 1991;260:G646–52.
107. Eades SC, Moore JN. Blockade of endotoxin-induced cecal hypoperfusion and ileus with an alpha 2 antagonist in horses. Am J Vet Res 1993;54:586–90.
108. King JN, Gerring EL. The action of low dose endotoxin on equine bowel motility. Equine Vet J 1991;23:11–17.
109. Bjarnason I, MacPherson A, Hollander D. Intestinal permeability: an overview. Gastroenterology 1995;108:1566–81.
110. Gisolfi CV, Summers RW, Schedl HP, et al. Human intestinal water absorption: direct vs. indirect measurements. Am J Physiol 1990;258:G216–22.
111. Roberts MC, Argenzio A. Effects of amitraz, several opiate derivatives and anticholinergic agents on intestinal transit in ponies. Equine Vet J 1986;18:256–60.
112. Hammer HF, Santa Ana CA, Schiller LR, et al. Studies of osmotic diarrhea induced in normal subjects by ingestion of polyethylene glycol and lactulose. J Clin Invest 1989;84:1056–62.
113. Lambert GP, Broussard LJ, Mason BL, et al. Gastrointestinal permeability during exercise: effects of aspirin and energy-containing beverages. J Appl Physiol 2001;90:2075–80.
114. Van Nieuwenhoven MA, Brummer RM, Brouns F. Gastrointestinal function during exercise: comparison of water, sports drink, and sports drink with caffeine. J Appl Physiol 2000;89:1079–85.
115. Hewetson M, Cohen ND, Love S, et al. Sucrose concentration in blood: a new method for assessment of gastric permeability in horses with gastric ulceration. J Vet Intern Med 2006;20:388–94.
116. Moses FM. The effect of exercise on the gastrointestinal tract. Sports Med 1990;9:159–72.
117. Bi L, Triadafilopoulos G. Exercise and gastrointestinal function and disease: an evidence-based review of risks and benefits. Clin Gastroenterol Hepatol 2003;1:345–55.
118. Neufer PD, Young AJ, Sawka MN. Gastric emptying during walking and running: effects of varied exercise intensity. Eur J Appl Physiol Occup Physiol 1989;58:440–5.
119. Schott HC 2nd, Hinchcliff KW. Treatments affecting fluid and electrolyte status during exercise. Vet Clin North Am Equine Pract 1998;14:175–204.
120. Noakes TD, Rehrer NJ, Maughan RJ. The importance of volume in regulating gastric emptying. Med Sci Sports Exerc 1991;23:307–13.
121. Moses FM, Ryan C, DeBolt J, et al. Oral–cecal transit time during a 2 hr run with ingestion of water of glucose polymer. Am J Gastroenterol 1988;83:1055.
122. Moses FM, Singh A, Villanueva V, et al. Lactose absorption and transit during prolonged high intensity running. Am J Gastroenterol 1989;84:1192.
123. Dainese R, Serra J, Azpiroz F, et al. Effects of physical activity on intestinal gas transit and evacuation in healthy subjects. Am J Med 2004;116:536–9.
124. Strid H, Simrén M, Störsrud S, et al. Effect of heavy exercise on gastrointestinal transit in endurance athletes. Scand J Gastroenterol 2011;46:673–7.
125. Rao SS, Beaty J, Chamberlain M, et al. Effects of acute graded exercise on human colonic motility. Am J Physiol 1999;276:G1221–6.
126. Tache Y, Martinez V, Million M, Wang L. Stress and the gastrointestinal tract III. Stress-related alterations of gut motor function: role of brain corticotropin-releasing factor receptors. Am J Physiol Gastrointest Liver Physiol 2001;280:G173–7.
127. van Wijck K, Lenaerts K, van Loon LJ, et al. Exercise-induced splanchnic

hypoperfusion results in gut dysfunction in healthy men. PLoS One 2011;6(7):e22366.
128. Marshall JC. The gut as a potential trigger of exercise-induced inflammatory responses. Can J Physiol Pharmacol 1998;76:479–84.
129. Wright H, Collins M, Villiers RD, et al. Are splanchnic hemodynamics related to the development of gastrointestinal symptoms in ironman triathletes? A prospective cohort study. Clin J Sport Med 2011;21:337–43.
130. Ahlborg G, Weitzberg E, Lundberg J. Metabolic and vascular effects of circulating endothelin-1 during moderately heavy prolonged exercise. J Appl Physiol 1995;78:2294–300.
131. McKeever KH, Antas LA, Kearns CF. Endothelin response during and after exercise in horses. Vet J 2002;164:38–46.
132. Ramaswamy CM, Eades SC, Venugopal CS, et al. Plasma concentrations of endothelin-like immunoreactivity in healthy horses and horses with naturally acquired gastrointestinal tract disorders. Am J Vet Res 2002;63:454–8.
133. van Nieuwenhoven MA, Brouns F, Brummer RJ. The effect of physical exercise on parameters of gastrointestinal function. Neurogastroenterol Motil 1999;11:431–9.
134. Gil SM, Yazaki E, Evans DF. Aetiology of running-related gastrointestinal dysfunction. How far is the finishing line? Sports Med 1998;26:365–78.
135. Fordtran JS, Saltin B. Gastric emptying and intestinal absorption during prolonged severe exercise. J Appl Physiol 1967;23:331–5.
136. Ashton T, Young IS, Davison GW, et al. Exercise-induced endotoxemia: the effect of ascorbic acid supplementation. Free Radic Biol Med 2003;35:284–91.
137. Baron P, Traber LD, Traber DL, et al. Gut failure and translocation following burn and sepsis. J Surg Res 1994;57: 197–204.
138. Pals KL, Chang RT, Ryan AJ, Gisolfi CV. Effect of running intensity on intestinal permeability. J Appl Physiol 1997;82: 571–6.
139. Cohen ND, Peloso JG. Risk factors for history of previous colic and for chronic, intermittent colic in a population of horses. J Am Vet Med Assoc 1996;208:697–703.
140. Cohen ND, Gibbs PG, Woods AM. Dietary and other management factors associated with colic in horses. J Am Vet Med Assoc 1999;215:53–60.
141. Hudson, JM, Cohen ND, Gibbs PG, et al. Feeding practices associated with colic in horses. J Am Vet Med Assoc 2001;219:1419–25.
142. Tinker MK, White NA, Lessard P, et al. Prospective study of equine colic risk factors. Equine Vet J 1997;29:454–8.
143. Traub-Dargatz JL, Kopral CA, Hillberg A, et al. Estimate of the national incidence of and operation-level risk factors for colic among horses in the United States, Spring 1998 to Spring 1999. J Am Vet Med Assoc 2001;219:67–71.
144. Brouns F, Beckers E. Is the gut an athletic organ? Digestion, absorption and exercise. Sports Med 1993;15:242–57.
145. Duren S. The gut during exercise. KER Equine Nutrition Conference 1997;39–43.
146. Meyer H. Influence of feed intake and composition, feed and water restriction, and exercise on gastrointestinal fill in horses.2. Eq Pract 1996;18:20–3.
147. Kronfeld DS. Body fluids and exercise: influences of nutrition and feeding management. J Equine Vet Sci 2001;21:417–28.
148. Argenzio RA, Lowe, JE, Pickard DW, et al. Digesta passage and water exchange in the equine large intestine. Am J Physiol 1974;226:1035–42.
149. Argenzio RA. Physiology of digestive, secretory, and absorptive processes. In: White NA, editor. The equine acute abdomen. Philadelphia: Lea & Febiger; 1990. p. 25–35.
150. Moore JN. A perspective on endotoxemia. AAEP Proceedings 2001;47:61–74.
151. MacKay R. Endotoxemia. In: Robinson NE, editor. Current therapy in equine medicine. Philadelphia: WB Saunders; 1992. p. 225–323.
152. Saunders PR, Santos J, Hanssen NPM, et al. Physical and psychological stress in rats enhances colonic epithelial permeability via peripheral CRH. Dig Dis Sci 2002;47:208–15.
153. Baker B, Gaffin SL, Wells M, et al. Endotoxaemia in racehorses following exertion. J S Afr Vet Assoc 1988;59:63–6.
154. Barton MH, Williamson L, Jacks S, et al. Effects on plasma endotoxin and eicosanoid concentrations and serum cytokine activities in horses competing in a 48-, 83-, or 159-km endurance ride under similar terrain and weather conditions. Am J Vet Res 2003;64:754–61.
155. Donovan DC, Jackson CA, Colahan PT, et al. Exercise induced alterations in pro-inflammatory cytokines and prostaglandin F2α in horses. Vet Immunol Immunopathol 2007;118:263–9.

Gastrointestinal diseases of athletic horses

47

Jorge Nieto

CHAPTER CONTENTS

Introduction

Moderate exercise and an active lifestyle have potential benefits to the gastrointestinal tract. Several studies in humans have shown an inverse relation between physical activity and the risk of gastrointestinal disease such as colon cancer, constipation, inflammatory bowel disease and irritable bowel disease.[1] However, strenuous exercise in human athletes has been associated with development of gastrointestinal disturbances, with symptoms reported to occur in up to 70% of endurance athletes during exercise.[2] Gastrointestinal bleeding, abdominal cramping, nausea and diarrhea have been described in marathon runners.[3,4] The gastrointestinal symptoms have been attributed to motility disorders, mechanical factors, altered secretion of neuroendocrine hormones and gastrointestinal ischemia.[5]

During exercise, splanchnic blood flow is redistributed to the working muscles and skin, at the expense of bowel perfusion. During high-intensity exercise, splanchnic blood flow may be reduced by up to 70%, and it has been estimated that gastrointestinal ischemia might be induced by a 50% reduction of splanchnic blood flow.[5] In addition, it has been reported that the use of some non-steroidal anti-inflammatory drugs (NSAIDs) may predispose to gastrointestinal problems related to marathon running.[4] Limited information exists regarding changes in blood distribution, motility, secretion and absorption through the gastrointestinal tract in horses during exercise. However, a study in ponies exercised on a treadmill, at an intensity of 75% of heart rate maximum, showed a significant reduction in blood flow (between 40 and 50%) to the large colon and cecum.[6] Therefore it is possible that some of the gastrointestinal clinical signs observed in horses during or after exercise may be due to the same proposed mechanism for human athletes.

Equine gastric ulcer syndrome

- The prevalence of gastric ulceration is high in athletic horses. Although racehorses in active training have the highest prevalence and severity of gastric ulceration, horses in other athletic disciplines are also commonly affected.
- The cause of gastric ulceration in horses is multifactorial.
- The diagnosis of gastric ulceration in horses is based on history, presence of clinical signs and confirmed by gastroscopy or response to therapy.
- The recommended treatments include the use of agents to decrease stomach acidity and management modifications.

Recognition

It has been estimated that approximately 2% of the human adult population suffers from gastroesophageal reflux disease (GERD). Signs and symptoms of GERD include acid reflux and heartburn. Up to 36% of healthy Americans suffer from heartburn at least once a month. GERD is a multifactorial disease that occurs when stomach acid and/or bile fluid flows back into the esophagus. With the availability of three-meter-long endoscopes veterinarians and owners became aware of the frequency and impact of gastric ulceration in adult horses in the 1990s. Gastric ulceration in horses more closely resembles GERD seen in man and is produced by exposure of the squamous mucosa to acid. In humans the majority of cases of gastric ulcers are caused by infection with *Helicobacter pylori*, a spiral-shaped, flagellated Gram-negative bacillus that colonizes the gastric mucosa of more than 50% of the human population. Although the majority of infected people are asymptomatic, in some individuals colonization produces gastric inflammation that can evolve to chronic gastritis, peptic ulceration and gastric cancer.[7] *Helicobacter* species have been isolated from feces and stomachs of healthy horses and horses with ulcers.[8] In addition, *Helicobacter* DNA has been found in the stomach and feces of adult horses and foals.[9,10] However, a clear and convincing association between *Helicobacter* colonization and gastric ulcers in horses has not been made. It has been the author's experience that in a small subpopulation of horses, gastric acid suppressant therapy fails to resolve gastric ulceration until parenteral antimicrobials (trimethoprim sulfa and metronidazole) are added to the treatment regimen. This anecdotal observation suggests that, in a small number of cases, bacteria may colonize ulcer beds, exacerbate ulceration and contribute to a failure to respond to routine treatments.

The term equine gastric ulcer syndrome (EGUS) was adopted to describe a group of diseases in foals and horses including erosions and ulcerations in the distal esophagus, non-glandular and glandular stomachs, and proximal duodenum of horses.[11] Equine gastric ulcer syndrome results from an unbalance between mucosal protective factors (mucus and bicarbonate production) and aggressive factors (HCl, pepsin and bile acids). In foals the disease is described in highly stressed newborn and in suckling foals.[12] In neonatal foals, due to other primary diseases, the signs may be subtle and ulcers can progress and occasionally perforate in the absence of overt clinical signs.[12] In suckling and early weanlings foals, lesions are found in the proximal duodenum and pylorus and may result in a functional obstruction causing delayed gastric emptying, requiring surgical bypass of the obstruction in some cases. In adult horses most of the ulcers are located on the squamous portion of the stomach, closer to the margo plicatus. Less commonly, the glandular portion of the stomach can also be affected. Glandular ulcers often are associated with clinical signs and the use of anti-inflammatory agents.

Physical examination

Clinical signs of gastric and duodenal ulceration in foals include bruxism, teeth grinding, inappetence, watery diarrhea and abdominal discomfort. Signs of EGUS in adult horses are subtle and not specific. Reported signs in adult horses include acute, chronic and recurrent abdominal pain, diarrhea or loose feces, weight loss, poor appetite, poor hair coat and body condition, obtundation, and decreased performance.[13,14] Horses with clinical signs have higher prevalence and severity of gastric ulceration.[14] In addition, 49% of horses presented to a referral center for abdominal pain had gastric ulceration; and the prevalence of ulceration in horses responding to medical treatment was higher compared to horses that required surgical treatment.[15]

Laboratory examination and diagnosis

Although the history, physical examination and laboratory findings may provide evidence in support of a diagnosis of gastric ulceration, endoscopic examination of the stomach is required for definitive diagnosis. With the availability of two- and three-meter endoscopes, gastric ulcers are now commonly diagnosed in foals and adult horses. Although a two-meter-long scope may reach the stomach of many adult horses, a three-meter-long scope is required to examine the lesser curvature, cardiac orifice, pyloric antrum and proximal duodenum. All feed and forage should be withheld for a minimum of 12 hours and water for 2–4 hours before endoscopy because the presence of feed material within the stomach will hamper complete examination. Distention of the stomach by insufflation with air may improve visualization by lowering the fluid level inside the stomach, exposing a bigger surface area. Feed material can easily attach to the mucosal wall, preventing evaluation of some areas. The use of tap water under pressure by using a 60 mL syringe or an automatic fluid pump attached to the biopsy port of the scope may assist with removal of the feed material. In an attempt to characterize and standardize the severity of gastric ulcers in horses the Equine Gastric Ulcer Council proposed an ulcer grading system[16] (Table 47.1; Fig. 47.1) that is commonly used by researchers and practitioners.

Observing a response to treatment with acid suppressant drugs may suggest the presence of gastric ulceration in horses with clinical signs. In horses with active abdominal pain, the use of lidocaine (20 mL) combined with an antacid (40 mL) administered orally by syringe may assist in the diagnosis if the colic subsides soon after administration of these agents.

Recently, a commercial two-part lateral flow immunoassay for the detection of blood in feces of horses became available. The tests use specific antibodies for the detection of equine albumin (source of blood caudal to the common bile duct) or equine hemoglobin (source of blood at any location of the GI tract). However the test has only a moderate negative (72%) and positive (77%) predictive value for the diagnosis of equine gastric ulcer disease.[17]

Treatment and prognosis

Therapy

The management of gastric ulceration should include, when possible, control or modification of risk factors. Gastric acidity is greatest when horses do not have access to feed material.[18] Therefore, continuous feeding or feeding several times a day may prevent or assist in gastric ulcer recovery. Allowing horses access to pasture grazing may also assist in the prevention of gastric ulcers, as one study showed that stall confinement is a risk factor for ulcer formation while turnout to pasture assists in resolution of ulceration.[19] High grain-concentrate diets increase plasma gastrin production and promote the production of volatile fatty acids in the stomach, which may contribute to ulcer formation.[20] Reducing the total amount of starch given each day as well as the amount provided in each meal may reduce EGUS prevalence. Alfalfa hay has been shown to increased gastric pH, due to the buffer capacity of its calcium and protein contents.[21] Therefore an alfalfa hay diet may buffer stomach acidity in horses. Other predisposing factors for ulcer formation include intensive exercise, transportation and the use of NSAIDs. Although limiting exercise may not be feasible, decreasing transportation and using agents to reduce gastric acid production in horses during active competition may be warranted. Avoiding or decreasing NSAID use, and using cyclooxygenase (COX)-2 specific anti-inflammatory drugs may also assist in the prevention or treatment of animals with gastric ulceration. However, management modifications are not always possible and often the treatment and prevention of gastric ulcers relies on agents to increase the gastric pH by reducing production of HCl. Medical treatment is recommended for horses with severe gastric ulcers, horses with clinical signs and horses under stressful conditions; in addition horses at risk of

Table 47.1 Grading system for gastric ulcers developed by the Equine Gastric Ulcer Council[16]

Grade 0	Intact epithelium, no hyperemia (reddening) or hyperkeratosis
Grade 1	Intact epithelium, areas of hyperemia or hyperkeratosis
Grade 2	Small, single or multifocal lesions
Grade 3	Large, single or multifocal lesions, or extensive superficial lesions
Grade 4	Extensive deep ulceration

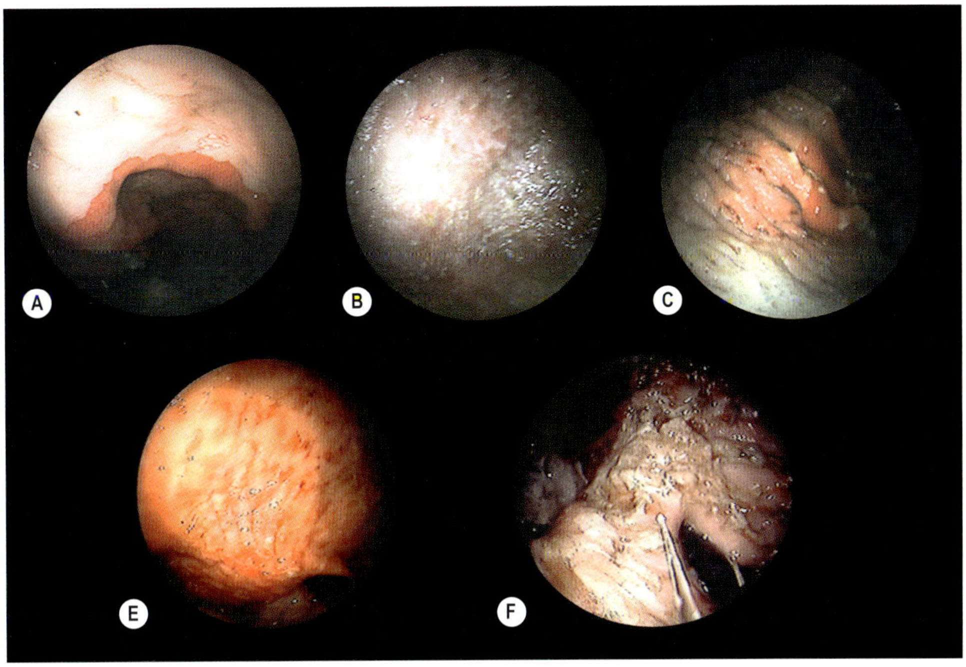

Fig 47.1 Endoscopic views of gastric lesions in horses to illustrate the grading system used to characterize lesion severity: **(A)** normal mucosa (grade 0); **(B)** intact epithelium, with hyperemia or hyperkeratosis (grade 1); **(C)** small, single or multifocal lesions (grade 2); **(D)** large, single or multifocal lesions or extensive superficial lesions (grade 3); **(E)** extensive deep ulceration (grade 4).

developing ulceration may be treated to prevent the development of ulcers. The initial recommended treatment time for most antiulcer medications is 28 days. Improvement of clinical signs should not be used to discontinue therapy, as clinical signs may improve or resolve faster than healing. If recheck endoscopy is available it may be used to evaluate improvement and adjust the length of treatment. The primary pharmacologic agents used for the treatment of gastric ulcers in horses include histamine type-2 receptor antagonists and proton pump inhibitors. Both drug types effectively decrease acid production and increase gastric pH in horses.[22,23] Proton pump inhibitors completely block gastric acid production by irreversible binding to the enzyme responsible for the terminal step in the acid secretory pathway. In horses the most commonly use histamine type-2 receptor antagonists are cimetidine and ranitidine and the most commonly use proton pump inhibitor is omeprazole. Omeprazole has a longer duration of action and can be administered once a day compared to ranitidine and cimetidine, which require administration three times a day. Two studies have compared omeprazole with cimetidine and ranitidine in racehorses in active training.[24,25] Both studies concluded that oral omeprazole once daily was more effective than either cimetidine[24] or ranitidine[25] in healing gastric squamous mucosal ulcers in racehorses.

Omeprazole is a pro-drug that is coverted into an active sulfonamide form by protonation. The active form of omeprazole binds irreversible with the hydrogen-potassium ATPase enzyme in the secretory canaliculi of parietal cells.[26] Omeprazole is commercially available for oral administration in a paste form and has been effective for the treatment (4 mg/kg) and prevention (2 mg/kg) of gastric ulceration in racehorses in active racing and training.[27] However the commercial paste is expensive and some compounding pharmacies manufacture paste or solution preparations that are considerable cheaper. A study in the author's laboratory compared the effects of the commercial paste vs a compounded suspension (both at a dose of 4 mg/kg BW) in racehorses in active exercise training. The compounded omeprazole suspension did not decrease the severity of gastric ulceration, whereas gastric ulcers resolved in horses that received the commercial paste (Fig. 47.2).[26] In addition, significantly lower blood omeprazole concentrations were detected in horses after administration of the compounded suspension (1.13 µg/mL peak concentration) compared to the commercial paste (2.85 µg/mL peak concentration). A different study comparing the commercial formulation with three generic compounded formulations found inconsistent results, with two of the three generic presentations failing to reduce the pH of gastric contents to a level considered necessary for ulcer healing (mean $pH < 4$).[28] Omeprazole is a lipophilic weak base that degrades rapidly in acidic aqueous solutions. The alkaline pH of the commercial paste (8.43,[26] 10.2[29]) is higher than the pH of some of the compounded products (3.41,[26] 5.1–5.7[28]) and it was hypothesized that the lower pH may be responsible for this lower efficacy.[26,28] The American Veterinary Medical Association established that compounding may only be performed when no approved use of an animal or human drug is available. In addition, compounding pharmacies are not regulated by the Food and Drug Administration; neither do the products require testing for strength or potency. Therefore veterinarians need to be careful when prescribing compounded medications.[29]

Prognosis

The prognosis for resolution of gastric ulcers is generally good with the implementation of appropriate medical therapy; however, recurrence rate can be high in performance horses. Alterations in diet (e.g. reduction in the amount of starch-rich feeds, increased forage including alfalfa), intermittent or prophylactic medical therapy, and other management strategies that target prevention of ulcer recurrence may be needed.

Etiology and pathophysiology

Relative to the size of the entire gastrointestinal tract, the stomach of the horse is small compared to other species. It is located in the dorsal part of the abdominal cavity and is divided in two parts: squamous (dorsal) and glandular (ventral) regions by the margo plicatus. The squamous region of the stomach is lined by non-glandular stratified squamous epithelium similar to the esophageal mucosa. It does not contain glandular structures and lacks effective protective mechanisms against acid injury. The primary barriers to acid in the squamous epithelium are the intracellular tight junctions and intracellular secretion of bicarbonate ions.[30] The ventral region of the stomach is lined by glandular epithelium that secretes HCl, pepsinogen, histamine, gastrin and serotonin. Acid is secreted in the glandular mucosa of the stomach by the parietal cells located in the oxyntic glands. Glands in this region also secrete mucus and bicarbonate that are important for mucosal defense against acid, pepsin and other corrosive agents.[31] Hydrogen ions are secreted into the gastric lumen by intracellular canaliculus located in the parietal cell. Acid secretion involves an elevation of intracellular calcium, follow by activation of protein kinase cascades, which trigger the translocation and insertion of the proton pump into the apical membrane of the cell.[32] The active transport of H^+ across the mucosal membrane is catalyzed by H^+, K^+-ATPase, and H^+ is pumped into the lumen in exchange for K^+. The more important regulators for gastric acid production are gastrin, acetylcholine and histamine (Fig. 47.3). Gastric releasing peptide stimulates G cells to produce gastrin; and somatostatin acts on the G cell to inhibit gastrin release. Gastrin acts on acid secretion directly on the parietal cell or indirectly on the enterochomaffin-like cells to produce histamine. Acetylcholine is produced by postganglionic cholinergic muscarinic nerves and also acts directly on the parietal cell or indirectly on the enterochomaffin-like cells. Histamine is produced by the enterochomaffin-like cells located in the lamina propria of the gastric gland and acts directly on the parietal cell.[32] The horse's stomach secretes acid even during the fasted state. Although the pH of gastric juice is acid, it has frequent periods of alkalinization (Fig. 47.4) due to the passage of duodenal fluid (bile and pancreatic secretions) through the pylorus into the stomach (Fig. 47.5).[31] Even under fasted conditions, periods of alkaline pH (6–7.5), lasting up to 5 min, can be seen periodically in horses.[31] Conjugated bile salts are normally maintained in their dissociated form in the intestine; however at the lower pH of the stomach, they may unionised and become lipid soluble, gaining access to the mucosa.[33] It is likely that, in addition to the damage caused by the acid to the mucosa, other factors such as pancreatic enzymes, and activation of pepsinogen and bile salts by acid, are also involved in the formation of gastric mucosal lesions in the stomach. While the squamous mucosa of the horse stomach has limited defense mechanism against corrosive agents, the glandular mucosa has a complex mechanism of protection.[34] Cells of the gastric glands secrete and form a mucosal barrier produced by a combination of mucus and bicarbonate. In addition, the gastric mucosa is also protected by prostaglandins that inhibit gastric acid production, increase mucus/bicarbonate secretion, stimulate mucosal repair, prevent swelling by stimulating sodium transport and produce vasodilation.[34]

Diets high in starch (gain and grain-concentrates) can produce ulcers in horses.[35] High concentrate diets are fermented in the stomach by resident bacteria, resulting in production of volatile fatty acids. The volatile fatty acids in a low pH environment have produced damage to the equine gastric squamous mucosa in vitro.[36]

Epidemiology

Risk factors identified for ulcer formation in horses include: history of colic, stress, poor hair coat, picky eater, straw being fed as the only forage, diets high in starch, transportation, stall confinement, intermittent feeding, intensive exercise, racing, illness, and use of

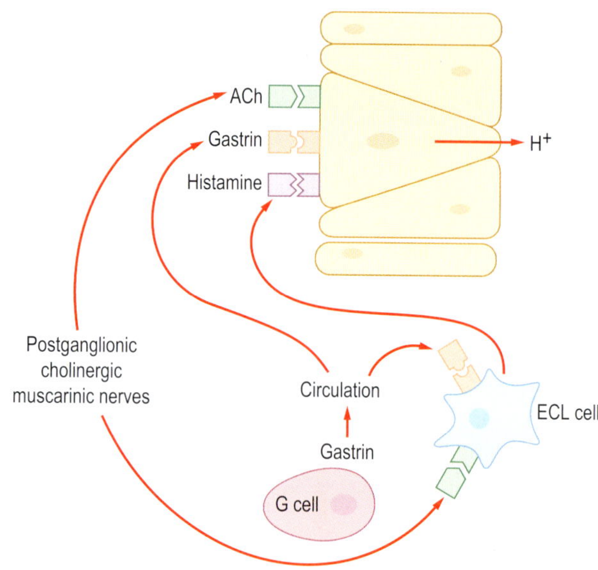

Fig 47.3 Diagram illustrating receptors in a parietal cell and regulators of acid secretion. Parietal cells contain receptors for gastrin, acetylcholine (ACh) and histamine. In addition, gastrin and ACh stimulate enterochromaffin-like cells (ECL cell) to release histamine.
Drawing by John Doval.

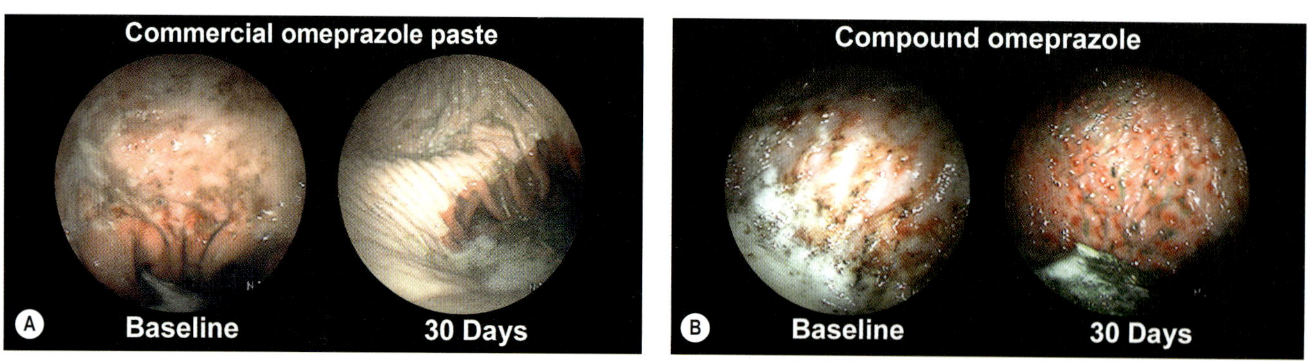

Fig 47.2 Photographs from the stomachs of two Thoroughbred racehorses in active race training. Horses were diagnosed with gastric ulceration by gastroscopy on day 0. They received a commercial omeprazole paste or a compounded omeprazole solution for 30 days. **(A)** Commercial omeprazole paste; **(B)** Compounded omeprazole suspension.

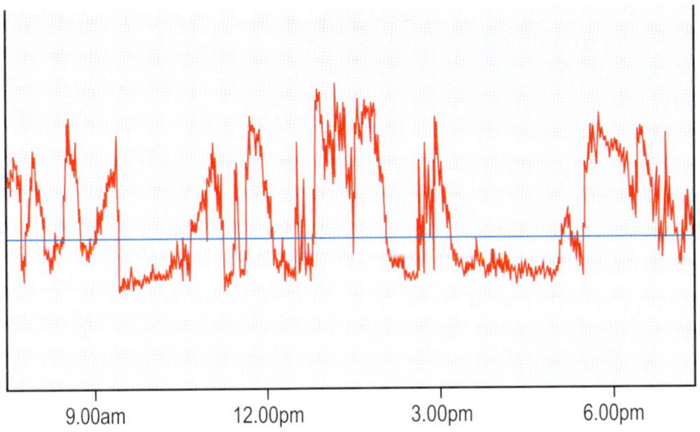

Fig 47.4 Figure showing a 12-hour continuous pH recording from the stomach of a healthy horse. The pH was recorded every second by using a three-meter-long electrode located at the level of the margo plicatus in a stabled horse with free access to grass hay. The horizontal blue line indicates a pH of 4.

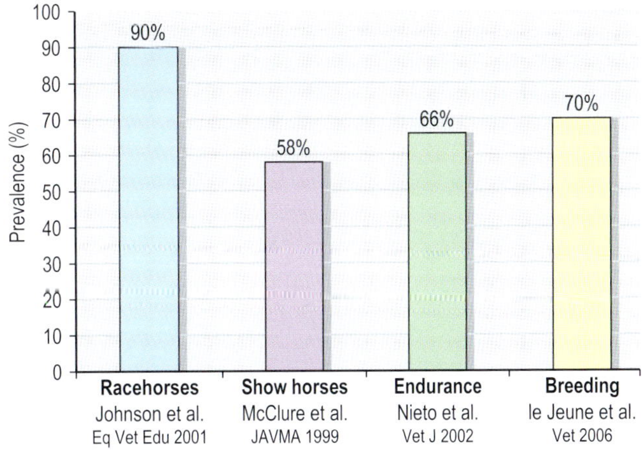

Fig 47.6 Graph showing the reported prevalence of gastric ulceration in different groups of horses.

From: Johnson et al. 2001,[42] McClure et al. 1999,[43] Nieto et al. 2002[26] and le Jeune et al. 2006.[44]

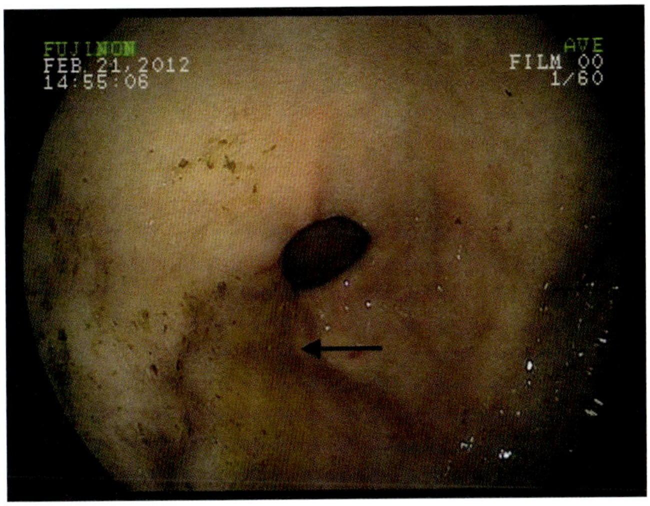

Fig 47.5 Endoscopic photograph of the pyloric region of a horse stomach. The arrow shows duodenal contents passing throughout the pylorus into the stomach. Note the hyperemia of the mucosa.

NSAIDs.[13,17,38] Racehorses in active training or racing are more predisposed to gastric ulceration.[39] The area more commonly affected with ulceration in the stomach of horses is the squamous region closer to the margo plicatus, likely because the mucosa in this area is close to the source of gastric acid and lacks effective protective mechanisms. Two recent studies in endurance horses have reported a higher prevalence of glandular lesions than has been reported for horses in other athletic disciplines.[37,40] In one of these reports, 27% of the horses had an active bleeding lesion in the glandular mucosa during an examination performed immediately after the end of an endurance race.[37] As the horses were not fasted before this examination it is possible that the actual prevalence and number of bleeding glandular mucosal lesions was higher than observed.

The presence of gastric ulceration is high in performance horses (Fig. 47.6). Reported prevalence of gastric ulceration is 80–90%[13,39,41,42] for Thoroughbred racehorses, 58% for show horses[43] and 66% for endurance horses.[37] However even pregnant and non-pregnant mares maintained on irrigated pastures have a high prevalence of squamous ulceration.[44] A study of Thoroughbred racehorses with no ulceration on arrival at the racetrack revealed that all the horses developed gastric ulceration after 4 to 9 weeks of active training. Even though the prevalence may be similar in different groups of horses, the severity is higher in racehorses in active training and racing. In addition, the severity is also higher in horses with clinical signs such as abdominal pain, poor performance or anorexia.[14,15]

Exercise has been suggested to play an important role in the formation of equine ulcers. Exercise has been shown to increase gastrin production in horses.[45] A study of horses exercised on a treadmill found increased abdominal pressure and decreased stomach volume during exercise, producing displacement of the acid contents in the lower part of the stomach to the squamous region and allowing excessive exposure of the proximal portion of the stomach to acidic gastric contents.[46]

The presence of gastric ulceration has been correlated with decreased performance in Thoroughbred racehorses on the basis of subjective assessment by the horse's trainers.[13] In one report of gastric ulceration in horses, poor exercise performance was the only abnormal finding.[47] The simulation of race training via regular intense exercise on a high-speed treadmill induces and maintains gastric ulceration in horses and has enabled evaluation of the effect of gastric ulceration on athletic performance.[48] Indices of exercise performance were evaluated in two groups of horses (ulcer vs no ulcers) before and after a gradual increase in exercise intensity for 56 days. At the end of the trial, horses without ulcers had a greater increased in oxygen consumption over time than did the horses with ulcers (Table 47.2).[48] Maximal oxygen consumption is a quantifiable and reproducible variable that indicates the limits of the cardiopulmonary system's ability to transport oxygen from the air to the tissues at a given level of physical conditioning and oxygen availability, and is frequently regarded as a primary correlate of flat racing performance. Although the exact mechanism(s) could not be determined, it was concluded that gastric ulceration adversely affects physiologic indices of performance in horses.

A study in horses after an endurance competition found active bleeding from the glandular mucosa.[37] Intense endurance exercise has been associated with gastrointestinal bleeding in human athletes.[3] A proposed mechanism for the gastrointestinal bleeding in endurance athletes includes the presence of intestinal ischemia caused by shunting of blood away from the splanchnic circulation followed by reperfusion injury, referred as ischemic enteropathy.[49] A similar mechanism may contribute to gastric injury and bleeding during strenuous exercise in horses but research is required to test this hypothesis. Horses on endurance races often are supplemented with oral electrolytes before, during, and after competition. A study giving oral hypertonic electrolytes to horses following the product insert recommendations (every hour for eight times) found an increase in ulcer number and severity in the non-glandular stomach.[50]

Right dorsal colitis (RDC)

- Right dorsal colitis is a protein-losing ulcerative disease affecting most commonly the right dorsal colon. The disease is associated with administration of NSAIDs and can affect horses, ponies and foals.
- Clinical signs are variable and include: lethargy, inappetence, colic, diarrhea and weight loss. Clinicopathologic findings include: anemia, hypoproteinemia, hypoalbuminemia and hypocalcemia.
- The diagnosis is based on clinical signs, history of NSAID administration, clinicopathologic abnormalities and ultrasound examination.
- Most horses can be treated medically by restricting NSAID use, diet modifications, reducing physiological stress and using selected medication. Refractory cases may require surgical intervention.

Recognition

Physical examination

The clinical presentation of RDC is non-specific and depends on the severity and duration of the disease. Reported clinical signs include inappetence, lethargy, signs of mild to severe colic, diarrhea or soft feces, dependant edema and weight loss.[51,52] Depending on the severity and the duration of disease, horses may be dehydrated and tachypneic. Weight loss may not be obvious in early cases.[51]

Laboratory examination

The most common clinicopathological abnormalities include mild anemia, hypoproteinemia, hypoalbuminemia and hypocalcemia.[53]

Table 47.2 Percentage change of physiologic indices of performance before and after 56 days' treadmill exercise training in 20 horses.[48] There was an incremental increase in exercise workload during the training protocol

VARIABLE	HORSES WITH ULCERS	HORSES WITHOUT ULCERS
Time to fatigue	18%	37%
Speed	–1%	3%
Stride length	2.3%	4.8%
VO_{2max}/M_b	6.7%	34.6%*
VCO_{2max}/M_b	8.5%	30.6%
Plasma lactate	2%	–11%

VO_{2max}/M_b = mass-specific maximal rate of oxygen consumption.
VCO_{2max}/M_b = mass-specific maximal rate of carbon dioxide consumption.
*Significant difference ($P < 0.05$) between groups.

Hypoproteinemia and hypoalbuminemia can be moderate to severe and are due to protein loss through the mucosa. Hypocalcemia likely reflects mucosal loss of protein-bound calcium and/or a decrease in calcium intake due to anorexia.[51] Values of peritoneal fluid usually are under reference values.

Diagnosis

A diagnosis of RDC can be challenging because of non-specific findings. The diagnosis is usually made by evaluation of the history, clinical signs and clinicopathologic data. Confirming the diagnosis requires visualization of the right dorsal colon by surgery, laparoscopy or necropsy (Fig. 47.7) or by observing a thickened right dorsal colon wall (>4 mm)[54] by ultrasonography through 11 to 15th intercostal spaces. However the technique lacks sensitivity because only a portion of the right dorsal colon can be imaged. The differential diagnoses for RDC include: gastric ulceration, other types of colitis, hepatic problems, inflammatory bowel diseases, tumors, parasitism, and bowel obstructions. A clinical report described the diagnosis of RDC by using ^{99m}Tc-HMPAO-labeled white blood cells in two horses. Scintigraphic evaluation of the colon of the horses 20 hours post-injection revealed a linear uptake of radiolabeled WBCs in the right cranioventral abdomen in the region of the right dorsal colon.[55]

Treatment and prognosis

Therapy

Surgical techniques for treating RDC include resection and bypass of colonic strictures, partial resections and bougienage of the affected segment.[51,56] However, the treatment of RDC is generally medical. As NSAID administration is proposed as an etiologic factor, avoiding the use of non-selective COX inhibitors is recommended. If NSAID treatment is necessary, the use of agents with a selective inhibition for the COX-2 isoenzyme (firocoxib) should be used. Dietary modifications are also recommended, such as feeding a pelleted low-bulk diet and eliminating or restricting roughage to minimize mechanical load on the colon. Administration of psyllium mucilloid has been recommended to promote the production of short-chain fatty acids that can promote healing of the affected mucosa. Studies in other species have shown that psyllium mucilloid increases the concentration of short-chain fatty acids that promote repair of colonic mucosa.[51] However it is unknown if psyllium promotes healing in horses with RDC. In addition it is unknown how much and for how long psyllium needs to be

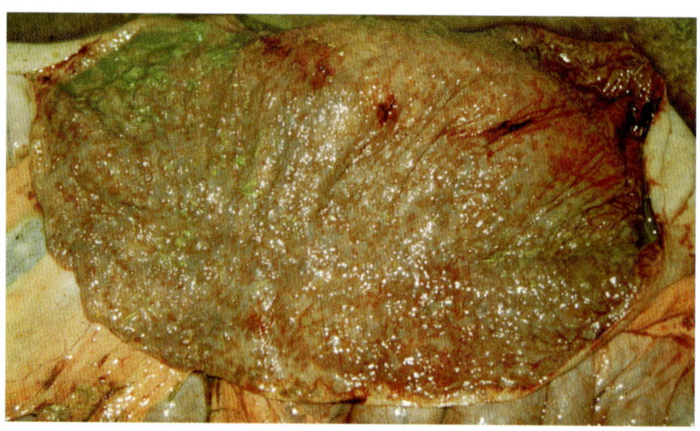

Fig 47.7 Picture of the large colon of a horse during a postmortem examination. Notice the severe and extensive areas of ulceration in the mucosa, induced by phenylbutazone toxicity.

administered in cases of RDC. The addition of oils (corn, linseed or fish) to the diet is advocated as a means to to increase the availability of prostaglandin (PG) E_2 and omega-3 fatty acids that may have anti-inflammatory effects.[51] The use of PGE_2 has been shown to prevent ulceration in the gastrointestinal tract of ponies after experimental administration of phenylbutazone (PBZ).[57] Misoprostol is a synthetic prostaglandin (PGE_1) that has been used in horses with RDC.[57] Although side effects in human are frequent and include nausea, abdominal pain and diarrhea, the author has only observed colic due to misoprostol in a small number of horses; colic resolved after discontinuation of misoprostol administration. As metronidazole has been used to treat humans with NSAID-associated enteropathies, it has been used in horses with RDC.[51] Horses with RDC will also require supportive therapy such as IV crystalloid fluids, correction of the colloid osmotic pressure and electrolyte administration. Serial monitoring of blood protein and albumin and thickness of the colon in horses with RDC is important, as not all cases respond to medical treatment and the treatment may take several weeks to show improvement.

Prognosis

The prognosis is guarded to fair, depending on severity.

Etiology and pathophysiology

Right dorsal colitis is a protein-losing ulcerative inflammatory bowel disease. Although the pathogenesis of RDC is unknown, it has been associated with the use of NSAIDs in horses, especially PBZ.[52] The principal pharmacological effect of NSAIDs arises from the inhibition of the COX enzymes, which convert polyunsaturated fatty acids to prostaglandins during the inflammatory process. Constitutively expressed prostaglandin E is important to maintain mucosal blood flow and promote mucosal repair of the gastrointestinal tract.[58] The proposed mechanism of damage to the colon is through hypoxia or ischemia of the mucosa as a consequence of decreased prostaglandin production.[52] Although doses of phenylbutazone higher than the clinically recommended (10 mg/kg s.i.d) have induced RDC in experimental horses, even lower doses (2 mg/kg s.i.d) have induced the disease in horses while water intake was restricted to half-maintenance requirements.[59,60]

Epidemiology

The condition can occur in horses of any breed, age, sex or activity; however, young performance horses appear to be predisposed.[51] Although most reported cases are associated with the use of prolonged or high doses of PBZ, the use of other non-selective NSAIDs (flunixin meglumine) has also been associated with RDC.[61] As previously mentioned, even short-term and appropriate doses of NSAIDs can induce the disease in susceptible horses. The cause for the predilection of NSAIDs to damage the right dorsal colon is not known. Though the term RDC refers to lesions in the right dorsal colon, administration of NSAIDs may produce lesions in all regions of the gastrointestinal tract.

Exercise-associated colic

- Colic is a common reason for elimination of horses from competition.
- Differential diagnoses of colic in horses during competition include: gastrointestinal pain, musculoskeletal pain, neurological diseases, hyperammonemia, pleuropneumonia and electrolyte imbalances.
- Equine athletes requiring abdominal surgery have a good prognosis to resume their athletic activities.

Recognition

Physical examination

Clinical signs of colic are variable and depend on the cause and the individual. Many problems in the equine athlete can manifest as non-specific pain that may resemble abdominal pain such as: muscle pain, neurological diseases, hyperammonemia, and pleuropneumonia. For that reason obtaining a detailed history, performing a complete physical examination and careful evaluation of all laboratory data are important in the assessment of performance horses presented with colic signs.

Diagnosis

Most types of colic in competition events are medical colics. The evaluation of horses with in this setting should include obtaining a complete history, performing a complete physical examination, passage of a nasogastric tube, performing a rectal examination, and evaluation of hydration status and electrolyte abnormalities. If the pain is severe or not responding to medical treatment, abdominal ultrasound and abdominocentesis may be required.

Treatment and prognosis

Therapy

Treatment goals in equine athletes with colic are to control pain, restore hydration, and correct electrolyte and acid–base imbalances. Dehydration and electrolyte abnormalities are more commonly seen in endurance and three-day event horses. The use of NSAIDs to control pain is not recommended until resolution of hypovolemia and/or dehydration. Alternatively, a low dose may be used initially in dehydrated horses. The preferred analgesic drugs in this circumstance are alpha-2 agonists and/or butorphanol. The IV route can be used for administration of fluid solutions or, in horses without evidence of gastric reflux, the oral route (via nasogastric tube) may be used. As exhausted horses often developed metabolic alkalosis, the use of crystalloid fluids with alkalinizing agents (lactate, acetate or gluconate) should be avoided. When fluids are given orally, balanced electrolyte solutions rather than plain water should be used to avoid exacerbation of electrolyte abnormalities. The decision to use drug therapy in horses at competition events needs to be done according to the severity of the problem, the organization ruling the competition and with owner consent.

Some equine athletes will require surgical treatment for resolution of the problem; however, with recent advances in diagnosis and surgical technique as well as intensive postoperative management, the outcome for equine athletes requiring emergency abdominal surgery seems to be favorable.

Prognosis

The prognosis is generally good for medical colic that develops in association with exercise. The prognosis for cases that require surgery will depend on the nature and severity of the intestinal insult.

Etiology and pathophysiology

Modern use of horses requires changes in feeding habits, from the original slow grazing of horses in pasture to less frequent feedings of concentrated diets. Horses performing physical activities commonly have restricted access to grazing and forage, while they receive large quantities of grain or gain-concentrate feeds and often have periods of feed deprivation. As previously described, periods of feed deprivation predispose horses to the development of gastric ulceration.[19] High-starch meals reduce gastric emptying rates[62] and therefore increase production of volatile fatty acids. Diffusion of volatile fatty acids across the squamous mucosa of the stomach may cause intracellular acidification and cell death.[36] Although in theory, adding oil to the diet may assist in the prevention of gastric ulceration by increasing prostaglandin synthesis and binding bile acids, inconsistent results have been reported.[63,64]

Exercise can be beneficial or harmful to the gastrointestinal tract, depending on the type and intensity of the exercise. While moderate aerobic exercise has been reported to be beneficial to the gastrointestinal tract of humans, intense and prolonged exercise can be detrimental.[1,2] Traveling and a new environment may also predispose some horses to colic by changing dietary management or introducing stressful situations.

Horses during or after exercise often show mild to severe signs of colic. Exercise in horses is associated with changes in several hormones that may affect absorption, secretion, perfusion and motility of the gastrointestinal tract.[65,66] Although the etiology of these types of colic is not completely known, decreases of water contents from the colon and reduction in motility may predispose these horses to impactions and ileus. Decreased perfusion to the bowel by shunting blood to other organs may also affect motility and produce ischemic pain. In addition electrolyte and acid base abnormalities contribute to the pathophysiology.

The amount of sweat produced by a horse depends on fitness, type and duration of exercise, and environmental conditions. Fluid losses by sweat production of 10 to 15 L/h have been reported under hot environmental conditions (see Chapter 41).[67] The sweat of horses is slightly hypertonic with respect to plasma and significant losses of Na^+, Cl^-, K^+, Ca^{2+} and Mg^{2+} can occur with prolonged exercise. During sweating, water is mainly lost from the extracellular fluid, causing a decrease in blood and plasma volumes and a perfusion reduction to several organs including the gastrointestinal tract. Water in the gastrointestinal tract accounts for 10% of the total body water and likely plays an important role in replacing plasma volume and electrolytes during long-distance rides.[67]

Epidemiology

Competition horses are at increased risk of gastrointestinal disease.[68] Regular exercise of horses at least once a week increases the odds (OR = 1.6) of developing colic compared to horses maintained on pasture at all times.[69] Eventing and race training have been found to be associated with a higher incidence rate of colic compared to non-competing animals.[70] Colic is a common reason for elimination of endurance horses during competition and decreased gastrointestinal sounds have been associated with an increased elimination rate.[71,72] A study that evaluated colic in 36 horses presented to referral centers after an endurance race competition reported a positive *Salmonella* culture in 8%.[71] The study evaluated horses from two referral practices. One of them (William R. Pritchard, Veterinary Medical Teaching Hospital at University of California) performs *Salmonella* cultures in all horses admitted with colic. The overall prevalence of *Salmonella* in horses presented for colic at the Veterinary Medical Teaching Hospital at University of California during the same time duration of the study was 0.95% (5713 colic cases, 54 positive *Salmonella* cultures; Jorge Nieto, unpublished data). The role of salmonellosis in the development of colic in endurance horses remains to be elucidated.

A study of horses that underwent colic surgery and were subsequently discharged from the hospital reported that a high proportion (86.1%) of animals resumed or started sporting activities. Hernia formation was the single significant predictor of reduced postsurgical athletic performance; however, the majority of horses (83%) achieved their presurgical level of performance.[73] When the owners were asked if they were satisfied with the outcome, 89.9% stated that they would recommend colic surgery. Equine athletes requiring surgical treatment for colic often can return to their previous level of activity.

Drugs used in performance horses that can produce colic-like symptoms

In the author's clinical practice (Veterinary Teaching Hospital at the University of California-Davis), horses have been presented because of development of abdominal pain after administration of fluphenazine, bisphosphonates and NSAIDs. Although fluphenazine and bisphosphonates do not have a direct effect on the gastrointestinal tract, their effects produce clinical signs that can be confused with abdominal pain.

Fluphenazine

Fluphenazine is a highly potent phenothiazine neuroleptic used in human medicine for the treatment of schizophrenia.[74] In horses, fluphenazine is used off-label for its anxiolytic and long-acting sedative effects. Clinical reports of adverse effects after a single or multiple doses of the long-acting fluphenazine decanoate or fluphenazine enanthate in horses have been published.[75–77] The clinical signs are consistent with extrapyramidal effects and include agitation, sweating, hypermetria, circling, severe pawing and striking, and swinging of the head and neck. The side effects have been observed after IM and IV administration. The death of a horse 92 hours after fluphenazine administration has been reported.[77] The horse developed severe respiratory distress; oxygen was administered through an intranasal catheter but the horse became recumbent, started paddling and was euthanized. The use of sedatives has little or no effect on the treatment of these animals. Reported effective treatments include the use of pentobarbital bolus (2 mg/kg, IV) or as continuous rate infusion (1 mg/kg/h) and anticholinergics drugs such as benztropine mesylate (0.018 mg/kg IV q 12 h; 0.035 mg/kg, PO, q 12 h) or diphenhydramine hydrochloride (0.67–1 mg/kg, IV).[75–77]

Bisphosphonates

Bisphosphonates are therapeutic agents, with strong affinity for bone, that markedly inhibit osteoclast activity.[78] Bisphosphonates are used in humans for the treatment of osteoporosis, malignant hypercalcemia and Paget's disease of bone.[79] According to their chemical structure, bisphosphonates are divided into non-nitrogen- and nitrogen-containing agents.[79] Tiludronate is a non-nitrogen-containing bisphosphonate licensed in Europe for use in horses with navicular disease, bone spavin and osteoarthritic lesions of the spine.[80–82] Zoledronic acid is a nitrogen-containing bisphosphonate that is 1000 more potent than non-nitrogen-containing bisphosphonates. Zoledronic acid has been used for the treatment of a number of orthopedic conditions in horses, including bone fragility syndrome, a debilitating condition that results in severe osteopenia.[83,84] As bisphosphonates reduce blood calcium levels, their use can result in severe hypocalcaemia. One horse presented to our hospital with signs of colic that developed after 9 days administration of zoledronic acid. The horse was pawing and sweating at the time of initial examination. Total blood Ca was 4.8 mg/dL (reference range 11.4–14.1 mg/dL), while ionized Ca was 0.6 mmol/L (reference value > 1.3 mmol/L). The horse responded to IV administration of calcium gluconate and crystalloid fluids (Fig. 47.8).

Non-steroidal anti-inflammatory drugs

NSAIDs are a class of frequently use therapeutic drugs with antipyretic, analgesic and anti-inflammatory properties. NSAIDs inhibit the COX enzymes, which convert polyunsaturated fatty acids to prostaglandins during inflammation.[85] The cyclooxygenases are membrane-bound proteins located on the surface inside of the endoplasmic reticulum and on the inner and outer membranes of the nuclear membrane.[85] Two COX enzymes have been described: COX-1 and COX-2. The constitutively expressed COX-1 is produced in most tissues and is involved in the production of prostaglandins that mediate physiologic housekeeping functions. By contrast, COX-2 is constitutively expressed in some tissues (brain, kidney and intestine) but in the majority of tissues its expression is induced in response to cytokines, mitogens or endotoxin.[86] Cyclooxygenases metabolize arachidonic acid for the synthesis of the various prostanoids such as prostaglandins PGD_2, PGE_2, PGF_2, prostacyclin, and thromboxane A_2.[87] Specific prostaglandins (PGE_2 and PGI_2) play a protective role in the gastrointestinal mucosa by reducing acid gastric secretion, increasing mucus production, vasodilation of mucosal blood vessels, and increasing duodenal bicarbonate secretion.[88]

The NSAID phenylbutazone is used in horses for the treatment of osteoarthritis and other musculoskeletal disorders.[89] Although PBZ is believed to be well tolerated by most horses, even recommended dosages have been reported to be associated with adverse effects, including anorexia, lethargy, gastrointestinal ulceration, right dorsal colitis, acute necrotizing enterocolitis, renal papillary necrosis and death.[90,91] The risk and severity of adverse effects may increase when PBZ is used in combination with another NSAID or in dehydrated animals.[92,93] Phenylbutazone is the most commonly used NSAID due to its efficacy, availability and affordability. The US Equestrian Federation allows the use of PBZ in horses (4 mg/kg, PO or IV) up to 12 hours prior to competition.[94] The International Equestrian Federation removed PBZ from the list of prohibited substances in 2010;[95] however, because of public concerns the decision was withdrawn. The mechanism of action of the most commonly used NSAID (PBZ, flunixin meglumine) is by blocking the function of COX-1 and COX-2 (i.e. non-selective COX inhibition). Clinicians prescribing NSAIDs for horses exposed to stressful conditions or for long periods of time should consider use of selective COX inhibitors. Selective COX-2 inhibitors still allow prostaglandin production by the COX-1 isoenzyme, and therefore are less harmful to mucosal heath. Firocoxib is an approved selective COX-2 inhibitor for use in horses by the American Quarter Horse Association and the United States Equestrian Federation.[94,96] Administration of firocoxib at the manufacturer's recommended dose for 30 days showed no adverse effect. In addition a study in horses with osteoarthritis showed that firocoxib and PBZ had comparable efficacy.[97]

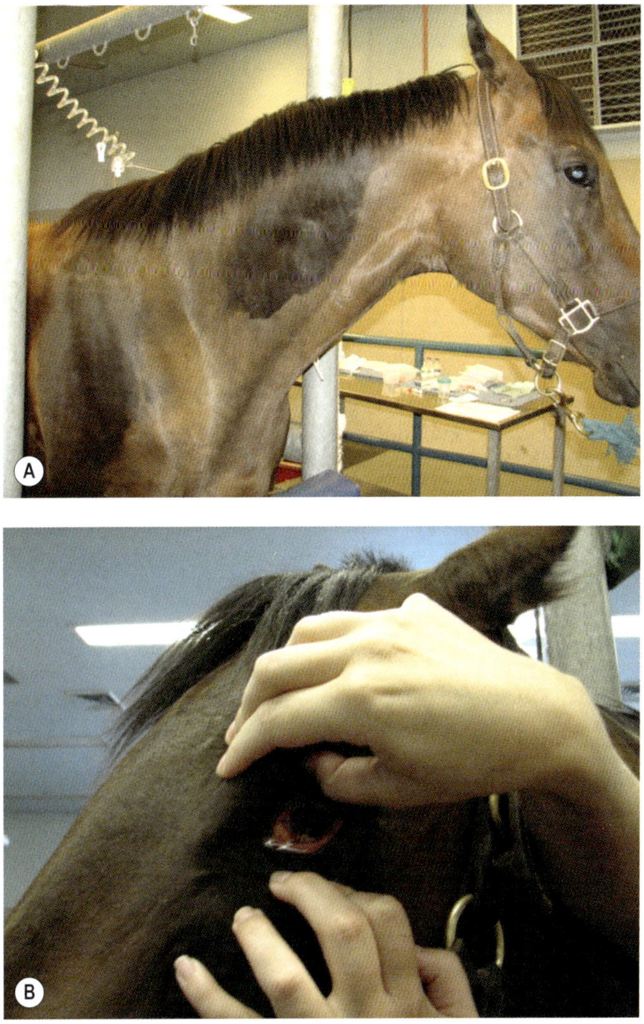

Fig 47.8 Picture of a horse with severe hypocalcemia, presented with signs of colic after 9 days of treatment with the bisphosphonate zoledronic acid. On arrival the horse was pawing, trembling and sweating **(A)**. Touching of the face elicited prolapse of the third eyelid **(B)**. The horse responded to IV administration of calcium gluconate. *Photos courtesy of Dr Monica Aleman.*

With thanks to Guy D. Lester, who created the original chapter in the first edition.

References

1. Martin D. Physical activity benefits and risks on the gastrointestinal system. South Med J 2011;104:831–7.
2. Moses FM. Exercise-associated intestinal ischemia. Curr Sports Med Rep 2005;4:91–5.
3. Fisher RL, McMahon LF Jr, Ryan MJ, et al. Gastrointestinal bleeding in competitive runners. Dig Dis Sci 1986;31:1226–8.
4. Smetanka RD, Lambert GP, Murray R, et al. Intestinal permeability in runners in the 1996 Chicago marathon. Int J Sport Nutr 1999;9:426–33.
5. Ter Steege RW, Geelkerken RH, Huisman AB, et al. Abdominal symptoms during physical exercise and the role of gastrointestinal ischaemia: a study in 12 symptomatic athletes. Br J Sports Med 2011.
6. Duren SE. The gut during excercise. In: Pagan JD, editor. Advances in equine nutrition I. Nottingham University Press; 1992–1997. p. 149–59.
7. Ruggiero P. *Helicobacter pylori* and inflammation. Curr Pharm Des 2010;16:4225–36.
8. Moyaert H, Pasmans F, Decostere A, et al. *Helicobacter equorum*: prevalence and significance for horses and humans. FEMS Immunol Med Microbiol 2009; 57:14–16.

9. Moyaert H, Haesebrouck F, Dewulf J, et al. *Helicobacter equorum* is highly prevalent in foals. Vet Microbiol 2009;133:190–2.
10. Contreras M, Morales A, Garcia-Amado MA, et al. Detection of *Helicobacter*-like DNA in the gastric mucosa of Thoroughbred horses. Lett Appl Microbiol 2007;45:553–7.
11. Andrews FM, Bernard W, Cohen H, et al. Recommendations for the diagnosis and treatment of equine gastric ulcer syndrom (EGUS). Eq Vet Edu 1999;1:122–34.
12. Lester GD. Gastrointestinal diseases of performance horses. In: Hinchcliff KW, Kaneps AJ, Geor RJ, editors. Equine Sports Medicine and Surgery. London: Elsevier Limited; 2004. p. 1037–48.
13. Vatistas NJ, Snyder JR, Carlson G, et al. Cross-sectional study of gastric ulcers of the squamous mucosa in thoroughbred racehorses. Equine Vet J Suppl 1999;34–9.
14. Murray MJ, Grodinsky C, Anderson CW, et al. Gastric ulcers in horses: a comparison of endoscopic findings in horses with and without clinical signs. Equine Vet J Suppl 1989;68–72.
15. Dukti SA, Perkins S, Murphy J, et al. Prevalence of gastric squamous ulceration in horses with abdominal pain. Equine Vet J 2006;38:347–9.
16. The Equine Gastric Ulcer Council. Recommendations for the diagnosis and treatment of equine gastric ulcer syndrome (EGUS). Eq Vet Edu 1999;11:262–72.
17. Videla R, Andrews FM. New perspectives in equine gastric ulcer syndrome. Vet Clin North Am Equine Pract 2009;25:283–301.
18. Murray MJ, Schusser GF. Measurement of 24-h gastric pH using an indwelling pH electrode in horses unfed, fed and treated with ranitidine. Equine Vet J 1993;25:417–21.
19. Murray MJ, Eichorn ES. Effects of intermittent feed deprivation, intermittent feed deprivation with ranitidine administration, and stall confinement with ad libitum access to hay on gastric ulceration in horses. Am J Vet Res 1996;57:1599–603.
20. Nadeau JA, Andrews FM, Patton CS, et al. Effects of hydrochloric, valeric, and other volatile fatty acids on pathogenesis of ulcers in the nonglandular portion of the stomach of horses. Am J Vet Res 2003;64:413–17.
21. Nadeau JA, Andrews FM, Mathew AG, et al. Evaluation of diet as a cause of gastric ulcers in horses. Am J Vet Res 2000;61:784–90.
22. Daurio CP, Holste JE, Andrews FM, et al. Effect of omeprazole paste on gastric acid secretion in horses. Equine Vet J Suppl 1999;59–62.
23. Murray MJ, Grodinsky C. The effects of famotidine, ranitidine and magnesium hydroxide/aluminium hydroxide on gastric fluid pH in adult horses. Equine Vet J Suppl 1992;52–5.
24. Nieto JE, Spier SJ, van Hoogmoed L, et al. Comparison of omeprazole and cimetidine in healing of gastric ulcers and prevention of recurrence in horses. Eq Vet Edu 2001;13:260–4.
25. Lester GD, Smith RL, Robertson ID. Effects of treatment with omeprazole or ranitidine on gastric squamous ulceration in racing Thoroughbreds. J Am Vet Med Assoc 2005;227:1636–9.
26. Nieto JE, Spier S, Pipers FS, et al. Comparison of paste and suspension formulations of omeprazole in the healing of gastric ulcers in racehorses in active training. J Am Vet Med Assoc 2002;221:1139–43.
27. Andrews FM, Sifferman RL, Bernard W, et al. Efficacy of omeprazole paste in the treatment and prevention of gastric ulcers in horses. Equine Vet J Suppl 1999;81–6.
28. Merritt AM, Sanchez LC, Burrow JA, et al. Effect of GastroGard and three compounded oral omeprazole preparations on 24 h intragastric pH in gastrically cannulated mature horses. Equine Vet J 2003;35:691–5.
29. American Veterinary Medical Association. Compounding AVMA policy/Veterinary Compounding. 2009.
30. Orlando RC. Esophageal epithelial defense against acid injury. J Clin Gastroenterology 1991;13(Suppl. 2):S1–5.
31. Merritt AM. Normal equine gastroduodenal secretion and motility. Equine Vet J Suppl 1999;7–13.
32. Johnson LR. Gastric secretion. In: Johnson LR, editor. Gastrointestinal physiology. 6th ed. St. Louis: Mosby, Inc.; 2001. p. 75–94.
33. Argenzio RA. Comparative pathophysiology of nonglandular ulcer disease: a review of experimental studies. Equine Vet J Suppl 1999;19–23.
34. Merritt AM. The Equine Stomach. In: AAEP 2003;75–102.
35. Coenen M. The occurrence of feed-induced stomach ulcers in horses]. Schweiz Arch Tierheilkd 1990;132:121–6.
36. Nadeau JA, Andrews FM, Patton CS, et al. Effects of hydrochloric, acetic, butyric, and propionic acids on pathogenesis of ulcers in the nonglandular portion of the stomach of horses. Am J Vet Res 2003;64:404–12.
37. Nieto JE, Snyder JR, Beldomenico P, et al. Prevalence of gastric ulcers in endurance horses–a preliminary report. Vet J 2004;167:33–7.
38. Luthersson N, Nielsen KH, Harris P, et al. Risk factors associated with equine gastric ulceration syndrome (EGUS) in 201 horses in Denmark. Equine Vet J 2009;41:625–30.
39. Hammond CJ, Mason DK, Watkins KL. Gastric ulceration in mature thoroughbred horses. Equine Vet J 1986;18:284–7.
40. Tamzali Y, Marguet C, Priymenko N, et al. Prevalence of gastric ulcer syndrome in high-level endurance horses. Equine Vet J 2011;43:141–4.
41. Bell RJ, Kingston JK, Mogg TD, et al. The prevalence of gastric ulceration in racehorses in New Zealand. N Z Vet J 2007;55:13–18.
42. Johnson JH, Vatistas NJ, Castro L, et al. Field survey of the prevalence of gastric ulcers in Thoroughbred racehorses and on on response to treatment of affected horses with omeprazole paste. Eq Vet Edu 2001;13:221–4.
43. McClure SR, Glickman LT, Glickman NW. Prevalence of gastric ulcers in show horses. J Am Vet Med Assoc 1999;215: 1130–3.
44. le Jeune SS, Nieto JE, Dechant JE, et al. Prevalence of gastric ulcers in Thoroughbred broodmares in pasture: a preliminary report. Vet J 2009;181:251–5.
45. Furr M, Taylor L, Kronfeld D. The effects of exercise training on serum gastrin responses in the horse. Cornell Vet 1994;84:41–5.
46. Lorenzo-Figueras M, Merritt AM. Effects of exercise on gastric volume and pH in the proximal portion of the stomach of horses. Am J Vet Res 2002;63:1481–7.
47. Franklin SH, Brazil TJ, Allen JK. Poor performance associated with equine gastric ulceration syndrome in four Thorougbred racehorses. Eq Vet Edu 2008;20:119–24.
48. Nieto JE, Snyder JR, Vatistas NJ, et al. Effect of gastric ulceration on physiologic responses to exercise in horses. Am J Vet Res 2009;70:787–95.
49. Bounous G, McArdle AH. Marathon runners: the intestinal handicap. Med Hypotheses 1990;33:261–4.
50. Holbrook TC, Simmons RD, Payton ME, et al. Effect of repeated oral administration of hypertonic electrolyte solution on equine gastric mucosa. Equine Vet J 2005;37:501–4.
51. Cohen ND. Right dorsal colitis. Eq Vet Edu 2002;14:212–19.
52. Galvin N, Dillon H, McGovern F. Right dorsal colitis in the horse: minireview and reports on three cases in Ireland. Ir Vet J 2004;57:467–73.
53. Bueno AC, Seahorn TL, Moore RM. Diagnosis and treatment of right dorsal colitis in horses. Comp cont educ pract vet 2000;22:173–81.
54. Reef VB. Adult abdominal ultrasonography. In: Equine diagnostic ultrasound. Saunders; 1998. p. 273–363.
55. East LM, Trumble TN, Steyn PF, et al. The application of technetium-99m hexamethylpropyleneamine oxime (99mTc-HMPAO) labeled white blood

cells for the diagnosis of right dorsal ulcerative colitis in two horses. Vet Radiol Ultrasound 2000;41:360–4.

56. Lane JK, Cohen JM, Zedler ST, et al. Right dorsal colon resection and bypass for treatment of right dorsal colitis in a horse. Vet Surg 2010;39:879–83.
57. Collins LG, Tyler DE. Experimentally induced phenylbutazone toxicosis in ponies: description of the syndrome and its prevention with synthetic prostaglandin E2. Am J Vet Res 1985;46:1605–15.
58. Blikslager AT. Cyclooxygenase-2 inhibitors in equine practice. Comp Cont Educ Pract Vet 1999;21:548–50.
59. Meschter CL, Gilbert M, Krook L, et al. The effects of phenylbutazone on the intestinal mucosa of the horse: a morphological, ultrastructural and biochemical study. Equine Vet J 1990;22:255–63.
60. MacAllister CG. Effects of toxic doses of phenylbutazone in ponies. Am J Vet Res 1983;44:2277–9.
61. Karcher LF, Dill SG, Anderson WI, et al. Right dorsal colitis. J Vet Intern Med 1990;4:247–53.
62. Metayer N, Lhote M, Bahr A, et al. Meal size and starch content affect gastric emptying in horses. Equine Vet J 2004;36:436–40.
63. Cargile JL, Burrow JA, Kim I, et al. Effect of dietary corn oil supplementation on equine gastric fluid acid, sodium, and prostaglandin E_2 content before and during pentagastrin infusion. J Vet Intern Med 2004;18:545–9.
64. Frank N, Andrews FM, Elliott SB, et al. Effects of dietary oils on the development of gastric ulcers in mares. Am J Vet Res 2005;66:2006–11.
65. Hall GM, Adrian TE, Bloom SR, et al. Changes in circulating gut hormones in the horse during long distance exercise. Equine Vet J 1982;14:209–12.
66. Nagata S, Takeda F, Kurosawa M, et al. Plasma adrenocorticotropin, cortisol and catecholamines response to various exercises. Equine Vet J Suppl 1999;30:570–4.
67. Flaminio MJ, Rush BR. Fluid and electrolyte balance in endurance horses. Vet Clin North Am Equine Pract 1998;14:147–58.
68. Archer DC, Proudman CJ. Epidemiological clues to preventing colic. Vet J 2006;172:29–39.
69. Cohen ND, Gibbs PG, Woods AM. Dietary and other management factors associated with colic in horses. J Am Vet Med Assoc 1999;215:53–60.
70. Tinker MK, White NA, Lessard P, et al. Prospective study of equine colic incidence and mortality. Equine Vet J 1997;29:448–53.
71. Fielding CL, Dechant JE. Colic in competing endurance horses presenting to referral centres: 36 cases. Equine Vet J 2011.
72. Fielding CL, Meier CA, Balch OK, et al. Risk factors for the elimination of endurance horses from competition. J Am Vet Med Assoc 2011;239:493–8.
73. Christophersen MT, Tnibar A, Pihl TH, et al. Sporting activity following colic surgery in horses: a retrospective study. Equine Vet J Suppl 2011;43(Suppl. 40): 3–6.
74. Altamura AC, Sassella F, Santini A, et al. Intramuscular preparations of antipsychotics: uses and relevance in clinical practice. Drugs 2003;63:493–512.
75. Kauffman VG, Soma L, Divers TJ, et al. Extrapyramidal side effects caused by fluphenazine decanoate in a horse. J Am Vet Med Assoc 1989;195:1128–30.
76. Brewer BD, Hines MT, Stewart JT, et al. Fluphenazine induced Parkinson-like syndrome in a horse. Equine Vet J 1990;22:136–7.
77. Baird JD, Arroyo LG, Vengust M, et al. Adverse extrapyramidal effects in four horse given fluphenazine decanoate. J Am Vet Med Assoc 2006;229:104–10.
78. Flanagan AM, Chambers TJ. Inhibition of bone resorption by bisphosphonates: interactions between bisphosphonates, osteoclasts, and bone. Calcif Tissue Int 1991;49:407–15.
79. Kimmel DB. Mechanism of action, pharmacokinetic and pharmacodynamic profile, and clinical applications of nitrogen-containing bisphosphonates. J Dent Res 2007;86:1022–33.
80. Gough MR, Thibaud D, Smith RK. Tiludronate infusion in the treatment of bone spavin: a double blind placebo-controlled trial. Equine Vet J 2010;42:381–7.
81. Coudry V, Thibaud D, Riccio B, et al. Efficacy of tiludronate in the treatment of horses with signs of pain associated with osteoarthritic lesions of the thoracolumbar vertebral column. Am J Vet Res 2007;68:329–37.
82. Denoix JM, Thibaud D, Riccio B. Tiludronate as a new therapeutic agent in the treatment of navicular disease: a double-blind placebo-controlled clinical trial. Equine Vet J 2003;35:407–13.
83. Katzman SA, Nieto JE, Arens AM, et al. Zoledronate for the treatement of equine bone fragility disorder: 10 cases. J Am Vet Med Assoc 2011;240:1323–8.
84. MacDonald MH, Nieto JE, Galuppo LD, et al. Clinical experience with the use of intravenous zoledronic acid in equine orthopedic practice. In: American College of Veterinary Surgeons Veterinary Symposium. Seatle WA; 2010. p. E43.
85. Blobaum AL, Marnett LJ. Structural and functional basis of cyclooxygenase inhibition. J Med Chem 2007;50:1425–41.
86. Smith WL, DeWitt DL, Garavito RM. Cyclooxygenases: structural, cellular, and molecular biology. Annu Rev Biochem 2000;69:145–82.
87. Little D, Jones SL, Blikslager AT. Cyclooxygenase (COX) inhibitors and the intestine. J Vet Intern Med 2007;21:367–77.
88. Martin GR, Wallace JL. Gastrointestinal inflammation: a central component of mucosal defense and repair. Exp Biol Med 2006;231:130–7.
89. Goodrich LR, Nixon AJ. Medical treatment of osteoarthritis in the horse – a review. Vet J 2006;171:51–69.
90. Lees P, Michell AR. Phenylbutazone toxicity in ponies. Vet Rec 1979;105:150–1.
91. Snow DH, Bogan JA, Douglas TA, et al. Phenylbutazone toxicity in ponies. Vet Rec 1979;105:26–30.
92. Gunson DE, Soma LR. Renal papillary necrosis in horses after phenylbutazone and water deprivation. Vet Pathol 1983;20:603–10.
93. Reed SK, Messer NT, Tessman RK, et al. Effects of phenylbutazone alone or in combination with flunixin meglumine on blood protein concentrations in horses. Am J Vet Res 2006; 67:398–402.
94. American Quarter Horse Association. Shows rules and regulations. In: Official Handbook of Rules and Regulations. AQHA, TX: 2008.
95. Federation Equestre Internationale. Veterinary Rules. Prohibited Substances List. 12th ed. 2010.
96. United State Equestrian Federation Rulebook. Drugs and Medications Guidlines. US Equestrian Federation, KY: 2007; p.2–3.
97. FDA US. Center for Veterinary Medicine. Freedom of information summary. EQUIOXX oral paste-0.82% firocoxib (w/w). NADA 2005;141–253.

section 9

Veterinary management of the performance horse

Veterinary aspects of training Thoroughbred racehorses

48

Christopher B. O'Sullivan Jonathan M. Lumsden

CHAPTER CONTENTS

Introduction

Providing optimal veterinary services to Thoroughbred racehorses requires an understanding of both the veterinary aspects of their care, and the dynamics and economics of the racing industry. The following chapter provides a demographic overview of Thoroughbred racing and in particular wastage. Commonly encountered diseases are discussed with an emphasis on the veterinary management and disease prophylaxis during both training and racing.

Demographics and wastage

Thoroughbred racing evolved in England over 200 years ago and now exists in over 50 countries.[1] A comparison of the size of Thoroughbred flat racing industries between some of the major racing countries based on foal crop, number of races and starters, prize money and betting turnover is illustrated in Table 48.1.

All facets of the Thoroughbred racing industry rely heavily on veterinary input, which extends from pre-conception to the end of a horses' athletic career. Termination of a racing career may result from veterinary advice pertaining to injury or disease, or be based on economic grounds and an assessment of athletic ability. Horses are typically retired to stud if they have accomplished a superior racing career that they are unlikely to better, or have genetic potential that would offset their future potential race earnings. Alternatively, other horses are routed to other athletic endeavors if they are functionally sound.

Horses have their first opportunity to race as 2 year olds and their competitive longevity is the result of a multitude of veterinary and specific industry-based factors. Generally the majority of the racing population is made up of horses aged 2 through 5 years of age. Sex distribution of the racing population commences with relatively equal proportions of males and females as yearlings and 2 year olds.[2,3] In subsequent racing years there is an attrition of females to breeding so that horses older than 4 years of age, are typically gelded males[2–4] (Fig. 48.1 and Fig. 48.2).

Age of first race start depends on athletic conformation, degree of maturity, genetics, aspirations and expectations of the owner and trainer, as well as race programming and prize money structure of the specific country. Attempts to judge musculoskeletal maturity and suitability for racing based on objective means such as physeal closure have been generally unsuccessful.[5]

The actual time of first race start is then dependent on the response to training, health, and soundness. Interestingly, in a study examining factors affecting early career wastage there was no correlation between sex and foaling date with time of first race start.[3] While concerns over racing 2-year-old horses exist, two studies

Table 48.1 A comparison of some key industry figures for international Thoroughbred flat racing among major racing countries, for the year 2000

COUNTRY	RACES	PURSES‡	AVERAGE PRIZE MONEY PER RACE	BETTING HANDLE‡	MARES	REG. FOALS	STARTS
United States	45,453	892,452,312	$19,721	11,321	36,503	24900*	364,910
Australia	18,802	444,399,966	$23,636	14,870	26,540	15,893	189,604
Japan	16,984	1,037,163,786	$61,067	33,722	9,378	7,064	180,266
Argentina	5,483	78,103,806	$13,368	202	13,479	8,761	60,196
Great Britain	6,270	98,629,353	$15,730	10,156	9,317	4,635	59,592
France	4,792	148,815,447	$31,054	12,598	7,770	4,984	54,939
Canada	4,376	110,713,003	$25,300	1,497	2,514	1,620	34,252
South Africa	3,901	38,004,055	$9,742	1,272	3,905	3,510	45,562
New Zealand	2,934	36,606,285	$12,477	358	7,893	4,161	32,387
Brazil	4,627	29,014,957	$6,271	219	3,510	2,826	36,989
Italy	3,938	59,844,309	$15,197	2,297	2,300	1,150	35,539
Turkey	4,272	106,241,395	$24,869	1,431	4,324	1,235	44,113
India	3,312	21,245,240	$6,415	478	4,056	1,902	22,463
Chile	4,872	28,712,338	$5,894	271	3,546	1,716	53,349
Germany	1,343	17,402,315	$12,958	129	1,800	977	13,354
Ireland	951	28,067,264	$29,514	4,322	13,763	7,550	11,309
Malaysia	731	12,375,466	$16,929	303	66	49	8,757
Hong Kong	769	108,662,421	$141,303	10,212	**	**	9,773
United Arab Emirates	334	44,478,570	$133,170	†	1	1	4,225
WORLD WIDE TOTALS AND AVERAGES	150,586	2,770,745,640	$18,400	**116,859**	170,850	102,930	1,415,956

Betting handle figures are for the year 2011 IN USD$ MILLIONS
Notes: US $ conversions of the Euro at 1.00 Euro = US $1.32
*Estimated figures
**No breeding industry
***Not reported
†No wagering
‡US Dollars in millions
Source: International Federation of Horseracing Authorities 2011 annual report.

found that horses who raced first as 2 year olds had greater numbers of career starts and raced longer than did horses that commenced racing at an older age.[2,3] This may in part be due to injury or disease that prevented these older horses competing as 2 year olds and which may have persisted further into their career.

Wastage refers to all losses occurring at any stage in the breeding, growth, training and racing of a racehorse. Wastage includes all losses in breeding, deaths at any stage, lost training days, un-raced horses and retirement. Considerable wastage occurs in the Thoroughbred racing industry as a whole from the time that the mare is covered to the commencement of racing by the progeny. A UK-based wastage study calculated 72.8% of mares each year fail to have progeny that will go on to race between 2 and 4 years of age.[6] In this study, the 1975 foal crop was followed and of those named and eligible for training only 50.6% raced as 2, 3, or 4 year olds; this result is confounded by horses reserved for National Hunt racing that did not race on the flat.[6] A more recent UK study following 1022 foals found 52% entered training at 2 years of age. Similar prospective studies of 353 and 553 yearlings sold at auctions in Australia revealed that approximately 50% of these horses raced as 2 year olds and that 75 to 80% of horses had raced by their 6-year-old seasons.[2,3]

Lameness, followed by respiratory disease, is the major cause of wastage for Thoroughbreds in race training, manifesting as lost or affected training days.[3,6–9] A UK wastage study found that 53% of horses showed lameness at some stage during a season and in 20% of cases the lameness was sufficient to prevent racing after injury.[6] A subsequent study identified lameness (67.6%) and respiratory disorders (20.5%) as the most common cause of lost training days.[7] Sore shins and inflammatory airway disease (IAD) were the most commonly encountered ailments in a UK study looking at failure to train and race.[10] Similarly a US-based study looking at 95 horses over an 81-day period reported musculoskeletal injuries altering training or racing schedules in 35–55% of horses and preventing training or racing for a period of time in 26–46% of horses.[11] A recent Australian wastage study of 2- and 3-year-old horses found that of lost or modified training days, 56% were due to lameness and 16% due to respiratory disease.[12] Similar findings have recently been reported out of New Zealand, identifying musculoskeletal (82%) and respiratory diseases (11%) as the major cause of involuntary time out of training.[9] A further reason horses may not race or race less than the average number of times is a 'lack of athletic ability'.[2,6]

Breakdowns, fatal musculoskeletal injuries and sudden death during racing and training have been a focus of many recent studies, most aimed at identifying risk factors in an attempt to minimize these injuries.[13–24] Regional differences exist with regard risk factors, prevalence and types of injuries between countries, states, regions and even individual tracks.[14–18] The rate of breakdown injuries during racing differs between countries, with rates of 2.2/1000, 2.9/1000 and 21/1000 starters in the USA, Australia and Japan, respectively.[13,14,19] These differences are difficult to interpret since they may in part be due to potential errors inherent with epidemiologic studies and different definitions of a breakdown.[17–20] Approximate risk of fatal or catastrophic musculoskeletal injury are 0.6/1000 starters in Australia and 1.4–1.7/1000 starters in the USA, while in the United Kingdom there are 0.8 deaths/1000 starters.[16,20–23] The reasons for differences in rates between countries are multifactorial, but dirt tracks, the presence of medications and longer races have all been implicated as possible factors factor contributing to a higher incidence of injury.[23–26] An Equine Injury Database™ was launched in 2008 with reported rates of fatality rates for 2008–2010 of 2.04–2.00/1000 starters.[27] Catastrophic life-threatening injuries appear more likely to occur when racing, whereas non-fatal injuries are more common in training, which may be a function of speed.[17,19] Breakdown injuries more commonly involve a forelimb than hindlimb, common sites of injury include fetlock and suspensory ligament, carpus, humerus, pelvis, tibia and superficial flexor tendon.[14,19,20,22] There is evidence that pre-existing lesions predispose to catastrophic injuries, highlighting the value of early identification of such lesions in preventing injury.[18,19,27–30]

A multitude of risk factors contributing to breakdown injuries have been identified, including track characteristics,[16,24,31] weather and season,[24] race distance, starting position and race quality.[20,32] Individual horse characteristics identified include racing frequency, training intensity, age at first start, duration of career, number of life time starts and the hoof or shoeing characteristics.[15,16,24,33,34] Causes of sudden death other than fatal musculoskeletal injuries that have been described include ruptured aorta, myocarditis, valvular insufficiency, sclerosis of the coronary arteries, severe pulmonary hemorrhage and disseminated massive hemorrhage.[35]

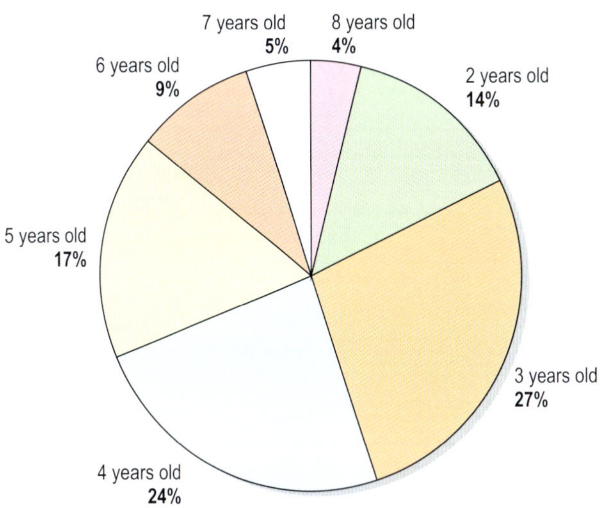

Fig 48.1 Age of racing Thoroughbreds.
Source of data VRC racing services.

Provision of services

A working relationship between the veterinarian and trainer is paramount to providing optimal services to a stable. Excellent communication is essential as is an appreciation of the trainer's perspective and recognition of the non-veterinary factors such as owner expectations and aims, economics and the trainer's previous personal

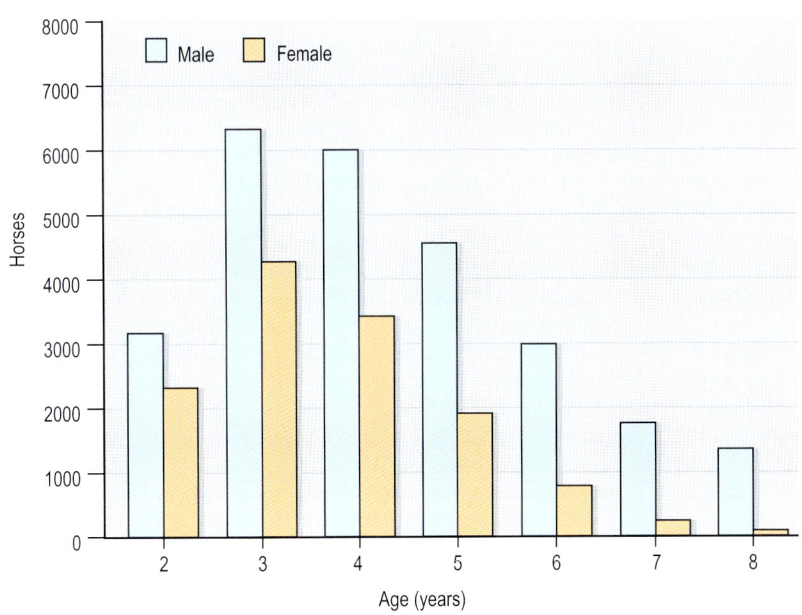

Fig 48.2 Age and sex of Thoroughbred race horses in Australia depicting the lower proportion of females at all ages.
Source of data VRC racing services.

experience. The veterinarian should also have knowledge of normal training techniques and schedules, which often differ between trainers. Veterinary services should be preventive as well as problem oriented and applied at both the individual-horse and whole-stable level. The level and extent of services provided on an ambulatory basis will be dictated by the ability to access a hospital or referral clinic.

The veterinarian–farrier relationship is important because of the prevalence and significance of hoof-related problems. Ideally management and prevention of hoof-related lameness should be a joint approach as opposed to demarcating and allocating 'foot' and 'non-foot' cases. Adequate diagnostics and an understanding of the principles involved in the application of physical and alternative therapies allow the veterinarian to appropriately prescribe and substantiate or refute their use.

Establishment of a complete and reliable recording system of disease, lameness and treatment is essential. Accurate recording of administered medications is important where withdrawal times prior to racing must be considered. The system must be easily accessible, efficient and permanent. Ensuring accurate identification of horses prior to treatment or procedures is paramount in a stable environment, particularly where there are large numbers of horses and staff involved. Similarly, clear instructions and great care should be taken when dispensing and administering medications that may be regulated by racing authorities.

The importance of a thorough clinical examination cannot be overstated. It is often easy to neglect the basics in the busy stable environment. A thorough relevant history and systematic clinical examination are the foundation of any accurate and efficient diagnosis, treatment and prognosis. Horses are often presented for a particular complaint but on closer inspection reveal multiple related and unrelated problems. It is also important to judge what can and cannot be done efficiently, adequately and practically at the racetrack/stable and what is better performed in the clinic setting.

Acquisition of racehorses involves selection of yearlings, 2 year olds and tried (older) horses. Economics and method of purchase by public auction or private treaty will determine the extent of veterinary pre-purchase examination. Limiting comments to lesions and conformational faults only, and their likely effects on future athletic soundness appears the most appropriate advice from a veterinary perspective.

General disease and injury management concepts

Prophylactic measures

Ligament, tendon and joint injuries may occur during breaking and pre-training and reports of swelling or lameness during this period warrants investigation. Subclinical conditions such as osteochondrosis may manifest during preliminary training and early identification may allow treatment with minimal impact on a horse's racing career.

Prophylactic measures to prevent and minimize problems are implemented as part of good stable management. Such measures include routine selection of horses for lameness and clinical examinations, vaccination and parasite prophylaxis programs. Feeding and training regimes are typically established by the trainers. Sound reasoning coupled with subtle diplomacy is required to obtain trainer compliance with regard to feed and work schedule related changes.

The veterinarian has an important role in advising trainers on the value of instructing stable hands and setting up reliable recording systems that ensure staff observe and report on their horses as they go about caring for and riding them. Feedback from stable staff is important at all levels including observations such as fecal amount and consistency, feed consumption, water intake, signs of colic, coughing or evidence of stable vices, all of which can be detected by educated grooms maintaining stalls. Regular assessment of body weights can be used as a monitor of fitness, disease or 'training off'. Recording rectal temperatures of horses with reduced feed intake, subdued demeanor or any other clinical signs of disease should be ingrained as an automatic process.

Daily tacking up can identify a variety of subtle changes including changes in gait as horses are walked out of stall, acquired swellings, skin conditions, nasal discharge and change in response to saddling or bitting. Riders, trainers and clockers can monitor for lameness and more subtle gait changes such as 'hanging on a rein', 'feeling rough' or repeatedly changing strides. Likewise other observations such as respiratory noise, altered breathing pattern or performance and poor recovery after exercise may all facilitate early identification of problems. The use of heart rate meters combined with global positioning system (GPS) data allows tracking of typical speed and heart rate curves and deviations from normal for individuals indicate need for closer veterinary investigation of musculoskeletal, respiratory or cardiovascular systems.

Routine 'trot-up' examinations are an efficient management tool for early detection of musculoskeletal disease and may consist of regular daily, weekly, pre-race or post-race evaluations. Ideally an environment is created where if there is any question as to what effect continued exercise will have on a horse, the trainer will be prompted to have the horse examined. Continuity and regular assessment of individual horses facilitates more specific treatment decisions and detection of subtle changes in gait or lameness. Such monitoring creates a rewarding environment for assessment of therapy, since race performance alone is not always an accurate determinant of therapeutic success.

General management of disease

Early detection and accurate diagnosis of disease coupled with appropriate therapy, rest periods and rehabilitation are all essential to maximize racing longevity. The goal of treatment should be a rapid return to soundness and functionality, without compromising long-term soundness and earning potential. The economic cost of unnecessary or incorrect therapy may be significant. Training alterations require additional considerations, including the impact on the animal's other body systems, particularly the musculoskeletal and cardiorespiratory systems. Furthermore, veterinarians should habitually establish appropriate 'informed consent' of trainers and owners since every treatment has a complication rate that may range from a mild injection site reaction to life-threatening colitis, sepsis or anaphylaxis. In this light, the veterinarian must also consider the risk of musculoskeletal injury with continued racing and training and, importantly, the associated risk to riders.

Medication of horses in training should include considerations of potential side effects as well as optimizing administration times in conjunction with training programs. There is often a compromise required between appropriate medication, required optimal rest and lost fitness. The final decision should be that of the trainer/owner, while the role of the veterinarian is to provide information regarding a disease and then provide a range of options for management, allowing the trainer to weigh up the cost benefits of therapy and modification of their training. Regulatory concerns and drug withdrawal times warrant careful consideration, particularly the use of oral preparations or 'in feed' drugs where stall contamination represents a particular concern.

Specific disease and injury management

The purpose of the following sections is to provide some general approaches to managing commonly encountered injuries and diseases of Thoroughbreds in race training. While different strategies are employed to address different pathology, some conceptual similarities exist with regard to the management of injured or diseased racehorses, particularly with respect to the effect of alterations in training.

Musculoskeletal diseases

Dorsal third metacarpal disease, carpal and fetlock joint disease and tendon or ligamentous injuries are the most common musculoskeletal problems leading to wastage.[7,12,23] Routine, diligent observation of subtle changes in symmetry and meticulous palpation combined with use of hoof testers and flexion tests aids early identification of the most likely site of lameness. Where possible, targeted diagnostic anesthesia and imaging is used which is both economical and time saving. Quality imaging modalities including radiography, ultrasonography and scintigraphy, are essential for accurate diagnosis, treatment and prognostication.

The presence of a secondary lameness is common and may go undetected without appropriate diagnostic anesthesia. Bilateral disease is commonly identified, particularly with carpal and fetlock injuries, tibial stress fractures and sites of osteochondrosis.[36–41] Lameness examinations can be aided in the fractious patient with a small dose of sedation.[42] Jogging in a circle or figure eight can also be useful for assessment of mild lameness and may help differentiate among sites of lesions causing lameness.

Exercise modification

Musculoskeletal diseases often require modifications to the training program, dictated by the disease or injury and the horse's level of fitness. Changing the typical training formula is achieved by alteration of distance and/or speed. Terminology differs geographically in describing the approximate speeds horses train and race and understanding local terminology allows assessment of the current work load and appropriate suggestions with regard to modifications. Speed and distance may be expressed in furlongs (220 yards or approximately 201 meters) (Table 48.2).

Trainers may have a variety of track surfaces available for training horses and advice with respect to training surface should be formulated based on knowledge of the local track characteristics, current track conditions and their contributions to injury risk. Traditionally turf has been associated with a lower risk of musculoskeletal injury than dirt, although confounding factors, primarily geographic, may contribute to this apparent lower risk.[16,24,43] Some specific injuries appear to have an association with particular track surfaces. There is an apparent increase in the incidence of proximal suspensory desmitis in horses working on deeper surfaces with wood chip, dirt and synthetic tracks having an increased incidence over turf. (PE Sykes 2002 pers comm). The incidence of dorsal third metacarpal disease is higher in horses training on dirt compared to wood fiber tracks.[44]

Track condition or rating, has been implicated to influence the risk of injury;[16,45,46] however, several large epidemiologic studies have found no association between track condition and injury rate.[20,24] The mechanical characteristics of dirt and turf tracks are determined in part by their structure, with moisture content being the major variable influenced by weather and track maintenence.[31,45,47,48] Injury risk is higher on turf tracks when the surface moisture content is low, resulting in a harder track and faster race times.[16,19] Dirt tracks, on the other hand, have been associated with injuries under a variety of conditions, typically when moisture content is either too low or high or surface is of inadequate depth or composition.[17,31,46] The mechanical characteristics of synthetic tracks, the majority of which have a wax component, are temperature dependent as well.[49] Synthetic tracks appear to potentially decrease the risks of fatal musculoskeletal injuries; however, they may contribute to an increased risk of other non-fatal injuries. The major contributor to track performance and safety is likely to be associated with good track maintenance regardless of the surface. Unleveled track surfaces and areas where track is compacted such as 'crossings' for horse and vehicular access and areas around starting chutes have been associated with increased risk of injury.[31,50] An inadequate banking or camber on turns may also contribute to injuries and alteration to track camber and surfaces have shown benefits in reducing injury rates in Thoroughbred and Standardbred racing.[51–53] Therefore considerations to track characteristics should be given, especially with advice regarding horses working at high speed or rehabilitating from injury.

Hill or incline work, either under saddle or on an inclined treadmill, allows work rate to increase while limiting speed.[54,55] Inclines modify the activity and loads on various muscles,[56] likely increasing the overall load on the hindlimbs that may be beneficial if attempting to strengthen the hind quarters, or being contraindicated in

Table 48.2 Common terminology and speeds associated with Thoroughbred flat work. A furlong is a measure of distance used in horse racing (1/8th mile, 220 yards approx. 200 m)

COMMON TERMS	APPROXIMATION TO RACE SPEEDS	SPEED (m/s)	TIME PER FURLONG
Trotting work (UK, Aust), jogging (USA)		Approx 4 m/s	
Slow work 'canter' '1/2 pace' (UK Aust), '*gallop*' (USA)	~50% race speed	Approx 8–12 m/s	18-second furlong (11 m/s)
¾ Pace work 'even time' (Aust, UK), '2-minute lick' (USA) Primarily aerobic	~75% race speed	Approx 13 m/s (2-minute mile)	15-second furlong
'Come or sprint home', *'gallop'* (Aust, UK) *'breezing'* (USA), home, finish or sprint Some anerobic contribution	Or 90–100% race speed	16–18 m/s	11–13-second furlong
Top race speeds		18 m/s	11-second furlong or better

horses with hindlimb injuries. Walking in waist deep water in a pool or on a submerged treadmill provides greater work to the advancing limb and may benefit attempts to improve extensor and particularly quadriceps strength.

Direction around turns (clockwise vs counterclockwise) influences limb-loading patterns with the lead limb subject to a greater load than the contralateral limb and this additional loading may predispose the lead limb to injury.[20,57] Typically in a counterclockwise racing direction the horse preferentially leads with the left forelimb on the turn, and for clockwise racing the right forelimb with most horses changing to the opposite lead at some stage during the straight.[58] Many injuries appear to have 'lead' or inside limb predilections dependent on the direction of racing such as dorsal third metacarpal disease,[59,60] superficial digital flexor tendonitis,[46] and antebrachiocarpal joint injuries, particularly the distal radius and proximal intermediate carpal bone.[58] 'Outside' limb injuries are commonly associated with the medial middle carpal joint.[58] Common musculoskeletal injuries associated with limb predilections may be minimized or prevented by training in both directions on turns. If introduced early in a training program it allows development of balance in both directions and minimizes repetitive loading of specified predilection sites.

Walking exercise can be provided by either hand walking, mechanical walkers, or treadmills. Often overlooked, walking is useful in horses that are temporarily out of work and beneficial in horses susceptible to 'tying-up' or with chronic joint complaints. Walking after high-intensity exercise improves recovery.[61] Ponying is useful for horses that do not settle at slow speeds or horses with back complaints, particularly wither or girth rubs. Some musculoskeletal back problems may be exacerbated, if the horse has tendency to track sideways.[62]

Swimming is a primarily aerobic exercise medium useful in reducing the effects of weight-bearing work and has been suggested to decrease the rate of musculoskeletal disease[63] (Fig. 48.3). While allowing non-weight-bearing joint motion, swimming does not stimulate appropriate bone responses or maintain joint ligament tone.[64] Potential complications of pools include infection of pre-existing wounds, interference injuries (higher risk in circular pools), exercise-induced pulmonary hemorrhage, colic and rarely drowning.[65] Swimming increases muscle activity in some selected muscle groups and therefore may be contraindicated in the presence of primary muscle injuries.[66]

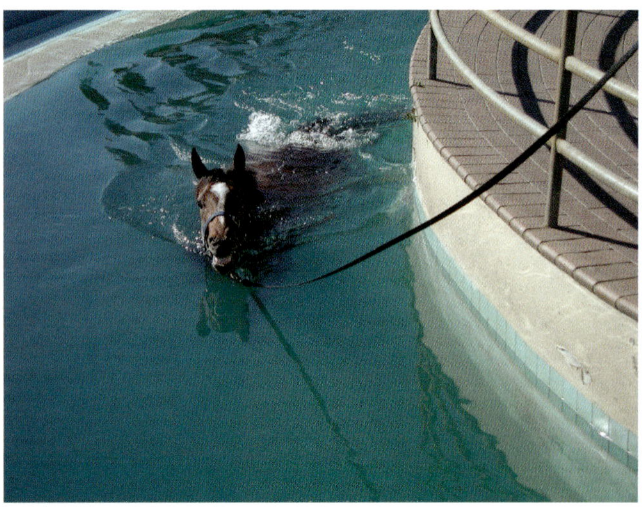

Fig 48.3 A Thoroughbred racehorse swimming in a circular pool.

The effect of complete cessation of exercise on a horse's level of cardiovascular fitness often depends on the horse's stage of training. Horses early in their training phase appear to lose significant amounts of aerobic fitness within 2 weeks, whereas horses more advanced in training are slower to detrain, losing fitness over 4–6 weeks.[67–69]

Bandages and bandaging

Support bandaging can be useful to minimize swelling and edema associated with acute pathology or intermittent limb edema. The effectiveness of lower limb athletic support bandages or boots in preventing injury and their effect on performance is unknown; studies in healthy human athletes indicate they can be performance impairing.[70] Studies of lower limb bandaging and athletic taping have had variable results in different studies: some have demonstrated a beneficial role through either reduced hyperflexion of the fetlock or reduced peak vertical forces,[71–73] while other studies have failed to demonstrate benefits of taping or bandages.[74] Support boots have been shown to reduce maximal extension of the fetlock at the walk and trot and may be beneficial reducing strain in the SDFT and suspensory ligament during rehabilitation.[74,75] Improperly applied bandages may contribute to pathology and any bandaging may be contraindicated at high speed due to effects on heat dissipation.[76,77] Work boots or padded bandages can be used to limit and reduce the severity of interference injuries.

Cold therapy

Cold therapy provides anti-inflammatory, analgesic effects and reduces cellular metabolic demands and should be considered in any acute or chronic injury.[78] Rapid icing of acute injuries is followed by intermittent icing for approximately 48–72 hours until inflammation is resolved; chronic injuries benefit from icing after every bout of high-intensity exercise.[55] Ice water slurries in large rubber boots are easy to apply, have the ability to include the carpus, and cool the limb more efficiently compared with commercial cold packs, reaching stable tissue temperatures in 10 minutes[79] (Fig. 48.4). Excessive icing can cause dermatitis and ice burns. Limiting 'icing' times to less than 30 minutes, applying multiple applications with durations of at least 20 minutes out of the ice and application of a barrier layer (Cling Wrap, UK; Saran Wrap, USA; Glad Wrap, Australia) seems to minimize this complication.

Joint diseases and injuries

Medical management of joint injuries and disease

Early and aggressive anti-inflammatory therapy is indicated with all joint injuries provided the diagnostic process is not compromised. Once the level of joint compromise is determined, appropriate specific treatment can be pursued. Joint inflammation can be controlled with systemic non-steroidal anti-inflammatories (NSAIDs) at recommended doses for 24–48 hours, combined with cold therapy and bandaging. Cessation of high-intensity exercise and the substitution of walking is indicated while the joint is acutely inflamed. Trotting and swimming can be used to maintain activity until the horse is able to return to its previous level of work intensity. Rapid resolution of synovitis and capsulitis is beneficial in avoiding capsular edema and capsular fibrosis that may lead to reduced range of joint motion.[80,81] Passive joint flexion may aid in maintaining range of joint motion.

Intra-articular medications (as discussed in chapter 23) are likely to be most efficacious if used in a planned manner with

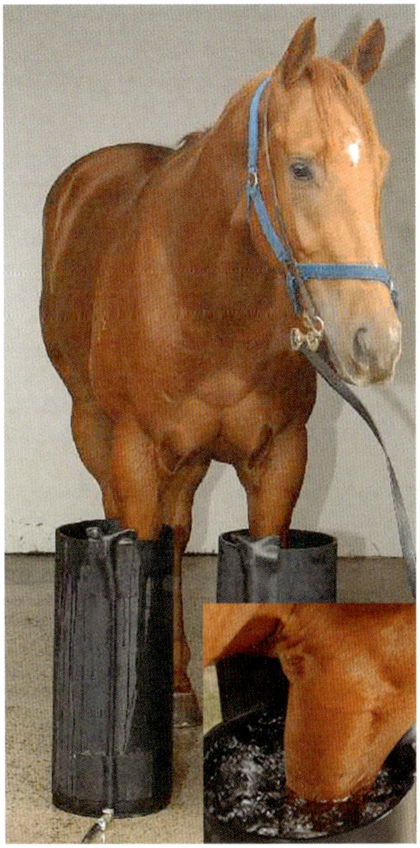

Fig 48.4 A Thoroughbred racehorse receiving cold therapy immersed in an ice slurry (inset) in large rubber turbulator boots. *Photo courtesy of Dr J. Walker.*

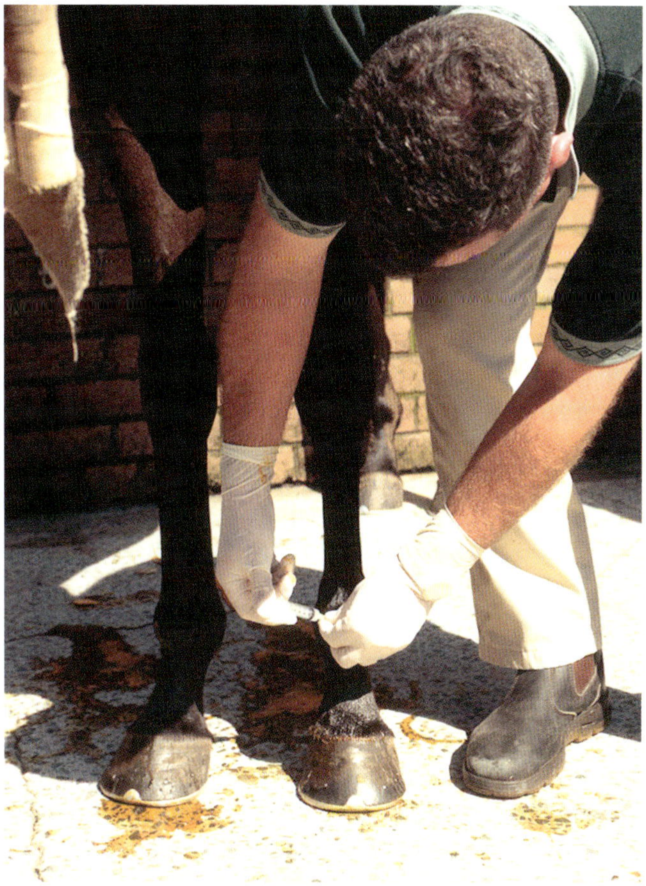

Fig 48.5 Intra-articular medication being administered via a dorsal approach to the left forelimb fetlock joint.

consideration given to the horses training and racing schedules. Maximal anti-inflammatory effect is likely to be gained by early treatment followed by cessation of high-intensity exercise. Joints that are chronically affected should be treated after exercise on a day of planned high-intensity fast work, allowing at least 3–5 days or longer of modified low-impact activity prior to racing. Medicating chronically inflamed joints prior to prolonged layoffs may be beneficial in assisting the resolution of synovitis and capsulitis. The majority of veterinarians use corticosteroids alone or in combination with hyaluronic acid as the mainstay and first choice intra-articular therapy in Thoroughbred racehorses.[82] Autologous conditioned serum is gaining popularity as a treatment, particularly in cases that either respond poorly to corticosteroid treatment or have a more chronic process requiring more regular and prolonged courses of therapy.[82–84]

Aseptic technique during intra-articular injections is essential and excessive ice therapy or the use of liniments or blisters should be avoided because the resultant dermatitis may compromise a suitable injection site (Fig. 48.5). Intermittent systemic anti-inflammatory therapy can be used in combination with long-term administration of disease-modifying osteoarthritic agents such as polysulfated glycosaminoglycans (PSGAGs), pentosan polysulfate, glucosamine and chondroitin sulfate.

Surgical management of joint injury and disease

The primary aim of surgery is to return the joint to non-painful function and limit the formation and progression of osteoarthritis. Surgery is occasionally indicated in order to salvage an animal for breeding or retirement. Before deciding if surgery is indicated, careful consideration must be given to the prognosis, expected rehabilitation time and economics. In many cases surgery assists the diagnostic process and may more accurately determine the prognosis and post-surgical management. Horses occasionally perform successfully with intra-articular lesions that may be addressed surgically, and weighing up the long-term benefits of surgery against the potential short-term economic losses can be difficult, particularly during the high earning stages of horse's careers. A good working relationship with a surgeon experienced in treating joint disease in Thoroughbred racehorses will facilitate the decision-making process. Importantly only horses not considered at risk of breakdown should continue to train and should be monitored for evidence of progression.

Osteoarthritis

Early osteoarthritis can be managed with medical therapy and rest when indicated. The progression of osteoarthritis is often difficult to accurately predict. Despite this, initial and subsequent joint radiography provides valuable assessment of disease progression, in conjunction with regular lameness examinations and assessment of response to therapy. Complete rest for long periods in older horses with osteoarthritis can often be contraindicated with regard to racing longevity, since retraining often places demands on the arthritic joints that they cannot accommodate. Alternatively, maintaining such horses in lower-intensity modified training regimens which include swimming, longer intervals between high-speed work combined with intermittent anti-inflammatory therapy, physical therapy and continual use of disease-modifying osteoarthritis agents may assist in prolonging their racing longevity. Advancing osteoarthritis requires continual monitoring, particularly for evidence of subchondral bone injury that may propagate to complete fracture. Eventually a stage is reached where the level of osteoarthritis becomes incompatible with safe and economic training and racing, and in these cases clinical findings combined with appropriate diagnostics support advice for retirement.

Bone-related injuries and diseases

Stress-related cortical bone injuries 'incomplete stress fractures' have been reported in a variety of bones including the third metacarpal bone, tibia, humerus, pelvis, sacrum, lumbar vertebrae and scapula. These manifestations of bone fatigue have been postulated in some instances as precursors to complete spontaneous fractures.[28,36,40,85–90] Similarly, exercise-induced subchondral bone injuries have been well documented in the third carpal bone and distal third metacarpal and metatarsal bones as well as other sites of osteochondral fractures, and have been proposed to be associated with cyclic loading and bone adaptation responses.[89,91,92]

Training modifications

Training protocols appear to directly influence bone-related injuries and disease.

Changes in training intensity induce bone adaptation via altered forces and fatigue damage, with initial bone weakening due to increased bone porosity.[93] The decreased mineral content is thought to significantly impact bone strength around 3 weeks after an alteration in training.[94,95] and may take up to 3–4 months or longer to replace the lost bone, during which time the bone is weaker.[94–96] It is the bone adaptation process itself that appears the more important component of bone weakening, rather than the fatigue damage.[97] Two-year-old horses appear to be at greatest risk of adaptive bone pathology as their skeleton models and remodels in response to race training. The lowest bone mineral density in these horses occurs at 2–3 months after entering race training.[96,98] Significant decreases in bone mineral content detrimental to bone strength occur during periods of inactivity,[99] and are likely a result of a decrease in bone strains leading to extensive bone remodeling and increased porosity.[93] A greater risk of bone fatigue-related injuries has been associated with return to work after periods of inactivity or lay-up.[90,100]

Since horses training at a slow speeds adapt their bones to that particular speed, the introduction of higher-speed pace work ('breezing') results in altered loads and bending forces requiring a further bone adaptation response, making bone susceptible to fatigue injury during this adaptation period.[93,101] A study examining gait and speed as risk factors for fatigue injury of the third metacarpal bone in 2-year-old Thoroughbred racehorses recommended training modifications to reduce the incidence of 'bucked shins' consisting of reducing the extent of the low-speed long-distance work and increasing the frequency of the short-interval high-speed work.[102] Therefore, allocating less training time to long-distance slow exercise and the introduction of earlier more frequent short distance fast exercise affords bone more time to adapt to race speeds.[90] Problems that may be encountered include the inability to control young poorly educated horses, and the uninvestigated effects of this training protocol on other structures, particularly tendons and ligaments. The most appropriate training regimens to obtain optimal remodeling and modeling responses of bone that will best accommodate forces associated with racing and training are yet to be determined.[103]

Dorsal metacarpal disease

Dorsal metacarpal disease manifesting as 'bucked or sore shins' is one of the most common causes of lost training days in 2-year-old Thoroughbreds; one survey reported it to affect 70% of Thoroughbreds, with increased risk of third metacarpal stress fracture within 6–12 months.[93,104,105] Deciding if affected horses can continue training will depend on severity of the condition as determined by regular palpation of shins, lameness examination and radiographic evaluation. Early identification of disease through palpation and detection of subtle lameness allows early treatment and the majority of horses to remain in training. Treatment should include immediate modifications to the training program and aggressive anti-inflammatory therapy. Monitoring the horse's gait during exercise and the level of pain on palpation of shins are useful in assessing the response to therapy. Swimming can be used to augment fitness, with the track regimen consisting of trotting and shorter distances of pace work regularly (for example, 1–2 furlongs every other day). Horses with more advanced dorsal metacarpal disease have marked pain, evidence of swelling or cortical lucency identified radiographically and should be removed from training on economic grounds for at least 6 weeks. They should be returned to training with suitable modifications to the training regimen as discussed above for horses with adaptive bone pathology. Recommended training schedules to avoid bucked shins and to manage horses with early evidence of bucked shins have been documented.[106]

Third metacarpal dorsal cortical stress fractures

Conservative management typically requires a minimum of 7 months rest with a variable degree of success in achieving healing.[107,108] Surgery offers an advantage with both lag screw fixation or the combination of osteostixis and positional screw fixation are reported to be more reliable than osteostixis alone, with healing and screw removal at 2 months after surgery, followed by resumption of training within 1 month of screw removal.[59,60,109]

Stress fractures at other sites

Stress fractures may be seen at a variety of sites (third metacarpal bone, tibia, humerus, pelvis, sacrum, lumbar vertebrae and scapula) and periods of reported rest for these fractures vary, so there is no clear consensus on an appropriate duration of stress fracture rehabilitation.[110] Provided the stress fracture is not at risk of propagation to a complete fracture, general recommendations include stall rest with hand walking (the horse should be offered about 10 minutes hand walking twice daily, doubling weekly) until the horse is sound at the trot in a straight line. The horse should be evaluated for lameness after 2–4 weeks, first at the walk and if appropriate at the trot. Once sound at the trot, access to a small yard (20 feet square) for a further month is followed by a month of pasture release prior to return to training. A more rapid rehabilitation plan can be instituted under direct veterinary supervision with gradual introduction to low-level trot work after the month of stall rest and walking; however, such a program requires regular lameness and radiographic evaluation to monitor healing and possibly follow-up scintigraphic evaluation. This protocol can minimize time of maximal exercise restriction, but return to high-speed training should be delayed for at least 3 months from time of stress fracture diagnosis. Stress reactions and non-adaptive exercise-induced bone remodeling can also be managed with a similar approach.

Subchondral bone injuries

Subchondral bone injury and associated osteoarthritis occurs primarily in the carpus associated with the third carpal bone and the fetlock joint in the palmar/plantar metacarpal/metatarsal condyles and proximal sesamoid bones.[85,89,111] The pathogenesis of these injuries is poorly understood but involves disease of both the articular cartilage and subchondral bone.[91,92,111] Subchondral epiphyseal bone changes have been identified as potential precursor to some slab fractures of third carpal bone and condylar fractures of the cannon bone.[85,90,113]

The diagnosis and management of subchondral bone diseases is problematic and both joint and bone disease issues should be addressed. Often radiographic findings are equivocal and in these cases scintigraphy can be a useful aid in diagnosis. Determining the degree of subchondral bone injury and collapse on radiographs alone can be difficult; computed tomography and MRI are superior to radiographs in detecting subchondral bone pathology.[113] Typically if subchondral bone damage is evident, prolonged periods of rest are usually required and surgery may be indicated particularly if disease is involving the carpus. Many advanced subchondral bone injuries carry a guarded prognosis for future athletic performance, due to chronic lameness.

Breakdown Injury

Major breakdown injuries in racing Thoroughbreds include severe bone and ligament injuries involving the fetlock (traumatic disruption of suspensory apparatus, condylar fractures and P1 fractures) and carpus (distal or proximal row slab fractures with unstable or collapsed carpus) as well as major fractures of the humerus, tibia and pelvis. Appropriate assessment and use of coaptation for transport of major musculoskeletal injuries has been well described elsewhere and is important knowledge for any racetrack veterinarian.[114] Appropriate first-aid measures prevent further osseous and cartilage injury; maintain skin cover and prevent further damage to blood supply that may ultimately determine the ability to salvage the animal. Removal of these patients from the racetrack environment allows appropriate diagnostics, communications and decision making to take place.

Tendon- and ligament-related injuries and diseases

The combination of training and aging may have a progressive detrimental effect on tendon strength. Micro-trauma due to accumulated submaximal strains results in alterations in tendon structure that decrease its ability to cope with cyclic strains and may ultimately result in injury.[115,116] There may be an 'optimal window' during growth and training for the development of tendon extracellular matrix that would best prepare the tendon for cyclic damage associated with race training; this timing and activity level is yet to be determined and excessive exercise at a young age may result in damage.[117] Prevention and early detection of lesions may become reality with further research into marker molecules that could allow identification of subclinical tendonitis.[118]

Tendon injuries

Superficial digital flexor tendon (SDFT) injuries are a substantial cause of wastage, with a reported incidence in racing Thoroughbreds of 8–43%, and are more prevalent in horses older than 2-years of age.[23,46,119–123] Astute observations of changes in flexor tendon profile, careful palpation and ultrasonography are the essential tools for the identification, assessment of severity, prognostication and monitoring of healing in tendon injuries.[119,120,124–126]

Clinically apparent swelling, heat and pain on palpation indicate the need for careful ultrasonographic evaluation. Re-evaluation of a tendon at 1–3 weeks after injury may provide a more accurate indication of lesion severity and is particularly important when a lesion is suspected but not well defined on the initial examination.[119,120,124,125] Peritendinous inflammation ('bandage bow') is typified by apparent tendon swelling with less intense pain on palpation when compared with tendonitis. Ultrasound confirmation of the diagnosis is required and treatment consists of aggressive anti-inflammatory therapy and cessation of pace work until all inflammation has resolved.[126,127] Slow resolution of inflammation or residual thickening should prompt follow-up ultrasonographic examination.

Ultrasonographic monitoring of healing allows alterations to be made in the rehabilitation program and examinations are advised prior to any major increase in the level of exercise intensity.[125,128,129] Clinical reassessment during rehabilitation is also important and changes should prompt ultrasonography. Blisters are not advised since they affect both the clinical and ultrasonographic assessment of a tendon and have no documented benefits.[122,130] The prognosis for SDFT injuries in the Thoroughbred is reported to range from 20–60% of horses returning to successful racing and up to 80% sustaining a re-injury.[120,131–134] Continuing to train with a mild lesion in a Thoroughbred racehorse results in progression to a more severe lesion. This is seldom economically or clinically successful and carries the risk of a catastrophic breakdown.

Controlled exercise rehabilitation programs may improve results with 71% of horses treated with a graded exercise program racing at least once compared with 25% of horses subjected to pasture rest alone.[135] The decision to embark on a rehabilitation program should take economics into consideration, particularly the costs and benefits.[125,128] Regardless of the level of rehabilitation undertaken, initial management involves cessation of training and aggressive anti-inflammatory therapy. The value of additional medical management procedures including intralesional or peritendinous sodium hyaluronate, polysulfated glycosaminoglycans and β-aminopropionitrile fumarate has not been well defined.[121,122] Similarly, regenerative medicine techniques including the use of stem cells, platelet-rich plasma and other growth factor based biologics have been widely used recently and have shown some promise; however, at this stage in flat racing Thoroughbreds, none have shown dramatic improvements over rest and rehabilitation alone.

Surgical intervention has been suggested to improve prognosis with tendon splitting in the acute phase often combined with superior check ligament desmotomy.[136,137] Superior check ligament desmotomy has a reported prognosis of 68–88% for returning horses to racing, with 52–56% racing at least 5 times after surgery.[123,138,139] These results are similar to reports of conservative therapy alone.[123,133] Furthermore, superior check desmotomy may increase the risk of suspensory ligament injury.[123] Regardless of additional therapies, the total time required prior to reintroduction to race training is 8–12 months; a worse prognosis is documented for horses rested for less than 6 months.[120,125,128]

Injuries of the suspensory ligament and its insertions

Training appears to have a strengthening effect on the suspensory apparatus with untrained horses more likely to experience ligament failure at smaller loads, whereas trained horses fail at greater loads with fracture of the proximal sesamoid bones.[140] The diagnostic approach is similar to that for tendon lesions although prognostication based on a lesion's ultrasonographic appearance is more difficult. Inferior ultrasonographic image quality compared to that obtained when imaging superficial digital flexor tendons and the presence of muscle fibers complicates both diagnosis and assessment of healing, particularly in the high suspensory area.[125,141] The prognosis for return to racing after suspensory desmitis has been reported to be relatively poor.[142]

Suspensory branch desmitis and sesamoiditis

Suspensory branch desmitis appears most prevalent in younger horses and particularly 2 year olds early in their career.[143–146] Desmitis of the suspensory branches may manifest with concurrent sesamoiditis, sesamoid fractures or splint bone lesions.[143,146] Sesamoiditis, on the other hand, is often identified prior to training and a range of severity exists and may progress with training.[144] Management of sesamoiditis is difficult and can be frustrating as recurrence with resumption of higher-intensity exercise is common. Initial therapy consists of local application of cold therapy, pressure bandaging and administration of systemic anti-inflammatory agents. Long-term rest up to 6 months is important to allow bone maturity and prevent fracture. Despite the benefits of long-term rest, the radiographic appearance of the lesions seldom makes an appreciable improvement. The long-term effect on the horse's career is not clear; however, it appears that the severity and presence of additional pathology such as enthesiophytes impact on both racing longevity and earning potential.[147,148]

Suspensory branch and body

Horses developing small lesions of the suspensory branch early in training often only require 4–6 months and have a fair to good prognosis. In contrast, lesions in older horses, more advanced lesions, or those slow to resolve ultrasonographically, have only a poor to fair prognosis and require prolonged periods of rest up to 12 months. A higher incidence of reoccurrence is seen in these horses, the desmitis behaving similar to that described in show and dressage horses.[149] Rehabilitation is similar as for tendons, with a graded exercise program and ultransonographic monitoring of healing combined with attention to foot balance, particularly avoiding excessive heel length. There are anecdotal reports of horses with mild lesions remaining in training and racing, particularly if speed work is limited to race starts only; however, there is a risk of progressive damage or complete failure.[149]

Lesions of the suspensory body are dealt with using similar methods as discussed for tendon injuries. The presence of concurrent splint bone lesions should be ruled out. Typically, management and the prognosis for return to racing is determined by the lesion severity and assessment of the healing response. At least 8–12 months is usually necessary prior to returning to training.

Proximal suspensory and its attachment

Lameness associated with the proximal suspensory ligament and its attachment is relatively common in Thoroughbred racehorses.[150] Diagnosis can be difficult because of the variety of ligament or bone lesions seen separately or together, with a wide range of clinical severity.[151] In addition, the intimate association of the carpometacarpal joint and proximal suspensory ligament limits the specificity of diagnostic anesthesia to identify lameness arising from the proximal suspensory area and the carpometacarpal and middle carpal joints.[146,149,152] Clinical differentiation of high suspensory pain and third carpal bone disease can be difficult.[149]

Horses identified with primary ligament lesions are managed similar to tendon injuries. Those with primary bone damage may have non-adaptive bone remodeling 'stress reaction', longitudinal or avulsion fracture of the palmar cortex of the third metacarpal.[153–155] Management of bone injuries has been discussed and typically at least 3–6 months is required depending on the specific lesion.

Nuclear scintigraphy may be particularly useful in assessing the relative contribution of bone and ligament pathology causing lameness. Mild lameness of short duration often responds to medical management. A combination of NSAIDs, infiltration of the proximal suspensory area with a corticosteroid, correction of dorsopalmar foot balance and modifications to training mimicking that advised for horses with a bone remodeling problems, have provided success in treating approximately half these cases. Horses are limited to a low-intensity workload until the lameness has resolved, typically within a 5-day period. Persistent lameness indicates the need for further diagnostics. Extracorporeal shock wave therapy may be useful for treatment of proximal suspensory ligament injury as well as having potential for treatment of other tendon, ligament or insertional injuries.[156,157]

Foot-related injuries and shoeing

The foot is a common site of lameness and poor foot conformation is a common Thoroughbred trait, particularly under run heels and long toes that may predispose to injury.[3,7,34,158,159] Foot balance in the dorsopalmar or plantar plane appears important. Excessive heel length or wedging and the resultant high hoof angles preferentially loads the suspensory ligament and SDFT, predisposing these structures to injury.[160–163] Suspensory apparatus failure has been associated with under run heels (difference in toe and heel angles) and low toe angles have been associated with an increased risk of catastrophic injury. Decreasing the difference between toe and heel angle and increasing the toe angle alone may reduce injury risk.[33,164,165] Toe grabs on shoes were banned based on their association with an increased incidence of injury.[34,165]

Overreach injuries are typically high impact, with deep tissue damage usually greater than is initially apparent. Rarely do they initially cause a significant lameness unless there is major tissue trauma. These injuries can become a site of lamina detachment and if overlooked result in pocketing of dirt and subsequent infection, manifesting as lameness 3–7 days after the initial injury (Fig. 48.6). Prevention of this sequelae requires excision of the separated tissue back to lamina attachment combined with bandaging while avoiding sand and dirt from gaining entry to the laminae–wall interface. Repetitively injured horses can be managed with 'bell boots' and shoeing changes.

Corns are a common cause of lameness and appear to be more commonly associated with flat sole, low heel and long toe conformations increasing weight-bearing in the caudal aspect of the foot.[166] Addressing foot balance combined with light paring of sole over the bruising and application of a seated out heart-bar shoe combined with 2–3 days low-intensity exercise is generally adequate to resolve lameness. In some cases it may be necessary to 'float' the affected heel off the shoe. Hoof treatments are initially aimed at reducing inflammation and softening the sole overlying the bruised area through localized poulticing coupled with anti-inflammatory agents. These modifications combined with low-impact work including walk, trot, swimming are undertaken until there is resolution of inflammation and lameness. Use of heart-bar or egg-bar shoes and correction of foot balance by removal of excess toe provides more support for the caudal third of the foot. Time is necessary for dissipation of interstitial fluid and re-cornification of the bruised solar tissue. Once the pain is resolved, hardening of the

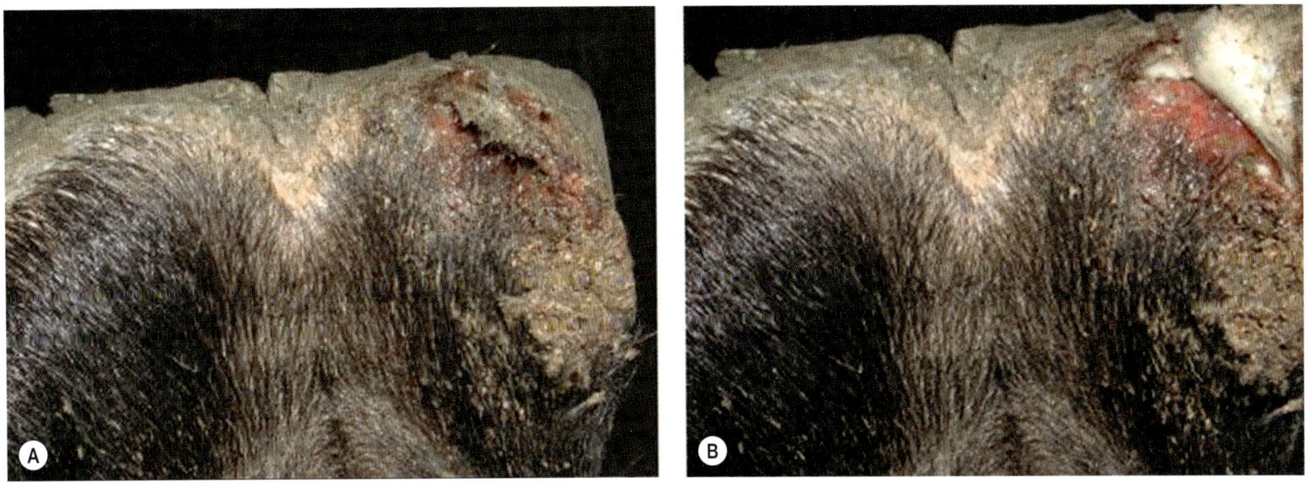

Fig 48.6 **(A)** Overreach injury to the lateral heel of a left forelimb above. **(B)** The lamina detachment that can be present with these injuries.

new sole can be achieved by applying diluted iodine solution (2%) or formalin (10%).

Quarter cracks are manifestations of shear forces within the hoof wall and laminae. Some cases may be associated with hoof imbalance and excessive wall length in the affected quarter.[167] Cracks may be identified prior to lameness, providing an opportunity to prevent crack propagation and lameness by corrective trimming/shoeing and modified exercise regimes. Depending on size, stability and the extent of propagation many smaller stable cracks can be debrided and patched. This combined with rasping of the quarter, attention to foot balance and application of a bar shoe all assist in stabilizing the crack.[168] Unfortunately many cracks in Thoroughbreds involve the heel or caudal aspect of the quarter and are not readily amenable to repair. These caudal cracks, and cracks with coronary band involvement often require stripping of the hoof wall to allow re-growth of stable horn tissue.

Pedal osteitis, pedal bone 'rim' fractures, sole bruises and other injuries secondary to solar concussion are often accentuated by exercise on sand tracks. Management includes sole pads, wide web seated out shoes and egg-bars shoes. Discrete sole lesions can be covered temporarily with a small welded plate to protect the area, while still allowing access of topical treatment.

High nails or 'nail presses' can be overlooked during lameness examinations. Nail and/or hematoma pressure may result in persistent lameness without evidence of infection. Evaluation of clinch heights and sequential application of hoof testers to each nail will facilitate their identification. If identified before the onset of infection the nail can be removed and iodine solution flushed down the nail hole to disinfect and facilitate drying. If infected, soaking the foot in Epsom salts, poulticing and debridement are indicated.

Interference injuries

Interference injuries can result from one or a combination of factors including conformation, shoeing, soundness and immaturity (Fig. 48.7). Identifying the cause of the interference is necessary in order to develop a plan aimed at resolving the problem. The presence of neurologic disease should be ruled out. If necessary, identification of the source of interference can be determined by applying chalk to the affected area to identify the limb and area causing the interference. Resolution requires ideal foot balance and in younger horses time is needed to learn and achieve balance on

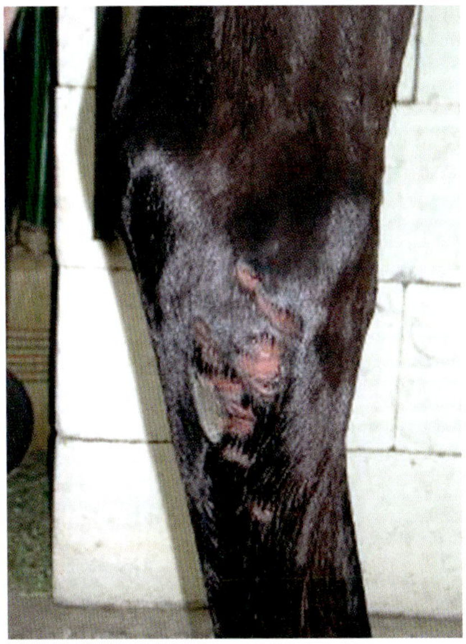

Fig 48.7 Multiple interference injuries on the medial aspect of this Thoroughbred's left hock. This type of interference is commonly referred to as 'hock hitting' or 'speedy cutting'.

the straight before high-speed work around turns is introduced. Protective bandaging and bell boots minimize trauma while attempts are made to resolve a problem. Lighter shoes, partial shoes ('tips') and 'safing'(rounding) of edges resolves many problems.

'Going down on bumpers' or 'running down behind' describes excoriation typically of the plantar fetlock in the hindlimbs and occasionally in the forelimbs (Fig. 48.8). This can be multifactorial and may be associated with fatigue, shoeing, or compensation for lameness. At times this may be severe and result in the removal of full-thickness skin cover. If no lameness problems are identified and if the problem continues with a temporary decreased intensity of training the application of wedged heels, extended heel or egg-bar shoes and correction of dorsoplantar foot balance can assist resolution. Recurrently injured horses often require taping of the fetlocks with protective padding such as orthopedic felt or other padding. All interference injuries should be treated as contaminated wounds with potential for infection.

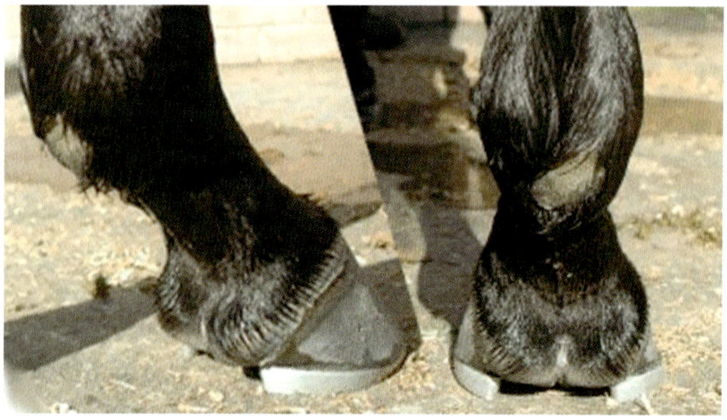

Fig 48.8 An example of 'running down behind' or 'going down on the bumpers' chronic excoriation seen here on the plantar aspect of the right hind fetlock in this Thoroughbred racehorse. Note also the slightly wedge-heeled shoe that has been applied in an attempt to reduce the ongoing trauma to the area.

Muscle-related injuries and disease

Recurrent exertional rhabdomyolysis (RER)

Most commonly seen in 2-year-old fillies RER is reported to affect approximately 5% of racing Thoroughbreds.[169,170] The quantitative correlation between muscle enzymes and severity of clinical signs is poor and elevation of muscle enzymes after exercise does not always indicate clinical rhabdomyolysis; conversely, clinically affected horses may have delayed peaks and more prolonged elevations of enzyme activity in serum.[169,171] Horses exhibiting elevated muscle enzymes and minimal clinical signs warrant further investigation and management changes, since the effect on ultimate performance is unknown.[171] Serial monitoring of muscle enzymes is a reasonable tool to determine responses to management changes and therapy. Cases responding poorly warrant further diagnostic evaluation.[171]

Management issues that can be manipulated include diet, exercise schedules and potential stressors.[172,173] Minimizing stressors by maintaining a regular daily work schedule and quieter stall location remote from major traffic areas in stable are recommended. Benefit can be gained from different exercise prior to track work, including extensive walking, swimming or 'ponying'. Tranquilization can also assist, with low doses of acepromazine (5–10 mg intramuscularly 60 minutes prior to work) effective in some cases. Reduction of the amounts of digestible carbohydrate in diet can be achieved by reduction of the quantity of grain or substitution of a less digestible carbohydrate source replacing oats with corn,[174] while adding fat to maintain dietary calories.[172] Dietary change may be more important in modulating the degree of nervousness and excitability rather than playing a direct role in the pathogenesis of the disease.[173] While the use of progestagens is often advocated, no association in elevation of muscle enzymes was seen in fillies associated with their estrous cycle; controlling estrus behavior may still act to minimize stress levels in some individuals.[169] Electrolyte, and vitamin E and selenium supplementation may also be of benefit.[171]

Working twice daily with one session only being light work avoiding 'days off' and substituting different forms of exercise on days that horses are not worked can all be effective managing difficult cases combined with reduction or complete removal of grain from diet on these rest days is indicated. A slow introduction of high-intensity work coupled with a gradual increase in carbohydrates which follows increased workloads limits subclinical elevations in muscle enzymes. Cases responding poorly to other management changes may respond to administration of muscle relaxants such as methocarbamol, dantrolene and phenytoin.[171,175] Use of oral branched-chain amino acid preparations prior to exercise has been reported anecdotally to reduce the magnitude of muscle enzyme elevations.

Treatment of acute cases includes immediate cessation of exercise and administration of polyionic fluids (either intravenous or oral, depending on severity) to achieve rehydration and promote diuresis, combined with administration of NSAIDs (flunixin meglumine or phenylbutazone). Acepromazine appears efficacious in calming these horses and may facilitate resolution of RER. Occasionally extremely uncomfortable horses may require α_2-agonists and opiates for analgesia.

Muscle strains and tears

Primary muscle injuries are difficult to verify as a source of lameness and usually require exclusion of skeletal lesions. Swelling, asymmetry and pain on deep palpation may be apparent in some cases. Measurement of muscle enzymes is of limited value as elevated enzyme levels are generally not a consistent finding with isolated muscle tears. Lameness is typically the most obvious at the walk and swing phase of the trot. Muscles commonly identified include semimembranosus, semitendinosus and brachiocephalicus. Accompanying bone lesions may be present and are seen most commonly at the tuber ischii with tears of the semimembranosus and semitendinosus. Muscle tears generally require a rest period of 2–3 weeks to resolve if no bony involvement is present;[172] more significant time appears required for tears of the brachiocephalicus, requiring 3–6 weeks of rest.

Back and wither injuries

Withers are a common site of injury due to saddle rubs or falls. These are susceptible to rubbing, hematoma formation and infection. They are best managed by avoiding saddle contact until completely healed and exercise may continue with use of military saddles or swimming and 'ponying'. Padding in most cases is inadequate due to the propensity to rub.

Diagnosis of back injuries and related pain is often difficult. Typically pain is muscular in origin and may be associated with an underlying lameness. The presence of bony pathology such as vertebral stress fractures and overriding spinous processes may be demonstrated with radiology or nuclear scintigraphy.[176,177] Treatment is directed at identifying the underlying cause coupled with temporary cessation of pace work, anti-inflammatories and local therapy.[178]

Infections of the musculoskeletal system

High-intensity exercise, close horse-to-horse and horse-to-handler interaction, confined surroundings and veterinary intervention contribute to Thoroughbred racehorses commonly experiencing a variety of musculoskeletal infections. Cellulitis is common and generally seen in the lower limb. Occasionally idiopathic peri-articular tarsal infections are seen.[179] Traumatic injury leading to osseous infection is common. Although rare, clinicians should be observant for signs of septic arthritis given the frequency of intra-articular therapy and the repercussions of this complication. There are rare reports of idiopathic synovial infections of horses in training.[180]

Successful treatment is facilitated by rapid identification and institution of appropriate antimicrobial therapy, adequate wound therapy, clean bandaging and avoiding areas of contamination, such as sand rolls, water activities, and the hands of the stable staff. Antibiotic selection should take into consideration the high concentrations of horses interacting in a common environs coupled with intense human contact and frequent use of antimicrobials. It is likely that individual racetrack environments will establish predominant pathogens with specific sensitivities akin to a hospital environment.

Respiratory diseases

Lower respiratory diseases

Respiratory disease is a major cause of wastage for horses in race training, and lower respiratory diseases in particular appear to contribute most significantly.[181–184] An appropriate diagnostic work-up consisting of a clinical examination and use of clinical pathology (hematology, transtracheal aspirate [TTA] and bronchoalveolar lavage [BAL]), endoscopy, ultrasonography and radiography, when indicated to allow appropriate management and prognostication.[185,186] In addition, assessment of the environment, stall or yard conditions including design, horse movements, bedding and feeding are important in the diagnosis and management of lower airway disease in the horse in training.

Coughing horses and inflammatory airway disease (IAD)

Horses suffering from IAD typically present as otherwise apparently healthy young horses usually 2–3 years old that have been in the stable environment for a couple of weeks or longer and present primarily for 'coughing'.[181–183,187–189] The presence of a nasal discharge may be variable. Endoscopic evaluation typically reveals a mucopurulent tracheal exudate containing elevated numbers of neutrophils. Although the severity of tracheal exudate has been correlated with lower airway inflammation, observing upper airway mucus may occur independently of lower airway inflammation; therefore its presence is not an indication for testing for lower airway inflammation.[190] Furthermore, neutrophil proportion of tracheal wash samples has been shown not to be as useful as visual assessment of tracheal mucus in identifying horses in training which require treatment and management for IAD.[191] Excessive coughing is stimulated by laryngotracheal palpation, auscultation with the aid of a rebreathing bag or passing an endoscope into the trachea.[181–183,187–189]

Historically, viral respiratory infections have been implicated as the major cause of lower respiratory disease in young racehorses.[192,193,194] Recent studies suggest a variety of pathogens, including bacteria, mycoplasma, endotoxin and non-infectious agents may contribute to IAD.[195–199] The role that bacteria isolated from transtracheal aspirates play in this syndrome is unclear. Their quantity, whether extra- or intracellularly located and species (*Streptococcus*, *Pasteurella* and *Bordetella* spp.) have all been considered as characteristic of IAD.[189] The role of antibiotics in treating IAD has yet to be established.

The environment appears to be an important component of IAD, triggering allergic or non-allergic airway inflammation.[187,200,201] Air quality improvements can be made by minimizing feed dust with low dust or wet feeds, soaking hay and feeding on the ground. Housing changes include improving ventilation by use of yards or pens and reviewing choice of bedding by avoiding straw and dusty beddings in favor of wood shavings or clean sand.[202] Minimizing noxious gases by regular stall cleaning and minimizing dust production by avoiding sweeping and mechanical 'blowers' in favor of hosing also improve air quality. Quarantine of cases may reduce risks if an infectious cause is suspected because of the sudden onset of multiple cases.

Pharmacologic therapy for IAD includes systemic or inhaled mucolytics, bronchodilators and corticosteroids. The presence of mast cells in BAL fluid may indicate the presence of immune-mediated airway disease. In such cases use of a short course of systemic corticosteroids and an inhaled mast cell stabilizer (sodium cromoglycate) may be indicated.[201,203,204]

Exercise-induced pulmonary haemorrhage (EIPH)

Exercise-induced pulmonary hemorrhage (EIPH) is thought to occur due to high transmural alveolar capillary pressures,[205,206] and numerous factors may contribute to the severity of hemorrhage including exercise intensity, distance, age, upper respiratory obstruction, heterogeneous ventilation, hemorrheological factors, small airway disease and lower airway inflammation.[207–212] Despite this, a recent study showed that age, sex, weight carried, track hardness, speed of racing or air quality did not have a strong association with development of EIPH.[213] The reported prevalence of EIPH depends on the criteria used, with epistaxis occurring in approximately 1–2% of race starters.[207,214] After high-intensity exercise (30–90 minutes) there is endoscopic evidence of EIPH in approximately 75% of horses.[207,208] Bronchoalveolar lavage (BAL) is a more sensitive means of documenting EIPH and has demonstrated its presence in nearly all racing Thoroughbreds. Furthermore, BAL may better correlate with severity and chonicity.[215]

Identification and appropriate treatment of IAD combined with the use of bronchodilators and furosemide prior to exercise are still the popular mainstays of EIPH therapy., Although efficacy in reducing EIPH has not been definitively demonstrated, pre-race administration of furosemide has been shown to decrease the incidence and severity of EIPH under race conditions.[216–217] Even in jurisdictions where furosemide is not allowed on race day it can be incorporated in the training program and used prior to high-intensity training. The furosemide dosage is typically (150–250 mg) given intravenously or intramuscularly 2–4 hours prior to work.[218,219] One study suggested administration 30 minutes prior to exercise was superior to administration at an earlier time of 240 minutes.[220]

The association with the high work intensity makes training modifications difficult; slower longer duration work may decrease severity of EIPH, since the disease has been documented with greater incidence in racing distances less than a mile.[212] Blood in the airway incites an inflammatory response and complete eythrophagocytosis takes up to 2 weeks.[221, 222] Management should be aimed at minimizing high-intensity exercise during the inflammatory period, and treating airway inflammation. Response to therapy can be assessed with a follow-up BAL. Investigation of the FLAIR™ nasal strip has shown potential benefits in upper airway mechanics and a reduction of EIPH; however, controversy (prohibited by some racing jurisdictions) and conflicting results exist with its use.[223–226]

Upper respiratory diseases

Upper respiratory diseases commonly manifest as poor performance, and in most cases are associated with abnormal upper respiratory noise. Upper airway abnormalities have a prevalence of approximately 6–10% in racing populations.[227–229]

Detailed investigation of an upper respiratory abnormality should include a thorough accurate history aimed at characterizing the noise and determining if there is an effect on performance. Historical information should also include detail of any previous upper airway surgical procedures or use of gear or tack to improve the observed problem. Track visits or the use of 'sound spectrum analysis' assist noise characterization.[230] Diligent and systematic clinical examination is indicated particularly with respect to palpation of the larynx, rostral nasal septum, jugular veins and assessment of facial symmetry, previous surgical scars and airflow from each nostril. Resting upper airway endoscopic examination should document nasal passages, nasopharynx, trachea and guttural pouches as well as laryngeal dynamic function induced by swallowing and nasal occlusion. Additional endoscopic evaluation may be obtained with the use of a custom-made 'epiglottic elevator' introduced via the contralateral nasal passage to examine the sub-epiglottic region.[231] Further diagnostics such as high-speed treadmill endoscopy, ultrasound, radiography and oropharyngeal examination may be indicated. The recent availability of over-ground dynamic video-endoscopic equipment has provided much needed visual documentation of upper airway function of racehorses exercising under their normal racetrack conditions.[232]

Over-ground dynamic respiratory endoscopy

The ability to image the upper airway of the racehorse during ridden exercise in the horse's normal working environment has greatly advanced veterinarians' ability to more readily and accurately replicate exercise-related dynamic upper airway obstructions. The ease of application, safety and tolerance by the horse in training of this instrumentation has allowed assessment of the influence of rider, tack, surface, head position and environment on upper airway conditions. Since the introduction of the first commercially available dynamic respiratory endoscope in 2008 providing diagnostic quality reproducible images, there are now several systems of varying quality, features and cost. The prevalence of upper airway performance limiting conditions, ease of application, reproducibility of diagnostic images and affordability has made this an invaluable tool to the Thoroughbred racetrack practitioner. The semi-rigid malleable insertion tube in conjunction with wireless telemetric video-endoscopic recording creates quality video recordings comparable to and in many cases superior to that obtained by treadmill video-endoscopy (Fig. 48.9 and Fig. 48.10). Essential to the clinical value of this diagnostic technique is reliable production of quality recordings, frame by frame (25 frames per second) analysis and control and documentation of the exercise protocol. There is little doubt that an established protocol, appropriate equipment preparation, maintenance, trained technical staff and experience are essential to achieve reliable quality recordings. These factors could be no more relevant than on the Thoroughbred racetrack where the environment and nature of the breed predisposes to an excitable patient and the need for efficiency. The over-ground examination requires clear communication with the trainer to coincide with the horses fast work. This individualized scheduling is essential to maximize the value of the examination and minimize the disruption to training schedules. Furthermore, the upper airway recording period of most interest is typically a brief period (30–60 second) of high-intensity exercise nearing the end of the exercise. If the recording does not produce diagnostic quality images, repeat examinations require scheduling to coincide with the horses' ongoing training/racing regime. Application of heart rate monitors and GPS systems are also easily adapted to the protocol and provide valuable information when assessing the exercise regime. In most horses, the

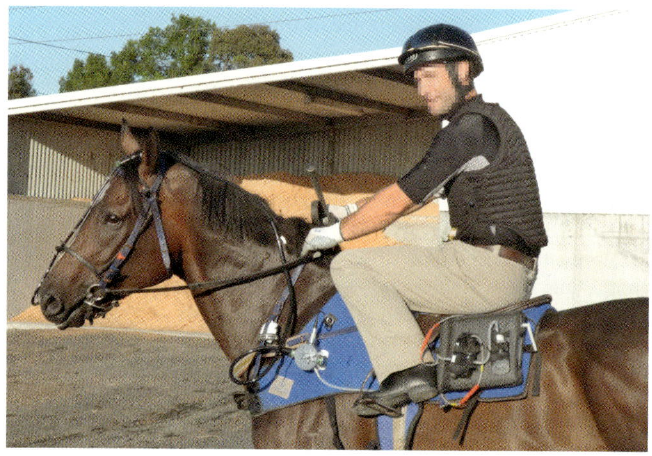

Fig 48.9 A horse with a fitted over-ground dynamic endoscopy unit that is head and saddle cloth mounted.

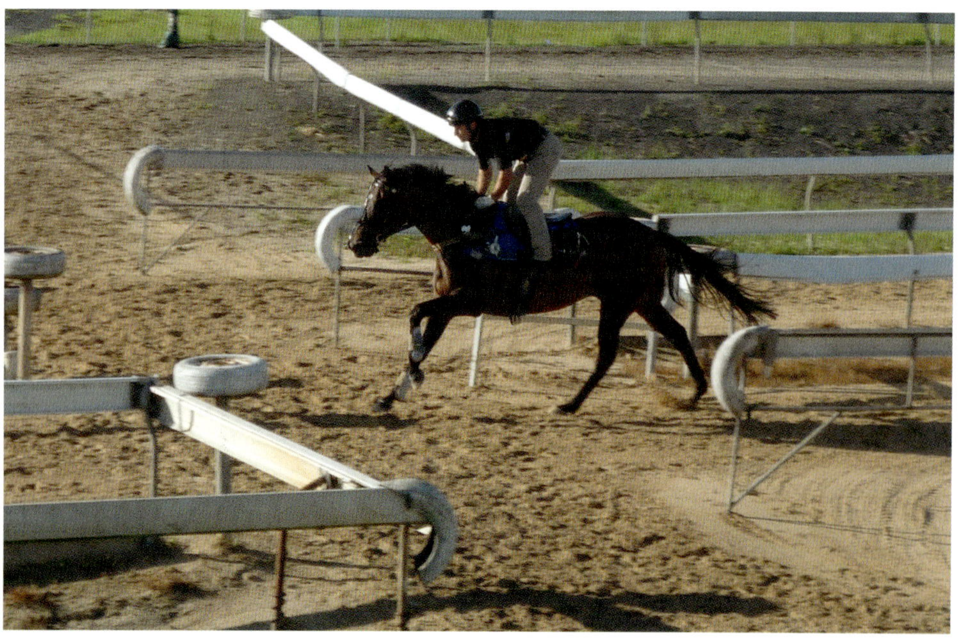

Fig 48.10 Exercising on racetrack with the over-ground dynamic endoscopy unit.

noise and poor performance is a race-related assessment; therefore, the goal of the exercise protocol is to replicate these conditions.[233] The chances of obtaining a definitive diagnosis from the examination are improved by emphasizing the need for trainers to replicate racing conditions as much as possible; this is often assisted by working the horse in company with another horse. The variability and tendency for training exercise regimes to not replicate the level of exertion reached during competitive racing has been associated with a lower sensitivity of over-ground endoscopy in diagnosing intermittent dorsal displacement of the soft palate versus endoscopy during high-speed treadmill strenuous exercise.[234] Accurately documenting sectional exercise times (200 m/furlong intervals) over the final 1000–1200 m is important to correlate frame-by-frame video findings with the stage of exercise and observations of the rider.

Left recurrent laryngeal neuropathy (RLN)

Once diagnosed, the prognosis and suitability for surgery should be carefully determined. Potential diagnostic oversights include previous surgery, arytenoid chondritis, fourth branchial arch defects and other upper airway or lower airway conditions such as IAD and EIPH in conjunction with RLN. Presence of these abnormalities will negatively impact on the surgical prognosis. Prior to considering surgical treatment there should be careful assessment of the horse's recent race record, including the distances over which it is racing. Many horses with early evidence of RLN are able to continue racing successfully over shorter distances. The level of arytenoid function at rest should be determined and graded using recognized laryngeal grading systems.[235,236] Horses with a history of exercise intolerance and/or noise during exercise and laryngeal function which reveals transient full abduction (grade IIIA Havermeyer) or less than full abduction (grade III/IV;[235] grade III B,C Havemeyer[236]) warrant endoscopic examination during exercise either over ground or on a high-speed treadmill.[235,237] This dynamic examination is important not only to determine the degree of left arytenoid cartilage abduction sustained during exercise but also to allow detection of additional upper airway obstructions occurring concurrently.[238] If arytenoid abduction at maximal exercise is judged better than would be obtained with surgery, continued training and racing with regular monitoring may be indicated; surgery may be required if there is progressive loss of function. Assessment of the dynamic function of the upper airway during exercise is invaluable in assessing the structures involved and their contribution to airway obstruction to determine the optimum treatment regime. Ultrasound examination of the laryngeal musculature (cricoarytenoideus lateralis m.) may also provide further clinical evidence of the likelihood of dynamic collapse during exercise. Prior to embarking on surgery, an assessment of the horse's athletic ability, distance of races and evaluation of other performance-limiting conditions may be better assessed by continued training and racing over 5–6 furlongs if the degree of airway compromise permits. That said, the previously held assessment that the racing outcome for horses after laryngoplasty was poorer for horses with grade III laryngeal function compared to that for horses with grade IV laryngeal function at the time of surgery has been shown to be unsubstantiated.[239] Prognosis for racehorses undergoing laryngoplasty has been reported to range from 40 to 85% for a successful outcome with horses able to return to training within 2 months. Despite the above-reported range, improved racing performance can be realistically expected in ~70% of racehorses when laryngoplasty is performed by experienced surgeons.[240–242] The most common postoperative complication after laryngoplasty is loss of abduction, with a loss of one grade or more reported to occur in approximately 50% of operated horses within 6 weeks of surgery.[243] Although follow-up endoscopic examination may reveal a loss of abduction postoperatively, the success or failure of the procedure should not be based on endoscopic assessment alone and should be assessed in conjunction with return to racing and dynamic exercising evaluation whenever possible. Retrospective performance analyzes of horses undergoing prosthetic laryngoplasty has shown that the degree of abduction does not reliably correlate with a successful surgical outcome.[241,244] Continued poor performance or respiratory noise after surgery is best evaluated by video endoscopic examination during exercise to accurately assess the exact cause of any ongoing airway obstruction and therefore determine the most appropriate management required. Complications of surgery, such as coughing and aspiration, may be managed by dampening feed, feeding at ground level and avoiding feeding prior to work. As the incidence of coughing in the immediate postoperative period is reported to be as high as 43%, these management procedures are recommended in all horses following surgery.[245] Horses showing persistent coughing either associated with eating or during exercise may require additional long-term medical management with mucolytics, antibiotics, intermittent use of anti-inflammatory throat sprays, and mucociliary transport mechanism stimulants. If the above management and time does not resolve persistent coughing, or if there is recurrent lower airway infection, suture removal may be indicated to prevent ongoing aspiration of saliva, water and feed material.

Neuromuscular pedicle grafting has been reported to provide a similar prognosis for successful return to racing compared to horses undergoing laryngoplasty, with 63% of unraced horses and 60% of horses which had raced prior to neuromuscular pedicle grafting winning at least one race after surgery. Despite this, of the horses that had raced prior to surgery ~40% had improved race performance after surgery.[245] Clinical and experimental evidence to date suggests this surgical procedure is best applied to horses identified with hemiparesis (grade III or less laryngeal function) and that are 2 years of age or younger due to the prolonged time required for re-innervation and the associated rehabilitation time (6–12 months). Laryngoplasty can be performed after neuromuscular pedicle grafting if re-innervation is unsuccessful, though horses that have had unsuccessful laryngoplasty are not candidates for re-innervation because of the associated disruption to the first cervical nerve and CAD fibrosis with laryngoplasty.[246–249] Other management options include racing in less competitive company and over shorter distances (5–6 furlongs; 1000–1200 m). Furthermore, permanent tracheostomy or temporary tracheotomy are both alternatives if sanctioned by racing authorities.

Intermittent dorsal displacement of the soft palate (IDDSP)

In the resting horse, diagnosis is tentatively based on a combination of appropriate history and endoscopic examination, subjective judgment of laryngopalatal instability and/or presence of soft palate or sub-epiglottic ulceration.[250] Careful questioning of riders provides valuable information; reports of 'gurgling type' noise particularly at the end of races or immediately after the winning post and poor performance in the final furlong is often reported. That said, ensuring history suggestive of IDDSP is a repeatable phenomenon is essential before embarking on exhaustive diagnostics and management changes. Evidence of epiglottic flaccidity, dysfunction or hypoplasia may further support the diagnosis of IDDSP, and warrants further investigation with radiography. Endoscopic examination of the guttural pouches is indicated to assess for the presence of inflammation or infection which may affect the pharyngeal branch of the vagal nerve coursing the ventral floor of the medial guttural pouch compartment. Although characteristic history and resting endoscopic findings may be useful, when used alone, these parameters have been shown to result in an inaccurate diagnosis in 35% of horses examined.[251] Dynamic exercising video-endoscopy of the upper airway either over ground or associated with high-speed treadmill exercise is essential for a definitive diagnosis of IDDSP. It is important to ensure that exercise protocols during over-ground dynamic endoscopic examinations replicate racing conditions as closely as possible to minimize the possibility of false-negative results. As important as definitively diagnosing IDDSP is the ability to document whether additional upper airway abnormalities are occurring concurrently.

Medical management may include continued training as the condition may resolve with increased fitness and weight loss, or rider and gear changes. Inexperienced riders can often encourage the likelihood of displacement by taking too heavy a 'hold' on the reins. Immature horses should be given time to mature, as many resolve their tendency for IDDSP. Gear changes including tongue ties, figure eight nosebands and a bit that secures the tongue (W bit, spoon bit or a 'Serena song' bit) used individually or combined can be effective. Analysis of racing records of a large number of Thoroughbred racehorses, with or without a definitive diagnosis of IDDSP, has revealed that use of a tongue tie has a beneficial effect on racing performance. Medical management of upper airway inflammation (pharyngitis) may be beneficial when neuritis of the pharyngeal branch of the vagus nerve accompanies upper airway inflammation.[252] Anti-inflammatory therapy, both systemic and local pharyngeal spray, may benefit these horses.[253,254] The laryngohyoid support device 'Cornell Collar' or 'Throat Support Device' is advocated as a non-surgical option to prevent IDDSP, by positioning the larynx in a more dorsal and rostral position. Despite promising experimental results the efficacy in resolving naturally occurring IDDSP is yet to be determined. The use of this device is associated with regulatory conditions in some countries and is not able to be used at all in others. When medical management fails, surgery is indicated and a variety of procedures have been described, including staphylectomy, sternothyrohyoideus myectomy, partial sternothyroidectomy, palatoplasty techniques and laryngeal tie-forward and epiglottic augmentation in the presence of epiglottic hypoplasia.[250,255] The surgical technique of choice remains controversial and is often individually surgeon preference driven. The laryngeal tie-forward procedure combining sternothyroideus myectomy and tenectomy appears to have gained most support recently for horses initially unsuccessfully managed conservatively, with only a short time out of training, approximately 2–3 weeks, required before resuming exercise.[255] Horses undergoing laryngeal tie-forward procedure are reported to be as likely to race postoperatively as matched controls and success rates as high as 83% have been reported in a small group of horses. The prognosis for horses improving their race performance regardless of the other types of surgery therapy pursued is reported to be approximately 60%.[250,255]

Arytenoid chondritis

Small mucosal lesions noted on the axial surface of arytenoids in the absence of arytenoid thickening are encountered infrequently and generally heal without complication, and without having effect on future racing performance.[256] They are typically seen in young Thoroughbreds in training or in yearlings around sale time. However, occasionally, they may progress or appear as localized granulomatous lesions which may occasionally be refractory to antibiotic and anti-inflammatory therapy, and require local excision. Rarely these mucosal lesions have been seen to progress to arytenoid chondropathy in yearlings, necessitating protracted antibiotic therapy or arytenoidectomy.[257] For this reason endoscopic monitoring of arytenoid mucosal lesions appears appropriate, and if indicated medical management consisting of cessation of high-intensity training, parenteral and topical antibiotics and anti-inflammatory agents.

Arytenoid chondropathy identified in the acute stages with only mild cartilage thickening may be managed with cessation of training and medical therapy, with a favorable prognosis for returning to racing in the short to medium term. Peri-arytenoid inflammation with minimal cartilage involvement may be arrested medically and may allow continued training if mucosa is intact and abductor function and airway are judged as adequate. Cases with minimal cartilaginous distortion, granulation tissue on the axial surface and complete arytenoid cartilage abduction capability may be managed with a combination of medical therapy, surgical debridement of granulation tissue and draining tract and short-term rest.[258,259] Horses failing to respond to the above approaches or those with moderate to severe cartilage thickening are candidates for partial arytenoidectomy. Partial arytenoidectomy is also indicated for horses with failed prosthetic laryngoplasty, particularly when failure is associated with postoperative infection. This procedure is associated with a convalescence period of 3–4 months. The reported success rate for horses returning to racing and attaining comparable preoperative earnings/start following partial arytenoidectomy is approximately 60%.[239,260,261] Compared to prosthetic laryngoplasty, a similar rate of return to racing is expected though postoperative earnings are likely to be lower.[261] Despite this, the likelihood of improved postoperative outcome can be managed by racing over shorter distances. Compared to horses having undergone prosthetic laryngoplasty, clinical indications are there is a lower incidence of horses requiring management for persistent coughing and aspiration following partial arytenoidectomy.

Other upper respiratory problems

Other regularly recognized upper respiratory problems that can be managed with minimal lost training time and while the horse remains in the stable include uncomplicated epiglottic entrapment and sub-epiglottic cysts. Problems that often require between 2 and 4 weeks out of training requiring surgery include alar fold flutter, axial deviation of aryepiglottic folds and atheromas. Pharyngeal collapse, fourth branchial arch defects, collapse of the apex of the corniculate process, septal abnormalities and advanced sinus cysts limiting airflow carry a poor prognosis for return to successful racing, even with appropriate surgery if indicated.

Gastrointestinal diseases

Parasite prophylaxis programs are best coordinated with the spelling facilities. Mouth cuts in the commissures are often encountered and may be overlooked in a horse 'hanging' on a rein. Management involves ruling out a musculoskeletal problem and minimization of the trauma by changing bits using topical medical therapies and changing to a thicker or rubber bit, using cheekers or ponying without bit until healed.

Gastric ulceration

Gastric ulceration in Thoroughbred racehorses is reported to affect 66–93% of the population, increasing to 80–100% for horses in advanced training or racing.[262–266] The disease most commonly manifests in racing Thoroughbreds as a decrease in feed intake, and conformation of ulceration is achieved via endoscopy, however a poor correlation exists between clinical signs and the severity of ulceration.[267] Risk factors include the stable environment, periods of no feed intake and administration of NSAIDs and corticosteroids.[263,264,268,269]

Feed management in horses with gastric ulceration should focus on regular feeding with multiple daily meals and constant access to hay in order to avoid any prolonged periods that horses are not eating.[268] Pharmacologic antiulcer therapy (H_2 blockers or proton pump inhibitors) in most cases improves appetite within 1–2 weeks of commencing therapy. Failure to improve may indicate need for further investigation and management changes. Since the prevalence of ulceration is high in the racing Thoroughbred population, and the severity of ulcers in our experience does not seem well correlated with clinical signs, a therapeutic trial may be indicated if gastric endoscopy is not available. Horses that respond to therapy should be maintained on therapy while in training, with omeprazole the preferred therapeutic.[270]

Colic

Typically the incidence of colic is low in racing populations. Swimming activity is noted occasionally to cause colic in some individual horses; in this capacity it is typically seen within 2 hours of a swimming episode.[271] The etiology of swimming-associated colic is undetermined but is typically associated with gaseous distension of the large bowel; usually, the majority respond to medical therapy, but a small number require surgical intervention. Individuals that seem predisposed to recurrent bouts require swimming to be removed from their training schedule.

Diarrhea

Severe enterocolitis needs to be recognized and treated immediately with aggressive medical therapy. Prophylaxis involves avoiding unnecessary use of antimicrobials. Use of specific antimicrobial agents appears to be associated with an increased frequency of enterocolitis. Inclusion of metronidazole in therapy may be indicated if diarrhea is associated with antimicrobial use. Concerns of potential salmonellosis warrants some form of isolation of these cases.

Cardiovascular diseases

Cardiovascular diseases, with the exception of atrial fibrillation, are relatively rare in racehorses. However, functional and anatomic cardiac abnormalities should not be overlooked as potential causes of poor performance.

Veins (septic and non-septic thrombophlebitis)

Typically associated with intravenous injections, thrombophlebitis can be very debilitating to a Thoroughbred racehorse. Once a vein is inflamed it should be avoided as a site of venipuncture, until inflammation is completely resolved. Cessation of high-intensity activity combined with hot packing and antimicrobials may hasten resolution. Progressive sepsis or thrombosis of both veins can become career threatening. The risks of thrombophlebitis may be decreased by use of a disposable 1.5-inch 18G catheter instead of a needle for administration of all agents that may incite an inflammatory response if delivered perivascularly.

Cardiac abnormalities

The most common indication for investigation of cardiac function in racing Thoroughbreds is poor or decreased performance. The most commonly identified pathologic arrhythmia is atrial fibrillation.[272] Atrial fibrillation is typically associated with a marked reduction in high-speed performance and may occur associated with a race or strenuous exercise. Atrial fibrillation may be paroxysmal, resolving within 24–48 hours of its identification after exercise and diagnosis may be difficult if the arrhythmia resolves before it is documented.[273,274] Cases with persistent atrial fibrillation require treatment to achieve conversion to a normal rhythm; the presence of pre-existing cardiac lesion as a contributing factor should be ruled out as this will negatively impact long-term athletic prognosis.[272,274,275]

Heart murmurs have been documented in a large portion of the population of racing Thoroughbreds; one study identified murmurs in 81% of 846 Thoroughbred racehorses and no association was found between racing performance and murmurs.[276] Investigation of cardiovascular function using Doppler echocardiography may be indicated if a murmur not typical of a functional systolic murmur is identified or in horses with poor performance not attributable to the respiratory or musculoskeletal systems. Documentation of apparently pathologic murmurs in young untrained horses warrants documentation and monitoring over time, since mitral and tricuspid regurgitant murmurs have been demonstrated to progress with training.[277]

References

1. Anon. www.horseracingintfed.com.
2. Bourke JM. Wastage in thoroughbreds. In: Proceedings Annual Seminar Equine Branch New Zealand Vet Association. 1995. p. 107–19.
3. Bailey CJ, Reid SW, Hodgson DR, et al. Factors associated with time until first race and career duration for Thoroughbred racehorses. Am J Vet Res 1999;60(10):1196–200.
4. Physick-Shead PW. Career profile of the Canadian Standardbred. Can J Vet Res 1986;50:449–56.
5. Gabel AA, Spencer CP, Pipers FS. A study of correlation of closure of the distal radial physis with performance injury in the standardbred. J Am Vet Med Assoc 1977;170(2):188–94.
6. Jeffcott LB, Rossdale PD, Freestone J, et al. An assessment of wastage in Thoroughbred racing from conception to 4 years of age. Equine Vet J 1982;14(3):185–98.
7. Rossdale PD, Hopes R, Wingfield Digby NJ, et al. Epidemiological study of wastage among racehorses 1982 and 1983. Vet Rec 1985;116:66–9.
8. Lindner A, Dingerkus A. Incidence of training failure among Thoroughbred horses at Cologne, Germany. Prev Vet Med 1993;15:85–94.
9. Perkins N. Wastage in NZ Thoroughbred racing industry: an epidemiological investigation. In: Proceedings Annual Seminar Equine Branch New Zealand Vet Association. 1999. p. 103–12.
10. Wilsher S, Allen WR, Wood JL. Factors associated with failure of Thoroughbred horses to train and race. Equine Vet J 2006;38(2):113–18.
11. Kobluck CN, Robinson RA, Clanton CJ, et al. Comparison on the exercise level and problem rate of 95 Thoroughbred racehorses. In Proceedings of the 36th Annual AAEP Convention. 1990. p. 471–5.
12. Bailey CJ, Reid SW, Hodgson DR, et al. Impact of injuries and disease on a cohort of two- and three- year old Thoroughbreds in training. Vet Rec 1999;23:487–93.
13. Haynes PF, Robinson RA. Racetrack breakdown pilot study summary. In: Proceedings of the 34th

Annual AAEP Convention. 1988. p. 673–6.
14. Bathe AP. 245 Fractures in Thoroughbred racehorses: results of a 2-year prospective study in Newmarket. In: Proceedings of the 40th Annual AAEP Convention. 1994. p. 175–6.
15. Estberg L, Stover SM, Gardner IA, et al. High-speed exercise history and catastrophic racing fracture in Thoroughbreds. Am J Vet Res 1996;57(11):1549–55.
16. Bailey CJ, Reid SW, Hodgson DR, et al. Flat, hurdle and steeple racing: risk factors for musculoskeletal injury. Equine Vet J 1998;30(6):498–503.
17. Kobluk CN. Epidemiologic study of racehorse injuries. In: White NA, Moore JN, editors. Current techniques in equine surgery and lameness. 2nd ed. Philadelphia: WB Saunders; 1998. p. 564–9.
18. Cohen ND, Mundy GD, Peloso JG, et al. Results of physical inspection before races and race-related characteristics and their association with musculoskeletal injuries in Thoroughbreds during races. J Am Vet Med Assoc 1999;215(5):654–61.
19. Ueda Y. Preventing accidents in racehorses: studies and measures taken by the Japan Racing Association. In: Report of the Committee on the Prevention of Accidents to Racehorses. Japan Racing Association; 1991.
20. Peloso JG, Mundy GD, Cohen ND. Prevalence of, and factors associated with, musculoskeletal racing injuries of Thoroughbreds. J Am Vet Med Assoc 1994;204(4):620–6.
21. McKee SL. An update on racing fatalities in the UK. Equine Vet Educ 1995;7:202–4.
22. Estberg L, Stover SM, Gardner IA, et al. Fatal musculoskeletal injuries incurred during racing and training in Thoroughbreds. J Am Vet Med Assoc 1996;208:92–6.
23. Wilson JH, Robinson RA, Jensen RC, et al. Equine soft tissue injuries associated with racing: descriptive statistics from American racetracks. In: Dubai International Equine Symposium Proceedings: 'The equine athlete: tendon, ligament and soft tissue injuries'. 1996;1:1–21.
24. Mohammed HO, Hill T, Lowe J. Risk factors associated with injuries in Thoroughbred horses. Equine Vet J 1991;23:445–8.
25. Dirikolu L, Woods WE, Boyles J, et al. Nonsteroidal anti-inflammatory agents and musculoskeletal injuries in Thoroughbred racehorses in Kentucky. J Vet Phamacol Ther 2009;32(3): 271–9.
26. Parkin TD, Clegg PD, French NP, et al. Race- and course-level risk factors for fatal distal limb fracture in racing Thoroughbreds. Equine Vet J 2004; 36(6):521–6.
27. http://www.jockeyclub.com/initiatives.asp.
28. Stover SM, Johnson BJ, Daft BM, et al. An association between complete and incomplete stress fractures of the humerus in racehorses. Equine Vet J 1992;24:260–3.
29. Stover SM, Ardans AA, Read DH, et al. Patterns of stress fractures associated with complete bone fractures in racehorses. In: Proceedings of the 39th Annual AAEP Convention. 1993. p. 131–2.
30. Poole RR, Meagher DM. Pathologic findings and pathogenesis of racetrack injuries. Vet Clin North Am Equine Pract 1990;6(1):1–30.
31. Clanton C, Kobluk CN, Robinson RA, et al. Monitoring surface conditions of a Thoroughbred racetrack. J Am Vet Med Assoc 1991;198:613–20.
32. Bailey CJ, Reid SW, Hodgson DR, et al. Risk factors associated with musculoskeletal injuries in Australian Thoroughbred racehorses. Prev Vet Med 1997;32:47–55.
33. Kane AJ, Stover SM, Gardner IA, et al. Horseshoe characteristics as possible risk factors for fatal musculoskeletal injury of Thoroughbred racehorses. Am J Vet Res 1996;57(8):1147–52.
34. Kane AJ, Stover SM, Gardner IA, et al. Hoof size, shape, and balance as possible risk factors for catastrophic musculoskeletal injury of Thoroughbred racehorses. Am J Vet Res 1998;59(12):1545–452.
35. Johnson B, Ardens A, Stover SM, et al. California racehorse postmortem program: A 4 year overview. In: Proceedings of the 40th Annual AAEP Convention. 1994. p. 167–9.
36. Mackey VS, Trout DR, Meagher DM, et al. Stress fractures of the humerus, radius and tibia in horses. Vet Radiol 1987;28:26–31.
37. McIlwraith CW, Yovich JV, Martin GS. Arthroscopic surgery for the treatment of osteochondral chip fractures in the equine carpus. J Am Vet Med Assoc 1987;191:531–40.
38. Kawcak CE, McIlwraith CW. Proximodorsal first phalanx chip fragmentation in 336 horses. Equine Vet J 1994;26(5):392–6.
39. Moore RM, Schneider RK. Arthroscopic findings in the carpal joints of lame horses without radiographically visible abnormalities: 41 cases (1986–91). J Am Vet Med Assoc 1995;206(11):1741–6.
40. Spike DL, Bramlage LR, Embertson R M, et al. Tibial stress fractures in 51 racehorses. In: Proceedings of the 42nd Annual AAEP Convention. 1996. p. 280–1.
41. Colon JL, Bramalge LR, Hance SR. Qualitative and quantitative documentation of the racing performance of 461 Thoroughbred racehorses after arthroscopic removal of dorsoproximal first phalanx osteochondral fractures 1986–1995. Equine Vet J 2000;32(6):475–81.
42. Buchner HH, Kubber P, Zohmann E, et al. Sedation and antisedation as tools in equine lameness examination. Equine Vet J 1999;(Suppl 30):227–30.
43. Wilson JH, Robinson RA. Risk factors for equine racing injuries. Comp Cont Educ Pract Vet 1996;18:682–90.
44. Moyer W, Spencer PA, Kallish M. Relative incidence of dorsal metacarpal disease in young Thoroughbred racehorses training on two different surfaces. Equine Vet J 1991;23(3):166–8.
45. Cheney JA, Shen CK, Wheat JD. Relationship of racetrack surface to lameness in the Thoroughbred racehorse. Am J Vet Res 1973;34(10):1285–9.
46. Rooney JR, Genovese A. survey and analysis of bowed tendon in Thoroughbred racehorses. J Eq Vet Sc 1981;1:49–53.
47. Zebarth BJ, Sheard RW. Impact and shear resistance of turf grass racing surfaces for Thoroughbreds. Am J Vet Res 1985;46(4):778–84.
48. Pratt GW. Racing surfaces a survey of mechanical behavior. In: Proceedings of the 13th Annual AAEP Convention. 1984. p. 321–31.
49. Peterson ML, Reiser RF, Kuo P, et al. Effect of temperature on race times on a synthetic surface. Equine Vet J 2010;42(4):351–7.
50. Kai M, Takahashi T, Aoki O, et al. Influence of rough track surfaces on compontents of vertical forces in cantering Thoroughbred horses. Equine Vet J 1999;(Suppl 30):214–17.
51. Fredrickson I, Dalin G, Drevmo S, et al. Ergonomic aspects of poor racetrack design. Equine Vet J 1975;7(2):63–5.
52. Oikawa M, Ueda Y, Inada J, et al. Effect of restructuring a racetrack on the occurrence of racing injuries in Thoroughbred horses. J Eq Vet Sci 1994;14:262–8.
53. Evans DL, Walsh JS. Effect of increasing the banking of a racetrack on the occurrence of injury and lameness in standardbred horses. Aust Vet J 1997;75(10):751–2.
54. Eaton MD, Evans DL, Hodgson DR, et al. Effect of treadmill incline and speed on metabolic rate during exercise in Thoroughbred horses. J Appl Physiol 1995;79(3):951–7.
55. Grant BD. Rest, exercise, and physical therapy programs. In: McIlwraith CW, Trotter GW, editors. Joint disease in the horse. Philadelphia: WB Saunders; 1996. p. 217–23.
56. Miyata H, Sugiura T, Kai M, et al. Muscle adaptation of Thoroughbred racehorses

trained on a flat or sloped track. Am J Vet Res 1999;60(12):1536–9.
57. Ratzlaff MH, Hyde ML, Grant BD, et al. Measurement of vertical forces and temporal components of the strides of horses using instrumented shoes. J Equine Vet Sci 1990;10:23–35.
58. Palmer S. Prevalence of carpal fractures in Thoroughbred and Standardbred racehorses. J Am Vet Med Assoc 1986;188:1171–3.
59. Cervantes C, Madison JB, Ackerman N, et al. Surgical treatment of dorsal cortical fractures if the third metacarpal bone in Thoroughbred racehorses: 53 cases (1985–9). J Am Vet Med Assoc 1992;200(12):1997–2000.
60. Dallap BL, Bramalage LR, Embertson RM. Results of screw fixation combined with cortical drilling for treatment of dorsal cortical stress fractures of the third metacarpal bone in 56 Thoroughbred racehorses. Equine Vet J 1999;31(3):252–7.
61. Hubbell JA, Hinchcliff KW, Muir WW, et al. Cardiorespiratory and metabolic effects of walking, standing and standing with a splint during the recuperative period from maximal exercise in horses. Am J Vet Res 1997;58(9):1003–9.
62. Ridgeway K, Harman J. Equine back rehabilitation. Vet Clin North Am Equine Pract 1999;15(1):263–80.
63. Misumi K, Sakamoto H, Shimazu R. The validity of swimming training for 2-year old Thoroughbreds. J Vet Med Sci 1994;56(2):217–22.
64. McIlwraith CW, Frisbie DD, Kawcak CE. Current treatments for traumatic synovitis, capsulitis, and osteoarthritis. In Proceedings of the 47th Annual AAEP Convention. 2001. p. 180–210.
65. F Walmsley E, Steel C, Haines G, et al. Colic after swimming exercise in racehorses: an investigation of incidence, management, surgical findings and outcome. Aust Vet J 2011;89(5):180–3.
66. Tokuriki M, Ohtsuki R, Kai M, et al. EMG activity of the muscles of the neck and forelimbs during different forms of locomotion. Equine Vet J 1999;(Suppl 30):231–4.
67. Knight PK, Sinha AK, Rose RJ. Effects of training intensity on maximal oxygen uptake. In: Persson SG, Lindholm A, Jeffcott LB, editors. Equine exercise physiology. vol 3. Davis, CA: ICEEP Publications; 1991. p. 77–82.
68. Art T, Lekeux P. Training induced modifications in cardiorespiratory and ventilatory measurements in Thouroughbred horses. Equine Vet J 1993;25:532.
69. Tyler CM, Golland LC, Evans DL, et al. Changes in maximum oxygen uptake during prolonged training, overtraining, and detraining in horses. J Appl Physiol 1996;81(5):2244–9.
70. Burks RT, Bean BG, Marcus R, et al. Analysis of athletic performance with prophylactic ankle devices. Am J Sports Med 1991;19:104–6.
71. Kobluk CN, Martinez del Campo L, Harvey-Fulton KA, et al. A kinematic investigation of the effect of a cohesive elastic bandage on the gait of the exercising Thoroughbred racehorse. Annu Proc AAEP 1988;34:135–48.
72. Crawford W, Vanderby R, Neirby D, et al. The energy absorbing capacity of equine support bandages. I. Comparison between bandages placed in various configurations and tensions. Vet Comp Othop Trauma 1990;1:2–9.
73. G Ramon T, Prades M, Armengou L, et al. Effects of athletic taping of the fetlock on distal limb mechanics. Equine Vet J 2004;36(8):764–8.
74. Smith RK, McGuigan MP, Hyde JT, et al. In vitro evaluation of nonrigid support systems for the equine metacarpophalangeal joint. Equine Vet J 2002;34(7):726–31.
75. Kicker CJ, Peham C, Girtler D, et al. Influence of support boots on fetlock joint angle of the forelimb of the horse at the walk and trot. Equine Vet J 2004;34(7):726–31.
76. Wilson AM, Goodship AE. Exercise-induced hyperthermia as a possible mechanism for tendon degeneration. J Biomech 1994;27(7):899–905.
77. Birch HL, Wilson AM, Goodship AE. The effect of exercise induced hyperthermia on tendon cell survival. J Exp Biol 1997;200(11):1703–8.
78. Porter M, Kobluk CN. Physical therapy and rehabilitation for equine athletes. In: White NA, Moore JN, editors. Current techniques in equine surgery and lameness. 2nd ed. Philadelphia: WB Saunders; 1998. p. 553–61.
79. Kaneps AJ. Tissue temperature response to hot and cold therapy in the metacarpal region of a horse. In: Proceedings of the 46th Annual AAEP Convention. 2000. p. 208–13.
80. Palmer JL, Bertone AL. Joint biomechanics in the pathogenesis of traumatic arthritis. In: McIlwraith CW, Trotter GW, editors. Joint disease in the horse. Philadelphia: WB Saunders; 1996. p. 104–19.
81. Pool RR. Pathologic manifestations of joint disease in the athletic horse. In: McIlwraith CW, Trotter GW, editors. Joint disease in the horse. Philadelphia: WB Saunders; 1996. p. 87–104.
82. Ferris DJ, Frisbie DD, McIlwraith CW, et al. Current joint therapy usage in equine practice: a survey of veterinarians 2009. Equine Vet J 2011;43(5):530–5.
83. Hraha TH, Doremus KM, McIlwraith CW, et al. Autologous conditioned serum: the comparative cytokine profiles of two commercial methods (IRAP and IRAP II) using equine blood. Equine Vet J 2011;43(5):516–21.
84. Textor J. Autologous biologic treatment of equine musculoskeletal injuries: platelet-rich plasma and IL-1 receptor antagonist protein. Vet Clin North Am Equine Pract 2011;27(2):275–98.
85. Young A, O'Brien TR, Pool RR. Exercise related sclerosis in the third carpal bone of the racing Thoroughbred. In: Proceedings of the 34th Annual AAEP Convention. 1988. p. 339–46.
86. Pilsworth, RC, Sheperd MC, Herinckx BM, et al. Fracture of the wing of the ileum, adjacent to the sacroiliac joint, in Thoroughbred racehorses. Equine Vet J 1994;26:94–9.
87. Seeherman HJ. Clinical applications of bone scanning. In: White NA, Moore JN, editors. Current techniques in equine surgery and lameness. 2nd ed. Philadelphia: WB Saunders; 1998. p. 592–605.
88. Stover SM. Stress fractures. In: White NA, Moore JN, editors. Current techniques in equine surgery and lameness. 2nd ed. Philadelphia: WB Saunders; 1998. p. 451–9.
89. Riggs CM, Whitehouse GH, Boyd A. Pathology of the distal condyles of the third metacarpal and third metatarsal bones of the horse. Equine Vet J 1999;31:140–8.
90. Shepherd MC. Stress fractures. Equine Vet Edu 2002;14(2):75–6.
91. Kawcak CE, McIlwraith CW, Norrdin RW, et al. The role of subchodral bone in joint disease: a review. Equine Vet J 2001;33(2):120–6.
92. Davidson EJ. Pathophysiology and clinical diagnosis of cortical and subchondral bone injury. In: Ross MW, Dyson SJ, editors. Diagnosis and management of lameness in the horse. 2nd ed. Missouri: Elsevier Saunders; 2011. p. 935–46.
93. Nunamaker DM. Metacarpal stress fractures. In: Nixon AJ, editor. Equine fracture repair. Philadelphia: WB Saunders; 1996. p. 195–9.
94. Rodan GA. Introduction to bone biology. Bone 1992;13:S3–6.
95. Anderson MW, Greenspan A. Stress fractures. Radiology 1996;199(1):1–12.
96. Riggs CM. Implications of bone adaptation in the Thoroughbred racehorse. In: Robinson NE, editor. Current therapy in equine medicine 4. Philadelphia: WB Saunders; 1997. p. 99–103.
97. Martin RB, Gibson VA, Stover SM, et al. Residual strength of equine bone is not reduced by intense fatigue loading: implications for stress fracture. J Biomech 1997;30(2):109–14.
98. Neilsen BD, Potter GD, Morris EL, et al. Changes in the third metacarpal bone

and frequency of bone injuries in young quarter horses during race training – observations and theoretical considerations. J Eq Vet Sc 1997;17(10):541–8.

99. Porr CA, Kronfeld DS, Lawrence LA, et al. Deconditioning reduces mineral content of the third metacarpal bone in horses. J Anim Sci 1998;76(7):1875–9.

100. Carrier TK, Estberg L, Stover SM, et al. Association between long periods without high-speed workouts and risk of complete humeral or pelvic fracture in Thoroughbred racehorses: 54 cases (1991–4). J Am Vet Med Assoc 1998;212(10):1582–7.

101. Nunamaker DM, Butterweck DM, Provost MT. Fatigue fractures in thoroughbred racehorses: relationship with age, peak bone strain and training. J Orthop Res 1990;8:604–11.

102. Boston RC, Nunamaker DM. Gait and speed as exercise components of risk factors associated with onset of fatigue injury of the third metacarpal bone in 2-year-old Thoroughbred racehorses. Am J Vet Res 2000;61(6):602–8.

103. Riggs CM. Fractures- A preventable hazard of racing Thoroughbreds. Vet J 2002;163(1):19–29.

104. Norwood GL. The bucked shins complex in Thoroughbreds. In: Proceedings of the 35th Annual AAEP Convention. 1989. p. 319–36.

105. Sullins K. Third metacarpal stress fractures. In: White NA, Moore JN, editors. Current techniques in equine surgery and lameness. 2nd ed. Philadelphia: WB Saunders; 1998. p. 460–3.

106. Nunamaker DM. The bucked-shin complex. In: Ross MW, Dyson SJ, editors. Diagnosis and management of lameness in the horse. 2nd ed. Missouri: Elsevier Saunders; 2011. p. 953–8.

107. Copelan RW. Incidence, location, and principles of treatment of stress fractures of the 3rd metacarpal bone. In: Proceedings of the 25th Annual AAEP Convention. 1979. p. 159–62.

108. Richardson DW. Dorsal cortical fractures of the equine metacarpus. Comp cont Educ pract Vet 1984;6:S248–265.

109. Jalim SL, McIlwraith CW, Goodman NL, et al. Lag screw fixation of dorsal cortical stress fractures of the third metacarpal bone in 116 racehorses. Equine Vet J 2010;42(7):586–90.

110. Pilsworth R, Shepherd M. Stress fractures. In: Robinson NE, editor. Current therapy in equine medicine 4. Philadelphia: WB Saunders; 1997. p. 104–11.

111. Pool RR. Pathologic manifestations of joint disease in the athletic horse. In: McIlwraith CW, Trotter GW, editors. Joint disease in the horse. Philadelphia: WB Saunders; 1996. p. 87–104.

112. De Haan CE, O'Brien TR, Koblik PD. A radiographic investigation of third carpal bone injury in 42 racing Thoroughbreds. Vet Radiol 1987;28: 88–92.

113. P O'Brien T, Baker TA, Brounts SH, et al. Detectjon of articular pathology of the distal aspect of the third metacarpal bone in throughbred racehorses: comparison of radiography, computed tomography and magnetic resonance imaging. Vet Surg 2011;40(8):942–51.

114. Bramlage LR. First aid and transportation of fracture patients. In: Nixon AJ, editor. Equine fracture repair. Philadelphia: WB Saunders; 1996. p. 36–42.

115. Patterson-Kane JC, Wilson AM, Firth EC, et al. Exercise-related alterations in crimp morphology in the central regions of superficial digital flexor tendons from young Thoroughbreds: a controlled study. Equine Vet J 1998;30:61–4.

116. Patterson-Kane JC, Firth EC, Parry DA, et al. Effects of training on collagen fibril populations in the suspensory ligament and deep digital flexor tendon of young Thoroughbreds. Am J Vet Res 1998;59(1):64–8.

117. Cherdchutham W, Meershoek LS, vanWeeren PR, et al. Effects of exercise on the biomechanical properties of the superficial digital flexor tendon in foals. Am J Vet Res 2001;62(12):1859–64.

118. Oikawa M, Goodship AE. Clinical and investigational advances in the prevention of tendonitis. Equine Vet J 1999;(Suppl 30):640–1.

119. Genovese RL, Rantanen NW, Simpson BS, et al. Clinical ewperience with quantitative analysis of superficial digiatal flexor tendon injuries in Thoroughbred and Standardbred racehorses. Vet Clin North Am Equine Pract 1990;6:129–47.

120. Genovese RL. Prognosis of superficial flexor tendon and suspensory ligament injuries. In: Proceedings of the 39th Annual AAEP Convention. 1993. p. 9–10.

121. Goodship AE. The pathophysiology of flexor tendon injury in the horse. Equine Vet Edu 1993;5:23–9.

122. Dowling BA, Dart AJ, Hodgson DR, et al. Superficial digital flexor tendonitis. Equine Vet J 2000;32(5):369–78.

123. Gibson KT, Burbridge HM, Pfeiffer DU. Superficial digital flexor tendonitis in Thoroughbred racehorses: outcome following non-surgical treatment and superior check desmotomy. Aust Vet J 1997;75(9):631–5.

124. Marr CM, CcMillan I, Boyd JS, et al. Ultrasonographic and histopahtological finding in equine superficial digital flexor tendon injury. Equine Vet J 1993;25(1):23–9.

125. Genovese RL, Reef VB, Longo KL, et al. Superficial digital flexor tendonitis–long term sonographic and clinical study of racehorses. In: Dubai International Equine Symposium Proceedings: 'The equine athlete: tendon, ligament and soft tissue injuries'. 1996. p. 187–205.

126. Reef VB. Musculoskeletal ultrasonography. In: Reef VB, editor. Equine diagnostic ultrasound. Philadelphia: WB Saunders; 1998. p. 39–186.

127. Romero JM, Dyson SJ. The diffusely filled limb. In: Robinson NE, editor. Current therapy in equine medicine 4. Philadelphia: WB Saunders; 1997. p. 23–7.

128. Gillis C. Tendon and ligament rehabilitation. In: Dubai International Equine Symposium Proceedings: 'The equine athlete: tendon, ligament and soft tissue injuries'. 1996. p. 417–21.

129. Marr CM. Advances in equine ultrasound. Vet Clin North Am Equine Pract 2001;17(2):305–17.

130. Rantanen NW. Principles of ultrasonographic examination of tendons and ligaments. In: Proceedings of the 39th Annual AAEP Convention. 1993. p. 9–10.

131. Silver IA, Brown PN, Goodship AE, et al. A clinical and experimental study of tendon injury, healing and treatment in the horse. Equine Vet J 1983;(Suppl 1): 1–43.

132. Bramlage LR. Superior check ligament desmotomy as treatment for superficial digital flexor tendonitis: initial report. In: Proceedings of the 32nd Annual AAEP Convention. 1986. p. 365.

133. Sawdon H, Yovich JV, Booth T. Superficial digital flexor tendonitis in racehorses. Long term follow up of conservatively managed cases. Aust Equine Vet 1996;14:21–5.

134. Genovese R, Longo K, Berthold B, et al. Quantitative sonographic assessment of superficial digital flexor injuries in Thoroughbred racehorses. In: Proceedings of the 43rd Annual AAEP Convention. 1997. p. 285–90.

135. Gillis CL. Rehabilitation of tendon and ligament injuries. In: Proceedings of the 43rd Annual AAEP Convention. 1997. p. 43:306–9.

136. Henninger RW. Superficial digital flexor tendinitis. In: White NA, Moore JN, editors. Current techniques in equine surgery and lameness. 2nd ed. Philadelphia: WB Saunders; 1998. p. 341–7.

137. Henninger RW, Bramlage LR, Schneider R. Short-term effects of superior check ligament desmotomy and percutaneous tenson splitting as a treatment for acute tendonitits. In: Proceedings of the 36th

Annual AAEP Convention. 1990. p. 539–40.

138. Bramlage LR, Rantanen NW, Genovese RL, et al. Long-term effects of surgical treatment of superficial digital flexor tendonitis by superior check desmotomy. In: Proceedings of the 34th Annual AAEP Convention. 1988. p. 655–66.
139. Fulton IC, MacLean AA, O'Reily JL, et al. Superior check ligament desomotomy for treatment of superficial digital flexor tendonitis in Thouroughbred and Standardbred horses. Aust Vet J 1994;71(8):233–5.
140. Buckowiecki CF, Bramlage LR, Gabel AA. In vitro strength of the suspensory apparatus in training and resting horses. Vet Surg 1987;16(2):126–30.
141. Wilson DA, Baker GJ, Pijanowski GJ, et al. Composition and morphologic features of the interosseous muscle in Standardbreds and Thoroughbreds. Am J Vet Res 1991;52(1):133–9.
142. Colbourne CM, Yovich JV. Suspensory ligament injuries in racing horses: ultrasonographic diagnosis and long term follow-up. Aust Equine Vet 1994;12(3):119–28.
143. O'Brien TR, Morgan JP, Wheat D, et al. Sesamoiditis in the Thoroughbred: a radiographic study. J Am vet Rad Soc 1971;12:75–87.
144. Hardy J, Marcoux M, Breton L. Clinical relevance of radiographic findings in proximal sesamoid bones of two-year-old standardbreds in their first year of training. J Am Vet Med Assoc 1991;198(12):2089–4.
145. Bertone AL. The fetlock. In: Stashak TS, editor. Adams' lameness in horses. 5th ed. Baltimore: Lippincott, Williams, Wilkinson; 2002. p. 768–82.
146. McIlwraith CW. Diseases of joints, tendons, ligaments and related structures. In: Stashak TS, editor. Adams' lameness in horses. 5th ed. Baltimore: Lippincott, Williams, Wilkinson, 2002. p. 459–644.
147. Spike DL, Bramlage LR, Howard BA, et al. Radiographic proximal sesamoiditis in Thoroughbred sales yearlings. In: Proceedings of the 43rd Annual AAEP Convention. 1997. p. 132–3.
148. Kane AJ, McIlwraith CW, Park RD, et al. 'The effect of radiographic changes in Thoroughbred yearlings on future racing performance.' In: Proceedings of the 46th Annual AAEP Convention. 2000. p. 370–4.
149. Dyson SJ, Arthur RM, Palmer SE, et al. Suspensory ligament desmitis. Vet Clin North Am Equine Pract 1995;11(2): 177–215.
150. Cowles RR. Proximal suspensory desmitis – a qualitative survey. In: Proceedings of the 46th Annual AAEP Convention. 2000. p. 143–4.
151. Dyson SJ. Proximal suspensory desmitis in the forelimb and the hindlimb. In: Proceedings of the 46th Annual AAEP Convention. 2000. p. 137–42.
152. Ford T, Ross M, Orsini P. A comparison of methods for proximal palmar metacarpal anesthesia in horses. Vet Surg 1988;18:146–50.
153. Bramlage LR, Gabel AA, Hackett RP. Avulsion fractures of the origin of the suspensory ligament of the horse. J Am Vet Med Assoc 1980;176(10 Pt1):1004–10.
154. Lloyd KC, Koblick P, Ragle C, et al. Incomplete palmar fractures of the proximal extremity of the third cetacarpal bone in horses: ten cases (1981–1986). J Am Vet Med Assoc 1988;192(6):798–803.
155. Ross MW, Ford TS, Orsini PG. Incomplete longitudinal fracture of the proximal palmar cortex of the third metacarpal bone in horses. Vet Surg 1988;17(2):82–6.
156. Boening KJ. Radial extracorporeal shock wave therapy for chronic insertional desmopathy of the proximal suspensory ligament. In: Proceedings of the 46th Annual AAEP Convention. 2000. p. 203–5.
157. McClure S. Extracorporeal shock wave therapy: What is it? What does it do to equine bone? In: Proceedings of the 46th Annual AAEP Convention. 2000. p. 197–9.
158. Cannon J. Common hoof conditions observed in racetrack practice. In: Proceedings of the 24th Annual AAEP Convention. 1979. p. 311–15.
159. Balch OK, Butler D, Collier MA. Balancing the normal foot: hoof preparation, shoe fit and shoe modifications in the performance horse. Equine Vet Educ 1997;9(3):143–54.
160. Stephens PR, Nunamaker DM, Butterweck DM. Applications of a Hall-effect transducer for measurement of tendon strain in horses. Am J Vet Res 1989;50:1089–95.
161. Denoix J. Functional anatomy of tendons and ligaments in the distal limbs. In: Dubai International Equine Symposium Proceedings: 'The equine athlete: tendon, ligament and soft tissue injuries'. 1996. p. 23–53.
162. Reimersma DJ, van dn Bogert AJ, Jansen MO, et al. Influence of shoeing on ground reaction forces and tendon strains in the forelimbs of ponies. Equine Vet J 1996;28:133–8.
163. Clayton HM. Effects of hoof angle on locomotion and limb loading. In: White NA, Moore JN, editors. Current techniques in equine surgery and lameness. 2nd ed. Philadelphia: WB Saunders; 1998. p. 504–9.
164. Kobluk CN, Robinson RA, Gordon BJ, et al. The effect of conformation and shoeing: a cohort study of 95 Thoroughbred racehorses. In: Proceedings of the 35th Annual AAEP Convention. 1989. p. 259–74.
165. Balch OK, Helman RG, Collier MA. Underrun heels and toe-grab length as possible risk factors for catastrophic musculoskeletal injuries in Oklahoma racehorses. In: Proceedings of the 47th Annual AAEP Convention. 2001. p. 334–5.
166. Barrey E. Investigation of the vertical hoof force distribution in the equine formlinb with an instrumented horseboot. Equine Vet J 1990; (Suppl 9):35–8.
167. Young J. Hoof balance: Methods and assessment. In: White NA, Moore JN, editors. Current techniques in equine surgery and lameness. 2nd ed. Philadelphia: WB Saunders; 1998. p. 510–12.
168. Goodness P. Composite repair of hoof injuries. In: White NA, Moore JN, editors. Current techniques in equine surgery and lameness 2nd ed. Philadelphia: WB Saunders; 1998. p. 516–18.
169. Frauenfelder HC, Rossdale PD, Ricketts SW. Changes in serum muscle enzyme levels associated with training schedules and the oestrus cycle in Thoroughbred racehorses. Equine Vet J 1986;18(5):371–4.
170. MacLeay JM, Sorum SA, Valberg SJ, et al. Epidemiologic analysis of factors influencing exertional rabdomyolysis in Thoroughbreds. Am J Vet Res 1999;60(12):1562–6.
171. Beech J. Chronic exertional rhabdomyolysis. Vet Clin North Am Equine Pract 1997;13(1):145–68.
172. Valberg SJ. Muscular causes of exercises intolerance in horses. Vet Clin North Am Equine Pract 1996;12(3):495–515.
173. MacLeay JM, Valberg SJ, Pagan JD, et al. Effect of diet on Thoroughbred horses with recurrent exertional rhabdomyolysis performing a standardized exercise test. Evj 1999;(Suppl 30):458–62.
174. Meyer H, Radicke S, Kienzle E, et al. Investigations on preileal digestion of starch from grain, potato and manioc in horses. J Vet Med A 1995;42:371–81.
175. Beech J, Fletcher JE, Lizzo F, et al. Effect of phenytoin on the clinical signs and in vitro muscle twitch characteristics in horses with chronic intermittent rhabdomyolysis and myotonia. Am J Vet Res 1988;49(12):2130–3.
176. Jeffcott LB. Historical perspective and clinical indications. Vet Clin North Am Equine Pract 1997;15(1):1–12.
177. Haussler KK, Stover SM. Stress fractures of the vertebral lamina and pelvis in thoroughbred racehorses. Equine Vet J 1998;11(1):374–81.

178. Marks D. Medical management of back pain. Vet Clin North Am Equine Pract 1999;15(1):17–194.
179. Pilsworth RC, Head MJ. A study of ten cases of focal peritarsal infection as a cause of severe lameness in the Thoroughbred racehorse: clinical signs, differential diagnosis, treatment and outcome. Equine Vet J 2001;33(4): 366–70.
180. Schneider RK, Bramlage LR, Moore RM, et al. A retrospective study of 192 horses affected with septic arthritis/ tenosynovitis. Equine Vet J 1992;24(6):436–42.
181. Burrel M. Endoscopic and virological observations on respiratory disease in a group of young Thoroughbred horses in training. Equine Vet J 1985;17:99–103.
182. MacNamara B, Bauer S, Iafe J. Endoscopic evaluation of exercise induced pulmonary hemorrhage and chronic obstructive pulmonary disease in association with poor performance in racing Standardbreds. J Am Vet Med Assoc 1990;196:443–5.
183. Sweeney C, Humber K, Roby K. Cytological findings of tracheobronchial aspirates from 66 Thoroughbred racehorses. Am J Vet Res 1992;53:1172–5.
184. Burrel MH, Wood JL, Whitwell KE, et al. Respiratory disease in Thoroughbred horses in training: the relationship between disease and viruses, bacteria and environment. Vet Rec 1996;139:308–13.
185. Cannon JH. Practical respiratory diagnosis. In: Dubai International Equine Symposium Proceedings: 'The diagnosis and treatment of respiratory disease'. 1997. p. 315–20.
186. A.Wisher S, Allen WR, Wood JL. Factors associated with failure of thoroughbred horse to train and race. Equine Vet J 2006;38:98–100.
187. Moore BR, Krakowka S, Robertson JT, et al. Cytological evaluation of bronchoalveolar lavage fluid obtained from Standardbred racehorses with inflammatory airway disease. Am J Vet Res 1995;56:562–7.
188. Christley RM, Hodgson DR, Rose RJ, et al. Coughing in Thoroughbred racehorses: risk factors and tracheal endoscopic and cytological findings. Vet Rec 2001;148:99–104.
189. Christley RM, Hodgson DR, Rose RJ, et al. A case-control studyof respiratory disease in Thoroughbred racehorse in Sydney, Australia. Equine Vet J 2001;33(3):256–64.
190. Koblinger K, Nicol J, McDonald K, et al. Endoscopic assessment of airway inflammation in horses. J Vet Intern Med 2011;25:1118–26.
191. Cardwell JM, Wood JL, Smith KC, et al. Descriptive results from a longitudinal study of airway inflammation in British National Hunt racehorses. Equine Vet J 2011;43:750–5.
192. Mumford JA, Rossdale PD. Virus and its relationship to the 'poor performance' syndrome. Equine Vet J 1980;12:3–9.
193. Christley RM, Hodgson DR, Rose RJ, et al. Attitudes of Australian veterinarians about the cause and treatment of lower respiratory tract disease in racehorses. Prev Vet Med 2000;46:149–59.
194. Berndt A, Derksen FJ, Robinson NE. Endotoxin concentrations within breathing zone of horses are higher in stables than on pasture. Vet J 2010;183:54–7.
195. Wood JL Burrell MH, Roberts CA, et al. Streptococci and *Pasteurella* spp. associated with disease of the equine lower respiratory tract. Equine Vet J 1993;25:314–18.
196. Wood JL, Chanter N. An outbreak of respiratory disease in horses associated with *Mycoplasma felis* infection. Vet Rec 1997;140:388–91.
197. Moore BR. Lower respiratory tract diseases. Vet Clin North Am Equine Pract 1996;12:457–72.
198. Wood JL, Newton JR, Chanter N, et al. A longitudinal epidemiological study of respiratory disease in racehorses: disease definitions; prevalence and incidence. In: Werney U, Wade JF, Munford Kaaden JO, editors. Equine infectious diseases VIII: Proceedings of the 8th International Conference of Equine Infectious Diseases. Newmarket: R&W Publications Ltd.; 1999. p. 64–70.
199. Chapman PS, Green C, Main JP, Cunningham FM, et al. Retrospective study of the relationsips between age, inflammation and the isolation of bacteria from the lower respiratory tract of Thoroughbred horses. Vet Rec 2000;146:91–5.
200. Moore BR, Krakowka S, McVey DS, et al. Inflammatory markers in bronchoalveolar lavage fluid of Standardbred racehorses with inflammatory airway disease: response to interferon alpha. Equine Vet J 1997;29:142–7.
201. Viel L. Lower airway inflammation in young performance horses. In: Robinson NE, editor. Current therapy in equine medicine 4. Philadelphia: WB Saunders; 1997. p. 426–7.
202. Clarke AF. Stable dust –threshold limiting values exposure variables and host risk factors. Equine Vet J 1993;25(3):172–4.
203. Thompson JR, McPherson EA. Prophylactic effects of sodium cromoglycate on chronic obstructive pulmonary disease in the horse. Equine Vet J 1981;13(4):243–6.
204. Derksen FJ. Inhalation therapy for the treatment of lower airway disease. In: Robinson NE, editor. Current therapy in equine medicine 4. Philadelphia: WB Saunders; 1997. p. 429–31.
205. West JB, Mathieu-Costello O. Stress failure of pulmonary capillaries as a mechanism for exercise induced pulmonary hemorrhage in the horse. Equine Vet J 1994;26:441–7.
206. Langesetmo I, Fedde MR Meyer TS, et al. Relationship of pulmonary arterial pressure to pulmonary hemorrhage in exercising horses. Equine Vet J 2000;32(5):379–84.
207. Pascoe JR, Ferraro GL, Cannon JH, et al. Exercise induced pulmonary hemorrhage in racing Thoroughbreds: a preliminary study. Am J Vet Res 1981;42:703–7.
208. Raphael CF, Soma L. Exercise induced pulmonary hemorrhage in Thoroughbreds after racing and breezing. Am J Vet Res 1982;46:1123–7.
209. Weiss DJ, Smith CM. Haemorrheological alterations associated with competitive racing activity in horses: implications for exercise induced pulmonary hemorrhage (EIPH). Equine Vet J 1998;30:7–12.
210. Pascoe JR. Exercise induced pulmonary hemorrhage. In: Robinson NE, editor. Current therapy in equine medicine 4. Philadelphia: WB Saunders; 1997. p. 441–3.
211. Roberts CA, Erickson HH. Exercise induced pulmonary hemorrhage workshop. Equine Vet J 1999;(Suppl 30):642–4.
212. Takahashi T, Hiraga A, Ohmura K, et al. Frequency of and risk factors for epistaxis associated with exercise induced pulmonary hemorrhage in horses: 251,609 race starts (1992–1997). J Am Vet Med Assoc 2001;218(9):1462–4.
213. Hinchcliff KW, Morley PS, Jackson MA, et al. Risk factors for exercise-induced pulmonary haemorrhage in thoroughbred racehorses. Equine Vet J 2010;42:228–34.
214. Bourke JM. Exercise induced pulmonary hemorrhage – the Australian situation. Proc 9th Int. Conf Racing Analysts and Veterinarians, New Orleans. 1992. p. 115–19.
215. Meyer TS, Fedde MR, Gaughan EM, et al. Quantification of exercise induced pulmonary hemorrhage with bronchoalveolar lavage. Equine Vet J 1998;30(4):284–8.
216. Gross DK, Morley PS, Hinchcliff KW, et al. Effect of furosemide on performance of Thoroughbred horses racing in the United States and Canada. J Am Vet Med Assoc 1999;215:664–9.
217. Hinchcliff KW. Effects of furosemide on athletic performance and

exercise-induced pulmonary hemorrhage in horses. J Am Vet Med Assoc 1999;215(5):630–5.

218. Manohar M, Hutchens E, Coney E. Pulmonary hemodynamics in the exercising horse and their relationship to exercise induced pulmonary hemorrhage. Br Vet J 1993;149:419–28.

219. Manohar M, Goetz TE, Sullivan E, et al. Pulmonary vascular pressures of strenuously exercising Thoroughbred horses after administration of phenylbutazone and frusemide. Equine Vet J 1998;30:158–62.

220. Lester G, Clarke C, Rice B, et al. Effect of timing and route of administration of furosemide in pulmonarly hemorrhage and pulmonary arterial pressure in exercising Thoruroughbred racehorses. Am J Vet Res 1999;60(1):22–8.

221. McKrane SA, Slocombe RF. Sequential changes in bronchoalveolar cytology after autologous blood inoculation. Equine Vet J 1999;(Suppl 30):126–30.

222. Erickson HH, Kindig CA, Poole DC. Role of the airways in exercise induced pulmonary haemorrhage. Equine Vet J 2001;33(6):537–9.

223. Geor RJ, Ommundson L, Fenton G, et al. Effects of an external nasal strip and frusemide on pulmonary hemorrhage in Thoroughbreds following high intensity exercise. Equine Vet J 2001;33(6):577–84.

224. Goetz TE, Manohar M, Hassan AS, et al. Nasal strips do not affect pulmonary gas exchange, anerobic metabolism, or EIPH in exercising Thoroughbreds. J Appl Physiol 2001;90(6):2378–85.

225. Kindig CA, McDonough P, Fenton G, et al. Efficacy of nasal strip and furosemide in mitigating EIPH in Thoroughbred horses. J Appl Physiol 2001;91(3):1396–400.

226. Holcombe SJ, Berney C, Cornelise CJ, et al. The effect of commercially available nasal strips on airway resistance in exercising horses. Am J Vet Res 2002;63(8):1101–5.

227. Raphel CF. Endoscopic findings in the upper respiratory tract of 479 horses. J Am Vet Med Assoc 1982;181(5):470–3.

228. Seeherman HJ. Left recurrent laryngeal neuropathy. In: Robinson NE, editor. Current therapy in equine medicine 4. Philadelphia: WB Saunders; 1997. p. 404–7.

229. Brown JA, Hinchcliff KW, Jackson MA, et al. Prevalence of pharyngeal and laryngeal abnormalities in Thoroughbred racing in Australia and their association with performance. Equine Vet J 2005;37(5):397–401.

230. Derksen FJ, Holcombe SJ, Hartmann W, et al. Spectrum analysis of respiratory sounds in exercising horses with experimentally induced laryngeal hemiplegia or dorsal displacement of the soft palate. Am J Vet Res 2001;62(5):659–64.

231. Blea JA, Arthur RM. How to evaluate and treat ulceration of the glosso-epiglottic fold (subepiglottic area) in the standing horse. Proc Am Ass Equine Practnrs 2003;49:295–300.

232. Desmaizieres LM, Serraud N, Plainfosse B, et al. Dynamic respiratory endoscopy without treadmill in 68 performance Standardbred, Thoroughbred and saddle horses under natural training conditions. Equine Vet J 2009;41(4):347–52.

233. Allen KJ, Franklin SH. Assessment of the exercise tests used during overground endoscopy in UK Thoroughbred racehorses and how these may affect the diagnosis of dynamic upper respiratory tract obstructions. Equine Vet J 2010;42(S38):587–91.

234. Allen KJ, Franklin SH. Comparisons of overground endoscopy and treadmill endoscopy in UK Thoroughbred racehorses. Equine Vet J 2010;42(3):186–91.

235. Rakestraw PC, Hackett RP, Ducharme NG, et al. Arytenoid cartilage movement in resting and exercising horses. Vet Surg 1991;20(2):122–7.

236. Dixon PM, Robinson NE, Wade JL, editors. Proc Havemeyer Workshop on Equine Recurrent Laryngeal Neuropathy. 96. Newmarket, UK: R & W Publications; 2004.

237. Hammer EJ, Tulleners EP, Parente EJ, et al. Videoendoscopic assessment of dynamic laryngeal function during exercised in horses with grade-III left laryngeal hemiparesis at rest: 26 cases (1992–1995). J Am Vet Med Assoc 1998;212(3):399–403.

238. Pollock PJ, Reardon RJM, Parkin TDH, et al. Dynamic respiratory endoscopy in 67 Thoroughbred racehorses training under normal ridden exercise conditions. Equine Vet J 2009;41(4):354–60.

239. WitteTH, Mohammed HO, Radcliffe CH, et al. Racing performance after combined prosthetic laryngoplasty and ipsilateral ventriculocordectomy or partial arytenoidectomy:135 Thoroughbred racehorses competing at less than 2400m (1997–2007). Equine Vet J 2009;41(1):70–5.

240. Tulleners EP, Stick JA. Laryngoplasty and repeat laryngoplasty. In: White NA, Moore JN, editors. Current techniques in equine surgery and lameness. 2nd ed. Philadelphia: WB Saunders; 1998. p. 137–42.

241. Russell AP, Slone DE. Performance analysis after prosthetic laryngoplasty and bilateral ventriculectomy for laryngeal hemiplegia in horses: 70 cases (1986–91). J Am Vet Med Assoc 1994;204(8):1235–41.

242. M. Hawkins JF, Tulleners EP, Ross MR, et al. Laryngoplasty with or without ventriculocordectomyfor treatment of left laryngeal hemiplegia in 230 race horses. Vet Surg 1997;26:484.

243. Dixon PM, McGorum BC, Railton DI, et al. Long-term survey of laryngoplasty and ventriculocordectomy in an older, mixed-breed population of 200 horses. Part 1. Maintenance of surgical arytenoid abduction and complications of surgery. Equine Vet J 2003;35:389–96.

244. Barakzai SZ, Boden LA, Dixon P. Postoperative race performance is not correlated with degree of surgical abduction after laryngoplasty in National Hunt Thoroughbred racehorses. Vet Surg 2009;38:934.

245. Fulton IC, Anderson BH, Stick JA, et al. Equine surgery. In: Auer JA, Stick JA, editors. 4th ed. Larynx: Elsevier Saunders; 2012. p. 592–623.

246. Fulton IC, Derksen FJ, Stick JA, et al. Treatment of left laryngeal hemiplegia in Standardbreds, using nerve muscle pedicle graft. Am J Vet Res 1991;52(9):1461–7.

247. Fulton IC. Treating equine laryngeal paralysis and paresis using a nerve muscle pedicle graft. In: Proceedings of the Veterinary Comparative Respiratory Society. Melbourne. 2000. Online: http://tvms.tufts.edu/vcrs/2000/present.htm.

248. Fulton IC, Stick JA, Derksen Fj. Laryngeal reinnervation in the horse. Vet Clin North Am Equine Pract 2003;19:189.

249. Fulton IC. Laryngeal re-innervation in the horse. In: Dixon PM, Robinson NE, Wade JL, editors. Proc Havemeyer Workshop on Equine Recurrent Laryngeal Neuropathy. 96. Newmarket, UK: R & W Publications; 2004. p. 60–2.

250. Robertson JT. Dorsal displacement of the soft palate. In: White NA, Moore JN, editors. Current techniques in equine surgery and lameness. 2nd ed. Philadelphia: WB Saunders; 1998. p. 131–5.

251. Lane JG, Bladon B, Litle Dm, et al. Dynamic obstructions of the equjine upper respiratory tract. Part 2. Comparison of endoscopic findings at rest and during high-speed treadmill exercise of 600 Thoroughbred racehorses.). Equine Vet J 2006;38:401–8.

252. Holcombe SJ, Derksen FJ, Stick JA, et al. Pathophysiology of dorsal displacement of the soft palate in horses. Equine Vet J 1999;(Suppl 30):45–8.

253. Tulleners E. Epiglottiditis. In: White NA, Moore JN, editors. Current techniques in equine surgery and lameness. 2nd ed. Philadelphia: WB Saunders; 1998. p. 135–7.

254. Holcombe SJ, Robinson NE, Jackson C, et al. Stabling, airway inflammation, and dorsal displacement of the soft palate in young horses. In: Proceedings of the 46th Annual AAEP Convention. 2000. p. 254–5.
255. Ducharme NG. Equine surgery. In: Auer JA, Stick JA, editors. 4th ed. Pharynx: Elsevier Saunders; 2012. p. 569–91.
256. Smith RL, Perkins NR, Firth EC, et al. Arytenoid mucosal injury in young Thoroughbred horses – investigation of a proposed etiology and clinical significance. N Z Vet J 2006;54:173.
257. Kelly G, Lumsden JM, Dunkerly G, et al. Idiopathic mucosal lesions of the arytenoid cartilages of 21 Thoroughbred yearlings: 1997-2001. Equine Vet J 2003;35(3):276–81.
258. Hay W, Tulleners E. Excision of intralaryngeal granulation tissue in 25 horses using a Nd:YAG laser (1986–1991). Vet Surg 1993;22:129–34.
259. Sullins KE. Minimally invasive laser treatment of arytenoid chondritis in 5 horses. In: Proceedings of the 47th Annual AAEP Convention. 2001. p. 120–2.
260. Tulleners EP, Harrison IW, Raker CW. Management of arytenoid chondropathy and failed laryngoplasty in horses: 75 cases (1979–1985). J Am Vet Med Assoc 1988;192(5):670–5.
261. Parente EJ, Tulleners EP, Southwood LL. Long-term study of partial arytenoidectomy with primary closure in 76 Thoroughbred racehorses (1992–2006). Equine Vet J 2008;40:214–18.
262. Hammond CJ, Mason DK, Watkins KL. Gastric ulceration in mature Thoroughbred horses. Equine Vet J 1986;18:284–7.
263. Murray MJ. Gastic ulceration in horses with colic: 91 cases (1987–90). J Am Vet Med Assoc 1992;195:1135–8.
264. Murray MJ, Schusser GF, Pipers FS, et al. Factors associated with gastic lesions in Thoroughbred racehorses. Equine Vet J 1996;28:368–74.
265. Johnson JH, Vatistas N, Castro L, et al. Field survey of the prevalence of gastric ulcers in Thoroughbred racehorses and on response to treatment of affected horses with omeprazole paste. Equine Vet Educ 2001;13:221–4.
266. Begg LM, O'Sullivan CB. The prevalence and distribution of gastric ulceration in 345 racehorses. Aust Vet J 2003;81(4):199–201.
267. Andrews FM, Nadueau JA. Clinical syndromes of gastric ulceration in foals and mature horses. Equine Vet J 1999;(Suppl 29):30–3.
268. Murray MJ, Eichorn ES. Effects of intermittent feed deprivation with ranitidine administration and stall confinement with ad libitum access to hay on gastric ulceration in horses. Am J Vet Res 1996;57: 1599–602.
269. Collier D. Gastric ulceration: a response to an unnatural environment. Equine Vet J 1999;(Suppl 29):5–6.
270. Vatistas NJ, Snyder JR, Neito J, et al. Acceptability of a paste formulation and efficacy of high dose omeprazole in healing gastric ulcers in horses maintained in race training. Equine Vet J 1999;(Suppl 29):71–6.
271. Walmsley E, Steele C, Haines G, et al. Colic after swimming exercise in racehorses: an investigation of incidence, management, surgical findings and outcome. Aust Vet J 2011;89(5):180–3.
272. Begg LM, Hutchins DR, Suann CJ. Atrial fibrillation. 11th annual ISPOR.
273. Holmes JR, Henigan M, Williams RB, et al. Paroxysmal atrial fibrillation in racehorses. Equine Vet J 1986;18(1): 37–42.
274. Mitten LA. Cardiovascular causes of exercise intolerance. Vet Clin North Am Equine Pract 1996;12(3):473–94.
275. Marr CM, Bowen M. Cardiology of the horse. 2nd ed. Saunders; 2010.
276. Kriz NG, Hodgson DR, Rose RJ. Prevalence and clinical importance of heart murmurs in racehorses. J Am Vet Med Assoc 2000;216(9):1441–5.
277. Young LE, Wood JL. Effect of age and training on murmurs of atrioventricular valvular regurgitation in young Thoroughbreds. Equine Vet J 2000;32(3):195–9.

Veterinary aspects of racing and training horses used for harness racing (trotters and pacers)

Anne Courouce-Malblanc Kenneth W. Hinchcliff

49

CHAPTER CONTENTS

The breed and racing

Origins of the breeds

Subsequent to their development in North America, Standardbreds and harness racing were exported to many countries. Competition in European countries is exclusively between trotters, whereas that in the remainder of the world is between either trotters or pacers.[1] Importantly, harness racing is about competition at a particular gait (either trot or pace) and less so about the breed, with many countries having indigenous breeds used for harness racing. Presently, at least 24 countries, including countries in Scandinavia, Europe, and Australasia have active organizations that promote Standardbred racing. The centers of Standardbred racing are the Mid-west and East Coast of the United States, eastern Canada, Scandinavia, France and Belgium, Australia and New Zealand. France is the only country which also has mounted trotters.

The Standardbred racehorse, sometimes referred to as the American trotter, originated in the United States and Canada in the early 1800s, with the breed society being formed in 1871.[2] Standardbred horses all trace their male lineage to Messenger, a Thoroughbred foaled in England in 1780 and exported to the United States. Messenger was the great-grandsire of Hambletonian 10 (1849–1876) to which all Standardbreds can trace their ancestry and to his four sons: George Wilkes, Dictator, Happy Medium and Electioneer.[3,4] However, while mainly derived from Thoroughbred stock, Morgan and Hackneys also contributed to the Standardbred gene pool.[2] The Standardbred name derived from the requirement that in order to be entered into the register of the new breed, trotters had to complete a mile in a prescribed (standard) time of 2 minutes 30 seconds and pacers in 2 minutes 25 seconds.

Although the Standardbred was derived from Thoroughbreds and in many respects resembles that breed, there are readily apparent differences. Standardbreds are often not as tall as are Thoroughbreds, being 15 to 16 hands at the withers, are more heavily muscled and tend to be longer in the body. A prominent aspect of many Standardbreds is the presence of a Roman nose and large head. The predominant colors are bay, brown and black, although gray horses do occur.

Standardbreds are divided into two groups based on gait while racing, although a small number (~2%) use both gaits at some stage in their racing career.[5] There is a strong influence of gait on breeding in that most horses race at the gait used by their sire. Approximately 20% of offspring sired by trotters register as pacers, while only 1% of offspring sired by pacers are registered as trotters.[6] The extent of the genetic difference between Standardbred trotters and pacers is as great or greater than that seen between some distinct horse breeds.[6]

The Standardbred (American trotter) is the origin of the Danish trotter, Romanian trotter, Swedish Standardbred trotter, and the Russian trotter.[2] The Coldblooded trotter of parts of Scandinavia is not related to the Standardbred, being derived from the Dole horse.[7] Trotters in Scandinavia derived approximately 94% of their genetic make-up from North American Standardbreds, with the remainder coming from French horses.[8] The principal breeds of horses used for harness racing include, in addition to those listed above, the French trotter, Italian trotter, Orlov trotter, Finnhorse, Icelandic toelter, Dole horse, and North-Swedish cold-blooded horses.[4]

In France, horses were first selectively bred for trotting races in the early to mid-1800s.The French trotter came from Norman stock crossed with English Thoroughbred and half-bred hunter types, Norfolk Roadster, and American Standardbred. The French trotter is sometimes referred to as a Norman trotter, due to the influence

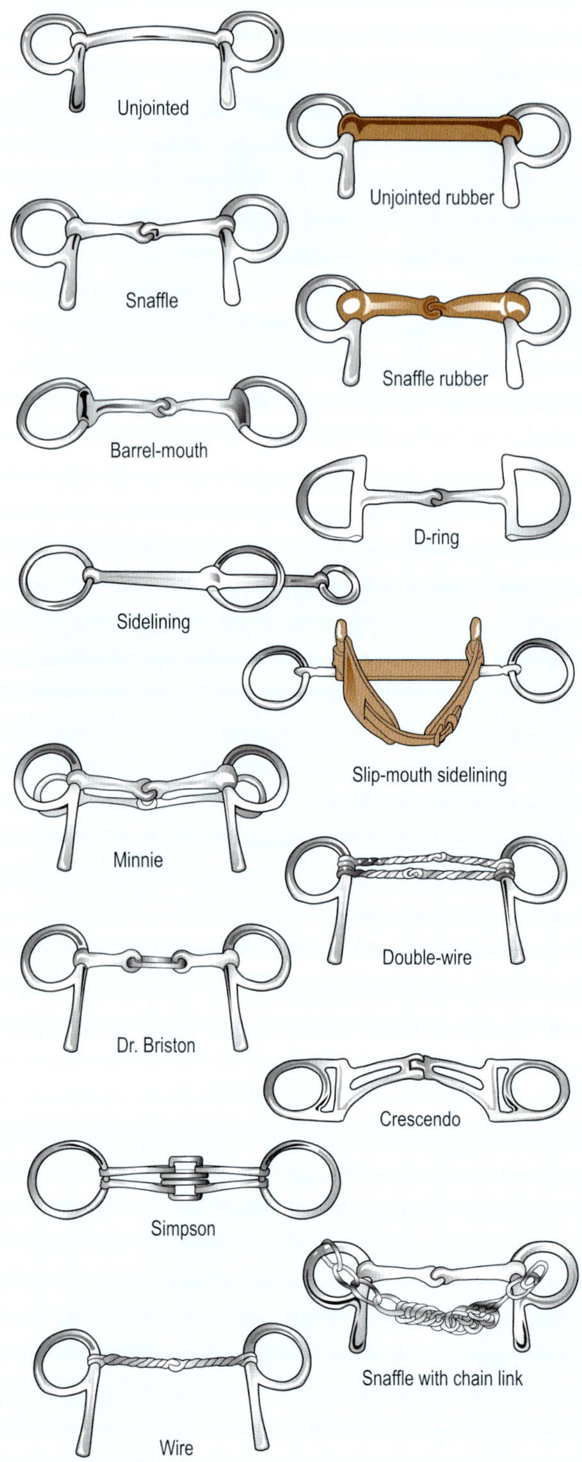

Fig 49.12. Bits used in Standardbred racehorses.
Redrawn with permission.[68] *Illustrations are copyrighted by the U.S. Trotting Association, and used here with the expressed permission of the copyright holder.*

initial preparation phase is similar to the foundation phase described above and consisted mainly of jogging the horses at a steady pace (see Table 49.3) for 5–6 weeks with one rest day per week. The midpreparation phase followed and signaled the start of fast work. Fast work normally involved the horses being harnessed-up into their hobbles and pulling the racing cart. The final preparation phase, which lasted about four weeks, then followed. In the racing or competition phase the majority of New Zealand trainers continued a similar pattern of training; however, about one-third of the trainers incorporated one or more 'strong' workouts (galloping rather than pacing in the cart).

The intensity of the fast work increased during training, but interestingly, the intensity of the jog work remained unchanged throughout training.[42] The speed at which horses were jogged remained at about 19 km/h whether they were in the initial preparation phase or the racing phase of training. The intensity of jog work described in the training program by Lovell (1994) was almost the same as that described by Sherman and Hopkins (1995). However, the horses in Lovell's program started with much less jog work, which was quickly increased to be approximately the same as that described by Shearman and Hopkins (1995) by week 5 of the program (Table 49.4). Both training programs introduced fast work at about the same time (week 5) and typically trained the horses with alternating fast and slow days. Lovell's program is slightly more scientific in that the work intensities are calculated from a standard fitness test, which he suggests should be carried out every two weeks or so. Basically the test uses heart rate measurements during a series of 1000 m trials at specific speeds to calculate the velocity at which the horse's heart rate reaches maximum. As the horse becomes fitter the speed at which it can travel at maximum heart rate increases, thereby allowing the adequate planning of appropriate training intensities. However, most trainers do not have access to heart rate monitors and therefore plan their training intensity around distance and time.

As the two training programs demonstrate, there is an increase in intensity of fast work approaching the final preparation and racing phases and a slight reduction in fast-work volume. The higher training intensities during these phases are designed to stress the horses in a way that is similar to the actual race. Neither training program actually asks the horses to complete time trials or to train at race pace for any length of time.

Interval and tapered training programs

Interval training attempts to improve performance by introducing training that is close to or even above race pace. Interval training for the racehorse has been discussed by Tom Ivers in his book *The Fit Racehorse.* In his book, Ivers outlines the general concept and proposed benefits of interval training and gives examples of structured interval training sessions.[43]

Interval training involves bouts of exercise alternated with periods of relief (or rest) and has been shown to be an effective way to train the appropriate energy systems in human and equine athletes.[44,45] Interval training decreases fatigue and allows for a greater amount of high-intensity work to be performed than if work was carried out in one continuous stretch. For example, suppose you exercised your horse continuously as hard as you could for three minutes, then on another occasion suppose you ran the horse intermittently, exercising the horse just as hard as you did continuously, but for only 30 seconds at a time with two minutes of rest between each run. If you repeat this six times, you would have completed the same amount of work but the degree of fatigue following the intermittent or interval exercise would be considerably less. After the continuous exercise, the horse would be extremely fatigued and tired compared

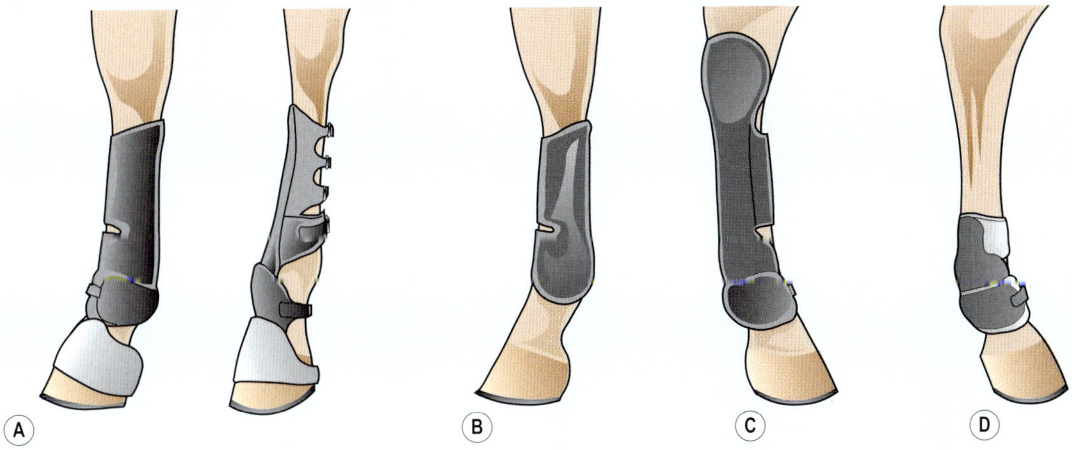

Fig 49.13 Protective boots worn on the hindlimbs by trotters.
Redrawn with permission.[68] Illustrations are copyrighted by the U.S. Trotting Association, and used here with the expressed permission of the copyright holder.

Table 49.3 Training phases for maiden pacers of a typical top trainer In New Zealand

TRAINING PHASE	TRAINING DAY	TYPE	DISTANCE (m)	SPEED (km/h)	INTENSITY (%)	DURATION (min:s)
Initial Preparation						
weeks 1–5	Mon–Sat	jog	12 400	19.6	44.9	38:20
	Sun	off				
Mid Preparation						
weeks 6–10	Mon, Wed, Fri	jog	11 900	19.1	43.7	37:40
	Tue, Thu, Sat	fast	4500	32.3	74.0	10:00
	Sun	off				
Final Preparation						
weeks 11–14	Mon, Wed, Fri	jog	12 800	19.5	44.6	39:20
	Tue, Thu, Sat	fast	3200	40.0	91.6	4:50
	Sun	off				
Racing						
two-weekly	Sat	race				
	Sun	off				
	Mon	jog	11 800	19.6	44.9	36:40
	Tue	jog	11 800	19.6	44.9	36:40
	Wed	jog	11 800	19.6	44.9	36:40
	Thu	fast	3000	41.6	95.3	4:30
	Fri	jog	11 800	19.6	44.9	36:40
	Sat	fast	3000	41.6	95.3	4:30
	Sun	off				
	Mon	jog	11 800	19.6	44.9	36:40
	Tue	fast	3000	41.6	95.3	4:30
	Wed	jog	11 800	19.6	44.9	36:40
	Thu	fast	3000	41.6	95.3	4:30
	Fri	jog	11 800	19.6	44.9	36:40
	Sat	race				

The means for 26 trainers (mid preparation phase) or 94 trainers (all other phases). Workout intensities are percentages of qualifying pace, which was calculated from the average qualifying time for a maiden pacer over 2400 m, which was 3:18 min:s. (From Shearman JP. Training of standardbred maiden pacers. Journal of Equine Veterinary Science 1995;16:116, with permission from Elsevier.)

Table 49.4 Suggested training for a mature Standardbred that has raced before but has been turned out for a prolonged rest

TRAINING PHASE	TRAINING DAY	TYPE	DISTANCE (m)	SPEED (km/h)	INTENSITY (%V_{HRmax})
Pretraining					
week 1	Mon–Tue	jog	5000	19.0	
	Wed–Sat	jog	6000	19.0	
	Sun	off			
week 2	Mon–Sat	jog	8000	19.0	
	Sun	off			
week 3	Mon–Sat	jog	10000	19.0	
	Sun	off			
week4	Mon–Fri	jog	13000	19.0	
	Sat	V_{HRmax}	4000	37.5	
	Sun	off			
Foundation training					
week 5	Mon, Wed, Fri	jog	10000	19.0	
	Tue, Thu	fast	2 x 1000		90%
	Sat	fast	3 x 1000		90%
	Sun	off			
week 6	Mon, Wed	jog	10000	19.0	
	Tue, Thu, Sat	fast	3 x 1000		90%
	Fri	V_{HRmax}	4000	37.5	
	Sun	off			
week 7	Mon, Wed, Fri	jog	10000	19.0	
	Tue, Thu, Sat	fast	3 x 1000		90%
	Sun	off			
week 8	Mon, Wed	jog	10000	19.0	
	Tue, Thu, Sat	fast	3 x 1000		90%
	Fri	V_{HRmax}	4000	37.5	
	Sun	off			
Racing					
week 9	Mon, Wed, Fri	jog	6-10000	19.0	
	Tue, Thu, Sat	fast	1 x 1600		90%
		fast	1 x 1600		first 1200 at 90% last 400 at 110%
	Sun	off			
week 10	Mon, Wed	jog	6-10000	19.0	
	Tue	fast	1 x 1600		90%
		fast	1 x 1600		first 1200 at 90% last 400 at 110%
	Thu	fast	1 x 1600		90%
		fast	1 x 1200		90%
		fast	1 x 400		110%
	Fri	V_{HRmax}	4000	37.5	
	Sat	fast	1 x 1600		90%
		fast	1 x 1600		800 at 90% next 400 at 110% last 400 in 30 s
	Sun	off			

V_{HRmax} is an exercise test, which uses four bouts of 1000 m at increasingly higher speeds to calculate the velocity at which the horse's heart rate reaches maximum. Overall, the horse covers 4000 m during this exercise test at an average speed of 37.5 km/h. Intensity is given as a percentage of the velocity reached at heart rate maximum during the V_{HRmax} test. Prior to all fast-work sessions and exercise tests, horses should be given a warm-up consisting of a jog for 3000 m at a speed of 19 km/h. (From Lovell D. Training Standardbred trotters and pacers. In: Hodgson DR, Rose, R., ed. The Athletic Horse: Principles and Practice of Equine Sports Medicine. Philadelphia: W.B. Saunders Company; 1994:399-408, with permission from Elsevier.)

to the horse after the interval training session. Essentially with interval training the recovery period allows for replenishment of stored energy in the muscles, removal of lactic acid and recovery from the exercise bout. Therefore the horse is less fatigued when it starts its next bout of exercise and the quality of training is better than if the horse completed the exercise continuously.

Normally, in training for middle to long-distance events, the exercise intensity is set around the anaerobic threshold to improve aerobic capacity without producing too much lactic acid and, consequently, fatigue. However, trainers should also think about training at intensities over the anaerobic threshold to help train the anaerobic energy system that is also required during a race. Shorter very high intensity sprint intervals may also help at improving speed.

When constructing an interval training program the following terms are used:

- *work interval* – the length of time the horse is exercising (sometimes expressed as the distance covered, e.g. 1000 m)
- *rest or relief interval* – the time between work intervals in a set. The relief interval may consist of light activity such as walking or mild to moderate exercise such as jogging
- *repetition* – the number of work intervals per set
- *sets* – a group of work and relief intervals.

An example of an interval training program can be seen in Table 49.5. In this program the recovery time has been set randomly at five minutes, during which time the horse walks. As can be seen from the table the trainer who developed this program considers that the interval training should only occur every four days.[44] Most interval training program allow more days between interval exercise bouts to allow for full recovery from the much higher stresses involved. Horses would normally be given slow work between the interval training days. Because of the high stresses involved, interval training is not recommended until a sound fitness base has been established.

Some trainers prefer to use heart rate measurements when programming exercise intensity for interval training rather than strict performance times, which can be influenced by track and weather conditions. If using the heart rate monitor, the aim at the start of interval training would be to get the horse's heart rate up to about 180–200 bpm (approximately anaerobic threshold). With a gradual increase in fitness this target can be progressively increased to a heart rate of about 200 bpm or more. In most cases, however, trainers will use the heart rate monitor to judge the recovery ability of the horses. A target of about 110–120 bpm after five minutes recovery indicates that the horse has recovered sufficiently to continue with the next bout of exercise. If the heart rate exceeds what is expected or takes much longer to recover than normal, it may be an indication that the previous exercise bout was too stressful and further work bouts should be abandoned. Unexpected high heart rates during training and recovery have also been suggested to be an early warning sign of physiological stress, possibly indicating low-grade lameness or musculoskeletal injury.

While the proposed benefits of interval training include the intense metabolic demands it produces, as well as the specific neuromuscular and fiber-type activation that is needed during a race, disadvantages include the time-consuming nature of the training compared to conventional training, and an increased risk of injury. Interval training was used in an attempt to increase time trial performance in a number of Standardbred racehorses over a prolonged period of time.[46] Horses were given a series of two-weekly taper training programs. The taper is a training technique used in human athletes to optimize performance by allowing adequate recovery from hard training prior to competition. During the second week of one of the taper programs (see taper 2 in Table 49.6) the researchers used a series of progressively shorter intervals to reduce duration but maintain adequate training intensity. There was a significant improvement in the horse's speed during the taper programs, (particularly taper 1), compared to the conventional training; however, there was also an increase in the number of injuries reported in the taper group using the interval training.[46] Also note that the high-intensity interval training days during taper 2 were not separated by recovery or rest days, possibly leading to inadequate recovery which may have caused the injury problems.

The main objective of any training program is to enhance performance while keeping the animal free from injury and disease. During training, stress in the form of exercise initiates changes within the horse's structural and biochemical make-up. These exercise-induced changes cause adaptation and improved performance if sufficient recovery is allowed. On the other hand, excessive stress due to inappropriate training or insufficient recovery produces maladaptation and poor performance.[45,47,48]

Overtraining syndrome (OTS)

Overtraining is a well-recognized phenomenon in both human and equine athletes and is an important cause of poor performance.[49] Humans affected by overtraining are excessively fatigued, have lower plasma lactate concentrations during exercise and have chronic depletion of muscle glycogen.[49] Racehorse trainers and veterinarians refer to affected horses as being 'stale', or 'sour'. The term OTS should be used for horses in heavy training losing performance without an obvious clinical reason and which is sustained for >2 weeks.[50] It is suggested that the diagnosis of overtraining syndrome is imprecise and that, in the absence of a scoring system to assess the psychological status of horses, the most effective method for diagnosis is the thorough assessment of the history and presenting complaint.[50] Signs of overtraining include:[47,49]

- decreased performance, such as slower split times
- unexplained poor performance or adverse persistent change in performance
- a decrease in body weight ≥6 kg
- reduced appetite
- decreased enthusiasm to train
- behavioral changes in which the horse might become moody and lethargic or nervous[51]
- increased heart rate during exercise and possibly slower recovery heart rate
- an increase in blood lactate concentration between 8 and 16% after pace and fast work[47] (this is not a consistent finding in studies of overtraining in horses[49])
- reduced plasma cortisol response to maximal exercise.[47,52]

There are not reliable changes in hemogram or leukogram of overtrained horses.[51] Changes in serum activity of muscle-derived enzymes are minor in overtrained horses and of limited diagnostic value.[51] Conversely, serum gamma-glutamyl transferase activity is markedly elevated in overtrained horses and can exceed 100 IU/L.[49,51]

The mechanism of overtraining in horses is poorly understood although it is hypothesized that disturbances of hypothalamic function are central to the disorder rather than a primary effect on muscle function.[53] Overtrained Standardbreds have abnormal pulsatile nocturnal growth hormone secretion which is speculated to be associated with longer phases of somatostatin withdrawal.[54] Standardized exercise tests are suggested to provide a way to detect subtle changes in hormonal responses in the individual, which could make an important contribution to the detection of early overtraining.[50,51] Red cell hypervolemia is not an underlying mechanism associated with overtraining,[55] and chronic muscle

Table 49.5 Sample interval training program for Standardbred horses

TRAINING LEVEL	DISTANCE (m)	REPETITIONS (NUMBER OF HEATS)	WORK INTERVAL TIME (min:s)	REST INTERVAL TIME (min:s)
1	600	2	0:56	5:00
2	800	2	1:15	5:00
3	1000	2	1:35	5:00
4	600	3	0:53	5:00
5	800	3	1:10	5:00
6	1000	3	1:28	5:00
7	1200	2	1:45	5:00
8	600	4	0:50	5:00
9	800	4	1:07	5:00
10	1000	4	1:25	5:00
11	1200	3	1:42	5:00
12	800	4	1:05	5:00
13	1000	4	1:23	5:00
14	1200	3	1:40	5:00
15	800	4	1:03	5:00
16	1000	4	1:20	5:00
17	1200	3	1:38	5:00
18	800	3	1:00	5:00
19	600	4	0:44	5:00
20	1000	2	1:18	5:00
21	800	2	0:58	5:00
22	600	3	0:42	5:00
23	1000	1	1:15	5:00
24	800	2	0:57	5:00
25	600	2	0:41	5:00

Aim: able to pace 1600 m in 1:57 (1000 m track).
Required base: at least 400 km in previous 84 days.
Frequency: every four days.
Rest-period criteria: heart rate 110 or less within 5 minutes of completing the interval.
Interval criteria: if time greater than 1.5 seconds outside scheduled time, session halted. Only proceed to next step if all criteria for previous level have been met.
(From Bayly WM. Training programs. The Veterinary Clinics of North America Equine Practice 1985;1:597-610, with permission from Elsevier.)

glycogen depletion is not a feature of the experimentally induced syndrome.[48]

Treatment and prevention of overtraining

The recommended treatment for overtraining is usually a dramatic reduction in the volume, intensity or frequency of workouts or an increase in the time between workouts. Fast workouts should be dropped and only light jogging continued. If the horse doesn't show improvement within 2–3 weeks, it should be spelled in the paddock and brought back up again after a few months' rest.

Prevention is preferred over treatment and the challenge for trainers is to detect the subtle changes in the horse's response and attitude to training that indicate too much training. Training logs with details of training volume, intensity and recovery should be kept, with regular changes in body weight, food intake and behavior noted. Regular weighing remains a cheap and easy way to monitor the effects of exercise training. Regular performance tests can also be helpful: for example, timing horses over set distances. As both the sprinting and staying ability of the horse are affected by overtraining, these performance tests should include a measurement of all-out speed and overall speed. If the horse takes longer to complete the test and seems tired, this might be an indication that more recovery is required. If time and equipment allows, a measurement of heart rate and blood lactate during and after exercise would also be useful. Above all, trainers need to be able to judge when the results of the training program are being threatened by too much exercise.

Veterinary problems of Standardbreds

Respiratory abnormalities

Whereas gait and respiration are linked in a 1 : 1 fashion in cantering or galloping horses, respiration is not linked to gait in pacing or trotting horses.[56,57] However, abnormalities of the respiratory tract are an important cause of poor performance or reduced racing frequency in Standardbreds. Standardbreds are afflicted with similar respiratory tract disease as are other racehorses, although their gait and associated tack makes problems such as dorsal displacement of the soft palate more problematic.

Upper airway abnormalities

Standardbreds in racing or training may develop a range of upper airway abnormalities including left laryngeal hemiplegia, dorsal displacement of the soft palate, and arytenoid chondritis. The characteristics of these diseases do not differ in any substantive way from those of other athletic horses, as discussed in Chapter 26. Dorsal displacement of the soft palate is a well-recognized syndrome in racing Standardbreds. Its apparent high prevalence in this breed may be related to their tendency to 'choke down' or excessively ventroflex the head during exercise. Treatments for intermittent dorsal displacement of the soft palate include application of a tongue-tie (Fig. 49.14), use of overcheck rein and bit, and surgical manipulation of the pharynx and associated musculature.

Lower airway abnormalities

Exercise-induced pulmonary hemorrhage occurs in Standardbreds, as in other athletic horses that compete at high speed. The prevalence of EIPH in Standardbred racehorses is assumed to be lower than in Thoroughbred racehorses, with 26–34% of horses reported

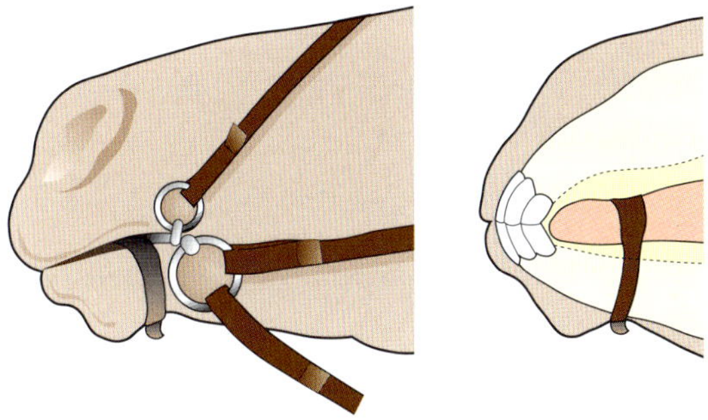

Fig 49.14 Tongue-tie used to prevent horses from 'choking down' during racing. The tongue-tie should not interfere with the driving bit or overcheck bit.

Redrawn with permission.[68] Illustrations are copyrighted by the U.S. Trotting Association, and used here with the expressed permission of the copyright holder.

Table 49.6 Two-week training cycles for the conventional and taper groups. Numbers in parentheses are training pace as percent of pace over the last 1200 m of the most recent 2400 m time trial

DAY	CONVENTIONAL TRAINING	TAPER 1	TAPER 2	TAPER 3
1	Rest	Jog 50 min (40%)	Fast 2400 m (89%)	Fast 3000 m (92%)
2	Jog 40 min (40%)	Fast 3000 m (90%)	Jog 50 min (50%)	Jog 50 min (50%)
3	Fast 2400 m (86%)	Jog 50 min (40%)	Fast 2400 m (89%)	Fast 3000 m (92%)
4	Jog 40 min (40%)	Fast 3000 m (90%)	Jog 50 min (60%)	Jog 50 min (50%)
5	Fast 2400 m (86%)	Jog 50 min (40%)	Fast 2400 m (89%)	Fast 3800 m (90%)
6	Jog 40 min (40%)	Fast 3800 m (90%)	Jog 50 min (60%)	Jog 40 min (50%)
7	Fast 3200 m (86%)	Jog 40 min (40%)	5 x 800 m intervals (100%)	Fast 1800 m (94%)
8	Jog 40 min (40%)	Rest	4 x 800 m intervals (100%)	Jog 30 min (50%)
9	Rest	Fast 1800 m (95%)	3 x 800 m intervals (100%)	Fast 1200 m (100%)
10	Fast 2400 m (86%)	Jog 30 min (40%)	2 x 800 m intervals (100%)	Jog 20 min (50%)
11	Jog 40 min (40%)	Fast 1200 m (100%)	1 x 800 m intervals (100%)	Fast 1200 m (100%)
12	Fast 2400 m (86%)	Jog 20 min (40%)	Walk	Walk
13	Jog 40 min (40%)	Walk	Walk	Walk
14	Time trial	Time trial	Time trial	Time trial

All fast work was completed with the horses harnessed up into their hobbles. Horses were only introduced to the above training programs after eight weeks of foundation training. As an example of intensity, the jog at 40% time trial pace was approximately 19 km/h. The relief period between interval repetitions was set at 5 minutes, during which the horses walked. (Reprinted from Shearman JP. Effect of tapered normal and interval training on performance of Standardbred pacers. Equine Vet J 2002;34:395, with permission from the Equine Veterinary Journal.)

to have blood in the trachea after racing.[58,59] However, these studies were based on a single examination and one[59] only reported as positive those horses with blood covering more than one-half of the tracheobronchial tree. When examined after each of 3 races, 87% of Standardbred racehorses have evidence of EIPH on at least one occasion,[60] suggesting that EIPH is as common in Standardbred racehorses as it is in Thoroughbred racehorses. Management of EIPH is discussed in Chapter 29.

Inflammatory airway disease is common in harness racehorses, is associated with altered physiological responses including lower V_4 and V_{200} and is considered to be a cause of reduced performance.[29] Inflammatory airway disease alters airway mechanics of Standardbred horses during hyperventilation at rest by increasing larger tidal volumes and lower respiratory frequencies, greater viscous lung resistance and dynamic work of breathing, changes which if present during exercise would impair performance.[29,61] A complete discussion of IAD is provided in Chapter 28.

Musculoskeletal disorders

(Adapted with permission from *Lameness in the Standardbred Horse* by F. Torre and M.W. Ross.[62])

The race track practitioner caring for Standardbred horses frequently deals with problems and lameness requiring prompt diagnostic and therapeutic aid, which in most cases must be compatible with the season racing activity and current drug use regulations.

Recognition of lameness

Lameness is the most important cause of poor racing performance in Standardbreds, as evidenced by 0.09 lameness events per horse-month in a group of 265 Danish trotters monitored prospectively.[63] A total of 84 lameness events occurred in 69 of the 265 horses during a five-month period compared with 16 adverse respiratory events and seven muscle events. Similar observations have been made in Thoroughbreds.

Risk factors for lameness in harness horses are not well recognized. There are variable effects of age, sex, stage of training, and/or trainer on the risk that a horse will become lame.[63,64] Increasing the banking of the track from 4.8 to 5.7 degrees decreased the incidence of major injury or lameness in trotters and pacers by 22%.[65]

Lameness severity can range from moderate to severe, being visible at a walk or trot in hand, to subtle or mild lameness seen only at speed or while racing. A 1- to 2-second increase in the time for a mile, generally reflected in a slower last quarter-mile time, accompanies many lameness problems but may be confused with other problems such as respiratory abnormalities or recurrent exertional rhabdomyolysis. Bilateral lameness may cause a reduction in race performance without other localizing signs. Lameness is a major cause of horses making breaks (breaking stride) at high speed, although shoeing (particularly in trotters) and equipment considerations are also important contributing factors.

Horses on a line (driver pulls harder on one line to keep a horse from bearing in or out), generally have ipsilateral lameness problems, although occasionally, horses with medial foot or carpal lameness can be on the contralateral line. If on a line at all, horses with hindlimb lameness are usually on the ipsilateral line. For instance, those with left hind lameness are usually on the left line. Horses on a shaft (rear of horse closer to one shaft) generally have contralateral hindlimb lameness. Occasionally, a horse with forelimb lameness (and 'hard on the line') will be on the opposite shaft (horse with right front lameness will be on left shaft). This is usually because the driver is pulling the horse hard enough with the right line to cause it to bend its hind end to the left. These horses are often affected with lameness in more than one limb. Horses with forelimb lameness are generally worse on turns, although foot soreness and splints worsen as the mile progresses. Horses with hock lameness may be worse going into a turn or while coming out of a turn, whereas those with metatarsophalangeal joint (MTPJ) lameness will be worse around turns. Horses with left hind lameness may be able to trot or pace the turns, but those lame in the right hind will be worse in turns. Pacers with hindlimb lameness and a history of being worse when on the pace than while on the trot are usually affected with stifle lameness. Track size varies in Standardbred racing and horses that are lame in the turns are usually worse on smaller tracks. However, racing is generally slower on smaller tracks, allowing lame horses, particularly those with soft-tissue injuries, to compete successfully.

Breed and gait differences

There is considerable difference regarding lameness distribution and prognosis in Standardbreds as compared with Thoroughbred racehorses. Gait difference between the breeds undoubtedly plays a role. The trot and pace are 2-beat gaits, and there is more equal distribution of load (and lameness) between the forelimbs and hindlimbs. Less rotational forces in certain joints of Standardbreds such as the carpus may reduce overload injury when compared with Thoroughbreds. Diseases such as suspensory disruption, catastrophic or incomplete fractures of the humerus, tibia, ilium, and third metacarpal/metatarsal, and bucked shins are much less common in Standardbreds. In general, Standardbreds (STB) have a better prognosis than Thoroughbreds for soft-tissue injuries such as suspensory desmitis and superficial digital flexor tendonitis. There appears to be differences in prognosis within the breed, and, in general, prognosis in trotters is worse than in pacers. Lameness in pacers can be difficult to see, particularly in the forelimb. Pacers can usually tolerate lameness better than trotters with the exception of some hindlimb problems such as stifle lameness.

Because many STB lamenesses are subtle, there is no substitute for evaluation of these horses at the track while jogging or training. It may be useful to sit behind the horse, particularly when evaluating subtle hindlimb lameness. Treadmill examination is useful in providing a consistent surface and speed for lameness evaluation but does not simulate turning or pulling weight. Unfortunately, lameness examinations cannot always be performed under ideal situations, and horses are commonly evaluated at a walk and trot in hand. Standardbreds evaluated at slow speed may not exhibit the same lameness as they do at high speed. Problems such as splints and foot soreness may only surface after training or racing, and examination at rest may be non-diagnostic. Care must be taken not to over-interpret subtle hindlimb lameness at a trot in hand. However, careful lameness examination can be useful, even in horses with subtle problems.

Lameness of the forelimb is slightly more common than that of the hindlimb, but there is a near equal distribution between hindlimb and forelimb lameness. Articular and periarticular injuries account for a majority of STB lameness, whereas long-bone abnormalities are less common. The carpus is the most common articular injury and is likely the most common source of lameness overall. The MTPJ is very important in hindlimb lameness, in fact nearly equal to that of the hock, and has been underemphasized.

Muscle diseases

Exertional rhabdomyolysis occurs in Standardbred racehorses. The disease occurs with an annual incidence of 6.4% in Swedish Standardbred trotters with females having 7.1 times the risk of males of developing the disease.[66] Nervous horses were 7.9 times more likely to develop the disease than were calm horses. The disease does not appear to be related to mutations in the R309H GYS1 gene in Standardbreds.[66]

Forelimb lameness

Front limb lameness in the racing Standardbred range from readily apparent lameness to subtle disturbances of gait. There are conditions in which the acute lameness requires immediate radiographic examination to rule out frequent injuries including sagittal fractures of proximal PI, proximal sesamoid fractures, pedal bone fractures, and less frequently injuries of the proximal metacarpal region. However, more commonly the complaint is a subtle to mild lameness which may be complicated by problems affecting the hindlimb. In such cases the clinician must investigate the horse's history, including the horse's gait, shoeing, recent performance, previous lameness, when the horse becomes lame (after the race, the next day), factors that exacerbate the lameness (e.g. training clockwise or counterclockwise, on turns or on the straight, at the beginning or at the end of the race), wrong postures (horse on a line, on a shaft), and efficacy of previous treatments.

Foot

The first step in diagnosis of lameness is a careful examination of the horse's conformation, especially foot conformation (club foot, toed-in, toed-out, hoof wall angle, lateral-medial balance, asymmetrical feet) and the presence of joint effusion, which is easily appreciated when affecting the fetlock and midcarpal joints. Joint distension is less obvious in the dorsal compartment of the coffin joint. The metacarpal region is frequently a site of visible abnormalities; enlargement of the body or branches of the suspensory ligament, bowed tendon, and constriction of the palmar annular ligament represent common findings.

Palpation detects areas of abnormal warmth and pain and allows evaluation of joint angles. The feet may have asymmetric warmth, increased digital pulse, and different responses to hoof testing. When possible, feet are first tested without removing the shoes, and ideally the horse should be kept shod until any examination of gait is completed. Lateral and medial quarters, lateral and medial middle sole, and lateral and medial toe are all tested. Compressing the frog rarely brings useful information, and squeezing the quarters may cause pain unrelated to primary lameness. The medial quarter is usually more sensitive and this finding must not be overinterpreted. Hoof or foot pain is a common occurrence, although it is often subtle.

Shoeing represents a source of useful information and should be discussed with the trainer to better understand the gait characteristics. For horses with a flat sole, overzealous padding may add to, rather than relieve, pressure on the sole. Wide web shoes with leather or rubber padding are useful in cases of pain originating from the distal interphalangeal (DIP) joint. Bar shoes are now less commonly used and may exacerbate coffin and fetlock joint problems, by limiting the natural slipping of the landing foot.

Corrective shoeing provides a solution for problems located in the hoof. This pain must be distinguished from problems related to osteoarthritis of the DIP joint. In this case, flexion of the distal limb frequently elicits pain. The final diagnosis of DIP osteoarthritis is the result of different investigations including history (the horse frequently gets worse at the end of the race and is on a line), conformation (foot smaller than the contralateral club foot), palpation (some pain may be elicited by deep palpation of the dorsal joint capsule, the dorsal wall and/or heels are warmer), diagnostic analgesia (being aware that this problem is not always resolved by intra-articular anesthesia and that the latter may abolish pain originating from the navicular area and from the sole), and exclusion of other sites of pain in the distal limb especially the fetlock.

Pastern and fetlock

Abnormalities of the fetlock account for approximately 40% of lameness events in a study of Danish trotters.[63] Radiographic examination often reveals a prominent osteophyte on the distal aspect of the middle phalanx associated with a variable degree of remodeling of the proximal aspect of the distal phalanx. Osteoarthritis of the DIP joint is frequently bilateral.

The metacarpophalangeal joint is frequently involved in front limb lameness. Survey radiographs may detect dorsoproximal fragmentation of the proximal phalanx and osteochondrosis of the proximal sagittal ridge on the dorsodistal metacarpus. These lesions are frequently diagnosed in yearlings and treated by arthroscopic surgery.

Acute synovitis of the metacarpophalangeal joint is observed in young horses when the training is intensified, especially on hard tracks. The horse appears moderately lame and sensitive to deep palpation of the dorsal joint capsule and to flexion test. Intra-articular anesthesia is usually diagnostic. In older horses, chronic thickening of the dorsal synovial pad (villonodular synovitis) is suspected when the lateromedial radiographic view shows flattening or osteolysis of the proximal aspect of the dorsal sagittal ridge and contrast radiography evidences a filling defect corresponding to the soft-tissue mass. Ultrasonography may be used to measure the thickness of the synovial pad.

The palmar aspect of the front limb fetlocks in Standardbreds is characterized by problems affecting the proximal sesamoid bones and adjacent soft tissues. Sesamoiditis in young horses has the typical radiographic feature of radiolucent lines in the palmar abaxial aspect of the bone. Scintigraphic findings are indicative of increased bone metabolism, but radiographic changes are only seen in 50% of Standardbreds with increased radioisotope uptake. In older horses, the radiographic changes include radiolucent lines in the proximal one-half of the bone, irregular palmar/abaxial radiographic outline, enthesophytes, and mineralization of the intersesamoidean ligament. When affecting the base of the sesamoid bone, the presence of enthesophytes is more properly considered distal sesamoidean desmitis.

Desmitis and tendonitis

The insertion of the suspensory branch on the proximal sesamoid bone becomes irregular, and ultrasonography provides the most accurate diagnostic tool. Suspensory branch desmitis is frequently associated with sesamoiditis. It may be caused by lateral-to-medial hoof imbalance, training over uneven track surfaces, strains, and fractures of the splint bone(s). Acute desmitis may be associated with metacarpophalangeal joint effusion. Ultrasonography is performed to assess the degree of ligament damage, with enlargement and loss of definition of the margins of the branch, focal hypoechoic areas, diffuse loss of echogenicity, and hyperechoic foci in horses with chronic desmitis being the most frequent findings. The corresponding splint bone may deviate abaxially, and radiographic monitoring may allow early diagnosis of secondary distal splint bone fracture.

Desmitis of the proximal insertion of the suspensory ligament is commonly diagnosed and carries a better prognosis than desmitis affecting the body or branches of the ligament. When the proximal aspect of the suspensory ligament is affected, the clinician must differentiate pain originating from the carpal joint and perform a local block (subcarpal block, axially to the origin of the splint bones, or direct infiltration over the proximal suspensory ligament). In cases of positive block, ultrasonography is used to assess damage to the suspensory ligament and bone remodeling of the palmar proximal metacarpus; a dorsopalmar radiographic view is used to assess the presence of palmar sclerosis of the third metacarpal (MCIII) in chronic cases.

Superficial digital flexor tendonitis represents a frequent indication for ultrasonographic examination of the distal limb of Standardbred racehorses. Most of the lesions are located in the middle and distal third of the tendon. A core lesion located in the palmarolateral border of the tendon characterizes over 30% of the lesions. Central core lesions are uncommon. Chronic recurrent lesions have the typical pattern of diffuse tendonitis. When the lesion affects the distal aspect of the tendon, the digital tendon sheath may be distended, and the typical notch of palmar annular ligament constriction is visible in the palmar outline.

Carpus

The midcarpal joint represents a predilection site of lameness in racehorses, especially young Standardbreds, and is a major cause of wastage in Standardbred racehorses.[64] Abnormalities of the carpus are a common cause of lameness in trotters – approximately 48% of lameness in one study of 265 horses examined over five months and 28% of 114 horses monitored over 12–18 months in another.[63,64] Typically, horses affected by midcarpal joint pain tend to trot with a wide-based gait, abducting the affected leg or legs in an attempt to minimize carpal flexion. Visual inspection reveals various degrees of joint effusion, especially on the dorsomedial aspect of the carpus. Palpation may elicit pain over the dorsal aspect of the carpus. The flexion test is positive and intra-articular analgesia abolishes the lameness in the majority of horses. A negative result from intra-articular analgesia does not necessarily exclude pain in this joint because subchondral bone damage under a relatively normal cartilage may cause pain that is difficult to abolish with intra-articular analgesia. With the exception of foals and yearlings, lesions are rarely located on the proximal front limb of Standardbreds, and nearly invariably lesions affecting the elbow and shoulder regions are the result of direct trauma.

Radiographic examination includes six basic views and a variable number of extra views: dorsopalmar (DP), flexed lateral-medial (LM), dorsolateral to palmaromedial oblique (DLPMO), dorsomedial to palmarolateral oblique (DMPLO), and 33° and 55° skyline views (dorsoproximal-palmarodistal skyline). The latter two views must be of excellent quality because it has been shown that a large number of injuries (especially affecting the third carpal bone) can be diagnosed only on the skyline view.

Treatment depends on the type and degree of injury. Young racehorses without radiographically visible abnormalities (a more sensitive diagnostic tool is represented by scintigraphy, which may reveal increased radionuclide uptake in the early phase of the disease) are best rested and treated with non-steroidal anti-inflammatory drugs, especially polysulfated glycosaminoglycans. Training modulation allows in most of the cases time for bone remodeling and prevents the progress of bone injuries.

Arthroscopic findings in horses with lameness located in the midcarpal joint but no radiographic findings include sinking and discoloration of articular cartilage, loss of articular cartilage in focal areas of the third and radial carpal bone, and rupture of the medial palmar intercarpal ligament. The devitalized cartilage is debrided and the underlying bone may be foraged using micropick technique, which augments cartilage repair. Rupture of the medial palmar intercarpal ligament is less common, and the treatment involves arthroscopic trimming and 4–6 weeks of rest followed by 4 to 6 weeks of walking exercise. The same postoperative protocol is used for routine arthroscopic surgery, whereas internal fixation of C3 slab fractures is followed by eight weeks of rest, radiographic control, and four weeks of walking exercise. There is usually no need for removal of the screw.

Hindlimb lameness

Careful palpation of all anatomic structures, including static flexion and extension of all joints, should be performed. Frequently overlooked sites of inflammation (in both the forelimb and hindlimb) include the dorsal aspect of the proximal phalanx (P-I, [incomplete midsagittal or dorsal frontal fractures]), proximal sesamoid bones (sesamoiditis, fractures, avulsion injury associated with the suspensory attachment), and carpus and proximal aspect of third metacarpal (MCIII) (avulsion or longitudinal fractures of MCIII, proximal suspensory desmitis, dorsomedial articular fracture, incomplete C-3 chip fractures), proximal plantar third metatarsal (MTIII) region (proximal and mid-body suspensory desmitis, pain along medial and lateral splint bones associated with hock lameness), and the metatarsophalangeal joint (MTPJ). In the hindlimb, it is easy to overlook subtle swelling of the suspensory origin and body, since these portions of the ligament are buried beneath the second and fourth metatarsal bones. Hoof tester examination should be performed in all horses since foot soreness is common. Foot soreness is less common in the hindlimb than in the forelimb, but does occur, as do osteoarthritis of the distal interphalangeal joint and navicular disease or fracture (rare). Secondary back, gluteal and trochanteric pain are common and treatment of these areas is often recommended along with therapy of concomitant hindlimb lameness. Back pain in Standardbreds is usually the result of muscle pain, rather than impingement or over-riding of dorsal spinous processes. Scintigraphic evaluation has failed to identify a single Standardbred racehorse with increased radioisotope uptake involving the dorsal spinous processes, whereas this scintigraphic abnormality is common in horses that are ridden.

Intra-articular and perineural analgesia is important in the diagnosis of Standardbred hindlimb lameness and many times is most reliably done at the track where horses can be moved and evaluated at speed. Care must be taken when incomplete fractures are suspected, particularly of the first phalanx (P-1) because the lesion can progress to a complete fracture. When performing the plantar digital block, the clinician must keep in mind that pain associated with proximal P-1 can be abolished. In these horses, the clinician inadvertently diagnoses a problem in the foot, when in reality the true source of pain is a midsagittal fracture of P-1. Because of the large number of Standardbreds with MTPJ lameness, basisesamoid or abaxial sesamoid nerve blocks are not useful. With these blocks, proximal diffusion of anesthetic occurs so frequently that misdiagnosis is common. I usually perform a plantar digital block, followed by a dorsal ring block, to desensitize the dorsal aspect of the foot. A low plantar perineural block is then performed. This technique is more successful in abolishing subchondral bone pain in the MTPJ than is the intra-articular technique, but all four nerves must be blocked (medial and lateral plantar nerve and medial and lateral plantar metatarsal nerves). Horses with incomplete fractures of MTIII, P-1, or the proximal sesamoid bones or those with non-adaptive remodeling may fail to respond or only partially improve with intra-articular analgesia but become completely sound with the low plantar block. A selective lateral plantar metatarsal block can be performed to identify those horses with stress reaction or non-adaptive remodeling of the distal aspect of MTIII. High plantar analgesia is often overlooked but is critical in the diagnosis of proximal suspensory desmitis or other avulsion injury associated with MTIII. Although all three compartments of the stifle joint should be independently blocked in horses suspected of lameness in this region, the medial femorotibial joint is most frequently affected.

The hind digits

The hind foot is much less commonly the cause of lameness than is the front foot, but is still the source of pain in many Standardbreds. Foot abscessation, quarter cracks, hoof avulsion, distal interphalangeal osteoarthritis, distal phalanx (P-III) fractures, and chronic 'foot soreness' from poor shoeing and balance occur. P-III fractures most commonly involve the left hind lateral and right hind medial wings of P-III, but this distribution is not as clear cut as in the forelimb. It is critical to separate pain originating from the foot from that of the metatarsophalangeal joint (MTPJ) and results of diagnostic analgesia need to be carefully interpreted. Anesthetic diffusion occurs when the posterior digital block is performed, and it is relatively common to desensitize structures in the pastern and MTPJ using this block. The most common diagnoses in horses, where inadvertent analgesia of the MTPJ occurs using posterior digital anesthesia, is midsagittal fracture of the proximal phalanx.

Interference is a common problem in trotters. Trotters that hike behind and have what appears to be unilateral hindlimb lameness can be lame in the ipsilateral forelimb. Foot or carpal lameness can cause shortening of the ipsilateral forelimb, causing interference and what appears to be ipsilateral hindlimb lameness. Superficial skin soreness or frank osteitis can result from interference, and trotters frequently 'make breaks' as the result of the problem. Corrective shoeing and the elimination of the primary source of pain are important.

Metatarsophalangeal joint

MTPJ is an important source of hindlimb lameness, and, in fact, many horses suspected of having tarsal or stifle pain will 'block out' with low plantar or intra-articular analgesia, if the techniques are routinely performed. One of the most common lameness conditions of the Standardbred racehorse is subchondral bone pain of the distal, plantarolateral aspect of MTIII. This is a form of stress or non-adaptive remodeling of MTIII, an early form of osteoarthritis, that is characterized by lameness most consistently abolished by low-plantar (or selective lateral plantar metatarsal) analgesia. Horses tend to have a 'stabby' hindlimb gait, will likely be on the contralateral shaft, be worse in the turns, and are often misdiagnosed as having tarsal pain. Intra-articular medication is usually ineffective and obvious signs of osteoarthritis such as effusion, a positive response to flexion, or other abnormalities found on palpation are usually absent. Radiographs are initially negative or equivocal, and the diagnosis is made with scintigraphy. Bone phase scintigraphic images reveal focal radiopharmaceutical uptake of distal, plantarolateral aspect of MTIII. A continuum of stress-related subchondral bone changes results in non-adaptive remodeling, sclerosis, and later areas of necrotic subchondral bone. In older horses, radiographic evidence of subchondral bone injury is seen, but in two and early three year olds, radiographic examination may be negative. Because this lesion is a result of a continuum of stress-related subchondral bone damage, management includes a reduction in stress. Modification in exercise intensity, corrective shoeing, swimming physiotherapy, and shock wave therapy has been used, but long-term rest may be best. Intra-articular medication, including corticosteroids, is not effective early in the disease process, presumably because pain originates from subchondral bone, and overlying cartilage damage is minimal. Later, when cartilage damage worsens and subchondral bone collapse occurs (radiolucent changes develop radiographically), injections decrease inflammation and lameness.

A common problem in Standardbreds is plantar process fragmentation of the proximal phalanx. Articular fragments, most commonly involving the medial aspect (can be biaxial and bilateral), can cause high-speed lameness and perhaps contribute to the development of OA in older horses. Large, abaxial, non-articular fragments can also cause lameness, but conventional surgical techniques are necessary for removal.

Fractures involving the MTPJ are more common in pacers than in trotters, with the exception of fractures of the proximal sesamoid bones. Midsagittal P-1 fractures are more common in the hindlimb than in the forelimb and can be difficult to diagnose. Pain from this fracture is often thought to originate from the foot because posterior digital analgesia abolishes lameness in some horses. Surgical fixation is recommended in horses with long or displaced fractures, but conservative management is successful in horses with short, midsagittal fractures. Dorsal frontal fractures of P-1 occur in pacers and in trotters, are more common in the RH, can be bilateral, and heal with conservative management. Fractures of MTIII condyles occur but are less common than in Thoroughbreds and are unusual in the trotter. Medial condylar fractures tend to spiral proximally, and horses are at risk for catastrophic injury either before surgical fixation or during anesthetic recovery. Lateral apical sesamoid fractures occur commonly. Lateral sesamoiditis causes lameness in two year olds trained in 2:15 to 2:18 for the mile, and prognosis is poor if substantial radiolucency exits.

Metatarsal region

The most common and important condition of the metatarsal region is suspensory desmitis. This is often a career-limiting or career-ending injury, particularly in the trotter. Proximal suspensory desmitis, avulsion fracture, or stress reaction/enthesopathy occur but can be difficult to diagnose, and high plantar analgesia is a must to differentiate pain from this areas from that of the MTPJ or tarsus.

Tarsus

Distal tarsitis remains the most common lameness of the tarsus. The disease involves OA of the DIT and TMT joints, but there is a significant periarticular soft-tissue component, likely caused by sliding or shear forces, and radiographs are often negative. Osteochondritis dissecans of the tarsocrural joint is the most common surgical condition of the tarsus, is likely hereditary in the breed, and causes effusion and high-speed lameness. Surgical removal of fragments is recommended in horses with clinical signs or those sold at public auction. Tarsocrural arthropathy, an insidious disease resulting in eventual severe lameness and widespread cartilage damage, is seen in older horses. Curb, a common soft-tissue lameness, is frequently tendonitis of the superficial digital flexor tendon rather than long plantar desmitis. Third and central tarsal bone slab fractures, enthesopathy at the attachment of the collateral ligament on the distal aspect of the calcaneus, occur occasionally.

Stifle

The most common condition of the stifle in Standardbreds is OA of the medial femorotibial joint. This condition is difficult to diagnose radiographically because, early on, the only sign is narrowing of the joint space seen on the caudocranial view. Effusion of the medial femorotibial joint is usually present but may be a subtle clinical finding. Intra-articular injections and corrective shoeing (aluminum shoe with a toe grab) usually help. Trotters appear able to race more successfully than do pacers with this problem. Osteochondritis dissecans and osseous cyst-like lesions occur and cause lameness.

The authors and editors gratefully acknowledge the contributions to this chapter of Michael Hamlin, a contributor to the previous edition.

References

1. Saastamoinen MT. Factors affecting age at onset of breaking, training, qualifying and first start in Finnish trotters. Acta Agriculturæ Scandinavica Section A, Animal Science 1991;41:137–45.
2. Porter V. Mason's world dictionary of livestock breeds, types, and varieties. 2002.
3. Greene C. Perspectives on bloodlines and breeding. In: Hoffman D, editor. The new care and training of the trotter and pacer. Columbus, OH: United States Trotting Association; 1996. p. 12–79.
4. Thiruvenkadan AK, Kandasamy N, Panneerselvam S. Inheritance of racing performance of trotter horses: An overview. Livestock Science 2009;124:163.
5. Physick-Sheard PW. Career profile of the Canadian Standardbred. I. Influence of age, gait and sex upon chances of racing. Can J Vet Res 1986;50:449–56.
6. Cothran EG, MacCluer JW, Weitkamp R, Bailey E. Genetic differentiation associated with gait within American Standardbred horses. Animal Genetics 1987;18:285.
7. Bjørnstad G, Roed KH. Breed demarcation and potential for breed allocation of horses assessed by microsatellite markers. Animal Genetics 2001;32:59.
8. Arnason T. Trends and asymptotic limits for racing speed in standardbred trotters. Livestock Production Science 2001;72: 135.
9. Reynaldo J-P. Le Trotteur Français. Editions Lavauzelle ed; 2007.
10. Records – pacers and trotters. Harness Racing Australia, 2011. (Accessed January 17, 2012, at http://www.harness.org.au/hra/annual/public/records.htm.)
11. Physick-Sheard PW. Career profile of the Canadian Standardbred. II. Influence of age, gait and sex upon number of races, money won and race times. Can J Vet Res 1986;50:457–70.
12. Tanner JC, Rogers CW, Firth EC. The relationship of training milestones with racing success in a population of Standardbred horses in New Zealand. NZ Vet J 2012;59:323.
13. Knight PK, Thomson PC. Age at first start and racing career of a cohort of Australian Standardbred horses. Aust Vet J 2011;89:325.
14. Wade CM, Guilotto E, Sigurdsson S, et al. Genome sequence, comparative analysis, and population genetics of the domestic horse. Science 2009;326:865.
15. Hill EW, Fonseca RG, McGivney BA, et al. MSTN genotype (g. 66493737C/T) association with speed indices in Thoroughbred racehorses. J Appl Physiol 2012;12:86–90.
16. Gómez MD. Genetic evaluation of racing performance in trotter horses by competitive models. Livestock Science 2011;41:1871–1413.
17. Tolley E, Notter D, Marlowe T. Heritability and repeatability of speed for 2- and 3-year-old standardbred racehorses. J Anim Sci 1983;56: 1294–305.
18. Tolley EA, Notter DR, Marlowe TJ. Heritability and repeatability of speed for 2- and 3-year-old standardbred racehorses. J Anim Sci 1983;56:1294–305.
19. Hintz RL. Genetics of performance in the horse. J Anim Sci 1980;51:582.
20. Miscellaneous statistics. In: Australian harness racing annual 2001. Melbourne: Australian Harness Racing Council; 2002. p. 163.
21. http://www.uet-trot.eu/pdf/en/stat06.pdf Accessed July 12, 2013.
22. Wastage in the Australian Standardbred. Harness Racing Australia, 1998. (Accessed January 19, 2012, at http://www.harness.org.au/hra/papers/WASTAGE2.HTM.)
23. Physick-Sheard P. Career profile of Canadian Standardbred. I. Influence of age, gait, and sex upon chances of racing. Can J Vet Res 1986;50:449–56.
24. Minkema D. Genetic studies on performance in Dutch trotters. Proc Int Symp Genet Horse Breeding 1975:24–32.
25. Physick-Sheard P. Career profile of the Canadian Standardbred II. Influence of age, gait and sex upon number of races, money won and race times. Can J Vet Res 1986;50:457–70.
26. Courouce A, Chatard JC, Auvinet B. Estimation of performance potential of standardbred trotters from blood lactate concentrations measured in field conditions. Equine Vet J 1997;29:365–9.
27. Leleu C, Cotrel C, Courouce-Malblanc A. Relationships between physiological variables and race performance in French standardbred trotters. Veterinary Record 2005;156:339.
28. Lindner AE. Relationships between racing times of Standardbreds and v4 and v200. J Anim Sci 2009;88:950.
29. Richard EA, Fortier GD, Pitel P, et al. Sub-clinical diseases affecting performance in Standardbred trotters: Diagnostic methods and predictive parameters. Vet J 2009;184:282.
30. Gauvreau GM, Staempfli H, McCutcheon LJ, et al. Comparison of aerobic capacity between racing standardbred horses. J Appl Physiol 1995;78:1447–51.
31. Buhl R, Ersboll AK, Eriksen L, Koch J. Changes over time in echocardiographic measurements in young Standardbred racehorses undergoing training and racing and association with racing performance. J Am Vet Med Assoc 2005;226:1881.
32. Kearns CF, McKeever KH, Kumagai K, et al. Fat-free mass is related to one-mile race performance in elite standardbred horses. Vet J 2002;163:260–6.
33. About Harness Racing. Horseman and Fair World, 2012. (Accessed January 19, 2012, at http://oddsonracing.com/about_racing.cfm.)
34. Vilar JM, Spadari A, Billi V, et al. Biomechanics in young and adult Italian standardbred trotter horses in real racing conditions. Vet Res Comm 2008;32:367.
35. Wilson BD, Neal RJ, Howard A, et al. The gait of pacers. 1: Minematics of the racing stride. Equine Vet J 1988;20:341–6.
36. Wilson BD, Neal RJ, Howard A, et al. The gait of pacers. 2: Factors influencing pacing speed. Equine Vet J 1988;20: 347–51.
37. Collier MA. Standardbred equipment. 2. A primer for veterinarians. Mod Vet Pract 1985;66.
38. Darish SM. Standardbred equipment. 1. A primer for veterinarians. Mod Vet Pract 1985;66.
39. Eaton MD. Energetics and performance. In: Hodgson DR, Rose, RJ, editors. The Athletic horse: Principles and practice of equine sports medicine. Philadelphia: W.B. Saunders Company; 1994. p. 49–61.
40. Hinchcliff KW, Lauderdale MA, Dutson J, et al. High intensity exercise conditioning increases accumulated oxygen deficit of horses. Equine Vet J 2002;34:9–16.
41. Lovell D. Training Standardbred trotters and pacers. In: Hodgson DR, Rose R, editors. The athletic horse: principles and practice of equine sports medicine. Philadelphia: W.B. Saunders Company; 1994. p. 399–408.

42. Shearman JP, Hopkins WG. Training of standardbred maiden pacers. J Equine Vet Sci 1995;16:116.
43. Ivers T. The fit racehorse. Cincinnatti, OH: Esprit Racing Team Ltd.; 1983.
44. Bayly WM. Training programs. The Veterinary Clinics of North America: Equine Practice 1985;1:597–610.
45. Tyler CM, Golland LC, Evans DL, et al. Changes in maximum oxygen uptake during prolonged training, overtraining, and detraining in horses. J Appl Physiol 1996;81:2244.
46. Shearman JP, Hamlin MJ, Hopkins WG. Effect of tapered normal and interval training on performance of Standardbred pacers. Equine Vet J 2002;34:395.
47. Hamlin MJ, Shearman JP, Hopkins WG. Changes in physiological parameters in overtrained Standardbred racehorses. Equine Vet J 2002;34:383.
48. McGowan CM, Golland LC, Evans DL, et al. Effects of prolonged intense training, overtraining and detraining on skeletal muscle metabolites and enzymes. Equine Vet J 2002;34:257.
49. McGowan CM, Whitworth DJ. Overtraining syndrome in horses. J Comp Exerc Physiol 2008;5:57–65.
50. Rivero JLL, van Breda E, Rogers CW. Unexplained underperformance syndrome in sport horses: Classification, potential causes and recognition. Equine Vet J 2008;40:611–18.
51. Tyler-McGowan CM, Golland LC, Evans DL, et al. Haematological and biochemical responses to training and overtraining. Equine Vet J 1999;31:621–5.
52. Golland LC, Evans DL, Stone GM, et al. Plasma cortisol and β-endorphin concentrations in trained and over-trained Standardbred racehorses. Pflügers Archiv 1999;439:11–17.
53. Wijnberg ID, van Dam KG, De Graaf-Roelfsema E, et al. (Over) training effects on quantitative electromyography and muscle enzyme activities in standardbred horses. J Appl Physiol 2008;105:1746–53.
54. de Graaf-Roelfsema E, Veldhuis PP, Keizer HA, et al. Overtrained horses alter their resting pulsatile growth hormone secretion. Am J Physiol 2009;297: R403–11.
55. Golland LC, Evans DL, McGowan CM, et al. The effects of overtraining on blood volumes in standardbred racehorses. Vet J 2003;165:228–33.
56. Cotrel C, Leleu C, Courouce-Malblanc A. Factors influencing variation in locomotor-respiratory coupling in Standardbred Trotters in the field. Equine Vet J 2006;38:562–6.
57. Evans DL, Silverman EB, Hodgson DR, et al. Gait and respiration in Standardbred horses when pacing and galloping. Res Vet Sci 1994;57:233–9.
58. MacNamara B, Bauer S, Iafe J. Endoscopic evaluation of exercise-induced pulmonary hemorrhage and chronic obstructive pulmonary disease in association with poor performance in racing Standardbreds. J Am Vet Med Assoc 1990;196:443–5.
59. Speirs VC, van Veenendaal JC, Harrison IW, et al. Pulmonary haemorrhage in standardbred horses after racing. Aust Vet J 1982;59:38–40.
60. Lapointe JM, Vrins A, McCarvill E. A survey of exercise-induced pulmonary haemorrhage in Quebec standardbred racehorses. Equine Vet J 1994;26: 482–5.
61. Pirrone F, Albertini M, Clement MG, et al. Respiratory mechanics in Standardbred horses with sub-clinical inflammatory airway disease and poor athletic performance. Vet J 2007;173: 144–50.
62. Torre F, Ross MW. Lameness in the standardbred horse. J Equine Vet Sci 2002;22:429–36.
63. Vigre H, Chriel M, Hesselholt M, et al. Risk factors for the hazard of lameness in Danish Standardbred trotters. Prev Vet Med 2002;56:105–17.
64. Steel CM, Hopper BJ, Richardson JL, et al. Clinical findings, diagnosis, prevalence and predisposing factors for lameness localised to the middle carpal joint in young Standardbred racehorses. Equine Vet J 2006;38: 152–7.
65. Evans DL, Walsh JS. Effect of increasing the banking of a racetrack on the occurrence of injury and lameness in standardbred horses. Aust Vet J 1997;75:751–2.
66. Isgren CM, Upjohn MM, Fernandez-Fuente M, et al. Epidemiology of exertional rhabdomyolysis susceptibility in standardbred horses reveals associated risk factors and underlying enhanced performance. PLoS ONE 2010;5:1–7.
67. Sylvester C. Training the trotter. In: Hoffman D, editor. The new care and training of the trotter and pacer. Columbus, OH: United States Trotting Association; 1996.
68. Haughton T. Choosing the right equipment. In: Hoffman D, editor. The new care and training of the trotter and pacer. Columbus, OH: United States Trotting Association; 1996.

Veterinary aspects of training event horses

50

Jonathan H. Foreman

CHAPTER CONTENTS

Definitions and background

Event horses are required to perform three sports in one: dressage, cross-country, and show jumping.[1] Events take place over one to three competition days. Complete three-day events (3DE) involve three tests on consecutive days: the Dressage Test on the first day, the Cross-Country Test (previously termed the Speed-and-Endurance Test) on the second day (Fig. 50.1), and the Jumping Test on the third day. The Dressage Test is intended to test obedience, balance, and suppleness in horses fit enough to gallop and jump Cross-Country the following day. Cross-Country is competed by galloping and jumping over 30–45 immovable obstacles with heights and spreads requiring speed, endurance, jumping scope, and courage on the part of both the horse and the rider (Fig. 50.1).[1] In the newer short format, the warm-up phases for Cross-Country are no longer a part of the formal judged competition. The reasoning behind the third day's test, show jumping, is to determine which horses are best able to compete effectively after the rigorous second day of the Cross-Country Test.

Internationally the sport is known as the Concours Complet d'Equitation Internationale (CCI, translated as 'complete equestrian competition').[1,2] International 3DE are ranked by the FEI as one (CCI*) through four-star (CCI****).[1] Annual CCI**** include Badminton and Burghley in the United Kingdom and Rolex Kentucky in the USA. The abbreviation CCIO designates an Official (Officiel) CCI to which national federations are invited to send selected representative teams and individuals, such as for the Olympic Summer Games or World Equestrian Games.[1]

One- and most two-day events are usually termed Horse Trials and involve a Dressage Test followed by an abbreviated form of the Cross-Country Test (Phase D only) and the Jumping Test, the latter two tests in no specified order.[1] The FEI recognizes international horse trials with the designation CIC (Concours Internationale de un jour, one- through three-star levels, Tables 50.1 and 50.2).[1] American events and horse trials are sanctioned by the United States

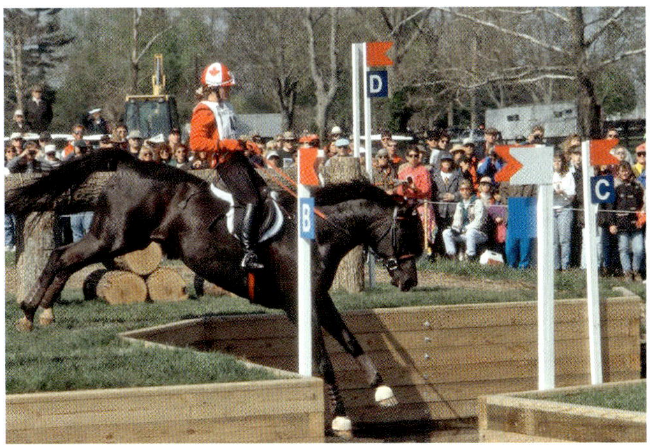

Fig 50.1 A Canadian horse and rider jumping down into a multi-element ditch complex during the Cross-Country Test at the Rolex Kentucky CCI****.

Table 50.1 Speeds, times, distances, number (#) of jumping efforts, and maximum fence heights, spreads, and drop heights required by FEI for sanctioned CCI and CIC Cross-Country Tests[4]

CCI CROSS-COUNTRY	CCI*	CCI**	CCI***	CCI****
Speed (m/min)	520	550	570	570
Time (min)	7–9	8–10	9–11	10–12
Distance (m)	3640–4680	4400–5500	5130–6270	5700–6840
Maximum # jumping efforts	30–32	35–37	38–40	42–45
CIC CROSS-COUNTRY	**CIC***	**CIC****	**CIC*****	**-**
Speed (m/min)	520	550	570	
Time (min)	4.5–6.0	5.0–6.5		5.5–7.0
Distance (m)	2400–3200	2800–3600	3200–4000	
Maximum # jumping efforts	29	32	36	
CCI TEST/CIC TEST	**CCI*/CIC***	**CCI**/CIC****	**CCI***/CIC*****	**CCI****/NO CIC******
Maximum fence height (m) – fixed	1.10	1.15	1.20	1.20
Maximum fence height (m) – brush	1.30	1.35	1.40	1.45
Maximum spread (m) – fence top	1.40	1.60	1.80	2.00
Maximum spread (m) – fence base	2.10	2.40	2.70	3.00
Maximum spread (m) – no height	2.80	3.20	3.60	4.00
Maximum drop height (m)	1.60	1.80	2.00	2.00

Table 50.2 Speeds, times, distances, number (#) of obstacles, number of jumping efforts, and maximum fence heights, spreads, and drop heights required by FEI for sanctioned CCI and CIC Jumping Tests[4]

CCI TEST/CIC TEST	CCI*/CIC*	CCI**/CIC**	CCI***/CIC***	CCI****/no CIC****
Speed (m/min)	350	350	375	375
Time (s)	60–78	69–86	72–88	80–96
Maximum distance (m)	600	600	600	600
Maximum # of obstacles	10–11	10–11	11–12	11–13
Maximum # jumping efforts	13	14	15	16
Maximum fence height (m)	1.15	1.20	1.25	1.25
Maximum fence spread (m) – oxer	1.35	1.40	1.45	1.45
Maximum fence spread (m) – triple bar	1.55	1.60	1.65	1.65

Equestrian Federation (USEF) and are ranked in increasing difficulty as Beginner Novice, Novice, Training, Preliminary (comparable to CCI*), Intermediate (CCI**), and Advanced (CCI***) (Table 50.3).[3] Combined Tests usually include only two of the three disciplines on a single day.[3]

Eventing began as a cavalry competition in northern Europe and made its first appearance as an Olympic sport in Stockholm in 1912. Over the years the sport has evolved through various iterations. In the older (now mainly abandoned) long format or 'classic' event, Cross-Country Day involved four phases.[4] Phase A was a trotting warm-up for Phase B, the Steeplechase, in which the horse galloped over brush fences at much faster paces (Table 50.1). Phase C was designed as a cool-down phase after Steeplechase. Phases A and C were known collectively as Roads and Tracks. After Phase C there was a mandatory veterinary inspection for 10–15 minutes (Phase X) to determine that the horse was sound and fit to continue. Phase

Table 50.3 Speeds, times, distances, and maximum fence heights, spreads, and number (#) of jumping efforts for United States Equestrian Federation events and horse trials[3]

TEST	NOVICE	BEGINNER NOVICE	TRAINING	PRELIMINARY	INTERMEDIATE	ADVANCED
Cross-Country Test						
Optimum speed (m/min)	300–350	350–400	420–470	520	550	570
Speed faults (m/min)	420	450	520	NA	NA	NA
Distance (m)	1400–2000	1600–2200	2000–2600	2200–3300	2600–3800	3200–4400
# jumping efforts	14–18	16–20	20–24	22–30	26–34	32–40
Maximum fence height (m) – fixed	0.79	0.90	1.00	1.10	1.15	1.20
Maximum fence height (m) – brush	0.91	1.10	1.20	1.30	1.35	1.40
Maximum spread (m) – fence top	0.84	1.00	1.20	1.40	1.60	1.80
Maximum spread (m) – fence base	1.22	1.50	1.80	2.10	2.40	2.70
Maximum spread (m) – no height	1.22	2.00	2.40	2.80	3.20	3.60
Maximum drop height (m)	1.01	1.20	1.40	1.60	1.80	2.00
Jumping Test						
Speed (m/min)	300	320	325	350	350	375
Maximum distance (m)	600	600	600	600	600	600
# jumping efforts	9–11	9–11	10–12	11–13	12–14	13–15
Maximum fence height (m)	0.79	0.90	1.00	1.10	1.20	1.25
Maximum fence spread (m) – oxer	1.05	1.15	1.25	1.35	1.45	1.50
Maximum fence spread (m) – triple bar	1.30	1.40	1.50	1.60	1.70	1.75

D was the Cross-Country Test itself over numerous immovable obstacles with heights and spreads increasing with increasing levels of difficulty (Fig. 50.1).[4] Prior to the 1960s, there was also a fifth phase on Cross-Country Day, Phase E, involving another warm-down Roads and Tracks phase after the Cross-Country phase. An additional rest stop (C Halt) became mandatory in long-format CCI*** and CCI**** in 1999. In 2002, the recommended distances for all phases were shortened and the speed required for Phase C was decreased to allow more walking for increased recovery from Phase B (Table 50.1).[4] These changes were made in response to a spate of recent fatal rider injuries and were based in part on the results of thermoregulatory research on Phases B and C performed prior to the 1996 Atlanta Olympic Summer Games.[5–23] That research demonstrated that shortening Phase B,[7–9] inserting two additional rest stops (C Halt) on Phase C,[9] and walking some (not all trotting) on Phase C[9] increased recovery under hot and humid conditions. Because a subcommittee of the International Olympic Committee in 2002 recommended abandoning eventing as an Olympic discipline, the short format was adopted for safety and financial concerns beginning with the Athens Olympics in 2004. The short format has now become the predominant form of 3DE throughout the world.

Equestrian sports governance

The Fédération Equestre Internationale (FEI) is the international governing body for nine equestrian sports, including dressage, show jumping, eventing, driving, vaulting, endurance, reining, para-dressage, and para-driving.[2] Each nation has its own national equestrian federation. Each national federation is a member of the FEI and governs competition at the national or regional level within that nation, whereas the FEI governs international competition. The national equestrian federation of the United States is the United States Equestrian Federation, formerly known for decades as the American Horse Shows Association (AHSA) and more recently known briefly as USA Equestrian. The International Olympic Committee (IOC) oversees Olympic competition. The FEI reports to the IOC for Olympic equestrian sports, including dressage, show jumping and eventing.

Demographics

At the introductory levels of eventing, innumerable different breeds are seen in competition, from ponies to Thoroughbreds and Warmbloods. National or regional influences are seen, particularly in the use of native Warmbloods, owing to their ready availability and popularity as sport horses in any given nation. The United States lags considerably behind in a native Warmblood or sport horse breeding and reward program compared to the European nations.

When the long format was the only format in 3DE, upper-level horses were primarily Thoroughbreds or Thoroughbred crosses. The Thoroughbred influence was necessary to have the inherent fitness and stamina required at the upper levels of long-format eventing. According to the World Breeding Federation for Sport Horses, in 1999–2000 all 10 of the Top 10 Sires of internationally ranked event horses were Thoroughbreds.[24] With less stamina required for the shorter distances in the newer short format, Warmbloods have now come to dominate the upper levels of eventing, particularly as they are better suited to achieve superior dressage scores. In 2011, the first 10 of the Top 100 Sires of event horses were Warmblood stallions, with 5 of the top 10 being Irish Sport Horses.[25] The 2011 FEI Top 10 Stud Book rankings for event horses were Selle Francais, Hanoverian, Irish Sport Horse, Holsteiner, Dutch Warmblood, Swedish Warmblood, Trakehner, British Sport Horse, Pferdezuchtverband Baden-Wuerttemberg, and Pferdezuchtverband Sachsen-Thüringen e.V.[25]

Five of the Top 10 Stud Books in eventing in 2011 were German Warmblood breeds.[25] Why have German breeds become so predominant in eventing compared to the previous dominance of Thoroughbreds? The diminution of the length and stamina required in Cross Country, combined with the German breeds' superior dressage movements, are the likely reasons. Gait and conformation analysis data on three-year-old dressage horses (n = 142) have shown German Warmbloods (Hanoverians [n = 31], Westphalians [n = 16], and Oldenburgers [n = 6]) to be biomechanically superior to both Selle Francais (n = 61) and purebred Spanish horses (n = 28) for use in competitive FEI dressage.[26] The superior stature and conformation of the German horses results in a longer stride length and decreased stride frequency. 'The German horses had gait characteristics more adapted to dressage competition,' the authors concluded.[26]

Three-day event horses may compete in CIC* or CIC** at five years old.[1] They must be at least six years old to compete in CIC***, CCI*, or CCI**.[1] Event horses must be at least seven years old to compete in CCI*** and CCI****.[1] They must be at least eight years old to compete in a Championship ('an official team competition…open to athletes from an unlimited number of nations') CCI****.[1]

Event horses have their most productive years at the upper levels at approximately 8–12 years of age. There are, however, always exceptions to be found, more often in older horses continuing to compete at upper levels than in younger horses competing precociously. Event horses can have difficulty remaining competitively sound later in life due to the rigorous galloping and jumping required. After their peak competitiveness has passed, many older horses ('school masters') are used further to teach younger riders to compete on safer mounts as they aspire to the higher levels of competition. While these older horses are often difficult to maintain completely sound, their experience and demeanor make them invaluable mounts for upcoming young riders. They also present common challenges to practicing veterinarians who are asked to help to maintain their soundness and fitness to compete despite their advancing ages.

Due to the collection, impulsion, bending, circling, and other movements required in dressage, common complaints in event horses include sore backs or hocks. Riders often complain of a horse's unwillingness to bend, perhaps worse in one direction than the other. Jumping and galloping Cross-Country (Fig. 50.1) also contribute to injuries sustained by event horses, as do the rigorous training regimens required to achieve sufficient fitness to compete at the upper levels. Bowed tendons and suspensory desmitis are common supporting leg lamenesses. Traumatic injuries are not uncommon during Cross-Country.

Veterinary services

Veterinarians are involved in eventing in various ways. Many are employed as primary health care providers on a daily basis. Others are secondary or tertiary health care providers, either in an elective or emergent manner. Elective referrals are often for more sophisticated diagnostic imaging techniques such as ultrasonography, scintigraphy, thermography, or magnetic resonance imaging of musculoskeletal injuries. Urgent referrals are sometimes necessary for all types of emergency conditions typical in any equine practice. Eventing competitors have embraced alternative therapies, either in lieu of or in addition to conventional therapeutic measures, in an effort to maintain soundness and maximize performance in these elite equine athletes.

Many practitioners also have contact with these horses only at competitions, as treating veterinarians (the conventional 'horse show veterinarian'), team veterinarians, drug testers, or official veterinarians. Treating and team veterinarians are also health care providers, but in the crucible of competition. Treating veterinarians often have contact with many of the same owners, riders, and horses over the course of a horse show circuit, and develop a valid long-term doctor–client–patient relationship. Team veterinarians function as treating veterinarians but for only one team, thus allowing more focused and intensive care for a more limited number of horses. The most difficult part of the team veterinarian's job is remembering the FEI Code of Conduct for the Welfare of the Horse,[27] which states that 'all those involved in international equestrian sport…acknowledge and accept that at all times the welfare of the horse must be paramount and must never be subordinated to competitive or commercial influences.'[27]

Drug testers and official veterinarians also have as their goal the welfare of the horse, but their responsibility is more regulatory than as health care providers. Drug testers or medication control personnel are responsible for collection of blood and urine samples and for establishing an appropriate chain of custody to establish the validity of any evidence of wrongdoing which they may have collected.[28] Official veterinarians are responsible for the health of all the horses competing at a show or event, and make decisions appropriate for that care under the rules of that competition. The competition's Organizing Committee, with the approval of the FEI and/or the national federation, selects a Veterinary Delegate for any FEI-sanctioned competition.[28] The national federation appoints the Foreign Veterinary Delegate for CCIOs, Regional Games, and Continental Games. The FEI appoints the Veterinary Delegate for FEI Championships and Olympic Games.[28] That Delegate is responsible to head the Veterinary Commission and is also responsible to the Ground Jury for veterinary matters. These responsibilities include: passport control; arrival examinations; control of veterinary practitioners within the stabling compound; recommendations to the Ground Jury about fitness to compete at official jogs or veterinary inspections (Fig. 50.2); and oversight of medication control.[28] Official veterinarians are sometimes at odds with treating or team veterinarians, but all should remember that the officials are ultimately responsible for the health, welfare, and safety of all the horses in the competition. The best relationships are those where the veterinary officials are somewhat flexible, within the rules, before the relationship becomes too adversarial. The treating veterinarians must also remember that the officials have as their primary mandate the welfare of the horse. These officials are often very experienced in their roles, and many have functioned as treating veterinarians in the past.

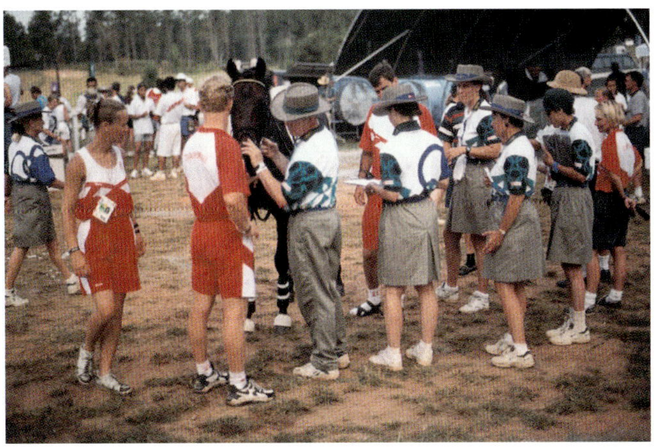

Fig 50.2 Professor Leo Jeffcott, Foreign Veterinary Delegate, taking a facial artery pulse while examining a Danish three-day event horse between Phases C and D at the 1996 Olympic Summer Games in Atlanta, Georgia.

Common diseases and conditions

Event horses may have all the same problems or internal diseases of any other horse. However, some conditions may be more common due to the type of activity in which they compete. As always, poor conformation may play a significant role in many unsoundnesses. For example, post-legged or straight hind leg conformation may predispose an event horse to hock or stifle lameness, as will sickle hocks or the cow-hocked conformation more common in some breeds.

Skeletal

Foot balance is of critical importance in event horses galloping over varying terrain with differing footing conditions, all possibly up, down, or sideways to the slope of the hills. Due to the repetitive stresses caused by jumping, event horses are predisposed to developing navicular disease. This predisposition is worsened by poor foot conformation, with under-run and contracted heels, common in many North American Thoroughbreds who are former racehorses. Sole bruises, pedal osteitis, and other foot conditions may also be seen due to poor foot conformation, the high training mileage required to keep event horses fit to perform, and the varying surfaces encountered in training and in competition. Event horses are somewhat more restricted in the use of corrective shoeing such as wedge shoes or bar shoes because they may be more prone to pulling or twisting them off while galloping and jumping Cross-Country. Event horses are often shod with threaded holes drilled into the heels of their shoes to allow heel caulks or studs of varying length to be changed before or even during the competition, depending upon the looseness and moisture content of the footing on the day of competition.

Due to the high velocities and jumping at speed required in eventing, supporting leg injuries such as bowed tendons or suspensory desmitis are common. These injuries are more common as event horses approach the upper levels where horses and riders must learn to negotiate larger fences at the required velocities. Fetlock synovitis or arthritis is seen secondary to extended dressage movements or galloping Cross-Country at upper levels, especially in former Thoroughbred racehorses converted to use as event horses.

Due to the stresses caused by the excessive hind limb reaching required in dressage ('impulsion'), hock pain and bone spavin are common maladies of event horses. Traumatic stifle injuries are more common in event horses as they progress up the ranks, owing to the greater height, spread, or drop of obstacles at the upper levels (Fig. 50.1, Tables 50.1–50.3).[29,30] These stifle injuries consist in increasing severity of dermal abrasions ('stifle rubs'), deeper soft-tissue or patellar desmitis injuries, or patellar fractures.[29,30]

Muscular

Exertional rhabdomyolysis (ER), myopathy, or tying-up is more common in event horses than in horses performing less strenuous activity. This condition may be related to hereditary Thoroughbred ER[31,32] but more commonly has no apparent hereditary component.[31] Unfitness and overheating seem to play important roles in the development of ER,[33–35] as may excessive dietary carbohydrate intake.[31,33] Diets higher in fat content have proven curative for many horses.[31] Up to 20% of the diet may be fed safely as fat, available in various commercial feed products.[34] One inexpensive and convenient manner of feeding more fat is to increase gradually the daily intake until as much as 2 cups (450–500 ml) of corn oil twice daily is top-dressed onto the horse's regular grain diet.[34]

Exertional rhabdomyolysis should be considered an emergency, whether it occurs during competition or training, and appropriate therapy should be instituted. Treatments should include cessation of exercise, provision of adequate cooling (oral water, water baths, shade, fans), administration of non-steroidal anti-inflammatory drugs (NSAIDs), acepromazine for tranquilization and peripheral vasodilatory effects, and eventually diuresis with fluids (40–60 L IV of isotonic fluid per 500-kg horse over 6–12 hours).

Heavier-bodied horses such as Warmbloods tracing some of their ancestry to draft breeds may be predisposed to development of polysaccharide storage myopathy (PSSM).[31,36] This condition manifests as poor performance, tying-up, muscle weakness, or shaking or shivering. Feeding more fat and less carbohydrate as energy sources is curative in many cases.[36]

Back soreness occurs in event horses, most commonly due to muscle soreness secondary to hindlimb lameness (primarily bone spavin). Back pain may also be secondary to poorly fitting or poorly stuffed saddles in some horses.[37] Less commonly, back pain in horses may be due to primary back disease (Fig. 50.3),[38] composed usually of overriding dorsal spinous processes, and sometimes of painful spinous processes without any actual overriding onto adjacent vertebrae. Thermography (Fig. 50.3A) and scintigraphy (Fig. 50.3B, C) may be important adjunctive diagnostic tools in evaluating back soreness.[39–41] Acupuncture with application of needles or cold laser can serve as both a diagnostic and therapeutic tool in back soreness.[42] Massage therapy may only be palliative but can serve to assist in improving performance if the horse feels better afterward, even if only temporarily. Chiropractic therapy is often used in horses with back soreness,[43] but may serve more to provide massage therapy than actual true chiropractic adjustment. Due to the size differences between patient and veterinarian, and the horse's large muscle masses, huge protected vertebral column, and flighty nature, some scientists argue that true chiropractic adjustment or manipulation of a horse's spine is virtually impossible in a standing athletic horse. Others feel just as strongly that spinal manipulation is possible and beneficial in athletic horses.[43]

Respiratory

Left laryngeal hemiplegia (LLH or 'roaring') is a common problem in event horses because of the need for horses of larger stature. Both Thoroughbred and Warmblood horses are more likely to be larger and thus are more likely to be roarers. Surgery is corrective of the hemiplegia but not necessarily of the audible noise. Ironically, the pre- or postoperative LLH noise is considered a fault in the American hunter show ring, so horses which develop LLH as hunters may actually undergo lifestyle changes and become jumpers or event horses. Other upper airway obstructions such as dorsally displaced soft palate or epiglottic entrapment may occur in horses competing in these sports but should not be considered to be more common than in other horse sports.

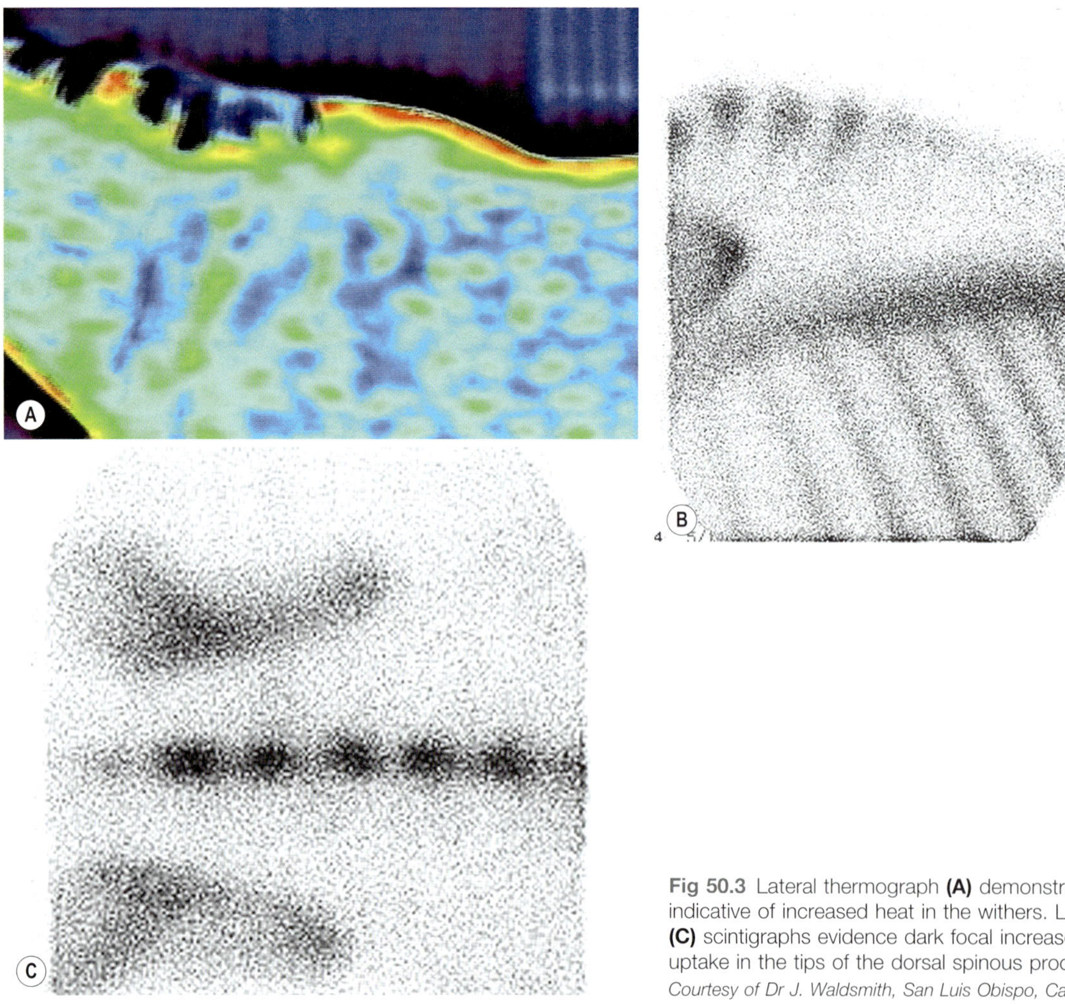

Fig 50.3 Lateral thermograph **(A)** demonstrates red-to-white areas indicative of increased heat in the withers. Lateral **(B)** and dorsal **(C)** scintigraphs evidence dark focal increased radiopharmaceutical uptake in the tips of the dorsal spinous processes of the withers. *Courtesy of Dr J. Waldsmith, San Luis Obispo, California.*

Sinus problems secondary to dental problems may be more common in these horses only because as they get older they may be more predisposed to cheek tooth problems. Guttural pouch disease and strangles are not common occurrences in these horses since these are typically diseases of younger, not older, horses.

Lower respiratory tract problems may be more common in these horses owing primarily to their age and the stress of transport.[44] Three-day events and horse trials are much more common in the mid-Atlantic region of the eastern USA, but the distances between horse shows for event horses are much greater in the midwestern and western USA. Pneumonia and pleuropneumonia in non-juvenile horses is clearly related to transport stress, particularly after transport greater than 500 miles.[45] Transport stress may be less of a factor in developing pleuropneumonia in European horses owing to the greater proximity of numerous competitions.

Exercise-induced pulmonary hemorrhage (EIPH) occurs in event horses during or after the Cross-Country Test (Fig. 50.4). Epistaxis is occasionally evident at the end of Cross-Country (Fig. 50.4) but endoscopy is not used routinely for diagnosis as it is in the racing industry. EIPH is not associated with exercise intolerance as commonly in event horses as it is in racehorses. The industry-wide North American prophylactic treatment with furosemide is not possible in event horses since it is prohibited due to concern over its dilution of urine and possible masking of positive tests for other prohibited substances.

Airway bronchoconstriction occurs sometimes in event horses. This constellation of diseases is known variably as recurrent airway disease (RAD), inflammatory airway disease (IAD), heaves, or chronic obstructive pulmonary disease (COPD) in more chronic cases. Eventing does not necessarily predispose these horses to allergic lung disease, but like many allergies it can be somewhat age-related in its onset and event horses tend to be older when they are at their prime competitive age. Management changes are critical but not curative since the allergy never disappears. Pasture turnout, wetting hay, and minimizing other dust exposure in bedding and diet minimizes allergen exposure and reduces the frequency and severity of exacerbations. Systemic treatment with corticosteroids and/or bronchodilators may be possible during training but is prohibited during competition.[28] Newer inhalation therapies may minimize the chances of a positive drug test but recent research with inhaled albuterol has shown that it is detectable in plasma for several hours after inhalation at therapeutic dosages.[46] Urine ELISA concentrations of inhaled albuterol are not detectable beyond 24 hours after administration, but those investigators recommended an additional 24 hours (48 hours total after the last dose) to avoid a positive urine test after use of the albuterol inhaler.[47] The best scheme should be to manage the disease as best as possible at home and to avoid therapy during competition while still maintaining exposure discipline even while away from home at a horse show or event.

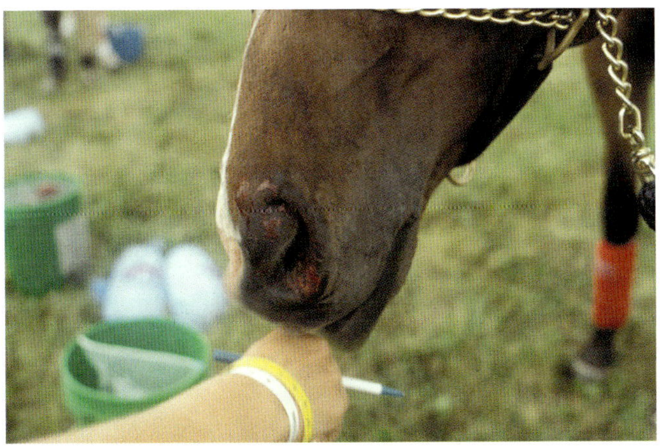

Fig 50.4 Epistaxis secondary to exercise-induced pulmonary hemorrhage in a three-day event horse during the Cross-Country Test at the 1999 North American Young Riders Championships in Wadsworth, Illinois.

Gastrointestinal

Dental problems in event horses may predispose them to misbehavior, head-shaking, or refusal to turn in the dressage ring or refusal of jumps in the Cross-Country Test or in stadium jumping. Sharp labial points may cause pinching of the cheek or even oral ulcers which result in oral soreness and sensitivity. Ill-fitting bits may cause similar problems in the rostral mouth area close to the first cheek teeth. Wolf teeth may interfere with proper bitting. Appropriate and regular dental care should be curative. The most common error is that the teeth feel properly floated on superficial examination of the rostral labial surfaces of the first cheek teeth, but caudal enamel hooks and/or buccal points may be present and may cause misbehavior even when not interfering with the bit. Proper and complete oral examination with a speculum and a light source should make the source of the problem evident.

Gastric ulcers may occur in event horses due to a number of factors. Dietary risk factors include high grain intake and minimal pasture exposure in some management situations.[48] Intense exercise and training stress may be ulcerogenic, as may transport stress. Minimizing stress is important whenever possible, and common anti-ulcer medications (omeprazole, cimetidine, ranitidine) are curative and legal under FEI Veterinary Regulations.[28]

Colic is another stress-related illness in event horses. Predisposing factors may include minimal pasture turnout, transport stress, changes in water and dietary intake at competitions, and stress of competition itself. Cross-Country exercise in particular may cause dehydration, especially at upper levels in conditions of high heat and humidity.[12–14,16,17,34] It has been estimated that as much as 10–15% of the horse's water content may be present in the large colon,[49] and this water reserve is the first source for the horse to mobilize in the face of dehydration. This increased colonic water resorption may result in dehydration of colonic contents and impaction colic. Treatment beyond oral and intravenous fluids and possibly mineral oil may require the horse to be removed from competition.[28]

Diarrhea is another transport, dietary, and competition stress-related illness which occasionally occurs in event horses. It should be considered an emergency, and is cause for withdrawal from competition and isolation from the general population within the home or competition stable.

Cardiovascular

Cardiovascular diseases are not common in event horses but may be important and performance-limiting when they occur. As elite athletes, these horses commonly have normal athletic arrhythmias such as second-degree atrioventricular block, sinus arrhythmia, wandering atrial pacemaker, or split first and/or second heart sounds. Murmurs should be considered pathologic when loud and systolic. Aortic insufficiency with minimal clinical implications may be ausculted in older horses as an acquired diastolic decrescendo murmur.

Atrial fibrillation (AF) occurs occasionally in event horses.[35] It is ausculted as an irregularly irregular arrhythmia and is heard most often after the Cross-Country Test. Typical idiopathic atrial fibrillation occurs as an exercise-induced arrhythmia for no apparent reason. Event horses may be more prone to atypical AF due to fluid and electrolyte loss, especially during conditions of increased heat and humidity (Fig. 50.5A).[35] For example, two horses of 99 starters during the 3DE in the 1996 Olympic Summer Games in Atlanta developed AF during the Cross-Country Test (Fig. 50.5A).[35] In these cases, isotonic fluids (60 L IV over 6–12 hours) were administered after exercise and were curative (Fig. 50.5B). Many horses have successfully completed the Jumping Test after developing transient fluid-responsive AF during or after the Cross-Country Test. Rest should be enforced after the competition is over, but the horse may be predisposed to subsequent episodes of AF, especially under adverse weather conditions resulting in increased fluid and electrolyte loss. Dietary supplementation of electrolytes, proper water intake, and appropriate fitness coming into the event may help to minimize the development of AF in future competitions.

Fatal arrhythmia and ruptured aorta[50] are two of the more common causes of sudden unexplained death in event horses. EIPH is rarely fatal in these horses (Fig. 50.4).

Neurological

Infectious neurological diseases (e.g. equine protozoal myelitis, West Nile virus, neurotropic equine herpesvirus-1) are not more common in event horses than in older horses performing in other sports. However, event horses occasionally sustain severe neurological trauma in jumping accidents during the Cross-Country Test (Figs 50.6 and 50.7). These severe somersaulting falls have become known recently in the sport as 'rotational falls.' They are often due to excessive speed as the horse approaches the fence, resulting in inaccurate jumping (Fig. 50.6A) or failure to jump at all on the approach side of the fence. The excessive speed causes the rider and the horse to have less time to make appropriate adjustments on approaching the fence, sometimes causing the horse to 'breast' the fence (hit it full force in the pectoral region, Fig. 50.6B) or to 'hang' one or both legs or shoulders on the approach side, causing it to flip or rotate over the fence. Other horses may leave 'too long' (Fig. 50.6A), causing the bascule or arc of the jump to fail to center over the jump and instead they begin their descent over or onto the jump itself. While frightening, these latter falls lead less commonly to rotation. In rotational falls, the sudden arrest of the horse's forward momentum (Fig. 50.6B) causes the horse to continue to rotate around itself until it is facing downward on the landing side of the jump (Fig. 50.6C), landing face first and causing its head and neck to sustain considerable potential trauma. Its momentum carries the rest of its hind quarters over its head and neck (Fig. 50.6D), resulting in the somersault or complete rotation so that it lands fully on its back, often on top of the rider.

Rotational falls often lead to skull fractures (Fig. 50.7), particularly of the basisphenoid area, with the rectus capitus muscle pulling downward on the basisphenoid area, resulting in fracture fragments moving with great velocity through the guttural pouch and causing considerable trauma. The fracture fragments can cause lacerations of vital structures within the guttural pouch and severe fatal hemorrhage from the internal carotid artery. Fractures of the cervical vertebrae may occur during rotational falls or especially at drop fences (Fig. 50.1) or water jumps where the horse's trajectory must carry it downward toward the ground. They invariably prove to be fatal to the horse. Riders can sometimes be injured severely in these rotational or drop jump falls.

Eventing organizations are making efforts to reduce the number of these fatal accidents through changes in qualification requirements, course designs and difficulty, and technological advancements in both rider equipment and jump design. 'Minimum eligibility requirements' have been promulgated by FEI to ensure that horse–rider pairs are appropriately qualified to compete at the proposed level.[1] One of the most innovative changes has been the development of breakaway jump technology in which Cross-Country jumps are designed to have some temporary feature which purposefully fails in order to dissipate the force of a horse jumping poorly or inaccurately. Frangible pins are the most common of these innovations (Fig. 50.8). These jump pins support the top rail of vertical Cross-County fences just as the rails in a Stadium Jumping course are supported by movable jump pins. The frangible pin is manufactured from much thicker aluminum metal than that used in traditional jump pins because the top Cross-Country rail is much heavier than in Stadium Jumping. The metal cylinder of the

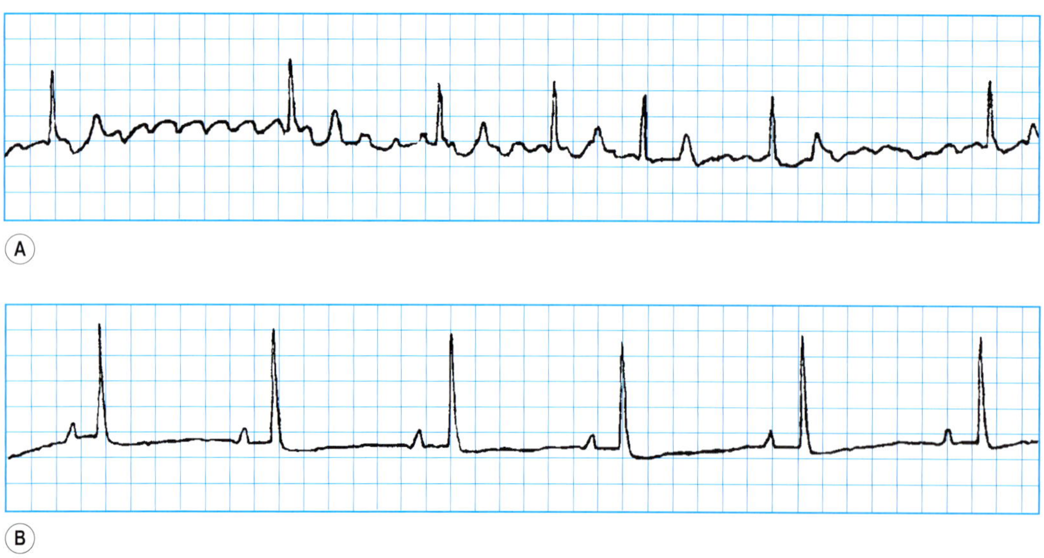

Fig 50.5 Electrocardiograms performed after the Cross-Country Test in a three-day event horse **(A)** documenting atrial fibrillation before treatment and **(B)** normal sinus rhythm after treatment with 60 L of lactated Ringer's solution IV at the 1996 Olympic Summer Games in Atlanta, Georgia.

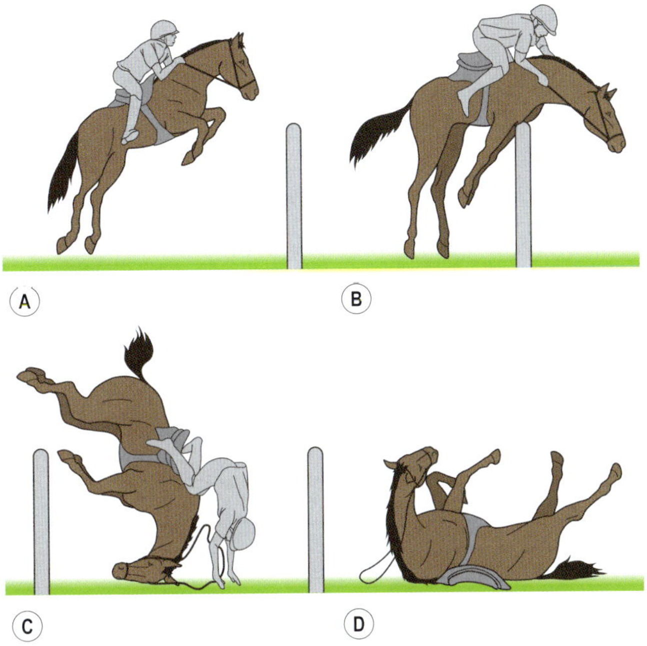

Fig 50.6 Schematic illustration of a horse approaching a Cross-Country jump and suffering a rotational fall. **(A)** The horse is approaching the jump with its carpi flexed and elevated in an appropriate jumping position but it has taken off 'too long,' leaving too much ground to cover in the air if it is to clear the top of the jump. **(B)** The horse's bascule (arc of jump) has descended to cause it to 'hang' its front limbs on the approaching side of the jump, causing a sudden stop to its flight and resulting in the start of a rotational fall. **(C)** The horse is now facedown and vertical on the descending side of the jump, causing its skull to strike the ground and its neck to begin to flex laterally, creating tremendous force and stress on the skull and cervical vertebrae. The rider is also in a precarious posture, facedown toward the ground where the rider often suffers cranial, cervical, or clavicular injury. **(D)** The horse's rotational momentum has continued so that it is now in dorsal recumbency, upside down. Its neck is raised, partially due to that same rotational momentum, and hopefully because at this point the horse may already be attempting to right itself by using its head and neck to leverage itself into a sternal or standing position. The rider in this illustration has luckily rolled free of the horse and did not suffer further injury from the horse landing on the rider.

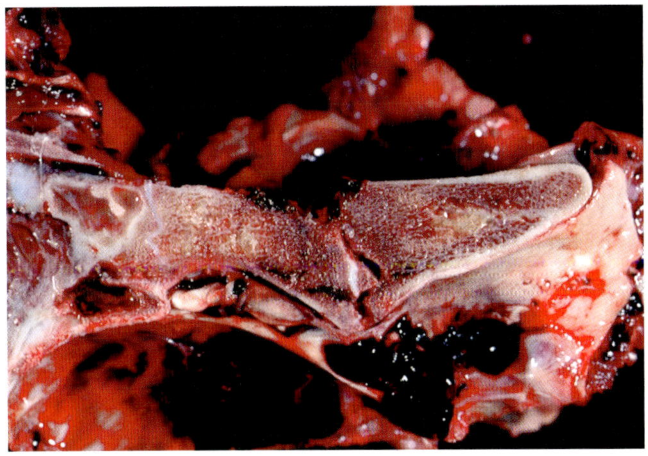

Fig 50.7 Photograph of a sagittally sectioned skull revealing a fracture at the basisphenoid/basioccipital junction. There is normally a suture present at that junction, and the fracture often occurs through this suture even in an aged horse. In this case the fracture has split through the suture but also has split out partially through the ventrum of the skull at the rostral aspect of the basoccipital bone.

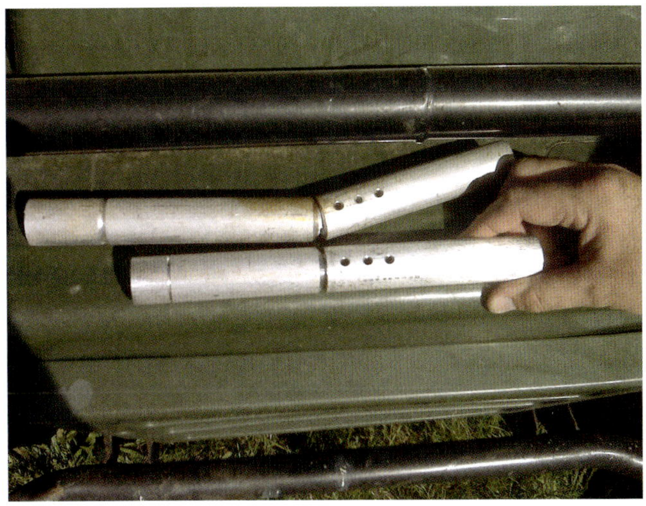

Fig 50.8 Frangible pins from a Cross-Country jump at the Rolex Kentucky CCI**** in Lexington, Kentucky in 2009. The bottom pin is a normal unused frangible pin. Note the thick circumferential score mark intended to create innate metal weakness to encourage and control the point at which the pin may fail when properly stressed. The top pin is partially fractured at the score mark after a horse descended forcefully on the supported rail. The pin was changed while there was a short hold on course so that the rail and the replacement pin would be in normal condition before the next horse approached the jump. *Courtesy of Dr Ryan Heaton, Fallbrook, California.*

frangible pin is scored to create a weakness in the metallic properties of the pin (Fig. 50.8). If the horse jumps poorly enough to exert sufficient downward force on the frangible pin, it fractures at the circumferential scoring mark and causes the pin to fail intentionally (Fig. 50.8), allowing the rail to drop and therefore to absorb and dissipate some of the force of the horse's downward fall. The horse may still fall but with less force; hopefully it will not fall in a rotational manner. The top rail must be tethered to the remainder of the jump with either rope or metal cable in order to keep the rail in close proximity to the base of the jump. This tethering keeps the rail from falling or rolling onto the horse or rider, who may have fallen on the landing side of the jump. Breaking a frangible pin or other breakable obstacle on Cross-Country also incurs additional penalty points to be added to the horse's total score.

Endocrine

Estrus behavior is the most common endocrine problem encountered in event horses. Cycling mares may act inappropriately during the dressage test when it is expected that they should be quiet and obedient. Altrenogest (Regu-Mate®) is prohibited under FEI rules without prior approval using FEI Equine Therapeutic Use Exemption (ETUE) Form 2.[28] Even though some riders or trainers believe it has a calming effect even in male horses, its use is prohibited in male horses, both in geldings or stallions. Judicious scheduling of competitions around heat cycles or neutering are other alternatives to hormonal control of estrous cycles.

Dermatological

Ringworm typically occurs in horses younger than those actively competing as event horses. Saddle-induced skin injuries are also rare as these riders usually take extra precaution to ensure that their saddles fit properly. Lacerations sustained during Cross-Country are common in event horses and pose particular problems since local anesthetics and sedatives are prohibited substances under all rules.[28] Permission may be obtained from the Veterinary Delegate and the Ground Jury for judicious use of small amounts of local anesthetic without sedation. Abrasions, or 'road rash' injuries, are also common from horses falling, slipping on wet grass or pavement, or rubbing their knees, hocks, or stifles over Cross-Country jumps. While the skin is raw and abraded, the concern in an unsound horse should be the probable underlying soft-tissue injury such as patellar ligament pain after a stifle rub. These skin and underlying injuries are of genuine concern to the riders since they may be sufficiently painful to cause a horse to be eliminated at the Horse Inspection on the morning after the Cross-Country Test and before the Jumping Test. They require considerable icing and other physical therapies. The use of alternative therapies no longer requires prior approval or documentation during FEI competition. However, shock wave therapy and cryotherapy are prohibited during competition or within 5 days prior to the first Horse Inspection of an FEI competition.[28]

Ocular

Ocular injuries are not common in these horses, and anterior uveitis is no more common than in other horses. Ocular disease should be investigated, however, as a possible problem whenever a horse suddenly becomes recalcitrant, unwilling to move forward or to jump as freely as usual.

Behavioral

Behavioral problems are sometimes the most difficult diagnoses, since the rider and trainer do not want to believe that something physical is not causing the horse's failure to perform. Perhaps a horse and rider are simply not suited to one another. If either member of the pair is too inexperienced ('too green'), they may not be able to compete effectively despite being completely healthy physically. Some riders, in their nervousness, make certain horses more nervous and skittish than other riders. Horses often 'go better' for the trainer than for the owner/rider, and that rider simply has a difficult time dealing with the fact that he/she does not ride as well as is necessary to get the best performance out of that horse. Tack and bit problems are relatively uncommon but may be the source for some misbehaviors, as may poor dentition. The recycled Thoroughbred racehorse is another problem, in that it often comes with poor foot conformation, other injuries such as bowed tendons, and racing-related inappropriate behavior for the show ring such as a frustrating willingness to be overly nervous and unwilling to quiet down at the appropriate time. Some veterinary practitioners feel that acupuncture may have a calming effect in nervous horses prior to competition (A. Young, personal communication, 2002).

Metabolic/heat-related

Anhydrosis is a rare problem but is sometimes seen in horses traveling to warmer climates from more temperate climates (e.g. from Chicago to Florida for the winter show circuit). Horses with anhydrosis fail to sweat effectively, although they may sweat in intermittent spotty patches but not diffusely as needed for proper thermoregulation. Diagnosis is by subcutaneous injection of epinephrine followed by a failure to sweat in the injected area. Therapy is primarily by heat management (ride in cooler climates and cooler times of the day, fans on the stall, frequent baths). One commercial product (OneAC®) has been touted as curative for many horses but controlled trials are not available.

Dehydration, fatigue, and heat-related illnesses are common in event horses, especially when competing in conditions of higher ambient heat and humidity.[5,7–9,10–17,19,34,35] The most difficult decision for the practitioner examining a hot sweaty horse is distinguishing between simple fatigue, exhaustion and/or possible heat stress, and heat stroke (Fig. 50.9).[35] Fatigued horses recover in 10–30 minutes with simple bathing and voluntary water ingestion. Exhausted horses, and those with possible heat stress as part of their exhaustion, do not recover as rapidly but are still willing to drink, move around gradually, and seem moderately alert eventually.[35] Horses with heat stroke are in shock and are profoundly depressed, unwilling to eat, drink, or walk, and do not recover without intensive care in the form of large volumes of intravenous fluids and repetitive external cooling.[35]

Cooling procedures for hot event horses have been the focus of considerable research over the last 20 years.[15,19,23,35] A number of different studies have shown that horses may be cooled actively with large volumes of ice-cold water placed repeatedly directly onto their backs and heavily exercised muscles (Fig. 50.10) without any complications such as overt tying-up or subclinical myopathy (manifested as increased plasma creatine kinase activity).[19,23,35] Use of this active cooling technique under conditions of adverse heat and humidity has been shown to accelerate the recovery of event horses.[19,23] Shade and fans may also be used to improve heat loss, minimize radiant heat gain, and speed recovery.[6,35] Use of a cooling blanket with special wicking material designed to improve cooling did not aid in cooling and was no better than ambient temperature-water bathing when compared to a positive control ice bath after treadmill-simulated eventing exercise.[51]

Horses will drink immediately after endurance exercise such as Steeplechase or Cross-Country, but only during approximately the first five minutes of recovery, so water or electrolyte water should be offered immediately.[52] If the horse fails to ingest water (i.e. it was not offered, or the horse was too exhausted to drink), water or electrolyte solutions may be administered orally via nasogastric tube (4–8 L of roughly isotonic fluid after exercise) with few complications once the horse has returned to its stall. Administration of intravenous fluids is indicated in horses with overt heat stroke, myopathy, and even simple fatigue and dehydration under severe climatic conditions (Fig. 50.9). Recommended volumes of isotonic fluid range from 10–30 L for simple fatigue and dehydration to 50–80 L over several hours' time for horses with more serious clinical problems.[35]

Prevention of heat-related illnesses is the purview of the treating veterinarian and should be undertaken aggressively to avoid problems during or after the competition. Horses' water intake should be monitored always, but especially after transport and when away from home. Body weight may be the best measure of monitoring hydration status if owners, riders, and grooms have access to a scale and are encouraged to use it.[7,17,53,54] Fluid-loading prior to competition has become more commonplace, especially prior to the Cross-Country Test.[15,35] Approximately 2–4 hours prior to competition, the horse may receive safely 4–8 L of oral electrolyte mixture in water (roughly isotonic) via nasogastric tube.[11,20–22] The only real risk from this procedure is iatrogenic epistaxis. For this reason, some riders or team veterinarians prefer to administer isotonic fluids (5–10 L) intravenously prior to exercise. Each rider must

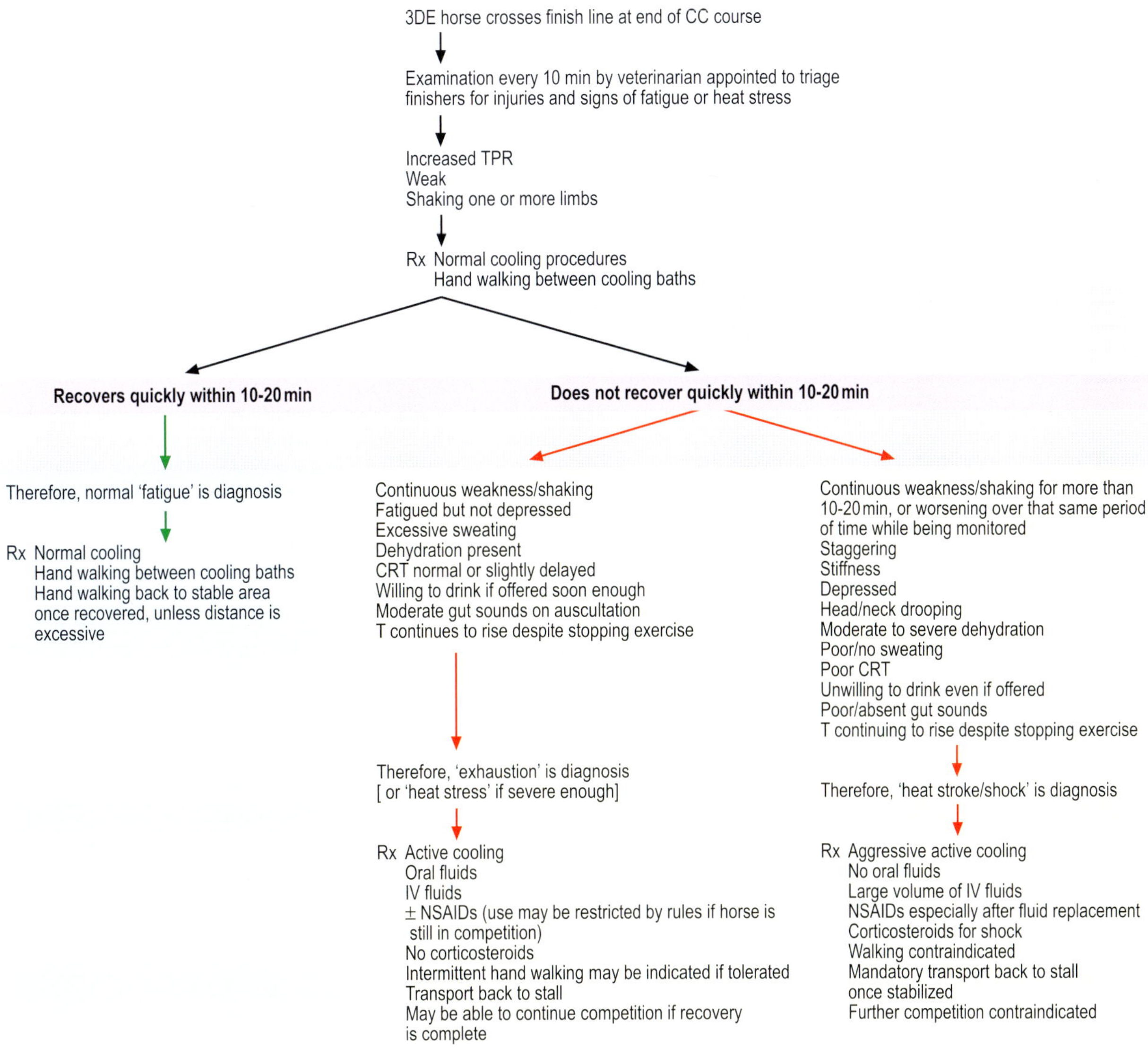

Fig 50.9 Decision-tree for distinguishing between simple fatigue, exhaustion and heat stress, and true heat stroke (3DE = 3-day event; CC = Cross-Country; TPR = temperature, pulse, respiratory rate; Rx = treatment; CRT = capillary refill time; NSAIDs = non-steroidal anti-inflammatory drugs).

also learn to be constantly aware of his/her horse's performance, strength, gait pattern, forwardness, and breathing patterns to be sensitive to the possibility that the horse is not feeling well, is 'not itself,' and may have some physical reason for performing poorly.[35] After exercise, proper active cooling techniques may assist in recovery and may help to prevent further possible heat-related illness (Figs 50.9 and 50.10).[6,15,19,23,35]

Medications during competition

The different governing bodies of equestrian sport retain the right to set their own drug rules and penalties for violations. Since 1992 FEI has maintained a zero tolerance policy toward nearly all drugs, including NSAIDs, in horses in competition. The inherent philosophy is that there should be a level playing field for all horse and rider pairs, and that to allow any performance-altering drugs to be present on the day of competition might allow one competitor to have an unfair advantage over his/her counterparts by having better medication, not necessarily a better horse. There are a few substances for which FEI has set maximum allowable limits, since they can be present in horses to a slight extent due to natural exposure through feedstuffs or other environmental contamination.[28] Those substances for which maximum thresholds have been established under FEI rules include: total carbon dioxide (36 mEq/L plasma), dimethyl sulfoxide (DMSO: 15 µg/ml in urine or 1 µg/ml in plasma), hydrocortisone (1 µg/ml in urine), salicylic acid (750 µg/ml in urine or 6.5 µg/ml in plasma), and the hormones boldenone, estranediol, and testosterone.[28] FEI rules allow the use during competition of most antibiotics, anthelminthics, vitamins, fluids and electrolytes, ranitidine, cimetidine, and omeprazole.[28]

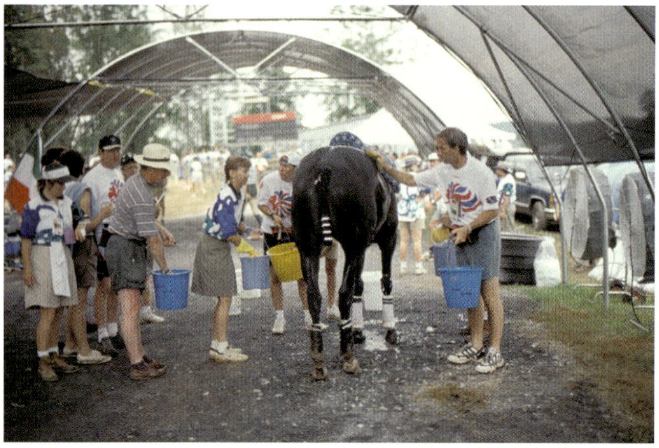

Fig 50.10 Active cooling performed on a British three-day event horse at the 1996 Olympic Summer Games in Atlanta, Georgia. The team veterinarian is observing the bathing of the horse and standing by to administer additional advice or treatment if necessary.

Prior to competition, a horse may require treatment for any of dozens of different medical or surgical problems. Regarding these varied situations, the FEI Veterinary Regulations state:

> *If a Horse must be treated with a Prohibited Substance prior to arrival at the Event (e.g. during transport), the Veterinary Commission/Delegate must be consulted by the Person Responsible as soon as possible upon arrival at the venue. On such occasions, a signed statement describing the reason for treatment, the active substance given, dose and the exact time of administration must be provided by the person who administered the treatment. This should be on ETUE 1…The Veterinary Commission/Delegate will carefully consider the lag time between the treatment and competition and any possible unfair advantage that the Horse may have as a result of the treatment. If satisfied that the Horse will not have an unfair advantage as a result of the treatment and that the Horse is fit to compete, the Veterinary Commission/Delegate is entitled to complete ETUE 1 retrospectively. Countersigning by the President of the Ground Jury is required.*[28]

Once the competition has begun,

> *When treatment with a Prohibited Substance is required, the Treating Veterinarian must consult with the Veterinary Commission/Delegate, prior to treatment, on the condition of the Horse, its fitness to compete and the preferred treatment. The Veterinary Commission/Delegate will examine the Horse and consider whether it is still fit to compete and whether it may have a possible unfair advantage as a result of the treatment. This must be carried out on a case-by-case basis. The welfare of the Horse must have absolute priority. If in agreement, ETUE 1 (VR Annex V) must be completed and countersigned by the President of the Ground Jury.*[28]

Three examples of entirely different clinical circumstances follow to illustrate common but complex interpretations of FEI medication rules. (1) A horse sustains an eye injury or corneal ulcer which requires local medication but which may not require any medication which might unlevel the playing field. To allow this horse to continue in competition, systemic flunixin meglumine should be avoided in this horse but might be used in a similar injury out of competition. (2) A horse sustains a small laceration which will not prohibit further competition but which requires suturing. Judicious use of a local anesthetic might be approved by the Veterinary Commission but sedation might not be approved prior to suturing. The local anesthetic will be in a small amount and should have no lasting consequence on the future of the competition. However, tranquilization might affect the competition since it might make an event horse performing a dressage test quieter, obviously depending upon the dose and drug used and its timing before the test. The legitimate use of the sedative or the local anesthetic to suture the laceration might also make it more difficult to detect a second dose given illicitly the following day. Finally, (3) a horse develops colic signs severe enough to require systemic use of an NSAID. This horse should be treated and removed from competition since it (a) has a medical problem severe enough to preclude it from further competition for medical reasons alone, and (b) has received one or more doses of an NSAID which might affect the outcome of the competition since the NSAID will also have musculoskeletal effects which might benefit the horse and create an unlevel playing field.

FEI Medication Control Programme statistics for 2011 documented that 8 of 13 banned substance violations were for anabolic or progesterone steroids.[55] The remainder were for morphine (2), paracetamol/acetaminophen (1), and the sedative/tranquilizers reserpine (1) and azaperone (1).[55] Overages of controlled medications (n = 39) included NSAIDs (22 total: phenylbutazone 10, oxyphenbutazone 6, salicylic acid 3, flunixin 2, dicolfenac 1); corticosteroids (dexamethasone 6, triamcinolone acetonide 2); acepromazine (3); local anesthetics (mepivacaine 2, procaine 1); bronchodilators (clenbuterol 1, theobromine 1); and ketamine (1).[55]

USEF rules are just as restrictive as those of the FEI for most forbidden substances such as stimulants or narcotics.[3] However, USEF rules are more liberal than FEI with respect to NSAIDs.[3] The philosophy simply put is that therapeutic medications allow some horses to continue to compete at an effective level over the course of a season or over the course of a long horse show. The rule specifically states, 'The full use of modern therapeutic measures for the improvement and protection of the health of the horse and/or pony is permitted…'[3] USEF rules prohibit the use of most drugs within 24 hours of competition. In a rule change which became effective 1 December 2011, only one of 7 approved NSAIDs may be detected legally in horses in USEF competition at any one time. Additionally, the single NSAID detected must be below a maximum permissible limit established by USEF. Those maximum allowable limits are set for plasma concentrations of phenylbutazone (15 μg/ml), flunixin (1 μg/ml), ketoprofen (0.25 μg/ml), meclofenamic acid (2.5 μg/ml), naproxen (40 μg/ml), diclofenac (0.005 μg/ml), and firocoxib (0.24 μg/ml).[3] Short- and long-acting tranquilizers and NSAIDs above the allowable limits are the most commonly detected foreign substances under USEF medication testing (S. Schumacher, personal communication, 2012).

Finally, there are innumerable unsanctioned or unrecognized horse shows which may not be subject to any drug testing by a governing body unless local law allows for testing. California law, for instance, allows state veterinarians from the California Drug and Food Administration to drug test any horse show in California, sanctioned or otherwise. Most European Union countries now have commonly restricted use of phenylbutazone in horses in general, although veterinarians in the United Kingdom have fought what they see as a restriction on their ability to practice freely to promote optimal health and pain relief in their equine patients.

Depending upon the governing body, the rider may also be subject to drug testing during a competition. Any competitor identified by the national federation as an international-level competitor is also subject to random, unannounced, out-of-competition drug testing by the national federation at any time.

References

1. Anonymous. FEI Rules for Eventing. Fédération Equestre Internationale, Lausanne, Switzerland, 2009 amended for 2012. www.horsesport.org, Accessed 24 January 2012.
2. Anonymous. FEI General Regulations, 23rd edition. 1 January 2009 amended for 2012. Fédération Equestre Internationale, Lausanne, Switzerland. www.horsesport.org, Accessed 24 January 2012.
3. Anonymous. United States Equestrian Federation 2012 Rulebook. United States Equestrian Federation, Lexington, Kentucky. http://www.usef.org, Accessed 24 January 2012.
4. Anonymous. FEI Rules for Eventing.Lausanne, Switzerland: Fédération Equestre Internationale; 2003. www.horsesport.org, 3 October 2002.
5. Andrews FM, Ralston SL, Williamson LH, et al. Weight loss, water loss and cation balance during the endurance test of a 3-day-event. Equine Vet J 1995;(Suppl 18):294–7.
6. Bradbury G, Allen AK. Equi-mist fan/mist system evaluation. In: Clarke AF, Jeffcott LB, editors. On to Atlanta '96. Guelph, Ontario, Canada: Equine Research Centre, University of Guelph; 1995. p. 75–8.
7. Foreman JH, Grubb TL, Benson GJ, et al. Physiological effects of shortening steeplechase in a 3-day-event. Equine Vet J 1995;(Suppl 20):73–7.
8. Foreman JH, Grubb TL, Benson GJ, et al. Acid-base and electrolyte effects of shortening steeplechase in a 3-day-event. Equine Vet J 1996;(Suppl 22):85–90.
9. Foreman JH. Modifications to the 1996 Olympic 3-Day-Events to optimise safety under hot and humid conditions. Pferdeheilkunde 1996;12:397–400.
10. Geor RJ, McCutcheon LJ, Ecker GL, et al. Thermal and cardiorespiratory responses of horses to submaximal exercise under hot and humid conditions. Equine Vet J 1995;(Suppl 20):125–32.
11. Geor RJ, McCutcheon LJ. Hydration effects on physiological strain of horses during exercise-heat stress. J Appl Physiol 1998;84:2042–51.
12. Harris PA, Marlin DJ, Mills PC, et al. Clinical observations made in nonheat acclimated horses performing treadmill exercise in cool (20°C/40% RH), hot, dry (30°C/40% RH) or hot, humid (30°C/80% RH) conditions. Equine Vet J 1995;(Suppl 20):78–84.
13. Harris PA, Marlin DJ, Scott CM, et al. Electrolyte and total protein changes in nonheat acclimated horses performing treadmill exercise in cool (20°C/40% RH), hot, dry (30°C/40% RH) or hot, humid (30°C/80% RH) conditions. Equine Vet J 1995;(Suppl 20):85–96.
14. Hinchcliff KW, Kohn CW, Geor R, et al. Acid:base and serum biochemistry changes in horses competing at a modified 1 Star 3-day-event. Equine Vet J 1995;(Suppl 20):105–10.
15. Jeffcott LB, Kohn CW. Contributions of equine exercise physiology research to the success of the 1996 Equestrian Olympic Games: A review. Equine Vet J 1999;(Suppl 30):347–55.
16. Kohn CW, Hinchcliff KW. Physiological responses to the endurance test of a 3-day-event during hot and cool weather. Equine Vet J 1995;(Suppl 20): 31–6.
17. Kohn CW, Hinchcliff KW, McCutcheon LJ, et al. Physiological responses of horses competing at a modified 1 Star 3-day-event. Equine Vet J 1995;(Suppl 20):97–104.
18. Kohn CW, Hinchcliff KW, McKeever KH. Effect of ambient temperature and humidity on pulmonary artery temperature of exercising horses. Equine Vet J 1999;(Suppl 30):404–11.
19. Kohn CW, Hinchcliff KW, McKeever K. Evaluation of washing with cold water to facilitate heat dissipation in horses exercised in hot, humid conditions. Am J Vet Res 1999;60:299–305.
20. Sosa Leon LA, Davie AJ, Hodgson DR, et al. Effects of oral fluid on cardiorespiratory and metabolic responses to prolonged exercise. Equine Vet J 1995;(Suppl 18):274–8.
21. Sosa Leon LA, Davie AJ, Hodgson DR, et al. The effects of tonicity, glucose concentration and temperature of an oral rehydration fluid solution on its absorption and elimination. Equine Vet J 1995;(Suppl 20):140–6.
22. Sosa Leon LA, Hodgson DR, Evans DL, et al. Effects of hyperhydration on cardiorespiratory and metabolic responses to exercise in horses during a simulated 2nd day of the 3-day-event. Pferdeheilkunde 1996;12:459–62.
23. Williamson L, White S, Maykuth P, et al. Comparison between post exercise cooling methods. Equine Vet J 1995;(Suppl 18):337–40.
24. Anonymous. World Breeding Federation for Sport Horses. www.wbfsh.org, 12 October 2002.
25. Anonymous. World Breeding Federation for Sport Horses. www.wbfsh.org, 23 January 2012.
26. Barrey E, Desliens F, Poirel D, et al. Early evaluation of dressage ability in different breeds. Equine Vet J 2002;(Suppl 34): 319–24.
27. Anonymous. FEI Code of Conduct for the Welfare of the Horse. Lausanne, Switzerland: Fédération Equestre Internationale; 2012. www.horsesport.org, 23 January 2012.
28. Anonymous. FEI Veterinary Regulations. Lausanne, Switzerland: Fédération Equestre Internationale; 2012.
29. Dyson S, Wright I, Kold S, et al. Clinical and radiographic features, treatment and outcome in 15 horses with fracture of the medial aspect of the patella. Equine Vet J 1992;24:264–8.
30. Dyson S. Stifle trauma in the event horse. Equine Vet Educ 1994;6:234–40.
31. Valberg SJ. Muscular causes of exercise intolerance in horses. Vet Clin North Am Equine Pract 1996;12:495–515.
32. MacLeay JM, Valberg SJ, Geyer CJ, et al. Heritability of recurrent exertional rhabdomyolysis in Thoroughbred racehorses. Am J Vet Res 1999;60:250–6.
33. MacLeay JM, Valberg SJ, Pagan JD, et al. Effect of diet on Thoroughbred horses with recurrent exertional rhabdomyolysis performing a standardized exercise test. Equine Vet J 1999;(Suppl 30):458–62.
34. Foreman JH. Metabolic causes of equine exercise intolerance. Vet Clinics North Am Equine Pract 1996;12:537–54.
35. Foreman JH. The exhausted horse syndrome. Vet Clin North Am Equine Pract 1998;14:205–19.
36. Valentine BA, Van Saun RJ, Thompson KN, et al. Role of dietary carbohydrate and fat in horses with equine polysaccharide storage myopathy. J Am Vet Med Assoc 2001;219:1537–44.
37. Harmon J. Tack and saddle fit. Vet Clin North Am Equine Pract 1999;15: 247–61.
38. Haussler KK. Osseous spinal pathology. Vet Clin North Am Equine Pract 1999;15:103–12.
39. von Schweinitz DG. Thermographic diagnostics in equine back pain. Vet Clin North Am Equine Pract 1999;15:161–77.
40. Weaver MP, Jeffcott LB, Nowak M. Radiography and scintigraphy. Vet Clin North Am Equine Pract 1999;15:113–29.
41. Zimmerman M, Dyson S, Murray R. Close, impinging and overriding spinous processes in the thoracolumbar spine: The relationship between radiological and scintigraphic findings and clinical signs. Equine Vet J 2012;44:178–84.
42. Klide AM, Martin BB Jr. Methods of stimulating acupuncture points for treatment of chronic back pain in horses. J Am Vet Med Assoc 1989;195:1375–9.
43. Haussler KK. Chiropractic evaluation and management. Vet Clin North Am Equine Pract 1999;15:195–209.
44. Kohn CW. Guidelines for horse transport by road and air. New York: American Horse Shows Association; 1999.
45. Austin SM, Foreman JH, Hungerford LL. Case-control study of risk factors for development of pleuropneumonia in horses. J Am Vet Med Assoc 1995;207: 325–8.
46. Kollias-Baker C, Stanley D. Detection of albuterol administered to performance horses with Torpex® (aerosol albuterol

sulfate) device. In: Torpex® (aerosol albuterol sulfate) technical research review. St. Joseph, Missouri: Boehringer Ingelheim Vetmedica, Inc.; 2002. p. 11–13.

47. Dirikolu L, Mollett BA, Troppmann A, et al. Apparent ELISA detection times for albuterol after administration with the Torpex® equine inhaler device. Vet Therapeutics 2002;3:297–307.
48. Murray MJ, Eichorn ES. Effects of intermittent feed deprivation, intermittent feed deprivation with ranitidine administration, and stall confinement with ad libitum access to hay on gastric ulceration in horses. Am J Vet Res 1996;57:1599–603.
49. Carlson GP. Hematology and body fluids. In: Gillespie JR, Robinson NE, editors. Equine Exercise Physiology 2. Davis, California: ICEEP Publications; 1987. p. 393–425.
50. Briggs K. Tragedy at 1998 Rolex Kentucky CCI***. The Horse; 1998, p. 59.
51. Foreman JH, Benson GJ, Foreman MH. Effects of a pre-moistened multilayered breathable fabric in promoting heat loss during recovery after exercise under hot conditions. Equine Vet J 2006;(Suppl 36):303–6.
52. Butudom P, Schott HC, Davis MW, et al. Drinking salt water enhances rehydration in horses dehydrated by frusemide administration and endurance exercise. Equine Vet J 2002;(Suppl 34):513–18.
53. Lawrence L, Jackson S, Kline K, et al. Observations on body weight and condition of horses in a 150-mile endurance ride. J Equine Vet Sci 1992;12:320–4.
54. Schott HC II, McGlade KS, Molander HA, et al. Body weight, fluid, electrolyte, and hormonal changes in horses competing in 50- and 100-mile endurance rides. Am J Vet Res 1997;58:303–9.
55. Anonymous. Prohibited substances detected in horses in 2011. Lausanne, Switzerland: FEI Veterinary Delegate Release, Fédération Equestre Internationale; 10 February 2012.

Veterinary aspects of training dressage horses

51

Emmanuelle van Erck-Westergren   Jonathan H. Foreman

CHAPTER CONTENTS

Definitions and background

The discipline of dressage consists of the execution of different movements and transitions which are considered to be the constituents of basic equitation for all equestrian disciplines. 'Dressage is considered the art of equestrian sport ... It is the highest expression of horse training.'[1] With adequate training, a horse will gain improved gymnastic skills enabling it to perform more sophisticated figures (Fig. 51.1).

Dressage is a test of obedience, balance and suppleness. 'The object of dressage is the harmonious development of the physique and ability of the horse. As a result it makes the horse calm, supple, loose and flexible but also confident, attentive and keen, thus achieving perfect understanding with his rider.'[1] The goal is that the horse 'gives the impression of doing of his own accord what is required of him. Confident and attentive, he submits generously to the control of his rider, remaining absolutely straight in any movement on a straight line and bending accordingly when moving on curved lines.'[1]

Dressage competitions are executed in a 60 m × 20 m rectangular arena, delimited by a low rail along which 12 lettered markers are placed symmetrically indicating where movements are to start or finish and where changes of pace or lead are to occur.[1] During a dressage competition, the ability of horse and rider to perform imposed figures and transitions is judged (Fig. 51.2). In all competitions, the horse must enter the ring and then stand square at a halt (and the rider must salute). Basic dressage gaits are walk, trot, and canter. The international standard requires that:

> *His walk is regular, free and unconstrained. His trot is free, supple, regular, sustained and active. His canter is united, light and cadenced. His quarters are never inactive or sluggish. He responds to the slightest indication of the rider and thereby gives life and spirit to all the rest of his body.*[1]

The basic gaits progress to more difficult movements at the upper levels such as extended trot or canter, counter canter, passage, pirouette, and piaffe. Except in a freestyle class, each horse and rider pair performs the same test in any given class or competition. In freestyle, the horse/rider pair performs a personalized sequence into which mandatory figures are integrated. In addition to technical skills, artistic qualities are also scored in freestyle dressage.

The judging of dressage competitions is based on overall harmony, level of difficulty, and specific technical criteria. One to five judges score each movement of the test and a composite score is calculated to determine the order of the final places. Dressage is scored by a subjective judging process. Collective marks are designed to summarize the performance of horse and rider and must reflect the qualities of the entire performance. They are derived from the observation of the judges of the separate test movements. The four collective marks include:

1. paces
2. impulsion
3. submission
4. the rider's influence: position, seat, and the correctness and effect of the rider's aids.

Significant variability in judging has been demonstrated, even at the Olympic level, suggesting that judges encounter difficulties in objective scoring and scores do not always align with overall performance.[2]

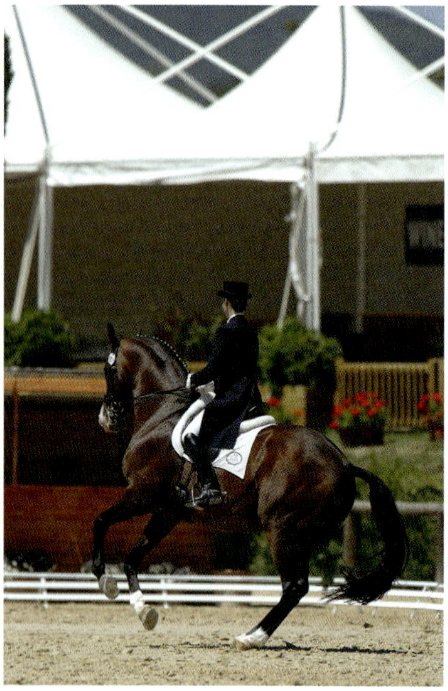

Fig 51.1 Dressage horse performing a canter pirouette. The pirouette is a turn of 360 degrees on the haunches around the inside hind leg. It is executed on two tracks with the inside hind leg describing a circle as small as possible. The horse is slightly bent in the direction of the turn and the poll remains the highest point during the entire movement.

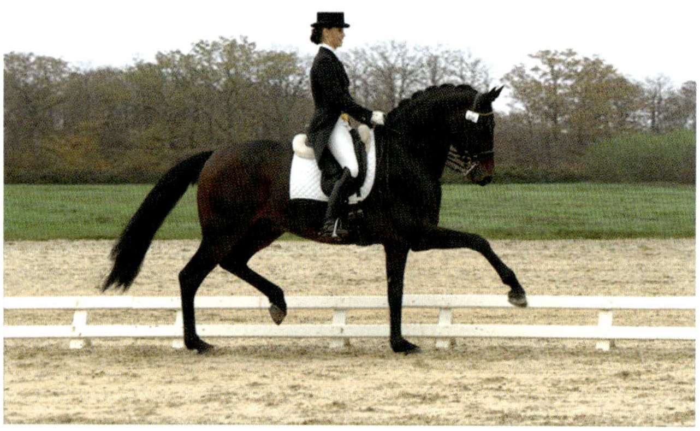

Fig 51.2. Dressage horse demonstrating a supple, sustained and balanced trot. Note the degree of fetlock extension. Hyperextension predisposes dressage horses to suspensory injuries.

Movements are judged on 'freedom and regularity of the paces; the harmony, lightness and ease of movements; the lightness of the forehand and the engagement of the hind quarters, originating in a lively impulsion; the acceptance of the bridle, with submissiveness throughout and without any tenseness or resistance.'[1] Rhythm, energy, balance, forward movement, and elasticity of the horse are qualities that are highly sought. Figures should be executed in an easy and fluent way, without abruptness or obvious tension between the horse and rider. The emphasis, at all times, is that the horse should be perceived as willing to perform the exercises and make difficult exercises appear easy. In the FEI guidelines, it is also stated that the aim should always be to demonstrate 'the harmony and willingness to perform, not force horses to show tricks.'[1]

Internationally the sport is known as the Concours de Dressage International (CDI).[1,3] International dressage competitions are ranked by the Fédération Equestre Internationale (FEI) as increasing in difficulty from one (CDI*) through three-star (CDI***). The abbreviation CDIO designates an Official (Officiel) CDI to which national federations are invited to send selected representative teams and individuals, such as for the Olympic Summer Games or World Equestrian Games.[3] Levels of increasing difficulty of FEI dressage competition include Prix St. Georges, Intermediate I, Intermediate II, Grand Prix, and Grand Prix Special.[1] Freestyle is also an FEI-sanctioned competition held at either the Intermediate or Grand Prix level. Competitions sanctioned by the United States Equestrian Federation (USEF) are progressively ranked as Training, First Level, Second Level, Third Level, Fourth Level, and Fifth Level (equivalent to international competition).[4] The standard for FEI championships and the Olympic Games consists of Grand Prix, Grand Prix Special, and Grand Prix Freestyle (Kur) tests.

In a rapidly growing sport, the FEI has taken an initiative to preserve unity in the basic principles, technical language, and guidelines for training and competing in dressage by publishing an *FEI Dressage Handbook*. This Handbook compiles guidelines related to judging, riding, and training. It also indicates the rules applied to competition, including authorized tack and riding practices.

A brief history of dressage

Horses have been used as mounts for the military since early history. The earliest work on training military horses for obedience and maneuverability was written by Xenophon, a Greek military commander. Through history, as the art of warfare evolved, lighter horses such as Arabians were bred to the heavy draught warhorses to improve their stamina and versatility. With these evolutions, dressage techniques became more sophisticated. During the Renaissance, European aristocrats participated in equestrian pageants to demonstrate the military skills of their mounts. Several prominent riding schools were later founded to perpetuate the art of dressage training (e.g. the Imperial Spanish Riding School of Vienna, and the French Cadre Noir). In 1912, dressage was introduced as an Olympic sport. At the time, only commissioned military officers were eligible to compete. The competition included tests of obedience and maneuverability that would later become known as dressage. In 1956, when many military cavalries were dismantled, the discipline was opened to civilians. Although women were not allowed to compete before 1964, over 80% of equestrian competitors today are female, with a substantial number competing into advanced age.[5]

Demographics

At the introductory levels of dressage, many breeds are seen in competition, from ponies to Thoroughbreds and Warmbloods. National or regional influences are seen, particularly in the use of native Warmbloods, owing to their ready availability and popularity as sport horses in any given nation.

At upper levels of competition, dressage horses are almost exclusively Warmbloods. In the origin of the Warmblood breeds, Arabian and Thoroughbred horses were bred to sturdier working breeds to lighten their conformation and improve their movement and stamina. The German Warmbloods are largely predominant at the upper levels, with five Germans studbooks represented in the World Breeding Federation for Sport Horses/FEI ranking of the top 10 breeds in dressage.[6] Of the 20 best internationally ranked individual horses, 15 are registered in German studbooks.[6] Gait and conformation analysis data on three-year-old dressage horses (n = 142) has shown German Warmbloods (Hanoverians [n = 31], Westphalians [n = 16], and Oldenburgers [n = 6]) to be biomechanically superior to both Selle Francais (n = 61) and purebred Spanish horses (n = 28) for use in competitive FEI dressage.[7] The superior stature and conformation of the German horses resulted in a longer stride length and decreased stride frequency. 'The German horses had gait characteristics more adapted to dressage competition,' the authors concluded.[7]

Studbooks operate a strict selection of their breeding mares and stallions to ensure a constant improvement of their dressage horses. Selection is based on conformation, performance, health, and offspring performance. The horses are requested to regularly participate in scheduled selection competitions. Veterinary examinations are compulsory to ensure the absence of heritable defects. To improve selection of the best breeders and maintain the quality of the horses produced with the increase in the trade of foreign semen, the results from performance tests and competitions of young horses are now used by major European Warmblood horse breeding associations for genetic evaluations.[8]

Selection according to conformation criteria is often more empirical and has shown a fairly low correlation with future performance.[9] However, it is of importance to the veterinary profession as it correlates with injury resistance.[10] Gait characteristics provide an early criterion for breeding in dressage breeding programs, but their implementation in practice is difficult as it requires the use of gait analysis techniques.[11] Behavior-related traits have also been examined as part of performance evaluations and may be partially predicted by personality traits analyzed earlier in life.[12]

The relationship between performance and particular traits such as ridden test scores has been scientifically studied. Specially designed young horse performance tests, including stallion tests, showed high heritabilities as well as high genetic correlations between analyzed traits and later competition results, thus proving their usefulness in predictability of dressage performance.[13] These performance test scores represent the main selection criteria in most modern breeding schemes of sport horses.[14]

Dressage horses may not compete under FEI rules until they are at least six years old.[1,3] Horses competing in the Olympic Games or World Equestrian Games must be at least seven years old.[3] Dressage horses may not compete in Grand Prix, Grand Prix Special, or Grand Prix Freestyle until they are at least seven years old.[1,3] In competitions, stallions usually perform better than geldings.

Dressage horses have their most productive years at the upper levels at approximately 8–12 years of age. In studies correlating performance with age, it has been demonstrated that dressage horses reach peak performance around the age of 10 years old.[15] Dressage is highly dependent on the human–equine interaction and mutual collaboration to compete successfully. The horse's individual qualities are intimately tied to rider's experience and equitation. At the elite level, dressage still reflects the rigorous demands of historical military cavalry training. Precision, obedience, stamina, versatility, and the competitive mindset of both rider and horse are unquestionable advantages to compete successfully. Mental skills of the rider, for instance, have been shown to have a positive effect on competitive dressage performance.[16]

Common diseases and conditions

Successful performance requires a healthy individual. The role of the veterinarian is to insure long-term health of the equine athlete. Early detection of subclinical disease is essential to limit the number of days out of training and to ensure a successful long-term career. Horses competing in dressage may have all the same problems or internal diseases of any other horse. However, some conditions may be more common due to the type of activity in which they compete, especially owing to the impulsion and extension required at the upper levels of dressage. Common complaints from dressage riders may include the horse not bending well, failing to canter on the correct lead, or cross- or counter-cantering by failing to change its lead behind after changing its lead correctly in front.

Skeletal

Poor conformation plays a significant role in many unsoundnesses. For example, post-legged or straight hind leg conformation can predispose a dressage horse to hock or stifle lameness, as will sickle hocks or the cow-hocked conformation which may be more common in some breeds. Due to the stresses caused by the bending and the excessive hindlimb reaching required in dressage ('impulsion'), hock pain and bone spavin are common maladies of dressage horses. See Figures 51.3A and B.

A recent survey of 11 363 registered members of British Dressage identified risk factors for lameness in dressage horses.[17] Owners reported in the 2005 survey that 33% of their dressage horses had been lame at some time during their career and 24% had been lame at some time in the last two years. Factors associated with occurrence of lameness in the previous two years included: age, height, indoor arenas, horse walkers, lunging, back soreness, arenas which became deeper when wet, and sand-based arenas.

Various types of arena surfaces may be associated with lameness problems. In the United Kingdom, survey results of dressage competitors and trainers indicate that wax-coated and mixed sand/rubber surfaces were less detrimental to soundness.[18] Woodchip surfaces were most often associated with lameness followed by sand alone, sand/PVC mixtures, and grass surfaces. Woodchips were associated with slipping and sand was associated with tripping during dressage exercises. The ideal surface was felt to have a limestone base; crushed concrete was to be avoided as a base material.

Forelimb problems in dressage horses may not be as common as hindlimb problems, but can still be of significance to individual horses. Forelimb problems can be caused or exacerbated by poor conformation. In one recent survey of foot conformation in 23 116 Dutch Warmblood horses (registered with the Royal Dutch Warmblood Studbook, KWPN), it was determined that competitive life was shorter for jumpers than for dressage horses.[19] 'Uneven feet' tended to shorten the competitive life of KWPN dressage horses and was associated significantly as a risk factor for lameness in elite jumpers.[19] Furthermore, foot conformation was found in 33 459 dressage horses and 30 474 show jumpers to be prevalent in 4.5–8% of KWPN horses annually from 1990–2002.[20] Improper hoof balance is not a rare problem and is best corrected with the farrier and veterinarian working together to achieve proper medial-to-lateral and left-to-right hoof balance. Corrective shoeing for poor forelimb foot conformation may be performed in dressage horses, but with some concern about shoe loss from overreaching from behind during extended trotting or cantering exercise.

Forelimb lameness in dressage horses may also be related to their lengthy extension at the upper levels of competition (Fig. 51.4). Fetlock synovitis or arthritis is seen secondary to extended movements at upper levels, especially in former Thoroughbred racehorses converted to use as dressage horses. Suspensory branch injuries can be common and may become chronic recurring causes of lost training time. Diagnosis is by palpation, flexion responses, local anesthesia to localize the lesion, and radiography and/or ultrasonography. Intra-articular or peri-ligamentous corticosteroid and/or hyaluronic acid injections are often used in the acute phases of distal forelimb

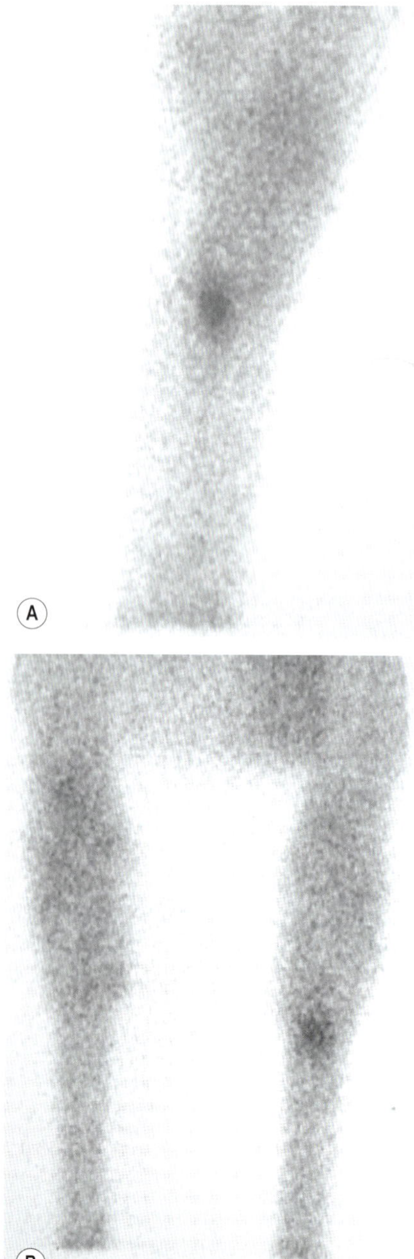

Fig 51.3 Right lateral **(A)** and plantar **(B)** scintigraphic views of a 13-year-old Thoroughbred dressage horse which had not been performing well for six weeks before its original presentation five months ago. On initial physical examination there was a suspicion of thickening of the high suspensory ligament region but it was normal on ultrasound examination. The horse was Grade +2/5 lame in the right hind limb and was made one grade worse with hock/stifle flexion and when lunging to the left (with the lame leg on the outside of the lunging circle). The original scintigraphic examination five months ago demonstrated moderate-to-severe focal uptake of radioisotope at the proximal plantar aspect of the third metatarsal near the tarsometatarsal joint on both the pool and bone phases. In these re-check views five months later, the lesion has become denser and more focal, despite months of stall rest and handwalking therapy. The prognosis is poor based on the severity of the lesion despite months of enforced rest.

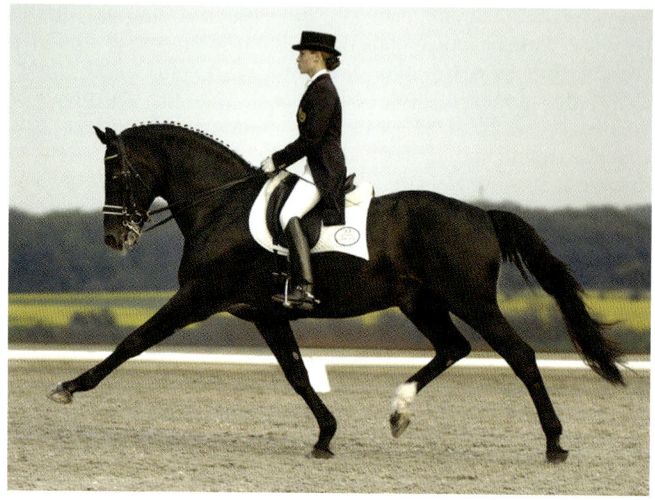

Fig 51.4 Dressage horse exhibiting hyperextension of the forelimb. He is also at a normal degree of poll flexion, required to be considered 'on the bit' but not 'behind' nor 'in front of the bit.'

injury to the fetlock, pastern, and coffin joints or the branches of the suspensory ligament. However, chronic corticosteroid use may be associated with iatrogenic calcification of ligament and joint capsule and counterproductive appearance of enthesiophytes (formation of a 'steroid arthropathy'). Progressive loading such as handwalking followed by walking with a rider on the back can be helpful eventually in the recovery from these injuries, but excessive turning such as may be done on a mechanical horse walker is to be avoided during recuperation.

Proximal suspensory ligament and check (accessory) ligament injuries require lengthy periods of recuperation. Local anesthesia of the joints and regions below the high metacarpus do not result in improvement. A positive response to a high palmar anesthetic block or to local anesthesia of the region around the head of the suspensory ligament is diagnostic. Intra-articular anesthesia of the middle carpal joint will also often result in improvement due to diffusion of local anesthetic out of the joint capsule and into the head of the suspensory ligament.[21] Ultrasound examination of the high suspensory and check ligament area may confirm the diagnosis by documentation of localized hemorrhage, edema, and fiber disruption. In horses which block out in this region but in which the high suspensory ligament does not reveal obvious ultrasonographic changes, a bone scan is indicated.[21] Proximal palmar stress injuries or stress fractures might be apparent on scintigraphic examination (as illustrated for plantar lesions in Figure 51.3). Follow-up scintigraphy might assist effectively in monitoring recovery, which may require six months or more for complete healing and soundness in the forelimb. Radiographs may confirm a classic 'gull-wing' appearance to the stress fracture which will manifest cortical and intramedullary calcification (callus formation) as the stress fracture begins to heal.[21]

Osteoarthritis of the medial aspect of the distal tarsal joints ('bone spavin') is common in dressage horses due to the excessive flexion and extension required for adequate impulsion to be competitive. Intra-articular corticosteroid administration is common for treatment of distal tarsal osteoarthritis. Repeated administration may be required every few months to maintain competitive soundness. In approximately 25% of horses, the distal intertarsal and tarsometatarsal joints intercommunicate, so anesthetic or corticosteroid injected into the easier site, the tarsometatarsal joint, will diffuse into the distal intertarsal joint and will require fewer injection sites to diagnose or medicate the horse.[22] Eventual fusion of the distal intertarsal and/or tarsometatarsal joints may result in soundness without further medication. For horses which tend to toe out behind ('cow-hocked'), squaring the toes and application of short lateral trailers on the shoes may assist in some correction of the conformation and limb flight. That correction may lead to less medial tarsal pain since straightening the breakover path minimizes undue stress on the dorsomedial aspect of the distal tarsal joints. Conversely, and seemingly contradictorily, in some horses with tarsal pain already shod with lateral trailers, removing the shoes with a lateral trailer may assist in recovery if the trailers are causing a sudden grip and stop of those feet, jolting the limbs acutely with each stride and exacerbating tarsal pain.

High hindlimb suspensory injuries can be difficult injuries for the horse to recover fully. They are often associated with the ipsilateral hind fetlock appearing to be dropped or hyperextended, with the fetlock on the injured limb hanging or sagging closer to the ground when weight-bearing. Lameness is exacerbated by tarsal/stifle flexion. Local anesthesia of the joints and regions distal to the proximal metatarsus do not result in improvement. A positive response to a high plantar anesthetic block or to local anesthesia of the region around the head of the suspensory ligament is diagnostic. Intra-articular anesthesia of the tarsometatarsal joint will also often result in improvement due to diffusion of local anesthetic out of the joint capsule and into the head of the suspensory ligament. As in the forelimb, ultrasonography should be diagnostic unless there is an avulsion stress fracture component to the lameness. Scintigraphy (Fig. 51.3) and radiography may be diagnostic in addition to ultrasonography in these horses. However, hindlimb high suspensory lesions carry a much poorer prognosis than the same injury in the forelimb (Fig. 51.3). Horses with hindlimb high suspensory injuries often respond initially to a lengthy period of recuperation, but return to even moderate work often results in exacerbation of the injury and an inability to continue to work soundly and safely.

Due to the collection, impulsion, bending, circling, and other types of movements required in dressage, sore backs are common complaints. Riders often complain of a horse's unwillingness to bend, perhaps worse in one direction than the other. The presence of a rider mounted on the dressage horse may influence the appearance of the lameness when the horse is trotting.[23] In particular, hindlimb lameness was more evident statistically when the horse was ridden as opposed to being jogged in hand.[23] In a recent Dutch study of 805 horses (70% dressage horses, 20% jumpers, 10% Standardbred trotters), 74% were found to be lame, with 32% of those lame horses also having back problems.[24] The authors concluded that 'there was a strong association between lameness and back problems and...there was a high prevalence of lameness among the horses with back problems.'[24] The result is that thoracolumbar and sacroiliac pain is common in dressage horses but often is due to muscle soreness secondary to other skeletal lamenesses.

In one study of risk factors for sacroiliac pain, dressage and showjumping horses were at significantly higher risk than other occupations.[25] Other factors associated with sacroiliac joint pain were taller and heavier horses and Warmblood breed horses (all of which certainly might characterize upper-level dressage horses). Conformation was not associated with sacroiliac pain but 'poor development of the epaxial muscles in the thoracolumbar region and asymmetry of the hindquarter musculature were common.'[25] Furthermore, 'in all horses restricted hindlimb impulsion was the predominant feature; invariably this was most obvious when the horse was ridden. Stiffness, unwillingness to work on the bit and poor quality canter were common.'[25] Demonstrable local pain on palpation was common. Scintigraphy documented lesions in 99% of horses with sacroiliac pain (73 of 74 horses examined). Response to local anesthesia was 100% in those horses in which injection was attempted (34 of 34 horses).[25]

Other factors associated with back pain include ill-fitting saddles,[26] inappropriate use of specific tack (e.g. side-reins, martingales) and asymmetrical equitation on the rider's part. The position of head and neck during work also has a significant influence on back movements and intervertebral motion. Thus bad equitation practices can predispose to back injury.[27,28] Among training techniques in dressage stirring considerable controversy is Rollkur or hyperflexion of the neck. During Rollkur, the neck is lowered and the poll is exaggeratedly flexed, bringing the bridge of the nose far behind the vertical line. Because this position cannot be sustained without forceful rider intervention, the FEI banned its use at CDIs.[29] The technique known as Low, Deep and Round (LDR), which achieves flexion without undue aggression is acceptable.

Primary back pathology has been described.[30,33] The most often cited type is over-riding spinous processes which may result in withers pain; local anesthesia may be diagnostic.[31] Local injections with corticosteroids or acupuncture may be palliative but surgery to prevent the impingement may be the only permanent solution.

Thermography has been used as a non-invasive method to assess changes in heat pattern which may be reflective of inflammation and pain in the back region.[32] Scintigraphy may also reflect local changes in the back which can be difficult to radiograph resolutely due to the thickness of the subject in that region.[25,31,33] Therapy for back pain should be directed at the primary lameness if present, such as management of distal tarsal pain (spavin). Once the primary lameness is alleviated, the secondary back pain often subsides. In the event of primary back pain, local solutions should be sought but many may be more palliative than curative. Successful management of back pain has been reported with use of acupuncture[34] and chiropractic manipulation[35] in addition to more conventional methods such as rest, massage, local heat, electrostimulation, and local injection.

Muscular

Exertional rhabdomyolysis (ER) is commonly termed myopathy or tying-up. It is a disease that is diagnosed in dressage horses and recognized as a cause of poor performance.[36] The prevalence of ER in Warmbloods is similar to that of racing breeds, although the more severe forms of ER are less frequently encountered.[37] Clinical expression of ER is highly variable and can manifest as excessive sweating, gluteal muscle or lumbar back pain, stiffness, or moderate lameness.[38] In more severe cases, muscle necrosis can occur and lead to myoglobinuria and subsequent renal failure.

The diagnosis of ER is based on history, clinical examination, including an attentive comparison of muscle masses, a lameness examination, and observation of increased activity of one or more plasma/serum muscle enzymes (CK, AST, LDH). Muscle atrophy and asymmetry of muscle masses are frequent features in chronic cases of ER. Definitive diagnosis can be made by observing a two-fold increase in CK levels 4–6 hours after 15 minutes of exercise. The post-exercise elevation in CK activity is often less dramatic than those encountered in Thoroughbred racehorses galloping in field settings.

Differential diagnosis between the different types of ER is based on muscle biopsy and/or genetic testing. Although perceived as invasive, muscle biopsies are usually well tolerated. In an epidemiological study based on clinical cases referred for histopathology of muscle samples, idiopathic exertional myopathy and polysaccharide storage myopathy (PSSM) were the most commonly diagnosed forms of ER in Warmbloods, followed by sporadic myopathy.[37] The genetically based PSSM has been shown to occur in dressage and showjumping breeds.[38] It has an autosomal dominant transmission.[39] Breeding horses with this disease results in at least a 50% chance that their offspring will be affected, regardless of the genetic status of the breeding partner.

In acute cases of ER, the horse should be restrained from walking and non-steroidal anti-inflammatory drugs (NSAIDs) should be administered to reduce pain. Sedation is necessary to rapidly alleviate anxiety and pain in more severe cases. Rehydration may be necessary and should be encouraged to promote diuresis, which is critical to dilute myoglobinuria and to try to prevent renal disease.

Effective management of ER-affected horses has been studied more in depth recently. For instance, the use of a low- starch, high-fat and high-fiber diet is effective in reducing the severity of ER.[40,41] There are several commercially available feeds that have been specifically formulated for sport horses with ER. However, adding high-quality, omega-3-enriched oil to the horse's regular diet is also a means of increasing energy provided by non-carbohydrate sources. Modification of the horse's working schedule is also essential to avoid recurrence of ER episodes. It usually requires daily turn-out and prolonged periods of warm-up.[42] The use of dantrolene sodium has been advocated,[43] but it is subject to doping regulation and has been banned from use in competition.

Prior to resuming training exercise after an episode of ER, the veterinarian should check that muscle enzyme activities have returned to normal and that the horse is comfortable and free of clinical signs. Muscle repair following injury depends on the severity and nature of the injury. Damage to the muscles after ER usually spares the basement membrane and often allows complete muscle regeneration.

Endocrine

Mares in their estrus cycle may exhibit inappropriate nervous behavior that can be deleterious to the quality of their performance during dressage competitions. As major competitions take place during the spring season, re-scheduling according to the mare's cycle can be difficult to achieve. The administration of altrenogest (Regu-Mate®) is advocated as hormonal control to mitigate estrus behavior. However, its use is restricted during competition and prior approval must be sought using FEI Equine Therapeutic Use Exemption (ETUE) Form 2, or equivalent. In some individual cases where altrenogest is highly effective, the calming effect could be considered detrimental for the mare's performance in competition. The use of this drug is prohibited in male horses, both in geldings or stallions.

Gastrointestinal

Regular oral and dental evaluation should be performed because any pain originating from the oral cavity may lead to defensive behavior, resistance to the rider's hand, head-shaking, or reluctance to work in dressage horses. The use of a bit is mandatory in dressage competitions. The appropriate selection of a bit is essential since an ill-fitted bit may cause excessive pressure or lesions over sensitive areas in the horse's oral cavity (bars, tongue, hard palate, or teeth). Inappropriate fitting of the bit or oral injuries can trigger defensive reactions or resistance to the action of the rein.[44] The presence of wolf teeth (PM 1) should also be checked as these might interfere with the bit and generate pain during exercise.

As in all horses engaged in a competitive career, gastric ulcers, colic, and diarrhea are stress-related disorders that regularly occur in dressage horses. These are secondary to various cumulative factors such as transport, intensive training, diet, and feeding practices. Gastric ulcers may be the most difficult condition to diagnose as clinical symptoms may be subtle and variable. Appetite and weight loss may be less common clinical signs than a failure to thrive at work or signs of discomfort when the horse is working. Some riders have described reluctance of the horse to leg yield. Although some were formerly prohibited, all common anti-ulcer medications (omeprazole, cimetidine, ranitidine) are now authorized under FEI Veterinary Regulations.

Respiratory

Competitive dressage at elementary and intermediate levels is only moderately aerobically demanding.[45] It could therefore be perceived that dressage horses can consequently tolerate mild degrees of respiratory impedance. However, the importance of appropriate poll flexion, as required in the discipline of dressage, has been shown to increase resistance to airflow in the upper respiratory tract.[46] Flexion at the poll contributes to increased work of breathing and can cause respiratory compromise in dressage horses with airway disease. Airway disease is probably largely underestimated in Warmbloods because it can develop subclinically and is not systematically accompanied by obvious, typical clinical signs such as cough or nasal discharge.[47] Dressage horses may have subclinical forms of both upper and lower airway disease that translate into apparent misbehavior, reluctance to work, or lameness as reported by the rider or trainer. Dressage horses with respiratory disease may be reluctant to flex their poll and may seek to extend their head and neck in an attempt to reduce airflow resistance and maximize ventilation.[48] Changes in behavior linked to respiratory airway disease can include abruptly head-jerking, head-shaking, yanking of the reins from the rider's hands, rearing, and failure to progress in training. The use of additional tack to force head flexion is often adopted in response to the horse's defensive attitude but further increases the horse's distress. Appropriate treatment results in improved behavior and yielding to the bit.[49]

Upper airway problems

Upper airway obstruction (UAO) has multiple causes, most of which remain undetectable or misdiagnosed upon resting examination.[50–53] Dynamic UAO is a common cause of respiratory noise during exercise and may lead to poor performance in racehorses.[52] However, in Warmbloods exercising at submaximal levels, UAO may occur without concomitant noise. Even in its complex forms, UAO is not systematically associated with a complaint of poor performance.[53] The generation of a respiratory noise represents a concern because it is a fault in the show ring in many disciplines (dressage, show hunters) and is a depreciating factor in the commercial value of many horses.

The recent advent of overground endoscopes has allowed the evaluation of upper airway mechanics under normal exercising conditions, particularly when the horse is being ridden in its normal manner and in its usual tack (Fig. 51.5). Overground endoscopy with a mounted rider may be a critical examination procedure for the diagnosis of upper airway conditions in dressage horses. A study comparing treadmill to track endoscopy in saddle horses showed that some conditions could not be elicited on a treadmill due to the absence of rider intervention.[54] In Warmbloods, the proportion of poorly performing horses in which a diagnosis of UAO was made was considerably higher when the horses were ridden (70%)[49] than when examined on a treadmill (21%).[55] Poll flexion and rider intervention are factors that have been shown to significantly influence the stability of the upper airway.[49]

Various interventions of the rider have been shown to cause alterations in upper airway morphology or stability.[49] These documented interfering interventions include: firm tightening of the reins; applying spurs to the thorax; abrupt transitions between gaits; working in tight circles; sudden changes in direction; excessive gathering of the horse, inducing increased vertical movement; and execution of dressage figures (pirouette, piaffé, and change of lead at the canter). The odds of developing UAO with the head flexed and with other forms of rider intervention are summarized in Table 51.1. Ninety percent and 81% of the horses developed UAO or worsened existing UAO with head flexion and rider intervention, respectively.[49] Head flexion and rider effect has a more significant influence on the development of UAO in dressage horses than in show jumpers. The positive predictive value (PPV) for head flexion was 86% for dressage versus 65% for show jumpers.[49] The PPV for other riding maneuvers was 83% for dressage versus 57% for show jumpers.[49] Other factors such as the bit or the use of martingales or side reins may also contribute to upper airway instability during ridden exercise.

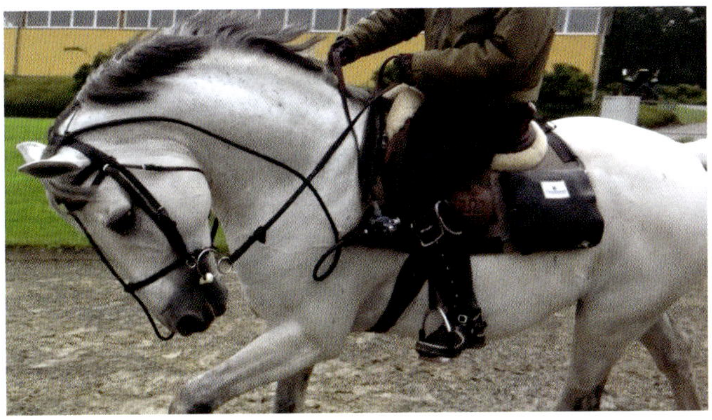

Fig 51.5 Horse being ridden with an overground endoscopy system in place. The endoscope is in the horse's nostril, runs dorsally over the face to the poll, and connects to the digital recording system housed in the pack on the rider's back. Research in field studies has shown that overground endoscopy is superior for non-racing performance horses in documenting unique airway dynamics as horses are ridden in their normal manner using their regular bit and bridle.[46] This strong degree of poll flexion can contribute to upper airway obstruction (Table 51.1) which may sometimes be diagnosed only through dynamic endoscopy, either on a treadmill or overground.

Dorsal displacement of the soft palate (DDSP) is one form of UAO diagnosed in dressage horses. It rarely generates a respiratory noise during exercise but can trigger coughing during exercise. Its prevalence is higher in dressage horses than in show jumpers, possibly because the more closed angle between head and neck in dressage (see Fig. 51.5) generates greater negative pressure in the nasopharyngeal region.[49,55–57] See Figure 51.6.

Recurrent laryngeal neuropathy (RLN) is a common cause of UAO in larger breeds of horses including the Warmblood breeds popular for dressage.[58] It is more frequently associated with respiratory noise during exercise than with poor performance in Warmbloods.[49] However, a mild degree of laryngeal dysfunction may progressively deteriorate over time, leading to sudden onset of an exercise-related respiratory noise and sometimes a concurrent reduced performance.[59] Studies have demonstrated that genetic factors play a significant role in the pathogenesis of RLN.[60–62] Because RLN may be hereditary, horses diagnosed with the disorder are excluded from many studbooks. Other UAO causing poor performance or exercise-induced respiratory noise described in dressage horses are palatal instability, epiglottic entrapment, and uni- or bilateral vocal cord collapse.

Underlying airway inflammation has been suggested as a possible predisposing factor to UAO. Pharyngeal instability is significantly affected by the presence of upper (pharyngeal) or lower airway inflammation.[49] In racehorses, only severe forms of pharyngeal lymphoid hyperplasia (PLH) or those associated with other respiratory disorders have been shown to generate upper airway dysfunction.[63–65] Lower airway inflammation can also impact upper airway stability by increasing respiratory impedance and work of breathing.[66,67] In contrast to pharyngeal instability, other forms of UAO are independent of inflammatory conditions.[49]

Lower airway disease

Several factors promote the occurrence of chronic inflammatory diseases in dressage horses, such as age (higher prevalence in older individuals) and environmental conditions. Dressage horses are often kept indoors in stables and have limited or no access to outdoor paddocks or pasture. This type of management encourages

Table 51.1 Effects of head flexion and other forms of rider intervention on dynamic upper airway obstruction (UAO) of 129 Warmbloods referred for upper airway endoscopy

DIAGNOSIS	HEAD FLEXION		RIDER INTERVENTION	
	ODDS RATIO	P (TWO-TAILED)	ODDS RATIO	P (TWO-TAILED)
Palatal instability	10.68*	<0.0001	6.56*	<0.0001
Dorsally displaced soft palate	1.98	0.239	2.41	0.082
Arytenoïd cartilage collapse	8.37*	0.0002	3.62*	0.0034
Vocal cord collapse	10.28*	<0.0001	9.11*	<0.0001
Axial deviation of the aryepiglottic folds	8.56*	0.027	3.63*	0.047
Multiple UAO	13.31*	<0.0001	10.83*	<0.0001

*Significant associations using logistic regression.
Modified from van Erck 2011.[49]

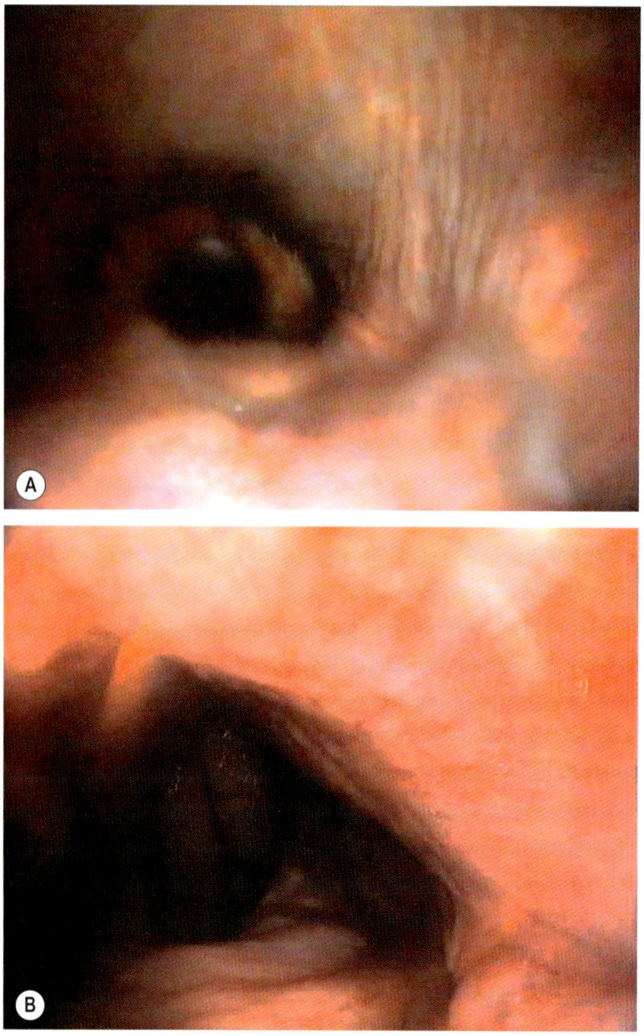

Fig 51.6 Image captured during overground endoscopy of the horse in Figure 51.5. The horse was referred for defensive behavior and cough, occurring only during exercise. Upper airway endoscopy during exercise shows that the horse had marked dorso-ventral collapse of the nasopharynx as soon as it was on the bit. Increased poll flexion led to repeated and prolonged dorsal displacement of the soft palate (DDSP), causing the horse to cough. No other noise was associated with the episodes of DDSP.

chronic respiratory inflammation.[68] Training, repeated transport, and co-mingling during competition may also promote the transmission of infectious diseases and lead to the development of lower airway inflammation such as recurrent airway obstruction (RAO) or inflammatory airway disease (IAD).[66]

Dressage horses affected by lower airway disease may not show significant respiratory signs but may not perform with their usual energy. The only indicators of IAD may include subtle changes in demeanor, misbehavior during exercise, coughing, or other mild respiratory signs.[48] In show horses, although IAD may not always seem overtly to affect performance,[69] it has been associated with a decreased willingness to perform.[70] Inflammatory airway disease is also detrimental to upper airway stability and may accelerate the onset of fatigue.[49]

Identifying inflammatory conditions of the lower airways is important in order to interrupt its progression and reduce the risks of athletic impairment. Diagnosis of IAD requires detection of mucus in the trachea and an increase in inflammatory cells in bronchial fluid. The presence of mucus in the trachea is regarded as a sign of IAD and tracheal endoscopy may be helpful.[69] A definitive diagnosis is obtained by the cytological analysis of a bronchoalveolar lavage (BAL), indicating an increase in one or more types of inflammatory cells: increased counts of neutrophils (>10%), mast cells (>2 %), and/or eosinophils (>2%).[66]

Recurrent airway obstruction is an inflammatory condition of the lower airways which is analogous to an allergic reaction. It is triggered by the inhalation of microscopic molds usually found in hay and straw in the indoor stable environment. Genetic factors play an important role in the pathogenesis of RAO but because the genes influencing the genetic susceptibility for RAO have not been identified, selection through breeding is difficult. Clinical manifestations of RAO may include nasal discharge, cough, marked abdominal expiration (increased expiratory effort), and respiratory distress. These signs are secondary to the pathological changes occurring in the airways which include excessive mucus accumulation, airway edema, and bronchoconstriction. The cytologic analysis of tracheal or bronchoalveolar lavage fluid allows evaluation of the severity of the disease process, analysis of the quality of the horse's environment, and determination of an appropriate course of therapy. Estimating the functional repercussions of the disease may also be indicated if permanent pathological sequelae are suspected.

Prevention remains the best method for the appropriate maintenance of a healthy lower airway. A dust-free and hygienic environment both at home and during shows limits risks of lower airway inflammation. Key prophylactic measures that can be implemented include the adoption of dust-free bedding and the use of silage or steamed hay and well-ventilated boxes. Because of doping issues, medical treatment is difficult leading up to and during competitions. Inhalation therapy represents a good option as the doses of medication delivered are much reduced compared to systemic administration and the resultant detection times are shorter. A special request needs to be addressed to the FEI officials before using an inhaling system at a show, even if the delivered substance is authorized.

Cardiovascular

Cardiovascular diseases are rarely encountered in dressage horses. Physiological arrhythmias and heart murmurs are regularly ausculted in high-level athletes.[71] It is critical to differentiate physiological from pathological conditions as the latter may affect performance, re-sale potential, and athletic longevity.

Valvular regurgitation is an age-related condition common in athletic horses. In a study of Warmblood horses, 10% of horses were reported as having performance affected by valvular regurgitation.[72] The study also looked into purchase practices and indicated that despite the presence of a heart murmur, 43% of affected horses were sold for the asking price but 36% were not sold because of the murmur.[72] The intensity of the associated heart murmur is not always proportional to the severity of the underlying condition. Doppler echocardiography is warranted to establish definitive diagnosis and to assess the severity of the disease.

When present, mitral regurgitation is the cardiac disorder most likely to lead to poor performance. As such, auscultation of a left-sided holo- to pansystolic murmur warrants further investigation. The intensity of the murmur does not always indicate severity of regurgitation. In addition to confirming the diagnosis, echocardiography allows assessment of the morphological and functional consequences. Sequential echocardiography allows the veterinarian to monitor progression over time and to give a more precise prognosis. Moderate-to- severe insufficiencies and intensive training are more likely to cause a more rapid progression of the condition. Atrial volume overload secondary to mitral regurgitation might predispose horses to atrial fibrillation.

Tricuspid regurgitation is a relatively common finding in equine athletes performing at higher level. It is often found in the absence of clinical signs and seldom has repercussions on the horse's ability to perform. However, horses with any signs of right-sided heart failure (peripheral edema, exercise intolerance, possibly combined with atrial fibrillation) should be evaluated carefully for tricuspid insufficiency.

Aortic insufficiency is common in middle-aged to older horses and hence will be found with some frequency in competitive Warmbloods. It is caused by a progressive thickening of the valves and is not always accompanied by a clinically audible murmur on auscultation. When audible, the associated murmur is a holodiastolic decrescendo murmur. Aortic regurgitation may predispose some horses to develop an arrhythmia during exercise, which may subsequently affect performance. The diagnosis of aortic valve regurgitation may need to be accompanied by an exercising ECG. Conversely, in most horses with aortic insufficiency, the condition is benign and not associated with clinical signs of any kind.

The occurrence of cardiac arrhythmias during exercise has been investigated in dressage horses competing normally at various levels.[73] Horses were considered clinically healthy based on general physical examinations. The only ancillary examinations performed were resting echocardiography and ECG, as well as exercising ECG. Isolated supraventricular and ventricular premature complexes occurred anecdotally during exercise in 6 of 27 and 1 of 27 horses, respectively. Normal sinus arrhythmia was often observed during post-exercise recovery. No significant associations were found between arrhythmia and age, gender, or presence of valvular regurgitation.[73]

Atrial fibrillation (AF) is commonly described as the most frequent cardiovascular cause of poor performance in equine athletes.[74] The prevalence of AF was reported to be around 2.5% in a mixed population of horses, with larger breeds being over-represented.[75] Some dressage horses have competed at international levels with sustained AF, probably because it is a submaximal, less aerobically demanding sport.[74] With AF, exercising horses usually have increased heart rates in order to compensate for a suboptimal diastolic filling, and thus these horses may fatigue prematurely. Development of ventricular tachycardia during exercise, secondary to AF, is a risk that may be fatal. Assessing ECG response to exercise in horses with AF is important to investigate and subsequently repeat if the horse is not defibrillated successfully.

Neurological

Infectious neurological diseases (e.g. Equine protozoal myelitis, West Nile virus, neurotropic equine herpesvirus-1) are not more common in dressage horses than in older horses performing in other sports.

Medications during competition

Medications allowed or disallowed during dressage competition are reviewed in Chapter 50.

References

1. Anonymous. FEI Rules for Dressage. 24th ed. Lausanne, Switzerland: Fédération Equestre Internationale; 2009 amended for 2012. www.horsesport.org, 24 January 2012.
2. Hawson LA, McLean AN, McGreevy PD. Variability of scores in the 2008 Olympic dressage competition and implications for horse training and welfare. Journal of Veterinary Behavior: Clinical Applications and Research 2010;5(4):170–6.
3. Anonymous. FEI General Regulations. 23rd ed. 1 January 2011 amended for 2012. Lausanne, Switzerland: Fédération Equestre Internationale; www.horsesport.org, 29 June 2012.
4. Anonymous. United States Equestrian Federation 2012 Rulebook. Lexington, Kentucky: United States Equestrian Federation; http://www.usef.org, 24 January 2012.
5. Meyers MC, Bourgeois AE, Leunes A, et al. Mood and psychological skills of elite and sub-elite equestrian athletes. Journal of Sport Behavior 1999;22.
6. Anonymous. World Breeding Federation for Sport Horses. www.wbfsh.org, 29 June 2012.
7. Barrey E, Desliens F, Poirel D, et al. Early evaluation of dressage ability in different breeds. Equine Vet J 2002;(Suppl. 34): 319–24.
8. Thorén Hellsten E, Viklund Å, Koenen EPC, et al. Review of genetic parameters estimated at stallion and young horse performance tests and their correlations with later results in dressage and show-jumping competition. Livestock Science 2006;103:1–12.
9. Koenen EPC, van Veldhuizen AE, Brascamp EW. Genetic parameters of linear scored conformation traits and their relation to dressage and show-jumping performance in the Dutch Warmblood Riding Horse population. Livestock Production Science 1995;43: 85–94.
10. Van Weeren PR, Crevier-Denoix N. Equine conformation: Clues to performance and soundness? Equine Vet J 2006;38:591–6.
11. Barrey E, Desliñes F, Blouin C, et al. Heritabilities of gait characteristics: Application for breeding in dressage. In: Lindner A, editor. Conference on Equine Sports Medicine and Science: The elite dressage and three-day-event horse. 2002. p. 91–5.
12. Visser EK, Van Reenen CG, Engel B, et al. The association between performance in show-jumping and personality traits earlier in life. Appl Anim Behav Sci 2003;82:279–95.
13. Wallin L, Strandberg E, Philipsson J. Genetic correlations between field test results of Swedish Warmblood riding horses as 4-year-olds and lifetime performance results in dressage and show jumping. Livestock Production Science 2003;82:61–71.
14. Giulotto E. Will horse genetics create better champions? Trends in Genetics 2001;17:166.
15. Stewart ID, Woolliams JA, Brotherstone S. Genetic evaluation of horses for performance in dressage competitions in Great Britain. Livestock Science 2010:128: 36–45.
16. Wolframm IA, Micklewright D. The effect of a mental training program on state anxiety and competitive dressage performance. Journal Vet Behavior: Clinical Applications and Research 2011:6:267–75.
17. Murray RC, Walters J, Snart H, et al. Identification of risk factors for lameness in dressage horses. Vet J 2010;184:27–36.
18. Murray RC, Walters J, Snart H, et al. How do features of dressage arenas influence training surface properties which are

potentially associated with lameness? Vet J 2010;186:172–9.
19. Ducro BJ, Gorissen B, van Eldik P, et al. Influence of foot conformation on duration of competitive life in a Dutch Warmblood horse population. Equine Vet J 2009;41:144–8.
20. Ducro BJ, Bovenhuis H, Back W. Heritability of foot conformation and its relationship to sports performance in a Dutch Warmblood horse population. Equine Vet J 2009;41:139–43.
21. Pleasant RS, Baker GJ, Muhlbauer MC, et al. Stress reactions and stress fractures of proximal palmar aspect of the third metacarpal bone in horses: 58 cases (1980–1990). J Am Vet Med Assoc 1992;201:1918–23.
22. Bell BTL, Baker GJ, Foreman JH, et al. In vivo investigation of communication between the distal intertarsal and tarsometatarsal joints in horses and ponies. Vet Surg 1993;22:289–92.
23. Licka T, Kapaun M, Peham C. Influence of rider on lameness in trotting horses. Equine Vet J 2004;36:734–6.
24. Landman MA, de Blaauw JA, van Weeren PR, et al. Field study of the prevalence of lameness in horses with back problems. Vet Rec 2004;155:165–8.
25. Dyson S, Murray R. Pain associated with the sacroiliac joint region: A clinical study of 74 horses. Equine Vet J 2003;35:240–5.
26. Harmon J. Tack and saddle fit. Vet Clin North Am Equine Pract 1999;15:247–61.
27. Álvarez CBG, Rhodin M, Bobbert MF, et al. The effect of head and neck position on the thoracolumbar kinematics in the unridden horse. Equine Vet J 2006;38:445–51.
28. Rhodin M, Álvarez CBG, Byström A, et al. The effect of different head and neck positions on the caudal back and hindlimb kinematics in the elite dressage horse at trot. Equine Vet J 2009;41: 274–9.
29. Anonymous. FEI Working Group Report on Stewards Guidelines. Lausanne, Switzerland: Fédération Equestre Internationale; 2010 (www.fei.org).
30. Haussler KK. Osseous spinal pathology. Vet Clin North Am Equine Pract 1999;15:103–12.
31. Zimmerman M, Dyson S, Murray R. Close, impinging and overriding spinous processes in the thoracolumbar spine: The relationship between radiological and scintigraphic findings and clinical signs. Equine Vet J 2012;44:178–84.
32. von Schweinitz DG. Thermographic diagnostics in equine back pain. Vet Clin North Am Equine Pract 1999;15:161–77.
33. Weaver MP, Jeffcott LB, Nowak M. Radiography and scintigraphy. Vet Clin North Am Equine Pract 1999;15:113–29.
34. Klide AM, Martin BB Jr. Methods of stimulating acupuncture points for treatment of chronic back pain in horses. J Am Vet Med Assoc 1989;195:1375–9.
35. Haussler KK. Chiropractic evaluation and management. Vet Clin North Am Equine Pract 1999;15:195–209.
36. Martin BB Jr, Reef VB, Parente EJ, et al. Causes of poor performance of horses during training, racing, or showing: 348 cases (1992–1996). J Am Vet Med Assoc 2000;216:554–8.
37. Piercy RJ, Rivero J-LL. Muscle disorders of equine athletes. In: Hinchcliff KW, Kaneps AJ, Geor RJ, editors. Equine Sports Medicine and Surgery. Edinburgh: Saunders, Elsevier; 2004. p. 77–110.
38. Quiroz-Roth E, Novales M, Aguilera-Tejero E, et al. Polysaccharide storage myopathy in the M. longissimus lumborum of showjumpers and dressage horses with back pain. Equine Vet J 2002;34:171–6.
39. McCue ME, Valberg SJ, Lucio M, et al. Glycogen synthase 1 (GYS1) mutation in diverse breeds with polysaccharide storage myopathy. J Vet Intern Med 2008;22:1228–33.
40. Valentine BA, Van Saun RJ, Thompson KN, et al. Role of dietary carbohydrate and fat in horses with equine polysaccharide storage myopathy. J Am Vet Med Assoc 2001;219:1537–44.
41. McKenzie EC, Valberg SJ, Godden SM, et al. Effect of dietary starch, fat, and bicarbonate content on exercise responses and serum creatine kinase activity in equine recurrent exertional rhabdomyolysis. J Vet Intern Med 2003;17:693–701.
42. Valberg SJ, Mickelson JR, Gallant EM, et al. Exertional rhabdomyolysis in quarter horses and thoroughbreds: one syndrome, multiple aetiologies. Equine Vet J 1999;(Suppl. 30):533–8.
43. McKenzie EC, Valberg SJ, Godden SM, et al. Effect of oral administration of dantrolene sodium on serum creatine kinase activity after exercise in horses with recurrent exertional rhabdomyolysis. Am J Vet Res 2004;65:74–9.
44. Cook WR, Mills DS. Preliminary study of jointed snaffle vs. cross under bitless bridles: Quantified comparison of behaviour in four horses. Equine Vet J 2009;41:827–30.
45. Williams RJ, Chandler RE, Marlin DJ. Heart rates of horses during competitive dressage. Comparative Exercise Physiology 2009;6:7–15.
46. Petsche VM, Derksen FJ, Berney CE, et al. Effect of head position on upper airway function in exercising horses. Equine Vet J 1995;(Suppl. 18):18–22.
47. Van Erck E, Art T. Clinical data on EIPH in horses from all equestrian disciplines and the relationship between EIPH, BALF cytology and respiratory function tests. Proc Havemeyer Foundation Workshop on Exercise-Induced Pulmonary Hemorrhage, San Diego, 2008. p. 9.
48. Platz C. Poor performance: The trainer's perspective (sport horse). Havemeyer Foundation Monograph Series No. 9. Inflammatory Airway Disease: Defining the syndrome. 2002.
49. Van Erck E. Dynamic respiratory videoendoscopy in ridden sport horses: Effect of head flexion, riding and airway inflammation in 129 cases. Equine Vet J Suppl 2011;40:18–24.
50. Parente EJ, Martin BB. Correlation between standing endoscopic examination and those made during high-speed exercise in horses – 150 cases. Proc Am Assoc Equine Practitioners 1995;41:170.
51. Ferrucci F, Zucca E, Croci C, et al. Rest and treadmill endoscopic findings in 87 race horses presented for poor performance. In: Lindner A, editor. The Elite Race and Endurance Horse, Conference on Equine Sports Medicine and Science (CESMAS). 2004. p. 133–6.
52. Tan RH, Dowling BA, Dart AJ. High-speed treadmill videoendoscopic examination of the upper-respiratory tract in the horse: The results of 291 clinical cases. Vet J 2005;170:243–8.
53. Lane JG, Bladon B, Little DRM, et al. Dynamic obstructions of the equine upper respiratory tract. Part 2: Comparison of endoscopic findings at rest and during high-speed treadmill exercise of 600 Thoroughbred racehorses. Equine Vet J 2006;38:401–8.
54. Van Erck E, Frippiat T, Dupuis M-C, et al. Upper airway dynamic endoscopy: Are track and treadmill observations comparable? Proc 4th World Equine Airways Symposium. Berne, Switzerland, 2009, p. 254.
55. Davidson EJ, Martin BB, Boston RC, et al. Exercising upper respiratory videoendoscopic evaluation of 100 non-racing performance horses with abnormal respiratory noise and/or poor performance. Equine Vet J 2011;43:3–8.
56. Franklin SH, Naylor JRJ, Lane JG. Videoendoscopic evaluation of the upper respiratory tract in 93 sport horses during exercise testing on a high speed treadmill. Equine Vet J 2006;(Suppl. 36):540–5.
57. Strand E, Fjordbakk CT, Holcombe SJ, et al. Effect of poll flexion and dynamic laryngeal collapse on tracheal pressure in Norwegian coldblooded trotter racehorses. Equine Vet J 2009;41:59–64.
58. Poncet PA, Montavon S, Gaillard C, et al. A preliminary report on the possible genetic basis of laryngeal hemiplegia. Equine Vet J 1989;21:137–8.
59. Dixon PM, McGorum BC, Railton DI, et al. Long-term survey of laryngoplasty and ventriculocordectomy in an older, mixed-breed population of 200 horses. Part 2: Owners' assessment of the value of surgery. Equine Vet J 2003;35: 397–401.

60. Ohnesorge B, Deegen E, Miesner K, et al. Laryngeal hemiplegia in Warmblood horses – a study of stallions, mares and their offspring. Zentralbl Veterinärmed A 1993;40:134–54.
61. Miesner K. Untersuchung über die abduktorische Funktionsstörung des Kehlkopfes beim Pferd: Genetische und umweltbedingte Einflussfaktoren sowie mögliche züchterische Massnahmen. Thesis of the Agricultural Faculty of the Friedrich-Wilhelms University, Bonn, Germany, 1996.
62. Dupuis MC, Zhang Z, Druet T, et al. Results of a haplotype-based GWAS for recurrent laryngeal neuropathy in the horse. Mamm Genome 2011;22:613–20.
63. Bayly WM, Grant BD, Breeze RG. Arterial blood gas tension and acid base balance during exercise in horses with pharyngeal lymphoid hyperplasia. Equine Vet J 1984;16:435–8.
64. Williams JW, Meagher DM, Pascoe JR, et al. Upper airway function during maximal exercise in horses with obstructive upper airway lesions. Effect of surgical treatment. Vet Surg 1990;19:142–7.
65. Bayly WM, Slocombe RF. Airflow mechanics in models of equine obstructive airway disease under conditions simulating exercise. Res Vet Sci 1997;62:205–11.
66. Couëtil LL, Rosenthal FS, DeNicola DB, et al. Clinical signs, evaluation of bronchoalveolar lavage fluid, and assessment of pulmonary function in horses with inflammatory respiratory disease. Am J Vet Res 2001;62:538–46.
67. Richard EA, Fortier GD, Denoix J-M, et al. Influence of subclinical inflammatory airway disease on equine respiratory function evaluated by impulse oscillometry. Equine Vet J 2009;41:384–9.
68. Robinson NE, Derksen FJ, Olszewski MA, et al. The pathogenesis of chronic obstructive pulmonary disease of horses. Br Vet J 1996;152:283–306.
69. Gerber V, Robinson NE, Luethi S, et al. Airway inflammation and mucus in two age groups of asymptomatic well-performing sport horses. Equine Vet J 2003;35:491–5.
70. Widmer A, Doherr MG, Tessier C, et al. Association of increased tracheal mucus accumulation with poor willingness to perform in show jumpers and dressage horses. Vet J 2009;182:430–5.
71. Young LE, Rogers K, Wood JL. Heart murmurs and valvular regurgitation in Thoroughbred racehorses: Epidemiology and associations with athletic performance. J Vet Intern Med 2008;22:418–26.
72. Verdegaal LJMM, Voorhout G, van Loon G, et al. Herzgeräusche als zufallsbefunde bei tierärtztlichen kauf- oder verfassungsuntersuchungen – Befundung und verlauf bei 77 klinisch gesunden pferden. Pferdeheilkunde 2002;18:263–72.
73. Barbesgaard L, Buhl R, Meldgaard C. Prevalence of exercise-associated arrhythmias in normal performing dressage horses. Equine Vet J 2010;42:202–7.
74. Young LE. Equine athletes: The equine athlete's heart and racing success. Exp Physiol 2003;88:659–63.
75. Else RW, Holmes JR. Pathological changes in atrial fibrillation in the horse. Equine Vet J 1971;3:56–64.

Veterinary aspects of training and racing endurance horses

52

Céline Robert

CHAPTER CONTENTS

Overview of the sport

Endurance riding is a competition to test the competitor's ability to safely manage the stamina and fitness of the horse over an endurance course in a competition against the track, the distance, the climate, the terrain and the clock.[1] Endurance is the fastest-growing FEI discipline. The worldwide increase in endurance riding has brought many veterinarians into contact with this equestrian discipline. The trend of faster speeds associated with less technically demanding competitions in international events in comparison to national events is well recognized.[2] This translates into much harder training of the horses than 15 years ago.

History and evolution

The origin of endurance is related to the historical needs of men to communicate and transfer information from one place to another in minimum time. Postal services in Europe and America illustrate this view of the history of endurance. The example of the famous Pony Express, a 1900-mile route, which connected St. Joseph (Missouri) to Sacramento (California), announced the beginnings of the discipline. As horses used to be the main form of transportation, it was natural to seek a horse that was fit and healthy and had the predisposition to long distances. American and European cavalry used endurance tests as part of their military training, as horses had to be fast and robust to travel long distances and conquer territories. The first endurance competitions occurred during the 19th century in Europe, Australia and the USA. Race conditions were very different from those we know today and the health of animals on arrival were not at all taken into account. In the 1900s, horses were still used in military activities that involved endurance exercise, notably the Brussels Ostend military raid of 1902, run over 132 km at 19 km/h average speed. The sport developed during the second part of the 20th century, with the famous 100-mile (160 km) Tevis Cup Ride that has been run every year since 1955, and the Florac race that was created in 1975 in France. In 1982 the FEI approved Endurance Riding as an official discipline and gradually the number of rides increased. In 1998, the World Championships were held in the United Arab Emirates (UAE). Thanks to the sponsorship of the UAE National Federation, 47 national federations came from all over the world to compete.[3] The sport has subsequently undergone tremendous growth internationally. Over the past 12 years, endurance has been the fastest-growing FEI discipline, with 879 international events held in 2010 as opposed to just 63 in 1999 (Fig. 52.1). One event can have several classes, which have specific criteria, such as distance and whether only young riders (aged ≤21 years) are allowed to participate.

An ongoing study[4] using the FEI database revealed that in 2008 there were 7017 starters at FEI rides of ≥100 km distance. Horses from nine countries, selected based on the anecdotally high number of endurance rides/riders and/or their tradition in endurance riding (Australia, France, Italy, South Africa, Spain, UAE, UK, Uruguay and USA), represented 61.7% of all starters. The greatest number of entries was recorded in the UAE (1497 in total), followed by France (1029) and Spain (408). The mean number of entries per class varied between 10.3 (South Africa) and 71.3 (UAE).

Endurance has developed into an extreme sport with longer distances traveled at higher average speeds. The horses are getting faster and lap times are decreasing rapidly. As an example, American rider Valerie Kanavy won the 1998 World Endurance Championships in Dubai, covering the 160-km course in 9:00:07 (h:min:s); her average speed of 17.77 km/h was a record at that time. The current world record was set in Abu Dhabi, UAE, in 2010. The 160 km were ridden in 6:21:12 (h:min:s) hours at an average speed of 25.18 km/h, which includes speeds during the race of up to 38 km/h.

Description of the sport

Typically, endurance rides are composed of both short-distance competitions (20–60 km) and long-distance competitions ranging from 80 to 480 km. Single day events are the most common (usually 40–160 km). FEI-recognized endurance rides must be over 80 km. For traditional 160-km races like Florac, the track stretches out over fresh ground and, while helping maintain the interest of the horses throughout, this presents a significant logistical challenge to the support crews and officials. In modern rides, the track often follows a 'clover-leaf' in which the loops return to a central base during the course of the race. Endurance events differ greatly from place to place, as the local topography determines whether it's 160 km of flat sand (Dubai), steep hills and deep canyon descents (Tevis Cup,

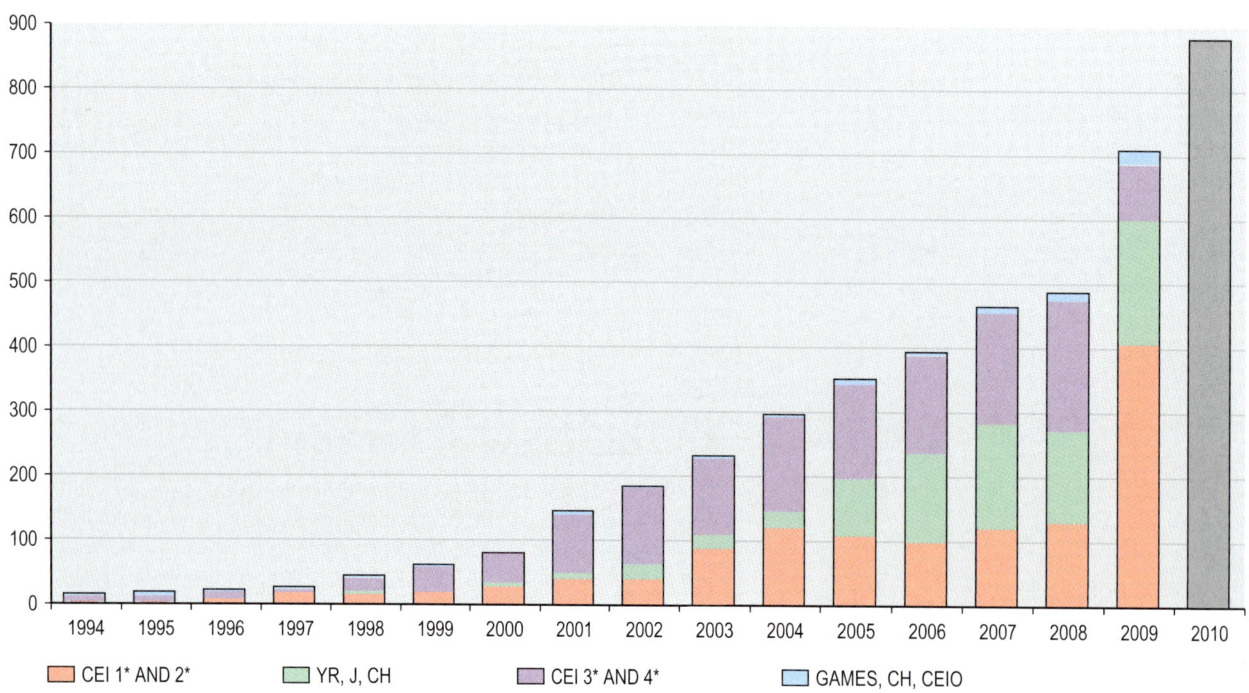

Fig 52.1 Evolution of the number of FEI-recognized endurance events since 1994.
Courtesy of www.fei.org

USA), miles of rolling hills (Newmarket, UK) or trails through forest (Compiègne, France).

The suitability of pure Arabians and Arabian crosses is well recognized for long-distance aerobic exercise. However, most endurance rides are open to horses of other breeds and in FEI Endurance Rules, any member of the Genus *Equus* counts as a 'horse'.[1] In a recent study[5], some breeds including Appaloosas, Missouri Fox Trotters, Tennessee Walking Horses, Quarter Horses, and Thoroughbreds, were all considered to be at higher risk for metabolic elimination, compared with Arabians. Previous studies[6,7] have found physiologic differences between Arabians and other breeds during race training. Arabians tend to be smaller and much thinner than their larger, more muscled Thoroughbred racing counterparts; they have a lower body mass index than Appaloosas and Quarter Horses; these factors likely favor thermoregulation during endurance exercise.

In endurance competition, the emphasis is placed on the horse finishing in good condition, rather than who finishes first. This explains the stringent rules with regards to veterinary checks throughout the race. The competition consists of a number of sections known as 'phases'. According to FEI rules, no phase may exceed 40 km and should, in principle, be not less than 20 km in length. At the end of each phase, there will be a compulsory halt for veterinary inspection. These halts are operated by establishing a vet gate with an inspection area that the competitors enter with the horse when they decide that the horse is ready to pass the veterinary inspection. However, before the scheduled presentation time has elapsed, the horse must demonstrate its fitness to continue which is assessed upon three criteria: pulse recovery, metabolic stability and gait. The time spent at each vet-gate prior to inspection by the vets is counted as part of the overall competition time and the aim is to determine whether the horse is fit to continue the ride. Veterinary inspection is followed by a compulsory rest period, or hold time that varies between 30 and 60 minutes, depending on the number of phases and length of the ride. An endurance ride is a competition against the clock. The combination that finishes the course in the shortest time will be classified as the winner of the competition after successfully completing all final Veterinary Inspections.[1]

The International Endurance Rides are divided into CEI (Concours de Raid d'Endurance International) and CEIO (Concours de Raid d'Endurance International Officiel). They are governed by the General Regulations, the Veterinary Regulations of the FEI and the rules for endurance events.[1] CEIs are divided into four different star levels. Characteristics of each type of CEI are described in Table 52.1.

Veterinarians and officials for endurance events

Unlike other equine disciplines, many veterinarians are present in endurance events. The Veterinary Commission has absolute control on all matters concerning horse safety, health and welfare. The Veterinary Commission is appointed by organizing committees; it is composed of a President of the Veterinary Commission, a Foreign Veterinary Delegate (for FEI-sanctioned endurance rides) and members whose number depends on the level of the race and the number of starters. One or more treating veterinarians are in attendance to provide emergency care at the event. Team Veterinarians are appointed by their national federation and are responsible for the health and welfare of team horses and, if requested, of individual competitor's horses. Individual competitor's private veterinarians can assume any function in the care of private competitors' horses. Finally, testing veterinarians are specifically responsible for carrying out medication control in certain geographical areas.[8]

The Veterinary Commission works in coordination with other officials. The Ground Jury will supervise all arrangements made by the Organizing Committee for the judging, veterinary control and timekeeping of the competition. The Technical Delegate must, in coordination with the Organizing Committee, check and approve, in advance, the layout of the course, the technical and administrative arrangements for the conduct of the event, for the examinations and inspections of horses, for the accommodation of horses and riders and for the stewarding of the event. He will supervise the briefing(s) and the conduct of all technical personnel. The Chief Steward is responsible for the organization of stewarding throughout the event.[1]

Veterinary controls

A series of veterinary inspections and examinations are established in the interest of the health, safety and welfare of the horse in the competition. Only competitors whose horses have passed all the inspections and examinations are entitled to be classified in the final list of results.

Table 52.1 Characteristics of the four levels of International Endurance Rides defined by the FEI

	1 STAR	2 STAR	3 STAR	4 STAR
Distance	80–119 km in 1 day	120–139 km in 1 day 70 km and 89 km over two days	140–160 km in 1 day 90–100 km over 2 days 70–80 km over 3 days or more	160 km in 1 day for Senior Chps 120–130 km in 1 day Junior and Young Rider Chps
Maximum heart rate at vet-gate	64 bpm within 20 minutes			
Maximum heart rate at final inspection	64 bpm within 30 minutes			
Horse age	at least 6 years	at least 6 years	at least 7 years	at least 8 years
Mandatory rest for horses	20 days			

Chps = Championship, bpm = beats per minute.

The first examination aims to establish the horses' identity (passports, registration documents, etc.) and to evaluate the general health of the horse, and in particular, to identify any contagious conditions. For most races, this examination is coupled with the first inspection that usually takes place on the day preceding the start of the competition.[8]

At the end of each phase, veterinary examination is conducted according to the same standards from the beginning of the ride to final inspection. It includes evaluation of heart rate, respiratory system, mucous membranes, gut sounds, soreness, lacerations or wounds, shoes and feet, gait and range of motion. Horses with abnormally high pulse rates, or pulse rates higher than the parameters defined in the schedule will not be allowed to continue in the competition (Table 52.1). Abnormalities in rate or character of breathing of such a nature as to endanger the safety of the horse, generally poor condition or abnormally high temperature will be cause for elimination. Any abnormal heart sounds, evidence of soreness, lacerations and wounds in the mouth, on the limbs and on the body, including girth and saddle galls, must be recorded. If participation in or continuation of the competition is bound to seriously aggravate any injury, the horse will not be allowed to continue. A recent study that evaluated performance and health indicators during a 160-km ride (elimination vs success) in 48 horses confirmed that this standardized veterinary examination allowed veterinarians to detect metabolically compromised horses.[9] At any inspection during the course, a horse with an irregularity of gait, which must be consistently observable through evaluation by trotting the horse on a loose lead in hand straight out and back, without prior flexion or deep palpation, will be removed from competition. An individual veterinary card issued before the first inspection is to be completed after each inspection.

If after passing the horse the examining veterinarian retains concerns about the horse's continuing ability, he may ask a competitor to present his horse for re-inspection during its hold time and 15 minutes prior to departure. This rule is in place to provide the benefit of the doubt for the opportunity to continue to the horse. When it is expected that the race is difficult (long distance, terrain, weather conditions), the Veterinary Commission, in consultation with the Ground Jury, may require horses to be presented for a compulsory recovery inspection at the last vet-gate, up to 15 minutes before that competitor's scheduled departure time from the vet-gate.

Physiology of endurance exercise

Metabolism

Endurance is an exercise at a moderate speed, over the long term.[10,11] The energy required for the effort mainly results from aerobic metabolism of fatty acids and glycogen in slow-twitch and intermediate contraction muscle fibers.[10] Aerobic capacity of a horse can increase with training, but is also influenced by breed; it seems to be lower in Andalusian when compared to Arabian and Anglo-Arabian horses.[12,13] Beyond a certain speed, there will be an increase in anaerobic metabolism.[10] This speed varies between 18 and 36 km/h depending on the horses and its state of physical conditioning.[11]

Thermoregulation

Endurance exercise leads to the generation of considerable intramuscular heat. Only about 20–25% of the energy expended by muscle metabolism is converted into mechanical work while the remaining 75–80% is dissipated as heat.[11,14–16] Horses competing in endurance rides produce a metabolic heat load that could raise core body temperature by 15°C/hour if mechanisms of heat dissipation did not exist.[17] Since core temperature increases only 1–3°C during the course of several hours ride,[14] it is clear that the majority of metabolic heat produced is dissipated.

Intramuscular heat must be shed to the external environment via shifts from muscle toward the skin with peripheral vasodilatation and increased skin temperature. The skin is then cooled by convection (wind currents), radiation (to a limited extent), and especially by the evaporation. In horses, heat dissipation occurs primarily by the production and evaporation of large volumes of sweat (65%), followed by respiratory evaporation (25%).[18,19] Sweat production has been estimated to reach 10 to 15 L/hour in endurance horses run at 16 km/h, but sweating rates may be up to 50% greater (and total sweat production may be 100% greater) when horses are exercised under hot and humid conditions.[18] Field studies of endurance rides have shown body mass losses (a reasonable reflection of fluid losses) ranging from 3 to 7% at the end of 80–160-km rides.[20,21]

Electrolyte losses

It is well known that equine sweat is hypertonic with respect to plasma osmolarity. Sweat contains relatively low levels of calcium, magnesium and phosphate but relatively high levels of sodium, potassium and chloride.[18] Sodium concentrations in sweat and plasma are equivalent.[10,22] In response to dehydration, Na^+ ions are reabsorbed in the kidney in exchange for K and H^+ ions. However, with substantial loss of Na^+ homeostasis is disturbed and the circulatory system is affected. This can be responsible for a decrease in blood pressure and increased capillary refill time and heart rate.[10] K^+ losses in sweat are very high; they are worsened by the mechanisms of renal sodium reabsorption. In addition, during the race, due to the elevation of blood cortisol levels related to stress, loss of K^+ in sweat and urine is increased. The loss of Cl^- ions in the sweat is the sum of losses in Na^+ and Cl^-. Cl^- is normally the primary ion reabsorbed by the kidneys. When the Cl^- concentration decreases, bicarbonate ions (HCO_3^-) are reabsorbed to maintain the anion gap within its normal range.[15] Calcium and magnesium contents in the sweat are greater than that of plasma. Sweating losses therefore can contribute to hypocalcemia and hypomagnesemia.

The practice of electrolyte administration by owners has significantly changed over the last 10-20 years; these practices may affect biochemical derangements currently identified on rides. Decreases in plasma $[Na^+]$, $[K^+]$, $[Cl^-]$ and $[Ca^{++}]$ are usually described at the end of the ride as compared with pre-ride values.[17,20,21,23] The magnitude of the fluid and electrolyte losses appears to be more marked in exhausted than in successful endurance horses.[24,25] Increasing speed, the presence of muddy terrain and increasing temperature contribute significantly to ion losses during endurance rides.[22,25]

Acid–base disorders

The endurance horse rarely develops metabolic acidosis. Aerobic metabolism associated with a moderate effort over the long term does not lead to a substantial increase in lactic acid levels nor a decrease in pH.[14] However, because of thermoregulatory mechanisms, the endurance horse may develop both metabolic and respiratory alkalosis.[15] In an attempt to maintain normal anion gap during exercise, bicarbonate is retained when potassium is unavailable for sodium exchange in the distal tubule, resulting in a metabolic alkalosis.[16,26,27] The increased respiratory effort to dissipate heat with concomitant loss of carbon dioxide results in some degree of respiratory alkalosis, particularly in hot environments.[15] A recent study[28] demonstrated that endurance horses frequently develop a complex acid–base imbalance characterized by mild strong ion alkalosis (due to hypochloremia), non-volatile buffer acidosis (due to increased plasma albumin concentration) and mild compensatory respiratory acidosis.

Substrate depletion

The capacity for endurance exercise is highly dependent on the availability of substrate for the synthesis of adenosine triphosphate (ATP), the body's energy currency. The endurance horse travels at speeds that can be maintained almost entirely by aerobic metabolism, with glucose and fatty acids the primary substrates for ATP re-synthesis in muscle. Glucose is derived from the breakdown of liver and muscle glycogen and de novo synthesis of glucose in the liver. Muscle glycogen is the primary carbohydrate reserve. Muscle glycogen is initially mobilized in slow-twitch fibers, followed by fast-twitch fibers.[15] Intramuscular glycogen depletion occurs with endurance exercise in horses.[29,30] Once glycogen has been fully depleted, there is little in the way of intracellular substrate for energy production, and muscular exercise often slows or stops. Free fatty acids derived either directly from muscle triglycerides or released from adipose tissue are an important source of energy for aerobic metabolism.[10,14,26] In the context of endurance exercise, the endogenous store of triglycerides is virtually inexhaustible. Their utilization allows a sparing of muscle glycogen reserves, a reduction in lactic acid accumulation and possibly help to delay the onset of fatigue.[14]

Oxidative stress

A number of studies have reported that exhaustive endurance races induce accelerated generation of reactive oxygen species (ROS). ROS result in lipid peroxidation, which induces adverse effects on the health status and performance of horses.[31,32] Both lipid peroxidation and Ca^{++} are important contributors to cell damage caused by physical injury or ischemia. Shortly after the onset of ischemia or physical injury, the extracellular Ca^{++} concentration falls dramatically, resulting in intracellular Ca^{++} accumulation, causing activation of some Ca^{++}-dependent enzymes that may damage the DNA and cleave structural proteins within the cell. Cells can tolerate mild oxidative stress and often respond by raising their level of antioxidant defenses. However, severe oxidative stress and high concentrations of free radicals may produce serious disturbances in cellular structure and metabolism.[32]

Specific diseases

Horses participating in endurance rides must maintain healthy homeostatic mechanisms while optimizing performance. These horses perform for hours over uneven terrain, and often in less than ideal environments (hot, humid weather; cold, chilling winds; rocky, mountainous country; and deep sand or mud). Mechanical problems that must be addressed include stresses applied to muscle, tendon, ligament, and bone that can cause lameness. Metabolic problems that must be overcome include fuel substrate depletion, dehydration, excessive hyperthermia, electrolyte loss, and body pH changes that can result in metabolic disease.[33]

Prevalence

A high elimination rate from endurance rides has been a regular matter for discussion in professional and public forums; moreover, in recent years, elimination rates seem to have increased.[4] Reported elimination rates range from 10% to 60% depending on the course and speed.[5,21,23,34–37] In both national and international venues, the primary reason for elimination from endurance competition is lameness. In a study based on records of all sanctioned 2007 endurance horse competitions (40 to 160 km) in the USA, the overall elimination proportion for the number of starts in the study was 18.9% (660/3493), with 147 horses eliminated for metabolic reasons and 312 horses eliminated for lameness.[5]

The largest and most recent study, based on 2008 FEI records for 9 countries from the 5 continents, confirms these tendencies.[4] Data for 4326 endurance ride starters were collected, of which 1991 finished the ride (46.0%). The most common reason for not completing the ride was elimination (45.9%), although 8.1% of all started horses were retired. The highest completion rates were recorded in Australia (63.9%), USA (63.6%) and South Africa (57.6%). There were 3 countries where fewer horses completed the ride than were eliminated: the UAE (34.1%), Uruguay (46.3%) and UK (43.2%). In agreement with results of previous studies,[38] lameness was the most frequent cause of elimination in all countries: eliminations for lameness represented 69.2% of all eliminations (31.8% of all entered horses). Eliminations for metabolic reasons accounted for 23.5% of all eliminations (10.8% of the starters). The ratio between elimination for lameness and metabolic reasons varied between countries, but lameness was at least twice as common as other reasons for elimination in all countries.[4]

Prevention and risk factors

While several epidemiological studies have been published investigating risk factors for wastage and/or injuries in Thoroughbred racehorses, there are few data available for endurance horses. The frequency of medical problems encountered in endurance events depends mainly on the temperature and humidity on race day. Under temperate conditions, medical problems are infrequent and represent about 20 to 25% of eliminations.[38] When the temperature exceeds 25 °C and humidity 70%, metabolic disorders may account for more than half of the causes of elimination. Multivariable analyzes performed on the 2008 FEI data revealed that the risk of elimination due to lameness or for metabolic reasons was significantly associated with country.[4] Several countries had increased risk for horses being eliminated for metabolic reasons compared with Australia, where the lowest elimination rate for metabolic reasons was recorded. If the number of entries was ≥80, then horses were at an increased risk of elimination for lameness ($OR = 1.60$, $P = 0.002$) than in rides where the number of entries was <80. The number of entries in the ride was also significantly associated with the risk of elimination due to metabolic reasons. No evidence was found for a significant effect of distance on elimination for either lameness or metabolic reasons.

AERC records from the ride year 2007 showed that the overall ride distance was associated with increased risk of elimination.[5] An interesting finding in that study was that abnormalities in capillary refill time, overall impression by the veterinarian, and gastrointestinal sounds prior to the start of competition were all associated with failure during the ride. Abnormalities in gait prior to the start of the ride were not identified as a risk factor for lameness elimination (or other type of elimination).

The welfare of endurance horses depends on the knowledge and skill of their riders and is protected through evaluation of horses by veterinarians before, during, and after these events. The philosophy of veterinary inspections is to pull any horse showing several signs of fatigue, but to let a horse with inconsistent lameness continue.[39] The cardiac recovery index used in the vet gates as a supplementary examination during the last phases of a ride; this method is useful for the early recognition of metabolic problems.[36,39,40] Equine welfare is further protected by standards set by the FEI. These standards include requiring horses to be fully mature before they are allowed to compete, requiring that horses be 'fit to continue' at all veterinary examination points, and requiring that horses not be under the influence of drugs or other performance-enhancing modalities during competition.[33]

Metabolic conditions

Pathophysiology and prevalence

Although musculoskeletal injuries may occur at any point along an endurance ride event, the most pressing emergency situations generally involve metabolic problems. Endurance rides combine a lengthy duration of continuous exercise with resultant loss of body fluids and electrolytes. Coupling this with additional demands placed on these horses from speed, challenging terrain, and possible adverse weather conditions, the most prevalent metabolic concerns fall under the umbrella of a complex known as exhausted horse syndrome (EHS). The fluid and electrolyte losses in EHS result in decreased fluid volume and increased blood viscosity, which can lead to inadequate tissue perfusion (Fig. 52.2). Renal hypoperfusion coupled with the adverse effects of circulating myoglobin (due to muscle injury) may lead to impaired renal function and occasionally to renal shutdown. Decreased substrate availability in muscle may lead to tying-up.[41] Decreased intestinal perfusion may contribute to, malabsorption of orally administered fluids and sometimes diarrhea. Fluid loss from diarrhea and endotoxemia may further compound the problem of dehydration, shock, and laminitis. Conversely, impaction of the large colon or caecum may occur due to the severity of the dehydration and the mobilization of water reserves from the colon in an attempt to maintain circulating blood volume.[15,16] The distal limbs may be most susceptible to the combined effects of dehydration and initiation of intravascular coagulation, leading to the development of laminitis. Substantial electrolyte losses may also promote neuromuscular irritability, with spontaneous muscular activity (muscle fasciculation), heart arrhythmias and synchronous diaphragmatic flutter.[15,16,42] Dehydration also compounds the problem of heat retention, because the horse has less extracellular fluid available to circulate heat to the skin surface and to make sweat in order to lose heat by evaporation[16], thus exacerbating the problem of overheating in exhausted horses.[15,41] In summary, a sick horse may be affected with myositis, synchronous diaphragmatic flutter, colic, and heat stress or prostration, and also has the potential to develop laminitis.[43] There are all degrees of metabolic compromise, ranging from very mild and barely detectable to extremely serious and life threatening. Dehydration can be severe enough to lead to hypovolemic and circulatory shock, resulting in a cascade of pathophysiologic events which may be irreversible, despite all attempts at therapy.[15]

There is little information available on the specific types of metabolic problems (and their outcomes). A recent study on 30 cases identified during the 2005 and 2006 Tevis Cup rides reported colic (40%), poor recovery (23%), myopathy (23%), synchronous diaphragmatic flutter (10%) and choke (3%).[44] In a study on 16 of the 20 CEI** and CEI*** events held in France in 2003, the proportion of horses requiring treatment varied between 4.2 and 16.4% depending on the ride.[45] On average 10.5% of the competitors received medical treatment for metabolic reasons. Metabolic eliminations and the need for treatment were more frequent in the latter stages of races (from the 3rd vet-check, e.g. 90 to 100 km). Of a total of 105 horses treated for metabolic disorders, diagnoses were dehydration and poor recovery (30.5%), colic (20.0%), exhaustion (15.2%), myopathy (19.0%), synchronous diaphragmatic flutter (7.6%), laminitis (4.8%) and heat exhaustion (2.9%). About two-thirds of treated cases were considered of mild or moderate severity. However, the other ones (corresponding to 3% of the competitors) were rated as marked or severe and potentially detrimental to the horse's athletic career.[45]

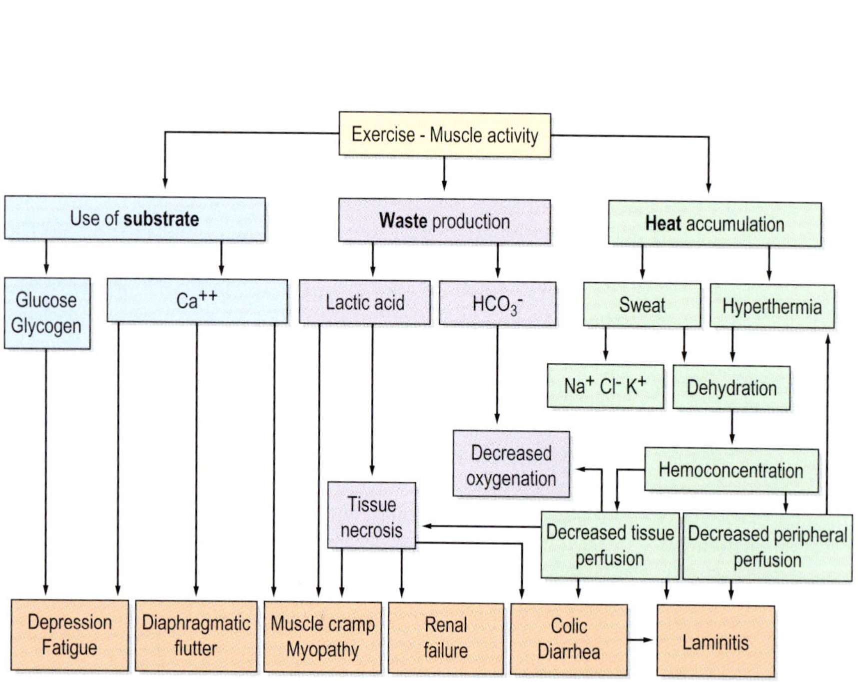

Fig 52.2 Schematic drawing of the possible succession of events leading to metabolic conditions of the endurance horse.

Exhausted horse syndrome (EHS)

Exhaustion is due to the compound effects of dehydration, electrolyte imbalances, heat accumulation, energy depletion and acid-base imbalance (i.e. base excess and alkalosis).[41,46,47] The onset or development of endurance fatigue is particularly sensitive to the effects of increased ambient heat and humidity.[15]

A horse at the initial stages of EHS may exhibit very subtle indications of any or all of the following signs: unstable heart rate, lack of impulsion, lack of attentiveness, lack of interest in food and water, glassiness of the eyes, increased skin tenting retention, increased jugular refill time, absent borborygmi, concentrated or absent urine.[41] A poor cardiac recovery (i.e. pulse fails to return toward normal after the cessation of exercise) should always alert the clinician to the possibility of EHS. One or more of the following clinical signs may be present: persistently elevated pulse (>60 beats/min after 30 min rest)[19] and respiratory (>40 breaths/min after 30 min rest) rates[19], depression, complete anorexia, unwillingness to continue exercise, elevated temperature, delayed capillary refill time and/or pale or marginated mucous membrane color, decreased pulse pressure and jugular distensibility, minimal but quite concentrated urine, dry feces.[15,19,43,46,47] Further signs may be atonic bowel, dilated anus, occasional colic, cardiac irregularities, muscle cramps with or without associated lameness, and synchronous diaphragmatic flutter.[15,43,46] Other less common signs include atrial fibrillation, diarrhea, rhabdomyolysis, recumbency and laminitis.[41]

Exhausted horses usually show a high degree of dehydration, with high packed cell volume, total protein, albumin and creatinine values, which could indicate a failure of compensatory fluid shift from the intracellular compartment in response to severe dehydration.[24,25,47] Hematology usually reveals increased RBC count, stress neutrophilia and lymphopenia. Most serum electrolytes are decreased (K^+, Cl^-, Ca^{++}, Mg^{++} and sometimes Na^+). Other changes include elevated CK, AST and LDH from muscular origin. However, electrolyte disturbances and laboatory evidence of muscle damage tend to be mild and do not necessarily aid in delineating sick horses from successfully completing horses.[25,44]

Diagnosis is based on the horse's history, clinical signs and laboratory findings. The most difficult task regarding EHS is recognition of the earliest stage of the condition. A severe case is easy to diagnose, but the goal of the endurance ride control veterinarian is to intervene in an impending EHS case while allowing well-adapted horses to continue performing. A hallmark of EHS is the horse's inability to replace fluid and electrolyte deficits by voluntary consumption of feed and water. Careful observation is essential in identifying the progression of clinical signs in horses that require aggressive therapy from those horses eating and drinking, which may equilibrate with non-invasive supportive care.[41] Treatment is based on replacing fluid, electolyte and substrate and returning the horse to a state of adaptative equilibrium (see below 'General considerations'). EHS usually responds to prompt vigorous treatment, but also can lead to death due to renal failure (especially if it is treated with customary doses of NSAIDs), hypovolemic shock, pulmonary edema, disseminated intravascular coagulation, diarrhea, or laminitis.[15,47]

Occasionally endurance horses will develop a post-exhaustion syndrome, which can be fatal. On the ride these horses show excessive fatigue and delayed recovery.[46] The condition of these horses seems to stabilize after treatment and they are generally permitted to depart. At home, they may remain, however, depressed and have little appetite. At presentation a few days later, they are severely depressed, weak, stiff, and reluctant to move. Clinical signs described above are still present: increased pulse and respiratory rates, dehydration, diminished gastrointestinal motility, and sometimes cardiac irregularities and/or severe, rapidly progressive laminitis. Major serum chemistry abnormalities are usually seen. The most consistent findings are elevated creatinine, bilirubin, liver (γGT) and muscle enzymes (CPK and AST) and marked hypochloremia and hypokalemia. Many of these horses die despite intensive supportive care.[46]

Synchronous diaphragmatic flutter (SDF)

SDF, commonly known as 'thumps', is the synchronous contraction of the diaphragm with the heart beat. This condition has been reported in horses with gastrointestinal disease, sepsis, lactation tetany, blister beetle toxicosis, endurance exercise, hypoparathyroidism, and alkalosis.[48]

Normally, half the blood calcium exists in the ionized, active form, while the other half is protein bound. Exercising horses can develop a state of alkalosis from hyperventilation,[48] massive chloride ion loss caused by prolonged sweating or inappropriate bicarbonate administration.[49] Alkalosis can result in hydrogen ion shifts and exposure of negative charges on serum protein molecules, which subsequently bind Ca^{++} and Mg^{++} resulting in a relative ionized hypocalcemia and hypomagnesemia with normal total Ca and total Mg values.[27,48,49] Lack of calcium allows sodium to diffuse spontaneously into the nerves, increasing nervous irritability and resulting in involuntary muscle contraction and fasciculation. Depolarization of the right atrium stimulates action potentials in the hyperexcitable phrenic nerve as it crosses over the heart.[48] This action will cause the diaphragm to contract, resulting in the abdominal muscles contracting in synchrony with the heart rate.[15,16,27]

SDF often occurs following a rest stop because, if the horse is rehydrated without electrolyte intake, the fluid replenishment further dilutes Ca^{++} and K^+ and exacerbates alkalosis. SDF is recognized by a twitching or convulsive motion in the flank area, almost like a hiccup, either unilaterally or bilaterally.[15] This abnormal diaphragmatic activity is in unison with the heart rate and not the respiratory rate.[15,27] Careful observation is necessary for appropriate diagnosis in the horse with an elevated respiratory rate as the horse recovers from exercise.[15] Other physical parameters may be within acceptable limits or the condition may occur as part and parcel to the exhaustion syndrome.[27] Blood analysis usually reveals low Ca^{++} values. In a recent study,[32] comparing blood values measured before the start of the race and at the 90-km check point in 9 horses eliminated for SDF and 9 finishers, there were no significant differences detected between the two groups for Na^+, K^+ and Cl^- concentrations whereas ionized calcium values were lower and lactate concentrations higher in SDF-eliminated horses. The increase in lipid peroxides and malondialdehyde between pre- and post-exercise values was also greater in SDF eliminated horses.[32]

The condition may resolve spontaneously with rest[50] or after the correction of electrolyte and acid–base imbalance and rehydration.[49] If the bowel is functional, treatment involves administration of oral fluids containing calcium and potassium.[27] Parenteral administration of balanced non-alkalizing fluids with calcium gluconate often speeds recovery.[27,50,51] However, hypocalcemic patients with concurrent hypomagnesemia are often refractory to calcium therapy unless the low serum magnesium concentrations are identified and corrected.[49] Intravenous administration of magnesium (as $MgSO_4$)[49] and dextrose-containing solutions[51] may therefore be necessary.

SDF is generally transient and not a life-threatening condition, but does indicate a metabolic imbalance, which if allowed to progress, may become dangerous. The development of SDF at any point in an endurance ride is ample reason for not allowing a horse to continue. Occasionally hypocalcemia causes tetany. The clinical signs of tetany are variable and may include stiff stilted gait, hindlimb ataxia, muscle fasciculation, trismus, dysphagia, salivation, anxiety, profuse sweating, tachycardia, cardiac dysrythmias, elevated body temperature, and in extreme situations convulsions, coma and death.

SDF is a recurrent problem in some horses.[51] Preventative measures should include electrolyte supplementation during the course of the event. Horses prone to development of SDF should have their dietary ratio of calcium and phosphorus adjusted around 1:2.[27] This adjustment precludes the feeding of alfalfa or other legume hay as the Ca/P ratio is deviated from the ideal depending on quality.[27,51] Some horses with chronic recurring SDF may have alterations of the phrenic nerve. Injury or scar tissue subsequent to pneumonia or pleuritis is a potential but unproven cause of refractory cases of SDF.[51] Anecdotally, osteopathic manipulations have also been reported to reduce the occurrence of SDF in some horses; in these cases, low cervical vertebral lesions or instabilities might be suspected.

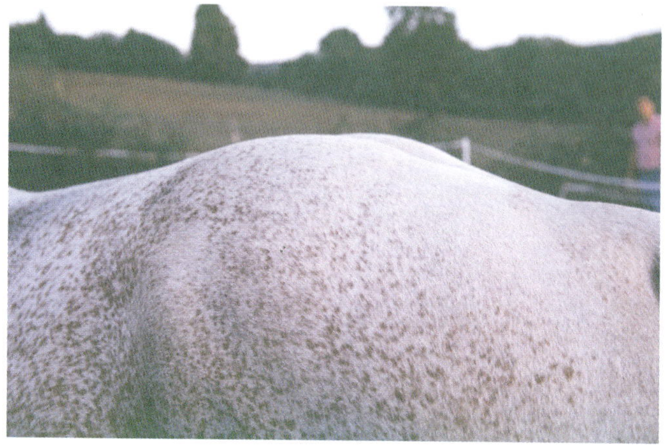

Fig 52.3 Typical appearance of the gluteal region in an endurance horse with myositis. The deformation usually appears within a few hours after the beginning of fluid therapy.

Exertional myopathy

Endurance horses appear to develop exertional myopathies (EM) in two circumstances: early after the start of the race (type A), or further into the race in conjunction with exhaustion (type B).[52] Type A myopathy usually occurs within the 5–20 minutes following commencement of exercise. EM is well documented in Thoroughbred and Standardbred racehorses, and often is associated with anxiety or improper feeding management.[2] Certain Arabian family lines also seem to be predisposed to recurrent EM. Polysaccharide storage disease has been anecdotally reported in Arabian horses.[52] Metabolic myopathy (type B) develops later in the ride, in conjunction with exhaustion due to electrolyte abnormalities, glycogen depletion, etc.,[14] and possibly compounded by abnormal muscle recruitment patterns that represent compensation for a newly developed unilateral lameness.[15] Exercise over difficult terrain and under cool, damp conditions also predisposes animals to EM.

Clinical findings vary from simple muscle soreness to paralytic myoglobinuria.[46] Affected horses are generally anxious, in pain, and exhibit tachycardia and tachypnea, reluctance to move, and gait abnormalities ranging from stiffness and shortened stride to significant lameness and recumbency.[14,53] Localized or more diffuse muscle cramping, hardening, stiffened, pain on palpation, and focal sweating are characteristic of exertional myopathy.[15] Muscle spasms may occur but are not consistently found.[46] Hindlimb and lumbar muscles are the most commonly affected (Fig. 52.3), but forearm or pectoral muscles may also be involved.[2,50] Myoglobinuria is observed in moderate to severe cases. The diagnosis of EM is based on clinical signs of muscle stiffness and pain after exercise in conjunction with elevations in serum creatine kinase (CK) and aspartate transaminase (AST) activities. The degree of elevation of muscle enzymes in serum is dependent on the severity of muscle damage as well as the length of time that has elapsed between the sample collection and the occurrence of muscle damage.[53] However, pain and muscle swelling are not associated with CK activities; in a recent study on 22 horses that successfully completed a 160-km ride, there was no concentration difference between finishers and non-finishers.[37]

Affected horses must be stopped and treated to relieve anxiety and muscle pain and replace fluid and electrolyte losses.[2,53] Severe rhabdomyolysis can lead to renal compromise because of the ischemic and combined nephrotoxic effects of myoglobinuria, dehydration, and non-steroidal anti-inflammatory drugs (NSAIDs). In mildly dehydrated horses, provision of free-choice electrolytes and water or administration of fluids through a nasogastric tube may be adequate. Horses with moderate to severe dehydration require IV administration of balanced polyionic electrolyte solutions. Hyperkalemia can occur with severe EM, necessitating the use of isotonic sodium chloride. If hypocalcemia is present, supplementation with calcium borogluconate is recommended.[53] In severely affected animals, regular monitoring of serum creatinine is advised to assess the extent of renal damage.

Tranquilizers such as acepromazine, xylazine, or detomidine with or without butorphanol provide excellent sedation and analgesia, and are safer compared to high doses of NSAIDs, considering the likelihood of significant concurrent dehydration.[2] Doses of flunixin meglumine and other toxic NSAIDs should be minimized in the face of dehydration. For severely affected horses, IV dimethyl sulfoxide (as a $<20\%$ solution) may be used as an antioxidant, anti-inflammatory agent, and osmotic diuretic;[53] in these horses, the administration of Dantrium (dantrolene sodium; 2–4 mg/kg orally) may also decrease muscle contractures and possibly prevent further muscle necrosis.

Horses that have had EM may recover without any further muscle problem. Others may have muscle fibrosis and loss of muscle mass, leading to gait abnormalities and disfigurement.[50] In severe cases the myocardium may be affected also with potentially life-threatening consequences.[16] EM is a syndrome with many causes.[53] Finding ways to reduce stress is recommended to help decrease episodes of myopathy in susceptible horses. Modification of diet and training regimens can also decrease the likelihood of recurrence. A nutritionally balanced diet with appropriate caloric intake and adequate vitamins and minerals are recommended (see Feeding management).

Colic

Although ileus has been hypothesized as the most likely cause for colic in endurance horses, gastric ulcerations and impaction have also been implicated.[54,55] In a retrospective study on 36 horses presented for colic within 48 h of an endurance ride in two equine referral centers in the USA, a diagnosis of open or ileus was made in the majority of horses (56%). During exercise there is re-distribution of blood flow away from abdominal viscera to the muscles and skin.[16,56] Reasons for ileus may include electrolyte derangements, dehydration leading to decreased intestinal perfusion and other unknown factors.[55] Exercise has also been shown to result in increased intra-abdominal pressure in horses which was postulated to have a role in the development of gastric squamous mucosal ulcers.[56] In one study of endurance horses, gastroscopy was performed after the horses completed 50-km and 80-km rides.[54] Twenty-seven percent of the horses had bleeding of the gastric glandular mucosa after the competition, a prevalence that is higher than in most other endoscopic reports on horses. The inference was that the gastric glandular mucosal bleeding may have been a sequel to the strenuous endurance rides. *Salmonella* infection may also represent a significant cause of colic in endurance horses.[55] In the study presented above, salmonellosis and enteritis (*Salmonella* negative) were recognized in 16% of the patients.

Most endurance horses with signs of colic during or post-ride have decreased gastrointestinal sounds on presentation. Abdominal ultrasonographic examination can be performed to identify signs consistent with exercise-induced ileus: distended and non-motile small intestine with a normal wall thickness.[46] Amounts of gastric reflux can be substantial.[55] As such, it is imperative that nasogastric reflux is checked in all endurance horses with colic.[47] Rectal examination has to be performed to minimize risk of rectal tearing that may be increased due to dehydration. Rectal examination usually reveals only hard and dry manure, sometimes distended intestine or nothing remarkable. Surgical lesions are uncommon despite significant abdominal pain,[44] and therefore medical management appears a viable option in most cases.[55]

Endurance horses pose unique challenges as they often have severe derangements of hydration and electrolyte parameters that may be related to the competition and not necessarily to the cause of colic.[55] Large amounts of IV fluids may be required to replace ongoing losses and deficits. If colic signs continue or recur, assessment for gastric reflux should be repeated because the volume of intestinal fluids can increase once the horse is rehydrated.[47] Usual medical treatment includes IV sedatives (detomidine or xylazine, butorphanol) and flunixin meglumine. Depending on race location and conditions, horses will receive treatment in the field or be presented to referral hospital for emergency medical care; in some cases hospitalization may be prolonged. However, colic in endurance horses appears to have an excellent prognosis. In the retrospective study on 36 horses presented in two equine referral centers, all horses survived but one.[55]

Metabolic encephalopathy

Central nervous system disorders can accompany metabolic disturbances in endurance horses. The exact origin of these disorders is unknown: hyperthermia, hypocalcemia, hyperammonemia, hypoglycemia and hyponatremia have been suspected. In a small case series of horses that developed neurologic abnormalities at the end of a CEI3*, all horses had shown discrete signs of poor performance on the loop prior to the onset of the problem: reduced speed on the track and increased recovery time at vet-gate presentation.[57]

Heat stroke occurs when the normal thermoregulatory processes fail. It is accompanied by clinically apparent disturbances in water and electrolyte balance and clotting mechanisms. The pulse becomes weak, with congested mucous membranes[19] and the horse shows signs of restlessness, dullness and incoordination.[46] It may be agitated and become violent or ataxic and collapse.[19] Respiratory rate can be elevated above the heart rate.[19]

Hyperammonemia-associated encephalopathy is usually secondary to intestinal disease or dysfunction.[58] The hypothesis is that an excessive production and absorption of ammonia associated with intestinal overgrowth of ammonia-producing bacteria would overwhelm normal liver metabolism causing ammonia toxicity and the encephalopathic signs.

Hypocalcemia frequently develops in endurance horses (see above) and commonly associated with SDF. Horses with hypocalcemia may also present other neuromuscular disorders (twitching, convulsions) and ataxia.

Sodium disorders, either hyponatremia or hypernatremia, may cause neurologic disorders in the horse; hyponatremia is the most frequent and may occur in adult horses with diarrhea or renal failure.[58] The origin of hyponatremia in endurance horses is hypotonic rehydration. Hypernatremia has been observed following oral electrolyte supplementation (equivalent to 180 g of NaCl and 60 g of KCl in a 450-kg horse) on an 80-km endurance ride.[59]

Severe hypoglycemia is rare in adult horses.[58] Endurance horses may develop during the ride following substrate depletion. The drop in blood glucose is probably gradual and rarely causes specific clinical signs.[57] However, hypoglycemia may contribute to signs of central nervous system abnormalities.[47]

Horses with metabolic encephalopathy show signs of disorientation, head pressing, blindness, depression or agitation, reduced consciousness, SDF, ataxia, muscle fasciculation, and sometimes seizures. Diagnosis is based on blood analysis investigating dehydration, electrolytes, acid–base balance, glucose and ammonia concentrations.

Initially, steps should be be taken to prevent further injury either to the horse or the public. The horse should be moved away from the vet-gate area. Sedation may be required in order to control propulsive walking or seizures (xylazine, detomidine, diazepam). A dosage that calms the horse but does not cause excessive lowering of the head is ideal, since lowering of the head might promote cerebral edema.[58] Subsequent treatment should be directed at correction of dehydration via IV administration of crystalloid fluids with added KCl (40 mEq/L) and calcium borogluconate. Hypertonic NaCl will more quickly reestablish intravascular volume than will an isotonic crystalloid; it will also help reduce neuronal cytotoxic edema and improve brain perfusion.[58] Other treatments may include diazepam or phenobarbital to control seizures,[47] corticosteroids, DMSO, diuretics, and 10% dextrose to correct hypoglycemia. Horses with central nervous signs may benefit from oxygen therapy. It is important to monitor serum electrolyte concentrations, acid–base status, glucose concentration and to correct any imbalances.[47]

Approximately half of affected horses are better within 12 hours with intensive care; major blood changes can persist for a few days. Some horses may become comatose and have a very guarded prognosis. Out of the four cases investigated one was euthanized, the three others recovered but only one continued his career in endurance races.[57]

Laminitis

The pathogenesis of laminitis associated with endurance exercise has yet to be clearly defined as is the case for the laminitis that develops in other circumstances.[60,61] Concussive exercise on hard ground at speed may result in physical tearing and deterioration of the laminae attachment of the hoof wall to the pedal bone within the hoof capsule (often referred historically as 'road founder'). Alternatively, the combined effects of dehydration, endotoxemia and intravascular coagulation in the distal limbs may contribute to the development of a form of 'metabolic' laminitis. Recent theories consider laminitis concomitant with other tissue inflammation as a good example of 'remote organ dysfunction' after a systemic inflammatory response.[61]

A survey among French endurance veterinarians in 2007 documented 16 cases of laminitis following 90- to 160-km endurance races.[62] All cases were observed in warm and humid conditions, supporting the hypothesis of an involvement of dehydration and metabolic disturbances in the development of laminitis. The ground conditions were hard or very hard (13/14), which favors a road founder component too. The proportions of horses from Arabian lineage (100%), of geldings (75%) and coated or fat horses (56%) were higher than those currently observed in French endurance horses.[45]

Laminitis can be observed in horses that finish the race (12/16 horses in the above study), but more often starts with reluctance to progress on the last loop and signs of fatigue leading to elimination at final vet examination (8/12). Prodromal signs usually appear within a few hours after competition (on average 13 h after the race [0–48 h] in the above study), i.e. earlier than the 24 to 60 hours of development reported for experimental models of laminitis.[63] However, delayed onset of laminitis up to 1 week after the ride has been observed. Laminitis may affect either all four feet or only the forelimbs. In the above study, laminitis affecting the forelimbs was diagnosed earlier (on average 8 h) than laminitis affecting the four feet (on average 19 h). Most cases were graded 3 (7/15) or 4 (5/15) on the Obel scale.

The challenge lies in the recognition of subtle clinical signs and the rapid implementation of a treatment to prevent disease progression. In the earliest stages, horses typically stand still, sometimes with a 'leaning back on the heels' stance; they are reluctant to move and exhibit a shortened stride. Horses also exhibit non-specific signs of metabolic disturbance: elevated heart rate, dehydration and reduced or absent gut sounds. The diagnosis of laminitis is based on the palpation of heat within the foot, increased digital pulse amplitude and localization of pain with hoof testers. Very rarely subsolar hematoma formation can cause acute lameness that mimics acute laminitis.[2]

Proactive measures aimed at preventing laminitis should be considered in all high-risk horses. Any horse that begins to shift weight or show signs of discomfort should be treated.[2,64] Distal limb cryotherapy has been demonstrated to be clinically and experimentally beneficial when initiated prior to or at the beginning of the prodromal stage of laminitis.[61] Medical therapy is aimed at preventing, limiting progression and reversing the underlying pathophysiological processes and controlling pain.[60] As for other metabolic problems in endurance horses, the priority is to correct water and electrolyte disorders using fluid therapy before administration of NSAIDs or acepromazine. Flunixin meglumine (0.25 mg/kg IV), phenylbutazone (2.2 to 4.4 mg/kg twice daily), acepromazine (0.025 mg/kg IM four times daily) and DMSO (1 g/kg IV diluted to 10% solution once or twice daily) are routinely used in various combinations.[64] Heparin may be used to both treat coagulopathy and prevent thrombus formation as well as for its anti-inflammatory properties; low-molecular-weight heparin is preferred as it does not cause equine RBC autoagglutination and has been reported to reduce the incidence and severity of laminitis in postoperative colic cases.[61] Acepromazine is the only drug demonstrated to increase digital blood flow in normal horses and can be used in treatment of the vascular component of laminitis. Other supportive care measures such as providing a deep bedding or sole/frog support are of course valuable in endurance horses.

The prognosis for horses with acute laminitis varies with the severity of the initial disease and the ensuing progression of lamellar injury, displacement of the distal phalanx, and distortion of the hoof capsule.[60] Horses without rotation or sinking are generally able to return to endurance competition. In the above study half the affected horses raced again, on average 13 months later.[62] Horses affected in all 4 feet were at five times increased risk ($P < 0.05$) to retire or to be subjected to euthanasia than horses affected in the forelimbs only.

General management of metabolic conditions

Emergency veterinary treatment is often required for endurance horses that have been removed from competition for metabolic derangements. Much of the treatment care of an endurance horse occurs in the 'field' with limited facilities or supplies,[43] but in some cases a horse must be shipped to a referral hospital for intensive and/or follow-up care or surgery. The organizing committee and the President of the Veterinary Commission must plan in advance for the management of sick horses. This includes the designation of a treatment veterinarian, provision of material and fluids in sufficient amounts, and arrangements with an equine referral facility with surgical capabilities. For high-level events, triage and emergency treatment facilities must be provided on site.[8]

Immediate care must include stopping exercise to minimize further damage. If the horse stops on the track, the trailer should be moved as close to the horse as possible rather than moving the horse to the trailer. In hot weather, the horse should be placed in the shade and cooled externally with large volumes of cold water over its entire body. If it is a cool day, the horse should be kept blanketed.

Correction of fluid and electrolyte disorders

Administration of fluids should be the first line of therapy and should precede the use of NSAIDs or phenothiazine-related tranquilizers. The latter have a vasodilatory effect and should not be used in dehydrated, fatigued horses.[65] Large volumes of intravenous fluids are necessary to restore fluid deficits and electrolyte balance.[43] Use of an aseptically placed intravenous jugular catheter (12-gauge) is recommended.[15,47] Both veins should be used in severely dehydrated horses.[19] The electrolyte deficits possible in an exhausted horse are enormous; there may be a salt deficit of 350 g. Therefore, the correction of dehydration should primary emphasize saline plus potassium replacement and secondarily emphasize the replacement of calcium, magnesium and glucose.[41] Sodium chloride or lactated Ringers solution (LRS) are suitable although NaCl may be preferred due to its acidifying properties. However, except in the severely compromised patients, it is suspected that the volume of mixed electrolyte solution administered is more important than its acidifying/alkalinizing nature.[15,41,47] Dextrose may be added to the fluids (to make a 5% dextrose solution) as an energy source if the horse is anorexic, hypoglycemic, or has neurologic signs.[47]

Controversy exists about the use of hypertonic solutions (HSS) in horses with dehydration.[47] The concern is that these animals may have clinically relevant intracellular fluids deficits and therefore should not be treated with a hyperosmotic agent. In a recent study, Fielding and Magdesian enrolled 22 horses disqualified for metabolic conditions at the 2009 Tevis Cup.[66a] Horses were separated into two groups. The group HSS received an initial bolus of 2 L of 7.2% NaCl solution and 5 L of LRS with 250 mL of 23% calcium gluconate solution simultaneously followed by additional LRS as deemed necessary by the treating veterinarian. The other group received LRS but not 7.5% NaCl. There was a greater increase in sodium and chloride concentrations in the HSS group and a larger decrease in PCV, TP, and albumin, which supports a greater expansion of plasma volume. A faster onset of urine production with HSS was observed, which could indicate improved renal perfusion. It was concluded that the administration for HSS appears to be safe in the treatment of endurance horses. However, it is extremely important that HSS administration is followed by either isotonic or hypotonic fluids.

Administration of fluids should be continued until reversal of clinical signs. Normally, once the fluid and electrolyte imbalances have been corrected, the other disorders (e.g. anorexia, colic, SDF) will resolve. Initial treatment usually includes rapid (30 to 40 ml/kg/h) infusion of 10 to 15 L of LRSS.[50] This is often sufficient to improve a horse's overall condition such that it will begin to eat and drink and further restore losses. However, some horses require 60 to 80 L LRS over 6–12 hours post-exercise.[16,47] The 22 horses enrolled in the above study[66b] received on average 20 L fluids. It is possible that overzealous fluid administration could lead to pulmonary or intestinal edema and this could have an effect on the development or persistence of intestinal ileus.

Oral fluid therapy may be considered in mildly affected patients. Fluids may be administered via nasogastric tube if the horse has normal gut sounds and no clinical evidence of colic.[43] The oral route has many advantages: large volumes can be given rapidly, they do not need to be sterile, and exact isotonicity is not required; and potassium and calcium can be given orally in large amounts without fear of cardiac or other complications.[43] Isotonic mixed electrolyte solutions may be administered at a rate of 4–8 L every 30–60 minutes.[19,46]

Sedation and pain control

Additional medical measures should also be taken to promote intestinal motility, renal function to manage pain, to counter possible endotoxemia, and to minimize the risk of laminitis. NSAIDs may be administered if the horse is in pain due to myopathy, laminitis or colic. However, NSAIDs should always be used cautiously as they may cause significant renal compromise in a hypovolaemic horse.[46,65] The dosages of NSAIDs should be reduced according to the degree of dehydration (Table 52.2); a prudent starting point is half or less of the usual recommended dosage.[41] Flunixin meglumine, which counters some of the effects of endotoxemia, may be beneficial. Corticosteroids may be indicated in horses with shock and possible pulmonary edema. It must be remembered that they may exacerbate impending laminitis.[15] If sedation is required, xylazine or detomidine should be considered.[46]

Table 52.2 Criteria for dehydration evaluation in endurance horses[46,50]

LEVEL OF DEHYDRATION	BODY WEIGHT LOSS	CLINICAL SIGNS
Mild	5–7%	Decreased urine output Dry mouth and mucous membranes Slight decrease in skin elasticity
Moderate	8–10%	Marked loss of skin elasticity Sunken eyes Weakness Increased heart rate, weak pulse
Marked	>10%	Profound depression Cold extremities Capillary refill time > 3 s Feces dry or absent Marked electrolyte disorders

Prognosis

The prognosis for horses requiring emergency veterinary treatment after being removed from endurance competition for metabolic reason appears to be good.[44] In a study on 100 horses treated for metabolic problems at 16 CEI events in France,[45] the average time until clinical improvement was two hours with recovery by 4.5 hours. Most horses (85%) were fully recovered by the following morning. Horses that develop metabolic problems should not be transported home until at least 24–48 hours after they have stabilized and treatment has stopped.[15] Moreover, any horse requiring intensive treatment at any CEI events must be given a mandatory rest period of 60 days before it is again eligible to participate in a CEI event.[1] Rest and restricted feed should be continued for several days, after which the horse can be slowly brought onto grain depending on its daily activity.

Arriving at an endurance competition with a horse that is truly fit and ready to compete is the best way to prevent exhaustion.[15] Providing a sufficient recovery time after transportation and before the race will help minimize travel-related dehydration and muscle fatigue. Adequate acclimatization is also necessary if the climate for competition is quite different from the horse's home climate. Finally, each rider must learn to be aware of how his horse feels underneath him to recognize early signs of fatigue and stop exercise before exhaustion.[15]

Musculoskeletal disorders

Lameness is by far the most common indication for elimination from endurance competition. Many causes of lameness in endurance athletes are transient, leading to elimination from competition on ride day, but resolving after rest with or without treatment. Often, the exact cause of lameness in these situations is not specifically determined as veterinary examination at vet-gates is not intended to accurately diagnose the cause of lameness (Fig. 52.4). Recurrent problems or significant acute injuries are more likely to result in a full diagnostic and therapeutic approach similar to that performed for any other sport horse.

Endurance horses suffer from lameness caused by proximal suspensory desmitis, which is by far the most common cause of unsoundness, followed by concussive foot problems and chronic osteoarthritis of the distal joints. Causes of lameness tend to vary somewhat in ranking from season to season and from one country to another. As the sport evolves, new types and incidence of injuries, more akin to those seen in flat racing, are being seen in endurance horses. In the Gulf countries, fractures related to stress pathology are increasingly diagnosed, the most common being localized to the metacarpophalangeal joint, but also in the humerus, pelvis and scapula.[2]

Injuries of the suspensory apparatus and its insertions

Suspensory ligament (SL) desmitis occurs most commonly on the forelimbs, affecting both the proximal area and branches. However, SL desmitis also occurs in the hindlimbs. The causes of SL desmitis

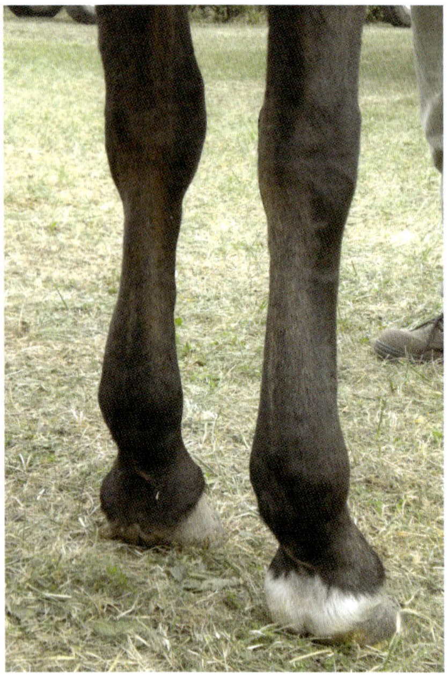

Fig 52.4 Swelling in the region of tendons and fetlock 12 hours after a 120-km endurance race.

likely relates to the requirement of horses to work in loose ground – the deep sand doesn't offer a steady support to the hooves during the landing phase – and also gallop at high speed on hard ground. On uneven terrain, any medial/lateral hoof imbalance would also predispose endurance horses to suspensory branch desmitis.[2]

Desmitis of the SL typically develops as an acute, often severe, traumatic injury in the later stages of the race when the horse becomes fatigued, but may occur in the earlier stages of a race in an unfit horse or a horse that had previous SL injury. It is also a common training injury.[64] Lameness may be sudden and severe or be more insidious in onset.[64] The diagnosis is based on palpation of the limb and is confirmed by ultrasonography. With branch lesions, usually one branch is affected; therefore, notable swelling may be evident on palpation compared to the opposite branch or leg.[2] In contrast, lesions of the proximal suspensory or body may be less obvious, and diagnosis is based on sensitivity to palpation, ultrasound and sometimes nerve blocks.[2,64] Proximal SL desmitis is characterized by loss of echogenicity of the dorsal-most fibers immediately distal to the carpometacarpal joint. Combining the use of diagnostic analgesia and ultrasonographic comparison between limbs can be helpful in determining the relevance of a lesion.[64] However there is often little correlation between ultrasonographic appearance of the SL, response to analgesia, ability to return to training, and incidence of recurrent lameness.

Treatment of an acute injury is based on NSAIDs after rehydration, ice therapy and bandage support. Misheff recommends extracorporeal shock wave therapy, rest, ensuring good foot balance, and a controlled rehabilitation and exercise program.[64] Ideally, activity should be limited to hand walking until no lameness is apparent at trot in hand on a hard surface, followed by a controlled and gradual increase in exercise with repeated ultrasonographic evaluations. The shoes used at return to training should have a wide toe and wide branch but narrow heels. In practice, riders will often let the horse rehabilitate at pasture until the following season. Clinical and ultrasonographic evaluations are necessary before a return to training. Local infiltration with corticosteroids may also be used. Newer treatment modalities used in other sport or race horses such as intraligamentous injection of platelet-rich plasma, autologous stem cells derived from fat or bone marrow, or surgical splitting or fasciotomy have not been evaluated in endurance horses.

Prognosis for return to function and rest period duration vary with clinical signs and lesion size. They are guided by improvement in lameness and ultrasonographic evaluation. Even if lameness with transient soreness and pain on palpation resolves without further problems, it can take 3–12 months rest and controlled activity before returning to normal training. Although other sport horses may be able to return to training sooner, elite endurance horses are not able to quickly recover and require a considerably longer period.[64] SL desmitis often occurs in conjunction with pathology of the fetlock joint, which must be managed simultaneously.

Tendonitis

Superficial digital flexor tendonitis (SDFT) is a common cause of lameness in endurance horses, especially in the forelimb. Deep digital flexor tendonitis (DDFT) occurs less commonly than SDFT, but appears to have a predilection for the hindlimb in endurance horses.[2] Conformation of Arabian horses with short tendons and high heels may be a predisposing factor. Slipping on the trail or poorly fitting limb protectors that become malpositioned during the ride can potentially result in SDFT. However, the causes for flexor tendonitis are more likely to be found in increasing speeds in both training and racing.

The acute form with obvious deformation and swelling may be observed at veterinary control points, the morning after the ride or after a hard training session. More subtle training injuries, wherein the SDFT may be warm and tender on palpation, occur relatively frequently. Lameness is often not apparent. Diagnosis is based on repeated ultrasonography, the ultrasonographic appearance of the tendon being often worse eight days after injury than it is initially.[64]

Endurance horses that sustain tendon injuries in training or competition are managed similarly to any athletic horse. As for other soft-tissue injuries, early ice therapy and NSAIDs after rehydration are warranted to reduce swelling and inflammation and to relieve pain. Rest duration, rehabilitation and prognosis depend on lesion severity and location. Surgical splitting of tendons with central core lesions, autogenous liquid bone marrow injection of split SDFT, and intralesional stem cells or platelet-rich plasma may be beneficial, but whether these therapies are more beneficial than rest alone is uncertain.[64]

Horses that sustain a rupture or partial rupture of the superficial digital flexor tendon have a poor prognosis for return to endurance competition. Horses with transient heat and tenderness but no swelling or fiber damage can usually be safely returned to training within 2–4 weeks after the resolution of clinical signs.[64] If the tendon is enlarged or if fiber separation has occurred, a substantially longer absence from training and competition is required. Endurance horses with SDFT have traditionally had a better prognosis for return to competition than horses that race over short distances at higher speeds.

Joint diseases and injury

Chronic osteoarthritis of the fetlock and hock are common in endurance horses. In a survey on 58 high-level endurance horses presented for pre-purchase examination, 30 and 12 horses showed radiographic changes in the front fetlock and distal part of the tarsus, respectively.[66b]

Osteoarthritis (OA) of the metacarpophalangeal (MCP) and metatarsophalangeal (MTP) joints and periarticular pathology are related to the chronic wear and tear associated with training and competing, and the fact that endurance horses may compete for several years.[64] Slipping on the trail can potentially result in soft-tissue injury of any joint, but especially the fetlock. Interference injury, especially of the medial part of the fetlock of the hindlimb, is common and, occasionally, lameness can result. The condition may be of sudden onset, in the evening or the day after the ride, or more chronic, resulting in intermittent lameness in training. Joint effusion associated with chronic or acute synovitis may be present, most often bilaterally. Front fetlocks are primarily affected. Flexion reveals pain and decreased range of motion. Clinical signs usually resolve after a few days of rest. However, synovitis will result in pain and intolerance to prolonged exercise. Diagnosis relies on radiography, intra-articular analgesia, ultrasonography or MRI. Radiological changes vary from very subtle to more obvious peri-articular modeling with osteophytes. Almost all endurance horses over 10 years of age have radiographic signs of fetlock joint disease. Ultrasonography may reveal hypertrophy of the dorsal synovial pads, thickening of the joint capsule, joint effusion, reduced cartilage thickness and other soft-tissue lesions. Management of fetlock OA in endurance horses is similar to that of any other athletic horse and may involve local therapy, judicious use of intra-articular corticosteroids and hyaluronan, rest periods and intravenous hyaluronan.[64] Horses should be shod with aluminum alloy in order to reduce show weight. Prognosis is guarded as fetlock OA is often responsible for recurrent lameness leading to repeated eliminations at vet controls.

OA of the distal tarsal joints usually affects both tarsometatarsal and intertarsal joints and is often bilateral, with one limb more affected than the other. Affected horses are positive to hindlimb flexion. Radiological signs typically include joint space narrowing and osteophyte formation but do not always correlate with clinical signs.[64] Tolerance of OA of the distal tarsal joints varies with horses. Even if it does not cause lameness in some horses, it may be responsible for recurrent myositis by compensatory phenomenon. Distal hock joint pain frequently occurs concurrently with paravertebral muscle pain and sore front feet: the 'terrible triad'. The best results are obtained when all three problems are treated simultaneously.[64] Intra-articular medication may be used in lame horses.

OA of the proximal or distal interphalangeal joint is generally poorly tolerated in the endurance horse and is rarely observed in high-level horses. In the aforementioned study of prepurchase radiographic files, only minor lesions were observed in four horses, a lower incidence when compared to a population of jumping horses.[66b] Palmar foot pain is less common in Arabian and Arabian crossbreeds than in larger breeds, but it does occur and can be an important cause of lameness. All forms of navicular disease can be observed in endurance horses.

Polysynovitis

Polysynovitis, defined as non-septic inflammation in two or more joints, can develop during or just at the end of the ride. Affected horses show effusion in several joints, most often the carpus, fetlocks, tarsus or stifle. The horse is reluctant to move and initial clinical signs may mimic laminitis; in addition, the two disorders may occur together with polysynovitis preceding the onset of laminitis. Prognosis is good except when the condition is complicated by laminitis. Clinical signs disappear within 24 hours with correction of metabolic disorders and NSAIDs treatment.

Foot-related injuries

Problems with the feet are a frequent cause of elimination from endurance competitions, as well as being a common cause of chronic or recurrent pain.[64] They are more regularly seen in the forelimb. Many lameness eliminations related to the feet are transient in nature: foot bruising, heel bulb trauma from overreaching, dislodged or sprung shoe.

Sole bruises are a common problem in horses traveling over hard ground.[14,64] This type of injury can be noticed after a certain distance of the trail has been covered. Horses show a bilateral lameness manifested as a shortened choppy gait. Lameness is often more pronounced on one limb. Application of a hoof tester around the solar margins of the foot elicits a painful response. Radiological abnormalities include loss of bone opacity at the margin of the distal phalanx and increased size and number of vascular channels.[64] Distal interphalangeal joint synovitis may occur concurrently. Management is aimed at protecting the solar margins and reducing concussion with the use of full padded shoes.[14]

Inflammation of the coronary band (coronitis) is frequently observed in the 24 hours after competition. It may be focal (usually dorsal) or all the way around and is usually painful on palpation. This usually does not progress to typical laminitis. The outer layer of hoof wall may peel away from the coronary band, but the horse is not lame, and there is no rotation of sinking of the distal phalanx. The episode is marked by a distinct defect in the hoof wall that usually grows out without further incident.[64]

Fractures

As endurance competition speeds have increased, musculoskeletal injuries that previously were thought to be more common to flat-racing horses are now seen in endurance horses. Thus, there is a growing number of fractures occurring during training and riding, especially in the Gulf countries. In the 2007–2008 season, the risk of fatal fracture in endurance horses was similar to that reported for flat racing. Although racing and training at lower speeds than Thoroughbred flat-race horses, endurance horses are at risk of exercise-associated bone pathology because of the long distances covered, some of which is completed at high speed.[2,65]

In the study of Misheff et al.,[65] from a total of 38 horses with 41 fractures, almost 75% of fractures involved either the proximal phalanx (mainly complete fractures) or third mecarpal/tarsal bone (lateral condylar fractures predominating). Fractures of the biaxial palmar eminence of the second phalanx, radius, humerus, scapular, third trochanter of the femur, ilium, and ischium were also recorded.

Most often, horses show acute, marked lameness during or shortly after training rides or races and diagnosis is is often confirmed at the venue by use of radiography. However, non-displaced fractures may not be diagnosed until several days after the fracture occurred. Radial, humeral or scapular fractures may result in chronic mild to moderate lameness and are diagnosed scintigraphically. The most unique pathology of endurance horses is bilateral forelimb fractures, which are often initially confused with back/pelvic injuries or acute laminitis.[65] That is why the bone on the contralateral limb should always be radiographed.

Depending on the severity of the fracture, but also on owner/trainer's preference, treatment may consist of surgical fixation with lag screw, casting only, or stable rest only, and sometimes euthanasia. Attending veterinarians at endurance rides should be prepared to provide appropriate stabilization in order to optimize chances for successful repair, e.g. splint materials should be available at endurance races. It is also important to not focus exclusively on the musculoskeletal injury because affected horses also may have metabolic compromise. If depleted, circulating fluid volume should be restored with fluid therapy prior to or simultaneous with the administration of NSAIDs. Before surgery, horses should be stabilized metabolically. In the case of non-displaced fractures, surgery may be performed the following day after overnight treatment with IV fluids.[65]

The prognosis for the horse to return to racing seems more guarded than the same injury in other disciplines. In the study of Misheff et al.,[65] of the 38 affected horses, 14 had raced again and two others were back in training. There seems to be a trend toward a lower number of individuals returning to their former level of athletic competition. The reasons for this are probably multifactorial and include the fact that in some cases a decision was made to retire the horse. A second factor is the presence of other areas of musculoskeletal pathology distant to the fracture site.

Back and wither injuries

Muscle pain affecting the back and skin sensitivity of the saddle and girth regions are common in endurance horses. They are likely related to rider imbalance or poor saddle fit. Additionally, compensatory back pain may develop secondary to lameness. These problems usually appear with more intense training and are often related to work overload. A horse that has strained or injured the paravertebral muscles appears stiff or rigid rather than lame, and instead of flexing and extending the spine normally when palpated, the horse tends to stiffen, squat, or crouch.[64] During the race, back injuries may lead to elimination during veterinary inspections. Treatment consists of removing the inciting cause when possible and reducing inflammation. Most horses respond to 2 weeks of reduced exercise in conjunction with NSAIDs and pulsed muscle massage. Injection of the paravertebral muscles with an anti-inflammatory agent can also be beneficial.

Nutrition and prophylactic measures

Sound nutritional management is crucial for optimal endurance exercise performance and prevention of metabolic problems. This includes consideration of diet composition, maintenance of optimal body condition, and strategies for provision of feed, electrolytes and water on race day.

Energy and protein requirements

As for all horses engaged in regular athletic activity, energy requirements depend on the intensity and duration of exercise, the type of terrain, the weight of the rider and tack, the ability of the rider, the fitness of the horse, and environmental conditions. Another consideration is the effect of the energy sources on substrate storage (particularly liver and muscle glycogen) and the ability to utilize fat during exercise.[67,68] Survey data from riders of top-level endurance horses in France suggest that average daily digestible energy intake is in the range of 21 Mcal for 440-kg horses,[69] which is low compared to other breeds or previous estimations on endurance horses (31 Mcal/day).[70] From a practical viewpoint, weekly assessment of body weight and/or body condition score (BCS) is necessary to determine the appropriateness of the feeding program; upward or downward adjustments are often needed for maintenance of constant bodyweight and condition. Indeed, there is evidence that body fatness, as reflected by BCS, may influence performance in endurance races.[9,35,71] Performance of horses with a low BCS (e.g. <3) may be limited by the supply of energy from fat reserves. However, over-conditioned horses (BCS >6) would be at a disadvantage due to carriage of excess weight and the insulating effects of subcutaneous adipose tissue. In general, feeding programs for endurance horses should target a BCS of approximately 4–4.5 on the 9-point scale.[70]

The precise protein requirements for endurance exercise are unknown. In the survey on French endurance horses, the overall protein content of the diet averaged 7.2% digestible protein, but ranged from 4.8% to 10.0% depending on the type of forage offered.[72] Higher protein diets may be undesirable because of the effects of excess dietary protein on heat production, acid–base balance, water requirements and, potentially, respiratory health.[73,74] There is evidence that dietary protein level alters urea metabolism in horses and then water requirements because of the need to increase urine production for clearance of endogenous urea loads.[73] Based on these considerations, it has been recommended that endurance horses should not be fed more than 2 g of digestible protein/kg BW/day (around 3–4 g crude protein depending on the feedstuffs).[70,74] The crude protein content of an endurance horse ration should not be higher than 12%.[67]

Feeding management during endurance training

Forage should be the foundation of any ration for horses, and the endurance horse is no exception. Most endurance horses have 12- to 24-hour pasture turnout. Ideally, an endurance horse's diet must provide 75% energy from hindgut fermentation.[75] It is recommended to feed endurance horses with at least 1.0 kg forage per 100 kg[67] and preferably 1.5 to 2.0 kg per 100 kg of body weight.[70] Grass hay is preferable to legume hay because of concerns regarding the effects of a higher protein diet. In the aforementioned survey on French horses the base of the diet was good-quality meadow hay (1.9 to 2.5 kg per 100 kg BW) regardless of the intensity of work.[69,72] Thus, forage represented more than 75% [52–93%] of total dry matter intake and supplied up to the 2/3 of the daily energy requirements. Feeding a high-fiber diet, would increase gastrointestinal tract fluid volume when compared to a low-fiber diet, which may be helpful in maintenance of hydration during exercise.[76] The horse's large intestine contains a fluid volume equivalent to 8–10% of bodyweight, with 10–20% of total body sodium, potassium and chloride, and there is some evidence that a portion of this fluid can be absorbed during prolonged exercise, thereby partially offsetting sweat fluid losses. Meyer and Coenen[76] observed that the quantity of sodium in the large intestine of hay-fed ponies was more than twice that of their grain-fed counterparts, while potassium was also greater.

Some type of supplemental energy concentrate is generally needed to meet energy requirements and maintain body weight during training and competition. Cereals or commercial concentrate feeds are commonly fed. The average quantity of concentrates fed to French endurance horses in training was 2.3 kg/day, which is low when compared to the amount fed to racehorses.[69,72] For 63% of the horses, a commercial concentrate was fed. The cereal grain most commonly used, either alone or mixed with commercial feed, was rolled barley. During high-level training periods, horses tended to have a little less forage and more concentrates, even though the total amount of energy per day did not significantly vary. The concentrates are generally provided in two meals a day. In order to prevent rapid fermentation of the starch provided by concentrates, it is advisable to limit the size of individual grain-based meals to no more than 1.5 kg (for a 450-kg horse).

Provision of a fat-supplemented diet is a popular dietary strategy in endurance horses, allowing a reduction in the level of starch feeding without compromising the caloric density of the ration.[67,77] Horses adapted to a fat-supplemented diet have increased capacity for the uptake and oxidation of fatty acids in muscle[78,79] and greater flexibility in the selection of substrate to meet energy demands.[68] Thus, fat supplementation enhances lipid oxidation and spares the use of endogenous carbohydrates during exercise. In horses adapted to a higher oil diet, an association of speed with less plasma acidity and urea was found in horses competing in 80-km races.[80] This suggests that fat adaptation and dietary protein restriction may improve performance. Supplemental fat or oil diets can be supplied using either commercial, fat-supplemented feed or supplemental vegetable oils as corn or soya oils.[75] Three to four weeks to adapt to a fat diet seems to be needed to see changes occur in the metabolic profile.[78] A suggested upper limit of oil supplementation is 100 g per 100 kg bodyweight per day or 10% of the total diet.[70] However, this level of fat supplementation appears to be considerably higher than that practiced by endurance owners and trainers; approximately 58% of the surveyed horses were fed vegetable oil, with an average amount of 15 g per 100 kg of body weight (maximum 46 g/100 kg of body weight).[72]

Vitamin and mineral supplementation should be adjusted according to the ration. Insofar as the forage is the foundation of the ration, it is essential to analyze the hay to better adjust the supplementation. Antioxidant supplementation is very popular in endurance as in other disciplines. All horses, but especially those in hard work, need vitamin E and selenium.[70] It is recommended to provide vitamin E at approximately 2000 IU per day and selenium at approximately 2 mg per day for a 450-kg horse.[81,82] In the total ration, selenium should not exceed 1 mg per 100 kg of body weight per day. Additional vitamin E is required if the horse is fed a vegetable oil–supplemented diet.[70] Selenium deficiency appeared uncommon (2%) in Californian endurance horses, even in non-supplemented horses.[83]

Endurance horses in regular training will require some form of electrolyte supplementation. As the sodium and chloride content of horse feedstuffs is low, salt supplementation is required to offset losses in sweat. In contrast, potassium losses in sweat are lower and forages tend to have a high content of potassium, which makes potassium balance less of a concern. One approach is to provide horses with free access to a salt block. However, it has been shown that there is great individual variation of voluntary sodium intake from a salt block.[84] Providing supplemental loose salt in the diet rather than salt blocks, e.g. 40–60 g/day of common salt, would be a better approach. At present, there are no data to support the concept of 'electrolyte loading' by feeding supplemental electrolytes for several days prior to competition. The additional electrolytes are quickly excreted within a few hours by the kidney.[77]

Feeding management before and during endurance races

There are several considerations regarding nutritional management before, during and after endurance races. Particularly important are the timing and composition of pre-race meals and strategies for electrolyte and water replacement during rides. However, horses are animals of routine and need a long time to adapt to any change in diet; changes in the ration in the days and to a lesser extent in the weeks before the race should therefore be avoided. In the aforementioned study of French horses, dry matter intake, fat percentage of the concentrates meal, total protein supply and protein/energy ratio did not change significantly throughout the training season.[69,72] Feeding of a high glycemic meal the night before a race to increase liver glycogen stores is hazardous and may increase the risk of exertional myopathy.

There has been considerable debate about when and what should be fed horses before they are exercised. There is evidence that the timing and composition of a meal consumed before exercise can influence metabolic response in horses.[70,85] Most notably, the hyperglycemia and insulinemia associated with the digestion and absorption of grain meals affect the mix of substrates utilized during exercise. Insulin is a potent inhibitor of lipolysis and fatty acid oxidation in skeletal muscle, and also promotes glucose uptake into muscle. Thus, hyperinsulinemia at exercise onset will suppress lipid oxidation and increase reliance on carbohydrate stores for energy transduction. For horses performing endurance exercise, this acceleration in carbohydrate oxidation associated with grain feeding may result in premature fatigue following carbohydrate depletion. For this reason, it is recommended that grain or concentrate meals should not be fed later than three hours pre-race.[70] On the other hand, studies in horses have demonstrated that limited forage meals consumed 2–3 hours before exercise have minimal effect on substrate availability and oxidation during sustained exertion, although large meals consumed near the start of exercise may result in a decrease in plasma volume as a result of fluid shifts into the gastrointestinal tract.[70] Such reductions in plasma volume could compromise cardiovascular and thermoregulatory function during exercise. In general, it seems reasonable to allow the consumption of small forage meals (1–2 kg, as fed) in the 1–3 h period pre-race.[67,70] According to our observations in the French endurance team, all horses were fed hay ad libidum the day before the ride and half of them received a small meal of concentrates about 2 hours before the start of the race.[69,72]

There is no consensus on what should be fed to endurance horses during a race. However, feed consumption at rest stops is important because appetite is an indicator of overall health, and feed intake may assist in the maintenance of normal gastrointestinal motility. Furthermore, the consumed feed may support energy supply and therefore could be important in sustaining work performance during the latter stages of races when endogenous fuel reserves are depleted.[67] The epinephrine peak induced by exercise decreases meal-induced hyperinsulinemia.[75,77] Therefore, the provision of small meals (1-2 kg of concentrate) at each vet-gate should not be responsible for metabolic problems.[73,77] In general, horses are offered their normal feed, but also other feedstuffs such as cereals, carrots and snacks to stimulate the appetite. The priority is to feed palatable feedstuffs, with secondary consideration given to the nutrient composition of the feed. Plain forage and water are also offered at rest stops.

After completion of the race, water should be offered immediately and in sufficient quantity (provide several buckets for the night) to allow the horse to compensate for water loss. The evening of the event, in France, trend and recommendations go to a distribution of hay without the addition of concentrates. The aim is not to overload the digestive system subsequent to dehydration, while promoting a gradual recovery by feeding a forage-based ration. Indeed, it is not feasible to replace the incurred energy deficit during the initial 12–24 h post-race period. Most endurance horses are given only light exercise (walking or pasture) for a few weeks post-race and this, combined with a return to the normal feeding pattern, will allow for replacement of lost body mass and energy reserves.[67]

Water and electrolyte replacement during endurance races

Water and electrolyte replacement are vitally important for mitigating risk of metabolic failure associated with dehydration and electrolyte imbalances. To investigate the value of electrolyte supplementation, a study of fluid and electrolyte balance was performed in endurance horses throughout training and the racing season.[86] It was demonstrated that fluid losses were adequately balanced by water intake; however, renal reabsorption of sodium and chloride were insufficient to compensate for electrolyte losses in sweat. These findings support the probable benefit of forced electrolyte supplementation in horses during endurance competition. Sodium and chloride should be the major components of an electrolyte supplement, although calcium and magnesium would be useful. Potassium supplementation is questionable, as moderate exercise can result in hyperkalemia; potassium-containing electrolyte formulations could exacerbate the hyperkalemia and, potentially, increase risk of cardiac arrhythmias and muscle cramping.[87]

A variety of strategies have been used with no consensus on the optimal method. Options include the administration of hypertonic electrolyte pastes before and during the race, the addition of electrolytes to meals offered at rest stops, and provision of hypotonic/isotonic electrolyte solutions for voluntary consumption. The optimal level of supplementation is also not known and likely varies between horses.

Many riders will administer an initial dose of electrolytes 2–3 h pre-race, with subsequent doses given at vet-gates. Most commercially available hypertonic electrolyte pastes contain salts (disodium phosphate, KCl, sodium citrate, $MgSO_4$, $CaCl_2$, calcium gluconate, magnesium gluconate, NaCl), vitamins (ascorbate mainly), glucose or molasses and glycine. These pastes normally restore the pre-ride levels of all electrolytes, except sodium, which is lost in much larger amounts.[77] Experimental studies have shown that hypertonic supplementation contributed to the restoration of electrolyte losses[88] and resulted in attenuated weight loss after exercise due to greater voluntary water intake during and after the ride.[59,85,89] However, this type of supplementation could cause the movement of water into the intestinal lumen with exacerbation of electrolyte imbalance. Hypertonic solutions may also promote the development of gastric ulcers,[90] anorexia,[84] or neuromuscular disorders.[87]

Another option is to offer horses a dilute salt water solution for voluntary consumption. As with the use of most commercially available hypertonic pastes, typical electrolyte intakes are low when compared to losses. Nonetheless, allowing horses to drink salt water during and/or immediately after exercise appears to enhance total fluid intake during the early recovery period and attenuate weight loss during exercise.[91–93]

Regular feeding is an important factor in relation to electrolyte intake and water balance. Forage present in the gut may hold ingested water for several hours as a reserve available for absorption during the race. It should also provide an adequate reserve for potassium. However, once the race starts, the ingestion of forage is often limited. From our study of top-level endurance horses, riders enhanced electrolyte recovery via regular feeding at vet-gates and only 21% of horses had a supply of electrolytes on race day.[68] So, it is probably unnecessary, and perhaps even unwise, to attempt to replace the entire estimated electrolyte deficit during the ride via oral electrolyte supplementation, because a substantial reserve of water and electrolytes is likely available in ingesta within the large intestine.[59]

Regardless of the method of electrolyte supplementation, fresh water should be offered at frequent intervals (every 30–40 min, particularly in hot weather) and water intake must be closely monitored, particularly with use of hypertonic electrolyte pastes. The administration of hypertonic electrolyte pastes is contraindicated in horses with a poor drinking response.[67]

Prophylactic measures

Parasite prophylaxis

A regular deworming program is essential for endurance horses as most of them are maintained in small paddocks and consequently at increased risk for parasite infestation. Ideally, the control program should be based on regular fecal egg counts and also fit with the competition schedule. It is also advisable to regularly collect feces from the paddocks to reduce the risk of re-infestation. In horses selected in the French team, the first deworming occurs early in the season, on average one week after return to training, and treats tapeworm.[72] Anthelmintics are then administered about every two months during the competitive season with at least one prophylactic treatment against small strongyles. A delay of 15 days to three weeks between deworming and races is advisable in case of adverse reaction.

Gastric ulceration

High prevalence of equine gastric ulcer syndrome (EGUS) has been reported in sport and race horses, including endurance horses. A prevalence of 66.6% was observed in a population of horses examined at the end of a 50- or 80-km ride.[54] In horses involved in high-level endurance competition (90–160-km ride), Tamzali et al.[94] found a 93% prevalence of gastric squamous ulcer disease, with severity of lesions being directly related to ride distance. Prevalence and score severity were significantly lower during inter-season than during the competition season. The differences between the two studies could be the attributable to the difference in training intensity and training duration. EGUS presenting clinical signs are non-specific and include poor appetite, weight loss or simply increased post-exercise recovery time. Presumably, as in racehorses, a poor correlation exists between clinical signs and the severity of ulcerations. If diagnostic endoscopy is not possible, a therapeutic trial may be indicated. Few modifications in housing and feeding management are possible in endurance horses, as most horses already live at pasture and are fed a hay-based diet. Usual anti-ulcer therapy may be routinely used during intense training periods in predisposed horses.

Vaccination

Currently, only vaccination against equine influenza is required to compete at FEI events.[8] The influenza immunization schedule is the same for all FEI disciplines and requires the last booster to be given within six calendar months + 21 days of arrival at the FEI event, with no vaccination within seven days of arrival at the FEI event. Therefore it is important to plan vaccinations to fit in with the competition schedule. Vaccination early in the season, a few weeks before the first race, usually covers the competitive season. However, vaccination every six months is recommended.[95]

Tetanus prophylaxis is of course essential in these horses often kept in pasture and that face all types of terrain during training or competition. Vaccinations against other diseases (rhinopneumonitis for instance) are recommended as endurance horses will meet many horses during competitions. It has been shown that both innate and acquired immunity were markedly altered after a 162-km endurance ride,[96] which may predispose endurance horses to the development of bacterial and viral infections.

General management of training and riding

It can take years for the combination of horse and rider to be ready to compete in a 160-km ride. The start of training is not very different from that practiced in other equestrian disciplines. However, a specific extensive preparation is essential to address the demands of long-distance rides, especially at high speed. Proper conditioning results in several physiologic changes that aid the prevention of exhaustion. In this way, the well-being of the horse can be maintained at all times.

Preliminary steps

It is essential to consider the strong temperament of the Arabian horse at each step of its training to ensure easy learning; thus, the horse will gradually and naturally get used to the external environment, to all the constraints of the sport, and especially stress associated with long-distance competitions.[97]

Outdoor work is the basis of endurance training. It must be practiced regularly, in accordance with the maturity of the horse. Until the age of five years, the duration of each ride should be limited to one hour. It will progressively increase up to 1.5–2 hours from six years of age. During the various workouts, a heart rate between 110 and 130 beats/minute seems reasonable for most horses. Such heart rates are easily obtained at active walk on hilly terrain, which stimulates aerobic metabolism and requires the same muscle work as gallop on flat terrain with lower risk for the musculoskeletal system.[97] Trot and canter can also be used on the flat for beginners.

Basic dressage training is essential for the physical preparation of endurance horses too. Schooling aims at teaching the horse to respect the aids, bringing him into balance through stretching exercises. It will develop a specific musculature and ensure a good attitude that will enable the horse to use its entire potential.[97]

Endurance training

The gradual transition of a leisure horse into a sport horse requires both physical and physiological body adaptations. Repetitive exercise results in a multitude of changes in the body, at cellular, tissue, organ and whole-organism levels.[98] Endurance conditioning based on the aforementioned notions will ensure adequate preparation for the competition effort. Distinct structures require different time for development: muscular and cardiorespiratory capacities develop in a shorter period of conditioning than do those of tendon, ligament, and bone.[14] Endurance conditioning increases plasma volume and thus makes more circulating fluid available for production of sweat for proper thermoregulation. With increased fitness, sweating begins earlier in exercise, and sweat is more dilute in electrolytes.[18] The endurance training also promotes economies of electrolytes with lower urinary and fecal losses.[84] Conditioning horses is also responsible for changes in digestion and substrate utilization.[80,99]

Endurance conditioning results in increased number of oxidative type II fibers and intramuscular capillary density.[100,101] These changes allow more work to be performed aerobically and delay the point in time at which glycogen is utilized inefficiently via anaerobic metabolism.[15] Training is also responsible for establishing a certain level of tissue strain and developing adaptation to it. Training contributes to developing flexibility, coordination, strength, and stamina to improve movement, save energy[14] and prevent musculoskeletal injuries. Such endurance conditioning allows the horse to progress from 40- to 140-km endurance rides.[97]

Resistance and speed training

With this more specific training, the horse will be able to address longer distance up to 160 km. Resistance training cannot be carried out without risk of accident if the endurance training step has not been completed or has been poorly conducted.[97] This training step requires experience and a deep knowledge and understanding between horse and rider. Resistance training is based on sessions of gallop lasting from one to three hours. This conditioning will facilitate the mobilization of fat reserves and increase the amount of glycogen in muscle influencing the metabolic characteristics of muscle; this will help to increase the workload/running speed before onset of substantial anaerobic metabolism (i.e. delays the onset of the lactate threshold).[70] The average speed during these training sessions varies from 300 to 500 meters/minute, depending on the fitness of the horse.[97] For high-level horses and to prepare for races on flat terrain, training speeds should reach the average speed of competition. With increasing racing speeds, it is necessary to train the horse at these higher speeds by introducing short-distance accelerations. However, because the incidence and frequency of trauma increase with speed, training speed should remain under 500 meters/minute.

Standard training programs

The art of training involves the judicious use of exercise of various intensities and durations in order to induce the optimal adaptations that will permit successful competition while preventing injury or occurrence of overtraining.[95,98] Training practices that may be recommended depending on the level of competition are presented in Box 52.1. Applying such training procedures will help a horse to progress towards the highest level.[97] However, experience and excellent horse riding technique are crucial for success and repetition of performance. Any exercise program should consider both the fitness and character of the horse to prevent overtraining. Overtrained horses usually display irritability, recalcitrance to work, restlessness, poor hair coat or poor appetite with weight loss. However, for training to be effective in inducing the desired conditioning there must be a degree of 'overreaching'.[95] Overreaching refers to the performance of an activity at a sufficient intensity and duration to induce some strain in the organism. Without this strain, there will be no conditioning effect.[95]

We had the opportunity to follow the senior national team for two consecutive seasons (2009 and 2010) and study the training practices of these elite horses.[72] During winter, all except young horses were in pasture 8–24 hours/day without workout. Detraining does not affect the horse's athletic capacity, and in the elite horses, which are very busy during the racing season, it has great benefit.[14] Conditioning usually began in February, depending on weather conditions. Between March and September, all horses had daily access to paddocks. Basal activity consisted of outdoor rides at a walk for a mean duration of two hours, two to three days a week. In half of the horses, training also included sessions at trot and canter, especially for horses trained in flat regions. In the final preparation phase, before the rides and championships, specific training sessions at canter were performed by all riders every 10 days on average. After a 160-km ride, horses were given 3–6 weeks' recovery. Indeed, horses need a few days of rest and appropriate diet to replace the energy expended during an endurance competition.[14] See Box 52.1.

Box 52.1 Practical considerations for conditioning endurance horses – training program proposed by Dr Jean-Louis Leclerc, coach of the French team 2006–2010

Training young horses
Standard outdoor rides at walk, trot and canter
Duration from 40 minutes to one hour
One or two schooling sessions per week

Conditioning for 40–60-km rides
For horses five years old or more
Regular outdoor rides mainly at active walk on hilly terrain + trot and gallop on good flat terrain
Duration from 1–1.5 hours
Keep schooling sessions outside the competition period
Long workouts at a slow pace for one or several consecutive days will help the horse to deal with the notion of working duration

Conditioning for 1* (90-km) endurance rides
Regular outdoor rides mainly at active walk on hilly terrain + trot and gallop on diverse terrain
Can be replaced by trotting sessions with phases of canter in flat regions
Minimum duration of 1.5 hours
3–5 days a week
Canter sessions of 20–30 minutes' duration can be gradually introduced once a week, speed remaining below 18 km/h on good flat terrain
Four weeks and 10–15 days before competition, the canter session shall be lengthened in two phases of 30–40 minutes' duration depending on the fitness of the horse. This work is performed on good flat terrain (racetrack, beach, soft trail ...) at 18 km/h average speed and below 20 km/h. Mean heart rate shall vary between 105 and 120 bpm. Any sudden increase in heart rate must lead to reduced exercise intensity. A 15 minute rest period is allowed between the two phases to water and feed the horse, and to examine the horse (as in vet-gates) to ensure that the exercise can be continued safely.

Preparation for 2* and 3* endurance rides
Working the horse 4–5 days a week is necessary to achieve this level of performance
To be effective, training must be planned in 2–3 consecutive working days followed by one day rest
During rest days, it is preferable to walk the horse for 1–1.5 hours in order to prevent muscle injury
Daily training program is similar to that planned for 90-km rides
Duration of training sessions should be increased from 1.5 to 2 hours, but not more to avoid overtraining
Very fit horses can be trotted on hilly terrain. Short bouts of gallops may also contribute to the consolidation of the osteoarticular system
During the weeks before competition, the schedule includes a training gallop of 1 hour at an average speed of 20 km/h on good terrain. Two accelerations at 25 and 30 km/h can be performed over the last three kilometers, i.e. the last seven minutes
Two-phases canter sessions (lasting 1 and 1.5 hour twice for 2* and 3*, respectively) can be introduced before competition in the same conditions as for 1* horses
Important point: a training program is not static and must be adapted to each horse and its progress during conditioning

Shoeing the endurance horse

Lameness in long-distance horses can be significantly exacerbated by poor hoof trimming and shoeing.[14] The importance of a properly trimmed, well-balanced, well-shod foot cannot be overemphasized, and a good farrier is an integral part of a successful endurance team.[64]

Problems encountered in hoof care of endurance horses are similar to those of hacking and trail horses, with the added difficulties of speed and very high mileage.[102] Ideal endurance shoeing combines many qualities, taking into consideration both the horse and the quality of the race tracks. The shoe should be strong and durable to hold for several hundred kilometers, and optionally offer a decent grip on asphalt or grass.[103] It should also be comfortable, shock absorbing and light to limit energy wastage[102] and reduce stress placed on the distal joints.

Unbalanced feet can predispose to abnormal loading of joints, ligaments, tendons, and bones, requiring compensatory movements.[14] A latero-medial trimming that respects the limb's conformation is vital to avoid problems with collateral ligaments of the distal limb joints.[64] The strength of the sole, the bars and the frog needs to be preserved. Most endurance horses are Arabians, with average-to-small hoof sizes[102] and vertical hoof wall. However, too much heel support should be avoided, as it will increase fetlock extension on deep ground.[102] Conversely, trimming and shoeing with a long shoe and low heel can lead to direct heel trauma, as well as increased strain on the sesamoid ligaments and digital flexor tendons.[64]

A wide range of shoe types are used in endurance horses (natural balance shoe, plastic shoe, full rolling shoe, etc.) but steel or aluminum sport shoes are the most commonly used. Most of the trainers and farriers agree upon aluminum and alloys that are light enough and allow the horse's own locomotion to shape the breakover to its own needs. However in some stables the ground is too abrasive for the horses to be shoed with aluminum or alloys. The fitting of the shoes must follow the natural anatomic shape of hoof and facilitate a breakover that will help locomotion. French toe rockering improves breakover and nail pitch, while relieving sole pressure by the shoe.[102] Shoes specifically designed for endurance are now found on the market, but a steel concave shoe with quarter clips or a parabolic shoe is a typical good working compromise. Antislip cones may be necessary for races but should be avoided whenever possible[103] as they may increase the risk for joint injury.

The use of sole protection against bruises, at least on the front feet, is usually recommended, as terrain can be quite variable.[102] As for the shoes, the use of pads and other sole protections depends on the trainer and the quality of the race tracks. A very large range of pads and other protections can be found. Blue polyurethane pads have long been the most used in endurance but present low shock-absorbing characteristics.[103] New pads, combining shock-absorbing and protective properties, have been specifically designed for endurance (Fig. 52.5). Hind feet, with their more concave soles, usually can be shod without pads.[102] Necessity for the use of filling products varies with the ground. In the desert, they are an absolute must because sand always get stuck and jammed between the pads and the sole and may cause overpressure on it. The filling products must be sufficiently soft not to put pressure on the sole but should hold enough to prevent the entry of sand.[103] Filling products without pads are now available. They can be added any time, whenever it's needed without pulling the shoe off.

Due to high wear, shoeing intervals can be quite short (from 3 to 5 weeks) in endurance horses. Nailing high and into solid wall

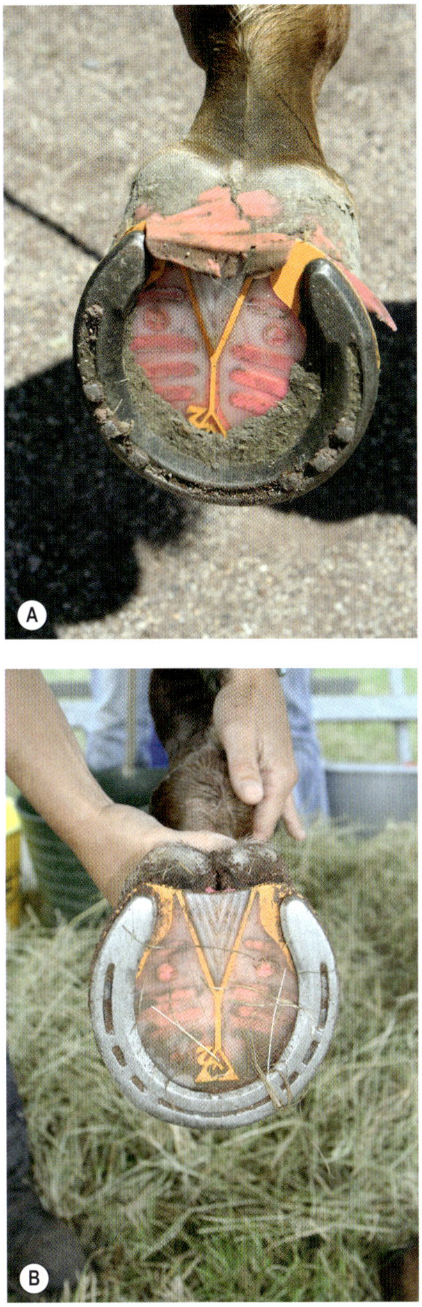

Fig 52.5 Standard shoeing in an endurance horse with alloy shoe, double density pad designed for endurance and resistant silicon packing **(A)**. Note changes in nails and shoe after the 120 km ride **(B)**.

may allow for reusing the same nail holes in the wall twice, thereby limiting the 'Swiss cheese' effect.[102] Shoeing programs must be established based on the date of the races, the last shoeing being done around 10 days before the race. Racing shoes should be relatively closely fit to decrease the risk of pulling-off as shoe loss during competition can be hard on the hoof and on the competitor's chances.[102] During the race, at each vet-gate, each shoe must be checked but not renewed if it has kept all its technical qualities. Unless damaged, the shoes should remain for the race. However, it is essential to have on-hand at least one ready-to-go spare pair of shoes in case of loss of shoe or excessive wear.

Fitness and poor performance investigation

Medical follow-up and poor-performance evaluation are commonly practiced. Major indications are poor recovery during the rides, performance lower than expected, repeated eliminations especially for metabolic reasons or evaluation of fitness level in the preparation for a special event or prepurchase examination.[104] The investigation of a poor-performing horse requires a complete and thorough evaluation of all body systems involved in exercise.[105] It begins with the collection of a detailed history. It is followed by a complete clinical medical and locomotor examination before any exercise. Common additional tests include blood sampling and upper and lower airway endoscopy with collection of respiratory samples.

Examining horses during and after exercise, either on a treadmill or in the field, is usually necessary to get a chance to identify the origin of poor performance. Thus, in a recent study of 27 endurance horses examined for loss of performance, the locomotor disturbances were not observed during the initial clinical examination, and appeared only during or at the end of the exercise.[106] Similarly, cardiac arrhythmias were detected from the continuous ECG recordings during the field test. Furthermore, suspected exercise-induced rhabdomyolysis was identified by severely increased plasma concentrations of muscular enzymes one hour after the field test in seven horses with no clinical sign of rhabdomyolysis and presenting normal CK, AST and LDH resting values.

Other additional tests may be performed according to the history of the horse, the results of pre-exercise and standardized exercise tests such as echocardiography, joint or tendon ultrasound, X-rays, gastroscopy and muscle biopsy.

Blood monitoring in endurance horses

Many blood parameters are modified by training, exercise or age and repeated blood tests are the basis of most follow-up programs. Serial samples will provide more information than a single analysis result. Some blood changes are specific to the endurance horse and must be considered.

Resting values

A low PCV, increased urea and total protein concentrations, and a high urine specific gravity are typical in horses trained for endurance.[107,108] In the follow-up of 8 horses during one endurance season, we observed that plasma urea, creatinine, TP and Na^+ concentrations increased during the first 8 weeks of training and PCV decreased during the second period of training.[86] During endurance training, re-absorption of osmotically active substances like urea and tubular conservation of electrolytes are part of the method of conserving water and sodium, inducing hypervolemia.[109] PCV, urea, TP and Na^+ concentration could therefore be considered as useful dynamic indicators in assessment of fitness and performance in endurance horses. Endurance training usually does not lead to major changes in serum $[Cl^-]$ and $[K^+]$.[6,86]

When monitoring horses selected in the national team, we observed that urea, total protein and alkaline phosphatase concentrations in blood samples taken at rest were higher than the reference values in, respectively, 100, 75 and 66% of the horses.[72] Training was associated with an increase in CK and sodium concentrations and a decrease in chloremia ($P < 0.05$). Monitoring of muscle enzymes appears useful because less well-trained horses usually have higher CK and ASTT values than fit horses. From our experience, a moderate increase in CK (<1.000 UI/L) or serum amyloid A values and marginally high or low leukocyte counts before exercise are often associated with increased recovery time and lower performance during rides. In a recent study, increased C-reactive protein concentrations were observed before the ride in 10 out of 17 endurance horses.[110]

Effects of exercise

Blood biochemical changes subsequent to races are fairly well known; however, the changes associated with a more moderate effort during or after standardized exercise tests are less well characterized. Patterns most frequently reported include increases in PCV, TP, plasma urea and creatinine concentrations and decreases in plasma [Na^+], [K^+], [Cl^-] and [Ca^{++}] at the end of the ride as compared with pre-ride values.[21,23,37,86,110] From our experience,[72] in fit endurance horses, signs of dehydration are significant only after strenuous exercise (more than two hours' duration in cool weather) while increases in total bilirubin, CK activity and serum amyloid A (SAA) concentrations appear to be proportional to the intensity of exercise. Accordingly, there are no significant changes in SAA or CK after limited distance rides but increases in both concentrations after long-distance rides.[110] However, it has been reported that increases in CK were not associated with the distance covered but with velocity and locomotion symmetry index at trot.[21,24,25] Since CK activity tend to rise and fall relatively quickly, this enzyme may be considered a good measure of training level and a horse's recovery from increased work. After exercise, there is typically leukocytosis and neutrophilia.[21,37,86,110] In the aforementioned study[106] the 27 poor-performing endurance horses were compared to 11 horses presented for simple athletic follow-up; no significant differences were found between groups for hematological data and most of the biochemical parameters analyzed at rest and after exercise. Only CK, potassium and SAA values were significantly higher, and monocyte counts and SOD values significantly lower, after standardized exercise tests in poor performers than in control horses.[106]

Blood lactate measurements are used regularly to assess the level of fitness in the sport horse.[111] As endurance exercise is primarily aerobic, lactate levels measured in endurance horses are normally quite low.[24,30] However, an experimental study has shown that a lactate-guided conditioning program could significantly enhance endurance performance over a six-week time period when the conditioning protocol was adjusted every two weeks based on improvement in VLA4 (the running speed at which blood lactate concentration reaches 4 mmol/L).[111]

Biomarkers

Recent studies have investigated the relationship of several potential biomarkers with performance in endurance horses. These studies were based on the concurrent analysis of a variety of blood biochemical, endocrine or antioxidant molecules and their association with training status and performance in long-distance exercise. The analysis of standard biochemical parameters usually fails to demonstrate an association between pre-race values and the outcome of the competition.[42,80,83,106,112,113] However, in a recent study on 20 Arabian endurance horses, SAA concentration appeared to be promising laboratory parameter as pre-ride values were a useful predictor of elimination during races. Specifically, none of the horses with SAA level higher than 1000 ng/ml completed the 120 or 160 km rides.[114] In another study, a higher concentration of thiobarbituric acid reactive substances (TBARS) before racing 80 or 160 km in distance was associated with reduced likelihood of completing the race and considered indicative of pre-existing oxidative stress.[113] In the same study, higher basal concentrations of inflammatory markers (TNF-α) and lower basal concentrations of anti-inflammatory markers (α-melanocyte-stimulating hormone) were associated with reduced performance.[115] Lower plasma calcium concentrations and elevation in lipid peroxidation products (lipid peroxide [LPO] and malondialdehyde [MDA]) were measured before and after a 120-km endurance ride in horses eliminated for synchronous diaphragmatic flutter; the authors concluded that Ca^{++} concentration may serve as a prognostic marker for endurance capacity in horses.[32]

Heart rate monitoring

Monitoring the heart rate is an objective method of evaluating the metabolic response to exercise, because the anaerobic threshold is reached around 150 beats per minute for the majority of horses.[14] It also permits the early recognition of exercise intolerance due to metabolic or orthopedic reasons. With knowledge of the heart rate, the horse's natural abilities and difficulties can be recognized and explored during conditioning or competition.[14] Resting heart rate in horses generally does not decrease with conditioning and low resting heart rates do not necessarily represent fitness. Athletic capacity is much more associated with maximal heart rate and stroke volume.[14] In race horses, the velocities at which heart rate reaches 200 bpm (V200) as well as VLA4 are used as indicators of fitness. However, most endurance horses do not reach a HR of 200 bpm nor a blood lactate concentration of 4 mmol/L. The velocity at which heart rate reaches 160 bpm (V160) appears easier to use.[106] Importantly, higher lactate concentrations and heart rates were reported in poor-performing endurance horses throughout both field tests and treadmill tests.[106]

Heart-rate recovery is also an important objective parameter for evaluation of fitness and exercise intolerance.[14] The faster the horse recovers the heart rate towards the normal range, the more efficient are body system activities during exercise performance. During rides, well-conditioned endurance horses are able to recover their heart rate to lower than 64 bpm within 5–10 minutes of arriving at the veterinary check point. Heart rates greater than 64 bpm at the 20–30-minute recovery time are reliably associated with dehydration, electrolyte depletion, muscle disorders, or pain. Low-grade lameness can sometimes be evidenced by increased heart rate and heart-rate recovery time too.[116] Elevations in the expected heart rate for determined exercise intensity may be detectable before lameness becomes visible. During standardized exercise tests, heart rates measured during recovery were significantly higher in poor performers than in control horses.[106]

Standardized exercise test

Poor performance investigation and standardized exercise tests (SET) in endurance horses are still uncommon. SET based on treadmill tests have been adapted from those applied in Standardbreds.[106] Horses need to be acclimatized to the treadmill by taking them through the different gaits and making sure they can reach adequate speed before attempting the test. After a warm-up consisting of five minutes at walk and five minutes at trot, the slope is set at a 4 percent incline and three steps are performed at speeds of 7.5, 8.2 and 9.0 m/s for three minutes each. The horse is allowed two minutes recovery at 3.5 m/s between each step and 10 minutes recovery at a walk at the end of the test. The entire test lasts approximately 30 minutes.

Field tests are more suited to endurance exercise and easier to implement in practice. They can be performed on a training track, a beach or a racetrack. The quality of the ground must be perfect, neither too firm nor too deep, to limit the risk of damage of the musculoskeletal system. Fraipont et al.[106] propose a warm-up phase of 10 minutes at walk and 10 minutes at trot, followed by three steps: a first step of a canter over 27 km at 6 m/s (22 km/h), followed by a second and a third steps run over 1500 m at 7.5 and 8.8 m/s (27 and 32 km/h), respectively. A recovery period at a slow trot over 700 m is allowed between each step and a recovery phase of 10 minutes at walk ends the test. The entire test lasts approximately two hours. For horses new in endurance (racing on 20 or 40 km), the first step is run over 6.5 km and 13 km, and the second and third steps over 1 km and 1.5 km, respectively.[106] Table 52.3 presents an adaptation of this SET protocol based on our own experience.[117]

During the field test, a GPS can be used to measure velocity and assist the rider in keeping a constant speed for each step. Ideally, it should be coupled with a telemetry ECG system to continuously monitor heart rate (HR) and possibly detection of cardiac arrhythmias. Venous blood samples are drawn at the end of each step (within 30 seconds) to measure total blood lactate concentrations. In fit endurance horses, blood lactate values remain lower than 2.5 or 3 mmol/L. Four derived parameters can be calculated from the measured variables, i.e. HR, speed and blood lactate concentration: the velocity at which blood lactate reached 4 mmol/L (VLA4), the velocities at which HRs reached 160 and 200 bpm (V160 and V200) and the HR corresponding to VLA4 (HR4). In healthy 160-km endurance horses, Fraipont et al. found average values VLA4 = 33.0 ± 6.1 km/h and V160 = 28.4 ± 1.5 km/h.[106]

It is very important to follow the recovery HR during the 30 minutes after stopping exercise. This can be done in different ways depending on the equipment available. You can measure the time required for the HR falls below 64, or record heart rate at 2, 5, 10 and 30 minutes post-exercise. A fit horse recovers (HR ≤ 64) in less than 10 minutes, and high-level horses often recover within 1–2 minutes. A rapid gait examination – like in vet-gates – should also be performed at the end of the test.

Subclinical diseases underlying poor performance

There are few data available on the causes of poor performance in endurance horses. In the study on 27 poorly performing endurance horses examined during a SET, a definitive diagnosis of subclinical disease was found in every horse.[106]

Respiratory problems were the most frequently encountered subclinical disorders with lower respiratory tract abnormalities (tracheal fluid neutrophilia, inflammatory airway disease, bacterial infection, exercise-induced pulmonary hemorrhage) being present in 85.2 percent of horses with decreased performance. Several factors inevitably promote the occurrence of inflammatory diseases, such as age (endurance horses are older) and environmental conditions. In Europe, endurance horses are often kept in 'traditional' environments, characterized by permanent outdoor pasture during spring and summer and collective indoor housing during autumn and winter. This type of management could encourage chronic inflammation. Intensive training, repeated transports and mingling during competitions may also promote the development and transmission of infectious diseases.[118] Endurance competition causes metabolic and hormonal alterations which disturb immunity, predisposing horses to infectious airway problems.[30,119] Investigation of the respiratory system performed on seven endurance horses before and after a 120-km endurance showed significant alterations of the respiratory function.[118] Competition caused an increase in pharyngitis and tracheal mucus scores, and significant neutrophilia in the tracheal wash. Post-competition tracheal wash samples contained a high amount of dust particles, including mold spores and pollen but also bacterial pathogens.

The other subclinical problems encountered were EM, locomotor disturbance and cardiac arrhythmias (ventricular premature complexes).[106] In this study, 66.7 percent of poorly performing horses had multiple concomitant problems as has been reported in previous studies in other sport horses.[105] Establishing that EM is a primary cause of poor performance is challenging when episodes of EM are intermittent. Persistent elevation in AST may indicate previous episodes of EM; however, if serum muscle enzymes are normal, an exercise challenge can be of value to detect underlying subclinical EM. If signs of stiffness develop during the test, exercise should be concluded. Small fluctuations in serum CK activity may occur with exercise because of enhanced muscle membrane permeability; however, most normal horses show little change in CK activity with this submaximal test and a three- to fourfold increase from basal CK activity is indicative of subclinical EM.[53]

Training programs that do not include enough rest days can also be implicated in exercise intolerance in endurance horses.[14] The condition is called overtraining syndrome (OTS) and involves metabolic, endocrine, and behavioral changes. OTS can have two forms: sympathetic and parasympathetic. The former is more common in racehorses and is characterized by the effects of catecholamines, with increased heart rate, decreased performance, irritability, increased catabolism of proteins, decreased renal perfusion, and increased cortisol levels. The parasympathetic form is more frequently seen in endurance horses and could be confused with a good conditioning stage: decreased heart rate and fast recovery rate followed by decreased performance, hypoglycemia due to absence of glucagon, adrenal failure, and immunosuppression. Blood analysis and clinical evidence of poor performance can indicate overtraining and support decisions to reevaluate the program. A long period of rest is mandatory for recovery and conditioning activities should be resumed gradually.[14]

Table 52.3 Duration of each step of standardized exercise test for endurance horses depending on the competitive level[117]

		COMPETITIVE LEVEL				
STEP	**SPEED**	**40 km**	**60 km**	**90 km**	**120 km**	**160 km**
1	20 km/h	15 min	30 min	45 min	1 hour	1.5 hour
2	25–27 km/h	1.000 meters			1.500 meters	
3	30–32 km/h	1.000 meters			1.500 meters	

References

1. Fédération Equestre Internationale. Rules for endurance events. 7th ed. effective 1 January 2009, Updates effective 1 January 2011. p. 28.
2. Holbrook TC. The endurance horse. In: Wiley-Blackwell, editor. Adam's and Stashak's lameness in horses. 6th ed. Chichester: UK; 2011. p. 1055–61.
3. Fédération Equestre Internationale. http://www.fei.org/
4. Nagy A, Murray JK, Dyson S. Elimination from elite endurance rides in nine countries: a preliminary study. Equine Vet J 2010;42(Suppl. 38):637–43.
5. Fielding CL, Meier CA, Balch OK, et al. Risk factors for the elimination of endurance horses from competition. J Am Vet Med Assoc 2011;239:493–8.
6. Muñoz A, Riber C, Santisteban R, et al. Effect of training duration and exercise on blood-borne substrates, plasma lactate and enzyme concentrations in Andalusian, Anglo-Arabian and Arabian breeds. Equine Vet J 2002;34(Suppl. 34):245–51.
7. Nielsen BD, Turner KK, Ventura BA, et al. Racing speeds of quarter horses, thoroughbreds and Arabians. Equine Vet J 2006;38(Suppl. 36):128–32.
8. Fédération Equestre Internationale. Veterinary regulations. 12th ed. effective 5 April 2010, Updates effective 1 January 2012, p. 90.
9. Barnes A, Kingston J, Beetson S, et al. Endurance veterinarians detect physiologically compromised horses in a 160 km ride. Equine Vet J 2010;42(Suppl. 38):6–11.
10. Smith CA. Electrolyte imbalances and metabolic disturbances in endurance horses. Comp Cont Ed Pract Vet 1985;7:575–82.
11. Feldman J. Principles of sport medicine for the endurance and eventing horse. J Equine Vet Sc 1994;14:331–2.
12. Castejón F, Rubio D, Tovar P, et al. A comparative study of aerobic capacity and fitness in three different horse breeds (Andalusian, Arabian and Anglo-Arabian). Zentralbl Veterinarmed A 1994;41:645–52.
13. Rivero JL, Ruz MC, Serrano AL, et al. Effects of a 3 month endurance training programme on skeletal muscle histochemistry in Andalusian, Arabian and Anglo-Arabian horses. Equine Vet J 1995;27:51–9.
14. Flaminio MJ, Gaughan EM, Gillespie JR. Exercise intolerance in endurance horses. Vet Clin North Am Equine Pract 1996;12:565–80.
15. Foreman JH. The exhausted horse syndrome. Vet Clin North Am Equine Pract 1998;14:205–19.
16. Hodgson DR. Metabolic problems seen in endurance races and cross-country competitions. Proceedings of the 9th International Congress of the World Equine Veterinary Association, Marrakech, Morocco, 22–26 January 2006. p. 285–8.
17. Schott HC 2nd, Hinchcliff KW. Treatments affecting fluid and electrolyte status during exercise. Vet Clin North Am Equine Pract 1998;14:175–204.
18. McCutcheon LJ, Geor RJ. Sweat fluid and ion losses in horses during training and competition in cool vs. hot ambient conditions: implications for ion supplementation. Equine Vet J 1996;28(Suppl. 22):54–62.
19. Conwell R. 2009 The exhausted/dehydrated/hyperthermic horse. Proceedings of the 48th British Equine Veterinary Association Congress, Birmingham, UK, 9–12 September 2009. p. 186–7.
20. Schott HC, McGlade KS, Molander HA, et al. Body weight, fluid, electrolyte, and hormonal changes in horses competing in 50- and 100-mile endurance rides. Am J Vet Res 1997;58: 303–9.
21. Barton MH, Williamson L, Jacks S, et al. Body weight, hematologic findings, and serum and plasma biochemical findings of horses competing in a 48-, 83-, or 159-km endurance ride under similar terrain and weather conditions. Am J Vet Res 2003;64:746–53.
22. Flaminio MJ, Rush BR. Fluid and electrolyte balance in endurance horses. Vet Clin North Am Equine Pract 1998;14:147–58.
23. Aguilera-Tejero E, Estepa JC, López I, et al. Plasma ionized calcium and parathyroid hormone concentrations in horses after endurance rides. J Am Vet Med Assoc 2001;219:488–90.
24. Castejón F, Trigo P, Muñoz A, et al. Uric acid responses to endurance racing and relationships with performance, plasma biochemistry and metabolic alterations. Equine Vet J 2006;38(Suppl. 36):70–3. http://www.ncbi.nlm.nih.gov/pubmed?db=pubmed&cmd=link&linkname=pubmed_pubmed&uid=17402394.
25. Muñoz A, Riber C, Trigo P, et al. Dehydration, electrolyte imbalances and renin-angiotensin-aldosterone-vasopressin axis in successful and unsuccessful endurance horses. Equine Vet J 2010;42(Suppl. 38): 83–90.
26. Rose RJ. Endurance exercise in the horse: a review. Parts I and II. Br Vet J 1986: 142:542–52.
27. Frazier DL. Synchronous diaphragmatic flutter. Proc Am Assoc Equine Pract 1991;37:833–4.
28. Viu J, Jose-Cunilleras E, Armengou L, et al. Acid-base imbalances during a 120 km endurance race compared by traditional and simplified strong ion difference methods. Equine Vet J 2010;42:76–82.
29. Snow DH, Baxter P, Rose RJ. Muscle fibre composition and glycogen depletion in horses competing in an endurance ride. Vet Rec 1981;108:374–8.
30. Jensen-Waern M, Lindberg A, Johannisson A, et al. The effects of an endurance ride on metabolism and neutrophil function. Equine Vet J 1999;31(Suppl. 30):605–9.
31. Marlin DJ, Fenn K, Smith N, et al. Changes in circulatory antioxidant status in horses during prolonged exercise. J Nutr 2002;132(Suppl. 2): 1622S–7S
32. Al-Qudah KM, Al-Majali AM. Higher lipid peroxidation indices in horses eliminated from endurance race because of synchronous diaphragmatic flutter (thumps). J Equine Vet Sc 2008;28: 573–8.
33. Frazier DL. Who speaks for the horse–the sport of endurance riding and equine welfare? J Am Vet Med Assoc 2000;216:1258–61.
34. Fregin GF. General discussion of physiologic observations recorded on 117 horses during 100-mile endurance rides. Proc Am Assoc Equine Pract 1979;25:315–21.
35. Garlinghouse SE, Burrill MJ. Relationship of body condition score to completion rate during 160 km endurance races. Equine Vet J 1999;31(Suppl. 30):591–5.
36. Robert C, Benamou-Smith A, Leclerc JL. Use of the recovery check in long-distance endurance rides. Equine Vet J 2002;34(Suppl. 34):106–11.
37. Schott HC 2nd, Marlin DJ, Geor RJ, et al. Changes in selected physiological and laboratory measurements in elite horses competing in a 160 km endurance ride. Equine Vet J 2006;38(Suppl. 36):37–42.
38. Burger D, Dollinger S. Raisons d'élimination, état de santé et carrière sportive des chevaux dans les raids d'endurance en Europe et dans les pays arabes: approche statistique. Prat Vet Equine 1998;30:91–7.
39. Slusher SH, Mackay-Smith MP. Endurance ride veterinary control. Proc Am Assoc Equine Pract 1991;37:793–805.
40. Robert C. (2005) How to recognise the exhausted horse before it's too late. In: Proceedings of 44th British Equine Veterinary Association Congress, Harrogate, UK, 14–17 September 2005. p. 90–1.
41. Tomlinson CM. Exhausted horse syndrome. Proc Am Assoc Equine Pract 1991;37:835–7.

42. Trigo P, Castejon F, Riber C, et al. Use of biochemical parameters to predict metabolic elimination in endurance rides. Equine Vet J 2010;42(Suppl. 38):142–6.
43. Loving NS. Emergency care at equine events: endurance. Proceedings of the 54th Annual Convention of the American Association of Equine Practitioners, San Diego, CA, USA, 8–10 December 2008.
44. Fielding CL, Magdesian KG, Rhodes DM, et al. Clinical and biochemical abnormalities in endurance horses eliminated from competition for medical complications and requiring emergency medical treatment: 30 cases (2005–2006). J Vet Emerg Crit Care (San Antonio) 2009;19:473–8.
45. Langlois C, Robert C. Epidemiology of metabolic disorders in endurance horses. Prat Vét Equine 2008;40: 51–60.
46. Sloet van Oldruitenborgh-Oosterbaan MM. Problems facing the endurance horse. In: Proceedings of 44th British Equine Veterinary Association Congress, Harrogate, UK, 14–17 September 2005. p. 75–7.
47. Whiting JM. The exhausted horse. In: Robinson NE, Sprayberry KA, editors. Current therapy in equine medicine. 6th ed. St Louis: Saunders; 2009. p. 926–9.
48. Toribio RE. Disorders of calcium and phosphate metabolism in horses. Vet Clin North Am Equine Pract. 2011;27:129–47.
49. Stewart AJ. Magnesium disorders in horses. Vet Clin North Am Equine Pract 2011;27:149–63.
50. Dwyer RM. The practical diagnosis and treatment of metabolic conditions in endurance horses. Equine Pract. 1986;8: 21–33.
51. Lewis LD. Feeding and care of horses for athletic performance. In: Feeding and care of the horse. 2nd ed. Victoria, Australia: Blackwell Publishing; 2005. p. 193–223.
52. Dowling PM. Metabolic disease and myopathies in endurance horses. Proceedings of the 18th American College Veterinary Internal Medicine, Seattle, 2000. p. 187–8.
53. Valberg SJ. Exertional rhabdomyolysis. Proceed. 52nd Annual Convention Am Assoc Equine Pract, San Antonio, TX, USA, 2006.
54. Nieto JE, Snyder JR, Beldomenico P, et al. Prevalence of gastric ulcers in endurance horses – a preliminary report. Vet J 2004;167:33–7.
55. Fielding CL, Dechant JE. Colic in competing endurance horses presenting to referral centres: 36 cases. Equine Vet J 2011.
56. Murray MJ, Pollmeir MG. Gastrointestinal disease and competition. Proceedings of the 9th Congress on Equine Medicine and Surgery in Geneva, Switzerland, December 2005.
57. Philippart M-A, Robert C. Neurological problems of metabolic origin in endurance horses. Prat Vet Equine 2008;40:59–68.
58. Divers TJ. Metabolic causes of encephalopathy in horses. Vet Clin North Am Equine Pract 2011;27:589–96.
59. Sampieri F, Schott HC 2nd, Hinchcliff KW, et al. Effects of oral electrolyte supplementation on endurance horses competing in 80 km rides. Equine Vet J 2006;38(Suppl. 36):19–26.
60. Parks A. 2009 Acute and chronic laminitis – An overview. Proceedings of the AAEP Focus Meeting on the Foot. Columbus, OH, USA. 21 July 2009.
61. Belknap JK, Faleiros RR, Moore RM. Update on equine acute laminitis. Proceedings of the 11th International Congress of the World Equine Veterinary Association, Guaruja, Brazil, 24–27 September 2009.
62. Courtois P-A, Ghyoros G, Robert C. (2008) La fourbure post-effort en endurance: résultats de l'enquête 2006–2007. Proceedings of the 38th Journées de l'AVEF, Reims, France, 9–11 October 2008.
63. Hood DM. Laminitis in the horse. Vet Clin North Am Equine Pract 1999;15:287–94.
64. Misheff MM. Lameness in endurance horses. In: Ross MW, Dyson SJ, editors. Diagnosis and management of lameness in the horse. 2nd ed. St Louis, MO: Elsevier Saunders; 2011. p. 1137–49.
65. Misheff MM, Alexander GR, Hirst GR. Management of fractures in endurance horses. Equine Vet Ed 2010;22: 623–30.
66a. Robert C, Coussedière M, Pélissier C. Prevalence of radiographic changes in the limbs of high level endurance horses – comparison with jumping horses. Proceedings of the 28th Congress of the European Association of Veterinary Anatomists, Paris, France, 29–31 July 2010, Anatomia Histologia Embryologia 39:319.
66b. Fielding CL, Magdesian KG. A comparison of hypertonic (7.2%) and isotonic (0.9%) saline for fluid resuscitation in horses: a randomized, double-blinded, clinical trial. J Vet Intern Med 2011;25:1138–43.
67. Geor RJ. Nutritional management of endurance horses. In: Proceedings of 44th British Equine Veterinary Association Congress, Harrogate, UK, 14–17 September 2005. p. 343–4.
68. Treiber KH, Geor RJ, Boston RC, et al. Dietary energy source affects glucose kinetics in trained Arabian geldings at rest and during endurance exercise. J Nutr 2008;138:964–70.
69. Mathews-Martin L, Leclerc J-L, Robert C. Feeding the endurance horse: current knowledge and observation of practices in the field. Prat Vet Equine 2011;43:39–48.
70. Harris P. Feeding management of elite endurance horses. Vet Clin North Am Equine Pract 2009;25:137–53.
71. Ménager S, Leclerc J-L, Robert C. (2010). Body measurements and performance in endurance horses: experimental determination of the optimal weight. Proceedings of the 28th Congress of the European Association of Veterinary Anatomists, Paris, France, Anatomia Histologia Embryologia 39:306.
72. Robert C, Mathews-Martin L, Leclerc J-L. High level endurance training: descriptive study based on the follow-up of the French team over seasons 2009 and 2010. Proceedings of the Equine NUtrition and TRAining Conference, Paris, France, 12–15 October 2011. Arno Lindner, p. 235–42.
73. Kronfeld D. Dietary fat affects heat production and other variables of equine performance, under hot and humid conditions. Equine Vet J 1996;28(Suppl. 22):24–34.
74. Graham-Thiers PM, Kronfeld DS, Kline KA, et al. Dietary protein level and protein status in Arabian horses during interval training and repeated sprints. J Equine Vet Sci 2000;20:516–21.
75. Spangfors P. Some aspects of feeding the endurance horse. In: Pagan JD, editor. Advances in equine nutrition. Nottingham: Nottingham University Press; 2000. p 341–9.
76. Meyer H, Coenen M. Influence of exercise on the water and electrolyte content of the alimentary tract. Proceedings of the 11th Conference of the Equine Nutrition and Physiology Symposium, 1989. p. 3–7.
77. Bergero D. New insights related to the nutritional management of endurance horses. Proceedings of the 2nd European Equine Nutrition and Health Congress, Lelystad, The Netherlands, 19–20 March 2004.
78. Dunnett C, Marlin DJ, Harris RC. Effect of dietary lipid on response to exercise: relationship to metabolic adaptation. Equine Vet J 2002;34(Suppl. 34):75–80.
79. Pagan JD, Geor RJ, Harris PA, et al. Effects of fat adaptation on glucose kinetics and substrate oxidation during low intensity exercise. Equine Vet J 2002;34(Suppl. 34):33–8.
80. Hoffman RM, Hess TM, Williams CA, et al. Speed associated with plasma pH, oxygen content, total protein and urea in an 80 km race. Equine Vet J 2002;34(Suppl. 34):39–43.
81. Hargreaves BJ, Kronfeld DS, Waldron JN, et al. Antioxidant status and muscle cell leakage during endurance exercise. Equine Vet J 2002;34(Suppl. 34):116–21.

82. Williams CA, Kronfeldt DS, Hess TM, et al. Antioxidant supplementation and subsequent oxidative stress of horses during an 80-km endurance race. J Anim Sci 2004;82:588–94.
83. Haggett E, Magdesian KG, Maas J, et al. Whole blood selenium concentrations in endurance horses. Vet J 2010;186:192–6.
84. Jansson A, Dahlborn K. Effects of feeding frequency and voluntary salt intake on fluid and electrolyte regulation in athletic horses. J Appl Physiol 1999;86: 1610–16.
85. Coenen M, Meyer H, Steinbrenner B. Effects of NaCl supplementation before exercise on metabolism of water and electrolytes. Equine Vet J 1995;(Suppl. 18):270–3.
86. Robert C, Goachet AG, Fraipont A, et al. Hydration and electrolyte balance in horses during an endurance season. Equine Vet J 2010;42(Suppl. 38):98–104.
87. Hess TM, Kronfeld DS, Williams CA, et al. Effects of oral potassium supplementation on acid-base status and plasma ion concentrations of horses during endurance exercise. Am J Vet Res 2005;66:466–73.
88. Sosa León LA, Hodgson DR, Carlson GP, et al. Effects of concentrated electrolytes administered via a paste on fluid, electrolyte, and acid base balance in horses. Am J Vet Res 1998;59: 898–903.
89. Düsterdieck KF, Schott HC 2nd, Eberhart SW, et al. Electrolyte and glycerol supplementation improve water intake by horses performing a simulated 60 km endurance ride. Equine Vet J 1999;31(Suppl. 30):418–24.
90. Holbrook TC, Simmons RD, Payton ME, et al. Effect of repeated oral administration of hypertonic electrolyte solution on equine gastric mucosa. Equine Vet J 2005;37:501–4.
91. Nyman S, Jansson A, Dahlborn K, et al. Strategies for voluntary rehydration in horses during endurance exercise. Equine Vet J 1996;28(Suppl. 22):99–106.
92. Schott HC 2nd, Düsterdieck KF, Eberhart SW, et al. Effects of electrolyte and glycerol supplementation on recovery from endurance exercise. Equine Vet J 1999;31(Suppl. 30):384–93.
93. Butudom P, Schott HC 2nd, Davis MW, et al. Drinking salt water enhances rehydration in horses dehydrated by frusemide administration and endurance exercise. Equine Vet J 2002;34(Suppl. 34):513–18.
94. Tamzali Y, Marguet C, Priymenko N, et al. Prevalence of gastric ulcer syndrome in high-level endurance horses. Equine Vet J 2011;43:141–4.
95. Mitchell RD. Maintenance care of the elite sport horse. Proceedings of the 11th International Congress of the World Equine Veterinary Association, Guaruja, Brazil, 24–27 September 2009.
96. Cywińska A, Wyszyńska Z, Górecka R, et al. The effect of the 162 km endurance ride on equine peripheral blood neutrophil and lymphocyte functions. Pol J Vet Sci 2010;13: 279–85.
97. Leclerc J-L. Training for endurance horses: traditional and evolving ideas. Prat Vet Equine 2009;41: 7–10.
98. Hinchcliff K. Introduction to the physiology of exercise. Proceedings of the 9th Congress on Equine Medicine and Surgery, Geneva, Switzerland, 15 December 2005.
99. Goachet AG, Varloud M, Philippeau C, et al. Long-term effects of endurance training on total tract apparent digestibility, total mean retention time and faecal microbial ecosystem in competing Arabian horses. Equine Vet J 2010;42(Suppl. 38):387–92.
100. Rivero JL. A scientific background for skeletal muscle conditioning in equine practice. J Vet Med A Physiol Pathol Clin Med 2007;54:321–32.
101. Hodgson DR, Rose RJ. Effects of a nine-month endurance training programme on muscle composition in the horse. Vet Rec 1987;121:271–4.
102. Castelijns H. If the shoe fits: preventive shoeing for different equestrian disciplines. Proceedings of the 10th Congress on Equine Medicine and Surgery, Geneva, Switzerland, 11–13 December 2007. p. 98–105.
103. Pélissier C. Shoeing for endurance horses: constraints and characteristics. Prat Vet Equine 2009;41:11–14.
104. Mackay-Smith MP. Prepurchase panel: the distance horse. Proc Am Assoc Equine Pract 1999;45, 22–3.
105. Martin BB Jr, Reef VB, Parente EJ, et al. Causes of poor performance of horses during training, racing, or showing: 348 cases (1992–1996). J Am Vet Med Assoc 2000;216:554–8.
106. Fraipont A, Van Erck E, Ramery E, et al. Subclinical diseases underlying poor performance in endurance horses: diagnostic methods and predictive tests. Vet Rec 2011;169:154.
107. Carlson GP. Blood chemistry, body fluids and hematology. In: Gillespie JR, Robinson NE, editors. Equine exercise physiology, vol. 2. Davis, CA: ICEEP Publications; 1987. p. 393–425.
108. Thomas DP, Fregin GF. Endurance training-induced hypervolemia in the horse. Med Sci Sports Exerc 1987;19:524–5.
109. McKeever KH, Schurg WA, Jarrett SH, et al. Exercise training-induced hypervolemia in the horse. Med Sci Sports Exerc 1987;19:21–7.
110. Cywińska A, Szarska E, Górecka R, et al. Acute phase protein concentrations after limited distance and long distance endurance rides in horses. Res Vet Sci 2012;93:1402–6.
111. Trilk JL, Lindner AJ, Greene HM, et al. A lactate-guided conditioning programme to improve endurance performance. Equine Vet J 2002;34(Suppl. 34): 122–5.
112. De Mello Costa MF, Anderson GA, Davies HM, et al. Circulating angiotensin converting enzyme in endurance horses: effect of exercise on blood levels and its value in predicting performance. Equine Vet J 2010;42(Suppl. 38): 152–4.
113. Muñoz A, Cuesta I, Riber C, et al. Trot asymmetry in relation to physical performance and metabolism in equine endurance rides. Equine Vet J 2006; 38(Suppl. 36):50–4.
114. Cywinska A, Gorecka R, Szarska E, et al. Serum amyloid A level as a potential indicator of the status of endurance horses. Equine Vet J 2010;42(Suppl. 38):23–7.
115. Holbrook TC, McFarlane D, Schott HC 2nd. Neuroendocrine and non-neuroendocrine markers of inflammation associated with performance in endurance horses. Equine Vet J 2010;42(Suppl. 38): 123–8.
116. Foreman JH, Lawrence LM. Lameness and heart rate elevation in the exercising horse. J Equine Vet Sci (Equine Sport Med) 1991;353.
117. Robert C, Leclerc J-L, van Erck-Westergen E, et al. Performance tests in endurance horses. Prat Vet Equine, 2011;43:23–6.
118. van Erck-Westergren E, Art T. Respiratory inflammation in endurance horses. Proceedings of the 4th World Equine Airways Symposium, Berne, Switzerland, 5–7 August 2009. p. 186–8.
119. Robson PJ, Alston TD, Myburgh KH. Prolonged suppression of the innate immune system in the horse following an 80 km endurance race. Equine Vet J 2003;35:133–7.

Veterinary aspects of competing and training polo horses

53

Aude Giraudet

CHAPTER CONTENTS

History

Originating from India,[1] where its name 'Pulu' came from, polo spread during the first millennium from India towards the Middle East, following the path of Mongol invasions. A 600-year-old polo field can still be seen in Ispahan, now a public park, where Shah Abbas the Great played polo. Discovered by British tea planters[2] in the region of Manipur (north-east of India) in the middle of the nineteenth century, polo was rapidly adopted by the British army and brought to England where the first match was played in 1869, from where it expanded to the USA, with the first match played in 1876, and where it became extremely popular. During these years, rules were progressively developed and adopted. Immigrants from the UK brought the game to Argentina,[3] the first match being held at the *estancia* of Negrete close to Buenos Aires in August 1875. Probably due to the unique feature of unlimited fields to play in association with a strongly developed equestrian culture and to the presence of horses suitable for the game, polo became extremely popular in a very short period of time in this country and remains today one of the Argentina's favorite sports. This country is today the undisputed leader of the game.

The first half of the 20th century was the peak period for modern polo. It was an Olympic sport from 1900 to 1936 and Argentina won the gold medal in 1924 and 1936.

Organization of the sport

Polo federation

In 1980, the Federation of International Polo[4] was created, and in 1987 the first world championship was held in Buenos Aires. Medium goal world championships are regularly organized throughout the world. FIP has more than 13 000 members worldwide (Table 53.1).

Each player is given a goal handicap by their national federation. The handicap reflects the level of the player (from -4 to10 goals). There are currently only eight players in the world who have a 10 goal handicap, all of them being Argentines.

When a team is assembled, the handicap of each team member is added to each other. The resulting team is classified as low goal (0–4), medium goal (6–14) or high goal (20 and above). In order to even the chances for a particular match, if two teams of different handicap are playing a handicap tournament, the team with the smallest handicap is awarded goals at the start of the game.

The calculation of these awarded goals is made by multiplying the difference between the two teams by the numbers of periods that will be played, then dividing the result by six. For instance, if two teams with a difference in handicap of four goals are opposed, the amount awarded to the team with the lower handicap is four times the number of periods, this being divided by six. For instance in a seven periods match, calculation will be as follow: $(4 \times 7)/6 = 4.66$. Any fraction is counted as a full goal. The final number of awarded goals in this example will be five.

Polo match rules

A match is composed of two teams of four players in each team.[4] A match is divided into 6–8 periods called *chukkers* of seven and a half minutes each, the clock being stopped every time the umpires intervene. Two umpires (mounted referees) will follow the game riding, while the *third man* attending the match from the side of the playground will help the umpires in case of disagreement or uncertainty between the mounted umpires, in which case the 'third man' has the casting vote, allowing a definitive decision.

Outdoor polo is usually played on a short-cut grass field, 275 m long by 180 m wide. Long sides are delimitated with long narrow boards that keep a rolling ball in the playing field while the short sides include a 7.5 m wide goal and are not boarded. Adjacent to each side of the fields are decelerating areas where horses can slow down and turn before returning to the game. Players use a stick to hit a 8.5 cm wooden or plastic ball; the aim of the game is for the ball to pass between the two posts delimitating the goals; there is no height limit to the goals.

Polo rules are complex, the aim being protection of both players and horses. When the ball travels, it creates a virtual line. No player can cross this line if this might endanger other players, including the one that has just hit the ball. In order to take the rolling ball, a player has to *follow the line*, and it might be necessary to *ride off* the line an opponent player to do so (Fig. 53.1). If the line is crossed, a penalty can be awarded to the opposing team. This rule has an immediate consequence on the horses. Polo horses have to accept contacts at rapid speed and be prepared to push an opponent's horse off the line of the ball (Fig. 53.2).

Doping regulation

After the accidental death of 21 polo horses that had suffered selenium intoxication[5] in 2009 in Florida, the USA started an official program of horse drug and medication testing. Doing so, they joined European countries, including the UK, Ireland and France, that had drug and medication testing programs underway for polo ponies. Doping control for polo horses is based around individual state regulations and is not mandated by the Federation of International Polo.

Table 53.1 Polo players' world repartition

	NUMBER OF PLAYERS	MAJOR COUNTRIES	
Europe	5097	England	2790
North America	3154	USA	3138
South America	4855	Argentina	3130

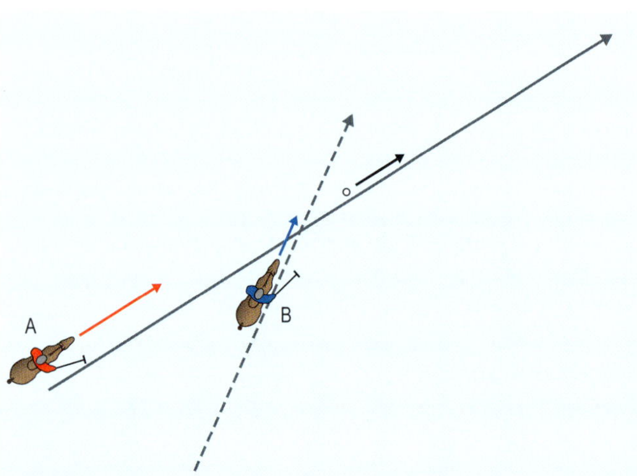

Fig 53.1 ''Foul'' penalty as player B crosses the line in front of player A, endangering him.

Match organization

Horses are equipped to allow the player the safest, most efficient game and to protect the horse. The mane is usually clipped, so the player's stick does not become entangled in the hair. The tail is braided and tied for the same purpose. All horses will wear a martingale (Fig. 53.3) to prevent the horse from raising its head while the player leans forward to hit the ball. As the horses are guided using one hand on the reins, the bits are strong. Several types of bits and bridles are used in various combinations.

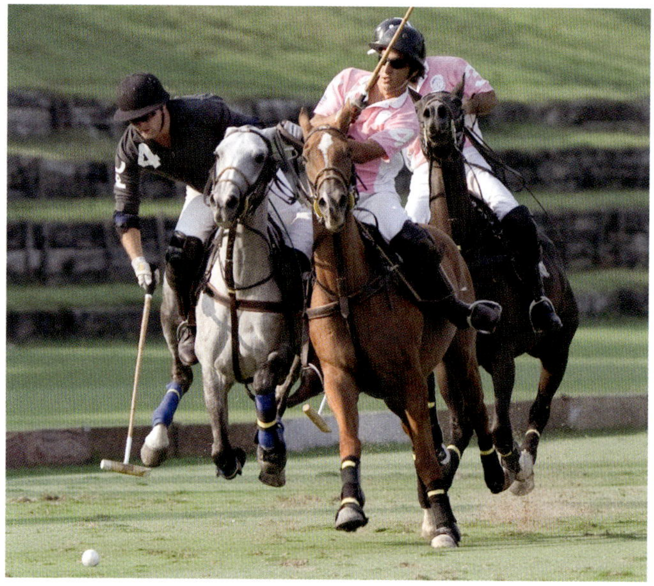

Fig 53.2 Two horses during a ride off.
Courtesy of www.argentinapolo.com, Hugues Denholm.

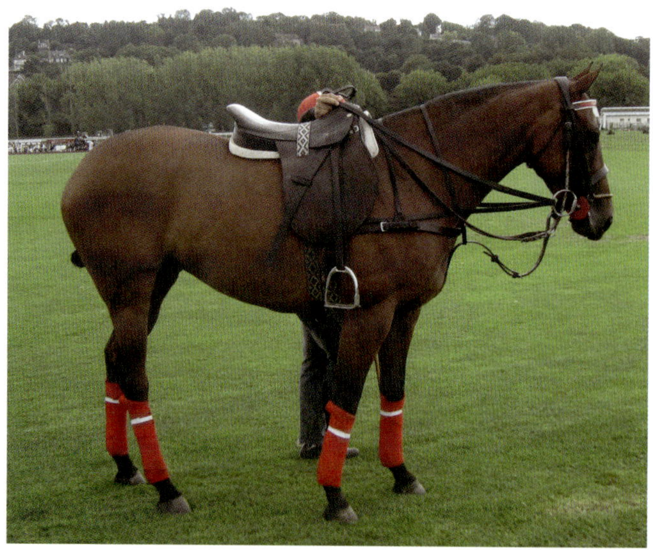

Fig 53.3 Horse ready to play with a martingale, a gag bit with rein and additional draw reins.

Saddles are secured with surcingles, so as not to slip when the player leans to the side. The legs of horses are protected from direct stick impact or from the ball with wraps (which are mandatory) and most of the horses have leg boots added to the wraps. Hoof boots are sometimes used on front feet to prevent injury from overreaching.

Management of horses during game

Close to the decelerating areas along the playing field are two places called *palenque* where each team gathers their equipment, staff and 10–20 horses for a single match. The caretakers are called *petiseros*. They groom, tack and warm up horses for the players. The players usually come back to the palenque to quickly change horse in between chukkers or even during a dull period of an ongoing chukker. Usually one or two petiseros attend one player during a match. One horse has always to be ready while the player is in action as a need for a change can happen at any time.

Usually when the horse is tacked, the warm-up phase lasts 3–5 minutes, consisting of cantering back and forth along the field; the horse then stands for a few minutes on the side on the field, waiting to be used in the game. When the player comes for a mount change, the horse that was playing has its girths slackened and is tied to its place in the palenque. There is no opportunity for active recovery because of the need to prepare the next horse. One particular horse can play two periods, but has to have at least one period of rest. It would be warmed up again before use, but usually for a slightly shorter time than for the first chukker.

Each horse does not necessarily have the same amount of playing time and workload during a match as this depends on its player's number and ability. Players' numbers indicate their role and place in the field. For example, player number one is supposed to play in the attack, player number four to play defense, players two and three will have to organize the game and are usually the ones with the higher handicap of the team. They also cover a larger field during the play and are more demanding on their horses.

Training of polo ponies (made pony)

After breaking and training for riding, a young horse must be *made pony* that is, to be able to play. This training includes two aspects:

- getting the horse fit enough to handle the very intense exercise they will have to do. This is progressively obtained with long sessions of slow canter or trot. Most of the time, one petiseros will ride one horse and lead as many as five horses during the training session. The mounted horse will canter while the led ones will trot. These sessions last from 45 minutes to one hour. This type of training is called *barrear*
- training the horse to abruptly accelerate, stop, and turn with as minimal as possible action of the rider. This will be obtained by individual training for each horse. They will be taught to *neck rein*: that is, to turn sharply with only light contact from the rein on the neck. Repeated rapid starts and stops will prepare the horse for the game. All this preparation is done by experienced petiseros. When the horse is sufficiently adapted to this type of exercise, the training will continue with the actual player practicing with a stick, mimicking the real game. This specific training is called *taquear*

Training matches[6] are occasionally organized to finalize the horse physical preparation as well as the player cohesiveness. Usually, the horse plays for six to seven months during spring, summer and early autumn. Then a period of full rest with the horses being most of the time in the field or at pasture will occur. This period allows many of the musculoskeletal injuries to heal and for the horse to recover.

An uninjured polo horse can play elite polo until about 12 years of age; then, in most cases it is used in lower polo games, which are less demanding on the musculoskeletal and cardiovascular systems.

Type of effort sustained

Exercise effort during a match and warm-up

There is a scarcity of scientific studies done on polo horses. Studies of other athletic horses are not directly applicable to polo horses as polo consists of short and fast running phases intercalated with rapid slow-down phases and sharp turns which are unlike any other equine sport. The typical effort is demonstrated in Figure 53.4.[7]

Warm-up period is usually less than five minutes, after which the horses then wait for about 10 minutes while the previous period is played. This very short, but rather intense, warm-up period for polo horses is not detrimental and actually allows the horse to reach a higher VO_{2max} in the following exercise.[8] Horses actually play for approximately 12 minutes, although this can vary depending on the player's position on the field and the rider's skill. The maximal speed reached during a game is 50 km/h (13.9 m/s).[7] Heart rates can be as high as 210–220 bpm.[7,10]

In total five studies have evaluated the effort produced by polo horses while playing. The first one held in 1985 worked on indoor polo horses;[9] all the other ones were carried out on non-elite and elite polo horses[6,7,10,11] playing outdoors. All five studies demonstrated the high intensity of the effort of polo horses during a match. Among other effort parameters, blood lactate concentrations were measured before and after a chukker in four studies.[6,7,9,11] In all these studies there was a significant increase in blood lactate concentrations during a chukker (Table 53.2). For instance, amongst horses playing outdoors, lactate concentrations from 9.2 to 18 mmol/L were measured and a marked elevation of the hematocrit of greater than 50% recorded, with the highest PCV being above 61%.[11] All of these parameters are consistent with maximal exercise. Interestingly, two studies[7,11] (B and D) carried on outdoor polo horses resulted in conflicting results. Although the lactate parameters followed a similar pattern for the two groups, the group of horses apparently having a more strenuous exercise (elevated mean heart rate post effort of 129 bpm compared to 80) showed an increase of hematocrit of 36%,[7] less intense than the 51% found in study B.[6] This discrepancy

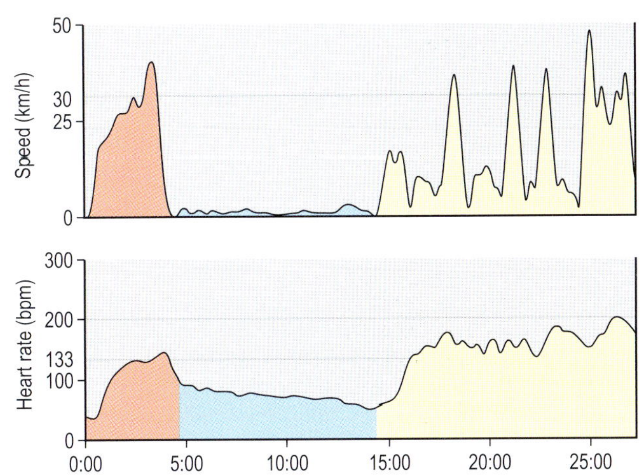

Fig 53.4 Simultaneous heart rate and speed of a horse during a chukker.

Table 53.2 Effort parameters from four studies on polo horses

	POLO TYPE	HR (bpm)	LACTATE (mmol/L)	HT INCREASE PRE- vs POST-EFFORT (%)
Study A[9]	Indoor medium	101 +/– 0.4	9.2 +/– 1.2	22
Study B[11]	Outdoor medium	80.2 +/– 1.91	10.24 +/– 0.4	51
Study C[6]	Elite outdoor	–	18.7 +/– 5.36	51
Study D[7]	Elite outdoor	129 +/– 18	10.34 +/– 4.7	36

HR: heart rate; HT = hematocrit.

could be due to the exact timing of heart rate measurement as heart rates of polo horses slow down very quickly after exercise;[10] this study focused on cardiovascular response of polo horses to exercise demonstrated a fall from 180 to 80 bpm in a five-minute period of time immediately after the effort. Elite horses involved in study B might have undergone a more strenuous effort than in study D but their heart rate post effort might have been monitored with a slightly delayed timing, allowing partial recovery.

When horses were monitored for heart rate and speed during a chukker[7] the synchrony of heart rate and the different accelerations the horse could be demonstrated, with a slight delay of 20 to 30 seconds between the fast boosts of gallop and heart rate rises.

Recovery immediately after completion of a chukker or match is usually passive and does not involve exercise. Blood lactate concentrations measured eight minutes after the end of the period revealed that the mean lactate after this short recovery period was only slightly lower than just after the effort (9.44 compared to 10.99 mmol/L).[12] Moreover, certain horses (four out of 22, 18%) had a rise in lactate concentration during this post-game phase. This has to be taken into account when horses are *doubled* in a game: that is, when a horse goes back to play after approximately 20 minutes' rest and a reduced second warm-up. Active recovery would probably be of benefit to these horses, although this not a traditional practice and would need additional grooms for the play.

Common medical conditions

EIPH

Exercise-induced pulmonary hemorrhage had been evaluated in polo horses.[13,14] Although experiencing intense effort, only 11% (three out of 27)[13] to 39% (11 out of 28)[14] of the polo horses had some evidence of blood in the trachea after exercise. None of these polo horses had blood at the nostril during or after competition and neither were they noticed to be underperforming. Nevertheless EPIH should be included in the differential diagnostic list of a poor-performing polo horse.

Diagnosis can be confirmed either by direct endoscopic evaluation of the trachea immediately after an intense effort or by performing a bronchoalveolar lavage in the hours to days after competition. Cytologic evaluation may reveal frank hemorrhage, if the horse was sampled quickly after the effort, with free red blood cells in the fluids. In case of delayed sampling, cytologic evaluation can confirm EIPH by the presence of hemosiderophages.

If EIPH is confirmed, it is necessary to explore any underlying disease that might contribute to EIPH; in particular, upper airway dysfunction, subclinical infection (viral or bacterial), and/or inflammatory airway disease need to be ruled out.

Management of EIPH as a single cause of poor performance is difficult and relapses often occur. Usual protocols include rest, corticosteroids and progressive exercise before resuming in full training (see Chapter 29).

Myositis

Rhabdomyolysis, diagnosed on clinical signs only, was retrospectively evaluated in polo horses in the USA and UK during a whole season. The mean incidence of exertional rhabdomyolysis[15] was 7.3%. Cases occurred in 82% of yards during a polo season. This incidence is higher than that described in racing Thoroughbreds.[16] The sex predisposition differs too, with fillies overrepresented in racing horses where males are three times less likely to develop rhabdomyolysis. In this single study,[15] the incidence among gelding polo ponies in the USA was 10% compared to a 1.5% among gelding polo ponies in England, and the incidence in females in both countries was close to 8%. Interestingly when considering only English horses, sex was approaching statistical difference, mares being more at risk of developing the disease than males. The difference between the two countries could not be elucidated from the management parameters that were analyzed.

When assessing genomes from various horses experiencing rhabdomyolysis due to polysaccharide storage myopathy, glycogen synthase 1 mutated gene was found in one polo horse.[17] This must be kept in mind when assessing a polo horse with recurrent bouts of rhabdomyolysis despite optimal management.

Considering the very intense type of exercise undertaken with a short warm-up period and no active recovery, the high incidence of rhabdomyolysis is not surprising. Diagnosis relies on detection of the classical clinical signs (stiffness, sudation, reluctance to move) in association with elevated serum activity of muscle-derived enzymes. Serial measurement of muscle enzyme activity in blood assists with assessing response to treatment and development of the disease.

Treatment will typically include:

- rest until complete assessment (biochemistry) is done
- fluid therapy with polyionic fluids (oral or IV in severe cases) to ensure hydration and to promote diuresis
- non-steroidal anti-inflammatory drugs for pain control
- acepromazine (tranquilizing effect and vasodilatory effect) might be used cautiously although opinions on its efficacy differ
- alpha-2 agonists, such as detomidine, romifidine or xylazine or opioids such meperidine, butorphanol, or morphine can be used if pain does not abate with the previously mentioned treatments.

See also Chapter 7 on muscle disorders of equine athletes.

Prevention and management of rhabdomyolysis are the same as for other equine athletes. Insuring a regular exercise schedule (ideally without 'off days') and modifying the feeding habit with minimized carbohydrates are pivotal preventive management.

Ligament injury and fetlock injuries

The suspensory ligament and insertions are subject to wer-and-tear lesions (chronic injury) as well as acute (traumatic) desmitis. Distal insertional desmitis appears to be one of most common polo injuries as it can be induced by the repeated torque forces applied to these structures.[18] Along with ligamentous injuries, chronic articular capsulitis might develop due to overtorsion, overextension or both of the joint. Figure 53.5 illustrates the forces exerted on the right front fetlock during an abrupt change of direction at high speed. This workload is accentuated by the special shoeing used when playing outdoors polo with the extra grip being on the hindlimb only. A biomechanical study demonstrated that the maximal turning speed of a horse is limited by the tendency of the horse's foot to slip on the ground.[19] Adding this extra grip on the ground allows the horse to turn faster but puts an extra load of work on the joint (Figs 53.5 and 53.6).

The result of repeated injury is that the fetlock will appear thickened with a diminished range of flexion and pain on the flexion test (Fig. 53.7) or tenderness and thickening of the distal insertion of the ligament might predominate. In acute cases, local edema accumulates around the injured ligament. Pain might not be obvious at rest, but will impair the horse from playing elite polo.

Diagnosis is essentially made after clinical and ultrasonographic evaluation. Chronic lesions will lead to change in the quality of collagen present (heterogeneous echogenicity and thickened structures will be visualized as well as focal calcification in chronic cases). Along with theses ligamentous lesions, on the suspensory branches insertion side, irregular bone surface is characteristic of chronic inflammation.

Treatment has evolved but still relies on classical local management:

- hydrotherapy and cold application, particularly just after the effort, may be helpful
- poultice application and leg wrap during resting periods
- non-steroidal anti-inflammatory drugs are commonly used (phenylbutazone, flunixin meglumine)
- regenerative medicine has been tried and shows some promise, although there is some debate about efficacy[20,21]
- shock waves therapy, particularly in cases of insertion desmitis, might ameliorate the prognosis.[22]

Direct trauma

Due to the many physical contacts, many types of musculoskeletal injuries occur during competition and need to be addressed individually. The most common injuries are mallet (stick) impacts on the horse's legs. Despite being protected, these regions are often injured. In acute cases, pain and edema is present; in more chronic ones, radiographic signs of bone remodeling will be present. Mallet injuries to proximal sesamoidean bones are particularly common and will impede the horse from playing for days.

The severity of any of this trauma should be evaluated by a complete clinical exam, including radiographic and ultrasonographic evaluation of the zone. Treatments of these traumatic injuries, depending on severity, include:

- protection of the zone
- immobilization if possible
- rest
- cold therapy (crushed ice or hosing)
- topical and/or general non-steroidal anti-inflammatory drugs.

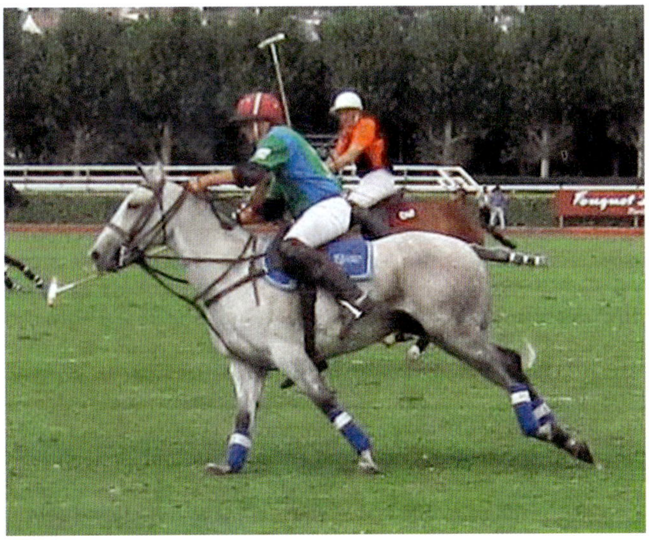

Fig 53.5 Polo horse changing course at high speed.

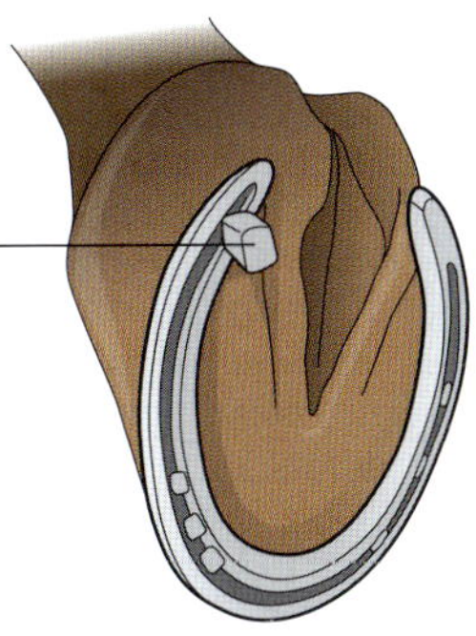

Fig 53.6 Typical hindlimb polo shoe.

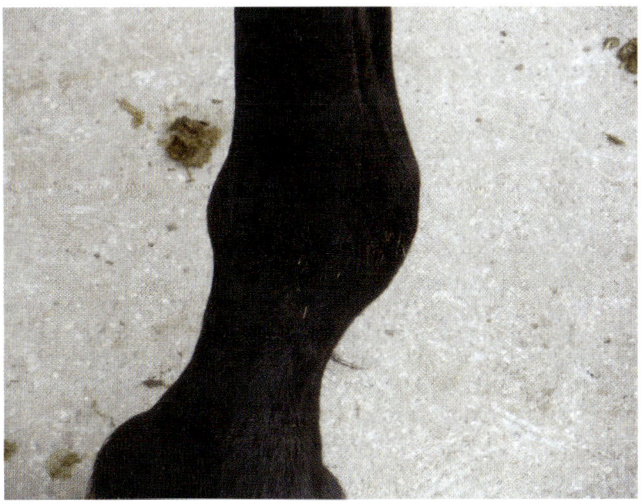

Fig 53.7 Thickened capsule and distended metacarpophalangeal joint in a polo horse.

References

1. http://www.argentinapolo.com/polohistory.html.
2. http://www.sportpolo.com/history/default.htm.
3. http://www.polodays.com/special.html.
4. http://www.fippolo.com/polo-basics/glossary.html.
5. Desta B, Maldonado G, Reid H, et al. Acute selenium toxicosis in polo ponies. J Vet Diagn Invest 2011;23(3):623–8.
6. Ferraz GC, Soares OA, Foz NS, et al. The workload and plasma ion concentration in a training match session of high-goal (elite) polo ponies. Equine Vet J 2010; Suppl 38:191–5.
7. Targa A. Etude des Paramètres de l'Effort chez le Cheval de Polo en Situation Réelle. Ecole Vétérinaire d'Alfort Thèse d'Ecole Vétérinaire d'Alfort France. 2009.
8. Mukai K, Hiraga A, Takahashi T, et al. Effects of three warm-up regimens of equal distance on VO_2 kinetic during supramaximal exercise in Thoroughbred horses. Equine Vet J 2010;Suppl 38:33–9.
9. Craig L, Hintz HF, Soderholm LV, et al. Changes in blood constituents accompanying exercise in polo horses. Cornell Vet 1985;75:297–302.
10. Marlin D, Allen C Cardiovascular demands of competition on low-goal (non-elite) polo ponies. Equine Vet J 1999;31(5):378–82.
11. Zobba R, Ardu M, Niccolini S, et al. Physical, hematological, and biochemical responses to acute intense exercise in polo horses. J Eq Vet Sciences 2011;31: 542–8.
12. Giraudet A. Personnal observation.
13. Voynick BT, Sweeney CR. Exercise-induced pulmonary hemorrhage in polo and racing horses. J Am Vet Med Assoc 1986;188(3):301–2.
14. Moran G, Carrillo R, Campos B, et al. Endoscopic evaluation of exercise induced pulmonary hemorrhage in polo ponies. Arch Med Vet 2003;35(1).
15. McGowan CM, Posner RE, Christley RM. Incidence of exertional rhabdomyolysis in polo horses in the USA and United Kingdom in the 1999/2000 season. Vet Rec 2002;150(5):535–7.
16. McGowan CM, Fordham T, Christley RM. Incidence and risk factors for exertional rhabdomyolysis in thoroughbred racehorses in the United Kingdom. Vet Rec 2002;151(21):623–6.
17. Stanley RL, McCue ME, Valberg SJ, et al. A glycogen synthase 1 mutation associated with equine polysaccharide storage myopathy and exertional rhabdomyolysis occurs in a variety of UK breeds. Equine Vet J 2009;41(6):597–601.
18. Marcella K. Polo Pony injuries. In Proceedings of the American Association of Equine Practionners, 1990, p. 647–60.
19. Tan H, Wilson AM. Grip and limb force limits to turning performance in competition horses. Proc R Soc B 2011;278:2105–11.
20. Argüelles D, Carmona JU, Climent F, et al. Autologous platelet concentrates as a treatment for musculoskeletal lesions in five horses. Vet Rec 2008;162(7): 208–11.
21. Herthel DJ. Enhanced suspensory ligament healing in 100 horses by stem cells and other bone marrow components. In Proceedings of the American Association of Equine Practionners, 2001, p. 319–21.
22. Crowe OM, Dyson SJ, Wrigh IM, et al. Treatment of chronic or recurrent proximal suspensory desmitis using radial pressure wave therapy in the horse. Equine Vet J 2004;36(4):313–06.

Veterinary aspects of training and competing western performance horses

54

Todd C. Holbrook

CHAPTER CONTENTS

Introduction

The western performance horse disciplines of cutting, reining, working cow horse, roping and barrel racing are widely popular in North America and some of these sports are experiencing rapid international growth. American Quarter Horses, often selectively bred for their respective sport, are the most commonly used, followed by Paint and Appaloosa horses. Agility is required for all western equestrian athletes to be successful as they must execute rapid acceleration, turning, deep stops and abrupt changes in direction. The equine veterinarian should be familiar with the demands placed upon these horses during training and competition of each specific discipline in order to provide optimal health care. This is especially true considering these athletes often present with complaints of reduced performance rather than overt lameness.

Overview of the sport

Demographics

The American Quarter Horse Association is the largest equine breed association in the world with over three million horses registered.[1] Reining became a sport recognized by the International Equestrian Federation (FEI) in 2000 and is one of the world's fastest-growing equestrian sports. The midwestern region of North America has the highest population of Quarter Horses (see Tables 54.1–54.3). Of the European countries, Italy and Germany have the highest number of registered Quarter Horses, yet the total number registered internationally comprises less than 5% of the population[1] (see Table 54.1). Annual purses associated with many of the western equestrian disciplines continue to increase steadily on a year-by-year basis. In the past decade, reining competition payouts increased over 150% from $4 966 323 in 2000 to $12 497 450 in 2010; annual purse statistics from this and other selected western events in 2011 are presented in Figure 54.1.[2,3] While many athletes compete well into their teenage years, horses actively competing in roping and barrel racing tend to be older, and may have trained or competed in other disciplines when younger. The cutting, reining, and cow horse industries have the most developed payout structures focused on age-categorized competitions most commonly referred to as futurities (for three year olds) and derbies (for 4–6 year olds). Training intensity is high, especially as two and three year olds. Rare elite athletes cross compete in both reining and reined cow horse events at the futurity and derby level. The phenotype of Quarter Horse utilized is somewhat sport dependent. Horses used for barrel racing often have more Thoroughbred influence in their pedigree and thus are taller with longer, less bulky muscles. Cutting horses tend to have the smallest frame of the western sport horses. Horses used for roping events differ somewhat based on their specific role; heeling horses tend to be smaller framed in comparison to heading horses.

Table 54.1 Top 10 countries outside of the United States for registered Quarter Horses

COUNTRY	HORSE POPULATION[1]		NEW REGISTRATION[2]	
	2011	CHANGE FROM PREVIOUS YEAR	2011	CHANGE FROM PREVIOUS YEAR
Mexico	35571	1056	1469	254
Germany	34776	894	1533	–150
Italy	23033	722	1288	96
France	7762	464	483	67
Austria	4680	247	278	41
Brazil	4535	726	126	–218
Venezuela	3898	208	264	20
Netherlands	3637	35	143	–26
Sweden	3056	167	153	–11

Table 54.2 Top 10 states/provinces in North America AQHA populations

STATE	HORSE POPULATION[1]		NEW REGISTRATION[2]	
	2011	CHANGE FROM PREVIOUS YEAR	2011	CHANGE FROM PREVIOUS YEAR
Texas	440872	–9762	15796	–1605
Oklahoma	179458	–4966	5875	–884
California	128203	–4296	3595	–322
Alberta	107645	842	3944	–293
Missouri	103781	–1812	2579	–333
Colorado	90443	–1407	2389	–309
Montana	88891	–1351	2570	–166
Nebraska	82201	–646	2935	–397
Kansas	80109	–2381	2364	–320
South Dakota	80005	–915	3213	–356

Table 54.3 Total AQHA population and registrations

	HORSE POPULATION[1]		NEW REGISTRATION[2]	
	2011	CHANGE FROM PREVIOUS YEAR	2011	CHANGE FROM PREVIOUS YEAR
United States	2635349	–59415	75225	–8534
Canada	242795	1419	8637	–823
International	147850	5950	7212	81
Grand Totals	3025994	–52090	91074	–9276

[1] Figures reflect elimination of all horses age 25 and over unless the owners(s) submitted documentation proving the horse is living.
[2] Reflects the number of American Quarter Horses registered during 2011 to residents within the state, province or country.

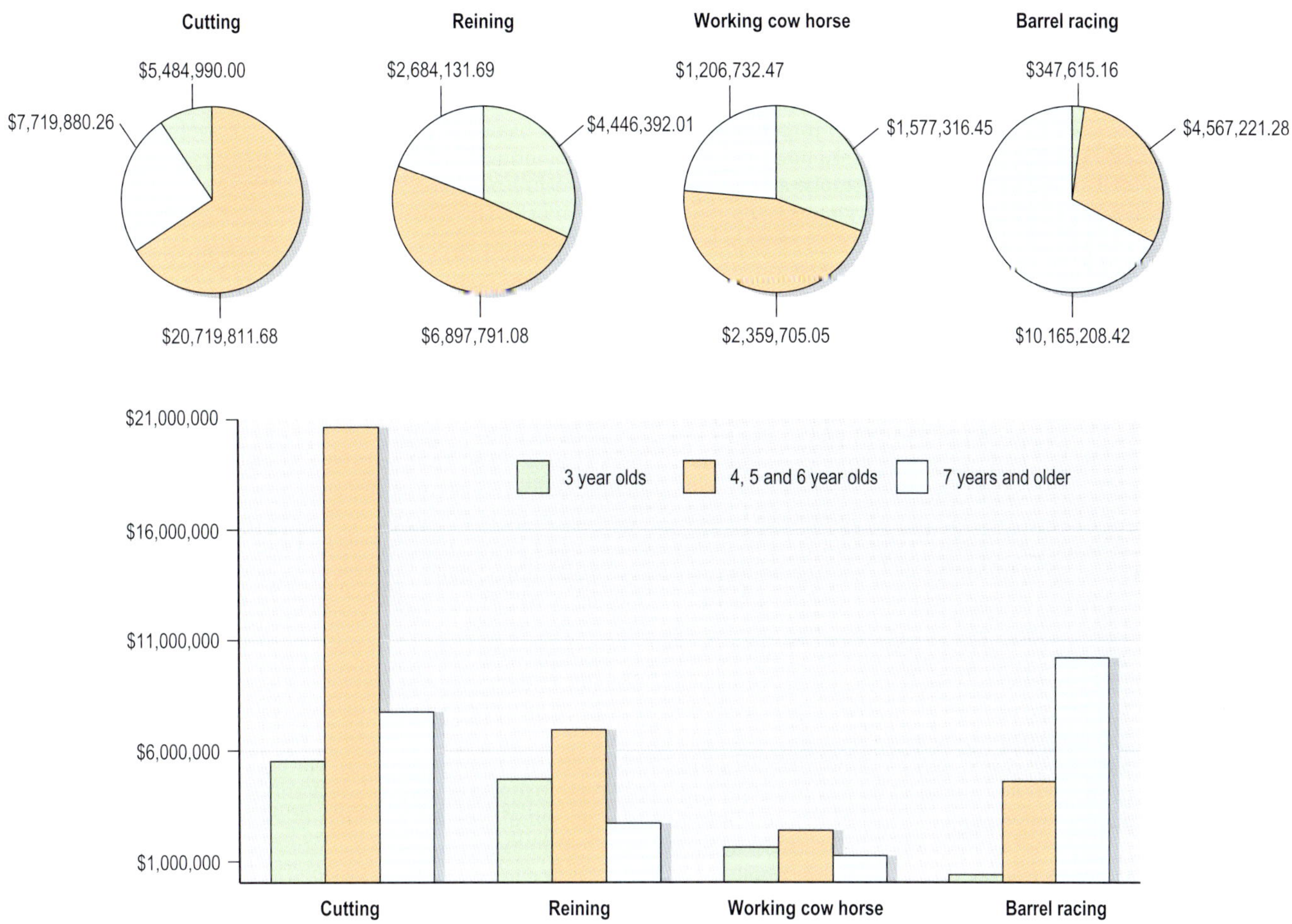

Fig 54.1 Performance earnings for barrel, cutting, reining and working cow horses during 2011 for age-specific events.

Wastage

While there is some welfare concern regarding the potential deleterious impact of intense early training on the young horse's musculoskeletal system, data to substantiate these concerns in western performance horses is lacking. Some sectors of the industry are skeptical that starting young horses a year later would decrease the incidence of athletic injury in the cutting industry.[4] Furthermore, research in young Thoroughbreds suggests that imposing controlled exercise at a very early age (three weeks to 18 months) is not detrimental to bone and joint development, and may in fact be beneficial.[5,6] A number of factors including athletic potential, injury, trainability, and economics can impact the successful development of a competitive western athlete. In contrast to the racing industry, there is a paucity of specific information regarding wastage due to athletic injuries in the western performance industry. Performance statistics from 2011 on offspring sired by the top 20 junior stallions in the cutting and reining industries indicates approximately 32% of performance-aged offspring become money earners.[7] While these statistics do not include non-money earning offspring that are shown, by extrapolation, this performance information is somewhat similar to findings in the Thoroughbred industry where approximately 27% of foals produced by Thoroughbred mares each year go on to race as two and four year olds.[8]

Training

Western performance horses are typically started under saddle as two and three year olds, regardless of discipline. It is not uncommon for those intended to compete in futurity events (reining, cutting, working cow horse) to be started lightly as a long yearling. Training regimens in elite futurity prospects are essentially continual through the horse's second and third years and this repetition and intensity predisposes these athletes to certain injuries.[9]

While training methods vary, most young western stock start in an O- or D-ring smooth or twisted snaffle bit with split reins. Training usually continues with this bit type for at least a year, and then the horse is typically transitioned to either a shank snaffle or hackamore before being moved to a bridle. Horses are initially ridden with two handed contact and, if applicable to the sport, later transitioned to respond to neck reining with one hand. As training progresses, more traditional unbroken mouthpiece bits with ports or spades are used with longer shanks for better control in horses required to stop abruptly. Gag bits are popular amongst barrel racing competitors. Barrel and rope horses are often ridden with closed reins and tie downs (standing martingale), as well as a breast plate and back cinch.

Young horses are usually started in the round pen for several days to weeks, followed by aerobic arena work for approximately 30–60 days prior to beginning more intense work. In the first 6–8 weeks horses are commonly worked briefly (15–30 minutes) 4–6 days a week. Much of this early activity is aimed at increasing suppleness, teaching the young horse to guide and respond appropriately to cues (bit and leg pressure). Early components of the stop and turnaround are typically introduced during this time period in relevant disciplines, while introduction to the rope and pulling weight, or turning around stationary objects is introduced in others. As aerobic fitness improves, repetition of maneuvers gradually increases, as can the duration of work. Typical time spent under saddle varies between 30 and 60 minutes daily, 5–7 days a week.

With the exception of barrel horse training, most western disciplines that use conventional motorized walkers only use them for walking exercise, and to cool out horses after work. In contrast, some barrel horse trainers use exercise walkers for aerobic conditioning (e.g. 45 minutes trotting 3 days a week). In these motorized exercise walkers the horse is not secured to the walker arm by the halter; thus they are allowed to move more naturally and can even be worked in tack.

Cutting and working cow horses are typically introduced to cattle during the first 60–90 days of training. Initially, they are usually worked on a single cow (or mechanical cow) in a large round pen, when they are taught to stop and turn, reciprocating the cow's movement around the outside wall of the pen and developing instinctive 'cow sense'. The duration of work on cattle tends to vary from 20 to 60 minutes dependent on the trainer and the individual horse's needs. Often longer periods of time may accrue under saddle, as horses are worked for brief periods of time on cattle interspersed with rest periods, when they are allowed to settle and taught to stand quietly before being asked to repeat the process. While somewhat trainer and discipline dependent, some horses may spend several hours a day saddled and tied out to the arena, a hitching post or mechanical walker.

All western athletes are gradually trained by repetition of event-specific maneuvers to increase precision and speed. Once a solid base of aerobic fitness is established after 30–60 days, anaerobic work is often gradually introduced with short episodes of high-intensity exercise 2–3 days a week. The activity utilized for this purpose varies with the different sports. Although limited research has been published on physiologic responses during western events, exercise associated with fast canter work (e.g. large fast circles), run downs, sliding stops and rollbacks, fast spins, intense cutting activity, and calf roping are all associated with heart rates typical of anaerobic work.[10–13] Most often anaerobic work is simply achieved as one executes these various maneuvers and repeats them at speed in the practice pen for the various sports. In contrast, some barrel horse trainers integrate fast speed work while exercising horses in fields or at local race tracks. Finished horses of all disciplines that are fit are typically worked for 30–45 minutes, 3–5 days a week to maintain fitness. Older weekend cutting horses, once trained and fit, may be worked on cattle less than once a week. Some trainers also utilize mechanical flags to assist training the stop and proper reaction timing. Roping horses and barrel racing horses that are transported by road almost every weekend to compete may receive minimal routine aerobic exercise between events to maintain fitness during the competition season.

Arena footing

With the exception of cutting pens, which are round and usually 125–175 feet in diameter for training cutters and working cow horses on cattle, most other disciplines utilize rectangular arenas 100–200 feet wide and 300–400 feet long for training. In light of the repetitive training methods necessary for development of competitive athletes, maintaining proper arena footing is extremely important to minimize lameness development. Firm ground may exacerbate lameness and progression of osteoarthritis associated with repetitive concussive forces during training. In contrast, deep footing may predispose to soft tissue injuries. Comparatively, cutting is typically performed in the deepest footing (4–6 inches deep) comprised primarily of sand with a more firm sand or clay base. In the author's experience, ground conditions are most variable at the smaller roping and barrel events. For sports other than cutting activity, quality arena footing often has a large sand component mixed with silt and clay; firmness varies, dependent upon the composition, density and depth of the top layer (3–4 inches). The density and depth of the top layer are primarily influenced by altering the moisture content and ground preparation. In both reining and working cow horse disciplines, sliding stops are a major component of competition. Therefore, footing in these two sports is especially critical. Outdoor arena footing for both of these sports typically has a firm packed base. Most commonly a clay base is used; limestone or granite screenings are used in some geographic regions, but these latter types are not preferable. The overlying footing component is often a less dense composition of sand, clay and silt. In the elite levels of cutting, reining and working cow horse competition, arena footing specialists are typically contracted for ground preparation at each major event. In the major cutting events, sand is the primary arena component with the footing being approximately 4.5 inches deep for futurity events and around 5 inches for older-aged events. In the events with pattern rein work, there is often a well-defined mixture of sand, clay and silt that is placed on the concrete arena floor to promote the sliding stop. The base is formed as this mixture is packed and the ground is worked with specialty drags. The top layer in optimal reining footing is uniformly approximately 2.5–3 inches deep, while footing for working cow horse competitions is slightly deeper. Certain portions of the arena for working cow horse competitions are prepared differently. The area for boxing may have additional sand and depth, while the footing at the fence often has higher moisture content and the base is sometimes scored to increase traction, making these arenas particularly difficult to maintain, according to arena specialist Bob Kiser.

Farriery and protective legwear

Maintenance of proper mediolateral balance and normal hoof pastern axis is critical as in other equine disciplines. Horses often remain unshod during early training, and on occasion even later during competition, in the front feet, if the individual has exceptional hoof quality and conformation. In general, cutting horses often have smaller feet. Currently, there appears to be a trend toward leaving aged event cutting horses barefoot as they often only train and compete in deeper sand footing. Steel keg shoes are also common, especially in older 'weekend cutters' as they often do ranch work in different footing at home (Grant Rezabek, personal communication, 2012). Roping and barrel horses are often shod with steel keg, rim, or natural balance shoes on the front feet and either keg or rim shoes on hind feet.[14–16] The front feet of reining horses are often shod with a squared or rounded toe, and the ground surface may be beveled around to the quarters or heels. The shoe is often set back at the toe to further enhance breakover, which is thought to promote front foot travel in the stop. Circumferential beveling may reduce medial and lateral torsional forces during the turn around. The hind feet of reining horses are shod with sliding plates which are flat, elongated, wide webbed steel shoes in which the nails are countersunk and the bottom of the shoe is polished with a grinder to increase the distance of the sliding stop. Typically, young reining horses have 'starting plates' ($\frac{3}{4}$ inch wide with short trailers) applied during the first 3–6 months of training. Over time, the width of the shoe (and length of trailer) is often increased; the toe is also commonly fashioned similar to a snow ski tip. In finished reining horses sliding plates most often range from 1 or 1¼ inches wide (Fig. 54.2). They can also be shod with a slightly longer toe and a lower angle thought to promote a longer sliding stop. Similar sliding plates are applied in working cow horses, calf roping horses and some heel horses to promote the sliding stop. Because more traction is required for working cow horses in the fence work, and in all of the aforementioned disciplines, the stop is most often shorter and deeper, the sliding plates used are not as wide and have shorter trailers than those applied to reining horses.

The form of leg protection utilized can vary, but most often some form of splint boot, usually neoprene, or a felt polo wrap is used for the front limbs of all western performance horses in training and competition. In reining horses that interfere at the carpus during the turnaround (spins), a variety of knee boots are used during training (Fig. 54.3). In addition, if the sliding stop is incorporated (reining, working cow horse, calf roping, heeling) some form of skid boot is usually applied to the hindlimbs. Most commonly this gear just protects the fetlock (Fig. 54.4A), while some reining horses that stop very deep may require skid boots that cover the hock to prevent excoriation (Fig. 54.4B). Bell boots are usually applied to the front feet for heel protection from hind foot interference, and protection of the coronet band which can be injured when horses step on themselves with the front feet during the turnaround. In those sports that do not require a sliding stop most often the hindlimb protective leg wear is similar to that applied to the forelimbs.

Common conditions in selected western disciplines

Reining

During competition, the reining horse performs one of 11 predetermined patterns that all have approximately 10 maneuvers in common.[17] These include four spins in each direction in which the horse rapidly pivots around the inside hind foot, large fast circles, and slow small circles, figure eights, flying lead changes, run downs, sliding stops, rollbacks, and the backup. This is a judged event that is typically completed in less than four minutes; credit is given for the degree of difficulty, and execution of the pattern in terms of smoothness, finesse, attitude, quickness, and speed control. The goal is to have a willingly guided horse whose every move is controlled by the rider with no apparent resistance. The sliding stop presumably increases stress on the back and hindlimbs, which may predispose to distal tarsitis, proximal suspensory desmitis, stifle and back injuries (Fig. 54.5). Acute avulsion fractures of the medial plantar process of P2 at the insertion of the superficial digital flexor tendon have also been associated with the stop.[18] Skin abrasions in the plantar fetlock and hock region can also occur if proper protective leg gear is not applied in deep stopping individuals. Lateral foot movement in the turnaround (spin) may predispose these athletes to quarter cracks, splints, soft tissue injuries of the digit (collateral ligaments) and coffin bone fractures. Interference injuries associated with the turnaround include coronary band trauma, accessory carpal bone and/or dorsomedial carpal trauma (Fig. 54.6). These athletes also seem to be predisposed to superficial digital flexor tendonitis and P2 fractures. Common performance complaints include not stopping well or 'holding the ground', falling out of lead, reluctance to take a lead or change leads, dropping a hip or shoulder, or problems in the turnaround (not holding a pivot foot). The diagnosis and treatment of common conditions is discussed in further detail below.

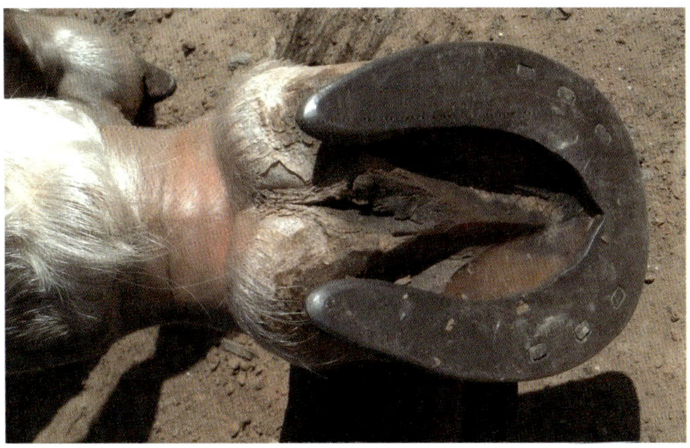

Fig 54.2 Typical sliding plate used on the hind feet of reining horses.

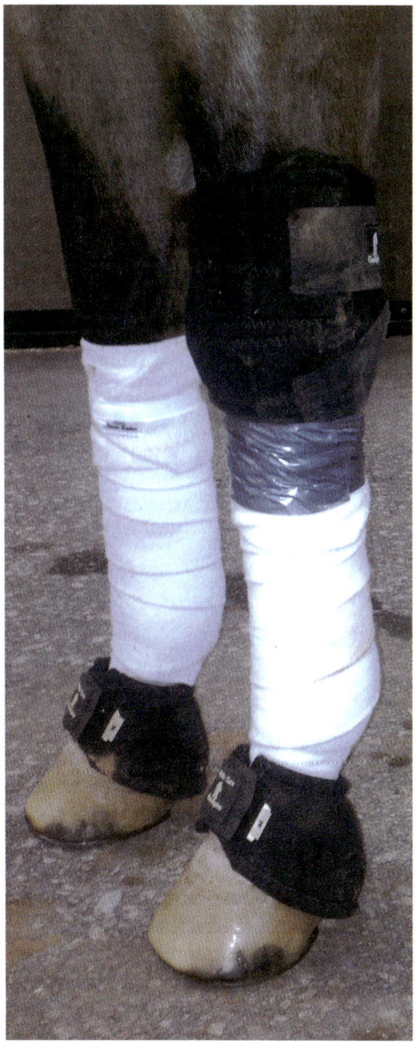

Fig 54.3 Protective knee boots are occasionally used in early training in certain individuals to prevent carpal interference injury during the turnaround.

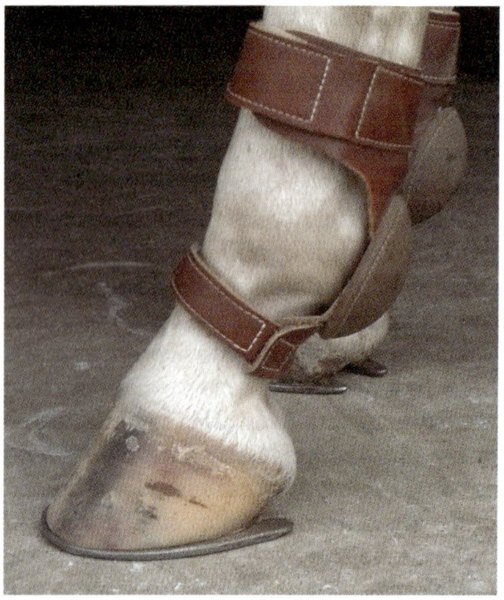

Fig 54.4A Skid boots are applied to the hind fetlocks of most reining horses, and often used in other sports that require the sliding stop (working cow horses, calf roping and heeling) to prevent friction-induced skin injury.

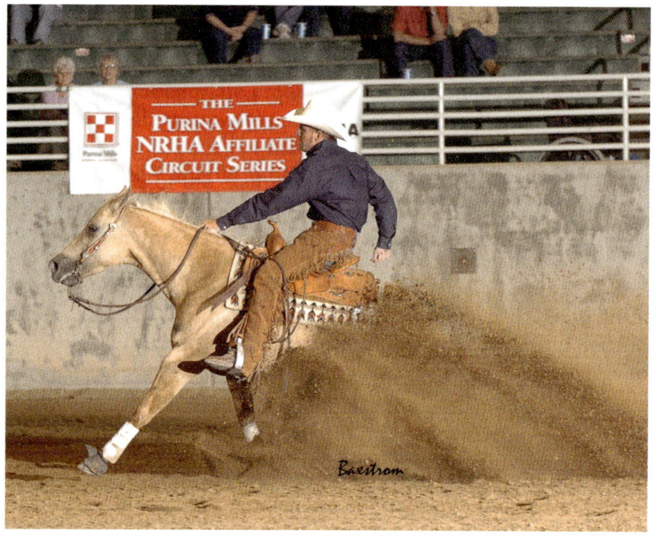

Fig 54.5 The sliding stop is one of the more demanding maneuvers performed by reining horses.

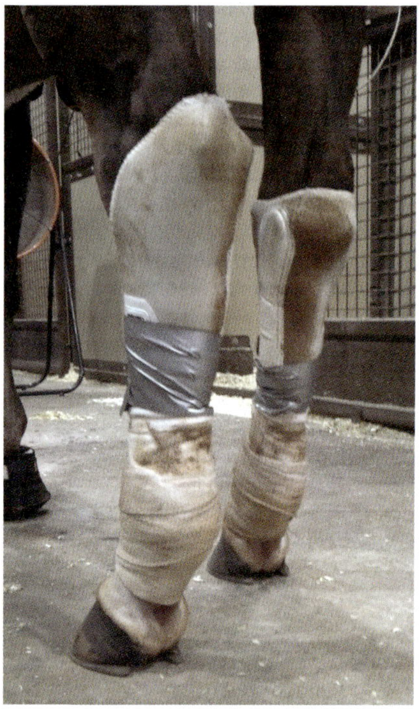

Fig 54.4B Protective boots are occasionally needed for the hock region in individual reining horses that stop very deep.

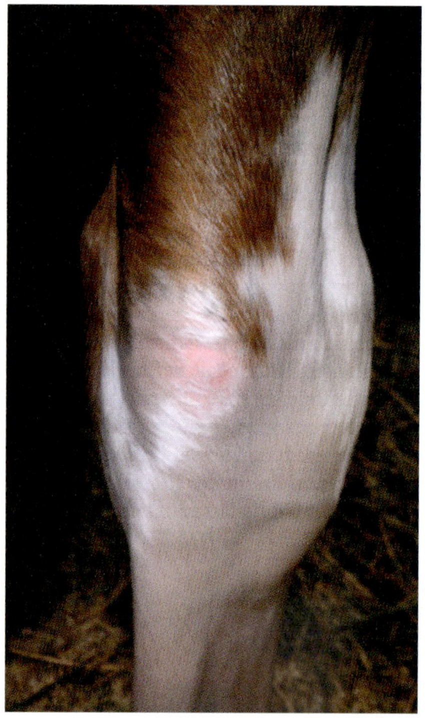

Fig 54.6 Interference injury to the accessory carpal bone region in reining horses can occur during the turnaround, most often in the early training period in two and three year olds.

Cutting

Cutting competition is judged in a 2.5 minute period during which time 2–3 individual cows are typically cut away from a herd of 20–60 cattle and worked. Once cut away from the herd, the rider drops the reins and the horse works the cow with minimal leg cues from the rider. These horses instinctively read the cows every movement and perform rapid stops and turns to mirror this movement and keep the cow cut out of the herd (Fig. 54.7).[19] The classic crouching stop and rapid turning that these athletes perform places increased stress, especially on the hindlimbs, which can predispose to hock, stifle, and back issues, but it is also stressful to the forelimbs. This activity and typical deep footing may also predispose these athletes to suspensory ligament desmitis.[20] Common complaints related to performance include not turning or stopping well and not holding the cow. The recognition and treatment of specific conditions are discussed in further detail below.

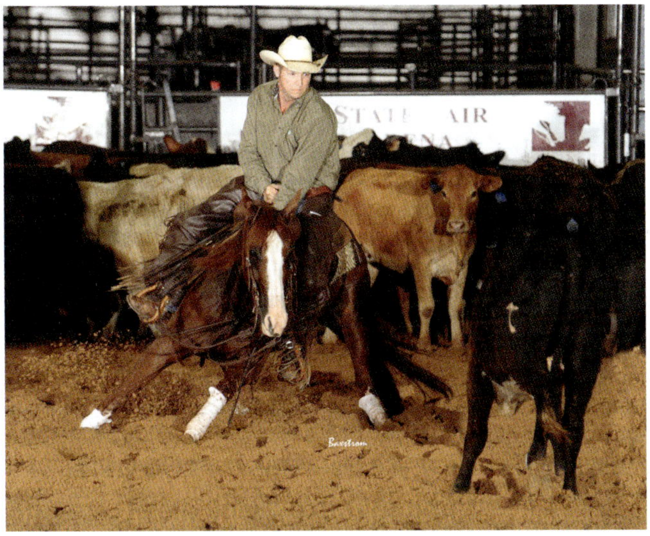

Fig 54.7 Cutting horse performing typical maneuvers in deep footing: note the position of the left hindlimb.

Working/reined cow horse

This discipline combines the aspects of cutting and reining with cow work requiring the horse to be shown in three different disciplines (herd work, rein work and cow work). The herd work is synonymous with cutting and is similarly judged in a 2.5 minute window of time as described above. In the rein work (also known as dry work) the horse completes an abbreviated reining pattern. During the first phase of the cow work the horse and rider work a single calf, mirroring its movement like cutting, demonstrating control over the calf. This is known as 'boxing' and is followed by taking the calf 'down the fence', also known as 'fence runs'. In this phase the rider drives the calf down the edge of the arena, usually at a gallop or lope, keeping it next to the fence. Once the calf passes the halfway mark on the fence the rider will step the horse just past the calf's head, causing it to reverse directions. The rider must complete a minimum of one turn in each direction. The last phase of the cow work is known as 'circling up'. In this portion the rider demonstrates control of the calf by loping the horse alongside the calf, driving it in a small circle. At least one circle must be completed in each direction.[21] Considering the similar demands placed on these athletes by the cutting and reining maneuvers they perform, many of the musculoskeletal issues common in reining and cutting horses also plague these athletes. The rapid turns at speed during fence work is a fairly unique stress of this sport. Injuries potentially associated with this activity include proximal P2 chip fractures at the dorsal aspect of the joint in the hindlimbs and soft tissue injuries at the insertion of the SDF branches in the forelimbs (Joe Carter, personal communication, 2012). Performance complaints may include similar issues described with both reining and cutting horses, and/or problems noted during the fence work. Conditions common to a variety of western athletes are discussed in more detail below.

Team roping and calf roping

The ultimate objective in roping events is to successfully rope the steer (or rope and tie the calf) in the fastest time. Team roping is composed of two competitors, a header positioned in the 'heading box' to the left of the chute, and a heeler positioned in the opposing 'heeling box' on the right. The header's job is to rope the horns or head of the steer, dally (wrap the rope around the saddle horn), and turn sharply left. In doing so, the heading horse drops its left shoulder and hip bracing with the right forelimb positioned laterally. This body position, coupled with the centrifugal force created as the 350–700 lb steer swings to the right on a tight rope, places increased stress on the right front limb and left hindlimb.[22] The heeler follows the steer initially on its right side. As the header sets up the steer, which swings it toward the right, the heeler drops behind the steer's left hip, positioned to catch the steer's hind feet. Once the steer's heels are caught, the heeler dallies. As the heel rope slack tightens, the header spins to the right and faces the steer, keeping his rope taught. Simultaneously, the heeler quickly stops his horse which stretches the steer between the roping team. The rapid stops required by a heel horse likely increases hindlimb stress. Top competitors can complete this task in less than 4 seconds. In both practice runs and competition, it is not uncommon for rope horses to complete multiple runs that can lead to fatigue.

Calf ropers start in the box to the right side of the chute. Once the calf is roped, the rider dismounts as the horse performs a sliding stop and the slack in the rope tightens. The horse works the rope, by backing up to tighten it as the roper runs down the rope to grab the calf by its flank, throwing the calf on its side; the roper then rapidly ties three of the calf's legs together. Competitive runs range from 8 to 9 seconds. Similar to heeling horses, these athletes likely have increased stress to the hindlimbs due to the sliding stop.

Common performance complaints in roping horses include reluctance to enter or stand quietly in the box, not holding the ground in a stop, not facing the steer well (heading), not working the rope (calf horses), and not 'making the corner' (turning left in heel horses).[23] Common causes of lameness in team roping horses include palmar foot pain, and distal tarsitis in both heading and heeling horses. Heading horses appear to be predisposed to carpitis and soft tissue injuries in the right forelimb (suspensory, distal sesmoidian ligaments, collateral ligaments, impar ligament and deep digital flexor tendon) as well as P2 fractures.[14,23] Calf roping horses are similarly predisposed to distal tarsitis, but also seem to be commonly affected with stifle injury, hindlimb proximal suspensory desmitis, fetlock osteoarthritis, fractures of P2 and the proximal sesamoids.[16] Specific conditions are described in further detail below.

Barrel racing

Futurity events in barrel racing are primarily focused on horses that are 4–5 years of age, with derbies for six and seven year olds. However, many barrel horses compete well into their teenage years in the non-age specific events. Barrel racing is a timed event where horses run a cloverleaf pattern around three 55 gallon barrels. The pattern varies in size dependent upon the arena dimensions. Most often the right barrel is turned first. All of the barrels are turned in a manner such that the horse's path is crossed as it completes a 360 degree turn around the barrel. The horses sprint toward the first barrel at full speed, rate, turn, and run to the second barrel, rate, turn, and run to the third barrel, rate, turn and sprint at full speed to the finish line.[24] A typical competitive run will range from 15 to 16 seconds in larger arenas. Common injuries in barrel horses include palmar foot pain, distal tarsitis, and suspensory ligament desmitis.[15] Common complaints by riders include reluctance to enter the arena, not turning a barrel well (especially the first), dropping a shoulder, knocking over, or running past the barrel, reduced speed after the last barrel, and slower times. Diagnosis and treatment of specific conditions are described in more detail below.

Specific veterinary conditions and their management

Musculoskeletal diseases

Rhabdomyolysis

In American Quarter Horses, Paints and Appaloosas there are currently two recognized forms of polysaccharide storage myopathy (PSSM). Type 1 is caused by an autosomal dominant genetic mutation that results in upregulation (approximately twofold) of muscle glycogen synthase enzyme (GYS1) activity.[25] Approximately 50% of PSSM cases in Quarter Horses and related breeds are due to the GYS1 mutation; the genetic basis of type 2 PSSM is currently not defined. [26] PSSM results in excessive glycogen storage and accumulation of abnormal polysaccharide in type 2 muscles.[27] Other studies indicate horses with PSSM have abnormally high insulin sensitivity, which results in increased glucose uptake and excessive glycogen storage.[27–29] The precise mechanism of exercise-induced myopathy in horses with PSSM is unknown. Some have hypothesized that there is a disruption in the conversion of glycogen to pyruvate and acetyl CoA which impairs the generation of citric acid cycle intermediates and energy, resulting in muscle damage.[30] The frequency and severity of muscle injury in horses with PSSM is influenced both by aerobic exercise frequency and diet. While the incidence of clinical myopathy in the individual western disciplines is unknown, the PSSM allele frequency ranges from 1.4 to 6.7 % in elite competitive subgroups of Quarter Horses. The allele prevalence was lowest in barrel racing horses (1.4%), followed by reining horses (4.3%), working cow horses (5.7%) and cutting horses (6.7%).[31]

In genetically susceptible individuals, PSSM is often precipitated upon returning to work following brief periods of rest during training. While the condition can be first recognized when horses start aerobic work under saddle, the average age at the development of clinical signs is six years.[32] Episodes are often recurrent, and the history may include complaints of reluctance to work, stop or turn, poor impulsion and collection, mild hindlimb lameness, and poor performance in general. On occasion, excessive work (especially in hot conditions) is associated with exercise-induced myopathy in horses without genetic predisposition. In these situations the clinical syndrome may be complicated by severe dehydration, electrolyte and acid–base derangements, and exhaustion.

Classically, the gluteal muscle groups of the hindlimbs and epaxial muscles of the lower back are affected and may be firm and swollen; however, other muscle groups may be involved. A shortened stride is usually obvious at the walk. Some horses are reluctant to move; other clinical signs may include sweating, tachycardia, tachypnea, spasmodic muscle contractures and fasciculations. Exertional myopathy associated with prolonged intense work can result in exhaustion and significant dehydration. Potential clinical signs include hyperthermia, lethargy, weakness, injected mucus membranes with a prolonged capillary refill time, and synchronous diaphragmatic flutter. Pigmenturia due to myoglobinuria is often present. Horses with severe myopathy may be recumbent and unable to rise. Although rare, life-threatening complications associated with severe rhabdomyolysis include renal failure and laminitis.

Although biochemical evidence of myopathy is expected following clinical episodes of PSSM, abnormal 'resting' creatine kinase (CK) and/or aspartate transaminase (AST) associated with recent work may be noted when examining horses with a history of poor performance. After a clinical episode, CK usually peaks 4–6 hours after the exercise bout, while AST peaks 12–24 hours later.[33,34] AST can remain elevated for as long as 10–14 days because of its long half-life.

Typically in Quarter Horses with a clinical suspicion of myopathy, hair roots or whole blood are submitted for genetic testing for type 1 PSSM. If this test is negative, a submaximal exercise test (SET) can be performed to support a diagnosis of exercise-associated myopathy. After obtaining a baseline serum sample, the horse is worked either on a lunge line or in round pen for 15 minutes at a trot with intermittent loping. In abnormal horses, this mild exercise bout can cause a threefold or greater increase in CK above baseline 4–6 hours after work; AST may increase by 50%. If the SET is suggestive of myopathy, a muscle biopsy can be obtained for histologic evaluation. The genetic basis of type 2 PSSM is currently unknown and the diagnosis is based on histology.[35]

Treatment of acute cases is dependent upon the severity of clinical signs and the presence of pigmenturia. Horses with mild signs that are not dehydrated and lack overt pigmenturia often recover with rest alone or combined with non-steroidal anti-inflammatory drug (NSAID) treatment. More severely affected horses with pigmenturia are often treated with intravenous balanced electrolytes to promote diuresis, as well as NSAIDs, and occasionally other medications (e.g. opioids and alpha-2 agonists) as indicated for analgesia. In severely dehydrated horses and those with significant pigmenturia, the dose, frequency and type of NSAID used should be considered in order to minimize the risk of nephrotoxicity. The prognosis for return to function is usually good; however, rarely, muscle atrophy can develop, which may negatively affect athletic function.

Many horses with PSSM can be managed with an athletic career if particular attention is paid to consistent exercise and strict dietary management. If possible, affected horses should have access to pasture turnout 12–24 hours a day. This may be difficult to achieve in certain sports as turnout may have deleterious seasonal effects on the hair coat which is not preferable in show horses, and some individuals may risk injury if turned out in sliding plates. In addition, routine daily exercise is important to maximize oxidative capacity in muscle.[32] Dietary management is also a necessity. Current recommendations include removing access to high non-structural carbohydrates (NSC), and feeding hay that is 12% or lower in NSC, with additional calories provided in the form of fat as 10–15% of daily digestible energy.[36,37]

Palmar heel pain

While palmar foot pain is common in all Quarter Horses, regardless of discipline, it is the most common cause of lameness in rope horses and barrel racing horses.[14,15,38] Common performance complaints in barrel horses include reluctance to enter the arena, failing to turn the barrels correctly (especially the first barrel), dropping a shoulder, or a decrease in the horse's speed. Performance issues in rope horses may include reluctance to enter the box and stand quietly, not running hard to the steer, and ducking in or out when turned sharply. Horses most often present with bilateral forelimb lameness. The lameness may be shifting in character, causing a shortened anterior stride phase, especially on firm ground.

A painful response to hoof testing over the frog and/or across the heels supports the diagnosis, and palmar digital nerve, navicular bursa and/or distal interphalangeal anesthesia is used to further localize the source of lameness. The source of pain may involve numerous structures in the heel region either separately, or in combination. These include the navicular bone, its fibrocartilagenous surface and bursa, collateral suspensory ligaments, distal sesmoidean impar ligament, the deep digital flexor tendon, as well as the collateral ligaments and distal interphangeal (DIP) joint. Diagnostic imaging modalities used to evaluate this region include radiography, magnetic resonance imaging (MRI), nuclear scintigraphy, computed tomography (CT) and ultrasonography. Compared to radiography, MRI has high sensitivity and specificity for confirming lesions within the navicular bone, suspensory ligaments, distal sesmoidean impar ligament, and deep digital flexor tendon.[39]

Treatment options will vary based upon the specific cause of heel pain. Maintenance of normal dorsopalmar and mediolateral hoof balance, and a straight hoof pastern axis should be a treatment goal in all horses. Specific shoeing strategies to manage palmar heel pain include enhancing breakover, heel elevation, and heel support. Shoes used to manage this condition include egg bar, natural balance, rockered or rail shoes with or without heel wedges. A variety of non-steroidal anti-inflammatory drugs can be used to reduce lameness during work. Other treatment options include injection of the DIP joint or navicular bursa with corticosteroids and sodium hyaluronate (HA) (Hylartin-V, Pfizer Animal Health, Fort Dodge, IA 50501), tiludronate (Tildren, CEVA Animal Health, Amersham, Buckinghamshire, HP7 9FB), shockwave therapy and chemical or surgical neurectomy. Prognosis appears to be dependent upon the lesion severity in the navicular bone and associated soft tissue structures.

Coronary band trauma and quarter cracks

Forelimb coronary band trauma can occur especially during early training in reining and reined cow horses learning to turn around, as well as heel bulb injuries from interference during sliding stops. The diagnosis and treatment of coronary band trauma is usually straightforward. The wound is cleaned and, if indicated, topical antiseptics/antimicrobials and a foot wrap are applied, plus or minus systemic NSAIDs. Typically, unless the trauma results in a full-skin thickness laceration, lameness is mild and training can continue without a period of rest. Bell boots are important to minimize coronary band trauma.

These same athletes appear to be predisposed to quarter cracks in the front feet potentially associated with hoof wall stress induced by rapid turning during intense work. They tend to be more common in horses with thin walls and flat feet in heavy work; mediolateral hoof imbalance may also predispose to their development (Mark Flarida, personal communication, 2012). Acute quarter cracks at the coronary band that involve the sensitive lamina can cause severe lameness. Secondary infection is common. Bleeding or drainage from the lesion can occur, especially after work. Treatment during the acute phase may include NSAIDs for pain management, as well as topical antiseptics and bandaging. Typically the shoe is removed, any mediolateral imbalance is corrected, and the crack is enlarged if drainage needs to be established. Once the infection is resolved, the crack can be stabilized, if indicated, using a number of methods including lacing and metal or acrylic patching. Often the heel is floated on the affected side followed by application of a bar shoe. Quarter cracks can become a chronic source of lameness and tend to be more difficult to manage in horses that must remain in training.

Pedal osteitis

Non-septic pedal osteitis may be more relevant in barrel racing and roping horses that tend to work on more inconsistent footing which is often too firm. It has also been recognized as a common condition in reining horses in Europe, and in reined cow horses.[18,40] The condition tends to cause chronic mild forelimb lameness which may be unilateral or bilateral. Pain upon application of hoof testers is typical in the toe region but some horses react across the entire sole. Radiographs are important to support the diagnosis and guide corrective shoeing. Demineralization and remodeling of the solar margin of the distal phalanx is typical; often the soles are thin and some individuals have an abnormally high palmar angle (Mike Schoonover, personal communication, 2012). Shoeing goals include increasing sole depth and avoiding sole pressure, maintaining an appropriate palmar angle and reducing concussion with rim pads or Equi-Pak soft pour-in pads (Vettec Inc. Oxnard, CA 93033). Intermittent NSAIDs are used for pain management. Exercising on proper footing to reduce concussion is also important.

Splints

During early training, medial forelimb splints are common in young horses, especially those with offset knees. Torsional forelimb forces associated with spins (reining horses) may predispose to their development. In the acute stage, the lameness is often mild and may be transient. Acute treatment may include rest, systemic NSAIDs, local treatment with: ice, corticosteroids: (perilesional infiltration or topically mixed with dimethyl sulfoxide), topical 1% diclofenac sodium, leg poultices and wraps. Lesions often remodel with continued training and are not usually a cause of chronic lameness. Chronic lameness can develop if lesions impinge upon the suspensory ligament.

Superficial digital flexor tendonitis

Tendonitis appears to occur more frequently in reining and working cow horses compared to the other western disciplines. It may be associated with intense training of the turnaround, and rundowns, especially if horses are worked to fatigue in deep footing. Acute onset of swelling and sensitivity at the site of injury is typical; sometimes this is noted prior to lameness. Ultrasonography is important for diagnosis as well as monitoring the response to treatment and assessing prognosis. Lesions appear to be more common in the middle to distal metacarpal region at the lateral or medial aspect of the tendon.[18] Acute treatment options include systemic NSAIDs, local application of ice, leg wraps, poultices, and local injection of corticosteroids. Rehabilitation involves an initial rest period followed by a controlled exercise program tailored to the individual based upon the ultrasonographic severity of the lesion. Additional treatment options include extracorporeal shock wave therapy (ESWT) and local injection of platelet-rich plasma or stem cells. Monitoring local heat and swelling coupled with periodic ultrasonographic reassessment is important during rehabilitation.

Suspensory desmitis

Suspensory ligament injuries are fairly frequent in western performance horses in both the front and hind limbs. Predisposing factors in the front limbs may include hindlimb lameness, intense work to fatigue especially in deep footing and mediolateral hoof imbalance. While branch lesions also occur, proximal suspensory desmitis (PSD) is more common in both the front and hind limbs. Pain may be induced by palpation, but heat and swelling are often not evident with proximal lesions. Other diagnostic tools include ultrasonography and radiology. Athletes that stop deep and use the hind quarters comparatively more (cutting, reining, working cow horses, calf roping, heeling and barrel racing) are likely predisposed to PSD of the hindlimbs. Lameness associated with hindlimbs PSD may be exacerbated by hock flexion; thus, peripheral nerve blocks may be needed to distinguish this condition from distal tarsitis. Therapy and rehabilitation for acute desmitis are similar to those described for tendonitis. Prognosis for hindlimb PSD is more guarded compared to forelimb proximal lesions. Non-responsive cases may benefit from surgical fasciotomy and resection of the deep branch of the lateral plantar nerve. Treatment of chronic PSD with minimal ultrasonographic fiber disruption may include local infusion of corticosteroids with or without pitcher plant extract for temporary analgesia (P-Bloc, *Sarracenia Purpurea* extract, Life Science Products, St. Joseph, MO 64506).

Hock lameness

Distal tarsitis (DT)

Osteoarthritis (OA) of the distal intertarsal (DIT) and tarsometatarsal (TMT) joints is the most common cause of reduced performance in cutting and reining horses, and the second most frequent cause of lameness in team roping and barrel racing horses.[14,15,20] Poor stopping, falling out of lead, or problems in the turnaround in reining horses, and late turning on a cow in cutting horses are common complaints. The condition is typically bilateral, but one leg may demonstrate a greater degree of lameness. Clinical diagnosis is supported by a positive response to upper hindlimb flexion and back soreness. Radiography may reveal evidence of OA; however, radiographs can be normal in horses with hock pain. Intra-articular anesthesia of the tarsometatarsal, distal intertarsal, and/or the proximal intertarsal (PIT) joints can be utilized if diagnostic confirmation is required. However, response to treatment with intra-articular (HA) with or without corticosteroids is often used to support the diagnosis in lieu of intra-articular anesthesia. This treatment, in conjunction with NSAIDs and limited exercise for 2–5 days, is often palliative if only the DIT and/or TMT joints are involved. The prognosis is more guarded if there is significant osteoarthritis in the PIT joint. The routine administration of systemic hyaluronate sodium (Legend, Bayer Healthcare LLC, Animal Health Division, Shawnee Mission, KS 66201) and/or polysulfated glycosaminoglycans (PSGAG) (Adequan IM, Luitpold Pharmaceutical Inc., Animal health Division, Shirley, NY 11967) may reduce the frequency of intra-articular medication. Surgical arthrodesis or alcohol-facilitated ankylosis of the DIT and TMT joints are treatment options in horses with advanced degenerative joint disease non-responsive to intra-articular corticosteroids.[41,42]

Hock osteochondrosis dessicans (OCD)

Tarsocrural joint effusion is typical; however, lameness is an inconsistent finding. Lesions may also be discovered on presale radiographs in the absence of effusion. Lesions at the distal intermediate ridge of the tibia (DIRT) followed by the lateral trochlear ridge of the tibiotarsal bone are the two most frequent anatomic sites of OCD in the hock. DIRT lesions are more common in two-year-old cutting horses than yearlings.[43] Flattening of the medial trochlear ridge was noted in approximately 12% of yearling and two-year-old cutting horses, but fragments at this location were uncommon.[43] Small non-displaced fragments may heal with conservative management, especially in weanlings that are not lame. Arthroscopic removal of displaced or large fragments is advised.

Stifle lameness

Performance deficits associated with stifle trauma or osteochondrosis may be noted prior to overt lameness. Complaints may include not holding the ground in stops in reining and cutting horses, or not planting a pivot foot when spinning in reining and reined cow horses, as well as problems turning in barrel horses. Subchondral cystic lesions (SCLs) of the medial femoral condyle are common, yet multiple etiologies ranging from osteoarthritis to soft tissue injuries (medial meniscus, medial collateral or cruciate ligaments) are possible. Acute lameness and effusion is typical with traumatic stifle injuries. Intra-articular anesthesia is used to localize the lameness. Imaging modalities often utilized include radiography and ultrasonography. Pain on palpation or limb manipulation may be present with certain acute soft tissue injuries (collateral ligament). Treatment options include: rest, intra-articular injection of HA and corticosteroids, arthroscopic debridement, stem cell and/or IRAP therapy.[44,45]

The prevalence of lesions in the stifle was approximately 44% in a recent review of radiographs in 458 yearling and two-year-old Quarter Horse cutting prospects. Flattening of the medial femoral condyle (MFC) was the most common radiographic lesion in the stifle; however its clinical relevance has recently been questioned.[43,46] Subchondral bone cysts (SBCs) of the MFC were also common in this study and occurred bilaterally over 50% of the time. SBCs in this location may cause effusion in the medial femorotibial joint, yet the severity of lameness can vary from mild to severe. Treatment options include corticosteroid injection into the cyst lining performed during arthroscopy or with ultrasonographic guidance. The overall success rate of this procedure is 90% and 67% in horses with unilateral and bilateral SBCs, respectively. However, discipline may influence the success rate of this procedure as only 55% of cutting horses returned to function, compared to 83% of reining horses.[47] Other surgical options for SBCs include arthroscopic debridement alone, or combined with: bone grafting, growth factor, chondrocyte or stem cell implantation.[48–50] Non-surgical treatment options include systemic and intra-articular joint therapy (PSGAG and HA) with or without intra-articular corticosteroids, and ESWT.

OCD lesions in the stifle are usually at the lateral femoral trochlear ridge; these may be asymptomatic and discovered on presale radiographs, or associated with lameness.[43] Stifle effusion is common, yet lameness can vary from subtle to obvious. Conservative management (rest) is considered in foals, or in individuals with mild radiographic lesions. Arthroscopic debridement is usually advised if the lesions are large, or the lameness is significant and fails to respond to conservative management. Medical treatment options include systemic and intra-articular joint therapy (PSGAG and HA) with or without intra-articular corticosteroids.

Lameness of the fetlock and pastern

Fetlock and pastern osteoarthritis

Osteoarthritis of the fetlock or pastern joints may affect any western athlete, but tends to be more frequently an issue in roping, barrel, reining, and reined cow horses. Joint effusion is usually notable with OA of the fetlock as the disease progresses. Ringbone in the front limb, associated with severe pastern OA, may be more frequent in aged roping and barrel racing horses, while it seems to more commonly affect the hindlimb in older reining horses. Radiography combined with peripheral or intra-articular nerve blocks are used to confirm the diagnosis. Medical treatment options include systemic and intra-articular joint therapy (PSGAG and HA) with or without intra-articular corticosteroids and intra-articular IRAP therapy. Surgical arthrodesis can be considered in horses with advanced pastern OA.

Fetlock osteochondrosis

Osteochondral fragments are fairly common in both the front and hind fetlocks. Lesions at the proximal caudal eminence of P1 may be associated with falling out of lead when the affected limb is on the outside of the circle in reining and working cow horses (Joe Carter, personal communication, 2012). Arthroscopic removal is indicated if associated with lameness or problems maintaining leads.

P2 fractures

Fractures of P2 appear to be a more common injury in heading and reining horses and can be catastrophic.[23] Reining horses also develop fractures of the medial plantar process associated with stopping and avulsion at the insertion of the medial branch of the SDF tendon, and the prognosis appears to be poor.[18]

Skin conditions

Fetlock and hock abrasions

Burns and abrasions of the skin at the plantar aspect of the fetlocks are most common in athletes that perform the sliding stop. Plantar hock lesions can also occur in very deep stopping horses. Protective skid boots are routinely used for prevention, while hock boots are occasionally needed in unique individuals.

Pastern dermatitis

Sweating due to frequent work, daily bathing, as well as the use of common protective leg wear amongst different horses may predispose to the development of pastern dermatitis commonly referred to as scratches, greasy heel, or mud fever. The dermatitis is typically confined to the caudal pastern region, but can occasionally extend proximally or distally. Clinical signs vary from several dry scabs, to deeper cracks in the creases of the caudal pastern, with or without exudation and edema which can cause prominent lameness. There are multiple potential etiologies for pastern dermatitis. Treatments include application of local astringents, antiseptics, antimicrobial ointments or sprays, corticosteroids, and systemic antimicrobials. Keeping the area clean and drying after bathing is important in healing and preventing recurrence.

Respiratory diseases

Upper respiratory diseases

Infectious respiratory disease in the western performance training industry, associated with the commingling of young horses in training barns, is not uncommon due to both viral (influenza and herpes) and bacterial (strangles) etiologies. A recent survey over a 24-month period investigating equine respiratory pathogens in the United States revealed some age- and breed-specific risk factors that are relevant to the industry. The largest age group represented in the study was horses 1–5 years of age. In this age group, the most prevalent cause of respiratory disease was equine influenza virus (61.7%), followed by EHV-1 (30.4%), EHV-4 (28.1%) and *Streptococcus equi* subspecies *equi* (18.4%).[51] While rhinovirus was not included as one of the pathogens screened for in the previous study, a two-year surveillance study in performance horses in Ontario revealed the two most common pathogens associated with acute signs of respiratory infection were EIV and rhinovirus. The average age of horses with clinical disease in this study was 3.2 years.[52]

Non-infectious upper respiratory diseases

Upper respiratory dysfunction leading to poor performance is most commonly implicated in barrel racing horses. The severity of left laryngeal hemiplegia (LLH), and significance of dorsal displacement of the soft palate (DDSP) may be better ascertained with dynamic upper airway endoscopy during a treadmill examination to determine if prosthetic laryngoplasty (for LLH), and/or treatment for DDSP is indicated. Upper airway obstruction that causes excessive respiratory noise can be an issue in horses that show in judged events which occasionally warrants surgical intervention.

Lower respiratory diseases

Exercise-induced pulmonary hemorrhage

Exercise-induced pulmonary hemorrhage (EIPH) is frequently diagnosed in barrel racing horses that present for the evaluation of poor performance. While the true prevalence and impact of EIPH on performance in this discipline is unknown, competitors are widely aware of the disease and frequently treat their horses in an attempt to prevent it. In one small study (20 barrel horses) the prevalence of EIPH was 70%.[53] A larger study in two-year-old racing Quarter Horses revealed a 65% prevalence of EIPH. The diagnostic (post-race endoscopy, bronchoalveolar lavage, transtracheal aspirate), and treatment (pre-race furosemide and FLAIR nasal strips (Flair LLC, Delano, MN 55328) options are similar to those used in racing Thoroughbreds, with the exception being the lack of medication restrictions at most barrel racing competitions. Despite these proven treatment options, widespread use and promotion of many other supplements as 'treatments' by riders is commonplace in the sport.

Inflammatory airway disease (IAD) and recurrent airway obstruction (RAO)

IAD and RAO are fairly common diagnoses in barrel racing and roping horses that present for poor performance unrelated to lameness. Interestingly, a recent study revealed Quarter Horses may indeed have a breed predisposition to lower airway inflammation.[54] Diagnostic confirmation is based upon lower airway cytology. In addition to environmental management to reduce exposure to dust during training, and exposure to hay mold, common treatment options include systemic and inhaled corticosteroids and bronchodilators. The absence of medication rules in many roping and barrel racing event venues enables treatment during competition in the majority of instances.

References

1. AQHA. 2011 Horse Statistics.pdf. AQHA.com: AQHA; 2012.
2. Timmons D. 2011 Year end performance earnings for 3, 4, 5, 6 and 7 year old and older horses in cutting, reining, working cow horse, and barrel horse competition. In: EquiStat, editor. Cowboy Publishing Group; 2012.
3. Staff Q. 2010 Annual Reining Statistics. Quarter Horse News. QuarterHorseNews.com: Morris Magazine Network; 2011.
4. Black JB, Frisbie D. Welfare concerns in the training and competition of the cutting, reining, and reined cow horse. In: McIlwraith CW, Rollin BE, editors. Equine Welfare. Oxford: Wiley-Blackwell; 2011. p. 302–17.

5. Kim W, Kawcak CE, McIlwraith CW, et al. Influence of early conditioning exercise on the development of gross cartilage defects and swelling behavior of cartilage extracellular matrix in the equine midcarpal joint. Am J Vet Res 2009;70: 589–98.
6. Kawcak CE, McIlwraith CW, Firth EC. Effects of early exercise on metacarpophalangeal joints in horses. Am J Vet Res 2010;71:405–11.
7. Tims K. Top Junior Reining and Cutting Sires (2011). QuarterHorseNews.com: Morris Magazine Network; 2012.
8. Jeffcott LB, Rossdale PD, Freestone J, et al. An assessment of wastage in thoroughbred racing from conception to 4 years of age. Equine Vet J 1982;78: 201–15.
9. Scott M. Musculoskeletal injuries in nonracing quarter horses. Vet Clin North Am Equine Pract 2008;24:133–52.
10. Rammerstorfer C, Potter GD, Brumbaugh GW, et al. Physiologic responses of acclimatized or non-acclimatized mature reining horses to heat stress: I. Heart rate, respiration rate, lactate, rectal temperature, cortisol and packed cell volume. J Equine Vet Sci 2001;21:431–8.
11. Gibbs PG, Potter GD, Nielsen BD, et al. Scientific principles for conditioning race and performance horses: Texas A&M University, Department of Animal Science, Equine Sciences Program, 1995.
12. Webb SP, Potter GD, Evans JW, et al. Physiological responses of cutting horses to exercise testing and to training. Equine Nutrition and Physiology Society 1988;261–5.
13. Kastner SB, Feige K, Weishaupt MA, et al. Heart rate and hematological responses of Quarter Horses to a reining competition. J Equine Vet Sci 1999; 19:127–31.
14. Dabareiner RM, Cohen ND, Carter GK, et al. Lameness and poor performance in horses used for team roping: 118 cases (2000–2003). J Am Vet Med Assoc 2005;226:6.
15. Dabareiner RM, Cohen ND, Carter GK, et al. Musculoskeletal problems associated with lameness and poor performance among horses used for barrel racing: 118 cases (2000–2003). J Am Vet Med Assoc 2005;227:1646–50.
16. Dabareiner RM. Calf roping and breakaway roping horses. In: Ross MW, J. Dyson S, editors. Diagnosis and Management of Lameness in the Horse. 2nd ed. St. Louis, Missouri: Elsevier Saunders; 2011.1075–6.
17. Committee. 2011 NRHA Pattern Book, NRHA.com, 2012.
18. Ferrero F. The European western performance horse In: Mike W, Ross SJD, editor. Diagnosis and Management of Lameness in the Horse. 2nd ed. St. Louis Missouri: Elsevier; 2011:1032–3.
19. Smith HA. Cutting. American Association of Equine Practitioners. 1997;31–4.
20. Jackman BR. Common lameness in the cutting and reining horse. In Depth: Lameness in the Western Performance Horse. American Association of Equine Practitioners; 2001. p. 6–11.
21. Unknown. NRCHA Rule book. NRCHA.com, 2012.
22. Galley R. The Team Roping Horse. American Association of Equine Practitioners Annual Convention 1997;40–5.
23. Galley RH. Injuries of the Team Roping Horse. American Association of Equine Practitioners Annual Convention 2001; 15–21.
24. Stricklin JB. Barrel Racing. American Association of Equine Practitioners Phoenix, AZ, 1997;37–9.
25. McCue ME, Valberg SJ, Miller MB, et al. Glycogen synthase (GYS1) mutation causes a novel skeletal muscle glycogenosis. Genomics 2008;91:458–66.
26. McCue ME, Valberg SJ, Lucio M, et al. Glycogen synthase 1 (GYS1) mutation in diverse breeds with polysaccharide storage myopathy. J Vet Intern Med 2008;22:1228–33.
27. De La Corte FD, Valberg SJ, MacLeay JM, et al. Glucose uptake in horses with polysaccharide storage myopathy. Am J Vet Res 1999;60:458–62.
28. Firshman AM, Valberg SJ, Karges TL, et al. Serum creatine kinase response to exercise during dexamethasone-induced insulin resistance in Quarter Horses with polysaccharide storage myopathy. Am J Vet Res 2005;66:1718–23.
29. Annandale EJ, Valberg SJ, Mickelson JR, et al. Insulin sensitivity and skeletal muscle glucose transport in horses with equine polysaccharide storage myopathy. Neuromuscul Disord 2004;14:666–74.
30. Borgia LA, Valberg SJ, McCue ME, et al. Effect of dietary fats with odd or even numbers of carbon atoms on metabolic response and muscle damage with exercise in Quarter Horse-type horses with type 1 polysaccharide storage myopathy. Am J Vet Res 2010;71:326–36.
31. Tryon RC, Penedo MCT, McCue ME, et al. Evaluation of allele frequencies of inherited disease genes in subgroups of American Quarter Horses. J Am Vet Med Assoc 2009;234:120–5.
32. Valberg SJ, McCue ME, Mickelson JR. The interplay of genetics, exercise, and nutrition in polysaccharide storage myopathy. J Equine Vet Sci 2011;31: 205–10.
33. Valberg SJ. Diagnostic Approach to Muscle Disorders. American Association of Equine Practitioners, San Antonio, TX, 2006;340–6.
34. Valberg SJ, Macleay JM, Billstrom JA, et al. Skeletal muscle metabolic response to exercise in horses with 'tying-up' due to polysaccharide storage myopathy. Equine Vet J 1999;31:43–7.
35. McCue ME, Armien AG, Lucio M, et al. Comparative skeletal muscle histopathologic and ultrastructural features in two forms of polysaccharide storage myopathy in horses. Vet Pathol 2009;46:1281–91.
36. Borgia LA, Valberg SJ, McCue ME, et al. Glycaemic and insulinaemic responses to feeding hay with different non-structural carbohydrate content in control and polysaccharide storage myopathy-affected horses. J Anim Physiol Anim Nutr (Berl) 2011;95:798–807.
37. Ribeiro WP, Valberg SJ, Pagan JD, et al. The effect of varying dietary starch and fat content on serum creatine kinase activity and substrate availability in equine polysaccharide storage myopathy. J Vet Intern Med 2004;18:887–94.
38. Lewis RD. Lameness in the Rodeo Horse. American Association of Equine Practitioners, San Diego, CA, 2001;1–5.
39. Martinelli MJ, Rantanen NW. Relationship between Nuclear Scintigraphy and Standing MRI in 30 Horses with Lameness of the Foot. American Association of Equine Practitioners Seattle, WA, 2005;359–65.
40. Snow VE. The reined cow horse. In: Mike W. Ross SJD, editor. Diagnosis and Management of Lameness in the Horse. 2nd ed. 2011. p. 1176–80.
41. Carmalt JL, Bell CD, Panizzi L, et al. Alcohol-facilitated ankylosis of the distal intertarsal and tarsometatarsal joints in horses with osteoarthritis. J Am Vet Med Assoc 2012;240:199–204.
42. Zubrod CJ, Schneider RK, Hague BA, et al. Comparison of three methods for arthrodesis of the distal intertarsal and tarsometatarsal joints in horses. Vet Surg 2005;34:372–82.
43. Contino EK, Park RD, McIlwraith CW. Prevalence of radiographic changes in yearling and 2-year-old Quarter Horses intended for cutting. Equine Vet J 2011:1–11.
44. Frisbie DD, Smith RK. Clinical update on the use of mesenchymal stem cells in equine orthopaedics. Equine Vet J 2010;42:86–9.
45. Frisbie DD, Kawcak CE, Werpy NM, et al. Clinical, biochemical, and histologic effects of intra-articular administration of autologous conditioned serum in horses with experimentally induced osteoarthritis. Am J Vet Res 2007;68: 290–6.
46. Barrett MF, McIlwraith CW, Contino EK, et al. Relationship between radiographic changes of the Medial Femoral Condyle and Performance in Quarter Horse Cutting Horses. American Association of Equine Practitioners, Baltimore, MD, 2010;30.

47. Wallis TW, Goodrich LR, McIlwraith CW, et al. Arthroscopic injection of corticosteroids into the fibrous tissue of subchondral cystic lesions of the medial femoral condyle in horses: a retrospective study of 52 cases (2001–2006). Equine Vet J 2008;40:461–7.

48. Ortved KF, Nixon AJ, Mohammed HO, et al. Treatment of subchondral cystic lesions of the medial femoral condyle of mature horses with growth factor enhanced chondrocyte grafts: A retrospective study of 49 cases. Equine Vet J 2011;44:606–13.

49. Howard RD, McIlwraith CW, Trotter GW. Arthroscopic surgery for subchondral cystic lesions of the medial femoral condyle in horses: 41 cases (1988–1991). J Am Vet Med Assoc 1995;206:842–50.

50. McIlwraith CW, Frisbie DD, Rodkey WG, et al. Evaluation of intra-articular mesenchymal stem cells to augment healing of microfractured chondral defects. Arthroscopy 2011;27:1552–61.

51. Pusterla N, Kass PH, Mapes S, et al. Surveillance programme for important equine infectious respiratory pathogens in the USA. Vet Rec 2011;169:12.

52. Diaz-Mendez A, Viel L, Hewson J, et al. Surveillance of equine respiratory viruses in Ontario. Can J Vet Res 2010;74: 271–8.

53. Biava JS, Gonçalves RC, Finger MA, et al. Exercise-induced pulmonary hemorrhage (EIPH) in Quarter Horses. World Equine Veterinary Association 2009;1.

54. Wasko AJ, Barkema HW, Nicol J, et al. Evaluation of a risk-screening questionnaire to detect equine lung inflammation: results of a large field study. Equine Vet J 2011;43:145–52.

Veterinary aspects of training the show jumping horse

55

Rachel C. Murray

CHAPTER CONTENTS

Introduction

The training of elite show jumping horses is driven by performance, both optimal short-term performance and longevity of high performance. The veterinarian is increasingly under pressure to assist in maintenance and improvement of performance, particularly at elite level where horses are sold for very large amounts and value of prize money is high. Although in the past there was a defined competition season, show jumping is now a year-round sport with indoor and outdoor shows, and elite horses travel internationally to compete in high-profile shows at all times of the year. At elite level, horses are transported considerable distances, often traveling directly from one show to another without returning home. There can be minimal time for recovery between events, or between traveling and events. As a result, veterinary support is often required in preparation for competitions, on the road or at competitions throughout the year.

Features of the sport

For both show hunter and show jumper classes, horses are required to jump a series of obstacles. For the show hunter the goal is the style and technique of jumping (including the approach), whereas for the show jumper the goal is to clear obstacles up to considerable heights, and style is less important. Jumps may be uprights or spread fences, and can be set as combinations of fences at defined distances apart that test the ability for the horse to shorten and lengthen its stride but still jump clear. For the show jumper, speed is also a factor in speed classes, during a jump off and often to stay within the set time for the round. Horses are therefore required to be able to jump fences at varying speeds, from a variety of angles, to shorten and lengthen their stride, accelerate and decelerate, and turn sharply, all of which place considerable strain on the tissues of the body. The type of injuries that jumping horses are at risk for reflects the strains that are experienced during competition and training.

Exercise demands

Show jumping is primarily a power sport, requiring a variety of skills in association with power and fitness. The cantering between fences has primarily aerobic demands, while each jumping effort significantly increases the heart rate above that needed for cantering between fences and appears to have additional anaerobic demands, particularly in horses with poor jumping fitness.[1,2] Show jumpers with efficient jumping technique, however, may use primarily aerobic metabolism. Fitness training therefore needs to improve aerobic capacity and power. Heart rate during show jumping has been reported as approximately 180–206 beats per minute during a jumping round.[1,3] In one study, jumping a spread fence during warm-up was associated with a higher heart rate than jumping an upright fence, which was suggested to result from a faster approach to a spread fence or increased power requirement. Heart rate tends to increase during the round to a maximum at the end, with heart rate recovery starting immediately at the end of the course.[1,2,4,5] Jumping a course has been associated with an increase in packed cell volume, consistent with splenic contraction.[2,5,6] Blood lactate concentrations of around 3–8 mmol/L have been reported after jumping.[1,3,7] Based on these lactate concentrations, active trotting recovery has been recommended to increase lactate clearance from muscles.[1] Less experienced horses tend to have higher blood cortisol concentrations, possibly indicating a higher level of exercise-associated stress when compared to more experienced horses.[7]

Biomechanics of jumping

To clear the jump, the horse's center of gravity is required to be raised high enough above the fence. The movement of the center of gravity and flight path is determined by the approach and take-off, which are critical in the success of the jump.[8] In the final approach stride, the forelimbs are required to brake and provide vertical forces for takeoff, so loading the support structures of the limb and extending the distal limb joints. The trailing forelimb experiences the highest peak vertical forces at take-off.[9]

The force for take-off is generated by muscular power in the hindlimbs, while the head and neck are raised to optimize power generation.[8,10,11] At take-off, there is flexion of the tarsal joints and extension of the metatarsophalangeal joints with a longer hindlimb stance duration than during a normal canter stride, allowing generation of large impulses (see Fig. 55.1). Frequently the hindlimbs may push off together, an equal distance from the fence. The higher the fence, the greater the vertical force required at take-off.[9] For spread fences, the hindlimb push off is greater than for an upright fence of the same height.[12] A successful jump needs high stride frequency into the fence and high acceleration pulse of the forelimbs and hindlimbs at take-off.[12] Faults are less likely to occur when take-off is further from the fence.[13]

On landing after a jump, there is a significant increase in the forelimb ground reaction force compared to normal canter.[9] The metacarpophalangeal and distal interphalangeal joint are hyperextended on landing, resulting in strains on the superficial and deep digital flexor tendons and the suspensory ligament (see Fig. 55.2). The superficial digital flexor tendons of the forelimbs undergo repetitive loading during jumping and considerable strain on landing, with relatively greater strain after jumping higher fences,[14] so it is likely that this potential overload predisposes the tendon to injury in elite horses jumping high fences. The deep digital flexor tendon plays an important role in stabilizing the distal interphalangeal joint, which is hyperextended on landing from a jump and therefore experiences considerable loading.[15] In the forelimb, landing puts greater strain on the trailing forelimb than the leading forelimb,[9] so a horse that with pain or less strength in the left forelimb, for example, may choose to approach and depart from the fence leading with the left forelimb. The departure stride is usually four time, with greater propulsive force generated by the trailing hindlimb.[9] Faults are less likely to occur when the trailing hindlimb lands closer to the fence.[13]

Individual horses have different jumping techniques. However, certain characteristics seem to be retained within an individual horse between a foal and a four year old.[16] Horses with greater jumping ability have been reported to show a lower displacement of the withers and tuber sacrale from the end of the last approach

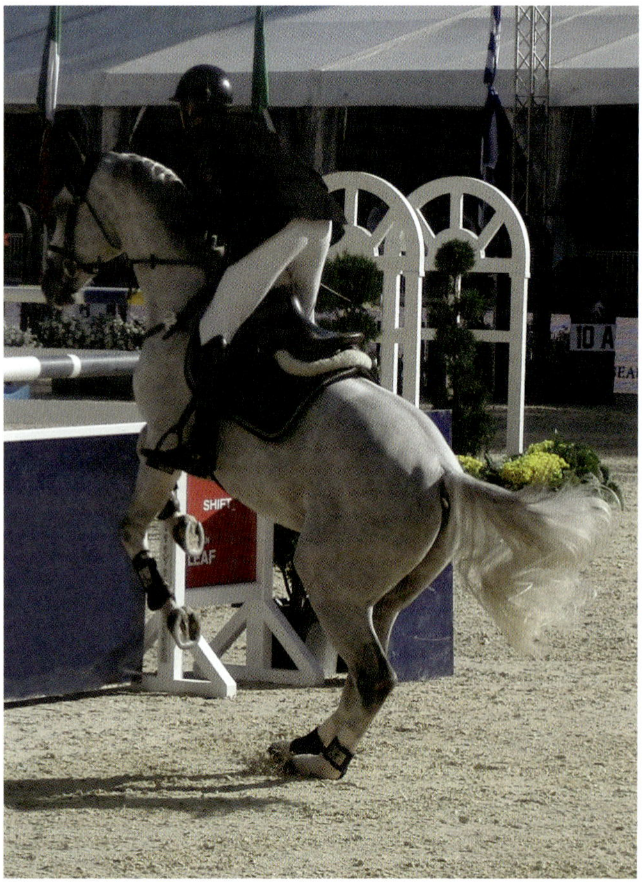

Fig 55.1 The take-off phase during jumping activity, showing the fetlock hyperextension and tarsal flexion required.

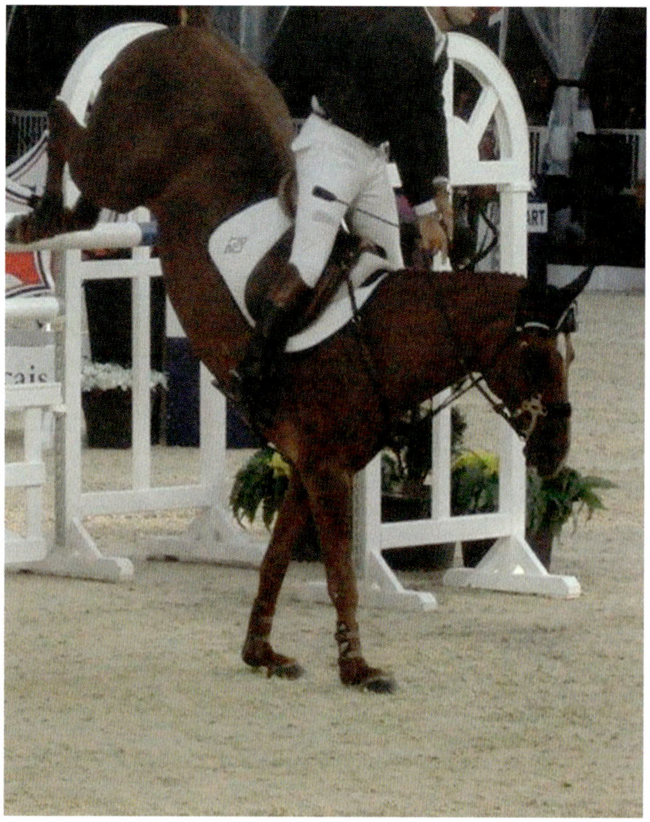

Fig 55.2 The landing phase of a jump, showing fetlock and carpal hyperextension, particularly in the trailing forelimb.

until the first departure stride during free jumping. Instead, they increase the flexion of the thoracolumbar and lumbosacral junctions during the hindlimb swing phase before take-off, indicating a more efficient jumping technique.[17]

Training influences the take-off and landing distance, bascule and height of the forelimbs above the fence.[18] Early jumping training has been shown to improve the efficiency of jumping by lower acceleration during the hindlimb push, lower velocity at take-off and less push forward of the center of gravity over a fence.[19] From an exercise physiology point of view, training increases aerobic capacity, and excitability and power output of the muscle by increasing the proportion of the oxidative muscle fibers.[10] Jumping training at an early age leads to increased adaptation of the middle gluteal muscle in particular.[10]

The rider has a large effect on the horse, exerting measurable effects on the horse's center of gravity, change in velocity and acceleration, and kinematics of the joints.[18,20] The combined weight of rider and saddle influences jumping kinematics.[21] Increased weight results in the leading forelimb landing closer to the fence, with increased extension of the fetlock and carpal joints, increasing the loading on the superficial digital flexor tendon and suspensory ligament. On the first departure stride, increased weight leads to increased stance duration in the hindlimbs and the head further in front of the vertical on landing.

Type of horse

Show jumping horses are increasingly Warmbloods, compared to historically where Thoroughbred and Thoroughbred cross horses predominated.[22,23] Currently, the trend appears to be for primarily lighter weight Warmblood horses, rather than the more traditional heavier weight type. There is some research indicating that locomotory muscles of good jumpers have a higher proportion of fast myosin heavy chains than less talented horses, particularly in the middle gluteal muscle.[3] Features of gait that are associated with better show jumping performance are a higher stride frequency and less deceleration in the last stride before jumping, suggesting more hindlimb power with less forelimb braking.[3]

Show jumping horses tend to be taller than in many other sports, giving the advantage of longer levers to jump and cover the ground.[23] Height at the withers is the conformational characteristic that has been most consistently connected with successful jumping performance.[8] Elite show jumpers are reported to have larger hock angles and smaller fetlock angles than other horses.[24] In a study that compared horses at elite and lower level, elite horses had lower bodyweight than the non-elite horses, indicating a higher fitness level.[22] Elite horses were older than non-elite animals, reflecting the time taken in the training and development of elite horses.[22] Jumping horses can start competing as four year olds, often in young horse classes. Performance ability and competition level increase to high-level performance from around nine years and to a peak at 12–13 years of age. Horses may continue competing into their late teens. Older, experienced horses may become schoolmasters for less experienced riders. These older horses may therefore have additional management requirements in order to maintain optimal performance, and close monitoring of tissues at increased risk of injury with age, especially the digital flexor tendons, is indicated.

Mares, geldings and stallions are used for show jumping. Results of one epidemiological study indicated that stallions were the most likely gender to go clear while mares were the most likely to have refusals.[25] Jumping horses are reported to have generally lower excitation levels and less interest in new objects than dressage horses,[26] which may relate to their initial selection or ongoing management.

In various countries, horses are bred specifically for jumping. Performance criteria that have been used for selection of breeding stock and their offspring include grading of jumping technique in young horse classes, success in classes at elite level and longevity of performance. Particular bloodlines within various breeds are considered to improve potential for high performance and longevity of performance. In Dutch and German Warmbloods, there was good heritability for free jumping technique, which tended to be higher than the heritability for jumping under the rider.[27] In French show jumpers, moderate heritability was shown for annual earnings and ranking records, while there was high heritability for performance tests in young horses using a subjective scoring of ability.[3] However, there was only low-to-moderate heritability for performance in Hungarian show jumping horses.[28] It is likely that this relates to the variations in training and performance between riders and trainers of different ability and experience. It is accepted that there are differences in riding technique and horse–rider harmony between experienced and novice riders. This has recently been quantified further,[29] illustrating the variation in jumping technique between riders of different ability and therefore the variable influence on the horse which impacts the horse's jumping performance.

Longevity of sport horses in jumping competition has been reported to be influenced by age of starting competition, with horses starting competition at four years of age being more likely to stay in competition longer than horses starting at six years of age. Less successful horses were less likely to stay in competition, and mares were more likely to be removed from competition than geldings with the same performance, potentially because they could be used for breeding.[30] In another epidemiological study, horses performance peaked at the age of 12–13 years and performance decreased with age in older horses.[25]

Nutrition

Nutrition of the show hunter and show jumper needs to be tailored to its level of work, stage in the season and temperament, along with its age and stage of training. For horses competing in more than one class in a day, or competing repeatedly over 3–4 days, it is important to consider energy reserves, both in relation to muscle glycogen depletion and replacement.[31,32] Forage is the primary component of the rations but concentrate feed is usually required to ensure that energy requirements are met. The quantity and composition (e.g. relative amounts of starch vs oil as sources of energy) can be tailored to individual temperament, workload and competition schedule. For horses at risk of gastric ulceration, access to forage and avoiding large starch-based meals (e.g. no more than 1.5 g starch/kg BW per meal) may be beneficial. For optimal performance, it is recommended that horses are not fed any large cereal-based meals less than 2–3 hours before exercise and they should certainly be avoided close to the time of jumping.[31,32] Large concentrate feeds can lead to a decrease in plasma volume, increase in blood insulin and decreases in blood glucose, which could reduce performance. However, giving access to small amounts of hay until the time of exercise may help to maintain gastrointestinal function and minimize risk of gastric ulceration.

Horse clothing/tack

The saddle acts to modify the interaction between rider and horse. The impact of saddle selection and fitting should not be underestimated by the veterinarian. A poorly fitting saddle can cause muscle pain and damage, potentially altering the gait, impacting on performance, and predisposing to other injury. Correct saddle fitting is therefore essential to the competitive jumper and should be taken into account when a veterinarian is involved with managing jumping horses. Ongoing maintenance of saddles is important during training of the developing horse and to maintain the competition horse, including altering of flocking or tree shape as the horse gains or loses muscle mass. Saddle design has changed over time to take into account the requirements of the jumping horse and rider. On landing over a jump, there is increased pressure under the front of the saddle with impact upwards from the forelimbs and downwards from the rider. Recently, some aspects of saddle design have been focussed on minimizing this impact with various modifications to improve performance including use of a double tree apparatus with an integrated shock absorber to absorb some of the energy and provide cushioning for rider and horse, which is claimed to reduce the impact on the horse's shoulder region by 30–50% on landing.

A variety of bits and bridle configurations can be used for show jumping. For the veterinarian involved in ongoing assessment of these horses, it is important to ensure that tack is fitted and used correctly so that injuries to the head and mouth are avoided. It is appropriate to examine the mouth and head on a routine basis in addition to the limbs and trunk.

There has been a recent trend for using tight or weighted boots, which are now affected by FEI regulations (a maximum weight of 500 g per limb is allowed for bandages or boots). Use of weighted boots has been shown to increase hindlimb elevation over a jump, which has been attributed to increased kinetic energy produced by the effect of the weighted boot on the hindlimb.[33] Use of weighted boots at walk has been suggested for increasing strength of lumbar musculature.[34] However, their use during jumping could potentially increase risk of injury to hindlimb structures or overstrain of the lumbar flexor musculature as a result of exaggerated movement.[33]

Studs, or shoe caulks, are frequently used in jumping horses to improve grip, particularly on slippery surfaces. Whether these are used, as well as the type and location of the studs within the shoes, tend to be based primarily on rider preference as there is limited scientific evaluation of stud use. Studs alter foot–ground interaction, significantly reducing slip, particularly in the trailing limb at canter.[35] Although considerable slip may be detrimental, a small amount of slip on landing after a jump or at each canter stride may be beneficial and is considered to be one mechanism by which energy is dissipated when the foot impacts the ground.[36] This varies on different surfaces and may be influenced by stud placement.[37] If energy dissipation is not achieved by slide, or alteration in ground surface, then the structures of the limb may experience abnormal forces which could potentially increase risk of injury.[38,39] Increased horizontal braking can create higher forces on the distal limb and more proximally within the limb, which could impact on laminar tearing, and increase risk of damage to subchondral bone, ligaments and tendons.[35] Studs may be placed in fore- or hindlimbs, and can be single or multiple at different locations within each foot. Hind limbs tend to slide more than forelimbs during braking, and the trailing forelimb in canter is affected most by use of studs, so it is important that the type and configuration of studs are selected for each limb. A single stud within the foot may allow rotation which is prevented by multiple studs, which allows some energy dissipation by rotational movement and allows the foot to turn on the floor, but leads to asymmetric loading of the structures of the limb. Placement of a medial stud increases the risk of tread injury if there is interference between limbs. The length, width and degree of taper of studs can be varied and will have different degrees of effect on foot–ground interaction. The long-term consequences of using studs on different surfaces and in different configurations are currently unknown but their potential contribution should be considered in relation to injury prevention and management.

Clinical evaluation of the jumping horse

As with examination of any patient, a detailed history is essential. In addition to standard queries, useful questions to the rider/trainer could include whether the horse has a preference for landing on a particular leading leg or prefers to take-off from the left or right, if the horse has become reluctant to jump a particular type of fence (such as combinations or spread fences), a reluctance to turn a particular way, refusing or rushing. Apart from a standard clinical examination, the horse should undergo dynamic evaluation in hand in a straight line and on the lunge on both hard and soft surfaces. Transitions between paces can be useful to detect subtle problems. For complete examination it is important to observe the horse ridden on the flat and over jumps. To determine the response to diagnostic analgesia in horses with subtle problems, evaluating ridden performance after diagnostic analgesia may be necessary.

For subtle problems and performance issues there is real value to assessment of the warm-up regime at a competition and the technique used in the course, so it can be advisable to either attend a competition or to get the rider to simulate a warm-up and competition round. This allows the veterinarian to assess whether there is adequate or excessive warm-up time or if there are excessive jumping efforts leading to fatigue in the ring.[40] Watching the warm-up technique can be useful in relation to symmetry of training direction, symmetry of approach and departure from a fence, and which lead the horse lands on after a fence. Evaluating how a rider presents the horse to a fence, and the rider position, can give a guide to the effort required by the horse. When presented to a fence at the optimal take-off point with a rider in balance, the horse has the best opportunity to minimize effort over the fence. If a horse is consistently presented too close or too far from the fence, or has to support a rider that is out of balance, the horse is likely to fatigue earlier or have to use active compensatory actions to clear the fence.

Subclinical lameness

Although injury or lameness may be clearly detectable, in some horses lameness may be subclinical, which can limit performance either by prevent the horse reaching a high competitive level or by leading to a decrease in performance (Box 55.1).[41,42] A horse with subclinical injury may alter its gait and movement to avoid discomfort or account for weakness, leading to an increased risk of secondary acute problems. For horses competing in international competitions, passing a veterinary inspection is a requirement, so supporting horses with potential low-grade problems may be required.

Specific injuries

Orthopedic problems

In a recent investigation of elite show jumping horses in four European countries, approximately 6% of days were lost to training and competing for health reasons, of which 78% were lost for orthopedic reasons.[43] These were considered primarily chronic overuse injuries,

Box 55.1 Possible signs of subclinical pain

1. Increased resistance, often on one rein only
2. Loss of rhythm or changing legs behind in canter
3. Reluctance to do a flying change one way
4. Unwillingness to use one canter lead into or after a fence
5. Resistance or refusal at a particular type of fence or combination
6. Rushing
7. Jumping to one side
8. Difficulty making distances in a combination
9. Reluctance to perform or reduced performance on a particular type of arena surface

although there were a smaller proportion of accidental injuries. In one study, the most frequent anatomical locations of injury in show jumping horses included the foot, digital flexor tendons and accessory ligament of the deep digital flexor tendon, suspensory ligament, back and pelvis, tarsus, fetlock and stifle.[22] Elite horses appear to be more at risk of injury to the superficial digital flexor tendon, the distal deep digital flexor tendon, and the accessory ligament of the deep digital flexor tendon than non-elite horses.

Foot pain

Like horses doing most sports, jumping horses are at risk of foot pain. This may be the result of trauma to the hoof capsule, including sole bruising or hoof cracks, which can be managed fairly simply. In the author's experience, evidence of laminar tearing is not unusual on magnetic resonance imaging examination of show jumping horses with low-grade or 'subclinical' foot pain, either alone or in conjunction with other causes of foot pain. This laminar tearing may be related to braking of the hoof against the ground surface (particularly where studs are used) while the forces of the limb continue to be applied to the distal phalanx, creating considerable forces at the laminar junction with the distal phalanx.

Alternatively, foot pain can result from damage to the osseous, ligamentar or tendonous tissues of the foot. Palmar foot pain occurs relatively frequently and may be related to navicular bone damage or a combination including injury to the deep digital flexor tendon, navicular bursa and navicular support ligaments.[44–46] Interestingly, in one study, non-elite horses had a greater risk of navicular bone/ligament injury than a comparative elite group, which could be because elite horses would not have reached elite status if they had been predisposed to this type of injury or disease.[22] Another explanation is that the forelimbs of non-elite horses experience greater load for a higher proportion of the stride than horses doing more advanced training. Damage to the deep digital flexor tendon within the hoof capsule is likely to present as foot pain and is likely to be predisposed by repeated hyperextension of the distal interphalangeal joint on landing. Damage to the collateral ligaments of the distal interphalangeal joint can be associated with twisting or asymmetric loading, which is likely to occur during a jumping round particularly at speed (see Fig. 55.3). This injury can be detected in some horses by use of ultrasonography, but magnetic resonance imaging is the best diagnostic technique.[44–47] Synovitis and osteoarthritis of the distal interphalangeal joint are common in jumping horses, particularly in the forelimbs, and may be found with or without other concurrent injury to the foot. Bone trauma or bruising is best detected and evaluated using magnetic resonance imaging.[46]

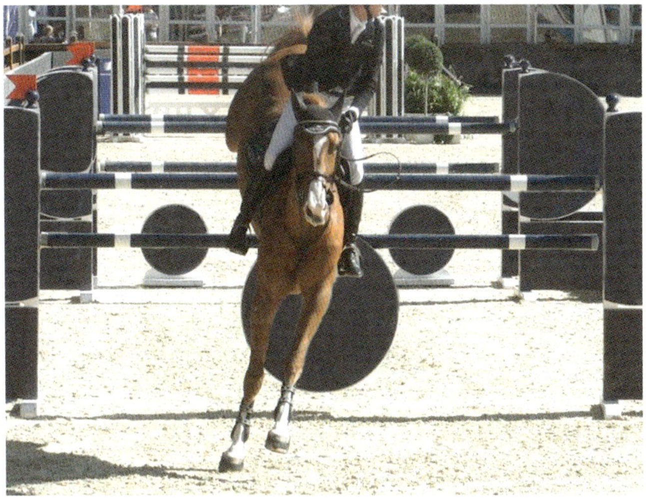

Fig 55.3 A horse turning upon landing from a jump during a speed class event. Note the loading of the limbs at an angle.

Digital flexor tendons

Compared to general purpose horses and horses doing other sports (except eventing), show jumping horses are at increased risk of injury to the forelimb superficial digital flexor tendon and distal deep digital flexor tendon.[22] In elite horses, degenerative change in the tendons with aging may contribute to this process. However, both epidemiological data and clinical impression supports an increased frequency of distal deep digital flexor tendon injuries in horses that jump.[42,48,49] This likely results from the strain on the superficial and deep digital flexor tendon on landing, and the increased strain with higher jumps.[9,14] Although superficial and deep digital flexor tendon injury occurs in both elite and non-elite show jumping horses, the risk appears greater in elite horses, which is probably related to the size of fences being jumped.[22] Injury to the accessory ligament of the deep digital flexor tendon is not uncommon in jumping horses, likely related to the strain on the deep digital flexor tendon during jumping, particularly on landing.

Suspensory ligament

Injury to the suspensory ligament can be a serious problem in jumping horses.[48] Either hindlimb or forelimb suspensory ligaments can be affected, and may initially present as poor performance or loss of power, particularly when both hindlimbs are affected. Proximal suspensory desmitis, midbody and branch injuries can occur, which can be evaluated ultrasonographically. Concurrent bone injury can be detected using scintigraphic or magnetic resonance imaging.

Tarsal pain

Distal tarsal pain occurs relatively frequently in jumping horses compared to racehorses or event horses.[22,23] The tarsus appears to be a risk site for both non-elite and elite horses. In the young or unfit horse, distal tarsal pain may be related to lack of muscle support resulting from poor muscle development or fatigue, leading to instability and joint strain. In the elite horse, tarsal pain could be associated with the tarsal compression required at take-off,[50] a hypothesis that is supported by observations of increased subchondral bone thickness in elite competition horses compared to general purpose horses, and by the radiopharmaceutical uptake pattern in the tarsus of elite show jumping where there is higher dorsal to plantar uptake ratio compared to general purpose horses.[51,52] It has also been shown that upper-level competition horses appear to have a different loading pattern through the tarsus compared with general purpose or racehorses, which might predispose to the pattern of injury seen.[52] Tarsal bone trauma has been reported in show jumping horses, detected using scintigraphic and magnetic resonance imaging.[53]

Fetlock injury

Synovitis and osteoarthritis of the metacarpophalangeal joint is common in the older show jumping horse. Thickening of the joint capsule may be beneficial in protecting the joint, but chronic capsulitis is associated with limited range of motion and resentment of flexion or manipulation of the joint. Radiography and diagnostic analgesia are useful in diagnosis.

Traumatic injury can occur due to interference by other limbs or impact with the jump. This may be superficial. However, bone injury can occur, including impact trauma to the dorsal aspect of the fetlock and pastern. Alternatively, bone injury in the fetlock joint can been seen in jumping horses associated with repetitive overloading and hyperextension of the joint.[54,55] The distal third metacarpal bone may be affected on the dorsal aspect of the parasagittal grooves located further palmar. Alternatively, or in addition, incomplete fracture or bone trauma to the sagittal groove of the proximal phalanx may occur unilaterally or bilaterally in show jumping horses. Magnetic resonance imaging and scintigraphic imaging are likely to provide most useful diagnostic information in horses with these problems.[54]

Stifle injury

Injury to the structures of the stifle joint is reasonably common in show jumping horses. In one study, competition jumping ponies were at higher risk of stifle injury that horses doing other sports.[22] In the young Warmblood jumper, stifle effusion and lameness seen early in training may be associated with osteochondrosis and/or subchondral bone cyst formation. Injury to the menisci and cruciate ligaments can be associated with considerable lameness, with chronic injury often leading to osteoarthritis. Trauma to the patella can occur from impact with a jump. Desmitis of the middle patella ligament seems most likely to occur in jumping horses[56] and in the author's experience can be associated with a history of entanglement with a fence.

Back pain

Back pain is common in show jumping horses and can be related to poorly fitting saddles, poor riding and training technique, muscle pain, or ligament /bone pathology. Impinging dorsal spinous processes may present as back pain or reduced performance with refusal at fences; the latter is potentially related to pain experienced at take-off and on landing when the back is extended. Pathology is likely to be observed radiographically. Scintigraphic imaging may be useful, but diagnostic local analgesia is generally required to confirm the clinical relevance.[57] Fracture of the dorsal spinous processes may occur if the horse falls over backwards. Osteoarthritis of the intervertebral facet joints can occur with or without osseous pathology, and can be associated with pain and poor performance.[58] Sacroiliac pain is relatively common in show jumping horses compared to horses doing some other sports, which may relate to turning during the course or jumping on a turn.[59] Most horses with chronic sacroiliac problems present with poor performance, but horses can show severe resistance and lameness. In addition to clinical examination, improvement following diagnostic local analgesia and altered radiopharmaceutical uptake on scintigraphic imaging can be useful in diagnosis.

Non-orthopedic health problems

Respiratory

Respiratory problems are reported to be the most frequent reason for poor performance in sport horses, following orthopedic problems. Upper airway obstruction may limit performance. Lower airway disease can be a problem in show jumping horses, primarily recurrent airway obstruction (RAO) or inflammatory airway disease (IAD). It has been shown that upper and lower respiratory disease are associated with poor willingness to perform in show jumpers, and this is most significant if there is increased tracheal mucus.[60] In one clinic seeing primarily show jumping horses with poor performance, it was reported that more than 50% of horses had evidence of lower airway disease, the majority of which were classified as RAO and IAD.[61] This finding is perhaps not surprising as many elite show jumping horses spend considerable time in environments unhealthy for the respiratory tract, including traveling long distances, staying in temporary stables at competitions, competing in indoor arenas and having limited access to turnout. Management of these horses should include the implementation of strategies that minimize access to respirable dust and molds, e.g. improving ventilation during travel and stabling, feeding dust-free forage, using low-dust bedding and by housing horses outside as much as possible. In an investigation of risk factors for injury in dressage horses, a respiratory problem increased risk of lameness by more than 4 times.[62] This association has not been investigated in jumpers, but a respiratory problem may increase fatigue and potential risk of injury.

Gastrointestinal problems

For horses that are on a competition schedule, risk of colic is potentially increased by traveling changes in feeding and routine which can occur during traveling and competing. It is important that horses traveling away to a competition are kept on the same feed and forage, so adequate home feed and forage should taken to the competition. If changes need to be made, risk of colic can be reduced by making any feed or forage changes more than 2 weeks prior to traveling or competing so that gut bacteria have time to become established. Changes in routine should be minimized as far as possible.

For some horses, changing to different water at a competition can reduce their water intake and increase risk of dehydration and impaction colic. Riders/grooms should be encouraged to monitor water intake and take action to encourage drinking. There are various strategies to increase water intake at a competition, which a veterinarian may be asked to advise on. Before traveling, training horses to drink away from home is useful; sometimes traveling with another horse that drinks easily encourages a reluctant horse to start drinking, and preparing by taking a source of home water to the competition is useful. Other strategies include adding salt to the feed, putting fruit juices into the water, putting sliced apples or carrots into the water bucket, and soaking hay and feeding it in water. The administration of oral (via nasogastric tube) or intravenous fluids may be necessary in horses that become dehydrated.

Gastric ulcers

Gastric ulcers have been increasingly recognized in horses undertaking a wide variety of sports, with an incidence of 40–60% reported in show jumping sport horses.[63,64] Competitive jumping horses are often in a potentially high stress environment, being on the road for large periods of time. The risk of gastric ulcer development may be increased by feeding a low-forage, high-concentrate diet, and by large amounts of starch (>1–2 g starch/kg bodyweight) being fed at one feed. Management of horses with a history of gastric ulceration should include dietary modification: i.e. increasing the proportion of forage in the ration; splitting the concentrate feed component of the ration into smaller meals. Ideally, definitive diagnosis is made by gastroscopy. However, response to treatment with omeprazole is often rapid and marked. Modifying management and removing risk factors for stress is required as far as possible, including turnout and feeding patterns. However, this can be difficult for horses in an ongoing competition schedule, so omeprazole treatment is often required on a longer-term basis for these horses, which is currently permitted under FEI regulations.

Cardiac

Heart murmurs may be of little or no clinical relevance in a horse that is currently successful in competition. However, if murmurs are detected at pre-purchase examination, or if murmurs are new or loud and there is evidence of poor performance or exercise intolerance, then further investigation may be indicated. In large, fit horses, localized murmurs associated with tricuspid regurgitation are unlikely to prevent athletic performance but should be investigated if there is poor performance. Aortic regurgitation is frequent in older horses and can progress to performance limitation. Mitral regurgitation is the most likely valvular condition to affect performance and progress to congestive heart failure, so should be investigated and monitored.[65]

Dysrhythmias may occur in show jumping horses but are of unknown significance. A study in normal show jumping horses reported a high prevalence of supraventricular premature complexes during warm-up and after exercise but no arrhythmias during the show jumping round, and that there were relatively few ventricular premature complexes.[4] Atrial fibrillation or sustained tachycardias or bradycardias are likely to be performance limiting.

Training for prevention of injury

Training is required to prepare the body for athletic activity. Too little training (demand) may prevent a horse from achieving its athletic potential, while too much training can exceed the capacity for adaptation, leading to overtraining injury and potentially irreversible damage. Training of the musculoskeletal system involves the translation of mechanical stimuli into altered composition/structure, leading to improved structural and material properties to withstand forces during peak loading. However, there is always a balance between optimal training for different body systems, balancing demands for cardiorespiratory fitness with loading of the musculoskeletal system. Training is focused on preparing the horse for jumping competition, taking into account the level at which it is training and competing because the demands of different levels of competition are different. However, repetitive training can be associated with overload injuries, so it is important to develop training regimens that maximize performance at specific competitions while reducing risk of injury during training.

Training program

A training program should include general fitness conditioning, skills training, and both muscle strength and endurance training. Training type needs to be balanced so that the horse is strong enough to perform the exercise required, fit enough to keep repeating it, and skilled enough to perform the exercise safely. Balancing these demands is important to avoid development of problems. For example, concentrating purely on skills training when the horse is not strong and fit enough to perform these skills can lead to resistance or altered gait, thereby risking injury or conflict behavior particularly if the movement keeps being repeated to 'improve' it. Concentrating only on strength training (e.g. for jumping) could allow the horse to jump high, but for only a few successful repetitions which is a problem if the horse needs to complete a long course. Alternatively, having the cardiovascular fitness to complete the galloping part of a course may not be adequate to perform successfully or avoid injury if there is inadequate muscle strength and endurance to achieve the height of the fences.

In principle, strength training requires small numbers of repetitions with increased loading, with adequate recovery period between sets. This increased loading could be based on height of fence, increased height of ground poles, or power of steps. Time for recovery between training sessions is necessary, so strength training is most appropriate only 2–3 times per week. Muscle endurance training needs to be balanced with increasing strength and includes higher numbers of repetitions at lower power. This can be done by repeating a specific movement (such as a jumping effort over a small fence, or raised poles) or by gradually increasing the length of time in a movement (e.g. more collected canter as required in a course). It is important to monitor the horse for muscle fatigue to avoid incoordination and potential injury.

Skills training involves the development of neural pathways, proprioceptive conditioning and flexibility. Building neural pathways requires many repetitions but these do not need to be at peak loading, e.g. jumping variable distance combinations over small fences until the horse learns how to cope before increasing the height of the fences. Proprioceptive conditioning includes use of poles, turns, bending in variable directions, slopes/inclines and variable surfaces, so hacking and turnout are useful. Gradually increasing flexibility demands during training can include smaller-diameter circles, bending both ways on circles, lateral work and collection/extension transitions, all of which may be useful training for the jumping horse.

General physiological/cardiorespiratory fitness training includes canter/gallop training with interval training, frequent transitions and hill work based on the requirements of the sport, where horses are required to accelerate and decelerate rapidly, and to perform at speed. This has to be balanced against the musculoskeletal demands and risks.

Core muscle stability and strength are essential requirements for the sport horse, as developing these muscles counteracts the weight of the rider, provides a stable point for limb attachment and stabilizes the joints of the back. Core muscle conditioning needs to be included in training programs and is important during rehabilitation following injury. Exercises performed from the ground are useful, triggering use of specific muscle groups, and have been shown to increase the size of the selected muscles. Feeding from the floor can be beneficial. Use of ground and raised poles in walk and trot, and training aids that improve posture can be included as part of a core muscle training program. Ridden work with the head low and including transitions, half halts, and grid work also can be useful for core muscle conditioning.

Rest and recovery time are essential during training. In a large epidemiological study of elite competition horses followed for a season, there was an average of 24% rest days (10–38)%.[43]

A rational training program is based on specific long- and short-term goals. Horses should be monitored carefully for stress, fatigue and illness and the schedule adapted as necessary. A training schedule can be tailored to peak at single or multiple events. Coming into a strenuous competition there can be value to tapering the volume (decreasing the total amount) of training beforehand, although maintaining the intensity (the quality) of the training to avoid pre-competition muscle glycogen depletion and fatigue but preparing proprioceptive, neural and muscular pathways.

Training session

Each training session should include warm-up, training period and cool-down parts. Warm-up has physiological benefits; allowing exercise to proceed more safely and efficiently. Warm-up should not be confused with stretching, which should generally be performed following warm-up or training. Warm-up can include three stages:

1. Passive warm-up, where the horse's body temperature is increased externally, using rugs or putting the horse into a warm environment.
2. General warm-up, which involves non-specific general movements to increase temperature, incorporating gentle movements such as energetic walk, short striding, slow trot, and slow canter on gentle turns with gentle flexions, at a moderately low heart rate.
3. Specific warm-up, which involves practicing the type of movements that the horse will be doing in the actual training session, potentially including jumping efforts.

Warm-up should take into account temperature and humidity. Cool down following hard training is important to return body temperature to normal and for muscle, cardiovascular and respiratory recovery.

At a competition, warm-up needs to balance the requirement for adequate physiological and psychological preparation with risk of muscular fatigue prior to performance. It would be usual to retain a similar passive and general warm-up to a training session but extend the specific warm-up prior to entering the arena at a competition. In a study comparing warm-up practices between lower level and intermediate-level show jumping, competitors warmed up significantly longer overall at intermediate- compared to lower-level competition. More jumping efforts and more successful jumping efforts were observed at intermediate- compared to lower-level competition.[66] However, the number of jumping efforts was small and at elite level it is likely that there is a threshold beyond which performance may be compromised by muscle fatigue.

References

1. Barrey E, Valette JP. Exercise-related parameters of horses competing in show jumping events ranging from a regional to an international level. Ann Zootech 1993;42:89–98.
2. Sloet van Oldruitenborgh-Oosterban MM, Spierenburg J, van den Broek ETW. The workload of riding-school horses during jumping. Equine Vet J 2006;(Suppl. 36):93–7.
3. Barrey E, Langlois B. How to breed the elite show jumper. In: Lindner A, editor. The elite show jumper. Proceedings of Conference on Equine Sports Medicine and Science; 2000. p. 13–24.
4. Buhl R, Meldgaard C, Barbesgaard L. Cardiac arrhythmias in clinically healthy showjumping horses. Equine Vet J 2010;42(Suppl. 38):196–201.
5. Lekeux P, Art T, Linden A, et al. Heart rate, haematological and serum biochemical responses to show jumping. In: Persson SGB, Lindholm A, Jeffcott LB, editors. Equine exercise physiology 3. Davis, California: IDEEP Publications, 1991. p. 385–90.
6. Art T, Amory H, Desmecht D, et al. Efect of show jumping on heart rate, blood lactate, and other plasma biochemical values. Equine Vet J 1990;(Suppl. 9): 78–82.
7. Sabev S. Effect of the jumping activity in the course of training exercise on the level of serum cortisol, blood lactate and heart rate in horses. Trakea Journal of Sciences 2011;9(1):78–82.
8. Clayton HM. Performance in equestrian sports. In: Back W, Clayton HM, editors. Equine locomotion. New York: Saunders; 2001.
9. Schamhardt HC, Merkens HW, Vogel V, et al. External loads on the limbs of jumping horses at take-off and landing. Am J Vet Res 1993;54(5):675–80.
10. Rietbroek NJ, Dingboom EG, Joosten BJ, et al. Effect of show jujping training on the development of locomotory muscle in young horses. Am J Vet Res 2007;68(11):1232–8.
11. Bogert AJ, van den Jansen MO, Deuel NR. Kinematics of the hindlimbs push-off in elite jumping horses. Equine Vet J 1994;23:80–6.
12. Barrey E, Galloux P. Analysis of the equine jumping technique by accelerometry. Equine Vet J Suppl 1997;23:45–9.
13. Deuel NR, Park J. Kinematic analysis of jumping sequences of Olympic show jumping horses. Equine Exerc Physiol 1991;3:158–66.
14. Meershoek LS, Schamhardt HC, Roepstorff L, et al. Forelimb tendon loading during jump landing and the influence of fence height. Equine Vet J Suppl 2001;33:6–10.
15. Meershoek LS, Schamhardt HC, Roepstorff L, et al. Joint moments in the distal forelimbs of jumping horses during landing. Equine Vet J Suppl 2001;33: 410–15.
16. Santamaria S, Bobbert MF, Back W, et al. Performance in equR. Evaluation of consistency of jumping technique in horses between the ages of 6 months and 4 years. Am J Vet Res 2004;65:945–50.
17. Cassiat G, Pourcelot P, Tavernier L, et al. Geiger Influence of individual competition level on back kinematics of horses jumping a vertical fence. Equine Vet J 2004;36:748–53.
18. Lewczuk D. The effect of training on linear jumping parameters in young stallions. Comp Exerc Physiol 2008; 4(3/4):159–65.
19. Santamaria S, Bobbert MF, Back W, et al. Effect of early training on the jumping technique of horses. Am J Vet Res 2005;66:418–24.
20. Powers P, Harrison A. Effects of the rider on the linear kinematics of jumping horses. Sports Biomech 2002;1(2): 135–46.
21. Clayton HM. Effect of added weight on landing kinematics in jumping horses. Equine Vet J 1997;(Suppl. 23):50–3.
22. Murray RC, Dyson SJ, Tranquille C, et al. Association of type of sport and performance level with anatomical site of orthopaedic injury diagnosis. Equine Vet J Suppl 2006;(36):411–16.
23. Dyson S. Lameness in the elite show jumper. In: Lindner A, editor. The elite show jumper. Proceedings of Conference on Equine Sports Medicine and Science; 2000. p. 211–20.
24. Holmström M, Magnusson LE, Philipsson J. Variation in conformation of Swedish warmblood horses and conformational characteristics of élite sport horses. Equine Vet J 1990;22(3): 186–93.
25. Marsalek M, Sedlackova M, Secka M. The influence of the age, sex and performance

level of horses on their success in the show jumping competition. J Central European Agriculture 2005;6(4):547–54.

26. Hausberger M, Muller C, Lunel C. Does work affect personality? A study in horses. PLoS ONE 2011;6(2):e14659.
27. Ducro BJ, Koenen EPC, van Tartwijk JMFM, et al. Genetic relations of movement and free-jumping traits with dressage and show-jumping performance in competition of Dutch Warmblood horses. Livestock Sci 2007;107: 227–34.
28. Posta J, Malovhr S, Mihok S, et al. Random regression model estimation of genetic parameters for show-jumping results of Hungarian Sporthorses. J Anim Breed Genet 2010;174:280–8.
29. Patterson M, Doyle J, Cahill E, et al. Quantifying show jumping horse rider expertise using IMUs. Conf Proc IEEE Eng Med Biol Soc 2010;2010:684–7.
30. Ricard A, Blouin C. Genetic analysis of the longevity of French sport horses in jumping competition. J Anim Sci 2011;89:2988–94.
31. Harris PA. Feeding before exercise and competition in the performance horse. Pferdeheilkunde 2006;22:542–8.
32. Harris P. Feeding the elite show jumper. In Lindner A, editor. The elite show jumper. Proceedings of Conference on Equine Sports Medicine and Science; 2000. p. 25–44.
33. Murphy J. Weighted boots influence performance in show-jumping horses. Vet J 2009;18:74–6.
34. Wennerstrand J, Johnston C, Rhodin M, et al. The effect of weighted boots on the movement of the back in the asymptomatic riding horse. Comp Exerc Physiol 2006;3:13–18.
35. Harvey AM, Williams SB, Singer ER. The effect of lateral heel studs on the kinematics of the equine digit while cantering on grass. Vet J 2012;192:217–21.
36. Pardoe CH, McGuigan MP, Rogers KM, et al. The effect of shoe material on the kinetics and kinematics of foot slip at impact on concrete. Equine Vet J 2001;(Suppl. 33):70–3.
37. Hernlund E, Egnevall A, Roepstorff L. Kinematic characteristics of hoof landing in jumping horses at elite level. Equine Vet J 2010;42(Suppl. 38):462–7.
38. Kane AJ, Stover SM, Gardner IA, et al. Horseshoe characteristics as possible risk factors for fatal musculoskeletal injury of thoroughbred racehorses. Am J Vet Res 1996;57:1147–52.
39. Hill AE, Stover SM, Gardner IA, et al. Risk factors for and outcomes of noncatastrophic suspensory apparatus injury in Thoroughbred racehorses. J Am Vet Med Assoc 2001;218:1136–44.
40. Benoit P, Mitchell RD. How to perform a specialized examination of the jumping sport horse. Proc AAEP 2006;52:597–9.
41. Dyson S. Lameness and poor performance in the sports horse: dressage, show jumping and horse trials (eventing). Proc AAEP 2000;46:308–15.
42. Dyson SJ. Lameness and poor performance in the sport horse: dressage, show jumping and horse trials. J Equine Vet Sci 2002;22(4):145–50.
43. Egenvall AA, Tranquille CA, Lönnell AC, et al. Days lost to training and competition in relation to amount of training in 263 elite showjumping horses in four European countries. Submitted.
44. Dyson S, Murray R. Use of concurrent scintigraphic and magnetic resonance imaging evaluation to improve understanding of the pathogenesis of injury of the podotrochlear apparatus. Equine Vet J 2007;39(4):365–9.
45. Dyson S, Murray R. Magnetic resonance imaging evaluation of 264 horses with foot pain: the podotrochlear apparatus, deep digital flexor tendon and collateral ligaments of the distal interphalangeal joint. Equine Vet J 2007;39(4):340–3.
46. Dyson SJ, Murray R, Schramme MC. Lameness associated with foot pain: results of magnetic resonance imaging in 199 horses (January 2001–December 2003) and response to treatment. Equine Vet J 2005;37(2):113–21.
47. Dyson SJ, Murray R, Schramme M, et al. Collateral desmitis of the distal interphalangeal joint in 18 horses (2001–2002). Equine Vet J 2004;36(2): 160–6.
48. Boswell RP, Mitchell RD, Ober TR, et al. Lameness in the show hunter and show jumper. In: Ross MW, Dyson SJ, editors. Lameness in the horse. 2nd ed. St Louis: Elsevier Saunders; 2011. p. 1096–112.
49. Dyson SJ, Murray R, Schramme M, et al. Lameness in 46 horses associated with deep digital flexor tendonitis in the digit: diagnosis using magnetic resonance imaging. Equine Vet J 2003;35:681–90.
50. Van Den Bogert AJ, Jansen MO, Deuel NR. Kinematics of the hind limb push-off in elite show jumping horses. Equine Vet J Suppl 1994;17:80–6.
51. Murray RC, Dyson SJ, Weekes JS, et al. Nuclear scintigraphic evaluation of the distal tarsal region in normal horses. Vet Radiol Ultrasound 2004;45(4):345–51.
52. Murray RC, Branch MV, Dyson SJ, et al. How does exercise intensity and type affect equine distal tarsal subchondral bone thickness? J Equine Vet Sci 2007;102(6):2194–200.
53. Murray RC, Werpy N, Audigie F, et al. The proximal tarsal region in Section C: Pathology. In: Murray RC, editor. Equine MRI. Oxford: Wiley Blackwell; 2011. p. 405–20.
54. Dyson SJ, Murray RC. Osseous trauma in the fetlock region of mature sports horses. Proc AAEP 2006;52:443–56.
55. Dyson S, Nagy A, Murray R. Clinical and diagnostic imaging findings in horses with subchondral bone trauma of the sagittal groove of the proximal phalanx. Vet Radiol Ultrasound 2011;52(6): 596–604.
56. Dyson SJ. Normal ultrasonographic anatomy and injury of the patellar ligaments in the horse. Equine Vet J 2002;34:258–64.
57. Zimmerman M, Dyson S, Murray R. Close, impinging and overriding spinous processes in the thoracolumbar spine: the relationship between radiological and scintigraphic findings and clinical signs. Equine Vet J 2012;44(2):178–84.
58. Girodroux M, Dyson S, Murray R. Osteoarthritis of the thoracolumbar synovial intervertebral articulations: clinical and radiographic features in 77 horses with poor performance and back pain. Equine Vet J 2009;41(2): 130–8.
59. Dyson S, Murray R. Pain associated with the sacroiliac joint region: a clinical study of 74 horses. Equine Vet J 2003;35(3):240–5.
60. Widmer A, Doherr MG, Tessier C, et al. Association of increased tracheal mucus accumulation with poor willingness to perform in show-jumpers an dressage horses. Vet J 2009;182:430–5.
61. Art T, Van Erck E. What do we know about the poor performance horse? In: Lindner A, editor. The acute poorly performing sports horse. Proceedings of Conference on Equine Sports Medicine and Science; 2008, p. 15–37.
62. Murray RC, Walters JM, Snart H, et al. Identification of risk factors for lameness in dressage horses. Vet J 2010;184(1):27–36.
63. McClure SR, Glickman LT, Glickman NW. Prevalence of gastric ulcers in show horses. J Am Vet Med Assoc 1999;215: 1130–3.
64. Mitchell RD. Prevalence of gastric ulcers in hunter/jumper and dressage horses evaluated for poor performance. In: Proceedings of 21st Annual Conference Association of Equine Sports Medicine, September 2001.
65. Patteson M. Prepurchase examination in horses: detection and significance of heart murmurs. In Pract 2010;32: 438–43.
66. Whitaker TC, Mills A, Duxbury LJ. Horse warm-up regimes at two different competitive levels of show jumping: a pilot study. Comp Exerc Physiol 2008;5(2):105–6.

Veterinary aspects of the aged equine athlete

56

Jo L. Ireland Catherine M. McGowan

CHAPTER CONTENTS

Introduction

Geriatric medicine has become increasingly important in equine sports medicine, although research regarding management, preventive health care and disease conditions in aging athletes is relatively limited. Between 10 and 26% of aged horses are used for competition,[1,2] participating in a wide range of non-racing disciplines, including dressage, eventing and showjumping. In certain disciplines, it takes many years of training to reach elite levels of competition, so management of the horse in its older years can become very important.

Definition and demographics of the aged equine athlete

The term 'geriatric', first used in human medicine in the early 1900s, describes the life stage characterized by progressive decline in physical condition, organ function, sensory function, mental function and immunity.[3] The age at which a horse is classified as geriatric or aged remains a subject for debate and can be defined in different ways, including chronological age, demographic age and physiological or functional age.[4] Physiological age considers the point at which peak physiological functions begin to decline and, while it varies between horses depending on their use, genetic and environmental factors, this is often considered to be reached at around 15–20 years of age.

There is limited available equine demographic information and few data providing population estimates and age distribution of horses. Anecdotally the life expectancy of horses is increasing and the proportion of aged animals in the equine population appears to be growing.[5] While equine demographic characteristics vary considerably between different countries, studies suggest that between 10 and 33% of the equine population could be classed as aged.[2,6–9]

Physiological alterations associated with aging

A common characteristic of aging body systems is progressive and irreversible change.[3] Age-associated physiologic deterioration occurs subsequent to damage caused by intrinsic living processes, environmental factors, and age-associated disease.[10] Factors influencing the rate of development of both normal aging and chronic diseases are often identical.[11] When assessing health and disease in the older patient it is important to recognize and distinguish between benign signs of aging, physiological changes with age which can predispose to disease and clinical signs of disease associated with aging. However, as many of these signs are non-specific, accurately making this distinction in aging horses can be difficult and changes frequently considered benign signs of senescence, such as musculoskeletal stiffness or reduced joint flexibility and exercise intolerance/fatigue,[5,12] are likely to represent clinical signs of disease.

Cardiorespiratory changes

As in other species, there appears to be a decline in cardiorespiratory capacity with increasing age in the horse. There is an age-related decline in maximal heart rate, maximal stroke volume and maximal oxygen uptake (VO_{2max}), which are reached at lower velocities in horses aged 20 years or greater (average 27 years) compared with young (average 7 years) and middle-aged (average 15 years) horses.[13,14] During incremental exercise tests, maximal velocity attained by old horses (>20 years) was lower than that of younger horses (8.7 ± 0.5 compared to 10.8 ± 0.5 m/s, respectively).[14] The velocity at which the onset of blood lactate accumulation is observed (blood lactate concentration of 4 mmol/L, VLa_4) was also lower in old mares (7.5 ± 0.4 m/s) compared with young mares (10.2 ± 0.7 m/s).[14]

Older horses without clinical respiratory disease have decreased pulmonary surfactant phospholipid content;[15] however, the importance of this age-related change in respiratory function in the development of disease has not yet been investigated. Healthy aged horses (average 27 years) have lower partial pressure of oxygen (PaO_2) and increased arterial blood pH compared to young horses (Table 56.1).[16] Increased alveolar to arterial PaO_2 gradient suggests impaired arterial blood oxygenation in aged horses; however, there were no significant alterations in acid–base balance compared to young horses.[16]

It is interesting to note that many of the age-associated reductions in cardiorespiratory capacity were not found until horses were greater than 20 years of age. Further, despite these reductions, older horses still showed improvements in maximal stroke volume and VO_{2max} after a training program.[13] This shows that training can partially reverse some of the decline in cardiovascular function older horses.

Thermoregulatory changes

Aged horses demonstrate decreased ability to thermoregulate during exercise. During submaximal exercise tests, aged mares reached a core temperature of 40°C significantly more rapidly compared to young mares, and the average heart rate of aged mares on reaching this core temperature was significantly greater than that of the young mares.[17] This reduction in thermoregulatory capacity is likely to be associated with the lower plasma volume, resting circulating blood volume and resting red cell volume in older compared to younger mares.[17]

Changes in the musculoskeletal system

Loss of muscle mass is common in geriatric humans; in elderly females, quadriceps cross-sectional area was a third smaller and voluntary isometric strength of the quadriceps muscles was significantly lower compared to young adult females.[18] There was a significant correlation between quadriceps size and strength, suggesting that weakness is predominantly due to reduced muscle mass.[18] In humans, reduced muscle strength with increasing age is considered to be a result of both loss and atrophy of muscle fibers, with a reduction in the proportion of type I fibers.[19] Similar changes in the profile of muscle fiber types have also been identified in aged horses, and can explain some of the lower exercise capacity seen in the older horse. The proportion of type I muscle fibers decreases and there are alterations in the activity of muscle enzymes, consistent with decreasing oxidative capacity of equine skeletal muscle, with increasing age.[20,21]

Post-mortem studies have identified age-related changes in articular calcified cartilage thickness, hyaline cartilage and subchondral bone thickness and bone density and micro-architecture.[22–24] Age-related degenerative changes in the surface of the navicular bone and the deep flexor tendon were found in older horses without a history of lameness and navicular disease.[25] Age-related changes have also been reported in components of articular cartilage. For example, non-enzymatic pentosidine cross-linking increases linearly with age, with a 10-fold increase between horses aged 5–30 years.[26] Another study found that while glycosaminoglycan content remained constant in samples taken from the metacarpophalangeal joints of horses ranging from three months to 31 years, there was a decline in hydration and cellularity of cartilage with increasing age, in addition to an age-related decrease in proteoglycan size through

Table 56.1 Arterial blood gas values, hematologic and serum chemistry values (mean ± standard error or standard deviation) of young and geriatric horses

	YOUNG HORSES	GERIATRIC HORSES	REFERENCES
pH	7.404 ± 0.005	7.428 ± 0.007*	16
PaO_2 (mmHg)	101.7 ± 1.6	90.2 ± 2.2*	16
$PaCO_2$ (mmHg)	43 ± 0.7	41.5 ± 1.0*	16
$P(A\text{-}a)O_2$ (mmHg)	7.2 ± 1.7	22.1 ± 2.5*	16
Mean cell volume (MCV) (fL)	47.8 ± 2.2	49.7 ± 2.2*	3
Mean cell volume (MCV) (fL)	43 ± 1	49 ± 2*	19
Mean cell hemoglobin (MHC) (pg)	16.3 ± 0.9	17.1 ± 0.8*	3
Lymphocytes ($\times 10^9$/L)	3.1 ± 1.1	2.2 ± 0.8*	3
$CD4^+/CD8^+$ cell ratio	4.07 ± 1.54	3.30 ± 1.31*	25
Ionized calcium (mEq/L)	3.00 ± 0.02	3.18 ± 0.05*	16
Ionized calcium pH corrected (mEq/L)	2.98 ± 0.03	3.14 ± 0.05*	16

*Significant difference between young and geriatric horses ($P < 0.05$).

the loss of glycosaminoglycan chains.[27] These changes may predispose older horses to osteochondral disease due to the cartilage becoming stiffer, more brittle, and more vulnerable to damage by mechanical loading.[26,27]

Hematological, biochemical and endocrine parameters

Some age-related differences in hematological parameters have been described in the horse, although, again, these are not usually evident until the horse is over 20 years of age. Clinically healthy aged horses have larger red blood cells (RBCs), with a higher erythrocyte mean cell volume (MCV)[28,29] and a higher mean cell hemoglobin concentration (MCH).[28] Increased MCH could reflect larger RBC size rather than a true increase in MCH concentration.[28] Anemia is not a feature of healthy aged horses until they are very old (≥30), and then reduced RBC count might be compensated for by an increased MCV or cell size.[30,31]

A proportion of aged horses do have decreased lymphocyte counts compared to younger adult horses and 17% horses aged 20 years and 13% of horses aged 30 years and older showed lymphocyte counts below the laboratory reference range.[28,31] This result is likely to be associated with immunosenescence in the older horse, which affects some horses to a greater degree than others (see below).

The effect of age on biochemical parameters in the horse is limited. Most studies have reported no significant differences in any of the biochemical parameters assessed between healthy young and aged horses.[28,29,32] Some minor variations in several biochemical parameters have been reported between different age groups of Arab mares.[33] They found a decrease in alkaline phosphatase (ALP) with increasing age, with the lowest mean values found in mares > 20 years of age. The same study also reported that phosphorus concentrations were below physiological levels in horses ≥14 years old and mean values for blood urea nitrogen (BUN) and creatinine increased with increasing age, although the highest mean creatinine found in the >20-year-old group was still within the laboratory reference range used.[33]

There are few endocrine changes in aged horses that can be clearly linked with performance. In a small study, thyroxine (T_4) and insulin-like growth factor (IGF)-I levels were significantly lower in older mares than younger mares, and further, certain IGF-binding proteins had lowest circulating concentrations in aged mares.[34] This led to research on the effects of exogenous administration of equine somatotrophin to aged horses on feed intake, body score, digestion, aerobic capacity, and immunocompetence.[35–37] Bodyweight, body condition scores, and feed intake were not affected by administration of equine somatotrophin to older horses.[36,37] However, greater muscle definition was reported in one study.[37] Daily administration of equine somatotrophin to older horses may improve nitrogen balance and fiber digestion.[37] Somatotrophin administration does not affect aerobic capacity (measured by VO_{2max}, maximum running velocity, or total running time) in older horses.[36] However, administration of equine somatotrophin to older horses appears to have a beneficial immune effect, by increasing the number of granulocytes, and the lymphoproliferative response to mitogens following treatment.[35]

Age-related immunological alterations: immunosenescence and inflamm-aging

Aging of the immune system, or immunosenescence, is defined as a decline in cell-mediated immunity, particularly with respect to lymphocyte number and function. Older horses have a reduced response to influenza vaccination, although the vaccine does confer some protection from clinical disease.[38,39] Compared to younger horses, healthy geriatric horses aged 20–30 years had impaired proliferation of lymphocytes in response to mitogen.[38] Peripheral blood mononuclear cells (PBMCs) demonstrate an age-related reduction in telomere length.[40] Horses > 20 years old had reduced cell counts of total lymphocytes, T cells, B cells and CD4+ and CD8+ T cells, with an increased CD4+: CD8+ cell ratio compared with younger horses.[41]

In contrast to immunosenescence, age-related increases in pro-inflammatory cytokines and other mediators result in a low-grade, chronic inflammatory state referred to as 'inflamm-aging'. Compared to younger horses, healthy aged horses (>20 years) have increased production of various inflammatory cytokines including interferon-γ (INFγ), interleukin (IL)-1γ, IL-6, IL-8, IL-15, IL-18 and TNFα gene expression and serum TNFα protein levels in peripheral blood compared to younger adult horses.[42,43] Furthermore, aged horses show an increased production of pro-inflammatory cytokines after infection with equine influenza[38] and stimulation with lipopolysaccharide.[42]

Common conditions affecting the aged equine athlete

The prevalence of owner-reported disease conditions increases with increasing horse age,[7,8] and increasing age is a risk factor for numerous different diseases including chronic laminitis,[44] strangulating lipoma,[45] recurrent airway obstruction (RAO),[46] left-sided valvular regurgitation,[47] ophthalmic lesions,[48] and neoplasia.[49] In large field-based studies where veterinary examinations have been performed on hundreds of aged horses 15 years and older, the most common conditions diagnosed were dental, musculoskeletal, respiratory, cardiac and endocrine disease.[32,50] Therefore it is likely that such conditions are more prevalent in aged sports horses compared to their younger counterparts.

Dental disease

While not considered a typical cause of poor performance dental disease is prevalent and can result in weight loss, pain and disease. Dental disease is the main oral disorder of horses, and is highly prevalent in aged horses.[32,50] Common dental conditions in aged horses include tooth loss, diastemata, periodontal disease and abnormalities of wear such as focal overgrowths, wave mouth, shear mouth and smooth mouth. Clinical signs of dental disease are frequently reported by owners of aged horses, yet the owner-reported prevalence of known dental problems is considerably lower.[51,52] Post-mortem studies have identified high levels of clinically important, non-diagnosed dental disorders in horses.[53,54] Together these data suggest dental disease, especially in the older performance horse, could be an important cause of poor performance.

In aged horses diastemata can develop secondary to acquired cheek teeth displacements, as a consequence of tooth loss or with lack of adequate compression of the narrow reserve crowns due to loss of angulation of the rostral and caudal cheek teeth.[55] Sharp transverse overgrowths or accentuated transverse ridges directly opposite diastemata will selectively widen them and compress food into them.[56] This can lead to painful and usually progressive secondary periodontal disease, which is a major factor in premature tooth loss in aging horses.[57] Periodontal disease has been reported to have a prevalence of over 30% in horses over 20 years of age presented for routine dental care.[58] In addition to premature tooth loss, this condition can cause pain, dysmastication and may predispose to displacement of cheek teeth.

Musculoskeletal disorders and lameness

Musculoskeletal disorders are amongst the most common reasons for referral[1] and a major reason for euthanasia in aged horses.[59] Owners of aged horses frequently report muscle stiffness and lameness as clinical signs, yet the owner-reported prevalence of musculoskeletal disease is considerably lower,[51,52] suggesting specific conditions might be undiagnosed.

Many of the non-traumatic musculoskeletal conditions seen in aged horses result from the culmination of years of athletic activity, confounded by the animal's individual conformational abnormalities.[60] However, rather than directly causing disease, it is possible that aging changes in the musculoskeletal system contribute to the development of orthopedic disease by increasing the effects of other risk factors including genetic factors, abnormal biomechanics and joint injury.[61]

Osteoarthritis

The most common musculoskeletal condition of aged horses is osteoarthritis, with 40% of diagnoses classified as degenerative disease (osteoarthritis or degenerative joint disease) in horses ≥20 years.[1] Osteoarthritis is also the most common owner-reported disorder in aged horses.[62] Although changes in exercise regimes might be required to manage the disease, many sports horses with osteoarthritis continue to perform in a wide range of athletic disciplines.[63]

While cartilage senescence contributes to the pathological changes in osteoarthritis, research studies in human patients investigating initial events, at both cellular and molecular level, which lead to these changes in the joint, have identified an inflammatory component with matrix degradation mediated by cells, cytokines and chemokines. Furthermore, age-related changes outside the joint, including sarcopenia and increased bone turnover, and within the joint, including changes in cells and extracellular matrix, likely increase the susceptibility of older adults to osteoarthritis and contribute to the development of the condition when other risk factors are also present.[64]

Presence of reduced flexibility of the joint and pain on flexion is commonly considered to indicate a clinically important underlying problem, most frequently osteoarthritis.[64] Measured using goniometry, range of motion in the tarsal and metacarpophalangeal joints is significantly lower in horses with owner-reported osteoarthritis.[50] The distal tarsal, metacarpophalangeal, proximal interphalangeal, carpal and stifle joints are the most frequently affected.[60] Pain management, control of inflammation, maintaining joint function and limiting disease progression are the primary aims of treatment.[63] Complementary and physical therapies may be indicated in addition to or in place of medications where drug restrictions are a concern.

Cardiac disorders

Cardiac murmurs are frequently detected as an incidental finding at veterinary clinical examination in horses of any age as many valvular insufficiencies are clinically well tolerated.[65] However, age has been identified as a significant risk factor associated with left-sided valvular regurgitation/insufficiencies (LSVR) such as aortic and mitral insufficiency.[47,66] The overall prevalence of cardiac murmurs in middle-aged and geriatric horses is approximately 20–30%.[32,47] The prevalence of LSVR increases with age, from 3.4% in horses aged <8 years to 13.5% in horses aged 15–23 years and to 14.8% in horses ≥24 years.[47]

There is no significant association between the presence of a heart murmur and reduced performance in young racehorses.[67] However, the effect of cardiac murmurs on performance in aged equine athletes has not been documented and there is a risk of progression to reduced cardiac output and ultimately congestive heart failure. Despite this risk, progression is reportedly rare in horses[68] and there was no significant difference in the mortality of horses with and without LSVR.[47]

Respiratory disease

Factors affecting the health of the lower respiratory tract can have a cumulative effect and over a lifetime older horses can be exposed to more pathogens and allergens that can ultimately lead to small airway disease and subclinical or clinical poor performance. In a referral hospital population, the third most commonly affected body system in aged horses was the respiratory system, accounting for 16% of all cases.[1] Recurrent airway obstruction (RAO) is the most prevalent respiratory disorder in aged horses, diagnosed in 6% within a referral hospital population.[1] Increasing age has been identified as a risk factor for RAO[46] and it has been suggested that the increasing risk of RAO in older animals can be due to repeated bouts of inflammation leading to progressive airway remodeling.[69]

While clinical signs of respiratory disease, such as coughing and nasal discharge, are frequently reported by owners of aged horses, the owner-reported prevalence of respiratory disease is considerably lower.[51,62] These findings suggest that clinical signs of respiratory disorders are prevalent in geriatric horses, but that respiratory disease is under-recognised or undiagnosed in a considerable proportion of affected animals. For information on the diagnosis and treatment of respiratory diseases please refer to Chapters 26-30.

Pituitary *pars intermedia* dysfunction (PPID)

Pituitary *pars intermedia* dysfunction (PPID) is a neurodegenerative disease associated with aging, affecting the *pars intermedia* of the pituitary gland.[70] PPID affects horses, ponies and donkeys, typically diagnosed in animals aged 18 to 23 years, with few cases reported in animals younger than 10 years, and is the most frequently diagnosed endocrine disorder of aged horses.[1,71] The prevalence of veterinary-diagnosed PPID increases significantly with increasing horse age.[72] Based on seasonally adjusted basal ACTH values, over 20% of horses 15 years and older have PPID.[72]

PPID is a slowly progressive disease with loss of dopaminergic inhibitory input to the melanotropes of the pituitary *pars intermedia*, leading to overproduction and elevated circulating levels of pro-opiomelanocortin (POMC)-derived peptides such as α-melanocyte stimulating hormone (α-MSH), β-endorphin, corticotrophin-like intermediate peptide (CLIP), and adrenocorticotrophic hormone (ACTH).[70] Clinical signs of PPID include hypertrichosis (commonly described as hirsutism), delayed or absent hair coat shedding, laminitis, lethargy, weight loss and altered fat distribution, epaxial muscle wasting, polyuria and polydipsia, hyperhidrosis or patchy sweating and increased susceptibility to infection.[71] The earliest clinical signs of PPID can be mild and non-specific including muscle wasting, leading to a 'poor topline' and relatively unapparent hair coat changes. Horses in the early stages of disease might not exhibit signs that are readily detectable by their owners as evidenced by the much lower owner-reported than veterinary diagnosis where the same horses have been studied.[72,73]

There are no studies examining the exercise capacity of PPID horses compared to aged or young horses; however, poor performance might be expected due the myopathy that has been found in horses with PPID.[74] Further, the lethargy purportedly associated with increased circulating β-endorphin levels[71] is likely to reduce willingness to exercise, even if not actual performance. It should be noted that uncomplicated cases of PPID do not have any hematological or biochemical changes that can be distinguished from age-matched controls.[72]

PPID is typically suspected on the basis of clinical signs, and confirmed using a basal ACTH test using seasonally adjusted reference ranges appropriate for both the laboratory and the latitude[72] or the dexamethasone suppression test.[71] As mentioned above, early clinical signs can be subtle and in the aged sports horse it is important to identify these signs early as treatment can be very effective.

Treatment

Pergolide mesylate, a dopamine agonist, is the treatment of choice for PPID and is now licensed for equine use in many countries (Prascend, Boehringer Ingelheim, Germany). Treatment must always be monitored and adjusted under veterinary management until the appropriate dose is achieved for the individual animal, but most horses will respond to a dose of 0.002 mg/kg per day. Up to 80% of horses will have a positive response to pergolide and many horses will continue or return to athletic function.[71,75,76] Unfortunately, drug use regulations in many areas have banned the use of pergolide in competing horses, which limits the use of pergolide as it must be administered daily.

Preventive health care and management for the aged equine athlete

Preventive health care strategies including exercise and nutrition, and routine preventive health care measures are important in reducing morbidity in elderly people, yet there is very limited published information regarding the role of management and routine health care in equine medicine. Reduced provision or frequency of preventive health care measures such as vaccination, dental care, farrier care and anthelmintic administration may occur in older horses[2,7,77] despite evidence to suggest they could be even more likely to require routine preventive health care. Veterinary assessments play an important role in any preventive health care program, yet a large proportion of aged horses do not receive regular veterinary visits.[7] Maintenance of the older equine athlete requires careful attention to preventive health care, in particular dental prophylaxis, hoof care, vaccination, anthelmintic administration and nutrition.

In summary, aged horses form a significant proportion of the non-racing performance horse population and maintaining performance in these horses is an important part of veterinary practice. There are a number of physiological alterations with age that predispose the older athletic horse to reductions in performance and subclinical or clinical disease and poor performance. However, with good preventive health care and continuation of an exercise training program, where possible, older horses can continue to perform well into their second decade and beyond.

With thanks to Laurie A. Beard, who created the original chapter in the first edition.

References

1. Brosnahan MM, Paradis MR. Assessment of clinical characteristics, management practices, and activities of geriatric horses. Journal of the American Veterinary Medical Association 2003;223:99–103.
2. Ireland JL, Clegg PD, McGowan CM, et al. A cross-sectional study of geriatric horses in the United Kingdom Part 1: Demographics and management practices. Equine Veterinary Journal 2011;43:30–6.
3. Fortney WD. Geriatrics and aging. In: Hoskins J, editor. Geriatrics and Gerontology of the Dog and Cat. 2nd ed. St. Louis, Missouri, USA: Saunders; 2004. p. 1–4.
4. Timiras PS. Old age as a stage of life: Common terms related to aging and methods used to study aging. In: Timiras PS, editor. Physiological Basis of Aging and Geriatrics. 4th ed. New York: Informa Healthcare USA; 2007. p. 3–10.
5. Hintz HF. The geriatric horse. Equine Practice 1995;17:8–10.
6. Mellor DJ, Love S, Gettinby G, et al. Demographic characteristics of the equine population of northern Britain. Veterinary Record 1999;145:299–304.
7. McGowan TW, Pinchbeck GL, Phillips C, et al. A survey of aged horses in Queensland, Australia. Part 1: Management and preventive health care. Australian Veterinary Journal 2010a;88:420–7.
8. Cole FL, Hodgson DR, Reid SWJ, et al. Owner-reported equine health disorders: results of an Australia-wide postal survey. Australian Veterinary Journal 2005;83:490–5.
9. Anon. USDA/APHIS Part 1: baseline reference of equine health and management, 2005. Fort Collins: National Animal Health Monitoring System; 2005. p. 1–60.
10. Masoro EJ. Physiology of aging. In: Fillit HM, Rockwood K, Woodhouse K, editors. Brocklehurst's Textbook of Geriatric Medicine and Gerontology. 7th ed. Philadelphia, USA: Saunders Elsevier; 2010. p. 51–8.
11. Fries JF. Aging, natural death and the compression of morbidity. New England Journal of Medicine 1980;303:130–5.
12. Codron E, Benamou-Smith A. Panorama of equine geriatrics. In: Proceedings of the 9th Congress of the World Equine Veterinary Association. 2006. Marrakech, January 22 to 26, 2006. p. 391–2.
13. Betros CL, McKeever KH, Kearns CF, et al. Effects of aging and training on maximal heart rate and VO2max. Equine Veterinary Journal Supplement 2002;34:100–5.
14. McKeever KH, Malinowski K. Exercise capacity in young and old mares. Am J Vet Res 1997;58:1468–72.
15. Christmann U, Hite RD, Witonsky SG, et al. Influence of age on surfactant isolated from healthy horses maintained on pasture. Journal of Veterinary Internal Medicine 2009;23:612–18.
16. Aguilera-Tejero E, Estepa JC, Lopez I, et al. Arterial blood gases and acid-base balance in healthy young and aged horses. Equine Veterinary Journal 1998;30:352–4.
17. McKeever KH, Eaton TL, Geiser S, et al. Age related decreases in thermoregulation and cardiovascular function in horses. Equine Veterinary Journal 2010;42 (Suppl. 38):220–7.
18. Young A, Stokes M, Crowe M. Size and strength of the quadriceps muscles of old and young women. European Journal of Clinical Investigation 1984;14:282–7.
19. Frontera WR, Hughes VA, Fielding RA, et al. Aging of skeletal muscle: a 12-year longitudinal study. Journal of Applied Physiology 2000;88:1321–6.
20. Kim J, Hinchcliff KW, Yamaguchi M, et al. Age-related changes in metabolic properties of equine skeletal muscle associated with muscle plasticity. The Veterinary Journal 2005;169: 397–403.

21. Lehnhard RA, McKeever KH, Kearns CF, et al. Myosin heavy chain profiles and body composition are different in old versus young Standardbred mares. The Veterinary Journal 2004;167:59–66.
22. Martinelli MJ, Eurell J, Les CM, et al. Age-related morphometry of equine calcified cartilage. Equine Veterinary Journal 2002;34:274–8.
23. Murray RC, Blunden TS, Branch MV, et al. Evaluation of age-related changes in the structure of the equine tarsometatarsal osteochondral unit. Am J Vet Res 2009;70:30–6.
24. Fürst A, Meier D, Michel S, et al. Effect of age on bone mineral density and micro architecture in the radius and tibia of horses: An Xtreme computed tomographic study. BMC Veterinary Research 2008;4:3 doi:10.1186/1746-6148-4-3.
25. Doige CE, Hoffer MA. Pathological changes in the navicular bone and associated structures of the horse. Canadian Journal of Comparative Medicine 1983;47:387–95.
26. Brama PA, TeKoppele JM, Bank RA, et al. Influence of site and age on biochemical characteristics of the collagen network of equine articular cartilage. American Journal of Veterinary Research 1999;60: 341–5.
27. Platt D, Bird JLE, Bayliss MT. Ageing of equine articular cartilage: structure and composition of aggrecan and decorin. Equine Veterinary Journal 1998;30: 43–52.
28. McFarlane D, Sellon DC, Gaffney D, et al. Hematologic and serum biochemical variables and plasma corticotropin concentration in healthy aged horses. American Journal of Veterinary Research 1998;59:1247–51.
29. Ralston SL, Nockels CF, Squires EL. Differences in diagnostic-test results and hematologic data between aged and young horses. American Journal of Veterinary Research 1988;49: 1387–92.
30. Satue K, Blanco O, Munoz A. Age-related differences in the hematological profile of Andalusian broodmares of Carthusian strain. Veterinarni Medicina 2009;54: 175–82.
31. Ireland JL, McGowan CM, Clegg PD, et al. A survey of health care and disease in geriatric horses aged 30 years or older. Vet J 2012;192(1):57–64.
32. McGowan TW. Aged Horse Health, Management and Welfare. PhD Thesis, School of Animal Studies: Faculty of Natural Resources, Agriculture and Veterinary Science, University of Queensland; 2009.
33. Gurgoze SY, Icen H. The influence of age on clinical biochemical parameters in pure-bred Arabian mares. Journal of Equine Veterinary Science 2010;30: 569–74.
34. Malinowski K, Christensen RA, Hafs HD, et al. Age and breed differences in thyroid hormones, insulin-like growth factor (IGF)-1 and IGF binding proteins in female horses. Journal of Animal Science 1996;78:1936–42.
35. McKeever KH, Malinowski K. Endocrine response to exercise in young and old horses. Equine Veterinary Journal Supplement 1999;30:561–6.
36. McKeever KH, Malinowski K, Christensen RA, et al. Chronic recombinant equine somatotrophin (eST) administration does not affect aerobic capacity or exercise performance in geriatric mares. Vet J 1998;155:19–25.
37. Ralston SL, Christensen RA, Malinowski K. Chronic effects of equine growth hormone (eGH) on intake, digestibility and retention of nutrients in aged mares. J Anim Sci 1996;74(Suppl 1):194.
38. Adams AA, Sturgill TL, Breathnach CC, et al. Humoral and cell-mediated immune responses of old horses following recombinant canarypox virus vaccination and subsequent challenge infection. Veterinary Immunology and Immunopathology 2011;139:128–40.
39. Muirhead TL, McClure JT, Wichtel JJ, et al. The effect of age on serum antibody titers after rabies and influenza vaccination in healthy horses. Journal of Veterinary Internal Medicine 2008;22: 654–61.
40. Katepalli MP, Adams AA, Lear TL, et al. The effect of age and telomere length on immune function in the horse. Developmental and Comparative Immunology 2008;32:1409–15.
41. McFarlane D, Sellon DC, Gibbs SA. Age-related quantitative alterations in lymphocyte subsets and immunoglobulin isotypes in healthy horses. American Journal of Veterinary Research 2001;62: 1413–17.
42. McFarlane D, Holbrook TC. Cytokine dysregulation in aged horses and horses with pituitary pars intermedia dysfunction. Journal of Veterinary Internal Medicine 2008;22:436–42.
43. Adams AA, Breathnach CC, Katepalli MP, et al. Advanced age in horses affects divisional history of T cells and inflammatory cytokine production. Mechanisms of Ageing and Development 2008;129:656–64.
44. Polzer J, Slater MR. Age, breed, sex and seasonality as risk factors for equine laminitis. Preventive Veterinary Medicine 1997;29:179–84.
45. Garcia-Seco E, Wilson DA, Kramer J, et al. Prevalence and risk factors associated with outcome of surgical removal of pedunculated lipomas in horses: 102 cases (1987–2002). Journal of the American Veterinary Medical Association 2005;226:1529–37.
46. Hotchkiss JW, Reid SWJ, Christley RM. A survey of horse owners in Great Britain regarding horses in their care. Part 2: Risk factors for recurrent airway obstruction. Equine Veterinary Journal 2007;39: 301–8.
47. Stevens KB, Marr CM, Horn JNR, et al. Effect of left-sided valvular regurgitation on mortality and causes of death among a population of middle-aged and older horses. Veterinary Record 2009;164:6–10.
48. Chandler KJ, Billson FM, Mellor DJ. Ophthalmic lesions in 83 geriatric horses and ponies. Veterinary Record 2003;153: 319–22.
49. Williams N. Disease conditions in geriatric horses. Equine Practice 2000;22:32.
50. Ireland JL, Clegg PD, McGowan CM, et al. Disease prevalence in geriatric horses in the United Kingdom: veterinary clinical assessment of 200 cases. Equine Vet J 2012;44:101–6.
51. McGowan TW, Pinchbeck GL, Phillips C, et al. A survey of aged horses in Queensland, Australia. Part 2: Clinical signs and owner perceptions of health and welfare. Australian Veterinary Journal 2010b;88:465–71.
52. Ireland JL, Clegg PD, McGowan CM, et al. Comparison of owner-reported health problems with veterinary assessment of geriatric horses in the United Kingdom. Equine Veterinary Journal 2012;44:94–100.
53. Kirkland KD, Maretta SM, Inoue OJ, et al. Survey of equine dental disease and associated oral pathology. Proceedings of the 40th Annual Convention of the American Association of Equine Practitioners, 1994. p. 119–120.
54. Brigham EJ, Duncanson GR. An equine post-mortem study: 50 cases. Equine Veterinary Education 2000;12:59–62.
55. Collins NM, Dixon PM. Diagnosis and management of equine diastemata. Clinical Techniques in Equine Practice 2005;4:148–54.
56. Dixon PM, Dacre I. A review of equine dental disorders. The Veterinary Journal 2005;169:165–87.
57. Klugh DO. Equine periodontal disease. Clinical techniques in Equine Practice 2005;4:135–47.
58. Wilson GJ, Liyou OJ. Examination of dental charts of horses presented for routine dentistry over a 12 month period. Australian Equine Veterinarian 2005;24:79–83.
59. Ireland JL, Clegg PD, McGowan CM, et al. Factors associated with mortality of geriatric horses in the United Kingdom. Prev Vet Med 2011;101:204–18.
60. Cary J, Turner T. Geriatric musculoskeletal disorders of the horse. In: Bertone J, editor. Equine Geriatric Medicine and Surgery. St Louis: W.B. Saunders; 2006. p. 217–21.
61. Loeser RF. Age-related changes in the musculoskeletal system and the

development of osteoarthritis. Clinics in Geriatric Medicine 2010;26(3):371–86.
62. Ireland JL, Clegg PD, McGowan CM, et al. A cross-sectional study of geriatric horses in the United Kingdom. Part 2: health care and disease. Equine Vet J 2011;43:37–44.
63. Malone ED. Managing chronic arthritis. Veterinary Clinics of North America: Equine Practice 2002;18:411–37.
64. Anderson SA, Loeser RF. Why is osteoarthritis an age-related disease? Best Practice and Research: Clinical Rheumatology 2010;24(1):15–26.
65. Marr CM, Bowen M. Cardiac disease in the geriatric horse. In: Bertone J, editor. Equine Geriatric Medicine and Surgery. St. Louis, Missouri: Saunders; 2006. p. 39–49.
66. Else RW, Holmes JR. Cardiac pathology in the horse: 1. Gross pathology. Equine Veterinary Journal 1972;4:2.
67. Young LE, Rogers K, Wood JL. Heart murmurs and valvular regurgitation in thoroughbred racehorses: epidemiology and associations with athletic performance. J Vet Intern Med 2008;22:418–26.
68. Davis JL, Gardner SY, Schwabenton B, et al. Congestive heart failure in horses: 14 cases (1984–2001). Journal of the American Veterinary Medical Association 2002;220:1512–15.
69. Lugo J, Harkema JR, deFeijter-Rupp H, et al. Airway inflammation is associated with mucus cell metaplasia and increased intraepithelial stored microsubstances in horses. Veterinary Journal 2006;172:293–310.
70. McFarlane D. Advantages and limitations of the equine disease, pituitary pars intermedia dysfunction as a model of spontaneous dopaminergic neurodegenerative disease. Aging Research Reviews 2007;6:54–63.
71. Schott HC. Pituitary pars intermedia dysfunction: equine Cushing's disease. Vet Clin N Am: Equine Pract 2002;18:237–70.
72. McGowan TW, Pinchbeck GL, McGowan CM. Prevalence, risk factors and clinical signs predictive for equine pituitary pars intermedia dysfunction in aged horses. Equine Vet J 2013;45:74–9.
73. Brosnahan MM, Paradis MR. Demographic and clinical characteristics of geriatric horses: 467 cases (1989–1999). Journal of the American Veterinary Medical Association 2003;223:93–8.
74. Aleman M, Watson JL, Williams DC, et al. Myopathy in horses with pituitary pars intermedia dysfunction (Cushing's disease). Neuromuscul Disord 2006;16(11):737–44.
75. Donaldson MT, LaMonte BH, Morresey P, et al. Treatment with pergolide or cyproheptadine of pituitary pars intermedia dysfunction (equine Cushing's disease). Journal of Veterinary Internal Medicine 2002;16:742–6.
76. Rohrbach BW, Stafford JR, Clermont RS, et al. Diagnostic frequency, response to therapy, and long-term prognosis among horses and ponies with pituitary par intermedia dysfunction, 1993–2004. J Vet Intern Med 2012;26:1027–34.
77. Mellor DJ, Reid SWJ, Love S, et al. Sentinel practice-based survey of the management and health of horses in northern Britain. Veterinary Record 2001;149:417–23.

57 Anesthesia of the equine athlete

John A.E. Hubbell

CHAPTER CONTENTS

Introduction

The initial question when discussing anesthesia of the equine athlete is 'Are there any horses that aren't athletes?' Compared with many other species, such as cows and cats, the answer is probably no. Having answered this initial question, there are suggestions in the literature that 'fit' horses, particularly 'fit' Thoroughbred horses, are more difficult to anesthetize than other horses.[1,2] Anecdotally, this increased level of difficulty seems to center on lower respiratory rates in 'fit' horses and issues of temperament. A search of the literature reveals few differences in respiratory and cardiovascular function in horses at rest, whether untrained, trained, or detrained. Training increases peak oxygen uptake without changing peak minute ventilation; thus the ratio of minute volume to oxygen uptake (the ventilatory equivalent for oxygen) decreases.[3] A reduction in the ventilatory equivalent indicates that a fit horse exchanges a smaller ventilatory volume to maintain a given oxygen uptake than the same horse when detrained. Further, the respiratory pattern in trained and untrained horses is similar, implying increased efficiency of oxygen extraction at the pulmonary level. This increased efficiency of oxygen extraction may partially account for the decreased respiratory rates observed in anesthetized 'fit' horses. Alveolar tensions of anesthetic gases rise at a slower rate in horses with slow respiratory rates, potentially delaying the attainment of brain anesthetic gas tensions sufficient for anesthesia. The potential decreases in respiratory function could be further exacerbated by the effects of anesthetic drugs and body position on the function of respiratory muscles and interruption of the normal, unique breathing strategy seen in this species.[4] Training does not alter resting heart rate, stroke volume, or cardiac output in the resting horses, but total red cell volume increases and plasma volume increases as much as 29%.[5–7] The increase in plasma volume may increase pre-load and enhance cardiac output in exercising 'fit' horses.[8] Other changes potentially pertinent to anesthesia include an apparent increase in muscle glycogen, muscle capillarization, and muscle mitochondrial density in 'fit' horses.[9]

History

These questions should be asked of the responsible party prior to anesthesia:

1. Has the horse been anesthetized previously? If so, what were the circumstances and were there any problems associated with the anesthetic period? Many athletic horses have been previously anesthetized, most without incident. Potential problems that could be uncovered by this question include untoward reactions to drug administration, excitement during induction or recovery, prolonged recovery, or rhabdomyolysis.
2. Is the horse tolerant of exercise? Horses that are intolerant of exercise may not tolerate anesthesia. Potential causes of exercise intolerance include ataxia, respiratory insufficiency, upper airway obstruction, and cardiac insuffciency, including atrial fibrillation or other arrhythmia, or rhabdomyolysis or other muscle diseases.
3. Has the horse recently experienced any respiratory disease? Anesthesia compromises resistance to respiratory disease in a number of ways including depression of mucociliary and

immune function, loss of the cough reflex, drying of the airway, and inhibition of nasal and laryngeal function. In normal animals these changes are short-lived, but in horses incubating respiratory disease, anesthesia may predispose to worsening signs and exacerbation of disease.

4. Does the horse make a respiratory noise at rest or during exercise? Anesthetic agents, notably the alpha$_2$-adrenoreceptor agonists, cause relaxation of the upper airway including the larynx.[10–12] This relaxation may augment a pre-existing condition resulting in partial or full respiratory obstruction. Such obstructions can be overcome with endotracheal intubation but may be problematic during recovery.
5. Has the horse ever tied up (rhabdomyolysis)? There is considerable evidence of genetic, gender, and breed predisposition for rhabdomyolysis.[13] Anesthesia can be a triggering event.
6. How does the horse react to new experiences? There is considerable variation amongst equines in their ability to adapt to new situations and experiences. Some horses are apparently calm despite being placed in stimulus-intensive environments while others become agitated without apparent provocation. The demeanor of the patient potentially affects the required doses of sedatives and may change preparations for anesthesia and recovery.
7. Is the horse receiving any medication? When was the last time the horse was medicated? Some individuals utilize long-acting tranquilizers and other drugs as part of their training regimens. The administration of drugs such as acepromazine, fluphenazine and reserpine can affect the required doses of anesthetic agents and the resultant pharmacologic response.

Physical examination

The physical examination is the centerpiece of pre-anesthetic data collection. The examination should focus on the cardiovascular, respiratory, neurological and musculoskeletal systems.

Cardiovascular system

The cardiovascular system is easily evaluated by palpating the pulse of a peripheral artery, checking the color of mucous membranes, measuring the capillary refill time, assessing skin turgor, and ausculting the heart. Normal pulse rates in quiet adult horses range from 25 to 45 beats per minute. Interruptions in the regular rhythm (pauses) are not uncommon in fit horses and are usually the result of sinus arrhythmias or second-degree atrioventricular blockade. A brief period of exercise should stimulate an increase in heart rate and resolve the arrhythmia. The most common pathologic arrhythmia in horses is atrial fibrillation.[14] Presumptive diagnosis of atrial fibrillation can be made on physical examination by palpating pulses of unequal strength occurring at irregular intervals and by ausculting variable-intensity heart sounds at varying intervals. An electrocardiogram should be obtained if pauses in the pulse rhythm do not respond to exercise or if there are pulses of variable intensity occurring at variable intervals. Heart murmurs can be ausculted in the majority of race horse.[15] Most are systolic murmurs, heard best at the heart base. Murmurs of grade II (out of VI) or less are interpreted as innocent flow murmurs if there is no other evidence of heart disease. Murmurs of potential significance include those that result from mitral valve insufficiency, aortic insufficiency or congenital ventricular septal defects, but they comprise less than 0.1% of the population. Additional information can be obtained via electrocardiography and echocardiography.

Transient periods of sinus tachycardia (heart rates greater than 50 beats/min) are not of concern but sustained tachycardia should be interpreted as an indicator of cardiovascular or metabolic disease. Atrial and, less frequently, ventricular premature contractions are observed in horses prior to surgery. Abnormal atrial and ventricular rhythm disturbances are a warning that there may be systemic illness, myocarditis, or associated cardiovascular compromise. Infrequent atrial or ventricular extra systoles (< 5/min when the heart rate is normal) without clinical evidence of cardiovascular compromise are tolerated in horses under general anesthesia. Horses with frequent ventricular premature contractions, paroxysmal ventricular tachycardia, or persistent ventricular tachycardia should not be anesthetized for elective procedures.

Respiratory system

Examination of the respiratory system is best accomplished in a quiet room or stall and is facilitated by stimulating the horse to breathe deeply. The lung fields over both sides of the thorax should be ausculted. Auscultation of the trachea may be useful in detecting the presence of mucopurulent material. Light squeezing of the trachea in a normal horse does not induce a cough but may produce a cough in a horse with upper respiratory tract infection.

Horses with suspect respiratory disease should receive a further diagnostic work-up, potentially including a complete blood cell count, plasma fibrinogen, tracheal wash and culture, and thoracic ultrasound and radiography. Horses with a history of severe respiratory tract infection may retain large quantities of mucopurulent material in the trachea and have abnormal respiratory sounds in the lung fields upon careful auscultation. Horses with respiratory tract infections should not be anesthetized for elective procedures because the added stress of surgery and general anesthesia predisposes to pneumonia and pleuritis.

Horses with respiratory stridor due to upper respiratory tract obstruction require special evaluation because sedation produces relaxation of the muscles of the upper airway which may worsen the stridor. Many normal horses make upper airway noises during recovery from general anesthesia because of congestion and edema of the nares and nasal turbinates. Horses with pre-operative stridor are more likely to do so. Nasal congestion is easily relieved by passing a 12 to 18 mm endotracheal tube into the nares past the site of the obstruction. Additional causes of stridor after anesthesia include dorsal displacement of the soft palate and partial or complete laryngeal paralysis.

The soft palate normally displaces dorsally with orotracheal placement of an endotracheal tube. When the endotracheal tube is removed the palate remains displaced until the horse swallows and the palate returns to its normal position below the epiglottis. An endotracheal tube can be used to stimulate swallowing if a horse makes a noise suggestive of dorsal displacement after removal of the endotracheal tube. The degree of obstruction of airflow should be evaluated by assessing the amount of airflow through the nostrils while noting the amount of effort (abdominal movement) required to produce airflow. A temporary tracheostomy may be required prior to induction or during recovery from anesthesia in horses with severe obstruction.

Nervous and musculoskeletal systems

The nervous and musculoskeletal systems should be examined to determine if the horse can see, ambulates normally, and bears weight on all four limbs. Horses that are blind in one eye may require special handling during induction and recovery. Slight gait deficits are usually inconsequential, but significant weakness, ataxia or lameness may pose problems during induction to and recovery from anesthesia. Simply walking the horse a short distance and circling it in a small circle provides a sufficient assessment of the horse's stability. Horses that are ataxic or not bearing weight on all four limbs may prove difficult to move while sedated. Thus they should be moved to the area of anesthetic induction prior to administering sedatives. Horses with central nervous system disease may need to be positioned in a specific recumbency (right lateral or left lateral) to facilitate return to standing.

Pre-anesthetic hematologic evaluation

The baseline hematologic evaluation of horses prior to anesthesia is dependent on the results of the physical examination but should include determination of the packed cell volume (PCV), total plasma solids, white blood cell count, and plasma fibrinogen. The PCV should be 55% or less to prevent blood sludging and achieve adequate tissue perfusion under anesthesia. Packed cell volumes less than 20% are associated with compromised oxygen delivery. Plasma protein levels below 3.5 g/dL are associated with the formation of peripheral and pulmonary edema because of inadequate plasma oncotic pressure. The hemogram of most horses in our referral hospital suggests mild leukocytosis with neutrophilia and lymphopenia that can be attributed to the effects of excitement and stress associated with transportation, hospitalization or pain. Total white blood cell (WBC) counts greater than 13 000/mL or less than 5500/mL are indications for further evaluation. Elective surgical procedures should be postponed in horses with abnormal WBC counts until the WBC count returns to normal. Plasma fibrinogen levels are used as an index of inflammation but are not specific to any disease. Plasma fibrinogen levels in excess of 300–400 mg/dL are considered abnormal and a reason to delay anesthesia. Preoperative serum chemistry and acid–base evaluations are not necessary unless specifically indicated. Muscle enzyme levels should be measured in horses with a history of rhabdomyolysis.

Pre-anesthetic medications

Pre-anesthetic medications in the horse include anticholinergics, tranquilizers/sedatives, and analgesics (Table 57.1). The administration of the anticholinergic agents atropine and glycopyrrolate is not recommended for routine use prior to anesthesia in horses. Anticholinergics decrease salivation and increase heart rate, but neither excessive salivation nor bradycardia is a frequent problem in the horse. The potential disadvantages (postoperative ileus, tachycardia, and increased myocardial oxygen consumption) are significant; thus anticholinergic administration should be limited to those cases where it is specifically indicated. Common cardiac arrhythmias that respond to anticholinergic agents include atrioventricular conduction disturbances, interference dissociation, and sinus bradycardia (heart rate less than 25 beats/min) with hypotension.

Sedatives and tranquilizers are used to produce a calm, tractable patient by decreasing excitement and unwanted behavior (movement) during induction and recovery. Sedatives and tranquilizers potentiate the action of anesthetic agents, so that the dose of the more potent agent can then be lowered, decreasing the potential for deleterious side effects including hypotension and hypoventilation. Horses that are weight bearing on all four limbs may benefit from intramuscular administration of sedatives because intramuscular administration produces a more prolonged effect than intravenous administration and potentially reduces the magnitude of the deleterious changes in cardiorespiratory function. Some drugs, particularly the phenothiazine tranquilizers (acepromazine), require up to 45 minutes to reach peak effect. Intravenous administration produces a quicker onset of action and an increased intensity of effect, but a shorter duration of effect, than does intramuscular administration. Ataxic or severely lame patients that are non-weight bearing on one limb should be moved to the induction area before administering the agent of choice.

Phenothiazine tranquilizers are used to produce calming by decreasing locomotor activity, reducing apprehension and increasing tractability. Phenothiazines should be avoided in horses that are severely stressed, have had excessive hemorrhage, or are hypovolemic because the drugs may cause excessive hypotension. Clinical

Table 57.1 Drug used for standing chemical restraint and as pre-anesthetics

DRUG	DOSE AND ROUTE	ONSET OF EFFECT	COMMENTS
Acepromazine	0.02–0.06 mg/kg, i.m., i.v.	30–40 min i.v., i.m.	Caution in stressed, hypotensive animals, potential for penile paralysis
Xylazine	0.5–1.0 mg/kg, i.v. 1.0–2.2 mg/kg, i.m.	3–5 min, i.v. 10–20 min, i.m.	Ataxia produced with head-down posture Begin with low dose and repeat as needed
Detomidine	0.01–0.02 mg/kg, i.v. 0.02–0.04 mg/kg, i.m.	4–6 min, i.v. 10–20 min, i.m.	Ataxia produced with head-down posture Begin with low dose and repeat as required Duration twice as long as xylazine Effective sublingually
Romifidine	0.08–0.16 mg/kg, i.v.	5–10 min, i.v. 10–20 min, i.m.	Less ataxia and less head down than xylazine or detomidine Duration similar to detomidine
Butorphanol	0.01–0.03 mg/kg, i.v.	3–5 min	Use in combination with a sedative or tranquilizer
Morphine	0.3–0.5 mg/kg, i.v.	3–5 min	Sedative with xylazine or detomidine before administering morphine Potential for excitement

doses usually produce minimal ataxia and weakness. The primary cardiovascular effect produced by phenothiazine tranquilizers is vasodilatation with resultant hypotension. The incidence of clinically significant hypotension following clinical doses of phenothiazines to normal horses is low, and horses that become hypotensive after phenothiazine administration usually respond to intravenous crystalloid administration. The risk of persistent paralysis of the retractor penis muscle should be noted before tranquilization of male horses, and the dose should be carefully limited to the minimum necessary to produce the desired effect.

Alpha$_2$ adrenoreceptor agonists produce sedation, muscle relaxation and analgesia when administered intravenously or intramuscularly to horses.[16–19] Horses that have received alpha$_2$ agonists assume a 'head-down' or 'sawhorse' stance and may frequently shift their weight from side to side (Fig. 57.1). Arterial blood pressure is initially increased due to drug-induced increases in peripheral vascular resistance. Hypertension may be sustained (20 to 60 minutes), particularly when detomidine or romifidine is used. Decreases in heart rate, sinus arrhythmia, and first- and second-degree atrioventricular blockade are common. These decreases in heart rate result in significant decreases in cardiac output, often to levels 50% of pre-drug values. Respiratory rate is usually decreased, but tidal volume increases. Relaxation of the muscles of the upper airway can predispose the horse to stridor. The administration of an alpha$_2$ agonist decreases salivation, gastric secretions, and gastrointestinal motility and increases urine volume. Other incidental effects of alpha$_2$ agonist administration include increases in intrauterine pressure, hyperglycemia and hypoinsulinemia.

Three alpha$_2$ agonists are approved for use in horses in the USA. Xylazine, a relatively short-acting alpha$_2$ agonist, has a rapid onset (1–3 minutes) and short duration of action (30–60 minutes) after i.v. administration. Xylazine is relatively non-specific, activating both alpha$_2$ and alpha$_1$ receptors. Detomidine, a more specific alpha$_2$ agonist, is approximately 100 times more potent than xylazine and has a duration of action at least twice as long. Romifidine is even more specific for alpha$_2$ receptors than detomidine and has a similar or longer duration of action depending on the dose. The degree of muscle relaxation and ataxia for a given level of sedation may be less with romifidine compared to xylazine or detomidine.

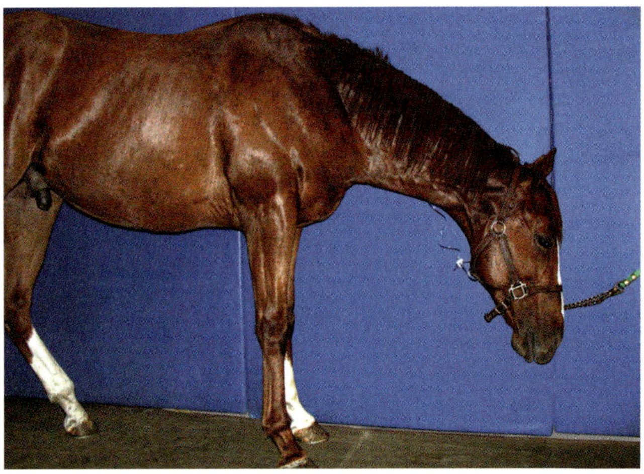

Fig 57.1 The posture of a horse after the administration of 1.0 mg/kg of xylazine intravenously. Note the ventral position of the head and neck, the relaxed facial muscles, and the unequal distribution of weight on the rear legs.

Sedative–opioid combinations are useful for standing procedures in the horse, producing sedation, analgesia, euphoria and a stuporous 'sawhorse' stance. Butorphanol and morphine are two drugs with opioid activity that have been used in combination with alpha$_2$ agonists to produce standing chemical restraint.[20,21] Opioids other than butorphanol are not routinely administered prior to anesthesia but can be used to supplement analgesia intraoperatively.

Many surgical procedures benefit from the administration of antibiotics pre-operatively. Antibiotics, particularly sodium or potassium penicillin, should be administered before anesthesia is induced because of their potential to cause hypotension during anesthesia.[22] Aminoglycoside antibiotics, including gentamicin, can cause neuromuscular weakness in some species, but this side effect is uncommon in horses. If antibiotics must be administered intraoperatively, cephalosporins, such as cefazolin, have been shown to produce minimal cardiovascular depression.[22]

Timing of anesthesia and animal preparation

Horses that are transported to the site of anesthesia should be given time to acclimate to the environment. Horses that are injured should be administered first aid, including splinting of the injury, to stabilize their condition. Superior anesthetic and surgical planning is possible if induction is not rushed. The author withholds food for 4 to 6 hours before anesthesia if possible in an attempt to reduce the amount of feed material in the upper gastrointestinal tract. The mouth should be rinsed prior to induction because foreign material left in the mouth could be pushed into the trachea during orotracheal intubation, leading to upper airway obstruction during or following anesthesia. A large-bore intravenous catheter should be placed in either jugular vein prior to induction of anesthesia. Pre-existing fluid deficits should be corrected prior to anesthesia. During anesthesia, 5–10 mL/kg/hour of balanced electrolyte solutions should be administered to promote perfusion, replace the lack of fluid intake, and replace insensible losses.

Induction of anesthesia

The smooth, safe and uneventful induction of anesthesia is dependent upon trained personnel, proper pre-medication of the animal, proper and timely administration of induction agents, appropriate equipment and facilities, and an atmosphere free of unnecessary stimuli that may excite the patient. Indoors, horses should be restrained against a solid wall with their hindquarters in a corner, if possible (Fig. 57.2). One assistant should be positioned at the horse's shoulder and another at the horse's hip. The anesthetist should administer the induction agent and hold the horse's head in a neutral posture until recumbency occurs. Some facilities utilize a 1.5 by 2.0 meter door securely mounted on a wall to facilitate restraint for induction (Fig. 57.3). Horses that must be anesthetized in the open benefit from having a head and tail rope applied before induction. As the horse begins to fall, it can be pulled to the appropriate side. Alternatively, the horse can be made to walk in small circles after the induction drugs are given. The horse will tend to fall toward the outside of the circle as the drugs take effect. The person holding the head should protect the head from sharp blows during the induction period and maintain control at all times.

Many drugs and drug combinations have been used to induce general anesthesia in horses (Table 57.2).[23] Most intravenous anesthetic techniques involve the combined use of dissociative anesthetics (ketamine, tiletamine–zolazepam) or thiobarbiturates

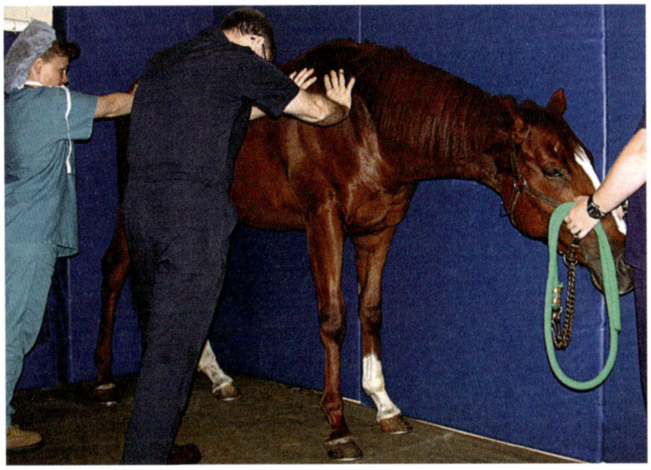

Fig 57.2 Correct placement of a horse for induction of anesthesia. The horse is positioned against a wall with its hindquarters in a corner. One attendant pushes on the point of the hip and another on the point of the shoulder. The attendant holding the head lifts the head as the anesthetic drugs take effect.

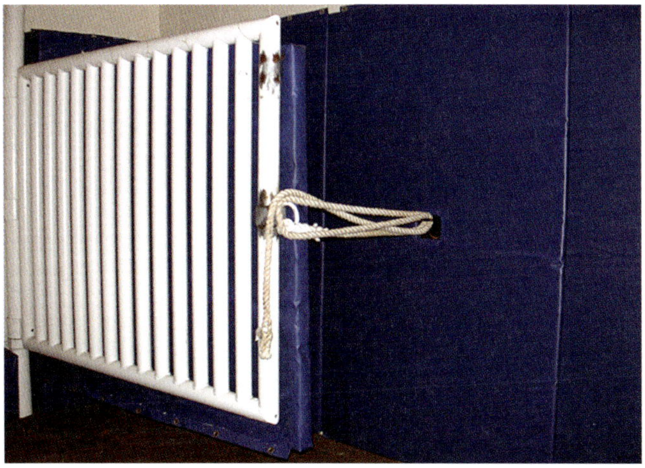

Fig 57.3 A padded door, firmly attached to a wall, can be used to control a horse's movement as anesthetic induction occurs.

Table 57.2 Drugs used for induction and maintenance of anesthesia in sedate horses

DRUG OR DRUG COMBINATION	DOSE	COMMENTS
Ketamine	1.5–2.0 mg/kg, i.v.	Horses must be maximally relaxed prior to administration. Relaxation can be produced with xylazine, diazepam or midazolam, or guaifenesin
Thiopental	4–6 mg/kg, i.v. with guaifenesin	Potential for apnea, particularly with increased doses
Guaifenesin	50–100 mg/kg, i.v. to effect	Primarily a muscle relaxant. Do not use alone. Use in sedate horses in combination with ketamine or thiopental
Diazepam or midazolam	0.06–0.1 mg/kg, i.v.	Primarily muscle relaxants. Use in sedate horses in combination with ketamine. Anticonvulsant
Tiletamine/zolazepam	0.7–1.0 mg/kg, i.v.	Horses should be fully sedated before administration. Produces 30 minutes of anesthesia with good muscle relaxation. Hypoventilation may occur
Tiletamine/zolazepam–ketamine–detomidine	Add detomidine (10 mg/mL, 1 mL) and ketamine (100 mg/mL, 4 mL) to 500 mg of tiletamine/zolazepam powder. Administer 1 mL/ 150 kg, i.v.	Administer to sedate horses. Small volume of drug required. Produces 30 to 40 minutes of anesthesia with good muscle relaxation. Hypoventilation may occur
'Triple Drip' mixture of guaifenesin (5%), ketamine (0.1%) and xylazine (0.05%)	2 mL/kg/h, i.v.	Not used for induction in adult horses. Used to extend xylazine–ketamine. Monitor ventilation and the degree of muscle relaxation

(thiopental) and muscle relaxants (guaifenesin, diazepam, midazolam). Horses that are non-weight bearing on one limb benefit from rapid induction techniques in order to minimize the period of ataxia that occurs as the drugs take effect. The administration of any drug or drug combination regimen designed to produce recumbency should always be preceded by the administration of sufficient doses of sedatives and/or tranquilizers to produce a calm, manageable patient.

Intravenous xylazine followed by intravenous ketamine produces 10 to 15 minutes of general anesthesia.[24] Xylazine–ketamine anesthesia produces recumbency with maintenance of reasonable cardiovascular function and acceptable respiratory depression. Recovery from anesthesia is relatively rapid and uneventful, with the horse rising to its feet 25 to 30 minutes after induction. Characteristically, an apneustic or breath-holding respiratory pattern occurs. The xylazine–ketamine technique has been modified in order to improve the quality of anesthesia. The addition of diazepam or midazolam and/or butorphanol to xylazine–ketamine improves muscle relaxation and analgesia with minimal cardiorespiratory depression and increases the duration of anesthesia to 20–25 minutes.[25,26] Alternatively, the proprietary combination of tiletamine and zolazepam can be administered after xylazine to produce intravenous anesthesia or to induce anesthesia prior to inhalant anesthesia.[27] Tiletamine–zolazepam is usually administered after sedation with an alpha$_2$ agonist and produces a longer duration of anesthesia than diazepam–ketamine. Thirty minutes of anesthesia is produced with the horse returning to standing posture within 60 to 75 minutes. The recovery from anesthesia after tiletamine-zolazepam anesthesia is not as controlled as recoveries from xylazine–ketamine anesthesia because of residual weakness, presumably produced by the zolazepam.

Horses that bear weight on all four limbs may benefit from the gradual administration of guaifenesin and guaifenesin drug combinations. Guaifenesin can be rapidly administered in 5% or 10% concentrations until the horse begins to show signs of muscle weakness and ataxia (weaving side to side, knees buckling). When sufficient muscle relaxation is present, ketamine or thiopental is administered to produce recumbency.[26] Guaifenesin combinations can also be used to extend the anesthetic period if inhalant administration is not possible or impractical.[28,29] Guaifenesin (5%) solution can be combined with xylazine (0.5 mg/mL) and ketamine (1–2 mg/mL) to produce a solution that is called 'Triple Drip'. The combination is administered to effect up to a rate of 2 mL/kg of bodyweight/hour, producing total intravenous anesthesia (TIVA) with excellent muscle relaxation and suitable analgesia. The quality of recovery is generally good if the anesthetic period is kept to less than one hour. 'Triple Drip' should not be used to produce anesthesia for greater than 90 minutes unless oxygen supplementation and respiratory support are provided. Midazolam has been investigated as a replacement for guaifenesin in 'Triple Drip' with seemingly equal efficacy.[30]

An endotracheal tube should be placed if the administration of inhalant anesthesia is anticipated or if oxygen supplementation is desired. Twenty to 30 mm (internal diameter) endotracheal tubes should be used in adult horses. A piece of plumber's pipe (5.0 cm in diameter) covered with non-slip tape is a useful bite block (Fig. 57.4). The tube is passed blindly while extending the head dorsally. Successful placement is confirmed by the minimal resistance to advancement when the tube is in the trachea and the passage of air with respiration.

Padding and positioning

Horses anesthetized and positioned on their side (lateral) or back (dorsal) recumbency are prone to myositis or neurogenic paralysis because of their great weight. Practical steps toward preventing these complications include the maintenance of adequate arterial blood pressure (mean arterial blood pressure greater than 60 mmHg), assuring proper ventilation and oxygenation, minimizing anesthetic duration, and padding and positioning the patient properly. All weight-bearing surfaces of the horse should be padded when the horse is recumbent, with particular attention paid to bony prominences (Fig. 57.5). A 2 m by 3 m foam rubber pad 20 cm thick works well for horses anesthetized and placed in lateral recumbency. Additional pads should be placed between the rear legs to support the upper leg.

Maintenance of anesthesia

Isoflurane and sevoflurane are the primary inhalant anesthetics used in the horse. Both drugs can safely be used to anesthetize horses, and the choice is left to personal preference and economic considerations.[31,32] Isoflurane and sevoflurane produce rapid induction and recovery from anesthesia.[33] Cardiac output is depressed with both drugs as are arterial blood pressures. Respiratory depression is significant with isoflurane and sevoflurane, with most anesthetized horses benefiting if controlled ventilation is employed. Horses anesthetized with isoflurane or sevoflurane usually benefit from the administration of a small dose of xylazine (0.1–0.2 mg/kg, i.v.) or detomidine (0.00–0.006 mg/kg, i.v.) during recovery from anesthesia.[34] Sedation allows additional time for exhalation of the inhalant agents, producing a more coordinated return to standing.

Monitoring anesthesia

Careful attention is paid to the cardiovascular system, the respiratory system, and ocular reflexes. Evaluations of these systems should be regularly recorded (every 5 minutes). As inhalant anesthesia deepens to surgical planes, the eye rotates medially; the eyelids

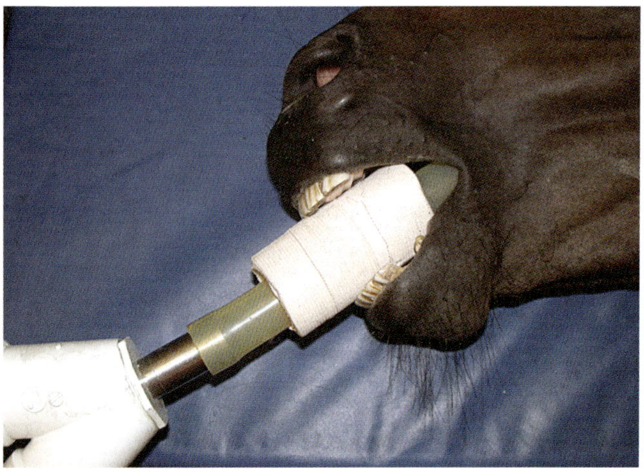

Fig 57.4 A 10 cm section of plumber's pipe is a useful speculum for endotracheal tube placement. The plastic pipe is covered with adhesive material to reduce slippage.

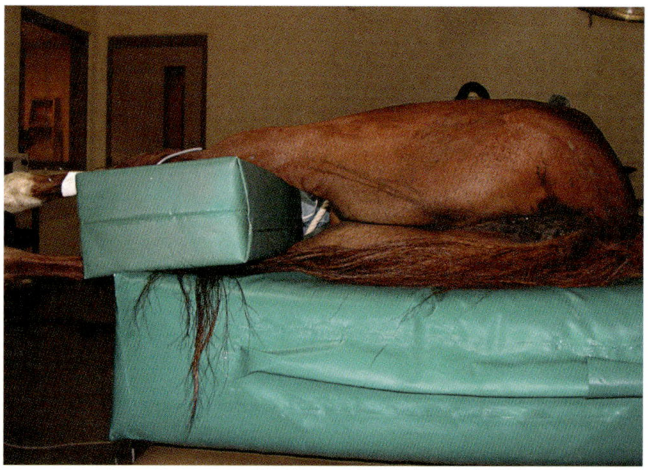

Fig 57.5 An appropriately padded anesthetized horse in right lateral recumbency. The weight of the left leg is supported by a pad placed between the hocks to reduce compression of the vessels of the right leg.

cease voluntary closure, and tear production decreases. Lateral nystagmus may continue until surgical anesthesia is reached. The palpebral reflex (eyelid closure following brushing of the lids) should decrease as anesthesia deepens, and is generally weak but present during surgical anesthesia. Corneal reflexes (closure of the eyelids in response to pressure on the cornea) should be present at all times during anesthesia. The anal reflex can be used to evaluate the depth of anesthesia if the head is covered; its absence indicates that the animal is too deeply anesthetized.

The heart rate in anesthetized horses normally ranges between 25 and 50 beats/min and does not usually change as the plane of anesthesia deepens or lightens. Anticholinergics should be given to increase rates when less than 25 beats/min. Heart rates in excess of 50 may indicate inadequate planes of anesthesia, hypotension, hypercarbia or hypoxemia. Directly measuring arterial blood pressure and recording the electrocardiogram accomplish more definitive monitoring of the cardiovascular system. The facial, transverse facial and dorsal metatarsal arteries are all easily palpated and catheterized (Fig. 57.6). Mean arterial blood pressure should range between 60 and 90 mmHg during anesthesia. A mean arterial blood pressure less than 60 mmHg is associated with post-anesthetic rhabdomyolysis and the loss of autoregulation of blood flow to vascular beds.[35] Mean arterial blood pressures greater than 90 mmHg are a sign of light anesthetic planes, and movement should be anticipated.

Hypotension is treated by decreasing the delivery of anesthetics (if possible), administering intravenous fluids, and administering vasoactive drugs. If the anesthetic plane is appropriate, the rate of fluid administration should be increased. The choice of fluid is determined by the horse's physical condition, acid–base, and electrolyte status. Hypotension that does not respond to fluid therapy is treated with vasoactive agents such as dobutamine or ephedrine. Dobutamine (1–5 μg/kg/min) is given by infusion and titrated to maintain the desired arterial blood pressure.[36] Signs of dobutamine overdose include tachycardia, hypertension, and supraventricular and ventricular premature arrhythmias. The infusion should be reduced or discontinued if signs of toxicity occur. Ephedrine administration increases arterial blood pressure and cardiac output.[37] Ephedrine (0.05–0.1 mg/kg) is given as an intravenous bolus and produces effects that persist for 20 to 30 minutes or longer. The administration of calcium solutions may produce increases in arterial blood pressure, particularly if ionized calcium levels are marginal or decreased. Alternatively, or in addition, co-infusions of lidocaine, ketamine, or alpha$_2$ agonists can be incorporated to permit a reduction in the requirement for the inhalant anesthetic, potentially supporting arterial blood pressure.[38,39]

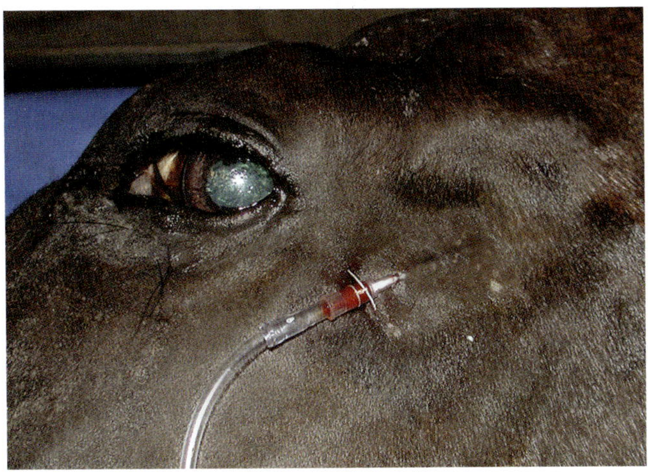

Fig 57.6 A 20-gauge over the-needle catheter placed in the transverse facial artery.

Respiration and oxygenation should be monitored by measuring ventilatory rate and measuring arterial blood gases and pH. Horses that are kept anesthetized for longer than 60 minutes can be expected to hypoventilate. If anesthetic durations of 60 minutes or greater are anticipated, intermittent positive pressure ventilation should be instituted, if possible, as soon as adequate arterial blood pressures are assured. Measurement of the end-tidal concentration of carbon dioxide in the expired airway gas can be used as an indirect assessment of arterial carbon dioxide tension, but the only consistent measurement of adequate ventilation and oxygenation is the measurement of arterial blood gases.[40] If spontaneous ventilation is inadequate, controlled ventilation should be instituted. Initial tidal volumes should be set at 12 to 18 mL/kg. Peak inspiratory pressure should be 20 to 30 cmH$_2$O. Respiratory rates should range from 5 to 8 breaths/min.

Horses that are being ventilated correctly ($PaCO_2$ of 40–50 mmHg) occasionally become relatively hypoxemic (PaO_2 less than 100 mmHg) during anesthesia. The cause of the hypoxemia is primarily attributed to mismatches of ventilation and perfusion that occur when horses are placed in lateral or dorsal recumbency.[41] Increasing cardiac output by the administration of fluids and drugs promoting cardiac contractility may help to prevent or reduce arterial hypoxemia. Positive end-expiratory pressure can be used to increase arterial oxygenation but this occurs at the expense of cardiac output because of limited venous return.[42] Intratracheal-tracheal albuterol can be used during anesthesia to increase oxygenation but the effect is inconsistent.[43]

The postoperative period

Recovery is the most difficult phase of equine anesthesia to control.[33,44] Optimally, horses should lie quietly for 20 to 35 minutes, roll to sternal recumbency and regain the standing position in one attempt. Horses attempting to rise too soon should be sedated with small doses of xylazine (0.2–0.4 mg/kg, i.v.) or detomidine (0.004–0.006 mg/kg, i.v.). If the horse has not attempted to rise one hour after the end of anesthesia, a handler should enter the recovery stall and stimulate the horse.

The most important feature of any area for recovery of anesthesia is a non-slip flooring surface. Horses exert considerable force as they rise and it is imperative that their feet do not slip as they place them to stand. There are a number of commercial surfaces available. The most consistent surfaces are wrestling or tumbling mats (Fig. 57.7). Three meter by four meter pads, 3 to 4 cm thick, work well. The mats compress as the horse rises, providing secure footing whether wet or dry. The recovery area should be quiet and have lights that can be dimmed. The walls should be padded with secure rings placed 2–3 meters from the floor to facilitate the use of ropes for assisting recovery. Ideally, a ceiling hook should be present for a hoist and sling. Two handlers should remain in the immediate area until the horse is standing. The horse can be helped to its feet by placing a head rope and tail rope (assisted recovery) and running the ropes through rings on opposite sides of the recovery stall (Fig. 57.8). The head and tail ropes are tightened for support as the horse rises to its feet, helping it to balance. More experienced handlers may prefer to remain in the recovery stall with the horse and simply grasp its halter or tail to steady it as it rises. If recovery is to occur out of doors, turf provides excellent footing for recovery and some padding should the horse fall.

Some horses become hypoxemic when they are disconnected from the anesthetic machine for recovery because of the sudden decrease in inspired oxygen concentration. Oxygen can be insufflated during the recovery period with a nasal oxygen catheter or demand valve.[45] For insufflation, oxygen flow rates should be set at a minimum of 15 L/min to effect a demonstrable change in arterial oxygen tension. More efficient methods of delivering oxygen can be achieved by using a demand valve, which supplies oxygen at high flow rates during the inspiratory phase of respiration (Fig. 57.9). Extubation is performed when the horse begins to swallow and attempts to chew. Prolonged anesthesia in dorsal recumbency can lead to congestion of the nasal folds and mucosa of the turbinates. Upper airway obstruction due to edematous nasal folds or turbinates can be relieved by manually holding the nasal cartilages open or by nasotracheal intubation if the obstruction is severe (Fig. 57.10). Rarely, laryngospasm or laryngeal paralysis occurs after the endotracheal tube is removed.

Horses that fail to rise within 90 minutes after the end of anesthesia should be evaluated for possible weakness, rhabdomyolysis or neuropathy. Postoperative weakness can result from lingering drug effects, hypotension, or electrolyte abnormalities (hypokalemia or hypocalcemia). Horses that attempt to stand but are non-weight bearing on one or more limbs should be evaluated for orthopedic injuries, rhabdomyolysis or neuropathy. Distinguishing rhabdomyolysis from neuropathy may be difficult in the horse recovering from anesthesia. Rhabdomyolysis most often affects the gluteal and the quadriceps muscles, whereas neuropathy affects the peroneal nerve supplying the extensors of the rear leg. Large quantities of myoglobin in the urine and the presence of swollen, hardened, affected muscles help differentiate rhabdomyolysis from

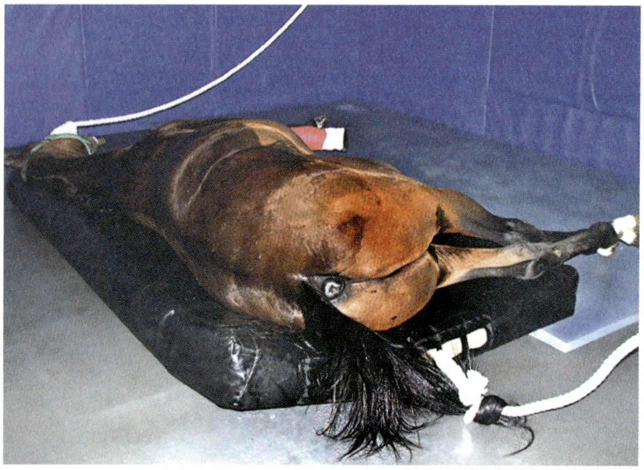

Fig 57.7 A horse resting on a 15 cm thick foam rubber pad in a recovery stall. A wrestling or tumbling mat is placed to provide good footing when the horse attempts to rise. Cotton ropes run from the halter and the tail to rings affixed to the walls of the recovery stall.

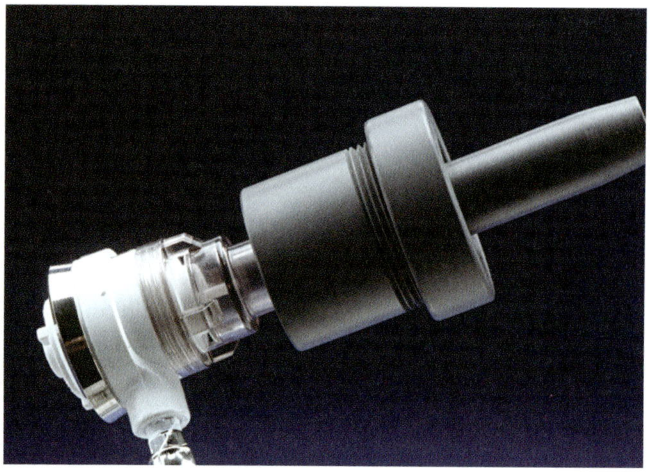

Fig 57.9 A demand valve is used to ventilate horses in recovery. Depression of the button on the end of the valve causes oxygen to flow. The button is depressed until a normal chest wall excursion is produced. The button is released and exhalation occurs.

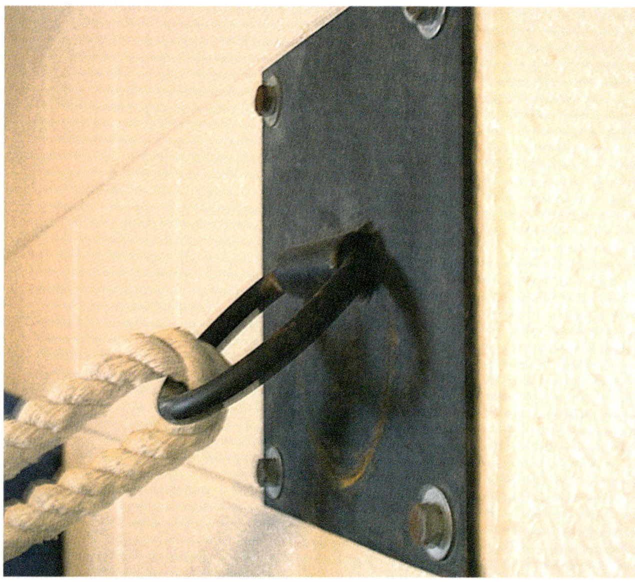

Fig 57.8 A cotton rope running through a ring affixed to a concrete block wall with expansion bolts. The rope is used to assist and control recovery from anesthesia.

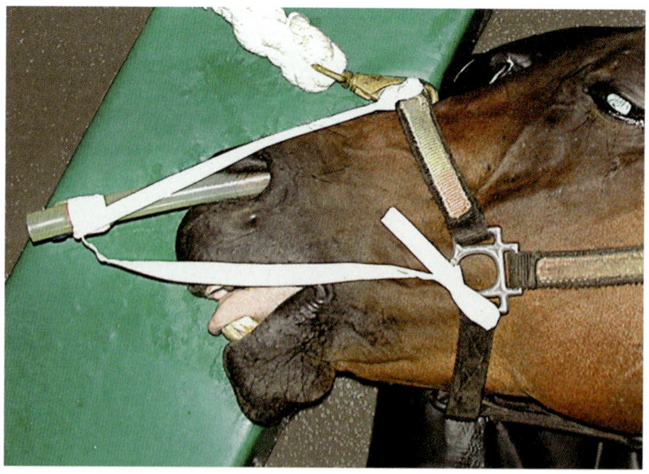

Fig 57.10 A 14 mm endotracheal tube placed in the ventral nasal meatus to facilitate respiration in the horse recovering from anesthesia. The tube is tied to the halter to ensure it can be retrieved after the horse stands.

neuropathy. Other conditions encountered in recovery include femoral and radial nerve palsy and paralysis. The incidence of these conditions is greatly reduced if appropriate padding and positioning are used. Horses that can stand on three legs have a good prognosis for recovery from rhabdomyolysis or neuropathy and generally respond to treatment within 72 hours. Horses that are bilaterally affected and unable to stand have a poorer prognosis.

Emergency sedation and anesthesia of the exhausted horse

Veterinarians and other personnel providing emergency care to horses injured while exercising are often faced with patients that are exhausted, excited, painful, and physically challenged (they may be recumbent or non-weight bearing on one or more limbs). This presentation, coupled with an animal whose evolutionary response to danger is flight, creates the potential for complicated patient management.

Horses that are injured when exercising may be unable to undergo the active 'cool-down' period that is usually incorporated into exercise regimens. This interruption delays the return of hemodynamics and acid–base values to pre-exercise levels.[46] Cardiac output remains increased when horses walk after exercise, leading to more rapid reductions in venous blood lactate concentrations and increases in serum bicarbonate concentration (Fig. 57.11). Most indices return to pre-exercise levels within 60 to 90 minutes whether the horses walk or stand stationary, but increases in rectal temperature persist.

Horses that are injured and cannot ambulate should have an intravenous catheter placed as soon as is practically possible. The early placement of a catheter allows replacement of lost fluids (perspiration, hemorrhage) and facilitates the delivery of sedatives, analgesics and anesthetic agents, if necessary. Injured horses, if agitated, may refuse to drink, thus delaying complete recuperation. The potential for the development of shock is common to most such situations. Volume replacement with balanced electrolyte solutions is of benefit regardless of the need for chemical restraint. Other supportive care may include non-steroidal anti-inflammatory drugs, antibiotics and oxygen administration.

The need to provide sedation and analgesia must be carefully assessed. First aid should include immobilization of the injury if possible and cessation of hemorrhage if present. Sedatives and tranquilizers can be safely administered to exhausted horses if indicated.[47] The doses required to produce full effects are approximately twice those needed in horses at rest, but unless the animal is completely uncontrollable, smaller doses should be given and repeated to effect.[48] Xylazine (2.2 mg/kg, i.v.) alone and in combination with acepromazine (0.04 mg/kg) administered to horses immediately after exercise produces heavy sedation with pronounced muscle relaxation sufficient for subsequent induction of anesthesia. Alternatively, detomidine (0.04 mg/kg, i.v.) can be used. The cardiorespiratory depression produced by the administration of these doses was qualitatively similar to that seen when standard doses are administered to horses at rest but does prolong recuperation and exercise-induced increases in body temperature (Fig. 57.12). If less pronounced sedation is desired, standard doses of detomidine (0.01–0.02 mg/kg, i.v.), xylazine (1 mg/kg, i.v.), or a combination of acepromazine (0.02 mg/kg, i.v.) and xylazine (1 mg/kg, i.v.) can be given and the response assessed in 2–5 minutes. The need for additional incremental doses is likely. The drugs should be repeated at a rate of one-half the standard dose to effect.

Calming and sedation should be produced before opioids or other analgesic agents are administered. Opioids (morphine, butorphanol, hydromorphone) carry the potential of producing excitement. This effect is most often seen in pain-free animals, but prior administration of a sedative or tranquilizer reduces its likelihood. Butorphanol (0.01–0.02 mg/kg) augments sedation and provides

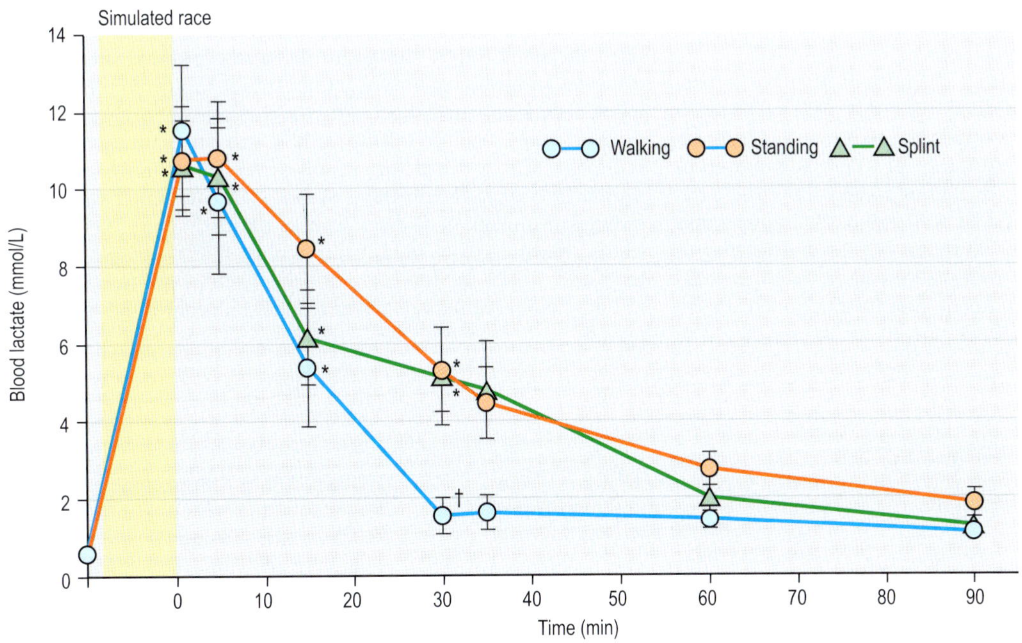

Fig 57.11 Blood lactate concentrations in horses recuperating from maximal exercise. The data represent mean ± standard error of the mean for six horses. *Indicates significant ($P < 0.05$) differences from baseline values within a trial. †Indicates significant ($P < 0.05$) differences from other groups at a given time.

Hubbell JAE, Hinchcliff KW, Muir WW, et al. Cardiorespiratory and metabolic effects of walking, standing, and standing with a splint during the recuperative period from maximal exercise in horses. Am J Vet Res 1997; 58:1007, with permission from the American Journal of Veterinary Research, http://avmajournals.avma.org/loi/ajvr.

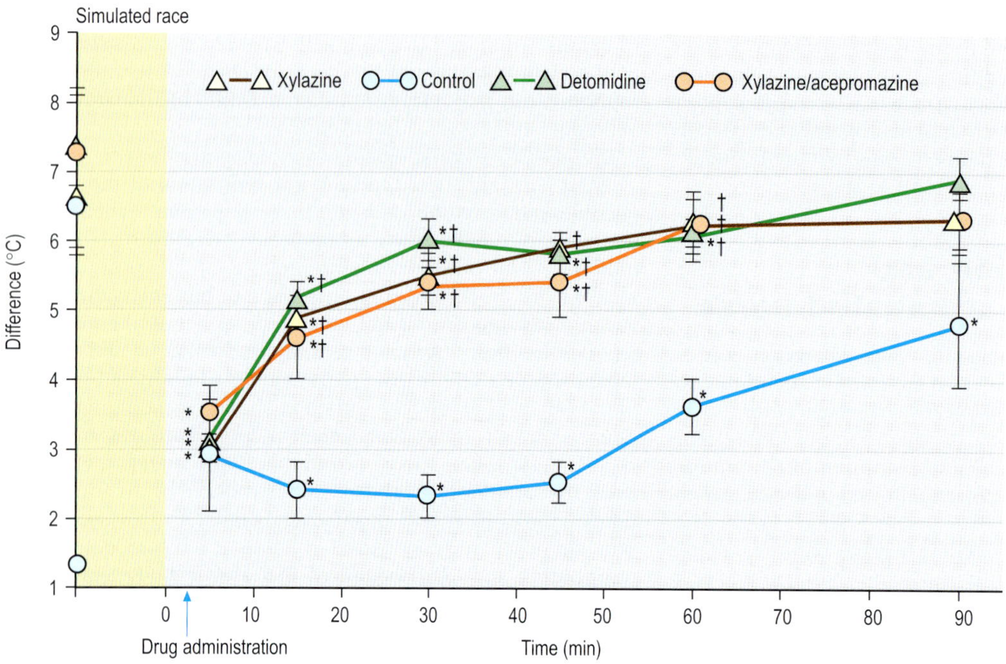

Fig 57.12 Mean blood temperature versus skin temperature difference for horses given various sedatives or saline solution immediately after maximal exercise on a treadmill. Error bars represent standard error. *Indicates significant ($P < 0.05$) differences from baseline value for that treatment. †Indicates significant ($P < 0.05$) differences from control values (i.e. the value obtained when horses were given saline solution). *Hubbell JAE, Hinchcliff KW, Schmall LM, et al. Cardiorespiratory and metabolic effects of xylazine, detomidine, and a combination of xylazine and acepromazine administered after exercise in horses. Am J Vet Res 1999; 60:1276, with permission from the American Journal of Veterinary Research, http://avmajournals.avma.org/loi/ajvr.*

analgesia of short duration. Morphine (0.05–0.1 mg/kg) can provide more profound analgesia. With larger doses, horses may head-press and try to move forward. Horses receiving morphine should be carefully monitored for 6 to 8 hours after administration because of the potential for hyperactivity due to residual opioid concentrations. Hyperactivity can be controlled with the administration of small doses of sedatives.

Anesthesia can be safely induced if sufficient sedation is produced.[49] Anesthesia is rarely indicated but can be utilized to facilitate removal of the horse from a public or precarious situation, to prevent further exacerbation of an injury, or to provide an opportunity for further diagnostic tests including radiography. The combinations of diazepam–ketamine or zolazepam–tiletamine cause anesthesia of 20 to 30 minutes' duration when administered to sedate horses. Alternatively, a combination of detomidine, ketamine, and zolazepam–tiletamine can be administered in a relatively small volume to produce anesthesia for 30 to 40 minutes. The proprietary combination of zolazepam-tiletamine (500 mg) can be reconstituted with 1 mL of detomidine (10 mg/mL) and 4 mL of ketamine (100 mg/mL) with the resultant solution administered to sedate horses at a rate of 1 mL/ 150 kg of body weight.[50] The cardiorespiratory effects of these combinations in exhausted horses are qualitatively similar to those seen when horses at rest are administered the same drugs. The return of exercise-induced increases or decreases in cardiorespiratory and metabolic indices to pre-exercise levels is delayed when short-term anesthesia is performed. Intravenous anesthesia can be safely extended with inhalant agents when indicated.[51] Larger ventilatory volumes may be required to maintain normal arterial partial pressures of carbon dioxide. Exercise-induced changes in metabolic indices such as pH and serum bicarbonate can be returned to normal if intravenous fluids are administered and 'light' anesthetic levels are utilized. Exercise-induced increases in body temperature may persist for the duration of the anesthetic period.

References

1. Short CE, Matthews NS, Tyner CL, et al. Special anesthetic considerations in the racing thoroughbred. Proc 2nd Int Cong Vet Anes 1985;137.
2. Hall LW. General anesthesia, fundamental considerations. Vet Clin North Am Equine Pract 1981;1:3–15.
3. Art T, Lekeux P. Training-induced modifications in cardiorespiratory and ventilatory measurements in Thoroughbred horses. Equine Vet J 1993;25:532–6.
4. Koterba AM, Kosch PC, Beech J, et al. Breathing strategy of the adult horse (*Equus caballus*) at rest. J Appl Physiol 1988;64:337–46.
5. Foreman JH, Bayly WM, Grant BD, et al. Standardized exercise test and daily heart rate responses of Thoroughbreds undergoing convention race training and detraining. Am J Vet Res 1990;51:914–20.
6. Snow DH, Mackenzie G. Some metabolic effects of maximal exercise in the horse and adaptations with training. Equine Vet J 1977;9:134–40.
7. McKeever KH, Schurg WA, Jarrett SH, et al. Exercise-training induced hypervolemia in the horse. Med Sci Sports Exerc 1987;19:21.
8. Kriz NG, Hodgson D, Rose R. Changes in cardiac dimensions and indices of cardiac function during deconditioning in horses. Am J Vet Res 2000;61:1553–60.
9. Snow DH, Valberg SJ. Muscle anatomy, physiology, and adaptations to exercise

and training. In: Hodgson D, Rose R, editors. The athletic horse: principles and practice of equine sports medicine. Philadelphia: WB Saunders; 1994. p. 145–79.

10. Lavoie JP, Pascoe JR, Kurpershoek CJ. Effects of xylazine on ventilation in horses. Am J Vet Res 1992;53:916–20.
11. Lavoie JP, Pascoe JR, Kurpershoek CJ. Effect of head and neck position on respiratory mechanics in horses sedated with xylazine. Am J Vet Res 1992;53:1652–7.
12. Lindegaard C, Husted L, Ullum H, et al. Sedation with detomidine and acepromazine influences the endoscopic evaluation of laryngeal function in horses. Equine Vet J 2007;39:553–6.
13. MacLeay JM, Sorum SA, Valberg SJ, et al. Epidemiological analysis of factors influencing exertional rhabdomyolysis in Thoroughbreds. Am J Vet Res 1999;60:1562–6.
14. Bonagura JD. Clinical evaluation and management of heart disease. Equine Vet Educ 1990;2:31–7.
15. Kriz NG, Hodgson DR, Rose RJ. Prevalence and clinical importance of heart murmurs in racehorses. J Am Vet Med Assoc 2000;216:1441–5.
16. Hoffman PE. Clinical evaluation of xylazine as a chemical restraining agent, sedative, and analgesic in horses. J Am Vet Med Assoc 1974;164:42–5.
17. Muir WW, Skarda RT, Sheehan W. Hemodynamic and respiratory effects of a xylazine–acepromazine drug combination in horses. Am J Vet Res 1979;40:1518–22.
18. Wagner AE, Muir WW, Hinchcliff KW. Cardiovascular effects of xylazine and detomidine in horses. Am J Vet Res 1991;52:651–7.
19. Freeman SL, Bowen IM, Bettshcart-Wolfensberger R, et al. Cardiovascular effects of romifidine in the standing horse. Res Vet Sci 2002;72:123–9.
20. Robertson JT, Muir WW. A new analgesic drug combination in the horse. Am J Vet Res 1983;44:1667–9.
21. Dyson DH, Pascoe PJ, Viel L, et al. Comparison of detomidine hydrochloride, xylazine, and xylazine plus morphine in horses: a double blind study. Equine Vet Sci 1987;7:211–15.
22. Hubbell JAE, Muir WW, Robertson JT, et al. Cardiovascular effects of intravenous sodium penicillin, sodium cefazolin, and sodium citrate in awake and anesthetized horses. Vet Surg 1987;16:245–50.
23. Matthews NS, Hartspeld SM, Cornick JL, et al. A comparison of injectable anesthetic regimens in horses. Vet Surg 1991;20:268–73.
24. Muir WW, Skarda RT, Milne DW. Evaluation of xylazine and ketamine hydrochloride for anesthesia in horses. Am J Vet Res 1977;38:195–201.
25. Butera TS, Moore JN, Garner HE, et al. Diazepam-xylazine-ketamine combination for short-term anesthesia in the horse. Vet Med Small Anim Clin 1978;73:490–9.
26. Brock N, Hildebrand SV. A comparison of xylazine-diazepam-ketamine and xylazine-guaifenesin-ketamine in equine anesthesia. Vet Surg 1990;19:468–74.
27. Hubbell JAE, Bednarski RM, Muir WW. Xylazine and tiletamine-zolazepam anesthesia in horses. Am J Vet Res 1989;50:737–46.
28. Greene SA, Thurmon JC, Tranquilli WJ, et al. Cardiopulmonary effects of continuous intravenous infusion of guaifenesin, ketamine, and xylazine in ponies. Am J Vet Res 1986;47:2364–7.
29. McCarty JE, Trim CM, Ferguson D. Prolongation of anesthesia with xylazine, ketamine, and guaifenesin in horses: 64 cases (1986–1989). J Am Vet Med Assoc 1990;197:1646–50.
30. Hubbell JAE, Aarnes TK, Bednarski RM, et al. Midazolam-ketamine-xylazine infusion for maintenance of total intravenous anesthesia in horses. Proc Am Assoc Equine Pract 2011;57:477.
31. Grosenbaugh DA, Muir WW. Cardiorespiratory effects of sevoflurane, isoflurane, and halothane anesthesia in horses. Am J Vet Res 1998;59:101–6.
32. Steffey EP, Howland D. Comparison of circulatory and respiratory effects of isoflurane and halothane anesthesia in horses. Am J Vet Res 1980;41:821–5.
33. Whitehair KJ, Steffey EP, Willits NH, et al. Recovery of horses from inhalation anesthesia. Am J Vet Res 1993;54:1693–702.
34. Matthews NS, Hartspeld SM, Mercer D, et al. Recovery from sevoflurane anesthesia in horses: comparison to isoflurane and effect of postmedication with xylazine. Vet Surg 1998;27:480–5.
35. Grandy JL, Steffey EP, Hodgson DS, et al. Arterial hypotension and the development of postanesthetic myopathy in halothane-anesthetized horses. Am J Vet Res 1987;48:192–7.
36. Swanson CR, Muir WW, Bednarski RM, et al. Hemodynamic responses in halothane-anesthetized horses given infusions of dopamine or dobutamine. Am J Vet Res 1985;46:365–70.
37. Grandy JL, Hodgson DS, Dunlop CI, et al. Cardiopulmonary effects of ephedrine in halothane-anesthetized horses. J Vet Pharmacol Ther 1989;12:389–96.
38. Schauvliege S, Marcilla MG, Verryken K, et al. Effects of a constant rate infusion of detomidine on cardiovascular function, isoflurane requirements and recovery quality in horses. Vet Anaes Analg 2011;38:544–54.
39. Villalba M, Santiago I, Gomez de Segura IA. Effects of constant rate infusion of lidocaine and ketamine, with or without morphine, on isoflurane MAC in horses. Equine Vet J 2011;43:721–6.
40. Cribb PH. Capnographic monitoring during anesthesia with controlled ventilation in the horse. Vet Surg 1988;17:48–52.
41. Nyman G, Hedenstierna G. Ventilation-perfusion relationships in the anaesthetized horse. Equine Vet J 1989;21:274–81.
42. Wilson DV, Soma LR. Cardiopulmonary effects of positive end-expiratory pressure in anesthetized, mechanically ventilated ponies. Am J Vet Res 1990;51:734–9.
43. Robertson SA, Bailey JE. Aerosolized salbutamol (albuterol) improves PaO_2 in hypoxaemic anaesthetized horses – a prospective clinical trial in 81 horses. Vet Anaes Analg 2002;29:212–18.
44. Hubbell JAE. Recovery from anaesthesia in horses. Equine Vet Educ 1999;11:160–7.
45. Mason DE, Muir WW, Wade A. Arterial blood gas tensions in the horse during recovery from anesthesia. J Am Vet Med Assoc 1987;190:989–94.
46. Hubbell JAE, Hinchcliff KW, Muir WW, et al. Cardiorespiratory and metabolic effects of walking, standing, and standing with a splint during the recuperative period from maximal exercise in horses. Am J Vet Res 1997;58:1003–9.
47. Hubbell JAE, Hinchcliff KW, Schmall LM, et al. Cardiorespiratory and metabolic effects of xylazine, detomidine, and a combination of xylazine and acepromazine administered after exercise in horses. Am J Vet Res 1999;60:1271–9.
48. Hubbell JAE, Hinchcliff KW, Schmall LM. Sedative administration to horses immediately after maximal exercise: determination of drug and dose. Proc Am Assoc Equine Pract 1997;43:279–84.
49. Hubbell JAE, Hinchcliff KW, Schmall LM, et al. Anesthetic, cardiorespiratory, and metabolic effects of four intravenous anesthetic regimens induced in horses immediately after maximal exercise. Am J Vet Res 2000;61:1545–52.
50. Muir WW, Gadawski JE, Grosenbaugh DA. Cardiorespiratory effects of a tiletamine/zolazepam-ketamine-detomidine combination in horses. Am J Vet Res 1999;60:770–4.
51. Rankin DC, Greene SA, Keegan RD, et al. Anesthesia of horses with a combination of detomidine, zolazepam, tiletamine, and isoflurane immediately after strenuous treadmill exercise. Am J Vet Res 1999;60:743–8.

Emergency procedures and first aid for the equine athlete

58

Joanne Hardy

CHAPTER CONTENTS

Introduction

The most commonly encountered emergencies in the athletic horse involve the musculoskeletal system. These include fractures, luxations, lacerations, puncture wounds, infection, and exertional rhabdomyolysis. Other injuries include head and ocular injuries. Although most of these conditions cannot be treated in the field, accurate identification and provision of appropriate emergency treatment are essential for a successful outcome.

Fractures and luxations

- A thorough physical examination is warranted for any athletic horse injury.
- Completion of physical examination can be complicated by the severity of the injury, and other factors such as anxiety, exhaustion, dehydration, and owner/trainer anxiety.
- The goals of initial coaptation of fractures are to relieve anxiety; prevent further injury; and allow safe transportation for additional evaluation.
- Emergency coaptation of unstable limbs should be performed before radiographic evaluation or transportation to a surgical facility.
- Appropriate transportation of the injured horse is important.

Initial assessment

History

Fractures or luxations should be suspected if a loud crack is heard, there is acute non-weight bearing lameness, the limb is misaligned, or the limb is visibly unstable.

Physical examination

Physical examination of the injured horse should be completed in the best possible setting to avoid further injury to the horse, or to bystanders. Help should be obtained to facilitate crowd control. A knowledgeable handler should be identified to help with horse restraint. While the veterinarian is examining the horse, the person responsible for making decisions on the patient should be sought, and emergency transportation (ideally, an equine ambulance) should be organized.

If the horse is recumbent, examination should be completed before attempting to stand the horse. If the horse is standing, examination should be completed before attempting to move the horse. Sedation and a twitch can be used to help restraint. For sedation, an alpha$_2$ agonist such as xylazine, or xylazine and acepromazine can be used. If sedation is needed immediately after maximal exercise, up to double the standard dosage regimen may be required to achieve effective sedation.[1] Butorphanol or detomidine should be reserved for horses that are not controlled with xylazine. It is important to remember that alpha$_2$ agonists will often cause the horse to lean forward, which may increase the weight on an injured forelimb and decrease the ability to manipulate the limb. Therefore the minimal effective dose should be used. In addition, heavy sedation will prolong the exercise-induced increase in body temperature, which may be significant in a hot humid environment. Active cooling by washing with cold water is an effective method of facilitating heat dissipation.[2] If the horse is recumbent and there is concern for a serious injury, general anesthesia should be induced and maintained until further assessment is made. General anesthesia can be safely induced in horses following maximal exercise using sedation with a combination of xylazine and acepromazine, followed by induction of anesthesia with ketamine and diazepam or tiletamine–zolazepam. The combination of guaifenesin and thiopental produces more hypotension and is less desirable.[3]

Once restraint is achieved, a brief assessment of circulatory status should be made, by evaluating heart rate, mucous membrane color, capillary refill time, and pulse quality. Identification of a heart rate of greater than 80 beats per minute accompanied by a delayed capillary refill time and poor peripheral pulse quality indicates the need for intravenous fluid support.

Once the general status of the patient has been assessed, location and assessment of the injury follows. It is useful to divide the limbs into four levels, which will help define the method of coaptation (Fig. 58.1).[4] Note that flexor tendon injuries located at the level of the metacarpus/metatarsus are considered level 1 injuries.

The presence of a fracture can be determined by: instability, crepitus, or abnormal motion. Luxations can be suspected when there is abnormal lateral-to-medial motion at the level of a joint, and can be confirmed with stress radiographs.

Special examination

Radiographic examination is indicated to confirm the presence of a fracture or luxation. If radiographic equipment is unavailable on site, external coaptation should be applied as if a fracture or luxation exists and the horse transported to a referral facility for further examination.

It is important to also remember that incomplete (hairline) fractures of the radius, tibia and other bones can be difficult to demonstrate radiographically, particularly in field conditions. Therefore, in the presence of severe lameness with pain localized to a long bone, external coaptation should be completed before transportation, to avoid catastrophic displacement of a fracture.

Laboratory examination

Laboratory determinations of biochemistry profile indices are more commonly available even in field situations. If available, parameters of hydration and electrolyte balance are useful to dictate fluid volume and type. In particular, measurement of lactate concentration using point-of-care equipment can provide a good evaluation of perfusion.[5]

Emergency treatment

Therapeutic aims

- Relieve anxiety
- Immobilize fracture or luxation for transportation
- Prevent further damage
- Provide safe transportation.

Therapy

The principles of emergency coaptation include:

- appropriate wound care before application of external coaptation

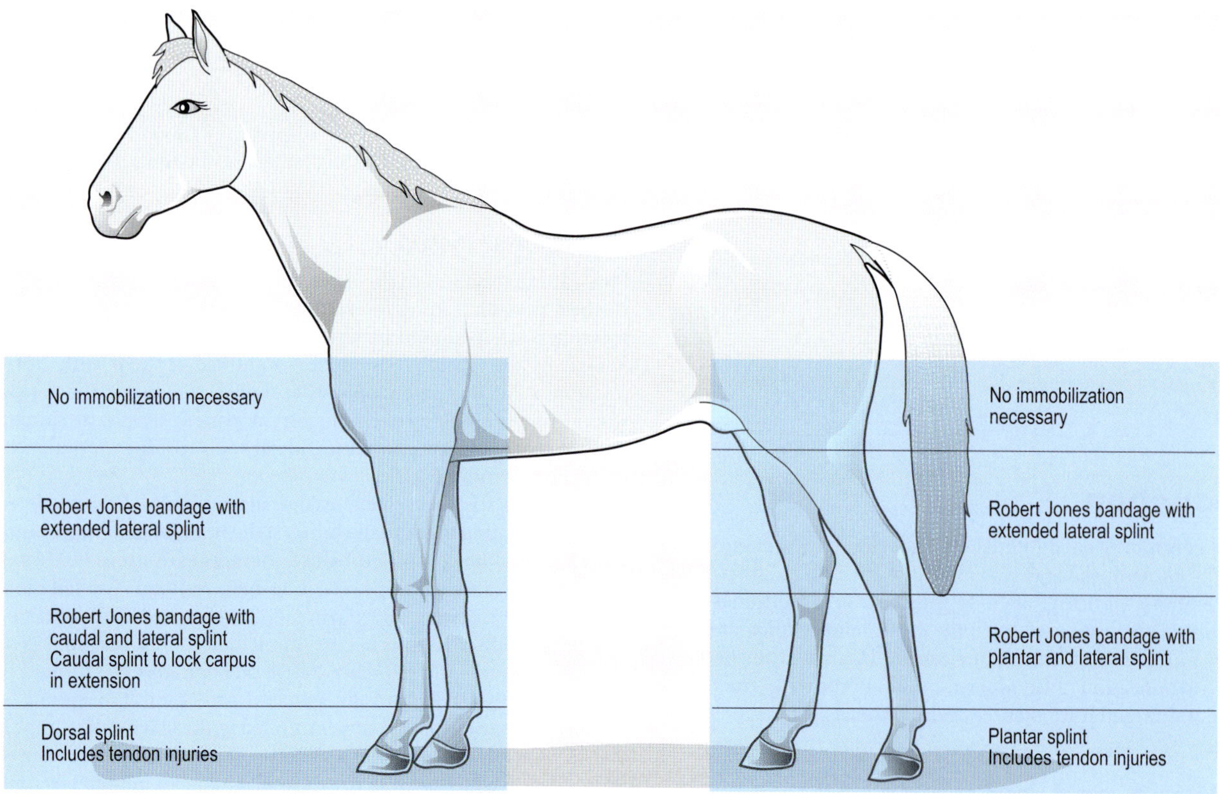

Fig 58.1 Classification of the level injury system used to understand methods of external coaption.
Nixon, A.J., (1996) Equine Fracture Repair, W.B. Saunders.

- provision of adequate padding to prevent skin abrasions
- immobilization of the joint below and above the area of injury
- prevention of latero-medial and cranio-caudal motion
- never ending a splint in the middle of a long bone segment, or at the end of a fracture line.

Bandage and splint application

Any wound should be carefully cleaned and debrided. An antiseptic ointment can be applied and held in place with conforming gauze. Cotton padding is applied to the entire length of the segment to be immobilized, and held in place with gauze followed by non-stretch bandage material. The bandage should be snug, to avoid loosening with packing of the cotton material. The splints are then applied and held in place, ideally with fiberglass casting tape. Whenever using casting tape, at least six layers should be applied. Casting tape is particularly useful if there is a luxation, as these can be difficult to keep stabilized. If unavailable, heavy tape can be used. It is important to make sure the splints are well padded to avoid the development of sores. See Box 58.1.

Classification of injuries

In order to facilitate emergency coaptation of unstable injuries, a classification system based on the location of the injury has been recommended (Fig. 58.1).[4] It is important to note that tendon lacerations located below the carpus/hock are considered level 1 injuries.

Immobilization of level 1 injuries

Level 1 injuries include phalangeal fractures, fetlock, pastern or coffin joint luxations, and severance of one or more flexor tendons. Although technically a level 1 injury, extensor tendon lacerations require a different mode of splint application and will be presented separately. Forelimb and hindlimb immobilization differ slightly, because of the presence of the reciprocal apparatus in the hindlimb.

Forelimb

In forelimb injuries, immobilization is best accomplished by aligning the cannon bone with the phalanges, to establish a straight column (Fig. 58.2). The horse will bear weight on its toe. To accomplish this goal, the forelimb is held above the carpus, bandaged, and the splint is applied on the cranial aspect of the distal limb, extending from the toe to the carpus. If there is latero-medial instability, a lateral splint can also be applied. Alternatively, the splint can be held in place using casting tape.

Hindlimb

In the hindlimb, the reciprocal apparatus prevents extension of the distal limb if the animal is non-weight bearing. Therefore the limb is best immobilized by applying the splint on the caudal aspect of the limb, from the toe to the point of the hock (Fig. 58.3). Again, if there is latero-medial instability, a lateral splint should also be placed or casting used to immobilize the splint. A cranial splint can also be placed; however, to facilitate placement, the limb can be pulled forward to straighten the fetlock.

Box 58.1 Materials needed for emergency coaptation of fractures or luxations

- Cotton padding
- Conforming gauze
- Non-elastic bandage
- Tape
- Casting tape
- Splints: PVC pipe material or 2″ × 4″ boards of different lengths

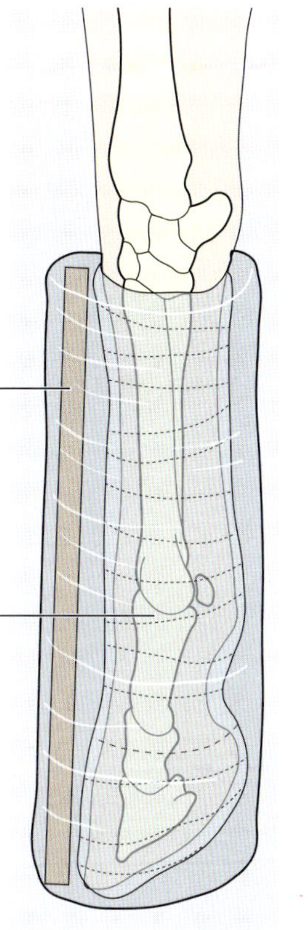

Fig 58.2 Application of a splint for level 1 injury of the forelimb.

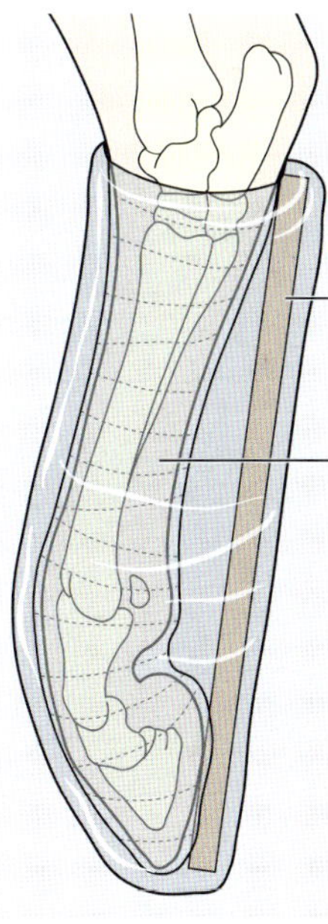

Fig 58.3 Application of a splint for level 1 injury in a hindlimb.

Use of the Kimzey[a] apparatus

A commercially available splint is available for level 1 injuries (Fig. 58.4). The advantages of this splint are that it is readily available, easy to apply and is effective in achieving immobilization. Two configurations are available: one with a slightly forward angled bar (for the forelimb) and one with a backward angle with the curve at the level of the fetlock (for the hindlimb). In the author's experience, the forward angle configuration is more effective for either fore- or hindlimb injuries. When used for prolonged immobilization, the stall should be deeply bedded to improve support of the foot. Alternatively, a heel piece can be welded onto the splint to increase weight-bearing surface area. Non-slip tape should be placed on the foot plate to make it less slippery, particularly on cement floors.

Extensor tendon injuries

With complete severance of both extensor tendons of the forelimb or hindlimb, the horse will knuckle over, which can cause injury to the dorsal aspect of the fetlock and further disruption of the wound. In this instance, external coaptation is needed to prevent knuckling over at the fetlock. A splint is applied to the cranial aspect of the fore- or hindlimb, with the hoof flat on the ground. Pulling the leg forward will facilitate application of a hindlimb splint.

[a]Kimzey Leg Saver, Kimzey Metal Products, Woodland, CA; www.kimzeymetalproducts.com.

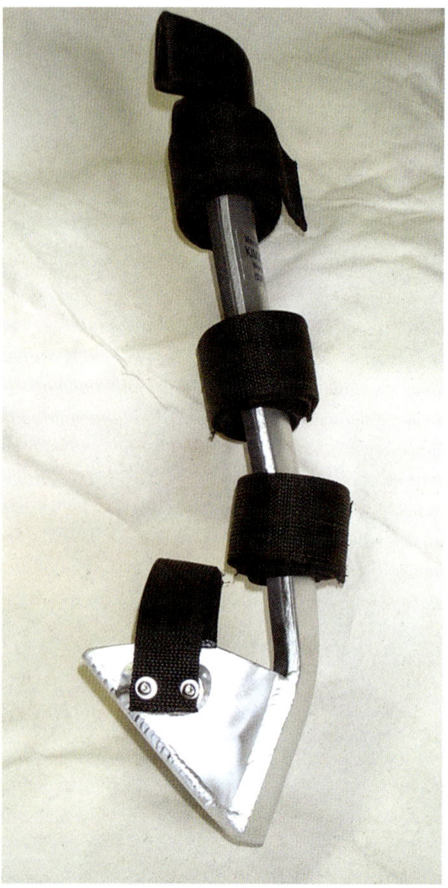

Fig 58.4 Illustration of the Kimzey Leg Saver. *John W. Kimzey, Kimzey Metal Products, CA.*

Immobilization of level 2 injuries

Examples of level 2 injuries include cannon bone fractures, wounds of the carpus or hock, olecranon fractures and radial nerve paralysis. Forelimb and hindlimb immobilization will again be discussed separately, because the angle of the hock requires a different splint configuration.

Forelimb

In level 2 injuries, two splints are needed, applied at 90-degree angle, with one splint lateral and one splint caudal. The splints need to extend from the hoof to the elbow (Fig. 58.5). For olecranon fractures and radial nerve paralysis, the goal of immobilization is to prevent tendon contracture and injury to the dorsal aspect of the limb. Only a caudal splint is needed for these types of injuries.

Hindlimb

As in the forelimb, two splints are needed, one applied laterally and the other applied caudally, from the hoof to the stifle. The angle of the hock makes it difficult to apply a caudal splint. Therefore the caudal splint can end at the point of the hock, rather than at the stifle (Fig. 58.6). Alternatively, if possible, a splint can be molded to the hock so it can be applied.

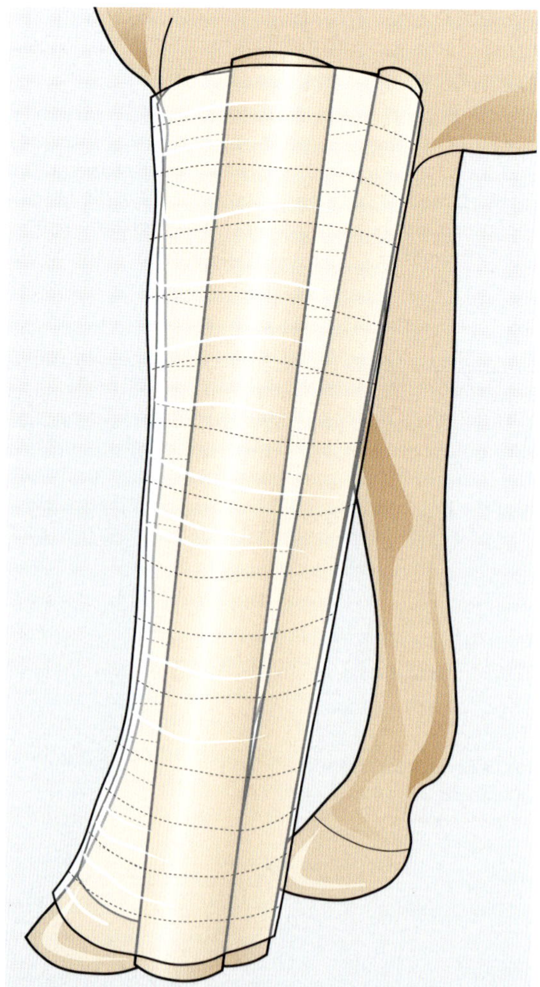

Fig 58.5 Application of splints for level 2 injury to the forelimb.

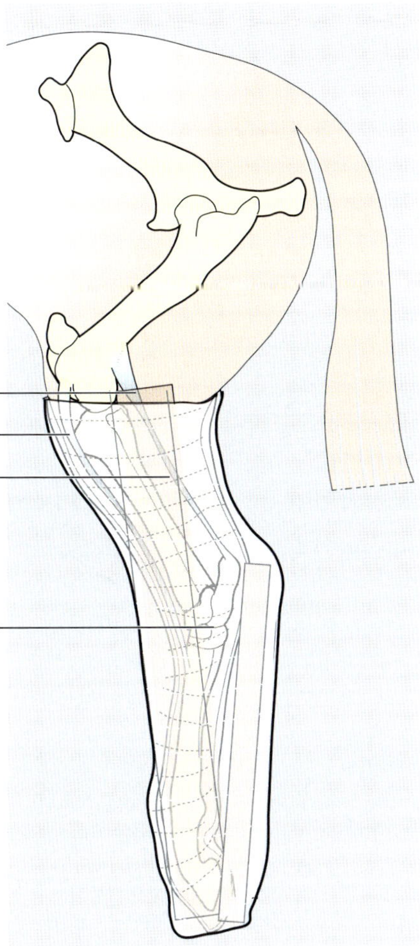

Fig 58.6 Application of a splint for level 2 injury in a hindlimb.

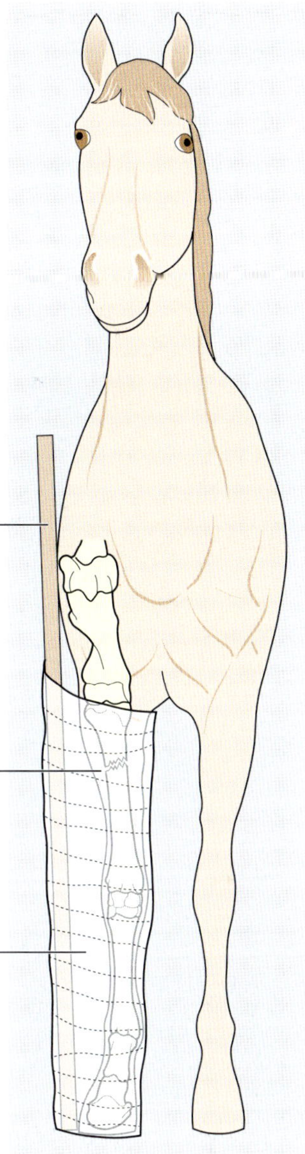

Fig 58.7 Application of splints for level 3 injury to the forelimb.

Immobilization of level 3 injuries

Level 3 injuries include fractures of the radius or tibia. With fractures at this level, the flexor muscles become abductors, resulting in displacement and comminution of the medial aspect of the limb. The medial aspect of both the radius and ulna does not include a muscle mass to help prevent penetration of the skin by fractured bone. Therefore the goal of external coaptation is to prevent abduction of the limb.

Forelimb

The splint is applied to the lateral aspect of the limb, and must extend from the hoof to the withers (Fig. 58.7). The tip of the splint can be taped around the chest for further stability.

Hindlimb

The splint is applied to the lateral aspect of the limb, extending from the hoof to the hip (Fig. 58.8).

Immobilization of level 4 injuries

Level 4 injuries include fractures of the scapula, humerus, femur or pelvis. External coaptation is not recommended for these injuries as these areas are not amenable to bandaging. Reliance on the hematoma and swelling around the injury for immobilization is needed. An immobilizing bandage should not be applied to the distal limb, as it will make it more awkward to move, and may increase motion at the fracture site. Increased motion at the fracture in return can result in severance of major vessels and significant and potentially fatal hemorrhage. If a fractured pelvis is present, the need for transportation should be discussed, as moving of the fracture segments can result in lacerations of major vessels. General anesthesia for pelvic fracture should be delayed for three to four weeks, to avoid fatal hemorrhage.

Guidelines for safe transportation

Before loading an injured horse, proper functioning of the vehicle should be assured. The horse should be stabilized, and the injury immobilized as best as possible before loading. All relevant paperwork (medical records, insurance information, contact numbers and map to referral facility) should be gathered, and the referral facility contacted.

The injured horse will need to negotiate loading and unloading a trailer with a potentially cumbersome splint applied to the injured leg. With a full leg splint, ambulation is facilitated by placing a rope around the pastern and pulling the leg forward synchronously with

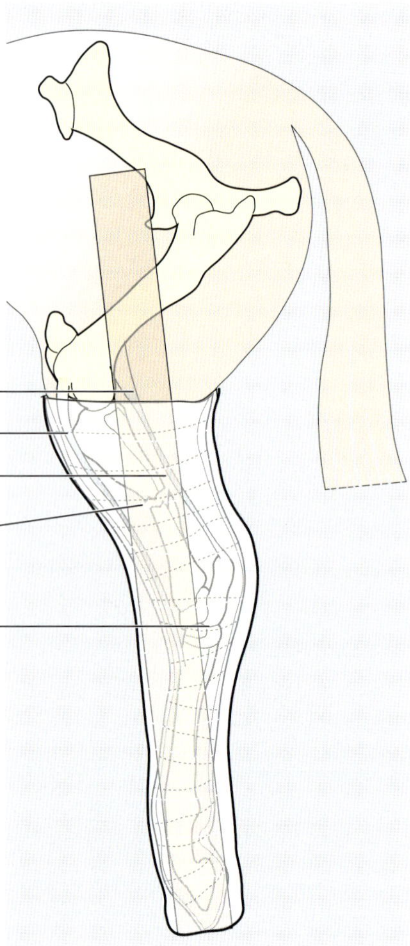

Fig 58.8 Application of a splint for level 3 injury in a hindlimb.

the horse attempting to move forward. Loading onto the trailer is facilitated by a low-angled ramp or by the use of a loading ramp. While in the trailer, the horse may lean on the wall and partitions to help reduce the load on the injured leg. It will be easier for the horse to travel with partitions in place rather than loose in a makeshift stall. A sling can be placed under the horse's abdomen to help the horse take weight off the injured limb. Many trailers today have standing stalls at 45-degree angles (slant load trailer), which helps horses balance during transport. If a regular straight-load trailer is used, the horse should face backward for a forelimb injury, and forward for a rear limb injury, to help cushion sudden stops. However, although this sounds good in theory, it may be difficult to load a horse backwards in a two-horse trailer, and undue stress to the injured horse should be avoided. Finally, providing hay will help relieve anxiety, and frequent stops should be made to check on the status of the horse and provide drinking water. If significant cardiovascular compromise exists, intravenous fluids can be administered while in transit.

If the horse is deemed severely injured and needs to remain recumbent, it can be pulled onto the trailer using a large tarp or blanket. A glide[b] is commercially available to help move recumbent horses. The horse should be kept sedated during transport, to avoid injuries. A head protector[c] or bandage can be used to protect the eye and head from self-induced trauma. Bandages should be applied to the lower limbs, also to avoid trauma caused by paddling.

[b] Large Animal Rescue Glide, www.rescueglides.com.
[c] Equine head protector, http://jupitervetproducts.com.

Wounds and lacerations

- First step: identification of all involved structures
- Control of hemorrhage
- Determine need for referral based on the presence of:
  - tendon injury
  - penetration of synovial structure
  - extensive degloving injury
  - severe blood loss
- Provide tetanus prophylaxis, analgesia, and appropriate antibiotic therapy
- In severe blood loss, provide cardiovascular support.

Assessment of wounds and lacerations

As with any condition, a general physical exam should be briefly completed before addressing the primary problem. If the wound is located on a limb, the presence and degree of lameness should be noted. The presence and severity of lameness is an important sign of a potentially more serious injury.

The wound is then evaluated for the following findings.

Location

Wounds in the following locations should be explored in detail for injury to important underlying structures:

- wounds over joints or tendon sheaths
- wounds over tendons, particularly flexor tendons
- wounds that have bone exposed, or that are down to bone.

Hemorrhage

The presence of severe hemorrhage may require hemorrhage control before further wound assessment is possible. Severe hemorrhage is best controlled using a pressure bandage applied directly over the bleeding area. Attempts to find the bleeding vessels are often not successful. It is important to remember that bleeding vessels are often satellite to sensory nerves and that attempts to grab a bleeding vessel with hemostats can lead to inadvertent pinching of a nerve and significant adverse reaction from the horse.

Wound configuration

Certain wound configurations may lead to significant damage to blood supply to the skin and subcutaneous tissues and will result in sloughing. Examples include an inverted 'V' configuration, or significant bruising or trauma to adjacent tissue.

Penetration of a body cavity

Wounds over the chest or abdomen have the potential for penetrating injuries to important organs. In the case of thoracic wounds, development of an open or closed pneumothorax can lead to severe respiratory distress. Any horse with chest trauma and respiratory distress should be evaluated for the presence of pneumothorax. Axillary wounds, even if they do not penetrate the chest, can aspirate air in the subcutaneous space leading to significant subcutaneous emphysema, which can lead to the development of pneumomediastinum and pneumothorax.

Determination of synovial structure involvement

The potential involvement of a synovial structure should be IMMEDIATELY determined. To evaluate penetration of a synovial structure the following steps can be followed:

- The horse is restrained and sedated as needed.
- A site of entry of the joint or tendon sheath remote from the wound is chosen.
- The site is clipped and prepared aseptically.
- Using sterile technique, saline or a balanced electrolyte solution is injected into the synovial structure, using an amount sufficient to achieve distention. The amount can vary from a few mL in the case of a distal tarsal joint injury to 100 mL or more for the femoro-patellar joint (Fig. 58.9).

It is also important to assess all possible joint compartments. The wound is observed for leakage of the injectate.

Determination of tendon involvement

Extensor tendon injury of the distal limbs will result in inability to appropriately place the hoof on the ground, resulting in the horse knuckling over. For this to occur, both tendons will have to be involved in proximal metacarpal/tarsal injuries.

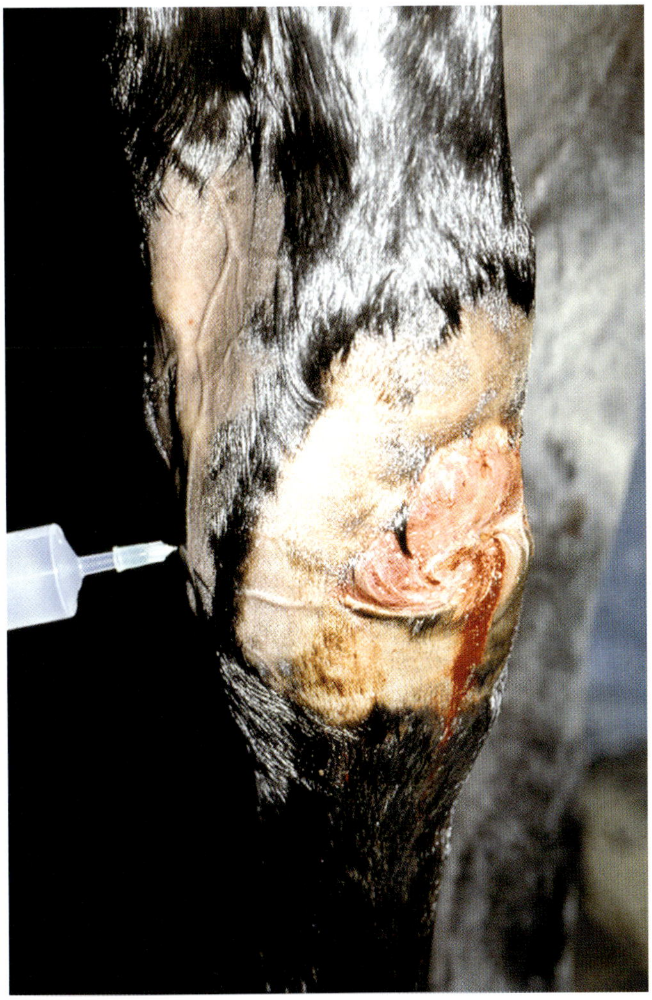

Fig 58.9 Injection of the middle carpal joint showing communication of the joint with a wound.

Flexor tendon injuries will result in hyperextension of the fetlock (superficial digital flexor), lifting up of the toe (deep digital flexor; Fig. 58.10) or complete dropping of the fetlock to the ground (severance of the suspensory ligament). In order to observe this the horse must bear weight on the limb at least transiently. Importantly, in the case of complete suspensory breakdown, there can be severe stretching of digital vessels, which can lead to thrombosis and avascular injury to the hoof. In complete breakdown injury, it is therefore critical to support the fetlock and not allow weight bearing until further stabilization can be performed.

Emergency treatment of limb wounds and lacerations

Wound care

The goal of initial wound care is to decontaminate the wound as much as possible, and prevent further contamination during transportation. Lavage with saline and sharp debridement of gross contaminants is used to accomplish this goal. Local antiseptics or antibiotics can be then packed in the wound to further decontaminate it.

Limb immobilization

Immobilization of the limb will be needed if there is injury to a supporting structure (bone or tendon) or significant instability (luxation). Please refer to the above section for a description of the appropriate method of immobilization.

Emergency treatment of wounds involving the chest or abdominal cavity

Pneumothorax

An open chest wound (Fig. 58.11) can result in the development of pneumothorax. Pneumothorax will cause respiratory distress manifested by a restrictive pattern of breathing. On auscultation, there will be absence of sound in the dorsal lung fields. Because of the incomplete mediastinum in horses, a unilateral chest wound can lead to bilateral pneumothorax.

An open pneumothorax is managed by providing a temporary seal over the chest wound. This is accomplished by bandaging the wound and applying an impervious airtight layer of a material such as plastic wrap (Fig. 58.12). The chest is then evacuated by inserting

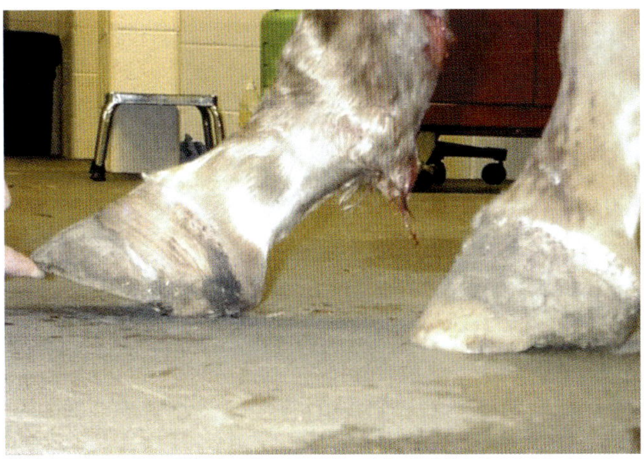

Fig 58.10 Hyperextension of the coffin joint in a horse with a completely severed deep digital flexor tendon.

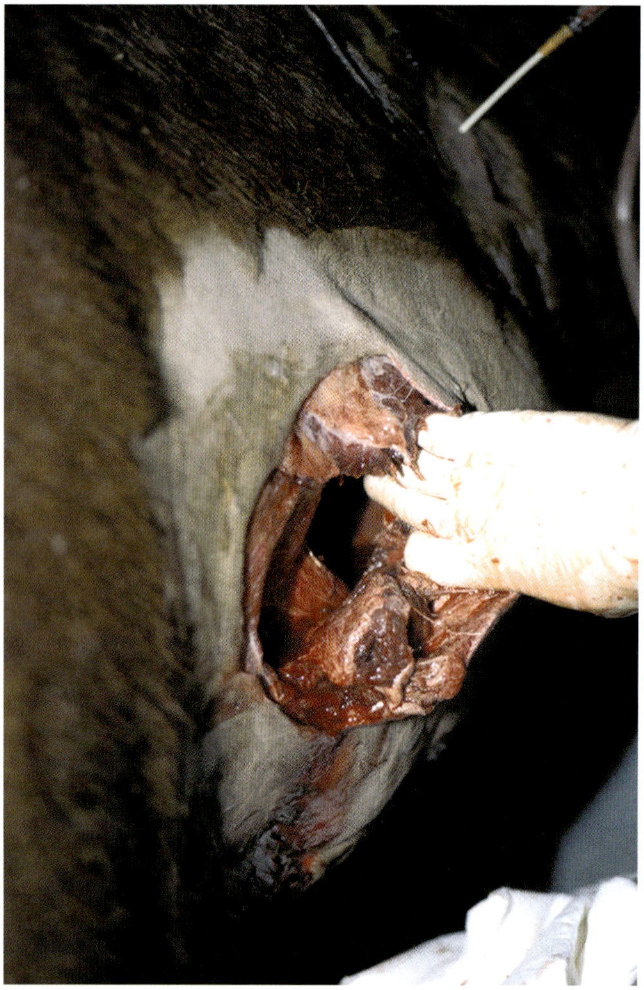

Fig 58.11 Open chest injury and pneumothorax in a horse. Note the placement of a 14-gauge catheter at the 12th intercostals space dorsally to evacuate air from the chest.

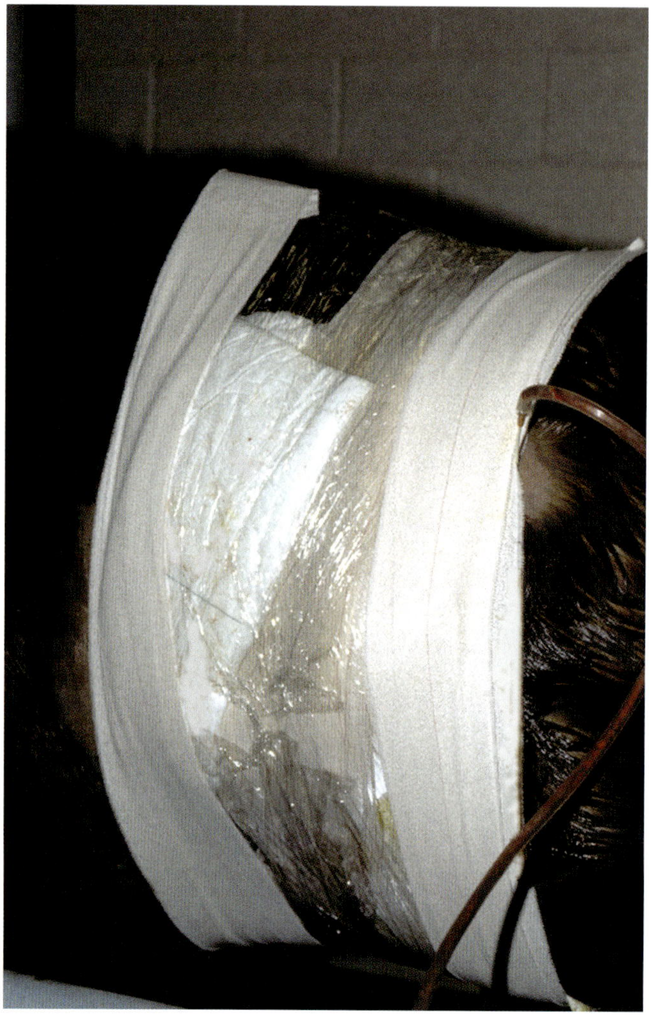

Fig 58.12 Application of an airtight bandage to a horse with an open pneumothorax.

a chest trocar, or if unavailable a 14-gauge catheter using aseptic technique in the dorsal aspect of the 12th to 15th intercostal space, and aspirating the air out of the chest. The use of a three-way stopcock will facilitate this procedure.

Penetrating abdominal wound

Penetrating abdominal wounds are serious and potentially fatal injuries. They can lead to penetration of a viscus, or development of peritonitis. If a penetrating wound is suspected, the wound should be cleaned, explored for the presence of a foreign body, and debrided. An abdominocentesis can be performed to detect fecal contamination indicative of a ruptured viscus. However, abdominocentesis may not be diagnostic in this early stage of peritoneal contamination, as indicators of peritonitis take several hours to develop. The wound can be bandaged, and broad-spectrum systemic antibiotics initiated. In the presence of a large wound, or if abdominal musculature is involved, the abdomen can be supported using an adhesive tape bandage or a commercially available abdominal support bandage.[d]

[d]Equine Hernia Belt, www.cmequineproducts.com.

Head injuries

Head injuries can result in severe central nervous system damage. Central nervous system (CNS) injury can be primary where contusions, lacerations and hemorrhage cause the acute damage, or secondary, when subsequent edema, reperfusion injury and necrosis result in worsening of the injury. Therapy for head injury is aimed at minimizing secondary CNS damage.

The causes of head injury in athletic horses include direct trauma from a fall, a blow to the head or falling over backwards onto the poll region. The associated injuries include basisphenoid fractures and avulsion of the ventral straight muscles of the head.

Basisphenoid fractures

The location of this injury can result in acute optic nerve damage, and cerebral signs. Temporary blindness can result. The diagnosis is made by radiography (Fig. 58.13), and treatment is targeted towards minimizing secondary brain damage, and supportive care.

Rectus and longus capitis muscle rupture

This injury occurs most commonly from falling over backwards. The muscles attach to the base of the cranium, and with injury,

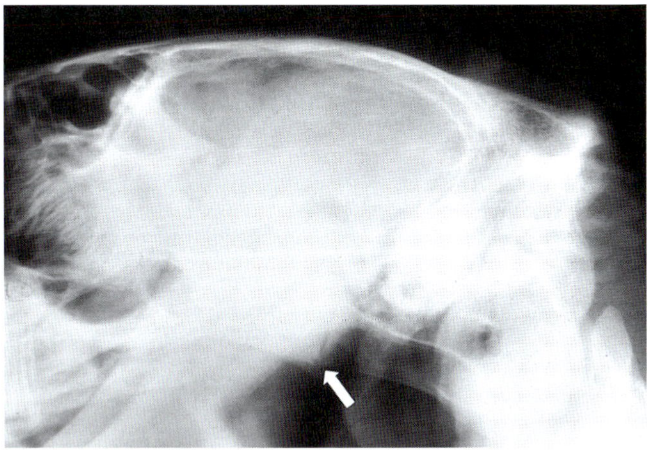

Fig 58.13 Lateral projection of the head of a horse with basisphenoid fracture (arrow).

hematoma, and even avulsion fractures of the muscular insertion, can result. Because of the location of these muscles within the guttural pouch septum, hematomas can rupture into the guttural pouch resulting in epistaxis. This epistaxis can be severe, and may require blood transfusion.

The diagnosis of this injury is made by endoscopy, where an epistaxis of guttural pouch origin is identified, in conjunction with a large hematoma in the guttural pouch septum. Radiographs are useful to demonstrate an avulsion fracture accompanied by a soft tissue opacity overlying the guttural pouches (Fig. 58.14).

Treatment is supportive, with anti-inflammatory drugs and edema-reducing agents.

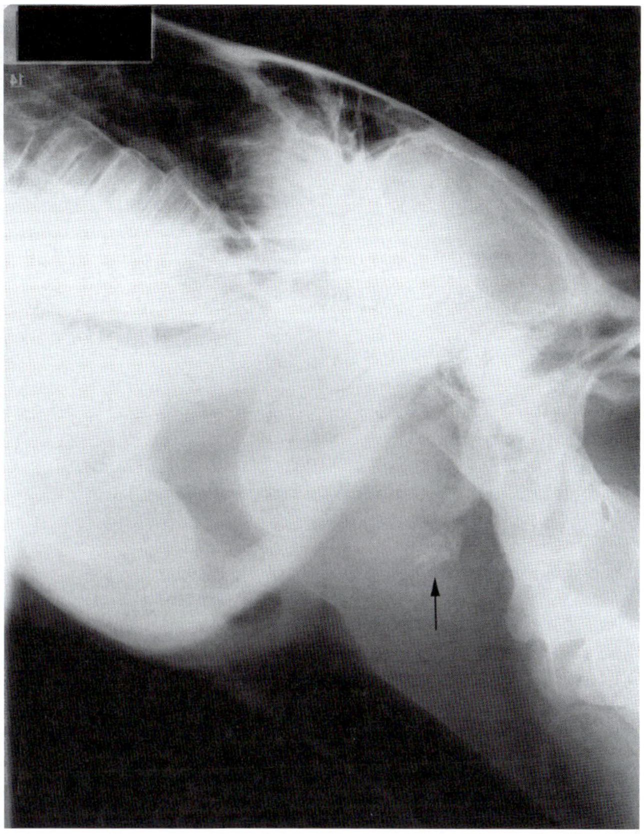

Fig 58.14 Lateral projection of the head of a horse with avulsion of the longus capitis muscle. Note the avulsion fractures located at the attachment of the longus capitis to the basisphenoid bone (arrow).

Treatment of acute head injuries

Horses with head injury can be severely ataxic, and need to be handled and moved with extreme caution. If the horse is down, a short-term general anesthesia is best used to move the horse to a referral facility for further evaluation.

Non-steroidal anti-inflammatory drugs (NSAIDs) are used to minimize inflammation. Although controversial, corticosteroids may be indicated if used in the immediate phase of injury. Dimethyl sulfoxide (DMSO) is often used to minimize secondary edema. If cerebrospinal fluid is seen exiting from a wound or from an ear canal, broad-spectrum antibiotic therapy should be initiated. If central nervous system edema is suspected, mannitol or 3% hypertonic saline can be administered. Magnesium has recently been proposed as another therapeutic agent for acute head injury.

Ocular injuries

Ocular injuries encountered in the athletic horse are traumatic in origin, and include periocular lacerations, corneal lacerations or foreign body penetrating injury, or direct blow to the eye with retinal detachment.

Evaluation of acute ocular injury includes evaluation of the different structures of the eye, as well as evaluation of cranial nerve function. Eyelids, conjunctiva, cornea, lens and fundic examinations can be performed to assess the degree of damage (Fig. 58.15). Vision can be assessed by the menace response, supplemented with obstacle course testing. Oculomotor, trochlear and abducent nerve function are assessed by the position of the eye, and pupillary light responses. Facial nerve and sympathetic innervation to the eye are assessed by eyelid tone, and position of the eyelashes.

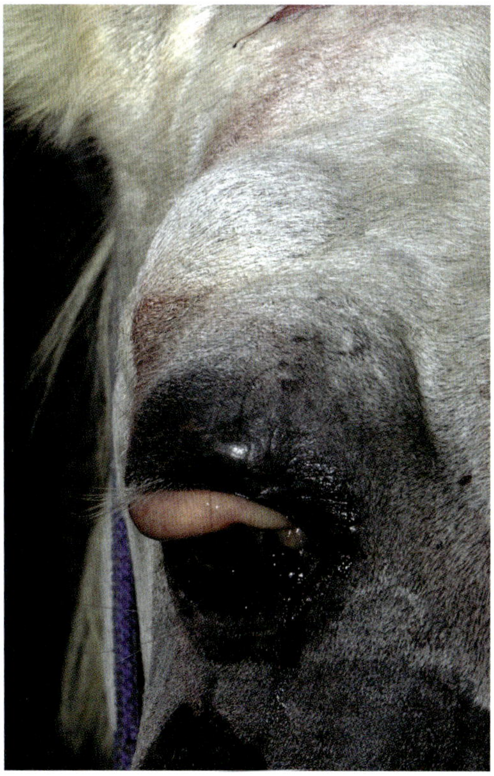

Fig 58.15 Horse with severe chemosis resulting from contact with an irritant.

Treatment of acute ocular injuries includes minimizing pain and inflammation, preventing infection, and preventing further injuries. If penetration by a foreign body is suspected, rapid surgical intervention is indicated to prevent further injury (Fig 58.16).

Anti-inflammatory drugs that are used to minimize pain and inflammation associated with ocular injuries include NSAIDs, DMSO, and topical osmotic agents. Pain from pupillary spasm can be minimized by dilating the pupil with atropine. Direct sunlight should be minimized by protecting the eye. Acute injuries can be associated with ulceration and secondary bacterial invasion. A broad-spectrum topical antibiotic can be used to prevent secondary infection of an ulcer.

Horses that are acutely blind will not negotiate their environment well. Further injury should be prevented by protecting the blind eye,[e] and by carefully handling the horse.

Acute rhabdomyolysis

Recognition

History and presenting complaint

Acute rhabdomyolysis (tying-up) is a generalized inflammation of skeletal muscles. Predisposing factors include genetics, intense exercise, exercise following a period of confinement, dietary practices, particularly the feeding of a high percentage of carbohydrate in the diet, general anesthesia, and sex (higher prevalence in females).

Physical examination

The manifestations of acute rhabdomyolysis (AR) will vary from mild stiffness to recumbency. The most common signs include a stiff gait with reluctance to move, tachycardia, tachypnea, focal or generalized sweating, hardness of large muscle groups such as the glutei, quadriceps and triceps, and muscle fasciculations. The urine will be dark to black as a result of myoglobinuria. Occasionally, particularly if the episode follows exertion, there will also be signs of endotoxemia (injected mucous membranes, poor peripheral pulse). Ileus, as manifested by absence of auscultable motility, presence of nasogastric reflux, and palpable small intestinal distention, can also be present, particularly if hypocalcemia is present.

Laboratory findings in AR include elevation in plasma muscle enzymes: early (within 6 hours) creatine kinase (CK) often reaching 50 000 to 100 000 units/dL followed by a later rise in aspartate aminotransferase (AST). Azotemia may be present, and may result from dehydration or from primary renal damage (acute tubular necrosis resulting from pigmenturia). Common electrolyte abnormalities include ionized hypocalcemia, and a metabolic alkalosis.

Treatment

Therapeutic aims

- Pain control
- Muscle relaxation
- Fluid support
  - correction of electrolyte abnormalities
  - prevention of acute renal failure.

Therapy

Acute rhabdomyolysis can be a very painful condition. Adequate fluid replacement should be ensured to prevent renal toxicity of some of these drugs. Drugs used for pain control include flunixin meglumine, phenylbutazone, and butorphanol. In severe cases, morphine can be added to the therapeutic regimen. If practical, lidocaine can be given as a constant rate infusion for additional pain relief.

Muscle relaxants are often added to, particularly when the large muscle groups are hard and painful. Methocarbamol, dantrolene, and guaifenesin are recommended, although efficacy is uncertain.

Acepromazine, a peripheral vasodilator, has been recommended to improve muscle blood flow. This should be used with caution in stallions, where it can result in priapism.

Fluid therapy is an essential part of the treatment of acute rhabdomyolysis. Renal tubular necrosis and subsequent renal failure can result from the combination of dehydration, pigmenturia, and nephrotoxicity of NSAIDs. Balanced electrolyte solutions are preferred. Calcium supplementation is indicated as low ionized calcium concentration is often present.

[e]Eye Saver, http://jupitervetproducts.com.

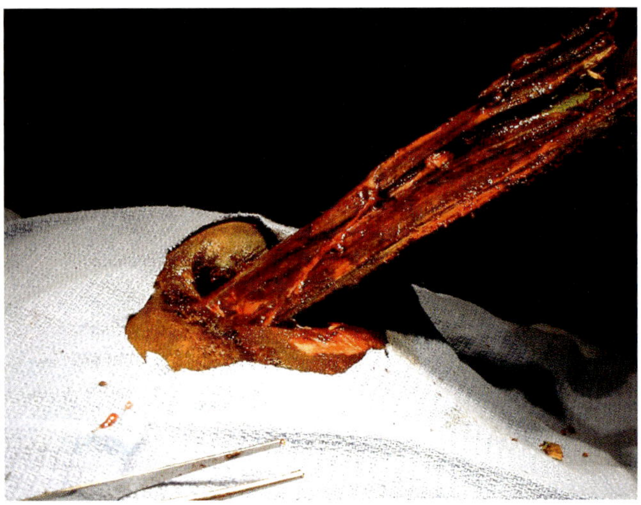

Fig 58.16 Horse presented with an injury to the right eye with a small piece of wood protruding from the ventral orbit. On surgical exploration, this large wood fragment was extracted from the orbit.

Emergency fluid therapy in the athletic horse

Injuries with blood loss, or horses suffering from exhaustion, acute rhabdomyolysis or overheating, are conditions that require emergency fluid replacement as part of their management. This section will discuss the basics of fluid therapy in shock states with emphasis on fluids used for resuscitation. Mention will be made of emergency treatment of the horse with an Hyperkalemic Periodic Paralysis (HYPP) event.

Designing a fluid therapy regimen

Fluids can be administered for maintenance purposes, when fluid intake is physically not possible or for replacement purposes when excessive losses have been incurred and/or ongoing losses are anticipated. In the athletic horse, replacement therapy is the mainstay of fluid therapy and will be discussed here. The first section will discuss the mathematics for fluid administration in horses, and the following section will outline the materials commercially available to achieve this goal.

Designing a replacement fluid therapy regimen requires the clinician to answer the following questions:

- What volume of fluids is required?
- What type of fluid is required?
- What route of administration is available/optimal?
- What will be the rate of administration?

Calculating the volume of fluid to give

The volume of fluid to give on a daily basis can be calculated using the equation in Box 58.2.

An estimate of dehydration can be made by using clinical, and if available, laboratory parameters, as outlined in Table 58.1. These numbers will be weighed in relation to the horse's clinical condition. For example, a nervous horse may have a transiently high heart rate in response to excitement, and a high hematocrit because of splenic contraction. The clinician will therefore have to use judgment in the interpretation of each parameter.

Ongoing losses can be the most difficult estimation, as losses through the gastrointestinal tract are difficult to measure. The equine gastrointestinal tract secretes and reabsorbs the equivalent of the extracellular volume (approximately 30% of body weight) on a daily basis. If ileus is present, the amount of reflux can be quantitated. If the large colon is not reabsorbing water, as in diarrhea, significant losses can occur. With severe diarrhea, approximately 50% of extracellular fluids can be lost on a daily basis.

The clinician must be aware that this calculation is a crude estimate, and volumes are then adjusted based on objective responses to fluid administration such as heart rate, pulse quality, capillary refill time (CRT), urine production, hematocrit, total protein (TP), and creatinine. These monitoring parameters will need to be repeated as often as dictated by the horse's clinical condition. With a horse in severe shock, monitoring cardiovascular parameters may need to be continuous, or at least every 15 minutes, until an improvement is noted. In a horse with severe ongoing fluid losses, cardiovascular parameters should be monitored at least every 4 hours, and laboratory parameters as frequently as four times a day until stabilized. Following these evaluations, an adjustment in the estimate of fluid requirements can be made.

Box 58.2

Total volume to give in the next 24 hours (in liters) =
Maintenance (60 mL/kg body weight/day)
+
estimate of dehydration (% of bodyweight)
+
ongoing losses

Deciding the type of fluids to give

Fluids available for administration in horses are of two categories: *crystalloids* are fluids containing substances that freely cross the capillary membrane; these include balanced electrolyte solutions, saline solutions, and dextrose solutions; and *colloids*, which are made up of fluids that are retained in the vascular space for a certain number of hours, because of their larger molecular size; these include plasma, albumin solutions, dextrans, and hydroxyethylstarch. Crystalloids are most commonly used for replacement fluid therapy in the athletic horse, whereas colloids are reserved for resuscitation purposes, and will be discussed in that section.

Crystalloids

There are two basic types of crystalloids available for horses: *balanced electrolyte solutions* (BES), which consist of electrolyte solutions in concentrations similar to plasma; and *saline solutions*, which contain only sodium chloride. Although considered a crystalloid, dextrose solutions are rarely used alone. Table 58.2 outlines the different composition of crystalloids commercially available for horses.

The decision to choose BES or saline is based, if available, on a serum chemistry profile. Saline is chosen if the sodium concentration is less than 125 mEq/L, or the potassium is greater than 5.9 mEq/L. Otherwise, a BES is used. If unavailable, a BES is safe, unless HYPP is suspected, in which case saline should be used. Several portable point-of-care monitoring devices that can measure blood gas and electrolytes are now available.[f]

Colloids

The addition of colloids to a fluid therapy regimen serves two purposes: address the problem of edema formation in hypoproteinemic states; or sustain the intravascular circulating volume. Selected products containing targeting antibodies are also available for the treatment or prevention of endotoxemia, *Rhodoccocus equi* pneumonia, and clostridial diseases. These products will not be discussed in this section. Colloidal solutions are available in two forms: natural or synthetic. Natural colloids are plasma, serum products or albumin. Table 58.3 summarizes the characteristics of each product. In general, plasma is selected when an increase in oncotic pressure is needed, but in addition, coagulation factors or specific

[f]IRMA Blood Analysis System, Diametrics Medical Inc., St-Paul, MN. www.diametrics.com.
I-Stat Portable Clinical Analyzer, I-Stat Corporation, East Windsor, NJ. www.istat.com.

Table 58.1 Physical and laboratory parameters used to estimate the percentage of dehydration in horses

% DEHYDRATION	HEART RATE (beats/min)	CRT (s)	PCV/TP (%/g/L)	CREATININE (mg/dL)
6	40–60	2	40/7	1.5–2
8	61–80	3	45/7.5	2–3
10	81–100	4	50/8	3–4
12	>100	>4	>50/>8	>4

CRT = capillary refill time; PCV = packed cell volume; TP = total protein.

Table 58.2 Composition of crystalloids commonly used for fluid therapy in horses

PRODUCT	APPROXIMATE pH	mOsmol/L	Na (mEq/L)	K (mEq/L)	Ca (mEq/L)	Mg (mEq/L)	Cl (mEq/L)	BUFFER (mEq/L)
Lactated Ringer's	6.5	273	130	4	3		109	Lactate 28
PlasmaLyte A	7.4	294	140	5		3	98	Acetate 27
PlasmaLyte 148	7.4	294	140	5		3	98	Gluconate 23 Acetate 27
PlasmaLyte 148	5.5	294	140	5		3	98	Gluconate 23 Acetate 27
5% Dextrose	4	252						Gluconate 23
0.9% NaCl	5	308	154				154	
7% NaCl		2400	1196				1196	
5% $NaHCO_3$	8	1190	595				595	
1.3% $NaHCO_3$		308	154				1541	

Table 58.3 Composition of colloids commonly used for fluid therapy in horses

CHARACTERISTICS OF COLLOID FLUIDS				
Characteristics	**5% albumin**	**Dextran 40**	**Dextran 70**	**Hetastarch**
Molecular weight (Da) weight average number-average range	69 000 69 000	40 000 25 000 10 000–80 000	70 000 39 000 15 000–160 000	450 000 70 000 10 000–3 400 000
Solvent		0.9% saline or 5% dextrose	0.9% saline or 5% dextrose	0.9% saline or BES
Concentration (%)	5	10	6	6
Half-life	14–16 days	2.5 h	6 h	25 h
Extravascular percentage (after 24 h)		22	33	39
Overall survival in blood		44 h	4–6 weeks	17–26 weeks
Colloid oncotic pressure (mmHg)	20	40	N/A	30

anticoagulants such as antithrombin are required by the disease process. Albumin solutions are not commonly used, as the intravascular half-life of albumin in states of compromised vascular permeability is short, and this solution does not have the added benefits of plasma. In addition, a commercial source for equine albumin solution is not always readily available. Synthetic colloids commonly used in horses include Dextran 70, pentastarch and hydroxyethylstarch (HES). Dextran 70 has fallen out of use as anaphylactic reactions have been reported, and the duration of effect on increasing colloid oncotic pressure is short relative to other products. Hydroxyethylstarch is the most commonly used product, but the dose should be limited to 10 mL/kg per day, as at higher doses it can affect coagulation. Pentastarch has not been as well investigated in horses; it has a narrower molecular weight range, and may be more efficacious at increasing colloid oncotic pressure, but the cost has limited its use. These products are used to increase plasma oncotic pressure, and their effect is best evaluated either by clinical response (decreased edema) or increased oncotic pressure (measured by colloid osmometry).[6,7] A refractometer cannot be used to monitor the effect of synthetic colloid administration.

Products used for resuscitation

The goal of fluid therapy in shock states is to rapidly expand circulating blood volume to improve perfusion and oxygen delivery. Isotonic crystalloids can serve this purpose, but must be administered at a rate of 60–80 mL/kg in the first hour (approximately one blood volume), for beneficial effects. Hypertonic solutions can be used to rapidly expand circulating volume by redistributing extravascular fluids into the vascular space, and provide faster restoration of intravascular volume deficits than isotonic solutions. Because of redistribution, the duration of effect of hypertonic solutions in horses is short, and additional isotonic fluid administration must follow their administration. Colloid solutions can be used to sustain the effect of hypertonic crystalloid solutions to several hours. For resuscitation, a combination of hypertonic saline and hetastarch would have the most beneficial and sustained effects. Table 58.4 lists the properties and dosages of fluids commonly used for resuscitation in the horse.

Materials for fluid therapy

The flow rate of fluids through an administration system is directly proportional to the diameter of the line and inversely proportional to the viscosity of the fluid and the length of the line. For routine use, 14-gauge catheters made of Teflon or polyurethane are used in adults. When gravity flow is used, a rate of 2–3 liters per hour can be achieved when fluids are approximately 10 feet higher that the jugular vein. For more rapid flow 10- or 12-gauge catheters with large-bore connecting sets can be used, but it should be remembered that 10-gauge catheters are more thrombogenic. Finally, both jugular veins can be cannulated for increased fluid administration and a pressure bag system or a pump can increase the rate of fluid flow. Peristaltic pumps can cause endothelial damage and increase the risk of thrombosis. See Box 58.3.

Epidemiology

Injuries occurring at equine athletic events are best documented in the Thoroughbred racing industry. Fatal musculoskeletal injuries are the most significant cause of death in horses during training or racing activities. In these horses, the injury is so severe as to warrant euthanasia, usually within 2 days of the injury. Forelimb sesamoid bone fracture, suspensory ligament rupture or third metacarpal fracture represent the most common training or racing-related injuries in Thoroughbred racehorses. Other fatal musculoskeletal injuries include carpal fractures, fractures of the scapula, tibia or pelvis, and first phalangeal fractures.[8] The influence of training intensity on the prevalence of injury is variable. In California, horses with intense racing schedules (35 furlongs of race in two months) were at greater risk of fatal musculoskeletal injury.[9] In contrast, Kentucky horses with injuries had less cumulative high-speed exercise in the months preceding the injury.[10] In one study, horses with toe grabs were at increased risk for fatal musculoskeletal injury, specifically suspensory apparatus failure or condylar fractures.[11] In one study, pre-race examination findings, particularly abnormalities of the suspensory ligament, were highly associated with an increased risk of injury during racing.[12] Table 58.5 describes the current recommended treatment, and prognosis of common injuries in the athletic horse.

Table 58.4 Fluid properties and dosages used for resuscitation in the horse

FLUID	PROPERTIES	DOSAGES
Lactated Ringer's	Crystalloid	Shock: 60 mL/kg
Hypertonic saline	Crystalloid	4 mL/kg rapidly; follow with isotonic fluids
Hetastarch	Synthetic colloid	4 mL/kg rapidly; do not exceed 10 mL/kg

Box 58.3 Materials needed for high-volume fluid therapy in field situations in horses

Catheters
- 12- or 14-gauge, cm
- Large-bore extension set

Administration set
- Coiled set
- Pressure bag

Fluids
- Balanced electrolyte solutions, 5 liters

Table 58.5 Selected traumatic injuries, recommended treatment and prognosis in adult horses

INJURY	RECOMMENDED TREATMENT	PROGNOSIS
Coffin bone fracture	Corrective shoeing or internal fixation	Extra-articular: good Articular: guarded
P2 fracture	Pastern arthrodesis	Good to guarded
P1 fracture	Internal fixation	Non-displaced: good Displaced or comminuted: guarded
Sesamoid fracture		
Apical	Surgical: extraction	Good
Midbody	Surgical: internal fixation	Guarded
Basilar	Medical or surgical	Guarded to poor
Comminuted/biaxial	Medical or surgical	Poor
Sagittal	Medical or surgical	Poor
Cannon bone fracture	Internal fixation	Guarded to poor depending on degree of comminution
Carpal fracture	Arthroscopic removal or internal fixation	Good for small fracture; guarded for large fracture; poor if carpal instability
Radius fracture	Hairline: stall rest Displaced: internal fixation	Hairline, non-displaced: good if no displacement occurs Displaced: grave

Continued

Table 58.5 Continued

INJURY	RECOMMENDED TREATMENT	PROGNOSIS
Olecranon fracture	Non-articular: stall rest Articular: internal fixation	Good unless extreme comminution or open
Humeral fracture	If >200 kg, stall rest If <200 kg, internal fixation	Guarded. Risk for contralateral laminitis if stall rest. Implant failure rate high with internal fixation
Scapular fracture		
Supraglenoid tubercle	Non-displaced: medical Displaced: surgical	Guarded
Body/neck	Surgical	Poor
Hock fractures		
Calcaneus	Large fragment: internal fixation Small or comminuted fractures: medical	Guarded Guarded
Tibial fracture	Hairline: stall rest Displaced: internal fixation	Hairline, non-displaced: good if no displacement occurs Displaced: grave
Femoral fracture	If >200 kg, stall rest If <200 kg, internal fixation	Guarded. Risk for contralateral laminitis if stall rest. Implant failure rate high with internal fixation
Patellar fracture	Fragmentation: arthroscopic removal Sagittal or comminuted fracture: internal fixation	Guarded to good Guarded
Luxations: hock, fetlock	Reduction and external immobilization	Good for light exercise if no articular injury

References

1. Hubbell JA, Hinchcliff KW, Muir WW, et al. Cardiorespiratory and metabolic effects of walking, standing, and standing with a splint during the recuperative period from maximal exercise in horses. Am J Vet Res 1997;58:1003–9.
2. Kohn CW, Hinchcliff KW, McKeever KH. Evaluation of washing with cold water to facilitate heat dissipation in horses exercised in hot, humid conditions. Am J Vet Res 1999;60:299–305.
3. Hubbell JA, Hinchcliff KW, Schmall LM, et al. Anesthetic, cardiorespiratory, and metabolic effects of four intravenous anesthetic regimens induced in horses immediately after maximal exercise. Am J Vet Res 2000;61:1545–52.
4. Bramlage L. Current concept of emergency first aid treatment and transportation of equine fracture patients. Compend Contin Educ Pract Vet 1983;5:S564–74.
5. Tennent-Brown BS. Interpreting lactate measurement in critically ill horses: diagnosis, treatment, and prognosis. Compend Contin Educ Vet 2012;34:E1–6.
6. Jones PA, Bain FT, Byars TD, et al. Effect of hydroxyethyl starch infusion on colloid oncotic pressure in hypoproteinemic horses. J Am Vet Med Assoc 2001;218:1130–5.
7. Jones PA, Tomasic M, Gentry PA. Oncotic, hemodilutional, and hemostatic effects of isotonic saline and hydroxyethyl starch solutions in clinically normal ponies. Am J Vet Res 1997;58:541–8.
8. Estberg L, Stover SM, Gardner IA, et al. Fatal musculoskeletal injuries incurred during racing and training in thoroughbreds. J Am Vet Med Assoc 1996;208:92–6.
9. Estberg L, Stover SM, Gardner IA, et al. Relationship between race start characteristics and risk of catastrophic injury in thoroughbreds: 78 cases (1992). J Am Vet Med Assoc 1998;212:544–9.
10. Cohen ND, Berry SM, Peloso JG, et al. Association of high-speed exercise with racing injury in thoroughbreds. J Am Vet Med Assoc 2000;216:1273–8.
11. Kane AJ, Stover SM, Gardner IA, et al. Hoof size, shape, and balance as possible risk factors for catastrophic musculoskeletal injury of Thoroughbred racehorses. Am J Vet Res 1998;59:1545–52.
12. Cohen ND, Mundy GD, Peloso JG, et al. Results of physical inspection before races and race-related characteristics and their association with musculoskeletal injuries in Thoroughbreds during races. J Am Vet Med Assoc 1999;215:654–61.

Reproductive management of the athletic horse

59

Laura C. Nath

CHAPTER CONTENTS

Introduction

Reproductive management of performance horses involves control of sex hormone related behavioral problems, management of mares and stallions to enhance their reproductive efficiency during and subsequent to their athletic careers and consideration of the effects of common practices on future reproductive function.

The mare

Normal estrus

The mare is seasonally polyestrus. The proportion of cycling mares is highest in the summer months in both the Northern and Southern Hemispheres. However, a small fraction of mares will continue to cycle throughout the year.[1,2] During winter, most mares are in a reproductively quiescent state, with small inactive ovaries. Winter anestrus is characterized by reduced pituitary production of follicle stimulating hormone (FSH) and luteinizing hormone (LH) and reduced secretion of hypothalamic gonadotrophin-releasing hormone (GnRH). After the winter solstice, increasing hours of daylight result in an increase in production and secretion of GnRH and a resultant increase in the pituitary hormones FSH and LH.[3] Most mares will enter a phase of transition between winter anestrus and normal cyclicity known as vernal transition. This phase is dominated by rises in FSH and waves of follicular development which are not accompanied by ovulation.[1,2] Vernal transition can persist for many weeks in which large follicles develop and the mare demonstrates fluctuations in sexual receptivity. Once the first ovulation occurs, mares usually resume normal cyclicity until the end of the physiologic breeding season. The characteristics of the autumnal transition from cyclicity to anestrus are similar to the vernal transition.

Estrus is the behavioral expression of sexual receptivity in the mare, and typically accompanies the follicular phase of the reproductive cycle.[4] Diestrus is the phase of the cycle in which the mare is not receptive, and typically accompanies the luteal phase of the cycle.[4] In normally cycling mares, each ovulation occurs approximately 21 days apart, and mares typically display estrus for 5–9 days, with ovulation occurring 1–2 days prior to the cessation of estrus.[2,4–6] Hormonal concentrations of estradiol and luteinizing hormone rise during estrus.[7] Serum progesterone concentration rises within 24–36 hours after ovulation and causes cessation of estrous behavior.[6] In the absence of progesterone, estradiol-17β is responsible for the behavioral and physiological changes that accompany estrus in mares.[4,8–10]

Rarely, seasonally anovulatory mares, ovariectomized mares and pregnant mares have been reported to show behavioral signs of estrus which is thought to arise from the effects of hormones secreted by the adrenal cortex.[11,12]

Suppression of estrus in mares

Owners or trainers might seek advice of a veterinarian in managing estrus in mares. Estrus is perceived to impede performance or disrupt training through the presence of back or hindquarter pain, increased aggression, ears back and tail swishing during riding or handling, submissive behavior or overt expression of estrus, such as winking, crouching and urinating.[13] It must be recognized that some problems which are perceived to be associated with estrus are not estrous behaviors. In some mares, problems attributed to the reproductive hormones are actually observed in the diestrous phase of the cycle.[14] In many situations, the manner in which the problem behavior is expressed is not specific to estrus and could be confused with other problems such as lameness, lack of training, or poor environmental enrichment. Behaviors which can easily be confused with estrus expression include submissive behaviors, urogenital discomfort and stallion-like behavior.[15] In estrus, mares usually express behaviors towards stallions, but these can also be directed at geldings. Typical signs include a relaxed, raised tail, ears neutral or forwards, leaning inwards, adoption of breeding posture, urinating and clitoral winking (see Fig. 59.1).[8] Submissive behaviors are distinct from estrous behaviors in that they typically involve leaning away from perceived threats, urinating and swishing the tail.

Some mares experience pain in the peri-ovulatory period, and this can range in intensity from mild discomfort on manual rectal palpation of the ovary, to back pain or overt colic.[8,16]

In women, changing levels of estrogen and progesterone within the menstrual cycle can influence non-reproductive body systems such as the musculoskeletal system. These effects include changes in pain perception, muscle recovery and tendon distensibility.[17–19] Therefore it is plausible that performance in mares could be affected by the stage of the reproductive cycle. Research looking specifically at this area in mares is lacking.

Mares presented for estrus-associated changes in behavior or athletic performance should be examined in order to confirm the diagnosis prior to initiating treatment. Historical details of interest would include a description of the perceived abnormality, the timing and duration of the abnormality, and any association with time of year. Most mares will cease cycling through the winter months, so abnormal behaviors observed during winter are unlikely to be associated with estrus. Signs might be more prominent in spring as mares are undergoing transition from winter anestrus to estrus.

The following procedures should be considered as part of a veterinary examination:

- general physical examination with particular consideration to ruling out other causes of a change in performance (musculoskeletal pain or disease involving another body system)
- observation of mare behavior when exposed to an intact stallion
- transrectal palpation and ultrasonographic examination of the genital tract at a time when the mare is showing behavior suggestive of estrus
- measurement of blood concentrations of reproductive hormones such as progesterone, estradiol, testosterone and inhibin. This is particularly important if a granulosa cell tumour is a differential diagnosis for behavioral problems.

Diagnostic confirmation is reliant on observing typical estrous behavior along with ultrasonographic and biochemical features consistent with estrus. Ultrasonographic features of estrus are described in detail elsewhere, but generally include the presence of one or more dominant follicles (>25 mm diameter) on the ovary, the absence of a functional corpus luteum on the ovary, and uterine edema with observation of uterine folding (see Figs 59.2 and 59.3).[4] Rectal palpation would be expected to reveal a soft cervix and this would also be visible on vaginal speculum examination. Reliably, progesterone will be <1 ng/ml in a mare in estrus and >1 ng/ml in diestrus. Blood concentrations for some hormones can vary widely depending on the assay used and the time of day the sample was taken. A concentration of estradiol in the range 20–45 pg/ml is consistent with estrus. An inhibin concentration >0.7 ng/ml or a testosterone concentration >100 pg/ml are consistent with a granulosa cell tumour.

Pharmacologic suppression of estrus

An ideal estrus control product should be highly effective at suppressing signs of estrus, easily administered, rapidly absorbed, require infrequent dosing and be safe for both animals and people.[20] It should have no residual effect on fertility, should not affect

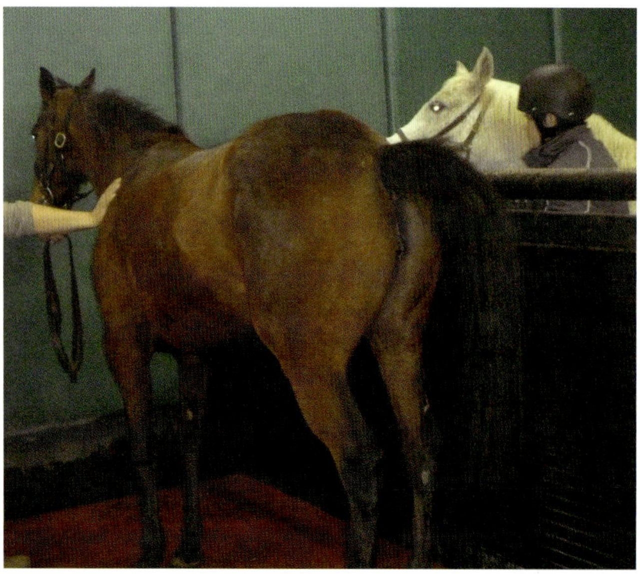

Fig 59.1 Mare in estrous displaying a typical posture. The ears are attentive, tail raised and hind end leaning in towards the stallion. Frequently, mares will also display clitoral winking and urinating.

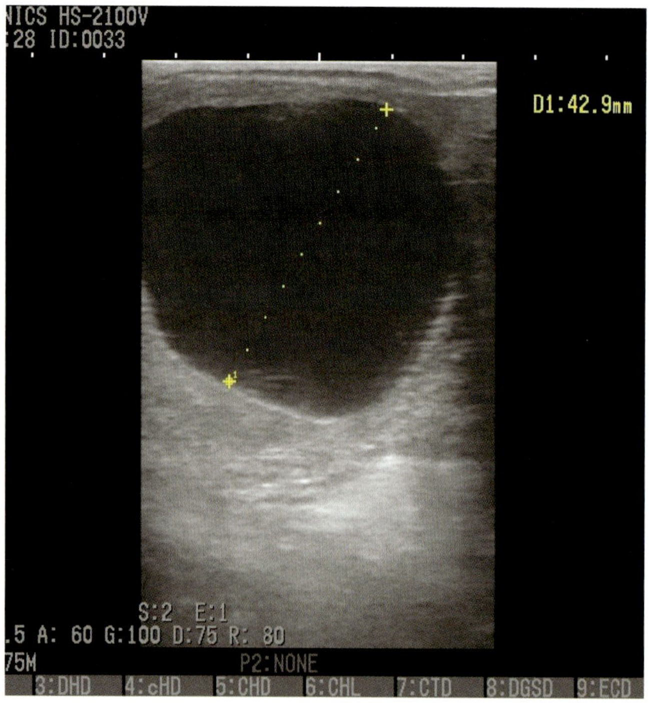

Fig 59.2 A large pre-ovulatory follicle measuring 42.9 mm in diameter.

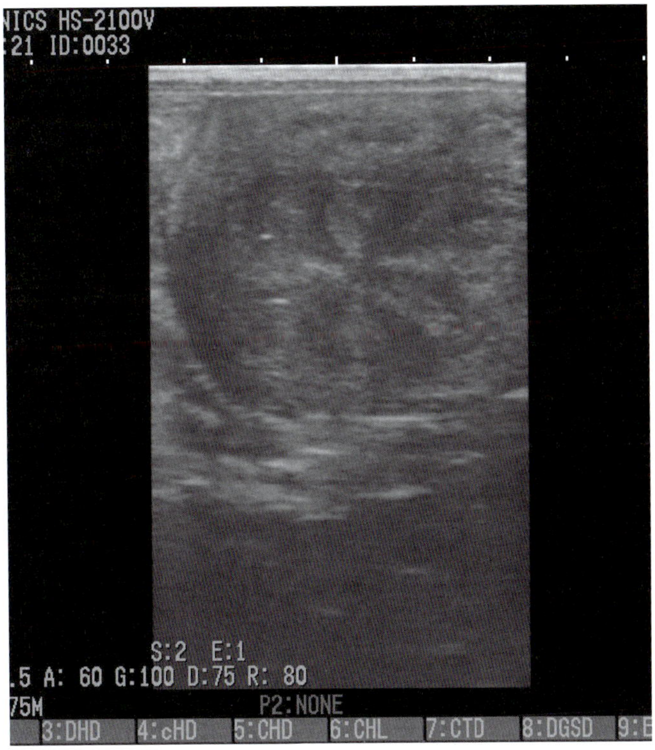

Fig 59.3 Typical appearance of the uterine horn of a mare in estrus. There is endometrial folding due to edema which gives the appearance of 'cut orange segments'or 'cycle spokes'.

performance, and should allow treated animals to begin a breeding career following withdrawal of treatment. There should ideally be no restriction on use of the product by rules controlling athletic horse events. The FEI publishes a list of prohibited or restricted substances at www.fei.org. Advice should be sought from other jurisdictions as to their rules for racing or competition as these can vary widely between countries and between different organizing bodies within the same country.

As described, ovarian function and expression of reproductive behavior are based on feedback mechanisms within the hypothalamo–pituitary–ovarian axis. Manipulation of the various points within this axis can allow for suppression of estrous behavior alone or both estrous behavior and ovulation. The primary methods for suppression of behavior include administration of exogenous progesterone or progestins, extending the duration of corpora lutea function, suppressing ovarian follicular activity and ovariectomy.[15]

Progestagens

Display of estrous behavior in mares is reliant more on the absence of progesterone than on the presence of estrogen.[8,10] Exogenous administration of efficacious progestagens inhibits estrous behavior and delays ovulation.[21,22] Natural progesterone and altrenogest are the progestagens with demonstrated efficacy.[23,24] Many other synthetic progestagens have been proven to not be effective in suppressing estrus or ovulation[21,22] or in maintaining pregnancy.[25–27] The failure of many synthetic progestagens to induce an effect in mares might be due to a lack of binding to progesterone receptors in this species.

Progesterone in oil administered daily at a rate of 100 mg or more is effective in suppressing behavioral signs of estrus in mares.[23] However, the requirement for daily intramuscular injection and the propensity of the formulation to induce injection site reactions renders it impractical for use in performance mares and fillies. Administration of a long-acting, compounded formulation of 1.5 g progesterone maintains serum levels of progesterone above 1.0 ng/ml, sufficient to suppress estrous behavior, for approximately 10 days[28] and a compounded formulation of 600 mg (BioRelease P4 LA300) maintained serum progesterone above 1.0 ng/ml for approximately 7 days.[29] Whilst these formulations show promise in that they alleviate the need for daily injection, consideration should be given to the potential for injection site reactions with repeated use in performance mares.[15,28] Progesterone implants designed for use in other species, such as Synovex S (Fort Dodge Animal Health) designed for use in steers, are unlikely to contain sufficient quantities of progesterone to suppress estrus in mares. The administration of 80 Synovex S pellets, a total dose of 2000 mg progesterone and 200 mg estradiol per mare, did not suppress estrus.[30] Intravaginal progesterone-releasing sponges are effective in suppressing behavioral oestrus in mares and have been used in breeding programs.[31–33] However, in addition to being unsightly and potentially uncomfortable, the devices would need to be replaced weekly and potentially harmful effects of a prolonged intravaginal device on future reproductive potential have not been investigated. Therefore these devices are not recommended for controlling estrous behavior in performance mares.

Altrenogest (Regu-Mate®, Intervet, Millsboro, DE) is a synthetic progestin registered for use in horses for suppressing estrus. It is likely to be the most commonly used pharmacological agent for this purpose across the world. Daily oral administration of altrenogest (0.044 mg/kg) to mares effectively inhibits behavioral estrus.[34] The threshold concentration of altrenogest required to suppress estrous behavior is lower than that required to suppress LH release and ovulation.[22] Continued expression of estrous behavior has been observed in mares treated with altrenogest and this therapeutic failure could be due to incorrect dosing (half-life is short and dosing needs to be at 24-hour intervals not 7 a.m. one day and 7 p.m. the next), failure in administration, errors in estrus detection, treatment during estrus and individual variability in responsiveness to the treatment.

In mares treated for 88 days, altrenogest effectively suppressed estrus with no evidence of adverse effects.[24] Mares receiving long-term altrenogest treatment demonstrated normal fertility when bred following withdrawal of the drug.[24] There is a risk that progestin therapy could promote uterine infection due to maintenance of a closed cervix. Consideration should be given to this potentially adverse effect when administering long-term progestin therapy.

The use of long-acting injectable altrenogest formulations has become popular in some countries for their ease of use and affordability. Several different formulations are available. The BioRelease MP 500 formulation, containing a total of 500 mg of altrenogest, provided the most prolonged suppression of estrus in one study.[22] Mares receiving BioRelease MP 500 ovulated a mean of 33.5 days after luteolysis was induced with prostaglandin $F_{2\alpha}$, compared to 8.8 days in control mares receiving 225 mg or 450 mg of altrenogest, respectively.[22] A further observation in this study was that several mares receiving BioRelease MP 500 did not show estrus at the time of ovulation and for variable periods up to 49 days after injection.[22] When considering the use of altrenogest in performance mares, trainers can be reassured that the product does not have any effect on body mass, condition score or dominance hierarchies, which was used as a model for aggression.[35] Of concern when handling oral formulations of altrenogest, is that the product is readily absorbed through human skin and there are anecdotal reports of the product interfering with the reproductive cycle and lactation in women. Therefore strict recommendations should be made for personnel to wear impervious gloves when handling the product.

Other synthetic progestagens infrequently administered to horses include medroxyprogesterone acetate (Depo-Provera, Pharmacia), hydroxyprogesterone caproate (also labeled as hydroxyprogesterone hexanoate), chlormadinone acetate, norgestomet and melengestrol acetate. Several studies have found medroxyprogesterone acetate ineffective for suppressing estrus[21,22] or for maintaining pregnancy after prostaglandin $F_{2\alpha}$-induced luteolysis.[25] Hydroxyprogesterone caproate/hexanoate failed to maintain pregnancy and did not block the return to estrus in pregnant mares without a functional corpus luteum.[25,26] Limited evidence suggests chlormadinone acetate ineffective for suppression of estrus in mares.[36] Norgestomet is also ineffective for suppressing estrus[37] or maintaining pregnancy.[25] Therefore, the use of these products at the dosages studied cannot be recommended for suppression of estrus in performance mares. Melengestrol acetate, administered orally at a dose rate of 15 or 20 mg once daily did not suppress estrus.[23] However, a more recent study suggested that at a dose rate of 100–150 mg orally once daily, this product could have an effect in mares.[38]

Caution is urged when considering the use of non-registered products in mares for estrus suppression. In most cases scientific assessment of these products has dismissed anecotal claims of efficacy, and there is little or no safety information available.

Pregnancy

Establishment of pregnancy prevents the secretion of prostaglandin $F_{2\alpha}$ from the endometrium, and thus a progesterone-secreting corpus luteum (CL) is maintained on the ovary. Maternal recognition of pregnancy in the mare is reliant on the presence of a mobile embryo within the uterus prior to day 14 post-ovulation. Prolonged luteal function can be maintained despite loss of the pregnancy if the embryo is terminated by manual crushing (via transrectal ultrasonography) on day 16–22 post-ovulation.[39] Following this procedure, the corpus luteum is maintained, and estrus suppressed for at least 60 days.[39] Although this method appears to be highly efficacious, it requires considerable investment in first establishing a pregnancy and might be considered unethical by some horse owners.

Intrauterine balls

Intrauterine balls, made of glass or polypropylene, can mimic the effect of an embryo in stimulating maternal recognition of pregnancy, suppression of prostaglandin $F_{2\alpha}$ and CL maintenance.[40,41] Using aseptic technique, a sterile glass ball (www.glassmarble.com) is manually placed through the cervix into the uterine body within 24 hours after ovulation, when the cervix should still be soft and open, but beginning to close. A 35 mm ball was retained in 12/12 mares, whereas a 25 mm ball was retained in only 6/12 mares.[41] Of 18 mares that retained the ball, estrus was suppressed in 7 (39%).[41] The duration of estrus suppression following placement of the ball ranged from 76 to 109 days.[41] This study also observed spontaneous prolonged luteal function, which is a well-recognized phenomena in mares, in 4/50 control cycles.[41] Removal of the glass ball is recommended when estrus suppression is no longer needed. The ball can be retrieved via a combination of per rectum and per vagina manipulation. Water-filled polypropylene intrauterine balls were also effective in prolonging the luteal phase in 9/12 mares.[40] Evidence suggests that placement of these intrauterine devices does not have an adverse effect on fertility.[40,41] However, there are anecdotal reports of the marbles fracturing in the uterus, with potentially severe consequences.[15] Placement of the intrauterine devices could be a relatively inexpensive, although somewhat unreliable, non-pharmacological method of long-term estrus suppression in mares.

Oxytocin

Administration of 60 IU oxytocin IM twice daily in early diestrus (days 7–14 after ovulation) induces a prolonged luteal phase and maintains serum progesterone above 1.0 ng/ml for greater than 30 days.[42] The exact mechanism behind the effectiveness of this protocol is not certain, but it is thought to block the oxytocin-induced prostaglandin $F_{2\alpha}$ release from the endometrium which normally induces luteolysis.[42] Vanderwall also reports that once-daily intramuscular administration of 60 IU oxytocin during this phase of the cycle is as effective as the twice-daily protocol first described.[15,42] Whilst the effect on estrus behavior was not studied directly, the endogenous progesterone levels maintained were high enough to suppress behavioral estrus. The researchers also suggested that the prolonged luteal phase could be terminated by the administration of prostaglandin $F_{2\alpha}$.[42] No adverse effects were observed in any of the mares receiving oxytocin for prolongation of the luteal phase. However, consideration should be given to the propensity of oxytocin to induce mild colic in horses,[43] and other effects on smooth and striated muscle. Notwithstanding, this protocol could be considered as a long-term method of suppressing estrus in performance mares.

Intrauterine oil

A recent study, designed to investigate the role of estrogen on maternal recognition of pregnancy, revealed that infusion of plant oil into the uterine lumen in late diestrus prolonged the luteal phase.[44] The effect was most reliable when performed on day 10 post-ovulation, and infusion of a 1 ml dose of either fractionated coconut oil with estradiol (10 mg/ml), fractionated coconut oil or peanut oil prolonged the luteal phase in 11/12 treated mares.[44] In mares which responded to the treatment, endogenous progesterone concentrations were maintained above 1 ng/ml for 30 days, at which point luteolysis was achieved by the administration of prostaglandin $F_{2\alpha}$. The mechanism by which plant oils suppressed luteolysis is not clear. The authors proposed that fatty acids present in the oil interrupted prostaglandin synthesis or release from the endometrium.[44] The failure of mineral oil to induce a similar response suggests that a physical effect of the oil in the endometrium was not responsible for prolonged luteostasis.[44] No adverse effects of the infusions was observed and this appears to be a promising method of suppressing estrus in mares.

hCG (diestrous ovulation)

A prolonged luteal phase can be achieved by the administration of 3000 IU hCG when a follicle >30 mm is observed in the diestrous phase of the cycle.[45] This protocol induces a diestrous ovulation and the resultant corpus luteum is too immature to respond to prostaglandin normally released from the endometrium in the absence of a pregnancy approximately 14 days after the estrous ovulation. However, this protocol relies on the development of a large follicle in diestrus, which occurs infrequently. Therefore it is likely to take several cycles before the protocol can be applied. For this reason, the administration of hCG to induce diestrous ovulation appears to be an impractical method for suppressing estrus in mares.

Follicular downregulation

Interestingly, follicular downregulation can be achieved through administration of a GnRH analogue, or through immunization against endogenous GnRH. Both of these methods result in a down-regulation of endogenous follicle stimulating hormone and consequently, a disruption of folliculogenesis. Administration of the GnRH analogue, deslorelin acetate (Ovuplant®; Peptech Animal Health, NSW, Australia; Fort Dodge Animal Health, Fort Dodge, IA) occasionally induces prolonged anovulatory periods in mares.[46,47] However, even the administration of multiple implants does not reliably prevent follicular activity. This method requires refining before it can be recommended for estrus suppression in mares.

A more reliable effect can be achieved through immunization against GnRH. Antibodies produced in response to the vaccine prevent endogenous GnRH from binding to receptors in the pituitary.[8] Consequently, there is a lack of follicular development and an induced state of anestrus.[8] A commercial vaccine registered as an aid in the control of estrus and estrus-related behavior in fillies and mares not intended for breeding is available in Australia (Equity®, Pfizer Animal Health). For primary vaccination it is recommended that initial vaccination is followed by a booster 4 weeks later. This protocol resulted in a reduction in 17β-estradiol and progesterone, and suppression of estrous behavior for at least three months following primary vaccination.[48] Other studies have confirmed that GnRH immunization effectively suppresses reproductive cyclicity.[49,50] However, some mares continue to demonstrate estrus behavior in the face of their anovulatory state.[49] In most treated mares, primary vaccination induces a response for approximately six months.[49,50] Of concern, is a report that mares retrospectively identified to have received the vaccine on at least two occasions during their racing careers, failed to cycle for consecutive seasons when they began their breeding careers.[51] This concession is suggested by the manufacturer's warning that the vaccine should not be used in horses intended for breeding. It does, however, present an efficacious means of suspending reproductive cyclicity in performance mares and fillies.

Ovariectomy

Bilateral ovariectomy is occasionally performed in performance mares to prevent behavioral estrus. However the procedure is not always successful in achieving this outcome, most likely because the behavior is not hormonal in origin.[8,52,53] Owners of mares with behavioral estrus problems reported the behavioral problems were alleviated after bilateral ovariectomy by colpotomy in 14/17 mares. Similar results were observed with an improvement in behavior in 19/23 mares after laparoscopic bilateral ovariectomy.[52] Careful case selection is required to maintain positive results with this treatment. If the problem behaviour is closely correlated with estrus (as confirmed by ultrasonographic examination of the ovaries) or absence of the problem behavior during winter anestrus, then the above studies suggest bilateral ovariectomy could be a viable, irreversible treatment. A positive response to reliable medical treatments such as progesterone, altrenogest or GnRH vaccination would give further support to a likely positive response to ovariectomy.

Anabolic steroids

Anabolic steroids remain in widespread use in many countries, despite regulations penalizing their detection. Steroids are likely to be administered to mares and fillies for their perceived effect in increasing condition.[54] Anabolic steroids administered to mares and fillies have a masculinization effect in appearance and behavior, which persists for several months following cessation of treatment.[55–58] Administration of anabolic steroids to mares commonly results in a dose-dependent reduction in ovarian size and cessation of estrous cyclicity, with a return to normal cycles occurring after the treatment is withdrawn.[55] Reduced fertility has been observed experimentally in mares receiving anabolic steroid treatment; however steroid treatment of mares during their racing careers did not appear to affect fertility when they commenced breeding.

Control of reproductive behavior in the stallion

The most important aspects of controlling behavior in stallions are sound training techniques and good handling and management.[59] Stallions that are not responsive to these methods might benefit from castration or pharmacologic modification of behavior. Veterinary interventions should always be combined with revised training, management and handling techniques when attempting to modify stallion behavior.

Surgical castration

A major indication for castration is to decrease or prevent aggressive or sexual behavior in male horses not intended for breeding.[60] Castration can be performed in the standing, sedated horse using local anesthesia or in recumbent horses under general anesthesia. Detailed descriptions of the procedure and options for anesthesia and restraint are provided elsewhere.[60–62] The choice of method and restraint are influenced by many factors including owner and veterinarian experience and preference, horse behavior and temperament, location of the testicles, weather, available equipment and facilities or surgical environment.

Most commonly, castration is performed when the horse is 1–2 years old.[60] Castrating at a very young age could present an increased risk for complication, as the inguinal rings are not yet adequately closed.[60] Reasons for delaying castration once it has become clear that the horse is not suitable for breeding are limited, but in some cases owners or trainers believe the horse will benefit from the ongoing effect of testicular hormones. In cattle and goats, castration results in slower daily weight gain and poorer feed conversion efficiency as compared to age-matched uncastrated controls.[63–66] Castration of male deer induces a change in muscle distribution, with increased hindquarter muscling and reduced forequarter muscling as compared to intact males.[67] In most domestic species, equivalent weights at slaughtering are achieved in castrated animals; however, there is a higher proportion of body fat as compared to intact males.[63–67] The influence of testosterone on growth potential or musculoskeletal development in male horses is not clear. Owners or trainers occasionally request castration in an attempt to reduce weight gain, which could aid in managing musculo-skeletal soundness. Children experience a pubertal growth spurt associated with a rise in circulating sex steroid concentrations.[68] It is not clear whether horses experience a similar pubertal growth phase and at what age this possibly occurs. Limited studies in dogs have not consistently identified a pubertal growth spurt.[69] In male dogs, prepubertal castration delays physeal closure and increases bone length.[69] The rate of radial distal physeal closure is not different between colts, geldings and fillies.[70,71]

Castration is effective in modifying male behavior, although geldings can continue to display aggression and male sexual behavioral traits including teasing, erection, mounting and copulation. There was no difference in manifestations of sexual or aggressive behavior in geldings castrated at less than two or greater than three years of age.[72] These findings indicate that circulating sex steroids are only partly responsible for sexual or aggressive behavior in male horses, and emphasize the need for effective training techniques and considered management and handling to minimize poor behavior in both stallions and geldings.

Pharmacologic modification of male behavior

Administration of progestagens is the most commonly used pharmacologic method for modifying male horse behavior.[59,73] The aim of progestagen administration is to downregulate the pituitary–gonadal axis and reduce circulating levels of testicular hormones,[59] thereby minimizing the influence these hormones have over male behavior. Anecdotal evidence suggests that progestagen administration to male horses suppresses sexual and aggressive behavior and has a general calming effect.[59] Treatment of stallions with 0.044 mg/kg altrenogest daily for 30 days did not affect sperm production or measures of sperm quality.[74] Nor was there any demonstrable change in most behavioral parameters, other than time to mount and ejaculate which was increased in altrenogest-treated stallions, but returned to normal length within 30 days of cessation of treatment.[74] Reductions in circulating concentrations of LH, testosterone, inhibin and estrogen conjugates were detected in altrenogest-treated stallions, all of which also returned to pre-treatment values within 30 days of cessation of treatment.[74] An increased dose of altrenogest (0.88 mg/kg), orally daily for 150 days, resulted in marked changes to fertility parameters, with reductions in libido, serum concentrations of testosterone and luteinizing hormone, total scrotal width, and sperm production and increased sperm abnormalities.[75] Similar results were observed in stallions treated at this dose (0.088 mg/kg) daily for only 8 weeks.[76] In addition, treatment at this dose for 240 days caused a reduction in sperm motility.[75] Adverse effects of progestagen treatment on sperm production are expected to be reversible; however, this has not been adequately investigated. Administration of progestagens at relatively high doses, compared to what is required in mares, could reduce aggressive and sexual behavior in stallions.[77]

Phenothiazine derivatives are occasionally used in stallions as aids for behavior modification.[59] They are no longer recommended for use in intact males because of the unsubstantiated but persisting perception of a small but important risk of penile paralysis and paraphimosis.[59]

Nutritional supplementation with L-tryptophan, a serotonin precursor, at a rate of 1–2 grams orally once or twice daily, could aid in modifying problem behavior and have a calming effect on stallions.[59] Under development is a calming pheromone which could also become useful as a long-term method of modifying problem behavior in stallions.[59]

Immunomodulation of male fertility and behavior

Similar to mares, the pituitary–gonadal axis in stallions can also be interrupted by downregulating GnRH production. This can be achieved through the administration of GnRH agonists, GnRH antagonists, or immunization against GnRH.[78] Of these available methods, immunization against GnRH appears to be the most practical. However, there is currently no vaccine registered for this purpose in male horses. Immunization of intact male horses against GnRH causes reduced serum testosterone concentration, scrotal width, sperm production and adversely affects sperm motility and morphology.[79] Young colts also show reductions in male sexual behavior and aggression, although these behavioral effects are less noticeable in mature stallions.[80,81] Treatment effects of these products appear to be reversible over time in most stallions.[79] However, as is the case in mares, the potential for some individuals to experience profound and prolonged pituitary downregulation after vaccination precludes the use of these agents in horses intended for breeding.

Combining breeding and athletic careers

Developments in assisted reproductive technologies have allowed increased flexibility in managing the breeding careers of mares and stallions while still performing as athletes.

Stallion

In all breeds except Thoroughbreds, there has been a progressive increase in the proportion of mares bred using chilled or frozen semen artificial insemination (AI). Advances in techniques for producing and managing chilled and frozen semen and improved pregnancy and foaling rates achieved with these techniques have increased the demand for such services. The capacity to store and transport semen allows for a stallion to commence a breeding career with relatively little disruption to athletic pursuits. Higher sperm production is observed in the natural breeding season, late spring to early autumn. However, good-quality semen can be collected from fertile stallions for processing at any time of year. The likely length of interruption to the stallion's athletic schedule varies depending on the procedures required. Evaluating a stallion for breeding soundness could take as little at 24 hours; however, considerable time can be lost if the stallion needs to be trained to mount a phantom mare, and breed an artificial vagina (sometimes greater than a week with training sessions taking place twice daily). Following this, stallions can be collected every other day for maximal harvest of sperm output. The number of insemination doses obtained per ejaculate will also vary depending on the individual stallion and the intended use of the semen. In general, a single ejaculate could provide 5–15 insemination doses. Therefore a freezing schedule typically lasts 2–4 weeks (after the stallion has been trained) to obtain approximately 50 insemination doses. Low-dose insemination techniques have also been developed to maximize the number of mares that can become pregnant when sperm numbers are limited. It is also important to mention that the techniques required, particularly for harvesting, managing and handling frozen semen, are highly specialized and better results will be obtained by experienced personnel dealing with such techniques on a regular basis. Training techniques providing clear distinction between performing and breeding may help to ensure that periodic breeding opportunities do not disrupt the stallion's athletic performance or general behavior.[82]

Individual stallion semen quality is one of the most important factors influencing the success of an artificial insemination program and a breeding soundness examination should be performed on any stallion being considered as a semen donor in an AI program. It has been estimated that 20% of stallions produce semen that freezes well, 60% produce semen that freezes adequately and 20% produce semen that freezes poorly.[83] The techniques required for chilling semen are less complicated, and for this reason a greater proportion of stallions will be suitable for breeding mares with chilled semen than frozen semen. Detailed descriptions of procedures and techniques involved in breeding soundness examination of stallions can be found elsewhere as well as discussion of factors influencing semen production and quality.[84,85]

It is particularly important to be aware of individual variability in fertility of thawed-frozen stallion semen, even in stallions that have excellent fertility when bred naturally or using chilled or fresh AI.[86] For an individual stallion, results of laboratory analysis of thawed-frozen semen give some indication of semen quality; however, often a test mating of a small number of mares (5–10) is required to prove fertility of the ejaculates. The accepted standard pregnancy rates with the use of frozen semen are 30–40% per cycle. This compares to 65–75% per cycle when using chilled AI or natural service.[87,88]

Mares

Developments in assisted reproductive technology have also had a dramatic impact on breeding options available to mares during their athletic careers.

Pregnancy

Impaired fertility in exercised mares appears to be mediated through altered hormonal profile,[89] reduced uterine blood flow as a result of redistribution to muscle, reduction of available glucose due to increased metabolic demands and exercise-induced rise in core body temperature.[90,91] Altered follicular dynamics, characterized by increased inter-ovulatory interval, increased number of dominant follicles, and a reduction in peak serum LH concentration, are observed in exercised mares.[89] Embryo recovery rates and embryo quality are poorer in exercised than non-exercised mares.[91,92] There is little information on the effect of different exercise levels in mares on risk of pregnancy loss. The first two-thirds of pregnancy in the mare are characterized by little or no increase in nutrient requirements or bodyweight over the non-pregnant state. Fetal heart rate does not demonstrate a change during moderate maternal exercise, which suggests that the fetus is not stressed by this activity.[93] Information in horses on the effect of pregnancy on performance are lacking. Studies in women report a progressive decline in all aspects of athletic performance during pregnancy.[94] A similar decline could be expected in mares and fillies.

Embryo transfer

Use and availability of embryo transfer (ET) in mares has expanded, particularly with the development of techniques for safe transport and storage of embryos. Embryo viability can now be maintained when transported from the site of collection to another facility for transfer or frozen storage. This removes the necessity for donor mares to be maintained at the same site as recipients and allows veterinarians with limited facilities to harvest embryos for transfer at a specialist facility. Embryo transfer techniques have changed little in the past decades and are described elsewhere.[95,96] Breed society restrictions vary, with most societies other than Quarter Horses restricting the number of foal registrations each year to one per mare.[96] Thoroughbred foals produced by embryo transfer are currently not registrable. Embryo transfer can allow multiple foals to be produced by performance mares whilst they continue to train and compete.[97] In seasonal sports such as polo, mares experiencing a break from competition can undergo several cycles at an embryo transfer facility, allowing multiple embryos to be harvested. The lack of a reliable, commercially viable method for superovulating donor mares continues to be a major limitation to embryo recovery rates.[96] Embryo harvest rates after a flushing procedure are excellent, such that it is assumed that any embryo present within the uterus will be recovered with standard techniques.[98] With good technique, attrition rates of embryos after harvest are small. Expected pregnancy rates in recipient mares at 12 days after ovulation following standard procedures are 90%, and at 30 days 85%.[98] When very small thawed-frozen embryos (morula or early blastocyst) are transferred, pregnancy rates in recipient mares are 60%.[96] However, attrition rates increase if the embryos are larger than this, with pregnancy rates in recipients of only 10–20% following transfer.[96]

The procedure for breeding embryo donor mares does not change from that used to establish pregnancy. Natural service or artificial insemination with either cooled or frozen semen can be employed. The highest embryo recovery rates are expected from mares bred with fresh or cooled semen and an embryo will be recovered from young fertile mares approximately 65–75% of the time using these techniques. Ultrasonography must be used to accurately record the day of ovulation to allow synchronization with a recipient mare and dictate the ideal day for the embryo flush procedure to be performed. The flush procedure is performed on day 6–8 after ovulation. If the embryo is to be frozen, the flush should be performed on day 6.[96] Mares are typically short-cycled with prostaglandin after the procedure, which allows for the procedure to be repeated in approximately 14–21 days and prevents inadvertent pregnancy in the donor mare.

Other assisted reproductive techniques

Standard in vitro fertilization procedures are not successful in horses; however, other assisted reproductive techniques such as intracytoplasmic sperm injection (ICSI) and oocyte transfer (OT) are available commercially at a limited number of equine facilities. Oocytes are generally collected by transvaginal ultrasound-guided follicular aspiration, from either immature or mature follicles.[96] In vivo matured oocytes are harvested a few hours prior to the expected time of ovulation. Pregnancy rates following in vitro maturation are poorer; however, this technique has the advantage of being able to be performed after the harvest of ovaries from recently deceased mares.[96] Oocyte harvest may be combined with intracytoplasmic sperm injection (ICSI) to circumvent the requirement for sperm capacitation and sperm motility. The use of ICSI or low-dose insemination with sex-sorted semen provides the added option of obtaining sex-selected offspring from mares during their competitive career.[99]

Reasonable pregnancy rates can be achieved by surgical transfer of invivo matured oocytes into the oviduct of a recipient mare.[96] The recipient mare can then be bred by either natural service or artificial insemination or spermatozoa can be directly transferred into the oviduct at the same time the oocyte transfer is performed.[96]

Other assisted reproductive techniques that can offer potential in future equine breeding programs include the freezing of oocytes, cloning and production of transgenic animals.[96]

Management of performance horses to optimize future reproductive potential

Wider consideration of the impact of treatments given to horses during their racing careers on future breeding potential is needed. The potential adverse responses to anabolic steroids and GnRH vaccine in particular, require attention. Anabolic steroids can interfere with estrous cyclicity in females and cause a reduction in testis size, sperm production and sperm quality in stallions.[55,100,101] Limited data in horses suggest that the effects of anabolic steroids are generally reversible following cessation of treatment. The long-term effect of administering many anabolic steroids in combination, or using these products outside the manufacturers' recommendations, remains unknown. Chronic misuse of anabolic steroids by human athletes can have serious and long-term effects on fertility and general health.[102]

In mares and fillies, careful application of a caslick surgery (suturing of the dorsal commissure of the vulval lips) can protect against adverse effects of chronic pneumovagina and improve fertility when mares are retired to stud. Conversely, suturing the vulval lips too far ventrally can interfere with urine flow and cause chronic reflux of urine into the anterior vagina. This can lead to chronic urine-induced inflammation involving the vagina, cervix and uterus.

In stallions, the general management, handling and discipline of reproductive behavior whilst in a performance career will influence expression of reproductive behaviors when the stallion commences a breeding career. Overzealous or inappropriate discipline can ruin the ability of a stallion to express reproductive behaviors and seriously damage his potential as a breeding prospect. Improper application of a stallion ring to prevent erections can cause penile scarring and interfere with the ability of the stallion to achieve and maintain a normal erection. Careful attention to the manner in which a stallion is introduced into a breeding program and consideration of his age, libido and the environment to which he is exposed are important to maintain his cooperation in the program.

The aspects of veterinary management pertaining to reproduction in performance horses involve not only control of reproductive behaviors but also mindfulness of the current and future reproductive potential of the horse. There are many methods available for suppression of reproductive behaviors in both female and male horses which allows for selection of the most appropriate method to suit both the client and the individual animal. Current practices need to be adapted to protect the breeding potential and maximize subsequent fertility of performance horses. Whilst the administration of various drugs such as anabolic steroids and GnRH agonists might be appropriate in some circumstances, their effect on the future reproductive potential of the horse must be considered. Application of assisted reproductive technologies can maximize reproductive potential by allowing for a greater number of foals to be produced from each animal. These technologies allow horses undertaking a performance career to concurrently commence breeding. With application of these technologies in the future, we could see mares and stallions competing against their own sons and daughters.

With thanks to Nigel R. Perkins, who created the original chapter in the first edition. The author also wishes to acknowledge the assistance of Oliver Pynn in acquiring images.

References

1. Dowsett KF, Knott LM, Woodward RA, et al. Seasonal variation in the estrous cycle of mares in the subtropics. Theriogenology 1993;39(3):631–53.
2. Ginther OJ. Occurrence of anestrus, estrus, diestrus, and ovulation over a 12-month period in mares. Am J Vet Res 1974;35(9):1173–9.
3. Hart PJ, Squires EL, Imel KJ, et al. Seasonal variation in hypothalamic content of gonadotropin-releasing hormone (GnRH), pituitary receptors for GnRH, and pituitary content of luteinizing hormone and follicle-stimulating hormone in the mare. Biol Reprod 1984;30(5):1055–62.
4. McCue PM, Scoggin CF, Lindholm ARG. Estrus. In: McKinnon AO, Squires EL, Vaala WE, et al, editors. Equine Reproduction. West Sussex: Blackwell Publishing; 2011. p. 1716–27.
5. Crowell-Davis SL. Sexual behavior of mares. Horm Behav 2007;52(1): 12–17.
6. Ginther OJ. Reproductive Biology of the Mare: Basic and Applied Aspects. Cross Plains, WI: Equiservices; 1992.
7. Medan MS. Plasma concentrations of Ir-inhibin, inhibin A, inhibin pro-alpha C, FSH, and estradiol-17 beta during estrous cycle in mares and their relationship with follicular growth. Endocrine 2004;25(1):7–14.
8. Pryor P, Tibary A. Management of estrus in the performance mare. Clin Tech Equine Pract 2005;4(3):197–209.
9. Asa CS, Goldfoot DA, Garcia MC, et al. The effect of estradiol and progesterone on the sexual behavior of ovariectomized mares. Physiol Behav 1984;33:681–6.
10. Munro CD, Renton JP, Butcher R. The control of oestrous behaviour in the mare. J Reprod Fertil 1979;(Suppl. 27): 217–27.
11. Asa CS, Goldfoot DA, Garcia MC, et al. Sexual behavior in ovariectomized and seasonally anovulatory pony mares (*Equus caballus*). Hormones Behav 1980;14:46–54.
12. Asa CS, Goldfoot DA, Ginther OJ. Assessment of the sexual behavior of pregnant mares. Hormones Behav 1983;17:405–13.
13. Jorgensen JJ, Vivrette S, Correa M, et al, editors. Significance of the estrous cycle on athletic performance in mares. 42nd Annual Convention American Association of Equine Practitioners 1996, Denver; 1996.
14. McDonnell SM. Estrous cycle-related performance problems. In: Robinson NE, editor. Current Therapy in Equine Medicine 3. 3rd ed. Philadelphia: Saunders; 1993. p. 635–6.
15. Vanderwall DK, Nie GJ. Estrus suppression. In: McKinnon AO, Squires EL, Vaala WE, et al, editors. Equine Reproduction. Chichester: Wiley-Blackwell; 2011. p. 1845–53.
16. Cox JH, DeBowes RM. Colic-like discomfort associated with ovulation in two mares. J Am Vet Med Assoc 1987;191(11):1451–2.
17. Bell DR, Myrick MP, Blackburn JT, et al. The effect of menstrual-cycle phase on hamstring extensibility and muscle stiffness. J Sport Rehabil 2009;18(4): 553–63.
18. Sarajari S, Oblinger MM. Estrogen effects on pain sensitivity and neuropeptide expression in rat sensory neurons. Exp Neurol 2010; 224:163–9.
19. Enns DL, Tiidus PM. The influence of estrogen on skeletal muscle. Sports Med 2010;40(1):41–58.
20. Shille V. Suppression or prevention of estrus in racing and sporting dogs. In: Bloomberg M, Dee J, Taylor R, editors. Canine Sports Medicine and Surgery. Philadelphia: Saunders; 1998. p. 309–12.
21. Gee EK, DeLuca C, Stylski JS, et al. Efficacy of medroxyprogesterone acetate in suppression of estrus in cycling mares. J Equine Vet Sci 2009;29(3): 140–5.
22. Storer WA, Thompson DL Jr, Gilley RM, et al. Evaluation of injectable sustained release progestin formulations for suppression of estrus and ovulation in mares. J Equine Vet Sci 2009;29(1): 33–6.
23. Loy R, Swan S. Effect of exogenous progestagens on reproductive phenomena in mares. J Anim Sci 1966;25:821–6.
24. Squires EL, Shideler R, Voss J, et al. Clinical applications of progestins in mares. Comp Contin Educ 1983;5: S16–22.
25. McKinnon AO, Lescun TB, Walker JH, et al. The inability of some synthetic progestagens to maintain pregnancy in the mare. Equine Vet J 2000;32:83–5.
26. McKinnon AO, Tarrida del Marmol Figueroa S, Nobelius AM, et al. Failure of hydroxyprogesterone caproate to maintain pregnancy in ovariectomised mares. Equine Vet J 1993;25:158–60.
27. McKinnon AO, Squires EL, Carnevale EM, et al. Ovariectomized

steroid-treated mares as embryo transfer recipients and as a model to study the role of progestins in pregnancy maintenance. Theriogenology 1988;29:1055–64.

28. Vanderwall DK, Marquardt JL, Woods GL. Use of a compounded long-acting progesterone formulation for equine pregnancy maintenance. J Equine Vet Sci 2007;27:62–6.
29. Staempfli SA, Clavier S, Thompson DL Jr, et al. Effect of a single injection of long-acting progesterone on the first ovulation in early and late spring transition mares. J Equine Vet Sci 2011;31:744–8.
30. McCue PM, Lemons SS, Squires EL, et al. Efficacy of Synovex-S implants in suppression of estrus in the mare. J Equine Vet Sci 1997;17:327–9.
31. Newcombe JR, Wilson MC. The use of progesterone releasing intravaginal devices to induce estrus and ovulation in anestrous Standardbred mares in Australia. Equine Pract 1997;19:13–21.
32. Grimmet JB, Hanlon DW, Duirs GF, et al. A new intra-vaginal progesterone-releasing device device (Cue-mare (TM)) for controlling the estrous cycle in mares. Theriogenology 2002;58:585–7.
33. Hanlon DW, Firth EC. The reproductive performance of Thoroughbred mares treated with intra-vaginal progesterone at the start of the breeding season. Theriogenology 2012;77:952–8.
34. Webel SK, Squires EL. Control of the oestrous cycle in mares with altrenogest. J Reprod Fertil Suppl 1982;32:193–8.
35. Hodgson D, Howe S, Jeffcott L, et al. Effect of prolonged use of altrenogest on behaviour in mares. Vet J 2005;169(1):113–15.
36. Neely DP, editor. Progesterone/progestin therapy in the broodmare. Proc Am Assoc Equine Pract 1988.
37. Wiepz GJ, Squires EL, Chapman PL. Effects of norgestomet, altrenogest, and/or estradiol on follicular and hormonal characteristics of late transitional mares. Theriogenology 1988;30:181–93.
38. Lopez-Bayghen C, Zozaya H, Ocampo L, et al. Melengestrol acetate as a tool for inducing early ovulation in transitional mares. Acta Vet Hung 2008;56:125–31.
39. Lefranc AC, Allen WR. Nonpharmacological suppression of oestrus in the mare. Equine Vet J 2004;36:183–5.
40. Rivera del Alamo MM, Reilas T, Kindahl H, et al. Mechanisms behind intrauterine device-induced luteal persistence in mares. Anim Reprod Sci 2008;107:94–106.
41. Nie GJ, Johnson KE, Braden TD, et al. Use of an intra-uterine glass ball protocol to extend luteal function in mares. J Equine Vet Sci 2003;23:266–73.
42. Vanderwall DK, Rasmussen DM, Woods GL. Effect of repeated administration of oxytocin during diestrus on duration of function of corpora lutea in mares. J Am Vet Med Assoc 2007;231:1864–7.
43. Meyer GA, Rashmir-Raven A, Helms RJ, et al. The effect of oxytocin on contractility of the equine oesophagus: a potential treatment for oesophageal obstruction. Equine Vet J 2000;32:151–5.
44. Wilsher S, Allen WR. Intrauterine administration of plant oils inhibits luteolysis in the mare. Equine Vet J 2011;43:99–105.
45. Hedberg Y, Dalin AM, Santesson M, et al. A preliminary study on the induction of dioestrous ovulation in the mare – a possible method for inducing prolonged luteal phase. Acta Vet Scand 2006;48:12.
46. Morehead JA, Blanchard TL. Clinical experience with deslorelin (Ovuplant™) in a Kentucky Thoroughbred broodmare practice (1999). J Equine Vet Sci 2000;20:358–402.
47. Johnson CA, Thompson DLJ, Kulinski KM, et al. Prolonged interovulatory interval and hormonal changes in mares following the use of Ovuplant™ to hasten ovulation. J Equine Vet Sci 2000;20:331–6.
48. Elhay M, Newbold A, Britton A, et al. Suppression of behavioural and physiological oestrus in the mare by vaccination against GnRH. Aust Vet J 2007;85(1–2):39–45.
49. Imboden I, Janett F, Burger D, et al. Influence of immunization against GnRH on reproductive cyclicity and estrous behavior in the mare. Theriogenology 2006;66(8):1866–75.
50. Tshewang U, Dowsett KF, Knott LM, et al. Preliminary study of ovarian activity in fillies treated with a GnRH vaccine. Aust Vet J 1997;75:663–7.
51. Robinson SJ, McKinnon AO. Prolonged ovarian inactivity in broodmares temporally associated with administration of Equity. Aust Eq Vet 2006;25:85–7.
52. Kamm JL, Hendrickson DA. Clients' perspectives on the effects of laparoscopic ovariectomy on equine behavior and medical problems. J Equine Vet Sci 2007;27(10):435–8.
53. Hooper RN, Taylor TS, Varner DD, et al. Effects of bilateral ovariectomy via colpotomy in mares: 23 cases (1984–1990). J Am Vet Med Assoc 1993;203:1043–6.
54. Pitts SC, Davis M. An evidence-based analysis of anabolic steroids as performance enhancers in horses. Equine Vet Educ 2007;19:388–91.
55. Skelton KV, Dowsett KF, McMeniman NP. Ovarian activity in fillies treated with anabolic steroids prior to the onset of puberty. J Reprod Fertil Suppl 1991;44:351–6.
56. Maher J, Squires EL, Voss J, et al. Effect of anabolic steroids on reproductive function of young mares. J Am Vet Med Assoc 1983;183:519–24.
57. Squires EL, Voss J, Maher J, et al. Fertility of young mares after long term anabolic steroid treatment. J Am Vet Med Assoc 1985;186:583–7.
58. Snow DH, Munro CD, Nimmo MA. Effects of nandrolone phenylpropionate in the horse: (2) general effects in animals undergoing training. Equine Vet J 1982;14:224–8.
59. McDonnell SM. Pharmacologic manipulation of stallion behaviour. In: McKinnon AO, Squires EL, Vaala WE, et al, editors. Equine Reproduction. West Sussex: Blackwell Publishing; 2011. p. 1415–18.
60. Blodgett G. Normal Field castration. In: McKinnon AO, Squires EL, Vaala WE, et al, editors. Equine Reproduction. West Sussex: Blackwell Publishing; 2011. p. 1557–61.
61. Pleasant R. Castration of the normal horse. In: Wolfe D, Moll H, editors. Large Animal Urogenital Surgery. Baltimore: Williams and Wilkins; 1999. p. 23–31.
62. Searle D, Dart A, Dart C, et al. Equine castration: a review of anatomy, approaches, techniques and complications in normal, cryptorchid and monorchid horses. Aust Vet J 1999;77:428–34.
63. Micol D, Oury MP, Picard B, et al. Effect of age at castration on animal performance, muscle characteristics and meat quality traits in 26-month-old Charolais steers. Livestock Sci 2009;120(1–2):116–26.
64. Bretschneider G. Effects of age and method of castration on performance and stress response of beef male cattle: A review. Livestock Prod Sci 2005;97(2–3):89–100.
65. Zamiri MJ, Eilami B, Kianzad MR. Effects of castration and fattening period on growth performance and carcass characteristics in Iranian goats. Small Rumin Res 2011;In press.
66. Steen RWJ, Kilpatrick DJ. Effects of plane of nutrition and slaughter weight on the carcass composition of serially slaughtered bulls, steers and heifers of three breed crosses. Livestock Prod Sci 1995;43(3):205–13.
67. Asher GW, Archer JA, Ward JF, et al. The effect of prepubertal castration of red deer and wapiti-red deer crossbred stags on growth and carcass production. Livestock Sci 2011;137:196–204.
68. Cutler G, Cassorla F, Ross J. Pubertal growth: physiology and

pathophysiology. Recent Prog Horm Res 1986;42:443–70.

69. Salmeri K, Bloomberg M, Scruggs S, et al. Gonadectomy in immature dogs: Effects on skeletal, physical and behavioural development. J Am Vet Med Assoc 1991;198:1193–203.
70. Uhlhorn H, Eksell P, Carlsten J. Scintigraphic characterization of distal radial physeal closure in young standardbred racehorses. Vet Radiol Ultrasound 2000;41(2):181–6.
71. Vulcano LC, Mamprim MJ, Muniz LMR, et al. Radiographic study of distal radial physeal closure in thoroughbred horses. Vet Radiol Ultrasound 1997;38(5): 352–4.
72. Line S, Hart B, Sanders L. Effect of prepubertal versus post pubertal castration on sexual and aggressive behaviour in male horses. J Am Vet Med Assoc 1985;186:249–51.
73. Goolsby HA, Brady HA, Prien SD. The off-label use of altrenogest in stallions: a survey. J Equine Vet Sci 2004;24:72–4.
74. Miller C, Varner DD, Blanchard TL, editors. Effects of altrenogest on behavior and reproductive function in stallions. Proc Am Assoc Equine Pract; 1997.
75. Squires EL, Badzinski SL, Amann RP, et al. Effects of altrenogest on total scrotal width, seminal characteristics, concentrations of LH and testosterone, and sexual behavior of stallions. Theriogenology 1997;48:313–28.
76. Brady H, Johnson N, Whisnant C, editors. Effects of oral altrenogest on testicular parameters and seminal characteristics in young stallions. Proc Am Assoc Equine Pract; 1997.
77. Johnson NN, Brady HA, Whisnant CS, et al. Effects of altrenogest on sexual/aggressive behavior, hormonal profiles, and testicular parameters in young stallions. Equine Vet J 1997;18: 249–53.
78. Stout TAE, Collenbrander B. Suppressing reproductive activity in horses using GnRH vaccines, antagonists or agonists. Anim Reprod Sci 2004;82–3:633–43.
79. Janett F, Stump R, Burger D, et al. Suppression of testicular function and sexual behavior by vaccination against GnRH (Equity™) in the adult stallion. Anim Reprod Sci 2009;115:88–102.
80. Dowsett K, Knott LM, Tshewang U. Suppression of testicular function using two dose rates of a water soluble gonadotrophin releasing hormone (GnRH) vaccine in colts. Aust Vet J 1996;74:228–35.
81. Malmgren L, Andresen O, Dalin A. Effect of GnRH immunisation on hormonal levels, sexual behaviour, semen quality and testicular morphology in mature stallions. Equine Vet J 2001;33:75–83.
82. McDonnell SM. Stallion sexual behaviour. In: Samper J, editor. Equine Breeding Management and Artificial Insemination. Philadelphia: Saunders; 2000. p. 53–61.
83. Sieme H. Freezing semen. In: McKinnon AO, Squires EL, Vaala WE, et al, editors. Equine Reproduction. Chichester, UK: Wiley-Blackwell; 2011. p. 2972–82.
84. Hurtgen J. Semen collection in stallions. In: Samper J, editor. Equine Breeding Management and Artificial Insemination. Philadelphia: Saunders; 2000. p. 91–108.
85. Magistrini M. Semen evaluation. In: Samper J, editor. Equine Breeding Management and Artificial Insemination. Philadelphia: Saunders; 2000. p. 81–90.
86. Samper J. Artificial insemination. In: Samper J, editor. Equine Breeding Management and Artificial Insemination. Philadelphia: Saunders; 2000. p. 109–31.
87. Allen WR, Brown L, Wright M, et al. Reproductive efficiency of Flatrace and National Hunt Thoroughbred mares and stallions in England. Equine Vet J 2007;39(5):438–45.
88. Nath LC, Anderson GA, Savage CJ, et al. Reproductive efficiency of Thoroughbred and Standardbred horses in North East Victoria. Aust Vet J 2010;88:169–75.
89. Kelley DE, Gibbons JR, Smith R, et al. Exercise affects both ovarian follicular dynamics and hormone concentrations in mares. Theriogenology 2011;76(4): 615–22.
90. Riemann M. Effects on the foetus of exercise in pregnancy. Scand J Med Sci Sports 2000;10:12–19.
91. Mortensen CJ, Choi YH, Hinrichs K, et al. Embryo recovery from exercised mares. Anim Reprod Sci 2009;110: 237–44.
92. Smith R, Vernon K, Gibbons J, et al. Exercise influences embryo quality in mares. Reprod Fertil Dev 2010;22:250.
93. Lehnhard R, Manso Filho H, Causey R, et al. Maternal and foetal heart rates during exercise in horses. Comp Exerc Physiol 2009;61:43–8.
94. Clapp J, Little K. Effect of recreational exercise on pregnancy weight gain and subcutaneous fat deposition. Med Sci Sports Exerc 1995;27:170–7.
95. McKinnon AO, Squires EL. Equine embryo transfer. Vet Clin North Am Equine Pract 1988;4:305–33.
96. McKinnon AO, Squires EL. Embryo transfer and related technologies. In: McKinnon AO, Pycock J, editors. Current Therapy in Equine Reproduction. St Louis: Saunders; 2007. p. 319–34.
97. Woods G, Steiner J. Embryo transfers from mares in athletic competition. Cornell Vet 1986;76:149–55.
98. Hartman DL. Embryo transfer. In: McKinnon AO, Squires EL, Vaala WE, et al, editors. Equine Reproduction. West Sussex: Wiley-Blackwell; 2011. p. 2871–9.
99. Lindsey A, Morris L, Allen WR. Hysteroscopic insemination of mares with low numbers of nonsorted or flow sorted spermatazoa. Equine Vet J 2002;34:128–32.
100. Squires EL, Todter G, Berndston W. Effects of anabolic steroids on reproductive capacity in young stallions. J Anim Sci 1982;54:576–82.
101. Garcia MC, Ganjam V, Blanchard TL. The effects of stanozolol and boldenone undecyclenate on plasma testosterone and gonadotrophins and on testis histology in pony stallions. Theriogenology 1987;28:109–19.
102. Parsinnen M, Seppala T. Steroid use and long term health risks in former athletes. Sports Med 2002;32:83–94.

Examination of the equine athlete prior to purchase

60

Brian H. Anderson Andrea Ritmeester Brendon Bell Andris J. Kaneps

CHAPTER CONTENTS

Introduction

- Aim and philosophy of the prepurchase examination.
- General approach and examination procedure.
- Special considerations and ancillary tests.
- Examination of different types of equine athlete.

A rigorous and thorough examination of the athletic horse by a veterinarian who understands and is familiar with the sporting endeavors of a particular athlete is a challenging and potentially troublesome task. With practice and diligence it can be a very rewarding professional and financial experience. In order to conduct such examinations proficiently, knowledge of the types of injuries and diseases affecting athletic horses and which may shorten or cause problems in a career should be understood. In this chapter the aim and philosophy of the prepurchase examination, general approach and examination procedure used, the use of special examination techniques and the differences in examination approach between various athletes will be discussed. The prepurchase examination of horses intended for breeding will not be discussed but has been reviewed elsewhere.[1,2]

Aim and philosophy

The selling and buying of athletic horses is essential for a vibrant and profitable equine industry. Breeders of horses strive to produce well-grown athletic individuals from superior blood lines in the hope of selling a product that will be successful on the racetrack, cross-country course or in the dressage arena. Horses are sold privately or at public auction sales. High-quality animals command high dollar prices from thousands to millions. Purchasers of high-quality animals want to ensure that their investment has a good chance of providing a successful return. Purchasers decide on the breeding, type and quality of the horse they desire and seek from the veterinarian an assurance that what they are about to buy does not have any problems currently or in the future that will inhibit the investment from performing up to expectation.

The ultimate decision on the purchase of any horse resides with the purchaser. As part of the decision-making process the veterinarian provides information to the purchaser on the health status of the horse. Successful athletes are seldom injury free and older athletes in particular have invariably suffered some 'wear and tear'. In the case of young unbroken athletes, a variety of congenital and acquired defects, which may interfere with an athletic career, might be present. For these reasons it should be understood by the purchaser that the veterinarian essentially conducts a risk assessment for the purchaser.

The aim of the examination of the equine athlete prior to purchase is to first identify, and second assess, the relative significance of factors of a veterinary nature, which at the time of examination might impair athletic performance in the occupation for which the horse is intended.[3] In addition, conditions that have the potential for impairment of athletic performance in the future should also be identified and an opinion of their significance made in light of the horse's intended use.[3,5]

The way in which the opinion of the examining veterinarian is presented to the purchaser has become very controversial. Unfortunately, it is a frequent perception by the purchaser that a veterinarian's examination prior to purchase provides a warranty that the prospective animal is free of all impediments currently and in the future and that such an examination in some way guarantees a risk-free purchase. This perception has been perpetuated to some extent by the use of the terms 'sound', 'suitable' or 'serviceable, all of which when used in the context of a prepurchase examination imply a degree of warranty. Using these terms when giving an opinion may leave the examining veterinarian legally vulnerable if the horse should prove to be unusable by the purchaser and they are not recommended.[6] Another reason why it is unwise to use such terminology is that in many instances a complete examination of the horse to be purchased is not possible. Providing an opinion on suitability or serviceability based on an incomplete examination is fraught with difficulties.

The veterinarian should confine his or her opinion to the functional significance of relevant examination findings.[7] A decision to purchase the horse or a decision on the suitability or serviceability of a horse for a specific intended purpose is a business judgment that is the sole responsibility of the purchaser and is made on the basis of a variety of factors, only one of which is the report provided by the examining veterinarian.[6,7]

It is common to find some clinical problems in athletic horses. Rather than take the easy road of advising against purchase where problems are recognized it is better to provide the purchaser with a balanced assessment of risk. Probably the most practical method is to assign a measure of likelihood or percentage chance that an abnormality or clinical finding will impair athletic performance.[4,8] In forming such an opinion the veterinarian draws on her or his own experience, the experience of others and the scientific literature. For example, recent evidence suggests that the presence of dorsal medial intercarpal disease identified on presale radiographs of the carpus of Thoroughbred yearlings is associated with a 20% chance of an affected horse not starting a race.[9]

It should be noted that the way in which the veterinary opinion is presented to the purchaser differs around the world. The variation often reflects the results of court decisions in cases of dispute and the establishment of legal precedent.[6] For example, the British Equine Veterinary Association recommends that the opinion given on examination for purchase be that a horse is 'suitable or unsuitable' for the purpose for which it is intended.[3] The equine industry accepts this method and the British legal system recognizes it as reasonable.[10]

Requirements for the prepurchase examination

In order to perform a successful prepurchase examination, a number of requirements should be met and include the following:[10]

- Clear communication with the purchaser or purchaser's agent, vendor or vendor's agent before, during and after the examination. This communication should be both verbal and in writing. The limitations of the veterinary examination should be discussed with the purchaser together with an explanation of how the examination findings will be reported. The results of the examination are privileged and confidential and are the property of the purchaser.
- If the vendor is a client of the veterinarian (current or past) this represents a potential conflict of interest. All parties should be consulted and if the examination is to go ahead this agreement should be made in writing (see Appendix at the end of this chapter). Part of this agreement should include full disclosure of relevant medical information by the vendor relating to the horse to be examined. It is strongly recommended not to proceed with the examination if the vendor refuses to provide this information to the purchaser or purchaser's agent (see Appendix).
- Written confirmation of what portions of the examination the purchaser requires (see Buyer's statement in Appendix at the end of this chapter). The requirement of additional ancillary tests should be indicated. Where regular examination procedures are unable to be performed (e.g. horse is not broken to lead) this should be detailed in the written report furnished to the purchaser. Other than for young stock, the horse should be in full athletic work and it is unwise to perform examinations on animals not in regular work because previous lameness or back problems may not be apparent.[8] These issues should be discussed carefully with the purchaser or purchaser's agent.
- A vendor's statement (see Appendix) should be completed in writing prior to examination of the horse.
- It is ideal although often not possible to have the vendor and purchaser present during the examination. A methodical and thorough examination process is required which includes examination before and after strenuous activity, preferably similar to that performed by the horse in its chosen occupation. Adequate personnel and conditions throughout this procedure are necessary.
- A thorough knowledge of the intended use of the horse. The veterinarian should have the skill necessary to differentiate normal and abnormal variations in physical and gait evaluations and be able to relate these to the horse's intended use so that an assessment on current and future performance can be made.
- Precise and detailed recording of examination findings.
- Be able to advise on the necessity of ancillary diagnostics and perform these or refer on for specialist examination.
- If the horse is to be insured or is being purchased for resale these issues should be discussed thoroughly with the purchaser. While some conditions identified during the examination will be acceptable risks for a certain intended use they may cause problems if the horse is to be insured or resold. For example, a distal intermediate ridge osteochondral fragment of the hock not resulting in clinical signs may be a low risk for purchase in a Thoroughbred yearling that is to be trained and raced by the buyer. If the purchaser, however, intends to condition the horse and sell it in a 'two year old in training sale' such a radiographic finding might deter a future purchaser. In addition, an insurance exclusion could be put in place on such a horse if the purchaser opted to surgically remove this fragment prior to further sale.

Examination procedure

Veterinarians use a variety of protocols for examination of the athletic horse prior to purchase.[6–8,11,12] Some veterinary societies recommend a standardized procedure that should be used by their members.[7,8,11,13] By following such methods a degree of protection is afforded the veterinarian in case of litigation and a standard method reduces the chances of missing problems. However, other veterinary associations such as the American Association of Equine Practitioners have not produced an official step-by-step protocol because of the legal ramifications that may arise if a veterinarian did not strictly adhere to the policy. In addition, by not using a standard protocol, veterinarians are free to adopt their own methods of examination.

One method used by the authors,[7] and one that has been well accepted in Australia, New Zealand and Great Britain, is based on a five-stage procedure and this is described below.

Stage 1. Preliminary examination

An accurate description of the horse is required. A vendor's/owner's statement should be completed (see Appendix). The current state of work should be noted and the resting examination conducted. This part of the examination is usually performed within the horse's stall or stable, the horse having been at rest for at least 30 min. Access to a dark area is useful for examination of the eyes. A nose to tail examination should be conducted and the hands passed over every part of the body. Each foot should be picked up, examined and a hoof tester applied. The limb joints are checked for effusion and flexed to detect pain or limitation of movement. The palmar/plantar flexor tendons, ligaments and soft tissues are evaluated for swelling, heat and pain. The accompanying checklist (see Appendix) should be followed precisely so that no part is overlooked. With experience the veterinarian develops an automatic inspection procedure. The horse is then brought out of the stable and inspected thoroughly from all sides. Conformation is evaluated with the horse standing on a level surface. At this stage if any obvious defect is present which would impair the function of the animal the examination is stopped with the consent of the purchaser. The premature termination of the examination and the reason is explained in the report.

Stage 2. Examination during walking, trotting, turning and backing

A competent attendant should handle the horse. The horse is walked 20 m away from the examiner and then back. The horse should be viewed from the front, back and sides. The horse is then trotted for 30–40 m and trotted back and then trotted in a circle both ways. The horse should be turned one way and then the other in tight circles and then backed a few paces. Coordination and proprioception are carefully assessed and to test for hindlimb strength a 'tail pull test' is used. Following this, a full series of flexion tests as outlined in the guidelines are performed. The significance and interpretation of flexion tests are controversial.[14] Force applied, duration of application, age and work history can all influence the outcome of these manipulations. Flexion tests should not be interpreted in isolation. Positive flexion tests without concurrent lameness or other clinical abnormalities may have little clinical significance.[15] In our hands flexion tests have proved useful as an indicator or 'warning' that further investigation may be required. More emphasis is placed on a positive response to flexion if a change in gait is maintained for more than 2–3 strides.[14]

The clinician should develop a consistent and repeatable technique and this is probably the best way of achieving reproducible results. If during this examination signs of lameness are present the examination may be terminated. Sometimes the purchaser wishes to continue with the examination – this is ill advised – but if the purchaser or vendor wishes to know the source of the lameness, the format, cost and person responsible for payment of this extra examination needs to be clarified.

Stage 3. Examination during and immediately after strenuous exercise

Within the confines of the animal's age, condition, training, fitness and only after the vendor's consent, exercise of sufficient intensity and duration should be performed so as to:

- induce rapid deep breathing so that unusual breathing sounds can be heard
- tire the animal so that strains and injuries and other exercise-related problems (e.g. epistaxis) may be revealed after a period of rest
- increase the action of the heart so that exercise-related cardiac abnormalities may be detected, e.g. atrial fibrillation.[7]

Examples of such exercise for the racehorse include a sufficient warm-up followed by a gallop for 400–600 m. The examiner should position himself or herself close to the horse to observe and listen to the breathing pattern. A normal horse has only a single respiratory sound heard on expiration. When an inspiratory sound is heard this typically is due to impaired arytenoid function (e.g. laryngeal neuropathy). Upper respiratory tract obstruction that results in loud inspiratory and expiratory sounds can be caused by conditions such as intermittent epiglottic entrapment, arytenoid chondritis or pharyngeal collapse. Excessive production of airway secretions and alar fold collapse are other possibilities. The horse should be pulled up as quickly as is safe and the breathing pattern closely observed to detect sounds of dorsal displacement of the soft palate, inspiratory noises typical of laryngeal neuropathy, abnormal nasal discharge and signs of respiratory distress. The horse should then have an endoscopic evaluation. Untrained animals, those too young or unable to be ridden should be lunged and the duration and intensity of exercise recorded.

Stage 4. Examination during the period after exercise

The animal should be allowed to 'cool down' quietly over a period such that respiratory and heart rates return to normal. A crude assessment of fitness and respiratory function can be made by evaluating heart and respiratory rate over this period. This period allows for any injuries or musculoskeletal problems to 'stiffen up' (e.g. osteoarthritic changes within the fetlock joints).

Stage 5. The final examination during walking, trotting, turning and backing

The horse is examined as in stage 2, paying careful attention to any signs of lameness. Lunging in the circle both ways for a few rounds is also advised. Hoof tester and flexion tests may be repeated if signs of lameness are present.

Avoiding problems in the prepurchase examination

Examination of claims made against veterinary surgeons relating to the prepurchase examination show they are of two broad types.[16]

In the first instance, the veterinarian is accused of not detecting an abnormality that subsequently becomes a problem. This most commonly relates to lameness occurring soon after purchase. A careful and thorough examination procedure should help reduce the chances of inadvertently making such errors. Testing for drug administration may also act as a deterrent to the use of agents that may hide lameness problems or help confirm the presence of such agents at the time of examination.

In the second instance the complaint is that the purchaser was not informed of a condition or abnormality (e.g. sarcoid) that could become a problem. To avoid this situation good communication before, during and after the examination with the purchaser is necessary. Most importantly the limitations of the examination procedure must be carefully discussed. Having a clear understanding of the expectations and intentions of the purchaser with respect to the future use and training of the horse is critical.

Another frequent problem is dissatisfaction expressed by the vendor. This may be that the veterinarian improperly discriminated against the horse in question by providing the purchaser with incorrect opinions regarding the significance of the clinical findings of the examination. Such examples include the diagnosis of lameness, response to flexion tests, significance of conformational defects and opinion on the significance of radiological findings. It must be remembered that the vendor is of course trying to sell the horse and a balanced opinion regarding any defect or abnormality present is naturally tainted by some bias.

Notwithstanding this, it behooves the examining veterinarian to confine his/her opinion to fact, which is supported by experience and knowledge of the scientific literature. A second opinion from a respected colleague may be very useful. Because opinions between veterinarians differ, it is best to confine any opinion given in terms of the degree of risk that any defect or abnormality may have currently or in the future on athletic performance. It is recommended that the veterinarian does not express his or her opinions relating to the outcome of the examination procedure to the vendor, although some veterinarian's believe otherwise.[17]

Special considerations and ancillary tests

Conformation assessment

The assessment of conformation is a very important part of the prepurchase examination. Many veterinarians believe that conformation, or more specifically, deficiencies in conformation, play a significant role in the maintenance of athletic soundness and contribute to the ability of elite performers. For example, it is well known that some conformational faults predispose athletic horses to injuries and lameness.[18–22] In addition, many astute observers of horses believe that the way horses are 'put together' has a major effect on how successful they are in various disciplines.[19,22] Unfortunately, objective scientific data to support these commonly held opinions is limited. Moreover, very talented individuals appear to compensate for deficiencies in conformation. It is probably true to say, however, that marked discrepancies from what is considered optimal conformation result in injuries that limit athletic performance. Limitations in the short term, especially in gifted individuals, can be overcome, but in the long term recurrent injury and lameness is more likely. Issues relating to the conformation assessment of various athletic horses are discussed below under the examination of each athlete. The reader is directed to more extensive recent reviews on the subject.[18–23]

Laboratory evaluation

Although a variety of laboratory evaluations may be useful as ancillary aids during the prepurchase examination,[24,25] drug testing and those tests required for insurance purposes or certification of disease status when horses are transported between states or countries are the most common. Blood tests such as evaluation of the hemogram, plasma fibrinogen and serum chemistry are not routinely performed but would be indicated to determine if observed clinical symptoms were significant, e.g. nasal discharge, cough, elevated rectal temperature or submandibular lymph node enlargement. The vendor's permission should be sought and, to avoid confusion with the interpretation of results, blood should be collected prior to exercise.

Because equine athletes are frequently medicated and because unscrupulous vendors might use drugs to mask musculoskeletal pain, many purchasers now request drug testing. Drug testing is thought to provide insurance against 'foul play' but the purchaser should be advised carefully as to the limitations associated with such testing. For instance, the range of drugs tested by some laboratories may be limited (e.g. only testing of non-steroidal anti-inflammatory agents), testing is expensive, results are not immediate, some drugs are difficult to detect (e.g. some intra-articularly injected agents) or are no longer traceable but still exert a pharmacologic effect. Therefore, a negative test is not always commensurate with an animal that has not been medicated. Blood is usually the fluid sampled but in fact urine, although more time-consuming to collect, is the preferred sample because many drug metabolites are concentrated in urine and many agents can be detected for extended intervals in urine.

The simple act of collecting a blood sample at the time of examination, especially if the vendor is advised in advance, can have a deterrent effect. Storing the blood at the veterinarian's practice to be analyzed at a later date at the discretion of the purchaser can potentially lead to problems relating to the 'chain of custody'. Instead we recommend the immediate analysis of blood collected for drug screening. In some countries (e.g. Britain and New Zealand) a standardized collection process is used[8] (see Appendix).

The Coggins test for equine infectious anemia (EIA) needs to be performed on horses that will travel interstate. For those horses imported into the USA and which might compete internationally, tests for piroplasmosis, dourine, glanders and EIA should be performed. When breeding stock are examined, tests for equine viral arteritis and contagious endometritis may be required.[8,24] In each case the client should be warned about the cost of such tests and the delays that testing might incur. Horses would ideally not be purchased until the results of such tests were known.

Examination of the cardiovascular system

During the clinical examination before and after exercise the cardiovascular system should be carefully examined. Chapter 32 discusses the evaluation of the cardiovascular system in detail. Principally the examiner determines if there is evidence of overt cardiac disease (elevated resting heart rate, elevated resting respiratory rate, distended jugular veins, dependent edema and exercise intolerance) cardiac murmurs or cardiac arrhythmias. Second, it is important to differentiate between physiologic cardiac murmurs and arrhythmias and those that are pathologic. Where there is doubt, an electrocardiographic examination and an echocardiographic examination may be required. It is advisable to seek specialist opinion in these areas. The following points should be kept in mind:[26]

- Physiologic murmurs (flow murmurs) are usually localized, of low intensity (grade 1 and 2), short in duration and sometimes musical. They are usually early to mid systolic, early diastolic or presystolic.

- Pathologic murmurs are often (but not always) louder, radiating and holo-pansystolic (mitral and tricuspid valve regurgitation) or holodiastolic (aortic valve regurgitation).
- Mild localized regurgitant murmurs may be associated with a low risk for athletic performance. Echocardiography is best.
- Sinus arrhythmia, sinus block and second-degree atrioventricular block are relatively common and of no clinical significance.
- Atrial fibrillation and premature beats (atrial premature complexes, ventricular premature complexes) are usually not acceptable in athletic animals. Exercise or 24-hour electrocardiographic examinations may be required to determine clinical significance.
- Imaging and the prepurchase examination.
- The most common ancillary diagnostic aid used to evaluate the musculoskeletal system in the prepurchase examination is radiography. Radiography was performed in 49% of all prepurchase evalutions in one review[27] and this was more likely if the examination was performed at a clinic. The principal indications or reasons for prepurchase radiography include:[28]
- Clinical examination findings indicating an abnormality that requires quantification/clarification (e.g. fetlock joint effusion with pain on flexion).
- Intended use of horse (e.g. dressage competitor versus low-level pleasure horse).
- In young unbroken horses or in horses unable to be rigorously exercised, or athletic horses that have been rested, survey radiographs may help identify clinically silent or quiescent lesions which may cause future problems when training starts or is recommenced.
- Client's instructions. Clients may instruct the examining veterinarian to perform a radiographic examination. The reasons for this can be many and include the desire to sell the horse in the future, previous bad experiences or because of advice from others.[28]
- A standard set of radiographs is required as part of the examination of Thoroughbred horses being exported for racing to some countries (e.g. Hong Kong and Macau).
- Purchase price.
- The routine use of radiography in the prepurchase examination can be problematic. Opinions differ as to the reliability of radiographs to be of predictive value for future athletic soundness.[28] Some veterinarians believe that radiography should be avoided if it will not influence the opinion given on clinical grounds. The added expense and the possibility that radiographs will only 'confuse the picture' especially if questionable changes are identified should also be considered. Regardless of these issues, radiographic lesions or changes can only be properly interpreted when combined with examination findings and clinical history. Radiographs by themselves may be meaningless. In addition, high-quality images with sufficient views are required.[29,30] The minimum number of radiographic views required to examine a specific anatomical site during prepurchase radiography are presented in Table 60.1.[28-30] The radiographs must be permanently marked with the name or number of the horse, date, name of the veterinarian or veterinary hospital and identification of the leg examined. A method for recognizing which oblique view has been taken (e.g. always placing markers on the lateral aspect of the film) is necessary. The radiographs belong to the veterinarian and are part of the animal's medical record and need to be kept for the period determined by the statute of limitations for the state or locality in which the veterinarian lives.

What are we looking for on prepurchase radiographs that may result in a reduced capacity to perform as an athlete?

When viewing radiographs during the prepurchase examination a thorough examination of each film is performed.[31] Significant radiographic abnormalities associated with the appendicular skeleton of the horse have been reviewed.[31] Any abnormalities should be described in terms of size, shape, position, density and relationship to adjacent structures. With respect to the athlete, however, there are a number of recognized conditions or anomalies observed on radiographs that carry a degree of risk for reduced athletic performance (Table 60.2).[28,29,31] The examiner should look carefully for the presence of developmental orthopedic disease (age, breed and joint specific), osteoarthritis or evidence of 'wear and tear', fracture and bone modeling. In young untrained animals developmental orthopedic disease must be conscientiously ruled out. In animals that have performed, especially older animals, osteoarthritis and 'wear and tear' injuries are important.

Table 60.1 Minimum recommended radiographic views for prepurchase radiography

Distal phalanx	
Lateromedial	LM
Dorsoproximal-palmaro (plantaro) distal oblique	Upright pedal or D45° Pr-Pa (PL) Di O
Dorsopalmar (plantar)	DPa (PL)
Navicular bone	
Lateromedial	LM
Dorsoproximal-palmaro (plantaro) distal oblique	Upright pedal or D60° Pr-Pa (PL) DiO
Palmaro (plantaro) proximal-palmaro (plantaro) distal oblique	Pa45° Pr-Pa (PL) Di O

Continued

Table 60.1 Continued

Pastern	
Specific views of the pastern can be taken. The horse should stand squarely on wooden blocks. However, for survey purposes the pastern is often included in views of the foot or the fetlock	
Lateromedial	LM
Dorsopalmar (plantar)	DPa (PL)
Dorsolateral – palmaro (plantaro) medial oblique	D45°L-Pa (PL) MO
Dorsomedial – palmaro (plantaro) lateral oblique	D45°M-Pa (PL) LO
Fetlock	
Lateromedial or flexed lateromedial	LM
Dorsoproximal palmaro (plantaro) distal oblique	D20-30° Pr-Pa (PL) Di O
Dorsoproximal lateral – palmaro (plantaro) distomedial oblique[a]	D5° or 10°Pr45°L-Pa (PL) Di MO
Dorsoproximal medial – palmaro (plantaro) distal lateral oblique[a]	D5° or 10°Pr45°M-Pa (PL) Di LO
Metacarpus/metatarsus	
Lateromedial	LM
Dorsopalmar (plantar) palmaro (plantaro)	DPa (PL)
Dorsolateral – palmaro (plantaro) medial obilque	D45°L-Pa (PL) MO
Dorsomedial – palmaro (plantaro) lateral oblique	D45°M-Pa (PL) LO
Carpus	
Lateromedial	LM
Flexed lateromedial	Flexed LM
Dorsopalmar	DPa
Dorsolateral – palmaromedial oblique	D50° or 60° L-Pa MO
Dorsomedial – palmarolateral oblique	D70° M-Pa LO
Flexed dorsoproximal – dorsodistal oblique	Flexed D 30° Pr-DdiO (skyline of C3)
Tarsus	
Lateromedial	LM
Dorsoplantar	DPL
Dorsolateral – plantaromedial oblique	D45° L-PL MO
Dorsomedial – plantarolateral oblique	D55° M-PL LO
Stifle	
Lateromedial	LM
Caudocranial	Cd Cr
Caudolateral – craniomedial oblique	Cd 30° L-Cr MO

[a]By angling the X-ray beam distally by 5° in the front fetlocks and 10° in the hind fetlocks the palmar or plantar aspect of the proximal phalanx can be clearly visualized to identify bone fragments at this site.

Table 60.2 Estimate of risk that various observed radiological changes result in reduced athletic performance[a,b]

REGION	RADIOLOGICAL DIAGNOSIS
Distal phalanx	• **Laminitis**[31] – high. • **Pedal osteitis complex/concussive trauma**[31]– moderate – manageable. • **Hoof imbalance** – low to moderate – manageable. • **Osteoarthritis (OA) distal interphalangeal joint**[31] – high. • **P3 Osseous cyst-like lesions**[31] – If communicate with joint risk is high. Upright pedal or D45° Pr-Pa (PL) DiO required. • **Ossification of hoof cartilages**[31] – low. • **Mineralized opacities adjacent to extensor process of P3**[28,31] – low, usually insignificant. • **Round smooth densities adjacent to palmar processes** – low, secondary centers of ossification or old fracture.[31,34]
Navicular bone	**Navicular syndrome** – controversial since radiological changes can be similar in sound and lame horses. Those most likely to be significant include:[28,29,31,35] • Increased number of enlarged synovial fossae. • Medullary sclerosis/loss in corticomedullary definition. • Medullary lucency. • Flexor cortex erosions/new bone formation. • Distal border fragments and palmar cortical thickening. • The above changes in combination with clinical findings are indicative of navicular disease/syndrome which represents a high risk for impairment in future athletic performance.
Pastern	• **DJD** – generally risk is high. Dorsal proximal P2 osteophytes may be incidental in Warmbloods.[8] • **Osseous cyst-like lesions (distal P1 or proximal P2)** – risk is high if communicate with proximal interphalangeal joint (especially if medial or lateral of midline) and if accompanying evidence of OA, low if isolated from joint. Centrally located cyst-like lesions in the distal aspect of P1 in yearling Thoroughbreds appear to have a low risk for future lameness unless they are large.[36] • **Osteochondral fragments palmar/plantar eminence of proximal P2** – risk is low–moderate.[37]
Fetlock	• **DJD**[31] – Generally risk is moderate–high in any performance horse. If supracondylar lysis and osteophyte formation on the sesamoid bones are present, risk is high. Reduced risk if only slight modeling, correlate with age, occupation and clinical findings. • **Palmar/plantar proximal P1 fragments** – origin may be proximal sesamoid bones or P1, can be articular or non-articular and could be avulsion fragments or OCD. Risk is considered low and articular fragments can be removed arthroscopically with a good prognosis. Little effect on ability to start a race (presale findings in Thoroughbred yearlings[9]) and little effect on racing performance in Standardbreds.[38] • **Ununited proximoplantar tuberosity** – suggested clinical significance 12.5%[39] when recognized in young animals. May heal back to parent bone in young animals. Correlate with exam findings. Evidence of periosteal proliferation, calcification of distal sesamoidean ligaments and articular involvement increases risk. • **Proximal dorsal P1 fragments** – possibly developmental in yearlings but most likely traumatic in adults. Risk is low if performance history is good and other signs of OA are absent. Correlate with age, occupation and exam findings. Prognosis following arthroscopic removal is very good.[9,29,31] In Thoroughbred yearlings hindlimb P1 fragments were associated with a reduced chance to race at two or three years.[9] and P1 fragments reduced yearling sales price in one study.[40] • **OCD** – distal MC3/MT3 and distal 2/3 of MC3/Mt3 sagittal ridge[9] – risk is variable. Large defects, those with fragments and those showing subchondral bone changes represent a moderate–high risk. Follow-up on yearling Thoroughbreds and Standardbreds showed these changes to have little effect on starting a race (Thoroughbred) or on racing career (Standardbred) – amenable to surgery with a reasonable prognosis.[9,29] Large lesions of the mid sagittal ridge (>10 mm long) in hind fetlocks in Thoroughbred yearlings were associated with reduced racing performance at two and three years.[41] • **Osseous cyst-like lesions of Mc3/Mt3 and proximal P1** – risk is high if communicate with articular surface. Some cysts, however, can be incidental findings.[29]

Continued

Table 60.2 Continued

REGION	RADIOLOGICAL DIAGNOSIS
Proximal sesamoid	• **Sesamoiditis**[31] – conflicting opinion and research evidence on risk. Proposed etiology varies between occupations.[31,42–45] Radiological changes include osteophytes, enthesophytes, osteolysis and enlarged vascular channels. If multiple changes then ultrasound of suspensory apparatus is warranted. Correlate with age, occupation, conformation (e.g. upright pasterns), exercise history and exam findings. Increased numbers of enlarged, irregular vascular channels especially if enthesophytes are present represent an increased risk.[9,45] Check for DJD of fetlock joint. In one study presale radiography of Thoroughbred yearlings showed >50% of proximal sesamoid bones had irregular vascular channels but this did not affect the ability of horses to start a race when two or three years old.[9] but in another study the presence of more than two irregularly shaped vascular channels was associated with less earnings and starts when two and three years of age.[46] Proximal sesamoid modeling in both front and hind fetlocks in Thoroughbred yearlings has been associated with reduced performance.[9,41] Young Standardbreds with sesamoid changes showed improvement over time and earnings as three- and four-year-old horses were not different to those horses without sesamoid changes.[44] • **Fractures**[43] – sesamoid fractures identified on presale radiographs of yearling Thoroughbreds did not appear to influence the ability to start a race at two or three years of age in one study.[9] In another study forelimb sesamoid fractures were associated with less chance of starting a race at two or three years.[41] These fractures (some of which may be separate centers of ossification), often occur when the horse is a foal and healing can result in a complete bony union.[43] An elongated or malshaped sesamoid bone can result if the fracture was displaced. Ability to start a race was not affected by these changes.[9] Hindlimb apical sesamoid fractures in particular appear to be low risk.[9] Fracture size, position and evidence of other changes should be evaluated in young horses to estimate risk. Prognosis is excellent for racing after arthroscopic removal of apical sesamoid fractures in weanlings or yearlings involving the hindlimbs and lateral forelimb but reduced for medial forelimb fractures.[47] In mature horses sesamoid fractures are often clinically significant and careful evaluation of the suspensory apparatus and fetlock joint is required.
Metacarpus/metatarsus	• **Exostoses/splints**[31] – active splints represent a short-term moderate–high risk for impaired athletic performance. Palmar soft tissues may require ultrasonography. • **Proximal MT3/MC3 sclerosis**[31] – may alert clinician to conduct an ultrasound of the proximal suspensory ligament but the presence of this change alone may have little clinical significance.
Carpus	• **DJD**[31] – generally risk is moderate–high for any performance horse. Mild changes, including mild articular osteophyte production, especially in the radiocarpal joint, have reduced risk. Assess with respect to age, conformation, occupation, work history and intended use. Smooth/mature non-articular enthesous bone formation on dorsal carpal bones – low risk.[28] Some third carpal bone sclerosis in racehorses is expected. Significant focal lucency and marked loss of trabecular pattern – high risk. Presale radiography of yearling Thoroughbred racehorses showed the presence of dorsal medial intercarpal disease reduced the chance of starting a race at age two or three by 20%.[9] A more recent study showed no affect on performance.[41] • **Dorsal proximal accessory carpal bone fractures** – Identified in yearling Thoroughbred presale radiographs and were shown to affect earnings potential as two and three year old racehorses. Prognosis is reduced if accompanied by mild dorsal peri-articular changes of the radiocarpal joint.[48] • **Osseous cyst-like lesions** – can affect any of the carpal bones, usually incidental findings.[28] Osseous cyst-like lesions of the radial carpal bone or distal radius may cause lameness – correlate with clinical signs.
Tarsus	• **OA (tarso-metatarsal and distal intertarsal joints)**[31] – Generally risk is moderate–high for any performance horse. Assessment of risk can be difficult based on radiographs alone because correlation between radiographic findings and lameness is poor. Therefore, clinical examination, age, occupation and exercise history is important. Smooth mineralized enthetic osteophytes on the dorsoproximal aspect of MT3 may be incidental findings without other articular changes – risk is low.[29] Thoroughbred yearlings with evidence of osteophyte or enthesophyte formation at the distal intertarsal or tarso-metatarsal joint margins were significantly less likely to start as two or three year olds (difference was 7%).[9] The presence of periarticular osteophytes dorsomedially in Icelandic Ponies had a 53% predictive value for lameness.[49] • **OCD**[31] – generally risk for affecting athletic performance is considered low–moderate but site, size, subchondral bone changes and other joint changes should be considered. Studies in conservatively treated Standardbred racehorses that were evaluated as young horses show racing performance to be similar to unaffected horses.[38,50] Other studies show mild reductions in earnings and numbers of starts (especially in two year olds).[51,52] Small or well-attached fragments are low risk but effusion and lameness may result (unpredictably) when workload increases.[28] Evidence of OCD of the tarsus had little effect on the ability of a Thoroughbred yearling to start as a two or three year old.[9,41] Success rates following arthroscopic surgery are good (75–80%).[53] • **Wedged, third and/or central tarsal bones** – represents a moderate–high risk for reduced athletic peformance and may predispose to fractures.[54] Check for associated OA.

Table 60.2 Continued

REGION	RADIOLOGICAL DIAGNOSIS
Stifle	• **OCD (osteochondritis dissecans)**[31] – most horses show clinical signs within the first two years of life. However, clinical signs can manifest at any age. In addition, radiographic changes may correlate poorly with intra-articular pathology. Therefore, clinical examination findings are most important and should be assessed together with site, size, subchondral bone change, presence of concurrent OA, age, occupation and exercise history to assess risk. Mild changes (flattening, irregularity) without effusion – low risk. Larger lesions have higher risk. Prognosis for successful athletic performance following arthroscopy for femoropatellar osteochondritis dissecans is 62–82%.[53,55] • **Subchondral cystic lesions (SCL)** – although some SCLs may be asymptomatic, all SCLs of the stifle (medial femoral condyle, proximal tibia) potentially have a moderate to high risk for affecting future athletic performance because the occurrence of associated lameness is unpredictable. Communication with the articular surface increases the risk. Interpretation of SCLs in asymptomatic yearling Thoroughbreds is problematic. One study showed no effect on racing performance between 2 and 4 years of age in horses with subchondral bone cysts (SBC) or subcondral cystic lesions.[56] In another study Thoroughbred yearlings with a SBC >6 mm deep had a reduced likliehood of starting a race at two and three years of age.[41] In addition, the results of surgical therapy can vary – arthroscopic debridement carries a 30–74% success rate for successful athletic performance.[57–59] Intra-lesional cortisone therapy in Thoroughbreds showed 81% of horses returned to athletic performance.[60] Shallow concavities of the distal medial femoral condyle without underlying subchondral changes on the articular surface are generally thought to be low risk.[28] • **DJD**[31] – risk is high and treatment only palliative.

[a]All conditions should be assessed in light of the clinical examination. Only rarely do radiographic lesions by themselves allow a complete assessment of risk. Assessment of risk has been generalized for each condition. However, each horse should be evaluated as an individual.
[b]Cited references describe aspects of the radiographic, radiological or clinical features of each condition.

Limitations and problems associated with prepurchase radiographs

Radiographic evaluation in the prepurchase environment has a number of limitations and these should be discussed with the purchaser. Routine radiographic views may not detect all lesions, apparently normal radiographs do not always exclude pathological processes (e.g. developing lesions may not be detected) and apparently abnormal findings may not have current or future clinical relevance. For example, Figure 60.1 shows a radiograph of a lateral-to-medial view of the left carpus of a four-year-old dressage horse. There are two, large, well-circumscribed lucencies in the accessory carpal bone. These are unlikely to be of clinical significance and the horse did not show any pain to palpation of the accessory carpal bone or lameness after carpal flexion. Another example of an obvious radiological lesion that is not necessarily clinically significant is shown in Figure 60.2. An old apical fracture of the medial proximal sesamoid bone in the right hind leg of this two-year-old Thoroughbred racehorse is present. The horse was purchased at a public auction sale as a yearling and has shown no lameness or clinical signs associated with this joint. The best way of deciding on current clinical significance of a radiographic change is to match it carefully with the physical examination. This is why a rigorous five-stage examination is useful.

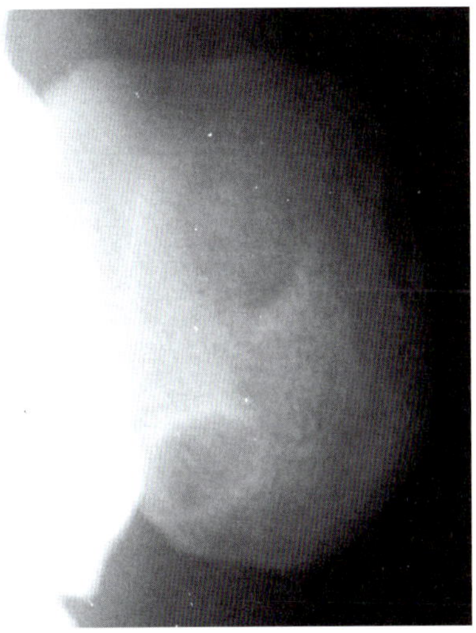

Fig 60.1 Lateral-to-medial view of the left carpus of a four-year-old dressage horse. Note the two, large, circular lucencies present in the accessory carpal bone. No clinical signs were associated with these findings.

More challenging is predicting the likelihood that radiographic changes will become a clinical problem when dealing with a young unproven animal that has not yet been subjected to training. Figure 60.3 shows a dorsolateral-palmaromedial oblique radiograph of the left carpus of a yearling Thoroughbred at a public auction sale. There is evidence of osteoarthritis with new bone formation on the dorsal medial surface of the radial carpal bone (carpitis change) and an osteophyte of the distal radial carpal bone. Because carpal disease is a common source of lameness in racing Thoroughbreds and these changes have been associated with reduced athletic performance,[9] a moderate to high risk for future lameness problems was attributed to this radiographic change. Recently, more objective information relating radiographic changes with future athletic performance has become available (see Table 60.2) to help veterinarians with risk assessment. If possible, however, rather than advising purely on radiographic changes it is better to use the combination of physical examination, conformation analysis, intended use and published information to provide the prospective purchaser with an opinion on the level of risk a particular radiographic change might pose.[32] The results from one recent study,[33] using the above method, showed that Thoroughbred yearlings who were categorized as low risk and started in a race within three years of sale were likely to earn more money than those categorized as high risk.

By giving purchasers an assessment of risk, rather than a 'pass or fail' opinion, the veterinarian can help facilitate a successful sale. However, the acceptance of risk by the purchaser can be variable and, depending on the experience of the purchaser, there is also a variable level of tolerance to faults or problems a horse may have. It may be advisable to seek more than one opinion on radiographic changes or send the films for review to a radiologist or surgeon.

Other imaging modalities

While not routine, ultrasonographic evaluation of the soft tissue structures distal to the carpus and hock has been performed with increasing frequency as part of the prepurchase examination in recent years. Common use of ultrasonography in equine practice, availability of good equipment and an expanded understanding of the importance of soft tissue musculoskeletal injury in athletic horses probably accounts for this. Indications for use include:[61]

- abnormalities identified during the clinical evaluation; careful palpation and comparison between limbs is required
- history of a previous injury
- at the purchaser's request or required by some jurisdictions, e.g. Hong Kong Jockey Club.

In addition, some veterinarians recommend ultrasonographic examination in circumstances when they suspect an injury could be present but which is not reported (e.g. event horses or racehorses that have been absent from competition for extended periods, were competing but have not competed recently, or where there is an unexplained reduction in work intensity).[8,61]

It is important that the veterinarian is familiar with the requirements for distal limb ultrasonography,[61,62] including equipment, scanning technique and permanent image recording. Image interpretation requires considerable experience. Acute and chronic tendon or ligament injury may have major consequences for future athletic performance. The site, severity, age and state of healing of any injury, together with the intended use of the horse, will determine the risk assessment for future problems in an individual case.

Nuclear scintigraphy is another imaging modality that could be utilized in the prepurchase examination.[29] It is not generally used and the potential use as a 'screening tool' in the context of a prepurchase examination would be problematic and is not recommended. An example of this is demonstrated in Figure 60.4. The prospective purchaser of an expensive elite eight-year-old dressage horse requested whole body scintigraphy. Intense bilateral uptake of radionuclide was identified within both tibiae. No hindlimb lameness was identified and radiographic examination indicated the most likely diagnosis to be bilateral enostosis-like lesions. Although the risk for future lameness associated with these lesions was considered low, lameness has been attributed to these changes

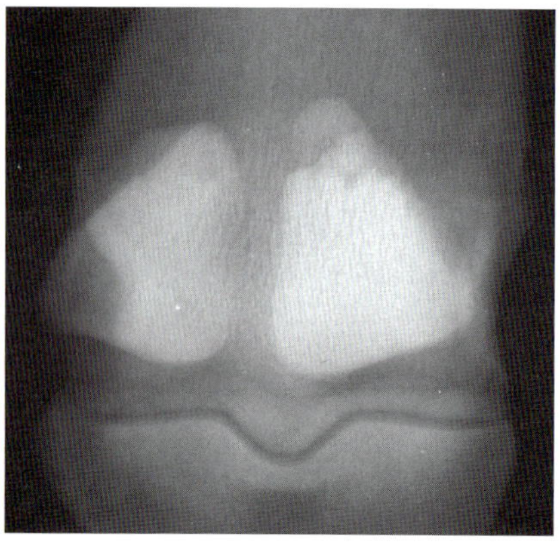

Fig 60.2 Dorsoplantar view of the right hind fetlock of a two-year-old Thoroughbred racehorse. Note the old apical fracture of the medial proximal sesamoid bone. No clinical signs were associated with this finding.

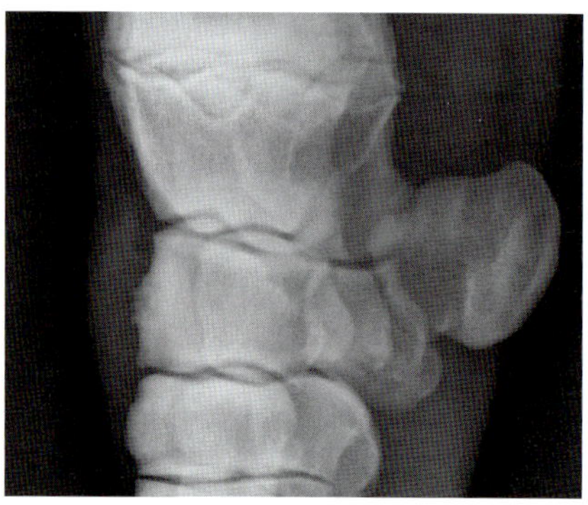

Fig 60.3 Dorsolateral-palmaromedial oblique radiograph of the left carpus of a yearling Thoroughbred. Note the new bone formation on the dorsal radial carpal bone and an osteophyte distally. These changes are consistent with osteoarthritis.

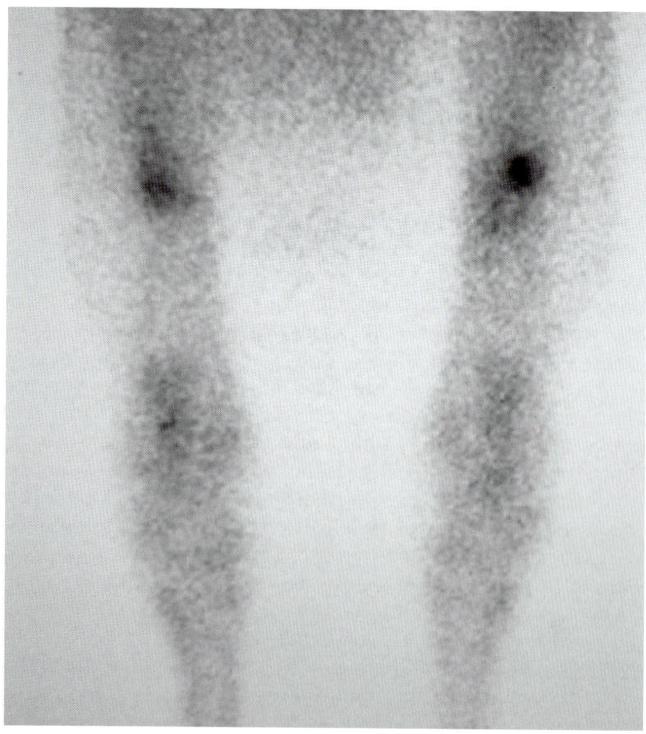

Fig 60.4 Scintigraphic image of the caudal aspect of the hindlimbs of an elite dressage horse. There is intense radionuclide uptake in both tibiae. The diagnosis was enostosis-like lesions (confirmed radiographically), which were not causing any lameness.

in some horses.[63] Regardless, in certain circumstances nuclear scintigraphy might be valuable and these include:

- assessing the current clinical significance of apparent radiological lesions or palpable osseous abnormalities
- assessing degree of healing of a previous injury, e.g. stress fracture of the pelvis or a dorsal metacarpal stress injury ('bucked shins')
- differentiating between chronic fractures and multipartite anomalies.[29]

Newer imaging modalities such as magnetic resonance imaging[64] and computed tomography could also be used in the prepurchase examination but the pros and cons would be similar to the use of nuclear scintigraphy.

Endoscopic examination of the upper respiratory tract and trachea

The use of endoscopy in the prepurchase examination is variable. Some veterinarians believe that endoscopy is only indicated if clinical examination findings determine that it would be useful (e.g. nasal discharge following exercise, abnormal respiratory noise heard at exercise). However, some abnormalities of the upper respiratory tract are not always associated with an abnormal respiratory noise, especially if the horse is not exercised fast enough. These might include ethmoid hematoma, mild arytenoid chondritis, some tumors, pharyngeal cysts and some epiglottic entrapments.[12] While dressage horses and showjumpers have competed successfully with significant laryngeal hemiplegia or other respiratory impediments, abnormal respiratory noise and reduced airflow may still affect performance and be of concern to rider and spectator. Endoscopy is recommended or indicated in the following situations:

- all racehorses should ideally be endoscoped before and after strenuous exercise
- equine athletes unable or unsuitable to be exercised strenuously. This includes yearlings at auction sales
- elite sport horses
- when abnormalities in the clinical evaluation are detected, e.g. abnormal respiratory noise at exercise, nasal discharge or cough, sinus swelling
- purchaser's request
- when purchase price demands a more comprehensive examination.[65]

A complete endoscopic examination of the upper respiratory tract and trachea is seldom performed. A methodical examination of both nasal passages, ethmoid turbinate areas, openings of the guttural pouches, pharynx, larynx and cervical trachea is usually sufficient. The examiner is looking for structural and functional abnormalities that would impair athletic performance, evidence of previous surgery or the origin of any observed nasal discharge or reason for cough.[65] It is important to document only that which was inspected and to record findings accurately. Use of a checklist is best.[65]

The limitations of the endoscopic examination should be made clear to the purchaser. A resting endoscopic examination is a static examination. There is therefore an inherent deficiency in the procedure to detect functional abnormalities that only become a problem when the horse is exercising at maximum intensity and when respiratory airflow is at a peak. Many of these abnormalities result in an abnormal respiratory noise at exercise. This is one reason why strenuous exercise is mandatory when examining the equine athlete for purchase. In the event an abnormal respiratory noise is heard at exercise but the resting examination is normal, videoendoscopy using an over-ground dynamic respiratory endoscope or during a treadmill exercise test is recommended.[66,67]

Conditions that may only be apparent during maximal exercise could include dynamic collapse of the arytenoid cartilage and vocal fold, intermittent dorsal displacement of the soft palate, dynamic collapse of the pharyngeal wall, intermittent epiglottal entrapment, dynamic axial collapse of the aryepiglottic folds, exercise-induced pulmonary hemorrhage and dynamic rostral displacement of the palatopharyngeal arch.

Difficulties arise when interpretation of laryngeal function is required and only a resting examination can be performed. Typically this occurs when scoping yearling Thoroughbred and Standardbred racehorses at sales. Laryngeal movement can be variable and a number of grading systems have been used to evaluate arytenoid abductor function.[65,68–71] Regardless of the system used most veterinarians agree that horses that cannot achieve full arytenoid abduction after swallowing or nasal occlusion are at a greater risk for reduced athletic performance due to dynamic collapse of the arytenoid cartilage and vocal fold. Indeed, when indices of racing performance were evaluated in Thoroughbred racehorses that had endoscopic evaluations at sale as yearlings were reviewed, horses that could not achieve full arytenoid abduction (grade 3 or 4) had significantly inferior racing performance compared with those that could.[68] Unfortunately, there are 'gray zones' and the interpretation and future effect on performance of laryngeal function typified by complete arytenoid abduction that is only maintained for a variable time (predominantly affecting the left arytenoid cartilage) is less clear.

One study[72] showed that Thoroughbred horses with this grade of laryngeal function had reduced earnings at age four while another study found no differences in performance between horses that had variable maintenance of arytenoid abduction vs horses with sustained arytenoid abduction.[73] Probably the best system is that used at auction sales in the United Kingdom where yearlings are trained to canter at the lunge. Evidence of a characteristic inspiratory noise at exercise and endoscopic evidence of impaired arytenoid abductor function is required for the horse to fail the conditions of sale and be returned to the vendor. An arbitration panel settles disputes. This system has been shown to be robust and accurate.[69] Unfortunately, the limitations of a static examination mean that some animals with clinically significant respiratory impairment at exercise will be missed. In addition, some animals with subclinical laryngeal neuropathy will progress to become clinically affected animals. Recent evidence suggests that progression of laryngeal neuropathy in non-affected or minimally affected horses may be as high as 15%. Very importantly, the progression may be rapid and can occur within weeks of purchase.[70] The use of laryngeal ultrasound to detect subclinical disease may be useful in the future.[74]

Examination of the Thoroughbred racehorse

Prepurchase examination of the Thoroughbred racehorse includes examination of yearlings at public auction sales, examination of young racehorses (two and three years of age) and examination of older proven racehorses. The aim of the prepurchase examination of yearlings is to identify athletic individuals who have optimal conformation and no evidence of existing cardiac abnormalities, orthopedic disease (primarily osteochondrosis), or upper respiratory tract abnormalities. The aim of the prepurchase examination of young or proven racehorses is similar but the emphasis is on identification of previous injuries or 'wear and tear' that will limit future successful performance. Apart from yearlings it is always best to perform a full five-stage evaluation as described earlier.

Prepurchase examination of yearlings at public auction sales

It is very important that the examining veterinarian be familiar with the conditions of sale for each sales company. Horses are auctioned with no warranty for use or soundness other than certain conditions listed in the conditions of sale.[75] The veterinarian must be familiar with certain diseases/disorders that if not declared prior to auction and identified after sale (within a specified time) may render the purchased horse returnable. These usually pertain to vices (windsucker), ataxia (wobbler), cryptorchidism, pregnancy and laryngeal hemiplegia. The process for arbitration of purchases in dispute is also in the conditions of sale. Drug testing is available at some sales. Conditions relating to endoscopic and radiographic examinations need to be carefully understood. These are printed in the sales catalog.

A description of the horse is not performed but the lot number (hip sticker) and presented animal should always be matched to the catalog description to ensure the correct horse is examined. It is preferable to work only for buyers with whom you have a relationship and whose requirements you understand. A limited examination is more commonly performed and accepted by buyers.[7] This is because the sales venue is a difficult environment to appraise animals carefully. Young excited horses with limited education can be difficult to examine. The combination of noisy surroundings, many other horses, poor lighting and crowds of people mean a complete examination is not possible. The examination generally includes:

- visual examination of the head, neck, body, external genitalia, fore- and hindlimbs
- palpation of the head, neck, body, fore- and hindlimbs and visible abnormality elsewhere on the body that is palpable; inspection of both eyes with a penlight
- auscultation of the heart (on both sides) and on some occasions the chest
- examination of conformation, limb movements during walking and coordination.

The veterinarian should make sure to:

- carefully inspect the feet and hoof pastern axis. 'Long toe-low heel', weak or collapsed heels, poor-quality hoof, contracted feet, clubfeet, markedly mismatched feet and overly small feet are undesirable and predispose to lameness. Horses with varus deformities of any joint seldom stay sound. Moderate to markedly 'offset knees', 'back in the knee', 'sickle hocks' or overly straight hocks may predispose to lameness and are undesirable.
- look for enlarged pasterns, sesamoid bones and flexor tendons.
- examine all joints for effusion. Osteochondrosis is suspected until proven otherwise.[76] Some mild effusion within carpal joints appears normal in yearlings and a variable fat pad in the stifle may mimic stifle effusion.
- horses that either cannot or have difficulty fully abducting both arytenoid cartilages are at high risk of performing poorly. Epiglottal entrapment, persistent dorsal displacement of the soft palate, arytenoid cartilage enlargement (chondritis), rostral displacement of the soft palate, subepiglottic cyst, cleft palate and marked hypoplasia of the epiglottis are all unacceptable conditions of the upper respiratory tract which will impair athletic performance. Conditions of sale at each sales venue will determine whether an animal is returnable or not.
- radiological lesions, which indicate a risk for future performance limitations, are listed in Table 60.2.

Examination of the mature horse

The examination procedure for prepurchase examinations of Thoroughbred racehorses is similar to other athletes. However, certain injuries in Thoroughbred racehorses result in reduced performance or may even prohibit successful athletic performance and are not tolerated as they might be in other equine athletes. Chronic foot problems, chronic osteoarthritic disease, subchondral bone injury, sesamoiditis, tendon/ligamentous injury and dynamic collapse of the arytenoid cartilages are conditions that have a high risk of reducing athletic performance. Chronic pulmonary hemorrhage and small airways disease are also responsible for poor performance. A recent review highlights foot, fetlock, carpal and suspensory ligament injuries as the most common orthopedic injury sites resulting in lameness in Throughbred racehorses.[77,78] Therefore, the veterinarian should focus on these areas during the examination procedure.

A buyer's statement should be completed and the veterinarian should discuss in detail with the potential purchaser what extra examinations are to be performed, e.g. endoscopy, radiography, ultrasonography, blood/urine tests. It should also be clear what the expectations for future training and racing will be. The vendor's statement should be completed and a full history relating to recent medication, training and racing should be attained.

A full five-stage examination is performed and endoscopy of the upper respiratory tract and trachea (preferably before and after exercise) and radiographs of the carpi, fetlocks and front feet are usually conducted. Other areas are radiographed if the clinical examination determines this would be beneficial. For stage 3 of the examination, the horse should be sufficiently warmed up and then galloped hard with the last 600 m in 39–40 seconds. The veterinarian should position him/herself so that any abnormal respiratory noise can be heard. The jockey should be asked to pull the horse up as quickly as is safe and canter back to the examiner. This is often the time when noises typical of dorsal displacement of the soft palate can be heard and as the horse slows and stops such noises can disappear. The trachea is auscultated for fluid and the chest is auscultated while the veterinarian listens carefully for disturbances in heart rhythm and heart sounds. The nostrils are checked for discharge (blood/mucus) and the mouth and lips checked for blood. The horse should have endoscopy performed as soon as possible and arytenoid function assessed and any pharyngeal or tracheal discharges identified and noted. After the horse has been hosed down an assessment is made of recovery with heart, respiratory rates and chest sounds noted at approximately 15 min intervals. The lower limbs are checked for interference injuries. The veterinarian should make sure of the following points:

- Evaluate conformation as for yearlings but pay close attention to the feet. Mild conformational flaws especially in the well-performed horse may have little significance. Conformational abnormalities play an important role in career longevity and they should be viewed with this in mind. It is interesting to note that a study of conformation of elite young Thoroughbred racehorses and sires showed that in the forelimbs most horses had mildly offset and valgus 'knees', were slightly 'over the knee', had slightly broken back hoof-pastern axes but had little deviation from the fetlock to the ground ('toe in or toe out'). In the hindlimbs being slightly 'cow hocked' and being 'toe out' was considered normal.[21]
- Acquired hoof deformities/injuries such as collapsed heels, shear heels, wry hooves, bruising and corns, medial-lateral hoof imbalance, broken hoof-pastern axes, mismatched feet,

poor shoeing and evidence of previous episodes of laminitis should be noted.

- Check for muscle asymmetry, especially differences in the gluteal musculature. Differences in height of the tuber sacrale if minor and unassociated with pain are often insignificant. Palpate the croup and back checking for pain and muscle spasm. 'Cycle the back' by inducing flexion and extension and assess lateral flexibility using a blunt probe that is run along the epaxial muscles on either side.[79]
- Look carefully for evidence of joint disease, pain/enlargement of the proximal sesamoid bones and ligamentous/tendinous thickening and sensitivity on palpation. Correlate findings with manipulative tests, radiographs and ultrasonographic examinations.
- Carefully record all findings and give opinions on current or future effects on performance in terms of an assessment of risk.

Examination of the Standardbred racehorse

When performing prepurchase examination on Standardbred racehorses, the use of the full five-stage examination is strongly advised. A number of purchasers request less extensive examinations and while this is appropriate, stages 1 and 2 should be considered a minimum examination as this allows for a detailed clinical examination and observation in motion. Beware of examination requests such as 'heart and wind only' or 'legs and heart' as use of these tailor-made types of examination allow for omission of important observations.

Clinical examination

Conformation

Limb conformational defects of particular importance to Standardbreds tend to center on the 'knees'. Pacers with 'toe out' conformation (viewed cranially/caudally when walking) may be at risk for interference due to knee strike at speed. Bench or offset knees are often associated with 'toe out' conformation and can also exacerbate knee strike. Horses with long pasterns and long toes/low heels are at risk for tendon injuries.

Skin conditions

Scars or excoriations on the side of the neck can be evidence of steering difficulties from the use of steering correction devices such as a pricker or boring pole.

Common injuries

Careful examination of the forelimb suspensory ligaments is advised as subtle evidence of previous desmitis may only show as a thickening of the width of the ligament. Non-weight-bearing palpation of the palmar flexor tendons in the pastern area may indicate previous 'low bows' (tendinitis) in a similar fashion to suspensory desmitis, as an increase in the width of the palmar flexor tendons. Any visible medial effusion of the intercarpal joint space warrants a suggestion for carpal radiography. Curbs (thickening at the plantar aspect of the tarsus) are common but are rarely of clinical concern. Partial (unicortical) or small midsagittal fractures of the dorsal first phalanx are common and deep palpation of the proximal dorsal cortex of P1 should be performed in all four limbs, particularly the hindlimbs. Any subtle visible bony thickening of proximo-dorsal P1 should warrant pastern radiographs. In such cases often only the lateral to medial projection shows evidence of periosteal disruption and new bone deposition on the proximal dorsal first phalanx indicative of this fracture. Hoof imbalances become more important in older Standardbreds; imbalance in younger horses is correctable and should be advised. Any effusion of the tibiotarsal joint would warrant radiographs to look for OCD, most commonly seen on the distal aspect of the distal intermediate ridge of the tibia. The interpretation of intermediate ridge OCD lesions if found is difficult as there is controversy about their clinical significance, especially with respect to performance. In young, unproven racehorses with intermediate ridge OCD lesions any tibiotarsal effusion may be significant to future performance, while in older proven racehorses with intermediate ridge OCD lesions, many can have adequate to date racing performances even in the face of moderate joint effusion. In a number of horses where routine hock radiographs are taken, intermediate ridge OCD lesions can show up as incidental findings.

Stage 3 exercise

Horses should be observed working under race condition where possible (e.g. fast working over 2000 m, coming home the last 400 m in 28 seconds). Working near race conditions allows for observation of respiratory noise while working, listening for knee strike and observing recovery rate post-exercise. At the end of the exercise phase is an ideal time for upper respiratory endoscopic examination if it is to be performed. Observation of laryngeal function shortly after work allows evaluation of the larynx while the horse still has an elevated respiratory effort during recovery and allows checking of the trachea for blood and mucopurulent discharge, often only seen post-exercise.

Ancillary tests

Electrocardiographic examination

An ECG examination as part of the prepurchase is commonly requested by Australian buyers primarily for a 'heart score' determination. Apart from the numerical heart score and assessment of T wave changes (so-called 'heart strain') the ECG does not add greatly to the prepurchase examination and its use is based mainly on purchaser's request.

Upper airway endoscopic examination

In the absence of someone reliable (bloodstock agent or prominent driver) having driven the Standardbred racehorse and consequently listened to the horse's respiratory noise under race-day conditions first hand, endoscopy is normally recommended as part of the prepurchase examination. Whilst laryngeal dysfunction is not as common in Standardbreds as Thoroughbreds, endoscopic examination is a reliable screening procedure for such problems. As mentioned previously, if a full five-stage examination is performed valuable information can be gained from examination of the tracheal lumen for blood and mucus after exercise ('hot scoping'). Luminal fluid may not be evident when examined without exercise ('cold scoping'). If a 'cold' endoscopic examination is performed (e.g. associated with a partial stages 1 and 2 examination) this should be stated in the report.

Radiography

The majority of Australasian Standardbreds examined prior to purchase are young, 'up and coming' horses with little hard racing experience. As such it is unusual to find many radiographic abnormalities indicative of chronic 'wear and tear'. For this reason recommendations on radiography are generally based on purchaser request and the personal preference of the examining veterinarian. It is common to find the presence of fetlock bony fragments (ununited plantar eminence of the proximal phalanx, and type I OCD fragments of the palmar/plantar aspect of the first phalanx),[38] especially when routine hindlimb fetlock radiographs are taken. As with distal intermediate ridge OCD the interpretation of such fetlock fragments with respect to future performance is very difficult. The majority of the fetlock fragments are incidental findings and do not appear to be of clinical significance. Interestingly, routine multiple joint radiographs are normally associated with the prepurchase examination of more expensive and often well-proven Standardbred racehorses. The interpretation of any such fetlock fragments must take into account that these horses have been performing well in the upper levels of competition and that it is most likely that these fragments have been present during their most recent performances and as such their clinical significance may be questionable. As with all radiographic findings their presence needs to be stated in the radiology report.

Examination of the proven racehorse

The prepurchase examination of the older proven racehorse follows the principles outlined above. In line with other breeds, the examination of proven animals compared with unproven ones requires special attention to signs and consequences of 'wear and tear'.

Hoof balance and shoeing abnormalities, e.g. long toes/low heels, should be looked for, as the chronicity of these is more important to the older racehorse. Deep digital palpation of the proximal row of carpal bones should be carried out to check for any withdrawal, which can indicate carpal disease and warrants radiography, especially skyline views. Another area deserving of careful deep digital palpation is the origin of the forelimb suspensory ligaments. Withdrawal to deep palpation in this area can be indicative of chronic suspensory origin desmitis. Especially scrutinize this area if there are any differences to palpation between the two front legs. Most racehorses are worked (stage 3) with knee boots on and it is worth examining these at the end of the exercise phase for evidence of brushing or knee strike.

In proven racehorses it is more common to undertake extensive radiographic examinations looking for signs of disease; knees and front fetlocks are normally requested.

Examination at yearling sales

Compared with Thoroughbreds, Standardbred yearlings tend to be less well handled and this limits the types of examinations possible at yearling sales. An abridged examination mostly centered on a basic clinical examination and determination of conformational defects is carried out. Base narrow conformation and toe out forelimb conformation on walking may predispose to knee strike. Bench/offset knees and 'back at the knee' are also looked upon as important knee conformational defects. Joint effusion (especially tibiotarsal) may indicate OCD. As is standard at yearling sales, endoscopy is often conducted and advised.

Examination of the sport horse prior to purchase

This section focuses on specific aspects pertaining to the examination of event horses, showjumpers and dressage horses prior to purchase. The majority of showjumpers and dressage horses competing internationally are Warmbloods, whereas most event horses competing at that level are Thoroughbreds, frequently ex-racehorses. Because these two types of horses are quite different, and present with their own unique conformational and soundness issues, they will be discussed separately.

Examination of the three-day event horse prior to purchase

Three-day eventing combines the disciplines of dressage, showjumping and cross-country, including a steeplechase and roads and tracks phase. Therefore, the event horse must primarily be a bold and clever jumper, with plenty of scope and speed. It is because of this that Thoroughbred horses tend to excel. However, in today's competitive environment, speed and braveness alone are no longer enough to succeed at the top level, and the horse must also have good basic gaits and a temperament suitable for dressage training, combined with a careful showjumping technique. Because the horses compete on extremely variable terrain and footing, three-day eventing places huge strains on the musculoskeletal system and horses with poor conformation are especially at risk of injury. The majority of injuries sustained by top-level event horses are repetitive strain injuries to soft tissues and joints, particularly to the superficial digital flexor tendons, and injuries resulting from direct trauma during the cross-country phase. Exertional rhabdomyolysis ('tying up') is also a common cause of failure to complete the event.

When examining a potential event horse prior to purchase it is important to obtain a thorough history pertaining to the horse's athletic endeavors up to the point of sale. Most horses being purchased for eventing are Thoroughbred horses that have finished their racing careers, and many racehorses are retired from racing due to injury. Therefore, if possible, the exact reason for the horse's retirement from the track should be ascertained. Although some racehorses are just too slow or are getting too old to continue racing competitively, many suffer from some kind of disability that has reduced their racing performance and may also affect their ability to become a top-class event horse. Superficial digital flexor tendinitis, dorsal carpal bone chip fractures and dorsoproximal first phalanx chip fractures are all common causes of lameness in racehorses that may result in their retirement from the racetrack. Similarly, a poor performer on the racetrack may suffer from respiratory problems such as left-sided laryngeal hemiplegia ('roaring') or exercise-induced pulmonary hemorrhage ('bleeding'). The owner's statement should include questions that specifically address these problems; i.e. whether the horse has ever been lame, whether it has ever bled from the nostrils and whether it has ever made an abnormal respiratory noise during exercise. If the horse has already competed as an event horse it is pertinent to determine how many events it has actually completed at what level, and the reasons for not completing events, such as being withdrawn from a competition due to unsoundness or exertional rhabdomyolysis.

After establishing a thorough history, a comprehensive clinical examination should be performed at rest with particular attention to conformation. Horses with poor foot conformation, very upright hoof-pastern axes, and horses that are back at the knees typically do not stand up well to top-level competition. In our experience Thoroughbred horses often have large front feet with flat soles, long toes and under-run heels. The long-toe, low-heel syndrome in particular appears to predispose these horses to chronic bruising and caudal heel pain when jumping large fences on hard ground, and foot-related lameness is one of the most common causes of event horses failing to complete the season. Synovial effusion, especially in the carpi and front fetlock joints, and a decreased range of joint motion with signs of resistance or pain on flexion should alert the veterinarian to the possibility of osteoarthritis subsequent to injury. The digital flexor tendons and suspensory ligaments should be carefully palpated for size and evidence of inflammation or pain, and an ultrasonographic examination of the tendons should be performed if there is any suspicion of previous injury. Following completion of the examination at rest the horse should be assessed while walking and trotting in hand on a hard, level surface (preferably concrete or asphalt), both before and immediately after flexion tests of the distal limbs and carpi in the front limbs, and full limb (spavin) tests in the hindlimbs. The horse should be ridden at a trot and canter on both reins in order to assess its paces and temperament, and if facilities permit the horse should be galloped a sufficient distance for the veterinarian to observe any abnormal respiratory noise and to evaluate heart rate, sound and rhythm following exercise. An endoscopic examination of the upper respiratory tract is usually performed immediately post-exercise to assess laryngeal function and examine for evidence of exercise-induced pulmonary hemorrhage. Once cooled off from the gallop the horse should be lunged at the trot on a 10-meter circle in both directions, preferably on a hard, level surface, to examine for low-grade lameness induced by exercise.

Given that many Thoroughbred horses are broken in and raced at a young age, most purchasers request radiographs to be taken of the most commonly injured areas, including the front feet, pastern and fetlock joints, the carpi and the hocks. Other areas may be subject to radiography if a problem is determined to exist based on the clinical examination, such as a painful splint bone exostosis or effusion in a hind fetlock joint. Commonly observed radiographic changes in Thoroughbred ex-racehorses being examined prior to purchase for eventing include evidence of pedal osteitis and chronic sesamoiditis, dorsoproximal first phalanx chip fractures, dorsal carpal osteophyte formation and/or chip fractures, and osteophyte formation on the dorsoproximal aspect of the third metatarsus at the level of the tarso-metatarsal joint space. Because radiographic evidence of pedal osteitis and sesamoiditis tends to persist throughout the horse's life we feel that they are generally not clinically significant provided that there is no evidence of ongoing pain or inflammation of these structures at the time of the examination. Traumatic chip fractures of the first phalanx and carpus usually result in the development of degenerative joint disease with ongoing exercise unless they are removed arthroscopically soon after forming; therefore, they must always be regarded with caution in horses expected to go on to athletic careers. Osteophyte formation on the dorsoproximal aspect of the third metatarsal bone seems to occur frequently in young Thoroughbred horses and can be present at a relatively early age. They are often bilateral and radiographically appear smooth-edged and of uniform density. In our experience, provided that the tarso-metatarsal joint space is uncompromised and well defined, and the horse exhibits no signs of lameness or abnormal response to hindlimb flexion tests, this specific radiographic change has not become clinically significant when the horses go on to become event horses. This is supported by the results of a retrospective study of equine prepurchase examinations performed between 1991 and 2000 at the University of California, Davis,[80] where 20/21 horses with significant radiographic changes in the distal intertarsal and tarsometatarsal joints were still able to compete at their expected level.

Examination of dressage horses and showjumpers prior to purchase

A good dressage horse must possess natural balance, elegance and athleticism, as well as power and a trainable mind. The majority of dressage horses competing internationally are Warmbloods with a high proportion of Thoroughbred blood, combining the athleticism of the Thoroughbred with the trainability of the Warmblood. Through training, the horse's center of gravity is shifted caudally by increasing the degree of flexion and loading of the hindlimbs, thereby freeing the forehand to create a more airborne, uphill type of movement. As well as the general increased loading of the hindlimbs, particularly the hock joints, the lateral movements required by the sport create a unique strain on the horse's back and additional twisting stress on the appendicular joints. Because the training of dressage horses predominantly involves repetitive exercises designed to maintain suppleness and increase muscle strength, these horses rarely suffer from acute traumatic injuries but more commonly from cumulative wear and tear lesions. This is exacerbated by the fact that it takes at least five years for a horse to be trained to Grand Prix level and most dressage horses continue to compete to an advanced age, often as old as 20 years.

As with top-level dressage horses, the majority of successful showjumpers are Warmbloods, as these are usually large, well-balanced, athletic individuals. The showjumper must be strong enough to jump large fences with precision and care, both from a virtual standstill and at speed, and supple enough to make sharp turns without losing impulsion. The stresses placed on the musculoskeletal system of elite showjumpers are huge, especially on the hocks and hindlimb suspensory apparatus during take-off and on the front feet and front limb suspensory apparatus at landing. Therefore, when examining dressage horses and showjumpers prior to purchase the veterinarian should pay specific attention to the front feet, pasterns, hocks, and the front and hind suspensory ligaments. The horse should be evaluated at rest, trotting freely in hand on a hard surface, and while ridden and lunged in both directions on a hard as well as a soft surface. It is important to remember when examining a dressage horse prior to purchase that a good rider is able to correct and hide a mild gait irregularity or lameness. Therefore the veterinarian should not just focus on the limbs but also look for changes such as increased resistance to bending in either direction or reluctance to accept the bit. It is useful to lunge the horse after it has been ridden to look for any differences in the gait that may be attributable to the rider.

Foot conformation is extremely important, as many Warmbloods have small feet relative to their bodyweight. Slight differences in the size and shape of the two front feet are common and not necessarily abnormal. However, marked asymmetry of the hooves is often an acquired condition as a consequence of a previous lameness (chronic under-loading of one foot relative to the other). The horse should be lunged or ridden in small circles on hard ground in both directions to exacerbate any low-grade, foot-related lameness. High suspensory (origin of suspensory) disease in the front limbs is very common both in dressage horses and in showjumpers. It results in a mild lameness that is typically observed most easily when the horse is circling in deep footing with the affected limb on the outside of the circle. Although most cases of front limb high suspensory disease resolve over time with the horse eventually returning to its previous level of competition, they can be very slow to heal. Hindlimb proximal suspensory ligament disease is a serious condition that frequently recurs with work. It tends to be associated with a straight hock conformation and is exacerbated by collection. Lesions of the suspensory body and branches are also common and are often the cause of retirement for showjumpers. Therefore it is important to carefully palpate the entire suspensory ligament for evidence of swelling, pain or inflammation. Digital flexor tendon sheath enlargement ('windgalls') that is bilaterally symmetrical is usually benign.

However, extreme unilateral distension is the result of chronic inflammation and is often associated with synovial proliferation and development of adhesions that may cause lameness. The thoracolumbar region should be carefully palpated because the back is prone to low-grade muscular injury and bony abnormalities such as impingement of the dorsal spinous processes that can cause recurrent discomfort. However, asymmetry of the tuber sacrale ('hunter's bumps') is common in showjumpers and is usually considered insignificant provided there is no evidence of lameness, loss of performance or palpable pain in the lumbosacral area.

Because the respiratory requirements for dressage horses and showjumpers are modest compared with those of three-day event horses, endoscopy may or may not be requested by the purchaser. Laryngeal hemiplegia is not usually performance limiting, but the noise produced may be disturbing to the purchaser, especially when the horse's head and neck are flexed. Most purchasers do request radiographs to be taken of the areas most commonly associated with decreased performance, including the front feet, pastern and fetlock joints, and the hocks.

Radiographs of the front feet and navicular bones do not correlate well with the presence of clinical signs and should be interpreted with caution, but certain radiographic lesions are a cause for concern. For example, in the dorsoproximal-palmarodistal oblique (upright pedal) view, up to seven conical nutrient foramina along the distal border of the navicular bone are considered normal. However, multiple enlarged or misshapen foramina and large central radiolucent areas (cysts) are almost always abnormal. It is interesting to note that larger breeds of horses such as Warmbloods tend to tolerate more extensive radiographic changes in the navicular bone and distal phalanx without an increased incidence of lameness compared to Thoroughbreds, which are less likely to be sound with similar changes.[80] Although many horses with mild navicular pain that are managed appropriately are acceptable for pleasure riding and lower levels of competition, the tendency to adopt a shortened stride is detrimental in a dressage horse and the pain associated with landing makes this condition incompatible with jumping big jumps. Ossification of the collateral cartilages ('sidebones') is frequently seen, especially in larger, heavier horses, but is rarely a source of lameness or related to any clinically significant foot abnormalities. Both front and hind proximal interphalangeal (pastern) joints often show slight bony modeling of the dorsoproximal articular margin of the second phalanx. Although these early radiographic changes are usually of no clinical significance, they can occasionally progress to proximal interphalangeal osteoarthritis ('ringbone'), especially in horses with short, upright pasterns. Small, smooth-edged radio-opaque bodies are often found at the dorsoproximal aspect of the first and third phalanges in Warmbloods. They are typically not considered clinically significant provided the joints are clinically normal and there is no radiographic evidence of osteoarthritis. Similarly, small smooth-edged osteophytes on the dorsoproximal aspect of the third metatarsal bone are frequently present without any compromise in performance. However, because osteoarthritis of the distal intertarsal and tarso-metatarsal joints is a common cause of lameness in dressage horses and showjumpers, any associated radiographic irregularity of the joint spaces and/or positive clinical response to hindlimb flexion tests should be viewed with extreme caution in a future performance horse.

Examination of the western performance horse prior to purchase

Western performance horses perform in a wide variety of disciplines, each of which places unique demands on the horse. Disciplines to be discussed include: reining and cutting, roping, barrel racing, and western pleasure. Close attention to conformation should be made in all western performance horse evaluations. Size of the hoof in relationship to body size, hoof balance, and hoof/pastern axis should all be closely evaluated. Abnormalities in these factors may predispose the horse to navicular syndrome and to osteoarthritis (OA) of the distal limb joints.[81] Upright rear limb conformation may predispose the horse to OA of the distal limbs and to bone spavin. The distal forelimbs should be evaluated closely for neurectomy scars, especially in middle-aged horses, because of the high incidence of heel pain in these horses.[82]

The genetic background of horses of the Quarter Horse breed should be scrutinized for presence of the hyperkalemic periodic paralysis (HYPP) gene. The American Quarter Horse Association registration certificate will designate if the horse has HYPP parentage or other genetic defects such as parrot mouth or cryptorchidism.[83]

Reining and cutting horses begin rigorous training as two year olds to prepare for futurity competitions that begin during their three-year-old season. These horses make rapid starts and stops, and abrupt changes in direction that will stress many of their musculoskeletal structures. Reining and cutting horses usually have a short and slight body style that allows for maximum agility. Areas of concern include: distal limbs (navicular region, distal interphalangeal and proximal interphalangeal joints), tarsal region, and stifles. Developmental orthopedic diseases such as osteochondrosis and flexural deformity must also be ruled out in young horses. Radiographic evaluations of the distal forelimbs, tarsi and stifles are commonly a part of the prepurchase examination.[84]

Roping horses need to make repeated short bursts of rapid acceleration and rapid stops. They have a more muscled and substantial body style compared with reining and cutting horses. Areas of concern on the prepurchase examination include the distal forelimbs (particularly the navicular region and the distal joints), and the tarsi. Rear limb tendinitis and suspensory desmitis commonly occur in this group of horses and these structures bear close evaluation.[84]

Barrel racing horses, and horses that compete in western performance games (gymkhana), place a premium on short bursts of speed and the ability to make short-radius, rapid turns. All the joints from the carpi and tarsi distal need close evaluation in these horses. Osteoarthritis, tendinitis and desmitis occur with high frequency in these athletes.

Western pleasure horses begin competition as three year olds so are in training at a young age. These horses work at very slow walk, trot and canter gaits in the ring. A premium is placed on a quiet disposition. Overt signs of displeasure by the horse such as tail wringing or excessive head and mouth movements are counted against the horse during competition. Areas of concern during prepurchase examination include the distal forelimbs, tarsi and back. Ring work at slow gaits predisposes some horses in this discipline to lower back pain. When possible, western pleasure horses should be evaluated under saddle to determine their responses during work.

References

1. Pycock JF. Evaluation of the reproductive system in stallions and mares for breeding purposes. In: Mair TS, editor. The pre-purchase examination. Suffolk: EVJ Ltd; 1998. p. 138–47.
2. Asbury AC. Medical evaluation of the reproductive system relevant to purchase. Vet Clin North Am Equine Pract 1992; 8(2):395–412.
3. Mantrell JAR. The aim of the pre-purchase veterinary

examination. Suffolk: EVJ Ltd; 1998. p. 9–13.

4. Beeman GM, Soule SG, Swanson TD. History and philosophy of the medical examination of horses for purchase. Vet Clin North Am Equine Pract 1992;8(2): 257–66.
5. Anderson GF. Evaluation of the hoof and foot relevant to purchase. Vet Clin North Am Equine Pract 1992;8(2):303–18.
6. Pascoe RR, Huntington PJ. A guide to examination of horses. 3rd ed. Artarmon: Australian Equine Veterinary Association; 1993. p. 6–9.
7. Goulden BE. Examination of horses. 2nd ed. Palmerston North: Equine Branch New Zealand Veterinary Association; 1997. p. 7.
8. Mitchell RD, Dyson SJ. Pre-purchase examination of the performance horse. In: Ross MW, Dyson SJ, editors. Diagnosis and management of lameness in the horse. St Louis: Saunders; 2003. p. 951–64.
9. Kane AJ, McIlwraith CW, Park RD, et al. The effect of radiographic changes in thoroughbred yearlings on future racing performance. Proc Am Assoc Equine Pract 2000;46:370–4.
10. Wilson HC. Legal aspects and do's and dont's. In: Mair T, editor. The pre-purchase examination. Suffolk: EVJ Ltd; 1998. p. 200–4.
11. Chandler N. The five stage prior to purchase examination. In: Mair TS, editor. The pre-purchase examination. Suffolk: EVJ Ltd; 1998. p. 20–4.
12. Marks D. Pre-purchase examination of jumpers and dressage horses. Proc Am Assoc Equine Pract 1999;45:4–12.
13. Sloet van Oldruitenborgh-Oosterbaan MM. Performance evaluation for the prepurchase examination: How is it done in the Netherlands. In: Lindner A, editor. Performance diagnosis and purchase examination of elite sport horses. CESMAS 2010. The Netherlands: Wageningen Academic Publishers; 2010. p. 141–6.
14. Starke SD, Willems E, Head M, et al. Proximal hindlimb flexion in the horse: Effect on movement symmetry and implications for defining soundness. Equine Vet J 2012;44(2012) 657–63.
15. Dyson SJ. Evaluation of the musculoskeletal system part 4: The use of flexion tests and small diameter lungeing. In: Mair TS, editor. The pre-purchase examination. Suffolk: EVJ Ltd; 1998. p. 95–100.
16. Schubert K. Veterinary Defence Society – experience of claims relating to prior to purchase examinations (PPEs). In: Mair TS, editor. The pre-purchase examination. Suffolk: EVJ Ltd; 1998. p. 205–10.
17. Soule GS. Pre-purchase examinations: An historical perspective and important things to consider. Proc Am Assoc Equine Pract 2009;55:286–91.
18. Ross MW. Conformation and lameness. In: Ross MW, Dyson SJ, editors. Diagnosis and management of lameness in the horse. St Louis: Saunders; 2003. p. 15–31.
19. Marks D. Conformation and soundness. Proc Am Assoc Equine Pract 2000;46: 39–45.
20. Stashak TS, Hill C. Conformation and movement. In: Stashak TS, editor. Adams' lameness in horses. 5th ed. Philadelphia: Lippincott Williams and Wilkins; 2002. p. 73–111.
21. Mawdsley A, Kelly EP, Smith FH, et al. Linear assessment of the Thoroughbred horse: an approach to conformation evaluation. Equine Vet J 1996;28(6): 461–7.
22. Holmstršm M, Magnusson L-E, Phillipsson J. Variation in conformation of Swedish Warmblood hoses and conformational characteristics of elite sport horses. Equine Vet J 1990;22:186.
23. Back W, Kawcak CE. The role of conformation on performance and predisposition to injury: is there a difference between thoroughbreds and warmbloods? In: Lindner A, editor. Performance diagnosis and purchase examination of elite sport horses. CESMAS 2010. The Netherlands: Wageningen Academic Publishers; 2010. p. 35–9.
24. Bousum P. Ancillary testing during the pre-purchase examination. Proc Am Assoc Equine Pract 1999;45:27–30.
25. McEwen JC. Drug testing, clinical pathology and other tests: routine medical control. In: Mair TS, editor. The pre-purchase examination. Suffolk: EVJ Ltd; 1998. p. 177–82.
26. Patteson M. Evaluation of the heart and cardiac disease. In: Mair TS, editor. The pre-purchase examination. Suffolk: EVJ Ltd; 1998. p. 117–25.
27. Dart AJ, Snyder JR, Pascoe JR, et al. Pre-purchase evaluation of horses: 134 cases (1988–1990). J Am Vet Med Assoc 1992;201(7):1061–7.
28. Phillips TJ. The use of radiography in the pre-purchase examination. In: Mair TS, editor. The pre-purchase examination. Suffolk: EVJ Ltd; 1998. p. 154–60.
29. Neuwirth L. Imaging and the pre purchase examination. In: White NA, Moore JN, editors. Current techniques in equine surgery and lameness. 2nd ed. Philadelphia: WB Saunders; 1998. p. 654–71.
30. Jackson MA, Vizard AL, Anderson GA, et al. Identification and prevalence of errors affecting the quality of radiographs submitted to Australian thoroughbred yearling sale repositories. Vet Radiol Ultrasound 2011;52(3):262–9.
31. Butler JA, Colles CM, Dyson SJ, et al. Clinical radiology of the horse. 2nd ed. Oxford: Blackwell Science; 2000.
32. Pilsworth R, Head M. Presales radiographic surveys in yearlings 1. Image interpretation and significance of lesions in the fetlock. In Practice 2010;32:174–83.
33. Abidin I, Anderson BH, Fulton IC, et al. Risk assessment for purchase of thoroughbred yearlings using radiographic evaluation. In Proceedings of the 29th Bain Fallon Conference 2007, Freemantle, WA, Australia.
34. Kaneps AJ, O'Brien TR, Redden RF, et al. Characterisation of osseous bodies of the distal phalanx of foal. Equine Vet J 1993;25:285–92.
35. Biggi M, Dyson S. Distal border fragments and shape of the navicular bone: Radiological evaluation in lame horses and horses free from lameness. Equine Vet J 2012;44(2012):325–31.
36. Vargus JV, Bramlage LR, Spike-Pierce DL. Racing prognosis of thoroughbred yearlings with subchondral bone lucencies in the proximal interphalangeal joint. Proc Am Assoc Equine Pract 2011;57:242.
37. Ruggles AJ. The proximal and middle phalanges and proximal interphalageal joint. In: Ross MW, Dyson SJ, editors. Diagnosis and management of lameness in the horse. St Louis: Saunders; 2003. p. 342–8.
38. Jorgensen HS, Proschowsky H, Falkronne J, et al. The significance of routine radiographic findings with respect to subsequent racing performance and longevity in Standardbred trotters. Equine Vet J 1997;29(1):55–9.
39. McIlwraith CW. Fetlock fractures and luxations. In: Nixon AJ, editor. Equine fracture repair. Philadelphia: WB Saunders; 1996. p. 153–62.
40. Preston SA, Zimmel DN, Chmielewski TL, et al. Prevalence of various presale radiographic findings and association of findings with sales price in Thoroughbred yearlings sold in Kentucky. J Am Vet Med Assoc 2010;236:440–5.
41. Jackson M, Vizard A, Anderson G, et al. A prospective study of presale radiographs of thoroughbred yearlings. RIRDC Publication No 09/082 July 2009.
42. Hardy J, Marcoux M, Breton L. Clinical relevance of radiographic findings in proximal sesamoid bones of two year old Standardbreds in their first year of race training. J Am Vet Med Assoc 1991; 198(12):2089–94.
43. Richardson DW. The metacarpophalangeal joint. In: Ross MW, Dyson SJ, editors. Diagnosis and management of lameness in the horse. St Louis: Saunders; 2003. p. 348–62.
44. Grondahl AM, Gaustad G, Engeland A. Progression and association with lameness and racing performance of radiographic changes in the proximal sesamoid bones of young Standardbred trotters. Equine Vet J 1994;26(2):152–5.
45. Spike DL, Bramlage LR, Howard BA, et al. Radiographic proximal sesamoiditis

in Thoroughbred sales yearlings. Proc Am Assoc Equine Pract 1997;43:132–3.
46. Spike-Pierce DL, Bramlage LR. Correlation of racing performance with radiographic changes in the proximal sesamoid bones of 487 thoroughbred yearlings. Equine Vet J 2003;35:350–3.
47. Schnabel LV, Bramlage LR, Mohammed HO, et al. Racing performance after arthroscopic removal of apical sesamoid fracture fragments in thoroughbred horses age <2 years: 151 cases (1989–2002). Equine Vet J 2007;39(1):64–8.
48. Higgins JL, Spike-Pierce DL, Bramlage LR. Racing prognosis of thoroughbred yearlings with dorsal proximal accessory carpal bone fragments. Proc Am Assoc Equine Pract 2010;56:402.
49. Bjšrnsdottir S, Axelsson M, Eksell P, et al. Radiographic and clinical survey of degenerative joint disease in the distal tarsal joints in Icelandic horses. Equine Vet J 2000;32(3):268–72.
50. Brehm W, Staecher W. Osteochondrosis (OCD) in the tarsocrural joint of Standardbred trotters – correlation between radiographic findings and racing performance. Proc Am Assoc Equine Pract 1999;45:164–6.
51. Laws EG, Richardson DW, Ross MW, et al. Racing performance of Standardbreds after conservative and surgical treatment for tarsocrural osteochondrosis. Equine Vet J 1993;25(3):199–202.
52. Beard WL, Bramlage LR, Schneider RK, et al. Post operative racing performance in Standardbreds and Thoroughbreds with osteochondrosis of the tarsocrural joint: 109 cases (1984–1990). J Am Vet Med Assoc 1994;204(10):1655–9.
53. McIlwraith CW. Clinical aspects of osteochondritis dissecans. In: McIlwraith CW, Totter GW, editors. Joint disease in the horse. Philadelphia: WB Saunders; 1996. p. 362–83.
54. Baird DH, Pilsworth RC. Wedge-shaped conformation of the dorsolateral aspect of the third tarsal bone in the Thoroughbred racehorse is associated with development of slab fractures in this site. Equine Vet J 2001;33(6):617–20.
55. Spike-Pierce DL, Bramlage LR. Ability to race of 518 thoroughbred weanlings and yearlings after arthroscopic debridement of femoropatellar osteochondritis dissecans. Proc Am Assoc Equine Pract 2009;55:456.
56. Whitman Jl, Morehead JP, Prichard MA, et al. Radiographic lucencies of the medial femoral condyle of thoroughbred sale yearlings: A preliminary investigation of the effect on race records. Proc Am Assoc Equine Pract 2006;52:416–19.
57. Howard RD, McIlwraith CW, Totter GW. Arthroscopic surgery for subchondral cystic lesions of the medial femoral condyle in horses: 41 cases (1988–1991). J Am Vet Med Assoc 1995;206(6):842–50.
58. Sandler EA, Bramlage LR, Embertson RM, et al. Correlation of lesion size with racing performance in thoroughbreds after arthroscopic surgical treatment of subchondral cystic lesions of the medial femoral condyle: 150 cases (1989–2000). Proc Am Assoc Equine Pract 2002;48:255–6.
59. Smith MA, Walmsley JP, Phillips TJ, et al. Effect of age at presentation on outcome following arthroscopic debridement of subchondral cystic lesions of the medial femoral condyle: 85 horses (1993–2003). Equine Vet J 2005;37(2):175–80.
60. Wallis TW, Goodrich LR, McIlwraith CW, et al. Arthroscopic injection of corticosteroids into the fibrous tissue of subchondral cystic lesions of the medial femoral condyle in horses: A retrospective study of 52 cases (2001–2006). Equine Vet J 2008;40 (5):461–7.
61. Dyson SJ. The use of musculoskeletal ultrasonography in the pre-purchase examination. In: Mair TS, editor. The pre-purchase examination. Suffolk: EVJ Ltd; 1998. p. 168–71.
62. Rantanen NW, Jorgenson JS, Genovese RL. Ultrasonographic evaluation of the equine limb: Technique. In: Ross MW, Dyson SJ, editors. Diagnosis and management of lameness in the horse. St Louis: Saunders; 2003. p. 166–88.
63. Dyson S. Enigma of enostosis-like lesions in the horse. Vet Rec 2011;168(12):324–5.
64. McClellan P, Charles B. Case 17. MRI cases in the standing sedated horse – Volume II. Hallmarq Veterinary Imaging 2008.
65. Lane JG. Endoscopy – what role of this technique in the veterinary examination of horses prior to purchase? In: Mair TS, editor. The pre-purchase examination. Suffolk: EVJ Ltd; 1998. p. 161–7.
66. Pollock PJ, Reardon RJM, Parking TDH, et al. Dynamic respiratory endoscopy in 67 thoroughbred racehorses training under normal ridden exercise conditions. Equine Vet J 2009;41(4):354–60.
67. Rosenstein DS, Stick JA. Diagnostic techniques in equine upper respiratory tract disease. In: Auer JA, Stick JA, editors. Equine surgery. 2nd ed. Philadelphia: WB Saunders; 1999. p. 314–26.
68. Stick JA, Peloso JG, Morehead JP, et al. Endoscopic assessment of airway function as a predictor of racing performance in Thoroughbred yearlings: 427 cases (1997–2000). J Am Vet Med Assoc 2001;219(7):962–7.
69. Lane JG. The examination of Thoroughbred yearlings for respiratory impediments at auction sales. In: Proceedings 15th Bain-Fallon Lectures, Australian Equine Veterinary Association; 1993. p. 235–48.
70. Dixon PM, McGorum BC, Railton DI, et al. Clinical and endoscopic evidence of progression in 152 cases of equine recurrent laryngeal neuropathy (RLN). Equine Vet J 2002;34(1):29–34.
71. Anderson BH. Recurrent laryngeal neuropathy – clinical aspects, endoscopy. In: McGorum B, Dixon P, Robinson E, Schumacher J editors. Equine respiratory medicine and surgery. Philidelphia: Elsevier; 2007. p. 483–96.
72. Garrett KS, Pierce SW, Embertson RM, et al. Endoscopic evaluation of arytenoid function and epiglottic structure in thoroughbred yearlings and association with racing performance at two to four years of age:2954 cases (1998–2001). J Am Vet Med Assoc 2010;236(6):669–73.
73. Hope J. Preliminary results of the endoscopy findings of the larynx and pharynx of horses at sales time. Website www.nzthoroughbred.com/ 24 May 2011.
74. Garrett KS, Woodie JB, Embertson RM. Association of treadmill upper airway endoscopic evaluation with results of ultrasonography and resting upper airway endoscopic evaluation. Equine Vet J 2011;43(3):365–71.
75. Martin BB, Kimmel JC, Cheney MW. The sales yearling. In: Ross MW, Dyson SJ, editors. Diagnosis and management of lameness in the horse. St Louis: Saunders; 2003. p. 836–7.
76. Ellis DR. Examinations at horse sales (Thoroughbreds). In: Mair TS, editor. The pre-purchase examination. Suffolk: EVJ Ltd; 1998. p. 37–42.
77. Arthur RM, Ross MW, Moloney PJ, et al. North American Thoroughbred. In: Ross MW, Dyson SJ, editors. Diagnosis and management of lameness in the horse. St Louis: Saunders; 2003. p. 868–79.
78. Pilsworth RC. The European Thoroughbred. In: Ross MW, Dyson SJ, editors. Diagnosis and management of lameness in the horse. St Louis: Saunders; 2003. p. 879–94.
79. Marks D. Orthopedic concerns in the pre-purchase examination. In: Robinson NE, editor. Current therapy in equine medicine. 5th ed. St Louis: Saunders; 2003. p. 493–9.
80. Hoogmoed LM, Snyder JR, Thomas HL, et al. Retrospective evaluation of equine prepurchase examinations 1991–2000. Equine Vet J 2003;35(4):375–81.
81. Turner TA. Shoeing principles for the management of navicular disease in horses. J Am Vet Med Assoc 1986;189:298–301.
82. Jackman BR, Baxter GM, Doran RE, et al. Palmar digital neurectomy in horses. 57 cases (1984–1990). Vet Surg 1993;22:285–8.
83. American Quarter Horse Association. Official handbook of rules and regulations. 2002;50:49.
84. Black JB. Purchase examination of the western show and performance horse. Proc Am Assoc Equine Pract 1999;45:1–3.

Appendix[7]

Buyer's statement

I,... (Buyer/Buyer's Agent),

request that the horse...undergo a prepurchase examination for use as a

....

This is to be undertaken by

Dr.. (Veterinarian)

....(Practice)

The recipient of this report is deemed to be aware that if some stages of the standard procedure recommended by the Equine Branch of the New Zealand Veterinary Association are not carried out, any information or opinion contained in this report is based on partial examination only. Some clinical signs of disease, injury or abnormality that may have manifested themselves in the full five stage examination may not be apparent in the restricted examination.

Where this examination and report are requested for the purpose of a business they are deemed to have been carried out upon the basis that the examining veterinarian's liability, howsoever arising, shall be no greater than a sum equivalent to 100 times the fee charged for the provision of this report. In addition, liability for consequential losses of any nature is also excluded.

This contract is governed by New Zealand law.

The Buyer/Buyer's Agent irrevocably agrees that the Courts of New Zealand will have exclusive jurisdiction to hear and determine all disputes under or in connection with this contract. The Buyer/Buyer's Agent further acknowledges that New Zealand is the forum conveniens for the hearing and determination for all disputes in connection with this contract.

Ownership of X-rays: The Buyer/Buyer's Agent acknowledges that any radiographs taken in the course of this examination are the property of the veterinary practice listed herein, but it is further acknowledged by the practice that copies of the radiographs will be supplied at the Buyer/Buyer's Agent's request and expense.

Reliance upon this report will constitute an acceptance of the limitations of liability referred to above.

In addition, the nature and extent of this report has been determined by particular request. In the circumstances the examining veterinarian disclaims any liability whatsoever to any party other than the party directly responsible for requesting and paying for the services rendered.

Please indicate with a tick which aspects of the examination for purchase you do/do not wish to have carried out.

(a) **Clinical Examination** (which is carried out in five stages)

Indicate with a tick please		YES	NO
Stage 1	Preliminary	☐	☐
Stage 2	During walking, trotting, turning and backing	☐	☐
Stage 3	During and immediately after strenuous exercise	☐	☐
Stage 4	During period after exercise	☐	☐
Stage 5	During walking, trotting, turning and backing	☐	☐

The Clinical examination will be carried out substantially in accordance with the standard procedure recommended by the Equine Branch of the NZ Veterinary Association (1997).

(b) Ancillary Examinations

Indicate with a tick please	YES	NO
Endoscopy	☐	☐
Radiography (tick areas to be radiographed):-	☐	☐

front feet ( ) front fetlocks ( ) hind feet ( )

carpi (knees) ( ) tarsi (hocks) ( ) hind fetlocks ( )

	YES	NO
Electrocardiography	☐	☐
Reproductive Examination	☐	☐

Other ancillary examinations (please specify) ....

....

....

I understand the horse's usual veterinary attendant is ....

(Veterinarian/Veterinarian's Practice)

Terms of payment. I understand that I will be responsible for payment for the examinations requested above.

Please note:- The certifying veterinarian takes no responsibility for, nor warrants the accuracy of, any information provided in the owner's statement including that given relating to the non-administration of drugs, freedom from vices, existing performance or suitability for intended use.

Signature .... (Buyer/Buyer's Agent)

Date ....

OWNER'S OR OWNER'S AGENT'S STATEMENT

Owner's Name ....

Address ....

Phone ....

Horse's Name .... Age ....

Sire .... Colour ....

Dam .... Sex ....

Breed ....

Agent's Name .... Phone ....

Address ....

How long have you been acquainted with this horse? ....

How long have you had this horse under your personal care? ....

Do you have knowledge of any?

1. Past or present disease? .... Has the horse ever bled from the nostrils? Yes/No
2. Lameness? .... Has the horse ever had signs of colic? Yes/No
3. Accidents? ....
4. Vices (stable or being ridden)? ....
5. Abnormalities? ....
6. Surgery? ....
7. Medications (particularly recent)? ....

Has this horse been recently examined by another veterinarian? ....

If so, for what purpose? ....

Use to which you understand the horse will be put? ....

Do you have any knowledge of past performance of this horse for the proposed use?

....

Is the horse in training/spelling? ....

How long has the horse been in training/spelling? ....

Who is the horse's usual veterinary attendant? ....

Signature of Owner or Owner's Agent ....

Veterinarian's record of the examination of a horse for sale

Veterinarian's Name: .... Practice Name ....

Address: ....

Horse's Name: ....

(Buyer/Buyer's Agent) ....

Description of horse said to be by .... out of ....

COLOUR	BREED OR TYPE	SEX	AGE	APPROX HEIGHT

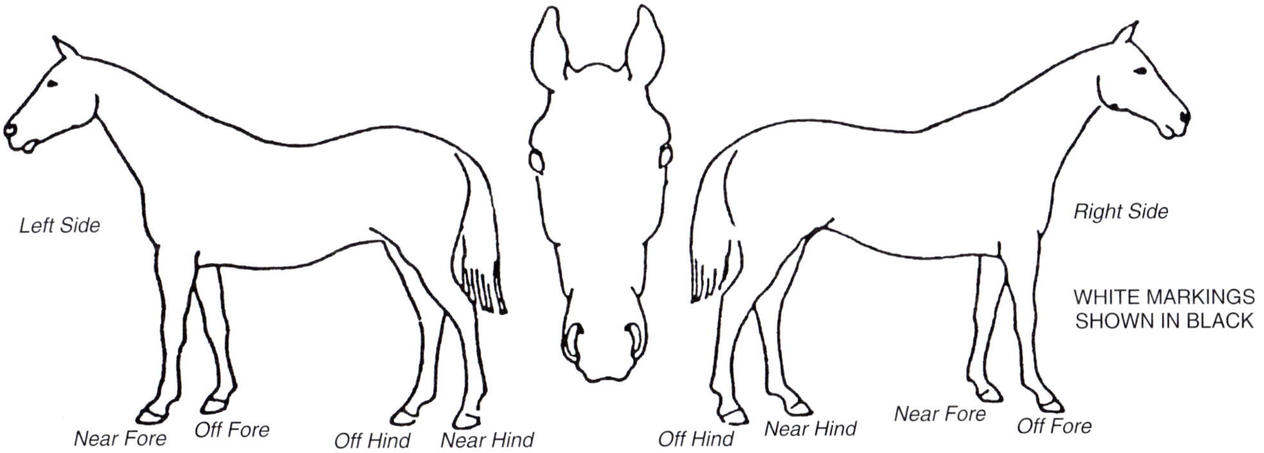

Markings: Head and Neck

Limbs: L.F ....

R.F ....

L.H ....

R.H ....

Body: ....

Brands: Left Shoulder .... Right Shoulder ....

Acquired Marks: ....

STAGE 1: – The Preliminary Examination – with the horse at rest in a stall and/or outside the stall. Complete the following with: N-Normal; AB-Abnormal; NE-Not Examined

GENERAL APPEARANCE
1. Physical Condition ......
2. Coat Condition ......

BILATERAL SYMMETRY
1. Head ......
2. Neck ......
3. Shoulders ......
4. Body ......
5. Pelvis ......
6. Legs ......

EYES
1. Symmetry ......
2. Reflexes ......
3. Lids ......
4. Mucous membranes ......
5. Cornea ......
6. Discharge ......
7. Examination with light ......

MOUTH
1. Lips ......
2. Tongue ......
3. Teeth ......
4. Approx age by teeth ......
5. Gums ......
6. Mucous membranes ......
7. Odour ......
8. Bite ......
9. Mandible ......

NASAL & PARANASAL
1. Symmetry ......
2. Air flow ......
3. Odour ......
4. Mucous membranes ......
5. Percussion ......
6. Discharge ......

EARS
1. Symmetry ......
2. Odour ......
3. Discharge ......

PHARYNX & LARYNX
1. Palpation ......
2. Auscultation ......

NECK
1. Symmetry ......
2. Jugular furrows ......
3. Thyroid ......
4. Trachea ......
5. Withers ......
6. Poll ......

CARDIOVASCULAR
Heart
1. Auscultation ......
   a. Resting rate ......
   b. Sounds ......

Pulse
   a. Resting rate ......
   b. Quality ......

PULMONARY
1. Resting rate ......
2. Auscultation ......
3. Percussion ......

DIGESTIVE
1. Auscultation ......
2. Inspection of faeces ......
3. Perineum ......
4. Rectal Temp. ......

GENITOURINARY
1. External genitalia ......
   a. Inspection ......
   b. Palpation ......

SKIN
1. Blemishes (saddle or girth sores etc) ......
2. Skin diseases ......
3. Hooves ......
4. Tail ......

NERVOUS SYSTEM
1. Inspection ......
2. Spine ......
3. Has horse been Denerved? ......

VICES
1. Cribbing ......
2. Aerophagia ......
3. Weaving ......
4. Head Shaking ......
5. Digging ......
6. Savaging ......
7. Other ......
8. Stable manners ......
9. Field manners ......

MUSCULOSKELETAL
Palpation & Manipulation of:
Left front leg
1. Chest & shoulder ......
2. Forearm ......
3. Carpus ......
4. Metacarpus – bone ......
   Metacarpus – tendon ......
5. Fetlock ......
6. Pastern ......
7. Foot – appearance ......
   – hoof tester ......
   – shoe type ......

Right front leg
1. Chest & shoulder ......
2. Forearm ......
3. Carpus ......
4. Metacarpus – bone ......
   Metacarpus – tendon ......
5. Fetlock ......
6. Pastern ......
7. Foot – appearance ......
   – hoof tester ......
   – shoe type ......

Left hind leg
1. Hip & thigh ......
2. Stifle ......
3. Tarsus ......
4. Metatarsus – bone ......
   Metatarsus – tendon ......
5. Fetlock ......
6. Pastern ......
7. Foot – appearance ......
   – hoof tester ......
   – shoe type ......

Right hind leg
1. Hip & thigh ......
2. Stifle ......
3. Tarsus ......
4. Metatarsus – bone ......
   Metatarsus – tendon ......
5. Fetlock ......
6. Pastern ......
7. Foot – appearance ......
   – hoof tester ......
   – shoe type ......

Flexion test results
–Left fore distal limb ....
–Right fore distal limb ....
–Left fore carpus ....
–Right fore carpus ....
–Left hind distal limb ....
–Right hind distal limb ....
–Left hind hock ....
–Right hind hock ....

Remarks:

....

....

....

STAGE 2 – Examination during walking, trotting, turning and backing

AT WALK

Symmetry of gait	.....
Stride	.....
Right fore leg	.....
Left fore leg	.....
Right hind leg	.....
Left hind leg	.....
Movement of head	.....

AT TROT

Symmetry of gait	.....
Stride	.....
Right fore leg	.....
Left fore leg	.....
Right hind leg	.....
Left hind leg	.....
Movement of head	.....
Turning	.....
Backing	.....

Remarks ....

STAGE 3 – Amination during and immediately after strenuous exercise

Type of Exercise (tick)

Walk	......
Lunge	......
Trot or pace	......
Canter	......
Gallop	......

During Exercise

Symmetry of gait	......
Stride	......
Breathing	......
Rhythm	......
Resp. noises	......

Immediately following Exercise

Respiratory System

Breathing

Rate	......
Rhythm	......
Sounds	......

Auscultation of

Pharynx	......
Thorax	......

Circulatory System

Mucous membranes	......
Heart	
Rate	......
Rhythm	......
Sounds	......

Remarks ....

STAGE 4 – Examination during the period after exercise

...... Minutes after

Exercise	......
Respiratory Rate	......
Rhythm	......
Lung sounds	......
Heart	
Rate	......
Rhythm	......
Sounds	......

...... Minutes after

Exercise	......
Respiratory Rate	......
Rhythm	......
Lung sounds	......
Heart	
Rate	......
Rhythm	......
Sounds	......

...... Minutes after

Exercise	......
Respiratory Rate	......
Rhythm	......
Lung sounds	......
Heart	
Rate	......
Rhythm	......
Sounds	......

Evidence of cuts or marks on limbs from fast exercise ....

Evidence of epistaxis..

Evidence of anal windsucking ....

Remarks ....

STAGE 5 – The final examination during walking, trotting, turning and backing

Walking

Symmetry of gait	......
Stride	......
Right fore leg	......
Left fore leg	......
Right hind leg	......
Left hind leg	......
Movement of head	......

Trotting

Symmetry of gait	......
Stride	......
Right fore leg	......
Left fore leg	......
Right hind leg	......
Left hind leg	......
Movement of head	......

Turning

On	
Right fore leg	......
Left fore leg	......
Right hind leg	......
Left hind leg	......

Backing

Hindlimb movements ......

Remarks: ....

....

....

Overall comments: ....

....

....

Date and Time of Examination ....

Address where Examination took place ....

Signed ....

International movement of athletic horses: quarantine and regulatory controls

61

Patricia M. Ellis Brian D. Stewart

CHAPTER CONTENTS

Introduction

The elite athletic horse of today is a global commodity. During the past decade, the volume of international movement of horses by air transport has grown dramatically.[1] Horses now travel for a diverse range of events including racing, dressage, eventing, show jumping, carriage driving and endurance riding in an ever-increasing number of countries. Traditionally most international events involving imported horses have been located in Europe and North America. New transport patterns are emerging with the advent of new competition venues in Eastern Europe, South America, the Arabian Peninsula, Asia and Africa[2] and the development of complex itineraries by horses visiting multiple countries to compete in races held within a relatively short period.[3]

The modern equine athlete can move vast distances rapidly and complete journeys well within the incubation period of most infectious diseases. History has shown that without adequate safeguards this can lead to explosive outbreaks of disease.[4-6] The increased volume of horse movement in a changing world trading environment poses significant quarantine challenges to regulatory authorities who must exclude foreign diseases from their countries without undue restriction to international trade.[2,7]

Governments and national authorities conducting international competitions have understandable concerns that:

- horses imported for a competition could bring in disease to the local population
- disease could occur in foreign horses due to exposure to a disease in the local horses
- a disease outbreak could result in cancellation of an important international event, especially if all horses (visiting and local) are held within the same competition venue
- prompt departure of foreign horses to their country of usual residency or next destination could be compromised by:
  - an outbreak of disease in the local population or in visiting horses
  - quarantine standards and management which do not meet the expectations of the horse's connections, the country of origin or country of next destination
  - inability to meet requirements for import to next destination
- horses returning from overseas could introduce disease into their country of normal residency.

Equine veterinarians in the private sector play an important role in the preparation of horses for export and in supervision of the health and welfare of horses during transport to and temporary residency in foreign countries. To avoid problems, unnecessary delays and loss of client goodwill, private sector veterinarians need to have a sound understanding of quarantine and regulatory requirements which allow horses to move safely between destinations.[8,9]

International spread of equine diseases

Economic, biological, political and ecological factors

A variety of factors have the potential to affect the global distribution and occurrence of equine diseases including:[10,11]

- international trade in horses and horse semen, the single most important factor
- changes in international trading policy as a result of multinational trade agreements
- emergence of previously undescribed pathogens such as contagious equine metritis and Hendra virus
- new variants of established pathogens
- climatic changes leading to altered migratory patterns of wild birds and extended insect vector ranges
- migration of reservoir and amplifying hosts such as birds and bats
- wind-blown carriage of insect vectors
- inadvertent introduction of exotic vectors such as ticks and mosquitos
- contaminated biological products and vaccines
- deliberate, illegal introduction of a foreign disease, e.g. bioterrorism.

Changes in agricultural practices can indirectly influence the distribution of arboviruses by favoring the expansion of vector habitats.[12] For example, increases in irrigated rice production and expansion of the pig breeding industry are thought to have contributed to expansion of the geographic range of Japanese encephalitis in the Asian region.

Disease and horse-related factors

Potential for disease spread by international movement is influenced by the epidemiology of the disease, the intended use of horses and whether horses are imported on a temporary or permanent basis.

The equine diseases most likely to be transferred across national borders are those characterized by an asymptomatic carrier state (e.g. equine infectious anemia, piroplasmosis, contagious equine metritis, equine viral arteritis, and dourine). The potential for their transfer is obviously greater if horses are imported on a permanent basis.[10,11] The latter three diseases are transmitted by the venereal route.

Horses imported on a temporary basis for competition or performance pose little risk of introducing diseases spread by the venereal route if they are prohibited from breeding during temporary residency. Likewise, if the arthropod vectors of a disease are not present in a country, temporary import of horses that would be otherwise ineligible (e.g. horses testing positive for piroplasmosis) under controlled conditions presents a much lower risk than horses imported on a permanent basis and released into the national herd.[13] In the latter case potential for iatrogenic spread by contaminated needles would be possible.

Horses imported to a country on a permanent basis pose a far greater threat of introducing disease than horses imported for a short-term stay under appropriate conditions of management. Competition horses imported for major races and events are registered animals, travel on passports and have a known residency, vaccination and disease testing history. They are kept under constant veterinary supervision before, during and after the event. During their brief residence, visiting horses have only limited exposure to the local horse population and are not used for breeding.[2,13]

Country factors

Evaluation of country factors, such as zoning and border controls, veterinary services, horse industry structure, disease control legislation, laboratory testing capacity and surveillance programs, are important inputs for assessing the likelihood of hazards being present in the horse population of an exporting country. Reliable and transparent information about the health status of a country's horses is critical for safe international movement.[14,15]

Border crossings can be more easily regulated in island countries such as Australia and New Zealand than in countries with land borders. Expansion of the European Union (EU) into Eastern Europe has created new disease control challenges as evidenced by the recent spread of equine infectious anemia from Romania to other EU member states.[16]

Impact of exotic disease outbreaks

An exotic disease outbreak can have a profound effect on the horse industry in an affected country and cause serious economic loss, disruption to normal activity and social distress.

Horses now travel from one hemisphere to another by air transport and complete their journeys within the incubation period of most major diseases. Spread of equine influenza, in particular, has increased since the introduction of air transport. In the past 30 years, the introduction of imported horses to susceptible indigenous populations has been responsible for explosive outbreaks of equine influenza including in South Africa (1986 and 2003), India (1987), Jamaica (1989), Hong Kong (1992), United Arab Emirates (1995/1996), Puerto Rico (1997), Philippines (1997), Japan (2007) and Australia (2007).[6,11]

Equine influenza was introduced to a naïve, unvaccinated South African horse population by imported horses from the USA in December 1986 and spread widely within a week. The explosive spread was aided by road transport of infected horses, lack of an all-in, all-out post-arrival quarantine policy and poor biosecurity by transport operators, horse trainers and veterinarians. The impact of the outbreak included extensive losses in State revenue due to cancellation of race meetings and subsequent loss of wagering taxes. Major horse events were canceled or had to be rescheduled. The horse industry also incurred significant costs arising from veterinary treatment of sick horses and the costs of compulsory vaccination.[4] The disease had a similar impact when it was reintroduced by imported horses in 2003, when once again there was a quarantine breakdown.[6]

Hong Kong suffered a similar fate in November and December 1992 when an outbreak of equine influenza, introduced by imported horses from UK or Ireland, led to a suspension of racing for one month. The outbreak resulted in the cancellation of seven race meetings, including an international event, with a potential loss of total betting turnover of nearly US$1 billion, over 15% of which would have been returned to the Hong Kong community by way of tax, duty and donations.[5,17]

Equine influenza was confirmed for the first time in the naïve Australian horse population in August 2007 and was introduced by horses imported from Japan. The incursion arose from a post-arrival quarantine breakdown but how equine influenza virus escaped from the government quarantine station was never established.[6] The outbreak sparked the single largest response to an animal disease emergency in Australia's history and provided an unprecedented challenge to Australia's emergency animal disease preparedness arrangements. Horse events and movements were disrupted for over six months. Eventually the disease was contained within certain areas in NSW and Queensland and eradicated but only after affecting nearly 10 000 properties and 76 000 horses.[18] Governments, the horse industry and dependent businesses suffered significant financial losses. Costs arising directly from the emergency response totaled $A97.7 million and over $A263 million was provided in government support and assistance packages to individuals and organizations. The economic impact on the horse industry and dependent business was probably billions of dollars but a lack of reliable data, particularly in the non-racing sector, made it difficult to quantify the losses.[19]

Disease outbreaks can also have profound human impact. During the Australian equine influenza outbreak, the psycho-social effects of the outbreak and the control response were measured using data collected by large online survey. Extremely high levels of non-specific psychological distress were reported by respondents, with 34% reporting high levels of psychological distress, compared to levels of around 12% in the general Australian population.[20]

Even diseases that do not infect horses can disrupt normal horse-related activity. The outbreak of FMD in the UK in 2001 had a devastating effect on the horse industry as well as on the farming community. Estimated horse industry losses reached £100 million per month in the first three months of the outbreak and the majority of horse-related sporting events were canceled.[21]

International regulatory framework

The World Trade Organization

The World Trade Organization (WTO)[22] deals with the global rules of trade between nations. Its main function is to ensure international trade flows as smoothly, predictably and freely as possible. Under the WTO Agreement on the Application of Sanitary and Phytosanitary Measures (the SPS Agreement), WTO member countries are required to base their sanitary import measures on science-based principles and guidelines, where they exist.[23] Sanitary measures relate to human and animal health and phytosanitary measures relate to plant health.

The WTO recognizes the World Organization for Animal Health, better known as the Office Internationale Epizooties (OIE), as the international reference organization for the animal health standards upon which import measures are based. Countries can legitimately adopt import restrictions more stringent than OIE standards if they can demonstrate a scientific need, which in practice means that quarantine conditions in excess of OIE standards should be based on a transparent risk analysis. The SPS Agreement also promotes recognition of the concept of disease-free zones and compartments within countries.

Office Internationale des Epizooties

The OIE, established in 1924, is the World Organization for Animal Health and is based in Paris. In 2011 the number of OIE member countries totaled 178, each of which is represented by a delegate to the World Assembly of Delegates (the decision-making body).[24] OIE's mission is to improve animal health and welfare and prevent the international spread of serious animal diseases.

OIE health standards relevant to the international movement of horses are the *Terrestrial Animal Health Code* and the *Manual of Diagnostic Tests and Vaccines for Terrestrial Animals*. Both are regularly updated as new scientific information comes to light.

OIE Terrestrial Animal Health Code

The *OIE Terrestrial Animal Health Code*[25] (the Code) is an essential reference for any official veterinarian involved in international trade. It is periodically updated and available online.

Volume I contains general provisions relating to:

- animal disease diagnosis, surveillance and notification
- risk analysis
- quality of veterinary services
- general recommendations for disease prevention and control
- trade measures, import/export procedures and veterinary certification
- veterinary public health
- animal welfare.

Volume II contains a chapter for each OIE listed disease and recommended wording for international veterinary certification relating to that disease. Criteria are presented which countries or zones must satisfy to be recognized as free from African horse sickness, equine influenza, dourine, glanders and VEE.

OIE Manual of Diagnostic Tests and Vaccines for Terrestrial Animals

The *OIE Manual of Standards for Diagnostic Tests and Vaccines for Terrestrial Animals*[26] (the 'Manual') is also available online. The purpose of the Manual is to foster harmonization of diagnostic methods for OIE listed diseases and other diseases of importance to international trade. Standards are described for laboratory diagnostic tests and for the production of veterinary vaccines. Specific chapters cover each of the diseases listed in the Code. Each disease chapter includes a well-referenced summary intended to provide information for veterinary officials and other readers who need a general overview of the tests and vaccines available for each disease. This is followed by a text giving greater detail for laboratory workers. The Manual also includes a list of OIE Reference Laboratories which have been designated by the OIE as centers of excellence in their particular field.

Diseases listed by OIE

The OIE maintains lists of notifiable diseases that member countries are required to monitor if they wish to take part in international trade. The most significant criterion for inclusion of a disease in the OIE list is its potential for international spread. Other criteria include zoonotic potential and capacity for significant spread within naïve populations.

Listed equine diseases include African horse sickness, contagious equine metritis, dourine, equine encephalomyelitis (Western), equine infectious anemia, equine influenza, equine piroplasmosis, equine rhinopneumonitis, equine viral arteritis, glanders, Venezuelan equine encephalomyelitis (VEE). Other significant diseases of horses such as equine encephalomyelitis (Eastern), Japanese encephalitis, screwworm, surra, vesicular stomatitis and West Nile fever are listed as multiple species diseases.

Reporting obligations are outlined Chapter 1.1 of the *Terrestrial Code*. Immediate reporting by veterinary authorities of member countries to OIE headquarters is required in the following epidemiological situations – the first occurrence of a listed disease; recurrence of a listed disease following a report declaring that an outbreak had ended; first occurrence of a new strain of a known pathogen; and any sudden and unexpected increase in distribution, incidence, morbidity or mortality of a listed endemic disease. Countries also now have to report immediately any emerging disease with significant morbidity or mortality or apparent zoonotic potential, even if unlisted.

In addition, each country maintains a schedule of diseases notifiable under its own animal health legislation, drawn from the above lists. Because some important diseases are not universally notifiable, the Thoroughbred industry has developed its own international reporting system through the International Thoroughbred Breeders Meeting. Quarterly disease reports are submitted to a collating center at the Animal Health Trust, Newmarket, England, and distributed to participating countries.[27]

Import risk analysis

Risk analysis is a valuable tool for decision making that can assist global movement of horses and open up new markets without compromising the health status of importing countries.

As mentioned earlier in this review, WTO Member Countries are encouraged to base quarantine conditions (SPS measures) on international standards, guidelines and recommendations or on a scientific assessment of risk. *The Terrestrial Code*[25] is the international standard referenced in the SPS Agreement and contains guidelines and principles for the conduct of import risk analyzes in Chapter 2.1.

The components of risk analysis are hazard identification, risk assessment, risk management and risk communication.[23] Briefly, the procedure should be science based and involves assessment and documentation of:

- potential exotic agents and pests of concern (hazards) that could be introduced by imported horses
- how exotic agents might be introduced into a country or zone by imported horses
- how horses in the importing country might be exposed to exotic agents thus introduced
- adverse health or environmental consequences resulting from exposure of domestic horses to such exotic agents.
- how identified risks can be best managed to protect the domestic horse population without having an unjustified effect on trade.

Risk communication involves exchange of information and opinions with potentially affected and interested parties at all stages of the process.

Risk analysis has already proved its value in overcoming potential barriers to the international movement of athletic horses testing positive for piroplasmosis. Government authorities in the USA and Australia used risk analysis as a decision-making tool when considering import of horses for the 1996 Olympic Games in Atlanta[28] and the 2000 Olympic Games in Sydney.[29] Temporary importation of horses serologically positive for equine piroplasmosis was allowed under specified conditions of management. An important legacy of the above risk analyzes is that subsequently a similar waiver allowed over 100 piroplasmosis-positive horses to compete in the 2010 World Equestrian Games in Kentucky, USA.[30]

Comprehensive risk analyzes of disease risks associated with import of live horses have been completed by New Zealand[13] and Australian veterinary authorities[31] and used as a basis for review of import standards. Both analyzes include sections relating to the temporary import of horses for racing and sporting events and recommended measures for their management.

Structured risk analysis, in compliance with OIE principles, provides countries importing horses with an objective and defensible method to assess risks associated with importation and to determine how those risks may be managed. Transparency is important. Exporting countries must be provided with clear and documented scientific reasons if import restrictions are imposed or if importation is refused. Transparent decisions also assure local horse industry organizations and other interested parties that all potential risks have been evaluated and are being managed appropriately.

Zoning and compartmentalization

Traditionally, the distribution of animal diseases has been viewed on a country-by-country basis, with the presence or absence of a particular disease anywhere within a country's borders serving to establish the status of the entire country. This conservative approach fostered an all-or-nothing standard of risk avoidance in quarantine policy development that precluded consideration of factors such as disease-free zones within a country.

The contemporary approach endorsed by the OIE recognizes that there are variations in the health status of animal populations, more often tied to climatological, geographical and biological factors and to husbandry systems than to national political boundaries. Generally, zoning is defined on a geographical basis, while compartmentalization applies to an animal subpopulation defined primarily by management and husbandry practices related to biosecurity. OIE guidelines relating to zoning and compartmentalization can be found in Chapter 4.3 of the *Terrestrial Code*.[25]

Application of the zoning concept to horse diseases was first prompted by outbreaks of AHS in previously free areas of Spain and Portugal in the years leading up to the 1992 Olympic Games in Barcelona. The *Terrestrial Code* was amended to provide for zoning in respect of AHS. Countries allowed horses to enter Spain on a temporary basis to compete in equestrian events at the Games despite the existence of an AHS-infected area in the south of Spain.[32]

Zoning is a valuable tool of trade for countries with significant endemic diseases of trade concern. South Africa's zoning of AHS enabled resumption of export of horses to member states of the European Union and a number of other countries, thus overcoming trade bans that had been in place for nearly 40 years.[33]

Recently a novel combination of OIE zoning and compartmentalization principles was used to establish an equine disease-free zone for the equestrian events of the 2010 Asian Games in Guangzhou, China.[34]

Role and responsibilities of government officials, shipping agents and veterinarians

Government officials, private practitioners and shipping agents all share responsibility for moving horses between countries and must communicate openly and frequently during the shipping process to avoid difficulties and delays.[9]

Government officials

The chief concerns for the veterinary authorities of any country hosting an international event are potential for spread of disease, animal welfare considerations and trade facilitation.[17]

Governments in importing countries have a primary responsibility to control the entry of foreign horses to protect the national horse population from exotic diseases. At the same time, they have to satisfy international obligations and facilitate trade. The importing country establishes import health requirements for horses by negotiation with their foreign counterparts, taking into account the disease status of the exporting and importing country and relevant international standards.[7,9,10]

An import permit may have to be obtained in advance of shipment for each consignment of horses. Often import conditions are attached to this permit. Import permits are used to ensure that only agreed and current conditions are used in trade, advance notice is given of consignments and that quarantine space is available for incoming horses (when appropriate).

The government of an exporting country is expected to act as the official independent agent of the importing country and is responsible for supplying or endorsing accurate official veterinary certification which satisfies all the health requirements of the importing country. If a problem arises with a shipment, officials in the exporting country cannot unilaterally alter agreed health conditions but must seek a dispensation from the country of destination.

Often shipments of horses transit other countries en route to their final destination. Governments in countries of transit may require that a transit permit be obtained in advance and/or that horses passing through meet the import requirements of the transit country in case a prolonged delay occurs due to mechanical failure of an aircraft.

Shipping agents

International transport of horses requires adequate lead time and considerable forward planning. Veterinarians approached for advice should recommend that clients engage a reputable and experienced shipping agent as the first step in commencing preparations for any international journey[8] as the key to success is often the competency of the shipping agent involved.[9]

A shipping agent acts as a representative of the owner and coordinates all facets of the shipping process from origin to destination. Shipping agents identify the most suitable and quickest route, prepare a travel plan, obtain all necessary permits and documentation, book road transport and air cargo space, liaise with airlines, provide shipping containers which conform to airline and welfare standards and supervise loading. They also interact with the quarantine and customs authorities of the countries of origin and destination and coordinate arrangements for and timing of any pre-export quarantine, premises certification, veterinary examinations, testing and vaccination necessary for the completion of the official export health certification. Agents may also supply experienced attendants to escort horses during the journey.[35]

Enquiries should also be made in advance about quarantine policy in the country of destination relating to the import of tack, horse feed, supplements and veterinary medications.[36]

An additional consideration which is sometimes overlooked is that quarantine protocols for return of horses to their country of normal residency should be investigated before horses depart to establish whether that country imposes any special conditions on the management of horses during temporary residency in a foreign country. For instance, to return directly within a specified time period, without additional testing, traveling horses may have to be isolated from other horses during a temporary absence.[36]

Equine veterinarians

In many countries, veterinarians in the private sector play a major role in the preparing horses for export. Their duties may include:

- collecting blood samples for laboratory testing
- conducting or supervising pre-export treatments and vaccinations, and
- providing certification about the health status of horses and the premises from which they originate.

Veterinarians engaged by clients or accredited by governments to perform export duties need to work closely with quarantine authorities and shipping agents. Contact must be made with government animal health officials at an early stage to obtain or confirm the current import requirements for the country of destination. The veterinarian must understand and fulfill these requirements exactly.[9]

Responsibilities include:

- being accredited for export duties (if appropriate)
- accurate completion of entries in horse passports and on other identification documents
- recording horse identification details (brands, markings, tattoos, microchip numbers) accurately by actual inspection of horses (rather than by copying other documents)
- confirming and recording the identity of each horse at the time of conducting any procedure so that any certification can be definitively linked to that animal
- collecting and submitting blood samples, performing inspections and administering vaccinations or treatments within the specified time frames
- labeling samples clearly and accurately
- transporting samples to the laboratory using correct techniques and appropriate storage conditions
- submitting samples to approved laboratories
- requesting the tests specified in the import conditions, and
- provision of conscientious certification about the health status of horses and premises.

Honest, accurate and reliable veterinary certification is the cornerstone of international movement.[15] Certification provided must be completed carefully and conscientiously and match the requirements of the importing country precisely. Even if some of the requirements appear unreasonable and raise difficulties for the client, the certifying veterinarian must ensure these requirements are met or contact a government official for guidance on interpretation of the wording. Conflict of interest should be avoided and integrity of certification must not be compromised because of commercial pressures. Veterinarians should never sign blank or incomplete certificates and should only certify those matters of which they have direct knowledge.

Misleading, inaccurate or false certification reflects adversely on the signing veterinarian and affects the reputation of the veterinary profession and government animal health services, nationally and internationally. Such certificates may result in loss of trade, spread of disease, financial loss to clients and exporters and litigation.

A useful guide to the ethical obligations and responsibilities of veterinarians involved in the preparation or certification of animals for export is presented in Chapter 5 of the *OIE International Animal Health Code*.[25]

Before departure, private veterinarians traveling internationally with horses should check whether the country of destination places any restrictions on import of veterinary medications and equipment or has any special registration requirements relating to veterinary practice by foreign veterinarians. Competition rules relating to prohibited substances and practices should also be ascertained.

Equine practitioners attending recently imported horses in quarantine stations must pay close attention to personal hygiene and comply with any operating procedures specified by quarantine management. Failure to implement appropriate biosecurity procedures by persons attending quarantined horses has resulted in quarantine breakdowns and disastrous equine influenza epidemics in South Africa (1986, 2003) and Australia (2007).[4,6]

Welfare legislation and standards

Welfare legislation governing international movement of horses varies from country to country.

Recommendations for the transport of horses by road, air and sea are presented in Chapter 7 of the *Terrestrial Code*.[25] The International

Air Transport Association (IATA) publishes Live Animal Regulations (LAR),[37] which provide guidelines for the safe and humane transport of animals by commercial airlines. The LAR contain useful information about the responsibilities of carriers and shippers, stocking density guidelines for horses, optimum temperature ranges, container standards and specific handling procedures for horses transported by air.

An increasing number of countries, including the European Union, have incorporated standards relating to animal welfare during transport into legislation.

Role of horse industry organizations

For maximum efficiency, measures to prevent international spread of equine diseases require industry participation and support[7,11] in addition to the efforts of government veterinary authorities. At international level, the umbrella bodies of the various sporting disciplines play an important role in setting international standards for the protection of the health and welfare of horses relevant to particular disciplines. The host nation of an international event has a responsibility to provide facilities and supervision which meet these standards.

When preparing for an international event, close and continued liaison between horse industry and quarantine officials is required from an early stage to negotiate and resolve the many quarantine issues which may arise.[17,36]

In some instances, the host organization may provide and manage quarantine facilities.[17] Convenient access to good training facilities is critical for the successful participation of foreign horses. If a country which quarantines or isolates imported horses after arrival wishes to host an international event, the responsibility for establishing an approved quarantine facility for foreign horses often rests with the organization conducting that event. Most government-operated quarantine premises do not have easy access to adequate training facilities where imported horses can maintain competitive fitness in isolation.[36]

Passports

The use of passports to assist the movement of competition horses across national boundaries is well established. Internationally accepted passports must meet certain criteria set by the OIE, international horse authorities and, in Europe, by the EU.[2]

Passports are intended to serve as a unique identification documents containing harmonized information about vaccinations and results of laboratory tests. They are issued by the relevant national horse industry organization of the country in which the horse is registered and should accompany a horse at all times. In some countries this is a legislative requirement.[2]

Vaccinations

In many jurisdictions, vaccination against equine influenza is compulsory for horses entering competitions or races and the vaccination status of all horses is regularly checked by horse industry officials.

It is important to establish before a horse departs on an international journey if local or foreign quarantine authorities impose any special requirements additional to or different from those known to apply to a specific discipline. For instance, because Australia is free from equine influenza, vaccination requirements for importation of horses to Australia are more stringent than those routinely required by racing authorities in Europe.[31,36] Likewise in some instances, sporting authorities conducting events in certain Asian countries require vaccination against Japanese encephalitis to protect visiting horses.[1]

Vaccination requirements can vary from country to country and between disciplines and hence will not be detailed in this review. The main point for veterinarians is that the vaccination requirements of quarantine authorities and sporting organizations for each consignment should be established well in advance of the proposed date of horse departure. The time frames specified by quarantine authorities for courses of vaccination are not arbitrary and must be respected.

Racing authorities

The International Federation of Horseracing Authorities (IFHA) is an umbrella body for the world's Thoroughbred racing authorities. The organization has developed an International Agreement on Breeding and Racing (IABR),[38] a series of recommended international guidelines which are agreed and endorsed (in whole or in part) by national racing authorities and carried forward into their own rules for racing and breeding. Of particular interest to veterinarians are Article 6 of the IABR which contains the template definition of a prohibited substance and Articles 22 to 25 which relate to the control of infectious diseases and management of foreign racehorses. Articles 22 to 25 contain general recommendations relating to passports, hygiene of transport vehicles and establishments, treatment procedures, veterinary inspections, vaccinations, health certificates and exchange of information about equine disease outbreaks.

The IFHA maintains an International Movement of Horses Subcommittee (IMHC). The role of the IMHC is to improve communication between countries conducting international races and to make recommendations about health issues that restrict trade. Significant expansion of international racing in recent years has resulted in logistical problems when horses compete in multiple countries within a short period of time before returning to their country of usual residency. Quarantine protocols vary from country to country and are usually developed to cater for direct movement to and from a specified country for competition. Complex itineraries cause logistical complications for racing authorities, government animal health services, connections of horses and shipping agents. Problems arise from variations between countries in quarantine requirements relating to health certification, minimum residency periods, testing, vaccination, housing and training during temporary residency and periods of quarantine or isolation.[3]

To address these problems and foster cooperation and international harmonization of health requirements, the IMHC developed detailed guidelines to facilitate the safe movement of registered racehorses competing on an international circuit. The guidelines were adopted by the IFHA in 2002 and are used as a basis for discussion by IFHA member countries with their government veterinary authorities. The guidelines are available online at http://www.horseracingintfed.com and are regularly reviewed and updated by the IMHC. The IMHC also collaborates with the OIE to ensure that international movement of horses is based on sound scientific principles.

Passports have been used for the identification of Thoroughbred horses for many years. Passports have to be endorsed for foreign travel by racing authorities before export and subsequently before the horse runs in a foreign country.

Federation Equestre Internationale

The Federation Equestre Internationale (FEI) is the international governing body of equestrian sport recognized by the International

Olympic Committee and is responsible for international administration of equestrian events in the disciplines of show jumping, dressage, eventing, driving, vaulting, reining and endurance riding. National Federations administer these disciplines at national level.[39]

The FEI has developed comprehensive rules and regulations to govern the above sports. Of particular relevance to equine veterinarians are the FEI Veterinary Regulations[40] which protects the health and welfare of horses competing in international events under FEI control. The Veterinary Regulations cover, inter alia, the duties of veterinarians, health and hygiene requirements and responsibilities, passport control, examinations and inspections of horses during events, control of prohibited substances and treatment of horses while under FEI control.

Horses are identified by a written description and a diagram in FEI passports. Compulsory microchipping of horses newly registered with the FEI came into effect on 1 January 2013. Only veterinarians approved by a National Federation (NF) are authorized to fill in the identification page of the passport and the description and diagram must be completed in accordance with FEI requirements for the identification of horses before an FEI passport is issued.[41] Some NFs have approved passport issuing organizations. In this case an FEI Recognition Card is added to the existing national passport which secures the horse 'registered' horse status. The vaccination section of the passport must be endorsed by a veterinarian and demonstrate that the horse has received a full course of equine influenza vaccinations in accordance with the requirements of FEI Veterinary Regulations. All horses registered with the FEI must also have a medication log book.[40]

The FEI collaborates closely with the OIE and plays an important role in negotiating expanded international movement of horses for competition in the Olympic disciplines,[39] a legacy which is of benefit to athletic horses of all breeds.

Overview of quarantine controls of major equine sporting nations

There are various internationally accepted risk management strategies which quarantine authorities use to reduce disease risks associated with importation of horses.[17] Individually, each may be not be perfect but, when used in combination, these measures can reduce the probability of importing an infected horse to a very low level, regardless of the starting probability. The combinations adopted vary from country to country depending on the country's health status and quarantine policy.

Certification of origin from a disease-free source

The risk of introducing a disease agent can be reduced by sourcing horses from a disease-free country, region, zone or premises. Alternatively, horses from an infected area may be required to be resident in an area free of the disease of concern for a specified period prior to exportation, a period long enough for that disease to be obvious if the horse is infected. Reliable and transparent information about the government veterinary services and disease surveillance programs in the country of export is obviously critical to the value of this strategy.

Separation and biosecurity

Separation of horses from other potentially infected horses (before export) and from susceptible horses (for a period after import), with appropriate biosecurity, reduces the risk of disease transmission and the likelihood that infected horses will remain undetected. It also provides an opportunity for observation, diagnosis and treatment (if appropriate) before imported horses are permitted to contact the domestic population. The risk of importing infected horses or releasing infected horses after arrival is thus reduced.

If suitable training and stabling facilities are available, separation need not disadvantage horses visiting for competition. At international race meetings in Asia[17] and Australia[36] temporary equine imports are isolated from resident horses and horses from countries not of equivalent health status except at the time of racing.

Separation from the host population and, if there are significant variations in health status, separation of temporary residents by region, ensures the success of international competitions. It is recommended as best health practice to prevent the spread of infectious diseases and also protects the health status of visiting horses, thus assisting their prompt and uneventful departure to their next destination.

Satisfactory arrangements to separate visiting horses from the domestic population can also give foreign animal health authorities confidence that their horses can visit safely even in the face of a local disease incident. For example, prompt action by racing and animal health officials in the USA salvaged European participation in an international race meeting at Arlington International Racecourse when an outbreak of equine viral arteritis occurred there in 1993.[42]

Diagnostic testing

Testing may be used to identify infected horses before or after export. The value of diagnostic tests in risk reduction depends on the availability and use of standardized tests of high sensitivity, the ability of a test to identify infected horses correctly. For example, a serological test may have a sensitivity of 99% in individual infected horses. Thus the probability of missing the disease when testing a single infected horse is 1%.

For import purposes, the negative predictive value of a test, the probability that a horse is not infected when a test result gives a negative result, is of paramount importance. Predictive values vary markedly according to the disease prevalence in the population from which the tested horse was drawn. As disease prevalence decreases, negative predictive value increases.[43] Reliable and transparent information about the prevalence of disease in the country of origin is critical for interpretation of test results.

When test results vary between different laboratories in different countries, trade problems can ensue.[10,44] Official approval of laboratories, adoption of OIE prescribed tests for international trade and use of the testing standards detailed in the *OIE Manual of Diagnostic Tests and Vaccines for Terrestrial Animals*[26] minimizes such problems.[10]

Rapid diagnostic tests are becoming more widely available. Commercially available influenza assay kits such as Directigen™ have been extensively used for both screening and diagnostic purposes in Hong Kong since 1998.[6] Realtime polymerase chain reaction (PCR) tests have become increasingly popular in diagnostics since the outbreak of equine influenza in Australia in 2007 and are extremely sensitive, more so than the commercially available kits.[45] All horses imported to Australia are now PCR tested for equine influenza before embarkation and after arrival.[31]

Vaccination

Vaccination against specific disease agents such as Japanese encephalitis can reduce the risk of disease in horses sourced from or imported into an infected region.[1] For other diseases, e.g. equine influenza, vaccination is of limited value as a risk management option. Equine influenza vaccination can prevent overt disease but a horse can still be infected and shedding virus at the time of import.[5,6,17,46]

Treatment

Treatment can be used to reduce the risk of importation of exotic parasites such as ticks. Insecticides may be applied to horses to minimize exposure to insect vectors during training sessions[31,36] and transport. Countries may also require horses to be treated for internal and external parasites before export.

Restrictions on destination, activity and season of import

An example of this strategy is avoidance of exposure to insect vectors by import into a vector-free zone[29] or, by only permitting importation during a season when insect vectors are not active. Another example is requiring competition horses not to breed or be resident on breeding premises during a period of temporary residency.

Protection of health status during international travel

Government authorities may require horses to travel on approved routes through approved countries and have no contact with other horses not of the same health status during transport. Special conditions may apply during transit of countries en route or if horses are trans-shipped from one aircraft to another during a transit. Conditions may be prescribed regarding cleaning and disinfection of horse transport vehicles and shipping containers, and protection of horses from insect vectors during transport.

Restrictions on duration of temporary residency

Visiting horses may only be permitted to remain in countries for a maximum specified period. The period may be set by the importing country or the country of usual residency, or both.

Contact information for major regulatory agencies

Each country has very specific quarantine conditions for temporary and permanent import of horses which are subject to change. Consequently, specific details cannot be given in this review and veterinarians should always seek advice from government officials or a reputable shipping agent before commencing preparation of horses for export. Many agencies now publish their quarantine conditions electronically. Readers are referred to contact information below.

Government animal health and quarantine authorities

Australia
Department of Agriculture, Fisheries and Forestry
GPO Box 858
Canberra ACT 2601
http://www.daff.gov.au/

European Commission
Agriculture and Rural Development
130 Rue de la Loi
B-1049 Brussels
Belgium
http://ec.europa.eu/agriculture/contact/index_en.htm

Hong Kong SAR, People's Republic of China
The Government of the Hong Kong Special Administrative Region
Agriculture, Fisheries and Conservation Department
5/F Cheung Sha Wan Government Offices
303 Cheung Sha Wan Road
Kowloon
Hong Kong
http://www.afcd.gov.hk/eindex.html

Singapore
Agri-Food and Veterinary Authority of Singapore
Regulatory Services Branch
5 Maxwell Road #02-00 Tower Block MND Complex
Singapore 069110
http://www.ava.gov.sg/

New Zealand
Ministry of Agriculture and Forestry
PO Box 2526
Wellington, 6140
http://www.maf.govt.nz/biosecurity-animal-welfare

Office International des Epizooties
12, rue de Prony
75017 Paris
France
http://www.oie.int/

United Arab Emirates
Ministry of Environment and Water
Animal Wealth Department
http://moew.gov.ae/portal/en/our-services/animal-wealth.aspx

United Kingdom
Department for Environment, Food and Rural Affairs
Nobel House
17 Smith Square
London SW1P 3JR
http://www.defra.gov.uk/animal-trade/

United States
United States Department of Agriculture
Animal and Plant Health Inspection Service Veterinary Services
National Center for Import and Export
International Health Standards Team
4700 River Road, Unit 33
Riverdale
Maryland, 20737
http://www.aphis.usda.gov/import_export/

World Trade Organization
Centre William Rappard
rue de Lausanne 154
CH-1211 Geneva 21
Switzerland
www.wto.org

Other organizations

Federation Equestre Internationale
HM King Hussein I Building
Chemin de la Joliette 8
1006 Lausanne
Switzerland
www.horsesport.org

International Air Transport Association
Cargo – Live Animals
PO Box 113
Montreal, Quebec
Canada H4Z 1M1
http://www.iata.org/workgroups/Pages/lapb.aspx

International Federation of Horseracing Authorities
46 place Abel Gance
92655 Boulogne Cedex
France
http://www.horseracingintfed.com

International harness racing organizations
http://www.harness.org.au/ausbreed/int_org.htm

With thanks to Keith L. Watkins, who co-created the original chapter in the first edition.

References

1. Herholz C, Fussel A-E, Timoney P, et al. Equine travellers to the Olympic Games in Hong Kong 2008: A review of worldwide challenges to equine health, with particular reference to vector-borne diseases. Equine Vet J 2008;40:87–95.
2. Sluyter FJH. Traceability of Equidae: a population in motion. Rev Sci Tech 2001;20:500–9.
3. Watkins KL, Devolz R, Ellis P, et al. Guidelines to facilitate the temporary movement of registered racehorses for international races. In: Hill DW, Hill WT, editors. Proceedings of the 14th International Conference of Racing Analysts and Veterinarians, Orlando, 2012. Newmarket, UK: R and W Publications; 2003. p. 280–96.
4. Guthrie AJ, Stevens KB, Bosman PP. The circumstances surrounding the outbreak and spread of equine influenza in South Africa. Rev Sci Tech 1999;18: 179–85.
5. Powell DG, Watkins KL, Li PH, et al. Outbreak of equine influenza among horses in Hong Kong during 1992. Vet Rec 1995;136:531–6.
6. Callinan I. Equine Influenza: The August 2007 outbreak in Australia. Commonwealth of Australia; 2008. Online. Available: http://www.equineinfluenzainquiry.gov.au/www/inquiry/equine.nsf/Page/Report Accessed 28 February 2012.
7. Timoney PJ. Equids and equine semen. International trade vs. disease control. In: Wernery U, Wade JF, Mumford JA, et al, editors. Equine Infectious Diseases VIII. Proceedings of the Eighth International Conference, Dubai, March 1998. Newmarket: R and W Publications; 1999. p. 328–31.
8. Cordes T, Mitchell R. Quarantine considerations and medical management of horses during international shipment. In: Robinson NE, editor. Current Therapy in Equine Medicine 4. Philadelphia: WB Saunders; 1997. p. 717–19.
9. Morgan AM. Regulatory aspects involved in the international movement of horses. In: Nakajima H, Plowright W, editors. Equine Infectious Diseases VII. Proceedings of the Seventh International Conference, Tokyo, 1994. Newmarket: R and W Publications; 1994. p. 336–8.
10. Timoney PJ. Factors influencing the international spread of equine diseases. Vet Clin North Am Equine Pract 2000; 16:537–51.
11. Timoney PJ. Infectious diseases and international movement of horses. In: Sellon DC, Long M, editors. Equine Infectious Diseases. Philadelphia: WB Saunders; 2007. p. 549–57.
12. Daniels P. Emerging arboviral diseases. Aust Vet J 2012;80:216.
13. Stone M. Import risk analysis: horses and horse semen. Wellington: Ministry of Agriculture and Forestry, New Zealand; 2000. Online. Available: http://www.biosecurity.govt.nz/files/regs/imports/risk/horse-ra.pdf 28 February 2012.
14. Ellis PM, Farr NH, Arab AA, et al. Demonstration of equine health status for international trading purposes: the United Arab Emirates strategy. In: Wernery U, Wade JF, Mumford JA, Kaaden OR, editors. Equine Infectious Diseases VIII. Proceedings of the Eighth International Conference, Dubai, March 1998. Newmarket: R and W Publications; 1999. p. 363–6.
15. Pastoret P-P, Chaisemartin D. The importance of governance and reliable veterinary certification. Rev Sci Off 2011;30:347–52.
16. DEFRA. Qualitative analysis of the risk of introduction of Equine Infectious Anaemia (EIA) into Great Britain from an EIA endemic area through temporary movement of UK origin horses. London, UK: DEFRA; 2011. Online. Available http://www.defra.gov.uk/animal-diseases/files/qra-eia-horse-movements-110624.pdf Accessed 5 March 2012.
17. Watkins KL. Endemic and exotic equine infectious diseases and their effect on international racing. In: Auer DE, Houghton E, editors. Proceedings of the 11th International Conference of Racing Analysts and Veterinarians, Queensland 1996. Newmarket: R and W Publications; 1996. p. 281–6.
18. Cowled B, Ward MP, Hamilton S, et al. The equine influenza epidemic in Australia: spatial and temporal descriptive analyzes of a large propagating epidemic. Prev Vet Med 2007;92:60–70.
19. Smyth GB, Dagley K, Tainsh J. Insights into the economic consequences of the 2007 equine influenza outbreak in Australia. Aust Vet J 2011;89(Suppl. 1): S151–18.
20. Taylor MR, Agho KE, Stevens GJ, et al. Factors influencing psychological distress during a disease epidemic: data from Australia's first outbreak of equine influenza. BMC Public Health 2008;8:347 Online. Available http://www.ncbi.nlm.nih.gov/pubmed/18831770 7 March 2012.
21. Jeffcott L. Foot and mouth disease in Great Britain. Where are we now? The Horse 2001;18(8):98.
22. World Trade Organization. Online. Available: http://www.wto.org/ 28 February 2012.
23. Murray N. International trade and the spread of animal diseases: assessing the risks. Veterinaria Italiana 2006;42: 319–36.
24. Office International des Epizooties. About us. Online. Available: http://www.oie.int 28 February 2012.
25. Office International des Epizooties. Terrestrial Animal Health Code. 20th ed. Paris: OIE; 2011. Online. Available: http://www.oie.int 28 February 2012.
26. Office International des Epizooties. Manual Diagnostic Tests and Vaccines for Terrestrial Animals. 6th ed. Paris: OIE; 2008. Online. Available: http://www.oie.int 28 February 2012.
27. Powell DG. The significance of surveillance and reporting on the prevention and control of equine diseases. Vet Clin North Am Equine Pract 2000;16:389–403.
28. Brooks LM. The equine piroplasmosis control programme at the 1996 Summer Olympic Games. In: Wernery U, Wade JF, Mumford JA, et al, editors. Equine Infectious Diseases VIII. Proceedings of the Eighth International Conference, Dubai, March 1998. Newmarket: R and W Publications; 1999. p. 371–5.
29. Martin R. Equine Piroplasmosis: the temporary importation of seropositive horses into Australia. Aust Vet J 1999;77: 308–9.
30. Allen AK. WEG veterinary review. The Horse December 2011:66.
31. Biosecurity Australia. Import risk analysis for horses from approved countries: final

report. Canberra: Biosecurity Australia; 2010.

32. Rodriguez M, Ladero JL, Castaño M, et al. African horse sickness in Spain: epizootiological and regulatory considerations. J Eq Vet Sci 1992;12:395–400.
33. Guthrie AJ. Regionalisation of South Africa for African horse sickness. In: Wernery U, Wade JF, Mumford JA, et al, editors. Equine Infectious Diseases VIII. Proceedings of the Eighth International Conference, Dubai, March 1998. Newmarket: R and W Publications; 1999. p. 376–9.
34. Murray G. The development of disease-free zones for equine diseases – including the example of China. Conf OIE 2009:125–30. Online. Available: http://www.oie.int/doc/ged/D9765.PDF 28 February 2012.
35. Santarelli JN. International movement: a shipper's perspective. In: Wernery U, Wade JF, Mumford JA, et al, editors. Equine Infectious Diseases VIII. Proceedings of the Eighth International Conference, Dubai, March 1998. Newmarket: R and W Publications; 1999. p. 336–8.
36. Ellis PM. Establishing a quarantine facility for imported racehorses. In: Auer DE, Houghton E, editors. Proceedings of the 11th International Conference of Racing Analysts and Veterinarians, Queensland, 1996. Newmarket: R and W Publications; 1996. p. 295–8.
37. International Air Transport Association. Live Animal Regulations. 38th ed. Montreal: International Air Transport Association; 2011.
38. International Federation of Horse Racing Authorities. International Agreement on Breeding and Racing. Online. Available: http://www.horseracingintfed.com/e-index.html 14 March 2012.
39. Sluyter F. International horse movement: health requirements versus impact on equestrian sport development. In: Wernery U, Wade JF, Mumford JA, et al, editors. Equine Infectious Diseases VIII. Proceedings of the Eighth International Conference, Dubai, March 1998. Newmarket: R and W Publications; 1999. p. 334–5.
40. Federation Equestre Internationale. Veterinary Regulations. 12th ed. Switzerland: FEI; 2010. Online. Available: http://www.fei.org/veterinary/veterinary-regulations 28 February 2012.
41. Federation Equestre Internationale. Identification of Horses. 5th ed. Switzerland: FEI; 2006. Online. Available: http://www.fei.org/sites/default/files/ID-e.print__1.pdf 28 February 2012.
42. Bork, RL. The Arlington experience. In: Powell DG, editor. Equine Infectious Disease – Developing an Action Plan. Kentucky: Maxwell H. Gluck Equine Research Centre; 1994. p. 13–14.
43. Smith RD. Veterinary Clinical Epidemiology: A Problem Orientated Approach. 2nd edn. Boca Raton, FL: CRC Press; 1995.
44. Edwards S, Castillo-Olivares J, Cullinane A, et al. International harmonisation of laboratory diagnostic tests for equine viral arteritis. In: Wernery U, Wade JF, Mumford JA, et al, editors. Equine Infectious Diseases VIII. Proceedings of the Eighth International Conference, Dubai, March 1998. Newmarket: R and W Publications; 1999. p. 359–62.
45. Elton D, Bryant N. HBLB's advances in equine veterinary science and practice – Facing the threat of equine influenza. Equine Vet J 2011;43:250–8.
46. Watson J, Daniels P, Kirkland P, et al. The 2007 outbreak of equine influenza in Australia: lessons learned for international trade in horses. Rev Sci Tech 2011;30:87–93.

section 10

Physical therapy and rehabilitation

Manual therapy and exercise for athletic horses

62

Lesley Goff

CHAPTER CONTENTS

Manual therapy

Background

Equine physiotherapy encompasses many forms of physical therapies, including manual therapy and exercise therapy. Research into the effectiveness of and the mechanisms of action of both manual therapy and exercise therapy for musculoskeletal disorders, especially back and neck pain, is quite extensive. Most of the research, however, is derived from the human field, as are other clinical techniques that have been developed for equine physiotherapy.

Manual therapy refers to the practice of passive or assisted movement techniques applied by the therapist to address pain and impairments in the articular, neural and muscle systems.[1] Manual therapy is applicable to the athletic horse when the animal's performance is affected by pain and impairment, and may include joint manipulation and mobilization to articular and neural tissue, and stretching and massage to soft tissues. Mobilization and manipulation are defined by the rate and depth of application of thrust to the joint, and in research they are often termed spinal manipulative therapy (SMT). There are various forms of massage techniques and stretching.

Exercise therapy in rehabilitation of the equine patient may include hydrotherapy, proprioceptive retraining and the implementation of neuromotor control concepts. Many equine exercise therapy strategies have, in a similar manner to manual therapy, been extrapolated from human evidence-based practice.

This section will endeavor to address the mechanism of action, efficacy, outcome measures and therapeutic applications of SMT, general massage and stretching techniques, as well as the principles and practice of equine exercise therapy for rehabilitation.

Mechanism of action

Manual therapy is well established clinically for the management of pain and impairment arising from the vertebral column in both man and the horse. Early beliefs regarding the mechanism of action for manual therapy on the spinal articular system included biomechanical effects of mobilization, and reduction in hypertonicity of paraspinal musculature. Evidence for these effects is not secure.[2] Contemporary research suggests the pain-relieving effect of manual therapy is due to neurophysiological mechanisms. Inhibitory pathways descending from higher centers in the central nervous system, and neural inhibitory systems at various spinal cord levels, are stimulated by afferent input from specific locally induced movements such as mobilization and manipulation.[3] This may result in hypoalgesia. There are also sympatho-excitatory effects associated with these techniques.[4] Mobilization to L4/5 vertebral level articulation resulted in side-specific sympathetic nervous system changes being recorded.[5]

Similar hypoalgesic effects to that seen in spinal manual therapy are imparted when mobilization is carried out to the extremity joints.[6] There is evidence that passive mobilization to the articulations of the knee in humans and rodents produces widespread and local hypoalgesic effects.[7]

Efficacy

Despite the fact that SMT is used clinically in horses and humans, views on the efficacy of SMT is mixed. Systematic reviews conclude that SMT used alone in man is not superior to other forms of treatment for acute or chronic low back pain.[8,9] In conclusions of a randomized trial,[10] SMT and motor control interventions both produced better short-term function than general exercise for back pain. However, this was not the case for medium or long-term effects. In another randomized clinical trial of individuals with chronic low back pain, supervised exercise was shown to be better than spinal manipulation or home exercises for trunk muscle function and patient satisfaction, but no different for pain, disability improvement in general health status and medication use.[11] For mechanical neck pain, manipulation or mobilization alone showed non-significant benefit on pain relief when assessed against placebo, control or other treatments.[12] Another group, however, showed short-term analgesic effect for neck pain following spinal mobilization or manipulation. Further, multimodal physical therapies that did not include manual therapy did not provide better pain relief than a control, whereas multimodal physical therapy that included spinal manual therapy provided pain relief that was better than a control.[13]

In the horse, high velocity, low amplitude thrusts directed perpendicularly to thoraco-lumbar vertebrae resulted in increased dorsoventral displacement of the trunk during passive spinal mobilization.[14] Gomez-Alvarez and colleagues[15] reported increases in spinal passive mobility after SMT, but these were decreased three weeks later compared to before treatment status.

Mobilization when used in combination with exercise has been shown to be useful for the extremity joints.[16] The selection of systematic reviews and randomized clinical trials quoted seem to favor manual therapy for the spine and extremities as part of multimodal intervention, especially when combined with exercise.

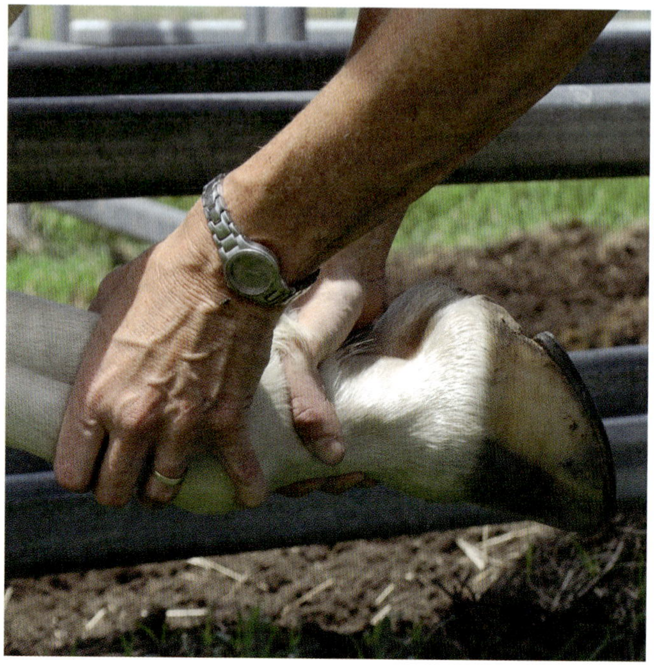

Fig 62.1 Mobilization technique for the left metacarpophalangeal joint. Therapist's left hand is stabilizing the distal metacarpal, whilst the right hand provides a rhythmical, cranially directed gliding movement of the proximal phalanx.

Indications and contraindications

In the athletic horse, back pain or sacroiliac pain is a common cause of poor performance.[17] Here, spinal mobilization techniques may be useful for short-term pain modulation of symptoms arising from the vertebral column. According to the evidence, combining SMT or manual therapy techniques with exercise will give the best outcomes. Exercise concepts in equine physiotherapy will be discussed further in this chapter.

A specific example where spinal manual therapy may be useful is where there is pain and dysfunction arising from the facet joints (single segment or group) in the thoracolumbar region of the horse's back. Local and specific passive movements applied to these segments can assist in restoring movement and function through hypoalgesia, followed by appropriate exercises to maintain this functional benefit. Examples where mobilization to extremities may be useful in the athletic horse is where there is injury to, or osteoarthritis in, the metacarpophalaneal joint. Mobilization, or articular gliding movements can be applied to the articulation between the metacarpus and the proximal phalanx (Fig. 62.1). These mobilizations do not reverse any degenerative changes that may be present,[18] but may induce hypoalgesia, therefore potentially allowing specific exercises to be effective at helping to restore function following the technique.

Spinal or extremity directed manual therapy is contraindicated if there is non-weightbearing lameness (fracture/ infection), osteomyelitis, ankylosis, bleeding disorders, ataxia +/− upper motor neurone signs.[18,19] SMT is also delivered with caution in cases where it is not yet established if back pain or poor performance is coming primarily from the vertebral column. Back pain is often secondary to another lameness, dysfunction or pathology in the horse's limbs, or may be associated with medical conditions such as exertional rhambdomyolysis and thrombosis of caudal aorta or iliac arteries.[17,20] The primary cause of the lameness must be diagnosed and treated by a veterinarian before the secondary back pain is addressed.

Massage

Background and mechanism of action

Massage is practiced widely amongst many professionals involved with management of sporting injuries in the equine field. As is the case for manual therapy, many of the massage techniques applied to horses have been derived from human clinical techniques. Types of massage techniques include petrissage, effleurage, tapotement and frictions. Massage can be considered a manual therapy, although the area to which it is delivered is less specific than SMT. There is limited data as to the possible mechanism of action of massage.[21] Proposed mechanisms include: increased muscle compliance, changes in circulation, hormone levels and psychophysiological parameters. However, this is all still inconclusive. Neurological effects may result from mechanical pressure via the increase or decrease of neural excitability as measured by the Hoffman reflex, but this has only been measured in petrissage.[21] The type of massage technique delivered may also affect the mechanism of action.

Efficacy

Despite its purported benefits and frequent use in the athlete, evidence for the efficacy of massage is scarce.[22] There is no clear evidence that massage can improve performance, enhance recovery or prevent muscular injury.[21] However, the large range of different massage techniques makes it difficult to combine results to get a good overall picture of massage.[21] A Cochrane database systematic review states that in humans massage may be beneficial for low back pain when combined with exercises and education.[23] A recent randomized controlled trial found that massage therapy may be effective for treating chronic back pain in people.[24] Randomized controlled trials have shown moderate levels of evidence for the use of massage to facilitate recovery from repetitive muscular contractions associated with strenuous exercise.[25] However, the overall consensus from the research is that further investigation using more standardized techniques and protocols is necessary to more conclusively demonstrate the efficacy of massage for musculoskeletal injury and sports performance.[22,25]

Indications

Although the efficacy of massage is inconclusive, due partly to poor study designs and lack of standardization, one cannot completely ignore the possible benefits of massage to the equine athlete. The muscular and fascial systems are extensive in the horse, therefore any one of a variety of massage techniques may have a beneficial effect, especially if incorporated into a multi-modal treatment plan.

Horses with pain and dysfunction in the epaxial musculature or the vast gluteal musculature may indeed benefit from massage techniques that could improve muscle compliance and decrease pain. An example is quoted by Hill and co-worker[26] where a goal of training young horses could be to create an earlier maximal protraction of the hindlimb, which may result in an increase in stride length. Massage (petrissage and effleurage) was applied to the caudal hindlimb muscles in eight horses and resulted in a significant increase in both passive and active hindlimb protraction.[26] Figure 62.2 shows application of a massage technique.

Deep friction massage has been proposed as an effective management for tendinopathy, which occurs frequently in the equine athlete; however, efficacy has not been confirmed as an isolated technique.[27]

Stretching

Background and efficacy

There are different types of stretching used in clinical practice, from sustained stretch, to eccentric loading stretch, and rhythmical stretching. There have been varied outcomes from research regarding the efficacy of stretching for athletic performance, and of course, much of the research is human-based. Despite the fact that the benefits of stretching on athletic performance are unclear, stretches are widely used in human and equine physiotherapy and rehabilitation.

There is suggestion that stretching before or after exercise can have negative effects on performance, especially in strength and power activities. Maximal isometric voluntary contraction (MVC) of a muscle was seen to be impaired following prolonged-hold (5 x 120 seconds) passive stretching to the plantar flexors.[28] Taylor and colleagues[29] surmise that the negative effects of stretching reported in research occurred because stretching routines studied were dissimilar to that practiced by athletes. These authors reported that the implementation of a dynamic sports-specific warm-up routine following the stretching negated the detrimental effects of stretching on jump height and sprint time, in human athletes.

Stretching may be beneficial for flexibility and reducing muscle soreness. Thirty seconds of therapist-applied passive stretch to hamstrings resulted in an increased in hamstring flexibility in healthy human subjects.[30] It has also been suggested that stretching may reduce the amount of muscle soreness felt following exercise[31] therefore making recovery easier. Eccentric loading stretch to the tendo-achilles in humans has found to be a successful treatment for mid-substance tendinopathy.[32]

A recent equine study looked at the effect of stretching on stride length and ROM in trot and found that stride length was not affected by stretch.[33] There were in fact some negative effects on range of joint motion following a more frequent stretching regime of six times per week. This may have implications on how frequently a stretching program should be carried out. Range of motion however, was measured with skin markers, thus results may have been affected by skin movements over the joints. It is clear that further research into the effects of stretching on equine athletic performance is required.

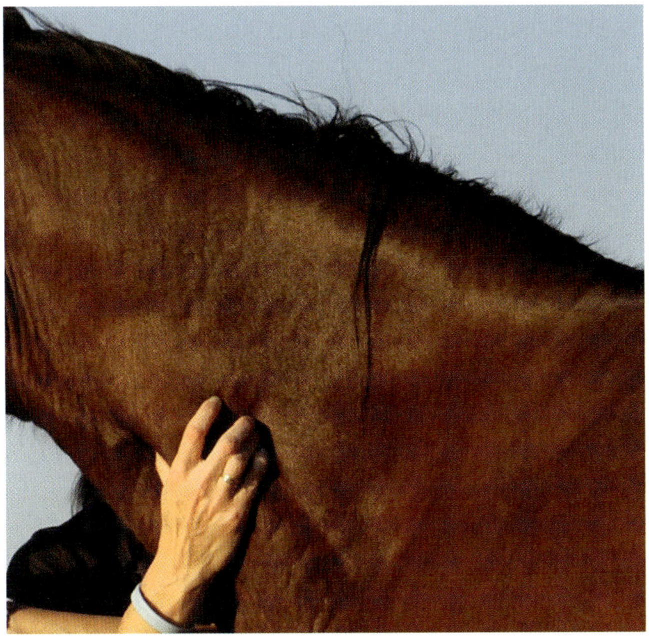

Fig 62.2 Massage technique (petrissage) to the left brachiocephalicus muscle.

Mechanism of action

Weir and colleagues[28] suggest that the effects of stretching are due to changes in the mechanical properties of muscles. In sustained static stretching, Kubo and co-workers[34] measured MVC after 10 minutes of static stretch to gastrocnemius and elongation of tendon via ultrasound. They found that there was no change in MVC, decreased viscosity of tendon, but that there was increased elasticity.

Another group of researchers[35] compared static stretching to dynamic stretching and concluded that both groups of stretch subjects showed increases in range of motion of plantar flexors, but the static stretch group significantly increased range of motion. This increase was attributed to reduced resistance of the muscle-tendon unit over range of motion, measured using electrodes. The dynamic stretch group showed little change in resistance over range of motion, but tendon stiffness had decreased significantly after stretching. The latter effect was measured using ultrasound. These authors concluded that in static stretching the muscle itself was affected, not the tendon, possibly due to an increase in the number of sarcomeres. Dynamic stretching was proposed to have more effect on the tendon, increasing both the storage and release capability of the tendon.

Indications and therapeutic application

It is possible that following exercise, stretching is the modality of choice to reduce muscle soreness and aid recovery in the equine athlete. Based on the research available, stretches of approximately 30 seconds, performed after exercise, may be useful for decreasing muscle soreness, and delivered three times per week may increase flexibility.

The nature of the stretch requires consideration when prescribing a stretching program. Based on the research of Mahieu and colleagues[35] static stretching is preferred for gaining a high range of motion. It is important however to keep in mind the range of motion requirements of the different equine sports. Dynamic stretching may be more beneficial if the stretch-shortening cycle intensity of the sport is high, and the tendon's capacity to store and release energy needs to be increased.

During gait, the equine muscle-tendon unit undergoes stretch-shortening cycles, that is eccentric exercise followed immediately by concentric exercise. In high intensity stretch-shortening cycles of the muscle-tendon unit, such as in showjumping, the tendon must be compliant enough to store and release a large amount of energy; the more elastic the tendon, the less likely the high stretch-shortening cycles would be to reach the maximum capacity of the tendon.[36] Therefore, the rationale for injury prevention in such a sport would be to increase the compliance of the muscle-tendon unit. In a low or moderate stretch-shortening cycle such as in trot, increased tendon compliance that may result from stretching may not be required as it is for high stretch-shortening cycle. This has been suggested in research.[36]

It is clear that more research on the effects of stretching on the equine athlete is required.

Outcome measures for manual therapy, massage and stretching

As the equine athlete cannot tell us of the outcome of interventions, outcome measures are often based on the observations of horse's function following treatment. However, assessments that are conducted 'in-field' may be difficult to perform with repeatability. Objective measurements provide a reproducible manner of assessing whether treatment has effected a change.

Examples of objective measurements for effects of manual therapy include use of goniometry, algometry, or even simply the use of tape measures. Ultrasonography can be used to objectively measure changes in tendon or ligament thickness in response to treatment, or muscle atrophy/hypertrophy in response to treatment. Video or photographs using grid lines as reference points enhances the objectivity of observational reassessment.

Equine studies have used algometry to assess whether there is a change in mechanical nociceptive threshold (MNT) in horses following manipulation of the spine[37]and soft tissue techniques.[38] Human and equine studies have also noted the high intra- and inter-observer reliability for using this non-invasive measurement tool.[39,40] Figure 62.3 shows an algometer being used to assess MNT over the middle gluteal muscle.

Goniometry has been used to measure joint range of motion in healthy Labrador retrievers and was found to be reliable and objective.[41] This measurement parameter has been shown to be a promising tool in documenting passive flexion of the equine fetlock, carpus and hock, if used by the same investigator[42] (Fig. 62.4). However, additional studies are needed for further validation of this assessment tool in the horse.

Tape measures can be used to measure limb circumference when looking for reduction in swelling or changes in muscle bulk, or to measure changes in distance between bony landmarks when assessing changes in joint range of motion. Bennell and co-workers[43] determined that both intra- and inter-observer reliability were excellent when measuring the distance between a lower limb bony landmark and a wall, using a tape measure. This measurement tool is simple to use providing the methods are documented.

Ultrasound has been used in human research to measure changes in muscle atrophy in the spine in low back pain.[44] Ultrasound has also been validated as a tool to assess symmetry of cross-sectional area of multifidus in the horse.[45] Ultrasound to measure changes in cross-sectional area of equine tendons has questionable inter-observer reliability, but acceptable intra-observer reliability.[46]

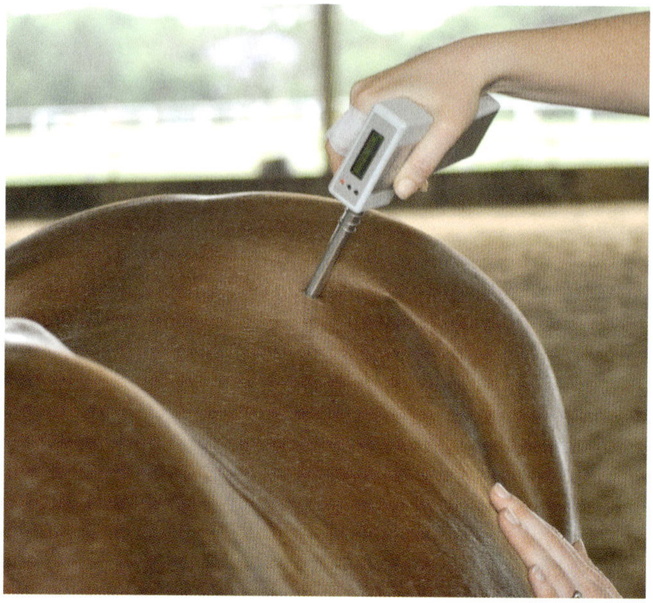

Fig 62.3 Algometer measuring the mechanical nociceptive threshold over the left epaxial musculature (iliocostalis).

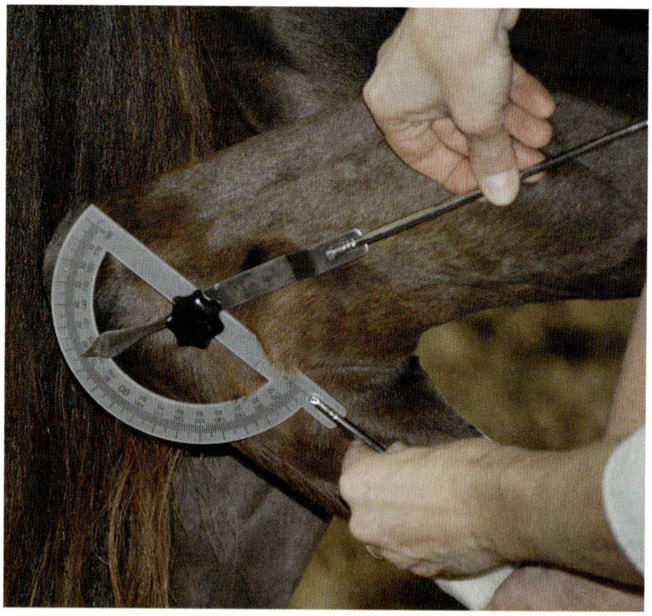

Fig 62.4 Goniometer measuring the passive flexion angle of the right hock.

In summary, manual therapy complements other physical therapeutic agents including specific therapeutic exercise, more general rehabilitative exercise and electrophysical agents. Physiotherapists often combine exercise therapy with passive joint mobilization to treat impairments related to joint function, and this is supported by research which suggests that the combination of manual therapy and exercise is most effective for back and neck pain,[13] as well as for osteoarthritis of the knee.[16] Exercise therapy includes specific therapeutic exercise as well as more general rehabilitative exercise, including aquatic therapy.

Exercise therapy

Exercise therapy is not specific to physiotherapy; it is implemented by many practitioners, individuals and trainers in rehabilitation and training of the sporting horse. This section will focus mainly on neuromotor control as this area has been investigated quite extensively by physiotherapists in both the human and equine physiotherapy fields, and there are implications for symptom management as well as further rehabilitation. There will be a less comprehensive reference to hydrotherapy, or water-based exercise.

Neuromotor control

Background

Neuromotor control concepts have been researched in physiotherapy and are derived from investigations related to back and neck pain and other musculoskeletal injuries in man. Neuromotor control can be defined as the unconscious muscular or motor response to an afferent signal concerning dynamic joint stability.[47] This motor response may entail both feedback and feed-forward components and is a major component of joint and postural stability.[48]

Recent research has shown that motor control concepts are applicable to horses with back pain, specifically through the initial research of Stubbs and colleagues.[49] It is well known that equine back and sacroiliac pain present as a range of clinical signs, but with poor performance being an outcome of such a dysfunction.[17] Stubbs and colleagues[49] have shown that sporting performance may be related to altered neuromotor control. This contributes to a functional instability between vertebrae, which may result in the recurrence of clinical signs that is noted to be common in the horse. It is thought that the stiffness of the epaxial muscles felt on palpation of a horse with back pain is associated with loss of function of the muscle multifidus, one of the deep stabilising muscles of the horse's vertebral column. Overactivity of the more superficial longissimus muscle group, which is suggested to be recruited to protect or 'splint' the vertebral column further when there is pain or dysfunction, is thought to be responsible for the apparent stiffness, and altered trunk and gait dynamics.[50] The compromise of more superficial musculature may increase the incidences of recurrence of symptoms of back pain.[51] These findings may explain the results of Gomez-Alvarez and co-workers[15] where they suggested recurrence of spinal dysfunction in horses could occur weeks after SMT intervention.

Stimulation of the dorsal sacroiliac joint capsule in pigs resulted in activity in the muscle multifidus, and stimulation of the ventral capsule resulted in activity in gluteal musculature.[52] These results suggest muscles around the sacroiliac joint in the quadruped may be important for neuromotor control in back and sacroiliac pain. This is particularly applicable to the equine athlete as it is well accepted that the pelvis and sacroiliac joint are the region via which all the propulsive forces are transmitted from the hindlimb, to the trunk.[17]

Following injury, damage to the connective tissue and sensory neural tissue in the joint capsules, ligaments, musculo-tendinous junction and muscle spindles causes altered proprioception.[53] Proprioceptive deficits have been identified in human musculoskeletal injuries and proprioceptive retraining, where appropriate, is an important part of rehabilitation.[54] Proprioceptive retraining for horses can involve the use of ground poles, tape, stretch rubber band or tubing and lightweight chains. Exercises that enhance proprioception can be used within a general sport-specific rehabilitation program.

Mechanism of action and efficacy

Specific evidence-based exercises that help restore neuromotor control have been developed for the clinical management of back pain in man, and these have been shown to reduce the risk of recurrence of symptoms.[44] Stubbs and colleagues[50] have developed dynamic mobilization exercises to target multifidus in the horse, and have shown a significant increase in multifidus bulk over a three-month period of delivering the exercises. It has been suggested that exercises such as these – which involved both movement and a static hold – have their effect by recruiting type II fibers which are selectively atrophied in the spinal muscles of back pain individuals.

The exercises proposed by Stubbs and colleagues[50] should assist in neuromotor control of the sacroiliac region as multifidus are continuous into the sacral spine. Specific atrophy of the gluteal musculature in the horse is apparent when sacroiliac joint dysfunction exists.[17] Therefore, exercises specific to the gluteal muscles are often used to help restore function in this case. There are no randomized trials or systematic reviews in the equine literature regarding specific neuromotor control exercises. However, as mentioned in the section on manual therapy, there is evidence to suggest that the combination of the specific exercises and manual therapy gives a good outcome in managing pain arising from the vertebral column.

Measurement outcomes

Ultrasound has been validated as a tool to assess symmetry of cross-sectional area of multifidus in the horse.[49] Ultrasound has also been utilized, but not validated when assessing the dorsal sacroiliac ligament[55] which is often asymmetrically atrophied in sacroiliac dysfunction in the horse.

Algometry has been validated as an assessment tool and could certainly be used here to assess mechanical nociceptive threshold following the implementation of a program to enhance neuromotor control.

Therapeutic protocol

Stubbs and colleagues[50] used a three-month program of cervical lateral bending exercises to stimulate multifidus along the entire length of the vertebral column. These exercises were performed five times in a session, five times per week. A horse that has had recurrent back pain, or poor performance related to back or sacroiliac pain, may benefit from a program similar to this. The horse may require manual therapy to provide some hypoalgesia prior to the implementation of the specific exercises. This would be follow the evidence that the combination of manual therapy and exercise provides a good outcome for back pain.

Taping can alter the timing of musculature around the human patella, as an adjunct to rehabilitation.[56] Taping is utilized in equine rehabilitation to enhance neuromotor control and can be used to facilitate the timing and activation of gluteal musculature, or abdominal musculature which is thought to assist in trunk dynamic function. In the horse, taping can be also utilized for its proprioceptive effects on distal limbs as well as trunk and pelvic musculature. The tape may be applied along the direction of the muscle fibers, to assist in facilitating muscle activity, or may be applied perpendicular to the direction of muscle fibers. The latter is thought to have more of an inhibitory effect on muscle activity, however, this is anectodal. Figure 62.5 shows taping designed to facilitate abdominal and pelvic musculature.

Other proprioceptive devices that can be used in rehabilitation include leg weights and light-weight tactile devices. Tactile stimulation of the hind pasterns during trot resulted in increased flight arcs of stifle, tarsal, metatarsal and distal interphalangeal joints.[57] This

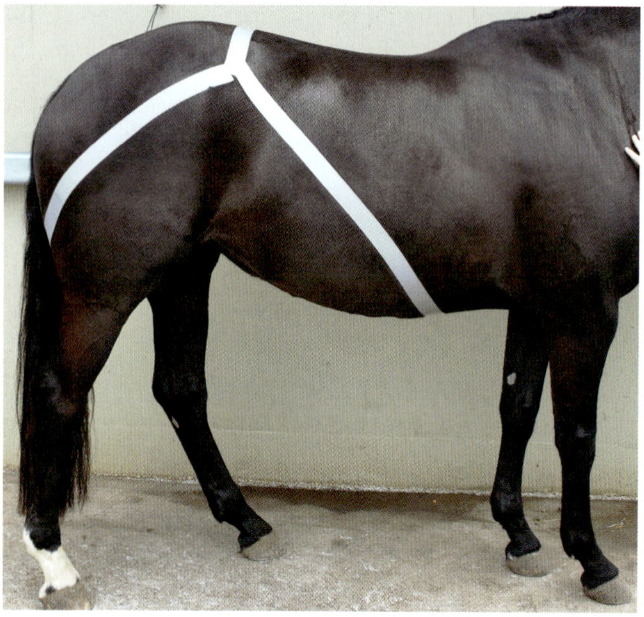

Fig 62.5 Taping to facilitate abdominal and pelvic musculature. The horse would be taped and then lunged or worked, to assess the effect of the tape on gait and movement.

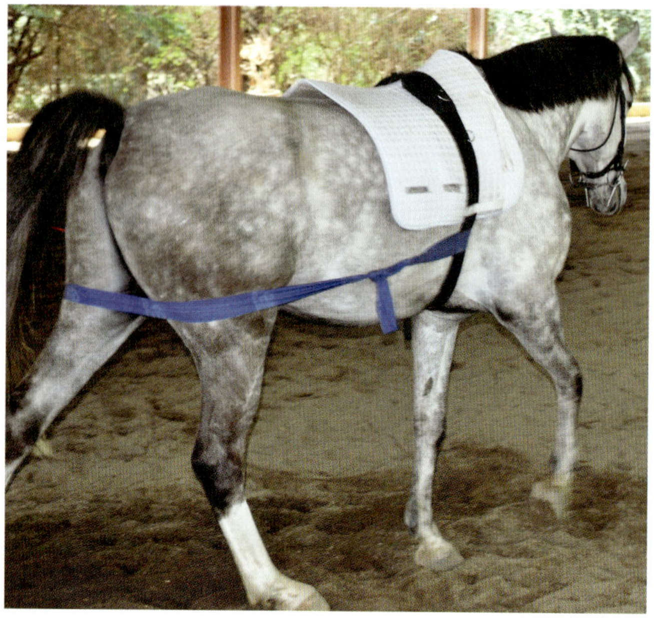

Fig 62.6 Use of stretch banding as a proprioceptive aid. The stretch band stimulates the receptors in the skin and muscle of the abdominal and posterior thigh regions. The horse would be lunged with the proprioceptive aids in situ, and the effect of the banding on gait and movement would be assessed.

type of proprioceptive intervention may help in rehabilitation of injuries that have resulted in altered use of the hindlimb during gait. The addition of 700 gram weights to the hind pasterns during trot was shown to increase concentric muscular activity across all hindlimb joints from the hip to the metatarsophalangeal joint, along with the increased flight arc.[58]

Stretch rubber band or tubing can be utilized as a proprioceptive device and can be integrated into a sport-specific exercise program. In Figure 62.6 the rubber banding is fixed to and passed behind the horse's pelvis. The tactile response of the horse to the rubber banding gave an impression of greater engagement of the hindlimbs and pelvis during exercise on the lunge.

The use of ground poles and obstacles stimulate proprioceptive awareness in the horse, and are useful in enhancing neuromotor control. Obstacles such as pedestals that the horse can walk up and over, or balance upon stimulate the propriceptive awareness, and assist in neuromotor control by encouraging the horse to engage abdominal and neck musculature to negotiate the obstacle.[53] Ground poles encourage the horse to contract the abdominal and hip flexor musculature, and may be used with the horse in-hand or ridden. Ground poles may be placed so that the horse can take equal length strides at the walk, and may be progressed, for example to raised cavaletti at a slow trot which encourages the horse to contract neck flexors and abdominals as well as engaging the limbs in order to stride over the cavaletti. Poles may be incorporated into sport-specific exercise, such as placed in a circle or a curve, or before small jumps. In-hand or ridden incline work encourages the horse to contract abdominal musculature and bring the hindlimbs under the body, especially in downhill work.[53]

Hydrotherapy

Background

Equine underwater treadmills, a cross between a treadmill and a swimming pool, are popular for training and rehabilitating horses from injury.[59] Due to some buoyancy, they are thought to allow the horse to exercise with reduced impact on the musculoskeletal system.[53] Underwater treadmill exercise programs, however, have a limited evidence base with respect to kinematics.

Borgia and co-workers[60] explored the potential benefits of the underwater treadmill for providing an increase in muscle oxidative capacity. It was thought that exercise in an underwater treadmill could increase the workload on a muscle without increasing exercise speed. The authors report that there was no skeletal muscle or cardiocirculatory training effect with four weeks of underwater treadmill training. It is to be noted, however, that the program followed was based on a set recommended by manufacturers for bowed tendon rehabilitation.

Water height can be raised and lowered in a underwater treadmill, however, it has been noted that there was no significant increase in heart rate with raising the level of the water from hoof or PIP height, to carpal or ulna height.[59] There was, however, an increased stride frequency and stride length recorded with the deeper water.

Swimming, the other form of water-based exercise popular in equine training and rehabilitation, requires the horse to be almost submerged, and is proposed to provide good cardiovascular conditioning as the horse has to work relatively hard to swim. In a report for the Australian Government Rural Industries Research and Development Corporation[61] it was concluded that horses in self-determined pace swimming gained no further cardiovascular changes than those achieved by standard on-land training programs. The authors suggest that programs directed at high intensity short sessions may have more benefits for improving fitness. Swimming, however, also provides an environment where there is less load on the musculoskeletal structures, compared to exercising on land, and therefore, may be useful for horses recovering from some musculoskeletal injuries. Swimming needs to be considered carefully for horses with neck or back pain, as they are required to hold their head high out of the water, therefore placing the thoracolumbar spine in extension.[53]

Therapeutic protocol

Both swimming and underwater treadmills provide exercise in environments that place less load on the musculoskeletal system than exercising on land. Therefore it makes sense that these modalities are good for the horse rehabilitating from musculoskeletal injury. Prescription of water treadmill for training effects in horses would seem unfounded, according to the literature.

It has been suggested that short-intensity swimming programs may have training effects. Therefore, horses involved in sports that place more demand on the cardiocirculatory system may benefit more from a swimming program along with the benefits of less stress on the limbs than on land. However, caution is required when considering swimming a horse with pain in the vertebral column.

Underwater treadmills provide a type of exercise that may be more beneficial to horses that are used for dressage and other sports that don't involve high speed. The gait assumed on a water treadmill is not dissimilar to the gait on land, so can be useful for providing exercise in rehabilitation without the concussive loads on the limbs that land exercise provides.[59]

References

1. Goff L. Manual therapy for the horse – a contemporary perspective. J Equine Vet Sci 2009;29:799–808.
2. Hearn A, Rivett D. Cervical SNAGS: a biomechanical analysis. Man Ther 2003;7:71–9.
3. Wright A. Hypoalgesia post manipulative therapy: a review of the potential neurophysiological mechanisms. Man Ther 1995;1:11–16.
4. Paungmali A, O'Leary S, Souvlis T, et al. Hypoalgesic and sympathoexcitatory effects of mobilization and movement for lateral epicondylalgia. Phys Ther 2003;83:374–83.
5. Perry I, Green A. An investigation into the effects of a unilaterally applied lumbar mobilization technique on peripheral sympathetic nervous system activity in the lower limbs. Man Ther 2008;13:192–9.
6. Paungmali A, O'Leary S, Souvlis T, et al. Naloxone fails to antagonize initial hypoalgesic effect of a manual therapy treatment for lateral epicondylalgia. J Manipulative Physiolog Ther 2004;27: 180–5.
7. Sluka K, Skyba D, Radhakrishnan R, et al. Joint mobilization reduces hyperalgesia associated with chronic muscle and joint inflammation in rats. J Pain 2006;7: 602–60.
8. Assendelft W, Morton S, Yu E, et al. Spinal manipulative therapy for low back pain. A metanalysis of the effectiveness relative to other therapies. Ann Intern Med 2003;138:871–81.
9. Rubenstein S, van Middelkoop M, Assendelft W, et al. Spinal manipulative therapy for chronic low-back pain: and update of a Cochrane review. Spine 2011;36:E825–46.
10. Ferreira M, Ferreira P, Latimer J, et al. Comparison of general exercise, motor control exercise and spinal manipulative therapy for chronic low back pain: a randomized trial. Pain 2007;131:31–7.
11. Bronfort G, Maiers M, Evans R, et al. Supervised exercise, spinal manipulation, and home exercise for chronic low back pain: a randomized clinical trial. Spine J 2011;11:585–98.
12. Gross A, Goldsmith C, Hoving J, et al. Conservative management of mechanical neck disorders: a systematic review. J Rheum 2007;34:1083–102.
13. Leaver A, Refshauge K, Maher C, et al. Conservative interventions provide short-term relief for non-specific neck pain: a systematic review. J Physio 2010; 5673–85.
14. Haussler K, Martin C, Hill, A. Efficacy of spinal manipulation and mobilisation on trunk flexibility and stiffness in horses: a randomized clinical trial. Equine Vet J 2010;42(Suppl.):S695–702.
15. Gomez-Alvarez C, L'Ami J, Moffatt D, et al. Effect of chiropractic manipulations on the kinematics of the back and limbs in horses clinically diagnosed back problems. Equine Vet J 2008;40:153–9.
16. Jansen M, Viechtbauer W, Lenssen A, et al. Strength training alone, exercise therapy alone, and exercise therapy with passive manual mobilisation each reduce pain and disability in people with knee osteoarthritis: a systematic review. J Physiother. 2011;57:11–20.
17. Jeffcott L, Dalin G, Ekman S, et al. Sacroiliac lesions as a cause of chronic poor performance in competitive horses. Equine Vet J 1985;17:111–18.
18. Haussler K. Review of manual therapy techniques in equine practice. J Equine Vet Sci 2009;29:849–69.
19. Goff L, Jull G. Manual therapy, Chapter 9. In: McGowan C, Goff L, Stubbs N, editors. Animal physiotherapy – assessment treatment and rehabilitation of animals. Oxford: Blackwell; 2007. p. 164–76.
20. Dyson S, Murray R. Pain associated with the sacroiliac joint region: a clinical study of 74 horses. Equine Vet J 2003;35:240–5.
21. Weerapong P, Hume P, Kolt G. The mechanisms of massage and effects on performance, muscle recovery and injury prevention. Sports Med. 2005;35: 235–56.
22. Brummit J. The role of massage in sports performance and rehabilitation: current evidence and future direction. N Am J Sports Phys Ther 2008;3:7–21.
23. Furlan A, Imamura M, Dryden T, et al. Massage for low-back pain. Cochrane Database Syst Rev 2008;8:CD001929.
24. Cherkin D, Sherman K, Kahn J, et al. A comparison of the effects of 2 types of massage and usual care on chronic low back pain: a randomized controlled trial. Ann Intern Med 2011;155:1–9.
25. Best T, Hunter R, Wilcox A, et al. Effectiveness of sports massage for recovery of skeletal muscle from strenuous exercise. Clin J Sport Med 2008;18:446–60.
26. Hill C, Crook T. The relationship between massage to the equine caudal hindlimb muscles and hindlimb protraction. Equine Vet J 2010;42(suppl): 683–7.
27. Joseph M, Taft K, Moscwa M, et al. Deep friction massage for the treatment of tendinopathy: a systematic review of a classic treatment in the face of a new paradigm of understanding. J Sport Rehabil 2011; 2011 Dec 30. [Epub ahead of print].
28. Weir D, Tingley J, Elder G. Acute passive stretching alters the mechanical properties of human plantar flexors and the optimal angle for maximal voluntary contraction. Eur J Appl Physiol 2005;93: 614–23.
29. Taylor K, Sheppard J, Lee H, et al. Negative effect of static stretching restored when combined with sport specific warm-up component. J Sci Med Sport 2009;12:657–61.
30. O'Hora J, Cartwright A, Wade C, et al. Efficacy of static stretching and proprioceptive neuromuscular facilitation stretch on hamstrings length after a single session. J Strength Cond Res 2011;25:1586–91.
31. Herbert R, de Noronha M, Kamper S. Stretching to prevent or reduce muscle soreness after exercise. Cochrane Database Syst Rev 2011;6:CD004577.
32. Verrall G, Schofield S, Brustad T. Chronic achilles tendinopathy treated with eccentric stretching program. Foot Ankle Int 2011;32:843–9.
33. Rose N, Northrop A, Brigden C, et al. Effects of a stretching regime on stride length and range of motion in equine trot. Vet J 2009;161:53–5.
34. Kubo K, Kanehisa H, Kawakami Y, et al. The influence of static stretching on viscoelastic properties of human tendon structures in vivo. J Appl Physiol 2001; 90:520–7.

35. Mahieu N, McNair P, De Muynck M, et al. Effect of static and ballistic stretching on the muscle-tendon tissue properties. Med Sci Sports Exerc 2007; 39:494–501.
36. Witvrouw E, Mahieu N, Danneels L, et al. Stretching and injury prevention: an obscure relationship. Sports Med 2004; 34:443–9.
37. Sullivan K, Hill A, Haussler K. The effects of chiropractic, massage and phenylbutazone on spinal mechanical nociceptive thresholds in horses without clinical signs. Equine Vet J 2008;40: 14–20.
38. Varcoe-Cocks K, Sagar K, Jeffcott L, et al. Pressure algometry to quantify muscle pain in racehorses with suspected sacroiliac dysfunction. http://www.ncbi.nlm.nih.gov/pubmed?term=varcoe-cocks Equine Vet J 2006;38:558–62.
39. Persson A, Brogardh C, Sjolund B. Tender or not tender: test-retest repeatability of pressure pain thersholds in the trapezius and deltoid muscles of healthy women. J Rehabil Med 2004;36:17–27.
40. Haussler K, Erb H. Mechanical nociceptive thresholds in the axial skeleton of horses. Equine Vet J 2006; 38:70–5.
41. Jaegger G, Marcellin-Little D, Levine D. Reliability of goniometry in labrador retrievers. Am J Vet Res 2002;63:979–86.
42. Liljebrink Y, Bergh A. Goniometry: is it a reliable tool to monitor passive joint range of motion in horses? Equine Vet J 2010;42(Suppl.):S676–82.
43. Bennell K, Talbot R, Wajswelner H, et al. Intra-rater and inter-rater reliability of a weight-bearing lunge measure of ankle dorsiflexion. Aust J Phys 1998;44: 175–80.
44. Hides J, Jull G, Richardson C. Long-term effects of specific stabilizing exercises for first-episode low back pain. Spine 2001; 26:E243–8.
45. Stubbs N, Riggs C, Clayton H, et al. Osseous spinal pathology and epaxial muscle ultrasonography in Thoroughbred racehorses. Equine Vet J 2010;42(Suppl.): S645–61.
46. Pickersgill C, Marr C, Reid S. Repeatability of diagnostic ultrasonography in the assessment of the equine superficial digital flexor tendon. Equine Vet J 2001;33:33–7.
47. Wyndow N, Cowan S, Wrigley T, et al. Neuromotor control of the lower limb in Achilles tendinopathy: implications for foot orthotic therapy. Sports Med 2010; 40:715–27.
48. Lam T, Anderschitz M, Dietz V. Contributions of feedback and feedforward strategies to locomotor adaptations. J Neurophysiol 2006;95: 766–73.
49. Stubbs N, Riggs C, Clayton H, et al. Osseous spinal pathology and epaxial muscle ultrasonography in Thoroughbred racehorses. Equine Vet J 2010;42(Suppl.): S654–66.
50. Stubbs N, Kaiser L, Hauptman J, et al. Dynamic mobilisation exercises increase cross sectional area of musculus multifidus. Equine Vet J 2011;43:522–9.
51. Hodges P, Hoorn W, Dawson A, et al. Changes in the mechanical properties of he trunk in low back pain may be associated with recurrence. J Biomech 2009;42:61–6.
52. Indahl A, Kaigle A, Reikeras O, et al. Sacroiliac joint involvement in activation of porcine spinal and gluteal musculature. J Spinal Disord 1999;12:325–30.
53. Paukelas R, Haussler K. Principles and practice of therapeutic exercise for horses. J Equine Vet Sci 2009;29:870–93.
54. Lim E, Tan M. Side-to-side difference in joint position sense and kinaesthesia in unilateral functional ankle instability. Foot Ankle Int. 2009;30:1011–17.
55. Goff L, Jasiewicz J, Jeffcott L, et al. Movement between the equine ilium and sacrum – in vivo and in vitro studies. Equine Vet J (Suppl.) 2006;36: 457–61.
56. Cowan S, Bennell K, Hodges P. Therapeutic patellar taping changes the timing of vasti muscle activation in people with patellofemoral pain syndrome. Clin J Sports Med 2002;12: 339–47.
57. Clayton H, White A, Kaiser L, et al. Himdlimb response to tactile stimulation of the pastern and coronet. Equine Vet J 2010;42:227–33.
58. Clayton H, Lavagnino M, Kaiser L, et al. Swing phase kinematic and kinetic response to weighting the hind pasterns. Equine Vet J 2011;43:210–15.
59. Scott R, Nankervis K, Stringer C, et al. The effect of water height on stride frequency, stride length and heart rate during water treadmill exercise. Equine Vet J 2010;42(Suppl.):S662–4.
60. Borgia L, Valberg S, Essen-Gustavsson B. Differences in the metabolic properties of gluteus medius and superficial digital flexor muscles and the effect of water treadmill training in the horse. Equine Vet J 2010;42(Suppl.):S665–70.
61. Davie A, Savage C, Fennell L. The effect of swimming training on the cardiac dimensions in Thoroughbred horses. RIRDC; 2008; publication no 08/156; PRJ 000842.

Equine rehabilitation: chiropractic treatment for athletic horses

63

Kevin K. Haussler

CHAPTER CONTENTS

Chiropractic treatment

Background

Chiropractic treatment is a form of manual therapy that is characterized by the use of high-velocity, low-amplitude thrusts typically applied to regions of stiffness, pain or muscle hypertonicity within the axial skeleton.[1] In humans, chiropractic care has primarily demonstrated clinical efficacy in treating acute and chronic neck and back pain.[2–4] Due to human applications and perceived therapeutic efficacy in treating musculoskeletal issues, chiropractic techniques have subsequently been applied to horses.[5] Equine chiropractic techniques within the United States were primarily developed and taught by Dr. Sharon Willoughby beginning in 1985. Since then, numerous veterinary chiropractic certification programs have been established worldwide. Currently, chiropractic evaluation and treatment techniques have been applied to sport horses for issues mostly related to poor performance and overt signs of back pain.[6,7]

Mechanism of action

The goal of chiropractic treatment is to restore normal joint motion, stimulate neurologic reflexes, and to reduce pain and muscle hypertonicity.[5] Multiple theories have been proposed and tested over the years to explain the pathophysiology of vertebral segment dysfunction and its interactions and influences on the neuromusculoskeletal system.[8,9] Chiropractic treatment is thought to affect mechanoreceptors (i.e., Golgi tendon organ and muscle spindles) to induce reflex inhibition of pain, reflex muscle relaxation, and to correct abnormal movement patterns.[10,11] The literature suggests that any stimulus that activates high-threshold receptors within the periarticular tissues has the potential to initiate unique neurologic reflexes associated with joint manipulation.[12] Alterations in articular neurophysiology from mechanical or chemical injuries can affect both mechanoreceptor and nociceptor function via increased joint capsule tension and nerve ending hypersensitivity.[13] Mechanoreceptor stimulation induces reflex paraspinal musculature hypertonicity and altered local and systemic neurologic reflexes. Nociceptor stimulation results in a lowered pain threshold, sustained afferent stimulation (i.e., facilitation), reflex paraspinal musculature hypertonicity, and abnormal neurologic reflexes.

It is likely that specific manual therapy techniques are inherently more effective than others in addressing each of these local, regional or systemic components.[14] The challenge is in choosing the most appropriate form of manual therapy or combination of techniques that will be efficacious for an individual patient with specific musculoskeletal disabilities. If soft tissue restriction and pain are identified as the primary components of a musculoskeletal injury, then massage, stretching and soft tissue mobilization techniques are indicated for increasing tissue extensibility.[15,16] However, if the musculoskeletal dysfunction is localized to articular structures, then stretching, joint mobilization and manipulation are the most indicated manual therapy techniques for restoring joint range of motion and reducing pain.[17,18]

Palpatory changes in osseous symmetry after manipulation often are associated with soft tissue alterations and not due to actual reductions of an articular misalignment or a 'bone out of place'.[19] The static position of the vertebral or sacroiliac joints in humans has been studied pre and post-manipulation by roentgen stereophotogrammetric analysis, which allows precise measurements of three-dimensional articular movement.[20] Static palpation changes have been noted pre and post-manipulation, however no changes have been reported with the roentgen stereophotogrammetric analysis. Therefore, soft tissue responses such as joint capsules, muscles, ligaments, tendons and postural neuromuscular reflex patterns should be the focus of future spinal manipulative studies and not articular malpositioning (i.e., bone out of place).[20]

Indications

Back pain is a common cause of poor performance in sport horses (see Chapter 21). Unfortunately, medical and surgical treatment options are often limited for affected horses. Manual therapy has the potential to provide important diagnostic and therapeutic approaches for addressing equine axial skeleton problems that are not currently available in veterinary medicine. Most of the current knowledge about equine manual therapies has been borrowed from human techniques, theories, and research and applied to horses. Therapeutic trials of joint mobilization or manipulation are often used because of limited knowledge about the effects of manual therapy in horses. The indications for joint mobilization and manipulation are similar and include restricted joint range of motion, muscle spasms, pain, fibrosis, or contracted soft tissues.[21] The principal indications for spinal manipulation are neck or back pain, localized or regional joint stiffness, poor performance, and altered gait that is not associated with overt lameness. Anecdotal evidence and clinical experience suggest that chiropractic is an effective adjunctive modality for the diagnosis and conservative treatment of select musculoskeletal-related disorders in performance horses. However, therapeutic trials of chiropractic manipulations are often used since we currently have limited formal research available about the effectiveness of chiropractic procedures in equine practice.

A thorough diagnostic workup is required to identify soft tissue and osseous pathology, neurologic disorders, or other lameness conditions that may not be responsive to manual therapy. Clinical signs indicative of a primary spinal disorder include localized musculoskeletal pain, muscle hypertonicity and restricted joint motion. This triad of clinical signs can also be found in a variety of lower limb disorders; however, they are most evident in horses with neck or back problems. Clinical signs indicative of chronic or secondary spinal disorders include regional or diffuse pain, generalized stiffness, and widespread muscle hypertonicity. In these cases, further diagnostic evaluation or imaging should be done to identify the primary cause of lameness or poor performance. Chiropractic treatment may help in the management of muscular, articular and neurologic components of select musculoskeletal injuries in performance horses. Musculoskeletal conditions that are chronic or recurring, not readily diagnosed, or are not responding to conventional veterinary care may be indicators that manual therapy evaluation and treatment is needed. Chiropractic treatment is usually more effective in the early clinical stages of disease processes versus end-stage disease where reparative processes have been exhausted. Joint manipulation is usually contraindicated in the acute stages of soft tissue injury; however, mobilization is safer than manipulation and has been shown to have short-term benefits for acute neck or back pain in humans.[22] Manipulation is probably more effective than mobilization for chronic neck or back pain and has the potential to help restore normal joint motion, thus limiting the risk of reinjury.[19]

Contraindications

Chiropractic treatment is not a 'cure all' for all joint or back problems and is generally contraindicated in the presence of fractures, acute inflammatory or infectious joint disease, osteomyelitis, joint ankylosis, bleeding disorders, progressive neurological signs, and primary or metastatic tumors.[21] Contraindications are often based on clinical judgment and are related to the technique applied and skill or experience of the practitioner.[21] Acute episodes of osteoarthritis, impinged dorsal spinous processes, and severe articular instability are often contraindications for manipulation. Inadequate physical or spinal examination and poorly developed manipulative skills are also contraindications for applying manual therapy.[23] All horses with neurologic diseases should be evaluated fully to assess the potential risks or benefits of joint mobilization or manipulation. Cervical vertebral myelopathy occurs because of both structural and functional disorders.[24] Static compression caused by vertebral malformation and dynamic lesions caused by vertebral segment hypermobility are contraindications for cervical manipulation; however, adjacent regions of hypomobile vertebrae may benefit from mobilization or manipulation to help restore joint motion and reduce biomechanical stresses in the affected vertebral segments. Serious diseases requiring immediate medical or surgical care need to be ruled out and treated by conventional veterinary medicine before any routine manual therapy is initiated, although manual techniques may contribute to the rehabilitation of most post-surgical cases or severe musculoskeletal injuries by helping to restore normal joint motion and function. Horses that have concurrent hock pain (e.g., osteoarthritis) and a stiff, painful thoracolumbar or lumbosacral vertebral region are best managed by addressing all areas of musculoskeletal dysfunction. A multidisciplinary approach entails combined medical treatment of the hock osteoarthritis and manual therapy evaluation and treatment of the back problem.

In humans, most adverse events associated with spinal manipulation are benign and self-limiting.[25] Mild adverse effects include transient stiffness or worsening of the condition that usually last less than one to two days and resolve without concurrent medical intervention. Severe complications following spinal manipulation are typically uncommon. Estimates of the incidence range from one in 200 000 to one per 100 million manipulations in humans.[22,26,27] The most common serious adverse events in humans are vertebrobasilar accidents, disk herniation and cauda equina syndrome.[28] Even though the complication rate of spinal manipulation is small, the potential for adverse outcomes must be considered because of the possibility of permanent impairment or death.[22] The benefits of chiropractic care in humans seem to outweigh the potential risks.[29] The risk of adverse effects associated with joint mobilization or spinal manipulation is unknown in horses. The apparent safety of spinal manipulation, especially when compared with other medically-accepted treatments for neck or low back pain in humans, should stimulate its use in the conservative treatment of spinal-related problems.[27,30] If an exacerbation of musculoskeletal dysfunction or lameness is noted after spinal manipulation, then a thorough re-examination and appropriate medical treatment should be pursued. If the condition does not improve with conservative care, referral for more extensive diagnostic evaluation or more aggressive medical treatment is recommended.

Therapeutic protocol

A thorough physical examination, coupled with orthopedic and neurologic evaluation, is used to identify common causes of lameness or neurological disorders. A detailed spinal examination helps to identify compensatory or concurrent musculoskeletal issues not readily diagnosed or treated with traditional medical or surgical approaches. The spinal evaluation focuses on evaluating and localizing segmental vertebral dysfunction, which is characterized by localized pain, muscle hypertonicity, and reduced joint motion. The challenge, as with any musculoskeletal injury, is to identify the specific musculoskeletal structures affected and quantify the associated disability or altered function present.

Manual palpation is used to localize and identify soft tissue and osseous structures for changes in texture, tissue mobility, or resistance to pressure.[31,32] The horse's response to being approached and its anticipation of palpation is often used as a behavioral indication of potential back pain or hypersensitivity. Soft tissue layers are evaluated from superficial to deep by increasing digital pressure and by focusing attention to specific tissues or structures with discrete palpatory movements. Shapes of structures, transitions between structures, and attachment sites are also palpated.[19] Soft tissue texture and mobility can be compared between the skin, subcutaneous tissue, thoracolumbar fascia, and muscle; similar to layers of an onion. Assessing patient response to palpation is especially important in evaluating tenderness or hypersensitivity.

The skin and subcutaneous tissues are gently mobilized by a firm, broad manual contact. Chronic scar tissue, adhesions, and fibrosis may produce pain or mechanical restrictions if affected tissues are restrained during locomotion or trunk movements. The superficial fascia is assessed for smoothness and uniform tonicity or compliance. The superficial fascia typically forms an external covering over muscles, whereas the deep fascia forms folds of connective tissue between muscle bellies and attaches to deeper osseous structures. The dense connective tissue that forms the deep fascia is systematically evaluated for masses, rents, scar tissue, and tonicity. Severe or deep trauma to the myofascial tissues (e.g., kicks, deep lacerations, abscesses, or hematomas) can produce residual fibrosis that limits adjacent muscular movements and fascial extensibility. The thoracolumbar fascia is the most prominent fascia of the trunk and is particularly evident at the thoracolumbar junction as it blends medially with the supraspinous ligament. In the lumbar region, the caudal aponeurotic portion of the thoracolumbar fascia attaches to the cranial aspect of the tuber sacrale and iliac wing, deep to the overlying middle gluteal muscle. The tendon of the thoracolumbar fascia is palpable cranial and medial to the tubera sacralia as it inserts on the second sacral spinous process in conjunction with the dorsal sacroiliac ligament.[33]

Muscle tone is an indirect measure of muscle activity or contraction. Muscle hypertonicity is the most commonly palpable abnormality in horses with acute or chronic back problems and can have either neural or myopathic origins.[34] Muscle hypertonicity may affect a small portion of a muscle (i.e., trigger point), an entire muscle belly, or a regional group of muscles. In general, localized muscle hypertonicity is considered indicative of an acute or primary back problem; whereas, regional or generalized longissimus muscle hypertonicity is often associated with chronic pelvic limb lameness or systemic disease.[34] Muscle fasciculations are usually indicative of profound muscle weakness, electrolyte imbalance or primary muscle pathology. However, muscles may also fasciculate at characteristic locations distant to an area of palpation, which is indicative of referred pain in humans. Referred pain is difficult to truly assess in horses due to the lack of verbal feedback.[35] Muscle spasms are characterized as an acute, severe form of muscle hypertonicity, with substantial pain, spasticity and loss of muscle function.

Osseous palpation involves evaluating bony structures for pain, morphology, asymmetries, and alignment. Individual cervical transverse processes, articular processes and thoracolumbar and sacral spinous processes are palpated for a painful response to firm digital pressure.[36] Typical signs of discomfort include avoidance reactions such as rapid elevation of the head, extension of the back, withers away from the applied pressure, or localized secondary muscle spasms indicative of local injury or impinged spinous processes. Paired bony pelvis prominences are palpated for dorsoventral and craniocaudal asymmetries and pain response to manual compression. Small amplitudes of unilateral or bilateral prominence of the tuber sacrale is common and is not considered clinically significant unless associated with clinical signs of localized pain or inflammation or positive findings on diagnostic imaging (e.g., scintigraphy). The apex of the second sacral spinous process is a reliable landmark used to evaluate relative dorsal or ventral tuber sacrale displacement. Fractures of tuber coxae typically produce palpable bony asymmetries and ventral displacement of fracture fragments, which are readily diagnosed on oblique radiographs of the pelvis.[37] The tail and caudal vertebrae are evaluated for tone, fractures and osseous deviations.

A complete musculoskeletal examination includes assessment of active and passive joint ranges of motion for all axial and appendicular articulations of interest. Active joint range of motion of the axial skeleton is evaluated during normal daily activities (e.g., lying to standing movements or locomotion) or during induced vertebral movements while using a carrot or other treat to produce active movements of the head, neck or trunk. Similar procedures can be used therapeutically as active stretching exercises to increase neck or trunk range of motion or for developing coordination and strength of the muscles responsible for trunk stabilization.[38] Normal vertebral movements consist of varying amounts and combinations of flexion, extension, left and right lateral bending, and left and right axial rotation. Abnormal active joint motion is characterized by weakness, incoordination, asymmetry, restricted, or excessive joint movements. The willingness, coordination and amount of vertebral segment motion are compared bilaterally and left-to-right range of motion asymmetries is documented. Local or regional causes of active vertebral movement restrictions or altered movement may include peripheral or central neuropathies, myopathies, intra-articular pathology (i.e., osteoarthritis), periarticular soft tissue adhesions, musculotendinous contractures, or protective muscle spasms.

Passive joint range of motion is evaluated by measuring the amount and characteristics of joint motion beyond the active range of joint motion. Assessing passive range of motion requires patient cooperation and muscular relaxation as each articulation is moved passively throughout its unique ranges and directions of motion. The goal of palpating joint movement is to evaluate the quality of joint motion, the initiation of resistance to motion and joint end feel, and the amplitude of joint motion present. Similar palpatory findings can be identified in soft tissues, such as skin, connective tissue, muscles or ligaments.[32] Passive joint range of motion is evaluated to detect whether a particular movement is normal, restricted or hypermobile. Passive joint mobility can be assessed either segmentally via palpation of individual vertebral motion segments or limb articulations or evaluated regionally via passive mobilization of vertebral regions or entire limbs. Causes of restricted articular movement include soft tissue (e.g., capsular fibrosis, muscle spasms or contractures) and osseous pathologies (e.g., malformations, osteoarthritis or ankylosis). Restricted vertebral segment motion can occur with or without localized muscle hypertonicity or pain.

Evaluation of passive joint range of motion within the axial skeleton begins at the head and continues to the tip of the tail. The occipitoatlantal (Occ-C1) articulation is evaluated in full ranges of flexion, extension and lateral bending for signs of pain or resisted motion. The atlantoaxial (C1-C2) articulation evaluated for altered or asymmetrical ranges of axial rotation. The intervertebral articulations of the second to seventh cervical vertebrae (C2-C7) are assessed individually for altered joint range of motion and joint end feel during combined lateral bending and rotation. Articulations of the mid-cervical region (C4-C6) are commonly restricted and painful in performance horses, presumably because of locally altered biomechanical influences. The individual spinous processes of the third to twelfth thoracic vertebrae (T3-T12) are manually deviated from midline, while monitoring for signs of reduced vertebral motion, localized or generalized pain response, and induced muscle hypertonicity. Horses with poorly fitting saddles (i.e., tree is too narrow) resent palpation and passive motion of the affected cranial thoracic vertebrae. The remaining thoracolumbar region (T13-L6) is evaluated in lateral bending and flexion and extension for similar signs of spinal dysfunction. Normal lateral bending range of motion is maximal at the mid-thoracic region and gradually diminishes toward the lumbosacral junction.[39] Conversely, flexion and extension are minimal within the thoracic region and gradually increase toward the lumbosacral junction, which is the site of maximal flexion and extension range of motion. Evaluation of segmental vertebral motion in flexion and extension requires the clinician to be on an elevated surface to induce ventrally-directed rhythmic oscillations over the individual thoracolumbar intervertebral articulations. Horses with impinged dorsal spinous processes strongly resent any induced extension of the affected vertebral segments. The pelvis and sacroiliac joints are evaluated for motion restrictions and pain during induced joint motion with directed ventrally forces applied over the tuber coxae or during abaxial compression of the tubera sacralia.

Outcome measures

Clinical signs indicative of a primary spinal disorder include localized musculoskeletal pain, muscle hypertonicity and restricted joint motion.[1] Therefore, outcome measures are often directed toward measuring these clinical signs or general performance or lameness parameters. Comparisons of the quality and quantity of passive range of motion, pain and muscle tone are evaluated pre- and post-treatment to assess potential therapeutic responses within vertebral motion segments.[40] Pilot work has demonstrated that manually-applied forces associated with chiropractic techniques are able to produced substantial segmental spinal motion.[41] Two randomized, controlled clinical trials using pressure algometry to assess mechanical nociceptive thresholds (MNTs) in the thoracolumbar region of horses have demonstrated that both manual and instrument-assisted spinal manipulation can reduce back pain (or increase MNTs).[36,42] Additional studies have assessed the effects of equine chiropractic techniques on increasing passive spinal mobility (i.e., flexibility) and reducing longissimus muscle tone.[43,44] The effect of manipulation on asymmetrical spinal movement patterns in horses with documented back pain suggest that chiropractic treatment elicits slight but significant changes in thoracolumbar and pelvic kinematics and that some of these changes are likely to be beneficial.[45,46]

Further research is needed to assess the effectiveness of specific chiropractic techniques or combined treatments for pain management and select lameness conditions. Currently there is no validated equine model for studying the effects of manual therapies which would allow characterization of the anatomic, biomechanical, neurophysiologic, pathophysiologic, cellular, or biochemical changes associated with soft tissue and joint mobilization or high-velocity thrusts.[12,18] Further understanding of the local and systemic effects of mobilization and manipulation on pain reduction and tissue healing is also needed. Additional studies are needed to determine the duration of the clinical effects of chiropractic treatment. Controlled trials using different forms of spinal manipulation (e.g., manual thrusts versus instrument-assisted thrusts versus manipulation under anesthesia) need to be done to determine which method is most effective for addressing specific disease processes. Studies are also needed to identify which specific clinical measures of back pain or performance are likely to benefit from the various forms of manual therapy, either individually or in combination. New methods of objectively measuring musculoskeletal dysfunction and further studies into the pathophysiology of chronic pain syndromes are needed to help assess the effectiveness of manual therapies on reducing morbidity and improving overall performance in equine athletes.

References

1. Haussler KK. Review of manual therapy techniques in equine practice. J Equine Vet Sci 2009;29:849–69.
2. Walker BF, French SD, Grant W, et al. A Cochrane review of combined chiropractic interventions for low-back pain. Spine (Phila Pa 1976) 2011;36:230–42.
3. Bronfort G, Haas M, Evans R, et al. Effectiveness of manual therapies: the UK evidence report. Chiropr Osteopat 2010;18:3.
4. Globe GA, Morris CE, Whalen WM, et al. Chiropractic management of low back disorders: report from a consensus process. J Manipulative Physiol Ther 2008;31:651–8.
5. Haussler KK. Chiropractic evaluation and management. Vet Clin North Am Equine Pract 1999;15:195–209.
6. Haussler KK. Current status of integrative medicine techniques used in equine practice. J Equine Vet Sci 2009;29:639–41.
7. Haussler KK. The role of manual therapies in equine pain management. Veterinary Clinics of North America: Equine Practice 2010;26:579–601.
8. Leach RA. Soft outcome measures of dysfunction. The chiropractic theories: Principles and clinical applications. 3rd ed. Baltimore, MD: Williams & Wilkins; 1994. p. 55–71.
9. Haldeman S. The evolution and importance of spinal and chiropractic research. J Manipulative Physiol Ther 1992;15:31–5.
10. Gatterman MI. Foundations of chiropractic. St. Louis: Mosby-Year Book, Inc.; 1995.
11. Cassidy JD, Lopes AA, Yong-Hing K. The immediate effect of manipulation versus mobilization on pain and range of motion in the cervical spine: a randomized controlled trial. J Manipulative Physiol Ther 1992;15:570–5.
12. Pickar JG, Bolton PS. Spinal manipulative therapy and somatosensory activation. J Electromyogr Kinesiol 2012.
13. Cameron MH. Physical agents in rehabilitation. Philadelphia: W.B. Saunders Company; 1999.
14. Triano J. The theoretical basis for spinal manipulation In: Haldeman S, editor. Principles and practice of chiropractic. 3rd ed. New York: McGraw-Hill; 2005. p. 361–81.
15. Lederman E. The biomechanical response. Fundamentals of manual therapy: physiology, neurology and psychology. St. Louis: Churchill Livingstone; 1997. p. 23–37.
16. Liptan GL. Fascia: A missing link in our understanding of the pathology of fibromyalgia. J Bodyw Mov Ther 2010;14:3–12.
17. Bronfort G, Haas M, Evans RL, et al. Efficacy of spinal manipulation and mobilization for low back pain and neck pain: a systematic review and best evidence synthesis. Spine J 2004;4:335–56.
18. Simmonds N, Miller P, Gemmell H. A theoretical framework for the role of fascia in manual therapy. J Bodyw Mov Ther 2012;16:83–93.
19. Liebenson C. Rehabilitation of the spine. 1st ed. Baltimore, MD: Williams & Wilkins; 1996.
20. Tullberg T, Blomberg S, Branth B, et al. Manipulation does not alter the position of the sacroiliac joint. Spine 1998;23:1124–9.
21. Scaringe J, Kawaoka C. Mobilization techniques In: Haldeman S, editor. Principles and practice of chiropractic. 3rd ed. New York: McGraw-Hill; 2005. p. 767–85.
22. Hurwitz EL, Aker PD, Adams AH, et al. Manipulation and mobilization of the cervical spine. A systematic review of the literature. Spine (Phila Pa 1976) 1996;21:1746–59; discussion 1759–60.
23. West DT, Mathews RS, Miller MR, et al. Effective management of spinal pain in one hundred seventy-seven patients evaluated for manipulation under anesthesia. J Manipulative Physiol Ther 1999;22:299–308.
24. Levine JM, Adam E, MacKay RJ, et al. Confirmed and presumptive cervical vertebral compressive myelopathy in older horses: a retrospective study

(1992–2004). J Vet Intern Med 2007; 21:812–19.

25. Rubinstein SM. Adverse events following chiropractic care for subjects with neck or low-back pain: do the benefits outweigh the risks? J Manipulative Physiol Ther 2008;31:461–4.
26. Thiel HW, Bolton JE, Docherty S, et al. Safety of chiropractic manipulation of the cervical spine: a prospective national survey. Spine 2007;32:2375–8; discussion 2379.
27. Oliphant D. Safety of spinal manipulation in the treatment of lumbar disk herniations: a systematic review and risk assessment. J Manipulative Physiol Ther 2004;27:197–210.
28. Stevinson C, Ernst E. Risks associated with spinal manipulation. Am J Med 2002;112:566–71.
29. Rubinstein SM, Leboeuf-Yde C, Knol DL, et al. The benefits outweigh the risks for patients undergoing chiropractic care for neck pain: a prospective, multicenter, cohort study. J Manipulative Physiol Ther 2007;30:408–18.
30. Dabbs V, Lauretti WJ. A risk assessment of cervical manipulation vs. NSAIDs for the treatment of neck pain. J Manipulative Physiol Ther 1995;18: 530–6.
31. Cauvin E. Assessment of back pain in horses. In Practice 1997;19:522–33.
32. Chaitow L. Palpation skills. New York, NY: Churchill Livingston; 1997.
33. Engeli E, Yeager AE, Erb HN, et al. Ultrasonographic technique and normal anatomic features of the sacroiliac region in horses. Vet Radiol Ultrasound 2006; 47:391–403.
34. Valberg SJ, Hodgson DR. Diseases of muscle. In: Smith BP, editor. Large Animal Internal Medicine. 3rd ed. St. Louis, MO: Mosby, Inc.; 2002. p. 1266–91.
35. Martin BB Jr, Klide AM. Physical examination of horses with back pain. Vet Clin North Am Equine Pract 1999;15:61–70.
36. Haussler KK, Erb HN. Pressure algometry: Objective assessment of back pain and effects of chiropractic treatment. Proc Amer Assoc Equine Practitioners 2003;49:66–70.
37. Dabareiner RM, Cole RC. Fractures of the tuber coxa of the ilium in horses: 29 cases (1996–2007). J Am Vet Med Assoc 2009;234:1303–7.
38. Stubbs NC, Clayton HM. Activate your horse's core: unmounted exercises for dynamic mobility, strength and balance. Mason, MI: Sport Horse Publications; 2008.
39. Townsend HG, Leach DH, Fretz PB. Kinematics of the equine thoracolumbar spine. Equine Veterinary Journal 1983;15:117–22.
40. Haussler KK. Equine chiropractic: general principles and clinical applications. Proc Amer Assoc Equine Practitioners 2000;46:84–93.
41. Haussler KK, Bertram JEA, Gellman K. In-vivo segmental kinematics of the thoracolumbar spinal region in horses and effects of chiropractic manipulations. Proc Amer Assoc Equine Practitioners 1999;45:327–9.
42. Sullivan KA, Hill AE, Haussler KK. The effects of chiropractic, massage and phenylbutazone on spinal mechanical nociceptive thresholds in horses without clinical signs. Equine Veterinary Journal 2008;40:14–20.
43. Haussler KK, Hill AE, Puttlitz CM, et al. Effects of vertebral mobilization and manipulation on kinematics of the thoracolumbar region. Amer J Vet Research 2007;68:508–16.
44. Wakeling JM, Barnett K, Price S, et al. Effects of manipulative therapy on the longissimus dorsi in the equine back. Equine and Comparative Exercise Physiology 2006;3:153–60.
45. Faber MJ, van Weeren PR, Schepers M, et al. Long-term follow-up of manipulative treatment in a horse with back problems. J Vet Med A Physiol Pathol Clin Med 2003;50:241–5.
46. Gómez Alvarez CB, L'Ami JJ, Moffat D, et al. Effect of chiropractic manipulations on the kinematics of back and limbs in horses with clinically diagnosed back problems. Equine Veterinary Journal 2008;40:153–9.

Physical treatment of the equine athlete

64

Anna Bergh

CHAPTER CONTENTS

Introduction

Sports medicine is a highly important area in the equine world, not only for elite sport horses, but also for the average horse in training. It includes different types of physical modalities for the treatment of musculoskeletal disorders. In this chapter, techniques such as thermotherapy, therapeutic ultrasound, extracorporeal shock wave therapy, electrical stimulation, laser therapy and magnetic field therapy will be described.

The techniques are described by providing background information, indications and contraindications, mechanism of action, a general description of treatment protocols, and finally a short overview of the outcome measures documented in the literature. There are very few validated treatment protocols for horses. Therefore, additional focus has been made to describe the mechanism of action. Techniques that lack clinical documentation might still be regarded as promising if there is a well-documented mechanism of action. The following information is mainly based on equine practice, but if there was a lack of scientific documentation regarding horses, examples are given from studies of other species. Therefore the text includes both case studies in horses and meta-analyzes in humans, studies that obviously do not have the same scientific nor clinical significance, but can be valuable to read.

Many therapies are claimed to stimulate the regeneration process, often by a reduction of inflammation and swelling, an increase in blood circulation and alleviation of pain. Depending on the aim of the treatment and its specific target tissue, its efficacy may be measured with a variety of assessment tools, often with higher intra-rater reliability than inter-rater reliability. For example, pain perception can be assessed with palpation[1], pain scales and questionnaires[2], muscle tenderness (mechanical nociceptive threshold) with an algometer[3,4], the degree of swelling and muscle bulk can be measured with diagnostic ultrasound, but also with simpler tools like measuring tape and calipers. The joint range of motion may be assessed with goniometer (Fig. 64.1).[5] Lameness can be evaluated by ordinary clinical lameness examination, but also with different forms of motion analyzes such as force plates, pressure mats, and high-velocity filming.[6]

Thermotherapy

Cryotherapy

Background

In sports medicine, cryotherapy is defined as the local use of cold to decrease tissue temperature, in order to prevent tissue damage and reduce pain, and in the end, hasten the recovery of the patient to resume normal functions.

Cryotherapy can be applied as ice packs (commercial ice/gel packs or self-made packages of ice/frozen vegetables), cold spray, ice massage, and cold water/ice immersion. Lately, the use of cold water immersion post-surgically has increased, in order to prevent an inflammatory reaction and formation of edema.

Indications and contraindications

Cryotherapy is used in acute soft tissue injuries to decrease blood supply, diminish rate of swelling, minimize production of irritants

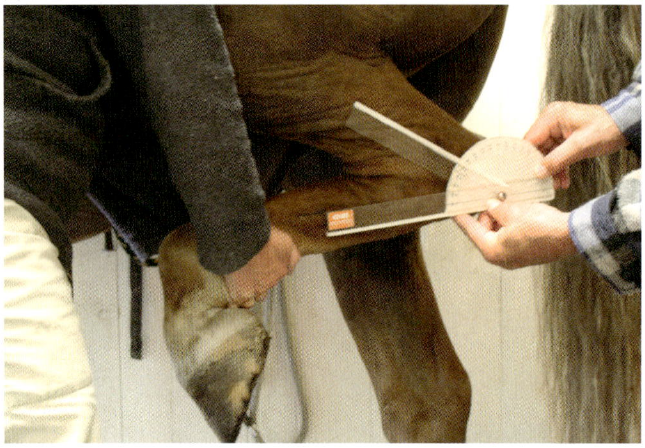

Fig 64.1 Goniometer used to measure tarsal joint range of motion. *Courtesy of Y. Liljebrink.*

and secondary cell necrosis, lessen inflammatory reaction, reduce muscle tension, and alleviate pain.[7,8]

Cryotherapy is also used in chronic injuries, such as soft tissue injuries and joint diseases, to alleviate pain, reduce muscle tension and decrease joint effusion and soft tissue swelling. Further, it is used to prevent post-exercise edema in limbs and joints to minimize an adverse secondary inflammatory response.

Cryotherapy is contraindicated for treatment of open wounds. Another limitation is treatment of areas with superficial nerves, insufficient blood circulation and impaired skin sensitivity. In humans, there are reports of adverse effects such as skin burns and cold-induced nerve palsy after 20 to 30 minutes of cooling.

Mechanisms of action

It is proposed that by decreasing tissue temperature, cryotherapy can reduce pain, tissue metabolism, muscle spasm, and minimize the inflammatory process, thereby stimulating tissue regeneration. Tissue temperature of 10–19 °C may be needed to optimize these therapeutic effects. However, temperatures below 10 °C may lead to tissue injury.[7,8]

After an injury, reduced hemorrhage and subsequent swelling is explained by a reduction in blood perfusion due to vasoconstriction. A significant decrease in soft tissue perfusion of the equine digit has been demonstrated scintigraphically in feet subjected to cryotherapy for 30 minutes.[9] It is well recognized that cryotherapy can prevent swelling from occurring, but it remains debatable whether it may help reduce edema that is already present.[7,8] A decrease in inflammation is also explained by decreased local metabolism and enzyme activity. It is suggested that tissue temperature needs to be around 10 °C for a period of about 15 min in order to reduce skin metabolic rates[11] and a joint temperature of 30 °C to slow the cartilage degrading enzymes.[12]

An analgesic effect is due to a reduction in nerve conduction velocity, and a reduction in muscle spasm caused by the influence on muscle spindle fiber activity.[13] It is shown that cold water immersion had the greatest effect on human tissue temperature and sensory nerve conduction.[14] Further, it is hypothesized that cryotherapy is working through the gate theory with intense stimulation of cold sensitive receptors at spinal level. There are also indications that cryotherapy reduces muscle force and affects proprioception, through a reduction in firing of muscle spindles and Golgi tendon organs. As a negative effect, it is recognized that collagen becomes less pliable with cold, along with a subsequent temporary reduction in mobility.[7]

Therapeutic protocol

Cryotherapy should be started immediately after the injury and continued until the response to trauma is stabilized, usually 24–72 hours. The general recommendation is that cold should be applied for at most 20 minutes, every two hours. Based on review articles in humans, recommendations range from 20 minutes 2–4 times per day, up to 30–45 minutes every two hours.[15] LaVelle & Synder suggest that 10 rather than 20 minute intervals achieve the same skin temperature, but with less 'hunting response' (an axonal reflex causing a secondary vasodilatation that is believed to occur after 20–30 minutes of cold treatment).[16] However, the question of a hunting response is still debated, and probably requires target areas that involve muscles. There are indications that cryotherapy does not create hunting responses in the treatment of equine distal limbs.[9,17,18] Using shorter repeated cold applications allows the skin temperature to return to normal between treatments, thus maintaining the low muscle temperature without endangering the skin.

In horses, the thermal response to cryotherapy has been studied in skin,[17,19] tendons[20,21] and hoof.[9,18] Cold water immersion is generally recommended at a temperature of 14–16 °C. Ice water immersion (0 °C) may be a more effective way of cooling the distal limb than cold packs, cooling splints and crushed ice. In humans, application of a pack of frozen peas produced skin temperatures adequate to induce skin analgesia in 10 minutes, and reduced metabolic enzyme activity to clinically relevant levels in 20 minutes. Finally, the application of cold should be monitored carefully to avoid ice burn. A damp barrier (like a wet towel) can be used between a contact cold source and the skin.

Outcome measures

There are studies in horses that support the clinical efficacy of cryotherapy. Studies indicate positive effects of 5–9 °C cold water treatment in horses with digital flexor tendon damage and suspensory ligament injury[22], as well as a positive effect on laminitis.[23] Another study showed a temperature decrease of 21 °C after the application of cold, reaching a minimum tissue temperature of 10 °C.[21] Finally, ice water immersion of the distal limb, at 3 °C for 48 hours, did not adversely affect the tissue.[18]

Most studies on cryotherapy in humans have used pain as an outcome measure. However, the efficacy of cold on relieving pain in clinical settings is uncertain. A Cochrane review reports that that ice alone seems to be more effective to reduce pain and swelling than control.[15] Further, the application of ice immediately before a rehabilitation program significantly decreased pain and increased weight bearing.[24] Ice therapy has showed benefit on pain relief, edema, joint motion and function, compared with control.[10]

Heat therapy

Background

Heat therapy is generally used to alleviate pain, reduce joint stiffness, muscle spasm and edema. It can be applied as *superficial heat*, affecting superficial tissues (heat wraps, hot packs, hot water bottles, warm water immersion, infrared light, electrically heated pads or blankets, high effect laser) and *deep heat*, which involves deeper layers of tissue like muscles (therapeutic ultrasound, high effect laser).

Indications and contraindications

Heat therapy is seldom applied in acute injuries, due to the vasodilatory effect and an increased risk of tissue swelling. Heat therapy is more commonly used for treatment of chronic tendinitis, joint diseases, joint stiffness and secondary muscle tenderness. It can also be used as a pre-treatment before passive joint motion or muscle stretching to increase the plasticity of connective tissue or as a comforting, sedative complementary treatment during general malaise.

Contraindications for heat therapy include infection, inflammation and neoplasia. As with cryotherapy, a contraindication is treatment of areas with insufficient blood circulation and impaired skin sensitivity. With a contact heat source, it is important to use enough insulation between the source and the skin. With infrared light and solariums, the animal should be placed at a safe distance from the heat emitting source and should not be close to something metallic that may hold excessive heat.

Mechanisms of action

It is proposed that by increasing tissue temperature, heat therapy can reduce pain, muscle spasm, joint stiffness and edema. The analgesic effect is explained by a direct influence on nerve conduction.[7,8] Although superficial heat may only reach the superficial parts of tissues (approximately 1 cm from the skin surface), there is a possibility that it affects superficial nerves and thus have both a sedative and pain-relieving effect explained by the gate control theory. A reduction in muscle spasm is explained by the influence of heat on muscle spindle fiber activity, breaking the pain-muscle spasm-pain cycle. It is claimed that temperatures over 42°C slow the signaling rate of muscle spindles, but increases the signaling of Golgi tendon organs.[7] Heat also reduces the viscosity of soft tissues and increases the elasticity of scar tissue, as well as reducing joint stiffness.[24]

Reduction of edema is explained by a vasodilatation effect, through spinal reflexes leading to a decreased smooth muscle tone of vessels. The increase in tissue temperature also creates an increase in metabolism. Enzymatic reactions are believed to increase with temperatures over 45°C, and a rise of 2–5°C is claimed to increase the action of phagocytic cells and cause an increase in blood flow with a reduction in swelling.[7,8,12]

Therapeutic protocol

Superficial heat can be applied with different types of heat packs covered in a moistened towel. The heat packs usually stay warm for approximately 30 minutes. Temperatures in superficial tissue can increase approximately 5°C after six minutes of superficial heat, and it takes approximately 15–30 minutes for deeper tissues to reach therapeutic levels. After approximately nine minutes of hot water hose therapy at a temperature of 38–41°C, the skin temperature over the equine metacarpal region was raised to 39.5–41°C and the subcutis to 39–40°C.[20] Further, tissue temperatures return to baseline approximately 15 minutes after end of treatment. As previously mentioned, heating of connective tissues before stretching facilitates joint motion. To maintain tissue flexibility the temperature must be raised to 40–45°C for 5–10 minutes. Thereafter, the tissue must be put under stress.[24]

The application of heat should be monitored carefully to avoid inflammatory reactions and burns. Contact heat sources warmer than 45°C should be wrapped in moist towels before application to the skin. Finally, the tissue temperature should be allowed to regain its normal temperature before new heat is applied, since there is an increased risk of burns with repeated heat administration.

Outcome measures

Studies in horses have shown a rise in tissue temperature after treatment with gel wraps, warm water hose and warm water bath.[9,17,20] A 25 % increase in blood flow was reported after a 30 minute, 47°C water bath.[9] A non-controlled study on 102 horses with various injuries reported a positive effect of dry whirlpool therapy, and that the temperature of the subcutis was raised 5°C.[25] In humans, there are no conclusive data on superficial heat therapy for either swelling or pain.[15]

Therapeutic ultrasound

Background

Therapeutic ultrasound has been used for injuries in the human musculoskeletal system since the 1950s. It is claimed to reduce pain and muscle spasms, and increase blood circulation and induce micro-massage at the cell-level, thus promoting tissue healing. However, there is an ongoing debate on its clinical efficacy.

The ultrasound machine contains a piezoelectric element which, when activated with an electric current, starts to vibrate. The vibration results in a sound wave, with a frequency dependent on the magnitude of the electric current. The sound waves are transmitted to the tissue through a transducer head that is put in contact with the skin of the horse. The wave is reflected in air-tissue interfaces, thus one needs an ultrasound coupling media between the transducer head and the skin. The absorption rate is higher in tissues that contain protein than fat. When the waves hit bone, they are reflected, which might lead to an increase in temperature and a pain reaction. The waves can either come in pulsations or continuously, thus emitting different levels of energy per unit of time.

Indications and contraindications

Therapeutic ultrasound is applied primarily in tendinitis, desmitis, sprains, lacerations, and myositis, but also in chronic conditions such as joint disease. Heating tissues prior to passive joint motion increases soft tissue extensibility facilitating treatment of contractures. Further, it is claimed to reduce adhesions, calcifications, and scar tissue, reduce nerve root irritation and speed bone healing. Besides these indications, therapeutic ultrasound can be used for phonophoresis, a means of delivering pharmaceuticals through the skin.

The contraindications for treatment are acute injuries and inflammatory disease, infection and neoplasia. Treatment should be avoided over areas with insufficient blood circulation, recent hemorrhaging, pregnant uterus, gonads, contaminated wounds and epiphyseal plates.

Therapeutic ultrasound has the potential to cause tissue damage if not handled properly, such as overheating and inflammation. Pain response to treatment can be observed as a withdrawal or stomping of the limb. Treatment of animals that are sedated or with impaired skin sensitivity should be restricted since they may not have a proper avoidance reaction. In humans, pain reactions, burns, and subperiosteal damage have been reported. The risk for so called 'standing waves' can be reduced by continually moving the transducer head.

Mechanisms of action

The mechanisms of actions for therapeutic ultrasound are divided into thermal and non-thermal effects.[26] The thermal effects include an increase in blood circulation,[27] and a direct influence on the nerve through a prolonged nerve transmission velocity.[7]

A non-thermal effect is explained by vibrations causing 'micro-massage at the cell level', which is thought to increase the cell membrane potential, permeability, and transport mechanisms. The vibrations are also believed to create micro-currents of liquid and cavitation (the formation of tiny gas bubbles in the tissues as the result of ultrasound vibration), which may cause tissue destruction.[7] The eventual effect of therapeutic ultrasound on bone healing is explained by an enhancement of the endochondral portion of fracture healing. Other proposed non-thermal effects are the acceleration of the inflammatory phase, stimulation of fibroblast proliferation and decreased pain.[7,27,28]

Therapeutic protocol

It is important that the electric apparatus and cords are functioning and protected from damage. Before using the ultrasound, one should make sure that it works properly by covering the transducer head with gel (or put it in a water bath) and increase the wattage to check if 'bubbles' are created. It is also important to calibrate the instrument regularly, since studies have shown a variability of 30% in output intensity.[28]

Treatment parameters

The settings of the apparatus often offer choice of frequency, intensity and duty cycle. The protocol should also include a specified treatment area, treatment duration, and speed of transducer head movement and treatment schedule.

The *frequency* determines the depth of wave penetration; 1 MHz heats to a depth between 2–5 cm, 2 MHz 1–3 cm and 3 MHz to 0.5–3 cm.

Intensity is the amount of energy delivered per unit area (W/cm^2). Intensity is set between 0.25–5 W/cm^{2}depending on treatment goals. The higher the intensity, the faster is the rise in tissue temperature. Higher intensities are used to heat tissues before motion treatment and lower, non-thermal intensities are often used when treating pain and muscle spasm.

The *duty cycle* can be set as either continuous or pulsed ultrasound; the thermal effects are reduced if the sound waves are delivered in pulses. The most commons ratio settings are 1 : 4, 1 : 5 or 1 : 1. The ratio 1 : 5 is often chosen when treating areas over superficial bone.

The *treatment area* should not exceed three times the transducer head area.

The *dosage* can be calculated as: energy (J =W/cm^2) x applicator size (cm^2) x time (sec).

Treatment times usually vary between 5–10 minutes.

Treatment regimes

Place the animal in a secure place. In order to create the best possible sound wave transmission, the hair should be clipped and a generous amount of acoustic gel applied between the transducer head and the skin. It is important that the ultrasound head is moved during treatment. It is possible to treat an area with an irregular surface by immersing area (such as a limb) into water.

In horses, treatment is usually performed at 1.5 W/cm^2 for 10 minutes, once or twice daily for 10–14 days. The thermal effects of ultrasound are difficult to predict because of the varying rates of absorption by different tissues. A lower temperature rise was seen in the treatment of dogs with an intact hair coat, compared to dogs with clipped hair. However, there was a great temperature increase within the hair. Temperature increase of 0.6–3.5 °C has been shown at 1–10 cm depth in canine muscles after treatment with 1–2 W/cm^2 and 1–3 MHz.[26]

Outcome measures

Lippiello and Smalley draw the conclusion that bone healing in equines was stimulated by ultrasound therapy.[29] There are divergent results from studies on muscle and tendon regeneration in horses and dogs.[30–34] In a clinical study without case controls, Lang treated 53 horses and 143 small animals. Based on owner evaluation, 63 % of the treatments were successful.[35] One study failed to demonstrate any positive effects of ultrasound therapy on the healing of surgically severed Achilles tendons in dogs (1 MHz, pulse ratio1 : 4, 0.7–1.0 W/cm2, 10 minutes, three times a week, 13 treatments). In human systematic reviews authors conclude that there is limited evidence to support the use of active ultrasound therapy for treating people with musculoskeletal disorders.[36,37]

Extracorporeal shockwave therapy (ESWT)

Background

Extracorporeal shock wave therapy (ESWT) was first used in human medicine as a treatment for urolithiasis. Since the early 1990s, it has been used in humans for the treatment of orthopedic disorders such as heel spurs or shoulder calcification. In veterinary medicine, extracorporeal shock wave therapy has mainly been used for treatment of bone and ligament injuries.

The most common means to create therapeutic shockwaves is via an electromagnetic source. The energy created is converted to shockwaves by an acoustic converter. This generates high-energy shockwaves (up to 100 MPa) of very short duration (5 μs) with a constant level of energy. Focused shockwave therapy consists of a targeting system, so that the treatment can be performed without damaging the surrounding tissue. Radial shock waves are most commonly created with a mechanical impulse device and are delivered to the surface of the horse.

Indications and contraindications

ESWT is commonly used in tendons, ligaments, navicular syndrome, osteoarthritis and osteoporosis of sesamoid bones. Dependent on the selected energy level, it is used in the treatment of bone tissue (either for stimulation of bone healing or removal of calcification), of soft tissues in close attachment of the bone (tendons and fascia) and in the treatment of pain.

Contraindications are infectious arthritis, neoplastic diseases, and acute unstable fractures. ESWT should not be administered over the lung field, head, heart, major blood vessels or pregnant uterus. Adverse reactions such as pain, increased lameness, hematoma and inflammation have been reported in horses. Studies on focused ESWT show a disorganization of collagen network in the treated normal tendon[38], as well as a potential to increase bone microcracking[39]. These studies recommend restricted exercise after treatment. However, other studies with ESWT on bone and bone-ligament interface showed no damage.

Mechanisms of action

The mechanism of action of ESWT is associated with the mechanical tension and pressure that the waves induce on tissue. Shockwaves release energy at the interfaces between tissues. It is proposed that ESWT increases blood circulation and stimulates the alignment of fibers in tendons and ligaments. Normal tendons treated with ESWT showed a transient stimulation of metabolism in tendinous structures, but six weeks after treatment the metabolism and level of glucosaminoglycans was lower than before treatment.[38,39] Shockwaves may affect sensory nerve fibers, resulting in an analgesic effect. No cutaneous analgesia or changes in measured gait analysis parameters were recognized following ESWT treatment of equine high palmar/plantar metacarpal/metatarsal pain, but reduced gait asymmetry was found at 72 hours following treatment.[40] One study reported a local cutaneous analgesic effect, but not a regional analgesic effect, when evaluated over 3–7 days after treatment.[41]

Therapeutic protocol

It is important to have the horse stand still during treatment, in order to conduct a precise treatment. ESWT may involve some discomfort, thus it is common to lightly sedate the horse during the treatment session. The treatment parameters include number of impulses, energy density, the pressure time, the peak pressure and the focal depth. The treatment protocol may entail up to 2000 impulses per session, with intensity of 0.10–1.8 mJ/mm^2 or according to the atmospheric pressure at the output probe, depending on the manufacturer's recommendation. Most treated injuries require 3–5 separate treatments with intervals of 1–2 weeks and specialized convalescence regimes.

Outcome measures

Studies on shockwave treatment of navicular disease and bone spavin have shown a reduction in lameness, from an acute improvement to improvement of longer duration.[42–48] A study on equine tendons does not support the treatment with ESWT on induced lesions in the accessory ligament of the deep digital flexor tendon,[47] nor in the superficial digital flexor tendinitis, but an increase in neovascularization was reported. Compared to control suspensory ligament, treated ligaments showed more small, newly formed collagen fibrils and greater expression of growth factors. A study on palmar heel pain showed no scintigraphic or radiographic changes after radial ESWT and the authors explain the eventual acute clinical benefit from treatment as analgesic effects rather than stimulation of local tissue metabolism.[48] This analgesic effect is discussed in a study describing a decrease in weight-bearing asymmetry after ESWT of horses with proximal suspensory ligament desmitis, however, there was no change in skin sensitivity after treatment.[41]

A study showed a positive effect on wound healing time, but not any significant changes in histology or immunohistochemical analyzes[49], nor difference in area of epithelialization and percentage of wound contraction. Further, studies have investigated the effect on bone healing.[50]

Neuromuscular electrical stimulation (NMES)

Background

In human medicine, the popularity of NMES reached its heights during the 1950s when researchers claimed that it could increase human muscle strength by 40%. There are different stimulator systems, with the common denominator of using superficial electrodes on the skin to induce muscle contractions.

Indications and contraindications

Muscle stimulators are generally used as supportive treatment for fractures, muscle sprains and contusions, following surgery and for muscle relaxation. It can be used in the treatment of tendon injuries to increase local blood circulation and thus promote healing. Further, it can be used for prevention; to increase muscle strength and endurance in healthy subjects and to prevent muscle atrophy during immobilization. It is called functional electrical muscle stimulation when used on denervated muscles.

Use of NMES is contraindicated when active motion is prohibited, and near neoplasia and skin infections. NMES should not be used in animals with seizures, over the heart and carotid sinuses, a pregnant uterus and areas with thrombophlebitis. It is important to remember that the rate of muscle fatigue is greater with NMES than with voluntary contractions. Reverse reactions such as pain and skin reactions from the stimulated area has been reported from human literature.

Mechanisms of action

The electric impulse stimulates the nerve to send an impulse to the muscle that causes a subsequent muscle contraction. The stimulation can either be peripheral on the motor axon branches or central through reflexive recruitment of spinal motor neurons.[51] The same motor units are repeatedly activated by the same amount of electrical current, and it is generally believed that NMES first recruits type II muscle fibers and then type I fibers, which is the reverse of the muscle recruitment pattern in a voluntary contraction.[52,53] However, there are discussions if the recruitment order mainly depends on the amount of electric current at the site of the motor nerve.[54]

The contraction leads to an increase in blood circulation[55], which might increase the rate of healing. It is generally believed that repeated muscle contractions will lead to an exhausted muscle with muscle relaxation as a result. The stimulation is also said to affect pain perception by secondary pain modulating pathways, for instance release of pain modulating substances.[56]

Therapeutic protocol

After the skin is shaved and the area cleaned, the two or more electrodes are placed on the skin over the selected muscle (Fig. 64.2). The electrodes should be flexible to follow the contour of the body; there are carbon-impregnated silicon rubber electrodes but also electrodes for single-use. The electrodes should have approximately the same size as the cross sectional area of the target muscle. Good electrode placement results in less discomfort during stimulation.

To improve transmission of the electrical current, gel is placed between the skin and the electrode. It is believed that the best muscle contraction is achieved if one of the electrodes is placed over a motor point, generally sited in the middle of the longitudinal axis of the muscles at the muscle-tendon junction. The identification of motor points is done by placing an electrode on the distal part of the muscle, while the other electrode is moved over the proximal part of the muscle and stimulating at 2 Hz and gradually increasing the stimulation intensity.

Treatment parameters

There are several parameters that can be altered; waveform (symmetrical, asymmetrical, biphasic), current intensity, amplitude, pulse duration, pulse frequency, ramp time, polarity and on/off time.

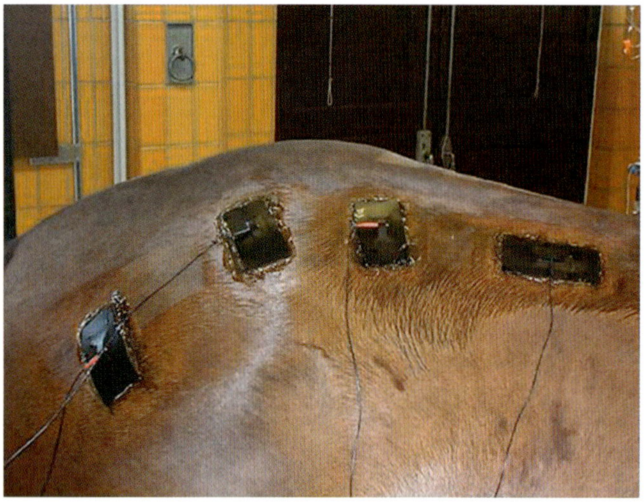

Fig 64.2 Neuromuscular electrical stimulation (NMES) device electrodes positioned on clipped and cleansed skin for stimulation of the gluteal and epaxial musculature.
Courtesy of A. Bergh.

The symmetrical biphasic *waveform* is generally the most comfortable setting.

The *intensity* of the current (mA) regulates the strength of the contraction. Stronger current recruits more muscle fibers at a greater distance from the electrode. The total intensity needed is dependent on each individual's capacitive resistance of the skin and by the Ohmic resistance from the hair and skin; the latter is reduced if the hair is clipped and the skin cleaned.

As the *pulse duration* (ms) increases, small pain fibers are recruited as well as larger muscle fibers. Studies have shown that humans prefer pulse duration of 300 ms during quadriceps muscle stimulation. Increasing the pulse amplitude and duration, and current density increases the maximum voluntary isometric torque, as well as the percentage of muscle group activated.[57] However; a rise of stimulus duration is connected to an increase in patient discomfort.

The *pulse frequency* affects the quality of the muscle contraction and the rate of muscle fatigue. Often a frequency of 20–60 Hz is chosen and maximal force of contraction generally occurs at 60–100 Hz. However, increasing the frequency also results in increased fatigue and discomfort. In humans, it is suggested that a frequency of 4–6 Hz reduces edema and improves circulation, 15 Hz is believed to stimulate muscle tone, 15–25 Hz improves endurance, 25 Hz affects bone healing and >30 Hz strengthens muscles.

A *ramp* up/down time is selected so that there is a gradual and comfortable increase/decrease of the muscle contraction. Generally a 2–4 s ramp up and 1–2 s ramp down time is selected.

The ratio of *on/off time* is dependent on the goals of treatment; strength training often uses a 1:4, 1:5 ratio, while endurance training uses 1:1 to 1:3 ratios. The treatment period in horses is generally between 15–30 minutes.

Based on human studies, it has been recommended to progressively increase the current intensity, and change the placement of the active electrodes in order to minimize the extent of muscle fatigue. In order to reduce discomfort, the stimulation should be delivered at low pulse amplitudes, pulse durations in the range 0.2–1 ms, stimulation train durations shorter than 2 s for stimulation over the nerve and longer than 2 s for stimulation over the muscle, and high pulse frequencies.[51]

Outcome measures

The effects of NMES on muscles are often assessed by muscle biopsies and ultrasound. Results from a study on healthy horses demonstrate that daily treatment with a NMES-protocol for five days a week over four weeks did not cause any significant changes in muscle fiber types and areas, glycogen content or enzyme activities.[58]

There are several studies on NMES and its effect on canine muscles. One study describes a better effect of 60 min NMES compared to 30 min (frequency of 50 Hz, with pulse duration of 300 milliseconds, and the on/off time was at a proportion of 1:2, 3–5 days a week for 60 days) evaluated with *m quadriceps femoris* morphometri.[59] Other studies have used NMES together with other modalities after muscle atrophy with positive results.[60] A study on the canine anterior cruciate ligament (ACL) shows less bony changes and larger thigh circumference.[61] Finally, one study describes the electrical impulse duration thresholds that evoke a maximal muscle contraction for 11 canine muscles.[62]

Human reviews report increased muscle strength due to NMES in athletic training, training during immobilization and pathology treatments.[63] The effect of NMES on healthy humans is equal to, but not superior to, voluntary strength training, and that the protocols with simultaneous voluntary muscle contractions seem to have more effect than electrostimulation alone. A study on 24 humans with back pain showed a larger reduction in pain with combined NMES/TENS treatment compared to placebo.[64]

Transcutaneous electrical nerve stimulation (TENS)

Background

As with NMES, there are a variety of systems using superficial electrodes on the skin to induce muscle contractions. However, TENS is primarily used to alleviate pain and to stimulate tissue healing by causing an increase in blood flow. The treatment is divided in high frequency TENS (100 Hz) without visible muscle contractions and low frequency TENS (4 Hz) with visible muscle contractions.

Indications and contraindications

TENS is generally used in animals with muscle tenderness and muscle spasm, to relieve both acute and chronic pain, and to stimulate wound healing. It can be used in both acute and chronic injuries; chronic pain as in arthritic conditions is often treated. Contraindications are impaired skin sensitivity and skin infections. In human medicine, adverse reactions like skin irritation, burn injuries and pain reactions are reported.

Mechanisms of action

High frequency TENS is claimed to reduce pain by the gate theory.[65] Low frequency TENS is claimed to alleviate pain through the release of pain modulating mediators like opioids and is therefore called 'acupuncture-like' TENS.[66] Muscle tension is reduced through repeated muscle contractions. There are several studies with conflicting results regarding the effect on blood circulation.[66–68]

Therapeutic protocol

TENS apparatus induces pulsations of direct current, transmitted to the body through two or several electrodes that are placed on the skin of the animal. The machine has controls for frequency, shape of pulsations, intensity of current and time. Just as with NMES, the skin needs to be shaved and cleaned, and a gel should be applied between the electrodes and the skin. The positioning of the electrodes is important; generally the electrodes are positioned over the source of pain, but can also be positioned on either side of the lesion, over nerve roots, over peripheral nerves, at motor points, at trigger points and at dermatomes. The intensity of electric current should be increased until the muscle flickers, and then a small reduction can be made.

The generally recommended protocols are to use approximately 130 Hz frequency to reduce pain by activation of the gate theory (acute pain and inflammation) and 2–5 Hz to activate the opioid system (chronic pain), with treatment times of 20–40 minutes. In humans, treatment periods differ between single sessions of 10–60 minutes, to weekly or twice weekly sessions of 20–60 minutes.[69] Some authors believe that 30–40 minutes of stimulation at least twice a day for a month may be needed to achieve significant pain relief.[70]

Outcome measures

There are no studies found on horses regarding the use of TENS. However, one study on dogs with mild osteoarthritis describes a pain relieving effect for 30–210 minutes after 70Hz TENS treatment, evaluated by force plate.[71] In humans, reviews indicate that for pain treatment, there are small differences in the efficacy of high and low frequency TENS. It is discussed if TENS is more efficient in soft tissue injuries than in osteoarthritis[69] and that there is insufficient evidence regarding its effect on acute pain.[72]

Laser therapy

Background

The word *laser* stands for *Light Amplification by Stimulated Emission of Radiation*. Laser light is created when energy from a power source excites a lasing medium, and energy is released as photons. Usually, a laser medium creates light with one wavelength. Different wavelengths are claimed to have different effects on living tissues, based on their absorption peaks and penetration depths. Laser light is highly synchronized (coherent) with high parallelism (collimated). The coherence and collimation will diminish when the light enters tissues.

Laser devices are categorized into surgical lasers and biostimulating lasers. They are also classified according to specific characteristics; laser medium, output effect and the risk for eye injury (class 1–4). In the following text, the focus will be on biostimulating lasers and not on lasers used for surgery or photodynamic therapy (used in cancer treatment).

Indications and contraindications

Laser therapy is generally used for wound healing, pain relief, reduction of inflammation, and treatment of injuries in the musculoskeletal apparatus. Examples of injuries treated include osteoarthritis, fractures, post-traumatic nerve degeneration, tendinitis and muscle sprains. Laser can also be used for acupuncture point stimulation.

Contraindications include treatment of horses with neoplasia and in those with impaired skin sensitivity (high effect laser) due to risks of burn injuries. Caution should also be taken when treating pregnant animals. Some laser light can cause eye injuries. The risk increases if there are reflecting materials near the treatment area. Class 1 and 2 includes low power lasers with no adverse effect on eyes and skin; class 3 A and B includes mid-power lasers, safe on skin but a risk for eye injury; class 4 includes high power lasers with a risk to both eyes and skin.

Mechanisms of action

Despite the frequent use of laser therapy, there is a lack of information of the precise mechanisms of action. Simplified, the photobiological effects of laser irradiation can be separated into three categories: photochemical (which is not yet universally accepted), photothermal and photomechanical (not applicable).[73]

Photochemical effect: Visible light is considered to cause electronic excitation of light sensitive molecules (photoacceptors, chromophores). The photon energy is converted into chemical energy in the cell, which is suggested to lead to changes in cell membrane permeability and normalization of cell functions, pain relief, and healing.[74] Photothermal effect results from transformation of absorbed light energy to heat, and are unlikely to apply to low level laser therapy, as temperatures are elevated by less than 1 °C.

The physiological effects of laser therapy include anti-inflammatory effects, more organized fibroblasts, increased cellularity, increased collagen formation, vasodilatation, increased concentration of capillaries, DNA synthesis, RNA production, and pain reduction through the influence of the pain gate and nerve velocity.[73–77]

Therapeutic protocol

The laser treatment parameters are wavelength, power, pulse rate, irradiated area, exposure time and treatment intervals. When treating animals, the depth of penetration through hair and pigment is an important issue. It is recommended that the irradiated area should be clipped and cleaned before treatment.[78] The laser dosimetric parameters are presented in Table 64.1.

In horses, treatment of soft tissues often has a dose of 2–8 J/cm^2 (lower range when acute injuries are treated), and 0.5–1 J/cm^2 if acupuncture points are treated. Skin lesions are generally treated with red light that will be absorbed in the skin, and deeper lesions can be treated with near infrared. When surgical lasers are used for biostimulation, the light beam is defocused and dosages between 10–100 J/cm^2 are used.

Outcome measures

It is difficult to present a consensus from existing laser therapy studies, as the treatment protocols often differ with the type of laser, various dosages, outcome measures and treated conditions.[75] Many studies focus on cellular responses[79] and most studies that investigate the clinical effect on horses are descriptive and not randomized controlled trials. Controlled trials on equine wounds treated with laser report varying degrees of success.[80,81] Other investigations suggest negative results regarding wound and tendon healing in horses.[82,83] Petermann used a pulsed laser system for the treatment of arthritis and tenosynovitis in horses, and reports a positive effect.[84] Other non-controlled studies report positive results from treatment with infrared laser on back pain and tendinitis in horses, as well as treatment of other injuries in the musculoskeletal apparatus.[85,86]

Studies have shown that defocused CO_2 laser therapy can increase temperature and blood circulation in skin and subcutis, but not in fetlock joints, and that treatment of aseptic fetlock arthritis was not statistically better than sham treatment at reducing the grade of lameness.[87,88] Another study reports an effect of defocused CO_2 laser treatment of traumatic arthritis superior to that of intra-articular injections of betamethasone in combination with sodium hyaluronate.[89]

In human medicine, no conclusions are drawn regarding the efficacy in skin disorders.[90] Meta-analyzes of the use of laser in musculoskeletal condition in humans have had diverse conclusions regarding the effectiveness for pain relief and quicker functional recovery.[91–93]

Magnetic field therapy

Background

Magnetic field therapy is available in two forms: pulsed electromagnetic therapy (PEMT) and static magnetic field therapy (SMFT). PEMT consists of pulsating/time variable magnets that are connected to an electrical source, which creates an electromagnetic field that changes polarity. SMFT magnets have permanent north and south poles, hence do not change polarity. The strength of the electromagnetic fields is measured in Tesla or Gauss (1 Tesla = 10000 Gauss) and frequency is measured in Hz. The magnetic field of the earth is about 50 μT.

Indications and contraindications

Common indications for magnetic field therapy are tendon and ligament injuries, laminitis, osteoarthritis and back pain. SMFT is generally used to increase blood circulation, thus promoting healing, and relieve pain. PEMT is generally used to alleviate pain, stimulate bone formation, and heal muscle- and tendon injuries, as well as stimulate neuronal regeneration. Magnetic field therapy is also used for prevention and as a comforting treatment; reducing muscle tension and calming the patient. Contraindications are acute infections, acute injuries, neoplasia, open wounds and pregnancy.

Mechanisms of action

Evidence for the scientific principles, biological mechanisms and clinical efficacy of magnetic therapy is limited. SMFT is proposed to have magnetic effects and PEMT to have electrical or ion flux effects.

Static magnets are believed to influence the blood circulation,[94] transport of ions over the cell membrane, which is supposed to increase cellular oxygen, fluid and gas circulation, and thus reduce inflammation and edema. It is suggested that magnetic fields selectively attenuate neuronal depolarization, especially in C-fibers, thus alleviating pain.[95]

It is believed that PEMT changes ion concentrations over the cell membrane, with secondary influence on nerve transmission and hormonal receptors. An increase in cell permeability is said to enhance the transportation of oxygen, nutrition, and waste products. It is also said to enhance the building of thymine in the nucleus of the cell, which can influence the genetic material. PEMT may influence the formation of cartilage and extracellular matrix during bone formation.[96,97]

Therapeutic protocol

The static magnets are often woven into blankets (Fig. 64.3), pads, and boots. The strength of the static magnets can vary between 10 gauss to 1000 gauss depending on manufacturer. In humans, SMFT is used from one hour once a week to several hours (22 hrs) a day for months.[98]

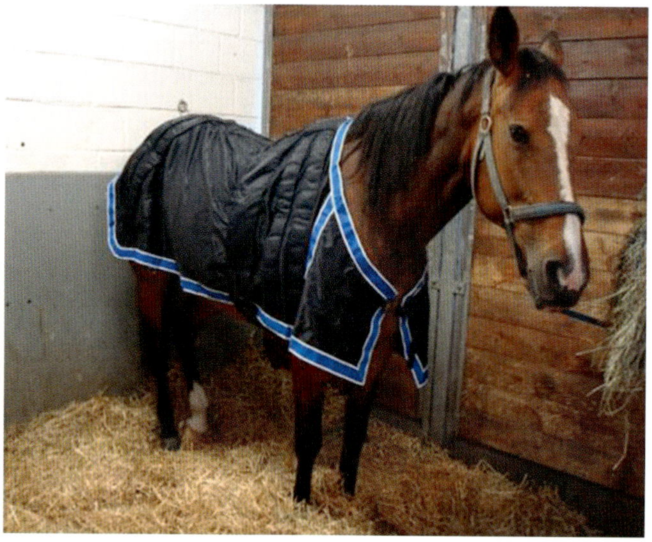

Fig 64.3 Blanket with self-contained static magnetic therapy devices. *Courtesy of A. Edner.*

Table 64.1 Dosimetric parameters of different laser irradiations

PARAMETER SYNONYM	COMMENTS	UNITS	LOW LEVEL LASER	HIGH POWER LASER
Power	Output 10^{-1}-hundreds of W	Power = energy/time (W = J/s)	W	10^{-3}–10^{-1} W
Intensity	Power density Irradiance	Intensity = power/area irradiated	W/cm^2	10^{-2}–10^{0} W/cm^2
Dose	Energy density Radiant exposure	Dose = power X irradiation time/area	J/cm^2	10^{-2}–10^{2} W
Pulse rate		Pulses/seconds	Hz	0 (cw) – 5000 Hz
Pulse duration		Time when laser light is emitted	s	1–500 ms
Pulse interval		Time when the laser is off between pulses	s	1–500 ms
Treatment time		Total time when the laser light is emitted	s	

The PEMT can consist of magnetic blankets or pads attached to an electrical source. The magnitude of the field is dependent on the intensity of the current that supplies the magnets. In humans, the treatment parameters in PEMT generally vary between 5–75 Hz, impulses of a few microseconds and an intensity of 30–500 mT.

Outcome measures

Review of the literature reveals inconsistent evidence regarding the use of magnetic fields. The effects of PEMT on bone and cartilage healing remain unclear.[96,97,99–101] In one study, the effect of electromagnetic field devices on healing of cannon bone osteotomies in horses was examined. The conclusion was that the electromagnetic devices did not have a local effect on the repair process of an acute, stable, osseous defect.[102]

The effect of magnetic field therapy on blood circulation has been reported. Results from a study on six horses suggest that SMFT with magnetic wraps for 48 hours does not increase blood flow to the portion of the metacarpus underneath the wrap.[103] Reviews discuss the applications of PEMT,[104] and one concludes that there is no evidence for changes in blood circulation in horses.[17] However, one report states that treatment with a 600 gauss static magnetic pad increased circulation and metabolic activity in equine limbs measured by scintigraphy.[101] Electromagnetic therapy once daily increased the concentration of blood vessels in equine superficial digital flexor tendon, but the maturation of the repair tissue was delayed in samples collected at 8 to 12 weeks.[105]

Meta-analysis of human studies suggests that there are no significant effects of static magnets for pain relief relative to placebo, besides limited evidence for the treatment of peripheral joint osteoarthritis.[98] However, there are indications that PEMT may improve activities of daily life in patients with osteoarthritis of the knee.[106] SMFT were no more effective than placebo in preventing delayed onset muscle soreness.[107]

The author and editors gratefully acknowledge the contributions to this chapter of Dr. Andris Kaneps, a contributor to the previous edition.

References

1. Ranner W, Gerhards H, Klee W. Diagnostic validity of palpation in horses with back problems. Berl Munch Tierarztl Wochenschr 2002;115(11–12):420–4.
2. van Loon JP, Back W, Hellebrekers LJ, et al. Application of a composite pain scale to objectively monitor horses with somatic and visceral pain under hospital conditions. J Equine Vet Sceince 2010;11(30):641–9.
3. Haussler KK, Erb HN. Mechanical nociceptive thresholds in the axial skeleton of horses. Equine Vet J 2006;38:70–5.
4. Love EJ, Murrell J, Whay HR. Thermal and mechanical nociceptive threshold testing in horses: a review. Vet Anaesth Analg 2011;38:3–14.
5. Liljebrink Y, Bergh A. Goniometry – is it a reliable tool to measure passive joint range of motion in horses? Equine Vet J 2010;42:676–82.
6. Keegan K. Gait Analysis for the Quantification of Lameness. In: Ross M, Dyson S, editors. Diagnosis and Management of Lameness in the Horse. 2nd ed. Saunders; 2010. p. 245–51.
7. Lehmann JF. Cryotherapy. In: Lehmann JF, editor. Therapeutic Heat and Cold. 4th ed. Baltimore: Williams & Wilkins; 1990.
8. Michlovitz SL, editor. Thermal agents in rehabilitation. 3rd ed. Philadelphia, PA: FA Davis; 1996.
9. Worster AA, Gaughan EM, Hoskinson JJ, et al. Effects of external thermal manipulation on laminar temperature and perfusion scintigraphy of the equine digit. NZ Vet J 2000;48:111–16.
10. Bleakley C, McDonough S, MacAuley D. The Use of Ice in the Treatment of Acute Soft-Tissue Injury. A Systematic Review of Randomized Controlled Trials. Am J Sports Med 2004;32.
11. Stålman A, Berglund L, Dungnerc E, et al. Temperature-sensitive release of prostaglandin E_2 and diminished energy requirements in synovial tissue with postoperative cryotherapy: a prospective randomized study after knee arthroscopy. J Bone Joint Surg Am 2011;2;93(21):1961–8.
12. Oosterveld FGJ, Rasker JJ. Effects of local heat and cold treatment on surface and articular temperature of arthritic knees. Arthritis Rheum 1994;37:1578–82.
13. Algafly AA, George KP. The effect of cryotherapy on nerve conduction velocity, pain threshold and pain tolerance. Br J Sports Med 2007;41:365–9.
14. Herrera E, Sandoval MC, Camargo DM, et al. Motor and sensory nerve conduction is affected differently by ice pack, ice massage and cold water immersion. Phys Ther 2010;90(4):581–91.
15. Brosseau L, Yonge KA, Welch V, et al. Thermotherapy for treatment of osteoarthritis. Cochrane Database Syst Rev 2004, Issue 4.
16. LaVelle BE, Synder M. Differential conduction of cold through barriers. J Adv Nurs 1985;10(1):55–61.
17. Turner TA, Wolfsdorf K, Jourdenais J, et al. Effects of heat, cold, biomagnets and ultrasound on skin circulation in the horse. Proc Am Ass Equine Practioners 1991;37:249–57.
18. Pollit CC, van Eps AW. Prolonged, continuous distal limb cryotherapy in the horse. Equine Vet J 2004;36:216–20.
19. Kasashima Y, Eto D, Kusano K, et al. Comparison of the method of cold therapy to equine limbs after training, with the aim of preventing tendinitis. J Equine Sci 2001;12:96.
20. Kaneps AJ. Tissue temperature response to hot and cold therapy in the metacarpal region of a horse. Proc Am Ass Equine Practnrs 2000;46:208–13.
21. Petrov R, McDonald MH, Tesch AM, et al. Influence of topical applied cold treatment on core temperature and cell viability in equine superficial digital flexor tendon. Am J Vet Res 2003;64:835–44.
22. Hunt ER. Response of twenty-seven horses with lower leg injuries to cold spa bath hydrotherapy. J Equine Vet Sci 2001;21:188–93.
23. van Eps AW, Pollitt CC. Equine laminitis model: Cryotherapy reduces the severity of lesions evaluated seven days after induction with oligofructose. Equine Vet J 2009;41.
24. McLean DA. The use of cold and superficial heat in the treatment of soft tissue injuries. Br J Sports Med 1989;23:53–4.
25. Watson JE, Harris JF, Henley EJ. In vivo temperature elevations using dry whirlpool therapy. Equine Pract 1984;6:11–14.
26. Steiss JE, McCauley L. Therapeutic ultrasound. In: Millis DL, Levine D, Amd RA, editors. Canine rehabilitation and physical therapy. Taylor: W.B Saunders, St Louis; 2004. p. 324–36.
27. Baker KG, Robertson VL, Duck FA. A review of therapeutic ultrasound: biophysical effect. Phys Ther 2001;81:1351–8.
28. Robertson VJ, Baker KG. A review of therapeutic ultrasound: effectiveness studies. Physic Therap 2001;81:1339–50.

29. Lippiello L, Smalley L. Densitometric assesment of equine bone repair following pulsed ultrasound therapy. Equine Pract 1991;4:17–24.
30. Morcos MB, Aswad A. treatment of two clinical conditions in racehorses by ultrasonic therapy. Equine Vet J 1978a; 10:128–9.
31. Bansal, BS, Sobti VK. Diatermi and ultrasonic therapy for various musculo-tendinous affections in dogs and horses. Indian Vet J 1990;67:352–5.
32. Keg PR. Experimentelle untersuchungen zur beurteilung der wirksamkeit von ultraschall bei der tendinnitis des pferdes. Pferdeheilkunde 1989;5: 285–9.
33. Morcos MB, Aswad A. Histological studies on the effects of ultrasonic therapy on surgically split flexor tendons. Equine Vet J 1978b;4:267–9.
34. Fernandes MAL, Alves GES, Souza, JCA. Clinical, ultrasonographic and histopathological studies of two protocols of ultrasonic therapy on experimental tendonitis in horses. Arquivo Brasileiro Med Vet Zootech 2003;55:27–34.
35. Lang DC. Ultrasonic treatment of musculoskeletal conditions in the horse, dog and cat. Vet Rec 1980;106:427–31.
36. van der Windt DA, van der Heijden GJ, van den Berg SG, et al. Ultrasound therapy for musculoskeletal disorders: a systematic review. Pain 1999;81: 257–71.
37. Rutjes AWS, Nüesch E, Sterchi R, et al. Therapeutic ultrasound for osteoarthritis of the knee or hip. Cochrane Db Syst Rev 2010, Issue 1.
38. Bosch G, de Mos M, van Binsbergen R, et al. The effect of focused extracorporeal shock wave therapy on collagen matrix and gene expression in normal tendons and ligaments. Equine Vet J 2009;41(4):335–41.
39. Da Costa Gomez TM, Radtke CL, Kalscheur VL, et al. Effect of focused and radial extracorporeal shock wave therapy on equine bone microdamage. Vet Surg 2004;33(1):49–55.
40. McClure SR, Sonea IM, Evans RB, et al. Evaluation of analgesia resulting from extracorporeal shock wave therapy and radial pressure wave therapy in the limbs of horses and sheep. Am J Vet Res 2005;66(10):1702–8.
41. Imboden I, Waldern NM, Wiestner T, et al. Short term analgesic effect of extracorporeal shock wave therapy in horses with proximal palmar metacarpal/plantar metatarsal pain. Vet J 2009;179(1):50–9.
42. Brown KE, Nickels FA, Caron JP, et al. Investigation of the immediate analgesic effects of extracorporeal shock wave therapy for treatment of navicular disease in horses. Vet Surg 2005;34(6): 554–8.
43. Dahlberg JA, McClure SR, Evans RB, et al. Force platform evaluation of lameness severity following extracorporeal shock wave therapy in horses with unilateral forelimb lameness. Am Vet Med Assoc 2006;229(1):100–3.
44. Crowe OM, Dyson SJ, Wright IM, et al. Treatment of chronic or recurrent proximal suspensory desmitis using radial pressure wave therapy in the horse. Equine Vet J 2004;36(4): 313–16.
45. Kawcak CE, Frisbie DD, McIlwraith CW. Effects of extracorporeal shock wave therapy and polysulfated glycosaminoglycan treatment on subchondral bone, serum biomarkers, and synovial fluid biomarkers in horses with induced osteoarthritis. Am J Vet Res 2011;72(6):772–9.
46. McCarrol GD, McClure S. Extracorporeal shock wave therapy for treatment of osteoarthritis of the tarsometatarsal and distal intertarsal joints of the horse. Proc Annu Conv Am Assoc Equine Pract 2000;46:200–2.
47. Waguespack RW, Burba DJ, Hubert JD, et al. Effects of extracorporeal shock wave therapy on desmitis of the accessory ligament of the deep digital flexor tendon in the horse. Vet Surg 2011;40(4):450–6.
48. Byron C, Stewart A, Benson B, et al. Effects of radial extracorporeal shock wave therapy on radiographic and scintigraphic outcomes in horses with palmar heel pain. Vet Comp Orthop Traumatol 2009;22(2):113–18.
49. Silveira A, Koenig JB, Arroyo LG, et al. Effects of unfocused extracorporeal shock wave therapy on healing of wounds of the distal portion of the forelimb in horses. Am J Vet Res 2010;71(2):229–34.
50. McClure SR, Van Sickle D, White MR. Effects of extracorporeal shock wave therapy on bone. Vet Surg 2004;33(1):40–8.
51. Maffiuletti NA, Minetto MA, Farina D, et al. Electrical stimulation for neuromuscular testing and training: state-of-the art and unresolved issues. Eur J Appl Physiol 2011;111:2391–7.
52. Delitto A, Robinson AJ. Electrical Stimulation of Muscle: Techniques and Applications. In: Clinical Electrophysiology. Baltimore: Williams & Wilkins; 1989.
53. Requena-Sánchez B, Padial Puche P, González-Badillo JJ. Percutaneous electrical stimulation in strength training an update. J Strength Cond Res 2005;19:438–48.
54. Bickel SC, Gregory CM, Dean JC. Motor unit recruitment during neuromuscular electrical stimulation: a critical appraisal. Eur J Appl Physiol 2011;111(10):2399–407.
55. Zicot M, Rigaux P. Influence of the frequency of neuromuscular electrical-stimulation of the leg on femoral arterial blood-flow. J Mal Vasc 1995;20 (1):9–13.
56. Hoffman P, Skarphedinsson JO, Delle M, et al. Electrical stimulation of the gastrocnemius muscle in the spontaneously hypertensive rat increases the pain threshold: role of different serotonergic receptors. Acta Physiol Scand 1990;138:125–31.
57. Han TR, Kim DY, Lim SJ, et al. The control parameters within the therapeutic range in neuromuscular electrical stimulation. Int J Neurosci 2007;117:107–19.
58. Bergh A, Nordlöf H, Essén-Gustavsson B. Evaluation of neuromuscular electrical stimulation on fibre characteristics and oxidative capacity in equine skeletal muscles. Equine Vet J 2010;42:671–5.
59. Raiser AG, Mazzanti A, Salbego FZ, et al. Different times of neuromuscular electrical stimulation medium frequency (kotz) in dogs. Cienc Rural 2011;41: 1593–9.
60. Ramos AT, Salbego FZ, Festugatto R, et al. Neuromuscular electric stimulation in dogs with induced muscle atrophy. Arq Bras Med Vet Zoo 2008;60: 76–82.
61. Johnson JM, Johnson AL, Pijanowski GJ, et al. Rehabilitation of dogs with surgically treated cranial cruciate ligament-deficient stifles by use of electrical stimulation of muscles. Am J Vet Res 1997;58:1473–8.
62. Sawaya SG, Combet D, Chanoit G, et al. Assessment of impulse duration thresholds for electrical stimulation of muscles (chronaxy) in dogs. Am J Vet Res 2008;69:1305–9.
63. Bax L, Staes F, Verhagen A. Does neuromuscular electrical stimulation strengthen the quadriceps femoris? A systematic review of randomised controlled trials. Sports Med 2005;35: 191–212.
64. Moore SR, Shurman J. Combined neuromuscular electrical stimulation and transcutaneous electrical nerve stimulation for treatment of chronic back pain: A double-blind, repeated measures comparison. Arch Phys Med Rehabil 1997;78 (1):55–60.
65. Shealy CN, Mortimer JT, Reswick J. Electrical inhibition of pain by stimulation of the dorsal column: preliminary clinical reports. Anesth Analg 1967;46:489–91.
66. Sluka KA, Walsh D. Transcutaneous electrical nerve stimulation: basic science mechanisms and clinical effectiveness. J Pain 2003;4:109–21.
67. Indergand HJ, Morgan BJ. Effects of high-frequency transcutaneous electrical nerve stimulation on limb blood flow

in healthy humans. Phys Ther 1994;74:361–7.
68. Cramp FL, McCullough GR, Lowe AS, et al. Transcutaneous electric nerve stimulation: the effect of intensity on local and distal cutaneous blood flow and skin temperature in healthy subjects. Arch Phys Med Rehabil 2002;83:5–9.
69. Nnoaham KE, Kumbang J. Transcutaneous electrical nerve stimulation (TENS) for chronic pain. Cochrane Db Syst Rev 2008, Issue 3. Art. No.: CD003222. DOI: 10.1002/14651858.CD003222.pub2.
70. Cheing G, Tsui A, Lo S, et al. Optimal stimulation duration of TENS in the management of osteoarthritic knee pain. J Rehabil Med 2003;35:62–8.
71. Levine D, Johnston K, Price N, et al. The effect of transcutaneous electrical nerve stimulation (TENS) on dogs with osteoarthritis of the stifle, in Proceedings. 32nd Vet Ortho Soc 2005.
72. Walsh DM, Hoew TE, Johnason MI, et al. Effectiveness of Transcutaneous Electrical Nerve Stimulation (TENS) treatment for acute pain in adults. Cochrane Db Syst Rev 2011, Issue 8.
73. Nussbaum EL, Baxter GD, Lilge L. A review of laser technology and tissue interactions as a background to therapeutic application of low intensity lasers and other light sources. Phys Ther Rev 2003;8:31–44.
74. Karu T. Photobiology of Low-Power laser therapy. New York: Harwood; 1989.
75. Schindl A, Schindl M, Pernerstorfer-Schön H, et al. Low-intensity laser therapy: a review. J Invest Med 2000;48:312–26.
76. Bjordal J, Couppe C, Chow R, et al. A systematic review of low-level laser therapy with location-specific doses for pain from chronic joint disorders. J Physiotherapy 2003;49:107–16.
77. Bjordal JM, Lopes-Martins RA, Joensen J, et al. A systematic review with procedural assessments and meta-analysis of low level laser therapy in lateral elbow tendinopathy (tennis elbow). BMC Musculoskelet Disord 2008;9:75.
78. Ryan R, Smith T. An investigation into the depth of penetration of low level laser therapy through the equine tendon in vivo. Ir J Vet 2007;60:295–9.
79. Collier MA, Haugland LM, Bellamy J, et al. Effects of holmium:YAG laser on equine articular cartilage and subchondral bone adjacent to traumatic lesions: a histopathological assessment. J Arthroscopic and Related Surg 1993;9:536–45.
80. Kaneps AJ, Hultgren BD, Riebold TW, et al. Laser therapy in the horse: histopathologic response. Am J Vet Res 1984;45(3):581–2.
81. Fretz PB, Li Z. Low energy laser irradiation treatment for second intention wound healing in horses. Can Vet J 1992;33:650–3.
82. Rupp S. Experimentelle untersuchung zur wirkung der Ga-Aslaserstrahlung (904nm) auf Sehnen-verletzungen beim pferd. Pferdeheilkunde 1991;1:135–42.
83. Petersen SL, Botes C, Oliveru A, et al. The effect of low level laser therapy (LLLT) on wound healing in horses. Equine Vet J 1999;31:228–31.
84. Petermann U. Laser acupuncture treatment of infected arthritis and tendosynovitis in horses. Prakt Tierarzt 1999;1.
85. McKibbin LS, Paraschak DM. A study of the effects of lasering on chronic bowed tendons at Wheatley Hall Farm Limited, Canada. Lasers Surg Med 1983;3:55–9.
86. Martin BB Jr, Klide AM. Treatment of chronic back pain in horses. Stimulation of acupuncture points with a low powered infrared laser. Vet Surg 1987;16(1):106–10.
87. Bergh A, Nyman G, Lundeberg T, et al. Effect of defocused CO_2 laser on equine tissue perfusion. Acta Veterinaria Scandinavica 2006;47 (1):33–42.
88. Bergh A, Nyman G, Roepstorff L, et al. Defocused CO_2 laser therapy in traumatic arthritis of the metacarpophalangeal joint: a randomized clinical study. Equine and Comparative Exercise Physiology 2006;3 (4):169–77.
89. Lindholm AC, Swensson U, Mitri NDE, et al. Clinical effects of betamethasone and hyaluronan, and of defocalized carbon dioxide laser treatment on traumatic arthritis in the fetlock joints of horses. J Vet Med A 2002;49:1–6.
90. Flemming K, Cullum N. Systematic reviews of wound care management (7): Low-level laser therapy, therapeutic ultrasound, electrotherapy and electromagnetic therapy for the treatment of chronic wounds. Health Technol Assess 2001;5(9):137–221.
91. Gam AN, Thorsen H, Lonnberg F. The effect of low level laser therapy on musculoskeletal pain: a meta-analysis. Pain 1993;53:63–6.
92. Brosseau L, Robinson V, Wells G, et al. Low level laser therapy (Classes III) for treating osteoarthritis. Cochrane Database Syst Rev 2007;(1):CD002046.
93. Yousefi-Nooraie R, Schonstein E, Heidari K, et al. Low level laser therapy for nonspecific low-back pain. Cochrane Database Syst Rev 2008;(2):CD005107.
94. McKay JC, Prato FS, Thomas AW. A literature review: The effects of magnetic field exposure on blood flow and blood vessels in the microvasculature. Bioelectromagnetics 2007;28:81–98.
95. Lednev VV. Possible mechanism of weak magnetic fields on biological systems. Bioelectromagnetics 1991;12:71–5.
96. Ryaby JT. Clinical effects of electromagnetic and electric fields on fracture healing. Clin Orthop 1998;355(Suppl):205–15.
97. Fini M, Giavaresi G, Nicolini A, et al. Effects of pulsed electromagnetic fields on articular hyaline cartilage: review of experimental and clinical studies. Biomed Pharmacother 2005;59:388–94.
98. Pittler MH, Brown EM, Ernst E. Static magnets for reducing pain: systematic review and meta-analysis of randomized trials. CMAJ 2007;177(7):736–42.
99. Bramlage L. The effect of a pulsating electromagnetic field on the acute healing of equine cortical bone. Proc 30th AAEP 1984;43–8.
100. Collier M. Radioisotope uptake in normal equine bone under the influence of pulsed electromagnetic field. Mod Vet Prac 1985;66:971–4.
101. Kobluk C, Johnston G, Lauper L. Scintigraphic investigation of magnetic field therapy on the equine third metacarpus. Vet Comp Orthop Traum 1994;7:9–13.
102. Sanders-Shamis M, Bramlage LR, Weisbrode SE, et al. A preliminary investigation of the effect of selected electromagnetic field devices on healing of cannon bone osteotomies in horses. Equine Vet J 1989;21:201–5.
103. Steyn PE, Ramey DW, Kirschvink J, et al. Effect of a static magnetic field on blood flow to the metacarpus in horses. J Am Vet Med Assoc 2000.
104. Auer JA, Burch GE, Hall P. Review of pulsing electromagnetic field therapy and its possible application to horses. Equine Vet J Oct 1983;15(4):354–60.
105. Watkins J, Auer JA, Morgan SJ, et al. Healing of surgically created defects in the equine superficial digital flexor tendon: Effects of PEMF on collagen-type transformation and tissue morphologic reorganization. Am J Vet Res 1985;46:2097–103.
106. Vavken P, Arrich F, Schefried O, et al. Effectiveness of pulsed electromagnetic field therapy in the management of osteoarthritis of the knee: a meta-analysis of randomised controlled trials. J Rehabil Med 2009;41:406–11.
107. Reeser JC, Smith DT, Fischer V, et al. Static magnetic fields neither prevent nor diminish symptoms and signs of delayed onset muscle soreness. Arch Phys Med Rehabil 2005;86:565–70.

Appendices

Appendix 1a.

Reference ranges for red cell variables in athletic horses

(Compiled by Janene Kingston and Kenneth W. Hinchcliff)

	RBC ($\times 10^{12}$/L)	Hb (g/L)	Hct L/L	MCV (fl)	MCH (pg)	MCHC (g/L)
Thoroughbreds						
Mixed aged and sex[1]	9.7 ± 1.3	134 ± 19	0.42 ± 0.05	43.8 ± 4.6	13.8 ± 1.8	315 ± 20
Untrained mares[2]	9.0 ± 1.3	148 ± 20	0.41 ± 0.06	45.3 ± 2.1	16.6 ± 0.8	361 ± 12
At rest[3]	9.5 ± 0.9	151 ± 12	0.42 ± 0.04	43.6 ± 2.2	15.7 ± 0.8	360 ± 13.4
1–3 h before racing[3]	10.8 ± 1.2	166 ± 13	0.47 ± 0.03	45.2 ± 3.3	15.9 ± 1.1	353 ± 12.1
Fit race horses[4]	8.85 ± 0.57	159 ± 11.4	0.43 ± 0.03	48.5 ± 3.1		
Colt stayers[5]	8.7–11.4	141–180	0.38–0.49	39.6–47.2	14.7–17.5	358–380
Colt sprinters[5]	7.8–10.6	124–170	0.32–0.47	40.1–47.0	14.8–17.4	355–380
Filly stayers[5]	8.2–11.4	135–174	0.36–0.47	39.5–46.6	14.5–17.1	355–379
Filly sprinters[5]	7.8–10.5	126–168	0.34–0.46	39.4–47.0	14.5–17.3	358–378
Jumpers[6]						
1 month training		158 ± 26	0.44 ± 0.06			
5 months training		131 ± 18	0.31 ± 0.05			
7 months training		140 ± 20	0.37 ± 0.06			
Standardbreds						
Mixed aged and sex[1]	8.7 ± 1.4	124 ± 19	0.39 ± 0.04	45.5 ± 4.1	14.3 ± 1.3	314 ± 24
In training[2]	8.8 ± 1.0	146 ± 17	0.39 ± 0.04	45 ± 2.4	16.6 ± 0.9	372 ± 12
Untrained[7]	7.8 ± 1.3	122 ± 1.5	0.35 ± 0.04			
3 weeks training[7]	7.2 ± 0.4	115 ± 5.1	0.32 ± 0.03			

	RBC (×10¹²/L)	Hb (g/L)	Hct L/L	MCV (fl)	MCH (pg)	MCHC (g/L)
7 weeks training[7]	7.2 ± 0.6	129 ± 8.9	0.33 ± 0.02			
6 weeks light training[8]		132 ± 3.2	0.36 ± 0.01			
12 weeks full training[8]		142 ± 3.9	0.38 ± 0.01			
7 weeks of training[9]	6.8 ± 0.2					
15 weeks of training[9]	9.8 ± 0.4					
28 weeks of training[9]	9.0 ± 0.1					
32 weeks of training[9]	8.8 ± 0.3					
Overtrained[9]	8.2 ± 0.2					
Quarter Horses						
Reining horses[10]	7.71 ± 0.60	129 ± 8.6	0.36 ± 0.02	45.3 ± 1.7	16.7 ± 0.65	370 ± 7.1
Polo horses						
5 months into season[11]		149 ± 3.0	0.39 ± 0.9			
Endurance horses						
Competing horses[12]			0.36 ± 0.03			
Competing horses[13]	7.94 ± 0.19	132 ± 4.1	0.37 ± 0.01	46.6 ± 0.92	16.1 ± 0.26	356.3 ± 4.5
Competing horses[14]			0.40 ± 0.04			
Arabian						
Mixed sexes[15]	8.41 ± 1.2	138 ± 21	0.39 ± 0.05	46.9 ± 1.9	16.4 ± 0.9	349 ± 10
4-year-old males[16]	7.1 ± 1.0	120 ± 7.0	0.43 ± 0.04	57 ± 8.0	17 ± 9.0	280 ± 40
Andalusian						
4-year-old males[16]	8.1 ± 1.1	119 ± 8.0	0.42 ± 0.06	52 ± 5.0	14.9 ± 2.0	270 ± 50
Lipizzan						
Stallions[17]	8.16 ± 0.06	135 ± 13	0.43 ± 1.3	52.7 ± 0.3	16.6 ± 0.94	314.8 ± 0.94
Mares[17]	7.53 ± 0.07	123 ± 12	0.43 ± 0.04	52 ± 0.39	16.4 ± 0.16	314 ± 0.86
Clydesdale						
70 geldings[18]	6.23–9.03	107.14.6	0.28–0.39	44.6		38.1
American miniature horse						
Mixed sex and age[19]	7.1 ± 1.2	126 ± 19	0.34 ± 0.05	48.4 ± 5.7		
Data are ranges or mean ± SD.						

References

1. Steel JD, Whitlock LE. Observations of the haematology of Thoroughbred and Standardbred horses in training and racing. Aust Vet J 1960;36:136–42.
2. Lumsden JH, Rowe R, Mullen K. Hematology and biochemistry reference values for the light horse. Can J Comp Med 1980;44:32–42.
3. Revington M. Haematology of the racing Thoroughbred in Australia 1: reference values and the effect of excitement. Eq Vet J 1983;15:141–4.
4. Snow DH, Ricketts SW, Mason DK. Haematological response to racing and training exercise in Thoroughbred horses, with particular reference to the leucocyte response. Eq Vet J 1983;15: 149–54.
5. Allen BV. Comparison of the haemogram between three-year-old Thoroughbred stayers and sprinters. Vet Record 1986;118:555–6.
6. Jablonska EM, Ziolkowska SM, Gill J, et al. Changes in some haematological and metabolic indices in young horses during the first year of jump-training. Eq Vet J 1991;23:309–11.
7. Rose RJ, Allen JR, Hodgson DR, et al. Responses to submaximal treadmill exercise and training in the horse:

changes in haematology, arterial blood gas and acid base measurements, plasma biochemical values and heart rate. Vet Record 1983;113:612–18.

8. Robertson ID, Bolton JR, Mercy AR, et al. Haematological and biochemical values in 12 Standardbred horses during training. Aust Eq Vet 1996;14:72–6.
9. Tyler-McGowan CM, Golland LC, Evans DL, et al. Haematological and biochemical responses to training and overtraining. Eq Vet J Suppl 1999;30: 621–5.
10. KŠstner SBR, Feige K, Weishaupt MA, et al. Heart rate and hematological responses of Quarterhorses to a reining competition. J Eq Vet Sci 1999;19:127–31.
11. Craig L, Hintz HF, Soderholm LV, et al. Changes in blood constituents accompanying exercise in polo horses. Cornell Vet 1985;75:297–302.
12. Carlson GP, Ocen PO, Harrold D. Clinicopathologic alterations in normal and exhausted endurance horses. Theriogenology 1976;6:93–104.
13. Rose RJ. Haematological changes associated with endurance exercise. Vet Record 1982;110:175–7.
14. Grosskopf JFW, Van Rensburg JJ, J. BH. Haematology and blood biochemistry of horses during a 210 km endurance ride. In: Snow DH, Persson SGB, Rose RJ, editors. Equine exercise physiology. Cambridge: Granta Editions; 1983. p. 416–24.
15. Jain NC. SchalmÕs Veterinary Hematology. Philadelphia, PA: Lea & Febiger; 1986.
16. Rubio MD, Munoz A, Santisteban R, et al. Comparative hematological study of two breeds of foals (Andalusian and Arab) subjected to exercise of progressive intensity. J Vet Med Sci 1995;57:311–15.
17. Cebulj-Kadunc N, Bozic M, Kosec M, et al. The influence of age and gender on haematological parameters in Lipizzan horses. J Vet Med A 2002;49: 217–21.
18. Geiser DR, Goble DO, Held JP. Normal hematology and serology of the Clydesdale draft horse. Eq Pract 1984;6:7–9.
19. Harvey RB, Hambright MB. Normal serum chemistry and hematology values of the American miniature horse. Eq Pract 1985;7:6–8.

Appendix 1b

Reference ranges for the leukogram of athletic horses

(Compiled by Janene Kingston and Kenneth W. Hinchcliff)

	WBC (×10⁹/L)	NEUTROPHILS (×10⁹/L)	LYMPHOCYTES (×10⁹/L)	MONOCYTES (×10⁹//L)	EOSINOPHILS (×10⁹//L)	PLATELETS (×10⁹//L)
Thoroughbreds						
Mixed aged and sex[1]	6.35–20.0	1.0–15.4	1.0–16.0	0.02–2.8	0–1.4	
Untrained mares[2]	8.1 ± 1.5	4.1 ± 1.0	3.4 ± 0.8	0.2 ± 0.1		239 ± 40
Six fit mature horses[3]						220 ± 40
At rest[4]	8.8 ± 1.3					
1–3 h before racing[4]	10.2 ± 1.7					
Fit race horses[5]	8.5 ± 1.9	5.3 ± 1.6	2.95 ± 0.98			
2-year-old in training[6]	6.8–11.1	3.2–6.5	2.3–5.0	0.21–0.90	0.08–0.46	
3-year-old in training[6]	6.6–11.0	3.3–6.4	2.1–4.8	0.32–0.97	0.07–0.36	
4-year-old in training[6]	5.8–10.4	3.2–6.3	1.9–3.7	0.30–0.98	0.03–0.34	
Colt stayers[7]	6.0–10.6	2.7–6.1	2.0–4.2	0.22–0.98	0.05–0.34	
Colt sprinters[7]	5.8–10.4	2.4–6.3	2.1–3.9	0.20–1.04	0.06–0.20	
Filly stayers[7]	6.4–10.6	2.9–6.3	2.1–4.6	0.21–1.01	0.04–0.32	
Filly sprinters[7]	6.7–10.8	2.6–6.7	2.1–4.5	0.24–0.96	0.06–0.22	

	WBC (×10⁹/L)	NEUTROPHILS (×10⁹/L)	LYMPHOCYTES (×10⁹/L)	MONOCYTES (×10⁹//L)	EOSINOPHILS (×10⁹//L)	PLATELETS (×10⁹//L)
Standardbreds						
Mixed aged and sex[1]	50.–17.5	1.6–14.3	0.3–10.8	0.05–1.6	0.02–1.6	
In training[2]	7.5 ± 1.3	3.8 ± 0.9	3.1 ± 0.7	0.2 ± 0.1	0.2 ± 0.2	139 ± 44
Untrained[8]	7.0 ± 1.3					
3 weeks training[8]	6.5 ± 0.7					
7 weeks training[8]	7.0 ± 0.7					
Mature racing horses[9]						157 ± 42
7 weeks of training[10]		3.8 ± 0.4	2.8 ± 0.1	0.37 ± 0.02	0.18 ± 0.03	
15 weeks of training[10]		4.7 ± 0.4	2.5 ± 0.2	0.43 ± 0.06	0.17 ± 0.03	
28 weeks of training[10]		4.8 ± 0.3	2.5 ± 0.2	0.45 ± 0.06	0.12 ± 0.01	
32 weeks of training[10]		5.0 ± 0.4	2.3 ± 0.2	0.43 ± 0.04	0.12 ± 0.02	
Overtrained[10]		4.7 ± 0.3	2.7 ± 0.2	0.49 ± 0.04	0.09 ± 0.01	
Quarter Horses						
Reigning horses[11]	7.5 ± 1.03	4.38 ± 0.51	2.89 ± 0.56	0.14 ± 0.17	0.10 ± 0.13	
Endurance horses						
Competing horses[12]	7.5 ± 1.2	4.5 ± 0.9	2.3 ± 0.6	0.33 ± 0.12	0.31 ± 0.2	
Competing horses[13]	8.73 ± 0.61	5.42 ± 0.78	2.82 ± 0.20	0.30 ± 0.06	0.46 ± 0.14	
Arabian						
Mixed sexes[14]	9.53 ± 2.35	4.75 ± 1.5	4.0 ± 1.3	0.42 ± 0.15	0.27 ± 0.11	
Lipizzan						
Stallions[15]	7.56 ± 0.13					
Mares[15]	7.48 ± 0.18					
Clydesdale						
70 geldings[16]	3.9–12.4	2.6–7.2	0.89–3.6	0–0.62	0–0.62	
American miniature horse						
Mixed sex and age[17]	10.0 ± 2.5	3.7 ± 0.8	5.9 ± 0.9	0.04 ± 0.08	0.3 ± 0.2	
Data are ranges or mean ± SD						

References

1. Steel JD, Whitlock LE. Observations of the haematology of Thoroughbred and Standardbred horses in training and racing. Aust Vet J 1960;36:136–42.
2. Lumsden JH, Rowe R, Mullen K. Hematology and biochemistry reference values for the light horse. Can J Comp Med 1980;44:32–42.
3. Bayly WM, Meyers KM, Keck MT, et al. Exercise-induced alterations in haemostasis in Thoroughbred horses. In: Snow DH, Persson SGD, Rose RJ, editors. Equine exercise physiology. Cambridge, UK: Granta Editions; 1983. p. 336–42.
4. Revington M. Haematology of the racing Thoroughbred in Australia 1: reference values and the effect of excitement. Eq Vet J 1983;15:141–4.
5. Snow DH, Ricketts SW, Mason DK. Haematological response to racing and training exercise in Thoroughbred horses, with particular reference to the leucocyte response. Eq Vet J 1983;15:149–54.
6. Allen BV, Kane CE, Powell DG. Leucocyte counts in the healthy English Thoroughbred in training. Eq Vet J 1984;16:207–9.
7. Allen BV. Comparison of the haemogram between three-year-old Thoroughbred stayers and sprinters. Vet Record 1986;118:555–6.
8. Rose RJ, Allen JR, Hodgson DR, et al. Responses to submaximal treadmill exercise and training in the horse: changes in haematology, arterial blood gas and acid base measurements, plasma biochemical values and heart rate. Vet Record 1983;113: 612–18.
9. Johnstone IB, Viel L, Crane S, et al. Hemostatic studies in racing Standardbred horses with exercise-induced pulmonary hemorrhage. Hemostatic parameters at rest and after moderate exercise. Can J Vet Res 1991;55:101–6.
10. Tyler-McGowan CM, Golland LC, Evans DL, et al. Haematological and biochemical responses to training and overtraining. Eq Vet J Suppl 1999;30: 621–5.
11. Kästner SBR, Feige K, Weishaupt MA, et al. Heart rate and hematological responses of Quarterhorses to a reining competition. J Eq Vet Sci 1999;19: 127–31.
12. Carlson GP, Ocen PO, Harrold D. Clinicopathologic alterations in normal and exhausted endurance horses. Theriogenology 1976;6:93–104.
13. Rose RJ. Haematological changes associated with endurance exercise. Vet Record 1982;110:175–7.
14. Jain NC. Schalm's veterinary hematology. Philadelphia, PA: Lea and Febiger; 1986.
15. Cebulj-Kadunc N, Bozic M, Kosec M, et al. The influence of age and gender on haematological parameters in Lipizzan horses. J Vet Med A 2002;49:217–21.
16. Geiser DR, Goble DO, Held JP. Normal hematology and serology of the Clydesdale draft horse. Eq Pract 1984;6:7–9.
17. Harvey RB, Hambright MB. Normal serum chemistry and hematology values of the American miniature horse. Eq Pract 1985;7:6–8.

Appendix 2

Reference ranges for serum biochemical variables in athletic horses

(Compiled by Janene Kingston and Kenneth W. Hinchcliff)

	Na mEq/L OR mmol/L	K mEq/L OR mmol/L	Cl mEq/L OR mmol/L	HCO3 mEq/L OR mmol/L	TOTAL CARBON DIOXIDE Mmol/l	TOTAL PROTEIN g/dL (g/L)	ALBUMIN g/dL (g/L)	GLOBULIN g/dL (g/L)	FIBRINOGEN mg/dL (g/L)	AST U/L	TROPONIN I[a]
Thoroughbreds											
Untrained mares (1)	138 ± 2.2	3.5 ± 0.5	99.5 ± 3.1			6.8 ± 0.4	3.2 ± 0.2	3.3 ± 0.4		165 ± 33.6	
Males (pre-race) (15)					31.1 (31.0–31.3)*	(68 ± 4)	(3.2 ± 2)	(33 ± 4)			
Females (pre-race) (15)					30.7 (30.6–30.9)*						
Race training, clinically normal (17)											≤ 0.15 μg/L
Standardbreds											
Racing (1)	140 ± 1.5	3.6 ± 0.4	99 ± 1.0			6.4 ± 0.5 (64 ± 5)	3.1 ± 0.2 (31 ± 2)	3.3 ± 0.5 (33 ± 5)		217 ± 140	
6 weeks light training (2)	140 ± 1.39	3.3 ± 0.3								336 ± 83	
12 weeks full training (2)	140 ± 1.73	3.2 ± 0.24								443 ± 280	
7 weeks of training (3)						6.7 ± 1.32 (67 ± 13.2)	3.2 ± 0.29 (32 ± 2.94)			299 ± 92	
15 weeks of training (3)						6.3 ± 0.8 (63 ± 8)	3.3 ± 0.17 (33 ± 1.7)			337 ± 140	
28 weeks of training (3)						6.7 ± 0.88 (67 ± 8.8)	3.4 ± 0.17 (34 ± 1.7)			401 ± 148	
32 weeks of training (3)						6.9 ± 0.88 (69 ± 8.8)	3.7 ± 0.17 (37 ± 1.7)			425 ± 144	
Trained, in stable (16)				30.2 +/– 1.2							
Overtrained (3)						6.7 ± 0.48 (67 ± 4.8)	3.7 ± 0.07 (37 ± 0.7)			645 ± 396	
After racing (18)											< 0.04ng/mL (95th percentile) and 0.06 ng/mL (99th percentile)
Performance horses											
Mixed breeds (4)	134–144	3.2–4.2	94–104			5.5–7.5 (55–75)	2.6–3.8 (26–38)	2.0–3.5 (20–35)	<400 <4	150–400	
Dressage horses											<0.022 μg/L
Endurance horses											

North America (5)	139.1 ± 2.5	3.6 ± 0.4	101.1 ± 2.4	[illegible]	[illegible] (70 ± 4.0)			
Australia (6)	134 ± 2.8	3.5 ± 0.3		26.9 ± 1.5	6.0 ± 0.7 (60 ± 7.0)	3.0 ± 0.4 (30 ± 4.0)	204 ± 107	
South Africa (7)	139 ± 3.4	3.3 ± 0.6			6.8 ± 0.3 (67.5 ± 3.3)			
North America, pre-race (19)								0.023 k 0.008 ng/ml.
Quarter horses								
Reigning horses (8)	143 ± 1.7	3.4 ± 0.8	100 ± 1.6					
Three-day event horses								
Australia (9)	136.8 ± 2.7	3.4 ± 0.8	99.5 ± 2.7		6.8 ± 0.5 (68 ± 4.7)	4.7 ± 0.3 (47.1 + 2.7)	174–401	
North America (10)	137.6 ± 4.4	3.6 ± 0.3	105 ± 5.3		6.5 ± 0.4 (65 ± 4.0)	4.0 ± 0.2 (40.1 ± 2.2)	333 ± 85	
Showjumpers								
In competition	138 ± 0.7	4.0 ± 0.1	105 ± 0.6	22.5 ± 0.9	6.7 ± 0.2 (67 ± 2.0)		105 ± 10	
Hunters/Thoroughbreds								
In training (11)							285 ± 42	
Heavy breeds								
English shire horses					7.2 ± 0.6 (72 ± 6.0)	2.8 ± 0.3 (28 ± 3.0)	172 ± 28	
Clydesdales	137.1 ± 5.2	3.6 ± 0.5	101.9 ± 4.6		7.2 ± 0.1 (72 ± 0.8)	3.6 ± 0.5 (36 ± 5.0)	234 ± 163	
Polo horses								
In competition (12)	136 ± 3.4	4.3 ± 0.8	98 ± 2.5	30.7 ± 1.7	7.3 ± 0.6 (73 ± 5.9)			
Driving horses and ponies								
Mixed breeds (13)	137 ± 2.0	3.4 ± 0.5	100 ± 2.0		6.5 ± 0.7 (64.5 ± 4.0)		179 ± 61	
American miniature horses								
Mixed sexes (14)	136 ± 2.2	4.3 ± 0.3			6.6 ± 0.6 (66 ± 6.0)		189 ± 33	

*mean and 95% confidence interval.
a. value depends on methodology and care should be taken in extrapolating these results to other horses using different methodology.
Lumsden JH, Rowe R, Mullen K. Hematology and biochemistry reference values for the light horse. Can J Comp Med 1980; 44: 32-42.

	CK U/L	LDH U/L	GLUCOSE mg/dL (mmol/L)	GGT U/L	SDH U/L	AP U/L	BLOOD UREA NITROGEN mg/dL (mmol/L)	CREATININE mg/dL (mmol/L)	TOTAL CALCIUM mg/dL (mmol/L)	IONIZED CALCIUM mg/dL (mmol/L)
Thoroughbreds										
Untrained mares (1)	44.5 ± 22.3	153 ± 36.7	94.9 ± 27.7 (5.27 ± 1.54)		1.8 ± 1.2	59 ± 16.7	49.6 ± 9.2 (17.7 ± 3.3)	1.3 ± 0.2 (115 ± 18)	11.9 ± 0.4 (2.89 ± 0.1)	
Standardbreds										
Racing (1)	38.5 ± 22.3	140 ± 33.5	81.9 ± 9.36 (4.55 ± 0.52)			45.6 ± 10.8	31.1 ± 4.8 (11.1 ± 1.7)	1.3 ± 0.2 (115 ± 18)	11.9 ± 0.52 (2.98 ± 0.13)	
6 weeks light training (2)	301 ± 177 (301 ± 177)			16 ± 5.9 (16 ± 5.9)						
12 weeks full training (2)	231 ± 104 (231 ± 104)			24 ± 12.5 (24 ± 12.5)						
7 weeks of training (3)	282 ± 216			20 ± 13.6						
15 weeks of training (3)	194 ± 40			40 ± 31.2						
28 weeks of training (3)	210 ± 69			35 ± 28.4						
32 weeks of training (3)	223 ± 64			51 ± 36.8						
Overtrained (3)	396 ± 524			70 ± 48						
Performance horses										
Mixed breeds (4)	100–30	<250	70–40 (4–8)	Oct–40		70–210	11.0–22.0 (4–8)	1.1–1.8 (108–132)	10.8–13.2 (2.7–3.3)	
Endurance horses										
North America (5)									12.2 ± 0.6 (3.04 ± 0.15)	
Australia (6)	80 ± 102	365 ± 140	98.2 ± 9.5 (5.45 ± 0.53)			159 ± 54		1.2 ± 0.2 (106 ± 17.7)	12.7 ± 0.7 3.17 ± 0.17	
South Africa (7)			68.4 ± 12.6 (3.8 ± 0.7)				15 ± 3 [illegible]		12.4 ± 0.4 [illegible]	

Quarter Horses										
Reigning horses (8)									11.39 ± 0.64 (2.99 ± 0.16)	
Three-day event horses										
Australia (9)	117–311		117 ± 12.6 (6.5 ± 0.7)			138–251	17 ± 3 (5.9 ± 1.1)	1.48 ± 0.19 (131 ± 16.4)	11.9 ± 0.64 (2.98 ± 0.16)	
North America (10)	218 ± 149		100.8 ± 7.2 (5.6 ± 0.4)				16.5 ± 1.4 (5.9 ± 0.5)	1.38 ± 0.25 (121 ± 21.7)	12.8 ± 0.8 (3.2 ± 0.2)	6.82 ± 0.4 (1.7 ± 0.1)
Showjumpers										
In competition	48 ± 4.0	375 ± 30							12.8 ± 0.28 (3.3 ± 0.1)	
Hunters/ Thoroughbreds										
In training (11)	115 ± 39	645 ± 168								
Heavy breeds										
English shire horses	58 ± 16			24.2 ± 6.0	0.8 ± 0.2	54 ± 11				
Clydesdales	56 ± 22		75.9 ± 19.2 (4.21 + 1.1)			91 ± 36	14.5 ± 3.2 (5.2 ± 1.14)	1.7 ± 0.3 (151 ± 26.5)	11.9 ± 1.1 (2.97 ± 0.27)	
Polo horses										
In competition (12)									12.9 ± 0.24 (3.21 ± 0.06)	
Driving horses and ponies										
Mixed breeds (13)	35 ± 9		97.2 ± 9.0 (5.4 ± 0.5)				15 ± 3 (5.5 ± 1.1)		12.0 ± 0.4 (3.0 ± 0.1)	
American miniature horses										
Mixed sexes (14)	273 ± 136		91 ± 12.4 (5.1 ± 0.7)	11 ± 4.4		181 ± 53	23.7 ± 3.8 (8.5 ± 1.4)	1.0 ± 0.2 (88.4 ± 17.7)	11.6 ± 0.4 (2.9 ± 0.1)	

References

1. Robertson ID, Bolton JR, Mercy AR, et al. Haematological and biochemical values in 12 Standardbred horses during training. Aust Eq Vet 1996;14:72–6.
2. Tyler-McGowan CM, Golland LC, Evans DL, et al. Haematological and biochemical responses to training and overtraining. Eq Vet J Suppl 1999;30: 621–5.
3. Rose RJ, Hodgson DR. Hematology and biochemistry. In: Hodgson DR, Rose EJ, editors. The athletic horse. Philadelphia, PA: WB Saunders; 1994. p. 64–78.
4. Carlson GP, Ocen PO, Harrold D. Clinicopathologic alterations in normal and exhausted endurance horses. Theriogenology 1976;6:93–104.
5. Rose RJ, Purdue RA, Hensley W. Plasma biochemistry alterations in horses during an endurance ride. Eq Vet J 1977;9: 122–6.
6. Grosskopf JFW, Van Rensburg JJ, J BH. Haematology and blood biochemistry of horses during a 210 km endurance ride. In: Snow DH, Persson SGD, Rose RJ, editors. Equine Exercise Physiology. Cambridge, UK: Granta editions; 1983. p. 416–24.
7. Kästner SBR, Feige K, Weishaupt MA, et al. Heart rate and hematological responses of Quarterhorses to a reigning competition. J Eq Vet Sc 1999;19:127–31.
8. Rose RJ, Ilkiw JE, Arnold KS, et al. Plasma biochemistry in the horse during 3-day event competition. Q Vet J 1980; 12:132–6.
9. Andrews FM, Geiser DR, White SL, et al. Haematological and biochemical changes in horses competing in a 3 Star horse trial and 3-day-event. Eq Vet J Suppl 1995:57–63.
10. Anderson MG. The influence of exercise on serum enzyme levels in the horse. Eq Vet J 1975;7:160–5.
11. Craig L, Hintz HF, Soderholm LV, et al. Changes in blood constituents accomanying exercise in polo horses. Cornell Vet 1985;75:297–302.
12. Snow DH. Haematological, biochemical and physiological changes in horses and ponies during the cross country stage of driving trial competitions. Vet Record 1990;126:233–9.
13. Harvey RB, Hambright MB. Normal serum chemistry and hematology values of the American miniature horse. Eq Pract 1985;7:6–8.
14. Cohen ND, Stanley SD, Arthur RM, et al. Factors influencing pre-race serum concentration of total carbon dioxide in Thoroughbred horses racing in California. Equine vet J 2006;38(6): 543–8.
15. Auer DE, Skelton KV, Tay S, et al. Detection of sodium bicarbonate administration (milkshake) to Standardbred horses. Aust Vet J 1993;70(9):336–40.
16. Begg, LM, Hoffman KL, Begg AP. Serum and plasma cardiac troponin I concentrations in clinically normal Thoroughbreds in training in Australia. Aust Vet J 2006;84(9):336–7.
17. Slack J, Boston RC, Soma L, et al. Cardiac Troponin I in Racing Standardbreds. J Vet Int Med 2012;26:12-02–1208.
18. Holbrook TC, Birks, EK, Sleeper MM, et al. Endurance exercise is associated with increased plasma cardiac troponin I in horses. Equine Vet J 2006;38:27–31.
19. Nostell K, Haggstrom J. Resting concentrations of cardiac troponin I in fit horses and effect of racing. J Vet Cardiol 2008;10:105–9.

Index

Note: Page numbers followed by 'f' and 't' refers to figures and tables respectively.

A

C

D

E

H

I

J

K

L

M

N

O

Q

R

T

U

V

W

X

Y

Z